7/08 £93-00 DC Retained 2019

WP
180
REF

Gynaecologic Surgical Procedures
Genital Diseases, Female / surgery

D1625630

WITHDRAWN

FOR
REFERENCE ONLY

NHS
Musgrove Park Hospital

Library Service
Musgrove Park Hospital

Library Service
Musgrove Park Academy
Musgrove Park Hospital
Taunton
Somerset
TA1 5DA

Tel: 01823 342433
Email: library@tst.nhs.uk

SWNHS
C20321714

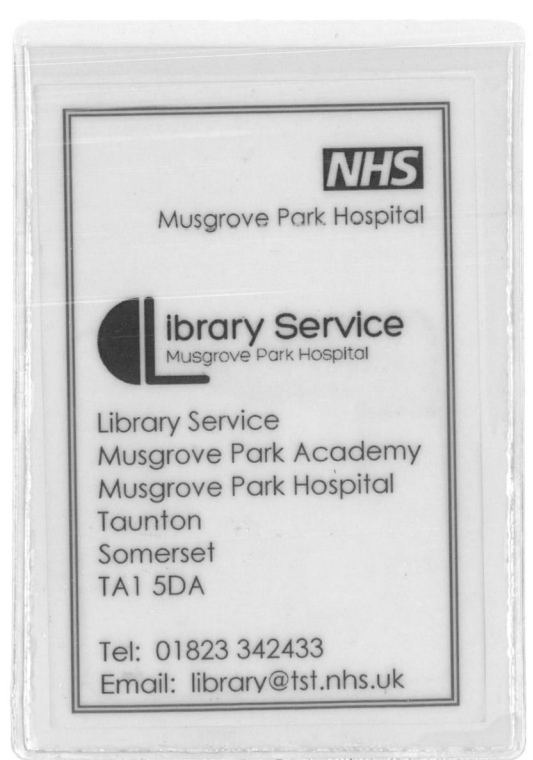

LIBRARY TAUNTON AND SOMERSET HOSPITAL

TENTH EDITION

TE LINDE'S OPERATIVE GYNECOLOGY

TENTH EDITION

TE LINDE'S OPERATIVE GYNECOLOGY

John A. Rock, MD
Senior Vice President, Medical Affairs
Dean, College of Medicine
Professor of Obstetrics and Gynecology
Department of Obstetrics and Gynecology
Florida International University
Miami, Florida

Howard W. Jones III, MD
Professor of Obstetrics and Gynecology
Director of Gynecologic Oncology
Vanderbilt University School of Medicine
Nashville, Tennessee

Wolters Kluwer Health | Lippincott Williams & Wilkins
Philadelphia • Baltimore • New York • London
Buenos Aires • Hong Kong • Sydney • Tokyo

Acquisitions Editor: Sonya Seigafuse
Managing Editor: Ryan Shaw
Project Manager: Rosanne Hallowell
Manufacturing Manager: Kathleen Brown
Marketing Manager: Kimberly Schonberger
Art Director: Risa Clow
Cover Designer: Larry Didona
Production Services: Aptara, Inc.

Tenth Edition
© 2008 by Lippincott Williams & Wilkins, a Wolters Kluwer business
530 Walnut Street
Philadelphia, PA 19106
LWW.com

© 2003 by Lippincott Williams & Wilkins. © 1997 by Lippincott-Raven. © 1992 by J. B. Lippincott Company.

All rights reserved. This book is protected by copyright. No part of this book may be reproduced in any form or by any means, including photocopying, or utilized by any information storage and retrieval system without written permission from the copyright owner, except for brief quotations embodied in critical articles and reviews.

Printed in China

Library of Congress Cataloging-in-Publication Data

Te Linde's operative gynecology.—10th ed. / [edited by] John A. Rock, Howard W. Jones III.
p. ; cm.
Includes bibliographical references and index.
ISBN-13: 978-0-7817-7234-1
ISBN-10: 0-7817-7234-6
1. Generative organs, Female—Surgery. I. Rock, John A. II. Jones, Howard W. (Howard Wilbur), 1942- III. Te Linde, Richard W. (Richard Welsley), 1894–1989. Te Linde's operative gynecology. IV. Title: Operative gynecology.

[DNLM: 1. Gynecologic Surgical Procedures. WP 660 T2721 2008]
RG104.T4 2008
618.1′45—dc22

2007046346

Care has been taken to confirm the accuracy of the information presented and to describe generally accepted practices. However, the authors, editors, and publisher are not responsible for errors or omissions or for any consequences from application of the information in this book and make no warranty, expressed or implied, with respect to the currency, completeness, or accuracy of the contents of the publication. Application of this information in a particular situation remains the professional responsibility of the practitioner.

The authors, editors, and publisher have exerted every effort to ensure that drug selection and dosage set forth in this text are in accordance with current recommendations and practice at the time of publication. However, in view of ongoing research, changes in government regulations, and the constant flow of information relating to drug therapy and drug reactions, the reader is urged to check the package insert for each drug for any change in indications and dosage and for added warnings and precautions. This is particularly important when the recommended agent is a new or infrequently employed drug.

Some drugs and medical devices presented in this publication have Food and Drug Administration (FDA) clearance for limited use in restricted research settings. It is the responsibility of health care providers to ascertain the FDA status of each drug or device planned for use in their clinical practice.

The publishers have made every effort to trace copyright holders for borrowed material. If they have inadvertently overlooked any, they will be pleased to make the necessary arrangements at the first opportunity.

To purchase additional copies of this book, call our customer service department at (800) 638-3030 or fax orders to (301) 223-2320. International customers should call (301) 223-2300.

Visit Lippincott Williams & Wilkins on the Internet: at LWW.com. Lippincott Williams & Wilkins customer service representatives are available from 8:30 am to 6 pm, EST.

9 8 7 6 5 4 3 2 1

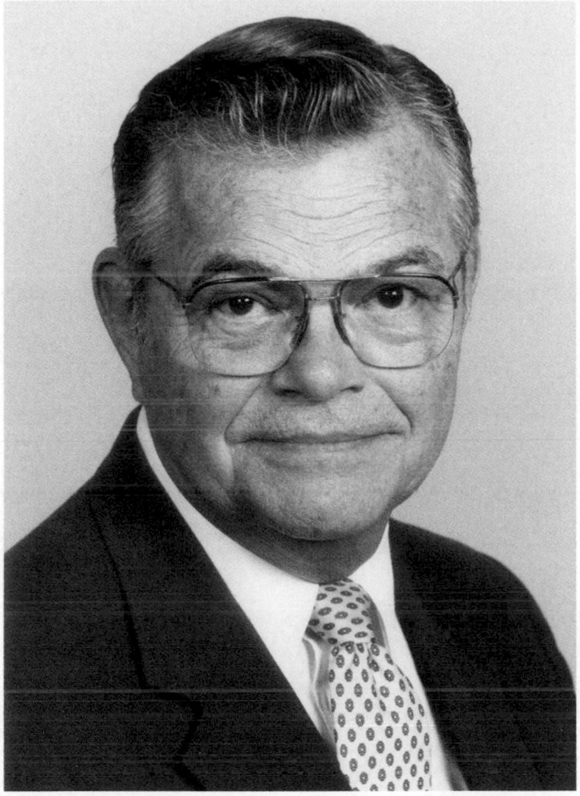

TO DR. GEORGE W. MORLEY

This tenth edition of *Te Linde's Operative Gynecology* is dedicated to our friend, admired and respected colleague, and contributor to previous editions of this book, Dr. George W. Morley, who passed away February 20, 2005 at age 81.

The last century was filled with spectacular progress in gynecologic surgery. Through his enthusiastic teaching, writings, mentoring to hundreds, compassionate and competent care of patients in the operating room and beyond, and especially his wise leadership of almost every national organization in gynecology and obstetrics, George was an active participant and contributor to this progress. Always totally loyal to his specialty, his institution, and the truth, he was fond of saying that we see farther by standing on the shoulders of giants who have gone before us. Now, we who knew George are able to see farther, do more, and do better for those we serve by having stood on his shoulders.

Dr. Te Linde and all the editors, authors, and publishers of *Te Linde's Operative Gynecology* since its beginning in 1946, are pleased and honored to dedicate this new edition to the memory of a gentle giant, George W. Morley, with our promise that the path of progress in gynecologic surgery will continue in this new century.

■ CONTENTS

SECTION V ■ SURGERY FOR BENIGN GYNECOLOGIC CONDITIONS

SECTION VI ■ SURGERY FOR OBSTETRICS

SECTION VII ■ SURGERY FOR CORRECTIONS OF DEFECTS IN PELVIC SUPPORT AND PELVIC FISTULAS

SECTION VIII ■ RELATED SURGERY

SECTION IX ■ GYNECOLOGIC ONCOLOGY

CONTRIBUTORS

Nadeem R. Abu-Rustum, MD
Associate Professor
Department of Obstetrics and Gynecology
Weill Medical College of Cornell University
Associate Attending Physician
Department of Surgery
Memorial Sloan-Kettering Cancer Center
New York, New York

Rony A. Adam, MD
Assistant Professor
Director, Division of Gynecologic Specialties
Department of Obstetrics and Gynecology
Emory University School of Medicine
Atlanta, Georgia

Michael P. Aronson, MD
Professor
Department of Obstetrics and Gynecology
University of Massachusetts Medical School
Director of Women's Health Services
Department of Obstetrics and Gynecology
University of Massachusetts Medical Center
Worcester, Massachusetts

Michael Baggish, MD
Chairman
Department of Obstetrics and Gynecology
Good Samaritan Hospital
Director of Obstetrics and Gynecology and Residency Training
TriHealth (Good Samaritan and Bethesda Hospitals)
Cincinnati, Ohio

Jack Basil, MD
Associate Director of Gynecologic Oncology
Department of Obstetrics and Gynecology
Good Samaritan Hospital
Cincinnati, Ohio

Alfred E. Bent, MD
Professor
Department of Obstetrics and Gynecology
Dalhousie University
Chief, Division of Gynecology
IWK Health Centre
Halifax, Nova Scotia, Canada

Eric J. Bieber, MD, MSHCM
Chair
Department of Obstetrics and Gynecology
Geisinger Health System
Danville, Pennsylvania
Chief Medical Officer
Geisinger Wyoming Valley
Wilkes-Barre, Pennsylvania

Lesley L. Breech, MD
Associate Professor
Department of Pediatrics and Obstetrics and Gynecology
University of Cincinnati College of Medicine
Chief, Pediatric and Adolescent Gynecology
Department of Pediatrics
Cincinnati Children's Hospital Medical Center
Cincinnati, Ohio

Gert H. Brieger, MD, PhD
Distinguished Service Professor
Department of History of Medicine
Johns Hopkins University School of Medicine
Baltimore, Maryland

Andrew I. Brill, MD
Director
Minimally Invasive Gynecology, Reparative Pelvic Surgery, and Surgical Education
California Pacific Medical Center
San Francisco, California

James J. Burke II, MD
Associate Professor and Director Gynecologic Oncology
Department of Obstetrics and Gynecology
Mercer University School of Medicine
Attending Gynecologic Surgeon
Department of Obstetrics and Gynecology
Memorial Health University Medical Center
Savannah, Georgia

Thomas W. Burke, MD
Professor
Department of Gynecologic Oncology
University of Texas
M.D. Anderson Cancer Center
Houston, Texas

Joseph Buscema, MD
Fellow
Department of Obstetrics and Gynecology
Johns Hopkins University School of Medicine
Baltimore, Maryland
Physician
Gynecologic Oncology and Obstetrics and Gynecology
Tucson, Arizona

William J. Butler, MD
Professor and Chairman
Department of Obstetrics and Gynecology
Mercer University School of Medicine
Director
Central Georgia Fertility Institute
Medical Center of Central Georgia
Macon, Georgia

David E. Carnovale, MD
Associate Professor
Clerkship Director
Mercer University School of Medicine
Department of Obstetrics and Gynecology
Director of Assisted Reproductive Technologies
Central Florida Fertility Institute
The Medical Center of Central Georgia
Macon, Georgia

Dennis S. Chi, MD
Associate Professor
Department of Obstetrics and Gynecology
Weill Cornell Medical College of Cornell University
Associate Attending Surgeon
Gynecology Service, Department of Surgery
Memorial Sloan-Kettering Cancer Center
New York, New York

Marta Ann Crispens, MD
Assistant Professor
Department of Obstetrics and Gynecology
Vanderbilt University Medical Center
Nashville, Tennessee

Mark A. Damario, MD
Associate Professor
Department of Obstetrics, Gynecology and Women's Health
University of Minnesota
Medical Director
Reproductive Medical Center
University of Minnesota Physicians
Minneapolis, Minnesota

John O. L. DeLancey, MD
Norman F. Miller Professor of Gynecology
Department of Obstetrics and Gynecology
University of Michigan Medical School
Fellowship Director, Female Pelvic Medicine and Reconstructive surgery
University of Michigan Health System
Ann Arbor, Michigan

Edie L. Derian, MD
Residency Program Director
Department of Obstetrics and Gynecology
Vice Chair
Department of Obstetrics and Gynecology
Geisinger Health Systems
Danville, Pennsylvania

James R. Dolan, MD
Division Director-Gynecologic Oncology
Department of Obstetrics and Gynecology
Advocate Lutheran General Hospital
Park Ridge, Illinois

Celia E. Dominguez, MD
Division of Reproductive Endocrinology and Infertility
Department of Obstetrics and Gynecology
Atlanta, Georgia

Alexander Duncan, MD
Assistant Professor
Department of Pathology and Laboratory Medicine/Hematology
Emory University School of Medicine
Director, Special Hemostasis Laboratory
Department of Laboratory Medicine
Emory Medical Labs
Atlanta, Georgia

Ruth M. Farrell, MD, MA
Assistant Professor of Surgery
Department of Obstetrics and Gynecology
Cleveland Clinic Lerner College of Medicine
Associate Staff
Department of Bioethics and Obstetrics and Gynecology
Cleveland Clinic Hospital Systems
Cleveland, Ohio

Sean L. Francis, MD
Assistant Professor
Department of Obstetrics and Gynecology
Medical College of Georgia
Section Chief, Urogynecology and Pelvic Surgery
Department of Obstetrics and Gynecology
MCG Health System
Augusta, Georgia

Donald G. Gallup, MD
Professor and Chair
Department of Obstetrics and Gynecology
Mercer University School of Medicine
Savannah, Georgia

John B. Gebhart, MD, MS
Assistant Professor-Division of Gynecologic Surgery
Department of Obstetrics and Gynecology
Chief
Division of Urogynecology
Mayo Clinic
Rochester, Minnesota

David M. Gershenson, MD
J. Taylor Wharton, MD Distinguished Chair in Gynecologic Oncology
Professor and Chairman
Department of Gynecologic Oncology
University of Texas MD Anderson Cancer Center
Houston, Texas

Victor Gomel, MD
Professor
Department of Obstetrics and Gynecology
Faculty of Medicine, University of British Columbia
Active Staff
Department of Obstetrics and Gynecology
BC Women's Hospital and Health Centre
Vancouver, British Columbia, Canada

Cornelia R. Graves, MD
Medical Director
Tennessee Maternal Fetal Medicine
Medical Director Maternal-Fetal Medicine
Baptist Hospital
Nashville, Tennessee

Victoria L. Green, MD, JD, MBA
Associate Professor
Department of Obstetrics and Gynecology
Emory University
Director, Gynecology Breast Clinic
Winship Cancer Institute at Grady Memorial Hospital; Avon Comprehensive Breast Center
Atlanta, Georgia

Heather M. Greene, BA
Research Coordinator
Department of Obstetrics and Gynecology
University of New Mexico Health Science Center
Albuquerque, New Mexico

W. David Hager, MD
Clinical Professor
Department of Obstetrics and Gynecology
University of Kentucky College of Medicine
Staff Director, U.K. Affiliated Residency Training Program
Department of Obstetrics and Gynecology
Central Baptist Hospital
Lexington, Kentucky

John S. Hesla, MD
Medical Director
Oregon Reproductive Medicine
Portland, Oregon

Mitchel S. Hoffman, MD
Professor and Director
Division of Gynecologic Oncology
University of South Florida
Medical Director
Gynecologic Oncology Program
Tampa General Hospital
Tampa, Florida

Ira R. Horowitz, MD, SM
Willaford Ransom Leach and Vice Chairman of Clinical Affairs
Director, Division of Gynecologic Oncology
Department of Obstetrics and Gynecology
Emory University School of Medicine
Chief Medical Officer
Department of Obstetrics and Gynecology
Emory University Hospital
Atlanta, Georgia

Fred Howard, MD
Professor
Department of Obstetrics and Gynecology
University of Rochester School of Medicine and Dentistry
Division Director, Gynecologic Specialities
Department of Obstetrics and Gynecology
Strong Memorial Hospital
Rochester, New York

Barry K. Jarnagin, MD
Associate Professor
Department of Obstetrics and Gynecology
Vanderbilt University School of Medicine
Nashville, Tennessee

Howard W. Jones, Jr., MD
Professor Emeritus
Department of Obstetrics and Gynecology
Eastern Virginia Medical School
Norfolk, Virginia
Professor Emeritus
Department of Obstetrics and Gynecology
Johns Hopkins University School of Medicine
Baltimore, Maryland

Howard W. Jones III, MD
Professor
Department of Obstetrics and Gynecology
Vanderbilt University School of Medicine
Director
Division of Gynecologic Oncology
Vanderbilt University Medical Center
Nashville, Tennessee

Thomas M. Julian, MD
Professor
Department of Obstetrics and Gynecology
University of Wisconsin
Madison, Wisconsin

Kenneth Kalassian, MD
Assistant Professor
Department of Pulmonary and Critical Care Medicine
Emory University
Medical Director
Department of Surgical Intensive Care Unit
Emory University Hospital
Atlanta, Georgia

Mickey M. Karram, MD
Professor of Obstetrics and Gynecology
Department of Obstetrics and Gynecology
University of Cincinnati
Director of Urogynecology and Reconstructive Pelvic Surgery
Department of Obstetrics and Gynecology
Good Samaritan Hospital
Cincinnati, Ohio

Steven D. Kleeman, MD
Assistant Professor
Department of Obstetrics and Gynecology
University of Cincinnati
Associate Director, Division of Urogynecology
Department of Obstetrics and Gynecology
Good Samaritan Hospital
Cincinnatti, Ohio

Melissa Kottke, MD
Clinical Instructor
Department of Obstetrics and Gynecology
Emory University
Atlanta, Georgia

S. Robert Kovoc, MD
J. D. Thompson Distinguished Professor of Gynecologic Surgery
Department of Obstetrics and Gynecologic
Emory University
Director, Emory Center for Pelvic Reconstructive Surgery and Urogynecology
Department of Gynecology and Obstetrics
Emory University Hospital
Atlanta, Georgia

John W. Larson, MD
Oscar I. and Mildred S. Dodek Professor and Chair
Department of Obstetrics and Gynecology
The George Washington University
Attending Physician and Chair
Department of Obstetrics and Gynecology
The George Washington University Hospital
Washington, DC

Raymond A. Lee, MD
Emeritus Professor
Division of Gynecologic Surgery
Department of Obstetrics and Gynecology
Consultant
Department of Obstetrics and Gynecology
Mayo Clinic
Rochester, Minnesota

Gary H. Lipscomb, MD
Professor
Department of Obstetrics and Gynecology
University of Tennessee Health Science Center
Chief of Gynecology
Department of Obstetrics and Gynecology
The Regional Medical Center
Memphis, Tennessee

Bhagirath Majmudar, MD
Associate Professor
Department of Obstetrics and Gynecology
Emory University School of Medicine
Surgical Pathologist
Pathology and Laboratory Medicine
Grady Memorial Hospital
Atlanta, Georgia

Sanford M. Markham, MD
Executive Associate Dean for Student Affairs
Professor of Obstetrics and Gynecology College of Medicine
Florida International University
Miami, Florida

John L. Marlow, MD
Clinical Professor
Department of Obstetrics and Gynecology
George Washington University School of Medicine
Washington, DC

Mark G. Martens, MD
Vice-President and Chief Medical Officer for Research
Planned Parenthood of Arkansas and Eastern Oklahoma
Tulsa, Oklahoma

G. Rodney Meeks, MD
Winfred L. Wiser Chain of Gynecologic Surgery
Director, Division of Gynecology
University of Mississippi Medical Center
Jackson, Mississippi

Luis E. Mendez, MD
Director of Gynecologic Oncology
Department of Obstetrics and Gynecology
Florida International University College of Medicine
Physician
South Florida Gynecologic Oncology
Coral Gables, Florida

Michael D. Moen, MD
Clinical Assistant Professor
Department of Obstetrics and Gynecology
University of Illinois
Director of Urogynecology
Department of Obstetrics and Gynecology
Advocate Lutheran General Hospital
Park Ridge, Illinois

Kelly L. Molpus, MD
Director of Gynecologic Oncology
Department of Obstetrics and Gynecology
Halifax Medical Center
Daytona Beach, Florida

Ana Alvarez Murphy, MD
Greenblatt Professor and Chair
Department of Obstetrics and Gynecology
Medical College of Georgia
Clinical Service Chief
Department of Obstetrics and Gynecology
MCG Health System
Augusta, Georgia

Lynn Parker, MD
Assistant Professor/Division Director of Gynecologic Oncology
Department of Obstetrics and Gynecology
University of Louisville Health Sciences Center
Louisville, Kentucky

Manuel Penalver, MD
Professor and Chairman
Department of Obstetrics and Gynecology
Florida International University College of Medicine
South Florida Gynecologic Oncology
Coral Gables, Florida

Herbert B. Peterson, MD
Professor
Department of Obstetrics and Gynecology
University of North Carolina School of Medicine
Chapel Hill, North Carolina

Marie Plante, MD
Associate Professor
Department of Obstetrics and Gynecology
Laval University
Chief, Division of Gynecologic Oncology
Department of Obstetrics and Gynecology
L'Hôtel-Dieude Québec
Quebec City, Quebec, Canada

Amy E. Pollack, MD, MPH
Adjunct Assistant Professor
School of Public Health
Columbia University
New York, New York

John A. Rock, MD
Senior Vice President, Medical Affairs
Dean, College of Medicine
Florida International University
Miami, Florida

William A. Rock, Jr., MD
Professor
Department of Pathology
University of Mississippi Medical Center
Medical Director, Clinical Laboratory
Department of Pathology
University Hospital and Clinics
Jackson, Mississippi

Robert M. Rogers, Jr., MD
Staff Gynecologist
Kalispell Regional Medical Center
Kalispell, Montana

Ted M. Roth, MD
Director, Bladder Control Center
Department of Women's Specialty Center
Central Maine Medical Center
Lewisten, Maine

Michel Roy, MD
Professor
Department of Gynecology
Laval University
Gynecologist and Oncologist
Department of Gynecology
CHUQ-Hotel-Dieu
Quebec City, Quebec, Canada

Eli A. Rybak, MD, MPH
Assistant Professor
Department of Obstetrics and Gynecology and Women's Health Fellow
Division of Reproductive Endocrinology and Infertility
Albert Einstein College of Medicine
Montefiore Medical Center
Bronx, New York

Joseph S. SanFilippo, MD, MBA
Professor
Department of Obstetrics and Reproductive Services
Vice Chair
Department of Reproductive Endocrinology and Infertility
University of Pittsburgh Physicians
Magee Womens Hospital
Pittsburgh, Pennsylvania

Howard T. Sharp, MD
Chief, General Division of Obstetrics and Gynecology
Department of Obstetrics and Gynecology
University of Utah School of Medicine
Salt Lake City, Utah

Bobby Shull, MD
Professor
Department of Obstetrics and Gynecology
Texas A & M University Health Science Center
Professor, Interim Chairman
Department of Obstetrics and Gynecology
Scott and White Memorial Hospital
Temple, Texas

Harriet O. Smith, MD
Director
Department of Gynecologic Oncology
University of New Mexico Health Science Center
Albuquerque, New Mexico

Richard M. Soderstrom, MD
Professor Emeritus
Department of Obstetrics and Gynecology
University of Washington School of Medicine
Seattle, Washington

Betty Ruth Speir, MD
Clinical Associate Professor
Department of Obstetrics and Gynecology
Clinical Professor
Department of General Surgery
University of South Alabama
Mobile, Alabama

John F. Steege, MD
Professor
Department of Obstetrics and Gynecology
University of North Carolina
Attending Physician
Department of Obstetrics and Gynecology
University of North Carolina Hospitals
Chapel Hill, North Carolina

Elizabeth L. Taylor, MD
Clinical Instructor
Department of Obstetrics and Gynecology
University of British Columbia
Active Staff
Department of Obstetrics and Gynecology
Vancouver General Hospital
Vancouver, British Columbia

Paul Underwood, Jr., MD
Professor
Department of Obstetrics and Gynecology
Medical University of South Carolina
Charleston, South Carolina

John R. Van Nagel, Jr., MD
Professor and Director
Division of Gynecologic Oncology
Department of Obstetrics and Gynecology
University of Kentucky Medical Center—Markey Cancer Center
Lexington, Kentucky

Edward Wallach, MD
J. Donald Woodruff Professor
Department of Obstetrics and Gynecology
Johns Hopkins University of Medicine
Lutherville, Maryland

Charles J. Ward, MD
Clinical Professor (Retired)
Department of Obstetrics and Gynecology
Emory University School of Medicine
Atlanta, Georgia
Clinical Risk Advisor
Department of Obstetrics and Gynecology
Rotunda Hospital
Dublin, Ireland

Jeffrey S. Warshaw, MD
Assistant Professor
Department of Obstetrics and Gynecology
University of Minnesota
Director
Department of Urogynecology
Hennepin County Medical Center
Minneapolis, Minnesota

Paul Michael Yandell, MD
Assistant Professor
Department of Obstetrics and Gynecology
Texas A & M Health Science Center and College of Medicine
College Station, Texas
Staff Member
Division of Female Medicine and Pelvic Reconstructive Surgery
Department of Obstetrics and Gynecology
Scott and White Hospital and Clinic
Temple, Texas

Mimi Zieman, MD
Clinical Associate Professor
Department of Obstetrics and Gynecology
Emory University
Atlanta, Georgia

Carl W. Zimmerman, MD
Professor
Department of Obstetrics and Gynecology
Vanderbilt University School of Medicine
Nashville, Tennessee

FOREWORD

Once again, the editors, authors, artists, and publishers have collaborated to produce a completely updated revision of *Te Linde's Operative Gynecology*, the most widely read textbook on this subject in the world. It has been translated into several foreign languages, and the eighth edition was the first to be translated into Chinese. This textbook is essential to the care of women with gynecologic disease.

There is a long history of publication of classic textbooks by distinguished members of the faculty of the Department of Gynecology and Obstetrics at Johns Hopkins. The list includes *William Obstetrics* and notable literary works of Kelly, Cullen, Novak, Wharton, Everett, Woodruff, Howard and Georgeanna Jones, Rock, and others. Many of these textbooks have been carried on in succeeding editions in the last 100 years. By describing and emphasizing "the Hopkins way" of caring for patients, these books have had great influence on the practice of gynecologists and obstetricians. *Te Linde's Operative Gynecology* is a prime example of this Hopkins tradition.

In the first edition in 1947, Dr. Te Linde wrote only about gynecologic operations that he had personal experience with, and advised subsequent editors to do the same. Since then, the subject of gynecologic surgery has become so large that it is no longer possible for any one or two gynecologic surgeons to be masters of the entire field, partly the result of development of subspecialties in gynecologic surgery. Therefore, it has been necessary to include authors other than the Hopkins authors who also qualify as experts in various aspects of the subject. The current edition includes 75 authors. This has resulted in a more complete national and even international presentation. This venerable textbook includes not only the usual and customary problems in gynecology that may require surgery for relief, but also the special, difficult, complicated, and unusual problems encountered occasionally.

The last century saw spectacular advances in the surgical treatment of gynecologic diseases. Consider that a tumor as common as uterine leiomyomata was a lethal disease in some women when the 20th century began. Because of the heroic surgical innovations of Howard Kelly and Thomas Cullen and others at Johns Hopkins and elsewhere, women who live in countries where modern gynecologic surgery is practiced no longer endure long suffering or die of this benign tumor. Similar advances have also been made in the management of cervical cancer, endometriosis, ectopic pregnancy, pelvic infections, uterine prolapse and vaginal relaxations, urinary incontinence, fistulas, infertility, congenital anomalies, etc. Throughout the century, progress in gynecologic surgery was chronicled by many textbooks. For example, Kelly's *Operative Gynecology* was the helpful companion of gynecologic surgeons in the first half of the 20th century, and *Te Linde's Operative Gynecology* served a similar function in the second half.

In addition to the scholarly work of the authors of chapters, one must also pay tribute to the brilliant artwork that has accompanied and explained the text. Originally, in Dr. Kelly's *Operative Gynecology*, the highest standard was set by the close collaboration, often in the operating room, between Dr. Kelly and his choice of Max Brodel as his personal artist. Their work together produced many masterpieces that are still outstanding teaching aides today. Brodel started the Hopkins School of Art in Medicine, and many of the graduates of this school, especially Leon Schlossberg, have contributed to every edition of *Te Linde's Operative Gynecology* and other texts. One cannot underestimate the value of their work in teaching gynecologic surgery. Because of the numerous illustrations, *Te Linde's Operative Gynecology* could qualify as an atlas of surgical technique, but it is much more.

Although an important part of the education and training of the gynecologic surgeon, *Te Linde's Operative Gynecology* cannot alone teach technical skills or substitute for spending years at the elbow of a seasoned, wise, and experienced mentor working in a proper health care facility, both of which are a necessary minimum in creating and maintaining an environment in which gynecologic surgery can be studied and learned and practiced. Proper technical skills are important in the successful performance of even the simplest operation. However, the most serious mistakes in the practice of gynecologic surgery may be made by those who know "how," but have not learned "when" and "why." The ability to perform a large number of gynecologic operations with a low morbidity and mortality rate, although desirable, is not *ipso facto* evidence that gynecologic surgery is being practiced correctly. The gynecologic surgeon must first study and understand the basic-science aspects of female reproductive organ function and the pathology, clinical manifestations, and psychosocial aspects of gynecologic disease. It takes time to evaluate patients properly, some moreso than others. This may be difficult in a busy gynecologic practice, but it is necessary in order that proper recommendations can be made for or against surgery. And, after one chooses the right patient for operation, one must choose the right operation for the patient. It is a mistake to do an abdominal hysterectomy when a vaginal hysterectomy would have significant advantages. One must select from a variety of operations available, and the one that most properly fits the needs of the individual patient depends upon many variables. It is a serious mistake to know only one operation and do it on every patient regardless of the circumstances. And remember always the admonition of John Burch that the golden rule of pelvic surgery is the conservation of useful function—for example, the conservation of normal ovaries at the time of hysterectomy in most premenopausal women.

When indicated, alternatives to surgical therapy should be offered. As an advocate for patients and as a guardian of professional integrity and responsibility, gynecologic surgeons must insist on working in a proper health care environment, evaluate the results of care carefully, and change indications for surgery and surgical techniques as warranted and based on valid data. New methods and innovations in surgical therapy must be subjected to proper analysis before adopted as standard practice. Arrangements should be made for long-term follow-up to determine the results of treatment. As Dr. Te Linde was fond of saying, "Never take a young gynecologic surgeon's opinion about the value of a new operation because he/she has not yet been able to follow patients long enough."

Although the decision to operate may at times seem complicated, it can be simplified. According to Dr. J.M.T. Finney, there are only three valid reasons to operate:

- To save life (as in ruptured ectopic pregnancy, cervical cancer, etc.)
- To relieve suffering (as in pain from endometriosis, urinary incontinence, etc.)
- To correct significant anatomical deformities (as in uterine prolapse, Meyer-Rokitansky-Kuster-Hauser Syndrome, etc.)

Now, modern gynecologic surgery can offer a fourth reason to operate:

- To allow the creation of life (as in tubal reconstructive surgery, various *in vitro* fertilization operations, etc.)

This is an indication that is unique to gynecologic surgery and a great gift to humankind.

If, in making the decision to operate, one cannot fit the patient into one of these categories, perhaps the decision is wrong and needs review, and even review by a consultant.

Te Linde's Operative Gynecology will help the gynecologic surgeon learn the important details of performing procedures correctly. More importantly, it will help the gynecologic surgeon learn how to evaluate patients correctly. Today, such great emphasis is placed on learning to use new technology and new instruments that basic fundamentals of clinical evaluation of the patient care are forgotten or ignored. The greatest improvements in the practice of gynecologic surgery will come from listening to the patient rather than mastering new technology. In my judgment, the absolutely most important chapter ever written about gynecologic surgery is Chapter 3 on Psychosocial Aspects of Pelvic Surgery, written first by Dr. Malcolm Freeman and now by Dr. Betty Ruth Speir. This chapter should be required reading for anyone practicing gynecologic surgery.

And what of the future? Gynecologic surgery is a dynamic field of medicine, always changing to benefit the health of women by curing or alleviating the symptoms of gynecologic disease. We can expect exciting new developments in the 21st century, although it will be difficult for the next century to exceed the fantastic progress made in the last century. Gynecologic surgery will change and benefit because the future of biomedical science is wide open. Incredible discoveries in the past 50 years will inevitably effect gynecologic surgery, discoveries including massive improvements in technology, new and better vaccines, stem-cell research, DNA research, nanoscience, etc. We can look forward to new developments such as the implantation of a tissue-engineered product which, once implanted, slowly disappears while the host replaces it with his or her own tissue. The knowledge and skills required of gynecologic surgeons will be completely different by the end of the 21st century.

In the current tenth edition, each chapter is well written, well illustrated, easy to read and understand, and comprehensive yet specific, with the most modern, up-to-date information. It is hard to imagine a more thorough review of gynecologic surgery. It is also hard to imagine anyone who plans to learn, practice, and teach gynecologic surgery without this textbook. It can be used as a ready reference, a ready consultant with ease. It can be considered as a partner or companion in practice.

All who contributed to this new edition of *Te Linde's* deserve our congratulations for a job well done. It will be a great help to those who work to improve and maintain the quality of life for women.

John D. Thompson, MD

PREFACE

The rapid pace of the introduction of new surgical techniques for the treatment of gynecologic disease has required the timely revision of *Te Linde's Operative Gynecology*. Until 1992 the text was revised every 7 to 9 years. Since then the interval to revision has significantly shortened to 4 to 5 years due to the rapid advances in the field of surgery. Dr. Richard Te Linde wrote the first edition. Today up to 72 contributors have shared their personal insights and surgical approaches for the treatment to improve the health of women. *Te Linde's Operative Gynecology* has been, and hopefully will continue to be, a major influence in maintaining and improving the quality of gynecologic surgery.

The tenth edition of *Te Linde's Operative Gynecology* presents the basic, sound principles for established gynecologic surgical technique. Major advances in the field of education of the gynecologic surgeon and the changing environment in which we practice gynecologic surgery are presented. John Deutsh, P. L. Malone, Leon Schlossburg, and others have contributed excellent medical illustrations throughout the last 10 editions. We appreciate the new medical illustrations prepared by Jennifer Smith in Chapters 17, Diagnostic and Operative Laparoscopy; 19, Control of Pelvic Hemorrhage; 23, Surgical Conditions of the Vulva; 32A, Abdominal Hysterectomy; 32C, Laparoscopic Hysterectomy; 34, Ectopic Pregnancy; 35A, Obstetric Problems; 36C, Paravaginal Defect Repair; 36D, Posterior Compartment Defects; 37, Stress Urinary Incontinence; 43, Intestinal Tract in Gynecologic Surgery; 50, Pelvic Exenteration; and 51, Surgical Reconstruction of the Pelvis in Gynecologic Cancer Patients; and by Joe Chovan in Chapter 18, Operative Hysteroscopy. The addition of color to the text offsets important figures and tables.

In view of the major focus on best surgical practices in surgical specialties, we have introduced a new section in each chapter that discusses the major take-home points. These best surgical practices present the opinion of the authors. Each clinical situation is unique, and readers should exercise their professional judgment accordingly. The information presented in the best practices is educational in nature and not a set of guidelines for use in any given situation. The authors, editors, and publisher are not responsible for errors or omissions or for any consequences from application of this or any other information in this book and make no warranty, expressed or implied, with respect to the contents of the publication.

Also new to this edition are definitions, which have been added as a part of the introduction of each chapter. The self-test questions in the Appendix have been revised and will allow the reader to "self test" after reviewing a specific topic. Perhaps more importantly, the editors have added for the first time a DVD of several surgical procedures previously introduced as "surgery in the retroperitoneal space," with accompanying text. Hopefully this will be a regular feature of future editions and will add an appreciation of the "Art of Surgical Techniques."

The authors wish to sincerely thank all the contributors and gratefully acknowledge the assistance of Barbara Schmitt, Lynne Black, Patsy Shepard, and the Lippincott Williams & Wilkins editorial team of Sonya Seigafuse, Ryan Shaw, Nicole Dernoski, Mark Flanders, and Rosanne Hallowell for their attention to details and hard work in the preparation of this book. As always, we are deeply indebted to those authors and editors who have labored to write the previous editions of this text. The current edition would not exist without their dedication. We owe a sincere debt of gratitude to Drs. Richard W. TeLinde, Richard F. Mattingly, and John D. Thompson.

John A. Rock, MD
Howard W. Jones, III, MD

SECTION I ■ GENERAL TOPICS AFFECTING GYNECOLOGIC SURGERY PRACTICE

CHAPTER 1 ■ OPERATIVE GYNECOLOGY BEFORE THE ERA OF LAPAROSCOPY: A BRIEF HISTORY

GERT H. BRIEGER AND HOWARD W. JONES, Jr.

Gynecology, spelled *gynaecology*, is defined by the Oxford English Dictionary as "that department of medical science which treats of the functions and diseases peculiar to women." The word was first used as such in the middle of the 19th century. In 1867, gynecology represented the physiology and pathology of the nonpregnant state. Although most histories of gynecology trace its roots back to antiquity, the field of medicine we call by that name today really has had a fairly recent origin. The successful removal of an ovarian tumor by Ephraim McDowell in 1809 was as rare an event as it was a spectacular one. In the preceding centuries, the history of gynecologic surgery was closely tied to the history of general surgery, and the obstacles that had to be overcome were the same. Infection, hemorrhage and shock, and pain were all effective barriers to any but emergency surgical procedures in the days before anesthesia.

"The history of gynecology," Howard Kelly wrote in 1912, "seems to me more full of dramatic interest than the evolution of any other medical or surgical specialty." Himself an accomplished historian of medicine, among his many other skills, Kelly noted that, "It was, notably, anesthesia which robbed surgery of its horrors, asepsis which robbed it of its dangers, and cellular pathology which came as a godsend to enable the operator to discriminate between malignant and non-malignant growths." Here, in a nutshell, we have the landmarks of much of the history of gynecology of the last 150 years. Ann Dally was correct when she noted that until recently, much of what has been written about the history of gynecology was written by gynecologists themselves, who picked their own heroes. With the rise of the new history of women and the social history of medicine since the 1970s, a much more balanced view has emerged.

There are many ways to approach the history of a medical and surgical specialty such as gynecology. The usual practice in textbooks that make an attempt to include some history is to tell the story in terms of who discovered what and who did which operation first. These facts are of interest but hardly constitute the history of the field. Besides the surgical operations of gynecology, the techniques devised, and the instruments to carry them out, there is much to be learned from the changing picture of diseases and their diagnoses; from the professionalization of the field, including the societies, journals, and textbooks that have been created; and from the education required to master the science and practice of operative gynecology. It is in these terms, rather than in tracing simply the great ideas and their creators, that this historical introduction proceeds.

Any major medical textbook can itself serve as a convenient window through which we can see history unfold. Robert Hahn has vividly described the changing world view of obstetrics by examining the succeeding editions of *Williams' Obstetrics* since its first edition in 1903. Likewise, the 50 years that have elapsed since the first edition of Richard Wesley Te Linde's *Operative Gynecology* provide an equal opportunity to describe the major developments in the companion field of gynecology.

BARRIERS TO SURGICAL PROGRESS

In ancient times, the lack of real anatomic knowledge was a barrier to the development of surgery. It is sometimes said that because the ancient Egyptians had effective techniques for the evisceration of bodies for mummification, they must have had a good knowledge of the body. However, removal of the internal organs during the embalming process was performed by technicians who did not concern themselves with the structure of the bodies they were preparing.

Anatomy was pursued in Alexandria during the Hellenistic period, but it had few, if any, practical applications until a later time. By the end of the 13th century, anatomic dissection again became more common, but often it was limited to one or two public dissections a year or the study of animals. Surgeons were responsible for the few autopsies that were performed to determine the cause of death. This was especially important if a crime was suspected or drowning had to be established.

Soranus, the Roman physician and writer who practiced in the reign of the Emperors Trajan (98–117) and Hadrian (117–138), is perhaps best known for his text entitled *Gynecology*. This book is somewhat mistitled because it is mostly devoted to what we would call obstetrics. Soranus wrote about prenatal and postnatal problems, as well as those associated with delivery itself. This ancient text has been translated and has an excellent introduction by Owsei Temkin. Recently, it has been reissued in a paperback edition.

Although Soranus's *Gynecology* still makes interesting reading, it hardly qualifies as an early text on the subject of operative gynecology. However, like other physicians of his time, Soranus clearly noted that the best midwife was one who was trained in all branches of therapy, "... for some cases must be treated by diet, others by surgery, while still others must be cured by drugs."

Although there were instances of anatomical study in earlier times, we generally begin the story with the work of Andreas Vesalius and the publication of his *De humani corporis fabrica* in 1543. Before this time, anatomic knowledge was not tied to the teaching and practice of medicine. The tradition of the surgeon-anatomists, of whom Vesalius was a stellar example, culminated in the late 18th century with the work of the English surgical teacher John Hunter (1728–1793) and his older brother William (1718–1783). It was William's classic book about the gravid uterus with its detailed engravings that shed new light on the structures of the female pelvis.

In the 19th century, for all types of surgery, the problems of pain, hemorrhage, and infection had to be solved before operations could be undertaken safely. The problems of surgical dressings and postoperative infections were generally a matter of trial and error. The Scottish surgeon and gynecologist Sir James Simpson (1811–1870) urged his surgical colleagues to perform their operations on the kitchen tables of their patients to avoid the dangers of hospital infections, or "hospitalism" as it came to be called.

In the 1840s, the Hungarian obstetrician Ignaz Semmelweis (1818–1865) showed clearly that puerperal fever could be prevented by disinfecting the hands of doctors before they examined their patients during the course of delivery. Despite good statistical evidence, his method of washing hands in chlorinated lime solution was not widely adopted. In fact, it met with outright resistance from most physicians. In this country, the Harvard anatomist and writer Oliver Wendell Holmes (1809–1894) met similar disbelief and resistance when he suggested in 1842 that it was the physicians themselves who were carrying the dreaded puerperal infections to their patients.

In the middle 1860s, Joseph Lister (1827–1912), while working in Glasgow, began experiments using carbolic acid, a phenol derivative, to clean the instruments, sutures, and dressings he was using in his operations. He based his work on an understanding of the germ theory of disease, which was then just in its infancy as a major theory of disease causation. Lister believed it was important to prevent the germs present in the air or on instruments and sutures from entering the wound, which would prevent the formation of the heretofore much desired laudable pus. Lister, too, met much opposition to his method of antisepsis. Partly because of the frequent changes in the system he was developing, which made it difficult for others to follow him, and because of the inadequate understanding of the germ theory by most surgeons, it took nearly two decades for antiseptic surgery to become routine. In Lister's case, as was also true for Holmes and Semmelweis, some of the resistance undoubtedly stemmed from the fact that doctors never like being told that what they are doing is actually causing harm to their patients.

Lister encountered a great deal of opposition, particularly in his own country. Lawson Tait (1845–1899), an active and polemical gynecologist who settled in Birmingham, was staunchly opposed to Lister's system of antisepsis. Tait paid much attention to general cleanliness when he was operating, and he actually achieved quite good results. However, his older colleague, Spencer Wells (1818–1897) of London, was a devoted follower of the antiseptic system in his many ovarian operations, perhaps because he had a clear grasp of the role of microbes. In 1864, the year before Lister began using carbolic acid in Glasgow and 3 years before he published his first results, Wells published a paper in the *British Medical Journal* entitled "Some Causes of Excessive Mortality after Surgical Operations." Wells clearly described the recent work on germs by Louis Pasteur (1822–1895) in France. There is no definite proof that Lister was aware of the paper, but it is hard to imagine that he did not know what was appearing in the national medical journal. Thus, gynecologists probably had a much greater hand in the development of safe surgery in the last century than is usually acknowledged.

BEGINNINGS OF GYNECOLOGIC SURGERY IN 19TH-CENTURY AMERICA

Opening the abdominal cavity to remove extrauterine pregnancies was successfully accomplished several times in the later 18th century but did not become routine until the advent of anesthesia and antisepsis/asepsis. Ephraim McDowell (1771–1830) (Fig. 1.1) made surgical history with his successful removal of a large ovarian cyst in his patient Jane Todd Crawford, who in 1809 rode 60 miles to her doctor's house in Danville, Kentucky, to undergo an untried operation without any assurance of cure and without the benefit of anesthesia. Although McDowell is often referred to as a backwoods physician, he was in fact a well-trained surgeon. His Edinburgh training probably gave him confidence in his diagnosis and courage to attempt a surgical cure rather than have his patient face certain death from her relentlessly growing tumor. During his study tour in Scotland, he probably heard that in the previous century, the popular surgical teacher John Hunter had suggested such an operation, believing that "women could bear spaying just as well as did animals."

The drama of McDowell's case is best described in the words of the surgeon himself:

> In December, 1809, I was called to see a Mrs. Crawford, who had for several months thought herself pregnant. She was affected with pains similar to labor pains, from which she could find no relief. So strong was the presumption of her being in the last stage of pregnancy, that two physicians, who were consulted on her case, requested my aid in delivering her. The abdomen was considerably enlarged, and had the appearance of pregnancy, though the inclination of the tumor was to one side, admitting of an easy removal to the other. Upon examination, per vaginum, I found nothing in the uterus; which induced the conclusion that it must be an enlarged ovarium. Having never seen so large a substance extracted, nor heard of an attempt, or success attending any operation, such as this required, I gave to the unhappy woman information of her

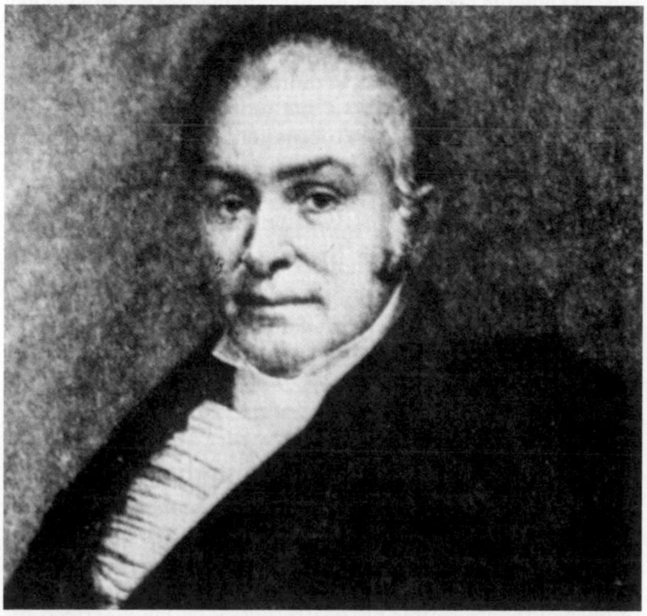

FIGURE 1.1. Ephraim McDowell (1771–1830). One of the earliest abdominal surgeons.

> dangerous situation. She appeared willing to undergo an experiment, which I promised to perform if she would come to Danville.... With the assistance of my nephew and colleague, James McDowell, M.D., I commenced the operation, which was concluded as follows: Having placed her on a table of the ordinary height, on her back, and removed all her dressing which might in any way impede the operation, I made an incision about three inches from the musculus rectus abdominis, on the left side, continuing the same nine inches in length, parallel with the fibers of the above named muscle, extending into the cavity of the abdomen, the parietes of which were a good deal contused, which we ascribed to the resting of the tumor on the horn of the saddle during her journey. The tumor then appeared in full view, but was so large that we could not take it away entire. We put a strong ligature around the fallopian tube near to the uterus; we then cut open the tumor, which was the ovarium and fibrinous part of the fallopian tube very much enlarged. We took out fifteen pounds of a dirty, gelatinous looking substance. After which we cut through the fallopian tube, and extracted the sack, which weighed seven pounds and one half. As soon as the external opening was made, the intestines rushed out upon the table; and so completely was the abdomen filled by the tumor, that they could not be replaced during the operation, which was terminated in about twenty-five minutes. We then turned her upon her left side, so as to permit the blood to escape; after which, we closed the external opening with the interrupted suture, leaving out, at the lower end of the incision, the ligature which surrounded the fallopian tube. Between every two stitches we put a strip of adhesive plaster, which, by keeping the parts in contact, hastened the healing of the incision. We then applied the usual dressing, put her to bed, and prescribed a strict observance of the antiphlogistic regimen. In five days I visited her, and much to my astonishment found her engaged in making up her bed. I gave her particular caution for the future; and in twenty five days, she returned home as she came, in good health, which she continues to enjoy.

McDowell's patient long outlived her surgeon. He did not publish his feat until 1816, by which time he had performed several more oophorectomies. McDowell is sometimes cited as a pioneer of early ambulation, unwitting as it was in his case. If his sturdy patient had not recovered so well, her failure would surely have been blamed on rising too early from her bed after such extensive surgery. McDowell also did not mention the intense drama of this Christmas day operation. When the townsfolk of Danville heard about his plan, they were incensed. They gathered in a tense group outside his house, with a rope slung over a tree, ready to lynch the surgeon if his "experiment" proved a failure. McDowell certainly had the nature of a true pioneer.

T. G. Thomas, in his 1876 centennial review of obstetrics and gynecology, reported that Alexander Dunlap of Springfield, Ohio, claimed he did his first ovarian operation in 1843. Dunlap said he sent the report of this case to a medical journal, which sent it back to him saying that they "could not publish the case of such an unjustifiable operation."

By 1876, Thomas wrote, "It is to estimate the amount of good this operation has bestowed upon humanity. Practised today in every civilized country in the world, yielding the statistics of seventy to seventy-five per cent of recoveries, and daily being improved in its various steps, it may well be regarded as one of the greatest surgical triumphs of the century."

In the middle decades of the 19th century, another American surgeon working in the South helped to popularize gynecologic surgery by another set of pioneering feats. James Marion Sims (1813–1883) told the dramatic tale of his development of a successful technique to repair vesicovaginal fistulas in his widely read autobiography *The Story of My Life*, which was published the year after his death (Fig. 1.2). He described his repeated attempts to achieve a permanent closure of these fistulas in a few of his young slave-women patients. Sims began

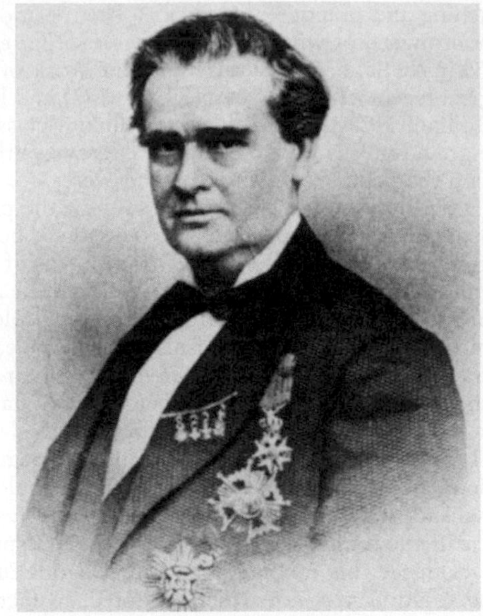

FIGURE 1.2. James Marion Sims (1813–1883).

his experiments in 1845 and continued them for 4 years. In these preanesthesia and preantiseptic days, Sims produced remarkable results. He had had no experience in pelvic surgery, and in fact claimed that he disliked it. It was his custom to turn away patients with pelvic disorders, referring them to other doctors in his Alabama neighborhood. Many of his planter friends owned slaves, some of whom suffered from vesicovaginal fistulas as a result of traumatic births. These wounds were considered incurable and made the young women unacceptable for household work. After several entreaties to help one of his planter friends who had such a slave, Sims began with a small group of women, operating on some of them repeatedly over the course of 4 years.

Sims's many failures only increased his determination to succeed. The colleagues who at first assisted him at the operations abandoned him, and his friends, he claimed, begged him to give up what was considered to be a hopeless effort. He trained other young slave patients to assist him, and on his 29th operation on one of the patients, he finally succeeded. In reviewing his work in 1852, Sims did cite several successful cases by other American surgeons between 1839 and 1849. He claimed originality for:

> 1st. for the discovery of a method by which the vagina can be thoroughly explored, and the operation easily performed [the Sims, or lateral, position]. 2nd. For the introduction of a new suture apparatus, which lies imbedded in the tissues for an indefinite period without danger of cutting its way out, as do silk ligatures. And 3rd. For the invention of a self-retaining catheter, which can be worn with the greatest comfort by the patient during the whole process of treatment.

The new "suture apparatus" used silver wire. This provided the breakthrough needed for the successful repair of vesicovaginal fistulae. Sims used silver in many of his other operations. In a 10th anniversary lecture at the New York Academy of Medicine in 1857, Sims somewhat immodestly told his august audience that the use of silver suture was one of the great achievements of 19th-century surgery. Sims wrote and spoke frequently about his development of a successful procedure for the definitive cure of vesicovaginal fistula, but never more eloquently than in his Anniversary Address in November

1857, in which he described his work with silver sutures over the previous 12 years. The audience included several past presidents of the academy and most of the distinguished colleagues at the Woman's Hospital. After four years of fruitless effort, Sims proclaimed a new dawn on 21 June 1849. Since that day, he claimed, he had used no other suture in any of his surgical work.

It is worth noting that Sims's early patients—the slave women of Montgomery, Alabama, and the poor Irish servant girls who were predominant patients of the Woman's Hospital in New York—were equally vulnerable, so it is not hard to see why some recent historians have been very critical of Sims and his coworkers. Yet with the advent of anesthesia and the use of antiseptic techniques, such surgery became increasingly routine. The repair of vesicovaginal fistulas and the removal of ovaries for a wide variety of indications were the beginning of the field of operative gynecology as it is known today. The story is, of course, not purely an American one. The English, French, and German contributions were important and can be found in any general history of medicine or of obstetrics and gynecology. In 1876, Sims became president of the American Medical Association, and in the same year, he and others founded the American Gynecological Association.

Even with the advent of effective and relatively safe anesthesia after 1846, it was several decades before surgeons were ready to increase the number of their operations. At midcentury and during the Civil War in the 1860s, surgery was generally confined to amputations after accidents; hernia repair when the intestine became incarcerated in the hernia sac, thus threatening life; an occasional ligation of a major vessel for aneurysm; and cystotomy for bladder stones. Therefore, Sims, operating in the 1840s, was truly a pioneer.

Also pioneers in the field of gynecologic surgery by midcentury were the Atlee brothers of Lancaster, Pennsylvania. They rediscovered oophorectomy, which was also being done in England by the 1860s, and were among the early leaders who performed myomectomy for fibroid tumors of the uterus.

Of semantic interest is the changing terminology for ovarian surgery. *Ovariotomy,* often used imprecisely to refer to removal of the ovary, actually was first used in that way in the 1850s by James Simpson and other British gynecologists. Ovariotomy means to cut into the ovary for removal of a cyst or tumor. In the 1870s, gynecologists such as Edmund Peaslee of New York, in his book on ovarian tumors, stated that *oophorectomy* was a more precise and distinctive term for removal of the ovary.

John Light Atlee (1799–1885) actively practiced medicine for 65 years, during which time he performed more than 2,000 operations and attended 3,200 births. John Atlee performed 78 ovarian operations between 1843 and 1883, with 64 recoveries and only 14 deaths. Thus, he validated McDowell's work of the early part of the 19th century. Atlee's younger brother, Washington Lemuel Atlee (1808–1878) (Fig. 1.3), also was involved in some of the ovarian cases, but deserves separate credit for being one of the first to successfully treat the problem of uterine leiomyomata.

The Atlee brothers were relatively conservative gynecologic surgeons. It was their careful approach coupled with their obvious successes that gave other surgeons increasing confidence to operate. Thus, they played an important role in the early stages of operative gynecology as it developed into the specialty it would become in the next generation. Ovariotomy, the most controversial of gynecologic procedures, was also the key to making it a surgical specialty. Indeed, some gynecologists claimed that operating for ovarian cysts and tumors laid the groundwork for all abdominal surgery in the last decades of the 19th century.

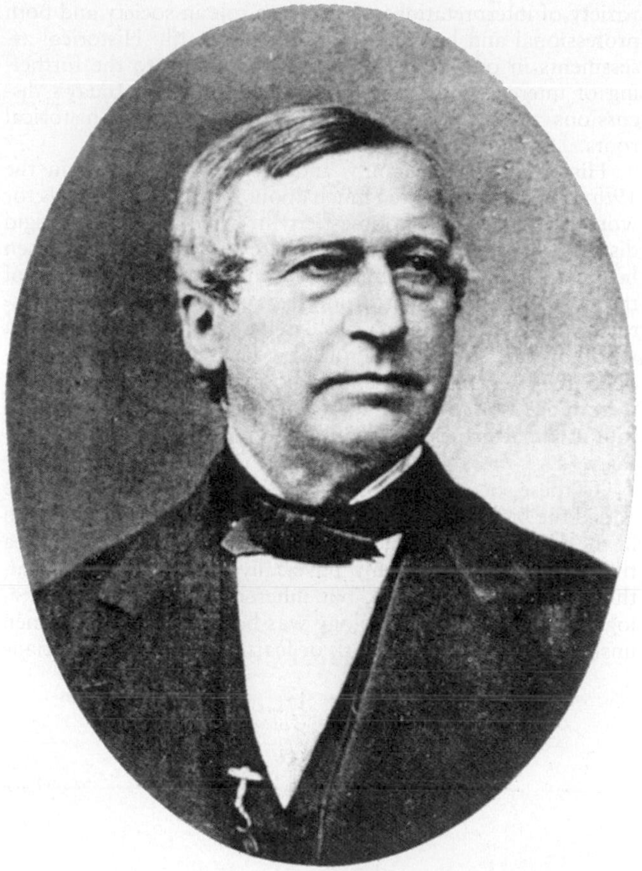

FIGURE 1.3. Washington Lemuel Atlee (1808–1878).

By the 1880s, the specialty of gynecology, or the science of women, as some historians have called it, was well on its way to being established as one of the subdivisions of medical labor. Ornella Moscucci, in her perceptive history of gynecology in Britain, quotes the eminent surgeon from Birmingham, Lawson Tait, in his aptly entitled book of 1889, *Diseases of Women and Abdominal Surgery:*

> The great function of woman's life has for years made her the subject of specialists, male and female, the obstetricians. The subsidiary relations of her special organs and the special requirements of her physique, based upon these, have necessitated the establishment of another class of specialist, the gynecologist.

WOMEN AS PATIENTS IN THE 19TH CENTURY

The growth of interest in women's diseases began long before the 19th century. In the Renaissance, for instance, the publication of a large, encyclopedic work entitled *Gynaecia*, by Caspar Wolf (1532–1601), and later similar collections represented what had been written since antiquity. The mere existence of such texts, however, does not mean that much attention was given to the treatment of women, except as it related to childbirth.

Any discussion of the treatment of women's diseases since the latter half of the 19th century must take into account a variety of interpretations of women's role in society and both professional and lay views of women's health. Historical assessments in our own time have contributed to the furthering of interest in the issues of women's health. Today's discussions are best understood in the light of their historical roots.

Historians of the family and the role of women in the 19th century have written much about the separate spheres for women and the cult of domesticity in which there was a rigid distinction between the home, where it was thought women belonged, and the economic world outside. Thus, the "cult of true womanhood," as historians have called it, made sharp distinctions between women's place in the family and the working world of men. As the social role of women was increasingly defined, they were, in a sense, held hostage in the home. Women were judged by the male world and themselves according to four cardinal virtues: piety, purity, submissiveness, and domesticity.

To these social distinctions between men and women were added the biologic differences. The biologic notions of women in the 19th century ranged widely, but they included the idea that women were not only physically weaker than men (although morally superior), but inherently diseased or pathologic. Their cyclical physiology was believed to make women unsuitable for sustained work or learning. Feminist historians of recent times have taken doctors of an earlier era to task for casting women as frail creatures entirely dependent on their biology, destined to be kept from the male world of education, politics, the professions, and any but domestic work. As Ornella Moscucci points out, however, the medical ideas about the social destiny of women were far more complex than has been assumed.

On both sides of the Atlantic, the view of Victorian women was influenced by the writings of eminent physicians. In Boston, a Harvard Medical School professor, Edward H. Clarke (1820–1877), wrote a book in 1873 entitled *Sex in Education; or, A Fair Chance for the Girls.* This book was widely reviewed and discussed. Similarly, Henry Maudsley (1835–1918) in England, an influential psychiatrist and medical teacher, also wrote about the supposed harm of higher education on the physiologic development of postpubescent girls. Clarke's book, which has become known as a uterine manifesto, clearly set the brain and the uterus in opposition. Higher education, Clarke claimed, might be good for developing the intellect, but that occurred at the expense of the reproductive organs, thus dooming the woman to a state of stunted womanhood and lifelong invalidism.

Sex in Education went through 17 printings and editions in the space of a few years. Because of its popularity and notoriety, it is worth citing one of Clarke's case reports:

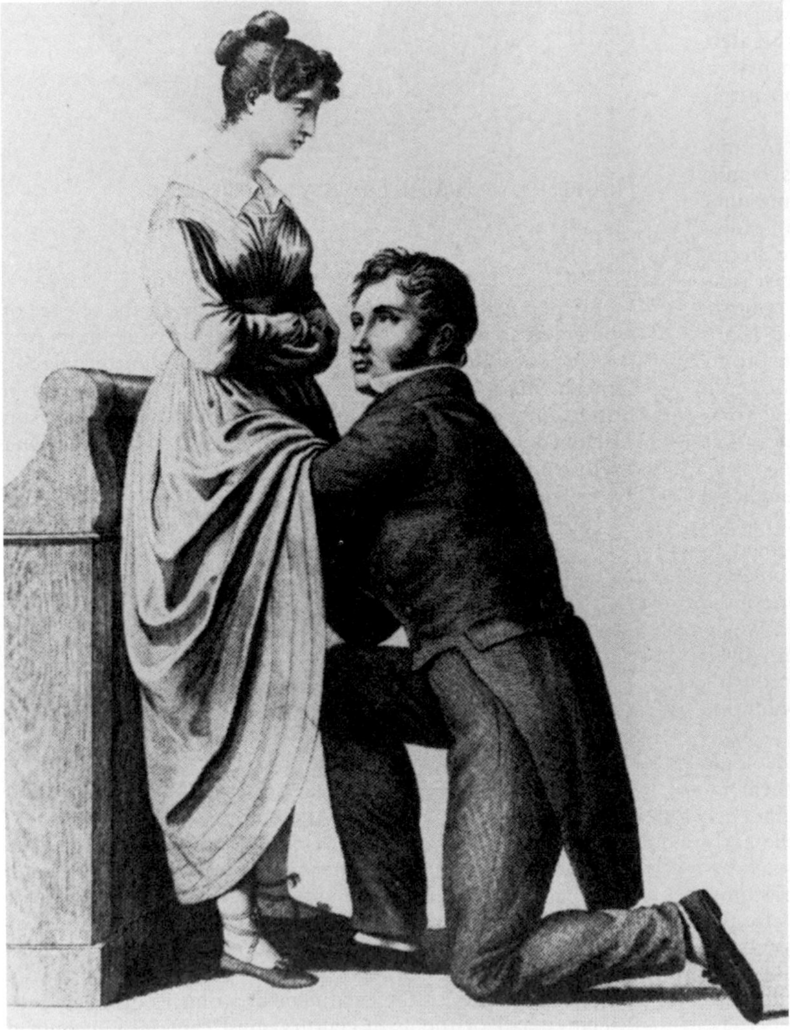

FIGURE 1.4. This famous illustration of "the touch" in a gynecologic examination is from a 19th-century French text frequently used in America. Note the avoidance of eye contact between doctor and patient and the dress shielding the woman's body from view. (From: Wertz RW, Wertz DC. *Lying-in: a history of childbirth in America,* expanded edition. New Haven, CT: Yale University Press, 1989:78, with permission.)

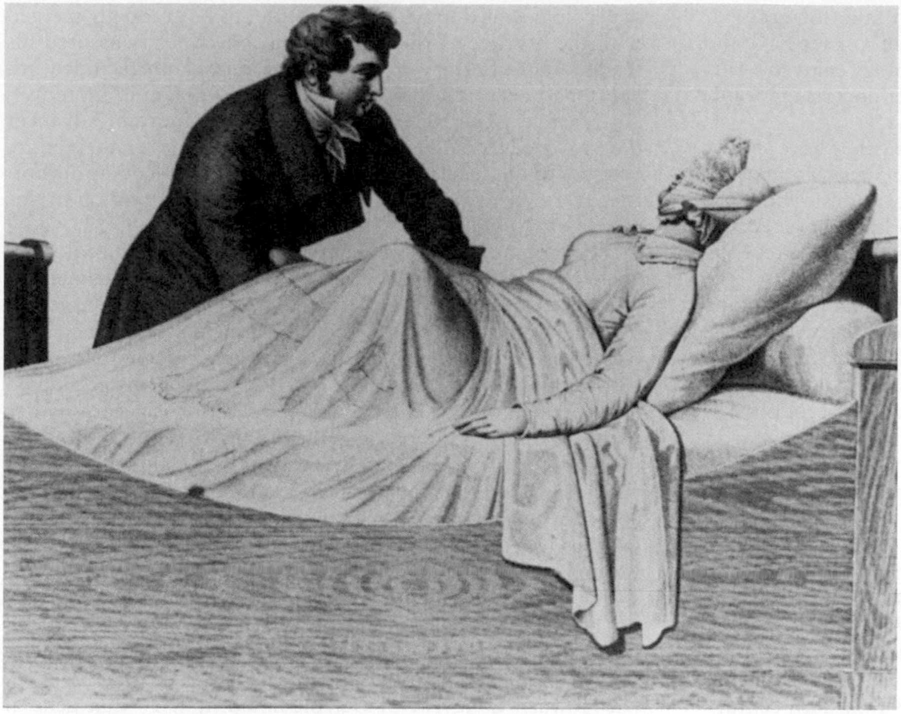

FIGURE 1.5. This 19th-century drawing illustrates another technique for preserving the patient's modesty: The doctor conducting a gynecologic examination looks directly into the woman's eyes to assure her that her private parts are safe from his gaze. (From: Wertz RW, Wertz DC. *Lying-in: a history of childbirth in America, expanded edition.* New Haven, CT: Yale University Press, 1989:84, with permission.)

> Miss D—went to college in good physical condition. During the four years of her college life, her parents and the college faculty required her to get what is popularly called an education. Nature required her, during the same period, to build and put in working order a large and complicated reproductive mechanism a matter that is popularly ignored—shoved out of sight like a disgrace. She naturally obeyed the requirements of the faculty, which she could see, rather than the requirements of the mechanism within her, that she could not see. Subjected to the college regimen, she worked four years in getting a liberal education. Her way of work was sustained and continuous, and out of harmony with the rhythmical periodicity of the female organization. The stream of vital and constructive force evolved within her was turned steadily to the brain, and away from the ovaries and their accessories. The result of this sort of education was, that these last-mentioned organs, deprived of sufficient opportunity and nutriment, first began to perform their functions with pain, a warning of error that was unheeded; then, to cease to grow; ... And so Miss D—spent the few years next succeeding her graduation in conflict with dysmenorrhea, headache, neuralgia, and hysteria.

Many writings in the 1870s and 1880s attempted to refute the medical notions of physicians such as Clarke and Maudsley. In this country, Mary Putnam Jacobi (1842–1906), a physician and future champion of women in higher education and the professions, submitted a prize-winning essay that refuted Clarke's contentions that work by the brain interfered with uterine function and the menses. In Britain, the pioneer woman-physician Elizabeth Garrett Anderson (1836–1917) claimed that it was boredom that caused the medical symptoms of middle-class women, not higher education.

By the middle of the 19th century, even the use of the speculum as a diagnostic instrument stirred controversy. The speculum was known to the ancients, but it fell into disuse by the early modern period. Early in the 19th century, Joseph Recamier (1774–1852) reintroduced it in Paris, and soon the speculum was routinely used in treating inflammatory disease. It was also used in the routine examination of prostitutes in France and England.

In the Victorian climate of concern about women and their diseases, as well as their moral sensibilities, vaginal examinations were not routine. When they were performed, great efforts were made to preserve the patient's privacy and dignity, as the accompanying illustrations show (Figs. 1.4 and 1.5). A battle over the morality of the use of the speculum also ensued. The speculum, opponents of its use believed, could lead to sexual stimulation and sexual excesses. The term "speculum rape" was used in the debates over the Contagious Disease Acts in England in the 1860s.

Meanwhile, the surgeons went about debating the advisability of oophorectomy. One of the most prominent proponents of ovarian surgery for symptoms not just associated with demonstrable ovarian disease was an American surgeon named Robert Battey (1828–1895) of Georgia. In 1872, he removed the ovaries of a 32-year-old woman who had claimed invalidism for 16 years. Battey reported that his patient was cured after the bilateral oophorectomy. (Cured of *what* remains the intriguing question.) In succeeding years, the Battey operation became popular with some surgeons. Battey himself tried a vaginal approach to the ovaries but soon reverted to abdominal section. He advocated bilateral removal of the ovaries, whether or not they revealed any sign of disease, to ameliorate menstrual difficulties or psychological symptoms.

With historical examples such as the Battey operation, it is no surprise that feminist historians today level charges of male physicians' exploitation of their female patients. One of the most drastic charges claimed that most of the gynecologic surgery of the late 19th century was a calculated plot against women, a tacit conspiracy between insecure husbands and anxious gynecologists.

Ann Douglas, a literary historian and feminist, was one of the earliest to invoke the notion of a conspiracy of male physicians to subject their female patients to mutilating, harmful, and unnecessary surgery. She simply dismissed 19th-century doctors as ignorant because they did not receive the kind of medical training we have now come to take for granted. However, because the physician of 1870 did not yet have the understanding of physiology or pathophysiology enjoyed by his colleagues a century later, calling most earlier doctors ignorant, callous, or worse was not warranted.

Those with a less conspiratorial view of history have shown that other views of both husbands and male physicians existed in the late part of the last century. The economist Thorstein Veblen, for instance, believed that nonworking wives served as status symbols for their husbands rather than as threats or temptations to eager surgeons.

Women learned and taught surgery, including gynecologic procedures, at the Women's Medical College of Pennsylvania from its founding in 1850. But it is also fair to say that there were few women actively practicing gynecologic surgery until well into this century. A notable exception was Mary Dixon Jones of Brooklyn, who by the 1890s had won respect from her male colleagues. Her story has recently been told by Regina Morantz-Sanchez, whose observations of Dixon Jones's career help us to understand how a woman made it in a man's world. Morantz-Sanchez, in her book about the libel trial of Dixon-Jones in the early 1890s, charts the development of gynecologic surgery as a specialty. Dixon-Jones was unusual because she was a successful woman-surgeon, but also because she was on the cusp of the developments in gynecology and its evolution from a field that viewed women in their social as well as their biological roles to a 20th-century surgical specialty that concentrated on the pathology of diseased organs and the most appropriate and effective surgical techniques.

Morantz-Sanchez nicely illustrates this evolution of gynecology by framing the developments by the textbooks of Thomas Addis Emmet and J. C. Skene of the 1880s, still using the language of women as "other" than men, with the 1909 text of Howard Kelly and Charles Noble, *Gynecology and Abdominal Surgery,* in which there is no discussion of women's social roles because the focus is on surgical technique. Thus, the language of medicine can be used to trace the changes in medicine itself.

THE RELATION BETWEEN SURGERY AND GYNECOLOGY

The complex relation between general surgery and gynecology played a continuing role in the professional definition of gynecology as a 20th-century specialty. Moreover, several important contributions to surgery, such as chloroform anesthesia, rubber gloves, and early ambulation, were influenced by gynecologists as well as surgeons. The latter two items are discussed subsequently.

By 1905, the Chicago gynecologist Franklin H. Martin (1857–1935) was convinced that the three closely allied fields—surgery, gynecology, and obstetrics—were making sufficient progress to warrant a new journal. There was a shared feeling, Martin wrote in the opening editorial of *Surgery, Gynecology, and Obstetrics,* "... that the field of the three allied specialties represented by its title is not over-cultivated, and that there is already a place for a creditable magazine representing in one publication these three divisions of surgery."

Another of the founding editors of the journal, the gynecologist J. Clarence Webster, wrote a provocative editorial in the first issue on "The Future of Gynecology." Webster firmly laid to rest an idea that had gained some acceptance by 1905—that gynecology was doomed to extinction, to be gradually merged with the practice of the general surgeon. Webster assured his readers that contrary to what some had claimed, much advance had occurred in the preceding decades, and, moreover, "... it is very evident that almost all the important advances have resulted from the work of men who have given their entire energies to the specialty. At the present day the leading authorities everywhere are those who still limit their attention to this sphere of work."

In a programmatic statement to the American Gynecological Society in 1920, Robert L. Dickinson (1861–1950) contended that gynecologists promote surgery. "But if we be just surgeons, by surgeons we may be displaced." In this presidential address to the society, Dickinson claimed that gynecologic procedures constituted one-fourth of all surgery, but this hardly accounted for the extent of the field, "... since operation is needed by less than one-tenth of the patients that come to the doctor for ailments peculiar to women (childbearing not included)." It was true, of course, that for much of the preceding century, gynecology was a medical rather than a surgical discipline, often taught in medical schools as part of the course on diseases of women and children.

In the early decades of the 20th century, the professional battles between the general surgeons (who increasingly dominated the field of abdominal surgery) and the gynecologists (who wished to lay claim to the same territory) waxed and waned. Dr. Howard Longyear of Detroit noted in 1917 that general surgeons tended to scorn the area of the pelvis, whereas this area was being increasingly perfected by gynecologists. These surgeons wanted to move upward in the body from surgery of the female genitalia and the pelvis to the abdomen. Longyear also noted that the Sims operation for vesicovaginal fistula did more to establish operative gynecology as a specialty than did any other single procedure or development.

The complex relations between surgery and gynecology also can be traced by following the name changes in the American Medical Association specialty section. In 1903, at its founding, it was called Section on Obstetrics and Gynecology. From 1912 until 1936, it was called Section on Obstetrics, Gynecology, and Abdominal Surgery. Then the name was changed once again, dropping the abdominal surgery component.

One area of joint progress forged by surgeons and gynecologists was the introduction of the use of rubber gloves, which helped to expand the work of all surgeons. The idea of using some form of protective covering for the surgeon's hands occasionally appeared in the medical literature in the early decades of the 19th century, but it was not until the end of the century that some of the associates of Dr. William S. Halsted (1852–1922) at the Johns Hopkins Hospital in Baltimore began to use gloves routinely. About two decades after their introduction, Dr. Halsted recalled the story:

> In the winter of 1889 and 1890—I cannot recall the month—the nurse in charge of my operating room complained that the solutions of mercuric chloride produced a dermatitis of her arms and hands. As she was an unusually efficient woman, I gave the matter my consideration and one day in New York requested the Goodyear Rubber Company to make as an experiment two pair of thin rubber gloves with gauntlets. On trial these proved to be so satisfactory that additional gloves were ordered. In the autumn, on my return to town, the assistant who passed the instruments and threaded the needles was also provided with rubber gloves to wear at the operations. At first the operator wore them only when exploratory incisions into joints were made. After a time the assistants became so accustomed to working in gloves that they also wore them as operators and would remark that they

seemed to be less expert with the bare hands than with the gloved hands.

I think it was Dr. Bloodgood, my house surgeon, who first made this comment and that he was the first to wear them invariably, when operating. . . . Dr. Hunter Robb in 1894, in his book on aseptic technic recommended that the operator wear rubber gloves. Dr. Robb was, at that time, resident gynecologist of the Johns Hopkins Hospital and had frequent opportunities to observe the technic of the surgical clinic.

Gynecologists were also closely involved in the form of postoperative care we have now come to take for granted: early ambulation after surgery. With the change from 2 or 3 weeks of enforced bed rest after surgery to active ambulation within a few hours of the operation, we have improved recovery, shortened hospital stays, and reduced costs, as well as postoperative complications. But like all new techniques or practices, early rising after surgery did not win rapid acceptance.

Ephraim McDowell's patient in 1809 not only was ambulant early, but also engaged in physical tasks such as making her own bed. Her surgeon clearly was not pleased with her activity, which was not in keeping with customary and usual practices of the day.

What we call early ambulation was not found again in the medical literature until the very last year of the 19th century, when Emil Ries, a professor of gynecology in Chicago, published a landmark paper, which soon disappeared from view. It was rediscovered four decades later. Ries noted in his 1899 paper that he wanted to change treatment radically by freeing patients from "... many irksome and disagreeable features of convalescence following vaginal and abdominal surgery." Ries found that his patients could be fed and allowed out of bed much sooner than was the usual custom. "Very soon I found," he wrote, "that the period for which it was advisable to confine such cases to bed could be counted by hours instead of days, so that of late I have allowed my patients to get up within twenty-four to forty-eight hours and to leave the hospital four to six days after their vaginal celiotomy." These patients, Ries also noted, did not have the listlessness or muscular weakness that was usually seen after 2 or 3 weeks in bed.

In the preoperative preparation of his patients, Ries also went against the usual custom of completely emptying the bowel. Most textbooks, he said, claimed that early action of the bowels helped to prevent peritonitis. However, in most patients with an empty intestinal tract, regular movements did not resume until after they were eating a regular diet. Ries maintained that cause and effect were confused because it was not movement of the bowels that prevented peritonitis, but freedom from inflammation that allowed the bowels to move.

At the meeting of the Southern Surgical and Gynecological Society in Baltimore in 1906, H. J. Boldt described 384 cases of early ambulation that he had accumulated since 1890. All recovered well. Ironically, Boldt reported, the most serious objection raised by his colleagues was that early ambulation increased the risk of thrombosis. This was clearly wrong, he said, from both a theoretic and an empirical point of view, because his patients had a better circulation from exercising.

Early ambulation was discussed repeatedly in the succeeding decade, but it received far from universal acceptance. Even Howard Kelly, the country's leading teacher of gynecology, noted in 1911 that great progress was made as a result of Boldt's and Ries's work, but that it was far from standard practice. Early ambulation really became a routine practice with the exigencies of World War II (which resulted in a shortage of hospital personnel) and with the work of Daniel J. Leithauser, a general surgeon from Detroit who rediscovered Boldt and Ries. Although doctors may not have prescribed early ambulation, as in the case of McDowell, patients probably were up and about far more often than we realize. Dr. Bert Dunphy of San Francisco told me that when he had a hernia repair while he was a house officer at the Peter Bent Brigham Hospital in 1938, his surgeon prescribed strict bed rest after the operation. Dunphy was up on the first day and thereafter and felt perfectly well, if a bit guilty.

GYNECOLOGY IN THE 20TH CENTURY AND DR. TE LINDE'S BOOK

In the 1890s, when Thomas Cullen (1868–1953) was a medical student in Toronto, he recalled that "... there were anteversions, anteflexions, retroversions, and retroflexions and that some of the displacements might be relieved by appropriate pessaries." Abdominal gynecologic operations, Cullen continued, "... were limited almost entirely to the removal of large ovarian cysts. An occasional myomatous uterus was removed, but the fatality in this class of cases was so high that the operation was rarely attempted." Cullen also said that he did hear of cancers of the uterus in his student days, but only cauterization or curettage was performed. Entire removal of the uterus was not yet being done.

By the turn of the 20th century, the leadership of gynecology in this country had clearly moved to the new Johns Hopkins Hospital, where Howard A. Kelly (1858–1943) (Fig. 1.6) began to train a series of young men who put gynecology on a strong academic footing in the next two generations. Kelly received both his bachelor's and medical degrees from the University of Pennsylvania. After his medical graduation in 1882, Kelly spent some time in Germany learning the latest surgical

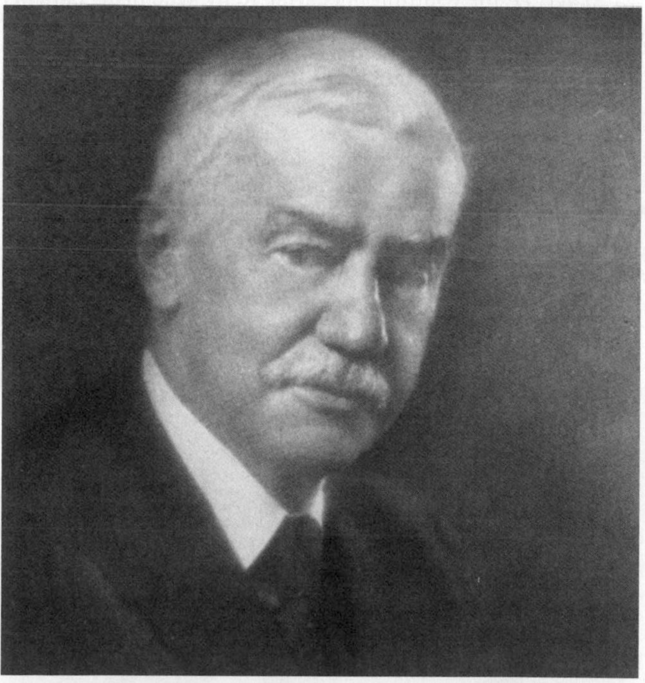

FIGURE 1.6. Howard A. Kelly (1858–1943). (From: Davis AW. *Dr. Kelly of Hopkins.* Baltimore: The Johns Hopkins Press, 1959, with permission.)

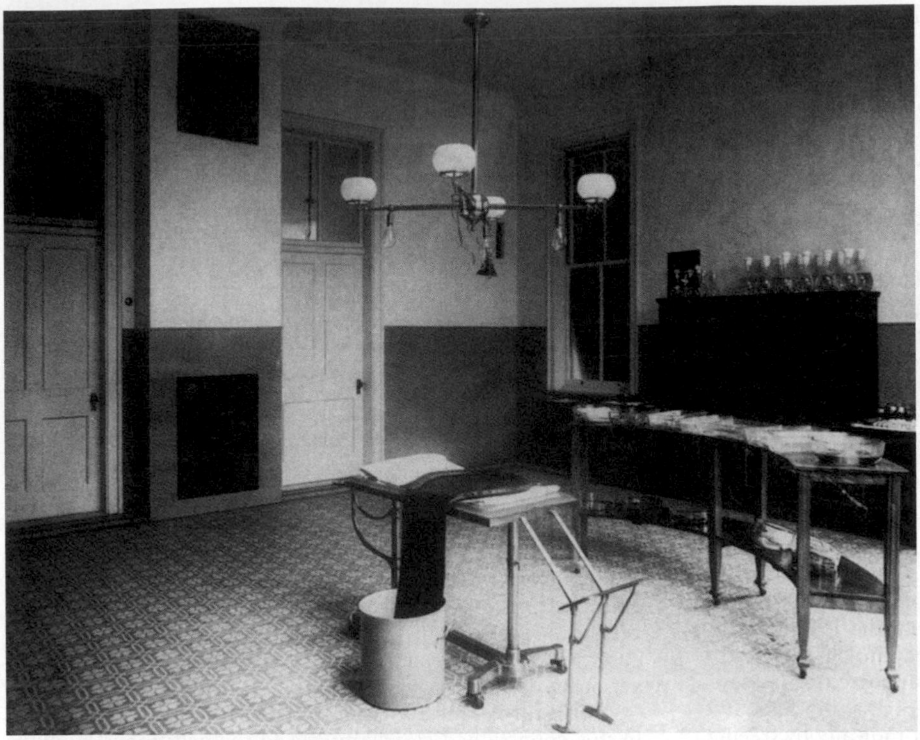

FIGURE 1.7. Dr. Howard A. Kelly's operating room at the Johns Hopkins Hospital. To the left is the door to the corridor. In the center is the door to the ether room. The rubber pad was used for drainage during irrigation of the abdomen. A similar pad was developed by Dr. Kelly for drainage of blood and amniotic fluid during and after a vaginal delivery.

and pathologic techniques. Back in Philadelphia at Kensington Hospital, he soon acquired a reputation as a brilliant operator. When his fellow Philadelphian William Osler became chief of medicine at the opening of the Johns Hopkins Hospital in 1889, he urged the trustees to hire Kelly as chief of obstetrics and gynecology.

At age 31, the youthful-appearing Kelly, who many patients thought was still a student or resident, initiated a residency program in gynecology with a strong link to the pathology department. Even more than half a century later, the leading texts in the field—*Eastman's (Williams') Obstetrics, Te Linde's Operative Gynecology,* and *Novak's Gynecologic and Obstetric Pathology*—were written by professors in Baltimore who had received their training at Hopkins with Kelly and his assistants.

Kelly soon found that his interests and skills were in gynecologic surgery; therefore, he turned the obstetric service over to J. Whitridge Williams (1866–1931), who became a leader in that field and the author of the most widely used textbook of the time. Kelly had a great interest in the female urinary system, realizing that the symptomatology of urinary tract disease is often intertwined with that of the reproductive organs. He invented the air cystoscope and devised ureteral catheters. He was the first to plicate the vesical sphincter for stress incontinence of urine. Physicians from all over the world came to Baltimore to watch him operate (Figs. 1.7 and 1.8).

Kelly's legendary operative skill was well described by Cullen, who later became one of Kelly's outstanding residents and successors to the chair at Hopkins. Kelly and Hunter Robb,

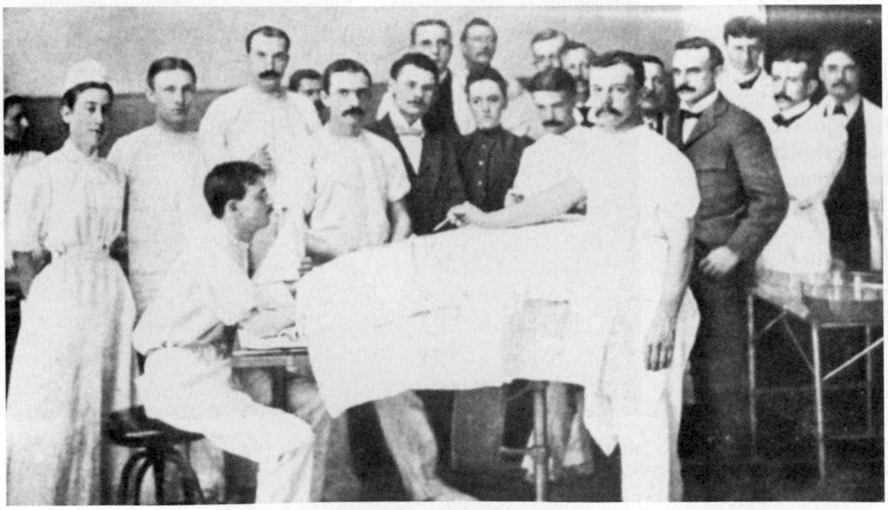

FIGURE 1.8. Howard Kelly operates. Grouped about the operating table, left to right, are Emma Beckwith, head nurse; Jay Durkee (*seated*); Thomas S. Cullen; Max Brödel (*center*); Elisabeth Hurdon; J. E. Stokes; and John G. Clark. (From: Davis AW. *Dr. Kelly of Hopkins*. Baltimore: The Johns Hopkins Press, 1959, with permission.)

his earlier resident, went to the Toronto General Hospital not long after Kelly became chief at Hopkins. Cullen was an intern in Toronto at the time and handled the instruments during an operation that Kelly and Robb had agreed to perform. Cullen's description speaks for itself:

> I turned around to thread a needle and when I turned back found to my amazement that the operator had the abdomen open. Operators in the General often took ten minutes to get that far. After cutting through the skin, fat and fascia they were apt to get lost in the muscles. Kelly and Robb working together used dissecting forceps as I had never seen them used. One man pulling each way, the cleavage between the muscles was seen at once and the opening in the abdomen could be completed without difficulty. I watched, fascinated, while Kelly went ahead and finished that operation and did the second, working with clock-like precision and at a speed I had not imagined possible. By the time he had finished, the course of my professional life was decided. Up to that afternoon I had intended to be a physician. From that afternoon I knew I had to be a surgeon.

Chance often determines the course of one's life, so it was fortunate for Cullen that he had to wait 6 months for his residency with Kelly to start. He used this time to begin the study of pathology with William H. Welch at Hopkins, and it was the close alliance of gynecology and pathology, begun by Kelly and continued by Cullen, that shaped the careers of many future gynecologists at Hopkins and elsewhere and determined the course of the field itself.

In 1898, Kelly published a two-volume textbook called *Operative Gynecology*, certainly the direct ancestor of the volume you have in your hands. Kelly wrote in the preface, "My aim in writing this book has been to place in the hands of the many friends who have from time to time visited me and followed my work, a convenient summary of the various gynecological operations I have found best in my own practice."

Although gynecology at the end of the last century was still a very young science, in Kelly's words, change was at hand: "Although I have spent several years in the preparation of my book, so rapid have been the changes in the gynecological field that I have found it necessary to rewrite some of the chapters two and even three times." A little more than a dozen years later, in the preface to his text entitled *Medical Gynecology*, Kelly reiterated the pace of the changes: "What a transformation two generations have witnessed in the field of gynecology! From modest beginnings, as a sort of minor specialty coupled with diseases of children and often professed by general practitioners with no special training, it has grown to the dignity of a major surgical specialty, so extensive that many gynecologists of today [1912] claim the entire field of abdominal surgery as their proper domain by right of discovery and conquest." This was also a time when radical or complete removal of tumors and repair of hernias became increasingly common. Kelly and his residents were pioneers in radical hysterectomy when Hugh Young of Hopkins introduced radical prostatectomy.

What imparted even greater value to all of Kelly's texts were the illustrations of Max Brödel, a German medical illustrator brought to Hopkins by Kelly (Fig. 1.9). Brödel's contributions to operative gynecology, including Te Linde's text 50 years after Kelly's, were portrayals of operative techniques, pelvic anatomy, and pathologic conditions. He set a standard for medical illustration never attained before or surpassed since.

As long ago as 1900, in his classic text, *Cancer of the Uterus*, Thomas Cullen, student of and successor to Kelly (Fig. 1.10), wrote that "The number of cases of cancer of the genital tract coming too late for operation is so appalling that the surgeon is ever seeking to devise ways and means by which the dread malady may be more generally detected at the earliest possible moment—at a time when complete removal of the malignant tissue is still possible. . . . But since it is the general practitioner who, as a rule, is the first consulted, upon him largely falls the responsibility of arriving at a timely diagnosis."

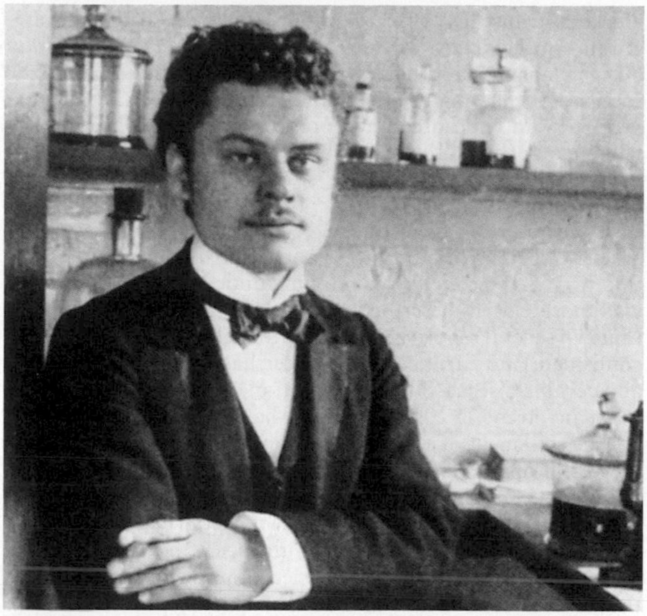

FIGURE 1.9. Max Brödel. (From: Robinson J. *Tom Cullen of Baltimore*. New York: Oxford University Press, 1949, with permission.)

One of the greatest advances in gynecology in this century has been the improvement in the early detection and cure rate of cancer of the uterine cervix that has resulted from the development of cytology and the recognition of carcinoma *in situ*. In 1943, George N. Papanicolaou (1883–1962) and

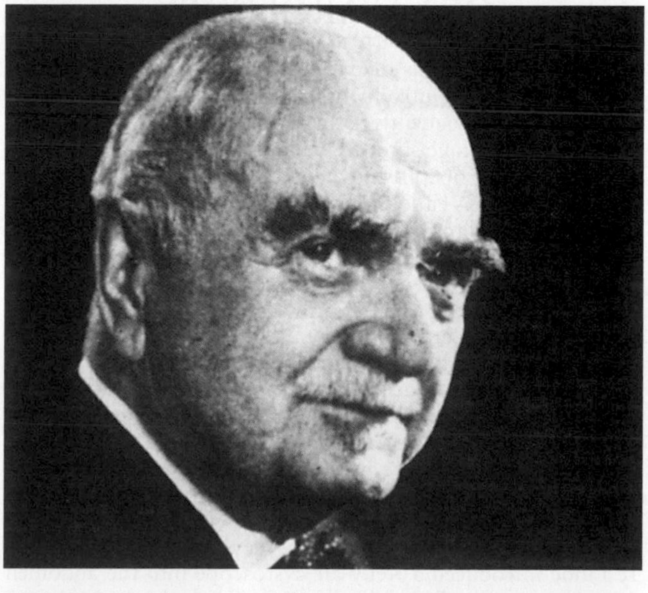

FIGURE 1.10. Thomas S. Cullen (1868–1953). (From: Robinson J. *Tom Cullen of Baltimore*. New York: Oxford University Press, 1949, with permission.)

Herbert Traut (1894–1963) published their seminal monograph entitled *Diagnosis of Uterine Cancer by the Vaginal Smear.* Papanicolaou had worked on this technique since the 1920s, but, like many other innovations in medicine, it took years to find widespread acceptance. Further publications by Papanicolaou and others, notably Ruth Graham, demonstrated beyond a doubt that cytologic studies could almost infallibly detect cervical cancer.

Cancer *in situ* was recognized early in the century by Cullen and in 1912 by J. Schottlander and F. Kermauner, but its relation to invasive cancer was not well understood. This relation was more clearly described in 1944 by G. A. Galvin and Te Linde in several reports. Since then, the relation has been amply confirmed, and early cervical cancer has become a detectable and curable disease. Since its inception by Hans Hinselmann in Germany in the 1920s, colposcopy has given a new dimension to the assessment of cervical carcinoma, making blind, random cervical biopsies unnecessary and providing more accuracy in finding and treating localized lesions.

By the early 1970s, the editor of a new journal, *Gynecologic Oncology,* pointed out that "... the scientific importance of gynecologic oncology may be gained from the observation that the tumors that we study and treat are prototypes for cancer in other areas of the body, for the histogenesis of the two principal uterine cancers is probably understood better than that of any other tumor in the body."

The immediate post–World War II years were a period of truly astounding medical developments and saw the explosive growth of medical research funding and new hospital construction. After 1945, penicillin became available for civilian use, and this was soon followed by other antibiotics. Hormone replacement became increasingly possible, and in 1946, the year that Richard Te Linde published the first edition of this textbook, Congress passed the Hill-Burton Act, making federal funds available to localities for the construction of new hospitals. These and other developments of the time greatly changed and expanded the work of medicine.

THE BEGINNING OF THE ERA OF LAPAROSCOPY

Although the emphasis of this historical chapter is on developments before the introduction of laparoscopy, the ability to visualize and subsequently to intervene by the less invasive laparoscopic technique surely represents an important milestone in the history of operative gynecology. The details of the history of the various endoscopic possibilities are discussed in the chapters devoted to these techniques, but a few general historical reflections may be in order at this point.

Laparoscopy seems to have been developed more or less independently in the United States and in various countries in Europe. In 1911, Bertram Bernheim, a general surgeon at Johns Hopkins, reported two cases in which, through a small abdominal incision, he introduced a proctoscope to examine the upper abdomen in a procedure he called organoscopy. The source of the illumination was an incandescent light on a band around his head. The experience must not have been satisfactory, as there were no follow-up reports.

In the mid-1930s at the same Johns Hopkins, in a trial of a small series of patients that was never published, Richard Te Linde introduced a Kelly air cystoscope into the abdomen through a small subumbilical incision with the patients in a deep Trendelenburg position. The Kelly air cystoscope was simply a 10-cm-long tube, which came in various diameters up to 2 cm, with a flange at the distal end and a suitable handle. It was routinely used at Hopkins to examine the bladder. The patient was in the knee-chest position for the cystoscopic examination. The bladder distended with air and when the obturator, which normally was also a part of the instrument, was removed. The light source was an incandescent bulb placed just above the patient's buttocks and a conical head mirror with a central hole to direct the light along the line of site. The illumination was very good with this technique. Although the pelvic organs could be seen with the introduction of the cystoscope into the abdomen, the area of inspection was so small that the concept was abandoned.

It is curious indeed that Te Linde apparently did not think of introducing the cystoscope through the posterior fornix with the patient in the knee-chest position, especially as this was the exact position used to cystoscope the bladder with the Kelly cystoscope and was a technique commonly and frequently used at Johns Hopkins during this era. At that time, female urology was part of the division of gynecology.

It remained for Albert Decker with T. H. Cherry to use the knee-chest position to introduce a lens cystoscope with a miniaturized incandescent bulb at the tip through the posterior fornix to visualize the pelvic organs. Thus, culdoscopy was born and was widely used in the United States during the era of 1950 to 1970, especially after the adoption of the fiberoptic cold light system, which gave far better illumination than the miniaturized incandescent bulb. During this era, it was not unusual at Johns Hopkins to have five or six patients per day listed in the operating room for a culdoscopic examination.

After about 1970, laparoscopy, with its fiberoptic cold light system, superseded the culdoscopic approach. About this time, operative laparoscopy blossomed, and one of the first widely used procedures was the ligation of the fallopian tubes by various techniques.

In Europe, in contrast to the United States, there was no great use of the culdoscope. The development of observational and operative laparoscopy continued uninterruptedly from about 1912, when, according to Cohen, the Swedish Hans Christian Jacobaeus described 109 laparoscopies in 69 patients using an electric cystoscope.

As previously mentioned, the historical details of procedures are included in the appropriate chapters. However, two general observations may be made.

First, developmental progress in endoscopy of the abdominal cavity has been a function of development of the physical sciences: optics, mechanics, electronics, etc. Thus, the current popular robotic laparoscopic procedures result not only from medical ingenuity but from the participation of the capitalistic industrial complex. The consequence of this is that the use of the laparoscopic instrumentation is greatly encouraged by commercial interests. The danger is—if there is a danger—that physicians may be unduly influenced by commercial as opposed to scientific priorities.

Second, the laparoscopic operative procedures have been widely adopted, often without randomized clinical trials to scientifically define and evaluate their role in operative gynecology.

These two points are made as an observation and not necessarily as a criticism, as the advantages of a shortened hospital stay and less patient discomfort are obvious. However, the fact is that there are few data on the short- and long-term results that are designed to evaluate results from laparoscopy with alternate procedures. The adoption of laparoscopic operative procedures progressed in spite of the recent emphasis on the importance of evidence-based medicine. Rock and Warshaw have elaborated on this aspect of operative laparoscopy.

Knowledge of the history of operative gynecology is not only of intrinsic interest but also allows us to appreciate our innovative predecessors and may stimulate some of us to be the subject of future historians.

OPERATIVE GYNECOLOGY, FIRST EDITION, 1946

Richard Wesley Te Linde was born in Wisconsin in 1894 and, except for the years that he attended a small liberal arts college in Holland, Michigan, he spent all his formative years in Wisconsin. When he was ready to go to medical school, he went to Madison, but in 1916, the University of Wisconsin had only a 2-year school. Te Linde completed the 2 preclinical years and then transferred to Johns Hopkins for the final 2 years. He graduated with the class of 1920 and spent the rest of his professional career associated with Hopkins, where he became chief of the gynecology division of the department of surgery and then chair of the separate department of gynecology in 1939. He held that post until his retirement in 1960, when the newly reunified department of obstetrics and gynecology was reestablished.

Just as his teacher Howard Kelly had felt the need to compile a textbook of operative gynecology half a century earlier, Te Linde believed that the many-sided specialty that gynecology had become by World War II required a new text. With Kelly's earlier text as a model, Te Linde wished to incorporate the vast changes that had occurred in the period separating the two books. During this 50-year span, there were changes in our knowledge of hormones, new surgical techniques, and the ability to visualize the abdominal and pelvic organs.

Te Linde chose the same simple title for his own text. Although Kelly's had been published by Appleton in New York, Te Linde chose Lippincott in Philadelphia. Gynecology, Te Linde wrote in the preface in 1946, was no longer to be considered simply a branch of general surgery. The gynecologist, he stressed, must still be a good surgeon but must also master the pathology of gynecologic disorders and the newly burgeoning field of endocrinology. New books were appearing in all these fields except gynecologic surgery, and it was this void that Te Linde wished to fill.

Te Linde wrote his text with the "... primary purpose of describing the technique of the usual and some of the rarer operative procedures. It also includes indications for and against operations as well as pre- and postoperative care of patients." Gynecologic pathology, Te Linde stressed in the Hopkins tradition, is the bedrock of good gynecologic surgery. "Without an understanding of it, surgery becomes merely a mechanical job, and errors in surgical judgment are inevitable." In the organization of his text and in the subsequent editions over the succeeding half century to the present edition, one can readily see important landmarks in the history of operative gynecology. Some of these were discussed in a previous section.

The 751-page first edition of 1946, all of it written by Te Linde, had a first printing of 5,000 copies, which quickly sold out. A second printing was equally successful. The reviews have always been laudatory. Of the sixth edition of 1985, edited by Richard Mattingly and John Thompson, the *Journal of the American Medical Association* reviewer ended by saying, " I cannot imagine any gynecologist who performs surgery doing without it, first as a primer and then as a reminder." By 1962, when the third edition appeared and Te Linde had retired from the chairmanship of his department, he decided that, like all the other major medical textbooks of the time, his book needed a group of authors to bring out new revisions. In the preface to that edition, he states that his book has never been simply a manual of surgical technique—that surgical philosophy is equally important. "What does it profit a woman if the operation is technically perfect and the procedure unnecessary or even harmful?" One reason unnecessary procedures still prevailed, Te Linde noted, was the lack of knowledge of gynecologic pathology, still the "bedrock upon which good surgery is done." Therefore, Te Linde justified including a considerable amount of pathology in his text. Pathology is what has differentiated gynecologic surgery from general surgery since Howard Kelly's years at the turn of the 20th century. Surgical texts, and by implication their surgical readers, have generally not devoted nearly as much attention to pathology as have gynecologists, some of whose leaders have actually been very well versed in pathology.

The fact that Te Linde could produce three editions, each larger than the first, is a testament to his broad knowledge of his field, his ability as a writer, and his stamina for hard work. He died in Baltimore in 1989 at the age of 95.

In the decades since the third edition of 1962, the world of medicine and the society in which it is practiced have seen much change. By the mid-1960s, when significant advances in the treatment of infections, malignancies, and hormonal disorders had become evident, these successes had an impact on gynecology just as they did in other areas of medicine. The reduction in mastoid infections, for instance, has changed the practice of the otolaryngologist considerably. In gynecology, the reduction in major pelvic inflammatory disease forced gynecologists to focus more of their attention on other disorders. Also affecting gynecologic surgery by the middle of this century were significant improvements in obstetric practices, which sharply reduced injuries to the bladder and rectum. Hysterectomies and suspensory operations were not performed for vague symptoms of illness as often as they had been.

We have also lived through social revolutions that have changed the way our society carries on its business and dispenses its social prerogatives. Especially prominent in the 1960s, a civil rights movement, greater concern for our environment, a resurgence of consumer rights, and a revitalized women's movement profoundly affected our social institutions, including medicine. Within medicine, no specialty has been more touched by these trends than obstetrics and gynecology.

The new feminism viewed abortion, childbirth, contraception, and gynecologic surgery as a means of social control of female patients by doctors, most of whom were men. The feminist movement challenged not only the domination of doctors but also the supposed benevolence of their knowledge and practices.

As the world has changed, so have our expectations. In the decades after the first edition of Te Linde's book appeared, when wonder drugs were touted as curing previously untreatable illnesses, the public began to expect much from its doctors, and we were not shy in claiming that ever-greater investments in medical research would lead to more cures. It is hardly surprising, then, that in these last few decades, as we began to spend increasing amounts of our gross national product for health, those who paid the bill became increasingly interested in seeing just what their money was actually buying. Like most other social institutions, medicine lost much of the autonomy it had for so long taken for granted. Although as a profession we did not always get all we wanted, we were for decades amazingly adept at preventing those things we did not want. Now that, too, has changed, as has the practice of medicine.

The division of labor in all areas of medicine grew as the 20th century progressed. In the last decades of the century, what used to be called general practice became the specialty of family practice. In the Anglo-American world of the late 20th century, both obstetrics and gynecology were caught in the middle of the battles between specialists and generalists. Likewise, they became involved in the tensions among primary, secondary, and tertiary medical care. Similar strife occurred in earlier centuries among those vying for a place and for status among physicians caring for women in childbirth and in disease. If one looks at the table of contents of this edition and compares it with a simpler period of half a century or a century ago, one will see what great breadth the field of operative gynecology continues to enjoy.

Bibliography

Anderson EG. Sex in mind and education: a reply. *Fortnightly Review* 1874;15:582.

Beacham WD. The American Academy of Obstetrics and Gynecology: first presidential address. *Obstet Gynecol* 1953;1:115.

Bernheim BM. Organoscopy. *Ann Surg* 1911;53:764.

Boldt HJ. The management of laparotomy patients and their modified after-treatment. *NY Med J* 1907;85:145.

Brieger GH. The development of surgery: historical aspects important in the origin and development of modern surgical science. In: Sabiston DC, ed. *Christopher's textbook of surgery*, 14th ed. Philadelphia: WB Saunders, 1991:1.

Brieger GH. Early ambulation: a study in the history of surgery. *Ann Surg* 1983;197:443.

Brunschwig A. Whither gynecology? *Am J Obstet Gynecol* 1968;100:122.

Cohen MR. *Laparoscopy, culdoscopy and gynecography*. Philadelphia: WB Saunders, 1970:112.

Cullen TS. *Cancer of the uterus: its pathology, symptomatology, diagnosis, and treatment*. New York: Appleton, 1900.

Cullen TS. The evolution of gynecology. *Ohio State Med J* 1924;20:484.

Cullen TS. The relation of obstetrics, gynecology and abdominal surgery to the public welfare. *JAMA* 1916;66:239.

Dally A. *Women under the knife: a history of surgery*. London: Hutchinson Radius, 1991.

Davis A. *Dr. Kelly of Hopkins*. Baltimore: The Johns Hopkins Press, 1959.

Decker A, Cherry TH. Culdoscopy: new method in diagnosis of pelvic disease—a preliminary report. *Am J Surg* 1944;64:40.

Dickinson RL. Original communications: a program for American Gynecology Society presidential address. *Am J Obstet Gynecol*, 1921;1:2.

Ehrenreich B, English D. *For her own good: 150 years of the experts' advice to women*. Garden City, NY: Anchor Press/Doubleday, 1978.

Gusberg SB. An introduction to volume 1. *Gynecol Oncol* 1972;1:i.

Hahn R. *Sickness and health: an anthropological perspective*. New Haven, CT: Yale University Press, 1995:209.

Halsted WS. The employment of fine silk in preference to catgut and the advantages of transfixing tissues and vessels in controlling haemorrhage. *JAMA* 1913;60:1119.

Harris S. *Woman's surgeon: the life story of J. Marion Sims*. New York: Macmillan, 1950.

Jacobi MP. *A question of rest for women during menstruation*. London: Smith & Elder, 1878.

Jones HW Jr, Jones GS, Ticknor WE. *Richard Wesley Te Linde*. Baltimore: Williams & Wilkins, 1986.

Kelly HA. Getting up early after grave surgical operations. *Surg Gynecol Obstet* 1911;13:78.

Kelly HA. *History of gynecology in America: a cyclopedia of American medical biography*, 2 vols. Philadelphia: WB Saunders, 1912:xxxix–xl.

Kelly HA. *Medical gynecology*. New York: Appleton, 1912.

Kelly HA. *Operative gynecology*. New York: Appleton, 1898.

Longo LD. The rise and fall of Battey's operation: a fashion in surgery. *Bull Hist Med* 1979;53:244.

Longyear HW. The relations of gynecology to general surgery, past and present. *JAMA* 1917;69:501.

Martin FH. Surgery, gynecology, and obstetrics. *Surg Gynecol Obstet* 1905;1:62.

Maudsley H. Sex in mind and on education. *Fortnightly Review* 1874;15:466.

McDowell E. Extirpation of diseased ovaria. *Eclectic Repertory* 1817;7:742. Reprinted in Brieger GH, ed. *Medical America in the nineteenth century*. Baltimore: The Johns Hopkins Press, 1972.

McGregor DK. *From midwives to medicine: the birth of American gynecology*. New Brunswick, MJ: Rutgers University Press, 1989.

Meigs JV. *Progress in gynecology: fifty years of surgical progress, 1905–1955*. Chicago: The Franklin H. Martin Memorial Foundation, 1955. Reprinted from Davis L, ed. *Surgery: gynecology and obstetrics with international abstracts of surgery*.

Morantz R. The lady and her physician. In: Hartman M, Banner L, eds. *Clio's consciousness raised: new perspectives on the history of women*. New York: Harper & Row, 1974:38.

Morantz-Sanchez R. *Conduct unbecoming a woman: medicine on trial in turn of-the-century*. New York: Oxford University Press, 1999.

Morantz-Sanchez R. Making it in a man's world: the late nineteenth-century surgical career of Mary Amanda Dixon Jones. *Bull Hist Med* 1995;69:542.

Moscucci O. *The science of woman: gynaecology and gender in England 1800–1929*. Cambridge: Cambridge University Press, 1990:30.

O'Dowd MJ, Philipp EE. *The history of obstetrics and gynecology*. New York: Parthenon Publishing Group, 1994.

Ricci JV. *The development of gynaecological surgery and instruments*. Philadelphia: Blakiston, 1949.

Ries E. Some radical changes in the after-treatment of celiotomy cases. *JAMA* 1899;33:454.

Robinson J. *Tom Cullen of Baltimore*. London: Oxford University Press, 1949.

Rock JA, Jeffrey RW. The history and future of operative laparoscopy. *Am J Obstet Gynecol* 1994:170:7.

Rock JA, Johnson TRB, Woodruff JD, eds. *The first 100 years: department of gynecology and obstetrics of the Johns Hopkins Hospital*. Baltimore: The Johns Hopkins University Press, 1991.

Russett CE. *Sexual science: the Victorian construction of womanhood*. Cambridge, MA: Harvard University Press, 1989.

Sims JM. On the treatment of vesico-vaginal fistula. *Am J Med Sci* 1852;23:59.

Sims JM. *Silver sutures in surgery.* The anniversary discourse, the New York Academy of Medicine. New York: S&W Wood, 1858.

Sims JM. *The story of my life*. New York: Appleton, 1884. Reprinted by Dacapo Press, 1968.

Simpson JY. *Hospitalism: its effects on the results of surgical operations*. Edinburgh: Oliver Boyd, 1869.

Speert H. *Obstetrics and gynecology in America*. Chicago: American College of Obstetricians and Gynecologists, 1980.

Temkin O, trans. *Soranus' gynecology*. Baltimore: The Johns Hopkins Press, 1956.

Thomas TG. A century of American medicine, 1776–1876: obstetrics and gynecology. *Am J Med Sci* 1876;72:138.

Webster JC. The future of gynecology. *Surg Gynecol Obstet* 1905;1:63.

Wells TS. Some causes of excessive mortality after surgical operations. *BMJ* 1864;2:384. See also Brieger G. American surgery and the germ theory of disease. *Bull Hist Med* 1966;40:135.

Wood AD. The fashionable diseases: women's complaints and their treatment in nineteenth century America. *J Interdisc Hist* 1973;4:25. Reprinted in Hartman M, Banner L, eds. *Clio's consciousness raised: new perspectives on the history of women*. New York: Harper & Row, 1974:1.

CHAPTER 2 ■ THE ETHICS OF PELVIC SURGERY

RUTH M. FARRELL, ELI A. RYBAK, AND EDWARD WALLACH

DEFINITIONS

Autonomy—The concept describing an individual's self-determination and the right to direct his or her own life through his or her own decisions, actions, and beliefs.

Informed consent—A process of communication between a physician and a patient that addresses the risks, benefits, and alternatives of a proposed medical intervention while meeting the core criteria of competence, exchange of information, understanding of exchanged information, and voluntary authorization.

Nonmaleficence—Literally translated as "do no harm," this concept describes the need to both prevent harm and refrain from harmful acts.

Beneficence—The duty to do good on the behalf of others through an active promotion of the good of the patient and shelter from harm.

THEORY AND PRACTICE OF ETHICS IN MEDICINE

The practice of medicine is governed by a system of beliefs that guide the actions of physicians and other health care professionals to act and make decisions that are regarded as ethically acceptable. Throughout the practice of medicine, different sets of standards and concepts of ethically acceptable behavior have existed as the predominant code for health care professionals. Codes such as those set by the Hippocratic oath served as the mainstay of professional behavior for centuries until a different system took its place in the first half of the 20th century. This transition is a reflection of changing societal values of health and well-being that evolved over time as a result of political, cultural, scientific, and technological advancement.

The field of bioethics emerged in the 1950s. Before that time, ethical principles of the Hippocratic oath were regarded as the ethical standards for medicine. The guiding principle of physician action was *primum non nocere*—first do no harm. In the Hippocratic tradition, the model of paternalism structured the therapeutic relationship. The physician was designated as the most qualified person to make decisions about treatment options for a patient. As such, it was the physician's judgment that determined what was to be considered as harm or benefit resulting from a medical procedure, not that of the patient or the patient's family. This was based on the belief that only an expert in science and medicine was qualified enough to make the best choice among treatment options for patients. During a time when medical therapies were limited and choices were few, this was not viewed as a problematic approach to patient care. However, as changes in society, science, and medicine unfolded, patients and the general public began to question these traditional views of the physician–patient relationship.

With the introduction of significant scientific and cultural revolutions that characterized the post–World War II period in the United States, these standards set by the Hippocratic oath were considered to be ineffectual to meet the growing demands of medicine and ethics. Movements advancing civil rights, women's issues, and the growing recognition of individual rights and autonomy dominated the social climate. Carried over into medicine and science, a new set of health care innovations introduced new moral debates to society and the medical profession about the purpose of medical care, the definition of health, and the ability of mankind to regulate the physiology of the human body. The birth control pill, organ transplant, and dialysis are just a few examples of the significant life-altering innovations of the time. The ethical questions raised in response to the cultural and scientific climate challenged the previous notions of ethical behavior of physicians. In particular, the notion that physicians were the most appropriate members in the therapeutic relationship to make choices for the patient was rejected. Decisions about the vast array of available medical therapies and choices seemed inherently incongruent with the concept of paternalism. With the rise in the importance of autonomy and individual rights, society campaigned to replace the paternalistic structure of medicine with a model that established the patient as the primary decision maker.

This movement resulted in the establishment of a system of principle-based ethics as the driving force behind modern medicine. In 1977, the Belmont Report outlined what these standards, also known as principles, should be. This massive effort to reshape modern bioethics resulted in the establishment of the following principles as the cornerstone of contemporary medical ethics: autonomy, beneficence, nonmaleficence, and justice.

Autonomy—The concept of autonomy embodies the ideal of self-determination—that a person shapes his or her own life through his or her own decisions, actions, and beliefs. As such, individuals have the right to make decisions about their lives that reflect their own beliefs of well-being and values. Inherent in the principle of autonomy is the requirement that others (i.e., physicians) must respect a patient's right of self-determination.

Nonmaleficence—Nonmaleficence, defined as "do no harm," has its origins in the original tenets of the Hippocratic oath. This principle encompasses both the need to prevent harm and to refrain from harmful acts.

Beneficence—The definition of the principle of beneficence is to do good on the behalf of others. In the case of the principle of beneficence, physicians are expected to actively promote the good of the patient, not just shelter him or her from harm. Though this may seem to be a subtle distinction from the principle of nonmaleficence, it is critical to the principle-based theory of ethics, as it requires the performance of positive acts to advance the well-being of others.

Justice—The principle of justice addresses the need to treat all persons fairly. In the case of health care, this pertains to both the physician–patient relationship and also the public health obligations of physicians in the allocation of scarce medical resources.

In this principle-based ethics model, all four core elements hold, in theory, equal importance. In many of the clinical situations that physicians routinely address, the solution to complex ethical dilemmas requires the balancing of these principles and, often times, a prioritization of one over the others. An example of this is in an emergent medical situation when the principle of beneficence may temporarily overrule autonomy. However these principles are weighted, they must, ultimately, must be used in a way that results in medical choices serving the good of the patient by reflecting his or her values and beliefs.

Though the system of principle-based ethics as established by the Belmont Report is the forerunner of ethical standards of behavior in modern medicine, other legitimate models of bioethical theory exist. They are broad in nature and are guiding principles, but all come from the view that the system of principle-based ethics does not offer enough to guide behavior in the complex setting of health care. Two examples of this are feminist ethics and casuistry. Feminist ethics is based on the notion that decisions are made in the context of relationships and personal virtues, such as compassion, friendship, and love. Principle-based ethics does not take these factors into consideration, neglecting the problems raised in a society in which men and women are not viewed as equals and, as a result, does not serve the true interests of the patient. A second example is casuistry, or case-based ethics. This theory is founded on the principle that moral lessons gained from the resolution of actual cases in medicine have more value than a set of theoretic and unchanging principles. Using this model, ethical reasoning results from weighing the outcomes of real cases as examples and forming a set of modifiable principles from those conclusions. These are just two examples of the diversity of ethical theories that guide medicine and serve as solutions to ethical puzzles that cannot be solved using the standard principle-based ethics commonly in place today.

The very nature of the field of obstetrics and gynecology sets the stage for a variety of ethical dilemmas. Issues surrounding the beginnings of human life and reproductive function naturally facilitate profound and often controversial questions and debate. In addition, the women's rights movement has raised other issues specific to the care of women, such as subjugation and control of women's bodies through society and medicine. Despite this broad range of issues, ethical discussions in obstetrics and gynecology are often perceived in terms of a single controversial issue: abortion. Yet the field of bioethics in women's health has a rich and broad set of important implications for the practice of medicine and the health of women. Recent advances in medicine and science have introduced novel therapeutic options to many of the conditions that gynecologists face on a daily basis, such as cervical cancer, fibroids, and infertility. Genetic and pharmaceutical therapies, new diagnostic modalities, and noninvasive surgical options set the stage for a multitude of multifaceted ethical questions and debates. This chapter will present some of the foundational concepts in bioethics and women's health that serve as a launching point for addressing the more complex and novel ethical issues as they arise in the present setting of medicine and the future.

THE PATIENT'S AUTONOMY AND INFORMED CONSENT

Autonomy is one of the four cornerstones of the physician–patient relationship. Informed consent is a mechanism whereby the autonomy of a patient is recognized, respected, and preserved in health care decisions. It is the result of a process whereby a patient makes a voluntary decision to proceed with a medical intervention with a good understanding of the nature and risks of the procedure, in addition to alternative therapies if the procedure is declined. The respect of informed consent has two purposes. On the one hand, the process of achieving informed consent respects and recognizes the patient's autonomy as a good in and of itself. On the other hand, patients benefit when they make decisions on their own behalf because they themselves are the most familiar with their own values, beliefs, and ideas of well-being and health. When patients make informed and voluntary decisions about their health care, they can make choices that meet their concept of good and beneficial.

The term *informed consent* has legal and ethical dimensions. Legally, informed consent can be viewed as an end point. The legal requirements of informed consent are met when the conversation between the physician and the patient is documented, either on an informed consent form or in the medical record. Often, getting a signature on a form is synonymous with achieving informed consent, but informed decision making goes well beyond the legal form. Ethically, informed decision making involves a process of communication between the physician and the patient, through which the patient is able to make an autonomous decision either to authorize the intervention (informed consent) or reject the intervention (informed refusal).

The legal and ethical dimensions of informed consent are often used interchangeably but can have very different meanings and implications. Unfortunately, the function and meaning of informed consent is often misinterpreted, and it is viewed primarily as a legal document with a patient's signature denoting full understanding and authorization. It is important to keep in mind that both the legal and ethical requirements of informed consent are essential in health care. However important legal documentation is, it should not be placed before the ethical duties to the patient. Legal documentation in a chart or on a form is not a substitute for the process of communication and autonomous decision making. It is important to keep in mind that not all legal documents with a patient's signature reflect that an adequate informed consent process has taken place.

A valid informed consent is both informed and autonomously authorized. To achieve this, the physician must ensure that five core components are met in the decision-making process: (i) competence, (ii) voluntariness, (iii) disclosure, (iv) understanding, and (v) authorization or refusal. These core components serve as a guide for physicians when discussing medical interventions with patients to ensure that a patient makes the most appropriate decision possible. Without satisfying all five of these core components, an adequate informed consent process has not been achieved.

Competence

In the usual clinical setting, other than situations involving formal psychiatric evaluation, the determination of competence tends to be more of a working judgment than a formal assessment. Often the terms *competence* and *decision-making capacity* are used interchangeably, although it should be understood that competence is a broader legal concept that speaks to the patient's ability to handle finances and other dimensions of his personal well-being. Beauchamp and Childress describe decision-making capacity as follows: "Although the properties most crucial to the determination of competence are controversial, in biomedical contexts a person has generally been viewed as competent if able to understand a therapy or research procedure, to deliberate regarding major risks and benefits, and to make a decision in light of this deliberation."

Disclosure

Autonomous decision making must be made in the context of information about the medical intervention. The physician must disclose sufficient information that allows the patient to make an informed decision reflecting his or her beliefs and values, including the risks, benefits, and alternatives of the proposed medical intervention. The core of ethical disclosure is about facilitating the patient's autonomous choice to accept or reject health care. Although there is no definitive rule about how much information should be given to the patient, a valid informed consent does not require that the patient be informed of every conceivable risk that could occur, no matter how remote or how trivial. Listing risks, either verbally or in writing, that do not have applicability to the patient, does not promote autonomy. Instead, a balance must be achieved between the patient and the physician to determine how much information and detail is necessary for the patient to make a meaningful decision.

Understanding

The patient must make a decision based on an understanding of the information provided. It is not sufficient to mention or list the possible risks to an intervention. The patient must comprehend the ramifications of these risks when considering whether to proceed with an intervention. The physician must be certain to convey information about the risks, including the possible procedures involved to address a bad outcome if it occurs. The patient should then be able to weigh the risks and the benefits of the procedure in his or her own terms.

Voluntariness

Ethically valid informed consent can only be obtained through the voluntary authorization by a patient for a medical intervention. It is not sufficient merely to meet the criteria of decision-making capacity, disclosure, and understanding. The patient must be able to use this information to formulate a decision that is not controlled by others. If a patient is manipulated or coerced into making a decision, then valid informed consent has not been achieved.

Authorization

The corollary of informed consent is informed refusal. Informed refusal is the decision of the patient to decline the proposed medical intervention. The respect for the patient's autonomy that is implicit in informed consent extends to the choice to refuse treatment, even when the decision is made against the recommendation of the physician. Informed refusal can be as minor as refusing a simple elective procedure to refusing lifesaving treatments. A patient may refuse treatment for a variety of reasons. One reason may be that the intervention or the outcome is misaligned with his or her concept of good. For example, a patient may refuse a medical therapy because he or she believes it to be harmful or incongruous with his or her personal beliefs.

A balance must be met between respect for the autonomy of the patient and the physician's duty to beneficence. It is the job of the physician to be as certain as possible that this decision is informed and consistent with the values and beliefs of the patient. In situations when the refusal may result in significant impairment, pain, or death, the physician should make every attempt to ensure that these decisions are consistent with the patient's beliefs and have been so over time. Physicians may still be considering their patient's best interest by giving preference to his or her spiritual or personal convictions over the medical good. Another important aspect of informed refusal is that it can occur either at the initiation of a treatment or later during the course of the treatment. This becomes apparent when a patient refuses to continue a treatment or undergo a similar or identical intervention. The willingness of the patient to undergo a therapy in the past does not mean that consent is implied in the future.

There are circumstances when a physician must proceed with a medical intervention without the informed consent of the patient. Generally, these circumstances involve emergent situations. For example, the patient may be suddenly incapacitated or unconscious and therefore incapable of providing any sort of autonomous authorization. Alternatively, the patient may be conscious and otherwise able to make decisions but, because of the emergent and critical nature of her condition, it is medically necessary to initiate an immediate intervention, and there is no time to engage in a discussion with the patient. In the first situation, there may be time to obtain authorization from an appropriate family member or designated medical decision maker. In the second situation (and sometimes in the first), there is no time, and the physician must make a decision on behalf of the patient. This decision should be made based on what is judged to be in the medical best interest of the patient and usually assumes most people would opt on the side of instituting lifesaving measures.

Informed consent plays a vital role in the practice of obstetrics and gynecology because this field of medicine pertains to the anatomy and function of the women's reproductive system and sexuality. Issues specific to women's health have been brought to the forefront because of concerns of historical control and subjugation of women and their bodies through society and medicine. In addition, there is a growing trend to recognize the vital role of relationships in a patient's medical decision making about reproductive issues. Patients rarely make decisions about their sexuality and reproduction in a vacuum but instead do so within the context of relationships with others, whether friends, partners, or families. It is critical to recognize these qualities inherent in obstetrics and gynecology when obtaining informed consent for a medical therapy or procedure to maximize the autonomous expression of the patient's personal preferences.

ETHICAL ISSUES IN SURGICAL TRAINING

Competence of the surgeon is a moral commitment to the patient, especially before undertaking a novel surgical procedure.

Adequate preparation in the basic and clinical sciences and training in surgical techniques must have been accomplished before any new surgical procedure is introduced into clinical medicine. An illustrative example of an overenthusiastic rush into a procedure was the sudden popularity of cardiac transplantation in the 1960s. The preparatory laboratory work in cardiac transplantation started in 1905, but the first successful replacement of the heart in a dog took place in 1960. Immune suppression, which is crucial to the procedure, was introduced in 1958, and longtime survival of grafts occurred by 1965. Christian Barnard reported the first successful human heart transplantation in December 1967 in South Africa. By the end of 1968, 101 human heart transplantations had been performed by 64 surgical groups in 22 countries. Most patients improved briefly and then died of rejection of the transplant or infections. In 2 years, the procedure was largely discredited, and it took more than 10 additional years to reestablish wide acceptance of the operation. This experience illustrates the need to limit difficult and complex procedures to specialized centers that have the resources and adequately trained surgeons to perform them.

This is equally true for complex pelvic surgery. The adoption of subspecialty boards by the American Board of Obstetrics and Gynecology, each with requirements for postresidency fellowship training and evaluation standards for certification, have helped to emphasize the need for specialized training in surgical techniques for pelvic surgeons. The rapid expansion of the use of laparoscopic surgery training procedures means the responsibility of providing future obstetricians and gynecologists who are technically skilled to serve society effectively and safely. In addition to underlying knowledge, clinical experience, training, and practice, the competent surgeon operates with the attentiveness and focus commensurate with the surgical theater. Indeed, legitimate concerns regarding the potential impairment of overfatigued house staff managing and operating on patients have facilitated changes in house staff work hours and training. Training programs are now charged with the simultaneous challenge of vigilantly protecting the welfare of their patients from potentially suboptimal care while ensuring that those surgeons, after completion of training, operate competently under emergent and suboptimal conditions.

Many surgeons trained before World War II participated in residency programs affiliated with large inner-city hospitals where patients without adequate resources or health insurance received care. It was accepted that these patients would receive treatment or even surgery by physicians-in-training (including senior medical students, interns, and residents), preferably under the supervision of skilled volunteers or paid clinical faculty and only when the trainee had reached the necessary level of competence. When health care became an entitlement under Medicare and Medicaid government-funded health insurance became more prevalent, many patients sought the services of private physicians. The so-called free care or resident services were often unable to recruit sufficient patients to provide adequate training for new surgeons. This was particularly true in pelvic surgery; given the choice, these patients sought refuge from the clinic, where privacy and dignity were hard to maintain, and fled in large numbers to private doctors' offices. Surgical teaching thereafter often involved the private patient, with the resident now performing complete procedures under the supervision and assistance of the patient's private doctor. The problem with this arrangement was that patients were either poorly informed or uninformed about the participation of physicians-in-training, and this often became apparent only when complications arose or the medical records were reviewed during litigation. Although patients are typically better informed now, it remains ethically necessary to inform them about teaching or training in each case so that objections can be dealt with before the planned procedure or other arrangements made. Most surgeons involved in teaching programs inform their patients that surgery demands a team effort and that residents may be involved in assisting or operating with them, but that, as the private surgeons of record, they not only will be present but also will be in charge and responsible for everything that takes place during the procedure. Teaching should not take place in the operating room without such a disclosure and the patient's informed consent. The resident's role, status, and experience should be clear to the patient. We are long past introducing medical students to patients as doctors rather than revealing their actual status.

Because of the limitation on the number of hours a doctor in training may work, producing competent surgeons today has become even more challenging than in the past. This situation has necessitated approaches to supplement and amplify the residency program specifically as it affects surgical training. Novel training methods designed to accelerate the learning curve have been devised. These are directed at familiarizing the trainee with instrumentation and the handling of surgical instruments, improving manual dexterity, sharpening hand-eye coordination, and heightening awareness of pelvic anatomy. In addition, decision-making skills and essentials of emergency management need to be developed during the course of residency training. One of the valuable approaches that has recently been resurrected is the animal surgical laboratory. Obviously, the size of structures in laboratory animals does not precisely simulate that in humans, and anatomic relationships do not reflect those of a human patient. Simulators for endoscopic surgical procedures use mannequins or human models. Fabricated pelvic models are also frequently used to heighten skills for practicing maneuvers for normal and operative delivery. These innovative exercises assist in preparing the student for experiences encountered in the operating room and may even succeed in refreshing the already practicing surgeon in performance of specific techniques. The final arbiter for gaining surgical skills is the surgical procedure itself, carried out in actual patients under the guidance and supervision of an accomplished surgeon who has the ability to communicate effectively about both the procedure and techniques. The only way to learn to manage surgical complexities adroitly is through personally encountering such complications while under the direct tutelage of a preceptor who has himself experienced these very complications. Simulated programs have also been developed that incorporate computerized lessons for improving history-taking skills and for simulating emergency management in the form of skill stations.

In addition to foundational medical and surgical knowledge, clinical experience, training, and practice, the competent physicians must act in a responsible and professional manner, whether in the clinical or surgical setting. Impairment of a physician's skills must be fully evaluated so that he may be given assistance to improve and injury to his patients is avoided. Health care institutions must have peer accessible mechanisms in place to facilitate this process.

EXAMINATION UNDER ANESTHESIA

An article published in the February 2003 edition of the *American Journal of Obstetrics and Gynecology* demonstrated that medical students were performing preoperative pelvic examinations on anesthetized patients without having obtained specific prior consent, and, because of public concern, both the American College of Obstetricians and Gynecologists (ACOG) and the Association of American Medical Colleges released statements emphasizing the predominance of patient autonomy and appropriate informed consent over the exigencies of medical education.

In actual practice, examination under anesthesia (EUA) is routinely performed only by members of the surgical team to enable better appreciation of the patient's pelvic anatomy. The surgical team typically numbers between one to four members; at its largest, it includes an attending surgeon, senior resident, junior resident/intern, and medical student. Although the major portions of the surgery are performed by the senior experienced surgeons, the junior assistants, such as the medical student, perform the essential and ancillary tasks of retraction, exposure, and minor suturing.

The ACOG statement issued in 2003 noted: "If a pelvic examination that is planned for an anesthetized woman undergoing surgery offers her no personal benefit and is performed solely for teaching purposes, it should be performed only with her specific informed consent, obtained when she has full decision-making capacity." One can legitimately argue that all surgeons and surgical assistants, including the medical student, require maximum appreciation of the surgical field to optimize their performances during the procedure. Accordingly, the pelvic examinations should not be construed as offering "no personal benefit" to the patient. Furthermore, the EUA should not be considered as separate from the rest of the procedure but as a necessity adjunct. This ability of the members of the house staff that provide intraoperative and postoperative assistance should not be curtailed by exclusion from an essential component of the gynecologic procedure.

At least three steps can be taken to ensure that the rights of the patient are respected while ensuring appropriate surgical care: (i) explicitly incorporating the EUA on the operative consent form, (ii) openly discussing with the patient the importance and participation of all team-members in the EUA, and (iii) ensuring an atmosphere of patient respect and dignity by agreeing in advance to a specific number of pelvic examinations.

MEDICAL LEGAL ASPECTS OF GYNECOLOGIC CARE

In addressing the issue of professional liability among obstetricians and gynecologists, the ACOG survey in 2003 indicated the mean number of claims among practicing obstetricians/gynecologists during their professional careers to date was 2.6. Of the respondents to the survey, 76% had experienced one or more claims.

Obstetricians and gynecologists pay among the highest premiums for professional liability insurance of all medical specialties. In many states, this factor has led to early retirement, elimination of obstetrical and/or surgical procedures from practice, or relocation to another state. Being named in a malpractice suit leads to endless hours of effort unrelated to medical practice, undesired anxiety, and, in some instances, withdrawal from practice. A number of factors contribute to the cost of insurance coverage. Obstetricians and gynecologists can exercise control over some of these factors to minimize the chances of being cited in a claim. Two simple principles are helpful in preventing a legal claim or in providing a defense should a claim be filed. These two concepts form the basis of all risk-management and loss-prevention strategies. Plaintiff and defense attorneys have reached consensus that two factors, documentation and communication, improve the odds that a lawsuit will not be filed or that a lawsuit, once filed, can be successfully defended.

By way of documentation, the following basic and simple initiatives should be a component of each physician's protocol for charting and record keeping.

1. Recording of date and time of each entry in the chart
2. Legible handwriting
3. Contemporary entry of all notes in the chart
4. Appropriate correction of inaccurate entries
5. Avoidance of conflict among physicians and nurses in the charting of patient information

The alacrity with which a physician responds to a patient's symptom or concerns can be established with certainty if notes are complete, properly dated, and timed. This chronology is instrumental in establishing a timeline for a patient's care and will be more credible in a courtroom or in a hearing than a plaintiff's client's recollection weeks or months after the fact. Because an adverse surgical outcome is not synonymous with negligence, expression of reasons for clinical judgment in choice of a diagnosis or treatment plan demonstrates that alternatives have been considered by the physician. The physician should document these alternatives in the chart and indicate that they were each discussed with the patient before treatment.

Entries in the chart should clearly demonstrate the course of care rendered and rationale underlying the choice of a specific treatment plan. These notes should be legible and interpretable by anyone who reviews the chart. An inability to read one's own handwriting can only negatively affect the physician's credibility. The time frame of management is crucial, and prompt recording of events will prevent doubt when events occurring before a complication are documented only after the complication has occurred. Notations regarding telephone conversations with consulting physicians or family members should also be entered in the chart with the date and time of contact. An incorrect entry in the chart should be corrected properly by striking out the erroneous entry and initialing and dating the changes. If a supplemental note is written, it should be listed as an addendum. A patient's chart should not be used as a vehicle for expressing opinions on the intelligence of or decision rendered by another health care provider or for the purpose of criticism.

When an unanticipated adverse event occurs, the insurance company or risk-management representative should be notified promptly. The communication of a physician with legal and/or insurance representatives and health care providers is important in anticipating legal problems. However, a cornerstone of medical care is the physician's sensitivity in communicating with the patient with understanding and compassion. She should be given ample time to ask questions, and these inquires should be answered truthfully. Breakdown of communications in the patient-physician relationship is a recurring theme in the pathway leading to litigation.

A physician may appear in court to testify in three possible scenarios: as a *defendant*, as a *material witness*, or as an *expert witness* on behalf of either the plaintiff or the defendant. Although each instance has its unique aspects, in all cases the physician will have an opportunity to prepare the testimony with the attorney who is trying the case. As a *defendant* at either a sworn deposition or in a courtroom, the physician will have received general and specific instructions from the attorney representing him/her with regard to how to respond to questions. Each response should be concise, to the point, and directed only at the specific question raised by the plaintiff's attorney. Most of all, the answers must be honest and forthright, as well as accurate with respect to the patient's clinical course and management as described in the medical records. The defendant should request the opportunity to view the medical record at any time should there be need to recall specific details such as dates, times, and sequences of events.

A physician may be called as a *material witness* because of his/her association with the specific case as a participant or observer, but not as a defendant. The same principles of deportment apply as for an appearance as a defendant. The material witness testifies on the facts of the case and should not express opinions that require personal expertise.

The physician who chooses to serve as an *expert witness* is called on to do so because of his/her personal experience and training with the particular clinical situation under consideration. The role of an expert witness carries with it significant responsibilities. First and foremost is the possession of knowledge, skills, and experience to fulfill this role. Second, the expert witness should be objective and unbiased, and able to discuss standards of care on a broad scale rather than be constrained by his/her personal approach. It is clearly unethical for an expert witness to lack the appropriate credentials and/or to misrepresent the standard of care reflected in the case for which he/she is testifying. Fundamentally, *standard of care* refers to a level of care that is generally thought to represent the norm. Standard of care rendered in specific conditions may differ from one locale or group of physicians to another, simply because standards are arbitrarily developed and not universally held. If an adverse event occurs, a distinction must be made between a bad outcome that is independent of the quality of rendered care and a bad outcome that is clearly due to negligence or to substandard care.

A number of safeguards exist to protect patients from faulty or unethical clinical practice. At the local level, hospital credentials committees, as required by the Joint Commission on Accreditation of Hospitals and Health Care Organizations, are given the responsibility for reviewing the credentials of applicants for initial and continuing staff privileges. This responsibility mandates attention to the volume of cases attended per annum and the quality of care rendered. Privileges can be curtailed for performance of specific procedures or may be suspended for practice in general in cases in which the physician provides inappropriate care or exhibits ethical infractions. The American Board of Obstetrics and Gynecology credentials specialists and subspecialists on the basis of training, experience, and performance on examinations. Over the past three decades, a periodic reexamination is required for maintenance of specialty certification. This maintenance-of-certification process involves evaluation of performance on didactic examinations and assessment of cognitive skills. Recently, the Accreditation Council for Graduate Medical Education or (ACGME) and the American Board of Medical Specialists (ABMS) have stressed the importance of education and achievement of six core competencies (patient care, medical knowledge, communication skills, professionalism, practice-based learning and improvement, and systems-based practice). In addition, certifying boards require proof of licensure in good standing for certification and recertification. State medical societies are empowered to review patients' complaints and charges of unethical behavior of licensees. The National Practitioners Data Bank receives and makes available data regarding infraction of practice standards. This device was established by Congress to prevent physicians with past disciplinary action and malpractice awards from relocating from one state to another without detection.

Unfortunately, there are too few safeguards aside from collegial observation that can monitor surgical technique and/or interaction with patients. The responsibility of the physician requires introspection and candor, especially when factors such as physical and mental impairment or substance abuse infringe on the physician's ability to practice safely and effectively. Professionalism is implicit in day-to-day behavior and self assessment. A recent publication that addresses the association of disciplinary action against physicians with unprofessional behavior in medical school emphasized the importance of professionalism as a core competency. The conclusion in the report was that disciplinary action among practicing physicians by state medical licensing boards correlated strongly with a history of unprofessional behavior in medical school. The strongest association was in those who had demonstrated irresponsible behavior or diminished ability to improve their behavior as students earlier on.

PRIVACY AND THE HEALTH PORTABILITY AND ACCOUNTABILITY ACT

In 1996, Congress passed the Health Insurance Portability and Accountability Act (HIPAA), establishing minimal national standards to ensure confidentiality of protected health information (also referred to as *individually identifiable health information*). This move was due, in part, to the mainstream use of electronic technology in health care, which promoted concern over patient confidentiality. The subsequent additions to the original HIPAA provisions included the Privacy Rules, extending jurisdiction to health plans, billing services, hospitals, and individual health care providers. At the time of compliance deadlines, all of these covered entities were required to implement the established standards to protect patients' individually identifiable health information. The caveat to the Privacy Rules was that the protection of patients' privacy could not negatively interfere with the quality of care or create unnecessary burdens to patient care.

Quoting from the guidelines published by the Centers for Disease Control and Prevention and the U.S. Department of Health and Human Services (DHHS), the HIPAA Privacy Rule:

- Gives patients more control over their health information;
- Sets boundaries on the use and release of health records;
- Establishes appropriate safeguards that the majority of health care providers and others must achieve to protect the privacy of health information;
- Holds violators accountable with civil and criminal penalties that can be imposed if they violate patients' privacy rights;
- Strikes a balance when public health responsibilities support disclosure of certain forms of data;
- Enables patients to make informed choices based on how individual health information may be used;
- Enables patients to find out how their information may be used and what disclosures of their information have been made;
- Generally limits release of information to the minimum reasonably needed for the purpose of the disclosure;

- Generally gives patients the right to obtain a copy of their own health records and request corrections; and
- Empowers individuals to control certain uses and disclosures of their health information.

The complexity of the HIPAA regulations has made their implementation challenging and controversial. Specific confusion regarding disclosures to family members abounds, particularly in cases when the patient has authorized his or her family to be an active participant in health care. This also arises among health care providers when seeking information about their patients to provide continuity of care. Ultimately, HIPAA does afford latitude for professional judgment as to the "best interests" of the particular patient, so long as the disclosures conform to the "minimum necessary standards." In addition, the Privacy Rule does not replace federal or state laws and makes an allowance for individual institutions to adopt more stringent policies to protect patients' privacy.

CONFIDENTIALITY

The foundation of the physician–patient relationship is trust. This is based on the premises that a patient has the right to privacy and respect of privacy allows for patients to disclose the necessary information to be assisted by their physician. This is particularly relevant in gynecology, in which patients share sensitive information with their physicians about intimacy and sexuality. For this reason, confidentiality is one of the most essential aspects to the successful therapeutic relationship.

It is the exception, more than the rule, for patient confidentiality to be violated. Tension and ambiguity, however, have long surrounded the parameters wherein breaches of patient confidentiality are justified. The Code of Ethics of the American Medical Association (AMA), revised in 1957, stated: "A physician may not reveal the confidences entrusted to him in the course of medical attendance, or the deficiencies he may observe in the character of patients, unless he is required to do so by law or unless it becomes necessary to protect the welfare of the individual or of the community." Exceptions to the breach of confidentiality include times when the withholding of information may harm a third party or threaten public health. Mandatory exceptions include cases of violence and violent crime and the negligence and abuse of individuals, including women, children, and the elderly. Some states also require mandatory reporting of infectious diseases that may pose a serious public health risk, such as certain sexually transmitted diseases and tuberculosis. A notable case of the need to violate patient confidentiality is *Tarasoff v. Regents of the University of California*. In this case, a court found the University of California negligent for failing to forewarn murder victim Tatiana Tarasoff and her family after Prosenjit Poddar confided in one of his therapists that he intended to kill her. Two months after the temporary detainment of Poddar for this initial threat, he acted on it by murdering Tarasoff. As the majority opinion in the 1976 Tarasoff case emphasized: "The protective privilege ends where the public peril begins."

Gynecologists are confronted with a variety of complex and difficult scenarios in the clinical and surgical arenas when it comes to maintaining or breaking patient confidentiality. In this setting, physicians must balance their legal obligations with their medical obligations of trust to the patient. Challenging and not uncommon conflicts of patient confidentiality occur in obstetrics. An example is when a woman seeks a termination or sterilization procedure while requesting confidentiality from her partner. Counseling such a patient, especially after having attained her trust and confidence, may help defuse the situation. Yet, physicians must keep their duty to the patient and her confidentiality in mind before acting in situations such as this. When in doubt, either over personal convictions or professional duties, a hospital ethics committee may be required to intervene. Ultimately, however, in the absence of a countervailing public health or legal mandate, the obligation of patient confidentiality predominates.

ETHICAL ISSUES IN RESEARCH ON HUMAN SUBJECTS

Although the Nuremberg medical war crimes trials of Nazi doctors and the ensuing Nuremberg Code in 1949 represent a landmark in research ethics involving human subjects, they made little impact on research practices in the United States. Biomedical research expanded exponentially after World War II without significant regulation or oversight. The Nuremberg Code established the need for the "voluntary consent of the human subject." It covered such other matters as the need to justify a study in terms of expected beneficial results and risks, avoiding harm and injury to subjects, freedom for the subject to withdraw, and obligation of the investigator to stop a study if continuation would likely cause injury, disability, or death.

In 1966, the U.S. Public Health Service introduced the requirement that all human subject research funded by the government must be peer reviewed by a local institutional review board. The objective was to protect the rights of the individuals involved and review the quality of the informed consent and the risks and benefits of the study. This regulation was the result of a growing awareness that these kinds of safeguards often were not followed even in the best academic institutions in the United States.

Indeed, in 1966, Dr. Henry K. Beecher, professor of anesthesia at Harvard University, published an article in the *New England Journal of Medicine* describing ethically troubling studies from prestigious institutions published in reputable journals. One disturbing publication described transplantation of a malignant melanoma from a terminally ill daughter to her consenting mother to look for tumor antibodies. The mother died of diffuse melanoma just more than a year later.

Several unethical studies reached the attention of the public during the 1960s and 1970s. In the Willowbrook study, for example, new residents on admission to an institution for the retarded were infected with hepatitis virus to study the course of the disease and search for a vaccine. Of highest notoriety was the Tuskegee study, which was organized by the U.S. Public Health Service to follow the natural history of syphilis in a cohort of 400 rural African American men. The lack of meaningful informed consent in 1932, when the study began, and the subsequent withholding of penicillin treatment until the study was exposed and halted in 1972 shocked the public and spurred Congress into action. The end result, as described above, was the issuance of the Belmont Report and its articulation of the prevailing principles of bioethics: autonomy, justice, and beneficence.

Federal regulations mandate the creation of ongoing institutional review boards (IRBs) with appropriate oversight of human subject research. Pursuant to the doctrine of autonomy, informed consent procurement is now a formalized process. In randomized controlled trials, potential participants must be notified of the risks, benefits, and alternatives to the care provided by the study. Beneficence and justice dictate that equipoise exists between the alternative treatments and between these treatments and the standard of care, and that potentially beneficial findings of the study will be meaningful and relevant for the study population.

This evolution of research ethics is important for students of surgery as well. Although federal regulations cover research funded by the government, their ethical underpinnings should apply to all research involving human subjects, regardless of the source of funding. Surgeons continually try to innovate and improve their skills and the procedures used, but they must be mindful of the possible need for antecedent work in basic science and the animal laboratory and the need for informed consent and peer review when significant deviation from standard practice is contemplated. In most instances, new surgical procedures should be developed in appropriately controlled research trials with all the safeguards needed for the protection of human subjects.

INFORMED REFUSAL AND THE JEHOVAH'S WITNESS PATIENT

Founded in the late nineteenth century, the Jehovah's Witness community is governed by the Watchtower Society, which issues doctrinal positions via its official journal, the *Watchtower*. On July 1, 1945, an article in that journal established the familiar Jehovah's Witness prohibition against blood transfusions. The biblical sources cited—Genesis 9:4, Leviticus 17:13–14, and Acts 15:19–21—are understood by conventional Judeo-Christian theology as proscriptions against consuming the blood of animals. Nevertheless, Jehovah's Witnesses forbid transfusions of whole blood or its constituents: plasma, packed red blood cells, platelets, and white blood cells. The penalty for transgression is severe: eternal damnation and, more immediately, social ostracism and "disfellowshipping" by other Witnesses. In the June 15, 2004, edition of the *Watchtower*, however, explicit clarifications were issued revealing that transfusion of fractionated components of plasma, packed red blood cells, platelets, and white blood cells were permissible and subject to the individual's discretion.

The wrenching ethical quandary arises when a Jehovah's Witness patient asserts her autonomy to refuse transfusion, thereby risking exsanguination during surgery or from medical conditions such as dysfunctional uterine bleeding. Could or should physician beneficence override a competent patient's refusal of treatment? When locked in conflict, which bioethical principle prevails: autonomy or beneficence? In these instances, it is also important for physicians to consider the concept of good and well-being from the perspective of the patient. Physicians often are in situations in which they cannot provide medical beneficence, but that does not prevent them from assisting in spiritual or emotional beneficence. In the case of a Jehovah's Witness, a physician may appeal to the principle of beneficence while withholding treatment at the request of a competent patient.

American courts have not reached consensus concerning the withholding of blood products for Jehovah's Witnesses, but several dominant trends appear. Surgeons who choose to respect the wishes of a competent Jehovah's Witness patient to refuse blood products in the face of imminent exsanguination are, in general, protected from wrongful death liability. Likewise, courts generally endorse a patient's right to refuse treatment. However, when the patient has dependents who would be otherwise abandoned, or in obstetric situations in which the fetal well-being will be placed in jeopardy, courts have intervened to order transfusions.

From an ethical perspective, a gynecologist contemplating a surgical procedure for a Jehovah's Witness should take the following steps to ensure that the patient and surgical team are prepared for the potential decision to withhold blood products:

- Extensive, confidential preoperative counseling to ascertain informed consent. Specifically, the surgeon should verify the patient's understanding and acceptance of Watchtower society doctrine, understanding of the potential repercussions of refusing transfusion, and awareness of the views of dissident Jehovah's Witnesses. This should be thoroughly documented in the chart. In cases in which the patient's decision-making capacity may be in question, the physicians should request additional professional input from a psychiatrist.
- Consultation, as needed, with the hospital ethics committee.
- Preoperative consultation with the anesthesiologist.

There are several prophylactic steps that can be taken to avoid the likelihood of a transfusion. These include preoperative iron and/or recombinant erythropoietin therapy and intraoperative use of vasopressin, volume expanders, hypotensive anesthesia, hypothermia, and ligation of major vessels

ADVANCED PLANNING AND END-OF-LIFE DECISION MAKING

Policies and regulations regarding death and dying have been set largely by the courts on a case-by-case basis when intractable controversies have arisen with doctors, patients, patients' families, or hospital administrators that must be resolved before a judge. The introduction of life-sustaining technology—such as the respirator that can keep the human body functioning biologically even in cases when the prospect of a return to normalcy is unlikely—has introduced a host of new dilemmas and questions about medical decisions at the end of life. When terminally ill patients, their families, and their health care teams all agree on the use and withholding of treatment at the end of life, there is usually no overt dilemma, except the question of the prudent use of scarce resources. When there is agreement among all parties, there is seldom a need to go to court, and courts discourage bringing these cases before them. When there is disagreement among the patient, the patient's family, the physician or team of physicians, and/or the hospital, the stage is set for conflict that often must be decided by an arbitrator. The courts have traditionally provided guidance in these types of cases. However, these rulings often are not universal and are influenced by contemporary public attitudes. Although not every case and its outcome are comparable, the general consensus is that the patient's autonomous choices are binding and that the ultimate goal of medicine is not to preserve life at any cost, but to relieve pain and suffering in keeping with the patient's wishes.

Since the development of these life-sustaining interventions, there have been several landmark cases: Karen Ann Quinlan, Nancy Cruzan, and Terri Schiavo. Each of these cases represents a different scenario in which physicians and family members struggle to make difficult decisions in surrogate for their loved one. The situation of Karen Ann Quinlan is one example of the type of disagreement that can occur between a patient's family and the providing health care institution. Karen Ann Quinlan was a 21-year-old woman who had been in a prolonged coma and sustained on a respirator. When the likelihood of recovery disappeared, her family's request to remove the respirator was challenged by the hospital. The courts ultimately ordered the removal of the respirator, and she died 10 years later.

In the case of Nancy Cruzan, a difficult decision had to be made when the wishes of the patient were unknown. Nancy Cruzan was in a prolonged coma, and her parents wanted to withdraw food and fluid. There was no record of her prior stated or documented wishes, and, as a result of a Missouri state law forbidding withdrawal without such evidence, this did not take place. The case was taken to the U.S. Supreme Court, who ultimately found the Missouri statute constitutional and, therefore, did not grant the request to the parents. This case is landmark because, in the course of handing down this decision, the U.S. Supreme Court established the right of competent patients to refuse any kind of treatment, also including life-sustaining treatment. In addition, the Supreme Court determined that no distinction was necessary between artificial feeding and other forms of therapy. Finally, evidence was found of Nancy Cruzan's prior wishes that she would not want to be kept alive in a permanent coma, and she was allowed to die after treatment was withdrawn.

The most recent case of Terri Schiavo is another example of the complexity of surrogate decision making. In contrast to the two previous cases, this one represents disagreement between the family members of the patient. On February 1990, Terri Schiavo suffered a myocardial infarction resulting in severe cerebral cortex injury leaving only minimal brain stem function intact. At the time of this initial event, Schiavo did not have a living will or written documentation of her medical care wishes. Her husband and parents worked together to care for her with the hope that she would recover all or part of her cerebral functions, having a feeding tube inserted and placing her in a skilled nursing facility. Eight years later, Terri's husband came to the conclusion that her status had not and would not improve. Stating that his wife had previously expressed her wishes to not live under such circumstances, he appealed to the courts to take on the role of the ward's surrogate to remove the feeding tube and allow her to die. A court order to remove the feeding tube in April 2001 was immediately followed by an appeal by her parents claiming that they had evidence that Schiavo would want to live. Furthermore, they believed that novel medical therapies would be able to improve Schiavo's condition and restore some of her ability to function. They based this on the belief that Schiavo was conscious and responsive and, given the ability to speak for herself, would express her desire to live.

In response to this new information, the court reversed its ruling and, 2 days later, the tube was reinserted. Over the course of 15 years, Schiavo's feeding tube was placed and removed a total of three times in response to different court rulings. After several attempts for appeal, the final ruling ordered the removal of the feeding tube in March 2005, and, less than 2 weeks later, Terri Schiavo passed away.

Many such cases did not deal directly with the issues pertaining to terminal illness, but they provided the moral and legal environment in which such requests can more readily be honored by the physician. Sufficient consensus among patient advocacy groups and professional medical organizations led to the Patient Self Determination Act, which was passed by Congress in 1990. This required hospitals to promote the use of advance directives by their patients to qualify for federal funds for Medicare and Medicaid. Almost every state in the country has enacted laws that allow for advanced-care planning to direct the care of and protect the rights of patients who are terminally ill and suddenly incapacitated. These are referred to as *advanced directives,* and they include a variety of different mechanisms whereby a patient can direct his medical care in the case of his sudden or gradual decline in decisional capacity. The different forms of advanced directives include:

Durable power of attorney for health care—This is a legal document in which a patient designates a specific individual to make health care decisions in the setting of loss of decisional capacity.

Living will—This is a legal document in which the patient describes his/her treatment preferences in the setting of loss of decision-making capacity, such as the continuation of nutrition, hydration, or ventilator support.

Health care proxy (attorney-in-fact for health care)—This is the individual designated by the patient to make surrogate decisions in the case of loss of decision-making capacity.

Do not resuscitate (DNR)—This is one type of advanced directive that specifically directs the withholding of lifesaving procedures in the case of cardiopulmonary arrest, such as cardiopulmonary resuscitation and defibrillation.

Gynecologists should familiarize themselves with different forms of advance directives and the applicable laws. They should also discuss these issues with their patients and their families to ensure that the best arrangement can be made. The ideal time to do this is preferably before such decisions are actually needed for implementation, such as before significant illness or surgery.

ETHICAL CHALLENGES SPECIFIC TO GYNECOLOGIC CARE

Several issues specific to the care of women and their reproductive health are ethical dilemmas unique to gynecology. These include abortion, examination under anesthesia before surgery, and assisted reproductive technologies. In each case, the nuances of addressing the health care issues of women requires additional consideration to ethical topics mentioned above.

Abortion

The termination of pregnancy is encountered in a variety of settings in obstetrics and gynecology. A patient may seek an abortion for a broad spectrum of circumstances, ranging from an unintended and undesired pregnancy (failure or nonuse of birth control, sexual assault, failure of emergency contraception), severe fetal anomalies (aneuploidy, congenital abnormalities incompatible with life), or threatened maternal health (preeclampsia, severe hyperemesis gravidarum, cardiomyopathy). Because of the many diverse clinical scenarios for the termination of a pregnancy, it benefits physicians to be aware of the issues surrounding abortion, whether or not they have personal objections to the procedure.

The core ethical and legal issues surrounding abortion include the right of the woman to control her own body and reproduction, the moral and legal status of the fetus, the rights and interests of the fetus to be protected from harm, and the degree to which outside parties such as national and state governments have authority in the protection or restriction of these rights. These issues tend to divide the general public and government into two polarized camps: prolife or prochoice. Because of the two extremes of positions that exist in the debate about abortion, very little headway has been made to find a common ground since the beginning of abortion law in the United States.

The two major legal cases that have shaped most abortion law in the United States in the past century are *Roe v. Wade* and *Planned Parenthood v. Casey*. Although these decisions do not encompass all laws pertaining to abortion, they are the two most well known and influential. In 1973, *Roe v. Wade* recognized the following rights: the fundamental right of privacy, protection of an individual's bodily integrity, and protection of an individual's decisional autonomy. The rights outlined in *Roe v. Wade* were weighed against the interests of the state in terms of the protection of a potential human life and the health of the mother. However, *Roe v. Wade* did not address questions such as the moral or legal status of the fetus. Under these three rights, the Supreme Court interpreted the Constitution as granting significant protections to an individual's right not to have a child. As such, a woman's choice to terminate a pregnancy was given to her and not to the government. At the same time, the Supreme Court recognized the states' interests in protecting both women's health and the potential life of the fetus, giving the individual states the authority to enact laws imposing strict safeguards and even restricting procedures.

Roe v. Wade also accomplished several other legal milestones. It set out to limit states' restrictions on a woman's right to terminate a pregnancy by instating a "strict scrutiny standard." By this standard, individual states that proposed laws such as mandatory husband consent requirements and mandatory waiting periods were determined to be unconstitutional. In addition, *Roe v. Wade* established a trimester framework for outlining the extent of the state's interests in abortion law. During the first trimester, the woman's interests had precedence above the interests of the state to protect the potential life. During the second trimester, a woman's privacy interests and the state's interest in the protection of the woman's life and the potential life of the fetus were balanced. After the time of viability, the state's interest in protecting the potential life had priority unless the life of the woman is at stake. Minors were also addressed under the Roe framework. Under *Roe v. Wade*, minors were required to inform or involve their parent or guardian in the decision to terminate the pregnancy. In cases when this was not possible, either because of fear of the consequences of disclosure or an unavailable guardian, minors were required to obtain a waiver of parental involvement mandate from the court, also known as a judicial bypass. Finally, *Roe v. Wade* placed federal and state limitations for the use of public funding of abortions for Medicaid patients.

Planned Parenthood v. Casey (1992) reaffirmed the central tenets of *Roe v. Wade* but changed the law significantly by removing the trimester framework based on the notion that it did not adequately recognize the state's interest in the potential life before viability. Under Casey, the states' interests take priority from the outset of pregnancy, not just during later gestations, and, as such, states were permitted to make laws to restrict abortion in the process of protecting their interests. These individual state-by-state laws were constitutional only if they met the "undue burden" standard. Under this, the state's restrictions could not place an undue burden on the woman to make a decision to terminate the pregnancy, such as a restriction that has the purpose or effect of placing a substantial obstacle in the path of a woman seeking an abortion of a nonviable fetus. Many states have interpreted "undue burden" in different ways, creating restrictions—such as increased parental involvement, mandatory waiting periods, and counseling biased toward continuing the pregnancy—that are deemed constitutional.

Abortion is one of the few medical procedures from which physicians may opt out in nonemergent situations because of ethical or religious objections. Under this situation, legislatures have recognized that professionals may legally refuse to provide abortion services. "Conscience" or "refusal" clauses make abortion services one of the few areas in which a physician legally may opt out of performing a medically indicated procedure because of personal objections; however, the scope of such rights to opt out differs from state to state. Legally, under the protections of conscientious objection, no physician is required to do a procedure if it is in conflict with his or her ethical, moral, or religious beliefs. This applies only in situations in which the patient's life is not at stake. In cases when the life of the woman is threatened by the ongoing pregnancy and no other providers are immediately available, a physician cannot refuse to treat the woman.

The statutes of conscientious objection do not exempt physicians from making a responsible, truthful, and timely referral to another practitioner or health care facility that provides the service or from rendering care in a life-threatening emergency when an alternate health care provider is not available. Failure to provide an appropriate referral can constitute malpractice (i.e., fall below the legal standard of care) and also may violate ethical standards of care. Many states have patient abandonment laws that put specific burdens on physicians to refer or transfer care of patients before terminating a relationship. At minimum, the physician is expected to guide the patient to valid resources to find an abortion provider.

The most recent debates about abortion pertain to the issues of partial birth abortion and RU-486. Partial birth abortion is a nonmedical term sometimes referring to a particular abortion procedure known as intact dilatation and extraction (intact D&X, or D&X)—a variant of the more common procedure known as dilatation and evacuation (D&E)—and including procedures that would be used for terminations in the early second trimester, beginning at 13 weeks of gestation. Many professional organizations for women's health have rebuked the validity of the partial birth bans. Legislation addressing partial birth abortion has been described by ACOG as "inappropriate, ill advised, and dangerous" because "intact D&X may be the best or most appropriate procedure in a particular circumstance to save the life or preserve the health of a woman, and only the doctor, in consultation with the patient, based upon the woman's particular circumstances, can make this decision." Arguments against partial birth abortion have been criticized for being simply a rhetorical strategy to place greater restrictions on the present abortion statutes. To date, all proposed bans on partial birth abortion have been deemed unconstitutional because it does not make exceptions for the health of the woman. The issue is still in question as an appeal to these rulings is expected.

A second area of controversy addresses new agents that facilitate access to abortion. In 2000, the Food and Drug Administration (FDA) approved mifepristone, also known as RU-486, for pregnancy termination. RU-486 had been established as a safe method of pregnancy termination in Europe for several years before it was marketed in the United States. However, the controversy that surrounded it delayed its introduction in this country by several years. Concerns about increased access and ease to abortion services fueled much of the debate. Despite this, RU-486 has been accepted as a safe and effective option to women considering termination of a pregnancy.

CONCLUSION

This chapter has presented a sample of the issues pertinent to the practice of gynecology. As a field that combines the challenges of medicine, surgery, and the complex issues specific to the care of women and their reproductive health, there are several other important ethical aspects that have not been addressed here. In addition, innovative technologies and therapeutic procedures present new dilemmas to the practicing physician on a regular basis. Physicians have many resources with which to approach some of the difficult questions that may arise in their own practices. Institution or individual practice ethics committees, oversight committees, and ethics consult services are available for multidisciplinary and peer review of challenging ethical cases. Physicians at all levels of practice should feel confident to turn to these mechanisms for guidance in the case of difficult ethical situations.

BEST SURGICAL PRACTICES

- Informed consent is a mechanism whereby the patient's autonomy is respected.
- Physicians are responsible for maintaining medical and surgical competence.
- The confidentiality of the patient should be protected. Only in special circumstances can it be overridden.
- Physicians should be familiar with the different forms of advance directives and discuss end-of-life decision making with their patients.
- Gynecologists should be aware that several issues specific to the care of women and their reproductive health present ethical dilemmas that are often unique to gynecology.

Bibliography

The American College of Obstetricians and Gynecologists Department of Professional Liability/Risk Management. *2003 ACOG survey on professional liability: national ACOG statistics*. Washington, DC: American College of Obstetricians and Gynecologists, 2004.

Beauchamp TL, Childress JF. *Principles of biomedical ethics*, 4th ed. New York: Oxford University Press, 1994.

Beecher HK. Ethics and clinical research. *N Engl J Med* 1966;274:1354.

The Belmont Report: Ethical principles and guidelines for the protection of human subjects of research. Washington, DC: Government Printing Office, 1979.

Department of Health, Education and Welfare, Ethics Advisory Board. *Report and conclusions: HEW support of research involving human in vitro fertilization and embryo transfer*. Washington, DC: Government Printing Office, 1979.

Faden RR, Beauchamp TL. *A history and theory of informed consent*. New York: Oxford University Press, 1986.

Gillon R. Refusal of potentially life-saving blood transfusions by Jehovah's Witnesses: Should doctors explain that not all JWs think it's religiously required? *J Med Ethics* 2000;26:299.

Gostin LO. Deciding life and death in the courtroom. *JAMA* 1997;278:1523.

HIPAA privacy rule and public health. Guidance from CDC and the U.S. Department of Health and Human Services. *MMWR Morb Mortal Wkly Rep* 2003 May 2;52 Suppl:1.

Hodgson CS. Disciplinary action by medical boards and prior behavior in medical school. *N Engl J Med* 2005;353:2673.

Jacox A, Carr DB, Payne R. New clinical-practice guidelines for the management of pain in patients with cancer. *N Engl J Med* 1994;330:651.

Jonsen AR. *The birth of bioethics*. New York: Oxford University Press, 1998.

King NMP. *Making sense of advance directives*. Dordrecht, The Netherlands: Kluwer Academic Publishers, 1993.

LaFollette H, ed. *Ethics in practice: an anthology*. Cambridge, MA: Blackwell, 1997.

Moreno-Hunt C, Gilbert WM. Current status of obstetrics and gynecology resident medical-legal education. *Obstet Gynecol* 2005;106:1382.

Papadakis MA, Teherani A, Banach MA, et al. Introduction. In Reich WT, ed. *The encyclopedia of bioethics*, revised ed. New York: Simon & Schuster Macmillan, 1995.

Papadakis MA, Teherani A, Ranach MA, et al. Disciplinary action by medical boards and prior behavior in medical school. *New England J. Med* 2005;25:2673.

Robertson JA. *Children of choice: freedom and the new reproductive technologies*. Princeton, NJ: Princeton University Press, 1994.

Rothman DJ. *Strangers at the bedside*. New York: Basic Books, 1991.

Ryan KJ. Abortion or motherhood, madness and suicide. *Am J Obstet Gynecol* 1992;160:1415.

Veatch RM. *Medical ethics*. Boston: Jones & Bartlett, 1989.

Wall LL, Brown D. Ethical issues arising from the performance of pelvic examinations by medical students on anesthetized patients. *Am J Obstet Gynecol* 2004;190:319.

CHAPTER 3 ■ PSYCHOLOGICAL ASPECTS OF PELVIC SURGERY

BETTY RUTH SPEIR

DEFINITIONS

Anxiety—A feeling of apprehension, uncertainty, and fear without apparent stimulus and associated with physiological changes (tachycardia, sweating, tremor, etc.).

Grief—The normal emotional response to an external and consciously recognized loss; it is self-limited, gradually subsiding within a reasonable time.

Insanity—Mental derangement or disorder. The term is a social and legal rather than medical one, and indicates a condition that renders the affected person unfit to enjoy liberty of action because of the unreliability of his behavior with concomitant danger to himself and others.

Regression—A return to a former or earlier state; a subsidence of symptoms or of a disease process; the turning backward of the libido to an early fixation at infantile levels because of inability to function in terms of reality.

PSYCHOLOGICAL ASPECTS OF PELVIC SURGERY

Neuroscientific research over the past decade continues to validate the oneness of the psyche and soma. Gynecological surgery does not simply alter the soma, but temporarily and sometimes permanently alters the psyche of the patient.

The modern gynecologist needs to be more than a skilled technician and must be willing and able to identify the potential psychological effects of the surgery performed and be prepared with the knowledge and skills to address these effects with the patient.

The technological revolution has presented today's surgeon with a vast array of sophisticated equipment. In capable hands, miraculous surgical feats can be performed on a woman's body, but at what cost to her psychological self? The removal or reconstruction of diseased or dysfunctional anatomy may set off a chain reaction of parallel events in a woman's psyche.

For a surgeon, the gynecologic operation may be an ordinary event of usually simple dimension. For the patient, each procedure is a unique experience. Her sense of well-being and health may be threatened. She may lose control over her body for some indefinite period of time. She may perceive the planned procedure as temporarily or even permanently affecting her sexual identity.

As complicated procedures become routine, the surgeon risks losing perspective about the impact of surgery on the life of the individual woman. The patient who experiences ablative genital (or breast) surgery is strongly influenced by her emotions. These vary in degree but are usually cumulative. As the patient passes through the presurgical, surgical, and postsurgical experiences, she may be stressed beyond her capacity to compensate. If help is not available to facilitate emotional healing and rehabilitation, permanent psychological damage may result.

The majority of women do heal and take up their lives, raise their children, work at their jobs, and relate well to their husbands or lovers. For them, the healing interval is relatively quick, and the stress is modest. Do not underestimate what can be learned from this segment of psychologically healthy women patients. In the 1940s, Abraham Maslow studied people with exceptional mental health to develop his hierarchy of needs theory. He discovered that these people's potential had never been weakened by negative thinking, destructive outlook, or destructive self-image. "The rest of us," he declared, "fixate at a lower level because someone or thing has implanted notions of limitations."

Once you become cognizant of the success statistics in your own patient population, you may discover why most women recover after gynecologic surgery to zestfully reembrace life, whereas others begin to slowly turn away from its possibilities.

It will never be enough for a surgeon to be a trained mechanic, able only to diagnose and repair. He or she must also be prepared to predict, recognize, and begin treatment of the psychological consequences of gynecologic disorders. This chapter is designed to help surgeons and other physicians better understand the female perspective and to use that knowledge to facilitate multidimensional healing.

ANKH

The ansate cross, Egyptian emblem of generation, symbol for life and soul and eternity, is a mark universally designated to depict femaleness (Fig. 3.2). By using this hieroglyph, modern scientists continue an ancient tradition of respect and reverence for women. Within the inner sanctum of every woman's mind lie symbols that are powerful and personal. These feminine identity markers are guarded and guided by her instincts, and no surgeon can successfully maneuver in this labyrinth of psychological and psychosexual emotion and cause no harm unless the female patient acts as a guide.

Egyptian writings from 2,000 years ago in the Kahan Papyrus depict the uterus as having an important and powerful effect on mental life, and current research tends to agree with the ancient scribes. The uterus has great symbolic value for many modern women, too. Beginning with the rite of passage called menstruation, a strong invisible bond is formed between a woman and her body. Her biological clock has been set. For the next 40 years or so, she will be reminded each month that

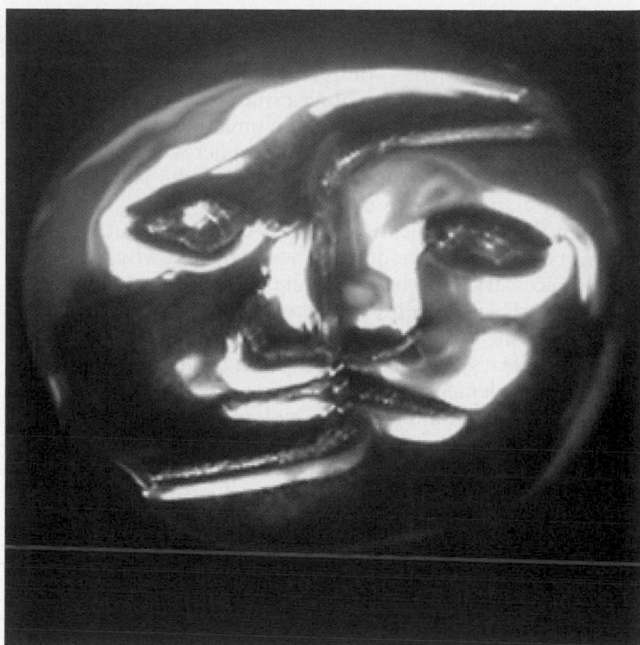

FIGURE 3.1. *Inseparable Psyche-Soma*: Sculpture by Jim Sardonis (http://www.sardonis.com).

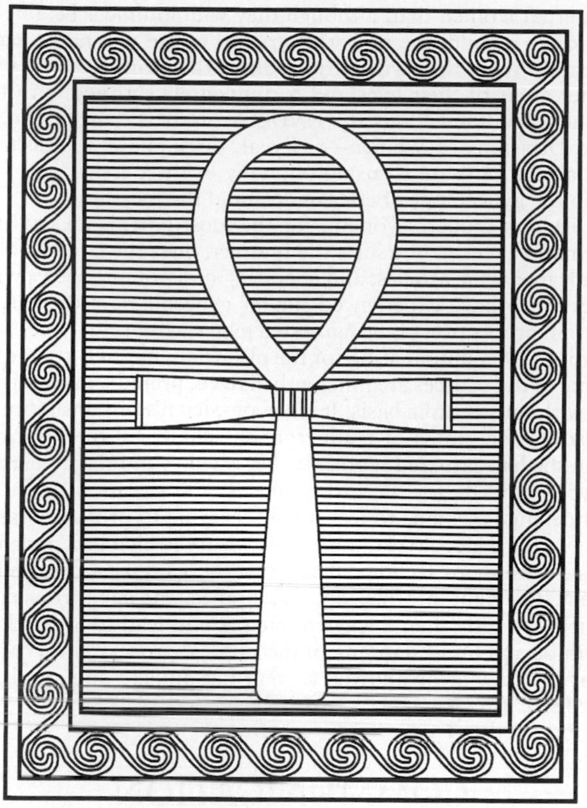

FIGURE 3.2. The ansate cross, or ankh amulet, is an ancient Egyptian symbol of life and sexuality.

she is a woman, and menstruation is regarded by many as palpable proof of their femininity.

Others believe that menstruation is part of a natural cleansing cycle that purges the body of poisons that accumulate during the month. They know from experience that the premenstrual symptoms of edema, bloating, headaches, and emotional tension will be washed away in the tide of their monthly flow.

For some, the rhythm of the menstrual cycle is used as a way to time and order their lives. Like the phases of the moon, this cycle bestows a sense of routine, regularity, and predictability that has emotional significance. With the onset of menstruation, a woman is forever changed. Surgical removal of any of the reproductive organs will change her again, but how?

The effect of a woman's menstrual cycle on many medical conditions is well documented. Medical suppression of ovulation is commonly used as a way to evaluate and treat such chronic conditions as migraine headache, epilepsy, asthma, rheumatoid arthritis, irritable bowel syndrome, and diabetes. Research at the National Institutes of Health and other leading institutions has shown "how nerves, molecules and hormones connect the brain and immune system, how the immune system signals the brain and affects our emotions, and documents how our brain can signal the immune system, making us more vulnerable to illnesses." What we have known intuitively is now understood scientifically. Hormones secreted during a woman's menstrual cycle affect her mood. Could the decline of these hormones during the natural aging process contribute to dementia? The future is alive with fascinating neuroscientific and neuroimmunomodulation elucidation, but today's woman is backlit by the skepticism of some scientists. Her concerns about her body and the way it will work after surgery are immediate and quite often heartrending.

A woman about to undergo a hysterectomy might wonder if her lover will be able to detect the absence of her uterus. After the surgery, will she be thought of as less of a woman? Will her partner abandon her for someone who is still complete, either in the sense of being able to offer the possibility of a child or complete in the sense of having experienced no unnatural surgical transformations?

Will orgasm be as pleasurable for her after the surgery? For many women, the uterus has symbolic significance as a sexual organ. The uterus contracts during orgasm. Some women perceive this as most pleasurable. If the patient believes the uterus is essential to sexual response, then, in fact, it often becomes so, and women with this mind-set may become sexually dysfunctional when it is removed.

Once the procedure is accomplished, will she still look and sound like a woman, or will she become noticeably more masculine? For others, the uterus is closely tied to feelings of attractiveness and sexual desirability. To a few women, removal of the uterus or ovaries or both constitutes a desexing, a permanent destruction of female identity and function. Sadly, certain members of the medical community as well as the feminist community perpetuate this notion and increase the attendant fear when they refer to women who must have their ovaries removed as *castrates*.

Some women become distressed when they learn they must deal with the certainty of absolute sterility. For those who choose motherhood, the uterus, ovaries, breasts, and vagina work in harmony with other factors to attract a necessary mate and get down to the business of creating new life. These organs become vital coconspirators in the sexual and reproductive aspects of a woman's life. Impending loss of these physical structures because of disease or dysfunction sometimes creates deep angst that must be resolved before surgery is attempted. Many women who have all the children they want and who do not wish to get pregnant again are still sometimes disturbed by the finality of the decision. The gynecologist should assure these maternal women that, although they will no longer be able to conceive a child, the powerful urge to create will never leave them. In time, they will learn to direct this primal energy into other areas of their lives and be immensely satisfied with the results. Studies such as the ENDOW Study: Ethnicity, Needs and Decisions of Women—a 5-year, three-phase, multicenter collaboration—are focusing on many of these issues and will help the gynecologist better understand the patient.

Today's modern woman, for the most part, is an avid information seeker. She surfs the Internet, buys the latest books, reads magazine articles, and conducts in-depth interviews with peers who have experienced similar gynecologic problems. A certain proportion of the harvested material is useful to her and perhaps even illuminating for the physician, but unfortunately, some of the sources are inherently flawed, prejudicial, illogical, or without scientific basis. It is the physician's responsibility to separate the grains of truth from the chaff. All the information she has gathered represents her attempt to prepare herself psychologically for the ordeal ahead, and she must never be condemned or made to feel small for trying to protect herself.

For the gynecologist, it is not necessary to change a patient's basic attitude or feelings. It is, however, vital to acknowledge them. The right information, reassurance, and support usually quickly modify many negative factors and lead to a healthier attitude and understanding of the surgical process. It is crucial that the patient be allowed to vent her anxiety and speak of her fears.

COMMUNICATION

Patients in General

Diplomats the world over understand the significance of effective communication. Indeed, the prospect for world peace depends on their ability to interact efficiently. A female patient's psychological bearing before, during, and after the gynecologic procedure can depend on the communication techniques used by her physician. You must establish rapport, speak of the real and present danger to her health, and then elaborate on your plans to protect her.

Whenever possible, provide pleasant surroundings where you and your patient can comfortably hold a private conversation. Push all other thoughts out of your mind. These few minutes belong exclusively to her, and the quality of the time you spend actively communicating will pay healthy dividends for you both.

Whether explaining the simplicity of a needle-directed breast biopsy or the intricacies of hysterectomy, you must be able to highlight the technical details of the procedure and its postsurgical realities in a nonthreatening but utterly truthful manner. Begin the presentation using simple but thorough explanations and examples of the procedures. Your patient will let you know how much information she can or wishes to process by the questions she asks.

Your patient needs confidence in your technical ability, and to know that her problem is being taken seriously and that you are qualified to competently help her cope with all of the ramifications of this new experience.

Dealing with the patient's feelings usually is not difficult if the surgeon accepts the viewpoint that many of the patient's emotions are part of the gynecologic situation. To the physician, the presurgical tension is predictable, familiar, transient, and simply comes with the territory, but to each new patient, it represents a dramatic and life-altering experience.

To interpret the patient's true feelings, simply listen to her. Listening well is both an art and a skill, and the surgeon who cares about the patient's complete health as well as her quick recovery works diligently to hone a sharp edge on this valuable tool. Listen, and you will hear the woman give a name to her most profound doubts and fears. Repeat her words so that you are absolutely certain you understand what she said and she is absolutely assured that you are listening to her.

Begin the communication process by finding out what the patient perceives will be done to her body and why the procedure is necessary. Find out what she believes the consequences of the surgery will be. How does she think the surgery will affect her life? As she discusses the implications of her decision, her knowledge, fears, and biases emerge. At this point, you should be able to supplement the patient's perspective with appropriate explanations about anatomy, physiology, and pathology. After this, it is time to describe in detail the usual preoperative, operative, and postoperative routines. Address the patient's questions and fears in as many ways as it takes for her to become confident that she understands what is about to happen to her.

Carefully explain what you are going to do to help her. If she wants to know, or needs to know, describe the common physical sensations, bandages, incisions, catheters, tubing, and medications that are associated with her particular procedure. Define the patient's role in her own convalescence and recovery. Give her a general timetable for how long she will feel discomfort, how long she will have to use pain medication, when she will be ambulatory, and finally, when she will be discharged from the hospital or outpatient center.

Relate the most common complications that might occur as the result of her surgery. Injuries that might affect the quality of her life, even temporarily, should never come as a postsurgical surprise, nor should they be glossed over during the signing of the consent forms. Iatrogenic injury remains the most common cause of lower urinary tract trauma. An understanding of the prevention, recognition, and treatment of urologic complications is important for every surgeon performing major pelvic surgery. Injury to a woman's genitourinary system may take 10 to 20 years to develop full-blown symptoms, about the same timeline as from multiple childbirths, but it remains a possibility. Physicians, however, disagree on whether to tell the patient that urinary incontinence after hysterectomy because of damage to the pelvic nerves or pelvic supportive structures could be a long-term adverse effect. Only 4% of the hysterectomies performed are for relief from symptoms of incontinence.

Complications such as the formation of adhesions may occur in as many as 55% of patients after gynecologic surgery. These adhesions can become a critical issue from a standpoint of reproductive potential. Their presence is also strongly associated with pelvic pain, abnormal bowel function, and small bowel obstruction.

The mentally competent patient has a moral, legal, and ethical right to make an intelligent informed decision and can only do it if she is privy to all of the available facts concerning her situation. It is essential that you involve her in the decision-making processes, because the more committed she is to the proposed treatment, the more involved she will become in her own preparation and rehabilitation. This point is supported by the findings of the ENDOW Study.

The art of touching, the therapeutic laying on of the hands, is important. Being lonely, frightened, and sick is a reason for the patient to be touched by her physician, especially if she seems particularly overwhelmed by her situation. To hold the patient's hand while talking to her or touch her shoulder is therapeutic. Even a comforting hug is appropriate if it fits the circumstances and the patient reaches out to you.

Before fetal monitoring, quality of labor was evaluated by sitting at the patient's bedside with the physician's hand on her abdomen to feel uterine contractions. Often, the presence of the physician and a warm hand on her abdomen made the patient relax, rest, and become calmer during active labor. Cancer patients, especially, on hearing bad news, need immediate human-to-human contact to stay grounded enough to face that terrible moment. The professional boundaries of roles, time, place and space, gifts and services, chaperoned examinations, physical contact, money and formal language were never intended to be an impermeable membrane separating a doctor's ability to administer human kindness. A healer's touch can often comfort a distressed patient when words are inadequate.

A patient's family is a vital part of her support system and can be a potent ally, or not, to the health care team. If your patient requests that family members be present during her consultation, allow it, but speak directly to her whenever possible.

Once the initial presurgical discussions are complete, your patient may need some time to digest all the new information she has received. After assimilation, allow her to contact you for clarification or to ask more questions. You should be available to her. You should instruct your personnel to facilitate her access to you. Too often, office personnel believe their role is to shield the physician from patients rather than to facilitate meaningful contact.

Patients from Other Cultures

Patients from other cultures abound in the United States and their numbers are increasing dramatically. These patients in many cases are often situated in dense clusters. Physicians in these areas are either multilingual or have assistants who are able to act as interpreters. However, no matter where your practice is located, chances are that at some point during your career as a physician, an individual from another culture will need your help.

Mull makes the following suggestions for communicating effectively with a person whose language you do not speak and whose culture is foreign to you: Make sure that your office staff are courteous and respectful. Show the genuine concern you feel. Be friendly and helpful to build rapport and develop a repertoire of knowledge. Familiarize yourself with the general principles of their traditional medicine. Whenever possible, have an interpreter present. Learn a few key phrases from their language, and use these for initial greeting and during examinations. Electronic linguistic assistants, such as the Franklin devices, are available in most languages. Include, at least in discussion, any family members your patient considers influential. Always ask what they have done to treat themselves. Have they consulted an influential family member? A healer? Have they used home or herbal remedies?

Physicians should be aware of common themes that exist in cross-cultural medicine, including:

- Fear of blood loss
- Fear of cold
- Tradition of male dominance
- Conservatism in sexual matters relative to teenage girls
- Poorly developed concept of preventive medicine
- Intolerance of side effects from medication
- Expectation of expeditious wellness
- Reluctance to discuss emotions with people who are not family members

Diaz-Gilbert cautions health care professionals to check their prejudices at the door and not to assume that a non–English-speaking person is uneducated. The following are some guidelines for effective communication with patients from other cultures:

- Allot extra time for the patient from another culture.
- Address every patient initially in English.
- Ask if the patient carries a bilingual dictionary.
- Gesture or write down simple words or phrases.
- Use visual cues, such as insurance forms, calendars, medication bottles, or anatomic sketches. If necessary, draw a picture to convey what you mean.

If the patient needs to perform a specific task, such as disrobing, carefully pantomime each step. Remain aware that direct eye contact, certain hand or finger gestures, and physical touch are offensive, disrespectful, or can be construed as sexually suggestive in certain cultures.

When a cultural language barrier exists, reliance on body language becomes crucially important. Work at learning to read it. These patients experience the same emotional responses to surgery and need the same education and reassurances. Having to use the services of a foreign doctor in an alien land makes the surgical process even more frightening for them.

PSYCHOLOGICAL PREPARATION FOR SURGERY

Massler and Devansan said there is an emotional response to any physical assault on the body. The magnitude of the response is expected to be proportional to the degree of emotional investment one has in the part of the body under siege. Among women, anatomic entities most vulnerable to this emotional reaction are the face, hair, breasts, genitalia, and abdominal wall.

Second only to cesarian birth, hysterectomy is the most frequently performed major surgical procedure done on reproductive-aged women. More than 600,000 women a year have a hysterectomy in the United States. Newer minimally invasive procedures have shortened hospital stays and have lessened visible disfigurement of the body. The majority recover quickly from the procedure and enjoy the new freedom that comes to an individual when a chronic health problem has been solved. Your patients, however, are not always older, wiser women, and they do not always recover quickly. If you know the signs to look for, you will be able to help that patient who is having a harder time adjusting to pelvic surgery, especially if it was a radical, life-threatening, or unexpected event.

In his book, *Matters of Life and Death,* Daniel Bruns writes, "Even the strongest person can be shaken by the horrors of some medical cures. Beyond this, life anxiety is even more common in persons with pre-existing emotional difficulties or characterological disorders. These persons may go through life like eggshells, intact and functioning, but with psychological fragility. When faced with an extreme life stressor, such a person may simply shatter." How will you, as the physician, recognize the vulnerable?

Roeske researched 13 factors related to poor prognosis for excellent mental health after hysterectomy. The following factors begin to define the patient who might react negatively to genital surgical stress:

1. Gender identity
2. Previous adverse reactions to stress

3. Previous depressive episodes
4. Family history of mental illness
5. History of multiple physical symptoms, especially lower back pain
6. Numerous hospitalizations or surgeries
7. Age less than 35 years at time of hysterectomy
8. Desire for a child or more children
9. Fear of loss of libido
10. Significant other's negative attitude toward procedure
11. Marital dissatisfaction or instability
12. Cultural or religious disapproval
13. Lack of vocation or hobbies

Barnes and Tinkham's research also indicates that patients tend to react to current stress in much the same way as they reacted to past crises and personal losses. Well-established patterns of behavior repeat themselves. By taking a patient's history, the surgeon can be forewarned about which patients are likely to have the most difficult time handling the emotional aspects of gynecologic surgery. Equipped with this information, the surgeon can prepare to offer extra support in the form of reassurance, educational information, and, if indicated or requested, the names of psychotherapists who are trained to deal with women's health issues.

COMMON EMOTIONAL RESPONSES TO SURGERY

Insecurity

Giving up control of one's body, even temporarily, is uncomfortable for all of us, but it is terrifying for people who feel generally insecure. One of the most common defense mechanisms against feelings of insecurity is to institute rigid controls over all aspects of life. These patients may have no control over getting sick. They will have little if any control during the surgical procedures. The postsurgical setting will be a hospital room where the staff tells the patient when to awake, take medicine, eat, bathe, walk, have visitors, and get blood drawn. The health care workers will probe such personal matters as urination, defecation, and passage of flatus. Anxiety, anger, and feelings of being assaulted combine with insecurity can produce an unhappy, fearful, and sometimes raging patient.

These feelings are greatly diminished when the patient believes the surgery will improve the quality of her life. There will eventually be relief of pain, removal of cancer, an end to heavy bleeding, restoration of fertility, or some other positive result. She will be better than she was before the surgery. The transition to becoming this healthier person is made easier when she trusts and believes in her physician.

Anxiety or Fear

Anxiety or fear associated with surgery is essentially universal. Most common is fear of the unknown or of what the patient imagines she will be forced to endure during hospitalization. Factual information about the surgical and recovery process and competent care by a compassionate hospital staff help to diminish this fear. Surgeons should assume responsibility for the behavior of the hospital staff toward their patients. When a patient reports ill treatment by any of the health care providers, the physician should deal with the situation personally to decrease the probability of a future recurrence of the offensive or thoughtless behavior.

Patients may fear the loss of economic competence. A woman who has worked for many years may lose her sense of usefulness when disabled for some variable length of time. Whether she plays a major or minor role, the contribution she makes to her family's economic stability will be important to her. Her identity and self-esteem derived from her job may also be threatened by the outcome of her surgery.

Fear of anesthesia is often a thinly disguised fear of dying as well as a fear of loss of control. It may be appropriate to confront the fear of dying directly so that the patient has the opportunity to express why she is afraid. Is the fear general or specific? Did a close relative suffer from the same affliction and die during or shortly after surgery? Does the patient have a strong intuitive feeling that something will go wrong? If so, ask her what you can do to modify the surgical situation. Determine whether the scheduled date of surgery or the particular hospital is significant. The fact that you consider her feelings an important issue and a normal part of the gynecologic disease process may be enough to calm her fears.

Regression and Dependency

In most people who are ill or who undergo surgery, regression to a more dependent state is fairly common. Dealing with a woman who is no longer self-sufficient or emotionally stable is difficult for the patient's family and friends. These members of her supporting cast are accustomed to her presurgical roles as wage earner, wife, mother, friend, cook, advisor, shopper, housekeeper, taxi driver, entertainer, and more. When she becomes ill and can no longer function to make their lives easier, family members and friends often become frustrated and angry. They may apply overt or subtle pressure to try to force the woman to exert herself and fulfill her usual roles. A change in roles is difficult, but often the illness teaches family and friends why this particular woman is valuable to them. Those who temporarily assume her normal duties or help her cope with the surgical experience, in many cases, discover strengths of hers of which they were previously unaware.

When the disease and prospect of surgery are new to the patient, all these factors, as well as a feeling of ill health, contribute to an emotional fragility that yields extremely labile emotions, including feelings of sadness, despondency, tearfulness, and irritability. The usual defense mechanisms are often temporarily weakened or destroyed. The woman is vulnerable to attack on all personal and professional fronts. She needs time with people she cares about, and she needs time alone to sort out her thoughts and emotions.

Grief

Grief is a normal, natural reaction to illness or loss of any kind and is essential to emotional healing. Recognizing the various stages of grief allows the surgeon to help the female patient understand what is happening to her.

Denial is the first and most primitive emotional response to loss and can take many forms. The patient may demonstrate denial by not going to the doctor when she finds a lump in her breast or when she notices abnormal bleeding. She may pretend the symptoms do not exist or are a temporary nuisance. Not remembering instructions the physician gave her could be a manifestation of denial. She may forget important facts or deny the seriousness of the problem. Denial allows people to function for a little while in a make-believe world. With this primitive mechanism, they survive emotional stresses they might otherwise be unable to handle.

Bargaining with a higher power is the second stage of grief. Many patients feel they have carte blanche to bargain when they are experiencing a loss. "Make this bad thing that has happened to me go away, and I swear, I will become a better person."

Guilt can surface before or after a loss. Most guilt feelings are completely inappropriate, in that the focus of the guilt rarely is directly related to the cause of the loss. When sick, many people feel that they are being punished for not being perfect. Explain to your guilt-ridden patients that their feelings are normal for the circumstances. Although guilt can sometimes deliver devastating, incapacitating blows, the good news is that it is usually transitory.

Depression comes in varying degrees to most people experiencing grief and is characterized by feelings of helplessness, hopelessness, and worthlessness. Other symptoms include middle-of-the-night insomnia, nightmares, loss of appetite or excessive eating, lethargy, difficulty making decisions, psychosomatic symptoms, and fatigue unexplained by activity.

Ask the patient if she has any of these symptoms. Postsurgical depression is common. Depressed patients usually admit that the sad feelings are routine and occur daily. When prolonged, they indicate the patient has been unable to work through the grief process. Something emotional has yet to be resolved.

Rage turned inward often manifests as depression. When the patient is able to identify what she is angry about, to ventilate the rage, the depression usually begins to lift. When she takes charge of her life again and makes decisions, even small ones, she begins to feel better, and feelings of helplessness, hopelessness, and worthlessness abate. However, when the depressed patient becomes suicidal, stringent intervention must occur. The suicidal patient presents serious challenges and so is discussed in specific detail later in this chapter.

The stage at which the patient ventilates her anger can be difficult for those providing care, but it should be accepted as healthy. The patient may go to extremes, writing letters to the newspaper or speaking of suing her physician. She may complain bitterly about the nursing staff and the hospital. Such actions are a form of protest at the stress that has been dealt to her body and mind. In most instances, this behavior means that the depression is lifting and the patient is beginning to move toward the resolution of her grief. The depressed patient should be encouraged to ventilate by talking, to establish an enjoyable form of physical exercise, and to begin to take charge of her own life.

Resolution and integration eventually occur. The stressful experience of loss finally becomes an accepted part of her life. The memory causes sadness and regret, but no longer the devastating immobilization found in the earlier stages of grief. Integration does not mean the experience is forgotten, only that it has less trauma associated with it. After integration, certain stimuli can provoke flashback grief. The painful emotional tapes begin to play again, but the patient learns that the bad time is a rerun and will not last long.

The stages of grief do not always occur in order. The patient may feel fragments of several of them at the same time. If a female patient's behavior seems bizarre, excessive, or out of the realm of what would usually be anticipated during her particular surgical experience, look for the role grief might be playing in her life.

PSYCHODYNAMICS SPECIFIC TO DIAGNOSIS AND SURGERY

Patient–Physician Bonding

Neither scalpel nor laser can divide the psyche and soma. As technical skills have improved and multiplied, comprehensive care of the gynecologic patient has declined. Increased emphasis on scientific and procedural care usually means less time in the consultation room and more time in the examining or procedure rooms. This is unfortunate for all concerned, because it takes time to explore the concepts, fears, and psychological well-being of the individual patient both before and after surgery.

It takes time to at least scan the books and magazines women read, to search the same Internet sites, to listen to the voices of their advocates, and essentially evaluate, critique, and learn from their sources of information. It is important to make the effort. Otherwise, you run the risk of being out of touch, or worse still, appearing arrogant and condescending. Women in general have a sixth sense about these attitudes, and women about to undergo surgery or those recovering from surgical trauma to their bodies are hypersensitive to all manner of psychological stimuli.

The medicolegal climate has also potentiated perioperative anxiety. When you inform your patient, as she prepares for surgery, that she can bleed to death, be subjected to blood transfusions, have an adverse reaction to anesthesia, or sustain bowel or urinary track injuries, you augment her innate fear of surgery. With strong pressure from extreme feminists groups on the patient to seek and maintain a controlling role in her life, over her destiny, and over the surgeon, it is more necessary than ever before that the pelvic surgeon take the time to explore the patient's psyche in the preoperative and postoperative periods to avoid undesirable psychological sequelae. Having personable, competent health care workers in your office who assist in preparing your patient for surgery is indispensable. Anatomic charts have become works of art and they, as well as videotapes and other teaching aids, are useful in explaining the technical details; however, despite all the educational tools and staff assistance, the most important person remains you, the doctor. Unless you sit and answer questions on a one-to-one basis, you are neglecting your responsibility to your patient.

Much of the time, the questions will deal with information the patient has gleaned from literature, popular talk shows, and the Internet. Some of the opinions she reads or hears will frighten her or make her suspicious, and a few patients may initially come to your office thinking of you as a potential enemy. A staunch feminist may express the belief that you are just another insistently prosurgical doctor out to hijack her womb and add it to your trophy collection.

Popular literature today often stresses sexism, ageism, and greed on the part of doctors. *The Silent Passage* and *Our Bodies, Ourselves* were among the first widely read books on which patients depended for their gynecologic information. In these, they read that "for well over a century in the United States, women's uteri and ovaries have been subject to routine medical abuse," and "one should not be railroaded into hysterectomy nor onto hormones." Hysterectomy is described as "devastating" surgery, and for some women, it certainly can be. These books found a wide audience and led to the publication of other books, which took an even more radical approach, all in the name of protecting women from castrating medical experts who might use their position of authority to hurt, not help, them.

The Ultimate Rape: What Every Woman Should Know about Hysterectomies and Ovarian Removal was inspired after the author underwent a hysterectomy. She suffered extreme physical and emotional trauma following the surgery, but when she reported this to her physicians, they advised her to go see a psychiatrist, because all her symptoms were in her head. The book's title is evidence of the rage she felt at their pronouncement. Now her voice is joined by others who believe that every woman has the right to be thoroughly informed about procedures and consequences before consenting to gynecologic modifications. And certainly, a woman should.

In *No More Hysterectomies,* touted as the first living textbook on the Web, the reader learns how the male-dominated medical profession and the insurance industry have sanctioned millions of unwarranted hysterectomies. One testimonial to the ideas presented in the book describes the current medical environment as a "woman's hormonal holocaust."

The enlightening news is that interest generated by these sources and their legions of followers has had a positive and direct effect on women's health research. Global studies are numerous and are concentrating on traditional as well as alternative methods of treatment for menopause, hysterectomy, hormone replacement therapy, cancer, endometriosis, fibroids, and dementia. For the first time in the history of medical science, ethnic research is being conducted on a large scale to determine how women in various cultures and with variances in their physiology react to menopause, gynecologic surgery, hormone therapy, and sexual function. The ENDOW Study has found ethnic/racial differences in women's perceptions of hysterectomy and their determinants in decision making regarding elective surgery. Negative connotations were found to be more prevalent among African American women, thus indicating a need for added support and information preoperatively. Future generations of women will reap the benefits from this research, but the overwhelming aura that prevails in today's gynecologic patient is one of confusion.

After reading just a sampling of the lay literature, some women feel that surgical removal of their female organs and commencement of hormonal therapy constitutes an unnatural, chemotherapy-like assault on their physical bodies. It is the task of the physician to admit into evidence the medical facts necessary to correct any gross misconceptions that could affect patient care. Sometimes it may seem as if the patient, armed with advice about natural remedies for her severe pelvic pain, heavy bleeding, or hot flashes, wants to drag you with her back into the Dark Ages. Be patient and also prepared, if necessary, to explain the medically sound benefits of life lived outside the cave.

Be compassionate. No matter how routine the job becomes, compassion is a vital requisite to becoming an exceptional communicator and healer. Empathy often follows experience, and those times when you are able to make a noticeably positive difference in your patient's life are inspirational. To try the one new thing that might help many patients in the future, it is necessary to earn the trust of a single patient in the present.

The days are gone when a doctor was considered omnipotent, when he, and rarely, she, received a hock of ham for the birth of a child, or had to tell a woman that she would have to live with the eventual hump on her back because it was a natural process of aging. Patients know about osteoporosis and heart disease and reproductive technology and brain neurotransmitters. The media have turned every living room into a medical school. Some patients present videos and clippings detailing current research and experimental treatments relative to their specific diagnoses. They know a little, and they want to know more. Many patients want to participate in their health care and absolutely should be encouraged to do so. Unlike the doctors of old, who, for the most part, had to contend with an uneducated populace, the modern physician must form a partnership with the modern patient. Mutual responsibility, respect, and trust eventually strengthen this bond. The cornerstone of the initial work is truth.

Use good judgment about when to tell all the facts, particularly those that point to a devastating diagnosis, but never lie. In 1961, 90% of physicians surveyed in a single large urban hospital stated that they withheld the diagnosis of cancer from their patients. Today, the position had been totally reversed, with 97% reporting that they reveal the true diagnosis of cancer.

Doctors, however, are not the only members of the team with ethical considerations. Patients also have the responsibility to tell the physician the truth relative to their symptoms, medications, allergies, past medical histories, and to relate any significant traumas or family history that could bear on their current situations.

Question your patient specifically about stressful life events. Did she respond to these in a positive or negative way? Of all inquiries, this is the most important indicator of how the patient will respond to any current stress. Once the physician knows the answer, psychological preparation for diagnosis or surgery can begin in earnest.

Researchers in the United Kingdom have compiled data from multiple trial studies confirming that psychological preparation for surgery is effective. The general hypothesis was that communication and counseling are important determinants of numerous factors, including the following:

- Accuracy of the diagnosis
- Effectiveness of disease management
- Disease or problem prevention
- Patient satisfaction
- Adherence to treatment
- Psychological well-being
- Patient understanding of procedures
- Professional satisfaction and levels of stress

Information about each of these parameters was compiled, and considerable evidence existed to support all the hypotheses. In review, Davis and Johnston reported that psychological preparation is effective in reducing negative effect, pain, medication, length of hospital stay, and in improving behavioral recovery and physiologic functioning.

Surgical Whispers

The surgeon should make it a point to be with the patient while anesthesia is administered. Knowing that you are there with her from the beginning will help her feel safe. At the end of each surgical procedure, whisper into your patient's ear, "You're going to be well very soon." You may be surprised to find she needs less pain medication and recovers quicker than patients without the benefit of this positive prophecy, because the mind itself is a powerful force, as evidenced by neuroscientific research. Dr. Esther M. Sternberg, director of integrative neural immune program and chief of the section on neuroendocrine immunology and behavior at the National Institute of Mental Health and National Institutes of Health, says that "with stress reduction endogenous opiates are produced that decrease pain. These come from the same cells in the hypothalamus that make the stress hormone CRH." Understanding these brain-immune connections will help the surgeon understand how his support and encouragement can decrease the patient's pain. Youngs and colleagues believe the surgeon or a familiar associate also should be present immediately after surgery to reassure the patient, orient her to her surroundings, and make certain she has adequate pain relief. Even if the patient appears unresponsive during the immediate postoperative phase, a familiar voice and reassuring word can be immensely beneficial.

Immediate Postoperative Care

Hospital stays are much shorter. Some outpatient hysterectomies are being performed. These factors are having a positive psychological effect on patients. A patient knows that she is getting well when she no longer requires needles and is able to ambulate and urinate without assistance. It has long been known that early ambulation significantly reduces morbidity as well as the incidence of phlebitis and pneumonia. As long as intravenous therapy and urethral catheterization are maintained, the patient remains immobile and consequently at higher risk for venous stasis, ileus, and pulmonary complications. The incidence of pulmonary embolus in the postoperative hysterectomy patient has decreased in the past decades with shortened stay and early ambulation.

Crisis Intervention

It is important to recognize a patient who is overwhelmed by stress. A stress crisis can occur during any phase between diagnosis and recuperation. A *crisis* has been described as an obstacle to important life goals that becomes insurmountable when the individual employs customary methods of problem solving. Kaplan highlighted the following four phases of crisis.

1. Arousal occurs, and attempts are made at problem solving.
2. Increased tension leads to distress and disorganization because arousal hinders rather than promotes coping behavior. Insomnia and fatigue frequently result.
3. Internal and external emergency resources are mobilized. Novel methods of coping are tried.
4. A state of progressive deterioration, exhaustion, and decompensation ensues as the problems drag on and on without resolution.

Dennerstein and van Hall report that the types of problems dealt with in crisis therapy include loss, change in status or role, interpersonal problems, and problems of choice between two or more alternatives. As an advocate, encourage your patient to communicate her feelings, to understand the problem enough to identify and define it, and then help her rehearse alternative ways of coping.

One of the best concepts to apply during any stressful situation is to give the assurance that this particular moment, no matter how painful, is temporary. The surgical procedure and all the stages of mending that follow will have a beginning, middle, and an end.

PSYCHOSEXUAL REHABILITATION

The goal of psychosexual rehabilitation after gynecologic or breast surgery is to restore sexual function, sexual identity, body image, and self-esteem. Most of the work must be done by the patient herself, but she may need assistance from her doctor and other health care providers because the experience is new to her. She has no gauge to measure what is normal for her particular situation and what is aberrant. You do.

She may expect too much too soon from herself, or she may head off in the opposite direction and begin to assume the role of invalid, but in most cases, she will be caught somewhere between these two extremes. Once she begins to exhibit her normal patterns of relating to others, you will know she has officially begun the process of genuine healing.

You will be able to tell when she enters the healing phase because she will become less dependent on you, the nurses, and even her family members. As her strength increases, she will want to resume her usual activities. The inevitable, normal, uncomfortable grief process will commence. Encourage the patient to talk about her feelings rather than repress them and begin to brood, because worry and rumination are forms of repetitive thought that are concomitant and predictive of depressed mood. Dreary thoughts fuel a depressed mood, turn it into something ugly and dangerous, and have the potential to cause long-term or permanent psychological damage.

The patient has the power within to effect change in herself. Family members and friends should be cautioned, at this point, to allow verbal ventilation. It's a form of healthy discontent that frequently provides the impetus to hurry and lose the sick image and begin to see herself well and strong again.

Cosmetics, dress, and grooming are important parts of the rehabilitation process. When a postoperative patient combs her hair, puts on lipstick, and demands her own nightgown instead of hospital garb, she has begun to heal. When a patient feels that the surgery was disfiguring, she needs to compensate by learning new ways to dress or groom. She needs to feel whole and complete and responsible again as quickly as possible.

The surgical patient begins to see herself as a sexual person when her sexual identity is validated by her sexual partner, friends, family, and even admiring strangers she passes on the street. The woman who has had a mastectomy or other body-altering surgery needs to know her partner still finds her attractive and desirable. Without this affirmation, she may have a great deal of trouble seeing herself as a sexual being. Some sexual partners cannot accept an incomplete person. This is another potential problem.

Some surgical procedures result in loss of vulva, clitoris, or vagina. Radical pelvic surgery can leave a woman with a colostomy or urinary diversion. A severely altered body image concurrent with loss of health and vigor poses a serious threat to a woman's self-esteem. The woman who has lost her sexual identity feels damaged beyond repair. Some report continuing pelvic pain without obvious structural cause. Interest in sex vanishes, and the patient may actually leave her sexual partner or force the partner to abandon her. As she terminates her sexual identity, she feels old before her time and begins to draw in the edges of her life. These women need intense psychosexual therapy if they are ever to heal emotionally. Table 3.1 outlines the major factors that occur with psychosexual dysfunction.

Most of the time, the mate or lover of the woman is caring and considerate of her. There is genuine concern for her health, hope for a quick recovery, and willingness to assume many aspects of her role until she is well. Often there is a deepening of affection between the couple as gifts of love and concern are given and received. That special someone is in the waiting room during the surgical ordeal and by the patient's bedside when she awakes. There are flowers and gifts and promises made and kept. There is an abundance of reciprocal love. Adjustment to new roles is relatively smooth, causing new bonds to form and old ones to strengthen.

TABLE 3.1

MAJOR FACTORS IN PSYCHOSEXUAL DYSFUNCTION

Symptomatic
Interpersonal (discord with significant other)
Organic (disease, malnutrition, malfunction of body organs)
Psychiatric (anxiety, depression, schizophrenia)
Alcohol or drug abuse
Iatrogenic (suggestions, medication, surgery)
Learned
Family (childhood negative sexual associations, experiences)
Religion (imposed prohibitions internalized)
Early unpleasant sexual experiences
Gynecologic disorders (damaged genitalia, loss of breasts, uterus)
Intrapsychic conflict
Failure to develop psychosexually
Restrictive childrearing
Religious influences

In other cases, the woman's partner becomes a bigger problem than her physical disability. It is possible her significant other constructed a fragile emotional bond with body parts rather than with the actual woman. If she had or has cancer, the partner may irrationally feel that the cancer is contagious. If she is receiving radiation treatment, he may feel that if he resumes sexual relations with her, he, too, might absorb radiation from her body and be burned. The couple may be accustomed to frequent sex, and any change in the woman's availability stresses the relationship. The fear of causing pain also has an inhibiting effect. Emotional isolation and loss of nurturing occur in both partners when the woman experiences physical disability. As surgeon to the postoperative patient, you are her first line of psychosexual defense, and yours will not be an easy job.

Depending on the study cited, sexual dysfunction exists in 23% to 43% of women and 31% of the men surveyed in the general population. One third of the women lacked sexual interest, one fourth were unable to experience orgasm in the menopause, one fifth reported lubrication difficulties, and another one fifth said they did not find sex pleasurable.

These figures come from members of the population willing to discuss sexual dysfunction. Many women and their physicians, who sometimes fear they are not qualified to help, are reluctant to speak of personal problems such as libido, arousal, coital pain, or past traumatic sexual events. Much of this reluctance can be overcome if the gynecologist knows what questions to ask when taking a sexual history, preferably during an initial or annual examination before any body-altering surgery.

Sexual Cycle Primer

Davis suggests that the physician ask the following open-ended questions to obtain a sexual history: Are you sexually active? Are you or your partner having any sexual difficulties at this time? Has there been any change in your sexual activity? Have you ever experienced any unwanted or harmful sexual activity? Another good question is: What sort of sexual problems do you have?

Even if the patient is initially reluctant to discuss such personal issues, she will have learned that you are willing to discuss them should the need arise. Davis also believes that a physician's confidence in dealing with sexual issues increase when the cycles of sexual response (desire, arousal, plateau, orgasm, and resolution) are learned and factors that affect them (psychological, environmental, and physiologic) understood.

Davis, in a sexual and sexual dysfunction tutorial, describes the following stages: desire, arousal, plateau phase, orgasm, and resolution phase.

Desire is the motivation and inclination to be sexual. It is dependent on internal (fantasies) and external sexual cues and also on adequate neuroendocrine functioning.

Arousal is characterized by erotic feelings and vaginal lubrication as blood flow increases to the vagina. In addition to feelings of sexual tension, the sexually excited woman may experience tachycardia, rapid breathing, elevated blood pressure, breast engorgement, muscle tension, nipple erection, and other physical signs of arousal such as a flush. This is the stage where the vagina lengthens, distends, and dilates, and the uterus elevates partially out of the pelvis.

During the *plateau phase,* sexual tension, erotic feelings, and vasocongestion reach maximum intensity. The labia become more swollen and turn dark red, and the lower third of the vagina swells and thickens to form the orgasmic platform. The clitoris becomes more swollen and elevated, and the uterus elevates fully out of the pelvis. Eventually, women reach the threshold point of orgasmic inevitability. *Orgasm* is a myotonic response mediated by the sympathetic nervous system and is experienced as a sudden release of the tension built up during previous phases. Women, unlike men, experience no refractory period but can experience multiple orgasms during a single cycle. They can also experience orgasms before, during, and after intercourse provided they receive enough clitoral stimulation.

The last phase is called the *resolution phase.* Women experience a feeling of relaxation and well-being. The body returns to a resting state. Complete uterine descent, detumescence of the clitoris and orgasmic platform, and decongestion of the vagina and labia take about 5 to 10 minutes.

Sexual adjustment is often significantly impaired in women after pelvic exenteration and gracilis myocutaneous vaginal reconstruction. Eighty-four percent of the patients in one of the few studies that exist resumed sexual activity within the first year after surgery. A modified version of the Sexual Adjustment Questionnaire was used and the responses outlined the most common problems patients face after the surgery: self-consciousness about a urostomy or colostomy, being seen nude by their partner, vaginal dryness, and vaginal discharge. It is hoped that future modifications in surgical technique, more realistic patient counseling, and aggressive postoperative support will minimize these problems in the future. Less serious matters can cause self-esteem and body image problems, too, if their aftermath includes or leads to bowel incontinence, urinary incontinence, vaginal vault prolapse, and scarring.

Bowel incontinence is rarely discussed even with a woman's physician because it is so embarrassing. Whether from obstetric injuries, injury to the anal muscles, infections, or diminished muscle strength from aging, once the cause and severity are determined, treatments can begin that include dietary changes, constipating medications, muscle strengthening exercises, biofeedback techniques, and sometimes, surgical repair of the muscle. Some or all of these remedies help the woman control the discharge of embarrassing gas or stool. It is most important to discuss possible remedies because many women feel there is nothing that can be done for them but the frightening colostomy, when in actual fact, colostomy is a procedure that is rarely required.

As many as 50% of all women experience occasional urinary incontinence. In an attempt to lessen the blow to a woman's ego and make the event more socially acceptable, manufacturers hire movie stars to make commercials about the effectiveness of diapers for grown women. Diapers do treat the symptoms and allow for more freedom of movement, but not in an intimate setting. For many years, gynecologists have instructed patients about Kegel exercises to tighten the muscles of the pelvic floor, but this may not be enough to stop the embarrassing leakage of urine. The patient needs to know that there are tests that can determine the exact cause of the problem, and treatment using bladder retaining therapy, medications, and surgery. Urinary incontinence may be more socially acceptable today, but it is never normal, no matter what the woman's age.

Both bowel and urinary incontinence can be caused by vaginal vault prolapse, and this condition must be ruled out because it drastically affects sexual functioning. The presence of a mass can cause painful intercourse, difficulty accepting penetration, and a great deal of psychological anxiety when the tissue can be seen in the vaginal opening. This condition, if left untreated, only worsens with time, but techniques that correct female organ–supporting defects in the pelvis can restore sexual functioning and with it, a woman's sense of vitality and feminine allure.

Patients who talk about their sex lives frequently describe four pleasures associated with sexuality. These universal elements are touching, genital caressing, orgasm, and gratifying a partner. When a patient is recovering from surgery or has experienced surgical loss of coital function, genital caressing as a receiver or giver can be satisfying. Once a woman learns early in life how to be orgasmic, she can often learn to be so again despite major genital loss, including her clitoris. When the ability to experience orgasm by one favorite means is destroyed by disease, the patient can be encouraged to experiment with alternative methods that do not conflict with her value system. Women who will never experience vaginal intercourse again can discover they are able, with education and imagination, to fulfill their feminine role as givers of pleasure if they choose to do so.

When a patient's psychosexual rehabilitation after surgery seems to be impaired and she fails to make steady progress toward resumption of her usual role, with appropriate self-esteem, energy, identity, and ability to handle stress, she should be offered help. Help should be offered as soon as she mentions the problem. Early intervention is often easy and brief. The surgeon should be the first person to help the patient, with counseling and, if necessary, suitable medications.

Hormonal Therapy

Hormone replacement therapy (HRT) remains a controversial issue. It is imperative that HRT be discussed preoperatively with the patient facing surgery and the loss of her ovaries. Initial misinterpretation of the results of the Women's Health Initiative Study (WHI) has created much fear and angst for both the gynecologist and the patient. The harmful effects were overestimated, and the media created undue alarm regarding breast cancer.

Pines, in careful evaluation of the data in the estrogen-progestin arm, shows the risk for breast cancer and cardiovascular events to be most minute, about 0.1% for every year of use. No risk was observed for women younger than 60 years of age. It must be remembered that the WHI study recruited women in their late 60s.

A 16-year study that involved 60,000 postmenopausal female nurses found that those who took hormone replacement therapy for 10 years reduced their risk of dying from all causes by 37%, with the most dramatic reduction being death from cardiac disease. After 10 years, the reduced risk for all causes was 16% because of the increased risk of dying from breast cancer. That risk rose to 43%, but the women who contracted breast cancer during the first 10 years had a lower death rate from the disease than women who had never taken hormones, probably because of early detection. Chances of early detection of breast cancer are probably better for hormone users because they receive regular check-ups.

In an extensive review of current literature on the subject, dubbed "the New Science of Estrogen," Hammond provides an overview of the risks and benefits of hormone replacement therapy and also includes information on therapeutic alternatives. Cardiovascular benefits of estrogen outweigh the risks. With combined estrogen-progestin therapy, studies have shown some increase in stroke and venous thromboembolism. Hammond feels that steroid hormonal therapy should be considered an integral part of the appropriate and necessary care of American women after menopause, and the anticipated reduction of cardiovascular disease and osteoporotic fractures by nearly 50% should be laudable goals for any health care system.

Statistics show overwhelmingly that cardiovascular disease (CVD)—not cancer—is the leading cause of mortality for postmenopausal women. In fact, one in two women will eventually die of heart disease or stroke, whereas only one in 25 women die of breast cancer. Although the incidence of heart disease, including coronary artery disease and stroke, is low in premenopausal women, heart disease is the most frequent cause of death in women older than the age of 50. Since 1984, the death rate from CVD in men has decreased, whereas the death rate for women has increased. Numerous epidemiologic studies support the long-term benefit of estrogen in preventing CVD. Observational studies, such as the Postmenopausal Estrogen/Progestin Intervention Study sponsored by the National Institutes of Health, revealed that HRT can increase high-density lipoprotein cholesterol and decrease low-density lipoprotein cholesterol. The Nurses' Health Study demonstrated a reduction in the risk of CVD of as much as 50% among current HRT users. Women who use estrogen have significantly less coronary artery stenosis than women who do not use it. Takahashi found that long-term HRT—for more than 2 years—may delay carotid intima-media thickness in healthy postmenopausal women.

Moreover, patients with the most advanced coronary artery disease experience the most benefit from HRT. Only 35% of women surveyed were aware of the connection between heart disease and menopause.

Current theories indicate that estrogen has extraordinarily complex biological effects that translate into a variety of actions in diverse tissues. There is growing scientific evidence that estrogen exerts its beneficial actions on tissues of the skeletal, urogenital, digestive, cardiovascular, ocular, and nervous systems.

Estrogen replacement therapy (ERT)/HRT is also first-line therapy for osteoporosis for most women, and treatment should begin as soon as possible after the menopause. Enough time has elapsed since the WHI media scare and cessation of estrogen therapy by users that a marked and rapid loss of bone density is being noted in those who stopped their replacement therapy. Yates and Barrett-Connor studied the association between hormone therapy (HT) cessation and hip fracture risk. Concurrent with WHI, women in National Osteoporosis Risk Assessment currently on HT had a 40% lower incidence of hip fracture compared with those who had never used HT. Women who stopped using HT more than 5 years earlier had similar hip fracture use to never users. Preliminary data suggest that even the elderly respond to estrogen replacement. However, there are therapeutic alternatives and lifestyle modifications (diet and routine exercise) that perimenopausal women must be counseled about to create a comprehensive preventive program. Such an effort can have a significant impact on long-term morbidity and mortality associated with osteoporosis.

Women have phenomenal memories because one of their jobs is to find every needle that gets lost in the proverbial haystacks of their homes. When they become less adept at remembering where they and other people put their things, they fear the worst—that they are losing their minds, and this fear is not illogical. Women compose 72% of the population older than the age of 85 years, and roughly half of this group has Alzheimer disease (AD). Not only do women constitute a greater proportion of this older population, but AD is expressed earlier in women than men. This may be related to the estrogen loss that occurs with menopause. Hammond cites a study that found women who took estrogen for more than 1 year experienced a dramatic delay in AD onset. But even the group of women who averaged only 4 months of estrogen therapy and most likely took the medication to control symptoms such as hot flashes experienced a delay in AD onset. It has been speculated that a brief exposure to estrogen influenced AD expression 20 to 30 years later by preventing an irreversible loss of neurons associated with the occurrence of hot flashes. Research is ongoing, but one study found that estrogen replacement therapy in postmenopausal women is associated with a 50% reduction in the risk of developing AD because it slows the decline of visual memory. The study by Lebrun and colleagues in clinical endocrinology supports findings that endogenous estrogens protect against cognitive decline with aging.

Colon cancer occurs more often in women than men and is a leading cause of cancer incidence and deaths in women. Even though mortality rates for colon cancer have decreased 25% among women in the last 20 years, it remains the third-leading cause of cancer deaths in this group. The concept that postmenopausal ERT may decrease the risk of colorectal cancer has received considerable attention, even though the hormone has no indication for this use. Multiple epidemiologic studies have been published that examined this relationship. The majority of these suggest an inverse, protective effect for estrogen, particularly with current use. Although the precise mechanism by which estrogen reduces colon cancer risk is unknown, it has been hypothesized that it affects bile acid metabolism or promotes tumor suppressor activity. The inclusion of estrogen as a measure to prevent colon cancer should be part of the discussions between menopausal women and their physicians. Counseling should include the American Cancer Society recommendations for annual digital rectal examination and fecal occult blood testing as well as a flexible sigmoidoscopy every 5 years or colonoscopy every 10 years.

Age-related macular degeneration (AMD) may be reduced by estrogen administration. This disease is the leading cause of legal blindness in the United States, accounting for as many as 60% of all new cases. There is no medical treatment, and surgical management in the form of photocoagulation is effective in only a small percentage of patients with the wet type of the disease. In the Rotterdam study, women who experienced menopause at an earlier age had a 90% increased risk of exhibiting signs of late AMD compared with those who experienced menopause at a later age. These data suggest that HRT reduces the risk of developing AMD.

Counseling women about replacement therapy must be combined with discussions about the importance of lifestyle changes, including:

- Normalization of weight
- Dietary intervention
- Smoking cessation
- Regular exercise
- Control of hypertension
- Control of diabetes
- Control of alcohol consumption
- Control of lipid elevations

Routinely, ERT/HRT counseling should go beyond simple symptom control to include both short- and long-term benefits, contraindications, common patient concerns, and misconceptions.

The contraindications to estrogen replacement that have been established by the Food and Drug Administration (FDA), include known or suspected pregnancy or breast cancer, estrogen-dependent neoplasia, undiagnosed abnormal genital bleeding, and active thromboembolic disorders. However, ongoing research suggests that some of these contraindications may not be absolute. In the meantime, all of the relative contraindications must be carefully discussed and weighed against the risk of not prescribing ERT/HRT. This is also a good time to discuss the common concerns and misconceptions that women have about estrogen, even if patients do not raise them. For example, many women are concerned that estrogen may bring on the return of monthly bleeding, restore fertility, or produce weight gain.

When bilateral oophorectomy is anticipated in a premenopausal patient, HRT should be discussed before surgery because one of the greatest fears of younger women is surgery-induced menopause. Patients should be told that estrogen therapy can be started immediately after surgery and that hot flashes and other menopausal symptoms can be avoided. The natural conjugated estrogens do not cause hypercoagulability and are safe during the immediate convalescent period.

Parker and colleagues, in a recent lead study in *Obstetrics and Gynecology,* recommend ovarian conservation until at least age 65 because of its benefit to long-term survival. With ovarian preservation, the need for exogenous hormones is delayed.

The long-term benefits of estrogen replacement therapy in preventing osteoporosis, cardiovascular disease, and colon cancer are well established. The health of the vagina and lower urinary tract is maintained. The *Journal of the British Menopause Society* says that various studies have demonstrated the efficacy of estrogen replacement in improving urinary and stress incontinence. The vagina lubricates more easily with sexual arousal, and intercourse is more comfortable with an estrogenic vaginal mucosa. Many women report an increased interest in and enjoyment of sex.

For women who do experience a loss of libido, even while taking estrogenic hormones, the new androgen therapies look promising as a way to improve sexual function and psychological well-being. Testosterone delivered via transdermal patches or gel bypasses the liver and has no negative effect on cholesterol. The skin serves as a constant reservoir; therefore, blood levels show fewer fluctuations.

However, there are physicians who believe that hormonal balances induced by prescription medications should only be offered for relief of extreme menopausal symptoms and only for a short while. The author of *Dr. Susan Love's Hormone Book* and *Dr. Susan Love's Breast Book* is one such physician. She is a staunch supporter of eating soybean products and using herbal remedies such as black cohosh to maintain estrogen levels, using of acupuncture and paced-respiration for hot flashes, exercising, and using vitamin and calcium supplements. But even she admitted in an interview, "If my symptoms [for menopause] worsen, I may feel that I want to take some kind of drug. I certainly would be open to that."

SPECIAL CASES

Every patient is special and deserves to be treated with compassion and sensitivity. Women in tumultuous life situations at the time of surgery present the greatest challenge.

The Teenager

Bluestein and Starling report that 1 million teenagers per year conceive. Of these million pregnancies, 400,000 end in abortion and 100,000 in miscarriage. Childbearing teenagers face a 60% excess in maternal mortality compared with adults and are most likely to suffer toxemia, anemia, hemorrhage, cervical trauma, cephalopelvic disproportion, excessive weight gain, and premature labor. These complications are due more to social and behavioral correlates than inherent adolescent aspects. Correlates include inadequate prenatal care, poor nutrition, substance abuse, and emotional distress.

One to two teenagers per 1,000 who have first trimester abortions experience fever, hemorrhage, and emergency abdominal surgical procedures. These numbers are lower than for older women, but the rate for cervical injury, which could affect future childbearing, is 5.5 per 1,000 teenagers, notably higher than the 1.7 to 3.1 per 1,000 for adults. Bluestein and Starling recommend the following communication techniques for the teenage patient: Guarantee confidentiality to build trust. Conduct the initial interview alone. Teenage girls may want to relate private information to the physician but not in the presence of a parent. Be patient. Gear communication to the patient's emotional and intellectual development. Be nonjudgmental. Gently explore the teenager's family and social environments. Will family members and friends support or harm your patient? Discuss the teenager's long-term plans. Be aware of ethnic differences in health-related matters.

Female patients who belong to local or national gangs come into the health care system with a unique set of problems and values. It is imperative that the surgeon not add to the patient's stress more than is absolutely necessary. Sometimes the simple act of being treated like a human being worthy of consideration is a novel and humbling experience.

The Senior Woman

It is easy to imagine a grandmother baking cookies or rocking a new baby in the family. Our culture makes it a little more difficult to imagine this same woman flushed and happy from an energetic romp in the sack with her favorite beau. Sex after age 60 is a reality for many women and men. These people enjoyed sex when they were young, they perfected it as the years flowed by, and the thought of doing without expression of the natural urges, even temporarily, is discomforting.

When an older woman faces gynecologic surgery, do not assume she is asexual. She may simply view her sex life as her private business and be loath to discuss it. Do not antagonize or humiliate the senior patient by assuming her sexuality is a thing of the past.

If the surgical procedure will affect her sexually, explain the consequences. Assure her that the surgery will leave her as whole and as functional as possible. Give this woman the opportunity to express her anxieties and to ask questions. If her mate or lover is present, include this person in the discussion. In the senior woman who has a large cystocele, rectocele, or uterine or vault prolapse, every effort should be made to avoid colpocleisis. Sacrospinous colpopexies and vaginal reconstructive surgery are indicated. The fact that a woman is older and sexually inactive at the time of surgery does not mean that she will never be active again. Much preparation and explanation must be given to evaluate and prepare her for the closing off of her vagina or its subsequent reconstruction should that become necessary.

Butler and colleagues advise that when taking a sexual history, ask if the symptoms started after a period of sexual activity. Excretory urogram and cystoscopy sometimes can be avoided with a diagnosis of postcoital cystitis and subsequent antibiotic treatment. A history of traumatic intercourse in the presence of an atrophic vagina may indicate a need for estrogen therapy and lubricants rather than dilation and curettage. Butler and colleagues also caution physicians not to assume an older woman is sexually inactive. They advise checking for sexually transmitted diseases in older women as you would in younger ones.

When surgery is indicated, perform it as if the senior woman was still young and had many years of sexuality ahead of her, because she probably does. If the surgery occurs in the genital area, do not shave her pubic hair. The procedure is archaic and microbiologically unnecessary if competent sterilization procedures are followed. As men age, they sometimes lose hair on the head. As women age, the pubic hair sometimes thins and once shaved, may never grow back.

Many older women have had to curb their sexual appetites to compensate for physiologic changes that have occurred in a mate. Removal of excessive vaginal mucosa during pelvic surgery compromises the vagina, which is already losing elasticity. This inhibits penetration during coitus and can cause painful intercourse. Be understanding and helpful if solutions are possible. If the dysfunction resulting from the surgery will be permanent, encourage the couple to experiment with various ways to please each other or seek the advice of a sex therapist who is knowledgeable about creative sexual play.

Butler and colleagues instruct physicians to educate themselves about the effects of medications on sexuality. More than 200 medications have sexual dysfunction as a side effect. Many are effective in lower doses that do not harm the libido or the patient's physical ability.

The positive benefits of a healthy sex life are multiple. Emotional intimacy and the ability to connect physically with another human being brings great joy and satisfaction. This need to connect intensifies rather than diminishes with age.

The Sexually Assaulted Patient

According to Federal Bureau of Investigation (FBI) statistics, reported rapes and sexual assaults in the United States are up nearly 5% since 2000. It is estimated that only about 16% of the rapes that occur are ever reported. One in three sexually assaulted victims is younger than the age of 12. Convicted rape and sexual assault offenders testify that two thirds of their victims are younger than 18. Two thirds of the victims older than 18 knew their attacker before the rape. A sad fact is that almost one fifth of the women who are raped before the age of 18 are raped again after the age of 18. Many require medical

TABLE 3.2

SYMPTOMS OF RAPE TRAUMA SYNDROME

Recurrent, painful recollections or dreams of the event
Suddenly acting or feeling as if the event were recurring
Demonstrations of fear, anger, or anxiety
Crying, restlessness, or tenseness
Controlled feelings masked by a false demeanor of calmness, composure, or subdued attitude
Matter-of-fact answering of questions
Inappropriate smiles or laughter
Inability to remember parts of the event because re-exposure to stimuli present during the traumatic moment reinvokes the associated pain
Decreased interest in important activities
Lack of future plans
Limited range of affect
Detachment toward others
Sleep disorders
Difficulty concentrating
Hypervigilance
Irritability
Angry outbursts

attention, as many as 22% suffer genital trauma, as many as 40% incur sexually transmitted disease, and 1% to 5% become pregnant as a result of the rape. Rape survivors are 13 times more likely than the general population to attempt suicide.

Most hospital emergency rooms have strict protocols to follow when treating sexually assaulted patients. The proper collection of evidence and initial treatment of injuries is a priority. The surgeon who repairs the gynecologic damage done to these female patients should be aware of the general characteristics of psychological trauma associated with rape.

The symptoms of rape trauma syndrome compiled by Blair and Warner can be found in Table 3.2. Many of these symptoms are the same as seen in posttraumatic stress disorder. These authors also outlined the following necessary skills that any caregivers attempting to help a sexually assaulted victim should possess:

- Understand rape and sexual assault
- Assess how the patient perceives the act
- Identify and reinforce patient's ability to cope
- Assist significant others
- Coordinate care and help if victim needs assistance
- Mobilize community resources

The rape patient, from the youngest child to the oldest adult, has survived the attack on her physical body. Most gynecologists are familiar with the legacy of these attacks (as many as 75% of patients seen with chronic pelvic pain were physically or emotionally abused). The assaulted patient now needs reassurance from her surgeon and other health care workers that she will also survive the damage done to her psyche.

The Cancer Patient

Bloch cautions physicians that the manner in which the diagnosis of cancer is disclosed to the patient can determine whether the patient lives or dies. It is imperative to instill hope and the desire to fight the disease. A diagnosis of cancer by telephone can be devastating and is viewed by many physicians and patients as a form of cruelty.

In her book *The Balance Within: The Science Connecting Health and Emotions,* Dr. Esther M. Sternberg presents evidence that the relief of stress can make you less vulnerable to illness. The cancer patient shares the same fears common to all surgical patients. She may be psychologically attached to the body part that must be removed. She may fear anesthesia, disfigurement, the unknown, the hospital experience and staff, debility, loss of economic competence, and sexual function.

In addition to the normal realm of anxiety associated with surgery, a diagnosis of cancer brings special stresses to a woman's life. Schain describes universal concerns experienced by people diagnosed with cancer no matter where in the body the cancer is located. These people fear death, postoperative adjuvant treatment, and recurrence.

The cancer patient is concerned about dying or being injured during the operation. Preoperative anxiety can manifest as anorexia, insomnia, tachycardia, fear, and panic. Acute depression is not uncommon and can lead to suicidal tendencies.

The patient is afraid of becoming unable to take care of her family members. Will she be sick for long? Who will raise her children if she dies? Who will care for her parents? Will her loved ones be supportive, or will they begin to back away from her? If the woman is alone, without mate or family, she fears becoming unable to care for herself.

The treating surgeon can ease some of the cancer patient's fear by free and open communication. Educate the patient about exactly what to expect, and offer reassurance if possible. Explain the procedure she is about to undergo and the positive benefits that you both hope will result.

Surgery and cancer in the urogenital region can be consciously or unconsciously interpreted as mutilation. The possibility of some degree of postoperative sexual dysfunction can create a fear of abandonment by the sexual partner. If possible, assure both the patient and her partner that they will continue to be able to bring joy, pleasure, and comfort to each other.

The psychological effect of cancer on a woman is largely determined by whether the malignancy is primary, recurrent, or terminal. The surgeon is usually the patient's first big gun aimed at the cancer and the patient's greatest hope for a complete cure. The surgeon most likely is the first physician to learn the stage of growth of the cancer, and the family will be waiting to hear the results of the surgical experience. How advanced is the cancer? What is the prognosis? What happens next?

If the news is good, the patient recovers and has routine checkups to monitor her health for the rest of her life. If the news is not good, the results should be revealed with as much sensitivity and hope as possible. No patient should ever be given an absolute death sentence.

The surgeon must wrestle with personal ethical and moral conflicts when the surgery for the cancer patient is palliative. Should procedures be performed that extend death and not life? If she is able, the patient herself must make the choice.

If the cancer patient elects to have the procedure, her care postoperatively may be shared by radiologists, chemotherapists, and others who specialize in cancer treatment. However, you as her gynecologist should maintain contact and assist in trying to get the patient well or at least enhance the quality of the remainder of her life. Meaningful psychosocial support should be based on established concepts of crisis intervention because cancer is a major life crisis. Counseling should be designed to support adaptive behaviors and feelings that reduce the psychological stress, restore and consolidate the patient's self-image, and normalize sexual functioning as quickly as possible. It is the surgeon's job to foster courage, not hope, in the terminal patient.

The Suicidal Patient

The World Health Organization (WHO) reports that suicide rates have increased 60% worldwide in the last 45 years, with 870,000 annual deaths. Approximately 30,000 people commit suicide each year in the United States. Cooper and colleagues studied more than 6,000 individuals and found that hopelessness ranked the highest of all symptoms associated with suicidal ideation in psychiatric patients and adolescents.

A surgeon probably will not know if a patient is contemplating suicide unless the patient admits to thinking about ending her life or unless a family member voices concern. Subtle warning signs include a chronic state of depression, lethargy, an inability to relate to others, weight loss or gain, lack of interest in life in general or the surgical procedure in question, a change in personal appearance, abnormal sleep patterns, or any strange behavior uncharacteristic of the particular patient. Many of these symptoms are normal for the presurgical and postsurgical patient, so it is easy to see how suicidal tendencies could hide within the maze.

To determine a patient's suicide potential, ask: Have you been troubled with thoughts of hurting yourself? Barbee advises physicians to ask directly: Have you ever thought of taking your own life? Do you feel like taking your life now? If the patient answers yes, the physician should find out if the patient has a simple, straightforward suicide plan that is likely to succeed.

A patient with low to moderate suicide potential is noticeably depressed but can identify some support system. There may be suicidal thoughts but no specific plan.

A patient with a high suicide potential feels profoundly helpless. Little or no support system seems to exist. Thoughts of suicide are frequent, and a plan exists that is likely to succeed.

The surgeon may be the first person to realize the patient is in emotional trouble and could be the only support system available if the patient has significantly withdrawn from others. Crisis therapy for the suicidal patient begins when the patient requests help or when someone recognizes her potential for self-destruction. By showing interest in her feelings and concern for her welfare, the surgeon initiates crisis intervention.

DEALING WITH DEATH

Death is a taboo subject for most physicians. Many doctors go to great lengths to avoid discussing the eventuality, and most are uncomfortable dealing with the emotional consequences of the death of a patient. To many physicians, death is viewed as a personal failure. Regardless of any internal attitudes, the surgeon is responsible for communicating the facts of the death to the family and for being the first person to help them cope with the loss of their loved one.

When a patient dies, explain to the family, to the best of your ability, exactly what happened. Assure them that everything medically possible was done. Ufema suggests the following guidelines to make the death experience as bearable as possible for all concerned:

- Ask about donations for transplantation.
- Provide an area where the family members can say goodbye.
- If it is true, tell the family members how the patient affected you personally.
- Transfer your protective feelings for the patient to the family members.
- Begin the grief process by saying, "Jane's body is ready for the morgue now. Would you like to say a final goodbye?"
- If family members want a lock of hair, allow them to take it.
- Give family members the patient's belongings.
- Provide an escort for any family member who is alone.
- Help the hospital staff cope with the loss.

Remember that it is permissible for the physician to show emotion with the family if the emotion is genuine. Someone is gone and will never see tomorrow.

FUTURE TRENDS

The new millennium was heralded with great joy and celebration. Its predominant theme was one of hope, and nowhere is this more evident than in the field of medicine, specifically for women's health issues. The hand that rocks the cradle now rules important aspects of the research world. During the next 20 years, 45 million women will enter menopause and live one third to one half of their lives postmenopausally. Research into improving the quality of their lives—and subsequently, all those they touch—has never been more important or timely.

As a multitude of women move through the life stages of maiden, mother, and crone, the health care they receive during one stage will be reflected in all those that follow. Boomer women, born between 1946 and 1964, will continue their legacy of reform by participating in medical clinical studies concerning endocrinology, gynecology, neurology, oncology, genetics, and finally, geriatrics. The daughters and sons they presented to the world will advance reproductive technology in all its genetic and social ramifications.

Robotic gynecological surgery, a recent gift of the technological world, is being performed. It is envisaged that most surgery in the future can and will be performed robotically. The systems currently in use are not intended to act independently from surgeons nor to replace them. They provide a means for the skilled surgeon to complete complex and advanced procedures with increased precision and with a minimally invasive approach. Medical students will soon be able to perfect their surgical techniques using cyberscalpels, simulated lifelike patient bodies, three-dimensional models, and long-distance mentors. The space industry has also yielded a smart surgical probe that will be used for breast biopsies. The small disposable needle with multiple sensors will be able to distinguish normal tissue from tumor tissue and greatly reduce the 18,000 breast biopsies per week now performed on women with suspicious lesions. Originally conceived as a robotic tool to aid astronaut/physicians during long-duration space flights, it has already found a medical application on Earth in neurosurgery.

Voice-activated language programs are making it possible to effectively communicate with multicultural patients and international colleagues. Advances in documentation techniques have made keeping and transferring accurate records less of a burden. More ethics classes will emerge to better prepare the medical student for the real-world challenges such as end-of-life issues, fiduciary responsibilities, confidentiality, informed consent, and religious or philosophical conflicts.

As surgeons, it will be your duty and privilege to witness, record, and practice the new knowledge and incorporate it with what is already known so that you can make a positive difference in the lives of women now living as well as those yet to be born.

CONCLUSION

Technology will never change the fact that women are emotional creatures by nature, even now that they have the choice whether to menstruate. Few experiences give women more satisfaction than sexuality and conception. Surgery on or near her reproductive tract is potentially fraught with emotional sequelae. The gynecologic surgeon's responsibility transcends a stunning performance in the surgical arena. Making appropriate decisions about the surgical procedure and considerately managing the patient's return to physical and psychological health are the hallmarks of an accomplished surgeon.

BEST SURGICAL PRACTICES

- The gynecologist shall treat the patient's psyche as well as her soma.
- Neuroscientific investigation has proven that stress contributes to unfavorable outcomes postoperatively.
- Preoperatively, the surgeon must make every effort to answer a patient's questions, allay her fears, and reduce her stress.
- Unanswered questions regarding the diagnosis, the intended procedure, possible complications, and postoperative sexuality are sources of stress.
- Cancer patients, young patients, patients living alone without family support, and patients with a language barrier should be considered special-needs patients. Extra time should be devoted to them.
- Personal communication on a one-to-one basis between the surgeon and patient should take place. Counseling by ancillary personnel and informative booklets should only be used adjunctively.
- A surgeon should try to be with the patient immediately before her surgery and during the induction of anesthesia.
- Be familiar with symptoms of depression and look for them during preoperative evaluation. Address potential problems before surgery, and make referrals when indicated.
- When oophorectomy is anticipated in a premenopausal patient, estrogen replacement therapy should be discussed and encouraged before surgery if there are no contraindications.
- Extra time spent listening, informing, and reassuring an anxious patient before surgery is often rewarded by a fast and uneventful recovery.

Bibliography

Abel G. *How to avoid being accused of sexual harassment.* The American Association of Sex Educators, Counselors, and Therapists (AASECT), 2000 Annual Conference, May 10–14.

Advincula AP, Falcone T. Laparoscopic robotic gynecologic surgery *Obstet Gynecol Clin North Am* 2004;31(3):599.

Andersen BL, Hacker NF. Psychosexual adjustment following pelvic exenteration. *Obstet Gynecol* 1983;61:331.

Andersen BL, Hacker NF. Psychosexual adjustment of gynecologic oncology patients: a proposed model for future investigation. *Gynecol Oncol* 1983;15:214.

Barbee MA. Recognizing suicide. *Nursing* 1993;(Oct):32N.

Barber CA, Margolis K, Luepker RV, et al. The impact of the Women's Health Initiative Study on discontinuation of postmenopausal hormone therapy: the Minnesota Heart Survey (2000–2002). *J Womens Health (Larchmt)* 2004;13(9):975.

Barnes AB, Tinkham CG. Surgical gynecology. In: Notman MT, Nadelson CC, eds. *The woman patient: medical and psychological interfaces.* New York: Plenum Press, 1978.

Blair TMH, Warner CG. Sexual assault. *Topics Emerg Med* 1992;(Dec):58.

Bloch R. Disclosing cancer diagnosis to a patient. *J Natl Cancer Inst* 1994;86:38.

Bluestein D, Starling E. Helping pregnant teenagers. *West J Med* 1994;161:140.

Boston Women's Health Collective (Author) Our bodies, ourselves Touchstone ISBN 0-7432-3611-5.

Bourla DH, Young TA. Age-Related Macular Degeneration: A Practical Approach to a challenging disease The Rotterdam Study. *J Am Geriatr Soc*, Volume 55, Number 6 July 2006.

Bowel incontinence (patient brochure). Arlington Heights, IL: American Society of Colon and Rectal Surgeons (ASCRS). ascrs@fascrs.org.

Brown J, Seeley D, et al. Correspondence re: urinary incontinence after hysterectomy. *Lancet* 2000;356:2012.

Bruns D. *Matters of life and death.* Greeley, CO: Health Psychology Associates.

Butler RN, Hoffman E, Whitehead DE, et al. Love and sex after sixty: how physical changes affect intimate expression. *Geriatrics* 1994;49:20.

Colditz GA. Estrogen, plus progestin therapy, and risk of breast cancer. *Clin Cancer Res* 2005;11(2 Pt. 2):909s.

Daly MJ, Sadock BJ, Kaplan HI, et al. Psychological impact of surgical procedures on women. In: Sadock BJ, Kaplan HI, Freedman AM, eds. *The sexual experience.* Baltimore: Williams & Wilkins, 1976:308.

Davis H, Johnston M. The effects of communication/counselling in medical practice: an evaluation. *J R Soc Med* 1994;87:429.

Dennerstein AO, Franz CP. *Conference report: third annual female sexual function forum: new perspectives in the management of female sexual dysfunction.* U.S. National Health and Social Life Survey and Kinsey Institute for Research on Sex, Gender, and Reproduction, Indiana University. Boston: October 26–29, 2000.

Dennerstein AO, Franz CP. New perspectives in the management of female sexual dysfunction. *Third Annual*

Dennerstein L, Wood C, Burrows, G. Hormone therapy: effects and side effects. In Dennerstein, L ed. Hysterectomy Melbourne: Oxford University Press 1982:107.

Derogatis LR. Breast and gynecologic cancers: their unique impact on body image and sexual identity in women. In: Vaeth JM, Blomberg RC, Adler L, eds. *Body image, self-esteem, and sexuality in cancer patients.* New York: Karger, 1980.

Diaz-Arrastia C, Jurnalov C, Gomez G, et al. Laparoscopic hysterectomy using a computer-enhanced surgical robot. *Surg Endosc* 2002;16(9): 1271.

Diaz-Gilbert M. Culturally diverse patients. *Nursing* 1993;(Oct):44.

Female Sexual Function Forum. U.S. National Health and Social Life Survey. Boston: October 26–29, 2000.

Freeman MG. Introduction to the sexual history. In: Walker HK, Hall WD, Hurst JW, eds. *Clinical methods*, 2nd ed. Boston: Butterworth, 1980.

Galovotti C, Richter DL. Talking about hysterectomy: the experiences of women from four cultural groups. *J Womens Health Gend Based Med* 2000;9(Suppl 2):S63.

Gross J. Our bodies, but my hysterectomy. *New York Times*, June 1994.

Hammond CB. Management of the menopausal woman. *Am J Manag Care* 2005;11(5):541.

Hammond CB. The Women's Health Initiative Study: perpectives and implications for clinical practice. *Rev Endocr Metab Disord* 2005;93.

Hammond C, Love S. *Controversies in hormone replacement therapy.* American College of Obstetricians and Gynecologists 46th Annual Clinical Meeting, 4th Scientific Session. New Orleans: May 9–13, 1998.

Hammond CB, Rackley CE, et al. Consequences of estrogen deprivation and the rationale for hormone replacement therapy. .*Am J Manag Care* 2000;6(14 Suppl):S746.

Health services research on hysterectomy and alternatives. Fact sheet. AHCPR Publication No. 97-R021. Rockville, MD: Agency for Health Care Policy and Research. http://ahrq.gov/research/hysterec.htm.

Hufnagel V. No more hysterectomies.

Kaplan HI, Sadock BJ. *Comprehensive textbook of psychiatry*, 5th ed. Baltimore: Williams & Wilkins, 1989:1563.

Kelley WE Jr. Robotic surgery: the promise and early development. *Laparoscopy and SLS Report* 2002;1:6.

Kritz-Silverstein D, Wingard DL, Barrett-Connor E, et al. Hysterectomy, oophorectomy, and depression in older women. *J Womens Health* 1994;3(4):255.

Lebrun CE, van der Schouw YT, de Jong FH, et al. Endogenous oesrogens are related to cognition in healthy elderly women. *Clin Endocrinol (Oxf)* 2005;63(1):50.

Lewis CE, Groff JY, Herman CJ, et al. Overview of women's decision making regarding elective hysterectomy, öophorectomy and hormone replacement therapy. *J Womens Health Gend Based Med* 2000:9(Suppl 2): S5.

Love S, Lindsey K. *Dr. Susan Love's hormone book*. New York: Random House, 1997.

Love S, Lindsey K, Williams M. *Dr. Susan Love's breast book*. Reading, MA: Addison Wesley Longman, 1990.

Margossian H, Falcone T. Robotically assisted laparoscopic hysterectomy and adnexal surgery. *J Laparoendosc Adv Surg Tech A* 2001;11(3):161.

Maslow A. A theory of human motivation. *Psychol Rev* 1984;50:370.

Massler DJ, Devansan MM. Sexual consequences of gynecologic operations. In: Comfort A, ed. *Sexual consequences of disability*. Philadelphia: George F. Stickley, 1978.

McCully KS, Jackson S. Hormone replacement therapy and the bladder. *J Br Menopause Soc* 2004;10(1):30.

Mericli M, Nadasy GL, Szekeres M, et al. Estrogen replacement therapy reverses changes in intramural coronary resostance arteries caused by female hormone depletion. *Cardiovasc Res* 2004;61(2):317.

Miller MM, Monjan AA, Buckholtz NS. Estrogen replacement therapy for the potential treatment or prevention of Alzheimer's disease. *Ann N Y Acad Sci* 2001;949:223.

Mull DJ. Cross-cultural communication in the physician's office. *West J Med* 1993;159:609.

Novack DH, Plumer R, Smith RL, et al. Changes in physician's attitude toward telling the cancer patient. *JAMA* 1979;241:897.

Parker WH, Broder MS, Liu Z, et al. Ovarian conservation at the time of hysterectomy for benign disease. *Obstet Gynecol* 2005;106(2):219.

Peters AAW, Trimbos-Kemper GCM, Admiraal C, et al. A randomized clinical trial on the benefit of adhesiolysis in patients with intraperitoneal adhesions and chronic pelvic pain. *BJOG* 1992;99:59.

Pines A. What is the actual lesson from the WHI study upon its completion? *Harefuah* 2004;143(10):722.

Plourde EL. *The ultimate rape: what every woman should know about hysterectomies and ovarian removal*. Irvine, CA: New Voice, 1998.

Prentice RL, Langer R, Stefanick ML, et al. Combined postmenopausal hormone therapy and cardiovascular disease: toward resolving the discrepancy between observational studies and the Women's Health Initiative clinical trial. *Am J Epidemiol* 2005;162(5):404.

Richter DL, Kenzig MJ, Greaney ML, et al. Physician-patient interaction and hysterectomy decision making: the ENDOW study. Ethnicity, Needs, and Decisions of Women. *Am J Health Behav* 2002;26(6):431.

Roeske NCA. Hysterectomy and other gynecologic surgeries: a psychological view. In: Notman MT, Nadelson CC, eds. *The woman patient: medical and psychological interfaces*. New York: Plenum, 1978.

Roovers JPWR, van der Vaart CH, et al. Correspondence re: urinary incontinence after hysterectomy. *Lancet* 2000;356:9246.

Schain WS. Sexual functioning, self-esteem and cancer care. In: Vaeth JM, Blomberg RC, Adler L, eds. *Body image, self-esteem, and sexuality in cancer patients*. New York: Karger, 1980.

Sheehy, G. The Silent Passage pocket Books, Simon and Schuster ISBN 0671567772.

Shelton AJ, Groff JY. Hysterectomy: beliefs and attitudes expressed by African-American Women. *Ethn Dis* 2001;11:732.

Sherwin BB. Estrogen and cognitive functioning in women. *Proc Soc Exp Biol Med* 1998;217:17.

Shute N. Menopause is no disease. Interview 3/24/97 with Susan Love. U.S. News & World Report. http://www.usnews.com.

Smart surgical probe licensed to fight breast cancer. NASA Ames Research Center. Moffett Field, CA: Computational Sciences Division. Press release, December 22, 2000.

Snyder H, Sickmund M. Juvenile offenders and victims: 1999 national report. Washington, DC: Office of Juvenile Justice and Delinquency Prevention, http://www.buildingblocksforyouth.org/justiceforsome/conclusion.html.

Sternberg E. *The balance within: the science connecting health and emotions*. New York: W. H. Freeman and Co., 2001.

Takahashi K, Tanaka E, Murakami M, et al. Long term hormone replacement therapy delays the age related progression of carotid intima thickness in healthy postmenopausal women Mauritas 2004 Oct 15;49 (2):170–7 (ISSN: 0378-5122).

Tjaden P, Thoennes N. *Tull report of the prevalence, incidence, and consequences of violence against women: findings from the National Violence Against Women survey*. Washington, DC: U.S. Department of Justice, Office of Justice Programs, National Institute of Justice, 2000.

Ufema J. Helping loved ones say goodbye. *Nursing* 1991;(Oct):42.

U.S. Public Health Service, The Surgeon General's call to action to prevent suicide Washington, DC 1999s.

Wagner JR, Russo P. Urologic complications of major pelvic surgery. *Semin Surg Oncol* 2000:18:216.

Warga C. *Menopause and the mind: the complete guide to coping with memory loss, foggy thinking, verbal confusion, and other cognitive effects of perimenopause and menopause*. New York: Simon & Schuster, 1999.

Warren MP, Halpert S. Hormone replacement therapy: controversies, pros and cons. *Best Prac Res Clin Endocrinol Metab* 2004;18(3):317.

WHO Health Statistics from the Americas, 2006 edition Suicide and intentional self-harm (E950-959); x60-x84) p 173.

Yates J, Barrett-Connor E, Barlas S, et al. Rapid loss of hip fracture protection after estrogen cessation: evidence from the national osteoporosis risk assessment. *Am J Obstet Gynecol* 2004;103(3):

Youngs DD, Ehrhardt AA, Wise TN. Psychological sequelae of elective gynecologic surgery. In: *Psychosomatic obstetrics and gynecology*. New York: Appleton-Century-Crofts, 1980:255.

CHAPTER 4 ■ PROFESSIONAL LIABILITY AND RISK MANAGEMENT FOR THE GYNECOLOGIC SURGEON

CHARLES J. WARD

DEFINITIONS

Ethical principles are the principles utilized to guide the medical profession in resolving conflicting obligations in health care. The five major ethical principles that are utilized are:

1. Autonomy—The moral right to bodily integrity and self-determination.

2. Beneficence—The duty to do good and be concerned for the medical well-being of the patient.

3. Nonmaleficence—The duty to refrain from harming the patient.

4. Justice—The right of the patient to be treated fairly and to a fair allocation of limited medical resources in the community.

5. Freedom—The ability to choose as well as to refuse treatment. Freedom also implies a lack of coercion, manipulation, or infringement on the patient's decision-making process.

Informed consent—A legal doctrine that requires physicians to obtain consent for treatment, whether it is diagnostic or therapeutic, medical or surgical, invasive or noninvasive.

Judgmental decision—A decision supported by either literature or common use that is generally defensible and not malpractice, even if the decision results in a less than desirous outcome.

Medical malpractice—Occurs when the treatment rendered is constituted to be below the degree of care exercised by physicians generally under the same or similar set of circumstances. A direct cause-and-effect relationship must exist between the breach in the standard of care and the outcome to constitute malpractice.

Maloccurrence—A poor clinical outcome that did not arise from a breach in the standard of care.

Standard of care—The degree of care exercised by physicians generally under the same or similar set of circumstances.

Risk management—Refers to those medical practices, protocols, and procedures that are designed to reduce patient injury and improve clinical outcomes.

In the new millennium, the gynecologic surgeon both in the United States and in Europe is not only faced with the constant threat of malpractice litigation but also with rapid advances in technology. These pressures require the need for continued education and training so that the surgeon practices within the current and evolving standard of care. This chapter outlines practical steps that should reduce the exposure to malpractice claims. It also discusses the litigation process and its emotional impact on the physician. This chapter is neither to be considered a substitute for legal counsel nor a source of legal advice. A bibliography is furnished for those who wish to explore this subject further.

The history of liability suits extends back to the 14th century. The first recorded malpractice suit in English law occurred in 1374. This case involved an action brought before the King's Bench against a surgeon, J. Mort. The plaintiff sustained an injury to the hand, and treatment of this injury left the hand maimed. The defendant surgeon was found not liable because of a legal technicality in the writ of complaint. But the rule was clearly laid down that if negligence were proven, the law would provide a remedy. The court further held that, "if the surgeon does well as he can and employs all his diligence to the cure, it is not right that he should be held culpable."

The civil liability of surgeons arises out of the rule laid down in 1534 by the English jurist Sir Anthony Fitzherbert, which stated, "it is the duty of every artificer to exercise his art right and truly as he ought."

The first recorded malpractice suit in the United States occurred in Connecticut in 1794 and was also against a surgeon. In this case, *Cross v. Guthrey,* the patient's husband sued the surgeon, Dr. Guthrey, after the patient died from postoperative mastectomy complications. The suit alleged that the doctor was guilty of negligence in operating on the plaintiff's wife

> . . . in the most unskillful, ignorant, and cruel manner, contrary to all the well-known rules and principles of practice in such cases, that the patient survived by but three hours, and that the defendant had wholly broken and violated his undertaking and promise to the plaintiff to perform said operation skillfully and with safety to his wife.

The jury found the surgeon liable and awarded damages of £40.

The 1970s and 1980s found the United States engulfed in a malpractice crisis. The malpractice trend has continued into the 21st century, both in the United States and Europe. The millennium continues to bring additional pressures to bear on the gynecologic surgeon. These pressures arise from areas such as the transformation of the practice from a fee-for-service (FFS) reimbursement to various managed care programs, third-party payer interventions, declining incomes yet increasing overhead costs, longer work hours, and sizable malpractice premiums. The 2003 survey of the American College of Obstetricians and Gynecologists (ACOG) membership revealed that nationally a 53% increase in malpractice premiums had occurred in the United States since the 1999 survey.

Because the obstetrician/gynecologist performs six of the 10 most common surgical procedures, it is not surprising to find this specialty to be the most frequently sued. The 2003 ACOG survey found that 76.3% of all fellows have been sued at least one time. The obstetrician/gynecologists surveyed had an average of 2.64 claims filed against them during their career. Even resident physicians in training reported that 29.6% had at least one professional liability claim filed against them during their training. Gynecologic care involved 38.3% of all the claims filed. Of the gynecologic claims, delay in or failure to diagnose was the most common allegation and accounted for 29% of gynecologic claims. Of these, failure to diagnose cancer accounted for 62.8% of the claims. Failure to diagnosis breast cancer was the most frequent type of cancer involved and accounted for 33% of the claims. The second most frequent claim involved failure to diagnose cervical cancer, which accounted for 7.4% of the claims. Failure to diagnose ovarian cancer accounted for 7.3% and was third in the failure to or delay in diagnosis of cancer claims. Major patient injury accounted for 25.4% of these claims. On average, four years elapsed from the onset of the claim to its closing. Of all the claims, 49.5% were dropped or settled without any payment on behalf of the physician. Obstetricians/gynecologists won 73.1% of those claims that were resolved by jury or court verdict, arbitration, or other alternative dispute resolution mechanism.

Contrary to popular impressions that "bad doctors" are the cause of most malpractice actions, studies have shown that physicians who possessed higher qualifications, were board certified, and had more experience were more likely to be sued. This is in part because of the fact that such physicians manage higher-risk patients; therefore, they are more likely to encounter adverse outcomes that can be a source of litigation.

Medical malpractice occurs when the treatment rendered is constituted to be below the degree of care exercised by physicians generally under the same or similar set of circumstances. Today most communities are held to a national standard of care that is defined as a duty to exercise the degree of care and skill expected of a reasonably competent practitioner in the same specialty acting under similar circumstances. *Maloccurrence*, or a poor outcome, is not malpractice unless the outcome arises from a direct effect of a breach of the standard of care. Substandard care per se does not always imply malpractice. There must exist a *direct cause-and-effect relationship* between the breach of the standard of care and the outcome to constitute malpractice.

RISK MANAGEMENT

Risk management refers to those medical practices and procedures that are designed to reduce patient injury and improve clinical outcomes. Risk management is an approach to the practice of medicine that minimizes the risk of lawsuits by practicing in a manner that reduces the possibility of human error, increasing the likelihood of obtaining desired results and providing a medical record that clearly outlines the treatment rendered, which in turn makes such a record very defensible. Risk management, whether in an office or hospital setting, must be a team effort. Each member of the health care team must understand that his or her actions can lead to liability for the others. This means that each member of the health care team must not only understand his or her responsibilities and duties, but also be capable of carrying out those responsibilities and duties.

Many hospitals now employ risk managers. Among their duties is the investigation of incident reports and adverse outcomes. The use of incident reports should be encouraged. An appropriate reply should be made to the author of such reports so that the author feels that they are not only contributing to the improvement of patient care but also that the hospital appreciates and considers their contributions. The risk manager should be able to establish appropriate targeted audits that help the institution identify its risks. With this knowledge, the staff and appropriate departments then can develop procedures and policies to correct the identified problems. Risk management should never be considered a punitive exercise, but rather an approach that will improve the quality of care rendered by all health care professionals.

Risk management cannot always prevent a lawsuit; however, frequently it can protect against a nonmeritorious claim or at least improve the outcome of a malpractice claim. Risk management also has been shown to decrease malpractice premiums in states where it was actively employed. The four cornerstones to solid risk management for the gynecologic surgeon are good surgical technique, appropriate knowledge of current developments and therapy, adequate documentation, and good patient communication. The former two are discussed throughout this book; the latter two are discussed in this chapter.

DOCUMENTATION

Documentation, or its absence, is a major problem in malpractice claims. The finest care given under the best of circumstances, if not documented, may be difficult if not impossible to defend in a court of law. Documentation should be made contemporaneously so that significant facts or incidents are not forgotten. Records should contain adequate documentation to provide sufficient reasons why a procedure was indicated or undertaken. Typed reports are preferred to handwritten reports because they are more legible and open to less question of interpretation. Physician notes should be factual, complete, and relevant. They should neither embellish nor appear grandiose. Only appropriate and widely accepted abbreviations are to be used. It is prudent to document both important negative findings and positive findings, especially in complicated cases. In court, those findings, positive or negative, not documented are often presumed to never have been established. Detrimental statements about the patient should be avoided, but it is prudent to document inappropriate patient behavior. This includes noncompliant behavior, such as failure to get requested tests or follow given advice. Broken or missed appointments also should be recorded. Medical records, especially operative notes, should avoid the words *unintentionally, inadvertently, accidentally, unfortunately*, and *unexplainable* because they imply negligent behavior. For example, in the case of ureteral injury, the surgeon can state that the ureter was cut, and the injury recognized and repaired. However, it is important to detail difficult dissections, the presence of extensive adhesions, or any event that makes a surgical case more difficult. It is always wise to outline a plan of therapy. The surgeon should be aware that *judgmental decisions*, supported by either literature or common use, are defensible and are not malpractice, even if they result in a less than desirous outcome.

There is a proper way to correct a record. Draw a single line through the error, but never obliterate the error. Write the correction either in the margin or on a separate page. Then date and initial the correction. Never change a record after a suit has been filed, because such behavior can lead to loss of credibility and generally makes a case indefensible.

OFFICE SETTING

The office frequently can be the catalyst of a malpractice claim. It can begin with the telephone, which some consider to be the most dangerous of liability risks. Misunderstanding and miscommunication easily can occur over the telephone. Improper telephone etiquette may change a disgruntled patient into an angry one who contemplates the instigation of a malpractice claim. Make sure that messages that require a reply by the physician are delivered in a timely manner and that the advice given is documented. Telephone calls of an urgent or emergency nature not only should be responded to in a timely manner, but also documented in the office chart with the date, time of call, time of response, and advice given. Prescription refills as well as patient instructions given over the telephone should be contemporaneously entered in the chart. Only standard abbreviations should be used in the medical chart. A protocol should be established to make sure that after-hour phone calls, problems, advice rendered, and prescriptions are documented in the patient's record.

Employees of the surgeon's office should be encouraged to provide a warm, courteous, and caring environment for patients who, for the most part, will be under considerable stress as they anticipate surgery or encounter the postoperative limitations that the surgery places on them.

New patients should be told of office policies regarding type of examination, laboratory work, and expected charges. This may be accomplished through written material. Owing to the time constraints that are often placed on the physician by managed care plans, the initial intake information is often obtained by forms filled out by the patient or a member of the office staff. The information should include not only the patient's symptom and pertinent history, but also her past medical, surgical, social, and family history. Drug allergies, identified risk factors, and current medications should be noted. The physician should review this information with the patient to clarify any questionable areas and be sure that the information is adequate for the appropriate management of the patient. Because the gynecologist is now taking care of an aging population, it is extremely important that the gynecologist be aware of all medications the patient is taking. This knowledge can decrease the risk of drug interactions and adverse reactions as new medications are added to the patient's regimen. In this regard, it would be prudent for the physician to have the names of the patient's current practitioners, so that the gynecologist can consult with them as needed. It also is prudent for the gynecologist to have access to a pharmacist, who may be more qualified to check for drug interactions, so that he or she can discuss any questions in this area when new medications are prescribed.

Appointments should be scheduled so that long delays are avoided, and overbooking should be discouraged. Remember that the patient's time is as valuable to her as yours is to you. Records should be kept of broken or missed appointments. This type of information is extremely helpful in establishing a noncompliant behavioral pattern. A protocol should be established for the follow-up on patients who fail to keep appointments.

The patient's confidentiality can be broken not only by employee gossip, but also by inadequate soundproofing in examination and consultation rooms. A simple test can be conducted by the surgeon by going into an examination room during working hours to see if he or she can hear conversation by the staff in the halls or other areas of the office. If such a problem exists, the staff should be made aware of it. Some simple solutions—such as background music and keeping up-to-date reading materials in the examination room to absorb the attention of patients awaiting the physician—may help to alleviate this potential breech of the patient's confidentiality.

A protocol should be in place so that reports, such as laboratory and x-ray studies, are seen and initialed by the physician before filing. Patients should be encouraged to call for the results of their tests (especially mammograms, because such results can be lost in the mail), but the physician may be held responsible for such reports. The patient can be made aware of this responsibility through verbal reminders as well as written notices posted conspicuously in the office.

Because the failure to diagnosis breast cancer is a leading cause of malpractice claims, it is prudent for the gynecologist to have a clear and sound approach to any patient who presents with a breast mass or symptom. Chapter 41 outlines the risk factors, diagnosis, and treatment of breast diseases. From a risk management approach, documentation is critical. It is prudent that the patient's medical record document the date the patient first noticed the change, the symptoms noted, and a detailed description of the physician's findings. Drawings of the mass showing the location and exact measurements of the change are most helpful. In some malpractice claims involving breast cancer, the patient has alleged that she told the gynecologist about breast symptoms on prior visits. Thus, it would be prudent for the gynecologist to document whether the patient had any breast symptoms or symptoms or complaints *on every visit.* Recommended referrals, as well as follow-up and return visits, should be recorded. A system of in-office chart follow-up for these high-risk patients is prudent. Reports of mammograms or other studies should exhibit evidence of review by the physician. If the patient fails to follow advice, the office records should note this, along with all attempts to contact the patient.

Billing and financial records have no place in the medical records. They must be kept separate. A confidential area should be made available for the patient to discuss the fees, insurance matters, or the bill. It is strongly advisable that the physician review every bill before it is turned over to a collection agency. The act of turning a bill over to a collection agency has been the start of many malpractice claims.

When records are requested, make sure to send only copies and only after the appropriate patient authorization has been obtained. Most states have laws that prohibit the transfer of records that deal with drug and alcohol abuse or mental illness without the express authorization of the patient. If the physician sends such information without proper authorization, a separate cause of action can be brought against the physician. Therefore, it is important to be aware of the individual state's laws. Always retain the original copy for as long as your state requires or the statute of limitation exists. Information of this nature usually can be obtained from the state medical board or medical society.

HOSPITAL SETTING

The hospital setting is the source of most events that lead to malpractice claims involving the surgeon. Patients entering the hospital are under considerable stress and may not comprehend the full scope of their therapy. Patients should be made aware that perfect outcomes cannot be guaranteed. They should be made to understand that the chance of an unfavorable outcome is not necessarily related to the quality of care but can occur virtually in any medical encounter. Results should never be guaranteed, but realistic expectations should be given, especially when performing corrective surgery, such as procedures for the treatment of urinary incontinence.

The hospital chart is an important vehicle for communicating significant information needed by the entire health team. Because what is not written in a medical record may be legally presumed to not have occurred, it is critical that the chart is complete, thorough, and that documentation be recorded contemporaneously. The chart should reflect the outline for the plan of management, both current and future, using only approved abbreviations. By clearly writing out the plan of management, especially in complicated cases, the entire health team is able to understand the approach to the treatment and respond in a positive and appropriate manner. Electronic medical records that contain the history, physical exam, physician progress notes, nursing notes, and lab and radiology reports, and that are readily accessible to the entire health care team have been shown to improve patient care.

Daily progress notes are generally advisable; however, more frequent notes are appropriate in complicated cases. Progress notes should be not only dated, but also timed. The timing of notes can be most beneficial from a risk management point of view. When a change in the patient's condition develops and the surgeon is notified of the patient's status, the response time may be critical in establishing the standard of care. The surgeon should develop the habit of timing all notes so that the habit becomes well established. Thus, the surgeon is less likely to forget to time a note in a critical situation.

Consultation should be encouraged, especially in complicated cases. Most patients appreciate this concern and understand that it is impossible with today's rapidly expanding advances in technology for one physician to have complete and superior knowledge in all situations. When consultation is obtained, to avoid confusion and lack of direction in the patient's therapy, one physician should be appointed to coordinate therapies and supervise critical orders.

The surgeon should carefully review all nursing notes on a daily basis. When there is a discrepancy between the observations of the physician and the nurse, the differences should be discussed. Then both parties should write clarifying notes that reflect the discrepancy in observations and its resolution in an appropriate chronological order.

The physician should review all laboratory reports. It is prudent to write progress notes about any significant or abnormal findings in the intended plan of action so that the subsequent members of the health team can understand the therapy and react in a positive manner.

MEDICATION ERRORS

Medication errors are a serious problem for the patient, surgeon, and hospitals. The Institute of Medicine has estimated that approximately one hundred thousand deaths occur annually in United States hospitals as a result of medical errors. The number of deaths from such errors has been compared with a jumbo jet crashing every day in the United States. These errors can arise from administering the wrong medication or giving the medication to the wrong patient, administering the incorrect dose, giving the medication at the incorrect time intervals, or failing to give the medication. Failure to be aware of patient allergies, age, weight, current medications, pregnancy status, and renal and hepatic status also contributed to these errors. Physician orders can be illegible, written incorrectly, or misinterpreted by nursing staff. Physicians should consider printing orders and sitting to write orders, as this has been shown to improve handwriting. One other solution to this problem—the use of computerized physician medication orders—has been shown to decrease prescription errors by 55% to 88%. Bar coding of drugs and blood products has also been shown to significantly decrease these errors. The nurse taking a verbal order from a physician should repeat the orders to the physician, because mistakes can be made when what is heard was not what was intended. For example, the nurse may misinterpret an order for 16 units of insulin as 60 units of insulin, thus it is prudent to say "one six" instead of 16 when giving a verbal numerical order. Never prescribe by ampules, vials, or volume, but rather by milligrams. Avoid the symbols < for less than and > for greater than, but rather write out the words for the symbols, as the symbols have been misinterpreted, leading to significant errors.

Abbreviations used in physician orders have led to many errors in interpretation. The Joint Commission on Accreditation of Healthcare Organizations (JCAHO) has issued a *minimum list of dangerous abbreviations* that must be on every hospital's *do not use list* to be in compliance with accreditation requirements (Table 4.1). These abbreviations should *not* be used in any of their forms, including upper- or lowercase or with or without periods. Other abbreviations that should be considered for prohibition are:

- *µg* (for microgram); use mcg
- *D/C* (for discharge); write out discharge
- *H.S.* (for half-strength); write out half-strength
- *c.c.* (for cubic centimeter); use mL
- *T.I.W.* (for three times a week); write out three or 3 times a week
- *Q.I.D.* (for four times a day); write out four or 4 times a day

It is imperative that derogatory remarks not be made in a patient's record. Physicians should never criticize the care rendered by another physician in front of the patient, nurse, or

TABLE 4.1

JCAHO FORBIDDEN ABBREVIATIONS

ABBREVIATION	POTENTIAL PROBLEM	PREFERRED TERM
U or u	Mistaken as zero, four, or cc	Write "unit"
IU	Mistaken as IV (intravenous) or 10 (ten)	Write "international unit"
Q.D. and QOD	Mistaken for each other; the period after the Q can be mistaken for an I	Write "daily" and "every other day"
Trailing zero (1.0 mg) or lack of leading zero (.1 mg)	Decimal point is missed or obscured (leading to a tenfold error)	Never write a zero by itself after a decimal point (1 mg) and always use a zero before a decimal point (0.1 mg)
MS, MSO4 and MgSO4	Confused for one another; can mean morphine sulfate or magnesium sulfate	Write "morphine sulfate" or "magnesium sulfate"

JCAHO, Joint Commission on Accreditation of Healthcare Organizations.

in an area where others may hear the discussion. There are proper avenues to take if one is dealing with an incompetent physician. To avoid breaching patient's confidentiality, idle discussions with other health care providers on elevators, in halls, or in the operating theater are to be avoided.

Follow-up and discharge care should be explained thoroughly to the patient. In an outpatient surgical center, at the time of discharge, many patients may still be under the influence of anesthesia or drugs that cloud their memories. Therefore, it is prudent not only to give verbal but also written discharge instructions. These instructions should cover medication, activity, diet, wound care, and follow-up appointments. The dose of any medication as well as the duration of its use should be noted clearly. Abbreviations that may not be understood by the patient are to be avoided. The physician's answering service and emergency phone numbers should be provided. A copy of the discharge instructions should be given to the patient, and one should be retained in the chart.

When a complication or less than desirous outcome occurs, the surgeon should promptly have a frank discussion concerning the matter with the patient and other significant family members. Spending the time and providing quality information in an honest and thorough manner is appreciated by the patient and the family and often diffuses a potential malpractice claim. Saying that you are sorry is not an admission of guilt. Most patients, when given a reasonable explanation of a less than desirable outcome, accept our human limitations, but disgruntled patients sue. It is important to convey the fact that medicine remains an art and is not an exact science.

Hospital rules and protocols are established to insure uniform quality of care. The physician or nurse's failure to comply with these rules and protocols can be interpreted as a violation of the standard of care. Therefore, it behooves all members of the health team to know and understand the appropriate rules and protocols. If the surgeon feels that he or she needs to alter a rule or protocol for a patient's benefit, he or she should document the reason contemporaneously in the hospital chart.

Surgeons must stay abreast of current technological advances; however, before using these advances, they must be adequately trained. A borderline skilled surgeon who is learning new procedures on private patients without the patient's knowledge or approval is not only risking a malpractice suit, but also may be accused of practicing under questionable ethical standards.

The resident or house officer adds another potential risk to malpractice exposure. All residents or house officers practice as trainees under the supervision of the training institution and the staff of the hospital. Those who supervise, be they attending, clinical faculty, or full-time faculty, are usually held accountable for residents' acts. Residents and house officers, however, also can be held accountable for their own actions. Thus, it is important for the surgeon in a supervisory role to not only review the chart, but also assess the patient. If the supervising physician disagrees with a resident's evaluation, a discrete discussion of the matter should be held with the resident. Then the surgeon and resident should document the appropriate findings and note the rationale behind his or her change in observations or therapy.

On initial contact with the patient, residents or house officers should convey the fact that they are trainees or residents, especially when training in a private hospital or facility. The patient has the right to refuse treatment by a resident, but most accept the advantage of such supervised training. It is prudent to document the acceptance or refusal of medical care from the resident or house officer, especially in an institution that is not directly connected with a medical school. When the patient is admitted to the hospital under the care of a resident, the resident should go over the reason for hospitalization. They should discuss the recommended therapy, appropriate alternatives, potential benefits, risks, and complications of the proposed therapy. The resident should only perform those procedures, without supervision, for which he or she has been fully trained. If a patient's condition requires more expertise than the resident possesses, the resident must inform the supervisory physician of the nature of the patient's condition and the need for procedures beyond the resident's expertise. If a complication arises, the resident, preferably in the presence of the attending physician, or a nurse, or other medical witness should take time to thoroughly and openly discuss the complication and its impact on the patient's subsequent treatment and hospital stay. This conversation should then be documented in the chart.

MANAGED CARE AND SOCIALIZED MEDICINE

Managed care was created in an effort to control the rapidly rising U.S. health care costs. The ideal goals of managed care were to reduce cost, improve clinical outcomes, and control the utilization of resources; however, these goals have not always been achieved. Managed care has become the dominant form of health care delivery in the United States and has had a tremendous impact on physicians as various types of managed care programs have rapidly replaced FFS. Managed care continues to evolve in an effort to meet the demands of the health care industry. At present, the major types of plans include: (a) health maintenance organization (HMO), which also includes independent practice associations (IPA); (b) preferred provider organizations (PPO); and (c) point-of-service (POS) plans.

HMO plans provide or arrange coverage of specific health-care services for a fixed prepaid fee. In-network providers required by the members then provide the service. In the IPA-type HMO, the plan contracts with individual physicians who maintain their own independent practice, offices, medical records, and staff but see HMO members.

PPO plans contract with independent providers who provide services at a discounted rate. Members in this plan generally use in-network providers but are permitted to use out-of-network providers as long as the member is willing to pay a higher out-of-pocket fee.

POS plans generally offer the cost control of an HMO plan with the choice of the FFS plans. This is accomplished by allowing members in the plan to choose from an HMO, PPO, or indemnity plan at the time the service is rendered. At present, POS plans have become the fastest growing managed care type plan.

In any managed care plan, financial conflicts can give rise to risks and liabilities for the physician not seen in an FFS form of medicine. Problems can potentially arise when a physician is paid through a capitation scheme or receives year-end bonuses or other monetary rewards for under utilization of services. In capitation, the physician receives a fixed dollar amount to cover the cost of health care services for enrolled members of the plan. This per capita rate is paid on a periodic basis whether the physician does or does not provide service to all members of the plan. This is intended to reduce overuse of services. Although this system of payment is a powerful incentive for the physician to manage patient care as efficiently as possible, conflicts can arise when services provided by the physician exceed the financial reimbursement from the plan. Such conflicts of interest can impair the physician's moral judgment, threaten the patient's health and well-being, and threaten the physician's professional credibility. The physician cannot jeopardize the patient's care because of financial constraint placed on him or her by the managed care plan. Physicians must make patient-care decisions based on what is best for the patient even if such decisions adversely affect the physician's financial status. The physician must discuss the appropriate alternatives to treatment that are available, even if the plan does not cover the cost of the preferred method of treatment, drug, test, or device. In such cases, the physician must become the patient's advocate and provide the care required to meet the patient's needs, even if the physician is not compensated for the care rendered. Legal precedents have established that the physician should act as a patient advocate in disputes over the financial cost of appropriate treatment and should attempt to convince the managed care plan administrators that the care is not only warranted, but that the care is the most appropriate for the patient's condition. Failure to practice within the standard of care because of the financial constraints of a managed care plan is never a defense should a malpractice suit arise from such an incident.

Under managed care plans in the United States and socialized medical plans in Europe, certain fundamental ethical values have become endangered owing to the financial constraints placed on the access to certain treatments, tests, or drugs, and the limitation to the availability of these treatments in a timely manner. These include fiduciary beneficence (the physician's obligation to act for the benefit of the patient), patient autonomy (the patient's right to make informed judgments regarding her care), and justice (the right to an adequate level of health care that is both available and accessible to all individuals). The physician must remain a strong advocate for the patient. The physician must have input into the decision-making process to be sure that resources are allocated in a proper and just way so that cost containment and economic efficiency are morally legitimate goals that enhance rather than undermine the quality of health care. Physicians must continue to inform the patient of the best treatment options available, whether or not these options are covered by the managed care plan or socialized medicine. They must remain a strong advocate for their patient's rights and should refuse to participate in medical plans or schemes that have policies that are deemed unethical.

COMMUNICATION

Good communication is a major key to preventing malpractice claims. It has often been stated that satisfied patients are less likely to sue, but disgruntled patients will sue. It has been shown that even physicians with borderline skills but excellent bedside manners are less likely to be sued than well-trained board-certified specialists who lack communication skills. Initial impressions usually are long lasting. Therefore, it is important on the first visit to convey the physician's philosophy and the nature of his or her practice. It is prudent to explain what the physician expects from the patient in this relationship because expectations and responsibilities exist for both the patient and physician. Patients are generally looking for a physician who is easy to talk to and will answer questions, be accessible, be fair, show respect, and provide good care for a reasonable cost. Inattention, indignation, and injury can be not only the cause for a suit, but in combination also dramatically increase the potential for a suit.

Surgeons should be aware that the majority of what a patient perceives is obtained through nonverbal communications. Patients generally retain only 30% of verbal communication. Body language, posture, and facial expressions all convey strong messages. For example, the surgeon who stands with his or her hand on the door and asks, do you have any questions, sends a strong message that he or she really does not have the time to answer questions; that his or her time is more important than the concerns of the patient. Simple things such as sitting in a relaxed position when the physician discusses a patient's condition or treatment generally convey a feeling of caring and concern. If notes or prescriptions are written in the examination room, the surgeon should make every attempt to face the patient while performing this task. The surgeon's back does not convey a sense of caring or concern.

In the hospital, the physician has to write daily progress notes and orders. The patient's bedside is an excellent place to write them. The surgeon then can explain the orders and therapy as they are written. Patients who are medicated have a slower reaction time and tend to easily forget things that are important to them. The silence that may ensue as the surgeon writes a note or thinks about the management gives the patient time to recall those important questions. This type of interaction builds trust and gives the patient the feeling that she is actively participating in her care and therapy.

Surgeons often do not realize the significant degree of stress a patient undergoes while she lies on the operating table before being anesthetized. The simple act of holding the patient's hand at this time can not only have a calming effect, but also demonstrate the physician's concern and care for the patient's well-being. In the office, little things such as warming speculums on a heating pad in the examination table drawer, providing adequate areas to dress and undress, and having mirrors in the examination room all help to convey a sense of caring for the patient's needs. During the preoperative visits, patients will often mention that their families and friends are praying for them. The surgeon may request that prayers are also offered to guide the surgeon's hands and judgment to bring about a cure from the malady requiring surgery. Some surgeons are known to offer a prayer at the start of an operation. Patients generally appreciate this expression of faith and humility. These gestures also tend to strengthen the patient surgeon bond.

Good communication encourages questions and involvement of family members, especially partners. Therefore, it is important that the physician, preferably, or a designated nurse or physician assistant take the necessary time to answer the patient's questions and address concerns in a setting where respect and confidentiality can be maintained easily. Beware of the patient with the "great expectation syndrome." Physicians have greatly oversold their abilities and have created false expectations that have led to unjustified expectations. If the surgeon feels that the patient expects more than he or she can reasonably provide, it is prudent to refer this patient to another physician.

When it becomes necessary to terminate the doctor–patient relationship, the surgeon must remember that this relationship is a contract, be it informal or implied, and certain steps are required to break the contract. The patient should be sent a letter by certified mail, return receipt requested. The letter should state a specific date for the termination to occur, usually 30 days from the date of mailing. The letter should contain a release for the patient's records. The patient should be instructed to sign and return the release before forwarding any of the patient's records. Always send a copy of the records, and never the original records, to the physician of her choice. The physician may include a list of other gynecologists in the patient's area or refer her to the local medical society for appropriate referral. These letters of termination need not go into great detail as to why the contract is being terminated. It is perfectly acceptable to say that, owing to a personality conflict, the surgeon does not feel that he or she can provide the quality of care the patient should receive. Thus, the physician is requesting that the patient seek care elsewhere. The physician is required to treat any emergency that might arise before the specified termination date.

Improper communication can result in physicians getting other physicians sued. Negative comments made about other physicians continue to be a major source of problems. As Walt Kelly's cartoon character Pogo once stated, "We have met the enemy and he is us." Nonprofessional opinions written in the medical record can open the treating surgeon, hospital, or other health care members to malpractice actions. Careless talk, second-guessing colleagues, and open debate, carried out in public areas, regarding the patient's treatment or status can all lead to unwarranted malpractice claims.

In situations involving multiple physicians, such as a group practice, communication between those physicians is extremely important. The medical records must be a complete and thorough source of this information. The records should reflect clear and factual accounts so that confusion does not arise regarding the patient's treatment or status. Lack of such communication can increase the risk of liability claims. In group practices, it is prudent to have set aside a specific time to discuss patients, especially those with complicated courses.

A physician should know his or her limitations and not let an inflated or unrealistic ego prevent appropriate consultations when the patient's condition may exceed his or her expertise. Continuous and appropriate communication with the consulting physicians ensures that the patient receives the highest quality of care, the goal all physicians strive to achieve.

INFORMED CONSENT

Informed consent is a legal doctrine that requires physicians to obtain consent for treatment, whether it is diagnostic or therapeutic, medical or surgical, invasive or noninvasive. Without informed consent, the physician can be held liable for violating the patient's rights regardless of whether the treatment was appropriate and rendered within the standard of care. Failure to obtain informed consent may result in the physician being accused of battery under common law.

Failure to provide informed consent was the primary charge in 2% of malpractice claims in the 2003 ACOG survey. This was a decrease from 5% recorded in the 1999 ACOG survey. The failure to provide adequate informed consent was found to be a secondary issue in almost one third of malpractice claims. Informed consent is an ongoing process that includes the exchange of information and the development of choices. Informed consent is a process of ongoing shared information. It provides for the development of choices and requires active participation from both the patient and the physician. Informed consent should never be confused with the mere signing of a consent sheet.

Since the 1948 Nuremberg Code, valid consent has consistently been described as having four characteristics: voluntary, competent, informed, and understanding. There are ethical considerations in the process of informed consent. The surgeon must respect the patient's *autonomy* or the patient's moral right to bodily integrity and self-determination. Respecting a patient's autonomy means that the gynecologist cannot impose treatments; however, it does not mean that the gynecologist must provide treatment if he or she feels that the treatment is inappropriate or may be harmful. Thus, *beneficence* or the principle that the physician has a duty to do good and be concerned for the medical well-being of the patient is also an important ethical principle in the process of informed consent. *Nonmaleficence* is the obligation to do no harm. Although there are subtle differences between the principles of beneficence and nonmaleficence, both principles play a role in almost every decision in the treatment of patients. The principle of *justice* is the most complex of ethical principles, because it requires the surgeon to not only treat the patient fairly but also consider the allocation of limited medical resources in the community.

The concept of *freedom*, a basic ethical element of informed consent, implies both an ability to choose as well as an ability to refuse treatment. Freedom also implies a lack of coercion, manipulation, or infringement on the patient's decision-making process. Recognition of different values, preferences, and alternatives is important in the process of free consent.

There may exist practical limitations to the informed consent process. These may include limitations of time, language barriers, ability to fully comprehend technical matters, and the communication abilities of the physician. These limitations, however, do not release the physician from the ethical requirements for reasonable communication. A physician's biases, the patient's rights, and confidentiality may also create problems while making ethical decisions. Conflicts of interest may arise. These conflicts may occur when the patient's well-being conflicts with managed care, physician's financial interests, treatment protocols, care plans, or practice guidelines. The American College of Obstetricians and Gynecologists has published excellent texts to address these concerns in detail.

Courts have recognized and states have adopted three different degrees of disclosure in informed consent. The first, *the professional or reasonable physician standard*, was prevalent before the 1970s. This degree of disclosure was based on the type and amount of information that a reasonable physician would tell the patient about the risks and benefits of a particular treatment. This paternalistic approach began to give way in the 1970s to the second type of disclosure, *the materiality or reasonable patient viewpoint standard*. This gave patients more input into the decision-making process. Under this standard, the physician had to disclose what a "reasonable person" would want to know under similar circumstances concerning the risks and benefits of a particular treatment. This concept is based on the patient's need rather than the professional perception of what the patient should know. The third, but not widely held, disclosure is *the subjective patient viewpoint*. Under this disclosure, physicians must disclose varying amounts of information based on the individual's personal needs and peculiar requirements. This form renders a standard extremely difficult for physicians to understand and apply.

The need for informed consent can be suspended in an emergency situation, but specific criteria must be met for a situation to be declared an emergency. The patient must be unconscious or incapacitated and suffering from a life-threatening or serious health-threatening condition requiring immediate medical treatment. It is important in these situations for the physician to document the following: a description of the patient's condition at the time of the emergency, the reason the emergency existed, and an explanation for the need for immediate attention.

Patients have the right to refuse treatment after receiving informed consent. Under these circumstances, for legal protection, the physician should document the reason the patient gave for refusal of the proposed treatment, the reason that the physician felt that the proposed treatment was indicated, and the possible jeopardy to the future health and well-being of the patient that might occur from the refusal of the treatment.

It would be prudent to have the patient sign a statement acknowledging the refusal for treatment and listing the potential adverse consequences that might occur. Another possible solution to informed refusal is to have the patient write a note in their own hand, in the clinical record, that not only states that she understands the consequence of refusal of treatment but goes on to list the potential adverse complications of her refusal, even listing death if that is appropriate. The patient should then sign her statement, and the physician and preferably a third party—such as a nurse, or preferably a family member—should witness the note.

The office setting provides the best environment for providing informed consent for several reasons. In this setting, the time for adequate consideration and adequate discussion is provided. Family members who have a definite influence on the patient's decision can attend or be encouraged to attend. If the physician lacks the ability or time to provide the necessary adequate informed consent, the physician can delegate this responsibility to a nurse practitioner or physician assistant who has been previously trained to provide informed consent and is able to answer the patient's questions. Pamphlets, audiovisual, and even interactive visuals can greatly assist in this process. Because people rarely retain more than 30% of verbal communications, the average patient leaves the physician's office having forgotten or not understanding most of what was shown and explained. Thus, the more the patient receives in writing or by audiovisual instruction, the better is her understanding.

Once the process of informed consent is complete, the physician can document the record to reflect when it took place, what was disclosed, that the patient had time to ask questions and have her questions answered to her satisfaction, and that the patient then requested the proposed treatment. Well-informed patients are more likely to overlook less than desirable outcomes and accept that medicine is still an art and not an exact science. Less-well-informed patients are more likely to have unrealistic expectations and sue when these expectations are not met. Therefore, the best protection to a malpractice claim may come from taking full advantage of the legal doctrine of informed consent.

The degree of disclosure in informed consent varies from state to state. Some states require elaborate consent, others much less. When a complication develops that was disclosed in the informed consent, however, there is no cause for legal action so long as the complication did not arise from a negligent act.

There is almost universal agreement that informed consent should encompass the following six areas:

1. Diagnosis
2. Nature and purpose of the procedure
3. Risks of the procedure
4. Likelihood of success
5. Reasonable alternatives
6. Prognosis if the treatment is refused

Figure 4.1 is a general surgical informed consent form meeting these requirements. There are several particular points to note. First, throughout the form, the words "I request" or "request for surgery" are included. These words are used to place greater emphasis on the patient's responsibility for her choice in selecting the proposed procedure. Next, a list of the "general risks of surgery" is provided. This list not only covers those risks that can arise from any surgical procedure but also the risks associated with anesthesia. In describing the risks and complications of the procedures, the words "may include but are not limited to such complications as" have been added and are used to indicate that the physician did not attempt to list every potential complication but rather those that a reasonable patient would expect to know before making a decision. In the section on alternative forms of treatment, the words "such as" indicate that only those alternatives considered to be appropriate need to be listed. Finally, space is provided to list any additional materials that the patient was given or might have reviewed in making her decision. If a claim arises, the physician can then explain to a jury the situation surrounding the alleged act of negligence and use the same material in his or her defense to show that a reasonable person was properly informed.

Figures 4.2 through 4.7 are informed consent forms covering the six most common gynecologic operative procedures. These forms describe each procedure in words that a patient can comprehend easily. A reading specialist has reviewed these informed consent forms and placed them in a language level of an individual with a sixth-grade education, which is generally that used by daily newspapers. Each of these forms covers the risks and complications as well as alternatives that apply to the specific procedure along with the "general risks of surgery."

Figure 4.2, the informed consent and request for dilatation and curettage, hysteroscopy, and cervical biopsy, lists the most common complication seen—namely, perforation of the uterus. It also notes that the procedure can have an adverse impact on subsequent pregnancies.

Figure 4.3, the informed consent and request for hysterectomy, covers complications seen, including injuries to the genitourinary tract, the most frequently seen complication. It also discusses the risk associated with blood transfusion.

Figure 4.4, the informed consent for laparoscopy-assisted vaginal hysterectomy or LAVH, goes over the complications of hysterectomy and the complications that laparoscopy may add to the procedure.

Figure 4.5, the informed consent and request for sterilization, clearly states that the procedure is not designed to be reversible. Many patients have a sterilization procedure performed in their twenties and, in this age of divorce and remarriage, later request that the sterilization be reversed. When the procedure cannot be reversed, patients may sue with a claim of "lost opportunities." This statement in the informed consent is designed to cover that particular area. Ectopic pregnancy, one of the known and accepted risks of any sterilization procedure, is clearly spelled out.

Figure 4.6, the informed consent and request for diagnostic and therapeutic laparoscopy, reviews the more commonly seen complications of injury to the gastrointestinal or genitourinary tracts and vascular injury. The form also notes the risk of exploratory laparotomy. This provides an opportunity for the physician to discuss this potential extension of a laparoscopy procedure so that the physician is not hesitant to proceed with laparotomy when the findings require that procedure.

Figure 4.7, the informed consent for repair of relaxation of pelvic organs and/or the correction of urinary incontinence problems, notes that recurrence of urinary incontinence is a potential complication. This is designed so that false expectations from the surgical procedure are not created.

These procedure-specific informed consent forms are detailed but have been found to be acceptable to patients. They also have made the defense of surgical complications much easier, especially when there is no negligence.

The legal requirements of informed consent vary from state to state and jurisdiction to jurisdiction. The surgeon should be aware of the degree of disclosure required, as well as any specific laws on informed consent that exist in his or her state. County or state medical societies are usually able to assist in providing this necessary information.

INFORMED CONSENT AND REQUEST FOR SURGERY

I, ______________________________, request Dr.____
and his/her associates / assistants to perform upon me (name of procedure):
____

Diagnosis and Procedure: The following has been explained to me in general terms and I understand that:

My condition has been diagnosed as: ____
The nature of the procedure is: ____
The purpose of this procedure is to: ____

General Risks of Surgery: As a result of the performance of this procedure there may be general risks involved such as: INFECTION, ALLERGIC REACTION, DISFIGURING SCAR, SEVERE LOSS OF BLOOD, LOSS OF FUNCTION OF ANY LIMB OR ORGAN, PARALYSIS, PARAPLEGIA OR QUADRIPLEGIA, BRAIN DAMAGE, CARDIAC ARREST, OR DEATH. In addition to these general risks, there may be other possible risks involved in this procedure. These risks and/or complications may include but are not limited to such complications as: ____

Likelihood of Success: The likelihood of success of the above procedure is: () Good () Fair () Poor

Prognosis: If I choose not to have the above procedure, my prognosis (future medical condition) is:
____

Alternative Forms of Treatment, such as: ______________________________
have been explained to me and I have chosen this surgical procedure as my method of treatment.

I understand and accept that during the procedure unexpected or unforeseen circumstances may make it necessary to do an extension of the original procedure or another procedure that is not named above. I request Dr. ______________________ and his/her associates or assistants of his/her choice to perform those procedures that they judge to be necessary.

BY SIGNING THIS FORM, I ACKNOWLEDGE THAT I HAVE READ OR HAD THIS FORM READ AND EXPLAINED TO ME AND THAT I FULLY UNDERSTAND ITS CONTENTS.

I HAVE BEEN GIVEN AMPLE OPPORTUNITY TO ASK QUESTIONS AND ANY QUESTIONS I HAVE ASKED HAVE BEEN ANSWERED OR EXPLAINED IN A SATISFACTORY MANNER. ALL BLANKS OR STATEMENTS REQUIRING COMPLETION WERE FILLED IN AND ALL STATEMENTS WITH WHICH I DISAGREE WERE MARKED OUT BEFORE I SIGNED THIS FORM.

I accept that medicine is not an exact science and understand that no guarantees can be given as to the results. Understanding these limitations, I request that Dr. ____________________ and his/her associates/assistants to proceed with surgery.

______________________________ ______________________________

Witness Person giving consent

Relationship to patient if not the patient ______________

Patient unable to sign because of:

Date: ______________
____

Additional materials used, if any, during the informed consent process for this procedure include: ______________
____
____

Date: ______________ Witness: ______________________________

FIGURE 4.1. Informed consent and request for surgery.

INFORMED CONSENT And REQUEST FOR DILATION & CURETTAGE, HYSTEROSCOPY, OR CERVICAL BIOPSY

I, ______________________________, request Dr.______________________________
and his/her associates / assistants to perform upon me (Circle procedure to be performed):

1. Dilation & Curettage--stretch open the canal of my uterus and scrape the lining of my uterus to obtain tissue for study.
2. Hysteroscopy--look inside my uterus with a small telescope and possibly remove any abnormal tissue, such as fibroid tumors, polyps, or scar tissue.
3. Cervical Biopsy--remove tissue from tip of my uterus for tissue study.

Diagnosis and Procedure: The following has been explained to me in general terms and I understand that:

My condition has been diagnosed as: ______________________________
The nature of the procedure is: ______________________________
The purpose of this procedure is to: ______________________________

General Risks of Surgery: As a result of the performance of this procedure there may be general risks involved such as: INFECTION, ALLERGIC REACTION, DISFIGURING SCAR, SEVERE LOSS OF BLOOD, LOSS OF FUNCTION OF ANY LIMB OR ORGAN, PARALYSIS, PARAPLEGIA or QUADRIPLEGIA, BRAIN DAMAGE, CARDIAC ARREST, or DEATH. In addition to these general risks, there may be other possible risks involved in this procedure. These risks and/or complications may include but are not limited to such complications as:

1. Perforation of my uterus (womb)--that is, one of the instruments might go through the wall of the uterus and make it necessary to do an immediate or future operation that could include the removal of my uterus and/or tubes and ovaries
2. Biopsy of my cervix--which may make it difficult for me to get pregnant or carry a pregnancy to term or 9 months
3. Injury to my cervix, uterus, tubes, and bowel--which could make necessary immediate and/or future surgical procedures

Likelihood of Success: The likelihood of success of the above procedure is: () Good () Fair () Poor

Prognosis: If I choose not to have the above procedure, my prognosis (future medical condition) is:
____

Alternative Forms of Treatment such as:

1. Office biopsy of the lining of my uterus (endometrial biopsy) or cervix (cervical biopsy)
2. Hormone therapy
3. Do-nothing and accept the consequences of my present condition

These alternative treatments have been explained to me, and I have elected this surgical procedure as my method of treatment.

I understand and accept that during the procedure unexpected or unforeseen circumstances may make it necessary to do an extension of the original procedure or another procedure that is not named above. I request that Dr. ______________________________ and associates or assistants of his/her choice to perform those procedures that they judge to be necessary.

BY SIGNING THIS FORM, I ACKNOWLEDGE THAT I HAVE READ OR HAD THIS FORM READ AND EXPLAINED TO ME AND THAT I FULLY UNDERSTAND ITS CONTENTS.

I HAVE BEEN GIVEN AMPLE OPPORTUNITY TO ASK QUESTIONS AND ANY QUESTIONS I HAVE ASKED HAVE BEEN ANSWERED OR EXPLAINED IN A SATISFACTORY MANNER. ALL BLANKS OR STATEMENTS REQUIRING COMPLETION WERE FILLED IN AND ALL STATEMENTS WITH WHICH I DISAGREE WERE MARKED OUT BEFORE I SIGNED THIS FORM.

I accept that medicine is not an exact science and understand that no guarantees can be given as to the results. Understanding these limitations, I request that Dr. ______________________ and his/her associates/assistants to proceed with surgery.

______________________________ Witness

______________________________ Person giving consent

Relationship to patient if not the patient ____________________

Patient unable to sign because of:

____

Date: ________________

Additional materials used, if any, during the informed consent process for this procedure include: ________________
____
____

Date: ______________________ Witness: ______________________________

FIGURE 4.2. Informed consent and request for dilation and curettage, hysteroscopy, or cervical biopsy.

INFORMED CONSENT And REQUEST FOR HYSTERECTOMY

I, ______________________________, request Dr.____
and his/her associates / assistants to perform upon me: (Circle procedure of choice)

1. Removal of uterus (womb)
2. Possible removal of tubes and/or ovaries
3. Possible removal of appendix

Diagnosis and Procedure: The following has been explained to me in general terms and I understand that:

My condition has been diagnosed as: ____
The nature of the procedure is: ____
The purpose of this procedure is to: ____

General Risks of Surgery: As a result of the performance of this procedure there may be general risks involved such as: INFECTION, ALLERGIC REACTION, DISFIGURING SCAR, SEVERE LOSS OF BLOOD, LOSS OF FUNCTION OF ANY LIMB OR ORGAN, PARALYSIS, PARAPLEGIA or QUADRIPLEGIA, BRAIN DAMAGE, CARDIAC ARREST, or DEATH. In addition to these general risks, there may be other possible risks involved in this procedure. These risks and/or complications may include but are not limited to such complications as:

1. Injury to bowel, bladder, or ureter, which could result in a fistula formation, an opening between bowel, bladder, ureter, and the vagina and/or skin
2. Need for a colostomy or a second operation to repair any of the above injuries
3. Possible need for hormones
4. Blood loss necessitating transfusion, which carries the risk of exposure to AIDS or the hepatitis virus
5. Pelvic pain due to adhesions, scar tissue, or residual ovary

Likelihood of Success: The likelihood of success of the above procedure is: () Good () Fair () Poor

Prognosis: If I choose not to have the hysterectomy, my prognosis (future medical condition) is:
____

Alternative Forms of Treatment such as:

1. Do nothing and accept the consequences of my present condition
2. Dilatation & Curettage procedure, laser treatment, or removal of fibroid tumors
3. Uterine artery embolization
4. Hormone therapy

These alternative treatments have been explained to me, and I have elected this surgical procedure as my method of treatment.

I understand and accept that during the procedure unexpected or unforeseen circumstances may make it necessary to do an extension of the original procedure or another procedure that is not named above. I request that Dr. ______________________________ and associates or assistants of his/her choice perform those procedures that they judge to be necessary.

BY SIGNING THIS FORM, I ACKNOWLEDGE THAT I HAVE READ OR HAD THIS FORM READ AND EXPLAINED TO ME AND THAT I FULLY UNDERSTAND ITS CONTENTS.

I HAVE BEEN GIVEN AMPLE OPPORTUNITY TO ASK QUESTIONS AND ANY QUESTIONS I HAVE ASKED HAVE BEEN ANSWERED OR EXPLAINED IN A SATISFACTORY MANNER. ALL BLANKS OR STATEMENTS REQUIRING COMPLETION WERE FILLED IN AND ALL STATEMENTS WITH WHICH I DISAGREE WERE MARKED OUT BEFORE I SIGNED THIS FORM.

I accept that medicine is not an exact science and understand that no guarantees can be given as to the results. Understanding these limitations, I request that Dr. ____________________ and his/her associates/assistants to proceed with surgery.

______________________________ ______________________________
Witness Person giving consent

Relationship to patient if not the patient ________________

Patient unable to sign because of:

Date: ______________

____

Additional materials used, if any, during the informed consent process for this procedure include: ____________
____
____

Date: ______________________ Witness: ______________________________

FIGURE 4.3. Informed consent and request for hysterectomy.

INFORMED CONSENT And REQUEST FOR LAPAROSCOPIC ASSISTED VAGINAL HYSTERECTOMY (LAVH)

I, ______________________________, request Dr.______________________________
and his/her associates / assistants to perform upon me: (Circle procedure of choice)

1. Removal of uterus (womb)
2. Possible removal of tubes and/or ovaries
3. Possible removal of appendix
4. Repair the following defects: ______________________________

Diagnosis and Procedure: The following has been explained to me in general terms and I understand that:

My condition has been diagnosed as: ______________________________
The nature of the procedure is: ______________________________
The purpose of this procedure is to: ______________________________

General Risks of Surgery: As a result of the performance of this procedure there may be general risks involved such as: INFECTION, ALLERGIC REACTION, DISFIGURING SCAR, SEVERE LOSS OF BLOOD, LOSS OF FUNCTION OF ANY LIMB OR ORGAN, PARALYSIS, PARAPLEGIA or QUADRIPLEGIA, BRAIN DAMAGE, CARDIAC ARREST, or DEATH. In addition to these general risks, there may be other possible risks involved in this procedure. These risks and/or complications may include but are not limited to such complications as:

1. Injury to blood vessels, bowel, bladder, ureter (tube that connects kidney to bladder) by way of puncture and/or burn
2. Injury to bowel, bladder, or ureter, which could result in a fistula formation, an opening between bowel, bladder, ureter,and the vagina and/or skin
3. Need for a colostomy or a second operation to repair any of the above injuries
4. Possible need for hormones
5. Blood loss necessitating transfusion, which carries the risk of exposure to AIDS or the hepatitis virus
6. Pelvic pain due to adhesions, scar tissue, or residual ovary
7. Embolism, which is the spreading of a gas or other fluid into other parts or organs of the body
8. Hernia in the incision site
9. Necessity for an exploratory laparotomy, which is the making of a larger incision through which the necessary surgery can be performed

Likelihood of Success: The likelihood of success of the above procedure is: () Good () Fair () Poor

Prognosis: If I choose not to have the hysterectomy, my prognosis (future medical condition) is:
____

Alternative Forms of Treatment such as:

1. Do nothing and accept the consequences of my present condition
2. Dilatation & Curettage procedure, laser treatment, or removal of fibroid tumors
3. Uterine artery embolization
4. Hormone therapy

These alternative treatments have been explained to me, and I have elected this surgical procedure as my method of treatment.

I understand and accept that during the procedure unexpected or unforeseen circumstances may make it necessary to do an extension of the original procedure or another procedure that is not named above. I request that Dr. ______________________________ and associates or assistants of his/her choice perform those procedures that they judge to be necessary.

BY SIGNING THIS FORM, I ACKNOWLEDGE THAT I HAVE READ OR HAD THIS FORM READ AND EXPLAINED TO ME AND THAT I FULLY UNDERSTAND ITS CONTENTS.

I HAVE BEEN GIVEN AMPLE OPPORTUNITY TO ASK QUESTIONS AND ANY QUESTIONS I HAVE ASKED HAVE BEEN ANSWERED OR EXPLAINED IN A SATISFACTORY MANNER. ALL BLANKS OR STATEMENTS REQUIRING COMPLETION WERE FILLED IN AND ALL STATEMENTS WITH WHICH I DISAGREE WERE MARKED OUT BEFORE I SIGNED THIS FORM.

I accept that medicine is not an exact science and understand that no guarantees can be given as to the results. Understanding these limitations, I request that Dr. ______________________ and his/her associates/assistants to proceed with surgery.

______________________________ ______________________________
Witness Person giving consent

Relationship to patient if not the patient ________________

Date: ________________ Patient unable to sign because of:

____

Additional materials used, if any, during the informed consent process for this procedure include: ______________
____
____

Date: ______________________ Witness: ______________________________

FIGURE 4.4. Informed consent and request for laparoscopic assisted vaginal hysterectomy (LAVH).

INFORMED CONSENT And REQUEST FOR STERILIZATION

I, ________________________________, request Dr.____

and his/her associates/assistants to perform upon me: (Circle procedure of choice)

1. Removal of a portion of the tubes through an incision in my lower abdomen
2. Laparoscopy ("band-aid" incision or incisions)
   a. Coagulation technique: ( ) Bipolar ( ) Unipolar
   b. Bands
   c. Clips
3. Hysteroscopy: insert a telescope-like instrument into my uterus (womb) and place ____________ into the opening of my tubes, inside the uterus, so that the openings will be blocked.

Diagnosis and Procedure: The following has been explained to me in general terms and I understand that:

This procedure is **NOT** designed to be reversible, and that I am intentionally giving up my ability to become pregnant.

The nature of the procedure is: ____

The purpose of this procedure is to: ____

General Risks of Surgery: As a result of the performance of this procedure there may be general risks involved such as: INFECTION, ALLERGIC REACTION, DISFIGURING SCAR, SEVERE LOSS OF BLOOD, LOSS OF FUNCTION OF ANY LIMB OR ORGAN, PARALYSIS, PARAPLEGIA or QUADRIPLEGIA, BRAIN DAMAGE, CARDIAC ARREST, or DEATH. In addition to these general risks, there may be other possible risks involved in this procedure. These risks and/or complications may include but are not limited to such complications as:

1. Failure to become sterile--that is, I could become pregnant either in my uterus (womb) or have an ectopic pregnancy (in my tube or other site)
2. Injury to bowel, bladder, ureter or blood vessel by way of burn and/or perforation, fistula formation (which is an opening that develops between the bowel, bladder, ureter and the vagina and/or or skin), requiring a second operation to repair the fistula
3. Major surgery--requiring colostomy or possible removal of uterus, tubes and/or ovaries
4. Necessity for an exploratory laparotomy (opening the abdomen) to either complete the laparoscopy procedure or repair any injury
5. Blood loss necessitating transfusion, which carries the risk of exposure to AIDS or the hepatitis virus

Likelihood of Success: The likelihood of success of the above procedure is: () Good () Fair () Poor

Prognosis: If I choose not to have the above procedure, my prognosis (future medical condition) is: ____

Alternative Forms of Treatment such as:

1 Diaphragm
2 Birth control pills
3 Intrauterine devices (IUD)
4 Barrier methods, (use of foams, condoms, etc.)
5 Rhythm method
6. Abstinence
7. Vasectomy (male sterilization)

These alternative treatments have been explained to me, and I have elected this surgical procedure as my method of treatment.

I understand and accept that during the procedure unexpected or unforeseen circumstances may make it necessary to do an extension of the original procedure or another procedure that is not named above. I request that Dr. ________________________________ and associates or assistants of his/her choice perform those procedures that they judge to be necessary.

BY SIGNING THIS FORM, I ACKNOWLEDGE THAT I HAVE READ OR HAD THIS FORM READ AND EXPLAINED TO ME AND THAT I FULLY UNDERSTAND ITS CONTENTS.

I HAVE BEEN GIVEN AMPLE OPPORTUNITY TO ASK QUESTIONS AND ANY QUESTIONS I HAVE ASKED HAVE BEEN ANSWERED OR EXPLAINED IN A SATISFACTORY MANNER. ALL BLANKS OR STATEMENTS REQUIRING COMPLETION WERE FILLED IN AND ALL STATEMENTS WITH WHICH I DISAGREE WERE MARKED OUT BEFORE I SIGNED THIS FORM.

I accept that medicine is not an exact science and understand that no guarantees can be given as to the results. Understanding these limitations, I request that Dr. ________________________ and his/her associates/assistants to proceed with surgery.

________________________________ ________________________________

Witness Person giving consent

Relationship to patient if not the patient ______________

Patient unable to sign because of:

Date: ______________ ________________________________

Additional materials used, if any, during the informed consent process for this procedure include: ______________

____

____

Date: ________________________ Witness: ________________________________

FIGURE 4.5. Informed consent and request for sterilization.

INFORMED CONSENT And REQUEST FOR LAPAROSCOPY

I, ______________________________, request Dr. ______________________________
and his/her associates/ assistants to perform upon me:

Laparoscopy--which involves inserting a telescope-like instrument into my abdomen through one or more small ("band-aid") size incisions to diagnose and/or repair any problems

Diagnosis and Procedure: The following has been explained to me in general terms and I understand that:

My condition has been diagnosed as: ______________________________
The nature of the procedure is: ______________________________
The purpose of this procedure is to: ______________________________

I understand that treatment may require the use of laser and/or electrocautery during the performance of this surgery.

General Risks of Surgery: As a result of the performance of this procedure there may be general risks involved such as: INFECTION, ALLERGIC REACTION, DISFIGURING SCAR, SEVERE LOSS OF BLOOD, LOSS OF FUNCTION OF ANY LIMB OR ORGAN, PARALYSIS, PARAPLEGIA or QUADRIPLEGIA, BRAIN DAMAGE, CARDIAC ARREST, or DEATH. In addition to these general risks, there may be other possible risks involved in this procedure. These risks and/or complications may include but are not limited to such complications as:

1. Injury to blood vessels, bowel, bladder, ureter (tube that connects kidney to bladder) by way of puncture and/or burn
2. Fistula formation, which is an opening between the bowel, bladder, or ureter and the vagina and/or skin, that requires a second operation to repair.
3. Colostomy
4. Embolism, which is the spreading of a gas or other fluid into other parts or organs of the body
5. Hernia in the incision site
6. Injury to the cervix, uterus, or tubes that might require additional surgery or might affect my ability to get pregnant or carry a pregnancy to full term (9 months)
7. Necessity for an exploratory laparotomy, which is the making of a larger incision through which the necessary surgery can be performed
8. Blood loss necessitating transfusion, which carries the risk of exposure to AIDS or the hepatitis virus

Likelihood of Success: The likelihood of success of the above procedure is: () Good () Fair () Poor

Prognosis: If I choose not to have the above procedure, my prognosis (future medical condition) is:
____

Alternative Forms of Treatment such as:

1. Do nothing and accept the consequences of my present condition
2. Performance of surgery through a larger incision in my abdomen
4. Drug therapy

These alternative treatments have been explained to me, and I have elected this surgical procedure as my method of treatment.

I understand and accept that during the procedure unexpected or unforeseen circumstances may make it necessary to do an extension of the original procedure or another procedure that is not named above. I request that Dr. ______________________________ and associates or assistants of his/her choice to perform those procedures that they judge to be necessary.

BY SIGNING THIS FORM, I ACKNOWLEDGE THAT I HAVE READ OR HAD THIS FORM READ AND EXPLAINED TO ME AND THAT I FULLY UNDERSTAND ITS CONTENTS.

I HAVE BEEN GIVEN AMPLE OPPORTUNITY TO ASK QUESTIONS AND ANY QUESTIONS I HAVE ASKED HAVE BEEN ANSWERED OR EXPLAINED IN A SATISFACTORY MANNER. ALL BLANKS OR STATEMENTS REQUIRING COMPLETION WERE FILLED IN AND ALL STATEMENTS WITH WHICH I DISAGREE WERE MARKED OUT BEFORE I SIGNED THIS FORM.

I accept that medicine is not an exact science and understand that no guarantees can be given as to the results. Understanding these limitations, I request that Dr. ____________________ and his/her associates/assistants to proceed with surgery.

______________________________ ______________________________
Witness Person giving consent

Relationship to patient if not the patient ____________________

Patient unable to sign because of:

Date: ______________

____

Additional materials used, if any, during the informed consent process for this procedure include: ______________
____
____

Date: ____________________ Witness: ______________________________

FIGURE 4.6. Informed consent and request for laparoscopy.

INFORMED CONSENT
And
REQUEST FOR REPAIR OF RELAXATION OF PELVIC ORGANS
And/Or
CORRECTION OF URINARY INCONTINENCE

I, ______________________________, request Dr.______________________________
and his/her associates/ assistants to perform upon me: (Circle procedure to be performed)

1. Anterior and/or posterior repair, that is, "tack up" the bladder and/or rectum
2. Enterocele repair, a repair to a hernia at the top of the vagina
3. Surgical correction of urinary incontinence problem by the following procedure(s) ______________________________

Diagnosis and Procedure: The following has been explained to me in general terms and I understand that:

My condition has been diagnosed as: ______________________________

The nature of the procedure is: ______________________________

The purpose of this procedure is to: ______________________________

General Risks of Surgery: As a result of the performance of this procedure there may be general risks involved such as: INFECTION, ALLERGIC REACTION, DISFIGURING SCAR, SEVERE LOSS OF BLOOD, LOSS OF FUNCTION OF ANY LIMB OR ORGAN, PARALYSIS, PARAPLEGIA or QUADRIPLEGIA, BRAIN DAMAGE, CARDIAC ARREST, or DEATH. In addition to these general risks, there may be other possible risks involved in this procedure. These risks and/or complications may include but are not limited to such complications as:

1. Injury to bowel, bladder, ureter (the tube from the kidney to the bladder) and urethra (tube from bladder to outside of body)
2. Fistula formation, an opening between the bowel, bladder, ureter and the vagina and/or skin, which would require a second operation to repair
3. Colostomy
4. Reoccurrence of my loss of control of urine
5. No improvement in my control of urine
6. Prolonged need of a catheter to drain my bladder
7. Discomfort with intercourse

Likelihood of Success: The likelihood of success of the above procedure is: () Good () Fair () Poor

Prognosis: If I choose not to have the above procedure, my prognosis (future medical condition) is: ______________________________

Alternative Forms of Treatment such as:

1. Exercise
2. Use of artificial supports (pessary)
3. Do nothing and accept my present condition and its potential risks

These alternative treatments have been explained to me, and I have elected this surgical procedure as my method of treatment.

I understand and accept that during the procedure unexpected or unforeseen circumstances may make it necessary to do an extension of the original procedure or another procedure that is not named above. I request that Dr. ______________________________ and associates or assistants of his/her choice perform those procedures that they judge to be necessary.

BY SIGNING THIS FORM, I ACKNOWLEDGE THAT I HAVE READ OR HAD THIS FORM READ AND EXPLAINED TO ME AND THAT I FULLY UNDERSTAND ITS CONTENTS.

I HAVE BEEN GIVEN AMPLE OPPORTUNITY TO ASK QUESTIONS AND ANY QUESTIONS I HAVE ASKED HAVE BEEN ANSWERED OR EXPLAINED IN A SATISFACTORY MANNER. ALL BLANKS OR STATEMENTS REQUIRING COMPLETION WERE FILLED IN AND ALL STATEMENTS WITH WHICH I DISAGREE WERE MARKED OUT BEFORE I SIGNED THIS FORM.

I accept that medicine is not an exact science and understand that no guarantees can be given as to the results. Understanding these limitations, I request that Dr. ____________________ and his/her associates/assistants to proceed with surgery.

______________________________ Witness

______________________________ Person giving consent

Relationship to patient if not the patient ____________________

Patient unable to sign because of: ______________________________

Date: ____________________

Additional materials used, if any, during the informed consent process for this procedure include: ______________________________

Date: ____________________ Witness: ______________________________

FIGURE 4.7. Informed consent and request for repair of relaxation of pelvic organs and/or correction of urinary incontinence.

LITIGATION PROCESS

The Claim

Several occurrences can forewarn a physician that a legal action may be impending. These include a complication or poor outcome, a disgruntled patient or dissatisfied family member, a request for medical records, or direct contact by the plaintiff's attorney. Under no circumstances should the physician ever discuss a potential case with the plaintiff's attorney unless he or she has been so advised by their attorney or insurance carrier claim investigator. Some plaintiff attorneys have been known to call a physician and ask for the physician's opinion about an alleged incident. The attorney may tape this conversation or later in a courtroom allege that on the date of such a contact the physician said something different from what the physician is now alleging occurred. This situation could possibly lead to the jury questioning a physician's credibility. Thus, it is best for the physician never to respond to a plaintiff's attorney except through his or her own defense team.

A lawsuit actually begins when a plaintiff's attorney files a formal Complaint or Declaration. This is a legal document that lists the allegations to support a claim of medical malpractice. Some states require that an affidavit from an expert witness supporting the contention of malpractice be filed with the Complaint or Declaration. Once the filing occurs, the court serves the defendant physician with a summons. The summons is attached to the complaint and may contain questions to be answered by the physician. Responses to the complaint must be filed within a specified period of time, usually within 20 to 30 days. The defendant physician must respond within that period of time or he or she can be found guilty by default. Thus, it is critical that the physician immediately contact his or her insurance carrier and/or attorney on receiving the summons. The physician should send the original summons by certified mail or hand deliver these documents to the insurance carrier. Keep a photocopy of the summons in a separate file. Most insurance carriers require that the physician notify them of any incidence that might result in a claim. Failure to do so could negate the physician's policy. It is prudent to know what the requirements of the insurance carrier are in this regard.

Once a suit has been filed, do not communicate with the patient, her family, or her attorney. When records are requested, be sure that a proper authorization from the patient has been received, and then send a complete copy of the chart. Never change or alter a record once the suit has been filed, because there are many methods by which a plaintiff's attorney can prove that records have been tampered with or altered.

Prepare a thorough chronological account of all events surrounding the incident. Include any oral communications that the physician had with the patient or her family. Gather all records, radiographs, laboratory tests, and consultant's reports, and maintain these documents along with the complaint in a separate file.

The physician's defense attorney will know all aspects of the law but may not be knowledgeable about the specific medical condition. Thus, it is imperative that the physician take an active role in educating the attorney in all medical aspects of the case, discussing not only the positive aspects of the therapy, but also any questionable areas. The defense attorney should thoroughly understand all medical aspects of the case and the physician's reasoning behind the particular treatment chosen. The physician should research literature for articles by authors who completely support the treatment rendered. The physician should help select expert witnesses who can support his or her views on the treatment that was rendered in the case.

During the discovery process, both parties submit questions called interrogatories that are to be answered under oath within a specific period of time. The defendant physician should help prepare answers to these interrogatories.

If a physician has only peripheral involvement in a case and receives a summons requesting records, it is prudent that he or she notify the insurance carrier as well as his or her attorney before any response is given. There are times when poorly worded answers result in the physician who has only a peripheral involvement being named in the actual suit. The physician should not take unnecessary chances, but rather exercise his or her legal right and have appropriate counsel before responding to any questions. The defendant physician should not discuss the suit with any other physicians unless so advised by his or her attorney or the insurance claims representative. Idle conversation in a surgical dressing room may be overheard by a physician who could become the plaintiff's expert. The only people with whom it is safe to discuss a case are the defense attorney and the insurance claims representative.

The Deposition

The deposition is a standard legal process that takes place as part of the discovery process. A deposition is taken under oath in the presence of a court reporter and is generally admissible during the trial phase of the lawsuit. The deposition is serious in that what a defendant physician states is cast in stone and if not properly articulated can end up as a millstone about the physician's neck. Thus, adequate preparation cannot be overemphasized. The physician should be familiar with all of the records, both office and hospital, including office and hospital protocols, rules, and regulations. The physician should insist on considerable preparation and education from the attorney about this important legal process before the deposition.

The deposition has many purposes, including to (a) discover facts, (b) lock in testimony, (c) narrow and clarify issues, (d) discover additional witnesses, and (e) provide an opportunity for settlement if appropriate. The deposition is primarily taken so that each side can learn the opinions, theories, and strategies of the physician, the opposing experts, and the other parties involved in the case. The opposing attorneys can thus prepare their cases for trial with the knowledge gained.

The demeanor of the physician is important. He or she should be professional, honest, and confident. Boredom, frustration, and hostility should not be shown. Anger can disrupt a physician's ability to concentrate, and under those circumstances, the physician may divulge things that should not be discussed. The physician should neither attempt to teach nor lecture during a deposition, remembering that the plaintiff already has an expert who stated that the physician committed malpractice. Therefore, any attempt to educate the lawyer is a frivolous and potentially dangerous act. During the deposition phase, the defendant physician is not acting as his or her own expert and thus should confine answers to short factual statements with no elaboration unless requested by further questioning. Answers should be specific and simple. Do not bring into a deposition any personal notes or records that include the physician's predeposition preparation. Such records are discoverable by the plaintiff's attorney if they are in the room. However, the physician should have a complete set of records to refer to. Never guess about an answer. If the physician does not understand the question, then simply state, "I do not understand the question," or "I do not know," or "I cannot recall." Avoid complex questions. Make the attorney break the questions down into simple ones by stating, "I do not understand the question. Would you please rephrase it?" Avoid repetitive questions by noting, "I have already answered that." When a question is asked, listen attentively, think, and organize your thoughts before responding. Then respond slowly, clearly, and as concisely as possible.

Given a hypothetical question, the physician should be sure the facts are consistent with his or her case and reply only as it applies to the case. If the hypothetical situation is not applicable to the physician's case, the physician should qualify the response and so state that the given facts are not applicable to the case. Again, remember that you are defending yourself and not acting as your own expert witness.

If the defense attorney objects to a question or the phrasing, do not answer the question until instructed to do so by the defense attorney. The physician should listen carefully to the objection raised by the defense attorney so that he or she can appropriately word the response. The physician should know the various alternative methods of therapy that might have been employed. The physician should have reasons why he or she selected the chosen therapy and be prepared to explain them in the courtroom. The deposition, however, is generally not the time to divulge any literature research that took place.

Avoid the word *authoritative*. Legally, it implies that every single statement in a book or journal is absolute fact. Because medicine is an art rather than an exact science, experts may have different opinions on the same subject. The physician can admit that a book is scholarly or written by intelligent, respected people, but should never concede that every statement in the text is absolutely correct, which would make such a text authoritative by legal definition.

Do not engage in bantering or make comments that could be overheard by the plaintiff's attorney during a recess or off-the-record moment. If the plaintiff's attorney overhears things stated during the recess, he or she has the right to come back on record and bring up such topics.

Do not accept the plaintiff's attorney's statement regarding prior testimony as being factual unless you are sure that the statements accurately reflect the stated facts. If you are not sure, state, "I do not know," or "I do not have sufficient information regarding that matter to be able to give an honest answer." Always request to see any unfamiliar documents, even your prior depositions, when questioned about these documents by the opposing counsel. Statements may be taken out of context and not truly reflect the intent of the author. When a deposition is over, the physician should politely excuse himself or herself, leave the room and wait for further instructions from the defense attorney. Prepare for a deposition as if it were a trial. Although the setting may be more casual and appear friendlier, your answers are given under oath and carry the same weight as if they were given before a jury in a courtroom.

After the deposition is completed, the physician is given an opportunity to read, sign, and correct his or her testimony. The physician has the right to correct the deposition, even change the meaning of an entire sentence, as long as this is accomplished during the specified time—usually 30 days. Because this is the only time the physician has the right to change his or her testimony, it is extremely important that the physician read and correct the deposition before it is used in legal proceedings.

The Trial

The trial is an adversarial experience during which allegations are made and facts are presented. In a courtroom, the plaintiff's attorney states his or her perception of the facts that are beneficial to the client. This perception may not always correlate with the defense's understanding of the facts. The jury, however, is instructed to judge a case by the facts as they understand them and not by what an attorney alleges. Often sharp, even bitter controversy develops over the interpretation of significant facts. Legal maneuvering can distort or even suppress the presentation of some facts. This is an emotionally draining experience.

Preparation for the trial is critical and should cover even demeanor and dress. Dress should be plain, conservative, and neat. Flashy or casual clothes project the wrong image. The physician wants to present himself or herself to the jury as a kind, considerate, compassionate person who projects warmth and sincerity, as well as being a voice of authority. The defendant physician should go to the court before the trial to become familiar with the surroundings. He or she may even want to sit in on a trial to get a feel for this new and foreign environment. The physician should discuss in great detail any questions that he or she has regarding the trial, its proceedings, or the defense. Listen to your attorney's advice! The more familiar a physician is with the court and its proceedings, the more confident and less frightened he or she will be as the trial proceeds.

There are several things a physician should do when called to the stand to testify. The physician should make and keep eye contact with the jury throughout the testimony. Physicians generally tend to focus their attention on the plaintiff's attorney as he or she asks questions; however, this is not helpful to the physician. Physicians are trained to read people's facial expressions. By maintaining eye contact with the jury, the physician can closely observe whether the jurors comprehend the testimony. If the physician feels that the jury does not understand an area of the testimony, he or she can elaborate further on a simpler level of explanation. Physicians must remember that the jury, not the plaintiff's attorney, reaches the verdict; therefore, it is critically important that the physician employ all of his or her talents to be sure that the jury understands the testimony. Be polite and humble. Important words in the courtroom are *Sir* and *Madam*. When a physician uses these words, they generate an air of humility that is pleasing to a jury. When a question is asked, be sure to take time to think before a response is given. Respond in nontechnical language that a 12-year-old child could understand. Listen carefully, and then speak clearly and audibly. Jurors like a physician who really tries to explain what he or she did step by step. Unlike during the deposition, in the courtroom the physician should be a teacher, using a blackboard or other audiovisual aids to explain complex issues. If the plaintiff's attorney tries to be overbearing and abrasive, react by being humble yet dignified. Repeat significant facts often so that the jury will remember them. Remember, people generally retain only 30% of verbal communication, so repetition is essential. The physician's body language, posture, and facial expressions also convey strong messages to the jury.

There are also several things a defendant physician should not do on the stand. Do not be arrogant, pompous, or overbearing. Never try to outsmart or manipulate the plaintiff's attorney; this is the way attorneys make their living. Never instigate a fight or argue with an attorney because it will cause you to lose dignity and respect in front of the jury. Even if the physician feels that the plaintiff's pain is of a mental or emotional nature and not physical, never belittle the patient's injury or pain. Remember that in the patient's mind, she is hurting, so show compassion and understanding. Never guess at an answer. If you do not know, then state, "I do not know," or "I do not recall." The physician should not worry if he or she misspeaks. The defense attorney, with further appropriate questions, generally is able to correct the mistake. Never get angry or show anger because anger breaks your concentration and often leads you to say things that should not be said.

The trial begins with opening statements. The plaintiff's attorney proceeds first because he or she has the burden to prove the existence of malpractice and causation of injury. Then the trial testimony phase begins. Again, the plaintiff's attorney begins with testimony and expert witnesses to try to establish that the defendant is negligent and the negligence caused the plaintiff's injury. During this initial presentation, the plaintiff's attorney has the right to (and frequently does) call the defendant physician to the stand. At this stage of the trial, the defendant's attorney cannot question or cross-examine the physician to clarify any response made by the physician, so it is extremely important that the physician take the time to understand the plaintiff's attorney's questions and then formulate and give a complete response so that the jury can understand the physician's position on the matter in question. Do not leave any questionable areas unexplained, because at this stage, the plaintiff's attorney is trying to establish points that are beneficial to their case. If the plaintiff's attorney asks a series of short questions that only require a yes-or-no answer and do not seem to give the physician time to explain his or her position completely, it is very important that the physician break such a sequence and take as much time as needed to clarify the answer. The physician can simply say to the plaintiff's attorney, "Sir or Madam, I did not finish my response to the last question."

During the testimony phase, the plaintiff's attorney usually employs one of four basic forms of attack on the defendant's reputation. The plaintiff's attorney may challenge the physician's competence, accuse the physician of being careless, or allege that the physician is not compassionate but rather an indifferent, uncaring, wealthy person. Finally, the attorney may attack the physician's credibility, especially if records were altered or if the physician contradicted testimony given under oath during the deposition. This is why it is so important for a physician to know exactly what he or she said in the deposition. The physician should outline the deposition, noting significant facts and any figures he or she might have used. Again, as in preparation for the deposition, the physician should have a thorough knowledge of the office and hospital records, including any rules, protocols, or policies that have any bearing on the case. Ignorance of any of these rules, protocols, policies, or records may provide all the evidence a plaintiff's attorney needs to raise a question of the physician's competence.

If at the end of the presentation the plaintiff has not produced sufficient evidence to establish the cause-and-effect relationship, the defense may request and be granted a directed verdict, and the suit is over.

Next, through testimony, expert witnesses, and medical documents, the defense tries to prove that the allegation of negligence is false and that the injuries were not a direct result of the defendant's actions. The defense attorney, on direct examination, will generally have the physician elaborate in detail those issues that are important to the defense, as such repetition is most helpful to the defendant physician. After the defense finishes its presentation, the plaintiff has the chance to rebut any new evidence brought out during this defense presentation.

Following this, each side presents closing arguments. During this phase, each side summarizes the major facts supporting their position. The plaintiff's attorney begins with his or her initial closing arguments. After the defense gives its closing arguments, the plaintiff's attorney responds with final closing arguments. In other words, the plaintiff's attorney has the last word before the jury. Once this is completed, the judge instructs the jurors on the applicable laws for the case. The jury is then given the case and retires to the jury room to begin deliberations. The formal decision or finding made by the jury or the judge is called the verdict.

It is important that the physician stay in the courtroom during the entire trial. The physician can help the defense attorney during the cross-examination of expert witnesses and reveal where the experts are inconsistent with known and accepted facts should this occur. The physician's very presence and demeanor can greatly influence the jury's perception. This can play a major role in the final outcome.

After the trial, an appeal process can be used in cases in which questions of law may be raised or awards appear to be excessive.

The 2003 ACOG survey revealed that obstetrician-gynecologists win 73.1% of the claims resolved by jury, court verdict, arbitration, or other alternative dispute resolution mechanism.

Emotional Impact

The practice of medicine in general, and of obstetrics and gynecology in particular, is filled with daily stresses uncommon to other professions. Physicians must deal with pain and suffering, problem patients, intense interpersonal relationships, and often unrealistic expectations. A relatively new—but unfortunately rather frequent—stress is the threat of malpractice litigation. The stress of a malpractice suit has been equated to the stress and emotional reaction one undergoes during the loss of a loved one. Unlike other professionals, a physician is unable to accept that a malpractice suit is part of the risk of doing business owing to the very nature of the doctor–patient relationship.

Part of the intense anger the physician experiences at the onset of a suit arises because of the shock that he or she experiences when a bond built on trust has been broken. The physician feels betrayed. The accusation of being incompetent or at least practicing one's job badly challenges the very core of one's professional integrity and stirs strong feelings of anger. This anger may be so intense that it spills out in all directions, frequently in an inappropriate manner that may strain many personal and professional relationships.

In a study conducted by psychiatrist Dr. Sarah Charles of physicians who had been sued, 96% of physicians reported not only emotional reactions, but also physical problems related to the suit. Eight percent had the onset of physical ailments, of which one fourth were life-threatening, such as coronaries, strokes, ulcers, and hypertension. Forty percent showed symptoms suggestive of major depressive disorders. Commonly experienced reactions were anger, mood changes, depression, tension, frustration, insomnia, fatigue, and alcohol and drug abuse. Fifteen percent of physicians lost confidence in themselves. Nineteen percent lost confidence in certain clinical situations. Fear is another common emotion experienced by sued physicians. They fear the loss of their patient's respect and confidence. They fear the loss of their own self-confidence, and, in this day of excess awards, they fear the loss of financial security. The physician's reputation, ego, and self-worth are challenged. Professional training demands that the physician hold his or her reactions in check. This training becomes counterproductive at the time of a malpractice suit.

The physician's marriage also is put under considerable stress. The spouse carries a great part of the emotional burden of litigation. There are many sleepless nights and interrupted plans as depositions and trials are scheduled, postponed, and rescheduled by a seemingly uncaring legal system. Mood changes and periods of irritability have to be handled by the spouse. These stressful situations can be the downfall of a weak or borderline marriage. Children are often disturbed by the knowledge that a parent is legally accused of malpractice. They may indeed feel that their parent has deceived or shamed them. Younger children especially may misunderstand the nature of the accusation and believe the allegations as fact, especially if the allegations are broadcast on radio, television, or in the newspaper. Physicians must take action to protect their mental health during this major period of stress, realizing that we live in a litigious environment and that the stress surrounding malpractice suits not only affects physicians, but also adversely affects all professions and occupations. Physicians need to discuss their feelings with their spouse, loved ones, mentors, or counselor.

Physicians and their spouses should become active in support groups. These groups have received the support of both the American College of Obstetricians and Gynecologists and American Academy of Pediatrics as outlined in their joint publication titled "Coping with Malpractice Litigations Stress." Such forums are not intended to provide psychiatric therapy, but rather are safe and informal groups where participants can share their common stresses and experiences in a sympathetic environment. The physician should not hesitate to seek counseling if the stress becomes so great that daily functions become impaired.

An open discussion with your children that shares their feelings and concerns, as well as yours, often relieves their anxiety. This type of communication often strengthens the family relationship and ultimately results in a positive effect from the terrifying ordeal of a malpractice suit.

BEST SURGICAL PRACTICES

- Risk management can lead to an improvement in clinical outcomes, reduce patient injury, reduce human errors, and provide better medical records, which not only assists the entire health care team in providing better care but can also assist the legal team in providing a better defense of an alleged medical malpractice claim.
- The cornerstones of risk management for the surgeon are good surgical technique, current knowledge and training in surgical advancements, good communication, and adequate documentation.
- Because patients rarely retain more than 30% of verbal communication, printed material can greatly assist the surgeon in providing adequate information about a surgical procedure or recommended treatment. Communication also is conveyed by body language; thus, it is prudent to sit in a relaxed posture when communicating with a patient, her significant other, or her family members.
- In the office, appropriate procedure and protocol manuals should exist that outline the duties of each employee and the proper procedure to handle phone messages, especially those of an urgent nature, so that not only a timely response occurs, but also instructions and medications are documented. The surgeon should periodically review his or her office procedures to insure that the patient's confidentiality is respected and that proper phone etiquette is maintained.
- Documentation that is contemporaneous, factual, complete, relevant, and preferably dictated and that uses approved abbreviations is essential in providing an appropriate medical record.
- Medical errors pose a serious threat to the patient's well-being. Using computerized orders, improving physician handwriting, using only standard approved abbreviations, and having all verbal orders read back to the surgeon by the nurse taking the orders have all been shown to reduce these errors.
- When multiple consultants are required to provide appropriate care, it is imperative that one of the consultants is designated to write critical orders, covering such things as fluids, medications, and important laboratory studies.
- Informed consent must respect the ethical principles of autonomy, beneficence, nonmaleficence, justice, and freedom. Informed consent must contain the diagnosis, nature, and purpose of the procedure; the risks; likelihood of success; and alternatives and prognosis if treatment is refused. Procedure-specific informed consent forms outline not only the risks that are specific to the procedure, but also the alternatives so that the patient is better informed. Informed consent is suspended in an emergency situation when the patient is unconscious or incapacitated. The surgeon should document the status of the patient and the fact that the situation is life-threatening and represents a serious threat to the patient's health. When a patient refuses appropriate treatment, the surgeon should document the potential risks or consequence of her refusal and preferably have the patient sign this documentation.
- In a managed care setting, the surgeon must be an advocate for the patient to insure that the patient does receive appropriate treatment even when the managed care plan may refuse to provide the best treatment for the condition being treated.
- Preparation for both a deposition and trial should consist of a review of the surgeon's office records, the hospital records, and the policies and procedure manuals for both the office and hospital. The surgeon should educate the defense team and be sure that the attorney has adequately prepared the surgeon for these legally challenging events. The surgeon should also review the literature, select articles that support his and/or her treatment, and help select expert witnesses that can be used by the defense.
- The litigation process can both be extremely stressful and have an impact on the surgeon's mental and physical health. Appropriate medical and emotional consultations may be required to get the surgeon through this adversarial process.

Bibliography

American College of Obstetricians and Gynecologists and the American Academy of Pediatrics, *Coping with malpractice litigations stress.* Washington, DC, December 1998.

American College of Obstetricians and Gynecologists. *Ethics in obstetrics and gynecology*, 2nd ed. Washington, DC: American College of Obstetricians and Gynecologists, 2004.

American College of Obstetricians and Gynecologists. *Informed refusal.* ACOG Committee Opinion 306. Washington, DC: American College of Obstetricians and Gynecologists, 2004.

American College of Obstetricians and Gynecologists. *Professional liability and its effects: report of a 1999 survey of ACOG's membership.* Washington, DC: American College of Obstetricians and Gynecologists, 1999.

American College of Obstetricians and Gynecologists. *Survey on professional liability*. Washington, DC: American College of Obstetricians and Gynecologists, 2003.
American College of Obstetricians and Gynecologists, Department of Professional Liability. *Coping with malpractice litigation stress*. Washington, DC: American College of Obstetricians and Gynecologists, 2005.
American College of Obstetricians and Gynecologists, Department of Professional Liability. *Risk management: an essential guide for obstetrician-gynecologists*. Washington, DC: American College of Obstetricians and Gynecologists, 2005.
Bates DW, Cohen M, Leape LL, et al. Reducing the frequency of errors in medicine using information technology. *JAMA* 2001;8:299.
Bates DW, Teich JM, Lee J, et al. The impact of computerized physician order entry on medication error prevention. *JAMA* 1999;6:313.
Beauchamp TL, Childress JF. *Principles of biomedical ethics*, 5th ed. New York: Oxford University Press, 2001.
Belli MM Sr, Carlova J. *Belli for your malpractice defense*, 2nd ed. Oradell, NJ: Medical Economics, 1989.
Berg JW, Appelbaum PS, Lidz CW, et al. *Informed consent: legal theory and clinical practice*. New York: Oxford University Press, 2001.
Burns CR. Malpractice suits in American medicine before the Civil War. *Bull Hist Med* 1969;43(1):41.
Charles SC. Coping with a medical malpractice suit. *West J Med* 2001;174:55.
Charles SC. The doctor-patient relationship and medical malpractice litigation. *Bull Menninger Clin* 1993;57:195.
Charles SC. How to handle the stress of litigation. *Clin Plast Surg* 1999;26:69.
Charles SC. The physician and malpractice litigation. *J Med Pract Manage* 1985;1(2):123.
Charles SC, Wilbert JR, Kennedy EC. Physician's self-reports of reactions to malpractice litigation. *Am J Psychiatry* 1984;141(4):563.
Chin S. Delay in gynecologic surgical treatment: a comparison of patients in managed care and fee-for-service plans. *Obstet Gynecol* 1999;93:922.
Crane M. Malpractice wars: our national survey confirms even the best doctors are targets. *Med Econ Obstet Gynecol* 1999;(August):29.
Danner D. *Medical malpractice: a primer for physicians*. Rochester, NY: The Lawyers Cooperative Publishing Co., 1988.
Elkins TE, Brown D. Informed consent: commentary on the ACOG Ethics Committee statement. *Womens Health Issues* 1993;3(1):31.
Emanuel EJ, Goldman L. Protecting patient welfare in managed care: six safeguards. *J Health Polit Policy Law* 1998;23(4):635.
Faden RR, Beauchamp TL. *A history and theory of informed consent*. New York: Oxford University Press, 1986.
Frisch PR, Charles SC, Gibbons RP, et al. Role of previous claims and specialty on the effectiveness of risk management education for office-based physicians. *West J Med* 1995;163:346.
Furrow BR, Greaney TL, Johnson SH, et al. *Health law*, 3rd ed. St. Paul, MN: West Group, 2000.
Furrow BR, Jost TS, Johnson SH, et al. *Health law cases, materials and problems*, 5th ed. St. Paul: West Publishing Corp, 2004.
Glabman M. The top ten malpractice claims [and how to minimize them]. *Hosp Health Netw* 2004;78:61.
Grubb A, Laing J. *Principles of medical law*, 2nd ed. London: Oxford University Press, 2004.
Gunderson M. Eliminating conflicts of interest in managed care organizations through disclosure and consent. *J Law Med Ethics* 1997;25:19.
Institute of Medicine. *Crossing the quality chasm: a new health system for the 21st century*. Washington DC: National Academy Press, 2001.
King JH. *The law of medical malpractice*. St. Paul, MN: West Publishing Co, 1986.
Kohn L, Corrigan J, Donaldson M, eds. *To err is human: building a safer health system. Report of the Institute of Medicine*. Washington DC: National Academy Press, 1999.
Lavery JP. The physician's reaction to a malpractice suit. *Obstet Gynecol* 1988;71:138.
Martin CA, Wilson JF, Fiebelman ND, et al. Physicians' psychologic reactions to malpractice litigation. *South Med J* 1991;84:1300.
Mohr JC. American medical malpractice litigation in historical perspective. *JAMA* 2000;283:1731.
Nora PF, ed. *Professional liability risk management: a manual for surgeons*. Chicago: Professional Liability Committee, American College of Surgeons, 1991.
Powers MJ, Harris N. *Clinical negligence*, 3rd ed. London: Butterworth, 2000.
Ransom SB, ed. *Practical strategies in obstetrics and gynecology*. Philadelphia: WB Saunders, 2000.
Rosenblatt R, Law S, Rosenbaum S. *Law and the American health care system*. New York: Foundation Press, 1997.
Rozovsky FA. *Consent to treatment: a practical guide*, 3rd ed. Gaithersburg MD: Aspen, 2004.
Sanbar SS. American College of Legal Medicine. *Legal medicine*, 6th ed. St. Louis: CV Mosby, 2004.
Sandor AA. The history of professional liability suits in the United States. *JAMA* 1957;163:459.
Strunk AL, Esser L. Overview of the 2003 ACOG survey of professional liability. *ACOG Clin Rev* 2004;9(6):13.
Studdert DM, Mello MM, Brennan TA. Medical malpractice. *N Engl J Med* 2004;350(3):283.
Terry K. Managed care. *Med Econ Obstet Gynecol* 2000;(May):17.
Walker LM. The income slide continues for ob-gyns. *Med Econ Obstet Gynecol* 2000;(October):63.
Ward CJ. Analysis of 500 obstetric and gynecologic malpractice claims: causes and prevention. *Am J Obstet Gynecol* 1991;165:298.
Ward CJ. Legal thoughts on malpractice claims: causes and prevention [comment]. *Am J Obstet Gynecol* 1992;167:295.
White AA, Pichert JW, Bledsoe SH, et al. Cause and effect analysis of closed claims in obstetrics and gynecology. *Obstet Gynecol* 2005;105:1031.
Wu AW, Cavanaugh TA, McPhee SJ, et al. To tell the truth. *J Gen Intern Med* 1997;12:770.

CHAPTER 5 ■ THE CHANGING ENVIRONMENT IN WHICH WE PRACTICE GYNECOLOGIC SURGERY

ERIC J. BIEBER AND EDIE L. DERIAN

DEFINITIONS

Institute for Healthcare Improvement (IHI)—A not-for-profit organization founded in 1991 dedicated to improving health care throughout the globe. Initiated the 100,000 lives campaign (www.ihi.com).

Institute of Medicine (IOM)—Not-for-profit organization chartered in 1970 as part of the National Academy of Sciences to provide unbiased, evidenced-based guidance to improve health in the United States (www.iom.com).

Pay for performance (P4P)—A broad construct that attempts to pay providers or health care organizations for achieving predetermined quality thresholds.

Hospitalist—Physician/providers who dedicate all or part of their practices to providing care specifically to patients within the hospital.

Computerized physician order entry (CPOE)—Use of a computer (especially within an electronic record interface) to perform electronic entry of medical orders for patients. Can occur in an inpatient or ambulatory setting.

100,000 lives campaign (100K)—An initiative from the IHI begun in 2005 to save 100,000 patients through dissemination of six quality initiatives in hospitals throughout the United States (www.ihi.com).

As gynecologic surgeons and care providers of women, we have witnessed major changes in our practices over the years. When we think back to our days as medical students and residents, even the youngest of us is able to appreciate the palpable differences that exist today: from how we manage our offices to how we approach diagnostic testing and treatment. Few of us appreciated how profound a role the computer would play in our daily practice or how this tool might empower us to provide the best possible care in each encounter. In this chapter, we will review the changes that are occurring in medical education from residency to postgraduate training. Issues regarding credentialing, especially as it relates to novel procedures, will be discussed. The importance of connectivity between services and the relevance of this in a time of multidisciplinary diagnosis and treatment will be reviewed. The electronic health record (EHR), its implementation and daily use, and its significant benefits and pitfalls will be reviewed in part.

The cornerstone of the modern practice of medicine continues to be the resounding theme of evidence-based medicine. Quality initiatives, including the Institute for Healthcare Improvement (IHI) recommendations, as well as many other proposals, have made attempts to promote the safest, most effective care of our patients. Additionally, pay-for-performance evaluations continue to be discussed; in some cases, they are actually included in pilot projects for surgical procedures. We are also being challenged to move from a time when surgical and other treatments were the mainstay of our practice to a new time of screening, prevention, and the promise of genomics. We discuss one of the latest trends: a move for at least some physicians, including obstetrician/gynecologists, to choose to function as hospital-based providers or hospitalists. Finally, we review the importance of evaluating evidenced-based methodologies for rating our literature.

CHANGES IN EDUCATION

One of the most significant changes in medical education has been the limitation of resident duty hours. Such regulation of work hours has been common in industries such as aviation, in which pilots and other crew are limited both in the number of hours worked as well as requirements for time off between work episodes. Although many gynecologists were trained in a time of every second or third night call, this is no longer acceptable or allowable. In July 2003, the Accreditation Council for Graduate Medical Education (ACGME) put into effect new requirements and regulations (www.acgme.org). These new regulations limit total duty hours to 80 hours per week when averaged over 4 weeks, limit in-house call to no more than every third night with 1 day off in 7, and limit continuous patient care hours to 30, with the last 6 hours to patient handoffs and educational activities, such as grand rounds. In addition, there must be 10 hours between shifts worked. New York led the way in creating legal mandates, but the ACGME and the various specialty resident review committees have quickly followed. This paradigm shift is a dramatic departure from times past, but recent data has suggested that decision making as well as technical skills may suffer with sleep deprivation. What is less clear is how this has affected actual patient care as well as resident experience.

Hutter and colleagues evaluated the impact of changing to the 80-hour workweek on surgical residents in Boston. They noted that after implementation of the 80-hour workweek, residents had lower burnout scores and less emotional exhaustion, whereas sleep and motivation to work were improved (Table 5.1). Objective quantitative measurement demonstrated no differences in the quality of patient care. In contrast, another pre- and postduty–hour implementation study from the surgery department of University of California Irvine did not show changes in measures of burnout. They did note a decrease in weekly work hours from 100.7 to 82.6 after implementation and found a significant decrease in formal educational time (Fig. 5.1). Of interest, time in the operating room, on clinical rounds, and in the clinic were not significantly different.

TABLE 5.1

SUMMARY OF MASLACH BURNOUT INVENTORY: HUMAN SERVICES SURVEY FOR THE SURGICAL RESIDENTS, BEFORE THE WORK-HOUR CHANGES (2003) AND 1 YEAR AFTER (2004)

Residents	Before	After	*P*
"Emotional exhaustion"	29.1 (high)	23.1 (medium)	0.02
"Depersonalization"	14.8 (high)	11.8 (high)	0.09
"Personal accomplishment"	37.8 (medium)	38.6 (medium)	0.57

Tabulated scores are listed as well as results, benchmarked to published cutoffs based on large national surveys (eg, "'low." "medium," and "high" groups), with the scale specific to medical workers.

From: Hutter MM, Kellogg KC, Ferguson CM, et al. The impact of the 80-hour resident workweek on surgical residents and attending surgeons. *Ann Surg* 2006;243:864, with permission.

In contrast to previous publications, a recent report from University of California San Francisco internal medicine residency did not demonstrate improvement in educational satisfaction with the onset of the new duty-hour regulations. Similarly, another obstetric and gynecologic survey pre- and postimplementation of duty hours at the University of Colorado demonstrated no differences in overall satisfaction with the residency. However, some key elements were found to be statistically elevated after implementation, including reading, reviewing literature, doing research, and some clinical aspects of training.

It is of interest that in the 2006 residency match, both general surgical as well as obstetric and gynecology slots were filled at a much higher percentage than previous years. Whether this is consistent with senior medical students sensing a change after the decrease in duty hours, thus creating a new perception of these "difficult" specialties, remains to be seen.

Less investigation has been performed on the impact of the duty-hour changes to medical students and how this might affect their learning. Brasher and colleagues used completed end-of-rotation evaluations pre- and postimplementation and found more negative comments after implementation, including decreased scores of residents as supervisors and teachers, and in teaching activities. What is less clear is this: As programs and residents have acclimated to these new standards, will there be adaptation as we get farther out from the change?

Obstetric residencies have responded to these directives and made significant changes in underlying residency structure. Nuthalapaty and colleagues, in querying obstetric residency programs, found that 98% reported changing their programs in response to the new regulations, 94% changed their on-call structure, 85% changed distribution of responsibility, and 80% modified how residents participate in rendering care to patients.

Outside this country, even more stringent regulations exist. For example, in Brazil, the Brazilian National Committee on Medical Residency created requirements in 1981 that limit maximum weekly work hours to 60, with 30 consecutive days of vacation each year and 10% of total hours mandated to be dedicated to education. Importantly, Brazil is not the most aggressive country to implement these changes; multiple countries around the globe have decreased duty hours to 48 to 56 hours per week. It is reasonable to ask the question: Have we seen the full evolution of these changes in the United States?

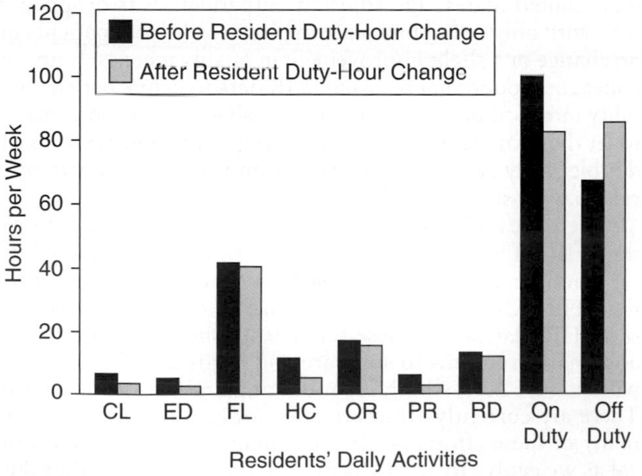

FIGURE 5.1. Residents' weekly activity 1 week before and 6 months after the introduction of duty-hour change. CL, clinic; ED, formal education; FL, floor work; HC, home call; OD, off duty; OR, operating room; PR, prerounds; RD, rounds. (From Gelfand DV, Podnos YD, Carmichael JC, et al. Effect of the 80-hour workweek on resident burnout. *Arch Surg* 2004;139:933.)

It has also been noted that in some cases, residents may work fewer hours than what might be seen in a private setting, in which every-other-night call may be commonplace. One article that questioned residents in internal medicine noted that at least half of residents believed sleep deprivation was a necessary foundation in residency training. A question for the future is whether regulations such as those that have been put in place for residents may also come to exist for all physicians. Certainly given the potential for significant manpower limitations in some specialties, as well as a trend away from rural- and toward hospitalist-type practices, this would be especially problematic and require significant redistribution of resources. There are additional issues with the duty-hour limitations, including the need to transition patient care from the previous on-call residents and the likelihood that some cases that are seen during the resident's call (especially from the emergency room) may come under the care of a different resident and result in a loss of continuity for both the resident and the patient. Although such changes have caused us to rethink classic patient flow in training programs, there is a need to learn how to appropriately transition care from one service to another. This will be critical as residents become attending physicians.

There remains limited information regarding real change in the quality of care rendered in this new paradigm. Indeed, the proponents for change would suggest the opposite: that a fresh team will deliver better care.

POSTGRADUATE TRAINING

Questions continue regarding how best to train clinicians in the postgraduate environment. Most find learning easy while in residency, with time often dedicated to didactic lectures. Few practicing physicians are afforded similar luxury, and yet significant technologic and medical advances continue throughout our careers. Given the limitations that state-by-state licensure imposes, as well as malpractice constraints, it is also difficult for physicians to cross state boundaries to learn novel surgical procedures and be tutored. Fortunately, there have also been advances in our ability to educate with Web-based or computer technology. The classic forum of the in-person lecture remains the gold standard for education. However, some institutions such as our own, have moved to Web-based programs to allow transmission of grand rounds or other educational forums in real time. This allows attendees to log on and participate regardless of their location, be it at home, in the office, or in the hospital. It also allows for lecturers to limit their time away from work as they may deliver their lecture from afar with remote transmission to multiple sites. In a time of shrinking grand-round budgets and limited external support for lectures, this may be one methodology for continuing to deliver state-of-the-art education to a diverse, ever-changing audience.

As we continue our transition from open surgery to minimal invasive surgery and now to robotic surgery, there continue to be questions regarding how to best credential surgeons on new technology. The issues discussed previously regarding limitations in postgraduate opportunities to mentor and train are the origin of some of these problems. How many preceptor cases are adequate for an individual surgeon to be able to demonstrate mastery? Unfortunately, most of us as educators realize there are profound differences between cases and surgeons. What one surgeon is able to master in 20 cases another may be able to conquer in five or fewer. At the writing of this chapter, most residents will garner adequate experience with minimal invasive techniques during their training, but few will master robotics during this time.

Previously, many gynecologic services existed in a silo, consulting other services only when specific situations existed. In the new practice of medicine, we are being faced with many multidisciplinary procedures requiring seamless transition between multiple providers and specialties to assure the best outcome. Uterine artery embolization would be one such example. Generally, gynecologists see the patient with symptomatic myomata, but on occasion, patients will self-refer to an interventional radiologist. In most cases, the interventionalist performs the procedure, but often this individual does not have admitting privileges. If the patient requires admission for pain management, the gynecologic service may be asked to admit and manage the patient. In addition, appropriate preoperative evaluation will need to be performed to decrease the risk of a failed or inappropriate procedure. Generally, all of the above are best accomplished in a setting where excellent communication exists between the services, and the patient seamlessly transitions through the treatment and is not held hostage to political or other logistic issues that often exist in the complicated systems we work within. This requires physicians and surgeons from multiple specialties to decide in advance how such programs should work and what each individual team member is responsible for providing. This often requires identification of specific team leaders (physician and nursing) from each discipline, as well as a specific leader who will have proximate authority to resolve issues that will predictably arise in such complex interactions. When services work in this manner, functioning at a high level, patient care is optimized. Because of the need to act across disciplines and in a teamlike manner, resident and even medical student curriculums have begun to emphasize the need to work as teams—a concept adopted long ago in the business world but adopted much more slowly in the world of independent thinking and functioning within medicine. In fact, team-building retreats are becoming departmental norms in many training programs around the country.

ELECTRONIC HEALTH RECORD

The advent of the electronic health record (EHR) has changed forever how medicine will be practiced. Most of us were trained in a time where orders and notes were written and charts were sent to a large repository (i.e., medical records). Many notes written by our colleagues were difficult to read or were unable to be located. Certainly, these were not often available in real time, across specialties or from home. Authentication of results was performed by hand and had to be reassociated with the correct chart, wasting significant time and resources that might be better directed. Prescriptions were written and handed to patients who then delivered them to a pharmacy. In a best-case scenario, writing was legible, charts were placed in their appropriate position within the repository, and the pharmacist could read the prescription. Unfortunately, often this was not the case.

In modern times, much of this has changed. Numerous opportunities exist with the EHR to overcome many of the technical issues associated with handwriting, but the opportunities go well beyond legibility. In addition, groups like the American Medical Informatic Association's College of Medical Informatics has called for integration of the EHR and personal health records (PHR) to provide the greatest value for our patients. Recent data have suggested other potential positive consequences of an EHR implementation. The Kaiser group reported that with an implementation of an EHR in the northwest United States, age-adjusted outpatient visits dropped by 9%, with only a slight increase in phone calls from patients but no change or a slight improvement in quality metrics. Embi and colleagues found that by using EHR data to define patient eligibility into a clinical trial and then causing an electronic prompt to let the provider know of patient eligibility, they were able to double study enrollment as well as improving physician referrals to their study.

There are multiple factors, which have made the adoption of the EHR difficult for some providers and groups. Likely highest amongst these is the cost to implement as well as maintain the EHR. Multiple third-party vendors exist that have various EHR platforms. These range from simple documentation and chart programs to software and hardware that integrates patient care across both inpatient and ambulatory platforms. There are currently efforts to standardize EHR language, but many of these efforts are in their infancy. It will become critical as we evolve to an all digital-based health record that these systems are able to communicate with one another, allowing patients to have their records available anywhere and anytime. Ford and colleagues evaluated EHR adoption rates in small physician groups of 10 or fewer partners. Using models, they projected the potential for broad adoption of EHR into the future. They suggest that it may take until 2024 for small

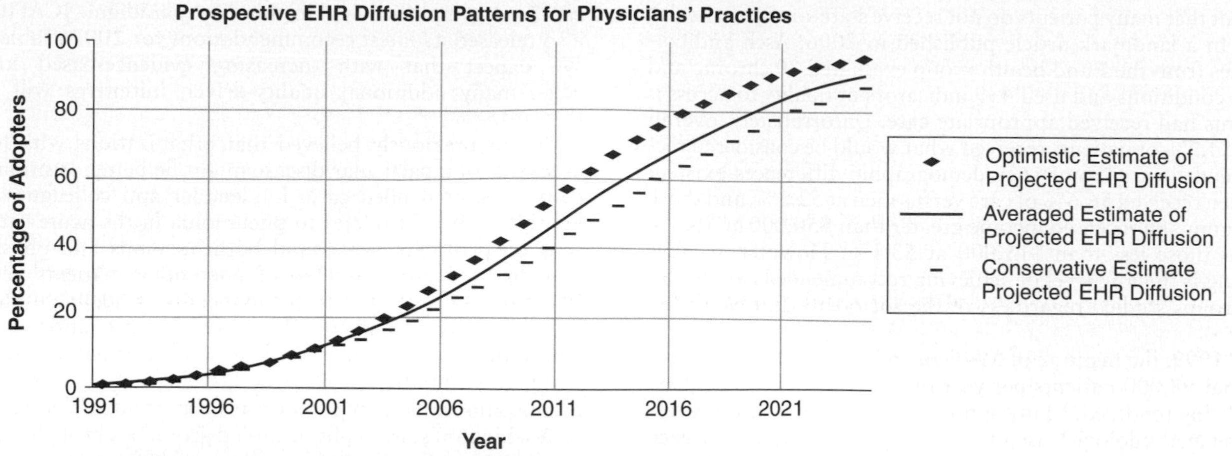

FIGURE 5.2. Three models of electronic health record (EHR) diffusion based on prior empirical estimates. (From Ford EW, Menachemi N, Phillips MT. Predicting the adoption of electronic health records by physicians: when will health care be paperless? *J Am Med Inform Assoc* 2006;13:106.)

groups to fully implement EHRs, which is much longer than is currently being called for by agencies interested in quality initiatives and cost containment (Fig. 5.2). Unfortunately, the health digital information superhighway appears to have a long way to go to be completed.

Baron and partners detail their personal experience as a small group of internists (four members) with implementing an EHR. They described alterations in work flow and the initial deterioration in their office environment for staff, patients, and physicians alike. However, they also state that in spite of the various limitations, "... none of us would go back to paper health records." They identified five key issues that are likely relevant for both small and large groups involved with implementing an EHR:

1. Financing of the EHR
2. Interoperability, standardization, and connectivity
3. Work-flow redesign issues
4. Technical support
5. Issues of change management

More recently, there have been questions regarding whether the EHR is really the panacea for moving medicine to Six-Sigma quality. Computerized physician order entry (CPOE) has been suggested as a key element in decreasing errors and improving quality. Several papers have recently addressed this issue with different conclusions. Upperman and colleagues evaluated the rates of adverse drug events (ADE) pre- and post-CPOE implementation. They noted an improvement in verbal order regulatory compliance, as well as an elimination of transcription errors after implementation. They also noted a statistical decrease in harmful ADEs and suggested that this improvement would result in one less harmful ADE for every 64 patient days. Han and colleagues noted a different experience when implementing a CPOE system in an academic tertiary-care children's hospital. Surprisingly, they noted that the mortality rate increased from 2.8% before CPOE implementation to 6.57% after, an increase that remained significant even after multivariate analysis. It is noteworthy that in this paper, the authors document that the CPOE training was given 3 months before implementation. They also note that the implementation itself occurred over a period of only 6 days for the entire pediatric hospital. This may be too long an interval from training and too short a period for implementation. It is interesting that two papers, both published from the same institution, could have such different conclusions.

Ash and colleagues have suggested that the mere implementation of an EHR is not in and of itself enough to insure that unexpected errors won't occur. They suggest that these errors fall into two broad categories: "those in the process of entering and retrieving information and those in the communication and coordination process that the patient care information system is supposed to support." The key for powering the CPOE and the EHR is likely through well-thought-out algorithms that allow us to take advantage of the computer's ability to maintain data while attempting to best understand what a particular patient needs, and while limiting changes in underlying clinical functionality, unless that change actually improves functionality.

There has also been a push to allow patients to have access to their records. This may allow patients to participate in their own care in a way not previously thought possible. Patients might be able to view data within the EHR for accuracy, reviewing such things as current or prior medications, allergies, etc. They could also be made aware of when lab test or studies are due or overdue, helping to improve compliance and screening. An even more novel concept that has been introduced by several groups is the ability of the patient to communicate with her care providers through Web-based messaging. Initially, providers were concerned regarding the potential for overuse or abuse, but Geisinger Health Systems now has almost 60,000 active users, and little evidence demonstrates this type of abuse. Indeed, in a time when it may be quite difficult to locate your patient during the course of a business day, asynchronous communication may be a preferable manner to communicate nonemergent information with patients. In addition, these data may be appropriately security encrypted at 128 bits and easily made part of the health record.

QUALITY INITIATIVES

Few clinicians would argue that quality is the most important parameter in health care today. Yet, it is becoming ever more evident that many patients do not receive state-of-the-art health care. In a landmark article published in 2006, Asch and colleagues from the Rand health group evaluated 30 chronic and acute conditions and used 439 indicators of quality to access if patients had received appropriate care. Unfortunately, overall only 54.9% of patients received what would be considered recommended care. Some sociodemographic differences existed: Women received 56.6% of care versus men at 52.3%, and those with annual household income greater than $50,000 at 56.6% versus those less than $15,000 at 53.1%. However, what is striking is the low level of achieving recommended care for all the groups studied regardless of the sociodemographic differences.

In 1999, the Institute of Medicine released a report suggesting that 98,000 patients per year die secondary to inadequate care being rendered. Many subsequent debates ensued regarding the methodologies used to attain these numbers. However, this report created a call to arms, challenging those individuals and organizations who provide care to improve the quality of care delivered to all patients. It has caused a number of initiatives from a broad base of organizations. In December 2004, the IHI, at its 16th Annual National Forum on Quality Improvement in Health Care, announced a goal to save 100,000 lives by 14 June 2006. The campaign invited all U.S. hospitals to join in implementing six broad initiatives that have demonstrated efficacy in well-performed clinical trials. These include:

1. Prevention of surgical site infections
2. Prevention of ventilator-associated pneumonia
3. Prevention of central line infections
4. Prevention of adverse drug events through medication reconciliation
5. Deployment of rapid response teams
6. Delivery of evidence-based care for acute myocardial infarction

What is particularly impressive about the IHI campaign is the extent of support across a broad range of disparate federal, state, political, and private organizations, including—but not limited to—the Center for Medicare and Medicaid Services (CMS), Veterans Health Administration, American Medical Association, American Nurses Association, Centers for Disease Control and Prevention, Joint Commission on Accreditation of Healthcare Organizations, the Leapfrog Group, and multiple others.

Recently, the IHI released information suggesting that these initiatives were able to save 122,300 patients. The challenge to implement the IHI recommendations as well as multiple other quality initiatives has caused a number of hospitals and large organizations to create chief quality officer (CQO) positions that are largely responsible for implementing and monitoring compliance to these programs. In essence, this may be the confluence of patient safety, performance improvement, utilization review, and other previous orphan committees.

Consistent with the IHI initiatives, other initiatives have come from CMS, including recommendations for optimization of diabetic patients. These include bundles of care much like the IHI central line bundle, in which appropriate care consists of all elements being appropriately performed or delivered within the correct time frame. Unfortunately, as the bundles become more complicated, it becomes more and more difficult for the provider to remember what has or has not been done. This may be yet another opportunity for the EHR to allow both the clinician and the patient to know what tests or interventions need to be performed, thus optimizing the encounter. Pilot trials are currently under way to evaluate what level of compliance can be accomplished within this new paradigm. JCAHO has also released its latest recommendations for 2007 (Table 5.2). We expect that with increasing evidence-based knowledge, many additional quality-driven initiatives will come forward.

It was previously believed that organizations with higher caseloads of a particular disease might be better positioned to deliver recommended care. Lindenauer and colleagues studied this tenet as it relates to pneumonia in the acute care setting. Surprisingly, they found both hospitals and physicians who had a higher caseload of pneumonia patients actually had reduced adherence to recommended guidelines—such as influenza and pneumococcal vaccine administration or early antibiotic administration—and had no better outcomes.

Quality initiatives are currently being led by a number of organizations, including some physician groups. For example, in Washington state, a physician-led group has brought all hospitals to the table to evaluate discrete performance measures regarding cardiac revascularization. Similarly, the California Perinatal Quality Care Collaborative in 1998 targeted improving antenatal steroid use as an initiative. They accumulated baseline data, developed educational materials, and broadly disseminated this information. They concluded that regional collaboration allowed an improvement from a baseline rate of administration of 76% to 86% postimplementation. Callcut and Breslin discuss how private groups, such as the Leapfrog Group, are playing an important role in moving the private regulatory movement forward and suggest that surgeons need to become more active participants in this process of reshaping and redefining our future.

How to best implement quality-improvement programs in a given setting is also continuing to be investigated. A recent evaluation of hospital quality-improvement implementation and subsequent impact on discrete patient safety metrics suggested that involvement by multiple units within a hospital might have a negative impact on results. Alternatively, having a higher percentage of physicians involved was associated with better scores on at least two of the four safety indicators. Interestingly, having a higher percentage of hospital staff or senior management involved had no impact on any of the indicators.

Most clinicians have not been trained in how to develop and implement quality-improvement programs. Curtis and colleagues have published a how-to paper that came out of an outcomes task force of the Society of Critical Care Medicine but has wide applicability to many areas of medicine (Table 5.3). The generalized lack of education and training in quality may explain some of the lethargy that Leape and Berwick allude to in their article "Five Years after *To Err Is Human:* What Have We Learned?". Table 5.4, which is presented in this same paper, suggests significant quality improvements that have been achieved by implementing discrete strategies in specific environments. If each of our organizations could fractionally achieve similar success, the impact on patient care might be quite remarkable. Leape and Berwick additionally call for the Agency for Healthcare Research and Quality (AHRQ) to act as the key entity to bring the various constituencies together and set goals that should be reached by 2010—a lofty proposal by anyone's standards, but well worth striving toward.

PAY FOR PERFORMANCE

The additional lingering question remains as to whether these measures will be subjected to pay for performance, with groups achieving higher levels of patient compliance being awarded higher levels of reimbursement. This is a marked change from

TABLE 5.2

2007 AMBULATORY CARE/OFFICE-BASED SURGERY NATIONAL PATIENT SAFETY GOALS

Goal 1	**Improve the accuracy of patient identification.**
1A	Use at least two patient identifiers when providing care, treatment, or services.
Goal 2	**Improve the effectiveness of communication among caregivers.**
2A	For verbal or telephone orders or for telephonic reporting of critical test results, verify the complete order or test result by having the person receiving the information record and read back the complete order or test result.
2B	Standardize a list of abbreviations, acronyms, symbols, and dose designations that are *not* to be used throughout the organization.
2C	Measure, assess, and, if appropriate, take action to improve the timeliness of reporting—and the timeliness of receipt by the responsible licensed caregiver—of critical test results and values.
2E	Implement a standardized approach to hand off communications, including an opportunity to ask and respond to questions.
Goal 3	**Improve the safety of using medications.**
3B	Standardize and limit the number of drug concentrations used by the organization.
3C	Identify and, at a minimum, annually review a list of look-alike/sound-alike drugs used by the organization, and take action to prevent errors involving the interchange of these drugs.
3D	Label all medications, medication containers (for example, syringes, medicine cups, basins), or other solutions on and off the sterile field.
Goal 7	**Reduce the risk of health care–associated infections.**
7A	Comply with current Centers for Disease Control and Prevention (CDC) hand hygiene guidelines.
7B	Manage as sentinel events all identified cases of unanticipated death or major permanent loss of function associated with a health care–associated infection.
Goal 8	**Accurately and completely reconcile medications across the continuum of care.**
8A	There is a process for comparing the patient's current medications with those ordered for the patient while under the care of the organization.
8B	A complete list of the patient's medications is communicated to the next provider of service when a patient is referred or transferred to another setting, service, practitioner, or level of care within or outside the organization. The complete list of medications is also provided to the patient on discharge from the facility.
Goal 11	**Reduce the risk of surgical fires.**
11A	Educate staff, including operating licensed independent practitioners and anesthesia providers, on how to control heat sources and manage fuels with enough time for patient preparation, and establish guidelines to minimize oxygen concentration under drapes.
Goal 13	**Encourage patients' active involvement in their own care as a patient safety strategy.**
13A	Define and communicate the means for patients and their families to report concerns about safety and encourage them to do so.

Note: Changes to the Goals and Requirements are indicated in **bold**. Gaps in the numbering indicate that the goal is inapplicable to the program or has been "retired," usually because the requirements were integrated into the standards.
From: http://www.jointcommission.org/PatientSafety/NationalPatientSafetyGoals/07_amb_obs_npsgs.htm, with permission.

being paid for delivery of units of health care or procedures in which disease states are being managed. As of 2004, almost 100 pay-for-performance initiatives had been started by a wide variety of sponsors, ranging from employers to the federal government. Epstein and colleagues, in an early article on the subject of paying for high quality care, called for several significant changes to facilitate adoption of pay-for-performance initiatives. These recommendations included an expansion in the scope of the efforts, as well as the amount of incentive available to the clinician or group; the importance of large groups such as CMS becoming involved; an expansion from the current small cadre of clinical indicators; an improvement in our ability to establish reliable metrics for evaluation of quality; and, finally, a call for investment in electronic infrastructure to facilitate all of the above.

A Cochrane systematic review of the subject of targeted payments to affect outcomes in primary care was unable to reach a conclusion because of limitations in prior study quality and power. Kouides and colleagues evaluated the use of financial incentives to increase rates of influenza vaccine administration and found that modest incentive increased an already high baseline administration rate. In another study on

TABLE 5.3

KEY STEPS FOR INITIATING, IMPROVING, EVALUATING, AND SUSTAINING A QUALITY IMPROVEMENT PROGRAM

Initiating or improving a quality improvement program

1. Do background work: Identify motivation, support team work and develop strong leadership.
2. Prioritize potential projects and choose the projects to begin.
3. Prepare for the project by operationalizing the measures, building support for the project, and developing a business plan.
4. Do an environmental scan to understand the current situation (structure, process, or outcome), the potential barriers, opportunities, and resources for the project.
5. Create a data collection system to provide accurate baseline data and document improvement.
6. Create a data reporting system that will allow clinicians and other stakeholders to see and understand the problem and the improvement.
7. Introduce strategies to change clinician behavior and create the change that will produce improvement.

Evaluating and sustaining a quality improvement program

1. Determine whether the target is changing with ongoing observation, periodic data collection, and interpretation.
2. Modify behavior change strategies to improve, regain, or sustain improvements.
3. Focus on sustaining interdisciplinary leadership and collaboration for the quality improvement program.
4. Develop and sustain support from the hospital leadership.

From: Curtis JR, Cook DJ, Wall RJ, et al. Intensive care unit quality improvement: a "how-to" guide for the interdisciplinary team. *Crit Care Med* 2006;34:211, with permission.

TABLE 5.4

CLINICAL EFFECTIVENESS OF SAFE PRACTICES

Intervention	Results
Perioperative antibiotic protocol	Surgical sites infections decreased by 93%
Physician computer order entry	81% Reduction of medication errors
Pharmacist rounding with team	66% Reduction of preventable adverse drug events
	78% Reduction of preventable adverse drug events
Protocol enforcement	95% Reduction in central venous line infections
	92% Reduction in central venous line infections
Rapid response teams	Cardiac arrests decreased by 15%
Reconciling medication practices	90% Reduction in medication errors
Reconciling and standardizing medication practices	60% Reduction in adverse drug events over 12 mo (from 7.6 per 1000 doses to 3.1 per 1000 doses)
	64% Reduction in adverse drug events in 20 mo (from 3.8 per 1000 doses to 1.39 per 1000 doses)
Standardized insulin dosing	Hypoglycemic episodes decreased 63% (from 2.95% of patients to 1.1%)
	90% Reduction in cardiac surgical wound infections (from 3.9% of patients to 0.4%)
Standardized warfarin dosing	Out-of-range international normalized ratio decreased by 60% (from 25% of tests to 10%)
Team training in labor and delivery	50% Reduction in adverse outcomes in preterm deliveries
Trigger tool and automation	Adverse drug events reduced by 75% between 2001 and 2003
Ventilator bundle protocol	Ventilator-associated pneumonias decreased by 62%

From: Leape LL, Berwick DM. Five years after *To Err Is Human:* what have we learned? *JAMA* 2005;293:2384, with permission.

immunizations, Fairbrother and colleagues evaluated use of cash bonus, enhanced fee for service, and feedback for improving baseline vaccination rates. They found only the bonus group statistically improved (increased by 25.3%), although they believed much of this effect was due to better documentation versus actual increased administration of vaccine. Roski and colleagues noted that in incentivized groups, documentation of tobacco use was markedly increased, as was accession to counseling programs; unfortunately, other important clinical end points were not different.

A more recent investigation evaluated a pay-for-performance initiative by PacifiCare Health Systems. Three quality measures were evaluated: cervical cancer screening, mammography, and HgbA1c. Unfortunately, only in the cervical cancer screening group was there an improvement after the intervention, and in spite of $3.4 million paid in pay-for-performance incentives, only nominal gains were made. Also, physicians with the highest initial baseline performance had the least improvement but were the recipients of the greatest portion of the paid bonus. This trial demonstrates the potential limitation of identifying discrete end points to reward heterogeneous groups of providers, all of whom start from different baseline levels of efficacy. Dudley has suggested that how an incentive is offered (i.e., reward or penalty) and factors such as what percentage of patients in a provider's panel incentives are applicable to may affect the success of these programs (Table 5.5). Rosenthal and colleagues, in evaluating multiple trials and multiple industries in which pay for performance has applicability, found little evidence that paying for quality is effective. They noted that even in other industries, results are inconsistent. They raise the concern that incentives may be too low, with limited penetrance within a given provider's or group's practice panel. An additional concern is making the target for incentive so much higher than baseline that the providers feel it is unachievable and therefore do not try. This is consistent with data from Beckman and colleagues, who interviewed providers in a pay-for-performance program. Interestingly, providers reviewed their personal profiles but did not always change their functional behaviors in response to the data.

A variation on pay-for-performance is where a provider being paid only if a certain outcome of a surgical procedure has been achieved and the entire care relative to the procedure is covered under one payment. These types of programs may have the greatest initial application in the area of cardiovascular surgery, for which outcome metrics of individual surgeons and hospitals have been reported for several years. In addition, there are well-defined clinical algorithms regarding "best practice." This may have driven the American Heart Association's Reimbursement Coverage and Access Policy Development Workgroup to publish a statement on pay-for-performance.

In addition to the previously noted problems with pay-for-performance programs, another limitation is that most programs to date have focused on single disease states or outcomes (such as immunization, or Pap test or mammogram compliance). In reality, many patients aged 65 or older have multiple medical problems, and treating single disease states in isolation may not lead to overall improved outcomes and enhanced quality. It is not surprising that 89% of Medicare's annual budget is consumed by patients with three or more chronic conditions. Boyd and colleagues evaluated current clinical practice guidelines (CPGs), which are often used in pay-for-performance programs, but which also focus on single disease states. In a hypothetical 79-year-old female patient with the common comorbities of chronic obstructive pulmonary disease, diabetes, osteoporosis, hypertension, and osteoarthritis, they found that following each CPG would lead to 12 prescribed medications and a potential outlay of $406 per month. There were also significant issues with the potential for drug-drug interactions if this "optimal" regimen was followed. They concluded that pay for performance based on CPGs for single disease states may create "perverse incentives" and actually decrease quality of care, and that significant effort should be placed on effectively treating the multiple chronic conditions that many of our patients have.

While these initiatives are in their infancy, there will likely be future pressures both at the state and federal level to achieve an ever-higher level of quality. In addition, pay-for-performance needs to evolve to incorporate these early findings into rationale paradigms for physicians, which align the needs of payers, providers, and our patients. It may also become quite difficult for groups and practices that do not have access to electronic data to be able to participate in such projects. Further incentives or underwriting installation of appropriate infrastructure will be critical.

TABLE 5.5

POTENTIAL DETERMINANTS OF THE EFFECTIVENESS OF A PAY-FOR-PERFORMANCE PROGRAM

Characteristics of the incentive	Enabling or inhibiting factors
The magnitude of the incentive	Environmental variables such as the general approach to payment—fee-for-service vs capitation—or accreditation requirements
The proportion of each provider's patients to whom the incentive applies	Organizational factors such as information technology
The cost of improving quality	Patient characteristics such as educational level

From: Dudley RA. Pay-for-performance research: how to learn what clinicians and policy makers need to know. *JAMA* 2005;294:1821, with permission.

HOSPITALISTS

In the last decade, there has been a move toward some practitioners working solely within the hospital setting to care for inpatients, a practice common outside the United States for decades. This started when data suggested that in some cases, patient care might be optimized and length of stay reduced by having a single individual responsible for overseeing a patient's stay in the hospital. Emergency department physicians have performed shift work for decades, but the change was most dramatic for hospitalists who are generally internists or family practitioners—fields that were more typically associated with primary care. With the advent of the resident 80-hour workweek, some services have been unable to be covered by residents, and again, the utility of a hospitalist coverage arrangement began to make sense.

Wachter and Goldman reviewed published studies and abstracts regarding hospitalist services and noted only 2 of 19 studies didn't demonstrate decreased length of stay (LOS). The range of LOS reductions was 7% to 27%, which even on the lower end often translate into significant savings to health care organizations. Several variations on the hospitalist model exist, including use of combinations of private staff, academic staff, and house staff. One study evaluated differences between community physicians, a private hospitalist service, and an academic hospitalist group within the same tertiary care hospital and found a 20% LOS and 10% cost reduction on the academic service versus 8% and 6% reductions for the private hospitalists and the community physicians, respectively. They did not note differences in mortality rates (either inpatient or 30-day) or readmission rates between the three groups. Another variation is to use the hospitalist to cover patients typically covered by surgical services. One trial evaluated use of a hospitalist in managing elderly hip fracture patients along with orthopedic surgeons. They noted decreased time to get patients to surgery, decreased length of hospitalization after surgery, and overall decreased LOS with no adverse impact on mortality or readmission. Another area of question has been how a hospitalist service might affect teaching and education for students and residents. Hauer and colleagues analyzed 1,587 house staff and student evaluations on internal medicine rotations during a 2-year period. They scored the hospitalist group (versus traditional attending physicians) higher in teaching effectiveness, knowledge, and feedback. More recently, the hospitalist trend in internal medicine and family practice has carried over to pediatric hospitals that have now created pediatric hospitalist services. Dwight and colleagues describe that with manpower reductions and limitations in house staff, amongst other issues, some Canadian hospitals have begun to successfully use a non-house-staff–based model effectively. Landrigan and colleagues performed a systematic review of the pediatric hospitalist literature, and consistent with nonpediatric hospitalist studies, these programs had an average LOS and cost decrease of 10%. They do note that many of the programs themselves do not generate adequate revenue to not lose money. An interesting article on keys to success for creating a pediatric hospitalist program suggests six key principles that may have broad applicability to establishment of similar programs in obstetrics and gynecology (Table 5.6).

Only recently has this trend carried over into obstetrics and gynecology. At this time, there are only a handful of hospitals in the country where "laborists" manage patients sent in from their colleagues, who are then only responsible for managing patients in the ambulatory setting. In a time when clinicians have become highly interested in balancing lifestyle and workplace activities, this concept may become more prevalent.

TABLE 5.6

SIX PRINCIPLES TO ESTABLISH A SUCCESSFUL PEDIATRIC HOSPITALIST PRACTICE

1. Voluntary referrals
2. Local design
3. Minimum physician-training requirements
4. Arrangement for appropriate follow-up
5. Communication among primary care physicians, subspecialists, and hospitalists
6. Data collection and outcome measures

Adapted from Percelay JM, Strong GB. American Academy of Pediatrics Section on Hospital Medicine. Guiding principles for pediatric hospitalist programs. *Pediatrics* 2005;115:1101.

RATING SCIENTIFIC EVIDENCE

It has become increasingly important for physicians to evaluate the adequacy of data to which we are constantly exposed. There has been a transition in articles published in the peer-reviewed literature over the last 10 years to a significant effort toward asking and answering questions in the most rigorous manner possible. Numerous methodologies exist for evaluating these trials, which place differing values on the quality, quantity, and consistency domains expressed within each report. Given the subtleties of these differing methodologies, a paper may be deemed to be stronger or weaker. AHRQ has reported on an evaluation of these various systems and describes the differences relative to the type of trial being evaluated (e.g., randomized control trial versus observational).

One of the most commonly used systems is seen in Table 5.7 and is described by the U.S. Preventive Services Task Force. This method describes the type of trial and gives a recommendation

TABLE 5.7

CLASSIFICATION OF REFERENCES AND RECOMMENDATIONS, ACCORDING TO THE U.S. PREVENTIVE SERVICES TASK FORCE

References	
Level I	Evidence obtained from at least 1 properly conducted randomized clinical trial
Level II-1	Evidence obtained from well-designed controlled study without randomization
Level II-2	Evidence from well-designed cohort or case-control studies, preferably from more than 1 center or research group
Level II-3	Evidence obtained from multiple time series with or without intervention
Level III	Opinions of respected authorities, based on clinical experience, descriptive studies, or reports of expert committees
Meta-analysis	A systematic structured process that is more than a literature review
Decision analysis	Use of mathematical models of sequences of several strategies to determine which is optimal
Cost-efficient analysis	Comparison of health care practice or techniques in terms of the relative economic efficiencies in providing health benefits
Recommendations	
Level A	Based on good and consistent scientific evidence
Level B	Based on limited or inconsistent scientific evidence
Level C	Based primarily on consensus and expert opinion
Level D	Fair evidence against the recommendation
Level E	Evidence against the recommendation

Adapted from American College of Obstetricians and Gynecologists. Reading the medical literature: applying evidence to practice. Washington DC: American College of Obstetricians and Gynecologists; 1998.

regarding the strength of the conclusion. It is relevant for us as practicing surgeons to be able to differentiate between data and reports that are merely interesting and those that should cause us to reevaluate our practice patterns. It is also important to understand not only what the grading system means but how the conclusions are reached for each of these unique systems. Because there are presently a number of systems and no one is universally used in journals or textbooks, this is an even greater challenge.

In a recent review of 55 American College of Obstetricians and Gynecologists practice bulletins, Chauhan and colleagues found that only 29% of 438 recommendations were level A (good and consistent evidence), whereas 33% of recommendations were level B (limited or inconsistent evidence) and 38% were level C (consensus and expert opinion). This is the quandary in medicine today: Evidence-based medicine is how all of us would like to practice, but unfortunately, all questions have not been answered to the extent needed. Because of this, panels of experts may by necessity have to revert to the best available data, which may be less than optimal. However, even in the field of medical ethics, there is an effort toward moving to formal tools for evaluating the validity of discussions and data. If the last 10 years is any indication to what will happen in the future, there will be an increasing number of randomized controlled trials that are well thought out and executed to aid us in determining how to best counsel our patients.

CONCLUSION

The examples illustrated in this chapter are but a small sampling of the numerous ongoing changes occurring daily. Many of these changes will likely affect our lives and practices—some more than others—but all are a radical departure from times not too distant. It will be interesting to evaluate how these changes evolve over editions of this textbook. Changes underscore the importance of lifelong education, not only in the functional practice of medicine but also in the art of the practice of medicine. It certainly makes our profession an exciting place to be—stay tuned!

BEST SURGICAL PRACTICES

- Resident education has been transformed to being less service oriented and more competency based. The 80-hour workweek has effected revolutionary changes in the mind-sets of today's trainees and the people who train them.
- Quality has always been important to physicians in theory, but new initiatives, such as the 100,000 lives IHI program, are making evidence-based practice a reality.
- The EHR is only in its infancy. This modality will alter every aspect of care delivered by physicians and effect communication between providers and their patients.
- By being dedicated providers for inpatients, hospitalists will render more efficient and timely care and therefore more effectively manage patients, with an eye to improving quality and decreasing error.
- Pay-for-performance is being investigated as a means to reward providers and health care organizations for optimizing predefined outcomes and quality metrics.

Bibliography

Accreditation Council Graduate Medical Education common program requirements. http://(www.acgme.org/dh_dutyhourscommonPR.pdf). Accessed 8/26/06.

Asch SM, Kerr EA, Keesey J, et al. Who is at greatest risk for receiving poor quality health care? *N Engl J Med* 2006;354:1147.

Ash JS, Berg M, Coiera E. Some unintended consequences of information technology in health care: the nature of patient care information system-related errors. *J Am Med Inform Assoc* 2004;11:104.

Baker G, Carter B. *Provider pay-for-performance incentive programs: 2004 national study results.* San Francisco: Med-Vantage, 2005.

Baron RJ, Fabens EL, Schiffman M, et al. Electronic health records: just around the corner? Or over the cliff? *Ann Intern Med* 2005;143:222.

Beckman H, Suchman AL, Curtin K, et al. Physician reactions to quantitative individual performance reports. *Am J Med Qual* 2006;21:192.

Boyd CM, Darer J, Boult C, et al. Clinical practice guidelines and quality of care for older patients with multiple comorbid diseases: implications for pay for performance. *JAMA* 2005;294:716.

Brasher AE, Chowdhry S, Hauge LS, et al. Medical students' perceptions of resident teaching: have duty hours regulations had an impact? *Ann Surg* 2005;242:548.

Bufalino V, Peterson ED, Burke GL, et al. American Heart Association's Reimbursement, Coverage, and Access Policy Development Workgroup. Payment for quality: guiding principles and recommendations: principles and recommendations from the American Heart Association's Reimbursement, Coverage, and Access Policy Development Workgroup. *Circulation* 2006;113:1151.

Callcut RA, Breslin TM. Shaping the future of surgery: the role of private regulation in determining quality standards. *Ann Surg* 2006;243:304.

Chauhan SP, Berghella V, Sanderson M, et al. American College of Obstetricians and Gynecologists practice bulletins: an overview. *Am J Obstet Gynecol* 2006;194:1564.

Curtis JR, Cook DJ, Wall RJ, et al. Intensive care unit quality improvement: a "how-to" guide for the interdisciplinary team. *Crit Care Med* 2006;34:211.

de Oliveira Filho GR, Sturm EJ, Sartorato AE. Compliance with common program requirements in Brazil: its effects on resident's perceptions about quality of life and the educational environment. *Acad Med* 2005;80:98.

Dudley RA. Pay-for-performance research: how to learn what clinicians and policy makers need to know. *JAMA* 2005;294:1821.

Dwight P, MacArthur C, Friedman JN, et al. Evaluation of a staff-only hospitalist system in a tertiary care, academic children's hospital. *Pediatrics* 2004;114:1545.

Embi PJ, Jain A, Clark J, et al. Effect of a clinical trial alert system on physician participation in trial recruitment. *Arch Intern Med* 2005;165:2272.

Epstein AM, Lee TH, Hamel MB. Paying physicians for high-quality care. *N Engl J Med* 2004;350:406.

Fairbrother G, Hanson KL, Friedman S, et al. The impact of physician bonuses, enhanced fees, and feedback on childhood immunization coverage rates. *Am J Public Health* 1999;89:171.

Ford EW, Menachemi N, Phillips MT. Predicting the adoption of electronic health records by physicians: when will health care be paperless? *J Am Med Inform Assoc* 2006;13:106.

Garrido T, Jamieson L, Zhou Y, et al. Effect of electronic health records in ambulatory care: retrospective, serial, cross sectional study. *BMJ* 2005;330:581.

Gelfand DV, Podnos YD, Carmichael JC, et al. Effect of the 80-hour workweek on resident burnout. *Arch Surg* 2004;139:933.

Giuffrida A, Gosden T, Forland F, et al. Target payments in primary care: effects on professional practice and health care outcomes. *Cochrane Database Syst Rev* 2000;(3):CD000531.

Goldfield N, Burford R, Averill R, et al. Pay for performance: an excellent idea that simply needs implementation. *Qual Manag Health Care.* 2005;14:31.

Goss JR, Maynard C, Aldea GS, et al. Clinical Outcomes Assessment Program. Effects of a statewide physician-led quality-improvement program on the quality of cardiac care. *Am Heart J* 2006;151:1033.

Halasyamani LK, Valenstein PN, Friedlander MP, et al. A comparison of two hospitalist models with traditional care in a community teaching hospital. *Am J Med* 2005;118:536.

Han YY, Carcillo JA, Venkataraman ST, et al. Unexpected increased mortality after implementation of a commercially sold computerized physician order entry system. *Pediatrics* 2005;116:1506.

Harris RP, Helfand M, Woolf SH, et al. Methods Work Group, Third U.S. Preventive Services Task Force. Current methods of the U.S. Preventive Services Task Force: a review of the process. *Am J Prev Med* 2001;20:21.

Hauer KE, Wachter RM, McCulloch CE, et al. Effects of hospitalist attending physicians on trainee satisfaction with teaching and with internal medicine rotations. *Arch Intern Med* 2004;164:1866.
Hutter MM, Kellogg KC, Ferguson CM, et al. The impact of the 80-hour resident workweek on surgical residents and attending surgeons. *Ann Surg* 2006;243:864.
Koch EG. Springtime for obstetrics and gynecology: will the specialty continue to blossom? *Obstet Gynecol* 2004;103:198.
Kohn KT, Corrigan JM, Donaldson MS. *To err is human: building a safer health system.* Washington, DC: National Academy Press, 1999.
Kouides RW, Bennett NM, Lewis B, et al. Performance-based physician reimbursement and influenza immunization rates in the elderly. The Primary-Care Physicians of Monroe County. *Am J Prev Med* 1998; 14:89.
Landrigan CP, Conway PH, Edwards S, et al. Pediatric hospitalists: a systematic review of the literature. *Pediatrics* 2006;117:1736.
Landrigan CP, Rothschild JM, Cronin JW, et al. Effect of reducing interns' work hours on serious medical errors in intensive care units. *N Engl J Med* 2004;351:1838.
Leach DC. Resident duty hours: the ACGME perspective. *Neurology* 2004;62:E1.
Leape LL, Berwick DM. Five years after *To Err Is Human:* what have we learned? *JAMA* 2005;293:2384.
Lindenauer PK, Behal R, Murray CK, et al. Volume, quality of care, and outcome in pneumonia. *Ann Intern Med* 2006;144:262.
Lund KJ, Teal SB, Alvero R. Resident job satisfaction: one year of duty hours. *Am J Obstet Gynecol* 2005;193:1823.
McCullough LB, Coverdale JH, Chervenak FA. Argument-based medical ethics: a formal tool for critically appraising the normative medical ethics literature. *Am J Obstet Gynecol* 2004;191:1097.
Nuthalapaty FS, Carver AR, Nuthalapaty ES, et al. The scope of duty hour-associated residency structure modifications. *Am J Obstet Gynecol* 2006;194:282.
Percelay JM, Strong GB. American Academy of Pediatrics Section on Hospital Medicine. Guiding principles for pediatric hospitalist programs. *Pediatrics* 2005;115:1101.
Phy MP, Vanness DJ, Melton LJ 3rd, et al. Effects of a hospitalist model on elderly patients with hip fracture. *Arch Intern Med* 2005;165:796.
Rosen IM, Bellini LM, Shea JA. Sleep behaviors and attitudes among internal medicine housestaff in a U.S. university-based residency program. *Acad Med* 2004;79:407.
Rosenthal MB, Frank RG. What is the empirical basis for paying for quality in health care? *Med Care Res Rev* 2006;63:135.
Rosenthal MB, Frank RG, Li Z, et al. Early experience with pay-for-performance: from concept to practice. *JAMA* 2005;294:1788.
Roski J, Jeddeloh R, An L, et al. The impact of financial incentives and a patient registry on preventive care quality: increasing provider adherence to evidence-based smoking cessation practice guidelines. *Prev Med* 2003;36:291.
Systems to rate the strength of scientific evidence. Prepared for ARHQ. http://www.ncbi.nlm.nih.gov/books/bv.fcgi?rid=hstat1.chapter.70996. Accessed 8/26/06.
Tang PC, Ash JS, Bates DW, et al. Personal health records: definitions, benefits, and strategies for overcoming barriers to adoption. *J Am Med Inform Assoc* 2006;13:121.
Upperman JS, Staley P, Friend K, et al. The impact of hospital-wide computerized physician order entry on medical errors in a pediatric hospital. *J Pediatr Surg* 2005;40:57.
Vidyarthi AR, Katz PP, Wall SD, et al. Impact of reduced duty hours on residents' educational satisfaction at the University of California, San Francisco. *Acad Med* 2006;81:76.
Wachter RM, Goldman L. The emerging role of "hospitalists" in the American health care system. *N Engl J Med* 1996;335:514.
Wachter RM, Goldman L. The hospitalist movement 5 years later. *JAMA* 2002;287:487.
Weiner BJ, Alexander JA, Baker LC, et al. Quality improvement implementation and hospital performance on patient safety indicators. *Med Care Res Rev* 2006;63:29.
Wirtschafter DD, Danielsen BH, Main EK, et al. California Perinatal Quality Care Collaborative. Promoting antenatal steroid use for fetal maturation: results from the California Perinatal Quality Care Collaborative. *J Pediatr* 2006;148:606.

CHAPTER 6 ■ TRAINING THE GYNECOLOGIC SURGEON

ROBERT M. ROGERS, JR.

DEFINITIONS

The competent surgeon—Definition yet to be determined.

Apprenticeship model—A teacher-oriented teaching model, usually without structure, purpose, or defined goals.

Learner-oriented model—A learner-oriented teaching model with structure as well as specific and directed objectives, using observational activities and developmental hands-on surgical skills, including sound clinical judgment. The program emphasizes competency-based training in primary care and basic surgical education.

Aims for health system improvement—Safety, effectiveness, patient-oriented care, timeliness, efficiency, and equitably, according to the Institute of Medicine.

Accreditation Council for Graduate Medical Education competencies for optimal patient care—ACGME has issued six competencies for resident physicians:

1. Patient care that is compassionate, appropriate, and effective for the treatment of health problems and the promotion of health.
2. Medical knowledge about established and evolving biomedical, clinical, and cognate sciences and the application of this knowledge to patient care.
3. Practice-based learning and improvement that involves investigation and evaluation of their own patient care, appraisal and assimilation of scientific evidence, and improvements in patient care.
4. Interpersonal and communication skills that result in effective information exchange and teaming with patients, their families, and other health professionals.
5. Professionalism as manifested through a commitment to carrying out professional responsibilities, adherence to ethical principles, and sensitivity to a diverse patient population.
6. Systems-based practice as manifested by actions that demonstrate an awareness of and responsiveness to the larger context and system of health care and the ability to effectively call on system resources to provide optimal care that is of optimal value.

The goal of a surgical residency is to prepare the resident surgeon for the independent practice of surgery. Societal and governmental pressures in the United States are now requiring the practitioner of surgery to be "competent" and accountable. However, the term *competent surgeon* has yet to be defined. Furthermore, the curricula and strategies to train the competent surgeon are not yet developed. The Residency Review Committee for Obstetrics and Gynecology structures and certifies "adequate" training for the gynecologic surgeon. Presently, the federal and state governments in the United States, as well as in other countries, are now questioning the quality of surgical education and the competency of practicing surgeons. This is true in all surgical specialties, including the training and practice of gynecologic surgery. Medicare and Medicaid payers are now demanding monitoring of quality indicators of surgical procedures and subsequent outcomes. Soon, these data on hospitals and individual surgeons will be translated into a pay-for-performance program. These data will also become available for public scrutiny. Unfortunately, the governmental laws, rules, and regulations concerning the practice of medicine and surgery are coming much faster than medical educators have time to study, develop, and validate the coming "competency-based" surgical training programs.

This chapter briefly discusses the present state of surgical training, the present-day problems that need to be addressed, and the pressures that are moving the development of training programs that will produce the "competent" gynecologic surgeons in the near future. Where have we been and where are we now? Where must we go and why? What are we to do? The interested reader will find more depth, other views, and further specifics on this topic in the references at the end of this chapter. In particular, the reader is referred to "Teaching and Evaluating Surgical Skills," edited by Rebecca G. Rogers, in *Obstetrics and Gynecology Clinics of North America,* June 2006.

WHERE HAVE WE BEEN AND WHERE ARE WE NOW?

For more than one hundred years, the apprenticeship model has been how gynecologic surgeons are transformed from medical students to resident gynecologic surgeons to independent practitioners. This system continues to be a "see one, do one, teach one" teaching model under the supervision of a surgical mentor. The surgical mentor predominantly teaches surgery based on his or her own personal experiences and much less on evidenced-based studies. The mentors in many surgical training programs today, as over the past century, have widely variable surgical skills and teaching styles. Thus, surgical instruction continues to be a "trial by exhaustion and humiliation, as well as a journey of harassment and abuse (Dunnington)." Surgical instructors have not been schooled in how to be effective mentors, how to teach surgery, and how to evaluate surgical skills. This is as true today as it has always been. Some instructors don't even allow the resident any hands-on surgical experience. They allow the resident to learn by assisting at the surgery. The apprenticeship model does not offer uniform caseloads with seasoned mentors to assure adequate experience in performing gynecologic surgery. The teaching of ethics, professionalism, patient care, medical knowledge, and leadership were and are rarely taught, except by the happenstance examples of the mentors.

Teaching in the apprenticeship model is teacher oriented rather than student oriented. Teacher-oriented teaching has been shown to be random, without structure and purpose or defined goals. The Residency Review Committee (RRC) for Obstetrics and Gynecology eventually established structure-and-process guidelines for surgical training in gynecology by defining the types of surgery with which the resident should be involved. Continuing today, the surgical skills and clinical judgment of the resident is subjectively determined by the individual residency program director. The newly graduated gynecologic resident has simply fulfilled a requirement of time served with no defined minimum requirements of acquired surgical skills and experience.

The educators and practitioners of clinical gynecology today have seen the significant inconsistencies and weaknesses of training gynecologic surgeons by the traditional apprenticeship model. In the past 15 to 20 years in the United States, various factors have arisen to further deteriorate the quality of surgical training. Observations within the ob/gyn residency programs themselves show several unfortunate trends. The two most crucial are the decreasing number and variety of gynecologic procedures and the exodus of many dedicated surgical instructors from academic centers to private practice or retirement. A third trend, being evaluated now, is the impact of the Accreditation Council for Graduate Medical Education (ACGME) restriction on resident duty hours in clinical training and on-call experience. However, Nuthalapaty and colleagues, in studying the new restriction on residents' working hours, report that "A reduction in resident participation in surgical care/procedures had a minimum prevalence of 38% across all clinical service types."

Surgical cases are moving out of the teaching centers to private surgical specialty centers. This is especially significant with minimally invasive procedures, such as operative laparoscopies for hysterectomy, midurethral slings for stress urinary incontinence, and operative hysteroscopy. More and more subspecialty gynecologic surgeons have opened private centers for operative laparoscopy and operative hysteroscopy to evaluate and treat many gynecologic problems, including the need for hysterectomies, infertility, pelvic pain, and urinary incontinence. This marketing by private gynecologic surgeons is in direct competition with the teaching centers for the same patient population. These private practitioners are not interested in teaching because the resident will "slow me down and increase my medical-legal liability." Historically, operative laparoscopy and laparoscopic hysterectomies among gynecologists primarily evolved in the private sector, not in the academic or teaching centers.

In addition, some traditional surgical diseases, often requiring hysterectomy and/or oophorectomy, are now increasingly managed medically without surgery or with minimally invasive procedures. Examples of such traditional surgical diseases are chronic pelvic pain, endometriosis, urinary incontinence, infertility, abnormal uterine bleeding, uterine fibroids, and ectopic pregnancy. Third-party payers have grasped hold of these medical and less invasive surgical therapies. They are more and more denying payments for the more invasive surgical procedures. These nonsurgical therapies significantly reduce financial costs for the third-party health care payers.

Because of financial pressures, there has been an exodus of many skilled surgeons and seasoned instructors to private practice or into health-related industries, such as pharmaceutical companies or surgical products companies. Some have become burned out and have chosen early retirement. Many medical doctors are now pursuing or have obtained degrees in business administration. Some have found other nonacademic pursuits with which to supplement their incomes. All these pursuits take time away from effective and dedicated resident teaching in gynecologic surgery.

Those clinical instructors who remain to teach residents no longer have dedicated time to teach. They have intense pressures upon them to generate within their departments the income to support not only themselves and their overhead costs, but also the many departmental activities and financial obligations. These pressures urge the attending surgeon to operate himself/herself as much as possible in order to speed the case along to get done and get the next case under way as soon as possible. The goal is to do as many surgical cases as possible in a day to generate more income. Obviously, the resident becomes a technical assistant with little opportunity for verbal and hands-on instruction. In addition, the attending surgeon perceives that he/she can perform the case faster and better with less medical-legal risk. However, this perception may not be true.

Also observed has been a shift in the learning environment of many residencies. In the past, the older gynecologic surgeons spoke of a sense of community, a sense of purpose, a sense of pride in their individual residency training programs. That sense of uniqueness in a residency program has disappeared with the departmental budget restraints and faculty turnover. Today, more residents appear to be overwhelmed by their patient responsibilities and lack real surgical training. There are presently no measurable standards by which to determine how well a gynecologic resident has been trained in various gynecologic surgical procedures. The surgical training method of apprenticeship with an individual mentor is no longer producing surgically qualified gynecologic surgeons. The role of "see one, do one, teach one" is wholly inadequate in this new era of laparoscopic surgery, operative hysteroscopy, and the expansion of surgical and medical knowledge needed to treat previous surgical gynecologic problems. The operating room cases available for resident training vary widely in complexity. They cannot be standardized for resident training. They may or may not be of sufficient difficulty and complexity for training, and they too often involve instructors who are not educated or experienced enough to do effective training in the operating room. In addition, the resident surgeon may be tired and stressed, and the surgical mentor may be uninterested in teaching and more interested in getting the case done quickly without undue teaching. Surgical training has become a game of chance, a hit-or-miss lucky draw of getting good training from a good mentor during good surgical cases.

In general within our specialty, the reality exists that the present resident in gynecologic surgery is now learning surgery with less surgical experience in the operating room with less experienced surgical instructors. Therefore, in general, the present-day gynecologic surgeon leaving residency is deficient in surgical experience, knowledge, and skill. As a result, some graduated residents continue their surgical training in postgraduate surgical fellowships or subspecialty fellowships, or join practices with experienced gynecologic surgeons who are willing to mentor them. This perception is now met head-on with continued reports of medical and surgical mistakes in U.S. hospitals and the ever-increasing costs for the delivery of health care. A true crisis in the quantity and quality of gynecologic surgical training is now fully upon us. As a specialty, our own observations of surgical teaching deficiencies have now been memorialized by governmental rules and regulations concerning the collection of surgical case data on complications and outcomes, and subsequent financial reimbursements.

WHERE MUST WE GO, AND WHY?

As a result of the societal and governmental outcry for top-quality medical and surgical care, the ACGME and the American Board of Medical Specialties (ABMS) have firmly moved to establish guidelines for the competency-based training for all physicians and surgeons. The former structure-and-process educational mandates are now being converted to competency-based educational programs. Unfortunately, the process toward competency-based training is neither well defined nor clear at this time. The steps in designing the new programs and curricula include a definition of competency, development of a competent educational process, reliable and valid tests of knowledge and performance, and continuing assessment and evaluation of the whole process from beginning resident to "competent" practicing surgeon. In 1999, the ACGME identified in principle six general competencies upon which all graduate medical education must be based: (i) patient care, (ii) medical knowledge, (iii) practice-based learning and improvement, (iv) interpersonal and communication skills, (v) professionalism, and (vi) systems-based practice. Few guidelines and definitions have been issued since. The RRC is struggling to define and implement these six core elements of a competent residency education. The timeline for implementation is ambitious and being pressured by the federal government payers and legislature. However, there is little to implement at this time. Current professional literature is beginning to generate some articles on developing and evaluating the outcomes of competency-based educational models. However, much remains to be accomplished.

Just as clinical and surgical care should be guided by evidence-based clinical studies, gynecologic surgical education should be guided by evidence-based educational studies. The studies will directly assist the RRC in establishing requirements for how best to teach a particular clinical or surgical skill or professional attribute, including techniques, decision making, and leadership qualities. Surgical teaching methods and outcomes need to be measured in a standardized manner. Surgical curricula need to be established and standardized to know what to teach and how to best teach the mandatory subject matter. The curriculum must include clear definitions of core knowledge, surgical skills preparation, judgment involved in preoperative evaluation, intraoperative performance, treatment of complications, and postoperative management. The professional attributes of ethical considerations and decision making; interpersonal communications with colleagues, coworkers, administrators, and especially patients; and leadership models must be integrated into the training curriculum with reliable measurable outcomes.

All this will not be possible without the education of dedicated surgical mentors who have been schooled and practiced in how to bring a young resident along the way from a student of surgery to a competent practicing surgeon. As mentioned, the old mentoring process was based on teacher-oriented teaching. The new mentors will focus on the learner-oriented teaching approach. As Reznick from the University of Toronto wrote in 1993:

> An important aspect of teaching operative skill is a realization that residents are adult learners. As such, teaching principles developed from adult learning theory will apply.
>
> Adult learning is enhanced by an approach that is self-directed and centered on the learner rather than on the teacher. Adult learning is facilitated by focusing on a problem or task. Abstract, subject-centered learning is less effective as a motivator. Adults come to an education activity, such as a surgical rotation, with a vast amount of past experience that must be recognized and utilized.

WHAT ARE WE TO DO?

As Roger C. Crafts said, "You will remember a little of what you hear, some of what you read, considerably more of what you see, but almost all of what you understand." This statement applies not only to the learning of scientific knowledge and principles, but also to the learning of technical skills and medical/surgical judgments. Studies of highly successful individuals, particularly with athletic or musical talents, indicate that their success is dependent on several factors. The first is, of course, individual motivation and talent. In the surgical field, obviously, hand–eye coordination and other psychomotor technical skills are inherent within the individual, yet they must be developed. Some 10% of medical students may not have the qualities to become competent surgeons. In addition, the successful resident has an inborn ability to face mistakes and failure with an eye to learning and improving rather than taking a guilty, defeatist attitude.

Second, the successful individual plans dedicated time for practice, practice, and more practice, yet in an effective and efficient, positive way. Complex procedures must be broken down into individual, practicable components with immediate feedback from a trained observer. As has been said, "Practice does not make perfect, perfect practice makes perfect." The repetitive performance of specific skills has been shown to be much more effective in surgical training than general training involving multitask procedures.

Third, the highest-performing successful individuals have clarity, purpose, and imagination in their chosen field. "The ability to improvise, to cope skillfully with novel situations, requires vision, which takes years to develop."

As emphasized, the training of the skilled and talented gynecologic surgeon must involve a skilled, caring, and interested mentor. The teaching quality of the surgical faculty does have an impact on positive student performance. This must also include a positive environment for immediate evaluation from both self and mentor. This environment many times is delicate and balances between confidence-building positive and self-defeating negative. Reznick writes:

> Surgical preceptors serve as extremely potent and influential role models. We do so in all the aspects of an operation, from our approach to tissue handling to our interpersonal relationships in the operating room. The second aspect is coaching. This role as a coach reminds us of a need to provide encouragement and discipline to the resident. In this way, we help create a scaffold upon which the resident can build.

Levels of resident surgical training include the use of the individual senses: hearing, seeing, and tactile feeling. In addition, individual surgical skills need to be practiced and then integrated into an operative framework. This framework enables the resident to perform a procedure step by step. However, fluidity of these skills, along with operative judgment, demands further refined practice and experience under close critical supervision. This final maturation process, called *automization,* not only involves psychomotor skill development, clinical judgment, excellence, and knowledge of the literature, but also involves the development of interpersonal skills with emphasis on managing the operating room team.

RESIDENTS AND SURGICAL EDUCATION

Learning through hearing involves carefully crafted, presented, and coordinated lectures, case presentations, and discussions. Observational activities include seeing videos, watching various surgical exercises on inanimate trainers, watching cadaveric dissections, and, of course, observing live surgical procedures. The development of hand–eye coordination and hands-on surgical skills involves the use of inanimate trainers, computer simulators, animal models, human cadaveric dissections, and, of course, surgery on actual patients under the careful tutelage of a surgical instructor and mentor. Obviously, the teaching and evaluation of surgical skills and clinical judgment before entering the live operating room presents several distinct ethical, medical-legal, and financial advantages.

Lectures and case discussions must include patient presentations; appropriate history taking; focused physical examinations; discussion of findings; medical or surgical options, including possible benefits; and possible risks and complications. An interactive teaching environment among teacher and students with feedback and explanations is more beneficial for learning. The modern gynecologic surgeon must not have the mind-set that "if you can cut it, you can cure it." Above all, the gynecologic surgeon must become an expert in the understanding, evaluation, and treatment options of gynecologic diseases and disorders. Auditory learning must include appropriate objectives, enthusiastic lecture presentations by the teacher, and appropriate postpresentation objective testing. Individual progress is best achieved when made accountable and measurable to the individual learner.

Likewise, observational learning when observing videos or surgery on animals, human cadavers, or live patients needs to be focused and broken down into individual surgical skills and decision components. The observations by the residents again must involve individual accountability and appropriate testing and measurement. Hands-on training must focus on specific and individual tasks within each complex surgical procedure.

Beginning exercises involve minimal equipment to practice knot-tying and the ergonomic use of surgical instruments. *Knot-tying boards* and *simple plastic trainers* are available from various surgical instrument companies. In addition, *video laparoscopic trainers* are also available for practicing more involved laparoscopic skills. Anastakis and colleagues showed "that both bench and cadaver training were superior to text learning and that bench and cadaver training were equivalent." A formal surgical training program within a residency does objectively improve the resident's surgical skills.

Animal models, particularly anesthetized pigs, allow the emerging gynecologic surgeon to get the actual feel of tissue dissections, see physiologic response, and experience a physical realism of operating on a live patient, especially with the immediate feedback of hemorrhage. However, the drawback of animal models is that the anatomy is often much different and the dimensions within the pelvis are much smaller than those in the human patient. However, the cost is much more affordable than present human cadaver courses and computer-simulated models, and the student has a real, physiologic hands-on operative experience. Other animal models may include various body parts of various animals to recreate the feel and texture of various human parts. However, to work on a live animal model, the technical support aspects can be complex, just as in the human model. The animal must be properly obtained, properly anesthetized in a properly prepared room with appropriate lighting, equipment, instrumentation, and technical and surgical support.

Advanced Surgical Training on Unembalmed Human Cadavers

A more advanced model for surgical training is the performance of dissection techniques and procedures on *unembalmed human cadavers*. This excellent model has been successfully used in teaching vaginal surgery, open laparotomy, hysteroscopy, and, of course, operative laparoscopy. We are fortunate in the United States to have the opportunity to have resident and postgraduate education courses using unembalmed cadavers. The use of human cadavers for postgraduate surgical education is not allowed or feasible in most countries of the world today. The human cadaver model is an excellent model on which to learn human pelvic anatomy, including the dimensions and relations of the various structures and tissues within the human body, proper dissection techniques, and the performance of various surgical procedures.

Even though the overhead financial cost of these courses is high, the intense and concentrated nature of the learning is well worth the expense in the minds of many individuals who have taken such training. The overhead expenses include the cost of administering the willed body programs in the various states; the immediate testing of the bodies for human immunodeficiency virus, hepatitis B and C, and syphilis; the proper handling of the bodies for cold preservation; the appropriate shipping, preparation of the body at the course site, and cost of technical support personnel in setting up the body at each workstation; and setting up the appropriate audiovisual equipment, instrumentation, and appropriate universal safety precautions. Teaching institutions interested in organizing such human cadaver teaching opportunities must inquire and coordinate their programs with their local medical school and state board of anatomic gifts. They must conform to the prevailing rules, regulations, and laws that control the use of these voluntarily willed bodies. Students and their instructors must be respectful, courteous, and appreciative of these individuals who allow their bodies to be used for their learning.

The participants in such a learning exercise must realize the purpose of this teaching is not only to appreciate and understand structural and pelvic support anatomy, but more importantly, to learn and practice proper tissue dissection techniques on human tissues. The practicing surgeon must be a master of the various tissue dissection skills and techniques to safely develop the surgical fields involved with the procedure. Further hands-on exercises in the cadaver allow each student to perform various gynecologic procedures. The purpose of cadaver learning is *not* to learn surgical instrumentation and basic skills, such as how to handle laparoscopic instruments and knot tying; these can be mastered with inanimate trainers. The purpose of cadaver learning is to learn dissectional surgical anatomy and to integrate surgical skills, already mastered, into an entire operative procedure. The goal of cadaver training is to significantly improve the operative experience of each participating surgeon. Ideally, operative procedures on his/her own patients will become safer (fewer operative complications), become more efficient (smoother dissections with less wasted motion and hesitation), have less blood loss (to obscure the field), and become more effective (better long-term results).

Teaching on human cadavers must have specific and directed objectives. Most gynecologic surgeons, when left to dissect a cadaver alone, do not have a clear understanding of the relevant anatomy and dissection techniques that need to be mastered. Dissection techniques must be taught in a specific and directed manner, likewise. The participant should already have the appropriate surgical skills to take full advantage of his or her learning on the cadaveric model. These skills can certainly be learned, as noted earlier, via training on the various inanimate trainers, animal models, and, eventually, the computer-simulated trainers.

All aspects of gynecologic surgery may be understood and practiced on the human cadaver. This includes dissection of the anterior abdominal wall; correlation with surgical incisions and laparoscopic trocar placement; and practicing of dissectional techniques, layer by layer within the pelvis itself, particularly in the retroperitoneal areas. The retroperitoneal areas include the presacral space; the pelvic brim area; the pelvic sidewall; the base of the broad ligament, where the ureter passes underneath the uterine artery; the paravesical space anteriorly; the pararectal space posteriorly; the vesicocervical and vesicovaginal spaces; the rectovaginal space, including the rectovaginal septum, and, of course, a thorough dissection and understanding of the anatomy of the retropubic space of Retzius. These dissections must be carried out carefully in a directed manner to find the structures contained within the dissection plane and to understand their relationships to other vital structures within the same and surrounding anatomic areas. Further dissections, whether open laparotomy or through the laparoscope, can also include appreciation of the various somatic nerves, such as the obturator nerve and even the femoral nerve in the iliopsoas groove. Other dissections can reveal the sacrospinous ligament; the sacral plexus of nerves, including the pudendal nerve and the sciatic nerve; the visceral innervation of the presacral space; the many components of the pelvic sidewall, including the inferior hypogastric plexus and its many branches; the cardinal ligament and uterosacral ligament complexes; and the various support tissues, such as the pubocervical fascia and rectovaginal septum.

Unembalmed cadavers also allow the opportunity to understand and perform vaginal surgery. This enables the student to dissect and to understand the structural and relational anatomy, and to perform procedures through the vagina for understanding of anterior vaginal wall prolapse or cystocele repair, apical prolapse or enterocele repair, and posterior wall prolapse or rectocele repair. Within the pelvic cavity, the various tissue layers—such as the peritoneum, visceral fascia, and anatomic structures—have the feel of the live patient, but neither bleed much nor cause undue anxiety during the learning of dissectional techniques. The operating gynecologist has the opportunity to practice surgical skills in a specific, focused manner, step by step, integrating all the steps to perform an entire procedure without the pressures of medical-legal considerations.

A less effective but still viable method of learning anatomy is on the embalmed cadaver, such as is found in medical schools. However, the opportunity to have the feel of live patient tissue is lost with the embalming process.

After these human cadaver specimens have been used for learning, these individual specimens are respectfully taken to a funeral home, where they are cremated. Their remains are returned to their home states and then to their families by the respective anatomic gifts registries. Again, we are appreciative for these individuals and their families who have voluntarily allowed their bodies to be used for anatomic and surgical training.

The program involving human cadavers must also have specific goals to allow the gynecologic resident and interested attending physician to develop a base of clinical and anatomic knowledge upon which to grow and develop as more experience is obtained in surgery. This core of knowledge and training in anatomy and surgical procedures is important so that the independent gynecologic surgeon can understand new techniques and surgical developments as the field of gynecology progresses in the future.

Computer-generated Simulators

Several computer companies are well on their way to developing effective *computer-based simulators* to train gynecologic surgeons, particularly involving open surgery, laparoscopic surgery, and hysteroscopic surgery. These computer-based simulators not only give the perception of operating on a "normal" patient but also allow for anatomic and pathologic variations within the practice patient. The computer provides a virtual attending mentor that offers immediate objective and nonjudgmental feedback. These computers are being programmed to allow for realistic haptics and the true feel of instrument motion and tissue pressure. The simulators provide skills maintenance, even with the decreasing caseload of major surgical procedures found in gynecologic residencies today. They are accessible for on-demand training 24 hours a day, every day of the week, 365 days of the year. The objective, unbiased, and nonjudgmental quantitative skills assessment motivates the individual because each resident is directly accountable for his or her own measured progress. Computer-based simulators allow for objective assessment of performance and outcome before the individual resident operates on a living patient.

The development of computer-based simulators by various research computer engineers is rapidly overcoming the challenges of computer costs, visual realism, anatomic realism, physical realism, haptic realism, and physiologic realism. Computer costs have decreased dramatically, thereby making this teaching modality much more affordable. Visual realism compares the look of the tissues on the computer screen with the real patient. Anatomic realism deals with the structural and relational anatomy within the field of operation. Physical realism deals with the size and feel of the instruments and tissues encountered. Haptic realism pertains to how things feel, like the feel of live surgery. The feel of mass, elasticity, gravity, and moving instruments is important in psychomotor development. Physiologic realism deals with possible hemorrhage at the surgical site; various movements of the patient, such as during respiration; and even pain perception by the poorly anesthetized patient. Visual realism and haptic realism allow the individual to practice hand-eye coordination. Issues of ethics, medical-legal concerns, and patient safety in teaching gynecologic surgery will be better solved as computer-based education becomes more affordable and more available.

Training in Laparoscopy

As a result of the need to train surgeons in complex laparoscopic procedures, various training formats have evolved in recent years in various countries around the world. Many of these training models are based on individual laparoscopic procedures (see Bibliography). However, in August 1998, Brill and Rogers published "A Comprehensive Program for Resident Training in Operative Laparoscopy," using an outline form. The thesis of this outline is that the basic laparoscopic anatomy, pathology, and fundamental technical and ergonomic skills—even for the most advanced laparoscopic procedures—can be found and practiced on the most readily available and basic of laparoscopic cases. Using plentiful cases such as laparoscopic sterilizations and diagnostic laparoscopic procedures, the resident gynecologic surgeon can be shown and taught basic laparoscopic techniques and maneuvers in preparation for performing more complex and advanced laparoscopic cases. Each surgical procedure is reduced to its fundamental technical and ergonomic components. These components can then be practiced on laparoscopic trainers and then on the simplest laparoscopic cases. These earliest and most available cases then provide most of the technical components required for the more advanced laparoscopic cases. They further state:

> At each level, proctoring in relevant anatomy can be used to unite process with specific procedures. We believe that the quality and durability of the learning process is dependent on proper sequencing and specific behavioral milestones: hearing, observation, comprehension, integration, sensation, and simulation with inanimate models, animal models, fresh cadaver dissection, and live patient surgery with preceptorship. Ultimately, development of necessary skills represents a balance between an individual's capacity for visual-motor processing, while referencing two-dimensional imaging, and level of conditioned responses obtained by simulation and practice.

PROPOSAL AND CONCLUSION

Millions of dollars are spent each year by commercial airlines and by the U.S. military in training aviation pilots using computer-modulated flight simulators, as well as actual training flights. Why has gynecologic surgical training lagged so far behind in the use of these modern modalities? Is a well-trained and seasoned surgeon not worth the expense to individuals in this society?

Julian and Rogers have again proposed a 5-year program for training competent obstetricians and gynecologic surgeons. The first year, PGY-1, consists of competency-based training in primary care medicine and basic surgical education. PGY-2, PGY-3, and PGY-4 consist of core education in obstetrics, gynecology, and their contained subspecialties. Importantly, for the more effective use of educational time in this era of limits on residents' work hours, the time to repetitively deliver hundreds of normal, spontaneous vertex vaginal deliveries needs to be rethought and revised. The PGY-5 year is a transition period from residency to independent practice. The fifth-year resident is a minimally supervised junior faculty member and assists in teaching, supervising, and evaluating the junior residents. The best way to learn and understand a clinical subject is to practice and teach. Concurrently, the resident will generate case lists and other experiences directly leading to board certification.

Julian and Rogers also propose the designation of several centers in the United States to develop and study the best methods to teach competency-based gynecologic surgery. Academic and practical input, as well as funding, from public and private payers of health care, from national foundations, and from specialty societies should be included in the process. The goal of these centers is the development of the best teaching methods for surgical training, as well as reliable competency criteria for learning evaluation. In turn, these centers will supply the RRC with an objective tested program to guide surgical training and establish criteria for program certification. It is in the financial and patient safety interests of the federal and state governments, as well as the private insurance payers, to fund this work in training competent surgeons, who will best use the limited funds available to care for the surgical needs of future society.

Also, with the loss of many skilled and seasoned educators from academic and teaching centers, the problem of dedicated and available educators must be immediately and directly addressed. The teachers themselves need to be mentored and trained, and must have financial incentives to be the best possible teachers. This is a proven business method of developing quality. The problem of dedicated and available surgical teachers must be addressed directly, not only by teaching institutions and the specialty, but most importantly, by the health care payers and the government policy makers. Postgraduate programs must be developed to increase the numbers of quality surgical instructors. These physicians should be getting PhDs in how to teach, not MBAs.

Testing of technical skills must be clearly addressed. The residents must be accountable for their own progress. Tests must be crafted so that they can measure their progress, both quantitatively and qualitatively. These tests must be feasible, reliable, and valid. Assessment and measurement leads to personal accountability, motivation to learn, and true measurable progress.

In addition, training of the individual gynecologic surgeon must not only emphasize individual skill development but should also include training in creating effective and harmonious surgical teams, particularly involving their administration and interpersonal relationships. Teamwork in the operating room is important to realize optimal performance. Until recently, there have been no tools to measure teamwork in the surgical setting. MaKary and coauthors have demonstrated that the Safety Attitudes Questionnaire can be used to measure teamwork, identify disconnects between or within disciplines, and evaluate interventions aimed at improving patient safety. Clearly, residents will participate as team members in the operating room. Using operating room briefings and debriefings as a means of improving teamwork communication will also optimize the student learning experience.

We need to train more effective and sensitive mentors. Mentors must provide each resident with a series of tasks and objectives to be achieved and reliably measured. The mentor must provide ongoing feedback in a positive and constructive manner. Without this continual feedback, deficiencies in an individual's training will not be corrected. The caring and effective mentor will have a professional yet personal relationship with the learner. The effective mentor in surgical education must be skilled in questioning, must ensure a comfortable environment for learning, and must be willing to question present surgical practices. "Without effective mentoring, students feel alone, perplexed, overwhelmed" with a decreased enthusiasm for learning (Dunnington).

Last, Resnick concludes:

> What makes an excellent operative teacher is adherence to basic, almost simple principals: treat residents as adult learners; set specific objectives; realize that operative skills are multidimensional; and be there, observe, be patient, provide feed-back, be positive, take the job seriously and structure the assessment process.

The proposed academic centers for developing excellence in surgical training will also teach motivated surgeons how to become enthusiastic, competency-based mentors. Seasoned surgical mentors who are well trained and dedicated will be the engines that power the overall progress to competency in modern surgical training and practice in the United States.

BEST SURGICAL PRACTICES

- Although the regulatory agencies have set the parameters for education in the surgical specialties, there is considerable latitude for optimization of the learning experience. Training of the individual gynecologic surgeon must not only emphasize individual skill development, but should also include training in creating effective and harmonious surgical teams, particularly involving their administration and interpersonal skills.
- The seasoned, well-trained, dedicated surgical mentor remains an important element that powers the overall progress to competency in modern surgical training and practice.

Bibliography

Accreditation Council for Graduate Medical Education. Outcome Project. ACGME, 1999.

Anastakis DJ, Regehr G, Reznick RK, et al. Assessment of technical skills transfer from the bench training model to the human model. *Am J Surg* 1999;177:167.

Bailit JL, Blanchard MH. The effect of house staff working hours on the quality of obstetric and gynecologic care. *Obstet Gynecol* 2004;103:613.

Blue AV, Griffith CH, Wilson J, et al. Surgical teaching quality makes a difference. *Am J Surg* 1999;177:86.

Brill AI, Rogers RM. A comprehensive program for resident training in operative laparoscopy. *J Am Assoc Gynecol Laparosc* 1998;5(3):223.

Brill AI, Rogers RM. A new paradigm for resident training [editorial]. *J Am Assoc Gynecol Laparosc* 1998;5(3):219.

Carraccio C, Wolfsthal SD, Englander R, et al. Shifting paradigms: from Flexner to competencies. *Acad Med* 2002;77:361.

Chou B, Handa VL. Simulators and virtual reality in surgical education. In Rogers RG, ed. Teaching and evaluating surgical skills. *Obstet Gynecol Clin North Am* 2006;33(2):283.

Coates KW, Kuehl TJ, Bachofen CG, et al. Analysis of surgical complications and patient outcomes in a residency training program. *Am J Obstet Gynecol* 2001;184:1380.

Crafts RC. *A textbook of human anatomy*, 3rd ed. New York: Churchill Livingstone, 1985:dedication page.

Cundiff GW. Analysis of the effectiveness of an endoscopy education program in improving residents' laparoscopic skills. *Obstet Gynecol* 1997;90:854.

Defoe DM, Power ML, Holzman GB, et al. Long hours and little sleep: work schedules of residents in obstetrics and gynecology. *Obstet Gynecol* 2001;97:1015.

Dunnington GL. The art of mentoring. *Am J Surg* 1996;171:604.

Fenner DE. Training of a gynecologic surgeon. *Obstet Gynecol* 2005;105:193.

Gawande AA. Creating the educated surgeon in the 21st century. *Am J Surg* 2001;181:551.

Goff BA, Lentz GM, Lee DM, et al. Formal teaching of surgical skills in an obstetric gynecologic residency. *Obstet Gynecol* 1999;93:785.

Gor M, McCloy R, Stone R, et al. Virtual reality laparoscopic simulator for assessment in gynaecology. *BJOG* 2003;110:181.

Hall LH. Surviving burnout [editorial]. *ACOG Clin Rev* 2006;11(3):1.

Haluck RS, Krummel TM. Computers and virtual reality for surgical education in the 21st century. *Arch Surg* 2000;135:786.

Hamdorf JM, Hall AC. Acquiring surgical skills. *Br J Surg* 2000;87:28.

Hasser CJ, Merril G. *Design of an endoscopy simulator*. Paper presented at: the 30th Annual Meeting of the American Association of Gynecologic Laparoscopists; November 18, 2001; San Francisco.

Institute of Medicine. Committee on Quality Health Care in America. *Crossing the quality chasm: a new health system for the 21st century*. Washington, DC: National Academy Press, 2001.

Julian TM. The training of gynecologic surgeons. *J Pelvic Med Surg* 2003;9:179.

Julian TM, Rogers Jr RM. Changing the way we train gynecologic surgeons. In Rogers RG, ed. Teaching and evaluating surgical skills. *Obstet Gynecol Clin North Am* 2006;33(2):237.

Lentz GM, Mandel LS, Goff BA. A six year study of surgical teaching and skills evaluation for obstetric/gynecologic residents in porcine and inanimate surgical models. *Am J Obstet Gynecol* 2005;193:2056.

Mandel LP, Lentz GM, Goff BA. Teaching and evaluating surgical skills. *Obstet Gynecol* 2000;95:783.

MaKary MA, Sexton JB, Freischlag JA, et al. Operating room teamwork among physicians and nurses: teamwork in the eye of the beholder. *J Am Coll Surg* 2006;202:746.

Nuthalapaty FS, Carver AR, Nuthalapaty ES, et al. The scope of duty hour-associated residency structure modifications. *Am J Obstet Gynecol* 2006;194:282.

Reznick RK. Teaching and testing technical skills. *Am J Surg* 1993;165:358.

Rogers RG, ed. Teaching and evaluating surgical skills. *Obstet Gynecol Clin North Am* 2006;33(2). Philadelphia: WB Saunders Co.

Rogers Jr RM, Julian TM. Training the gynecologic surgeon. *Obstet Gynecol* 2005;105:197.

Rosser JC, Rosser LE, Savalgi RS. Objective evaluation of a laparoscopic surgical skill program for residents and senior surgeons. *Arch Surg* 1998;133:657.

Royal Australian College of Obstetricians and Gynaecologists. *Guidelines for training in advanced operative laparoscopy*. East Melbourne: Royal Australian College, 1993.

Royal College of Obstetricians and Gynaecologists. *Working party report of the RCOG Working Party on Training in Gynaecological Endoscopic Surgery*. London: RCOG Press, 1994.

Royal College of Obstetricians and Gynaecologists Working Party. *Implementation of the recommendations of the Working Party in Gynaecological Endoscopy Surgery*. London: RCOG Press, 1994.

Society of Obstetricians and Gynaecologists of Canada. *Guidelines for training in operative endoscopy in the specialty of obstetrics and gynaecology*. Toronto: Society of Obstetricians and Gynaecologists of Canada, 1992.

Sorosky JI, Anderson B. Surgical experiences and training residents: perspective of experienced gynecologic oncologists. *Gynecol Oncol* 1999;75:222.

SECTION II ■ PRINCIPLES OF ANATOMY AND PERIOPERATIVE CONSIDERATIONS

CHAPTER 7 ■ SURGICAL ANATOMY OF THE FEMALE PELVIS

JOHN O. L. DELANCEY

DEFINITIONS

Urinary trigone—The urinary trigone is a triangular visible area in the bladder, the apices of which are the ureteral orifices and the internal urinary meatus. This is a layer of smooth muscle connecting the ureters and the urethra, the edges of which are visible cystoscopically and when the bladder is open.

Urethra and vesicle neck—The urethra is that portion of the lower urinary tract outside of the bladder that the urethral lumen traverses. That portion of the urethra lumen that is surrounded by the bladder vasculature is referred to as the vesicle neck.

Endopelvic fascia—The endopelvic fascias are those tissues outside of the muscularis of the pelvic organs that attach these organs to the pelvic sidewall. There is also some extension of loose areolar tissue over the surfaces of the organ. The surgical fascia used by gynecologists during pelvic reconstructive surgery, however, is primarily composed of the muscularis of the vaginal wall.

Pelvic spaces—The space between the bladder and the anterior portion of the pelvic walls is the perivesical space or space of Retzius. The space between the lower urinary tract and the genital tract is the vesicovaginal or vesicocervical space. This is bounded laterally by the "bladder pillars," which is the region in which the tissues that go to the vagina separate from those that go to the bladder base. The rectovaginal space lies between the posterior vaginal wall and the anterior surface of the rectum, and lies primarily above the top of the perineal body.

Pelvic diaphragm—The term *pelvic diaphragm* refers to the levator ani muscle and its covering fasciae, both the superior fascia and the inferior fascia. The term *pelvic floor* refers to all of the supportive structures that are involved with pelvic organ support. Sometimes the term *pelvic floor* and *pelvic diaphragm* can be used interchangeably, especially in the British literature.

VULVA AND ERECTILE STRUCTURES

The bony pelvic outlet is bordered by the ischiopubic rami anteriorly and the coccyx and sacrotuberous ligaments posteriorly. It can be divided into anterior and posterior triangles, which share a common base along a line between the ischial tuberosities. The tissues filling the anterior triangle have a layered structure similar to that of the abdominal wall (Table 7.1). There is a skin and adipose layer (vulva) overlying a fascial layer (perineal membrane) that lies superficial to a muscular layer (levator ani muscles).

Subcutaneous Tissues of the Vulva

The structures of the vulva lie on the pubic bones and extend caudally under its arch (Fig. 7.1). They consist of the mons, labia, clitoris, vestibule, and associated erectile structures and their muscles. The mons consists of hair-bearing skin over a cushion of adipose tissue that lies on the pubic bones. Extending posteriorly from the mons, the labia majora are composed of similar hair-bearing skin and adipose tissue, which contain the termination of the round ligaments of the uterus and the obliterated processus vaginalis (canal of Nuck). The round ligament can give rise to leiomyomas in this region, and the obliterated processus vaginalis can be a dilated embryonic remnant in the adult.

The labia minora, vestibule, and glans clitoris can be seen between the two labia majora. The labia minora are hairless skin folds, each of which splits anteriorly to run over, and under, the glans of the clitoris. The more anterior folds unite to form the hood-shaped prepuce of the clitoris, whereas the posterior folds insert into the underside of the glans as the frenulum.

Unlike the skin of the labia majora, the cutaneous structures of the labia minora and vestibule do not lie on an adipose layer but on a connective-tissue stratum that is loosely organized and permits mobility of the skin during intercourse. This loose attachment of the skin to underlying tissues allows the skin to be easily dissected off the underlying fascia during skinning vulvectomy in the area of the labia minora and vestibule.

In the posterior lateral aspect of the vestibule, the duct of the major vestibular gland can be seen 3 to 4 mm outside the hymenal ring. The minor vestibular gland openings are found along a line extending anteriorly from this point, parallel to the hymenal ring and extending toward the urethral orifice. The urethra bulges slightly around the surrounding vestibular skin anterior to the vagina and posterior to the clitoris. Its orifice is flanked on either side by two small labia. Skene ducts open into the inner aspect of these labia and can be seen as small, punctate openings when the urethral labia are separated.

Within the skin of the vulva are specialized glands that can become enlarged and thereby require surgical removal. The holocrine sebaceous glands in the labia majora are associated with hair shafts, and in the labia minora they are freestanding. They lie close to the surface, which explains their easy recognition with minimal enlargement. In addition, lateral to the introitus and anus, there are numerous apocrine sweat glands, along with the normal eccrine sweat glands. The former structures undergo change with the menstrual cycle, having increased secretory activity in the premenstrual period. They can become chronically infected, as in hidradenitis suppurativa, or neoplastically enlarged, as in hidradenomas, both of which may require surgical therapy. The eccrine sweat glands present in the vulvar skin rarely present abnormalities, but on occasion they can form palpable masses as syringomas.

TABLE 7.1

LAYERS OF THE ANTERIOR TRIANGLE OF THE PERINEUM

- Skin
- Subcutaneous tissue
  - Camper's fascia
  - Colles fascia
- Superficial space
  - Clitoris and its crura
  - Ischiocavernous muscle
  - Vestibular bulb
  - Bulbocavernous muscle
  - Greater vestibular gland
  - Superficial transverse perineal muscle
- Deep space-perineal membrane
  - Compressor urethrae
  - Urethrovaginal sphincter

The subcutaneous tissue of the labia majora is similar in composition to that of the abdominal wall. It consists of lobules of fat interlaced with connective tissue septa. Although there are no well-defined layers in the subcutaneous tissue, regional variations in the relative quantity of fat and fibrous tissue exist. The superficial region of this tissue, where fat predominates, has been called Camper's fascia, as it is on the abdomen. In this region, there is a continuation of fat from the anterior abdominal wall, called the digital process of fat.

In the deeper layers of the vulva, there is less fat, and the interlacing fibrous connective tissue septa are much more evident than those in Camper's fascia. This more fibrous layer is called Colles fascia and is similar to Scarpa's fascia on the abdomen. Its interlacing fibrous septa of the subcutaneous tissue attach laterally to the ischiopubic rami and fuse posteriorly with the posterior edge of the perineal membrane (i.e., urogenital diaphragm). Anteriorly, however, there is no connection to the pubic rami, and this permits communication between the area deep to this layer and the abdominal wall. These fibrous attachments to the ischiopubic rami and the posterior aspect of the perineal membrane limit the spread of hematomas or infection in this compartment posterolaterally but allow spread into the abdomen. This clinical observation has led to the consideration of Colles fascia as a separate entity from the superficial Camper fascia, which lacks these connections.

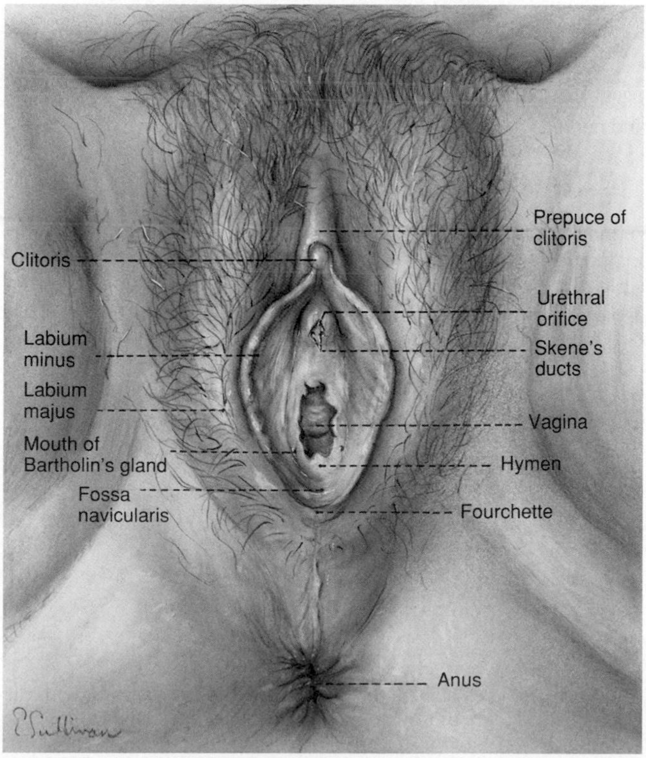

FIGURE 7.1. External genitalia.

Superficial Compartment

The space between the subcutaneous tissues and perineal membrane, which contains the clitoris, crura, vestibular bulbs, and ischiocavernous and bulbocavernous muscles, is called the superficial compartment of the perineum (Fig. 7.2). The deep compartment is the region just above the perineal membrane; it is discussed later.

The erectile bodies and their associated muscles within the superficial compartment lie on the caudal surface of the perineal membrane. The clitoris is composed of a midline shaft (body) capped with the glans. This shaft lies on, and is suspended from, the pubic bones by a subcutaneous suspensory ligament. The paired crura of the clitoris bend downward from the shaft and are firmly attached to the pubic bones, continuing dorsally to lie on the inferior aspects of the pubic rami. The ischiocavernous muscles originate at the ischial tuberosities and the free surfaces of the crura to insert on the upper crura and body of the clitoris. A few muscle fibers, called the superficial transverse perineal muscles, originate in common with the ischiocavernous muscle from the ischial tuberosity and lie medial to the perineal body.

The paired vestibular bulbs lie immediately under the vestibular skin and are composed of erectile tissue. They are covered by the bulbocavernous muscles, which originate in the perineal body and lie over their lateral surfaces. These muscles, along with the ischiocavernous muscles, insert into the body of the clitoris and act to pull it downward.

The Bartholin greater vestibular gland is found at the tail end of the bulb of the vestibule and is connected to the vestibular mucosa by a duct lined with squamous epithelium. The gland lies on the perineal membrane and beneath the bulbocavernous muscle. The intimate relation between the enormously vascular erectile tissue of the vestibular bulb and the Bartholin gland is responsible for the hemorrhage associated with removal of this latter structure.

The perineal membrane and perineal body are important to the support of the pelvic organs. They are discussed in the section on the pelvic floor.

Pudendal Nerve and Vessels

The pudendal nerve is the sensory and motor nerve of the perineum. Its course and distribution in the perineum parallel the pudendal artery and veins that connect with the internal iliac vessels (Fig. 7.3). The course and division of the nerve are described with the understanding that the vascular channels parallel them.

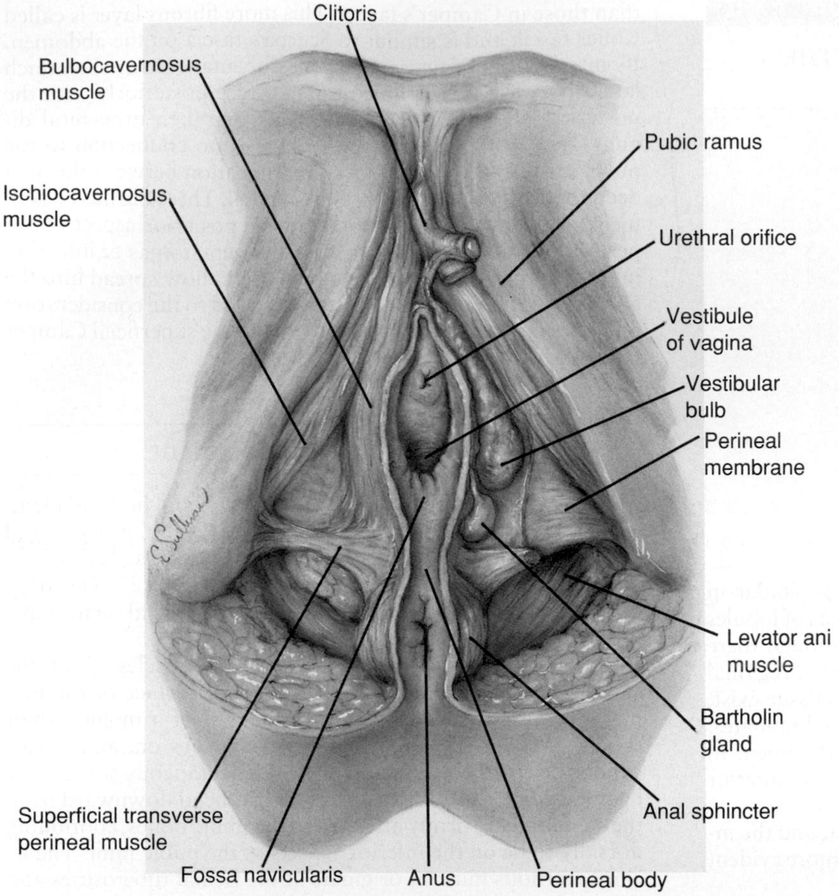

FIGURE 7.2. Superficial compartment and perineal membrane.

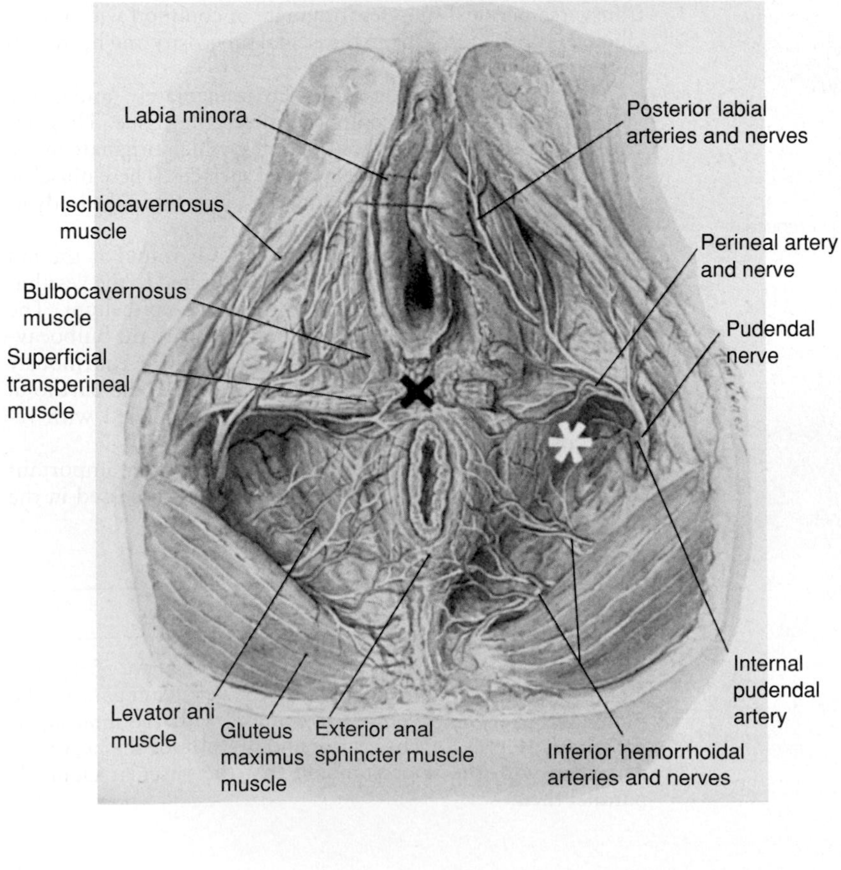

FIGURE 7.3. Pudendal nerve and vessels, with the position of the ischiorectal fossa (*asterisk*) and the perineal body (*cross*) indicated. (From: Anson BJ. *An atlas of human anatomy.* Philadelphia: WB Saunders, 1950, with permission.)

The pudendal nerve arises from the sacral plexus (S2–S4), and the vessels originate from the anterior division of the internal iliac artery. They leave the pelvis through the greater sciatic foramen by hooking around the ischial spine and sacrospinous ligament to enter the pudendal (Alcock's) canal through the lesser sciatic foramen.

The nerve and vessels have three branches: the clitoral, perineal, and inferior hemorrhoidal. The clitoral branch lies on the perineal membrane along its path to supply the clitoris. The perineal branch (the largest of the three branches) enters the subcutaneous tissues of the vulva behind the perineal membrane. Here it supplies the bulbocavernous, ischiocavernous, and transverse perineal muscles. It also supplies the skin of the inner portions of the labia majora, labia minora, and vestibule. The inferior hemorrhoidal branch goes to the external anal sphincter and perianal skin.

Lymphatic Drainage

The pattern of the vulvar lymphatic vessels and drainage into the superficial inguinal group of lymph nodes has been established by both injection studies and clinical observation. It is important to the treatment of vulvar malignancies; an overview of this system is provided here. This area is described and illustrated in more detail in Chapter 33.

Tissues external to the hymenal ring are supplied by an anastomotic series of vessels in the superficial tissues that coalesce to a few trunks lateral to the clitoris and proceed laterally to the superficial inguinal nodes (Fig. 7.4). The vessels draining the labia majora also run in an anterior direction, lateral to those of the labia minora and vestibule. These lymphatic channels lie medial to the labiocrural fold, establishing it as the lateral border of surgical resection.

Injection studies of the urethral lymphatics have shown that lymphatic drainage of this region terminates in either the right or left inguinal nodes. The clitoris has been said to have some direct drainage to deep pelvic lymph nodes, bypassing the usual superficial nodes, but the clinical significance of this appears to be minimal.

The inguinal lymph nodes are divided into two groups—the superficial and the deep nodes. There are 12 to 20 superficial nodes, and they lie in a T-shaped distribution parallel to and 1 cm below the inguinal ligament, with the stem extending down along the saphenous vein. The nodes are often divided into four quadrants, with the center of the division at the saphenous opening. The vulvar drainage goes primarily to the medial nodes of the upper quadrant. These nodes lie deep in the adipose layer of the subcutaneous tissues, in the membranous layer, just superficial to the fascia lata.

The large saphenous vein joins the femoral vein through the saphenous opening. Within 2 cm of the inguinal ligament, several superficial blood vessels branch from the saphenous vein and femoral artery. They include the superficial epigastric vessels that supply the subcutaneous tissues of the lower abdomen; the superficial circumflex iliac vessels that course laterally to the region of the iliac crest; and the superficial external pudendal vessels that supply the mons, labia majora, and clitoral hood.

Lymphatics from the superficial nodes enter the fossa ovalis and drain into one to three deep inguinal nodes, which lie in the femoral canal of the femoral triangle. They pass through the fossa ovalis (saphenous opening) in the fascia lata, which lies approximately 3 cm below the inguinal ligament, lateral to the pubic tubercle, along with the saphenous vein on its way to the femoral vein. The membranous layer of the subcutaneous tissues spans this opening as a trabeculate layer called a fascia cribrosa, pierced by lymphatics. The deep nodes are found under this fascia in the femoral triangle.

The femoral triangle is the subfascial space of the upper one third of the thigh. It is bounded by the inguinal ligament, sartorius muscle, and adductor longus muscle. Its floor is formed by the pectineal, adductor longus, and iliopsoas muscles. The femoral artery bisects it vertically between the anterosuperior iliac spine and pubic tubercle. The femoral vein lies medial to the artery; the femoral nerve is lateral to it.

As these vessels pass under the inguinal ligament, they carry with them an extension of the transversalis fascia, which is the extraperitoneal connective tissue deep to the rectus abdominis muscle called the femoral sheath. These sheaths extend about 2 to 3 cm below the inguinal ligament before fusing with the vascular adventitia. Besides the two parts of the femoral sheath that accompany these vessels, a third portion—the femoral canal—can be found in the space medial to the vein. The abdominal opening of this is the femoral ring. The femoral canal contains the deep inguinal lymph nodes. Lymph channels from these nodes pierce the membrane filling the femoral ring to

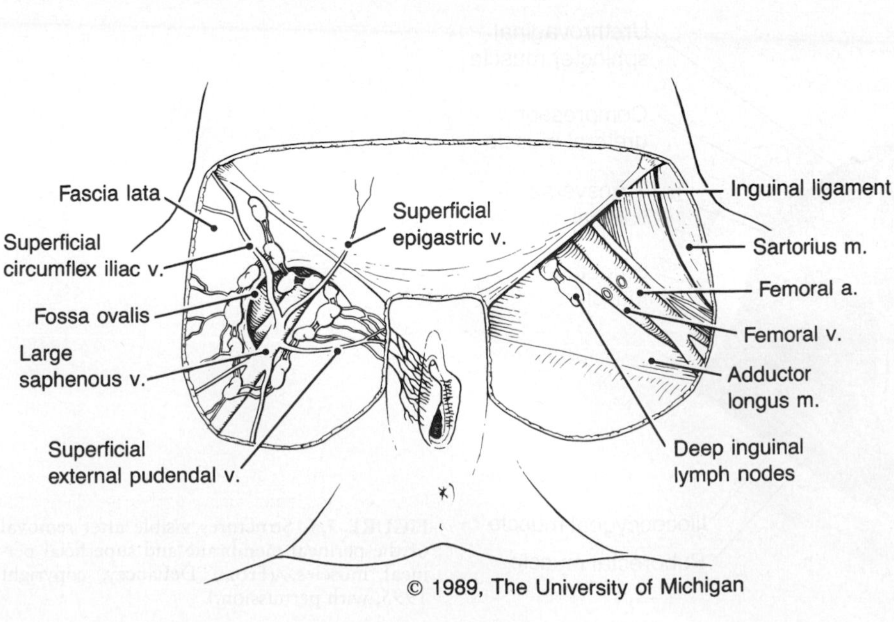

FIGURE 7.4. Lymphatic drainage of the vulva and femoral triangle. Superficial inguinal nodes are shown in the right thigh, and deep inguinal nodes are shown in the left thigh. Fascia lata has been removed on the left.

communicate with the external iliac nodes. Also within this region, the femoral vessels give rise to the deep external pudendal vessels. The external pudendal vessels run deep to the femoral vein over the pectineal muscle to pierce the fascia lata. Here they become subcutaneous and form anastomoses with branches of the internal pudendal vessels as well as the deep femoral and lateral circumflex femoral arteries.

THE PELVIC FLOOR

When humans assumed the upright posture, the opening in the bony pelvis came to lie at the bottom of the abdominopelvic cavity. This required the evolution of a supportive system to prevent the pelvic organs from being pushed downward through this opening. In the woman, this system must withstand these downward forces but allow for the passage of the large and cranially dominant human fetus. The supportive system that has evolved to meet these needs consists of a fibromuscular floor that forms a shelf spanning the pelvic outlet and that contains a cleft for the birth canal and excretory drainage. A series of visceral ligaments and fasciae tethers the organs and maintains their position over the closed portions of the floor. The floor consists of the levator ani muscles and perineal membrane. The openings in these structures for parturition and elimination have required the development of ancillary fibrous elements that are concentrated over open areas in the muscular floor to support the viscera in these weak areas. This section discusses the structures of the pelvic floor; the fibrous supportive system is described in the section on the pelvic viscera and cleavage planes and fascia.

Perineal Membrane (Urogenital Diaphragm)

The perineal membrane forms the inferior portion of the anterior pelvic floor. It is a triangular sheet of dense, fibromuscular tissue that spans the anterior half of the pelvic outlet (Fig. 7.2). It was previously called the urogenital diaphragm, and this change in name reflects the appreciation that it is not a two-layered structure with muscle in between, as was previously thought. It lies just caudal to the skeletal muscle of the striated urogenital sphincter (formerly the deep transverse perineal muscle). Because of the presence of the vagina, the perineal membrane cannot form a continuous sheet to close off the anterior pelvis in the woman, as it does in the man. It does provide support for the posterior vaginal wall by attaching the perineal body and vagina and perineal body to the ischiopubic rami, thereby limiting their downward descent. This layer of the floor arises from the inner aspect of the inferior ischiopubic rami above the ischiocavernous muscles and the crura of the clitoris. The medial attachments of the perineal membrane are to the urethra, walls of the vagina, and perineal body.

Just cephalad to the perineal membrane lie two arch-shaped muscles that begin posteriorly to arch over the urethra (Fig. 7.5). These are the compressor urethral and the urethrovaginal sphincter. They are a part of the striated urogenital sphincter muscle in the woman and are continuous with the sphincter urethrae muscle. They act to compress the distal urethra. Posteriorly, intermingled within the membrane are skeletal muscle fibers of the transverse vaginal muscle and some smooth muscle fibers. The dorsal and deep nerve and vessels of the clitoris are also found within this membrane and are described later.

The primary function of the perineal membrane is related to its attachment to the vagina and perineal body. By attaching these structures to the bony pelvic outlet, the perineal membrane supports the pelvic floor against the effects of increases in intraabdominal pressure and against the effects of gravity. The amount of downward descent that is permitted by this mechanism can be assessed by placing a finger in the rectum, hooking it forward, and pulling the perineal body downward. If the perineal membrane has been torn during parturition, then an abnormal amount of descent is detectable, and the pelvic floor sags and the introitus gapes.

Perineal Body

Within the area bounded by the lower vagina, perineal skin, and anus is a mass of connective tissue called the perineal body (Fig. 7.3). The term *central tendon of the perineum* has also

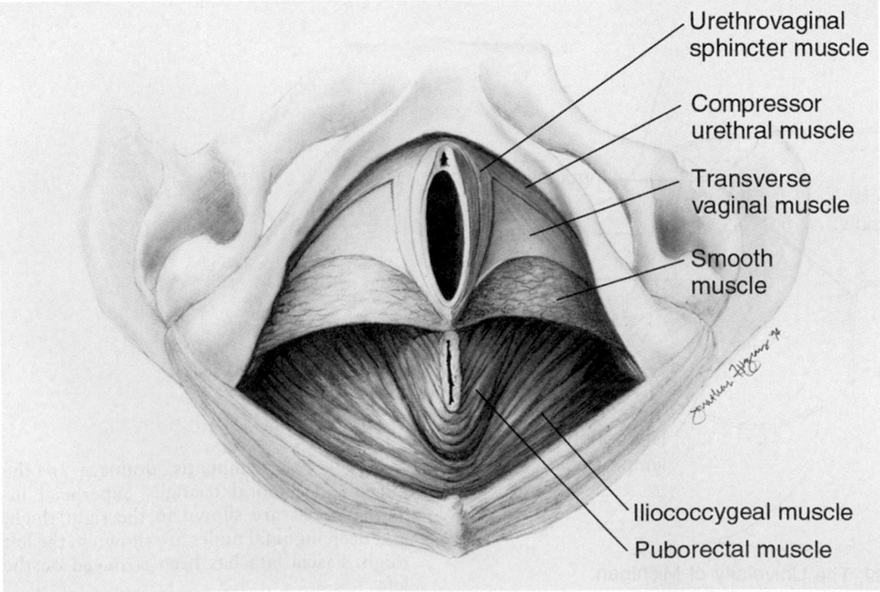

FIGURE 7.5. Structures visible after removal of the perineal membrane and superficial perineal muscles. (From: DeLancey, copyright 1995, with permission.)

been applied to this structure and is descriptive, suggesting its role as a central point into which many muscles insert.

The perineal body is attached to the inferior pubic rami and ischial tuberosities through the perineal membrane and superficial transverse perineal muscles. Anterolaterally, it receives the insertion of the bulbocavernous muscles. On its lateral margins, the upper portions of the perineal body are connected with some fibers of the pelvic diaphragm. Posteriorly, the perineal body is indirectly attached to the coccyx by the external anal sphincter that is embedded in the perineal body, and it is attached at its other end to the coccyx. These connections anchor the perineal body and its surrounding structures to the bony pelvis and help to keep it in place.

Posterior Triangle: Ischiorectal Fossa

In the posterior triangle of the pelvis, the ischiorectal fossa lies between the pelvic walls and the levator ani muscles (Fig. 7.3). It has an anterior recess that lies above the perineal membrane. It is bounded medially by the levator ani muscles and anterolaterally by the obturator internus muscle. The main portion of the fossa is lateral to the levator ani and external anal sphincter, and it has a posterior portion that extends above the gluteus maximus. Traversing this region is the pudendal neurovascular trunk.

Anal Sphincters

The external sphincter lies in the posterior triangle of the perineum (Fig. 7.6). It is a single mass of muscle, which has traditionally been divided into superficial and deep portions. The subcutaneous portion lies attached to the perianal skin and forms an encircling ring around the anal canal. It is responsible for the characteristic radially oriented folds in the perianal skin. The superficial part attaches to the coccyx posteriorly and sends a few fibers into the perineal body anteriorly and forms the bulk of the anal sphincter seen separated in third-degree midline obstetric tears. The fibers of the deep part generally encircle the rectum and blend indistinguishably with the puborectalis, which forms a loop under the dorsal surface of the anorectum and which is attached anteriorly to the pubic bone (Fig. 7.6).

The internal anal sphincter is a thickening in the circular smooth muscle of the anal wall. It lies just inside the external anal sphincter and is separated from it by a visible intersphincteric groove. It extends downward inside the external anal sphincter to within a few millimeters of the external sphincter's caudal extent. The internal sphincter can be identified just beneath the anal submucosa in repair of a chronic fourth-degree laceration of the perineum as a rubbery white layer that is often erroneously been referred to as fascia during obstetrical repair of 4th degree laceration. The longitudinal smooth muscle layer of the bowel, along with some fibers of the levator ani, separates the external and internal sphincters as they descend in the intersphincteric groove.

Levator Ani and Pelvic Wall

Unfortunately, the extreme abdominal pressures generated during embalming greatly distort the levator ani muscles by forcing them downward. Most anatomy atlases therefore fail to give a true picture of the horizontal nature of this strong supportive shelf of muscle. Examination of the normal standing patient is the best way to appreciate the nature of this closure mechanism, because the lithotomy position causes some relaxation of the musculature. During routine pelvic examination of the nullipara, the effectiveness of this closure can be appreciated, because it is often difficult to insert a speculum if the muscles are contracted and not relaxed.

The opening between the bones and muscles of the pelvic wall is spanned by the muscles of the pelvic diaphragm: the pubococcygeal, iliococcygeal, puborectal, and coccygeal muscles (Fig. 7.7). The most medial of these muscles is the puborectal–pubococcygeal complex. The pubococcygeal portion of these muscles has an insertion into the anococcygeal raphe and the superior surface of the coccyx, whereas the puborectal portion represents those inferior fibers that pass behind and insert

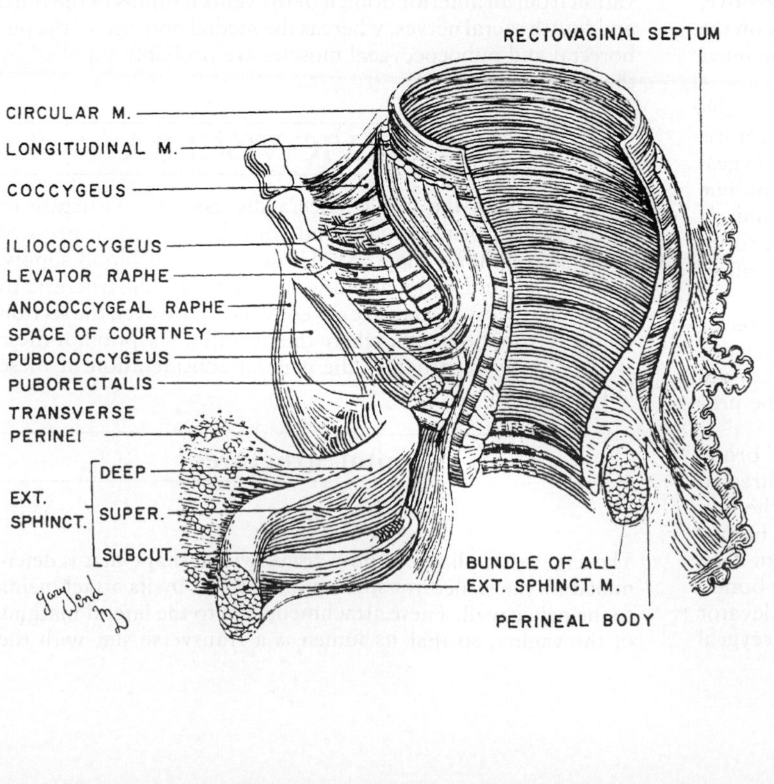

FIGURE 7.6. Semidiagrammatic dissection of the anorectal region in the woman with the external sphincter cut in the anterior midsagittal plane and reflected posteriorly (mucosa removed). The origin of the anterior muscle-bundle is clarified, and the remaining anterolateral portions of the external sphincters are interdigitated into the transverse perinei. (From: Oh C, Kark AE. Anatomy of the external anal sphincter. *Br J Surg* 1972;59:717–772, with permission.)

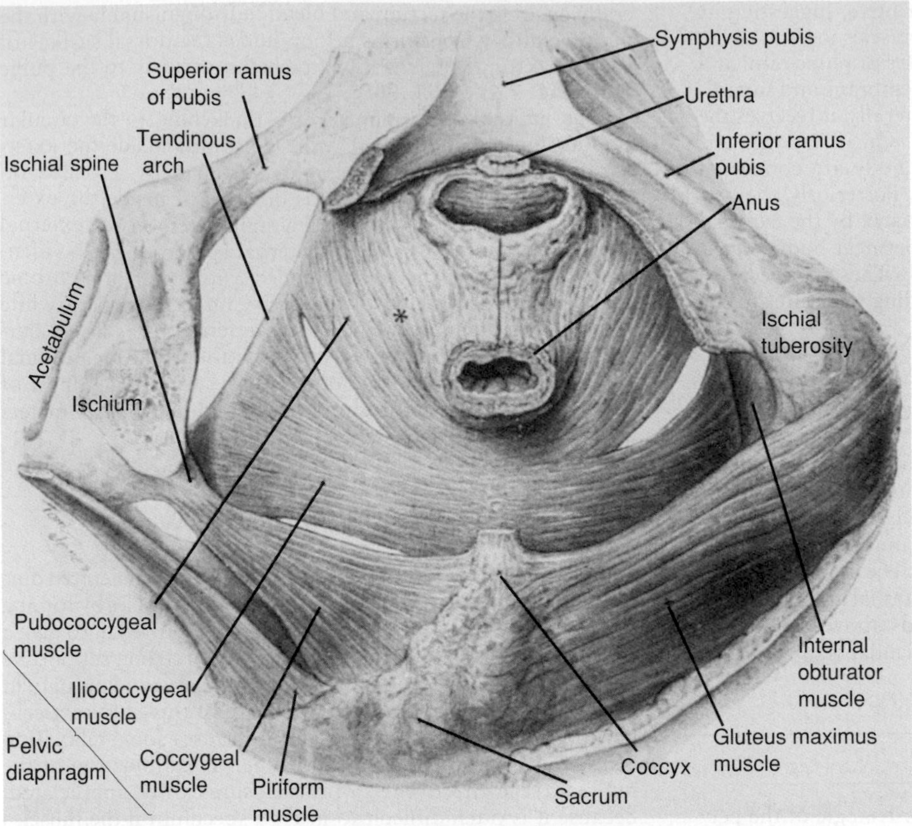

FIGURE 7.7. Anatomy of the pelvic floor. The asterisk indicates the puborectalis portion of the pubococcygeal muscle. (From: Anson BJ. *An atlas of human anatomy.* Philadelphia: WB Saunders, 1950, with permission.)

into the rectum. Both portions arise from the inner surface of the pubic bones and pass the urethra without attaching to it. Some fibers attach to the lateral vaginal wall and external anal sphincter and form a sling around the rectum before returning to a similar course on the other side. The pubococcygeal portion passes posteriorly from its origin ventral to the iliococcygeal muscle, where its fibers insert between the internal and external anal sphincter muscles in the intersphincteric groove, and form a sling behind the rectum. A few fibers also run on the cephalic surface of the iliococcygeal muscle to reach the inner surface of the sacrum and the coccyx.

The iliococcygeal muscle arises from a fibrous band overlying the obturator internus called the arcus tendineus levatoris ani. From these broad origins, the fibers of the iliococcygeal muscle pass behind the rectum and insert into the midline anococcygeal raphe and the coccyx. The coccygeal muscle arises from the ischial spine and sacrospinous ligament to insert into the borders of the coccyx and the lowest segment of the sacrum.

These muscles are covered on their superior and inferior surfaces by superior and inferior fasciae. When the levator ani muscles and their fasciae are considered together, they are called the pelvic diaphragm, not to be confused with the urogenital diaphragm (perineal membrane).

The muscle fibers of the pelvic diaphragm form a broad U-shaped layer of muscle with the open end of the U directed anteriorly. The open area within the U through which the urethra, vagina, and rectum pass is called the urogenital hiatus. The normal tone of the muscles of the pelvic diaphragm keep the base of the U pressed against the backs of the pubic bones, keeping the vagina and rectum closed. The region of the levator ani between the anus and coccyx formed by the anococcygeal raphe (see previous discussion) is clinically called the levator plate. It forms a supportive shelf on which the rectum, upper vagina, and uterus can rest. The relatively horizontal position of this shelf is determined by the anterior traction on the fibrous levator plane by the pubococcygeal and puborectal muscles and is important to vaginal and uterine support.

The iliococcygeal and coccygeal muscles receive their innervation from an anterior branch of the ventral ramus of the third and fourth sacral nerves, whereas the medial portions of the puborectal and pubococcygeal muscles are probably supplied by the pudendal nerve.

THE PELVIC VISCERA

This section on the pelvic viscera discusses the structure of the individual pelvic organs and considers specific aspects of their interrelations (Fig. 7.8). Those aspects of blood supply, innervation, and lymphatic drainage that are idiosyncratic to the specific pelvic viscera are covered here. However, the section on the retroperitoneum, where the overall description of these systems is given, provides the general consideration of these latter three topics.

Genital Structures

Vagina

The vagina is a pliable hollow viscus with a shape that is determined by the structures surrounding it and by its attachments to the pelvic wall. These attachments are to the lateral margins of the vagina, so that its lumen is a transverse slit, with the

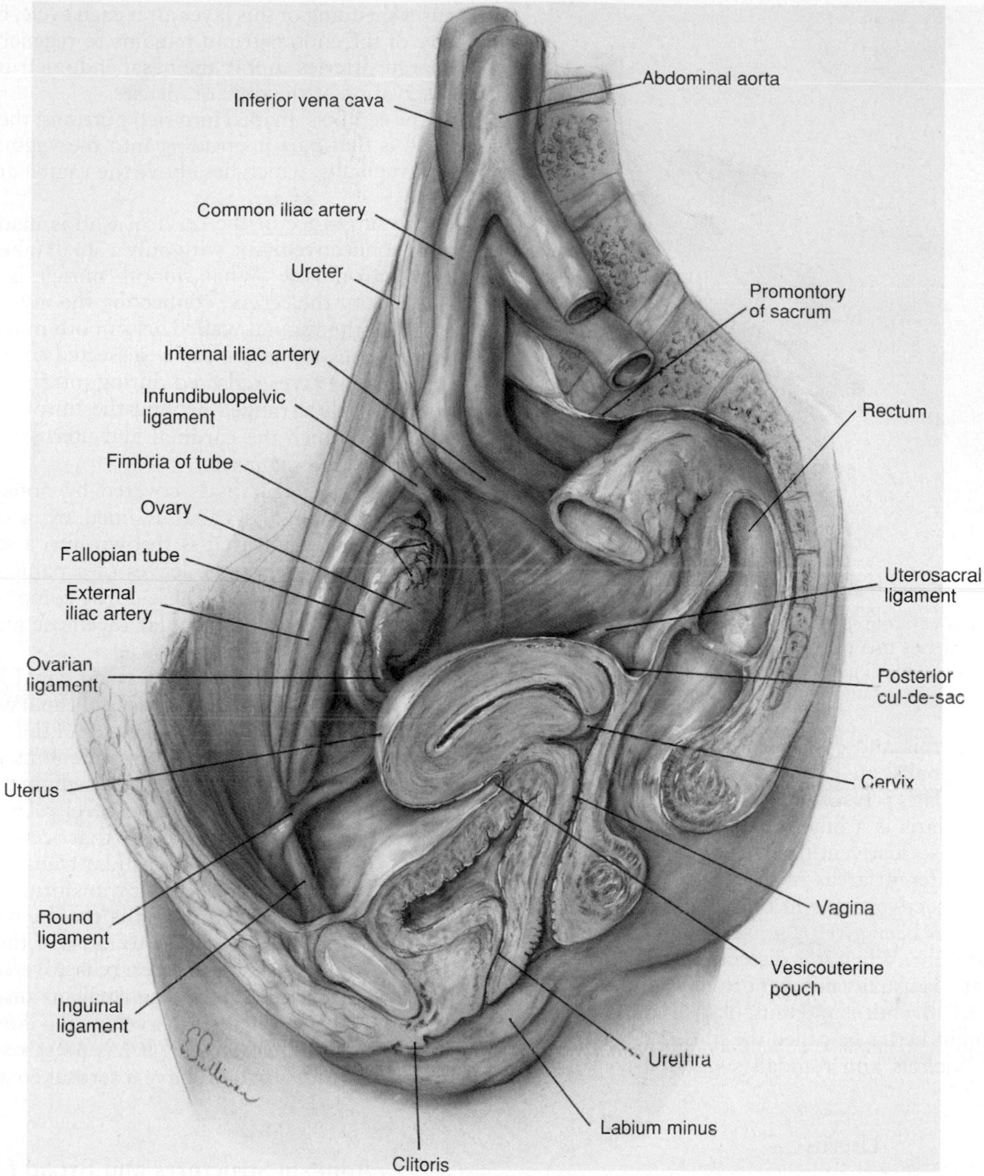

FIGURE 7.8. The pelvic viscera.

anterior and posterior walls in contact with one another. The lower portion of the vagina is constricted as it passes through the urogenital hiatus in the levator ani. The upper part is much more capacious. The vagina is bent at an angle of 120 degrees by the anterior traction of the levator ani muscles at the junction of the lower one third and upper two thirds of the vagina (Fig. 7.9). The cervix typically lies within the anterior vaginal wall, making it shorter than the posterior wall by about 3 cm. The former is about 7 to 9 cm in length, although there is great variability in this dimension.

When the lumen of the vagina is inspected through the introitus, many landmarks can be seen. The anterior and posterior walls have a midline ridge, called the anterior and posterior columns, respectively. These are caused by the impression of the urethra and bladder and the rectum on the vaginal lumen. The caudal portion of the anterior column is distinct and is called the urethral carina. The recesses in front of and behind the cervix are commonly called the anterior and posterior fornices of the vagina, and the creases along the side of the vagina, where the anterior and posterior walls meet, are called the lateral vaginal sulci.

The vagina's relations to other parts of the body can be understood by dividing it into thirds. In the lower third, the vagina is fused anteriorly with the urethra, posteriorly with the perineal body, and laterally to each levator ani by the "fibers of Luschka." In the middle third are the vesical neck and trigone anteriorly, the rectum posteriorly, and the levators laterally. In the upper third, the anterior vagina is adjacent to the bladder and ureters (which allow these latter structures to be palpated on pelvic examination), posterior to the cul-de-sac, and lateral to the cardinal ligaments of the vagina.

The vaginal wall contains the same layers as all hollow viscera (i.e., mucosa, submucosa, muscularis, and adventitia). Except for the area covered by the cul-de-sac, it has no serosal covering. The mucosa is of the nonkeratinized stratified squamous type and lies on a dense, dermislike submucosa. The similarity

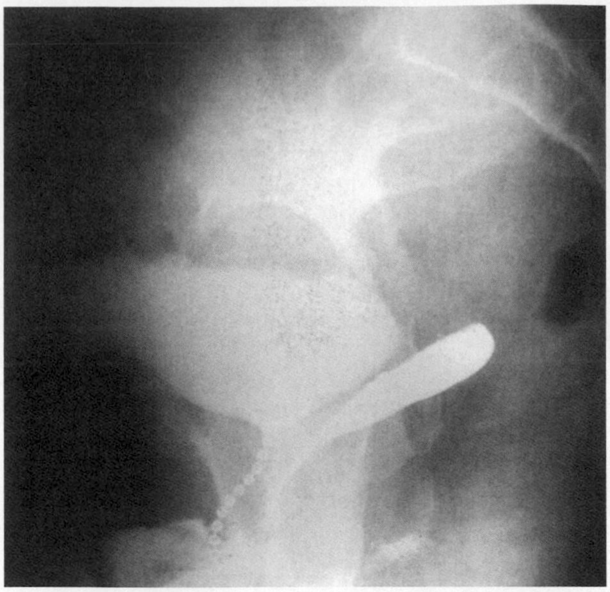

FIGURE 7.9. Bead chain cystourethrogram with barium in the vagina showing normal vaginal axis in a patient in the standing position.

of these layers to dermis and epidermis has resulted in their being called the "vaginal skin."

The vaginal muscularis is fused with the submucosa, and the pattern of the muscularis is a bihelical arrangement. Outside the muscularis there is an adventitia that has varying degrees of development in different areas of the vagina. This layer is a portion of the connective tissue in the pelvis called the endopelvic fascia and has been given a separate name because of its unusual development. When it is dissected in the operating room, the muscularis is usually adherent to it, and this combination of specialized adventitia and muscularis is the surgeon's "fascia," which might better be called the fibromuscular layer of the vagina, as Nichols and Randall suggested in *Vaginal Surgery*.

Uterus

The uterus is a fibromuscular organ with shape, weight, and dimensions that vary considerably, depending on both estrogenic stimulation and previous parturition. It has two portions: an upper muscular corpus and a lower fibrous cervix. In a woman of reproductive age, the corpus is considerably larger than the cervix, but before menarche, and after the menopause, their sizes are similar. Within the corpus, there is a triangularly shaped endometrial cavity surrounded by a thick muscular wall. That portion of the corpus that extends above the top of the endometrial cavity (i.e., above the insertions of the fallopian tubes) is called the fundus.

The muscle fibers that make up most of the uterine corpus are not arranged in a simple layered manner, as is true in the gastrointestinal tract, but are arranged in a more complex pattern. This pattern reflects the origin of the uterus from paired paramesonephric primordia, with the fibers from each half crisscrossing diagonally with those of the opposite side.

The uterus is lined by a unique mucosa, the endometrium. It has both a columnar epithelium that forms glands and a specialized stroma. The superficial portion of this layer undergoes cyclic change with the menstrual cycle. Spasm of hormonally sensitive spiral arterioles that lie within the endometrium causes shedding of this layer after each cycle, but a deeper basal layer of the endometrium remains to regenerate a new lining. Separate arteries supply the basal endometrium, explaining its preservation at the time of menses.

The cervix is divided into two portions: the portio vaginalis, which is that part protruding into the vagina; and the portio supravaginalis, which lies above the vagina and below the corpus.

The substance of the cervical wall is made up of dense fibrous connective tissue with only a small (about 10%) amount of smooth muscle. What smooth muscle is there lies on the periphery of the cervix, connecting the myometrium with the muscle of the vaginal wall. This smooth muscle and accompanying fibrous tissue are easily dissected off the fibrous cervix and form the layer reflected during intrafascial hysterectomy. It is circularly arranged around the fibrous cervix and is the tissue into which the cardinal and uterosacral ligaments and pubocervical fascia insert.

The portio vaginalis is covered by nonkeratinizing squamous epithelium. Its canal is lined by a columnar mucus-secreting epithelium that is thrown into a series of V-shaped folds that appear like the leaves of a palm and are therefore called plicae palmatae. These form compound clefts in the endocervical canal, not tubular racemose glands, as formerly thought.

The upper border of the cervical canal is marked by the internal os, where the narrow cervical canal widens out into the endometrial cavity. The lower border of the canal, the external os, contains the transition from squamous epithelium of the portio vaginalis to the columnar epithelium of the endocervical canal. This occurs at a variable level relative to the os and changes with hormonal variations that occur during a woman's life. It is in this active area of cellular transition that the cervix is most susceptible to malignant transformation.

There is little adventitia in the uterus, with the peritoneal serosa being directly attached to most of the corpus. The anterior portion of the uterine cervix is covered by the bladder; therefore, it has no serosa. Similarly, as discussed in the following, the broad ligament envelops the lateral aspects of the cervix and corpus; therefore, it has no serosal covering there. The posterior cervix does have a serosal covering.

Adnexal Structures and Broad Ligament

The fallopian tubes are paired tubular structures 7 to 12 cm in length (Fig. 7.10). Each has four recognizable portions. At the uterus, the tube passes through the cornu as an interstitial portion. On emerging from the corpus, a narrow isthmic portion begins with a narrow lumen and thick muscular wall. Proceeding toward the abdominal end, next is the ampulla, which has an expanding lumen and more convoluted mucosa. The fimbriated end of the tube has many frondlike projections to provide a wide surface for ovum pickup. The distal end of the fallopian tube is attached to the ovary by the fimbria ovarica, which is a smooth muscle band responsible for bringing the fimbria and ovary close to one another at the time of ovulation. The outer layer of the tube's muscularis is composed of longitudinal fibers; the inner layer has a circular orientation.

The lateral pole of the ovary is attached to the pelvic wall by the infundibulopelvic ligament and the ovarian artery and vein contained therein. Medially, it is connected to the uterus through the uteroovarian ligament. During reproductive life, it measures about 2.5 to 5 cm long, 1.5 to 3 cm thick, and 0.7 to 1.5 cm wide, varying with its state of activity or suppression, as with oral contraceptive medications. Its surface is mostly

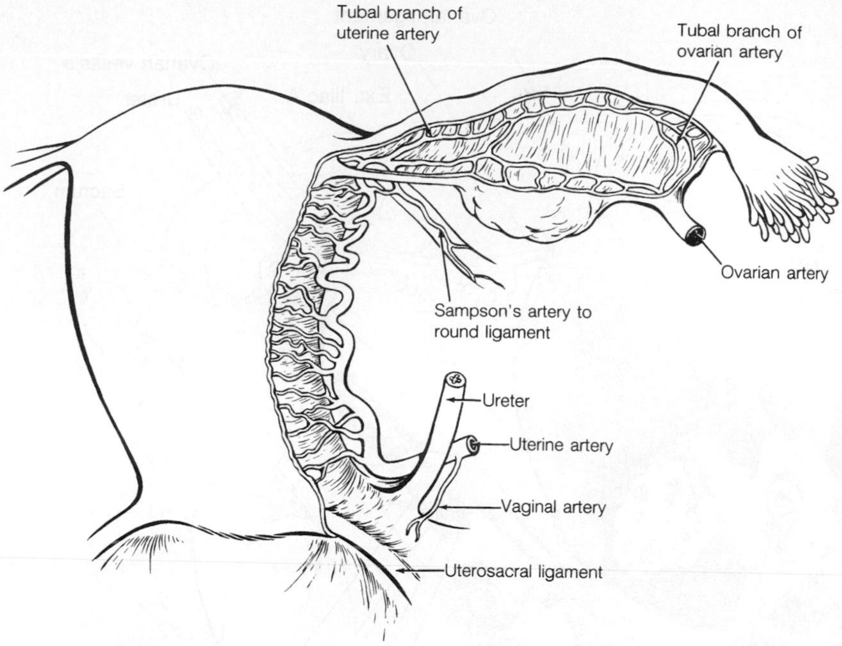

FIGURE 7.10. Uterine adnexa and collateral circulation of uterine and ovarian arteries. The uterine artery crosses over the ureter in the cardinal ligament and gives off cervical and vaginal branches before ascending adjacent to the wall of the uterus and anastomosing with the medial end of the ovarian artery. Note the small branch of the uterine or ovarian artery that nourishes the round ligament (Sampson artery).

free but has an attachment to the broad ligament through the mesovarium, as discussed in the following.

The ovary has a cuboidal to columnar covering and consists of a cortex and medulla. The medullary portion is primarily fibromuscular, with many blood vessels and much connective tissue. The cortex is composed of a more specialized stroma, punctuated with follicles, corpora lutea, and corpora albicantia.

The round ligaments are extensions of the uterine musculature and represent the homolog of the gubernaculum testis. They begin as broad bands that arise on each lateral aspect of the anterior corpus. They assume a more rounded shape before they enter the retroperitoneal tissue, where they pass lateral to the deep inferior epigastric vessels and enter each internal inguinal ring. After traversing the inguinal canal, they exit the external ring and enter the subcutaneous tissue of the labia majora. They have little to do with uterine support.

The ovaries and tubes constitute the uterine adnexa. They are covered by a specialized series of peritoneal folds called the broad ligament. During embryonic development, the paired müllerian ducts and ovaries arise from the lateral abdominopelvic walls. As they migrate toward the midline, a mesentery of peritoneum is pulled out from the pelvic wall from the cervix on up. This leaves the midline uterus connected on either side to the pelvic wall by a double layer of peritoneum.

Within the upper layers of these two folds, called the broad ligaments, lie the fallopian tubes, round ligaments, and ovaries (Fig. 7.11). The cardinal and uterosacral ligaments are at the lower margin of the broad ligament. These structures are visceral ligaments; therefore, they are composed of varying amounts of smooth muscle, vessels, connective tissue, and other structures. They are not the pure ligaments associated with joints in the skeleton.

The ovary, tube, and round ligament each have their own separate mesentery, called the mesovarium, mesosalpinx, and mesoteres, respectively. These are arranged in a constant pattern, with the round ligament placed ventrally, where it exits the pelvis through the inguinal ligament, and the ovary placed dorsally. The tube is in the middle and is the most cephalic of the three structures. At the lateral end of the fallopian tube and ovary, the broad ligament ends where the infundibulopelvic ligament blends with the pelvic wall. The cardinal ligaments lie at the base of the broad ligament and are described under the section on supportive tissues and cleavage planes.

Blood Supply and Lymphatics of the Genital Tract

The blood supply to the genital organs comes from the ovarian arteries and uterine and vaginal branches of the internal iliac arteries. A continuous arterial arcade connects these vessels on the lateral border of the adnexa, uterus, and vagina (Fig. 7.10).

The blood supply of the upper adnexal structures comes from the ovarian arteries that arise from the anterior surface of the aorta just below the level of the renal arteries. The accompanying plexus of veins drains into the vena cava on the right and the renal vein on the left. The arteries and veins follow a long, retroperitoneal course before reaching the cephalic end of the ovary. They pass along the mesenteric surface of the ovary to connect with the upper end of the marginal artery of the uterus. Because the ovarian artery runs along the hilum of the ovary, it not only supplies the gonad but also sends many small vessels through the mesosalpinx to supply the fallopian tube, including a prominent fimbrial branch at the lateral end of the tube.

The uterine artery originates from the internal iliac artery. It usually arises independently from this source but can have a common origin with either the internal pudendal or vaginal artery. It joins the uterus near the junction of the corpus and cervix, but this position varies considerably, both with the individual and the amount of upward or downward traction placed on the uterus. Accompanying each uterine artery are several large uterine veins that drain the corpus and cervix.

On arriving at the lateral border of the uterus (after passing over the ureter and giving off a small branch to this structure), the uterine artery flows into the side of the marginal artery that

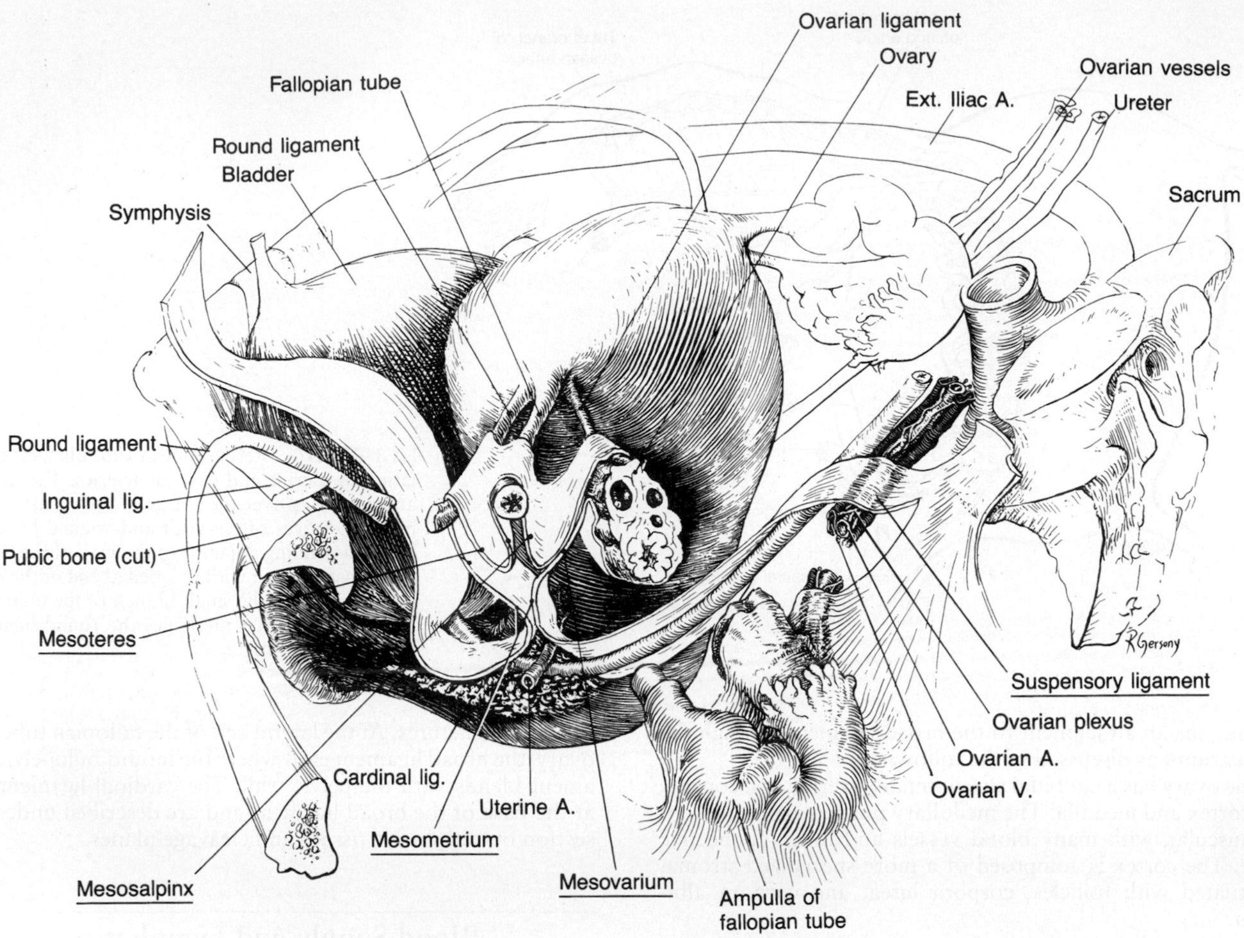

FIGURE 7.11. Composition of the broad ligament.

runs along the side of the uterus. Through this connection, it sends blood both upward toward the corpus and downward to the cervix. Because the marginal artery continues along the lateral aspect of the cervix, it eventually crosses over the cervicovaginal junction and lies on the side of the vagina.

The vagina receives its blood supply from a downward extension of the uterine artery along the lateral sulci of the vagina and from a vaginal branch of the internal iliac artery. These form an anastomotic arcade along the lateral aspect of the vagina at the 3- and 9-o'clock positions. Branches from these vessels also merge along the anterior and posterior vaginal walls. The distal vagina also receives a supply from the pudendal vessels, and the posterior wall has a contribution from the middle and inferior hemorrhoidal vessels.

Lymphatic drainage of the upper two thirds of the vagina and uterus is primarily to the obturator and internal and external iliac nodes, and the distal-most vagina drains with the vulvar lymphatics to the inguinal nodes. In addition, some lymphatic channels from the uterine corpus extend along the round ligament to the superficial inguinal nodes, and some nodes extend posteriorly along the uterosacral ligaments to the lateral sacral nodes. These routes of drainage are discussed more fully in the discussion of the retroperitoneal space.

The lymphatic drainage of the ovary follows the ovarian vessels to the region of the lower abdominal aorta, where they drain into the lumbar chain of nodes (paraaortic nodes).

The uterus receives its nerve supply from the uterovaginal plexus (Frankenhäuser ganglion) that lies in the connective tissue of the cardinal ligament. Details of the organization of the pelvic innervation are contained in the section on retroperitoneal structures.

Lower Urinary Tract

Ureter

The ureter is a tubular viscus about 25 cm long, divided into abdominal and pelvic portions of equal length. Its small lumen is surrounded by an inner longitudinal and outer circular muscle layer. In the abdomen, it lies in the extraperitoneal connective tissue on the posterior abdominal wall, crossed anteriorly by the left and right colic vessels. Its course and blood supply are described in the section on the retroperitoneum.

Bladder

The bladder can be divided into two portions: the dome and base (Fig. 7.12). The musculature of the spherical bladder does not lie in simple layers, as do the muscular walls of tubular viscera, such as the gut and ureter. It is best described as a meshwork of intertwining muscle bundles. The musculature of the

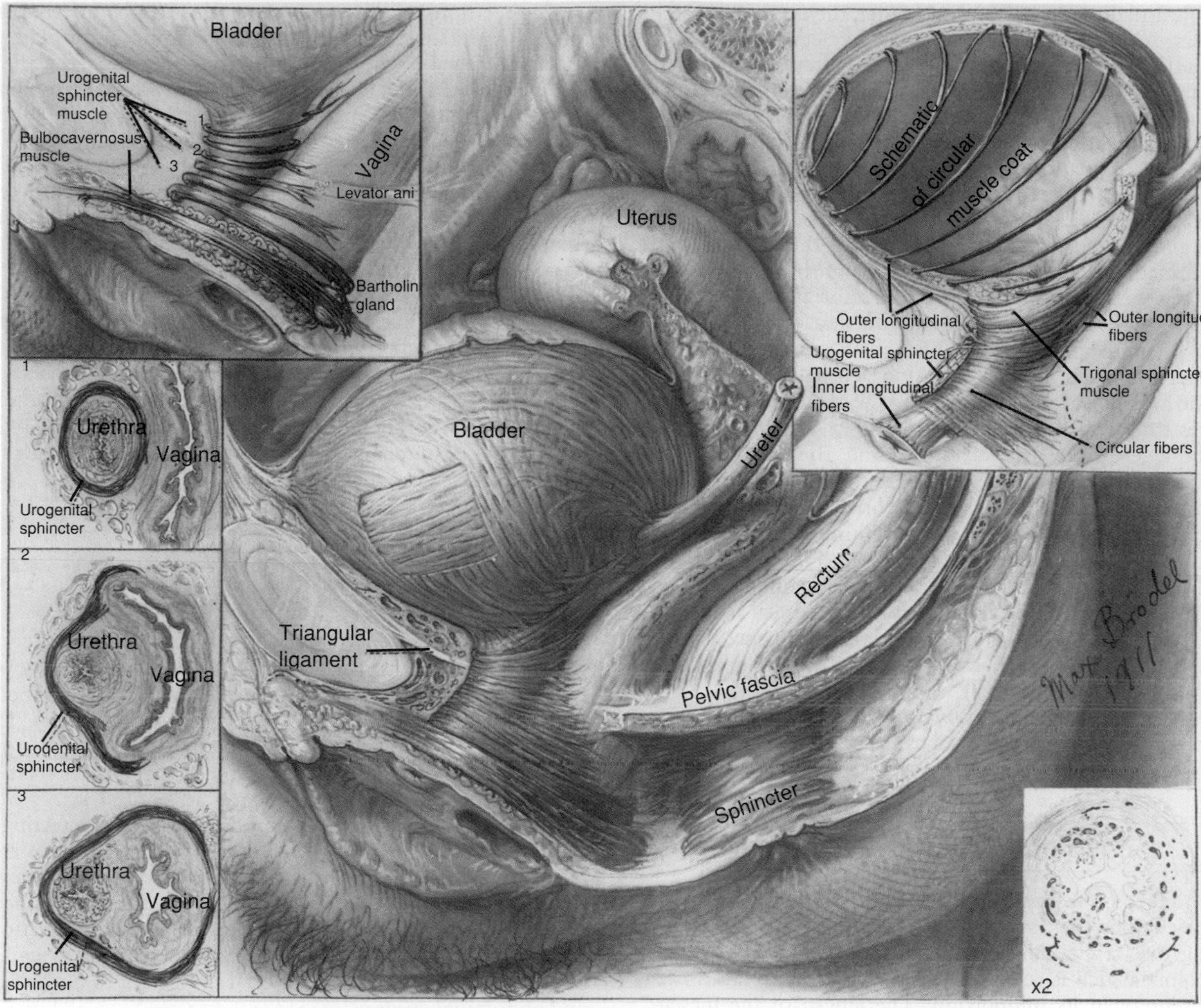

FIGURE 7.12. Lateral view of the pelvic organs showing the urethra and bladder. **Inset 3:** Two portions of the striated urogenital sphincter muscle, namely, the urethrovaginal sphincter and the urethral sphincter. The compressor urethra is not seen. (From: The Brödel Collection, Department of Art as Applied to Medicine, Johns Hopkins Medical Institution, Baltimore, MD, with permission.)

dome is relatively thin when the bladder is distended. The base of the bladder, which is thicker and varies less with distention of the dome, consists of the urinary trigone and a thickening of the detrusor, called the detrusor loop. This is a U-shaped band of musculature, open posteriorly, that forms the bladder base anterior to the intramural portion of the ureter. The trigone is made of smooth muscle that arises from the ureters that occupy two of its three corners. It continues as the muscle of the vesical neck and urethra. There it rests on the upper vagina. The shape of the bladder depends on its state of filling. When empty, it is a somewhat flattened disk, slightly concave upward. As it fills, the dome rises off the base, eventually assuming a more spherical shape.

The distinction between the base and dome has functional importance, because they have differing innervations. The bladder base has α-adrenergic receptors that contract when stimulated and thereby favor continence. The dome is responsive to β or cholinergic stimulation, with contraction that causes bladder emptying.

Anteriorly, the bladder lies against the lower abdominal wall. It lies against the pubic bones laterally and inferiorly and abuts the obturator internus and levator ani. Posteriorly, it rests against the vagina and cervix. These relations are discussed further in consideration of the pelvic planes and spaces.

The blood supply of the bladder comes from the superior vesical artery, which comes off the obliterated umbilical artery and inferior vesical artery, which is either an independent branch of the internal pudendal artery or arises from the vaginal artery.

Urethra

The urethral lumen begins at the internal urinary meatus and has a series of regional differences in its structure. It passes through the bladder base in an intramural portion for a little less than a centimeter. This region of the bladder, where the urethral lumen traverses the bladder base, is called the vesical neck.

The urethra itself begins outside the bladder wall. In its distal two thirds it is fused with the vagina (Fig. 7.12), with which it shares a common embryologic derivation. From the vesical neck to the perineal membrane, which starts at the junction of the middle and distal thirds of the bladder, the urethra has several layers. An outer, circularly oriented skeletal muscle layer (urogenital sphincter) mingles with some circularly oriented smooth muscle fibers. Inside this layer is a longitudinal layer of smooth muscle that surrounds a remarkably vascular submucosa and nonkeratinized squamous epithelium that responds to estrogenic stimulation.

Within the submucosa is a group of tubular glands that lie on the vaginal surface of the urethra. These paraurethral (or Skene's) glands empty into the lumen at several points on the dorsal surface of the urethra, but two prominent openings on the inner aspects of the external urethral orifice can be seen when the orifice is opened. Chronic infection of these glands can lead to urethral diverticula, and obstruction of their terminal duct can result in cyst formation. Their location on the dorsal surface of the urethra reflects the distribution of the structures from which they arise.

At the level of the perineal membrane, the distal portion of the urogenital sphincter begins. Here the skeletal muscle of the urethra leaves the urethral wall to form the urethrovaginal sphincter (Fig. 7.5) and compressor urethrae (formerly called the deep transverse perineal muscle). Distal to this portion, the urethral wall is fibrous and forms a nozzle for aiming the urinary stream. The mechanical support of the vesical neck and urethra, which are so important to urinary continence, is discussed in the section of this chapter devoted to the supportive tissues of the urogenital system.

The urethra receives its blood supply both from an inferior extension of the vesical vessels and from the pudendal vessels.

Sigmoid Colon and Rectum

The sigmoid colon begins its S-shaped curve at the pelvic brim. It has the characteristic structure of the colon, with three tenia coli lying over a circular smooth muscle layer. Unlike much of the colon, which is retroperitoneal, the sigmoid has a definite mesentery in its midportion. The length of the mesentery and the pattern of the sigmoid's curvature vary considerably. It receives its blood supply from the lowermost portion of the inferior mesenteric artery: the branches called the sigmoid arteries.

As it enters the pelvis, the colon straightens its course and becomes the rectum. This portion extends from the pelvic brim until it loses its final anterior peritoneal investment below the cul-de-sac. It has two bands of smooth muscle (anterior and posterior). Its lumen has three transverse rectal folds that contain the mucosa, submucosa, and circular layers of the bowel wall. The most prominent fold, the middle one, lies anteriorly on the right about 8 cm above the anus, and it must be negotiated during high rectal examination or sigmoidoscopy.

As the rectum passes posterior to the vagina, it expands into the rectal ampulla. This portion of the bowel begins under the cul-de-sac peritoneum and fills the posterior pelvis from the side. At the distal end of the rectum, the anorectal junction is bent at an angle of 90 degrees where it is pulled ventrally by the puborectalis fibers' attachment to the pubes and posteriorly by the external anal sphincter's dorsal attachment to the coccyx.

Below this level, the gut is called the anus. It has many distinguishing features. There is a thickening of the circular involuntary muscle called the internal sphincter. The canal has a series of anal valves to assist in closure, and at their lower border the mucosa of the colon gives way to a transitional layer of non–hair-bearing squamous epithelium before becoming the hair-bearing perineal skin.

The relations of the rectum and anus can be inferred from their course. They lie against the sacrum and levator plate posteriorly and against the vagina anteriorly. Inferiorly, each half of the levator ani abuts its lateral wall and sends fibers to mingle with the longitudinal involuntary fibers between the internal and external sphincters. Its distal terminus is surrounded by the external anal sphincter.

The anorectum receives its blood supply from a number of sources (Fig. 7.13). From above, the superior rectal (hemorrhoidal) branch of the inferior mesenteric artery lies within the layers of the sigmoid mesocolon. As it reaches the beginning of the rectum, it divides into two branches and ends in the wall of the gut. A direct branch from the internal iliac artery arises from the pelvic wall on either side and supplies the rectum and ampulla above the pelvic floor. The anus and external sphincter receive their blood supply from the inferior rectal (hemorrhoidal) branch of the internal pudendal artery, which reaches the terminus of the gastrointestinal tract through the ischiorectal fossa.

PELVIC CONNECTIVE TISSUE AND CLEAVAGE PLANES

The pelvic viscera are connected to the lateral pelvic wall by their adventitial layers and thickenings of the connective tissue that lie over the pelvic wall muscles (Fig. 7.14). These attachments, as well as the attachments of one organ to another, separate the different surgical cleavage planes from one another. These condensations of the adventitial layers of the pelvic organs have assumed supportive roles, connecting the viscera to the pelvic walls, in addition to their role in transmitting the organs' neurovascular supply from the pelvic wall. They are somewhat like a mesentery that connects the bowel, for example, to the body wall. It has a supportive function as well as a role in carrying vessels and nerves to the organ. An understanding of their disposition is important to both vaginal and abdominal surgery.

The tissue that connects the organs to the pelvic wall has been given the special designation of *endopelvic fascia*. It is not a layer similar to the layer encountered during abdominal incisions (rectus abdominis "fascia"). It is composed of blood vessels and nerves, interspersed with a supportive meshwork of irregular connective tissue containing collagen and elastin. These structures connect the muscularis of the visceral organs to pelvic wall muscles. In some areas, there is considerable smooth muscle within this tissue, as is true in the area of the uterosacral ligaments. Although surgical texts often speak of this fascia as a specific structure separate from the viscera, this is not strictly true. These layers can be separated from the viscera, just as the superficial layers of the bowel wall can be artificially separated from the deeper layers, but they are not themselves separate structures.

Pelvic Connective Tissue

The term *ligament* is most familiar when it describes a dense connective tissue band that links two bones, but it also describes ridges in the peritoneum or thickenings of the endopelvic fascia. The ligaments of the genital tract are diverse. Although they share a common designation (i.e., ligament), they are composed of many types of tissue and have many different functions.

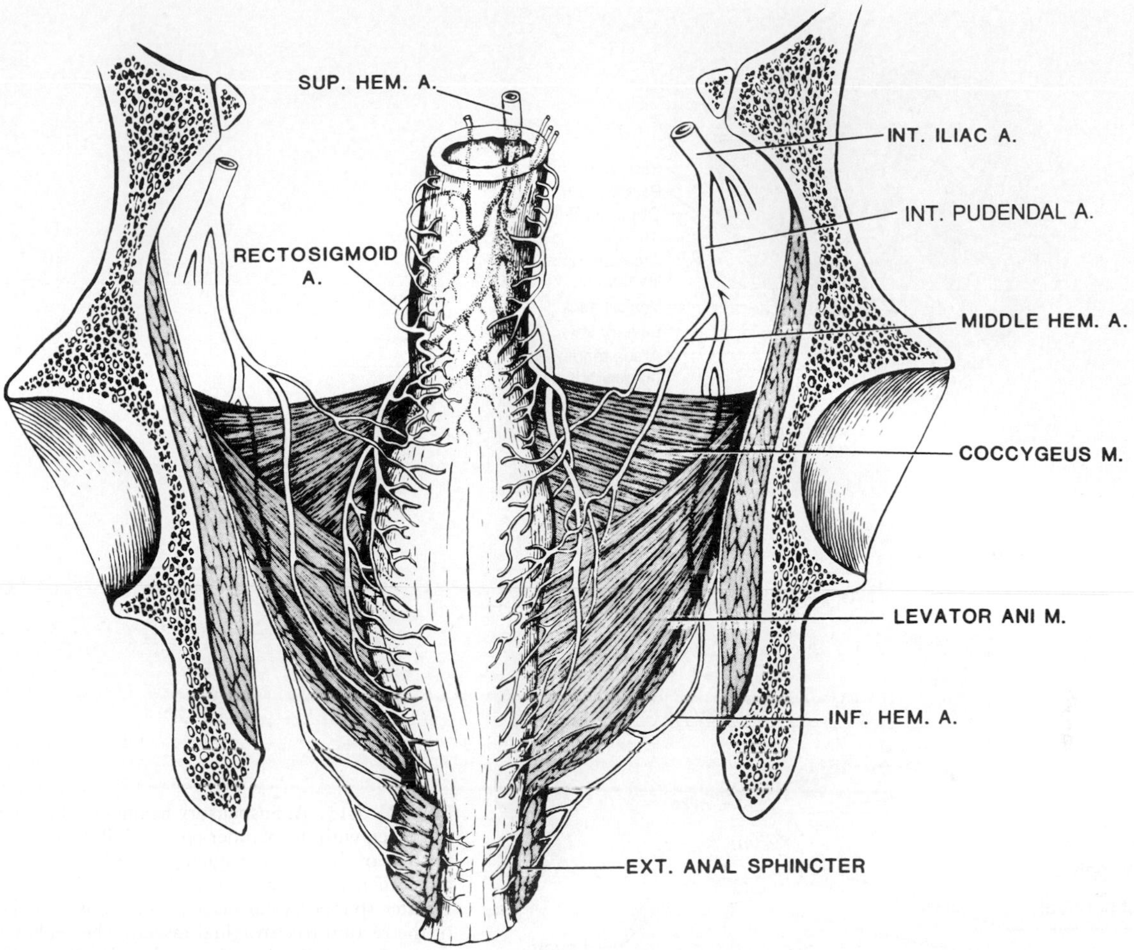

FIGURE 7.13. Rectosigmoid colon and anal canal, showing collateral arterial circulation from superior hemorrhoidal (inferior mesenteric), middle hemorrhoidal (hypogastric or internal iliac), and inferior hemorrhoidal (internal pudendal) arteries.

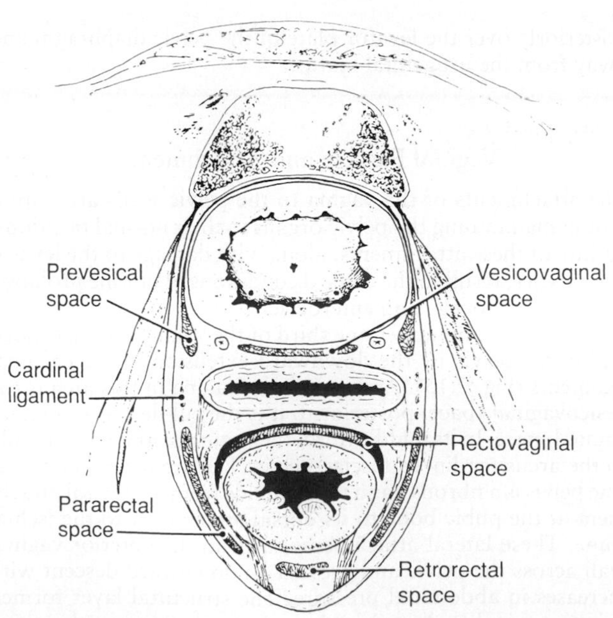

FIGURE 7.14. Cross section of the pelvis showing cleavage planes.

Uterine Ligaments

The broad ligaments are peritoneal folds that extend laterally from the uterus and cover the adnexal structures. They have no supportive function and were discussed in the section on the pelvic viscera.

Within the broad ligament, beginning just caudal to the uterine arteries, there is a thickening in the endopelvic fascia that attaches the cervix and upper vagina to the pelvic side walls (Fig. 7.15), consisting of the cardinal and uterosacral ligaments (parametrium). The term *uterosacral ligaments* refers to that portion of this tissue that forms the medial margin of the parametrium and that borders the cul-de-sac of Douglas. The term *cardinal ligament* is used to refer to that portion that attaches the lateral margins of the cervix and vagina to the pelvic walls. The cardinal and uterosacral ligaments, therefore, are simply two parts of a single body of suspensory tissue. The term *parametrium* refers to all of the tissue that attaches to the uterus (both cardinal and uterosacral ligaments), and the term *paracolpium* refers to the portion that attaches to the vagina (cardinal ligament of the vagina). The uterosacral ligament portion of the parametrium is composed predominantly of smooth muscle, the autonomic nerves of the pelvic organs, and some

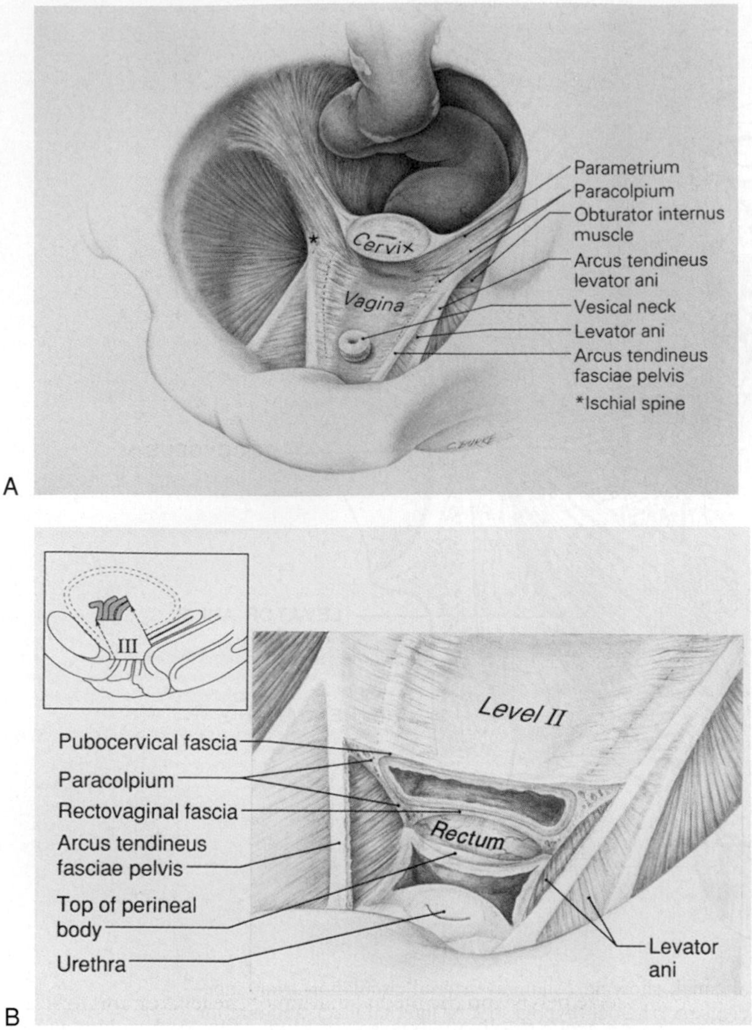

FIGURE 7.15. A: Suspensory ligaments of the female genital tract seen with the bladder removed. B: Close-up of the lower portion of the middle vagina (level II) shows how the lateral attachments of the vagina result in an anterior layer under the bladder (pubocervical fascia) and a posterior layer in front of the rectum (rectovaginal fascia). The cephalic surfaces of the transected distal urethra and vagina (level III) are shown. (From: DeLancey JOL. Anatomic aspects of vaginal eversion after hysterectomy. *Am J Obstet Gynecol* 1992;166:1717, with permission.)

intermixed connective tissue and blood vessels, whereas the cardinal ligament portion consists primarily of perivascular connective tissue and the pelvic vessels. Although they are often described as extending laterally from the cervix to the pelvic wall, in the standing position they are almost vertical as one would expect for a suspensory tissue. Near the cervix, they are discrete, but they fan out in the retroperitoneal layer to have a broad, if somewhat ill-defined, area of attachment over the second, third, and fourth segments of the sacrum. These ligaments hold the cervix posteriorly in the pelvis over the levator plate of the pelvic diaphragm.

The cardinal ligaments lie at the lower edge of the broad ligaments, between their peritoneal leaves, beginning just caudal to the uterine arteries. They attach to the cervix below the isthmus and fan out to attach to the pelvic walls over the piriformis muscle in the area of the greater sciatic foramen. Although when placed under tension they feel like ligamentous bands, they are composed simply of perivascular connective tissue and nerves that surround the uterine artery and veins. Nevertheless, these structures have considerable strength, and the lack of a separate "ligamentous band" in this area does not detract from their supportive role. They provide support not only to the cervix and uterus but also to the upper portion of the vagina (paracolpium) to keep these structures positioned posteriorly over the levator plate of the pelvic diaphragm and away from the urogenital hiatus.

Vaginal Fasciae and Attachments

The attachments of the vagina to the pelvic walls are important in maintaining the pelvic organs in their normal positions. Failure of these attachments, along with damage to the levator ani muscles, result in the clinical conditions of uterine prolapse, cystocele, rectocele, and enterocele.

The cervix and upper one third of the vagina are suspended within the pelvis by the downward extension of the cardinal ligaments (Fig. 7.15). Anterior to the vagina in this area is the vesicovaginal space; posterior to it is the cul-de-sac and rectovaginal space. In its middle third, the vagina is attached laterally to the arcus tendineus fasciae pelvis. The arcus tendineus fasciae pelvis is a fibrous band that extends from its ventral attachment at the pubic bone to its dorsal attachment to the ischial spine. These lateral attachments suspend the anterior vaginal wall across the pelvis and prevent its downward descent with increases in abdominal pressure. The structural layer formed by the vaginal wall and its lateral attachments to the arcus tendineus is clinically referred to as the pubocervical fascia.

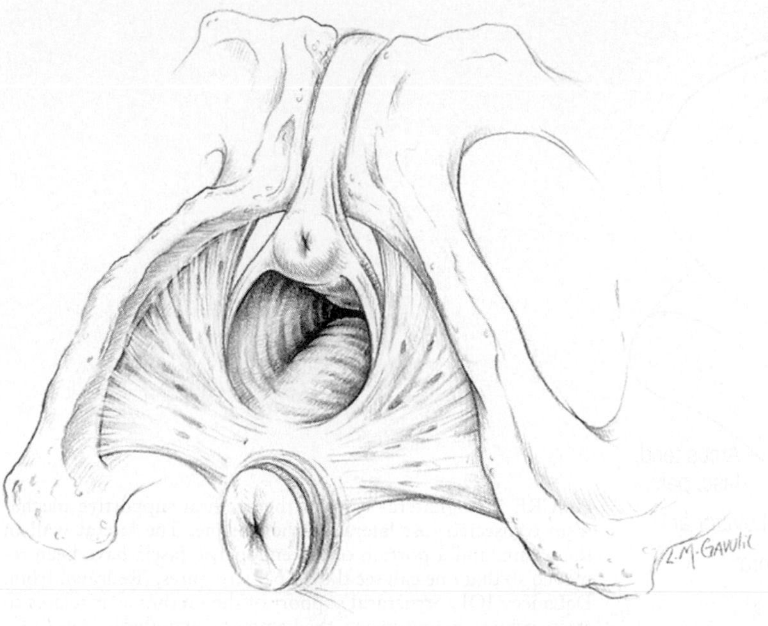

FIGURE 7.16. The peripheral attachments of the perineal membrane to the ischiopubic rami and direction of tension on fibers uniting through the perineal body. (From: DeLancey JOL. Structural anatomy of the posterior compartment as it relates to rectocele. *Am J Obstet Gynecol* 1999;180:815–823, with permission.)

Support of the posterior vaginal wall prevents the rectum from bulging forward in the clinical condition known as rectocele. This support varies in different levels of the vagina. In the distal 2 or 3 cm of the posterior vaginal wall, attachments of the perineal body to the ischiopubic rami hold the perineal body in place and prevent protrusion of the distal rectum (Fig. 7.16). In the midvagina above this, the vagina is attached laterally to the fascia covering the inside of the levator ani muscles (Fig. 7.17). This connection prevents the middle of the posterior vaginal wall from moving forward and downward during increases in abdominal pressure. The combination of these attachments results in a structural layer that has been referred to by the term *fascia of Denonvilliers*. Detailed histologic studies of this area, however, have failed to reveal a separate layer in the midline between the muscularis of the vagina and the rectovaginal space except in the distal vagina, where the dense connective tissue of the perineal body separates these structures.

Urethral Supports

The support of the proximal urethra is important in the maintenance of urinary continence during times of increased abdominal pressure. The distal portion of the urethra is insepa rable from the vagina because of their common embryologic derivation. These tissues are fixed firmly in position by connections of the periurethral tissues and vagina to the pubic bones through the perineal membrane (Fig. 7.18). A hammocklike layer composed of the endopelvic fascia and anterior vaginal wall provides the support of the proximal urethra. This layer is stabilized by its lateral attachments both to the arcus tendineus fasciae pelvis and the medial margin of the levator ani muscles. The arcus tendineus fasciae pelvis is a fibrous band stretched from a ventral attachment at the lower portion of the pubic bones about 1 cm above the lower margin of the pubic bones and 1 cm from the midline to the ischial spine. The muscular attachment of the endopelvic fascia allows contraction and

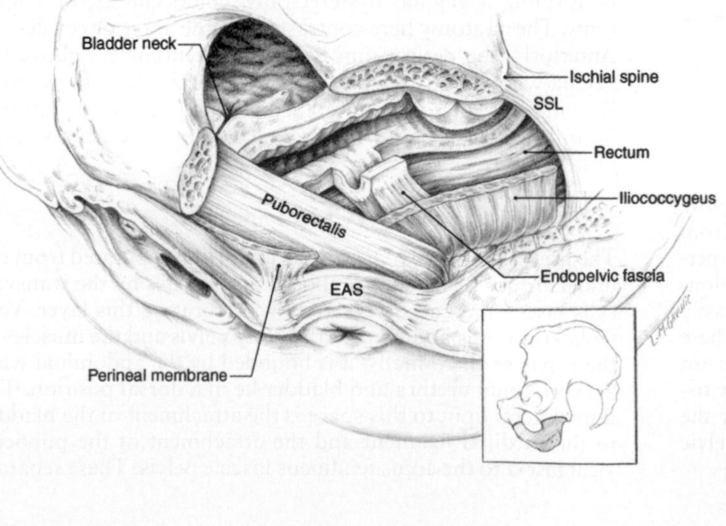

FIGURE 7.17. Lateral view of the pelvic organs after removal of the left ischial bone and ischial tuberosity. The bladder, vagina, and cervix have been cut in the sagittal plane to reveal their lumens. The rectum has been left intact. A strip of the posterior/lateral vaginal wall with its attached endopelvic fascia are shown, indicating their position relative to the levator ani muscle and this fascia's course and attachment. The two portions of the levator ani muscle (puborectalis and iliococcygeus) are visible. The ischial spine and the intact sacrospinous ligament are above the level of the removed ischial tuberosity. The left half of the perineal membrane (urogenital diaphragm) is shown just caudal to the puborectalis portion of the levator ani muscle after its detachment from the inferior pubic ramus that has been removed. (From: DeLancey JOL. Structural anatomy of the posterior compartment as it relates to rectocele. *Am J Obstet Gynecol* 1999;180:815–823, with permission.)

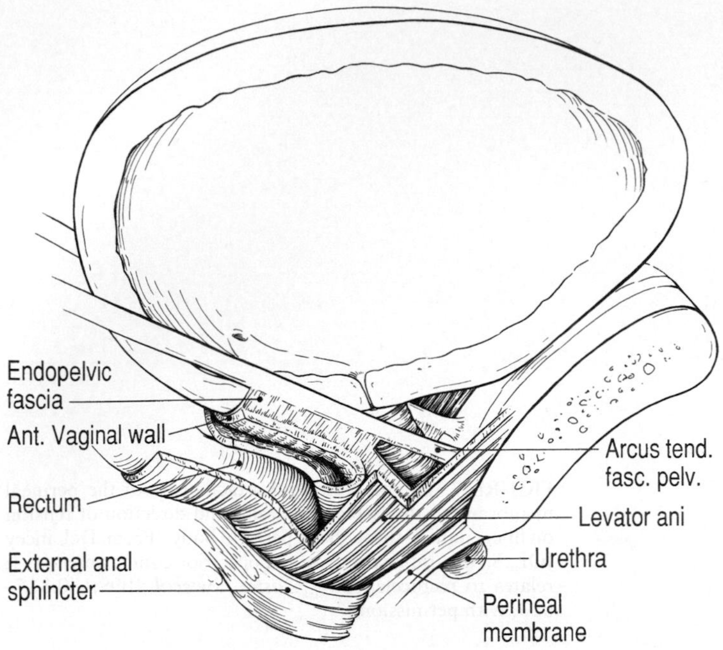

FIGURE 7.18. Lateral view of the urethral supportive mechanism transected just lateral to the midline. The lateral wall of the vagina and a portion of the endopelvic fascia have been removed so that one can see the deeper structures. (Redrawn from: DeLancey JOL. Structural support of the urethra as it relates to stress urinary incontinence: the hammock hypothesis. *Am J Obstet Gynecol* 1994;170:1713, with permission.)

relaxation of the levator ani muscles to elevate the urethra and to let it descend.

During increases in abdominal pressure, the downward force caused by increased abdominal pressure on the ventral surface of the urethra compresses the urethra closed against the hammocklike supportive layer, thereby closing the urethral lumen against the increases in intravesical pressure. The stability of the fascial layer determines the effectiveness of this closure mechanism. If the layer is unyielding, it forms a firm backstop against which the urethra can be compressed closed; however, if it is unstable, the effectiveness of this closure is compromised. Therefore, the integrity of the attachment to the arcus tendineus and the levator ani is critical to the stress continence mechanism.

The muscular attachment is responsible for the voluntary control of vesical neck position visible during vaginal examination or fluoroscopy when the pelvic muscles are contracted and relaxed. Relaxation of these muscles with descent of the vesical neck is associated with the initiation of urination and contraction with arrest of the urinary stream. The limit of downward vesical neck motion is determined by the connective tissue elasticity in the attachments to the arcus tendineus fasciae pelvis.

Cul-de-sacs, Cleavage Planes, and Spaces

Each of the pelvic viscera can expand somewhat independently of its neighboring organs. The ability to do this comes from their relatively loose attachment to one another, which permits the bladder, for example, to expand without equally elongating the adjacent cervix. This allows the viscera to be easily separated from one another along these lines of cleavage. These surgical cleavage planes are called spaces, although they are not empty but rather are filled with fatty or areolar connective tissue. The pelvic spaces are separated from one another by the connections of the viscera to one another and to the pelvic walls.

Anterior and Posterior Cul-de-sacs

Properly termed the *vesicouterine and rectouterine pouches,* the anterior and posterior cul-de-sac separate the uterus from the bladder and rectum.

The anterior cul-de-sac is a recess between the dome of the bladder and the anterior surface of the uterus (Fig. 7.19). The peritoneum is loosely applied in the region of the anterior cul-de-sac, unlike its dense attachment to the upper portions of the uterine corpus. This allows the bladder to expand without stretching its overlying peritoneum. This loose peritoneum forms the vesicouterine fold, which can easily be lifted and incised to create a bladder flap during abdominal hysterectomy or cesarean section. It is the point at which the vesicocervical space is normally accessed during abdominal surgery.

The posterior cul-de-sac is bordered ventrally by the vagina anteriorly, the rectosigmoid posteriorly, and the uterosacral ligaments laterally. Its peritoneum extends for approximately 4 cm along the posterior vaginal wall below the posterior vaginal fornix where the vaginal wall attaches to the cervix. This allows direct entry into the peritoneum from the vagina when performing a vaginal hysterectomy, culdocentesis, or colpotomy. The anatomy here contrasts with the anterior cul-de-sac. Anteriorly, the peritoneum lies several centimeters above the vagina whereas posteriorly, the peritoneum covers the vagina. Keeping this anatomic difference in mind facilitates entering both the anterior and the posterior cul-de-sacs during vaginal hysterectomy.

Prevesical Space

The prevesical space of Retzius (Fig. 7.14) is separated from the undersurface of the rectus abdominis muscles by the transversalis fascia and can be entered by perforating this layer. Ventrolaterally, it is bounded by the bony pelvis and the muscles of the pelvic wall; cranially, it is bounded by the abdominal wall. The proximal urethra and bladder lie in a dorsal position. The dorsolateral limit to this space is the attachment of the bladder to the cardinal ligament and the attachment of the pubocervical fascia to the arcus tendineus fasciae pelvis. These separate

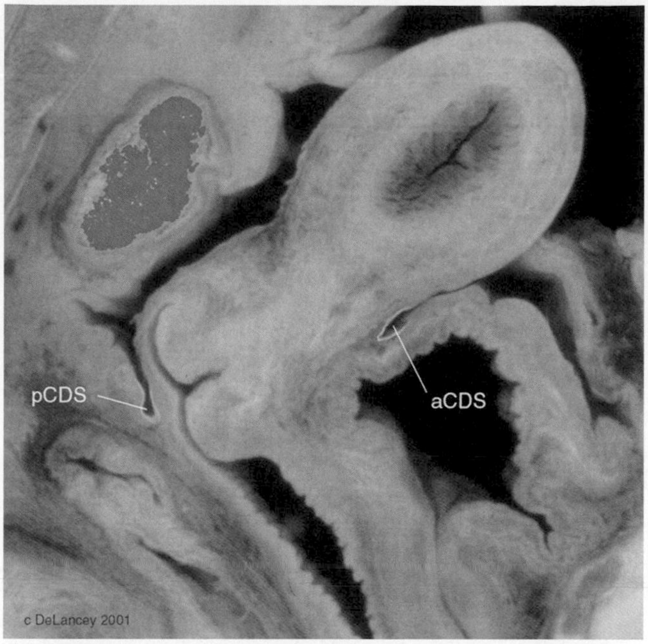

FIGURE 7.19. Sagittal section from a 28-year-old cadaver showing the anterior cul-de-sac (aCDS) and the posterior cul-de-sac (pCDS). Note how the posterior cul-de-sac peritoneum lies on the vaginal wall, whereas the anterior cul-de-sac lies several centimeters from the depth of the peritoneum in this area. (Peritoneum digitally enhanced in photograph to aid visibility.) (From: DeLancey, copyright 2001, with permission.)

this space from the vesicovaginocervical space. This lateral attachment is to the arcus tendineus fasciae pelvis, which lies on the inner surface of the obturator internus and pubococcygeal and puborectal muscles.

Important structures lying within this space include the dorsal clitoral vessels under the symphysis at its lower border and the obturator nerve and vessels as they enter the obturator canal. A branch to the obturator canal often comes off the external iliac artery and lies on the pubic bone; therefore, dissection in this area should be performed with care (Fig. 7.20). Lateral to the bladder and vesical neck is a dense plexus of vessels that lie at the border of the lower urinary tract. They are deep to the pubovesical muscle, and although they bleed when sutures are placed here, this venous ooze usually stops when the sutures are tied. Also within this tissue, lateral to the bladder and urethra, lie the nerves of the lower urinary tract. The upper border of the pubic bones that form the anterior surface of this region has a ridgelike fold of periosteum called the iliopectineal line. This is sometimes used to anchor sutures during urethral suspension operations.

Vesicovaginal and Vesicocervical Space

The space between the lower urinary tract and the genital tract is separated into the vesicovaginal and vesicocervical spaces (Fig. 7.14). The lower extent of the space is the junction of the proximal one third and distal two thirds of the urethra, where it fuses with the vagina, and it extends to lie under the peritoneum at the vesicocervical peritoneal reflection. It extends laterally to the pelvic side walls, separating the vesical and genital aspects of the cardinal ligaments.

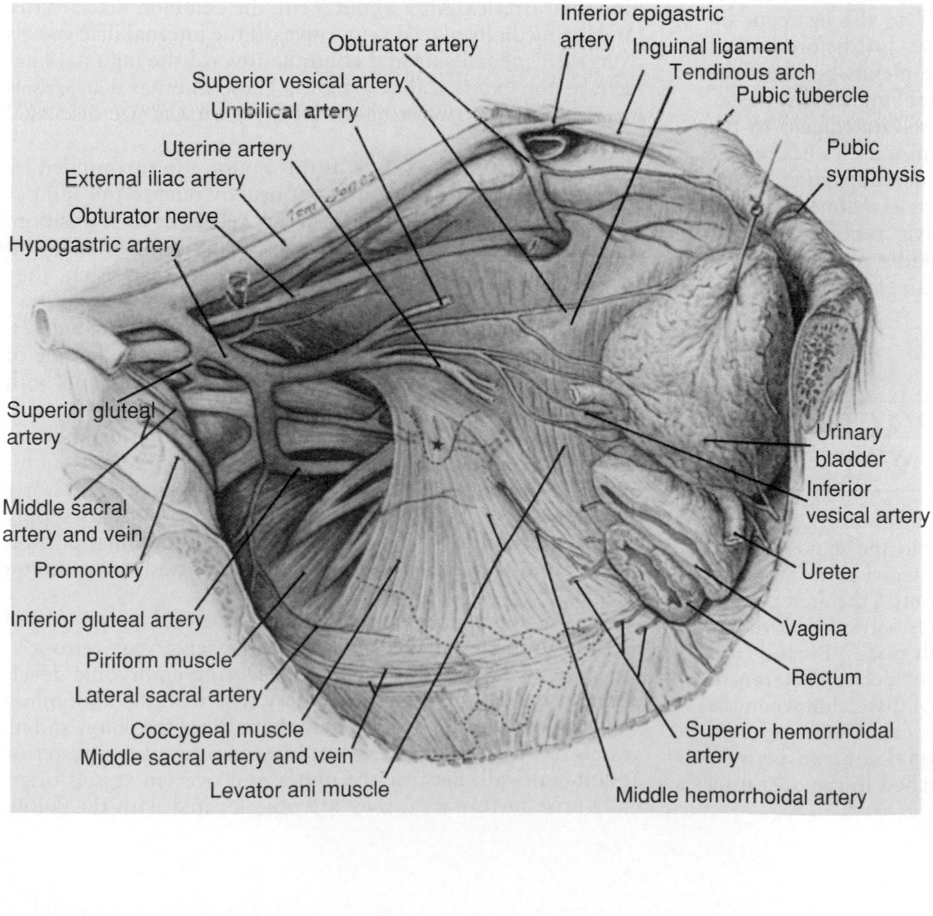

FIGURE 7.20. Structures of the pelvic wall. (From: Anson BJ. *An atlas of human anatomy.* Philadelphia: WB Saunders, 1950, with permission.)

Rectovaginal Space

On the dorsal surface of the vagina lies the rectovaginal space (Fig. 7.14). It begins at the apex of the perineal body, about 2 to 3 cm above the hymenal ring. It extends upward to the cul-de-sac and laterally around the sides of the rectum to the attachment of the rectovaginal septum to the parietal endopelvic fascia. It contains loose areolar tissue and is easily opened with finger dissection.

At the level of the cervix, some fibers of the cardinal-uterosacral ligament complex extend downward behind the vagina, connecting it to the lateral walls of the rectum and then to the sacrum. These are called the rectal pillars. They separate the midline rectovaginal space in this region from the lateral pararectal spaces. These pararectal spaces allow access to the sacrospinous ligaments (mentioned afterward). They also form the lateral boundaries of the retrorectal space between the rectum and sacrum.

Region of the Sacrospinous Ligament

The area around the sacrospinous ligament is another region that has become more important to the gynecologist operating for problems of vaginal support. The sacrospinous ligament lies on the dorsal aspect of the coccygeal muscle (Fig. 7.20). The rectal pillar separates it from the rectovaginal space.

As its name implies, the sacrospinous ligament courses from the lateral aspect of the sacrum to the ischial spine. In its medial portion, it fuses with the sacrotuberous ligament and is a distinct structure only laterally. It can be reached from the rectovaginal space by perforation of the rectal pillar to enter the pararectal space or by dissection directly under the enterocele peritoneum. This area is covered in more detail in Chapter 35.

Many structures are near the sacrospinous ligament, and their location must be remembered during surgery in this region. The sacral plexus lies immediately to the ligament on the inner surface of the piriformis muscle. Just before its exit through the greater sciatic foramen, the plexus gives off the pudendal nerve, which, with its accompanying vessels, passes lateral to the sacrospinous ligament at its attachment to the ischial spine. The nerve to the levator ani muscles lies on the inner surface of the coccygeal muscle in its midportion. In developing this space, the tissues that are reflected medially and cranially to gain access contain the pelvic venous plexus of the internal iliac vein, as well as the middle rectal vessels. If they are mobilized too vigorously, they can cause considerable hemorrhage.

RETROPERITONEAL SPACES AND LATERAL PELVIC WALL

The retroperitoneal space of the posterior abdomen, presacral space, and pelvic retroperitoneum contain the major neural, vascular, and lymphatic supply to the pelvic viscera. These areas are explored during operations to identify the ureter, interrupt the pelvic nerve supply, arrest serious pelvic hemorrhage, and remove potentially malignant lymph nodes. Because this area is free of the adhesions from serious pelvic infection or endometriosis, it can be used as a plane of dissection when the peritoneal cavity has become obliterated. The structures found in these spaces are discussed in a regional context, because that is the way they are usually approached in the operating room.

Retroperitoneal Structures of the Lower Abdomen

The aorta lies on the lumbar spine slightly to the left of the vena cava, which it overlies. The portion of this vessel below the renal vessels is encountered during retroperitoneal dissection to identify the paraaortic lymph nodes (Fig. 7.21). The renal blood vessels arise at the second lumbar vertebra. The ovarian vessels also arise from the anterior surface of the aorta in this region. In general, the branches of the vena cava follow those of the aorta, except for the vessels of the intestine, which flow into the portal vein, and the left ovarian vein, which empties into the renal vein on that side.

Below the level of the renal vessels and just below the third portion of the duodenum, the inferior mesenteric artery arises from the anterior aorta. It gives off ascending branches of the left colic artery and continues caudally to supply the sigmoid through the three or four sigmoid arteries that lie in the sigmoid mesentery. These vessels follow the bowel as it is pulled from side to side, so that their position can vary, depending on retraction.

Inferiorly, a continuation of the inferior mesenteric artery forms the superior rectal artery. This vessel crosses over the external iliac vessels to lie on the dorsum of the lower sigmoid. It supplies the rectum, as described in the section concerning that viscus.

The aorta and vena cava have segmental branches that arise at each lumbar level and are called the lumbar arteries and veins. They are situated somewhat posteriorly to the aorta and vena cava and are not visible from the front. When the vessels are mobilized, as is done in excising the lymphatic tissue in this area, they come into view.

At the level of the fourth lumbar vertebra (just below the umbilicus), the aorta bifurcates into the left and right common iliac arteries. After about 5 cm, the common iliac arteries (and the medially placed veins) give off the internal iliac vessels from their medial side and continue toward the inguinal ligament as the external iliac arteries. These internal iliac vessels lie within the pelvic retroperitoneal region and are discussed afterward.

The aorta and vena cava in this region are surrounded by lymph nodes on all sides. Surgeons usually refer to this lumbar chain of nodes as the paraaortic nodes, reflecting their position. They receive the drainage from the common iliac nodes and are the final drainage of the pelvic viscera. In addition, they collect the lymphatic drainage from the ovaries that follows the ovarian vessels and does not pass through the iliac nodes. The nodes of the lumbar chain extend from the right side of the vena cava to the left of the aorta and can be found both anterior and posterior to the vessels.

The ureters are attached loosely to the posterior abdominal wall in this region, and when the overlying colon is mobilized, they remain on the body wall. They are crossed anteriorly by the ovarian vessels, which contribute a branch to supply the ureter. Additional blood supply to the abdominal portion comes from the renal vessels at the kidney and the common iliac artery.

This region can be exposed either by a midline peritoneal incision to the left of the small bowel mesentery or, retroperitoneally, by reflection of the colon. During embryonic development, the colon and its mesentery fuse with the abdominal wall. A cleavage plane exists here that allows the colon and its vessels to be elevated to expose the structures of the posterior abdominal wall. Because the ureter and ovarian vessels originally arise in this area, they are not elevated with the colon.

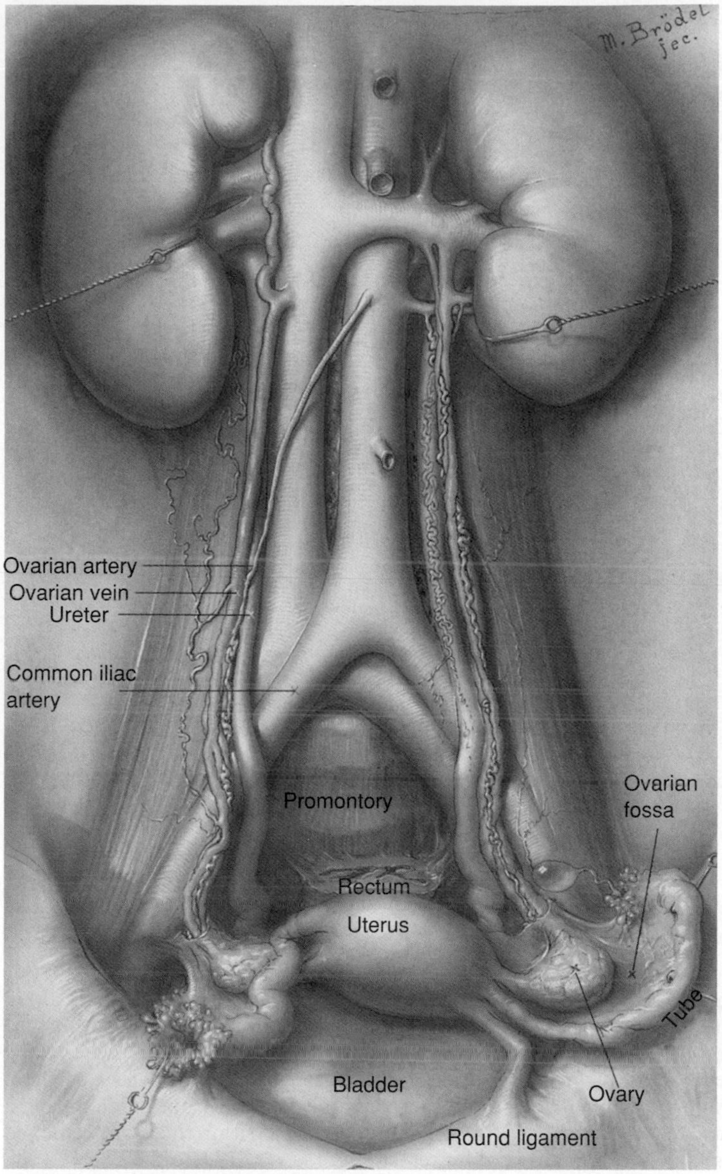

FIGURE 7.21. Structures of the retroperitoneum. Note the anomalous origin of the left ovarian artery from the left renal artery rather than from the aorta. (From: The Brödel Collection, Department of Art as Applied to Medicine, Johns Hopkins Medical Institution, Baltimore, with permission.)

Presacral Space

The presacral space begins below the bifurcation of the aorta and is bounded laterally by the internal iliac arteries (Figs. 7.22 and 7.23). Lying directly on the sacrum are the middle sacral artery and vein, which originate from the dorsal aspect of the aorta and vena cava (and not from the point of bifurcation, as sometimes shown). Caudal and lateral to this are the lateral sacral vessels. The venous plexus of these vessels can be extensive, and bleeding from it can be considerable.

Within this area lies the most familiar part of the pelvic autonomic nervous system, the presacral nerve (superior hypogastric plexus). The autonomic nerves of the pelvic viscera can be divided into a sympathetic (thoracolumbar) and parasympathetic (craniosacral) system. The former is also called the adrenergic system, and the latter is called the cholinergic system, according to their neurotransmitters. α-adrenergic stimulation causes increased urethral and vesical neck tone, and cholinergic stimulation increases contractility of the detrusor muscle. Similarly, adrenergic stimulation in the colon and rectum favors storage, and cholinergic stimulation favors evacuation. β-adrenergic agonists, which are used for tocolysis, suggest that these influence contractility of the uterus. As is true in the man, damage to the autonomic nerves during pelvic lymphadenectomy can have a significant influence on orgasmic function in the woman.

How these autonomic nerves reach the organs that they innervate has surgical importance. The terminology of this area is somewhat confusing, because many authors use idiosyncratic terms. However, the structure is simple: It consists of a single ganglionic midline plexus overlying the lower aorta (superior hypogastric plexus) that splits into two trunks without ganglia (hypogastric nerves), each of which connects with a plexus of nerves and ganglia lateral to the pelvic viscera (inferior hypogastric plexus).

The superior hypogastric plexus lies in the retroperitoneal connective tissue on the ventral surface of the lower aorta and

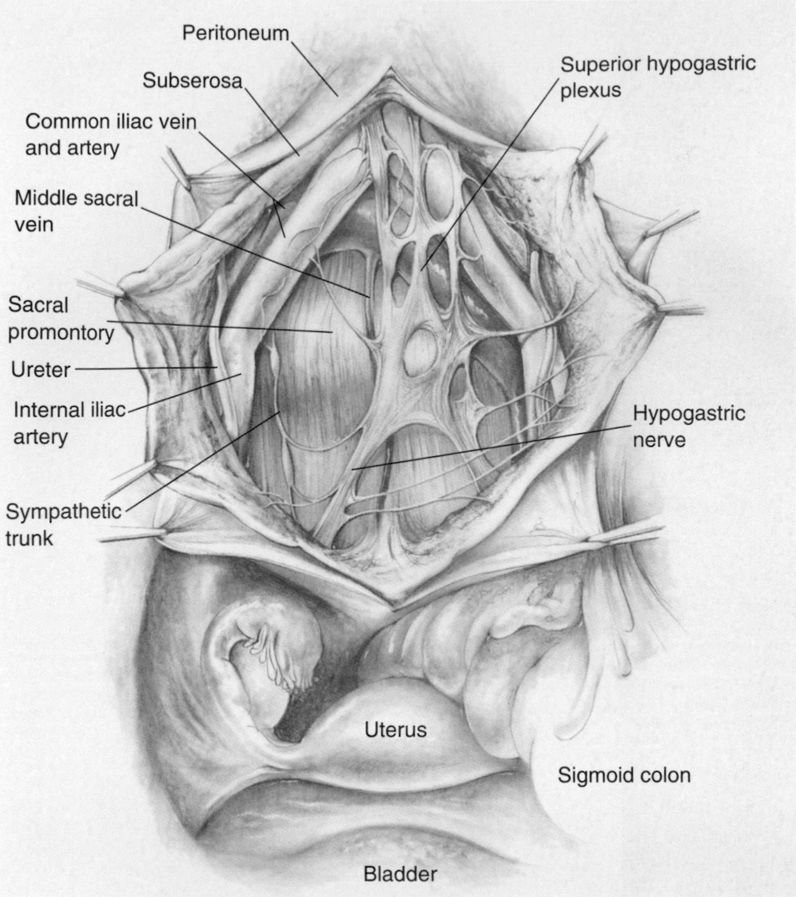

FIGURE 7.22. Presacral nerve plexus, showing passage of sympathetic trunk over bifurcation of aorta. Observe the division of the trunk into left and right presacral nerves. (Redrawn from: Curtis AH, Anson BJ, Ashley FL, et al. The anatomy of the pelvic autonomic nerves in relation to gynecology. *Surg Gynecol Obstet* 1942;75:743, with permission.)

receives input from the sympathetic chain ganglia through the thoracic and lumbar splanchnic nerves. It also contains important afferent pain fibers from the pelvic viscera, which makes its transection effective in primary dysmenorrhea. It passes over the bifurcation of the aorta and extends over the proximal sacrum before splitting into two hypogastric nerves that descend into the pelvis in the region of the internal iliac vessels. The hypogastric nerves end in the inferior hypogastric plexus. The hypogastric plexuses are broad expansions of the hypogastric nerves. Their sympathetic fibers come from the downward extensions of the superior hypogastric plexus and pelvic splanchnic nerves from the continuation of the sympathetic chain into the pelvis. Parasympathetic fibers come from sacral segments 2 through 4 by way of the pelvic splanchnic nerves (nervi erigentes) to join these ganglia. They lie in the pelvic connective tissue of the lateral pelvic wall, lateral to the uterus and vagina.

The inferior hypogastric plexus (sometimes called the pelvic plexus) is divided into three portions: the vesical plexus anteriorly, uterovaginal plexus (Frankenhäuser ganglion), and the middle rectal plexus. The uterovaginal plexus contains fibers that derive from two sources. It receives sympathetic and sensory fibers from the tenth thoracic through the first lumbar spinal cord segments. The second input comes from the second, third, and fourth sacral segments and consists primarily of parasympathetic nerves that reach the inferior hypogastric plexus through the pelvic splanchnic nerves. The uterovaginal plexus lies on the dorsal (medial) surface of the uterine vessels, lateral to the sacrouterine ligaments' insertion into the uterus. It has continuations cranially along the uterus and caudally along the vagina. This latter extension contains the fibers that innervate the vestibular bulbs and clitoris. These nerves lie in the tissue just lateral to the area where the uterine artery, cardinal ligament, and uterosacral ligament pedicles are made during a hysterectomy for benign disease, and within the tissue removed during a radical hysterectomy.

The location of the sensory fibers from the uterine corpus in the superior hypogastric nerve (the presacral nerve) allows the surgeon to alleviate visceral pain from the corpus by transecting this structure. It does not provide sensory innervation to the adnexal structures or to the peritoneum and is therefore not useful for alleviating pain in those sites. Another important way in which the autonomic nervous system is involved is through damage to the inferior hypogastric plexus during radical hysterectomy. The extension of the surgical field lateral to the viscera interrupts the connection of the bladder and sometimes the rectum to their central attachments.

The ovary and uterine tube receive their neural supply from the plexus of nerves that accompany the ovarian vessels and that originate in the renal plexus. These fibers originate from the tenth thoracic segment, and the parasympathetic fibers come from extensions of the vagus.

As the lumbar and sacral nerves exit from the intervertebral and sacral foramina, they form the lumbar and sacral plexuses. The lumbar nerves and plexus lie deep within the psoas muscle on either side of the spine. The sacral plexus lies on the piriformis muscle, and its major branch, the sciatic nerve, leaves the pelvis through the lower part of the greater sciatic foramen. The

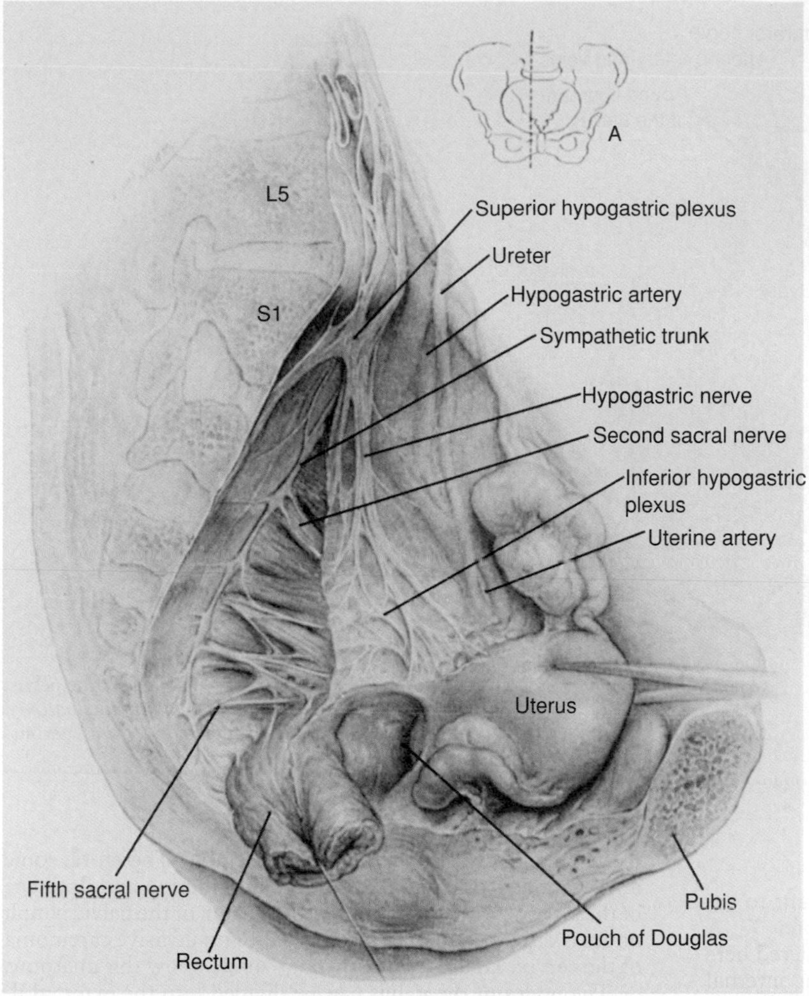

FIGURE 7.23. Nerves of the female pelvis. (From: Anson BJ. *An atlas of human anatomy.* Philadelphia: WB Saunders, 1950, with permission.)

sacral plexus supplies nerves to the muscles of the hip, pelvic diaphragm, and perineum, as well as to the lower leg (through the sciatic nerve). The femoral nerve from the lumbar plexus is primarily involved in supplying the muscles of the thigh.

Pelvic Retroperitoneal Space

Division of the internal and external iliac vessels occurs in the area of the sacroiliac joint. Just before passing under the inguinal ligament to become the femoral vessels, the external iliac vessels contribute the deep inferior epigastric and deep circumflex iliac arteries. There are no other major branches of the external iliac artery in this region.

Internal Iliac Vessels

Unlike the external iliac artery, which is constant and relatively simple in its morphology, the branching pattern of the internal iliac arteries and veins is extremely variable (Figs. 7.24 and 7.25). A description of a common variant is included here. The internal iliac artery supplies the viscera of the pelvis and many muscles of the pelvic wall and gluteal region. It usually divides into an anterior and posterior division about 3 to 4 cm after leaving the common iliac artery (Table 7.2). The vessels of the posterior division (the iliolumbar, lateral sacral, and superior gluteal) leave the internal iliac artery from its lateral surface to provide some of the blood supply to the pelvic wall and gluteal muscles. Trauma to these hidden vessels should be avoided during internal iliac artery ligation as the suture is passed around behind vessels.

The anterior division has both parietal and visceral branches. The obturator, internal pudendal, and inferior gluteal vessels primarily supply muscles, whereas the uterine, superior vesical, vaginal (inferior vesical), and middle rectal vessels supply the pelvic organs. The internal iliac veins begin lateral and posterior to the arteries. These veins form a large and complex plexus within the pelvis, rather than having single branches, as do the arteries. They tend to be deeper in this area than the arteries, and their pattern is highly variable.

Ligation of the internal iliac artery has proved helpful in the management of postpartum hemorrhage. Burchell's arteriographic studies showed that physiologically active anastomoses between the systemic and pelvic arterial supplies were immediately patent after ligation of the internal iliac artery (Fig. 7.25). These anastomoses, shown in Table 7.2, connected the arteries of the internal iliac system with systemic blood vessels either directly from the aorta, as is true for the lumbar and middle sacral artery, or indirectly through the inferior mesenteric artery, as with the superior hemorrhoidal vessels. These *in vivo* pathways were quite different from the anastomoses that had previously been hypothesized on purely anatomic grounds.

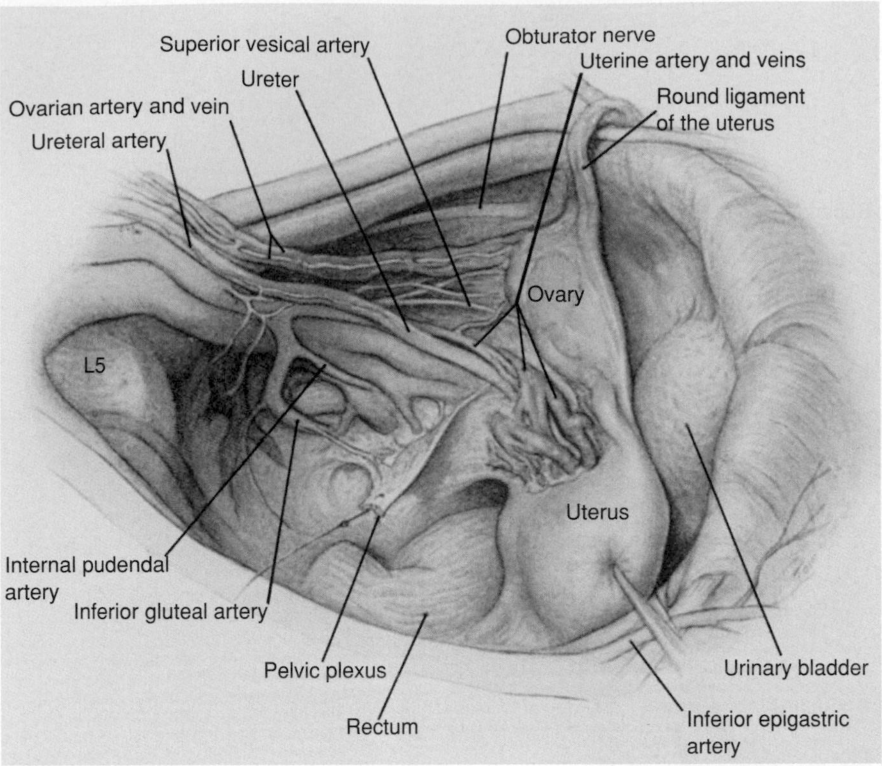

FIGURE 7.24. Arteries and veins of the pelvis. (From: Anson BJ. *An atlas of human anatomy.* Philadelphia: WB Saunders, 1950, with permission.)

Pelvic Ureter

The course of the ureter within the pelvis is important to gynecologic surgeons and is fully considered in Chapter 37. A few of the important anatomic landmarks are considered here (Fig. 7.24). After passing over the bifurcation of the internal and external iliac arteries, just medial to the ovarian vessels, the ureter descends within the pelvis. Here it lies in a special connective tissue sheath that is attached to the peritoneum of the lateral pelvic wall and medial leaf of the broad ligament. This explains why the ureter still adheres to the peritoneum and does not remain laterally with the vessels when the peritoneal space is entered.

The ureter crosses under the uterine artery ("water flows under the bridge") in its course through the cardinal ligament. There is a loose areolar plane around it to allow for its peristalsis here. At this point it lies along the anterolateral surface of the cervix, usually about 1 cm from it. From there it comes to lie on the anterior vaginal wall and then proceeds for a distance of about 1.5 cm through the wall of the bladder.

During its pelvic course, the ureter receives blood from the vessels that it passes, specifically the common iliac, internal iliac, uterine, and vesical arteries. Within the wall of the ureter, these vessels are connected to one another by a convoluted vessel that can be seen running longitudinally along its outer surface.

Lymphatics

The lymph nodes and lymphatic vessels that drain the pelvic viscera vary in their number and distribution, but they can be organized into coherent groups. Because of the extensive interconnection of the lymph nodes, spread of lymph flow, and thus malignancy, is somewhat unpredictable. Therefore, some important generalizations about the distribution and drainage of these tissues are still helpful. Distribution of the pelvic lymph nodes is discussed further in Chapter 46 on invasive carcinoma of the cervix. Figures 46.22 through 46.25 show this anatomy.

The nodes of the pelvis can be divided into the external iliac, internal iliac, common iliac, medial sacral, and pararectal nodes. The medial sacral nodes are few and follow the middle sacral artery. The pararectal nodes drain the part of the rectosigmoid above the peritoneal reflection that is supplied by the superior hemorrhoidal artery. The medial and pararectal nodes are seldom involved in gynecologic disease.

The internal and external iliac nodes lie next to their respective blood vessels, and both end in the common iliac chain of nodes, which then drain into the nodes along the aorta. The external iliac nodes receive the drainage from the leg through the inguinal nodes. Nodes in the external iliac group can be found lateral to the artery, between the artery and vein, and on the medial aspect of the vein. These groups are called the anterosuperior, intermediate, and posteromedial groups, respectively. They can be separated from the underlying muscular fascia and periosteum of the pelvic wall along with the vessels, thereby defining their lateral extent. Some nodes at the distal end of this chain lie in direct relation to the deep inferior epigastric vessels and are named according to these adjacent vessels. Similarly, nodes that lie at the point where the obturator nerve and vessels enter the obturator canal are called obturator nodes.

The internal iliac nodes drain the pelvic viscera and receive some drainage from the gluteal region along the posterior division of the internal iliac vessels as well. These nodes lie within the adipose tissue that is interspersed among the many branches of the vessels. The largest and most numerous nodes lie on the lateral pelvic wall, but many smaller nodes lie next to the

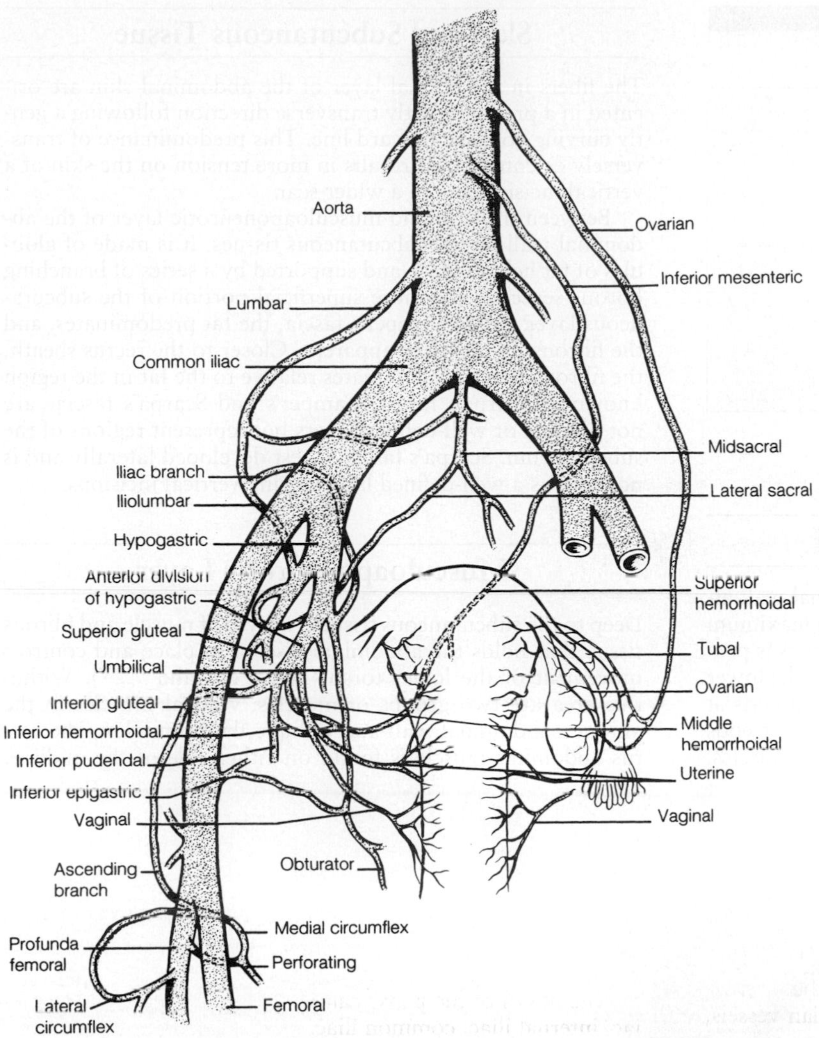

FIGURE 7.25. Collateral circulation of the pelvis.

viscera themselves. These nodes are named for the organ by which they are found (e.g., parauterine).

Not only is it difficult in the operating room to make some of the fine distinctions mentioned in this anatomic discussion, but also there is little clinical importance in doing so. Surgeons generally refer to those nodes that are adjacent to the external iliac artery as the external iliac group of nodes and to those next to the internal iliac artery as the internal iliac nodes. This leaves those nodes that lie between the external iliac vein and internal artery, which are called interiliac nodes.

The direction of lymph flow from the uterus tends to follow its attachments, draining along the cardinal, uterosacral, and even round ligaments. This latter connection can lead to metastasis from the uterus to the superficial inguinal nodes, whereas the former connections are to the internal iliac nodes, with free communication to the external iliac nodes and sometimes to the lateral sacral nodes. The anastomotic connection of the uterine and ovarian vessels makes lymphatic connections between these two drainage systems likely and metastasis in this direction possible.

The vagina and lower urinary tract have a divided drainage. Superiorly (upper two thirds of the vagina and the bladder), drainage occurs along with the uterine lymphatics to the internal iliac nodes, whereas the lower one third of the vagina and distal urethra drain to the inguinal nodes. However, this demarcation is far from precise.

The common iliac nodes can be found from the medial to the lateral border of the vessels of the same name. They continue above the pelvic vessels and occur around the aorta and the vena cava. These nodes can lie anterior, lateral, or posterior to the vessels.

TABLE 7.2

COLLATERAL CIRCULATION AFTER INTERNAL ILIAC ARTERY LIGATION

Internal Iliac Systemic
Iliolumbar
Lateral sacral
Middle hemorrhoidal
Lumbar
Middle sacral
Superior hemorrhoidal

TABLE 7.3

TABLE OF ABDOMINAL WALL LAYERS

Skin
Subcutaneous layer
  Camper's fascia
  Scarpa's fascia
Musculoaponeurotic layer
  Rectus sheath—formed by conjoined aponeuroses of the external oblique muscle
Internal oblique muscle: fused in lower abdomen
Transverse abdominal muscle
Transversalis fascia
Peritoneum

THE ABDOMINAL WALL

Knowledge of the layered structure of the abdominal wall allows the surgeon to enter the abdominal cavity with maximum efficiency and safety. A general summary of these layers is provided in Table 7.3. The abdomen's superior border is the lower edge of the rib cage (ribs 7 through 12). Inferiorly, it ends at the iliac crests, inguinal ligaments, and pubic bones. It ends posterolaterally at the lumbar spine and its adjacent muscles.

Skin and Subcutaneous Tissue

The fibers in the dermal layer of the abdominal skin are oriented in a predominantly transverse direction following a gently curving concave upward line. This predominance of transversely oriented fibers results in more tension on the skin of a vertical incision and in a wider scar.

Between the skin and musculoaponeurotic layer of the abdominal wall lie the subcutaneous tissues. It is made of globules of fat held in place and supported by a series of branching fibrous septa. In the more superficial portion of the subcutaneous layer, called Camper's fascia, the fat predominates, and the fibrous tissue is less apparent. Closer to the rectus sheath, the fibrous tissue predominates relative to the fat in the region known as Scarpa's fascia. Camper's and Scarpa's fasciae are not discrete or well-defined layers but represent regions of the subcutaneum. Scarpa's fascia is best developed laterally and is not seen as a well-defined layer during vertical incisions.

Musculoaponeurotic Layer

Deep to the subcutaneous tissue is a layer of muscle and fibrous tissue that holds the abdominal viscera in place and controls movement of the lower torso (Figs. 7.26 and 7.27). Within this area are two groups of muscles: vertical muscles in the anterior abdominal wall and oblique flank muscles. The rectus abdominis muscle is found on either side of the midline,

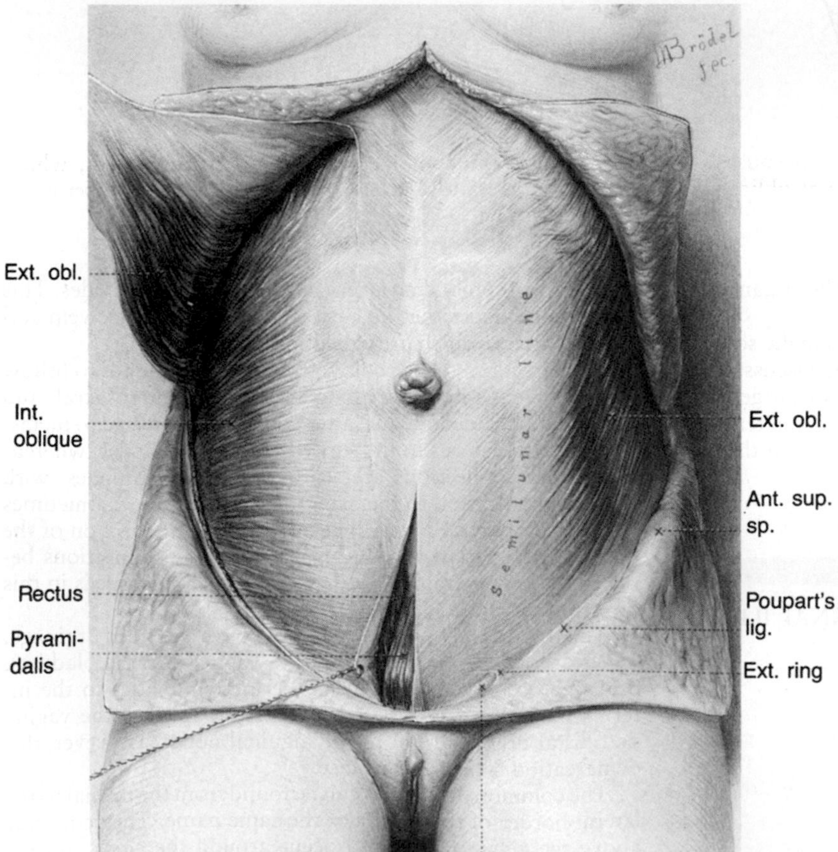

FIGURE 7.26. External oblique, internal oblique, and pyramidal muscles. (From: Kelly HA. *Gynecology.* New York: Appleton, 1928, with permission.)

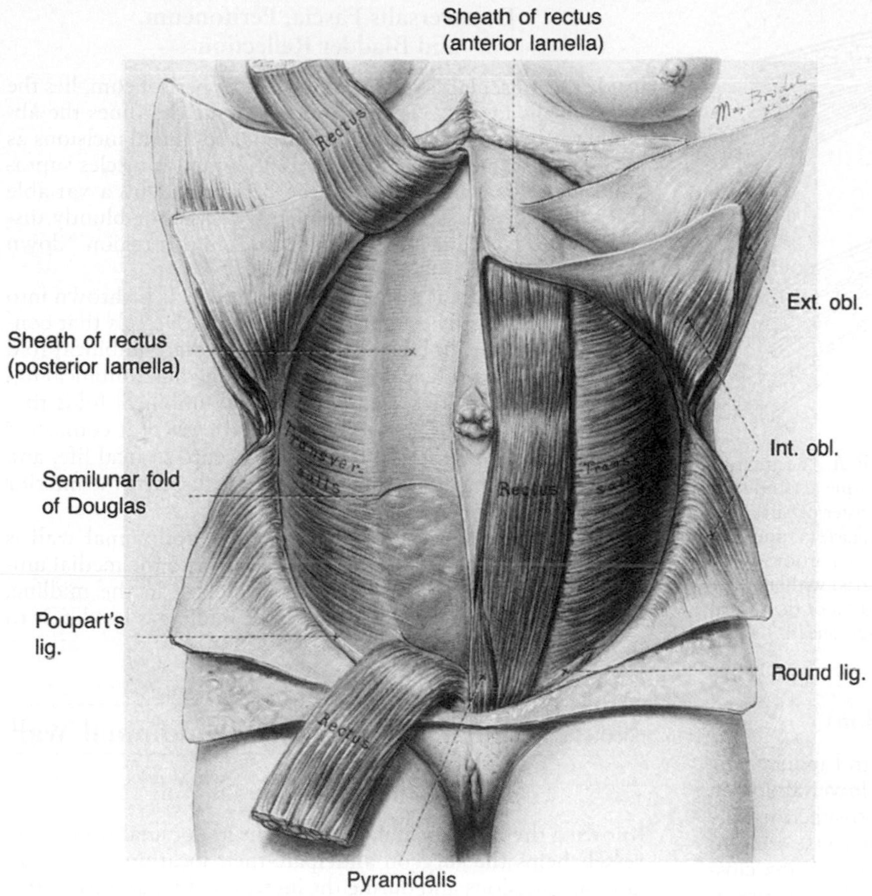

FIGURE 7.27. Transverse abdominal and rectoabdominal muscles. (From: Kelly HA. *Gynecology.* New York: Appleton, 1928, with permission.)

and the pyramidalis muscle is located just above the pubes. Lateral to these are the flank muscles: the external oblique, internal oblique, and transverse abdominal. The broad, sheet-like tendons of these muscles form aponeuroses that unite with their corresponding member of the other side, forming a dense white covering of the rectus abdominis muscle properly called the rectus sheath (rectus "fascia").

Rectus Abdominis and Pyramidal Muscles

Each paired rectus abdominis muscle originates from the sternum and cartilages of ribs 5 through 7 and inserts into the anterior surface of the pubic bone. Each muscle has three tendinous inscriptions. These are fibrous interruptions within the muscle that firmly attach it to the rectus abdominis sheath. In general, they are confined to the region above the umbilicus, but they can be found below it. When this happens, the rectus sheath is attached to the rectus muscle there, and these two structures become difficult to separate during a Pfannenstiel incision.

The pyramidal muscles arise from the pubic bones and insert into the linea alba in an area several centimeters above the symphysis. Their development varies considerably among individuals. Their strong attachment to the midline makes separation of their attachment here difficult by blunt dissection.

Flank Muscles

Lateral to the rectus abdominis muscles lie the broad, flat muscles of the flank. The aponeurotic insertions of these muscles join to form the conjoined tendon, or rectus sheath, which covers the rectus abdominis. Because of its importance, it is discussed separately subsequently.

The most superficial of these muscles is the external oblique. Its fibers run obliquely anteriorly and inferiorly from their origin on the lower eight ribs and iliac crest. Unlike the external oblique muscle's fibers, which run obliquely downward, the fibers of the internal oblique muscle fan out from their origin in the anterior two thirds of the iliac crest, the lateral part of the inguinal ligament, and the thoracolumbar fascia in the lower posterior flank. In most areas, they are perpendicular to the fibers of the external oblique muscle, but in the lower abdomen, their fibers arch somewhat more caudally and run in a direction similar to those of the external oblique muscle.

As the name *transversus abdominis* implies, the fibers of the deepest of the three layers have a primarily transverse orientation. They arise from the lower six costal cartilages, the thoracolumbar fascia, the anterior three fourths of the iliac crest, and the lateral inguinal ligament. The caudal portion of the transverse abdominal muscle is fused with the internal oblique muscle. This explains why, during transverse incisions of the lower abdomen, only two layers are discernible at the lateral portion of the incision.

Although the fibers of the flank muscles are not strictly parallel to one another, their primarily transverse orientation and the transverse pull of their attached muscular fibers place vertical suture lines in the rectus sheath under more tension than transverse ones. For this reason, vertical incisions are more prone to dehiscence.

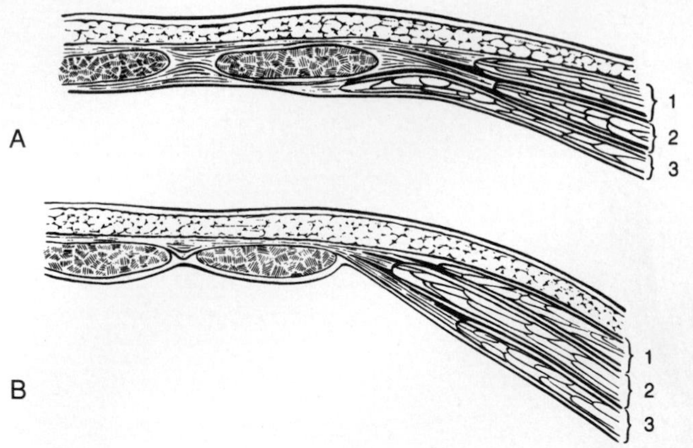

FIGURE 7.28. Cross section of lower abdominal wall. **A:** The anterior fascial sheath of the rectus muscle from external oblique (*1*) and split aponeurosis of internal oblique (*2*) muscles. The posterior sheath is formed by aponeurosis of the transverse abdominal muscle (*3*) and split aponeurosis of the internal oblique muscle. **B:** Lower portion of the abdominal wall below arcuate line (linea semicircularis) with absence of a posterior fascial sheath of the rectus muscle and all of the fascial aponeuroses (*1,2,3*) forming the anterior rectus muscle sheath.

Rectus Sheath (Conjoined Tendon)

The line of demarcation between the muscular and aponeurotic portions of the external oblique muscle in the lower abdomen occurs along a vertical line through the anterosuperior iliac spine (Fig. 7.28). The internal oblique and transverse abdominal muscles extend farther toward the midline, coming closest at their inferior margin, at the pubic tubercle. Because of this, fibers of the internal oblique muscle are found underneath the aponeurotic portion of the external oblique muscle during a transverse incision. In addition, it is between the internal oblique and transverse abdominal muscles that the nerves and blood vessels of the flank are found and their injury avoided.

In forming the rectus sheath, the conjoined aponeuroses of the flank are separable lateral to the rectus muscles but fuse near the midline. As they reach the midline, these layers lose their separate directions and fuse. Many specialized aspects of the rectus sheath are important to the surgeon. In its lower one fourth, the sheath lies entirely anterior to the rectus muscle. Above that point, it splits to lie both ventral and dorsal to it. The transition between these two arrangements occurs midway between the umbilicus and the pubes and is called the arcuate line. Cranial to this line, the midline ridge of the rectus sheath, the linea alba, unites these two layers. Sharp dissection is usually required to separate these layers during a Pfannenstiel incision. A vertical peritoneal incision cuts the posterior sheath.

The lateral border of the rectus muscle is marked by the semilunar line of the rectus sheath. Above the arcuate line, this is the level at which the anterior and posterior layers of the sheath split. Below it the transversalis fascia fuses with the sheath. The semilunar line is not always where the three layers of flank muscles join. During a transverse lower abdominal incision, the external and internal oblique aponeuroses are often separable near the midline.

The inguinal canal lies at the lower edge of the musculofascial layer of the abdominal wall. Through the inguinal canal, in the woman, the round ligament extends to its termination in the labium majus. In addition, the ilioinguinal nerve and the genital branch of the genitofemoral nerve pass through the canal.

Transversalis Fascia, Peritoneum, and Bladder Reflection

Inside the muscular layers, and outside the peritoneum, lies the transversalis fascia, a layer of fibrous tissue that lines the abdominopelvic cavity. It is visible during abdominal incisions as the layer just underneath the rectus abdominis muscles suprapubically. It is separated from the peritoneum by a variable layer of adipose tissue. It is frequently incised or bluntly dissected off the bladder to take the tissues in this region "down by layers."

The peritoneum is a single layer of serosa. It is thrown into five vertical folds by underlying ligaments or vessels that converge toward the umbilicus. The single median umbilical fold is caused by the presence of the urachus (median umbilical ligament). Lateral to this are paired medial umbilical folds that are raised by the obliterated umbilical arteries that connected the internal iliac vessels to the umbilical cord in fetal life, and the corresponding lateral umbilical folds caused by the inferior epigastric arteries and veins.

The reflection of the bladder onto the abdominal wall is triangular in shape, with its apex blending into the medial umbilical ligament. Because the apex is highest in the midline, incision in the peritoneum lateral to the midline is less likely to result in bladder injury.

Neurovascular Supply of the Abdominal Wall

Vessels of the Abdominal Wall

Knowing the location and course of the abdominal wall blood vessels helps the surgeon anticipate their location during abdominal incisions and during the insertion of laparoscopic trocars (Fig. 7.29). The blood vessels that supply the abdominal wall can be separated into those that supply the skin and subcutaneous tissues and those that supply the musculofascial layer.

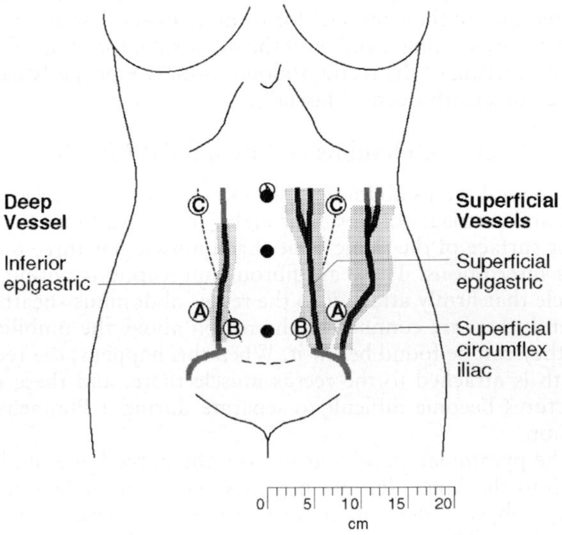

FIGURE 7.29. Normal variation in epigastric vessels. A, B, and C designate safe spots for laparoscopic trocar insertion. Dotted lines indicate lateral border of rectus muscle. (From: Hurd WW, Bude RO, DeLancey JOL, et al. The location of abdominal wall blood vessels in relationship to abdominal landmarks apparent at laparoscopy. *Am J Obstet Gynecol* 1994;171:642, with permission.)

Although there is only one set of epigastric vessels in the subcutaneous tissues (superficial epigastric), there are both superior and inferior epigastric vessels in the musculofascial layer, so care must be taken in using these terms to avoid confusion.

The superficial epigastric vessels run a diagonal course in the subcutaneum from the femoral vessels toward the umbilicus, beginning as a single artery that branches extensively as it nears the umbilicus. Its position can be anticipated midway between the skin and musculofascial layer, in a line between the palpable femoral pulse and the umbilicus. The external pudendal artery runs a diagonal course from the femoral artery medially to supply the region of the mons pubis. It has many midline branches, and bleeding in its territory of distribution is heavier than that from the abdominal subcutaneous tissues. The superficial circumflex iliac vessels proceed laterally from the femoral vessels toward the flank.

The blood supply to the lower abdominal wall's musculofascial layer parallels the subcutaneous vessels. The branches of the external iliac, the inferior epigastric, and the deep circumflex iliac arteries parallel their superficial counterparts (Fig. 7.29). The circumflex iliac artery lies between the internal oblique and transverse abdominal muscle. The inferior epigastric artery and its two veins originate lateral to the rectus muscle. They run diagonally toward the umbilicus and intersect the muscle's lateral border midway between the pubis and umbilicus. Below the point at which the vessels pass under the rectus, they are found lateral to the muscle deep to the transversalis fascia. After crossing the lateral border of the muscle, they lie on the muscle's dorsal surface, between it and the posterior rectus sheath. As the vessels enter the rectus sheath, they branch extensively, so that they no longer represent a single trunk. The angle between the vessel and the border of the rectus muscle forms the apex of the Hesselbach triangle (inguinal triangle), the base of which is the inguinal ligament.

Lateral laparoscopic trocars are placed in a region of the lower abdomen where injury to the inferior epigastric and superficial epigastric vessels can occur easily. The inferior epigastric arteries and the superficial epigastric arteries run similar courses toward the umbilicus. Knowing the average location of these blood vessels helps in choosing insertion sites that will minimize their injury and the potential hemorrhage and hematomas that this injury can cause. Just above the pubic

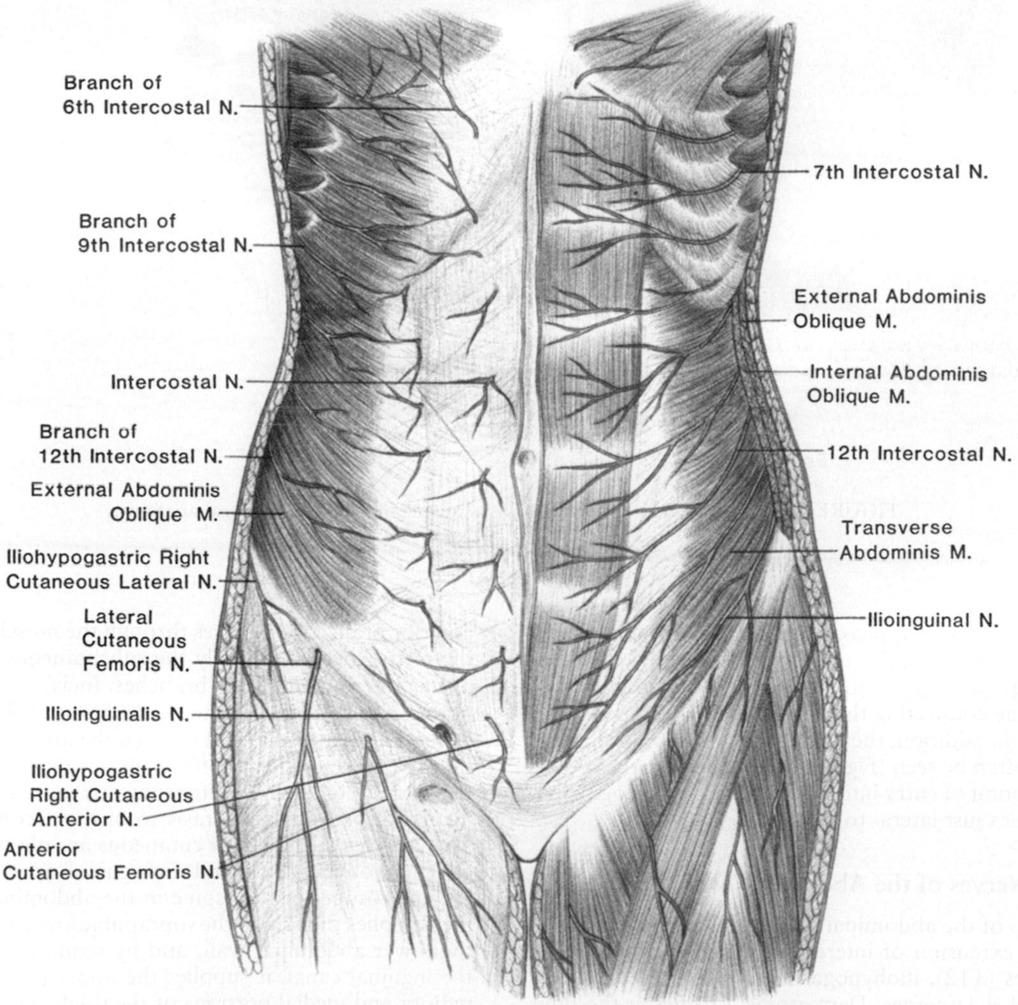

FIGURE 7.30. Nerve supply to the abdomen. **Right:** Deep innervation of T6BT12 to the transverse abdominal, internal oblique, and rectal muscles. **Left:** Superficial distribution, including cutaneous nerves, after penetration and innervation of the external oblique muscle and fascia. Innervation of the groin and thigh also is shown.

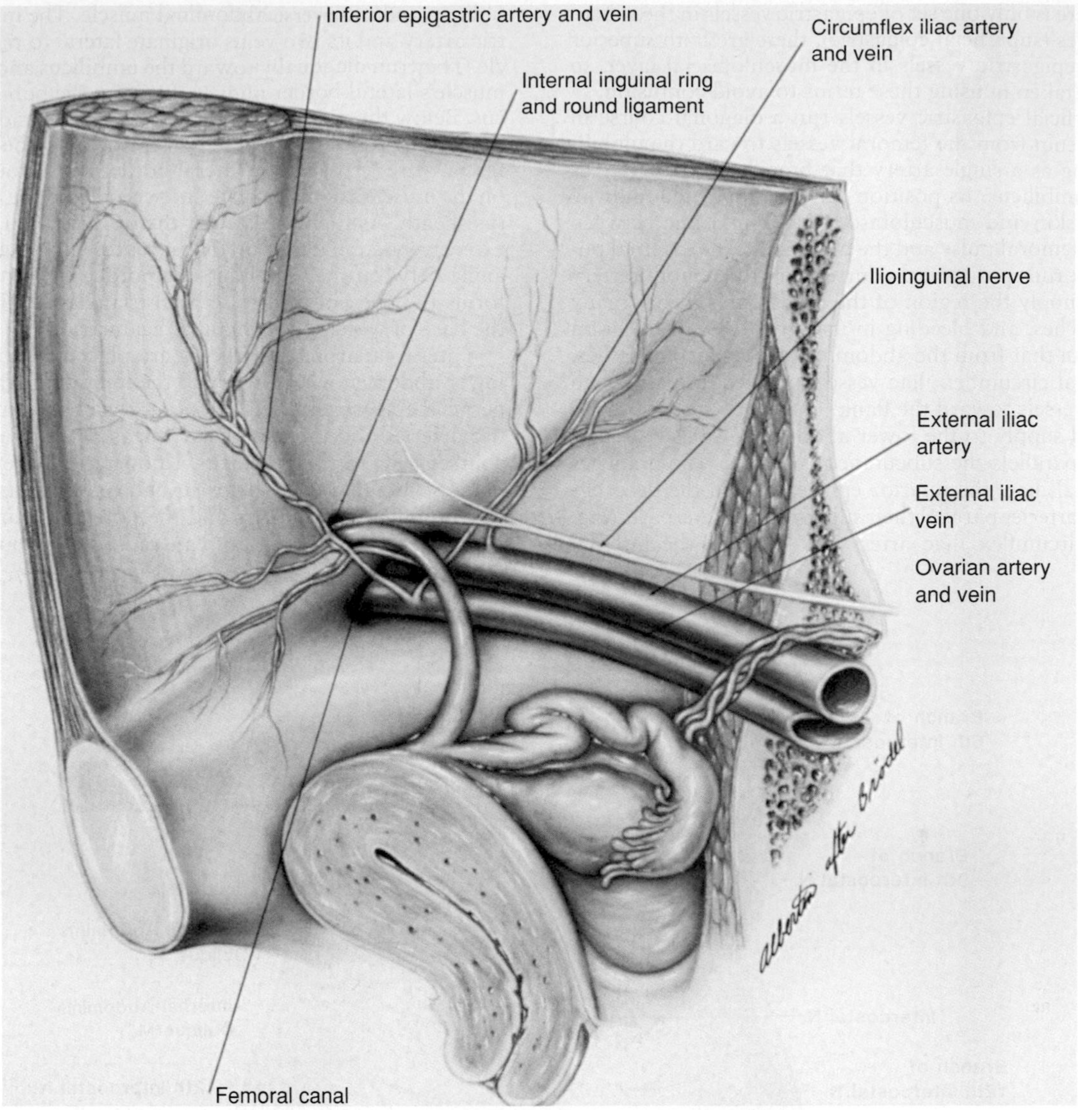

FIGURE 7.31. Sagittal view of female pelvis, showing inguinal and femoral anatomy.

symphysis, the vessels lie approximately 5.5 cm from the midline, whereas at the level of the umbilicus, they are 4.5 cm from the midline (Fig. 7.30). Therefore, placement either lateral or medial to the line connecting these points minimizes potential vascular injury. In addition, the location of the inferior epigastric vessel can often be seen (Fig. 7.31) by following the round ligament to its point of entry into the inguinal ring, recognizing that the vessel lies just lateral to this point.

Nerves of the Abdominal Wall

The innervation of the abdominal wall (Fig. 7.30) comes from the abdominal extension of intercostal nerves 7 through 11, subcostal nerves (T12), iliohypogastric nerves (T12 and L1), and ilioinguinal (L1) nerves. Dermatome T10 lies at the umbilicus.

After giving off a lateral cutaneous branch, each intercostal nerve pierces the lateral border of the rectus sheath. There it provides a lateral branch that ends in the rectus muscle. The anterior branch then passes through the muscle and perforates the rectus sheath to supply the subcutaneous tissues and skin as the anterior cutaneous branches. Incisions along the lateral border of the rectus lead to denervation of the muscle, which can render it atrophic and weaken the abdominal wall. Elevation of the rectus sheath off the muscle during the Pfannenstiel incision stretches the perforating nerve, which is sometimes ligated to provide hemostasis from the accompanying artery. This may leave an area of cutaneous anesthesia.

The iliohypogastric and ilioinguinal nerves pass medial to the anterosuperior iliac spine in the abdominal wall. The former supplies the skin of the suprapubic area. The latter supplies the lower abdominal wall, and by sending a branch through the inguinal canal, it supplies the upper portions of the labia majora and medial portions of the thigh. These nerves can be entrapped in the lateral closure of a transverse incision and may lead to chronic pain syndromes.

The genitofemoral (L1 and L2) and femorocutaneous (L2 and L3) nerves can be injured during gynecologic surgery. The genitofemoral nerve lies on the psoas muscle (Fig. 7.31), where pressure from a retractor can damage it and lead to anesthesia in the medial thigh and lateral labia. The femoral cutaneous nerve can be compressed either by a retractor blade lateral to the psoas or by too much flexion of the hip in the lithotomy position, causing anesthesia over the anterior thigh.

BEST SURGICAL PRACTICES

- Important anatomic relationships of the ureter include the following:
  - The ureter lies medial to the ovarian vessels at the bifurcation of the internal and external iliac arteries entering the pelvic brim.
  - The ureter courses under the uterine artery approximately at 1.5 cm lateral to the cervix.
  - The ureter lies directly on the anterior vaginal wall very near the place where the vagina is detached from the cervix during the hysterectomy.
- Branches of the ilioinguinal and iliohypogastric nerves run in the region of the abdominal wall involved in lower abdominal transverse incision and can be involved with nerve entrapment syndromes after these incisions.
- Support of the pelvic organs comes from the combined action of the levator ani muscles that close the genital hiatus and provide a supportive layer on which the organs can rest and by the attachment of the vagina and uterus to the pelvic sidewalls.
- The internal iliac vessels supply the pelvic organs and pelvic wall and gluteal regions. The complexity of these multiple branches varies from individual to individual, but the key feature is the multiple areas of collateral circulation that come into play immediately after internal iliac artery ligation so that blood supply to the pelvic organs has diminished pulse pressure but continues to have flow even after the ligation.
- The blood supply to the female genital tract is an arcade that begins at the top with input from the ovarian vessels, lateral supply by the uterine vessels, and distal supply by the vaginal artery. There is an anastigmatic artery that runs along the entire length of the genital tract. For this reason, ligation of any single one of these arteries does not diminish flow to the uterus itself.

Bibliography

Anson BJ. *An atlas of human anatomy*. Philadelphia: WB Saunders, 1950:241.

Burchell RC. Arterial physiology of the human female pelvis. *Obstet Gynecol* 1968;31:855.

Campbell RM. The anatomy and histology of the sacrouterine ligaments. *Am J Obstet Gynecol* 1950;59:1.

Cox HT. The cleavage lines of the skin. *Br J Surg* 1941;29:234.

Curry SL, Wharton JT, Rutledge F. Positive lymph nodes in vulvar squamous carcinoma. *Gynecol Oncol* 1980;9:63.

Dalley AF. The riddle of the sphincters. *Am Surg* 1987;53:298.

Daseler EH, Anson BJ, Reimann AF. Radical excision of the inguinal and iliac lymph glands. *Surg Gynecol Obstet* 1948;87:679.

DeLancey JOL. Anatomic aspects of vaginal eversion after hysterectomy. *Am J Obstet Gynecol* 1992;166:1717.

DeLancey JOL. Correlative study of paraurethral anatomy. *Obstet Gynecol* 1986;68:91.

DeLancey JOL. Structural anatomy of the posterior compartment as it relates to rectocele. *Am J Obstet Gynecol* 1999;180:815.

DeLancey JOL. Structural aspects of the extrinsic continence mechanism. *Obstet Gynecol* 1988;72:296.

DeLancey JOL. Structural support of the urethra as it relates to stress urinary incontinence: the hammock hypothesis. *Am J Obstet Gynecol* 1994;170:1713.

DeLancey JOL, Toglia MR, Perucchini D. Internal and external anal sphincter anatomy as it relates to midline obstetric lacerations. *Obstet Gynecol* 1997;90:924.

Fernstrom I. Arteriography of the uterine artery. *Acta Radiol* 1955;122 (Suppl):21.

Fluhmann CF, Dickmann Z. The basic pattern of the glandular structures of the cervix uteri. *Obstet Gynecol* 1958;11:543.

Forster DS. A note on Scarpa's fascia. *J Anat* 1937;72:130.

Funt MI, Thompson JD, Birch H. Normal vaginal axis. *South Med J* 1978;71:1534.

Goerttler K. Die architektur der muskelwand des menschlichen uterus and ihre funktionelle bedeutung. *Morph Jarb* 1930;65:45.

Goff BH. The surgical anatomy of cystocele and urethrocele with special reference to the pubocervical fascia. *Surg Gynecol Obstet* 1948;87:725.

Hudson CN. Lymphatics of the pelvis. In: Philipp EE, Barnes J, Newton M, eds. *Scientific foundations of obstetrics and gynecology*, 3rd ed. London: Heinemann, 1986:1.

Huffman J. Detailed anatomy of the paraurethral ducts in the adult human female. *Am J Obstet Gynecol* 1948;55:86.

Hughesdon PE. The fibromuscular structure of the cervix and its changes during pregnancy and labour. *J Obstet Gynaecol Br Commonw* 1952;59:763.

Huisman AB. Aspects on the anatomy of the female urethra with special relation to urinary continence. *Contrib Gynecol Obstet* 1983;10:1.

Hurd WW, Bude RO, DeLancey JOL, et al. The location of abdominal wall blood vessels in relationship to abdominal landmarks apparent at laparoscopy. *Am J Obstet Gynecol* 1994;171:642.

Hutch JA. *Anatomy and physiology of the bladder, trigone and urethra*. New York: Appleton-Century-Crofts, 1972.

Klink EW. Perineal nerve block: an anatomic and clinical study in the female. *Obstet Gynecol* 1953;1:137.

Krantz KE. The anatomy of the urethra and anterior vaginal wall. *Am J Obstet Gynecol* 1951;62:374.

Krantz KE. Innervation of the human uterus. *Ann N Y Acad Sci* 1959;75:770.

Kuhn RJ, Hollyock VE. Observations on the anatomy of the rectovaginal pouch and septum. *Obstet Gynecol* 1982;59:445.

Lawson JON. Pelvic anatomy. I. Pelvic floor muscles. *Ann R Coll Surg Engl* 1974;54:244.

Lawson JON. Pelvic anatomy. II. Anal canal and associated sphincters. *Ann R Coll Surg Engl* 1974;54:288.

Milley PS, Nichols DH. The relationship between the pubo-urethral ligaments and the urogenital diaphragm in the human female. *Anat Rec* 1971;170:281.

Milloy FJ, Anson BJ, McAfee DK. The rectus abdominis muscle and the epigastric arteries. *Surg Gynecol Obstet* 1960;110:293.

Morley GW, DeLancey JOL. Sacrospinous ligament fixation for eversion of the vagina. *Am J Obstet Gynecol* 1988;158:872.

Muellner SR. Physiology of micturition. *J Urol* 1951;65:805.

Nesselrod JP. An anatomic restudy of the pelvic lymphatics. *Ann Surg* 1936;104:905.

Nichols DH. Sacrospinous fixation for massive eversion of the vagina. *Am J Obstet Gynecol* 1982;142:901.

Nichols DH, Milley PS, Randall CL. Significance of restoration of normal vaginal depth and axis. *Obstet Gynecol* 1970;36:251.

Nichols DH, Randall CL. *Vaginal surgery*, 3rd ed. Baltimore: Williams & Wilkins, 1989.

O'Connell HE, Hutson JM, Anderson CR, et al. Anatomical relationship between urethra and clitoris. *J Urol* 1998;159:1892.

Oelrich TM. The striated urogenital sphincter muscle in the female. *Anat Rec* 1983;205:223.

Oh C, Kark AE. Anatomy of the external anal sphincter. *Br J Surg* 1972;59:717.

Oh C, Kark AE. Anatomy of the perineal body. *Dis Colon Rectum* 1973;16:444.

Parry-Jones E. Lymphatics of the vulva. *J Obstet Gynaecol Br Emp* 1963;70:751.

Plentl AA, Friedman EA. *Lymphatic system of the female genitalia*. Philadelphia: WB Saunders, 1971.

Ramsey EM. Vascular anatomy. In: Wynn RM, ed. *Biology of the uterus*. New York: Plenum Press, 1977:60.

Range RL, Woodburne RT. The gross and microscopic anatomy of the transverse cervical ligaments. *Am J Obstet Gynecol* 1964;90:460.

Reiffenstuhl G. The clinical significance of the connective tissue planes and spaces. *Clin Obstet Gynecol* 1982;25:811.

Ricci JV, Lisa JR, Thom CH, et al. The relationship of the vagina to adjacent organs in reconstructive surgery. *Am J Surg* 1947;74:387.

Ricci JV, Thom CH. The myth of a surgically useful fascia in vaginal plastic reconstructions. *Q Rev Surg Obstet Gynecol* 1954;2:253.

Richardson AC, Edmonds PB, Williams NL. Treatment of stress urinary incontinence due to paravaginal fascial defect. *Obstet Gynecol* 1981;57:357.
Roberts WH, Habenicht J, Krishingner G. The pelvic and perineal fasciae and their neural and vascular relationships. *Anat Rec* 1964;149:707.
Roberts WH, Harrison CW, Mitchell DA, et al. The levator ani muscle and the nerve supply of its puborectalis component. *Clin Anat* 1988;1:256.
Roberts WH, Krishingner GL. Comparative study of human internal iliac artery based on Adachi classification. *Anat Rec* 1967;158:191.
Sampson JA. Ureteral fistulae as sequelae of pelvic operations. *Surg Gynecol Obstet* 1909;8:479.
Sato K. A morphological analysis of the nerve supply of the sphincter ani externus, levator ani and coccygeus. *Acta Anat Nippon* 1980;44:187.
Schreiber H. Konstruktionsmorphologische Betrachtungen uber den Wandungsbau der menschlichen Vagina. *Arkiv fur Gynaekologie* 1942;174(B43):222.
Skandalakis JE, Gray SW, Rowe JS. *Anatomical complications in general surgery.* New York: McGraw-Hill, 1983:297.
Stulz P, Pfeiffer KM. Peripheral nerve injuries resulting from common surgical procedures in the lower portion of the abdomen. *Arch Surg* 1982;117:324.
Tobin CE, Benjamin JA. Anatomic and clinical re-evaluation of Camper's, Scarpa's and Colles' fasciae. *Surg Gynecol Obstet* 1949;88:545.
Uhlenhuth E, Nolley GW. Vaginal fascia, a myth? *Obstet Gynecol* 1957;10:349.
Zacharin RF. The anatomic supports of the female urethra. *Obstet Gynecol* 1968;32:754.

CHAPTER 8 ■ PREOPERATIVE CARE

SANFORD M. MARKHAM AND JOHN A. ROCK

DEFINITIONS

Preoperative care—The patient management period during which time gynecologic pathology, defects, and injury are assessed and diagnosed; an accurate decision is made for a surgical intervention; the patient is appropriately appraised of the problem and need for surgery as well as options available; and necessary preoperative evaluation and preparation is accomplished.

Preoperative evaluation—The assessment of a patient before surgery for the purpose of detecting factors that could affect surgical outcome and may include, in addition to a thorough physical examination, laboratory testing, imaging procedures, and consultations.

Preoperative physical examination—A complete physical examination of the whole body with special emphasis directed toward the breast, abdomen, and the pelvis and rectum.

Preoperative laboratory and imaging assessment—An assessment that is limited to those tests that are statistically of importance in detecting factors that could/would alter surgical outcome and are selected based on the patient's individual history and physical examination and not on a predetermined panel for all patients.

Preoperative gynecologic surgery assessment category—A complexity categorization of gynecologic surgical cases for purposes of selecting necessary preoperative testing and predicting surgical outcome. Categories include uncomplicated gynecologic pathology with an uncomplicated medical/surgical status, complicated gynecologic pathology with uncomplicated medical/surgical status, and uncomplicated or complicated gynecologic pathology with a complicated medical/surgical status.

The preoperative care and management of women has proven to be a critical factor in achieving anticipated and successful outcomes of both emergent and scheduled gynecologic surgical procedures. Although the importance of a thorough history and physical examination remain key elements in the preoperative evaluation of all gynecologic patients, the use of "routine" preoperative laboratory evaluation and imaging procedures have undergone considerable change since prior editions of this textbook. This is because of the impact of recent patient care outcome reviews that have focused on indicated preoperative testing compared with "routine" testing. *Cost-effectiveness* and *evidence-based medicine* are terms that are now commonly used by both the medical professionals and by managed care organizations (MCOs) when ordering and approving preoperative laboratory assessment and imaging tests. This approach makes essential the understanding of what constitutes necessary and essential preoperative testing based on current evidence from both prospective and retrospective studies.

A thorough review of medical sources does not yet provide sufficient controlled trial data to make evidence-based decisions on most preoperative laboratory and imaging testing for gynecologic surgery. The Cochrane Library contains recent controlled trial studies on individual gynecologic surgical procedures, but it does not currently contain controlled trial studies that relate to cost-effectiveness of any gynecologic preoperative testing or procedures. However, significant other case series data do exist that support the need for minimal preoperative testing in the uncomplicated gynecologic patient as well as specific preoperative testing and imaging for the complicated case.

This chapter is designed to provide to gynecologic surgeons an in-depth understanding of the essential features of preoperative care from the preoperative examination in the office, or emergency room, to the time of surgery. Included are suggestions relating to appropriate preoperative testing and evaluation based on the experience of gynecologic surgeons and anesthesiologists. Also included are accumulated data that demonstrate the benefits of preoperative evaluation to patient care. Foremost, it is essential to keep in mind that each woman must be considered individually, based on her medical findings and needs, and that no suggestions can be completely adapted to all women preparing for gynecologic surgery.

IMPORTANCE OF PREOPERATIVE CARE

Successful surgical outcomes of operative gynecologic procedures occur as the result of several factors in addition to good surgical skills and techniques. These factors include:

1. An appropriate preoperative evaluation (the ability to accurately assess and diagnose gynecologic pathology, defects, and injury)
2. An appropriate patient selection (the ability to determine when surgical intervention is a necessary course of action)
3. An appropriate discussion with the patient regarding the benefits and risks of the surgery (the ability to communicate to the patient both short- and long-term complications in a manner that can be understood)
4. An ability to work with MCO organizations in terms of obtaining preoperative approval and complying with individual health care plan guidelines

Once a gynecologic pathology or defect has been detected and surgical intervention is thought to be the appropriate course of action, surgical planning should be instituted. In nonemergent cases, this planning should include a specific time for preoperative evaluation. The purpose of the preoperative evaluation is to accomplish the following tasks as described by Fischer: (a) decrease surgical morbidity, (b) minimize expensive delays and cancellations on the day of surgery, (c) evaluate and optimize patient health status, (d) facilitate the planning of anesthesia and perioperative care, (e) reduce patient anxiety through education, and (f) obtain informed consent. Although these objectives were presented in the context of accomplishing the tasks in a setting of a preoperative evaluation clinic, they are equally applicable to surgical planning in smaller communities where preoperative evaluation clinics are not available, provided that the major components of the operating team, specifically the gynecologist, anesthesiologist, and consultants are available.

The importance of effective preoperative evaluations should not be underestimated. Many studies have repeatedly shown that preoperative patient conditions are significant predictors of postoperative morbidity. It is essential that all women undergoing preoperative assessment have a complete history and thorough physical examination as a key element in their workup. This examination is of importance to determine factors that could affect surgical outcome. When medical status questions arise that cannot be answered by the gynecologist, then laboratory testing and imaging procedures, as well as consultations, become essential to promote optimal outcomes.

In the past, preoperative testing developed around the use of a history and physical examination. Batteries of "routine" individual and multiphasic laboratory tests and imaging procedures were used to detect subclinical or presymptomatic medical problems that might affect the outcomes of the surgical procedure. Additionally, it was felt that less than desirable outcomes of gynecologic surgical procedures could be minimized through the use of a wide battery of tests to prove or disprove normalcy before surgery. It was also felt that this reduction in less-than-desirable outcomes might also provide some legal protection.

Unfortunately, the use of multiple "routine" tests has resulted in considerable additional costs for surgery and has created a problem as to what should be done when preoperative test results are found to be unexpectedly abnormal. It has been reported that data from the last two decades indicate 60% to 70% of laboratory tests ordered preoperatively are not required based on a review of the history and/or physical examination. Other studies suggest that only 1% or less of routinely ordered preoperative tests revealed abnormalities that might have influenced perioperative management. Furthermore, between 30% and 60% of all unexpected abnormalities detected by preoperative laboratory tests were not actually noted or investigated before surgery. This fact alone suggests that not only does the ordering of multiple "routine" tests not provide legal protection but quite possibly it also sets up an opportunity for increased legal liability. Finally, the cost of accomplishing these unnecessary preoperative "routine" tests adds many millions of dollars to health care costs each year without any proven benefit to patient care.

Using this information and applying it to the preoperative assessment of gynecologic surgery patients in the future, a preoperative evaluation should strive to answer the following three questions as outlined by Roizen.

1. Is the patient in optimal health?
2. Can, or should, the patient's physical or mental condition be improved before surgery?
3. Does the patient have health problems or use any medications that could unexpectedly influence perioperative events?

Therefore, all preoperative assessment and care should be directed toward answering these questions, using only those preoperative testing modalities that are expected to give information that leads to answers, as opposed to the random "routine" batteries of tests used in the past.

Additionally it is most important to dedicate a portion of the preoperative care time to a discussion with the patient of options for management of her gynecologic problem, including both short- and long-term potential complications. All patients must be given sufficient medical information to allow them to make an educated decision about whether to proceed with the planned surgery. Examples of gynecologic issues that suggest the need for informed decisions include the recently reported significant increase in urinary incontinence following hysterectomy (60%) or the higher than previously reported failure rate of tubal sterilization (CREST [Collaborative Review of Sterilization] study: 10-year accumulative failure rate of 18.5 per 1,000), or the common recurrence of abnormal uterine bleeding leading to a subsequent hysterectomy in women with a history of abnormal uterine bleeding controlled by oral contraceptive pills who elect to undergo a tubal sterilization (relative risk 1.8). Not only is the discussion time useful in fostering a good physician–patient relationship, but it becomes extremely important if outcomes of surgery are less than expected, particularly if the discussion was documented in the patient's record.

HISTORY AND PHYSICAL EXAMINATION

History

Preoperative care of a patient always begins by carefully taking a complete history and doing a thorough preoperative examination. For the surgeon, the process of the history and the physical examination are fundamental to good surgical results. The physical and mental preparation of the patient are key to patient satisfaction after surgery. It is essential that the operating gynecologist personally take the history. This personal contact with the patient is of value to both the patient and surgeon. During this time, the gynecologist can gain an individual perspective of not only the gynecologic problems but also the patient's general status. The patient can, in turn, ask direct questions relating to the surgical procedure as well as express her concerns. This interchange gives the surgeon a unique impression of the problem and allows the surgeon to better assess the pathology or defect that requires surgery. This also places the gynecologist in a much better position to arrive at an accurate diagnosis, determine the essential preoperative testing that will be needed, and select the most appropriate surgery to manage the problem.

Good history taking and a thorough physical examination require time and patience, neither of which is easily available given the expanded demands of gynecologic practice. However, the reward for the gynecologist who takes the time to listen to the patient and accomplish a complete physical examination is the avoidance of unnecessary surgery. Unnecessary operations, particularly for patients already troubled by some difficult problem of life, may prove to be unsuccessful in relieving the patient's symptoms and also concentrate attention unnecessarily on the pelvic organs. If the condition is not urgent, do not make a firm decision regarding recommendation for major pelvic surgery on the first consultation.

Emergent and urgent conditions, by necessity, require a different approach of rapid assessment and action. In most gynecologic cases, however, the patient is counseled on the need for surgery only after all physical and psychological aspects of her case are thoroughly evaluated. The surgeon who does not ask questions and offer explanations, and who does not carefully consider choices, usually has less than desirable outcomes.

A patient's history should be concise, but accuracy should not be sacrificed for the sake of brevity. It has become a common practice to use a preprinted form or a computer template, if using electronic medical records, when obtaining a history. Unfortunately, no medical form is applicable to every case. Maximum efficiency can be achieved by using a standard patient-completed history form (Fig. 8.1) along with a physician-completed history and physical examination form or electronic record template (Figs. 8.2 and Fig. 8.3). The physician can use the patient-completed form to efficiently assimilate the information and direct the history and physical examination process. The physician's history and physical examination form serve as a structured reminder of the essentials of the history-taking process as well as summarize the patient's medical history to facilitate the decision to accomplish surgery. The electronic record template can be tailored to include subsections of any portion of the history or physical examination. These forms additionally serve as a record for Current

B-1b DEPARTMENT OF OBSTETRICS AND GYNECOLOGY
Patient Self History

DATE
HOSP. NO.
NAME
BIRTH DATE
ADDRESS

● File most recent sheet of this number ON BOTTOM ●

IF NOT IMPRINTED, PLEASE PRINT DATE, HOSP. NO., NAME AND LOCATION

The University of Iowa Hospitals and Clinics requests this information for the purpose of providing patient care. Some questions may seem personal or appear to have no relationship to your care, but your responses are important. This information will help your health care providers to better understand how your health problems are affecting your daily life, and to find out how they can best help to improve your overall health. Your responses will be held in strict confidence. If you have questions or concerns about information on the form, please talk with your health care provider. If you choose not to respond to these items, patient care may be compromised/influenced.

GYNECOLOGIC/OBSTETRIC HISTORY

1. Age ________
2. When was the first day of your last period? ______/______/______
3. Date of most recent pelvic exam? ______/______/______ normal / abnormal (please circle)
4. Date of most recent Pap smear? ______/______/______ normal / abnormal (please circle)
5. Date of most recent mammogram? ______/______/______ normal / abnormal (please circle)
6. ☐ No ☐ Yes Have you ever been told you had an abnormal Pap smear? If *yes*, when? ________
   If treated, what kind of treatment was done? ________
7. How old were you when you first started your periods? ________
8. Usually, your periods come (came) every ________ days, and last(ed) ________ days.
9. Are/Were your periods usually: ☐ Regular ☐ Irregular ☐ Light ☐ Moderate ☐ Heavy ☐ Very painful ☐ A little painful ☐ Painless
10. ☐ No ☐ Yes Do you have bleeding between periods? (If *yes*, describe) ________
11. Describe any problems you are currently having (or had) with your periods.
12. ☐ No ☐ Yes Do you need a birth control method today? (For gynecology appointment only)
    (If *no*, move on to question 14)
13. Which method do you want today? ________
14. List current/past birth control methods below:

Methods used	Year started	Year quit	Problems	Reason you stopped using this method

15. Total number of pregnancies ________ Number of living children ________ Age at first pregnancy ________

Year	Length of pregnancy	Losses	Delivery	Complications: Mother	Complications: Baby
	D-Around due date P-Premature L-Late	A-Abortion M-Miscarriage S-Stillbirth E-Ectopic/(Tubal)	V-Vaginal CS-C-section	DM-Diabetes BP-Blood Pressure BL-Bleeding S-Seizures	J-Jaundice BD-Birth Defect MR-Mentally Retarded B-Breech
1.					
2.					
3.					
4.					
5.					
6.					
7.					
8.					

16. ☐ No ☐ Yes ☐ Undecided Are you trying to become pregnant? (For gynecology appointment only)
17. ☐ No ☐ Yes ☐ Undecided Is it possible you want to have children in the future? (For gynecology appointment only)
18. ☐ No ☐ Yes Have you had any difficulty becoming pregnant?
    If *yes*, describe ________
19. ☐ No ☐ Yes Are you currently breast feeding?

76339/4-97 THE UNIVERSITY OF IOWA HOSPITALS AND CLINICS

B -1b | C LABORATORY | D X-RAY EXAM | E CONSULTATION | F SPEC. EXAM | G THERAPY | H PATHOLOGY | I DIAGNOSIS

FIGURE 8.1. Patient history (Hx) form. (From: University of Iowa Hospitals and Clinics, with permission.)

B-1b PATIENT SELF HISTORY P. 2 **Pt. Name** ________ **Hosp. No.** ________

20. Have you had any of the following? Please give approximate dates.

Dates	No	Yes		Dates	No	Yes	
____	☐	☐	Vaginal infection	____	☐	☐	Genital herpes
____	☐	☐	Vaginal itching/dryness/discharge/odor	____	☐	☐	Gonorrhea
____	☐	☐	Unusual vaginal bleeding	____	☐	☐	Chlamydia
____	☐	☐	Pain/bleeding with intercourse	____	☐	☐	Syphilis
____	☐	☐	Hot flashes	____	☐	☐	Genital warts
____	☐	☐	Uterine fibroids	____	☐	☐	HIV / AIDS
____	☐	☐	Involuntary loss of urine	____	☐	☐	Group B Strep
____	☐	☐	Bladder/kidney infection	____	☐	☐	Partner with any of the above infections
____	☐	☐	Pelvic inflammatory disease				

MEDICAL/SURGICAL HISTORY

21. Have you **ever had** or do you **currently have** any of the following?

No	Yes		No	Yes	
☐	☐	Diabetes	☐	☐	Blood transfusions (year ____)
☐	☐	High blood pressure	☐	☐	Blood diseases
☐	☐	Chest pain/heart attack	☐	☐	Sickle cell disease
☐	☐	Rheumatic fever	☐	☐	Trauma (such as fractures, concussion)
☐	☐	Heart murmur	☐	☐	Surgery(s) (If yes, what kind?)
☐	☐	Blood clots (in your lungs, brain or heart)			________ date ____
☐	☐	Stroke			________ date ____
☐	☐	Anemia	☐	☐	Hospitalization in the last 5 years?
☐	☐	Kidney/Bladder problems			For what reason: ____
☐	☐	Epilepsy/Convulsions			For what reason: ____
☐	☐	Hepatitis/Jaundice	☐	☐	Gall bladder problems
☐	☐	Liver problems	☐	☐	Stomach problems/vomiting
☐	☐	Varicose veins	☐	☐	Blood in stools
☐	☐	Thyroid problems	☐	☐	Constipation/Diarrhea
☐	☐	Tuberculosis	☐	☐	Cancer (If yes, what kind?)
☐	☐	Lived with someone who had Tuberculosis			________ date ____
☐	☐	Asthma	☐	☐	Physical abuse
☐	☐	Depression	☐	☐	Alcohol dependency
☐	☐	Mental illness and/or suicide attempts	☐	☐	Drug dependency
☐	☐	Breast disease	☐	☐	Intravenous drug use
☐	☐	Migraine headaches	☐	☐	Sexual abuse
☐	☐	Frequent headaches			

IMMUNIZATION HISTORY

☐No	☐Yes	☐Not sure	Have you had the Chicken Pox (Varicella-zoster)?
☐No	☐Yes	☐Not sure	Are you immune to rubella (German measles)?
☐No	☐Yes	☐Not sure	Have you had a hepatitis B vaccination? (3 shots)?
☐No	☐Yes	☐Not sure	Have you had a tetanus shot in the last 10 years?
☐No	☐Yes	☐Not sure	Have you had a recent skin test for TB?

FAMILY HISTORY

22. ☐No ☐Yes Are you adopted? *If yes, skip and go on to next section (General).*

23. Has anyone in your family had trouble with the following [include mother (M), father (F), brother (B), sister (S), grandfather (GF), grandmother (GM), aunt (A), uncle (U), son (SN), or daughter (D)]. (Place the appropriate initials in any categories that apply.)

No	Yes		Who	No	Yes		Who
☐	☐	Breast cancer	____	☐	☐	Birth defects	____
☐	☐	Female organ cancer	____	☐	☐	Multiple gestation (twins, triplets)	____
☐	☐	Other cancer	____	☐	☐	Mother used DES (a medicine	
		If yes, what? ____	____			to prevent miscarriage)	____
☐	☐	Diabetes	____	☐	☐	Hereditary disease	____
☐	☐	Stroke	____			If yes, what? ____	
☐	☐	High blood pressure	____				
☐	☐	Heart attack	____	☐	☐	Cystic Fibrosis	____
☐	☐	High cholesterol	____	☐	☐	Sickle cell disease	____
☐	☐	Osteoporosis (bone thinning)	____	☐	☐	Pre eclampsia (high blood pressure in pregnancy)	____

FIGURE 8.1. (*Continued*)

Procedural Terminology (CPT) coding documentation, as well as for later clinical research. Experience has shown that important omissions are much less frequent when information is compiled on a standard form. Care should be taken, however, to not allow such a form to restrict the accurate recording of the present illness. Forms always can be expanded to document an event in the patient's history that might have an important bearing on the present illness.

A few points should be stressed concerning proper gynecologic history taking. The menstrual history must be accurate and detailed. The clue to a correct diagnosis of the gynecologic condition for which surgery is being considered often appears in the pattern of menstrual irregularity, whether the menstrual disturbance results from an organic lesion or a dysfunctional cause. In fact, differentiation between dysfunctional and early organic disease is one of the most common and difficult clinical distinctions that must be made before surgery. Accurate dates of the last and previous menstrual periods are of major importance. When there is a discrepancy between menstrual dates and pelvic findings in a patient of reproductive age, pregnancy

B-1b DEPARTMENT OF OBSTETRICS AND GYNECOLOGY
Patient Self History
Page 3

DATE
HOSP. NO.
NAME
BIRTH DATE
ADDRESS

● File most recent sheet of this number ON BOTTOM ●

IF NOT IMPRINTED, PLEASE PRINT DATE, HOSP. NO., NAME AND LOCATION

CURRENT MEDICATION HISTORY

24. Please list medications used during the last three months on a routine basis

Name of Medication	Date started	Currently Taking Yes	No	Reason for Taking Medication

25. List any allergies to medications/Latex/Iodine ____________

GENERAL HEALTH QUESTIONS

26. ☐ No ☐ Yes Are you concerned about your eating habits?
27. ☐ No ☐ Yes Are you concerned with your weight?
28. ☐ No ☐ Yes Do you currently use WIC (Women's, Infant's and Children's Nutrition program)?
29. ☐ No ☐ Yes Are you currently using vitamins (or prenatal vitamins)?
30. ☐ No ☐ Yes Do you drink caffeine (like coffee, colas)?
    If *yes*, how many cups per day? ____________
31. ☐ No ☐ Yes Do you exercise regularly?
32. ☐ No ☐ Yes Have you been taught how to do self breast exam?
33. ☐ No ☐ Yes Do you examine your breasts monthly?
34. ☐ No ☐ Yes Have you had your cholsterol checked?
    Year/Results ____________
35. ☐ No ☐ Yes Do you smoke cigarettes?
    If *yes*, # ________ packs per day for ________ years.
36. ☐ No ☐ Yes Do other people in your house smoke?
    If *no*, are you an ex-smoker ☐ No ☐ Yes Quit ________ years ago.
37. ☐ No ☐ Yes Do you drink alcohol?
    If yes, how many drinks, glasses of wine, or beers do you have in one week?
    (Circle one) 1-2 drinks 3-6 drinks 7-25 drinks over 25 drinks
38. If you had a baby before, how did you adjust emotionally after delivery of other children?
    ☐ No problem ☐ Crying, Mood swings ☐ Depressed ☐ Never been pregnant
39. If pregnant, how has your mood been so far during pregnancy?
    ☐ No problem ☐ Have felt depressed, sad, blue or anxious for more than two weeks at a time?
    ☐ Never been pregnant
40. How much help/support do you get from others in your house for day to day activities (for example, housework and childcare)?
    ☐ A lot of help ☐ Some help ☐ Little, if any

PLEASE CHECK ANY OF THE FOLLOWING TOPICS TO RECEIVE MORE INFORMATION:

☐ birth control methods
☐ safer sex practices
☐ depression
☐ stress/anxiety reduction
☐ nutritional counseling
☐ weight control
☐ mammograms
☐ sexually transmitted disease
☐ getting pregnant and having a healthy baby
☐ sexual abuse, incest, or rape
☐ osteoporosis (bone thinning)
☐ cholsterol
☐ other ____________
☐ stopping smoking
☐ substance abuse
☐ menopause
☐ sexual problems
☐ incontinence (loss of urine)

Patient Signature ____________ Date: ____________

THE UNIVERSITY OF IOWA HOSPITALS AND CLINICS

FIGURE 8.1. (*Continued*)

should be suspected and a pregnancy test accomplished. A discrepancy between menstrual dates and pelvic findings in a patient with suspected pregnancy requires a serum quantitative human chorionic gonadotropin (hCG) testing to identify appropriate progression of the pregnancy, along with a pelvic ultrasound when the pelvic examination and hCG test results are at odds.

Good gynecologic history taking can also provide valuable clues relating to findings in the physical examination. In a woman younger than 50 years of age with a history of maternal diethylstilbestrol (DES) exposure, attention should be paid to the potential presence of a variety of anatomical defects of the müllerian duct system such as a "T-shaped" uterus, vaginal adenosis, or cervical defects ("cock's comb" cervix). A documented history of Type II herpes simplex viral infection of the lower genital tract has long-term implications for future recurrences and symptomatology. Of equal importance in postmenopausal women is obtaining an accurate date of the menopause. Some women are now cycling well into their fifties. Variations in vaginal bleeding in these patients may be of far different significance than vaginal bleeding in a woman 10 to 15 years postmenopausal.

B-1b PATIENT SELF HISTORY P. 4 **Pt. Name** ____________________ **Hosp. No.** __________

It is extremely important that we be able to contact you so that we may notify you of test results, return appointments, or schedule changes. So that we may efficiently do this and maintain confidentiality for you, please check the boxes below that apply to you.

_____ You may send letters to my home.

_____ You may phone me at home and leave messages. My phone number is __________

_____ You may phone me at home, but leave no messages.

_____ You may phone me at work and leave messages. My work phone number is __________

_____ You may phone me at work, but leave no messages.

_____ You may phone me at a number other than home or work. Phone number __________

May we leave messages at this number? ______

Whose number is this? __________

_____ An alternative address that would allow mail to get to me is __________

____

The best time of day to phone me is __________

Other comments __________

____

Patient Signature ____________________ Date __________

FIGURE 8.1. (Continued)

The patient's reproductive history is also of great importance, particularly a history of previous pregnancies and complications of pregnancy such as dystocia, cesarean section, postpartum infection, abortion, urinary tract infections, excessive infant size, vaginal lacerations, deep vein thrombophlebitis, and pulmonary embolization. A well-taken marital history may reveal dyspareunia and/or unsatisfactory sexual relations, which may explain some symptoms that resemble organic pelvic disease.

Because the symptoms of urinary tract disease so closely resemble those of reproductive tract disease, a urologic history is important, along with laboratory investigation of the urinary tract before a final diagnosis is determined and a decision made regarding surgery. Too often the symptoms of urinary frequency, urgency, and dysuria have been diagnosed as a mechanical support defect of the urinary bladder and treated by surgical repair with plication of the bladder neck, although the real problem of chronic urinary tract infection or neurogenic dysfunction of the bladder remains undiagnosed. Put in another way, a disorder of the lower urinary tract can produce symptoms suggestive of reproductive tract disease and vice versa. For this reason, basic urologic training is advocated for every gynecologist. The gynecologist who is adept with a urologic workup, including cystoscopy and cystometrics, can evaluate a case better than one who must depend entirely on consultation and urology reports.

B-1b CLINICAL NOTES
GENERAL GYNECOLOGIC EVALUATION/
PRE-OP SURGERY EVALUATION
Department of Obstetrics and Gynecology

● File most recent sheet of this number ON BOTTOM ●

DATE
HOSP. NO.
NAME
BIRTH DATE
ADDRESS
SS #
IF NOT IMPRINTED, PLEASE PRINT DATE, HOSP. NO., NAME AND LOCATION

	Date of last visit:	(See last clinical note if seen less than 12 months ago)
Informant		Relation to Patient:
Cc:		
HPI:		LMP
PMHx	Illnesses:	Operations:
		Hx. of Gyn Surgeries
	Medications:	
		Hx. of Hormone Replacement Therapy:
	Allergies:	Method of contraception:
		Hx. of STDs
Habits:	Tobacco: Alcohol:	Street Drugs:
FHx:		
Social Hx	Marital History: Education:	Occupation(s):
Health	Pap smear HX:	Mammogram HX:
Behaviors		
	Performs Self Breast Exam:	Cholesterol level:
	Immunizations: Last Tetanus Toxoid (Yr.)	Rubella titer: Immune Nonimmune Unknown
	Hepatitis B (Yr.)	
	Influenza (Yr.)	

B -1b | C LABORATORY | D X-RAY EXAM | E CONSULTATION | F SPEC. EXAM | G THERAPY | H PATHOLOGY | I DIAGNOSIS

75790/3-97 THE UNIVERSITY OF IOWA HOSPITALS AND CLINICS

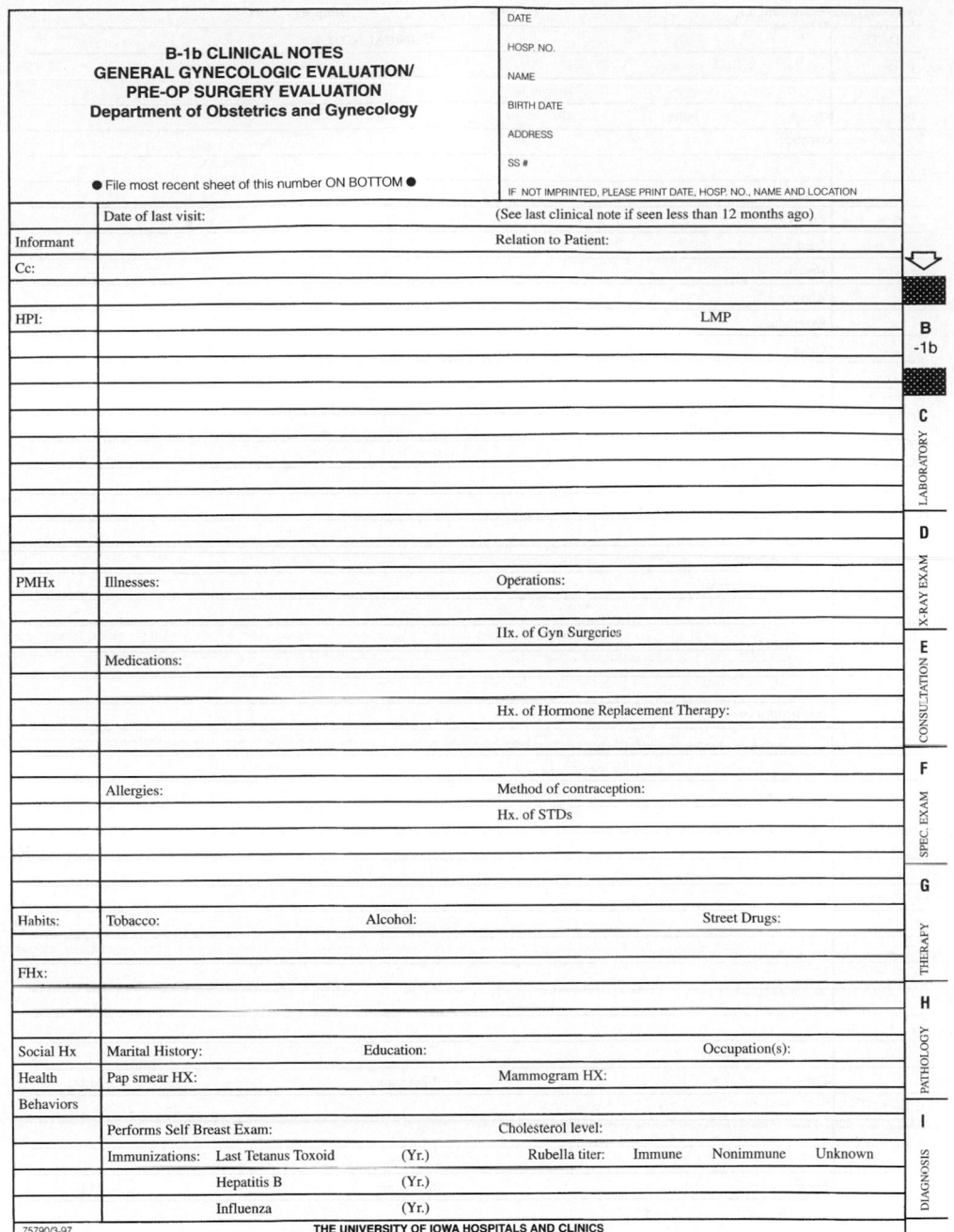

FIGURE 8.2. Physician's history (Hx) and physical examination (PE) form. (From: University of Iowa Hospitals and Clinics, with permission.)

Symptomatology of gastrointestinal tract disease can also mimic disease of the reproductive tract. Thus, a proper gastrointestinal tract history along with appropriate laboratory investigation make a significant contribution toward arriving at a correct diagnosis and treatment plan before gynecologic surgical intervention. Constipation, irritable bowel syndrome, colitis, Crohn's disease, and diverticulitis can cause abdominal and pelvic pain that is not dissimilar to the pain of endometriosis, pelvic adhesions, or ovarian neoplasms. Therefore, basic gastrointestinal training is also advocated for all gynecologists. The gynecologist experienced in accomplishing sigmoidoscopy is better prepared to assess gynecologic cases being considered for surgery than the gynecologist who lacks such experience.

Because abnormal uterine bleeding can result from a variety of endocrine and metabolic disorders, a history of hypothyroidism, hyperprolactemia, insulin metabolism errors, as well as other endocrine and metabolic defects in the patient and in her family are of considerable importance in assessing and treating menorrhagia and metrorrhagia. A positive history followed by appropriate endocrine testing can give physicians significant insight into the etiology of the problem and allow

Gynecology Evaluation (cont'd.) Pt. Name Hosp. #

DATE	CLINICAL NOTES
ROS	
PE	Temp: Pulse: BP:
	HEENT
	Neck
	Lungs
	Cardiac
	Breasts
	Abdomen
	Extremities
	Other
	Pelvic - External Genitalia
	Bartholin/Urethra/Skene
	Vagina
	Cervix
	Uterus
	Adnexa
	Rectovaginal
LABS	
	IMPRESSION:
	PLAN:
	Date:________ Signature:________ M.D.
	Date:________ Signature:________ M.D.

FIGURE 8.2. *(Continued)*

them to institute proper management without always requiring surgery.

Musculoskeletal and neurologic defects of the low back, pelvis, and hips can result in pain similar to that found in gynecologic pathology and disease. Therefore, an orthopedic and neurologic history is an important addition to a thorough gynecologic history.

Finally, the common use of herbal therapy and dietary supplements have resulted in some unanticipated problems during surgery. For this reason, a gynecologic history is not complete without inquiring as to the use of herbs and dietary supplements. Experience has shown that garlic, ginger, ginkgo, and ginseng can potentiate an anticoagulant effect, and bilberry, dandelion, and garlic can potentiate hypoglycemia. Other herbs, such as ephedra, guarana, and ginseng, can potentiate stimulants, and valerian, kava, and St. John's wort can potentiate sedation. Knowledge of herbal and dietary supplement use in the preoperative period allows time to discontinue the therapy before surgery and thus avoid a potential adverse reaction.

General Health Examination

Experience has shown that the obstetrician/gynecologist often is the only physician to whom a patient consults, particularly if the symptoms of her problem seem to involve the reproductive tract. As such, preoperative care requires a complete

B-1b Admission H/P—Obstetrics/Gynecology (Copy—Discard Confidentially)—*Final*

Outpatient Visit
ETC—ETC Emerg Trmt Ctr

File most recent confidentially discard previous versions of the same visit print date/time

|Date of Service
|Hospital #
|Name
|Birth Date/Age/Sex
|IDX #

CHIEF COMPLAINT

HISTORY OF PRESENT ILLNESS

PAST OBSTETRICAL HISTORY

GYNECOLOGICAL HISTORY

FAMILY HISTORY

SOCIAL HISTORY

PAST MEDICAL HISTORY

MEDICATION LIST as of
No medications on the active list

MEDICATION NOTES

ALLERGY NOTES

REVIEW OF SYSTEMS

PHYSICAL EXAM

RESULTS REVIEWED

IMPRESSION

PLAN

PROCEDURE NOTE

PAIN MONTTORING

COUNSELING/COORDINATION OF CARE

UNSTRUCTURED DOCUMENTATION

STAFF PHYSICIAN COMMENTS

REVIEWERS/CONTRIBUTORS
Final Reviewer:
Other Contributor:

Document Dictated/Initiated

FIGURE 8.3. Physician's electronic record template history and physical form. (From: University of Iowa Hospitals and Clinics, with permission.)

physical examination and not just a focused examination on the lower abdomen and pelvis. This complete physical examination should include blood pressure assessment, weight and height measurement, temperature recording, thyroid and neck examination, auscultation of the heart and lungs, examination of the breasts, neurologic and orthopedic assessment, and examination of the abdomen and pelvis. During the physical examination, particular attention should be given to evidence of abnormal sexual development; abnormal growth of hair on the face, chest, abdomen, extremities, back, and pubic regions; and to sexual ambiguity of the external and internal female genitalia. In addition, it is the responsibility of the gynecologist to carry out a critical evaluation of cardiac and pulmonary function before the accomplishment of any surgery. The need for additional medical and/or anesthesia consultation must be determined before surgical scheduling to complete the preoperative care assessment.

In any patient who presents with gynecologic disease and has symptoms remotely suggestive of urinary tract infection and/or disease, a meticulously collected, midstream clean-catch, or catheterized urine specimen should be examined and cultures obtained. Past data have suggested that complications of a single catheterization in terms of urinary tract infection or significant bacteriuria is minimal, whereas the complication of performing a gynecologic surgery in the presence of an undetected preexisting urinary tract infection offers a somewhat higher risk. Doing a transurethral catheterization in gynecologic patients with urinary tract symptoms is not considered to be a hazard to the normal bladder and can provide valuable information for the total assessment of gynecologic symptoms.

Gynecologic Examination

The gynecologic examination includes a thorough inspection and palpation of the breasts, abdomen, pelvis, and rectum. Ample time should be dedicated to this portion of the preoperative evaluation because defects detected during this examination affects surgical planning. This examination should be completed by the gynecologist performing the surgery rather than by other physicians or staff. In some institutions, however, a gynecologic team approach is used in the preoperative care process, and in such cases, the operating gynecologist may not always be the preoperative evaluation gynecologist. In this situation, the evaluating and the operating surgeon together must review the completed preoperative evaluation and plan, along with the patient's concerns and wishes. The operating surgeon must then make time before the surgery to meet the patient, review the plan of management with her, and respond to all of her questions.

Breast Examination

The breasts are inspected for symmetry, size, condition of the nipples, the presence of gross lesions, and the presence of discharge. Normal breast tissue, which feels rather shotty to the fingertips, is often erroneously suspected to be tumorous by the patient and is sometimes even misjudged by the physician who is unfamiliar with the proper method of breast palpation. The breasts are examined in both the upright and supine positions for symmetry, contour, and a palpable mass. The supine shoulder of the breast being examined should be raised slightly to bring the lateral aspect of the breast tissue level with the remaining portion of the breast. The arm is then raised above the head to flatten the breast against the thoracic cage. This action permits easy examination of the full thickness of the breast tissue. Examination using the flat ventral surface of the fingers and palm almost always allows identification of an existent significant lesion. Any suspicious lesion is evaluated by mammography, ultrasonography, aspiration, and/or biopsy to confirm or discount the existence of significant breast pathology. The nipples and adjacent areolar tissue are gently compressed to detect the presence of discharge or secretion (galactorrhea).

Cytologic examination of breast secretions has been reported in the past to be useful in the diagnosis of very early breast carcinoma before the clinical detection of a gross lesion. Current imaging techniques, along with fine needle biopsy, offer diagnostic accuracy before abnormal breast secretion is usually experienced, however. Nonetheless, the observation of bilateral secretion showing only the presence of fat cells on an unstained microscopic examination is reassuring and can be accomplished in an office setting. Minimal galactorrhea is not uncommon, particularly in parous women and those in early pregnancy. Other causes of galactorrhea must be considered and include prolactin-secreting tumors of the pituitary, dopamine-agonist medications, birth control pills, and primary hypothyroidism. In these cases, galactorrhea is usually found to be bilateral. Unilateral secretion should be evaluated by placing a drop of the secretion on a slide and sending the slide to cytology for examination and diagnosis. The importance of a thorough breast examination is not only to detect a previously undiagnosed breast pathology but also to detect other medical problems (galactorrhea) that could affect the outcome of a planned gynecologic surgery.

Abdominal Examination

Examination of the abdomen requires both visual inspection and palpation. Percussion and auscultation also may be useful. Bulging of the flanks suggests free abdominal fluid, but thin-walled ovarian cysts and irregularly shaped uterine leiomyomas can give a similar clinical picture. Although large ovarian cysts and leiomyomas most often cause protrusion of the anterior abdominal wall, there are a number of confusing exceptions. Palpation for a fluid wave in the lateral quadrants of the abdomen is useful. Percussion for areas of flatness or tympany and for shifting dullness can help determine whether distention is due to intraperitoneal fluid or to intestinal gas. Auscultation is especially useful to differentiate between a large tumor, a distended bowel, or an advanced pregnancy as the cause of abdominal enlargement. When physical findings are conflicting or inconclusive, imaging procedures such as abdominal-pelvic ultrasound, abdominal computed tomography scan, or magnetic resonance imaging are quite helpful in completing the assessment of an abnormal abdominal examination.

Areas of tenderness and acute pain should be noted, along with the consistency of the pain and whether the pain is experienced with palpation and/or rebound. Location may give some insight into the abdominal organ or tissues involved. Palpation tenderness is more commonly related to pathology of a specific organ, whereas rebound tenderness would suggest peritoneal involvement.

Pelvis and Rectum Examination

An accurate evaluation of the female reproductive tract is essential to establish the underlying cause of gynecologic symptoms. Although a detailed description of a pelvic examination is not provided in this chapter, it is important to stress a few of the steps necessary for proper evaluation of the female pelvis. Before an adequate pelvic examination can be performed, the bladder must be emptied by voiding. A clean-catch specimen is obtained for complete urinalysis and for culture and antibiotic sensitivity studies, if indicated. On the other hand, reports of urinary incontinence require examination with a full bladder in the lithotomy and in the erect position to demonstrate stress incontinence of the urethral sphincter. Inspection of the vulva for gross lesions includes examination of the Bartholin and Skene glands for evidence of cyst formation and purulent exudate as sources of gynecologic infection. Particular attention is given to the mons pubis and labia majora and minora for subtle changes in skin pigmentation, for vesicle formation, and for small, raised lesions that may be evidence of viral or bacterial infection or of early neoplasia. The outlet is closely inspected for relaxation of the anterior and posterior vaginal walls and for uterine descensus now referred to as pelvic organ prolapse. The vaginal mucosa is observed for any visible lesions, evidence of infection, and for estrogen effect. The patient is asked to bear down and cough without the use of a tenaculum to demonstrate the degree of relaxation of the anterior and posterior vaginal walls and the extent of uterine descensus. The urethra is compressed along its entire length to assess the possibility of a suburethral diverticulum, which often is manifested by a purulent discharge from the urethral meatus or a tender suburethral mass.

The cervix is evaluated for abnormal gross pathology, particularly ulceration, neoplastic growths, inflammation, and abnormal discharge. A Papanicolaou smear is obtained by a combined sampling of cells taken from the portio of the cervix by means of a flat stick, and from the endocervical canal by means of a small circular brush or by use of a cervical broom for liquid-based assessment. This type of combined cytologic smear or liquid-based cytology is extremely valuable in detecting cervical and endocervical lesions and is always a part of a complete gynecologic examination. Pelvic surgery always should be preceded by a recent cytologic study of the cervix. Patients with abnormal Papanicolaou smears showing repeated mild dysplasia, moderate to severe squamous cell dysplasia (CIN II–III), or high-risk human papillomavirus (HPV) should be evaluated by colposcopy, and suspicious lesions should be biopsied. Abnormal smears showing glandular cell dysplasia require both an endocervical and endometrial evaluation, such as an endocervical curettage and endometrial biopsy, before proceeding to pelvic surgery. A negative Papanicolaou smear does not, however, exclude the possibility of a cervical, endocervical, or endometrial neoplasm. False-negative cervical smears have been reported. Because 80% to 90% of all preclinical malignancies of the cervix demonstrate no significant gross lesion, it is impossible to be certain of the condition of the cervix without a Papanicolaou smear or a colposcopy and a colposcopically directed cervical biopsy if lesions are identified. The use of 3% acetic acid or Lugol's (strong iodine solution) staining of the cervix may be beneficial in identifying lesions for biopsy. Some pathologists, however, caution against the use of Lugol's because of the effect that it has on cervical cells, which sometimes interferes with an accurate pathological assessment.

The uterus is examined bimanually by the abdominal-vaginal route for position, size, mobility, irregularity, and tenderness to motion. Both adnexal regions are evaluated vaginally and by rectovaginal examination. The rectal examination should never be omitted from the routine pelvic examination. Rectal examinations provide information that cannot be obtained through the vaginal examination alone. The rectal examination provides insight into the competence of the anal sphincter as well as the presence of lesions of the anal canal and lower rectum. The rectal and vaginal examinations together are an effective method for detecting pelvic pathology and are especially useful for evaluating the broad and uterosacral ligaments, cul-de-sac of Douglas, uterus, and adnexa. The index finger is inserted into the vagina while the middle finger is inserted into the rectum to a higher level than is possible with the vaginal index finger (Fig. 8.4). This method offers the most effective opportunity of evaluating the ovaries, posterior cul-de-sac, and posterior aspect of the broad ligament. When pelvic findings are doubtful or inconclusive, imaging techniques may be helpful in determining the preoperative diagnosis. When imaging techniques are inconclusive or unavailable, however, a more adequate examination may be performed under general anesthesia before a final decision for or against gynecologic surgery

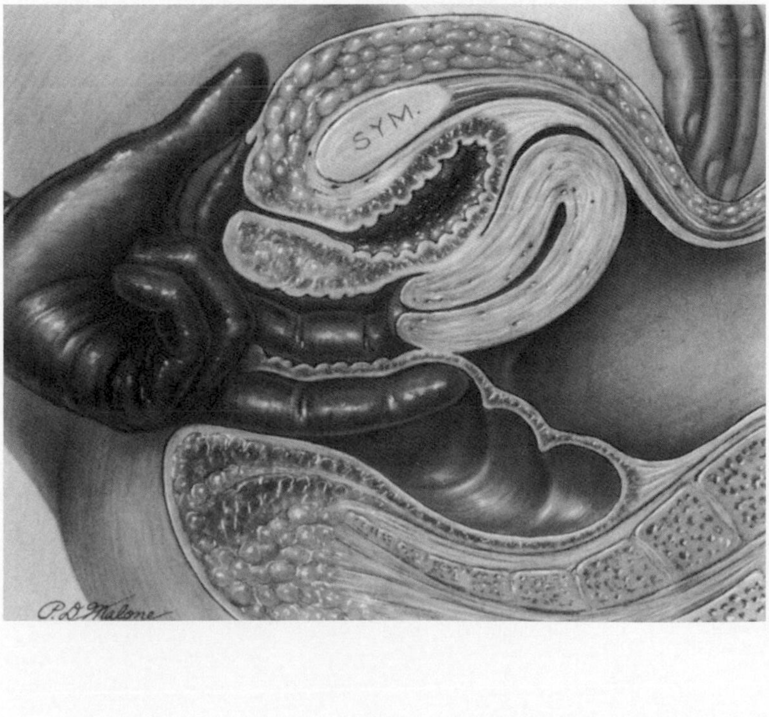

FIGURE 8.4. Rectovaginal-abdominal examination.

is made. Indeed, a complete pelvic examination always should precede any gynecologic surgery, whether it be major or minor. The pelvic organ findings of this examination should be described carefully in the operative note for future reference. Suspected pelvic pathology frequently can be ruled in or out after a thorough preoperative pelvic examination, and needless laparotomy or laparoscopy can be avoided. The most common area of clinical confusion occurs in determining the presence of an ovarian cyst, which can be confused with bowel, bladder, or uterine leiomyomas. If a normal ovary is palpated and a cyst not identified by imaging techniques such as pelvic ultrasound, an unnecessary operative procedure frequently can be spared.

LABORATORY ASSESSMENT

Before the era of evidence-based medicine, most patients undergoing gynecologic surgery were assessed by a thorough history and physical examination followed by a battery of laboratory tests, the purpose of which was to detect a medical disease or defect that could adversely affect surgical outcome. These tests were accomplished on almost all patients, irrespective of age or concurrent medical or surgical pathologies, and might include (a) blood count with hemoglobin and hematocrit, (b) urinalysis, (c) coagulation studies, (d) chemistry panel, (e) chest x-ray, and (f) electrocardiogram. This relatively universal use of "routine" preoperative testing has not proven to be beneficial in terms of good patient care and, additionally, it has added significantly to the high cost of medical care. In one study, an average of 72.5% of preoperative tests ordered by surgeons were considered unnecessary based on a review of the patient's history and physical examination. This same study suggested a medical care savings of between $4 billion and $10 billion per year in the United States by eliminating these unnecessary tests with no adverse effect on outcome.

Over the last 10 to 15 years, data have surfaced allowing gynecologists to better assess needed preoperative tests from those that in the past were labeled "routine" tests. Because of information such as this, and because of pressures from MCOs, the volume of preoperative testing has been reduced. With this reduction in the ordering of unnecessary tests, however, comes a reduction in the ordering of necessary tests. This finding emphasizes the need to accurately differentiate between indicated preoperative testing and the past practice of routine blanketed testing of gynecologic patients preparing for surgery. A large portion of the remainder of this chapter focuses on the best-case series data to help guide the gynecologist when ordering appropriate preoperative tests based on the individual patient's history and physical examination.

Key to the understanding of appropriate preoperative testing is an understanding of (a) the risk category of the patient and (b) the degree of complexity of the planned surgery. The risk category of any preoperative gynecology patient may be divided into one of six different classes as established by the American Society of Anesthesiologists (Table 8.1). The degree of complexity of the planned surgery may be divided into one of three separate types as identified by Roizen and colleagues (Table 8.2). Preoperative testing should be planned around the assessed risk of the patient based on her age, history and physical

TABLE 8.1

CLASSIFICATION OF PHYSICAL STATUS, ESTABLISHED BY THE AMERICAN SOCIETY OF ANESTHESIOLOGISTS

Class	Description
P1	A normal healthy patient
P2	A patient with mild systemic disease
P3	A patient with severe systemic disease
P4	A patient with severe systemic disease that is a constant threat to life
P5	A moribund patient who is not expected to survive without the operation
P6	A declared brain-dead patient whose organs are being removed for donor purposes

From: ASA Manual for Anesthesia Department Organization and Management, American Society of Anesthesiologists, Park Ridge, IL, 2003–04, with permission.

TABLE 8.2

TYPES OF SURGICAL PROCEDURES FOR WHICH ANESTHESIA MAY BE ADMINISTERED

Type	General Definition	Special Examples
Type A	*Minimally invasive* procedures that have little potential to disrupt normal physiology and are associated with only rare periprocedural morbidity related to anesthesia. These procedures rarely require blood administration, invasive monitoring, and/or postoperative management in critical care setting.	Cataract extraction, diagnostic arthroscopy, postpartum tubal ligation
Type B	*Moderately invasive* procedures that have a modest or intermediate potential to disrupt normal physiology. These procedures may require blood administration, invasive monitoring, or postoperative management in a critical care setting.	Carotid endarterectomy, transurethral resection of the prostate, and laparoscopic cholecystectomy
Type C	*Highly invasive* procedures that typically produce significant disruption of normal physiology. These procedures commonly require blood administration, or postoperative management in a critical care setting.	Total hip replacement, open aortic aneurysm, aortic valve replacement, and posterior fossa craniotomy for aneurysm

From: Roizen MF, Foss JF, Fischer SP. Preoperative evaluation. In: Miller RD, ed. *Anesthesia*, 5th ed. Philadelphia: Churchill Livingstone, 2000:843, with permission.

examination, and the degree of complexity based on the invasiveness of the proposed surgery. Current data as well as experience suggest that, rather than a routine set of tests, all preoperative testing should be inextricably related to the type and complexity of the proposed gynecologic surgery and to the presence of the confounding medical or surgical condition.

Asymptomatic Patients

In an extensive review of currently available evidence on the value of routine preoperative testing in healthy or asymptomatic patients, Monro and colleagues (1997) found that there were no controlled trials assessing the value of basic tests previously thought to be essential in presurgical evaluation and care. These tests included chest x-ray, electrocardiogram, blood counts and hemoglobin, coagulation studies, blood chemistries, and urinalysis. The authors further noted that all currently available evidence on preoperative testing of healthy or asymptomatic patients came only from case series studies. After reviewing all of the available case series data, they concluded that the power of preoperative tests to predict adverse postoperative outcomes in asymptomatic patients is either weak or nonexistent.

Conclusions such as this have resulted in (a) a marked reduction in the recommendation of routine testing and (b) the suggestion that the amount of routine testing of preoperative healthy asymptomatic patients be related to the patient's age. Currently, in this category of patients, it has been recommended that a hemoglobin or hematocrit be accomplished on all patients older than the age of 6 months; an electrocardiogram (ECG) on all patients older than the age of 40; and a blood urea nitrogen (BUN) test and a glucose test on all patients older than the age of 65. Additionally, a pregnancy test should be accomplished on all reproductive-age women who are at risk of early pregnancy (sexually active, no contraception, or questionably effective contraception) (Table 8.3).

Symptomatic Patients and Patients with Medical or Surgical Pathologies or Defects

Women considered for gynecologic surgery who are symptomatic and/or have other medical or surgical pathologies or defects must be considered in a different light from asymptomatic, healthy women during their preoperative evaluation and testing. Preoperative testing should be accomplished to determine the current status of medical or surgical pathologies and provide data on the potential effect that the compounding problem will have on the outcome of the proposed surgery. This would allow, if possible, for necessary medical correction or improvement of the problem before surgery in an attempt to minimize adverse outcomes of surgical intervention.

Despite the lack of an evidence-based preoperative evaluation plan to guide preoperative testing, experience supports adopting a diagnosis-based preoperative testing protocol when planning any gynecologic surgery. A number of diagnosed-based or clinical condition-based protocols have been suggested. Because the diagnosed-based preoperative testing evaluation recommended by Fischer (1999) considers both clinical outcomes as well as cost-effectiveness, it is most appropriate in the preoperative evaluation of gynecologic patients who are other than healthy and asymptomatic (Table 8.4). This approach links necessary preoperative laboratory and imaging testing with concurrent medical disease—including cardiovascular, pulmonary, and endocrine pathologies—as well as with malignancies and the use of many common drug therapies.

TABLE 8.3

RECOMMENDED PREOPERATIVE TESTING FOR HEALTHY ASYMPTOMATIC GYNECOLOGIC PATIENTS

Above Age 6 Months[a]	Above Age 40[a]	Above Age 65[a]
Hct or Hbg	Hct or Hbg ECG	Hct or Hbg ECG BUN/glucose
All Women in Reproductive Age, Sexually Active, Questionable Contraception		
Pregnancy test		

[a]Recommendation of MF Roizen, Preoperative evaluation. In: Miller RD, ed. *Anesthesia*, 5th ed. Philadelphia: Churchill Livingstone, 2000:854, with permission.

PREOPERATIVE EVALUATION: OVERVIEW

The outcome of pelvic surgery depends largely on four preoperative factors:

1. The skill and judgment of the gynecologic surgeon
2. The ability to surgically correct the gynecologic abnormality or disease process
3. The severity, stability, and reversibility of concurrent medical/surgical pathologies
4. The availability of experienced support professionals for consultation as indicated, specifically from anesthesia, medicine, and surgery

Preoperative evaluation and care of the women undergoing gynecologic surgery must include not only a thorough physical assessment but also correction or stabilization of any concurrent medical or surgical pathologies that could adversely affect the surgical outcome. A skilled and appropriate gynecologic surgical procedure can have an undesirable outcome because of an unstable condition or incompletely prepared patient.

For this reason, when the preoperative history, physical examination, or laboratory testing reveals instability of the cardiovascular, pulmonary, renal, or hematologic systems, a consultation should be considered. The intent is to achieve maximal stabilization before surgery. If the patient can not be stabilized, then delaying or postponing the surgery must be considered based on the risk and benefit of the surgical procedure for the patient. A preoperative diminished cardiac, pulmonary, or renal reserve; a blood coagulopathy; or dehydration and/or hypovolemia can play a critical role in the outcome of the surgery.

Particular attention must be given to the senior gynecologic patient. Not only does this group of women represent the fastest-growing segment of gynecologic patients, but they also are more frequently prone to have other medical issues that can affect the outcome of gynecologic surgery. The U.S. Department of Health and Human Services (DHHS) has recently noted that the U.S. population older than the age of 65 was growing faster than the population as a whole. They stated that currently 13 out of every 100 Americans are 65 years of

TABLE 8.4

DIAGNOSED-BASED PREOPERATIVE TESTING

Preoperative Diagnosis	ECG	CXR	Hct/Hb	CBC	Lytes	Renal	Glucose	Coag	LFTs	Rx Levels	Ca+
Cardiac disease											
MI history	X				±						
Stable angina	X				±						
CHF	X	±				±					
HTN	X	±			X[a]	X					
Chronic atrial fib	X									X[b]	
Periph vascular disease	X										
Valvular heart disease	X	±									
Pulmonary disease											
Emphysema	X	±								X[c]	
Asthma											
Chronic bronchitis	X	±		X							
Diabetes	X				±	X	X				
Hepatic disease											
Infectious hepatitis								X	X		
Alcohol/drug induced								X	X		
Tumor infiltration								X	X		
Renal disease			X		X	X					
Hematological disorders				X							
Coagulopathies				X				X			
CNS disorders											
Stroke	X			X	X		X			X	
Seizures	X			X	X		X			X	
Tumor	X			X							
Vascular/aneurysms	X		X								
Malignancy				X							
Hyperthyroidism	X		X		X						X
Hypothyroidism	X		X		X						
Cushing's syndrome				X	X		X				
Addison's disease				X	X						
Hyperparathyroidism	X		X		X						X
Hypoparathyroidism	X										X
Morbid obesity	X	±					X				
Malabsorption/poor nutrition	X			X	X	X	X	±			
Select drug therapies											
Digoxin (Digitalis)	X				±					X	
Anticoagulants			X					X			
Dilantin										X	
Phenobarbital										X	
Diuretics					X	X					
Steroids				X			X				
Chemotherapy				X							
Aspirin/NSAID											
Theophylline										X	

X = Obtained.
± = Consider.
[a]Patients on diuretics.
[b]Patients on digoxin.
[c]Patients on theophyilline.
From: Fischer SP. Cost-effective preoperative evaluation and testing. *Chest* 1999; 115:98S, with permission.

age or older, and in 2030 this number will increase to 20 out of 100. They additionally noted that there were significantly more women than men in this older population, with women composing 59% of the group aged 65 years and older and 71% of those aged 85 years and older. DHHS data from 2004 indicated that women born in 2002 will live to an age of 79.9 years. Additionally, if a women reached age 65 in 2002, she can expect to live an additional 19.5 years, and if she reached age 75 in 2002, she can expect to live an additional 12.4 years. Considerable data as well as experience have shown that this group of senior gynecologic patients has significantly greater health care problems and therefore will require a greater effort in the preoperative evaluation in terms of laboratory evaluation and consultation.

With this increase in concurrent medical and surgical problems, and the resulting increase in operative risks of gynecologic surgery in the senior population, it is important to note that chronologic age, by itself, is not always an accurate indicator of organ function. Atheromatous changes of the cardiovascular system are uncommon in women until well past menopause. This biologic phenomenon is just one of the many factors that promote female (compared with male) longevity. As a consequence of increased longevity, a high percentage of women are in the postmenopausal period of their life when gynecologic disease becomes more prevalent and surgery becomes more necessary. In spite of the increased concurrent medical and surgical problems and greater operative risks, excellent surgical skills, meticulous medical control of concurrent disease, and anesthesia carefully attuned to the physiologic requirements of the senior gynecologic patient have kept the risk of surgery at a level not much greater than that for the premenopausal patient. Age alone should therefore not be a contraindication for surgery.

Guidelines for the preoperative evaluation of the gynecologic patient may be divided into three separate areas.

1. Uncomplicated gynecologic pathology with an uncomplicated medical/surgical status
2. Complicated gynecologic pathology with uncomplicated medical/surgical status
3. Uncomplicated or complicated gynecologic pathology with a complicated medical/surgical status

The following preoperative evaluation recommendations are made based on the most current data from case series studies, evidence-based medical data, and consensus opinions of gynecologic preoperative care.

Preoperative Evaluation, Uncomplicated Gynecologic Pathology, Uncomplicated Medical/Surgical Status

A gynecologic patient who has an uncomplicated gynecologic pathology and no concurrent medical or surgical conditions that would affect surgical outcome should undergo the following preoperative evaluation.

1. Thorough history
2. Complete physical examination
3. Hematocrit or hemoglobin if older than 6 months of age
4. Electrocardiogram if older than 40 years of age
5. Blood urea nitrogen and glucose if older than 65 years of age
6. Pregnancy test if in the reproductive age, sexually active, and not on contraception or if using questionably effective contraception
7. Sexually transmitted diseases testing (chlamydia, gonococcus, syphilis, hepatitis, and human immunodeficiency virus [HIV]) with suspected or documented exposure
8. Blood type and screen if the potential exists for more than minimal surgical blood loss

Preoperative Evaluation, Complicated Gynecologic Pathology, Uncomplicated Medical/Surgical Status

A gynecologic patient who has a complicated gynecologic pathology and no concurrent medical or surgical conditions that would additionally affect surgical outcome should undergo the following preoperative evaluation (complicated gynecologic pathology includes past abdominal/pelvic surgery with evidence of or anticipation of pelvic adhesive disease, tumors, or cysts of a size making surgery more difficult or complicated; suspected or proven cancerous lesions; concurrent infection of the reproductive tract; or active or chronic bleeding from the reproductive tract, resulting in a demonstrated or highly probable hematologic instability).

1. Thorough history
2. Complete physical examination
3. Laboratory testing listed under uncomplicated gynecologic pathology
4. Complete blood cell (CBC) count with suspected or evidence of pelvic infection, hemorrhage, or anemia
5. Prothrombin time (PT), activated partial thromboplastin time (APTT), and either a platelet function analysis (PFA-100) or a bleeding time with hemorrhage or anemia
6. Liver function tests and renal tests with any suspected hepatic or renal pathology
7. Type and cross match in an anticipated high blood loss surgery, otherwise only a type and screen
8. Anesthesia consultation

Preoperative Evaluation, Uncomplicated or Complicated Gynecologic Pathology, Complicated Medical/Surgical Status

A gynecologic patient who has either an uncomplicated or complicated gynecologic pathology and a concurrent medical or surgical problem offers the greatest risk for gynecologic surgery (concurrent medical or surgical problem includes cardiac, pulmonary, vascular, renal, intestinal, endocrine, neurologic, and orthopedic pathologies, as well as use of medications for these defects). These patients should undergo the following preoperative evaluation:

1. Thorough history
2. Complete physical examination
3. Laboratory testing listed under uncomplicated gynecologic pathology
4. Laboratory testing listed under complicated gynecologic pathology
5. Prothrombin time (PT) and an International Normalized Ratio (INR) in women with a history of venous thrombosis or pulmonary embolism on warfarin
6. Factor V Leiden, prothrombin 20210A gene mutation, antithrombin, lupus anticoagulant, and antiphospholipid antibodies in women with a suspected thrombophilia
7. Liver function tests, renal function tests, electrolyte and/or blood sugar tests in women with renal, liver, or intestinal disease; on diuretics; with an unexplained fever; with endocrine disease, including diabetes, hypoglycemia, parathyroid disease, or adrenal and pituitary disease; or with a recent history of radiation or chemotherapy
8. Electrocardiogram with suspected or known cardiac pathology
9. Anesthesia consultation
10. Medicine, cardiology, pulmonary medicine, endocrinology, urology, and surgery consultation as indicated

PREOPERATIVE MANAGEMENT AND PREPARATION

Preoperative care includes not only preoperative evaluation and laboratory testing, but also any medical or gynecologic evaluation and treatment in the months preceding the surgical procedure to help achieve maximal physical status. Achieving this goal is rewarded by a less complicated surgical procedure with better outcomes. Examples of this medical or gynecologic management include a number of treatments. Ovarian suppression through the use of a gonadotropin-releasing hormone agonist in the 2 to 3 months before surgery has proven to be beneficial in hysteroscopic resection of uterine submucous leiomyomas larger than 2 cm in size and in myomectomies when the uterine volume is equivalent to or larger than a 12-week pregnant uterus size. A similar suppression is also useful in decreasing the thickness of the endometrial lining in an endometrial ablation, although an endometrial suction curettage can achieve a somewhat similar result. Perioperative antibiotic treatment of postmenopausal women undergoing reparative surgery for genital prolapse can be beneficial in reducing recurrent cystitis but has not been shown to significantly alter the outcome of surgery.

Use of preoperative vaginal estrogen cream starting 4 to 6 weeks before surgery may help in controlling uropathogens as well as thickening the vaginal mucosa, which results in an easier dissection of the vagina and in reducing postoperative morbidity. Routine preoperative endometrial sampling before hysterectomy has not been found to be cost-effective unless there is suspicion of endometrial pathology, such as manifested by abnormal perimenopausal or menopausal bleeding or the presence of abnormal glandular cells on Papanicolaou test. In the latter case, endocervical sampling additionally is necessary.

Another area of preoperative planning requiring an experienced decision by the gynecologist and possibly the anesthesiologist is the regulation of medications taken by the patient before surgery. When and how to modify insulin in diabetic women, surgery on women taking anticoagulants, and continuation or discontinuation of birth control pills are some examples of issues that must be addressed in the preoperative period and conveyed to the patient in a manner that she understands. Because of the uniqueness of each patient, it is not possible to provide a table of preoperative medication managements that can be applied to every patient. However, some general suggestions serve as guidelines in the preoperative management of the more common concurrent diseases.

Preoperative insulin control in patients with diabetes is thought to be essential to achieve good surgical outcome. Older animal data have shown a relationship between hyperglycemia and wound healing with reduced tensile strength and wound failure. Experience has suggested a similar relationship in the gynecologic patient. It is therefore important to comanage each diabetic woman undergoing gynecologic surgery with her primary care physician or internist to achieve this optimal control, and once achieved, to continue the insulin regime right up to the time of surgery. Every attempt should be made to schedule the diabetic patient's surgery as a first morning case to minimize the time period between the patient's last oral intake and the onset of the surgical procedure. A protocol for patient preoperative management of insulin regulation may be found in Table 8.5. Some patients may present with an insulin pump, in which case a decision will need to be made regarding continuing the pump at a basal rate and transitioning to an intravenous (IV) infusion, or discontinuing the pump after a subcutaneous injection of a long-acting insulin. Planning for complex insulin preoperative management should be accomplished in conjunction with the patient's medical physician and with anesthesia. Patients who are scheduled for gynecologic surgery who are on Coumadin (warfarin), heparin, or low-molecular-weight heparin (LMWH) represent another preoperative management issue. A number of options are available for converting the patient from warfarin to heparin. Experience has suggested that stopping the warfarin 5 days before the planned gynecologic surgery and converting to low-dose heparin 5,000 U subcutaneously every 12 hours 4 days preoperatively provides satisfactory anticoagulation protection. As an alternative, it has been recommended by some anesthesiologists that heparin be instituted only when the INR for prothrombin falls below 2. The low-dose heparin can be continued postoperatively until the patient is back on oral feeding, at which time the warfarin can be reinitiated. It is further suggested that these women use elastic stockings or intermittent pneumatic compression (IPC) hose at the beginning of the surgery and continue with this mechanical support through to the point of full postoperative ambulation.

TABLE 8.5

RECOMMENDATION FOR PREOPERATIVE INSULIN MANAGEMENT: CLASSIC "NONTIGHT CONTROL" REGIMEN OF ROIZEN

1. Day before surgery: Patient should be given nothing by mouth after midnight; a 13-ounce glass of clear orange juice should be at the bedside or in the car for emergency use.
2. At 6 a.m. on the day of surgery, institute intravenous fluids using plastic cannulae and a solution containing 5% dextrose, infused at a rate of 125 mL/h/70 kg body weight.
3. After institution of intravenous infusion, give one-half the usual morning insulin dose (and usual type of insulin) subcutaneously.
4. Continue 5% dextrose solutions through operative period, giving at least 125 mL/h/70 kg body weight.
5. In recovery room, monitor blood glucose concentration and treat on a sliding scale.

Roizen MF. Anesthetic implications of concurrent diseases. In: Miller RD, ed. *Anesthesia*, 5th ed. Philadelphia: Elsevier, 2000:903, with permission.

Another preoperative medication issue involves the continuation or discontinuation of oral contraceptive pills before gynecologic surgery. Studies in the 1970s suggested a relationship between use of preoperative oral contraceptive pills and intraoperative or postoperative venous thrombosis. For this reason, in the past it has been the practice to discontinue oral contraceptive pills 2 to 4 weeks before surgery and convert to mechanical contraception. This practice, however, is unsupported by any current prospective controlled studies and places the patient at risk for unwanted pregnancy as well as menstrual irregularities. Therefore, routine discontinuation of oral contraception before gynecologic surgery is not recommended, but instead mechanical venous support, such as elastic stockings or IPC, be used at the time of surgery.

The immediate preoperative preparation of the patient includes the preoperative examination by the gynecologic surgeon and the anesthesia assessment in the anesthesia preoperative clinic or by an individual anesthesiologist. In most cases, the assessment for anesthesia risks is accomplished before the day of surgery. If significant anesthesia risk is present, such as cardiovascular or pulmonary pathology, this allows time for relevant information to be obtained, additional testing accomplished, other consultation carried out, and treatment instituted in an attempt to have the patient in optimal condition on the day of surgery. In some cases involving low-risk ambulatory procedures, however, the anesthesia assessment is accomplished on the day of surgery. Experience suggests that an open dialog between the gynecologic surgeon and the anesthesiologist regarding the planned surgery is an essential element in achieving a successful outcome with the lowest patient risk.

Most gynecologic surgical patients are admitted on the day of surgery. Because of this, preoperative guidelines and instructions for patient activity and actions at home are important and need to be made clear to every patient. The goal is to have the patient rested and in the optimal physical condition with an empty stomach and reduced contents in the lower gastrointestinal tract at the time of surgery. There is no evidence to support the idea that marked reduction of activity on the day before surgery is beneficial; however, it would be reasonable to recommend planning activities so that the patient is not overstressed. Food intake on the day before surgery need not be restricted except for the evening meal before the morning of surgery, which should be light and easily digestible. An overloaded intestinal tract during surgery is particularly hazardous not only because it poses an anesthetic risk but also because it increases postoperative nausea and gas formation. The patient should be instructed to not eat or drink after midnight on the evening before surgery unless the surgery is scheduled for the late afternoon. Some exceptions to this rule might occur with the taking of indicated medications with water. Such an exception should be discussed between the gynecologist and the anesthesiologist in the preoperative evaluation sessions. Women who are scheduled for a late afternoon surgery may have a light breakfast of a liquid diet if taken no fewer than 6 hours preoperatively.

Women undergoing major abdominal surgery in which bowel entry or injury is anticipated (or is a high probability) should undergo a complete bowel prep. This complete bowel preparation should consist of the single use of a commercially available cleansing preparation such as GoLYTELY or NuLYTELY (Braintree Laboratories, Inc., Braintree, MA). This impression is not universally supported, however. A 2005 Cochrane Review of bowel preparation before colon surgery failed to demonstrate convincing evidence that mechanical or complete bowel preparation reduced the rates of common complications. Nevertheless, a cleansing preparation continues to be standard of care in gynecologic surgeries involving bowel resection or repair. In all other major abdominal cases, the lower colon should be cleansed by a preoperative enema the evening before surgery. If the colon is not completely emptied, then a repeat enema may need to be given before performing the operation, allowing adequate time for evacuation. The patient needs to be given careful instructions for the use of enemas at home and the possible need for a repeat enema in the hospital before surgery. This issue is often overlooked in preoperative care and results in a more difficult surgical procedure because of space limitation and a less comfortable patient in the postoperative period. An adequate night's rest before surgery is also important for the patient. In some cases, the use of a mild sedative may be considered.

Preoperative prophylactic broad-spectrum antibiotics or surgical antimicrobial prophylaxis has frequently been used in gynecologic surgery on the basis of the potential for vaginal flora contamination of the operative field and because of the close proximity of the rectum and intestinal tract. Data do not support the routine use of preoperative broad-spectrum antibiotics in uncomplicated, noninfected gynecologic laparoscopic or hysteroscopic surgery. Data, as presented in the 2005 Compendium of the American College of Obstetricians and Gynecologists, do, however, support the use of preoperative broad-spectrum antibiotics in vaginal hysterectomy or abdominal hysterectomy. In these procedures, the occurrence of postoperative cuff cellulitis and pelvic abscess has been significantly reduced with use of a preoperative antibiotic. First-, second-, or third-generation cephalosporins (e.g., cefazolin, cefotetan, or cefotaxime, 2 g IV) are effective as a prophylactic coverage. As an alternative, metronidazole 500 mg IV may be utilized. When used, the prophylactic antibiotic should be given as a single dose approximately 1 to 2 hours before beginning surgery and may be repeated if the operation lasts longer than 3 hours or if there is significant blood loss (in excess of 1,500 mL). If the preoperative examination and testing identifies vaginal infections such as bacterial vaginosis, treatment before surgery with metronidazole 500 mg orally 2 times a day for 7 days, or metronidazole intravaginal gel (0.75%) one 5-g applicator intravaginally daily for 5 days, or clindamycin vaginal cream (2%) one 5-g applicator intravaginally daily for 7 days should be accomplished. In like manner, any sexually transmitted disease discovered during preoperative examination and testing should be fully treated before surgery.

Infections occurring after surgery in the female reproductive tract arise from the introduction of normal vaginal flora into the surgical field. Surgery on the reproductive tract accomplished through a bacteriologically contaminated field (e.g., the vagina) seeds bacteria into the pedicles and surgical margins of pelvic tissues and provides an excellent nidus for infection in devitalized tissue beds. Therefore, pelvic surgery provides an ideal condition for aerobic (principally polymicrobial rather than monomicrobial) infections. Tissue destruction and sutures lower the tissue oxidation-reduction (redox) potential. Lower tissue oxygen levels enhance the growth of facultative anaerobes that normally inhabit the vagina. As tissue hypoxia progresses, primary anaerobic bacteria survive and proliferate. Therefore, the more common postoperative infection in the vaginal vault, although initially polymicrobial, usually can be prevented with the use of the preoperative prophylactic antibiotic when the vaginal apex has been opened during a vaginal or abdominal hysterectomy.

Although prophylactic antibiotics are effective in reducing the incidence of postoperative infectious morbidity, they should never be used as a substitute for the time-honored principles of adequate hemostasis and gentle handling of tissue. Despite Wangensteen's disparaging statement that "antibiotics will turn a third-class surgeon into a second-class surgeon, but will never turn a second-class surgeon into a first-class surgeon," current data suggest that even in the hands of a highly skilled surgeon, prophylactic preoperative antibiotics offer improved outcomes in gynecologic pelvic surgery such as vaginal and abdominal hysterectomy.

Preoperative Procedures in the Operating Suite

Just before surgery, the patient is brought to the operating theater and transferred either directly to the operating table in the operating room or to an operating table in the anesthesia room adjoining the surgical suite. Preoperative preparation includes any trimming of pubic hair, preparation of abdominal and vaginal skin, and placement of a catheter, if indicated. Preoperative shaving of pubic and abdominal hair before gynecologic surgery is generally not recommended; in fact, preoperative shaving is associated with a significantly higher surgical site infection (SSI) rate, particularly if completed the night before the operation. These guidelines note studies showing SSI rates of 5.6% in patients who had hair

TABLE 8.6

RECOMMENDATIONS FOR PREOPERATIVE PREPARATION OF THE PATIENT TO PREVENT SURGICAL SITE INFECTIONS

1. Whenever possible, identify and treat all infections remote to the surgical site before elective operation, and postpone elective operations on patients with remote site infections until the infection has resolved.
2. Do not remove hair preoperatively unless hair at or around the incision site will interfere with the operation.
3. If hair is removed, remove immediately before the operation, preferably with electric clippers.
4. Adequately control serum blood glucose levels in all diabetic patients, and particularly avoid hyperglycemia perioperatively.
5. Encourage tobacco cessation. At a minimum, instruct patients to abstain for at least 30 days before elective operation from smoking cigarettes, cigars, pipes, or other form of tobacco consumption.
6. Do not withhold necessary blood products from surgical patients as a means to prevent surgical site infections.
7. Require patients to shower or bathe with an antiseptic agent on at least the night before the operative day.
8. Thoroughly wash and clean at and around the incision site to remove gross contamination before performing antiseptic skin preparation.
9. Use appropriate antiseptic agent for skin preparation.
10. Apply preoperative antiseptic skin preparation in concentric circles, moving toward the periphery. The prepared area must be large enough to extend the incision or create new incisions or drain sites, if necessary.
11. Keep preoperative hospital stay as short as possible while allowing for adequate preoperative preparation of the patient.
12. No recommendation to taper or discontinue systemic steroid use (when medically permissible) before elective operation. (unresolved issue)
13. No recommendation to enhance nutritional support for surgical patients solely as a means to prevent surgical site infection. (unresolved issue)
14. No recommendation to preoperatively apply mupirocin to nares to prevent surgical site infection. (unresolved issue)
15. No recommendation to provide measures that would enhance space oxygenation to prevent surgical site infections. (unresolved issue)

From: Hospital Infection Control Practices Committee, Centers for Disease Control and Prevention (CDC). *Am J Infect Control.* Philadelphia: Elsevier 1999;27:266–267, with permission.

removed by shaving compared with 0.6% in those who had no hair removed. Furthermore, shaving the night before surgery resulted in a significantly higher rate of SSI than shaving just before the operative procedure (7.1% versus 3.1%). Experience has shown that in some gynecologic procedures, removal of pubic and abdominal hair is useful, and in these situations, hair clipping is recommended immediately before the surgery.

After hair trimming and catheterization, the patient is usually sufficiently anesthetized for a careful bimanual pelvic examination, at which time the surgeon can obtain very valuable information not easily obtainable when the patient is awake. Detection of reduced mobility, identification of cysts or masses not previously known, and determination of the position of pelvic organs not appreciated in past examinations may persuade the gynecologist to alter the planned surgical approach or incision type. After the pelvic examination, the perineum and vagina are cleansed, followed by the abdominal preparation.

The pelvic cleansing should be accomplished before all pelvic or abdominal surgery. There is always the possibility that findings at the time of operation may make a total abdominal hysterectomy advisable, even when the preoperative plan did not include such an extensive procedure. It is extremely disconcerting to find that a total abdominal hysterectomy must be performed at the time of a laparotomy if the vagina is not properly prepared. For this reason, it is strongly recommended that preoperative vaginal preparation be accomplished as a routine procedure. To clean the perineum and vagina, the vulva and perineum are first scrubbed by a nurse or surgical assistant with a sponge soaked in surgical soap or a povidone-iodine solution using a gloved hand. Before this preparation, Kelly pads should be placed under the buttocks and low back to catch wash and preparation solutions, and the perineum and vulva washed and wiped free of gross contamination (mucus, blood, bowel content). These pads should be removed before draping the patient to prevent contaminated fluids and concentrated iodine wash solutions from pooling and remaining under the buttocks during the operative procedure. After the perineal and vulvar preparation, the vagina is next scrubbed with a soapy sponge or a povidone-iodine sponge stick held in the gloved hand. After the vaginal scrub, the nurse or operative assistant inserts his or her fingers in the vagina and spreads the fingers to enlarge the vaginal outlet. At the same time, the perineum is depressed to allow the soapy water or povidone-iodine solution to run out of the vagina. This solution is then flushed away with sterile water poured into the vagina. After this, the remaining cleanup is accomplished with a sterile sponge on a sponge forceps, which is used several times to clean the vagina with an appropriate antiseptic solution.

After the vaginal, vulvar, and perineal cleanup, the abdomen is prepared with a 5-minute scrub using a povidone-iodine or similar solution or with a three- to four-round application of a povidone-iodine gel sponge stick. Particular attention should be paid to cleansing the umbilicus with a Q-tip/cotton swab applicator. The surgically prepared area should extend superiorly from the inferior rib cage to the midthigh inferiorly. The lateral margins of the skin preparation should extend to the anterior iliac crest and the anterior axillary line. The actual skin washing and preparation should be accomplished using concentric circles moving toward the periphery. To additionally protect the incision from contamination, many surgeons use a clear plastic adhesive (3M Steri-Drape Ioban 2 or similar product) placed over the skin at the site of the incision.

The Hospital Infection Control Practices Advisory Committee of the Centers for Disease Control and Prevention has published Guidelines for Prevention of Surgical Site Infection (1999), which are important in gynecologic surgery and should be noted (Table 8.6).

Universal Precautions for the Prevention of Seropositivity for Acquired Immunodeficiency Syndrome

Because surgeons are at risk for acquiring seropositivity for the acquired immunodeficiency syndrome (AIDS) through contamination from body fluids and blood products, certain precautions should be taken at the time of surgery. In 1988, the Centers for Disease Control published a document recommending that blood and other body fluid precautions be consistently used for all patients, regardless of their blood-borne infectious status. This extension of blood and other body fluid precautions to all patients is referred to as Universal Blood and Fluid Precautions, or simply Universal Precautions. Under universal precautions, blood and body fluids of all patients are considered potentially infectious for human immunodeficiency virus (HIV), hepatitis B virus (HBV), and other blood-borne pathogens.

Universal precautions are intended to prevent parenteral, mucous membrane, and nonintact skin exposure of the surgeon to blood-borne pathogens. Immunization with HBV vaccine is also recommended as an important adjunct to the universal precautions for surgeons who are exposed to the risks. Protective barriers reduce the risk of exposure of the surgeon's skin or mucous membrane to potentially infectious materials. In the operating room, protective barriers include gowns, gloves, masks, and protective eyewear. Masks and protective eyewear or face shields reduce the incidence of contamination of mucous membranes of the mouth, nose, and eyes. Gloves reduce the incidence of contamination of the hands, but they cannot prevent penetrating injuries, such as puncture by a needle or other sharp instrument. Special care must be taken to prevent any injury by needles, scalpels, or other sharp instruments or devices. Should a contamination occur in spite of these precautions, immediately and thoroughly wash the hands and other skin surfaces that have been contaminated and institute the medical institution's policy on rapid antigen testing to determine if the surgeon should consider prophylaxis for HIV.

SUMMARY

Gynecologic surgery encompasses a wide variety of surgical procedures from minimally invasive operations to radical and extensive dissections of pelvic pathology. No matter what the extent of the procedure, all gynecologic surgery should be considered to have three separate parts: (a) the preoperative care and management phase, (b) the surgical procedure itself, and (c) postoperative care and the management phase. Each part is inextricably related to the others, and each part is vital in the overall outcome of the gynecologic pathology being managed. Preoperative care and management sets the stage for a successful surgical procedure. Best outcomes are linked to a patient being in optimal physical and medical status before surgery. The preoperative process begins with an accurate diagnosis and an appropriate decision to operate. The preoperative evaluation serves to assess the patient's overall medical status and specific gynecologic problem by a thorough history, a complete physical examination, and the ordering of appropriate laboratory testing to support the safety of the planned procedure. The preoperative evaluation additionally serves to identify other pathologies and problems that could interfere with optimal surgical outcome and to implement corrections before surgery. Suggestions for accomplishing a thorough history and physical examination have been outlined in this chapter. Preoperative testing should be based on the patient's age, history, physical examination, and the degree of complexity of the proposed surgery. Suggestions for appropriate testing for both uncomplicated and complicated gynecologic patients have been made. Additional suggestions for management of gynecologic patients in the immediate preoperative period have also been made. Finally, of great importance is the open dialog between the gynecologic surgeon and the anesthesiologist regarding surgical planning, with consultation of other specialists when complicated medical or surgical issues are present. As a result of these actions and efforts, the gynecologic surgeon and the patient arrive in the operating room with little doubt as to the pathology, the overall medical status, and the plan for surgical correction.

BEST SURGICAL PRACTICES

- Successful surgical outcomes of operative gynecologic procedures occur as a result of several factors, including (a) appropriate preoperative evaluation, (b) appropriate patient selection, (c) appropriate discussion with the patient regarding the benefits and risks of surgery, and (d) ability to work with managed care organizations so as to obtain required approvals.
- Preoperative patient conditions are significant predictors of postoperative morbidity. It is essential that all women undergoing preoperative assessment have a complete history and thorough physical examination as a key element of their workup.
- Key to the understanding of appropriate testing is an understanding of (a) the risk category of the patient and (b) the degree of complexity of the planned surgery.
- A close dialog should exist between the gynecologic surgeon and the anesthesiologist as well as with other medical/surgical specialties providing consultative support for the patient.

Bibliography

American College of Obstetricians and Gynecologists Practice Bulletin. *Compendium 2005. Antibiotic prophylaxis for gynecologic procedures.* Washington, DC: ACOG, 2001;23:294.

Bonnar J. Can more be done in obstetric and gynecologic practice to reduce morbidity and mortality associated with venous thromboembolism? *Am J Obstet Gynecol* 1999;180:784.

Brown JS, Sawaya G, Thom DH, et al. Hysterectomy and urinary incontinence: a systematic review. *Lancet* 2000;356:535.

Centers for Disease Control. Universal precautions for prevention of transmission of human immunodeficiency virus, hepatitis B virus, and other bloodborne pathogens in healthcare settings. *MMWR Morb Mortal Wkly Rep* 1988;37:377.

Centers for Disease Control and Prevention. Hospital Infection Control Practices Advisory Committee. Guidelines for prevention of surgical site infections, 1999. *Am J Infect Control* 1999;27:250.

Chen BH, Giudice LC. Dysfunctional uterine bleeding. *West J Med* 1998; 169:280.

The Cochrane Database of Systemic Reviews. Mechanical bowel preparation for elective colorectal surgery. *Cochrane Database Syst Rev* 2005;1:1.

Eagle KA, Brundage BH, Chaitman BR, et al. Guidelines for perioperative cardiovascular evaluation for noncardiac surgery. Report of the American College of Cardiology/American Heart Association Task Force on Practice Guidelines (Committee on Perioperative Cardiovascular Evaluation for Noncardiac Surgery). *J Am Coll Cardiol* 1996;27:910.

Fischer SP. Cost-effective preoperative evaluation and testing. *Chest* 1999; 115:96S.

Flanagan K. Preoperative assessment: safety considerations for patients taking herbal products. *J Perianesth Nurs* 2001;16:19.

Glister BC, Vigersky RA. Perioperative management of type 1 diabetes mellitus. *Endocrinol Metab Clin North Am* 2003;32:411.

Golub R, Cantu R, Sorrento JJ, et al. Efficacy of preadmission testing in ambulatory surgical patients. *Am J Surg* 1992;163:565.

Goodson WH, Hunt TK. Studies of wound healing in experimental diabetes mellitus. *J Surg Res* 1977;22:221.

Greene GR, Sartwell PE. Oral contraceptive use in patients with thromboembolism following surgery, trauma, or infection. *Am J Public Health* 1972;62:680.

Hammond CB. *Therapeutic options for menopausal health.* Monograph. Durham, NC: Duke University School of Medicine, 2000.

Hillis SD, Marchbanks PA, Ratliff Taylor S, et al. For the U.S. Collaborative Review of Sterilization Working Group. Tubal sterilization and long-term risk of hysterectomy: findings from the United States Collaborative Review of Sterilization. *Obstet Gynecol* 1997;89:609.

Jacobs LG, Nusbaum N. Perioperative management and reversal of antithrombotic therapy. *Clin Geriatr Med* 2001;17:189.

Kramarow E, Lentzner H, Rooks R, et al. *Health, United States, 1999, with health and aging chartbook.* Hyattsville, MD: National Center for Health Sciences, U.S. Department of Health and Human Resources, 1999.

Kaplan EB, Sheiner LB, Boeckmann AJ, et al. The usefulness of preoperative laboratory screening. *JAMA* 1985;253:3576.

Macario A, Roizen MF, Thisted RA, et al. Reassessment of preoperative laboratory testing has changed the test-ordering patterns of physicians. *Surg Gynecol Obstet* 1992;175:539.

Masukawa T, Levinson EF, Forst JK. The cytologic examination of breast secretions. *Acta Cytol* 1966;10:261.

Mittendorf R, Aronson MP, Berry RE, et al. Avoiding serious infections associated with abdominal hysterectomy: a meta-analysis of antibiotic prophylaxis. *Am J Obstet Gynecol* 1993;169:1661.

Monro J, Booth A, Nicholl J. Routine preoperative testing: a systemic review of the evidence. *Health Technol Assess* 1997;1:1.

Narr BJ, Hansen TR, Warner MA. Preoperative laboratory screening in healthy Mayo patients: cost-effective elimination of tests and unchanged outcomes. *Mayo Clin Proc* 1991;66:155.

Ross AF, Tinker JH. Anesthesia risk. In: Miller RD, ed. *Anesthesia*, 3rd ed. New York: Churchill Livingstone, 1990:715.

Roizen MF. Anesthetic implications of concurrent diseases. In: Miller RD, ed. *Anesthesia*, 5th ed. Philadelphia: Churchill Livingstone, 2000:903.

Roizen MF. More preoperative assessment by physicians and less by laboratory test [editorial comment]. The value of routine preoperative medical testing before cataract surgery. *N Engl J Med* 2000;342:168.

Roizen MF, Foss JF, Fischer SP. Preoperative evaluation. In: Miller RD, ed. *Anesthesia*, 5th ed. Philadelphia: Churchill Livingstone, 2000:824.

Scher KS. Studies on the duration of antibiotic administration for surgical prophylaxis. *Am Surg* 1997;63:59.

Tan MW, DeBerry M, Teasdale TA. Comprehensive preoperative geriatric assessment. *J Okla State Med Assoc* 2004;97:498.

U.S. Department of Health and Human Services. *Health, United States, 2004.* Table 27. Life expectancy at birth, at 65 years of age, and at 75 years of age. DHHS Publication No. 2004–1232. 2004:143.

Velanovich V. Preoperative laboratory screening based on age, gender, and concomitant medical diseases. *Surgery* 1994;115:56.

Vessey MD, Doll R, Fairbairn AS, et al. Postoperative thromboembolism and the use of oral contraceptives. *Br Med J* 1970;3:123.

Vogt AW, Henson LC. Unindicated preoperative testing: ASA physical status and financial implications. *J Clin Anesth* 1997;9:437.

Watts SA, Gibbs NM. Outpatient management of the chronically anticoagulated patient for elective surgery. *Anaesth Intensive Care* 2003;31:145.

Westhoff C, Davis A. Tubal sterilization: focus on the U.S. experience. *Fertil Steril* 2000;73:913.

CHAPTER 9 ■ POSTANESTHESIA AND POSTOPERATIVE CARE

ALEXANDER DUNCAN, IRA R. HOROWITZ, AND KENNETH KALASSIAN

DEFINITIONS

Hospital-acquired pneumonia (HAP)—Pneumonia that develops 48 hours or more after hospital admission because of organisms that were not incubating at the time of admission.

Hypoxic pulmonary vasoconstriction—Local reflex in the lung that diverts blood away from poorly oxygenated regions.

Low-molecular-weight heparin (LMWH)—Product that acts by inhibiting factor Xa.

Tissue plasminogen activator (t-PA)—Compound used for nonsurgical thrombolysis.

Venous thrombotic event—A venous thromboembolism that includes vascular clotting, such deep vein thrombosis, pulmonary embolism, and arterial thrombosis.

Virchow's triad—Factors that increase risk of vascular thromboembolism, e.g., hypercoagulability, stasis, trauma to vessels.

V/Q abnormalities—Ventilation/perfusion abnormalities, including increased shunting to increased dead space in the lung.

Postoperative complications are the most important factors in defining the outcome of the first 72 hours following a patient's surgical procedure. It is critical to monitor basic physiological parameters—such as renal, cardiovascular, and respiratory functions—and laboratory tests to optimize and sustain recovery from surgery and anesthesia.

Postoperative morbidity can be minimized by an appropriate preoperative assessment of the surgical patient. This should include emphasis on identifying the patient at risk for venous thromboembolic complications and administering prophylactic anticoagulation. Optimized nutritional status and support has also been shown to improve wound healing and decrease the postoperative recovery time.

POSTOPERATIVE VASCULAR COMPLICATIONS

About 2 million venous thrombotic events, or venous thromboembolisms (VTEs), occur in the United States each year. About 500,000 of these events are deep vein thrombosis (DVT) in the hospital, and as many as 200,000 are pulmonary embolisms (PEs). Twenty-five percent of PEs are fatal, and VTE has been recognized as the biggest preventable cause of morbidity and mortality in U.S. hospitals. Ten percent of hospital deaths in the United States are due to PE, and some patient groups, including gynecological patients, have a higher-than-usual risk for VTE, with a general incidence of about 15% to 20%. The risk of fatal postoperative PE among these patients is closer to 40%.

PE has few defining characteristics, but the onset of respiratory distress compounded by hypotension, chest pain, and cardiac arrhythmias can be harbingers of impending death and are complications that convert an otherwise successful surgery into a postoperative fatality. Only 70% of patients who die of a PE have it considered in their differential diagnosis.

Modern diagnostic studies have provided more accurate information about the frequency of vascular complications and can identify those patients who are at risk of an embolic event. Pre- and postoperative prophylaxis with heparin or low-molecular-weight heparin (LMWH), and concomitant use of embolic stockings and intermittent pneumatic compression stockings have significantly reduced the risk of PE in the moderate and high-risk patients. Clarke-Pearson and colleagues, using univariant and regression analysis, designed a prognostic model to evaluate the risk of postoperative VTE for an individual patient. In a group of 411 gynecology patients, the prognostic factors they identified included type of surgery, age, leg edema, non-Caucasian ethnicity, severity of varicose veins, previous radiotherapy, and a prior history of DVT.

More than 130 years ago, Rudolph Virchow conceptualized the factors leading to postoperative thrombosis. These included venous stasis, changes in the blood constituents, and impaired function of the vessel wall. The blood clotting process is complicated (Fig. 9.1), but it is initiated by the actions of tissue factor (TF) in factor VII after injury to vessels exposes the subendothelium and promotes platelet adhesion and aggregation to form a primary platelet plug. The process is completed by the actions of multiple components and factors in the blood that generate thrombin, the potent rate-regulating enzyme, which then interacts with fibrinogen and factor XIII to form an insoluble clot (Fig. 9.2).

When patients have cancer or sustain venous damage from the surgical procedure, such as occurs with skeletonization of the pelvic vasculature, the up-regulation of thrombin generation has more profound effects. TF, fibrin, and thrombin all have angiogenic properties that can interfere with tissue properties by degrading matrix metalloproteinases, promoting cell migration, and enhancing metastasis. Tumors also up-regulate the production of TF and plasminogen activator inhibitor-1 (PAI-1), again promoting the generation of procoagulant activity. This multifactorial activity helps to explain the high incidence of VTE in the gynecological cancer patient.

These tumorigenic effects on coagulation occur in addition to the typical acute postsurgical reaction of any of the hemostasis proteins. These include increases in fibrinogen, factor V, factor VIII, and von Willebrand's factor, which promotes platelet adhesion and function. There is usually an increase in

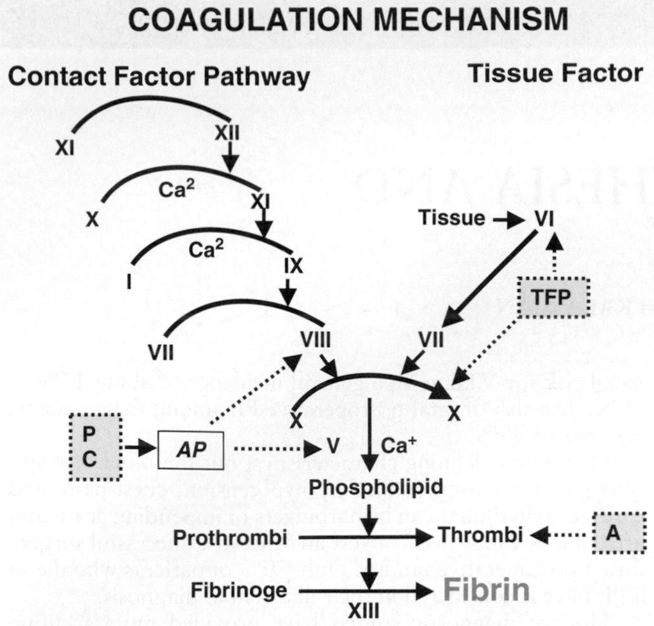

FIGURE 9.1. Formation of venous thrombus following various surgical procedures with the activation of clotting factors and aggregation of platelets. AP, activated protein, PC, protein C, TFP, tissue factor peptide.

platelet number in the postoperative period, and the normal fibrinolytic response is blunted by the increase in PAI-1 and thrombin activatable fibrinolysis inhibitor (TAFI). Essentially, the fibrinolytic system is nonfunctional for several days following surgery, which most likely limits the ability of plasmin to impede healing the wound by preventing degradation of fibrin.

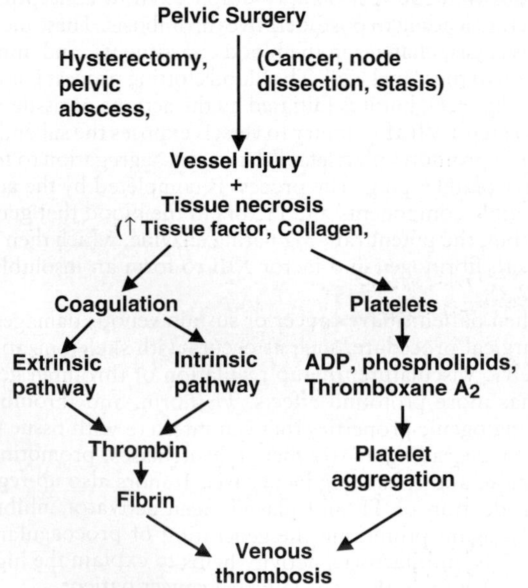

FIGURE 9.2. Schematic representation of the cascade clotting mechanism, illustrating the role of extrinsic and intrinsic factors. Increases in tissue thromboplastinlike substance and collagen-activated factor XII initiate the formation of fibrin through the extrinsic and intrinsic pathways, principally by the activation of factor X. ADP, adenosine diphosphate.

Venous stasis is thought to be the cornerstone of postoperative thrombosis. Venous stasis in the pelvis and lower extremities results in platelet activation, promoting the adhesion of platelets to the endothelial cells lining the vessel, which are already stressed in a procoagulant mode. This results in conditions that encourage the development of a thrombus. These physiological changes in venous hemodynamics occur in the pre-, peri- and postoperative periods. Doran has shown that venous return from the lower extremities is decreased by half during surgical procedures because of the impact of muscle relaxation from anesthetic agents. Scanning using I^{125} fibrinogen has demonstrated that venous thrombosis is initiated during the surgery in 50% of patients who subsequently manifest a DVT. Lower-extremity blood flow has been shown to decrease to about 75% of the normal drainage flow in the immediate postoperative period. This is an important reflection of Virchov's triad on the role of adequate vessel flow. This reduction in flow persists for about 14 days after surgery because of the loss of muscle-pumping function in the legs. The major site of thrombus formation is the soleal venous sinuses of the calf, a portion of the venous arcade that joins the posterior tibial and peroneal veins draining the soleal muscle. Thrombi from these sinuses often occur posterior to valves located at the junction where these sinuses drain into the collecting veins. Thrombi often occur in these sinuses and in valve cusps in bedridden patients.

Another contributing factor to venous stasis during prolonged surgery is the use of tight packing of the intestines in the upper abdomen with obstruction of the underlying vena cava. The type and length of operation are directly related to the incidence of postoperative VTE, as outlined in Table 9.1.

Diagnosis of Venous Thromboembolism

The traditional clinical methods used to diagnose venous thrombosis of the lower extremities are of limited value, with error rates approaching 50% for both false-negative and false-positive rates. Most of the diagnostics problems occur because of the insidious nature of venous thrombosis in the lower extremity, which takes place in the soleal veins. Modern imaging methods have evolved considerably in recent years, ranging from I^{125} fibrinogen scanning to venography to Doppler duplex ultrasound and impedence plethysmography. Although venography remains the gold standard, compression ultrasonography is widely used, having a good negative predictive value (98%) for proximal DVT and slightly lower (96%) for calf DVT. However, it is still inferior to venography, which remains the reference source (Table 9.2).

Venography

The venogram has had the most extensive and rigorous use in clinical practice of all imaging techniques. However, it is not routinely used because it is invasive, uses contrast dye, has limitations, and provides an increased risk in many patients who have renal compromise.

I^{125}-Labeled Fibrinogen Scanning

This technique was first developed in the 1960s and used widely for many years. It involves the intravenous injections of isotope-labeled fibrinogen, which is expected to be incorporated into the evolving thrombus and can be imaged by a scintillation scanner. Because of the use of isotopes, it is technically cumbersome and rarely used, despite many large studies

TABLE 9.1

LEVELS OF THROMBOEMBOLISM RISK IN SURGICAL PATIENTS WITHOUT PROPHYLAXIS

Level of risk examples	Calf DVT, %	Proximal DVT, %	Clinical PE, %	Fatal PE, %	Successful prevention strategies
Low risk Minor surgery in patients <40 yr with no additional risk factors	2	0.4	0.2	0.002	No specific measures Aggressive mobilization
Moderate risk Minor surgery in patients with additional risk factors; nonmajor surgery in patients aged 40–60 yr with no additional risk factors; major surgery in patients <40 yr with no additional risk factors	10–20	2–4	1–2	0.1–0.4	LDUH q12h, LMWH, ES, or IPC
High risk Nonmajor surgery in patients >60 yr or with additional risk factors; major surgery in patients >40 yr or with additional risk factors	20–40	4–8	2–4	0.4–1.0	LDUH q8h, LMWH, or IPC
Highest risk Major surgery in patients >40 yr plus prior VTE, cancer, or molecular hypercoagulable state; hip or knee arthroplasty, hip fracture surgery; major trauma; spinal cord injury	40–80	10–20	4–10	0.2–5	LMWH, oral anticoagulants, IPC/ES + LDUH/LMWH, or ADH

Modified from Gallus et al. and International Consensus Statement.
Source: Geerts WH, Heit JA, Clagett GP, et al. Prevention of venous thromboembolism. [Sixth ACCP Concensus Conference on Antithrombotic Therapy] *Chest* 2001;119(Suppl 1):132S–175S.

validating its use in the 1970s and 1980s and a high correlation to venography.

Impedance Plethysmography

Impedance plethysmography (IPG) is based on the principal of electrical resistance in specific areas of the body. When there is resistance to blood flow that is due to a thrombus, there is marked reduction in the electrical resistance over that vessel. IPG is most useful in proximal venous thrombosis, but is relatively poor in visualizing thrombi below the knee because of the small caliber and slow flow rates through the soleal sinuses. The technique is only about 50% accurate compared with venography in detecting DVT below the popliteal vessels.

Huisman and colleagues evaluated 471 outpatients clinically suspected of acute onset DVT. Four sequential IPGs were obtained on days 1, 2, 5, and 10 of the study. Of the 137 patients with abnormal results, 117 (85%) had abnormal results on day 1, with the other 20 patients becoming positive by day 10. When compared with venography, serial IPG had a specificity of 92% and a sensitivity of 100%. The use of serial testing clearly improved the ability to diagnose DVT. Another similar study by Vaccaro and associates involving 252 patients using single-test IPG gave a sensitivity of 84% and a specificity of 78%, confirming the superiority of the serial testing protocol. Given the short length of hospital stays now, it is unlikely that serial IPG would be possible despite its high correlation with venography.

Doppler Ultrasound

The use of Doppler ultrasound, often with computer color enhancement, has become the most widely used imaging technique for diagnosis of DVT. Its major physiological use is in the measurement of flow velocity in larger blood vessels. In this technique, a reflected sound signal is converted to both an audible form and visual image on a computer screen. In the presence of a thrombosis, there is a decrease in the reflected signal that can be heard or, more likely, can be visualized. Most modern ultrasound machines use color enhancement to identify arteries (red) and veins (blue). This technique is again very useful to identify DVTs in the iliac, femoral, or popliteal veins, but again, its sensitivity falls off markedly when applied to the small vessels in the calf, usually to less than 60%.

Real-Time Ultrasound

Real-time ultrasound has been compared with venography, and in a study by Aitken and associates, it demonstrated a sensitivity of 94% and a specificity of 100% in a small study of 46 patients. In a slightly larger study of 121 patients by Appelman and colleagues, the sensitivity was found to be 96%, and specificity was 97%.

TABLE 9.2

DIAGNOSIS OF DEEP VENOUS THROMBOSIS (DVT)

Method	Sensitivity and specificity	Indication and comments
Clinical history and physical examination		Classic symptoms often absent in proven DVT <60% with suggestive symptoms proven to have DVT Absence of symptoms does not exclude pulmonary embolism
D-dimer ELISA (plasma)	Sensitivity 97% Specificity: poor	Useful to exclude the diagnosis if D-dimer (ELISA) is <500 mug/mL Many conditions increase D-dimer levels (false-positive results)
B-mode compression ultrasonography ± Doppler	Symptomatic proximal DVT: Sensitivity 93%–97% Specificity 98% Asymptomatic DVT: Sensitivity 38%–59% Specificity: high	Noninvasive test First-line modality for confirming diagnosis in symptomatic patients Not useful for screening of asymptomatic patients Compression component best for thigh DVT
Impedance plethysmography	Symptomatic DVT: Sensitivity 90% Specificity 95% Asymptomatic DVT: Sensitivity 22% Specificity 98%	Noninvasive test Limited to *serial* examination in symptomatic patients with proximal DVT Insensitive to calf-vein thrombi and nonocclusive thrombi
MR venography	Proximal DVT: Sensitivity 100% Specificity 96% Calf-vein DVT: Sensitivity 87% Specificity 97%	Noninvasive but expensive Ability to screen for DVT in asymptomatic patients Can also image lungs for pulmonary embolism in same setting
Contrast-enhanced CT venography	Distal and proximal DVT: Sensitivity 100% Specificity 96%	Noninvasive test Superior to venography in evaluating the great vessels Expensive Less contrast than conventional venography Can image lungs for pulmonary embolism in same setting
Ascending contrast venography phlebography	Reference standard	Invasive test Reference standard but expensive Risk for contrast nephropathy and allergic reactions Risk for thrombogenicity (usually superficial veins) Negative test does not exclude pulmonary embolism Equivocal results in recurrent DVT

Source: De Wet CJ, Pearl RG. Venous thromboembolism: deep-vein thrombosis and pulmonary embolism. *Anesthesiol Clin North Am Clin* 1999; 17(4):895–922.

Compression Ultrasound

This technique has been used in some large DVT trials, such as the PREVENT trial, but there have been few studies directly comparing it with venography. In a recent small study by Tomzowski and colleagues involving 160 medically ill patients, 12 patients had venographically proven DVT. Compression ultrasound technique had a sensitivity of 28% and a specificity of 98%, but despite the small numbers of venographically confirmed patients, the method performed poorly, having both false-positive and -negative findings.

Duplex Doppler Ultrasound

This is a combination technique using real-time and Doppler methods in a procedure known as B mode or duplex Doppler imaging. It allows a radiologist to visualize the vessel and identify any thrombus in it. In a study by Langsfeld and colleagues, 431 patients were examined; 86 patients had a DVT. This gave a sensitivity of 100%, but two false positives dropped the specificity to 78%. Technical issues may have given one incorrect result, the second patient was pregnant, and the study was considered falsely positive because of aortocaval compression from the pregnant uterus.

In a study by Kristo and associates comparing duplex Doppler, venography, and single bilateral IPG, the respective sensitivities and specificities were as follows, respectively: ultrasound, 92% and 100%; venography, 100% and 75%; and IPG, 50% and 83%. *For many reasons, duplex B mode imaging has become the noninvasive imaging method of choice, essentially replacing venography as the "practical" gold standard.*

Light Reflection Rheography

Light reflection rheography (LRR) uses infrared light directed at the skin. The backscattered rays are quantitated, which allows an estimation of blood volume. A decreased venous emptying rate of 0.35 is considered positive for DVT. In a study in patients with gastrointestinal problems in which 69 limbs were tested by venography and LRR, the sensitivity for LRR was 96%, the specificity was 83%, the positive predictive value was 79%, and the negative predictive value was 97%.

LRR could prove to be a low-cost, sensitive tool for DVT detection. Further studies are needed to determine if the technique fulfills its early promise. However, in one study of 411 asymptomatic pregnant women in second and third trimesters who did not have DVT, the use of LRR denoted a significant false-positive rate of 25% and an inadequate study rate of 19%. This gave an overall specificity of only 45%, indicating that LRR is not for use in DVT diagnosis in pregnant women.

Radioisotope Imaging

Various imaging methods have been tried using radioisotopes to try to detect thrombi in both arteries and veins by labeling components of the clotting system, such as platelets or fibrinogen. These components would be incorporated into the developing thrombus, and the focused radioactivity would then allow "visualization" by a detector. Radioactive-tagged antibodies to both platelets and factors have also been used for DVT diagnosis.

$Indium^{111}$-labeled platelets have demonstrated good success with high sensitivity and specificity. The same is true for $fibrinogen^{125}$- and $technetium^{99m}$-labeled platelets.

Although all of these radioisotope-labeled methods have some proponents, the advances in computer and ultrasound methods will probably outweigh significant development of radioisotopic methods for routine clinical VTE diagnosis.

Indirect Computed Tomography Venography

The new and evolving technique of indirect computed tomography (CT) venography, using intravenous contrast medium injection followed by CT scanning of the limbs or chest, has a high potential for detecting DVT or PE. Some early studies have indicated detection of thrombi at least to calf level and perhaps lower. There are few studies comparing CT venography and CT pulmonary angiography. A recent study by Nchimi evaluated 1,408 patients with both techniques for PE detection and included lower-extremity DVT as a secondary finding. They found that in 48% of patients with DVT, the upper end of the thrombus was between the ankle and the knee. Comparing the two techniques, CT venography detected 17% more VTE than CT pulmonary angiography.

Magnetic Resonance Imaging/Magnetic Resonance Imaging Venography

The use of magnetic resonance imaging (MRI) techniques with or without contrast media is another new approach to VTE detection. There are several different technologies using MRI, but all basically use the differences in signal intensities to distinguish flowing blood from stagnant blood (i.e., clot). Although there have been few large scale studies published, the major advantage of MRI is that no contrast medium is required, allowing the technique to be used in pregnant women. One study by Carpenter and colleagues indicated no statistical differences between contrast venography and MRI in DVT diagnosis. MRI is still in its infancy for DVT diagnosis, but it is likely that continued improvements in computer software will provide for the advancement of MRI as a tool for VTE diagnosis.

Nonimaging Methods

The use of laboratory tests as a means of exclusion of VTE has gained momentum in the last decade. The use of the *automated quantitative D-dimer assay* has gained widespread acceptance, especially in emergency rooms, to exclude DVT. In a study by Wells and associates comparing IPG and D-dimer with contrast venography, the combination of IPG and a negative (normal) D-dimer test gave a negative predictive value of 97%. In this same study, the combination of positive IPG and positive D-dimer had a positive predictive value of 93% for any DVT and 90% for proximal DVT.

The use of an appropriate D-dimer assay in isolation has been shown to have about 95% negative predictive value for exclusion of DVT. Despite numerous studies, there is still no proven consistent correlation between a positive D-dimer assay and venous thrombosis.

Because the diagnosis of PE can be difficult in many older patients, especially those with heart failure or other cardiovascular complications, some preliminary studies have been done using combinations of D-dimer, B-type natriuretic peptide (BNP), and cardiac troponins to determine if a better distinction can be made between a PE and an underlying cardiac complication. These studies are likely to be the forerunners for other combinations of lab tests to identify more specific negative or even positive predictive markers for VTE.

Risk Factors for Vascular Complications

Several clinical factors are known to identify the patient with an increased risk for VTE (Table 9.3). The most prevalent and important include age >40 years, obesity >20% above ideal weight, prolonged surgery, and immobility in the pre-, peri-, and postoperative periods. Pelvic malignancy, prior VTE, known thrombophilia risk, severe diabetes, heart failure, prior radiation therapy, and chronic obstructive pulmonary disease all increase the VTE risk.

Age

An autopsy study by Sevitt and Gallagher demonstrated that DVT was most prevalent in patients older than 60 years. Several studies have shown a linear risk of fatal PE with increasing age. Approximately 10% of hospitalized patients' deaths are due to PE, and only about 35% of these are diagnosed ante mortem. Contributing factors include degenerative changes in the vascular tree, increases that occur in the concentration of many coagulation factors, and, possibly, increased platelet adhesiveness.

Immobility

Prolonged inactivity in the preoperative patient promotes an impairment of venous flow in the lower extremities. Many diagnostic techniques also produce a decrease in muscle tone with a secondary decrease in venous flow. These hemodynamic changes promote sludging of red cells and activation of platelets, setting the stage for VTE during the operative period. This is one of the main risk factors described by Virchow for the etiology of thrombosis.

Studies done using I^{125} fibrinogen scanning pre- and immediately postsurgery have indicated that in 50% of patients who subsequently developed VTE, the initiation of clot formation occurred during the surgical procedure. This is amplified

TABLE 9.3

PROFILE OF PATIENT AT HIGH RISK FOR VENOUS THROMBOSIS

Factor	Condition
Age	<40 Major surgery
Age	>60 Nonmajor surgery
Obesity	
Moderate	75–90 kg or >20% above ideal weight
Morbid	115 kg or >30% above ideal weight with reduced fibrinolysin and immobility
Immobility	
Preoperative	Prolonged hospitalization; venous stasis
Intraoperative	Prolonged operative time; loss of pump action of calf muscles; compression of vena cava
Postoperative	Prolonged bed confinement; venous stasis
Trauma	Damage of wall of pelvic veins
Radical pelvic surgery	
Malignancy	Release of tissue thromboplastin[a]
Activation of factor X; reduced fibrinolysin	
Radiation	Prior radiation therapy
Medical diseases	Diabetes mellitus
Cardiac disease; heart failure	
Severe varicose veins	
Previous venous thrombosis with or without embolization[a]	
Chronic pulmonary disease	
Molecular hypercoagulable state	

[a] Highest risk.

during prolonged anesthesia, with generalized muscle relaxation further promoting venous stasis in the lower extremities, which compounds the thromboembolic risk. For this risk, the judicious use of prophylactic anticoagulation in the high-risk patient should include the operative phase and continue at a minimum until the patient is fully ambulatory.

Postoperative immobility also promotes VTE risk by continuing venous stasis, and studies have shown that 66% of patients who develop a DVT do so in the first 48 hours after surgery. Other compounding issues include sitting with legs crossed or dangling over the bed or the exaggerated Fowler position. These positions all produce impairment of lower extremity venous return. Postoperative patients should be ambulated early and aggressively; if ambulation is not possible, they should have their legs elevated to 15 degrees above the horizontal.

Other Factors

Other factors include *previous VTE, varicose veins, severe diabetes, cardiac failure, chronic obstructive pulmonary disease,*

TABLE 9.4

RISK OF THROMBOEMBOLISM

Deficiency/dysfunction
Antithrombin
Protein C
Protein S
Heparin cofactor II
Factor V Leiden
Prothrombin variant 20210A
Antiphospholipid antibodies
Lupus anticoagulant
Anticardiolipin
Hyperhomocystinuria
Dysfibrinogenemia
Decreased levels of plasminogen
Decreased levels of plasminogen activators
Heparin-induced thrombocytopenia

and *underlying thrombophilia.* Given the high incidence of factor V Leiden (5%) and the G20210A prothrombin gene mutations (3%) in the Caucasian populations, which are well-recognized risk factors for venous thrombosis (Table 9.4), these genetic risk factors are common enough to make a major contribution to preoperative thrombosis, even in the patient with no prior VTE history.

Underlying malignancy is a huge contributor to risk, most likely because of the significant up-regulation of TF that is known to occur with many malignancies. Up-regulation of TF increases thrombin generation by several mechanisms and promotes platelet activation and angiogenesis, as discussed earlier.

A review of these risk factors clearly identifies the high-risk VTE patient, and it is essential that these surgical risk variables are identified and understood in designing appropriate thromboprophylaxis and monitoring parameters to prevent venous thrombosis.

Prophylaxis

Prevention remains the most effective tool in the treatment of VTE. Between 5% and 45% of gynecological surgery patients develop DVT in their legs; of these, 20% have popliteal or femoral involvement; and of these, 40% will progress to PE with its high mortality. It is imperative that methods for prophylaxis are planned and implemented before surgery (Table 9.5).

At the sixth American College of Chest Physicians (ACCP) Consensus Conference, Geerts and colleagues—in a review of PE in 7,000 gynecologic surgery patients in prospective clinical trials—reported a reduction in the rate of fatal PE of 75% using thromboprophylaxis (Table 9.6).

Low-Dose Unfractionated Heparin

Low-dose unfractionated heparin (UFH) has been the mainstay of prophylactic treatment for many years, with numerous prospective randomized clinical trials validating a risk reduction in DVT incidence from 35% to 45% to about 7% in the high-risk patient. In one large study by Kakkar and colleagues (Table 9.7) incorporating 4,000 patients at multiple centers, patients were randomized to 5,000 units USP calcium heparin subcutaneously starting 2 hours before surgery and subsequently every 8 hours thereafter for the next 7 days. The

TABLE 9.5

AGENTS USED IN VENOUS THROMBOEMBOLISM

Agent	Mechanism of action	Comments
Heparin	Combines with AT-III and neutralizes activated factors: IIa (thrombin activity) Xa (responsible for thrombin generation) XIIa, XIa, IXa	Prevention and treatment of venous thromboembolism Risk of heparin-induced thrombocytopenia Requires monitoring (aPTT) when used for treatment
LMWH Ardeparin Dalteparin Enoxaparin	Combines with AT-III and prevents thrombin generation through its anti-factor Xa effect	Prevention and treatment of venous thromboembolism Risk of heparin-induced thrombocytopenia No anti-IIa activity (if molecular weight <5.6 kDa) aPTT does not reflect anticoagulation state More predictable pharmacokinetic profile Renal failure and dehydration increase effective plasma concentration
Heparinoid Danaparoid	Same as LMWH High anti-Xa/IIa ratio	Prevention and treatment of venous thromboembolism Similar to LMWH but may be used for anticoagulation when heparin-induced thrombocytopenia is present
Direct thrombin inhibitors and hirudin	Directly inhibits thrombin activity	Prevention and treatment of venous thromboembolism May be used for heparin-induced thrombocytopenia
Plasminogen activators: Nonselective Streptokinase Urokinase	Activates plasminogen, which leads to the formation of plasmin, which dissolves fibrin clot (no effect on polymerized fibrin clot) Also degrades fibrinogen, which leads to fibrinogen degradation products and decreases in plasma fibrinogen	Treatment of life-threatening DVT or pulmonary embolism High risk of bleeding Many contraindications such as recent surgery or trauma
Thrombus-selective tissue plasminogen activator	Activates fibrin-bound plasminogen Degrades fibrinogen (to a lesser extent)	
Warfarin	Inhibits correct synthesis of vitamin K–dependent coagulation factors (II, VII, IX, X) These factors cannot bind calcium and therefore remain inactive Inhibits protein C (vitamin K–dependent)	Long-term treatment and prevention of venous thromboembolism Contraindicated in pregnancy (teratogenic) High risk of bleeding Requires anticoagulation monitoring Numerous drug interactions
Inferior vena caval filters	Trap larger emboli	Used as prevention of pulmonary embolism when anticoagulation fails or is contraindicated Used prior to pulmonary embolectomy or pulmonary endarterectomy
External pneumatic leg compression	Prevents venous stasis Stimulates fibrinolytic system	Used as prophylaxis for DVT Possibly contraindicated in peripheral arterial disease

Source: De Wet CJ, Pearl RG. Venous thromboembolism: deep-vein thrombosis and pulmonary embolism. *Anesthesiol Clin North Am* 1999,17(4):895–922.

reduction in VTE between the control group (25%) and the treatment group (8%) was highly significant. The most important finding was the decrease in fatal PE from 16 patients in the control group to two in the treatment group confirmed by autopsy.

Because there is no change in the activated partial thromboplastin time (APTT) because of the low level of subcutaneous heparin, there was no increase in postoperative bleeding. This is because the main impact of the low-dose heparin is exerted via antithrombin through factor Xa, as well as directly on thrombin. There is also a secondary effect in which heparin releases tissue factor pathway inhibitor (TFPI), which also helps to down regulate factor Xa by forming a complex involving TF:F Xa:F VIIa:TFPI.

These studies, as well as those shown in Table 9.8, clearly validate the efficacy of low-dose UFH in reducing VTE in

TABLE 9.6

PREVENTION OF DEEP VENOUS THROMBOSIS (DVT) AFTER GYNECOLOGIC SURGERY[a]

Regimen	No. of trials	No. of patients	Incidence of DVT, %	95% CI	Relative % reduction
Untreated control subjects	12	945	16	14–19	—
Oral anticoagulants	5	183	13	8–18	22
IPC	3	253	9	6–13	44
LDUH	11	1,092	7	6–9	56
ES	1	104	0	0–3	"99"

[a]Pooled data from randomized trials that used routine FUT as the primary outcome.
Source: Geerts WH, Heit JA, Clagett GP, et al. Prevention of venous thromboembolism. [Sixth ACCP Consesus Conference on Antithrombotic Therapy] *Chest* 2001;119(1)Suppl:132S–175S.

surgical patients using an initial dose of 5,000 units 2 hours before surgery, and then 5,000 units every 12 hours for the next 5 days. For the truly high-risk patient, such as those with a prior VTE or multiple risk factors, 5,000 units every 8 hours should be used.

Low-Dose Unfractionated Heparin/Dihydroergotamine

The combination of low-dose UFH and dihydroergotamine (DHE) treatment was shown to work well by adding the known effect of DHE as a selective venous vasoconstricting agent to the anticoagulant properties of UFH. The data in Table 9.9 support the use of this treatment modality, but none of these products are now sold in the United States.

Dextran 70/Dextran 40

In 1972, Bonnar and Walsh described the use of dextran 70 to prevent thrombosis after pelvic surgery. A subsequent study by Bernstein and colleagues involving radical hysterectomy patients using dextran 70 as prophylaxis showed a decrease in DVT incidence from 33% to 5%. Dextran works by interfering with platelet function, interacts with factor V and VIII, and inhibits fibrinolysis. Despite some comparable studies between dextran and low-dose UFH, the Sixth ACCP Consensus Conference in 2001 recommended against using dextran products in VTE prophylaxis.

TABLE 9.7

PULMONARY EMBOLISM AND DEEP VENOUS THROMBOSIS IN PATIENTS ON LOW-DOSE HEPARIN AND IN CONTROLS

	Low-dose heparin	Control
Number of patients	2,045	2,076
Number of deaths from all causes	80	100
Deaths caused by pulmonary embolism (verified at autopsy)	2	16
Deep venous thrombosis	8%	25%

Source: Kakkar W, Corrigan TP, Fossard DP. Prevention of postoperative pulmonary embolism by low dose heparin. *Lancet* 1975;2:45.

Low-Molecular-Weight Heparins

LMWHs act by primarily inhibiting factor Xa with a small component of activity against thrombin. They now have become the mainstay of prophylaxis treatment and are continuing to replace all other forms of drug therapy. The drugs have a longer half-life than UFH and are much more biopredictable. If LMWH levels are measured in patients using an anti-Xa assay, there is a remarkable homogeneity of response. This has led the U.S. Food and Drug Administration (FDA) to recommend against the need to monitor when used LMWHs are for VTE prophylaxis. There are currently four LMWH drugs available in the United States (Fragmin, Lovenox, Innohep, and Arixtra). They are subtly different in molecular weights and in manufacturing processes, but in essence, they are almost identical in clinical efficacy. They are not, however, dosed in the same way, some using milligrams and other units, or even units per kg. Pharmacists can provide accurate dosage information about any of the products available.

Multiple studies reported in the literature essentially show equivalence or better for the LMWHs compared with UFH in the prevention of VTE, but almost all of these show a much lower bleeding risk for the LMWH treatment groups, even with hard data for bleeding risk being quantitated by transfusion requirements. LMWHs have also been compared with dextran and used in combination with DHE with good outcomes, but the reality is that *in normal clinical practice, LMWHs by themselves provide adequate protections with minimal complications.* One other advantage of the LMWH preparations is their much lower incidence of heparin-induced thrombocytopenia (HIT) when used as *de novo* therapy. However, if a patient has had HIT in the past, these preparations should not be used because there is about a 90% cross-reactivity between UFH and LMWH for the antibody causing HIT. The one exception to this is Arixtra, the synthetic factor Xa inhibitor, which has not been shown to cause clinical HIT to date.

It is highly likely, given the once-per-day dosage requirement and the lack of HIT risk, that LMWHs will continue to dominate in uses for thromboprophylaxis in VTE.

Compression Modalities

As long ago as 1944, Stanton et al. used static compression to decrease venous stasis by decreasing the luminal diameter of the veins, increasing blood flow velocity. In the mid-1970s, Sigel

TABLE 9.8

RESULTS OF PROPHYLACTIC TREATMENT OF VENOUS THROMBOSIS AFTER GYNECOLOGIC SURGERY[a]

				Venous Thrombosis (%)					
Investigators	Year	Type of surgery	Number of patients	Control	Heparin	LMWH	Dextran	AC	Pneumatic calf compression
Bonnar et al.	1973	Simple hysterectomy	260	15.0	—	—	0.1	—	—
		Radical malignant	62	33.0	—	—	5.0	—	—
Ballard et al.	1973	Major gynecologic, age 40	110	29.0	3.6	—	—	—	—
McCarthy et al.	1974	Major gynecologic	130	—	10.9	—	16.2	—	—
Baertschi et al.	1975	Major gynecologic	458	—	2.3	—	—	4.7	—
Gjonnaess and Abildgaard	1976	Major gynecologic, age 50	95	8.0	2.0	—	—	—	—
Adolf et al.	1978	Major gynecologic	454	29.3	7.0	—	—	—	—
Taberner et al.	1978	Major gynecologic	146	23.0	6.0	—	—	6.0	—
Clarke-Pearson et al.	1983a	Gynecologic malignant	185	12.4	14.8	—	—	—	—
Clarke-Pearson et al.	1984	Gynecologic malignant	107	34.6	—	—	—	—	12.7
Borstad et al.	1992	Major gynecologic malignant	141	—	0.00	0.00[b]	—	—	—

[a]Detected by ^{125}I-labeled fibrinogen scan.
[b]One patient had pulmonary embolism 3 days after discontinuation of LMWH.
AC, anticoagulants; LMWH, low-molecular-weight heparin.

and colleagues showed an increase in blood velocity of 20% using graduated compression stockings but a 200% increase in velocity using intermittent sequential compression.

Mittelman and colleagues showed that uniform intermittent calf compression was not as effective as intermittent sequential compression at increasing thigh blood flow. This is another example of a component of Virchow's triangle, namely, stasis being involved in the VTE protection mechanism.

It is possible that another component of the triad—the coagulation system—is also influenced by intermittent pneumatic compression (IPC) because several groups have shown that it stimulates fibrinolysis, perhaps by increasing prostacyclin production. Prostacyclin is a potent natural vasodilator and antiplatelet agent released from endothelial cells. Guyton and colleagues found increased quantities of 6-keto prostaglandin $F_{1\alpha}$ in patients undergoing IPC compared with controls. The 6-keto prostaglandin $F_{1\alpha}$ is a specific breakdown product of prostacyclin. Frango and associates have shown a 16-fold increase in prostacyclin production in cultured endothelial cells submitted to pulsatile shear stress compared with a twofold increase with contact shear stress.

Graduated Compression Stockings Initial studies evaluating antiembolic stockings proved inconclusive and relied on several different methods to diagnose VTE, which compounded the uncertainty. Sigel and colleagues designed a compression thromboembolism deterrent (TED) hose with graduated pressures of 18, 14, 12, 10, and 8 mm Hg from the ankle to the upper thigh. Scurr and associates evaluated TED hose in a study of 75 patients older than 40 years undergoing major abdominal

TABLE 9.9

THROMBOSIS PREVENTION WITH DIHYDROERGOTAMINE MESYLATE PROPHYLAXIS[a]

Treatment and dose	Numbers of patients treated	Patients with DVT	Patients without DVT	P Value[b]
DHE/heparin sodium, 5,000 IU	214	18 (8.4%)	196 (91.6%)	—
DHE/heparin sodium, 2,500 IU	226	32 (14.2%)	194 (85.8%)	.0396
Heparin sodium, 5,000 IU	222	32 (14.4%)	190 (85.6%)	.0341
DHE mesylate, 0.5 mg	110	18 (16.4%)	92 (83.6%)	.0263
Placebo	108	22 (20.4%)	86 (79.6%)	.0024

DHE, dihydroergotamine mesylate; DVT, deep venous thrombosis.
[a]All treatment modalities administered 2 hours before surgery and every 12 hours postoperatively for 5 days.
[b]*P* level compares with DHE–heparin sodium, 5,000 IU.
Source: Sasahara AA, DiSerio FJ, Singer JM, et al. Dihydroergotamine-heparin prophylaxis of postoperative deep vein thrombosis: a multicenter trial. *JAMA* 1984;251:2960.

surgery in which only one leg had TED hose applied. Using I^{125} fibrinogen scanning as the diagnostic tool, 19 patients had DVTs in the control leg, and only 1 had a DVT in the TED hose leg. A subsequent similar study by Inada and colleagues found a DVT frequency of 14.5% in the control leg and only 3.6% in the TED leg. Malignancy is a powerful predisposition to VTE secondary to stasis and TF production by the tumor. In a study by Allan and associates assessing the efficacy of TED stocking in patients undergoing abdominal surgery for malignant and benign diseases, the incidence of DVT in the benign disease group was 24.5% in the control limb and 6.1% in the TED limb. However, in the malignant disease group, the incidence of VDT was only slightly increased in the control limb at 27.9%, but the incidence of DVT in the TED limb was significantly higher at 11.5%, clearly amplifying the impact of the tumor on the DVT risk. The Sixth ACCP Consensus Conference suggested that TED hose with early ambulation was an acceptable and effective means of VTE prophylaxis in the low-risk gynecology surgery patient.

External Intermittent Pneumatic Compression. These techniques also promote increased blood flow in the lower extremities that is due to decreased stasis and improved fibrinolysis. Nicolaides and colleagues compared intermittent sequential pneumatic compression, nonsequential (one chamber) pneumatic compression, and UFH in the prevention of DVT. Using pressures of 35, 30, and 20 mm Hg sequentially for 12 seconds at the ankle, calf, and thigh, they observed a 240% increase in peak blood velocity. In contrast, using the single-chamber device at 35 mm Hg, the increase was only 180%. The intermittent sequential device was more effective than the single-chamber device and was as effective as 5,000 units of UFH every 12 hours in preventing DVT. In addition, the intermittent sequential device increased the time interval for clot formation proximal to the calf compared with UFH. In another study, the same authors compared electrical calf stimulus, low-dose UFH, intermittent sequential compression, and TED hose in 150 patients older than 30 years undergoing major abdominal surgery. The incidence of proven DVT was 18%, 9%, and 4%, respectively.

In a similar study in patients undergoing surgery for gynecological malignancy comparing no thromboprophylaxis to nonsequential external compression, the control group had a VTE frequency of 34.6%. In the compression treatment group, the VTE incidence was reduced to 12.7%. Diagnostic tools for VTE were IPG and I^{131}.

Treatment of Venous Thrombosis

The initial treatment of VTE in most hospitals still involves the use of intravenous UFH, although some LMWHs are approved for treatment of VTE. Given the potential variability of the hypercoagulable state in these patients, constant intravenous infusion UFH still remains the easiest drug to use. Most patients are now treated using a weight-based heparin nomogram and are given a loading dose of 80 units/kg to a maximum of 10,000 units. They are maintained on a constant infusion of 18 units/kg, and the first APTT or factor Xa assay should be done at 4 to 6 hours after the initiation of therapy. Because of the large thrombus burden these patients may have, they can clear or use UFH at an accelerated rate; thus, they are often undertreated. Patients with malignancies will typically require higher-than-average doses until the cancer has been surgically removed or treated. Care must be taken to reduce the infusion, or these patients are susceptible to bleeding that is due to heparin overtreatment. There is little place for intermittent bolus treatment with UFH in modern anticoagulation practice.

If the APTT is used to monitor efficacy of UFH therapy, it should be used in conjunction with the laboratory heparin monitoring nomogram. Because APTT reagents can vary widely between institutions, the old concept of using a ratio of 1.5 to 2 times some poorly defined control APTT value is completely outmoded and can lead to erroneous and inadequate anticoagulation therapy.

Standard clinical practices—such as leg elevation to minimize or treat leg edema after a DVT—are still appropriate. Patients should probably not be aggressively mobilized as long as they have significant leg edema. Most patients will require 5 to 7 days of UFH or LMWH treatment, and the modern trend is to rapidly introduce oral anticoagulation, usually within 24 to 48 hours after initiation of heparin therapy. This will not always be possible in this population, but any UFH or LMWH treatment should be continued until the international normalized ratio (INR) is in the therapeutic range of 2 to 3 for several days. Oral anticoagulation is usually continued for 3 to 6 months or longer, depending on the circumstances and any other complicating factors (i.e., prior VTE or congenital thrombophilia).

The patient who is found to have an asymptomatic DVT of the lower extremity poses a dilemma for some physicians. Some feel that this is not a significant risk and should not be treated, but the risk of thrombus extension into the proximal and popliteal veins remains high and is a possibility. Although this is still a small risk for most patients, the longer-term complications of postphlebitic syndrome from the damaged valves in those veins can produce significant morbidity for such patients, leading to chronic leg edema and venous stasis ulceration. For that reason, most practitioners would elect to anticoagulate women with asymptomatic DVT. With the onset of widespread DVT prophylaxis in many hospitals, the problem of whether to treat asymptomatic DVT may become moot.

POSTOPERATIVE PULMONARY COMPLICATIONS

Postoperative pulmonary complications (PPCs) after abdominal surgery remain an important cause of increased morbidity, mortality, and resource use. Atelectasis, pneumonia, and pulmonary thromboembolic disease following abdominal surgery continue to occur frequently despite continuing advances in anesthetic, surgical, and postoperative treatment. The incidence of PPCs has surpassed that of postoperative cardiac complications, and PPCs have a greater impact on postoperative outcomes. Gynecologic surgery is increasingly performed in patients with advanced age, multiple comorbid conditions, and increased risk for the development of PPCs. Risk factors for PPCs in patients undergoing a gynecologic surgery procedure vary among studies, but are consistent with other patient groups undergoing abdominal surgical procedures (Table 9.10). The most important PPCs in terms of incidence, morbidity, mortality, and resource use are atelectasis, pneumonia, respiratory failure, and pulmonary thromboembolic disease.

An understanding of the physiology that predisposes to PPCs, the risk factors for their development, and the preventive

TABLE 9.10

RISK FACTORS FOR POSTOPERATIVE PULMONARY COMPLICATIONS IN GYNECOLOGIC SURGERY PATIENTS

Age >60 years
Cancer
Congestive heart failure
Smoking within 8 weeks of surgery
Upper abdominal incision
Vertical incision
Incision length >20 cm

and therapeutic measures to minimize and treat them are of critical importance to all gynecologic surgeons.

Perioperative Respiratory Physiology

Effects of Anesthesia

General anesthesia results in important alterations in respiratory physiology (Table 9.11). Anesthetic agents influence not only the ventilatory response to oxygen and carbon dioxide but also the pattern of respiration. Inhalational agents and intravenous agents both result in a reduction of the ventilatory response, but differ in their effects on respiratory pattern. The classic breathing pattern produced by inhalational anesthetics is a rhythmic, rapid, and shallow pattern of respiration with no intermittent sighs, whereas intravenous anesthesia is associated with slow, deep respirations. Little metabolism of inhalational anesthetics occurs during surgery, with most of the anesthetic agents stored in the tissues, such as muscle and fat.

At the conclusion of anesthesia, most of the stored anesthetic agent is eliminated via the lungs. As a result of tissue stores, significant concentrations of the anesthetic agent may be present well into the recovery phase, particularly after high anesthetic doses, long anesthetic times, or the presence of cardiopulmonary disease. This prolonged anesthetic effect can lead to clinically significant respiratory depression in the postoperative period.

The number of functional alveolar units participating actively in gas exchange is directly related to the functional residual capacity (FRC). General anesthesia is associated with a reduction in FRC by approximately 16%. This reduction occurs irrespective of the anesthetic techniques used. The cause of the reduction in FRC is multifactorial and includes cranial movement of the diaphragm, chest wall relaxation with reduction in thoracic volume, reduction in respiratory compliance, and shift of central blood volume from the thorax into the abdomen. Reduction in FRC can have marked adverse effects on perioperative gas exchange, especially the development of hypoxemia.

Atelectasis is defined as the absence of gas from a part or the whole of the lungs that is due to the failure of expansion or resorption of gas from the alveoli. It occurs in the dependent areas of the lungs within 5 minutes of anesthetic induction in a patient with healthy lungs. Atelectasis may be caused by compression, gas resorption, or surfactant impairment. Compression occurs when the distending pressure in the alveolus is reduced to a level that causes the alveolus to collapse. In the setting of general anesthesia, compression occurs mainly as result of impairments in diaphragmatic position and function. In addition to the cephalad movement of the diaphragm that is due to relaxation from anesthesia as described above, increased intraabdominal pressure from bowel edema, peritoneal fluid, and hematoma forces the diaphragm cephalad and contributes substantially to compressive atelectasis. The contractile function of the diaphragm is not altered as a result of an effect of anesthesia itself because diaphragmatic dysfunction, which almost always presents after upper abdominal surgery, does not arise after lower abdominal surgery.

Other factors contributing to postanesthesia pulmonary complications include reabsorption atelectasis, hypoxic pulmonary vasoconstriction, and ventilation/perfusion abnormalities.

Although most gynecological surgery is done in the pelvis, upper abdominal operations are sometimes done by gynecologic oncologists, and extension of the surgical incision and operative procedure into the upper abdomen produce increased respiratory effects. Respiratory muscle dysfunction is the major effect of upper abdominal surgery on respiratory physiology (Table 9.12). Tidal breathing depends on inspiratory muscle function, especially the function of the diaphragm. Other accessory muscles of respiration are recruited when work of breathing increases, such as when diaphragmatic dysfunction is present, during states of increased oxygen consumption, and in the presence of cardiopulmonary disease. In addition to breathing, respiratory muscles play an integral role in the generation of cough and act as stabilizers of the thorax and abdomen. Upper abdominal surgery may affect each of these respiratory muscle functions by several different mechanisms.

An important change following upper abdominal surgery is a shift in respiratory pump function from the diaphragm to accessory inspiratory and expiratory muscles of respiration. This

TABLE 9.11

EFFECTS OF ANESTHESIA ON RESPIRATORY PHYSIOLOGY

Reduced ventilatory response to oxygen and carbon dioxide
Rhythmic rapid shallow breathing pattern
Reduced functional residual capacity
Diaphragmatic dysfunction
Atelectasis
Ventilation-perfusion mismatching
Blunting of hypoxic pulmonary vasoconstriction
Impairment in mucociliary clearance

TABLE 9.12

EFFECTS OF UPPER ABDOMINAL SURGERY ON RESPIRATORY PHYSIOLOGY

Reduction in lung volumes: residual volume, total lung capacity, functional residual capacity, and vital capacity
Reflex inhibition of phrenic nerve activity resulting in decreased diaphragmatic function
Increased neck and intercostal inspiratory accessory muscle use
Tonic and phasic contraction of abdominal expiratory muscles

results in a rapid shallow breathing pattern of respiration. The contractile function of the diaphragm is impaired by inhibition of phrenic nerve output by stimulation of visceral and somatic nerve pathways during manipulation of the abdominal viscera and the peritoneum. The less efficient accessory muscles of inspiration, such as the intercostals and neck muscles, assume an increased share of the respiratory effort. Tonic and phasic contraction of the expiratory abdominal muscles also occurs. The net effect on respiratory mechanics is a reduction in lung volumes, including the FRC (which leads to atelectasis), V/Q abnormalities, and hypoxemia. These changes may be aggravated by hypoventilation that is due to the residua of general anesthesia, postoperative sedative-hypnotic therapy, and pain. In addition to a submaximal voluntary activation of inspiratory muscles, pain may also have a direct effect, through unknown mechanisms, on inspiratory muscle function.

Atelectasis

Clinically significant atelectasis occurs in 15% to 20% of patients undergoing abdominal surgery. The pathophysiologic effects of atelectasis include decreased respiratory compliance, increased pulmonary vascular resistance, predisposition to acute lung injury, and hypoxemia. Atelectasis may also be a precursor to more serious PPCs, such as postoperative pneumonia. The definition of atelectasis is not uniform across clinical studies, with most investigations incorporating a global definition of a PPC that includes atelectasis. However, generally accepted criteria for the diagnosis of atelectasis include impaired oxygenation in a clinical setting where atelectasis is likely, unexplained temperature of greater than 38°C, and chest radiographic evidence of volume loss or new airspace opacity. Risk factors implicated in the development of atelectasis after abdominal surgery include advanced age, obesity, intraperitoneal sepsis, prolonged anesthesia time, nasogastric tube placement, and smoking.

The risk of atelectasis may be reduced by a number of interventions (Table 9.13). Preoperative smoking cessation is effective if it is started well in advance of surgery (6–8 weeks before operation). If smoking cessation is attempted in close proximity to a planned surgical procedure, the improvement in mucociliary clearance in combination with reduced cough may lead to a secretion burden that paradoxically increases the risk of PPCs. Atelectasis is effectively prevented and treated by deep breathing exercises and mobilization. Voluntary lung inflation exercises enable redistribution of gas into areas of low compliance. Mechanical aids, such as incentive spirometry, have not been shown to be superior to properly performed deep breathing maneuvers. Effective deep breathing exercises require the patient to be conscious and cooperative. Chest physiotherapy is extremely labor intensive and has potential disadvantages in that it may exhaust the patient, cause pain, induce bronchospasm, and cause transient hypoxemia. Because chest physiotherapy has never been shown to be superior to deep breathing exercises in preventing or treating atelectasis, it is not recommended after abdominal surgery. Continuous positive airway pressure reduces the incidence of significant postoperative hypoxemia and may reduce rates of pneumonia and intubation. However, the cost, complexity, and potential complications of continuous positive airway pressure limit the practicality of routine application of this technique to patients undergoing abdominal surgery.

Although evidence suggests that effective postoperative pain control reduces PPC, there is inconclusive evidence as to whether postoperative epidural analgesia is superior to patient-controlled analgesia. Both modalities, however, appear to be superior to on-demand narcotic analgesia in reducing PPCs. Laparoscopic procedures reduce postoperative pain scores, as well as have less adverse effect on postoperative respiratory muscle function. Through these mechanisms, atelectasis is reduced with a laparoscopic as opposed to open abdominal surgical procedure. Irrespective of the procedure used, postoperative gastric decompression should be used selectively rather than routinely for postoperative nausea, symptomatic abdominal distention, or inability to tolerate oral intake. Routine nasogastric tube use significantly increases rates of atelectasis without reducing risk of aspiration in comparison with selective decompression.

TABLE 9.13

PREVENTION AND TREATMENT OF ATELECTASIS

Smoking cessation 8 weeks before elective surgery
Laparoscopic procedure
Deep breathing exercises
Mobilization
Adequate analgesia (epidural or patient-controlled analgesia preferred)
Selective gastric decompression

Postoperative Pneumonia

Hospital-acquired pneumonia (HAP) is defined as pneumonia that develops 48 hours or more after hospital admission because of an organism that was not incubating at the time of hospitalization. HAP after abdominal surgery has a high attributable mortality, increases hospital length of stay and cost, and has lasting effects on patient-centered outcomes. Hospital length of stay is increased by approximately 11 days, and hospital charges are increased by 75%. HAP is also associated with a fourfold increase in risk of discharge to a skilled nursing facility. Women have a risk of developing HAP after abdominal surgery that is twice that of men.

HAP is caused by a wide spectrum of bacterial pathogens and is occasionally due to viral or fungal pathogens in immunocompetent patients (Table 9.14). Common pathogens

TABLE 9.14

COMMON PATHOGENS CAUSING HOSPITAL-ACQUIRED PNEUMONIA

Early onset (≤4 days)
Streptococcus pneumoniae
Methicillin-sensitive *Staphylococcus aureus*
Hemophilus influenzae
Escherichia coli
Klebsiella pneumoniae
Enterobacter species
Proteus species
Serratia marcescens
Late onset (≥5 days)
All of the above plus:
Pseudomonas aeruginosa
Multidrug-resistant *Klebsiella pneumoniae*
Acinetobacter species

TABLE 9.15

RISK FACTORS FOR MULTIDRUG-RESISTANT PATHOGENS CAUSING HOSPITAL-ACQUIRED PNEUMONIA

Immunosuppressive disease or therapy
Home infusion therapy
Chronic dialysis
Home wound care
Residence in a nursing home or extended care facility
Antimicrobial therapy in the preceding 90 days
Current hospitalization of 5 days or more
Hospitalization for 2 days or more in the preceding 90 days
High frequency of antibiotic resistance in the community, hospital, or patient care unit

include the aerobic Gram-negative bacilli and *S. aureus* species. Early-onset HAP, defined as occurring within the first 4 days of hospitalization, is usually associated with a better prognosis and is more likely to be caused by antibiotic-susceptible pathogens. Late-onset HAP (occurring on or after 5 days of hospitalization) is more likely to be caused by multidrug-resistant (MDR) pathogens, which are associated with increased morbidity and mortality. The risk of HAP that is due to MDR pathogens is related to characteristics of the patient, the health care environment, and the prescribed medical treatment (Table 9.15).

Bacterial colonization of the lower respiratory tract under conditions that promote bacterial invasion is necessary for HAP to develop. Sources of colonization include air, water, equipment, fomites, and direct transfer from health care providers. Among conditions that promote invasion are severity of underlying illness, comorbid conditions, prior exposure to antimicrobials, and exposure to invasive devices, such as nasogastric tube. Risk of colonization may be modified by several means (Table 9.16). Infection control procedures, including guidelines for alcohol-based hand disinfection and appropriate barrier precautions, should strictly be observed. Early removal of invasive devices, in particular nasogastric tubes, and avoidance of endotracheal intubation when noninvasive ventilation is feasible, will reduce the risk of HAP. As one of the mechanisms for initial colonization of the lower respiratory tract includes microaspiration of gastrically residing bacteria, measures to minimize aspiration and to reduce gastric bacterial overgrowth are important preventive measures. All patients should be maintained in a least a semirecumbent position with the head elevated to 30 to 45 degrees. Restriction of the use of stress ulcer prophylaxis to patients who meet criteria (i.e., receiving mechanical ventilation or coagulopathy/therapeutic anticoagulation) is critical in controlling a possible risk factor for HAP. Implementation of a restrictive red blood cell transfusion strategy, in patients without evidence of active bleeding, is proven to reduce infectious complications of all kinds, including HAP. Adherence to such a strategy not only reduces infectious complications but reduces overall in-hospital mortality and may reduce recurrence of malignancy. In patients younger than age 55 and with an APACHE II score less than 25, a hemoglobin target of 7.0 should be adopted, with a hemoglobin target of 9.0 reserved for patients who do not meet these criteria. Strict control of hyperglycemia has been widely adopted as a means of reducing morbidity and mortality, including the risk of infection. Although the optimal glucose target and the means of achieving that target remain controversial, an attempt to limit capillary blood glucose to less than 150 mg/dL in both diabetic and nondiabetic patients appears warranted.

TABLE 9.16

INTERVENTIONS TO DECREASE RISK FOR HOSPITAL-ACQUIRED PNEUMONIA

Strict adherence to infection control procedures
Early removal of invasive devices
Semirecumbent positioning of the patient
Restriction of acid suppression therapy
Restrictive red blood cell transfusion strategy
Strict control of hyperglycemia

The clinical definition of HAP includes a new opacity on chest radiograph (posterior-anterior and lateral views preferred) plus two of the following: fever greater than 38°C, leukocytosis or leukopenia, and purulent respiratory secretions. The diagnosis of HAP should be supported by sampling of lower respiratory tract secretions, with either an endotracheal aspirate or a bronchoscopic specimen, before the initiation of empiric antibiotic therapy. The initial step in choosing antibiotic therapy for suspected HAP is determination of the patient's risk of infection with an MDR pathogen (Fig. 9.3). One of the consequences of increasing antimicrobial resistance is an increased probability of inappropriate initial empiric treatment. Inappropriate or delayed empiric treatment results in a substantial excessive attributable mortality and hospital length of stay. Prompt institution of appropriate empiric therapy based on risk stratification for the presence of a possible MDR pathogen is crucial to improving patient outcome in HAP.

Initial therapy should be administered intravenously, with a switch to the enteral route of administration in selected patients with a good clinical response and a functional gastrointestinal tract. Combination therapy should be used initially if patients are at high risk of being infected with a MDR pathogen. Monotherapy is appropriate for those patients deemed to be low risk. Duration of therapy should be based on clinical response and may often be safely terminated before the traditional 14- to 21-day treatment period, provided the etiologic pathogen is not *Pseudomonas aeruginosa*. Clinical improvement usually takes 48 to 72 hours, and therapy should not be changed during this time unless there is a rapid clinical decline. The responding patient should have therapy tailored to the most focused regimen possible on the basis of microbiologic studies. The nonresponding patient should be evaluated for drug-resistant organisms, complications of pneumonia (e.g., parapneumonic effusion or empyema), extrapulmonary sites of infection, or noninfectious causes of symptoms and signs of pneumonia (e.g., drug fever with drug-induced lung injury).

Respiratory Failure

Respiratory failure denotes either the inability to maintain normal tissue oxygen transport or the normal excretion of carbon dioxide. Clinically, respiratory failure is usually diagnosed by levels of arterial PO_2 and PCO_2, although the levels that constitute the threshold for respiratory failure are arbitrary. An arterial PO_2 of less than 60 mm Hg or an arterial PCO_2 of greater than 45 mm Hg generally indicates significant

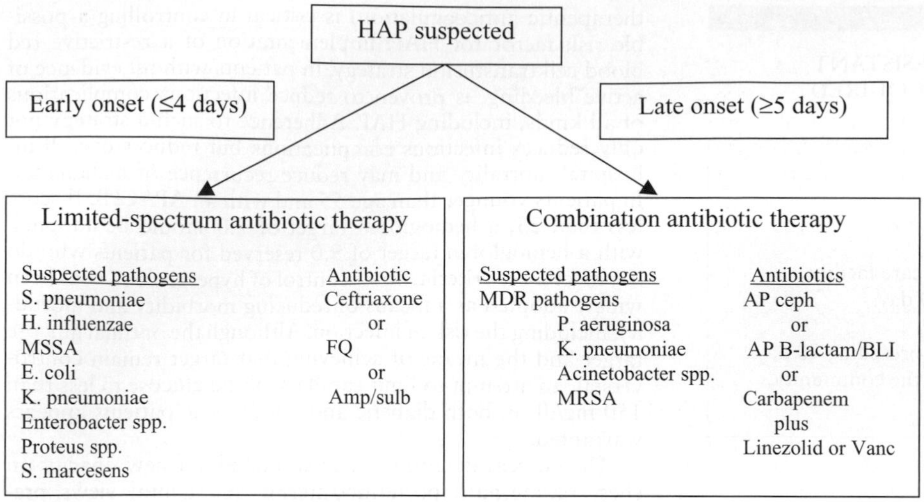

MSSA = Methicillin S. Aureus, FQ = Fluoroquinolone, Amp/sulb = Ampicillin/sulbactam, MDR = Multidrug-resistant, MRSA = Methicillin-resistant S. Aureus, AP ceph = Anti-pseudomonal cephalosporin, Anti-pseudomonal B-lactam/B-lactamase inhibitor, Vanc = vancomycin

FIGURE 9.3. Algorithm for initiating empiric antibiotic therapy for hospital-acquired pneumonia (HAP).

respiratory compromise in patients without preexisting lung disease. The diagnostic and therapeutic approach to the patient with respiratory failure is dictated by the underlying mechanism of abnormal gas exchange (Table 9.17).

Five basic pathophysiologic mechanisms cause acute hypoxemic respiratory failure. These include *hypoventilation*, *V/Q abnormalities* (shunt and dead space), *venous admixture* (reduction in saturation and PO_2 of mixed venous blood), *diffusion limitation*, and *low inspired fraction of oxygen*. Hypoventilation is usually due to depression of respiratory drive at the level of the central nervous system as a result of drug therapy or the residua of anesthesia as described above. V/Q abnormalities, primarily shunt, are the most common cause of hypoxemic respiratory failure and result from such conditions as atelectasis, pneumonia, pulmonary edema, and pulmonary thromboembolic disease. Venous admixture in a patient with preexisting normal lung function usually occurs as a result of a low cardiac output state such as seen in an acute coronary syndrome or early severe sepsis before volume resuscitation. Diffusion limitation and low inspired fraction of oxygen are uncommon causes of hypoxemia in the absence of chronic lung disease and high altitude, respectively.

The spectrum of causes of hypoxemia often can be narrowed according to the appearance of the chest radiograph. A simplified approach to chest radiographic interpretation for other than the pulmonary or critical care medicine specialist involves classifying the pulmonary parenchyma as generally white or black (normal). The causes of a white chest radiograph include atelectasis, pneumonia, pulmonary edema, and acute lung injury. Further characterization of a white chest radiograph includes the description of the radiographic opacities as diffuse or localized. Diffuse infiltrates are commonly associated with hydrostatic pulmonary edema that is due to cardiac pump failure, nonhydrostatic pulmonary edema that is due to lung injury from a variety of causes (e.g., aspiration or pancreatitis), or atypical pneumonias that are rarely hospital acquired (e.g., influenza, *Mycoplasma,* or *Chlamydia* pneumonia). Focal infiltrates are suggestive of atelectasis or pneumonia. The causes of a black or a normal chest radiograph include pulmonary thromboembolic disease, microatelectasis, exacerbation of underlying obstructive lung disease, intracardiac or pulmonary ateriovenous right-to-left shunt, and a low cardiac output state. In the case of a black or white chest radiograph, information obtained from the history and physical examination may be crucial for determining the nature of further diagnostic testing to pinpoint the etiology of respiratory failure.

Ventilatory failure, the inability to maintain an appropriate arterial PCO_2, is caused by three major mechanisms: insufficient respiratory drive, excessive respiratory workload including increased dead space, or respiratory pump dysfunction. Insufficient ventilatory drive is usually due to drug therapy or the residua of anesthesia as stated above, but may also be due to a primary central nervous system disorder (such as stroke, intracranial hemorrhage and obesity-hypoventilation syndrome) or to toxic-metabolic encephalopathy as a result of a wide variety of underlying conditions. Increased ventilatory workload may result from increased CO_2 production, increased dead space, altered respiratory mechanics (increased airway

TABLE 9.17

PATHOPHYSIOLOGIC MECHANISMS OF HYPOXEMIC RESPIRATORY FAILURE AND VENTILATORY FAILURE

Hypoxemic respiratory failure	Ventilatory failure
Hypoventilation	Insufficient respiratory drive
V/Q abnormalities (shunt, dead space)	Excessive respiratory workload
Venous admixture	Respiratory pump dysfunction
Diffusion limitation	
Low inspired fraction of oxygen	

resistance or decreased pulmonary compliance), or compensation for metabolic acidosis.

Increased CO_2 production is a by-product of overall increases in metabolism. Fever, delirium with marked agitation, severe sepsis, overfeeding, and hyperthyroidism would be examples of clinical states associated with increased CO_2 production. Increased dead space is a hallmark of severe chronic obstructive pulmonary disease; in patients with normal lung function, increased dead space is usually due to either pulmonary thromboembolic disease or a change in respiratory pattern. Rapid shallow breathing as a result of the physiologic changes induced by anesthesia, and upper abdominal surgery produces an increase in the proportion of ventilation to the anatomic dead space and a decrease in effective alveolar ventilation. In addition to anesthesia and upper abdominal surgery as causes of respiratory pump dysfunction in the postoperative patient, any other cause of respiratory muscle weakness may result in ventilatory failure. Endocrine disorders, such as myasthenia gravis or hypothyroidism, as well as electrolyte abnormalities, such as hypophosphatemia, are examples of conditions that could significantly contribute to respiratory muscle weakness and pump dysfunction.

Treatment of acute respiratory failure depends on the underlying cause and is best accomplished in an appropriately monitored environment, such as the intensive care unit with the aid of a specialist in critical care medicine, as mechanical support of ventilation—via either conventional endotracheal intubation/mechanical ventilation or noninvasive positive pressure ventilation—may be necessary (Fig. 9.4). Management of mechanical ventilation and its consequences has acquired a level of complexity that mandates subspecialist care and is beyond the scope of this chapter.

POSTOPERATIVE CARE OF THE URINARY BLADDER

The most common postoperative problem in the female bladder is atony caused by overdistention and the reluctance of the patient to initiate the voluntary phase of voiding. After abdominal/pelvic surgery, the patient is often unwilling to contract the abdominal muscles to produce sufficient intraabdominal pressure against the dome of the bladder to initiate the voiding reflex. After anterior colporrhaphy, spasm, edema, and tenderness of the pubococcygeal muscles may obstruct the process of voiding. The operative trauma from plication of the pubovesicocervical fascia causes edema of the urethral wall and submucosa, especially at the urethrovesical junction, thus contributing to the urinary obstruction.

For spontaneous voiding to occur, the parasympathetic function of the bladder detrusor must be coordinated with the voluntary motor function of the abdominal wall and the levator muscles. In the past, it was customary to insert an indwelling urethral catheter for 5 or more days after vaginal plastic surgery. Although this technique is still used in many clinics, a suprapubic catheter has proved to be an effective alternative. The suprapubic technique was developed and introduced to the gynecologic literature in 1964. When inserted at the time of surgery, the suprapubic Silastic tube eliminates the necessity for repeated bladder catheterization until spontaneous voiding occurs. Although used preferentially after anterior vaginal colporrhaphy, suprapubic bladder catheterization also is useful when the need for prolonged bladder drainage is anticipated, such as after radical Wertheim hysterectomy. A suprapubic catheter also can be inserted when a Marshall-Marchetti-Krantz urethral suspension is performed.

The procedure for suprapubic bladder drainage is performed either before or after the operative procedure. Catheter placement consists of insertion of a 12F Silastic (silicone) catheter into the bladder through a needle trocar (Fig. 9.5). A 12F pigtail (Bonnano) Teflon catheter and other modifications also have been used by many surgeons. The bladder is filled with 300 mL of sterile water, and the needle trocar is inserted through the surgically cleaned anterior abdominal wall about 2 cm above the symphysis pubis. When the stylet is removed from the trocar, clear fluid should pass from the bladder under pressure. About 10 cm of the suprapubic catheter is threaded through the trocar, after which the trocar is removed by sliding it over the indwelling tube. The opposite end of the Silastic catheter is connected to a sterile 1-L drainage bottle or to a sterile closed drainage urinometer bag. The tubing should be filled with fluid at all times and should be anchored to the skin with silicone paste or sutured to the skin to avoid accidental removal. A two-way stopcock is inserted between the catheter and drainage tubing for easy opening and closing of the system. The system is not irrigated unless there is plugging of the bladder catheter and failure of drainage.

Alternatively, at the Emory University Hospital, a Foley catheter is placed through the abdominal wall. After placing a Kelly clamp through the urethra and elevating the dome of the bladder, an incision is made in the abdominal wall superior to the Kelly clamp. A 14F Foley catheter is then pulled into the bladder and connected to gravity drainage. If a suprapubic urethropexy is performed, a 2- to 3-cm opening is made in the dome of the bladder, and the bladder is inspected to ensure that no sutures penetrated the mucosa. The Foley catheter is placed in the bladder and sutured in place with a no. 2.0 absorbable purse-string suture. Using the preceding techniques for insertion of a suprapubic Foley catheter, we have decreased the frequency of catheter obstruction. Seven to 10 days postoperatively, the suprapubic catheters are clamped and postvoid residuals are evaluated. Patients with more than 100 mL of residual urine after spontaneous voiding require an extended period of catheterization. If the urinary residual is less than 100 cc on two successive voidings of more than 200 cc each, the suprapubic catheter can be removed. In many patients who require prolonged catheterization following radical hysterectomy or pelvic support surgery, intermittent self-catheterization using a clean but not sterile technique has become favored by many gynecologists. We believe, as do other authors, that prophylactic antibiotics given during the use of an indwelling bladder catheter are ineffective in preventing urinary tract infection. Although urinary tract symptoms may be delayed with the use of prophylactic antibiotics, it is our experience that the incidence of infection is unchanged and that a subsequent urinary tract infection may result from resistant organisms that are more difficult to treat later. Therefore, we prefer to treat only patients who have significant bacteriuria and pyuria, which includes about 10% to 15% of the patients with suprapubic drainage.

POSTOPERATIVE GASTROINTESTINAL TRACT MANAGEMENT

Dysfunction of the gastrointestinal tract remains a challenge in postoperative management. Each patient should be treated as an individual and not placed on a standard protocol for

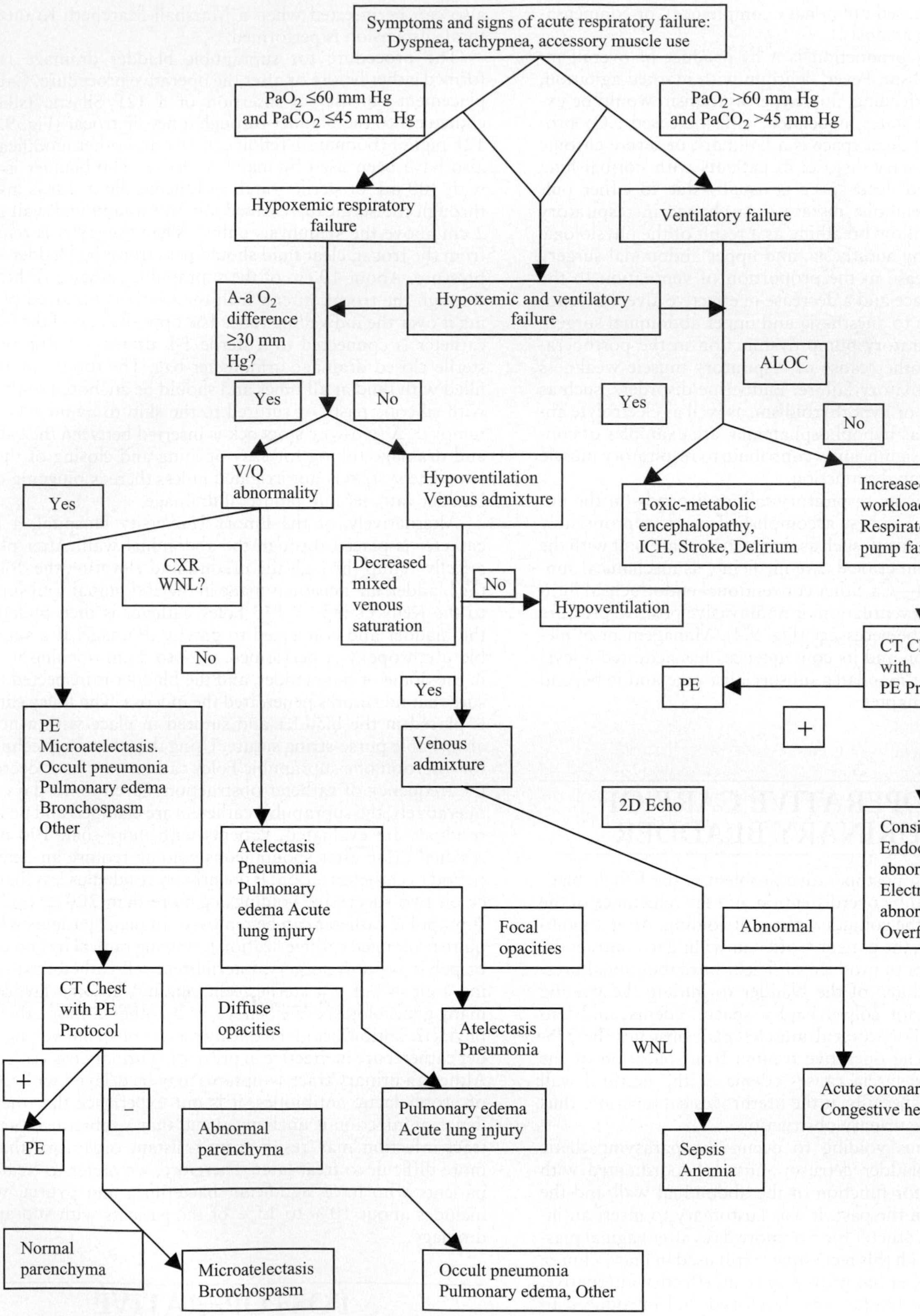

FIGURE 9.4. Algorithm for the evaluation of respiratory failure. ALOC, altered level of consciousness; CT, computed tomography; CXR, Chest X-ray; ICH, intracranial hemorrhage; PE, pulmonary embolism; WNL, within normal limits.

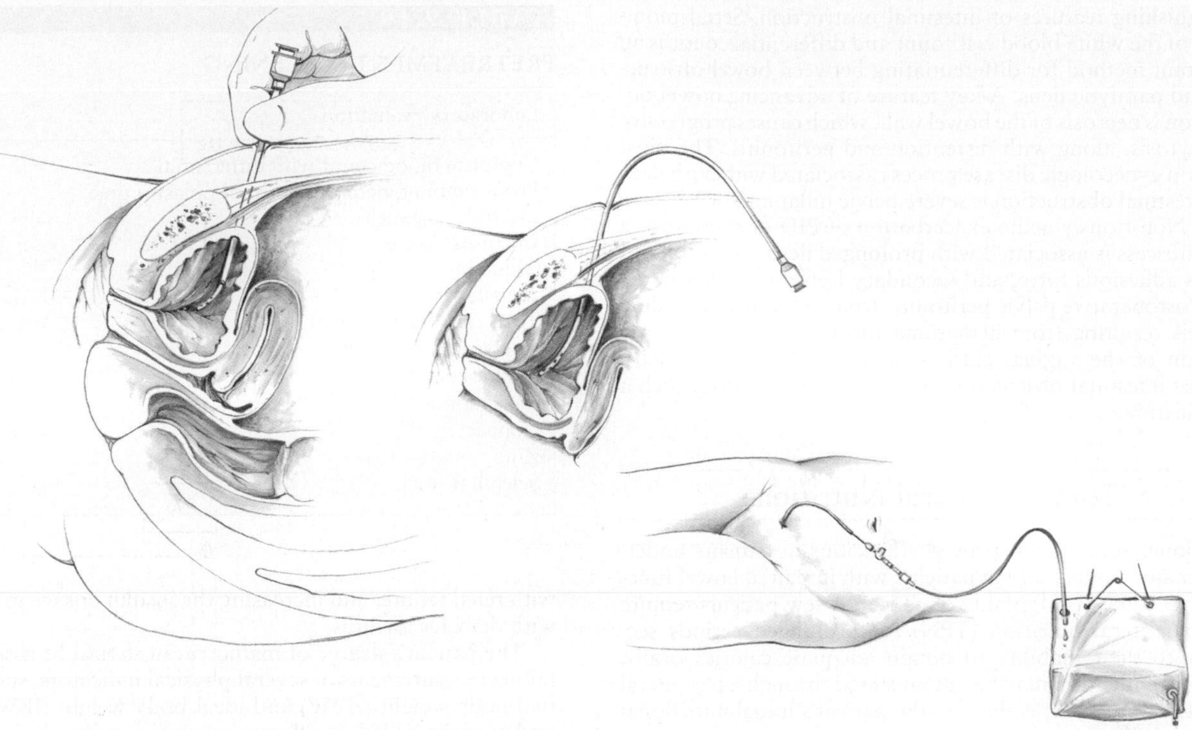

FIGURE 9.5. Method of inserting a suprapubic tube into the bladder through a needle, with resultant drainage into a bottle. Suprapubic catheterization avoids the trauma to the urethra caused by repeated catheterization of an indwelling catheter.

advancing diets. Patients who have had uncomplicated surgery may be given a regular diet on the first postoperative day if bowel sounds are present, if abdominal examination reveals no distention, and if the patient is no longer nauseated from her anesthesia. Seriously ill or malnourished patients or patients requiring extensive bowel surgery may benefit from preoperative and postoperative parenteral nutrition.

It is important to differentiate between postoperative ileus and postoperative obstruction (Table 9.18) if proper therapy is to be initiated promptly with beneficial results. The distinction may be difficult. This is because partial bowel obstruction is often accompanied by a secondary ileus as part of the clinical picture. Only by close clinical monitoring of the bowel sounds, serial abdominal radiographic studies, and frequent white blood cell counts can one clearly separate these two postoperative complications. Adynamic ileus is the more common clinical entity, a fact that may mislead the surgeon into a false sense of security unless he or she remains acutely aware of the

TABLE 9.18

DIFFERENTIAL DIAGNOSIS BETWEEN POSTOPERATIVE ILEUS AND POSTOPERATIVE OBSTRUCTION

Clinical feature	Postoperative ileus	Postoperative obstruction
Abdominal pain	Discomfort from distention but not cramping pains	Cramping progressively severe
Relation to previous surgery	Usually within 48–72 h of surgery	Usually delayed, may be 5–7 d for remote onset
Nausea and vomiting	Present	Present
Distention	Present	Present
Bowel sounds	Absent or hypoactive	Borborygmi with peristaltic rushes and high-pitched tinkles
Fever	Only if related to associated peritonitis	Rarely present unless bowel becomes gangrenous
Abdominal radiographs	Distended loops of small and large bowels; gas usually present in colon	Single or multiple loops of distended bowel (usually small bowel) with air–fluid levels
Treatment	Conservative with nasogastric suction, enemas, cholinergic stimulation	Conservative management with nasogastric decompression Surgical exploration

distinguishing features of intestinal obstruction. Serial monitoring of the white blood cell count and differential count is an important method for differentiating between bowel obstruction and paralytic ileus. A key feature of advancing bowel obstruction is necrosis of the bowel wall, which causes progressive leukocytosis, along with distention and peritonitis. The most common gynecologic disease process associated with both ileus and intestinal obstruction is severe pelvic inflammatory disease (PID). Notoriously acute exacerbation of PID or rupture of a pelvic abscess is associated with prolonged ileus. Occasionally, fibrous adhesions form, and secondary bowel obstruction occurs. Postoperative pelvic peritonitis from any cause, including cellulitis resulting from hematoma formation and secondary infection of the vaginal cuff, is often associated with ileus, whereas intestinal obstruction only rarely results from such a complication.

Total Parenteral Nutrition

Nutritional support has proved efficacious in patients undergoing major surgery and in patients with impaired bowel function, inadequate oral intake, or cancer. A few patients require total parenteral nutrition (TPN) for prolonged periods secondary to their inability to obtain adequate calories orally. Parenteral nutrition may be administered through a peripheral or central access, depending on the patient's initial nutritional status and the time required on TPN.

Hospitalized patients may require TPN for disease processes such as gastrointestinal tract obstruction, prolonged ileus, short-bowel syndrome, radiation enteritis, intraabdominal abscess, pancreatitis, regional enteritis, and enterocutaneous fistula. A patient with any condition that prevents oral intake of adequate amounts of food for more than 7 to 10 days probably requires central parenteral nutrition. Because it is much easier to maintain an adequate nutritional state than to improve a poor one, the decision to use TPN should not be delayed.

TPN is not without complications. Many of these pertain to the need for central venous access. Catheter tip infection is one of the more frequently encountered problems. Meticulous aseptic technique when placing the central venous catheter and adherence to aseptic technique when using the catheter minimizes the risk of infection. Antibiotic-coated central venous catheters have been around for more than a decade and are coming more into favor as compelling data surface suggesting decreased infection rates with their use. At the Emory University Hospital, central venous catheters coated with chlorhexidine and silver sulfasalazine are being used. Other potential problems with central venous catheters include catheter or air embolism and pneumothorax or hemothorax. TPN itself can cause fluid overload, electrolyte abnormalities, or metabolic disturbances.

Patient Evaluation

A complete medical history and physical examination must be obtained before parenteral nutrition is initiated. Particular attention should be paid to identifying patients with cardiovascular or renal disease, hyperlipidemia, diabetes, and thyroid disease. TPN modification can include decreasing or eliminating fat emulsion in patients with severe cardiovascular disease or hyperlipidemia, administering low-nitrogen TPN to patients with renal failure, and increasing the insulin dosage in patients with diabetes mellitus.

The patient's degree of malnutrition should be assessed by taking measurements of several physical indicators, such as actual body weight (ABW) and ideal body weight (IBW), usual body weight (UBW; preillness), creatinine to height index, triceps skin fold thickness (TSFT), and arm circumference (AC). The arm muscle circumference (AMC) is calculated and used as an index of nutritional status.

$$AMC = AC - (TSFT \times 3.14)$$

Fat stores are reflected in the triceps skin fold measurement, whereas somatic proteins are evaluated by measuring muscle mass, such as the AMC. The Frisancho standards (1984) are used to interpret body weight (kg), triceps (mm), and bone-free arm muscle area (cm^2). Patients found to be in the 5th to 10th percentiles are severely malnourished and require an anabolic environment. Weight loss is considered significant when the $(UBW - ABW)/UBW \times 100$ is $>10\%$. Weight loss during starvation occurs at a rate of 0.4 kg/d. Survival also is compromised when the ABW falls below the 70th percentile of the IBW. In addition to the preceding physical measurements, a thorough evaluation of chemical indicators is required (Table 9.19) before initiating TPN. Extensive monitoring is required while the patient is receiving TPN (Table 9.20).

TABLE 9.19

PRETREATMENT SCREENING

Laboratory evaluation
Complete blood count with differential
Prothrombin time/partial thromboplastin time
Electrolytic panel
Chemistry panel
Albumin
Transferrin
Total lymphocyte count
Triglycerides
Magnesium
Phosphorus
Copper
Zinc
Selenium

TABLE 9.20

TREATMENT MONITORING

Test	Frequency
Electrolyte panel	Twice weekly
Chemistry panel	Weekly
Magnesium	Weekly
Transferrin	Weekly
Triglycerides	Monthly, or as needed
Zinc	Monthly, or as needed
Copper	Monthly, or as needed
Selenium	Monthly, or as needed

TABLE 9.21

DESIGN OF PARENTERAL NUTRITION PROGRAMS: EXAMPLES

Nonobese patient weighing 60 kg; assume basal Harris-Benedict equation estimate of daily caloric requirements of 1,250 kcal/d

Patient characteristics

1. Euvolemic, normal urine output, and no unusual gastrointestinal losses; therefore, appropriate initial estimate of daily fluid requirement is 30 mL/kg body weight
2. Moderately stressed with normal renal and hepatic function; therefore, appropriate to provide 1.2 g protein per kg body weight
3. Nonobese; therefore, appropriate to provide Harris-Benedict estimate plus 20% for calories, i.e., 1,250 kcal plus 20% = 1,500 kcal

Program design

1. Fluid requirement: 30 mL × body weight; 30 × 60 = 1,800 mL
2. Caloric requirement: Harris-Benedict estimate plus 20%; 1,250 kcal + 250 kcal = 1,500 kcal
3. Protein requirement for moderately stressed patient: 1.2 g/kg body weight; 60 × 1.2 = ~70 g protein. 70 g protein × 4 kcal/g protein = 280 kcal
4. Fat requirement: 30% of total calories; 30% × 1,500 kcal = 450 kcal
5. Carbohydrate requirement: caloric requirement minus the sum of protein and fat calories; 1,500 − (280 + 450 kcal) = 770 kcal. 770 kcal carbohydrate ÷ kcal/g carbohydrate (3.4) = ~225 g carbohydrate
6. Therefore, consider the following parenteral nutrition formula: 1.5 L amino acids, 5% dextrose, 15%; plus 250 mL of 20% fat emulsion, which provides 1,750 mL, 1,565 kcal, 75 g protein, 225 g carbohydrate, and 500 fat calories. Note that 5% amino acids equals 50 g protein per liter
7. If institution uses three-in-one admixture (amino acids plus dextrose plus fat in one container) and stock solutions of 10% amino acids, 70% dextrose, and 20% lipid, a comparable parenteral nutrition program would be 1.5 L amino acids, 5%; dextrose, 15%; fat, 3.5%

Similar patient characteristics except patients volume-expanded

1. Consider the following fluid-restricted parenteral nutrition formula: 1 L of amino acids, 7%; dextrose, 20%; plus 250 mL 20% fat emulsion, which provides 1,250 mL, 1,460 calories, 70 g protein, 200 g carbohydrate, and 500 fat calories

McMahon MM. Parenteral nutrition. In: Goldman L, Ausiello D, eds. *Cecil textbook of medicine.* 22nd ed. Philadelphia: WB Saunders Company, 2004.

The physical and chemical measurements of malnutrition are subject to many influences during illness and should be treated as confounding variables. For example, albumin values less than 3.2 g/dL are frequently used to indicate malnutrition. Starker and colleagues observed that in hospitalized patients, albumin and body weight measurements in conjunction provided better indications of sodium balance and extracellular fluid volume. In addition, albumin serum levels are required for maintenance of the intravascular colloid oncotic pressure and as a carrier protein.

The half-life of albumin is 20 days and thus reflects a depletion of visceral proteins of at least 3 weeks' duration. Transferrin, with a half-life of 8 to 9 days, provides the clinician with a measurement of recent protein status changes. Because transferrin is required to bind Fe^{2++}, its level is affected by intravascular iron status and can increase during pregnancy, in patients with hepatitis, and in patients receiving estrogen supplementation. Serum protein content can be reduced in protein-losing enteropathy, nephropathy, chronic infections, uremia, and during catabolism. Transferrin reflects recent losses and remains a better indicator of protein status and change than albumin. Total lymphocyte counts of less than 1,500 mL are indicative of an immunocompromised patient. Immunologic skin testing for recall antigens and total lymphocyte counts have been correlated with both nutritional status and morbidity and mortality. Its usefulness in the assessment of nutritional status is limited to confounding variables such as cancer, side effects of cancer treatment protocols, stress of trauma or surgery, and infection. Phosphorus and the trace elements are thoroughly evaluated before initiating TPN and during TPN because they are often depleted with many disease states and are required when alimenting (Tables 9.7, 9.8, 9.9, and 9.19–9.22).

Nutritional Requirements

TPN consists of six components: carbohydrates, fat, protein, electrolytes, vitamins, and trace elements. The Harris-Benedict basal energy expenditure (BEE) accounts for two thirds of the total daily energy requirements, with the remaining one third obtained from protein. Daily requirements for protein are between 1.5 and 2.5 g/kg/day. Patients receiving TPN who are

TABLE 9.22

TRACE MINERALS

	Deficiency		Toxicity	
Minerals and levels	Symptoms	Etiology	Symptoms	Etiology
Zinc, 55–150 mg/dL	Diarrhea, mental depression, alopecia, night blindness, dermatosis, impaired taste, hypogonadism, impaired wound healing	Gastrointestinal (failure of ingestion, absorption, retention) Large wounds Protein-energy malnutrition Cancer	Vomiting Diarrhea Neurologic damage ("zinc shakes")	Increased ingestion from galvanized containers Metal fume fever
Selenium, 90–150 μg/dL (synergism with vitamin E)	Myositis with muscle weakness Cardiomyopathy with arrhythmias and congestive heart failure	Unsupplemented TPN	Liver cirrhosis Alopecia Pathologic loss of nails Dermatitis	Increased ingestion (rare)
Chromium, 50–200 μg/d	Neuropathy Encephalopathy New insulin–dependent diabetes mellitus	Unsupplemented TPN Increased renal loss secondary to injury Gastrointestinal losses	Respiratory Lung cancer	Workers manufacturing products containing hexavalent chromium
Phosphorus, 3.0–4.5 mg/dL	Nausea, vomiting, anorexia, dysarthria, paresthesia, hemolytic anemia, peripheral neuropathy, respiratory depression, congestive heart failure, renal glycosuria	Gastrointestinal (failure of ingestion, absorption, retention) Cellular anabolism Respiratory or metabolic alkalosis $Al(OH)_3$ antacids Alcoholism	Neurotoxicity secondary to compensatory hypocalcemia	Renal failure Hypoparathyroidism
Magnesium, 136–145 mEq/L	Nausea, vomiting, muscle weakness, lethargy, tetany, muscle tremor, personality changes	Gastrointestinal (failure of ingestion, absorption, retention) Cellular catabolism, acidosis, K^+ depletion Glomerular dysfunction	Hyporeflexia, lethargy, respiratory depression, cardiac arrest	Magnesium supplementation in patients with renal compromise
Copper, 70–155 μg/dL	Hypochromic anemia not responsive to iron, neutropenia	THAS without copper or high amino acids Gastrointestinal (failure of ingestion, absorption, retention) Pregnancy, lactation (increased requirements) Renal losses	Jaundice—hepatic necrosis Intravascular hemolysis Gastric hemorrhage Tremors, choreoathetoid movements, dementia, rigidity, dysarthria	Iatrogenic Wilson's disease Absorption of copper nitrate salves in burn patients

THAS, total hyperalimentation solution; TPN, total parenteral nutrition.

severely malnourished and stressed require larger amounts of protein daily.

The basal energy expenditure (BEE) is calculated as follows.

$$\text{BEE (kcal/d)} = 655 + 9.56(\text{wt}) + 1.85(\text{ht}) - 4.68(\text{age})$$

Height is in cm; weight is in kg

Once the patient has reached the estimated daily calorie goal, a 24-hour nitrogen balance study is performed by obtaining a 24-hour urine collection and an A.M. electrolyte panel. If a large quantity of fluid from the nasogastric tube, ileostomy, fistula, or wound is present, this also should be collected and sent for nitrogen measurements.

$$N_2\text{ (g) balance} = N_2\text{ (g) in} - N_2\text{ (g) out}$$

Adding 4 to the N_2 out value accounts for nitrogenous losses in the stool and skin. This does not include an estimate of the losses from the gastrointestinal tract and wound, as previously described.

N_2 (g) balance = N_2 (g) in × [N_2 (g) out + 4]
N_2 (g) out = urine volume (mL) × urine urea N_2 (mg/dL)
N_2 (g) in = amino acids per day/6.24
6.24 = g protein/g nitrogen

Patients with normal renal and liver function are started on standard total hyperalimentation solution THAS (Table 9.19). Each liter provides a total of 1,020 kcal, including 41 g of amino acids and 250 g of dextrose. The osmolality of this solution is 1,850 mOsm, which therefore necessitates a central venous access. The calories-to-nitrogen ratio of this solution is 157:1 and is optimal in nonstressed patients. The addition of lipids also is effective in promoting a positive nitrogen balance. The total daily sodium concentration should be equivalent to that of normal saline (150 mEq/L). This can be altered to accommodate patients who require sodium restriction or loading. Table 9.23 outlines the recommendation for daily electrolyte requirements. It should be noted that acetate serves as a precursor to bicarbonate, because the latter is not compatible in the THAS solution. Multivitamins are added daily to 1 L of THAS, whereas trace elements are divided equally in the volume to be infused during a 24-hour period. The recommended daily allowances for both fat- and water-soluble vitamins are outlined in Table 9.24.

Blood glucose levels in patients receiving TPN should be between 100 and 200 mg/dL. A minimum of 10 IU should be added to each liter when required. This permits about 50% to adhere to the plastic tubing. This can be supplemented with subcutaneous doses of regular insulin to obtain the desired blood glucose level. About one half to two thirds of the previous day's requirements are added in divided doses to the THAS solutions.

Intravenous lipids provide a nonprotein source of energy and serve as a source of essential fatty acids. Ten percent fat emulsions (550 kcal/500 mL) and 20% fat emulsions (1,000 kcal/500 mL) are commercially available. In patients receiving standard TPN, 500 mL of 10% fat emulsion are infused twice weekly at a rate of 42 mL/h. However, when fat emulsion is used with peripheral THAS, the patient requires 2 L of peripheral THAS and 1 L of 10% fat emulsion daily. Twenty percent fat emulsions also can be used for calories in patients with glucose intolerance or patients who require a decreased protein-calorie percentage.

Patients deficient in fatty acids present with dermatitis, hemolytic anemia, thrombocytopenia, elevated liver enzymes, and poor wound healing.

TABLE 9.23

DAILY ELECTROLYTE REQUIREMENTS FOR PARENTERAL NUTRITION

Electrolyte	Dosage (mEq/d)
Sodium	60–150
Potassium	60–240
Phosphate	30–45
Calcium	10–15
Magnesium	8–26
Acetate	80–120
Chloride	60–150

To improve glucose tolerance, the first liter should be started at a rate of 42 mL/h. On the second day, the solution can be increased to 84 mL/h; on day 3, it can be increased to 124 mL/h. If the patient is unable to tolerate this schedule, increments can be decreased to 21 mL/h each day. Treatment monitoring is outlined in Table 9.20. Total nitrogen balance should be recalculated if there is a marked change in the patient's condition or in the parenteral nutrition administered.

Recent data in the surgical literature suggest that supplementing TPN with glutamine dipeptides improves nitrogen balance, preserves intestinal permeability and absorption, and improves recovery of lymphocytes. These authors also demonstrated a shorter hospital stay in postoperative patients receiving glutamine dipeptide-enriched TPN compared with controls receiving TPN alone.

Initiating Total Parenteral Nutrition

Safe venous access is required for initiating TPN. A reliable intravenous catheter should be placed into a large central vein with the catheter tip located so that blood flow dilutes the highly concentrated nutritional fluids. The insertion site also should allow easy fixation of the catheter at the entrance site, minimum catheter movement during body movements, and easy dressing changes. A subclavian vein approach satisfies the requirements for safe catheter placement, but neither internal jugular vein nor antecubital fossa placement is optimal. The internal jugular vein should be used only if the subclavian approach has failed. Movement of the head and neck results in an increased incidence of occluding venous access when the internal jugular vein has been cannulated.

Anatomy of Infraclavicular Subclavian Vein

In 1952, Aubaniac, a French physician, was among the first to advocate use of the subclavian vein for intravenous infusions. Wilson and colleagues cannulated the superior vena cava through a percutaneous puncture of the subclavian vein. They reported a high percentage of successful cannulations and a low incidence of complications.

As Figure 9.6 shows, the subclavian vein is located within the costoclavicular-scalene triangle, which is bounded anteriorly by the medial end of the clavicle, posteriorly by the upper surface of the first rib, and laterally by the anterior scalene muscle. The anterior scalene muscle separates the subclavian vein from the subclavian artery, which lies beneath and along the lateral aspect of the muscle. The subclavian vein is covered by 5 cm of the clavicle medially and joins the internal jugular vein near the medial border of the anterior scalene muscle to form the innominate vein. The innominate vein descends behind the sternum and joins with the opposite innominate vein to form the superior vena cava. The subclavian vein, which is about 3 or 4 cm long, continues as the axillary vein below the clavicle en route to the axilla. Several other significant structures occupy this region. The phrenic nerve courses across the anterior surface of the anterior scalene muscle near its attachment to the first rib and courses medially to lie posterior to the subclavian vein. It can be injured if the posterior wall of the vessel is penetrated. The internal thoracic nerve and apical pleura are in contact with the posterior surface of the subclavian vein at its junction with the internal jugular vein. The roots of the brachial plexus formed by the fifth, sixth, seventh, and eighth cervical and first thoracic nerves lie lateral to the anterior scalene muscle on the lateral side of the subclavian artery. If a cannulating needle is directed too far laterally, the brachial nerve plexus could be injured or the subclavian artery could be

TABLE 9.24

RECOMMENDED DIETARY ALLOWANCES[a]

Patient parameters						Fat-soluble vitamins				
Age (years) or condition	Weight[b] (kg)	(lb)	Height[b] (cm)	(in)	Protein g	Vitamin A >mg RE[c]	Vitamin D IU[d]	Vitamin E IU[e]	Vitamin K >mg	Ascorbic acid (C) mg
Females 11–14	46	101	157	62	46	800	400	12	45	50
15–18	55	120	163	64	44	800	400	12	55	60
19–24	58	128	164	65	46	800	400	12	60	60
25–50	63	138	163	64	50	800	200	12	65	60
51+	65	143	160	63	50	800	200	12	65	60

[a] The allowances, expressed as average daily intakes over time, are intended to provide for individual variations among most normal persons as they live in the United States under usual environmental stresses. Diets should be based on a variety of common foods in order to provide other nutrients for which human requirements have been less well defined.
[b] Weights and heights of Reference Adults are actual medians for the US population of the designated age, as reported by NHANES II. The median weights and heights of those under 19 years of age were taken from Hamill PV et al. *Am J Clin Nutr* 1979;32:607–629. The use of these figures does not imply that the height-to-weight ratios are ideal.
[c] Retinol equivalents. 1 retinol equivalent = 1 mg retinol or 6 mg β-carotene.
[d] As cholecalciferol. 10 mg cholecalciferol = 400 IU of vitamin D.
[e] α-Tocopherol equivalents. 1 mg d-α-tocopherol = α-TE = 1.49 IU.
Source: National Academy of Sciences. *Recommended Dietary Allowances*, 10th ed. Washington, DC. National Academy Press, 1989.

punctured. The thoracic duct on the left side and the lymphatic duct on the right cross the anterior scalene muscle on either side of the thorax to enter the superior aspect of each subclavian vein near its junction with the internal jugular vein. These lymphatic vessels are rarely encroached on during subclavian catheterization.

Subclavian Catheter Placement

As illustrated in Figure 9.7A, the subclavian catheter is inserted with the patient in the supine position, with the foot of the bed elevated 6 to 12 inches to increase the pressure in the subclavian vein and produce venous distention. After meticulous aseptic preparation of the skin with povidone-iodine (Betadine), the skin and subcutaneous tissues are infiltrated with a 1% solution of lidocaine (Xylocaine) if the patient is awake. The point of needle insertion is about 1 cm below the junction of the inner and middle third of the clavicle. Most central venous catheter units include an external introducer catheter (Teflon) and an internal (silicone) infusion catheter. The outer Teflon sheath accommodates a no. 12 needle, which fits snugly into and protrudes beyond the end of the Teflon catheter. The needle and sheath are introduced into the skin with the shaft of the needle held almost parallel with the anterior chest wall (Fig. 9.7A). The needle is directed medially and advanced along the undersurface of the clavicle. It is not necessary to scrape the

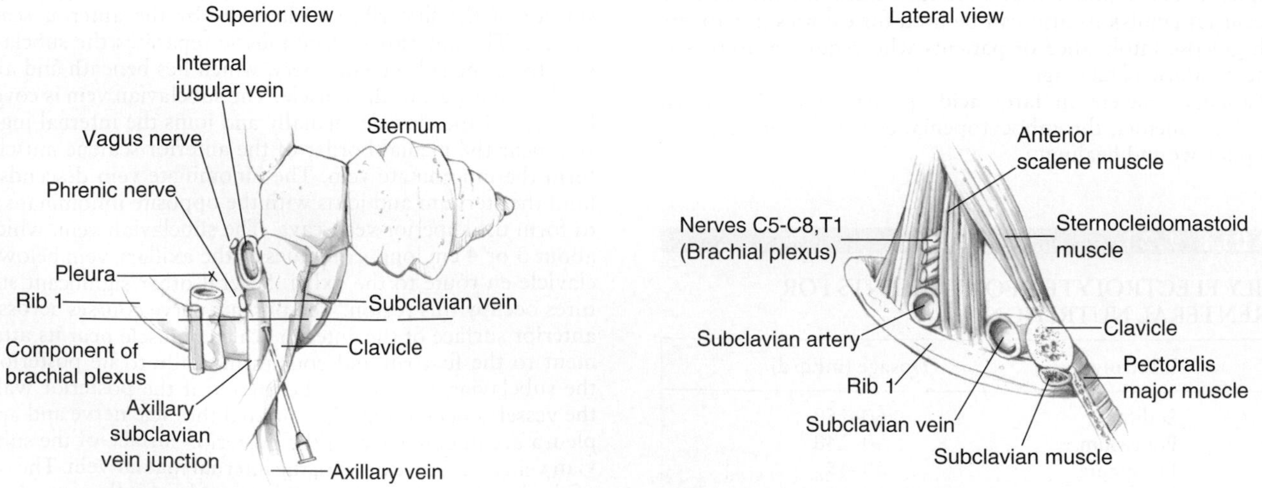

FIGURE 9.6. Anatomic relations of the subclavian vein. The broken line represents the location of the transverse section for lateral view. (Adapted from: Moosman DA. The anatomy of infraclavicular subclavian vein catheterization and its complications. *Surg Gynecol Obstet* 1973;136:71, with permission.)

Water-soluble vitamins						Minerals						
Thiamine (B_1) mg	Riboflavin (B_2) mg	Niacin (B_3) mg	Pyridoxine (B_6) mg	Folate >mg	Cyanocobalamin (B_{12}) >mg	Calcium mg	Phosphorus mg	Magnesium mg	Iron mg	Zinc mg	Iodine >mg	Selenium >mg
1.1	1.3	15	1.4	150	2	1,200	1,200	280	15	12	150	45
1.1	1.3	15	1.5	180	2	1,200	1,200	300	15	12	150	50
1.1	1.3	15	1.6	180	2	1,200	1,200	280	15	12	150	55
1.1	1.3	15	1.6	180	2	800	800	280	15	12	150	55
1	1.2	13	1.6	180	2	800	800	280	10	12	150	55

posterior surface of the clavicle to ensure that the pleura is protected from puncture. By applying suction constantly, the needle passes beneath the skin and immediately aspirates dark red blood, which confirms entry into the vein. If the vein is not entered, the needle is withdrawn and readvanced in a similar manner but in a slightly more cranial or caudal direction. As soon as a free flow of blood is obtained, the introduced Teflon sheath is advanced far enough to be certain that it is securely placed within the vein. The sheath is held in place by the connector, the finger is placed over the end of the needle to prevent air embolism, and the internal needle is replaced (Fig. 9.7B) by the silicone infusion catheter that accompanies the central venous pressure kit (Fig. 9.7C). A thin wire stylet inside the infusion catheter allows the catheter to be advanced easily; occasionally, the stylet must be withdrawn slightly to advance the catheter as far as possible into the innominate vein and superior vena cava. The silicone infusion catheter is advanced until the attached connector can be securely wedged into the connector of the Teflon sheath (Fig. 9.7C). After the infusion catheter is connected to an intravenous fluid line, the Teflon

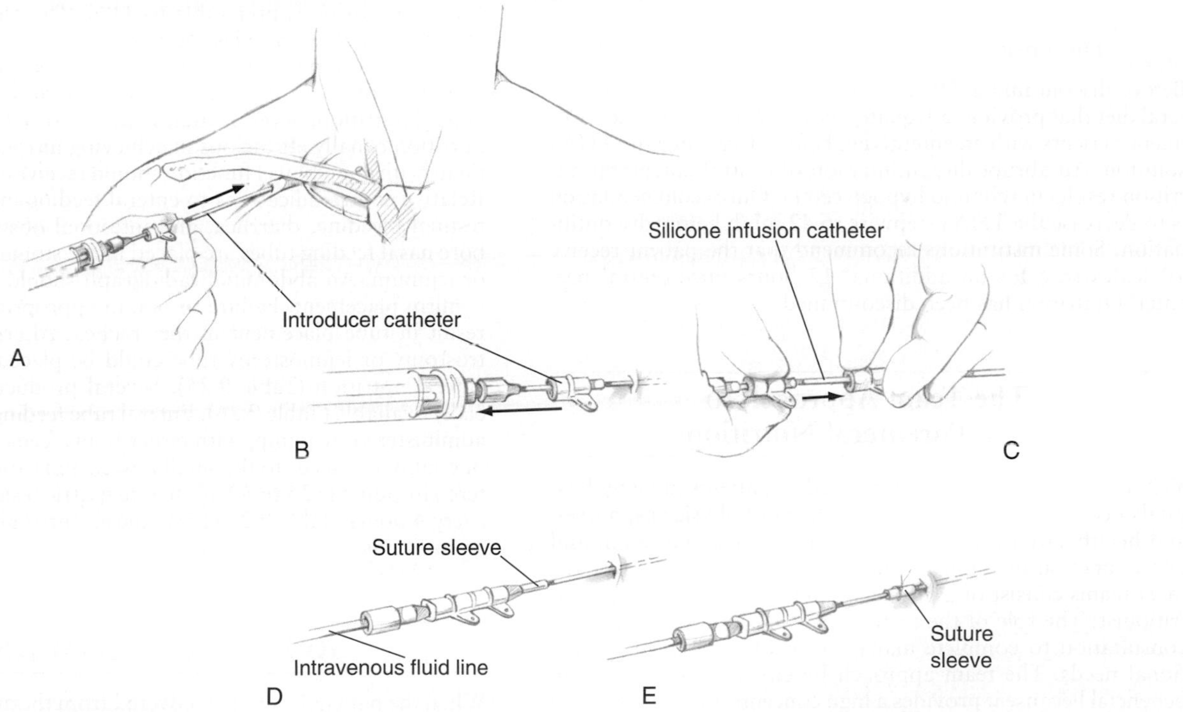

FIGURE 9.7. Insertion of subclavian catheter for monitoring central venous pressure. **A:** After locally anesthetizing the puncture site, the needle with overlying introducer catheter is directed medially between the first rib and the clavicle at the junction of the middle and inner third of the clavicle. The needle is held parallel to the anterior chest wall and advanced along the undersurface of the clavicle. Entry into the vein is evident with aspiration of blood in the attached syringe. **B:** The needle and syringe are removed from the Teflon sheath, and a finger is held over the end of the open catheter to prevent entry of air. **C:** The silicone infusion catheter is inserted through the introducer catheter until the two connectors meet and lock firmly. **D:** The intravenous fluid line is connected to the silicone infusion catheter. **E:** The suture sleeve is advanced to the skin surface, where the catheter is sutured firmly to the skin.

sheath is carefully withdrawn from the vein, remaining partially in the subcutaneous tissue while leaving an ample length of the infusion catheter in the vena cava (Fig. 9.7D). A suture sleeve on the introducer sheath is slid down to the puncture site and sutured to the skin (Fig. 9.7E). The tip of the catheter is preferably positioned in the superior vena cava and should not be advanced into the right atrium or ventricle, where it could cause accidental trauma to the heart wall or cardiac arrhythmias. To ensure its continued sterility and proper function, the subclavian vein catheter should not be used to replace fluids or withdraw blood for laboratory studies, if it is at all possible to avoid these uses. A central venous line for hyperalimentation is an exception to this rule. The dressing should be changed daily, and the catheterization site cleaned with povidone-iodine or a similar antimicrobial solution.

Cardiac and Respiratory Insufficiency

Patients with congestive heart failure require decreased sodium and decreased total fluid volume. The best solution can be prepared from the most concentrated solutions of glucose, amino acid, and fat available. Fluid-restricted solutions also may be beneficial for patients with respiratory failure, who should receive less total glucose in favor of more fat because the respiratory quotient (CO_2/O_2) of glucose (1.00) is greater than that of fat (0.70) and because excess glucose will increase the load of CO_2 the lungs must excrete. Excessive total caloric intake resulting in fat synthesis from glucose substrate may severely compromise respiratory function because large amounts of CO_2 are released (respiratory quotient 8.0).

Discontinuing Total Parenteral Nutrition

Before discontinuing TPN, the patient should tolerate an enteral diet that provides adequate calories. It is permissible to aliment patients with an enteral diet before decreasing the THAS solution. An abrupt discontinuation of central parenteral nutrition results in rebound hypoglycemia. Our recommendation is to decrease the THAS stepwise to 42 mL/h before discontinuation. Some institutions recommend that the patient receive 10% dextrose for an additional 12 hours once central parenteral nutrition has been discontinued.

The Team Approach to Total Parenteral Nutrition

TPN can now be safely administered to patients in many hospitals because of the existence of a team of physicians, nurses, and health care professionals. Although the composition and exact function of the team members vary between hospitals, most teams consist of a physician, nurse, pharmacist, and nutritionist. The role of the team varies in each institution from consultation to complete management of the patient's nutritional needs. The team approach by either method is highly beneficial because it provides a high concentration of personnel with knowledge, expertise, and interdisciplinary communication at the patient's bedside. Team members can provide continuing education on nutrition therapy, continuously audit and collect quality control data, and investigate ways to improve the safety and efficacy of TPN as a treatment modality. Most teams operate with a standardized protocol that covers patient assessment, catheter insertion techniques, solutions used, and monitoring functions performed.

TABLE 9.25

PROTOCOL FOR ENTERAL TUBE FEEDING

Nasogastric route: Use small-bore, flexible tube (8F preferred); obtain radiograph after placement to confirm position.
Elevate head of bed at least 30 degrees.
Use feeding pump for continuous feeding.
Begin with full-strength formula at 25–30 mL/h and, if tolerated, increase by 25–30 mL/h at 12-h intervals until desired total volume is reached.[a]
Check gastric residuals every 4 h; if greater than 100 mL, hold feeding, and repeat at hourly intervals until residuals are less than 100 mL before resuming feeding.
Irrigate with 30–50 mL of water after each residual check or after any medications are given. (If patient requires additional free water, use greater volumes of water for irrigation.)
If patient experiences diarrhea or intestinal cramping, slow rate of feeding or decrease concentration of formula.

[a]When using hypertonic formulas or feeding into the jejunum with a nasojejunal or jejunostomy tube, diluting the formula to one-half or three-quarter strength may improve tolerance initially. The concentration then can be increased after the desired volume is reached.

Enteral Nutrition

Enteral nutrition is preferable to TPN. The old adage "if the gut works, use it," applies for several reasons. Ease of administration, economic considerations, and decreased number of complications are all advantages of enteral feeding over parenteral nutrition. Several studies have shown TPN and enteral nutrition equally efficacious in achieving nitrogen balance. Patients with good bowel function should receive enteral feedings. Relative contraindications to enteral feeding include gastrointestinal bleeding, diarrhea, and intestinal obstruction. Small-bore nasal feeding tubes are placed in the stomach, duodenum, or jejunum. An abdominal radiograph should be obtained to confirm placement. Failure to obtain appropriate studies may result in tube placement in the trachea. Alternatively, a gastrostomy or jejunostomy tube could be placed for long-term enteral nutrition (Table 9.25). Several products are commercially available (Table 9.26). Enteral tube feedings are routinely administered by pump, with either bolus feeds to the stomach or continuous feeds to the small bowel, and should be administered by pump at 25 to 30 mL/h with gastric residuals evaluated every 4 hours. Table 9.27 shows the essential and nonessential amino acids.

ROUTINE ORDERS

When the patient has fully recovered from the anesthetic and is ready for return to the nursing floor and routine postoperative care, we have found the basic postoperative orders shown in Figure 9.8 to be useful. They are only a general outline. This list should be expanded to include the special needs of each postoperative patient.

It is imperative that each patient be evaluated before being transferred from the recovery room. If the patient is not ready for transfer, additional efforts are made to stabilize the patient

TABLE 9.26

COMMONLY USED ADULT COMMERCIAL ENTERAL FEEDING FORMULAS[a]

	Category formulation			
Polymeric balanced	**1.0 kcal/mL**	**1.2 kcal/mL**	**1.5 kcal/mL**	**2.0 kcal/mL**
≤16% protein	Ensure, Resource, Isocal, Osmolite, Nutren 1.0		Nutren 1.5, Ensure Plus, Resource Plus, Boost Plus, Comply	Nutren 2.0, Deliver, Magnacal
17%–20% protein	Osmolite HN, Isocal HN, Ensure HN, Ultracel, Jevity		Ensure Plus HN	TwoCal HN
≥20% protein	Sustacal, Replete, Promote, Protain XL (22%), Isosource VHN (25%)		TraumaCal	
Modified-conventional				
≤16% protein	Peptamen, Reabilan, Vivonex Plus, Criticare HN			
17%–20% protein	Vital HN, Reabilan HN, Alitra Q			
Peptide based	Peptamen (16%), Reabilan (12.5%), Criticare HN (14%), Peptamen VMP (25%), Reabilan HN (17.5%), Alitra Q (21%), Vital HN (16%), SandaSource Peptical (20%)		Crucial (25%)	
Elemental	Tolerex (8%), Vivonex T.E.N. (15%), Vivonex Plus (18%)			
Modified-disease specific (% protein)[b]				
Critical care	Immun-Aid (32%), Impact (22%), Impact/Fiber (22%)	Perative (20%)		
Glucose intolerance	Glytrol (18%), Choice dM (17%), Glucema (16.7%), Diabeta Source (20%)			
Hepatic	Travasorb Hepatic (11%), Hepatic-Aid (15%)	Hepatic Aid II (15%)	Nutrahep (11%)	
Malabsorption renal			Lipisorb (17%), Travasorb Renal (7%)	Renal Cal (6–9%), Amin-Aid (4%)
Pulmonary			NutriVent (18%), Respalor (20%), Pulomocare (16.7%)	
Modular supplements				
Protein	Casec, ProMod			
Carbohydrate fat	Moducal, Polycose Microlipid, MCT oil			

MCT, medium chain triglyceride.
[a]This table includes only a partial listing of commercial products.
[b]Manufacturers market these products as disease specific. The author's use of this designation is intended neither to endorse the manufacturer's claims of special efficacy in the diseases specified nor to deny that the polymeric-balanced or modified-conventional formulas might be appropriate or even superior in these conditions.
Rombeau JL. Enteral nutrition. In: Goldman L, Ausiello D, eds. *Cecil textbook of medicine.* 22nd ed. Philadelphia: WB Saunders Company, 2004.

or transfer her to an intensive care bed. On transferring, the frequency of physicians' rounds should be based on the severity of the patient's condition. All patients should be evaluated on the evening of surgery and appropriate documentation made in the chart. A thorough evaluation of the vital signs, catheter drainage (nasogastric, peritoneal, and Foley), and pulmonary status is required, and abdominal examination is performed. Each physician has a desired protocol for postoperative management. The routine orders outlined in this chapter provide the clinician with a framework to design patient care plans that address the individual patient's requirements. Laboratory and radiographic evaluation of the postoperative patient also is tailored to the individual patient. Unfortunately, many physicians are predominantly concerned with quantitative test values. However, it is just as important to develop a close rapport with the patient, the patient's family, and the nursing staff. Only through good communication can the gynecologic surgeon deliver optimum medical care.

TABLE 9.27

AMINO ACIDS

Essential	Nonessential
Arginine	Alanine
Histidine	Asparaginine
Isoleucine	Aspartic acid
Leucine	Cysteine
Lysine	Glutamic acid
Methionine	Glutamine
Phenylalanine	Glycine
Threonine	Proline
Tryptophan	Serine
Valine	Tyrosine

BEST SURGICAL PRACTICES

- Approximately 500,000 hospitalized patients develop DVT and approximately 200,000 PE.
- Ten percent of hospital deaths in the United States are secondary to a PE.
- Tumors up-regulate the production of TF and PAI-1, which promotes coagulation and VTE.
- Anti–factor Xa assay can be used to monitor patients who are anticoagulated with LMWHs.
- General anesthesia is associated with a reduction of FRC by approximately 16%.
- Atelectasis occurs in 15% to 20% of patients undergoing abdominal surgery.
- An arterial PO_2 of less than 60 mm Hg or an arterial PCO_2 of greater than 45 mm Hg indicates significant respiratory compromise in patients without preexisting lung disease.
- Increased CO_2 production is a by-product of increased metabolism (i.e., fever, marked agitation, severe sepsis, overfeeding and hypothyroidism).
- During stress, urinary nitrogen levels may increase greater than or equal to 20 g in 24 hours, corresponding to a loss of 600 g of hydrated body protein.

BASIC POSTOPERATIVE ORDERS

Patient's Name: ______________.

1. Admit to Unit #____
2. Diagnosis:
3. Allergies:
4. Condition:

5a. Vital signs:
____ q 15 minutes until stable
____ q 2 hours for 24 hours
____ q 8 hours, if stable

5b. Notify House Officer (H.O.) if
BP < 90/60, > 160/100
Pulse <60, >120
Temp >38.0°C

6. Activity:
____ Bed rest
____ Ambulate
____ Other (specify)
7. Diet:
____ NPO
____ Other (specify)
8. Intravenous fluids:
9. Incentive inspirometer q 2 hours while awake
10. Encourage deep breathing
11. Drains:

Type	Location	Drainage
____ Nasogastric	____ Stomach	____ Low/intermittent suction
____ Peritoneal	____ Pelvis	____ Bulb suction
____ Foley catheter	____ Bladder	____ Gravity

12a. Fluid intake and output chart.
12b. Notify H.O. if urine output <30 cc/h.

13. Pain medication: Specify
(a) route of administration
(b) dosage
14. Antiemetic medication: Specify
(a) route of administration
(b) dosage
15. Antibiotics
16. Venous thrombosis prophylaxis
17. Other medications
18. Catheterize q 6 hours, or sooner, if bladder is full and patient unable to void.

FIGURE 9.8. Sample of basic postoperative orders.

Bibliography

Adolf J, Buttermann G, Weidenbach A, et al. Optimization of postoperative prophylaxis of thrombosis in gynecology. *Geburtshilfe Frauenheilkd* 1978;38:98.

Aitken AGF, Godden OJ. Real-time ultrasound diagnosis of deep vein thrombosis: a comparison with venography. *Clin Radiol* 1987;38:309.

Allan A, Williams JT, Bolton JP, et al. The use of graduated compression stockings in the prevention of postoperative deep vein thrombosis. *Br J Surg* 1983;70:172.

Almond DJ, Guillou PJ, McMahon MJ. Effect of i.v. fat emulsion on natural killer cellular function and antibody-dependent cell cytotoxicity. *Hum Nutr Clin Nutr* 1985;39:227.

American Thoracic Society. Guidelines for the management of adults with hospital-acquired, ventilator-associated, and healthcare-associated pneumonia. *Am J Respir Crit Care Med* 2005;171:388.

Apelgren KN. Triple lumen catheters: technological advance or setback? *Am Surg* 1987;53:113.

Appelman PT, DeJong TE, Lampmann LE. Deep venous thrombosis of the leg: US findings. *Radiology* 1987;163:743.

Askanazi J, Carpentier YA, Elwyn DH, et al. Influence of total parenteral nutrition on fuel utilization in injury and sepsis. *Ann Surg* 1980;191:40.

Askanazi J, Elwyn DH, Silverberg PA, et al. Respiratory distress secondary to a high carbohydrate load. *Surgery* 1980;87:596.

Aubaniac R. L'injection intraveineuse sous claviculaire: advantages et technique. *Presse Med* 1952;60:1456.

Auler JO Jr, Miyoshi E, Fernandez CR, et al. The effects of abdominal opening on respiratory mechanics during general anesthesia in normal and morbidly obese patients: a comparative study. *Anesth Analg* 2002;94(3):741.

Baertschi U, Schaer A, Bader P, et al. [A comparison of low dose heparin and oral anticoagulants in the prevention of thrombo-phlebitis following gynaecological operations (author's translation).] [German] *Geburtshilfe und Frauenheilkunde* 1975;35(10):754.

Baker JP, Detsky AS, Wesson DE, et al. Nutritional assessment: a comparison of clinical judgment and objective measurements. *N Engl J Med* 1982;306:969.

Ballantyne JC, Carr DB, deFerrantis S, et al. The comparative effects of postoperative analgesic therapies on pulmonary outcome: cumulative meta-analyses of randomized, controlled trials. *Anesth Analg* 1998;86(3):598.

Ballantyne JC, Carr DB, Chalmers TC, et al. Postoperative patient-controlled analgesia: meta-analyses of initial randomized control trials. *J Clin Anesth* 1993;5(3):18.

Ballard RM, Bradley-Watson PJ, Johnstone FD, et al. Low doses of subcutaneous heparin in the prevention of deep vein thrombosis after gynaecological surgery. *J Obstet Gynaecol Br Commonw* 1973;80:469.

Barbul A, Fishel RS, Shimazu S, et al. Intravenous hyperalimentation with high arginine levels improves wound healing and immune function. *J Surg Res* 1985;38:328.

Bearman GM, Munro C, Sessler CN, et al. Infection control and the prevention of nosocomial infections in the intensive care unit. *Semin Respir Crit Care Med* 2006;27(3):310.

Bistrian BR, Blackburn GL, Hallowell E, et al. Protein status of general surgical patients. *JAMA* 1974;230:858.

Bjornson HS, Colle R, Bower RH, et al. Association between microorganism growth at the catheter site and colonization of the catheter in patients receiving total parenteral nutrition. *Surgery* 1982;92:20.

Blackburn GL, Bistrian BR, Maini BS, et al. Nutritional and metabolic assessment of the hospitalized patient. *J Parenter Enteral Nutr* 1977;1:11.

Blackburn GL, Etter G, Mackenzie T. Criteria for choosing amino acid therapy in acute renal failure. *Am J Clin Nutr* 1978;31:1841.

Bluman LG, Mosca L, Newman N, et al. Preoperative smoking habits and postoperative pulmonary complications. *Chest* 1998;113(4):883.

Bohner H, Kindgen-Milles D, Grust A, et al. Prophylactic nasal continuous positive airway pressure after major vascular surgery: results of a prospective randomized trial. *Langenbecks Arch Surg* 2002;387(1):21.

Bonnar J. Venous thromboembolism and gynecologic surgery. *Clin Obstet Gynecol* 1985;28:432.

Bonnar J, Walsh J. Prevention of thrombosis after pelvic surgery by British Dextran 70. *Lancet* 1972;1:614.

Bonnar J, Walsh J, Haddon M, et al. Coagulation system changes induced by pelvic surgery and the effect of dextran 70. *Bibl Anat* 1973;12:351.

Borstad E, Urdal K, Handeland G, et al. Comparison of low molecular weight heparin vs. unfractionated heparin in gynecological surgery: II. Reduced dose of low molecular weight heparin. *Acta Obstet Gynecol Scand* 1992;71:471.

Bower RH, Talamini MA, Sax HC, et al. Postoperative enteral versus parenteral nutrition: a randomized controlled trial. *Arch Surg* 1986;121:1040.

Brenner DA. Total parenteral nutrition at home. *Outpatient Ther Med* 1987;2:1.

Brooks-Brunn JA. Postoperative atelectasis and pneumonia: risk factors. *Am J Crit Care* 1995;4(5):340; quiz 350.

Brooks-Brunn JA. Risk factors associated with postoperative pulmonary complications following total abdominal hysterectomy. *Clin Nurs Res* 2000;9(1):27.

Brun-Buisson C, Brochard L. Corticosteroid therapy in acute respiratory distress syndrome: better late than never? *JAMA* 1998;280:182.

Bullock TK, Price SA, et al. A retrospective study of nosocomial pneumonia in postoperative patients shows a higher mortality rate in patients receiving nasogastric tube feeding. *Am Surg* 2004;70(9):822.

Carpenter JP, Holand GA, Baum RA, et al. Magnetic resonance venography for the detection of deep venous thrombosis: comparison with contrast venography and duplex Doppler ultrasonography. *J Vasc Surg* 1993;18:734.

Celli BR, Rodriguez KS, Snider GL. A controlled trial of intermittent positive pressure breathing, incentive spirometry, and deep breathing exercises in preventing pulmonary complications after abdominal surgery. *Am Rev Respir Dis* 1984;130:12.

Chastre J, Fagon JY, Bornet-Lecso M, et al. Evaluation of bronchoscopic techniques for the diagnosis of nosocomial pneumonia. *Am J Respir Crit Care Med* 1995;152(1):231.

Chory ET, Mullen JL. Nutritional support of the cancer patient: delivery systems and formulations. *Surg Clin North Am* 1986;66:1105.

Christenson M, Hitt JA, Abbott G, et al. Improving patient safety: resource availability and application for reducing the incidence of healthcare-associated infection. *Infect Control Hosp Epidemiol* 2006;27(3):245.

Chumillas S, Ponce JL, Delgado F, et al. Prevention of postoperative pulmonary complications through respiratory rehabilitation: a controlled clinical study. *Arch Phys Med Rehabil* 1998;79(1):5.

Clarke-Pearson DL, Coleman RE, Siegel R, et al. Indium 111 platelet imaging for the detection of deep venous thrombosis and pulmonary embolism in patients without symptoms after surgery. *Surgery* 1985;98:98.

Clarke-Pearson DL, Coleman RE, Synan IS, et al. Venous thromboembolism prophylaxis in gynecologic oncology: a prospective controlled trial of low-dose heparin. *Am J Obstet Gynecol* 1983;145:606.

Clinical Nutrition Cases. Is chromium essential for humans? *Nutr Rev* 1988;46:17.

Cook D, Guyatt G, Marshall J, et al. A comparison of sucralfate and ranitidine for the prevention of upper gastrointestinal bleeding in patients requiring mechanical ventilation. Canadian Critical Care Trials Group. *N Engl J Med* 1998;338(12):791.

Delafosse B, Bouffard Y, Viale JP, et al. Respiratory changes induced by parenteral nutrition in postoperative patients undergoing inspiratory pressure support ventilation. *Anesthesiology* 1987;66:393.

DeWet CJ, Pearl RG. Venous thromboembolism: deep-vein thrombosis and pulmonary embolism. *Anesthesiol Clin North Am* 1999;17(4):895.

Dinsmore RE, Wedeen V, Rosen B, et al. Phase-offset technique to distinguish slow blood flow and thrombus on MR images. *AJR Am J Roentgenol* 1987;148:634.

Dodek P, Keenan S, Cook D, et al. Evidence-based clinical practice guideline for the prevention of ventilator-associated pneumonia. *Ann Intern Med* 2004;141(4):305.

Doran FSA. Prevention of deep vein thrombosis. *Br J Hosp Med* 1971;6:773.

Duggan M, Kavanagh BP. Pulmonary atelectasis: a pathogenic perioperative entity. *Anesthesiology* 2005;102(4):838.

Fabregas N, Ewig S, Torres A, et al. Clinical diagnosis of ventilator associated pneumonia revisited: comparative validation using immediate post-mortem lung biopsies. *Thorax* 1999;54(10):867.

Fagevik Olsen M, Wennberg E, Johnsson E, et al. Randomized clinical study of the prevention of pulmonary complications after thoracoabdominal resection by two different breathing techniques. *Br J Surg* 2002;89(10):1228.

Flanders SA, Collard HR, Saint S. Nosocomial pneumonia: state of the science. *Am J Infect Control* 2006;34(2):84.

Ford GT, Rosenal TW, Clergue F, et al. Respiratory physiology in upper abdominal surgery. *Clin Chest Med* 1993;14(2):237.

Frango JA, Eskin SG, McIntire LV. Flow effects on prostacyclin production by cultured human endothelial cells. *Science* 1985;227:1477.

Gazzaniga AB, Day AT, Sankary H. The efficacy of a 20 per cent fat emulsion as a peripherally administered substrate. *Surg Obstet Gynecol* 1985;160:387.

Geerts WH, Heit JA, Clagett G, et al. Prevention of venous thromboembolism (Sixth ACCP Consensus Conference on Antithrombotic Therapy). *Chest* 2001;119(1 Suppl):132S.

Gjonnaess H, Abildgaard U. Bleeding in gynecological surgery: influence of low dose heparin. *Int J Gynaecol Obstet* 1976;14:9.

Greene KE, Peters JI. Pathophysiology of acute respiratory failure. *Clin Chest Med* 1994;15(1):1.

Groeben H. Epidural anesthesia and pulmonary function. *J Anesth* 2006;20(4):290.

Gumpton DP, Khayat A, Scheiber H. Endogenous plasminogen activator and venous flow: therapeutic implications. *Crit Care Med* 1987;15:122.

Gumpton DP, Khayat A, Scheiber H. Pneumatic compression stockings and prostaglandin synthesis: a pathway to fibrinolysis? *Crit Care Med* 1985;13:266.
Hall JC, Tarala R, Harris T, et al. Incentive spirometry versus routine chest physiotherapy for prevention of pulmonary complications after abdominal surgery. *Lancet* 1991;337(8747):953.
Hall JC, Tarala R, Tapper J, et al. Prevention of respiratory complications after abdominal surgery: a randomised clinical trial. *BMJ* 1996;312(7024):148; discussion 152.
Hall JC, Tarala RA, Hall JL. A case-control study of postoperative pulmonary complications after laparoscopic and open cholecystectomy. *J Laparoendosc Surg* 1996;6(2):87.
Hauser CJ, Shoemaker WC, Turpin I, et al. Oxygen transport responses to colloids and crystalloids in critically ill surgical patients. *Surg Gynecol Obstet* 1980;150:881.
Haydock DA, Hill GL. Improved wound healing response in surgical patients receiving i.v. nutrition. *Br J Surg* 1987;74:320.
Hebert PC, Wells G, Blajchman MA, et al. A multicenter, randomized, controlled clinical trial of transfusion requirements in critical care. Transfusion Requirements in Critical Care Investigators, Canadian Critical Care Trials Group. *N Engl J Med* 1999;340(6):409.
Hedenstierna G, Rothen HU. Atelectasis formation during anesthesia: causes and measures to prevent it. *J Clin Monit Comput* 2000;16(5–6):329.
Heird WC, Grundy SM, Hubbard VS. Structured lipids and their use in clinical nutrition. *Am J Clin Nutr* 1986;43:320.
Hilgard P. Experimental vitamin K deficiency and spontaneous metastases. *Br J Cancer* 1975;35:391.
Hodgkinson CP, Hodari AA. Trocar suprapubic cystostomy for postoperative bladder drainage in the female. *Am J Obstet Gynecol* 1966;96:773.
Hoover JC, Ryan JP, Anderson EJ, et al. Nutritional benefits of immediate postoperative jejunal feeding of an elemental diet. *Am J Surg* 1980;139:153.
Huisman MV, Buller HR, Ten Cate JW, et al. Serial impedance plethysmography for suspected deep venous thrombosis in outpatients. The Amsterdam General Practitioner Study. *N Engl J Med* 1986;314:823.
Inada K, Koike S, Shirai N, et al. Effects of intermittent pneumatic leg compression for prevention of postoperative deep venous thrombosis with special reference to fibrinolytic activity. *Am J Surg* 1988;155:602.
Ireton-Jones CS, Turner WW Jr. The use of respiratory quotient to determine the efficacy of nutrition support regimens. *J Am Diet Assoc* 1987;87:180.
Jourdain B. Role of quantitative cultures of endotracheal aspirates in the diagnosis of nosocomial pneumonia. *Am J Respir Crit Care Med* 1995;152(1):241.
Kakkar W, Corrigan TP, Fossard DP. Prevention of postoperative pulmonary embolism by low dose heparin. *Lancet* 1975;2:45.
Knill RL. Control of breathing: effects of analgesic, anaesthetic and neuromuscular blocking drugs. *Can J Anaesth* 1988;35(3[Pt 2]):S4.
Kollef MH. Inadequate antimicrobial treatment: an important determinant of outcome for hospitalized patients. *Clin Infect Dis* 2000;31(Suppl 4):S131.
Konrad F, Schreiber T, Grunert A, et al. Measurement of mucociliary transport velocity in ventilated patients: short-term effect of general anesthesia on mucociliary transport. *Chest* 1992;102(5):1377.
Kristo DA, Perry ME, Kollef MH. Comparison of venography, duplex imaging and bilateral impedance plethysmography for diagnosis of lower extremity deep vein thrombosis. *South Med J* 1994;87:55.
Laghi F, Tobin MJ. Disorders of the respiratory muscles. *Am J Respir Crit Care Med* 2003;168(1):10.
Langsfeld M, Hershey FB, Thorpe L, et al. Duplex B-mode imaging for the diagnosis of deep venous thrombosis. *Arch Surg* 1987;122:587.
Lawrence VA, Hilsenbeck SG, Mulrow CD, et al. Incidence and hospital stay for cardiac and pulmonary complications after abdominal surgery. *J Gen Intern Med* 1995;10(12):671.
Lawrence VA, Dhanda R, Hilsenbeck SG, et al. Risk of pulmonary complications after elective abdominal surgery. *Chest* 1996;110(3):744.
Lawrence VA, Cornell JE, Smetana GW. Strategies to reduce postoperative pulmonary complications after noncardiothoracic surgery: systematic review for the American College of Physicians. *Ann Intern Med* 2006;144(8):596.
Lazo-Langner A, Goss GD, Spaans JN, et al. The effect of low-molecular weight heparin on cancer survival: a systematic review and meta-analysis of randomized trials. *J Thromb Haemost* 2007;5:729.
Leiter LA, Marliss EB. Survival during fasting may depend on fat as well as protein stores. *JAMA* 1982;248:2306.
Magnusson L, Spahn DR. New concepts of atelectasis during general anaesthesia. *Br J Anaesth* 2003;91(1):61.
Malhotra A. Intensive insulin in intensive care. *N Engl J Med* 2006;354(5):516.
McAlister FA, Bertsch K, Man J, et al. Incidence of and risk factors for pulmonary complications after nonthoracic surgery. *Am J Respir Crit Care Med* 2005;171(5):514.
McCarthy TG, McQueen J, Johnstone FD, et al. A comparison of low dose subcutaneous heparin and intravenous dextran 70 in the prophylaxis of deep venous thrombosis after gynaecological surgery. *J Obstet Gynaecol Br Commonw* 1974;81:486.
McMahon MM. Parenteral nutrition. In: Goldman L, Ausiello D, eds. *Cecil textbook of medicine*. 22nd ed. Philadelphia: WB Saunders Company, 2004.
Mirtallo JM, Schneider PT, Mauko K, et al. A comparison of essential and general amino acid infusions in the nutritional support of patients with compromised renal function. *J Parenter Enteral Nutr* 1982;6:109.
Mittleman JS, Edwards WS, McDonald JB. Effectiveness of leg compression in preventing venous stasis. *Am J Surg* 1982;144:611.
Moller AM, Vilebro N, Pedersen T, et al. Effect of preoperative smoking intervention on postoperative complications: a randomised clinical trial. *Lancet* 2002;359(9301):114.
Moore FD. Energy and the maintenance of the body cell mass. *J Parenter Enteral Nutr* 1980;4:228.
Moosman DA. The anatomy of infraclavicular subclavian vein catheterization and its complications. *Surg Gynecol Obstet* 1973;136:71.
Morgan G, Mikhail M, Murray M. *Clinical anesthesiology*. 4th ed. New York: McGraw-Hill;2006:127.
Morlion BJ, Stehle P, Wachtler P, et al. Total parenteral nutrition with glutamine dipeptide after major abdominal surgery: a randomized, double-blind, controlled study. *Ann Surg* 1998;227:302.
Moudgil R, Michelakis ED, Archer SL. Hypoxic pulmonary vasoconstriction. *J Appl Physiol* 2005;98(1):390.
Nagendran J, Stewart K, Hoskinson M, et al. An anesthesiologist's guide to hypoxic pulmonary vasoconstriction: implications for managing single-lung anesthesia and atelectasis. *Curr Opin Anaesthesiol* 2006;19(1):34.
Nchimi A. Incidence and distribution of lower extremity deep venous thrombosis at indirect computed tomography venography in patients suspected of pulmonary embolism. *Thromb Haemost* 2007;97:566.
Nelson R, Edwards S, Tse B. Prophylactic nasogastric decompression after abdominal surgery. *Cochrane Database Syst Rev* 2005(1):CD004929.
Nicolaides AN, Fernandes IF, Pollock AV. Intermittent sequential compression of the legs in the prevention of venous stasis and postoperative deep venous thrombosis. *Surgery* 1980;87:69.
Nourdine K, Combes P, Carton MJ, et al. Does noninvasive ventilation reduce the ICU nosocomial infection risk? A prospective clinical survey. *Intensive Care Med* 1999;25(6):567.
Padberg FT, Ruggiero J, Blackburn GL, et al. Central venous catheterization for parenteral nutrition. *Ann Surg* 1981;193:264.
Pappachen S, Smith PR, Shah S, et al. Postoperative pulmonary complications after gynecologic surgery. *Int J Gynaecol Obstet* 2006;93(1):74.
Platell C, Hall JC. Atelectasis after abdominal surgery. *J Am Coll Surg* 1997;185(6):584.
Quality A.f.H.R.a., Nationwide Inpatient Sample. 2000.
Rayburn W, Wolk R, Mercer N, et al. Parenteral nutrition in obstetrics and gynecology. *Obstet Gynecol* 1986;41:200.
Reilly JJ, Gerhardt AL. Modern surgical nutrition. *Current Problems in Surgery* 1985;22:1.
Richards MJ, Edwards JR, Culver DH, et al. Nosocomial infections in medical intensive care units in the United States. National Nosocomial Infections Surveillance System. *Crit Care Med* 1999;27(5):87.
Rombeau JL. Enteral nutrition. In: Goldman L, Ausiello D, eds. *Cecil textbook of medicine*. 22nd ed. Philadelphia: WB Saunders Company, 2004.
Rose D, Yarborough MF, Canizaro PC, et al. One hundred and fourteen fistulas of the gastrointestinal tract treated with total parenteral nutrition. *Surg Gynecol Obstet* 1986;163:345.
Rucquoi M. Respiratory dead space and anesthesia. *Acta Anaesthesiol Belg* 1988;39(3 Suppl 2):29.
Sanders RA, Sheldon GF. Septic complications of total parenteral nutrition: a five year experience. *Am J Surg* 1976;132:214.
Sandstedt S, Lennmarken C, Symreng T, et al. The effect of preoperative total parenteral nutrition on energy-rich phosphates, electrolytes and free amino acids in skeletal muscle of malnourished patients with gastric carcinoma. *Br J Surg* 1985;72:920.
Sasahara AA, DiSerio FJ, et al. Dihydroergotamine-heparin prophylaxis of postoperative deep vein thrombosis: a multicenter trial. *JAMA* 1984;251:2960.
Sevitt S, Gallagher NG. Venous thrombosis and pulmonary embolism: a clinical pathological study in injured and burned patients. *Br J Surg* 1961;48:475.
Shils ME, Young VR, eds. *Modern nutrition in health and disease*. 7th ed. Philadelphia: Lea & Febiger, 1988.
Shulman SM, Chuter T, Weissman C. Dynamic respiratory patterns after laparoscopic cholecystectomy. *Chest* 1993;103(4):1173.
Siafakas NM, Mitrouska I, Bouros D, et al. Surgery and the respiratory muscles. *Thorax* 1999;54(5)458.
Stanton JR, Freis ED, Wilkins RW. Acceleration of linear flow in deep veins with local compression. *J Clin Invest* 1944;28:553.
Starker PM, Gump FE, Askanazi J, et al. Serum albumin levels as an index of nutritional support. *Surgery* 1982;91:194.
Starker PM, LaSala PA, Askanazi J, et al. The influence of preoperative total parenteral nutrition on morbidity and mortality. *Surg Gynecol Obstet* 1986;162:569.
Stella MH, Knuth SL, Bartlett D Jr. Respiratory response to mechanical stimulation of the gallbladder. *Respir Physiol Neurobiol* 2002;130(3):285.
Taberner DA, Poller L, Burslem RW, et al. Oral anticoagulants controlled by the British: comparative thromboplastin versus low-dose heparin in prophylaxis of deep vein thrombosis. *Br Med J* 1978;1:272.

Tablan OC, Anderson LJ, Besser R, et al. Guidelines for preventing health-car–associated pneumonia, 2003: recommendations of CDC and the Healthcare Infection Control Practices Advisory Committee. *MMWR Recomm Rep* 2004;53(RR-3):1.

Thompson DA, Makary MA, Dorman T, et al. Clinical and economic outcomes of hospital acquired pneumonia in intra-abdominal surgery patients. *Ann Surg* 2006;243(4):547.

Tobin WR, Kaiser HE, Groeger AM, et al. The effects of volatile anesthetic agents on pulmonary surfactant function. *In Vivo* 2000;14(1):157.

Tomkowski WZ, Davidson BL, Wisniewska J, et al. Accuracy of compression ultrasound in screening for deep venous thrombosis in acutely ill medical patients. *Thromb Haemost* 2007;97:191.

Torosian MH, Daly JM. Nutritional support in the cancer-bearing host: effects on host and tumor. *Cancer* 1986;58(Suppl 8):1915.

Tracey KJ, Legaspi A, Albert JD, et al. Protein and substrate metabolism during starvation and parenteral refeeding. *Clin Sci* 1988;74:123.

Trousseau A. *Phlegmasia alba dolens: clinique medicale de l'Hotel Dieu de Paris*, vol. 3. London: New Sydenham Society, 1868:695.

Vaccaro P, Van Aman M, Miller S, et al. Shortcomings of physical examination and impedance plethysmography in the diagnosis of lower extremity deep venous thrombosis. *Angiology* 1987;38:232.

van den Berghe G, Wouters P, Weekers F, et al. Intensive insulin therapy in the critically ill patients. *N Engl J Med* 2001;345(19):1359.

Vamvakas EC, Blajchman MA. Deleterious clinical effects of transfusion-associated immunomodulation: fact or fiction? *Blood* 2001;97(5):1180.

Vassilakopoulos T, Mastora Z, Katsaounou P, et al. Contribution of pain to inspiratory muscle dysfunction after upper abdominal surgery: a randomized controlled trial. *Am J Respir Crit Care Med* 2000;61(4 Pt 1):1372.

Vernet O, Christin L, Schutz Y, et al. Enteral versus parenteral nutrition: comparison of energy metabolism in lean and moderately obese women. *Am J Clin Nutr* 1986;43:194.

Vinton NE, Laidlaw SA, Ament ME, et al. Taurine concentrations in plasma and blood cells of patients undergoing long-term parenteral nutrition. *Am J Clin Nutr* 1986;44:398.

Virchow R. *Handbuch der speciellen Pathologie and Therapie*, vol II. Erlangen and Stuttgart: F Enke, 1854.

Walder B, Schafer M, Henzi I, et al. Efficacy and safety of patient-controlled opioid analgesia for acute postoperative pain: a quantitative systematic review. *Acta Anaesthesiol Scand* 2001;45(7):795.

Wells PS, Byill-Edwards P, Stevens P, et al. A novel and rapid whole-blood assay for D-dimer in patients with clinically suspected deep vein thrombosis. *Circulation* 1995;91:2184.

Young GP, Thomas RJS, Bourne DWF, et al. Parenteral nutrition. *Med J Aust* 1985;143:597.

CHAPTER 10 ■ WATER, ELECTROLYTE, AND ACID–BASE METABOLISM

JACK B. BASIL

DEFINITIONS

Anion gap—A concept used to estimate anion and cation levels in serum and conditions that influence them. It is estimated by subtraction of the sum of the chloride and bicarbonate anions from the sodium cations

$$(Na^+ - [Cl^- + HCO_3^-].$$

Extracellular fluid (ECF)—The compartment outside of cells that contains approximately one third of the volume of body water.

Henderson-Hasselbach—An equation for stating the expression for the dissociation constant of an acid. This equation may be expressed in terms of the bicarbonate, where

$$pH = 6.1 + \log HCO_3^-/\alpha(Paco_2)$$

where $\alpha = 0.03$mM/L/mm Hg at 38°.

At normal blood pH 7.4, the ratio of HCO_3^- to $\alpha(Paco_2)$ is 20 to 1.

Metabolic acidosis—Acidosis resulting from increase in acids other than carbonic acid.

Metabolic alkalosis—Alkalosis in which plasma bicarbonate is increased and there is a rise in plasma concentration of CO_2.

Oncotic pressure—The total influence of the protein on the osmotic activity of plasma water.

Osmotic pressure—The pressure that develops when two solutions of different concentrations are separated by a semipermeable membrane.

Respiratory acidosis—Acidosis secondary to pulmonary insufficiency resulting in retention of carbon dioxide.

Respiratory alkalosis—Alkalosis with an acute reduction of plasma with a proportionate reduction in plasma CO_2.

Proper management of fluids and electrolytes in the gynecologic surgical patient is of extreme importance. Gynecological surgical patients can differ in age, baseline nutritional status, and in the complexity of medical problems that they possess. The stresses of surgery and the bodies' complex responses to that stress need to be understood to best care for these patients. The tendency to standardize postoperative care for all patients should be avoided.

The human body is about 60% water by weight (Table 10.1). An exchange of approximately 2 liters of fluid per day exists normally. This is a balance between an intake of 1,500 mL orally and 500 mL from foodstuffs, and an output of between 750 and 1,500 mL of urine, 500 mL in insensible losses, and 300 mL in stool. Thus, total body water, body weight, osmolality, and oncotic pressure are critical concepts if one is to understand water metabolism. Comprehension of renal physiology, electrolytes, and acid–base metabolism is also important. This chapter discusses these concepts in detail.

RENAL PHYSIOLOGY

Blood enters the glomerulus by way of afferent arterioles. The filtration process begins with the filtrate passing into Bowman's space. Filtration depends on hydrostatic pressure, which forces the filtrate out of the capillary, and oncotic pressure, which holds the filtrate in. The oncotic pressure in the glomerulus usually is negligible, resulting in net flow into Bowman's space. The filtrate then passes into the proximal tubule, where an isoosmotic solution of sodium bicarbonate, glucose, water, and amino acids is absorbed. The filtrate (urine) enters the descending portion of the loop of Henle, where it becomes hyperosmotic secondary to absorption of water into the interstitium. As urine flows up the ascending limb, sodium and chloride are absorbed, making the urine more dilute. Urine then enters the distal convoluted tubule, where active absorption of sodium occurs with exchange of potassium. Under the control of antidiuretic hormone (ADH), water is absorbed from the urine (in the collecting tubule and duct) into the interstitium, causing concentration of urine. Hydrogen ions secreted from tubular cells into the lumens of the tubules help maintain pH balance. Carbonic anhydrase in the renal tubular cells causes the transformation of water and carbon dioxide to bicarbonate and free hydrogen ion (Fig. 10.1). In acidotic states, bicarbonate is reabsorbed into the bloodstream, and hydrogen ions are excreted into the tubular lumen. In alkalotic states, the opposite occurs.

OSMOTIC FORCES (OSMOLALITY AND OSMOTIC PRESSURE)

If a solute is added to pure water, then the presence of the second molecular species interferes with the normal activity of water molecules. As a result, water diffuses more slowly through the solution, and the solution has a higher boiling point and lower freezing point. These effects of solute on the colligative properties of water are related principally to the number of molecules present per unit volume rather than to the specific kind of molecule or the total weight of solute present. The determination of osmolality is a measure of the number of molecules in the solution that is effective in reducing the concentration and, therefore, the chemical properties of water. The slower rate of diffusion of water caused by the solute accounts for the fact that water diffuses from zones of low osmolality (high water concentration) to zones of high osmolality (low water concentration). The hydrostatic pressure that must be applied

TABLE 10.1

BODY WATER COMPARTMENTS IN HEALTH

Parameter	Total body water	Intra-cellular water	Extra-cellular water[a]
Total body water (%)	100	67	33
Body weight (%)	60	40	20
Actual volume in a 60-kg person (L)	36	24	12
Osmolality (mOsm/kg of water)	290	290	290

[a]The intravascular water space is about one fourth of the extracellular water space. The intravascular volume is substantially larger than the intravascular water space because of the additional space occupied by blood cell and plasma proteins. The intravascular volume (blood volume) is about 7% of body weight or slightly more than 4 L in a 60-kg person.

to the zone of high osmolality to oppose exactly osmotic pressure is equal to the osmotic pressure between the zones of high and low osmolality. The effect of solute concentration on the freezing point vapor pressure of water is the basis for the clinical measurement of osmolality in body fluids.

The osmolality of normal extracellular fluid (ECF) is determined almost entirely by sodium and its accompanying anions. Under certain conditions, other substances (e.g., glucose, mannitol, alcohol, urea) can accumulate and contribute highly to plasma osmolality. Increased blood levels of glucose can artificially lower the serum concentration of serum sodium and thus serum osmolality. Serum sodium is lowered by 1.6 mEq/L for every increase in serum glucose of 100 mg/dL. The contribution

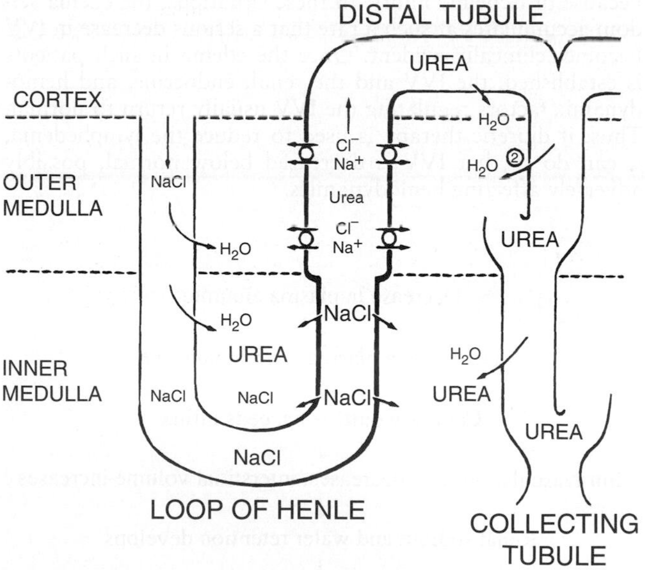

FIGURE 10.1. Passive model of the concentrating mechanism in the inner medulla. Arrows indicate movements of water (H_2O), sodium chloride (NaCl), and urea between the tubule and the interstitium. In the vasa recta, there is perfect exchange between the two limbs. (From: Jamison RL, Buerkert J. The urinary concentrating mechanism. *N Engl J Med* 1976;295:1059, with permission.)

of each of these solutes to plasma osmolality can be directly determined in the clinical laboratory by measuring freezing point depression or by calculation. Calculation of plasma osmolality (P_{osm}) from the known concentration of solutes is as follows:

$$\begin{aligned} P_{osm} = {} & 2 \times [\text{Na}]\ \text{mEq/L} + \text{glucose mmol/L} \\ & + \text{urea mmol/L} \\ & + \text{osmolar concentration of other solutes} \end{aligned}$$

For normal plasma:

$$\begin{aligned} P_{osm} = {} & 2 \times 140\ \text{mEq/L} \\ & + (900\ \text{mg glucose/L}(180\ \text{mg glucose/mOsm}) \\ & + \text{other solutes (negligible in normal plasma)} \\ = {} & 290\ \text{mOsm/L} \end{aligned}$$

Most laboratories use different units, and the formula can be shortened to:

$$\begin{aligned} & P_{osm} + 2 \times \text{Na}^+\ (\text{mEq/L}) + \text{glucose (mg/dL) } 18 \\ & + \text{BUN (mg/dL) } 2.8 = \text{mOsm/L} \end{aligned}$$

The osmolalities of intracellular fluid (ICF) and ECF are equal because cell walls (except for the collecting duct of the kidney) are always freely permeable to water. Potassium is the major intracellular cation and is found in concentrations of about 150 mEq/L of cell water. Thus, potassium and its accompanying anions—principally phosphate and protein—account for almost all of the osmolality of ICF. In health, Na^+ is excluded from cells and K^+ is maintained in cells in most cases because of the cellular Na^+-K^+ pump.

ONCOTIC FORCES (ONCOTIC PRESSURE AND COLLOID OSMOTIC PRESSURE)

Just as crystalloids in solution, such as Na^+, Cl^-, and urea, reduce the concentration of water, so do colloids, such as albumin and globulins. In biologic solutions, however, the contribution of proteins in lowering the effective concentration of water is far less than that of crystalloids, because there are far fewer protein molecules than crystalloid molecules. One gram of albumin (molecular weight [MW] 68,000) theoretically yields 0.015 mOsm ([1,000 mg/68,000 mg mmol/L] × 1 mOsm mmol/L), whereas 1 g of sodium chloride theoretically yields 34.3 mOsm ([1,000 mg/58.5 mg mmol/L] × 2 mOsm mmol/L). Thus, gram for gram, sodium chloride is theoretically 2,300 times more effective in increasing the osmolality of a solution than albumin. The oncotic pressure of solutions is expressed in millimeters of mercury (mm Hg) for the same reason that osmotic forces are expressed in units of hydrostatic pressure.

Although oncotic forces are small in relation to osmotic forces, they are important in biologic systems because plasma proteins are selectively retained in the intravascular space. Thus, the effective concentration of water and electrolytes is selectively reduced in the intravascular space compared with the interstitial space. All other things being equal, this results in diffusion of water and electrolytes from the interstitial to the intravascular space. At the capillary level, however, where these oncotic forces are at work, the capillary blood hydrostatic pressure opposes an inward diffusion of water and electrolytes. At the arterial end of the capillary, the effect of capillary blood hydrostatic pressure (~35 mm Hg) pushing fluid outward is greater than the effect of capillary blood oncotic pressure (equivalent to 25 mm Hg), causing outward diffusion of fluid. Therefore, net outward movement of water and electrolytes occurs. At the venous end of the capillary, the capillary blood oncotic pressure (equivalent to ~25 mm Hg) exceeds capillary blood hydrostatic pressure (now ~15 mm Hg); therefore, net inward movement of water and electrolytes occurs. In health, the rate of fluid outflow from the arterial end of the capillary equals the rate of uptake at the venous end of the capillary.

REGULATION OF WATER AND ELECTROLYTE DISTRIBUTION BETWEEN INTRACELLULAR AND EXTRACELLULAR COMPARTMENTS

Osmotic forces regulate the distribution of water between ECF and ICF. Under all steady-state conditions, ECF osmolality equals ICF osmolality. The implications of these principles when water or solute is added to body fluids are discussed in the following sections.

Effect of Addition of Water on Extracellular and Intracellular Fluid Volume and Osmolality

The ingestion of water or the intravenous (IV) infusion of water, as 5% solution of dextrose in water (D_5W), results in expansion of all body fluid compartments. Because the osmolality of all body compartments is the same, the water is distributed in the body water compartments in proportion to their size. For example, 1,000 mL of D_5W is infused into a normal 60-kg person with a plasma osmolality of 290 mOsm/L and a serum sodium level of 140 mEq/L. Assuming that no excretion of water occurs, the change in volume of the body water compartments (Table 10.1) when complete mixing has occurred is as follows: The ICF is increased by about 666 mL, and the ECF is increased by about 333 mL. The intravascular water, which is 25% of the ECF, is increased by only about 83 mL. Plasma osmolality decreases by about 2%. This is sufficient to completely suppress ADH release and cause a maximum water diuresis in a normal person.

Effect of Addition of Solute on Extracellular and Intracellular Fluid Volume and Osmolality

If solutes that penetrate cells slowly (e.g., glucose) are ingested, infused, or actively excluded from cells (e.g., Na^+), water is obligated to remain with these solutes in the ECF so that conditions of osmotic equilibrium between ICF and ECF are met. If these solutes are given in isotonic solutions (i.e., if the osmolality of the solution equals that of body fluids), conditions of osmotic equilibrium are met without shifts of water between ICF and ECF. Thus, the ECF is selectively expanded. On the other hand, if these solutes are ingested without water or given as hypertonic solutions, ECF osmolality rises as these solutes move into the ECF, and water diffuses from ICF to ECF until osmolality in the two compartments is equal. Thus, the ECF expands as the ICF contracts.

Although certain other solutes, such as urea and ethyl alcohol, increase plasma osmolality, they do not affect the steady-state distribution of water between ECF and ICF because these solutes readily penetrate cells and rapidly distribute throughout the body water space. Nevertheless, in non–steady states, such as rapid removal of urea by hemodialysis, transient redistribution of water between ECF and ICF does occur. Such shifts of fluid in brain tissue can lead to significant changes in brain function.

Regulation of Water and Electrolyte Distribution between the Intravascular and Interstitial Compartments

As discussed, the regulation of fluid and electrolyte transfer at the capillary level is determined by the balance among oncotic forces, hydrostatic forces, and capillary permeability to plasma proteins. These forces can be perturbed in the following ways.

Hypoalbuminemia results in a fall in plasma oncotic pressure, a rise in the effective concentration of water and electrolytes into the intravascular space, and, all other things being equal, net movement of water and electrolytes into the interstitial space. As a consequence, intravascular volume (IVV) decreases, and the kidney responds by retaining sodium and water in an attempt to restore IVV to normal. If the hypoalbuminemia is sufficiently pronounced (≤2.5 g/dL) and the expected renal retention of sodium and water occurs, edema develops before a new equilibrium between outflux and influx of fluid at the capillary level is achieved.

The sequence of events that leads to edema formation is depicted in Figure 10.2. The stimulus to renal sodium and water retention in hypoalbuminemia is a decrease in IVV. In many hypoalbuminemic patients, the retention of sodium and water does not completely restore IVV to normal. In fact, in some patients with marked hypoalbuminemia, massive edema (expansion of the interstitial volume) may be present, yet the IVV may be dangerously low, even to the point of shock.

Marked edema also can develop in the presence of extensive lymphatic obstruction, distal to a venous obstruction, or because of ischemic injury. In these situations, the edema seldom accumulates at such a rate that a serious decrease in IVV becomes clinically evident. Once the edema in such patients is established, the IVV and the renal, endocrine, and hemodynamic factors regulating the IVV usually return to normal. Thus, if diuretic therapy is used to reduce the lymphedema, it can do so, but IVV is decreased below normal, possibly adversely affecting hemodynamics.

Decrease in plasma albumin
↓
Decrease in plasma oncotic pressure
↓
Capillary outflux exceeds influx
↓
Intravascular volume decreases, interstitial volume increases
↓
Renal sodium and water retention develops
↓
Edema develops when a large interstitial fluid volume is needed to raise interstitial pressure enough to prevent the excessive capillary outflux caused by hypoalbuminemia

FIGURE 10.2. Sequence of events leading to edema formation in hypoalbuminemia.

REGULATION OF WATER AND SODIUM EXCHANGES WITH THE EXTERNAL ENVIRONMENT

The following discussion focuses on the normal response of the kidney to perturbations of sodium or water balance because an examination of the state of renal sodium and water excretion often is key to the understanding of the pathogenesis of a disorder of fluid and electrolyte balance and usually provides the basis for planning appropriate fluid and electrolyte therapy.

Water Balance

Water balance equals water intake minus water output. Sometimes it is assumed that the measurement of fluid intake and output, as it is performed clinically, is a measure of water balance. The difficulty in assessing the state of water balance based on the measurement of intake and output is indicated in Table 10.2, which lists all the sources of intake and output of water from the body. It is evident from this table that only a few of the important components of water balance are included in the measurement of intake and output. For this reason, some serious disturbances of water balance may not be reflected in the intake and output record. Fortunately, the accurate measurement of water balance does not require that special techniques be used to measure the various sources of intake and output of water from the body. Instead, in most clinical situations, changes in water balance can be assessed simply by following changes in body weight. In the management of a compromised postoperative patient, it is imperative to follow daily weights.

In most clinical situations, changes in water balance occur secondarily to changes in sodium balance. For example, in the pathogenesis of fluid retention in congestive heart failure (CHF), the primary event is positive sodium balance because of a decreased renal capacity to excrete sodium. The ingested water is retained as a secondary event to maintain plasma osmolality at some level set by the thirst mechanism. If sodium had not been retained, water would not have been retained. For this reason, the key to preventing fluid retention in such patients is the regulation of sodium intake and output, not water intake.

Less commonly, a change in water balance is the primary event, and changes in sodium balance are secondary to the change in water balance. To recognize such situations, it is necessary to understand the normal renal response to primary changes in water balance. Because the capacity of the kidneys to concentrate and dilute the urine is commonly evaluated by measurement of the specific gravity of urine, it is first necessary

TABLE 10.2

COMPONENTS OF WATER BALANCE[a]

Sources	Measured clinically	Comments
Water intake		
Oral intake of liquids, intravenous fluids	Yes	
Water in solid food	Rarely	Water content of solid food in diet of normal adult averages 800–1,000 mL/d.
Metabolic water	No	The average adult forms about 200–300 mL of water daily by oxidation of carbohydrate and fat to water and CO_2
Water absorbed by way of respiratory tract during use of gases hydrated by ultrasonic nebulizer	No	Up to 350 mL of water can be absorbed daily at respiratory volumes of 10 L/min.
Water output		
Sensible losses		
Urine	Yes	Output variable in health, depends on water intake. Usual range is 600–2,500 mL/d. With renal insufficiency and loss of renal concentrating capacity, urine flow rate depends principally on rate of solute excretion.
Sweat	No	In hot environments, several liters of water can be lost daily.
Stool	Rarely	A normally formed stool contains 80–100 mL of water. Diarrheal stools are principally water: diarrheal losses can be quantitated by collecting and weighing the feces.
Other sensible losses		
Gastric drainage, transudation from skin, etc.	Variable	
Insensible losses		
Evaporation from skin	No	Normally 450 mL is lost daily. In an average-sized adult with fever, losses increase about 10% per degree Fahrenheit.
Evaporation from lung surfaces	No	Normally 450 mL is lost daily. Losses increase by 50% with doubling of ventilatory rate.

[a]Water balance = water intake − water output.

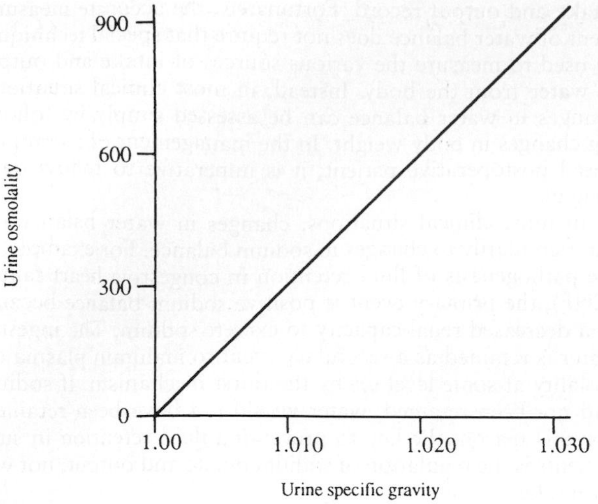

FIGURE 10.3. Approximate relation between specific gravity and osmolality in normal urine.

to consider the relation between urine osmolality (U_{osm}) and specific gravity.

$$\text{specific gravity} + W_s/WH_2O$$

where:

WH_2O = weight of an equal volume of water; and
W_s = weight of the solution.

On the average, in normal urine, a linear relation exists between urine osmolality and specific gravity, as shown in Figure 10.3. This relation is disturbed when molecules that have molecular weights much higher than the predominant normal urinary solutes are excreted in large amounts. Thus, in the presence of large numbers of molecules with high molecular weight, specific gravity is no longer a reliable index of osmolality. The normal, predominant urinary solutes are sodium, potassium, chloride ions, and urea, which have molecular weights of 23, 39, 35, and 60, respectively. The commonly encountered urinary solutes that cause large increases in specific gravity but small increases in urine osmolality are glucose (MW 180), mannitol (MW 181), dextran (MW 20,000 to 40,000), iodine-containing radiographic contrast (MW 600 to 800), and protein (but only with heavy proteinuria). If these substances are absent, urine specific gravity can be relied on to reflect urine osmolality. If these substances are present, urine osmolality must be measured directly to determine the true extent to which the kidneys have concentrated or diluted the urine.

Normal Renal Response to Water Deprivation

The permeability of the collecting duct to water is markedly increased when ADH is released. Thus, as the tubular fluid enters the collecting duct, water diffuses from the collecting duct into the hypertonic medullary interstitium, resulting in a marked reduction in urine volume and a marked increase in urine osmolality. In health, the osmolality of the medullary interstitium is 900 to 1,200 mOsm/L. Thus, in states of maximum water conservation, the urine osmolality approaches 900 to 1,200 mOsm/L. In such circumstances, urine flow rates approximate 0.5% or less of the normal glomerular filtration rate (GFR), resulting in urine flow rates of about 20 mL/h, or 500 mL/d, when kidneys function normally. Elderly people are unable to concentrate their urine, with maximum osmolalities among the aged often below 800 mOsm/L.

Normal Response to Water Loading

The administration of water or hypotonic solutions results in a reduction in the osmolality of body fluids. A 2% reduction in plasma osmolality (e.g., plasma osmolality from 290 to 284 mOsm/L, serum sodium from 140 to 137 mEq/L) is sufficient to completely suppress ADH secretion. In an average, healthy adult, the ingestion of 1 L of water is more than enough to elicit such a response and to cause the formation of a maximally dilute urine. When ADH secretion is inhibited and renal function is normal, urine specific gravity usually is less than 1.005, urine osmolality is less than 100 mOsm/kg, and urine flow rates approach 15% to 20% of the GFR (i.e., 10 to 15 mL/min, 600 to 900 mL/h). Elderly patients also cannot dilute their urine as well as young persons, with the minimum osmolality being 200 mOsm/L or slightly higher.

Sodium Balance

Sodium balance equals sodium intake minus sodium output. The components of sodium balance are shown in Table 10.3. From this table, it is evident that the kidneys play the central role in the regulation of sodium balance by adjusting sodium excretion to match sodium intake. Unless there are abnormal losses of sodium through the skin or gut, sodium balance can be assessed simply by determining dietary sodium intake and by measuring the urinary excretion of sodium. These measurements usually are not necessary because if the patient has free access to water and an intact thirst mechanism, water is ingested and retained in proportion to the level of sodium retention. Thus, changes in sodium balance are reflected by changes in body weight. Occasionally, the measurement of urine sodium excretion is useful. For example, when body weight and serum sodium concentration are stable and there are no abnormal extrarenal sodium losses, the measurement of the 24-hour urinary excretion of sodium accurately reflects sodium intake.

Normal Renal Response to Sodium Restriction and Sodium Loading

When sodium intake is abruptly reduced from a normal level (e.g., 170 mEq/24 h) to a very low level (e.g., 10 mEq/24 h), it takes 3 or 4 days until maximal renal sodium conservation occurs. During this period of adjustment, renal sodium output exceeds intake, and water is lost with sodium in isosmotic proportion from the ECF. One to two liters of ECF usually is lost in the change from a normal to a very low sodium intake. Thus, normal people come into balance on a low sodium intake, but the ECF volume then may be regulated at a suboptimal level. This is potentially dangerous because the patient may be vulnerable to the potential hypotensive effects of anesthesia or additional volume losses that can occur during surgery.

The normal renal response to salt loading is analogous to that of salt restriction in that it takes several days for the renal excretion of sodium to increase in response to the higher level of sodium intake. Thus, when balance is finally achieved, ECF volume is being regulated at an expanded level, which can be

TABLE 10.3

COMPONENTS OF SODIUM BALANCE[a]

Sources	Comments
Sodium intake	
Dietary	Normal adults intake of salt is about 10 g NaCl daily (~170 mEq Na^+ and Cl^- or 4 g Na^+). Restricted dietary salt intake usually is 2 g sodium (87 mEq NaCl) daily
Parenteral	1,000 mL normal saline (0.9% saline) = 9 g NaCl = 155 mEq Na^+ + 155 mEq Cl^-
Sodium output	
Urine	Variable. In health, reflects intake, since virtually all ingested NaCl is excreted in urine
Skin	Negligible except with sweating. Sweat contains 50–60 mEq Na^+/L and several liters of sweat may be lost each day in hot environments.
Gastrointestinal secretion	
Normally formed stool	Na^+ ~1 mEq/24 h
Diarrheal stool	
Secretory (infectious)	Na^+ ~130 mEq/L
Fermentative (malabsorption)	Na^+ ~50 mEq/L
Vomitus or gastric aspirate	
Normally acid gastric juice	Na^+ ~40 mEq/L
Achlorhydria	Na^+ ~130 mEq/L
All other secretions (bile, pancreatic juice, small bowel secretions)	Na^+ ~130 mEq/L

[a]Sodium balance = sodium intake – sodium output.

undesirable. For example, a patient with underlying heart disease who achieves sodium balance on a high intake of sodium chloride is more vulnerable to the development of CHF if additional fluids are administered.

CLINICAL ASSESSMENT OF DISORDERS OF WATER AND ELECTROLYTE METABOLISM

Disorders of ECF electrolyte composition may be detected by measurement of the serum electrolyte concentrations. Identification of the process (or processes) behind the disturbance of electrolyte composition and the planning of subsequent therapy are critically dependent on the clinician's ability to accurately assess whether the disturbance in ECF electrolyte composition is associated with volume expansion, volume contraction, or a normal volume.

In the evaluation of a patient's ECF volume status, it must be kept clearly in mind that the critical volume is that portion of the IVV that is effective in determining the filling pressure of the ventricles and, hence, the cardiac output. Hereafter, this theoretic volume is referred to as the effective IVV.

In light of this definition, the most effective IVV is that which maintains an optimal cardiac output and thus maximizes tissue perfusion. Although the actual IVV and the effective IVV are the same in many clinical situations and can be expected to change in direct proportion, in a number of important clinical states, the actual IVV is different from the effective IVV. For example, in acute metabolic acidosis, increased venoconstriction can develop, resulting in an abnormal increase in central venous pressure (CVP) and cardiac output. Under this circumstance, the actual IVV could be less than normal, whereas the effective IVV is greater than normal. That is, because of the increase in venous tone, an IVV that is lower than normal can maintain a normal effective IVV.

Acute changes in venous tone induced by drugs (e.g., morphine, furosemide, norepinephrine), changes in acid–base status, and the presence of bacterial endotoxin also can disrupt the normal relation between the actual IVV and the effective IVV.

The most reliable clinical means for assessing the status of the effective IVV is the pulmonary capillary wedge pressure. This measurement is an estimate of the pulmonary capillary pressure, which is a measure of the filling pressure of the left ventricle. Factors that increase pulmonary capillary wedge pressure tend to increase cardiac output by increasing capillary outflux. When effective IVV is considered within these constraints, it becomes clear that under virtually any physiologic or pathophysiologic circumstance, an optimal effective IVV is one that results in a pulmonary capillary wedge pressure that is high enough to promote optimal cardiac output but low enough to prevent pulmonary edema.

Fortunately, in most clinical situations, it is not necessary to resort to measuring pulmonary wedge pressure to assess whether a disturbance of ECF composition is associated with an effective IVV that is abnormally high, abnormally low, or normal. Instead, an accurate assessment of the effective IVV usually can be made by a careful clinical assessment using the criteria listed in Table 10.4. This table lists the bedside and laboratory means to assess volume status according to whether the findings are consistent with an effective IVV that is less than normal or an effective IVV that is nearly normal or expanded.

Also shown in Table 10.4 are the conditions under which the given means for evaluating the IVV must be qualified (i.e., the conditions that may render the meaning of the finding indeterminate with respect to the evaluation of IVV). For example, the relation between an increase in weight and a change in IVV is rendered indeterminate if, at the same time, the patient has

TABLE 10.4

ASSESSMENT OF EFFECTIVE INTRAVASCULAR VOLUME (IVV)

Suggestive evidence	Qualifying conditions[a]
Significantly decreased effective IVV	
History of fluid and electrolyte deprivation or loss (eg., vomiting, diarrhea)	Difficulty in establishing by history whether the magnitude of loss or deprivation is sufficient to result in negative balance of water and electrolytes
Decrease in body weight below normal not explained by inadequate caloric intake	None
Blood pressure less than usual for patient with orthostatic hypotension	1. Patient receiving methyldopa (Aldomet), prazosin (Minipress), minoxidil (Loniten), or other drugs that interfere with vascular α-receptors 2. Autonomic insufficiency as in diabetics, quadriplegics, and after prolonged bed rest
Elevated serum creatinine associated with concentrated urine (U_{osm}/P_{osm} >1.5), and Na^+ conservation: (U_{Na} <20 mEq/L) or $\%E/F_{Na}$ <1%	Decreased renal perfusion owing to: (a) severe hepatic failure (hepatorenal syndrome); (b) severe cardiac failure. Acute, high-grade urinary tract obstruction (see text)
Low central venous pressure or pulmonary capillary wedge pressure	See text
Decreased tissue turgor	See text
Hematocrit above normal	Presence of conditions that may cause erthrocytosis
Nearly normal or expanded effective IVV (i.e., absence of significant intravascular volume depletion)	
Hypertension with patient in sitting or standing position and no orthostatic fall in blood pressure	None
Presence of cardiac failure: Left ventricular failure: audible third heart sound or pulmonary edema	Patients with markedly reduced cardiac output and very large left ventricles may have decreased effective IVV despite an audible third heart sound
Right ventricular failure: peripheral edema with increased venous pressure (neck vein distention, increased intravenous pressure)	Right ventricular failure but normal left ventricular function (see text)
Increase in weight above normal not explained by increased caloric intake	1. Significant hypoalbuminemia 2. Development of third spaces (e.g., ascites, bowel obstruction)
Increased central venous pressure	See text
Increased pulmonary capillary wedge pressure	See text
Edema, ascites, or pleural effusion	See text
Hematocrit less than normal	Presence of conditions that can cause loss, destruction, or decreased production of red blood cells

$\%E/F_{Na}$, percentage of excretion of filtered sodium (see text).
[a]Qualifying conditions are circumstances that can render the meaning of the finding indeterminate with respect to the evaluation of the effective IVV.

developed a third space, as in bowel obstruction. In this instance, the entire weight gain could be caused by the accumulation of fluid outside the IVV. Thus, the finding of weight gain in this setting cannot be used as evidence of an increase in effective IVV.

I suggest that the evaluation of effective IVV, using the criteria in Table 10.4, be approached in the following manner. First, whenever a finding can be significantly qualified, it should not be used in arriving at a final decision. Second, as many independent means as practical should be used to assess the effective IVV to minimize the effect of possible error on the final decision. The greater the number of independent, unqualified findings that agree in favor of a given clinical decision, the more likely it is that the decision is correct. If such a systematic approach to clinical decision making is used, it should be possible to arrive at an accurate evaluation of volume status in most circumstances.

DATABASE FOR ASSESSMENT OF EFFECTIVE INTRAVASCULAR VOLUME

Body Weight

All patients should be weighed on admission to the hospital and then periodically during their hospital stay. In patients undergoing surgery, or in whom problems in fluid and electrolyte balance are anticipated, weight must be measured daily.

Alterations in body weight are the result of changes in body water content plus solid tissue content (fat, protein, bone). Gains or losses of solid tissue are almost always related to changes in caloric intake and seldom exceed 0.25 kg/24 h. For example, a patient who takes no calories for 24 hours is forced to consume her endogenous stores of fat and protein to meet the energy requirements for continued life. The complete oxidation of fat yields 9 cal/g, and protein yields 4 cal/g. It can be readily calculated that the complete oxidation of 0.25 kg of solid tissue (in starvation, a mixture of about 87% fat, 13% protein) yields enough calories to meet basal daily energy needs. Thus changes in weight exceeding 0.25 kg/24 h are almost always attributable to changes in water balance. Although the relation between body weight and effective IVV can be variable, usually the relation between changes in body weight and IVV can be correctly assessed by the application of the two guidelines. The first is that a decrease in body weight below normal (for the patient), and not explained on the basis of inadequate caloric intake, can be assumed to be accompanied by a decrease in IVV. The second is that an increase in body weight above normal not explained by increased nutrition can be assumed to be accompanied by an increase in IVV except when the weight gain develops in association with the following conditions.

- Significant hypoalbuminemia: serum albumin less than 2.5 g dL
- Venous obstruction or congestion
- Development of third spaces (e.g., obstructed or ischemic bowel)

Under these three general conditions, an increase in body weight may not reflect an increase in the effective IVV.

Renal Function

Creatinine, a byproduct of muscle energy metabolism, is produced at a constant rate that is related to muscle mass. Normal men produce 20 to 25 mg/kg (ideal body weight)/24 h, and women produce 15 to 20 mg/kg (ideal body weight)/24 h. Nearly all of the creatinine produced is excreted by glomerular filtration. Therefore, changes in the concentration of serum creatinine reflect changes in the GFR, and the clearance of creatinine (Ccr) is an index of the GFR.

$$Ccr = U_{cr}V/S_{cr} \sim GFR$$

where:

$Scr =$ serum creatinine;
$Ucr =$ urinary creatinine concentration;
$V =$ urine volume per unit time.

Thus, by rearranging this equation:

$$S_{cr} \sim U_{cr}V/GFR$$

Normally, as muscle mass (which is proportional to $U_{cr}V$) increases, the GFR increases proportionately less. Therefore, on the average, children have lower serum creatinine values than do adults, and large adults have higher serum creatinine levels than do small adults. Because of these considerations, a single range of serum creatinine values cannot be applied to everyone. The suggested normal ranges of serum creatinine for adults, according to ideal body weight, are shown in Table 10.5. Creatinine clearance for men can be estimated, using the formula derived by Cockcroft and Gault, from the patient's age, body weight, and serum creatinine level as follows.

$$C_{cr} \text{ in mL/min} = \frac{[(140 - \text{age}) \times \text{weight in kg}]}{[72 \times S_{cr} \text{ in mg/dL}]}$$

This result multiplied by 0.85 provides a better estimate for women because of their relatively smaller muscle mass. Azotemia is arbitrarily defined here as a serum creatinine level greater than the upper limit of normal for body size, as shown in Table 10.5. The blood urea nitrogen level is influenced by dietary protein intake, tissue metabolism, and urine flow rate, in addition to GFR, and should not be relied on to assess changes in GFR.

TABLE 10.5

NORMAL RELATION BETWEEN BODY SIZE AND SERUM CREATININE LEVEL

Ideal body weight	Expected range of serum creatinine level[a] (mg/dL)
<55 kg (120 lb)	0.6–1.0
55–80 kg (120–175 lb)	0.8–1.2
>80 kg (175 lb)	1.0–1.4

[a] Autoanalyzer picric acid method.

The following guidelines are suggested for the evaluation of the IVV in light of the state of renal function. The azotemia can be assumed to result from decreased renal perfusion if the serum creatinine level is elevated, the urine is concentrated ($U_{osm}:P_{osm}$ ratio greater than 1.5; specific gravity higher than 1.015), and renal sodium conservation is present (U_{Na} level <20 mEq/L) on a random and untimed urine sample. The fractional excretion of sodium is based on serum and random urine concentrations of sodium and creatinine. If below 1%, azotemia can be attributed to decreased IVV, unless the patient has severe liver or cardiac disease.

$$\%E/F_{Na} = \text{percentage of fractional excretion of filtered sodium (excreted } Na^+) \times 100/(\text{filtered } Na^+)$$

where:

$S_{cr} =$ serum creatinine concentration in mg/dL;
$S_{Na} =$ serum Na^+ concentration in mEq/L;
$U_{cr} =$ urine creatinine concentration in mg/dL; and
$U_{Na} =$ urinary Na^+ concentration in mEq/L.

If severe cardiac failure and severe liver failure (hepatorenal syndrome) can be excluded, the decreased renal perfusion can be assumed to be caused by a decreased effective IVV.

Edema, Ascites, and Pleural Effusion

Effective IVV is increased when edema, pleural effusion, or ascites occurs in the setting of CHF. Increased effective IVV cannot be assumed in the presence of edema, ascites, or pleural effusion if there is significant hypoalbuminemia or venous obstruction, or if the accumulation of fluid is in a relatively small area of capillary injury (e.g., pleural effusion caused by pulmonary infarction).

Tissue Turgor

Tissue turgor is a function of the elasticity of the solid components of tissue and the degree of distention of the tissues by interstitial fluid. If tissue is depleted of interstitial fluid, it becomes less elastic (i.e., it less readily returns to its original shape after being deformed). Skin turgor is best assessed on the forehead and anterior chest. In patients less than 50 years of age, the turgor of the dorsum of the hand also can be used. In older patients, the elasticity of the solid components of tissue is decreased, and the turgor of the skin becomes unreliable in interpreting changes in interstitial volume.

Central Venous Pressure

The measurement of CVP is a relatively simple but useful means for monitoring cardiac function and cardiovascular status. For the valid measurement of CVP, the catheter must be placed in the large intrathoracic veins near the right atrium (as assessed by chest radiograph), and the catheter must be patent (as assessed by the cyclic variation of CVP with ventilatory movements: decreased CVP during inspiration, increased CVP during expiration).

In normal adults, CVP is about 5 to 12 cm H_2O. CVPs below 3 cm H_2O are commonly seen in children and young adults who have no evidence of a decreased effective IVV. In older adults and elderly persons, CVP of less than 3 cm H_2O can be assumed to reflect a significant decrease in effective IVV.

CVP is an index of the filling pressure of the right atrium, which, in turn, is an index of the filling pressure of the right ventricle. In uncomplicated circumstances, expansion of the IVV results in increased CVP, whereas contraction of the IVV results in decreased CVP. CVP cannot be used to assess the adequacy of left ventricular function in patients in whom left ventricular function may be impaired relative to right ventricular function. CVP also is unreliable when lung disease is present, because it is commonly falsely elevated. In such patients, left ventricular function can be monitored by observing for signs and symptoms of left ventricular failure (dyspnea, development of an audible third heart sound, or pulmonary edema), or by direct measurement of pulmonary capillary wedge pressure. Under normal circumstances, the pulmonary capillary wedge pressure is about equal to the CVP plus 6 mm Hg.

Pulmonary Capillary Wedge Pressure

Technical refinements of the Swan-Ganz catheter make it possible to measure pulmonary artery systolic and diastolic pressure, CVP, pulmonary wedge pressure, and cardiac output using the thermodilution technique with the same catheter. This permits a definitive assessment of the volume status of the patient, because it can be determined whether the cardiac output is appropriate for a given pulmonary wedge pressure. Specific guidelines for the interpretation of the relation between pulmonary wedge pressure and cardiac output are discussed in the following sections.

Patients with Normal Volume Status

Pulmonary wedge pressure can be expected to be between 8 and 12 mm Hg in a patient with a normal cardiopulmonary system and a normal effective IVV. Cardiac output is normal. Pulmonary wedge pressure can be less than 8 mm Hg without indicating volume contraction; in this circumstance, the cardiac output is normal despite the unusually low pulmonary wedge pressure.

Patients Who Are Volume Contracted

Patients who have a normal cardiopulmonary system but who are significantly volume depleted usually have a pulmonary wedge pressure below 8 mm Hg and their cardiac output is less than normal. In patients with chronic pulmonary hypertension (e.g., those with chronic left ventricular failure), a higher than normal pulmonary wedge pressure is needed to drive a satisfactory cardiac output. Thus, in such patients, pulmonary wedge pressure can be above the normal range but be inappropriately low for the patient. This situation can be identified by showing that: (a) cardiac output is less than normal, despite the elevated pulmonary wedge pressure; (b) volume infusion causes an increase in cardiac output toward a more favorable range; and (c) despite further increase in pulmonary wedge pressure with volume expansion, pulmonary function does not deteriorate. (Pa_{O_2} does not decrease, Pa_{CO_2} does not increase, and pulmonary compliance does not worsen.)

Patients Who Are Volume Expanded

In patients with a normal cardiopulmonary system, pulmonary wedge pressure usually is above 18 mm Hg when volume expansion is substantial. Cardiac output is above normal. If cardiac function is impaired, cardiac output will be inappropriately low for the level of pulmonary wedge pressure.

When a given pulmonary wedge pressure is being interpreted, the serum albumin level also should be taken into consideration, because this opposes the effect of capillary hydrostatic pressure to cause migration of fluid from the capillary lumen to the interstitial space. Thus, at any given elevated pulmonary wedge pressure, pulmonary edema develops more rapidly in a patient who is hypoalbuminemic than in one who has a normal serum albumin concentration. In some patients, it is not possible to obtain a reliable pulmonary wedge pressure. In most of these patients, the pulmonary artery diastolic pressure is a good estimate of the pulmonary wedge pressure. If pulmonary hypertension is present, then pulmonary vascular resistance is increased; thus, pulmonary artery diastolic pressure may not be a good index of the pulmonary wedge pressure. In such patients, it is important to be able to obtain a wedge pressure. Finally, in patients who are being ventilated with high levels of positive end-expiratory pressure, pulmonary wedge pressure may become an unreliable index of left atrial filling pressure because the high intrapulmonary pressures may cause obstruction of the catheter orifice. Patients must be briefly taken off the ventilator for accurate measurements. Other circumstances in which pulmonary artery wedge pressure measurements may be inaccurate include the presence of mitral stenosis or pulmonary venous obstruction.

Blood Pressure

The following guidelines are suggested for the evaluation of the effective IVV from measurement of blood pressure.

1. A nearly normal or expanded effective IVV can be assumed in patients with hypertension that is demonstrated in the sitting or standing position.
2. Effective IVV may be decreased in patients who previously were hypertensive but who have become normotensive.
3. Effective IVV may be decreased in patients who develop orthostatic hypotension (a drop in systolic pressure greater than 10 mm Hg in changing from the supine to the sitting or standing position).

Orthostatic hypotension also can be present, in the absence of volume contraction, as a result of prolonged bed rest, during the use of such antihypertensive agents as methyldopa (Aldomet) or of vasodilators (Prazosin, Minoxidil). If the pulse rate does not rise as blood pressure falls when a patient stands, autonomic neuropathy should be considered as a cause of postural hypotension.

Systemic Vascular Resistance

Other measurements of hemodynamic importance derived from Swan-Ganz readings include calculations of resistance across the pulmonary and systemic vascular beds. The calculations are as follows:

$$PVR = \frac{P_{PA}\,P_{PAW} \times 80}{QT}$$

$$SVR = \frac{PSA - PRA \times 80}{QT}$$

where:

P_{PA} = mean right atrial pressure;
P_{PAW} = mean pulmonary artery wedge pressure;
PVR = pulmonary vascular resistance;
PSA = mean systolic arterial pressure;
QT = cardiac output in liters per minute; and
SVR = systemic vascular resistance.

Normal values are 50 to 150 dyne-s/cm for pulmonary vascular resistance and 800 to 1,200 dyne-s/cm for systemic vascular resistance. Pulmonary vascular resistance is elevated in hypovolemic shock, cardiogenic shock, pulmonary embolism, or airway obstruction; it is diminished in septic shock. Systemic vascular resistance is elevated in hypovolemic shock, cardiogenic shock, pulmonary embolism, and sometimes in right ventricular infarct and cardiac tamponade; it is decreased in end-stage liver disease and septic shock.

CLINICAL ASSESSMENT OF DISORDERS OF EXTRACELLULAR FLUID COMPOSITION

Hyponatremia

The schema for the evaluation of a hyponatremic patient depends on the assessment of volume status. That is, it must first be determined whether the patient's hyponatremia is associated with an effective IVV that is decreased, normal, or increased. Once this is decided on the basis of the assessment of IVV, a further separation, based only on the state of renal sodium and water excretion, is made. Each of the final categories contains relatively few diagnostic possibilities, and the presence or absence of each of these conditions in a given patient usually can be readily determined. The scheme for the evaluation of a hypernatremic patient is analogous, except that it depends on the assessment of the state of renal water excretion.

Clinical Assessment

In the discussion that follows, only patients with true hyponatremia are considered (i.e., hyponatremia in which serum osmolality is decreased in proportion to the reduction in serum sodium concentration, after appropriate correction for any elevation in the plasma urea nitrogen). By making this distinction, hyponatremia caused by accumulation of ECF solutes such as glucose or mannitol can be excluded. In this type of hyponatremia, the decreased concentration of ECF sodium is the result of the shift of water from cells to the ECF in response to the osmotic gradient caused by the accumulation of the solute. As a consequence, the hyponatremia is associated with an increased plasma osmolality. These patients also can be readily identified either by the presence of hyperglycemia sufficient to explain the decrease in serum sodium concentration or by a history of administration of large amounts of mannitol (0.100 g in adults), usually in the presence of a decreased capacity to excrete mannitol (decreased GFR).

Also to be excluded are patients with spurious hyponatremia that results from the abnormal accumulation of plasma lipids or proteins. In such circumstances, the concentration of sodium in plasma water is normal; however, the concentration of sodium expressed per liter of whole plasma is reduced because an abnormally large volume of whole plasma is occupied by the lipids or proteins, which do not contain plasma water and electrolytes. Thus, when aliquots of hyperlipemic or hyperproteinemic plasma are analyzed, a lower amount of sodium is determined to be present in a given volume of whole plasma. Plasma osmolality, however, is normal because lipids and proteins do not contribute importantly to plasma osmolality (see section on osmotic forces). Patients with spurious hyponatremia can be readily identified by the presence of markedly elevated total serum protein levels (e.g., multiple myeloma) or grossly lipemic serum. The distinction can be readily made if lipemic serum is subjected to centrifugation and the lipoprotein layer is removed before evaluation, if flame photometry is being used for measurement of serum Na^+. Spurious hyponatremia is no longer a consideration in most laboratories, because serum Na^+ concentration is determined by ion-specific electrodes, and increased levels are not affected by lipemic serum. Symptoms of hyponatremia include increased tendon reflexes, lethargy, mental confusion, and muscle twitching, which are followed by convulsions, coma, and possibly death if levels fall beneath 115 mEq/L.

Hyponatremia and Volume Depletion Associated with Renal Sodium Wasting

The normal renal response to volume depletion and hyponatremia is the virtual elimination of sodium from the urine (Fig. 10.4; see section on Sodium Balance). Thus, the presence of an excessive amount of urinary sodium under these conditions indicates that renal sodium loss is the cause or a major contributing factor to the state of sodium depletion. A spot urine sodium concentration greater than 40 mEq/L, a %E/FNa above 1%, or a urinary sodium excretion rate greater than intake indicates such renal sodium wasting. The conditions discussed in the following sections are associated with hyponatremia, IVV depletion, and renal sodium wasting.

Chronic Renal Disease. All types of renal disease can be associated with renal salt wasting. In adults with such a disorder, the serum creatinine level is virtually always above 2 mg and usually much higher before a significant salt leak develops. These azotemic patients usually require 85 to 170 mEq of sodium daily (5 to 10 g of sodium chloride) to maintain salt balance at a normal effective IVV. Thus, if sodium intake is decreased in azotemic patients by anorexia or vomiting, or if additional sodium losses occur (e.g., diarrhea or diuretic therapy), the inability of the diseased kidneys to conserve sodium and water normally may rapidly lead to the development of significant sodium and water deficits. Water intake usually continues; therefore, sodium balance is more adversely affected than water balance. As a consequence, the patient becomes volume contracted with hyponatremia. With the onset of CHF or the nephrotic syndrome, the salt leak of chronic renal failure usually disappears, and salt intake must be restricted.

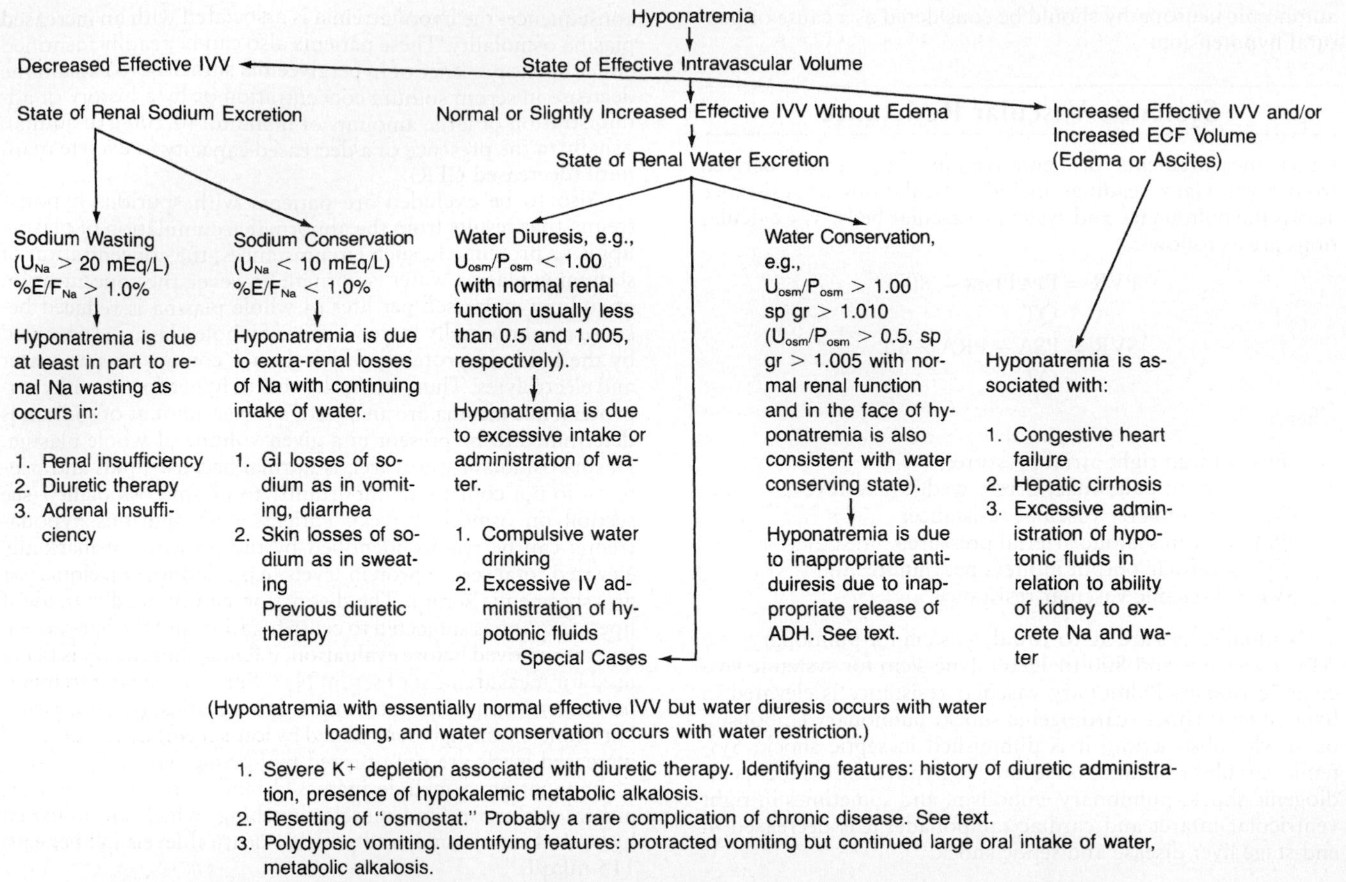
Hyponatremia
Decreased Effective IVV
State of Effective Intravascular Volume
State of Renal Sodium Excretion
Normal or Slightly Increased Effective IVV Without Edema
Increased Effective IVV and/or Increased ECF Volume (Edema or Ascites)
State of Renal Water Excretion
Sodium Wasting (U_{Na} > 20 mEq/L) $\%E/F_{Na}$ > 1.0%
Hyponatremia is due at least in part to renal Na wasting as occurs in:
1. Renal insufficiency
2. Diuretic therapy
3. Adrenal insufficiency
Sodium Conservation (U_{Na} < 10 mEq/L) $\%E/F_{Na}$ < 1.0%
Hyponatremia is due to extra-renal losses of Na with continuing intake of water.
1. GI losses of sodium as in vomiting, diarrhea
2. Skin losses of sodium as in sweating
Previous diuretic therapy
Water Diuresis, e.g., U_{osm}/P_{osm} < 1.00 (with normal renal function usually less than 0.5 and 1.005, respectively).
Hyponatremia is due to excessive intake or administration of water.
1. Compulsive water drinking
2. Excessive IV administration of hypotonic fluids
Water Conservation, e.g., U_{osm}/P_{osm} > 1.00 sp gr > 1.010 (U_{osm}/P_{osm} > 0.5, sp gr > 1.005 with normal renal function and in the face of hyponatremia is also consistent with water conserving state).
Hyponatremia is due to inappropriate antiduiresis due to inappropriate release of ADH. See text.
Hyponatremia is associated with:
1. Congestive heart failure
2. Hepatic cirrhosis
3. Excessive administration of hypotonic fluids in relation to ability of kidney to excrete Na and water
Special Cases
(Hyponatremia with essentially normal effective IVV but water diuresis occurs with water loading, and water conservation occurs with water restriction.)
1. Severe K^+ depletion associated with diuretic therapy. Identifying features: history of diuretic administration, presence of hypokalemic metabolic alkalosis.
2. Resetting of "osmostat." Probably a rare complication of chronic disease. See text.
3. Polydypsic vomiting. Identifying features: protracted vomiting but continued large oral intake of water, metabolic alkalosis.

FIGURE 10.4. Approach to the assessment of a hyponatremic patient. This approach considers only patients with true hyponatremia (i.e., in nonazotemic patients, serum osmolality is reduced in proportion to the decrease in serum sodium). Thus, patients are excluded who have lowered concentrations of serum sodium because of hyperlipidemia, hyperproteinemia, or the abnormal accumulations of solutes in the extracellular fluid, such as glucose or mannitol. ADH, antidiuretic hormone; $\%E/F_{Na}$, fractional excretion of sodium; GI, gastrointestinal; IVV, intravascular volume.

Diuretic Therapy. The diuretics include thiazide agents or loop diuretics, such as furosemide, bumetanide, and ethacrynic acid. Diuretics induce a renal salt-wasting state, and if the urinary output of sodium exceeds intake, sodium depletion ensues. Rarely, diuretics cause hyponatremia without evidence of volume depletion if severe potassium depletion has resulted from their use (Fig. 10.4).

Adrenal Insufficiency (Addison's Disease). Destruction of the adrenal gland or sudden withdrawal of chronic, daily glucocorticoid therapy results in inadequate adrenal function. The lack of mineralocorticoid causes wasting of renal salt but retention of renal potassium and leads to sodium depletion. The lack of glucocorticoid results in a decreased capacity to excrete a water load and leads to hyponatremia but not to volume depletion or hyperkalemia.

Hyponatremia and Volume Depletion Associated with Renal Sodium Conservation

A spot urine sodium concentration of less than 20 mEq/L or a $\%E/F_{Na}$ below 1% in a hyponatremic, volume-contracted patient is evidence of normal renal sodium conservation and indicates that the cause of the sodium depletion is nonrenal in origin or that it occurred during previous diuretic therapy. The fact that the serum sodium concentration is lower than normal indicates that water balance is less negative than sodium balance. The conditions discussed in the following sections can result in volume depletion and hyponatremia as a result of extrarenal losses of sodium.

Gastrointestinal Losses. If losses of fluid from the upper gastrointestinal tract (e.g., vomiting, gastric aspiration) cause the hyponatremia, and if the gastric juice is normally acid, metabolic alkalosis is present. If diarrheal losses cause the hyponatremia, metabolic acidosis may be present. In patients with gastric achlorhydria, upper gastrointestinal losses also can lead to metabolic acidosis.

Losses of Sodium from the Skin. Sweat contains about 50 mEq/L of sodium and is a hypotonic fluid. If sweat losses are not replaced, then hypernatremia can develop. In most situations, the water losses from the skin are replaced more adequately than the sodium losses. Thus, most patients with significant sodium losses that are due to sweating become hyponatremic. Skin losses of fluid and electrolytes also can occur after burns or other skin injuries. These are isotonic losses of sodium and lead to hyponatremia if the water losses are more adequately replaced than the sodium losses.

Losses of Sodium from Prior Diuretic Therapy. The natriuretic action of most diuretics lasts less than 24 hours. Hyponatremia is made worse if water intake is excessive.

Hyponatremia and Normal Volume Status Associated with Water Diuresis

In a patient with normal renal function who has become hyponatremic as a result of the administration or ingestion of excessive amounts of water, intravascular and ECF volume are normal to slightly expanded, and high rates of urine flow in association with maximally, or nearly maximally, dilute urine can be expected (see section on Water Balance). In a patient with preexisting renal functional impairment, water loading also increases urine flow rate and dilution of the urine; however, maximally dilute urine cannot be formed. Hyponatremia secondary to water loading may occur in compulsive water drinkers, who usually are severely neurotic or psychotic, or after excessive IV administration of hypotonic fluids. Many of these patients also have high levels of ADH for various reasons (e.g., drugs, psychosis). Without this elevation of ADH, presuming normal renal function, consumption of 20 L of water a day would be necessary for development of frank hyponatremia.

Hyponatremia and Normal to Slightly Elevated Volume Status Associated with Water Conservation

As discussed, it is appropriate to observe a brisk water diuresis in a patient with normal renal function who is hyponatremic and has evidence of normal or slightly elevated IVV without edema. When high flow rates of hypotonic urine are not observed, the patient is exhibiting an inappropriate antidiuresis. This may result from the inappropriate release of ADH, although other mechanisms also can be involved (e.g., decreased renal blood flow, certain drugs). Another characteristic of such patients is that administered sodium is promptly excreted in the urine, perhaps because of the effect of atrial natriuretic factors. On the other hand, when sodium intake is curtailed, renal sodium conservation is observed. These patients also exhibit normal adrenal and renal function, and are not edematous. The syndrome of inappropriate antidiuresis has been associated with various clinical states, including malignant tumors (e.g., in the lung or pancreas), central nervous system (CNS) disorders (e.g., head trauma, meningitis), infections (e.g., tuberculosis, bacterial pneumonias), the postoperative state, hypopituitarism, and myxedema, as well as with many drugs (Table 10.6). Infusion of oxytocin to induce uterine contraction also can cause hyponatremia because of the antidiuretic effects of oxytocin.

Within the category of hyponatremia associated with normal IVV are three special categories. The feature that sets these apart is that patients may exhibit evidence of water conservation when water is withdrawn or an appropriate or nearly appropriate water diuresis when water is administered. That is, it appears that osmoregulation has been reset to "defend" a lowered plasma osmolality. The first special category includes patients who have an unusual response to diuretic therapy, characterized by hyponatremia, severe potassium depletion, and metabolic alkalosis. Despite the hyponatremia and normal IVV, exchangeable sodium is nearly normal, suggesting intracellular movement of sodium. Potassium replacement must be accomplished before specific treatment of hyponatremia. The second category involves patients with an unusual manifestation of a chronic illness, such as pulmonary tuberculosis, that resets the osmostat. The third category includes patients with sodium depletion resulting from any cause in whom the decrease in effective IVV is minimized by excessive water intake and retention. This effect of excessive water intake can occur in any of the causes of sodium depletion.

TABLE 10.6

ANTIDIURETIC DRUGS

Sulfonylureas (chlorpropamide, tolbutamide)
Cytotoxic agents (vincristine, cyclophosphamide)
Nicotine
Morphine
Barbiturates
Carbamazepine
Psychotropics (tricyclics)
Clofibrate
Isoproterenol
Nonsteroidals
Salicylates
Acetaminophen
Vasopressin
Oxytocin

Hyponatremia Associated with Increased Effective Intravascular Volume or Increased Extracellular Fluid Volume (Edema or Ascites)

Congestive Heart Failure. When hyponatremia develops spontaneously in the course of chronic CHF (i.e., is not the result of excessive water administration or diuretic therapy), it usually is indicative of severe cardiac insufficiency and has a poor prognosis. The cause of the hyponatremia in such patients has been ascribed to a decreased capacity to increase renal free water clearance perhaps because of (a) increased fractional reabsorption of glomerular filtrate proximal to the renal diluting sites of the distal nephron and (b) an elevated ADH level.

Cirrhosis of the Liver. Patients with cirrhosis and ascites have a decreased capacity to excrete a water load, possibly because of the same mechanisms at work in patients with CHF.

Excessive Administration of Hypotonic Fluids. This usually is an iatrogenic situation and must be especially guarded against in postoperative patients whose ADH levels are elevated because of stress, pain, hypovolemia, or drugs, as well as in elderly patients who are unable to maximally dilute their urine.

Hypernatremia

All patients with hypernatremia are volume contracted, except those in whom the disorder develops as a result of excessive administration of hypertonic saline or sodium bicarbonate and the rare patients with essential hypernatremia (Fig. 10.5). The following discussion considers only the first group of patients; the latter section on treatment discusses all forms of hypernatremia. Patients with hypernatremia usually have CNS deficits, and they may also have confusion and neuroseizures. Autopsy findings often reveal hemorrhages or thromboses of brain tissue.

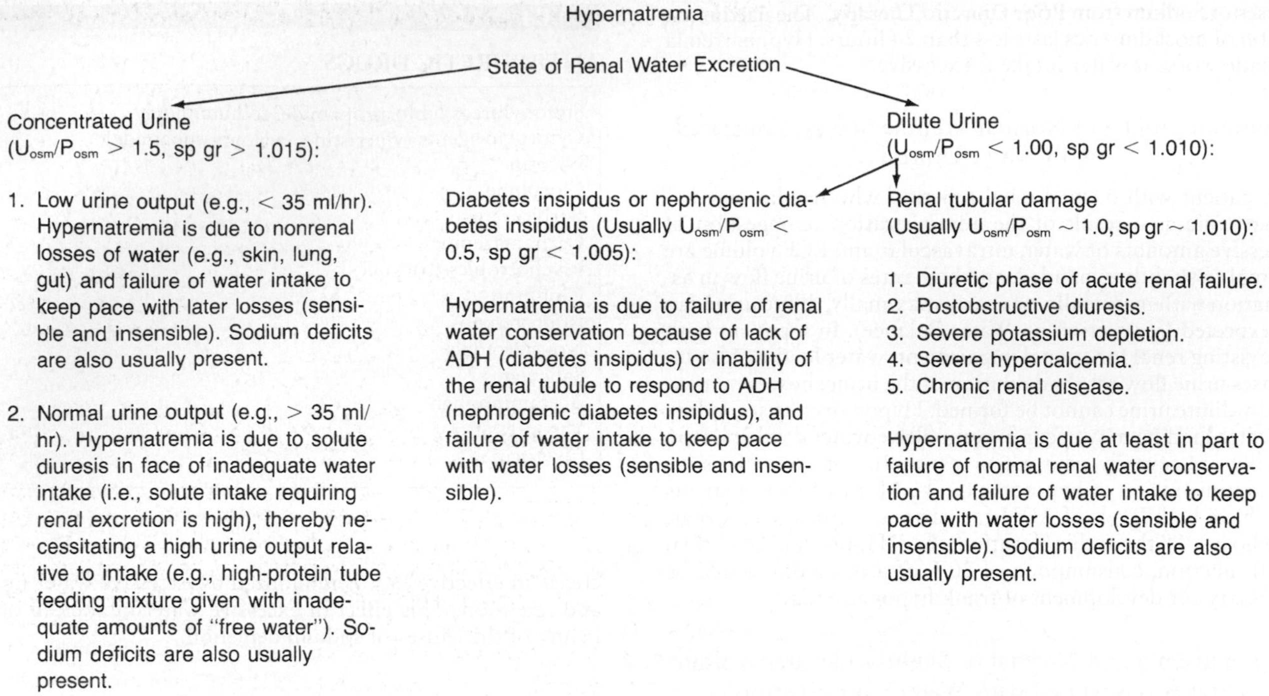

Hypernatremia
State of Renal Water Excretion
Concentrated Urine
(U_{osm}/P_{osm} > 1.5, sp gr > 1.015):
1. Low urine output (e.g., < 35 ml/hr). Hypernatremia is due to nonrenal losses of water (e.g., skin, lung, gut) and failure of water intake to keep pace with later losses (sensible and insensible). Sodium deficits are also usually present.
2. Normal urine output (e.g., > 35 ml/hr). Hypernatremia is due to solute diuresis in face of inadequate water intake (i.e., solute intake requiring renal excretion is high), thereby necessitating a high urine output relative to intake (e.g., high-protein tube feeding mixture given with inadequate amounts of "free water"). Sodium deficits are also usually present.
Dilute Urine
(U_{osm}/P_{osm} < 1.00, sp gr < 1.010):
Diabetes insipidus or nephrogenic diabetes insipidus (Usually U_{osm}/P_{osm} < 0.5, sp gr < 1.005):
Hypernatremia is due to failure of renal water conservation because of lack of ADH (diabetes insipidus) or inability of the renal tubule to respond to ADH (nephrogenic diabetes insipidus), and failure of water intake to keep pace with water losses (sensible and insensible).
Renal tubular damage
(Usually U_{osm}/P_{osm} ~ 1.0, sp gr ~ 1.010):
1. Diuretic phase of acute renal failure.
2. Postobstructive diuresis.
3. Severe potassium depletion.
4. Severe hypercalcemia.
5. Chronic renal disease.
Hypernatremia is due at least in part to failure of normal renal water conservation and failure of water intake to keep pace with water losses (sensible and insensible). Sodium deficits are also usually present.

FIGURE 10.5. Approach to the assessment of a hypernatremic patient. This approach does not consider patients with hypernatremia secondary to excessive administration of hypertonic saline. ADH, antidiuretic hormone.

Hypernatremia Associated with Formation of Concentrated Urine

The normal renal response to decreased intake of water or increased extrarenal losses of water is the formation of maximally concentrated urine (see section on Water Balance). In most clinical situations in which hypernatremia is the result of water depletion, the expected renal response is a U_{osm}:P_{osm} ratio greater than 1.5 and a specific gravity above 1.015. Thus, the finding of hypernatremia with evidence of renal conservation of water indicates that the hypernatremia is caused by excessive nonrenal losses of water or solute diuresis.

Excessive Nonrenal Water Loss. Hypernatremia typically develops in patients with accelerated rates of nonrenal water loss owing to a hot environment, fever, or hyperventilation and in whom water losses are not replaced because the patient cannot perceive or communicate thirst. Despite the hypernatremia, sodium deficits usually are present because initially, as water deficits develop, renal sodium excretion increases to maintain normal plasma osmolality and serum sodium concentration. When more than about 15% of ECF volume is lost, renal conservation of sodium occurs; if the water losses continue, hypernatremia develops. The presence of volume deficits is indicated by the signs of IVV depletion, as previously described. Urine flow rate usually is less than 35 mL/h.

Solute Diuresis. The amount of water that must accompany the excretion of a given amount of solute in the urine is determined by the osmolality of the renal medullary interstitial fluid (with which the collecting duct fluid must equilibrate) and the plasma level of ADH activity (which determines the permeability of the collecting duct to water and, therefore, the rate at which water moves from the collecting duct to medullary interstitial fluid to achieve osmotic equilibrium). Hypernatremia results if water intake does not keep pace with renal water losses, because although renal sodium excretion also is increased in solute diuresis, renal sodium reabsorption is affected proportionately less than water reabsorption. Large amounts of mannitol infused intravenously or high-protein mixtures fed by nasogastric tube (each gram of protein yields 8 mOsm as urea, phosphate, and potassium) can cause a solute diuresis sufficient to cause hypernatremia if water intake is inadequate. In solute diuresis, urine volume usually is greater than 35 mL/h.

Hypernatremia Associated with Formation of Dilute Urine

The finding of hypernatremia in combination with isotonic or hypotonic urine indicates that, at least in part, the hypernatremia results from failure of normal renal conservation of water. Failure to concentrate the urine under these conditions may result from the lack of ADH (hypothalamic–pituitary diabetes insipidus) or impaired renal tubular function that interferes with the development of a hypertonic medullary interstitium (renal tubular damage).

Central diabetes insipidus or nephrogenic diabetes insipidus should be suspected immediately in a patient with hypernatremia when the urine is very dilute (a U_{osm}:P_{osm} ratio <0.5, or specific gravity <1.005).

In patients with renal tubular damage, the ability to concentrate and dilute the urine is decreased. As a result, under all conditions, the urine is isotonic or nearly isotonic with plasma. Hypernatremia can supervene when water losses exceed sodium losses and water intake does not keep pace with water losses. Despite the hypernatremia, significant sodium deficits usually are present because renal sodium wasting also usually is a feature of these disorders. The following sections are examples of clinical situations in which renal tubular damage can be associated with hypernatremia.

Diuretic Phase of Acute Renal Failure. Occasionally, in a patient recovering from acute renal injury, tubular function is more severely affected than glomerular function. Thus, an inordinately large fraction of the glomerular filtrate escapes reabsorption, resulting in high urine flow rates. The period of inappropriate diuresis can persist for a few days to several weeks.

Postobstructive Diuresis. The sudden release of chronic urinary tract obstruction often is followed by several days or weeks in which urine flow rates are abnormally high. Short-lived nephrogenic diabetes insipidus develops in some patients.

MANAGEMENT OF WATER AND ELECTROLYTE BALANCE

Water requirements should be carefully monitored, especially in hospitalized patients. Patients with known fluid deficits or excesses should be approached as demonstrated in Tables 10.7 and 10.8. Maintenance requirements can be calculated from two simple formulas.

TABLE 10.7

GENERAL GUIDELINES FOR PLANNING FLUID AND ELECTROLYTE THERAPY IN COMPLICATED CASES

Volume-contracted patients (from water and electrolyte loss)

Deficit Replacement

Moderate volume contraction (e.g., decreased effective IVV causing azotemia but not hypotension). Plan to replace deficits in about 24 h (e.g., 0.9% saline at 200–250 mL/h). If patient is hypernatremic, 0.9% and 0.45% saline can be alternated.

Severe volume contraction (e.g., decreased effective IVV causing hypotension). Give 0.9% saline as rapidly as practicable until the hypotension is corrected.

Estimate maintenance needs and add this amount to the fluids used to correct the preexisting water and electrolyte deficits.

For patients with normal renal function and no abnormal losses:

Maintenance	*Equivalent Intravenous Fluid Orders*
Water: 2,500–3,000 mL/24 h	Alternate:
Sodium: 150 mEq/24 h	5% dextrose in 0.45% saline with
Potassium: 40 mEq/24 h	5% dextrose in 0.25% saline
	Each day add:
	Multivitamins to first liter
	Potassium chloride 20 mEq to first and second liters
	Infuse at 100–125 mL/h

Nutrition (Short Term)

At least 400 carbohydrate calories/24 h

For patients with acute renal failure with no urine output and no abnormal losses:

Maintenance	*Equivalent Intravenous Fluid Orders*
Water: 600 mL/24 h	600 mL 20% glucose in water and multivitamins per 24 h
Sodium: 0	
Potassium: 0	

Nutrition (Long Term)

At least 400 carbohydrate calories/24 h

See Table 8.8. if patients have abnormal losses of water and electrolytes.

Monitor patient frequently:

- Weigh daily.
- Measure serum creatinine and electrolyte levels daily or more frequently if necessary.
- Measure CVP or pulmonary wedge pressure in complicated cases. If patient has normal cardiopulmonary function, CVP is sufficient. If cardiac disease or pulmonary hypertension is suspected, pulmonary wedge pressure measurement is preferred.
- Evaluate water and electrolyte needs daily or more frequently in patients with high rates of abnormal losses.

Volume-expanded patients (increased effective IVV)

Correct volume excess:

- Mild (e.g., simple edema): Decrease NaCl intake.
- Moderate (e.g., mild pulmonary vascular congestion): Induce diuresis with diuretic and allow the sodium and water losses to go unreplaced.
- Severe volume excess (e.g., severe pulmonary edema): Steps 1 and 2 and phlebotomy or ultrafiltration (if the patient is anemic) and/or digitalis, vasodilators, if heart disease is present.

Estimate ongoing losses (as above) and begin replacing when volume excesses have been corrected.

Monitor patient frequently.

CVP, central venous pressure; IVV, intravascular volume.

TABLE 10.8

MAJOR SOURCES, LOSS RATES, AND REPLACEMENT FLUIDS IN ABNORMAL WATER AND ELECTROLYTE LOSS

Sources	Rate of loss	Replacement fluid
Fever	Insensible water losses (normally 450 mL/24 h from skin and 450 mL/24 h from lung) increase by about 10% per degree Fahrenheit or 20% per degree Celsius for each degree of temperature above normal.	Replace with 5% dextrose in water
Hyperventilation	Doubling alveolar ventilation (i.e., 50% reduction in $Paco_2$) increases insensible water losses from lung by 50%. Thus, the increase in alveolar ventilation required to reduce $Paco_2$ from 40 to 20 mm Hg increases insensible loss from lung from 450 to 675 mL/24 h.	Replace with 5% dextrose in water
Gastric fluid	Rates of loss from nasogastric suction usually are 1–2 L/24 h but can be much greater. Normal composition of gastric juice is about H^+ 100 mEq/L; sodium 40 mEq/L; potassium 10 mEq/L; and chloride 150 mEq/L.	Replace with 0.45 normal saline and potassium chloride (usually 20–40 mEq/L) as needed[a]
Diarrheal fluid	Losses can vary from trivial to several liters daily. In adults, diarrheal fluid usually resembles extracellular fluid except that the bicarbonate concentration is higher (about 30–50 mEq/L) and chloride concentration is lower (about 80 mEq/L). Potassium concentration is variable (10–40 mEq/L)	Replace with 0.45 normal saline and 50 mEq of sodium bicarbonate/L and potassium chloride (usually 20 mEq/L), as needed[a]
Urine in acute renal failure	Because of tubular injury, urine sodium concentration usually is between 40 and 80 mEq/L and is largely independent of urine flow rate.	Replace with 0.45 normal saline and potassium chloride, as needed[a]

[a]The rate of potassium replacement usually is determined by the serum potassium concentration rather than the rates of potassium loss. For example, even though a patient in acute renal failure may be losing 30 mEq/24 h potassium in the urine, it may not be necessary to replace this amount, since potassium may be entering the extracellular fluid at an even faster rate because of catabolism of cellular proteins. On the other hand, the potassium losses in gastric fluid may amount to only 10 to 20 mEq/24 h, yet far greater amounts of potassium may have to be administered to maintain a normal serum potassium level, since gastric aspiration may lead to metabolic alkalosis, causing renal potassium wasting and extensive diffusion of potassium into intracellular fluid.

The first is the 4–2–1 rule (Table 10.9). A more simplified method of calculation using this formula in adults would be to administer 60 mL/h of fluid for the first 20 kg of body weight. Subtract 20 from the patient's weight (in kg), and add this difference to calculate the hourly rate. For example, a patient who weighs 65 kg has a maintenance requirement of 105 mL/h.

The second method is to calculate the body surface area and multiply by 1,000. A patient with a body surface area of 1.5 m^2 would require 1,500 mL of fluid daily.

TABLE 10.9

MAINTENANCE REQUIREMENTS BY 4-2-1 RULE[a]

Body weight category	Fluid rate (mL/kg)	Weight category (kg)	Fluid (mL/h)
0–10	4	10	40
11–20	2	10	20
21 +	1	40	40

[a]Patient weighs 60 kg. Fluid requirement would be 100 mL/h.

Intraoperative Fluid Administration

The guidelines for fluid replacement during the perioperative period are dictated by (maintenance) basal requirements, deficits, intraoperative losses, and third-space losses. The basal requirement has been discussed. Deficits include actions of general or spinal anesthesia on effective blood volume, intestinal losses (bowel obstruction or diarrhea), perspiration, and blood loss. In some cases, a CVP or Swan-Ganz catheter may be needed to assess IVV.

Intraoperative losses of fluid occur through several routes. Evaporation from peritoneal surfaces occurs, but quantifying it is difficult. The most obvious source of fluid loss, blood loss, is first assessed by looking into the suction canister. Fluid from irrigation should be subtracted. A soaked lap pad contains about 50 mL of blood, and a 4 × 4 pad contains about 5 mL. These are crude approximations. For instance, a moistened lap pad absorbs less than a dry one. Most researchers recommend a replacement rate of 3 to 1 for blood loss using crystalloid suspension and 1 to 1 using colloid suspension. While anesthetized, patients experience third-space loss. This phenomenon is the movement of isotonic fluid from the intravascular space to the interstitial space. A replacement of 2 to 4 mL/kg/h is usually adequate to accommodate third-space losses. Actual total intraoperative losses may be difficult or impossible to monitor

TABLE 10.10

COMPOSITION OF PARENTERAL FLUIDS[a]

Solutions	Cations				Anions		
	Na	K	Ca	Mg	Cl	HCO_3	Osmolality (mOsm)
Extracellular fluid	142	4	5	3	103	27	280–310
Lactated Ringer solution	130	4	3	—	109	28[b]	273
0.9% sodium chloride	154	—	—	—	154	—	308
D_5 45% sodium chloride	77	—	—	—	77	—	407
D_5W	—	—	—	—	—	—	253
3% sodium chloride	513	—	—	—	513	—	1,026

[a]Electrolyte count in mEq/L.
[b] Present in solution as lactate that is converted to bicarbonate.

during long and difficult surgical procedures. Monitoring of vital signs and urine output (optimal, 0.5 mL/kg/h) is extremely important. Sometimes invasive monitoring can be used to guide the clinician.

Crystalloid solutions contain only sugars and electrolytes (Table 10.10). Lactated Ringer solution is usually used because its composition more closely resembles the extracellular component than does normal saline. Generally, solutions that contain less sodium than lactated Ringer solution does should not be used in the perioperative setting. Although D_5W solutions have an osmolality greater than 250, they are unsuitable as routine perioperative replacement because the sugar is metabolized. Normal saline is another popular crystalloid solution. It is preferred over lactated Ringer solutions in the perioperative period when the patient is hyponatremic or if brain injury is present. Hypertonic saline is rarely used in the perioperative setting. Because water tends to follow sodium, its theoretic advantage is that water is drawn into the intravascular space from the interstitial space; hence, smaller volumes of hypertonic solution than isotonic solution are needed to provide the same intravascular expansion. Crystalloid solutions are preferentially used over colloid solutions for perioperative fluid replacement.

Colloid solutions include albumin, hetastarch, and dextran. Blood is also a colloid but is discussed in another chapter. Colloids are used primarily when patients have a low colloid oncotic pressure or when large amounts of crystalloids have been infused. For example, if a patient has suffered a significant protein loss from ascites secondary to pelvic malignancy, colloids should be used early in the fluid replacement process. If a patient's blood pressure becomes difficult to maintain after infusion of sufficient crystalloid, colloids should be used.

Albumin, hetastarch, and dextran are three commonly used colloid solutions. Albumin is the most popular of the colloid solutions. It is a blood product but has the advantage of complete absence of infectious agents. In addition, it is treated with heat, eliminating the possibility of transmission of hepatitis or human immunodeficiency virus (HIV). It comes in 5% and 25% concentrations. Hetastarch consists of large polymer molecules and comes in a solution of saline. It is synthetic; therefore, its use does not affect the blood supply. There is no risk for viral transmission. Hetastarch is metabolized by the kidney and so must be used judiciously in those who have renal disease. Other disadvantages include potential volume overload, dilution hypoproteinemia, and decreased coagulation. The half-life of hetastarch can be as long as 13 days. Dextran is similar to hetastarch in mode of action. Additional problems with this substance are interference with cross matching and histamine release. Dextran and hetastarch should be carefully monitored. Usually no more than 1,500 mL of hetastarch or 1,000 mL of dextran should be infused during a 24-hour period.

In summary, crystalloids should be used primarily for perioperative volume replacement. Colloid solutions should be used under the following conditions:

1. Large amounts of crystalloid are needed to maintain normal hemodynamics.
2. Assessment of circulatory status is difficult.
3. The patient has an elevated pulmonary capillary wedge pressure.
4. The colloid pressure is below 12.

Colloid oncotic pressure may be difficult to ascertain in a routine clinical setting; therefore, total protein or albumin levels can be used to give a rough approximation of colloid pressure. If blood loss is more than 25% of total blood volume (in an otherwise healthy patient), transfusion of red cells must be considered. Hemoglobin concentrations can help. If the patient is elderly or suffers from lung, heart, or renal disease, then the transfusion trigger point is higher.

Experience has shown that hemoglobin levels between 7 and 8 are generally well tolerated in healthy adults. Primate experiments have demonstrated adequate perfusion of tissues with hemoglobin levels of 5 as long as the blood pressure, urine output, and pulse are satisfactory.

Correction of Volume Deficits

Estimating the Magnitude of Sodium or Water Deficits

If the patient has been weighed daily, the magnitude of the water deficit owing to external losses of water can be estimated from the decrease in body weight. The coexisting sodium deficits can be estimated by examining the weight deficits in light of the serum sodium concentration. For example, if the patient has acutely lost 3 kg and the serum sodium concentration is within 10% either way of normal serum sodium concentration (i.e., 126 to 154 mEq/L), little error is incurred by assuming that the patient has lost 3 L of ECF (i.e., isotonic saline); therefore, replacement therapy should be about 3 L of 0.9% saline (155 mEq/L). Using an equivalent amount of lactated Ringer solution offers no advantage, because the kidneys adjust electrolyte excretion to make up for small differences between the composition of the ECF and the isotonic saline.

In patients in whom sodium and water deficits cannot be documented by changes in body weight, or in whom the losses are from the IVV into internal third spaces, approximate but useful guidelines are available to estimate the magnitude of the IVV deficit. These guidelines are as follows.

1. A loss equivalent to 15% of ECF volume (about 2 to 3 L in the average adult) results in a decrease in tissue turgor, but blood pressure and renal function, as judged by serum creatinine level, usually are normal.
2. Losses of sodium and water in excess of 15% of ECF volume usually are accompanied by decreased tissue turgor, orthostatic or frank hypotension, and significant elevation of serum creatinine level.

Correction Rates and Criteria for Assessment

Sodium and water losses great enough to result in hypotension represent a medical emergency, and rapid IV administration of isotonic saline is indicated until the hypotension is reversed. Thereafter, the rate of IV therapy is guided by the adequacy of the IVV as assessed by other criteria, particularly the measurement of blood pressure and pulse in the supine and sitting positions, urine flow rate, and CVP or pulmonary wedge pressure. In patients with less severe degrees of volume depletion, salt and water deficits often can be corrected by increasing oral intake. Salt can be added to food (the salt packets commonly present on hospital trays provide slightly more than 1 g of sodium chloride), or plain sodium chloride tablets can be given, with unrestricted water allowance, letting the patient's thirst mechanism dictate water intake. As a guide to the amount of sodium chloride that should be added to the diet to restore the deficits, 1 L of ECF contains 140 mEq of sodium, or about 9 g of sodium chloride. The adequacy of replacement therapy can be assessed over the ensuing days by measurement of change in body weight and blood pressure and by the decrease in serum creatinine level.

Correction of Volume Excess

Expansion of effective IVV sufficient to precipitate pulmonary edema is a medical emergency and requires the usual treatment of pulmonary edema, including placement of the patient in the sitting position or elevation of the head of the bed and administration of oxygen, vasodilators—such as nitrates, hydralazine, or angiotensin-converting enzyme inhibitors (e.g., captopril, enalapril, lisinopril)—digitalis, and loop diuretics, as needed. If the pulmonary edema does not improve, then phlebotomy may be required to relieve the vascular congestion. If the volume excess is less severe (e.g., simple edema), the problem usually can be controlled by decreasing salt intake, adding a diuretic drug, or both. The effectiveness of treatment can be guided by the decrease in body weight and periodic measurement of serum electrolyte and creatinine levels.

Correction of Hyponatremia

The approach to the correction of hyponatremia depends on (a) whether the patient has significant CNS symptoms as a result of the hyponatremia (coma or seizures) and (b) the cause of the hyponatremia. If the patient has coma or seizures as a result of hyponatremia, the serum sodium level is commonly below 125 mEq/L and the reduction usually has occurred rapidly, over a few hours to days. In these situations, regardless of the cause of the hyponatremia, the serum sodium level should be rapidly raised toward normal by the IV administration of 3% saline. The serum sodium level should be raised to 125 mEq/L at a rate of 1 to 2 mEq/h. The rate of replacement can be slowed once the serum sodium level reaches 125 mEq/L, because neurologic symptoms are rare above this concentration. Rapid elevation of the serum sodium concentration to normal or hypernatremic levels must be avoided, because it may cause central pontine myelinolysis. The correction using 3% saline (513 mEq/L) can be calculated as follows:

$$\text{volume TBW} = 0.6\text{H total body weight in kg}$$
$$\text{volume TBW} \times (\text{desired } [Na^+] - \text{actual } [Na^+]) = \text{total } Na^+ (\text{mEq})$$

where:

$[Na^+]$ is expressed in mEq/L; and TBW = total body water.

The total amount of sodium required can then be replaced at a rate of 2 mEq/h using hypertonic saline. For example, if a 71-kg woman with neurologic symptoms has a serum sodium level of 113 mEq/L, correction to a serum sodium level of 125 mEq/L can be achieved as follows:

$$\text{volume TBW} = 0.6 \times 71 = 42.6$$
$$42.6 \times (125 - 113) = 511 \text{ mEq } Na^+$$

Therefore, this patient requires 1 L of 3% saline to raise her serum sodium level by 12 mEq. The liter of hypertonic saline is administered over 6 to 12 hours. Serum electrolyte levels should be checked every few hours and rates of replacement readjusted as necessary. The infusion of hypertonic saline results in diffusion of water from ICF to ECF until isosmotic conditions are restored. This results in reduction of cell volume and an increase of ICF osmolality toward normal as well as in an expansion of ECF volume. The expansion of the ECF by the hypertonic saline may precipitate or worsen CHF. Therefore, patients who receive hypertonic saline should be carefully observed for signs of pulmonary edema and, if such signs are present, vigorously treated with a loop diuretic.

Hyponatremia Associated with Volume Depletion

The administration of isotonic saline in amounts sufficient to replace existing sodium deficits usually results in complete correction of the hyponatremia, as discussed, in connection with the treatment of volume depletion, because restoration of effective IVV toward normal allows a water diuresis. If specific disease states, such as adrenal insufficiency or diarrhea, are associated with the development of the hyponatremia and volume depletion, these also require treatment.

Hyponatremia Associated with Normal Intravascular Volume

If the hyponatremia is associated with excessive intake of water, restricting water intake to normal corrects the problem. If the hyponatremia is owing to an inappropriate antidiuresis, water intake must be restricted below normal—for example, to about 800 mL of measured liquid intake daily in an average-sized adult (Table 10.2). This usually results in negative water balance, a fall in body weight, and a rise in serum sodium concentration toward normal. Excess total body water can be calculated as follows:

$$\text{actual TBW} = 0.6 \times \text{total body weight in kg}$$
$$\frac{\text{actual serum } [Na^+] \times \text{actual TBW}}{\text{desired serum } [Na^+]} = \text{desired TBW}$$
$$\text{actual TBW} - \text{desired TBW} = \text{excess TBW in L}$$

where:

$[Na^+]$ is expressed in mEq/L.

If a specific cause for the inappropriate antidiuresis can be identified, it should be eliminated (Table 10.6).

Hyponatremia Associated with Expanded Intravascular Volume and Extracellular Fluid

The spontaneous development of hyponatremia in the course of severe congestive heart or liver failure is an ominous sign. The hyponatremia usually does not cause any clinical symptoms, and although it can be successfully treated by water restriction, clinical improvement usually does not follow. Furthermore, during such treatment, patients complain bitterly of thirst. Thus, water restriction sufficient to raise the serum sodium concentration to normal is not indicated. Water intake should be restricted, however, to prevent the serum sodium concentration from decreasing to less than 120 mEq/L in an effort to prevent possible CNS symptoms of hyponatremia.

Correction of Hypernatremia

Hypernatremia Secondary to Water Depletion

The amount of water needed to correct the serum sodium concentration toward normal is given in the following equation:

$$\text{actual TBW} = 0.6 \times \text{total body weight in kg}$$
$$\text{actual serum } [Na^+] \times \text{actual TBW}$$
$$\text{desired serum } [Na^+] = \text{desired TBW}$$
$$\text{desired TB} - \text{actualTBW}$$
$$= \text{water necessary to lower serum } [Na^+]$$

where:

$[Na^+]$ is expressed in mEq/L.

The rate of correction usually is 1 to 2 mEq/h. This deficit usually would be corrected with administration of hypotonic fluid over 24 to 48 hours along with the water and electrolytes needed to maintain day-to-day water and electrolyte balance. The underlying cause of the hypernatremia also must be corrected if possible.

Hypernatremia Secondary to Excessive Administration of Hypertonic Saline

In the rare instance of hypernatremia secondary to excessive administration of hypertonic saline, which occurs when intraamniotic infusion of hypertonic saline is used to induce abortion, hypernatremia is owing solely to positive sodium chloride balance. Therefore, treatment involves simply inducing a state of negative sodium chloride balance while maintaining a slightly positive water balance. If the hypernatremia is associated with impairment of CNS function (Na^+ usually exceeds 160 mEq/L), 2 to 3 L of 5% solution of glucose in water should rapidly be given IV, along with sufficient furosemide to induce a urine flow rate of about 10 to 20 mL/min. About 100 mg of IV furosemide is an appropriate initial dose. This results in the excretion of urine containing about 140 mEq/L of sodium and chloride and 10 mEq/L of potassium. If, at the same time, only the water and potassium are replaced (e.g., replacement of each 1,000 mL of urine with 1,000 mL of 5% solution of glucose in water plus 10 to 20 mEq of potassium chloride, given IV), the patient is selectively depleted of sodium chloride, and plasma electrolytes can be restored to normal within several hours. During this period of correction, serum and urine electrolyte levels must be monitored frequently to assess the adequacy of IV replacement therapy, particularly the rate of potassium administration.

POTASSIUM METABOLISM

Disorders of potassium metabolism frequently coexist with disorders of sodium and water balance. For example, sodium and potassium losses often accompany gastrointestinal losses of water and electrolytes. The recognition and management of potassium depletion under these circumstances were discussed earlier in connection with the management of disorders of sodium and water balance. Even small movements of potassium into and out of cells can cause significant changes in the serum potassium since more than 90% of potassium resides intracellularly. It also is important to recognize disorders in which disturbances of potassium balance are the primary abnormality or the major feature of the electrolyte disturbances.

Hyperkalemia

Hyperkalemia is defined as a serum potassium level greater than 5 mEq/L. Serum potassium levels between 5 and 6 mEq/L usually cause little or no functional abnormality, but such levels indicate that an abnormality of potassium regulation is present. This sign should be heeded and its cause investigated, because further small elevations in serum potassium concentration can seriously impair cardiac and skeletal muscle function. At a serum potassium level of 6 or 7 mEq/L, the electrocardiogram (ECG) begins to show tall, peaked T waves, and skeletal muscle weakness may be present. At a serum potassium level greater than 7 mEq/L, severe ECG abnormalities may be present, including complete suppression of atrial activity and an idioventricular rhythm that can then lead to ventricular tachycardia and fibrillation. Profound skeletal muscle weakness leading to respiratory arrest also may develop. If serious hyperkalemia is suspected, an ECG should be obtained immediately along with a blood specimen for potassium measurement. The ECG findings establish whether life-threatening hyperkalemia is present. Table 10.11 lists the principal clinical conditions associated with hyperkalemia.

Pseudohyperkalemia can result from hemolysis of red blood cells as a result of the mechanical trauma of venipuncture. Such pseudohyperkalemia should be readily recognized, because both potassium and hemoglobin are released by the damaged cells. If the serum potassium level has been significantly raised by *in vitro* hemolysis, the serum is visibly pink because of the presence of free hemoglobin. Patients with extraordinarily high white blood cell counts or platelet counts also can exhibit pseudohyperkalemia as the result of excessive traumatic *in vitro* lysis of these cells. Pseudohyperkalemia can be avoided by drawing venous blood samples under low pressure into a heparinized syringe.

Management

Life-Threatening Hyperkalemia. ECG shows sine waves or loss of atrial activity and a broad QRS complex. Serum potassium level usually is higher than 7 mEq/L.

1. Infuse 10 mL of 10% calcium gluconate intravenously over a few minutes with ECG monitoring to observe for reversal of ECG changes toward normal. The same infusion of 10 mL of 10% calcium gluconate can be repeated once. Calcium ion directly antagonizes the effects of potassium on

TABLE 10.11

CAUSES OF HYPERKALEMIA

Cause	Effect
Excessive intake of potassium Transfusion of blood stored for prolonged periods	Shortened life span of stored RBCs after transfusion leads to excessive release of RBC potassium to ECF. Plasma potassium of stored blood also is increased (30 mEq/L) after 14 days of storage.
Excessive oral or intravenous intake of potassium	Acute ingestion of 500 mEq potassium chloride can cause fatal hyperkalemia with normal renal function. If renal function is impaired, even normal potassium intake can cause severe hyperkalemia.
Excessive release of intracellular stores of potassium Chemotherapy of malignancies Catabolism of hematomas Rhabdomyolysis Succinylcholine action on muscle Sepsis with excessive catabolism of muscle protein Acute digitalis poisoning Familial hyperkalemic periodic paralysis Intravenous hypertonic glucose or mannitol Intravenous arginine	The potential for any of these conditions to cause serious hyperkalemia is greatly increased when they coexist with impaired renal function.
Metabolic acidosis	H^+ displaces K^+ from intracellular sites, causing increased diffusion of K^+ into ECF.
Impaired renal capacity to excrete potassium Grossly reduced glomerular filtration rate	Almost all of filtered potassium is reabsorbed. Excreted potassium represents almost exclusively potassium secreted by the tubules. Nevertheless, grossly reduced glomerular filtration rate is associated with grossly reduced tubular function and hence the tendency to hyperkalemia.
Impaired tubular function Hyperkalemic renal tubular acidosis	Some patients with normal or mildly reduced glomerular filtration rate can have substantial impairment of potassium secretion (e.g., lupus patients with interstitial nephritis, mild obstructive uropathy)
Decreased aldosterone secretion Addison's disease Primary hypoaldosteronism	Alosterone is necessary for normal potassium and H^+ secretion and normal Na^+ absorption in the distal renal tubule.
Hyporeninemic hypoaldosteronism	Common in patients with diabetes mellitus or obstructive uropathy.
Drugs that suppress angiotension formation β-blocking agents (e.g., propranolol) Prostaglandin synthetase inhibitors (e.g., indomethacin, ibuprofen) Angiotensin-converting enzyme inhibitors (e.g., captopril, enalapril, lisinopril)	Angiotensin II causes aldosterone secretion; β-blockers and nonsteroidal antiinflammatory drugs directly suppress angiotensin formation by suppressing renin production. Captopril prevents angiotensin II formation by blocking conversion of angiotensin I.
Drugs that interfere with renal potassium secretion	Spironolactone competitively inhibits the action of aldosterone. Triamterene and amiloride block potassium secretion even in the absence of aldosterone.
Ureteral implantation into jejunal loop	Increased reabsorption of potassium from jejunum causes predisposition to hyperkalemia.

ECF, extracellular fluid; RBCs, red blood cells.

myocardial metabolism. The onset of action is a few minutes. If the patient is taking digitalis, consider not giving the calcium, and proceed on to the next step.

2. Infuse 50 g of glucose, 10 units of regular insulin, and 50 mEq of sodium bicarbonate. The onset of action is about 15 minutes. Additionally, an IV infusion of glucose, insulin, and sodium bicarbonate (e.g., 500 mL of 10% dextrose in water plus 15 units of regular insulin plus 50 mEq of sodium bicarbonate) may be started. Infuse over several hours. This maneuver causes potassium to move intracellularly. The amount of glucose infused must be altered or omitted in hyperglycemic diabetic patients.
3. Nebulized albuterol at a dose of 10 to 20 mg is recommended. The peak action is approximately 90 minutes.
4. As soon as practical, give sodium polystyrene sulfonate (Kayexalate) by mouth, nasogastric tube, or retention enema (e.g., 20 to 50 g of Kayexalate every 2 to 4 hours). An equal number of grams of sorbitol should be given if the Kayexalate is administered into the upper gastrointestinal tract. Sorbitol, a sugar that is poorly absorbed from the intestine, causes an osmotic diarrhea and prevents concretions of Kayexalate from forming within the gut. Kayexalate is an ion-exchange resin that removes potassium by binding potassium and releasing sodium into body fluids.

5. Hemodialysis may be required in patients in whom these measures fail.

Moderate Hyperkalemia. ECG shows only peaked T waves; serum potassium level usually is below 7 mEq/L.

1. Reduce potassium intake (normal potassium intake is 60 to 100 mEq/24 h). Reducing dietary potassium to 50 to 60 mEq/24 h usually is sufficient to correct mild hyperkalemia.
2. Kayexalate may be needed periodically to control the serum potassium level.
3. Correct metabolic acidosis if present.
4. Stop administration of medications that can contribute to hyperkalemia, such as angiotensin-converting enzyme inhibitors, nonsteroidal antiinflammatory drugs, and potassium-sparing diuretics.

Hypokalemia

Hypokalemia is defined as a serum potassium level below 3.5 mEq/L (Table 10.12). Significant symptoms usually do not result from hypokalemia unless the serum potassium level is less than 3 mEq/L. An important exception is in patients who are receiving digitalis preparations. In such patients, hypokalemia, or

TABLE 10.12

CAUSES OF HYPOKALEMIA

Cause	Comments on pathogenesis
Decreased potassium intake	With 0 mEq potassium intake, stool potassium is about 10 mEq/2 h, urinary potassium is <30 mEq/24 h or is <20 mEq/L.
Excessive renal losses of potassium	Urinary potassium usually greater than 30 mEq/24 h or 20 mEq/L.
Diuretic therapy	All diuretics except for spironolactone, triameterene, and amiloride cause renal potassium wasting. *Mechanism*: Diuretics cause increased sodium delivery to distal tubular sites where sodium is reabsorbed in exchange for potassium or hydrogen ion.
Diuretic phase of acute tubular necrosis and other causes of osmotic diuresis	*Mechanism*: Same as above.
Metabolic alkalosis	*Mechanism*: Renal tubular cell potassium concentration increased resulting in enhanced potassium secretion.
Gentamicin or amphotericin B nephrotoxicity	Renal tubular damage presumably causes increased back flux of potassium into renal tubules in the case of amphotericin.
Increased renal mineralicorticoid effects	Increased activity of distal tubular site, which reabsorbs sodium in exchange for potassium or H^+.
Mineralocorticoid therapy (DOCA, 9 α-fluodrocortisone)	
Primary aldosteronism	
Secondary aldosteronism (e.g., cirrhosis of the liver, renal artery stenosis, malignant hypertension)	
Cushing's syndrome	
Excessive licorice or chewing tobacco (glycyrrhizic acid)	
Bartter's syndrome	
Renal tubular acidosis	*Mechanism*: Distal: Possibly increased renal potassium secretion in exchange for sodium at the distal tubular site because of decreased availability of H^+ for secretion Proximal: Increased bicarbonate excretion leads to increased renal potassium excretion.
Excessive gastrointestinal losses of potassium	
Vomiting, gastric drainage, diarrhea, laxative abuse	Renal potassium excretion also increased in the case of vomiting or gastric drainage.
Villous adenoma of rectum	Loss of potassium-rich mucus per rectum
Shift of potassium from the extracellular to the intracellular fluid	
Correction of metabolic acidosis	H^+ leaves cells, K^+ enters cells during correction of metabolic acidosis.
Correction of hyperglycemia	K^+ enters cells with glucose to provide cation to balance anion that forms during metabolism of glucose
Hypokalemic periodic paralysis	Unexplained familial disorder
Miscellaneous	
Ureterosigmoidostomy	Colonic secretion of HCO_3^- and K^+ with absorption of Na^+ and Cl^- results in hypokalemic metabolic acidosis.

even low-normal serum potassium levels, can increase myocardial irritability and lead to serious arrhythmias. In addition to increasing myocardial irritability, hypokalemia can cause profound muscle weakness and ileus. Chronic severe hypokalemia also can cause metabolic alkalosis and decreased capacity to concentrate the urine. The ECG in hypokalemia often shows U waves, although this finding is not diagnostic of hypokalemia.

Management

Mild Asymptomatic Hypokalemia. This usually can be corrected simply by eliminating the cause of the potassium wasting or by increasing potassium intake. If the hypokalemia is caused by diuretic therapy, potassium depletion usually can be avoided by administering spironolactone or triamterene. Potassium supplementation also can be used, but if the patient is on a low sodium chloride intake, the potassium supplement must be given as potassium chloride. The use of other, more palatable potassium salts (e.g., gluconate, citrate, acetate) and all forms of potassium in food is much less effective in correcting hypokalemia, and this treatment is used primarily in patients on a normal sodium chloride intake.

Severe or Symptomatic Hypokalemia. This usually requires IV administration of potassium chloride. In general, the use of IV solutions that contain more than 40 mEq/L of potassium should be avoided, because infusing high concentrations of potassium can cause hyperkalemia or cardiac disturbance. In correcting even severe potassium deficits, it is seldom necessary to infuse more than 120 to 160 mEq/24 h of potassium chloride. When higher rates are used, frequent monitoring of the patient's ECG and serum potassium level is essential. Intravenous replacement of potassium should never run at a rate of greater than 10 mEq/h. The oral route of potassium replacement should be used whenever possible.

Calcium

Approximately 99% of body calcium is contained in bone. Up to 40% of the extracellular calcium that circulates in the bloodstream is bound to plasma proteins. However, the unbound or ionized form of calcium is the form that exerts physiologic activity. Total calcium is a measure of both the bound and unbound or ionized form. Serum albumin levels affect the total serum calcium, as albumin is the plasma protein to which the majority of calcium is bound.

$$\text{corrected calcium in mg/dL} = \text{measured calcium} + [(4 - \text{albumin in g/dL}) \times 0.8]$$

Ionized or unbound calcium can be measured if specifically requested. Its concentration is affected by the serum pH. With alkalosis when the pH is increased, a decrease in ionized calcium results from the increased protein binding of calcium. Conversely, with acidosis, a decrease in protein binding causes an increase in ionized calcium.

The homeostasis of calcium is quite complex, and calcium serves many important functions. Calcium plays a role in regulation of muscle contraction and nerve conduction. Additionally, it functions in the coagulation cascade. The majority of calcium is stored in bone; however, calcium is under the control of several other organ systems, including the integument, endocrine, and renal. Parathyroid hormone (PTH) appears to be the major hormone effecting calcium homeostasis. Vitamin D must be present, however, for it to exert its maximal effect. PTH causes the following.

- Mobilization of calcium and phosphorus from bone
- Increased renal tubular reabsorption of calcium
- Increased intestinal absorption of calcium
- Decreased renal tubular reabsorption of phosphorus

Hypocalcemia

Clinical manifestations of hypocalcemia (defined as a calcium level below 8 to 8.5 mg/dL) are characterized by neuromuscular irritability. Symptoms can include numbness, muscle cramping, paresthesias, Chvostek (twitching of facial muscles) and Trousseau (carpal spasm) signs, tetany, and seizures. Patients can also experience psychosis and memory loss. On physical examination, patients may have hyperactive deep tendon reflexes. ECG findings of hypocalcemia include a prolonged QT interval, which can lead to heart block or ventricular fibrillation. Causes of hypocalcemia are shown in Table 10.13.

Treatment of hypocalcemia should be directed at its underlying cause. A low total calcium level with a normal ionized calcium level signifies a low level of plasma proteins. These patients usually are asymptomatic, and calcium replacement in this setting usually is not necessary.

For patients with acute symptomatic hypocalcemia, calcium gluconate or chloride should be given intravenously. These may cause a local cellulitis or tissue necrosis if infiltration occurs. If infiltration occurs, especially with the chloride solution in emergent situations, 10 mL of 10% calcium gluconate can be administered intravenously over 15 minutes. In addition, 10 to 20 mL of calcium gluconate can be placed in 1 L of D_5W and administered over 24 hours. If the serum albumin level is below 2 mg/dL, then it may be prudent to replace albumin, especially if the urine output is low. Because albumin is heat treated, there is no risk of hepatitis or HIV exposure. In cases of symptomatic hypocalcemia, magnesium levels must be checked and corrected if necessary. In those patients with metabolic acidosis and hypocalcemia, the hypocalcemia should be treated initially followed by the correction of the acidosis.

Long-term treatment of hypocalcemia involves adequate nutritional supplementation of calcium, vitamin D, or both. If the serum phosphorus level is high, hypoparathyroid disease must be suspected and the patient treated accordingly. If the serum phosphorus is normal or low, then primary bone disease (hungry bone) must be considered. It is imperative that magnesium levels be checked because replenishment of calcium cannot be accomplished in a patient who is hypomagnesemic.

Hypercalcemia

The clinical manifestations of hypercalcemia usually are seen when the total serum calcium is greater than 12 mg/dL. Common presenting symptoms include weakness, fatigue, nausea, vomiting, constipation, polyuria, polydipsia, lethargy, and confusion. Psychiatric disturbances and coma can be seen in severe

TABLE 10.13

CAUSES OF HYPOCALCEMIA

Deficiency or absence of parathyroid hormone
Vitamin D deficiency—decreased intestinal absorption
Septic shock—suppression of parathyroid hormone products
Renal failure—decreased 1:25 dihydroxycholecalciferol
Hypomagnesemia—decreased parathyroid hormone release and decreased organ response to calcium
Hyperphosphatemia

cases of hypercalcemia. ECG changes include prolongation of PR and QRS intervals with a shortening of the QT interval. Complete heart block and cardiac arrest can occur in profound hypercalcemia. Additional laboratory abnormalities can include elevations in serum amylase and creatinine levels. The phosphorus level is critical in establishing the cause of hypercalcemia. A phosphorus level below 3.5 mg/dL suggests hyperparathyroidism, whereas an elevated phosphorus level suggests an underlying malignancy.

Hypercalcemia, unlike many other electrolyte disturbances, is rarely iatrogenically induced. There are several causes of hypercalcemia. The majority of hospitalized patients with hypercalcemia have an underlying malignancy, whereas the most common etiology of hypercalcemia in the ambulatory setting is hyperparathyroidism. Additional causes of hypercalcemia include thiazide diuretics, lithium, vitamin D intoxication, hyperthyroidism, and sarcoidosis. In the setting of gynecology, hypercalcemia is most often seen with malignancy. In patients with cancer, hypercalcemia results from increased bone resorption and decreased renal excretion. Metastasis to the bony skeleton causes an increase in osteoclastic activity that increases bone resorption. Some gynecologic tumors, however, may cause hypercalcemia by production of a substance similar to PTH, causing bone resorption without evidence of bony metastasis.

Volume expansion is crucial in the treatment of acute hypercalcemia. Replacement with normal saline solution decreases calcium reabsorption in the proximal renal tubule, thus improving renal function. Initial IV fluid therapy should be aggressive, with rates of 250 to 500 mL/h, as most patients are volume contracted. Addition of loop diuretics such as furosemide may aid in increasing urinary calcium excretion, but caution must be used because these drugs may result in volume contraction and hypokalemia. After initial volume is restored, 3 to 6 L/d of normal saline solution should be given. Close monitoring of daily patient weights, intake and output, and frequent monitoring of serum electrolytes is necessary in patients with hypercalcemia.

Bisphosphates are commonly used for the treatment of hypercalcemia. This class of drugs inhibits osteoclast precursors and induces osteoclast cytotoxicity, thereby decreasing serum calcium levels. Etidronate disodium (Didronel) is given at a dose of 7.5 mg/kg IV over 2 hours daily for 3 to 7 days. Alternatively, pamidronate (Aredia) is given as a single dose of 60 to 90 mg IV over 4 to 24 hours. Peak onset of action with these medications is usually seen in 48 to 96 hours and may last 2 to 3 weeks. The single dose of 90 mg IV of pamidronate is recommended for severe cases of hypercalcemia because of its effectiveness.

Zoledronic acid (Zometa) is a new-generation, nitrogen-containing bisphosphonate that has been shown to be superior to pamidronate at inhibiting the induction of hypercalcemia of malignancy. Zometa can be given over 5 minutes in a 4-mg dose for the initial treatment of hypercalcemia and an 8-mg dose for relapsed or refractory hypercalcemia. The duration of response with zoledronic acid is approximately 32 days with a 4-mg dose and 43 days with a 8-mg dose compared with 18 days with a 90-mg dose of pamidronate.

Calcitonin increases renal excretion of calcium and inhibits osteoclastic activity. In patients with hypercalcemia, calcitonin can be given at a dose of 4 to 8 IU/kg intramuscularly (IM) or subcutaneously (SC) every 6 to 12 hours. Commercial calcitonin preparations are generally from salmon. It has a rapid onset of action, and serum calcium levels may decrease within several hours. Its effect usually subsides after several days but may be potentiated by concomitant glucocorticoid administration. Calcitonin has minimal side effects. Tachyphylaxis is seen with calcitonin, limiting its repeated usage and causing it to be less consistently effective compared with other available hypercalcemic treatments.

Glucocorticoids decrease the intestinal absorption of calcium, promote urinary excretion of calcium, and may lower calcium levels by a direct cytolytic effect on some tumor cells. Lowering of serum calcium levels with glucocorticoids may take 5 to 10 days. Dosages may vary from 20 to 100 mg of oral prednisone or its IV equivalent per day. Side effects limit the long-term use of glucocorticoids for hypercalcemia.

Another potent inhibitor of bone resorption is gallium nitrate. Its onset of action is usually seen in 1 to 2 days, with a peak at 5 to 10 days after administration. Gallium nitrate is administered in a dose of 100 to 200 mg/kg per day for 5 days in a continuous drip. It is important to maintain a saline diuresis of at least 2 L/d during this therapy. Side effects are relatively uncommon, but renal toxicity may be seen. Gallium nitrate in early studies was significantly more effective than calcitonin with or without the addition of corticosteroids. Its obvious disadvantage over the biphosphates is that it requires continuous IV infusion over 4 or 5 days.

Oral and IV phosphorus has been used successfully to treat hypercalcemia. It has fallen out of favor, however, because it causes decreased excretion of calcium from the kidneys. Intravenous phosphorus can also lead to soft-tissue deposition of calcium compounds and renal failure. It was used in patients with serum phosphorus levels less than 3 mg/dL and normal renal function. For patients with extremely high calcium levels and severe symptoms (e.g., coma, arrhythmia), renal dialysis may be necessary for rapid correction of hypercalcemia.

Plicamycin (Mithramycin) is an antibiotic that blocks bone resorption, thus lowering serum calcium. The recommended dose of plicamycin in the treatment of hypercalcemia is 25 mg/kgIV over 4 to 6 hours and may be repeated every 24 to 48 hours. Its onset of action is relatively quick, and peak action is usually noted in 2 to 3 days. Side effects can be severe and include nausea, vomiting, bleeding, thrombocytopenia, renal failure, and hepatotoxicity. These side effects are more common with repeated doses of plicamycin. Because of these side effects, plicamycin usually is reserved for hypercalcemia of malignancy or hypercalcemia refractory to other therapies.

Magnesium

Magnesium has several functions in the human body. Its primary role is in neuromuscular function, but it also serves as an enzyme cofactor in protein and carbohydrate metabolism. The majority (60%) of magnesium in the body is contained within the bone. Most of the remainder is found intracellularly, with only about 1% found in the extracellular fluid. Normal serum magnesium levels are between 1.2 and 2.2 mEq/L. Magnesium metabolism depends on potassium and calcium levels. The kidney serves as the organ primarily responsible for magnesium homeostasis. Magnesium is filtered at the glomerulus and reabsorbed in the ascending loop of Henle and to a lesser degree in the proximal and distal tubules.

Hypomagnesemia

Hypomagnesemia is more common than hypermagnesemia. Hypomagnesemia results from decreased gastrointestinal absorption with conditions such as chronic diarrhea, malabsorption syndromes, and nasogastric suction. Increased renal and gastrointestinal losses from osmotic diuresis, hypercalcemia, and medications such as cisplatin, diuretics, and aminoglycosides also can cause hypomagnesemia. Hypomagnesemia can result from decreased intake in malnutrition. For example, 10% to 15% of hospitalized patients and more than half of patients in intensive care units exhibit low magnesium levels. Lastly, patients with heavy alcohol use may have hypomagnesemia.

Symptoms and signs of hypomagnesemia are usually nonspecific but may be manifested by neuromuscular excitability. Hypomagnesemia is often seen in combination with hypokalemia, hypocalcemia, and metabolic alkalosis. Neurologic abnormalities include weakness, dizziness, lethargy, confusion, tremors, fasciculations, and seizures. Typical ECG findings are prolonged PR and QT intervals; however, atrial and ventricular arrhythmias can result.

The treatment of hypomagnesemia involves the replacement of magnesium. Mild or chronic cases may be treated with oral magnesium supplements. Oral repletion is also preferred in asymptomatic patients. This is accomplished by giving 240 mg of elemental magnesium one to four times a day. Diarrhea is the most common side effect. For severe or acute cases, IV magnesium is indicated. Obstetricians and gynecologists are familiar with the 4-g magnesium load mixed with 50 mL of D_5W to infuse over 30 minutes. Deep tendon reflexes should be evaluated frequently because hyperreflexia suggests hypermagnesemia. Long-term oral therapy can be provided with magnesium oxide, 300 mg/d. Patients should receive proper nutritional counseling and be warned to avoid alcohol. Any underlying medical disorder that may contribute to magnesium losses should be treated. Hydration status should be evaluated because overhydration can lead to mild forms of hypomagnesemia. Gastrointestinal tract losses and alcohol consumption also should be addressed in the evaluation of this disease process.

Hypermagnesemia

Hypermagnesemia is rare and usually iatrogenic. Causes of hypermagnesemia include therapy with magnesium-containing antacids or laxatives or secondary to administration of parenteral hyperalimentation. Often hypermagnesemia is seen in patients with some degree of renal insufficiency. Lastly, it can be seen in preeclamptic or preterm labor patients treated with IV magnesium.

Mild to moderate hypermagnesemia usually is asymptomatic, but patients with severe cases may present with several symptoms. Clinical manifestations are normally seen if magnesium levels are greater than 4 mEq/L. Signs and symptoms include nausea, vomiting, weakness, lethargy, and somnolence. A prolonged PR interval, widening of the QRS complex, and increased T-wave amplitude can be seen with levels greater than 5 mEq/L. Areflexia occurs at levels above 6 to 7 mEq/L. Respiratory arrest, bradycardia, and hypotension can be seen when levels are higher than 10 to 11 mEq/L. Finally, cardiac arrest can occur when serum magnesium is above 14 mEq/L.

Discontinuation of magnesium intake is the primary therapy for symptomatic hypermagnesemia. Patients with severe cases should be given 10% calcium gluconate, 10 to 20 mL IV over 10 minutes. The calcium therapy antagonizes the effects of magnesium and is cardioprotective. Supportive therapy and mechanical ventilation may be necessary in those with respiratory failure. Hemodialysis may be required in patients with hypermagnesemia and renal insufficiency.

Phosphorus

As with magnesium, the majority of phosphorus is contained with the bony skeleton and the intracellular space, and only 1% is found in the extracellular fluid. As a result, serum phosphate levels may not accurately reflect total body phosphate stores. A normal range for serum phosphorus is 3 to 4.5 mg/dL. Phosphorus serves as an important energy source by means of high-energy phosphates. It is a key component to protein and lipid structure, and is a vital component for carbohydrate metabolism.

Hypophosphatemia

Causes of hypophosphatemia defined as a serum phosphate below 2.5 mg/dL include a redistribution of phosphate into the cells, a decrease in intestinal absorption, or an increase in renal excretion. Several causes of hypophosphatemia are listed in Table 10.14. Most patients with mild hypophosphatemia are asymptomatic. Moderate to severe hypophosphatemia causes neuromuscular abnormalities, including weakness, rhabdomyolysis, paresthesias, confusion, seizures, and coma. Erythrocyte, leukocyte, and platelet dysfunction also can be seen because of a depletion of cellular adenosine triphosphate (ATP) and 2,3-diphosphoglycerate.

Most patients with serum phosphate levels between 1 and 2.5 mg/dL usually are asymptomatic. Treatment is aimed at correcting the underlying cause. In cases of chronic hypophosphatemia, oral repletion can be instituted at a dose of 500 to 1,000 mg of elemental phosphorus two to three times per day, and the most common side effect is diarrhea. This can be given in the form of sodium/potassium phosphate tablets called Neutra-Phos or Neutra-Phos K (each contains 250 mg of elemental phosphorus). Parenteral administration of phosphorus is indicated when serum phosphorus levels are below 1 mg/dL. Infusion at a dose of 2.5 to 5 mg elemental phosphorus/kg given every 6 hours is recommended. When the serum levels are greater than 1.5 to 2 mg/dL, patients may be switched to oral supplements. Care must be taken to avoid hyperphosphatemia. Also, concomitant calcium supplementation often is needed to prevent hypocalcemia. Serum magnesium, calcium, and potassium levels should be monitored closely.

Hyperphosphatemia

Hyperphosphatemia is relatively rare and is seen with either an increased endogenous or exogenous phosphorus load or with a decrease in renal clearance of phosphorus. Renal failure is the most common cause of hyperphosphatemia.

TABLE 10.14

CAUSES OF MODERATE TO SEVERE HYPOPHOSPHATEMIA (<1.5 mg/dL)

Respiratory alkalosis
Malabsorption
Vitamin D deficiency
Hyperalimentation
Treatment of diabetic ketoacidosis
Hyperparathyroidism
Excessive alcohol use

TABLE 10.15

PRIMARY DISORDERS OF ACID–BASE REGULATION

Acid-base disturbance	Primary (initiating) event	Secondary (compensatory) event	Resultant change in blood H^+ and pH
Metabolic acidosis	↓ HCO_3^-	↓ Pco_2^-	H^+ ↑, pH ↓
Metabolic alkalosis	↑ HCO_3^-	↑ Pco_2 (Minimal and only with severe increase in HCO_3^-)	H^+ ↓, pH ↑
Respiratory acidosis			
Acute (24 h)	↑ $Paco_2$	Negligible ↑ HCO_3^-	H^+ ↑, pH ↓
Chronic (3-7 days or longer)	↑ $Paco_2$	Important ↑ HCO_3^-	
Respiratory alkalosis	↓ $Paco_2$	↓ HCO_3^-	H^+ ↓, pH ↑

Elevated phosphorus levels also may be seen secondary to rhabdomyolysis, tumor lysis syndrome, hypoparathyroidism, and respiratory or metabolic acidosis. Clinical manifestations include numbness, tingling, muscle cramps, paresthesias, and tetany and are caused by hypocalcemia. Hyperphosphatemia causes hypocalcemia by decreasing calcium absorption from the gastrointestinal tract.

Addressing the underlying cause is the cornerstone of management for hyperphosphatemia. In acute cases, saline diuresis can be used in patients with normal renal function. Additionally, administration of glucose and insulin causes a shift in phosphorus from extracellular fluid to the intracellular space. Dialysis may be required if renal failure is present. Oral phosphate binders such as calcium carbonate can be used in patients with chronic hyperphosphatemia.

ACID–BASE METABOLISM

Chemicals that are able to provide a hydrogen ion (H^+) such as HCl and H_2CO_2 are defined as acids. Bases are defined as chemicals with the ability to accept a (H^+) and include OH^- and HCO_3^-. The acidity of a solution is governed by the concentration of hydrogen ions it contains. The pH of a system is defined as the negative logarithm of hydrogen ions within that system expressed in moles per liter (mol/L). The normal pH of human ECF ranges from 7.35 to 7.45.

Buffer Systems

In order for optimal cellular function to occur within the body, the pH must remain in this range. Humans have the ability to absorb excess acids or alkali in circumstances of abnormal pH. The lungs correct for acid–base disorders in an acute setting until the kidneys can compensate. In acidotic states, patients will hyperventilate to decrease CO_2 levels in the blood. Conversely, in alkalotic states, patients will hypoventilate, driving up the level of CO_2 in the blood. Renal function will gradually compensate by retaining or releasing bicarbonate and hydrogen ions. The most important human buffer system is the bicarbonate system. It is the principal extracellular buffer. This buffer system is described by the Henderson-Hasselbach equation.

$$pH = 6.1 + \log (HCO_3^-)(@[Paco_2])$$

where:

6.1 = pK; @ = 0.03 mmol/L/mm Hg at 38°C (solubility coefficient).

Organic phosphates, bicarbonate, and peptides are the major intracellular buffers.

Table 10.15 shows the directional changes in acid–base parameters for the primary acid–base disorders. If the kidney detects a respiratory acidotic state, CO_2 and H_2O in renal tubule cells are converted by carbonic anhydrase to carbonic acid (H_2CO_3). This dissociates into H_2CO_3, which is secreted back into ECF, and H^+, which is exchanged for sodium from the renal tubule. This in effect causes excretion of the hydrogen ion into the urine, where it is buffered with ammonium and phosphate ions or acted on by carbonic anhydrase (in the tubule) to ultimately form CO_2 and H_2O. The CO_2 is absorbed back into the cell, where more bicarbonate can be generated to buffer ECF acidosis. If a patient has a respiratory alkalosis, available levels of CO_2 are low, causing a decrease in hydrogen excretion. Figure 10.6 shows the expected range of arterial pH, $Paco_2$, and bicarbonate concentrations for primary acid–base disturbances. Figure 10.7 shows a simplified means of determining the acid–base status of patient given pH and $Paco_2$. A line is drawn between the pH and $Paco_2$ lines and extended to the line marked "fixed acids." If the patient has a pH of 7.1 and a $Paco_2$ of 70, she has a respiratory acidosis, because the line

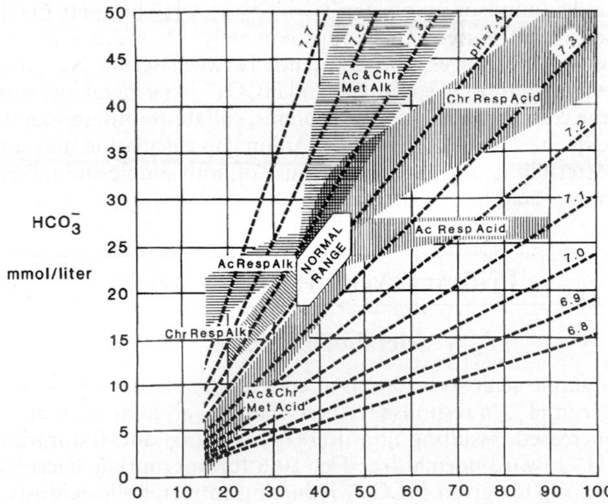

FIGURE 10.6. Range of arterial blood pH, Pco_2, and bicarbonate concentrations in the primary acid–base disturbances. The width of the bands indicates the 95% confidence limits of the range of variable. (From: Arbus GS. An in vivo acid–base nomogram for clinical use. *Can Med Assoc J* 1973;109:291, redrawn and expanded to include chronic respiratory alkalosis, with permission.)

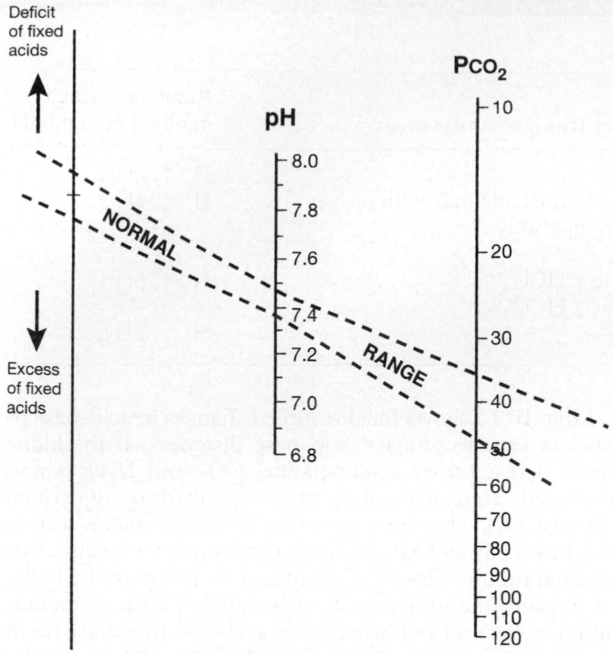

FIGURE 10.7. Normogram for acid–base disturbance.

drawn falls within the normal range of fixed acids. If, however, she has a pH of 7 and a $Paco_2$ of 38, she would have a pure metabolic acidosis with no compensation. A pH of 7.5 with a $Paco_2$ of 27 characterizes a patient with respiratory alkalosis with metabolic compensation.

Anion Gap

The definition of anion gap is = $\{Na^+\} - [\{Cl^-) + HCO_3^-]$. The normal anion gap is approximately 12 ± 2 mEq/L. In most circumstances, the difference between serum Na^+ and the combination of serum Cl^- and HCO_3^- is a general measure of the combination of serum proteins, sulfate anions, inorganic phosphates, and organic acids. Anion gap calculation may aid in determining the underlying cause of both simple and mixed forms of acid/base disturbances.

Primary Acid–Base Disorders

Metabolic Acidosis

Metabolic acidosis begins as a reduction in plasma HCO_3 and a rise in H^+. In response to these changes, alveolar ventilation is increased, resulting in a decrease in $Paco_2$ and restoration of H^+ toward normal (see Fig. 10.6 for appropriate decrease in $Paco_2$ for given HCO_3^- reduction in metabolic acidosis). Metabolic acidosis can be divided into normal anion gap and increased anion gap acidosis. Table 10.16 shows the major causes of metabolic acidosis.

Increased Anion Gap. Renal failure, either acute or chronic, can result in an increased anion gap metabolic acidosis resulting from the kidneys' inability to excrete inorganic acids, such as phosphate and sulfate. Organic acid accumulation also results in an increased anion gap metabolic acidosis. In the case of lactic acidosis, cellular respiration is disturbed. This occurs as a result of anaerobic glycolysis in muscle, red blood cells, and other tissues. Conditions such as shock, hypoxemia, and septicemia can produce lactic acidosis by causing inadequate oxygen delivery to tissues. Conditions such as diabetic ketoacidosis, alcoholic ketoacidosis, and starvation cause an accelerated rate of organic acid production by lipolysis and ketogenesis. Ingestion of substances such as salicylates, methanol, ethylene glycol, and paraldehyde can result in an increased anion gap metabolic acidosis.

TABLE 10.16

MAJOR CAUSES OF METABOLIC ACIDOSIS

Increased Anion Gap
Accumulation of Acids
Alcoholic ketoacidosis
Diabetic ketoacidosis
Lactic acidosis
Starvation
Salicylate ingestion
Methanol ingestion
Ethylene glycol ingestion
Paraldehyde ingestion
Reduced Excretion of Acids
Renal failure
Normal Anion Gap
Excessive Bicarbonate Loss
Diarrhea
Ureterosigmoidostomy
Proximal renal tubular acidosis
Small bowel or pancreatic drainage
Carbonic anhydrase inhibitors
Excessive Acid Production
Ammonium chloride
Arginine HCl
Lysine HCl
Hyperalimentation-containing acids
Decreased Renal Bicarbonate Production
Distal renal tubular acidosis
Hyporeninemic hypoaldosteronism

Normal Anion Gap. Normal anion gap metabolic acidosis occurs with abnormal increases in net bicarbonate losses. This can occur when the kidney fails to reabsorb bicarbonate in proximal renal tubular acidosis. The administration of carbonic anhydrase inhibitors can also cause normal anion gap metabolic acidosis. Excessive diarrhea or small bowel/pancreatic drainage can cause bicarbonate losses from the gastrointestinal tract. Hyperchloremic acidosis occurs when the kidney fails to regenerate bicarbonate in conditions such as distal renal tubular acidosis and hyporeninemic hypoaldosteronism. Lastly, administration of acid salts can result in chloremic acidosis.

MANAGEMENT

The treatment for metabolic acidosis depends on the severity of acidosis and the underlying cause. A clinical manifestation of metabolic acidosis is hyperventilation. In the surgical patient, metabolic acidosis is commonly due to hypoxia secondary to inadequate tissue perfusion and subsequent accumulation of lactic acid. Volume resuscitation, including blood transfusion, will correct many of these cases of metabolic acidosis. Volume resuscitation and insulin are recommended to correct diabetic ketoacidosis. Patients with this form of metabolic acidosis will often require 4 to 5 liters of intravenous fluid on diagnosis. Regular insulin can be given with a loading dose of 15 to 20 IU, followed by a continuous insulin infusion at 5 to 10 IU/h. In cases of renal tubular acidosis, bicarbonate therapy, thiazide diuretics, and a low salt diet are used for correction.

In cases of acute, severe acidosis (pH <7.1, bicarbonate <10), patients will become dyspneic with depressed cardiac function and mental status changes. It may be necessary to administer intravenous bicarbonate to these patients. In general, the serum bicarbonate concentration should not be acutely raised to levels greater than 15 to 18 mEq/L. Too-rapid correction requires infusion of large amounts of sodium bicarbonate, which can cause overexpansion of the ECF and CHF. Finally, rapidly restoring the plasma bicarbonate level to normal may produce alkalosis because of persistence of a low Pa_{CO_2}. That is, if plasma bicarbonate is rapidly restored to normal or above in the treatment of metabolic acidosis, alveolar ventilation frequently persists at elevated levels for an additional 24 to 48 hours. Thus, the low P_{CO_2} with normal plasma bicarbonate level can result in severe alkalosis, which, in turn, can cause cardiac arrhythmias, tetany, and seizures.

Metabolic Alkalosis

Metabolic alkalosis occurs when extracellular bicarbonate concentration is increased and renal excretion of this excess bicarbonate is decreased. This cascade may begin with the loss of a hydrogen ion. The major causes of metabolic alkalosis are listed in Table 10.17.

One of the most common causes of metabolic alkalosis is vomiting or gastric suction. Volume contraction ensues, and bicarbonate is saved in the kidney. Profound potassium depletion can also increase renal reabsorption of bicarbonate and cause a metabolic alkalosis. Diuretics cause a metabolic alkalosis by inducing a sodium chloride excretion without bicarbonate, excretion of potassium, and secondary aldosteronism.

Figure 10.8 depicts the normal handling of HCl and $NaHCO_3$ produced by the gastric mucosa. The initial reactants ($NaCl + H_2CO_3$, step 1) are the same as the final products ($NaCl + H_2CO_3$, step 4). Thus, gastric acid secretion normally has no net effect on acid–base regulation. If the gastric HCl is lost from the body and is not replaced, metabolic alkalosis will ensue (Fig. 10.9).

Mineralocorticoid excess in conditions such as hyperaldosteronism, Bartter syndrome, Liddle syndrome, and Cushing syndrome can cause metabolic alkalosis. The mechanism for alkalosis in these conditions is an increase in bicarbonate via the kidneys. Hypercalcemia can result in an increase in proximal tubular reabsorption of bicarbonate leading to metabolic

Step 1 HCl is formed and enters gastric fluid
Step 2 $NaHCO_3$ is formed and enters body fluids
Step 3 HCl moves to duodenum and reacts with $NaHCO_3$ (from bile or pancreatic fluid)
Step 4 NaCl and H_2CO_3 are formed

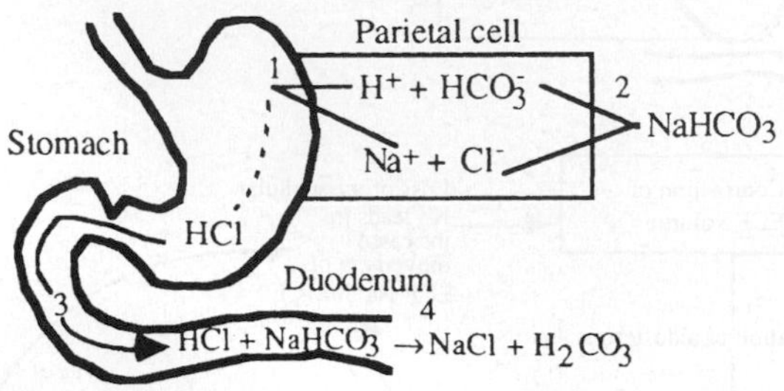

Summation: No net effect on acid-base balance since:
One H^+ and one HCO_3^- are formed in Steps 1 and 2.
One H^+ and one HCO_3^- are destroyed in Step 4.

FIGURE 10.8. Normal disposal of hydrochloric acid and sodium bicarbonate formed by gastric mucosa.

alkalosis. Lastly, massive alkali administration in the form of massive blood and/or platelet transfusion or $NaHCO_3$ ingestion can lead to metabolic alkalosis.

Management

Metabolic alkalosis can have serious consequences, such as tetany, major motor seizures, production of hypokalemia and cardiac arrhythmias (particularly in patients receiving digitalis), suppression of alveolar ventilation, and decrease in cerebral blood flow. Furthermore, the presence of metabolic alkalosis often is a sign that the patient is significantly volume contracted. For these reasons, it is important to treat metabolic alkalosis and its underlying causes. Effective treatment consists of replacing sodium, potassium, and chloride deficits as they occur, as discussed. Rarely, it is necessary to treat metabolic alkalosis with IV infusion of hydrochloric acid, ammonium chloride, arginine hydrochloride, or a carbonic anhydrase inhibitor (acetazolamide). This form of treatment is necessary in patients who cannot undergo the sodium bicarbonate diuresis necessary to correct the metabolic alkalosis. This inability usually is the result of severely impaired renal or cardiac function.

TABLE 10.17

MAJOR CAUSES OF METABOLIC ALKALOSIS

Extracellular volume depletion
Mineralocorticoid excess
Increased renal acid excretion
Massive alkali administration

Respiratory Acidosis

Inadequate alveolar ventilation leads to respiratory acidosis. Acutely, this can occur with depression of the medullary respiratory center by sedating drugs or narcotics, impaired respiratory excursion of the thorax by paralysis or trauma, and by airway obstruction. Chronic respiratory acidosis can be seen in conditions such as emphysema, severe kyphoscoliosis, and extreme obesity with Pickwickian syndrome.

Management

The treatment for respiratory acidosis is to increase alveolar ventilation (by endotracheal intubation, mechanical ventilation, or bronchodilation). Within minutes, severe respiratory acidosis can be reversed with adequate ventilation.

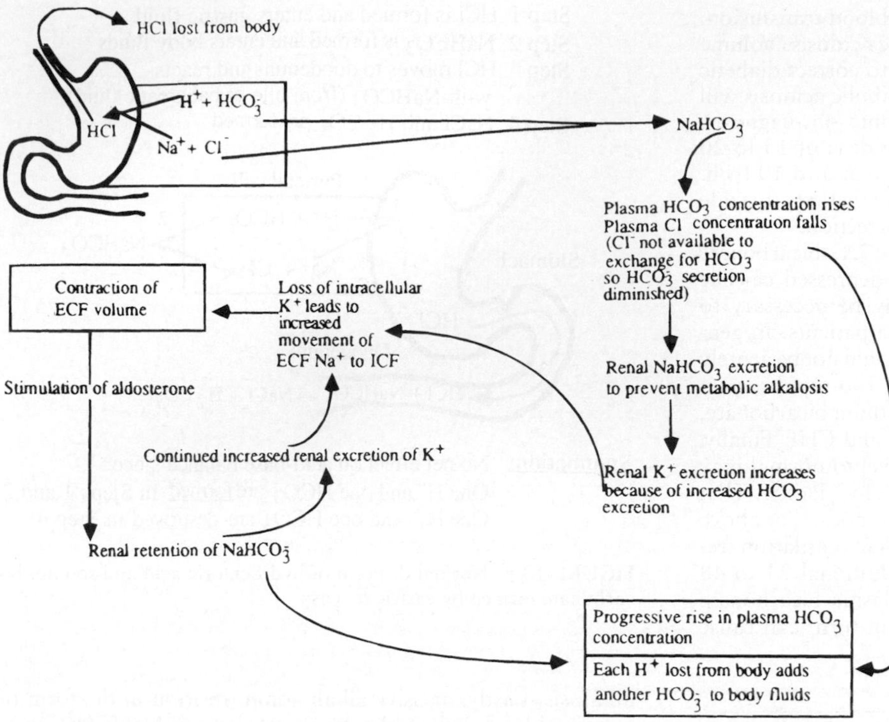

FIGURE 10.9. Pathogenesis of metabolic alkalosis from loss of gastric hydrochloric acid.

In patients with chronic respiratory acidosis, severe posthypercapnic alkalosis develops if the $PaCO_2$ is rapidly restored to normal and the patient is unable to initiate and sustain a bicarbonate diuresis. This inability usually results from sodium chloride or potassium chloride deficits. If sodium chloride or potassium chloride is provided to correct volume contraction and intracellular potassium deficits, a bicarbonate diuresis ensues, and correction of metabolic alkalosis is achieved.

Respiratory Alkalosis

Respiratory alkalosis occurs when hyperventilation decreases PCO_2, resulting in an increase in pH. Hyperventilation may be secondary to conditions such as pulmonary embolism and CHF, which can cause hypoxia. Fever, sepsis, salicylate toxicity, and hepatic failure all can increase alveolar ventilation and cause respiratory alkalosis. This condition can also be iatrogenically induced by mechanical ventilation. Chronic hyperventilation can be seen in pregnancy, exposure to high altitudes, and underlying pulmonary disease.

Management

The symptoms of acute respiratory alkalosis (e.g., paresthesia, lightheadedness, tetany) can be rapidly controlled by raising $PaCO_2$ to normal (e.g., by rebreathing into a paper bag). If the patient is being supported on a ventilator, the dead space can be increased, or tidal volume and respiratory rate can be decreased while oxygenation is maintained. Definite treatment consists of removing the cause of hyperventilation. Respiratory alkalosis also can cause tetany and seizures and predispose to cardiac arrhythmias (by causing an intracellular shift of potassium), particularly in patients receiving digitalis. If the patient is septic, aggressive measures should be taken to alleviate this. She should be treated with appropriate antibiotics and adequate volume replacement. Surgery may be necessary if the patient has an abscess.

Mixed acid–base disturbances can commonly be seen in severely ill patients. Anion gap measurements and careful evaluation of compensatory changes in the pH, HCO_3^-, and PCO_2 are necessary in the workup and management of these patients. The treatment of mixed acid–base disturbances is aimed at the underlying disease process.

BEST SURGICAL PRACTICES

- Maintenance fluids in a hospitalized patient should be calculated by one of two formulas. The 4–2–1 rule recommends administering 60 mL/h of fluid for the first 20 kg of body weight, then subtracting 20 from the patient's weight in kg and adding this difference to calculate the hourly rate. The alternative method for calculating maintenance fluids is to take the body surface area and multiply by 1,000 to come up with the daily fluid requirement in mL.
- The initial step in correcting either hyponatremia or hypernatremia is an accurate assessment of the patient's volume status (decreased, normal, or increased).
- In severe life-threatening hyperkalemia (ECG showing sine waves and broad QRS complexes), patients should first receive 10 mL of calcium gluconate IV for cardioprotective purposes. These patients should then receive an amp of D50, 10 units of regular insulin, and 50 mEq of sodium bicarbonate. Subsequently, these patients should then receive 20 to 50 g of Kayexalate every 2 to 4 hours and infusions of glucose and insulin.
- In the treatment of severe hypokalemia, potassium should never run at a rate greater than 10 mEq/h, and solutions should not contain more than 40 mEq/L of potassium.

- Magnesium metabolism is closely related to potassium and calcium levels. In cases of symptomatic hypocalcemia, magnesium and potassium must be checked and corrected accordingly.
- For any acid–base disturbance, it is important to elucidate the underlying cause for both the diagnosis and treatment to be effective and successful

ACKNOWLEDGMENT

This chapter is based on material from *Water, Electrolyte, and Acid–Base Metabolism* by Claire M. Fritsche, Lee A. Hebert, and Jacob LeMann Jr., which appeared in the seventh edition of *Te Linde's Operative Gynecology.*

Bibliography

Agus Z. Hypomagnesemia. *J Am Soc Nephrol* 1999;10(7):1616.

Altura BT, Brust M, Bloom S, et al. Magnesium dietary intake modulates blood lipid levels and atherogenesis. *Proc Natl Acad Sci USA* 1990;87:1840.

American Diabetes Association. Magnesium supplementation in the treatment of diabetes. *Diabetes Care* 1992;14:1065.

Aono T, Kurachi K, Miyata M, et al. Influence of surgical stress under general anesthesia on serum gonadotropin levels. *J Clin Endocrinol Metab* 1976;42:144.

Arbus GS. An in vivo acid–base nomogram for clinical use. *Can Med Assoc J* 1973;109:291.

Arieff AI. Hyponatremia, convulsions, respiratory arrest, and permanent brain damage after elective surgery in healthy women. *N Engl J Med* 1986;314:1529.

Arieff AI, deFronzo RA. *Fluid, electrolyte and acid–base disorders*. New York: Churchill Livingstone, 1985.

Ayus JC, Krothapalli RK, Arieff AI. Treatment of symptomatic hyponatremia and its relation to brain damage: a prospective study. *N Engl J Med* 1987;317:1190.

Beutler B, Cerami A. Cachectin and tumor necrosis factor as two sides of the same biological coin. *Nature* 1986;320:584.

Bilezikian JP. Management of acute hypercalcemia. *N Engl J Med* 1992;326:1196.

Breen P. Arterial blood gas and pH analysis: clinical approach and interpretation. *Anesthesiol Clin North Am* 2001;19(4):885.

Brown JM, Grosso MA, et al. Cytokines, sepsis and the surgeon. *Surg Gynecol Obstet* 1989;169:568.

Claes Y, Van Hemelrijck J, Van Gerven M, et al. Influence of hydroxyethyl starch on coagulation in patients during the perioperative period. *Anesth Analg* 1992;75:24.

Claybaugh JR, Share L. Vasopressin, renin, and cardiovascular responses to continuous slow hemorrhage. *Am J Physiol* 1973;224:519.

Cockcroft DW, Gault MH. Prediction of creatinine clearance from serum creatinine. *Nephron* 1976;16:31.

Cohen JJ, Kassirer JP. *Acid base*. Boston: Little, Brown, 1982.

Dacey M. Endocrine and metabolic dysfunction syndromes in the critically ill: hypomagnesemic disorders. *Crit Care Clin* 2001;17(1):155.

Epstein FH. Signs and symptoms of electrolyte disorders. In: Maxwell MH, Kleeman CR, eds. *Clinical disorders of fluid and electrolyte metabolism*. New York: McGraw-Hill, 1980.

Fisken RA, Heath DA, Somers S, et al. Hypercalcemia in hospital patients: clinical and diagnostic aspects. *Lancet* 1981;1:202.

Fuss M, Cogan E, Gillet C, et al. Magnesium administration reverses the hypocalcaemia secondary to hypomagnesemia despite low circulating levels of 25-hydroxyvitamin D and 1,25-dihydroxyvitamin D. *Endocrinology* 1985;22:807.

Golzarian J, Scott WH. Hypermagnesemia induced paralytic ileus. *Dig Dis Sci* 1994;39:1138.

Harrington JL. Metabolic alkalosis. *Kidney Int* 1984;26:88.

Heinsimer JA, Lefkowitz RJ. Adrenergic receptors: biochemistry, regulation, molecular mechanisms and clinical indications. *J Lab Clin Med* 1982;100:641.

Kapoor M, Chan G. Fluid and electrolyte abnormalities. *Crit Care Clin* 2001;17(3):503.

Kendler KS, Weitzman RE, Fisher DA. The effect of pain on plasma arginine vasopressin concentrations in man. *Clin Endocrinol* 1978;8:89.

Klahr S. *The kidney and body fluids in health and disease*. New York: Plenum, 1984.

Klee GG, Kao PC, Heath H III. Hypercalcemia. *Endocrinol Metab Clin North Am* 1988;573:600.

Knochel JP. Neuromuscular manifestation of electrolyte disorder. *Am J Med* 1982;72:521.

Lennon EJ, Lemann J Jr. Fluid and electrolyte balance. In: Te Linde RW, Mattingly RF, eds. *Operative gynecology*, 6th ed. Philadelphia: JB Lippincott, 1985.

Leone BJ, Spahn DR. Anemia, hemodilution, and oxygen delivery. *Anesth Analg* 1992;75:651.

Levi M, et al. Disorders of phosphate and magnesium metabolism. In: Coe FC, Favus MJ, eds. *Disorders of bone and mineral metabolism*. New York: Raven, 1992:587.

Major P, Lortholary A, Hon J, et al. Zoledronic acid is superior to pamidronate in the treatment of hypercalcemia of malignancy: a pooled analysis of two randomized, controlled clinical trials. *J Clin Oncol* 2001;19(2):558.

Martinez F, Lash R. Intensive care unit complications: endocrinologic and metabolic complications in the intensive care unit. *Clin Chest Med* 1999;20(2):401.

Matthay MA. Invasive hemodynamic monitoring in critically ill patients. *Clin Chest Med* 1983;4:233.

Maxwell MH, Kleeman CR, Narins RG. *Clinical disorders of fluid and electrolyte metabolism*, 4th ed. New York: McGraw-Hill, 1987.

Narins RG. Therapy of hyponatremia: does haste make waste? *N Engl J Med* 1986;314:1573.

Narins RG, Emmett M. Simple and mixed acid–base disorders: a practical approach. *Medicine* 1980;59:161.

Ponce SP, Jennings AE, Madias NE, et al. Drug-induced hyperkalemia. *Medicine* 1985;64:357.

Riggs JE. Neurologic manifestations of electrolyte disturbances. *Neurol Clin* 2002;20(1):227.

Roacha E, Silva M, Velasco IT, et al. Hypertonic saline resuscitation: saturated salt-dextran solutions are equally effective, but induce hemolysis in dogs. *Crit Care Med* 1990;18:203.

Robertson G, Aycinesa P, Zerbe R. Neurogenic disorders of osmoregulation. *Am J Med* 1986;2:339.

Schrier RW. Pathogenesis of sodium and water retention in high-output and low-output cardiac failure, nephrotic syndrome, cirrhosis and pregnancy. *N Engl J Med* 1988;319:1065.

Schrier RW, ed. *Renal and electrolyte disorders*, 2nd ed. Boston: Little, Brown, 1980.

Skillman JJ, Lauler DP, Hickler RB, et al. Hemorrhage in normal man: effect of renin, cortisol, aldosterone, and urine composition. *Ann Surg* 1967;166:865.

Slotman GJ, Burchard KW, et al. Thromboxane and prostacyclin in clinical acute respiratory failure. *J Eur Res* 1985;39:1.

Spiegel A. The parathyroid glands: hypercalcemia and hypocalcemia. In: Goldman L, ed. *Cecil textbook of medicine*, 21st ed. Philadelphia: WB Saunders 2000:1399.

Steiner RW. Interpreting the fractional excretion of sodium. *Am J Med* 1984;77:699.

Waters J, Miller L. Cause of metabolic acidosis in prolonged surgery. *Crit Care Med* 1999;27(10):2142.

Williams SE. Hydrogen ion infusion for treating severe metabolic alkalosis. *BMJ* 1976;2:1189.

Ziegler, R. Hypercalcemic crisis. *J Am Soc Nephrol* 2001;12(17 Suppl):S3.

CHAPTER 11 ■ POSTOPERATIVE INFECTIONS: PREVENTION AND MANAGEMENT

W. DAVID HAGER AND JOHN W. LARSEN

DEFINITIONS

Bacteremia—Infection of the bloodstream can complicate any pelvic infection, but is seen more frequently in association with abscesses, peritonitis, and septic pelvic thrombophlebitis.

Cuff cellulitis—A soft tissue infection of the surgical margin in the upper vagina where the uterus was removed.

Drug fever—Elevated temperature that is due to an allergic reaction to medications.

Febrile morbidity—A temperature of 38°C (100.4°F) or greater recorded on two occasions, at least 6 hours apart, more than 24 hours after the surgical procedure.

Necrotizing fascitis—A severe synergistic bacterial infection of the fascia, subcutaneous tissue, and skin that is usually caused by group A hemolytic streptococci, often in combination with other bacteria.

Surgical wound class—The surgical wound infection rate per 100 operations in the United States by wound class is 2.1% for clean, 3.3% for clean-contaminated, 6.4% for contaminated, and 7.1% for dirty or infected cases.

Urinary tract infection—The criterion for defining a urinary tract infection (UTI) is more than 100,000 colonies/mL of a single pathogen from a clean catch urine and more than 10,000 colonies/mL from a catheterized specimen.

Vaginal cuff hematoma/cuff abscess—A walled-off collection of blood originating from an oozing vascular pedicle or along the vaginal cuff. If the collection becomes infected, it is an abscess.

Wound cellulitis—Soft-tissue infection localized to the skin and adipose tissue above the fascia that is characterized by erythema, warmth, and swelling, as well as tenderness.

Wound seroma—A collection of serous fluid beneath the skin surface.

Infection complicating surgical procedures has been the consternation of gynecologists since the first operations were performed. Even when medical and surgical care are beyond reproach, infectious morbidity can complicate the postoperative course. Unfortunately, using antibiotics prophylactically at the time of surgery does not eliminate this risk of infection.

It is imperative that the gynecologic surgeon understand basic infectious disease concepts to treat infected patients appropriately. Diagnosis and treatment are not guess work but depend on understanding basic principles.

An understanding of bacteria that are a part of the normal vaginal flora enables the gynecologist to recognize the pathogenic bacteria that contribute to postoperative infection. Certain risk factors play a role in increasing postoperative infection rates. Knowledge of these factors can enable the surgeon to take action to alter those risks. There are various types of postoperative infection, each with its own unique time of onset and usual bacterial etiology. Knowledge about likely causes of a disorder can facilitate decision making when an antibiotic is empirically selected to treat the patient.

Appropriate patient evaluation, including proper culturing techniques, is critical to this diagnostic process. Steps to prevent infection must become routine with every surgeon on every case. These steps are necessary not only for the operator, but also for all personnel participating in the surgical and medical treatment of the patient. These steps are described later in this chapter.

FEBRILE MORBIDITY

In the evaluation of patients who have an elevated temperature in the postoperative period, it is important to recognize that all febrile morbidity is not infectious morbidity. Treating a fever without a definite cause of infection may do more harm than good.

Several different definitions of febrile morbidity have been used, and this may create confusion for the surgeon. The most frequent definition is a temperature of 38°C (100.4°F) or greater recorded on two occasions, at least 6 hours apart, more than 24 hours after the surgical procedure. This excludes a fever during the first 24 hours. Operative site infections during this time are unusual unless there is preexisting infection at the operative site or gross contamination of the site. Some investigators have used a definition of a single temperature elevation of 39°C (101°F) or greater recorded on any occasion in the postoperative period as indicative of febrile morbidity. We prefer the former definition.

Regardless of the choice of definition of febrile morbidity, it is important to treat infection and not fever. Fever may trigger sensitivity to the possibility of infection, but a positive culture or the presence of definite clinical criteria should be present before a diagnosis is made and treatment initiated.

INCIDENCE

In evaluating the incidence of postoperative infection in published studies, it is important to consider whether infectious morbidity or febrile morbidity was used to define infection, what the socioeconomic status of the population studied was, whether antibiotic prophylaxis was used, and whether there were other confounding variables that might have influenced infection rates (e.g., multiple surgical procedures, experience of the surgeon, or site of the study).

Prospective studies report the incidence of acute pelvic infection after abdominal hysterectomy to be 3.9% to 50%. The range for infection after vaginal hysterectomy is 1.7% to 64%. The incidence of septic pelvic thrombophlebitis (SPT) after gynecologic procedures is 0.1% to 0.5%.

VAGINAL FLORA

The most frequent source of bacteria that cause postoperative pelvic infection among women is the vagina. The vagina is colonized by large numbers of a variety of bacteria that normally exist in a symbiotic relationship. Several factors influence the vaginal flora, including age, sexual activity, stage of the menstrual cycle, use of antibiotic or immunosuppressive agents, and any invasive procedure.

Mean bacterial counts in vaginal secretions are 10^8 to 10^9 bacteria/mL, with three to six different species present. The most frequent aerobic bacteria are *Lactobacilli* sp, *Gardnerella vaginalis, Staphylococcus epidermidis, Corynebacterium* sp, *Enterococcus faecalis* species of *Streptococcus*, and *Enterobacteriaceae*. Anaerobes outnumber aerobes and include *Peptostreptococcus* sp, *Peptococcus* sp, *Prevotella bivia, Prevotella disiens,* and members of the *Bacteroides fragilis* group (Table 11.1). These same bacteria are frequently isolated from sites of pelvic infection among women who have undergone gynecologic surgery. This indicates, as Schottmueller proposed at the turn of the century, that pelvic infections are principally a result of endogenous sources of bacteria. The concepts of antibiotic prophylaxis and antiseptic douching before surgery or preoperative placement of antiseptic gel are related to reducing these large numbers of bacteria. Although investigators have found that colonization rates change in relation to the stage of the menstrual cycle, no data have supported the concept that timing of gynecologic surgery in relation to menses alters infection rates.

Surgery itself alters the numbers and types of bacteria in the vagina and cervix. After vaginal and abdominal hysterectomy, the number of lactobacilli decreases, and the number of facultative Gram-negative rods, *B fragilis* group species, and enterococci increases. Preoperative hospitalization before surgery on a gynecologic ward also alters the vaginal flora in a direction toward more virulent organisms.

TABLE 11.1

BACTERIA COMPOSING NORMAL VAGINAL FLORA

Aerobes	Anaerobes
Staphylococcus aureus	*Peptostreptococcus* sp
Staphylococcus epidermidis	*Peptococcus* sp
Group B streptococcus	*Bacteroides* sp
Streptococcus sp	*Fusobacterium* sp
Enterococcus faecalis	*Prevotella bivia*
Lactobacilli	*Prevotella disiens*
Corynebacterium sp	*Bacteroides fragilis* group
Escherichia coli	
Klebsiella sp	
Gardnerella vaginalis	

RISK FACTORS FOR INFECTION

Several factors may increase the infectious morbidity of postoperative patients (Table 11.2). Of all the factors mentioned, the most basic appears to be immunocompromise. Anything that plays a role in altering the host's own defense mechanisms can result in a greater chance of infectious morbidity.

Some risk factors can be controlled by the surgeon, whereas others cannot be influenced by the surgeon or operative team and must be dealt with as they occur. Lower socioeconomic status is a risk factor for infection in gynecologic surgery. Although economic status is convenient for epidemiologic studies, the clinical effect is believed to be a result of inadequate nutrition and poor hygiene. Obesity is another risk factor for infection, probably reflecting poor hygiene, altered nutrition, risk of diabetes, and prolonged operative time. These result in altered wound healing and greater possibilities for infection.

When a hysterectomy is performed through an infected operative site, there is an increased risk of postoperative infection. Likewise, contamination of the operative field by break in sterile technique or injury to the bowel promotes infection. Young age has been considered a risk factor for posthysterectomy infection, although the exact reason is unclear. This increased risk in younger patients may result from the presence of more virulent bacteria in the vagina or increased vascularity and difficulty in obtaining adequate hemostasis. Other factors are not as clear-cut and may result from interacting effects. For example, duration of surgery is considered to be a risk for infection in most studies, but this actually may reflect experience of the operating surgeon, complexity of the case, or a greater chance of inadequate hemostasis. Lack of adequate hemostasis increases the risk of undrained collections of blood and creates an ideal culture medium for contaminating bacteria. Low hemoglobin and hematocrit levels, preoperatively or postoperatively, have been mentioned as factors in increased rates of postoperative infection, especially of abdominal incisions. No data, however, have indicated that raising the volume of red blood cells decreases the rate of infection. Leaving an excessive amount of devitalized tissue (e.g., large, ligated pedicles) can predispose to a greater risk of infection. Pedicles should

TABLE 11.2

RISK FACTORS FOR POSTOPERATIVE INFECTION

Altered immunocompetence
Premenopausal age
Obesity
Radical surgery
Bacterial vaginosis
Prolonged preoperative hospitalization
Excessive intraoperative blood loss
Hematoma or serous fluid collection
Operator inexperience
Lower socioeconomic status
Prolonged operative time
Poor nutrition
Excessive devitalized (necrotic) tissue
Foreign bodies
Diabetes mellitus
Systemic disease
Failure to use prophylactic antibiotics
Surgery in an infected operative site

be trim and dry, dead space should be closed, and hemostasis obtained.

Failure to use antibiotic prophylaxis in situations in which they have been shown to be beneficial may be a risk for pelvic infection. Prophylactic antibiotics should be used according to the accepted protocol for that procedure. The use of a vaginal cuff drain has been shown to have a significant beneficial effect on decreasing morbidity but has fallen out of favor because of the simplicity and effectiveness of antibiotic prophylaxis.

Bacterial vaginosis, characterized by increased vaginal concentrations of certain anaerobic and facultative bacteria, has been shown to increase the relative risk of postoperative infection in gynecologic procedures. The presence of increased concentrations of pathogenic bacteria adjacent to the site of incision in the vagina allows for ascending spread of these organisms in a susceptible host. Although treatment of bacterial vaginosis in pregnant women may decrease their risk of preterm delivery and preterm, premature rupture of membranes, no studies have shown a decreased rate of postoperative infection in bacterial vaginosis–positive women treated before gynecologic surgery.

ETIOLOGY

All women have bacteria colonizing the vagina in greater or lesser numbers. Women without symptoms have a mean of 4.2 species present. It is these same bacteria normally existing in a symbiotic relationship that ultimately can invade tissue altered by surgery, leading to clinical infection. The virulence of the bacteria and the volume inoculated are countered by the host's immune defense mechanisms and may be aided by prophylactic antibiotics to combat the occurrence of infection.

The bacteria listed in Table 11.3, which are responsible for postoperative infection after gynecologic surgery, are the same organisms that can be recovered from vaginal cultures of women before hysterectomy, according to Hemsell. The volume of bacteria present and their proximity to the operative site promote a polymicrobial infection in women who experience posthysterectomy infectious morbidity. Aerobic bacteria may initiate the infectious process; as tissue is devitalized and the oxidation reduction potential is altered, anaerobes proliferate and add to the tissue damage. Large, necrotic tissue pedicles and undrained collections of blood are ideal sites for infection to occur. Once the infection has begun, the body's host immune defense mechanisms initiate an inflammatory response and attempt to wall off and localize the infection. Infected hematomas and abscesses can result.

TABLE 11.3

PATHOGENS RESPONSIBLE FOR INFECTIONS AFTER GYNECOLOGIC SURGERY

Aerobic gram-positive cocci
Staphylococcus aureus
Staphylococcus epidermidis
Streptococcus viridans group
Group B streptococci
Streptococcus faecalis
Aerobic gram-negative bacilli
Escherichia coli
Proteus mirabilis
Klebsiella sp
Gardnerella vaginalis
Anaerobes
Peptostreptococcus sp
Peptococcus sp
Prevotella bivia
Prevotella disiens
Bacteroides melaninogenicus
Bacteroides capillosus
Bacteroides fragilis group
B fragilis
B ovatus
B thetaiotaomicron
B distasonis
B vulgatus
Clostridium perfringens
Fusobacterium sp

CATEGORIES OF INFECTION

Not all women who have temperature elevation after gynecologic surgery are infected, and not all of those who are infected have the same clinical syndrome. It is important to categorize the infectious process because treatment can vary accordingly.

Cuff Cellulitis

Cuff cellulitis is an infection of the surgical margin in the upper vagina where the uterus was removed. Symptoms and signs of infection usually begin late in the hospital course or even after discharge from the hospital. These patients' immediate postoperative course may have been completely benign. There is always an element of induration, erythema, and edema in the vaginal cuff immediately after hysterectomy. If the patient becomes infected, she will often have initial symptoms of lower abdominal pain, pelvic pain, back pain, fever, and abnormal vaginal discharge. Examination may reveal persistent hyperemia, induration, and tenderness of the vaginal cuff and possibly purulent discharge along with fever. The parametrial and adnexal areas are nontender. The white blood cell count usually is mildly to moderately elevated.

Gram-positive aerobes, facultative Gram-negative aerobes, and obligate anaerobes can all contribute to the cause of cuff cellulitis. Single- or multiple-agent broad-spectrum coverage is effective in treating this infection, although single agents usually are preferred to reduce costs and the likelihood of an allergic reaction.

Infected Vaginal Cuff Hematoma or Cuff Abscess

Hysterectomy can result in small amounts of oozing from vascular pedicles or along the vaginal cuff. This bleeding may result in a walled-off collection of blood called a hematoma. If this localized mass above the vaginal cuff becomes infected, an abscess may result. Bacteria, especially anaerobes, flourish in this environment.

Women with a vaginal cuff abscess present with fever that is usually early in the postoperative period. Other symptoms include chills, pelvic pain, and rectal pressure. Clinical findings include temperature elevation; lower abdominal and vaginal cuff tenderness; the presence of a tender, fluctuant mass near the cuff; and, occasionally, purulent drainage from the cuff. The pain and tenderness is often more predominant on one side.

An infected cuff hematoma actually can present later in the postoperative course than an abscess and usually is associated with a drop in the hemoglobin and hematocrit levels. The hematoma may not be readily palpable but can be delineated on pelvic ultrasound or computed tomographic (CT) scan.

Postoperative Ovarian Abscess

The patient who develops fever and abdominal and pelvic pain late in the postoperative hospital course or after hospital discharge may have a pelvic abscess, possibly of ovarian origin. If there is a sudden increase in abdominal or pelvic pain, a rupture may have occurred. A ruptured abscess should be managed as a surgical emergency with a laparotomy and excision or drainage of the infected mass. The inciting site for an ovarian abscess is a place of recent follicle expulsion or a site of surgical trauma to an ovary in a premenopausal woman. Ovaries should not be aspirated or probed at the time of hysterectomy for fear that bacteria from the vagina may penetrate the ovary and initiate infection. Once again, anaerobes are the predominant bacteria in an ovarian abscess.

If an ovarian abscess is suspected, then a CT scan should be ordered. The CT scan not only identifies the size and location of the abscess but also allows for visualization and evaluation of the ureters, bladder, and colon. A pelvic ultrasound also may be useful to localize the abscess. Many abscesses respond to broad-spectrum antibiotic therapy; but if a tender, fluctuant mass persists, drainage is necessary. A radiologic interventionist may be able to accomplish percutaneous drainage with a needle or catheter using CT or ultrasound guidance, or colpotomy drainage may be possible. For colpotomy drainage to be accomplished safely, the abscess must be fluctuant, fixed in the cul-de-sac, and dissecting the upper third of the rectovaginal septum. With either approach, a closed-suction drain should be placed to ensure complete and continued evacuation during the next 2 to 3 days.

Septic Pelvic Thrombophlebitis

Septic pelvic thrombophlebitis (SPT) complicates gynecologic surgery in 0.1% to 0.5% of procedures. It is usually a diagnosis of exclusion, made when a postoperative patient with febrile morbidity does not respond to appropriate parenteral antibiotic therapy in the absence of an undrained abscess or infected hematoma. The development of SPT is enhanced by venous stasis (e.g., obesity, diabetes), vascular injury, or bacterial contamination of pelvic vessels.

Two forms of SPT have been described. The classic form is seen in association with abdominal surgery. This form occurs 2 to 4 days after surgery and is characterized by fever, tachycardia, gastrointestinal distress, unilateral abdominal pain, and, in 50% to 67% of cases, a palpable abdominal cord resulting from acute thrombus formation. The enigmatic form complicates parturition or pelvic surgery and is characterized by spiking temperatures despite clinical improvement on antibiotics; tachycardia during the temperature spikes; and small, diffusely scattered thrombi in small pelvic vessels. Pelvic findings are minimal in both forms. The diagnosis often may be confirmed by CT scan or magnetic resonance imaging.

The traditional mainstay of treatment for SPT is anticoagulation with heparin for 7 to 10 days. Some experts recommend changing antibiotics or extending coverage before heparin is considered. All patients should be treated with antibiotics effective against heparinase-producing *Bacteroides* sp. Long-term anticoagulation is not required unless septic pulmonary emboli have occurred. Lysis of fever may occur 24 to 48 hours after starting heparin, yet other cases may require much longer for complete resolution. Treatment should be continued until the patient is afebrile for 48 hours and clinically well.

Osteomyelitis Pubis

Osteomyelitis pubis rarely complicates gynecologic procedures adjacent to the symphysis pubis, such as retropubic urethral suspension, radical vulvectomy, or pelvic exenteration. Direct or contiguous seeding of the periosteum from pelvic bacteria results in a delayed-onset infection 6 to 8 weeks after the original procedure. Patients report pain and tenderness along the symphysis pubis, especially with ambulation. Low-grade fever, an elevated erythrocyte sedimentation rate, and a moderate leukocytosis have been reported, as well as positive cultures from blood or the bone itself. Aggressive antibiotic therapy covering *Staphylococcus aureus* and facultative Gram-negative bacilli is essential for adequate recovery. If the response is not adequate, surgical debridement of the pubis is necessary.

Wound Infection

Surgical wound infection is possible with any transabdominal gynecologic procedure, but especially with those that are contaminated. Extensive study of the epidemiology of wound infections resulted in a classification of operative wounds in relation to contamination and increasing risk of infection (Table 11.4). Because the vagina is entered during hysterectomy, even an uninfected hysterectomy is classified as a clean-contaminated operation. Fortunately, prophylactic antibiotics and minimally invasive, laparoscopic procedures have greatly reduced the risk of severe, surgical wound infections.

The rates of wound infection according to case classification of the operative wound are summarized in Table 11.5. Culver and colleagues, using the National Nosocomial Infections Surveillance System, reported the percentage of operations in the United States by wound class and the surgical wound infection rate per 100 operations to be 2.1% for clean, 3.3% for clean-contaminated, 6.4% for contaminated, and 7.1% for dirty or infected cases. The more contaminated the operative site, the greater is the risk of wound infection. Fortunately, despite polymicrobial contamination by bacteria from the vagina when it is entered at the time of hysterectomy, prophylactic antibiotics, adequate host resistance, and good surgical technique result in most patients avoiding wound infection.

The Centers for Disease Control and Prevention (CDC) definitions of surgical wound infection were modified by Horan et al. This system divides infections into two major categories: (a) an organ/space surgical site infection (SSI), and (b) superficial and deep incision infection. An SSI may be in any anatomic area that was opened or manipulated during a surgical procedure other than the incision itself. This would include most of the infections that develop after hysterectomy. It must develop within 30 days of the procedure and be accompanied by one of the following: diagnosis by a surgeon or attending

TABLE 11.4

CLASSIFICATION OF OPERATIVE WOUNDS IN RELATION TO CONTAMINATION AND INCREASING RISK OF INFECTION

Clean
Elective, primarily closed and undrained
Nontraumatic, uninfected
No inflammation encountered
No break in aseptic technique
Respiratory, alimentary, genitourinary tracts not entered
Clean-Contaminated
Alimentary, respiratory, or genitourinary tract entered under controlled conditions and without unusual contamination
Appendectomy
Vagina entered
Genitourinary tract entered in absence of culture-positive urine
Minor break in technique
Mechanical drainage
Contaminated
Open, fresh traumatic wounds
Gross spillage from gastrointestinal tract
Entrance of genitourinary tract in presence of infected urine
Major break in technique
Incisions in which acute nonpurulent inflammation is present
Dirty or Infected
Traumatic wound with retained devitalized tissue, foreign bodies, fecal contamination, or delayed treatment, or wounds from a dirty source
Perforated viscus encountered
Acute bacterial inflammation with pus encountered during operation

Source: Altemeier WA, Burke JF, Pruitt BA, et al. *Manual on control of infection in surgical patients,* 2nd ed. Philadelphia: JB Lippincott, 1984:28, with permission.

physician; an abscess or other evidence of infection identified during reoperation or by radiologic or histopathologic examination; aseptically obtained organ/space fluid or tissue, the culture of which resulted in bacterial isolates; or purulent drainage from a drain placed through a stab wound into the organ/space.

TABLE 11.5

SURGICAL WOUND INFECTION RATES IN 84,691 OPERATIONS BY TRADITIONAL WOUND CLASSIFICATION SCORE

Wound class	Operations (%)	Surgical wound infection rate (per 100 operations)
Clean	58	2.1
Clean-contaminated	36	3.3
Contaminated	4	6.4
Dirty or infected	2	7.1

Source: Culver DH, Horan TC, Gaynes RP. Surgical wound infection rates by wound class, operative procedure and patient risk index. *Am J Med* 1991;91:152S, with permission.

Wound Cellulitis

Abdominal wound infections are categorized by their location and severity. The least severe are localized to the skin and adipose tissue above the fascia. Wound cellulitis is characterized by erythema, warmth, and swelling, as well as tenderness. If there is no purulent drainage, antibiotic therapy alone with a cephalosporin or augmented penicillin often is effective. *Staphylococcus aureus,* coagulase-negative staphylococci, and streptococci cause most of these infections.

Wound Seroma

A collection of serous fluid beneath the skin surface is a seroma. A small amount of serous drainage may be managed with limited opening of the incision, drainage, and cleansing. Larger collections may require more extensive incision and drainage.

Deep Wound Infection

When purulent drainage is noted, the wound should be opened widely to allow drainage and removal of necrotic tissue. The incision should be probed gently to evaluate fascial integrity. If the fascia is intact, healing is hastened by mechanical debridement followed by loose, wet-to-dry packing with gauze moistened with saline; dilute hydrogen peroxide (1:1 mixture with saline) or Dakin's solution, 0.5%. Povidone-iodine is to be discouraged because it does not promote the development of granulation tissue. An antibiotic effective against anaerobes must be used.

Evisceration of bowel may occur if the infection involves the fascia. This is a surgical emergency requiring identification of the defect, freshening of the fascial edges, placement of intraabdominal and subcutaneous closed suction drains, and reinforced closure of the fascia. Some surgeons would leave the skin open for delayed closure; others would close it primarily.

Necrotizing Fascitis

This severe complication results from synergistic bacterial infection of the fascia, subcutaneous tissue, and skin. This rapidly progressive infection is characterized by cyanosis of the skin and frequently blistering necrosis. It is most commonly caused by group A, beta-hemolytic streptococci, but may be a polymicrobial, synergistic infection with anaerobic bacteria or *Clostridium perfringens.* It is seen more frequently in diabetic and immunocompromised patients. Patients present with severe pain in the area of involvement; clinical signs of sepsis; and a viscous, cloudy, malodorous drainage. The wound edges may be purple or even necrotic. If gangrene occurs in the area of fascitis, bullae of the skin and crepitus in the subcutaneous tissue may be seen. Treatment includes antibiotics effective against streptococci and anaerobes, plus prompt and extensive resection of the tissue involved.

Urinary Tract Infection

Infection of the lower urinary tract is a frequent complication of gynecologic surgery. The patient may have low-grade fever, dysuria, frequency, and urgency, but in many situations has no symptoms. The criterion for defining a urinary tract infection

(UTI) is more than 100,000 colonies/mL of a single pathogen from a clean catch urine and more than 10,000 colonies/mL from a catheterized specimen. Appropriate sterile technique for insertion and management of indwelling catheters is important in preventing UTI. In general, urethral catheters should be removed as soon as possible after surgery unless the surgery has involved the bladder itself. Treatment of a documented UTI should be with an appropriate oral or parenteral antibiotic. The quinolone antibiotics offer the broadest spectrum of coverage for empiric treatment of urinary pathogens, although resistance to these agents develops quite rapidly.

Bacteremia

Infection of the bloodstream can complicate any pelvic infection, but is seen more frequently in association with abscesses, peritonitis, and SPT. Antibiotics effective against the isolated organism should be used. Treatment beyond 5 to 7 days usually is not necessary to eradicate the offending pathogen. Antibiotics can be stopped when the patient has no clinical evidence of infection and has been afebrile for 24 to 48 hours.

Drug Fever

This diagnosis should be considered when appropriate parenteral antibiotics have been used and there are no localizing signs of infection and no undrained collection of fluid. Fevers are usually steady but can fluctuate. Many patients exhibit an eosinophilia. The antibiotic(s) should be discontinued.

EVALUATION OF THE PATIENT WITH SUSPECTED INFECTION

Fever is the most common sign of postoperative infection, but it is important to remember that fever is not always, or indeed not usually, caused by infection in the postoperative patient (Table 11.6). In a large study of 537 women who underwent major gynecologic surgery, Fanning et al. found that 39% developed postoperative fever, but only 17 patients (8%) actually had a documented infection. Other signs and symptoms of postoperative infection can include erythema, induration, and/or tenderness around the incision, drain, or intravenous infusion site; leg pain; tenderness or swelling; costovertebral angle (CVA) tenderness; cough; or dysuria. When any of these or other signs or symptoms alerts the surgeon to the possibility of a postoperative infection, an appropriate workup is indicated. A diagnosis of infection should be made or at least a high probability of infection should be present before antibiotics are started.

TABLE 11.6

FEVER EVALUATION IN GYNECOLOGIC PATIENTS

History
Time of onset
Surgical procedure
Risk factors
Antibiotic prophylaxis
Symptoms
Ancillary illnesses
Physical Examination
Upper respiratory
Lower respiratory
Gastrointestinal
Urinary tract
Wound
Pelvis
Laboratory
Complete blood cell count with differential
Catheterized urinalysis
Chemistry panel
Cultures
Urine
Blood
Surgical site

History

Careful history taking often can be the source of helpful clues to the cause of postoperative infection. The time of onset of the complicating infection is important. Ledger emphasized that the interval between surgery and the onset of fever is helpful in determining the cause of infection. For example, Garibaldi and colleagues suggested that most cases of early postoperative fever are not infectious in origin. Possible noninfectious causes include pulmonary atelectasis, hypersensitivity reactions to antibiotics or anesthetics, pyrogenic reactions to tissue trauma, or hematoma formation. Infectious causes of early postoperative fever include aspiration pneumonia, group A α-hemolytic streptococcal wound infection, or surgery in a previously infected site (e.g., pelvic inflammatory disease or recent D&C or cone biopsy). Other important aspects of history include the surgical procedures performed (e.g., abdominal versus vaginal approach, whether ovaries were invaded), risk factors encountered (pelvic abscess, bowel injury), use of antibiotic prophylaxis, symptoms, and whether the patient had any ancillary illnesses (smoking history, history of cardiac valvular disease, immunosuppression).

Physical Examination

Gynecologic surgeons tend to focus on the pelvis as the source of all postoperative infections. Instead, a comprehensive evaluation of the entire patient should be carried out. The upper respiratory tract should be examined to rule out otitis, pharyngitis, and bronchitis and the lower respiratory tract to rule out pneumonia. The gastrointestinal tract should be checked to evaluate bowel function, distention, and tenderness. Breast examination is usually only important in postpartum patients. The urinary tract should be evaluated, and the possibility of pyelonephritis must be considered. Intravenous access, especially central lines or other indwelling foreign bodies, should be carefully inspected and palpated for evidence of infection. The surgical wound must be examined carefully, and if the site of infection has not been identified or symptoms suggest a pelvic infection, a pelvic examination should be carried out. The pelvic examination should evaluate the vaginal cuff for discharge, erythema, and induration. Palpation for tenderness and for masses should be done and cultures obtained if pus is identified.

Laboratory and Imaging Evaluation

In recent years, it has become clear that a routine postoperative "fever workup"—including a variety of studies, such as a complete blood count, urine analysis, chest x-ray, and multiple cultures—is largely unrewarding in identifying the site of postoperative infections. A careful history and physical examination are the best guides to which laboratory tests, if any, are indicated. In a retrospective review of 257 patients who underwent major gynecologic surgery, Lyon et al. found that a urine culture was positive in only 9% of the patients who were cultured and less than 2% of all febrile patients. Fewer chest x-rays were ordered, and they were almost always negative, with only 1.5% of all febrile patients having a significant finding. Similar results were described by Fanning et al., who also noted that none of the 77 blood cultures in their series of 211 febrile postoperative patients was positive.

In a follow-up study, Schwandt et al. outlined a protocol for evaluating postoperative gynecological patients as follows: (a) record temperatures every 4 hours; (b) for temperatures greater than 38°C (100.4°F), evaluate the patient by history and physical examination; (c) when no significant signs or symptoms are identified, order no tests, and observe the patient. Antibiotics are not started at this point. The authors felt that this protocol of selectively ordering lab tests to evaluate a postoperative fever did not compromise patient care and saved considerable resources. Similar findings also have been reported in a retrospective review by McNally et al.

Although current practice discourages the use of "routine" testing to evaluate a postoperative fever, the clinician must be sensitive to special circumstances, unusual signs or symptoms, or persistent fever or other warning signs. Special circumstances could include a patient who was at high risk for infection because of immunosuppression, gross bacterial contamination at surgery, infection already present before surgery, or patient in such a frail or unstable condition that any postoperative infection could be fatal. Unusual signs or symptoms, which include evidence of necrotizing fasciitis or gas-forming organisms and, most common of all, persistence of fever or other signs or symptoms of infection, definitely warrant a more exhaustive evaluation and, in most cases, prompt aggressive therapy.

A complete blood count with differential usually is indicated, and electrolytes, renal function tests, and liver-associated tests may be useful if sepsis is anticipated, prior damage to these organs exists, and/or antibiotics excreted or metabolized by these organs may be used. Acute pancreatitis can be ruled out by a normal serum amylase and lipase.

Blood cultures are not frequently indicated; but in patients with high fever, those with persistent fever despite antibiotics, or those who are immunocompromised, they may be useful. This is particularly true when patients have indwelling central lines for longer than a few days, especially if these lines have been used for several functions (blood transfusions, antibiotics, electrolytes, etc.), and/or the patient had bacteremia that could seed the tip of the line. In these cases, at least one culture should be taken through the central line catheter. Other cultures of pus from an abdominal incision, the vaginal cuff, an undrained collection, or a drainage tube occasionally may be helpful in a patient who is not responding to antibiotics or in whom an unusual infection (actinomyces) is suspected. A sputum Gram stain and culture is rarely useful but should be considered in a symptomatic, immunosuppressed patient who could have tuberculosis, coccidioidomycosis, or some other atypical pneumonia.

A number of different imaging techniques may be useful in special circumstances. A CT scan of the abdomen/pelvis should identify an abscess. In many cases, CT-guided percutaneous catheter drainage in combination with intravenous antibiotics is the treatment of choice. Renal function always should be satisfactory before administering intravenous contrast for a CT or intravenous pyelogram. Ultrasound can be used to scan the abdominal incision and pelvis for an abscess or hematoma. Ultrasound of the heart can diagnose valvular vegetations associated with bacterial endocarditis. It also is useful for evaluation of the leg vein for venous thrombosis. Pelvic or abdominal vein thrombosis can be diagnosed easily in most cases using CT scanning. Radioactive-tagged white blood cell scans can be useful for localizing occult infections, but these have largely been replaced by CT scans.

TREATMENT

The following factors must be considered when making antibiotic choices for the treatment of postoperative infections.

1. Pelvic infections are polymicrobial in etiology.
2. The most frequent causative organisms are aerobic, Gram-positive cocci (streptococci, *S. epidermidis*, *S. aureus*), facultative Gram-negative rods (*Escherichia coli*, *Klebsiella* sp, *Enterobacter* sp), anaerobic cocci (peptostreptococci), and anaerobic rods (*Prevotella* sp, *Bacteroides* sp, *B. fragilis*).
3. Enterococci may occasionally cause sepsis or be a sole isolate but usually accompany other bacteria and are not principal pathogens.
4. The choice of an antibiotic is made empirically before culture results are available.
5. The timing of onset of the infection may be an indicator of a pathogen group.
6. Resistance to frequently used antibiotics is developing.
7. Single agents may be as effective as multiple agents in treating postoperative infections.

The polymicrobial nature of postoperative pelvic infections results in about 20% aerobic Gram-positive cocci, 20% Gram-negative rods, and 60% anaerobes. Infections that occur in the first 24 hours after surgery usually are caused by Gram-positive cocci or occasionally by facultative Gram-negative rods. Infections that occur after the first 48 hours more frequently have an anaerobic component. The effect of timing should be considered in making the initial choice of an antibiotic because an extended-spectrum penicillin or cephalosporin may be the best choice in early-onset infections (Table 11.7).

The gold standard for treating gynecologic postoperative infections has been gentamicin, 2 mg/kg loading dose, followed by 1.5 mg/kg maintenance dose for patients with normal renal function, plus clindamycin, 900 mg administered parenterally every 8 hours. Unfortunately, increasing resistance among anaerobic rods to clindamycin is altering the effectiveness of this regimen. The fear of nephrotoxicity or ototoxicity when gentamicin is used for short treatment courses in young, healthy women has not been borne out. Aminoglycoside serum levels may be obtained if the treatment is expected to last more than 72 hours. The addition of ampicillin to the previous combination extends the spectrum of coverage to include enterococci.

To overcome the resistance of anaerobes to clindamycin, metronidazole may be used in combination with an aminoglycoside, ampicillin, or both. Metronidazole in combination with levofloxacin, 500 mg daily, is also used frequently. The dose of metronidazole is 500 mg every 6 hours. The oral

TABLE 11.7

TREATMENT CHOICES FOR GYNECOLOGIC INFECTION

Postoperative infection	Recommended regimen	Failures	Penicillin allergy
Mild to moderate	Extended-spectrum penicillin or cephalosporin (e.g., piperacillin/tazobactam, 4.5 g/6 h; [this dose goes with pip/tazo] ticarcillin/clavulanic acid, 3.1 g/4–6 h; metronidazole 500 mg/6 h and levofloxacin 500 mg/d ceftriaxone, 2 g followed by 1 g/24 h; cefoxitin, 2 g/6 h; cefotetan 2 g/12 h; cefotaxime, 1 g/8 h [IV doses]).	Clindamycin/gentamicin or metronidazole/gentamicin	Clindamycin/gentamicin
Severe	Clindamycin/gentamicin or metronidazole/gentamicin (e.g., clindamycin, 900 mg/8 h or metronidazole, 500 mg/6 h plus gentamicin, 2 mg/kg followed by 1.5 mg/kg/8 h or a single daily dose of 5 mg/kg [ampicillin, penicillin, or vancomycin may be added to cover enterococci]).	Add ampicillin to clindamycin/gentamicin; imipenem	Clindamycin/gentamicin
Pelvic abscess	Meropenem 500 mg–l g/IV q8h; clindamycin/gentamicin; metronidazole/gentamicin	Evaluate need for surgical drainage	NA
Septic pelvic thrombophlebitis	Meropenem 500 mg–l g/IV q8h; or metronidazole plus heparin		NA

NA, not applicable.

absorption of this antibiotic is such that blood levels are equivalent to parenteral administration. Metronidazole is only effective against anaerobes and has minimal to no aerobic spectrum.

Investigators have studied various extended-spectrum penicillins and cephalosporins as single agents for the treatment of mild to moderately severe postoperative pelvic infections. These agents have an extended spectrum of *in vitro* antibacterial activity and β-lactamase stability. Single agents—such as cefoxitin, cefotetan, cefuroxime, ticarcillin/clavulanic acid, and piperacillin/tazobactam—avoid the problems of admixture with multiple agents and the potential for aminoglycoside toxicity. In our experience, persistence of infections despite these single agents usually is caused by anaerobic infection.

If an abscess is present and medical management is used to attempt to eradicate it or allow for stabilization before drainage is undertaken, meropenem, a carbapenem, is an excellent choice in a dose of 500 mg given IV every 6 to 8 hours. Metronidazole is a good option when anaerobes are suspected. If the patient has evidence of clinical improvement and decrease in size of the abscess, antibiotics should be continued; if there is no improvement by 48 to 72 hours, surgical drainage is indicated.

Parenteral antibiotics should be continued until the patient is afebrile and clinically well for 24 to 48 hours. At that point, antibiotics may be discontinued and the patient discharged. Several studies show no benefit to the continuation of oral antibiotics after successful parenteral therapy or observing the patient for an additional 24 hours in the hospital.

If there is not a good response to appropriate antibiotic therapy within 72 hours, the patient should be completely reevaluated. After another review of the history and physical examination, imaging studies should be considered. Perhaps a chest x-ray may indicate new consolidation or an abdominal and pelvic CT scan may identify a collection or abscess or even septic thrombophlebitis. If a fever persists, antibiotics may be discontinued, and the patient recultured before new antibiotics are started. SPT should be considered.

PREVENTION OF INFECTION

In this modern era of antibiotics, we have become somewhat lax in our efforts to prevent infection because we assume that if infection occurs, we can easily and effectively treat it. This ignores the potential for morbidity in the patient and the tremendous economic burden imposed by postoperative infections. In a 5-year study of wound infections after abdominal hysterectomy, Kandula and Wenzel found that women with infections were hospitalized an average of 3.55 days longer, resulting in a significant financial impact. It is important to implement specific strategies aimed at preventing postoperative infection and to use these with every patient. In doing so, a significant number of infections can be prevented. Identifying risk factors is important preoperatively. Major risks are obesity, bacterial vaginosis, radical surgery, and excessive blood loss (>1,000 cc).

Some guidelines apply to all situations, and some are specific to certain types of infection. Careful hand washing, avoiding contact with septic patients before proceeding to the operating

TABLE 11.8

RECOMMENDATIONS FOR HAND WASHING

In the absence of a true emergency, personnel should always wash their hands:

- Before performing invasive procedures (Chlorhexidine gluconate 1% solution and ethyl alcohol 61% has been used to replace water-aided hand scrubs with soap in many institutions. We recommend that the initial scrub of the day be with traditional washing for 5 minutes).
- Before taking care of particularly susceptible patients, such as patients who are severely immunocompromised and newborns
- Before and after touching wounds, whether surgical, traumatic, or associated with an invasive device
- After situations during which microbial contamination of hands is likely to occur, particularly those involving contact with mucous membranes, blood, body fluids, secretions, or excretions
- After touching inanimate sources that are likely to be contaminated with virulent or epidemiologically important microorganisms
- After taking care of an infected patient or one who is likely to be colonized with microorganisms of special clinical or epidemiologic significance, such as multiple-drug resistant bacteria
- Between contact with different patients in high-risk units

Most routine, brief patient care activities involving direct patient contact, other than those described, do not require hand washing.

Most routine hospital activities involving indirect patient contact do not require hand washing.

Source: Garner JS, Favero MS. Guideline for hand washing and hospital environmental control, 1985. In: *Guidelines for the prevention and control of nosocomial infections.* Washington, DC: US Department of Health and Human Services, PB82–9234401, 1985:7, with permission.

room, avoiding consecutive contact with patients without hand washing, and minimizing the operating room exposure for infected personnel are a few of the seemingly obvious precautions that frequently are violated.

The skin is colonized with bacteria, some of which are transient and reside on the integument for only a short time, and some of which are resident and are present continuously. One can effectively remove the transient microflora with routine hand washing with soap. The resident organisms require antimicrobial products for their inhibition of growth or elimination. It is not just the surgeon but also nursing personnel who can be the vectors of bacteria. Hand washing thus becomes the most important means of preventing the spread of infection (Table 11.8).

Prevention of Postoperative Pneumonia

All patients who undergo general endotracheal anesthesia are at risk for retention of pulmonary secretions, alveolar collapse, and in turn, atelectasis and possibly pneumonia. Atelectasis is frequently a cause of immediate postoperative fever. To help prevent this complication, all patients undergoing surgery, and especially those with chronic obstructive airway disease, should be encouraged to discontinue or decrease smoking and have any upper respiratory infections treated before operation. Postoperatively, coughing, deep breathing, and devices to encourage alveolar expansions should be used. Adequate analgesia to control pain that interferes with respiratory effort should be administered. Early ambulation should be encouraged.

Prevention of Urinary Tract Infection

UTIs can complicate gynecologic surgery because of the proximity of the urethra to the operative site in the vagina. This effect is augmented by the placement of an indwelling urinary catheter. To limit UTIs, appropriate placement and management of catheters is essential. Personnel should be instructed in the proper sterile placement of catheters, maintained as a closed drainage system without traction on the device. Catheters should be placed only when necessary and should be removed as soon as feasible. Routine culture of terminal urine specimens when catheters are removed has not proven cost-effective in our institution.

Prevention of Operative Site and Wound Infections

Other Considerations

Multiple studies have demonstrated that antibiotic prophylaxis significantly reduces infectious morbidity following both vaginal and abdominal hysterectomy. These results do not mean that the important surgical principles that have been shown to reduce morbidity can be ignored, but the use of prophylactic antibiotics in many gynecologic surgical procedures has reduced the incidence of postoperative surgical site infections from 30% to 50% to about 15% in most series.

Theory of Antibiotic Prophylaxis

At the time of hysterectomy, vaginal or cervical bacteria are inoculated into the surgical site, and it is hypothesized that antibiotics in these tissues at this time augment host defense mechanisms to reduce the incidence of clinical infections. For antibiotic prophylaxis to work effectively, several important criteria must be fulfilled. First, the operative procedure must have a significant risk of bacterial contamination and, in the absence of prophylactic antibiotics, an appreciable incidence of operative site infection. Hysterectomy or other gynecologic procedures involving the cervix, vagina, or vulva all qualify for the criterion. Second, the prophylactic antibiotic administered should be effective against expected pathogens and have a low rate of side effects. Third, the antibiotic should not be one that would be routinely used therapeutically. Although many antibiotic regimens have proven effective in prospective, randomized trials for gynecologic surgery, the cephalosporins have emerged as the generally recommended antibiotic because of their effectiveness, low incidence of side effects, and low cost. Finally, for effective antibiotic prophylaxis, the tissue levels of the chosen antibiotic need to be optimal at the time bacterial contamination of the surgical site occurs. This means that the antibiotic needs to be administered shortly before the start of surgery, usually at the time the patient is brought into the operating room and anesthesia is induced.

Choice of Antibiotics for Prophylaxis

As noted, the antibiotic selected for a given procedure should be effective, have few side effects, be administered in a way that results in a minimal risk of antibiotic-resistant infections, and be inexpensive. In a metaanalysis of 25 prospective, randomized trials of prophylactic antibiotics for abdominal hysterectomy, Mittendorf et al. reported a reduction of serious postoperative infections from 21.1% to 9%. The most commonly used antibiotic for hysterectomy is cefazolin, because it meets the preceding criteria and has a relatively long half-life of 1.8 hours. Recommended prophylactic antibiotic regimens for various gynecologic procedures are listed in Table 11.9.

Cephalosporins generally should not be given to patients with a history of penicillin allergy. Metronidazole and clindamycin have been particularly effective when anaerobic contamination is anticipated in penicillin-sensitive patients.

In women with damaged or artificial heart valves or others at increased risk for bacterial endocarditis, combination antibiotics such as ampicillin (2 g) and gentamicin (1.5 mg/m^2) are recommended. If the patient is allergic to penicillin, vancomycin (1 g over 1 to 2 hours) is substituted for ampicillin. Unlike prophylactic antibiotics given for operative site infections when only a single dose is administered, it is recommended that a second dose be given 6 hours later.

Adverse Reactions

Although reactions to cephalosporins occur from 1% to 10%, severe side effects such as anaphylaxis have been reported in only about 0.02% of patients. The majority of reactions are skin rashes and urticaria, which usually are resolved by the time the patient has recovered from anesthesia postoperatively. Diarrhea secondary to pseudomembranous colitis associated with β-lactam antibiotics has been reported in up to 15% of patients, but it is probably not so common in women receiving only a single prophylactic dose. Although the induction of bacterial resistance to commonly used antibiotics has been a theoretical concern, this has not been a clinical problem when prophylactic antibiotic use is limited to a single dose of common cephalosporins. More potent "big gun" antibiotics should be reserved for specific indications and not used in a prophylactic setting to avoid induction of resistant organisms.

Surveillance for nosocomial infections must be carried out by the hospital infection control program so that surgeons are aware of their individual rates of postoperative infection. Several studies have shown that surgeon-specific wound infection rates can be reduced effectively by such reporting mechanisms.

The classic work of Cruse and Foord helped to delineate specific factors that influence wound infection rates. Others have added to this work so that preoperative and intraoperative management routines can be recommended even though they have not all been confirmed in controlled trials. Preoperative hospitalization should be limited as much as possible. Same-day admission is not just cost-effective for third-party payers, it makes good sense from an infection control perspective. Hair removal should be avoided unless there is an abundance of hair at the operative site. Using a depilatory or clipping the hair is suggested if removal is necessary. Patients should be discouraged from shaving themselves at home before admission.

Because bowel entry is a major cause of contamination and subsequent wound or surgical site infection, having the bowel prepared whenever possible bowel involvement is suspected is beneficial. The Condon bowel prep includes adequate use of a cathartic plus oral neomycin and erythromycin in three doses the day before surgery. The use of a povidone-iodine douche or insertion of gel has been recommended for the night before admission or the day of surgery. Although this practice has been recommended for many years, and povidone-iodine solution and gel have been demonstrated to decrease vaginal bacterial counts to undetectable levels 10 minutes after application, the bacterial flora gradually return to approximately one half pretreatment levels in 2 hours. The benefit of vaginal cleansing with an antiinfective agent the night before, or even immediately before surgery, has not been evaluated in a prospective, randomized trial.

TABLE 11.9

ANTIMICROBIAL PROPHYLACTIC REGIMENS BY PROCEDURE

Procedure	Antibiotic	Dose
Vaginal/abdominal	Cefazolin	1 or 2 single dose IV
Hysterectomy[a]	Cefoxitin	2 g single dose IV
	Cefotetan	1 or 2 single dose IV
	Metronidazole	500 mg single dose IV
Laparoscopy	None	—
Laparotomy	None	—
Hysteroscopy	None	—
Hysterosalpingogram	Doxycycline[b]	100 mg twice daily/5 d orally
IUD insertion	None	—
Endometrial biopsy	None	—
Induced abortion/D&C	Doxycycline	100 mg orally 1 h before procedure and 200 mg orally after the procedure
	Metronidazole	500 mg twice daily orally for 5 d
Urodynamics	None	—

D&C, dilation and curettage; IV, intravenously; IUD, intrauterine device.
[a]A convenient time to administer antibiotic prophylaxis is just before induction of anesthesia.
[b]If hysterosalpingogram demonstrated dilated tubes. No prophylaxis indicated for a normal study.
Source: ACOG Practice Bulletin 2001;23:269, with permission.

Bacterial vaginosis has been found to be a risk factor for postoperative infection when present before surgery in women undergoing hysterectomy. In a prospective study of 175 women who underwent major gynecologic surgery, Lin et al. found a 36% incidence of postoperative febrile morbidity in patients who had bacterial vaginosis preoperatively and only a 20% incidence of fever among the women who had a lactobacillus-predominant vaginal flora ($p = 0.045$). Although some data support the benefit of treating pregnant women with bacterial vaginosis to decrease the rates of preterm labor, premature rupture of the membranes, and intraamniotic infection, no data have shown a beneficial effect of preoperative treatment of hysterectomy patients. In light of the obstetric data, some gynecologists recommend screening hysterectomy patients preoperatively and treating those who are infected with metronidazole because anaerobes play such a significant role in postoperative gynecologic infections.

All gynecologists should employ careful hand-washing techniques or Avagard use preoperatively and when seeing patients. Appropriate gowns and eye coverings should be worn. Wearing double gloves is an effective way to decrease the chances of percutaneous injury. Careful surgical technique is essential to minimize postoperative infections. Adequate hemostasis should be obtained whenever possible. The amount of dead space should be limited. Large areas of necrotic tissue should be excised, and vascular pedicles should be short. Closing the subcutaneous space has no benefit, and using suture there can actually increase the rate of superficial wound infection. If the case is dirty, consideration should be given to delayed wound closure. If drains are used, they should be closed-suction drains, not gravity drains. Draining the subcutaneous space often is helpful in large patients to eliminate serous and bloody fluid.

UNIVERSAL PRECAUTIONS

The epidemics of acquired immunodeficiency syndrome and hepatitis B viral infection have brought to light the risks of lethal infection of the surgeon or other members of the operative team by blood or tissue fluids in association with surgery. Believing that all at-risk situations can be identified by history, physical examination, or laboratory data is naive and dangerous. To overcome this prevalent thought, universal blood and body fluid precautions were developed. This concept treats all patients' blood and certain other body fluids capable of transmitting blood-borne pathogens as potentially infectious. Universal precautions include the following requirements: (a) the use of gloves when touching blood and body fluids, mucous membranes, or broken skin, or when handling items or surfaces soiled with blood or body fluids; (b) the use of masks and eye protection during procedures that can generate splashing or droplets in the air; (c) the use of a gown or plastic apron if splashing of blood is anticipated; (d) careful hand washing if hands are contaminated with blood or body fluids; (e) extraordinary care in handling needles or other sharp objects, and proper disposal of sharp objects in puncture-resistant containers; (f) the availability of emergency resuscitation devices to minimize the need for emergency mouth-to-mouth resuscitation; and (g) the exclusion from patient care of personnel with exudative lesions or weeping dermatitis until these conditions are resolved.

Assuming that every patient is potentially infected, using specific protocols for the safe use of invasive procedures and taking steps to avoid any and all risk-taking behavior by medical personnel can help to prevent nosocomial infections.

Multiple studies have shown that double gloving significantly reduces the risk of blood contamination to the surgeon and other members of the operative team. In a large study from Finland, Laine and Aarnio reported a 7.4% glove perforation rate for single gloves in 1,020 surgeon uses. When double gloves were used, the inner glove was perforated in only 0.52% of 1,148 uses. Overall, someone in the surgical team had a glove perforation during 18.9% of the operative procedures, and the literature quotes rates of up to 61% in orthopedics and trauma surgery. The most common site of perforation is the index finger of the left hand of the surgeon; but all members of the team are at risk, and gloves can be torn in clamps or retractors as well as punctured by needlestick injuries. Manufacturing defects in the gloves themselves are uncommon but do occur and may go unnoticed until blood is seen on the finger or hand. Although double gloving does reduce dexterity and tactile sensation, it also reduces the potential for blood contamination almost 10-fold. It is a good general practice and always should be used in high-risk situations.

BEST SURGICAL PRACTICE

- Major risks factors for postoperative infection include immunocompromise, obesity, bacterial vaginosis, prolonged surgery, radical surgery, and excessive blood loss (>1,000 cc).
- Prophylactic antibiotics have been shown to reduce infectious morbidity for most major gynecologic surgery, including hysterectomy. For antibiotic prophylaxis to work effectively, several important criteria must be fulfilled: (a) the operative procedure must have a significant risk of bacterial contamination; (b) the prophylactic antibiotic administered should be effective against expected pathogens and have a low rate of side effects; (c) the antibiotic should not be one that would be routinely used therapeutically; and (d) the tissue levels of the antibiotic need to be optimal at the time surgery occurs.
- Infections that occur in the first 24 hours after surgery usually are caused by Gram-positive cocci or occasionally by facultative Gram-negative rods. Infections that occur after the first 48 hours more frequently have an anaerobic component. Pelvic infections are polymicrobial in etiology: 20% anaerobic Gram-positive cocci, 20% Gram-negative rods, and 60% anaerobes.
- Rather than routine "fever workup" for postoperative fever evaluation, a careful history, and physical examination are the best guides to which laboratory tests, if any, are indicated. Possible noninfectious causes of early postoperative fever include pulmonary atelectasis, hypersensitivity reactions to antibiotics or anesthetics, pyrogenic reactions to tissue trauma, or hematoma formation.
- To manage deep wound infection, the incision should be probed gently to evaluate fascial integrity. If the fascia is intact, healing is hastened by mechanical debridement followed by loose, wet-to-dry packing with gauze moistened with saline; dilute hydrogen peroxide (1:1 mixture with saline) or Dakin's solution, 0.5%. Povidone-iodine is to be discouraged because it does not promote the development of granulation tissue.
- Evisceration of bowel may occur if a postoperative wound infection involves the fascia. This is a surgical emergency requiring identification of the defect, freshening of the fascial edges, placement of intraabdominal and subcutaneous closed suction drains, and reinforced closure of the fascia.

Some surgeons would leave the skin open for delayed closure; others would close it primarily.

The use of universal precautions to minimize the risk of the surgeon, surgical team, or health care worker acquiring a potentially fatal human immunodeficiency or hepatitis B viral infection from the patient is strongly encouraged. Although high-risk patients may be identified, all patients pose a risk to the surgeon.

Bibliography

American College of Obstetricans and Gynecologists. Bulletin-74 ACOG, 2006. *Antibiotic prophylaxis for gynecologic procedures.* Washington, DC: ACOG, 2006:1216.

Brough SJ, Hunt TM, Barrie WW. Surgical glove perforations. *Br J Surg* 1988;75:317.

Brown CEL, Lowe TW, Cunningham FG, et al. Puerperal pelvic thrombophlebitis: impact on diagnosis and treatment using x-ray computed tomography and magnetic resonance imaging. *Obstet Gynecol* 1986;68: 789.

Centers for Disease Control and Prevention. Public Health Service guidelines for the management of health-care worker exposure to HIV and recommendations for postexposure1prophylaxis. *MMWR Morb Mortal Wkly Rep* 1998;47(RR-7):1.

Centers for Disease Control and Prevention. The 2002 USPHS/IDSA Guidelines for Preventing Opportunistic Infections among HIV-Infected Persons. *MMWR Morb Mortal Wkly Rep* 2002;51(RR-8):xx.

Classen DC, Evan RS, Pestotnik SL, et al. The timing of prophylactic administration of antibiotics and the risk of surgical-wound infection. *N Engl J Med* 1992;326:281.

Condon RE, Schulte WJ, Malongoni MA, et al. Effectiveness of a surgical wound surveillance program. *Arch Surg* 1983;118:303.

Cruse PJE, Foord R. The epidemiology of wound infection: a 10 year prospective study of 62,939 wounds. *Surg Clin North Am* 1980;60:27.

Cuchural GJ, Tally FP, Jacobus NV, et al. Susceptibility of the *Bacteroides fragilis* group in the United States: analysis by site of isolation. *Antimicrob Agents Chemother* 1988;32:717.

Culver DH, Horan TC, Gaynes RF. Surgical wound infection rates by wound class: operative procedure and patient risk index. *Am J Med* 1991;91:152S.

Dellinger EP, Gross PA, Barrett TL, et al. Quality standard for antimicrobial prophylaxis in surgical procedures. Infectious Disease Society of America [review]. *Clin Infect Dis* 1994;18:422.

DeSouza MV. New fluoroquinolones: a class of potent antibiotics. *Mini Rev Med Chem* 2005;5:1009.

Dinsmoor MJ. Imipenem-cilastatin. *Obstet Gynecol Clin North Am* 1992; 19:475.

Donowitz GR, Mandell GL. Beta lactam antibiotics. *N Engl J Med* 1988; 318:490.

Duff P. The aminoglycosides. *Obstet Gynecol Clin North Am* 1992;19:511.

Duff P. Prophylactic antibiotics for hysterectomy. In: Mead PB, Hager WD, Faro S, eds. *Protocols for infectious diseases in obstetrics and gynecology*, 2nd ed. Malden, MA: Blackwell Scientific, 2000;476.

Eason E, Wells G, Garber G, et al. Antisepsis for abdominal hysterectomy: a randomized controlled trial of povidone-iodine gel. *BJOG* 2004;111: 695.

Evaldson GR, Frederici H, Jullig C, et al. Hospital-associated infections in obstetrics and gynecology: effects of surveillance. *Acta Obstet Gynecol Scand* 1992;71:54.

Fanning J, Neuhoff RA, Brewer JE, et al. Frequency and yield of postoperative fever evaluation. *Infect Dis Obstet Gynecol* 1998;6:252.

Fille M, Mango M, Lechner M, et al. *Bacteroides fragilis* group: trends in resistance. *Curr Microbiol* 2006;52:153.

Gallup DC, Gallup DG, Nolan TE, et al. Use of a subcutaneous closed drainage system and antibiotics in obese gynecologic patients. *Am J Obstet Gynecol* 1996;175:358.

Garibaldi RA, Brodine S, Mutsumiya S, et al. Evidence for the noninfectious etiology of early postoperative fever. *Infect Control* 1985;6:273.

Garner JS, Favero MS. Guideline for hand washing and hospital environmental control, 1985. *Guidelines for the prevention and control of nosocomial infections.* Washington, DC: US Department of Health and Human Services, 1985:7.

Grossman JH, Adams RL. Vaginal flora in women undergoing hysterectomy with antibiotic prophylaxis. *Obstet Gynecol* 1979;53:23.

Hager WD, Pascuzzi M, Vernon M. Efficacy of oral antibiotics following parenteral antibiotics for serious infections in obstetrics and gynecology. *Obstet Gynecol* 1989;73:326.

Hager WD, Rapp RP. Metronidazole. *Obstet Gynecol Clin North Am* 1992;19:475.

Haley RW, Culver DH, White JW, et al. The efficiency of infection surveillance and control programs in preventing nosocomial infections in US hospitals. *Am J Epidemiol* 1985;121:182.

Harris WJ. Early complications of abdominal and vaginal hysterectomy. *Obstet Gynecol Surv* 1995;50:795.

Hemsell DL. Gynecologic postoperative infections in obstetric and gynecologic infectious disease. In: Pastorek JG, ed. *Obstetric and gynecologic infectious disease.* New York: Raven Press, 1994; 141.

Hemsell DL, Bowden RE, Hemsell PG, et al. Single-dose cephalosporin for prevention of major pelvic infection after vaginal hysterectomy: cefazolin vs. cefoxitin vs. cefotaxime. *Am J Obstet Gynecol* 1987;156:1201.

Hemsell DL, Johnson ER, Bowden RE, et al. Ceftriaxone and cefazolin prophylaxis for hysterectomy. *Surg Gynecol Obstet* 1985;161:197.

Hemsell DL, Johnson ER, Heard MC, et al. Single-dose piperacillin vs. triple-dose cefoxitin prophylaxis at vaginal and abdominal hysterectomy. *South Med J* 1984;82:438.

Hemsell DL, Nobles B, Heard MC. Recognition and treatment of posthysterectomy pelvic infections. *Infect Surg* 1988;7:47.

Hoyme UB, Tamimi HK, Eschenbach DA, et al. Osteomyelitis pubis after radical gynecologic operations. *Obstet Gynecol* 1984;63:475.

Jaffe TA, Nelson RC, DeLong DM, et al. Practice patterns in percutaneous image-guided intraabdominal abscess drainage: survey of academic and private practice centers. *Radiology* 2004;233:750.

Jenson SL, Kristensen B, Fabrin K. Double gloving as self protection in abdominal surgery. *Eur J Surg* 1997;163:163.

John JF. What price success? The continuing saga of the toxic therapeutic ratio in the use of aminoglycoside antibiotics. *J Infect Dis* 1988;158:1.

Kamat AA, Brancazio L, Gibson M. Wound infection in gynecologic surgery. *Infect Dis Obstet Gynecol* 2000;8:230.

Kandula PV, Wenzel RP. Postoperative wound infection after total abdominal hysterectomy: a controlled study of the increased duration of hospital stay and trends in postoperative wound infection. *Am J Infect Control* 1993;21:201.

Korn AP, Gullon K, Hessol N, et al. Does vaginal cuff closure decrease the infectious morbidity associated with abdominal hysterectomy? *J Am Coll Surg* 1997;185:404.

Laine T, Aarnio P. How often does glove perforation occur in surgery? Comparison between single gloves and a double-gloving system. *Am J Surg* 2001;181:564.

Lars P, Naver S, Gottrup F. Incidence of glove perforations in gastrointestinal surgery and the protective effect of double gloves: a prospective, randomised, controlled study. *Eur J Surg* 2000;166:293.

Larsen JW, Hager WD, Livengood CH, et al. Guidelines for the diagnosis, treatment and prevention of postoperative infections. *Infect Dis Obstet Gynecol* 2003;11:65.

Leaper D, Ayliffe GA, Gilchrist B. Postoperative wound infection. *J Wound Care* 1996;5:330.

Lin L, Song J, Kimber N, et al. The role of bacterial vaginosis in infection after major gynecologic surgery. *Infect Dis Obstet Gynecol* 1999;7: 169.

Lyon DS, Jones JL, Sanchez A. Postoperative febrile morbidity in the benign gynecologic patient. *J Reprod Med* 2000;45:305.

Mage G, Masson FN, Canis M. Laparoscopic hysterectomy. *Curr Opin Obstet Gynecol* 1995;7:283.

McNally CG, Krivak TC, Alagoz T. Conservative management of isolated post hysterectomy fever. *J Reprod Med* 2000;45:572.

Mead PB, Hager WD, Faro S. *Protocols for infectious diseases in obstetrics and gynecology*, 2nd ed. Malden, MA: Blackwell Scientific, 2000.

Monif GR, Thompson JL, Stephens HD, et al. Quantitative and qualitative effects of povidone-iodine liquid and gel on the aerobic and anaerobic flora of the female genital tract. *Am J Obstet Gynecol* 1980;137:432.

Ong CT, Kuti JL, Nicolau DP. Pharmacodynamic modeling of imipenem-cilastatin, meropenem and piperacillin-tazobactam for empiric therapy of skin and soft tissue infections: a report from the OPYAMA program. *Surg Infect* 2005;6:419.

Persson E, Bergstrom M, Larsson PG, et al. Infections after hysterectomy: a prospective, nation-wide Swedish study. *Acta Obstet Gynecol Scand* 1996;75:757.

Peters WA. Bartholinitis after vulvovaginal surgery. *Am J Obstet Gynecol* 1998;178:1143.

Rhomberg PR, Fritsche TR, Sader HS, et al. Clonal occurrences of multidrug-resistant Gram-negative bacilli: a report from the meropenem yearly susceptibility test information collection program in the United States (2004).

Diagn Microbiol Infect Dis 2006;54:249–257. http://www.dmidjournal.com/medline/record/MDLN.16466890.

Sawyer RG, Pruett TL. Wound infections. *Surg Clin North Am* 1994;74:519.

Schwandt A, Andrews SJ, Fanning J. Prospective analysis of a fever evaluation algorithm after major gynecologic surgery. *Am J Obstet Gynecol* 2001;184:1066.

Shapiro M, Munoz A, Tager IB, et al. Risk factors for infection at the operative site after abdominal or vaginal hysterectomy. *N Engl J Med* 1982;307:1661.

Solomkin J, Teppler H, Graham DR, Gesser RM, et al. Treatment of polymicrobial infections: *post hoc* analysis of three trials comparing ertapenem and piperacillin-tazobactam. *J Antimicrob Chemother* 2004;53(suppl S2):51.

Soper DE. Bacterial vaginosis and postoperative infections. *Am J Obstet Gynecol* 1993;169:467.

Thomason JL, Gelbart SM, Scaylione NJ. Bacteria vaginosis: current review with indications for asymptomatic therapy. *Am J Obstet Gynecol* 1991;165:1210.

CHAPTER 12 ■ SHOCK IN THE GYNECOLOGIC PATIENT

HARRIET O. SMITH AND HEATHER M. GREENE

DEFINITIONS

Cardiogenic shock—Shock in which there is intrinsic pump failure.

Class I hypovolemia—Blood losses of less than 15% of the total blood volume with no measurable changes in blood pressure, resting pulse, or respiratory rates.

Class II hypovolemia—1,000 mL of blood loss, consistent with tachycardia; however, resting blood pressure is generally preserved.

Class III hypovolemia—Blood loss equivalent to 30% to 40% of plasma volume marked by insufficient perfusion, tachycardia, tachypnea, severely diminished urinary output, and cold clammy skin.

Class IV hypovolemia—Acute blood loss of more than 2,000 mL or more than 40% of circulating volume, which is immediately life threatening.

Distributive shock—Shock in which total body water is normal or slightly decreased but is pooled into the interstitial fluid compartment, resulting in intravascular volume depletion.

Extracardiac obstructive shock—Shock in which the heart is intrinsically normal and total volume is adequate, but mechanical factors interfere with pump performance.

Hypovolemic shock—Shock in which there is an inadequate circulating blood volume resulting from hemorrhage or acute volume depletion.

Infection—A pathologic process caused by the invasion of normally sterile tissue or fluid or body cavity by pathogenic or potentially pathogenic microorganisms.

Neutropenic fever—Presence of three oral temperatures of 38°C (100.4°F) or a single temperature higher than 38.5°C (101.3°F) coexistent with a low absolute neutrophil count (ANC, less than 500/mm^3).

Septic shock—Sepsis with hypotension that persists despite adequate fluid resuscitation, leading to derangements in cellular and organ system function.

Systemic inflammatory response syndrome—Presence of a early hyperdynamic phase of shock but no site of infection can be found.

Shock states are among the most formidable conditions that the gynecologist is likely to encounter. The morbidity and economic impact of shock are enormous, considering the costs of primary treatment, the management of multiorgan failure syndrome, and providing care for long-term disabilities that may result from partial or total loss of organ function. In the United States annually, septic shock alone affects 100,000 to 300,000 patients at an annual cost of $5 billion to $10 billion. Although recent studies indicate improvements in survival, 50% to 60% of those affected with septic shock will not survive despite aggressive therapy and significant expenditure. In obstetrics, two of the three most common causes of maternal mortality are complications from hemorrhage and sepsis. Therefore, it is critical for the practicing obstetrician-gynecologist to understand the pathogenesis, clinical signs and symptoms, and management of shock because prompt recognition and early intervention significantly reduces morbidity and mortality.

Although shock can be defined as a condition in which tissue perfusion is incapable of sustaining aerobic metabolism, in practical terms shock is best defined as an acute clinical syndrome characterized by hypoperfusion and severe dysfunction of organs vital for survival. These manifestations result from an acute generalized disturbance in the normal cardiovascular circulation. Cardiac output and circulatory blood volume may be compromised by direct myocardial injury or from hypovolemia. Clinical manifestations include mean arterial hypotension and circulatory collapse. Severe hypovolemia can occur as a direct result of uncontrolled hemorrhage or, as in septic shock, may result from the pathological redistribution of circulating volume.

CLASSIFICATION AND ETIOPATHOGENESIS

Based on the underlying cause, shock can be divided into four main categories (Table 12.1):

1. *Hypovolemic shock*, in which there is an inadequate circulating blood volume resulting from hemorrhage or acute volume depletion
2. *Distributive shock*, in which total body water is normal or slightly decreased, but is "pooled" into the interstitial fluid compartment, resulting in intravascular volume depletion
3. *Cardiogenic shock*, in which there is intrinsic pump failure
4. *Extracardiac obstructive shock*, in which the heart is intrinsically normal and total blood volume is adequate, but mechanical factors interfere with pump performance

Often, shock results from more than one of these circulatory disturbances, and the apparent cause of persistent cardiovascular dysfunction can change with time and intervening therapy. For example, septic shock is generally considered the result of tissue hypoperfusion; however, endotoxins and mediators released from injured cells have additional direct myocardial depressant effects. Thus, the cardiac presentation is similar for both hypovolemic shock and cardiogenic shock from intrinsic cardiac disease. Cardiogenic shock is characterized by a low systolic blood pressure (<80 mm Hg) associated with a severely reduced cardiac index (usually <1.8 L/min/m^2) and a high left ventricular filling pressure (usually >18 mm Hg). Pulmonary edema may be present or absent. Extracardiac

TABLE 12.1

CLASSIFICATION OF SHOCK STATES

Classification	Conditions encountered in gynecology and obstetrics
Hypovolemic	
Hemorrhagic	Obstetric hemorrhage, ectopic pregnancy, acute operative blood loss, retroperitoneal bleeding, trauma
Nonhemorrhagic	Vomiting, diarrhea, acute drainage of ascites, renal losses (diuretics, postobstructive diuresis, acute tubular necrosis), peritonitis
Distributive	Sepsis, anaphylaxis, preeclampsia, advanced ovarian cancer with ascites and/or pleural effusions, intestinal obstruction, adrenal insufficiency, cerebral or spinal cord injuries, toxic/pharmacologic (vasodilators, benzodiazepines), endocrinologic
Cardiogenic	Myocardial infarction, myocarditis, pharmacologic/toxic depression (anthracycline, β-blockers, calcium channel blockers), cardiomyopathies, mechanical valve failure, arrhythmias
Extracardiac obstructive	Massive pulmonary embolism, cardiac tamponade, constrictive pericarditis, coarctation of the aorta, severe pulmonary hypertension, mediastinal tumors, tension pneumothorax, positive-pressure ventilation
	Mixed sepsis, neurogenic shock, anaphylaxis, toxin poisoning, drug overdose, amniotic fluid embolism

obstructive shock is characterized by the inability of the ventricle to fill during diastole, which severely reduces stroke volume and cardiac output. In the gynecologic patient, massive pulmonary embolus is the most common example.

Regardless of the precipitating event, hypotension results from an inadequate circulatory volume caused by cardiac insufficiency, loss of sympathetic tone, inadequate plasma volume, or a combination of these factors (Fig. 12.1). Prolonged hypotension and organ hypoperfusion leads to cellular injury that, if left unchecked, culminates in cardiovascular collapse and death or organ system failure. Because the most common types of shock encountered in obstetrics and gynecology are from hypovolemia (usually, resulting from hemorrhage) or sepsis, this chapter will focus on the recognition and management of these forms of shock.

Hypovolemic Shock

Hypovolemic shock may be subdivided into four classes based on presenting signs and symptoms (Table 12.2). This classification schema is useful for understanding the pathophysiologic mechanisms responsible for the changes in clinical presentation with progressively greater increments of blood loss and for estimating initial crystalloid or blood requirements. The clinical manifestations of hemorrhagic shock can vary greatly, depending on the rate and the total volume lost, and red cell loss as measured by hemoglobin and hematocrit which do not take into account total or plasma volume. Therefore, these patients may be hypovolemic, euvolemic, or hypervolemic. Recent studies of acute hypovolemic anemia using tagged red blood cell (RBC) studies have found that in the first few hours after surgery, the hematocrit is transiently *elevated* by as much as 5% because of failure of the plasma volume to correct in accordance with blood loss. When the rate of loss has been gradual, as might be found with an unruptured ectopic pregnancy or a retroperitoneal bleed, plasma refill and other compensatory mechanisms can ensure an adequate circulating plasma volume, and the resuscitative requirements can be severely underestimated. Once initial fluid resuscitation is begun, close observation and frequent reassessment are required as these patients remain at risk for circulatory collapse.

Class I hypovolemia is associated with losses of less than 15% of the total blood volume (Table 12.2); usually, there are no measurable changes in blood pressure, resting pulse, or respiratory rates. Transcapillary refill and other compensatory mechanisms usually restore plasma volume within 24 hours. With class II hypovolemia, or up to 1,000 mL blood loss, the most consistent clinical finding is tachycardia. The increase in heart rate is often associated with a narrowed pulse pressure (the difference between systolic and diastolic pressures). The resting blood pressure, however, is generally preserved by compensatory mechanisms, including the renin-angiotensin system and the hypothalamic–hypophyseal–adrenal system. In response to a decrease in wall tension or sodium, or sympathetic activation, the juxtaglomerular cells release renin into plasma. Renin converts angiotensinogen into angiotensin I, an inactive polypeptide, which is metabolized in the liver to angiotensin II, a potent vasoconstrictor that stimulates aldosterone secretion from the renal cortex. Aldosterone, along with the pituitary release of antidiuretic hormone, promotes sodium and water retention. These mechanisms increase venous return and, consequently, stroke volume, cardiac output, and blood pressure. Thus, oliguria is a common manifestation of hypovolemic shock. In response to hypovolemia, norepinephrine and epinephrine are locally and systemically released. Catecholamine-mediated effects are inotropic and chronotropic, resulting in increased cardiac output. Venoconstriction enhances venous return, which also increases stroke volume and cardiac output. In response to the catecholamine–mediated increase in peripheral vascular resistance, the diastolic blood pressure is increased, which leads to a narrowed pulse pressure. Typically, the resting blood pressure is normal; however, when blood pressure and pulse are recorded in the standing, sitting, or reclining position, postural hypotension is usually observed. This is the major clinical distinction between class I and class II hypovolemic shock. As long as these compensatory mechanisms remain intact, shock is almost always eventually reversible, hence the frequently used descriptive term *early* shock.

Although patients with losses of 20% to 30% of their blood volume may ultimately require RBC replacement for immediate resuscitation, crystalloid is usually adequate. Crystalloid replacement is guided by the 3:1 rule: 300 mL crystalloid per 100 mL of blood (plasma volume) loss. In normal adults, approximately two thirds of the total body water is intracellular, and the remaining one third in the extracellular fluid compartment is disproportionately distributed between the interstitial and intravascular compartments in a 3:1 ratio. Colloid oncotic pressure, the effective osmotic pressure between the intravascular and interstitial compartments, is dependent on

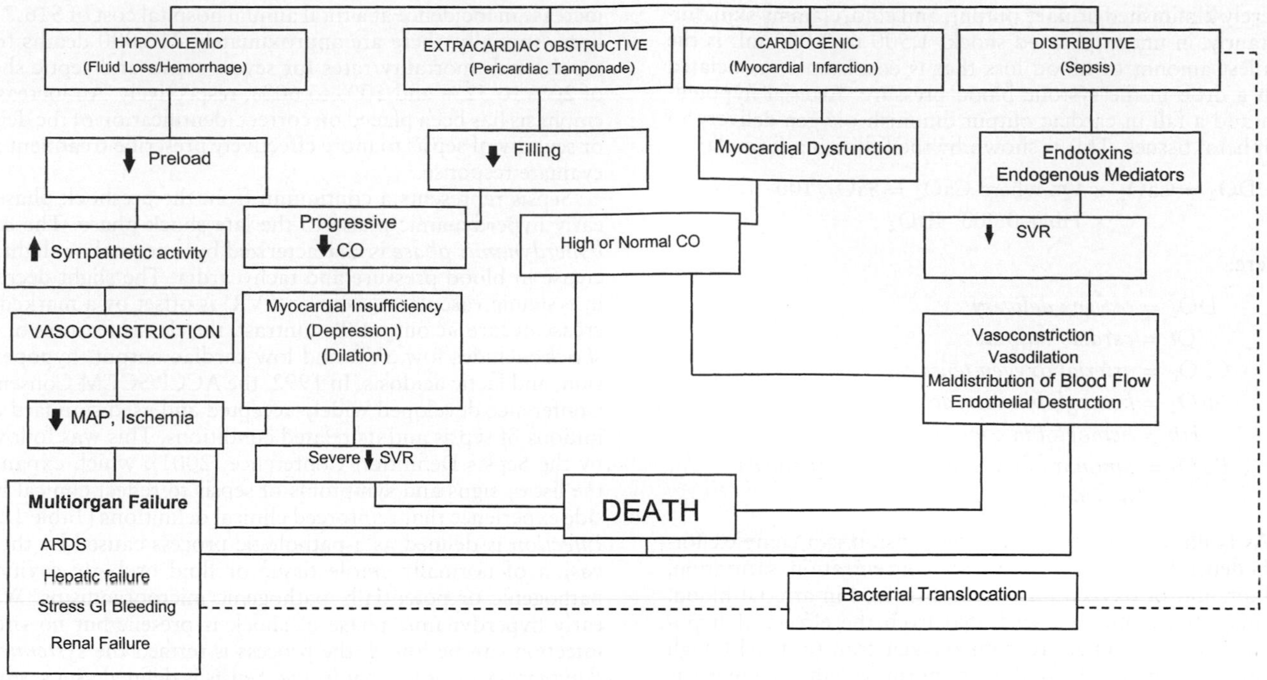

FIGURE 12.1. Pathogenesis of human shock. CO, cardiac output; MAP, mean arterial pressure; SVR, systemic vascular resistance; ARDS, adult respiratory distress syndrome; GI, gastrointestinal. (Adapted from Hollenberg SM, Parrillo JE. Shock. In Fauci AS, Martin JP, Braunwald E, et al., eds., *Harrison's principles of internal medicine,* vol. 1. New York: McGraw-Hill; 1997:217.)

transcapillary hydrostatic and oncotic pressures, and the relative permeability of capillary membranes that divide these spaces. Because of these forces, within 24 hours of intravenous crystalloid administration, approximately two thirds will disperse into the interstitial compartments.

Although the principal determinant of oxygen delivery is hemoglobin, tissue oxygenation remains adequate as long as intravascular volume is adequate, and cardiac output appropriately increases despite major reductions in hemoglobin (<7 g/dL). This is because oxygen delivery is not dependent on hemoglobin concentration alone. However, in class III hypovolemic shock (Table 12.2), which is associated with a blood loss equivalent to 30% to 40% of the plasma volume, the physiologic compensatory mechanisms previously described begin to fail. Patients almost always present with classic signs of insufficient perfusion, including marked tachycardia, tachypnea,

TABLE 12.2

CLASSIFICATION OF HYPOVOLEMIC SHOCK[a]

	Class I	Class II	Class III	Class IV
Blood loss (mL)	<750	750–1,500	1,500–2,000	>2,000
Blood volume (%)	<15	15–30	30–40	>40
Heart rate (beats/minute)	<100	>100	>120	>140
Blood pressure	Normal or increased	Normal (+ tilt[b])	Decreased (mean arterial pressure <60 mm Hg)	Decreased
Pulse pressure	Normal	Decreased	Decreased	Decreased
Capillary refill	Normal	May be delayed	Usually delayed	Always delayed
Respirations (breaths/min)	Normal 14–20	Mildly increased 20–30	Moderate to marked tachypnea 30–40	Marked tachypnea; respiratory collapse >35
Urinary output (mL/h)	>30	20–30	5–15	Essentially anuric
Mental status	Normal or anxious	Anxious	Confused	Lethargic, obtunded

[a]In a 70-kg, nonpregnant adult.
[b]Measure heart rate and blood pressure in standing, sitting, and recumbent positions with 5 minutes between measurements to permit equilibration. Orthostatic change (+ tilt) is a postural increase in pulse of 10 to 15 beats/minute or a drop in systolic blood pressure of at least 10 mm Hg.
Adapted from *Advanced trauma life support® student manual.* Chicago: American College of Surgeons, 1997, second impression 1999:9.

severely diminished urinary output, and cold, clammy skin. Importantly, in uncomplicated shock, 1,500 to 2,000 mL is the smallest amount of blood loss that is consistently associated with a drop in the systolic blood pressure. Arterial hypotension and a fall in cardiac output diminish oxygen delivery to peripheral tissues. This is shown by the following formula:

$$DO_2 = CaO_2 \times Qt, \text{ where } CaO_2 = SaO_2/100 \cdot 1.39 \times Hb + 0.003 \cdot PaO_2.$$

Where:

DO_2 = *oxygen delivery;*
Qt = *cardiac output;*
CaO_2 = *arterial oxygen tension;*
SaO_2 = *hemoglobin saturation;*
Hb = *hemoglobin concentration; and*
PaO_2 = *amount of oxygen physically dissolved in arterial blood.*

As is illustrated, arterial oxygen tension is a complex formula dependent on the hemoglobin concentration, saturation, and amount of oxygen physically dissolved in arterial blood. Anemia effects must be separated from the effects of hypovolemia, as both interfere with oxygen transport. Although the lower limit of tolerated acute normovolemic anemia has not been established, most normal individuals tolerate Hb of 7 g/dL, partially as a result of improved O_2 delivery facilitated by increase in 2,3-diphosphoglycerate levels in RBCs.

Tissues that can maintain their oxygen consumption accomplish this by increasing their *oxygen extraction*, the ratio of oxygen consumption to oxygen delivery. This results in an increase in the arterial and venous oxygen difference and a reduction in the mixed venous oxygen tension. Eventually, under conditions of increased oxygen demand (stress, sepsis) or insufficient oxygen delivery (severely reduced cardiac output, hypovolemia, and profound anemia), these compensatory mechanisms fail, and tissue hypoxia and lactic acidosis ensue. Cerebral and cardiac functions are maintained by diverting blood flow from the skin, muscles, gastrointestinal tract, and kidneys. Complicated shock associated with loss of compensatory physiologic mechanisms is often called *intermediate shock*. In this phase, reversibility is dependent on prompt crystalloid and blood product replacement to avoid irreversible ischemia of vital organs.

Class IV hypovolemic shock, defined as an acute blood loss of more than 2,000 mL, or more than 40% of the circulating volume, is immediately life threatening. Survival depends on rapid transfusion of blood and crystalloid and immediate surgical intervention before cardiac and cerebral circulation fail, resulting in ischemia in these organs. When vital organs fail, total cardiovascular collapse, coma, and eventually death or multiorgan failure is likely. The transition between the intermediate stage of shock and *irreversible shock* (*late shock, cold shock*) is dependent on the duration and severity of the hypovolemia; however, once cellular injury has occurred within the brain and cardiac muscle, shock is almost always irreversible and fatal.

Septic Shock

Over the past several decades, the incidence of sepsis—the precursor to septic shock and multiorgan failure—has increased. In the United States alone, sepsis and septic shock affect an estimated 750,000 patients per year with an expected 1.5% annual increase in incidence at a total annual hospital cost of $16.7 billion. Annually, there are approximately 215,000 deaths from sepsis, with mortality rates for severe sepsis and septic shock of 20% to 52% and 50% to 60%, respectively. An increasing emphasis has been placed on correct identification of the degree or severity of sepsis to more effectively prescribe treatment and evaluate response.

Sepsis represents a continuum from the preshock phase or early hyperdynamic phase to the late shock phase. The *early hyperdynamic phase* is characterized by a normal or slight decrease in blood pressure and tachycardia. The slight decrease in systemic vascular resistance (SVR) is offset by a marked increase in cardiac output. In contrast, the classic features of *late shock* includes low SVR and low cardiac output, hypoperfusion, and lactic acidosis. In 1992, the ACCP/SCCM Consensus Conference developed widely accepted and used standard definitions of sepsis and its related conditions. This was followed by the Sepsis Definition Conference (2001), which expanded the list of signs and symptoms of sepsis to reflect clinical bedside experience that reinforced clinical definitions (Table 12.3). *Infection* is defined as a pathologic process caused by the invasion of normally sterile tissue or fluid or body cavity by pathogenic or potentially pathogenic microorganisms. When early hyperdynamic phase of shock is present but no site of infection can be found, the process is termed the *systemic inflammatory response syndrome*. *Sepsis* is defined as a systemic response to infection manifested by two or more of the following: fever or hypothermia, tachycardia, tachypnea, and an elevated or severely depressed white blood cell count. *Septic shock* is sepsis with hypotension that persists despite adequate fluid resuscitation, leading to derangements in cellular and organ system function. Although helpful in differentiating categories of sepsis, Levy and colleagues note that these definitions do not allow for precise classification and staging of patients with this condition. Therefore, a rudimentary stratification scheme termed Predisposing Factors, Infection, Response, and Organ Dysfunction (PIRO) was developed to classify patients in terms of their predisposing conditions, the nature of the insult (which in the case of sepsis is the infection), and the nature and magnitude of host response and the degree of concomitant organ dysfunction (Table 12.4).

Microbial factors contribute to outcome in patients with severe sepsis. Hospital-acquired bacteremia has increased coincident with the rise in predisposing risk factors: an aging population with underlying systemic disease (diabetes mellitus, cirrhosis, malignancy, lymphoproliferative disorders), invasive devices, burns, prolonged or indiscriminate use of broad–spectrum antibiotics, aggressive cytotoxic chemotherapy, and use of corticosteroids and other immunosuppressive agents. Most nosocomial infections are associated with the use of invasive devices: 83% of pneumonias in mechanically ventilated patients, 97% of urinary tract infections in catheterized patients, and 87% of bloodstream infections in patients with central intravenous lines. Although sepsis can be caused by fungi and viruses, Gram-positive bacteria and Gram-negative bacteria are the most common isolates from patients with severe sepsis. Gram-negative organisms used to account for more than half of all episodes of bacteremia, but recent studies indicate that mortality caused by Gram-positive bacteremia now equals or exceeds that of Gram-negative bacteremia. Staphylococci, mainly *Staphylococcus aureus* or coagulase-negative staphylococcus, and streptococci such as *Streptococcus pneumoniae* are the most frequent microbes involved. In obstetrics and gynecology, Gram-positive aerobes account for 31% of bacteremic episodes, and Gram-positive anaerobes, mainly group B streptococcus and *Peptococcus*, 18% of septic

TABLE 12.3

CLINICAL DEFINITIONS OF INFECTION SYNDROMES

Infection	Microbial phenomenon characterized by an inflammatory response to the presence of microorganisms or the invasion of normally sterile host tissue by those organisms.
Bacteremia	Presence of viable bacteria in the blood.
Systemic inflammatory response syndrome	Systemic inflammatory response to a variety of clinical insults. The response is manifested by two or more of the following conditions: temperature >38°C or <36°C; heart rate >90 beats/min; respiratory rate >20 breaths/min or $Paco_2$ <32 mm Hg; or WBC >12,000/μL, <4000/μL, or more than 10% immature (band) forms.
Sepsis	The systemic response to infection. This response is manifested by two or more of the following conditions as a result of infection: temperature >38°C or <36°C; heart rate >90 beats/min; respiratory rate >20 breaths/min or $Paco_2$ <32 torr (<4.3 kPa); WBC >12,000 μL or <4,000 μL, or more than 10% immature (band) forms.
Severe sepsis[a]	Sepsis associated with organ dysfunction, hypoperfusion, or hypotension. Hypoperfusion and perfusion anomalies may include but are not limited to lactic acidosis, oliguria, or an acute alteration in mental status.
Septic shock	Sepsis with hypotension despite adequate fluid resuscitation, along with the presence of perfusion abnormalities that can include, but are not limited to, lactic acidosis, oliguria, or an acute alteration in mental status.
Patients who are on inotropic or vasopressor agents may not be hypotensive at the time that perfusion abnormalities are measured.	
Hypotension	A systolic blood pressure of <90 mm Hg or a reduction of >40 mm Hg from baseline, in the absence of other causes of hypotension.
Multiple organ dysfunction syndrome	Presence of altered organ function in an acutely ill patient such that homeostasis cannot be maintained without intervention.

WBC, white blood cell count; bpm, beats per minute.
[a]Sepsis with organ system dysfunction.
Adapted from the American College of Chest Physicians/Society of Critical Care Medicine Consensus Conference. Definitions for sepsis and organ failure and guidelines for the use of innovative therapies in sepsis. *Crit Care Med* 1992;20:866.

episodes; Gram-negative microbes are responsible for 41% of all septic episodes. The most commonly isolated Gram-negative bacteria are *Escherichia coli*, *Klebsiella pneumoniae*, and *Pseudomonas aeruginosa*, with *Escherichia coli* predominating. Less frequent isolates include *Enterobacter aerogenes Acinetobacter*, *Proteus*, *Serratia*, *Aeromonas*, *Xanthomonas*, *Citrobacter*, *Achromobacter*, *Salmonella*, and *Shigella* sps.

The Gram-negative bacterial cell wall consists of an inner and outer cell membrane, the latter of which contains lipopolysaccharide (LPS), or bacterial endotoxin. LPS consists of three principal regions: the O antigen, the R core antigen, and lipid A, which is responsible for toxicity. The lipid A portion of the LPS molecule mediates the binding of CD14 and Toll-like receptors (TLRs—specifically TRL4) and perhaps other receptors with lipopolysaccharide-binding protein (LBP). This coupling enables LPS to bind to mammalian cells. Depending on the involved cell type, LPS-LBP-CD14-TRL4 receptor binding induces the release of a variety of mediators. These include cytokines, interferon–λ, prostaglandins, prostacyclins, thromboxane A_2, leukotrienes, complement protein fragments (especially C3a, C5a), platelet-activating factor (PAF), and catecholamines. Peptidoglycan and lipoteichoic acids of Gram-positive bacteria, certain polysaccharides, extracellular enzymes, and toxins are also able to induce intracellular responses similar to those of LPS (Fig. 12.2). The inflammatory cytokines interact by way of autocrine, paracrine, and endocrine mechanisms to stimulate leukocytes and vascular endothelial cells to release other cytokines, express cell–surface adhesion molecules, and increase production of arachidonic metabolites. Biologically, their effects appear to be synergistic. Tumor necrosis factor (TNF)–α in particular plays an early, critical role in cellular activation and the propagation of the inflammatory response. TNF–α levels are elevated in severe sepsis, myocardial infarction, adult respiratory distress syndrome, and multiorgan failure and correlate with increased mortality rates. In contrast, interleukin (IL)-1 levels are only slightly increased in humans with severe sepsis and do not appear to correlate with severity or outcome. However, plasma concentrations of IL-6 in plasma levels can discriminate among patients who survive or die from severe sepsis/septic shock. In women with pelvic inflammatory disease (PID), cervical as well as systemic IL-6 levels are increased, and correlate with higher erythrocyte sedimentation rate and white blood cell counts. These data suggest that measurements of specific inflammatory cytokines such as IL-6 may eventually be used to evaluate response to therapy in patients with PID.

Hemostatic defects are common in sepsis and result from vascular endothelial cell injury thought to be caused by endotoxins and phospholipid-derived mediators. The net coagulation defects in sepsis are predominantly procoagulant and override the anticoagulant effects that concomitantly occur. Prostaglandin E_2 and prostacyclin are potent vasodilators, whereas thromboxane A_2 is a potent vasoconstrictor that, together with PAF, promotes platelet aggregation. Blood coagulation results from activation of the intrinsic, extrinsic, and common pathways, culminating in the generation of thrombin. Thrombosis is enhanced by impairment of antithrombin III and tissue plasminogen activator, as well as by plasminogen activator inhibitor–1, released by stimulated monocytes. Neutrophils, attracted by the injured vascular epithelium, release prostacyclins that inhibit thrombin formation and elastases—free oxygen radicals, proteases, and leukotrienes that are responsible for fibrinolysis. Microcirculation is further impaired by the resulting microthrombi and the cytotoxic effects of cytokines released by inflammatory cells

TABLE 12.4

THE PIRO SYSTEM FOR STAGING SEPSIS

Domain	Present	Future	Rationale
Predisposition	Premorbid illness with reduced probability of short-term survival; cultural or religious beliefs, age, sex	Genetic polymorphisms in components of inflammatory response (e.g., TLR, TNF, IL-1, CD14); enhanced understanding of specific interactions between pathogens and host diseases	Premorbid factors impact on the potential attributable morbidity and mortality of an acute insult; deleterious consequences of insult heavily dependent on genetic predisposition (future)
Insult infection	Culture and sensitivity of infecting pathogens; detection of disease amenable to source control	Assay of microbial products (LPS, mannan, bacterial DNA); gene transcript profiles	Specific therapies directed against inciting insult require demonstration and characterization of the insult
Response	SIRS, other signs of sepsis, shock, CRP	Nonspecific markers of activated inflammation (e.g., PCT or IL-6) or impaired host responsiveness (e.g., HLA-DR); specific detection of target of therapy (e.g., protein C, TNF, PAF)	Both mortality risk and potential to respond to therapy vary with nonspecific measures of disease severity (e.g., shock); specific mediator-targeted therapy is predicated on presence and activity of mediator
Organ dysfunction	Organ dysfunction as a number of failing organs or composite score (e.g., MODS, SOFA, LODS, PREMOD, PELOD)	Dynamic measures of cellular response to insult-apoptosis, cytopathic hypoxia, cell stress	Response to preemptive therapy (e.g., targeting microorganism or early mediator not possible if damage already present; therapies targeting the injurious cellular process require that it be present)

PIRO, Predisposing Factors, Infection, Response, and Organ Dysfunction; TLR, Toll-like receptor; TNF, tumor necrosis factor; IL, interleukin; LPS, lipopolysaccharide; SIRS, systemic inflammatory response syndrome; CRP, C-reactive protein; PCT, procalcitonin; HLA-human leukocyte antigen-DR; PAF, platelet-activating factor; MODS, multiple organ dysfunction syndrome; SOFA, sepsis-related organ failure assessment; LODS, logistic organ dysfunction system; PEMOD, pediatric multiple organ dysfunction; PELOD, pediatric logistic organ dysfunction.
From: Levy MM, Fink MP, Marshal JC, et al. 2001 SCCM/ESICM/ACCP/ATS/SIS International Sepsis Definitions Conference. *Crit Care Med* 2003;31 (4):1250, with permission.

attracted to the damaged endothelium. This effect has been proposed as a possible mechanism for persistent organ system dysfunction. Thrombocytopenia is common. Although fulminate disseminated intravascular coagulation can eventually develop, the coagulation profile is usually consistent with compensated intravascular coagulation with fibrinolysis. That is, fibrinogen levels are normal or slightly decreased, prothrombin time (PT) and partial thromboplastin time (PTT) are within the normal range, and the D-dimer assay is only weakly positive.

Regardless of whether the initial insult is infection, pump failure, or hypovolemia, a major feature of the systemic inflammatory response is the rapid loss of lean body mass associated with net nitrogen losses (20 to 30 g/d). The primary sites of total protein catabolism are the skeletal muscle, connective tissue, and gut mucosa. Hepatic uptake of amino acids is increased, with a concomitant increase in the synthesis of acute-phase proteins. Energy expenditure is often 1.5 to 2 times the basal rate and is increased in proportion to the degree of injury by a process known as aerobic glycolysis. The net result is a significant increase in the production and release of lactate and pyruvate from muscles, wounds, and monocytes. Hepatic gluconeogenesis is increased, as well as glycogenolysis. As hypoperfusion worsens, lactic acid is generated by hypoxic tissue, resulting in metabolic acidosis. Initially, a blood gas analysis usually demonstrates a respiratory alkalosis, but a metabolic acidosis of multifactorial origin eventually develops. The decreases in bicarbonate are often in excess of the measured increase in lactic acid. Hyperglycemia can occur, especially in diabetic patients; however, impaired gluconeogenesis and excessive insulin release can lead to profound hypoglycemia. Lipolysis and ketogenesis are also increased, and in the absence of nutritional support, long-chain fatty acid deficiency develops.

In patients who develop irreversible organ failure, the systemic inflammatory response is maintained long after the initial injury and response have abated. Although the mechanisms for this process are poorly understood, undetected microcirculatory dysfunction may be a critical factor. More likely, at some critical point, the perpetuation of cellular and organ system hypermetabolism becomes independent of host regulatory mechanisms.

At the cellular level, differences in ionic composition between the cellular and extracellular compartment are normally maintained by semipermeable membranes, energy–dependent cell transport mechanisms, transmembrane differences in

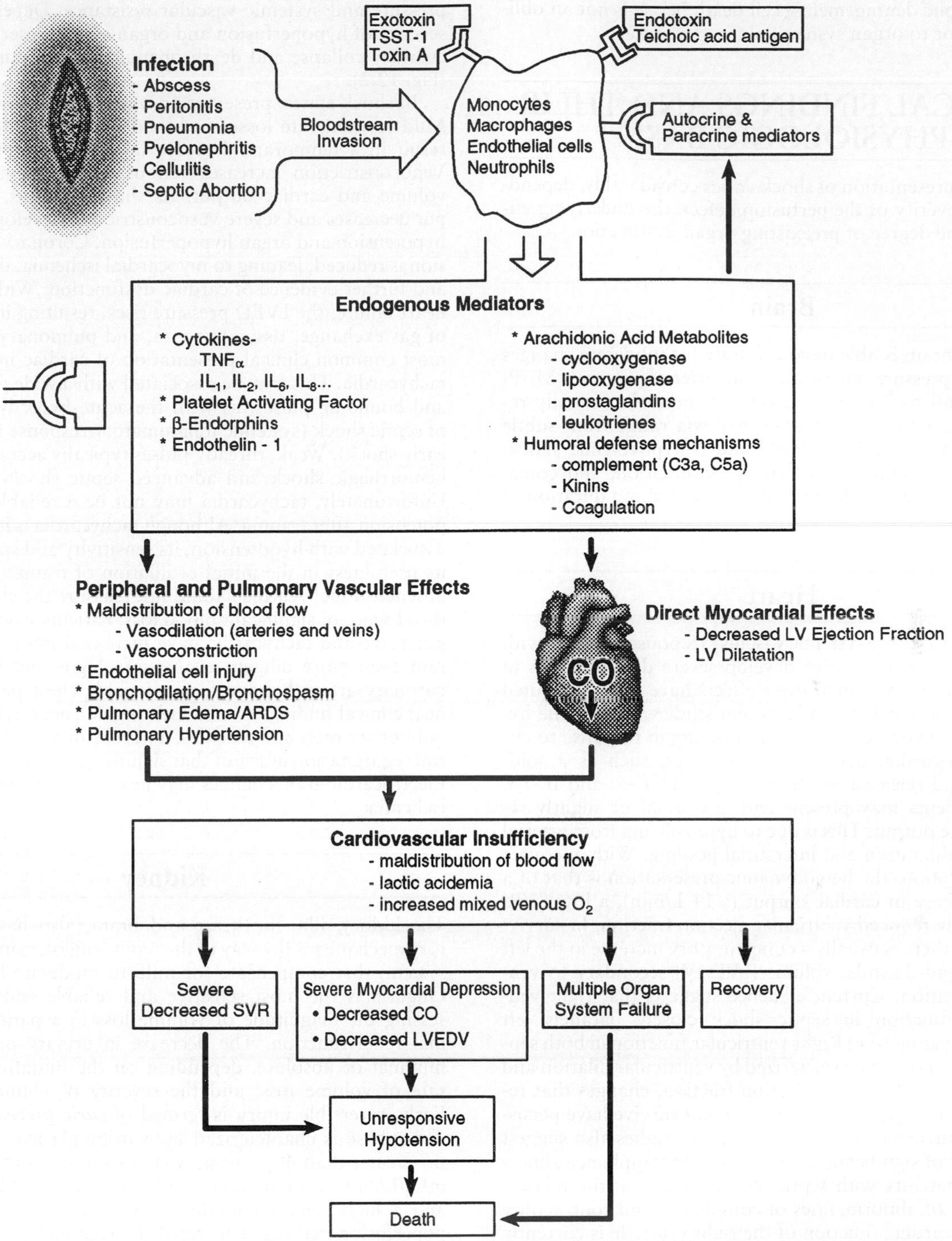

FIGURE 12.2. Pathogenesis of human septic shock. TSST, toxic shock syndrome toxin-1; TNF, tumor necrosis factor; IL, interleukin; ARDS, adult respiratory distress syndrome; LV, left ventricle; SVR, systemic vascular resistance; CO, cardiac output; LVEDV, left ventricular end-diastolic volume. (Adapted from Parillo JE. Pathogenetic mechanisms of septic shock. *N Engl J Med* 1993;328:1471; and Cunnion RE, Parillo JE. Myocardial dysfunction in sepsis: recent insights. *Chest* 1989;95:941.)

electrical potential, particle charge, and oncotic pressure. With the development of metabolic acidosis, coupled with a decreased production of intracellular cyclic adenosine triphosphate (the energy substrate for cell transport), the normal ionic composition within cells that is critical for mitochondrial function can no longer be maintained. There is an influx of sodium and water and an efflux of potassium, resulting in gradual hemoconcentration and hyponatremia. Although irreversible cellular injury and, ultimately, cell death can result from organ system dysfunction caused by these metabolic derangements, cell death per se is not an obligate precursor to organ system failure or demise.

CLINICAL FINDINGS AND THEIR PHYSIOLOGIC BASIS

The clinical presentation of shock varies considerably, depending on the severity of the perfusion defect, the underlying etiology, and the degree of preexisting organ dysfunction.

Brain

Because the brain is able to compensate for moderate changes in perfusion pressure, unless the mean arterial pressure (MAP) falls below 60 to 70 mm Hg, cerebral perfusion usually remains intact. Symptoms of brain hypoxia range from subtle changes in mental acuity (class I and II hypovolemic shock; Table 12.2) to confusion, lethargy, obtundation, and coma. Mental status changes depend on the severity and duration of hypovolemia.

Heart

In addition to a severe systemic vascular response, patients with sepsis and septic shock also develop severe derangements in cardiac function. Although these effects have been attributed to global myocardial ischemia, recent studies support the hypothesis that myocardial depression occurs in response to circulating myocardial depressant substances, such as a soluble compound released by the pancreas, TNF-α, and IL-1β. Initially, patients may present with a normal or slightly reduced cardiac output. This is due to hypovolemia from arterial and venous dilatation and interstitial pooling. With adequate fluid resuscitation, the hemodynamic presentation is that of a marked increase in cardiac output (>11 L/min), a low SVR, and a severely reduced ventricular ejection fraction. In surviving patients, there is usually a compensatory increase in the left ventricular end-diastolic volume (LVEDV) secondary to ventricular dilatation. Current evidence suggests that right ventricular dysfunction in septic shock closely parallels left ventricular dysfunction. Right ventricular function in both sepsis and septic shock is characterized by ventricular dilation and decreased right ventricular ejection fraction, changes that resolve in 7 to 14 days. Patients who do not survive have persistent right ventricular dysfunction. Several studies also suggest the existence of significant right ventricular compliance abnormalities in patients with septic shock. However, the relative contribution of abnormalities of compliance and contractility to impaired cardiac function of the right ventricle is currently unknown.

The initial cardiac effects of septic shock include decreased contractility and, in survivors, compensatory ventricular dilatation. Because stroke volume is maintained and tachycardia is pronounced, cardiac output is almost always dramatically increased. In this setting, cardiac output is a poor measure of myocardial performance. In the recovery phase, the SVR returns to normal over 24 hours or so, and the cardiac index drops to near normal levels. In septic shock fatalities, little or no initial reduction in stroke volume or increase in LVEDV was found, suggesting that ventricular dilatation is absent in these patients, which accounts for the lack of compensatory increase in stroke volume or cardiac output needed to maintain arterial pressure and systemic vascular resistance. Depending on the severity of hypoperfusion and organ system reserve, cardiocirculatory collapse and death or multiorgan failure may ensue (Fig. 12.2).

In shock states, preservation of cardiac function is critical. Mild to moderate losses in blood volume (up to 1,500 mL) result in a temporary decrease in cardiac output and SVR. Venoconstriction increases venous return, enhancing stroke volume and cardiac output. As shock worsens, cardiac output decreases and severe vasoconstriction develops, leading to hypotension and organ hypoperfusion. Coronary artery perfusion is reduced, leading to myocardial ischemia, dysrhythmias, and further evidence of cardiac dysfunction. With progressive heart failure, the LVED pressure rises, resulting in impairment of gas exchange, tissue hypoxia, and pulmonary edema. The most common clinical presentation of cardiac involvement is tachycardia. This may be associated with a wide pulse pressure and bounding pulses, as with the acute hyperdynamic phase of septic shock (systemic inflammatory response syndrome, or early shock). Weak, thready pulses typically accompany severe hemorrhagic shock and advanced septic shock (late shock). Unfortunately, tachycardia may not be a reliable sign of hypotension after trauma. Although tachycardia is independently associated with hypotension, its sensitivity and specificity limit its usefulness in the initial evaluation of trauma victims, and absence of tachycardia should not reassure the clinician about the absence of significant blood loss. Patients who are both hypotensive and tachycardic have increased mortality and warrant even more diligent evaluation. Signs and symptoms of coronary artery hypoperfusion include chest pain and dyspnea; clinical findings can include jugular neck vein distention, pulmonary rales and crackles, a new S_3 or S_4 gallop, and a mitral regurgitation murmur that signifies papillary muscle injury. Electrocardiogram changes may be consistent with myocardial ischemia.

Kidney

The kidney, like the heart and brain, also has autoregulatory mechanisms (by way of the renin–angiotensin–aldosterone system) that compensate for mild to moderate hypovolemia. Oliguria is the most sensitive and reliable end point in assessing the magnitude of volume loss in a patient with normal renal function. The decrease in urinary output can be minimal or absolute, depending on the initiating insult, the rate of volume loss, and the severity of volume depletion. Early, reversible injury is termed *oliguric prerenal azotemia*. This phase is characterized by a urine-plasma creatinine ratio greater than 40, a urine sodium excretion of less than 20 mEq/L/24 h, a fractional excretion of sodium of less than 1%, and a high urine osmolality (>500 mOsm). Prolonged hypoperfusion can result in renal damage and acute renal failure. Oliguric acute renal failure is characterized by a urine–plasma creatinine ratio of less than 20, an elevated urinary sodium (>40 mEq/L/24 h), a fractional excretion of sodium of more than 1%, and a decrease in the ability to concentrate urine. In this phase, urine osmolality is generally less than 350 mOsm.

In contrast to early hypovolemic shock, in the acute phase of septic shock, the renal-vascular response is one of marked oliguria in association with reduced renal blood flow. Kidney failure develops despite relative conservation of the mean arterial pressure and an intravascular volume that is normal or slightly reduced. Depending on the severity of the perfusion defect and the redistribution of blood flow, the resulting perfusion defect can be partial or total, and tubular or cortical necrosis, or both, can result.

Skin and Mucous Membranes

When the skin is poorly perfused, its temperature falls and its color changes, so that it is cold to the touch and pale, dusky, or mottled in appearance. When hypoxemia is pronounced, the skin may become frankly cyanotic. Sympathetic stimulation results in increased sweat gland secretion; consequently, the skin may be moist, cold, or clammy. With mild hypovolemia, capillary refill, which is clinically assessed by compressing and then releasing pressure on the fingernail beds, remains normal. However, with losses of 30% or more of the circulating volume, patients nearly always demonstrate a positive capillary refill test (>2 seconds). The lips and oral cavity may appear dry or chapped. The conscious patient usually experiences intense thirst.

Lung

The pulmonary vasculature is particularly susceptible to injury. Clinical manifestations include dyspnea, progressive hypoxemia, diffuse bilateral pulmonary infiltrates, and reduced compliance, a condition is referred to as adult respiratory distress syndrome (ARDS). The combination of ARDS and Gram-negative sepsis is particularly ominous, because nearly 50% of patients diagnosed with sepsis develop acute lung injury/ARDS, contributing to mortality rates of 80% to 90%. ARDS results from increased pulmonary capillary permeability and the accumulation of extravascular lung water. Inflammatory cells spill into the alveoli, destroying the delicate type I alveolar cells. This is followed by proliferation of type II pneumocytes, thickening of the alveolar–capillary membranes, and subsequent fibrosis. Clinically, ARDS is characterized by intrapulmonary shunting, widening of the alveolar-arterial oxygen gradient, and reduced pulmonary compliance and functional residual capacity. Radiographic findings are consistent with pulmonary edema, despite a normal or low pulmonary capillary wedge pressure (PCWP). Arterial Pao_2 remains low (<65 mm Hg), even with supplemental oxygen, and assisted mechanical ventilation is often required.

Liver

In sepsis, the liver plays a critical role in host defense response. Kupffer cells are important for bacterial scavenging, inactivation of bacterial products, and proinflammatory cytokine production and clearance. Cytokine receptor–mediated responses within hepatocytes include gluconeogenesis, amino-acid uptake, and increased synthesis of coagulant and complement factors and protease inhibitors. Paradoxically, the acute phase protein response also contributes to a procoagulant state, inhibiting the production and function of protein C. Primary hepatic dysfunction refers to sepsis-induced derangements that fairly rapidly results in disseminated intravascular coagulation and bleeding. Reduced perfusion appears to be the most important initiating event. Secondary hepatic dysfunction is a more frequent, silent, and at times imperceptible dysfunction that probably results from spillover of bacterial, endotoxin, and inflammatory mediators. At this juncture, most of the liver's function is clinically intact. Liver dysfunction associated with multiorgan failure is characterized by elevated bilirubin levels, rarely exceeding 10 mg/dL, approximately 80% of which is conjugated. Hyperbilirubinemia results from the breakdown of RBCs and from hepatocellular dysfunction. Although alkaline phosphatase often is 1 to 3 times that of normal, more dramatic elevations may be observed, especially in the elderly. Patients with hepatic failure secondary to sepsis continue to demonstrate progressively worsening abnormalities in glucose, fat, and amino acid metabolism. The amino acid profile is typically one of decreased branched chain and increased aromatic amino acids.

Gastrointestinal Tract

Gastrointestinal failure presents as gastrointestinal stress bleeding, which is characterized clinically by "coffee-ground" staining of gastric aspirates, or frank, bright red bleeding. In addition to blood loss, the resulting mucosal injury increases the likelihood of translocation of bacteria to the blood and liver. *Bacterial translocation*—the movement of viable organisms from the gut lumen across intact epithelium into the mesenteric lymph nodes, liver, spleen, lungs, or the systemic circulation—has been postulated as a potential source of bacteria and sepsis. Normally, the gastrointestinal mucosa serves as an important mechanical barrier to systemic contamination by intraluminal microbes. The normal gut flora consists predominantly of anaerobic bacteria that displace more pathogenic organisms such as *Escherchia coli* and *Candida albicans* away from the gastrointestinal mucosa, a host defense mechanism termed *colonization resistance*. The source of Gram-negative bacteremia after trauma and hypovolemic shock is thought to be from mucosal endothelial cell injury or from bacterial translocation. The microvascular circulation of the mesenteric villi appears to be highly susceptible to mesenteric ischemia, leading to further endothelial cell injury. As with the kidney and lung, inflammatory cells are attracted to the site of endothelial cell injury. Cytokines and oxygen free radicals are released that promote additional injury that may result in mucosal ulceration or bleeding, or both.

Summary of Shock Presentation

Clinical signs and symptoms and systemic manifestations are frequently subdivided into early, usually reversible manifestations (Table 12.5) and late findings (Table 12.6). In early stages, the clinical findings of hypovolemic and septic shock differ, but are usually reversible, whereas the clinical features are essentially the same for late or irreversible shock. When diagnosis or intervention is delayed or insufficient, shock can become irreversible, resulting in permanent organ dysfunction or death. The patient may enter a chronic condition of continued malfunction of one or more organ systems—despite adequate volume restoration, the absence of persistent infection, and other identifiable insults (Fig. 12.1)—termed *multiorgan failure syndrome*. Multiorgan failure, depending on the number of organ systems involved, carries a mortality of 30% to 100% and is the most common cause of death from shock. In addition to continued central nervous system, cardiac, and renal dysfunction, organ system failure in its classic presentation usually involves the lungs first (24 to 72 hours after the original injury), then the liver (5 to 7 days), followed by the gastrointestinal tract (10 to 15 days) and kidneys (11 to 17 days). However, many variations in clinical presentation are seen. For example, patients

TABLE 12.5

PRESENTING FEATURES OF SHOCK: EARLY SIGNS AND SYMPTOMS

	Hypovolemic (hemorrhagic) shock		Septic shock	
Organ system	Symptom or sign	Cause	Symptom or sign	Cause
Central nervous	Mental status changes[a]	Decreased cerebral perfusion	Subtle mental changes, septic encephalopathy	Decreased cerebral perfusion Cytokine-induced endothelial cell damage results in a leaky blood-brain barrier.
Circulatory				Subtle mental changes, septic encephalopathy
Heart	Tachycardia, rapid thready pulse	Adrenergic stimulation increases contractility, increasing cardiac output and SVR. Cardiac output decreases with depressed contractility, decreasing SVR.	Tachycardia; bounding pulse	Myocardial ischemia, depressed cardiac function, cardiac output may be increased or decreased[a]; decreased SVR
Systemic	Normotensive or hypotensive[a], decreased JVD[a]; narrow pulse pressure	Decreased SVR and venous return secondary to volume loss Sympathetic stimulation increases vascular tone.	Normotensive or slightly hypotensive; widened pulse pressure	SVR decreased from reduced circulatory volume from extravascular pooling
Renal	Oliguria[a]	Decreased perfusion from decreased circulating volume	Oliguria	Afferent arteriolar vasoconstriction
Respiratory	Normal or tachypneic[a]	Sympathetic stimulation, acidosis	Tachypnea	Pulmonary edema, acidosis, muscle fatigue
Skin	Cold, clammy	Vasoconstriction, sympathetic stimulation	Warm	Increased cardiac output, peripheral vasodilation, febrile response
Other			Fever or hypothermia	Infection, endotoxins, cytokines

SVR, systemic vascular resistance; JVD, jugular neck vein distension.
[a]Variable in severity, depending on the rate and volume of loss.

can develop acute tubular necrosis without other organ system dysfunction.

Febrile Neutropenia

Neutropenic fever is clinically defined by three oral temperatures of 38°C (100.4°F) or a single temperature higher than 38.5°C (101.3°F) coexistent with a low ANC (less than 500/mm^3). Over the past several decades, bacteremia in febrile neutropenic patients has shifted from Gram-negative to Gram-positive organisms secondary to more frequent use of indwelling catheters, which are particularly at risk for Gram-positive colonization from skin flora. Other contributing factors include use of prophylactic antibiotics, the type of chemotherapy given, and regional climactic conditions. In the early 1970s, the empirical use of intravenous broad-spectrum antibiotics in febrile neutropenic patients significantly reduced infection-related mortality; patients were typically hospitalized and treated until their ANC had recovered and they were afebrile for at least 24 hours. However, in nearly half of neutropenic patients who receive standard antibiotic therapy, no bacterial infection is identified. Recent estimates indicate that cancer patients account for 126,209 severe sepsis cases annually in the United States—16.4 cases per 1,000 people per year. Severe sepsis is associated with 8.5% of all cancer-related deaths at a cost of 3.4 billion dollars per year; the overall mortality rate for febrile neutropenia is approximately 6%. Costs of hospitalization, risks of exposure to nosocomial infections, emergence of drug resistance, and variable compliance with antibiotic regimens formed the basis for stratification of febrile neutropenic cancer patients into high- and low-risk groups. Individual studies and systematic reviews indicate that low-risk patients with neutropenic fever may be treated safely with oral antibiotics. A metaanalysis of neutropenic patients (1980–1994) found that antibiotic prophylaxis significantly reduced the risk of death over placebo or no treatment (RR 0.67, 95% CI 0.55, 0.81) and that oral fluoroquinolone prophylaxis significantly reduced mortality (RR 0.52, 95% CI 0.35, 0.77). Despite this, quinolone prophylaxis increases the risk for harboring antibiotic-resistant organisms. A subsequent metaanalysis of the Cochrane Database of Systemic Reviews found that adding anti–Gram-positive therapy did not adversely affect survival. Overuse of Gram-positive coverage has led to the emergence of resistant enterococci and, more recently, *S. aureus* species. Because of concerns regarding the spread of vancomycin resistance, its empirical use in this setting is specifically discouraged. In one recent study, in select low-risk

TABLE 12.6

PRESENTING FEATURES OF SHOCK: LATE SIGNS AND SYMPTOMS

	Hypovolemic shock or septic shock	
Organ system	Symptom or sign[a]	Cause
Central nervous	Disorientation, obtundation	Hypoxia, worsening cerebral edema
Circulatory		
Heart	Cardiac dysfunction, tachycardia, and other arrhythmias	Irreversible ischemia, decreased cardiac index, decreased ejection fraction
Systemic	Jugular neck vein distention may be increased or decreased; normotension or progressive hypotension	Right heart failure, extravascular pooling
Renal	Oliguria progressing to anuria	Acute renal failure
Respiratory	Tachypnea	Adult respiratory distress syndrome
Skin	Cold, clammy	Vasoconstriction, sympathetic stimulation
Other	Lactic acidosis Coagulopathy, thrombocytopenia, depressed platelet function	Anaerobic metabolism, hepatic dysfunction; endothelial cell injury, platelet deposition, vascular thrombosis; hepatic dysfunction

[a] Variable in severity, depending upon the rate and volume of loss.

febrile neutropenic patients (no clinical evidence of infection, IL-8 <60 ng/L), withholding empiric antibiotic therapy did not increase adverse events and resulted in cost savings of $572 per patient. In hospitalized febrile neutropenic patients with hematological malignancies, piperacillin-taxobactam was found to be more effective and cost-efficient than ceftriaxone plus gentamicin. The specific management of neutropenic patients must be based on the underlying malignancy, prior prophylactic therapy, institutional/community drug-resistance patterns, and patient risk factors.

MANAGEMENT OF SHOCK

For the gynecologist who infrequently encounters a moribund, unstable patient in shock, it may be useful to remember to restore *ORDER*. The mnemonic, *ORDER*, outlined in Table 12.7, provides the appropriate sequence of resuscitative priorities. After immediate resuscitative measures are initiated, it is highly recommended that continued management of all but the least complicated cases be carried out in a modern critical care unit. A team approach with the benefit of staff trained in intensive care medicine can greatly improve the likelihood of survival, as well as significantly reduce morbidity. General guidelines for managing shock are provided in Table 12.8.

Oxygenate

For patients with minimal or no respiratory distress, oxygen delivery at 1 to 6 L/min by nasal cannula may be sufficient. When respiratory distress is evident, oxygen delivery by face mask at the recommended flow rate (8–10 L/min) will increase the inspired oxygen concentrations to 80% to 100% with an oxygen reservoir, compared with 40% to 60% without a reservoir. For patients who are disoriented or obtunded, tiring, or unable to maintain sufficient arterial oxygenation ($Pa{O_2}$ <60 mm Hg), the airway must be protected. Immediate endotracheal intubation with positive pressure ventilation should be instituted. Oxygenation in patients with increased compliance and high intrapulmonary shunt fractions (e.g., ARDS, pulmonary edema) can be improved by the addition of positive end-expiratory pressure (PEEP) at physiologic or low levels (5–15 cm H_2O). Because high levels of PEEP can reduce venous return and, consequently, reduce cardiac output, patients needing higher levels may benefit from invasive hemodynamic monitoring to determine the "best" PEEP to optimize oxygen delivery.

Restore Circulating Volume

Initial fluid therapy should consist of a 1- to 2-liter fluid challenge with an isotonic electrolyte solution, preferably Ringer's lactate. Normal or half normal saline solution can also be infused; however, prolonged use of these infusions increases the risk of hyperchloremic acidosis if renal function is impaired. Because severe hypernatremia increases the risk of brain dehydration or death, hypertonic saline is not recommended except under special circumstances and is not part of the initial management. Albumin and other colloidal solutions (high– or low–molecular-weight dextran, polyethyl starches) have been advocated to restore and maintain circulation under the premise that these agents are more likely to remain in the intravascular

TABLE 12.7

RESUSCITATIVE PRIORITIES IN THE MANAGEMENT OF OVERT SHOCK: RESTORE ORDER

O:	*Oxygenate* (assure adequate airway, tidal volume, 6–8 L/min of oxygen by closed mask, nasal catheter, or endotracheal tube)
R:	*Restore circulatory volume* (one or more intravenous lines, assess volume loss and replace with crystalloid; administer whole blood or packed red blood cells; with severe hemorrhage or disseminated intravascular coagulation, replace clotting factors as indicated; sterile packing until hemodynamic stability is restored; central venous monitoring; obtain cultures if indicated with intravenous access)
D:	*Drug therapy* (pharmacologic support of blood pressure, antibiotics, miscellaneous agents for specified conditions)
E:	*Evaluate response to therapy* (identify etiology of shock; volume replacement based on right heart catheterization or central venous monitoring; reevaluate hemoglobin, coagulation profiles, serum chemistries [potassium, phosphate, acid–base, PaO_2, creatinine]; modify treatment plan/pharmacologic therapy; obtain culture results; radiographic studies—abdominal films, chest x-ray, CT scan, ventilation–perfusion scan, as indicated by suspected underlying condition)
R:	*Remedy the underlying cause* (surgical control of bleeding using selective interventional embolization or surgery; antibiotic therapy based on culture results)

Adapted from Cavanagh D, Marsden DE. Hemorrhagic shock in the gynecologic patient. *Clin Obstet Gynecol* 1985:28:383.

TABLE 12.8

GENERAL GUIDELINES FOR MANAGING SHOCK

Cardiovascular/hemodynamic	
Blood pressure	Maintain systolic blood pressure at least 90 mm Hg; mean arterial pressure at least 60 mm Hg
Pulmonary capillary wedge pressure	14–18 mm Hg
Central venous pressure	12–15 cm H_2O
Oxygen delivery	Maintain hemoglobin over 8 g/dL; 10 g/dL in patients with cardiac compromise
Oxygen saturation	Arterial oxyhemoglobin saturation least 92% (pulse oximetry saturation does not reflect arterial PaO_2 with significant hypotension or compromised peripheral perfusion)
Cardiac index	>4 L/min/m^2 (septic shock) >2.2 L/min/m^2 (other shock states)
Pulmonary	Normalize alveolar-arterial gradient (PaO_2 >30 mm Hg or SaO_2 >55%)
Blood gases	Maintain: PaO_2 80–100 mm Hg; $PaCO_2$ 30–35 mmHg; pH >7.35[a]
Renal	Maintain urine output of 20–30 mL/h (0.5 mL/kg/h); normalize blood urea nitrogen, creatinine
Hepatic	Bilirubin <3 mg/dL
Mental status	Restore/maintain orientation
Coagulation studies	Normalize
Serum lactate level	Should be 2.2 mMol/L; suspect tissue hypoperfusion when elevated

[a] Mild acidosis is preferable to alkalosis to maximize oxygen dissociation at the cellular level.

Adapted from Jimenez EJ. Shock. In: Civetta JM, Taylor RW, Kirby RR, eds. *Critical care,* 3rd ed. Philadelphia: Lippincott-Raven Publishers, 1997:89; and Hollenberg SM, Parrillo JE. Shock. In Fauci AS, Martin JP, Braunwald E, et al., eds. *Harrison's principles of internal medicine,* vol. 1. New York: McGraw-Hill; 1997:220.

compartment. In trauma and perioperative patients, hypoalbuminemia of some degree is almost universal, and results from crystalloid administration, increases in capillary permeability, and sequestration of albumin in the interstitial compartment. Albumin has been used in edematous patients based on rationale that edema fluid may be "pulled" into the intracellular compartment and excreted. This practice is not supported by scientific data and may actually be harmful. Colloids can eventually "leak" across damaged pulmonary capillary epithelium, promoting the development of pulmonary edema. Metaanalyses of albumin administration versus crystalloid infusion found a 4% to 6% increase in the risk for death in those patients who received albumin. However, as shown by Sort et al., albumin may be lifesaving in selected clinical settings, specifically patients with cirrhosis and spontaneous bacterial peritonitis. The choice of fluid replacement also has considerable cost implications, because colloid is more expensive than crystalloid administration and more expensive than hydroxyethyl starch.

In most cases, hemorrhagic shock should be managed initially by inserting one or two large-bore (14- or 16-gauge) angiocatheters for volume replacement. Central venous catheterization is *not* recommended for most patients. Central venous access will not improve the rate of fluid administration and carries the risk of pneumothorax and other potentially life-threatening complications. Central circulation can also be improved by elevating the feet or by placing the patient in the Trendelenburg position. Blood can be drawn for initial laboratory assessment at the time that intravenous access is obtained and should include a complete blood count with differential and platelets, electrolytes, blood urea nitrogen (BUN), creatinine, calcium, magnesium, glucose, phosphate, and, where indicated, serum human chorionic gonadotropin-β, liver function studies, clotting profiles, serum lactate, and blood cultures.

In patients with distributive shock, or shock following ischemic injury from severe or prolonged hypovolemia, damage to the capillary endothelium results in increased capillary permeability and greater interstitial losses, and larger volumes of fluid are required to restore circulatory volume than may be apparent by clinical estimation of the plasma volume. For example, 6 to 7 liters of fluid may be required for what appears to be 1 to 1.5 liters of plasma volume depletion. Most of these patients have some degree of cardiac dysfunction and are at high risk for lung injury from injudicious volume expansion. Because central venous pressure and PCWP are often discordant, right heart catheterization has been advocated after immediate fluid resuscitation. Additional volume replacement or pressure support may then be based on determinations of the pulmonary artery mean and occlusive pressures, cardiac output, cardiac index, and SVR. Mixed venous oxygen content can be also obtained to estimate oxygen delivery at the cellular level. For patients with pulmonary injury, shunt fractions and alveolar-arterial oxygen differences can be calculated and used to guide ventilatory and RBC transfusion requirements. Connors and colleagues, in a prospective study of 52 critically ill patients with multiorgan system disease, found that clinical estimates of volume status are significantly different from estimates based on right heart catheterization parameters; in this study, major changes in therapy (altering the rate of fluid administration, or starting or stopping a pressor agent, or both) occurred in 48.4% of cases after catheterization.

Many cardiologists and critical care physicians believe that therapy guided by pulmonary artery catheterization (PAC) leads to improved patient outcomes. However, the "routine" use of Swan-Ganz catheters in patients with sepsis is controversial. One or more randomized controlled clinical trials could clarify this issue; however, attempts at randomized controlled trials have failed, mostly because of physician biases for or against their use. In the absence of controlled trials, observational studies permitting, placement of right heart catheters at the discretion of the physician are being used in an attempt to clarify the risk/benefit ratio. These studies are inherently biased because the more critically ill the patient is, the more likely she is to undergo right heart catheterization, and the more likely she is to die, independent of this intervention—a selection bias termed *confounding by indication.* In one observational study of 5,735 critically ill patients in five teaching hospitals, PAC use was found to be associated with increased mortality and cost with no clear benefit. A PAC Consensus Conference concluded that there is insufficient evidence to support the routine use of PACs in septic patients, but PAC improves outcome in patients with myocardial infarction complicated by cardiogenic shock and right ventricular infarction. In patients with respiratory failure (i.e., ARDS versus pulmonary edema), determinations of pulmonary artery mean and occlusive pressures, cardiac output, cardiac index, and systemic vascular resistance may be useful to determine the underlying cause and to guide fluid therapy, but it is uncertain that using PACs in this setting improves survival.

Specific blood component therapy has virtually replaced whole blood transfusion as the standard of care. Packed red blood cells (PRBC) have a volume of 200 to 250 mL and a hematocrit of 70%. Combined with normal saline, PRBCs are the component of choice for hemorrhagic shock. Loss of approximately 20% of blood volume is equivalent to 1,500 mL blood loss and in a normal 70-kg individual is not associated with a significant reduction in oxygen-carrying capacity or ventricular-filling pressures when adequate crystalloid resuscitation is given. Because the oxygen-carrying capacity is met in most healthy patients with a hemoglobin of 7 g/dL, empiric transfusion for moderate anemia (8 to 10 mg/dL) is no longer recommended. Nevertheless, because most of the oxygen transported in the blood is by hemoglobin, correction of anemia is an important component in optimizing oxygen delivery at the cellular level (Table 12.8). In general, these recommendations regarding RBC transfusion have been derived from the management of trauma victims that were in normal health before an acute event. In critically ill patients and those with significant underlying cardiac disease, RBC transfusions have been used liberally to maintain hemoglobin levels between 10 and 12 g/dL to reduce the potential adverse effects of oxygen debt.

The importance of weighing the benefits of RBC transfusion against potential adverse effects has received considerable attention. Current estimates of the risk per unit of blood in the postnucleic acid testing era are 1 in 872,000 to 7 million and 1 in 4–8 million for hepatitis C virus and human immunodeficiency virus (HIV), respectively. Other risks of contamination include human T-cell lymphotrophic virus (1/250,000–2,000,000), acute hemolytic reactions (1/250,000–1,000,000), delayed hemolytic (1/1,000), and transfusion-related lung injury (1/5,000). Currently, bacterial contamination of platelets poses the greatest risk of transfusion transmitted disease. Of 4 million platelet units transfused annually in the United States, as many as 4,000 are bacterially contaminated, resulting in 333 to 1,000 cases of severe sepsis. Concern for infectious risks (HIV, hepatitis), shortages, and expense led many governmental agencies and advisory boards, including the American College of Obstetricians and Gynecologists, to adopt lower thresholds for empiric transfusion. In a multicenter, randomized controlled clinical trial of critically ill patients, there were no differences in mortality rates when hemoglobin levels were maintained between 7 and 9 mg/dL compared with scheduled transfusions to maintain levels between 10 and 12 mg/dL, and mortality rates among younger (<55 years) and less acutely ill patients were significantly lower for those who were not transfused. The immunomodulation effects of blood transfusion—immune suppression, allograph tolerance, and the potential development of autoimmune diseases—probably occurs secondarily to exposure and sensitization of leukocytes. Immunosuppression may contribute to postoperative infection in transfused patients and may increase recurrence for some solid tumors. Despite these risks, the benefit of leukocyte reduction of cellular blood components is unproven. Because the cost of universal leukodepletion is in excess of $500 million, this practice is unlikely to be adopted without proven benefit.

Preoperative autologous donation, the practice of donating blood before surgery, accounted for 6% of blood transfused blood in 1992 but has declined to about 2%. Preoperative autologous transfusions are also more costly than allogeneic blood transfusion. HIV and hepatitis C transmission risks, which spawned the wide acceptance of this practice, have dramatically declined in recent years, and autologous blood donation may actually be harmful to patients and include bacterial contamination, volume overload, administration error/ABO incompatibility, and perioperative anemia, necessitating allogeneic transfusion. This practice is also wasteful, as up to half of the blood donated for this purpose in the United States is ultimately discarded. Advantages include the prevention of transfusion-transmitted disease, red cell alloimmunization, and transfusion reaction. To transfuse preoperative autologous blood during shock, acute normovolemic hemodilution entails the removal of whole blood from a patient immediately before surgery, and volume is restored with crystalloid or colloid. After major bleeding is controlled, the blood is infused. Relative contraindications include infection, malignancy, and contaminants (amniotic fluid/gastrointestinal contents/ascites/pus) within the operative field. Despite this, both acute normovolemic hemodilution and cell salvage can be used in women undergoing cesarean section who are at risk for profound hemorrhage (placenta percreta) who will not accept blood products.

A higher threshold for blood transfusion is warranted in patients with renal, coronary artery, and/or chronic obstructive lung disease because of the associated increased risk for myocardial infarction and perioperative death. Most experts recommend maintaining hemoglobin levels above 10 g/dL in these patients. Survival is also improved in cervical cancer patients undergoing chemoradiation therapy by maintaining the hemoglobin concentration above 12 g/dL.

Epoetin alfa (Procrit; Ortho Biotech Inc., Raritan, NJ) is currently approved in the United States for the treatment of anemia in patients with nonmyeloid malignancies who receive concomitant chemotherapy. In cancer patients receiving chemotherapy, epoetin alfa 10,000 U and increased to 20,000 U three times weekly, depending on hemoglobin level after 4 weeks, improved patient-reported functional capacity and quality of life independent of response to chemotherapy. Epoetin alpha has become a valuable alternative to transfusion in patients with inflammatory diseases that reduce erythropoiesis (e.g., renal failure, carcinoma) or who refuse blood products. Its use can reduce the need for transfusion when given preoperatively to anemic patients. Epoetin alpha is not effective without appropriate iron intake, preferably given with vitamin C, to enhance absorption. Although there are no adverse effects recorded in cancer patients, two recent trials have shown lower survival rates in patients treated with epoetin alpha instead of transfusion. Further studies are needed to address the presence of erythropoietin on tumor cells and its impact on tumor progression, especially in this clinical setting. Red-cell substitutes are in various stages of clinical development and may become lifesaving alternatives in military and trauma settings or for patients who refuse other options.

When blood loss exceeds 25% of the blood volume, whole blood—or, in the presence of bleeding consistent with coagulopathy, PRBCs and fresh frozen plasma (FFP) in a 4:1 ratio—has been the standard of care until recently. However, 4–5 platelet concentrates, or 1 unit of single-donor apheresis platelets, or 1 unit of whole blood provides a quantity of factors similar to 1 U FFP (except for factor V and VIII) and is usually sufficient for hemostasis. True dilutional coagulopathy does not occur until greater than 100% of blood volume has been replaced. Therefore, it is recommended that coagulation profiles be obtained in patients with microvascular bleeding and transfusion with FFP not be given unless the PT/PTT is greater than 1.5 times normal values or, in absence of lab determinants, only for massively transfused patients with ongoing microvascular bleeding or when warfarin therapy must be given. Cryoprecipitate is concentrated FFP in a small volume of 10 to 15 mL (1 bag per 5 kg in a 70-kg individual). Because cryoprecipitate is pooled factor components from multiple donors, risk of infection is significantly increased. Cryoprecipitate should be reserved for patients with deficiencies in factor VIII, von Willebrand factor, fibrinogen factor XIII, and/or fibronectin who fail desmopressin acetate. When disseminated intravascular coagulation is suspected based on massive transfusion and the persistence of significant oozing/bleeding, FFP instead of cryoprecipitate is the component of choice. To avoid the risks of hemolysis, agglutination, and clotting, all blood products should be administered through filtered lines with normal saline without electrolyte or drug additives. To prevent hypothermia, warming of blood products is indicated when the volume infused exceeds 50 mg/kg/h.

When transfusion is massive (10 U PRBCs in 24 h), platelets in addition to packed cell transfusion are needed. One unit of platelet concentrate will increase the count by 5,000 to 10,000/μL. Preoperative platelet and intraoperative platelet counts of 50,000/μL or less are indications for platelet transfusion when major surgery or further bleeding is anticipated. Platelet transfusions may also be indicated for platelet dysfunction. FFP is indicated for patients with disseminated intravascular coagulation, severe liver disease, or massive transfusion and for specific clotting disturbances when the factor concentrate is not available. FFP is not indicated for volume expansion or nutritional support and should not be given empirically with PRBC transfusions.

Drug Therapy

Pharmacologic Support of Blood Pressure

Inotropic agents and vasopressors recommended in the management of hypotensive shock are outlined in Table 12.9. Except for the newer agents (inamrinone, milrinone acetate), all of these sympathomimetic agents have both inotropic and vasoconstrictive effects. Because of their cardiotropic effects, dopamine hydrochloride and dobutamine hydrochloride are the preferred agents in the initial treatment of shock. Epinephrine and norepinephrine, which are potent vasoconstrictors, are usually reserved for refractory hypotension. It is important to bear in mind that these vasoactive drugs are not indicated until adequate volume replacement has been given and are seldom of benefit in the management of hemorrhagic shock. Use of vasopressors in the face of inadequate volume resuscitation can worsen preexisting ischemia, increasing cellular and organ system injury. The judicious use of sympathomimetic agents after sufficient hydration may be useful to correct inadequate cardiac function and persistent hypoperfusion.

Because they reduce myocardial oxygen requirements and improve myocardial performance, vasodilators (nitroglycerin, nitroprusside) are generally preferred in the management of patients with cardiogenic shock who have mean arterial pressures higher than 70 mm Hg. Vasodilators are not indicated in the setting of hypovolemic and septic shock associated with low arterial pressures secondary to peripheral vasodilatation. Under these circumstances, vasodilators would serve to further reduce venous return and may intensify hypotension and further reduce coronary artery perfusion.

Dopamine is the preferred catecholaminergic agent in the management of the hypotensive patient whose MAP is less than 60 mm Hg. Dopamine stimulates dopaminergic, α-adrenergic, and β-adrenergic receptors in a dose-dependent fashion. At low doses (1–3 μg/kg/min), dopamine stimulates cerebral, renal, and mesenteric dopaminergic receptors, resulting in vasodilatation and an increase in urinary output. At moderate doses (2–10 μg/kg/min), both α-adrenergic and β-adrenergic receptors are stimulated, but the β_1-adrenergic effects predominate. The β_1-adrenergic cardia effects are inotropic, increasing myocardial contractility, sinoatrial rate, and impulse conduction, thereby increasing cardiac output. Myocardial oxygen consumption is also increased, with no compensatory increase in coronary artery blood flow. In a patient with myocardial ischemia, these effects can compromise cardiac function. At higher rates of infusion, there is some stimulation of the α-adrenergic receptors, resulting in vasoconstriction and a rise in blood pressure. At doses above 20 μg/kg/min, the α-adrenergic effects predominate, resulting in renal, mesenteric, and peripheral arterial vasoconstriction. Dopamine has little β_2-adrenergic activity (i.e., systemic vasodilator effects).

Dobutamine is a direct-acting inotropic agent with both β_1-adrenergic and β_2-adrenergic effects, and is the pharmacologic treatment of choice in patients with cardiogenic shock. Stimulation of the β_2-adrenergic receptors effectively reduces afterload, and thus pulmonary congestion, without increasing oxygen consumption or causing clinically significant tachycardia, which is a frequent and undesirable side effect of dopamine in this clinical setting. Because cardiogenic and septic shock can

TABLE 12.9

PHARMACOLOGIC SUPPORT OF THE CARDIOVASCULAR SYSTEM

		Adrenergic effects				
Agent	Usual dose range	α	β	Dopamine	Peripheral vascular effects	Clinical setting
Inotrophic agents						
Dopamine	1–2 μ/kg/min	+	+	+++	Vasodilation (+)	Oliguria, hypotension
	2–10 μ/kg/min	++	++	+++	Vasoconstriction (++)	Hypotension, bradycardia
	10–30 μ/kg/min	+++	++	+++	Vasoconstriction (+++)	Hypotension, bradycardia
Dobutamine	2.5–15 μg/kg/min (usual); 2–30 μg/kg/min	+	+++	0	Vasodilation (++)	Cardiogenic shock; cardiac pulmonary edema with marginal blood pressure
Isoproterenol	1–10 μg/min	0	+++	0	Vasodilation (++++)	Refractory bradycardia, refractory torsade de pointes
Vasopressors						
Phenylephrine		+++	0	0	Vasoconstriction (+++)	Distributive shock, when no cardiac effect desired
Levarterenol (norepinephrine)	2–20 μg/min (usual); 0.5–89 μg/min	+++	++	0	Vasoconstriction (++++)	Initial emergency treatment of hypotension of any cause
Epinephrine	0.5–1 mg (1:10,000)	+	++	0	Vasoconstriction (++++)	Cardiac arrest
	1–200 μg/min	++	+++		Vasodilation (+++)	Severe hypotension and bradycardia
	0.3–0.5 mg subcutaneous (1:1,000)					Anaphylaxis
Inamrinone (formerly, amrinone)	Load: 0.75 mg/kg IV bolus, then 5–10 μg/kg/minute (up to 40 μg/kg/minute)	Direct myocardial effect, at least in part secondary to inhibition of cardiac cyclic AMP		0 0 0	Vasodilation (++)	Congestive heart failure, cardiogenic shock, usually used combined with dobutamine
Milrinone lactate	Load 50 μg/kg over 3 min; then 0.375–0.75 μg/kg/min	Direct myocardial effect, at least in part secondary to inhibition of cardiac cyclic AMP		0 0 0	Vasodilation (++)	Congestive heart failure, cardiogenic shock, usually used combined with dobutamine
Metaraminol bitartrate	Load: 0.5–5 mg, then 15 to 100 mg infusion	+++	+	0	Vasoconstriction (++++)	Reversal of hypotension from spinal anesthesia; adjunctive treatment for hypotension from hemorrhage, drug reactions, and brain trauma or tumor

IV, intravenous; AMP, adenosine monophosphate phosphodiesterase.

be associated with myocardial depression, an elevated LVEDL, and an abnormally high PCWP, dobutamine may be preferred or needed in addition to dopamine. Used together at moderate doses, dopamine and dobutamine can maintain arterial pressure with less of an increase in pulmonary artery occlusive pressure or pulmonary congestion than when dopamine is used alone. Inamrinone is a phosphodiesterase inhibitor with positive inotropic and vasodilator activity. Its effects are not blocked by use of α-, β-, cholinergic-, or ganglionic-blocking agents. In part, inamrinone acts by inhibiting myocardial cyclic adenosine monophosphate phosphodiesterase (AMP) activity, thereby increasing cardiac cyclic AMP levels. Inamrinone improves lung compliance in mechanically ventilated patients with severe cardiogenic pulmonary edema and is currently recommended in the setting of severe acute congestive heart failure with a systolic blood pressure greater than 100 mm Hg. Inamrinone and milrinone are synergistic with dobutamine, and these agents are often used together for acute refractory congestive heart failure and cardiogenic shock.

Isoproterenol is a synthetic sympathomimetic amine with nearly pure β-adrenergic effects. Although its potent inotropic and chronotropic properties increase cardiac output, isoproterenol increases tachycardia and oxygen consumption and can induce or exacerbate myocardial ischemia. Isoproterenol is seldom used to treat shock. The vasopressors (phenylephrine, norepinephrine, and epinephrine) are used for refractory shock. Although epinephrine and norepinephrine have both β- and α-adrenergic effects, they differ in that epinephrine has more potent α-adrenergic activity. These potent agents increase blood pressure predominantly by increasing systemic and peripheral vascular resistance and must be used with great caution in patients with shock because they may induce or exacerbate myocardial ischemia.

Antibiotic Therapy

Antibiotic therapy should be initiated immediately, as soon as samples of blood and other suspected sites of infections have been obtained for culture. The agents selected should be based on the likely pathogens at the probable site of infection, recent antibiotic use, and the patterns of antimicrobial resistance within the hospital or community (Table 12.10). Empiric broad-spectrum therapy should cover both Gram-positive and Gram-negative organisms; anaerobic coverage is also indicated when a pelvic source is suspected (tuboovarian abscess or septic abortion). Initially, these agents should be given at maximum doses, with dose modification for impaired renal function. Acceptable regimens include an extended-spectrum penicillin (azlocillin, mezlocillin, piperacillin) or third-generation cephalosporin (cefotaxime, ceftazidime) combined with an aminoglycoside. Extended-spectrum penicillins combined with aminoglycoside therapy may be more effective than cephalosporin-aminoglycoside combinations for Gram-negative sepsis, and in the absence of a penicillin allergy, broad-spectrum β-lactam antibiotic–β-lactamase inhibitor combinations, such as ticarcillin–clavulanate, may be preferable. If *Pseudomonas aeruginosa* is suspected, coverage must include two agents: an aminoglycoside with either an appropriate third-generation cephalosporin (ceftazidime) or a β-lactam antibiotic β-lactamase inhibitor combination, or a carbapenem, or a fluoroquinolone, to prevent the rapid development of resistance.

Anaerobic coverage may consist of clindamycin or metronidazole (Flagyl), although dose modifications are required for hepatic failure. Because of the emergence of clindamycin-resistant *B. fragilis*, β-lactam antibiotic–β-lactamase inhibitor combinations and metronidazole are better agents for the empiric treatment of *B. fragilis*; clindamycin can be substituted after drug sensitivity is verified. The only available coverage for methicillin-resistant *Staphylococcus aureus* is vancomycin, which requires dose adjustments in patients with renal compromise. When the suspected source of infection is a peripheral or central venous access site, vancomycin may be added to cover for *Staphylococcus* spp., pending culture results.

Empiric broad-spectrum antibiotic therapy should be replaced with specific therapy as soon as possible because of the significant adverse effects. These include disruption of the normal gut mucosal barrier that increases the risk for opportunistic infections including yeast sepsis (*C. albicans*), enterococcus infection, and pseudomembranous enterocolitis. *Clostridium difficile*–induced colitis (CDIC) is a gastrointestinal disorder that results from colonization by and overgrowth of *C. difficile*, a Gram-positive, spore-forming anaerobic bacillus. Exposure to oral antibiotic therapy is the most common predisposing factor; an association with clindamycin use is well established, but anyone colonized with *C. difficile* who receives antibiotic therapy is at risk. Associated medical comorbidities include advanced age and diabetes, recent bowel preparation, admission to an intensive care unit, and chemotherapy. *C. difficile* infection usually presents with mild to moderate diarrhea, sometimes associated with lower abdominal cramping; systemic symptoms are usually absent. The laboratory diagnosis is made by stool culture.

Severe colitis without pseudomembrane formation is associated with profuse, debilitating diarrhea, abdominal pain, and distension. Systemic manifestations include fever, nausea, anorexia, malaise, and dehydration, and leukocytosis and fecal leukocytes are commonly found. Pseudomembranous colitis is characterized by worsening symptoms, and proctosigmoidoscopy reveals characteristic adherent yellow plaques. When colitis is life-threatening, patients appear acutely ill, with abdominal tenderness and distension, fever, tachycardia and hypotension, or shock. The development of a paralytic ileus and colonic dilatation can result in a paradoxical decrease in diarrhea. When *C. difficile* infection is suspected, antibiotic therapy should be discontinued, or agents less likely to disrupt the normal colonic microflora—such as aminoglycosides and aztreonam should be given. Antidiarrheals decrease gastrointestinal peristalsis and increase the duration of toxin exposure and should be avoided. Oral metronidazole is the drug of choice; oral vancomycin is reserved for patients who cannot tolerate or do not respond to metronidazole. Metronidazole—but not vancomycin—can be used intravenously in patients who cannot tolerate oral intake. Patient with systemic manifestations require aggressive replacement of fluid and electrolytes and may require surgical intervention.

Reports of increasing resistance in *Bacteroides* group isolates and the impact of these antibiotics on the incidence of *C. difficile* have raised additional concerns regarding the use of quinolones in the treatment of anaerobic infections. Quinolones remain an effective therapy for infections caused by enteric Gram-negative and -positive bacteria and are an important alternative to β-lactam antibiotics. Advantages include spectrum of activity, pharmacokinetic profile, and once-daily oral administration. Quinolones available for clinical use have been classified into four generations, mainly based on their spectrum of activity. The second generation (fluoroquinolone) has a fluorine substitute at position 6, which markedly increases activity against Gram-negative organisms. Of the fluoroquinolones, the two most widely used are ciprofloxacin and ofloxacin; ciprofloxacin is the most active against *P. aeruginosa* and a valuable alternative in patients with impaired

TABLE 12.10

EMPIRIC ANTIBIOTIC SELECTION

	Suspected source of sepsis				
	Lung	Abdomen	Skin/soft tissue	Urinary tract	Central nervous
Major community-acquired pathogens	*Streptococcus pneumoniae*[a] *Hemophilus influenzae* *Legionella* species *Chlamydia pneumoniae* *Pneumocystis carinii*	*Escherichia coli* *Bacteroides fragilis*	Group A streptococcus *Staphylococcus aureus* *Clostridium* species Polymicrobial enteric Gram-negative rods *Pseudomonas aeruginosa* anaerobes staphylococci	*Escherichia coli* *Klebsiella* species *Enterobacter* species *Proteus* species	*Streptococcus pneumoniae*[a] *Neisseria meningitidis* *Listeria monocytogenes* *Escherichia coli* *Haemophilus influenzae*
Empiric antibiotic therapy	Macrolide and third-generation cephalosporin or levofloxacin	Imipenem-cilastatin; pipercillin–tazobactam ± aminoglycoside	Vancomycin ± imipenem-cilastatin; pipercillin-tazobactam	Ciprofloxacin ± aminoglycoside	Vancomycin + third-generation cephalosporin; meropenem
Major nosocomial pathogens[b]	Aerobic Gram-negative bacilli	Aerobic Gram-negative rods Anaerobes *Candida* species	*Staphylococcus aureus* Aerobic Gram-negative rods	Aerobic Gram-negative rods Enterococci	*Pseudomonas aeruginosa* *Escherichia coli* *Klebsiella* species Staphylococci species
Empiric antibiotic therapy	Cefipime; imipenem-cilastinin plus aminoglycoside	Imipenem-cilastatin ± amphotericin B	Vancomycin + cefipime	Vancomycin + cefipime	Cefipime or menopenem + vancomycin

[a]Empiric antibiotic selection for invasive pneumococcal disease should be based on known antibiotic susceptibility patterns in the community. High-level penicillin resistance among pneumococcal isolates is increasing, as has resistance to third-generation cephalosporins and quinolones.
[b]Empiric antibiotic selection for hospital-acquired sepsis should be based on antibiotic resistance patterns for bacteria from each specific institution or intensive care unit. Antibiotic regimen may be modified 48–72 hours later, based on culture and antibiotic susceptibility.
Adapted from Simon D, Trenholme G. Antibiotic selection for patients with septic shock. *Crit Care Clin* 2000;16:217.

renal function. Ciprofloxacin is preferable against Gram-negative bacteria, whereas moxifloxcin should be used to target Gram-positive organisms. Levofloxacin and ofloxacin show an intermediate response to Gram-positive bacteria, and norfloaxcin is an intrinsically weak fluoroquinolone against Gram-positive organisms. The emergence of drug resistance has limited their potential against *S. aureus*. Quinolones are not recommended for children or breast-feeding and pregnant women and should be used with caution in the elderly.

Necrotizing fasciitis is a rare, potentially fatal infection of the subcutaneous tissue associated with progressive destruction and necrosis of fascia and fat. Culture results can differentiate between two distinct types: type 1, caused by mixed anaerobes and facultative bacteria (Enterobacteriaceae and non–group A streptococci); and type 2, associated with group A streptococcus alone or in association with *Staphylococcus* spp. Risk factors include diabetes mellitus, peripheral vascular disease, intravenous drug use, obesity, underlying malignancy, malnutrition, renal failure, and trauma. The portal of entry is usually an open wound. Diabetes mellitus is a major predisposing factor. Cutaneous manifestations of streptococcal necrotizing fasciitis include diffuse swelling of the affected area followed by the appearance of bullae filled with clear fluid, which rapidly take on a purplish or violaceous color. Without intervention, the lesions evolve into frank cutaneous gangrene, sometimes with myonecrosis. The inflammatory process advances along fascial planes, and systemic symptoms ensue, which can include shock, multiorgan failure, and coagulopathy. It can be difficult to distinguish between cellulitis, surgical wound infections, and necrotizing fasciitis. In addition to antibiotic therapy, infected wounds must be inspected and debrided until viable margins are obtained. Repeat debridement is often necessary. Initial antibiotic therapy is empiric and should consist of a combination of a β-lactam plus a β-lactamase inhibitor, plus clindamycin. Specific therapy directed at the offending organisms should be given, once identified by Gram stain or culture.

Additional Therapies

Recombinant Human-activated Protein C (Drotrecogin Alfa)

Drotrecogin alfa activated (DTAA), also known as activated protein C, is an endogenous protein that promotes fibrinolysis and inhibits thrombosis and inflammation and is important modulator of coagulation and inflammation associated with severe sepsis. DTAA is converted from its inactive precursor protein by thrombin coupled to thrombomodulin. The conversion of DTAA is impaired during sepsis as a result of the down-regulation of thrombomodulin by inflammatory cytokines. DTTA administration of 24 μg/kg of body weight per hour for 96 hours has been shown to reduce coagulopathy and inflammation, decreasing mortality rates in patients with severe sepsis by 6.1% to 13.8%. DTTA has also been proven to decrease mortality by 15.5% in older (75+ years of age) patients. DTTA, now approved by the FDA, is marketed with the brand name Xigris (Eli Lilly and Company) and is the first therapeutic intervention specifically indicated for severe sepsis. DTAA therapy is relatively cost-effective when targeted to patients with severe sepsis of greater severity of illness and a reasonable life expectancy if they survive the episode of sepsis. However, the cost is high and accounts for about 9% of the average total cost of hospitalization per patient treated. Adverse effects include increased risk of bleeding or intracranial hemorrhage in patients treated with anticoagulant therapy, oral anticoagulants, glycoprotein IIb-IIIa inhibitors, and low-molecular-weight heparins. Further research is needed to determine if DTAA therapy is cost-effective for patients with sepsis and less severe illness.

Intensive Insulin Therapy

Patients with severe sepsis and septic shock may develop complications associated with hyperglycemia and insulin resistance, which may increase their risks of severe infections, septicemia, and death. Recent studies have examined the effects of blood glucose normalization with intensive insulin therapy among patients with severe sepsis and septic shock. Maintaining a blood glucose level at 4 to 6.1 mmol/L compared with 10 to 11.1 mmol/L reduced the episodes of septicemia by 46% and lowered the mortality rates in patients with bacteremia from 29.5% to 12.5%.

Adrenal Replacement Therapy

The role of corticosteroid therapy in shock has recently been reevaluated. Patients with severe sepsis may develop either systemic inflammatory response syndrome (SIRS)-induced glucocorticoid receptor resistance or relative adrenal insufficiency. The prevalence of adrenal insufficiency in septic shock has been reported to be about 50%. Consequently, it has been assumed that corticosteroids could be used as antiinflammatory agents, but short courses of high-dose corticosteroids do not appear to reduce mortality from severe sepsis and septic shock. However, one intravenous dose of stress dose hydrocortisone has been shown to improve vasopressor activities in septic shock, and prolonged therapy with low-dose hydrocortisone was associated with reversal of shock state. Benefits included improvement in systemic hemodynamics, a reduction in the duration of vasopressor use, and improvement in mortality rates without altering the risks for gastroduodenal bleeding, superinfection, or hyperglycemia. Therefore, hydrocortisone (or equivalent) therapy at a dose of 200 to 300 mg is indicated in patients with septic shock immediately after they undergo an adrenocorticotropin hormone test and should be continued for 5 to 11 days when absolute or relative adrenal insufficiency is present.

Antacids

The risks of stress ulceration of the gastric mucosa can be significantly reduced by the use of oral antacids, intravenous H_2-blocking agents, or oral sucralfate. A recently described predisposing risk factor for Gram-negative pneumonia and sepsis is a reduction in gastric acidity from the routine use of antacids or H_2-blockers, such as cimetidine and ranitidine, to prevent stress-induced bleeding. Driks and associates, in a prospective randomized trial, found that the use of sucralfate, which provides equivalent prophylaxis against stress bleeding without reducing gastric acid levels, was associated with approximately half of the rate of pneumonia found with H_2-blockers or antacid use. Evidence that sucralfate is preferable to antacids or H_2-blockers is far from conclusive. Nevertheless, one of these agents should be used to protect the gastrointestinal tract from stress ulceration.

Nutrition

Malnutrition in intensive care unit (ICU) patients has been associated with increased morbidity, mortality, and length of hospitalization that is due to increased ventilator dependency, higher rates of infection, and impaired wound healing. As many as 40% of adult patients at the time of their hospital admission are affected by poor nutrition. Nutritional support should be based on laboratory assessment of preexisting nutritional status (albumin, transferrin, thyroxine-binding prealbumin, somatomedin-C). When total parenteral nutrition (TPN) is used, the usual rule of thumb is to provide between 25 and 35 nonprotein kcal/kg/d fairly equally distributed between fat and carbohydrate. Optimal assessment of caloric requirements in the patient with shock requiring mechanical ventilation is especially important. Although underfeeding can compromise pulmonary status, increased CO_2 production from excessive carbohydrate loads can exacerbate hypercapnia and complicate weaning efforts. Intralipid therapy should be used judiciously in neutropenic and immunosuppressed patients because of its depressive effects on mononuclear and polymorphonuclear monocytes, and increased risks for infection. The goal of amino acid therapy is to reduce catabolic expenditure, and usually, 1 to 1.5 g/kg is sufficient. Electrolytes, BUN, creatinine, glucose, liver function studies, calcium, magnesium, and phosphate levels should be monitored as frequently as clinically indicated to adjust carbohydrate, lipid, or protein loads and to correct specific electrolyte deficits. Trace elements (zinc, copper, chromium, and manganese) should be provided. Recent reports suggest that outcomes can be improved by providing oral glutamine to patients with systemic inflammatory response syndrome. Glutamine is a nonessential amino acid that is unstable in aqueous solutions and cannot be provided by standard TPN solutions. Special attention to nutritional needs should be provided for older, critically ill patients. It is estimated that 12% to 50% of acute inpatients 65 years of age and older are malnourished as assessed by measurements such as body mass index (BMI), biochemical indices (serum albumin, prealbumin, and transferring), and clinical parameters. Reasons for this include poor dentition, loss of appetite, and in the postoperative period, the inability to actually chew and swallow food. Although often not considered by the operating surgeon, oral health and hygiene seriously affect perioperative and overall health. A number of pathogens associated with gingivitis include *P. gingivalis*, *S. sobrinus*, and *S. aureus*, all three of which have been associated with an increased risk for aspiration pneumonia. In general, enteric'rather than parenteral—nutrition is preferred, even in critically ill ICU patients, because enteric nutrition is less likely to be associated with hepatobiliary dysfunction, metabolic derangements, or infection complications, and it is less expensive.

Other Therapies

Kerver and colleagues demonstrated that antibiotic prophylaxis with oral tobramycin, amphotericin B, and polymyxin E in critically ill patients requiring ventilatory support significantly reduced the incidence of nosocomial infection rates and their associated mortality. Prophylactic use of nystatin "swish and swallow" with 5 to 10 mL of nystatin (100,000 U/mL) has been found to reduce the incidence of systemic candidiasis as well as local wound infections. Hypothermic patients should be treated with warming therapy by elevating the room temperature, using radiant heat, or using convective warming therapy.

Critically ill patients with acute renal failure may benefit from continuous renal replacement therapies such a hemofiltration or hemoultrafiltration. These systems are unique in that they can be used in patients with hemodynamic instability. The use of high-permeability membranes in these systems allows the removal of measurable quantities of cytokines, although plasma levels do not seem to be affected by this process. At least theoretically, highly permeable membranes may have a limited capacity to remove molecules involved in the pathogenesis of sepsis. Continuous plasma filtration absorption (CPFA) is a modality of blood purification in which plasma is separated from whole blood and circulated in a sorbent cartridge. Its rationale is an attempt to remove molecules that are not removed by hemofiltration or other hemodialysis techniques. In an initial trial, CPFA was associated with increased systemic vascular resistances and significant reductions in the use of vasopressors. This suggests that CPFA may prove superior to conventional hemofiltration in patients with acute renal failure.

Evaluate Response to Therapy

Once oxygenation and restoration of the intravascular volume have been completed, it is important to reassess the patient's response to therapy (Table 12.11). Thorough investigation to determine the underlying cause should be performed so that definitive therapy may be implemented. In managing the patient with septic shock, right heart catheterization with hemodynamic monitoring, if not previously initiated, may be considered (Table 12.9), especially in those patients who have not responded to resuscitative efforts or who have evidence of pulmonary edema, myocardial infarction, or congestive heart failure. Arterial blood gases should be obtained to affirm adequate ventilation. Electrolyte, coagulation, and complete blood count results should now be available, and deficits may be corrected based on specific laboratory findings. In the face of specific organ system dysfunction, such as renal or hepatic failure, doses of antibiotics, vasopressors, and fluid support should be modified. Gastrointestinal losses should be replaced based on the electrolyte and acid–base composition of the site of loss.

Hyponatremia usually results from excessive crystalloid replacement, although renal losses can be increased secondary to a high protein intake, hyperglycemia, diuretic therapy, or acute failure. Symptoms can include coma or seizures, but hyponatremia is generally asymptomatic unless severe (serum sodium <125 mEq/dL). The management of mild, asymptomatic hyponatremia associated with an expanded intravascular volume is fluid restriction. Severe hyponatremia should be corrected by raising the serum sodium level to a minimum of 125 mEq/L. Hypernatremia is usually secondary to insufficient volume replacement and can be corrected using isotonic crystalloid solution, such as half normal saline.

Hypokalemia usually occurs secondary to diuretics, digitalis, β-antagonists, aminoglycosides, some penicillins, and gastrointestinal losses. Intravenous replacement may be safely accomplished with 20 to 40 mEq of potassium per liter of isotonic solution. In the intensive care setting, severe, life-threatening hypokalemia may be treated by giving intravenous KCl at a rate of 20 mEq per hour in as little as 25 to 50 mL of compatible solution. Hyperkalemia can develop secondary to renal failure, excessive potassium administration, tissue destruction, and acidosis, which shifts intracellular potassium into the extracellular fluid compartment. Shifting potassium into the intracellular compartment by infusing insulin with glucose (10 U regular insulin after 1 ampule of 50% glucose), or insulin with sodium bicarbonate or with albuterol is effective treatment. For life-threatening hyperkalemia (serum potassium >7 mEq/L), calcium gluconate, 10 mL of 10% solution, can be given intravenously over 2 to 5 minutes, followed by a second dose if needed. Finally, calcium exchange resins, such as sodium polystyrene sulfonate (15–30 g in 50–100 mL of 20% sorbitol), bind potassium in exchange for sodium within the gastrointestinal tract and are commonly used in patients with chronic renal failure.

Metabolic acidosis usually is satisfactorily corrected with appropriate ventilatory, electrolyte, and crystalloid

TABLE 12.11

EVALUATION OF RESPONSE TO INITIAL ATTEMPTS AT FLUID RESUSCITATION[a]

	Rapid response	Transient response	No response
Vital signs	Return to normal	Transient improvement; recurrence of decreased blood pressure or increased heart rate	Persistent tachycardia, hypotension, altered mental status
Estimated blood loss (%)	Minimal (10–20)	Moderate and ongoing (20–40)	Severe (>40)
Need for more crystalloid	Low	High	High
Blood preparation	Low	Moderate to high	Immediate
Need for operative intervention	Possibly	Likely	Very likely

[a]2000 mL Ringer's lactate solution in adults, 20 mg/kg in children.
Adapted from American College of Surgeons,. *Advanced trauma life support® student manual.* Chicago: American College of Surgeons, 1997, second impression 1999:9.

administration. The routine use of bicarbonate is not recommended for mild to moderate metabolic acidosis (pH 7.25–7.34). Bicarbonate use may shift the oxygen–hemoglobin dissociation curve and reduce oxygen delivery at the cellular level. Furthermore, excessive alkalinization can induce tetanus, seizures, and cardiac arrhythmias, and increase lactate production. When acidosis is severe (pH <7.2), intravenous bicarbonate is given by slow infusion (1–3 ampules of 7.5% $NaHCO_3$ [44.6 mEq/ampule] in 500–1000 mL D_5W), with the dose based on calculation of the total deficit. Approximately one half of the deficit can be replaced in 3 to 4 hours. No further replacement is necessary once the pH is 7.2 or greater. Serum potassium and calcium levels should concomitantly be monitored, because these shift into the intracellular space as the acidosis is corrected, resulting in hypokalemia or hypocalcemia.

Remedy the Underlying Cause

Although some causes of bleeding—such as a retroperitoneal hematoma developing after hysterectomy—can resolve without surgical intervention, all patients with continued intraabdominal bleeding and bleeding associated with persistent hemodynamic instability despite appropriate colloid and blood product replacement require immediate surgical intervention. Vaginal or other lacerations, if present, should be repaired. If the underlying case is septic abortion, prompt evacuation of the uterine contents is indicated as soon as adequate serum and tissue levels of broad-spectrum antibiotics are reached. Nonhemorrhagic causes of hypovolemic shock should be identified, and specific therapy should be directed at the underlying cause.

Investigational Agents

Several studies have looked at the clinical use of antibodies that would effectively neutralize bacterial endotoxin and mitigate its effects. Polyclonal antiserum directed against a mutant strain (J-5) of *E. coli* was the first of these agents subjected to clinical trial. In 1982, Ziegler and colleagues found that in subgroups of patients with Gram-negative bacteremia with or without shock, immunization was associated with a significant reduction in mortality. However, immunization provided protection only for patients with Gram-negative bacteremia or septic shock associated with Gram-negative septicemia and did not benefit patients with sepsis or shock from other causes. J-5 antiserum did not become available for clinical use because it is difficult to manufacture and, because pooled donor serum is required, it carries the risk of blood-borne infections.

The use of monoclonal antibodies has also been investigated. The first of these, immunoglobulin (Ig)G antibody purified from pooled plasma obtained from volunteers immunized with *E. coli,* did not demonstrate a significant difference in survival in patients with profound septic shock. Two additional monoclonal antibodies to endotoxin have subsequently been developed with more optimistic results. One of these, E5, an IgM antibody with reactivity to lipid A, was developed from murine splenocytes immunized with J-5 mutant *E. coli* cells. A second, HA-1A, a human monoclonal IgM antibody that binds to the lipid A domain of endotoxin, was also developed from J-5 mutant cells. Both of these monoclonal antibodies were able to improve survival and mitigate organ system dysfunction in patients with Gram-negative sepsis. Antibodies to TNF-α and a recombinant form of IL-1 receptor antagonist (a naturally occurring protein that binds to IL1 receptors), were especially intriguing, because it was anticipated that they could be used for patients with inflammatory response syndrome in the absence of an identifiable infection. In a pilot clinical trial, Vincent and colleagues found that anti-TNF antibody improved left ventricular function in 10 patients with septic shock; however, only 3 of the 10 patients survived. More recent trials using cytokine antagonists—including PAF- and TNF-α receptor antagonists—in the treatment of shock have demonstrated little benefit.

The high mobility group box protein 1 (HMGB1), a proinflammatory cytokine that plays a vital role as a delayed and potent mediator of local and systemic inflammation, has also been investigated. Secreted by macrophages and monocytes or passively released from necrotic cells of any tissue type, high levels of HMGB1, like TNF-α, have been shown to increase the sensitivity of animals to endotoxins, and HMGB1 levels are significantly increased in patients with severe sepsis. Administration of neutralizing anti-HMGB1 antibodies, recombinant HMGB1 A box protein, and ethyl pyruvate in septic animals has been shown to decrease mortality. Unlike TNF-α and other previously described cytokine targets, HMGB1's delayed kinetics may provide a greater temporal treatment window for neutralization therapy.

Other cytokines of recent interest in antiinflammatory and immunomodulatory therapies include granulocyte colony stimulating factor (G-CSF) and granulocyte-macrophage colony stimulating factor (GM-CSF). G-CSF differs from GM-CSF in its specificity of action on developing and mature neutrophils, effects on neutrophils kinetics, and toxicity profile. Recombinant GM-CSF has toxicity profile consistent with the priming of macrophages for increased formation and the release of inflammatory cytokines, whereas recombinant G-CSF induces the production of antiinflammatory factors such as IL-1 receptor antagonist and TNF receptors, and is protective against endotoxin- and sepsis-induced organ injury. G-CSF and GM-CSF can augment the functional antimicrobial activities of neutrophils in addition to up-regulating multiple antimicrobial mechanisms in monocytes and macrophages, enhancing pathogen eradication. In one study, pretreating animals with G-CSF effectively prevented the overactivation of Kupffer cells by both Gram-negative and Gram-positive bacterial substances. Although most clinical studies have examined G-CSF and GM-CSF therapy in neutropenic patients, further trials in are needed to identify the subset of patients who may benefit from G-CSF and/or GM-CSF therapy.

Polymorphisms present in cytokine genes may influence concentration of inflammatory and antiinflammatory cytokines produced in a patient's response to infection, suggesting that genetic factors significantly contribute to a patient's overall outcome when infected with inflammatory and infectious diseases. Recent studies have also discovered inflammatory responses associated with neutrophil defects, including alterations in pattern recognition in molecules such as CD14 and TLRs. An increased understanding of genetic influence on susceptibility to inflammatory responses may lead to individualized therapy directed at patients that may be at greater risk for hyper- or hypoinflammatory response to infection.

Nitric oxide (NO) and reactive oxygen species exert multiple modulating effects on inflammation and play a key role in the regulation of immune responses. Low concentrations of nitric oxide produced by constitutive and neuronal nitric oxide synthases inhibit adhesion molecule expression, cytokine and chemokine synthesis, and leukocyte adhesion and transmigration. Large amounts can be toxic and proinflammatory. Actions of nitric oxide are dependent on the cellular context, concentration, and initial priming of immune cells. The effects of both nitric oxide and superoxide in immune regulation are exerted through multiple mechanisms, which include interactions with diverse cell signaling pathways. Consequently, nitrous oxide has both proinflammatory and antiinflammatory effects, and both enhances and reduces platelet activation and function. Drugs that interfere with nitrous oxide, including statins, angiotensin receptor blockers, NAD(P)H oxidase inhibitors, and NO-aspirin agents, are beginning to be introduced in the treatment of inflammation and sepsis.

SUMMARY

The management of patients with systemic inflammatory response syndrome and shock states remains one of the most formidable challenges facing the practicing gynecologist. However, with early recognition, prompt intervention, and continued aggressive surveillance, a satisfactory outcome is achievable in most cases. Thus, caring for the patient in shock, although challenging, may well be rewarding.

BEST SURGICAL PRACTICES

- Management of shock requires restoration of ORDER: *oxygenation,* with ventilatory support, if needed; *restore* circulating volume with crystalloid and, if needed, blood products; *drug therapy,* with antibiotics or pressors; *evaluation* of response to therapy; and *remedy* the underlying cause.
- Regardless of the precipitating event, the severity of hypovolemia can be estimated using guidelines established by the American College of Surgeons. Initially, crystalloid replacement should be initiated to replace volume.
- Blood product use should be based severity of anemia, symptoms, and ongoing blood loss. In asymptomatic patients without significant cardiopulmonary or renal disease, there is no "transfusion trigger," for which blood replacement is essential.
- Critical care multidisciplinary teams with training and experience to address respiratory, nutritional, and other aspects of care have significantly reduced both mortality and morbidity from shock states.
- When a patient presents with septic shock, broad-spectrum antibiotic therapy directed against Gram-positive, Gram-negative, and anaerobic organisms should be initiated after cultures are obtained. Attempt to identify the etiology; sources such as abscesses should be drained, and infected wounds should undergo debridement. Subsequent antibiotic therapy should be guided by culture results. Indiscriminate use of antibiotics has led to drug resistance; empiric use of agents such as vancomycin is discouraged because of the development of methicillin resistant staphylococcus infections.

Bibliography

Aderem A. Role of Toll-like receptors in inflammatory response in macrophages. *Crit Care Med* 2001;29(7 Suppl):S16.

Alderson P, Bunn F, Lefebvre C, et al. Human albumin solution for resuscitation and volume expansion in critically ill patients. *Cochrane Database Syst Rev* 2004(4):CD001208.

Alexander SL, Ernst FR. Use of drotrecogin alfa (activated) in older patients with severe sepsis. *Pharmacotherapy* 2006;26(4):533.

Ali S, Roberts PR. Nutrients with immune modulating effects: what role should they play in the intensive care unit? *Curr Opin Anaesthesiol* 2006;19(2):132.

Allon M, Copkney C. Albuterol and insulin for treatment of hyperkalemia in hemodialysis patients. *Kidney Int* 1990;38(5):869.

American College of Chest Physicians/Society of Critical Care Medicine. Consensus Conference. Definitions for sepsis and organ failure and guidelines for the use of innovative therapies in sepsis. *Crit Care Med* 1992;20(6):864.

American College of Obstetricians and Gynecologists. *Blood component therapy.* ACOG technical bulletin no. 199. Washington, DC: 1995.

American College of Obstetricians and Gynecologists. *Septic shock.* ACOG technical bulletin no. 204. Washington, DC: ACOG, 1995.

American College of Surgeons. *Advanced trauma and life support student manual,* 8th ed: Chicago: American College of Surgeons, 2004.

American Society of Anesthesiologists. Practice guidelines for blood component therapy: a report by the American Society of Anesthesiologists Task Force on Blood Component Therapy. *Anesthesiology* 1996;84(3):732.

Andersson U, Tracey KJ. HMGB1 in sepsis. *Scand J Infect Dis* 2003;35(9):577.

Angus DC, Linde-Zwirble WT, Lidicker J, et al. Epidemiology of severe sepsis in the United States: analysis of incidence, outcome, and associated costs of care. *Crit Care Med* 2001;29(7):1303.

Annane D, Aegerter P, Jars-Guincestre MC, et al. Current epidemiology of septic shock: the CUB-Rea Network. *Am J Respir Crit Care Med* 2003;168(2):165.

Annane D, Bellissant E, Bollaert PE, et al. Corticosteroids for treating severe sepsis and septic shock. *Cochrane Database Syst Rev* 2004(1):CD002243.

Badr KF. Sepsis-associated renal vasoconstriction: potential targets for future therapy. *Am J Kidney Dis* 1992;20(3):207.

Barr J, Hecht M, Flavin KE, et al. Outcomes in critically ill patients before and after the implementation of an evidence-based nutritional management protocol. *Chest* 2004;125(4):1446.

Bates DW, Sands K, Miller E, et al. Predicting bacteremia in patients with sepsis syndrome. Academic Medical Center Consortium Sepsis Project Working Group. *J Infect Dis* 1997;176(6):1538.

Baumgartner JD, Glauser MP, McCutchan JA, et al. Prevention of gram-negative shock and death in surgical patients by antibody to endotoxin core glycolipid. *Lancet* 1985;2(8446):59.

Bellomo R, Farmer M, Boyce N. Combined acute respiratory and renal failure: management by continuous hemodiafiltration. *Resuscitation* 1994;28(2):123.

Bernard GR, Vincent JL, Laterre PF, et al. Efficacy and safety of recombinant human activated protein C for severe sepsis. *N Engl J Med* 2001;344(10):699.

Billiar TR, Curran RD. Kupffer cell and hepatocyte interactions: a brief overview. *JPEN J Parenter Enteral Nutr* 1990;14(5 Suppl):175S.

Bisno AL, Stevens DL. Streptococcal infections of skin and soft tissues. *N Engl J Med* 1996;334(4):240.

Blanco JD, Gibbs RS, Castaneda YS. Bacteremia in obstetrics: clinical course. *Obstet Gynecol* 1981;58(5):621.

Bochud PY, Glauser MP, Calandra T. Antibiotics in sepsis. *Intensive Care Med* 2001;27(Suppl 1):S33.

Bone RC, Fisher CJ Jr, Clemmer TP, et al. A controlled clinical trial of high-dose methylprednisolone in the treatment of severe sepsis and septic shock. *N Engl J Med* 1987;317(11):653.

Burke DJ, Alverdy JC, Aoys E, et al. Glutamine-supplemented total parenteral nutrition improves gut immune function. *Arch Surg* 1989;124(12):1396.

Busch CJ, Wanner GA, Menger MD, et al. Granulocyte colony-stimulating factor (G-CSF) reduces not only gram-negative but also gram-positive infection associated proinflammatory cytokine release by interaction between Kupffer cells and leukocytes. *Inflamm Res* 2004;53(5):205.

Carlson DL, Willis MS, White DJ, et al. Tumor necrosis factor-alpha induced caspase activation mediates endotoxin-related cardiac dysfunction. *Crit Care Med* 2005;33(5):1021.

Carrico CJ, Meakins JL, Marshall JC, et al. Multiple-organ-failure syndrome. *Arch Surg* 1986;121(2):196.

Cerra FB. Hypermetabolism-organ failure syndrome: a metabolic response to injury. *Crit Care Clin* 1989;5(2):289.

Chapnick EK, Abter EI. Necrotizing soft-tissue infections. *Infect Dis Clin North Am* 1996;10(4):835.

Connors AF Jr, Speroff T, Dawson NV, et al. The effectiveness of right heart catheterization in the initial care of critically ill patients. SUPPORT Investigators. *JAMA* 1996;276(11):889.

Cunneen J, Cartwright M. The puzzle of sepsis: fitting the pieces of the inflammatory response with treatment. *AACN Clin Issues* 2004;15(1):18.

Cunnion RE, Parrillo JE. Myocardial dysfunction in sepsis: recent insights. *Chest* 1989;95(5):941.

Dalen JE, Bone RC. Is it time to pull the pulmonary artery catheter? *JAMA* 1996;276(11):916.

Deitch EA. The role of intestinal barrier failure and bacterial translocation in the development of systemic infection and multiple organ failure. *Arch Surg* 1990;125(3):403.

Deitch EA, Shi HP, Lu Q, et al. Serine proteases are involved in the pathogenesis of trauma-hemorrhagic shock-induced gut and lung injury. *Shock* 2003;19(5):452.

Demetri GD, Kris M, Wade J, et al. Quality-of-life benefit in chemotherapy patients treated with epoetin alfa is independent of disease response or tumor type: results from a prospective community oncology study. Procrit Study Group. *J Clin Oncol* 1998;16(10):3412.

Desai MH, Rutan RL, Heggers JP, et al. Candida infection with and without nystatin prophylaxis: an 11-year experience with patients with burn injury. *Arch Surg* 1992;127(2):159.

Dhainaut JF, Marin N, Mignon A, et al. Hepatic response to sepsis: interaction between coagulation and inflammatory processes. *Crit Care Med* 2001; 29(7 Suppl):S42.

Driks MR, Craven DE, Celli BR, et al. Nosocomial pneumonia in intubated patients given sucralfate as compared with antacids or histamine type 2 blockers: the role of gastric colonization. *N Engl J Med* 1987;317(22): 1376.

Estella NM, Berry DL, Baker BW, et al. Normovolemic hemodilution before cesarean hysterectomy for placenta percreta. *Obstet Gynecol* 1997;90(4 Pt 2): 669.

Friedman G, Silva E, Vincent JL. Has the mortality of septic shock changed with time? *Crit Care Med* 1998;26(12):2078.

Gafter-Gvili A, Fraser A, Paul M, et al. Meta-analysis: antibiotic prophylaxis reduces mortality in neutropenic patients. *Ann Intern Med* 2005;142(12 Pt 1): 979.

Gallup DG, Nolan TE. The gynecologist and multiple organ failure syndrome (MOFS). *Gynecol Oncol* 1993;48(3):293.

Goldie AS, Fearon KC, Ross JA, et al. Natural cytokine antagonists and endogenous antiendotoxin core antibodies in sepsis syndrome. The Sepsis Intervention Group. *JAMA* 1995;274(2):172.

Goodnough LT. Autologous blood donation. *Crit Care* 2004;8(Suppl 2):S49.

Goodnough LT, Brecher ME, Kanter MH, et al. Transfusion medicine. First of two parts—blood transfusion. *N Engl J Med* 1999;340(6):438.

Goodnough LT, Shander A, Brecher ME. Transfusion medicine: looking to the future. *Lancet* 2003;361(9352):161.

Gorschluter M, Hahn C, Fixson A, et al. Piperacillin-tazobactam is more effective than ceftriaxone plus gentamicin in febrile neutropenic patients with hematological malignancies: a randomized comparison. *Support Care Cancer* 2003;11(6):362.

Grange CS, Douglas MJ, Adams TJ, et al. The use of acute hemodilution in parturients undergoing cesarean section. *Am J Obstet Gynecol* 1998; 178(1 Pt 1):156.

Grogan M, Thomas GM, Melamed I, et al. The importance of hemoglobin levels during radiotherapy for carcinoma of the cervix. *Cancer* 1999;86(8):1528.

Gutierrez G, Reines HD, Wulf-Gutierrez ME. Clinical review: hemorrhagic shock. *Crit Care* 2004;8(5):373.

Guzik TJ, Korbut R, Adamek-Guzik T. Nitric oxide and superoxide in inflammation and immune regulation. *J Physiol Pharmacol* 2003;54(4):469.

Hardee ME, Arcasoy MO, Blackwell KL, et al. Erythropoietin biology in cancer. *Clin Cancer Res* 2006;12(2):332.

Hebert PC, Wells G, Blajchman MA, et al. A multicenter, randomized, controlled clinical trial of transfusion requirements in critical care. Transfusion Requirements in Critical Care Investigators, Canadian Critical Care Trials Group. *N Engl J Med* 1999;340(6):409.

Higgins TL, Steingrub JS, Tereso GJ, et al. Drotrecogin alfa (activated) in sepsis: initial experience with patient selection, cost, and clinical outcomes. *J Intensive Care Med* 2005;20(6):339.

Hollenberg SM, Kavinsky CJ, Parrillo JE. Cardiogenic shock. *Ann Intern Med* 1999;131(1):47.

Jimenez EJ. *Critical care*, 3rd ed. Philadelphia: Lippincott-Raven Publishers; 1997.

Kerver AJ, Rommes JH, Mevissen-Verhage EA, et al. Prevention of colonization and infection in critically ill patients: a prospective randomized study. *Crit Care Med* 1988;16(11):1087.

Klastersky J, Glauser MP, Schimpff SC, et al. Prospective randomized comparison of three antibiotic regimens for empirical therapy of suspected bacteremic infection in febrile granulocytopenic patients. *Antimicrob Agents Chemother* 1986;29(2):263.

Krishnagopalan S, Kumar A, Parrillo JE, et al. Myocardial dysfunction in the patient with sepsis. *Curr Opin Crit Care* 2002;8(5):376.

Kumar A, Thota V, Dee L, et al. Tumor necrosis factor alpha and interleukin 1beta are responsible for in vitro myocardial cell depression induced by human septic shock serum. *J Exp Med* 1996;183(3):949.

Levy MM, Fink MP, Marshall JC, et al. 2001 SCCM/ESICM/ACCP/ATS/SIS International Sepsis Definitions Conference. *Crit Care Med* 2003;31(4): 1250.

Lindholm MG, Kober L, Boesgaard S, et al. Cardiogenic shock complicating acute myocardial infarction; prognostic impact of early and late shock development. *Eur Heart J* 2003;24(3):258.

Luyer MD, Jacobs JA, Vreugdenhil AC, et al. Enteral administration of high-fat nutrition before and directly after hemorrhagic shock reduces endotoxemia and bacterial translocation. *Ann Surg* 2004;239(2):257–264.

Madjdpour C, Heindl V, Spahn DR. Risks, benefits, alternatives and indications of allogenic blood transfusions. *Minerva Anestesiol* 2006;72(5):283.

Manns BJ, Lee H, Doig CJ, et al. An economic evaluation of activated protein C treatment for severe sepsis. *N Engl J Med* 2002;347(13):993.

Marsden DE, Cavanagh D. Hemorrhagic shock in the gynecologic patient. *Clin Obstet Gynecol* 1985;28(2):381.

Maupin RT. Obstetric infectious disease emergencies. *Clin Obstet Gynecol* 2002;45(2):393.

McIntyre L, Walley KR. Importance of underlying mechanism and genotype on outcome of sepsis trials. *Crit Care Med* 2001;29(3):677.

Mekontso-Dessap A, Brun-Buisson C. Statins: the next step in adjuvant therapy for sepsis? *Intensive Care Med* 2006;32(1):11.

Napolitano LM. Immune stimulation in sepsis: to be or not to be? *Chest* 2005;127(6):1882.

Napolitano LM. Perioperative anemia. *Surg Clin North Am* 2005;85(6):1215.

Nathan L, Peters MT, Ahmed AM, et al. The return of life-threatening puerperal sepsis caused by group A streptococci. *Am J Obstet Gynecol* 1993;169(3):571.

Nijhuis CO, Kamps WA, Daenen SM, et al. Feasibility of withholding antibiotics in selected febrile neutropenic cancer patients. *J Clin Oncol* 2005;23(30):7437.

Oberholzer A, Souza SM, Tschoeke SK, et al. Plasma cytokine measurements augment prognostic scores as indicators of outcome in patients with severe sepsis. *Shock* 2005;23(6):488.

Parker MM, Ognibene FP, Parrillo JE. Peak systolic pressure/end-systolic volume ratio, a load independent measure of ventricular function, is reversibly decreased in human septic shock. *Crit Care Med* 1994;22(12):1955.

Parrillo JE. Pathogenetic mechanisms of septic shock. *N Engl J Med* 1993;328(20):1471.

Parrillo JE, Burch C, Shelhamer JH, et al. A circulating myocardial depressant substance in humans with septic shock: septic shock patients with a reduced ejection fraction have a circulating factor that depresses in vitro myocardial cell performance. *J Clin Invest* 1985;76(4):1539.

Parrillo JE, Parker MM, Natanson C, et al. Septic shock in humans: advances in the understanding of pathogenesis, cardiovascular dysfunction, and therapy. *Ann Intern Med* 1990;113(3):227.

Paul M, Borok S, Fraser A, et al. Additional anti-Gram-positive antibiotic treatment for febrile neutropenic cancer patients. *Cochrane Database Syst Rev* 2005(3):CD003914.

Priest BP, Brinson DN, Schroeder DA, et al. Treatment of experimental gram negative bacterial sepsis with murine monoclonal antibodies directed against lipopolysaccharide. *Surgery* 1989;106(2):147; discussion 54.

Pulmonary Artery Catheter Consensus conference: consensus statement. *Crit Care Med* 1997;25(6):910.

Raghavan M, Marik PE. Anemia, allogenic blood transfusion, and immunomodulation in the critically ill. *Chest* 2005;127(1):295.

Ramphal R. Changes in the etiology of bacteremia in febrile neutropenic patients and the susceptibilities of the currently isolated pathogens. *Clin Infect Dis* 2004;39(Suppl 1):S25.

Rangel-Frausto MS, Pittet D, Hwang T, et al. The dynamics of disease progression in sepsis: Markov modeling describing the natural history and the likely impact of effective antisepsis agents. *Clin Infect Dis* 1998;27(1): 185.

Reed RL 2nd. Antibiotic choices in surgical intensive care unit patients. *Surg Clin North Am* 1991;71(4):765.

Reviewers CIGA. Human albumin administration in critically ill patients: systemic review of randomized controlled trials. *BMJ* 1988;317:235.

Richards MJ, Edwards JR, Culver DH, et al. Nosocomial infections in combined medical-surgical intensive care units in the United States. *Infect Control Hosp Epidemiol* 2000;21(8):510.

Richter HE, Holley RL, Andrews WW, et al. The association of interleukin 6 with clinical and laboratory parameters of acute pelvic inflammatory disease. *Am J Obstet Gynecol* 1999;181(4):940.

Ronco C, Brendolan A, Dan M, et al. Adsorption in sepsis. *Kidney Int Suppl* 2000;76:S1485.

Rosenthal RA. Nutritional concerns in the older surgical patient. *J Am Coll Surg* 2004;199(5):785.

Roumen RM, Hendriks T, Wevers RA, et al. Intestinal permeability after severe trauma and hemorrhagic shock is increased without relation to septic complications. *Arch Surg* 1993;128(4):453.

Safdar A, Rolston KV. Vancomycin tolerance, a potential mechanism for refractory gram positive bacteremia observational study in patients with cancer. *Cancer* 2006;106(8):1815.

Samama CM, Bastien O, Forestier F, et al. Antiplatelet agents in the perioperative period: expert recommendations of the French Society of Anesthesiology and Intensive Care (SFAR) 2001—summary statement. *Can J Anaesth* 2002;49(6):S26.

Sands KE, Bates DW, Lanken PN, et al. Epidemiology of sepsis syndrome in 8 academic medical centers. *JAMA* 1997;278(3):234.

Schiffer CA, Anderson KC, Bennett CL, et al. Platelet transfusion for patients with cancer: clinical practice guidelines of the American Society of Clinical Oncology. *J Clin Oncol* 2001;19(5):1519.

Sevransky JE, Levy MM, Marini JJ. Mechanical ventilation in sepsis-induced acute lung injury/acute respiratory distress syndrome: an evidence-based review. *Crit Care Med* 2004;32(11 Suppl):S548.

Shah MR, Hasselblad V, Stevenson LW, et al. Impact of the pulmonary artery catheter in critically ill patients: meta-analysis of randomized clinical trials. *JAMA* 2005;294(13):1664.

Sharma S, Kumar A. Septic shock, multiple organ failure, and acute respiratory distress syndrome. *Curr Opin Pulm Med* 2003;9(3):199.

Shoemaker WC, Appel PL, Kram HB. Hemodynamic and oxygen transport effects of dobutamine in critically ill general surgical patients. *Crit Care Med* 1986;14(12):1032.

Shoemaker WC, Appel PL, Kram HB, et al. Comparison of hemodynamic and oxygen transport effects of dopamine and dobutamine in critically ill surgical patients. *Chest* 1989;96(1):120.

Simon D, Trenholme G. Antibiotic selection for patients with septic shock. *Crit Care Clin* 2000;16(2):215.

Snyder HS. Lack of a tachycardic response to hypotension with ruptured ectopic pregnancy. *Am J Emerg Med* 1990;8(1):23.

Sort P, Navasa M, Arroyo V, et al. Effect of intravenous albumin on renal impairment and mortality in patients with cirrhosis and spontaneous bacterial peritonitis. *N Engl J Med* 1999;341(6):403.

Sprung CL, Caralis PV, Marcial EH, et al. The effects of high-dose corticosteroids in patients with septic shock: a prospective, controlled study. *N Engl J Med* 1984;311(18):1137.

Sprung CL, Peduzzi PN, Shatney CH, et al. Impact of encephalopathy on mortality in the sepsis syndrome. The Veterans Administration Systemic Sepsis Cooperative Study Group. *Crit Care Med* 1990;18(8):801.

Stein GE, Goldstein EJ. Fluoroquinolones and anaerobes. *Clin Infect Dis* 2006;42(11):1598.

Tachi M, Hirabayashi S, Harada H, et al. Pathophysiology and treatment of streptococcal toxic shock syndrome. *Scand J Plast Reconstr Surg Hand Surg* 2002;36(5):305.

Tracey KJ, Cerami A. Tumor necrosis factor: an updated review of its biology. *Crit Care Med* 1993;21(10 Suppl):S415.

Tsalis KG. Comment to: Septic shock: current pathogenetic concepts from a clinical perspective. *Med Sci Monit* 2006;12(4):LE4.

Tslotou AG, Sakorafas GH, Anagnostopoulos G, et al. Septic shock; current pathogenetic concepts from a clinical perspective. *Med Sci Monit* 2005;11(3):RA76.

Valeri CR, Dennis RC, Ragno G, et al. Limitations of the hematocrit level to assess the need for red blood cell transfusion in hypovolemic anemic patients. *Transfusion* 2006;46(3):365.

Van Bambeke F, Michot JM, Van Eldere J, et al. Quinolones in 2005: an update. *Clin Microbiol Infect* 2005;11(4):256.

van Deventer SJ. Cytokine and cytokine receptor polymorphisms in infectious disease. *Intensive Care Med* 2000;26(Suppl 1):S98.

Varlotto J, Stevenson MA. Anemia, tumor hypoxemia, and the cancer patient. *Int J Radiat Oncol Biol Phys* 2005;63(1):25.

Vidal L, Paul M, Ben-Dor I, et al. Oral versus intravenous antibiotic treatment for febrile neutropenia in cancer patients. *Cochrane Database Syst Rev* 2004(4):CD003992.

Vincent JL, Abraham E. The last 100 years of sepsis. *Am J Respir Crit Care Med* 2006;173(3):256.

Vincent JL, Bakker J, Marecaux G, et al. Administration of anti-TNF antibody improves left ventricular function in septic shock patients: results of a pilot study. *Chest* 1992;101(3):810.

Vincent JL, Navickis RJ, Wilkes MM. Morbidity in hospitalized patients receiving human albumin: a meta-analysis of randomized, controlled trials. *Crit Care Med* 2004;32(10):2029.

Waikar SS, Chertow GM. Crystalloids versus colloids for resuscitation in shock. *Curr Opin Nephrol Hypertens* 2000;9(5):501.

Wang H, Bloom O, Zhang M, et al. HMG-1 as a late mediator of endotoxin lethality in mice. *Science* 1999;285(5425):248.

Waters JH, Biscotti C, Potter PS, et al. Amniotic fluid removal during cell salvage in the cesarean section patient. *Anesthesiology* 2000;92(6):1531.

Waterstone M, Bewley S, Wolfe C. Incidence and predictors of severe obstetric morbidity: case control study. *BMJ* 2001;322(7294):1089; discussion 93.

Wiernik A, Jarstrand C, Julander I. The effect of intralipid on mononuclear and polymorphonuclear phagocytes. *Am J Clin Nutr* 1983;37(2):256.

Williams MD, Braun LA, Cooper LM, et al. Hospitalized cancer patients with severe sepsis: analysis of incidence, mortality, and associated costs of care. *Crit Care* 2004;8(5):R291.

Winter WE 3rd, Maxwell GL, Tian C, et al. Association of hemoglobin level with survival in cervical carcinoma patients treated with concurrent cisplatin and radiotherapy: a Gynecologic Oncology Group Study. *Gynecol Oncol* 2004;94(2):495.

Wu WC, Rathore SS, Wang Y, et al. Blood transfusion in elderly patients with acute myocardial infarction. *N Engl J Med* 2001;345(17):1230.

Young MJ, Woolliscroft JO, Billi JE. Steroids and septic shock. *Infect Surg* 1987;7:173.

Yu DT, Black E, Sands KE, et al. Severe sepsis: variation in resource and therapeutic modality use among academic centers. *Crit Care* 2003;7(3):R24.

Ziegler EJ, Fisher CJ Jr. , Sprung CL, et al. Treatment of gram-negative bacteremia and septic shock with HA-1A human monoclonal antibody against endotoxin: a randomized, double-blind, placebo-controlled trial. The HA-1A Sepsis Study Group. *N Engl J Med* 1991;324(7):429.

Ziegler EJ, McCutchan JA, Fierer J, et al. Treatment of gram-negative bacteremia and shock with human antiserum to a mutant *Escherichia coli*. *N Engl J Med* 1982;307(20):1225.

CHAPTER 13 ■ WOUND HEALING, SUTURE MATERIAL, AND SURGICAL INSTRUMENTATION

GARY H. LIPSCOMB

DEFINITIONS

Healing by primary intention—Wound healing that occurs if the wound layers are reapproximated following injury.

Healing by secondary intention—Wound healing that occurs if wounds are left open after injury and allowed to close spontaneously from the formation of granulation tissue.

Healing by third intention—Wound healing that occurs when the wound is closed after an initial period of delay of several days; also referred to as *delayed primary closure.*

Absorbable sutures—Sutures that lose the majority of their tensile strength before 60 days when implanted in body tissues.

Non-absorbable sutures—Sutures that maintain the majority of their tensile strength before 60 days when implanted in body tissues.

Knot-pull tensile strength—Breaking strength of a suture when tied around a plastic tube using a surgeon's flat knot and stressed from either end.

WOUND HEALING

Ideally, organic tissue lost by destruction or injury would be replaced with tissue identical in form and function. This process is known as *regeneration*. Although tissue regeneration does occur in lower animals (e.g., salamanders), humans have lost this ability for the most part. With the exception of the epidermis of the skin, mucosa of the intestinal tract, and liver, damaged human tissue heals by the laying down of collagen, a repair process better known as *scarring*. This process is responsible for emergently sealing the wound and ultimately providing long-term structural support for the injured organ, but is unable to reproduce other functions of the replaced tissue. As a result, the healing process also leads to disease if an organ becomes unable to function properly owing to extensive replacement of functioning tissue by nonfunctioning scar. Heart failure following a massive myocardial infarction is an example. In other cases, the healing process itself directly produces disease (e.g., postoperative adhesion formation following surgical procedures or tubal occlusion after pelvic inflammatory disease).

Physiology of Wound Healing

The healing of a wound involves several distinct biological processes: (a) inflammation, (b) epithelialization, (c) fibroplasia, (d) wound contraction, and (e) scar maturation. Although considered distinct, these processes do not occur in a strict sequence but often simultaneously with each other. These repair mechanisms are also nonspecific. They are activated whether a wound is made with a surgical scalpel and sutured closed or by trauma and then allowed to heal without surgical closure. However, the nature of the wound influences the degree to which each individual process is involved, and this in turn can affect the ultimate success of the repair.

Inflammation

The inflammatory phase of healing is the initial response to any injury involving more than an epithelial surface. This phase can be divided into two separate but simultaneously occurring responses: a vascular and a cellular response. Both are initiated by amines, most notably histamine, as well as the kinins and proteolytic enzymes released by the injured tissue. Immediately after injury, a transient vasoconstriction of the local vasculature lasts for 5 to 10 minutes. Vasoconstriction is followed by vasodilatation and an increase in vascular permeability. Edema caused by the escape of plasma through altered vessel walls becomes clinically apparent at this point.

The cellular response is characterized by the migration of leukocytes into the injured area. Although the agents responsible for this active migration of leukocytes remain unclear, chemotactic factors are thought to play a major role. Initially, the polymorphonuclear leukocytes and monocytes in the wound are present in the same concentration as in the systemic circulation. As a result, polymorphonuclear leukocytes predominate for the first 3 days. Because polymorphonuclear leukocytes are relatively short-lived compared with monocytes, the latter stages of the inflammatory phase are characterized by a predominance of monocytes that transform into macrophages. These leukocytes actively phagocytize bacteria, foreign proteins, and necrotic debris. As polymorphonuclear leukocytes die, their intracellular enzymes and debris are released into the wound and become part of the wound exudate. These released enzymes also facilitate the breakdown of material not phagocytized by the leukocytes. This accumulated exudate or pus develops even in the absence of bacteria. Even when this exudate is sterile, the presence of proteolytic enzymes, including collagenase, can interfere with epithelialization and fibroplasia, and thus, interfere with continued wound healing. Poor wound healing, however, is more common in wounds contaminated with bacteria and foreign material. In these cases, the inflammatory response may persist for long periods of time.

Epithelialization

By virtue of their exposed location, the epithelial surfaces of the gastrointestinal, urogenital, and respiratory tract as well as the skin itself are continually subjected to the physical and chemical trauma associated with the activities of daily living. As a result, these surfaces are constantly replacing damaged or destroyed cells through a process known as *epithelialization*. Epithelialization occurs by migration and subsequent maturation of immature epithelial cells from the deeper basal layers of surrounding areas. If the cellular damage is confined entirely to the epithelium, the healing response is merely an exaggerated form of the basic normal replacement process.

If an injury involves the supporting connective tissue beneath the epithelium, however, the other components of the healing processes, in addition to epithelialization, become involved. If the injury severs blood vessels, the vessels retract, and the process of hemostasis is initiated. If bleeding is not too severe, a blood clot soon forms. This clot subsequently contracts, dehydrates, and becomes a scab. Within 12 hours, basal cells from the surrounding epithelial surfaces begin migrating onto the injured surface. Epithelial cells move beneath the scab, detaching it from the wound and sealing the surface. In incised and sutured wounds, epithelialization generally produces a watertight seal within 24 hours of injury. This new layer of epithelial cells is initially thin and poorly attached to the underlying surface, rendering it susceptible to injury from even minor trauma. Final epithelial healing is accomplished by differentiation and maturation of the migrated cells and by scar formation through fibroplasia.

Fibroplasia

The process by which wounds regain strength is termed *fibroplasia*. Fibroplasia results in the production of the collagen necessary to form a fibrous scar and ultimately determines the final strength of the healed wound. This process begins with the differentiation of mesenchymal cells into fibroblasts. Fibroblasts then migrate into the wound, apparently along fibrin strands produced during clot formation. Once at the injury site, fibroblasts proliferate and manufacture the glycoproteins and mucopolysaccharides that make up the ground substance of connective tissue. Ground substance is an amorphous matrix that is believed to induce aggregation of collagen subunits and influences the final orientation of the fibers.

Once the ground substance is produced, fibroblasts begin to synthesize the basic building block of collagen-tropocollagen. Tropocollagen is a stiff elongated macromolecule of three helically intertwined chains of amino acids consisting of two identical $\alpha 1$ chains and one $\alpha 2$ chain. Within the ground substance and at the proper pH, osmolality, and temperature, tropocollagen molecules polymerize into collagen fibrils by forming covalent bonds with their neighbor. These fibrils bond with other fibrils to form collagen bundles. It is not until 4 to 5 days after injury that the wound produces enough collagen to result in a measurable increase in wound tensile strength. Before this time, the wound is held together only by fibrous adhesion. This time frame between wounding and an increase in tensile strength originally was referred to by Howes and Harvey as the "lag period" of wound healing.

Wound Contraction

The manner in which tissue heals is dependent on whether tissue integrity is simply interrupted (as in a surgical incision) or tissue is removed (as in an avulsion injury). In both types of injury, tissue seals itself, begins to reepithelialize, and synthesizes collagen for structural support. However, when large amounts of tissue are missing, the edges of the wound must be brought closer together so that the previously noted tissue responses can repair the defect. This process is known as *contraction*. Contraction of wound margins begins about 5 days after injury and corresponds with the fibroplasia phase of healing. Because this process can be inhibited by cytochrome poisons, such as potassium cyanide, and by smooth muscle relaxants, older theories attributing wound contraction to passive collagen changes have been discarded. Instead, wound contraction appears to be an active process produced by contractile proteins within the fibroblasts. If the area is too large for contraction to bring the edges together, the wound remains covered with granulation tissue, or if small enough, it is covered with epithelium only. Epithelialization of such a wound prevents weeping, but without the normal underlying supporting stroma, it remains too fragile to provide lasting protection. Pathologic progression of skin contraction ultimately may result in restriction of joint or limb mobility. This deformity is termed *contracture* and should not be confused with contraction.

Scar Maturation

The bulky scar formed during the fibroplasia phase consists of randomly oriented soluble collagen fibers. This scar has little tensile strength. During scar maturation, the disordered fibers are replaced with fibers arranged in a more orderly fashion, producing a denser and stronger scar. Collagen fibers also continue to form covalent bonds within fibrils as well as between adjacent fibrils and fibers, resulting in a continued increase in wound tensile strength over time. This maturation process may continue for years.

During scar maturation and remolding, the breakdown of old disordered collagen slightly exceeds production of new organized collagen fibers. The resulting new scar is softer and less bulky than the original scar but also is stronger because of its more organized and extensively cross-linked nature. However, if collagen production exceeds breakdown, then a keloid or hypertrophied scar results.

Surgical Wound Healing

Depending on the manner of wound closure, three types of surgical wound healing are recognized: primary, secondary, and third intention. Figure 13.1 illustrates these types of wound healing.

Primary Intention

Healing occurs by primary intention if the wound layers are reapproximated following injury. This apposition of tissue layers allows healing to occur in a minimum of time, with no separation of wound edges and with minimum scar formation. This is the desired mode of healing for surgical incisions.

Secondary Intention

It has been known for centuries that a wound has a higher resistance to infection when left open rather than closed. This was demonstrated experimentally in dogs by Bilroth, who applied dressings soaked in liquid feces and pus to wounds. Wounds left open remained healthy in appearance, whereas those that were subsequently closed became infected. As a result, contaminated or infected surgical wounds often are left unapproximated and allowed to close spontaneously. This type of wound healing is referred to as healing by secondary intention. This healing

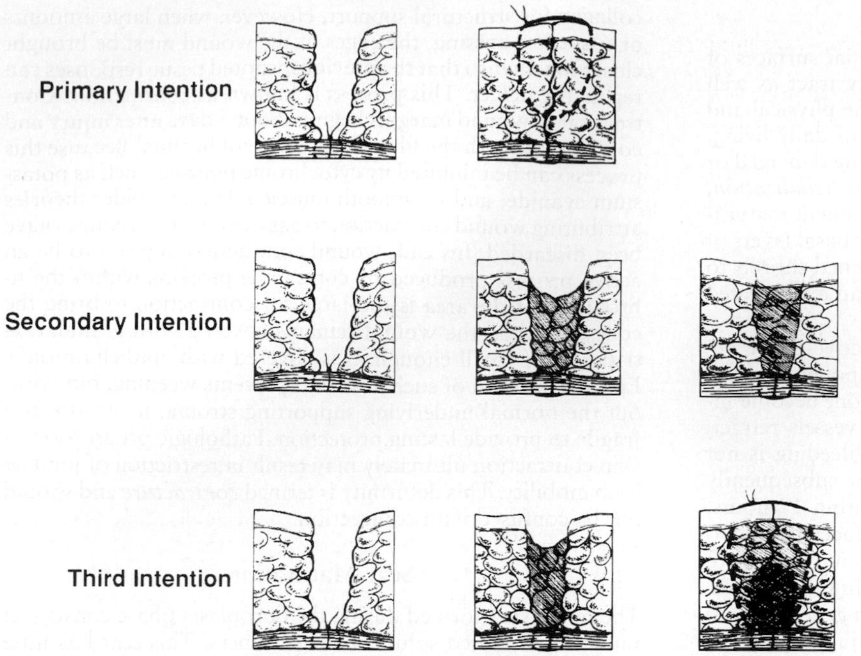

FIGURE 13.1. Types of wound healing.

process obviously is more complicated and prolonged than that of primary intention. The wound eventually heals by a combination of contraction and the formation of granulation tissue with the wound gradually filling in from the raw surfaces. This type of healing is slow and frequently characterized by formation of excessive scar tissue. Granulation tissue from the healing wound also may protrude above the wound margin during this process. This can prevent final epithelialization of the surface and require further treatment for complete healing.

Third Intention

Wound healing by third intention, also known as *delayed primary closure,* refers to the technique of wound closure after a period of delay. This method often is used after postoperative wound breakdown or as an alternative to healing by secondary intention of wounds that should not be closed primarily, such as grossly contaminated or infected wounds. The timing of closure is important. After delays of 7 to 8 days, the wound edges become increasingly difficult to approximate because of the increasing collagen content. Edlich and colleagues have suggested that closure on or after the fourth day appears to be ideal. This concept also is supported by Lowery and Curtis, who showed that wounds closed after a delay of between 3 and 6 days have the lowest infection rates. Furthermore, studies by Fogdestam revealed that wounds closed during this time frame also have greater wound strength at 20 days than wounds closed primarily.

Methods of Wound Closure

Wound dehiscence with evisceration is a serious complication of abdominal surgery. This complication is associated with prolonged morbidity and high mortality. Published mortality figures range from 18% to 35%, with a mean of 20%. Wound dehiscence occurs in 0.5% to 5% of all abdominal surgeries, but is less frequent (0.1% to 0.7%) with gynecologic abdominal procedures. Potential reasons for the decreased rate of dehiscence associated with gynecologic surgery include the use of transverse incisions, healthier patients, lower infection rates, and a lower rate of bowel enterotomies.

Traditionally, gynecologic surgeons have been taught that vertical incisions are associated with a greater likelihood of dehiscence than transverse incisions. Critical review of the earlier data supporting this conclusion reveals that significant confounding variables often were ignored. In general, vertical incisions often were performed emergently on sicker patients or those who had other risk factors for dehiscence, such as cancer. Transverse incisions typically were performed on relatively healthy patients undergoing elective surgery. At least two randomized studies by Greenall and colleagues and Stone and associates have shown no difference in hernia formation or dehiscence between vertical and transverse incisions.

Proper suture selection is critical in preventing wound dehiscence. The wound may break down if the suture has too little initial tensile strength or if the suture is absorbed too quickly before the wound regains enough strength to resist normal stress. The suture also is only as strong as the knots placed in it. If the knot is tied using an improper technique or too few knots are placed, the knot can slip and the suture line fail. The issues involved with proper suture selection and knot security are discussed in detail later in this chapter. Proper surgical technique is one of the most critical factors in preventing wound dehiscence. Several studies have indicated that the most common cause of wound dehiscence is intact sutures pulling through fascia. Animal studies have confirmed that incisions closed with wide loose fascial bites have greater tensile strength than those closed using smaller fascial bites. Sanders and DiClementi also have shown that tightly tied fascial sutures result in fascial necrosis beneath the sutures. Thus, the old adage that one should "approximate and not strangulate fascia" is well taken.

Although the use of loose, wide fascial bites appears to reduce the likelihood of suture pull-through, the optimum distance sutures should be placed from the fascial edge is unknown. However, data obtained by Campbell and colleagues can provide some guidelines. When the pull-out force and pull-out energy of sutures placed in cadaver fascia were plotted against bite size, bites of 0.9 cm yielded the maximum pull-out force, but maximum pull-out energy was obtained with bite sizes of 1.2 to 1.5 cm. Unfortunately, it is unknown whether pull-out energy or pull-out force is more clinically relevant.

Tera and Aberg, working with human cadavers, have shown that the strength of a sutured midline incision is approximately doubled if sutures are placed lateral enough to include the edge of rectus muscle. Normally a bite of approximately 1.5 to 2 cm is required to include rectus muscle in a midline closure. From these studies, it appears that fascia sutures should be placed at least 1.0 cm from the fascia edge and that bites of 1.5 cm or larger are probably preferable.

The use of large tissue bites may be responsible, in part, for the success of mass closure techniques, such as retention sutures, or the Smead-Jones closure, in which wide sutures are passed through fascia, muscle, and peritoneum. The Smead-Jones mass closure consists of a combination "far" mass closure bite at least 2.5 cm from the fascial edge on each side of the incision with a second "near" bite through the fascial edge. This far-far/near-near technique is considered the gold standard for vertical closure because it has been shown consistently to be more secure than simple layered closure.

Unfortunately, the Smead-Jones technique is time consuming and requires a large number of sutures. One solution to this problem has been the use of a continuous running mass closure. In gynecologic surgery, abdominal incisions traditionally have been closed in layers with interrupted sutures. The belief that interrupted sutures provide greater wound security than a continuous suture is not well documented, and there are several well-performed studies using both general surgery and gynecologic oncology patient populations showing continuous closure to be comparable to Smead-Jones closure provided that adequate tissue bites are taken. A recent metaanalysis of available randomized trials suggests that a continuous technique also is associated with decrease in subsequent ventral hernia formation. The continuous technique is not only the most rapid of all the mass closure methods, it also is more rapid than traditional interrupted layer techniques. One theoretical advantage of a continuous suture line is that any stress on the incision is distributed along the entire suture line and not confined to one loop of suture, thereby potentially decreasing the likelihood of suture pullout.

Mass closure techniques classically have used a nonabsorbable permanent suture. The use of nonabsorbable sutures occasionally produces painful palpable knots or results in the formation of suture sinuses. The development of slowly absorbed synthetic sutures has allowed the use of these sutures for running continuous closures, thus avoiding the potential complications of nonabsorbable sutures. Several studies are now available showing excellent results using a continuous absorbable suture line for fascial closure even in high-risk patients. Although the use of continuous polyglycolic acid and polyglactin 910 sutures to close vertical midline incisions has been discouraged by some surgeons, others have obtained good results in patients at low risk for dehiscence. Since these initial studies, other synthetic absorbable sutures (polydioxanone and polyglyconate) that retain their tensile strength much longer than polyglycolic acid and polyglactin 910 have become available. Because of this delayed loss of tension strength compared with other absorbable suture material, polydioxanone and polyglyconate sutures are especially well suited for continuous fascial closure and should be considered the absorbable sutures of choice for mass closure of patients at high risk for dehiscence.

The manner in which the incision is made also may influence the dehiscence rate. Although no good data are available, it has been suggested that the shearing produced when scissors are used to incise the fascia results in increased fascia necrosis and an increased breakdown rate when compared with incisions produced by a scalpel. Likewise, the use of electrosurgery to incise the fascia has been implicated by some data to result in an increase in the dehiscence rate. These factors are magnified if the fascia then is closed improperly. Because such fascia necrosis generally occurs only at the cut edge of the fascia, the use of generous fascia bites during fascial closure probably is more important in preventing fascial dehiscence than the manner of opening the fascia.

SUTURE MATERIAL

It is unknown when humankind first learned to use strings or animal sinews to ligate bleeding vessels or approximate tissue. Any material used for this purpose is commonly referred to as *suture,* whereas the act of reapproximating tissue with suture is known as *suturing*. The first recorded use of suture and suturing dates to the 16th century B.C. in the Edwin Smith papyrus, the oldest record of a surgical procedure. Over the centuries, many different materials have been used as sutures. These materials include metals (gold, silver, and tantalum wire), plant material (linen and cotton), and animal products (horsehair, tendons, intestinal tissue, and silk).

The United States Pharmacopeia (USP) is the official compendium that defines the various classes of suture as well as sets standards for dimensions and minimum tensile strength for each class of suture marketed in the United States. Most sutures today significantly exceed the minimum tensile strength required by the USP (Table 13.1).

TABLE 13.1

U.S. PHARMACOPEIA–REQUIRED KNOT-PULL TENSILE STRENGTH (LB)

	Absorbable sutures		Nonabsorbable sutures		
Size	Natural	Synthetic	Class I	Class II	Class III
4-0	1.7	2.4	1.3	1.0	1.8
3-0	2.7	3.9	2.1	1.5	3.0
2-0	4.4	6.2	3.2	2.3	4.0
1-0	6.1	8.8	4.8	3.2	7.5
1	8.4	11.6	6.0	4.0	10.5

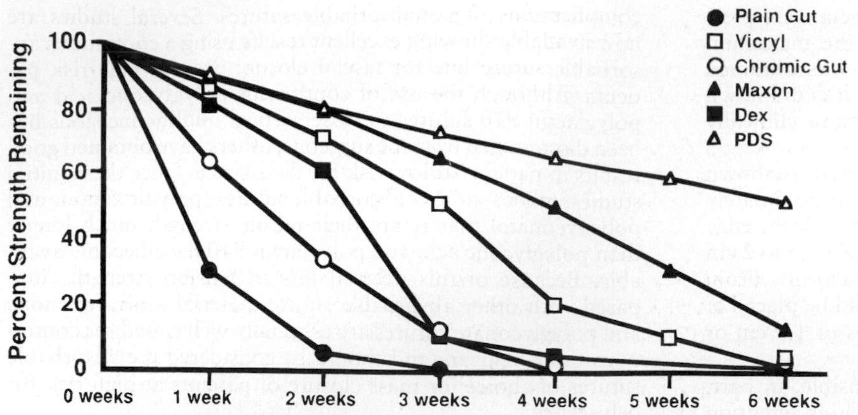

FIGURE 13.2. Percentage of *in vivo* tensile strength of absorbable sutures remaining at various postoperative times.

Sutures are divided into size categories based on diameter as defined by the USP. Sutures progressively larger than 0 are numbered in increasing numerical order; that is, 1, 2, etc. Sizes progressively smaller than 0 are indicated by an increasing number of zeros; that is, 0, 00, 000. The smaller the suture, the more zeros. For simplicity, the smaller numbers often are written numerically as 1–0, 2–0, etc., where the first numeral refers to the number of zeros.

The USP characterizes sutures based on their rate of absorption by bodily tissues. Sutures initially are classed as either absorbable or nonabsorbable. Absorbable sutures lose the majority of their tensile strength before 60 days when implanted in body tissues. Absorbable sutures are further subdivided by the USP into natural and synthetic sutures. Figure 13.2 illustrates the percentages of tensile strength remaining for common absorbable sutures at various postoperative time intervals.

Nonabsorbable sutures are defined as sutures that maintain the majority of their tensile strength for more than 60 days in body tissue. These sutures are further subdivided by the USP into three classes: class I is composed of silk or synthetic fibers; class II is composed of cotton or linen fibers or coated natural or synthetic fibers, with the coating forming a casting of significant thickness but not contributing appreciably to strength (these coatings typically are added to improve handling characteristics or resist degradation); and class III sutures are composed of monofilament or multifilament metal wire.

Natural Absorbable Sutures

Plain and Chromic Catgut

One of the oldest suture materials is plain catgut. Catgut consists of highly purified strands of collagen obtained from the submucosa of animals. Despite its name, catgut normally is obtained from sheep or cattle intestines. The name is believed to have originated from the Arabic term *kitgut,* which referred to the strings of a musical instrument known as a kit. Kitgut was made from sheep intestines and probably served as a readily available source of suture material. Over the years, the term has evolved into *catgut.*

Because plain catgut is a foreign protein, it elicits a marked inflammatory response in tissue. It is rapidly degraded by proteolytic enzymes released by white blood cells. This suture loses more than 70% of its tensile strength in 7 days and is totally digested by 70 days. Plain gut is used in tissue in which strength is needed for very short periods of time. It is ideal for Pomeroy tubal ligations because it dissolves rapidly and thus allows the severed ends to fall apart. Less rapidly absorbed sutures, particularly permanent suture, are associated with higher failure rates, probably because of fistula formation.

Chromic gut is treated with chromic acid salts that bind to the antigen sites in the collagen. The resulting suture elicits less inflammatory response and subsequently is more resistant to degradation. Chromic catgut maintains more than half of its tensile strength at 7 to 10 days, with some measurable strength up to day 21. It is suitable for tissue in which long-term strength is not needed. Examples of such tissue include serosal, visceral, and vaginal tissues. This suture should not be used in skin because the inflammatory response can cause scarring, and the suture often serves as a nidus for infection. Because natural absorbable sutures are degraded by the proteolytic enzymes released by inflammatory cells, these sutures lose strength more rapidly in infected tissue. Because catgut is derived from animal intestines, primarily cow and sheep, there has been increasing concerns over the possibility of theoretical infection with transmissible spongiform encephalopathies (TSE), such as "mad cow." Intestines are currently classified as tissues of medium infectivity with regard to TSE. Furthermore, because all inactivation processes for TSE cause severe changes to catgut, it is not possible to apply these methods to these sutures to eliminate infectious agents. Risk management is only possible by restricting sources to TSE-free herds. Because of these concerns, catgut sutures have been taken off the market in many countries of Europe as well as Japan. Where available, catgut has become progressively more expensive. Because the primary advantage of catgut over many of the synthetics has been cost, many believe use of catgut sutures will soon become obsolete.

Synthetic Absorbable Sutures

Polyglycolic Acid and Polyglactin 910

During the 1970s, two synthetic absorbable sutures (polyglycolic acid and polyglactin 910) became available in the United States. These sutures were designed to be stronger, longer-lasting, and less reactive than catgut. Both sutures are composed of braided filaments of a synthetic polymer. Polyglycolic acid (Dexon: Sherwood/Davis & Geck, St. Louis, MO) is a copolymer of glycolic acid, whereas polyglactin 910 (Vicryl: Ethicon, Somerville, NJ) is a copolymer of lactic and glycolic acid. The two sutures have very similar biologic properties.

Breakdown is by hydrolysis rather than digestion by proteolytic enzymes. The result is minimal inflammatory reaction and a constant absorption rate. There essentially is no loss in tensile strength in the first 7 to 10 days after implantation. Approximately 50% to 60% of tensile strength remains after 14 days, 20% to 30% after 21 days, and almost no tensile strength at 28 days. The initial tensile strength of both these sutures is significantly greater than catgut suture of equal size. In fact, the tensile strength of the synthetic absorbable sutures is almost equal to the tensile strength of a catgut suture one size larger.

One disadvantage of the synthetic absorbable sutures is that they do not handle as well as catgut suture. To counter this difficulty, manufacturers have attempted to enhance the handling qualities of their products by offering versions with various surface coatings or variations with finer and more tightly woven filaments. Although these refinements improve handling characteristics, they increase the tendency of knots to slip. As a result, additional throws may be needed when using these versions of polyglycolic acid or polyglactin 910.

These sutures can be used in most situations in which chromic catgut would be used and have replaced catgut almost entirely for many surgeons. Because they retain tensile strength longer than natural absorbable sutures, they are acceptable for fascial closure in patients at low risk for fascial dehiscence.

Polyglyconate and Polydioxanone

Sutures of polyglycolic acid and polyglactin are by necessity composed of braided filaments because the inherent rigidity of the polymers produces a monofilament suture too stiff for general surgical use. A newer class of polymers allow the production of pliable monofilament sutures. This type of suture is represented by polyglyconate (Maxon) and polydioxanone (PDS). Although subtle differences exist between the two sutures, they are similar enough to consider them together when discussing the biologic properties of this suture class.

The initial tensile strength of these monofilament sutures is comparable to that of the multifilament absorbable sutures. However, this class of suture undergoes absorption at a much slower rate than other absorbable sutures. As a result, tensile strength is maintained for a longer period of time. More than 90% of initial tensile strength is maintained by the end of the first postoperative week, 80% at 2 weeks, 50% at 4 weeks, and 25% at 6 weeks. As with the other synthetic sutures, inflammatory response is minimal. An additional advantage is that these monofilament sutures lack interstices that could serve as a nidus for bacterial infection. As a result, chronic inflammation is rarely seen with this class of monofilament sutures. In comparison, infected absorbable braided sutures have been shown experimentally by Buckall to contain bacteria even after 70 days of implantation.

Because of their delayed absorption profile, both polyglyconate and polydioxanone are excellent choices for fascial closure. Because these sutures are composed of only one fiber, care must be taken to insure that the strand is not inadvertently damaged by instruments, needles, or other sharp-edged material. Such damage may not be easily recognized in the operating room but can seriously weaken a monofilament suture and may result in suture line disruption postoperatively. This precaution is even more critical when a continuous suture line is used.

Poliglecaprone 25 and Polyglactin 910 (Rapide)

With recent advances in polymer chemistry, it is now possible to manufacture the synthetic equivalent of surgical gut. First introduced in 1993, poliglecaprone 25 (Monocryl) has the absorption similar to chromic catgut. Unlike natural collagens, poliglecaprone 25 produces highly uniform and predictable absorption patterns. Like the other synthetic sutures, poliglecaprone 25 is absorbed by hydrolysis and thus does not induce the inflammatory response of catgut. This monofilament suture retains approximately 50% to 60% of its original tensile strength at 7 days postoperatively, 20% to 30% at 14 days, and by 21 days has lost essentially all tensile strength. This particular suture has the advantages of chromic catgut suture, but without many of the disadvantages (i.e., intense inflammatory response and somewhat unpredictable absorption rate). Although it is similar to chromic catgut in tensile strength and actually maintains its tensile strength longer than chromic catgut, it is not recommended by the manufacturer for use for fascial closure or in any tissue in which approximation under stress is required.

Polyglactin 910 Rapide (Vicryl Rapide) is identical in chemical structure to polyglactin 910 but is of lower molecular weight. The result is a braided suture with performance characteristics similar to plain catgut. Absorption is rapid, with 70% of tensile strength lost in the first 7 days. After 10 to 14 days, essentially no strength remains. It is intended for use in the superficial soft tissue where only short-term support is needed. It can be used for skin closure because of its rapid absorption and minimal inflammatory response. The sutures typically begin to fall off at 7 to 10 days. Because sutures remaining in skin longer than 7 days may cause scarring, any suture remaining at this time can be wiped off with sterile gauze or, if necessary, cut. This suture is an excellent choice for first- and second-degree episiotomy and vaginal laceration closure. Because of the intense inflammatory response produced, gut sutures are associated with more significantly postepisiotomy pain than synthetic sutures, whereas long-delayed absorbable synthetic sutures are associated with the presence of unabsorbed suture and knots after the postpartum period. Although this suture does not meet USP strength requirements for synthetic absorbable sutures, its tensile strength exceeds the tensile strength specifications for similar size natural collagen suture.

Nonabsorbable Sutures

By definition, nonabsorbable sutures are suitably resistant to the action of living mammalian tissue. These sutures, however, are not completely resistant to absorption. Over time, these sutures also lose tensile strength and in the case of natural fiber sutures eventually are completely absorbed or digested. Despite beliefs to the contrary, the initial tensile strength of many nonabsorbable sutures is less than comparable-size absorbable suture (Table 13.1). Nonabsorbable sutures, however, have the advantage of maintaining tensile strength for long periods of time. Disadvantages of nonabsorbable sutures include the potential suture-related pain, palpable sutures, and occasionally the formation of suture sinuses.

Natural Nonabsorbable Sutures

Modern nonabsorbable natural fiber sutures are composed of either surgical silk or cotton. Silk suture is one of the best handling sutures. The handling and knot-tying characteristics of silk suture remains the standard against which other sutures are judged. This suture has little "memory"; that is, it does not tend to return to its original form after being bent or twisted. As a result, it handles well, ties easily, and possesses excellent knot security. Silk suture loses more than half of its tensile strength after 1 year of implantation and frequently cannot be found after 2 years. In this respect, it can be viewed as a delayed absorbable suture. Because silk is a foreign animal protein, it initiates the greatest inflammatory response of the nonabsorbable sutures. The multifilament nature and the capillary action of this suture makes it unsuitable in contaminated tissue or in tissues in which the potential for infection is high.

Cotton is the other natural nonabsorbable natural suture material still available today. It is rarely used in modern surgical practice. Cotton is the weakest of the nonabsorbable sutures. Cotton loses 50% of its original tensile strength within 6 months of implantation, but still has 30% to 40% remaining at the end of 2 years. Unlike silk, which loses tensile strength when exposed to moisture, wet cotton is 10% stronger than dry cotton. Because wet cotton also is easier to handle, it is commonly moistened before use.

Synthetic Nonabsorbable Sutures

A wide variety of nonabsorbable synthetic sutures exist. Nylon is a synthetic polyamide polymer derived from coal, air, and water. It is available both as a braided polyfilament suture (Neurolon, Surgelon) and as a monofilament suture (Dermalon, Ethilon). Monofilament nylon has slightly greater tensile strength than braided nylon, but braided nylon handles better and has better knot security than the monofilament nylon suture. Monofilament nylon suture incites less inflammatory reaction and is less prone to infection than the braided nylon sutures. However, because nylon is relatively inert, all types of nylon suture produce minimal tissue reaction. Nylon undergoes slow hydrolysis in tissue over extended periods of time. It loses approximately 15% to 20% of tensile strength each year.

Polyester sutures are produced only in braided forms. Most differences in the properties of these sutures are determined by whether they are coated and by the type of coating. The uncoated forms (Mersilene, Dacron) generally offer the best knot security. As with synthetic absorbable suture, coatings can improve the handling characteristics of the polyester sutures. Knot security of coated polyester sutures is generally poorer than that of uncoated sutures. Coatings currently used include polytetrafluoroethylene, also known as Teflon (Polydek, Ethiflex, and Tevdek) polybutilate (Ethibond), and silicone (Ti-Cron).

Polypropylene (Prolene, Surgilon) is a monofilament suture composed of a linear hydrocarbon polymer. It has the least tissue reactivity of all nonabsorbable sutures. Although polypropylene has a high memory, it also exhibits a small degree of plasticity. If it is tied carefully and the knots set firmly, a flattening occurs where the strands cross. This flattening helps lock the knot and thus provides somewhat greater knot security than is possible with many other monofilament nonabsorbable sutures. As with the absorbable monofilament sutures, the same precautions to prevent damage to the suture must be observed with the monofilament nonabsorbable sutures.

Metal Sutures

Although silver wire was used by Sims for closure of vesicovaginal fistulas, metal sutures are rarely used in gynecologic surgery today. Historically, metal sutures have been used in infected sites or for repair of wound dehiscence and evisceration. Stainless steel once was used routinely by the military for closure of battle wounds of the abdomen. Metal sutures have the highest tensile strength of all suture material. They are also particularly nonreactive. Metal sutures, however, are difficult to handle, require the use of special instruments, and tend to puncture gloves and tissue. With the availability of other nonabsorbable suture materials that also offer high tensile strength and low reactivity but are easier to handle, little reason exists to use these sutures in gynecologic surgery today.

Choice of Suture for Fascial Closure

Tensile strength is critical, although many factors are important in choosing a suture for fascial closure. As noted, the most common cause of dehiscence is sutures pulling through fascia. Because a fascial closure can only be as strong as the weakest component, suture for fascial closure should maintain a tensile strength greater than that of the fascia through the critical healing period. Because the incidence of wound infection is related to the amount of suture material placed in the wound, it would also seem reasonable to use the smallest suture able to provide this necessary tensile strength.

All sutures marketed in the United States must meet minimum tensile strength requirements as defined by the USP. The tensile strength measurement required by USP is knot-pull tensile strength. In measuring knot-pull tensile strength, the suture is tied around a plastic tube using a flat surgeon's knot with one end held in place and the opposite end attached to a tensilometer. Although these data are easily obtained from the various suture manufacturers and are frequently used in suture advertisements, knot-pull tensile strength is not particularly applicable to actual surgical situations. A more useful measurement of strength is obtained using the knotted loop model as suggested by Herman. In this model, a loop is formed by tying a suture around a glass rod using sufficient square knots to prevent slippage. The rod is removed and the loop placed over two right angle rods gripped in the jaws of a tensilometer. The jaws are then separated at a constant rate until breakage occurs. This model stresses the material and the knot more comparably to actual *in vivo* situations and also allows estimation of knot security. Assuming no slippage at the knot, tensile strength calculated using the knotted-loop model is approximately twice the knot-pull tensile strength.

The force required to pull a loop of suture through intact fascia (pull-out force) is frequently cited as 8.3 pounds. This figure is derived from work on the fascia of dogs by Howes and Harvey in 1929 and does not necessarily apply to humans. Fortunately, several studies are now available that have measured the strength of human fascia (Campbell et al., Tera and Aberg, Boerema). Two of these studies, by Campbell and colleagues and Tera and Alberg, were performed using human cadavers. The third study by Boerema measured the pull-out force of fascia at the time of surgery on living patients. All three produced data that indicated the pull-out force for human fascia was approximately 15.2 to 24.2 pounds.

Fascial incisions regain their strength slowly, achieving approximately 10%, 25%, 30%, and 40% of original strength by postoperative week 1, 2, 3, and 4, respectively (Fig. 13.3). The point at which fascia has regained enough strength to resist the stress of daily activities is unknown. Some estimation of this time frame can be obtained from available data on fascial dehiscence. The majority of fascial dehiscence occurs between 2 and 12 days postoperatively, with a mean occurring around day 7 to 8. Dehiscence rarely occurs after postoperative day 12 but has been reported up to day 18. This would suggest that in most patients, fascia has regained enough strength by 2 weeks after surgery to resist reasonable stresses, but that in a limited number of patients, fascia may not regain sufficient strength to prevent dehiscence until 3 weeks postoperatively.

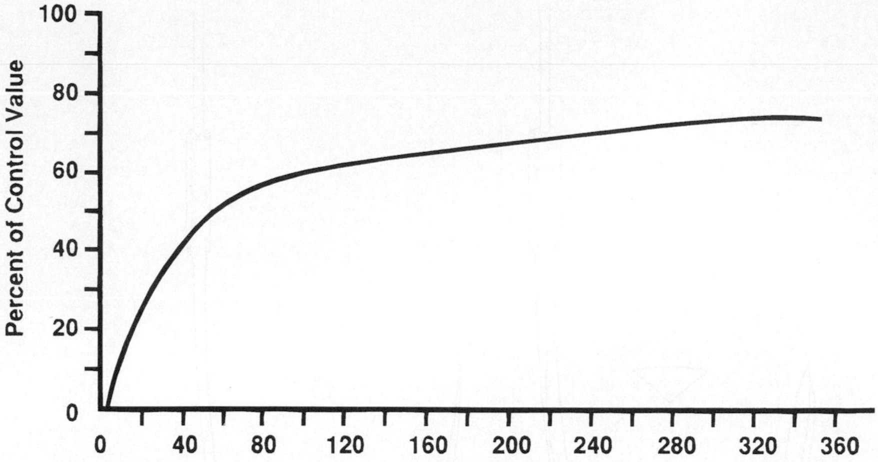

FIGURE 13.3. Fascial tensile strength after surgery. (Adapted from Howes EL, Sooy JW, Harvey SC. The healing of wounds as determined by their tensile strength. *JAMA* 1929; 92:42.)

Using the fascia pull-out data, tensile strength as measured by the knotted-loop model following various lengths of implantation in animals, and dehiscence data, the appropriate size absorbable suture for fascial closure can now be estimated. As can be seen in Figure 13.4, both 1 and 0 polydioxanone and polyglyconate retain tensile strength greater than the fascial pull-out force for 4 to 6 weeks, but polyglycolic acid sutures of the same size maintain adequate tensile strength only for 7 to 14 days. Based on this model, a 1 or 0 polydioxanone or polyglyconate suture appears to be the most appropriate absorbable suture for fascial closure. Unfortunately, although these types of data are theoretically appealing, there are little clinical data to support these conclusions. It must be realized that in most healthy patients, fascial dehiscence does not occur, even when rapidly absorbed sutures are used. Before the development of the synthetic absorbable sutures, 1 and 0 chromic catgut sutures were frequently used for fascial closure. In fact, based on a survey of ob/gyn residency programs, chromic catgut still was being used for fascial closure in 16.1% of vertical fascial incisions and 23.4% of transverse fascial incisions as of 1979. Although fascial dehiscence in healthy patients remained uncommon after fascial closure with chromic catgut, dehiscence rates of up to 11% were reported for other patient populations. Likewise, polyglycolic acid and polyglactin 910 sutures have been used for fascial closure with good success, even in patients at risk for dehiscence.

Surgical Needles

Needles are necessary to carry suture material through tissue. The specific needle required for a procedure is determined by the tissue type, its location and accessibility, and the surgeon's personal preference. All surgical needles have three basic components: the eye, the body, and the point.

The eye of the needle is the point of attachment for suture. Eyes may be classed as closed, French, or swaged. Closed eyes are similar to those on household sewing needles, whereas French eye needles have a slit with ridges inside the slit to catch and hold the suture. Swaged or eyeless needles have the suture mechanically attached to the end of the needle to form a continuous unit. Eyed needles have several disadvantages over swaged needles, including difficulties with threading and the need to pull a double loop of suture through the tissue. Swaged needles are available with either the suture permanently attached or attached in such a manner that it can be removed from the

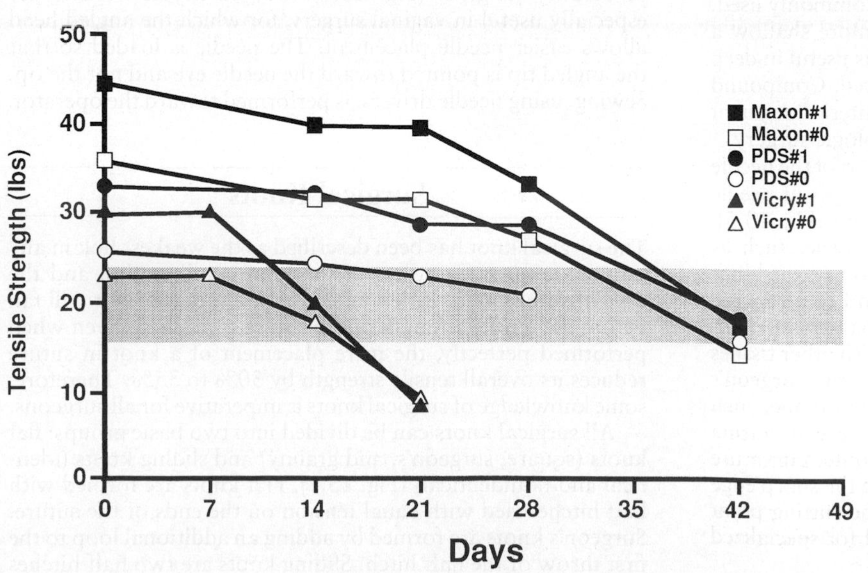

FIGURE 13.4. The tensile strength of various implanted suture materials over time and the point at which tensile strength is less than fascial pull-out strength (14.5 to 24.2 lb).

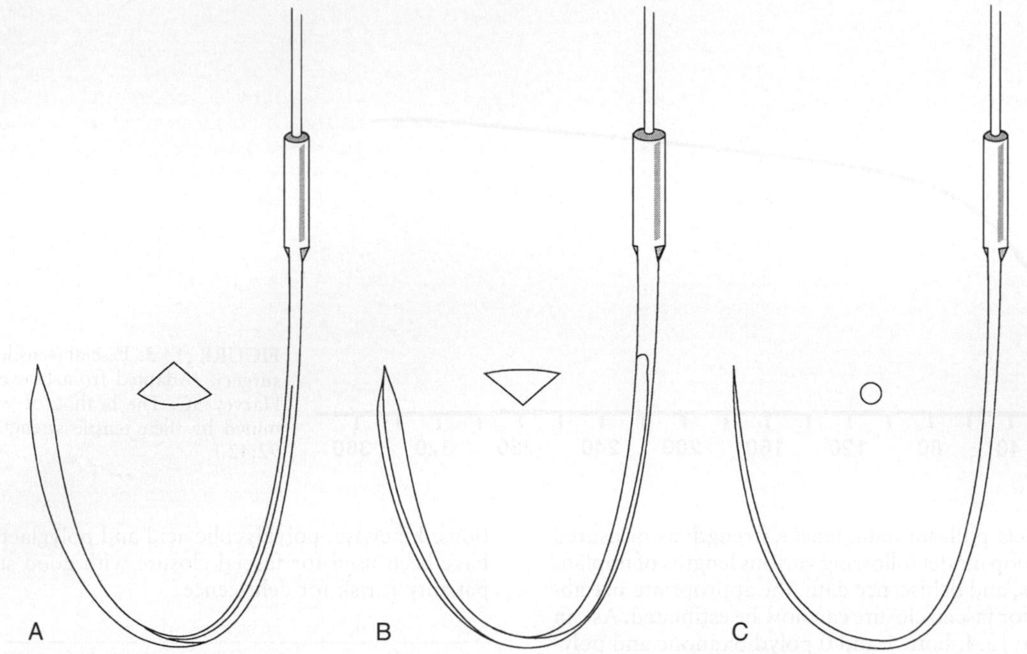

FIGURE 13.5. Common points and body shapes for curved needles.

needle by a slight straight tug on the suture. These controlled-release needles, also known as "pop-off" needles, increase the speed at which interrupted sutures can be placed.

The shape of the body or shaft of a needle determines how easily the needle performs in different applications (Fig. 13.5). The longitudinal shape of the body may be straight, half-curved, curved, or compound. Straight needles are used commonly when tissue is easily accessible. This type of needle is rarely used by gynecologists except for skin closure. Half-curved, or ski, needles may be used to close skin, but have primarily been used in gynecology to facilitate laparoscopic suturing. Curved needles require less space for maneuvering than other needles, thus are ideally suited for most surgical procedures. Curved needles are commonly named based on the percentage of a circle they complete; that is, a $^1/_2$ circle needle is one half of a full circle. Curved needles are available in various curvatures, with the $^3/_8$ circle the most commonly used. The less of an arc the needle completed, the more shallow a bite the needle takes. For example, a $^5/_8$ needle is useful in deep wounds in which a deep, narrow bite is required. Compound curve needles were originally developed for anterior segment ophthalmic surgery and are not used in gynecologic surgery.

The point of the needle begins at the widest part of the needle body and extends to the extreme tip. The two types of needle points are the cutting point and the tapered point (Fig. 13.5). Tapered points are used in easily penetrated tissue, such as bowel or peritoneum. A variation of the taper point is the blunt point, which has a rounded blunt tip at the end of a tapered shaft. This needle tip was designed for use in friable tissue, but has been advocated by some surgeons for use with other tissues because of its reduced likelihood to penetrate the surgeon's gloves or skin. Cutting needles are used in tough tissue, such as skin. The most common cutting needle is the reverse cutting needle. Its sharp edge is on the outside of the outer curvature of the needle. Conventional cutting points have the sharp edge on the inside of the curvature. Variations of the cutting point include spatula and lancet points and are used for specialized applications such as ophthalmology.

Needle Holders

Straight needles can be held and pushed through tissue with the fingers. Straight needles can be used only to sew in a straight line, and only then when the tissue is easily accessible. When straight needles are used, sewing is done in a direction away from the operator.

In the depths of a wound, curved needles are needed. A needle holder is required when curved needles are used. All needle holders have a broad head with a variety of surfaces to prevent the needle from slipping or rotating. Needle holders may be large and heavy, or small and delicate, depending on the size needle to be used. Many needle holders have ring finger grips and locking mechanisms. Two common types of basic needle holders used in gynecology are Wagensteen (straight) or Heaney (angled) (Fig. 13.6). Curved needle holders are especially useful in vaginal surgery, for which the angled head allows easier needle placement. The needle is loaded so that the angled tip is pointed toward the needle eye and not the tip. Sewing, using needle drivers, is performed toward the operator.

Surgical Knots

The surgical knot has been described as the weakest link in any knotted suture, regardless of the knot configuration and the type of suture used. If tied improperly, a surgical knot will fail before the tensile strength of the suture is reached. Even when performed perfectly, the mere placement of a knot in suture reduces its overall tensile strength by 30% to 35%. Therefore, some knowledge of surgical knots is imperative for all surgeons.

All surgical knots can be divided into two basic groups: flat knots (square, surgeon's, and granny) and sliding knots (identical and nonidentical) (Fig. 13.7). Flat knots are formed with half hitches tied with equal tension on the ends of the suture. Surgeon's knots are formed by adding an additional loop to the first throw of the half hitch. Sliding knots are two half hitches

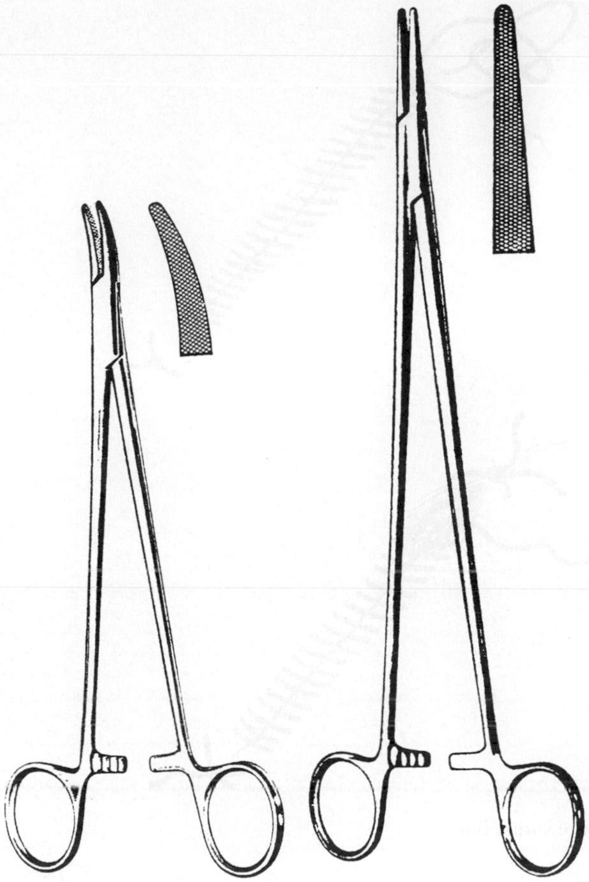

FIGURE 13.6. Needle holders. (Courtesy of Zinnati Surgical Instruments, Inc., Chatsworth, CA.)

either nonidentical (square knot) or identical (granny knot), tied with greater tension on one segment than the other.

The term *sliding knot* suggests the tendency of the knot to slip compared with the flat, but this is not completely true. Simple sliding knots of two or three throws do slip often and should not be used as surgical knots. Brouwers and colleagues have shown, however, that flat knots with only two throws also tend to slip rather than break.

The flat square knot is the most secure of all the surgical knots and theoretically the most desirable knot for tying suture.

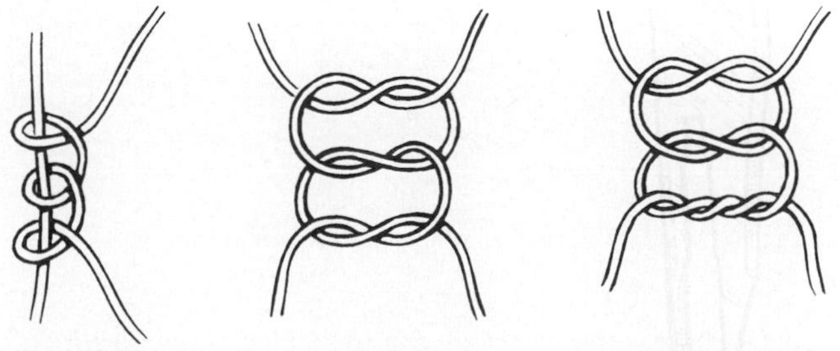

FIGURE 13.7. Flat and sliding knots.

However, according to a study by Trimbos, sliding knots are used more commonly by gynecologists than are square knots. It has been shown also that many surgeons actually tie sliding knots despite being convinced they tie flat knots. Sliding knots frequently are used in actual surgical practice for two reasons. The crossing of the surgeon's hands needed to tie square knots unavoidably releases tension on the knot, and this can lead to knot slippage. The tying of deep ligatures is most easily performed by keeping constant tension on one suture. Thus, sliding knots may be preferable to square knots in certain situations. Whichever knot is used, the operator should be aware of the knot being used and the number of throws needed to obtain maximum knot capacity.

The number of throws required for knot security is frequently debated. Too few throws and the knot is weaker than the suture; additional throws above that needed to equal the sutures tensile strength adds unneeded suture to the wound and may increase the infection rate. When flat square knots are used, Brown has shown that maximum knot-holding capacity was achieved with four throws in all noncoated suture tested. In fact, three throws were sufficient to achieve maximum knot-holding capacity except for sutures composed of nylon (both monofilament and braided). The addition of coating to improve handling characteristics also decreases knot security. In a 1983 study, Rodeheaver and colleagues showed that coated suture required two additional flat throws to equal the maximum knot-holding capacity of uncoated suture. In a similar study by Van Rijssel and colleagues, the knot-holding capacity of a sliding knot with one extra throw equaled that of square knots in smaller gauge (3-0) suture. In larger sutures (0), square knots remained stronger than sliding knots with an extra throw, but sliding knots with more than five throws were not tested. From these studies, it appears that a surgical knot of four to six throws is adequate for most sutures. The exact number of throws required, of course, depends on the type of suture and whether a flat or sliding knot is formed.

It is common practice for some surgeons to leave suture tails long to prevent knot disruption should the knot slip. As might be expected, the usefulness of this practice is dependent on the type of suture involved. It has been shown that any knot slippage in nylon, polydioxanone, and polypropylene sutures results in total knot disruption. In other sutures (polyglyconate and polyglactin), initial knot slippage is followed by knot recomposition. The reconstituted knot remains intact until greater force is applied. A long suture tail is only helpful in preventing knot disruption in this latter class of suture.

Knot security is of utmost importance when using a continuous suture line. It is common practice for many surgeons to form the terminal knot in a continuous suture line by tying the ending single strand to the last loop of suture. This "loop-to-strand" knot is a potentially weak configuration. Unless multiple square knots are used, the single strand may slip from the knot when placed under tension. As a result, the entire suture line disrupts. At reoperation, the strand may appear broken but, in fact, one of the three terminal knot ends has slipped through what appears to be an intact knot (Fig. 13.8). A safer method for tying continuous suture is to run two sutures to the midpoint of the incision and tie the two single strands to each other, thus avoiding the "loop-to-strand" knot.

SURGICAL INSTRUMENTATION

A multitude of surgical instruments are designed to perform one unique function or slightly improve on the performance

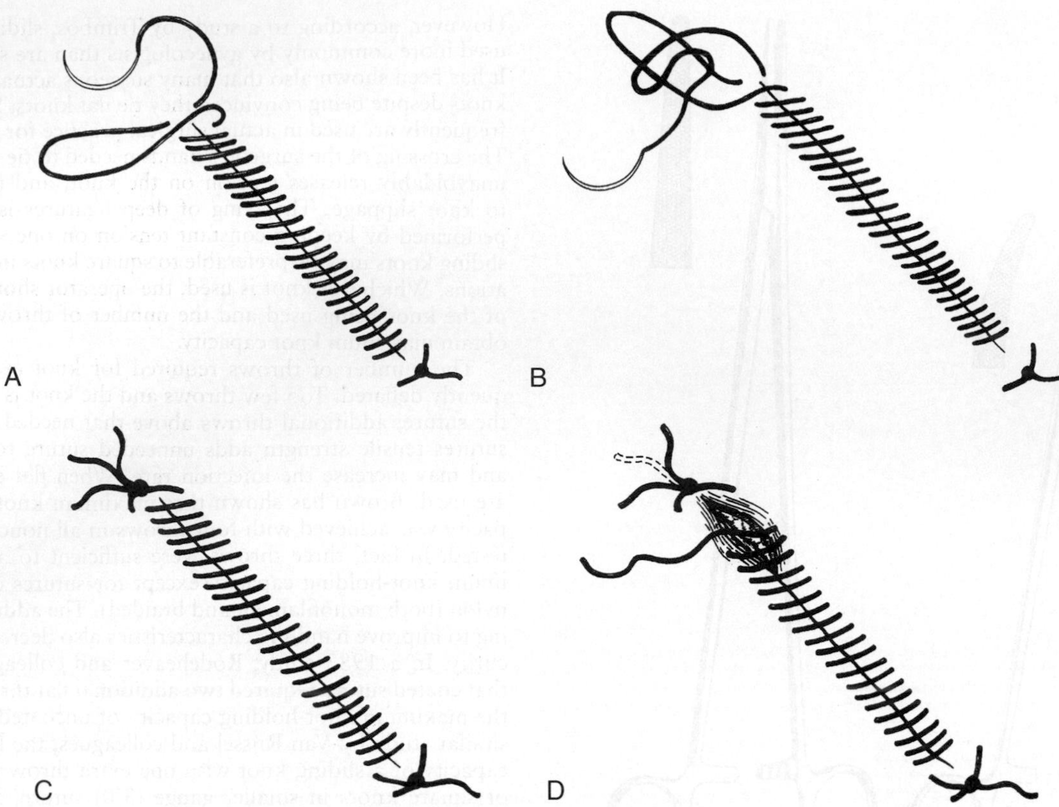

FIGURE 13.8. Development of suture line.

of another instrument. This section is not intended to be a comprehensive list of all instruments available, but a review of the basic surgical instrumentation needed for most common gynecologic procedures.

Scalpel

The scalpel is the first instrument used in most surgeries and remains the best instrument for dividing tissue with minimal trauma to surrounding tissue. Scalpel blades come in various sizes and shapes to allow performance of different tasks (Fig. 13.9). The basic scalpel blade has a straight ribbed back and an oval cutting surface. This basic blade is commonly available in sizes 10, 15, 20, and 22. The 10 scalpel blade is the most versatile and the most commonly used size. The smaller blades are used for fine dissection and when precise turns are required in making the incision—that is, plastic surgery—although the larger blades are used to rapidly perform an incision. Blades such as the 11 and 12 are designed for specific purposes. The 11 blade is bayonet-shaped and used to perform stab incisions for drains and in draining abscesses. The 12 blade is hook-shaped

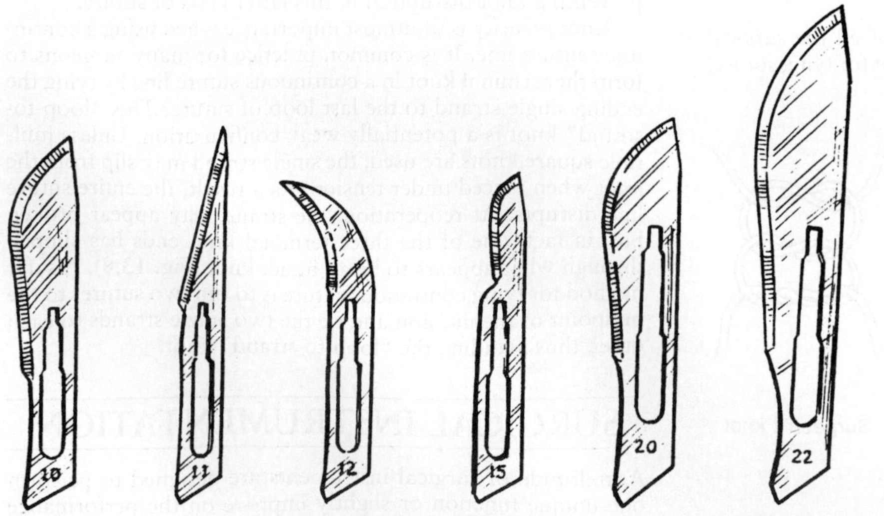

FIGURE 13.9. Surgical scalpel blades.

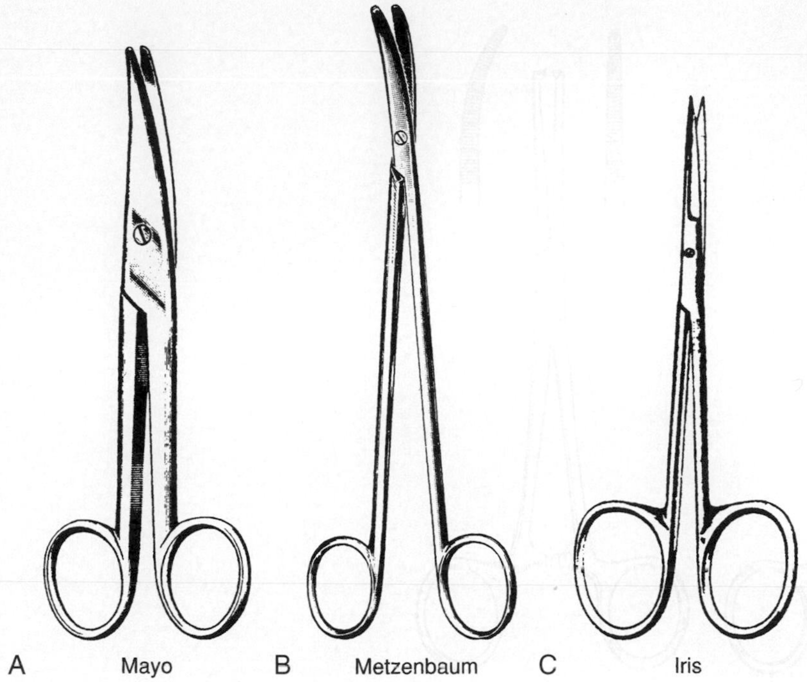

FIGURE 13.10. Surgical scissors. (Courtesy of Zinnati Surgical Instruments, Inc., Chatsworth, CA.)

and was originally used for myringotomies. It is infrequently used by gynecologists.

Scissors

The scissors are the second most commonly used instrument to divide tissue. In addition to cutting, scissors also can be used for blunt dissection by opening the scissors after the tips have been inserted into a tissue plane. The basic scissors designs used in gynecology surgery are the Mayo, Metzenbaum, and Iris scissors. All come in both straight and curved versions (Fig. 13.10). Curved scissors allow horizontal cutting deep in a wound and thus improve visibility. Curved scissors also are used to cut tissue in a smooth curve, such as for incising the vaginal cuff in an abdominal hysterectomy.

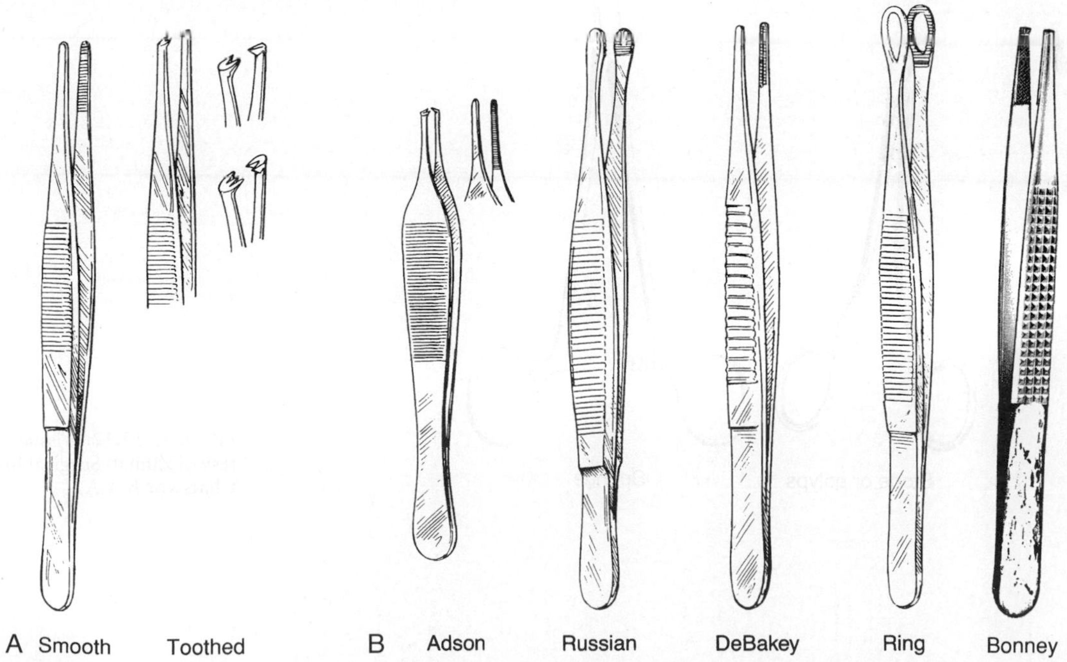

FIGURE 13.11. Tissue (thumb) forceps. (Courtesy of Zinnati Surgical Instruments, Inc., Chatsworth, CA.)

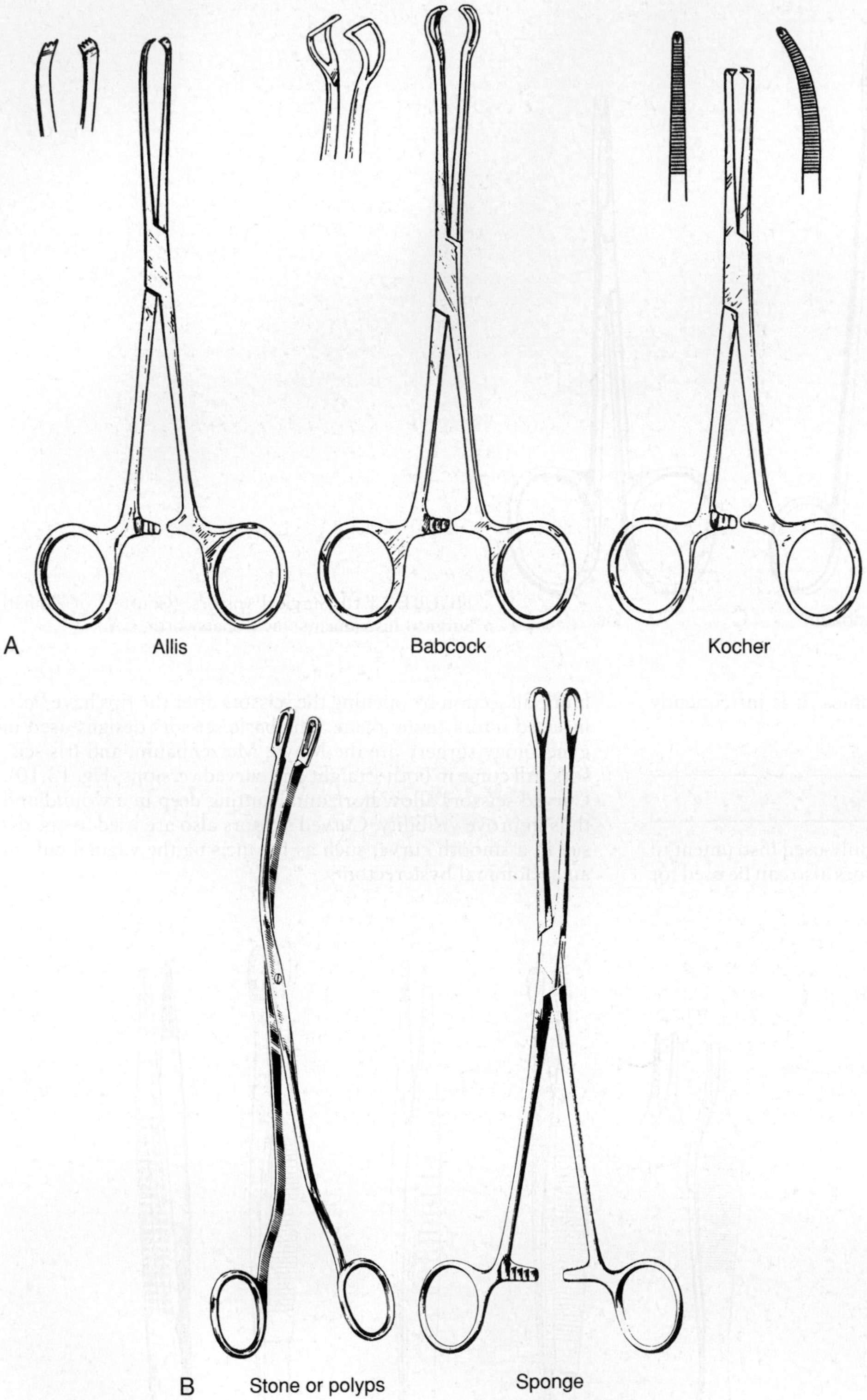

FIGURE 13.12. Tissue clamps. (Courtesy of Zinnati Surgical Instruments, Inc., Chatsworth, CA.)

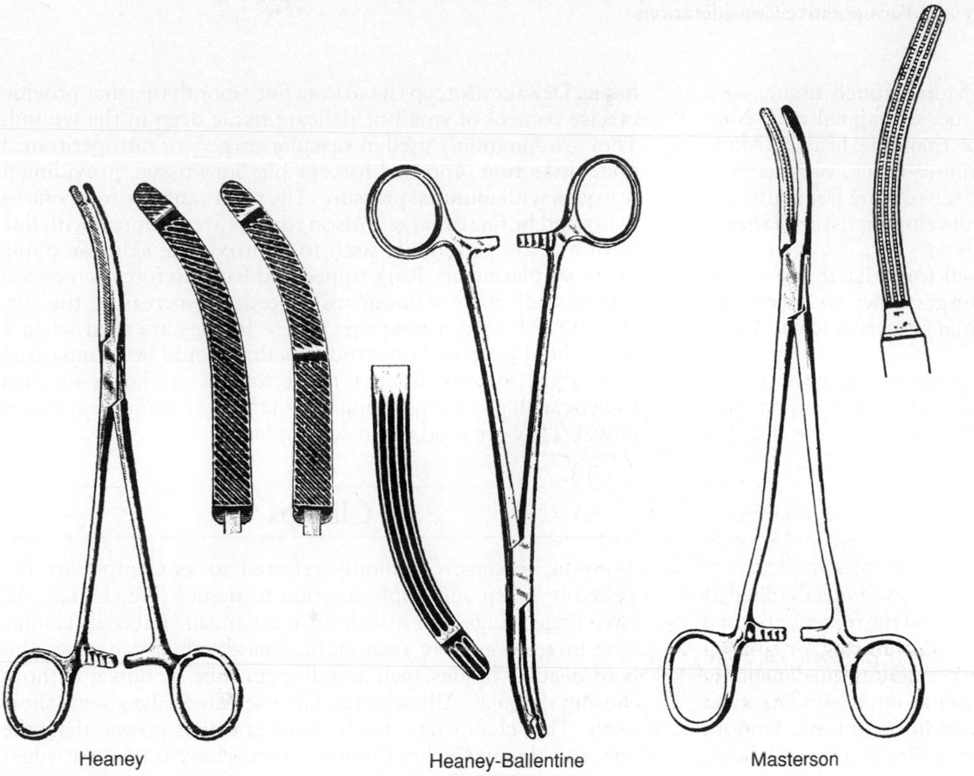

FIGURE 13.13. Hysterectomy clamps. (Courtesy of Zinnati Surgical Instruments, Inc., Chatsworth, CA.)

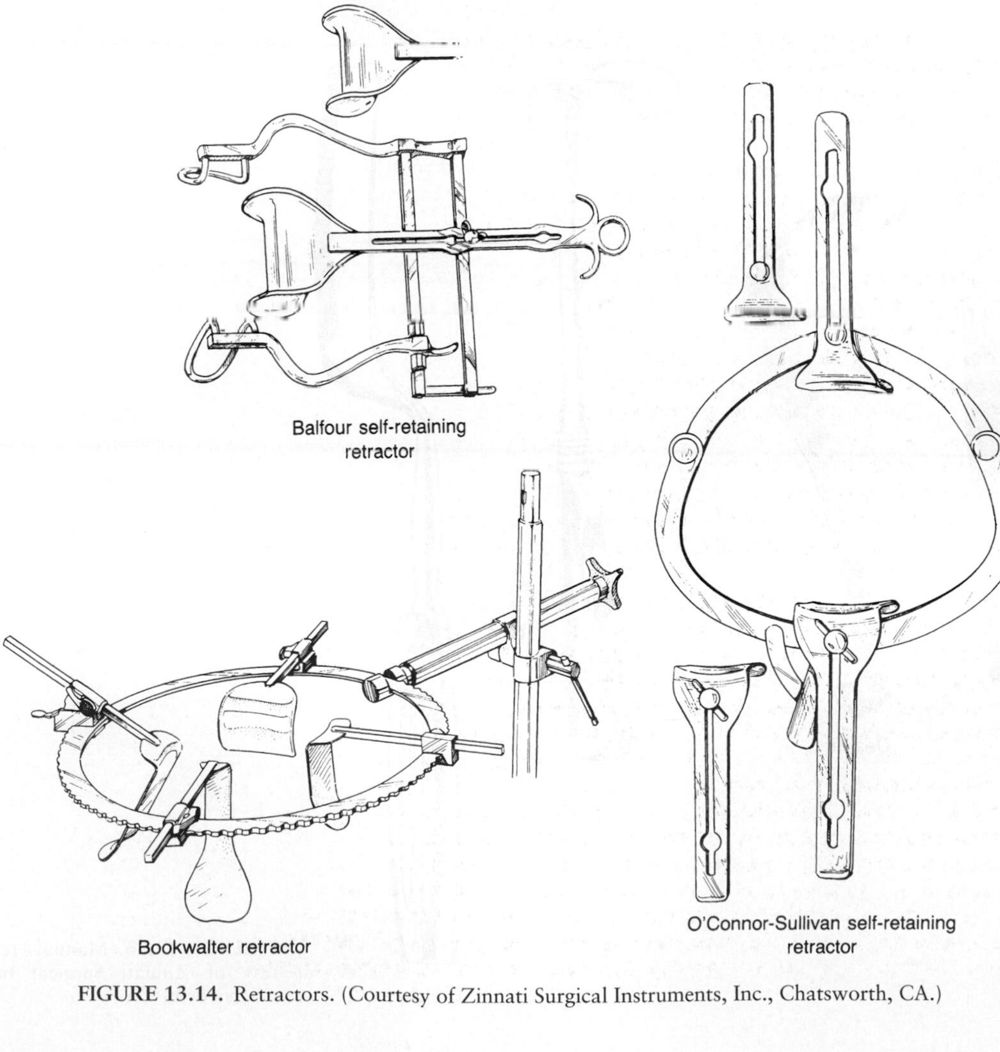

FIGURE 13.14. Retractors. (Courtesy of Zinnati Surgical Instruments, Inc., Chatsworth, CA.)

Mayo scissors are used when dividing tough tissue, such as the rectus fascia, parametrial tissue, or vaginal cuff. Metzenbaum scissors are more delicate than the heavier Mayo scissors and are used for cutting thinner tissue, such as peritoneum and adhesions. Metzenbaum scissors are frequently use for retroperitoneal dissection or for developing tissue planes in adhered or distorted tissue.

Iris scissors are small scissors used for delicate dissection. Originally designed for ophthalmic surgery, they are used in gynecology for precise vulvar and vaginal surgery, such as fistula repair or colporrhaphy.

Suture scissors are used only to cut suture and never tissue. Suture scissors are general-purpose scissors with blunt ends to avoid the possibility that the tips will injure structures distal to the suture.

Tissue Forceps

Tissue or thumb forceps consist of two strips of metal joined at one end (Fig. 13.11). The opposable ends of the forceps are used to grasp and hold tissue during dissection, suturing, or cutting. These ends are of varying shapes and configuration, depending on the purpose for which the forceps are intended. The most common alteration to the ends is the addition of teeth. Smooth forceps without teeth are used when handling friable or delicate tissue. DeBakey forceps have long fine smooth tips that provide precise control of small or delicate tissue deep in the wound. They are commonly used in vascular surgery or retroperitoneal node dissection. Toothed forceps bite into tissue, providing a firm grip with minimal pressure. The teeth can vary from one to many and be fine or large. Adson forceps are equipped with fine teeth and are commonly used to approximate skin for staple or suture placement. Ring-tipped and Russian forceps increase the grasping force without using teeth by increasing the surface area of the grasping tips. These forceps are used when a secure hold is needed on structures that would be traumatized by toothed forceps. Bonney tissue forceps are heavy-toothed forceps with serrations along the shaft for maximum gripping power. They are used when sewing fascia.

Clamps

Grasping forceps, commonly referred to as clamps, are designed to grasp and apply traction to tissues (Fig. 13.12). All have finger rings and a locking mechanism. Babcock clamps have no teeth and are atraumatic. These clamps can grasp and hold delicate tissues such as fallopian tube or bowel without causing damage. Allis clamps have serrated edges with short teeth. This clamp has much more grasping power than the Babcock clamp. Kocher/Oschner clamps have transverse ridges

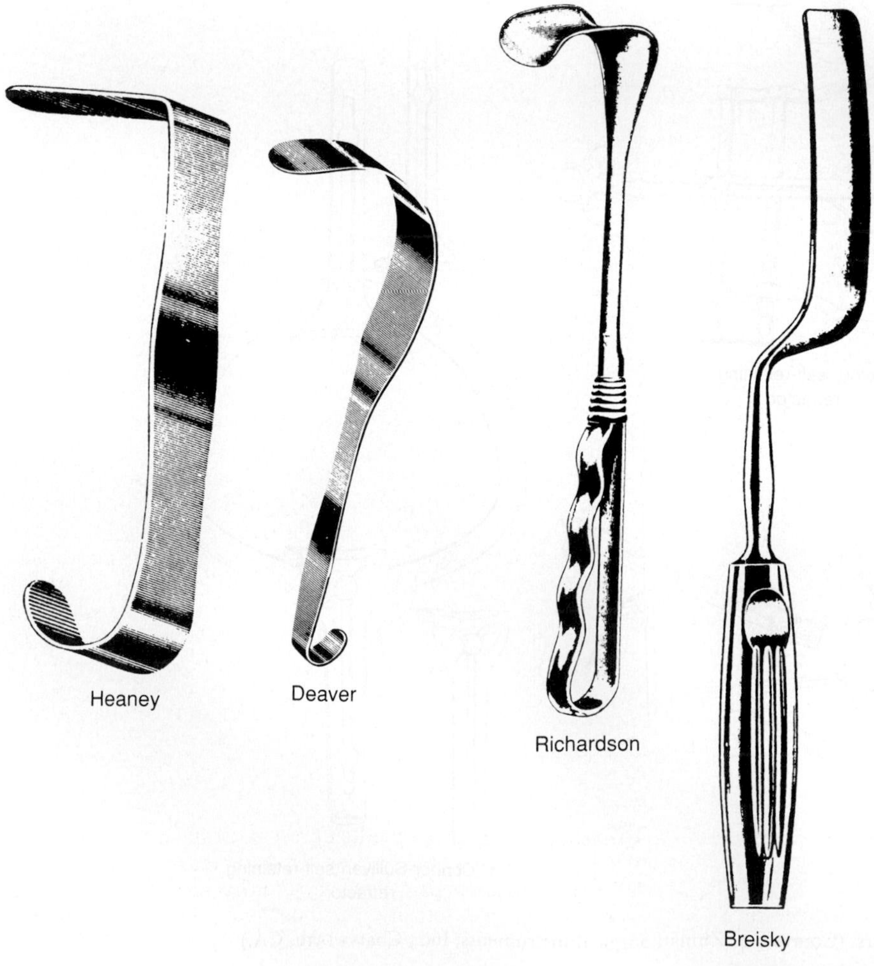

FIGURE 13.15. Manual retractors. (Courtesy of Zinnati Surgical Instruments, Inc., Chatsworth, CA.)

along the shaft and interlocking teeth at the tip. Because of their design, tissue within the clamp is unlikely to slip. These clamps are frequently used to grasp heavy tissue such as fascia and occasionally as hysterectomy clamps. Ring forceps can be used like ring-tipped tissue forceps, but more commonly are used to hold folded sponges. In this fashion, they can be used to retract tissue, sponge fluid or blood, or apply solutions to the skin in preparation for surgery. Renal stone forceps were designed to remove stones from the renal pelvis but are commonly used by the gynecologic surgeon to explore the uterine cavity for polyps or retained tissue. When used in this capacity, they are inserted, opened, rotated 180 degrees, closed, and withdrawn.

Heaney, Heaney-Ballentine, and Masterson clamps are the commonly used clamps for clamping the parametrial and paracervical tissue during hysterectomy (Fig. 13.13). Hysterectomy clamps are heavy crushing clamps with ridged shafts. The classic clamps (Heaney, Heaney-Ballentine) also have toothed tips. The more recent Masterson clamp lacks a toothed tip and was designed to generate the least amount of crushing force.

Retractors

Retractors are used to hold tissue out of the operative field to improve exposure during surgical procedures (Fig. 13.14). Retractors are either held by an assistant (manual retractors) or use counterpressure from other tissue (self-retaining retractors) to hold themselves in place.

Self-retaining retractors frequently are used to hold the sides of the incision apart during gynecologic surgery. Gynecologists seem to favor the O'Conner-O'Sullivan retractor when performing pelvic surgery. General surgeons, on the other hand, prefer the Balfour retractor. The O'Conner-O'Sullivan is a circular retractor with four blades, two permanently attached lateral retractors to retract the sidewalls, and a removable upper and lower blade to retract the bowel and bladder, respectively. This retractor is available with large or small lateral blades, whereas the removable blades come in several sizes. The Balfour retractor also has two lateral blades but only one additional retractor blade. This blade normally is employed as an upper blade with a manual retractor used for bladder retraction if needed. However, if the bowel is carefully packed away with laparotomy packs, the third blade can be used as a bladder retractor. All blades of the Balfour retractor are removable and available in different sizes.

The Bookwalter retractor is the most versatile of retractors, providing excellent exposure to the operative field. It consists of a circular metal ring to which a wide variety of retractors can be attached at any point. Its best use is during radical pelvic surgery or when operating on massively obese patients. In extremely obese patients, it may necessary to attach the Bookwalter retractor to the operating table.

Manual retractors allow maximum flexibility in providing exposure (Fig. 13.15). They can be used alone or as a supplement to self-retaining retractors. Common manual retractors include the Heaney, Deaver, and Richardson retractors. Specialized retractors include the Briesky-Navratil (used during sacrospinous vault suspension), Army-Navy, and Parker retractors (used for skin and subcutaneous tissue).

Dilators

Dilators are metal or plastic cylinders used to dilate the cervical os to sufficient size to admit other surgical instruments (Fig. 13.16). Dilators may have tapered (Hank and Pratt) or rounded (Hegar) tips. Dilators with tapered tips require less force to perform dilatation than dilators with rounded tips. The sizes are measured either by diameter or by circumference. The unit of measurement for diameter is millimeters, whereas the unit of measurement for circumference is in French calibration. The relationship of the two measurements can be calculated by the formula for the circumference of a circle where the diameter times pi (3.14) equals the circumference. For comparison purposes, approximately 3 French equals 1 mm of diameter.

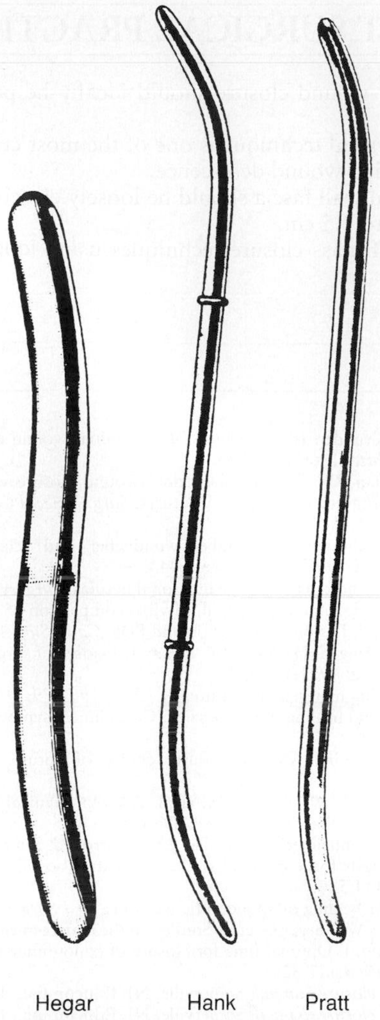

FIGURE 13.16. Common cervical dilators. (Courtesy of Zinnati Surgical Instruments, Inc., Chatsworth, CA.)

CONCLUSION

This chapter has attempted to present an introduction to the mechanisms of wound healing, wound closure, suture material, and instrumentation. It is hoped that this chapter will be a useful resource not only for those embarking on a surgical career but also for experienced surgeons as well.

BEST SURGICAL PRACTICES

- Secondary wound closure should ideally be performed on day 4.
- Proper surgical technique is one of the most critical factors in preventing wound dehiscence.
- Abdominal wall fascia should be loosely closed with suture bites of 1 to 1.5 cm.
- The use of mass closure techniques using long-delayed or permanent suture to close fascia is recommended to reduce fascial dehiscence.
- The use of catgut sutures has been limited in many countries because of increasing concerns over the possibility of theoretical infection with transmissible spongiform encephalopathies (TSE), such as "mad cow" disease.
- Suture knots produced by tying a loop of suture to a single strand are less secure than those tied using a strand to strand. This is particularly critical when using monofilament suture.

Bibliography

Alexander HC, Prudden JF. The causes of abdominal wound disruption. *Surg Gynecol Obstet* 1966;124:1223.

Archie JP, Feltman RW. Primary abdominal wound closure with permanent, continuous running monofilament sutures. *Surg Gynecol Obstet* 1981;153: 721.

Bilroth T. Beobachtungs-studien über wundfieber und accidentelle wund-krankheiten. *Arch Klin Chir* 1866;6:443.

Boerema I. Cause and repair of large incisional hernias. *Surgery* 1971;69:111.

Bourne RB, Bitar H, Andreae PR, et al. In-vitro comparison of four absorbable sutures: Vicryl, Dexon Plus, Maxon and PDS. *Can J Surg* 1988;31:43.

Brouwers JE, Oosting H, Haas D, et al. Dynamic loading of surgical knots. *Surg Gynecol Obstet* 1991;173:443.

Brown RP. Knotting material and suture. *Br J Surg* 1992;79:399.

Bryant WM. Wound healing. In: Bekiesz ed. Ciba clinical symposia. *Ciba-Geigy* 1977;29:2.

Buckall TE. Abdominal wound closure: choice of suture. *J R Soc Med* 1981;74:580.

Campbell JA, Temple WJ, Frank CR, et al. A biomechanical study of suture pullout in linea alba. *Surgery* 1989;106:888.

Corman ML, Veidenheimer MC, Coller JA. Controlled clinical trial of three suture materials for abdominal wall closure after bowel operations. *Am J Surg* 1981;141:510.

Douglas DM. The healing of aponeurotic incisions. *Br J Surg* 1952;40:79.

Edlich RF, Rogers W, Kasper G, et al. Studies on the management of the contaminated wound. I. Optimal time for closure of contaminated open wounds. *Am J Surg* 1969;117:323.

Ethicon. *Wound closure manual.* Somerville, NJ: Ethicon Inc., 1985.

Ethicon. *Wound closure manual.* Somerville, NJ: Ethicon Inc., 1994.

Fagniez PL, Hay JM, Lacaine F, et al. Abdominal midline incision closure. *Arch Surg* 1985;120:1351.

Fogdestam I. A biomechanical study of healing rat skin incisions after delayed primary closure. *Surg Obstet Gynecol* 1981;153:191.

Gallup DG, Talledo EO, King LA. Primary mass closure of midline incisions with a continuous running monofilament suture in gynecologic patients. *Obstet Gynecol* 1989;73:675.

Greenall MJ, Evans, Pollack AV, et al. Midline or transverse laparotomy? A random controlled clinical trial. *Br J Surg* 1980;67:180.

Greenburg AG, Salk RS, Peskin GW. Wound dehiscence: pathology and prevention. *Arch Surg* 1979;114:143.

Hartko WJ, Ghanekar G, Kemmann E. Suture materials currently used in obstetric-gynecologic surgery in the United States: a questionnaire survey. *Obstet Gynecol* 1982;59:241.

Herman JB. Tensile strength and knot security of surgical suture materials. *Am Surg* 1971;37:209.

Higgins GA, Antkowiak JG, Esterkyn SH. A clinical and laboratory study of abdominal wound closure and dehiscence. *Arch Surg* 1969;98:421.

Hodgson NC, Malthaner RA, Ostbye T. The search for an ideal method of abdominal fascial closure: a metaanalysis. *Ann Surg* 2000;231:436.

Hoffman MS, Villa A, Roberts WS, et al. Mass closure of the abdominal wound with delayed absorbable suture in surgery for gynecologic cancer. *J Reprod Med* 1991;36:356.

Howes EL, Harvey SC. The strength of the healing wound in relation to the holding strength of the chromic catgut suture. *N Engl J Med* 1929;200:1285.

Hunter J. *Treatise on blood, inflammation and gunshot wounds.* London: Nichol, 1794:216.

Katz AR, Mukherjee DB, Kagnanov AL, et al. A new synthetic monofilament absorbable suture made from polytrimethylene carbonate. *Surg Gynecol Obstet* 1983;161:213.

Kim YB, DuBeshter, Nilaoff JM. Continuous single-layer closure of midline abdominal incisions in high-risk gynecologic patients. *J Gynecol Surg* 1992;8:15.

Knight CD, Griffen FD. Abdominal wound closure with continuous monofilament polypropylene suture. Experience with 1000 cases. *Arch Surg* 1983; 118:1305.

Lichtenstein IL, Herzoikoff S, Shore JM, et al. The dynamics of wound healing. *Surg Gynecol Obstet* 1970;130:685.

Lowery KF, Curtis GM. Delayed suture in the management of wounds: analysis of 721 traumatic wounds illustrating the influence of time interval in wound repair. *Am J Surg* 1950;80:280.

Orr JW, Orr P, Barrett JM, et al. Continuous or interrupted fascial closure: a prospective evaluation of No. 1 Maxon in 402 gynecologic procedures. *Am J Obstet Gynecol* 1990;163:1485.

Paterson-Brown S, Dudley HAF. Knotting in continuous mass closure of the abdomen. *Br J Surg* 1986;73:679.

Peacock EE. Wound healing. In: Schwartz SI, Shires GT, Spenser FC, et al., eds. *Principles of surgery*. 3rd ed. New York: McGraw-Hill, 303.

Ray JA, Doddi N, Regula D, et al. Polydioxanone (PDS), a novel monofilament synthetic absorbable suture. *Surg Gynecol Obstet* 1981;151:497.

Reul GJ. The role of sutures in the complications in vascular surgery and their relationship to pseudoaneurysm formation. In: Bernham VM, Town JB, eds. *Complications in vascular surgery*. New York: Grune & Stratton; 1981:615.

Rodeheaver GT, Tacker JG, Edlich RF. Mechanical performance of polyglycolic acid and polyglactin-910 synthetic absorbable suture. *Surg Gynecol Obstet* 1981;153:835.

Rodeheaver GT, Tacker JG, Edlich RF, et al. Knotting and handling characteristics of coated synthetic sutures. *J Surg Res* 1983;35:525.

Sanders RJ, DiClementi D. Principles of abdominal wound closure: II. Prevention of dehiscence. *Arch Surg* 1977;112:1188.

Sanders RJ, DiClementi D, Ireland K. Principles of abdominal wound closure: I. Animal studies. *Arch Surg* 1977;112:1184.

Sanz LE. Sutures: a primer on structure and function. *Contemp Obstet Gynecol* 1990;33:99.

Sanz LE. Wound management: technique and suture material. In: Sanz LE, ed. *Gynecologic surgery*. Oradell, NJ: Medical Economics; 1988:21.

Sanz LE, Patterson JA, Kamath R, et al. Comparison of Maxon suture with Vicryl, chromic catgut, and PDS sutures in fascial closure in rats. *Obstet Gynecol* 1988;71:418.

Sloop RD. Running synthetic absorbable suture in abdominal closure. *Am J Surg* 1981;141:572.

Stone HH, Hoefling SJ, Strom PR, et al. Abdominal incisions: transverse vs vertical placement and continuous vs interrupted closure. *South Med J* 1983;76:1106.

Stone IK, Fraunhofer, Masterson BJ. The biomechanical effects of tight suture closure upon fascia. *Surg Obstet Gynecol* 1986;163:448.

Tera H, Aberg C. Tissue strength of structures involved in musculo-aponeurotic layer sutures in laparotomy incisions. *Acta Chir Scand* 1976;142:349.

Trimbos JB. Security of various knots commonly used in surgical practice. *Obstet Gynecol* 1984;64:274.

Trimbos JB, Van Rijssel EJC, Klopper PJ. Performance of sliding knots in monofilament and multifilament suture material. *Obstet Gynecol* 1986;68:425.

The United States Pharmacopeia, 23th rev. Taunton, MA: Rand McNally; 1994.

Van Rijssel EJC, Trimbos JB, Booster MH. Mechanical performance of square knots and sliding knots in surgery: a comparative study. *Am J Obstet Gynecol* 1990;162:93.

Wasiljew BK, Winchester DP. Experience with continuous absorbable suture in the closure of abdominal incisions. *Surg Obstet Gynecol* 1982;154:375.

Wilhelm DL. Inflammation and healing. In: Anderson WA, Kissane JM, eds. *Pathology*. 7th ed. St Louis: CV Mosby, 25.

SECTION III ■ PRINCIPLES OF GYNECOLOGIC SURGICAL TECHNIQUES AND MANAGEMENT OF ENDOSCOPY

CHAPTER 14 ■ INCISIONS FOR GYNECOLOGIC SURGERY

JAMES J. BURKE II AND DONALD G. GALLUP

DEFINITIONS

Arcuate line—The demarcation above which the posterior lamella of the internal oblique aponeurosis fuses with the aponeurosis of the transversalis muscle and passes posterior to the rectus muscles. Below this line, the aponeurosis of the internal oblique passes anterior to the rectus muscles.

Cherney incision—A transverse abdominal incision in which the rectus muscles are transected at their insertion on the pubic symphysis. The fascia may or may not be dissected free from the rectus muscles. Entry into the peritoneum may be vertical or transverse.

Dehiscence—Disruption of a surgical wound, either superficial or deep. Superficial dehiscence is separation of the skin and subcutaneous tissue because of seroma, hematoma, or abscess formation. Fascial dehiscence describes the separation of the fascia without extrusion of the bowel.

Evisceration—Disruption of the fascia with extrusion of the bowel through the wound.

Gridiron incision—A muscle splitting, oblique incision, useful for a transperitoneal or extraperitoneal approach to pelvic organs, similar to a McBurney's incision.

Hernia—A late complication of wound disruption. A fascial disruption occurs with protrusion of the peritoneum, bowel, and omentum. The skin and subcutaneous tissue are intact.

Langer lines—The natural, anatomic tissue lines on the abdominal skin.

Linea alba—Where the aponeurosis of the internal and external oblique muscles insert, anterior to the rectus musculature.

Maylard incision—A transverse abdominal incision in which the rectus muscles are transected after ligation of the inferior epigastric vessels. The fascia is not dissected free of the rectus muscles. The peritoneum is usually entered in a transverse fashion.

Panniculectomy—Surgical removal of the pannus, excess skin, and subcutaneous fat, which hangs like an apron from the abdomen. Removal facilitates gynecological surgery.

Pfannenstiel incision—A commonly used transverse abdominal incision in which the rectus muscles are not cut and the fascia is dissected superiorly and inferiorly along the rectus muscles. The peritoneum is usually entered vertically.

Schuchardt incision—An incision made in the vagina, along the sulcus of the vagina from the lateral fornix to the introitus and through the perineum. This incision can increase room in the vagina so as to aid in difficult vaginal surgeries.

Smead-Jones closure—An interrupted closure of the anterior abdominal wall using a far-far, near-near approach. The closure includes all of the abdominal wall structures on the far-far portion and only the fascia on the near-near portion.

One of the lasting marks of any abdominal surgery, and most noticeable to the patient, is the scar made by the incision. In selecting an incision, the gynecologist must take into consideration the underlying pathology prompting the surgery, the suspicion of malignancy, the absence or presence of upper abdominal disease, and the underlying comorbid state of the patient. Although there are many types of incisions for gynecological surgery, selection of any incision must be highly individualized. However, selection of an incision should not be dictated by patient choice to preserve cosmesis if it may compromise the surgical approach. Conversely, unduly large or poorly positioned incisions may increase the likelihood of infection, herniation, or dehiscence, as well as unsightly cosmesis. During the surgical consenting process, the patient should be counseled on the location of the incision, the rationale for the particular incision, and any possible complication that may arise from the planned incision. In gynecologic oncology patients, the need for urinary diversion, colostomy, or an extraperitoneal approach to node-bearing areas will dictate the type of incision to be made. This chapter presents the classic incisions used by gynecologists to perform most gynecologic surgery. In addition, incisions used for gynecologic oncology will be shown. Finally, discussion and management of common complications associated with abdominal incisions will be presented.

ANATOMY OF THE ANTERIOR ABDOMINAL WALL

To avoid injury to vessels and nerves and to close any incision with minimal chance of dehiscence, abdominal wall anatomy should be thoroughly understood. The abdominal wall protects the visceral organs and vasculature within the abdominal cavity. Cephalad, the anterior abdominal wall extends to the costal margins and the xiphoid process. The costal cartilages of the seventh, eighth, ninth, and tenth ribs form a portion of the cephalad boundary. Lateral boundaries include the iliac crests; inferiorly, the abdominal wall is delineated by the inguinal ligaments, the pubic crests, and the superior border of the symphysis pubis. The principal anatomic structures of the abdominal wall include the overlying skin, subcutaneous tissue, muscles, fascia, and the nerves and vascular supply to these structures. Many factors—such as age, muscle mass and tone, obesity, intraabdominal pathology, previous pregnancies, and posture—can result in variation in the contour of the abdominal wall. These variations in contour affect abdominal wall topography and may present problems in the correct choice and placement of incisions.

Skin and Lymphatics

The skin contains small vessels, lymphatics, and nerves. A minimal loss of skin sensation can result from any abdominal incision. Numbness below a transverse incision frequently occurs. As stated in the discussion on nerve supply, laterally extended transverse abdominal incisions can result in numbness of the skin on the anterior thigh.

The lymphatic drainage of the upper abdominal wall passes directly to the axillary lymph nodes. The lymphatic drainage of the lower abdomen passes to the inguinal nodes and then to the iliac chain. Some lymphatics around the umbilicus drain toward the liver through the falciform ligament. When an incision is placed transversely in the lower abdomen, lymphatic drainage of the abdominal wall above the incision site is interrupted. Some tissue swelling may develop temporarily until collateral lymphatic drainage can be established. Patients should be counseled about this possible swelling before undergoing surgery.

In 1861, Langer, working with cadavers, described cleavage lines of the skin that pull the skin edges apart when cut across. These have become known as Langer lines (Fig. 14.1). These lines usually run horizontally across the abdomen. A vertical incision in the skin of the abdomen cuts perpendicular to Langer lines, whereas a horizontal incision cuts parallel to them. Thus, transverse incisions heal with a relatively fine scar, and vertical incisions can heal with a broad scar, particularly in the lower abdomen.

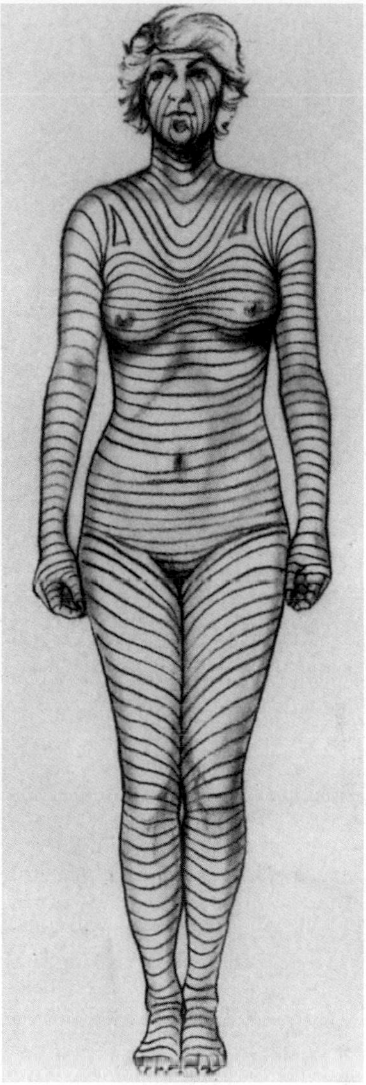

FIGURE 14.1. Langer lines run horizontally across the lower abdomen. A transverse incision cuts parallel to the Langer lines and usually heals with a fine scar.

Muscles and Fascia

The abdominal muscles assist in respiration, defecation, urination, coughing, and childbirth by increasing intraabdominal pressure. They work synergistically with the muscles of the back to flex, extend, and rotate the trunk and pelvis. There are two groups of muscles that form the musculature of the anterior abdominal wall. The flat muscles include the external oblique, the internal oblique, and the transversalis. Their fibers basically run diagonally or transversely. The second group, composed of the rectus muscles and the paired pyramidalis muscles, have fibers that run vertically (Fig. 14.2). The recti, with their thin investing fascia, are muscles of locomotion and posture. The paired pyramidalis muscles arise from the crest of the pubic symphysis and insert into the lower linea alba. Preservation of the pyramidalis muscles is not essential when making incisions. The integrity of the anterior abdominal wall is not associated with this second group of muscles.

A cross section of the lower abdominal wall shows that the fascia of the abdominal muscles envelop the anterior and posterior surfaces of the rectus muscles and anchor the external oblique, internal oblique, and transversalis muscles to the vertical (rectus) muscles (Fig. 14.3). There is excellent fascial support anteriorly and posteriorly to the rectus muscles above the arcuate (semicircular) line. In this location, the fascial aponeurosis of the external oblique and the split fascial aponeurosis of the internal oblique fuse together anterior to the rectus muscle and insert in the midline (linea alba). Above the arcuate line, the posterior lamella of the internal oblique aponeurosis fuses with the aponeurosis of the transversalis muscle, passes posterior to the rectus muscle, and inserts in the midline. The lower half of the lower abdominal wall is weakened below the arcuate line, at a level about horizontal to the anterior superior iliac spine, where the posterior division of the rectus sheath disappears. In this location, the divided lamella of the internal oblique muscle combines and passes anterior to the rectus muscle. From this lower portion of the lower abdominal wall to the pubic rami, only the attenuated transversalis fascia and the peritoneum lie adjacent to the posterior surface of the muscle. It is in this weakened section of the lower abdomen that most incisional hernias occur after pelvic surgery through lower midline incisions. In the lower abdomen, the force required to approximate edges of a vertical incision is 30 times greater than the force required to approximate edges of a transverse incision.

The external oblique muscle and its aponeurosis form the most anterior layer of the flat muscles. The external oblique muscle originates from the lower eight ribs. Superiorly, the fibers of this muscle run transversely; inferiorly, they assume an oblique downward course. A portion of the muscle gives rise to a broad fibrous aponeurosis, which courses medially, anterior to the rectus muscle. The next posterior fanlike muscle is the internal oblique, which originates primarily from the iliac crest,

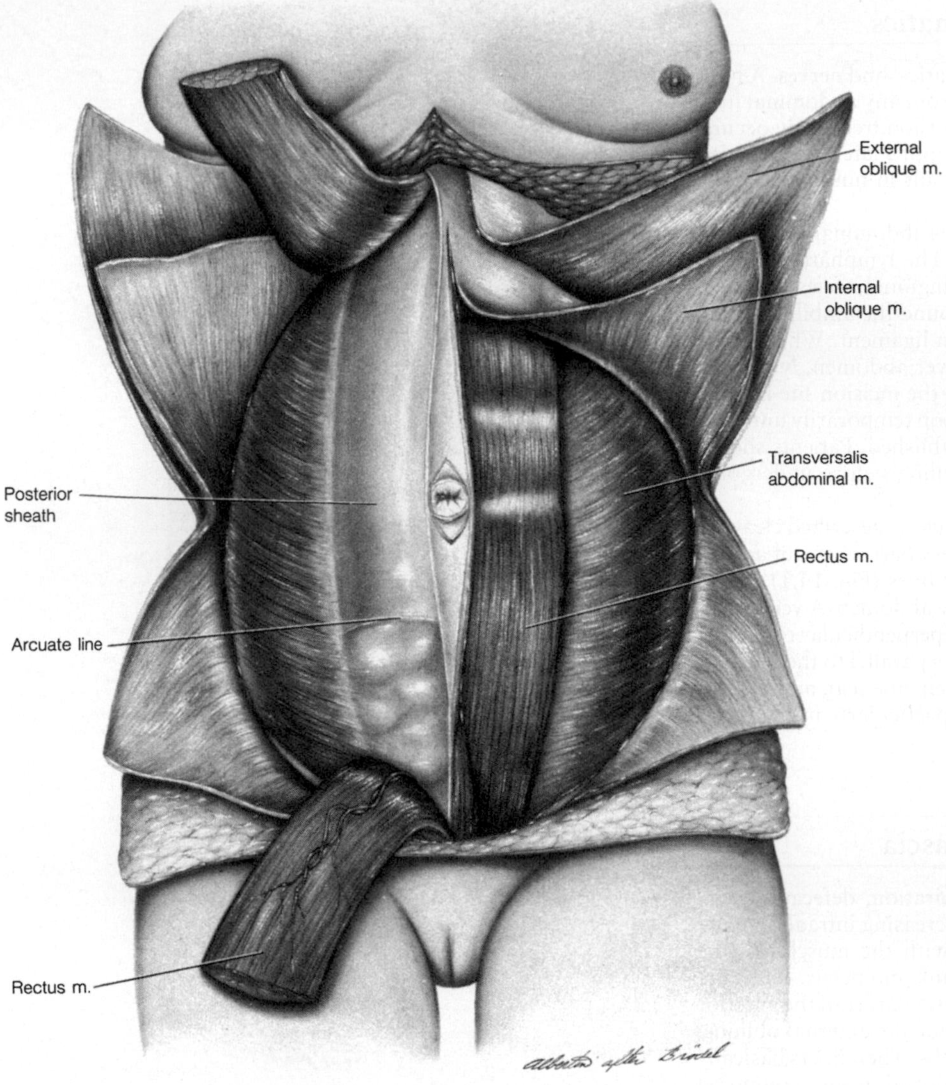

FIGURE 14.2. Musculature of the abdominal wall (*left*), showing reflection of external and internal oblique muscles along with anterior division of rectus sheath, which exposes the transversalis and rectus muscles. Tendinous inscriptions in rectus sheath are visible above the umbilicus. The rectus muscle has been reflected (*right*) to demonstrate the posterior rectus sheath and the abrupt cessation of the posterior lamella of the internal oblique at the linea semicircularis (*arcuate line*). Below the *arcuate line*, the intestines are separated from the abdominal wall by the peritoneum and the attenuated fascia of the transversalis muscle.

the thoracolumbar fascia, and the inguinal ligament. The midportion of the muscle runs an upward oblique course and gives rise to the aponeurosis of the internal oblique. As noted, at the lateral border of the rectus musculature, the aponeurosis splits and forms a sheath around the rectus muscle, rejoining medial to the rectus to help form the linea alba. The third flat muscle, the transverse abdominis, arises from the lower six costal cartilages, thoracolumbar fascia, and internal lip of the iliac crest. It has a truly transverse course. Above the midway point between the umbilicus and pubis, the aponeurosis of this muscle passes behind the rectus muscle and contributes to the posterior rectus sheath. Below this point, the aponeurosis passes anterior to the rectus muscle, contributing to the anterior rectus sheath. Medial to the rectus muscle, the fascia of all three flat muscles insert to form the linea alba.

The major functions of the flat muscles are to assist with respirations and to assist in increasing intraabdominal pressure. Each time these muscles contract, they pull at the linea alba. Because the linea alba represents the insertion of six major abdominal muscles (three on each side), cutting it, as with lower midline incisions, actually interrupts the major portion of the insertion of these six muscles. Thus, contractions of these muscles in the postoperative period can result in considerable tension on a suture line in the linea alba and can cause considerable discomfort.

The rectus abdominis muscle arises from the pubic crest. It courses superiorly and inserts into the xiphoid process with the upper attachments being three times as broad as its pubic insertion. It has three or four fibrous insertions. One is at the level of the umbilicus; two are usually halfway between the umbilicus and the insertions, superiorly and inferiorly. Of note, the fibrous insertions are tightly adherent to the anterior rectus sheath. These limit the retraction of the muscle when it is cut. Thus, when performing a transverse-muscle cutting incision, it is not necessary to reapproximate the rectus muscle. The pyramidalis, a triangular muscle, usually lies anterior to the rectus and arises from the anterior portion of the symphysis, inserting into the inferior portion of the linea alba. The midportion of this muscle usually has an avascular raphe, which can easily be incised for adequate exposure of the Retzius space.

Blood Supply

The abundant blood supply to the anterior abdominal wall comes from several sources. The main arterial supply consists

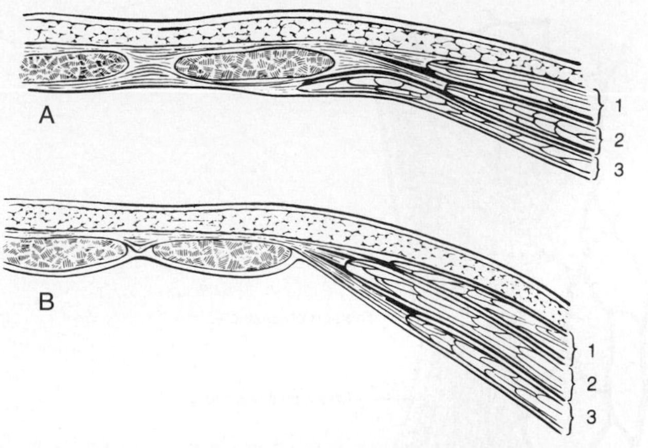

FIGURE 14.3. Cross section of lower abdominal wall. **A:** The anterior fascial sheath of the rectus muscle from external oblique muscle (*1*) and split aponeurosis of internal oblique muscle (*2*). The posterior sheath is formed by aponeurosis of transversalis muscle (*3*) and split aponeurosis of internal oblique muscle. **B:** Lower portion of abdominal wall below arcuate line (linea semicircularis) with absence of a posterior fascial sheath of the rectus muscle and all of the facial aponeuroses (*1–3*) forming the anterior rectus sheath.

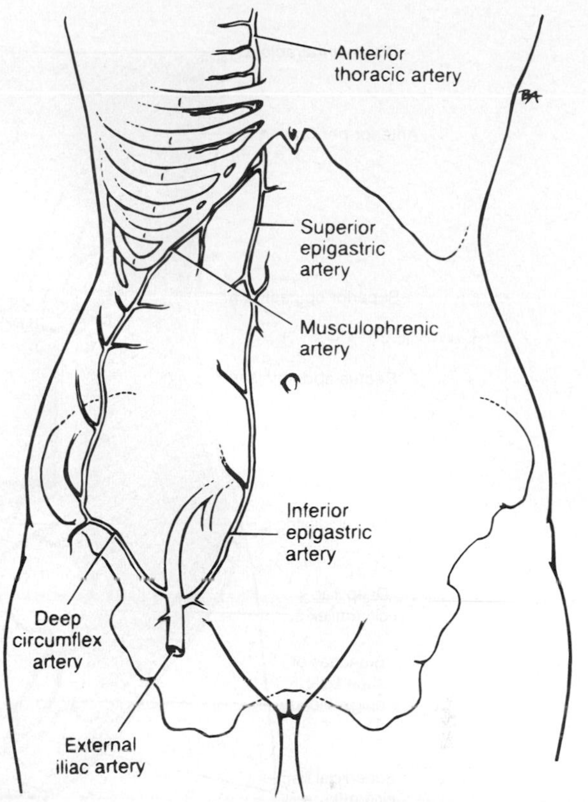

FIGURE 14.4. The major arterial blood supply of the anterior abdominal wall consists of four major vessels. Two lateral and two medial contribute to the rich anastomosis. (From Gallup DG. Opening and closing the abdomen and wound healing. In: Gershenson D, Curry S, DeCherney A, eds. *Operative gynecology.* 1st ed. Philadelphia: WB Saunders, 1993:127, with permission.)

of the superior epigastric, musculophrenic, deep circumflex iliac, and inferior epigastric vessels. The medial abdominal wall receives blood from the epigastric arteries, whereas the lateral wall is supplied by the musculophrenic and deep circumflex iliac arteries. The lateral wall is also supplied by the lower intercostal and lumbar arteries (T8 to T12 and L1). This freely anastomosing vascular system provides one continuous arterial and venous channel on both sides of the anterior abdominal wall, extending from the subclavian artery and vein (cephalad) to the external iliac vessels (caudad) (Fig. 14.4). Because of the rich anastomosis, vascular deficiency is usually not a complication of abdominal wall surgery. The linea alba is relatively bloodless. The limited vascular supply in this area of fascial fusion can impair wound healing when lower midline incisions are used. Thus, a secure closure is mandatory to avoid incisional hernias or eviscerations.

Conversely, the epigastric vessels are subject to injury, particularly when a muscle-splitting incision is used. Also, the deep circumflex or musculophrenic vessels can be injured when an extraperitoneal approach is chosen.

The superior epigastric artery is a continuation of the internal thoracic (mammary) artery. It enters the sheath of the rectus from behind the seventh costal cartilage and descends posterior to the rectus. It has multiple branches in the substance of the rectus muscle and anastomosis to the inferior epigastric artery. In the upper abdomen, cephalad to the umbilicus, the main branch of the artery tends to lie posterior to the midportion of the rectus muscle (Fig. 14.5). The inferior epigastric artery arises from the external iliac artery near the midinguinal point. It continues in a cephalad course along the posterior lateral portion of the rectus muscle and has an anastomosis with the superior epigastric arteries. The lower a transverse incision is made, the more lateral the inferior epigastric arteries are encountered. Bleeding from branches of the inferior epigastric vessels beneath the rectus muscle can dissect cephalad or caudad along the entire length of the posterior sheath. Below the arcuate line, bleeding can dissect laterally and inferiorly along the retroperitoneal planes and spaces, resulting in extensive hematomas of the abdominal wall and pelvis. Such bleeding can produce confusing acute abdominal signs in the postoperative patient, and large quantities of blood may be lost in these loose tissues and spaces.

The musculophrenic artery, arising from the internal thoracic, courses along the costal margin, behind the cartilages. It has an anastomosis with the deep circumflex artery, which originates from the external iliac at about the same level as the inferior epigastric artery. The deep circumflex courses behind the inguinal ligament and along the iliac crest, eventually piercing the transversus muscle and digitating between that muscle and the internal oblique. Before its anastomosis with the musculophrenic, it can be relatively large. Care must be taken when these muscles are incised laterally.

The venous drainage of the abdominal wall accompanies the arteries. The veins of the abdominal wall may be dilated in patients with obstruction of blood flow through the liver and porta hepatis.

Innervation

The nerve supply to the anterior abdominal wall is easily damaged by some incisions. The anterior abdominal wall is supplied by the thoracoabdominal nerves, the iliohypogastric nerves, and the ilioinguinal nerves. The thoracoabdominal nerves, which are the seventh to eleventh intercostal nerves, leave the intercostal spaces and travel caudad and anterior between the

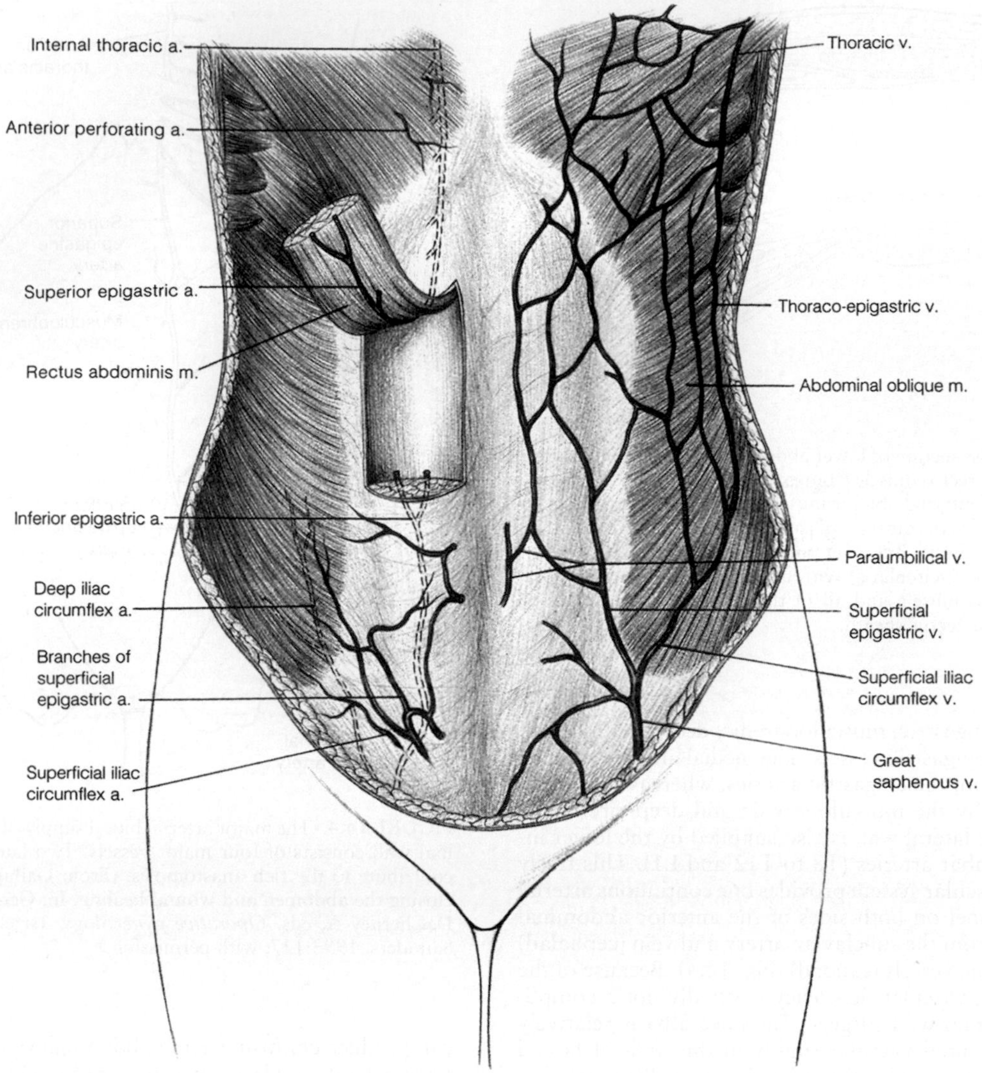

FIGURE 14.5. Arterial and venous circulation of abdominal wall. The superior and inferior epigastric arteries provide a rich arcade for the rectus muscles, arising superiorly from the internal thoracic artery and inferiorly from the external iliac artery. The venous system has a similar origin, with the exception that the superficial inferior epigastric vein communicates with the saphenous vein of the leg.

transversus and internal oblique. They supply these muscles and the external oblique. They enter the sheath of the rectus, and their branches supply the rectus and the overlying skin. Most of the nerves are supplied by several trunks. Any one nerve in the anterior abdominal wall contains fibers from the last two to three intercostal nerves. When an incision is made lateral to the midline, a transverse type is least likely to cause injury to nerves. In the upper abdomen, an obliquely caudad and laterally directed incision is least likely to cause significant nerve injury. In the lower part of the abdomen, an obliquely directed cephalad and laterally directed incision is relatively nerve sparing.

A vertical incision that passes lateral to the rectus muscle or through the muscle itself can denervate medially lying tissue. Depending on the length of the incision, atony or atrophy of the muscle can occur. A midline incision in the linea alba or a transverse incision (even through the rectus muscle), however, does not interfere with motor innervation of the abdominal musculature.

A minimal loss of skin sensation can result from abdominal incisions and is unavoidable in most cases. The iliohypogastric and ilioinguinal nerves are sensory in function (Fig. 14.6). Injury to the former, when wide transverse incisions are used, can result in sensation changes in the skin over the mons, whereas injury to the latter can result in sensation changes to the labia majora. A widely placed transverse incision can result in numbness of the skin over the upper anterior thigh. Both nerves are chiefly derived from the first lumbar nerve root. Although they lie for a distance between the internal oblique and the transversus, they do not enter the rectus sheath. They do not supply the external oblique or the rectus muscle. Both nerves supply the lower fibers of the internal oblique and transversus. If damage occurs to these nerves at the level of the anterosuperior iliac spine, these muscle fibers are denervated. A weakening

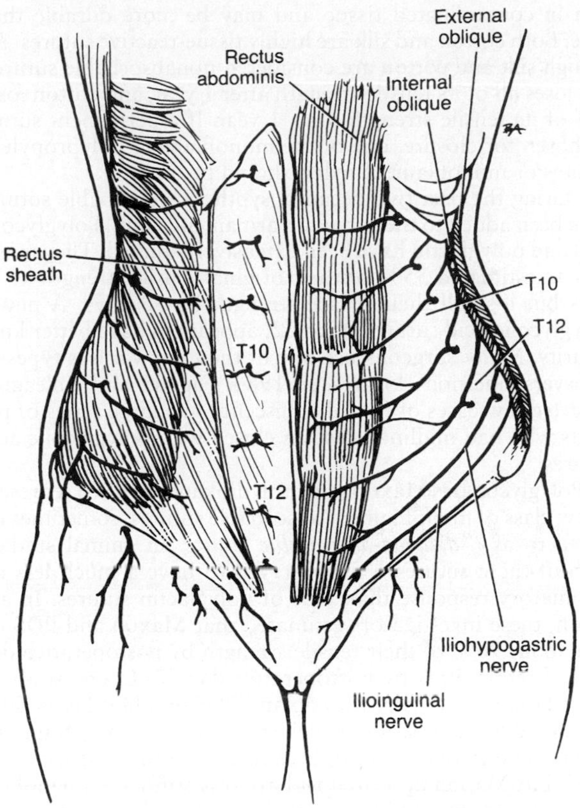

FIGURE 14.6. Major innervation of the anterior abdominal wall. The iliohypogastric nerves and ilioinguinal nerves supply the sensory innervation of the lower abdominal wall. (From Gallup DG. Opening and closing the abdomen and wound healing. In: Gershenson D, Curry S, DeCherney A, eds. *Operative gynecology.* 1st ed. Philadelphia: WB Saunders, 1993:127, with permission.)

of the normal canal-controlling mechanism can occur, predisposing the patient to an inguinal hernia.

PHYSIOLOGY OF WOUND HEALING

Wound complications are a psychological and economic problem for the patient and include infections, dehiscence, and evisceration, as well as late-occurring problems such as incisional hernias and wound sinus formation. Factors negatively affecting proper wound healing include diabetes, malnutrition, prior irradiation or chemotherapy, older patient age, alcoholism, preoperative shaving the evening before the operation (instead of clipping of hair), longer duration of preoperative hospitalization, longer duration of the operation, use of Penrose-type drains brought out through the incision, ascites, malignancy, immunosuppression (including long-term corticosteroid therapy), and obesity. In addition, factors affecting wound disruption that usually occur in the absence of infection include choice of suture material, closure technique, occurrence of excessive coughing caused by pulmonary disease, retching and vomiting, and intestinal obstruction.

The four phases of wound healing are inflammation, migration, proliferation, and maturation. Breaks in the normal cycle of wound healing can occur anywhere, depending on preexisting conditions. Increases in fibroblasts during the proliferation phase, which occurs from day 5 through day 20, provide most of the strength to the wound. By day 21, most wounds have regained almost 30% of their original tensile strength. Any wound contamination or the presence of foreign bodies can cause chronic inflammation, wound sinuses, delayed incisional herniae, or the early postoperative problems of infection and dehiscence.

The risks of wound infections are directly related to the classification of wounds (Table 14.1). Obviously, few surgeons would primarily close a dirty wound. Many of the abdominal procedures performed by gynecologists include a hysterectomy.

TABLE 14.1

WOUND CLASSIFICATION

Class	Category	Definition	Wound infection rate(%)
I	Clean	Wounds are made under ideal operating room conditions. The procedures are usually elective, and no entry is made into the oropharyngeal cavity or lumen of the respiratory, alimentary, or genitourinary tract. Inflammation is not encountered, and no break in technique occurs. The wounds are always primarily closed and seldom drained. Almost 75% of all operations are included in this group.	<5
II	Clean-contaminated	Wounds occur from entry into the oropharyngeal cavity, respiratory, alimentary, or genitourinary tract without significant spillage. Clean wounds are included in this category when there is a minor break in surgical technique. These procedures include about 16% of all operations.	2–10
III	Contaminated	This category includes open, fresh, and traumatic wounds; operations with a major break in sterile technique; and incisions encountering acute, nonpurulent inflammation, such as in cholecystitis or cystitis.	15–20
IV	Dirty	Old (>4 h) traumatic wounds, perforated viscera, or operations involving clinically evident infections are included in this category. Wounds containing foreign bodies or devitalized tissue are also considered dirty.	>30

Whenever the vagina is entered, the procedure is then classified as a clean-contaminated procedure with attendant risk.

SUTURES

Suture choice is basically a surgeon's prerogative, but the characteristics of suture material intended for fascial closure should be well known to the surgeon. Additionally, suture choice should be based on the patient's condition, the type of incision, and the strength and reaction of the suture (Table 14.2). In general, the ideal suture material should have the following characteristics: knot security, inertness, adequate tensile strength, flexibility, ease in handling, smooth passage through tissue, nonallergenicity, resistance to infection, and absorbability at a predictable rate. Neither plain catgut nor chromic catgut maintains tensile strength during the critical time of wound healing. They should not be used for fascial closure of the abdominal wall, irrespective of the type of incision used. Estimation of tensile strength of chromic suture after 14 days is 34%, whereas plain gut has none.

In general, sutures are classified as nonabsorbable if they maintain tensile strength for more than 60 days. In the permanent suture group, monofilament sutures yield less inflammation than that of polyfilament sutures. Wire has been the traditional suture used by surgeons for decades in high-risk patients, particularly when infection was an associated operative finding. However, wire is difficult to tie and breaks easily if bent sharply. If placed too closely to the incisional edges, it may cut through tissues. In some patients, wire can cause a prickling sensation. Also, wire ends may penetrate the surgeon's gloves, exposing the surgeon to body fluid–borne pathogens. Furthermore, in animal models, both monofilament nylon and monofilament polypropylene sutures have elicited less infection in contaminated tissue and may be more durable than wire. Both cotton and silk are highly tissue-reactive sutures. Although silk and cotton are considered nonabsorbable sutures, silk loses all of its tensile strength after 1 year, and cotton loses half of its tensile strength after 1 year. If a permanent suture is chosen for closure, one of the monofilament polypropylene sutures or monofilament nylon should be used.

During the past two decades, synthetic absorbable sutures have been added to the surgeon's armamentarium. Polyglycolic acid and polyglactin have been extensively studied. They maintain an estimated 55% of their original tensile strength at 14 days but lose all their tensile strength by 30 days. A newer polyglycolic acid suture, Dexon 2, appears to have better knot security. Many surgeons use one of these for various types of transverse incision closures. In 1984, Fagniez and colleagues reported few cases of fascial dehiscence in a large series of patients who had midline incisions closed with polyglycolic acid sutures.

Polyglyconate (Maxon) and polydioxanone (PDS) represent a new class of monofilament absorbable sutures, sometimes referred to as a *delayed-absorbable suture.* In animal studies, both of these sutures were observed to have a much less inflammatory response than that of polyglactin sutures. In addition, these investigators estimated that Maxon and PDS retain about 90% of their tensile strength by postoperative day 14 and retain 50% by postoperative day 30. In one study of degradation patterns of Maxon and PDS in rabbit fascia, PDS was noted to be superior. Rodeheaver and associates found no significant difference in knot-breaking strength in these two sutures, but Maxon appeared to have less stiffness in handling. Another study in rabbits also revealed the tensile strength superiority of Maxon and PDS compared with polyglycolic acid and polyglactin. In this study, Maxon was thought to have the best knot security. These investigators also observed that the most

TABLE 14.2

COMMONLY USED SUTURES FOR GENERAL CLOSURE

Suture type	Tissue reaction	Relative strength	Knot security
Absorbable			
Monofilament			
Plain gut	4	1	2
Chronic gut	3	2	3
Polydioxanone (PDS)	1	4	2
Polyglyconate (Maxon)	1	3	2
Polyglecaperone 25 (Monocryl)	1	2	2
Vicryl Rapide	2	2	2
Braided			
Polyglycolic acid (Dexon, Dexon 2)	2	3	2
Polyglactin 910 (Vicryl)	2	3	2
Poly (L-actide/glycolide) (Panacryl)	2	3	3
Nonabsorbable			
Monofilament			
Polypropylene monofilament (Surgilene, Novofil, Prolene)	1	4	1
Stainless-steel wire (Flexon)	1	4	4
Nylon (Dermalon, Ethilon, Surgilon)	1	3	2
Braided			
Natural (silk, cotton)	4	2	3
(Dacron, Mersilene, Ti-Cron, Ethibond, Tevdeck)	2	3	3

Scale on 1, least; 4, most.

consistent knot security was achieved when six square knots were used. Alternatively, two surgeon's knots and two square knots can be used. Our clinical impression is that there is little difference in suture handling and knot security when Maxon and PDS II are compared. When wound healing is anticipated to take longer than 2 weeks, particularly for fascial closure of midline incisions, one of these two delayed-absorbable sutures should be highly considered. In addition, usage of one of these sutures should be considered in the presence of infection or contamination.

Finally, knot security will depend on suture size and the tissue needing approximation. Although sliding knots, also known as *nonidentical sliding knots,* can be safely used for pelvic viscera, sutures used to close abdominal wall fascia should be tied with square knots. Sometimes it is convenient to tie a loop-to-strand knot as a way of terminating a continuous suture, rather than tying a single-strand to single-strand knot. Hurt and colleagues eloquently conducted a safety evaluation of tying a loop-to-strand knot with a monofilament suture, poliglecaprone (Monocryl®). In these experiments, the authors used 0-0 and 2-0 gauge suture, randomly comparing single-strand with single strand, square knots with loop-to-strand, square knots with loop-to-single strand, nonidentical sliding knots. A total of 40 knots were tied in each group and evaluated by tensiometry. The major outcome studied was the proportion of knots becoming untied in each group. The authors found that when monofilament sutures were tied loop-to-single strand with nonidentical sliding knots, 85% and 55%, respectively, of 0-0 and 2-0 gauge sutures untied. None of the single-strand to single-strand square knots untied, and 15% and 5%, respectively, of the 0-0 and 2-0 gauge sutures, tied loop-to-single strand with square knots, untied. Although these conditions were carefully controlled and were conducted *ex vivo,* care must be taken to lay down square knots (six throws) while tying monofilament suture in a loop-to-single strand fashion. Van Rissel and colleagues observed poor knot performance when a surgeon's knot plus two square knots was made with monofilament sutures. We have not noticed this problem with knots tied similarly.

DRAINS

Sometimes, drainage of the abdominal cavity is appropriate after an operation for a tuboovarian abscess or some other type of pelvic infection. In addition, intraperitoneal drainage may be helpful for oozing peritoneal surfaces after complicated hysterectomies or other pelvic surgery. Although used in the past for prevention of lymphoceles or ureteral fistulae, retroperitoneal drains are not routinely used after radical pelvic surgery.

The use of prophylactic drains in the subcutaneous space or "wet" subfascial space remains controversial. Some investigators suggest that the lowest clean-wound infection rate is found in patients who have no drains. However, use of a closed drainage system for large potential spaces (for example, in dissection of a large incisional hernia or when mesh or a fascial or myocutaneous graft is used) should be considered. Drainage may also be necessary to prevent subsequent hematoma formation when persisting defects in blood coagulation result in persistent "oozing." As discussed later, two published series on pelvic-abdominal surgery in obese patients indicate an advantage with the use of subcutaneous drains. On the other hand, Scott and coworkers operated on 56 patients whose panniculi measured 6 to 11 cm in thickness. They used systemic and oral antibiotics, transverse incisions, copious lavage, and tape to close the skin. No drains were used, and only one patient had a wound infection. Few randomized prospective studies with adequate statistical power to answer the question of whether or not to drain exist. In some series, only patients at high risk for wound infection were drained subcutaneously or subfascially, which clearly results in noncomparable groups for evaluation because of selection bias. Farnell and associates, in a prospective study, analyzed 3,282 incisions of the wound varieties listed in Table 14.1. When patients with clean-contaminated or contaminated wounds received subcutaneous closed-drainage systems, alone or with antibiotics or saline irrigation, no significant advantage was noted compared with primary closure without drainage. However, a trend favoring subcutaneous drainage and antibiotic irrigation was seen in patients with contaminated wounds.

Although the adage "the solution to pollution is dilution" is used quite often during wound irrigation, irrigation with bactericidal agents may be detrimental. In one study, irrigating solutions *in vitro* and in laboratory animals—such as 1% povidone-iodine, 0.25% acetic acid, or 0.5% sodium hypochlorite—were shown to have cytotoxic effects when applied to human fibroblasts. In the same study, hydrogen peroxide did not retard wound healing but had minimal bactericidal potency.

Drains can be classified into two basic categories: passive and active. The former function primarily by overflow, sometimes being assisted by gravity. The latter are connected to some type of suction device. The use of passive drains in wounds may be one reason that wound drainage has been associated with increased infection rates. The two types of passive drains used—whether Penrose or cigarette (a Penrose drain with gauze placed inside it to enhance capillary activity), if used at all—should never be brought out through the incision because of the risk of wound infection or seroma formation. We prefer a closed drainage system such as a Jackson-Pratt or a Blake. Both have small reservoir systems (100 mL) that are relatively easy for paramedical personnel to manage on the ward. In our experience, the Blake drain, with its longitudinal ridges, offers less chance of obstruction from small tissue fragments or clots than does the Jackson-Pratt drain. However, no large prospective, randomized trials comparing these systems have been done.

In patients who undergo a clean-contaminated procedure without prophylactic antibiotics, closed-suction drainage of the wound may be beneficial. When antibiotics are used, prophylactic drainage may not be advantageous, with exception of its use in obese patients. To avoid clot formation and subsequent obstruction, the drain is placed on suction early, usually while completing closure of the incision. In addition, the nursing staff should be instructed to "strip" the drain catheter each shift while the drain is in place. Drains in the subfascial or subcutaneous space should be removed, not advanced, when the drainage is less than 50 mL per 24 hours, usually by postoperative day 2 or 3.

PREVENTION OF WOUND COMPLICATIONS

Wound infection, dehiscence, and evisceration usually occur early in the postoperative period, whereas suture sinuses and incisional hernias are late manifestations of impaired primary wound healing. Management of these problems is discussed later in this chapter.

The usual rate of significant wound infections is 5% or less for all abdominal operations and is related to many factors, including surgeon experience, the population operated on, the procedure performed, and the comorbid condition of the patient. Large series, such as those by Cruse and Foord, have added to current knowledge about wound infections and their causes. Preoperative showering with hexachlorophene lowered the infection rate in clean wounds (1.3%) compared with the rate with no showering (2.3%). In addition to others, Cruse and Foord also observed that clip preparation of abdominal and/or pubic hair versus shave preparation the evening before surgery resulted in fewer wound infections. Truthfully, the only reason to remove hair is to prevent interference with wound approximation in some incisions. Other methods of hair removal, including the use of depilatories, have been advocated by some surgeons, but they are relatively expensive. In the series reported by Seropian and Reynolds, the wound infection rates for depilatory preparations versus no hair removal were equal (0.6%). We prefer to use an electric clipper, clipping the hair, in the operating room, when it is necessary to remove pubic hair.

Skin preparations and draping do not need to be complex. Recently, a randomized, controlled trial by Ellenhorn and colleagues compared iodophor scrub-and-paint skin preparation with iodophor paint only in 234 patients. The patients underwent abdominal surgeries in a comprehensive cancer center and were matched for age, the presence of diabetes, and obesity. The primary end point—rate of wound infection—was identical between the two groups, with each group having a wound infection rate of 10%. The authors suggest that the traditional scrub-and-paint method of skin preparation could be replaced by the paint-only technique, saving cost and time in the operating room. Obviously, patients that have sensitivities to iodine compounds will need skin preps with other agents. In another study of 2,253 consecutive general surgical procedures, the use of disposable gown and drape systems, rather than reusable cotton material, reduced postoperative infection incidence from 6.4% to 2.3%. Plastic adhesive drapes have been shown to be disadvantageous in preventing wound infections and may actually increase infection rates if the adhesive loosens and the drape detaches from the skin. As shown in earlier studies, operative procedures that exceeded 90 minutes had much higher infection rates than did shorter-length procedures. This study from Duke University also revealed a relatively higher wound infection rate in women older than 60 years of age compared with men.

Newer antiseptic scrub techniques have been developed, including povidone-iodine (Betadine), 4% chlorhexidine gluconate (Hibliclens), and 3% hexachlorophene (pHisoHex). Of the three, Hibliclens produced the best immediate and persistent reduction in normal hand flora. A 3-minute skin preparation is adequate. Furthermore, the time-honored 10-minute scrub of the surgeon's hands is unnecessary. Galle and coworkers observed no difference in infection rates between a 5-minute versus a 10-minute scrub time. A lesser time obviously decreases total operative time and water usage.

Incisions of the skin should not be made with cautery. In one study, Kenady found the wound infection rate doubled when a Bovie device was used compared with a knife. Discarding the skin knife has not been shown to reduce wound infection rates, but instead leaves an extra "sharp" on the operative field that may injure the health care team. In a randomized prospective study, the rate of postoperative wound infections was not significantly different after the use of one or two scalpels for the incision (Hasselgren et al., 1984). The same scalpel can be safely used for superficial and deep incisions. The incision should be made in a bold strike to minimize dead space. In general, subcutaneous sutures should be avoided because the subcutaneous tissue does not provide support. In some patients, a fine (4-0) running polyglycolic acid suture in the subcutaneous layer may diminish tension from the approximated skin edges. Chromic catgut should never be used to close the fascia and should not be used in subcutaneous closure. In general, delayed closure should be used for contaminated or dirty wounds. Alternatively, intermittent staples can be placed in the skin with intervening saline moistened "wicks" into the subcutaneous spaces. When a bacteria-containing organ is opened (the unprepped bowel or abscessed gynecological organs) and delayed closure is not used, copious saline irrigation of all layers for closure should be instituted. In addition, a monofilament delayed or nonabsorbable suture should be used in the closure. Systemic antibiotics can help control wound infections when pelvic infection is encountered. To be of benefit, they should be administered at least 30 minutes before the skin incision and readministered if the operation is prolonged. Currently, first- and second-generation cephalosporins are the most popular antibiotics used in the prophylactic setting.

ABDOMINAL INCISIONS

In general, abdominal incisions used for most gynecologic procedures can be divided into transverse or vertical incisions. For extraperitoneal incisions and access to organs not associated with the female genital tract, modifications of oblique incisions are sometimes used. Because of the ease and rapid entry, the abdomen was originally routinely opened by a longitudinal incision in the linea alba. One of the first successful abdominal operations was performed by McDowell in 1809. In the early days of abdominal surgery, transverse incisions were generally avoided because they were more time-consuming. Also, an unfounded fear was that transection of the rectus muscle would leave a defect because of retraction of the muscle. As previously stated in the section on anatomy, the adherence of the recti to the anterior rectus fascia by several transverse inscriptions prevents retraction. In the late 1800s and early 1900s, several transverse incisions were developed, such as the Küstner, Pfannenstiel, Maylard, and Cherney incisions. Most of the transverse incisions used for pelvic surgery are identified by the name of the surgeon who first described them, whereas the few vertical abdominal incisions have no such eponyms.

Transverse Incisions

Transverse incisions for pelvic surgery are attractive because they produce the best cosmetic results. Additionally, low transverse incisions are as much as 30 times stronger than midline incisions, are less painful, and result in less interference with postoperative respirations. Wound dehiscence is allegedly more common with vertical incisions. The older literature suggests that wound evisceration was three to five times more common and hernia occurrence was two to three times more common when vertical incisions were used compared with transverse incisions. Many earlier studies reported an increased incidence of eviscerations with midline incisions that could be associated with inappropriate closures. More recent studies, however, have shown no difference in the risk of wound dehiscence or even a slight advantage for midline incisions. A large study, completed at Hutzel Hospital in Detroit by Hendrix and colleagues, found that there was no difference in fascial dehiscence between transverse (Pfannenstiel) and vertical incisions.

Transverse incisions have certain associated disadvantages. They are relatively more time-consuming and relatively more hemorrhagic. Occasionally, nerves are divided, and division of multiple layers of fascia and muscle can result in formation of potential spaces with subsequent hematoma or seroma formation. Ability to explore the upper-abdominal cavity adequately is compromised with most low transverse incisions.

Pfannenstiel Incision

Most surgeons would agree that the Pfannenstiel incision provides the best wound security of all gynecologic incisions. The cosmetic results are excellent, but exposure is limited. Thus, it should not be used for patients with known gynecologic malignancies. It should not be used when pelvic exposure is needed in operating on patients with nonmalignant conditions, such as severe endometriosis or large leiomyomas with distortion of the lower uterine segment, or when reoperating on a patient for hemorrhage.

The original, true Pfannenstiel incision is described as a transverse incision that is slightly curved (concavity upward) and may be made at any level suitable to the surgeon (Fig. 14.7A). It is usually 10 to 15 cm long and extends through the skin and subcutaneous fat to the level of the rectus fascia. The rectus fascia is incised transversely on either side of the linea alba, which is cut separately, joining the two lateral incisions but leaving the rectus fascia intact across the midline (Fig. 14.7B). The rectus sheath is separated from the underlying muscle by inserting the fingers on either side of the cut edge of the sheath and pulling the fascia in opposite directions, with one hand toward the head and the other hand toward the feet. This maneuver frees the fascia from the anterior surface of the rectus muscle as far as desired between the symphysis and the umbilicus (Fig. 14.7C). The rectus muscles are then separated in the midline, and the peritoneum is opened vertically (Fig. 14.7D). This procedure avoids the necessity of dissecting the subcutaneous fat away from the anterior rectus fascia, as is done in the Küstner incision. It separates the perforating nerves and small blood vessels that enter the fascia from the underlying muscles and nourishes the fascia, although it possibly weakens the incision.

If the Pfannenstiel incision is extended laterally beyond the edge of the rectus muscles and into the substance of the external and internal oblique muscles, injury to the iliohypogastric or ilioinguinal nerves can occur, with resulting neuroma formation. In addition, closure of this extended fascial incision can entrap these nerves in either the closing suture or surrounding scar tissue. To avoid these nerve injuries in laterally extended incisions, including a Cherney or Maylard incision, the lateral extensions should have sutures placed only in the external oblique fascia.

The incision may be wet and require subfascial drainage. The fascia can be closed with a running technique in patients with clean wounds or clean-contaminated wounds. Polyglycolic acid, polyglactin 910, or one of the delayed-absorbable sutures can be used. In assessing the use of running versus interrupted polyglycolic acid sutures in midline incisions, Fagniez and colleagues observed no difference in fascial dehiscence in a randomized prospective trial of 3,135 patients.

Subcutaneous sutures are usually unnecessary (unless they are being used as tension-releasing sutures for the skin closure), and the skin is closed with a subcuticular suture (preferably monofilament), reinforced surgical tape (e.g., Steri-Strips), skin glue, or staples.

Küstner Incision

Some surgeons advocate a Küstner incision, incorrectly referred to as a modified Pfannenstiel incision. The slightly curved transverse skin incision begins below the level of the anterior superior iliac spine and extends just below the pubic hairline, through subcutaneous fat, down to the aponeurosis of the external oblique muscle and the anterior sheath of the recti in the same manner as all other transverse incisions (Fig. 14.8A). The superficial branches of the inferior epigastric artery and vein may be encountered in the subcutaneous fat at the lateral margin of the incision. When encountered, they can be ligated or sealed with Bovie cautery. The fascia is cleaned superiorly and inferiorly until a sufficient area is exposed from the region of the umbilicus to the symphysis to permit an adequate vertical incision in the linea alba. Excessive separation of the fat from the fascia in the lateral margins of the incision is unnecessary and can provide sites for small postoperative hematomas. Separation of the rectus muscles and entrance into the peritoneum are performed in the same manner in the ordinary midline incision (Fig. 14.8B). Because of the importance of obtaining adequate hemostasis in the subcutaneous fat of the skin flaps, this incision is definitely more time-consuming than the low midline incision or the Pfannenstiel incision. It offers little or no advantage, and its extensibility is severely limited. If this incision is used, strong consideration of subcutaneous, closed-suction drainage should be given.

Cherney Incision

The Cherney differs from the muscle-dividing Maylard incision by the location of transection of the recti. In both incisions, the skin and fascia are divided transversely as with a Pfannenstiel, but Cherney advocated freeing the rectus muscles at their tendinous insertion into the symphysis pubis. The recti are then retracted cephalad to improve exposure. The transverse Cherney incision is about 25% longer than a midline incision from the umbilicus to the symphysis.

The Cherney incision provides excellent access to the space of Retzius for urinary incontinence procedures. It provides excellent exposure of the pelvic side wall when needed—that is, in patients who require hypogastric artery ligation. Occasionally, the surgeon who uses a Pfannenstiel incision finds the incision inadequate for exposure for hemostasis or not large enough to expose areas of associated abnormal conditions. Under these circumstances, the safe approach is not to transect the rectus muscles halfway but to perform a Cherney incision. Partial incision of the rectus muscle can lead to injury to the inferior epigastric vessels. Also, if conversion to a Maylard is attempted after a previous Pfannenstiel, the anterior rectus sheath will have already been widely separated from the rectus muscles. The ends of the muscle are likely to retract and will not reunite when the edges of the aponeuroses are later reapproximated. In this situation, it may be necessary to reapproximate the rectus muscle ends with horizontal mattress sutures.

Even if the peritoneum is opened, the space of Retzius can be bluntly dissected (Fig. 14.9). The inferior epigastric vessels, which course more laterally in the caudad portion of the abdominal wall, are identified. The pyramidal muscles are sharply dissected. The fibrous tendinous rectus muscles are then dissected sharply from their insertion into the symphysis pubis (Fig. 14.10). Bleeding is negligible in this area, and the inferior epigastric vessels do not need to be ligated. The peritoneal incision can be extended laterally about 2 cm cephalad to the bladder while the vessels are visualized.

As stated earlier, transverse incisions, particularly the Cherney and the later-described Maylard, can result in nerve injury. The femoral nerve is particularly at risk when a self-retaining retractor with deep lateral blades is used in these widely extended incisions. If a self-retaining retractor is used with either of these incisions, the lateral blades should be only deep enough to fit under the edges of the incision. They should not rest on the psoas muscle.

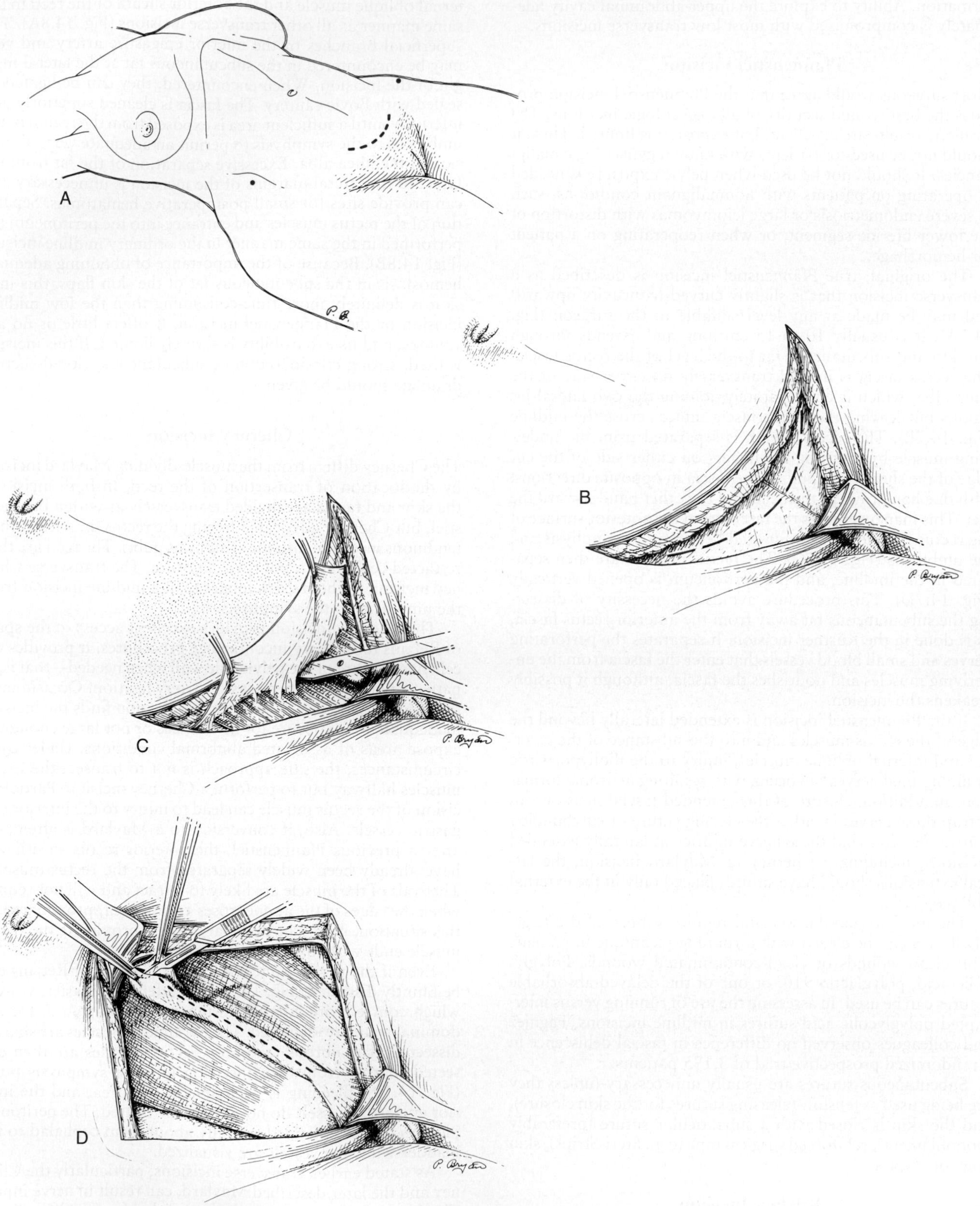

FIGURE 14.7. **A:** The skin incision for a Pfannenstiel incision is elliptical just above the symphysis pubis. **B:** The skin, subcutaneous fat, and fascia of the abdominal wall are incised transversely. **C:** The fascia is separated from the rectus muscle superiorly, inferiorly, and laterally. Small perforating vessels require ligation or coagulation. **D:** The rectus muscles are separated, and the peritoneum is incised in the midline.

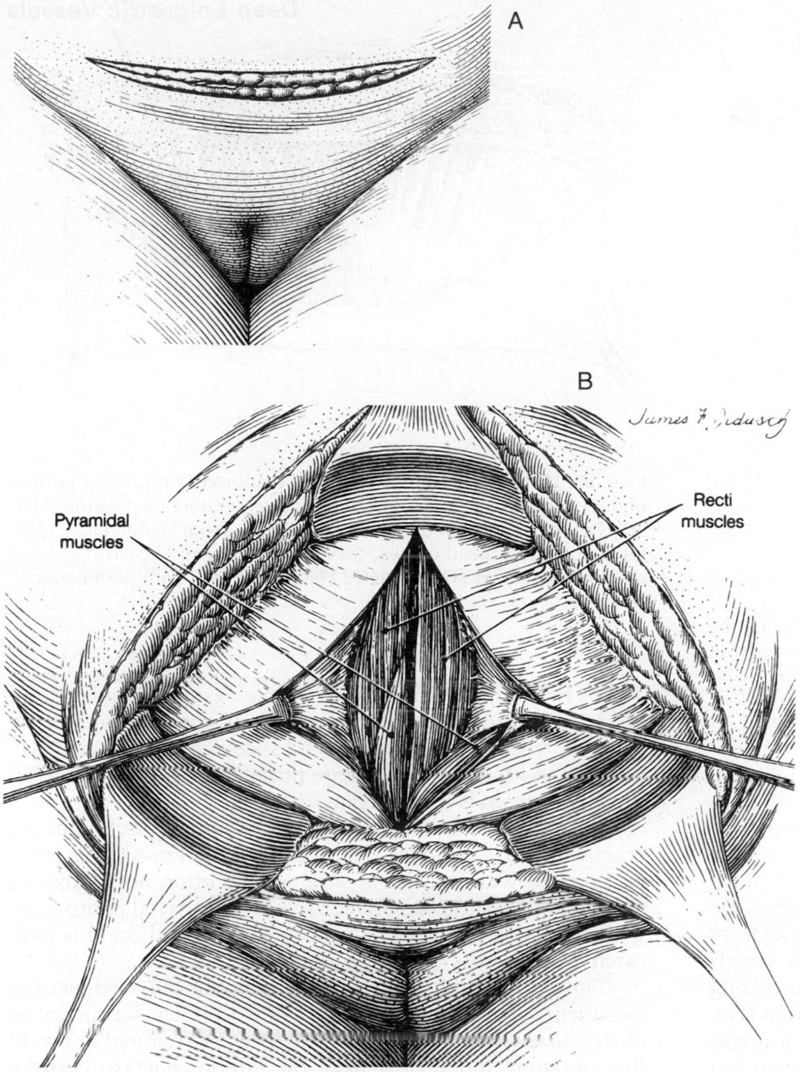

FIGURE 14.8. Küstner incision. A: Skin incision just below hairline. B: Midline incision through fascia, exposing rectus and pyramidalis muscles. The rectus muscles are retracted laterally, and the peritoneum is incised in the midline.

In closing a Cherney incision, we prefer to close the peritoneum separately with a running polyglycolic acid suture. Drainage of the subfascial space may be necessary. The ends of the rectus tendons are united to the inferior portion of the lower flap of the rectus sheath with five or six interrupted delayed-absorbable or permanent sutures in horizontal mattress configuration (Fig. 14.11). To avoid osteomyelitis, the rectus muscles should not be sutured to the periosteum of the symphysis pubis. Fascial closure is then accomplished with a running continuous suture of delayed-absorbable suture, as in the Pfannenstiel. Although the lines of tension favor transverse incisions as opposed to vertical incisions, running sutures should be placed at least 1.5 cm from the fascial edge and 1.5 cm from one another. The remainder of the closure is similar to the Pfannenstiel closure, depending on the surgeon's preference.

Maylard Incision

The Maylard incision is a true transverse muscle-cutting incision in which all layers of the lower abdominal wall are incised transversely. This incision was originally described by Ernest Maylard in 1907. The incision provides excellent pelvic exposure and is used by many surgeons for radical pelvic surgery, including radical hysterectomy with pelvic lymph node dissection and pelvic exenteration. Although we prefer midline incisions for patients with suspicious adnexal masses, young patients with adnexal masses that are questionable for malignancy by radiographic and serological studies may be candidates for this cosmetic incision. Patients must be informed that if malignancy is found, the transverse incision will take the form of a "hockey stick" (i.e., a J-shaped incision; see Incisions for Extraperitoneal Approaches), or a separate upper-abdominal incision will be used to evaluate the upper-abdominal cavity and retroperitoneal paraaortic nodes.

The Maylard-Bardenheuer incision has been modified in several aspects since its original description. Before the skin incision is made, a series of three to four perpendicular markings with a sterile marking pen are made across the planned line of the incision. These markings help in later approximation of the skin edges. The transverse skin incision is made about 3 to 8 cm above the symphysis, depending on the indications for surgery and patient age and weight. The skin incision should never be made in a deep skin crease or beneath a large panniculus. The fascia is incised transversely, and the aponeurosis is not detached from the underlying muscle.

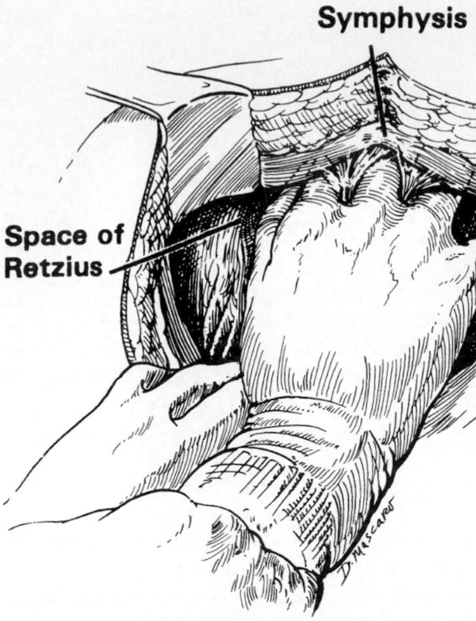

FIGURE 14.9. Developing the space of Retzius. The weight of the hand of the operator easily separates the bladder from the overlying symphysis in the relatively bloodless midline. (From Gallup DG. Opening and closing the abdomen. In: Phelan JP, Clark SL, eds. *Cesarean delivery.* New York: Chapman & Hall, 1988:449, with permission.)

After a transverse fascial incision lateral to the borders of the rectus muscles, the inferior epigastric vessels, lying on the posterior lateral border of each muscle, are identified. (Some surgeons suggest preservation of these vessels even when the rectus muscles are transected.) The vessels are teased away from their attachments by using a gentle finger dissection. The vessels are ligated before incising the rectus muscles to avoid tearing of the vessels, vessel retraction, and hematoma formation (Fig. 14.12). The fingers of the surgeon tease the overlying rectus muscle from the peritoneum, and the muscles are sectioned between the fingers by using a Bovie cautery.

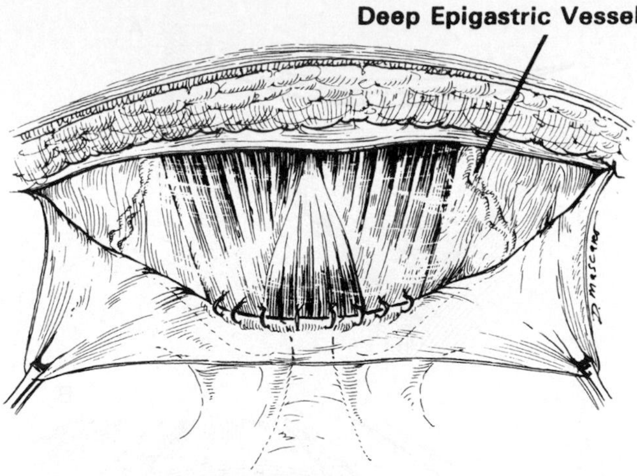

FIGURE 14.11. Reuniting of the rectus tendons to the inferior portion of the lower flaps. The deep inferior epigastric vessels are positioned laterally in the caudad portion of the abdomen. (From Gallup DG. Opening and closing the abdomen. In: Phelan JP, Clark SL, eds. *Cesarean delivery.* New York: Chapman & Hall, 1988:449, with permission.)

For better approximation of the muscles during closure, we prefer to suture the underlying muscle to the overlying fascia before entering the peritoneum. A 2-0 delayed-absorbable "U" suture is used, and the knots are placed anterior to the fascia. The peritoneum is incised transversely.

Closure of the fascia is similar to the running technique for other transverse incisions. The muscles do not need to be reapproximated with individual sutures (exception noted above), although some surgeons prefer to close the parietal peritoneum with a running polyglycolic suture. A subfascial drain is indicated if hemostasis is not absolute (Fig. 14.13).

Caution should be exercised in using the Maylard incision in patients with impaired circulation to the leg secondary to obstruction of the common iliac arteries or terminal aorta. In this situation, blood flow from the inferior epigastric artery may provide the only additional collateral circulation to the

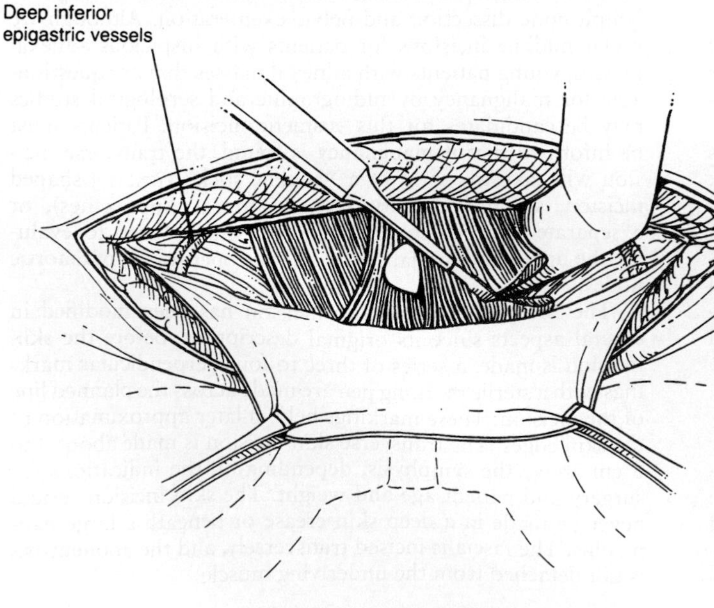

FIGURE 14.10. The finger of the operator is placed posterior to the rectus muscle, and with gentle traction, the muscle is pulled cephalad. The rectus muscle can then be dissected from its insertion at the symphysis by the Bovie device. The peritoneal incision can then be extended laterally, avoiding the inferior epigastric vessels, which are positioned laterally. (From Gallup DG. Abdominal incisions and closures. In: Gallup DG, Talledo OE, eds. *Surgical atlas of gynecologic oncology.* Philadelphia: WB Saunders, 1994:43, with permission.)

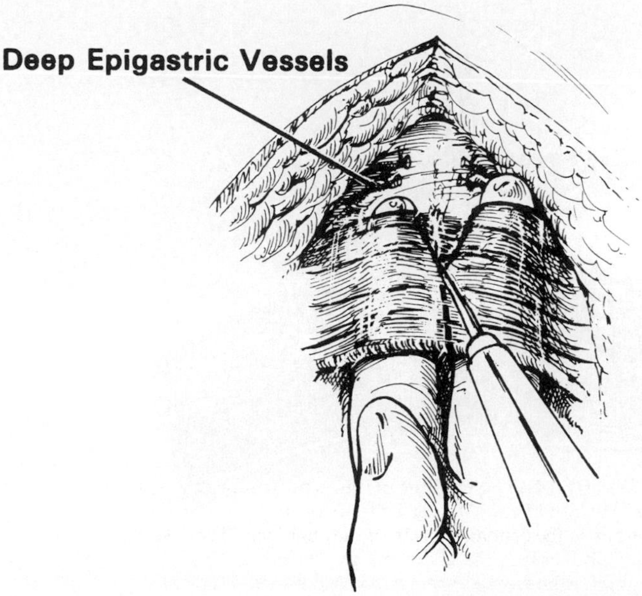

FIGURE 14.12. Maylard incision. The rectus muscles are incised with a knife or a Bovie device. The hand of the surgeon is withdrawn as the muscle is cut. The inferior epigastric vessels were previously isolated, sectioned, and ligated. (From Gallup DG. Opening and closing the abdomen. In: Phelan JP, Clark SL, eds. *Cesarean delivery.* New York: Chapman & Hall, 1988:449, with permission.)

lower extremity. Ligation of this artery could result in lower-extremity ischemia and a real vascular surgical emergency. In the gynecologic patient with clinical evidence of impaired circulation in the lower extremity, a midline incision should be used.

Vertical Incisions

Generally, vertical incisions afford excellent exposure. They can be easily extended and provide rapid entry to the abdominal cavity. Whether midline or paramedian, the resulting scar may be wide.

Midline (Median) Incision

As stated in the section on anatomy, the midline incision is the least hemorrhagic incision, as well as the incision that affords rapid entry into the abdominal/pelvic cavity. Exposure is excellent, and minimal nerve damage occurs. However, dehiscence and hernias are said to be more common, particularly in the area inferior to the arcuate line. Abdominal wound disruption is one of the most serious postoperative problems associated with gynecologic surgery. The "burst abdomen," or evisceration, seen more frequently in general surgery patients, occurs with a frequency of 0.3% to 0.7% in gynecologic patients and is associated with a mortality of 10% to 35%. The type of incision is only one factor associated with evisceration, and wound infection is present in more than half the cases. Use of chromic catgut for fascial closure is associated with a higher incidence of dehiscence compared with that for any other class of suture. Mechanical factors—such as wound hematomas, paroxysmal coughing associated with chronic lung disease, and gastrointestinal problems (retching, vomiting, ileus)—can lead to evisceration. Newer closure techniques have been shown to have lower wound infection, dehiscence, and hernia rates and are discussed later in the chapter.

The midline incision is the most easily mastered gynecologic incision because the fascial area is relatively bloodless and the rectus muscles are usually separated in parous women. If the patient has a prior midline incision, the surgeon should incise the peritoneum more cephalad to the earlier incision to avoid injury to possibly adherent bowel. In patients undergoing radical pelvic surgery or surgery for deep-seated, adherent pelvic masses, we prefer to develop the space of Retzius to allow extension of the incision between the pyramidal muscles, providing better exposure in the deep pelvis. In nulliparous women, the midline separation between the rectus muscles may not be obvious. In such cases, the pyramidalis muscles are useful landmarks in directing the surgeon to the midline. Because this incision can easily be extended, the midline incision is the most versatile of all incisions used by gynecologists.

Hemostasis from incision of more anterior layers should always be complete before the peritoneum is entered (usually done with the scalpel) (Fig. 14.14). Once the abdomen is

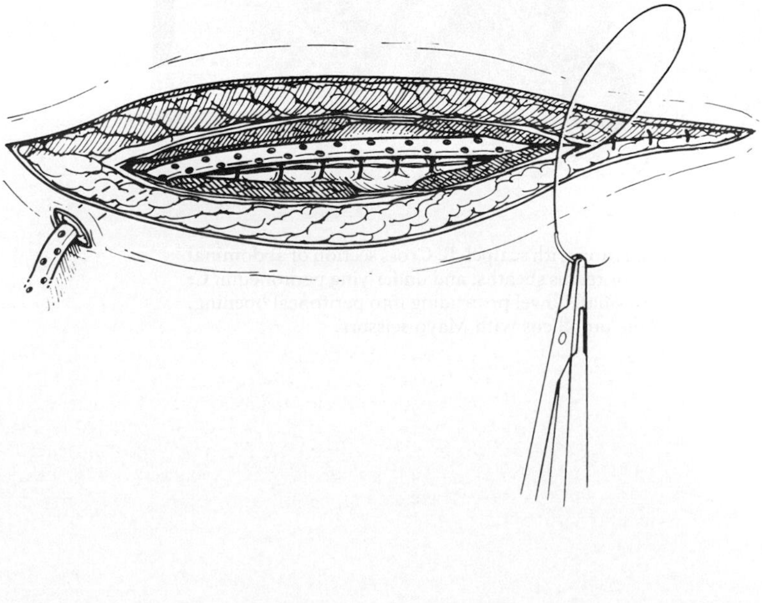

FIGURE 14.13. The peritoneum has been closed with 2-0 polyglycolic acid sutures. A closed drainage system is used if hemostasis is not absolute. A running delayed-absorbable suture is used, placing the bites about 1.5 cm from the fascial edge. (From Gallup DG. Abdominal incisions and closures. In: Gallup DG, Talledo OE, eds. *Surgical atlas of gynecologic oncology.* Philadelphia: WB Saunders, 1994:43, with permission.)

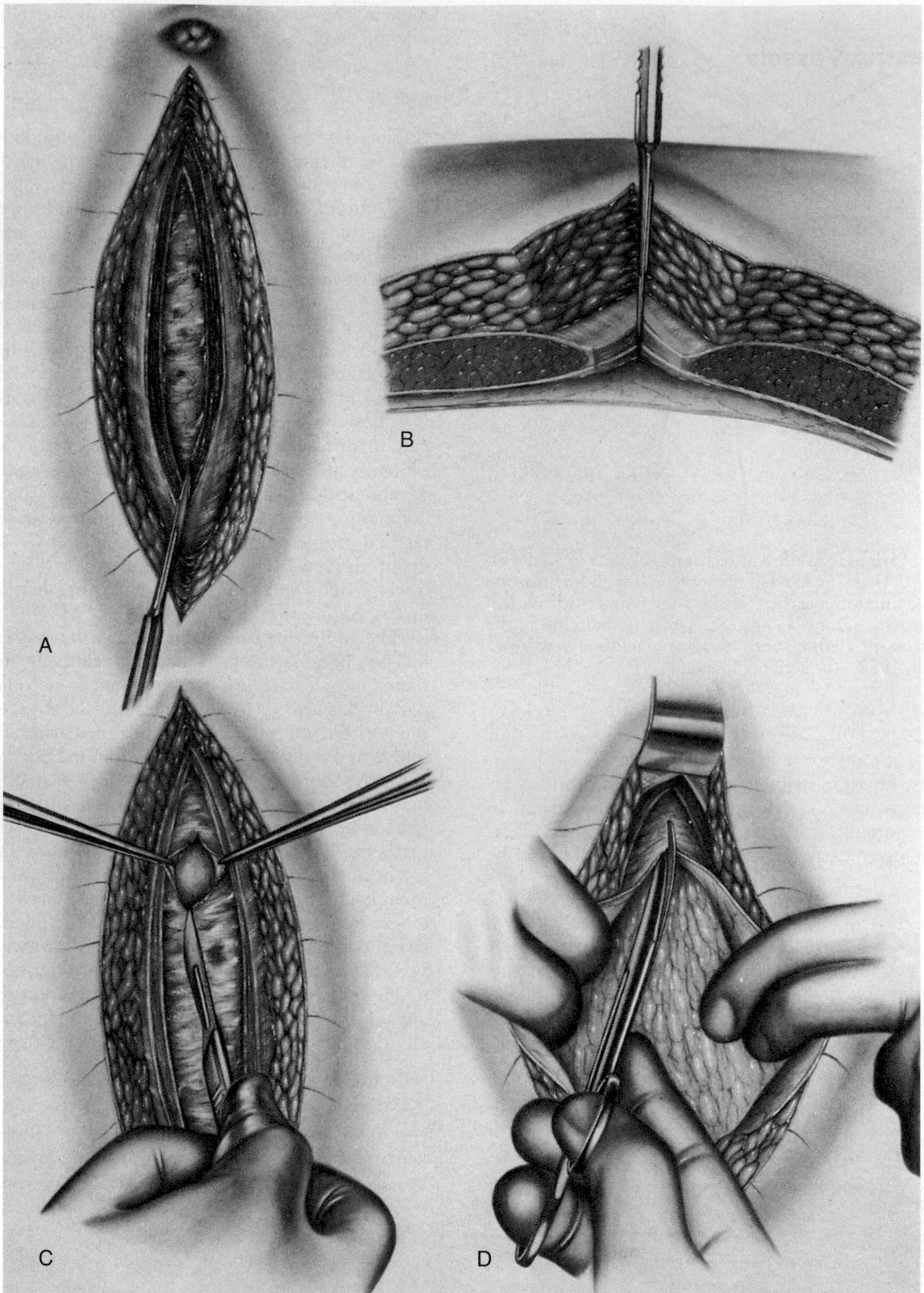

FIGURE 14.14. **A:** Cutting of linea alba in low midline incision with scalpel. **B:** Cross section of abdominal wall showing skin, subcutaneous fat, anterior and posterior rectus sheaths, and underlying peritoneum. **C:** Opening of peritoneum with knife, and demonstration of small bowel protruding into peritoneal opening. **D:** Enlargement of peritoneal opening to the region of the umbilicus with Mayo scissors.

explored (in a repetitive systematic fashion), the bowel must be carefully packed out of the pelvis. Seldom are more than two or three moist laparotomy packs needed to accomplish exposure of the pelvis. If more packs are required or there is a struggle to pack the upper abdominal contents cephalad, anesthesia may be inadequate. The more packs used, the more likely the small-bowel terminal nerve endings will be damaged, resulting in postoperative adynamic ileus. Use of more modern table-fixed retractors, such as the Bookwalter retractors, not only improves exposure in vertical and transverse incisions but also limits the use of excessive packs.

Paramedian Incision

Paramedian incisions have been advocated over midline incisions because of alleged greater strength. In a prospective study, Guillou and coworkers found no significant difference in respiratory complications, wound infection, and dehiscence when comparing midline, medial paramedian, and lateral paramedian incisions. None of the patients with lateral paramedian incisions developed an incisional hernia. The incidence of hernia in midline and medial paramedian incisions was the same. In a randomized prospective study, however, Cox and colleagues found 22 incisional hernias in patients with midline incisions compared with two hernias in the patients who had paramedian incisions. Like the midline or median incision, the paramedian incision has excellent extensibility and exposure, particularly on the side of the pelvis where the incision is made. For example, a left paramedian incision can be useful when operating for disease that involves the sigmoid colon and/or the left pelvic sidewall.

Although advantageous in some situations, paramedian incisions have many potential problems, including increased infection rates, increased intraoperative bleeding, increased operating time, and the possibility of nerve damage with resultant atrophy to the rectus muscle. Long paramedian incisions can increase pain with respiration during the immediate postoperative period. If a paramedian incision is placed parallel to a previous midline incision, or vice versa, the blood supply between the two incisions can be inadequate, resulting in tissue slough, delayed healing, and/or incisional herniae formation.

Closure of Vertical Incisions

Although closure of transverse incisions (discussed previously) raises little controversy because of the inherent relative strength of the incision, the closure of vertical incisions is controversial. Three general comments about closure can be made:

1. Paramedian incisions, because of their location, may require layered closure. However, we tend to use a mass running closure with a looped delayed-absorbable suture. No data exist to guide closure technique in these incisions.
2. With the advent of modern suture materials and knowledge about suturing techniques, retention sutures are rarely needed, except in some cases of evisceration.
3. With midline incisions, rectus muscles should not be sutured together unless there is sufficient diastasis to cause symptoms.

In closing midline incisions, some surgeons prefer a layered closure (Fig. 14.15). However, two metaanalyses (Weiland et al. and Hodgson et al.) have shown that mass closures are superior to layered closures with respect to postoperative incisional herniae, wound dehiscence, suture sinuses, infection, and wound pain. If a layered closure is used, sutures should always be loosely tied because the major cause of wound evisceration is too many sutures placed too closely together, placed too close to the fascial edge, and tied too tightly (remember, "approximate; not strangulate"). Often, at reoperation for evisceration, the sutures and knots are intact, but the suture has simply torn through the fascia. To avoid wound disruptions in high-risk patients, several investigators have advocated a Smead-Jones closure technique (Fig. 14.16). This is a far-far, near-near mass closure technique. The first (far-far) bite includes both the fascia and peritoneum on each side, and only the anterior fascia is included in the near-near bite. The widely spaced initial pass takes the tension off the healing incision, and the carefully placed near-near bites approximate the fascial edges to allow good healing without intervening fat or muscle. A No. 1 nylon or No. 1 polypropylene suture is used, with the key to the success of this closure being widely spaced far-far bites (at least 1.5 to 2 cm from the fascial edges). The main disadvantage to the Smead-Jones closure is that it is time-consuming.

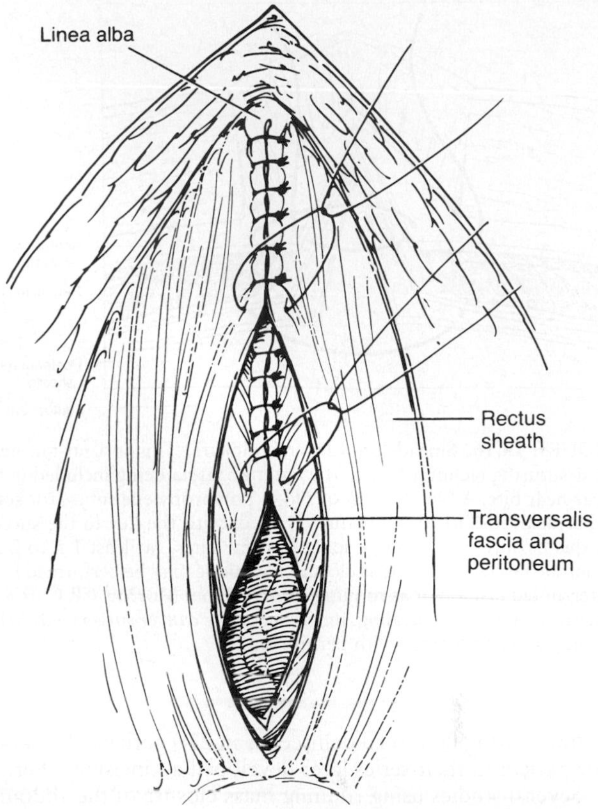

FIGURE 14.15. Layered closure of a midline incision. The peritoneum can be closed with a continuous 2-0 absorbable suture. The posterior and anterior fasciae can be closed with interrupted No. 0 delayed-absorbable suture. Figure-of-eight sutures also work for fascial closure. (From Gallup DG. Opening and closing the abdomen and wound healing. In: Gershenson D, Curry S, DeCherney A, eds. *Operative gynecology.* 1st ed. Philadelphia: WB Saunders, 1993:127, with permission.)

In 1976, Jenkins proposed that bursting of an abdominal wound can be prevented by using wide bites of nonabsorbable continuous suture through fascia, muscle, and peritoneum. Some investigators, particularly those who perform general surgery, have advocated a single-layer running mass-closure technique as an expedient, yet safe, technique for closing the abdomen. A study performed by Gallup and colleagues reported the use of this technique in high-risk patients in 1989,

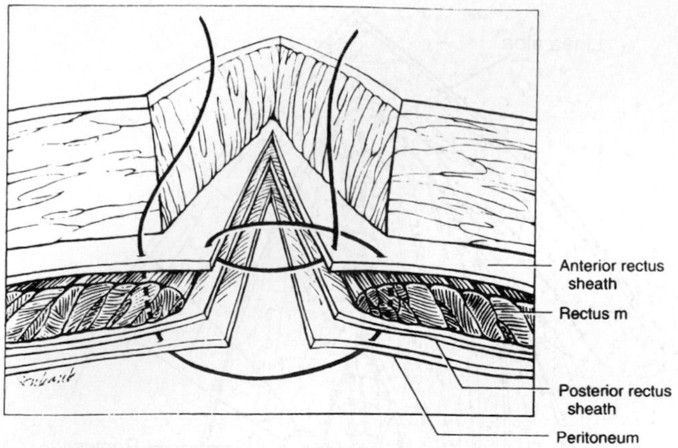

FIGURE 14.16. Smead-Jones layered closure. This is a far-far, near-near suturing technique, with the anterior fascia being included in the near-near bite. A No. 1 nylon or No. 1 polypropylene suture (or some other delayed-absorbable suture) is used, with the key to the success of this closure being widely spaced far-far bites. (at least 1.5 to 2 cm from the fascial edges). This closure technique may be performed in an interrupted fashion or as running suture. (From Morrow CP, Curtin JP. Incisions and wound healing. In: *Gynecologic cancer surgery.* Churchill Livingstone, 1996:152, with permission.)

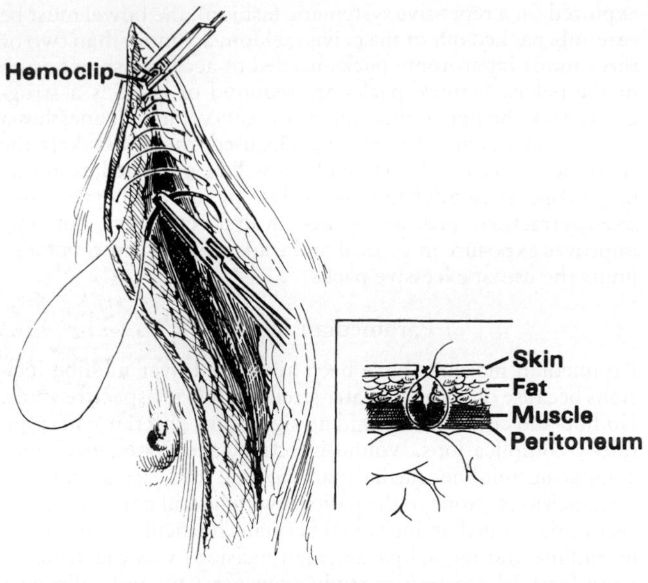

FIGURE 14.17. Closure of a midline incision using a No. 2 polypropylene, running mass closure. The anterior fascia, muscle, posterior fascia, and peritoneum are included in the bites (*inset*), which are taken 1.5 to 2 cm from the fascial edge and about 1 cm apart. With permanent polypropylene suture, a hemoclip can be used on the short end to avoid suture unraveling. (From Gallup DG. Opening and closing the abdomen. In: Phelan JP, Clark SL, eds. *Cesarean delivery.* New York: Chapman & Hall, 1988:449, with permission.)

demonstrating no fascial dehiscence in 210 patients. However, one patient in their series later developed an incisional hernia.

Several studies using running mass closure of the abdomen have been published and are listed in Table 14.3. These studies show a fascial dehiscence rate of 0.4% with this closure technique. The patient with the fascial dehiscence reported by Sutton and Morgan eviscerated after the closure suture was transected by a Kevorkian curette during wound debridement. In a randomized prospective study, Stone and colleagues found no difference in dehiscence rates between interrupted and mass closures.

Gallup and colleagues closed the midline incisions in their study with a continuous No. 2 polypropylene suture, placing the bites 1.5 to 2 cm from the fascial edge and including all anterior abdominal wall layers (the peritoneum, if easily located, the fascial layers, and the intervening muscle) (Fig. 14.17). One suture should be started from each end of the incision, tying the ends in the middle and securing the suture with three square knots (six throws). In the original series, a small hemoclip was placed above each knot to prevent unraveling. These caveats must be kept in mind with this closure technique: (a) a double-strand suture should never be tied to a single strand, and (b) the sutures should not be pulled too tightly, as this distributes tension unequally over the incision and negates the major advantage of this closure. Not all investigators include the peritoneum in the closure, but they still report excellent results. As shown by Ellis and Heddle in 1977, closure of the peritoneum as a separate layer appears to play no significant role in wound healing when midline incisions are used.

One problem with the use of large-bore, permanent suture for mass closure is occasional, late-occurring wound sinus

TABLE 14.3

CLOSURE WITH RUNNING SUTURES IN MIDLINE INCISIONS

Investigators	Patients	Material	Patients with fascial dehiscence
Archie and Feldman 1981	120	MFPP (No. 1)	1
Murray and Blaisdell 1978	255	PGA (No. 1)	1
Shepherd et al. 1983	200	MFPP (No. 2)	0
Knight and Griffen 1983	419	MFPP (No. 1)	4
Gallup et al. 1989	210	MFPP (No. 2)	0
Montz et al. 1991[a]	231	MFPG (0)	0
Sutton and Morgan 1992[b]	154	MFPB (0)	1
TOTALS	1589		(0.4%)

MFPP, monofilament polypropylene; PGA, polyglycolic acid; MFPG, monofilament polyglyconate; MFPB, monofilament polybuster.
[a]Looped suture with running Smead-Jones technique.
[b]Looped suture.

formation. However, with the development of monofilament (delayed) absorbable sutures (Maxon and PDS), the risk of wound sinus formation is significantly reduced. Again, Gallup and colleagues changed their running closure technique to avoid this problem of sinus formation by using No. 1 Maxon suture. This suture was selected because of its relatively easier handling and knot security. The closure technique (running mass closure) was similar to the closure with polypropylene suture; however, seven throws were used for each knot, and each knot was buried. Most of the 285 patients with midline incisions closed with the No. 1 Maxon were at high risk for wound disruption. Of these, seven developed superficial wound infections, one developed a ventral hernia, and one had an evisceration on postoperative day 4. At reexploration of this last patient, the central knot of the intact suture had untied, and later questioning of the surgeons revealed that only four throws had been used per knot. Montz and colleagues also reported no eviscerations or hernias in their series. Most of the recent running mass closure articles, however, have no long-term follow-up to assess later hernia formation.

Oblique Incisions

Oblique incisions can be used for a transperitoneal or an extraperitoneal approach.

Gridiron (Muscle-Splitting) Incision of McBurney

The McBurney incision is an excellent choice for an uncomplicated appendectomy and can be used for the extraperitoneal drainage of an abscess from pelvic inflammatory disease. In pelvic inflammatory disease, when drainage becomes necessary for an indolent broad ligament abscess that does not respond to antibiotics and does not point into the cul-de-sac for drainage, drainage through a gridiron incision is most effective. The incision is constructed as for an appendectomy, except that it is made a little lower, and the peritoneal cavity is not entered. Similarly, if drainage of the pelvis is required during a pelvic laparotomy, the drain should not exit through the midline incision, but rather through a small gridiron (stab-wound) incision in the lower abdomen. In treating a large tuboovarian abscess that extends out of the pelvis and does not respond to antibiotic therapy, extraperitoneal drainage through a McBurney incision is also possible by approaching the abscess laterally. This permits entrance into the site of infection without soiling the peritoneal cavity.

The gridiron incision is made obliquely downward and inward over the McBurney point (Fig. 14.18A). The location can be varied when the incision is performed for appendectomy during pregnancy or when it is used for abscess drainage, as mentioned above. The incision in the skin can be made at a lower level to preserve the cosmetic appearance of the abdominal wall. The incision is carried through the skin and subcutaneous fat to the external oblique muscle. The fibers of the muscle are separated in the direction in which they run (Fig. 14.18B). The internal oblique and the transverse abdominis are separated in the line of their fibers (Fig. 14.18C). At this point, the internal oblique and the transversus abdominis course in the same direction and are closely fused. Retractors are avoided, if possible. Instead, the peritoneum should be gently reflected away from the abdominal wall inferiorly and the abscess entered beneath the round ligament for extraperitoneal drainage. Thickened indurated tissue may make this step difficult. If the parietal peritoneum is adherent to the peritoneal surface of the abscess, drainage still may be possible without transversing free space in the peritoneal cavity. The surgeon should avoid contaminating the peritoneal cavity with pus, if possible.

The gridiron incision can be used in the left lower quadrant to drain an abscess on the left side of the pelvis as well as to perform sigmoid colostomy. Closure is depicted in Figure 14.18D–E and is best made with a delayed-absorbable suture.

Rockey-Davis Incision

An alternative to the McBurney incision is the Rockey-Davis (or Elliot) incision. It is a transverse incision placed at the junction of the middle and lower thirds of a line extending from the anterosuperior iliac spine to the umbilicus. Medially, the incision extends to the border of the rectus muscle. The aponeurosis of the external oblique muscle is split in the line of its fibers. The internal oblique and transversus muscle fibers can be separated by blunt finger dissection. The peritoneum is incised transversely. This incision has provided satisfactory exposure to pathology in either lower-abdominal quadrant. A similar incision made lower on the abdomen preserves the cosmetic appearance of the abdominal wall.

Incisions for Obese Patients

Obesity, especially when the condition is morbid (>130% of ideal body weight or body mass index >30 kg/m^2), presents problems with incision placement and closure. Obesity is a recognized high-risk factor for wound infections and complications. Pitkin observed a 4% wound complication rate in nonobese women undergoing abdominal hysterectomy compared with a 29% rate in obese patients. Krebs and Helmkamp reported a wound infection rate of 24% in massively obese patients when a periumbilical transverse incision was used. Because muscle cutting may be needed for this transverse incision, entry time can be lengthy and the resulting incision relatively bloody. If any transverse incision is chosen for obese patients, it should be far removed from the anaerobic moist environment of the subpannicular fold (Fig. 14.19).

In 1977, Morrow and colleagues suggested modifications of preoperative care, intraoperative techniques, and postoperative care in obese gynecologic patients and observed only a 13% wound infection rate. Gallup subsequently modified Morrow's techniques. He operated on a group of 97 mostly high-risk obese patients and then compared them with obese patients not operated on by the modified protocol. The wound infection rate in obese patients not operated on by protocol was 42% compared with a 3% rate in protocol-operated obese patients.

Gallup's original protocol, which we still use for obese patients on our service, has only been modified by fascial closure techniques. All patients have careful cleansing of the umbilicus and undergo preoperative showering. Minidose subcutaneous heparin, 5,000 to 8,000 U, is administered 2 hours before surgery and every 12 hours after surgery, continuing until the patient is fully ambulatory. Alternatively, low-molecular-weight heparin may also be used. In addition, sequential compression devices are used in these high-risk patients. Prophylactic antibiotics are routinely given, and clip preparation of abdominal hair (rather than shaving) is used. The midline incision is made by first retracting the panniculus caudad, below the inferior margins of the symphysis, to avoid an incision in the anaerobic subpannicular fold (Fig. 14.19). The skin incision is a periumbilical incision because it is usually extended around the umbilicus. The fascial incision is always extended to the symphysis.

Once the uterus and other organs are removed, the pelvic peritoneum is not reapproximated. However, the vaginal cuff is closed. Fascia may be closed with a Smead-Jones or running

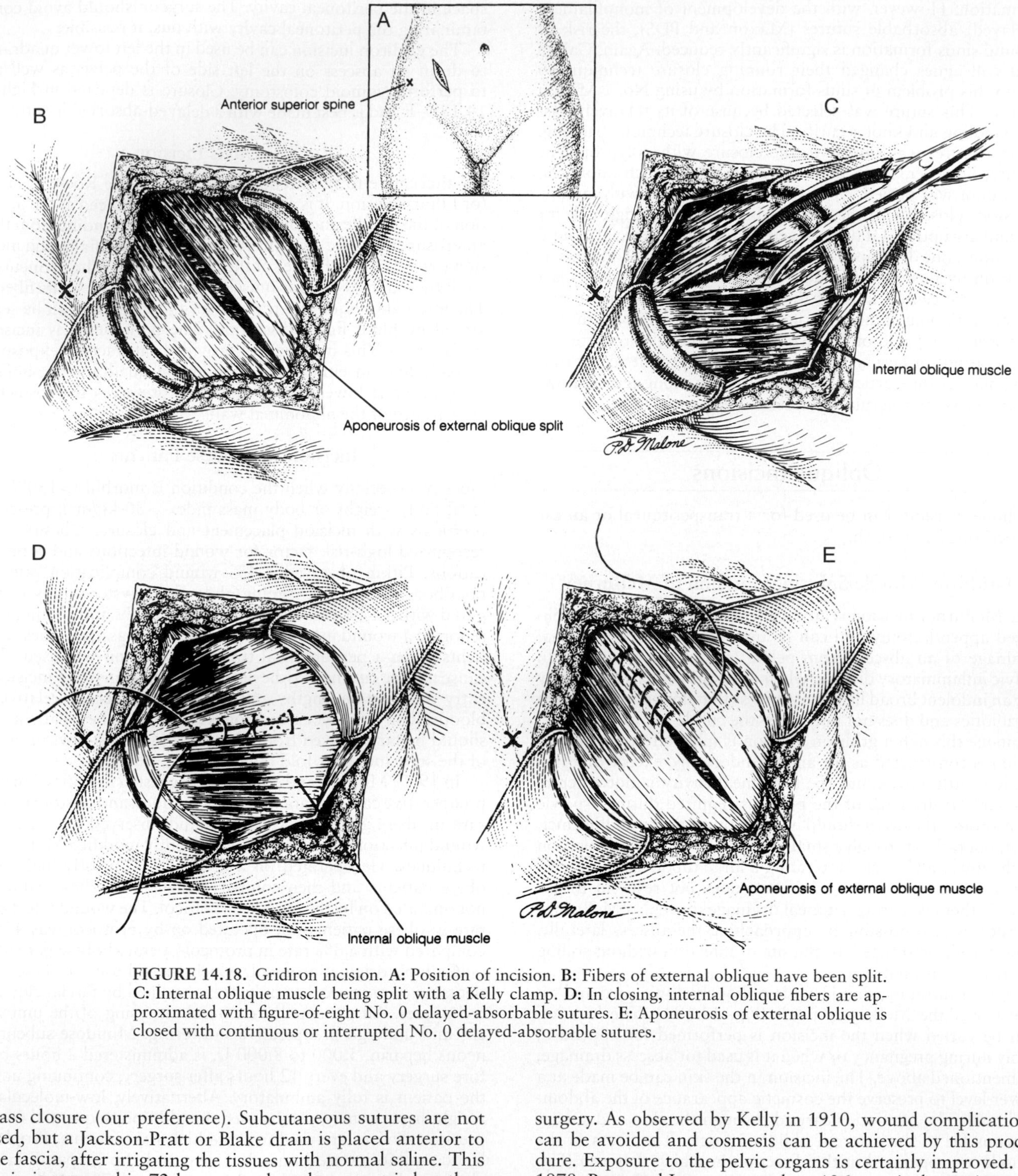

FIGURE 14.18. Gridiron incision. **A:** Position of incision. **B:** Fibers of external oblique have been split. **C:** Internal oblique muscle being split with a Kelly clamp. **D:** In closing, internal oblique fibers are approximated with figure-of-eight No. 0 delayed-absorbable sutures. **E:** Aponeurosis of external oblique is closed with continuous or interrupted No. 0 delayed-absorbable sutures.

mass closure (our preference). Subcutaneous sutures are not used, but a Jackson-Pratt or Blake drain is placed anterior to the fascia, after irrigating the tissues with normal saline. This drain is removed in 72 hours or when the output is less than 50 mL per 24 hours. The skin is closed with staples, which are left in place for 2 weeks. Unless small bowel surgery has been done, a nasogastric tube is rarely needed. Gallup's relatively low wound infection rate in obese patients supports this type of operative management.

Panniculectomy and Abdominoplasty

An alternate surgical approach in the massively obese patient is to remove the large panniculus before the intended pelvic surgery. As observed by Kelly in 1910, wound complications can be avoided and cosmesis can be achieved by this procedure. Exposure to the pelvic organs is certainly improved. In 1978, Pratt and Irons reported on 126 panniculectomies, and 85 of these were performed to facilitate exposure to the surgical field. The average hospital stay was only 14 days, but 34.5% of the patients had some degree of morbidity. In the series by Voss and colleagues, 5 of 76 (6.6%) patients undergoing panniculectomy and hysterectomy developed pulmonary embolism. In another series, investigators encountered excessive blood loss and acknowledged the need for transfusion in combined surgery. More recently, several series have noted the relative safety of combining abdominoplasty with other surgical

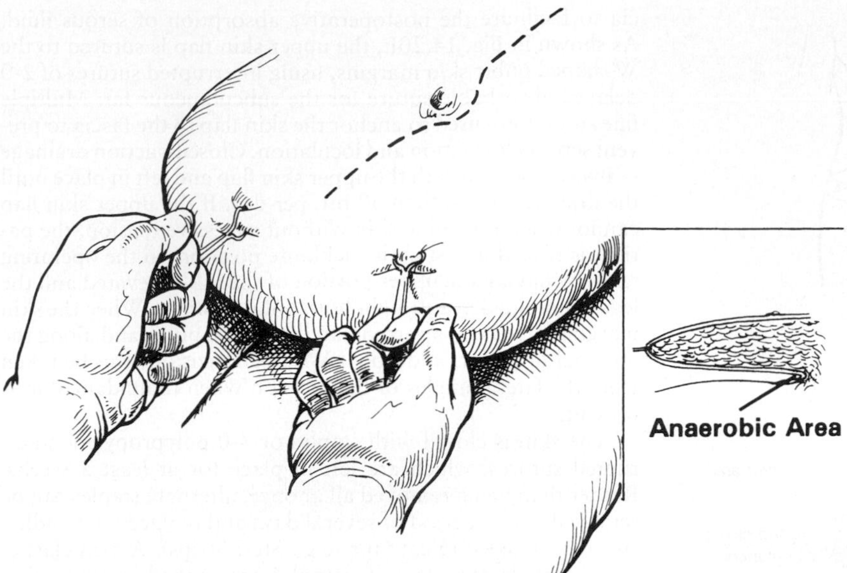

FIGURE 14.19. Midline incision in an obese patient. The panniculus is retracted inferiorly, and the incision avoids the moist anaerobic environment (*inset*) beneath the subpannicular fold. (From Gallup DG. Opening and closing the abdomen. In: Phelan JP, Clark SL, eds. *Cesarean delivery.* New York: Chapman & Hall, 1988:449, with permission.)

procedures. Hopkins and colleagues performed a retrospective review of patients who underwent panniculectomy at the time of gynecological surgery. They identified 78 patients (average weight 278 lb) on whom the procedure was performed. Their infection rate was a laudable 2.6%, with an equally impressive average blood loss of 71 mL. Four of the patients had minimal incisional separations.

As more sophisticated monitoring, better antibiotics, better suture material and techniques, and a safer blood supply have become more available, selective use of combined gynecologic procedures and plastic surgical removal of the panniculus is increasing. In a study of patients who had a mean weight of 261 lb, Morrow et al. found no operative mortality and a mean hospital stay of 8.2 days. Only 11% of the patients required transfusion. The investigators in this series emphasized that the panniculectomy should be performed initially to improve exposure.

Although removal of a large panniculus results in better exposure, patient selection for this potentially morbid procedure should be carefully considered. Also, the patient must be counseled and must be strongly motivated to lose weight and change her nutritional habits. If the patient is not committed to these lifestyle changes, it seems impractical to perform an extensive abdominoplastic procedure and incur the associated morbidity. If the surgical procedure is not urgent, an alternative would be to defer the procedure until the patient has achieved 40% to 50% of the planned weight loss.

Patients who have large diastasis recti in association with the panniculus are also candidates for this procedure, at which time plication of the rectus fascia should be performed, either directly or using a "vest-over-pants" layered technique. In many instances, the rectus abdominoplasty is as much a cosmetic and therapeutic benefit to the patient as is the panniculectomy. When both anatomic conditions exist, the panniculectomy alone does not give a satisfactory surgical result.

Of the various operative techniques available for panniculectomy and abdominoplasty, the elliptical transverse incision, originally described by Kelly, has proved to be the procedure of choice. Two modifications of the transverse panniculectomy can be useful. The most common procedure includes an elliptical "watermelon" incision (Fig. 14.20A), extending from the lateral aspect of the lumbar regions to about 3 to 4 cm above the umbilicus. If the patient requests the preservation of the umbilicus, it can be excised and transplanted to the upper pedicle of skin. However, as shown by Cosin and colleagues, this transplantation can lead to increased wound complications. Inferiorly, the transverse incision follows the concave skinfold that separates the overhanging panniculus from the suprapubic skin. The underlying fat is excised deeply in a slightly wedged manner, with the deep portion of the fat extending outward and slightly beyond the skin margin to avoid ischemia of the skin edge. Meticulous attention must be given to absolute hemostasis (a time-consuming procedure) to avoid postoperative hematoma formation and infection. The excessive use of cautery, which produces a favorable environment for bacterial growth in devitalized tissue, should be avoided. The lateral angles of the incision may require separate "V" incisions to avoid the unsightly folds of redundant fat (Fig. 14.20B). When these V-shaped wedges are closed, the angle of the incision is converted into a Y-shaped configuration, which eliminates the excessive skin in the lateral aspects of the abdominal wall. After the removal of the large panniculus, the abdomen can be opened either transversely or vertically. A vertical incision has been advocated to improve exposure. If an abdominoplasty is required to approximate widely separated rectus muscles, a midline incision is necessary. In this way, a tight closure of the rectus fascia or a vest-over-pants repair, as shown in Figure 14.20D–E, gives additional strength to the abdominal wall. If the rectus fascia is of poor quality and does not provide adequate support to the abdominal wall, a mesh graft can be inserted at the completion of the procedure, either anterior or posterior to the rectus muscle (discussed below). If the fascia of the rectus sheath can be plicated in the midline, wide plication and anchoring of the medial margins of the rectus muscle can be used to close the diastasis, resulting in a firm abdominal wall.

A second type of transverse panniculectomy is a "W" technique, initially described by Regnault in 1975 and shown in Figure 14.20C. The incision is outlined before the operative procedure in the form of a "W" over the symphysis pubis, inside the hairline. The incision is started in the center of the mons pubis and extended laterally and downward on each side to the

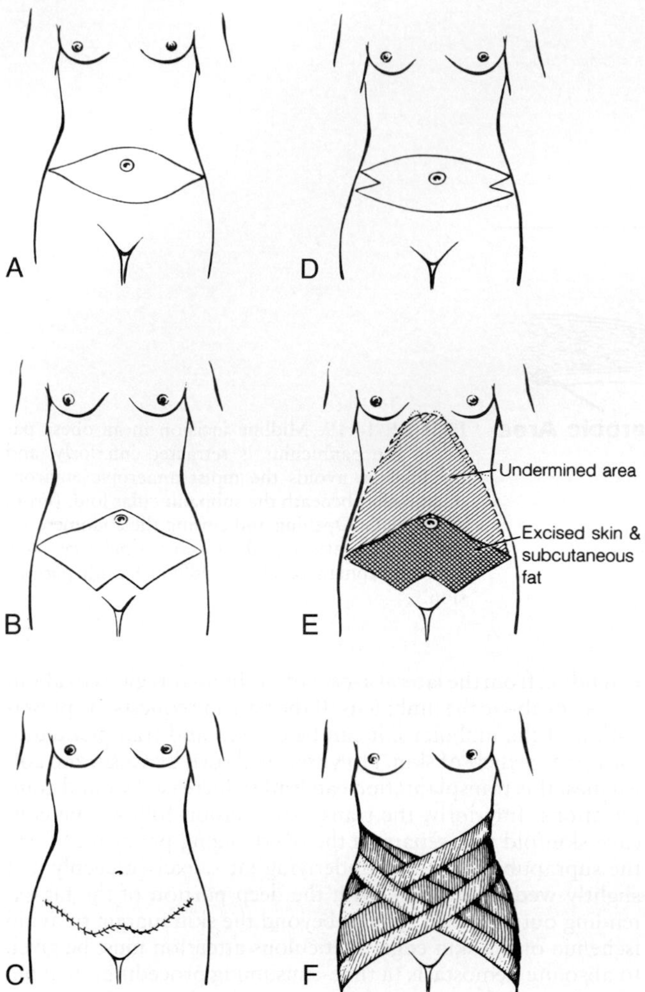

FIGURE 14.20. Panniculectomy incisions. **A:** Elliptical transverse incision extending from region of iliac crest passes above and below umbilicus. **B:** V-shaped incision in lateral angles eliminates folds of skin in abdominal wall. **C:** W-shaped incision over the mons pubis extends along the inguinal ligament to the iliac crest. **D:** The upper incision passes above the umbilicus. Wide mobilization of the upper skin flap is carried to the sternum and rib margins. **E:** After removal of panniculus and skin, the upper skin flap is sutured without tension to the lower skin margin. **F:** A firm elastic dressing is crisscrossed over the abdominal wall for abdominal support and prevention of seroma formation.

inguinal fold near the external inguinal ring. The line then follows above the inguinal ligament in the panniculus skin crease to the region of the iliac crest on each side of the pelvis. The upper margin of the incision is drawn above the umbilicus to the upper margin of the redundant fat. If the umbilicus is to be relocated, the new umbilical site is drawn in the upper skin flap before the incision is made, and the umbilicus is transposed to the upper skin flap after the incision is closed.

In closing the W-shaped incision of Regnault after the abdominal or pelvic operation is completed, the upper flap of the abdominal skin is mobilized superficial to the fascia as far as necessary to the region of the xiphoid process and to the inferior margin of the costochondral junctions of the rib cage (Fig. 14.20D). A thin layer of fat is left attached to the fascia to facilitate the postoperative absorption of serous fluid. As shown in Fig. 14.20E, the upper skin flap is sutured to the W-shaped pubic skin margins, using interrupted sutures of 2-0 delayed-absorbable suture for the subcutaneous fat. Multiple fine sutures are used to anchor the skin flap to the fascia to prevent seroma formation and loculation. Closed-suction drainage is always used beneath the upper skin flap and left in place until the drainage is less than 50 mL per day. If the upper skin flap cannot reach the pubic skin without excessive tension, the patient is placed in a slightly jackknife position on the operating table by having the upper portion of the table elevated and the legs maintained in a straight horizontal position. When the skin margins have been approximated over the pubis and along the inguinal ligament, additional V-shaped incisions can be taken from the lateral angles of the incision when redundant skin is present.

The skin is closed with staples or 3-0 polypropylene interrupted sutures, which are left in place for at least 2 weeks. Rather than being removed all at once, alternate staples can be removed over a period of several days and replaced with adhesive reinforced surgical tape (e.g., Steri-Strips). A firm elastic-based tape dressing (e.g., Elastoplast) is applied under tension over the abdominal wall in a crisscross manner, beginning at the rib cage and extending to the thighs (Fig. 14.20F). This abdominal support relieves tension on the suture line and also prevents seroma and hematoma formation beneath the skin flaps. Another technique is to use an abdominal binder (or multiple binders placed end to end) to support the anterior abdominal wall and prevent seroma and hematoma formation.

INCISIONS FOR EXTRAPERITONEAL APPROACHES

Although controversial as a routine surgical procedure, the value of a staging laparotomy to assess paraaortic lymph nodes in patients with advanced stage (IIB to IV) cervical cancer has been studied extensively over the past two decades. As the stage of disease increases, the incidence of positive paraaortic nodes is progressively higher and has prompted organizations such as the Gynecologic Oncology Group to require paraaortic node sampling before placing patients with advanced cervical cancer on some phase III studies. Serious bowel complications have been observed in cervical cancer patients who have had operative evaluation through a transperitoneal approach followed by radiotherapy. When extraperitoneal approaches to evaluate paraaortic lymph nodes are compared with transperitoneal approaches before radiation therapy, more serious, later-occurring small bowel problems are associated with the latter approach (Wharton et al., 1977). To avoid these complications, an extraperitoneal approach has been advocated by means of bilateral superior groin incisions, a unilateral J-shaped incision, or an upper-abdominal incision.

We use the J-shaped incision or the "sunrise" incision for staging. If bulky pelvic nodes are evident or paraaortic nodes contain metastases, these can be removed without entering the peritoneum and may improve patient response to therapy (Downey et al., 1989). Irradiation with concurrent chemotherapy can then be safely used, starting almost immediately.

J-Shaped Incision

A modification of the extraperitoneal inguinal incision (a modified Gibson incision) was described in the gynecologic

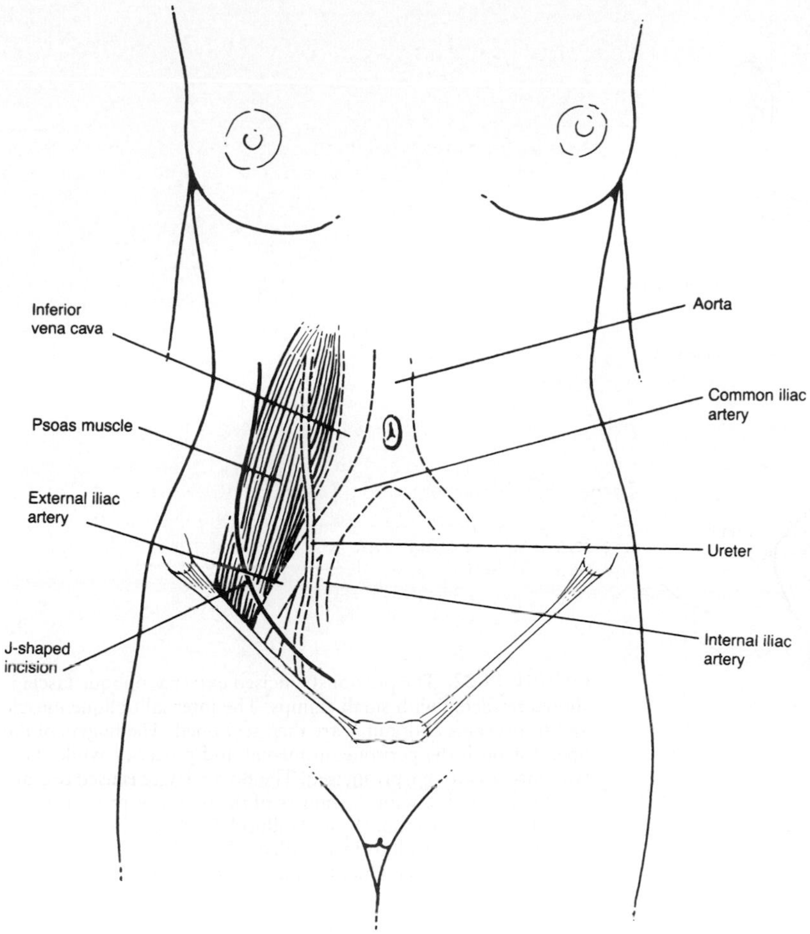

FIGURE 14.21. J-shaped incision on the right is shown in relation to deeper structures, the ureter, iliac vessels, and great vessels. It is initiated about 3 cm cephalad to the umbilicus and is carried inferiorly parallel to the round ligament. (From Gallup DG. Abdominal incisions and closures. In: Gallup DG, Talledo OE, eds. *Surgical atlas of gynecologic oncology.* Philadelphia: WB Saunders, 1994:43, with permission.)

literature by Berman and colleagues in 1977. These investigators prefer to make the skin incision on the left, because the left paraaortic lymphatic channels are lateral and posterior to the aorta. They believe that it is technically more feasible to dissect the precaval nodes from a left-sided incision if a single incision is to be used for extraperitoneal paraaortic node sampling. We prefer to make the incision on the right, as discussed later.

Access is gained by a vertical incision, starting just cephalad to the umbilicus and 3 cm medial to the right iliac crest. Caudad to the crest, the incision is carried medially, about 3 cm cephalad and parallel to the inguinal ligament (Fig. 14.21). The fascial layers are incised separately (Fig. 14.22). Exposure of the extraperitoneal space is achieved by rolling the peritoneum medially and cephalad (Fig. 14.23). The round ligament and inferior epigastric vessels can be ligated and transected to improve exposure. The paraaortic area is exposed by blunt dissection, and node sampling is performed by removing the precaval fat pad over the vena cava. With a Deaver retractor on the medial and cephalad portion of the incision, paraaortic nodes can be sampled to the level of the inferior mesenteric artery, directly anterior and lateral to the aorta.

In the left-sided approach, left paraaortic node dissection is more easily accomplished. Berman and colleagues described lifting the peritoneum from the underlying vena cava to resect the precaval fat pad. They cautioned that gentle traction must be used when dissecting the precaval nodes to avoid injury to the inferior mesenteric vessels and also suggested that the table should be tilted toward the patient's right to facilitate dissection.

The inferior vena cava lies relatively posterior to the aorta, and we have experienced technical difficulties in removing precaval nodes through a left-sided approach. In a later updated report from the same institution, Ballon and associates observed that 2 of 95 patients had avulsion of the inferior mesenteric artery (repaired without sequelae). In addition to the relative difficulty in sampling right-sided nodes, the lower portion of a J-shaped incision lies in future radiation fields in some patients.

Sunrise Incision

Because there is a delay in initiation of irradiation by some radiation oncologists when a midline incision is used for staging, Gallup and colleagues have subsequently used a supraumbilical incision to remove paraaortic nodes extraperitoneally. In this small reported series, the mean number of paraaortic nodes removed was 12.2, and the mean operating time was 111 minutes. All but 2 of 20 patients underwent external-beam irradiation within 2 weeks of the operative procedure (Fig. 14.24).

The sunrise skin incision is initiated in a transverse manner about 4 to 6 cm cephalad to the umbilicus (Fig. 14.25). It is carried laterally in a downward fashion to the level of the iliac

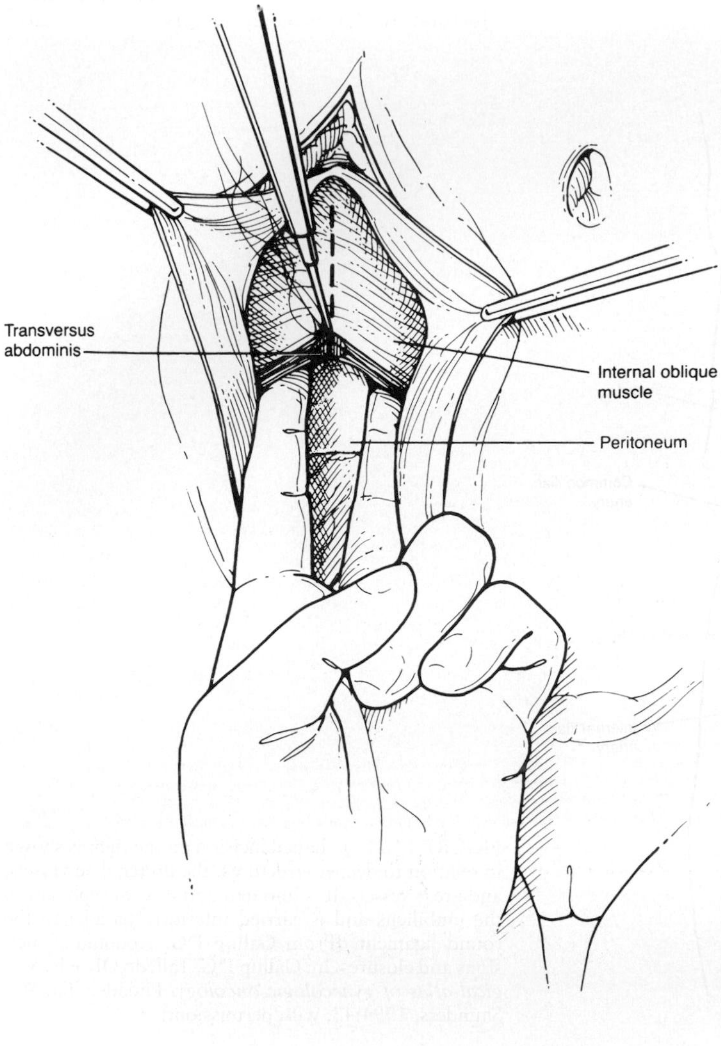

FIGURE 14.22. The previously incised external oblique fascia is shown retracted with small clamps. The internal oblique muscle and transversus abdominis are then sectioned. The fingers of the operator push the peritoneum medial and posterior while these two muscles are sharply incised. The Bovie device is used to transect these muscles, with the fingers of the operator protecting the underlying peritoneum. (From Gallup DG. Abdominal incisions and closures. In: Gallup DG, Talledo OE, eds. *Surgical atlas of gynecologic oncology.* Philadelphia: WB Saunders, 1994:43, with permission.)

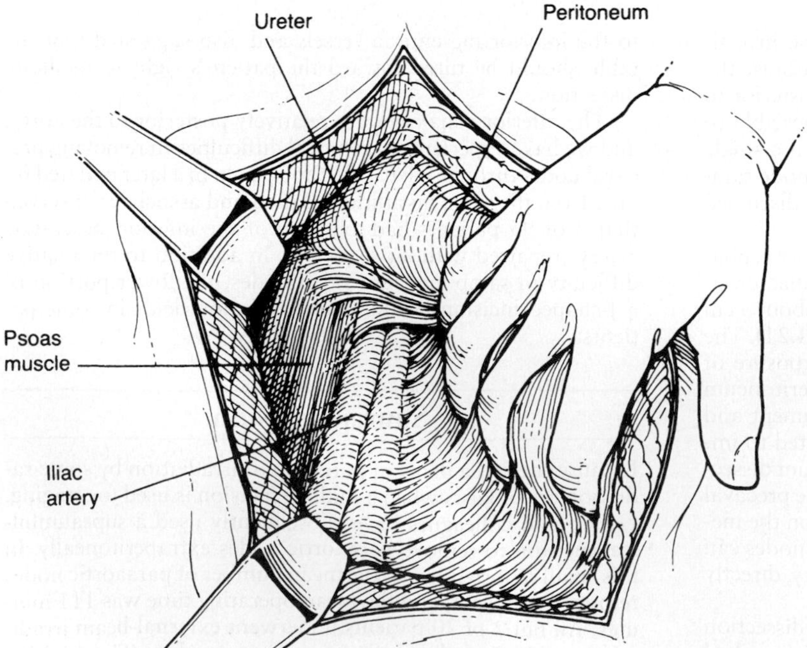

FIGURE 14.23. With the round ligament sectioned, the peritoneum is bluntly dissected by the hand of the operator. The psoas muscle is palpated, as is the external iliac artery lying medial to the psoas. The peritoneum is gently swept from lateral and caudad to medial and cephalad. This maneuver easily exposes the psoas muscle and the pelvic vessels. The ureter remains on the medial left of the retracted peritoneum. (From Gallup DG. Abdominal incisions and closures. In: Gallup DG, Talledo OE, eds. *Surgical atlas of gynecologic oncology.* Philadelphia: WB Saunders, 1994:43, with permission.)

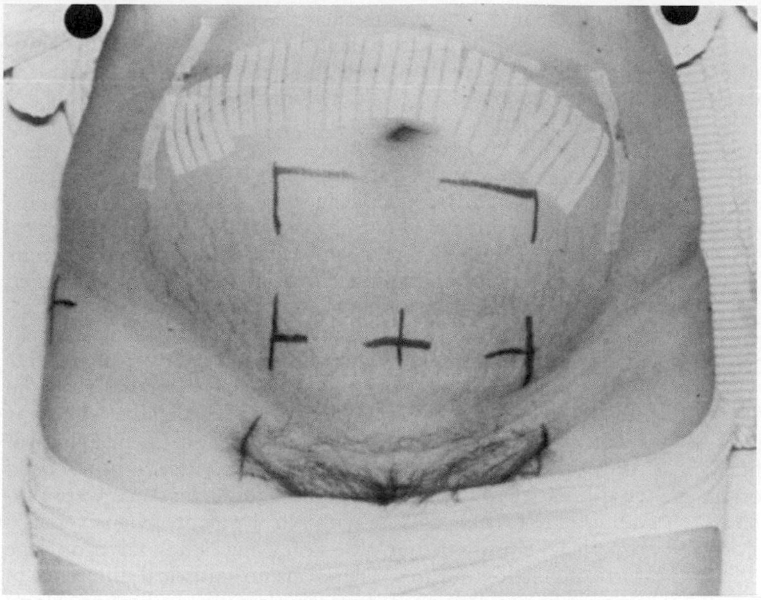

FIGURE 14.24. The sunrise incision made 3 days before this illustration shows Steri-Strips approximating the skin. The radiation field in this postoperative patient has been outlined for early irradiation after a staging procedure for carcinoma of the cervix. (From Gallup DG. Opening and closing the abdomen and wound healing. In: Gershenson D, Curry S, DeCherney A, eds. *Operative gynecology.* 1st ed. Philadelphia: WB Saunders, 1993:127, with permission.)

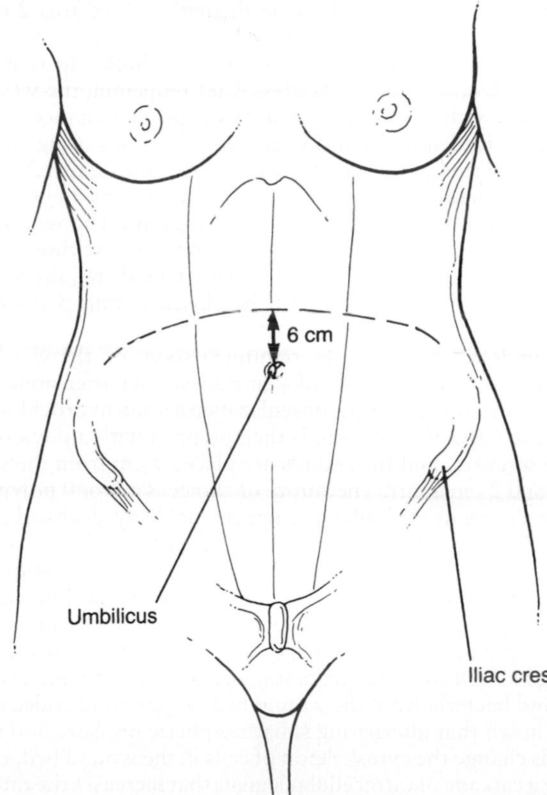

FIGURE 14.25. For an extraperitoneal approach to paraaortic nodes, we prefer to use the sunrise incision. In the center, this incision is about 6 cm above the umbilicus. The incision is carried laterally and downward to the level of the iliac crests. In the event of palpable bulky disease in the lower common iliac or pelvic nodes, the incision can be extended caudad to remove the nodes. (From Gallup DG. Abdominal incisions and closures. In: Gallup DG, Talledo OE, eds. *Surgical atlas of gynecologic oncology.* Philadelphia: WB Saunders, 1994:43, with permission.)

crests. Preoperatively, the site of the supraumbilical incision can be estimated and varied by placing a radiopaque object at the level of the umbilicus during intravenous contrast computed tomography (CT) to estimate the level of the bifurcation of the aorta. In thin patients, a unilateral incision, usually performed on the right side, can be used, and adequate exposure to both sides of the aorta can be obtained. In the event of bulky disease in the lower common iliac or pelvic nodes, the incision can be extended in a caudad fashion to remove these nodes. The advantage of pelvic node debulking in cervical cancer patients, who were later irradiated, has been reported by Downey and associates.

Once the skin and subcutaneous tissue are incised, the fascia is also incised transversely. After the rectus muscles are dissected free from their attachments to the anterior fascia, they are transected with a Bovie device. In relatively obese patients, the left rectus is also transected for adequate exposure to the left paraaortic nodes. Because the deep epigastric vessels lie posterior to, and in the center of, the rectus muscle at this level, the vessels do not need to be isolated separately. Any bleeding can be controlled with ligation or cautery. With the rectus transected, the transversus abdominis muscle is located on the right and is incised with scissors or cautery. The peritoneum is retracted medially and cephalad by the hand of the surgeon. The incision into the transversus is extended more inferiorly and laterally to complete the transection of this muscle without entering the peritoneum. The fingers of the surgeon stretch the wound to ensure adequate exposure.

The surgeon's hand is inserted deep into the incision until the psoas and external iliac vessels are palpated. The peritoneum is bluntly dissected from caudad and lateral to cephalad and medial, separating it from the underlying common iliac vessels until the great vessels are exposed. This maneuver is similar to that illustrated in Fig. 14.23, except the peritoneum is swept more cephalad. If the peritoneum is entered during any of these maneuvers, it should be closed immediately. A self-retaining retractor can be inserted to retract the right ureter and ovarian vessels to avoid injury. The precaval nodes, located within the fat pad over the vena cava, are then resected in the usual manner by using vascular clips and scissors and a "clip-cut" technique.

In thin patients, the paraaortic nodes lateral and anterior to the aorta can be removed through a right abdominal approach. If exposure is limited, however, the left rectus muscle can be transected and the peritoneum mobilized from the left side as previously described.

When node dissection is completed, a closed drainage system (Jackson-Pratt or Blake) may be brought out cephalad to the incision through a stab wound. If both spaces are opened, the drains are placed bilaterally in the extraperitoneal spaces, with the fascia and skin closed in the usual manner.

DELAYED PRIMARY CLOSURE AND SECONDARY CLOSURE

The value of delayed primary wound closure in managing possible contaminated wounds has been recognized by military surgeons for many years. In 1968, Grosfeld and Solit reported that patients with perforating appendicitis had a reduction in wound infection rates from 34.1% to 2.3% when delayed closure was used. Similarly, in a high-risk group of patients—which included patients with obesity, cancer, possible contamination from above-and-below procedures, infection, and bowel content contamination—Brown and colleagues found a marked reduction in wound infection rates when delayed primary closure was used compared with immediate closure in matched patients. The infection rate for the former group was 2.1%; for the latter, 23.3%. Possible candidates for such a closure include patients with suppurative appendicitis, ruptured tuboovarian abscess, extensive bowel injury in the unprepared bowel, or diverticulitis with contamination. Delayed closure can also be of value in select patients who have groin incisions associated with radical vulvectomy procedures.

After closure of the fascia, the wound is irrigated with copious amounts of saline. Some investigators prefer to then spray the wound with a combined broad-spectrum antibiotic spray. Vertical interrupted mattress sutures of No. 3 nylon or No. 3 monofilament polypropylene are placed 2 to 3 cm apart. They are loosely tied over dilute povidone-iodine dressing gauze. The wound dressing sponges are changed two to three times a day with a wet-to-dry technique, using sterile saline or 0.1% Dakin's solution (sodium hypochlorite). Some surgeons use bridges, consisting of rolled gauze on the lateral borders of the incision, to support these sutures. In 4 to 5 days, depending on the appearance of granulation tissue in the subcutaneous tissues, the previously placed sutures are tied to approximate the skin edges. Tincture of benzoin is placed at the lateral edges of the closed incision, and Steri-Strips are used to approximate uneven skin edges.

Alternatively, the skin edges of the incision can be closed with widely spaced staples, "wicking" the intervening spaces with saline-soaked gauze (e.g., Nu-gauze or Kerlex strips). Once adequate granulation tissue is present, the skin edges can be reapproximated with nonabsorbable monofilament sutures and local lidocaine at the patient's bedside before discharge from the hospital.

Superficial separation of layers anterior to the fascia is usually associated with wound infections, seromas, or hematomas. Many centers suggest opening the wound, usually the entire length; obtaining appropriate cultures for antibiotic choice; and allowing healing by second intention, with once- or twice-daily wound-dressing changes. Although most cleansing in a second-intention scenario is accomplished by home health care personnel, patients are inconvenienced by this method. A trend in many centers and practices has been to perform delayed closure after a period of 2 to 5 days. In 1988, in a prospective randomized study, Hermann and associates found that secondary closure, performed 2 days after wound drainage had ceased, resulted in a significant reduction in healing time when compared with healing by second intention.

In a larger series of patients on an obstetrics and gynecology service, Walters and colleagues found a similar advantage in delayed closure of wounds. In 35 patients who underwent reclosure, 85.7% had their wounds successfully closed. Patients in this study had abdominal incisions that had been opened owing to infection, hematoma, or seroma. The fascia was intact in all patients, and all patients had wound debridement and cleansing for a minimum period of 4 days. All patients in this series had reclosure performed in the operating room and received three doses of cefazolin. The closure was done by an en bloc technique, using No. 2 monofilament nylon sutures. In a series from the University of Mississippi (Dodson et al.), patients with extrafascial wound dehiscence were randomized to en bloc closure with No. 1 polypropylene versus a superficial closure through the skin using No. 2 polypropylene vertical mattress sutures. There was no statistical difference in the number of days needed to complete wound healing. However, the en bloc group required longer time for closure, and these patients experienced more pain. Of note, none of these patients received prophylactic antibiotics, and all wounds were reclosed under local anesthesia in the patient care area 2 to 6 days after reopening the wound.

Our technique for reclosing wounds is similar to that reported by Dodson and associates. After reopening the wound in patients with extrafascial dehiscence, the subcutaneous tissues are debrided daily, and wet-to-dry dressings using sterile saline are placed in the wound two to three times daily. Antibiotics are generally not used unless the patient has a concomitant infection (e.g., cellulitis or cuff infection). The wound is closed when a healing bed of granulation tissue without exudate or necrotic debris is present. Many wounds require sharp debridement, but most can still be closed within 5 days of reopening.

Wounds are closed in the treatment room on the ward or in the office with local 1% lidocaine anesthesia after premedication with 50 mg of intramuscular meperidine hydrochloride or similar narcotic. The skin is then prepped with a povidone-iodine solution, and the sutures are placed 1 cm from the skin edges and 2 cm apart. The suture of choice is a No. 0 polypropylene suture or a similar permanent or delayed absorbable suture. We leave the sutures in for 2 weeks.

An alternative to secondary closure is the utilization of vacuum-assisted closure device (VAC). This method utilizes a pump, a spongelike material and alternating negative pressure, and rest periods to pull the edges of the wound together, optimizing blood flow, reducing tissue edema, and removing excess fluid and bacteria from the wound bed. Venturi and colleagues have shown that alternating subatmospheric pressure and rest periods change the cytoskeleton of cells in the wound bed, triggering a cascade of intracellular signals that increases the rate of cell division and subsequent formation of granulation tissue.

COMPLETE WOUND DEHISCENCE AND EVISCERATION

Technically, wound dehiscence means separation of all layers of the abdominal incision, but wound dehiscence has been subdivided based on the layers of tissue that have separated. Incomplete or partial dehiscence (superficial dehiscence) means separation of the skin and all tissue layers posterior to the skin, sometimes including the fascia. However, if the disruption includes the peritoneum, the disruption is called a complete dehiscence. Should the intestine protrude through the wound, the term *evisceration* (also a burst abdomen) is used. The frequency of fascial dehiscence ranges between 0.3% and 3% of all cases of pelvic surgery.

Evisceration is one of the most feared and dangerous postoperative complications. The mortality rate associated with evisceration has been to be reported as high as 35% and is usually associated with other complications, such as sepsis. However, Helmkamp's 10-year study noted a mortality rate of only 2.9% in 70 cases, which may reflect improved supportive care available for these patients in recent years. Evisceration is less likely to occur in gynecology patients than in general surgery patients.

Older studies reported that the type and location of the incision and the type of suture used were major causative factors in evisceration. However, many of the predisposing factors for complete wound disruption or evisceration are metabolic and include malnutrition, poorly controlled diabetes, corticosteroid use, and older age. Mechanical factors associated with dehiscence and evisceration include obesity, intraabdominal distention (including rapid postoperative reaccumulation of ascites), infection, retching, and coughing. In addition, any process that can impair wound healing, such as radiotherapy or chemotherapy, can contribute to an increased risk for wound disruption. As noted, complete wound dehiscence and evisceration are usually problems associated with tissue failure and not suture failure. Rollins and associates noted that about half of their patients with serious wound complications had prior abdominal or pelvic surgery. In the series reported by Jurkiewicz and Morales, 88% of eviscerated wounds had tearing of suture through the fascia, with knots and suture intact. Thus, large loose sutures with secure knots are always preferable to tight strangulating sutures that cause ischemia of the incision margin.

Eviscerations usually occur from day 5 to 11 after operation, with a mean of about 8 days. One of the early signs of complete dehiscence and impending evisceration is the seepage of serosanguineous pink discharge from an apparently intact wound. It can be present for several days before evisceration occurs. Although occult hematomas are usually the cause of such discharge, these wounds need to be examined carefully by probing with a cotton-tipped swab to assess the integrity of the fascial closure. Frequently, the patient is conscious of something giving way, "tearing" or "popping" immediately before the burst abdomen becomes clinically apparent.

With few exceptions, complete dehiscence or eviscerations should be closed as soon as they are recognized. In case of evisceration, when a delay of several hours is anticipated because of a recent meal, the bowel can be replaced by using sterile gloves, gently packing it in place with lap pads soaked in saline, and securing it with an abdominal binder. Broad-spectrum antibiotics should be initiated, and baseline blood counts and serum electrolyte studies should be obtained.

Closing an evisceration should be performed in the operating room (never on the floor) and always under general anesthesia so that the extent of the dehiscence may be determined. Necrotic tissue clots and suture material should be removed, and aerobic and anaerobic cultures should be obtained. The bowel and omentum should be inspected and thoroughly

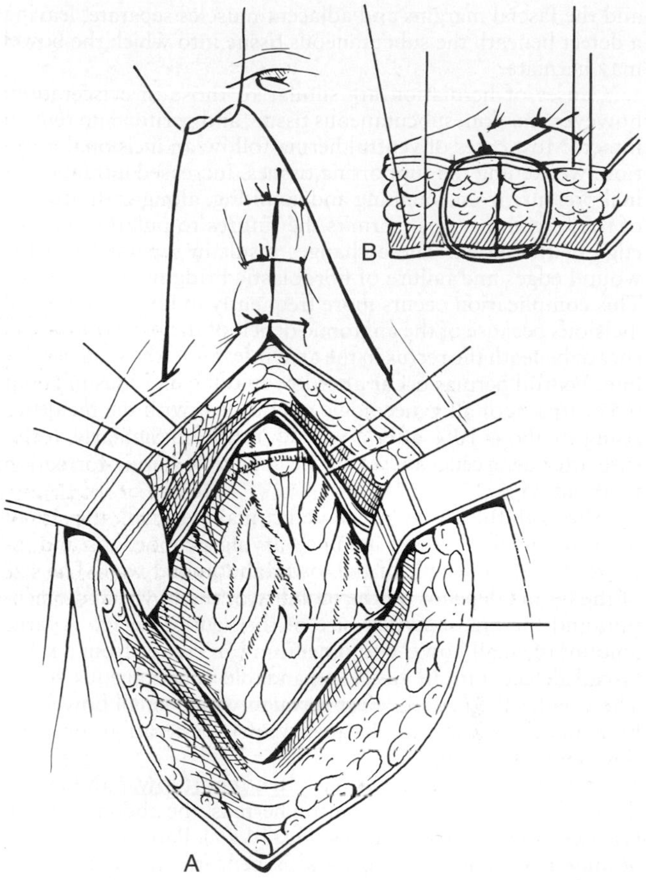

FIGURE 14.26. **A:** Secondary closure of an evisceration with through-and-through silver wire and preferably No. 2 polypropylene sutures. **B:** All layers are incorporated.

cleansed with several liters of warm normal saline. If the fascial margins can be located and are not ragged, a Smead-Jones closure (Fig. 14.16) with large-bore polypropylene or nylon can be used. The subcutaneous tissue and skin are packed open for later delayed closure or VAC placement.

If the wound edges are ragged or the patient's condition is poor, a through-and-through retention suture of No. 2 nylon or polypropylene is used. The sutures are placed at least 2.5 to 3 cm from the skin edges and are passed through all layers. To allow for edema, they are placed 2 cm apart (Fig. 14.26). To prevent inclusion of the underlying intestine in a suture, all sutures are held up before the first one is tied. Skin edges unopposed between the through-and-through sutures can be approximated with interrupted 3-0 polypropylene. The through-and-through sutures should be left in place for 3 weeks. A nasogastric tube should be used in the immediate postoperative period to avoid abdominal distention, and broad-spectrum antibiotics should be continued and modified according to culture results.

INCISIONAL HERNIA

Incomplete healing of an operative wound will result in an incisional hernia. In this situation, the peritoneum remains intact, and the fascial margins and adjacent muscles separate, leaving a defect beneath the subcutaneous tissue into which the bowel may herniate.

Causes of herniation are similar to those of evisceration; however, the skin, subcutaneous tissue, and peritoneum remain intact. Most cases of ventral hernia follow an incisional infection, weakening the supporting tissues. Increased intraabdominal pressure from coughing and vomiting, along with necrosis of the fascial margins, permits the sutures to pull through the edge of the fascia. These changes result in separation of the wound edges and failure of fibroblastic bridging of the fascia. This complication occurs more frequently in lower-abdominal incisions because of the anatomic deficit of the posterior fascial sheath beneath the rectus in the area inferior to the semicircular line. Ventral hernias occur after low midline incisions in about 0.5% to 1% of all gynecologic operations, with the incidence rising to about 10% after a wound infection. Similarly, reclosure after dehiscence increases the chance of hernia formation to about 25%.

Although the initial fascial defect may be small, the size of the resultant hernia can assume varying proportions and involve the entire length of the lower-abdominal wall. The size of the hernia depends on the mobility of the bowel and omentum and the final aperture size of the ventral defect. A large amount of small bowel and omentum can escape from a small fascial defect into an easily expandable subcutaneous space. The smaller the fascial defect through which small bowel can herniate, the greater the frequency of incarceration, obstruction, and infarction.

Patients with ventral hernias often report lower-abdominal discomfort, and with large ventral hernias, the abdominal wall is distended to varying degrees (Fig. 14.27). Patients with large hernias may note bowel peristalsis beneath the skin and report that the bulge becomes smaller when they are in a recumbent position. The hernia is more noticeable during coughing and straining and can increase in size over time because of enlargement of the hernial ring or incorporation of additional segments of bowel into the hernial sac. Rarely, a ventral hernia produces acute symptoms of visceral torsion, incarceration, and infarction. Repair of the hernia is preferably done on an elective basis.

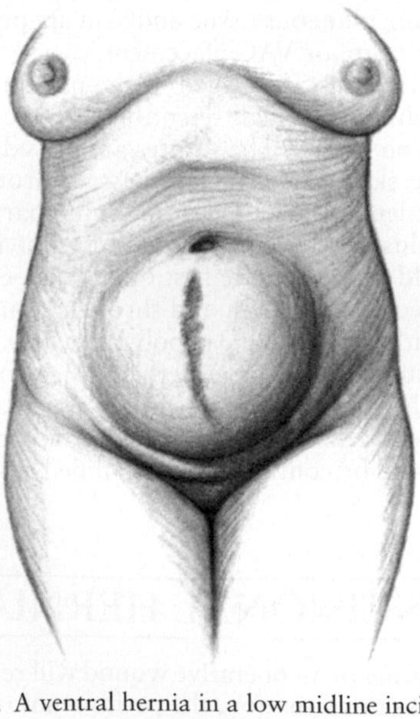

FIGURE 14.27. A ventral hernia in a low midline incision.

Surgical Management of Small Hernias

The principles of ventral hernia repair include (a) dissection of the hernia sac from the subcutaneous fat, rectus fascia, and peritoneal margin; (b) excision of the redundant hernia (peritoneal) sac; and (c) closure of the abdominal wound, using a layer-for-layer closure, an overlap repair of the rectus fascia, or the placement of a synthetic mesh prosthesis.

The low midline incisional scar is excised, and the underlying subcutaneous fat is mobilized free from the adjacent hernia sac. Sharp dissection is used to separate the skin and underlying fat widely from the margins of the hernia sac (Fig. 14.28A). The surgeon should defer opening the sac until the boundaries of the hernia have been delineated and dissected, because this aids in identifying the various tissue planes. To identify the margins of the fascial ring, it is advisable to open the sac and separate any underlying bowel from the peritoneal surface of the sac (Fig. 14.28B). Loops of small bowel and adherent omentum frequently obscure the true identity of the sac, and many pockets of the peritoneal lining are formed by fibrous bands that anchor the bowel to the peritoneum. After releasing the omentum and bowel, with particular attention given to hemostasis, it is important to determine whether the hernia defect can be adequately closed with the adjacent fascia before excising the line of the sac. If adequate fascial tissue remains after the dissection, either a layer-for-layer or an overlap fascial closure should be done. If inadequate fascia is available to close, the defect must be bridged with a synthetic mesh. However, most incisional hernias can be closed without the use of a mesh support. When there has been failure of an initial hernia repair, when the hernia defect is so large that the edges cannot be adequately approximated, or when the tissues of the abdominal wall are attenuated, the use of synthetic mesh is strongly advised.

The layer-for-layer closure is accomplished after closure of the peritoneum as the initial layer. The fascial margins of the anterior rectus sheath are then sutured with nonabsorbable or delayed absorbable suture (Fig. 14.28C). Interrupted far-near, near-far pulley sutures (modified Smead-Jones) that include the inner margin of the abdominal musculature are placed to avoid subsequent pull-through of the suture from the edge of the incision. These sutures serve as internal stay sutures and increase the tensile strength of the wound while healing takes place.

When there is adequate fascial margin of good strength, a vest-over-pants closure gives extra support to the defect and produces a double-layer closure of the fascia (Fig. 14.28D). The surgeon should separate the peritoneum and posterior rectus sheath from the hernia margins to permit an overlap of the anterior fascia. The peritoneum is closed separately with a continuous suture of No. 2-0 delayed-absorbable suture of polyglactin material. The anterior rectus sheath of the hernia margins is separated widely on each side of the wound. Horizontal mattress sutures of a permanent suture (such as polypropylene) are placed 3 to 4 cm distant from the fascial edge and pass through the free margin of the opposite fascia before returning to the distal portion of the anterior fascia. The sutures are held untied until all sutures have been placed. When the sutures are tied, the free fascial margin is drawn firmly beneath the opposite fascial layer, producing a double support to the hernia closure. The

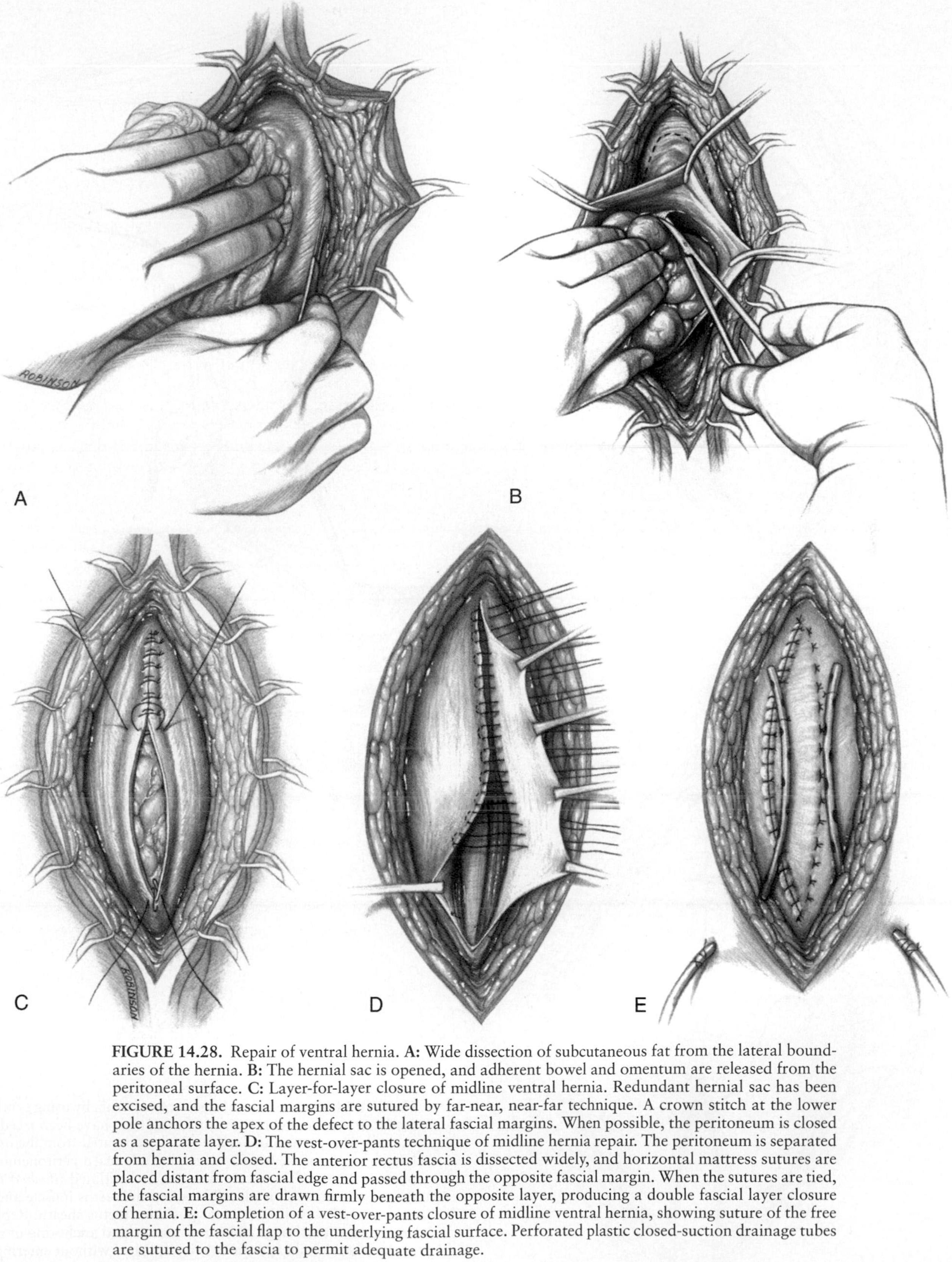

FIGURE 14.28. Repair of ventral hernia. **A:** Wide dissection of subcutaneous fat from the lateral boundaries of the hernia. **B:** The hernial sac is opened, and adherent bowel and omentum are released from the peritoneal surface. **C:** Layer-for-layer closure of midline ventral hernia. Redundant hernial sac has been excised, and the fascial margins are sutured by far-near, near-far technique. A crown stitch at the lower pole anchors the apex of the defect to the lateral fascial margins. When possible, the peritoneum is closed as a separate layer. **D:** The vest-over-pants technique of midline hernia repair. The peritoneum is separated from hernia and closed. The anterior rectus fascia is dissected widely, and horizontal mattress sutures are placed distant from fascial edge and passed through the opposite fascial margin. When the sutures are tied, the fascial margins are drawn firmly beneath the opposite layer, producing a double fascial layer closure of hernia. **E:** Completion of a vest-over-pants closure of midline ventral hernia, showing suture of the free margin of the fascial flap to the underlying fascial surface. Perforated plastic closed-suction drainage tubes are sutured to the fascia to permit adequate drainage.

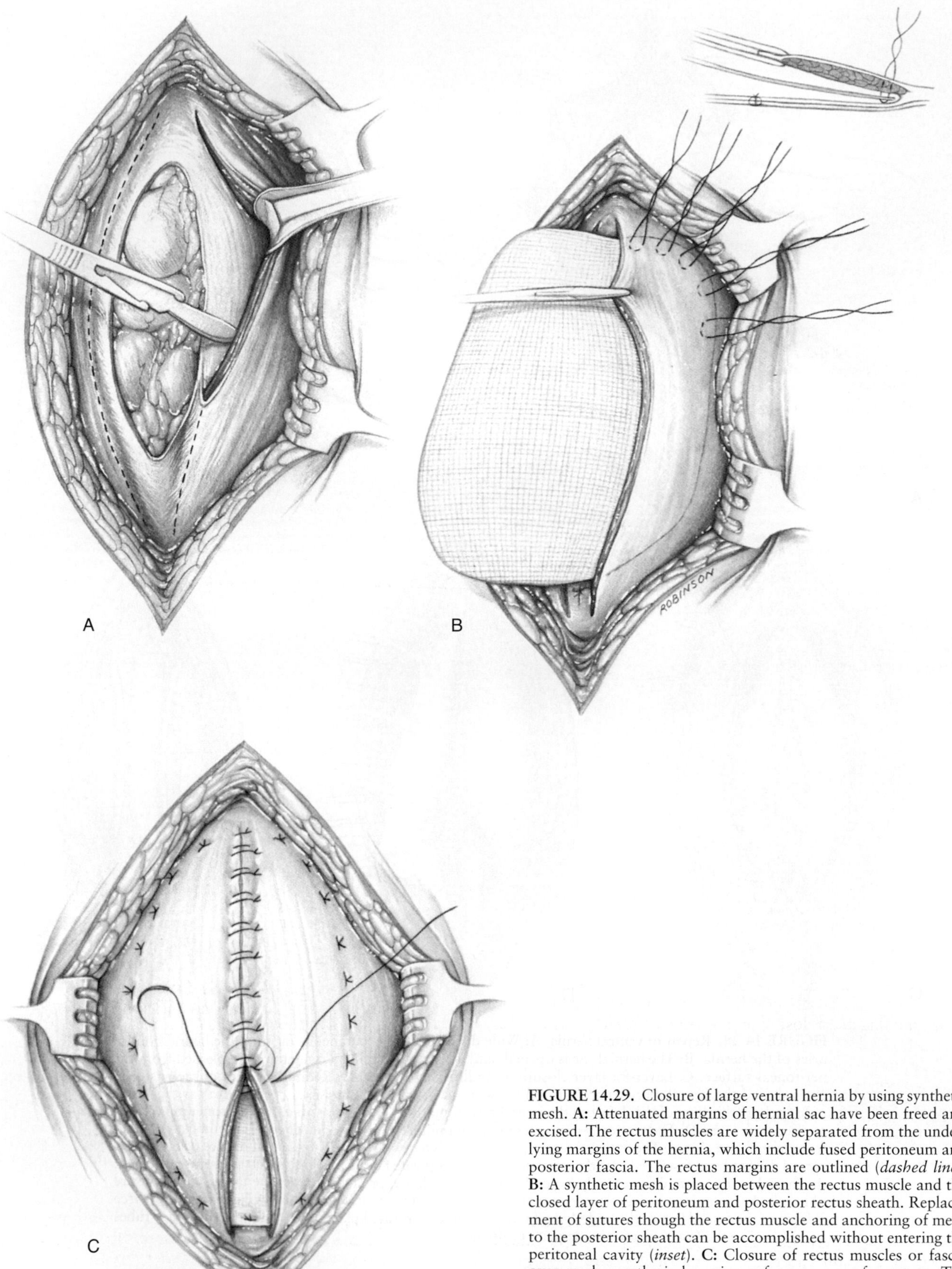

FIGURE 14.29. Closure of large ventral hernia by using synthetic mesh. **A:** Attenuated margins of hernial sac have been freed and excised. The rectus muscles are widely separated from the underlying margins of the hernia, which include fused peritoneum and posterior fascia. The rectus margins are outlined (*dashed line*). **B:** A synthetic mesh is placed between the rectus muscle and the closed layer of peritoneum and posterior rectus sheath. Replacement of sutures though the rectus muscle and anchoring of mesh to the posterior sheath can be accomplished without entering the peritoneal cavity (*inset*). **C:** Closure of rectus muscles or fascia over mesh prosthesis by using a far-near, near-far suture. The margins of the mesh show the width of the permanent hernial support.

remaining free fascial margin is sutured to the fascial surface (Fig. 14.28E) to complete the double-layer closure.

When closure of the fascial margins is complete, Jackson-Pratt or Blake drains can be inserted beneath the skin flaps for subsequent drainage (Fig. 14.28E). Penrose drains should not be used. The drains should exit through a separate stab incision in the skin several centimeters away from the primary incision.

Surgical Management of Large Hernias

In repairing a ventral hernia with a large fascial defect and poor abdominal tissue, it may be necessary to reinforce the hernia defect with a synthetic mesh. When using mesh, it is important to dissect the hernia sac as previously described and to define the layers of the abdominal wall carefully (Fig. 14.29A). Because of the placement of a foreign body in the abdominal incision, meticulous hemostasis and aseptic technique are essential. The implanted mesh must completely bridge the entire defect, with adequate margins for suturing to the adjacent rectus muscles.

After the hernia sac is removed and the margins of the fascial defect are freed, the rectus muscle is released from the underlying posterior fascial sheath and peritoneum (Fig. 14.29A). The fascia and peritoneum beneath the rectus muscle should be dissected widely around the margins of the defect to permit closure of the peritoneum without tension. A large piece of mesh is then inserted between the rectus muscle and the closed peritoneum (Fig. 14.29B). Lateral sutures are placed to anchor the mesh to the fascia so that the mesh does not buckle when the overlying rectus muscles are approximated in the midline. Nonabsorbable sutures are used to anchor the mesh to the rectus abdominis muscle. Closure of the rectus fascia over the mesh is then attempted, using the far-near, near-far closure technique (Fig. 14.29C).

If the rectus muscles or fascia cannot be approximated in the midline without undue tension, several other approaches may be used to repair these large herniae. These surgical techniques use a series of relaxing incisions in the anterior abdominal wall fascia to allow the surgeon to reapproximate the fascial edges over the defect. Again, when using these techniques, careful attention to hemostasis is paramount. In the fascial partition method, the subcutaneous tissue is widely dissected, anterior to the rectus fascia and lateral to the rectus musculature. Parasagittal incisions (Fig. 14.30A) are then made in both the external oblique fascia (several centimeters lateral to the rectus musculature) and transverse abdominis fascia (just lateral to the rectus musculature—care must be taken not to injure the inferior epigastric vasculature in this region) to mobilize tissue lateral to the fascial defect. The fascia may then be closed with either running mass closure or interrupted Smead-Jones sutures (Fig. 14.30B).

The sliding myofascial flap uses relaxing incisions in the external oblique fascia only (Fig. 14.31A). These relaxing incisions are made lateral to the rectus musculature, from the level of the lowest rib to the inguinal ligament. Further dissection laterally is completed with a combination of blunt and sharp dissection and carried as far as possible (Fig. 14.31B). Once adequately mobilized, the peritoneum and fascia are closed in a Smead-Jones fashion (Fig. 14.31C).

Should the subcutaneous tissues be "wet," a closed-suction drainage system may be placed longitudinally on either side of the fascial incision and the subcutaneous fat and skin closed separately. Suction is applied to the drainage tubes to give negative pressure beneath the skin and prevent elevation of the skin flaps by serum or blood. The drains may be removed by day 5 but must be left in place until there has been complete cessation of incisional drainage.

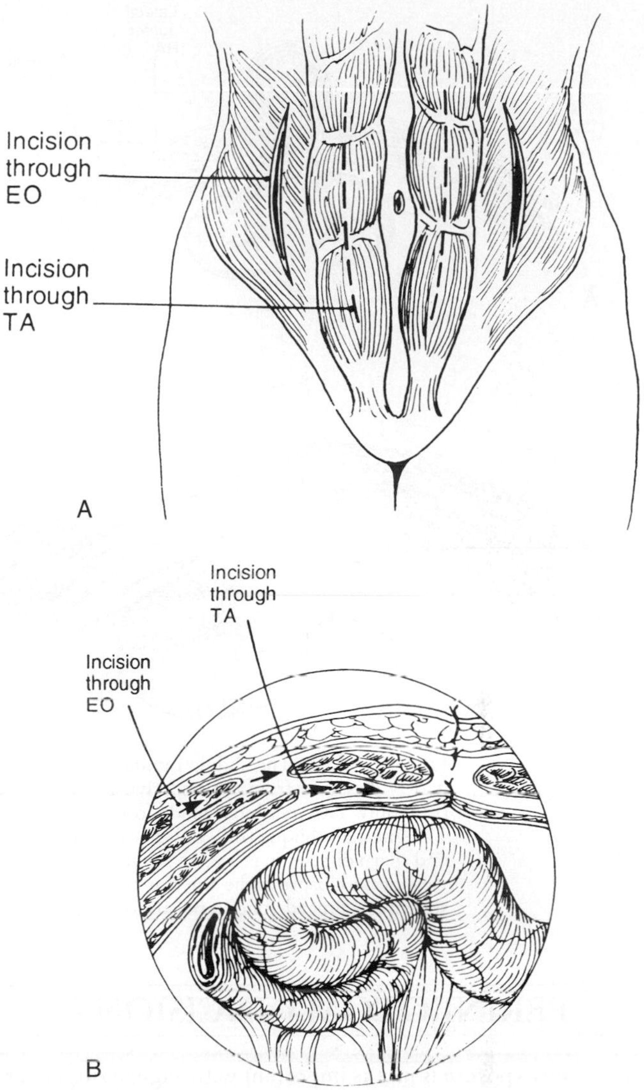

FIGURE 14.30. In the fascial partition method, relaxing incisions are made that allow wide mobilization of the fascia. **A:** Parasagittal relaxing incisions are placed through the external oblique (EO), lateral to the rectus muscles. The *dotted line* denotes similarly placed incisions in the transverse abdominis (TA) muscles. **B:** This cross-sectional view demonstrates location of the incisions with a closure of either an interrupted or Smead-Jones type.

Postoperatively, the patient is ambulated on the day after surgery, without prolonged bed rest. The abdominal incision should be protected from excessive strain (e.g., coughing) by use of an elastic abdominal binder. If the bowel becomes distended, the use of nasogastric tube decompression should be considered (but is rarely needed). Prophylactic antibiotics are used perioperatively to prevent secondary infection in the operative site and are particularly useful in patients in whom mesh has been used for closure of a large hernia defect. Alternatively, many incisional hernias are being repaired by general surgeons using a laparoscopic approach rather than reincision.

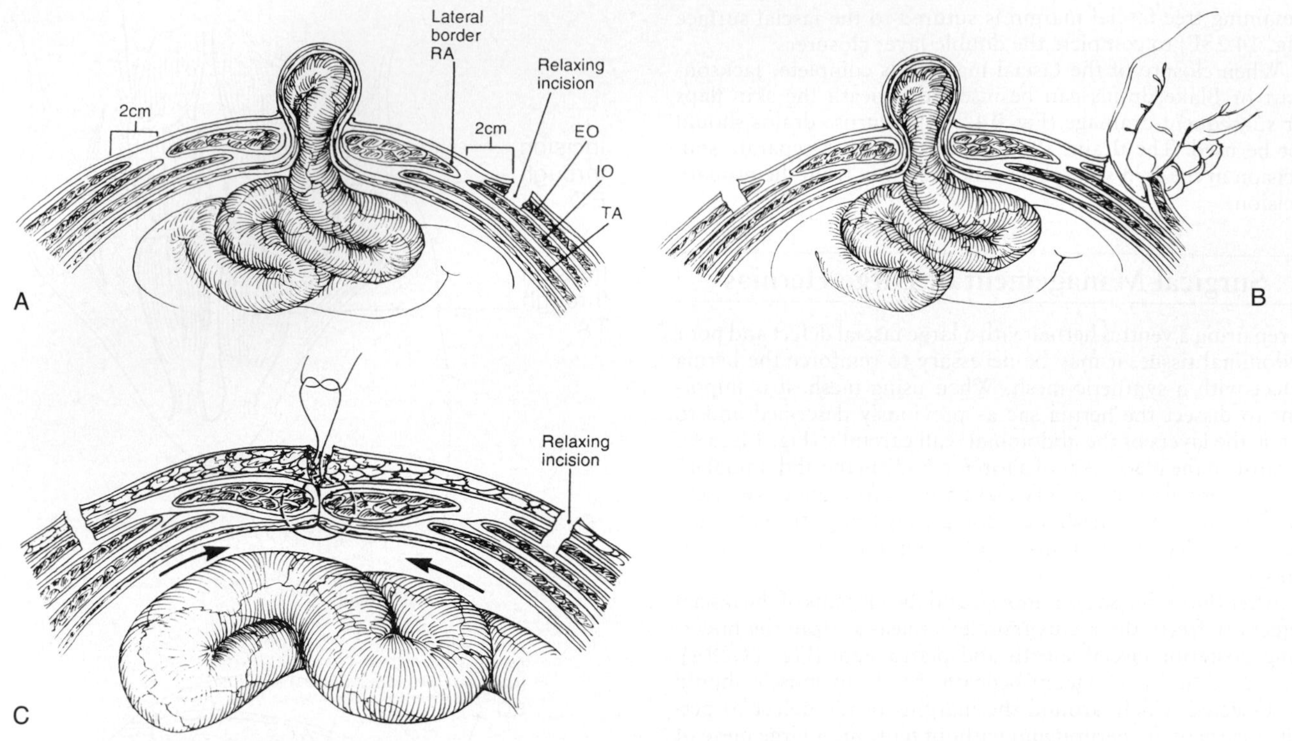

FIGURE 14.31. The sliding myofascial flap. **A:** Initially, the subcutaneous tissues must be sharply and widely dissected from the underlying fascia. A vertical relaxing incision is made in the external oblique (EO) only. This incision is made from the level of the lowest ribs to just cephalad to the inguinal ligament. The internal oblique (IO) and the transverse abdominis (TA) are not incised. **B:** A combination of blunt and sharp dissection is used to separate the EO from the IO as far laterally as possible. **C:** A cross-sectional view of the closure of the anterior abdominal wall after performing the sliding myofascial flap. The closure shown is a Smead-Jones type, although an interrupted mass closure may be used.

PERINEOTOMY INCISIONS

Adequate exposure is just as important with vaginal surgery as it is with abdominal surgery. When exposure is not adequate with abdominal operations, the incision is extended, or some other measure is used to improve exposure. Certain measures also can improve exposure with vaginal operations. A tight vaginal introitus may restrict exposure of the upper vagina but can be enlarged at the beginning of the operation by making a midline or mediolateral episiotomy incision. A mediolateral incision can be made on one or both sides of the vaginal introitus. If a midline episiotomy is made and closed transversely, the vaginal introitus can be made larger than before, if that is deemed advisable. These incisions can be closed with 2-0 or 3-0 delayed-absorbable suture.

Sometimes the entire vagina is small in caliber because of virginity or nulliparity, atrophic shrunken vaginal mucosa, previous colporrhaphy, or previous irradiation or disease. The vaginal vault may be fixed in a relatively high position, with relatively little descensus. Because adequate exposure through the vagina may be impossible, some operations may require an abdominal approach. On the other hand, required exposure may be obtained by making a Schuchardt incision. The entire vagina can be enlarged with this incision, achieving remarkable improvement in exposure of the upper vagina. Therefore, a patient whose problem might otherwise have necessitated an abdominal approach can have the advantage of a perfectly satisfactory vaginal operation if a Schuchardt incision is made.

According to Speert (1958), Langenbeck made a deep relaxing incision into the perineal body in attempting vaginal hysterectomy for uterine cancer in 1828. Similar incisions were used by Olshausen in 1881 and Duhrssen in 1891. Karl Schuchardt described his incision in 1893:

> to make more accessible from below a uterus whose mobility is limited.... With the patient in the lithotomy position and her buttocks elevated, a large, essentially sagittal incision is made, somewhat convex externally, beginning between the middle and posterior third of the labium majus, ... extending posterior toward the sacrum, and stopping two fingerbreaths [*sic*] from the anus. The wound is deepened only in the fatty tissue of the ischiorectal fossa, leaving the funnel of the levator ani muscle, the rectum behind it, and the sacral ligaments intact. Internally, the sidewall of the vagina is opened into the ischiorectal fossa and the vagina divided in its lateral aspect by a long incision extending up to the cervix. There thus results a surprisingly free view of all the structures under consideration.

The incision is ordinarily made on the patient's left side by a right-handed operator (Fig. 14.32). A left-handed operator may find it technically easier to make the incision on the patient's right side. Bilateral incisions have been advocated in extreme cases. The side on which the incision is made may be dictated by the location of the pathology to be removed. Injection of the tissues to be incised with sterile saline solution can be helpful, especially beneath the vaginal mucosa in the line of the incision. The assistant pulls upward to the left with the index finger placed as deep as possible in the vagina just to the left of the urethra. The operator makes countertraction

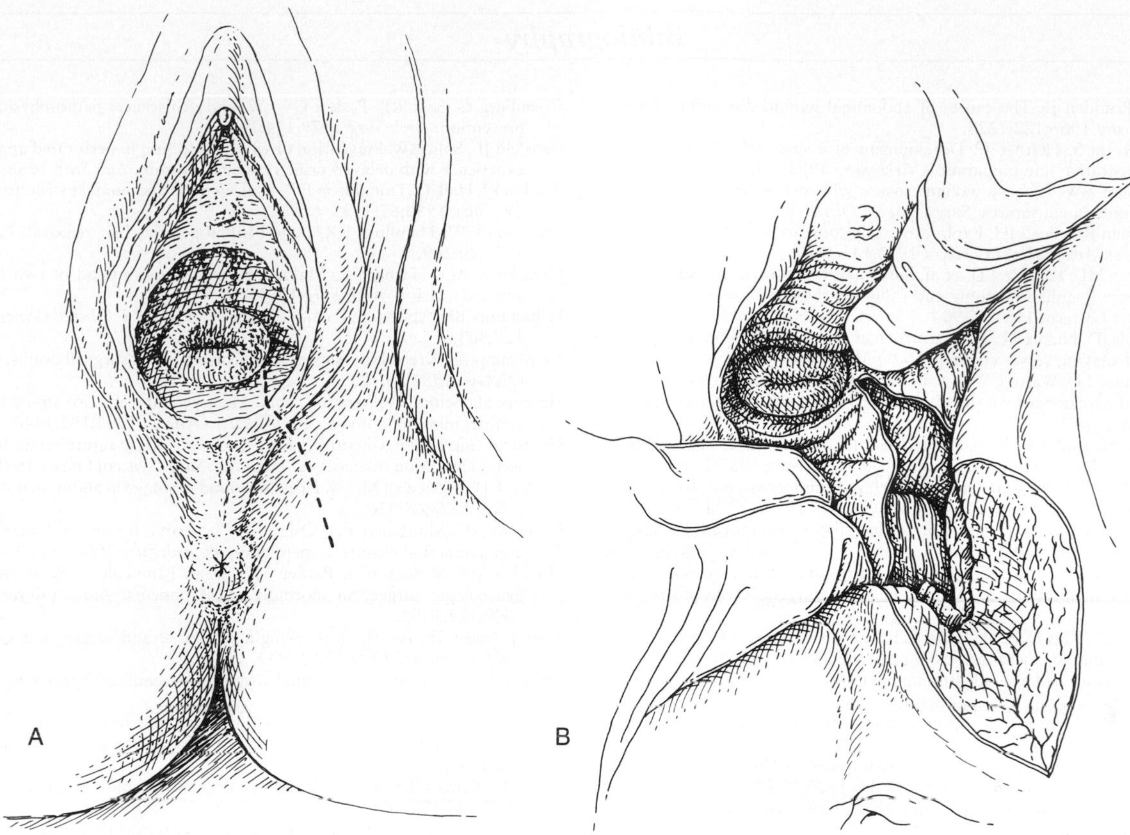

FIGURE 14.32. **A:** The Schuchardt incision begins at the 4-o'clock position in the vaginal introitus and extends into the buttock and up the posterolateral wall of the vagina to the cervix. **B:** The ischiorectal fossa fat is exposed. The puborectalis muscle is divided. The left paravesical and pararectal spaces can be exposed through the incision.

by placing two fingers in the vagina and pulling downward to the right. This pull and counterpull in opposite directions stretches the left vaginal wall. The incision is made with the electrosurgical unit beginning at the 4-o'clock position at the introitus and extending downward in the skin of the buttock to the level of the anus. The incision is then carried upward through the vaginal mucosa into the upper third of the vagina. As the incision is deepened, the fingers of the operator's left hand are used to displace the rectum medially to protect it from injury. The ischiorectal fossa fat is visible below the puborectalis muscle, which is incised with the electrosurgical knife (Fig. 14.32). If necessary, the left paravesical space can be developed. For the best possible exposure, the apex of the vaginal incision should intersect any incision made around the cervix, achieving hemostasis by coagulation or ligation.

At the end of the operation, the Schuchardt incision is closed with 2-0 and 3-0 delayed-absorbable sutures, attempting to reapproximate the puborectalis muscle edges and to obliterate the dead space in the ischiorectal fossa. Drainage of these incisions is usually not necessary.

The Schuchardt incision most often is used for extensive vaginal hysterectomy for early invasive cervical cancer. We also have used it when performing extensive dissections to remove endometriosis in the vaginal vault, to gain better exposure for difficult vaginal hysterectomy or vesicovaginal fistula repair, to repair injuries to the lower ureter, to remove organized hematomas just above the puborectalis muscle, to drain lymphocysts vaginally, or to remove benign cystic teratomas in the lower presacral area behind the rectum. It can convert a technically difficult, complicated, and dangerous vaginal operation into one that is simple, easy, and safe. It is difficult to understand why perineotomy incisions are so quickly performed for obstetric operations and so reluctantly for gynecologic operations.

BEST SURGICAL PRACTICES

- During counseling for surgery, location of the incision, rationale, and any potential complications must be presented to the patient.
- Fascial closures (of midline and some transverse incisions) should be accomplished with delayed absorbable monofilament suture. Plain catgut or chromic catgut should *never* be used for fascial closures.
- Closed drainage systems (i.e., Jackson-Pratt or Blake) should be used when drains are considered. Passive drains, such as Penrose drains, should not be used.
- To prevent surgical site infections, hair removal should be done by clipping and *not* by shaving.
- Monofilament sutures should be tied with either three square knots (six throws) or one surgeon's knot and two square knots (four throws).
- For superficial dehiscence, consider delayed closure or vacuum-assisted device closure over secondary-intention closure with wet to dry dressing changes for improved patient healing. Delayed closure in the office may be less expensive and more convenient for the patient compared to VAC.

Bibliography

Alexander HC, Prudden JF. The causes of abdominal wound disruption. *Surg Gynecol Obstet* 1966;122:1223.

Alexander JW, Aerni S, Plettner JP. Development of a safe and effective one-minute preoperative skin preparation. *Arch Surg* 1985;120:1367.

Archie JP, Feldman RW. Primary wound closure with permanent continuous running monofilament sutures. *Surg Gynecol Obstet* 1981;153:721.

Averette HE, Dudan RC, Ford JH. Exploratory celiotomy for surgical staging of cervical cancer. *Am J Obstet Gynecol* 1972;133:1090.

Ballon SL, Berman ML, Lagasse LD, et al. Survival after extraperitoneal pelvic and paraaortic lymphadenectomy and radiation therapy in cervical carcinoma. *Obstet Gynecol* 1981;57:90.

Balthazar ER, Colt JD, Nicols RL. Preoperative hair removal: a random prospective study of shaving versus clipping. *South Med J* 1982;75:799.

Berman ML, Lagasse LD, Watring WG, et al. The operative evaluation of patients with cervical carcinoma by an extraperitoneal approach. *Obstet Gynecol* 1977;50:658.

Bourne RB, Bitar H, Andrese PR, et al. In-vivo comparison of four absorbable sutures: Vicryl, Dexon Plus, Maxon and PDS. *Can J Surg* 1988;31:43.

Brown SE, Allen HH, Robins RN. The use of delayed primary wound closure in preventing wound infections. *Am J Obstet Gynecol* 1977;127:213.

Cherney LS. A modified transverse incision for low abdominal operations. *Surg Gynecol Obstet* 1941;72:92.

Cosin JA, Powell JL, Donovan JT, et al. The safety and efficacy of extensive abdominal panniculectomy at the time of pelvic surgery. *Gynecol Oncol* 1994;55:36.

Cox PJ, Ausobsky JR, Ellis H, et al. Towards no incisional hernias: lateral paramedian versus midline incisions. *J R Soc Med* 1986;79:711.

Cruse PJE. Infection surveillance: identifying the problem and the high-risk patient. *South Med J* 1977;70[Suppl 1]:40.

Cruse PJE, Foord R. A five year prospective study of 23,649 surgical wounds. *Arch Surg* 1973;107:206.

Cruse PJE, Foord R. The epidemiology of wound infection: a 10-year prospective study of 62,939 wounds. *Surg Clin North Am* 1980;60:27.

Daversa B, Landers D. Physiologic advantages of the transverse incision in gynecology. *Obstet Gynecol* 1961;17:305.

Dineen P. A critical study of 100 conservative wound infections. *Surg Gynecol Obstet* 1961;113:91.

Dodson MK, Magann EF, Sullivan DL, et al. Extrafascial wound dehiscence: deep en bloc closure versus superficial skin closure. *Obstet Gynecol* 1994;83:142.

Dougherty SH, Simmons RL. The biology of surgical drains. *Curr Probl Surg* 1992;9:648.

Downey GO, Potish RA, Adcock LL, et al. Pre-treatment surgical staging in cervical carcinoma: therapeutic efficacy of pelvic lymph node dissection. *Am J Obstet Gynecol* 1989;160:1055.

Edlich RF, Panek RH, Rodeheaver GT, et al. Physical and chemical configuration of suture in the development of surgical infection. *Ann Surg* 1973;177:679.

Ellenhorn JDI, Smith DD, Schwarz RE, et al. Paint-only is equivalent to scrub-and-pain in preoperative preparation of abdominal surgery sites. *J Am Coll Surg* 2005;201:737.

Ellis H, Heddle R. Does the peritoneum need to be closed at laparotomy? *Br J Surg* 1977;64:733.

Fagniez P, Hay JM, Lacaine F, et al. Abdominal midline incisions closure: a randomized prospective trial of 3,135 patients, comparing continuous vs. interrupted polyglycolic acid sutures. *Arch Surg* 1984;120:1351.

Farnell MB, Worthington-Self S, Mucha P Jr, et al. Closure of abdominal incisions with subcutaneous catheters. *Arch Surg* 1986;126:641.

Fletcher HS, Joseph WL. Bleeding into the rectus abdominis muscle. *Int Surg* 1973;58:97.

Galle PC, Homesley HD, Rhyne AL. Reassessment of the surgical scrub. *Surg Gynecol Obstet* 1978;147:214.

Gallup DG. Extraperitoneal and transperitoneal approaches for removal of retroperitoneal pelvic and paraaortic lymph nodes. In: Thompson JP, Rock JA, eds. *Te Linde's operative gynecology updates*. 8th ed. Philadelphia: JB Lippincott Co, 1993:1.

Gallup DG. Modification of celiotomy techniques to decrease morbidity in obese gynecologic patients. *Am J Obstet Gynecol* 1984;150:171.

Gallup DG, Jordan GH, Talledo OE. Extraperitoneal lymph node dissections with use of a midline incision in patients with female genital cancer. *Am J Obstet Gynecol* 1986;155:559.

Gallup DG, King LA, Messing MJ, et al. Paraaortic lymph node sampling by means of an extraperitoneal approach with a supraumbilical transverse "sunrise" incision. *Am J Obstet Gynecol* 1993;169:307.

Gallup DG, Nolan TE, Smith RP. Primary mass closure of midline incisions with a continuous polyglyconate monofilament absorbable suture. *Obstet Gynecol* 1990;76:872.

Gallup DG, Talledo OE, King LA. Primary mass closure of midline incisions with a continuous running monofilament suture in gynecologic patients. *Obstet Gynecol* 1989;73:67.

Greenburg G, Salk RP, Peskin GW. Wound dehiscence: patho-physiology and prevention. *Arch Surg* 1979;114:143.

Grosfeld JL, Solit RW. Prevention of wound infection in perforated appendicitis: experience with delayed primary wound closure. *Ann Surg* 1968;168:891.

Guillou PJ, Hall TJ, Donaldson DR, et al. Vertical abdominal incisions: a choice? *Br J Surg* 1980;67:359.

Hamilton HW, Hamilton KR, Lone FJ. Preoperative hair removal. *Can J Surg* 1977;20:269.

Hasselgren AO, Harbery E, Malmer H, et al. One instead of two knifes for surgical incision. *Arch Surg* 1984;118:917.

Helmkamp BF. Abdominal wound dehiscence. *Am J Obstet Gynecol* 1977; 128:803.

Helmkamp BF, Krebs HB, Amstey MS. Correct use of surgical drains. *Contemp Ob/Gyn* 1984;23:123.

Hendrix SL, Schimp V, Martin J, et al. The legendary superior strength of Pfannenstiel incision: a myth? *Am J Obstet Gynecol* 2000;182:1446.

Hermann GG, Bagi P, Christofferson I. Early secondary suture versus healing by second intention of incisional abscesses. *Surg Gynecol Obstet* 1988;167:16.

Higson RH, Kettlewell MGW. Parietal wound drainage in abdominal surgery. *Br J Surg* 1978;65:326.

Hodgson NC, Malthaner RA, Ostbye T. The search for an ideal method of abdominal fascial closure: a meta-analysis. *Ann Surg* 2000;231(3):436.

Hopkins MP, Shriner AM, Parker MG, et al. Panniculectomy at the time of gynecologic surgery in morbidly obese patients. *Am J Obstet Gynecol* 2000;182:1502.

Hurt J, Unger JB, Ivy JJ, et al. Tying a loop-to-strand suture: is it safe? *Am J Obstet Gynecol* 2005;192:1094.

Jenkins TPN. The burst abdominal wound: a mechanical approach. *Br J Surg* 1976;63:873.

Jurkiewicz MJ, Morales L. Wound healing, operative incisions, and skin grafts. In: Hardy JD, ed. *Hardy's textbook of surgery*. Philadelphia: JB Lippincott Co, 1983:108.

Keill RH, Keitzer WF, Henzel J, et al. Abdominal wound dehiscence. *Arch Surg* 1973;106:573.

Kelly HA. Excision of the fat of the abdominal wall: lipectomy. *Surg Gynecol Obstet* 1910;10:229.

Kenady DE. Management of abdominal wounds. *Surg Clin North Am* 1984; 64:803.

Knight CD, Griffen FD. Abdominal wound closure with a continuous monofilament polypropylene suture. *Arch Surg* 1983;118:1305.

Krebs HB, Helmkamp F. Transverse periumbilical incision in the massively obese patient. *Obstet Gynecol* 1984;63:241.

Krupski WC, Sumchai A, Effeney DJ, et al. The importance of abdominal wall collateral blood vessels. *Arch Surg* 1984;119:854.

Küstner O. Der suprasymphysare kreuzschnitt, eine methode der coeliotomie bei wenig umfanglichen affektioen der weiblichen beckenorgane. *Monatsschr Geburtsh Gynakol* 1896;4:197.

Langer K. Cleavage of the cutis (the anatomy and physiology of the skin): presented at the Meeting of the Royal Academy of Sciences, April 25, 1861. *Clin Orthop* 1973;91:3.

Lineweaver W, Howard R, Soucy D, et al. Topical antimicrobial toxicity. *Arch Surg* 1985;120:1985.

Macht SC, Krizek TJ. Sutures and suturing: current concepts. *J Oral Surg* 1978;36:240.

Maylard AE. Direction of abdominal incision. *Br Med J* 1907;2:895.

McBurney C. The incision made in the abdominal wall in cases of appendicitis, with a description of a new method of operating. *Ann Surg* 1894;20:38.

McDowell E. Three cases of extirpation of diseased ovaria: 1817. *Am J Obstet Gynecol* 1995;172:1632.

McMinn RMH, Hutchings RJ, Logan BM. *Color atlas of applied anatomy*. Chicago: Mosby Year Book, 1984:110.

Mead PB. Managing infected abdominal wounds. *Contemp Ob/Gyn* 1979;14:69.

Mendenez MA. The contaminated wound. In: O'Leary JP, Waltering EA, eds. *Techniques for surgeons*. New York: John Wiley and Sons, 1985:36.

Metz SA, Chegini N, Masterson BJ. In vivo tissue reactivity and degradation of suture materials: a comparison of Maxon and PDS. *J Gynecol Surg* 1989;5:37.

Montz FJ, Creasman WT, Eddy G, et al. Running mass closure of abdominal wounds using an absorbable looped suture. *J Gynecol Surg* 1991;7:107.

Morris DM. Preoperative management of patients with evisceration. *Dis Colon Rectum* 1982;25:249.

Morrow CP, Hernandez WL, Townsend DE, et al. Pelvic celiotomy in the obese patient. *Am J Obstet Gynecol* 1977;127:335.

Moss JP. Historical and current perspective on surgical drainage. *Surg Gynecol Obstet* 1981;152:517.

Mowat J, Bonnar J. Abdominal wound dehiscence after cesarean section. *Br Med J* 1971;2:256.

Moylan JA, Kennedy B. The importance of gown and drape barriers in the prevention of wound infection. *Surg Gynecol Obstet* 1980;151:465.

Murray DH, Blaisdell FW. Use of synthetic absorbable sutures for abdominal and chest wound closures. *Arch Surg* 1978;113:477.

Nelson JH, Boyce J, Macasaet M, et al. Incidence, significance, and follow-up of para-aortic lymph node metastases in late invasive carcinoma of the cervix. *Am J Obstet Gynecol* 1977;128:336.

Olson M, O'Connor MO, Schwartz ML. A 5-year prospective study of 20,193 wounds at Minneapolis VA Medical Center. *Ann Surg* 1984;199:253.

Parsons L, Ulfelder H. *Atlas of pelvic surgery*. 2nd ed. Philadelphia: WB Saunders, 1968:156.

Peterson AF, Rosenberg A, Alatary SO. Comparative evaluation of surgical scrub preparation. *Surg Gynecol Obstet* 1978;146:63.

Pfannenstiel JH. Uber die vortheile des suprasymphysaren fascienguerschnitt fur die gynaekologischen koeliotomien. *Samml Klin Vortr Gynaekol (Leipzig) Nr 268,* 1900;97:1735.

Pitkin RM. Abdominal hysterectomy in obese women. *Surg Gynecol Obstet* 1976;142:532.

Postlethwait RW. Long-term comparative study of nonabsorbable sutures. *Ann Surg* 1970;171:892.

Pratt JH. Wound healing: evisceration. *Clin Obstet Gynecol* 1973;16:126.

Pratt JH, Irons B. Panniculectomy and abdominoplasty. *Am J Obstet Gynecol* 1978;132:165.

Rees VL, Coller FA. Anatomic and clinical study of the transverse abdominal incision. *Arch Surg* 1943;47:136.

Regnault P. Abdominoplasty by the W technique. *Plast Reconstr Surg* 1975; 55:265.

Richards PC, Balch CM, Aldrete JS. Abdominal wound closure. *Ann Surg* 1983; 197:238.

Rodeheaver GT, Powell TA, Thacker JG, et al. Mechanical performance of monofilament synthetic absorbable sutures. *Am J Surg* 1987;154:544.

Rollins RA, Corcoran JJ, Gibbs CE. Treatment of gynecologic wound complications. *Obstet Gynecol* 1966;28:268.

Sanz LE, Smith S. Mechanism of wound healing, suture material, and wound closure. In: Buchsbaum HJ, Walton LA, eds. *Strategies in gynecologic surgery*. New York: Springer Verlag, 1986:53.

Sanz LE, Patterson JA, Kamath R, et al. Comparison of Maxon suture with Vicryl, chromic catgut, and PDS sutures in fascial closure in rats. *Obstet Gynecol* 1988;71:918.

Savage RC. Abdominoplasty combined with other surgical procedures. *Plast Reconstr Surg* 1982;70:437.

Schuchardt K. Eine neue Methode der Gebarmutterexstirpation. Sentralbl Chir 1893;20:1121.

Scott HW, Law HD, Sandstead HH, et al. Jejunoileal shunt in surgical treatment of morbid obesity. *Ann Surg* 1970;171:770.

Seropian R, Reynolds BM. Wound infections after preoperative depilatory versus razor preparation. *Am J Surg* 1971;121:251.

Shepherd JH, Cavanagh D, Riggs D, et al. Abdominal wound closure using a nonabsorbable single-layer technique. *Obstet Gynecol* 1983;61:248.

Shull BL, Verheyden CN. Combined plastic and gynecologic procedures. *Ann Plast Surg* 1988;20:252.

Speert H. *Obstetric and gynecologic milestones*. New York: Macmillan, 1958:630.

Stone HH, Hester TR. Topical antibiotic and delayed primary closure in the management of contaminated surgical incisions. *J Surg Res* 1972;12:70.

Stone HH, Holfling SJ, Strom PR, et al. Abdominal incisions, transverse vs. vertical placement and continuous vs. interrupted closure. *South Med J* 1983;76:1106.

Sutton G, Morgan S. Abdominal wound closure using a running, looped monofilament polybuster suture: comparison to Smead-Jones closure in historical controls. *Obstet Gynecol* 1992;80:650.

Thompson JB, Maclean KF, Collier FA. Role of the transverse abdominal incision and early ambulation in the reduction of postoperative complications. *Arch Surg* 1949;59:1267.

Thorek P. *Anatomy in surgery*. 3rd ed. New York: Springer-Verlag, 1985:368.

Tollefson DG, Russell KP. The transverse incision in pelvic surgery. *Am J Obstet Gynecol* 1954;68:410.

van Rissel EJC, Trimbos BJ, Booster MH. Mechanical performance of square knots and sliding knots in surgery: a comparative study. *Am J Obstet Gynecol* 1990;162:93.

Voss SC, Sharp HC, Scott JP. Abdominoplasty combined with gynecologic surgical procedures. *Obstet Gynecol* 1986;67:181.

Venturi ML, Attinger CE, Mesbahi AN, et al. Mechanisms and clinical applications of the vacuum-assisted closure (VAC) device: a review. *Am J Clin Dermatol* 2005;6(3):185.

Wallace D, Hernandez W, Schlaerth JB, et al. Prevention of abdominal wound disruption utilizing the Smead-Jones closure technique. *Obstet Gynecol* 1980;56:226.

Walters MD, Dombroski RA, Davidson SA, et al. Reclosure of disrupted abdominal incisions. *Obstet Gynecol* 1990;76:597.

Weiland DE, Bay RC, Del Sordi S. Choosing the best abdominal closure by meta-analysis. *Am J Surg* 1998;176(6):666.

Weiser EB, Bundy B, Hoskins WJ, et al. Extraperitoneal versus transperitoneal selective paraaortic lymphadenectomy in the pre-treatment surgical staging of advanced cervical carcinoma: a Gynecologic Oncology Group study. *Obstet Gynecol* 1989;33:283.

Wharton JT, Jones HW, Day TG, et al. Preirradiation celiotomy for invasive carcinoma of the cervix. *Obstet Gynecol* 1977;49:333.

CHAPTER 15 ■ PRINCIPLES OF ELECTROSURGERY AS APPLIED TO GYNECOLOGY

RICHARD M. SODERSTROM AND ANDREW I. BRILL

DEFINITIONS

Active electrode monitoring—Technique of placing a sleeve around the electrode to detect stray energy and to carry the induced energy to ground. Stray energy generally occurs from breaks in insulation or capacitive coupling.

Ammeter—Device that measures the amount of current flowing through a conductor at a specific moment.

Ampere—Quantity of electrons that move through a conductor over time (coulombs per second).

Bipolar—Type of electrode or electrical delivery system in which the active and passive electrodes are of similar sizes and, thus, similar current densities. The bipolar generators are usually calibrated against a 100-V load of resistance.

BLEND—Term used when the electrical current is interrupted between 20% and 50% of the time.

Capacitance or capacitive coupling—Ability of two conductors to transmit or receive electrical flow while separated by an insulator; one conductor carries the active current and induces a separate current in the nearby conductor. In general, it occurs in monopolar circuits consisting of two metal plates or tubes separated by air or another insulator. It does not occur during bipolar electrosurgery.

COAG—Term used to describe an interrupted electrical current. In some generators, the period of interruption of current flow can be adjusted from 10% to 50%. At the same power settings, the voltage of the waveform is always higher than it is with CUT waveforms.

Coulomb—Measure of a quantity of electrons.

Current (power) density—Surface area of an electrode in contact with tissue during electrical flow. The smaller the spot of contact, the greater is the heat effect for the same amount of time, increasing by the square root of the area of contact.

Current rate (amperes)—Flow rate of a quantity (coulombs) of electrons.

CUT—Term used when referring to a continuous or undamped electrical current. At the same power settings, the voltage of the waveform is always lower than it is with COAG waveforms or BLEND.

Desiccation—Act of coagulating tissue after making contact with an active electrode. Either CUT or COAG waveforms may be used, but CUT waveform is preferable. Intracellular temperature stays below 100°C, which leads to cell shrinkage and dehydration.

Direct coupling—Occurs when two conductive materials in the same circuit touch during electrical activation or are close enough that arcing can occur. A break in the insulation of an electrode that allows sparking to tissue is an example of direct coupling.

Edge density—Affinity of electrons to concentrate at the edges of flat or irregularly shaped electrodes as they exit the electrode. This feature enhances the cutting ability of blade-shaped electrodes.

Electricity—Movement of electrons between two oppositely charged poles, positive and negative.

Electrocautery—Transfer of energy by heat, such as a hot wire. Electrons do not move into the affected tissue; only heat is transferred.

Electrosurgery—Transfer of energy from an electrosurgical generator to tissue by means of energy packets (electrons).

Energy (joules)—Quantity of work produced over time. Energy (joules) equals work (watts) multiplied by time (seconds).

Faradic effect—Electrical stimulation of muscle responding to a frequency of electrical current that is less than 100,000 cycles per second.

Fulguration—Intentional application of sparks to tissue surface to coagulate surface bleeding. The COAG waveform is preferable.

Heat (thermal energy)—Produced as electrons move from the low resistance of an electrosurgical probe to the high resistance of tissue. This energy may boil (vaporize) or denature (coagulate) tissue, depending on the extent and rapidity with which heat is generated.

Hybrid laparoscopic trocar sleeve—Conductive trocar sleeve used in laparoscopy that is covered by an outer nonconductive locking sleeve.

Impedance (ohms)—Resistance to flow of electrons through a conductor. Although resistance refers to direct current through a uniform wire, such as copper, it is generally substituted for impedance. Impedance is correctly applied with changes in voltage (alternating or fluctuating), frequency (modulating or demodulating), or tissue type (lipid membranes, soft tissue, fibrous tissue, fat, muscle, bone, or artificial appliances). It can measure the combination of tissue resistance and capacitance. Impedance in human tissue is generally 100 to 1,000 V; in the fallopian tube, it is 400 to 500 V.

Isolation ground circuitry—Safety feature that uses transformers not in contact with the parent generator so that the induced electrical flow "floats" its own separate circuit. If a break in the floating circuit occurs, all energy within that circuit stops and does not seek ground.

Kilohertz (kHz)—Measure representing 1,000 cycles of radio waves per second.

Monopolar—Type of electrode or electrical system in which the active electrode is small (high current density) and the passive electrode is large (low current density). Most monopolar generators are calibrated against a 500-V load of resistance.

Open circuit—State in which a generator is activated before the active electrode touches tissue. This promotes higher voltage, especially in the COAG mode, than activating the generator after touching the tissue. Open circuitry is used to start fulguration.

Patient return electrode (grounding pad)—Large conductive pad (low current density) placed on the patient to complete an electrosurgical pathway.

Return-electrode monitoring—Dual-padded patient return-electrode system designed to monitor irregular separation of the ground pad.

Sparking (arcing, fulguration)—Result of electrical flow through gas (air, argon).

Vaporizing—Raising the cellular temperature rapidly above 100°C, which causes cell rupture, releasing steam.

Voltage (volts)—Force (pressure) driving current.

Watts (work)—Amount of work produced by electron flow (current). Work (watts) equals force (volts) multiplied by current rate (amperes).

Waveform—Oscillation characteristic of an alternating electrical current from positive to negative.

Waveform frequency—Number of oscillations of an alternating electrical current, usually between 350,000 and 4 million cycles per second in electrosurgery.

Usually, little attention is paid to the applied principles of electrical physics when surgeons receive their formal training. Most training programs consider electrosurgery a skill acquired by the student through hands-on exposure, and the average faculty knowledge in the biophysical principles of electrosurgery is awarded through a "grandfather" process of credentialing. As a result, many myths about the risks of electrosurgery have been perpetuated during the past decades. Furthermore, the absence of fundamental knowledge handicaps the potential to transform science into art. The modern electrosurgical generator (ESU) is a finely tuned solid-state instrument that offers many versatile variables for the contemporary surgeon to harness, allowing he or she to deliver controlled energy to tissue in either a discrete or broad manner to obtain a specific effect and outcome.

HISTORY OF ELECTROSURGERY

Dating back to antiquity, applying heat to wounds has been a part of the medical armamentarium. Neolithic skulls unearthed in France revealed evidence of thermal cauterization. Hippocrates used heat to destroy growths and to treat phthisis and epilepsy; his aphorism that fire succeeds when other methods fail influenced medicine and surgery for centuries. Albucasis in 980 B.C. described using a hot iron to stem bleeding; as opposed to the controlled delivery of energy by modern electrosurgery, this approach using direct thermal transfer is true cautery.

Electrosurgery is often erroneously referred to as *electrocautery*. Because the mechanisms of action and possible outcomes including potential risks of these two methods are quite different, it is important to separate these hemostatic techniques with correct knowledge and terminology. *Surgical diathermy*, a term commonly used outside the United States, literally means "through heating." This is not a feature of monopolar techniques, whereas it may be applicable to certain aspects of bipolar electrosurgery.

Most historians credit Arsenne d'Arsonval, in 1893, as the first to use high-frequency alternating currents for medical therapy. In 1907, Riviere described "white coagulation" at low voltages without a spark. In 1925, Ward showed that a continuous sine waveform from a vacuum-tube oscillator was most effective for tissue cutting and that an interrupted sine waveform from a spark-gap oscillator produced more effective tissue coagulation. Harvey Cushing, a neurosurgeon, and William T. Bovie, a physicist, were the most effective promoters of electrosurgery, using it with success during brain surgery to control hemorrhage. Cushing and Bovie published their results in 1928, describing the three distinct effects of electrosurgery: desiccation, cutting, and coagulation. Since then, manufacturers of electrosurgical units have provided medicine with an array of electrosurgical generators, each improving, with time, in output characteristics and safety features.

In the early 1970s, electrosurgery was the main energy source used during laparoscopy, and it was used with great efficacy, even though most procedures were typically sterilization and simple adhesiolysis. Anecdotal reports of bowel injuries presumed to be secondary to "sparking" of monopolar energy prompted several investigators to develop bipolar instrumentation, as they asserted these tools would reduce the bowel injuries caused by the monopolar technique. By 1980, bipolar electrosurgery had become a standard part of the surgical armamentarium of most laparoscopic surgeons. In parallel, laser instrumentation specifically designed for endoscopic procedures became available, and postgraduate education in their application became commonplace, temporarily relegating electrosurgery as a backup method. Despite the early promises of laser surgery, surgical injuries formerly attributed to monopolar electrosurgery have persisted; no study to date has demonstrated a reduction in laparoscopic complications, especially bowel injuries, in step with changes from bipolar electrosurgery to laser technology.

Near the end of the 1980s, general surgeons recognized the advantages of laparoscopic surgery, especially for cholecystectomy, and quickly became frustrated by several limitations of contemporary lasers, returning to electrosurgical generators for comparatively more versatility and power. The manufacturers responded quickly with the production of solid-state generators specifically designed for endoscopic use. Each energy source capable of destroying tissue can, in specific circumstances, lead to a surgical complication that may be unique to that energy source. But a watt is a watt, and when the output of energy of any source is matched for power density, power output in wattage, and for the same amount of time (joules), the same tissue injury occurs. Although many hazards attendant to an energy source such as electrosurgery can be reduced and managed, not all can be eliminated. Surgeons are expected to be familiar with their surgical tools and appreciate the variables inherent in each technology.

BASIC ELECTRICAL DEFINITIONS

Electrons are particles of energy that, when pushed (or passed) through human tissue perform work, thereby creating heat and necrosis. *Voltage* is the pressure force required to push electrons. The standard unit of measure of this electrical pressure is 1 V. Thus, in drawing the analogy of electricity to water, an electron is to a molecule of water what voltage is to water pressure.

Whereas volume of water may be measured in cubic centimeters, the volume of electrons is measured in *coulombs*. If

TABLE 15.1

ELECTROPHYSICS DEFINITIONS EQUATED TO A HYDRAULIC ANALOGUE

Electrical concept	Electrical unit	Equation	Hydraulic analogue
Energy	Joule	—	Energy
Charge	Coulomb	(6.3 × 1,018 electrons)	Volume (mass)
Power	Watt	Joules/second	Power
Voltage	Volt	Joules/coulomb	Pressure difference
Current	Ampere	Coulombs/second	Flow
Impedance	Ohm	Volts/ampere	Resistance

we push a volume of water through a conduit at a given pressure during a specific period, we create *current*. In electricity, current (measured in *amperes*, or coulombs per second) means the passage of a given quantity of electrons through a conductor during a given period of time. With water or electricity, as resistance increases, the flow of current decreases (given constant pressure or voltage). The difficulty of pushing the electrons through tissue or other material can be defined as resistance (impedance) and is measured in *ohms* (Ω).

Electrical power (*watts*) is the energy produced. The electrical power may be defined as pressure times current, volts times current, or volts times electron flow per second. (Ohm's law: electric current is directly proportional to voltage and inversely proportional to resistance; $I = E/R$). The total energy consumed during a period of time is measured in *joules* (Table 15.1). For a complete list of terms used in electrosurgery, see Definitions.

FUNDAMENTALS OF ELECTROSURGERY

Electrocautery is not electrosurgery; it is a term frequently misused when physicians actually mean electrosurgery. *Electrocautery* involves use of a direct electrical current to heat a metal conductor with a high resistance, which makes the metal physically hot. Tissue is then directly heated or cauterized by touching the hot metal object to tissue. In contemporary surgery, few instruments employ the principles of electrocautery, because it affords no precise control over thermal effects. *Electrosurgery* involves manipulating electrons through living tissue by using a high-frequency alternating current with enough current concentration (current density) to create heat within a tissue cell to destroy tissue. *Electrosurgical generators* are machines that produce an alternating current of electricity at a frequency that does not stimulate muscle activity (500,000 to 3 million cycles per second). Whereas direct current flows in one direction only, alternating current flows to and fro, first increasing to a maximum in one direction and then increasing to a maximum in the other direction. This *sinusoidal waveform* can be interrupted or varied, which create different surgical effects.

The output waveform of alternating current has a negative and a positive excursion, or peak. As it passes through each cell, the electrolytic polarity is agitated, creating cellular heat (Fig. 15.1). Thus, as opposed to direct heating by electrocautery, thermal effects of electrosurgery are a secondary thermodynamic phenomenon. The measurement from zero polarity to positive or negative polarity is called the *peak voltage* of the waveform (the relation is the same for peak current). The measurement from plus peak to negative peak, which is twice peak voltage, is called *peak-to-peak voltage*. For historical reasons alone, a pure *CUT* current is a simple sinusoidal (undamped, uninterrupted, or nonmodulated) waveform that is produced by continuous output (Fig. 15.2), whereas a waveform produced by highly interrupted (modulated or damped) output is called *COAG* current (Fig 15.3).

When there is a continuous current or waveform, the peak voltage need not be as high as with the COAG waveform to create the same wattage (i.e., power is conserved regardless of the degree of current interruption). However, when a coagulation effect must be enhanced, the interrupted COAG waveform is preferable and is created by pushing higher energy bursts of electrons through the tissue. The cooling effect of the current off time between bursts facilitates the coagulation effect. For an instant, with the interrupted waveform, a comparatively higher peak voltage than the uninterrupted waveform is present within the electrical circuit. Most electrosurgical generators also provide BLEND current, which does not result from combined CUT and COAG waveforms, as is commonly thought. Rather, the BLEND current is a waveform that is interrupted at variable intervals, delivering variable degrees of coagulating and cutting properties (Fig. 15.4). The degree to which the BLEND mode cuts or coagulates depends on the relative time interval that the current is on or off. Thus, one of the tissue effects of electrosurgery depends on the various modes of delivering electric current (Fig. 15.5).

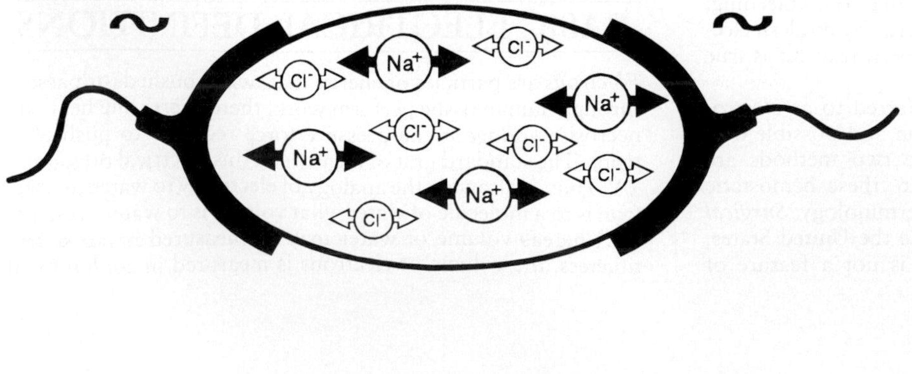

FIGURE 15.1. The sine wave of negative or positive polarity of an alternating current creates intracellular heat as it passes through each cell.

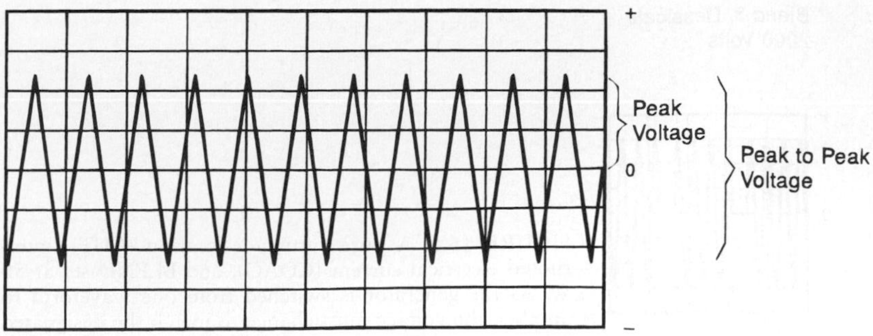

FIGURE 15.2. An undamped (or CUT) waveform is a continuous delivery of energy.

MONOPOLAR ELECTROSURGERY

As electrons, pushed with a given voltage, are concentrated in one specific location, heat within the tissue increases rapidly. This concentration is defined as *current density.* The traditional diathermy generator, an example of equipment using this principle, is familiar to many physicians. Electrons are passed through the body by applying two large metal conductors or plates, of equal size, on opposite sides of the tissue to be heated. The electrons are pushed through the plate called the *active electrode* and then received on the other plate, the *return (neutral) electrode* or ground plate, as they pass through a myriad of circuits through the interposed tissues. Once the electrons enter the body (conductor), they are dispersed through the tissue toward the pathways of least resistance to the return electrode. Because current is dispersed over the entire surface area of both plates (low current density), any generated heat is of low intensity and below the burn threshold. However, if either plate is significantly reduced in size, current density (and thus heat) is correspondingly increased and a burn may then occur (Fig. 15.6).

Thus, an active electrode that concentrates current of high current density creates a burn where current enters the body; similarly, a burn will occur if this current is conducted out the body via a return electrode of small contact area (high current density).

Like water, electrons flow through the path of least resistance. If tissue resistance is high but the corresponding voltage pressure is low, the current may cease to flow or may search out alternate pathways with lower resistance. When the voltage is increased, the electrons have more "push" to find an alternate pathway, such as through a vital structure where the current is concentrated, or they might seek out an alternate return electrode, like a cardiac monitor electrode. Therefore, the surgeon should use the lowest voltage necessary to accomplish a given task and must ensure that the dispersive electrode is in good contact with the patient and broad enough to reduce current density far below the level of tissue burning. Contemporary electrosurgical generators with isolated ground circuitry systems and/or return-electrode sentinel systems preclude alternate pathways and are preferable when an ineffective or incomplete return path is present.

ELECTROSURGICAL GENERATORS

Significant differences exist among electrosurgical generators. In general, instrumentation set by a number dial is calibrated to peak voltage rather than power output, as is typically found in generators that have a digital liquid-crystal display window showing the output in watts. To determine the wattage output with dial-a-number generators, the operator must refer to an output graph found in the manufacturer's manual; some generators have these output curves imprinted on the top of

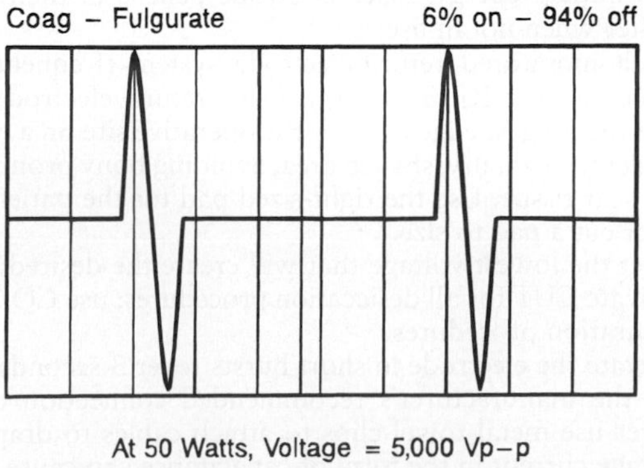

FIGURE 15.3. The damped or interrupted waveform (or COAG) delivers energy less than 10% of the time.

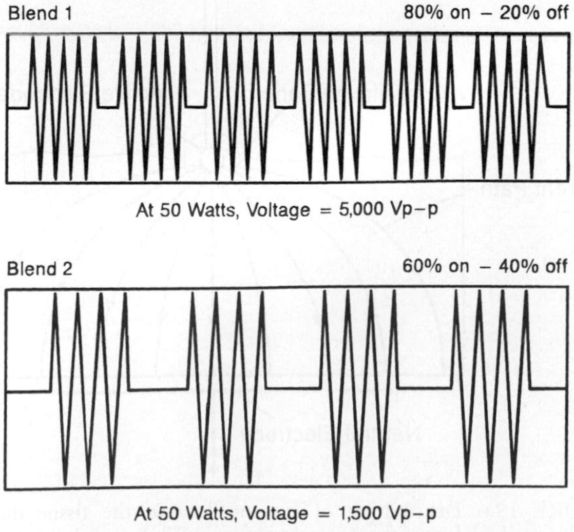

FIGURE 15.4. BLEND settings can vary as to the percentage of time the generator delivers the energy.

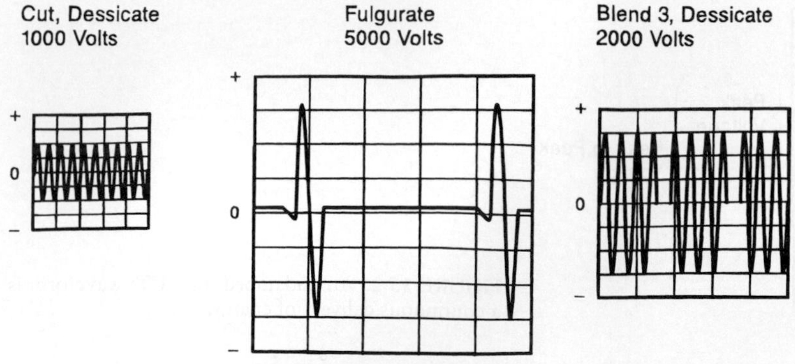

FIGURE 15.5. A pure cutting/desiccation (CUT), interrupted electrical current (COAG), and BLEND set at 50 W. As the generator is switched from one waveform to another, the voltage must change to match the designated power output. The voltage increases from CUT to BLEND to COAG.

the generator box (Fig. 15.7). The power output set by the manufacturer is the power available at the start of the electrosurgical process; however, this power output decreases as tissue impedance progressively increases during the heating of cellular fluids. Hence, the power output measurement of each generator is calibrated against a fixed resistance. For monopolar use, most generators are calibrated against a 500-V load; for bipolar use, the load is usually set at 100 V (Fig. 15.8). Each electrosurgical generator has its own power output characteristics; the proper settings can be found with attention to the manual and with experience.

For general surgical use, most generators can produce a maximum of 8,000 V in the COAG mode. An 8,000-V pressure can push electrons 3 mm through room air under certain atmospheric conditions, which means that arcing to distant tissue is improbable; most of the time, electrosurgical generators are used in the 1,000- to 3,000-V range. The waveform frequency is set above 350,000 cycles per second to prevent muscle stimulation. At frequencies below 100,000 cycles per second, tetanic muscle contraction can occur, which is known as the *faradic effect* and is undesirable. The higher the frequency of the generator output, the more "leakage" of current occurs, which can enhance the induction of current on nearby conductors by capacitance, potentially harmful during certain endoscopic procedures.

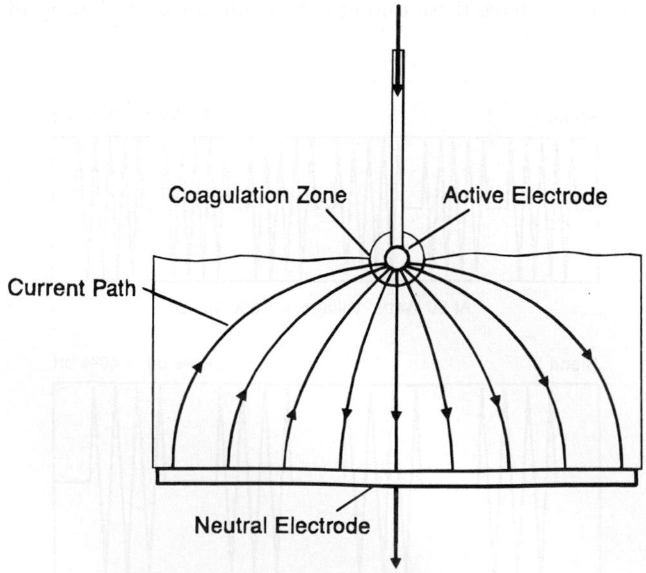

FIGURE 15.6. Distribution of current flow in the tissue during monopolar high frequency surgical technique. When one electrode pole is reduced in size, the tissue in contact with the smaller electrode is heated rapidly because of a high current (power) density.

Most contemporary generators offer an *isolated ground circuitry* system to reduce the risk of monopolar energy seeking an alternative pathway to ground; older-model generators are known as *ground-referenced generators.* With an isolated or "floating" ground system, the electricity delivered to the patient and returned to the generator is created by an induction of current in transformers that are insulated or isolated from the frame of the generator. When a break in the circuit occurs, the electrons do not seek ground, and thus, no current flows. This also reduces the risk of an aberrant burn to the surgeon, unless the surgeon is leaning against the patient, thus becoming part of the isolated circuit.

Return-electrode safety systems use disposable return electrodes (called *ground pads*), which are usually composed of two conductive pads placed side by side. Built-in monitors, through low-impedance feedback to the generators, measure pad-to-skin contact stability and power-density contact by measuring the balance of contact between the two adjacent pads. If there is an imbalance or poor contact to the patient leading to higher current density, an alarm sounds, and the generator output is automatically terminated. The return electrode should be oriented so that each pad is at equal distance from the operating site and in close proximity and the largest edge faces the operative site.

The basic principles of safety during electrosurgery include the following:

1. Avoid arcing electrosurgical energy to a hemostat during coaptive coagulation: Always touch the hemostat first, and then initiate energy. Place electrode pencils in their safety holster when not in use.
2. Use a monitored return-electrode system (frequently referred to as a REM system). Place return electrode pads with the longest edge close to the operative site on a nondependent, clean, dry, shaved area, avoiding bony prominence and scar tissue. Use the right-sized pad for the patient, but never cut a pad to size.
3. Select the lowest voltage that will create the desired effect. Activate CUT for all desiccation procedures; use COAG for fulguration procedures.
4. Activate the electrode in short bursts (over 3 seconds).
5. Use the manufacturer's recommended connection cables. Never use metal towel clips to attach cables to drapes, as leakage current in the form of capacitance can cause a skin burn.
6. Inspect instrument insulation before each use.

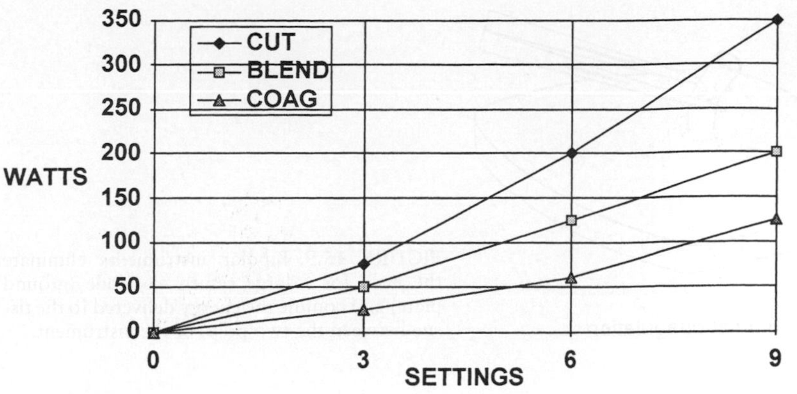

FIGURE 15.7. The characteristics of the monopolar power output curves in a generator with dial settings to a maximum of 350 W against a 500-V load. The power in each waveform chosen is different for the same setting.

7. If the patient has a pacemaker, get advice from the pacemaker representative before using monopolar energy. Consider using bipolar electrosurgery.
8. If the usual power settings are inadequate, do not increase the power until the circuit is checked, especially the contact of the return electrode.

BIPOLAR ELECTROSURGERY

As mentioned earlier, in monopolar electrosurgery, a ground plate or return (dispersive) electrode carries the flowing electrons back to the generator after they have passed through the patient. The electrons are first focused by the active or efferent electrode to a point of high current density generating temperatures sufficient to burn tissue, and then dispersed over the larger surface area of the return electrode, where any thermal effects are well below the threshold for burning.

The bipolar system incorporates an active (efferent) electrode and a return (afferent) electrode into a two-poled instrument, such as forceps or scissors. This eliminates the need for a ground plate, allowing the instrument to produce a high current density at each pole of the forceps (Fig. 15.9). This permits a discrete amount of desiccation that is confined primarily to the shape and size of the forceps in contact with the tissue, and eliminates the chance of stray or alternate pathways.

Although these advantages over monopolar electrosurgery seem obvious, several restrictions unique to bipolar electrosurgery need to be appreciated. First, the load of impedance (tissue resistance) used to calibrate power output is usually several times lower than that with monopolar modes in contemporary generators. In a generator that has an output-selection knob measuring volts rather than watts, the bipolar output of energy is many watts less than the same setting in the monopolar side of the generator. In generators that read power output in watts, the impedance load is three to five times less than the load used to calibrate monopolar output, so the tissue effect may be much less than the same output reading for monopolar. Therefore, in most situations, bipolar applications are limited to a discrete area held between the forceps or scissor poles, with a restricted power output but with high power density. For sterilization procedures, the manufacturer's advice should be followed because each instrument can differ in design and ability to desiccate completely. With bipolar electrosurgery, only a CUT or continuous waveform should be used.

BIOPHYSICAL BEHAVIOR OF ELECTROSURGERY

Electrosurgery may be used to cut (*vaporize*), or to coagulate deeply (*desiccate*) or superficially (*fulgurate*). These terms are frequently interchanged but stand for specific electrosurgical end points that should be familiar to the surgeon. As mentioned earlier, at the end of an electrode, the tissue effect depends on the shape and size of the electrode, the frequency and degree of current modulation, the peak voltage, and the current coupled against output impedance. The tissue may be cut in a smooth deliberate fashion without arcing, or it can be burned and charred by carbonization.

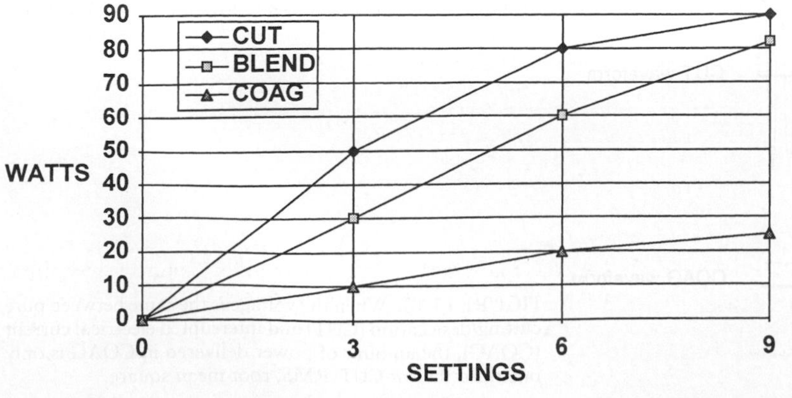

FIGURE 15.8. The characteristics of bipolar power output curves in a generator with dial settings to a maximum of 100 W against a 100-V load. Note that the power in each waveform chosen is different for the same setting.

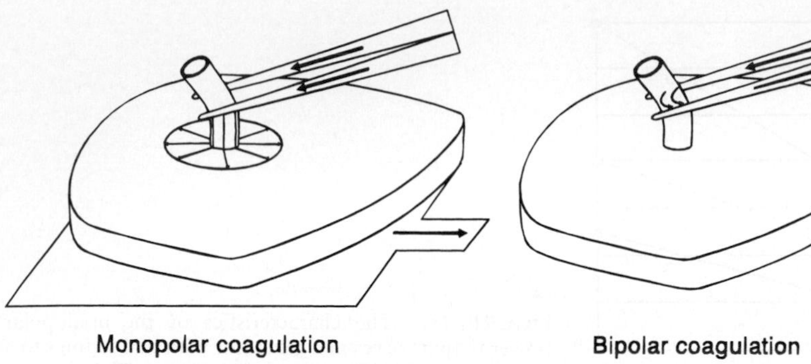

FIGURE 15.9. Bipolar instruments eliminate the need for a large return electrode (ground plate) and confine the energy delivered to the tissue between the two poles of the instrument.

Electrocoagulation may be performed in many different forms, from slow delicate contact coagulation (*desiccation*) to the charring effects of the spray coagulation mode (*fulguration*), at times leading to carbonization. The temperature differences can vary from 45°C to more than 500°C.

The essential characteristic of CUT waveforms is that they are continuous sine waves—that is, if the voltage output of the generator is plotted over time, a pure CUT waveform is a continuous sine wave alternating from positive to negative at the operating frequency of the generator, 500 to 3,000 kHz. The COAG waveform consists of short bursts of high-voltage radiofrequency sine waves. With the sine wave frequency of 500 kHz, the COAG bursts occur 31,250 times per second. The important feature of the COAG waveform is the pause between each burst. First, suppose that a COAG waveform had the same peak voltage as the CUT waveform. The average power delivered (heat per second) would be less because the COAG is turned off most of the time (Fig. 15.10). Then suppose that the COAG waveform had the same average voltage as the CUT waveform and thus could deliver the same heat per second. Because the COAG is turned off most of the time, it can only produce the same average voltage as the CUT by having large peak voltages and currents during the periods when the generator is on (Fig. 15.11).

A high-voltage COAG waveform can spark to tissue without significant cutting effect because the heat is more widely dispersed by the long sparks and because the heating effect is intermittent. The temperature of the water in the cells does not get high enough to flash into steam. In this way, the cells are dehydrated slowly yet are not torn apart to form an incision. Because the high peak voltage is a quality of the COAG waveform, it can drive a current through high resistances. In this way, it is possible to fulgurate long after the water is driven out of the tissue and to actually char it to carbon.

Coagulation is a general term that includes both desiccation and fulguration. Fulguration can be contrasted with desiccation in several ways. First, sparking to tissue with fulguration *always* produces necrosis anywhere sparks land. This is not surprising, because each cycle of voltage produces a new spark, and each spark has an extremely high current density. In desiccation, the current is no more concentrated than the area of contact between the electrode and the tissue (Fig. 15.12). As a result, desiccation may or may not produce necrosis, depending on the current density. For an equal level of current flow, fulguration is always more efficient at producing surface necrosis; however, the depth of tissue injury is superficial compared with that of contact desiccation. With fulguration, the sparks jump from one spot to another in a random fashion, and the energy is "sprayed" rather than concentrated (Fig. 15.13).

In general, fulguration requires only one fifth the average current flow of desiccation. For example, if a ball electrode is pressed against moist tissue, the electrode begins in the desiccation mode, regardless of the waveform (Fig. 15.12). The initial tissue resistance is low, and the resulting current is high, typically 0.5 to 0.8 A (average). As the tissue dries out, resistance rises until the electrical contact is broken. Because moist tissue is no longer touching the electrode, sparks jump to the nearest areas of moist tissue in the fulguration mode, as long as the voltage is high enough to make a spark. Eventually, the resistance of desiccated tissue stops the flow of electrons, self-limiting the depth of coagulation.

Electrosurgical electrodes can be sculpted to perform certain tasks. A needle electrode, a knife, a wire loop, or even a scissors can be shaped and sized to a specific duty. When the

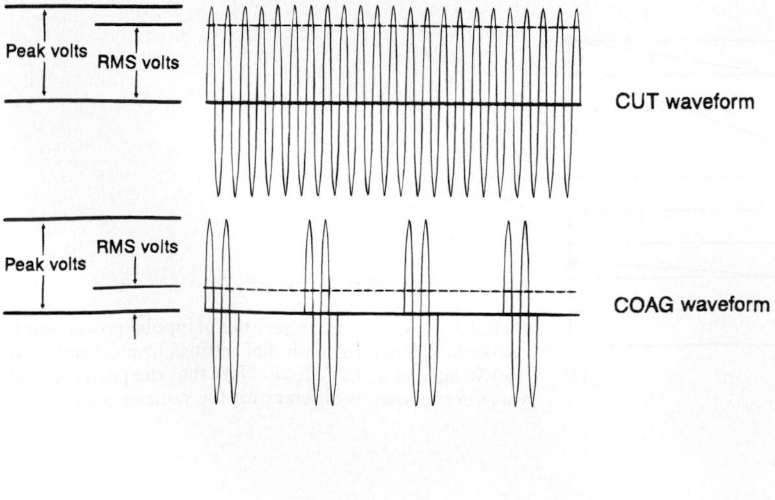

FIGURE 15.10. When the voltage is the same between pure cutting/desiccation (CUT) and interrupted electrical current (COAG), the amount of power delivered in COAG is only one third that of CUT. RMS, root mean square.

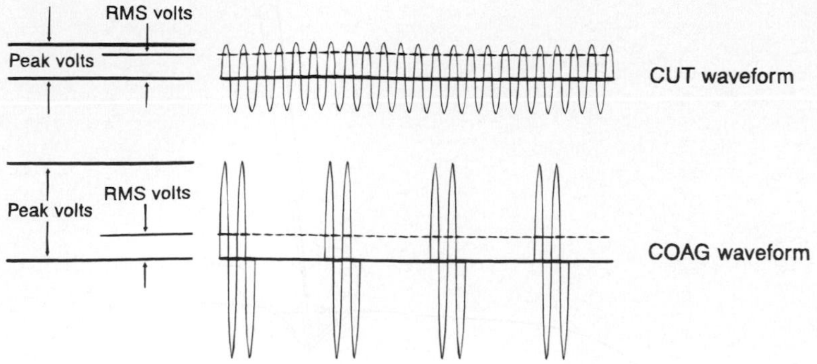

FIGURE 15.11. When the power settings are equal between pure cutting/desiccation (CUT) and interrupted electrical current (COAG), the peak voltage of COAG is about three times higher than that of CUT. RMS, root mean square.

waveform variables are added, cutters can be made to coagulate, and coagulators can be made to cut. The faster an electrode passes over or through tissue, the less is the coagulation effect, leading to more cutting. If the power setting and the electrode size remain constant, more desiccation of the adjacent tissue occurs the slower the electrode is passed through the tissue (Fig. 15.14). The more broad the electrode is, the less cutting and more coagulation effect there are (Fig. 15.15). If the electrode is touched to the tissue before keying the generator, desiccation occurs, but with more lateral charring in the COAG mode than in the CUT mode. There is a point at which the desiccation effect is limited in depth by the impedance to flow at a fixed power setting. Interwoven into these acts are the output intensity and output impedance characteristics of the different electrosurgical generators. If a constant voltage can be maintained at a given power setting, which is variable as tissue resistance changes, lateral thermal damage is controlled, giving the surgeon a predetermined surgical effect. By using "smart" generator technology that integrates feedback from the output electrode, newer generators output a constant voltage to control the depth of coagulation independent of the cutting rate.

INCISIONS

High electrical current that is delivered with a fine electrode of small surface area yields a high power density, which generates intense intracellular heat, causing the intracellular water to boil and thereby literally exploding or vaporizing the cell. Steam vapor occupies six times the volume of liquid water. The vaporization of the cell dissipates heat, a cooling effect that reduces thermal damage to adjacent tissue. This cooling effect, however, allows for little heat transfer to deeper tissue, resulting in minimal or no coagulation effects when electrosurgery is used at the CUT mode. To further enhance the vaporizing effects of the CUT waveform, the electrode should be activated just before touching the tissue (Fig. 15.16). The low-voltage sparks, by their high power density, produce a plume of steam and carbon particles between the electrode and the impacted tissue through which the current is rapidly conducted. This highly focused electrical energy yields the maximum power density, resulting in the most efficient cutting effects and the least thermal damage. Therefore, to incise tissue, CUT current should be used with a small or thin electrode that is activated just before making contact with the target tissue. The electrode "glides" on a layer of steam as the sparks do the cutting.

Because speed of passage and electrode size and shape determine the heat effect on tissue to be incised and the degree of lateral thermal spread, the amount of desired thermal effect decides what electrode to use and how fast the incision should be made. In addition, the chosen waveform can play a role. To compound the decision, the natural resistance of the tissue (e.g., fat has high impedance) to be incised should be considered.

In cutting or vaporization, the voltage must exceed about 200 peak V to ionize the air between the electrode and tissue for sparking. Although most choose a scalpel to incise the skin, a knife or needle electrode can mimic the incision if the surgeon

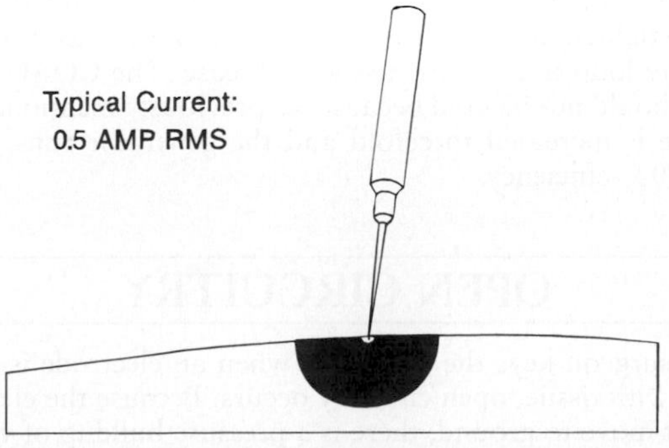

FIGURE 15.12. Desiccation occurs by touching the tissue before keying the generator, which creates deep penetration of heat and minimal charring of the surface tissue.

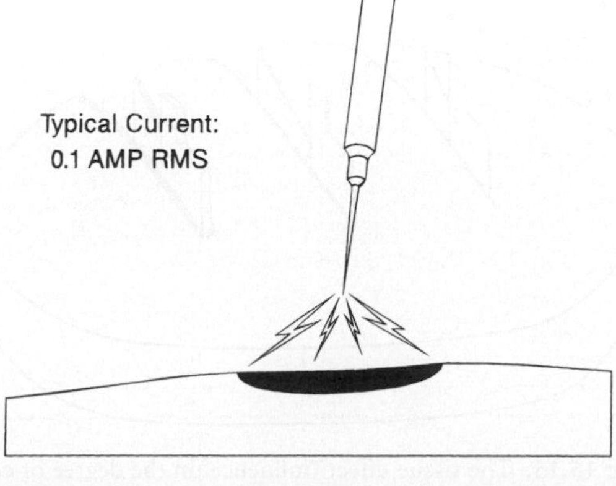

FIGURE 15.13. Fulguration sprays spark to the surface of tissue, causing a rapid surface char with minimal heating of the deeper layers.

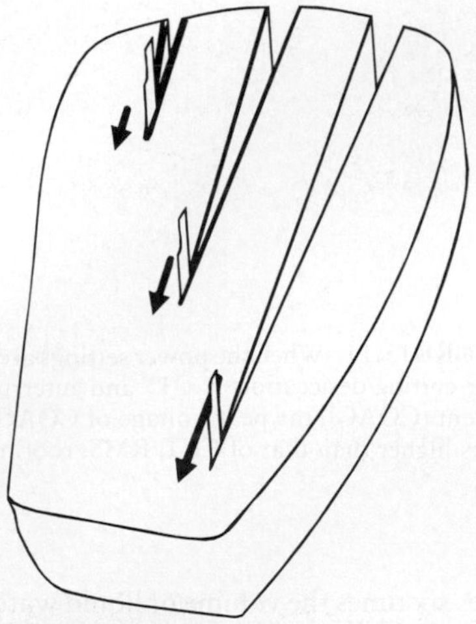

FIGURE 15.14. The tissue effect (influence on the degree of coagulation) of increasing the speed of passage of a cutting electrode of the same size and at the same depth of cut.

applies the principle of speed of passage and waveform. With either electrode, the speed of passage is coupled with a CUT waveform. Because a needle electrode has the highest power density, if the speed of passage is swift and the waveform is set at pure CUT, no visible desiccation of tissue occurs, but like a knife, the skin bleeds with minimal coagulation effect. A slow deliberate sweep of the electrode causes some desiccation effect, and the skin may blister and heal poorly. For that reason, only the experienced electrosurgeon should cut the skin with an active electrode.

As an example, abdominal fat, which has a high intrinsic impedance, can be readily cut using a blade electrode with a COAG waveform because of the high current density at the edge of that electrode. Small bleeders at the edge of the incision are simultaneously fulgurated. As larger vessels are exposed, such as the superficial epigastrics, the blade can then be rotated 90 degrees to desiccate these structures before incision, using its broad surface and lower current density. Thus, manipulating a particular electrode with a certain waveform can produce a spectrum of desired thermal end points.

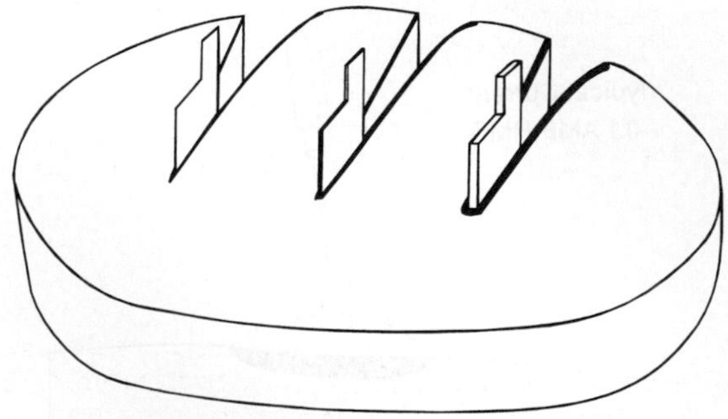

FIGURE 15.15. The tissue effect (influence on the degree of coagulation) of increasing the size of a cutting electrode if the speed and depth of cut are constant.

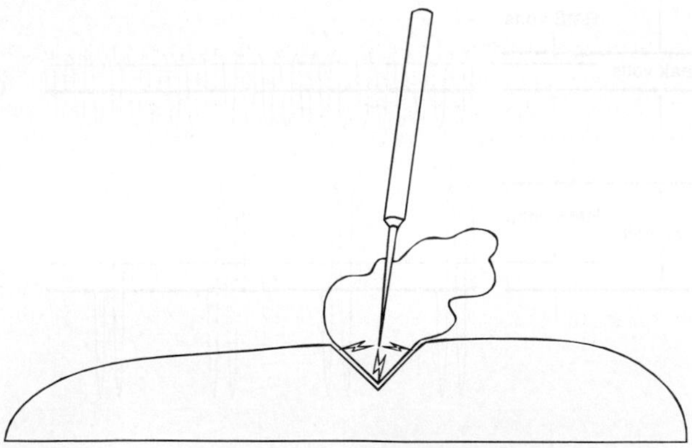

FIGURE 15.16. Electrosurgical cutting. Because of the continuous flow of low-voltage energy in the pure cutting/desiccation (CUT) mode, the high power density of each spark vaporizes the cells into steam. The cutting effect is enhanced by allowing a needle or blade electrode to glide along the layer of steam, letting the sparks do the cutting.

DESICCATION TECHNIQUE

The most common desiccation maneuver used in surgery is the coaptation of blood vessels. Coaptive coagulation involves clamping a bleeding vessel with a conductive clamp and applying a current to coagulate and promote a collagen weld of the vessel. To prevent overdesiccation of surrounding tissue, the low-voltage, uninterrupted waveform (CUT) should be applied. It is important that the generator not be activated until the electrode is in contact with tissue. With monopolar energy, deep desiccation of the tissue in the grasp of the instrument, such as a hemostat, is uniform throughout the thickness of the tissue; with bipolar energy, the output characteristics are such that the surface is heated first, leaving the center of the tissue mass to be heated last. For this reason, many recent models of bipolar electrosurgical generators are preset in the CUT mode and have a current flow meter (ammeter) to ensure that desiccation is complete. If the tissue is too thick, the bipolar current may cease to flow before deep desiccation is complete; thus, if the tissue coagulated is cut, it may bleed briskly.

CUT techniques can be used to amputate large tissue pedicles with either monopolar or bipolar modes provided that the amount of energy is sufficient. The monopolar snare-electrode, common to intracolonic surgery, can be used to amputate an ovarian pedicle with ease and with minimal lateral spread if the power setting is kept low. In addition, time must be allowed to first desiccate the tissue to be cut. Then, by increasing the pressure to tighten the snare, the cutting effect of the waveform and the wire loop transect the tissue with ease. The COAG waveform should not be used because, as previously mentioned, the voltage is increased threefold and the generator runs at less than 10% efficiency.

OPEN CIRCUITRY

If the surgeon keys the generator when an electrode is not in touch with tissue, open circuitry occurs. Because the electrons cannot move to ground, there is a pressure buildup of voltage output by the generator. An analogy would be holding a finger over the end of a garden hose with the faucet valve completely open. When the finger is released from the end of the hose, for a moment the water pressure buildup projects the water well beyond the point of projection when the current flows continuously under steady pressure.

In general, open circuitry should not be used except to initiate a fulguration of tissue or to start an incision. A common accident that occurs during routine surgery is when the surgeon keys the generator before touching a hemostat for coaptation of a blood vessel. Because of the high voltage created by open circuitry, especially in the COAG mode, the voltage drives the energy through the surgical glove of the person holding the hemostat. Before this was understood, the glove was usually blamed as being defective.

FULGURATION TECHNIQUES

The fulguration or COAG waveform is frequently used at the wrong time and for the wrong reasons. The generator manufacturers introduced terms that at the outset seemed to simplify the output waveform choices available to surgeons. For the most part, however, the assigned labels COAG and CUT have confused the surgeon about the science of their purposes. If the surgeon coapts tissue with a grasping electrode, either waveform begins to desiccate tissue. If, however, the tissue shrinks away from the electrode contact point, sparking (fulguration) occurs, creating surface char that acts as an insulator, preventing deeper desiccation.

If an electrode is held off the surface of the tissue and the generator is activated, sparking to tissue occurs, sending each spark in a random fashion to char the surface only because the char acts as an insulator. Surface charring is desirable to stop surface oozing, such as muscle bleeding of a venous nature. Because blood is saline rich, a bloody field is hard to coagulate because of ready conduction and diffusion of current density. Irrigating with a nonelectrolyte solution or removing the blood from the bleeders by using suction improves the task. For arterial vessels larger than 1 to 2 mm, fulguration is usually not effective, and desiccation, staples, or ligatures are usually required.

Because the tissue effect of fulguration is due to the high power density of each spark, the effect of a single spark is probably the same, independent of voltage (at least within the voltage range of current generators). Thus, during fulguration techniques, the higher output settings can be used with more efficiency, reducing the chance of touching the electrode to the tissue, which might cause an undesirable desiccation effect. It is this feature of fulguration that encouraged the development of the argon beam coagulator.

ARGON BEAM COAGULATOR

The argon beam coagulator is a monopolar electrode device that is housed inside a cannula through which argon gas is dispelled at 12 L per minute for open laparotomy and 4 L per minute for laparoscopy (Fig. 15.17). The ionization properties of argon gas flowing over the electrode enhance the distance the spark can travel to complete the circuit to the tissue surface. Because the electrons prefer to stay in the stream of argon gas rather than pass through room air or carbon dioxide (CO_2), each having a higher resistance to electron flow, the collimation or parallel alignment of the sparks leaves a more uniform surface coagulation effect. These properties create a bright bluish hue to the sparks, which makes them easy to see and aim at the bleeding surface. The gas, expelled under pressure, blows the pooled blood away from the surface bleeders, making coagulation more discrete and efficient. Flooding the field with glycine while fulgurating the tissue adds another dimension to efficient surface coagulation (see below). To create the planned fulguration effect, the wand must move like a paintbrush to prevent deep tissue damage.

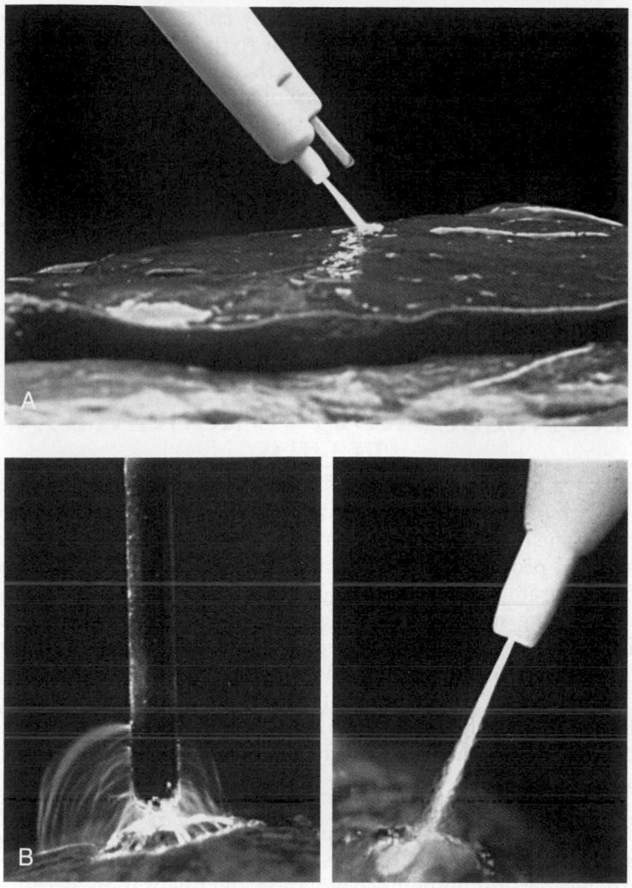

FIGURE 15.17. The argon beam coagulator enhances the electrosurgical technique of fulguration by injecting argon gas over a monopolar electrode inside of a narrow cannula. The ionization characteristics of the gas lengthen the distance a spark can be maintained. Because electrons choose to flow the path of least resistance, they stay collimated in the flow of gas, so the enhanced flow of sparks can be directed with efficiency. The ionized gas has its own unique blue hue that makes the sparks easily visible for accurate fulguration. **A:** The argon beam coagulator at work. **B:** Sparking effect of standard electrode (L) compared with argon beam coagulator (R). (From Valleylab, Inc., Boulder, CO, with permission.)

ELECTROSURGERY DURING PREGNANCY

No data indicate that using electrosurgical techniques in a pregnant patient has any untoward effect on the fetus at any stage of development. Owing to the dispersion effect, the fetus, bathed in electrolyte-rich amniotic fluid, is protected from any concentration of electrical current. Just as the output frequency of all electrosurgical generators is above the faradic effect (the level that stimulates muscle contraction) for adult electrosurgery, the same is true for the fetus.

During a cesarean section, the only concern is the accidental touching of an activated electrode to the fetus, which causes tissue heating. This does not mean that the usual technique of making an incision in the uterus would preclude using an electrosurgical incision, but rather that a "backstop" under the incision line, between the amniotic membrane and the muscle wall, should be in place. Although using a nonconductive material, such as a plastic suction tip, may seem wise, a metal ribbon retractor also can be used because it has a large surface area serving to diffuse the current density. Caution should be exercised when using the gloved finger of the surgeon as a backstop because if open circuitry is used, the voltage may create a hole in the glove.

NONELECTROLYTE IRRIGATION FLUIDS

As with operative hysteroscopy and cystoscopy, nonelectrolyte fluids, such as glycine and sorbitol, can be used during other surgical procedures to facilitate electrical energy to desiccate or fulgurate tissue. Blood does not mix well with these fluids, leaving streamers that can be easily seen in these media. Electricity seeks out the electrolytic-rich blood, and its ability to coagulate is enhanced because the energy is not dispersed, as it would be in an electrolyte-rich irrigant, such as lactated Ringer solution. This is particularly helpful during microsurgical procedures and during surface fulguration of broad oozing surfaces.

Rather than delivering the fluid under great pressure as is typically done with laparoscopic irrigation-aspiration systems, a slowly applied low-pressure flooding of the field helps identify bleeders for pinpoint coagulation and fulguration. Because flooding has a cooling effect on all fluids, the power requirements may be significantly higher than dry-surface coagulation. Coagulation of submerged tissue may impair the surgeon's field of view with bubbles as hydrogen gas and other combustibles are released from the cellular vaporization. To prevent risk of hypoosmolality from excess intravascular absorption of electrolyte free media, residual nonelectrolyte fluids should be removed from the peritoneal cavity.

BIPOLAR VESSEL SEALING

The latest advance in bipolar electrosurgery is the introduction of three novel ligating-cutting devices that minimize thermal damage by delivering electrical energy as high current and low-voltage output. These electrosurgical instruments deliver radiofrequency energy to cut, vaporize, coagulate, and seal over a wide range of tissue conditions, providing surgeon-controlled tissue effects. Tonal feedback from a dedicated generator confirms complete desiccation of the tissue bundle, after which the pedicle is sequentially cut by advancing a centrally set mechanical blade within laparoscopic devices. By directly responding to incremental increases in tissue resistance during tissue desiccation, total energy delivery is dramatically less than conventional bipolar systems. Consequently, sticking and charring to surrounding tissue are reduced, and lateral thermal spread is minimized.

Relying on the breakthrough discovery that vessel wall fusion can be achieved using electrical energy to denature collagen and elastin in vessel walls to reform into a permanent seal with high tensile strength, the LigaSure Vessel Sealing Device (Valleylab, Boulder, CO) is available for laparoscopic use in 5 mm and 10 mm and for laparotomy or vaginal surgery in 7-inch Pean-style and 9-inch Heaney-style clamps. Using a solid-state feedback technology, the type of tissue held in the forceps is diagnosed, and the appropriate amount of energy is delivered to effectively seal arterial blood vessels, veins, and lymphatics up to 7 mm in size. The vessel to be sealed is grasped in the jaws of the instrument, and a calibrated force is applied to the tissue while temperature generation is minimized.

The second device, by PK Technology (ACMI-Gyrus, Minneapolis, MN), uses advanced solid-state generator software to deliver pulsed energy with continuous feedback control. The cycle stops once it senses that tissue response is complete, and the cool-down phase ensures that the collagen and elastin matrix reforms without tissue fragmentation. Instruments are available as both 5-mm and 10-mm laparoscopic PK cutting devices and 9.75-inch Heaney-style open forceps for laparotomy or vaginal surgery.

A third device, the EnSeal Laparoscopic Vessel Fusion System (SurgRx, Inc., Palo Alto, CA) is a 5-mm laparoscopic bipolar instrument with a set of "smart electrode" plastic jaws embedded with nanometer-sized spheres of nickel that conduct a locally regulated current. Tissue temperatures never exceed 120°C because of the progressive generation of resistance in the plastic jaws. With this device, desiccation is facilitated by simultaneously advancing a mechanical blade that both cuts and squeezes the tissue bundle to eliminate tissue water.

Because the proximity of the distal tines of a conventional bipolar grasper precludes the capability to generate a spark sufficient to cut an interposed tissue pedicle, laparoscopic scissors and shears depicted as bipolar cutting devices are actually mechanical cutting devices that provide desiccation at the edge of the jaws. True electrosurgical cutting is possible using bipolar instrumentation with the advent of recent technology that integrates a low-voltage, impedance-feedback generator paired with two novel electrodes. The 5-mm PK Cutting Electrode (Gyrus-ACMI, Boston, MA) consists of a retractable active needle electrode paired with a return electrode collar near the distal tip. Tissue cutting is generated when both electrodes are placed in contact with tissue and then drawn across the tissue surface during activation. A 5-mm cutting-coagulation spatula electrode (Gyrus-ACMI, Boston, MA) has multiple conductive surfaces that can be manipulated and keyed to either cut or coagulate tissue. Because the PK electrosurgical generator produces a low-voltage output, the high impedance posed by very desiccated or fatty tissues may preclude vaporization by either of these newer bipolar electrodes.

APPLIED PHYSICS IN LAPAROSCOPY

Because the tissue effect of electrophysics depends on the size and shape of each electrode, the chosen waveform, and the power output, the challenge facing the laparoscopist is to properly match and mix the electrodes and generators. For instance, because of the difference in the power density of the forceps as they grasp the tissue, a 5-mm grasping forceps desiccates tissue much slower than does a 3-mm forceps of similar design. A knife electrode can be used to incise tissue, yet when coagulation is needed, the surgeon can place the flat side of the electrode on the tissue and, with a CUT waveform, desiccate the tissue. Regardless of the waveform, a ball-shaped electrode desiccates when pressed against tissue, but if the surgeon holds the ball electrode away from an oozing surface and delivers a high-voltage coagulation waveform, the bleeding area can be fulgurated without deep tissue penetration.

As one electrode is changed to another, the surgeon should adjust the generator output to match the task at hand. This is especially important when needle electrodes are used after a more blunt electrode. If not, the tissue touched by the high current density of the needle electrode can be severely damaged, and passive heat transfer can destroy the needle electrode.

When bipolar instruments are used, if a COAG waveform is used, a sticking phenomenon is common; as a general rule, an uninterrupted or CUT waveform should be used with bipolar instruments. During tubal sterilization with bipolar forceps, if the COAG waveform is used, tubal coagulation may be incomplete as current flow is prematurely terminated by the rising impedance from surface char. The same problem can happen when blood vessels surrounded by fat (e.g., mesenteric vessels) are coagulated with a bipolar instrument using a COAG waveform; here, cutting a presumptively desiccated vessel may lead to bleeding from a still patent lumen. When using an uninterrupted waveform, an in-line ammeter can be a valuable accessory, particularly for tubal sterilization, to ensure that all of the tissue between the forceps has been coagulated before transection.

As with laser surgery, during operative laparoscopy, smoke accumulation can occur, especially when fulguration techniques are used; for the most part, desiccation techniques create steam. Smoke can be reduced or eliminated by irrigating the field to be coagulated with glycine or sorbitol rather than with saline or lactated Ringer solution because the energy can be applied during tissue submersion. If the surgeon floods the field as electrical energy is being delivered, the energy is not dispersed within the solution, as it is with electrolyte-rich fluids; in a liquid media, smoke does not develop.

In the early 1980s, it was thought that the occasional bowel perforation after a laparoscopy was the result of sparking or arcing to the bowel when electrodes were used. Because the physics of fulguration do not allow an arc to be maintained in one spot, it is now understood that at the worst, only a surface charring of the bowel could occur. To burn a hole in the bowel, the electrode must touch the bowel during the delivery of electroenergy and remain in contact with the bowel wall long enough to coagulate deep into the bowel wall. For this reason, it is best to disconnect electrodes from the generator when they are not needed for energy delivery. To prevent accidentally touching the bowel with an active electrode, the surgeon should withdraw the laparoscope from the operating field to maximize the panoramic view before keying the generator.

CAPACITANCE IN MONOPOLAR ELECTROSURGERY

Capacitance is a physical property of monopolar energy whereby two conductors in close proximity, each insulated from one another, can induce an electrical current from one to the other (Fig. 15.18), which can then be released or discharged. The amount of this induced transfer of energy is influenced by the length of the conductors (the longer the distance, the more effect), the distance between the conductors (the shorter the distance, the more the effect), the character of the waveform (COAG waveform increases the effect), and the frequency of the waveform (the higher the frequency of the generator, the more the capacitance effect). The operating laparoscope becomes a capacitor when monopolar energy with a high-voltage interrupted current is transmitted through a long insulated electrode, especially if the electrosurgical generator emits high-frequency cycles. Because the operating channel is eccentrically located in the shell of the laparoscope, thus in close proximity, the induced current in the shell can be 50% to 80% of that current flowing through the active electrode into the laparoscope shell (Fig. 15.19).

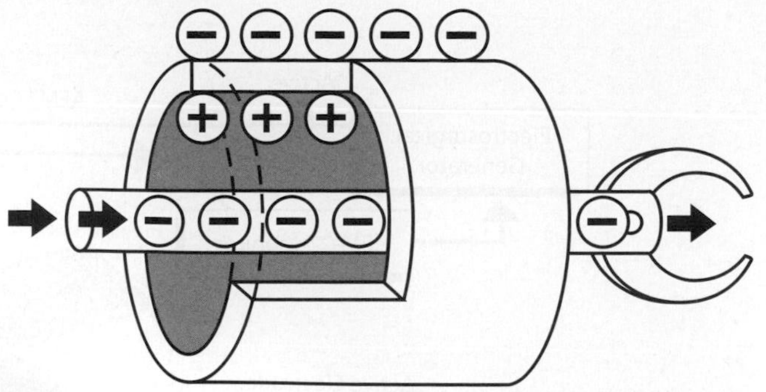

FIGURE 15.18. Capacitance is the induction of electrical current between two conductors separated by insulation; one conductor carries the active current and induces, by high-frequency radio waves, a separate current in the nearby conductor.

If a metal trocar sleeve is used to transport the operating laparoscope into the abdomen, the induced current is quickly transferred through the metal sleeve, through the patient from the umbilicus, and finally to the return electrode. Because the current (power) density is broad (low) where the trocar sheath contacts the abdominal wall, no harmful heating occurs. If the trocar sheath is nonconductive (e.g., fiberglass) or radiolucent, or if a plastic securing collar is used (with either a metal or nonconductive trocar sleeve), the current remains isolated, and the laparoscope cannot deliver the induced energy via the umbilicus to the return electrode. In this scenario, if a vital structure, such as bowel, touches the laparoscope or cannula (especially

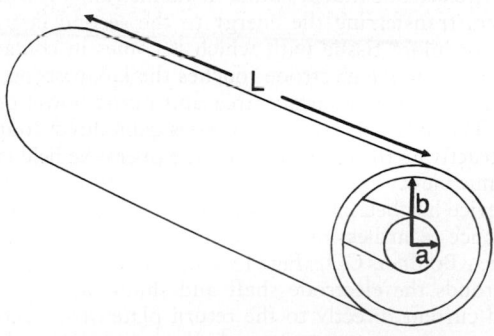

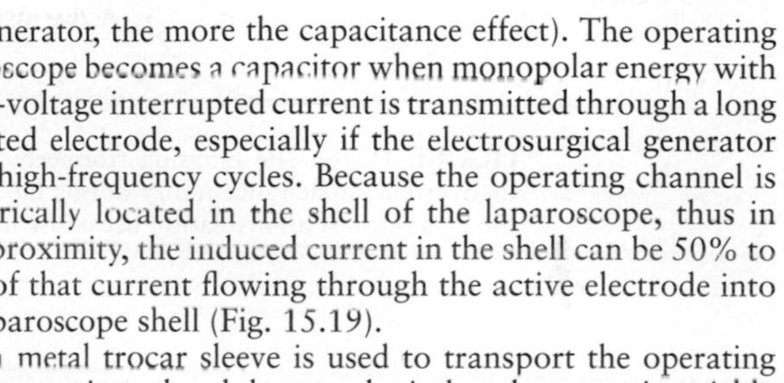

$$\text{Capacitance:} \quad C = \frac{2\pi\, \varepsilon_0\, K\, l}{L_N\left(\frac{b}{a}\right)}$$

FIGURE 15.19. Part of the formula that increases the capacitance effect in endoscopic surgery is the length (L) of the capacitor plus the diameter of the electrode (a), divided by the distance of separation or insulation (b).

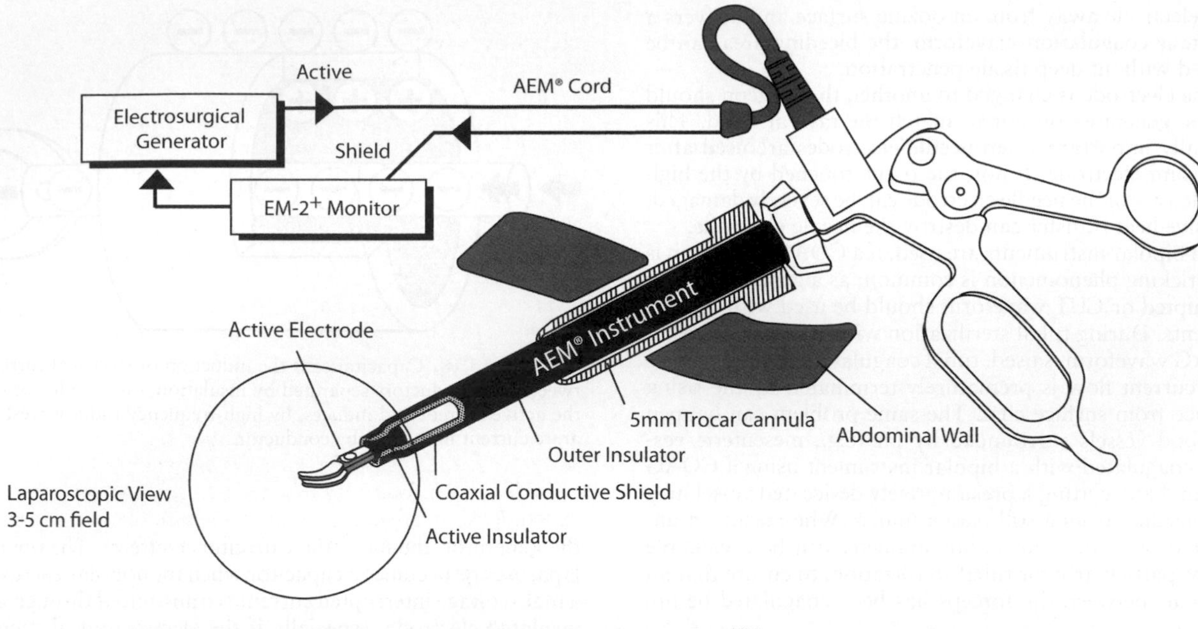

FIGURE 15.20. The Encision (formerly known as Electroshield™) device eliminates the threat of an inadvertent capacitance injury during laparoscopy by returning the capacitance-induced current back to the generator. If an insulation breakdown occurs, it alerts the surgeon.

a small portion of its surface) while energy is being activated, the energy induced into the laparoscope can burn the organ; typically, this may occur outside of the view of the laparoscopist. This same problem can occur when a secondary trocar sleeve is made of metal and uses a plastic securing collar (*hybrid laparoscopic trocar sleeve*) if that sleeve is used to transport a monopolar electrode. In this situation, the metal trocar sleeve becomes an active electrode by the capacitance effect. The best way to reduce this risk is to use all-metal trocar sleeves and metal securing collars; the next best way is to use all-plastic sleeves and collars. *Never mix plastic with metal.*

Unintended electrical injuries also can result from *direct coupling* or insulation failure. Direct coupling occurs when the active electrode touches other metal instruments within the abdomen, transferring the energy to the second instrument, which can injure tissue with which it comes in contact. For example, the active electrode touches the laparoscope, which then touches a small surface area and burns bowel or other organs. The only way to avoid injuries from direct coupling is never to activate the electrode until the operative field is in full panoramic view.

A device has been manufactured that eliminates the risk of capacitance regardless of the type of trocar sleeve used (Encision, Inc., Boulder, CO) (Fig. 15.20). The device is a cannula that shrouds the electrode shaft and shunts all capacitance-coupled current directly to the return plate of the generator, thereby avoiding transmission to biologic tissue. In addition, if there is a break in the insulation of the active electrode, which could promote direct coupling of the primary current to other metal instruments or adjacent tissue, this device alerts the surgeon with an audible alarm. Insulation failures occur when the insulation shield of the electrode is compromised from high voltage, abuse, poor handling, or mechanical accidents. The defect in the insulation, often too small to be recognized, can divert the full current from the generator to unintended tissue proximal to the end of the electrode. Sometimes the defect is on the part of the electrode that is within the trocar sleeve.

NUANCES OF ELECTROSURGERY TECHNIQUES

Before taking any electrosurgical action to control bleeding, accurately determine the source of bleeding and its proximity to vital anatomy. Identify the bleeders by combining mechanical tamponade with active hydrolavage. If the bowel, bladder, or ureter is in close proximity to the bleeder, mobilize that structure sufficiently before applying energy.

Because the output voltage of COAG current is very high, contact coagulation is generally limited to superficial layers because of the accelerated buildup of tissue resistance from rapid desiccation and carbonization. Conversely, electrode contact using the lower-voltage CUT current heats tissue more gradually, leading to deeper and more reliable penetration.

Coaptive sealing of the uterine and ovarian vessels using any type of monopolar current may be ineffective if the blood flow remains uninterrupted. Unless a vessel is sufficiently squeezed before electricity is applied, current density is dramatically reduced by conduction in blood, as any heat is dissipated by convection. Bipolar cautery is recommended for these longer pedicles.

Preferentially use BLEND or COAG current for a wider zone of hemostasis during incision of vascular tissues and to facilitate dissection of tissues with greater impedance, such as fatty or desiccated pedicles and adhesions. On the other hand, it is more prudent to use the lower-voltage CUT current via the edge of an electrode whenever lateral thermal spread may pose extra liability to adjacent tissues.

If bleeding in the vicinity of the bowel, bladder, or ureter cannot be controlled with pressure alone, carefully direct short bursts of noncontact COAG current with a broad-surface electrode to attain hemostasis with the least-possible amount of electrosurgical penetration. Still, visceral bleeding is best controlled by mechanical means, using the patience of pressure or suture ligation.

Although the flow of current is restricted to the tissue between the poles during bipolar electrosurgery, this does not eliminate the risk of thermal injury to tissue that is distant from the site of directed hemostasis. As current is applied between the poles, the intervening tissue gradually desiccates until it becomes thoroughly dehydrated. Desiccation is complete when the tissue whitens and visible steam emission stops. If the application of current continues, the heat spreads well beyond the electrical limits of the instrument. Unwanted thermal damage can be minimized by terminating the flow of current at the end of the visible vapor phase, applying current in a pulsatile fashion to permit tissue cooling, and securing pedicles by a stepwise process that alternates between partial desiccation and incremental cutting. Because the rate of temperature generation is a direct function of the volume of tissue being desiccated, thermal spread can also be reduced by using the sides or tips of a slightly open forceps to press or lift, rather than coapt for hemostasis.

As with contact monopolar coagulation, tissue between the electrodes of a bipolar instrument may become adherent during desiccation. Repeated attempts to shake the tissue free may lead to traumatic avulsion of a key vascular pedicle. A stuck vascular pedicle can usually be unglued by energizing the opened device while immersed in a conductive irrigant, such as saline. Once the solution is boiled by the high current density between the electrodes, the mechanical action of bubbling is usually sufficient to atraumatically free the pedicle.

ELECTROPHYSICS APPLIED TO OPERATIVE HYSTEROSCOPY

With endometrial ablation, the resectoscope cutting loop and a roller electrode or coagulating loop are used. Some surgeons shave the endometrial lining with the cutting loop electrode; others desiccate the endometrial lining with the roller ball or bar. A few surgeons shave first and then "paint" the shaved myometrium with the roller electrode or coagulation loop. Unfortunately, studies on the tissue effects of different techniques, electrodes, and waveforms are few in number. Even the pressure applied to the endometrial surface changes the current (power) density; the more the pressure, the broader is the contact surface of the electrode, creating a decreased current density. Because the speed of passage of the electrode unique to each surgeon is another variable, only the outcome statistics can be evaluated with any reasonable scrutiny. Some surgeons exclusively use a COAG waveform at 30 W; others have reported success using a CUT waveform at 100 W.

Typically, endomyometrial resection is accomplished using a pure interrupted CUT waveform while dragging the wire loop in a slow deliberate motion to a depth of 4 mm through the tissue, providing some coagulation effect in addition to the cutting. By using the CUT waveform, bubble formation on the anterior surface of the endometrial cavity is less than that in the coagulation mode. The same waveform with a light contact of the coagulation loop electrode set at 100 W is used during the painting phase. Unlike the roller-ball or roller-bar electrode, which can trap dead tissue in its axle and increase the impedance of electron flow, the coagulation loop electrode avoids that impedance. By not rolling, the surface of the electrode in contact with tissue stays clean, much like an eraser cleans itself. If the roller electrode is a bar or barrel, either slow the rolling motion or increase the power output because of lower current density. At the end of the ablation procedure, some surgeons switch to a COAG waveform at 75 W. With the increased peak voltage of this waveform, skipped areas are sought out by the electrons under higher pressure, ensuring complete surface coagulation.

Monopolar resectoscopic surgery is uniquely associated with accidental burns to the vagina and perineum. Because the inner and outer sheaths of the resectoscope are separated by air, which is an insulator, current can be induced into the outer sheath by capacitive coupling. Insulation breaches can divert the direct current from the proximal electrode to the outside sheath. Episodes of relatively high current density on touching small areas of genital tissue with the outer sheath can be sufficient to burn tissue. From investigations using *in vitro* anatomical surrogates, these injuries occur from defects in electrode insulation, especially when interrupted COAG current is used and the cervix is overdilated and is in contact with less than 2 cm of the outer sheath of the resectoscope. Resectoscopic monopolar electrode injury and subsequent current diversion can be promulgated by the high electrical force created by open circuit activation as well as prolonged activation along already desiccated tissue.

BIPOLAR HYSTEROSCOPIC SURGERY

Departing entirely from monopolar electrosurgery, a new family of instrumentation has been recently introduced that uses bona fide bipolar technology to attain the desired electrosurgical effect. The primary advantage of bipolar electrosurgery stems from the isolation of the electrical circuit between a set of closely separated active electrodes. Nevertheless, performance is like a monopolar device, providing tissue vaporization and desiccation while retaining all of the inherent safety features of bipolar electrosurgery.

The VersapointTM system (Gynecare/Ethicon, Somerville, NJ) consists of a dedicated bipolar electrosurgical generator and a variety of specialized hysteroscopic and resectoscopic bipolar electrodes for different tissue end points, including 1.6-mm flexible coaxial electrodes with variable tip geometry and vaporizing and cutting loop electrodes for resectoscopic surgery. A key feature of the system is its ability to adjust automatically to a default power setting for each type of electrode, which can then be adjusted by the surgeon The patient contact end of each electrode consists of two poles separated by a ceramic insulator, referred to as the *return* and *active tip*. The active tip electrode is fabricated in a range of configurations and sizes to produce tissue effects ranging from tissue vaporization to desiccation. To function, both electrodes have to be simultaneously immersed in isotonic saline. The VERSAPOINT generator varies the output power in response to local impedance changes at the active electrode. A high-impedance vapor pocket is created that surrounds and insulates the active electrode from completing the circuit through the normal saline until tissue contact is made. Once contact occurs, current flows through the tissue, and by seeking the path of least resistance, returns through the saline to the proximal return electrode and finally back to the generator.

BIPOLAR ENDOMETRIAL ABLATION

The NovaSure Global Endometrial Ablation System consists of a single-use, three-dimensional bipolar device and radiofrequency generator that enables a controlled endometrial ablation in an average of 90 seconds without the need of a hysteroscope or hysteroscopic skills (Fig. 15.21). The device is inserted transcervically into the uterine cavity; the sheath is retracted by deploying a fan-shaped bipolar electrode that conforms to the uterine cavity. Unlike the balloon concept of other devices designed for endometrial ablation, vacuum is used to ensure good electrode tissue contact. This also allows removal of blood, endometrial debris, and steam, eliminating any uncontrollable steam ablation effect. Any type of "pretreatment" of the endometrium is not necessary.

The electrode consists of a conformable bipolar metallized porous fabric mounted on an expandable frame. An integral component of the handheld endometrial device is an intrauterine measuring device to evaluate uterine cavity width. Once the length is evaluated by sounding, the values are keyed into the generator, which automatically calculates the needed output power to ensure a confluent area of ablation within the uterine cavity.

A perforation detection system is an integral part of the NovaSure System. Delivered at a slow flow rate and pressure, CO_2 pressure is monitored within the uterine cavity, with the generator sensing a maintained pressure over a known period of time. Once the proper pressure is maintained, confirming good uterine wall integrity, the generator proceeds with the ablation in an automatic or semiautomatic mode.

Using a constant power output generator, the maximum power delivered is 180 W. The depth of ablation is controlled by

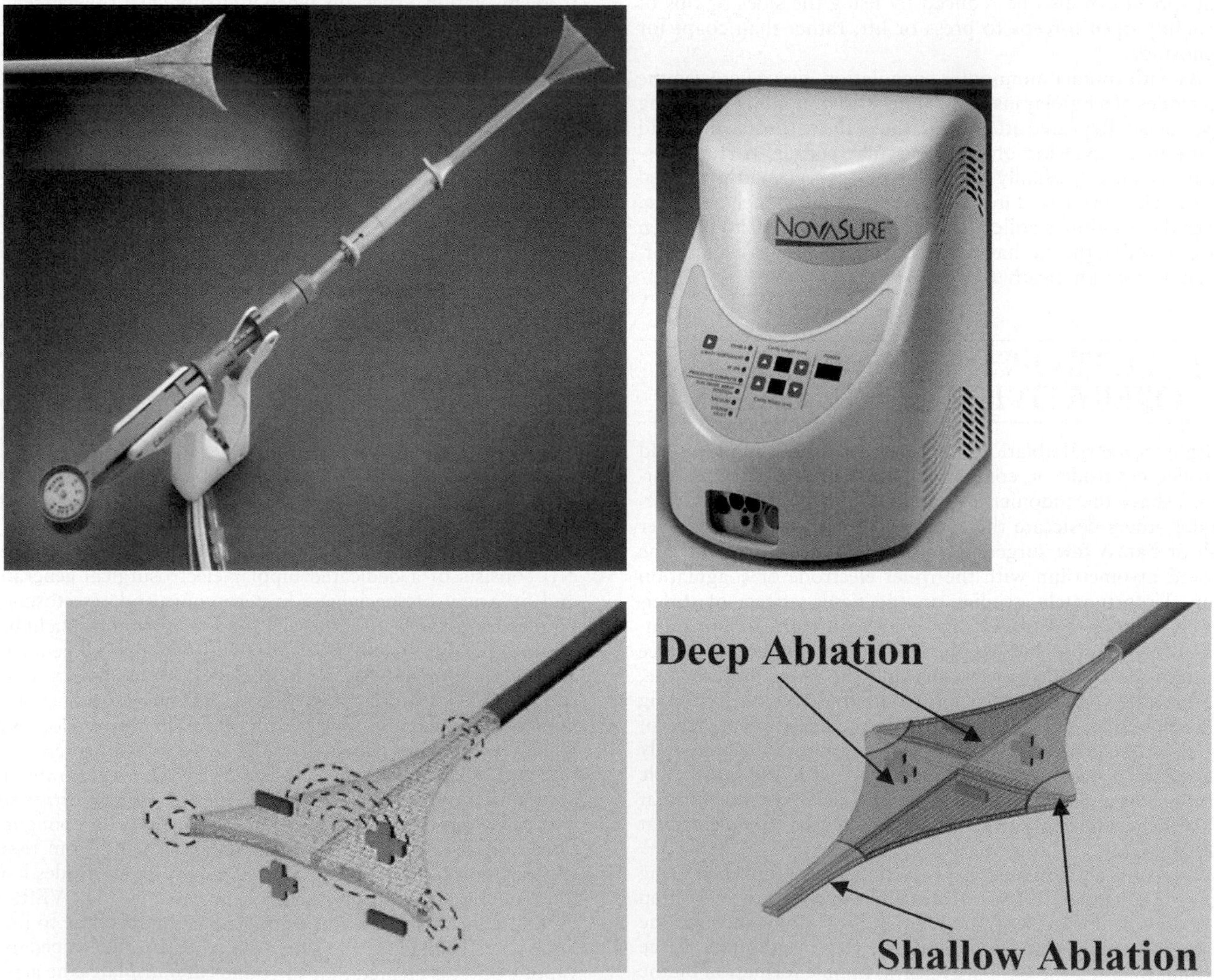

FIGURE 15.21. The NovaSure Global Endometrial Ablation System is a bipolar device for endometrial ablation using a metallized mesh electrode, vacuum for firm tissue contact, and a controlled generator designed to create a shallower depth of desiccation at the cornual area and lower uterine segment, with a deeper ablation in the uterine midbody.

monitoring tissue impedance during the procedure. A shorter center-to-center distance between electrodes provides a shallower depth of desiccation at the cornual area and lower uterine segment, and a deeper ablation in the uterine midbody. Once the tissue impedance reaches 50 ohms, or after 2 minutes, the NovaSure Global Endometrial Ablation System terminates the process.

APPLIED PHYSICS IN LOOP ELECTRODE EXCISION PROCEDURES

For almost half a century, circular and other shaped wire electrodes have been available for use as biopsy tools in dermatology and gynecology. In gynecology, these loops were used for cervical and hot-cone biopsies. After such biopsies, anecdotal case histories of severe scarring led gynecologists to choose nonelectrical methods of cervical biopsy by the 1950s. Although the rate was not established, infertility after hot-cone cervical biopsy occurred because of cervical stenosis.

Today, a renewed interest in electrosurgical wire loop biopsy has surfaced in the form of loop electrode excision procedure (LEEP), also referred to as large loop excision of transformation zone (LLETZ). As an outpatient procedure, LEEP or LLETZ surgery offers a one-time approach to a pesky problem plus an adequate and complete biopsy specimen. Made popular by British and French gynecologists, this excisional approach to cervical dysplasia gives a histologic confirmation of the treatment of the entire lesion, unlike the limited sampling of the lesion by colposcopic-directed biopsy followed by cryosurgery or laser ablation.

The long-term results after cervical healing are not available. No publication has evaluated different electrode loops matched with different electrosurgical generators, exploring their thermal effects on the tissue left behind the remaining viable cervix. Performing LEEP procedures is a complete exercise in the applied principles of electrosurgery. The following features of LEEP procedures should be appreciated:

Electrode size: The thinner the wire, the higher the power density, giving a better cutting effect. Electrode wires thicker than 0.20 mm in diameter can cause deep coagulation, up to a 10-mm depth, depending on speed of excision and waveform.

Waveform: There is an increasing depth of coagulation as the waveform is blended from a pure damped waveform to a 50:50 ratio of undamped-to-damped waveform.

Power density: In addition to the diameter or gauge of the wire used, the size and depth of the biopsy must be considered. As the electrode loop sinks deeper into the cervical tissue, the power density, as measured by the length and total surface area of wire loop penetrating the cervical tissue, decreases rapidly, losing the cutting effect created by a high power density. To compensate for this change, the operator must increase the power output from the generator during the incision process *or* increase the speed of the electrode incision process. If the power output is adequate (usually at 60 W) but the loop is passed through the tissue at a slow pace, deep coagulation of the cervix may occur. When possible, it is preferable to use a generator with a low-output impedance because this keeps the energy fluctuations created by different tissue densities to a minimum. Several generators that are especially helpful in LEEP procedures have been designed. They control the flow of energy through a low-impedance feedback by controlling voltage; the effect is much like a speed-control device in an automobile. If a constant voltage can be maintained at a given power setting that changes as tissue resistance changes, lateral thermal damage is controlled, giving the surgeon a predetermined surgical effect. Using constant voltage controls the depth of coagulation independent of the cutting rate.

Speed of incision: The more rapid the passage of the wire through the cervical tissue, the cleaner the incision, with less thermal artifact in the excised specimen. Conversely, the slower the passage, the more thermal damage to the adjacent tissue, resulting in better coagulation of the cone bed but more tissue necrosis and postoperative scarring. The loop wire should be rigid; a loop that bends or flexes reduces the speed of incision, leading to deep coagulation even when a pure cutting waveform is used. It appears that tungsten wire, because of its rigid characteristics (especially at higher temperatures), is preferred over stainless-steel wire, unless the yoke of the loop electrode handle can be shaped so that the stainless-steel wire remains rigid.

Because the vaginal fluids are rich in electrolytes, the vagina and cervix should be rinsed with a nonelectrolytic fluid before biopsy; the acetic acid solution used during colposcopy is adequate. The generator should be keyed or activated *before* the electrode touches the tissue, and the energy should be delivered in a continuous mode until the biopsy is complete. If the operator turns the energy off during the excisional biopsy, deep coagulation will occur when the generator is restarted, and the power may be insufficient to cut the tissue.

Care should be taken to not touch the metal speculum with the active electrode. Because the surface area of the metal speculum (in contact with the patient) is large, the current density is too low to cause a burn, but the effective high-frequency energy delivered through the speculum is altered to a much lower frequency, which may stimulate involuntary muscle contractions of the patient. This is not painful, but it is startling and disconcerting to both patient and operator. Thus, the use of an insulated metal speculum is preferable.

It is better to cut and excise with minimal coagulation during the biopsy process and then use fulguration, not desiccation, to control spot bleeding. Use a large ball electrode held close to, yet off of, the bleeding site, and switch to a damped (coagulation) waveform with high-voltage output. If the operative field is obscured with electrolyte-rich blood, reduce the amount of blood by blotting with a dry swab or with suction during the fulguration process. As an alternative, slow irrigation with a nonelectrolytic solution (e.g., sterile or distilled water) also allows effective spot fulguration with the ball electrode.

Again, with LEEP or LLETZ procedures, it is best to choose a rigid loop electrode with a steady pace of transfer through the tissue to be excised. Choose an uninterrupted waveform with minimal, if any, higher-voltage characteristics. A pure CUT waveform delivered through an electrode, transecting tissue at a slower rate, creates some coagulation effect. The latter may be preferable to a partially interrupted waveform (BLEND) passed through a loop electrode that may "stall" because of inadequate power as it tries to pass through the cervical tissue.

COMPLICATIONS DURING ELECTROSURGERY

The most common complication during electrosurgery is a return-electrode burn that is due to improper application of the electrode. Because these burns account for two thirds of electrosurgical accidents, each manufacturer provides specific recommendations for skin preparation and site application. Alternate site burns, such as to cardiac monitor leads, usually result from improper grounding, use of too much power, and high-voltage application.

Intraoperative complications during laparotomy are rare. Following the principles of electrosurgery should prevent such occurrences.

With laparoscopy, claims of sparking to adjacent organs causing burns or perforation can be refuted if one understands the principle of fulguration. Because human tissue cannot maintain an arc as metal can, the tissue effect is one of surface charring without the consequences of deep penetration. An exception is the use of the argon beam coagulator, which if held in one spot can cause deeper penetration than that of the random scatter of high-voltage fulguration. Although capacitance, described above, can lead to a serious injury when monopolar electrosurgery is used, the variables that must be present are such that the incidence is uncommon. Although monopolar electrosurgery can be used safely, the surgeon must have a thorough grasp of electrosurgical principles. Bipolar energy, with its reduced power output, can give a false sense of security. If one studies the energy physics of each tool, the adage "a watt is a watt is a watt" rings true.

With operative hysteroscopy, uterine perforation with the active electrode is the most common electrosurgical complication. Using proper technique with the admonition of never activating the electrode during a forward motion will largely eliminate perforation injuries. Understanding the tissue effect of different-shaped electrodes, coupled with the principle of using the lowest power necessary to perform the task, will also reduce complications.

SUMMARY

Electrosurgery provides the surgeon with a wide range of options: type of current, power level, monopolar or bipolar systems, and electrodes of various shapes and sizes. With the proper equipment and a basic understanding of the electrosurgical principles, the reproductive surgeon can use electrosurgery in many useful ways. Faulty or improper equipment or a lack of understanding by the surgeon can result in poor surgical outcome and unnecessary complications. Just as physicians are expected to understand and prescribe drugs in a precise and logical manner, so should they have a working knowledge of the energy sources they choose to use in surgery.

BEST SURGICAL PRACTICES

- Electrosurgery creates a desired tissue effect by delivering high-frequency alternating current with different electrodes that manipulate electrons to sufficient concentration (current density) in living tissue.
- The electrosurgical generator produces sinusoidal waveforms, variants of current, and voltage as either a continuous (undamped) output current called CUT, a moderately interrupted (damped) output called BLEND, or a highly interrupted (damped) output called COAG. In most circumstances, the CUT waveform should be used to cut and desiccate tissue, reserving the COAG waveform for surface fulguration to control small open bleeders and for superficial coagulation.
- Whereas each waveform is associated with specific tissue effects, these behaviors can be altered by the shape and size of the electrode via the manipulation of current density. All of these tissue effects are also influenced by the electrode velocity through the tissue. Prudent electrosurgical techniques integrate these variables, depending on the desired result.
- The lower-voltage CUT waveform should be used to incise tissue and for coaptive sealing of larger blood vessels. The higher voltage of the COAG current produces rapid tissue desiccation and carbonation, resulting in increased tissue resistance limiting coagulation to superficial small vessels. The BLEND current may provide a satisfactory combination for cutting through fatty tissues, such as the subcutaneous tissue or omentum.
- Coaptive sealing of the uterine and ovarian vessels using any type of monopolar current may be ineffective if the blood flow remains uninterrupted. Unless a vessel is sufficiently squeezed before electricity is applied, current density is dramatically reduced by conduction in blood, as any heat is dissipated by convection. Bipolar cautery is recommended for these larger pedicles.
- Fundamental principles to reduce risk during electrosurgery include:
  - When coaptively desiccating tissue with a hemostat, always touch the hemostat first, and then initiate the energy.
  - Place electrode pencils in their safety holster when not in use.
  - With monopolar systems, use a monitored return-electrode system (frequently referred to as a REM system). Place return electrodes close to the operative site on a clean, dry, shaved area, avoiding bony prominence and scar tissue.
  - Activate CUT for all desiccation-coagulation procedures; use COAG for fulguration procedures.
  - Activate the electrode in short bursts (about 3 sec). Use the manufacturer's recommended connection cables. Inspect instrument insulation before each use. If the usual power settings seem inadequate, do not increase the power until the circuit is checked, especially the return electrode.
  - Select the lowest voltage that will create the desired effect. Consider using bipolar methods. Bipolar systems deliver current as an uninterrupted CUT waveform calibrated against a lower resistance than monopolar systems. As such, it is wise to use a current flow meter to confirm complete desiccation of tissue, especially during tubal sterilization. In some tissues, the thermal effect will be limited such that monopolar application will be preferable.
  - The degree of thermal necrosis on tissue that is electrically incised is dependent on the velocity of passage as well as electrode size and shape and the electrosurgical waveform.
  - As one electrode is changed to another, the surgeon should adjust the generator output to match the task at hand.
  - The most common complication during electrosurgery is return-electrode burns, owing to improper application of the electrode. Prophylactic measures include proper skin preparation and site application. Alternate site burns, such as to cardiac leads, usually result from improper grounding, use of too much power, and high-voltage application.
- Nuances of Electrosurgery Techniques
  - Before taking any electrosurgical action to control bleeding, accurately determine the source of bleeding and its proximity to vital anatomy. Identify the bleeders by combining mechanical tamponade with active hydrolavage. If the bowel, bladder, or ureter is in close proximity to the

bleeder, mobilize that structure sufficiently before applying energy.

- Because the output voltage of COAG current is very high, contact coagulation is generally limited to superficial layers. That is because of the accelerated buildup of tissue resistance from rapid desiccation and carbonization. Conversely, electrode contact using the lower-voltage CUT current heats tissue more gradually, leading to deeper and more reliable penetration.
- Preferentially use BLEND or COAG current for a wider zone of hemostasis during incision of vascular tissues and to facilitate dissection of tissues with greater impedance, such as fatty or desiccated pedicles and adhesions. On the other hand, it is more prudent to use the lower-voltage CUT current via the edge of an electrode whenever lateral thermal spread may pose extra liability to adjacent tissues.
- If bleeding in the vicinity of the bowel, bladder, or ureter cannot be controlled with pressure alone, carefully direct short bursts of noncontact COAG current with a broad-surface electrode to attain hemostasis with the least-possible amount of electrosurgical penetration. Still, visceral bleeding is best controlled by mechanical means, using the patience of pressure or suture ligation.
- Although the flow of current is restricted to the tissue between the poles during bipolar electrosurgery, this does not eliminate the risk of thermal injury to tissue that is distant from the site of directed hemostasis. As current is applied between the poles, the intervening tissue gradually desiccates until it becomes thoroughly dehydrated. Desiccation is complete when the tissue whitens and visible steam emission stops. If the application of current continues, the heat spreads well beyond the electrical limits of the instrument. Unwanted thermal damage can be minimized by terminating the flow of current at the end of the visible vapor phase, applying current in a pulsatile fashion to permit tissue cooling, and securing pedicles by a stepwise process that alternates between partial desiccation and incremental cutting. Because the rate of temperature generation is a direct function of the volume of tissue being desiccated, thermal spread can also be reduced by using the sides or tips of a slightly open forceps to press or lift, rather than coapt for hemostasis.
- As with contact monopolar coagulation, tissue between the electrodes of a bipolar instrument may become adherent during desiccation. Repeated attempts to shake the tissue free may lead to traumatic avulsion of a key vascular pedicle. A stuck vascular pedicle can usually be unglued by energizing the opened device while immersed in a conductive irrigant, such as saline. Once the solution is boiled by the high current density between the electrodes, the mechanical action of bubbling is usually sufficient to atraumatically free the pedicle.

Bibliography

Brill AI. Energy systems for operative laparoscopy. *J Am Assoc Gynecol Laparosc* 1998;5(4):333.

Brill AI. Energy systems for operative hysteroscopy. *Obstet Gynecol Clin North Am* 2000;27(2):317.

Brill AI, Feste JR, Hamilton TL, et al. Patient safety during laparoscopic monopolar electrosurgery: principles and guidelines. Consortium on Electrosurgical Safety During Laparoscopy. *JSLS* 1998;2(3):221.

Luciano AA, Frishman GN, Kratka SA, et al. A comparative analysis of adhesion reduction, tissue effects, and incising characteristics of electrosurgery, CO_2 laser, and Nd-Yag laser at operative laparoscopy. *J Laparoendosc Surg* 1992;2:305.

Luciano AA, Whitman GF, Maier DB, et al. A comparison of thermal injury, healing patterns and postoperative adhesion formation following CO_2 laser and electromicrosurgery. *Fertil Steril* 1987;48:1025.

McCarus SD. Physiologic mechanism of the ultrasonically activated scalpel. *J Am Assoc Gynecol Laparosc* 1996;3(4):601.

Miller CE. Total laparoscopic hysterectomy using ultrasound energy. In: Sutton C, Diamond M, eds. *Endoscopic surgery for gynecologists*. 2nd ed. London: WB Saunders Company; 1988.

Miller CE. Use of the harmonic scalpel in endometriosis surgery. In: Sutton C, Jones K, Adamson GD, eds. *Modern management of endometriosis*. London: Taylor & Francis; 2005.

Munro MG. Mechanisms of thermal injury to the lower genital tract with radiofrequency resectoscopic surgery. *J Minim Invasive Gynecol* 2006; 13(1):36.

Odell RC. Biophysics of electrical energy. In: Soderstrom RM, ed. *Operative laparoscopy: the master's techniques*. New York: Raven Press; 1993:35.

Pearce JA. *Electrosurgery*. London: Chapman & Hall; 1986.

Reich H, Vancaillie TG, Soderstrom RM. Electrical techniques. In: Martin DC, ed. *Manual of endoscopy*. Baltimore: Port City Press; 1990:105.

Voyles CR, Tucker RD. Education and engineering solutions for potential problems with monopolar electrosurgery at laparoscopy. *Am J Surg* 1992; 164:57.

CHAPTER 16 ■ APPLICATION OF LASER GYNECOLOGY

JOHN MARLOW

DEFINITIONS

Cervical conization—Operation that removes a volume of tissue from the central longitudinal axis of the cervix, including the external os and a length of the canal.

CW—Continuous wave delivery with nonvarying laser energy oscillating constantly.

Laser—Light amplification by the stimulated emission of radiation.

Nd:YAG—Neodymium-doped yttrium aluminum garnet laser.

NHZ—Nominal hazardous zone. Zone of potential hazardous reflection of laser.

Power density—Concentration of laser energy at the impact site formula: PD = 1 W × 100/spot size mm^2

Pulsed laser—Laser energy delivered in the form of a single pulse or train of pulses.

Q-switched laser—Laser mode with reduction of pulse time and significant increase in peak power.

TEM—Transverse electromagnetic mode. Laser energy distribution in beam.

LASER HISTORY

The term *laser* is an acronym for *l*ight *a*mplification by *s*timulated *e*mission of *r*adiation. In 1917, Albert Einstein predicted and described the process of stimulated emission of radiation, but it was not until 1953 that Charles Townes and coworkers produced a device called a maser, which amplified microwaves by stimulated emission of radiation. In 1958, Schawlow and Townes published a hypothesis that described the laser in general terms. In 1960, Maiman constructed the first working laser, which consisted of a ruby crystal having a wavelength of 690 nanometers (nm). It was stimulated to emit laser energy by pumping with light from a xenon flash lamp. The carbon dioxide (CO_2) laser generating energy at a wavelength of 10,600 nm was developed by Patel in 1964 at the Bell Laboratories. It was used for the first time in experimental surgery in 1965. In 1973, laser was first used in gynecology by Kaplan and colleagues, who reported CO_2 laser vaporization of infected cervical tissue. Since that time, a large number of reports of CO_2 laser for lower reproductive tract surgery have accumulated. During the late 1970s, the CO_2 laser was coupled to the laparoscope, and the first successful operative laser laparoscopies were performed.

Other lasers have proved useful in gynecologic surgery. Some have wavelengths that are conducted by quartz fibers. In 1963, the neodymium-aluminum-garnet (Nd:YAG) laser was developed, and in 1984, the frequency-doubled YAG wavelengths of KTP 532 became available for clinical trials. Each of these fiber-optic lasers is used successfully in gynecology, particularly in the field of operative endoscopy, where fiber-optic delivery simplifies the application of the laser energy.

Any surgical procedure that requires cutting, coagulating, or removing tissue can be performed by laser. The effectiveness of laser energy relates to its ability to be delivered to tissue using microscopes and endoscopes. Laser surgery can vaporize tissue layer by layer, without touching it, with minimal thermal damage and optimal clinical results.

LASER PHYSICS

Stimulated Emission

Laser light is extremely bright, of similar color and direction, and is most often described in terms of its wave characteristics or wavelength. Wavelength is the distance between two successive crests or troughs, and wavelength determines the color of the light. Wavelengths are usually measured in microns or nanometers (nm). One micron equals 1/1,000 mm, and 1 nm equals 1/1,000,000 mm. Electromagnetic waves are often referred to as light, although visible light occupies only a small portion of the electromagnetic spectrum. CO_2 laser energy in the far infrared portion of the spectrum, although invisible to the eye, may therefore be correctly thought of as light energy (Table 16.1).

An atom is composed of a positively charged nucleus surrounded by electrons that orbit this nucleus. Each electron orbit can be described in terms of energy levels. As orbital distance from the nucleus increases, energy level increases. As described by the laws of quantum mechanics, when an electron moves from a higher-energy orbit to a lower-energy orbit, the atom loses a specific amount of energy in the form of a photon, which also has a specific wavelength.

Lasers contain what is referred to as an active lasing medium: a collection of atoms or molecules that are housed in an optically resonant cavity. This cavity, often cylindrical, is designed so that light of a specific wavelength will resonate between the closed ends of the cavity, much as sound will resonate in a properly constructed chamber. The active medium is stimulated, or "pumped," by an external energy source, such as electricity or light, which stimulates the active lasing medium to higher energy levels. As decay back to resting energy levels occurs, photons of energy are released into the optical cavity. Electrons that are still in excited higher orbital energy levels can also be stimulated by bombardment with these newly released photons so that they undergo identical decay and emit an identical photon. This is called *stimulated emission,* because one photon has stimulated the production of another photon.

TABLE 16.1

LASER COLORS AND WAVELENGTHS

Name	Color	Wavelength (nm)
Alexandrite	Red or near infrared	755/798
Argon	Blue-green	488/515
CO_2	Infrared	10,600
Diode	Red-orange	750/950
Dye laser	Yellow-green-red	577/630
Erbium YAG	Mid infrared	
Eximer	Ultraviolet	193/351
KTP-YAG	Green	532
Krypton	Green-yellow	532/568
Helium neon	Red	632
	Green	543
	Yellow	594
	Orange	612
HolmiumYAG	Mid infrared	2150
Gold vapor	Red	630
Krypton	Red, yellow, green	647
Nd:YAG	Near infrared	1,064
Ruby	Deep red	694
Copper vapor/green, yellow		

The optical cavity of the laser tube is closed at each end by a mirror. One of these mirrors is totally reflective, but the other is semitransparent. Although photon direction in the tube is random, a certain number of photons will be emitted in the axis of the optical cavity. The others are focused by the mirrors so that most are resonating or bouncing back and forth along the axis of the cavity. Some of these photons emerge through the semitransparent mirror and are emitted from the laser as the monochromatic parallel coherent laser beam. Coherent means that the waves are all in phase or perfectly aligned. The laser thus creates a light that travels in a tight beam over long distances.

Laser power is measured in terms of watts, and laser energy is expressed in terms of joules. One joule equals 1 W of power applied for 1 second. Lasers are named for the active medium contained in their optical cavities. Many different lasers have been constructed for diverse uses. In gynecologic surgery, the CO_2 and YAG lasers are the most commonly used. Despite many efforts, fiber-optic delivery systems have never been satisfactorily adapted to CO_2 laser energy. However, other lasers produce wavelengths that are conducted along quartz fibers. The use of the fiber is of great advantage in endoscopic surgery because it can be passed down the channel of an operative telescope, suction irrigator probe, or other hollow channel within the instrument.

Power Density and Transverse Electromagnetic Mode

When laser energy passes from the laser, the photons are coherent and parallel and theoretically could travel in space in this form to infinity. This changes when laser light is focused through a lens or directed into a quartz fiber. CO_2 laser energy is usually focused by a lens to a relatively small spot: the focal point of that lens. Focal spot size varies directly with the focal length of the lens. In surgical usage, however, additional lenses or mechanical devices allow the surgeon to change the spot-size diameter with ease. For any given power setting of the CO_2 laser, the concentration or density of the power is greater as the spot size becomes smaller, and conversely, as the spot size (tissue impact area) is enlarged, the power density decreases. By focusing or defocusing the laser energy, it is used as a cutting or coagulating tool. The concentration of laser energy at its focal point is referred to as its *power density* (PD) and is expressed as watts per square centimeter. A simplified formula for power density is watts per square mm calculated by the formula PD = power in watts × 100/area of spot size in mm squared. Because the calculation of power density is relatively complicated, most surgeons prefer to note the power setting on the laser and the effective spot size used for surgery. Obviously, the biologic effect and type of surgical injury are varied by changing spot size.

Although the photons of laser light are parallel, laser energy is not completely uniform throughout the cross-sectional diameter of the beam (Fig. 16.1). The term *transverse electromagnetic mode* (TEM) refers to the energy distribution of the cross-sectional diameter. For example, in most CO_2 surgical lasers, the energy distribution is greatest at the center of the beam and decreases toward the periphery. If one graphs the energy distribution of the cross-sectional beam diameter of the CO_2 laser, the resultant curve is bell-shaped. This Gaussian distribution does not hold true in fiber-optic lasers, YAG, potassium-titanyl-phosphate (KTP), and argon, in which energy distribution tends to be more uniform. However, when energy from these lasers enters a quartz fiber, conduction alters parallelism, and beam divergence of approximately 15 degrees occurs at the fiber tip. Thus, laser energy emerging from a fiber-optic conductor is not coherent, and the greatest concentration

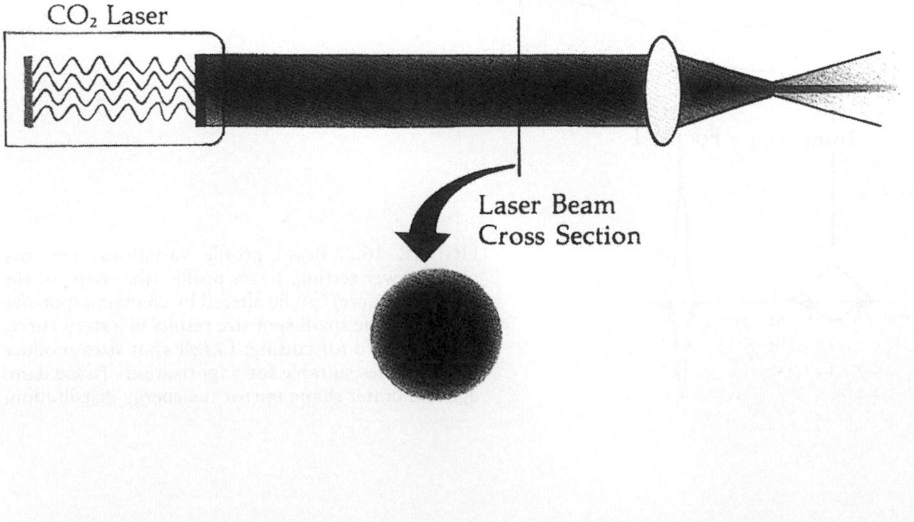

FIGURE 16.1. Transverse electromagnetic mode. Laser energy distribution is not uniform throughout the cross section of the beam. Energy concentration is highest at the beam center and decreases toward the periphery.

of this energy exists at the fiber–air or tissue interface where the spot size is smallest—that is, the same diameter as the conductor.

Time Dependence of Lasers

The effect of lasers on tissue is dependent on the duration that the tissue is exposed to laser energy. In continuous wave (CW) mode delivery, the laser oscillates constantly and delivers nonvarying power to the tissue. A pulsed laser can deliver energy in the form of a single pulse or a train of pulses. The duration of a pulse is typically less than 0.25 second. Pulsing the laser to the tissue for a short duration is useful to control the delivery and power of the beam. Significantly higher power density can cut tissue with minimal coagulation necrosis at the margins. A *Q-switching laser* is a laser that reduces its pulse time and significantly increases its peak power. In this mode, laser radiation is released in a short burst of laser light with high peak power. When the shutter of the optical cavity is rapidly opened, the laser energy is discharged in an extremely short period of time (10^{-6}–10^{-9} seconds). Laser energy of 10^7 watts can be obtained using this mode. A Q-switched laser pulse is used when it is critical to minimize adjacent tissue effects, for example, in laser surgery to the eye. Pulsing lasers at extremely high peak power (e.g., 500–2500 pulses/second) permit cutting tissue with lower water content.

MEDICAL LASERS AND TISSUE INTERACTION

CO_2 Laser

Laser energy interacts with tissue causing biologic, photochemical, or thermal reactions. The laser energy is absorbed, scattered, or affected by the thermal conductivity and local circulation of the tissue. The primary tissue effect of the surgical lasers used in gynecology is thermal. The beam profile for any given power setting can be altered by changing the spot size diameter (Fig. 16.2). Soft tissue is about 80% water by volume. CO_2 laser is highly absorbed by water, limiting its penetration to the surface of the tissue, where it can be monitored visually. Deep penetration of this laser energy into tissue is minimal as long as intracellular and extracellular water remains to be vaporized. When heat is delivered by the laser beam, the tissue's temperature is elevated. The area of laser impact has a shape reflecting the laser beam's intensity profile. When tissue temperature is elevated to 57°C, irreversible damage to the cell's proteins occurs, and the cell dies. Between 57°C and 100°C, there will be tissue death without vaporization. Above 100°C, vaporization occurs, with conversion of the fluid content of tissue to vapor and the other cellular components being converted to smoke. This product is referred to as the *laser plume*. When the plume is evacuated, it debrides the area and effectively removes the tissue. Additional tissue damage results from lateral conduction of heat away from the laser impact site. The amount of damage caused by heat conduction is directly proportional to the amount of time spent in lasing.

There are three zones of laser tissue damage that may be defined: (i) the area vaporized, (ii) the area of tissue death that results from the heated tissue short of vaporization, and (iii) the area of tissue damage caused by conduction of the heat away from the lased site (Fig. 16.3). Knowledge of beam geometry also plays a role in achieving a specific laser surgical effect. For example, a sharply focused laser beam with power settings of 15 to 25 W and a spot diameter of 0.2 mm produces a high power density up to 50,000 to 80,000 W/cm^2. This laser beam configuration produces narrow tissue vaporization comparable to an incision made by a scalpel (Fig. 16.4). Defocusing the beam enlarges the spot, and using the same settings, power density is reduced to 500 to 1,000 W/cm^2. This technique is used to treat a thin surface rapidly. The proper power setting and spot diameter combine to determine effect on the tissue. The surgeon can view the process through an operative microscope with little fear of deep thermal damage. This margin of safety has contributed to the popularity of CO_2 laser surgery.

There are several advantages of CO_2 laser over a knife and electrosurgical instruments. Laser surgery is performed with no contact to the tissue. No bacteria is transferred from the surgical instrument to the tissue. The laser beam sterilizes the operative field as it vaporizes it. Because it removes tissue with vaporization and evacuation, the suctioned plume allows the tissue base to heal without a devitalized tissue covering. Postoperative pain is reduced because nerve endings are sealed by the

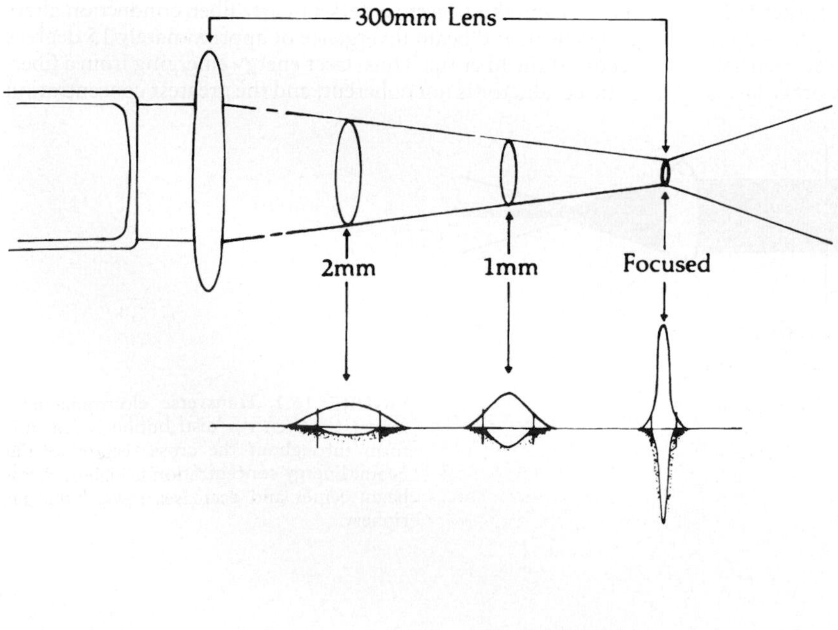

FIGURE 16.2. Beam profile variations. For any given power setting, beam profile (the shape of the Gaussian curve) can be altered by changing spot-size diameter. The small spot size results in a steep curve, which is used for cutting. Larger spot sizes produce flatter curves suitable for vaporization. Tissue damage and crater shape mirror the energy distribution.

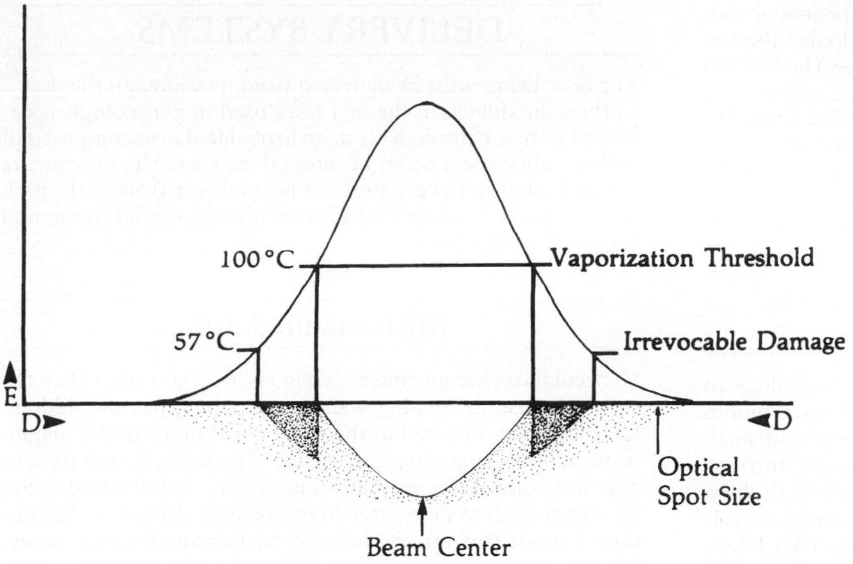

FIGURE 16.3. Beam profile and tissue damage. Laser wounds produce three zones of tissue damage: the vaporization crater, the area of tissue necrosis caused by heating tissue to temperatures between 57° and 100°C, and the area of damage resulting from heat conduction. Higher power settings produce more rapid vaporization of tissue and lessen secondary thermal damage.

beam. Coagulating lasers can be used in patients with bleeding disorders. The laser can be delivered for easy access to confined areas with a clear field of view.

Helium Neon

The helium neon laser (HeNe) is a gas laser with a wavelength of 633 nm in the red portion of the visible spectrum. It is a low-powered laser with output ranging from 1 to 100 mW. It is used in many common tools, including bar-code scanners. The most popular HeNe lasers produces red light. Other colored helium neon lasers include green with a wavelength of 543 nm, yellow at 594 nm, and orange at 612 nm.

Helium neon laser is used as an "aiming beam" for lasers that have nonvisible wavelengths, such as carbon dioxide. When HeNe laser is aligned with the nonvisible laser, it defines the laser's impact site for the surgeon. This alignment of these two laser beams is checked before treatment begins.

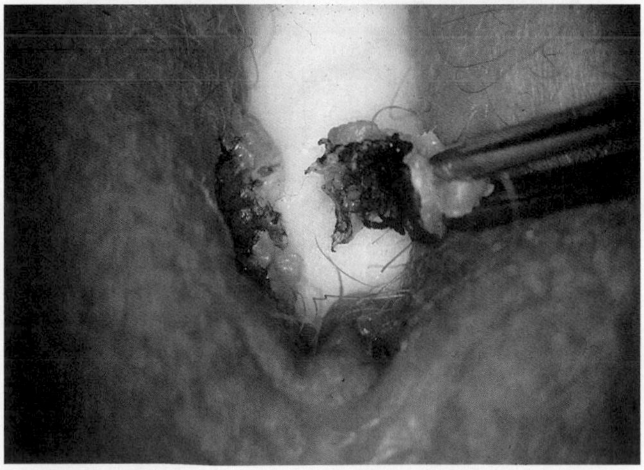

FIGURE 16.4. Carbon dioxide laser used as a cutting tool. Excisional biopsy of the vulva using a freehand delivery with a spot size of 0.2 mm and a power density of 50,000 watts per square centimeter. Water-soaked cotton acts as a backstop.

Neodymium YAG

YAG laser energy is able to penetrate tissue to a much greater depth. Unlike CO_2 laser, the neodymium-doped yttrium aluminum garnet (Nd:YAG) laser is poorly absorbed by water. The YAG is often used in a liquid medium. Because it penetrates water so well, the YAG is not a good laser for vaporization. It is an effective coagulator, however, as it passes deeper into tissue before absorption occurs.

YAG energy scatters in tissue, so thermal damage is greater than with CO_2 laser. It is absorbed with a power density that is maximum below the tissue surface. This limits the ability to visually monitor the YAG laser's depth of penetration and stresses the importance of the surgeon to understand the physics of each laser. YAG laser can be transmitted through quartz fibers and fluids. The depth of penetration provides excellent hemostasis. Goldrath and colleagues in 1981 recognized this and used Nd:YAG laser for the first hysteroscopic endometrial ablations. This laser is also used for removal of hair and vascular lesions in a Q-switched delivery.

Argon, KTP-YAG

The argon laser produces a blue-green light that has two distinct bands at 488 nm and 515 nm, whereas KTP-YAG is located at 532 nm on the electromagnetic spectrum. These are referred to as *colored lasers* because they are in the visible spectrum. These lasers can be transmitted through water or quartz fibers of 200 to 600 micron diameter. Hemoglobin and other deeply colored pigments absorb their wavelengths and are responsible for their use in vascular and pigmented lesions. Penetration into skin, typically 1 to 2 mm, is affected by the concentration of skin pigments. Argon, KTP-YAG lasers produce a moderate scatter 100 times that of CO_2 laser. This results in an excellent hemostasis. Because of the scatter, they have minimal cutting ability. The depth of tissue injury is roughly correlated with the laser power settings.

The KTP-532 laser derives its name from the potassium (K), titanyl (T), and phosphate (P) crystal used to double the frequency and halve the wavelength of the YAG laser. The 532-nm wavelength is emerald green. Its tissue effects are very similar to those produced by the argon laser. The KTP-532 is used to vaporize or to coagulate, and energy emerging from the end of the fiber can be used to cut tissue. Their greatest application has been in endoscopic surgery, because the delivery systems for their energy can be passed down the operative channel of an endoscope.

Holmium YAG

This laser's wavelength is 2,100 nm. It is used in urology to disintegrate renal stones and ablate obstructing tissue within the prostate. It can be delivered through both large and small fibers. The smaller fiber of 200 microns gives access through flexible ureteroscopes to reach the lower pole of the kidney. It is pulsed at 350 to 700 microseconds at repeating intervals of 5 to 20 Hz to disintegrate the stones. The Ho-YAG laser's depth of penetration in tissue is 0.4 mm. Like CO_2 laser, this laser is absorbed at the superficial layers of tissue. Vaporization speed, coagulation depth, and hemostasis can be precisely controlled. These properties can be particularly useful in gynecologic endoscopy. Laser treatment can be delivered through small channels to areas of difficult access. Of equal interest is its ability to limit the lateral spread of the thermal energy. The risk of injury to bowel, ureters, blood vessels, and nerves because of any lateral thermal spread is reduced.

Dye Lasers

Argon-pumped rhodamine-B-dye lasers are tuned to produce a specific wavelength of light. They are delivered to cells that have been sensitized with hematoporphyrin derivatives (HPDs). Certain HPD drugs concentrate in malignant tissue and are activated by specific laser wavelengths. This results in a cytotoxic effect on the tumor. The release of singlet oxygen results in the death of the cancer cells. The U.S. Food and Drug Administration has approved specific HPDs for use in cancer therapy, and it is currently in use in oncologic centers.

Aesthetic surgery

Aesthetic surgery for women is the newest use of lasers by some gynecologic surgeons. The applications include hair removal, vein treatment, and epithelial resurfacing. Some of the lasers used are listed in Table 16.2.

TABLE 16.2

LASER USED IN AESTHETIC SURGERY

Carbon dioxide 1,064 nm
Erbium–YAG 2,940 nm
Diode 810 nm 100 msec long pulse 595
Alexandrite 755 nm Q-switched for blue, black green tattoo removal
Ruby long pulse 694 nm Q-switched
Nd:YAG 1,064nm long pulse, Q-switched, frequency doubled 532 nm for red or orange ink tattoo removal

DELIVERY SYSTEMS

The laser beam must be delivered from its source to the tissue. Carbon dioxide laser, the first laser used in gynecology, is delivered to tissue through air in an articulated arm composed of hollow tubes and a series of internal mirrors. The mirrors are precisely aligned to keep the laser beam directed along the path of the arm. At the distal end a lens made of a special compound focuses the laser beam.

Micromanipulator

Gynecologists became interested in laser surgery after they observed its use in treating vocal cord papillomas in children. CO_2 laser was directed to the vocal cord tumor under magnification of an operating microscope. The delivery unit used to aim and control the laser beam is called a micromanipulator. This system allows the surgeon to precisely deliver the laser to the tissue. It was attached to the microscope for easy access by the surgeon. The beam was reflected to the tissue by a mirror controlled by a joystick. After observing the effective use with this instrumentation on children's vocal cord papillomas, surgeons adapted the system to gynecology. They substituted a colposcope for the operating microscope and used it to treat the cervix and vulva (Fig. 16.5). Micromanipulators can be fitted with focusing lenses similar to a zoom lens of a camera. This allows the spot to be varied in size without changing the optical focus for the surgeon.

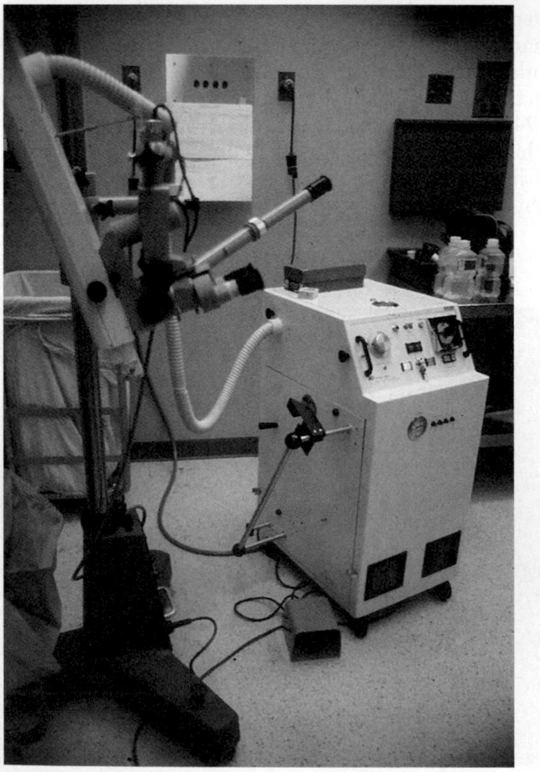

FIGURE 16.5. First laser instrument used in gynecology. A micromanipulator is attached to a colposcope for carbon dioxide laser treatment of the cervix, vagina, and vulva. 1978. Photo courtesy of Columbia Hospital for Women, Washington, DC.

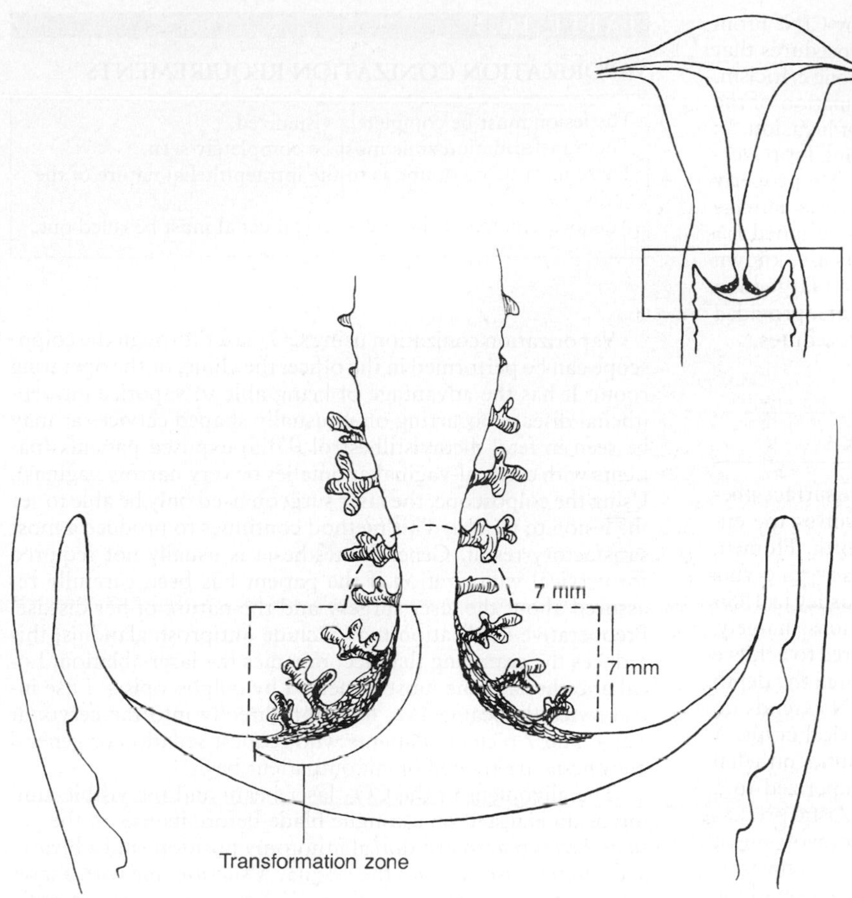

FIGURE 16.6. Cervical vaporization defect. After the cervix has been vaporized to the approximate depth, an additional 3 mm of endocervical canal is vaporized to avoid endocervical prolapse and to ensure that the new squamocolumnar junction is just inside of the external os.

Laser Hand Piece

As CO_2 laser became popular in the 1980s, other delivery systems were developed, including the freehand mode. This system is composed of a focusing lens contained within a metal tube that is held in the hand. The lens typically has a short focal length, capable of producing a very small 0.2-mm spot size. With this narrow beam, the laser is used as a cutting instrument. By pulling the hand piece away from the tissue, the surgeon creates a larger spot size used for vaporizing tissue. Cutting and coagulating external genital surgery became its principal application (Fig. 16.6).

ENDOSCOPY

The next advancement was the use of lasers in laparoscopy. CO_2 laser was delivered through large channels in a single puncture operative laparoscope. The large channels were necessary to transmit the beam and avoid reflections from the channel walls. Rigid wave guides were introduced that could also be used through ancillary 3 mm or larger channels.

FIBER OPTICS

As fiber lasers including Nd:YAG and KTP became available, they were also delivered through small channels. Fiber delivery is less cumbersome and produces less plume and more hemostasis. It requires smaller channels. The aiming beam is easily seen. This mode of delivery is especially useful in hysteroscopy because fiber lasers could be used through fluid distending media. Neodymium and holmium YAG are delivered through optical quartz fibers 100 to 600 microns in diameter. At the tip of the fiber, the beam diverges, so power density is greatest just off the tip of the fiber. The beam also can also be defocused by moving the tip of the fiber farther away from the target tissue.

LASER SURGERY OF THE LOWER REPRODUCTIVE TRACT

The first use of lasers in gynecology was to treat cervical intraepithelial neoplasia (CIN) and visible condylomata of the lower reproductive tract. The precise cutting and ablative properties of CO_2 laser prompted an interest in this surgery. It was successfully used in the 1980s, and CO_2 laser was enthusiastically received by many gynecologists. Colposcopy provided an accurate means of identifying the location and size of the lesions, and CO_2 laser provided unparalleled precision to treat these conditions. Micromanipulator delivery is most popular, although another alternative is using the laser hand piece while visualizing the surgical field through a colposcope.

CIN, later also referred to as squamous intraepithelial lesions (SILs), has been treated successfully by either *in situ* destruction or excision. In 1968, Palucek and Townsend reported a series in which cryosurgery was used to destroy CIN. From the beginning, however, the use of destructive procedures that did not produce a pathologic specimen evoked strong criticism, fearing that lack of a complete pathologic examination of the target tissue could result in a missed diagnosis of invasion. In the late 1960s, Cartier in Paris developed a cutting loop electrode with a wire diameter of 200 micron that, when properly used, produced only a very small amount of thermal damage in the excised specimen. A larger wire loop was designed for excisional cervical surgery in the United States. Its use, known as a loop electrode excision procedure (LEEP) or a large loop excision of transformation zone (LLETZ) procedure, provided a tissue specimen as an alternative to ablation procedures.

Laser Surgery of the Cervix

Although CIN has been described as a noninvasive surface phenomenon, it is well known that the process involves the endocervical crypts. The work of Te Linde, Danforth, Flumen, Burghardt, and others pointed out that the endocervical crypts were involved in CIN, but it was Anderson and Hartley in 1980 who really emphasized the therapeutic implications; namely, adequate depth of destruction or excision is required to achieve satisfactory results. Anderson and Hartley measured the depth of crypt involvement and found that 99% of CIN extends no further than 4 mm from the surface into the cervical crypt. A logical assumption can then made. If an area of intraepithelial neoplasia on the cervix was either excised or vaporized to a depth greater than 4 mm, virtually all of the neoplastic process would be treated. This concept of depth-of-crypt involvement is extremely important to the surgeon, for it dictates a measurable depth of destruction to be achieved by vaporization of the transformation zone if a surgical specimen is not to be removed by conization (Fig. 16.6).

It follows that if the lesion of intraepithelial neoplasia is visualized in its entirety (i.e., if the borders of the lesion are clearly seen on the cervix, and the lesion does not extend up into the canal), then it can be biopsied and correctly diagnosed as intraepithelial neoplasia. This assumption provides the justification for all nonexcisional, ablative procedures used to destroy cervical intraepithelial disease. Laser ablation—by virtue of its ability to be delivered under colposcopic magnification and applied according to a patient's specific, unique anatomy—is a valuable tool.

Vaporization Conization

Cervical conization has been defined as an operation that removes a volume of tissue from the central longitudinal axis of the cervix; this includes the external os and a certain length of endocervical canal. The actual shape of the volume of tissue removed should be determined by the distribution of the lesion and not by some preconceived geometric shape. *Conization*, then, is a generic term, and does not necessarily imply that a perfect cone-shaped defect has been produced in the cervix. Cones can be asymmetric and are short, long, thin, cylindrical, or any other shape that accomplishes the intended goal of complete removal of the lesion and the tissue at risk. A number of techniques have been used to perform conization operations. In laser surgery, the end result is the same. If the CIN lesion cannot be entirely visualized or a neoplasm cannot be properly diagnosed for any reason, the CIN should not be treated by an ablative procedure. The requirements for vaporization conization are listed in Table 16.3.

TABLE 16.3

VAPORIZATION CONIZATION REQUIREMENTS

The lesion must be completely visualized.
The transformation zone must be completely seen.
There must be no doubt as to the intraepithelial nature of the disease.
Adenocarcinoma of the endocervical canal must be ruled out.

Vaporization conization using CO_2 laser through the colposcope can be performed in the office, the clinic, or the operating room. It has the advantage of being able to vaporize intraepithelial disease occurring on unusually shaped cervices as may be seen in fetal diethylstilbestrol (DES)-exposed patients (patients with cervical-vaginal anomalies or very narrow vaginas). Using the colposcope, the laser surgeon need only be able to see the lesion to treat it. This method continues to produce a most satisfactory result. General anesthesia is usually not required for cervical vaporization if the patient has been carefully reassured about the laser surgery and the nature of her disease. Preoperative medication may include antiprostaglandins; this reduces the cramping that accompanies the laser ablation. Local anesthesia is the most preferred by colposcopists. I use intracervical lidocaine 1%, injection directly into the cervix at 12, 4, and 7 o'clock. Patients who request sedation or general anesthesia are treated on an outpatient basis.

The alignment of the CO_2 laser beam and the visible aiming beam is tested on a tongue blade before its use on the patient. She is placed in a dorsal lithotomy position, and a bivalve speculum is inserted into the vagina. A suction line with a laser filter is attached to the speculum. This is necessary to maintain a clear view of the operative site. Paper drapes and flammable material are avoided because of the risk of fire. Wet towels are placed at the margins of the operative field. No special prep is necessary. The cervix is cleaned with a 4% acetic acid solution, and the lesion to be treated is identified. The margin of the transformation zone is outlined by a series of vaporization craters, using short bursts of laser energy (Fig. 16.7). The entire transformation zone is included in the area to be vaporized. The dots are connected so that the area to be treated is completely outlined. A spot size of 2 mm is used for the vaporization operation. An experienced laser surgeon may use a higher power setting and be able to direct the laser more rapidly, shortening the operative time. Lower power settings mean greater ease of vaporization and very accurate observation of the depth of the defect. The vaporization is carried to 7 mm (Fig. 16.8). The depth can be measured with a calibrated measuring device. Often, the cervix and the area of the external os are not flush, and an accurate measurement of depth of vaporization may be difficult. For this reason, it seems more accurate to divide the cervix into sections and then destroy the tissue section by section. In this way, part of the normal cervical anatomy is preserved throughout the operation, and even though the topography of the cervix may change, the exact depth of destruction can always be measured for each section. The margin peripheral to the transformation zone is treated for a distance of 2 to 5 mm.

Cervical stenosis can occur following ablative treatment. In a series of cervical stenosis patients reported by Valle and colleagues, Marlow successfully treated cervical stenosis with CO_2 and YAG lasers. Lasers have also been used to successfully treat stenosis in other organs. Laser surgery is preferred because of the minimal damage to adjacent tissue. Urologists

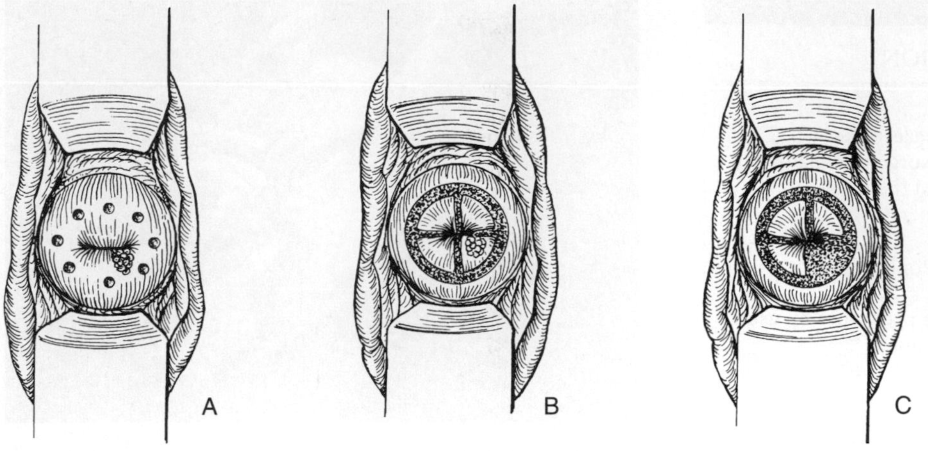

FIGURE 16.7. Cervical vaporization for cervical intraepithelial neoplasia. The cervix is reexamined with the colposcope and the margin of the vaporization conization is outlined by a series of vaporized tissue craters (A), the craters are connected and the cervix is divided into four quadrants (B), and the tissue is vaporized quadrant by quadrant to a depth of 7 mm (C).

treat narrowing of the prostatic urethra with holmium YAG laser. Oncologists treat obstructive stenosis of the esophagus with photodynamic therapy.

Bleeding is usually not encountered during vaporization procedures; however, if bleeding does occur, a wet cotton-tipped applicator is used to tamponade the vessel. The power density is then lowered by defocusing the beam or by slightly reducing the power, and the bleeding point is coagulated by using a rapid circular motion to surround the vessel. If bleeding is not controlled with this technique, other forms of hemostasis should be considered.

Excision Laser Conization of the Cervix

The goals of excisional conization are to produce a conization biopsy specimen that is adequate for pathologic examination and, if possible, excise all disease. The indications for laser excisional conization are the same as for cold-knife conization:

1. The lesion extends into the canal and cannot be entirely seen.
2. The entire transformation zone cannot be visualized.
3. Abnormal cytology is noted in the absence of a positive colposcopy.
4. There is positive endocervical curettage.
5. Invasive cancer cannot be ruled out by biopsy.

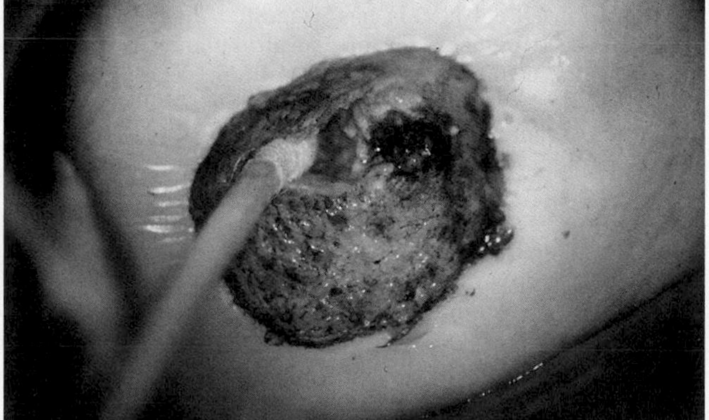

FIGURE 16.8. The end result of a vaporization cone performed in the office under local anesthesia. The endocervical canal is exposed with a cotton applicator for examination. A wet applicator is used within the canal to limit the laser beam from vaporizing the upper canal. Note the lack of bleeding.

The average excisional conization penetrates the cervical stroma more deeply than the vaporization conization, and the patient may experience more discomfort, as well as more bleeding, with this procedure. Although excisional conization can be satisfactorily performed with local anesthesia, I do not hesitate to perform this procedure on an outpatient basis under general anesthesia. The surgeon determines the size of the cone to fit the patient and lesion. A weighted speculum is placed in the vagina, and the anterior lip of the cervix is grasped with an atraumatic tenaculum. The cervix is painted with 4% acetic acid, and the patient is recolposcoped. The borders of the lesion are carefully noted. Following a tongue blade test of the beam, I use CO_2 laser settings of 25 to 50 W and the smallest spot size of 0.5 to 1 mm. Smoke evacuation is carried out with a filtered suction. Gentile traction with a laser conization hook allows the surgeon to tailor the cone shape to the distribution of the lesion or transformation zone. A water-soaked small cotton applicator can be inserted into the canal as a backstop to prevent deeper incision in the upper canal.

Excisional conization of the cervix by LEEP has provided an alternative procedure to laser with shorter operating time and reduced instrumentation expenses.

Laser Combination Procedures

One application of CO_2 laser is the combination cone. The central lesion in the cervix is removed by LEEP or knife conization. This is followed by laser vaporization of intraepithelial disease extending to the vagina. Large areas of intraepithelial neoplasia and multifocal lesions that involve much of the cervix and then extend into the vagina or even involve the vulva can be treated by this combination laser procedure. Peripheral portions of the lesion should be previously biopsied and proven to be benign. Thus, the indications for both excisional and vaporization have been met, and a conservative procedure has been performed. Combination procedures are the most conservative procedures possible because the operation is microsurgical and tailored to destroy the smallest amount of tissue.

Postoperative Instructions

Patients undergoing laser surgery to the cervix usually require very little postoperative care. The patient is seen in

TABLE 16.4

ADVANTAGES OF LASER CONIZATION

There is less bleeding than with a scalpel.
There is less tissue damage than with the electric cautery.
The procedure has advantages over cryosurgery in that it can be done with much more precision, and the results are better for lesions of all sizes.
Morbidity is low.
All types and extents of intraepithelial neoplasia can be treated.
The most conservative procedures can be performed by using combinations of vaporization and excision.

postoperative follow-up in 2 to 4 weeks. Coitus is avoided for at least 4 weeks. Temperature elevations above 38°C and bleeding heavier than her normal menses are reported. About 15% of these patients will have some small amount of vaginal bleeding. Excessive bleeding is encountered in only about 2% of the patients. The patient is allowed to return to work within 48 hours. The very definite advantages associated with laser are listed in Table 16.4.

Results of Laser Surgery of the Cervix

Baggish and Dorsey reported a series of more than 4,000 cases of CIN treated by laser with an overall success rate between 96% and 97%. In those patients monitored by colposcopy, cytology, and biopsy for 1 year or more, vaporization procedures and excision conization procedures seem to produce about the same cure rate. In addition, cure rates do not vary when degree of CIN is taken into consideration. Persad and colleagues reported 1,126 patients with CIN treated over 13 years by laser with no evidence of recurrence or persistence in 92%. The median follow-up was 60 months. Other authors, such as Burke and colleagues, Reid (1987), and Wright, report success rates between 95% and 98%.

Laser Surgery of the Vulva

Unlike the cervix, the vulva is often the site of multifocal disease. There is no doubt that the concepts of accurate identification of disease and proper depth of destruction must also be applied to the therapy of vulvar intraepithelial neoplasia (VIN). Vulvar laser surgery should be done with the aid of the colposcope, and I usually prefer to use the micromanipulator. It is also imperative that the surgeon performing laser surgery on the vulva or the vagina has a working knowledge of vulvovaginal histology and of the variations in thickness of normal and abnormal neoplastic vulvovaginal epithelium.

Vulvar skin is composed of two layers, epidermis and dermis (Fig. 16.9). The margin between epidermis and dermis is an irregular one because of the rete ridges. Between the rete ridges are projections of dermis known as *dermal papillae.* The dermis can be divided into two layers: the superficial papillary layer and the deeper reticular layer. There are also skin appendages, such as pilosebaceous follicles, eccrine sweat glands, and apocrine glands, which project deep into the dermis. VIN, as well as human papillomavirus (HPV), may involve skin appendages and epidermis. Although the thickness of the epidermis may be a fraction of a millimeter, the dermis may measure 7 to 8 mm in thickness, and skin appendages may penetrate the full thickness. It is the goal of the laser surgeon to remove the

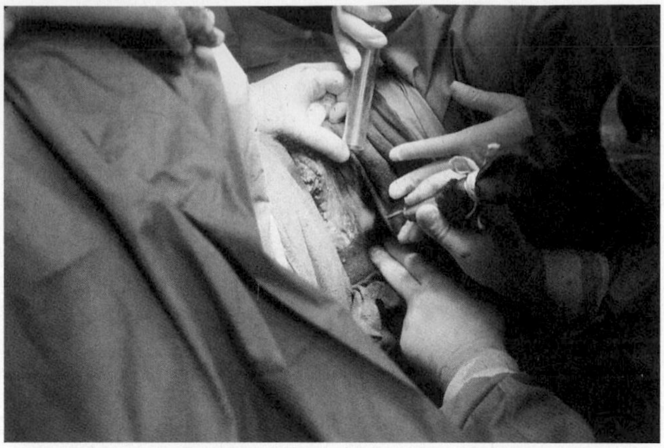

FIGURE 16.9. Vulvectomy using freehand CO_2 laser in operating room. The laser can be used to cut or vaporize tissue. Smoke evacuation tube is held directly over the laser site to remove any laser plume. Wet towels placed at margins to prevent combustion of drapes. The laser arm is covered with a sterile drape.

involved epidermis and a portion of the skin appendage that may also be involved in the disease process.

When the epidermis is removed by the plastic surgeon's knife in obtaining a split-thickness graft, or when the epidermis is removed by the laser surgeon during a vaporization procedure for intraepithelial neoplasia, the donor site or the vaporization site heals without replacement by a skin graft because the remaining skin appendages located in the dermis have not been completely destroyed. Each skin appendage serves as a source of squamous epithelium, so that when reepithelialization takes place, the process proceeds from the skin appendages. On the other hand, if the entire thickness of the dermis is taken and the skin appendages are completely destroyed, the operative site must be grafted or closed. It is important for the surgeon to review vulvar biopsies to judge the extent, if any, of disease into the skin appendages.

Unlike cervical vaporization, the depth of vaporization on the vulva cannot be measured. The expert laser microsurgeon is able to recognize the depth of ablation and can remove epidermis so accurately that the papillary dermis is not entirely destroyed. The papillary dermis can be identified at colposcopic magnifications. Reid (1991) has suggested that four surgical planes can be recognized. The first surgical plane represents the epidermis down to the basement membrane. The second surgical plane is described as extending into the papillary layer of the dermis so that the laser surgeon removes both the epidermis and the papillary dermis. The third surgical plane reaches well into the reticular dermis and uncovers the coarse collagen bundles that can be seen through the colposcope as grayish white fibers. The fourth surgical plane involves complete removal of the skin right down to the underlying subdermal fat. If this level is reached, healing must take place from the periphery, or a graft must be supplied.

Condylomata Accuminata

The human papillomavirus involves the epidermis and may also involve the superficial portions of skin appendages. One of the common mistakes of the novice surgeon is to go too deeply into the dermis in an attempt to destroy condylomas. Although only the warty lesion itself plus the surrounding epidermal margin need to be destroyed, a power density that is sufficient to accomplish this maneuver without creating excessive carbonization at the impact site must be used. Power densities below 600 W/cm^2 cause excessive carbonization, and irradiance of the carbonized surface of the vulva will raise laser-impact-site temperatures to more than 600°C. The power densities that I like to use are between 600 and 1,500 W/cm^2, and a 2- to 3-mm focal spot size with a power setting of 15 to 30 W will accomplish this. Each condylomata should be identified and the laser beam directed this target. Laser vaporizes the condylomata rapidly with the beam. The char and debris are wiped away, and the proper surgical level is colposcopically identified. Vaporization is taken to the papillary dermis (second surgical plane). Cold normal saline is used to cool the vulvar skin, because cooling helps reduce the heat diffusion and, therefore, the resultant tissue injury lateral to the laser impact site.

Vulvar Intraepithelial Neoplasia

It is impossible to colposcopically differentiate between some forms of HPV lesions that occur on the vulva and significant VIN. Therefore, it is extremely important to obtain a biopsy specimen of the vulva in as many areas as necessary to correctly identify the pathology before laser surgery. Local or general anesthesia may be used for vulvar laser surgery. In the case of multiple lesions or very large areas of involvement, general anesthesia is more practical (Fig. 16.9). Despite extensive vulvar laser surgery, patients usually are allowed to return home on the day of the operation.

When laser surgery is used, the vulva is recolposcoped, and 4% acetic acid is applied to demonstrate areas and borders of neoplastic or viral involvement. The larger areas are outlined in the manner described for CIN. If a lesion is large, it may be divided into smaller areas for lasing, because this provides a more accurate approach. As soon as the laser beam is passed over the surface of the tissue, all landmarks disappear. Proper identification and marking of the limits of the disease by the laser is a highly necessary step in treatment. A spot size of 2 to 3 mm and a power setting of 15 to 50 W may be used, depending on the surgeon's skill in manipulating the beam and spot size. Although destruction must be carried to the third surgical plane (i.e., the reticular dermis), the first step in vulvar laser surgery always involves identifying the papillary dermis. When the tiny micropapules of this layer are seen, the laser surgeon again ablates through this most superficial dermis, wiping away char and identifying the underlying reticular dermis. Often intermittent pulses of laser energy can improve surgical control of the laser beam. Instead of reducing the power of the beam, it is possible to use the mechanical timer on the laser console to reduce exposure by delivering one-tenth-second to one-twentieth-second bursts of laser energy. This technique allows the surgeon time to react to the microsurgical review of the tissue and more easily control the rate of energy delivery, thus too-deep penetration, char, and residual thermal damage are also reduced to a minimum.

Postoperative Care

If the lasing has been extensive, a Foley catheter may be required to avoid the immediate discomfort caused by urinary salts on the denuded vulvar surface. Catheters can be placed either through the urethra or suprapubically. Suprapubic drainage avoids the deposit of urinary salts on the wound, reducing pain and possible infection.

Customarily, an antibacterial cream or ointment, such as sulfadine cream or bacitracin ointment, is applied to the lased tissue to protect the raw surface from agglutination and to help prevent superficial infection. The patient must be given instructions to keep the vulvar folds separated, and the application of this medication helps in this respect. An ice pack is placed on the vulva when the patient leaves the operating room. Sitz baths begin the first day after laser surgery and are continued two times a day until the patient is no longer uncomfortable and the vulvar area is well on the way to reepithelialization. The patient is seen in a week to ensure there is no agglutination of vulvar folds.

Results of Vulvar Laser Surgery

The results of laser surgery on the vulva have been quite satisfactory, and there are some definite advantages to using the CO_2 laser for this disease as opposed to using conventional skinning vulvectomy. These again include accurate ablation of relatively large areas and a more controlled depth of removal because of colposcopically identifiable tissue planes (Fig. 16.10). Rapid healing usually occurs because of relatively little residual thermal damage. In Dorsey's series of more than 100 patients with intraepithelial neoplasia, 1-year cure rates have been more than 90%. Other lower reproductive tract laser surgeons report similar figures. One of the greatest benefits of vulvar laser surgery is that normal vulvar anatomy, particularly the labia minora and clitoris, is maintained (Fig. 16.11). This may not be possible when skinning vulvectomy is performed.

Laser Surgery of the Vagina

Vaginal intraepithelial neoplasia (VAIN) and associated HPV infections are among the most difficult lower reproductive tract intraepithelial neoplasias to treat for a number of reasons:

1. The vagina has a large surface area, which is difficult to visualize colposcopically.
2. There are many rugae and folds in the vagina.
3. The angle of the vaginal axis makes it difficult to treat by perpendicular beam impact.
4. The vaginal fornices are difficult to stabilize because they are quite distensible, and the cervix may hide portions of the fornix.
5. The colposcopic appearance of VAIN varies greatly and often goes unrecognized even by the expert colposcopist.

VAIN does not demonstrate mosaic patterns except in areas of adenosis. Often one sees coarse punctation, but the lesion may vary in color from a pale grayish white to the intense whiteness produced by hyperkeratosis. Often the lesions are multifocal and the borders are usually distinct, although the lesions may be somewhat serpiginous. VAIN may appear as an iodine-free zone. In the postmenopausal patient, it is helpful to treat the patient with topical estrogen for 2 weeks before examination for optimal accuracy of the iodine test.

The laser microsurgeon must be particularly aggressive in obtaining adequate biopsy specimens for VAIN. If the patient has had a hysterectomy, the lateral fornix may contain a dimple that must be everted for adequate visualization and biopsy. A laser hook or skin hook can be used to evert this area and stabilize the tissue so that appropriate biopsy can be obtained. The surgeon should be certain of the noninvasive nature of the disease before vaporization is performed.

Technique for Laser Vaporization Of Vain

The squamous epithelium of the mucous membrane of the vagina rests on a basement membrane. Below this is the lamina propria of the vagina, and this layer corresponds to the dermis of the vulvar skin. Below the lamina propria is a layer of muscle,

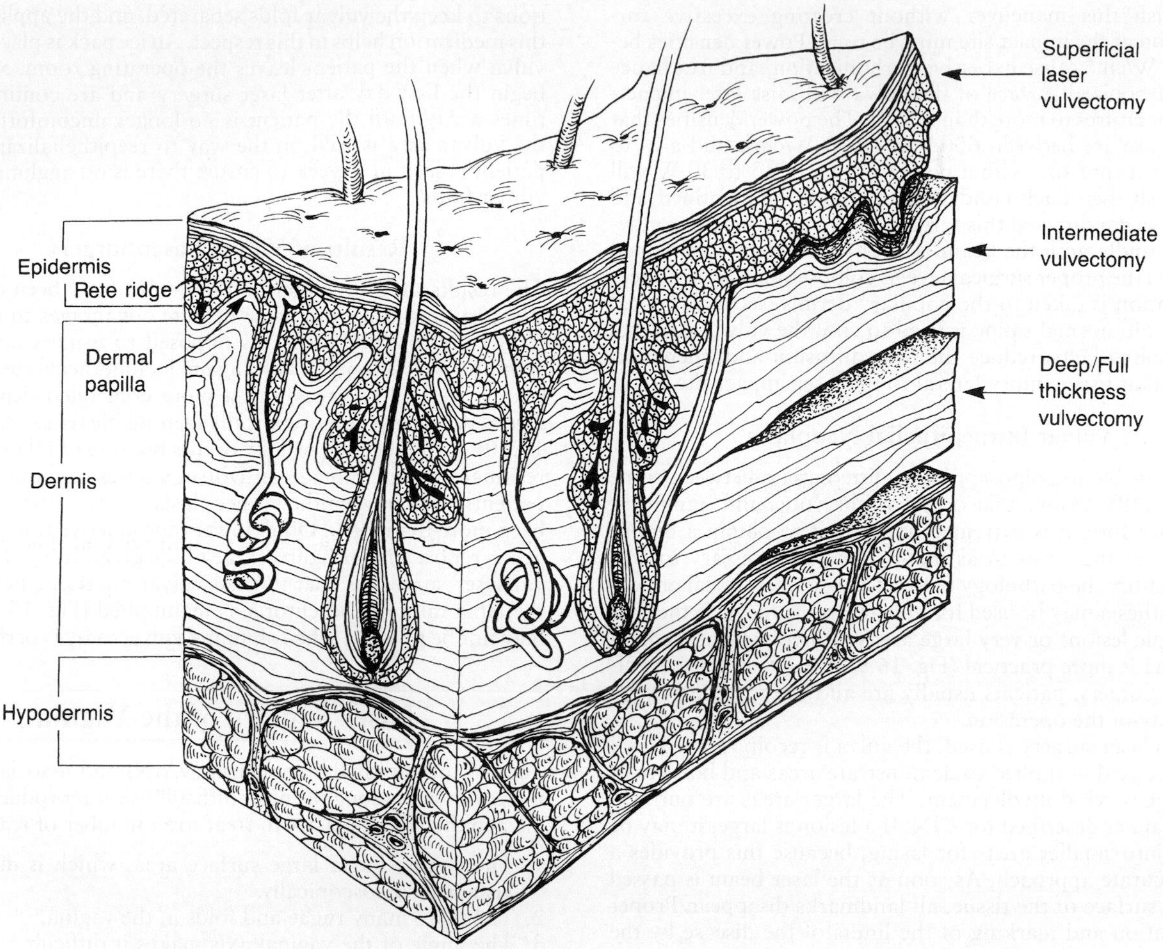

FIGURE 16.10. Vulvar skin. Vulvar skin is composed of epidermis and dermis plus the skin appendages. Complete removal of the epidermis and partial removal of the dermis still results in reepithelialization of the wound because of squamous recolonization from the skin appendages.

loose connective tissue, and fat. When the vaginal epithelium is destroyed, there must be visual identification of the underlying lamina propria because, as in the case of the vulva, it is impossible to accurately measure the depth of destruction in this very irregular area. Because the vaginal squamous epithelium is only a fraction of a millimeter thick and there are no skin appendages in the vagina, ablation is a superficial operation.

Exposing the vaginal epithelium by manipulating the speculum for diagnosis and laser treatment is painful for most patients. The surgeon often cocks the speculum to one side and shoots through the open sides to manipulate the target into a position that is perpendicular to the laser beam. The vaginal rugae must also be ironed out to ensure even laser energy application. All of this is most uncomfortable. For this reason, most patients with VAIN require general anesthesia on an outpatient basis.

The micromanipulator is preferred for laser VAIN treatment because it eliminates bulky and unnecessary instrumentation from the vagina. A spot size of 2 mm and power settings of 15 to 30 W are used. Large areas are subdivided so that more accurate ablation can be performed. The laser beam is rapidly passed over the area, and the epidermis is lifted away from the underlying lamina propria. A wet sponge or cotton swab is used to wipe away char and coagulated epithelium. Often the surgeon will find that the tops of rugae have been removed, but the troughs or valleys in between still contain viable dysplastic epithelium. With proper use of the speculum and other instruments, this problem is easily overcome. Adequate margins of 5 mm or more are used.

Postoperative Care for Vaginal Laser Surgery

Much of the discomfort encountered in postoperative vaginal laser surgery stems from laser wounds in the vaginal introitus. Because VAIN and VIN are so often multifocal diseases, many of these patients will have had extensive laser surgery of the entire lower reproductive tract. In addition to sitz baths and protective vulvar creams, we also use daily vaginal applications of either estrogen or sulfa cream or of some other bacteriostatic preparation. With extensive laser treatment, vaginal walls can touch each other. The patient should also be examined at intervals to make sure that vaginal coaptation is not occurring. Vaginal healing usually takes place from the periphery of the wound because of the lack of skin appendages in vaginal mucosa. If the laser surgeon has been thorough and the denuded area is large, healing is often delayed, and granulation tissue may result. This granulation tissue can be removed and the wound then treated with silver nitrate.

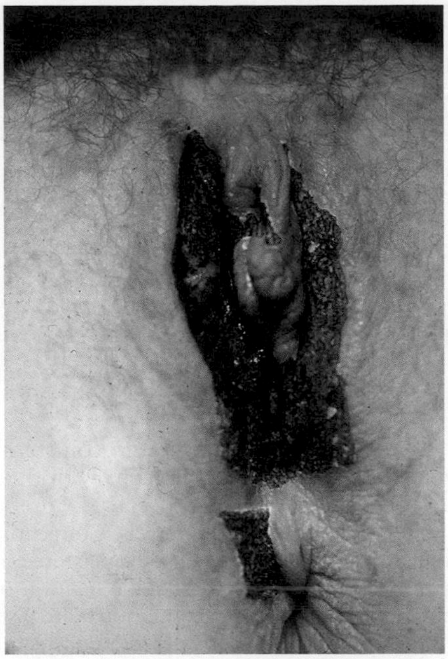

FIGURE 16.11. Laser surgery to vulva for multifocal VIN. Treatment is tailored to intraepithelial lesion's distribution. Normal clitoral and perianal tissue is preserved.

Results of Laser Vaporization of VAIN

Dorsey reported more than 80 patients treated with CO_2 laser for VAIN with a recurrence rates for multifocal HPV-associated VAIN of 30% within the first year. Patients with unicentric VAIN had a better than 90% chance of cure with one laser surgery. Townsend and colleagues have reported very satisfactory cure rates in the laser therapy of this disease.

Indications for Laser Surgery and HPV Infection

Although 1-year cure rates produced by laser surgery for lower reproductive tract intraepithelial neoplasia have been very satisfactory, particularly in cervical cases, the persistence or recurrence of wart virus lesions has been discouraging to patients and physicians alike. Our inability to cure HPV manifestations has led many laser surgeons to question the indications for laser surgery for this disease. Most agree that intraepithelial neoplasia should be treated; however, disagreement concerning the advisability or necessity of therapy for minor HPV infection prevails. For example, patients who have evidence of HPV infection found on a cytologic smear or who have a whitish change in the vaginal introitus after application of acetic acid are dubious candidates for laser surgery. Because recurrence or persistence of subclinical HPV is so common, a more logical approach is to monitor these patients carefully but not subject them all to surgery unless significant change occurs.

Anal Intraepithelial Neoplasia

Because of the high frequency of multifocal disease, colposcopic examination is not complete without inspection of the perianal tissue and the anal canal. The same techniques that were described earlier are used for the diagnosis and treatment of intraepithelial neoplasia and HPV in this region. An anoscope is used to inspect the anal canal. The surgeon should be careful to avoid lasing hemorrhoids with CO_2 laser because of its poor hemostasis with large vessels. A theoretic hazard of laser surgery in this region is the ignition or possible explosion of methane gas from the bowel. Some surgeons insert a wet gauze sponge in the rectum to keep stool out of the field. I have never experienced this complication.

TABLE 16.5

LASER LAPAROSCOPY PROCEDURES

Procedure	Percentage
Fulguration or excision of endometriosis	68
Lysis of adhesions	62
Ovarian cystectomy	31
Division of uterosacral ligaments	30
Presacral neurectomy	10
Salpingo-oophorectomy and variations	22
Removal of ectopic pregnancy	10
Myomectomy	4
Neosalpingostomy	4
Laparoscopically assisted vaginal hysterectomy	18
Retropubic urethropexy	10
Sacral colpopexy	3

INTRAABDOMINAL LASER SURGERY

Intraabdominal laser surgery has provided a significant and useful new tool for surgery in gynecology. It is unique and offers an alternative to the knife and electrosurgical instruments. Its use in the abdomen began in the late 1970s, and by the first part of the 1980s, there were substantial number of reports from both Europe and the United States dealing primarily using CO_2 laser. Numerous reports attested to the efficacy of laser in both reproductive and reconstructive surgery (Table 16.5).

The advantages of laser surgery in the abdomen include precision, limited adjacent tissue damage, rapid healing, minimal scarring, and the ability to treat areas of difficult access from a remote site. An example of the minimal trauma of laser on tissue is the research work of Bern, who demonstrated the ability to remove intracellular chromosomal material with the carbon dioxide laser without destroying the cell. Extensive studies of laser energy in basic science preceded its use in

TABLE 16.6

INFERTILITY LASER PROCEDURES

Adhesiolysis
Fenestration of paraovarian and polycystic cysts
Vaporization of endometriosis
Fimbrioplasty
Neosalpingostomy
Resection of ectopic pregnancy
Tubal anastomosis
Tubal implant
Myomectomy
Metroplasty

TABLE 16.7

MICROSCOPIC DELIVERY

Advantages
Greatest magnification
Spot-size control
Ease of deep pelvic surgery
Instrument-free field
Constant focus
Remote control
Disadvantages
Delivery angle restricted
Difficult to change spot
Larger spot size with a greater margin of injury

clinical medicine. This pool of knowledge of lasers exceeds any other surgical tool in use today. Before a surgeon attempts laser surgery in the abdomen, it is essential that he or she be completely trained and skilled in the same procedures without the laser. The delivery of laser under microscopic control was used first in open abdominal infertility surgery (Table 16.6). Microscopic delivery provides the greatest magnification of the surgical field for laser use. The optimum focal distance of the lens is 300 to 350 mm to provide room between the patient and the microscope. The greatest precision is obtained when the laser beam focus and microscopic focus are the same. Control of the laser is in the micromanipulator, so no instrument need be in the field. The angle with which the laser beam can be delivered, however, is limited to the viewing angle of the microscope. The advantages and disadvantages of the microscopic delivery are listed in Table 16.7. Free hand delivery offers an alternative without this limitation (Table 16.8).

Today the major interest in gynecologic surgery has shifted to the endoscopic delivery of the laser beam.

GYNECOLOGIC LASER LAPAROSCOPY

Laparoscopy was introduced in the late 1960s with unipolar electrical instruments for tubal sterilization. During the 1970s, Semm described the techniques of laparoscopic vessel ligation and tissue suturing, and in 1978, Bruhat used the CO_2 laser with an operative laparoscope to treat ectopic pregnancy. The

TABLE 16.8

FREE HAND DELIVERY

Advantages
Can be used without magnification
Develops smallest spot size possible
Multiple angle of delivery possible
Focus and defocus is easy
Highest power density for minimal tissue injury
Disadvantages
Cumbersome equipment
Shallow depth of focus
Difficult to maintain precise focus
Handpiece must be in field

TABLE 16.9

METHODS FOR ACHIEVING LAPAROSCOPIC HEMOSTASIS

Unipolar electrocoagulation
Bipolar electrocoagulation
Laser coagulation
Extracorporeal ligatures
Extracorporeal sutures
Intracorporeal sutures
Endocoagulation (Semm)
Hemoclip

ability to cut and vaporize tissue, and to control bleeding as well, provided gynecologic laser surgeons with the tools necessary to do complicated surgical procedures. Laser alone may not result in hemostasis with large vessels. Conventional methods for achieving hemostasis must also be mastered by the laser laparoscopist (Table 16.9). These include ligation of vascular pedicles and electrical surgical coagulation. The laser is a surgical tool and should not be considered a complete system of laparoscopy by itself. It should be viewed as an instrument that forms a part of our laparoscopic armamentarium.

The CO_2 laser can be connected to an operative laparoscope through a laser coupler that transmits the beam through a focusing lens and then down a special channel in the laparoscope. Interchangeable lenses provide focal lengths commensurate with the length of the laparoscope. Focal spot sizes produced by these systems are usually a bit less than a millimeter in diameter. The CO_2 laser is an excellent laser for laparoscopic usage because it cuts quickly, produces very little thermal damage, and can be used for vaporization, coagulation, or excision. It is very safe in the hands of a knowledgeable surgeon because of its almost complete absorption at the surface of the tissue containing water. The mirrors in the CO_2 laser arm must be very carefully aligned. The fiber-optic laser's energy through flexible small quartz fibers simplifies its use in endoscopic surgery. The deeper penetration of these wavelengths, however, must always be kept in mind.

The blue or green aiming beams of these lasers are more easily seen against the reddish background of the abdominal organs than is the helium–neon beam. The quartz laser fibers will pass through an 18-gauge or smaller needle, so hand pieces designed for suction and irrigation also may have a central channel that accommodates the fiber. This enables the surgeon to use suction, irrigation, and laser energy through one hand piece, and these hand pieces fit easily through a 5-mm trocar sheath. The disadvantages of fiber-optic lasers are that they do not cut quite as well as CO_2 lasers and are less safe because of their penetration of both tissue and water.

The safe and effective use of the laser in laparoscopy has been demonstrated by Daniell and Brown, Daniell and Herber, Feste, Martin, Kelly and Roberts, Baggish, Dorsey, and Nezhat and colleagues. Laser laparoscopy has translated into shorter hospital stays, recduced costs, and less scarring. The disadvantages of laser laparoscopy include the expense of the equipment, outdating of instrumentation, and requirement for special training and maintenance.

YAG laser energy was first used through the laparoscope in 1982. Some laser surgeons consider the delivery of YAG energy by bare fiber too dangerous for use in the abdominal cavity because of the deep penetration of the YAG beam and danger of injury to organs below the surface.

Technique

Under general intubation anesthesia, the patient is placed in a modified lithotomy position so that the thigh is almost level with the patient's abdomen. This enables the surgeon to direct the laparoscope cephalad. This maneuver may be important not only for exploration but also for operating at the pelvic brim. If the hip is flexed and the thighs are elevated, the scope and perhaps the accessory instrumentation cannot be manipulated freely because they will be in contact with the patient's thighs. After preparation and draping, an intrauterine manipulating device is placed into the uterus for two purposes: to elevate or maneuver the uterus during surgery without having to use intraabdominal instruments for this task and to perform chromopertubation when necessary. If adhesions are suspected to the laparoscopy trocar insertion site, I prefer to use a technique demonstrated by Professor Palmer of Paris. Using his technique, the insertion site is selected in the midclavicular line, two finger widths below the left costal margin. The insufflation needle is attached to syringe half filled with normal saline. After inserting the needle through the abdominal wall, an aspiration is performed to rule out vessel or bowel perforation. If the aspiration is negative, the normal saline is injected and should have minimal resistance. Resistance indicates that the needle tip is not within the abdominal cavity. If this test is negative, the gas insufflation is initiated. A low opening pressure confirms correct needle placement within an open space in the peritoneum. Next, the laparoscopic trocar is inserted at the needle site. Additional trocars are inserted under direct vision.

Irrespective of the type of laser used, a superior suction-irrigation device that does not obstruct is needed. The new rapid-fill automatic insufflators are highly desirable because they can be set to maintain a constant intraabdominal pressure and will deliver a flow of CO_2 and simultaneously record intraabdominal pressure. A high-intensity light source is also of great importance. A video camera is attached to the laparoscope, and the operative endoscopy is performed while the surgeon views the video monitor (Fig. 16.12). The advantage of video usage is that the entire operating room becomes a team. The assistant is always aware of the progress of the operation, and the surgeon is able to stand erect while inspecting all parts of the abdominal cavity.

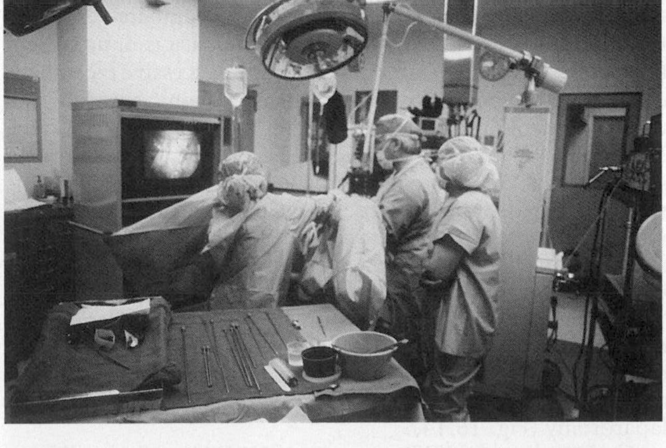

FIGURE 16.12. Operating room during laser laparoscopy. Video monitor is placed opposite surgeon for viewing by the entire operating team, including referring physician observers.

Most of our advanced operative laparoscopic procedures require three trocars. The laparoscope is most commonly inserted in the umbilicus margin. Ancillary trocars are placed according the pathology found, the procedure planned, and access by the surgical team. They are inserted under direct vision to avoid abdominal wall and deep pelvic vessel injury. The anterior pelvis should be inspected before the trocar insertion to identify the bladder margin if possible and avoid injury to this organ. Transillumination of the anterior abdominal wall helps to identify large vessels and rectus muscle margins.

I prefer to use 5-mm trocars and a 5-mm 30-degree laparoscope for diagnostic use. The 30-degree laparoscope allows the surgeon to see the undersurface of the abdominal wall better. For operative laparoscopy, trocars of larger diameters are selected depending on the intended use such as the need for specimen pouches. Laparoscopic needle holders and curved needles can be passed without difficulty through larger sleeves.

After the trocars and instruments have been inserted, the laser source is attached to the laparoscope or ancillary instrument. Calibration of the laser is tested. I prefer 10 W for 0.1-second settings for this. Beam alignment, aiming beam, spot size, power setting, and continuous or pulsed delivery is tested on a tongue blade. Suction, filtration of the plume, and irrigation systems are prepared.

Power setting and timing mode for the surgery to be performed is selected. Pulsed delivery is used where a precise tissue effect is important. If the aiming beam is difficult to see within the pelvis, decreasing the laparoscopic light may be helpful. The operative site is inspected and a suction device positioned in close proximity to maintain visibility if significant plume is anticipated. Adequate backstops for the laser beam are checked is CO_2 is used. Care is taken not to laser tissue if it is covered with a layer of water because this will result in the fluid boiling and unnecessary thermal damage.

Carbon Dioxide Adhesiolysis

Laparoscopy has greatly increased our capacity to identify postoperative and postinflammatory pelvic adhesions. Endometriosis is the third common cause of adhesions. Laparoscopy is used to diagnose endometriosis at early stages before the development of dense adhesions. Advanced endometriosis is associated with vascular adhesions that can be treated with laser. Omentum adhesions to the anterior abdominal wall are handled rapidly and efficiently with laser through an operative laparoscope alone without insertion of other trocars. Bowel adhesions prove a more difficult problem. A pulsed laser can be used if a backstop can be manipulated between loops of bowel, or if the loop of bowel can be held gently apart so the laser energy is directly applied to the adhesion without fear of bowel damage. Laser adhesiolysis must consider vital structures such as bowel, ureters, and major blood vessels that may be attached or in close proximity. Filmy adhesions can be vaporized and divided with low power density and pulsed for precise control. With appropriate technique, the adhesion can be vaporized without damage to underlying structures such as tube, ovary, or bowel. Thick adhesions between delicate structures such as tube and ovary may be lased with intermediate power density and spot size.

The proper power density must be selected for each laser procedure. In general, power densities used in intraabdominal laser surgery are relatively low. Because CO_2 laser energy continues to travel once it cuts through the target tissue, the surgeon must select an appropriate backstop (Fig. 16.13). Various rods are available to use as both dissecting tools and laser

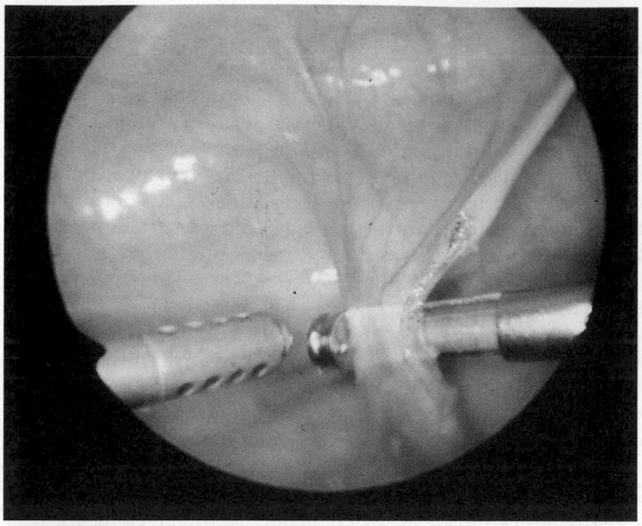

FIGURE 16.13. Laparoscopy laser lysis of adhesions. The laser beam is delivered within the hollow ancillary probe to the pelvic adhesion. The distal end probe acts as a backstop and limits the laser vaporization to the tissue within the window of the probe. Note the second probe in close proximity to maintain clear visibility.

backstops. Glass, Pyrex, and quartz rods should be avoided because they may shatter under the intense heat of the laser. Water that is pooled or injected retroperitoneal serves as an excellent backstop for CO_2 laser. Titanium with dulled surfaces or blackened rods can also be used. Constant irrigation with body-temperature physiologic solutions washes away any char that may accumulate.

Although CO_2 laser is superb for coagulating small bleeders, vessels larger than 0.5 mm in diameter may be difficult to coagulate. If it is not immediately apparent that the laser is achieving hemostasis without significant damage to tissue, conventional methods of hemostasis, such as electrosurgical coagulation or suturing, should be used. A filtered evacuation system to remove the laser plume is needed to maintain a clear field of view.

Surgery using laser energy has been compared with mechanical and electrosurgical devices. Evaluation of a single instrument's use must consider multiple other variables such multiple disease classifications, individual surgeon's skill, absence of long-term follow-up, and the use of concomitant multiple adjuvant therapies. This makes evidence-based comparisons difficult if not impossible.

Laser Surgery of the Fallopian Tube

Laparoscopic tuboplasty using electrosurgical instruments was reported in 1980 by Gomel and others with successful outcomes. The ability to diagnose and treat tubal obstruction during the same procedure was attractive and spurred interest in laparoscopic tuboplasty. The shortened recovery period and the potential shortened time to conception was also attractive. Steptoe and Edwards successfully introduced *in vitro* fertilization in 1978 with the term cesarean delivery of Louise Brown, who weighed 5 pounds, 12 ounces. For the 20% of couples with tubal obstruction, the expansion of assisted reproductive technology (ART) has significantly reduced the number of tubal surgeries done for fertility. There remains a group of patients who for some reason may benefit from laparoscopic surgery on the tube. Examples include patients with pain associated with tubal disease and patients who chose not to use ART. They can select laser tubal surgery with its unique capabilities. The success of this procedure is related to the preoperative integrity of the tube. The technique involves using an atraumatic grasping tool to stabilize and expose the tube. Any obstruction site including the fimbria is identified. The central site of distal obstruction can be identified by observing the vascular distribution. The tube is gently distended by intrauterine injection of dilute indigo-carmine solution. The use of a backstop is not necessary. As the laser incises the distal tube, the lumen is immediately identified as the dye appears. Three or four radial incisions are made in the closed tube with a small spot-size laser beam so that satisfactory eversion of mucosa can be accomplished without suturing. The defocused laser beam is applied to the outside of the fimbria. Heat and the resultant contraction of desiccated tissue cause the eversion of the fimbria. Flowering of the tube is accomplished using a spot size of 3 to 5 mm and a low power setting of 2 to 5 W of CO_2 laser. This technique was first described by Bruhat and is referred to as Bruhat's procedure.

Laser Myomectomy

The indications for a laparoscopic myomectomy are the same as the indications for myomectomy in general. Significant size, rapid growth, selected cases of infertility or pressure symptoms, and heavy bleeding have all been acceptable indications for surgical intervention. Pedunculated leiomyomas can be easily removed at laser laparoscopy, but intramural myomas that are deeply imbedded in the myometrium may pose a real challenge.

Laparoscopic myomectomy is a controversial procedure because of the need to perform careful uterine reconstruction if the patient desires future childbearing. This operation should not be attempted by any laparoscopist who is not familiar with advanced laparoscopic suturing techniques or ability to close the myometrium in layers.

An injection of a dilute solution of vasopressin is made to the margins of the leiomyoma and the surrounding myometrium. Lower abdominal accessory trocars are used according to the size and location of the fibroids. Incisions to remove the fibroids are made away from the ovaries and tubes if possible to reduce postoperative adhesions to these structures. Lateral forceps are used to grasp the myometrium, and this is gently stripped away from the underlying myoma, much in the way that an orange is peeled. Laser is used to coagulate vessels on the surface of the leiomyoma and, as the base is approached, to coagulate and cut vessels in that area. If excessive bleeding is encountered, bipolar coagulation or endoscopic suturing will usually control the bleeding. Constant traction is placed on the leiomyoma as it is being removed through a midline site. A small myoma corkscrew instrument can be used through this trocar to stabilize and exert the necessary traction. Larger intramural leiomyomas 6 to 8 cm in size may require morcellation using a morcellator or minilaparotomy. The specimen can also be removed through colpotomy by morcellation.

Myomectomy must be carefully performed, and hemostasis must be complete at the end of the procedure. The possibility of excessive blood loss during this operation is always present, and both patient and surgeon must be prepared for immediate laparotomy (Fig. 16.14).

Carbon dioxide, KTP, argon, and YAG lasers have all been used for myomectomy. Closure of the myometrial defect is accomplished using continuous layers of absorbable sutures. An

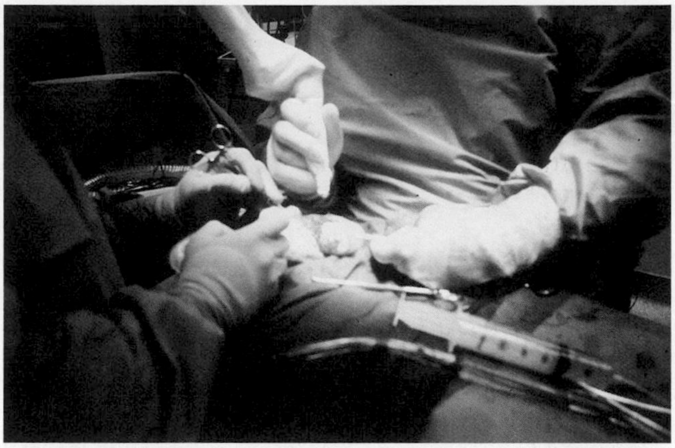

FIGURE 16.14. Open free-hand laser myomectomy. Retractor surfaces are covered with wet towels to prevent reflection of the laser beam.

adhesion reducing barrier is applied to cover the incision at the end of the surgery.

Laser Surgery for Endometriosis

Laparoscopy provides a diagnostic and therapeutic surgical procedure for endometriosis. Continued monitoring and management also uses laparoscope.

Small implants of mild-to-moderate endometriosis can be effectively vaporized, coagulated, or excised with either the CO_2 or the fiber-optic laser. Even small endometrial implants are surrounded by subclinical endometriosis, so a margin of vaporization or coagulation may be needed around the endometrial implant. Dense adhesions associated with advanced endometriosis can also be treated, including those located over the ureter. Cases of severe endometriosis involving the ureter and bladder may require preoperative cystoscopy and placement of ureteral catheters. It is usually easier to visualize the ureter at the bifurcation of the common iliac artery as it passes into the pelvis. The ureter is then traced down to the cardinal ligament, where it is more difficult to identify. The ureter can be moved beneath the peritoneum by manipulating the ureteral catheter so that its position is more easily seen. Illuminated ureter catheters have also been used to identify its tract. Injection of the irrigating fluid retroperitoneally into the broad ligament or the lateral pelvic side wall will provide a watery backstop that helps with periurethral dissection and safety, particularly if CO_2 energy is used. This is not protective for fiber-optic laser energy. Hydrodissection can separate the ureter from the implant so that excision with scissors is safely expedited.

Ovarian endometriosis, the second most common site, can benefit from the precision of laser surgery. Damage to the deeper stroma of the ovarian cortex is minimized using a pulsed laser delivery. The technique involves first inspecting the operative site and adjacent vital structures. The ovary is maneuvered for optimum exposure. This may require lysis of adhesions between the ovary and lateral pelvic walls. Any lesion that can be seen through the laparoscope can be treated with the laser using the operative laparoscope. Carbon residual following treatment is irrigated with a physiologic Ringer's lactated solution.

Martin has emphasized the importance of excision and histologic confirmation of suspected endometriosis lesions. The peritoneum adjacent to the lesion is incised, and the opening is enlarged. Blunt dissection is performed, using a probe or with the aid of the irrigating fluid. Forceps are used to elevate the peritoneum, and the laser is used to complete the excision. Small blood vessels, usually encountered in this type of dissection, are sealed by laser. Results of reported early series of endometriosis treated laparoscopically have been compiled by Martin and Diamond. These compare favorably to results produced by conventional surgery at laparotomy (Table 16.10). More recent reports with controlled, randomized trials of CO_2 laser laparoscopy for the treatment of endometriosis and pelvic pain have continued to emphasize favorable outcomes.

Ovarian Cystectomy

Resection of an ovarian cyst at laparoscopy is controversial. Some surgeons are concerned that spillage of an undiagnosed malignant ovarian tumor can result in the spread of the cancer. On the other hand, gynecologic oncologists are increasingly using laparoscopy in the evaluation and treatment of pelvic cancers. Although rare, most ovarian malignancies are not discovered when they are at an early stage. On the other hand, practicing gynecologists are commonly presented with ovarian cysts for treatment. The vast majority of young women with persisting cystic adnexal masses will not have ovarian cancer. If a concern for possible ovarian cancer develops, laparoscopy provides access for histologic diagnosis. The cystic masses should always be first evaluated by noninvasive means, such as pelvic ultrasound, magnetic resonance imaging, or computed tomography. Appropriate ovarian tumor markers are also available. Symptomatic paraovarian cysts can be drained easily with laser. No direct contact with the cyst is necessary unless the surgeon desires to create an enlarged window or obtain tissue for histology. Unilocular, symptomatic, persisting ovarian cysts with benign imaging profile and thin walls are best suited for laparoscopy. The surgeon can encounter cysts whose contents, if spilled, can stimulate adverse peritoneal response. This group of cysts include mucinous cystadenomas and dermoids. A means for copious irrigation with a physiologic solution should be available. To avoid recurrence, ovarian endometriomas should be excised rather than vaporized. Suturing the ovary in most cases is avoided because it is rarely needed and it can result in adhesions to the ovary. Daniell published a small series of patients with polycystic ovaries unresponsive to hormone treatment that were able to achieve ovulation following laser surgery to the subcapsular cysts.

Uterosacral Ligament Surgery

Pain stimuli originating from the cervix are transmitted through the sacral sympathetic chain. From there they are conducted through the uterosacral ligaments to the sacral sympathetic plexus by way of nerve roots S2, S3, and S4. This plexus is concentrated within the uterosacral ligament at its attachment to the back of the cervix. Severance of the uterosacral was first reported by Doyle in 1963. He reported relief of pelvic pain in 86% of 235 patients. Feste reported relief of dysmenorrhea in 78% of the women who underwent CO_2 laser division of the uterosacral ligaments and who were monitored for 5 years. Lichten in 1987, in a well-controlled series, reported a success rate of more than 80% in patients followed for more than a year. Dorsey reported 60 patients undergoing uterosacral ligament division for either primary dysmenorrhea or

TABLE 16.10

CO_2 LASER LAPAROSCOPY FOR ENDOMETRIOSIS

	Patients		Minimal or Mild		Moderate		Severe or Extensive	
Investigator	Number	Pregnant	Number	Pregnant	Number	Pregnant	Number	Pregnant
ENDOMETRIOSIS IN ALL PATIENTS								
Kelly and Roberts, 1983	10	6 (60%)	3	3 (100%)	7	3 (43%)	0	0 (0%)
Feste, 1983	140	82 (59%)	106	62 (58%)	31	18 (58%)	3	2 (67%)
Daniell, 1985	48	26 (54%)	24	16 (67%)	15	7 (47%)	9	3 (33%)
Martin and Diamond, 1986	115	54 (47%)	56	23 (41%)	45	22 (49%)	14	9 (64%)
Davis, 1986	64	37 (58%)	31	20 (65%)	26	15 (58%)	7	2 (29%)
Nezhat, 1986	102	65 (64%)	24	18 (75%)	51	32 (63%)	27	15 (56%)
Adamson, 1986	156	86 (55%)	133	77 (58%)	20	7 (33%)	3	0 (0%)
Bowman, 1986	35	18 (51%)	19	12 (63%)	13	4 (31%)	3	2 (67%)
Donnez, 1987	70	40 (57%)	42	26 (62%)	21	11 (52%)	7	3 (43%)
Paulsen, 1987	431	225 (52%)	257	144 (56%)	174	81 (47%)	0	0 (0%)
Gast, 1988	122	57 (47%)	105	49 (47%)	17	8 (47%)	0	0 (0%)
Nezhat, 1989	243	168 (69%)	39	28 (72%)	86	60 (70%)	118	80 (68%)
TOTALS	1,536	864 (56%)	839	478 (57%)	506	268 (53%)	191	116 (61%)
ENDOMETRIOSIS AS AN ISOLATED FACTOR								
Feste, 1985	60	42 (70%)	44	3 (70%)	14	10 (71%)	2	1 (50%)
Martin, 1985	34	23 (67%)	13	9 (69%)	11	6 (55%)	10	8 (80%)
Nezhat, 1986	102	65 (64%)	24	18 (75%)	51	32 (63%)	27	15 (56%)
Adamson, 1986	60	39 (65%)	47	31 (66%)	11	7 (61%)	2	0 (0%)
Paulsen, 1987	228	169 (74%)	140	109 (78%)	88	60 (68%)	0	0 (0%)
Gast, 1988	27	7 (26%)		NA		NA	0	0 (0%)
Nehat, 1989	243	168 (69%)	39	28 (72%)	86	60 (70%)	118	80 (68%)
TOTALS	754	513 (68%)	307	226 (74%)	261	175 (67%)	159	104 (65%)

NA, not available.
Adapted from: Martin DC, Diamond MP. Operative laparoscopy: comparison of lasers with other techniques. *Curr Probl Obstet Fertil* 1986;9:564.)

dysmenorrhea associated with endometriosis. Significant pain relief occurred in 70% of the women monitored over the course of the year. The uterosacral ligament can sometimes be confused with the ureter, so the latter structure must always be positively identified. The ureter is identified at the bifurcation of the common iliac artery and traced into the pelvis to a point at which it disappears in the cardinal ligament. At the same time that the uterosacral ligament is identified, the division is planned close to its insertion into the uterus. Uterosacral ligaments vary tremendously in size and structure. The division should begin at the posterior cervical wall. Lateral to the uterosacral ligament lies a branch of the uterine artery as well as the ureter, so one should stay medial. Power settings of 20 W may be used on the CO_2 laser; on fiber-optic lasers, 10 to 15 W will suffice (Fig. 16.4).

Tubal Pregnancy

Laparoscopic laser surgery for tubal pregnancy was reported by Bruhat in 1978. Ampullary ectopic pregnancies are usually intramural rather than intraluminal, and this is the perfect setting for a laser incision. A dilute solution of vasopressin can be delivered percutaneously to the tube, and the laser is used for the linear salpingostomy. Hemostasis is achieved by any of the lasers, however, bipolar coagulation may be necessary for very active bleeding. Usually the pregnancy is extruded from the tube as the incision is made. Gentle traction with an atraumatic forceps or with an irrigation stream is helpful. It is not necessary or desirable to curette the tube in an effort to remove the contents. It is always necessary to monitor any conservatively treated tubal pregnancy with postoperative human chorionic gonadotropin (hCG) titers to rule out persistent trophoblastic disease.

Partial salpingectomy is sometimes necessary. This may be particularly true for isthmic tubal pregnancies. Pregnancies in this region of the tube are usually intraluminal, and although they are not encountered as frequently as are ampullary pregnancies, segmental rupture may occur earlier, and recanalization of the tube is infrequent. For this reason, excision of the segment may be desirable. This can be performed by coagulation on either side of the ectopic pregnancy and then excision with laser or laparoscopic scissors. Bipolar coagulation may be necessary because of the bleeding despite the use of vasopressin. The ability to diagnose ectopic pregnancy early with sensitive hCG tests and sonograms has decreased the incidence of ruptured ectopic pregnancies. This has also resulted in an increase use of nonsurgical treatment of early unruptured ectopic pregnancy.

Salpingectomy is used when the tube is destroyed or when future pregnancy is not desired.

It is essential to follow any conservatively treated tubal pregnancy with postoperative hCG titers to rule out persistent trophoblastic disease.

Salpingo-Oophorectomy and Laparoscopically Assisted Hysterectomy

These procedures are now well known to most laparoscopic surgeons, and we have found the laser to be of assistance in their performance. These operations involve securing large vascular pedicles. Laser energy, usually delivered through the operative laparoscope, has been used mainly for:

- Dividing large pedicles that have either been coagulated with bipolar forceps or suture ligated
- Accomplishing division of adhesions, ablating endometrial implants, and performing other tasks related to removal of the specimen
- Dividing the peritoneum over the bladder, mobilizing the bladder off of the cervix finding uterosacral ligaments, and entering the vagina from above all of these specifically in laparoscopically assisted hysterectomy

Laser through the operative laparoscope allows for rapid and safe performance of these steps without the need for constantly introducing or removing instruments through the trocar sleeves.

HYSTEROSCOPIC LASER SURGERY

Nd:YAG Laser

The first endometrial ablation series by Goldrath and colleagues in 1981 used fiberoptic YAG laser for the energy source. Because of its ability to penetrate tissue, the YAG represents an ideal laser for endometrial ablation. Myometrium is normally about 2 to 3 cm in thickness except at the cornu, where it may be significantly less. Endometrial thickness can usually be measured in terms of a few millimeters. Because YAG laser energy delivered by the unclad laser fiber penetrates about 4 mm, the YAG can be used to effectively coagulate the endometrium and the inner layers of the myometrium. The risk of damage to tissues outside the myometrium is minimal.

The YAG laser is a very effective coagulating tool, and where properly used for endometrial ablation, it gave good results. Fiber laser ablation has the advantage of being able to be delivered through small caliber hysteroscopes. The width of laser beam from the fiber, however, is narrow: less than 1 mm in diameter. The treatment of the entire uterine chamber with YAG resulted in a prolonged operative time.

All patients who are candidates for endometrial ablation should have an examination of the endometrium to rule out malignancy or premalignant lesions. Atypical adenomatous hyperplasia should not be ablated. Patients can be given medication to suppress the endometrium. Note that one of the advantages of hysteroscopic laser surgery is that normal saline distending medium avoids the dangers associated with vascular absorption of nonionic solutions used in electrosurgery. Controlled close-loop distending systems improve visualization, even in the presence of active bleeding. An effort is made to destroy all endometrium in the uterine cavity. Care is taken in proximity to the internal os of the fallopian tubes, considering the thinning of the wall at that point and the deep penetration of YAG laser. In the lower endometrial cavity, the laser treatment is extended to the internal cervical os. Laser ablation of the endocervix is avoided to reduce the risk of stenosis, hematometria, and postoperative bleeding.

Garry and associates have reported a series of more than 600 endometrial ablations accomplished with laser without complications and with an overall success rate of more than 80%.

Continuous-flow resectoscopes with rollerball, loop, or electrosurgical tips are faster and easier to use than the fiber-optic laser. Global endometrial ablation techniques have replaced the fiber lasers for most with a few selected indications. However, the original endometrial ablations techniques are used as the gold standard for effectiveness comparisons.

Other hysteroscopic surgeries that have used laser include metroplasty, division of uterine septa, destruction of intrauterine synechiae, and excision of submucous leiomyomas. Small caliber hysteroscopes can be used with fiber laser because of their small operative channels, an advantage when the uterine cavity or cervical canal is very narrow.

Laser Metroplasty

Any of the fiber-optic lasers can be used for division or removal of uterine septa and synechiae. It should be emphasized that when septa are divided, concomitant laparoscopy should be performed to ensure that perforation does not occur.

Pedunculated myomas may be removed by laser division of the pedicle. Deeper submucous myomas are more easily handled by resectoscopic surgery.

LASER SAFETY

It is important that surgeons, nurses, and all those associated with laser surgery have an understanding of the potential health and safety hazards associated with the use of medical laser systems and the precautions needed to use them safely. Laser injury and potential hazards can be considered related to the organ systems at risk. The eye is considered to be the organ most vulnerable to damage by laser. The eye collects and concentrates light energy on the retina. It has a natural protective mechanism in the lid and tearing reflexes. However, many lasers are extremely intense and are delivered so rapidly that injury can occur. Lasers in the visible and near infrared bands will be transmitted through the eye to the retina. With sufficient intensity, they can cause visual loss. Laser light cannot damage a tissue unless the light energy can reach and be absorbed in that tissue. Injury to the cornea and lens may occur with lasers in specific spectral bands in the ultraviolet and infrared spectrum. The laser energy necessary to injure the cornea is much greater that that required to injure the retina. Protective measures for eye protection include spectacles, goggles, or coverall goggles to filter out the specific laser wavelength while transmitting visible light. Colposcopes and operative lenses of laparoscopes shield the laser surgeon's eyes from CO_2 laser injury when delivered through these systems. The fiber-optic lasers that penetrate water and clear glass also penetrate the eye. In endoscopic surgery, special glasses or filters specific for the laser are used for protection. The optical filter is coupled to the eyepiece of the telescope and can be activated when the surgeon steps on the foot switch. As a general rule, eye protectors are required for work with class 4 lasers. Any surgical lasers with an average power exceeding 0.5 W are class 4. Most surgical lasers are class 4.

Skin is considerably less vulnerable to laser injury than the eye. Skin injury can also occur from ignition of flammable material by the laser beam. Laser hazards to operating room personnel and patient includes accidental exposure from misdirection of the laser beam. The risk of this happening can be reduced by using the "standby" mode when not actually operating. Surgeons are not highly susceptible to laser injury. However, when using handheld laser delivery systems, one should remember that the surgeon's hand is the closest to the laser target and subject to reflection from adjacent surgical instruments. Fortunately, most reflected beams are highly divergent because the beam is normally focused. The zone of potential hazardous reflection is referred to as a nominal hazard zone (NHZ). Service personnel may encounter laser beams that are unfocused and concentrated. Electrical hazards of laser equipment are similar to other types of electrical or electronic equipment. There is no unique electrical safety problem associated with laser use. Biomedical engineer and technicians should have no difficulty providing guidance for the control of any electrical hazards from laser equipment.

Vaporization of tissue produces smoke with potential health hazards. Careful evacuation and filtration of the laser plume will reduce any hazard of laser smoke inhalation. The evacuation of the plume is most effective if the tip of the tube is within 2 cm of the tissue being treated. It is important to remove smoke from the closed abdominal cavity during laparoscopic surgery. This allows the surgeon to see clearly as well as removing it from inhalation by the operating room personnel. Special high-efficiency masks provide additional respiratory protection. Warning or indicator signs are required by ANSI Z-136–1986 for class 4 laser treatment controlled areas. Sliney and Trokel have provided an excellent reference text concerning medical lasers and their safe use.

SUMMARY

I have used laser surgery in gynecology for more than 32 years. Over this period, many applications of laser have been recognized and defined, as outlined in this chapter. Numerous skilled surgeons throughout the world have contributed to its literature. Lasers are unique and useful tools in the hands of trained surgeons. They are not a magic wand that can be used to accomplish all surgical tasks. The introduction of lasers to gynecologic surgery occurred at a time when laser use in the military, aerospace, and everyday life was highly publicized. This focus of attention was responsible, in part, for laser's introduction to gynecology. The initial popularity of laser surgery in turn stimulated the development of more sophisticated electrosurgical instruments. This has resulted in the improvement of the tools using electrosurgical energy. The techniques for laser surgery performed by experienced gynecologists are presented in this chapter. The long-term benefits and future use of lasers in gynecology will require carefully designed and randomized studies.

BEST SURGICAL PRACTICES

- Understand the physics and tissue effects of the laser you are using.
- Implement precautions needed for laser safety.
- Set the time the laser is exposed to tissue for the optimum effect.
- Biopsy tissue before coagulation or vaporization if intraepithelial stage is in doubt.
- Select appropriate backstops if laser beam can continue through the tissue being treated.

Bibliography

Adamson GD, Lu J, Subak LL. Laparoscopic CO_2 laser vaporization of endometriosis compared with traditional treatments. *Fertil Steril* 1988;50:704.

American College of Obstetricians and Gynecologists Committee on Gynecological Practice. *Report on carbon dioxide laser*. Washington, DC: ACOG, April 1994.

Anderson MC, Hartley RB. Cervical crypt involvement by cervical intraepithelial neoplasia. *Obstet Gynecol* 1980;55:546.

Apfelberg DB, Mittleman H, Chadi B. Carcinogenic potential of in vitro carbon dioxide laser exposure of fibroblast. *Obstet Gynecol* 1989;61:493.

Baggish MS. Management of cervical intraepithelial neoplasia by carbon dioxide laser. *Obstet Gynecol* 1982;60:479.

Baggish MS. Status of the carbon dioxide laser for infertility surgery. *Fertil Steril* 1983;40:442.

Baggish MS, Chong AP. Carbon dioxide laser microsurgery of the uterine tube. *Obstet Gynecol* 1981;58:111.

Baggish MS, Chong AP. Intraabdominal surgery with the CO_2 laser. *J Reprod Med* 1983;28:269.

Baggish MS, Dorsey JH. CO_2 laser for the treatment of vulvar carcinoma in situ. *Obstet Gynecol* 1981;57:371.

Baggish MS, Dorsey JH. The laser combination cone. *Am J Obstet Gynecol* 1985;151:23.

Baggish MS, Barbot J, Valle RF. *Diagnostic and operative hysteroscopy: a text and atlas.* Chicago: Yearbook Medical Publishers, Inc.; 1989.

Baggish MS, Sze E, Badawy S, et al. Carbon dioxide laser laparoscopy by means of a 3.0 mm diameter rigid waveguide. *Fertil Steril* 1988;50:419.

Bellina JH. Microsurgery of the fallopian tube with the carbon dioxide laser: analysis of 230 cases with a two-year follow-up. *Lasers Surg Med* 1983;3:555.

Bellina JH, Hemmings R, Voros JI, et al. Carbon dioxide laser and electrosurgical wound study with an animal model: a comparison of tissue damage and healing patterns in peritoneal issue. *Am J Obstet Gynecol* 1984;158:327.

Bellina JH, Voros JI, Fick AC, et al. Surgical management of endometriosis with the carbon dioxide laser. *Microsurgery* 1984;5:197.

Bern MW. Directed chromosome loss by laser microirradiation *Science* 1974;22: 700–705.

Bruhat MA, Mage G. Use of CO_2 laser in salpingotomy. In: Kaplan I, ed. *Laser surgery III*. Jerusalem: Jerusalem Academic Press, 1979:271.

Bruhat MA, Mage G, Pouly SL, *Operative laparoscopy* Medsil: McGraw-Hill Publishers, New York; 1991.

Bruhat MA, Maahes H, Mage G, et al. Treatment of ectopic pregnancy by means of laparoscopy. *Fertil Steril* 1980;33:411.

Burke L, Covell L, Antonioli D. Laser therapy of cervical intraepithelial neoplasia: factors determining success rate. *Lasers Surg Med* 1980;1:113.

Buttram VC Jr. Evolution of the revised American Fertility Society classification of endometriosis. *Fertil Steril* 1985;43:347.

Byrne MA, Taylor-Robinson D, Wickenden C, et al. Prevalence of human papillomavirus types in the cervices of women before and after laser ablation. *BJOG* 1988;95:201.

Cartier R. Colposcopie pratigue laboratoire. Cartier. 1984.

Choe JK, Dawood MY, Andrews AH. Conventional versus laser reanastomosis of rabbit ligated uterine horns. *Obstet Gynecol* 1983;61:689.

Chong AP. Infertility amenable to laser surgery. *Basic Adv Laser Surg Gynecol* 1985;279:296.

Chong AP, Baggish MS. The use of carbon dioxide laser in tubal surgery. *Int J Fertil* 1983;28:24.

Daniell JF, Brown DH. Carbon dioxide laser laparoscopy: initial experience in experimental animals and humans. *Obstet Gynecol* 1982;59:761.

Daniell JF, Miller N. Polycystic ovaries treated by laser vaporization. *Fertil Steril* 1989;51:232–236.

Daniell JF, Herbert CM. Laparoscopic salpingostomy utilizing the CO_2 laser. *Fertil Steril* 1984;41:558.

Daniell JF, Pittaway DE. Use of the CO_2 laser in laparoscopic surgery: initial experience with the second puncture technique. *Infertility* 1982;5:15.

Daniell JF, Kurtz B, Gurley L. Laser laparoscopic management of large endometriomas. *Fertil Steril* 1991;55:692.

David SS. Microsurgical management of distal tube disease. In: Reyniak JV, Lauersen NH, eds. *Principles of microsurgical techniques in infertility*. New York: Plenum; 1982:161.
Davis GD, Brooks RA. Excision of pelvic endometriosis with the carbon dioxide laser laparoscope. *Obstet Gynecol* 1988;72:816.
Department of Health, Education and Welfare/Food and Drug Administration Report on Laser Products. *Federal Register* 40(148): part II, July 1975.
Diamond E. Microsurgical reconstruction of the uterine tube in sterilized patients. *Fertil Steril* 1977;28:1203.
Diamond NP, Daniell JF, Martin DC, et al. Tubal patency in pelvic adhesions at early second look laparoscopy following intraabdominal use of the carbon dioxide laser: initial report of the Intraabdominal Laser Study Group. *Fertil Steril* 1984;42:717.
Dlugi AM, Saleh WA, Jacobsen G. KTP/532 laser laparoscopy in the treatment of endometriosis associated infertility. *Fertil Steril* 1992;57:1186.
Dorsey JH. The evolution of operative colposcopy. *Colpos Gynecol Laser Surg* 1986;2:65.
Dorsey JH. Indications and general techniques for lasers in advanced operative laparoscopy. *Obstet Gynecol Clin North Am* 1991;15:555.
Dorsey JH. Marsupialization techniques with the CO_2 laser: methods and case reports. *Colpos Gynecol Laser Surg* 1986;2:113.
Dorsey JH. Recurrent cervical intraepithelial neoplasia (CIN) and the endocervical button. *Colpos Gynecol Laser Surg* 1984;1:221.
Dorsey JH. The role of lasers in advanced operative laparoscopy. *Obstet Gynecol Clin North Am* 1991;15:545.
Dorsey JH, Baggish MS. Initiating a CO_2 laser program. *Basic Adv Laser Surg Gynecol* 1985;373:381.
Dorsey JH, Sharp HT. *Laparoscopic surgery and ovarian disorders: diagnosis and management of ovarian disorders*. New York: Igaku-Shoin; 1995: 350.
Doughtery TJ, Kaufman JE, Goldfarb A, et al. Photoradiation therapy for the treatment of malignant tumors. *Cancer Res* 1978;38:2628.
Doyle JB: Paracervical uterine denervation for relief of pelvic pain. *Clin Obstet Gynecol* 1963;6:742.
Fayez JA, Collazo LM, Vernon C. Comparison of different modalities of treatment for minimal and mild endometriosis. *Am J Obstet Gynecol* 1988;159:927.
Feste JR. CO_2 laser laparoscopy: CO_2. In: Keye WR Jr, ed. *Laser surgery in gynecology and obstetrics*. Chicago: YearBook Medical Publishers; 1990.
Feste JR. Laser laparoscopy: a new modality. *Fertil Steril* 1984;41:74S.
Fluhman GG. Involvement of clefts and tunnels in carcinoma-in-situ of the cervix uteri. *Am J Obstet Gynecol* 1962;83:1410–1419.
Fuller TA, Nadkarni VJ, et al. Carbon dioxide laser fiber optics. *Bio-Laser News* 1985;4:1.
Garry R, Shelley-Jones D, Mooney P, et al. Six hundred endometrial laser ablations. *Obstet Gynecol* 1995;85:24.
Giles JA, Gafar A. The treatment of CIN: do we need lasers? *BJOG* 1991;98:3.
Goldrath M, Fuller T, Segal S. Laser photovaporization of endometrium for the treatment of menorrhagia. *Am J Obstet Gynecol* 1981;140:14
Gomel V. Causes of failure of reconstructive infertility microsurgery. *J Reprod Med* 1980;24:239.
Gordon HK, Duncan ID. Effective destruction of cervical intraepithelial neoplasia (CIN) 3 at 100°C using the Semm cold coagulator: 14 years' experience. *BJOG* 1991;98:14.
Gordts S, Boeckx W, Brosens I. Microsurgery of endometriosis in infertile patients. *Fertil Steril* 1984;42:520.
Grosspietzsch R, et al. Experiments on operative treatment of tubal sterility by CO_2 laser technique. *Proceedings of the Third International Congress on Laser Surgery Tel-Aviv*, 1979:256.
Gurgan T, Urman B, Aksu T, et al. Laparoscopic CO_2 laser uterine nerve ablation for treatment of drug-resistant primary dysmenorrhea. *Fertil Steril* 1992;58(2):422.
Hagen B, Skjeldestad FE. The outcome of pregnancy after CO_2 laser conization of the cervix. *BJOG* 1993;100:717.
Helkjaer PE, Eriksen PS, Thomsen CF, et al. Outpatient CO_2 laser excisional conization for cervical intraepithelial neoplasia under local anesthesia. *Acta Obstet Gynecol Scand* 1993;72:302.
Hoffman MS, Pinelli DM, Finan M, et al. Laser vaporization for vulvar intraepithelial neoplasia III. *J Reprod Med* 1992;37:135.
Hulka JF, Omran K, Bergen GS. Classification of adnexal adhesions: a proposal and evaluation of its prognostic value. *Fertil Steril* 1978;30:661.
Jordan JA. Laser treatment of cervical intraepithelial neoplasia. *Obstet Gynecol* 1979;34:831.
Kaplan I, Goldman J, Ger R. The treatment of erosions of the uterine cervix by means of the CO_2 laser. *Obstet Gynecol* 1973;41:795.
Kelly RW. Laser surgery for adhesions. *Basic Adv Laser Surg Gynecol* 1985;323:329.
Kelly RW, Diamond MP. Intra-abdominal use of the carbon dioxide laser for microsurgery. *Obstet Gynecol Clin North Am* 1991;15:537.
Kelly RW, Roberts DK. Experience with the carbon dioxide laser in gynecologic microsurgery. *Am J Obstet Gynecol* 1983;146:586.
Keye WR Jr. *Laser surgery in gynecology and obstetrics*. Chicago: Yearbook Medical Publishers Inc.; 1990.
Keye WR Jr, Hansen LW, Astin M, et al. Argon laser therapy of endometriosis: a review of 92 consecutive patients. *Fertil Steril* 1987;47:208.
Klink F, Grosspietzsch F, Klitzing LV, et al. Animal in vivo studies and in vitro experiments with human tubes for end-to-end anastomotic operation by a CO_2 laser technique. *Fertil Steril* 1978;30:100.
Krebs HB. The use of topical 5-fluorouracil in the treatment of genital condylomas. *Obstet Gynecol Clin North Am* 1987;14(2): 559.
Larsson G, Alm P, Grundsell H. Laser conization versus cold knife conization. *Surg Gynecol Obstet* 1982;154:59.
Lomano JM. Ablation of the endometrium with the Nd:YAG laser: a multi-center study. *Colpos Gynecol Laser Surg* 1986;4:203.
Lomano JM. Photocoagulation of early pelvic endometriosis with the Nd:YAG laser through the laparoscope. *J Reprod Med* 1985;30:2.
Lopes A, Morgan P, Murdoch J, et al. The case for conservative management of "incomplete excision" of CIN after laser conization. *Obstet Gynecol* 1993;49:247.
MacLean AB, Murray EL, Sharp F, et al. Residual cervical intraepithelial neoplasia after laser ablation. *Lasers Surg Med* 1987;7:278.
Mage G, Canis M, Pouly JL, et al. CO_2 laser laparoscopy: a ten-year experience. *Eur J Obstet Gynecol Reprod Biol* 1988;28:120.
Mage G, Chany Y, Bruhat MA. Intraabdominal conservative surgical treatment for endometriosis by CO_2 laser. *Contrib Gynecol Obstet* 1987;16:297.
Mage G, Pouly JL, Bruhat MA. Laser microsurgery of the oviducts. *Basic Adv Laser Surg Gynecol* 1985;299:321.
Maiman TH. Stimulated optical radiation in the ruby. *Nature* 1960;157:493.
Marlow JL. Laparoscopy. In: Coppleson ed. *Gynecologic oncology: fundamental principles and clinical practice*. London: Churchill Livingston; 1981.
Marlow JL. Lasers in intra-abdominal gynecologic surgery. In: Fuller ed. *Surgical lasers: a clinical guide*. New York: Macmillan Publishing Company; 1987.
Martin DC. Laparoscopic and vaginal colpotomy for the excision of infiltrating cul-de-sac endometriosis. *J Reprod Med* 1988;33:806.
Martin DC. Laser techniques for pelvic adhesions. *Basic Adv Laser Surg Gynecol* 1985;331:340.
Martin DC, Diamond MP. Operative laparoscopy: comparison of lasers with other techniques. *Curr Probl Obstet Gynecol Fertil* 1986;9:564.
Murdoch JB, Morgan PR, Lopes A, et al. Histological incomplete excision of CIN after large loop excision of the transformation zone (LLETZ) merits careful follow up, not retreatment. *BJOG* 1992;99:990.
Mylotte MJ, Allen JM, Jordan JA. Regeneration of cervical epithelium following laser destruction of intraepithelial neoplasia. *Obstet Gynecol Surv* 1979;34(11):859.
Nezhat C, Crowgey SR, Garrison CP. Surgical treatment of endometriosis via laser laparoscopy and video laparoscopy. *Contrib Gynecol Obstet* 1987;16:303.
Nezhat C, Winer WK, Nezhat F, et al. Smoke from laser surgery: is there a health hazard? *Lasers Surg Med* 1987;7:376.
Nezhat CR, Nezhat FR, Luciano AA, et al. *Operative gynecologic laparoscopy: principals and techniques*. New York: McGraw–Hill; 1995.
Ott DE. Carboxyhemoglobinemia due to peritoneal smoke absorption from laser tissue combustion at laparoscopy. *J Clin Laser Med Surg* 1998;16: 309.
Palmer R. La coeleoscopic gynecologique. *E.M.C. Gynecologie Fascicule* 1965;71:A.10.
Patel CKN. High-power carbon dioxide lasers. *Sci Am* 1968;219:23.
Pegues RF, Dorsey JH. Gynecologic laparoscopy. *Complications Laparosc Surg* 1995;12:313.
Persad VL, Perotic MA, Guijon FB. Management of cervical neoplasia: a 13 year experience with cryotherapy and laser. *Journal of Lower Genital Tract Disease* 2001;5(4):199.
Pittaway DE, Maxson WS, Daniell JF. A comparison of the CO_2 laser and electrocautery on postoperative intraperitoneal adhesion formation in rabbits. *Fertil Steril* 1983;40:366.
Polanyi TG, Bredemeir HC, Davis TW. A CO_2 laser for surgical research. *Med Biol Eng* 1970;8:541.
Reid R. Laser surgery of the vulva. *Obstet Gynecol Clin North Am* 1991;15:491.
Reid R. Physical and surgical principles governing expertise with the carbon dioxide laser. *Obstet Gynecol Clin North Am* 1987;14:513.
Rettenmaier MA, Berman ML, DiSaia PJ, et al. Photoradiation therapy of gynecologic malignancies. *Gynecol Oncol* 1984;17:206.
Rock JA, Katayama KP, Martin EJ, et al. Pregnancy outcome following uterotubal implantation: a comparison of the reamer and sharp wedge excision techniques. *Fertil Steril* 1979;31:634.
Schawlow AL. Advances in optical lasers. *Sci Am* 1963;209:36.
Schawlow AL, Townes CH. Infrared and optical masers. *Physiol Rev* 1958;112:1940.
Semm K. New methods of pelviscopy for myometry, ovariectomy, tubectomy, and adenectomy. *Endoscopy* 1979;2:85.
Semm K. Tissue punches and loop ligation: new aids for surgical-therapeutic pelviscopy. *Endoscopy* 1978;10:119.

Sesti F, DeSantis L, Farne C, et al. Efficacy of CO_2 laser surgery in treating squamous intraepithelial lesions. *J Reprod Med* 1994;39:441.

Sliney DH, Trokel SL. *Medical lasers and their safe use.* Springer-Verlag, 1993.

Spitzer M, Krumholz BA. Photodynamic therapy in gynecology. *Obstet Gynecol Clin North Am* 1991;15:649.

Steptoe P, Edwards R. Birth after reimplantation of a human embryo. *Lancet* 1978;2(8085):366.

Surrey MW, Hill DL. Treatment of endometriosis by carbon dioxide laser during gamete intrafallopian transfer. *J Am Coll Surg* 1994;179:440.

Sutton CJG, Ewen SP, Whitelaw N, et al. Prospective, randomized, double-blind, controlled trial of laser laparoscopy in the treatment of pelvic pain associated with minimal, mild, and moderate endometriosis. *Fertil Steril* 1994;62: 699.

Sutton CJG, Pooley AS, Ewen SP, et al. Follow-up report on a randomized controlled trial of laser laparoscopy in the treatment of pelvic pain associated with minimal to moderate endometriosis. *Fertil Steril* 1997;68:1070.

Tadir Y, Kaplan I, Zuckerman Z, et al. New instrumentation and technique for laparoscopic carbon dioxide laser operations: a preliminary report. *Obstet Gynecol* 1984;63:582.

Thompson AD, et al. Investigation of laser cervical cone biopsies negative for premalignancy or malignancy. *Journal of Lower Genital Tract Disease* 2002;6(2):84.

Townes, Schawlow. Infrared and optical mases. *Phys Rev* 1958;6(112):1940–1949.

Townsend DE, Richart RM. Cryotherapy and CO_2 laser management of CIN, a controlled comparison. *Obstet Gynecol* 1983;61:75.

Townsend DE, Smith LH, Kinney WK. Condylomata acuminata: roles of different techniques of laser vaporization. *J Reprod Med* 1993;38:362.

Trofatter KF Jr. Interferon. *Obstet Gynecol Clin North Am* 1987:569.

Turner RJ, Cohen RA, Voet RL, et al. Analysis of tissue margins of cone biopsy specimens obtained with "cold," CO_2 and Nd:YAG lasers and a radio frequency surgical unit. *J Reprod Med* 1992;37:607.

Ueki M, Kitsuki K, Miksaki O, et al. Clinical evaluation of contact Nd:YAG laser conization for cervical intraepithelial neoplasia of the uterus. *Acta Obstet Gynecol Scand* 1992;71:465.

Valle RF, Sankpal R, Marlow JL, et al. Cervical stenosis: a challenging clinical entity. *J Gynecol Surg* 2002;18:129.

Vergote IG, Makar AP, Kjorstad KE. Laser excision of the transformation zone as treatment of cervical intraepithelial neoplasia with satisfactory colposcopy. *Obstet Gynecol* 1992;44:235.

Woodruff JD, Paurstein CJ. *The fallopian tube.* 1st ed. Baltimore: Williams & Wilkins, 1969:336.

Wright VC. Laser vaporization of the cervix for the management of cervical intraepithelial neoplasia. *Basic Adv Laser Surg Gynecol* 1985;207: 215.

Wright TC, Cox JT, Massad LS, et al. 2001 consensus guidelines for the management of women with cervical intraepithelial neoplasia. *J of Lower Genital Tract Disease* 2003;7(3):154.

CHAPTER 17 ■ DIAGNOSTIC AND OPERATIVE LAPAROSCOPY

HOWARD T. SHARP, SEAN L. FRANCIS, AND ANA ALVAREZ MURPHY

DEFINITIONS

Aqua dissection—The use of fluid, most often sterile water or saline, under force, to separate one anatomical plane from another. The laparoscopic motorized irrigation is an excellent tool for performing aqua dissection.

Chromopertubation—A procedure in which a colored dye is passed through the fallopian tubes to confirm that they are patent.

Colpotomy—A surgical incision in the vagina. The *-tomy* part of the word is from the Greek word *tome,* meaning cutting.

High definition—A term initially introduced in the 1930s to define the then-new technology that replaced the experimental systems that ranged from 15 lines to about 220 lines of resolution. High-definition television (HDTV) is now defined as resolution 1,080 or 720 lines. HD is broadcast digitally and consequently produces a more vivid and realistic picture.

Morcellate—To divide into small portions.

Reposable—A trocar/sleeve kit in which disposable trocars are used with reusable sleeves in an effort to reduce the cost of disposable products while ensuring sharp, undamaged instruments more commonly found in the disposable kits.

Veres needle—A spring-loaded needle designed to allow entry into body cavities without trauma to underlying organs during laparoscopy.

Laparoscopic surgical advances have accelerated remarkably over the past decades. What was initially a primitive tool for diagnostic purposes and simple procedures such as tubal sterilization has evolved into a more coordinated system for the repair or removal of diseased abdominal and pelvic organs. As operative laparoscopy has become more complex and technology has continued to advance, new challenges and complications have been recognized. The proper use of equipment and techniques can greatly add to patient safety and satisfaction. To this end, the purpose of the chapter is to review contemporary equipment, commonly used surgical techniques, and strategies to avoid and manage complications associated with laparoscopic surgery.

HISTORY

The first description of endoscopy is attributed to Phillip Bozzini in 1805, as he attempted to view the urethral mucosa with a simple tube and candlelight. Hysteroscopy was the first gynecologic endoscopic procedure performed when Pantaleoni used a cystoscope to identify uterine polyps in 1869. Laparoscopy was first performed by Jacobaeus of Sweden in 1910, wherein a Nitze cystoscope, composed of a candle and a hollow tube, was used to illuminate the peritoneal cavity. Kalk of Germany was instrumental in developing laparoscopy into a diagnostic and surgical procedure in the early 1930s. By the end of the 1930s, laparoscopy was being used in the diagnosis of ectopic pregnancy and the performance of tubal sterilization. Raoul Palmer of France reported the use of gaseous distention with lithotomy Trendelenburg positioning in 1947. The use of "cold light" and fiberoptics were landmark innovations credited to Fourestier, Gladu, Valmiere, and Kampany and Hopkins, respectively. Monopolar electrosurgery for tubal sterilization was popularized in the 1960s. Semm of Germany reported advanced operative laparoscopic procedures such as salpingectomy, myomectomy, oophorectomy, ovarian cystectomy, and salpingostomy in the 1970s. These pioneers of endoscopic surgery and many others have laid the crucial groundwork that has enabled modern gynecologic surgeons to perform advanced operative laparoscopy on a routine basis, with a variety of energy systems under increasingly ergonomic and efficient conditions.

INDICATIONS FOR LAPAROSCOPY

Diagnostic Laparoscopy

Laparoscopy can provide valuable clinical information in a number of circumstances. It can aid in the evaluation of patients with acute pelvic and abdominal pain, including ovarian torsion, ovarian cyst rupture, ectopic pregnancy, appendicitis, and pelvic inflammatory disease. In the evaluation of less emergent conditions, such as chronic pelvic pain and infertility, it is useful to identify pelvic adhesions, endometriosis, hernias, uterine fibroids, and adnexal masses. Before performing diagnostic laparoscopy, a thorough history, detailed physical examination, and appropriate imaging studies should be completed.

Operative Laparoscopy

Most surgeries traditionally performed by the abdominal or vaginal approach can now be performed laparoscopically. Studies are still needed to better define which advanced procedures are most appropriate to perform laparoscopically from an economic and safety vantage point. Operator experience is a critical factor that must be considered. Commonly performed laparoscopic procedures include adhesiolysis, treatment of endometriosis, tubal sterilization, ovarian cystectomy, oophorectomy, salpingectomy, salpingostomy, and hysterectomy. More advanced procedures include repair of pelvic organ prolapse, tubal reanastomosis, myomectomy, radical hysterectomy, and lymphadenectomy.

EQUIPMENT

Contemporary laparoscopy equipment consists of an imaging system comprising a telescope (laparoscope) and video camera system, an insufflation or abdominal wall lift system, and specialized surgical instruments. Digitization and robotics are areas that continue to evolve.

Imaging Systems

Imaging systems consist of a laparoscope, light source, fiberoptic cord, camera unit, and monitors. High-definition digital cameras are now available that are compatible with the increased resolution capabilities of high-definition flat screen monitors. Most imaging systems are also equipped with a printer, video recorder, or DVD recorder for documentation.

The laparoscope in its basic form is a telescope. Laparoscopes range from 1.8 mm to 12 mm in diameter, with a distal end (objective) available in varying viewing angles (Fig. 17.1). The 0-degree deflection-angle telescope is most commonly used and provides a straightforward view, whereas a 30-degree fore-oblique lens allows for visualization in a large frontal view but must be continuously directed to maintain field orientation. Operative laparoscopes are equipped with a central channel that allows laser, electrosurgical, or mechanical instruments to be introduced into the abdomen. Light is introduced through the laparoscope with a fiberoptic cable powered by a light source. It is important that the light source have sufficient power to deliver adequate light through the fiber-optic cable. Ideally, high-intensity light sources that use xenon or halogen are used. Though a significant amount of original light is lost from the original hot light source, the fiber-optic cable is able to transmit enough heat to burn paper drapes as well as patient's skin; therefore, caution should be used to avoid inadvertent contact with drapes or the patient.

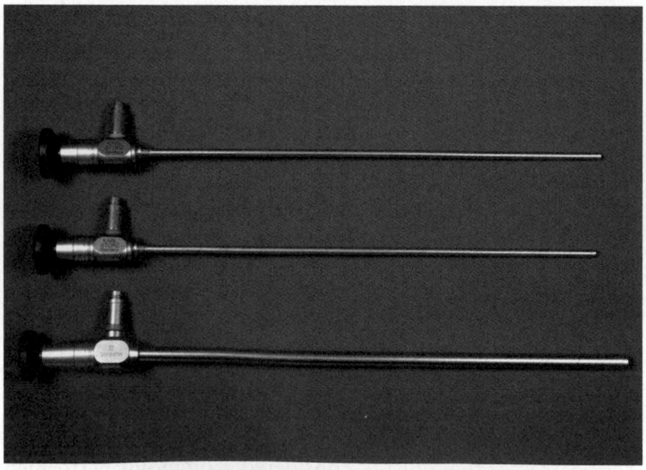

FIGURE 17.1. Telescopes used in laparoscopy. *Top,* 5-mm, 0-degree viewing angle laparoscope. *Middle,* 5-mm, 30-degree viewing angle laparoscope. *Bottom,* 10-mm, 0-degree viewing angle laparoscope.

The camera unit consists of a camera head, cable, and camera control. The camera head attaches to the eyepiece of the laparoscope and captures images transmitted by the laparoscope. Camera/laparoscopes are now available as combined, fused units that are fully autoclavable, with push-button zoom and auto-focus features. The basis of laparoscopic cameras is the solid state silicon computer chip or charge-coupled device (CCD). This is composed of silicon elements, which emit an electric charge when exposed to light. Each silicon element contributes one pixel unit to the image produced. The image resolution is dependent on the number of pixels on the chip. Most laparoscopic cameras have 250,000 to 380,000 pixels. Three-chip CCDs provide better image clarity but are more expensive, as they have a separate chip for each primary color, as opposed to the single chip CCD. High-resolution color monitors with 700 lines are needed to provide optimal visualization. High-definition digital cameras used with high-definition flat panels can be used with up to 1,100 lines of resolution. Newer developments include the use of voice-activated, wireless systems designed to provide central control over operating room devices using either a microphone or a movable touch-pad screen.

Insufflation and Abdominal Lifting Systems

Insufflation systems allow gas to fill the abdominopelvic cavity to optimize visualization. Insufflators are designed to deliver gas at low rates during initial Veres needle insertion, but are also able to provide high flow rates when gas is lost to maintain a relatively constant set intraabdominal pressure during surgery. Insufflation may be achieved with a Veres needle or the Hassan trocar, filtered tubing, an insufflator, and gas tanks. Insufflation tubing with a 0.3-micron filter is recommended to prevent intraperitoneal contamination with bacteria, microparticles, and debris from the insufflator and gas tank. A Veres needle is often used to create a pneumoperitoneum, although other methods, such as direct trocar insertion and open laparoscopy, will be discussed. The Veres needle is available in reusable or disposable models containing a springloaded tip that retracts as it pierces the abdominal wall, allowing a blunt tip to engage on entry to the peritoneal cavity (Fig. 17.2). This is designed to avoid damaging bowel or other intraabdominal organs. Though filtered room air has been used, carbon

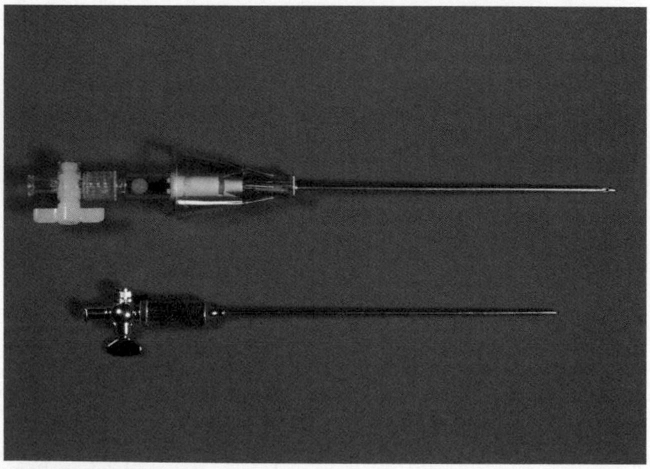

FIGURE 17.2. Disposable (*top*) and reusable (*bottom*) Veres needle.

dioxide is most commonly used today. Carbon dioxide has the advantage of being rapidly absorbed by blood. However, it is converted to carbonic acid on moist peritoneal surfaces, which can cause pain. For this reason, nitrous oxide or helium are preferred by some, especially in cases using local anesthesia or conscious sedation. Some have advocated the use of heated or hydrated gas to prevent hypothermia during laparoscopy. Insufflators that contain a heating unit have little or no effect on temperature by the time the gas has traveled 50 to 100 cm in tubing. In longer surgeries, prevention of hypothermia is better achieved by using a heated body surface blanket or the Insuflow device (Lexicon), which delivers heated and hydrated gas. Gasless laparoscopy can also be performed with the use of a mechanical lifting arm that attaches to a fanlike retractor along the peritoneal surface of the abdominal wall, obviating the need for gas distension. Some favor this approach in patients with cardiopulmonary risk factors.

Surgical Instrumentation

Trocars and sleeves are used to pierce the abdominal wall for placement of the laparoscope and surgical instruments (Fig. 17.3). Trocar sleeves range from 2 to 15 mm in diameter and are available as reusable, disposable, and reposable systems. Disposable systems consist of completely disposable trocars and sleeves. They offer the advantage of consistent sharpness but are more expensive. Reusable trocars offer the advantage of being the most cost-effective, but they must be maintained for sharpness. Reposable systems are composed of a disposable bladed or nonbladed trocar with a reusable sleeve. All are acceptable for use. Most sleeves contain a Luer-lock port that attaches to insufflation tubing. Trocar tips may be pyramidal, conical (reusable), bladed, blunt tipped, or have optical access (disposable). Conical and blunt-tipped trocars have the advantage of making smaller fascial defects but require greater force to place. Optical access trocars such as Optiview (Ethicon) and Visiport (U.S. Surgical) enable the surgeon to visualize the layers of the abdominal wall during placement. Expandable trocar sheaths are available that are initially placed through the abdominal wall with a Veres needle and then expanded to accept a 5- to 12-mm port (Step port, InnerDyne). These offer the advantage of creating smaller abdominal wall defects and thereby reducing the risk of hernia formation and injury to the inferior epigastric vessels.

Ancillary instruments may be placed through secondary trocar sleeves to aid in diagnostic and operative laparoscopy (Figs. 17.4 and 17.5). These include blunt probes; a variety of graspers, including toothed and atraumatic graspers; scissors; needle drivers; knot pushers; biopsy forceps; suction-irrigators; energy delivery tools; specimen retrieval bags; and tissue morcellators. A uterine manipulator may be used to improve access to the uterus, fallopian tubes, ovaries, and the posterior and anterior cul-de-sacs. These are available in reusable and disposable models. Some manipulators are inserted in a fixed position and allow limited uterine mobility, whereas others are hinged and allow the uterus to be moved anteriorly, posteriorly, and laterally. Many of these also offer the ability to perform chromotubation for evaluation of fallopian tube patency.

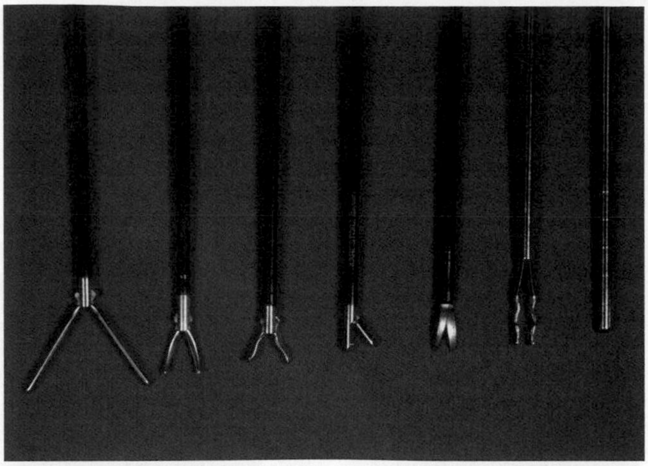

FIGURE 17.4. Ancillary instruments for laparoscopic surgery. Shown from left to right: bowel grasper, Maryland dissector, atraumatic forceps, biopsy forceps, scissors, Kleppinger bipolar forceps, blunt measuring probe.

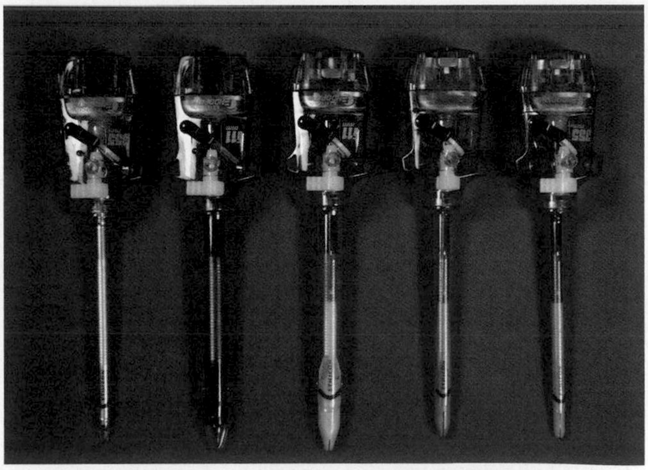

FIGURE 17.3. Trocars and sleeves. Shown from left to right: blunt-tipped, optical-access trocars are shown in 5- and 11-mm sizes. Bladed trocars are seen in 11-, 8-, and 5-mm sizes.

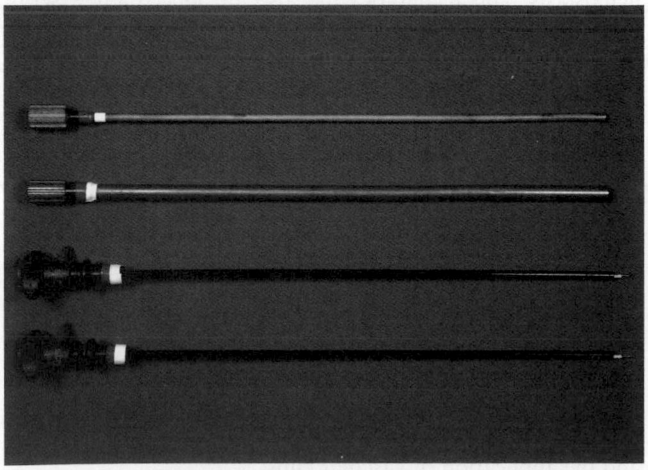

FIGURE 17.5. Suction irrigator sleeves. From top to bottom: 5-mm sleeve, 10-mm sleeve, 5-mm sleeve with monopolar L-hook, 5-mm sleeve with monopolar needle point.

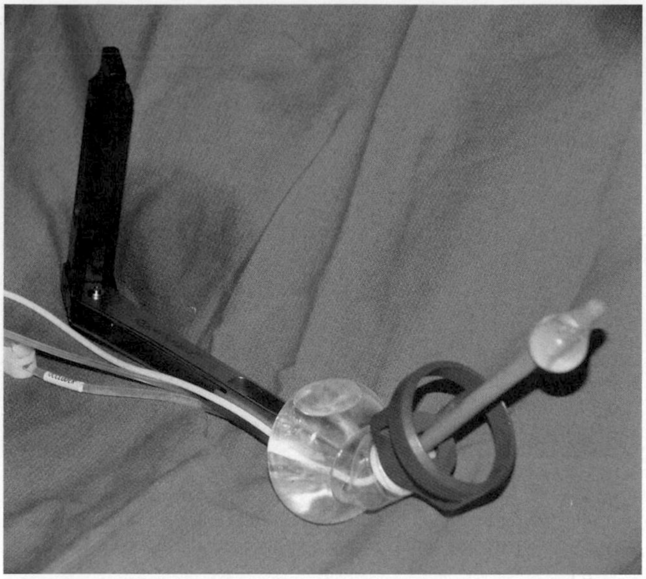

FIGURE 17.6. KOH manipulator.

More advanced manipulators, such as the KOH Colpotomizer (CooperSurgical) (Fig. 17.6), provide a stainless-steel cup that engulfs the cervix, allowing the surgeon to cut against it when resecting the uterus and cervix from the vagina during a laparoscopic hysterectomy. The same device also provides a balloon that is inflated to prevent the pneumoperitoneum from escaping through the vagina once the incision has been made on the vaginal cuff. Though this instrument can significantly facilitate the hysterectomy, it is more expensive than other manipulators, and the time required to insert it can potentially contribute to the overall anesthesia time.

Energy and Hemostasis

The application of energy systems to laparoscopy has expanded laparoscopic surgeons' ability to perform complex surgeries with the capability to rapidly divide tissues and maintain hemostasis. This technology has also introduced a new set of complications, such as unrecognized bowel burns from inadvertent direct and capacitative coupling. In an effort to reduce risks associated with monopolar electrosurgical devices, several options are available. One is the use of endomechanical energy; a second is the use of bipolar electrosurgery, laser, or ultrasonic energy; and a third is the gaining of a better understanding of electrosurgical principles. Though our understanding of laparoscopically applied electrophysics has improved, gynecologic surgeons often have no formal electrosurgical training or credentialing in contrast to the once-common laser safety courses. Electrosurgery and laser principles are explained in Chapters 15 and 16.

Endomechanical Energy

Endomechanical energy can be used for tissue division and hemostasis in a number of ways, including suturing, stapling, and the application of vascular clips.

Suture. The simplest laparoscopic ligature to apply is the pretied loop, available as a slip knot on a push rod that is

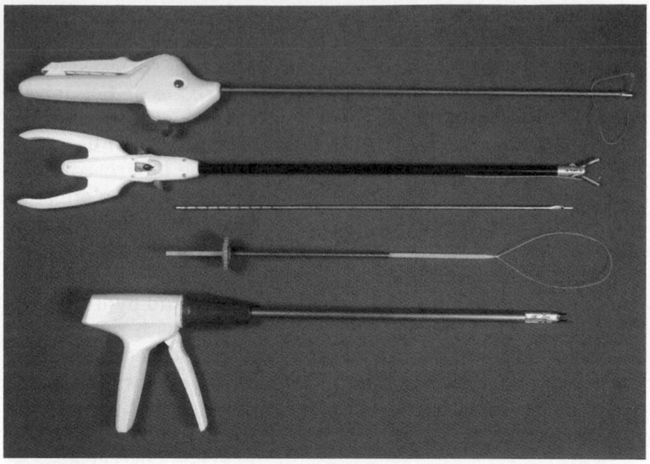

FIGURE 17.7. Laparoscopic suturing/hemostasis devices. From top to bottom: Suture Assistant (Ethicon), Endostitch (U.S. Surgical), closed tipped knot pusher (Ranfac), Endo-loop (U.S. Surgical), LigaClip (Ethicon).

used to push a suture loop around a tissue pedicle for hemostasis (Fig. 17.7). The Roeder loop, which was modified by Kurt Semm for laparoscopic use, can also be tied in the operating room using standard suture. Laparoscopic suturing can be performed using stock suture, ideally 36 to 48 inches in length (Fig. 17.8). Needle drivers are used to drive needles through tissue, and knots may be tied outside the laparoscopic port (extracorporeal knot) or within the body (intracorporeal knot). Extracorporeal knots are usually performed as sliding square knots, pushed through the trocar sleeve to the tissue by multiple passes of a knot pusher, which serves as the surgeon's finger (Fig. 17.9). Intracorporeal knots are tied within the abdomen by looping the suture material around the laparoscopic needle holders using the same technique as an "instrument tie" (Fig. 17.10). Laparoscopic suturing requires considerable practice to confidently load the needle into the needle driver and place sutures accurately. To this end, the Endostitch (U.S. Surgical) was developed, wherein the needle is preloaded and the suture is passed through tissue up to 2 cm thick by closing a handle and a toggle switch (Fig. 17.7). The endostitch is a 10-mm instrument with jaws measuring 4 mm wide and 2 cm long. Other automated products are also available, including the Suture Assistant (Ethicon Endosurgery) (Fig. 17.7) and the Lapra-ty (Ethicon Endosurgery). In an effort to accommodate surgeons desiring to use the laparoscopic needle driver and suture, companies such as Cook produce self-righting needle drivers, which are intended to automatically fix the needle at a perpendicular or oblique position to the needle driver. Such devices facilitate suturing laparoscopically.

Staplers. The endo-GIA, originally designed for gastrointestinal anastomosis, is used in gynecologic laparoscopy as a stapling device for securing and dividing tissue. When the jaws of the instrument are closed over tissue and as the grip is fired, six staggered rows of staples, 3 cm in length and 1 cm in width, are placed. A knife blade simultaneously divides the tissue, leaving three rows of staples on each side of the incision.

Vascular Clips. Endoscopic vascular clips may be used to achieve hemostasis for bleeding vessels or pedicles (Fig. 17.7). These offer the advantage of being used near vital structures,

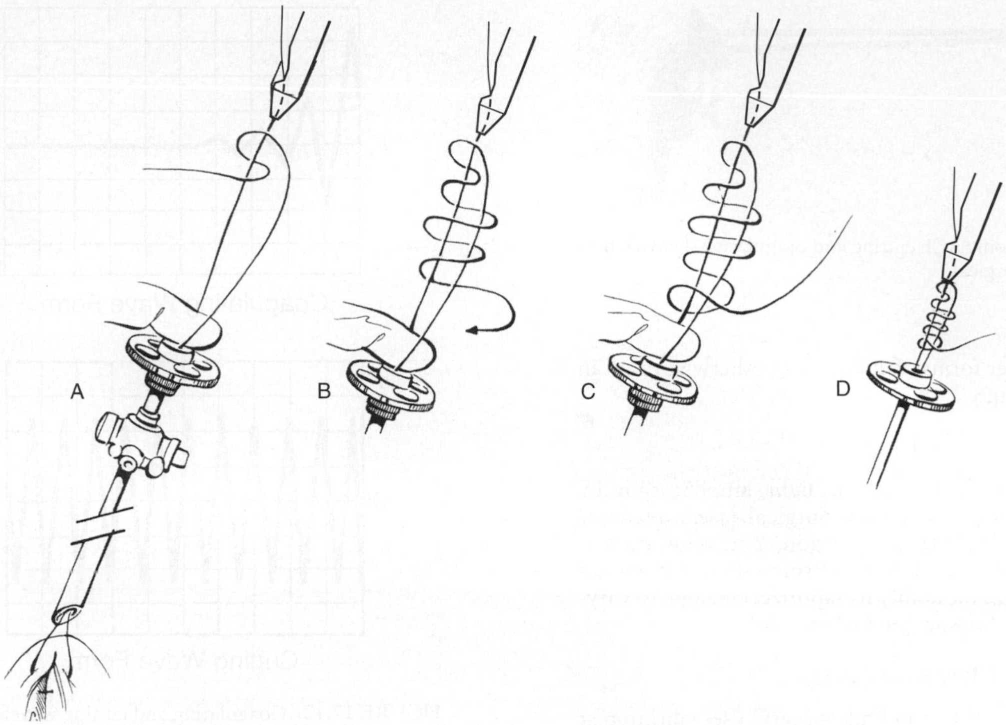

FIGURE 17.8. Extracorporeal knot tying with slip knot. **A:** With both suture ends outside the body, the suture is cut below the needle. A single throw is made. **B:** With the free end of the suture, three revolutions are made around both suture strands. **C:** The tail of the suture is inserted through the lowest loop. **D:** The tail is pulled to tighten the knot, the suture is cut above the knot, and the slip knot is pushed with a closed-nose knot pusher to the desired position. (Modified from Murphy AA. Operative laparoscopy. *Fertil Steril* 1987;47:1.)

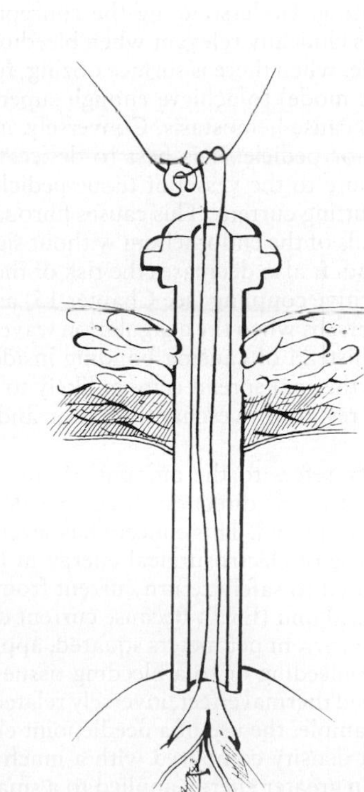

FIGURE 17.9. Extracorporeal knot tying with the Clarke knot pusher. (Modified from Hulka JF, Reich H. *Textbook of laparoscopy.* 2nd ed. Philadelphia: WB Saunders; 1994:202.)

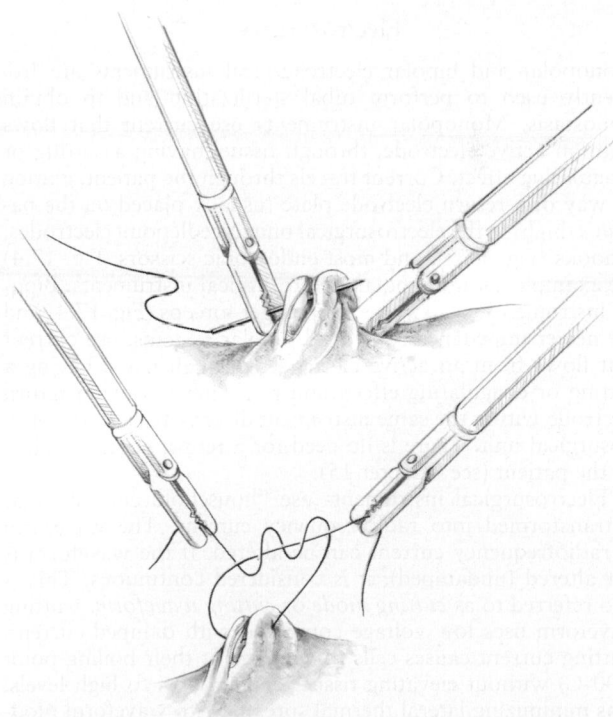

FIGURE 17.10. Intracorporeal knot tying. **A:** The needle is passed through the tissue. **B:** A surgeon's knot is made with the instruments and pulled tight.

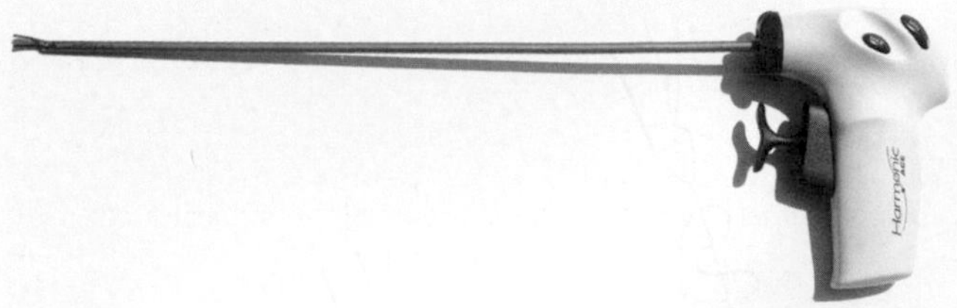

FIGURE 17.11. Harmonic ACE cutting and coagulating shears. Courtesy of Ethicon Endosurgical.

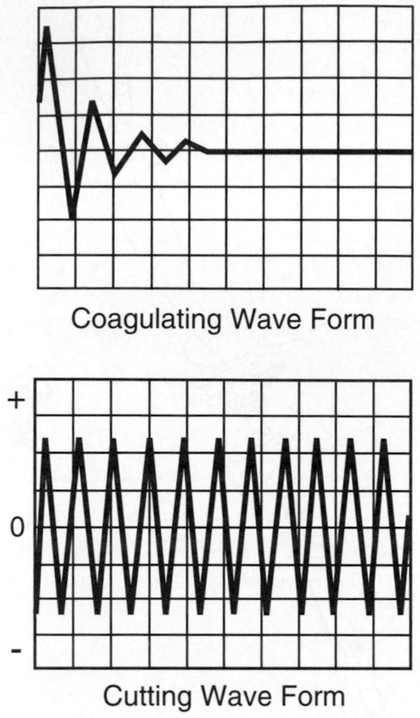

FIGURE 17.12. Coagulating and cutting waveforms.

where the use of other forms of energy may otherwise result in lateral thermal damage.

Laser Energy

The term *laser* is an acronym for light amplification by spontaneous emission of radiation. Surgical lasers available for gynecologic use include CO_2, argon, potassium-titanyl-phosphate (KTP), and neodymium:yttrium-aluminum-garnet (Nd-YAG). These have the ability to vaporize, cut, and, to varying degrees, coagulate tissue (see Chapter 16).

Ultrasonic Energy

The Harmonic Scalpel (Ethicon Endosurgery) uses vibration at the rate of 55,000 cycles per second as an energy source to break hydrogen bonds in tissue, resulting in cutting or coaptation of vessels. The Harmonic Scalpel is available as a 5-mm rounded "scalpel" with a blunt or hooked edge or as a 5- to 10-mm "shear" or Harmonic Ace (Fig. 17.11), which can be used to grasp tissue. This modality results in minimal lateral thermal spread of energy, and there is no risk of electrical injury.

Electrosurgery

Monopolar and bipolar electrosurgical instruments are frequently used to perform tubal sterilization and to obtain hemostasis. Monopolar instruments use current that flows from an active electrode, through tissue, having a cutting or coagulating effect. Current travels through the patient, exiting by way of a return electrode plate (usually placed on the patient's thigh) to the electrosurgical unit. Needlepoint electrodes, L-hooks (Fig. 17.5), and most endoscopic scissors (Fig. 17.4) are examples of monopolar electrosurgical instruments. Bipolar instruments, such as the Kleppinger forceps (Fig. 17.4) and the newer impedance-controlled bipolar systems, use current that flows from an active electrode, through tissue having a cutting or coagulating effect, and returning through a return electrode within the same instrument directly back to the electrosurgical unit. There is no need for a return electrode plate on the patient (see Chapter 15).

Electrosurgical instruments use "household current" that is transformed into radiofrequency current. The waveform of radiofrequency current can be altered. If the waveform is not altered (undamped), it is considered continuous. This is also referred to as *cutting mode* or *cutting waveform*. Cutting waveform uses low voltage compared with damped current. Cutting current causes cells to vaporize at their boiling point (100°C) without elevating tissue temperatures to high levels, thus minimizing lateral thermal spread. With waveform modification, current can be interrupted (damped) to varying degrees (Fig.17.12). These modifications refer to blend 1 (80% on, 20% off), blend 2 (60% on, 40% off), blend 3 (50% on, 50% off), and coagulation (6% on, 94% off). As a result of current interruption (coagulation), bursts of energy with higher voltage (5,000 V) and therefore lower current, given a constant wattage (watts = voltage × current), will occur. This results in denaturation and charring (fulguration) to cause hemostasis with minimal cutting. Understanding the concepts of cutting and coagulation is clinically relevant when bleeding is encountered. For example, when there is surface oozing, fulguration is used (coagulation mode) to achieve enough superficial lateral thermal spread to cause hemostasis. Conversely, in the case of a bleeding vessel or pedicle, it is best to desiccate the vessel by applying pressure to the vessel or tissue pedicle with a tissue grasper and cutting current. This causes fibrous bonding of the dehydrated cells of the endothelium without significant lateral thermal spread. It also decreases the risk of thermal bowel injury from capacitive coupling (see Chapter 15) as lower voltage is used. Conversely, when the coagulation waveform is used in this scenario, instead of causing bonding inside the vessel, superficial lateral thermal spread is more likely to occur along the tissue surface, resulting in eschar formation and subsequent bleeding.

Current density refers to the amount of current flow per cross-sectional area in the direction of current flow described in amps per meters squared. This concept has several direct applications to the use of electrosurgical energy in laparoscopy. This principle is used to safely return current from the patient to the electrosurgical unit (ESU). Because current density is described in terms of current per meters squared, applying energy to a small area of bleeding or to a bleeding tissue pedicle will result in an intended thermal effect, inversely related to the electrode size. For example, the use of a needlepoint electrode will have high-current density compared with a much larger spatula tip, resulting in greater energy applied to a small surface in the former. The current density principle is used to allow current to exit the body without causing injury, as it exits through the relatively large surface area of the return electrode, usually placed on the patient's thigh. This does not cause an exit site burn because of low current density. Exit site burns have typically occurred when part of the return electrode has peeled away from the patient, resulting in a smaller area of surface contact, thus creating high current density at the exit site.

Bipolar instruments have undergone significant transformation in recent years. Simple bipolar systems, such as the ESU with a Kleppinger forceps, have evolved to devices that provide bipolar energy that senses tissue impedance to perform controlled energy delivery. These devices, such as Enseal (Surgrx), Plasma Kinetic dissection forceps (Gyrus Medical), and Ligasure (Valleylab), use pressure and pulsed current to seal vessels with minimal lateral thermal spread. These devices can seal vessels up to 7 mm in diameter.

Robotics

In 1994, the first U.S. Food and Drug Administration–approved robotic surgical device called AESOP (Automatic Endoscopic System for Optimal Positioning, Computer Motion, Inc.) was introduced. With this system, the surgeon can control the orientation of the laparoscope through voice commands. The da Vinci Robotic Surgical System (Intuitive Surgical) and Zeus Robotic Surgical System (Computer Motion) allow the surgeon to operate from a remote station with hand controls that can provide increased dexterity and minimize fatigue, tremors, or incidental hand movement. These systems are being used in surgical centers but have not gained universal adoption because of technical training and cost limitations. The optimal application for these devices is continuing to be defined.

POSITIONING THE PATIENT FOR LAPAROSCOPIC SURGERY

The patient should be placed on the operating table in the low lithotomy position with the buttocks at or slightly over the table's edge to allow placement and use of an intrauterine manipulator and to have access to the perineum if needed during surgery. The patient's thighs should be in the same plane as the abdomen to allow freedom of motion for laparoscopic instrumentation. When the knees are bent and elevated above the plane of the abdominal wall, it is difficult to gain access to the upper abdomen and pelvic brim without bumping into the legs because of the fulcrum effect of instruments placed into lower ports. Stirrups should have ample padding to support the lower leg without creating pressure points. Particular attention should be given to preventing injury to the peroneal nerve, which is especially vulnerable to compression injury. It is preferable to use a stirrup that can be elevated without undraping the patient so that a high lithotomy position can be used for easier vaginal access if needed. To avoid stretch injury to the femoral, sciatic, or obturator nerves, the thigh should be flexed no more than 90 degrees, and the hips should be abducted no more than 45 degrees.

Surgical Suite

Efficient orientation of the surgical suite is critical for efficient laparoscopic surgery. In general, a right-handed surgeon stands on the patient's left side with the surgical assistant on the patient's right; however, some surgeons prefer the patient's right side. The monitor is usually placed between the patient's legs if only one is available. In the case of two monitors, these are usually placed near the patient's lower legs. Newer surgical suites have done away with towers and have ceiling-mounted, movable flat screens, which are highly ergonomic. The insufflation monitor is usually placed across from the surgeon so intraabdominal pressure can be viewed. Insufflation tubing, light cords, electrosurgical cords, and suction-irrigation tubing should be out of the surgeon's path if perineal access is necessary. Knowledgeable operating room personnel are likewise critical to the laparoscopic mission. The scrub technician usually stands caudad to the surgical assistant. A circulating technician assists in troubleshooting equipment and obtaining supplies and equipment.

ENTERING THE ABDOMINAL CAVITY

The abdominal cavity may be initially entered at the umbilicus or alternative sites by Veres needle, open laparoscopy, or direct trocar insertion.

Umbilical Site Veres Needle Technique

When the umbilical site and Veres needle technique is used, the Veres needle is first placed into the abdominal cavity to establish a pneumoperitoneum, and a trocar is subsequently placed into the pneumoperitoneum. A metaanalysis of methods used to establish pneumoperitoneum compared open access (Hasson-type) with closed access (needle/trocar), and two types of closed access techniques (direct trocar versus needle/trocar). It was noted that deaths were only reported in the needle/trocar group. However, because of the rarity of death as an outcome, the statistical risk could not be compared meaningfully. The metaanalysis was underpowered to adequately compare the two closed techniques. Therefore, the question of which technique for initial port placement is safest has not been definitively answered to date.

A scalpel is used to make a small skin incision in accordance with the size of the trocar to be placed at the umbilicus. The umbilicus should be elevated and the scalpel held parallel to the long axis of the patient to avoid incidentally lacerating the great vessels, which lie in close proximity to the umbilicus. Having the anesthesiologist decompress the stomach with a nasogastric tube will decrease the risk of inserting the Veres needle or trocar into an overdistended stomach. The patient's abdomen should be relaxed by neuromuscular blockade if general anesthesia is being used to allow adequate elevation for Veres needle and trocar insertion. The patient should be lying in a flat or neutral position on the operating table because the use of Trendelenburg positioning may cause the trajectory of the Veres needle or trocar to be closer to the great vessels rather than the pelvic cavity. In the thin patient, the Veres needle or trocar should be directed toward the hollow of the sacrum to avoid the great vessels (Fig. 17.13). In the obese patient, the aorta is typically above the level of the umbilicus; therefore, the Veres needle or trocar may be inserted vertically (90 degrees to the long axis of the patient), as long as the abdominal wall has been elevated adequately (Fig. 17.14). Placing the Veres needle close to the base of the umbilicus takes advantage of the thin natural confluence of tissue planes at the umbilicus. Separate clicks can be heard or felt as the needle traverses the rectus fascia and then peritoneum.

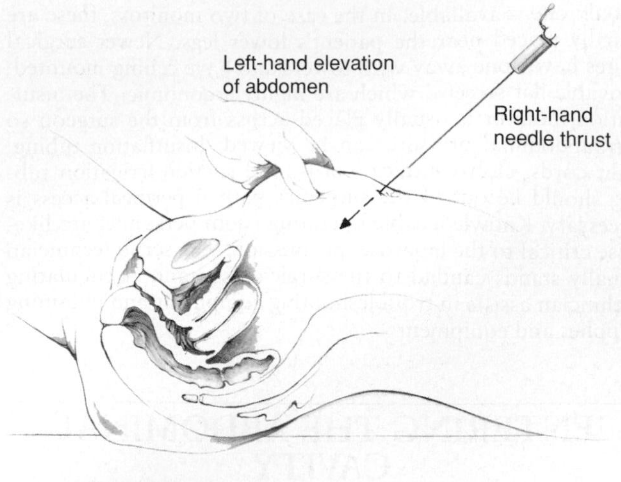

FIGURE 17.13. Insertion of the Veres needle.

Correct placement of the Veres needle into the abdominal cavity can be assessed by several techniques. The hanging drop technique is used by placing a small amount of sterile saline in the top of the Veres needle to verify a negative intraabdominal pressure as it descends into the abdominal cavity. Alternatively, the syringe barrel test can be performed by watching the column of saline descend the barrel of a syringe attached to the Veres needle. Aspiration of a syringe attached to the Veres needle can test for blood or gastrointestinal contents. Low-flow insufflation should be performed at a flow rate of approximately 1 L/ min until further signs of intraabdominal needle placement are confirmed, such as low intraabdominal pressure (<10 mm Hg) or loss of dullness to percussion over the right upper quadrant. If the "intraabdominal" pressure reading is higher than 10 mm Hg, the probability of extraperitoneal insufflation is high, and the approach should be reassessed. A prospective, observational study of four tests to ascertain Veres needle placement compared the double click test, the hanging drop test, the aspiration test, and the initial five insufflation pressures in 345 women. High insufflation pressures were the most sensitive for preperitoneal insufflation. High-flow insufflation may be used in the presence of reassuring signs of correct needle placement. During insufflation, intraabdominal pressures should not exceed 20 to 25 mm Hg to avoid interfering with diaphragmatic excursion and central venous return from caval compression. After an adequate pneumoperitoneum has been established,

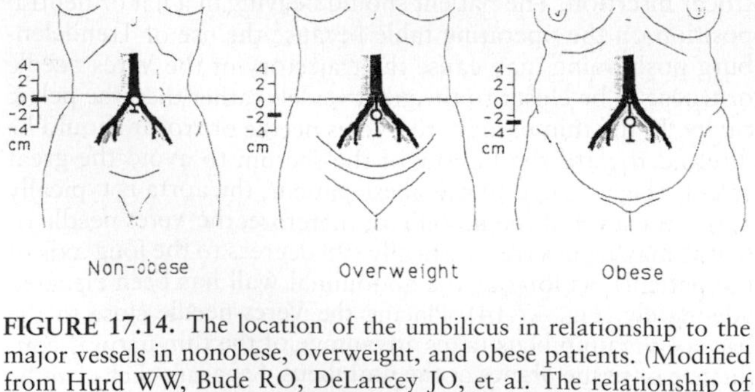

FIGURE 17.14. The location of the umbilicus in relationship to the major vessels in nonobese, overweight, and obese patients. (Modified from Hurd WW, Bude RO, DeLancey JO, et al. The relationship of the umbilicus to the aortic bifurcation: implications for laparoscopic technique. *Obstet Gynecol* 1992;80:48.)

ranging from 1 to 5 liters depending on body habitus, a trocar is inserted at the umbilicus, paying attention to the angle of insertion based on body habitus, as discussed. Once the trocar is placed, the bladed or central portion is removed, and the laparoscope is placed through the trocar sleeve to ensure correct placement before attaching the insufflation tubing to the trocar sleeve.

Alternates to Umbilical Entry

When Veres needle insufflation is not successful, or in patients who are at risk for adhesions near the umbilicus, placing the Veres needle at a site other than the umbilicus is usually successful. Two commonly used sites are Palmer's point and the left ninth intercostal space. Palmer's point is located 3 cm from the midline and 3 cm below the left rib cage. The needle is directed 15 degrees cephalad after the skin has been stretched caudally. If the ninth intercostal space is used, the Veres needle should be placed between the ninth and tenth rib, grazing the top of the tenth rib. This grazing minimizes the risk of damaging the intercostal neurovascular bundle. The rib cage provides a natural elevation of a space devoid of bowel regardless of patient weight. There is a remote chance of pneumothorax with this technique. Before performing either of these techniques, palpation for splenomegaly should be performed. After Veres needle placement, a 5-mm trocar is usually placed at Palmer's point.

Open Laparoscopy

Hasson described the technique of open laparoscopy in 1971 as a way of avoiding blind trocar placement. A small incision is made at the umbilicus. Allis clams are used to grasp the fascia, which is incised, and the peritoneum is entered directly. A Hasson-type cannula is used that can be anchored to sutures in the rectus fascia. In a review of more than 5,000 cases over nearly three decades, this technique has been shown to be associated with a low complication rate.

Direct Trocar Insertion

Direct trocar placement has also been described by placing the trocar through the umbilicus initially, rather than using the Veres needle.

SECONDARY TROCAR PLACEMENT

One or two secondary ports are usually adequate for most laparoscopic procedures. More complicated surgeries may require up to five. These may be placed lateral to the inferior epigastric artery or in the midline above the bladder. The size and number of trocars will depend on the procedure and equipment to be used. A 2- to 5-mm trocar may be used for diagnostic laparoscopy to maneuver pelvic organs for adequate visualization. Most instruments for tissue manipulation will fit through a 5-mm port. Some energy delivery systems and tissue retrieval systems require the use of larger ports (8 to 15 mm). Anticipating the need for larger ports can lead to significant cost savings when disposable trocars are used.

The placement of lateral trocars can be associated with injury to the inferior epigastric artery. Before lateral trocar placement, this vessel can usually be seen along the anterior abdominal wall as it branches off the external iliac artery. Insertion of a spinal needle through the anterior abdominal wall at the intended site of trocar insertion can help find a safe trajectory away from the inferior epigastric artery. If the vessel can not be seen, a safe location can usually be found by measuring 5 cm superior to the pubic symphysis and 8 cm lateral. Secondary trocars should be inserted in a controlled fashion, under direct vision. Placement of suprapubic secondary trocars should be placed well above the bladder. Two finger breadths measured above the pubic symphysis has been standard terminology for midline trocar placement. Because of the significant differences in finger widths among surgeons, and considering the increased risk of bladder injury using the suprapubic location, it is also worth placing a spinal needle through the anterior abdominal wall in the midline to ensure that the port is well above the bladder. If the patient has had a prior laparotomy, the bladder may be tented superiorly, and it may be necessary to place the trocar higher.

TISSUE REMOVAL

Small tissue fragments, such as peritoneal biopsy specimens, may be removed through 5-mm trocar sleeves. Large, dense specimens, such as leiomyoma fragments, require larger ports (10 to 15 mm). Fluid-filled specimens, such as ovarian cysts, may be placed in a plastic specimen removal bag (Fig. 17.15) and drained while in the bag to avoid spillage (Endocatch, U.S. Surgical Corp., Endopouch, Ethicon Inc.). Posterior colpotomy can also be performed for specimen removal. Colpotomy may be performed vaginally, as one would when performing vaginal hysterectomy or laparoscopically. Laparoscopic colpotomy is performed by first inserting a lubricated sponge stick into the posterior vaginal fornix for cul-de-sac elevation. An incision is then made between the uterosacral ligaments into the posterior vaginal fornix, using the sponge stick as a backstop. Laser, unipolar scissors, or the Harmonic Scalpel may be used as an energy source. An endoscopic specimen bag may be removed through the colpotomy incision. A wet lap pad may be placed vaginally to allow optimal pneumoperitoneum for laparoscopic closure of the colpotomy, or the colpotomy may be closed vaginally. Alternatively, morcellation may be performed with a handheld morcellator or an electromechanical morcellator (Fig. 17.16). For safety reasons, it is important that the tip of the morcellator be in view at all times. Keeping the cutting tip elevated and parallel with the abdominal wall adds to visualization and decreases the risk of inadvertently injuring bowel and other vital structures, as severe injuries have been reported, including injury to the pancreas. The specimen should be drawn up into the morcellator rather than pushing the morcellator into the specimen.

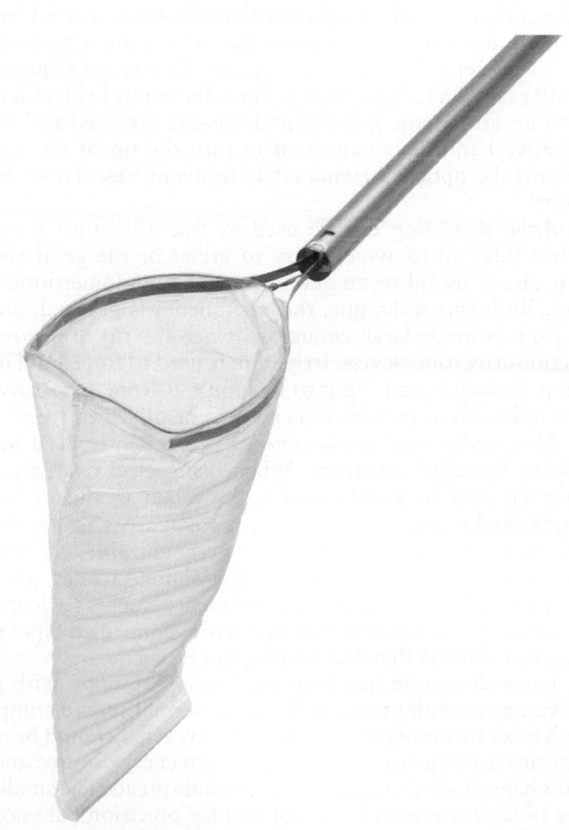

FIGURE 17.15. Endopouch specimen removal bag. Courtesy of Ethicon Endosurgical.

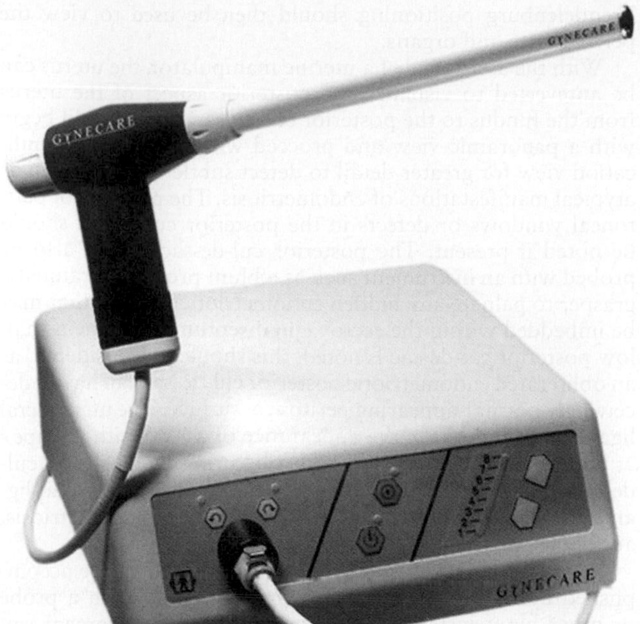

FIGURE 17.16. Endoscopic morcellator. Courtesy of Gynecare Inc.

DIAGNOSTIC LAPAROSCOPY

A systematic approach to diagnostic laparoscopy, like checklists for pilots, can help ensure thoroughness in what is regarded as a routine surgery. After insertion of the laparoscope, the abdomen should be carefully examined, particularly the area in the trajectory of the Veres needle or trocar, to ensure that inadvertent bowel or vascular damage was not caused.

Trendelenburg positioning should then be used to view the pelvic cavity and organs.

With the assistance of a uterine manipulator, the uterus can be anteverted to visualize the posterior aspect of the uterus from the fundus to the posterior cul-de-sac. This should begin with a panoramic view and proceed with a closeup magnification view for greater detail to detect subtle findings, such as atypical manifestations of endometriosis. The presence of peritoneal windows or defects in the posterior cul-de-sac should be noted if present. The posterior cul-de-sac should also be probed with an instrument such as a blunt probe or atraumatic grasper to palpate any hidden endometriotic nodules that may be imbedded within the rectovaginal septum. Anytime a shallow posterior cul-de-sac is noted, this should be considered, as an obliterated endometriotic posterior cul-de-sac can have a deceivingly normal-appearing peritoneal surface. The uterosacral ligaments should have the appearance of a "V" with the apex at the cervix. If peritoneal fluid is obscuring the posterior cul-de-sac, the fluid should be removed by suction. The broad ligaments should be inspected for the presence of endometriosis, adhesions, or fibroids.

The ovaries should be viewed globally. This can be accomplished by simply flipping the ovary superiorly with a probe or other blunt instrument, or the uteroovarian ligament can be grasped with an atraumatic grasper from the contralateral port and rotated by twisting the grasper clockwise for the left ovary and counterclockwise for the right ovary. This provides an excellent view of the undersurface of the ovary that can be easily held in place for inspection of the ovarian fossa and pelvic sidewall. With the ovary lifted up away from the sidewall, the transperitoneal course of the ureter can usually be seen. The ureter is optimally visualized by looking for peristalsis as it crosses the common iliac artery at the pelvic brim. One advantage of identifying the ureter early during surgery is that the peritoneal surface can become edematous as the case proceeds, likely from prolonged carbon dioxide exposure and manipulative contact. The fallopian tube should be handled with care. Fallopian tube forceps are available that allow the tube to be grasped at the mesosalpinx while surrounding the tube. The proximal portion of the tube should be examined for nodules, which may be indicative of salpingitis isthmica nodosa. The fimbria should be examined delicately, looking for any sign of phimosis. Anterior to the fallopian tubes, the round ligaments should be viewed and traced laterally to identify the presence of hernia. The anterior cul-de-sac is best seen by using the uterine manipulator to place the uterus in a retroverted position. In this position, the anterior surface of the uterus and the bladder parietal peritoneum can be seen well. The anterior abdominal wall should be viewed for the presence of endometriosis or hernia.

The appendix should be viewed, looking for any sign of inflammation, endometriosis, or fecalith. This is best performed by using an atraumatic bowel grasper. The upper abdomen should also be inspected, taking note of the liver, gallbladder, and diaphragmatic surfaces. If needed, the large and small intestine can also be inspected by "running" the bowel with two atraumatic bowel graspers. A panoramic, 360-degree evaluation is helpful to ensure that no upper abdominal adhesions have been missed that may have caused the intestine to be adherent to the anterior abdominal wall. It is possible in the presence of such adhesions to place a trocar through and through the intestine unknowingly. This condition can be ruled out by placing the laparoscope through one of the lower ports for visualization of the umbilical port. Chromopertubation may be performed by instilling a diluted indigo carmine solution through the uterine manipulator. Lack of spill may be due to obstruction, tubal spasm, or leakage from the cervix. It is therefore important to have a tight uterine cannula seal at the cervix.

OPERATIVE LAPAROSCOPIC PROCEDURES

Adhesiolysis

Pelvic adhesions have been associated with infertility and chronic pelvic pain. It should be recognized that chronic pelvic pain is often a complex condition, and in the absence of gastrointestinal obstructive symptoms, adhesiolysis is usually often not curative of pain. To better understand the nature of symptomatic adhesion, pain mapping under conscious sedation may be a useful technique. In performing adhesiolysis, optimal results depend on the use of microsurgical technique, gentle tissue handling, and meticulous hemostasis with minimal tissue fulguration. Adhesiolysis can be performed by a number of techniques, including blunt and sharp dissection, electrodissection, aquadissection, and laser dissection.

Blunt dissection is the most rudimentary form of adhesiolysis. Although not recommended, this technique is usually used in treating thin, avascular adhesions. Virtually any type of laparoscopic instrument can be used to place traction on an adhesion to cause separation. If bleeding or significant resistance is encountered, this technique should be abandoned.

Sharp dissection is the preferred method for dealing with all adhesions, especially thick avascular adhesions. The advantage of sharp dissection over electrodissection is the decreased risk of inadvertent electrosurgical injury. This is performed in a similar fashion to laparotomy. The adhesion is held on tension with an atraumatic grasper, and scissors are used to lyse the adhesive band. It is important to turn the tip of the scissors toward the optical viewing angle to avoid vascular or bowel injury.

Aqua dissection can be used to free adhesions from the pelvic sidewall to avoid injury to ureter or the great vessels. It is also a useful technique in removing endometriotic nodules. With this technique, the peritoneum is grasped, and an incision is made large enough to place the tip of a powered suction-irrigation device. Irrigation is used to force fluid under the peritoneum, causing it to balloon out from deeper tissues. The adhesion or peritoneum can then be dissected free.

Monopolar and *bipolar energy* is frequently used to lyse thicker vascular adhesions. When using electrosurgery, care must be used to avoid injury to bowel. It is always best to start from known to unknown. As known areas are freed from adhesions, unknown areas become recognizable. Monopolar instruments, like scissors and needlepoint electrodes, are ideal for these adhesions. Bipolar instruments, such as Kleppinger forceps, bipolar scissors, or newer tissue-controlled bipolar energy instruments that seal vessels, can be used.

Laser dissection has been used in laparoscopy with great success as a result of minimal lateral thermal spread compared with most forms of electrosurgery. However, it should be noted that this form of energy is indeed still an energy source and obtains hemostasis through lateral thermal spread. The small spot size of laser makes this a useful tool for precision adhesiolysis. The CO_2 laser has a depth of penetration of 0.1 mm and is excellent for cutting. With the adhesion on tension, the CO_2 laser is introduced through the operating channel of the laparoscope or through a secondary port.

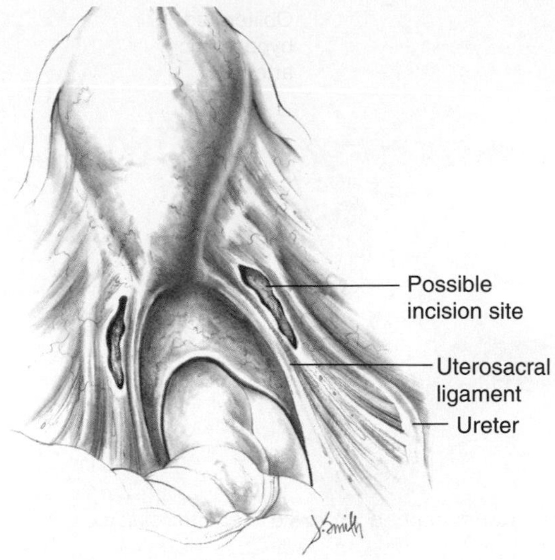

FIGURE 17.17. Pelvic sidewall dissection. The peritoneum has been incised so that the retroperitoneal structures can be visualized.

The Harmonic Scalpel is used with a technique similar to both bipolar dissection (laparosonic coagulating shears and Harmonic ACE) and monopolar dissection (scalpel tip), depending on which tip is used. This technique does not use electrosurgery. These have the advantage of limited lateral thermal spread, similar to the newer bipolar electrosurgical instruments.

Sidewall and Retroperitoneal Space Dissection

It is often necessary to identify the course of ureter and iliac vessel in cases of pelvic sidewall adhesions or endometriosis. If the ureter is able to be identified at the pelvic brim but then is obscured by adhesions, endometriosis, or an ovarian mass along its caudad course, the peritoneum overlying the sidewall can be grasped and opened with scissors (Fig. 17.17). A Maryland dissector can be used to gently spread the peritoneum to view the ureter. If the anatomy is distorted, it may be necessary to start the dissection at the pelvic brim or by opening the round ligament. If the round ligament is to be opened, it should be divided with an energy source as lateral as possible, and a blunt grasper can be used to dissect the retroperitoneal space, watching for the ureter on the medial leaf of the broad ligament and avoiding the iliac vessels. Developing the pararectal space can help to define anatomic landmarks to avoid inadvertent vascular or ureteral injury. Once the ureter and uterine artery are located, adhesions can be lysed with an energy system of the surgeon's choice.

Posterior Cul-de-sac Dissection

When endometriosis or pelvic adhesions partially or completely obliterate the posterior cul-de-sac and are associated with pelvic pain or infertility, a surgical approach is usually indicated. Cul-de-sac obliteration secondary to endometriosis often involves deep fibrotic endometriosis that may involve the rectum, rectovaginal septum, or uterosacral ligaments. Dissection of the posterior cul-de-sac may be necessary and can be performed laparoscopically by skilled surgeons. The goal is to lyse adhesions, excise large or deep endometriotic lesions, and resect or vaporize small superficial lesions.

The patient should undergo a bowel prep before surgery. A uterine manipulator is used to antevert the uterus, and a rectal probe is placed in the rectum to delineate and retract the rectum posteriorly. A sponge stick placed in the vagina can further delineate the rectum from the vagina (Fig. 17.18). The anterior rectum is carefully dissected from the posterior aspect of the uterus or vagina with scissors, laser, harmonic scalpel, or tissue-controlled bipolar energy system. The use of monopolar and traditional bipolar energy can result in significant thermal injury to the rectum. Aquadissection may also be useful. Dissection should continue until the loose areolar tissue of the rectovaginal space is reached. If a ureter is near the site of dissection, the position of the ureter should be confirmed before any dissection takes place. The fibrotic endometriosis can then be excised from the posterior vagina or uterosacral ligaments. If endometriosis extends to the vaginal mucosa, this is excised, and the posterior vagina is closed vaginally or laparoscopically. Palpation of the endometriotic nodule before and after removal is helpful to ensure complete excision.

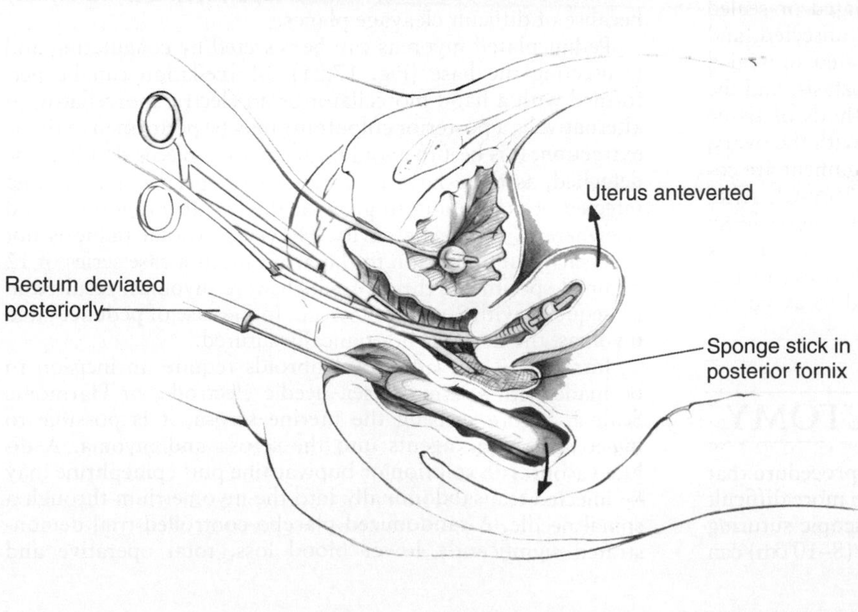

FIGURE 17.18. Dissection of the posterior cul-de-sac. Instruments in the uterus, posterior fornix of the vagina, and rectum help define the anatomy.

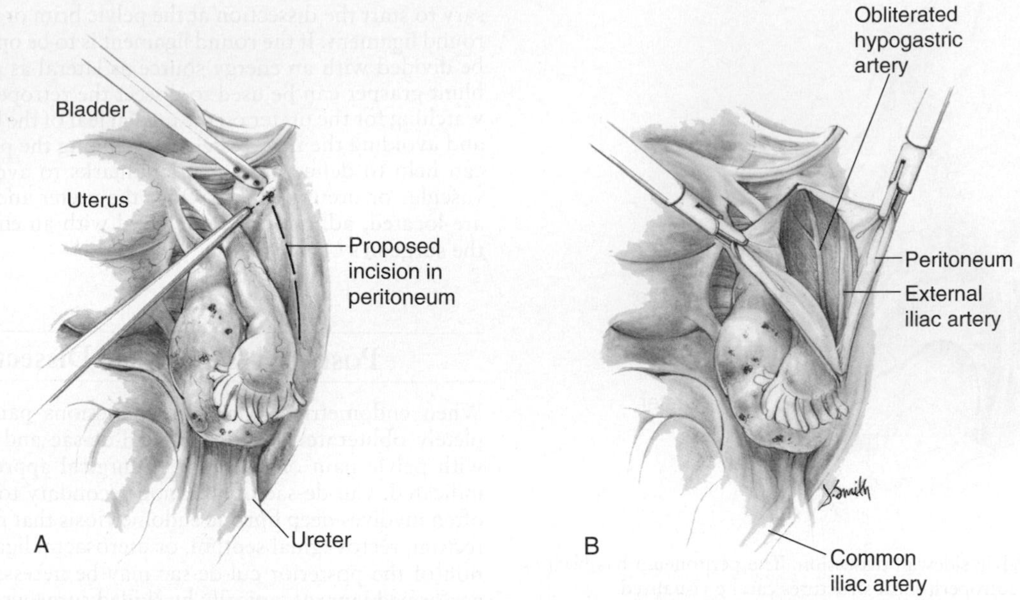

FIGURE 17.19. Dissecting the retroperitoneal space. **A:** The peritoneum overlying the pelvic sidewall is incised. **B:** The peritoneum is opened and the ureter and vessels identified.

Oophorectomy and Salpingo-oophorectomy

Several techniques for laparoscopic oophorectomy or salpingo-oophorectomy have been described. One procedure involves the placement of three loop ligatures around the ovary and adnexa. Before placement of the loops, the structures must be free of adhesions. Incisions in the mesosalpinx are sometimes necessary to facilitate placement. The ovary or adnexa is cut distal to the three loops. Small bleeding points can be coagulated on the stump, but care must be taken not to coagulate the suture.

Alternatively, the peritoneum is opened, and the ureter is identified (Fig. 17.19A,B). Lactated Ringer solution or saline can be injected into the retroperitoneal space to push the ureter away from the site of coagulation and increase the margin of safety. The uteroovarian ligament is coagulated or sealed with bipolar energy or ultrasonic energy and transected, and the infundibulopelvic ligament is then coagulated or sealed and transected. Pedicles are examined for hemostasis, and the ovary is removed by one of the described methods of tissue removal. If the fallopian tube is to be removed with the ovary, the proximal fallopian tube and uteroovarian ligament are coagulated or sealed before transection (Fig. 17.20A–C). After transection of the infundibulopelvic ligament, the mesosalpinx is coagulated or sealed and cut in the same manor that is used for salpingectomy. Laparoscopic stapling devices can also be used on the pedicles, but care must be used to avoid the ureter.

LAPAROSCOPIC MYOMECTOMY

Laparoscopic myomectomy is a heterogeneous procedure that can range from a simple procedure to one of the more difficult laparoscopic surgeries requiring expert laparoscopic suturing skills. For example, large pedunculated fibroids (8–10 cm) can be detached in a few minutes. Large intramural fibroids may take several hours to remove and repair in the hands of expert laparoscopic surgeons. Two case-control studies comparing open with laparoscopic myomectomy have both demonstrated significantly longer mean operating room time and shorter hospital stays with the laparoscopic group. The use of a preoperative gonadotropin-releasing hormone (GnRH) agonist may be considered in patients who are anemic. A prospective randomized study using leuprolide acetate in patients undergoing laparoscopic myomectomy also demonstrated significantly lower blood loss and operative times in the treatment group. The authors of this study noted increased operative time in the subset of markedly hypoechoic fibroids because of increased fibroid softness. Other studies have shown longer operative times and a higher conversion to laparotomy rate associated with the use of GnRH agonists in laparoscopic myomectomy because of difficult cleavage planes.

Pedunculated myomas can be resected by coagulating and transecting the base (Fig. 17.21). Morcellation can be performed with a hand morcellator or an electric morcellator, or alternatively, a posterior colpotomy may be performed to tissue extraction. It is best to avoid losing myoma pieces that become detached, as there have been reports of specimens becoming infected or continuing to grow at the trocar incision site and elsewhere in the pelvic cavity. However, loss of tissue is not necessarily an indication for laparotomy, as a case series of 12 retained specimens, three of which were myomas, resulted in no sequelae with 2-year follow-up. In the case of pedunculated myomas, the defect is not typically sutured.

Intramural and subserosal fibroids require an incision to be made with scissors, laser, needle electrode, or Harmonic Scalpel. Before incising the uterine serosa, it is possible to inject hemostatic agents into the serosa and myoma. A dilute vasopressin solution or bupivacaine plus epinephrine may be injected transabdominally into the myometrium through a spinal needle. A randomized placebo-controlled trial demonstrated significantly lower blood loss, total operative and

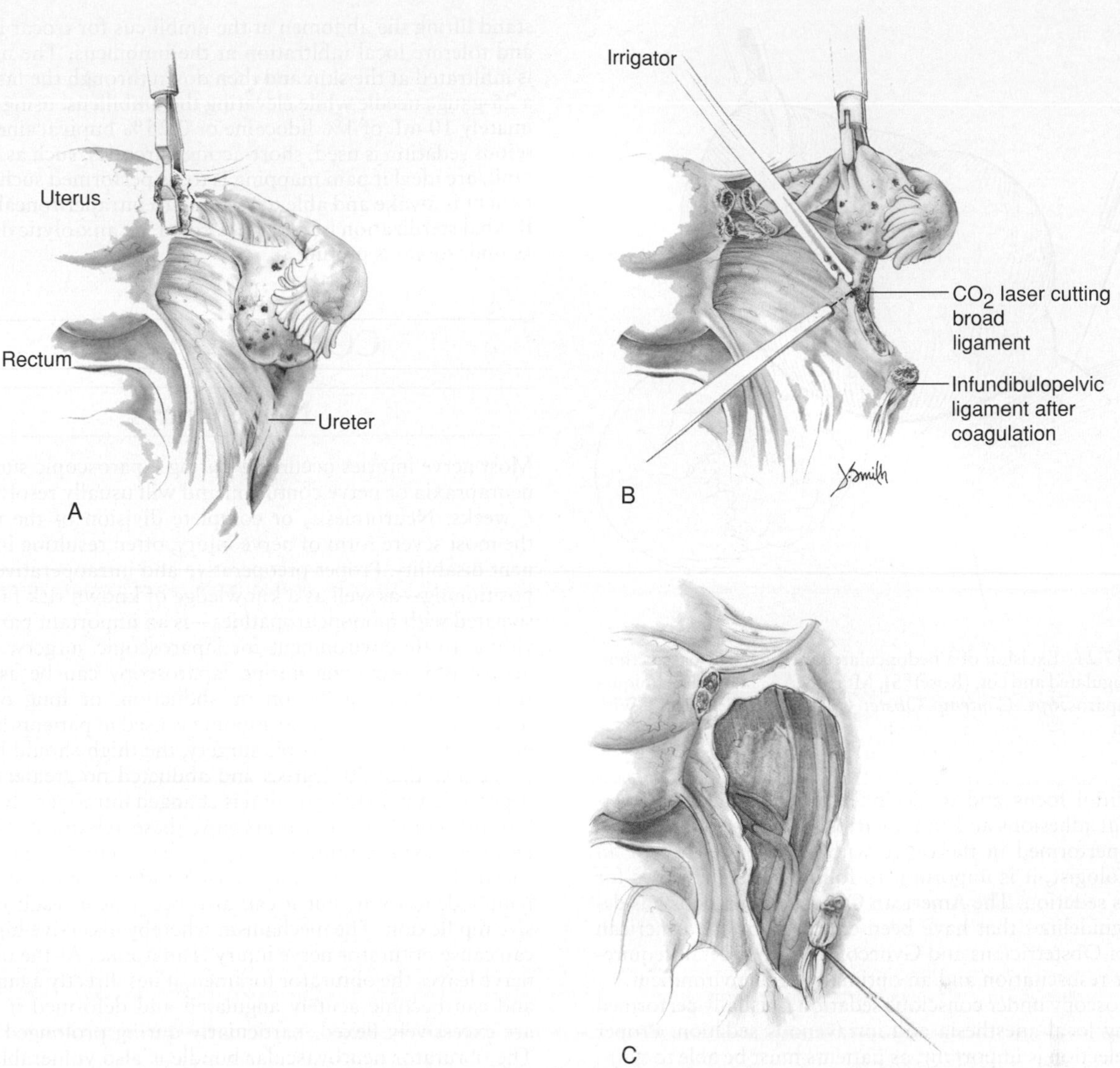

FIGURE 17.20. Oophorectomy with the use of bipolar coagulation. **A:** The uteroovarian ligament is coagulated then transected. **B:** The infundibulopelvic ligament is coagulated with bipolar forceps, then cut. **C:** An endoloop may be placed on the infundibulopelvic ligament after transaction for added hemostasis.

enucleation time, and degree of surgical difficulty associated with bupivacaine plus epinephrine compared with saline. When the whorled white appearance of the myoma is seen, the edges of the uterine serosa are held open with atraumatic graspers, and a corkscrew retractor is screwed into the myoma. Using upward traction with the corkscrew retractor, the myoma is peeled away from the uterine corpus (Fig. 17.22). Hemostasis is achieved with electrosurgery or Harmonic Scalpel. The defect is sutured closed in two or three layers, depending on the depth of the defect, using a delayed absorbable suture as described previously. Another option is to perform uterine closure through a minilaparotomy if the fundus or area to be sutured is able to be delivered through a small incision. Uterine rupture has been reported in patients undergoing laparoscopic myomectomy, and pregnancy should be monitored with the same caution given to patients who have undergone abdominal myomectomy. It is not known whether laparoscopic repairs are equivalent to repair by laparotomy.

LAPAROSCOPY USING LOCAL ANESTHESIA OR CONSCIOUS SEDATION

Laparoscopy can be performed under conscious sedation in the operating room or in a nonhospital environment, such as physician's office, using conscious sedation or local anesthesia without the assistance of an anesthesiologist. Microlaparoscopy is often used with 2- or 3-mm instrumentation. Local anesthesia and conscious sedation has long been used to perform tubal ligation. The use of microlaparoscopic instrumentation has assisted in performing laparoscopy under conscious sedation in the office setting for pain mapping in chronic pelvic pain patients. Pain mapping may be useful in patients with chronic pelvic pain of uncertain etiology, as this enables the patient to participate in the evaluation of the pelvis while searching

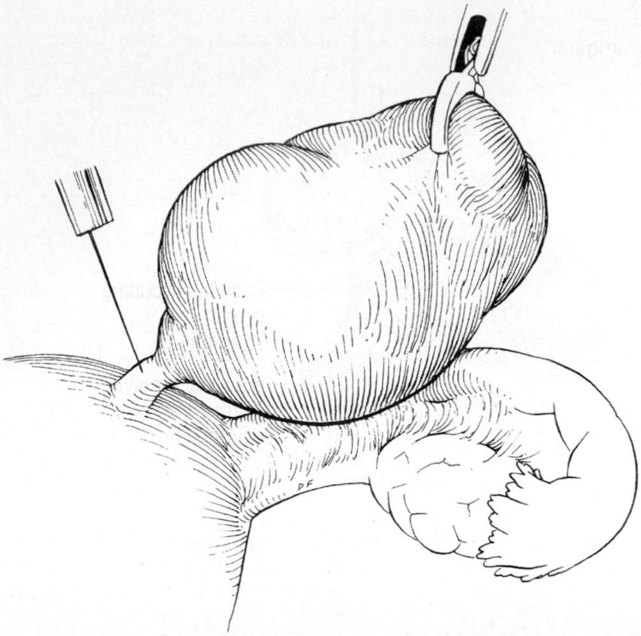

FIGURE 17.21. Excision of a pedunculated myoma. The base is thoroughly coagulated and cut. (Roseff SJ, Murphy AA. Helpful techniques in laser laparoscopy. *Contemp Obstet Gynecol* 1988;32:168.) With permission.

for a painful focus and to decipher between incidental versus painful adhesions and endometriosis. If conscious sedation is to be performed in the office without the presence of an anesthesiologist, it is important to follow state guidelines for conscious sedation. The American College of Surgeons has developed guidelines that have been endorsed by the American College of Obstetricians and Gynecologists that detail requirements for resuscitation and an optimally safe environment.

Laparoscopy under conscious sedation is usually performed combining local anesthesia and intravenous sedation. Proper patient selection is important, as patients must be able to withstand lifting the abdomen at the umbilicus for trocar insertion and tolerate local infiltration at the umbilicus. The umbilicus is infiltrated at the skin and then down through the fascia with a 25-gauge needle while elevating the umbilicus, using approximately 10 mL of 1% lidocaine or 0.25% bupivacaine. If conscious sedation is used, short-acting narcotics, such as remifentanil, are ideal if pain mapping is to be performed such that the patient is awake and able to respond to intraperitoneal stimuli. If tubal sterilization is to be performed, an anxiolytic drug such as midazolam is useful.

COMPLICATIONS

Nerve Injury

Most nerve injuries occurring during laparoscopic surgery are neurapraxia or nerve contusion and will usually resolve within 6 weeks. Neurotmesis, or complete division of the nerve, is the most severe form of nerve injury, often resulting in permanent disability. Proper preoperative and intraoperative patient positioning—as well as a knowledge of known risk factors associated with mononeuropathies—is an important part of providing a safe environment for laparoscopic surgery. Femoral neuropathy occurring during laparoscopy can be associated with excessive hip flexion or abduction, or long operating times. When lithotomy positioning is used in patients undergoing vaginal or laparoscopic surgery, the thigh should be flexed no greater than 90 degrees and abducted no greater than 45 degrees. If a patient's position is changed intraoperatively from low lithotomy to high lithotomy, these relationships should be maintained. Obturator neuropathy is most commonly associated with direct injury during radical pelvic surgery or lymphadenectomy, but it can also occur as a result of excessive hip flexion. The mechanism whereby excessive hip flexion can cause obturator nerve injury is anatomic. As the obturator nerve leaves the obturator foramen, it lies directly against bone and can become acutely angulated and deformed if the hips are excessively flexed, particularly during prolonged surgery. The obturator neurovascular bundle is also vulnerable during

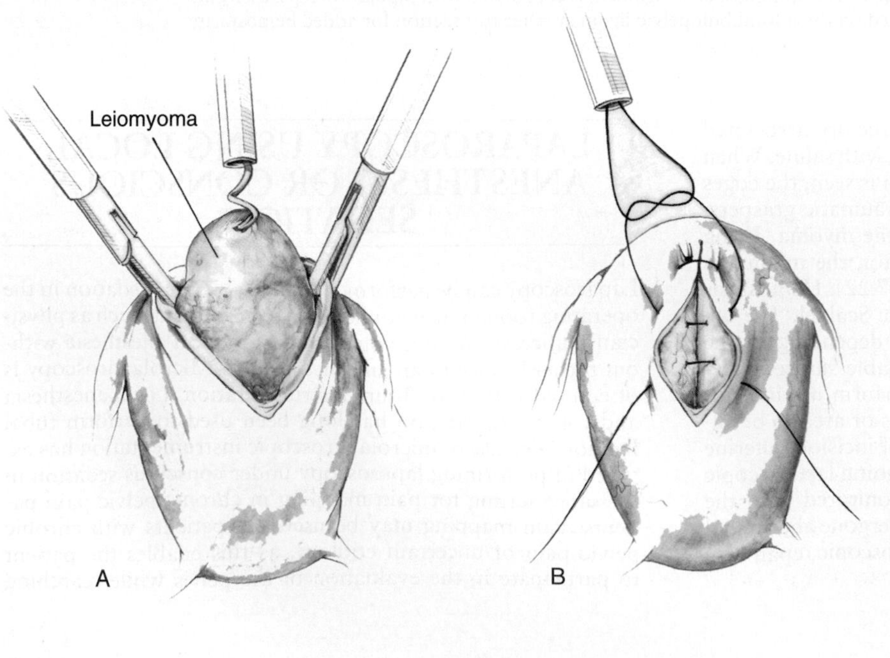

FIGURE 17.22. Myomectomy. **A:** The leiomyoma is grasped with forceps or a corkscrew and is dissected from the myometrium with careful blunt and sharp dissection. **B:** The defect, if large, is closed with sutures in two layers.

laparoscopic retropubic dissection, particularly during the paravaginal repair of lateral defects of the anterior vaginal wall. Surgeons who operate in these spaces should be well versed in the anatomy of the obturator nerve. The iliohypogastric and ilioinguinal nerves can be injured from lateral trocars with subsequent suture ligature and fibrotic entrapment. Care should be taken to avoid extreme lateral trocar placement; however, there is considerable anatomic variation in the course of these nerves, and injury can not always be avoided. Sciatic neuropathy during laparoscopic surgery can be a result of tension caused by nerve stretching. Injury to the sciatic nerve has been reported in procedures lasting as short as 35 minutes in free-hanging stirrups. The peroneal division of the sciatic nerve is under the least amount of tension when the knee and hip are flexed, as the nerve is fixed at the sciatic notch and the fibular head. Tension along the nerve is increased with hip flexion when the knee joint becomes straightened or externally rotated. Patients at increased risk of sustaining sciatic nerve injury are long-legged, obese, or short in stature. In hanging-type stirrups, long-legged or obese patients have a tendency for external hip rotation, and shorter patients have less flexion at the knee. In such cases, stirrups that support the ankle and calf may be more appropriate.

Vascular Injuries

Of all the injuries associated with laparoscopy, vascular injuries are the most acutely life threatening, particularly in the case of injury to the aorta, vena cava, or iliac vessels. Injury can occur during Veres needle placement, trocar insertion, or during tissue dissection. Injury to the great vessels requires immediate laparotomy, manual compression, repair, and usually transfusion. Injury to smaller vessels can usually be rendered hemostatic with the use of bipolar electrosurgery, hemostatic clips, or laparoscopic suturing techniques. Injury to the inferior epigastric vessels can occur during placement of the lateral trocar. The inferior epigastric artery can usually be seen before lateral trocar placement as it branches off the external iliac artery running cephalad along the abdominal wall peritoneum. If it is injured, a bipolar forceps can be placed through the contralateral port in an attempt to coagulate. Alternatively, several endoscopic fascial closure devices are now available that allow a suture to be passed through the fascia and peritoneum that can result in vascular occlusion. Hemostasis can usually be immediately achieved by placing a 30-cc Foley catheter through the trocar site with the aid of an 8-inch clamp and inflating the balloon for tamponade. This injury can also be managed by enlarging the trocar site by a few centimeters to visualize, clamp, and ligate the bleeding vessel.

Gastrointestinal Injury

Gastrointestinal injury is the most lethal injury associated with laparoscopy, with a mortality rate reported as high as 3.6%. Injury may occur from Veres needle placement, trocar insertion, adhesiolysis, tissue dissection, devascularization injury, or thermal injury. As a general rule, Veres needle injury needs no repair as long as the puncture is not associated with bleeding or a subsequent rent from additional tissue manipulation. In the case of colonic puncture without tearing, nonoperative management with antibiotics, copious irrigation, and suction has been suggested. There has been little evidence-based literature published about stomach injury during laparoscopy, but it is estimated that gastric perforation occurs approximately 1 in 3,000 cases. Risk factors for stomach injury include a history of upper abdominal surgery and difficult induction of anesthesia, as a gas-distended stomach can distend to below the level of the umbilicus. Orogastric or nasogastric suction before Veres needle or trocar placement can help lower this risk. Trocar injury to the stomach requires repair by laparoscopy or laparotomy. The defect may be oversewn with a delayed absorbable suture in layers, and the abdominal cavity should be irrigated and suctioned, being sure to remove any food particles as well as gastric juices. Nasogastric suction is usually maintained postoperatively until normal bowel peristalsis occurs.

Veres needle and trocar injury to the small intestine may not be obvious because of small bowel redundancy and a tendency for small bowel to fall out of view. Furthermore, a through-and-through trocar injury may be hidden from laparoscopic view. Potential injury should be investigated when multiple anterior abdominal wall adhesions are present. A lower quadrant secondary port can be used to view the umbilical port site. If there are no abdominal wall adhesions but a bowel injury is suspected, the bowel should be run with laparoscopic bowel graspers or manually by standard laparotomy until an injury is satisfactorily ruled out. A full-thickness injury to the small bowel of 5 mm or greater should be repaired in two layers with an interrupted layer of 3-0 delayed absorbable suture to approximate the mucosa and muscularis, and a serosal layer of 3-0 interrupted silk suture placed perpendicular to the long axis of the intestine to avoid stricture formation. This is usually performed by laparotomy or by minilaparotomy at the umbilical site, where the injured bowel loop is pulled through to the skin surface and repaired. Laparoscopic repair has also been reported as effective by surgeons with advanced gastrointestinal surgical skills. If the laceration to the small bowel exceeds one half of the luminal diameter, segmental resection is recommended.

Trocar injury to the colon is reported to occur with a frequency of approximately 1 per 1,000 cases. Undetected injury to the large intestine can be associated with significant morbidity compared with injury to the small intestine and stomach because of the high concentration of coliform bacteria in the large intestine. Therefore, if injury to the colon is suspected, the area should be inspected carefully using atraumatic bowel graspers, or laparotomy may be performed. The management of large intestinal injuries depends on size, site, and length of time from injury to diagnosis. In general, once the diagnosis of colonic injury is made, broad-spectrum antibiotics should be administered, and consultation should be sought with a surgeon who has experience with bowel injury. In the case of a small rent with minimal soilage, the defect can be closed in two layers with copious irrigation. When a larger injury has occurred and the bowel has not been prepared with a mechanical or antibiotic regimen, or when the injury involves the intestinal mesentery, a diverting colostomy is usually necessary. In the case of delayed (postoperative) diagnosis, a diverting colostomy should be performed. If injury to the rectosigmoid colon is suspected, filling the posterior cul-de-sac with normal saline and performing proctosigmoidoscopy, or injecting air into the rectum through a catheter-tipped bulb syringe and looking laparoscopically for bubbles, may aid in detection (flat tire test).

Thermal injuries are histologically different from traumatic injuries and therefore must be treated differently. Thermal bowel injuries can be differentiated histologically from traumatic injury by the presence of coagulation necrosis and the absence of capillary ingrowth and white cell infiltrate in the former. Because of this coagulation necrosis, thermal injuries require wide resection even though the bowel may still have a normal appearance adjacent to the injury, as it may take days for the extent of the injury to become apparent.

Trocar Site Hernia

In a retrospective review of more than 3,500 laparoscopies in 1993, the frequency of incisional hernias was reported to be 0.17%. The fascia should be closed in trocar sites that are 10 mm and larger. Although there are case reports of hernia occurring at 5-mm trocar sites, closing 5-mm trocar sites usually requires enlarging the skin incision or using laparoscopic fascial closure devices, which may not be warranted in this rare possibility. Closing the fascia may not entirely prevent hernia formation. A survey of more than 3,200 gynecologists noted that 18% of hernias occurred despite fascial closure and appeared to be related to the number of laparoscopies performed rather than the length of the surgeon's career. Trocar site hernias can present as occult or incarcerated hernias. A defect is usually palpable over the trocar site incision with Valsalva, or a mass can be seen. If the patient presents with signs of bowel obstruction, the bowel must be inspected carefully, and if there is evidence of necrosis or vascular compromise, the bowel should be resected.

Urinary Tract Injury

Bladder injury during laparoscopy is estimated to occur 1 in 300 cases. Higher injury rates have been reported with laparoscopic hysterectomy and bladder neck suspension. Risk factors for bladder injury include a distended bladder during suprapubic trocar insertion; previous surgery causing distortion to bladder anatomy, causing it to be pulled cephalad with the parietal peritoneum; and endometriosis obliterating the anterior cul-de-sac. Inserting a Foley catheter into the bladder before trocar placement and using lateral trocar sites will lessen the risk of bladder injury. In cases when a midline, suprapubic trocar is used, and the superior aspect of the bladder cannot be deciphered, filling the bladder with 300 mL of water or saline through a Foley catheter will define the bladder margins. Intraoperative signs of bladder injury include clear fluid in the operative field, visible bladder laceration, and gas distention of the Foley bag. To adequately make the diagnosis, the bladder wall can be inspected directly, or methylene blue or indigo carmine, diluted with 200 to 300 mL of sterile normal saline, may be instilled retrograde through the Foley catheter. Intentional cystotomy or cystoscopy may be performed for inspection in the case of doubt and to inspect the extent of the injury to ensure that there is no ureteric involvement.

Recommendations for repair of bladder injuries have been reviewed in a consensus statement of the International Society of Urology (Société Internationale d'Urologie). In the acute setting, bladder injuries can be treated with catheter drainage alone if the injury is small, uncomplicated, and isolated. A cystogram should be performed on the 10th day of drainage, and more than 85% of bladder injuries will be healed. A surgical repair should be performed if the Foley catheter is unable to provide adequate drainage because of blood clots or persistent extravasation, or if there is concomitant injury to the urethra or ureter. Cystotomy closure should be performed using a watertight, multilayered repair with absorbable suture. Laparoscopic repair may be performed in the case of a small injury with adequate surgical expertise and adequate exposure, as long as the ureters and bladder neck are not compromised.

According to a nationwide Finnish record linkage study, although the overall complication rates for laparoscopy are decreasing, the rate of ureteral injury has remained steady at 1%, with the greatest risk associated with laparoscopic hysterectomy. A review of the world literature through 2003 concluded that laparoscopically assisted vaginal hysterectomy was the most frequently performed surgery associated with ureteral injury. The usual time to diagnosis in postoperative patients with ureteral injury is typically between 2 and 7 days but has been reported as late as 33 days after surgery. Patients often present with symptoms of abdominal pain, fever, hematuria, flank pain, or peritonitis. Leukocytosis is a common finding. Management of ureteral injury should be undertaken in collaboration with a surgeon trained in ureteral injury repair. In the majority of cases, percutaneous or cystoscopic stenting techniques can be used. Laparotomy is usually performed for end-to-end anastomosis or reimplantation of the ureter into the bladder, but in experienced hands, repair may be performed laparoscopically. The literature is growing in favor of intraoperative diagnostic cystoscopy after complex vaginal, laparoscopic, and abdominal pelvic surgery in an effort to avoid delayed diagnosis of injuries to the urinary tract. It appears that cases in which the diagnosis is delayed are most likely to result in the greatest morbidity and legal repercussions.

CONCLUSION

Laparoscopy has become a mainstay of gynecologic surgery. Laparoscopic technology continues to evolve, requiring continual education and research. The main benefits of laparoscopic surgery have been shorter hospitalization, improved cosmesis, and, in some cases, improved safety and cost. Evidence-based surgical studies are difficult to perform but will be required to fully understand the role of each laparoscopic procedure in terms of long-term outcomes and cost.

BEST SURGICAL PRACTICES

- A good laparoscopic surgeon should know his or her limitations and not hesitate to call for help.
- Conversion to laparotomy is not considered failure.
- Careful selection of patients is the first key to success in any surgery.
- Preparation is essential in laparoscopic surgery and may include a "pilots checklist" and/or "dress rehearsal" to avoid being caught with too few or wrong-size trocar ports.
- "Shortcuts" modifying a surgical procedure in an effort to facilitate one's laparoscopic abilities "change" the procedure. Once the surgical technique has been changed, success rates obtained from literature or prior experience can not be attributed to the new procedure.
- Careful positioning of the patient can help avoid nerve injuries.
- Traction-countertraction and exposure are important in open and laparoscopic surgery. To maximize these, an additional trocar port is often helpful.
- Consider intraoperative cystoscopy with indigo carmine in complex pelvic surgery.
- Understand your energy source—e.g., monopolar, harmonic.

Bibliography

Batres F, Barclay DL. Sciatic nerve injury during gynecologic procedures using the lithotomy position. *Obstet Gynecol* 1983;62:92S.

Gomez RG, Ceballos L, Coburn M, et al. Consensus statement on bladder injuries. *BJU Int* 2004;94:27.

Grainger AH, Soderstrom RM, Schiff SF, et al. Ureteral injuries at laparoscopy: insights into diagnosis, management and prevention. *Obstet Gynecol* 1990;75:839.

Harkki-Siren P, Sjoberg J, Kurki T. Major complications of laparoscopy: a follow-up Finnish study. *Obstet Gynecol* 1999;94:94.

Hershlag A, Loy RA, Lavy G, et al. Femoral neuropathy after laparoscopy: a case report. *J Reprod Med* 1990;35:575.

Irvin W, Andersen W, Taylor P, et al. Minimizing the risk of neurologic injury in gynecologic surgery. *Obstet Gynecol* 2004;103:374.

Kadar N, Reich H, Liu CY, et al. Incisional hernias after major laparoscopic gynecologic procedures. *Am J Obstet Gynecol* 1993;168:1493.

Krebs HB. Intestinal injury in gynecologic surgery: a ten-year experience. *Am J Obstet Gynecol* 1986:155:509.

Levy BS, Soderstrom RM, Dail DH. Bowel injuries during laparoscopy. *J Reprod Med* 1985;30:660.

Loffer F, Pent D. Indications, contraindications and complications of laparoscopy. *Obstet Gynecol Surv* 1975;30:407.

Montz FJ, Holschneider CH, Munro MG. Incisional hernia following laparoscopy: a survey of the American Association of Gynecologic Laparoscopists. *Obstet Gynecol* 1994;84:881.

Nezhat C, Nezhat F, Ambrose W, et al. Laparoscopic repair of small bowel and colon: a report of 26 cases. *Surg Endosc* 1993;7:88.

Nezhat C, Seidman D, Nezhat F, et al. The role of intraoperative proctosigmoidoscopy in laparoscopic pelvic surgery. *J Am Assoc Gynecol Laparosc* 2004;11:47.

Nezhat CH, Seidman DS, Nezhat F, et al. Laparoscopic management of intentional and unintentional cystotomy. *J Urol* 1996;156:1400.

Oh BR, Kwon DD, Park KS, et al. Late presentation of ureteral injury after laparoscopic surgery. *Obstet Gynecol* 2000;95:337.

Ostrzenski A, Radolinski B, Ostrzenska KM. A review of laparoscopic ureteral injury in pelvic surgery. *Obstet Gynecol Surv* 2003;58:794.

Palter SF, Olive DL. Office microlaparoscopy under local anesthesia for chronic pelvic pain. *J Am Assoc Gynecol Laparosc* 1996;3:359.

Pellegrino MJ, Johnson EW. Bilateral obturator nerve injuries during urologic surgery. *Arch Phys Med Rehabil* 1988;69:46.

Spinelli P, Di Felice G, Pizzetti P, et al. Laparoscopic repair of full-thickness stomach injury. *Surg Endosc* 1991;5:156.

Taylor R, Weakley FL, Sullivan BH. Non-operative management of colonic perforation with pneumoperitoneum. *Gastrointest Endosc* 1978;24:124.

Tulikangas PK, Gill IS, Falcone T. Laparoscopic repair of ureteral injuries. *J Am Assoc Gynecol Laparosc* 2001;8:259.

Van Der Voort M, Heijnsdijk EA, Gouma DJ. Bowel injury as a complication of laparoscopy. *Br J Surg* 2004;91:1253.

Wang PH, Lee WL, Yuan CC, et al. Major complications of operative and diagnostic laparoscopy for gynecologic disease. *J Am Assoc Gynecol Laparosc* 2001;8:68.

Wu MP, Lin YS, Chou CY. Major complications of operative gynecologic laparoscopy in southern Taiwan. *J Am Assoc Gynecol Laparosc* 2001;8:61.

CHAPTER 18 ■ OPERATIVE HYSTEROSCOPY

MICHAEL S. BAGGISH

DEFINITIONS

Hysteroscopy—Direct visual inspection of the cervical canal and uterine cavity through a rigid, flexible, or contact hysteroscope.

Index of refraction—The bending of light caused by the ratio of its velocity in room air to its velocity within an optical fiber.

Resectoscope—A specialized electrosurgical endoscope that consists of an inner and outer sheath equipped with a 30° telescope. The inner sheath has a common channel for the telescope fluid medium and electrode.

Uterine synechiae—Adhesions that form between the anterior and posterior walls of the uterus as a result of trauma or infection in a milieu of estrogen deprivation.

INTRODUCTION

Hysteroscopy has become a standard part of the gynecologic surgeon's armamentarium and is now routinely taught as part of residency training curriculums and postgraduate seminars. As gynecologists have grown better acquainted with the benefits and techniques of operative hysteroscopy, and as hysteroscopy increasingly has become the method of choice for treatment of intrauterine pathology, the number of complications has also risen. Most of these complications are caused by operator error and inexperience.

Hysteroscopic procedures were first described by Panteleoni in 1869, but the technique did not excite substantial interest within the specialty until the late 1970s. There has been concern that hysteroscopy performed as a routine office procedure to diagnose the causes of abnormal uterine bleeding might spread undiagnosed endometrial carcinoma transtubally. The most vocal opponents of hysteroscopy have continued to perform dilatation and curettage (D&C) rather than hysteroscopy to diagnose, among other things, endometrial carcinoma. However, Roberts and colleagues documented the presence of malignant cells in inferior vena cava blood immediately after vigorous curettage of the endometrium, and the disparaging rhetoric against hysteroscopy seems to have little basis in fact. Indeed, during the mid-1980s, hysteroscopy replaced blind D&C as the standard procedure for precise diagnosis of intrauterine pathology.

The advantages of hysteroscopy as an accurate diagnostic technique are that it not only allows direct visual observation and accurate localization of pathology but also provides a means to sample the site most likely to yield positive results. During the 1980s, 1990s, and early 2000s, gynecology has shifted heavily toward endoscopy as a specialty.

The philosophy of least-invasive surgery is driven by the positive outcomes of shortened hospital stays and diminished recovery times and by good performance in a competitive free-market environment. Operative hysteroscopy has, in many instances, superseded even laparoscopy in meeting these strategic criteria. Hysteroscopy generally is a low-risk technique that uses the endocervical canal, the natural passageway of the body, to gain entry into the intrauterine environment. Refinements of optical and fiber-optic light instrumentation and of operative accessories allows high-resolution and excellent visual documentation by hysteroscopy, and tremendous advances still are being made. Nonhysteroscopic techniques to treat intrauterine septa and adhesions are obsolete. Ablation or resection of the endometrium is considered an acceptable alternative to hysterectomy for the management of abnormal uterine bleeding. Submucous myomata no longer require hysterectomy because they can be satisfactorily managed conservatively by operative hysteroscopy. Cornual and interstitial tubal obstruction also are now managed hysteroscopically. Office-based, low-skill techniques for rapidly managing abnormal uterine bleeding by means of thermal catheters are now a reality. Hysteroscopy in the 21st century has finally found its proper niche, and every gynecologist is required to learn the skills of hysteroscopy, just as every urologist surely must be an accomplished cystoscopist.

Learning how to perform an adequate hysteroscopy and then becoming competent to do hysteroscopic surgery are practice, skill-related techniques. Older methods of acquiring endoscopic skills focused on course attendance, preceptorship, and practice. During the late 1990s and continuing to the present time, simulators have been developed to facilitate hand-eye coordination exercises. Several of the computer-based models with advanced interactive graphics provide sophisticated models for the student to shave myomas, ablate endometrium, and pass cannulas into tubal ostia (Fig. 18.1A).

However, the most basic skill levels a hysteroscopist must attain are the ability to insert the scope safely into the uterine cavity followed by satisfactory distension of the cavity to obtain clear visualization of that cavity. The preceding are not taught by simulation and must be learned *in vivo*. Without this skill set, hysteroscopy cannot be successfully performed.

INSTRUMENTATION

Telescopes

The 4-mm telescope (lens) gives the sharpest, clearest image in addition to a small outside diameter (Fig. 18.1B). The most desirable optics provide a large field that subtends an angle of approximately 105 degrees (Fig. 18.1C). However, 3-mm diameter telescopes, which have greatly improved optics, provide comparable views. These contemporary 3-mm-diameter telescopes coupled to endoscopic video systems with zoom lenses are highly satisfactory for office hysteroscopy, as well as for operative hysteroscopy. Telescopes are usually available with a 0-degree straight-on or a 30-degree fore-oblique view

(Fig. 18.1D). The major advantage of the 0-degree lens is that it allows the operator to see operative devices as a relatively distant panorama, whereas this view is lost when 30-degree lens is used. The telescope has three parts: the eyepiece, the barrel, and the objective lens (Fig. 18.1E). Surrounding the optics are numerous small-diameter incoherent fiber-optic bundles that provide intense cold illumination to the operative field. Although a few manufacturers provide focusing telescopes that permit contact hysteroscopy, the standard telescope has fixed optics. The contact hysteroscope is a highly specialized device used largely in research settings. Although magnifying hysteroscopes reached a peak of popularity in the 1980s, their full practical value has not been realized.

Light Generators

The quality and power of light delivered to the telescope depend on the wattage and characteristics of the remote light generator and the type and structural integrity of the connecting fiber-optic light cable. Three general types of light generators are available: tungsten, metal halide, and xenon. The simplest and cheapest generator is the tungsten generator, which produces an orange-yellow light; the xenon white light is a powerful generator that provides the best shower for video imaging (Fig. 18.2A). The xenon light generator is well worth the additional cost because of its superior color and intensity (Fig. 18.2B–D).

Fiber-optic light cables must be intact to convey the optimal light from the generator to the telescope. Broken fibers can be easily identified by viewing the stretched-out cable against a dark background and looking for light emitting through the sides of the cable. The liquid cable conducts light effectively and, when combined with a xenon generator, provides superior light.

Diagnostic and Operative Sheaths

A diagnostic sheath is required to deliver the distending medium into the uterine cavity. The telescope fits into the sheath and is secured by means of a watertight seal that locks into place. The sheath is 4 to 5 mm in diameter, depending on the outer diameter of the telescope, with a 1-mm clearance between the inner wall and the telescope, through which either carbon dioxide or liquid distending medium is transmitted (Fig. 18.1C). Medium instillation into the sheath is controlled by means of an external stopcock. Even the 5-mm instrument allows easy access through the narrow endocervical canal past the point of maximal constriction (i.e., the internal os). Therefore, diagnostic hysteroscopy usually can be performed without cervical canal dilatation. If the hysteroscope is inserted into the canal under direct vision (as it should be), and if the axis of the cervical and uterine canal are carefully followed until the corpus is reached, there should be no risk of perforation. Imprecise or loose coupling between the telescope and sheath will result in leakage of the medium at that interface.

Operative sheaths have a larger diameter than do diagnostic sheaths (Fig. 18.3A–C). They range in size from 7 to 10 mm and average 8 mm in diameter. The operative sheath allows space for instillation of the medium, for the 3- to 4-mm telescope, and for the insertion of operating devices. The operating channel is sealed with a rubber nipple or gasket to prevent leakage of the distending medium. The standard operating sheath consists of a single common cavity shared by the medium, telescope, and

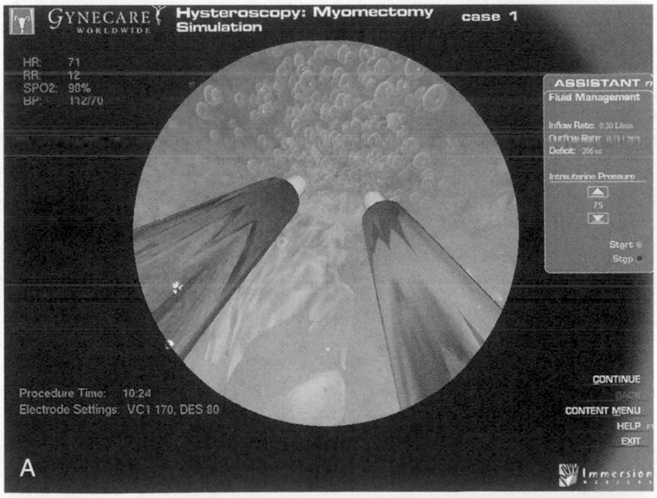

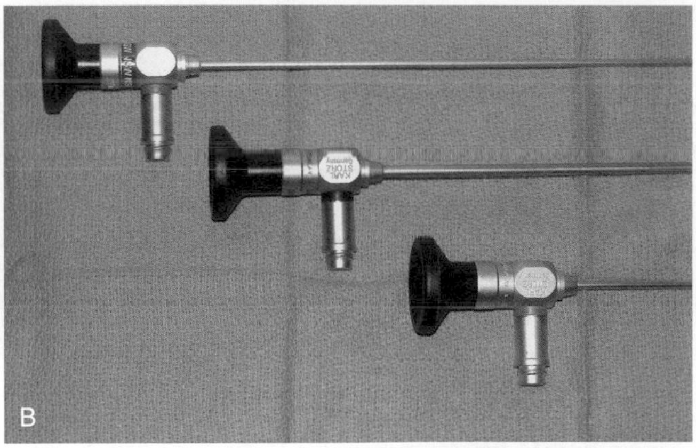

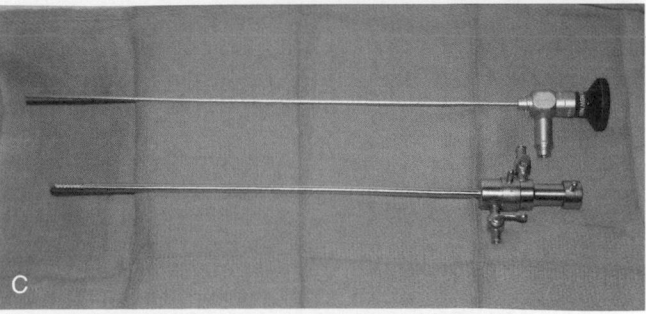

FIGURE 18.1. A: Computerized simulation permits the gynecologist to interact by manipulating a resectoscope and resecting a virtual submucous myoma. (From Baggish MS, Valle RF, Guedj H. *Hysteroscopy: visual perspectives of uterine anatomy, physiology and pathology.* Philadelphia; Lippincott, Williams & Wilkins, 2007, with permission.) B: Three 4-mm (outer and diameter) telescopes are shown here. *Top* is a 30-degree, *middle* is a 70-degree, and *below* is a 0-degree telescope. (From Baggish MS, Valle RF, Guedj H. *Hysteroscopy: visual perspectives of uterine anatomy, physiology, and pathology.* Philadelphia: Lippincott, Williams & Wilkins, 2007, with permission.) C: Telescopes must couple to a 5-mm sheath to be practically functional. The distention liquid or gaseous medium gains access to the uterine cavity via the sheath.

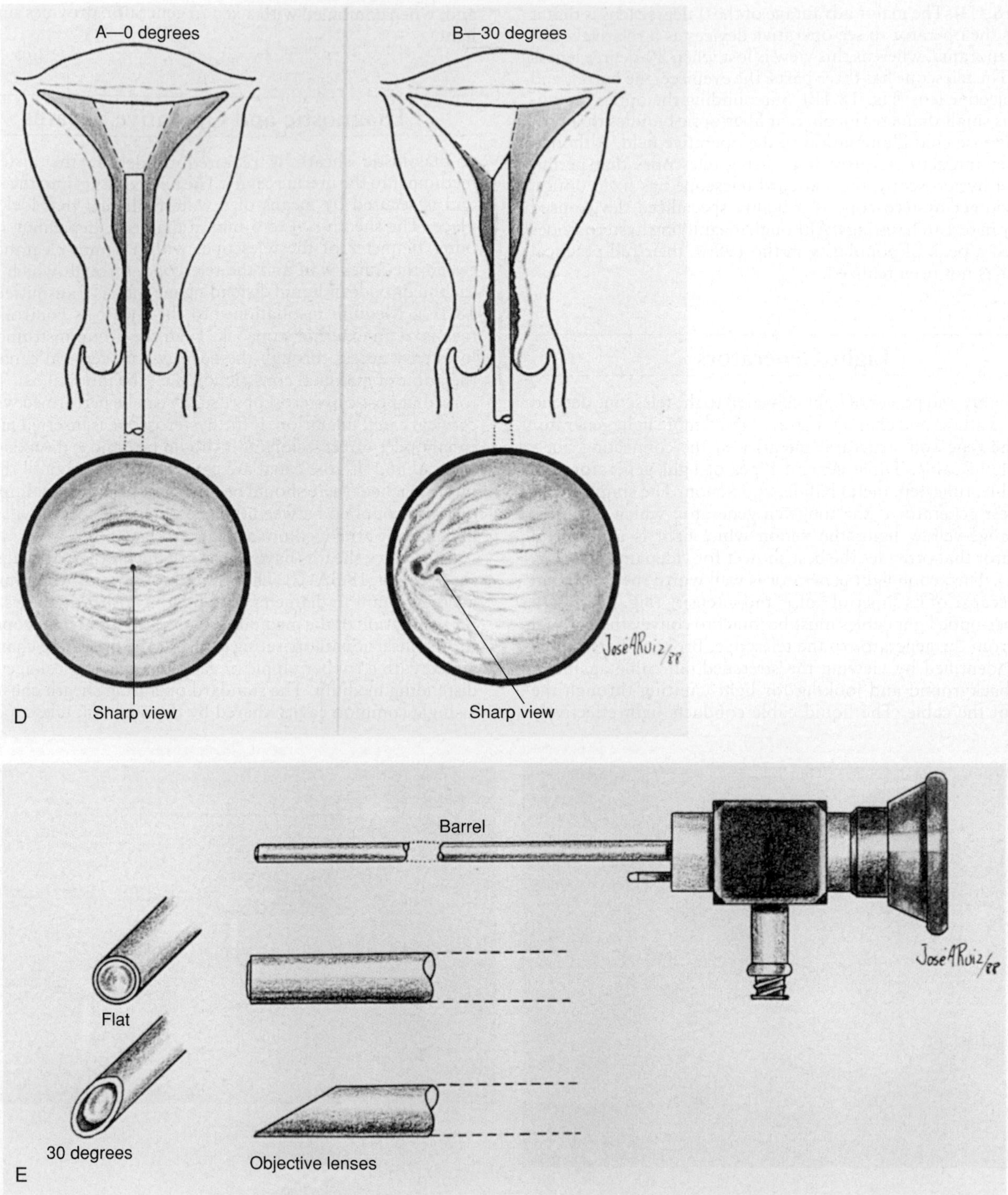

FIGURE 18.1. (*Continued*) **D:** Telescopes are available with either straight-on (0 degrees) or fore-oblique (30 degrees) viewing objective lenses. **E:** A telescope can be conveniently subdivided into three parts: eyepiece, barrel, and objective lens. (From Baggish MS, Barbot J, Valle RF. *Diagnostic and operative hysteroscopy.* Chicago: Mosby-Year Book, 1989, with permission.)

operating tools. The major disadvantages of this type of sheath are that the uterine cavity cannot be flushed with the distending medium, and the operative tools cannot be accurately placed and manipulated within the cavity (Fig. 18.4A). Hysteroscopes with isolated channels overcome the problems inherent to the common cavity sheath (Fig. 18.4B). The dual operating channels permit flushing of the cavity and precise placement of operating accessories. The most recently introduced isolated-channel sheath consists of a double-flushing sheath (Fig. 18.4C) that permits media instillation by way of the inner sheath and media return by way of the perforated outer sheath. The constant flow of the fluid medium in and out of the cavity creates a

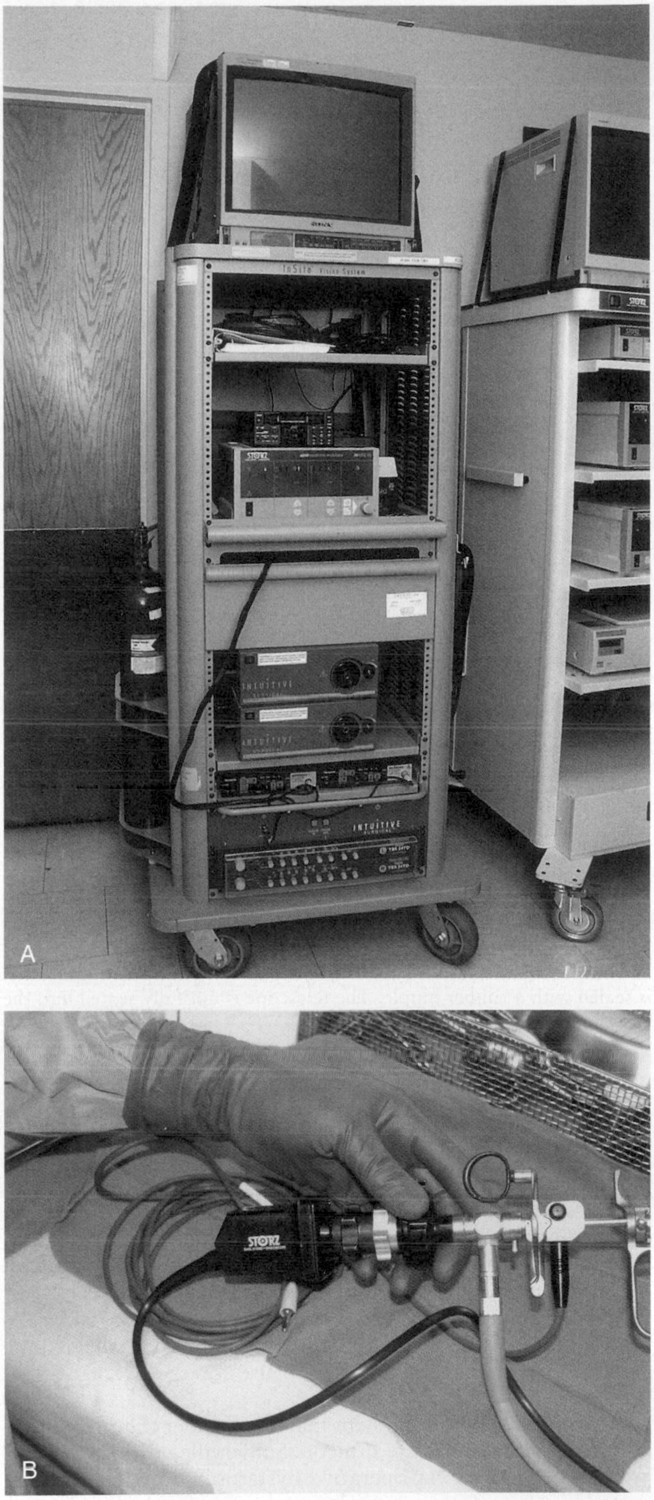

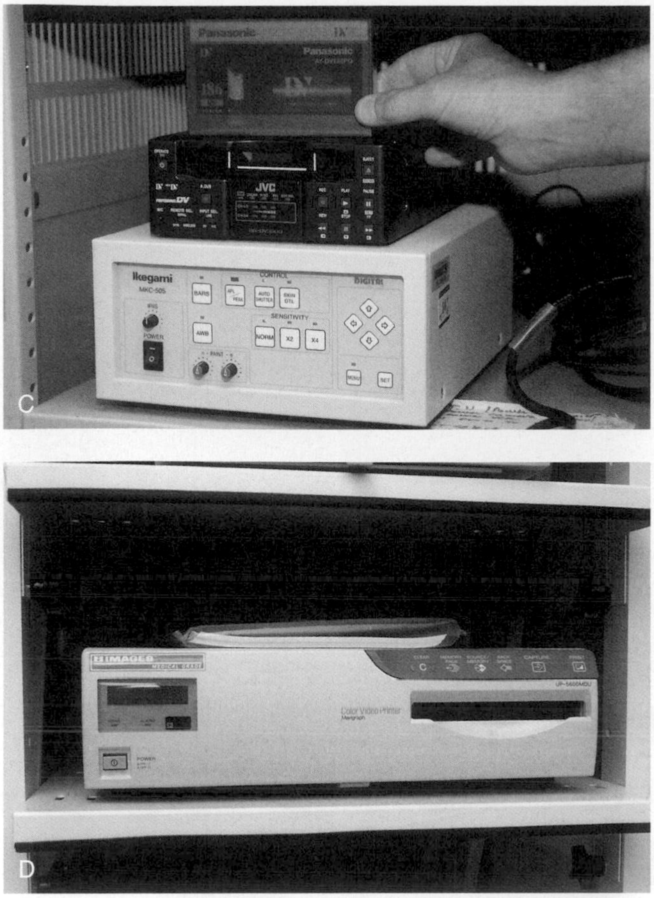

FIGURE 18.2. **A:** This surgical cart is adaptable for either the office or the operating room. It contains a TV monitor, light source, recording unit, television control unit, and electrosurgery generator. The light is a xenon source, which provides clear white light. **B:** The most advanced high-definition recording devices rely on digital technology. A digital recorder is shown here. (From Baggish MS, Valle RF, Guedj H. *Hysteroscopy: visual perspectives of uterine anatomy, physiology, and pathology.* Philadelphia: Lippincott, Williams & Wilkins, 2007, with permission.) **C:** This three-chip video camera is attached to the hysteroscopic telescope. It transmits a three-chip color image. **D:** The digital printer produces four prints per sheet of paper. The image printer is activated by a button on the endoscopic video camera.

very clear operative field. The single isolated operating channel has a diameter sufficiently large (3 mm) to permit an entirely new generation of larger, sturdier operating tools to be used (Fig. 18.4D). The new sheath combines the advantages of the resectoscope with the facility of the operating hysteroscope.

The resectoscope is a specialized electrosurgical (monopolar or bipolar) endoscope that consists of an inner sheath and outer sheath (Fig. 18.5A). The outer sheath is for fluid return as described above. The inner sheath has a common channel for the telescope, fluid medium, and electrode (Fig. 18.5B). The double-armed electrode is fitted to a trigger device that pushes the electrode out beyond the sheath and then pulls it back within the sheath (Fig. 18.5C). The operating tools consist of three basic electrodes: a ball, barrel, and cutting loop (Fig. 18.5 D–G). Most resectoscopes are equipped with a 30-degree telescope. The lens is angled toward the electrode to

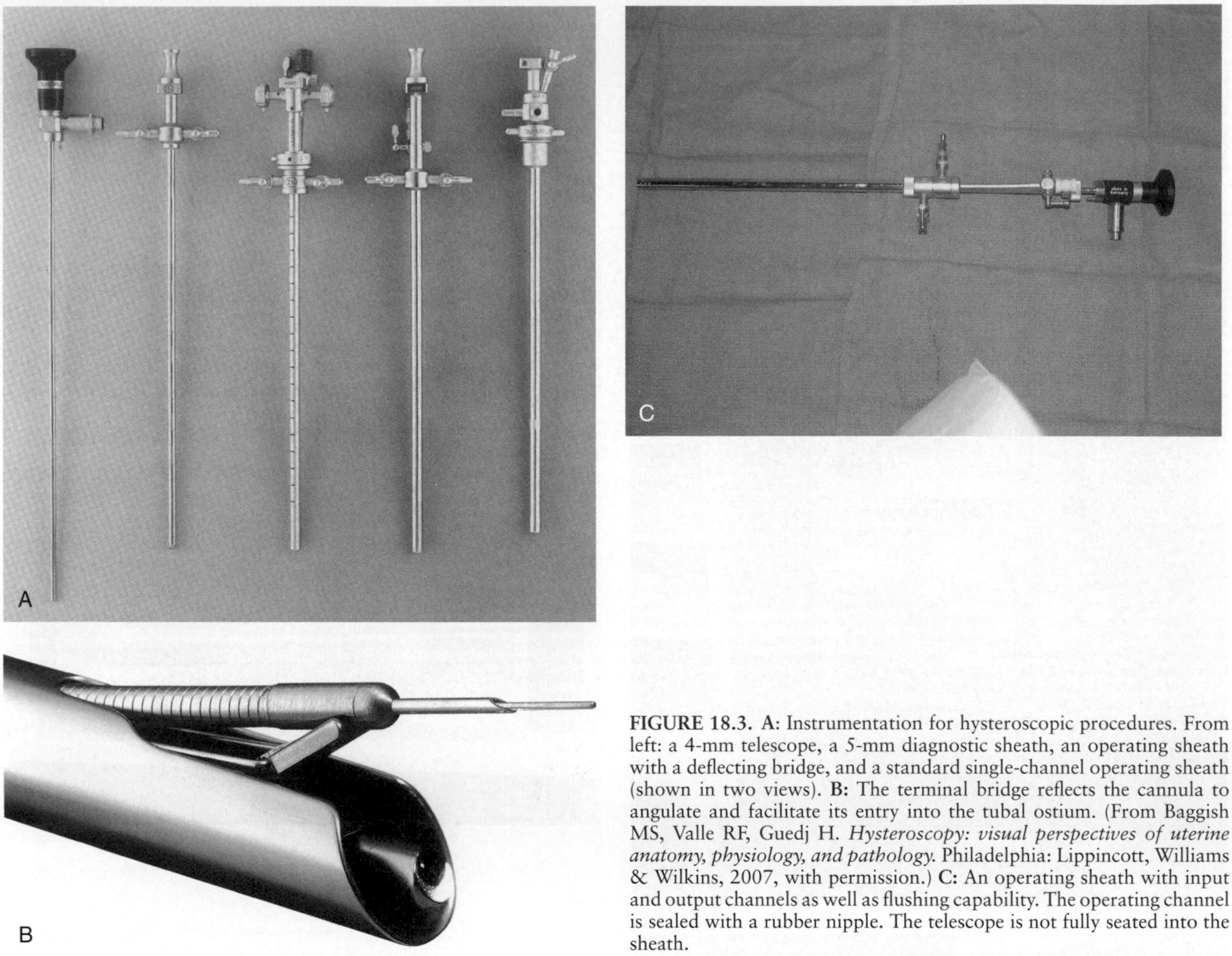

FIGURE 18.3. A: Instrumentation for hysteroscopic procedures. From left: a 4-mm telescope, a 5-mm diagnostic sheath, an operating sheath with a deflecting bridge, and a standard single-channel operating sheath (shown in two views). B: The terminal bridge reflects the cannula to angulate and facilitate its entry into the tubal ostium. (From Baggish MS, Valle RF, Guedj H. *Hysteroscopy: visual perspectives of uterine anatomy, physiology, and pathology.* Philadelphia: Lippincott, Williams & Wilkins, 2007, with permission.) C: An operating sheath with input and output channels as well as flushing capability. The operating channel is sealed with a rubber nipple. The telescope is not fully seated into the sheath.

permit a clear view of the near operative field. Vision of the electrode is lost when the electrode is fully extended outward. Most operating sheaths measure 8 mm or more outer diameter. Dilatation is usually required for insertion. Contemporary small diameter resectoscope uses a 3-mm telescope and a 7- to 7.5-mm sheath.

ACCESSORY INSTRUMENTS

During the late 1990s, many new accessory devices appeared on the market. The standard accessories are the 7F (i.e., 2.3 mm) alligator grasping forceps, biopsy forceps, and scissors. The small size of these fragile semirigid instruments is a disadvantage, and excessive torque at the junction of the shaft and handle frequently leads to breakage. However, flexible devices are less likely to fracture and are equally as facile compared with the semirigid variety. Development of the large isolated-channel sheath has made the use of totally flexible 3-mm operating instruments feasible. The scissors and graspers are substantially heavier and almost indestructible (Fig. 18.6A–C).

A variety of monopolar and bipolar electrodes are also now available for operative hysteroscopy. Monopolar balls, needles, shaving loops (3 mm), and ridged (vaporizing) loops can be inserted through the large operating channel (Fig. 18.7A,B). Bipolar needles for myolysis, as well as bipolar ball and cutting loop electrodes, have been manufactured (Fig. 18.7C), together with bipolar scissors and needles.

The hysteroscopic sheath has an advantage over the resectoscopic sheath, allowing insertion of an aspirating cannula (2.3 or 3 mm), which permits the operator to selectively clear the field of bubbles and debris that cannot be removed by the way of the return second sheath (Fig. 18.8). Nevertheless, the resectoscope is generally easier to use for the average gynecologist.

A complete bipolar system marketed under the trade name of Versapoint (Gynecare, Ethicon, Somerville, NJ) permits cutting and ablation via operative hysteroscopes or via a dedicated bipolar resectoscope. The mechanism for the bipolar current flow through the electrode is illustrated in Figure 18.9A. The electrodes measure 5F diameter (i.e., 2 mm) and therefore can be accommodated by standard and isolated hysteroscopic channels (Fig. 18.9B). The biggest advantage of this bipolar technology is the same that exists for the neodymium-doped yttrium-aluminum-garnet (Nd-YAG) laser; that is, saline may be used as the distending medium for the operative hysteroscopy. This obviates the risk of hyponatremia (see sections on media and complications).

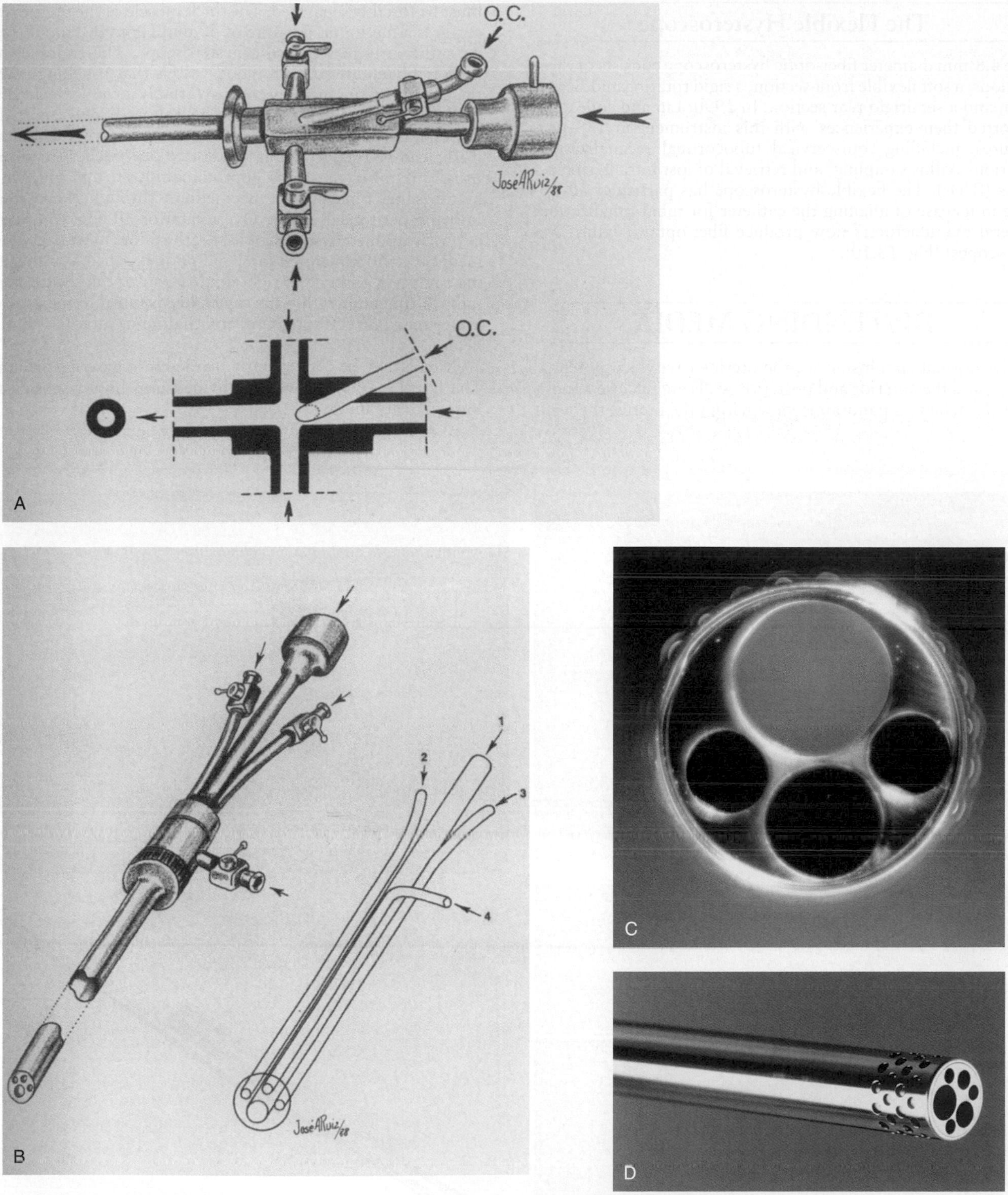

FIGURE 18.4. A: A single-channel operating sheath consists of a single cavity that the telescope, distending medium, and operating instruments share. O.C., operating channel. **B:** A dual-channel operating sheath is constructed with *(1)* isolated channels for a telescope, *(2* and *3)* two operating devices, and *(4)* distending medium. **C:** The terminal portion of the second generation isolated-channel hysteroscope shows the channel for the 4-mm optic (*top*) and a 3-mm operating channel for a variety of large accessory instruments (*bottom*). The two channels at either side are the fluid intake channels. **D:** The double sheath mechanism of the isolated-channel hysteroscope. The perforations in the outer sheath are for fluid return. The uterus is continuously flushed. (A and B: From Baggish MS, Barbot J, Valle RF. *Diagnostic and operative hysteroscopy*. Chicago: Mosby-Year Book, 1989, with permission; C and D: From Bryan Corporation, Woburn, MA, with permission.)

The Flexible Hysteroscope

The 4.8-mm diameter fiber-optic hysteroscope consists of three sections: a soft flexible front section, a rigid rotating middle section, and a semirigid rear section. In 1990, Lin and colleagues reported their experiences with this instrument in 153 procedures, including transcervical tubocornual recanalization, chorionic villus sampling, and retrieval of lost intrauterine devices (IUDs). The flexible hysteroscope has particular advantage in its ease of aligning the catheter for tubal canalization. Several manufacturers now produce fiber-optic (flexible hysteroscopes) (Fig. 18.10).

DISTENDING MEDIA

Under normal circumstances, the uterine cavity is a potential space, and the anterior and posterior walls are in close apposition. To achieve a panoramic view within the uterus, the walls must be forcibly separated. The thick muscle of the uterine wall requires a minimum pressure of 40 mm Hg to distend the cavity sufficiently to see with a hysteroscope. The endometrium is so richly endowed with blood vessels that touching it with the sheath of the hysteroscope invariably produces bleeding. The walls of the uterus must be held more widely apart during operative hysteroscopy. Although a variety of distending media can be used to attain the desired degree of distention, it usually requires pressures approximating 70 mm Hg, which at the same time propel the medium through the oviducts into the peritoneal cavity. Overdilatation of the cervix with a loosely applied hysteroscopic sheath results in leakage of the medium, suboptimal pressure, and poor expansion of the uterine cavity. In contrast, a tight application of the sheath maintains the medium within the cavity, keeps intrauterine pressure above mean arterial pressure, and maintains a clear operative field.

Media may be conveniently divided into gaseous or liquid. The latter may be further subdivided into high-viscosity and low-viscosity fluids.

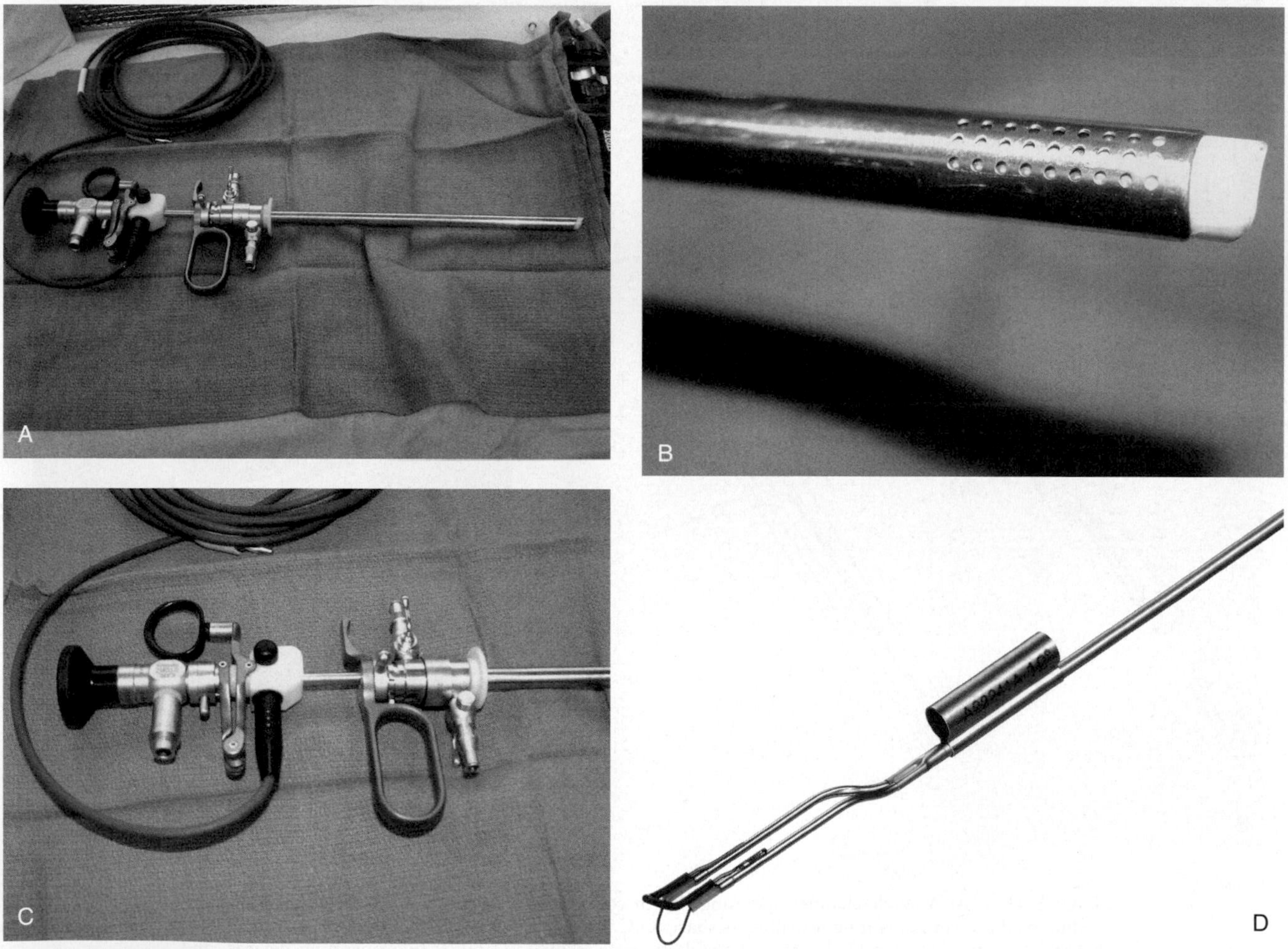

FIGURE 18.5. **A:** The resectoscope shown here is equipped with fluid entry and exit ports. A flushing sheath as the trigger mechanism is pulled back the electrode extends out from the terminal portion of the sheath. **B:** The terminal portion of the sheath shows the output external sheath. Fluid enters through the inner sheath (terminus white). **C:** A 30-degree telescope couples to the sheath. The electric cord carries current, which is transmitted to the electrode. **D:** The cutting loop electrode is the instrument for shaving submucous myomas.

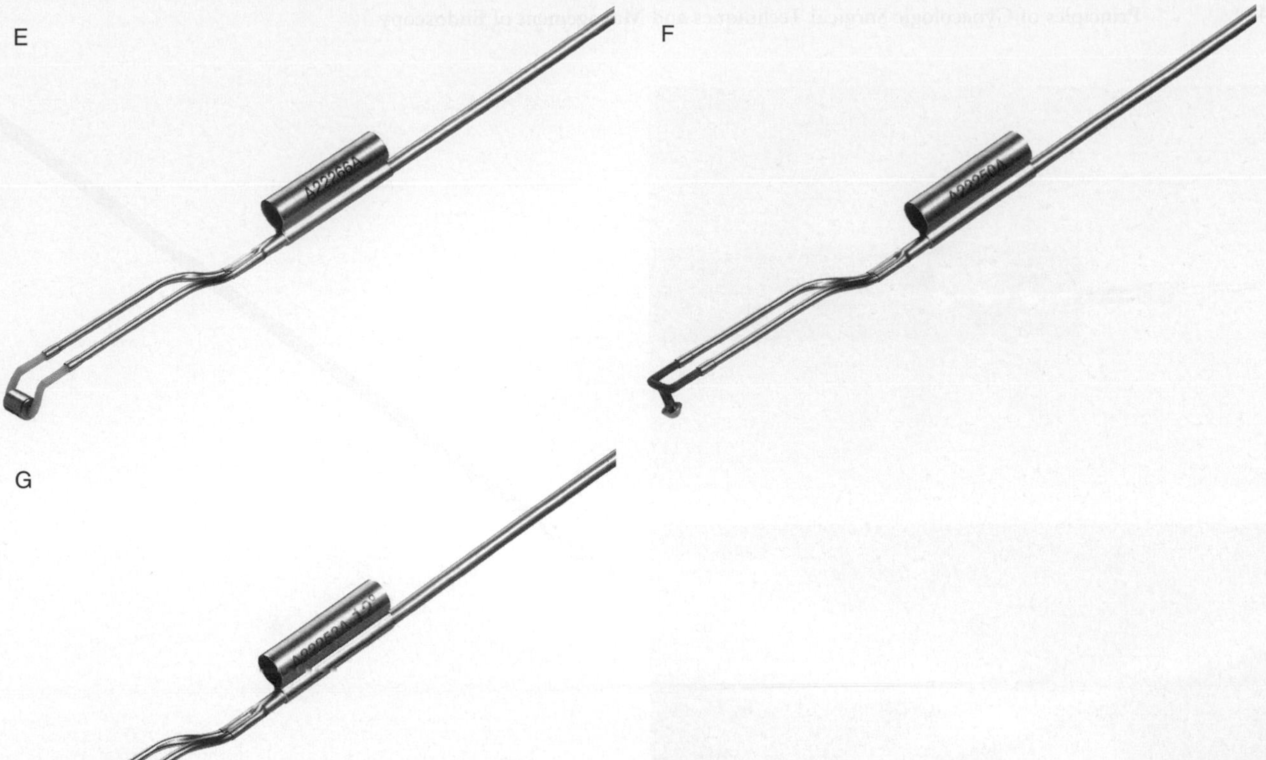

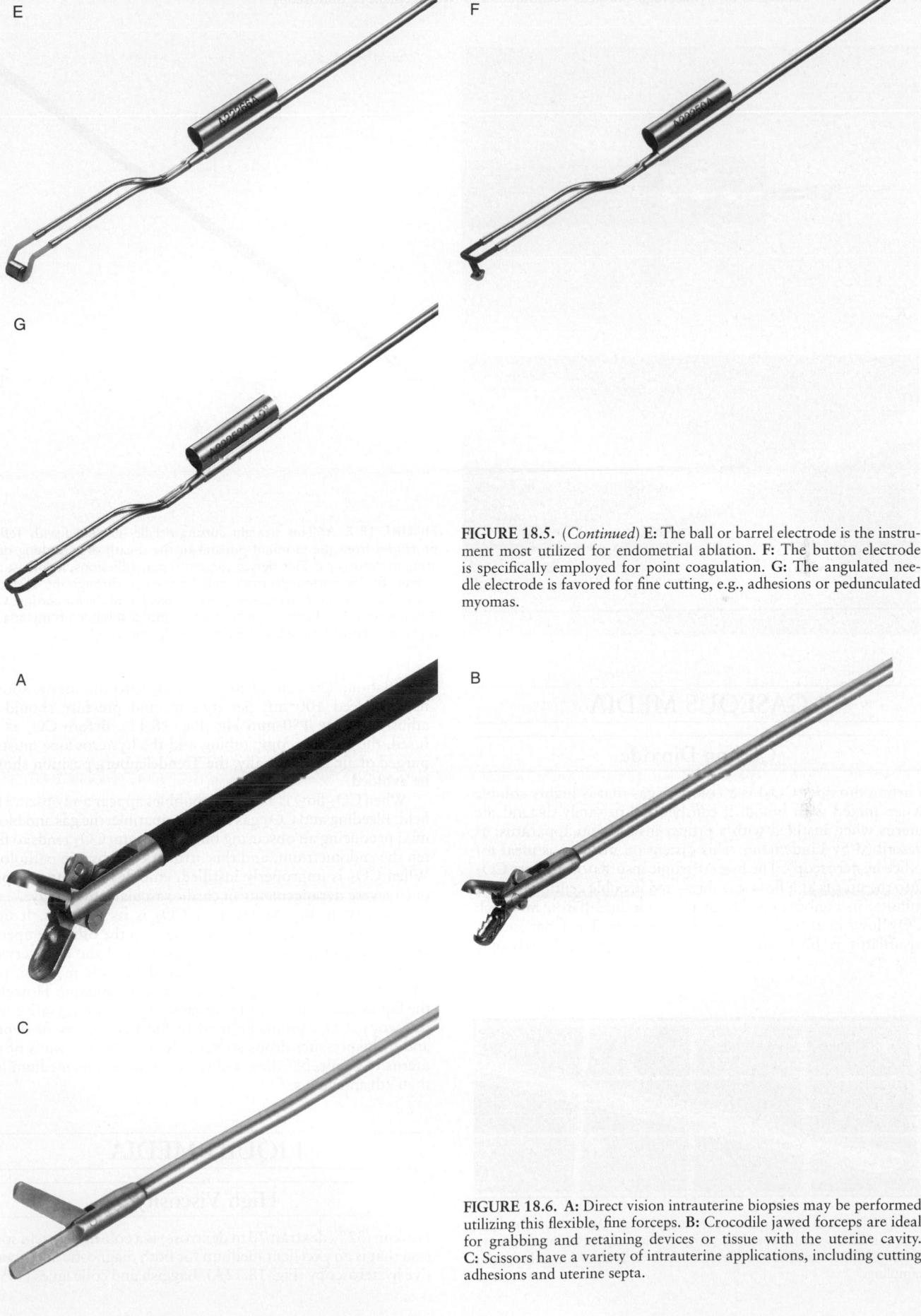

FIGURE 18.5. (*Continued*) **E:** The ball or barrel electrode is the instrument most utilized for endometrial ablation. **F:** The button electrode is specifically employed for point coagulation. **G:** The angulated needle electrode is favored for fine cutting, e.g., adhesions or pedunculated myomas.

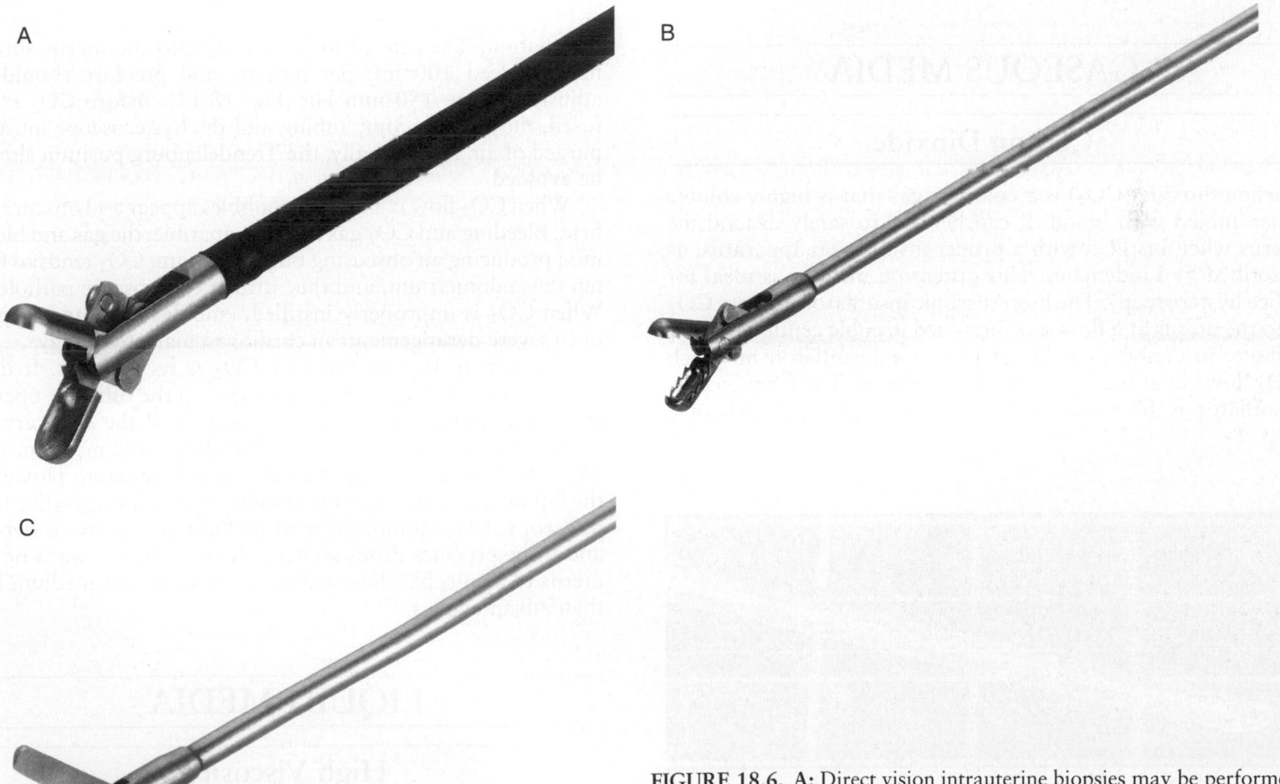

FIGURE 18.6. **A:** Direct vision intrauterine biopsies may be performed utilizing this flexible, fine forceps. **B:** Crocodile jawed forceps are ideal for grabbing and retaining devices or tissue with the uterine cavity. **C:** Scissors have a variety of intrauterine applications, including cutting adhesions and uterine septa.

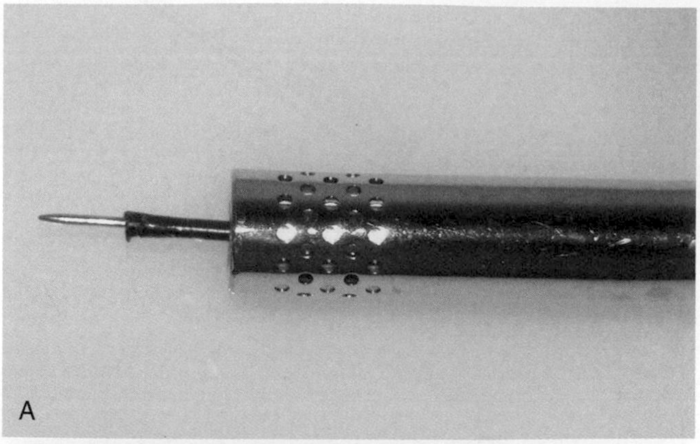

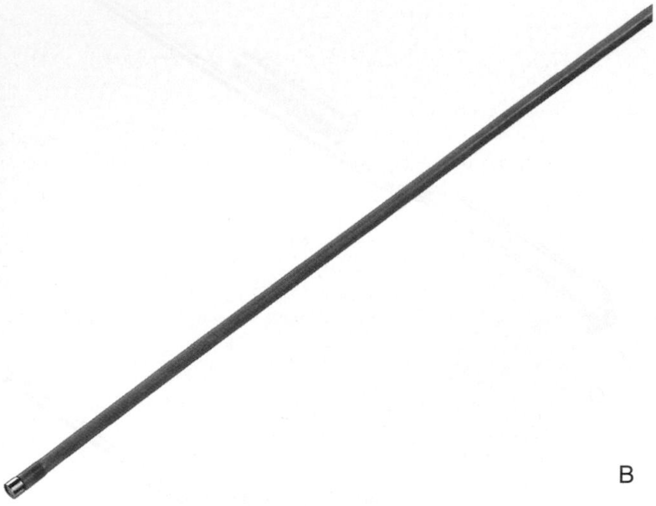

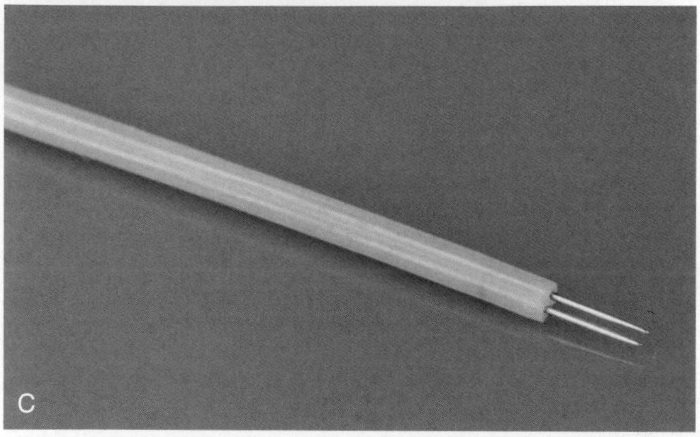

FIGURE 18.7. A: This straight cutting needle (insulated with Teflon) protrudes from the terminal portion of the sheath of a flushing operating hysteroscopy. This device can cut septa, adhesions, myomas, and polyps. **B:** The button electrode may be inserted through the operating channel and used for coagulation indications but never for cutting. **C:** A 3-mm bipolar needle that can be inserted into a submucous myoma for myolysis. (From Unimed, Largo, FL, with permission.)

GASEOUS MEDIA

Carbon Dioxide

Carbon dioxide (CO_2) is a colorless gas that is highly soluble when mixed with blood. It can be used to safely distend the uterus when instilled with a proper insufflation apparatus, as described by Lindemann. This distension medium is ideal for office hysteroscopy. The hysteroscopic insufflator delivers CO_2 into the uterus at a flow rate measured in cubic centimeters per minute, in contrast to the laparoscopic insufflator, in which CO_2 flows in at the rate of liters per minute. The laparoscopic insufflator is both unsuitable and unsafe for hysteroscopic insufflation. The rate of flow of CO_2 into the uterus should never exceed 100 mL per minute, and pressure should be adjusted below 150 mm Hg (Fig. 18.11). Before CO_2 is infused, the hysteroscopic tubing and the hysteroscope must be purged of air. Additionally, **the Trendelenburg position should be avoided.**

When CO_2 flow is excessive, bubbles appear and obscure the field. Bleeding and CO_2 gas are incompatible; the gas and blood mix, producing an obscuring bubbling foam. CO_2 tends to flatten the endometrium, and this artifact can obscure pathology. When CO_2 is improperly instilled, emboli form and can produce severe derangements in cardiovascular physiology.

The best feature in favor of CO_2 is its neatness. It does not foul instruments, it does not mess up the office or operating room, and it allows entry evaluation of the endocervical canal. CO_2 is therefore an excellent diagnostic medium, perhaps the best, according to Siegler and Kemmann. However, the liquid media are superior in most aspects for operative hysteroscopy. CO_2 cannot be used to flush the cavity of debris, and if the pressure drops sufficiently to allow the walls of the uterus to coapt, bleeding will ensue, making this medium less than advantageous.

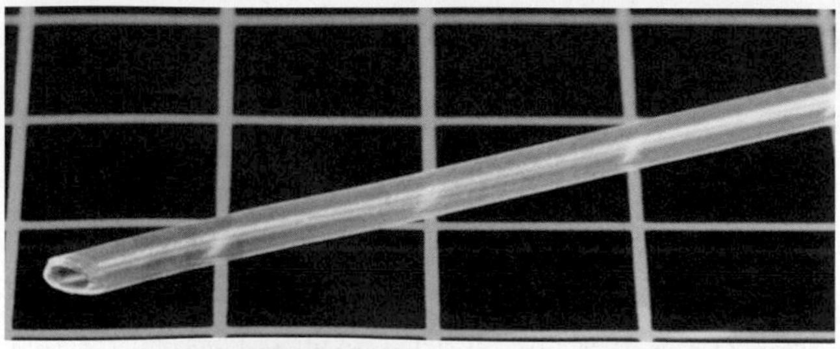

FIGURE 18.8. A 9F aspirating cannula (Cook OB/GYN). The cannula can be inserted through the large 3-mm channel of the operating hysteroscope for aspiration of either debris or fluid, or for endometrial sampling.

LIQUID MEDIA

High Viscosity

Hyskon (32% dextran 70 in dextrose) is a colorless, viscid solution that is an excellent medium for both diagnostic and operative hysteroscopy (Fig. 18.12A). Baggish and colleagues (1992)

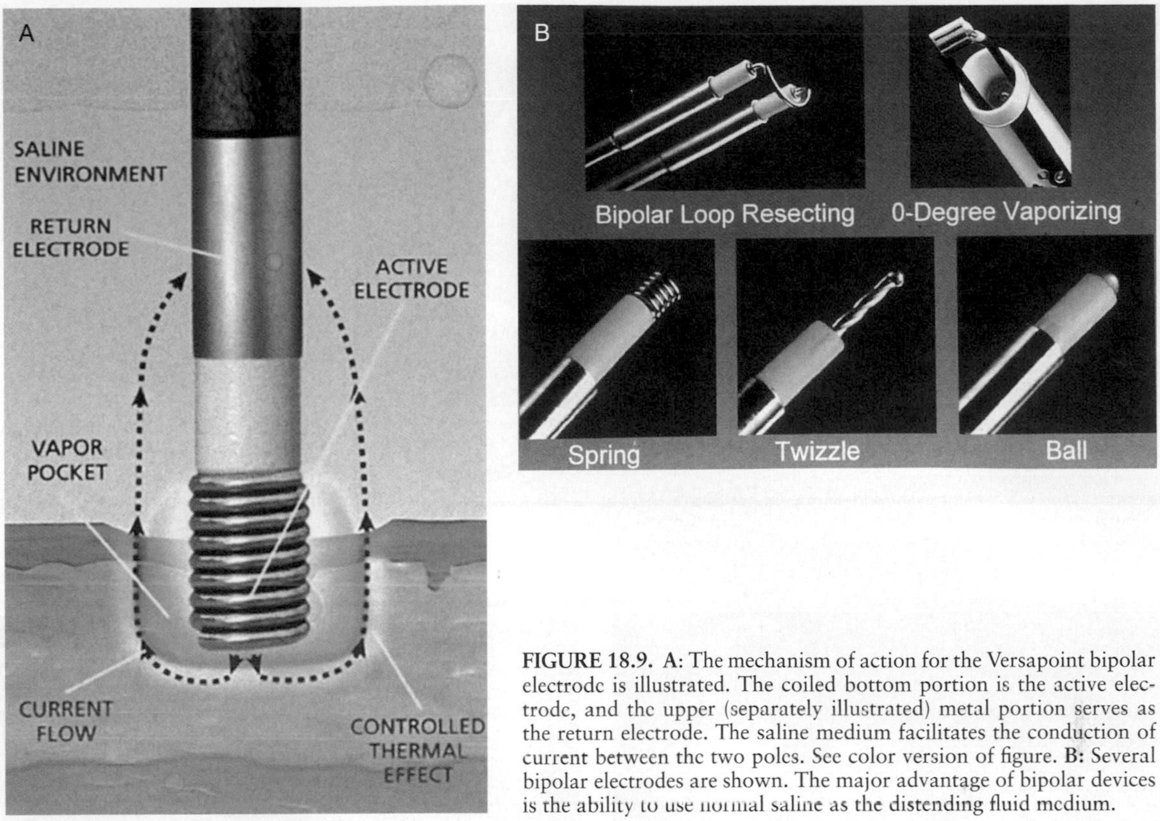

FIGURE 18.9. A: The mechanism of action for the Versapoint bipolar electrode is illustrated. The coiled bottom portion is the active electrode, and the upper (separately illustrated) metal portion serves as the return electrode. The saline medium facilitates the conduction of current between the two poles. See color version of figure. **B:** Several bipolar electrodes are shown. The major advantage of bipolar devices is the ability to use normal saline as the distending fluid medium.

published data on blood levels of Hyskon attained during a variety of operative procedures. Hyskon blood levels were not directly correlated with either the volume of instilled medium or the operative time. The blood levels did correlate with the degree of uterine damage created. The mean intrauterine pressure measured during Hyskon infusion was 76 mm Hg. Ruiz and Neuwirth monitored Hyskon reactions in nearly 2,000 hysteroscopies and reported a rate of pulmonary edema of 0.11% and anaphylactoid reaction of 0.05%. Although no significant correlation between volume and reaction was demonstrated, the investigators cautioned that when more than 500 mL of Hyskon were instilled, the incidence of pulmonary edema increased to 1.4%. They recommended that 500 mL represent the upper limits for Hyskon infused during a single case. Hyskon is a safe medium and has properties that other media do not share. A major advantage of Hyskon is its immiscibility with blood, which permits excellent visualization, even during active bleeding, and permits the surgeon to pinpoint the site of bleeding.

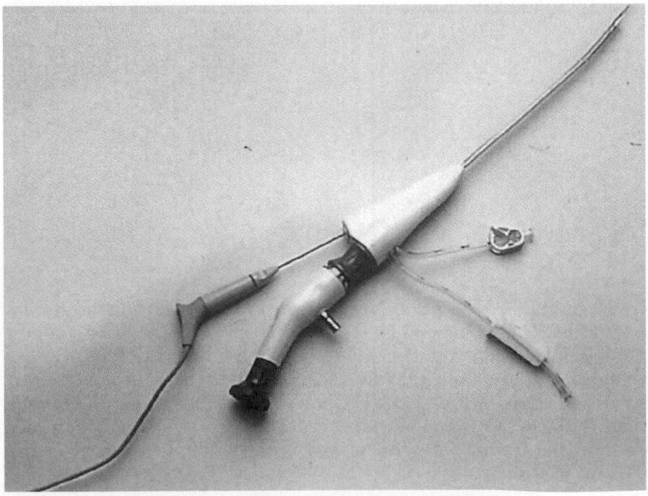

FIGURE 18.10. Flexible fiber-optic hysteroscopes can be manipulated to turn at virtually any angle.

Because Hyskon is so viscid, it is difficult to instill during diagnostic hysteroscopy when the 5-mm sheath with the 1-mm clearance between the lens and sheath is used. Up to 650 mm Hg pressure may be required to push it through the sheath-lens interface. With the addition of a simple hand pump (Cook OB/GYN, Spencer, IN), a 60-mL syringe of Hyskon is easy to instill and is ideal for diagnostic office hysteroscopy (Fig. 18.12B,C). Most diagnostic hysteroscopies can be satisfactorily completed with less than 100 mL of Hyskon, whereas most operative procedures usually require 200 to 500 mL of Hyskon (Fig. 18.12B). Interestingly, Hyskon interaction with heat induced by Nd-YAG laser at about the 100°C level appears to complement the thermal action of the laser.

A disadvantage of Hyskon is that dried residue tends to harden and clog hysteroscopic sheath channels. This clogging is easily prevented by immediately flushing the scope and sheath with hot water after completion of the surgery.

As we have mentioned, two types of Hyskon reactions have been reported. The rare idiosyncratic anaphylactoid reaction should be managed like any acute allergic reaction. The second reaction is caused by excessive vascular uptake of dextran, which allows a more general manifestation of its physiologic actions, including fibrinoplastic action, stearic exclusion,

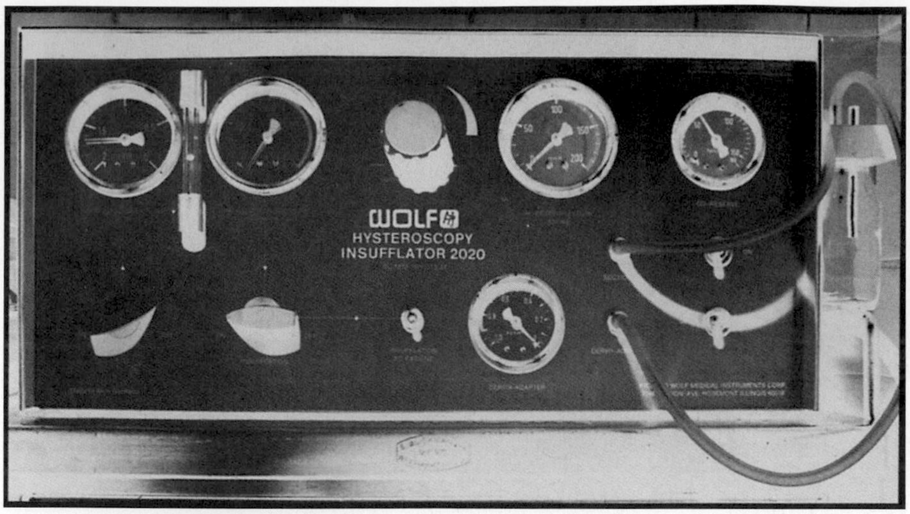

FIGURE 18.11. CO_2 must be infused by a special insufflator that measures flow rate (not to exceed 100 mL per minute) and uterine pressure (not to exceed 150 mm Hg).

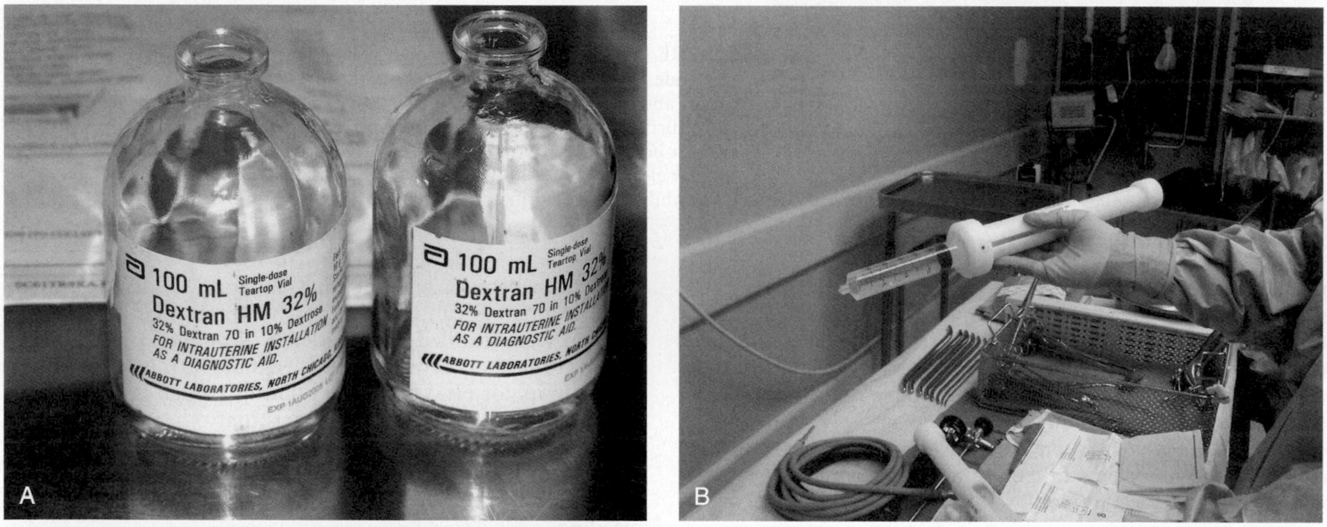

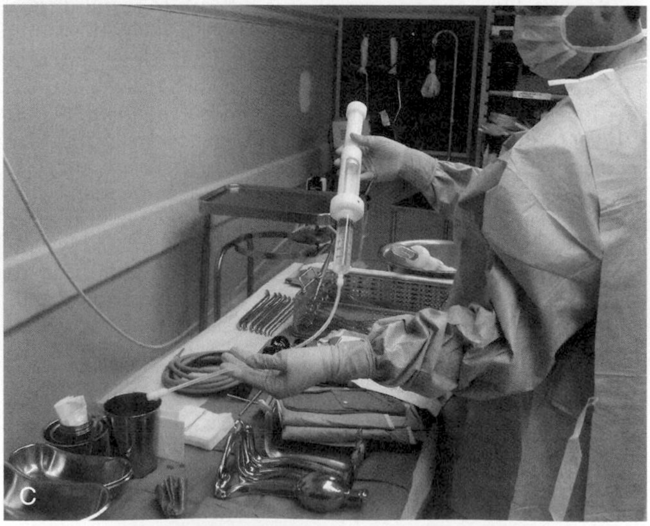

FIGURE 18.12. **A:** The author's favorite medium for viewing the uterine cavity in the clearest fashion is 32% dextran 70, Hyskon. The medium is nonmiscible with blood. **B:** A simple Hyskon Pump (Cook OB/GYN). This syringe driver allows Hyskon to be administered through even a diagnostic sheath with ease. **C:** Hyskon is pumped through the 60-mL syringe to the hysteroscopic sheath by means of special tubing that Luer locks into the syringe on one end and onto the intake channel of the sheath on the other end.

alteration of platelet adhesiveness, and interference with von Willebrand's factor (factor VIIIR). The end result is a bleeding diathesis. The osmotic activity of dextran is such that for each gram of Hyskon instilled into the vascular space, 20 mL of interstitial water will be pulled into the circulation; 100 mL of Hyskon (32% dextran) will expand the plasma volume by 32 g × 20 mL or a total of 640 mL.

As the volume of intravascular Hyskon increases, a critical level is reached, and pulmonary edema occurs. Finally, dextran 70 (Hyskon) is a mixture of macromolecules ranging from 25 to 125 kd. Although the lower-weight molecules are rapidly excreted, the larger molecules can interfere with glomerular filtration and will remain in the bloodstream for 4 to 6 weeks, as detailed in the report by Mishler. Seven case reports of Hyskon-related pulmonary edema were published between 1985 and 1990. The pathogenesis of the Hyskon reaction has been incorrectly described as an example of noncardiogenic pulmonary edema, and this incorrect description has unfortunately been propagated from report to report. No evidence whatsoever supports this hypothesis. The Hyskon-induced pulmonary edema reaction is fully understood, and its actions are cardiogenic, as described earlier. Hyskon can be used universally with electrosurgical devices, lasers, and conventional equipment.

Low Viscosity

Several general statements regarding low viscosity fluid safety may be considered here. Low-viscosity fluids must be continuously flushed through the uterine cavity if a clear view is to be obtained. This means that delivered fluid must be continuously circulated out of the cavity and clean fluid constantly added to make up for the deficit to maintain uterine distension. A standard diagnostic sheath does *not* allow for flushing; therefore, if a low-viscosity fluid is used for distension, the view will be suboptimal because the inevitable ooze of blood will mix with the distending fluid, creating a colored fluid through which the operator will see the field.

The safest distending medium will be isoosmolar—i.e., the electrolyte content will amount to 300 mOsm. Additionally, the sodium content of the fluid should approximate 140 mEq/L. Ergo, the ideal low-viscosity fluid medium is 0.9% sodium chloride.

Regardless of the type of medium infused, the surgeon is responsible for monitoring the infused volume and reconciling that volume with the collected volume. Positive infusion differences require that the procedure be stopped when deficits range from 500 mL (hypoosmolar) to 1,000 mL (isoosmolar). Clearly, the surgeon and the anesthesiologist must communicate because fluid overload scenarios will usually necessitate the anesthesiologist helping to manage the ensuing pathophysiology. Additionally, intravenous fluids infused by the anesthesia team will add to the increased circulatory volume. The gynecologist should be aware that most anesthesiologists infuse lactated Ringer solution, which in itself can create hyponatremia.

Finally, any fluid including physiologic salt solutions can and will produce pulmonary edema when excessive volumes are administered via the hysteroscope because the pressure gradient to maintain uterine distension is 60 to 70 mm Hg and subendometrial venous pressure is 4 mm Hg. Inevitably, fluids will diffuse into the venous circulation.

Low-viscosity distention media may be delivered by hanging the usual 2- to 3-L bag or bottle of fluid 6 to 8 feet above the operating table, permitting the fluid to infuse by gravity feed. A newer technology for instilling low-viscosity fluid is by rotary pump. The newest pumps weigh the fluid in real time and give the surgeon a constant readout of flow rate and total volume of fluid infused (Fig. 18.13A).

Normal Saline, Ringer Lactate

Normal (physiologic) saline (0.9% sodium chloride) is perhaps the safest of any hysteroscopic media. The worst results of excessive vascular absorption are fluid overload and pulmonary edema, which are managed by diuresis and support. The medium is readily available in 3-L sterile bags that can be mounted on an intravenous pole or given via an infusion pump. Garry and colleagues (1992) reported excellent safety results and precise maintenance of uterine pressure by using a pump delivery system, which was combined with one of the operating channels of the dual-channel operating sheath to provide an outflow tract and thus a constant flow rate through the uterine cavity (Fig. 18.13B–D).

Unfortunately, because saline is an efficient conductor of electrons, it does not permit a current density that is high enough for tissue action when using a monopolar system. Saline is therefore not suitable for monopolar electrosurgery, although it is effective when the Nd-YAG laser, the KTP/532 laser, bipolar electrodes, and mechanical devices such as scissors are the hysteroscopic accessories of choice.

In contrast with the Hyskon medium, saline leaks easily out of the uterus. Constant infusion and high flow rates are required to maintain distension. This medium also mixes easily with blood, which further necessitates constant flow of the medium through the operative field for flushing. The large volumes of fluid required make this medium less than ideal for office use.

The best drape for the operating room is the urologic pouch (tucked under the buttocks) with a plastic reservoir pocket into which the outflow fluid may be collected and quantified to determine the fluid deficit (i.e., the difference between instilled fluid and returned fluid). The surgeon should be given a running account by a nurse or surgical assistant of the volume of fluid instilled (i.e., liters of fluid hung on intravenous pole minus volume of return fluid). Whenever any significant fluid deficit is calculated, the procedure should be discontinued and scheduled for completion at a later date. For purposes of this chapter, a significant overload of isotonic sodium chloride could be quantitated to 1.5 to 2 L.

Glycine 1.5% and Sorbitol 3%

Glycine (1.5%) and sorbitol (3%) solutions were first used in urologic surgery, principally for male patients. They were adopted later by gynecologists for use with monopolar electrosurgical devices (e.g., the resectoscope). Both glycine and sorbitol are used for hysteroscopic distension, but both have significant disadvantages inherent to their composition. Clearly, better and safer alternatives exist for uterine distention. Both solutions are hypoosmolar (sorbitol, 178 mOsm/L; glycine, 200 mOsm/L). When delivered by a high-pressure infusion pump, glycine has been reported to cause disturbances in oxygenation and coagulation. However, the principal hazard of these media relates to their vascular absorption and the creation of an acute hyponatremic, hypo-osmolar state. A fluid deficit equal to or greater than 500 mL should alert the surgeon to a likelihood of hyponatremia and hypoosmolality. Two reports have presented data concerning significant complications secondary to hyponatremia. In one series of four women, two died (50% mortality); in the other, one of four women died (25% mortality). Absorption of hypo-osmolar solutions produces a gradient between the circulating blood and the brain cells. The brain cells respond by pumping cation out to

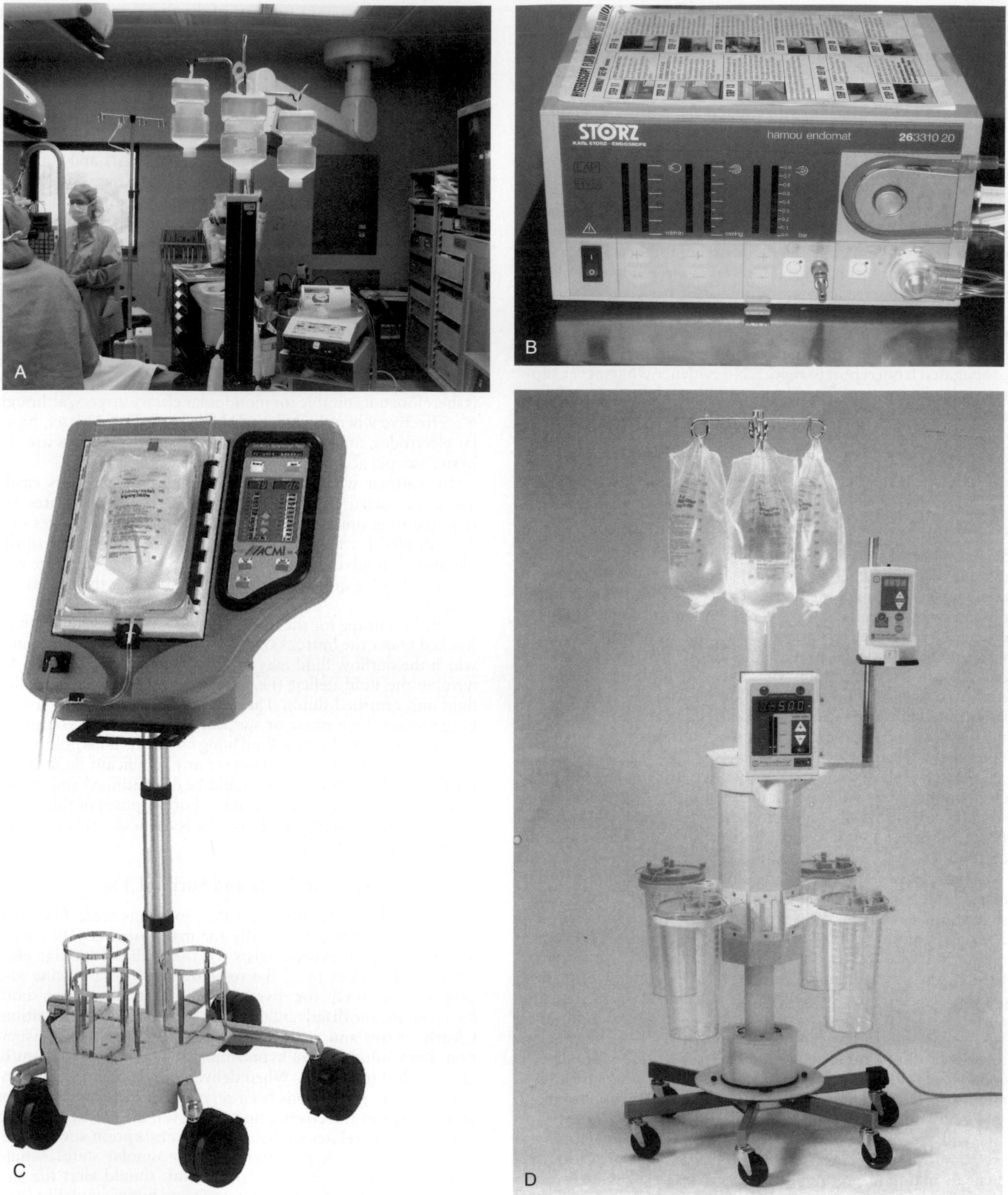

FIGURE 18.13. A: This fluid instillation stand is equipped to handle four 3-liter bottles or bags. The height is easily adjusted to provide a head of pressure to infuse into the uterus. **B:** The advantage of this pump relates to its ability to provide a constant flow of low-viscosity fluid and to maintain sufficient pressure to keep the uterine walls distended. **C:** This pump delivery system not only delivers fluid but also weighs each bag and continuously calculates fluid volume infused and volume collected. **D:** This apparatus is very similar to the technology shown in Figure 13C but permits the usage of multiple bags of fluid.

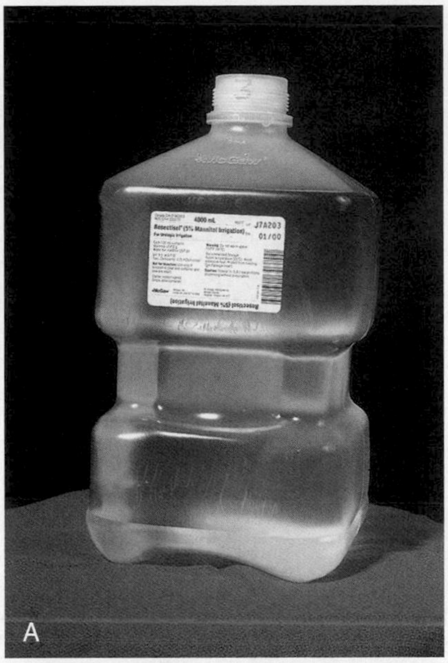

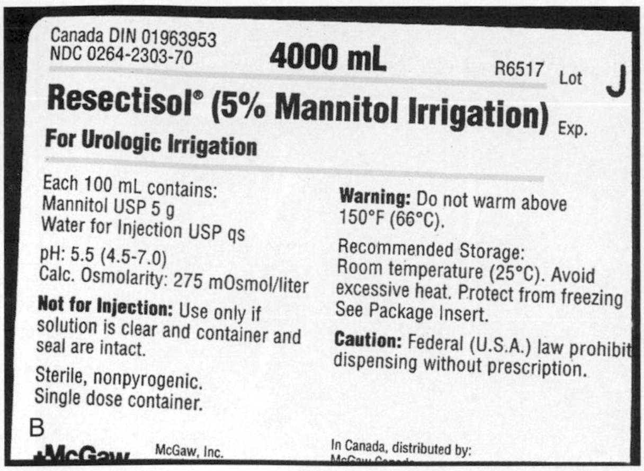

FIGURE 18.14. **A:** A 4-L bottle of sterile 5% mannitol solution for infusion into the uterus. **B:** Magnified view of the label detailing the content of the solution. Note the osmolarity is 275 mOsm/L.

diminish the positive infusion of water into the brain. Unfortunately, the cation pumping mechanism of the brain is deficient in women, secondary probably to the actions of progesterone, and women are at significantly greater risk for the development of life-threatening cerebral edema when a hypoosmolar state exists. When sorbitol or glycine are used as uterine distension media, we refer the reader to the papers of Arieff and Ayus and those of Baggish for a detailed discussion of the treatment of acute severe hyponatremia.

Minimally, preoperative, intraoperative, and 4-hour postoperative serum sodium determinations should be requested on a stat basis. A fact that all hysteroscopists should bear in mind is the consistent overfilling of the medium bags by the manufacturer. Typically, the bags have 150 mL more fluid than indicated.

5% Mannitol and 2.2% Glycine

Mannitol (5%) and glycine (2.2%) are safer than the former two solutions because they may be used with electrosurgical devices and are approximately isoosmolar. Mannitol has an osmolality of 285 mOsm and is an osmotic diuretic (Fig. 18.14A,B). Its optical characteristics are equivalent to glycine and sorbitol; however, it is an infinitely safer medium. In a study of 181 hysteroscopic examinations using isotonic 2.2% glycine, although there was a mean decrease in sodium of 9 mmol/L in patients absorbing 1,000 mL, the serum osmolality remained normal with no significant adverse sequelae.

As already noted above, regardless of the medium used, the exact volume of fluid infused (taking into account bag overfilling) must be accurately measured and recorded. In a similar fashion, the operating room nurse must empty collection canisters to accurately measure the medium return volume; less compulsion about these measurements is unacceptable.

DIAGNOSTIC HYSTEROSCOPY TECHNIQUES

Diagnostic hysteroscopy can be performed in an office setting under local anesthesia. The injection of lidocaine 1%, 10 to 15 mL, directly into the cervix produces excellent anesthesia for this easy operation, and discomfort for the patient can be diminished by ibuprofen (Motrin), 600 to 800 mg, administered 30 minutes before the procedure. Patients who require cardiac prophylaxis (e.g., prolapsed mitral valve) should be covered by appropriate antibiotics. Patients should be given suitable information for informed consent.

Accurate knowledge of the position of the uterus is critical to facilitate the examination. The best view of the uterus is obtained during the proliferative phase of the menstrual cycle. The patient is placed in the dorsal lithotomy position. The perineum and vagina are gently swabbed with povidone-iodine or another suitable antiseptic solution. A Sims retractor is placed in the posterior vagina and retracted downward (Fig. 18.15A). The edge of the cervix comes into view and is grasped with a single toothed tenaculum (Fig. 18.15B). A suitable telescope is selected and checked by the operator for clarity of the eyepiece and objective lens. If necessary, the lens is cleansed with a soft saline-soaked or water-soaked sponge. The light generator is switched on, and the fiber-optic cable is attached to the telescope. The telescope is inserted into the diagnostic sheath, and the selected medium is flushed through the sheath to expel any air within the sheath (Fig. 18.16A,B). At Good Samaritan Hospital in Cincinnati, 60 mL of Hyskon, delivered by a Cook OB/GYN handheld pump, is routinely used for office hysteroscopy. Typically, one full syringe of this medium is ample for completion of a diagnostic examination of the uterus. The flow of Hyskon starts as the hysteroscope is engaged into the external os of the cervix.

If CO_2 is the selected medium, the flow rate is adjusted to deliver 30 mL per minute. The hysteroscope is engaged into the external cervical os. As the endoscope is advanced, the gas separates the walls of the endocervix, allowing an excellent view of the endocervical folds and crypts. The internal os is seen above as the endoscope is manipulated along the axis of the canal and through the os under direct vision. Flow is adjusted to a rate 60 mL per minute when the isthmus is entered (Fig. 18.17A,B).

Routine dilatation of the cervix should be avoided because even careful and gentle insertion of cervical dilators will traumatize the endocervix and endometrium. Typically, the

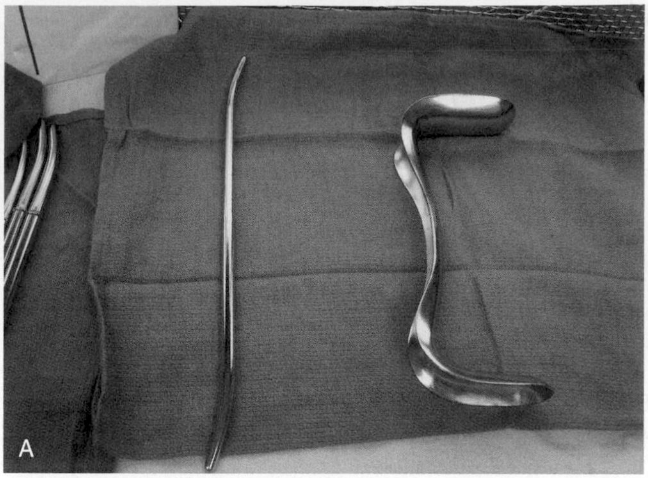

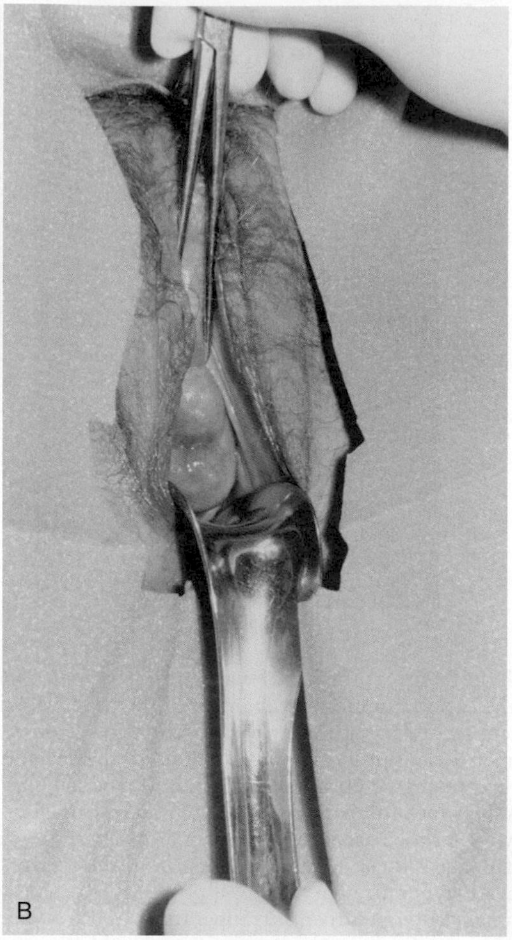

FIGURE 18.15. **A:** The Sims retractor is the instrument of choice for retracting the posterior vaginal wall. On the left of the Sims retractor is a Pratt dilator, which is used to atraumatically and gradually dilate the cervix for entry of the hysteroscope. **B:** The Sims retractor is most convenient for retraction of the posterior vaginal wall. This brings the edge of the cervix into view, and it can be easily grasped with the single-toothed tenaculum. This provides an excellent view for office and operative hysteroscopy.

endocervical canal shows longitudinal folds, papillae, and clefts. The vascular pattern of the normal endocervix reveals branching treelike vessels. These are especially well observed with a focusing hysteroscope. The internal os appears as a narrow constriction at the top of the endocervical canal. The isthmus is a cylindrical extension above the os. The corpus is a capacious cavity above the isthmus. The central point of müllerian duct fusion is seen projecting down from the fundus. The cornua occupy either side of this fused area. The tubal ostia are visible at the upper extremities of the fundal cornua and show great variation in their appearance and angle of entry into the uterine cavity. The uterine mucosa (endometrium) is smooth and pink-white in color during the proliferative phase. The gland openings appear as white-ringed elevations surrounded with netlike vessels. During the secretory phase of the cycle, the endometrium is lush and velvety; it protrudes into the cavity irregularly and can be easily mistaken for small polyps. The hue of secretory endometrium is

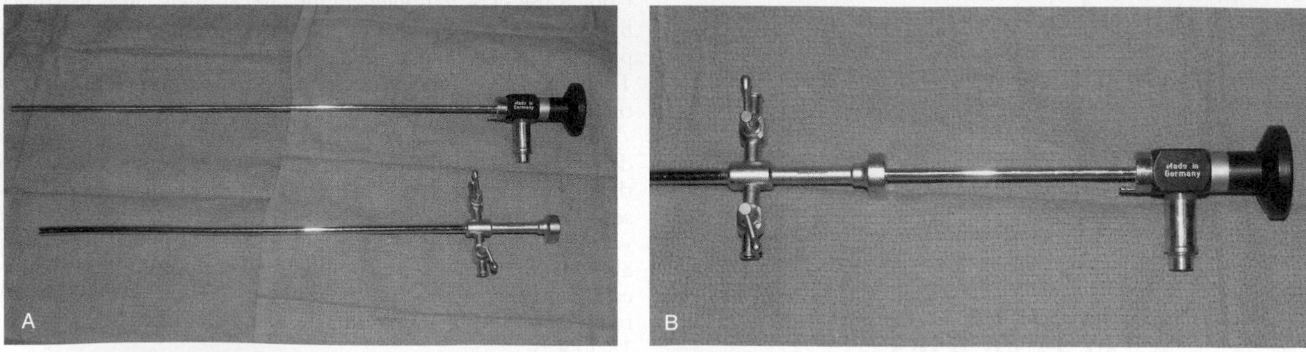

FIGURE 18.16. **A:** The diagnostic lens (telescope) and its 5-mm outer diameter diagnostic sheath are excellent instruments for office or surgicenter outpatient hysteroscopy. **B:** Close-up showing 0-degree 4-mm telescope engaging into the diagnostic sheath.

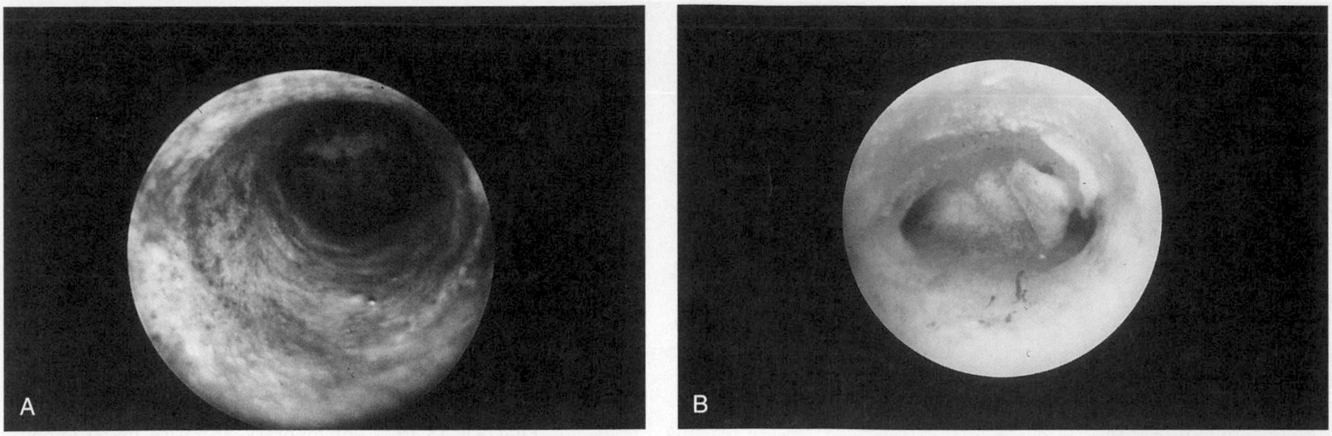

FIGURE 18.17. A: This view is taken within the distended cervix looking upward into the dark corpus. **B:** The hysteroscope's objective lens is just above the internal os. The panoramic cavity is seen. The recesses to the right and left are the cornu.

magenta. The interior of the cavity, particularly when liquid media are used, first appears cloudy, with fine debris floating in the medium.

When CO_2 is the distending medium, the endometrium is artificially flattened. Although the cornua are easily recognized, the tubal ostia may not be seen during the latter phase of the menstrual cycle. The thickness of the endometrium can be easily appreciated by placing pressure on the telescope and pushing on the posterior wall of the uterus. This maneuver creates a groove in the endometrium.

OPERATIVE HYSTEROSCOPY TECHNIQUES

The telescope is inserted into the operative or resectoscope sheath. If the operative sheath is used, a proper nipple is selected and attached to the opening of the operating channel (Fig. 18.18A,B). The sheath is flushed with the distending medium, and light cable is attached. Careful dilatation with Pratt dilators should be performed until the operative sheath negotiates a tight passage through the cervix. With the medium flowing, the hysteroscope can be inserted into the uterine cavity under direct vision or coupled to the television camera. The uterine cavity is scanned, and the operator mentally notes landmarks (e.g., the tubal ostia, depth of the cornua, the location and attachments of the lesion, the proximity of the internal cervical os). The flow of the debris with the liquid medium will also help the operator locate the tubal ostia. If there is difficulty viewing the cavity clearly, the hysteroscope has probably been inserted too deeply, and the telescope has come in contact with the uterine wall. When the view is blocked, the most prudent first maneuver is to **pull the instrument back with the medium flowing into the uterus.**

After a clear view is obtained, the operating device (e.g., electrode or scissors) is inserted into the cavity and advanced to make contact with the endometrium for relative calibration and spatial orientation within the cavity. The knowledgeable and skilled endoscopist at this point inserts an aspirating cannula to further clear the cavity of debris. The cavity can

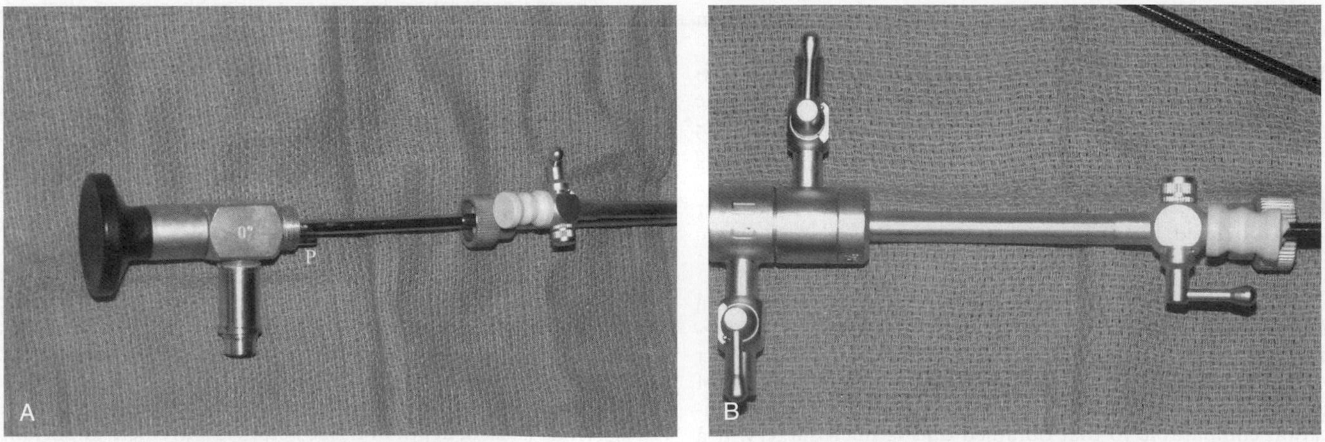

FIGURE 18.18. A: The telescope is secured by means of a water-tight pin and screw mechanism. A gray nipple gasket covers entry into the operating channel. **B:** Close-up of operating sheath. A flexible instrument has been inserted via the gray nipple into the operating channel. The two stopcocks are for (*1*) infusion of the distending medium and (*2*) return and jettison of circulating fluid. Note all stopcocks are opened.

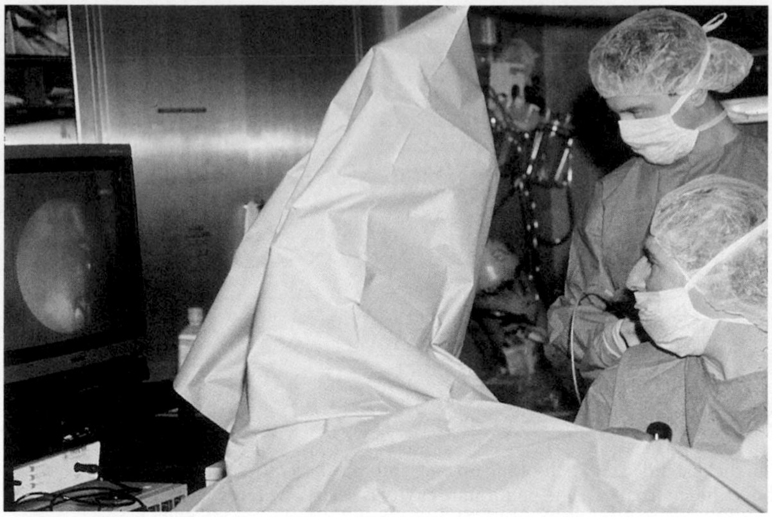

FIGURE 18.19. Contemporary operative hysteroscopy is performed with a microchip video camera attached to the eyepiece of the telescope. The operator and assistants all view the field by way of a high-resolution video monitor.

also be further distended with a constant flow sheath by closing off the return valve stopcock. The valve is then opened, and the cavity is flushed clear. No operative procedure can even be performed unless an absolutely unobstructed view is obtained.

In certain cases, it is advantageous to perform a simultaneous laparoscopy to permit an assistant to view the serosal surface of the uterus to provide some additional insurance against inadvertent perforation. Laparoscopy is recommended during the cutting of septa, during lysis of uterine adhesions, and during excisions for large submucous myomata.

Most experienced hysteroscopic surgeons use the endoscopic microchip camera coupled directly to the telescope. The current state of the art technology employs digital cameras and digital recorders. Performance of hysteroscopic surgery by video monitoring has the following advantages (Fig. 18.19):

1. Some camera lenses permit sufficient magnification of the operative field for the image to fill the entire video monitor screen.
2. The video camera eliminates one source of operator fatigue by allowing the endoscopist to sit upright rather than hunched over.
3. An image projected clearly on the video screen helps residents, nurses, and students maintain interest throughout the procedure; enables them to learn more about the technique; and allows them to render better assistance than is possible with conventional procedures.
4. The risk of an eye injury and the need for protective eyewear are obviated.

Endoscopic video camera lenses range in focal length from 25 to 38 mm. A 28- to 30-mm lens provides satisfactory magnification. The operator should first view the cavity by direct vision and should then attach the camera to the eyepiece of the lens. The view with the coupled camera provides magnification comparable to that obtained during microsurgery. If a video recorder is available, a permanent record of the procedure can be captured on tape. A xenon light generator provides the best illumination for video techniques, although less expensive light sources may be satisfactory when coupled to newer cameras, which are highly light sensitive.

LASERS AND ELECTROSURGICAL DEVICES

The Nd-YAG laser, which works by thermal energy, is the preferred laser for hysteroscopic surgery. Electrosurgical devices exert their tissue actions in a similar fashion: Light energy from lasers is transformed to thermal energy by electron flow (Fig. 18.20A). Lasers and electrosurgical devices both produce coagulation at 60°C to 70°C and vaporization at 100°C (Table 18.1), and both require sufficient power density to exert the desired action. Similar tissue actions can be produced by raising the power density or by keeping the power constant and increasing the tissue exposure time. A 1-mm laser fiber delivering 30 watts of power to tissue will create a power density of 3,000 W/cm^2. A 3-mm ball electrode will need to generate 300 W of power to create a similar power density (Fig. 18.20B).

The Nd-YAG laser beam can be transmitted equally well with any distending medium, whereas monopolar electrosurgical devices operate most effectively in an electrolyte-free medium.

Uterine perforation by either a laser fiber or an electrode is much more serious than perforation by scissors or another mechanical device because the thermal energy can inflict great damage to surrounding structures (e.g., bowel or bladder). The injury may not attain its maximum damage until 2 or 3 days after surgery. Therefore, either laparoscopy or laparotomy is indicated in such cases to determine the extent of injury.

The surgeon must be familiar with the physics governing the actions of lasers or electrosurgical tools and with the tissue actions exerted by these energized devices. A knowledgeable surgeon would not use a ball device to cut or a loop electrode to coagulate tissue. Proper selection of wattage depends on disease pathology and location. High power applied for a long period of time is risky, is inappropriate, and will inevitably lead to unwanted tissue injury.

Regardless of whether a laser, resectoscope, or handheld electrode is used, depth of tissue action is extremely important; transmural injury is possible at high-power densities or with prolonged exposure. One must keep in mind that the thickness of the distended uterine wall (0.5 to 1 cm) is considerably less than that of the nondistended uterine wall (1.5 to 2 cm) (Fig. 18.21A,B).

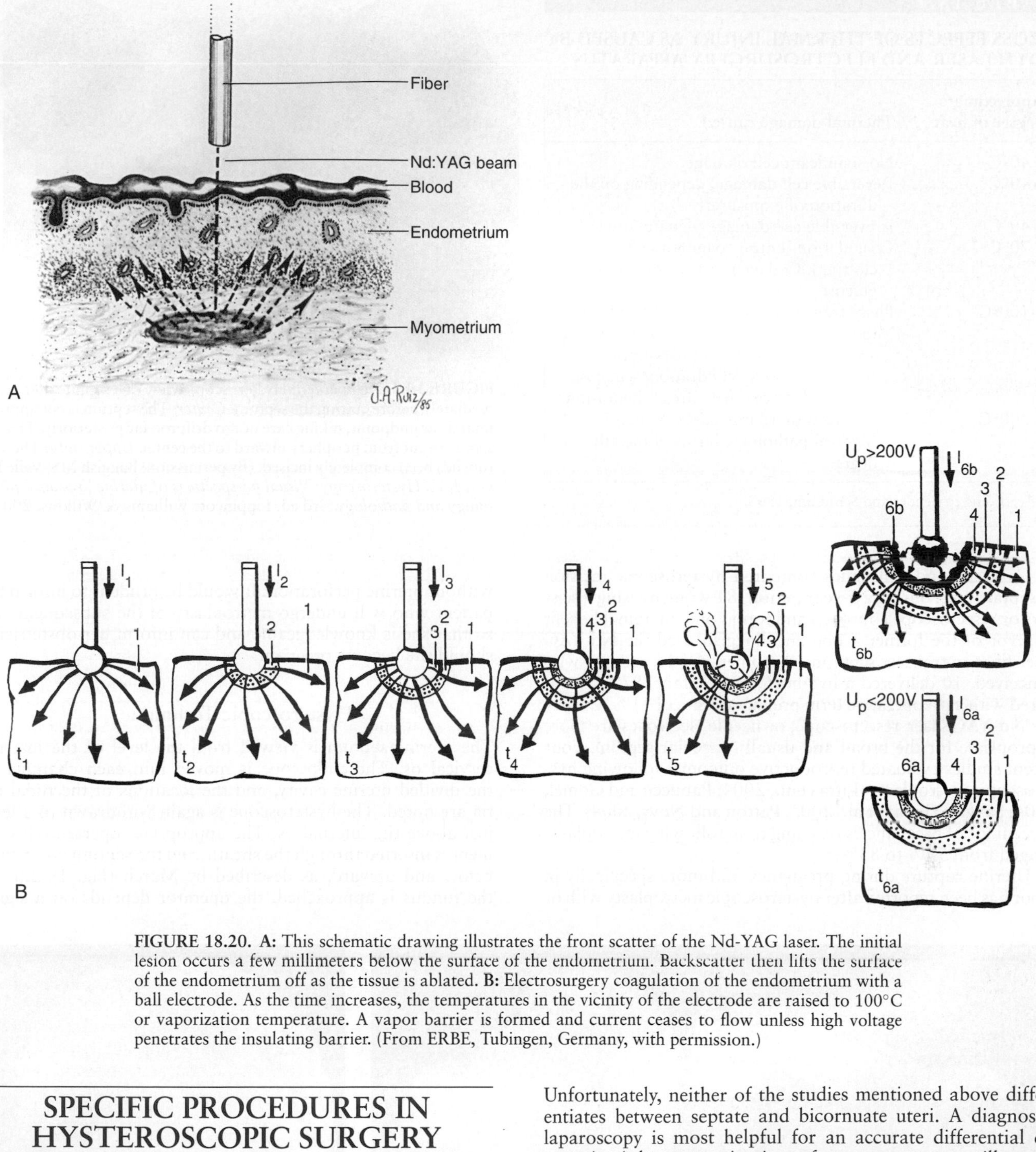

FIGURE 18.20. A: This schematic drawing illustrates the front scatter of the Nd-YAG laser. The initial lesion occurs a few millimeters below the surface of the endometrium. Backscatter then lifts the surface of the endometrium off as the tissue is ablated. B: Electrosurgery coagulation of the endometrium with a ball electrode. As the time increases, the temperatures in the vicinity of the electrode are raised to 100°C or vaporization temperature. A vapor barrier is formed and current ceases to flow unless high voltage penetrates the insulating barrier. (From ERBE, Tubingen, Germany, with permission.)

SPECIFIC PROCEDURES IN HYSTEROSCOPIC SURGERY

Septate Uterus

Modern hysteroscopy has rendered the correction of septate uterus relatively simple and straightforward by the transcervical route, as documented by DeCherney and associates (1986) and by March and Israel (1987). Uterine septa are a treatable factor contributing to pregnancy wastage usually secondary to premature labor and late second-trimester abortion. The diagnosis of a uterine septum is usually made at hysterosalpingography or during a diagnostic hysteroscopy. Unfortunately, neither of the studies mentioned above differentiates between septate and bicornuate uteri. A diagnostic laparoscopy is most helpful for an accurate differential diagnosis. A laparoscopic view of a septate uterus will reveal a wide but otherwise normal fundus, whereas the bicornuate uterus typically appears heart shaped. Alborzi and associates (2003) in a small study reported that sonohysterography is sufficiently accurate to differentiate bicornuate from septate uterus, thereby eliminating the need for diagnostic laparoscopy. A bicornuate uterus, if pregnancy wastage is demonstrated, should be treated by a Jones or Strassman procedure. A septate uterus should be treated hysteroscopically. The standard technique, reported by March and colleagues (1978), is to cut the septum with scissors under direct hysteroscopic view.

TABLE 18.1

GROSS EFFECTS OF THERMAL INJURY AS CAUSED BY BOTH LASER AND ELECTROSURGERY APPARATUS

Approximate degree of heat	Thermal damage caused
<40°C	No significant cell damage.
>40°C	Reversible cell damage, depending on the duration of exposure.[a]
>49°C	Irreversible cell damage (denaturation).[a]
>70°C	Coagulation (Latin: coagulation 5 clotting). Collagens are converted to glucose.
>100°C	Phase transition from liquid to vapor of the intracellular and extracellular water. Tissue rapidly dries out (dessication) (Latin: *ex sico* 5 dehydration). Glucose has an adhesive effect after dehydration.
>200°C	Carbonization (Latin: *carbo* 5 coal). Medical pathologic burns of the 4th degree.

[a]According to Bender and Schramm, 1968.

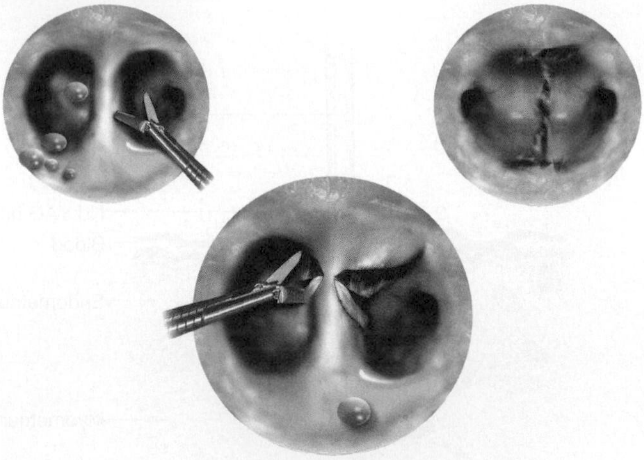

FIGURE 18.22. *Upper left:* Hysteroscopic view of a septate uterus immediately before cutting the septum. *Center:* The septum is cut approximately at midpoint, taking care not to drift too far posteriorly. Thicker septa are cut from periphery inward to the center. *Upper right:* The septum has been completely incised. (By permission: Baggish MS, Valle RF, Guedj H. *Hysteroscopy: Visual perspectives of uterine anatomy, physiology and pathology.* 3rd ed. Lippincott Williams & Wilkins, 2007.)

Cararach and colleagues compared hysteroscopic incision of septate uteri during a 5-year period (81 women) using a scissors or resectoscope approach and found only marginal benefit in favor of the former. Choe and Baggish used the Nd-YAG laser fiber to transect septa in 14 women. Of 13 patients who conceived, 10 delivered a live-born, term infant (87%), compared with a preoperative term pregnancy rate of 11%. Clearly the Nd-YAG laser, resectoscope, or needle electrodes are more appropriate for the broad and usually vascular septum. Four recent studies evaluated reproductive outcomes following hysteroscopic metroplasty (Litta et al., 2004; Pabuccu and Gomel, 2004; Saygili-Yilmaz et al., 2003; Patton and Novy, 2004). The percentage of pregnancies reaching term following metroplasty ranged from 50% to 83%.

Uterine rupture during pregnancy and more specifically in labor has been reported after hysteroscopic metroplasty with or without uterine perforation. It would be prudent to inform the patient who will undergo metroplasty of the subsequent risk so that she is knowledgeable and can inform her obstetrician should she become pregnant.

Hysteroscopic Technique

The uterine septum is viewed from the level of the internal cervical os. The endoscope is moved into each chamber of the divided uterine cavity, and the locations of the tubal ostia are noted. The hysteroscope is again withdrawn to a level just above the internal os. The appropriate operating instrument is inserted through the sheath, and the septum is cut from below and upward, as described by March (Fig. 18.22). As the fundus is approached, the operator depends on a signal

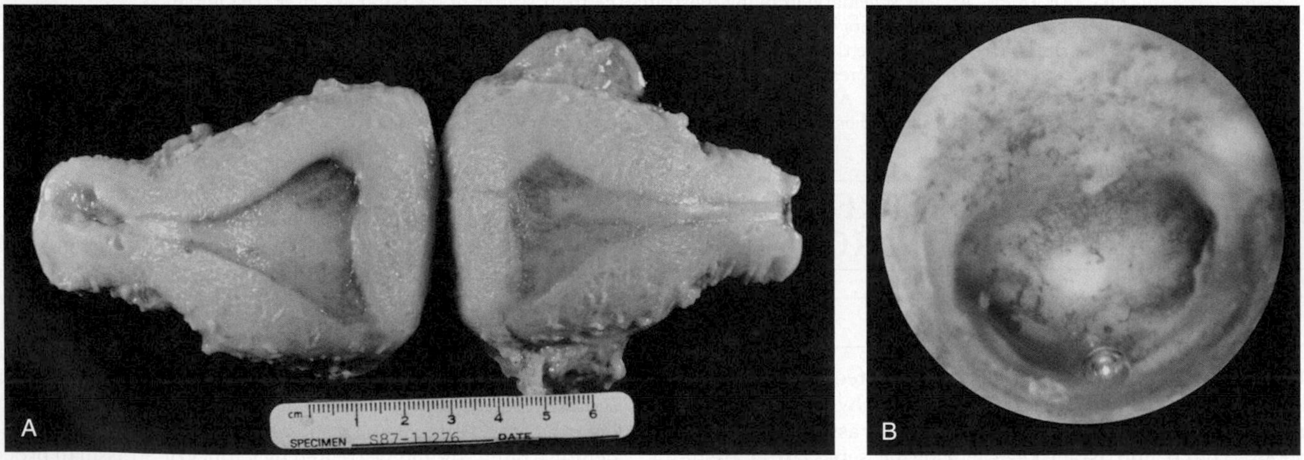

FIGURE 18.21. A: A uterus that is removed at hysterectomy shows the thick walls of the myometrium. These walls average approximately 1.5 cm in thickness, with the exception of the cornu, where the myometrium is thinner. **B:** The uterus is distended with the liquid medium. The walls of the uterus are now much thinner, averaging 0.5 to 1 cm in thickness.

from the assistant to indicate when the quality of the hysteroscope light demonstrates transmission through the intact uterine wall. A dialog between the hysteroscopist and laparoscopist prevents perforation. A new technique permits the operator to scan the uterus ultrasonographically to determine whether the myometrium has been entered and to monitor the amount of space existing between the operating device and the serosal surface of the uterus. It is not necessary to excise the septum completely; incising the septum is quite adequate. Transection eliminates the septum and unites the uterus into a single cavity. We take the opportunity here to stress an important technical point. The surgeon should be aware of the common tendency of the cutting instrument to drift posteriorly and should clip the septum squarely in the middle. When the drift goes unnoticed, the operating instrument invariably cuts into the myometrium and causes pulsatile bleeding. Similarly, correcting the septum too perfectly at the level of the fundus will result in deep penetration into the myometrium and subsequent hemorrhage (Fig. 18.23A–C). If a multichannel hysteroscope is used, a 3-mm ball electrode may be used to coagulate the bleeding vessel. The double-needle bipolar electrode is a safe alternative method for electrocoagulation.

If bleeding does ensue, a Foley catheter with a 10-mL balloon is inserted into the endometrial cavity at the terminus of the operation and inflated to 5 to 6 mL. The pressure exerted by the bag on the uterine walls is sufficient to control the bleeding promptly. The bag is deflated 6 to 12 hours postoperatively and is removed if no further bleeding ensues. Overinflation of a catheter bag can lead to uterine rupture; therefore, one should add increments of water, 1 to 2 mL at a time, to the catheter bag until bleeding ceases. Patients are usually advised to take 2.5 mg of estrogen daily by mouth for 30 days after surgery. Antibiotics are not routinely administered.

Uterine Synechiae

Adhesions form between the anterior and posterior walls of the uterus as a result of trauma or infection in a milieu of estrogen deprivation. Classically, this problem follows an abortion or postpartum hemorrhage, for which a vigorous curettage has been performed to control the bleeding, as reported by March and associates. Friedler and associates report the incidence of adhesions after one abortion to be 16.3%. This figure rises to 32% after three or more abortions. The severity of adhesions also typically rises as the number of abortions increase. Guida and associates reported a significant reduction in the formation of adhesions following sundry hysteroscopic operations via the postoperative instillation of hyaluronic

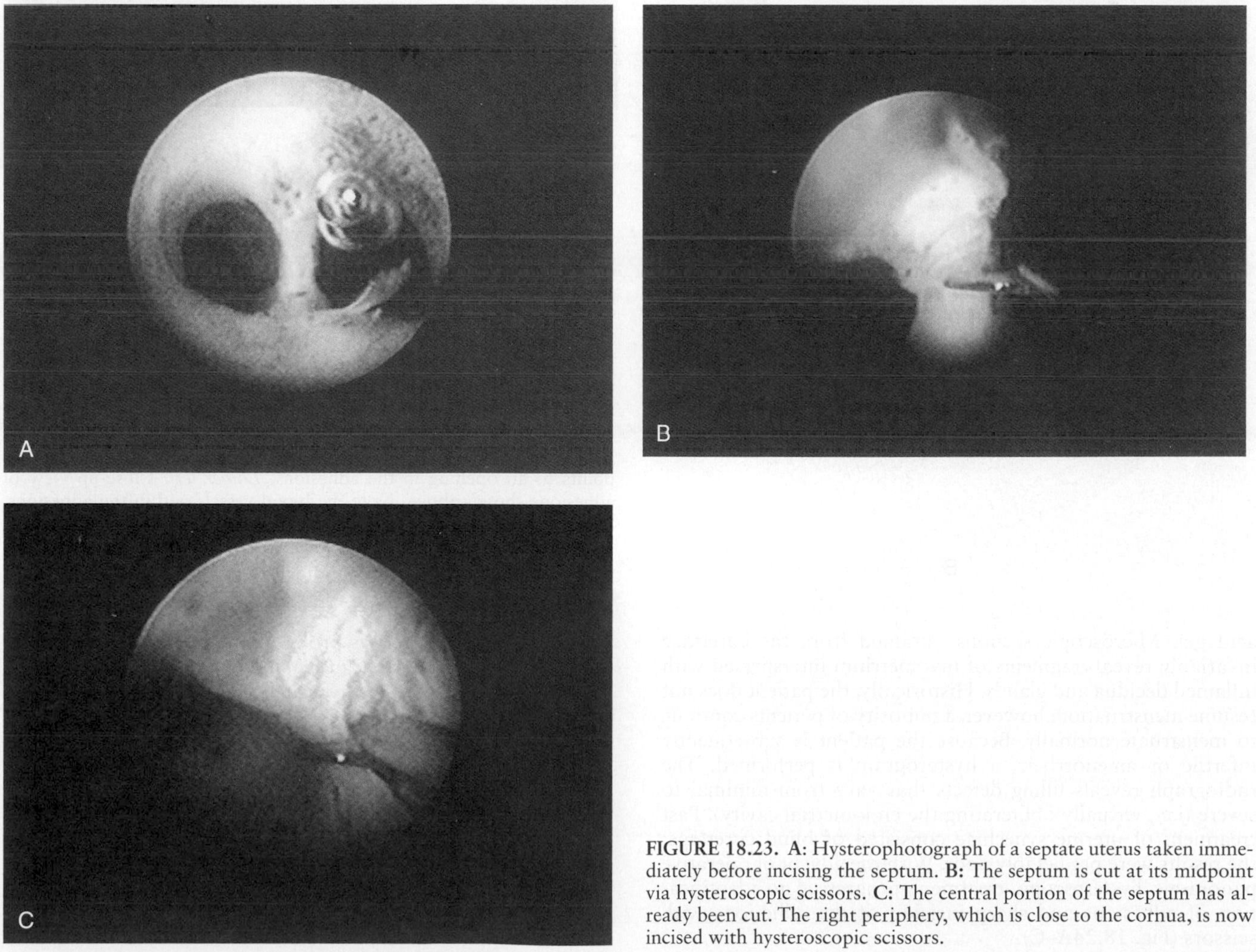

FIGURE 18.23. A: Hysterophotograph of a septate uterus taken immediately before incising the septum. **B:** The septum is cut at its midpoint via hysteroscopic scissors. **C:** The central portion of the septum has already been cut. The right periphery, which is close to the cornua, is now incised with hysteroscopic scissors.

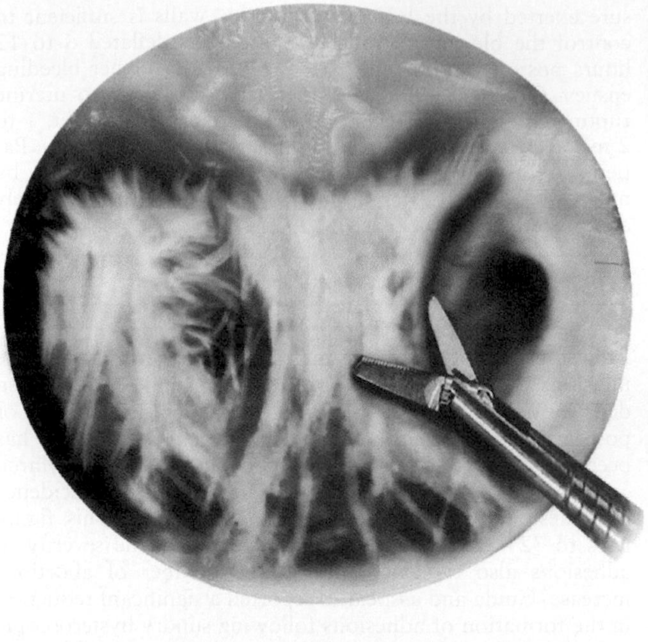

A

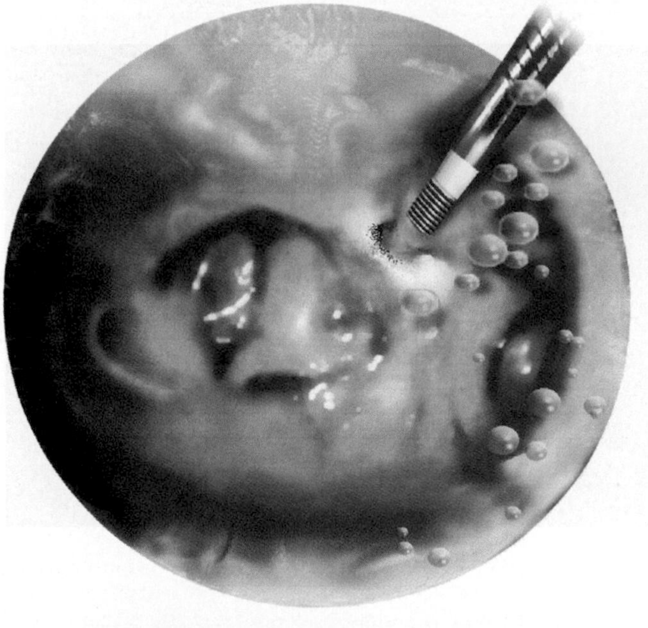

B

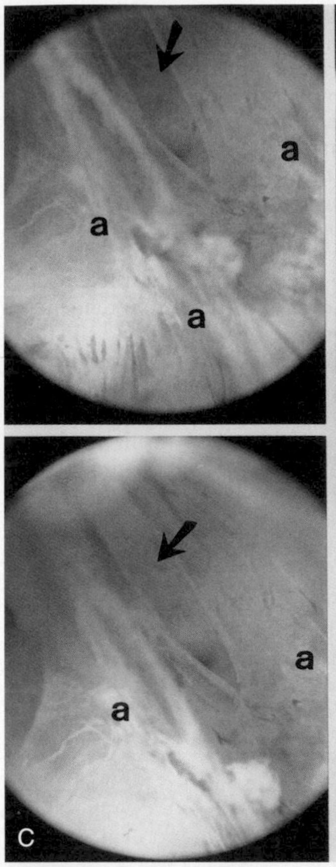

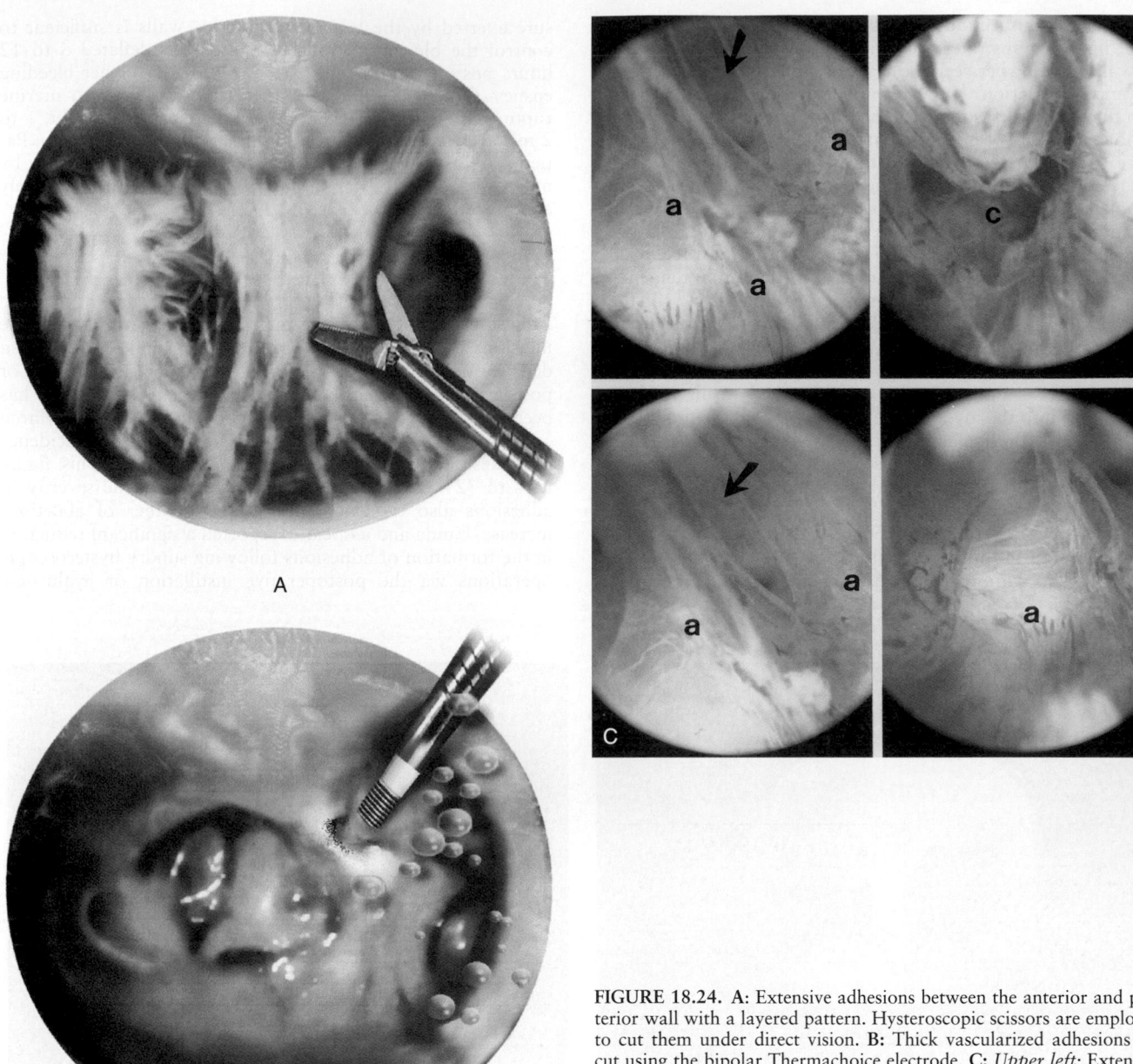

FIGURE 18.24. **A:** Extensive adhesions between the anterior and posterior wall with a layered pattern. Hysteroscopic scissors are employed to cut them under direct vision. **B:** Thick vascularized adhesions are cut using the bipolar Thermachoice electrode. **C:** *Upper left:* Extensive diaphragm-like adhesions cover the cavity of the uterus (*a*). The arrow points to an opening in the adhesions. *Lower left:* Close-up view of adhesions shown above. Note the blood vessels within the adhesions. *Lower right:* Following the incisions into the adhesions shown on the left, another layer was encountered (*upper right*). The latter was cut, exposing the main uterine cavity (*c*).

acid gel. Microscopic sections obtained from the curettage invariably reveal fragments of myometrium interspersed with inflamed decidua and glands. Historically, the patient does not resume menstruation; however, a minority of patients continue to menstruate normally. Because the patient is subsequently infertile or amenorrheic, a hysterogram is performed. The radiograph reveals filling defects that vary from minimal to severe (i.e., virtually obliterating the endometrial cavity). Past treatment of uterine synechiae consisted of blind curettage; the results were predictably poor. With the advent of operative panoramic hysteroscopy, treatment progressed to identification of adhesions and sharp incision of the adhesions with scissors (Fig. 18.24A–C).

Adhesiolysis surgery is probably the most difficult of hysteroscopic operations. Because numerous vascular channels are opened up, the risk of intravascular absorption of the medium is high. Rock and colleagues reported a technique of laparoscopically injecting the uterus with leukomethylene blue dye to help identify the junction at which the anterior and posterior walls were adhered. Capella-Allouc and associates reported 31 cases of severe adhesions that underwent hysteroscopic lysis ranging over 1 to 4 operations. The number of subsequent pregnancies after treatment was 43%, and the live birth rate was 32%. A report from Belgium (2004) of 46 women with Ashermann disease, of whom one third had severe adhesions, described live births as greater than 40%.

Hysteroscopic Technique

A thorough diagnostic hysteroscopy is performed to assess the degree of adhesion formation and deformity of the cavity. Small openings in the curtain of adhesions in which there are flow patterns of tiny blood fragments and tissue debris are helpful and should be sought out, as are any normal anatomic landmarks. Photographs, videotapes, and detailed drawings are helpful reminders in planning the strategy for cutting these adhesions.

Simultaneous laparoscopy is prudent measure to prevent perforation of the uterus. Flexible or semirigid scissors, the resectoscope, Versapoint, and the Nd-YAG laser are the operating instruments of choice, although some operators use the monopolar needle electrode at 40 to 50 W of cutting power, blend 1 or 2. The laser is initially set to deliver 30 to 50 W of power. The medium is instilled into the cavity by way of an operating sheath. Continuous maintenance of distention is one key to success. Filmy and central adhesions should be cut first, always following the fluid flow. Marginal and dense adhesions should be tackled last, always cutting from below and moving upward. A second key to success is to maintain the hysteroscope in midchannel relative to the uterine walls. The cavity can usually be restored to reasonably normal architecture. Bleeding is not uncommon during this operation, particularly when cutting marginal adhesions, because the border between adhesion and myometrium is blurred. Hyskon provides an advantage here.

The patient should be placed on conjugated estrogens, 2.5 mg daily, during postoperative recovery. Placement of an IUD within the cavity to keep the walls from adhering is clearly not based on scientific fact but has been used for so many years that it is standard postoperative measure.

Cannulation of Fallopian Tube

Novy and associates described a technique for passing a special catheter into the tubal ostium and through the obstructed interstitial portion of the tube. The procedure was successful in 92% of the cases. Dumesic and Dhillon reported a tubal cannulation procedure in which they used a flexible guiding insert to facilitate passage of the cornual cannulation catheter. These techniques are useful for treating interstitial obstruction secondary to cellular debris and tubal spasm. The obvious advantage of this cannulation technique is its usefulness in treating cases that might otherwise require tubocornual anastomosis. Pregnancy rates range from 25% to 54% in 6 months.

Hysteroscopic Technique

A 5.5F Teflon cannula with a metal obturator (Cook OB/GYN) is introduced through the operating channel of the hysteroscopic sheath. The obturator is removed. A 3F catheter with a guide cannula wire is introduced into the 5.5F cannula by way of a Y-adapter on the end of the cannula, engaged into the tubal ostium, and gently advanced into the tube. When the cornual portion of the tube is negotiated or when resistance is encountered, the guide wire is withdrawn, and leukomethylene blue or indigo carmine dye injected through the 3F catheter. Simultaneous laparoscopy allows one to see the dye exit the fimbriated end of the tube and confirm patency. Alternatively, one can place a radiologic plate beneath the patient and inject opaque dye (Fig. 18.25).

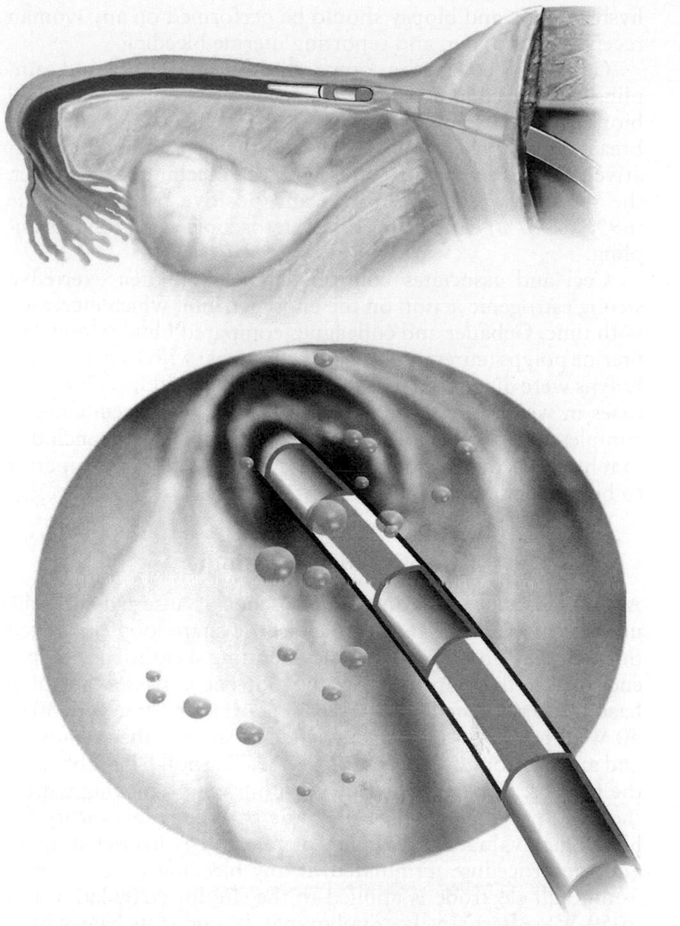

FIGURE 18.25. An inner guide wire is inserted via direct hysteroscopic view into the tubal ostium and advanced. An outer cannula is then advanced over the guide wire. Methylene blue may be injected to demonstrate tube patency to an assistant viewing from above via laparoscopy. (By permission: Baggish MS, Valle RF, Guedj H. *Hysteroscopy: Visual perspectives of uterine anatomy, physiology and pathology.* 3rd ed. Lippincott Williams & Wilkins, 2007.)

Uterine Polyps

Functional and nonfunctional polyps produce intermenstrual bleeding, as reported by Barbot. Functional polyps tend to be smaller than nonfunctional polyps. If a hysterogram is performed, then a focal filling defect will be seen. Diagnosis is directly and readily made by hysteroscopy. Polyps protrude into the endometrial cavity. A functioning polyp has a lining identical to the surrounding endometrium. The nonfunctioning polyp presents as a white protuberance covered with branching surface vessels; thick-walled vessels are usually seen within the depths of the polyps. Polyps are relatively easy to diagnose and similarly to treat.

Endometrial polyps secondary to tamoxifen therapy in women undergoing treatment for breast cancer is a problem for which hysteroscopy may prove to be indispensable. Taponeco and colleagues reported on 414 breast cancer patients who underwent hysteroscopy (334 treated with tamoxifen and 80 controls). Significant differences were found in malignant (7.8%) and atypical (9%) hyperplastic polypi between the treated group versus controls (0 cases). The authors recommended that hysteroscopy and biopsy should be performed on any woman receiving tamoxifen and reporting uterine bleeding.

Garuti and colleagues compared the accuracy of blind sampling of the endometrium versus hysteroscopically directed biopsies in postmenopausal women receiving tamoxifen for breast cancer. The authors reported that sensitivity and negative predictive value of 100% with each technique. However, the specificity (80% vs. 68%) and positive predictive value (69% vs. 43%) were better for hysteroscopic versus blind sampling.

Ceci and associates confirmed that tamoxifen exerted a strong estrogenic action on the endometrium, which increased with time. Gebauer and colleagues compared blind removal of uterine polyps (curettage and polyp forceps) with hysteroscopy. Polyps were diagnosed in 43% of cases by curettage. Out of 45 cases in which polyp forceps removed the polyp remnants or complete polyps remained in 31 cases. The authors concluded that hysteroscopically controlled polyp extraction was superior to blind techniques.

Hysteroscopic Technique

A multichannel operating hysteroscope is inserted into the uterine cavity, and a retractable electric snare loop is inserted through the 3-mm channel of the operating sheath. The polyp is encircled by the loop such that the loop encompasses the polyp base as it is tightened. The polyp is cut off at the base with 30 to 40 W of power for cutting current. The snare is then removed, and an alligator jaw forceps is inserted. The polyp is grabbed by the forceps. The hysteroscope is withdrawn, removing with it the freed polyp, which is sent to the pathology laboratory for histologic evaluation. The site of removal is inspected again and the procedure terminated. If any bleeding is observed, a 3-mm ball electrode is applied to the site for coagulation (40 to 50 W). Alternatively, a polyp may be cut at its base with a needle electrode or laser fiber. The polyp may also be shaved by means of the resectoscope (Fig. 18.26).

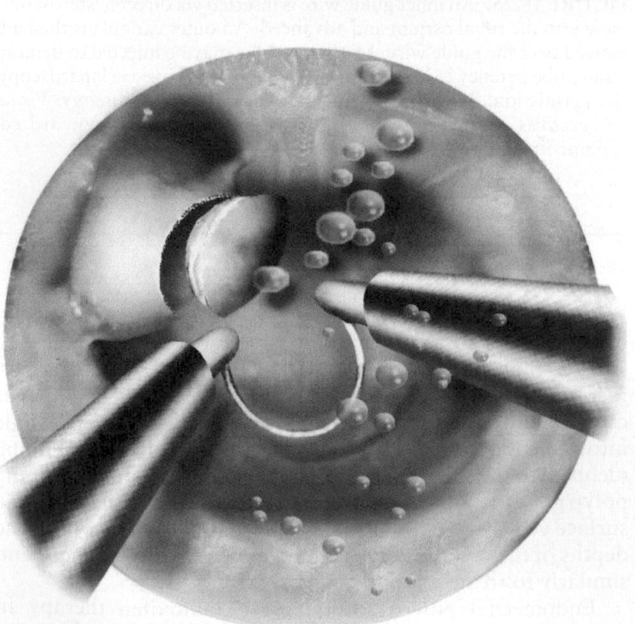

FIGURE 18.26. A functioning polyp on the right corpal wall of the uterus is resected by means of a resectoscopic loop electrode. Note that the technique is the same as the one employed for shaving a submucous myoma. (By permission: Baggish MS, Valle RF, Guedj H. *Hysteroscopy: Visual perspectives of uterine anatomy, physiology and pathology.* 3rd ed. Lippincott Williams & Wilkins, 2007.)

Myomata Uteri

Submucous myomas characteristically appear as white spherical masses covered with a network of fragile thin-walled vessels when viewed by hysteroscopy. Myomas typically are sessile or pedunculated. A hysterogram shows a filling defect that is not dissimilar to that produced by a polyp. Unfortunately, blind D&C is a grossly inaccurate method of diagnosing this disorder. Although subserous and intramural myomas rarely produce alarming symptoms, even when they attain relatively large size, smaller lesions in the submucous location invariably cause considerable bleeding. Additionally, submucous myomas are commonly associated with chronic endometritis, which interferes with implantation of the fertilized ovum and become a contributing factor to subfertility.

In the past, a diagnosis of submucous myoma was usually followed by a recommendation for hysterectomy. Today, hysteroscopic surgery offers a therapeutic alternative to that radical approach. Various regimens of drug therapy (e.g., danazol [Danocrine] and gonadotropin-releasing hormone [GnRH] analogs such as leuprolide acetate [Lupron] or goserelin acetate [Zoladex]) have been recommended as supplementary preoperative medical therapy. The general plan is to treat symptomatic patients for 2 to 3 months preoperatively to reduce the size and vascularity of the lesion during surgery. All patients should be given detailed information concerning the need for typing and holding of blood and the possibility of hysterectomy if intractable bleeding occurs.

Valle (1990) reported data on 59 cases of abnormal bleeding, dysmenorrhea, and infertility that were diagnosed as submucous myomas. Hysteroscopy eliminated or markedly decreased bleeding in 52 of these cases. Baggish and Sze treated 71 patients with symptomatic myomas and four patients with incidental submucous myomas. The treatment methods used with the multichannel hysteroscope were Nd-YAG laser (n = 41), monopolar loop (n = 6), monopolar needle (n = 6), bipolar needles (n = 10), and electrosurgery or scissors and laser (n = 12). As with Valle's series, results were excellent; 65 of 75 (87%) returned to normal menses postoperatively. Barbot and Parent (personal communication, 1994) performed resectoscopic myomectomies in 825 women, of whom 83% were relieved of abnormal bleeding and suffered no recurrence.

Litta et al described a technique of not only resecting the submucous component but continuing hysteroscopic resectoscopic cutting into the myometrium to remove more myomatous tissue. We do not resect into the myometrium because the risks of severe hemorrhage, perforation, and subsequent dehiscence are increased.

Emanuel and colleagues reported 285 women who underwent hysteroscopic resection of submucous myomas. The median follow-up was approximately 4 years (1–104 months), and 85.5% of the operated patients required no further surgery.

Clark and associates treated 37 women using the bipolar Versapoint electrode via ablation or excision. Improvement of bleeding symptoms was reported in 78% of the patients, and 92% were satisfied with the treatment. No significant complications were reported.

Hysteroscopic Technique

Several variations of hysteroscopic procedures are now available to manage submucous myomas. Current resectoscopic techniques differ little from those described by Neuwirth (1978) and by DeCherney and Polan. However, the resectoscopic instrumentation has vastly improved compared with those earlier instruments. Self-flushing sheaths, straight and offset cutting loops, and diminished-diameter, low-profile scopes are among these recent improvements. In addition, electrosurgical generators have been modernized and are safer devices than instruments from the 1970s and 1980s (Fig. 18.27). Under video control, the resectoscopic technique consists of progressive shaving of the myoma and harvesting the pieces of tissue for subsequent histologic evaluation. For fundal myomas, the straight electrode is the most effective device, whereas the angulated electrode is preferred for lesions located on the anterior or posterior walls (Fig. 18.28A). (The electrode should be activated only while returning toward the hysteroscope, never while advancing outward away from the lens.) The greatest disadvantage to this technique centers on the needs to repeatedly remove the shaved nuggets of tissue (Fig. 18.28B).

The four Nd-YAG laser techniques described by Baggish and associates (1999) use power levels of 30 to 60 W. The first uses a hysteroscopic needle inserted through the operating channel, through which about 5 to 10 mL of 1:100 vasopressin solution (1 mL vasopressin in 99 mL sterile water) is injected into the myoma. The conical, sculpted, 1-mm laser fiber is brought into contact with the myoma to cut across its base. Scissors can be combined with the laser to free the myoma from its base. The myoma is extracted intact by way of the cervical canal. This technique is useful for myomas up to 3 cm in diameter. The second Nd-YAG technique uses a 1-mm ball of sculpted fiber that is drawn over the myoma multiple times for ablation of the myoma until it is level and flat in relation to the surrounding endometrium. This technique is used for 1- to 2-cm myomas. The third technique is similar to that used with the resectoscope. Layer upon layer of the myoma is sliced off until the base is reached. The fourth technique is used for a large (2- to 5-cm) lesion. The laser is used to devascularize the myoma by making multiple punctures into its substance. The large myoma can then be quartered with laser and extracted piece by piece (Fig. 18.29). These same laser techniques can be performed with monopolar and bipolar electrosurgical electrodes to either resect or ablate myomas.

Other electrosurgical techniques may be employed in conjunction with the large isolated-channel, flushing hysteroscope. Three-mm needles, shaving loops, and bipolar electrodes may be used to perform all of the optional operations described above for the resectoscope and laser. The fine-needle electrode can be substituted for laser fiber to excise pedunculated or section sessile myomas. The 3-mm retractable cutting loop can perform shaving procedures in a fashion similar to that of the resectoscope loop. The bipolar needles can be plunged many times into the substance of the submucous myoma of any size to coagulate the interior of the myoma (myolysis).

If postoperative bleeding occurs, a 10-mL Foley balloon is placed in the cavity and blown up to 5 mL for 6 to 12 hours. If the cavity is large, a 30-mL balloon inflated with 10 to 15 mL of water can be used. We prefer to do a simultaneous laparoscopy when large myomas (3- to 5-cm) are resected and extracted. Regardless of myoma size, a simultaneous laparoscopy should be performed whenever concern for perforation exists. The central fundal myoma is associated with the greatest risk of uterine perforation.

Reports caution that uterine rupture can occur during pregnancy after hysteroscopic myomectomy. This is particularly the case when the operator attempts to resect the intramural portion of the submucous myoma.

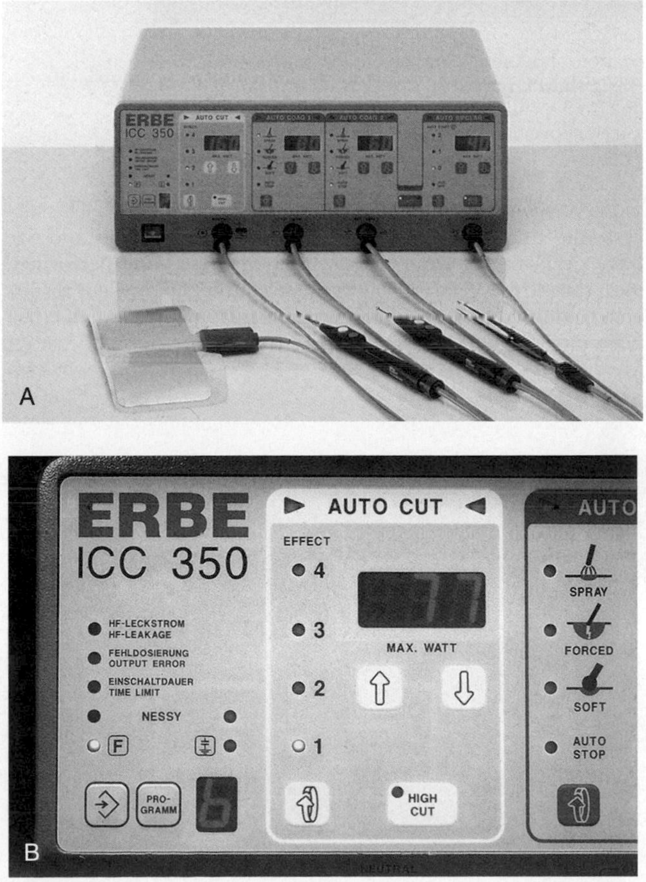

FIGURE 18.27. A: A modern, state-of-the-art, computerized, constant-voltage electrosurgical generator. This apparatus is divided into cut, coagulation, monopolar, and bipolar functions. It incorporates numerous and sophisticated safety features. **B:** Close-up of the electrosurgical generator panel. The high cut feature is for bipolar cutting (vaporization).

Endometrial Ablation

More than 600,000 hysterectomies are performed annually in the United States, although the advent and growth of integrated health care will target this largely elective operation for reduction because of its substantial cost. The numbers will be further reduced because 40% of hysterectomies are unnecessary and 20% show no pathology; hence, cheaper alternatives are continuously sought. According to a recent study of hysterectomy by the New York State Department of Health, 30,065 hysterectomies were performed in that state during 1986, 10% of which were performed for the principal diagnosis of disorders of menstruation. A very large recent study from the United Kingdom (2005) observed that 16,100 out of a total of 37,298 hysterectomies were performed for dysfunctional uterine bleeding. Endometrial ablation or resection is the hysteroscopic alternative to hysterectomy as treatment for abnormal uterine bleeding. Two earlier reports by Droegemueller and colleagues describe blind procedures such as cryocoagulation that were used in an attempt to control dysfunctional uterine bleeding by creating physical destruction of the endometrium without sacrificing the uterus. Unfortunately, either the techniques themselves were associated with significant side effects or the endometrium promptly regenerated.

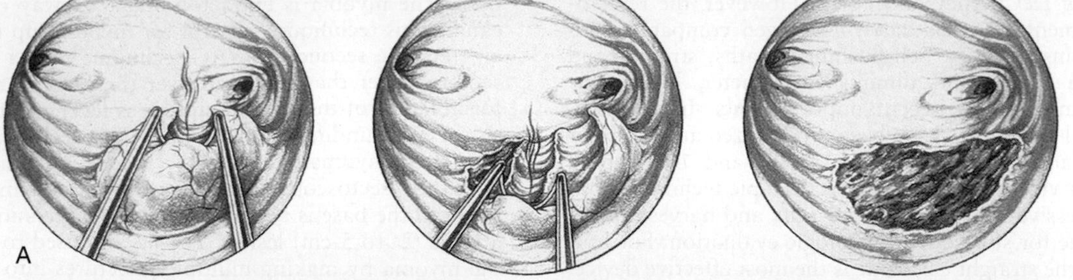

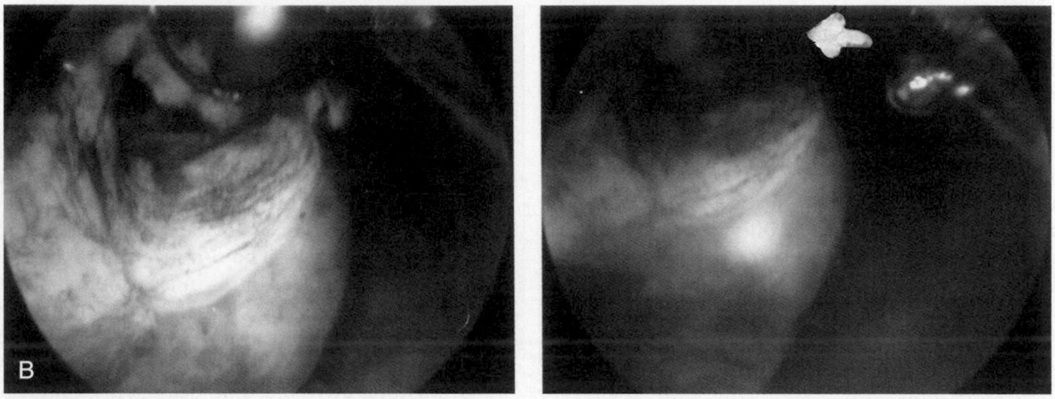

FIGURE 18.28. **A:** The shaving technique for the elimination of a submucous myoma is shown using an angulated loop electrode via the resectoscope. (From Baggish MS, Barbot J, Valle RF. *Diagnostic and operative hysteroscopy.* 2nd ed. St. Louis: Mosby-Year Book, 1999, with permission.) **B:** A chunk of tissue has been cut out of this myoma. The resectoscopic loop is seen above (*left*). The picture to the right shows the loop extended farther into the cavity (*arrow*).

Since the first practical method of hysteroscopic ablation was described in 1981, several thousand cases have been performed by a variety of techniques, including the Nd-YAG laser, the resectoscopic roller ball or loop, and, most recently, the long hysteroscopic ball electrodes. Garry and associates (1995) reported 600 endometrial laser ablations performed on 524 women. No major operative morbidity was reported. The success rate (mean age, 43 years) was 83.4%. Baggish and Sze have performed 568 ablations; 401 of these were performed with the Nd-YAG laser, 167 by electrosurgery. Excellent results were obtained in 89% of the women treated, and amenorrhea was achieved in 58%. Again, no major operative complications

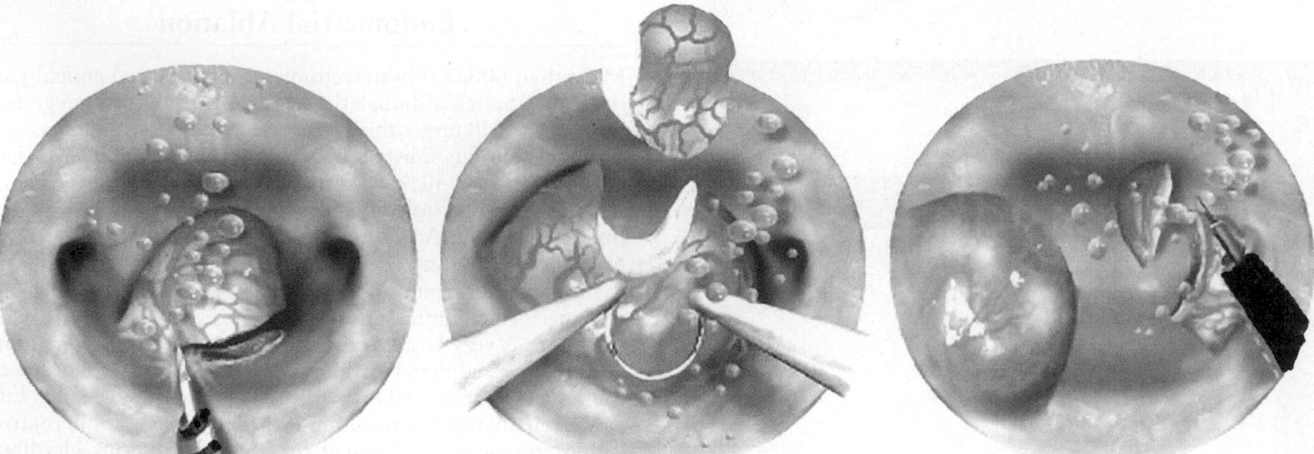

FIGURE 18.29. **A–C:** Several techniques and instruments may be used to deal with submucous myomas. **A:** shows a laser fiber within an irrigation cannula cutting a myoma at its base. **B:** shows an electrode shaving a myoma. **C:** shows an electrosurgical needle cleaving a piece of a submucous myoma. (By permission: Baggish MS, Valle RF, Guedj H. *Hysteroscopy: Visual perspectives of uterine anatomy, physiology and pathology.* 3rd ed. Lippincott Williams & Wilkins, 2007.)

were observed. Magos and co-workers reported 250 cases of endometrial resection with a 92% improvement in abnormal bleeding. However, data obtained from the Royal College of Obstetricians and Gynaecologist's Mistletoe (Minimally Invasive Surgical Technique Laser, Endothermal or Endoresection) Study in 1997 revealed a 6.4% rate of significant complications associated with endometrial resection alone and a rate of 11.4/1,000 with emergency hysterectomy. This compares with complication rates of 2.7% and 2.1% for laser and roller ball, respectively. The latter two techniques had emergency hysterectomy rates of 1.3/1,000 (i.e., 11 times less than endometrial resection).

Two large controlled, randomized studies compared hysterectomy with hysteroscopic ablation/resection. Dwyer and colleagues prospectively compared 100 cases of endometrial resection and 100 cases of abdominal hysterectomy for menorrhagia. Postoperative morbidity, length of hospital stay, time to return to work, normal daily activities, and sexual intercourse were significantly lower for the endometrial resection group. Dysmenorrheic premenstrual symptoms were significantly higher in the endometrial resection group. Pinion and associates randomized 204 patients to abdominal or vaginal hysterectomy ($n = 99$), endometrial laser ablation ($n = 53$), or endometrial resection ($n = 52$). Women treated by ablation or resection had less morbidity and a shorter recovery time. After 12 months, 89% of the hysterectomy group and 78% of the hysteroscopy group were very satisfied with the effect of surgery; 95% in the first group and 90% in the second reported acceptable improvement in symptoms. Equal numbers in each group stated that they would recommend the same operation to others. Mints and colleagues reported on 104 premenopausal women who underwent endometrial resection (1990–1995) with a mean follow-up period of 29 months: 21% reported amenorrhea postoperatively; 51% described minimal bleeding; 11% reported the postoperative onset of dysmenorrhea; and 12.5% underwent subsequent hysterectomy. Seidman and associates reported higher rates of amenorrhea in women older than 45 years of age. Lefler reported a telephone survey following resectoscopic resection followed by ball electrode ablation for 109/117 women. He reported 55% amenorrhea, 19% reduced menses, and 16% subsequent hysterectomy rate. Sowter and colleagues performed a metaanalysis about preoperative administration of agents producing endometrial atrophy before hysteroscopy surgery. The use of GnRH analogues was associated with shorter operative times, greater rates of amenorrhea, and reduced dysmenorrhea. GnRH produced more consistent atrophy than danazol or progestogens. Several published reports confirm the cost-effectiveness and efficacy of endometrial ablation for the control of abnormal uterine bleeding compared with hysterectomy. Hidlebaugh and Orr evaluated the long-term economic aspects of hysteroscopic ablation versus hysterectomy for dysfunctional uterine bleeding. Long-term direct and indirect costs of ablation were $5,959 versus $11,777 for hysterectomy.

Hysteroscopic Technique

All patients who might be candidates for endometrial ablation should have been managed first by hormonal treatment in an attempt to control the abnormal uterine bleeding. If this strategy

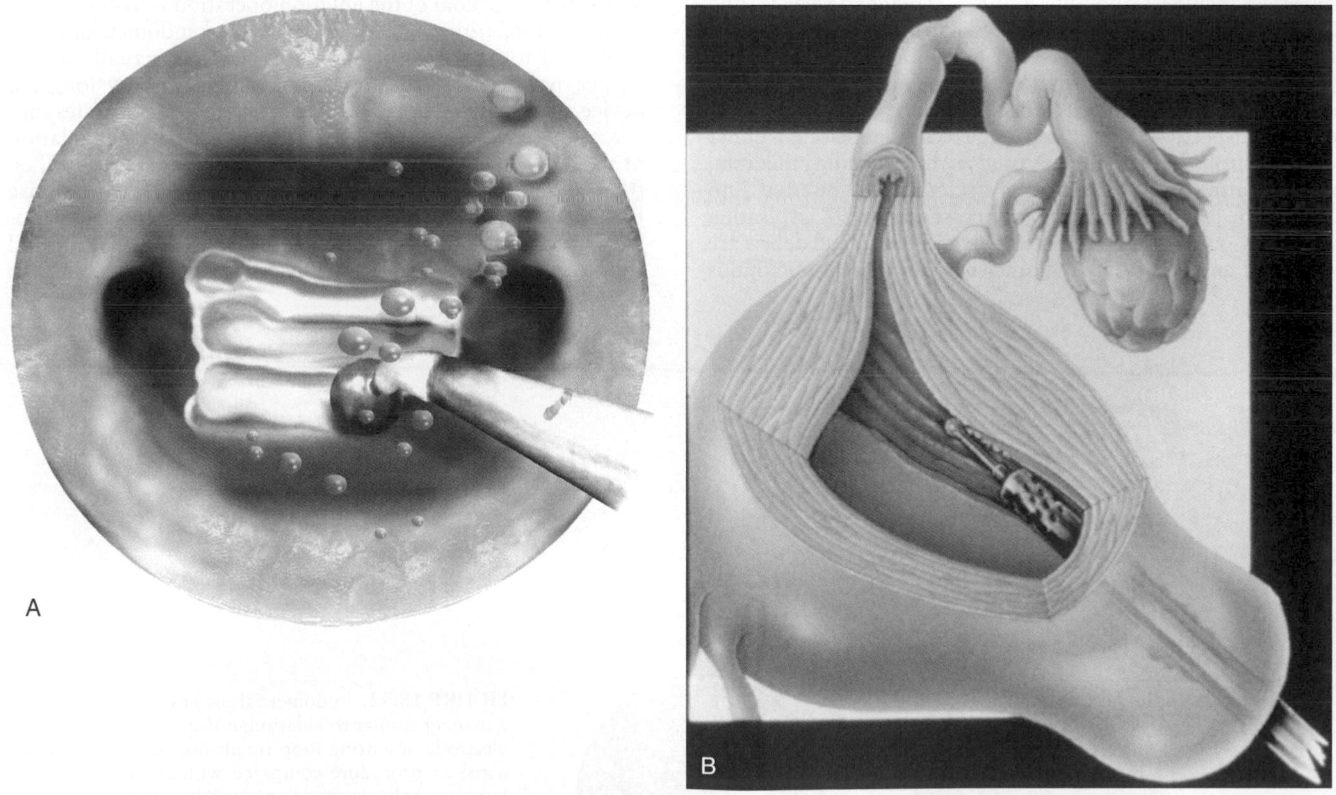

FIGURE 18.30. A: The ball electrode is dragged from side to side via moving the entire hysteroscope, thereby ablating the uterine fundus. **B:** The anterior and posterior walls are ablated by dragging the energized ball electrode from above downward. This creates 2- to 3-mm furrows in the endometrium. Conduction heat damage can extend another 1 to 2 mm. (By permission: Baggish MS, Valle RF, Guedj H. *Hysteroscopy: Visual perspectives of uterine anatomy, physiology and pathology.* 3rd ed. Lippincott Williams & Wilkins, 2007.)

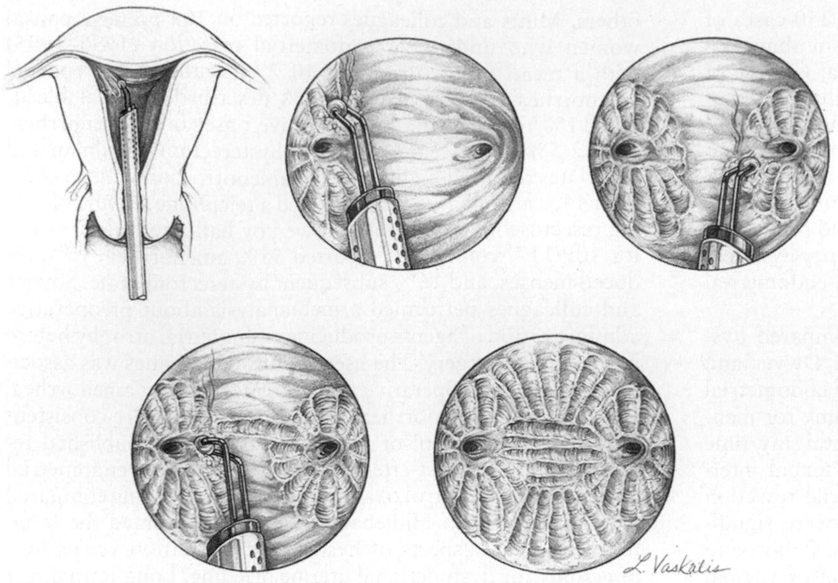

FIGURE 18.31. The resectoscope with ball electrode attached is inserted into the uterine cavity. Initially, the cornu and fundus are carefully ablated, taking care to keep dwell time low to reduce the risk of deep heat-conduction injury. Next, the anterior wall is ablated, followed by the posterior wall. (By permission: Baggish MS, Valle RF, Guedj H. *Hysteroscopy: Visual perspectives of uterine anatomy, physiology and pathology.* 3rd ed. Lippincott Williams & Wilkins, 2007.)

fails, and if the woman does not desire to bear children, then she is a candidate for endometrial ablation. A preoperative diagnostic hysteroscopy, endometrial sampling, or both should be performed to exclude endometrial carcinoma or atypical hyperplasia, and all pertinent hematologic studies and consultations should be performed. All patients are pretreated to atrophy the endometrium. The drugs available to accomplish this effect include Danocrine, Lupron, Zoladex, Megace, and Depo-Provera. It is our experience that the best endometrial suppression is seen after 6 weeks of drug therapy.

A simultaneous laparoscopy is not performed during endometrial ablation unless a perforation or other transmural injury is suspected. Depending on the technique selected, either 5% mannitol or 0.9% saline is used as the distending medium. The operating hysteroscope or resectoscope is inserted into the uterine cavity. With the hysteroscope, a 9F aspirating cannula (Cook OB/GYN) is inserted, and blood and debris are evacuated until the cavity is clear. We prefer to treat the fundus by dragging the laser fiber or the ball electrode from side to side (cornu to cornu) (Fig. 18.30A). The anterior and lateral walls are ablated next, before the posterior wall. Ablation should not be extended below the internal os into the cervix (Fig. 18.30B). Power settings for the electrosurgical generator range from 50 to 150 W, depending on the size of the ball, barrel, or loop electrode (Figs. 18.31 and 18.32). Laser power is set at 40 to 60 W. The goal of the ablation operation is to destroy the visible endometrium, including the cornual endometrium, to a depth of 1 to 2 mm. The conduction heat will actually spread deeper, usually to 3 to 5 mm, depending on how long the device remained on the tissue. This penetration translates into extensive superficial myometrial destruction and coagulation of the radial branches of the uterine cavity (Fig. 18.33). When the endometrium sloughs, regeneration is prevented because basal and spiral arterioles do not survive the 100°C heat exposure. Over a period of 6 to 8 weeks, the uterine walls scar and shrink. Subsequent sampling or hysteroscopy is possible after

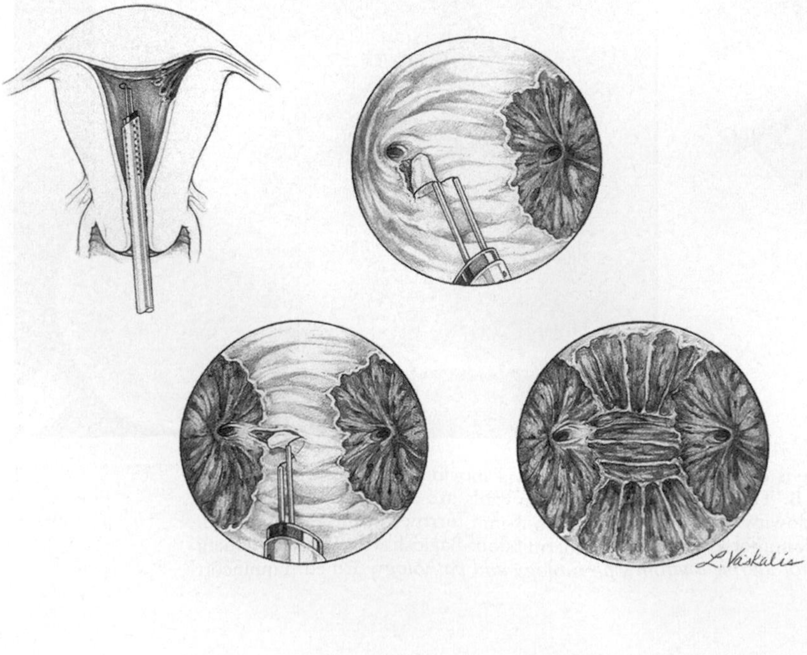

FIGURE 18.32. Endometrial resection is performed in a manner similar to ablation; however, instead of a ball electrode, a cutting loop is substituted. This is clearly a riskier procedure compared with ablation by either laser or ball electrode, particularly relative to deep myometrial resection with the accompanying risks of hemorrhage and/or perforation. (By permission: Baggish MS, Valle RF, Guedj H. *Hysteroscopy: Visual perspectives of uterine anatomy, physiology and pathology.* 3rd ed. Lippincott Williams & Wilkins, 2007.)

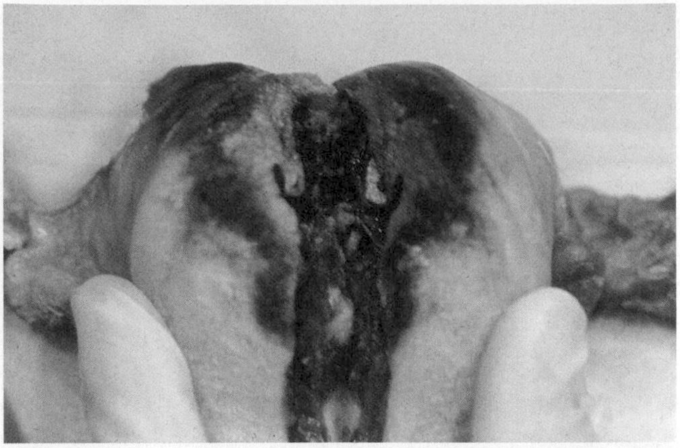

FIGURE 18.33. The uterus was removed 5 days after a Nd-YAG laser ablation. Note the extensive laser injury involving about half the thickness of the myometrium. Laser penetration depends not only on power but also on the length of time the laser beam remains in contact with the tissue.

endometrial ablation. The mean duration of the operation is about 30 minutes. Patients usually are sent home on the day of surgery. The operation is usually completed with little or no blood loss (Fig. 18.34A–C).

Nonhysteroscopic Minimally Invasive Techniques for Endometrial Ablation

Although these new techniques are not hysteroscopic in the strictest sense, they are nonetheless closely related and should be included in this chapter. The basis for these methods encompass the following logic:

1. Removal of the skill factor as a variable for endometrial ablation
2. Elimination of requirement for a distending medium
3. Reduction in the time required to perform the operation
4. Equivalency of efficacy compared with hysteroscopic ablation
5. Performance in an office setting

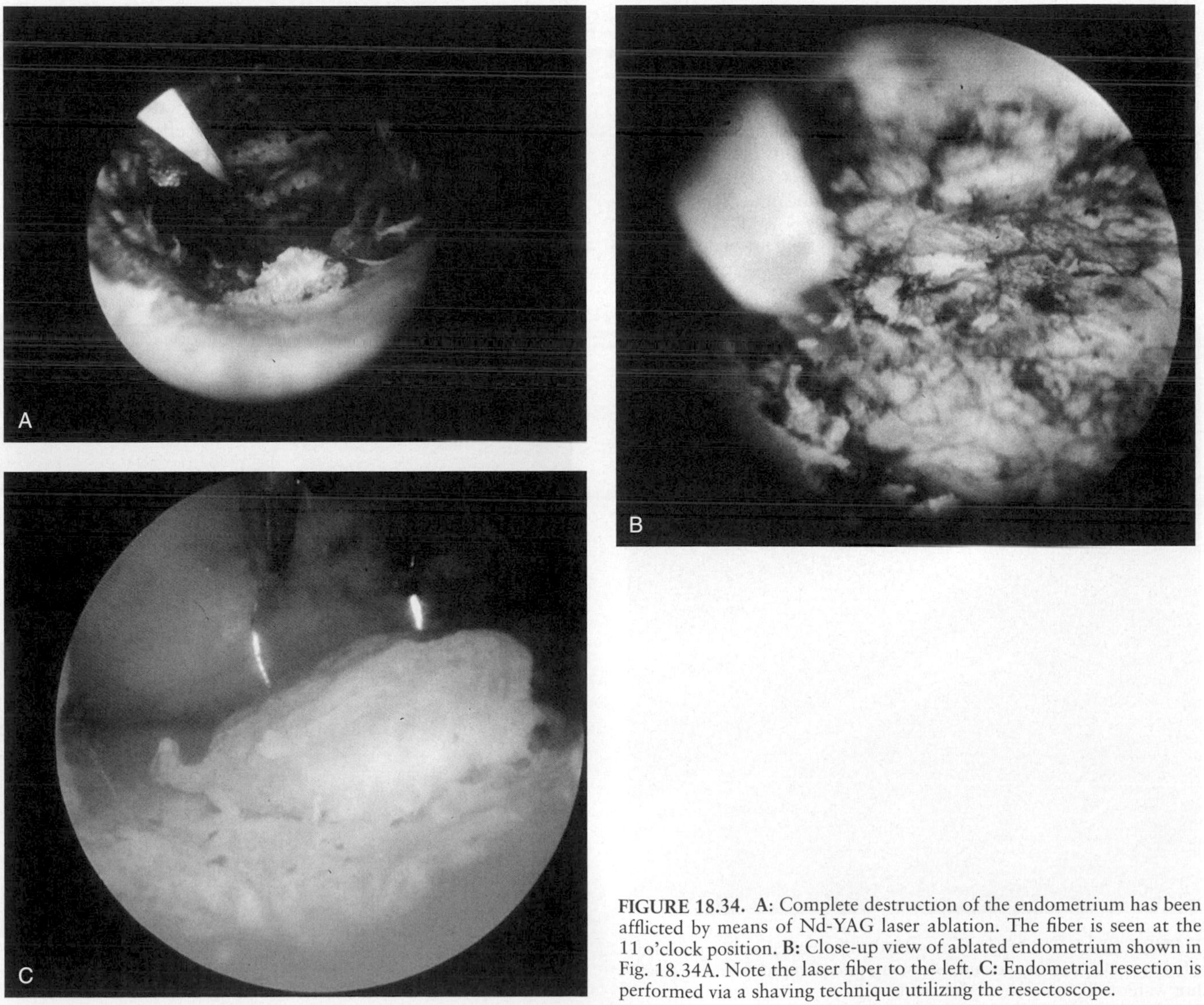

FIGURE 18.34. A: Complete destruction of the endometrium has been afflicted by means of Nd-YAG laser ablation. The fiber is seen at the 11 o'clock position. **B:** Close-up view of ablated endometrium shown in Fig. 18.34A. Note the laser fiber to the left. **C:** Endometrial resection is performed via a shaving technique utilizing the resectoscope.

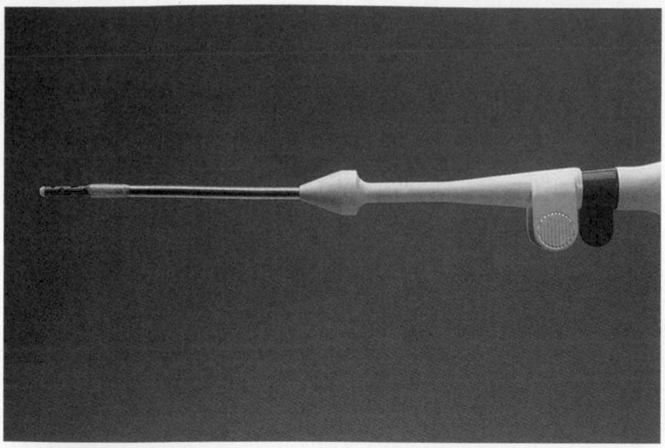

FIGURE 18.35. Innerdyne (Tyco) "Enable" cannula. The terminal mushroom fitting and the acorn seal the cervix and isolate the corpal cavity from the cervical canal. The apparatus contains an *in situ* heater and thermistors.

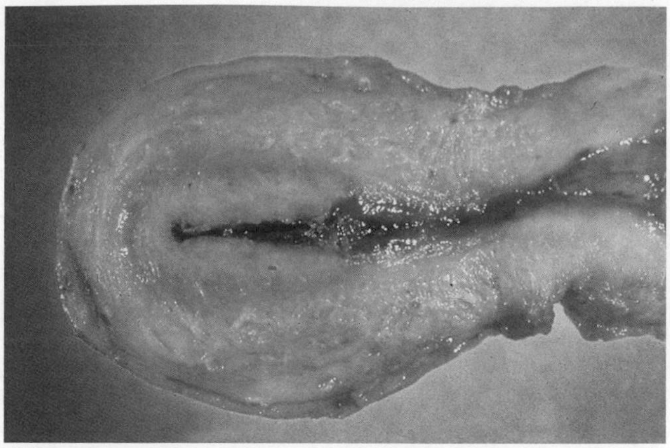

FIGURE 18.37. Hemiresection of a uterus removed at hysterectomy after "Enable" 15-minute ablation. Notice the brown, "cooked" appearance of the endometrium. See color version of figure.

The first practical technique described by Phipps and colleagues used a microwave technique of heating the endometrium by a probe inserted into the uterine cavity, exposing the endometrium to temperatures of 60°C to 65°C for 15 minutes. Thijssen reported a large multicenter study using the technique. The report described a number of serious complications, including fistula formation and third-degree burn injuries. Several techniques using balloons containing hot water, balloons covered with monopolar electrodes, computerized continuously circulating *in situ* hot saline, and cryosurgical and photochemical techniques have been reported (Figs. 18.35 to 18.37). One of the first devices approved for the marketplace was the Thermachoice balloon apparatus (Ethicon Inc., Somerville, NJ), which was developed by Neuwirth. A cannula fitted with a thermal balloon is placed in the uterine cavity (Fig. 18.38). Sterile water distends the balloon and is heated *in situ* to 80°C to 90°C. Thermistors mounted on the balloon give a continuous readout of temperature within the uterine cavity. NaDH diaphorase staining showed destruction to a depth of 3.3 to 5 mm. The published data show efficacy to be lower than that for hysteroscopic ablation and cost to be no less than that for hysteroscopic ablation. The dream of an office-based procedure has not yet been realized.

Since the publication of the last edition of this book, several additional ablation devices have obtained approval

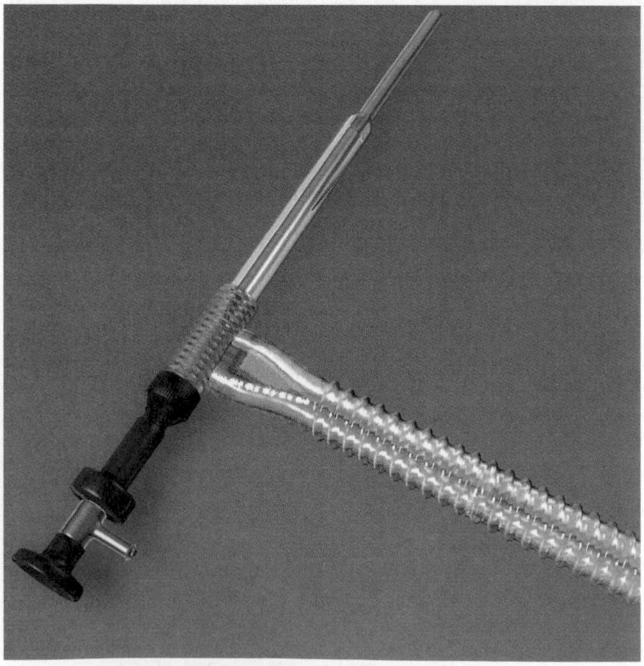

FIGURE 18.36. The HTA System (Hydrothermablator, Boston Scientific) uses a hysteroscope and reservoir system to pump and circulate hot water (saline) in the uterine cavity.

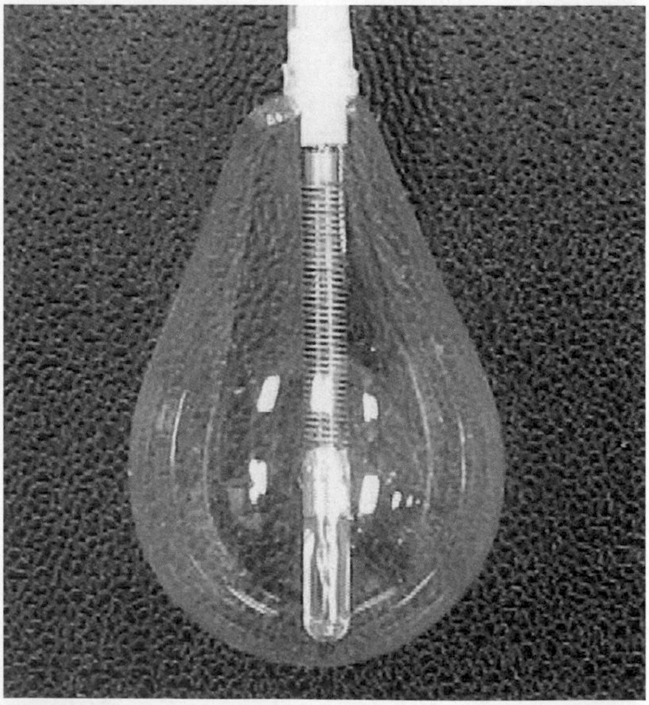

FIGURE 18.38. Close-up view of inflated thermal balloon. Note the *in situ* coil, which heats the water within the balloon.

from the U.S. Food and Drug Administration, including HTA system (Hydro-Therm Ablation), Cavaterm, Novasure, and microwave. Cooper and colleagues published data comparing the Novasure device versus roller-ball ablation. Abbott and associates compared the Cavaterm and Novasure devices at 6 and 12 months relative to accomplishing amenorrhea/hypomenorrhea in menorrhagic women and found comparable results between the two systems. Glasser and Zimmerman evaluated the HTA system in women with irregular cavities (12- to 20-month follow-up). Corson compared the HTA system in 187 cases with resectoscopic ball ablation in 89 cases. Success rates were 77% for HTA and 82% for roller ball. Amenorrhea at 12 months was observed in 40% HTA and 51% roller ball. Loffer and Grainger reported 5-year follow-up data comparing the Thermachoice uterine balloon with roller-ball ablation for control and abnormal (dysfunctional) uterine bleeding; 255 cases were treated, follow-up was available for 147 cases, and 25 cases required additional therapy to control the bleeding. Fifty-eight balloon treated and 59 roller-ball treated reported normal or less bleeding (out of 147 interviewed cases). Baggish and Savells recently published data (2007) on complications with the HTA, Novasure, Thermachoice microwave devices.

Miscellaneous Procedures

Intrauterine Device Removal

Although the number of IUD insertions has diminished over recent years, the gynecologist is occasionally called on to search for and remove a device with an indicator string that is not seen in the cervix. In such circumstances, the operating hysteroscope is a vital tool with which to locate the device and remove it under direct vision, according to Valle and colleagues. The hysteroscope is inserted, and the device is viewed. If a string is seen, an alligator-jaw forceps is inserted, and the string is grasped. The hysteroscope is withdrawn, pulling the device through the uterine cavity and the cervix to the exterior. If the IUD is embedded, then a rigid grasping forceps is required. The IUD is located, and the large jaws of the rigid instrument grab the extruded portion of the IUD itself. Strong pressure is exerted on the jaws as the sheath of the hysteroscope is slowing withdrawn from the uterus, into the cervix, and out of the vagina.

Biopsy of Intrauterine Lesions

When a tumor is suspected, the operative hysteroscope is inserted into the cavity, a 9F biopsy forceps is directed to the tumor site, and multiple biopsy specimens are obtained in a fashion analogous to that used with colposcopic biopsies. A 9F plastic cannula is inserted by way of the operating channel, and strong suction is applied to the mouth of the cannula by means of a 30-mL syringe. The cannula is removed, and the contents are flushed out with saline into a bottle of fixative. Similarly, a 9F curette can be inserted under direct vision. Alternatively, a diagnostic hysteroscope can be inserted into the uterus. The site of pathology is noted. The endoscope is withdrawn, a Novak curette is inserted into the cavity, and biopsy specimens are taken at the previously located site. Finally, the hysteroscope is pulled back to the level of the internal cervical os, a small Novak curette is inserted alongside the hysteroscope, and a directed biopsy specimen is obtained.

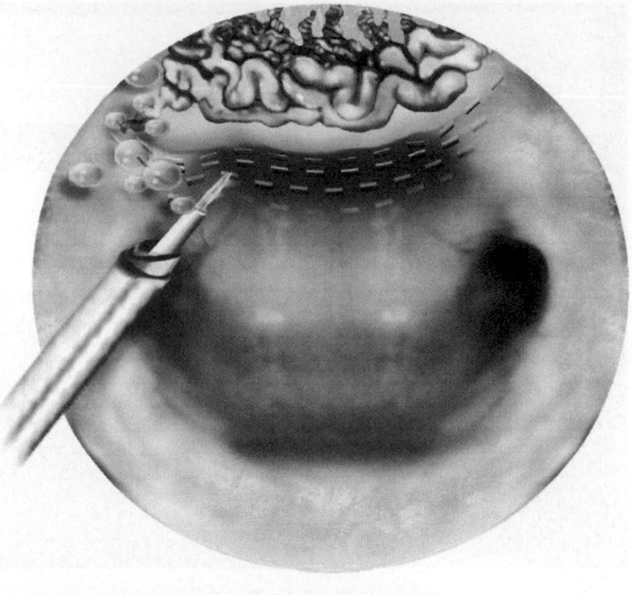

FIGURE 18.39. A vascular malformation is illustrated here. Large, coiled, abnormal vessels are seen in the myometrium. The dotted lines indicate the pulsatile downward movement of the anterior wall that is produced by the vascular malformation. A Nd-YAG laser fiber is in position to coagulate the vessels by a "front-scatter" laser action.

Hemangiomas and Arteriovenous Malformations

Hemangiomas and arteriovenous malformations can be diagnosed by their characteristic hysteroscopic appearance and by a history of massive unresponsive bleeding. Historically, women with these conditions are young and of low parity. Hysteroscopic examination shows the subsurface of the endometrium to be covered with irregular bluish-purple vessels that form an abnormal tangle of distended channels that differ markedly from the normal fine-capillary net pattern. The abnormal channels are not unlike the vessels that cover the surface of submucous myomas. The Nd-YAG or holmium YAG laser fiber is inserted through the operating channel, and the fiber is held several millimeters above the vascular abnormality at a power up to 50 to 60 W. The laser is discharged without touching the vessels or the surface of the endometrium (Fig. 18.39). The laser energy causes the vessels to collapse and coagulate and the surface to blanch white. The endometrium neighboring the abnormality is also treated and coagulated. The fiber is then withdrawn, the field is aspirated clear, and the hysteroscope is withdrawn. Similar treatment is repeated two to three times at 1-month intervals or until all evidence of the abnormality is obliterated. Alternatively, angiomas may be managed via invasive radiologic techniques (e.g., embolization).

COMPLICATIONS

Unfortunately, accurate data concerning complications are hard to obtain, although one simple fact is clear: As greater numbers of gynecologists have begun to perform operative hysteroscopy, the rate of complications has increased. Voluntary surveys are worthless. Only state-mandated reports, such as those that are required for laparoscopic cholecystectomy in New York, have rendered any useful information. The exception to this is an excellent report by Smith and colleagues, which details complications encountered by 42 gynecologists

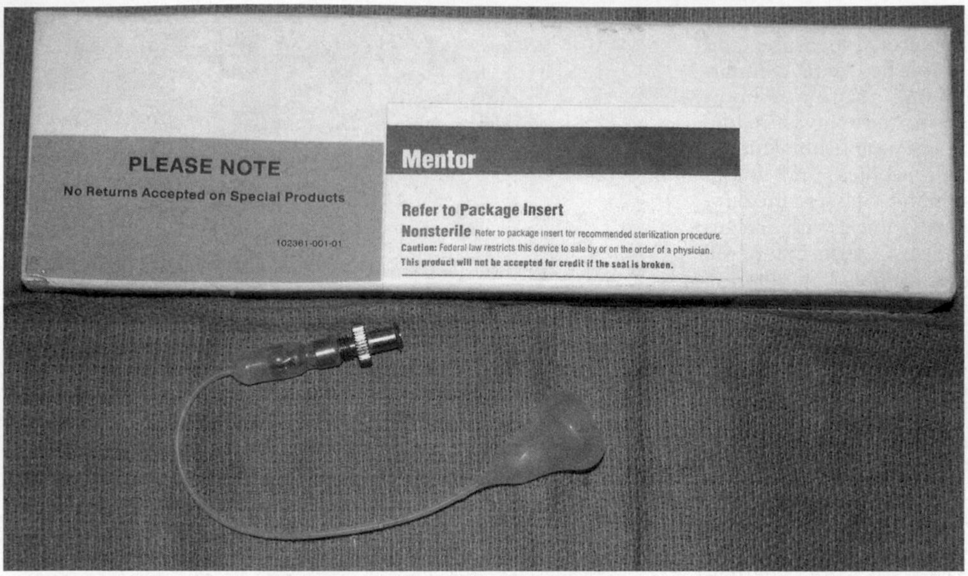

FIGURE 18.40. This specially designed balloon may be placed within the uterine cavity, inflated to tamponade the uterine wall. The intrauterine pressure will usually control bleeding. A 10-mL Foley catheter (balloon inflated to 5 mL) may be used for this same purpose.

performing 257 endoscopic procedures (operative laparoscopy and hysteroscopy) in 218 patients (mean 5.4 case per surgeon) over a period of 15 months at the Swedish Hospital Medical Center in Seattle. Of 43 endometrial ablations, perforation was observed in three, fluid imbalance in two, and technical failure to complete in two. Myomectomy was performed in 30 and ablation plus myomectomy in 13. Perforation occurred in two, fluid imbalance in four, and fistula, sepsis, or both in three. Lysis of septa or synechiae was performed in 14 women, with perforation or hemorrhage in six patients. The overall complication rate ranged from 12% to 43%.

Aydeniz and colleagues reported on complications associated with a multicenter experience of 21,676 operative hysteroscopies. MacLean-Fraser and associates evaluated the complication rates in 875 women who underwent endometrial ablation between 1990 and 2000. Significant complications occurred in 9.3% repeat ablations and 2% of primary ablations. Jansen and colleagues, using data from 82 hospitals, prospectively tracked intra- and postoperative complications in 13,600 cases. A total of 38 complications (0.28%) were identified. The most frequent surgical complication was perforation and entry related.

Similarly, the Mistletoe data cited in the Endometrial Ablation section are useful accurate data relative to endometrial ablation/resection complications.

Propst and colleagues reviewed data on 925 women who had hysteroscopies. Excessive fluid absorption was the most common complication. Myomectomy and resection of uterine septum had greatest odds for complication (odds ratio [OR] 7.4).

Intraoperative and Postoperative Bleeding

The most common complications inherent to hysteroscopic surgical procedures are intraoperative and postoperative bleeding. Generally speaking, intraoperative bleeding can be managed by aspirating the blood and by increasing the pressure of the distending medium so that it exceeds arterial pressure and compresses the walls of the uterus sufficiently to stop bleeding. Then the bleeding vessel may be coagulated with a 3-mm ball electrode with the use of forced coagulation at 30 to 40 W of power or by multiple jabs with bipolar needles at 20 to 30 W of power with the generator set for automatic bipolar. If the counterpressure of the medium is relaxed (at the termination of the procedure) and bleeding continues, then control is best obtained by inserting an intrauterine balloon initially inflated to 2 to 5 mL. If this pressure does not promptly stop the bleeding, then a larger balloon can be distended to 10 mL until the bleeding has stopped (Fig. 18.40). More distension may be required for larger uteri. Care must be taken because overinflation of an intrauterine balloon can itself rupture the uterus. The balloon remains in place for 6 to 8 hours, is partially deflated for 6 hours, and, finally, is totally deflated before removal. When the bleeding is pulsatile, the source is arterial rather then venous. If this type of bleeding is not immediately controlled by balloon compression, then hysterectomy will usually be required. Delayed postoperative bleeding is most commonly associated with endometrial slough (after ablation), chronic endometritis, or spontaneous extrusion and expulsion of the intramyometrial portion of a previously resected submucous myoma (Figs. 18.38 and 18.39). Bleeding-clotting studies should be obtained in cases of late postoperative bleeding, particularly if these studies were not performed preoperatively in women with a diagnosis of abnormal uterine bleeding (preoperative endometrial ablation or myomectomy).

A French group (2003) prospectively studied a decade of operative hysteroscopies (2116 cases). Thirteen cases of major bleeding were reported, with six requiring intrauterine catheter placements. The highest-risk procedure for associated hemorrhage was hysteroscopic adhesiolysis.

Uterine Perforation

Uterine perforation can occur during any operative hysteroscopy procedure but is most common during septum resection, myomectomy operations, and adhesion takedown. The best insurance against this complication is simultaneous laparoscopy. Among novice operators, perforation can occur even during insertion of the hysteroscope. With appropriate care, this sort of perforation should not happen, because the cervix and internal os should be negotiated under direct vision, and the cavity should likewise be entered under direct vision. Examination under anesthesia is also simple and lets the operator know the direction of the uterine axis.

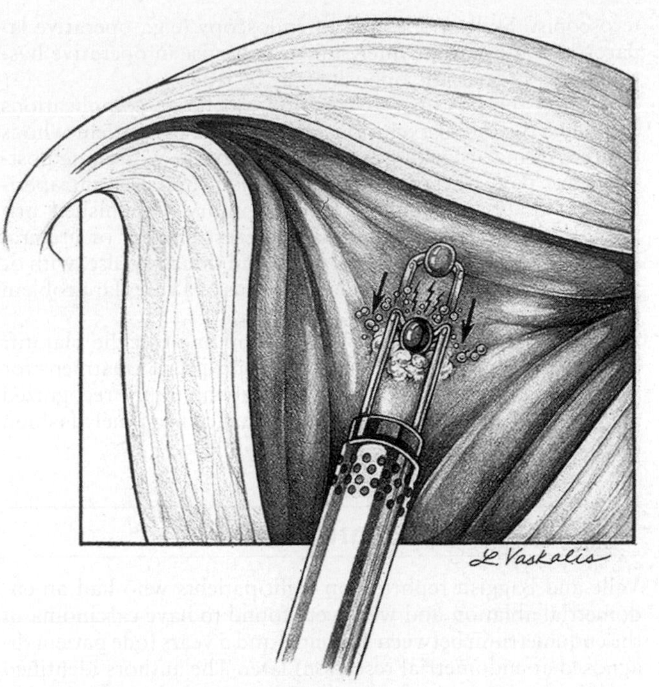

FIGURE 18.41. The operator should never apply power to an energy device while advancing the electrode. The power can safely be applied as the electrode returns toward the sheath. (By permission: Baggish MS, Valle RF, Guedj H. *Hysteroscopy: Visual perspectives of uterine anatomy, physiology and pathology.* 3rd ed. Lippincott Williams & Wilkins, 2007.)

As we noted above, the most dangerous perforations are those associated with lasers and electrosurgical devices. The risk of this type of injury can be reduced by not activating the energy device during a thrusting or forward movement. The foot pedal is activated only during the return phase of the laser fiber or electrosurgical electrode. If a perforation does happen with an energy device, then laparotomy is required to ensure that no injury has been inflicted on the intestine, bladder, or ureter (Fig. 18.41).

A risk of perforation is associated with the septum transection in its final phase at the level of the uterine fundus because the operator may have some difficulty determining where the septum ends and the myometrium begins. This risk is constant regardless of the cutting instrument used. The operator rapidly becomes aware that uterine perforation has occurred because distention becomes difficult to maintain and the flow of the distending medium exits at the perforation site. An alert assistant viewing by laparoscope should warn the hysteroscopist of impending perforation the moment an increasing intensity of light transmission through the thinning uterine wall is observed. If perforation is unnoticed and if simultaneous laparoscopy is not performed, a serious complication is even possible with a nonenergy instrument, but this is far less common than those occurring with lasers or electrodes. Nevertheless, if a perforation is suspected, that patient should be carefully observed in the hospital. Injuries to the iliac vessels can occur as the result of uterine perforation. An unexplained falling blood pressure, together with medium leakage, should alert the surgeon to this possibility. Perforation of the uterus during hysteroscopy can place a woman at an increased risk for uterine rupture during a future pregnancy (Fig. 18.42).

Poor Visibility in the Operative Field

Inability to see the operative field is a common problem. The usual cause of this problem is deep insertion of the hysteroscope so that the telescope lies directly in contact with the endometrium. The surgeon will see nothing but a red blur. The natural tendency is to push the hysteroscope deeper in. This strategic mistake invariably leads to perforation. Another cause of visibility problems is blood within the uterine cavity secondary to dilatation. The fastest way to deal with a bloody cavity is rapid flushing with the hysteroscopic medium combined with aspiration using a cannula placed into the cavity via the operating channel.

Overdilatation of the cervix is an equally common mistake that results in excessive leakage of distending medium and an inability to maintain distension, with the resultant inability to perform the operative hysteroscopy. Blood and debris can cloud

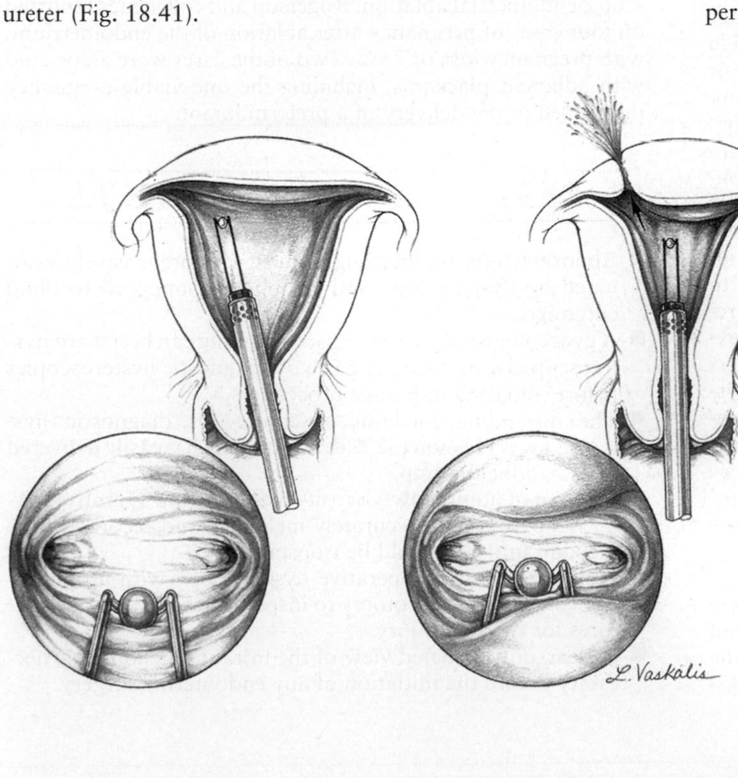

FIGURE 18.42. Perforation should be immediately suspected when the endometrial cavity depressurizes and collapses around the hysteroscope, creating a compromised view of the cavity. (By permission: Baggish MS, Valle RF, Guedj H. *Hysteroscopy: Visual perspectives of uterine anatomy, physiology and pathology.* 3rd ed. Lippincott Williams & Wilkins, 2007.)

the field to such a degree that accurate operative endoscopy is impossible. Overdilatation is a less common occurrence when Hyskon is selected as the distending medium. If the operator cannot clearly see the field, it is better to discontinue the procedure rather than press on and risk a catastrophic error. It is easy to become disoriented in the uterine cavity if normal anatomic landmarks cannot be recognized.

Gas Embolus

CO_2 embolism can occur during diagnostic or operative laparoscopy. This will happen if an inappropriate method (e.g., laparoscopic insufflator) is used to infuse CO_2 into the uterus. However, this complication may occur when a proper CO_2 hysteroscopic insufflator is used. The diagnosis is made by the presence of a cog-wheel murmur accompanied by a rapid fall in expired CO_2.

Brundin and Thomasson observed 70 women during CO_2 hysteroscopy and reported the presence of the mill (cog)-wheel murmur in seven (10%). When the hysteroscopy was stopped, the murmur disappeared. Corson and colleagues infused CO_2 gas directly into the circulation of ewes. At 90 cc per minute, the P_{CO_2} dropped; however, at lower flow rates, only transient drops in P_{CO_2} were observed. The investigators concluded that CO_2 clearance is very efficient owing to its high solubility in blood.

Air embolism is exceedingly dangerous and has been reported to occur during hysteroscopy. Corson and colleagues and Perry and Baughman have reported this type of complication. These investigators recommended avoiding the Trendelenburg position, purging air from all tubing and sheaths, and careful dilatating to avoid opening venous channels. Baggish and Daniell reported air embolism that resulted in death secondary to the use of gas-cooled coaxial Nd-YAG laser fibers.

Infection

The endometrium seems to be peculiarly resistant to infection, and infection is an unlikely complication associated with or coming after hysteroscopy. Hysteroscopy should be avoided in the presence of gross cervical infection, uterine infection, or salpingitis. Infection is otherwise uncommon after even extensive intrauterine surgery (e.g., adhesiotomy or myomectomy). Prophylactic antibiotics should be administered only when indications exist such as a history of rheumatic carditis, congenital heart defect, or prolapsed mitral valve, or in cases of suspected chronic endometritis (submucous myoma or imbedded IUD). Baggish and colleagues (1999) observed only 13 infections out of 5,000 cases that could be casually related to the hysteroscopic operation. Salat-Baroux and associates reported seven mild infections out of 4,000 hysteroscopic examinations. On the other hand, McCausland and co-workers reported three cases of tuboovarian abscess after operative hysteroscopy. Agostini and associates reported 30 infections associated with 2,116 operative hysteroscopies. Eighteen of these infections were cases of endometritis.

Operator Technique

The most serious complications happen because of operator error. Most often, these are the result of inexperience and are avoidable. Difficult cases beyond the capabilities of the primary care gynecologist should be referred to the expert hysteroscopist. Skill in one area of endoscopy (e.g., operative laparoscopy) does not confer similar expertise in operative hysteroscopy. Indeed, the opposite may be truer.

During the postoperative period, operative complications should be the initial exclusion diagnosis for any patient who is not recovering according to the usual pattern. Worsening postoperative pain, fever, nausea, distension, and free intraperitoneal air are the signals of bowel injury. Diminished urinary output, fever, and distension suggest bladder or ureteral trauma. Falling blood pressure and rapid thready pulse, with or without distension, should raise concerns of a vascular problem and third-space hemorrhage.

Most negligence cases adjudicated in favor of the plaintiff have involved delayed initiation of appropriate treatment for an operative complication. Cases involving injury recognized at the time of surgery and correctly managed in a timely fashion do not usually become medicolegal problems.

Cancer after Ablation

Valle and Baggish reported on eight patients who had an endometrial ablation and who were found to have carcinoma of the endometrium between 5 months and 5 years (one patient diagnosed at endometrial resection) later. The authors identified risk factors for carcinoma in all patients, including obesity, hypertension, and diabetes. Additionally, five out of eight showed hyperplasia on preoperative biopsy. The investigators considered that women with abnormal uterine bleeding who fall into the high-risk category might be better served by hysterectomy rather than by endometrial ablation.

The risk of leiomyosarcoma is less than 1%. Nevertheless, any myoma or part of a myoma that is excised should be sent to the pathology laboratory for evaluation. This, of course, includes resectoscopic fragments.

Pregnancy after Hysteroscopic Ablation

Fortunately, this is not a common complication after hysteroscopic endometrial ablation. Rogerson and colleagues reported on four cases of pregnancy after ablation of the endometrium, with pregnancy loss of 75%. Two of the cases were associated with adherent placentas, including the one viable pregnancy that ended in the delivery of a preterm infant.

BEST SURGICAL PRACTICES

- Abnormal uterine bleeding is most comprehensively evaluated by hysteroscopy and sampling as opposed to blind curettage.
- A gynecologist or gynecologist in training can best learn hysteroscopy by performing 25 to 50 diagnostic hysteroscopies before initiating operative procedures.
- The distending medium of choice for diagnostic hysteroscopy is Hyskon (32% dextran), which is easily delivered via a handheld pump.
- Infusion of liquid, low-viscosity media during operative hysteroscopy must be accurately measured and recorded. The medium infused should be isoosmolar.
- Perforation during operative hysteroscopy with an energy device requires laparotomy to inspect intraabdominal structures for thermal injury.
- A clear, unobstructed view of the intrauterine milieu is necessary before the initiation of any endouterine surgery.

Bibliography

Aberdeen Endometrial Ablation Trials Group. A randomized trial of endometrial ablation versus hysterectomy for the treatment of dysfunctional uterine bleeding: outcome at four years. *BJOG* 1999;106:360.

Abbott J, Hawe J, Hunter D, et al. A double-blind randomized trial comparing the Cavaterm and the Novasure endometrial ablation systems for the treatment of dysfunctional uterine bleeding. *Fertil Steril* 2003;80:203.

Agostini A, Cravello L, Desbriere R, et al. Hemorrhage risk during operative laparoscopy. *Acta Obstet Gynecol Scand* 2002;81:878.

Agostini A, Cravello L, Shojai R, et al. Postoperative infection and surgical hysteroscopy. *Fertil Steril* 2002;77:766.

Alborzi S, Dehbashi S, Parsanezhad ME. Differential diagnosis of septate and bicornuate uterus by sonohysterography eliminates the need for laparoscopy. *Fertil Steril* 2002;78(1):176.

Arieff AI, Ayus C. Endometrial ablation complicated by fatal hyponatremic encephalopathy. *JAMA* 1993;270:1230.

Aydeniz B, Gruber IV, Schauf B, et al. A multicenter survey of complications associated with 21,676 operative hysteroscopies. *Eur J Obstet Gynecol Reprod Biol* 2002;104:160.

Baggish MS. Contact hysteroscopy: a new technique to explore the uterine cavity. *Obstet Gynecol* 1979;54:350.

Baggish MS. Hysteroscopic media: a two-edged sword [Editorial]. *J Gynecol Surg* 1992;8:197.

Baggish MS. A new laser hysteroscope for Nd-YAG endometrial ablation. *Lasers Surg Med* 1988;8:248.

Baggish MS, Baltoyannis P. New techniques for laser ablation of the endometrium in high risk patients. *Am J Obstet Gynecol* 1988;159:287.

Baggish MS, Barbot J, Valle RF. *Diagnostic and operative hysteroscopy: a text and atlas*. Chicago: Mosby-Year Book, 1989.

Baggish MS, Brill AI, Rosenzweig B, et al. Fatal acute glycine and sorbitol toxicity during operative hysteroscopy. *J Gynecol Surg* 1993;9:137.

Baggish MS, Dauauluri CH, Rodriguez F, et al. Vascular uptake of Hyskon (dextran 70) during operative and diagnostic hysteroscopy. *J Gynecol Surg* 1992;8:211.

Baggish MS, Dorsey JH. Contact hysteroscopic evaluation of the endocervix as an adjunct to colposcopy. *Obstet Gynecol* 1982;60:107.

Baggish MS, Paraiso MF, Breznock EM, et al. A computer controlled, continuously circulating, hot irrigating system for endometrial ablation. *Am J Obstet Gynecol* 1995;173:1842.

Baggish MS, Ringgenberg E, Sze EHM. Adenocarcinoma of the corpus uteri following endometrial ablation. *J Gynecol Surg* 1995;11:91.

Baggish MS, Sze EHM. Experience with 568 endometrial ablation procedures. *J Gynecol Surg* 1996;174:908.

Baggish MS, Sze EHM, Morgan G. Hysteroscopic treatment of symptomatic submucous myomata uteri with the Nd-YAG laser. *J Gynecol Surg* 1989;5:127.

Baggish MS, Savells H. Complications associated with minimally invasive nonhysteroscopic endomontrial ablatie techniques *J Gynecol Surg* 2007;23:7.

Barbot J. Hysteroscopy for abnormal uterine bleeding in diagnostic and operative hysteroscopy. In: Baggish MS, Barbot J, Valle RF, eds. *Diagnostic and operative hysteroscopy: a text and atlas*. Chicago: Mosby-Year Book; 1989:147.

Barbot J, Parent B, Doeler B. Hysteroscopic de contact et cancer de pendometre. *Acta Endosc* 1978;8:17.

Barbot J, Parent B, Dubuisson JB. Contact hysteroscopy: another method of endoscopic examination of the uterine cavity. *Am J Obstet Gynecol* 1980;136:721.

Brink DM, DeJong P, Fawcus S, et al. Carbon dioxide embolism following diagnostic hysteroscopy. *BJOG* 1994;101:717.

Brundin J, Thomasson K. Cardiac gas embolism during carbon dioxide hysteroscopy: risk and management. *Eur J Obstet Gynecol Reprod Biol* 1989;33:241.

Burnet, JE. Hysteroscopy-controlled curettage for endometrial polyps. *Obstet Gynecol* 1964;24:621.

Bustos-Lopez H, Baggish MS, Valle RF, et al. Assessment of the safety of intrauterine instillation of heated saline for endometrial ablation. *Fertil Steril* 1998;65:155.

Cameron IM, Mollison J, Pinion SB, et al. A cost comparison of hysterectomy and hysteroscopic surgery for the treatment of menorrhagia. *Eur J Obstet Gynecol Reprod Biol* 1996;70:87.

Capella-Allouc S, Morsad F, Rongieres-Bertrand C, et al. Hysteroscopic treatment of severe Asherman's syndrome and subsequent fertility. *Human Reprod* 1999;14:1230.

Cararach M, Penella J, Ubeda A, et al. Hysteroscopic incision of the septate uterus: scissors versus resectoscope. *Hum Reprod* 1994;9:87.

Ceci O, Bettocchi S, Marello F, et al. Hysteroscopic evaluation of the endometrium in postmenopausal women taking tamoxifen. *J Am Assoc Gynecol Laparosc* 2000;7:185.

Choe JK, Baggish MS. Hysteroscopic treatment of septate uterus with neodymium-YAG laser. *Fertil Steril* 1992;57:81.

Clark TJ, Mahajan D, Sunder P, et al. Hysteroscopic treatment of symptomatic submucous fibroids using a bipolar intrauterine system: a feasibility study. *Eur J Obstet Gyn Reprod Biol* 2002;100:237.

Cooper J, Gimpelson R, Laberge P, et al. A randomized, multicenter trial of safety and efficacy of the NovaSure system in the treatment of menorrhagia. *J Am Assoc Gynecol Laparosc* 2002;9:418.

Corson, SL. A multicenter evaluation of endometrial ablation by Hydro ThermAblator and rollerball for treatment of menorrhagia. *J Am Assoc Gynecol Laparosc* 2001;8:359.

Corson SL, Brooks PG, Soderstrom RM. Gynecologic endoscopic gas embolism. *Fertil Steril* 1996;65:529.

Corson SL, Hoffmann JJ, Jackowski J, et al. Cardiopulmonary effects of direct venous CO_2 insufflation in ewes. *J Reprod Med* 1988;33:440.

Creinin M, Chen M. Uterine defect in a twin pregnancy with a history of hysteroscopic fundal perforation. *Obstet Gynecol* 1992;79:879.

DeCherney AH, Cholst I, Naftolin F. The management of intractable uterine bleeding utilizing the cystoscopic resectoscope. In: Siegler AM, Lindeman HJ, eds. *Hysteroscopy: principles and practice*. Philadelphia: JB Lippincott; 1984:140.

DeCherney AH, Polan MI. Hysteroscopic management of intrauterine lesions and intractable uterine bleeding. *Obstet Gynecol* 1983;61:392.

DeCherney AH, Russell JB, Graebe RA, et al. Resectoscopic management of mullerian fusion defects. *Fertil Steril* 1986;45:726.

Droegemueller W, Greet BE, David JR, et al. Cryocoagulation of the endometrium at the uterine cornua. *Am J Obstet Gynecol* 1978;131:1.

Droegemueller W, Greet BE, Makowski E. Cryosurgery in patients with dysfunctional uterine bleeding. *Obstet Gynecol* 1971;38:256.

Dumesic DA, Dhillon SS. A new approach to hysteroscopic cannulation of the fallopian tube. *J Gynecol Surg* 1991;7:7.

Dwyer N, Hutton J, Stirkat GM. Randomized controlled trial comparing endometrial resection with abdominal hysterectomy for surgical treatment of menorrhagia. *BJOG* 1993;100:237.

Edstrom K, Fernstrom I. The diagnostic possibilities of a modified hysteroscopic technique. *Acta Obstet Gynecol Scand* 1970;49(4):327.

Emanuel MH, Wamsteker K, Hart AA, et al. Long-term results of hysteroscopic myomectomy for abnormal uterine bleeding. *Obstet Gynecol* 1999;93:743.

Fisher JC. Principles of safety in laser surgery and therapy. In: Baggish MS, ed. *Basic and advanced laser surgery in gynecology*. Norwalk, CT: Appleton-Century-Crofts; 1985:85.

Friedler S, Margalioth EJ, Kafka I, et al. Incidence of post-abortion intrauterine adhesions evaluated by hysteroscopy: a prospective study. *Hum Reprod* 1993;8:442.

Gabriele A, Zanetta G, Pasta F, et al. Uterine rupture after hysteroscopic metroplasty and labor induction. *J Reprod Med* 1999;44:642.

Garry R, Hasham F, Kokri MS, et al. The effect of pressure of fluid absorption during endometrial ablation. *J Gynecol Surg* 1992;8:1.

Garry R, Shelley-Jones D, Mooney P, et al. Six hundred endometrial laser ablations. *Obstet Gynecol* 1995;85:24.

Garuti G, Cellani F, Colonnelli M, et al. Hysteroscopically targeted biopsies compared with blind samplings in endometrial assessment of menopausal women taking tamoxifen for breast cancer. *J Am Assoc Gynecol Laparosc* 2004;11:62.

Gebauer G, Hafner A, Siebzehnrubl E, et al. Role of hysteroscopy in detection and extraction of endometrial polyps: results of a prospective study. *Am J Obstet Gynecol* 2002;186:1104.

Glasser MH, Zimmerman JD. The Hydro ThermAblator system for management of menorrhagia in women with submucous myomas: 12- to 20-month follow-up. *J Am Assoc Gynecol Laparosc* 2003;10:52.

Goldenberg M, Zolti M, Seidman DS, et al. Transient blood oxygen desaturation, hypercapnia and coagulopathy after operative hysteroscopy with glycine used as the distending medium. *Am J Obstet Gynecol* 1994;170:25.

Goldrath MH. Vaginal removal of the pedunculated submucous myoma: the use of laminaria. *Obstet Gynecol* 1987;70:670.

Goldrath MH, Fuller T, Segal S. Laser photovaporization of endometrium for the treatment of menorrhagia. *Am J Obstet Gynecol* 1981;140:14.

Gonzales R, Brensilver JM, Rovinsky JJ. Post-hysteroscopic hyponatremia. *Am J Kidney Dis* 1994;23:735.

Guida M, Acunzo G, DiSpiezio Sardo A, et al. Effectiveness of auto-crosslinked hyaluronic acid gel in the prevention of intrauterine adhesions after hysteroscopic surgery: a prospective, randomized, controlled study. *Hum Reprod* 2004;19:1461.

Halverson LM, Aserkoff RD, Oskowitz SP. Spontaneous uterine rupture after hysteroscopic metroplasty with uterine perforation. *J Reprod Med* 1993;38:236.

Hamou JE. Hysteroscopic et microhysteroscopic avec un instrument nouveau: le microhysteroscope. *Endosc Gynecol* 1980;2:131.

Hamou JE. Microhysteroscopy: a new procedure and its original application in gynecology. *J Reprod Med* 1981;26:375.

Harris WJ. Uterine dehiscence following laparoscopic myomectomy. *Obstet Gynecol* 992;80:545.

Hidlebaugh DA, Orr RK. Long-term economic evaluation of resectoscopic endometrial ablation versus hysterectomy for the treatment of menorrhagia. *J Am Assoc Gynecol Laparosc* 998;5:351.

Howe RS. Third trimester uterine rupture following hysteroscopic uterine perforation. *Obstet Gynecol* 1993;81:827.

Jansen FW, Vredevoogd CB, van Ulzen K, et al. Complications of hysteroscopy: a prospective, multicenter study. *Obstet Gynecol* 2000;96:266.

Jones HW, Seegar-Jones G. Double uterus as an etiological factor in repeated abortion: indications for surgical repair. *Am J Obstet Gynecol* 1953;65:325.

Kivnick S, Kanter MH. Bowel injury from rollerball ablation of the endometrium. *Obstet Gynecol* 1992;79:833.

Lefler HT Jr. Long-term follow-up of endometrial ablation by modified loop resection. *J Am Assoc Gynecol Laparosc* 2003;10:517.

Lin BL, Iwata Y, Liu KH, et al. Clinical application of a new Fujinon operating fiberoptic hysteroscope. *J Gynecol Surg* 1990;6:81.

Lin JC, Chen YO, Lin BL, et al. Outcome of removal of intrauterine devices with flexible hysteroscopy in early pregnancy. *J Gynecol Surg* 1993;9:195.

Lindemann HJ. The use of CO_2 in the uterine cavity for hysteroscopy. *Int J Fertil* 1972;17:221.

Lindemann HJ, Mohr J. CO_2 hysteroscopy, diagnosis and treatment. *Am J Obstet Gynecol* 976;124.

Litta P, Pozzan C, Merlin F, et al. Hysteroscopic metroplasty under laparoscopic guidance in infertile women with septate uteri: follow-up of reproductive outcome. *J Reprod Med* 2004;49(4):274.

Lobaugh ML, Bammel BM, Duke D, et al. Uterine rupture during pregnancy in a patient with a history of hysteroscopic metroplasty. *Obstet Gynecol* 1994;83:838.

Loffer FD, Grainger D. Five-year follow-up of patients participating in a randomized trial of uterine balloon therapy versus rollerball ablation for treatment of menorrhagia. *J Am Assoc Gynecol Laparosc* 2002;9:429.

Lomano JM. Photocoagulation of the endometrium with the Nd-YAG laser for the treatment of menorrhagia: a report of 10 cases. *J Reprod Med* 1986;31:26.

MacLean-Fraser E, Penava D, Vilos GA. Perioperative complication rates of primary and repeat hysteroscopic endometrial ablations. *J Am Assoc Gynecol Laparosc* 2002

Magos AL, Baumann R, Lockwood GM, et al. Experience with the first 250 endometrial resections for menorrhagia. *Lancet* 1991;337:1074.

March CM. Hysteroscopy for infertility in diagnostic and operative hysteroscopy. In: Baggish MS, Barbot J, Valle RF, eds. *Diagnostic and operative hysteroscopy: a text and atlas*. Chicago: Mosby-Year Book; 1989:136.

March CM, Israel R. Gestational outcome following hysteroscopic lysis of adhesions. *Fertil Steril* 1981;36:455.

March CM, Israel R. Hysteroscopic management of recurrent abortion caused by septate uterus. *Am J Obstet Gynecol* 1987;156:834.

March CM, Israel R, March AD. Hysteroscopic management of intrauterine adhesions. *Am J Obstet Gynecol* 1978;130:65.

McCausland VM, Fields GA, McCausland AM, et al. Tubo-ovarian abscess after operative hysteroscopy. *J Reprod Med* 1993;38:198.

Mints M, Radestad A, Rylander E. Follow up of hysteroscopic surgery for menorrhagia. *Acta Obstet Gynecol Scand* 1998;77:435.

Mishler JM. Synthetic plasma volume expanders—their pharmacology, safety, and clinical efficacy. *Clin Haematol* 1984;13:75.

Neuwirth RS. Endometrial ablation using a thermal balloon system. *Contemp Obstet Gynecol* 1995;40:35.

Neuwirth RS. Hysteroscopic management of symptomatic submucous fibroids. *Obstet Gynecol* 1983;62:509.

Neuwirth RS. Hysteroscopic resection of submucous leiomyoma. *Contemp Obstet Gynecol* 1985;25:103.

Neuwirth RS. A new technique for and additional experience with hysteroscopic resection of submucous fibroids. *Am J Obstet Gynecol* 1978;131:91.

Neuwirth RS, Amin HK. Excision of submucous fibroids with hysteroscopic control. *Am J Obstet Gynecol* 1976;126:95.

Neuwirth RS, Duran AA, Singer A, et al. The endometrial ablater: a new instrument. *Obstet Gynecol* 1994;83:792.

Novy MJ, Thurmond AS, Patton P, et al. Diagnosis of cannula obstruction by transcervical fallopian tube cannulation. *Fertil Steril* 1988;50:434.

Overton C, Hargreaves J, Maresh M. A national survey of complications of endometrial destruction for menstrual disorders: the Mistletoe study. *BJOG* 1997;104:1351.

Pabuccu R, Gomel V. Reproductive outcome after hysteroscopic metroplasty in women with septate uterus and otherwise unexplained infertility. *Fertil Steril* 2004;81(6):1675.

Pantaleoni D. On endoscopic examination of the cavity of the womb. *Med Press Circ* 1869;8:26.

Patton PE, Novy MJ. The diagnosis and reproductive outcome after surgical treatment of the complete septate uterus duplicated cervix and vagina septum. *Am J Obstet Gynecol* 2004;190:1669.

Perlitz Y, Rahav D, Ben-Ami M. Endometrial ablation using hysteroscopic instillation of hot saline solution into the uterus. *Eur J Obstet Gynecol Reprod Biol* 2001;99:90.

Perry CP, Daniell JF, Gimpelson RJ. Bowel injury from Nd-YAG endometrial ablation. *J Gynecol Surg* 1990;6:199.

Perry PM, Baughman VL. A complication of hysteroscopy: air embolism. *Anesthesiology* 1990;73:546.

Phipps JH, Lewis BV, Robert T, et al. Treatment of functional menorrhagia with radio-frequency endometrial ablation. *Lancet* 1990;335:374.

Pinion SB, Parkin DE, Abramoukh DR, et al. Randomized trial of hysterectomy, endometrial laser ablation, and transcervical endometrial resection for dysfunctional uterine bleeding. *BMJ* 1994;309:9793.

Porto R, Gaujoux J. Une nouvelle methode d'hysteroscopic instrumentation et technique. *J Gynecol Obstet Biol Reprod (Paris)* 1972;7:691.

Propst AM, Liberman RF, Harlow BL, et al. Complications of hysteroscopic surgery: predicting patients at risk. *Obstet Gynecol* 2000;96:517.

Quinones RG. Hysteroscopy with a new fluid technique. In: Siegler AM, Lindemann HJ, eds. *Hysteroscopy: principles and practice*. Philadelphia: JB Lippincott Co; 1984:41.

Reed TP, Erb RA. Hysteroscopic tubal occlusion with silicone rubber. *Obstet Gynecol* 1983;61:388.

Roberts S, Long L, Jonasson O. The isolation of cancer cells from the bloodstream during uterine curettage. *Surg Gynecol Obstet* 1960;111:3.

Rock JA, Singh M, Murphy A. A modification of technique for hysteroscopic lysis of severe uterine adhesions. *J Obstet Gynecol* 1993;9:191.

Rogerson L, Gannon MJ, Donovan PJ. Outcome of pregnancy following endometrial ablation. *J Gynecol Surg* 1997;13:155.

Romer T. Benefit of GnRH analogue pretreatment for hysteroscopic surgery in patients with bleeding disorders. *Gynecol Obstet Invest* 1998;45[Suppl 1]:12.

Ruiz JM, Neuwirth RS. The incidence of complications associated with the use of Hyskon during hysteroscopy: experience in 1793 consecutive patients. *J Gynecol Surg* 1992;8:219.

Salat-Baroux J, Hamou JE, Maillard G, et al. Complications from microhysteroscopy. In: Siegler A, Lindemann H, eds. *Hysteroscopy*. Philadelphia: JB Lippincott Co; 1984.

Saygili-Yilmaz E, Yildiz S, Erman-Akar M, et al. Reproductive outcome of septate uterus after hysteroscopic metroplasty. *Arch Gynecol Obstet* 2003;268:289.

Schmitz MJ, Nahhas WA. Hysteroscopy may transport malignant cells into the peritoneal cavity: case report. *Eur J Gynaecol Oncol* 1994;15:121.

Seidman DS, Bitman G, Mashiach S, et al. The effect of increasing age on the outcome of hysteroscopic endometrial resection for management of dysfunctional uterine bleeding. *J Am Assoc Gynecol Laparosc* 2000;7:115.

Siegler AM, Kemmann EK. Hysteroscopic removal of occult intrauterine contraceptive device. *Obstet Gynecol* 1975;46:604.

Siegler AM, Kemmann EK. Hysteroscopy: a review. *Obstet Gynecol Surg* 1975;30:567.

Singer A, Almanza R, Gutierrez A, et al. Preliminary clinical experience with a thermal balloon endometrial ablation method to treat menorrhagia. *Obstet Gynecol* 1994;83:732.

Smith DC, Donohue LR, Waszak SJ. A hospital review of advanced gynecologic endoscopic procedures. *Am J Obstet Gynecol* 1994;170:1635.

Sowter MC, Singla AA, Lethaby A. Pre-operative endometrial thinning agents before hysteroscopic surgery for heavy menstrual bleeding. *Update in Cochrane Database Syst Rev* 2002;(3):CD001124;PMID:12137619.

Strassman EO. Plastic unification of double uterus. *Am J Obstet Gynecol* 1952;64:25.

Sullivan B, Kenney P, Seibel M. Hysteroscopic resection of fibroid with thermal injury to sigmoid. *Obstet Gynecol* 1992;80:546.

Taponeco F, Curcio C, Fasciani A, et al. Indication of hysteroscopy in tamoxifen treated breast cancer. *J Exp Clin Cancer Res* 2002;21:37.

Tapper AM, Heinonen PK. Experience with isotonic 2.2% glycine as distension medium for hysteroscopic endomyometrial resection. *Gynecol Obstet Invest* 1999;47:263.

Thijssen RFA. Radio-frequency induced endometrial ablation: an update. *BJOG* 1997;104:608.

Valle RF. Hysteroscopic evaluation of patients with abnormal uterine bleeding. *Surg Gynecol Obstet* 1981;153:521.

Valle RF. Hysteroscopic removal of submucous leiomyomas. *J Gynecol Surg* 1990;6:89.

Valle RF. Hysteroscopy for gynecologic diagnosis. *Clin Obstet Gynecol* 1983;26:253.

Valle RF, Baggish MS. Endometrial carcinoma after endometrial ablation: high-risk factors predicting its occurrence. *Am J Obstet Gynecol* 1998;179:569.

Valle RF, Sciarra JJ. Hysteroscopy: a useful diagnostic adjunct in gynecology. *Am J Obstet Gynecol* 1975;122:230.

Valle RF, Sciarra JJ, Freeman DW. Hysteroscopic removal of intrauterine devices with missing filaments. *Obstet Gynecol* 1977;49:55.

Vilos GA. Intrauterine surgery using a new coaxial bipolar electrode in normal saline solution (Versapoint): a pilot study. *Fertil Steril* 1999;4:740.

Vilos GA, Vilos EC, Pendley E. Endometrial ablation with a thermal balloon for the treatment of menorrhagia. *J Am Assoc Gynecol Laparosc* 1996;3:383.

Yaron Y, Shenhav M, Jaffa AJ, et al. Uterine rupture at 33 weeks gestation subsequent to hysteroscopic uterine perforation. *Am J Obstet Gynecol* 1994;170:786.

Zikopoulos KA, Kolibianakis EM, et al. Live delivery rates in subfertile women with Asherman's syndrome after hysteroscopic adhesiolysis using the resectoscope or the Versapoint system. *Reprod Biomed Online* 2004;8:720.

CHAPTER 19 ■ CONTROL OF PELVIC HEMORRHAGE

HOWARD W. JONES III AND WILLIAM A. ROCK, JR.

DEFINITIONS

Autologous blood transfusion—A transfusion done with the patient's own blood. Blood is usually drawn 2–4 weeks before anticipated surgery and stored. It, or the components, can be transfused if the patient requires a blood transfusion during surgery. This minimizes the risk of a transfusion reaction.

Hemostatic clips—Small V-shaped clips of stainless steel, titanium, or plastic that can be applied on small vessels or tissue for hemostasis.

Homologous blood transfusion—Transfusion of blood or blood products from another human being.

Parachute pack—Sometimes called an umbrella pack. A towel or large sheet is inserted through the vagina into the pelvis, and it is then filled from below with gauze packing. The edges are twisted together, and the pack is pulled down against the pelvic floor to control deep pelvic bleeding after pelvic exenteration.

Peanut dissector—A long clamp with a small cotton bud placed in the tip of the jaws. It is a useful tool for blunt pressure dissection of small spaces.

Total blood volume—About 8% of total body weight or between 4.5 and 5.0 liters in the average woman. Acute blood loss of 25% of total blood volume (about 1,500 cc) produces symptoms of tachycardia, hypotension, and decreased urine output. Transfusion should be considered when operative blood loss exceeds 15% of total blood volume. This can be roughly calculated by multiplying the patient's weight in kilograms by 10 (750 cc for a 75-kg woman).

The prevention and control of bleeding are fundamental to the success of any operation. Preoperative, intraoperative, and postoperative hemorrhage are potential complications in every patient undergoing gynecologic surgery. Preoperative hemorrhage is encountered in a variety of circumstances, such as in women with intraperitoneal bleeding from a ruptured tubal pregnancy or in patients taking heparin who have intraperitoneal hemorrhage associated with ovulation. Intraoperative hemorrhage can result from vascular injury, and postoperative bleeding is often a carryover from failure to control bleeding during surgery that was not apparent when the abdomen was closed because of reflex vasoconstriction or hypotension.

A knowledge of the normal coagulation mechanism and potential abnormalities of this important system is important for every surgeon. Preoperative evaluation will minimize the risks of abnormal surgical bleeding. Surgical techniques and operations are designed to control bleeding and avoid hemorrhage; but, from time to time, every surgeon is confronted with heavy and uncontrolled bleeding during an operation. The surgeon who has the knowledge and experience in these difficult situations will not only have the skills required, but also will exhibit the leadership and confidence necessary to direct the whole operative team so that control of bleeding can be accomplished promptly and effectively.

Many benign gynecologic conditions are associated with an increase in menstrual blood loss (menorrhagia), an increase in the duration of menstrual flow (metrorrhagia), an increase in the frequency of menstrual periods (polymenorrhea), or combinations of all three. Repeated small menstrual hemorrhages, such as those that occur with menorrhagia, will reduce the iron stores in the body over time. The daily dietary intake of iron usually is sufficient to replace the iron lost with normal menstruation, but it is inadequate to replace the increased loss of iron associated with heavy menstruation. In gynecologic patients with a history of heavy or prolonged menstrual blood loss, it is a good idea to check the hematocrit or hemoglobin before setting a date for elective surgery. Preoperative iron supplementation is indicated in these women because a good hemoglobin level and adequate iron stores are the first step in managing perioperative hemorrhage. Transfusion before elective gynecologic surgery is rarely if ever indicated in women with chronic blood loss anemia. Menstrual blood loss may be controlled with hormonal therapy while surgery is delayed and iron supplementation given to enable the patient to replete her own hemoglobin stores.

The preoperative use of epoetin alfa (recombinant erythropoietin) for correction of preoperative anemia has been used successfully in orthopedics. Its application in gynecologic surgery remains unclear. It is probably most applicable in gynecologic patients with chronic renal failure, nonmyeloid (hematopoietic) leukemia, or human immunodeficiency virus (HIV). Occasionally, other forms of anemia will be encountered that require a more extensive evaluation and treatment before elective surgery. On the other hand, some women who present with acute blood loss from a ruptured ectopic pregnancy or malignancy may require urgent transfusion even as preparations are being made for surgical intervention.

FUNDAMENTAL CONCEPTS OF NORMAL COAGULATION

Every surgeon should understand at least the basic mechanisms of normal hemostasis that can be relied on when surgical injury to tissue is inflicted. Bleeding during gynecologic surgery usually results from cutting or lacerating small or large vessels, but occasionally it may result from or be complicated by some preexisting or intraoperative defect in the clotting mechanism. The surgeon should be able to recognize when normal hemostasis is interdicted so that available remedies to protect against or remedy excessive bleeding can be found. Hemostasis is a complex, intricate, integrated, complementary, and countervailing system that maintains a delicate balance between normal coagulation and hypocoagulation or hypercoagulation. Unusual clinical situations can arise that require hematologic consultation for resolution. A specialist in coagulation disorders can provide invaluable assistance in the diagnosis and treatment of many rare disorders of coagulation.

The following is a discussion of the principles and concepts of normal hemostasis, abnormal hemostasis (congenital and acquired), and management techniques.

Effective hemostasis is the result of all aspects of the coagulation system functioning together to stop bleeding. Coagulation is the working interrelation of five aspects of a complex biochemical and vascular system that causes the formation and dissolution of the fibrin platelet plug. These five components are (a) vasculature, (b) platelets, (c) plasma clotting proteins, (d) fibrinolysis and clot inhibition, and (e) the hypercoagulable response. How these five components interrelate in the normal setting must be understood before one can appreciate how the five relate to bleeding or abnormal clotting in disease states.

Vasculature

The vasculature presents an endothelial-lined flexible conduit through which red cells, white cells, platelets, and all of the plasma proteins flow. At the interface between the flowing blood and vessel wall are several inhibitory biochemical systems that prevent the generation of the platelet–thrombin clot. The antiplatelet substance prostacyclin, produced in the vessel wall, inhibits platelet adhesion to the vessel wall. The surface antithrombin III–heparan sulfate complex inhibits deposition of thrombin and fibrin.

A tear in the vessel wall removes the endothelial cell layer, exposing the basement membrane, smooth muscle, collagen, and supporting adventitia. These substances are biochemical activators of platelets and have their own thromboplastic activity, which initiates fibrin generation and deposition. Therefore, the disruption in the vessel wall removes the protective covering of the endothelial cells, exposing platelet clumping and clot-initiating substances that produce a platelet–fibrin mass that will plug the tear in the vessel wall. A disease or medication that interferes with or intensifies this process can cause bleeding or inappropriate clotting. The vessel wall is diagrammed in Figure 19.1.

Congenital diseases associated with inadequate connective tissue and vascular dysfunction associated with bleeding are rare. The more frequently seen conditions are hereditary hemorrhagic telangiectasia, Ehlers-Danlos syndrome, and Marfan syndrome, which are characterized by defects in the quality of collagen. Defective collagen is responsible for poor clot formation and platelet activation at the injured site. No disease is known to be associated with excessive inappropriate clotting related to the vasculature as a structure. The congenital diseases closest to that definition are a predisposition to atherosclerosis owing to abnormalities in lipid metabolism, such as hypercholesterolemia, homocystinemia, and diabetes mellitus.

Acquired diseases of the vessel associated with bleeding include deficiencies in vitamin C; Cushing syndrome; acute and chronic inflammatory diseases, such as infectious vasculitis and immune vasculitis; pyrogenic purpura; embolic purpura; and anaphylactoid reactions from drugs. Myeloproliferative disorders, such as multiple myeloma and Waldenström macroglobulinemia, produce abnormal proteins that interfere with vascular function and therefore permit bleeding.

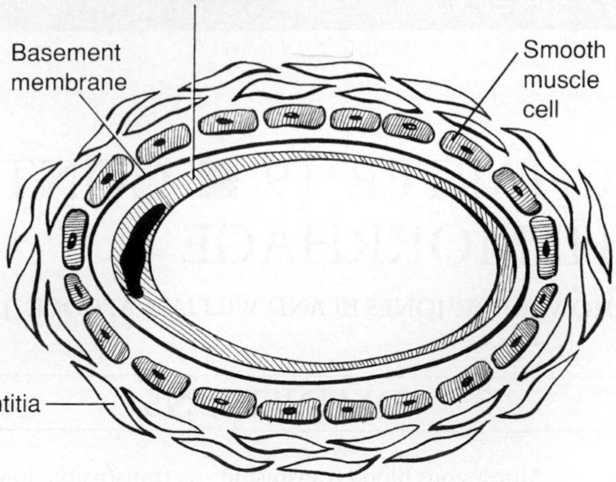

FIGURE 19.1. Vessel cross section.

Routine laboratory assessment of vascular function is extremely primitive. The capillary fragility test, the only routinely available test used to assess vascular function, has limited value. It is sensitive to only the severest vascular structure abnormalities. More in-depth studies include vascular biopsies and skin window testing procedures, which are research procedures. There are no routinely available methods for assessing increased vascular activity in the area of inappropriate clotting.

Platelet Function

Platelets are disk-shaped fragments of the large multinucleated megakaryocytes released from the bone marrow on a daily basis (normal count is 150 × 10^3/mL to 400 × 10^3/mL) (Fig. 19.2). Their life span is 8 to 10 days. These microscopic fragments have a well-defined substructure that can be directly correlated with platelet function.

The surface activation of the receptor sites on the platelet causes it to change first to a sphere and finally to a spiderlike structure, with pseudopods in all directions. This release reaction is the summation of biochemical and structural changes in the platelet, which are characterized as follows: The surface receptor sets up a biochemical chain reaction, resulting in the generation of thromboxane A_2. This causes contraction of the protein thrombosthenin, which causes the ejection of the platelet contents. Of great importance are the dense granules with nonmetabolic adenosine diphosphate (ADP). ADP is a potent platelet-aggregating agent that, in a dominolike sequence, stimulates more platelets, generating a large platelet plug.

The congenital diseases associated with poor platelet function are divided into four types of dysfunction: (a) adhesion to collagen, (b) adhesion to subendothelium, (c) release reaction defects, and (d) ADP aggregation defects. With the exception of von Willebrand disease, a defect in the adhesion to subendothelium, all the congenital defects are rare and not essential to this discussion. von Willebrand disease (Table 19.1) is a classically autosomal, dominantly inherited disorder resulting from absence, decreased production, or abnormal function of a large multimeric protein synthesized by megakaryocytes and vascular endothelium. This protein is responsible for the proper binding of platelets to the collagen surface exposed in

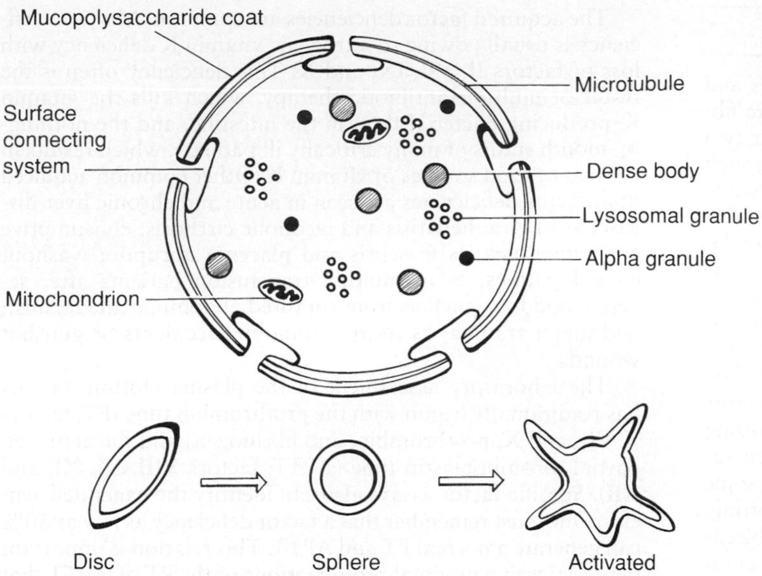

FIGURE 19.2. Platelet cross section.

vascular trauma. Its absence results in the failure of platelets to bind normally to disruptions in the vasculature, preventing formation of the platelet plug necessary for normal hemostasis. The condition remains undetected in most patients until some form of vascular trauma occurs or surgery is performed. In addition, such patients are particularly sensitive to aspirin or other antiplatelet medications and bleed excessively in surgery while taking this kind of medication. von Willebrand disease is the most common congenital platelet disorder and is the disease most likely to go undetected until surgery. This disorder is particularly dangerous because, in its milder forms, a history of bleeding in surgery is negative and the preoperative coagulation screen is normal. Acquired defects in platelet function are much more common and can be classified into two groups: (a) those that are the result or consequence of a disease, such as renal failure, myeloproliferative disorders (polycythemia vera, chronic myelogenous leukemia), and increased fibrin split products in consumptive coagulopathies; and (b) those that are iatrogenic, such as defects caused by medications (aspirin, nonsteroidal antiinflammatory drugs, antibiotics, antihistamines, tricyclic antidepressants, dextran) and cardiopulmonary bypass surgery.

Congenitally increased platelet function has not been described. Acquired disorders associated with increased platelet function, however, are common. The stress of routine surgery or trauma (fractured hip, femur, or pelvis) can create a hypercoagulable state with thrombocytosis and increased platelet activity.

The laboratory assessment of platelet function has been expanded from the research laboratory and is more readily available to the surgeon. The routine analysis of platelet function should begin with a platelet count and PFA-100. In special cases, platelet adhesion and platelet aggregation are useful in identifying the inadequate or overstimulated platelet. In addition, biochemical markers for increased platelet use or turnover can be demonstrated with platelet factor IV and β-thromboglobulin assays. Studies by Gewirtz and colleagues confirm previous studies that the bleeding time is not a good prediction of surgical bleeding.

TABLE 19.1

MORE COMMONLY SEEN RARE CONGENITAL CLOTTING DISORDERS

Name	Incidence (per million)	Treatment
Factor VIII (classic hemophilia A, sex-linked)	60–80	FVIII concentrate
Factor IX (classic hemophilia B, sex-linked)	15–20	FIX concentrate
von Willebrand disease (dominant; autosomal)	5–10	Cryoprecipitate (DDAVP), factor VIII concentrate with von Willebrand factor

DDAVP, Deamino-D-arginine vasopressin.
The remainder of the known congenital clotting factors are very rare and occur with such low frequency that their discussion, diagnosis, and management can be found elsewhere. (See Harker LA. *Hemostasis manual,* 2nd edition. Philadelphia: FA Davis;1974; Corriveau DM, Fritsma GA. *Hemostasis and thrombosis.* Philadelphia: JB Lippincott Co;1988; Triplett DA, ed. *Laboratory evaluation of coagulation.* Chicago: ASCP Press;1982.)

Plasma-Clotting Proteins

Plasma-clotting proteins are a group of serine proteases and cofactors that interact in a synergistic system to generate fibrin. The activation of the clotting system can be initiated in two ways: either by contact activation with factor XII or through thromboplastin activation of factor VII. The clotting cascade is diagrammed in Figure 19.3. As we will see later in the discussion of fibrinolysis and antithrombin systems, anticoagulation forces are initiated at the inception of clotting. The tear in the vessel wall, described earlier, begins the orderly activation of the plasma-clotting system. The fibrin contribution to the platelet–fibrin plug is initiated with the activation of factor XII by collagen and of factor VII by tissue juice (thromboplastin). Any congenital or acquired disorder of the clotting factors can lead to inadequate or no generation of fibrin. Each clotting factor has a different role and significance in the overall generation of fibrin. This also is true with abnormal increases in some clotting factors that are associated with inappropriate clotting.

The congenital-factor deficiencies associated with bleeding are either relatively common or rare. The relatively common group includes hemophilia A (factor VIII deficiency) and hemophilia B (factor IX deficiency). Both are seen in the male and rarely in the female disorders with sex-linked inheritance patterns. The rare group includes all the remaining factors that have an autosomal recessive inheritance pattern or a dominant pattern with variable penetrance.

The acquired factor deficiencies are common. Multiple deficiency is usually owing to iatrogenic vitamin K deficiency with loss of factors II, VII, IX, and X. This deficiency often is the result of multiple-antibiotic therapy, which kills the vitamin K–producing bacterial flora in the intestine, and the nothing-by-mouth status of many critically ill patients, which results in the loss of food sources of vitamin K. Other common acquired multifactor deficiencies are seen in acute and chronic liver disease, as in viral hepatitis and alcoholic cirrhosis; consumptive coagulopathies, as in sepsis and placenta abruptio; washout coagulopathies, as in multiple-transfusion patients after severe blood loss (such as from ruptured abdominal aneurysms); and major trauma, as from automobile accidents or gunshot wounds.

The laboratory assessment of the plasma clotting factors has traditionally begun with the prothrombin time (PT; factors V, VII, and X, prothrombin, and fibrinogen) and the activated partial thromboplastin time (APTT; factors VIII, IX, XI, and XII). Specific factor assays also can identify the exact deficiencies. One must remember that a factor deficiency as low as 30% can generate a normal PT and APTT. This relation is important in investigating minimal prolongations of the PT or APTT that appear insignificant but could be hiding a moderately severe deficiency. The tissue factor pathway inhibitor modulates activated factors X and VIII but is not apparently significant in disease.

The sensitivity of the PT and APTT reagents is essential to the appreciation of the proper use of these tests as preoperative

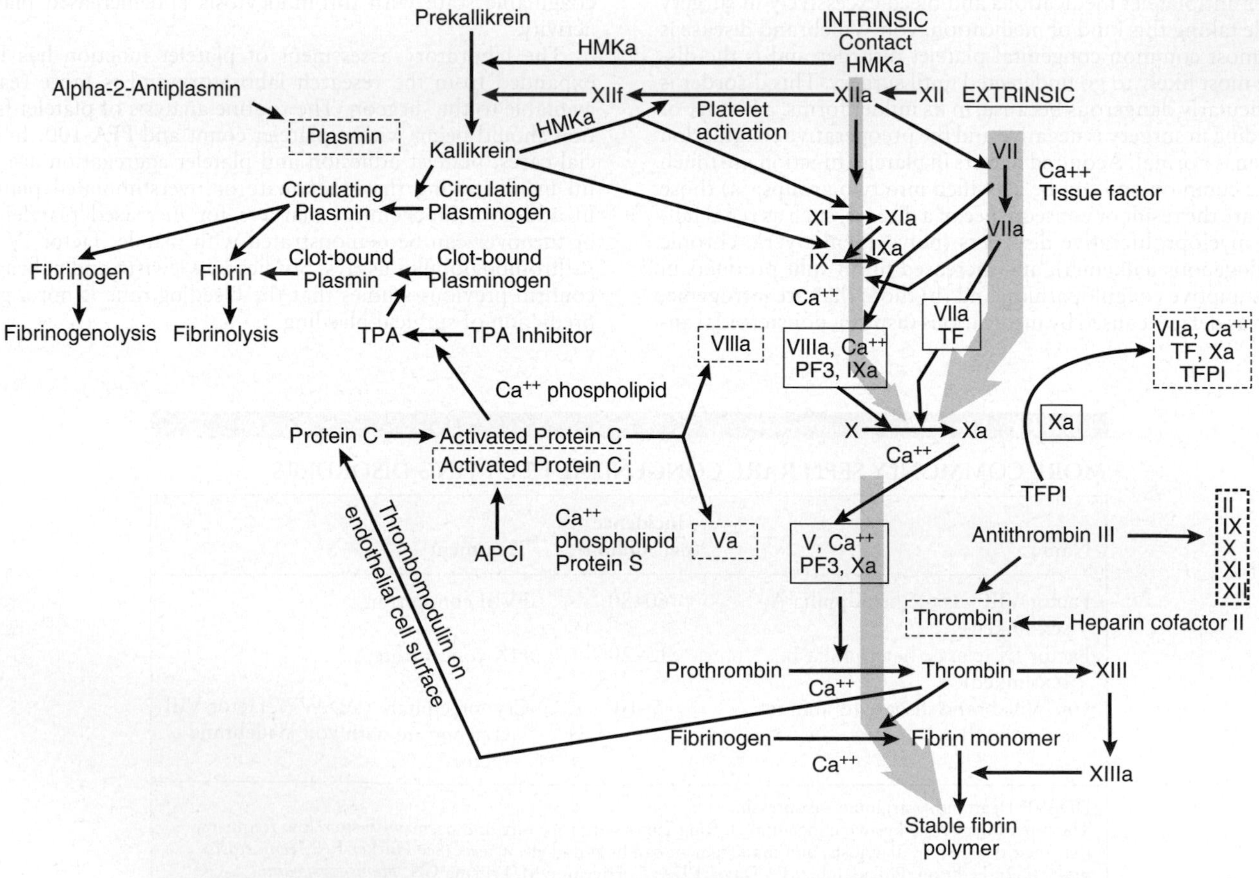

FIGURE 19.3. Coagulation system. Dashed boxes indicate destruction of factors. APC1, activated protein C1; HMKa, high-molecular-weight kininogen; PF3, platelet factor 3; TPA, tissue plasminogen activator; TF, tissue factor; TFPI, tissue factor pathway inhibitor.

TABLE 19.2

THERAPEUTIC RANGES FOR THE INTERNATIONAL NORMALIZED RATIOS

Condition	Therapeutic ranges
Prophylaxis for venous thromboembolism in high-risk surgery and in hip surgery	2.0–3.0
Treatment of venous thrombosis and pulmonary embolism	2.0–3.0
Prevention of systemic embolism	
Tissue heart valves	
Acute myocardial infarction	
Valvular heart disease	
Atrial fibrillation	
Bileaflet mechanical value in aortic position	
Treatment for mechanical prosthetic heart valves (high risk)	2.5–3.5
Prevention of recurrent systemic embolism	
Prevention of recurrent myocardial infarction	

From: Hirsh J, Dalen JE, Anderson DR, et al. Oral anticoagulants: mechanism of action, clinical effectiveness, and optimal therapeutic range. *Chest* 2002;119:8S.

screening tests or in monitoring warfarin and heparin anticoagulant therapy. Recent publications from Europe and the United States stress the importance of and need for a standardized prothrombin reagent system in the United States. The lack of sensitivity of the rabbit brain thromboplastin used in the United States has led to the overcoumarinization of some patients. The original value of 2.0 to 2.5 times the control was based on the more-sensitive human thromboplastin. Current recommendations have lower ratios (Table 19.2). These ratios are applicable only in stable, coumarinized patients. Studies of different APTT reagents have revealed a similar variability of sensitivity to heparin.

Fibrinolysis

The activation of the fibrinolytic system begins with the activation of the plasma substrate plasminogen. This substrate is converted by naturally occurring activators such as urokinase, kallikrein, and clot-activated proteases to the active enzyme plasmin. Plasmin is the active enzyme that if free or clot-bound lyses fibrin clots and destroys fibrinogen. This enzyme is modulated by α_2-antiplasmin and antitrypsin, which destroy the active enzyme plasmin.

This enzymatic conversion of fibrinolysis normally is initiated by clot formation or by a direct activator such as urokinase or tissue plasminogen activator (tPA). tPA released from the endothelium activates tissue plasminogen and is neutralized by plasminogen activator inhibitor-1 (PAI-1). Sometimes direct activation is seen in liver disease and during extracorporeal bypass. This activation also can be secondary to disease, as in a consumptive coagulopathy—such as bacterial sepsis—or a large abdominal aneurysm.

Hypercoagulable State

With physiologic stress, such as emotional stress and surgical stress, there is a response of fright or flight. This response to stress is evident in the coagulation system. The plasma-clotting proteins, such as fibrinogen and factor VIII, increase, and the platelet count and stickiness can increase as well. This normal response is important in ensuring hemostasis at the time of increased need. When this process is exaggerated, uncontrolled, or unmodulated, inappropriate clotting can occur, which produces venous and arterial clots and all their sequelae. In gynecologic surgery, the normal physical hypercoagulable state, as well as the inappropriate state, must be understood to appreciate the diagnosis, intervention, and management of postoperative vascular occlusive complications. Virchow, in 1845, was the first to conceptualize the triad of blood flow, vessel wall, and content of blood itself as a basis for inappropriate clotting. An understanding of the relation of the three parts is essential to explain what has occurred in the problem patient.

CONGENITAL CAUSES OF INAPPROPRIATE CLOTTING

The congenital etiology of inappropriate arterial and venous clotting has long been ill defined. Only recently has it been more completely elucidated (Tables 19.3 and 19.4). Procoagulants, when increased on a congenital basis, have been associated with a propensity to generate clots. These procoagulants include fibrinogen and factor VIII; however, they are not present frequently enough to warrant testing every suspect case. Naturally occurring inhibitors of clotting are defined as those factors that actively destroy clotting factors or substrates as they are formed. The more common of these rare deficiencies are antithrombin III, protein C, protein S, factor V Leiden (R506Q),

TABLE 19.3

RISK FACTORS FOR ARTERIAL THROMBOSIS

Inherited
Elevated cholesterol, triglycerides, lipoprotein (a), decreased high-density lipoprotein
Diabetes
FVII polymorphism
Hyperhomocysteinemia
Methylenetetrahydrofolate reductase mutation C677T
PLA_2 glycoprotein IIb/IIIa
Gender, male > female
Acquired
Antiphospholipid antibodies
Lupus anticoagulant
Hypertension
Diet with increased fat
Infection: chlamydia, cytomegalovirus
Heparin-induced thrombocytopenia
Social class, body mass index
Mixed hereditary/acquired
Factor VIII
Fibrinogen
FVII
Homocysteine
C-reactive protein
Von Willebrand factor

From: Triplett DA. Thrombophilia: laboratory evaluation. *ASCC Clinical Laboratory News* 2002;28:12.

TABLE 19.4

RISK FACTORS FOR VENOUS THROMBOSIS

Inherited
Common
Factor V Leiden (R506Q)
Factor II mutation (G21201A)
Factor VIII
Rare
Antithrombin III deficiency
Protein C deficiency
Protein S deficiency
PAI-1 polymorphism
Dysfibrinogenemia
Factor XII deficiency
Prekallikrein (Fletcher factor) deficiency
Plasminogen deficiency
Tissue plasminogen activator deficiency
Acquired
Surgery and trauma
Prolonged immobilization
Older age
Cancer
Myeloproliferative disorders
Previous venous thrombosis
Pregnancy/puerperium
Contraceptives/hormone replacement
Activated protein C resistance not due to FV Leiden
Antiphospholipid syndrome
Mild-to-moderate hyperhomocysteinemia
Obesity/metabolic syndrome

From: Seligsohn U, Lubetsky A. Genetic susceptibility to venous thrombosis. *N Engl J Med* 2001;344:1222.

factor II mutation (G21201A), PAI-1 polymorphisms 4G/5G, and methylenetetrahydrofolate reductase mutations (C677T, A1298C).

IMPAIRED FIBRINOLYSIS

A congenital decrease in the plasma substrate plasminogen results in inadequate fibrinolysis of thrombi. This deficiency can be qualitative and quantitative, with similar effects.

A congenital decrease in tPA that normally is released from the vascular endothelium is associated with impaired fibrinolysis. An abnormal increase in plasminogen activator inhibitor also will reduce the level of tPA, resulting in inappropriate clotting, elevated PAI-1 secondary to obesity, metabolic syndrome, or acute phase reactions.

The decrease or absence of Fletcher factor (prekallikrein) and factor XII also can result in impaired fibrinolysis because of a decrease in activation of circulating plasminogen at the time of clot activation.

ACQUIRED CAUSES OF INAPPROPRIATE CLOTTING

The number of acquired causes of inappropriate clotting is much greater than the number of congenital causes and is expanding every day because the same chemistry found in the congenital mechanism can be identified as a deficiency in an ongoing disease process. These include such risk factors as an elevated factor VIIIc, fibrinogen, metastatic cancer, myeloproliferative disorders, and diabetes/metabolic syndrome.

Iatrogenic causes of inappropriate clotting are common findings in the hospital setting and generate great concern. Such causes include the postsurgical state, medication, vascular prosthetic devices, and immobilization for any reason.

As a physiologic acute-phase response to surgical stress, an exaggerated outpouring of clotting factors and platelets in combination with a decrease in physiologic inhibitors can result in clot formation. This often occurs in deep leg veins, particularly in association with venous stasis.

Prosthetic devices such as grafts, shunts, and artificial heart valves can provide a clottable surface that will form a nidus for initial thrombosis quickly followed by further clot formation, resulting in obstruction or embolization.

The vascular component of acquired thrombotic disease has only recently been described in detail. It appears that decreased blood flow through a vein can decrease the contact between thrombin and thrombomodulin, diminishing the contact with protein C and predisposing the vein to thrombosis. However, the arterial side with high blood flow rates has a rich capillary bed with greater contact with protein C, lysing clots more efficiently. Local thrombus formation can be generated by direct mechanical disruption of the vascular endothelium, traumatic damage to the vessel wall, infectious or chemical damage to the vessel wall, and vasculitis.

PREOPERATIVE COAGULATION ASSESSMENT FOR SURGICAL PATIENTS

For the preoperative evaluation, gynecologic patients must of necessity be divided into two categories: those having routine or elective surgery and those having emergency surgery.

Elective Surgery

The elective gynecologic surgical patient must be evaluated in two ways: general medical history and specific nature of the surgery. The medical history taken at bedside, with review of the medical chart when available, is an excellent place to begin. Table 19.5 highlights the most important positive and negative findings to be identified.

Preoperative coagulation screening is of limited value without complete knowledge of the patient's past and current

TABLE 19.5

PERTINENT MEDICAL HISTORY TO SCREEN FOR COAGULATION PROBLEMS

History of spontaneous bruising or bleeding
History of unusual bruising or excessive bleeding after surgery
Family history of bruising or bleeding after surgery
Medication associated with bruising or bleeding
Current medication within past week
Previous coagulation testing
Current coagulation testing

TABLE 19.6

TESTS TO INDICATE COAGULATION STATUS

Test	Reference range[a]	Level of alarm	Significance
Hematocrit (%)	37–47	25	Tissue anoxia
White cell count (mL)	4×10^3–12×10^3	3×10^3–25×10^3	Susceptibility to infection, leukemia
Platelet count (mL)	140×10^3–400×10^3	100×10^3–700×10^3	Bleeding, myeloproliferative disorder
Fibrinogen (mg/dL)	150–400	100	Bleeding, liver disease, intravascular consumption
Prothrombin time (s)	10–13	14	Bleeding factor deficiency
Activated partial thromboplastin time (s)	28–38	40	Bleeding factor deficiency, inhibitor
PFA-100	Collagen–epinephrine	Prolonged closure time	Screen for medication effect
Bleeding time (will not predict surgical bleeding)			

[a]Reference ranges may vary in each laboratory, reflecting method, instrumentation, and reagents.

history. It does not replace a good history and physical examination. One should not expect this screening to reveal the estimated blood loss in a routine surgical procedure. It is essential, however, for resolving and eliminating risk factors that can affect postoperative bleeding (Tables 19.6 and 19.7).

Risk factors such as unknown history or known history in an emergency surgical procedure; positive personal or family history of bleeding or bleeding with or without surgery; and known history of taking medications that can affect coagulation, such as antiplatelet medication, acquired vitamin K deficiency (nothing-by-mouth status with long use of antibiotics), and fibrinolytic therapy (decreased fibrinogen), are assessed by preoperative screening.

A preoperative coagulation screen is not usually indicated unless the medical history and physical examination reveal suspicious or explained findings that suggest a risk of surgical bleeding. These findings might include a history of unexplained surgical bleeding, family history of bleeding, bleeding after medication, or evidence of bruising or bleeding on examination, to mention only a few.

The risk of blood-borne infections and adverse reactions is always present, but the documented need for blood as a lifesaving substance will validate the decision. When blood is transfused when indicated but is not justified in writing, this lifesaving substance becomes a liability to all who use it. The routine preoperative orders for blood require knowledge of the specific needs of the patient and the surgeon's usual transfusion requirements for a specific surgical procedure. For the routine gynecologic procedure, such as simple hysterectomy in an otherwise healthy woman, a type and antibody screen are appropriate. With the type and antibody screen, the patient's blood is screened for unexpected antibodies. No specific blood units are set aside, but blood is available from the general inventory in an emergency. If an unexpected antibody is identified, the blood bank should notify the ordering physician and set aside 2 U of antigen-negative cross-matched compatible blood for use in an emergency situation.

In an emergency, the blood bank can release blood immediately (with a type and match to follow) with a 99.99% safety factor when the previous screen for unexpected antibodies was negative. Additionally, when the surgeon can wait 10 to 15 minutes, an immediate spin cross match can be performed to further verify ABO compatibility between donor and recipient. The value of the type and antibody screen is in monetary savings for the patient, and there is no undue or unnecessary risk to the patient.

In more complex procedures, such as pelvic exenteration for cancer, where there usually is significant blood loss, a type and cross match for the average number of units used is appropriate. With extremely difficult procedures or other complicating diseases, additional blood, fresh-frozen plasma, and platelets may be required during the procedure and should be requested preoperatively.

Ideal or time-proven guidelines are difficult to establish for every operative case. Each surgical experience will benefit the surgeon, and over time he or she will establish usual transfusion requirements for both type and antibody screen, as well as type and cross match. The hospital quality assurance program, in planning with the transfusion service or blood bank and transfusion committee, should establish guidelines to assist the surgeon in identifying the usual blood transfusion needs. The use of either Guidelines for Transfusion Therapy (Boral) or Maximal Surgical Blood Order Schedule (Judd) is helpful in developing hospital guidelines.

TABLE 19.7

COAGULATION PROFILES

Brief coagulation profile	Complete coagulation profile
CBC (includes WBC differential)	CBC (includes WBC differential)
Platelet count	Platelet count
Prothrombin time	Prothrombin time
Partial activated Thromboplastin time	Partial activated Thromboplastin time
	Fibrinogen
	PSA-100

CBC, complete blood count; WBC, white blood cell.

Emergency Surgery

As the emergency procedure is begun, decisions regarding blood replacement must be made. A direct approach to blood replacement therapy and the complications of such therapy depends on a clear understanding of the following concepts.

1. As bank blood replacement with just packed red cells corrects the blood loss problem, it may create an acquired bleeding disorder, thrombocytopenic hemophilia. Platelets and fresh-frozen plasma may be indicated.
2. The patient's bleeding potential is dynamic and will change rapidly and frequently with the loss of blood and replacement therapy.
3. Direct monitoring before, during, and after surgery offers the best chance to diagnose and manage the bleeding. Direct monitoring also allows formulation of plans and adjustment of the replacement therapy program.

COMPONENT THERAPY FOR REPLACEMENT BEFORE SURGERY

With surgery planned, the preoperative data can be evaluated. Assuming the patient does not have hemophilia, von Willebrand disease, severe liver disease, or liver failure, a prolonged PT and APTT may suggest a less common acquired or congenital bleeding disorder. (The blood sample must be properly drawn and mixed well and must not be taken from an A-line containing heparin or from an infusion site.) Assistance from a clinical pathologist or hematologist should be requested if an intrinsic bleeding disorder is suspected.

COMPONENT THERAPY FOR REPLACEMENT DURING SURGERY

According to Schifman and Steinbronn, when intraoperative blood loss exceeds 15% of the patient's estimated blood volume, the surgeon should consider red blood cell transfusion to replace the acute blood loss. As a general rule, 15% of an adult's blood volume equals the patient's weight (in kilograms) times 10. For example, for a 50-kg woman (110 lb), 15% of blood volume is (50 × 10) 500 mL; for a 75-kg woman (165 lb), 15% of blood volume is (75 × 10) 750 mL; for a 100-kg woman (220 lb), 15% of blood volume is (100 × 10) 1,000 mL. The patient's estimated blood volume, the estimated intraoperative blood loss, the anticipation of additional blood loss, the presence of preoperative anemia, and the risk of hypoxic complications must all be taken into consideration when deciding whether to transfuse.

When massive blood replacement therapy is under way, intraoperative monitoring of coagulation at 2-hour intervals, or after every 10 U of blood transfused, usually is sufficient. One should remember that a patient bleeding during a surgical procedure has a higher demand for clotting factors and platelets than does a patient at bed rest. In many oncology cases in which the patient is undergoing chemotherapy, a platelet count of 50,000/mL is adequate; in a surgical case in which the patient is bleeding, a 50,000/mL platelet count is not adequate to achieve a good platelet plug. The use of blood and blood components in the management of massive bleeding that is due to a major vessel rupture has the following objectives:

1. To maintain sufficient blood volume and circulating red cells to sustain life
2. To replace blood sufficiently to achieve adequate coagulation and hemostasis, assuming there was extensive loss of plasma-clotting factors and platelets
3. To avoid falling so far behind in replacement that management involves not only bleeding from a vascular tear but also bleeding at the microvascular level because of insufficient clotting factors and platelets

Each of these objectives requires repeated assessment of the patient throughout the surgical procedure. Careful monitoring by established routine policies often is the best way to handle a crisis situation created by massive bleeding.

Formulas for blood transfusion that are applied ritualistically without the benefit of laboratory data may resolve the need to treat but do not answer the needs of the patient. The formulas described below are designed to initiate the marshaling of blood bank resources. They do not replace the thoughtful analysis of laboratory data coupled with the selection of a specific blood component to correct a specific deficit. The following guidelines are recommended for component therapy in clinical situations requiring massive blood replacement to maintain normal hemostasis.

For every 6 to 8 U of packed red blood cells, 2 U (500 mL) of fresh-frozen plasma should be given. The size and age of the patient affect blood replacement. If the patient's blood volume can accommodate an additional 500 mL of fresh-frozen plasma, this amount should be transfused and the PT and APTT monitored.

Platelets should be given when the platelet count falls below 100,000/mL in massive hemorrhage. (Measurement error of a platelet count can be as high as 62,000/mL in a bleeding patient.) When a long surgical procedure is anticipated, or when more than 6 U of blood are given, 6 U of platelets in a volume of 300 mL should be given toward the end of the surgical procedure or when surgical hemostasis is achieved. This amount should be administered once to provide a maximum bolus effect. Because platelets are often difficult to obtain, their use should be reserved until near the end of the procedure. Otherwise, they may be lost and therefore unavailable when needed because of continued blood loss and replacement during extensive surgical repair. Pooling and transporting the platelets can take up to an hour, so the blood bank should be given sufficient notice to have them available in surgery when needed. In assessing the patient's coagulation status, it should be remembered that clotting factors are constantly changing. Six units of platelets will achieve maximum bolus effect in an average patient (3 U in a child or small adult) and will also enable evaluation of platelet use. A platelet count of 40,000 to 60,000/mL should be expected in a 70-kg person after transfusion of 6 U of platelets. Monitoring the platelet count after transfusion and for the next several hours will reveal the success of replacement, consumption, and life of the platelets.

When the PT and APTT are prolonged (more than 14 seconds and 40 seconds, respectively) after replacement therapy, intrinsic disease must be considered initially, if only to be ruled out later. A borderline hemophiliac or patient with liver disease may manifest excessive bleeding after stress, trauma, or blood replacement because of the increased coagulation needs. A mild hemophilia or liver disease is rare as an unknown, but it is possible. Therefore, administration of fresh-frozen plasma in these 2-U (500-mL) doses should begin to correct the deficiencies caused by massive red blood cell replacement. If oozing continues despite the rapid transfusion of 6 U of fresh-frozen plasma, a clotting problem or other ongoing bleeding disorder should be suspected and additional support sought.

When the fibrinogen level falls below 100 mg/dL, transfusion of 20 U of cryoprecipitate will provide about 150 mg/dL fibrinogen in a 70-kg person. A low fibrinogen level is rare because fibrinogen is stable and present in fresh-frozen plasma. Liver disease or intravascular consumption must be suspected if the fibrinogen level is initially less than 100 mg/dL and remains low throughout surgery and recovery. The 20 U of cryoprecipitate will achieve therapeutic levels quickly and permit monitoring over several hours.

The goals of intraoperative monitoring are as follows:

- To assess changes in the coagulation mechanism resulting from blood loss and replacement therapy
- To identify the coagulation components affected and determine the correct components to initiate therapy
- To determine the success of replacement component therapy in an extensive operative procedure
- To enable selection of components to achieve the following values: PT less than 14 seconds, APTT less than 40 seconds, fibrinogen more than 100 mg/dL, and platelets more than 80×10^3/mL. If surgical hemostasis appears to have been achieved from a technical viewpoint and bleeding is present but mild, one can "wait to see" for 2 hours. If bleeding is profuse and worsening, 2 to 4 U of fresh-frozen plasma and a 6- to 10-U dose of platelets are given, and then packed red cells are given as needed. The patient is monitored when the transfusion is completed. Laboratory monitoring is repeated after 1 to 2 hours, whether the patient is bleeding or not, to determine the success of replacement.

COMPONENT THERAPY FOR POSTOPERATIVE REPLACEMENT

The presurgical and intrasurgical alarm levels for hematocrit, platelet count, PT, APTT, fibrinogen, and clot retraction also apply postoperatively, and a comparison of these values provides an accurate assessment of the bleeding patient. Significant clinical bleeding with good postoperative coagulation values suggests surgical bleeding. When laboratory values are abnormal, however, further surgery can be delayed until an attempt at aggressive specific component therapy is made. We have found that when abnormal coagulation studies exist, the following causes predominate, in order of frequency (most frequent first):

1. Low platelet count owing to transfusion of only packed red cells or fresh-frozen plasma
2. Prolonged PT and APTT owing to replacement with packed red cells without fresh-frozen plasma. In administering aggressive replacement therapy, it should be remembered that some patients have a meager blood volume. Careful monitoring of venous and arterial pressure, as well as cardiac output, should be considered in blood component therapy. Often a slower rate of administration can achieve hemostasis without cardiovascular overload. In rare cases, phlebotomy may be required to create needed space for transfusion. If nearly normal coagulation values are achieved but bleeding continues, surgical causes for bleeding should be considered.
3. Low fibrinogen level owing to dilution with plasma expanders or concurrent development of a disseminated intravascular coagulation

The goals of postoperative monitoring are as follows:

- To determine whether a coagulopathy was created by blood replacement and to determine current status
- To determine the success of specific component therapy and identify the need for additional components
- To enable the surgeon to distinguish surgical from nonsurgical bleeding

The routine use of postoperative monitoring, whether the patient is bleeding or not, will achieve these goals. As the surgeon reviews the results of each case, he or she will develop a valuable assessment of the patient's usual postoperative coagulation states. With this knowledge, the unexpected is recognized and resolved in a more timely manner.

RISKS OF BLOOD TRANSFUSION

Transfusions of whole blood were given sporadically before 1900, usually to treat specific diseases rather than to replace lost blood volume. Indeed, heavy bleeding was thought to be beneficial and therapeutic for many diseases. Even as late as World War I, the importance of blood loss and replacement was not recognized, because shock was thought to be owing to toxins released from traumatized tissue. It was the work of Cannon and Bayliss in 1919 and of Blalock in 1930 that proved that the important factors in shock were the loss of circulating blood volume and the decreased return of venous blood to the right heart.

Landsteiner discovered the four major blood groups in 1900. Banking and storage of donated blood became possible with refrigeration and the addition of sugar and later sodium citrate as an anticoagulant. In World War II, a remarkable program was organized to collect and store large quantities of type O (so-called universal donor) blood for shipment to U.S. military hospitals throughout the world. Many lives were saved by the use of this banked blood to treat the shock associated with battle casualties. This experience firmly established the need for blood banks and the importance of blood transfusions in combatting hypovolemic shock from hemorrhage before, during, and after surgery.

To be safe, homologous blood must be collected from carefully selected volunteer donors and properly matched to the potential recipient. Although many lives have been saved by properly administered transfusions, gynecologic surgeons must be aware of the potential hazards of perioperative transfusions. The risks of red blood cell transfusion were reviewed by a National Institutes of Health and Food and Drug Administration Consensus Development Conference on Perioperative Red Cell Transfusion and published in 1988. The following excerpt is taken directly from their report.

In deciding whether to use red blood cell transfusion in the perioperative period, the need for possibly improved oxygenation must be weighed against the risks of adverse consequences, both short term and long term. The disadvantages are of two general types: transmission of infection and adverse effects attributable to immune mechanisms.

Any infectious agent that is present in the blood of a donor at the time of donation is potentially transmissible to a susceptible recipient. The consequence may be seen as clinical morbidity and mortality after an incubation period characteristic of the agent or recognized only by serological or other types of laboratory testing. If the agent produces chronic infection, clinical mortality may not be seen until years after the transfusion (Table 19.8).

TABLE 19.8

BLOOD TRANSFUSION RISKS

Disease or situation	Risk
Viral infection	
HIV	1:1.9 million
HTLV	1:250,000–1:2.0 million
Hepatitis B	1:180,000
Hepatitis C	1:1.6 million
Bacterial contamination	
Platelet packs (stored at room temperature)	1:12,000
Packed or whole red blood cells	1:5 million
Fatal red-cell hemolytic reaction	1:250,000–1:1.1 million
Delayed red-cell hemolytic reaction	1:1,000–1:1,500
TRALI	1:5,000
Febrile red-cell nonhemolytic reaction	1:100
Allergic (urticarial reaction)	1:100
Anaphylactic reaction	1:150,000

HIV, human immunodeficiency virus; HTLV, human t-cell lymphotrophic virus; TRALI, transfusion-related acute lung injury. From: Zoon KC. Ten years after: what has been achieved by Consent Decrees: the FDA view. Paper presented at: Fifth Annual FDA and the Changing Paradigm for Blood Regulation; January 16–18, 2002; New Orleans, LA; Schreiber GB, Busch MP, Kleinman SH, et al. The risk of transfusion-transmitted viral infections: the retrovirus epidemiology donor study. *N Engl J Med* 1996;334:1685; Dziecxkowski JS, Anderson KC. Transfusion biology and therapy. In: Fauci AS, Martin JB, Braunwald E, et al., eds. *Harrison's principles of internal medicine.* 14th edition. New York: McGraw-Hill;1998:718; Goodnough LT, Breacher ME, Kanter MH, et al. Transfusion medicine: first of two parts—blood transfusion. *N Engl J Med* 1999:340;438.

In modern blood banking practice, bacterial contamination of red blood cell units is rare. For practical purposes, the transmissible agents of greatest concern are viruses.

- Cytomegalovirus infection occurs with moderate frequency among those recipients without prior infection. Most of these infections are asymptomatic, except among immunocompromised people. The use of the newer leukocyte reduction filters ($<5 \times 10^6$) is under extensive clinical study and application as an alternative to cytomegalovirus-negative blood.
- Human T-cell lymphotropic viruses occur with low but not negligible frequency among donor populations in the United States. It is not known whether transfusion-transmitted infection with these viruses among adults results in T-cell leukemia/lymphoma and/or neurological disease several to many years later.
- On rare occasions, other microbial agents—including paroviruses, malaria, *Toxoplasma,* Epstein-Barr virus, and *Babesia*—cause infection and disease.

It is known for the human hepatitis viruses that the incidence of infection in recipients increases with the number of donor exposures. This relationship is probably true for other transfusion-transmitted infections. If homologous transfusion is to be used, therefore, the number of units administered should be kept to a minimum.

HIV, about which there is the greatest public concern, presently poses only a remote hazard because of donor selection and laboratory screening procedures. The consequences of HIV infection are rarely seen until 2 or many more years have elapsed, but ultimately morbidity and mortality are extremely high.

Immunologic consequences also complicate homologous red blood cell transfusion. Hemolytic and nonhemolytic reactions are largely caused by alloimmunization to red blood cell and leukocyte antigens. Compatibility testing virtually has eliminated immediate hemolytic transfusion reactions; when they occur, they are largely owing to human error. Nonhemolytic febrile reactions occur in 1% to 2% of recipients owing to sensitization to leukocyte antigens. This may be reduced by the use of leukocyte reduction filters ($<5 \times 10^6$).

Although blood transfusions are and will remain an essential component of perioperative gynecologic care, an awareness of their associated risks is important in every patient before electing their use. There is every reason to carefully consider the risk:benefit ratio of giving "just one bottle of blood." Indeed, it is the rare clinical situation in which this action can be justified.

The growing public concern about transfusion-associated infections should make gynecologic surgeons aware of the importance of being selective in their use of transfusion therapy. The public has been greatly sensitized by the transfusion-associated transfer of acquired immunodeficiency syndrome (AIDS). The most common transfusion-related viral infection, however, is non-A, non-B hepatitis, which accounts for 90% to 95% of cases of previous transfusion-acquired hepatitis and possibly as many as 3,000 deaths per year in the United States. Ultimately, on further testing, many of these cases will be found to have hepatitis C. When mortality or significant morbidity occurs with blood transfusion, the gynecologic surgeon must be able to show that the transfusion was indicated.

There are alternatives to blood and blood component transfusion that may be considered in critically ill patients such as those with sepsis and deseminated intravascular coagulation. The drug activated protein C, drotrecogin alfa (Xigris), is recombinant human activated protein C (drotrecogin alfa, activated). It is used in replacement therapy in sepsis and holds a great promise in the management and survival in sepsis. By replacing this essential naturally occurring anticoagulant, there is reversal of the bleeding and thrombosis seen with sepsis. Its specific application in septic gynecological surgical patients has not been reported in any large study.

Recombinant activated FVII (NovoSeven) has been clinically demonstrated to successfully manage patients with FVIII and FIX inhibitors. It has also been used in management of bleeding in cardiovascular surgery, liver failure, and Coumadin overdose, and disseminated intravascular coagulation. It has significantly reduced the use of blood components in these disorders, and although expensive, it has the potential to greatly improve the outcomes with these disorders.

By reducing the need for blood and blood components with the use of activated protein C, drotrecogin alfa, and recombinant activated FVII, one can reduce the infectious disease exposure of blood, as well as the generation of allogenic antibodies. Not only may there be improved survival, but also there should be a substantial reduction of blood and blood components used in the treatment of similar complications in gynecological surgery.

According to Friedman and colleagues, in every age range the mean hematocrit of men is higher than that of women. Women adapt to this relative state of anemia physiologically by a variety of mechanisms. Their red blood cells have a greater capacity than those of men to release oxygen. The erythrocyte oxygen dissociation curve of women is right-shifted when compared with that of men. Levels of 2,3,-diphosphoglycerate, adenosine triphosphate (ATP), and glucose-6-phosphate are higher in the red blood cells of women than in those of men. Because of these physiologic adaptations, Friedman and colleagues suggest that a lower hematocrit support level to govern the blood transfusion of female surgical patients be considered.

There are a variety of methods to support circulating volume, but there is no available material to support oxygen transport. Future research may be successful in developing modified hemoglobin solutions and perfluorochemical emulsions for oxygen transport, but there currently is no substitute for red blood cells for this purpose.

In a comprehensive discussion of perioperative interventions to decrease transfusion of allogeneic blood products, Ereth and associates suggest that an increased awareness of transfusion-related morbidity from allogeneic blood products has resulted in increased development and application of alternatives to allogeneic transfusion. As an indication of what can be accomplished, a program instituted by the Transfusion Committee of the Methodist Hospital of Indianapolis modified transfusion practice in the hospital by establishing new transfusion guidelines based on national standards rather than on local practices and by implementing educational and monitoring systems. As reported by Rosen and colleagues, over a 3-year period, the total decrease in donor exposures for patients was 42,072. Overall savings amounted to $1,627,348. This program was able to effect substantial cost and patient risk reductions, even though hospital services involving blood transfusion increased. A comprehensive update titled "Transfusion Medicine in Obstetrics and Gynecology" was published recently by Santoso and associates.

AUTOLOGOUS BLOOD TRANSFUSION

Blood collected from a patient for retransfusion at a later time into the same patient is called autologous blood. Autologous blood transfusions have been endorsed by the Council on Scientific Affairs of the American Medical Association and by the Committee on Hospital Transfusion Practice of the American Association of Blood Banks. If established guidelines are followed, autologous blood is the safest type of blood for transfusion. It does not eliminate all risks associated with red blood cell transfusion, because there is still the possibility of a hemolytic reaction caused by the rare clerical error or bacterial contamination. It does eliminate the risk of alloimmunization and the risk of transferring such infections as hepatitis, malaria, cytomegalovirus, and AIDS. In patients with rare blood types who have antibodies to common blood antigens, it may be the only blood available for transfusion. Autologous blood transfusion is acceptable to most Jehovah's Witnesses who have a religious objection to transfusion with homologous blood or blood products. The use of autologous blood decreases the need for banked blood, which may then be reserved for other purposes. Given the improved safety of allogeneic transfusions today, the increased protection afforded by donating autologous blood is limited and may not justify the increased cost. This choice may be presented to the patient who has concerns about blood transfusion.

Intraoperative Autologous Transfusion

The frequency of autologous transfusion has increased appreciably in the past decade, especially for cardiovascular operations. Keeling and colleagues reported on the use of the Haemonetics Cell Saver for autologous intraoperative transfusion in 725 consecutive general hospital patients. Seventy-five percent were cardiovascular patients, but a variety of other patients, including gynecology/obstetric patients, were represented.

A general subject review of intraoperative autologous transfusion was published by Popovsky and associates in 1985. These investigators stated that although the technology of the earlier experiences was comparatively crude and associated with technical problems and complications, better methods have been developed in recent years to eliminate problems in the operation and maintenance of the machinery and to make intraoperative autologous transfusion safe. Our experience in gynecologic surgery reported by Shapiro and Toledo, although limited at this point to a series of 25 myomectomy operations, has demonstrated to our satisfaction that intraoperative autologous transfusion is convenient to use and does not in any way interfere with the performance of the procedure.

The Haemonetics Cell Saver operates by retrieving blood from the operative site by suctioning it into a double-lumen catheter, in which it is immediately anticoagulated with heparin. It is then collected in a cardiotomy reservoir, where a filter removes gross debris. The blood is then pumped to a spinning centrifuge bowl, where the red blood cells are separated, washed with normal saline solution, and then concentrated to a hematocrit of about 50%. The supernatant waste that is subsequently collected contains saline, anticoagulant, activated coagulation factors, platelets, leukocytes, free hemoglobin, and other small debris. The washed packed red blood cells are pumped into a reinfusion bag. The blood is then directly transfused to the patient through a filter. The reagents and the collecting system are sterile and disposable. The entire process takes 8 to 10 minutes to process about 250 mL of packed cells. The machine is maintained and operated by a trained technician.

At least until additional data are available to the contrary, intraoperative autologous transfusion is contraindicated in patients with malignant disease and in patients with bacterial contamination of blood in the operative field. Although the addition of antibiotic agents to the cell-washing system can reduce or eliminate contaminating bacteria, some bacteria with the potential of causing systemic infection if retransfused may remain. There is a theoretical concern that malignant cells contained in retransfused blood may be responsible for generalized seeding of the malignant process. Although there are no data to support or deny this position—for medicolegal reasons at least—intraoperative autologous transfusion should be considered contraindicated in a patient with cancer unless the need is desperate. It is difficult to distinguish the hematologic changes induced by intraoperative autologous transfusion from the changes induced by hemorrhage and massive transfusion with homologous blood. Guidelines for the use of component therapy are the same for both groups.

Merrill and colleagues reported the use of intraoperative autotransfusion in 38 patients with ruptured ectopic pregnancy. Transfusion-related morbidity occurred in six patients; two patients developed clinical coagulopathy, two patients developed pulmonary edema, and two patients developed minor transfusion reactions from concomitantly used bank blood. The total amount of retransfused blood was 49,475 mL, or 59% of the total amount of blood administered. This saved about 90 U of banked blood.

It must be remembered that both autologous (intraoperative) and homologous blood are essentially packed red blood cells. One risk with autologous blood transfusions is forgetting that only the patient's packed cells are transfused. The patient still will need fresh-frozen plasma and platelets when massive transfusion of autologous blood is used.

Predeposit Autologous Blood Transfusion

Because blood transfusion is so rarely required in gynecologic surgery for benign disease, predeposit of autologous blood for intraoperative transfusion is rarely indicated. However, certain patients may strongly desire this approach if there is any possibility of requiring a transfusion; in some patients with malignant disease or other extensive surgery, the risk of transfusion may be significant. Experience has shown that autologous blood can be collected and stored as whole blood, red blood cells, plasma, or platelets for retransfusion into the same patient during surgery if needed or at some other time. Donation can be scheduled at weekly intervals up to 3 days before surgery. Oral iron therapy is administered, and the hematocrit and hemoglobin levels must not be low. The American Association of Blood Banks' standards for elective preoperative autologous blood donation include the following guidelines:

- A hemoglobin of no less than 11 g/dL or a packed cell volume of no less than 34%
- Phlebotomy no more frequently than every 3 days and not within 72 hours of surgery

If a patient's condition is stable enough to allow elective surgery, then preoperative donation for autologous transfusion is not contraindicated. Mann and associates studied the safety of autologous blood donation before elective surgery for a variety of potentially high-risk patients. Of 300 patients in the study, 46 were at least 70 years old. Four percent of patients experienced a minor reaction to blood donation. This method of providing autologous blood should have applicability in gynecologic surgery. Experience suggests that it should be encouraged when practical.

The number of centers providing autologous blood transfusion programs will probably continue to increase as a result of AIDS and public knowledge of the possibility of spread of this disease by homologous blood transfusion, even though rare. Programs encouraging selected patients to donate their own blood before surgery are becoming increasingly popular, despite the numerous logistical problems that must be solved. Only 2% of the blood collected in the United States is for predeposit autologous transfusion.

Much of gynecologic surgery is elective, and many patients are comparatively healthy. Elective gynecologic surgery often is scheduled 3 to 4 weeks in the future. During this time, many patients can have blood predeposited for use during operation. Only about 2% of patients undergoing elective hysterectomy require blood transfusion, depending on the skill of the operator and the extent and nature of the gynecologic pathology. Routine predeposit of autologous blood is not recommended for hysterectomy for benign disease.

Goodnough and colleagues have found that the administration of recombinant human erythropoietin increases the amount of autologous blood that can be collected before surgery. The volume of red cells donated by patients treated with erythropoietin during the study was 41% greater than that donated by patients given placebo.

BASIC SURGICAL PRINCIPLES TO AVOID EXCESSIVE BLEEDING IN PELVIC SURGERY

It is easier to stay out of trouble than to get out of trouble! A good knowledge of the surgical anatomy is the basis for avoiding hemorrhage. A well-planned surgical procedure with good exposure, precise placement of the clamps, skillful dissection technique, and careful suture placement are all important. In addition to good technical ability, surgical judgment is a key ingredient to a consistently excellent surgical outcome. Should the densely adherent bladder be dissected a little more before clamping across the vagina? Should the endometriosis in the posterior cul-de-sac be dissected free from the sigmoid colon or just cauterized? These decisions occur constantly during any operation, and the surgeon who knows the patient, the disease entity being treated, the technical details of the planned surgical procedure, and his or her own technical abilities can confidently make these judgments that will result in a successful surgical outcome and avoid complications such as intraoperative hemorrhage.

Among the many contributions to surgery made by William S. Halsted, first chief of surgery at Johns Hopkins Hospital, was a surgical technique that emphasized meticulousness in dissection, gentleness in the handling of tissues, accuracy in hemostasis, precision in wound approximation, and absolute asepsis. This meticulous technique has become widely known in the United States as the Halstedian technique. It promotes good tissue healing by reducing tissue damage and wound infection. The accuracy of dissection, hemostasis, and tissue approximation is emphasized rather than speed, but wasting time with unnecessary hesitation, indefiniteness, and indecision can increase blood loss and the risk of infection. The experienced surgeon will be able to finish the operative procedures in a deliberate, purposeful, timely, and precise manner. The speed with which the dissection is performed should be varied from one phase of the operation to the other, but the operation should progress in an orderly manner. For example, the incision can be fashioned with some haste, but dissection around deep pelvic veins must be performed with great caution to avoid injury and bleeding. Although shorter operative procedures are generally associated with less blood loss and lower rates of infection, the pace of the procedure should be governed by the difficulty of the surgery and the skill and experience of the surgeon. Too much haste will sooner or later result in excessive blood loss or injury to adjacent organs or structures, which will ultimately prolong the operation. Technical aspects of surgical technique, including good exposure, gentle handling of tissues, accurate clamp placement, and good suture technique—which includes secure knot tying—are all important characteristics that will minimize blood loss and contribute to a successful and well-executed operative procedure.

It is impossible to place too much emphasis on the need for **optimum exposure** to limit blood loss. During vaginal operations, a contracted pelvic outlet will limit exposure for vaginal hysterectomy. A leiomyomatous uterus may require morcellation to allow sufficient exposure for safe vaginal removal. A Schuchardt incision may be required to improve exposure during vaginal operations. If exposure is inadequate, bleeding from vessels in the upper broad ligament may not be controllable from below, and an abdominal incision may be necessary to achieve final hemostasis from above. When hemorrhage is a problem during vaginal or laparoscopic surgery, the question always arises, "When should the operation be converted to an open abdominal procedure so that improved exposure and better access can be used to control the bleeding?" The answer to this question will vary depending on a variety of circumstances, but good exposure will go a long way toward solving many surgical difficulties. During abdominal operations, the exposure achieved will depend on the choice of incision, the method of retracting, the placement and intensity of the lights, and the presence of willing and skilled assistants. *Suction should be available* to keep the field as free of blood as possible and is preferred over sponges for two reasons. First, sponges can cause damage to delicate serosal surfaces. Second, a determination of the amount of blood lost can be more accurate if the largest percentage has actually been suctioned into a calibrated bottle and measured. One can then add to this exact amount an estimate of the amount of blood lost on the drapes, sponges, and lap packs. The record of the amount of blood lost should be as accurate as possible and can be of great value in making correct decisions subsequently about the patient's care, especially regarding the need for blood replacement in case there is a suspicion of hypovolemia. Good lighting of the surgical field is important. In addition to the standard surgical lights, we have found that a *headlight* worn by the surgeon and/or the assistants is very useful in providing excellent lighting deep in the pelvis. There are also *lighted retractors,* which may be helpful in some vaginal surgery.

For pelvic laparotomy, the patient usually is placed in a modest Trendelenburg position. In this position, the packs required to keep the intestines displaced in the upper abdomen tend to stay in place better, thereby enhancing exposure. An anesthetic or muscle relaxant is needed to keep the patient from pushing her bowels into the operative field, especially when the dissection is tedious, and good exposure is mandatory for safe performance of the operation. A retractor with an upper blade or blades to retract the intestines out of the pelvis is very useful and reduces the requirement for Trendelenburg positioning and anesthetic muscle relaxation.

It usually is possible, and always desirable, to keep the number of clamps in the operative field to an absolute minimum. If the field is cluttered with clamps, the operators cannot see as well to operate. The length of the instruments must vary, depending on the thickness of the abdominal wall, the depth of the pelvis, and other variables. Pedicle clamps, tissue forceps, dissecting scissors, needle holders, and all other instruments must be longer for operations on obese patients and for extensive operations in a deep pelvis. The handles of the instruments must come all the way out and above the level of the incision so as not to interfere with the operator's view of the pelvis. There is an unfortunate tendency for gynecologic surgeons to use instruments that are too short. The operator must stand high enough to see down into the pelvis. The patient's abdominal wall should be at about the level of the operator's umbilicus, not too high or too low.

Cushing, a neurosurgeon, introduced the *hemostatic silver metal clip* in 1911 to occlude cranial vessels inaccessible to ligation. More recently, clips have been made of stainless steel, tantalum, and the new synthetic absorbable nonopaque polydioxanone polymer. The latter has the advantage of not causing the streaked artifact of metal clips when subsequent computed tomography (CT) of the pelvis is performed. Clips cause little tissue reaction, usually are easily and rapidly applied, and provide secure control of bleeding vessels in relatively inaccessible places in the pelvis where ligation would be more difficult. A small vessel can be quickly occluded with a clip even before the vessel is cut, thus keeping the field dry and the tissues to be dissected free of blood staining. Clips are especially useful in retroperitoneal dissections. They are available in several sizes. Disposable applicators loaded with multiple clips are available, obviating the need for reloading and facilitating rapid use. If appropriately used, clips can reduce blood loss, facilitate dissection, and reduce operating time.

Working with Bovie, Cushing also pioneered the use of *electrosurgery* for hemostasis. Modern electrosurgical units are radiofrequency generators that supply 500,000 to 2 million Hz of alternating current to the tip of the electrode. The best techniques for use of electrosurgical equipment and important safety information are well discussed in Chapter 15, but several points should be emphasized. An electrosurgical instrument can be used to coagulate small vessels or to cut through fat or muscle. If a "blend" cut is used, small vessels will be coagulated as the instrument divides the tissue.

The needlepoint electrode can be used for precise incisions with minimal tissue injury from collateral thermal effect. Superficial coagulation of small vessels can be achieved by holding the electrode close to the tissue, pressing the "coagulation" button, and allowing the sparks to jump to the tissue surface. The blood should not be allowed to pool. Dry surfaces are much more effectively coagulated with the electrosurgical instrument. If bleeding is brisk, the vessel is grasped with a fine-pointed clamp or forceps, and hemostasis can be achieved by touching the metal clamp with the tip of the electrosurgical instrument and apply the "cutting" current. This may seem paradoxical, but the "cutting" current actually results in a deeper tissue effect in these circumstances, leading to better sealing of large vessels. Bipolar electrodes built into tissue forceps are also very effective for coagulating smaller vessels during tedious dissections. Experience in the use of electrosurgery will result in maximum efficiency with minimum tissue damage and a shorter operating time.

With a thorough knowledge of pelvic anatomy, the surgeon should emphasize the **development of pelvic planes and spaces**. This will avoid unnecessary bleeding and allow more accurate placement of clamps on vessels. Certain parts of the dissection can be delayed until later, especially if they are not needed now and blood loss is likely to be increased. For example, when abdominal hysterectomy is performed, dissection of the bladder away from the cervix and vagina may be associated with blood loss and should not be performed at the beginning of the operation. Exposure of the anterior lower uterine segment and cervix is not required until the uterine vessels and broad ligament need to be clamped. Until then, there is no need to start this potentially bloody dissection.

In the early days of abdominal pelvic surgery, postoperative hemorrhage was common because an effective technique of hemostasis was not known. The usual method of performing abdominal hysterectomy involved use of a ligature en masse around the lower uterus. This mass ligature saved time and was used to occlude both uterine and ovarian vessels simultaneously. The uterine corpus with adnexa attached was simply amputated above the ligature. The stump thus formed was such a large mass of tissue that it could not be safely returned to the peritoneal cavity because of the danger of intraperitoneal bleeding. Therefore, sometimes the stump was fixed extraperitoneally in the incision so that it was available for hemostatic clamping if the need arose. It was not until 1889 that Stimson published a technique for secure individual ligation of the uterine and ovarian vessels that was responsible for significantly reducing the incidence of postoperative hemorrhage. Kelly published a similar technique with illustrations in 1891. The technique of ligating large tissue pedicles with large sutures has been suggested for some types of total laparoscopic hysterectomy in recent years. In our opinion, mass ligation of such large pedicles is a step backward that will, sooner or later, lead to significant hemorrhage.

In abdominal operations today, all major vascular pedicles should be individually ligated, twice if technically feasible. Delayed-absorbable sutures should be used and the knots firmly tied. Vascular pedicles should be small and the vessels skeletonized as much as possible so that a secure ligature with little extraneous tissue can be accomplished. A vascular pedicle where the tip of the clamp is free, such as the infundibulopelvic ligament, should always be ligated first with a free tie to occlude the vessels. The pedicle is then secured with a transfixion suture ligature placed between the previous free tie and the clamp. This technique avoids hematoma formation and the rare occurrence of a traumatic arteriovenous fistula. If a suture ligature is to be held long for traction or later identification, there is a danger that it will become loosened or be pulled off, with a resulting hematoma or bleeding. Sutures used to ligate vessels should usually be cut and rarely held for traction for that reason. During vaginal hysterectomy, the upper broad ligament containing the uteroovarian ligament and the fallopian tube should be doubly clamped. The lateralmost clamp is replaced by a free tie completely around the pedicle. Tied tightly, this ligature compresses the vessels in the pedicle so that the most medial clamp (the one closest to the uterus) can then be replaced with a suture ligature placed through the pedicle, passed around the tip of the clamp both ways, and tied tightly around the pedicle. This is one vascular ligature that can be held long for identification and traction with minimal risk of bleeding.

"The finer the suture, the finer the surgeon" is an aphorism that is associated with meticulous surgical technique. The aphorism is good advice, up to a point. The newer delayed-absorbable sutures are strong, and smaller-gauge sutures are strong enough to ligate vessels. However, it is dangerous to use fine suture to ligate large pedicles. The suture may break or cut through the tissue if there is too much tension on the pedicle. Fine needles with small sutures are useful for controlling localized venous or arterial bleeding, but larger suture with bigger bites are less likely to pull through infected or malignant tissue. Proper suture selection for the specific technique and patient is an important part of obtaining the best result from any given surgical procedure.

INTRAOPERATIVE MEASURES TO CONTROL PELVIC HEMORRHAGE

Despite adequate technical skills and careful dissection, serious hemorrhage can suddenly complicate almost any operative procedure. These occasions call for a maximum use of a surgeon's knowledge, technical ability, and leadership to produce a happy outcome. The first task is to control the hemorrhage. *A finger should immediately be placed on the bleeding point for prompt, atraumatic control with pressure.* When the blood has been suctioned out and the fingertip exposed, it may be gently rolled off the bleeding point while a fine-tipped clamp of adequate length is poised to clamp the bleeding vessel and suction is ready to provide exposure. In most instances, this will adequately control the hemorrhage, although it is often necessary to place another clamp, clip, or suture adjacent to the first clamp to control the other side of the lacerated vessel or other nearby bleeders. It is most important to avoid placing too many clamps in the area because this will obscure the bleeding site and cause additional trauma to the vessels. Multiple sutures and/or clips may also cause more bleeding and can injure adjacent structures, such as the ureter, bladder, pelvic vessels, and nerves. Cautery should not be used to attempt to control significant bleeding. It will only cause increased bleeding and more tissue injury.

If an immediate attempt to control the hemorrhage by simple means is unsuccessful, the *bleeding should be controlled again with pressure*, either with a fingertip, a sponge forceps, or occasionally by packing. The surgeon should step back, take a deep breath, and carefully consider the situation. *The anesthesiologist should be made aware of the hemorrhage and consulted* about the patient's stability, blood loss up to this point, availability of blood for transfusion, intravenous lines, and so forth. The anesthesiologist will play an important role in fluid and blood replacement, monitoring coagulation factors and ensuring perfusion of vital organs. Therefore, it is important that he or she be fully aware of the situation and an active participant in such decisions as how long to safely continue surgery. The anticipated difficulty in controlling the hemorrhage must be honestly evaluated, and the patient's overall condition and the planned operative procedures should be considered and discussed with the surgical team. If *additional suction or instruments* are needed, they should be requested. If *additional or more experienced assistants* or additional scrub and/or circulating nurses are needed, they should be requested. Would it be helpful to have your partner, a gynecologic oncologist, a urologist, a general surgeon, or a vascular surgeon scrub in? They are probably not immediately available, so it is important to request their help sooner rather than later.

If the patient is stable and any necessary equipment—such as a second suction, deeper retractors, or hemoclips—has been readied, it is reasonable to reconsider the anatomy, obtain good exposure, and have another try at controlling the bleeding. If you are lucky, the 10 minutes or so that the hemorrhage has been controlled by pressure will result in a substantial reduction in the bleeding. Perhaps the vessel or bleeding site can be more clearly seen and controlled with a clamp and a few small sutures or a clip or two. Arterial bleeding in the pelvis usually is easily controlled. The vessels have thick walls and are not easily torn further. Blood spurting from the vessel leads to its easy identification. If the artery can be clamped, it usually can be ligated, a clip can be applied, or both. If an artery has mostly retracted from view with only one small edge still visible, that edge may be grasped with a clamp and gently twisted, thus decreasing the amount of bleeding sufficiently to allow clipping or ligation. *Venous hemorrhage in the pelvis may be a much more difficult problem.* Such bleeding can vary in magnitude from a trivial ooze to life-threatening hemorrhage. Pelvic veins can be fragile, tortuous, hidden from view, and distended. Blood returning through the lacerated vein can come from multiple deeper sources that are unavailable for ligation. Placing clamps and sutures blindly is dangerous and can even make the problem worse. Electrocoagulation of a laceration in a large vein should not be attempted because it will inevitably result in a larger hole that will be even more difficult to secure. Sometimes the best procedure is to hold a finger or a pack against the bleeding site for a minimum of 5 minutes, after which the bleeding may stop or decrease so that the bleeding vessel can be identified and controlled with a clip or a suture. Digital pressure to control venous bleeding takes advantage of the fact that the pressure in pelvic veins is very low. The initial use of digital pressure also is less likely to cause further tearing and trauma to the vein. Sometimes additional careful dissection in the area is required to free the vessel above and below, to allow more precise ligation or clipping. A long, finely pointed instrument is used to clamp the vessel, and clips are placed on each side. If the vessel can be sufficiently liberated, another instrument is gently slipped beneath the first one so that its point is free. Then a fine ligature is placed around the clamp. If necessary, clips can also be placed on each side of the tie.

If the bleeding has still not been controlled at this point or if bleeding cannot be controlled by pressure on the bleeding site, consultation should be requested to get additional help or expertise. By this time, the surgeon may feel frustrated, and it is important to maintain control of the operation and the surgical team. Blood and clotting factors should be replaced as discussed earlier in this chapter, the patient kept warm, and the whole situation reevaluated with input from all members of the team. The surgeon must maintain a positive outlook and exert good judgment and leadership. Good leadership involves using the skills and ideas of each member of the surgical team. Good judgment involves knowing which ideas to use, when to use them, and when to ask for help.

Special Techniques

Diffuse venous oozing, which may be associated with malignancy, inflammation, or extensive lysis of adhesions, can usually be controlled by electrosurgery (sometimes on the "spray" mode) or packing for 5 to 15 minutes. When these techniques are not effective, various **hemostatic agents** may be considered. Most of the studies on these agents have been done on animals, and there is very little literature comparing these agents with each other in human subjects.

Older agents such as *oxidized, regenerated cellulose* come in a thin, pliable, woven sheet (Surgicel NuKnit®, Johnson & Johnson, USA) or a soft, multiple-layered, fuzzy pad that can be separated into thin sheets or used as a pliable pad (Surgicel Fibrillar®, Johnson & Johnson, USA). *Absorbable, gelatin foam* pads (Gelfoam®, Pharmacia and Upjohn, USA) are also available in several sizes, and can be cut to fit. These stiff sponges are about 4 mm thick and can be applied dry or moistened with saline to make them pliable. Both of these sheets or pads can be applied to an oozing surface and covered with a pressure pack for 5 minutes or so, during which time clot formation will, it is hoped, form on the cellulose or gelatin matrix. The patient must have normal clotting factors for these products to work.

Microfibrillar collagen "flour" (Avitene®, Davol, USA or InStat®, Johnson & Johnson, USA) is a soft, granular material that can be placed on a semidry surface or into a small crevice for hemostasis. This bovine collagen material can be applied directly and compressed against an area of a small bleeding vessel. It acts as a fibrin nidus to accelerate thrombus formation on the surface of the vessel. It will only control bleeding from a small arteriole or venule. Caution must be exercised in the use of this material because it can produce secondary fibrosis in the pelvis and even a persistent palpable mass. There have been reports of retroperitoneal fibrosis and ureteral obstruction secondary to the use of this material.

In one case of severe bleeding from deep pelvic veins, we were successful in finally controlling the bleeding with multiple layers (sandwiches) of Gelfoam and Avitene cut to appropriate size from sheets and stacked one on top of the other. If coagulation factors have been depleted because of multiple transfusions, the Gelfoam can be soaked in thrombin. When the material is applied, the field should be as dry as possible. Constant pressure can be applied by placing sutures that can be tied on top of the sandwiches. There is a new commercial product made of absorbable collagen sponge coated with human coagulation factor and thrombin that sounds very good, but it is not yet U.S. Food and Drug Adminstration (FDA) approved for use in the United States (TachoSil®, Nycomed, Denmark).

Malviya and Deppe have reported the successful use of *fibrin glue*, a biodegradable tissue adhesive and sealant and topical hemostatic agent, to control life-threatening hemorrhage in one obstetric and two gynecologic patients. The fibrin glue (Tisseal®, Baxter Pharma, USA or Crosseal®, Ethicon, USA) is prepared from equal amounts of cryoprecipitate (highly concentrated human fibrinogen) and bovine thrombin. It imitates the last stages of physiologic coagulation at the local site. It is available as a spray applicator or in a dual syringe set. This technique has been used successfully in microvascular, cardiovascular, and thoracic surgical procedures and has recently been reported in controlling hemorrhage in liver transplantation. Schwartz and colleagues compared spray on fibrin sealant to standard techniques for hemostasis in 121 patients undergoing liver resection. Time to achieve hemostasis and postoperative complications were significantly less in the patients randomized to fibrin sealant. This technique should be helpful in extensive pelvic dissections for gynecologic cancer, especially to control low-pressure pelvic vein bleeding that is not controllable by other standard measures.

Gynecologic surgeons usually do not have the luxury of using *tourniquets* to control bleeding. There are, however, two special procedures in which tourniquets have been used to advantage. These are myomectomy and uterine unification operations. The tourniquet is fashioned in the manner used by vascular, thoracic, and trauma surgeons to occlude major vessels. A vesiloop or a small Silastic pediatric catheter can be used for this purpose. A tourniquet loop can be placed around the uterine isthmus through a small hole made in the broad ligament just lateral to the uterine vessels. Loops also can be placed around both infundibulopelvic ligaments through the same hole in the broad ligament. When these are snugged down tightly and held with a Kelly clamp, the entire circulation to the uterus can be occluded. A sterile Doppler probe can be used to ensure that arterial pulsations have disappeared completely. This technique can reduce blood loss to a minimum in these two procedures. Similarly, vessel loops or "bull dog" vascular clips can be used above and below the defect when repairing a sizable hole in the wall of a large vein or artery that cannot be sacrificed.

Unnecessary bleeding in the area of dissection stains tissues, obscures visibility, restricts technical freedom, and gradually adds up to a significant amount of blood loss that may require replacement. Reducing the circulation to the operative field by deliberate induction of hypotension is a safe and effective anesthetic technique in properly selected patients. *Hypotensive anesthesia* is not recommended for most routine gynecologic surgery. The technique requires planning and cooperation between the surgeon and the anesthesiologist. It has been used for radical pelvic surgery in the past, but is rarely used today.

Hypogastric Artery Ligation

One of the methods of controlling severe pelvic hemorrhage is ligation of both hypogastric arteries. In 1893 at the Johns Hopkins Hospital, Howard Kelly performed bilateral hypogastric artery ligation to control hemorrhage during hysterectomy for uterine cancer. Hypogastric artery ligation was later introduced by Mengert and colleagues and was then extensively investigated by Burchell. Burchell demonstrated that the pulse pressure in the artery just distal to the point of ligation was decreased significantly (77%) on the same side. If both hypogastric arteries are ligated, the pulse pressure is decreased by 85%. This reduction in pulse pressure presumably allows blood clots to form at the site of bleeding from damaged vessels. Blood flow in vessels distal to the point of ligation is decreased by only 48%.

Because it is important to preserve some of the collateral circulation to the pelvis—including the lumbar, iliolumbar, middle sacral, lateral sacral, superior and middle hemorrhoidal, and gluteal arteries—it is important to ligate the anterior division of the hypogastric artery distal to the posterior parietal branch, as demonstrated in Figure 19.4. In ligating the hypogastric artery, the peritoneum is opened over the external iliac artery from the round ligament to the infundibulopelvic ligament. The ureter is left attached to the medial peritoneal reflection to avoid disturbing its blood supply. The hypogastric artery is gently cleaned off with a fingertip or the tip of the suction. The hypogastric vein is also identified on the pelvic sidewall, if possible; but as long as the artery is well visualized and separated from the sidewall, it is not necessary to dig around risking more bleeding to isolate the hypogastric vein. The posterior branch of the hypogastric artery must be clearly identified before double ligation of the anterior division is performed. Nonabsorbable suture is passed around the artery with a right-angle clamp and tied. A second free-tie suture is placed distal to the initial ligature to avoid recanalization. Transfixion or division of the vessel is not recommended in this procedure. The hypogastric arteries should be ligated bilaterally, if possible, to obtain the best results. When possible, we believe that the arterial branch closest to the bleeding point should be ligated. Because the uterine artery is the first visceral branch of the hypogastric artery, it may be feasible to identify this artery and ligate it separately if the bleeding is from the uterus. This may be a somewhat more difficult procedure than ligating the entire anterior division of the hypogastric artery and should not be attempted in the face of massive pelvic bleeding, distorted pelvic anatomy, or shock.

When massive bleeding is present but the uterus has not been removed (as may occur in certain obstetric operations), it is important to ligate both ovarian arteries also. This procedure is easily accomplished by extending the lateral peritoneal incision up to the infundibulopelvic ligaments. The ureter must be identified. The artery should be ligated with a single, permanent ligature, but the artery should not be cut. This avoids the need for multiple ligatures and the risk of retraction and retroperitoneal bleeding of the vessel. A single hemoclip also can be placed on each ovarian artery as a quicker and easier method of occlusion. Care should be taken to avoid injury to the ovarian vein. If there is difficulty in distinguishing the artery from the ovarian vein, ligation of both the ovarian artery and vein within the infundibulopelvic ligament is acceptable. Even though ligating both the arterial and venous circulation to the ovary leads to a high incidence of postoperative cystic enlargement of the ovary, this complication is preferable to the risk of recurrent pelvic bleeding when the ovarian arteries are not ligated.

As an alternative to ligating the ovarian artery in the infundibulopelvic ligament, Cruikshank and Stoelk have described a technique of ligating this artery at the point of its anastomosis with the uterine artery in the medial mesosalpinx. This point of ligation allows maintenance of the blood flow to the tube and ovary but occludes the ovarian artery

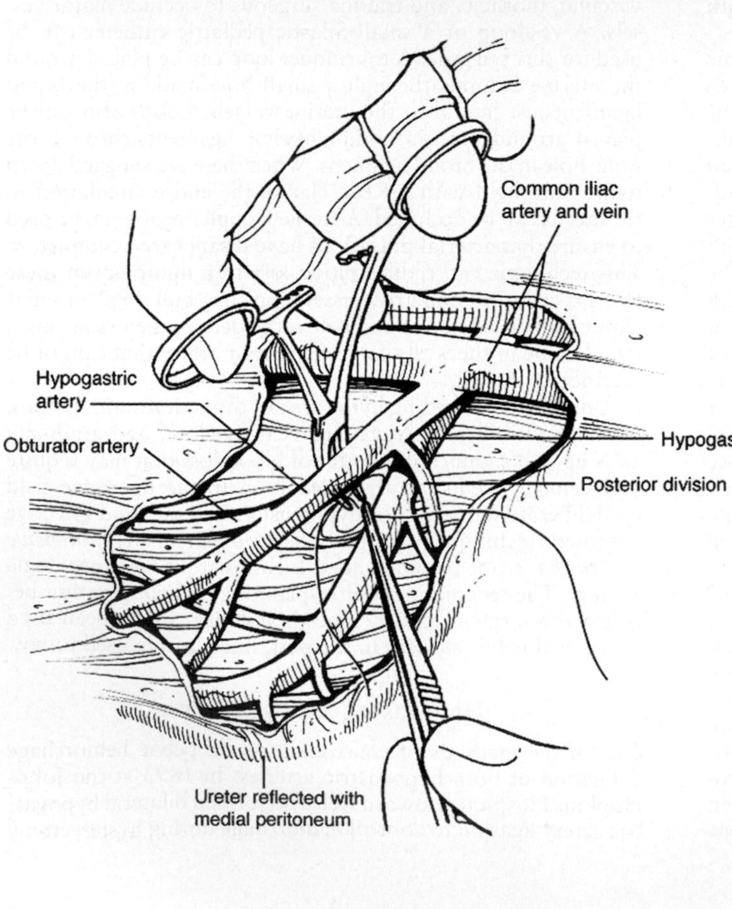

FIGURE 19.4. Ligation of the right hypogastric artery. The clamp is passed laterally to medial and the ligature is placed around the anterior division of the hypogastric artery. Note the ureter is attached to the peritoneum, which is reflected medially.

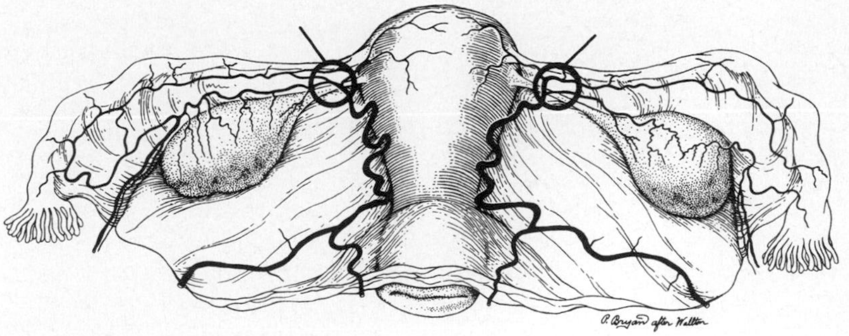

FIGURE 19.5. In addition to ligation of the anterior division of the hypogastric artery, the blood flow to the uterus through the ovarian artery can be ligated in the medial mesosalpinx without interfering with the blood flow to the tube and ovary.

blood flow to the uterus (Fig. 19.5). Because this technique allows uninterrupted blood supply to the ovaries, it is probably preferable.

For post–cesarean delivery hemorrhage, Fehrman has recommended bilateral ligation of the uterine arteries as primary treatment. When this method was used in 66 patients, only 6 required hysterectomy to achieve hemostasis. If bilateral uterine ligation is not effective in controlling the uterine bleeding, Fehrman recommends supplementary ligation of the round ligaments and the ovarian ligaments at their junction with the uterine corpus. He also believes that bilateral uterine artery ligation is a more effective treatment for life-threatening uterine hemorrhage than is bilateral hypogastric artery ligation.

The vaginal artery can originate as a separate branch from the hypogastric artery. Uncontrollable bleeding from the vagina may not be stopped by hysterectomy or by ligation of the uterine arteries. Hypogastric artery ligation is required.

Pregnancy after Hypogastric Artery Ligation. Amazingly, there are many reports of full-term deliveries after bilateral hypogastric artery ligation with and without bilateral ovarian artery ligation. This is ample testimony to the abundant collateral blood supply to the uterus that can develop over time. According to Burchell, the blood flow to the pelvis is reduced by as much as 50%, and yet there remains an adequate reserve to nourish a future term pregnancy. Ischemic necrosis of pelvic tissues does not occur unless additional collateral pathways are destroyed.

The collateral circulation of the female pelvis is extensive and provides a variety of intercommunicating sources of arterial blood from various sites along the arterial tree. These collateral vessels anastomose with the hypogastric artery and the blood supply to the uterus through a number of circuitous arterial pathways in the pelvis. During a difficult hysterectomy, the collateral circulation can create problems in achieving adequate hemostasis. Therefore, it is important to have a clear understanding of the various extrapelvic arteries that communicate with the pelvic circulation.

Packing Techniques

In rare cases, standard techniques of pressure, clipping, ligation, or application of hemostatic agents is unsuccessful for controlling bleeding. Several techniques may be considered in these cases. Trauma surgeons will occasionally pack persistent venous bleeding and close the abdomen when the procedure has been prolonged and/or the patient is unstable. The patient is then reoperated on in 24 to 48 hours when coagulation factors and blood volume have been normalized and everyone is refreshed. In some cases, the packing can be brought out through a large, hollow, soft rubber drain placed in a separate incision in the abdominal walls. The packing can then be removed through the drain in 48 hours under a light general anesthesia without opening the abdomen. If bleeding persists, it can sometimes be controlled by vascular embolization by the interventional radiologist.

Some surgeons have found the *parachute pack*, or umbrella pack, to be useful as a last-ditch effort to control persistent venous bleeding from the pelvic floor muscles after pelvic exenteration. This area is very deep in the pelvis, and exposure may be unsatisfactory from either above or below. This technique involves the formation of a large pack of loose gauze within an outstretched, opened piece of gauze or plastic sheet. The center of the sheet is inserted through the vagina and positioned in the pelvic cavity from above. The pack is then stuffed from below with one or more gauze packing rolls or "fluffs" (Fig. 19.6A). When an adequate volume has been obtained, the corners of the sheet are twisted together, and the stuffed ball of packing is pulled down against the pelvic floor, compressing the vessels of the pelvic floor muscles and paravaginal tissues (Fig.19.6B). Downward traction is maintained by clamping the twisted sheet at the vaginal introitus with several sturdy clamps. These are padded with gauze or foam rubber as they rest tightly against the perineum. The handles should be taped shut, but may be reclamped from time to time to maintain pressure on the towel as it stretches. The pack can be left in place with perineal traction for 24 to 48 hours until the bleeding has ceased. It is removed vaginally by first withdrawing the internal gauze and then the outside bags, sheet, or towel.

Potentially Troublesome Anatomic Locations

Iliac Vessels

One of the most dangerous places in the pelvis to dissect is in the region of the bifurcation of the common iliac artery and vein. This is the "axilla" of the pelvis, where many lymph nodes that drain the cervix are found. The hypogastric vein and its branches are at risk of injury when dissecting between the distal common iliac artery and the psoas muscle and deeper in the area of lumbosacral nerve trunks. When the surgeon pulls on surrounding areolar tissue, a relatively loose and thin-walled vein may inadvertently be torn or pulled into the dissecting scissors. The vein wall may not be distinct, especially when the tissue is bloodstained. One is wise to proceed cautiously. Furious hemorrhage threatening exsanguination can result from laceration of either the external iliac vein or the hypogastric vein where they join together, or from laceration of their major branches in the area. On the medial side of these veins, the lateral sacral veins disappear into the sacral foramina. Fatal hemorrhage can result from laceration of these vessels. If they are torn where they enter the foramina, they cannot be

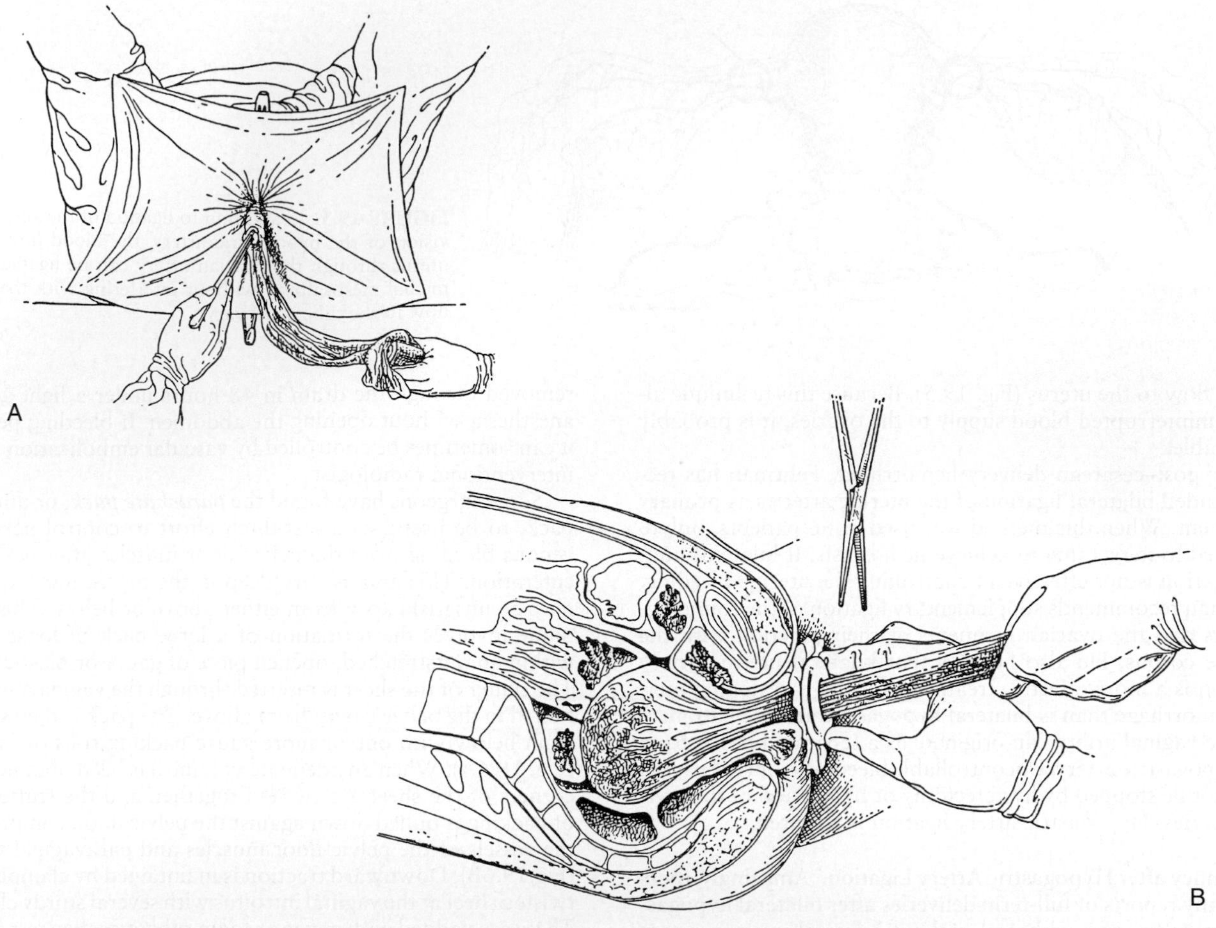

FIGURE 19.6. A and B: The parachute pack can be used to control bleeding from the deep pelvic veins after pelvic exenteration. A plastic sheet or towel is packed with gauze rolls through the vaginal or perineal opening. The ball of gauze packing is then pulled down to exert pressure against the vessels of the pelvic floor.

clamped and ligated. They cannot be clipped. They are kept open by their attachment to the walls of the foramina. Extreme measures may be required to control such bleeding. One can try to pack the foramen with bone wax, but this usually is not successful. Alternatively, multiple layers (sandwiches) of absorbable gelatin sponge (Gelfoam) and microfibrillar collagen (Avitene) can be held in place with a strong pressure pack for 20 minutes and, perhaps, ultimately the packing can be fixed with sutures. This area deserves its reputation as the "corona mortis" of the pelvis.

Obturator Fossa

Numerous variations in the branches of the hypogastric artery and vein are encountered in dissecting the obturator fossa, especially in the floor of the fossa. The "web" of paracervical tissue separating the paravesical and pararectal spaces contains branches of the hypogastric artery and vein. These vessels must be carefully ligated with clips or sutures during a radical hysterectomy. The dissection can be carried to the depths of the paravesical space and pararectal space by carefully ligating or clipping each vessel encountered. The obturator artery and vein are usually found just below the obturator nerve. In a radical hysterectomy or even a pelvic exenteration, these vessels are usually not disturbed. If injured, they may be ligated or clipped. If these vessels are allowed to retract through the obturator foramen into the upper thigh without being ligated, bleeding into the thigh may be a significant problem.

Pararectal Space

When dissecting in the pelvis, one should avoid making a deep, narrow hole with a bottom that cannot be exposed in case a deep vein might be lacerated. For example, development of the pararectal space must be done carefully because of the danger of injuring the internal iliac veins against the pelvic sidewall. The space is developed between the ureter and the hypogastric artery. The dissection is directed posteriorly at first but soon changes to a more caudal direction. Failure to make this directional change can result in laceration and bleeding from veins in the bottom of the space. If development of the pararectal space is difficult, such as after pelvic radiation therapy, the paravesical space should be opened, then the cardinal ligament or "web" can be taken down bit by bit, starting with the uterine vessels at their origin or insertion into the internal iliac vessels. As clips or small clamps are used to take down the cardinal ligament, the pararectal space gradually is opened inferiorly, with the ureter identified medially and the iliac veins visualized laterally. The pararectal space can be expanded with sharp dissection or with pressure from a small cotton bud in the tip of a long clamp (we call it a "peanut dissector" because the cotton bud is about the size of a small peanut). It should not be forced.

Aortic Area

The removal of lymph nodes around the aorta and vena cava can result in serious hemorrhage from either vessel if not done carefully and with adequate exposure. An abdominal incision that provides sufficient exposure for a routine pelvic operation is not ordinarily sufficient for dissection around the aorta and vena cava unless the incision is extended. A laceration in the aorta must be repaired. The aorta cannot be ligated without serious consequences. Although the vena cava usually can be ligated without serious problems, a laceration in the vena cava should be repaired. Bleeding is controlled by placing a finger over the laceration and gaining the necessary exposure by retraction and suctioning. Continuous no. 5–0 Prolene suture on a small vascular needle is used to close the laceration from side to side as the finger is slowly withdrawn. The same technique can be used to repair lacerations in other large veins, such as the common and external iliac veins. These two veins usually can be ligated with no untoward results, but we prefer to repair the laceration if possible, and it usually is possible. Lacerations of the common and external iliac arteries must always be repaired. These vessels cannot be ligated without serious consequences. If the laceration is not repairable, the artery should be replaced.

Presacral Space

In the presacral region, bleeding usually can be avoided by choosing a plane of dissection that is superficial to the anterior sacral artery and vein. The retrorectal space is easily entered and developed inferiorly to the tip and lateral margins of the sacrum without appreciable bleeding, provided the dissection is carefully made with the hand and in the correct plane superficial to the presacral fascia and the vessels that overlie the periosteum of the sacrum. Timmons and colleagues and Khan and associates have recommended using metal thumbtacks to control presacral hemorrhage when the usual methods fail. Sterilized metal thumbtacks are placed directly over the bleeding point in the presacral fascia and pushed all the way into the sacrum with the thumb. We have used a combination of bone wax and thumbtacks with success. Bleeding from the veins can be aggravated by imprecise use of clips, ligatures, or cautery. Packs, hemostatic agents, and thumbtacks may be preferable in controlling the bleeding in this area.

POSTOPERATIVE BLEEDING

With normal hemostasis and proper surgical technique, postoperative hemorrhage is a rare occurrence. Every patient, however, should be carefully monitored postoperatively for signs of occult bleeding. The intensity and duration of the monitoring will depend on the type of surgery and the medical condition of the patient. In addition to measuring the vital signs such as pulse, blood pressure, and urine output, the abdominal incision and/or the perineum should be inspected for bleeding. Any sign of restlessness in the patient may be an indication of blood loss. A hematocrit can be checked if there is a suspicion of postoperative bleeding or anemia. Because the risk of postoperative hemorrhage is so low in routine, uncomplicated gynecologic surgery, many experts do not recommend routinely checking the hematocrit or hemoglobin postoperatively; but a hematocrit 8 to 12 hours postop may be helpful for radical surgery, patients with intraoperative hemorrhage, or patients who were not "dusty dry" when the abdomen was closed.

Occult intraperitoneal bleeding is one of the most serious postoperative complications after abdominal or vaginal surgery. It may not become evident in the recovery room. There may be no vaginal bleeding, the patient's vital signs may be stable for 12 to 18 hours after the operation is completed, and then suddenly severe hypotension, tachycardia, tachypnea, restlessness, and abdominal distention lead to a diagnosis of intraperitoneal hemorrhage that has actually been developing slowly since surgery. In most cases, a small vessel has been slowly bleeding. Only after a significant blood loss has occurred do changes in the vital signs or symptoms of abdominal distention alert the clinician to a problem. In retrospect, subtle signs of hypovolemia usually have been present. Persistent low blood pressure, low urine output, and a restless, uncomfortable patient will alert the vigilant recovery room or ward staff that a problem is present; the surgeon should be notified. Once again, a surgeon with good leadership and team-building skills should educate nurses and other caregivers responsible for the postoperative care of the patient to be observant for these findings, and they should be encouraged to call too soon rather than too late with any concerns about the patient's postoperative course.

The diagnosis of intraperitoneal bleeding in the postoperative patient can be difficult. Peritoneal signs are subtle and can be masked by incisional pain and analgesic medications. Unfortunately, the initial examination of the abdomen may be quite benign. The peritoneal cavity has an enormous capacity for occult blood loss without appreciable abdominal distention. As much as 3,000 mL of blood (about 65% of the total blood volume of a 70-kg person) can be hidden in the peritoneal cavity, with only a 1-cm increase in the radius of the abdomen. Occult intraperitoneal hemorrhage is even more serious when one considers that the postoperative patient may not have had replacement of all the blood that was lost at the initial operation and may already be hypovolemic when she reaches the recovery room. *Abdominal ultrasound* is a rapid, noninvasive, readily available method of confirming the diagnosis of intraperitoneal bleeding. A rapid, low-tech method of testing for intraperitoneal blood is to insert a long 18-gauge spinal needle into the abdominal cavity in one of the lower quadrants under local anesthesia. This is definitely not a "noninvasive" technique and may not demonstrate intraperitoneal bleeding unless the abdomen is grossly distended. If a patient has experienced an unexpected drop in hematocrit postoperatively but is very stable, an abdominal and pelvic CT scan is another good way to identify (or rule out) intraabdominal hemorrhage or a hematoma (Fig. 19.7).

Sometimes it is difficult for the surgeon who performed the original operation to convince himself or herself that bleeding is persistent and intervention is urgently needed. A consult with a colleague is often helpful. There may be a temptation to blame the coagulation system and look for some defect in clotting factors. A routine coagulation profile, ordered at the first suspicion, or even simple observation of clot formation in a tube of blood at the bedside will eliminate this possibility. However, the experienced surgeon knows that the most common reason for intraperitoneal blood and postoperative shock is loss of surgical hemostasis—a vessel has become disligated. The question now becomes: Should the patient be immediately operated on again to identify and control the bleeding or taken to the radiology suite in an attempt to control the bleeding by embolization? Both techniques are highly effective, and we have generally used the stability of the patient as a guide. For instance, if the patient is unstable with a rapid pulse, falling

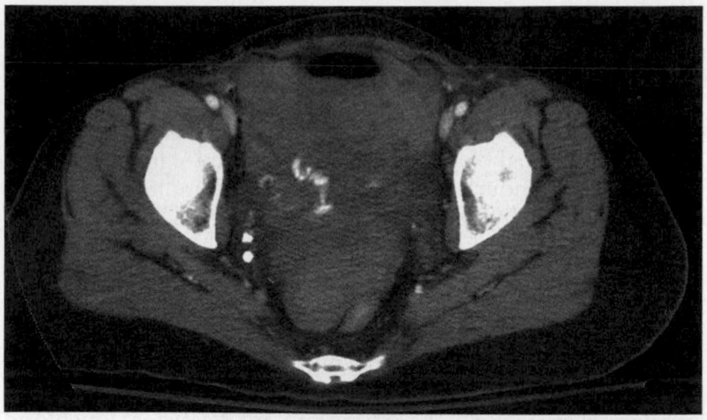

FIGURE 19.7. Axial CT image of the pelvis in a 52-year-old woman who is 5 hours postop from a vaginal hysterectomy. Note the extravasation of contrast from an arterial injection into the right internal iliac artery.

blood pressure, and/or low urine output, or if the interval since surgery is short, suggesting fairly rapid hemorrhage, we would prefer to quickly return to the operating room where we have a team of anesthesiologists and other personnel to monitor the patient, assist with blood replacement, and treat hemorrhagic shock. On the other hand, if the patient is reasonably stable and bleeding does not appear too brisk based on time from surgery and the volume of blood in the abdomen or retroperitoneal space by ultrasound estimate, then it is reasonable to try to identify the bleeding artery and embolize it by transcatheter interventional radiological techniques.

Whichever plan is selected, one or more large-bore intravenous lines should be started, and fluid replacement should begin with packed red blood cells ordered and started as indicated and available. A Foley catheter should be inserted and urine output monitored. Broad-spectrum antibiotics should be started. If the patient is not in the recovery room, she should be transferred there or to a monitored bed with easy access to the operating room. Preop labs should be obtained, and the operating room and anesthesia service should be notified, as well as the interventional radiology team if appropriate.

Arterial Embolization

In 1969, Nusbaum and colleagues described arterial embolization to control bleeding from esophageal varices by selectively cannulating the superior mesenteric artery and infusing small doses of vasopressin into terminal vessels. The subsequent use of particulate matter to achieve hemostasis within bleeding viscera developed rapidly. Selective angiographic arterial embolization has been used to control hemorrhage after abdominal and vaginal hysterectomy and other gynecologic operations, hemorrhage from cervical cancer and gestational trophoblastic disease, postpartum hemorrhage, hemorrhage from abdominal pregnancy, and retroperitoneal hemorrhage. Experience has shown that selective pelvic artery embolization is a comparatively simple and safe procedure. Dramatic results can be seen. Clinical success rates of more than 90% are routinely reported when embolization is used for postsurgical and posttraumatic hemorrhage. Therefore, embolization rather than surgical ligation is appropriately selected as the primary procedure to control bleeding in patients who are stable or who cannot tolerate another operation.

The method of intravascular embolization is quite simple, although it requires the expertise of a skilled interventional radiologist. Percutaneous catheterization of the femoral artery under local anesthesia provides direct access in a retrograde manner to the hypogastric artery (Fig. 19.8). The brachial artery can also be used for access to the vascular system. If prior hypogastric artery ligation has obstructed this pathway, arteriography of the pelvic vasculature through one of the collateral arteries usually localizes the specific bleeding vessel or vessels, although with greater difficulty. The site of bleeding can be accurately identified with angiography and fluoroscopy if the rate of bleeding is 2 to 3 mL per minute or more. The hypogastric artery or the specific collateral vessel is cannulated for injection (Fig. 19.9A–C). A variety of materials can be used for embolization, including small pieces of Gelfoam, metal coils, small Silastic spheres, autologous clot, subcutaneous tissue, and other hemostatic materials. Gelfoam is one of the most practical and easily injected materials. It is sterile, is nonantigenic, remains in the vessel for 20 to 50 days, and forms a fibrin mesh framework on which blood clots can develop. Its immediate effect is to obstruct the distal artery or arteriole and reduce pulse pressure in the bleeding vessel, thereby permitting clot formation and cessation of bleeding. Material is injected under angiographic observation. When it becomes evident by repeat angiography that the bleeding vessel has been occluded, the catheter is removed and the patient is carefully monitored for evidence of further bleeding.

After embolization, patients usually have no complications or evidence of the effects of local ischemia. Those who have not had a hysterectomy will resume normal menstruation. Some patients will exhibit evidence of a mild postembolization syndrome, including pain, fever, leukocytosis resulting from

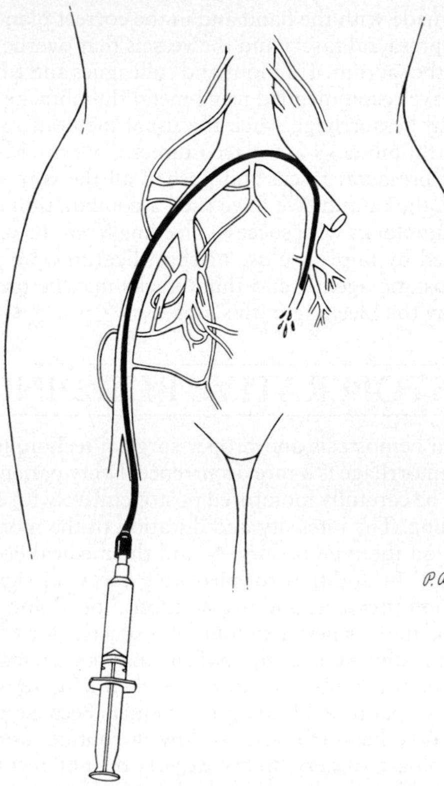

FIGURE 19.8. The femoral artery can be catheterized under local anesthesia to provide access to the hypogastric artery and its branches.

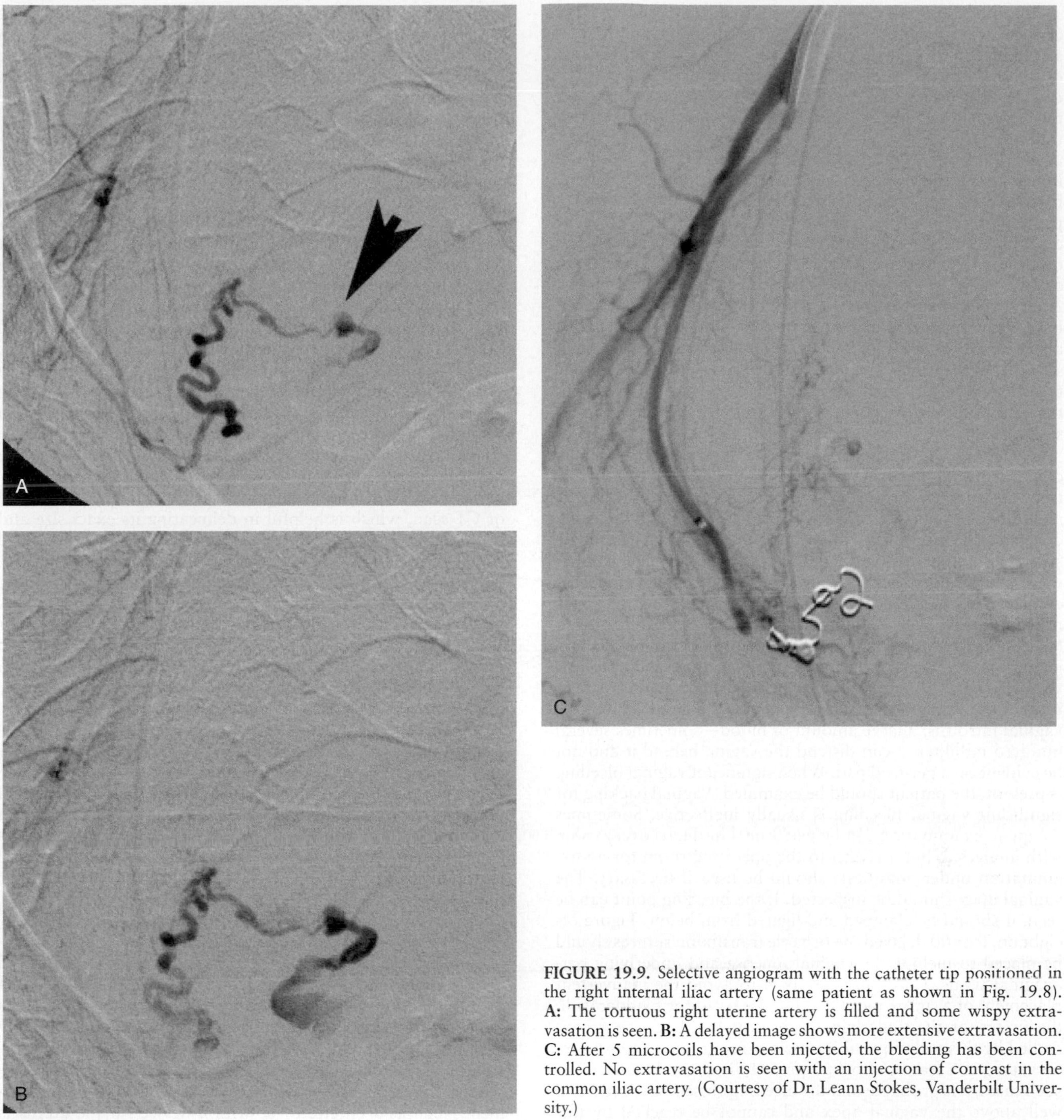

FIGURE 19.9. Selective angiogram with the catheter tip positioned in the right internal iliac artery (same patient as shown in Fig. 19.8). **A:** The tortuous right uterine artery is filled and some wispy extravasation is seen. **B:** A delayed image shows more extensive extravasation. **C:** After 5 microcoils have been injected, the bleeding has been controlled. No extravasation is seen with an injection of contrast in the common iliac artery. (Courtesy of Dr. Leann Stokes, Vanderbilt University.)

vascular thrombosis, and tissue necrosis. A few isolated cases of more serious problems have been reported, including bladder necrosis, vesicovaginal fistula, neuropathies, and renal toxicity from the contrast medium. The overall complication rate should be less than 10%.

Reoperation

If reoperation is selected, the patient should be as stable as possible, with blood running or at least available in the room. Two suctions should be ready and an adequate staff and assistants involved. If the patient has previously had an abdominal operation, the incision should be reopened. A preoperative ultrasound or CT scan should have identified the bleeding as intraperitoneal or retroperitoneal. The previous procedure should be mentally reviewed to identify any possible ligatures that were tentative or any troublesome bleeding sites that may have continued to bleed. When the abdomen is opened, the clots should be evacuated and a search instituted for the bleeding sites, starting with the most likely locations. Care should be taken when removing clots from the pelvic area.

Bleeding sites should be carefully ligated, sutured, or clipped. It is not unusual to reopen the abdomen and find no active bleeding sites. This is somewhat disconcerting because of the concern that the problem will repeat itself after the abdomen is again closed. Every attempt should be made to get the pelvis and abdomen completely dry before closing a second time.

During reoperation, patients are at increased risk of ureteral injury. In addition to exercising care in clamping and ligating bloodstained tissue with distorted anatomy, it may be wise to prove ureteral integrity at the end of the operation. This can be done by injecting 5 mL of indigo carmine dye intravenously and observing efflux of dye from each ureteral orifice through the cystoscope or by opening the bladder dome (see Chapter 38). After reoperation, patients are also at increased risk of developing postoperative complications such as pulmonary atelectasis, abdominal distention from ileus, postoperative infection, incisional complications, and coagulation disorders from multiple transfusions. The anticipation of these complications allows the adoption of measures to prevent or manage them correctly should they occur.

Postoperative hemorrhage from the vaginal vault usually comes from the vaginal artery in the lateral vaginal fornix or from one of its branches. Most often, the lateral vaginal angle, including the vaginal artery, is not properly secured or becomes disligated. To prevent such bleeding, the lateral vaginal angle stitch should be anchored in tissue lateral to the angle so that the angle cannot slip out. This stitch should not be held because traction will loosen it. Excessive vaginal bleeding may be noted in the recovery room or after the patient has returned to her room. Every attempt should be made to establish an objective measurement of the amount of blood lost and to follow vital signs and changes in hematocrit values. One must realize that the vagina is a distensible organ. If a clot occludes the vaginal introitus, a large amount of blood—sometimes several hundred milliliters—can distend the vagina behind it and not be evident on a perineal pad. When significant vaginal bleeding is present, the patient should be examined. Vaginal packing for significant vaginal bleeding is usually ineffective. Sometimes adequate examination can be performed in the recovery room with analgesia, but a return to the operating room for an examination under anesthesia should be used if necessary. The vaginal apex should be inspected. If the bleeding point can be seen, it should be clamped and ligated from below. Figure-of-eight no. 0 or 00 delayed-absorbable transfixion sutures should be placed to include the vaginal mucosa and underlying paravaginal tissue. Care must be taken to avoid the inadvertent placement of a suture into the musculature of the bladder wall, the ureter, or the underlying rectum. If bleeding is not controlled by this technique, it is unwise to continue to add suture on suture in a frantic effort to control the vaginal bleeding. In such cases, it is probable that the bleeding vessels have retracted well above the vaginal apex and cannot be reached by this approach.

If surgical hemostasis cannot be achieved transvaginally, laparotomy may be necessary. A vaginal pack will not control significant bleeding from the vaginal vault that has already required a return to the operating room, although a temporary pack may slow the blood loss while the patient is prepared for laparotomy. In some patients, the hemorrhage will be delayed until 10 to 14 days after surgery, when the sutures lose their tensile strength. Posthysterectomy disruption of the vaginal vault with hemorrhage also can result from coitus.

Bleeding from anterior and posterior colporrhaphy usually is from veins that have not been secured. In this situation, a fairly tight vaginal pack effectively compresses these vessels and controls the bleeding. It seldom is necessary to reexplore an anterior or posterior colporrhaphy to locate and ligate a specific bleeding vessel. The patient will feel an uncomfortable sensation of urgency of urination that will be relieved when the pack is removed in 24 to 48 hours. A Foley catheter will be needed while the pack is in place.

A *postoperative pelvic hematoma* can cause serious morbidity, especially if it is large and becomes infected. Hematomas can develop above the vaginal vault, along the pelvic sidewall, in the retroperitoneum extending up to the kidneys, in the paravesical space, in the abdominal wall, and in the ischiorectal fossa and vulva. A hematoma in the ischiorectal fossa and on the vulva may be obvious on examination when the patient reports discomfort in the area. If it is below the puborectalis muscle attachment to the vagina, it will not dissect into the pelvis above but will be limited to the perineum and buttocks. A pelvic hematoma may be recognized in a patient whose postoperative discomfort and anemia exceed what is normally expected, whose temperature is progressively increasing, and whose postoperative abdominal distention is slow to resolve. If a patient is on anticoagulant therapy, even simple coughing can spontaneously cause a tremendous postoperative pelvic hematoma. Abdominal and pelvic examinations may reveal a mass. A definitive diagnosis can be made by ultrasound or CT scan, which is helpful in delineating its exact size and location. An extended, morbid, and complicated postoperative course may be alleviated if a large hematoma can be drained. Sometimes simple drainage through the vaginal vault can be accomplished by probing with a uterine dressing forceps. A small Penrose drain can be inserted through the drainage tract and left in place for a day or so. If drainage cannot be achieved in this simple way, drainage with guidance of CT or through an abdominal incision may be necessary. In our experience, if a large hematoma can be drained, the patient's recovery will be expedited. But in some cases, drainage is difficult or contraindicated and infection is not present. In such a patient, it may be preferable to allow the hematoma to gradually resolve over a few months. Unfortunately, sometimes a hematoma will not resolve completely, and residual fibrosis will persist and continue to cause pain. We have removed large pieces of an organizing hematoma as late as 1 year after operation. For these reasons, we prefer to drain pelvic hematomas initially whenever possible.

There are a few other special circumstances. *Hemorrhage after uterine curettage* is extremely rare, even with perforation of the uterus. The perforation is usually caused by the uterine sound and occurs through the corpus. Under most circumstances, the curettage should be stopped and the patient's vital signs checked for several hours. It is extremely unlikely that any problem will develop, and overnight hospital admission as a precautionary measure may be unnecessary. However, if the perforation was caused by a wide, blunt instrument (such as a curette or a suction device), if the uterus is pregnant or contains cancer, or if fatty tissue appears in the curettage specimen, then overnight observation should be considered and the patient closely observed for intraperitoneal bleeding or a broad ligament hematoma. Ultrasound, CT scan, or laparoscopy also may be performed in high-risk cases to assess the damage and determine if a hematoma or active bleeding is present. A misdirected curette can lacerate the uterine artery and vein, with subsequent intraperitoneal bleeding or broad ligament hematoma formation. In such cases, laparotomy or laparoscopy should be considered to evaluate and control the bleeding and evacuate the hematoma. A hysterectomy may or may not be necessary, depending on the damage to the uterus.

Hemorrhage from cervical conization can occur in the first 24 hours or 7 to 14 days later, when cervical sutures lose their tensile strength. If the patient is bleeding heavily at any time after conization, the cervix should be inspected. Measures to control the bleeding include resuturing, cautery, and Monsel's solution. If bleeding is not profuse, Monsel's solution, Gelfoam, and/or a small pack can be tried. In taking the conization specimen, one must be certain that the apex of the cone intersects the endocervical canal. If the cervical incision is misdirected to one side or the other, the uterine vessels are in danger of laceration. Serious hemorrhage or broad ligament hematoma may result. To prevent this problem, the cervix should first be sounded to ascertain the direction of the endocervical canal and the incision planned accordingly.

SUMMARY

Careful preoperative evaluation of the patient and thoughtful preoperative planning on the part of the surgeon and surgical team will help prevent or minimize significant operative blood loss. However, intraoperative or postoperative hemorrhage does occur from time to time and represents a significant challenge to the technical skill and the emotional control of the surgeon. He or she must take charge of the situation, organize a plan to control the bleeding, instruct and motivate the other members of the surgical team, and, finally, execute the technical steps necessary to obtain hemostasis. Each part of this approach is important. We hope that the ideas and techniques discussed in this chapter will make the reader more prepared to meet this challenge.

BEST SURGICAL PRACTICES

- Preparation to prevent and control operative bleeding starts before the surgical procedure. The patient should be thoroughly evaluated for risk factors that may increase the possibility of hemorrhage. Congenital and acquired coagulation disorders need to be diagnosed by a careful and thorough history and appropriate lab tests. The problem to be treated surgically should be thoughtfully considered and the surgical approach devised, adjusted, or modified to suit the patient, her lesion, and the abilities of the surgical team. Preoperative consultations with other specialists should be sought if indicated. The medical conditions of the patient should be optimized.
- The possibility and risks of blood transfusion should always be discussed with the patient as part of informed consent before surgery. The risk of a febrile reaction to transfusion is approximately 1%. Transmission of hepatitis B via transfusion occurs about 1 in every 180,000 transfusions, whereas the risk of HIV transmission with modern blood banking procedures is approximately 1 in 1.9 million.
- During the operative procedure, the surgical approach should be well planned, and possible problems and their management should be considered. Good exposure, proper use and awareness of the anatomy, and careful dissection, clamping, and suturing are all important technical skills that will reduce the risk of uncontrolled hemorrhage. Finally, and perhaps most importantly, good surgical judgment must be used to reduce risk and obtain the best outcome for the patient.
- When life-threatening intraoperative hemorrhage occurs, the surgeon should control the bleeding by pressure and organize and lead the operative team in the complex task of identifying and controlling the hemorrhage. This is one of the most challenging of all emergencies and requires leadership, judgment, knowledge, and technical skill.
- When intraoperative blood loss exceeds 15% of the patient's blood volume (about 500–1,000 mL), transfusion should be considered. The patient's medical history, her vital signs, the probability of additional blood loss, and response thus far will all determine how quickly transfusion is initiated. Packed red blood cells or other appropriate blood components should be used for transfusion rather than whole blood.
- Hematocrit and coagulation factors—as well as serum calcium, electrolytes, and glucose—should be followed every 120 minutes or after 10 U of transfusion. Although it is best to use actual serum levels of coagulation factors, as a rough guide, after every 6 to 8 U of packed red cells, 2 U of *fresh frozen plasma* should be given. If fibrinogen levels fall below 100 mg/dL, 20 U of *cryoprecipitate* should be given. A bolus of *6 U of platelets* should be given if the platelet count falls below 100,000 and the patient is actively bleeding.
- The pelvic surgeon should be able to use special techniques such as packing, thrombotic agents, and hypogastric artery ligation and know their indications for the control of pelvic hemorrhage.
- Postoperative bleeding may be difficult to diagnose. Attentive and well-trained recovery room and ward nursing personnel are essential. Abdominal and pelvic ultrasound and/or CT scanning are very helpful in making the diagnosis of postoperative bleeding and localizing the site of bleeding.
- Embolization of arterial bleeders by interventional radiology techniques and reoperation are both effective techniques to manage postoperative hemorrhage. When the patient is relatively stable and an experienced interventional radiology team is available, embolization is generally preferred today because it is associated with less morbidity.

Bibliography

Abbas FM, Currie JL, Mitchell S, et al. Selective vascular embolization in benign gynecologic conditions. *J Reprod Med* 1994;39:492.

Albala DM, Lawson JH. Recent clinical and investigational applications of fibrin sealant in selected surgical specialties. *J Am Coll Surg* 2006;202:685.

Alvarez M, Lockwood CJ, Ghidini A, et al. Prophylactic and emergent arterial catheterization for selective embolization in obstetric hemorrhage. *Am J Perinatol* 1992;9:441.

Amrein PC, Ellman L, Harris WH. Aspirin-induced prolongation of bleeding time and perioperative blood loss. *JAMA* 1981;245:1825.

Arepally GM, Ortel TL. Clinical practice: heparin-induced thrombocytopenia. *N Engl J Med* 2006;355:809.

Baggaley RF, Boily MC, White RG, et al. Risk of HIV-1 transmission for parenteral exposure and blood transfusion: a systematic review and meta-analysis. *AIDS* 2006;20:805.

Barrett NA, Kam PC. Transfusion-related acute lung injury: a literature review. *Anaesthesia* 2006;61:777.

Behnam K, Jarmolowski CR. Vesicovaginal fistula following hypogastric embolization for control of intractable pelvic hemorrhage. *J Reprod Med* 1982;27:304.

Berkowitz RL, Bussel JB, McFarland JG. Alloimmune thrombocytopenia: state of the art 2006. *Am J Obstet Gynecol* 2006;195:907.

Bernard GR, Vincent JL, Laterre PF, et al. Efficacy and safety of recombinant human activated protein C for severe sepsis. *N Engl J Med* 2001;344:699.

Bertina RM, Koeleman BPC, Koster T, et al. Mutation in blood coagulation factor V associated with resistance to activated protein C. *Nature* 1994;369:64.

Bickell WH, Wall MJ, Pepe PE, et al. Immediate versus delayed fluid resuscitation for hypotensive patients with penetrating torso injuries. *N Engl J Med* 1994;331:1105.

Blajchman MA. The clinical benefits of the leukoreduction of blood products. *J Trauma* 2006;60:S83.

Burchell RC. The umbrella pack to control pelvic hemorrhage. *Conn Med* 1968;32:734.

Carless PA, Henry DA. Systematic review and meta-analysis of the use of fibrin sealant to prevent seroma formation after breast cancer surgery. *Br J Surg* 2006;93:810.

Chung AF, Menon J, Dillon TF. Acute postoperative retroperitoneal fibrosis and ureteral obstruction secondary to the use of Avitene. *Am J Obstet Gynecol* 1978;132:908.

Ciavarella S, Reed RL, Counts RB, et al. Clotting factor levels and the risk of diffuse microvascular bleeding in the massively transfused patient. *Br J Haematol* 1987;67:365.

Clark SL, Phelan JP, Yeh SY, et al. Hypogastric artery ligation for obstetric hemorrhage. *Obstet Gynecol* 1985;66:353.

Cruikshank SH, Stoclk EM. Surgical control of pelvic hemorrhage: bibteral hypogastric artery ligation and method of ovarian artery ligation. *South Med J* 1985;78:539.

Cushing H. The control of bleeding in operations for brain tumors: with description of silver "clips" for occlusion of vessels inaccessible to the ligature. *Ann Surg* 1911;54:1.

Dagi RF. The management of postoperative bleeding. *Surg Clin North Am* 2005;85:1191.

Dahlback B, Carlsson M, Svensson PH. Familial thrombophilia due to a previously unrecognized mechanism characterized by poor anticoagulant response to activated protein C: prediction of a cofactor to activated protein C. *Proc Natl Acad Sci U S A* 1993;90:1004.

DeBernardo RL Jr, Perkins RB, Littell RD, et al. Low-molecular-weight heparin (dalteparin) in women with gynecologic malignancy. *Obstet Gynecol* 2005;105:1006.

Dehaeck CMC. Transcatheter embolization of pelvic vessels to stop intractable hemorrhage. *Gynecol Oncol* 1986;24:9.

Dodd RY. The risk of transfusion transmitted infections. *N Engl J Med* 1992;327:419.

Dubay ML, Holshausen CA, Burchell RC. Internal iliac artery ligation for postpartum hemorrhage: recanalization of vessels. *Am J Obstet Gynecol* 1980; 136:689.

Edmunds LH, Addonizio VP. Massive transfusion. In: Colman RW, Hirsh J, Marder VJ, et al, eds. *Hemostasis and thrombosis: basic principles and clinical practice.* 2nd ed. Philadelphia: JB Lippincott Co;1987:913.

Ereth MH, Oliver WC, Santrach PJ. Perioperative interventions to decrease transfusion of allogenic blood products. *Mayo Clin Proc* 1994;69:575.

Esmon NL, Owen W, Esmon C. Isolation of a membrane bound cofactor for thrombin catalyzed activation of protein C. *J Biol Chem* 1982;257:859.

Etchason J, Petz L, Keeler E, et al. The cost effectiveness of pre-operative autologous blood donations. *N Engl J Med* 1995;332:719.

Evans S, McShane P. The efficacy of internal iliac artery ligation in obstetric hemorrhage. *Surg Gynecol Obstet* 1985;160:250.

Fehrman H. Surgical management of life threatening obstetric and gynecologic hemorrhage. *Acta Obstet Gynecol Scand* 1988;67:125.

Ferraris VA, Swanson E. Aspirin usage and perioperative blood loss in patients undergoing unexpected operations. *Surg Gynecol Obstet* 1983;156:439.

Gewirtz AS, Miller ML, Keys TF. The clinical usefulness of the preoperative bleeding time. *Arch Pathol Lab Med* 1996;120:353.

Given FT, Gates HS, Morgan BE. Pregnancy following bilateral ligation of the internal iliac (hypogastric) arteries. *Am J Obstet Gynecol* 1964;89:1078.

Haas S. The use of a surgical patch coated with human coagulation factors in surgical routing: a multicenter postauthorization surveillance. *Clin Appl Thromb Hemost* 2006;12:445.

Harima Y, Shiraishi T, Harima K, et al. Transcatheter arterial embolization therapy in cases of recurrent and advanced gynecologic cancer. *Cancer* 1989;63:2077.

Harker LA. *Hemostasis manual.* 2nd edition. Philadelphia: FA Davis Co; 1974.

Hillyer CD, Emmens RK, Zago-Novaretti M, et al. Methods for the reduction of transfusion-transmitted cytomegalovirus infection: filtration versus the use of seronegative donor units. *Transfusion* 1994;34:929.

Hirsh J, Dalen JE, Deykin D, et al. Oral anticoagulants: mechanism of action, clinical effectiveness, and optimal therapeutic range. *Chest* 1992;102[Suppl]:3125.

Hirsh J, Deykin D, Poller L. "Therapeutic range" for oral anticoagulant therapy. *Chest* 1986;89[Suppl]:11.

Hong YM, Loughlin KR. The use of hemostatic agents and sealants in urology. *J Urol* 2006;176:2367.

Johnson H, Knee-Ioli S, Butler TA, et al. Are routine preoperative laboratory screening tests necessary to evaluate ambulatory surgical patients?. *Surgery* 1988;104:639.

Judd WB. Pretransfusion testing in clinical laboratory medicine. In: McClatchey KD, ed. *Clinical laboratory medicine.* Baltimore: Williams & Wilkins;1994:1733.

Kanji S, Devlin J, Piekos K, et al. Recombinant human activated protein C, drotrecogin alfa (activated): a novel therapy for severe sepsis. *Pharmacotherapy* 2001;21:1389.

Kaplan EB, Sheiner LB, Boeckmann AJ, et al. The usefulness of preoperative laboratory screening. *JAMA* 1985;253:3576.

Kelly HA. Ligation of both internal iliac arteries for hemorrhage in hysterectomy for carcinoma uteri. *Bull Johns Hopkins Hosp* 1894;5:53.

Kelly HA. Ligature of the trunks of the uterine and ovarian arteries as a means of checking hemorrhage from the uterus and broad ligaments in abdominal operations. *Johns Hopkins Hosp Rep* 1891;2:220.

Ketchum L, Hess JR, Hiippala S. Indications for early fresh frozen plasma, cryoprecipitate, and platelet transfusion in trauma. *J Trauma* 2006;60:S51.

Khan FA, Fang DT, Nivatvongs S. Management of presacral bleeding during rectal resection. *Surg Gynecol Obstet* 1987;165:275.

Lattouf JB, Beri A, Klinger CH, et al. Practical hints for hemostasis in laparoscopic surgery. *Minim Invasive Ther Allied Technol* 2007;16:45.

Lee VS, Tarassenko L, Bellhouse BJ. Platelet transfusion therapy: platelet concentrate preparation and storage. *J Lab Clin Med* 1988;111:371.

Leonard F, Lecuru F, Rizk E, et al. Perioperative morbidity of gynecological laparoscopy: a retrospective monocenter observational study. *Acta Obstet Gynecol Scand* 2000;79:129.

Levy GG, Nichols WC, Lian EC, et al. Mutations in a number of the ADAMTS gene family cause thrombotic thrombocytopenic purpura. *Nature* 2001;413:488.

Lovisetto F, Zonta S, Rota E, et al. Use of human fibrin glue (Tissucol) versus staples for mesh fixation in laparoscopic transabdominal preperitoneal hernioplasty: a prospective, randomized study. *Ann Surg* 2007;245:222.

MacLennan S, Williams LM. Risks of fresh frozen plasma and platelets. *J Trauma* 2006;60:S46.

Madjdpour C, Heindl V, Spahn DR. Risks, benefits, alternatives and indications of allogenic blood transfusions. *Minerva Anestesiol* 2006;72:283.

Madjdpour C, Spahn DR, Weiskopf RB. Anemia and perioperative red blood cell transfusion: a matter of tolerance. *Crit Care Med* 2006;34:S102.

Malviya VK, Deppe G. Control of intraoperative hemorrhage in gynecology with the use of fibrin glue. *Obstet Gynecol* 1989;73:284.

Mannucci PM. Desmopressin (DDAVP) in the treatment of bleeding disorders: the first 20 years. *Blood* 1997;90:2515.

Mannucci PM, Tenconi PM, Gastaman G, et al. Comparison of four virus-inactivated plasma concentrates for treatment of severe von Willebrand disease; a cross-over randomized trial. *Blood* 1992;79:3130.

Mannucci PM, Tripodi A. Laboratory screening of inherited thrombotic syndromes. *Thromb Haemost* 1987;57:247.

Mengert WF, Burchell RC, Blumstein RW, et al. Pregnancy after bilateral ligation of the internal iliac and ovarian arteries. *Obstet Gynecol* 1969;34:664.

Mintz PD, Henry JB, Boral LI. The type and antibody screen: symposium on blood banking and hemotherapy. *Clin Lab Med* 1982;2:169.

Mitty HA, Sterling KM, Alavarez M, et al. Obstetric hemorrhage: prophylactic and emergency arterial catheterization and embolotherapy. *Radiology* 1993;188:183.

Morgan CH, Penner JA. Bleeding complications during surgery: part I. Defects of primary hemostasis and congenital coagulation. *Lab Med* 1986;17:207.

Morgan CH, Penner JA. Bleeding complications during surgery: part II. Acquired hemorrhagic disorders. *Lab Med* 1986;17:262.

Moscardo F, Perez F, de la Rubia J, et al. Successful treatment of severe intra-abdominal bleeding associated with disseminated intravascular coagulation using recombinant activated FVII. *Br J Haematol* 2001;114:174.

Muto A, Nishibe T, Kondo Y, et al. Sutureless repair with Tachocomb sheets for oozing type postinfarction cardiac rupture. *Ann Thorac Surg* 2005;79:2143.

Nordestgaard AG, Bodily KC, Osborne RW, et al. Major vascular injury during laparoscopic procedures. *Am J Surg* 1995;169:543.

Ozier Y, Schulmberger S. Pharmacological approaches to reducing blood loss and transfusions in the surgical patient. *Can J Anaesth* 2006;53:S21.

Papp Z, Toth-Pal E, Papp C, et al. Hypogastric artery ligation for intractable pelvic hemorrhage. *Int J Gynaecol Obstet* 2006;92:27.

Pearl ML, Braga CA. Percutaneous transcatheter embolization for control of life-threatening pelvic hemorrhage from gestational trophoblastic disease. *Obstet Gynecol* 1992;80:571.

Perioperative Red Cell Transfusion. *NIH Consens* Dev. Conf. Consensus Statement 1988;7:1–19.

Poller L, Hirsh J. Special report: a simple system for the derivation of international normalized ratios for the reporting of prothrombin time results with North American thromboplastin reagents. *Am J Clin Pathol* 1989;92:124.

Poon MC. Use of recombinate FVIIa in hereditary bleeding disorders. *Curr Opin Hematol* 2001;8:312.

Prati D. Transmission of hepatitis C virus by blood transfusions and other medical procedures: a global review. *J Hepatol* 2006;45:607.

Rao LM, Rapaport SI. Factor VIIa catalyzed activation of factor X independent of tissue factor: its possible significance for control of hemophilic bleeding by infused factor VIIa. *Blood* 1990;75:1069.

Repine TB, Perkins JG, Kauvar DS, et al. The use of fresh whole blood in massive transfusion. *J Trauma* 2006;60:S78.

Rock WA Jr, Meeks GR. Managing anemia and blood loss in elective gynecologic surgery patients. *J Reprod Med* 2001;46:507.

Rodgers CRP, ed. A critical reappraisal of the bleeding time. *Semin Thromb Hemost* 1990;16:1.

Rohrer MJ, Michelotti MC, Nahrwold DL. A prospective evaluation of the efficacy of preoperative coagulation testing. *Ann Surg* 1988;208:554.

Rosen NR, Bates LH, Herod G. Transfusion therapy: improved patient care and resource utilization. *Transfusion* 1993;33:341.

Santoso JT, Saunders BA, Grosshart K. Massive blood loss and transfusion in obstetrics and gynecology. *Obstet Gynecol Surv* 2005;60:827.

Santoso JT, Lin DW, Miller DS. Transfusion medicine in obstetrics and gynecology. *Obstet Gynecol Surg* 1995;50:470.

Schafer M, Lauper M, Krahenbuhl L. Trocar and Veress needle injuries during laparoscopy. *Surg Endosc* 2000;15:275.

Schwartz M, Madariago J, Hirose R, et al. Comparison of a new fibrin sealant with standard topical hemostatic agents. *Arch Surg* 2004;139:1148.

Shah HN, Hegde S, Shah JN, et al. A prospective, randomized trial evaluating the safety and efficacy of fibrin sealant in tubeless percutaneous nephrolithotomy. *J Urol* 2006;176:2488.

Shinagawa S, Nomura Y, Kudoh S. Full-term deliveries after ligation of bilateral internal iliac arteries and infundibulopelvic ligaments. *Acta Obstet Gynecol Scand* 1981;60:439.

Sieber PR. Bladder necrosis secondary to pelvic artery embolization: case report and literature review. *J Urol* 1994;151:422.

Simon PH, Conner C, Delcour C, et al. Selective uterine artery embolization in the treatment of cervical pregnancy: two case reports. *Eur J Obstet Gynecol Reprod Biol* 1991;40:159.

Sitges-Serra A, Insenser JJ, Membrilla E. Blood transfusions and postoperative infections in patients undergoing elective surgery. *Surg Infect (Larchmt)* 2006;7(Suppl 2):S33.

So-Osman C, Nelissen RG, Eikenboom HC, et al. Efficacy, safety and user-friendliness of two devices for postoperative antologuous shed red blood cell re-infusion in elective orthopaedic surgery patients: a randomized pilot study. *Tranfus Med* 2006;16:321.

Sproule MW, Bendomir AM, Grant KA, et al. Embolisation of massive bleeding following hysterectomy, despite internal iliac artery ligation. *BJOG* 1994;101:908.

Stimson LA. On some modifications in the technique of abdominal surgery, limiting the use of the ligature en masse. *Trans Am Surg Assoc* 1889;7:65.

Strumper-Groves D. Perioperative blood transfusion and outcome. *Curr Opin Anaesthesiol* 2006;19:198.

Svensson PJ, Dahlback B. Resistance to activated protein C as a basis for venous thrombosis. *N Engl J Med* 1994;330:517.

Swanson K, Dwyre DM, Krochmal J, et al. Transfusion-related acute lung injury (TRALI): current clinical and pathophysiologic considerations. *Lung* 2006;184:177.

Thompson JD. Anemia due to gynecologic disease: its correction by the use of iron orally. *South Med J* 1957;50:679.

Timmons MC, Kohler MF, Addison WA. Thumbtack use for control of presacral bleeding, with description of an instrument for thumbtack application. *Obstet Gynecol* 1991;78:313.

Traver MA, Assimos DG. New generation tissue sealants and hemostatic agents: innovative urologic applications. *Rev Urol* 2006;8:104.

Werner EJ, Broxson EH, Tucker EL, et al. Prevalence of von Willebrand disease in children: a multiethnic study. *J Pediatr* 1993;1123:893.

Winslow RM. Current status of oxygen carriers (blood substitutes): 2006. *Vox Sang* 2006;91:102.

Yamashita Y, Harada M, Yamamoto H, et al. Transcatheter arterial embolization of obstetric and gynaecological bleeding: efficacy and clinical outcome. *Br J Radiol* 1994;67:530.

Yugi H, Mizui M, Tanaka J, et al. Hepatitis B virus (HBV) screening strategy to ensure the safety of blood for transfusion through a combination of immunological testing and nucleic acid amplification testing—Japanese experience. *J Clin Virol* 2006;36(Suppl 1):S56.

Rao LR, Rapaport SI, [illegible] VP. [illegible] activation of factor X independent of [illegible] tissue factor: its possible significance for control of [illegible] blood [illegible] by tissue factor pathway inhibitor. Blood 1995;[illegible]:1065.
Redmond B, Lefkus R, Kumar D, et al. Efficacy of fresh whole blood in massive transfusion. [illegible]
Rock WA Jr, Meyer FK, Martin [illegible] and blood loss in elective gynecologic surgical patients. [illegible]
Rodig? [illegible]. A critical reappraisal of the bleeding time. [illegible]
[illegible] A comprehensive evaluation of the effects [illegible]
Rosen [illegible] H, Rowe [illegible] transfusion in [illegible] surgical patients [illegible]
Sandberg? [illegible] Blood loss and transfusion [illegible]
[illegible] Transfusion practice [illegible] and [illegible]
[illegible] C, [illegible] Coagulation [illegible] Vox Sang [illegible]
[illegible] Comparison of [illegible] blood [illegible]
[redacted]
[illegible] blood [illegible]
[illegible] tranexamic acid for reduction of blood loss [illegible]
[illegible] blood transfusion and [illegible]
McCrory? [illegible] Efficacy, safety and [illegible] of two devices for postoperative salvage [illegible] blood [illegible] in [illegible] orthopedic [illegible] a randomized pilot study. Transfus Med 2006;16:321.
[illegible] Pulmonary? embolization in massive blood transfusion [illegible] Br J [illegible] 1969;[illegible]
[illegible] Current understanding in the technique of abdominal surgery [illegible] the use of the [illegible] Trans Am Surg Assoc 1897?
[illegible] Perioperative blood transfusion and outcomes [illegible]
[illegible] Blood transfusion in [illegible] patient [illegible] N Engl J Med 1994;[illegible]
[illegible] Transfusion-related acute lung injury [illegible] clinical and pathophysiologic considerations [illegible]
[illegible] devices in [illegible] for the use of [illegible]
[illegible] of [illegible] blood [illegible]
[redacted]
[illegible] the effects of [illegible] on [illegible] and [illegible]
[illegible] MJ, [illegible] et al. Transfusion and [illegible] blood [illegible]

SECTION IV ■ SURGERY FOR FERTILITY

CHAPTER 20 ■ THE IMPACT OF ASSISTED REPRODUCTIVE TECHNOLOGY ON GYNECOLOGICAL SURGERY

HOWARD W. JONES, Jr.

DEFINITIONS

Conceptus—The derivates of a fertilized oocyte at any stage of development from fertilization to birth, including extraembryonic membranes; the preembryo, embryo, or fetus; the products of conception; and all structures that develop from the zygote, both embryonic and extraembryonic. This term is commonly interchanged with the term *preembryo* during *in vitro* fertilization treatment.

Controlled ovarian hyperstimulation—Pharmacologic stimulation of the ovaries, generally with gonadotropins and/or clomiphene citrate, with the objective of multifollicular recruitment and hence retrieval of multiple oocytes.

Cryopreservation—Maintaining the viability of cells or tissue by storing at very low temperatures; freezing.

Developmental states—*Preembryo:* The conceptus during early cleavage stages until development of the embryo. The pre-embryonic period ends at approximately 14 days after fertilization with development of the primitive streak. *Morula:* The 16-cell stage upward until blastocyst formation; the stage commonly observed between 72 and 96 hours postinsemination. Some authors believe that the term *morula* is inappropriate for mammals. *Blastocyst:* The conceptus in the postmorula stage possessing a fluid-filled cavity. Attached to the inner surface of the trophoblast is an inner cell mass from which the embryo develops. *Embryo:* The stage of the organism after development of the primitive streak; persists until major organs are developed. Once the neural groove and the first somites are present, the embryo is considered formed. In the human, the embryonic stage begins at approximately 14 days postfertilization and encompasses the period when organs and organ systems are coming into existence.

Embryo transfer—Replacement of embryos after *in vitro* fertilization either transcervically or via cannulation of the fallopian tubes.

***In vitro* fertilization**—An assisted reproductive technique wherein oocytes are retrieved from the ovaries and fertilized extracorporeally with subsequent embryo replacement.

Natural cycle *in vitro* fertilization—*In vitro* fertilization after retrieval of preovulatory oocyte(s) from unstimulated ovaries.

Oocyte—The female gamete from inception of the first meiotic division until fertilization. In oogenesis, a cell that develops from an oogonium. *Metaphase II oocyte:* An oocyte with chromosomes at MII; characterized by the presence of a first polar body. A fully mature oocyte. A secondary oocyte. *Metaphase I oocyte:* An oocyte with chromosomes at MI; characterized by the absence of both a first polar body and a germinal vesicle. An oocyte at an intermediate stage of maturation. *Prophase I oocyte:* An oocyte with chromosomes at PI; characterized by a germinal vesicle.

Oocyte retrieval—Harvest of oocytes from the ovaries, either with laparoscopic- or ultrasound-guided follicular aspiration.

Ovarian reserve—Biologic age of an individual's oocyte. Diminished ovarian reserve, which may be reflected by an elevated early follicular phase follicle-stimulating hormone and/or estradiol level, correlates with reduced chances for success after *in vitro* fertilization.

Prezygote—The penetrated oocyte that displays pronuclei and the second polar body; a pronuclear stage conceptus. The stage of development before syngamy. Some authors refer to this stage as an *ootid*. Pronuclei are commonly observed 10 to 20 hours after insemination.

Zygote—The one-cell stage after pronuclear membrane breakdown before first cleavage. This stage is characterized by maternal and paternal chromosomes assuming positions on the first cleavage spindle, thus the lack of a nucleus. Commonly observed 18 to 24 hours after insemination. *Syngamy:* The union of two gametes in fertilization to form a zygote. The process or reorganization and pairing of maternal and paternal chromosomes in the zygote after pronuclear membrane breakdown.

ASSISTED REPRODUCTIVE TECHNOLOGY AND THE EXPECTATIONS OF PREGNANCY

By law, *in vitro* fertilization (IVF) centers are required to report their results annually to the Centers for Disease Control and Prevention (CDC). At this writing, results for 2003 are available. The number of reported cycles in the United States was 112,872 with 35,785 live births, for a live birth rate of 31.7%.

However, the results are very much age related. This is best seen in the 91,522 cycles using fresh, nondonor eggs (the other cycles used frozen or donor eggs/preembryos). Thus, for those younger than age 35, there is a 37% chance of a live birth, but at age 41 to 42, the expectation is 11%, and older than 42, it is but 4% for a single cycle of treatment.

These are the results against which surgical results must be judged. However, the judgment is not easy—indeed, a sophisticated comparison is impossible. This is because the IVF CDC data are cycle based, and reported surgical data are patient based on results after a certain interval, usually about 2 years (i.e., about 24 cycles). Furthermore, surgical results are seldom satisfied by age. In addition, surgical results are often stated as pregnancy rates rather than live birth rates.

For many conditions discussed herein, the IVF single cycle live birth rate exceeds the 24-month surgical pregnancy rate.

ASSISTED REPRODUCTIVE TECHNOLOGY AND ENDOMETRIOSIS

In patients who have pain and endometriosis, there can be little doubt that surgical ablation of all visible lesions is an attractive therapeutic option.

Our concern here is with those patients who are infertile and have no other factor than endometriosis. What is the relative role of IVF and/or surgery in such situations?

There has been some discussion as to whether infertility can be explained on the basis of endometriosis per se. This observer is persuaded that endometriosis per se can be closely associated with infertility. The possibility of pregnancy with a viable delivery per menstrual cycle of exposure is referred to as fecundity. Normal fecundity is in the 20% to 25% range. In the patient with endometriosis and infertility, monthly fecundity ranges from 2% to 10%.

To be sure, even though pregnancy may follow removal of all viable endometriosis in patients with endometriosis as a single factor, fecundity remains below normal. In a study by Rock and colleagues, the postoperative fecundity rate was found to be but 3.2%.

The issue of the usefulness of surgery for endometriosis was prospectively tested by a Canadian collaborative group who studied the outcome in 341 patients with early disease followed for 36 weeks after laparoscopy. For those who had ablation, the fecundity rate was 4.7%, compared with 2.4% in the diagnosed but untreated group.

Thus, surgery seems to be marginally helpful in the therapy of infertility that is due solely to endometriosis. The problem may well be that in peritoneal endometriosis, many lesions are not visible to the naked eye and therefore not available to treatment,

Contrariwise, IVF works very well in this circumstance. For example, Suzuki and colleagues studied the outcome from IVF in 248 cycles comparing the outcome in (a) 80 cycles with ovarian endometriomas, (b) 248 cycles with endometriosis without ovarian endometriomas, and (c) 283 cycles without endometriosis but with tubal infertility. The pregnancy rates were—and these can be considered fecundity rates—25.3%, 22.3%, and 23.9%, respectively.

It is true that patients with advanced endometriosis—especially with endometriomas, which destroy ovarian tissue—will make follicular aspiration difficult. In this circumstance, the IVF pregnancy outcome is diminished.

There are, of course, nonsurgical options for therapy, but if the primordial goal is pregnancy, there seems little doubt that the treatment of choice for patients with endometriosis is IVF.

ASSISTED REPRODUCTIVE TECHNOLOGY AND TUBAL INFERTILITY

In an ideal world, in cases of tubal infertility, the relative roles of surgery and/or assisted reproductive technology (ART) could be evaluated by a prospective randomized trial. Such a trial has not, nor is never likely, to be done.

Indeed, no prospective trial exists comparing open surgery with laparoscopic surgery in the treatment of tubal disease. Nevertheless, on the basis of experience and nonrandomized surgical end results, it seems to be agreed that if any surgical treatment is to be done for tubal disease, it should be done by the laparoscopic route.

Thus, it is necessary, on the basis of experience and nonrandomized surgical end results, to evaluate the relative roles of surgery and ART in the treatment of infertility that is due to tubal malfunction. Interestingly enough, during the last decade, there have been far fewer end results reports from laparoscopic treatment for tubal disease than appeared in the latter decades of the 20th century. This certainly signifies that IVF has become the treatment of choice for most patients with tubal obstruction. Indeed, some authors have flat out stated that surgery has a very limited place in the treatment of tubal infection causing infertility.

After an extensive review, Sacks and Trew concluded that surgery may be an option for selected patients with some types of tubal disease. They pointed out, however, that if tubal surgery is to be done, it must be restricted to specialized centers with sufficient volume and experience to produce consistent and satisfactory results. It may be added that patients considered for tubal surgery should not be older than the early 30s to allow for IVF if the surgery fails and that *there must be no other infertility factor.*

Proximal Tubal Obstruction

This is a tricky diagnosis. There is a high false-positive rate—i.e., tubal obstruction may seem to be diagnosed by hysterosalpingogram or even hydrotubation only to discover that soon after the procedure, these patients have a spontaneous pregnancy.

Debris that can be removed by catheterization—or even a hysterosalpingogram or hydrotubation that seems to fail—seems to be sufficient to explain such clinical puzzles. If the isthmic end of the tube is clear and the proximal obstruction is just distal to the isthmus, and if the remainder of the tube appears normal, such lesions are very likely to be due to a polyp or salpingitis isthmica nodosa. For such patients in a specialized center, a pregnancy rate in the 50% to 60% range has been reported. For all other circumstances with proximal tubal obstruction, and especially where experienced care is unavailable, IVF is the preferred therapy.

Distal Tubal Disease

There are innumerable classifications of distal tubal disease that is due to an inflammatory process. However, the experienced clinician clearly understands what is meant by mild tubal disease. These cases can be considered for surgery *if all other ancillary criteria are met*. Thus, the peritubal adhesions must be delicate and easily lysed by laparoscopic surgery. The tube must be normal, or at the most only slightly enlarged and not thickened or subject to hydrosalpinx. The endosalpinx, if visible, must not appear to be edematous or dusky.

If an experienced reparative surgeon is available, laparoscopic treatment may give an expectation of pregnancy in the range of 50% over two years.

Hydrosalpinx

A specialized situation exists with hydrosalpinx. Suheil Musher in 1994 was the first to recognize that patients with hydrosalpinx did not do as well with *in vitro* fertilization as compared with those without hydrosalpinx. He reported this from the Jones Institute by studying 188 patients with hydrosalpinx and found that there was an 18% pregnancy rate, compared with a 31% rate for those patients who had had bilateral salpingectomy. This observation has been verified many times, even with more contemporary IVF techniques and with prospective randomized trials.

Thus, for patients who are to have IVF and who have a hydrosalpinx, the removal of the tube or tubes is required. Interestingly enough, proximal tubal occlusion seems to work as well as salpingectomy. Significantly, a study in the United Kingdom showed that only 28% of those clinics surveyed had a protocol or guidelines for the treatment of patients with hydrosalpinx. Thus, it seemed that the deleterious effect of hydrosalpinx on results from IVF and the treatment of such a situation is not practiced as widely as it should be.

The question further arises as to whether tubal disease of an inflammatory nature short of hydrosalpinx is detrimental to the results with IVF. The answer is no. Thus, to enhance IVF, no tubal surgery is required except for hydrosalpinx.

ASSISTED REPRODUCTIVE TECHNOLOGY AND UTERINE FIBROIDS

Long before the days of ART, the relation of fibroids to infertility was vigorously debated. On one hand, there were certainly patients who at delivery were found to have fibroids that were surely there at conception. On the other hand, every gynecologist of experience with infertility patients has identified individuals whose only finding was a fibroid, the removal of which was followed by a term delivery.

Attempts to quantify and characterize these observations are elusive largely because the size and localization of fibroids are of infinite variety. In pre-ART days, there were a number of studies reporting pregnancy rates of more or less 50% after myomectomy in patients with infertility when the fibroid was the only determined abnormality. Just before the ART era, the author reported one such series and reviewed others. Among 42 patients, there was a 45% term delivery rate within 2 years. For the 19 patients younger than age 30, the pregnancy rate was an interesting 76%.

Such studies do not impress those who emphasize evidence-based medicine by prospective two-arm studies, but those with experience, including the author, are persuaded that in some patients, fibroids can be the only cause of infertility.

There is much speculation about why fibroids cause infertility. It is understandable that lesions that distort the endometrial cavity and therefore presumably the overlying endometrium can cause the mischief. However, in the study referred to above, there were patients with normal endometrial cavities with intramural and/or subserous fibroids, the removal of which was followed by pregnancy.

Thus, going into the days of ART, many observers, including this one, were persuaded that fibroids per se were sometimes the cause of infertility.

In the era of ART, the clinical problem takes a special twist. Specifically, what is the proper clinical action when a patient is required to have ART for whatever reason only to find that she also has fibroids? The author, prejudiced from the days before ART, is persuaded that removal of the fibroid before proceeding with ART is the proper course of action.

Fortunately, in the ART era, there are studies directed to exactly this point. Bulletti and colleagues studied a group of patients who underwent surgical removal of myomas before *in vitro* fertilization (Group A) and found that such patients had a cumulative success rate of 33%. On the other hand, patients who underwent *in vitro* fertilization without previous surgery had a 15% clinical pregnancy rate and a 12% delivery rate. The authors were persuaded of the beneficial effects of surgical removal of fibroids before undergoing ART procedures. Benecke and associates studied the impact of intramural leiomyomas on pregnancy outcome as compared with the control group. They found a significant negative impact on implantation rates in the intramural myoma group versus the control group. The implantation rate in the myoma group was 16.4% versus 27.7% in the control group; the delivery rates 31.2% in the myoma group and 40.9% in the control group. They concluded that patients with intramural fibroids have a lesser expectation of pregnancy with the ART technology. Gianaroli and colleagues studied 129 IVF intracytoplasmic sperm injection cycles in 75 patients with one or more intramural or submucosal fibroid and compared them to 127 patients without fibroids. In the fibroid group, the implantation rate was significantly lower than in the study group, 18% as compared with 26.5%. And finally, Surrey and associates were interested in whether postmyomectomy patients had a different pregnancy rate from those patients with a normal uterus from the start. Their findings were that the IVF–embryo transfer results were similar in the two groups, and they concluded that precyclic resection of appropriately selective, clinically significant myomas results in IVF results that are similar to patients who do not have fibroids.

The results of these studies, as well as clinical experience, clearly suggest that patients who require IVF and who are found to have fibroids would benefit from the removal of those fibroids. The only possible exception could be for very young patients—that is, younger than age 30—who when properly informed are prepared to have a trial of IVF with the understanding that if it fails, myomectomy would be desirable before a subsequent IVF trial.

ASSISTED REPRODUCTIVE TECHNOLOGY AND THE INDICATION FOR HYSTERECTOMY

Before the era of ART, it was standard practice to totally remove the uterus if adnexal ablation was required, for whatever cause. This was to prevent future mischief from diseases of the uterus, especially carcinoma of the cervix or corpus.

This has changed. The uterus, if otherwise free of disease, can be left in patients requiring bilateral oophorectomy who wish to retain their reproductive potential using a donor egg or perhaps even cryopreserved oocytes or preembryos. Generally speaking, donor eggs are used only for those within the reproductive age, but donor-egg children have been reported in women in their 50s.

ASSISTED REPRODUCTIVE TECHNOLOGY AND THE PRESERVATION OF FERTILITY AFTER OVARIAN DESTRUCTION

The first decade of the 21st century has witnessed for the first time the possibility of preserving reproduction by the host's own genome after removal of the host ovary or its destruction by radiation or chemotherapy. This goal can be achieved if bits of ovarian tissue, oocytes, or fertilized eggs are cryopreserved or vitrified before the ovary is exposed to the procedure that would result in this destruction. It should be emphasized that although all procedures above have been implemented, such procedures must be considered experimental until more data accumulate and the efficiency and safety have been established. The purpose of this section is not to discuss technological details but simply to provide the gynecological surgeon with the possibilities that should be offered to appropriate patients to preserve their reproductive potential in spite of therapy which of itself would destroy any remaining ovarian tissue. It should also be pointed out that this discussion is limited to situations in which ART technology involving cryopreservation or vitrification is involved. It, therefore, does not discuss patients in whom it is possible to preserve a small portion of ovarian tissue in borderline ovarian tumors, for instance, or other situations whereby ovarian tissue can be preserved *in situ*.

To be a candidate for ovarian or oocyte harvest before treatment that will eliminate the oocytes, the patient must be relatively young, as oocytes degenerate in number and quality with age. Stating an exact age is difficult, as patients vary in regard to ovarian reserve. Indeed, a test of ovarian reserve may be in order to offer some patients more precise information. Such a test can be done by evaluating basal estradiol 17-β (E_2) and follicle-stimulating hormone, as well as by challenge tests designed to evaluate ovarian reserve. Generally speaking, patients older than age 35 become poor candidates unless tests indicate a robust ovarian reserve. Furthermore, such testing and the harvest of eggs or ovarian tissue requires time, and all concerned must evaluate the delay in terms of its effect on the prognosis as far as tumor therapy is concerned. It goes without saying that those offered cryobanking should have a reasonable prognosis for their malignancy and that the gonadotropic stimulation—if used and if it causes a rise in E_2—would not have an adverse stimulatory action on the neoplasm under treatment.

This entire matter has been reviewed by the Practice Committee of the American Society for Reproductive Medicine.

There are three options for cryobanking.

Cryopreservation of Fertilized Eggs

Cryopreservation of fertilized eggs is a routine procedure in contemporary IVF programs. This is by far the most efficient cryobanking option. There are realities. Results are highly individualistic. However, for a patient with average ovarian reserve, there should be adequate surviving fertilized eggs to expect a pregnancy rate of about 40% following a single cycle of egg harvest. The number of harvested fertilized oocytes is the key, and if time is available to harvest eggs from more than one cycle, the pregnancy rate would be substantially increased. The feasibility of this must be obviously individualized.

Cryopreservation of Mature Oocytes

At the moment, cryopreservation of immature oocytes rather than mature (M2) oocytes is not to be considered, as this involves not only cryopreservation but the maturation of the immature oocyte *in vitro*, which itself is extremely inefficient. However, cryopreservation of mature oocytes either by standard slow freezing or by vitrification with fast freezing and with subsequent thawing, fertilization, and live-born children has been reported.

At the moment, this is far less efficient than the cryopreservation of fertilized eggs. With few exceptions, this procedure is in the case-report mode. However, a few active centers have quantified their data. Boroni and colleagues cryopreserved 927 oocytes from 146 patients with a thaw survival rate of 74.1%. There was a 90.2% fertilization rate. They reported 18 clinical pregnancies, for a 9.7% pregnancy rate per transfer and a 12.3% pregnancy rate per patient among those patients who had had more than one transfer. Thus, the procedure has but a modest clinical efficiency.

Cryopreservation of Ovarian Tissue

Cryopreservation of bits of ovarian tissue with later transplantation has shown maintenance of ovarian function in mice, sheep and subhuman primates. Indeed, a viable sheep from such a procedure has also been reported.

Schnorr and colleagues reported the restoration of ovarian function in the monkey by subcutaneous forearm transplantation, and Oktay and associates have reported the same in the human. With the same technique, a single pregnancy followed by a miscarriage was reported by the same group.

The first human live birth after freeze-thawing and autotransplantation of ovarian cortical tissue was reported by Donnez and colleagues in 2004. The patient at age 25 was treated by chemotherapy for Hodgkin's lymphoma. Before treatment, five biopsy samples were removed from the left ovary. At age 32, after chemotherapy—which caused the patient to be amenorrheic—the thawed fragments of ovary were returned to the ovary. Periods resumed, and 9 months after the transplant, a spontaneous pregnancy occurred. A healthy live-born girl was born at term.

A second live birth was reported from Israel in a patient treated for non-Hodgkin's lymphoma. In this particular case, IVF was required. Other live-born children using this technique will undoubtedly be reported.

At this writing, it would seem that oocyte cryopreservation is more efficient than ovarian tissue cryopreservation if preembryo cryopreservation is not feasible. However, the circumstances surrounding a particular patient may require one or another of the techniques quite aside from their intrinsic efficiency.

BEST SURGICAL PRACTICES

- In patients whose infertility is probably due to asymptomatic endometriosis, surgery can be marginally helpful, but postoperatively the fecundity of these patients is far below normal.
- In patients with infertility who require IVF and who have asymptomatic inflammatory damage to the fallopian tubes,

no surgical procedure is required unless the patient has one or both hydrosalpinges.

- In patients who require a bilateral adnexectomy for whatever reason, it may be desirable to not remove a residual normal uterus so that reproductive potential with cryopreserved or donor elements is maintained.
- Before removing normal ovarian tissue in patients whose reproductive goal has not yet been realized, it is necessary to consider whether her reproductive potential can be maintained by assisted reproductive technology.
- The uterus, if otherwise free of disease, can be left behind in patients requiring bilateral oophorectomy who wish to retain their reproductive potential using a donor or cryopreserved oocytes or preembryo.
- Those offered cryobanking should have a reasonable prognosis for their malignancy and that the gonadotropic stimulation—if used and if it causes a rise in E_2—would not have an adverse stimulatory action on their neoplasm under treatment.
- Oocyte cryopreservation is more efficient than ovarian tissue cryopreservation if preembryo cryopreservation is not feasible.
- If the primary goal is pregnancy, the treatment of choice for patients with endometriosis is *in vitro* fertilization.

Bibliography

Aboulghar MA, Mansour RT, Serour GI, et al. The outcome of in vitro fertilization in advanced endometriosis with previous surgery: a case-controlled study. *Am J Obstet Gynecol* 2003;188:371.

Aubard Y, Piver P, Cogni Y, et al. Orthotopic and heterotopic autographs of frozen-thawed ovarian cortex in sheep. *Hum Reprod* 1999;14:2149.

Babaknia A, Rock JA, Jones Jr HW. Pregnancy success following abdominal myomectomy for infertility. *Fertil Steril* 1978;30:644.

Benecke C, Kruger TF, Siebert TI, et al. Effect of fibroids on fertility in patients undergoing assisted reproduction: a structured literature review. *Gynecol Obstet Invest* 2005;59:225.

Borini A, Sciajno R, Bianchi V, et al. Clinical outcome of oocyte cryopreservation after slow cooling with a protocol utilizing a high sucrose concentration. *Hum Reprod* 2006;21:512.

Bulletti C, Ziegler DE, Levi Setti P, et al. Myomas, pregnancy outcome, and in vitro fertilization. *Ann N Y Acad Sci* 2004;1034:84.

Candy CJ, Wood MJ, Whittingham DG. Restoration of a normal reproductive life-span after grafting of cryopreserved mouse ovaries. *Hum Reprod* 2000;15:1300.

Centers for Disease Control and Prevention. 2003 Assisted Reproductive Technology (ART) Report: Section 1—Overview.

Donnez MM, Dolmans MM, Demylle D, et al. Live birth after orthotopic transplantation of cryopreserved ovarian tissue. *Lancet* 2004;364:1405.

Dubuisson JB. Are there still indications for tubal surgery in infertility? *Presse Med* 1998;27:1793.

Dyer SJ, Tregoning SK. Laparoscopic reconstructive tubal surgery in a tertiary referral centre: a review of 177 cases. *S Afr Med J* 2000;90:1015.

Gianaroli L, Gordts S, D'Angelo A, et al. Effect of inner myometrium fibroid on reproductive outcome after IVF. *Reprod Biomed Online* 2005;10:473.

Gosden RG, Baird DT, Wade JC, et al. Restoration of fertility to oophorectomized sheep by ovarian autographs stored at –196 degrees C. *Hum Reprod* 1994;9:597.

Hammadieh N, Afnan M, Evans J, et al. A postal survey of hydrosalpinx management prior to IVF in the United Kingdom. *Hum Reprod* 2004;19:1009.

Johnson NP, Mak W, Sowter MC. Surgical treatment for tubal disease in women due to undergo in vitro fertilization. *Cochrane Database Syst Rev* 2001;3:CD002125.

Johnson NP, Sadler L, Merrilees M. IVF and tubal pathology—not all bad news. *Aust N Z J Obstet Gynaecol* 2002;42:285.

Kassabji M, Sims JA, Butler L, et al. Reduced pregnancy outcome in patients with unilateral or bilateral hydrosalpinx after in vitro fertilization. *Eur J Obstet Gynecol* 1994;56:129.

Kyono K, Fuchinoue K, Yagi A, et al. Successful pregnancy and delivery after transfer of a single blastocyst derived from a vitrified mature human oocyte. *Fertil Steril* 2005;84:1017.

Marcoux S, Maheux R, Berube S. Laparoscopic surgery in infertile women with minimal or mild endometriosis. Canadian Collaborative Group on Endometriosis. *N Engl J Med* 1997;337:217.

Meiro D, Levron J, Eldar-Geva T, et al. Pregnancy after transplantation of cryopreserved ovarian tissue in a patient with ovarian failure after chemotherapy. *N Engl J Med* 2005;353:318.

Nackley AC, Muasber SJ. The significance of hydrosalpinx in *in vitro* fertilization. *Fertil Steril* 1998;96:373–384.

Oktay K, Buyuk E, Veeck L, et al. Embryo development after heterotopic transplantation of cryopreserved ovarian tissue. *Lancet* 2004;363:837.

Oktay K, Karlikaya G. Ovarian function after transplantation of frozen, banked autologous ovarian tissue. *N Engl J Med* 2000;342:1919.

Practice Committee of the American Society for Reproductive Medicine, Birmingham, Alabama. Endometriosis and infertility. *Fertil Steril* 2004;81:1441.

Practice Committee of the American Society for Reproductive Medicine, Birmingham, Alabama. Ovarian tissue and oocyte cryopreservation. *Fertil Steril* 2004;82:993.

Rock JA, Guzick DS, Sengos C, et al. The conservation surgical treatment of endometriosis: evaluation of pregnancy success with respect to the extent of disease as categorized using contemporary classification systems. *Fertil Steril* 1981;35:131.

Sacks G, Trew G. Reconstruction, destruction and IVF: dilemmas in the art of tubal surgery. *BJOG* 2004;111:1174.

Schnorr J, Oehninger S, Toner J, et al. Functional studies of subcutaneous ovarian transplants in non-human primates: steroidogenesis, endometrial development, ovulation, menstrual patterns and gamete morphology. *Hum Reprod* 2002;17:612.

Stadtmauer LA, Riehl RM, Toma SK, et al. Cauterization of hydrosalpinges before in vitro fertilization is an effective surgical treatment associated with improved pregnancy rates. *Am J Obstet Gynecol* 2000;183:367.

Strandell A, Lindhard A, Waldenstrom U, et al. Hydrosalpinx and IVF outcome: a prospective, randomized multicentre trial in Scandinavia on salpingectomy prior to IVF. *Hum Reprod* 1999;14:2072.

Surrey ES, Minjarez DA, Stevens JM, et al. Effect of myomectomy on the outcome of assisted reproductive technologies. *Fertil Steril* 2005;83:1473.

Surrey ES, Schoolcraft WB. Laparoscopic management of hydrosalpinges before in vitro fertilization-embryo transfer: salpingectomy versus proximal tubal occlusion. *Fertil Steril* 2001;75:612.

Suzuki T, Izumi S, Matsubayashi H, et al. Impact of ovarian endometrioma on oocytes and pregnancy outcome in in vitro fertilization. *Fertil Steril* 2005;83:908.

Tjer GC, Chui TT, Cheung LP. Birth of a healthy baby after transfer of blastocysts derived from cryopreserved human oocytes fertilized with frozen spermatozoa. *Fertil Steril* 2005;83:1547.

CHAPTER 21 ■ RECONSTRUCTIVE TUBAL SURGERY

VICTOR GOMEL AND ELIZABETH TAYLOR

DEFINITIONS

Falloposcopy—A transvaginal endoscopic procedure to examine the fallopian tubes, especially the intramural and isthmic segments.

Fimbrial phimosis—Agglutination of the fimbriae.

Fimbrioplasty—The reconstruction of the fimbriae or tubal infundibulum.

Hysterosalpingography (HSG)—An X-ray based contrast test to assess the uterine cavity and the fallopian tubes.

Hydrosalpinx—A distally occluded tube, usually secondary to infection, which distends with accumulation of serous fluid.

Pelvic inflammatory disease (PID)—An inflammatory disorder of the uterus, fallopian tubes, and adjacent pelvic structures usually secondary to a sexually transmitted infection.

Salpingoovariolysis—The division and/or excision of periadnexal adhesions with the aim of restoring normal anatomy.

Salpingoscopy—An endoscopic examination of the ampullary portion of the tubal lumen.

Salpingostomy—The creation of a new stoma in a tube with a completely occluded distal end.

Tubal cannulation—The passage of a flexible guide wire and narrow-gauge cannula through the proximal tubal ostia along the length of the tube.

Tubotubal anastomosis—The surgical approximation of tubal segments after tubal sterilization or excision of an occluded or diseased portion of tube.

The physiologic functions of the human oviduct include proovarian sperm transport to the site of fertilization; ovum pickup and prouterine transport of the ovum; ampullary retention of the ovum (approximately 72 hours); provision of a suitable environment for fertilization to occur and for the zygote to survive; and eventually, transport of the zygote from the ampulla to the uterine cavity. Alterations in any of these functions (caused by either damage to the ciliated epithelium or tubal distortion or occlusion) can result in tubal implantation (owing to the lack of transport of the zygote to the uterus) or infertility (owing to the prevention of sperm meeting the oocyte).

TUBAL FACTOR INFERTILITY

Much of the increase in the incidence of both infertility and tubal pregnancy in the past three decades has been the result of tubal damage after sexually transmitted pelvic infections. The most commonly isolated organisms are *Chlamydia trachomatis*, *Neisseria gonorrhoeae*, and *Mycoplasma hominis*. These organisms appear to account for most primary invasions; however, in 15% to 60% of cases of acute pelvic inflammatory disease (PID), aerobic or anaerobic bacteria, or both, can also be identified. The clinical picture can vary from an almost asymptomatic condition to a life-threatening event. Patients with a more severe clinical appearance often have both aerobic and anaerobic infection.

The classic clinical picture of PID, which includes pain, fever, and lower genital tract infection, occurs in less than 50% of affected patients. Gomel reported (1983a) that more than half of the patients who were investigated for infertility and were found to have a hydrosalpinx gave no previous history of acute PID. This observation has since been confirmed. Indeed, the wide variation in the clinical presentation makes the diagnosis problematic.

It has been estimated that acute PID occurs at a rate of 10 cases per 1,000 women per year in the age group 15 to 39 years, and at a rate of 20 cases per 1,000 women in the age group 15 to 24 years. Just as there is difficulty in diagnosing PID, there is difficulty in ascertaining the trend in its incidence. Chlamydia, the most frequently isolated organism in PID, is increasing. Since 1984, the rate per 100,000 population has increased annually.

The infertility rate after a single episode of PID correlates with the degree of residue of tubal damage. Tubal infertility also increases with recurrent episodes of PID. Infertility occurred in 8% of patients with one episode, 20% with two episodes, and 40% in those with three or more episodes of PID. Further, up to two thirds of cases of tubal-factor infertility and one third of cases of ectopic pregnancy may be attributable to *C. trachomatis* infection.

Reconstructive tubal surgery, by open access, was at one time the only treatment option for infertile women with damaged fallopian tubes. This is no longer the case. Improvement in the outcomes, simplification of the techniques, and much wider availability of *in vitro* fertilization (IVF) and assisted reproductive technology (ART) provide such couples with a realistic therapeutic alternative. In addition, tubal cannulation has been shown to have a role in women with apparent cornual occlusion. Furthermore, it has been demonstrated that many tubal reconstructive procedures can be performed by laparoscopic access. Thorough investigation of both the male and female partners will aid in the selection of the most appropriate treatment option.

INVESTIGATION

The investigation of the infertile couple should be concluded rapidly, accurately, and inexpensively, with as little invasion as possible. In addition, the emotional needs of the couple must be recognized and addressed. This chapter will discuss only investigations specific to tubal and peritoneal factors of infertility.

Tubal Insufflation

Tubal insufflation is a tubal patency test that is now rarely performed. The test was first described by Rubin in 1920, and although there have been modifications of the original technique, the test rightfully bears his name: Rubin's test. The procedure uses an endocervical cannula connected, by rubber tubing, to a mercury manometer and a source of carbon dioxide (CO_2). The rate of gas flow through the system is gradually increased to about 30 to 60 mL per minute. The cervix can be submerged in sterile water in the upper vagina to detect any leakage of the gas from the cervical canal. Tubal patency can be determined by one or more of the following: a written record of the rise and rapid fall of the gas pressure, auscultation of the lower abdomen for the gas passing through the tubes into the peritoneal cavity, or direct visualization of the pressure changes on a mercury manometer. Although normal fallopian tubes demonstrate patency by the rapid escape of gas at pressures below 100 mm Hg, the test is still considered in the normal range if patency is demonstrated below 180 mm Hg. A negative Rubin's test cannot be interpreted as conclusive for tubal obstruction. A study by Sweeney and Gepfert documented this fact by reporting an ultimate pregnancy rate of 50% in patients whose tubal insufflation test had recorded pressures greater than 180 mm Hg. The use of a smooth-muscle relaxant (such as inhaled amyl nitrate) or a mild sedative (such as Valium, 10 mg) before any tubal function test may be helpful in decreasing tubal spasm.

As with hysterosalpingography, which is discussed next, Rubin's test should be performed before ovulation, about the tenth day of the cycle.

Hysterosalpingography

Hysterosalpingography (HSG) is a contrast study of the uterine cavity and fallopian tubes. It is a simple, inexpensive, safe, and rapid diagnostic procedure that, when performed properly, provides valuable information about the uterine cavity and tubal architecture.

Contraindications to HSG include pregnancy, uterine bleeding, lower genital tract infection, PID, and allergy to the contrast material. In women with a history of recurrent PID, or with any suggestion of a recent exacerbation, there is a significant risk of reactivation of quiescent PID. This occurs in about 3% of such patients. To combat this risk, some centers prophylactically administer antibiotics. During the preliminary history and physical examination, the physician must search for possible contraindications and screen for and treat any lower genital tract infections.

Technique

HSG must be timed to occur between the complete cessation of menstruation and ovulation. This will avoid the risk of disturbing a luteal phase pregnancy. Such timing also avoids radiation exposure to the oocyte that will resume meiosis after the luteinizing hormone surge. Administration of a nonsteroidal anti-inflammatory before the procedure reduces the patient's discomfort and diminishes errors associated with hysterosalpingography. The latter is especially applicable to errors regarding cornual occlusion. This has been clearly demonstrated in a study by Lang and Dunaway.

An oil-soluble or water-soluble contrast medium can be used. A recent Cochrane metaanalysis concluded that use of an oil-soluble media increases subsequent pregnancy rates when compared with intervention (odds ratio 3.30; 95% CI 2.00–5.43), however there was no significant difference in the odds of pregnancy with oil-soluble versus water-soluble media (odds ratio 1.49; 95% CI 0.95–1.54). Water-soluble media are most widely used, however, as pelvic granuloma formation has been reported after use of oil-soluble media. Further, patients tolerate the water-soluble media better, and water-soluble media coat the surfaces without sticking to them, producing sharp and finely shaded images and greater visual detail of the lesions. These characteristics enable better assessment of the intraluminal architecture (Fig. 21.1). The contrast material is eliminated within 30 minutes.

After the patient has emptied her bladder, she is placed on the radiographic table. A bivalve speculum is inserted into the vagina, and the cervix and upper vagina are washed with an antiseptic solution. The appropriate cannula, which is filled with contrast material and emptied of any air, is attached to the cervix in such a way as to ensure a tight seal. The speculum is removed before the injection of contrast material. Removal of the speculum is important (especially if the metal variety is used), not only to decrease the patient's discomfort, but also to avoid obscuring the cervical canal and vaginal fornices on the x-ray film.

HSG must be performed under fluoroscopic control with use of an image intensifier. With the syringe attached to the cannula, the contrast material is injected very slowly to avoid discomfort, contraction of the uterus, spasm of the uterotubal junction, and obscuring of the lesions with a large quantity of contrast material. Films are taken to record salient features as they appear on the monitor. An average of three to five films are taken. Preliminary films are of limited value; they can be

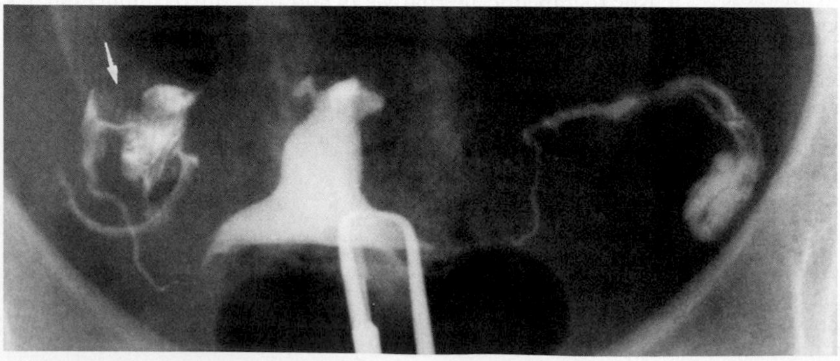

FIGURE 21.1. Hysterosalpingogram. Early film demonstrates a normal uterus and a left hydrosalpinx. On the right there is an ampullary defect (*arrow*) at the site of a previous tubal pregnancy, which was treated with parenteral methotrexate administration.

used to identify misplaced intrauterine contraceptive devices or areas of pelvic calcification. Such information can also be gained by examining the first film.

As the contrast material is injected slowly and intermittently, the endocervical canal, isthmus, and uterine cavity are visualized. To straighten the uterus, firm traction is maintained on the cervix. A film is taken at this point. It is essential to obtain films early during the procedure to record any intrauterine lesions and details of the intratubal architecture. Such details are obscured by larger amounts of contrast material in the uterus, tubes, and peritoneal cavity. Another film is taken when the contrast material starts to escape into the peritoneal cavity (Fig. 21.1). Injection of medium is continued slowly until tubal patency is unquestionably established. Manipulation of the uterus with the cannula may be necessary to display specific tubal segments. A film is obtained when abnormal findings are encountered. In certain cases, a true lateral film may provide useful information. When taking this exposure, the traction on the cervix is temporarily released to obtain information regarding the position of the uterus, the location of intrauterine lesions, and the course and configuration of the tubes.

The last phase of the procedure includes a delayed fluoroscopic examination and a film taken 10 to 20 minutes (when water-soluble contrast material is used) after removal of the cannula. This examination and film may yield information about the external contour of the internal genitalia, the shape of the ovarian fossa, and the presence of periadnexal adhesions.

With adherence to proper technique, complications are rare. Major complications include PID, uterine perforation, bleeding from the tenaculum site, and intolerance to iodine, especially if intravasation of contrast occurs.

HSG performed using water-soluble media provides precise information about the uterus and oviducts that can assist in patient management. Abnormal uterine findings include fusion anomalies, T-shaped uterus, submucous fibroids and endometrial polyps, intrauterine synechiae (Fig. 21.2), and other less commonly identified lesions, such as adenomyosis. Tubal abnormalities that can be observed are listed in Table 21.1 (Figs. 21.3–21.6).

It must be noted that HSG has limitations: (a) it often does not indicate the exact nature of intrauterine lesions, (b) it is associated with false-positive results with regard to cornual occlusion, and (c) it has a low positive predictive value in the diagnosis of periadnexal adhesions and endometriosis. For these reasons, laparoscopy and—when necessary—hysteroscopy are undertaken to elucidate the diagnosis. Indeed, HSG and laparoscopy are complementary, not competitive, procedures in the investigation of infertility associated with tubal and peritoneal factors.

In many instances, HSG demonstrates the presence of severe tubal damage or conditions deemed inoperable. Severe intratubal adhesions and distal tubal occlusion in association with cornual lesions, such as salpingitis isthmica nodosa, are examples of contraindications of reconstructive surgery. In such instances, the couple may be advised of the significance of the findings, and IVF may be recommended as primary treatment, without recourse to laparoscopy.

Selective Salpingography and Tubal Cannulation

Selective salpingography is the injection of a contrast medium directly into the uterine tubal ostium with the use of a special radiopaque cannula inserted through the cervix. The increased pressure generated by the direct injection helps to overcome obstructions associated with mucous plugs or minor synechiae. Selective salpingography is technically possible in approximately 90% of available tubes.

Cannulation of the tube requires the use of a special flexible guide wire and narrow-gauge cannula. This cannulation system is introduced through the larger cannula, which is used for selective salpingography.

If HSG demonstrates a cornual or proximal tubal obstruction (Fig. 21.7), selective salpingography with or without tubal cannulation (Fig. 21.8) should be the next step; this is ideally performed in the same setting. These techniques are useful in differentiating true from false cornual occlusion. The benefits of this approach have been shown for apparent cornual spasm, obstructions caused by amorphous material (tubal plugs), and tubal synechiae. Indeed, half of tubes that were proximally blocked at selective salpingography were found to be normal after tubal catheterization in the largest series reported to date. It is doubtful that these techniques have a real therapeutic effect on occlusions that are due to obliterative fibrosis, chronic follicular salpingitis, salpingitis isthmica nodosa, or endometriosis.

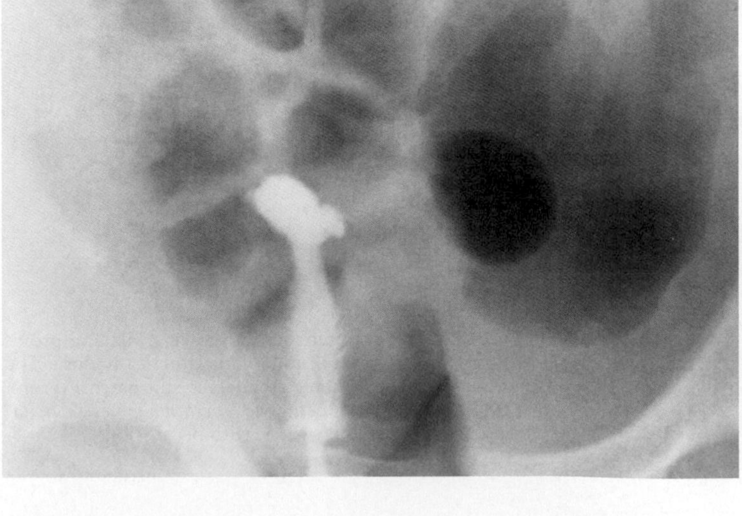

FIGURE 21.2. Hysterosalpingogram in a patient with Asherman syndrome. Contrast material outlines the cervical canal and a part of the lower uterine cavity, the remainder of which is obliterated by synechiae. (From: Gomel V, Taylor PJ. *Diagnostic and operative gynecologic laparoscopy.* St Louis: Mosby; 1995, p. 106, with permission.)

TABLE 21.1

ABNORMALITIES OF THE OVIDUCT

Abnormalities of the oviduct		
Abnormality	**Signs**	**Comments**
TUBOCORNUAL REGION		
Failure of contrast to enter tube	Simple obstruction	May be owing to tubal spasm; may be unilateral or bilateral
Salpingitis isthmica nodosa (SIN)	Appears as a simple obstruction or as spicules of contrast radiating from tubal lumen	May be unilateral or bilateral
Endometriosis	Similar to SIN, usually with more pronounced punctate pattern	May be unilateral or bilateral
Polyps	Small globular or elongated vacuoles surrounded by contrast medium	
ISTHMUS		
Occlusion	Contrast outlines portion of the isthmic segment	Most commonly owing to prior surgical sterilization or tubal pregnancy; less commonly to SIN; and uncommonly to tuberculosis and endometriosis
AMPULLA		
Intraluminal adhesions	Patchy filling defects	Caused by endosalpingeal infection
Tubal pregnancy	Obstruction, stenosis, round defect, occasionally calcification	
INFUNDIBULUM		
Hydrosalpinx	Obstruction usually bilateral	Most common type of occlusion
Phimosis of distal tubal ostium	Intraluminal retention of contrast medium and slow intraperitoneal spill from stenosed tube	Both conditions are usually sequelae of pelvic inflammatory disease
INTRAPERITONEAL SPREAD		
Adhesions	Localized pooling and loculation of contrast medium around distal end of oviducts	

(Modified from: Gomel V, Taylor PJ. *Diagnostic and operative gynecologic laparoscopy.* St Louis: Mosby; 1995:105.)

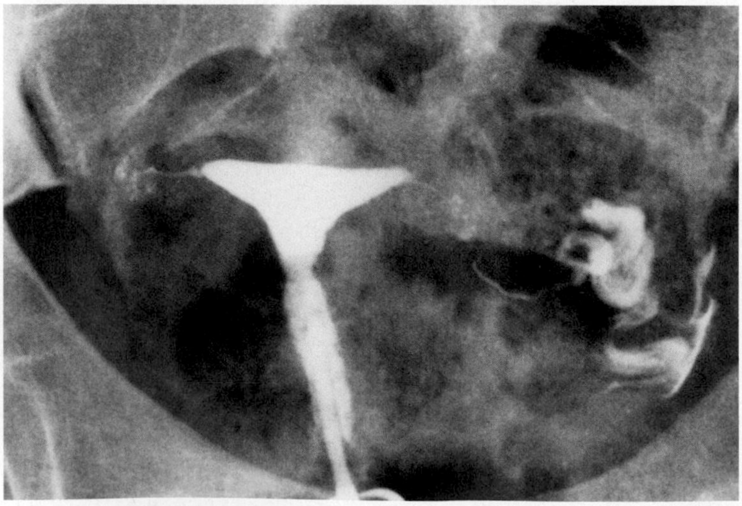

FIGURE 21.3. Hysterosalpingogram showing bilateral proximal isthmic lesions typical of salpingitis isthmica nodosa. The right tube is occluded, whereas the left is still patent. (From: Gomel V, Taylor PJ. *Diagnostic and operative gynecologic laparoscopy.* St Louis: Mosby; 1995, with permission.)

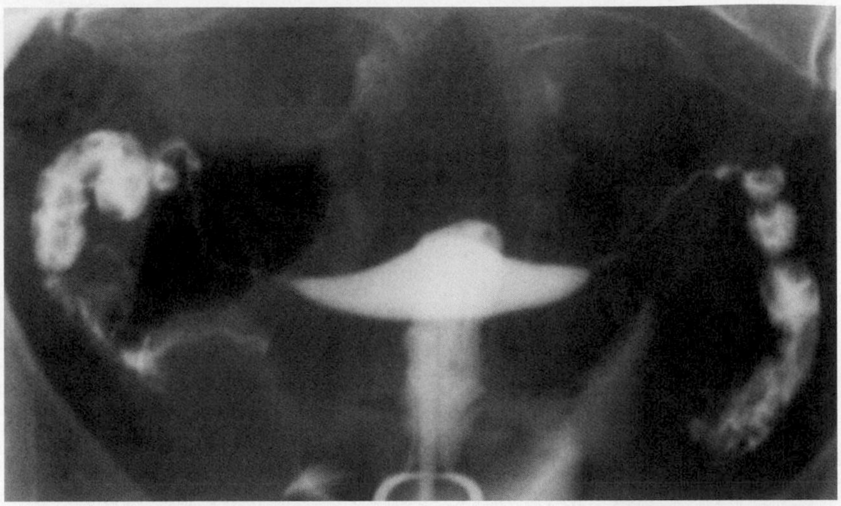

FIGURE 21.4. Hysterosalpingogram. Both tubes exhibit extensive intratubal adhesions. (From: Gomel V, Taylor PJ. *Diagnostic and operative gynecologic laparoscopy.* St Louis: Mosby; 1995, p. 106, with permission.)

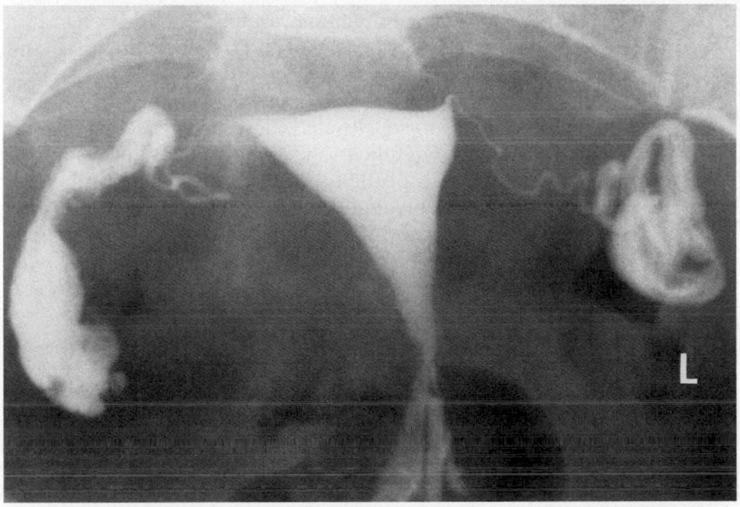

FIGURE 21.5. Hysterosalpingogram showing bilateral hydrosalpinx. The longitudinal epithelial folds are preserved in the left tube. (From: Gomel V, Taylor PJ. *Diagnostic and operative gynecologic laparoscopy.* St Louis: Mosby; 1995, p. 106, with permission.)

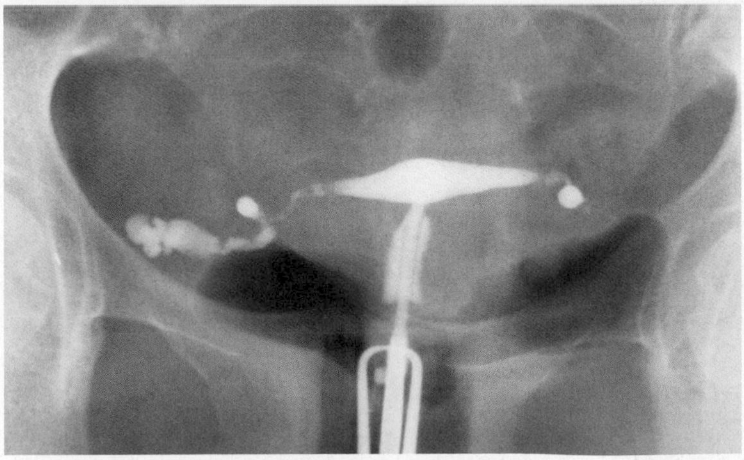

FIGURE 21.6. Hysterosalpingogram. The tubes exhibit findings typical of a prior tuberculous salpingitis. (From: Gomel V, Taylor PJ. *Diagnostic and operative gynecologic laparoscopy.* St Louis: Mosby; 1995, p. 108, with permission.)

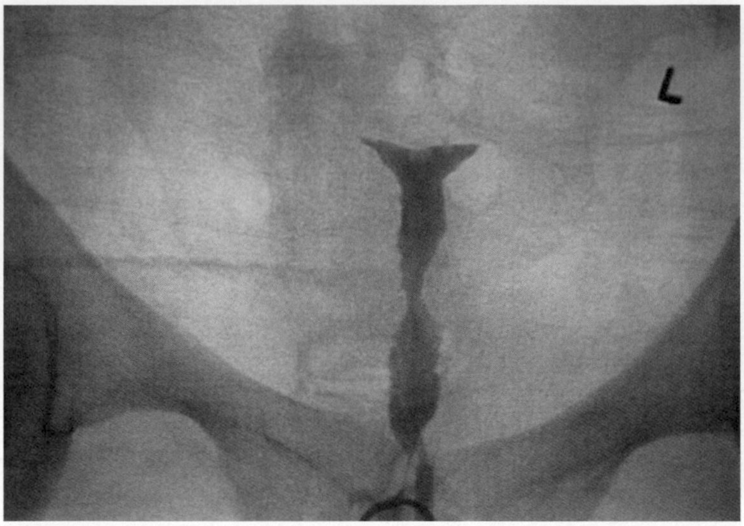

FIGURE 21.7. Hysterosalpingogram showing bilateral cornual occlusion. (From: Gomel V, Taylor PJ. *Diagnostic and operative gynecologic laparoscopy.* St. Louis: Mosby, 1995, p. 109, with permission.)

Salpingoscopy

Salpingoscopy is the endoscopic examination of the ampullary portion of the tubal lumen. This can be accomplished with a rigid or flexible hysteroscope during either laparoscopy or laparotomy. If the distal tube is totally occluded (hydrosalpinx), it is necessary to make a small opening at the fimbriated end to permit the introduction of the scope. The tubal lumen is visualized while distended with physiologic solution injected through the outer sheath of the rigid hysteroscope or the channel of the flexible hysteroscope. The distal end of the tube must be appropriately manipulated to bring it into the axis of the scope. Salpingoscopy permits direct assessment of the tubal epithelium. The findings have been classified into five grades. Grade 1 refers to normal mucosal architecture. Grade 2 refers to tubes that demonstrate variable degrees of flattening of both major and minor mucosal folds, which are largely preserved. Grade 3 refers to tubes that demonstrate focal adhesions between mucosal folds. Grade 4 refers to tubes with extensive intraluminal adhesions or disseminated flattened epithelial areas. Grade 5 refers to tubes that are rigid and hollow with a complete loss of epithelial folds. Findings at salpingoscopy appear to be predictive and prognostic of pregnancy outcome, as demonstrated by Henry-Suchet et al., Brosens and Puttemans, Bowman and Cooke, Marana et al., and Marchino et al.

Microsalpingoscopy has been used to examine the integrity of the tubal mucosa more closely. Microsalpingoscopy uses an endoscope that has magnification capability enabling visualization of individual cells of the tubal epithelium. The epithelium is stained with concentrated methylene blue solution injected through the cervical cannula. It is then assessed under magnification. The level of staining of the nuclei of the tubal cells is inversely proportional to functional integrity of the mucosa. This technique is at present investigational; thus, its value remains to be determined.

Falloposcopy

Falloposcopy is a transvaginal microendoscopic technique aimed at exploring the entire length of the tube, especially the intramural and isthmic segments. A linear eversion catheter system has been used to perform falloposcopy without the need for preliminary hysteroscopy and anesthesia. The patient requires

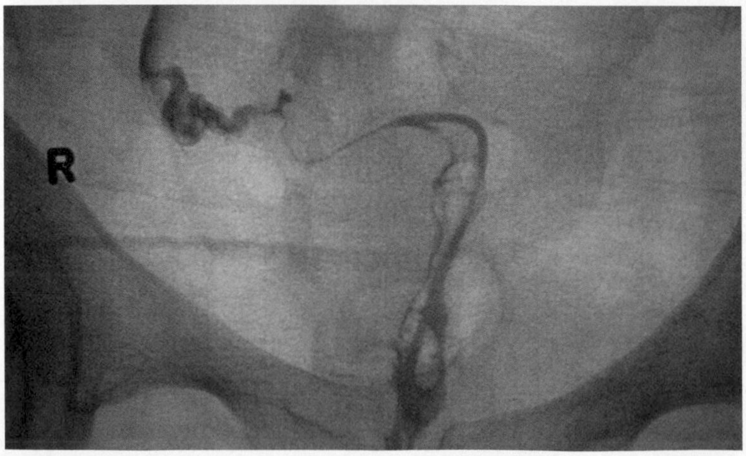

FIGURE 21.8. Tubal cannulation (same patient as in Fig. 21.7). The occlusion has been relieved, and the tube has opacified. (From: Gomel V, Taylor PJ. *Diagnostic and operative gynecologic laparoscopy.* St. Louis: Mosby; 1995, p. 109, with permission.)

premedication to decrease the discomfort associated with the procedure.

The system includes a linear eversion catheter with an outer plastic polymer body 2.8 mm in diameter and a sliding stainless-steel inner body 0.8 mm in diameter, containing a 0.48-mm fiber-optic endoscope. The tip of the outer catheter is angulated so it can be directed toward the uterotubal junction. Once the tubal ostium is identified, the tip of the catheter is held against the ostium. The pressure within the eversion catheter is increased, and the membrane of the eversion catheter is introduced into the fallopian tube for a short distance. The endoscope is pushed down the lumen to the tip of the introduced catheter. The image obtained is displayed on a high-resolution color monitor. The eversion catheter and the endoscope it houses are advanced in the described manner, slowly and gradually, with the endoscope always maintained within the inverting membrane to prevent the tip of the endoscope from piercing the tubal wall.

Falloposcopy may be used as a means of tubal catheterization and has the added benefit of permitting assessment of the lumen of the tube, especially its intramural and isthmic segments. In 1992, Kerin proposed a classification based on a scoring system that takes into account the degree of tubal patency, tubal dilatation, epithelial and vascular changes, intratubal adhesions, and other abnormal findings.

This technique, which requires expensive disposable equipment, did not gain clinical acceptance. Technical improvements, amelioration of the image quality, and parallel reduction in cost may trigger reassessment of the cost-effectiveness of this procedure in the future.

Tests Designed to Assess Tubal Function

Salpingography, salpingoscopy, and falloposcopy are designed to assess tubal morphology.

Procedures designed to assess function are being developed. Early attempts at using radioactive microspheres as oocyte surrogates to evaluate egg transport did not appear to be clinically valuable. Uher and colleagues have introduced biodegradable microspheres into the pouch of Douglas by either cul-de-sac puncture or laparoscopy. These microspheres, which were recognizable by fluorescence, were collected in a cervical cup 24 hours later. Microspheres were present in the cup in 66% of 69 patients with unexplained infertility and in 100% of 20 patients with male factor infertility.

Radionuclide Hysterosalpingography

Radionuclide HSG is a scintigraphic procedure designed to evaluate the spontaneous proovarian transport of microspheres in the genital tract. A solution containing ^{99m}Tc-labeled albumin microspheres is squirted toward the external cervical os of the cervix and upper vagina. The subsequent transport of the microspheres through the cervix, uterus, and tubes is monitored by a gamma camera equipped with a pinhole collimator. The pro-ovarian transport of microspheres depends on both the anatomic patency and the functional integrity of the uterus and oviducts. This test is designed to assess primarily the sperm transport function of the uterus and tubes. This technique is still experimental but preliminary work indicates it is not predictive of fertility potential, and so this technique may have only limited use in the future.

Laparoscopy

Laparoscopy permits direct visualization of the peritoneal cavity, pelvis, and internal reproductive organs. It can also test tubal patency with the use of concomitant chromopertubation. Laparoscopy is an invasive procedure that usually requires a general anesthetic. It is the most accurate way to identify periadnexal adhesive disease and endometriosis.

There are those who argue in favor of an immediate laparoscopy bypassing HSG. An analysis of 18 published series demonstrates good congruence between laparoscopic and HSG findings. These collected data indicate that the sensitivity and specificity of HSG are approximately 76% and 83%, respectively. These studies represent a selected population of patients in whom the prevalence of tubal occlusion was 38%. This prevalence figure falls to 10% in studies of large numbers of unselected patients, which reflects more accurately the general population. If the sensitivity and specificity figures reported above are applied to a hypothetical group of patients with a 10% rate of tubal occlusion, 3% of those with a normal HSG will have an abnormal laparoscopy. Thus, the laparoscopy will be normal in about 97% of patients. These data support delaying endoscopy for 4 to 6 months in those with an apparently normal HSG, except in women of older reproductive age.

Based on the preceding information, a well-performed HSG should be the preliminary investigation for tubal factor infertility. This approach permits the identification of (a) uterine anomalies and lesions; (b) cornual occlusion or lesions, even in the presence of cornual patency; (c) distal tubal occlusion; and (d) assessment of intratubal architecture. This information is of paramount importance to the surgeon at the time of laparoscopy, especially if the condition is amenable to laparoscopic surgery, which should be performed during the same time. Indeed, with the advanced imaging techniques and newer therapeutic modalities available today, laparoscopy solely for the purpose of diagnosis should be rarely required.

Laparoscopic Survey

A thorough laparoscopic survey will identify any adhesions, along with their extent and nature; reveal the presence of endometriosis, its extent, and other abdominal and pelvic lesions; and permit assessment of the uterus, ovaries, and tubes. The information yielded by the prior HSG and this survey enable the surgeon to undertake reconstructive laparoscopic surgery and to recommend surgery by open access or the use of assisted reproductive technologies. These will be discussed later (see Selection of Treatment).

A bimanual pelvic examination is performed on the anesthetized patient. The cervix is then exposed, and a uterine cannula is attached to the cervix. In addition to permitting intraoperative chromopertubation, the cannula enables manipulation of the uterus and enhances laparoscopic visualization.

Once the laparoscope is inserted, the entire peritoneal cavity is inspected. Inspection commences in the upper abdomen and includes the liver and the undersurface of the diaphragm, which are inspected in a clockwise fashion. Particular attention is then focused on the lower abdomen and pelvis. To improve access to the pelvis, the patient is placed in the Trendelenburg position. The bowel is displaced upward, initially by manipulating the uterus and thereafter by using the probe inserted through a second puncture, usually placed suprapubically in the midline, or in one of the lower quadrants.

A general panoramic inspection of the pelvis is performed with the laparoscope at some distance from the pelvic organs.

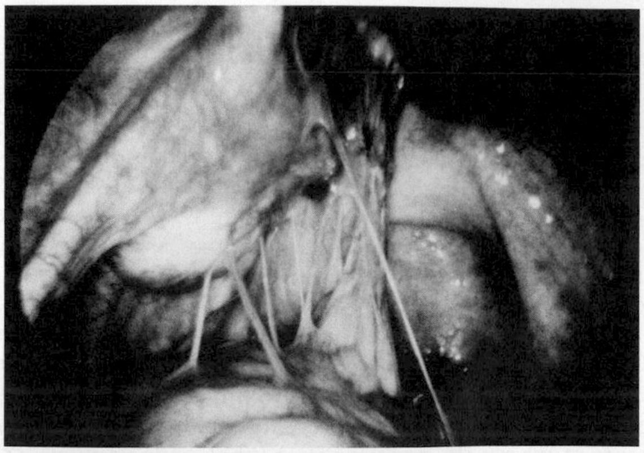

FIGURE 21.9. Laparoscopy. Periadnexal adhesions cover and fix the distal half of the fallopian tube. See color version of figure.

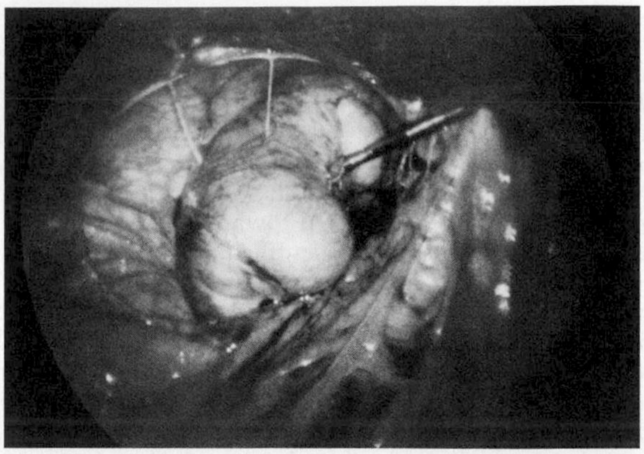

FIGURE 21.10. Laparoscopy. Thin-walled dilated hydrosalpinx with extensive pelvic and periadnexal adhesions. See color version of figure.

This permits a general impression to be formed. Subsequently, a systematic survey is performed. The laparoscope is advanced; appropriate manipulation of the uterus, with the cervical cannula, and of the suprapubic probe enhances visibility of specific organs. The uterus is assessed, along with its anterior surface, the vesicouterine pouch, and the dome of the bladder.

The uterus is then moved into anteversion. The fundus and the posterior surface of the uterus, the uterosacral ligaments, and the pouch of Douglas are thoroughly inspected. If fluid is present in the pouch, its nature is noted. It will be necessary to aspirate the fluid to inspect the underlying peritoneal surfaces. To aspirate the fluid, the probe is replaced by a suction cannula, which can also be used as a manipulating probe. The aspirated fluid can be sent for microbiologic or biochemical studies as deemed necessary. The cul-de-sac and the lateral peritoneal surfaces are inspected for any scarring or evidence of endometriosis.

The extent and type of pelvic and periadnexal adhesions are noted (Fig. 21.9). Each tube and ovary and the respective pelvic side walls are thoroughly scrutinized. Once the anterior surface of the ovary is inspected, the ovary is elevated and flipped upward with the probe, exposing its posterior surface, the fossa ovarica, and the pelvic sidewall down to the level of the uterosacral ligament, which are assessed. The tube is inspected from the proximal to the distal end. Attention is paid to any evidence of fusiform swelling at the uterotubal junction (which is usually caused by salpingitis isthmica nodosa or endometriosis) and the presence of fimbrial phimosis or frank distal tubal occlusion (hydrosalpinx) (Fig. 21.10). The ovarian fimbrial relation is assessed, and the fimbriae are viewed en face. Once the other adnexa are similarly assessed, chromopertubation is performed by injection of dilute indigo carmine or methylene blue solution through the uterine cannula. The passage of the dye solution is followed through the tube, and the nature of the spill is examined by viewing the fimbriae to determine the presence of prefimbrial phimosis or fine fimbrial adhesions that may impede ovum pickup.

Abdominal, pelvic, and periadnexal adhesions may impede laparoscopic access to the pelvis and the adnexa, in which case, preliminary adhesiolysis may be necessary.

SELECTION OF TREATMENT

Two treatment options for achieving pregnancy are available to the infertile woman with damaged fallopian tubes: reconstructive surgery and IVF. Surgery and IVF must not be regarded as competitive treatments but rather as complementary treatments necessary to achieve the desired goal. The choice of treatment is ideally dependent on various considerations, both technical and nontechnical.

Technical Considerations

In vitro fertilization is the only treatment option for women with inoperable fallopian tubes and tubal disease coincident with another important fertility factor, such as male factor infertility. In many instances, reconstructive tubal surgery should be the first treatment option. Specifically, patients with a tubopelvic factor whose surgical treatment will improve their fertility or increase the success rate of an IVF cycle tubal surgery should be offered reconstructive tubal surgery. IVF may be attempted if reconstructive tubal surgery proves unsuccessful.

The provision of accurate information regarding both IVF and tubal surgery is essential in the decision-making process of the couple. The couple must be given the live birth rate per cycle of IVF, the cumulative birth rate after multiple cycles of treatment, and the potential complication rates, including multiple pregnancy, abortion, and ectopic pregnancy. In addition, the effect of frozen embryo replacement on the cumulative pregnancy rate must be considered in the analysis. Similar information must also be provided regarding reconstructive tubal surgery. It is imperative that such figures reflect the experience of the center in which treatment will be performed and not those reported in international journals. However, in this chapter, by necessity, figures derived from the world literature will be used.

In Vitro Fertilization and Embryo Transfer

Data collected prospectively for ART treatments during the year 2003 from 399 programs in the United States provided the following outcome data, which were tabulated by the Centers for Disease Control and Prevention (CDC). There were 112,872 cycles of ART in 2003. Of these cycles, 91,032 (74%) were standard IVF cycles (fresh, nondonor gametes), and of these standard IVF cycles started, 79,602 (87.4%) had oocyte retrieval and 74,295 (81.6%) progressed to embryo transfer. Overall, the live birth rate per cycle initiated was 28.3%, and the live birth rate per embryo transfer was 34.7%. In cycles that resulted in a clinical pregnancy, 82.2% resulted in a live birth. Of live births, 65.8% were singleton births and 34.2% multiple births.

Of note, the number of ART cycles performed in the United States has almost doubled from 64,036 cycles in 1996 to 122,872 in 2003. The number of live babies delivered in 2003 (48,756) was almost two and a half times higher than in 1996 (20,659). The explanation for this increase is most certainly multifactorial. One important factor is the improved success rate of ART in the last decade. Whereas in 1992 the live-birth rate per cycle initiated was 14.5%, this rate in 2003 was 28.3%.

Intracytoplasmic sperm injection (ICSI) represents a very important progress in ART, especially in the treatment of male infertility. In 2003, 56% of ART cycles used ICSI for fertilization of eggs, representing an increase from previous years. This increase largely reflects the expanding use of ICSI to couples not diagnosed with male factor infertility. In male factor infertility, the use of ICSI is associated with a success rate that almost equals that of standard IVF in the absence of male factor (Table 21.2).

The outcome of both standard IVF and ICSI is adversely affected by the age of the female partner. In standard IVF, with couples who had no associated male factor infertility, the live birth per oocyte retrieval rates based on the age of the female partner were as follows: 34 years or less, 42.6%; 35 to 37 years, 35.9%; 38 to 40 years, 26.2%; 41 to 42 years, 16.1%; and more than 42 years, 6.0%. The live birth per oocyte retrieval rates for IVF using ICSI in couples that had male factor infertility were approximately the same for each group, demonstrating a similar decline with increasing age. These rates were 41.8%, 35.0%, 24.1%, 13.5%, and 4.2%, respectively. This trend is also observed in couples with and without male factor infertility (Table 21.2).

Success with transfer of cryopreserved embryos has improved significantly. Frozen embryos were used in approximately 14% of all ART cycles performed in 2003 (17,517 cycles). The rate of live birth per transfer was 27% as compared with 34.7% for fresh embryo transfer. So, although replacement of frozen embryos improves the cumulative success rate for a couple, the overall net effect remains limited because not all of the cycles provide spare embryos, and not all of the frozen embryos withstand the thawing process.

IVF and embryo transfer is not risk free, especially in stimulated cycles. Although uncommon, ovarian hyperstimulation, bleeding, and infection can occur. Pregnancies resulting from IVF have an abortion rate of about 16%. The overall tubal pregnancy rate is approximately 1% to 2% of ART cycles. A study from our center demonstrated a tubal pregnancy rate of 2.6% (of clinical pregnancies) among IVF patients without tubal factor infertility. However, this rate was 12% in patients with prior tubal disease (these are the patients who must choose between IVF and tubal surgery).

ART procedures are associated with a significant increase in the rate of multiple pregnancy (relative risk [RR] >20). The CDC Assisted Reproductive Technology report for 2003 indicated that of the resulting live births, only 65.8% were singleton; 31.0% were twins, and 3.2% were triplets or higher order. This high rate of multiple births has a tremendous personal and social impact. Perinatal morbidity and mortality are markedly increased in pregnancies complicated by multiple gestation. The cost, both emotionally and financially, of caring for premature or abnormal children is great. It is important to note that monofetal pregnancies also are associated with elevated risk as compared with non-ART singleton pregnancies; more than 10% of monofetal births are preterm, and the perinatal mortality rate (about 19 per 1,000) is higher than non-ART singleton pregnancies. Indeed, an important study from Sweden that compared the obstetric outcomes of babies conceived with IVF (n = 5,856) to all babies born in the general population during a span of 13 years (1982–1995) demonstrated the following: Children resulting from an IVF conception had increased rates of low birth weight (RR = 5), major malformations (RR = 1.4), cerebral palsy (RR = 4), and death (RR = 2). Such elevated personal and societal costs must be considered when embarking on any ART procedure.

Reconstructive Surgery

The overall risks of reconstructive tubal surgery are small and include the recognized complications of anesthesia and surgery. Surgery, if successful, offers multiple cycles in which to achieve conception and the opportunity to have more than one pregnancy. The abortion rate subsequent to reconstructive tubal surgery is not increased over that of the normal population. The live birth and ectopic pregnancy rates depend on the specific nature of the tubal disease and the extent of tubal damage.

After thorough investigation of the couple, a decision must be made regarding whether to proceed with reconstructive

TABLE 21.2

CDC 2003 ASSISTED REPRODUCTIVE TECHNOLOGY REPORT

Live births per oocyte retrieval in ART cycles 2003					
	Age (years)				
	<35	35–37	38–40	41–42	>42
Male factor infertility					
IVF	42.6%	35.9%	26.2%	16.1%	6.0%
IVF with ICSI	41.8%	35.0%	24.1%	13.5%	4.2%
No male factor infertility					
IVF	42.6%	35.9%	26.2%	16.1%	6.0%
IVF with ICSI	37.8%	32.2%	21.8%	11.0%	4.2%

ART, assisted reproductive technology; IVF, *in vitro* fertilization; ICSI, intracytoplasmic sperm injection.

surgery. The preceding arguments and results yielded by IVF must be taken into consideration in this decision-making process. In addition, the results achieved by the center in which the patient will be treated must be considered. The results are dependent on the proper selection of patients and the technical expertise of the team and the surgeon.

Nontechnical Considerations

The nontechnical considerations include age, cost, and the wishes of the couple. Female fecundity is adversely affected by age. Fecundity begins to decline at about 31 years of age. This trend has been observed both in "normal" couples and in those with unexplained infertility. This decline becomes more evident after 37 years of age.

In women of advanced reproductive age, the marked decline of fecundity rate per cycle of IVF must be weighed against the fact that reconstructive surgery offers multiple cycles during which conception can occur. Therefore, although the younger woman may consider surgery first and IVF thereafter (if this becomes necessary), those between 37 and 40 years of age may be advised to consider IVF first.

Health insurance coverage and the cost of the procedure, depending on the jurisdiction, and the resources of the couple play important roles in the decision-making process. Another often underestimated potential factor is the economic impact of a multiple pregnancy, which occurs much more frequently with IVF.

The perceptions and wishes of the couple regarding treatment options depend on many influences, including their own values and ethical views. There may be disagreement between partners. The physician should provide detailed information for the couple as clearly and accurately as possible and should abstain from interfering with their decision making except to clarify misunderstandings and misinterpretations. The physician must advise against active treatment when the prognosis is poor because treatment with essentially no chance of success cannot be justified.

Selection

Periadnexal adhesive disease may be the only apparent lesion or may be present in addition to tubal occlusion. The tubes may be occluded at their outer end or proximally as the end result of disease processes, or the tubes may have been interrupted by a previous sterilization.

If periadnexal adhesive disease is the sole lesion, laparoscopic salpingoovariolysis, performed preferably at the time of the initial diagnostic laparoscopy, is the approach of choice. For patients who have undergone this procedure, the reported intrauterine pregnancy rates range from 51% to 62%, and the ectopic pregnancy rates range from 5% to 8%.

Agglutination of the fimbriae (fimbrial phimosis) necessitates a fimbrioplasty, which can also be performed laparoscopically. This condition often coexists with periadnexal adhesions, which are dealt with first. The reported intrauterine pregnancy rates after laparoscopic fimbrioplasty range from 40% to 48%, and the ectopic pregnancy rates range from 5% to 6%.

Distal tubal occlusion (hydrosalpinx) can be treated surgically. Indeed, removal or proximal occlusion of a hydrosalpinx is recommended before IVF. A recent Cochrane metaanalysis confirms the earlier work of Strandell *et al* in demonstrating that the odds of ongoing pregnancy and live birth (OR 2.13, 95% CI 1.24–3.65) were increased after laparoscopic salpingectomy for unilateral or bilateral hydrosalpinges before IVF.

In major published series, the live birth rates after microsurgical salpingostomy range from 20% to 37%, and ectopic pregnancy rates range from 5% to 18%. The improved results achieved with the use of microsurgical techniques are much less impressive with salpingostomy than with other tubal procedures. Furthermore, salpingostomy, performed by laparoscopic access, yields almost similar results to those achieved by open access.

The factors that affect the outcome of salpingostomy include distal ampullary diameter, tubal wall thickness, nature of the tubal endothelium, extent of adhesions, and type of adhesions. These prognostic factors have been quantified in a numerical scoring system (approved by the American Fertility Society in 1988). In cases deemed favorable (mild), the reported live birth rates after microsurgical salpingostomy range from 40% to 60%. This rate drops to less than 20% in cases considered unfavorable (severe). In such cases, IVF may be the initial treatment of choice. If surgery is the initial treatment of choice, the decision of whether to proceed with an immediate laparoscopic salpingostomy or undertake reconstructive microsurgery must depend on local experience and success rates with both approaches.

In cases of proximal tubal occlusion, selective salpingography or transcervical fallopian tube cannulation may be useful in elucidating false-positive results obtained by HSG and in overcoming obstruction associated with a mucous plug or synechiae. True pathologic tubal occlusion resulting from salpingitis isthmica nodosa, endometriosis, or extensive postinflammatory fibrosis may be treated by microsurgical tubocornual anastomosis using a minilaparotomy as access. The reported live birth rates after such procedures range from 33% to 56%, and ectopic pregnancy rates range from 5% to 7%.

Because in the vast majority of cases of reversal of tubal sterilization the available tubal segments are normal, the outcome of a microsurgical anastomosis is an anatomically and physiologically normal, albeit shortened, fallopian tube. In our institution, the intrauterine pregnancy rate in those less than 35 years of age at the time of reversal is approximately 70%, with most pregnancies occurring within 18 months of surgery; in those 35 years or more, it is 55%. The ectopic pregnancy rate is approximately 2%.

Repair of Fimbriectomy

Surgical correction of a Kroener's sterilization (fimbriectomy) is possible, but the outcome depends on the remaining ampullary length. Live birth rates of about 30% have been reported when more than 50% of the ampulla has been preserved. Tubal length, in such cases, can be determined by HSG, and in the absence of sufficient ampullary length, IVF should be recommended as the initial treatment. Fortunately, this type of sterilization is now rarely performed.

Summary

The choice of the primary treatment and any subsequent treatment depends on a careful consideration of both nontechnical and technical factors. These must be individualized for each patient. Information about success and complication rates of the available treatment options must accurately reflect local experience. Active involvement of the couple in the decision-making process is more likely to result in resolution of the conflict of infertility if treatment proves unsuccessful.

MICROSURGERY

Microsurgery has been defined as "surgery under magnification." In fact, magnification is only a single facet of microsurgery, which embraces a broad concept of tissue care designed to minimize tissue damage.

The basic principles of microsurgery include the following:

- Using a technique designed to minimize tissue injury. In addition to delicate handling of tissues and judicious use of electrical or laser energy, frequent intraoperative irrigation with heparinized lactated Ringer solution is performed to keep serosal surfaces moistened and prevent desiccation.
- Preventing foreign body contamination of the peritoneal cavity.
- Obtaining meticulous pinpoint hemostasis while minimizing adjacent tissue damage.
- Identifying proper cleavage planes.
- Completely excising abnormal tissues.
- Precisely aligning and approximating tissue planes.
- Using magnification, which permits prompt identification of abnormal morphologic changes, recognition and avoidance of surgical injury, and application of the preceding principles with the use of fine microsurgical instruments and suture materials.
- Performing a thorough pelvic lavage at the close of the procedure to remove from the peritoneal cavity any blood clots, foreign body, or debris that may be present.

Thus, microsurgery is a surgical attitude as much as a technique.

In the late 1960s, Swolin used magnification with electrosurgery for the reconstruction of distal tubal occlusion. In addition, he strived to reduce peritoneal trauma and kept the operative site wet by frequent irrigation. Magnification, including the use of an operating microscope, and microsurgical techniques were subsequently expanded and used in the correction of pathologic cornual and midtubal occlusions and in reversal of sterilization. This approach permitted us to perform tubocornual anastomosis as opposed to a tubouterine implantation in cases of pathologic corneal occlusion. Such an anastomosis in such cases preserves tubal integrity and thus is a more physiological approach to tubal reconstruction.

Microsurgery, in fact, finds its ultimate application in tubal anastomosis. The use of magnification, microsurgical instruments, and sutures enables the recognition of subtle abnormalities (even in the presence of tubal patency), the excision of abnormal tissues, and the correct alignment of the tubal segments and precise apposition of each layer. Indeed, the application of microsurgery has significantly improved the outcome of such procedures. However, in the treatment of distal tubal occlusion, any improvement attributable to the use of microsurgical techniques has been modest, despite the reduction in postoperative adhesions and improved tubal patency rates.

The introduction of microsurgery into gynecology has yielded benefits much greater than simple improvement in the outcome of certain fertility operations. It created a great awareness of the effects of peritoneal trauma and the resulting postoperative adhesions. It also promoted the use of conservative approaches that are now considered standard care for women undergoing surgical treatment for benign gynecologic disease. These are additional and important reasons to continue to teach reconstructive infertility surgery.

Thus, microsurgery is a surgical philosophy, a delicate surgical approach designed to minimize peritoneal trauma and tissue disruption and to prevent postoperative adhesions while increasing the accuracy of the procedure and improving the outcome.

Microsurgical techniques are equally applicable to both laparotomy and laparoscopic access. We demonstrated the applicability of microsurgical techniques by laparoscopy for adhesiolysis, salpingo-ovariolysis, fimbrioplasty, and salpingostomy as early as the mid-1970s. Microsurgical techniques must be used in all reproductive operations, irrespective of the mode of access. This is especially important today because most such procedures are performed by laparoscopy and minilaparotomy.

The laparoscope provides a degree of magnification. It is also possible to bring the distal end of the laparoscope close to the area of interest and achieve excellent visibility and illumination. There are microsurgical advantages inherent to laparoscopic access. Operating within a closed peritoneal cavity eliminates the need to use packs and prevents the introduction of foreign materials such as lint and talcum powder. The pressure effect of the pneumoperitoneum diminishes venous oozing and permits spontaneous coagulation of minor vessels. It is possible to perform intraoperative irrigation to expose any bleeding vessels and keep tissues moistened. Fine electrodes can also be used to achieve precise electrosurgical hemostasis. Like microsurgery, laparoscopic procedures are performed with few instruments. The instrument manufacturers have at last recognized the need for proper microsurgical instruments for laparoscopy; they are now readily available. We must stress, however, that the large volume of insufflation necessary in operative laparoscopy causes desiccation of the mesothelial cells that line the peritoneum. This phenomenon, which may enhance formation of postoperative adhesions, can be largely prevented by the use of warmed humidified gas, which can be accomplished with the introduction of a special apparatus into the CO_2 line. There is also evidence that CO_2 pneumoperitoneum alters the protective mechanisms of cells against free radicals. This increases with the duration of the pneumoperitoneum, insufflation pressure, and flow rate. This deleterious effect may be partly overcome by frequent irrigation with lactated Ringer solution. Experimental data in animals suggest that the addition of a small percentage of oxygen to the pneumoperitoneum reduces these local effects, as well as the systemic effects of carbonemia and acidosis.

Major Equipment and Surgical Instruments

The major equipment includes an electrosurgical generator suitable for both general and microsurgical work and, depending on the access mode used, either an operating microscope or appropriate laparoscopic equipment.

Most of the good modern electrosurgical generators can be used for both general and microsurgical work. Such generators are now standard equipment in most operating rooms.

When access to the pelvis is achieved by laparotomy or minilaparotomy, magnification is obtained by the use of an operating microscope or loops. Loops provide low levels of fixed magnification. It is difficult to work with loops that provide magnification greater than 4 times. They are suitable for use only in simple short procedures and are quite helpful when used to divide adhesions or excise endometriotic lesions located deep in the pelvis.

Magnification is best obtained with an operating microscope that provides magnification ranges from 2 times to 40 times; coaxial illumination of a constant visual field enables precise focusing and change of the level of magnification. In gynecologic microsurgery, an objective lens with a focal

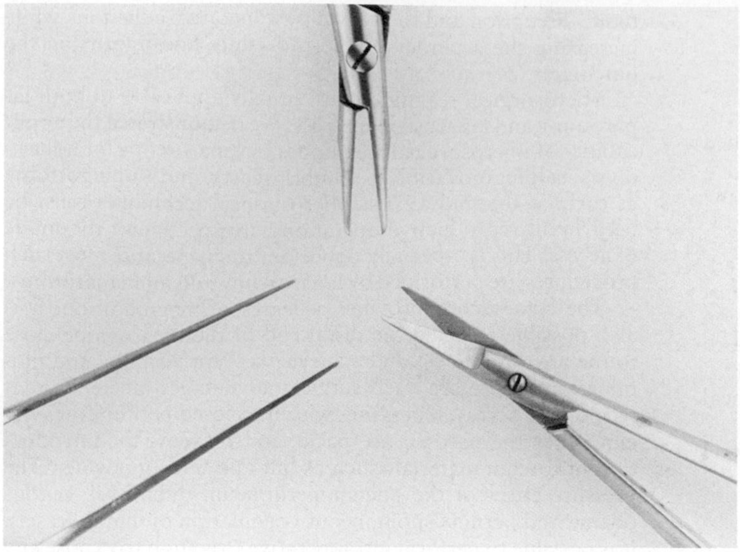

FIGURE 21.11. The working tips of the principal microsurgical instruments: plain forceps, scissors, and needle holder.

distance of 250 to 300 mm allows for a suitable working distance under the lens. The microscope can be mounted on the floor or ceiling. Focusing, varying the level of magnification, and other functions of the microscope can be manual or motorized. The latter version is preferable because changes can be readily accomplished through controls on a foot pedal while the surgeon's hands remain in the operative field. Most modern operating microscopes are equipped with beam splitters, which permit the fitting of two pairs of binoculars so that both the surgeon and the assistant can simultaneously view the operative field. A miniature television camera can also be fitted to the same beam splitter, which enables the operating room personnel to follow the surgery on the monitor and allows video recordings of the procedure to be made.

When laparoscopic access is used, a good laparoscope equipped with a high-resolution mini TV camera and monitor is required. The laparoscope does not offer the stereoscopic vision and the excellent depth of field that the operating microscope provides. Nonetheless, first generations of three-dimensional laparoscopic equipment and magnification devices have been produced. Progress is under way.

Good microsurgical instruments are now available from many manufacturers. Their shape is obviously different for open and laparoscopic procedures. However, their functions are similar. The basic microsurgical instruments are few and include plain and toothed platform microforceps, microscissors, microneedle holder, and straight scissors and/or a microblade to transect the tube (Fig. 21.11). The forceps have rounded tips with a shaft designed so that they, like the scissors and needle holder, have good ergonomics and can be used comfortably. Teflon-coated probes with variable rounded tips are used for retraction.

Electromicrosurgery requires the use of a true insulated microelectrode of 100 or 150 microns in diameter with a free pointed conical tip. The microelectrode is connected to the handle of the electrosurgical unit with an adaptor. A rocker switch mounted on the handle allows delivery of current in cutting, coagulating, or blend modes. Irrigation can be performed with an appropriate laparoscopic irrigator. For open procedures, a device with a fingertip control (Gomel irrigator, Fig. 21.12) is commercially available and enables accurate irrigation.

Immediate Preoperative Preparation

Before the induction of anesthesia, the surgeon must ensure that all necessary equipment and instruments are present and in working order. After the induction of anesthesia, the patient's bladder is catheterized with a Foley catheter, which is connected to continuous drainage. If intraoperative chromopertubation is required, either a pediatric Foley catheter or an appropriate uterine cannula is introduced through the cervix and fixed in

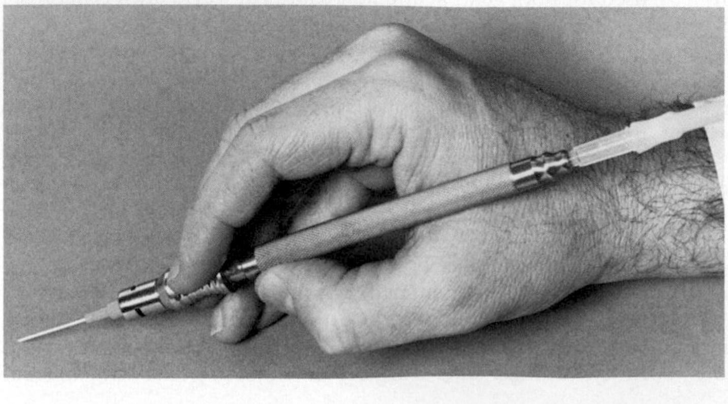

FIGURE 21.12. The Gomel microsurgical irrigator. An intravenous cannula has been attached to the tip of the irrigator. Fingertip control of the sliding valve permits one to initiate or stop irrigation.

place. The catheter or cannula is connected either directly or by means of an extension tube to a syringe filled with dilute dye solution.

When open surgical access is used, anteversion and elevation of the uterus can be achieved either by selecting a suitable uterine cannula or by packing the vagina. With the latter option, a pediatric Foley catheter should first be placed in the uterine cavity if intraoperative chromopertubation is desired.

Surgical Access

As indicated earlier in the text, many reconstructive tubal operations can be performed by laparotomy, minilaparotomy, or laparoscopic access. The selection of the specific access route depends on the nature of the lesion, the type of procedure required, and the skill of the surgeon. The aim is to select the access route that will yield the best outcome for the patient.

Many reconstructive operations, especially those for distal tubal disease, can be efficiently performed by laparoscopic access. Because of the advantages inherent in undertaking such a procedure at the time of the initial diagnostic laparoscopy, it is preferable that a surgeon trained in this type of surgery perform the initial laparoscopy.

Access by Laparoscopy

Once a proper pneumoperitoneum is obtained, the principal trocar and cannula are inserted (usually intraumbilically), the trocar is removed, and the laparoscope is introduced through the cannula. The details of performing a laparoscopy will not be described in this chapter. A thorough laparoscopic survey is performed as described earlier in this text, and the nature and extent of the tubal and pelvic lesions is assessed. The information yielded by the prior HSG, complemented by the laparoscopic findings and the status of the other fertility parameters, permits the surgeon to select the therapeutic approach that is best for the patient.

The laparoscopic survey requires the establishment of a secondary portal for the introduction of a probe or other appropriate instrument. This ancillary portal is placed suprapubically in the midline or in one of the lower abdominal quadrants. The undertaking of reconstructive surgery will necessitate the establishment of additional portals of entry. These are placed, depending on the clinical findings and the procedure to be performed, at sites that permit easy access to the operative field.

Abdominal Incision Minilaparotomy

In reconstructive tubal surgery, a transverse suprapubic incision is the type used most often. Since 1985, we have used a small, minilaparotomy, suprapubic transverse or vertical (if a midline or paramedian scar is present) incision to gain access to the pelvis. The length of this minilaparotomy incision is usually 5 to 6 cm. The prior pelvic findings and especially the depth of the patient's subcutaneous adipose layer determine the length of the incision. The site of the proposed incision is infiltrated with a long-acting anesthetic agent, such as 0.25% bupivacaine (Marcaine) solution. A transverse suprapubic incision is made and extended down to the fascia. The subcutaneous fat is dissected over the fascia, in the midline upward and downward. The fascia is then incised vertically in the midline. The recti muscles are separated in the midline, and the peritoneum is incised vertically, with the incision curbed laterally at the lower end to avoid the bladder. The subcutaneous tissues are reinfiltrated with the same solution before closure of the skin incision. Thereafter, a bilateral ilioinguinal nerve block is established. The small size of the incision; the lack of bowel manipulation, along with gentle handling of tissues during the procedure; and the use of local anesthesia reduce postoperative discomfort and analgesia requirements. This approach permits prompt mobilization of the patient and discharge from the hospital or surgical center within 4 to 24 hours. Most of our patients are discharged on the same day. These patients return to normal activity almost as rapidly as those who have had their procedures performed laparoscopically.

It is essential that the surgical personnel thoroughly wash their gloves after they have been put on and again before making the peritoneal incision. Once the peritoneal cavity is entered, a wound protector is introduced through the incision, and a small Dennis-Brown retractor is applied. A disposable device, Protractor, combines the functions of wound protector and retractor, providing circumferential retraction with maximal exposure for the incision size. This device is preferable because it is easy to use and enhances access through minilaparotomy. Pads soaked in heparinized (5,000 U/L) lactated Ringer solution can be introduced into the pouch of Douglas to further elevate the uterus and isolate the bowel already displaced by a mild (10- to 15-degree) Trendelenburg tilt.

Once the surgical site is well exposed, the operating microscope is positioned. Although the operating microscope can be draped, we have not found this to be necessary, particularly if foot pedals control the microscope. Intraoperative irrigation is performed with heparinized lactated Ringer solution in an intravenous bag that is elevated and connected with intravenous tubing to a Gomel microsurgical irrigator (Fig. 21.12). This enables periodic irrigation of the exposed peritoneal surfaces and ovaries to prevent desiccation and to visualize individual bleeders.

Pelvic Lavage

At the close of a reconstructive procedure, irrespective of the type and the mode of access, the operative site is inspected to ensure that complete hemostasis has been achieved. Any bleeding vessels are electrodesiccated. A thorough pelvic lavage is then performed with the irrigation solution until the fluid remains clear. Pelvic lavage serves to remove from the peritoneal cavity any blood clots or other debris that may be present.

When laparoscopic access is used for the procedure, underwater examination of the operative site may be performed. When the irrigation fluid remains clear, the pneumoperitoneum pressure is reduced, and the region is inspected with the distal end of the laparoscope under the surface of the fluid. This permits prompt recognition of any small bleeding vessels, which can be desiccated with use of a microelectrode or microbipolar forceps.

Once the irrigation fluid is completely suctioned out of the pelvis, some investigators leave varying amounts of physiologic solution in the peritoneal cavity to reduce postoperative adhesions. We use 200 to 300 mL of lactated Ringer solution. Hyskon, which was in vogue for many years, is no longer used. There are promising new products designed to prevent adhesion formation that are easy to apply by both open and laparoscopic access; these are currently undergoing clinical trials. The topic of ancillary measures for adhesion prevention is outside the purview of this chapter and will not be discussed further.

SURGICAL TECHNIQUE

In this chapter, the following procedures will be discussed: salpingo-ovariolysis, fimbrioplasty, salpingostomy, tubotubal anastomosis to repair midtubal disease or to reverse a prior sterilization, tubocornual anastomosis to treat proximal tubal disease, and other procedures performed rarely in unusual circumstances.

The techniques used in these procedures are essentially the same irrespective of the access route.

Whereas procedures for distal tubal disease are very amenable to laparoscopic access, anastomotic procedures are technically more difficult to accomplish by this route. Isthmic–isthmic and isthmic–ampullary anastomosis (usually used for sterilization reversal) have been performed with varying degrees of accuracy through laparoscopic access, but accomplishing other types of anastomoses (especially tubocornual) through this mode of access is much more difficult.

With microsurgical procedures, our aim has always been to keep the techniques as simple as possible in order that the results will be reproducible not only by surgical virtuosi but also by all physicians who practice in this field.

Our more recent technical modifications, including access through minilaparotomy incision and the use of a Protractor, were the result of the same thought process. Although we remain enthusiastic proponents of laparoscopic access, we do not let this enthusiasm blind us to the possibility that some procedures may still be performed better by improvements in traditional methods.

Salpingo-Ovariolysis

Pelvic and periadnexal adhesions usually are the sequelae of PID. These adhesions may be broad or shallow; they are usually not too vascular and extend from one structure to another. In so doing, they tend to leave a space or potential space between the involved structures, an aspect that facilitates adhesiolysis (Fig. 21.13). Dense cohesive adhesions often result from prior surgery. In this case, adjacent structures are intimately conglutinated. The adherent area is devoid of the superficial mesothelial layer of peritoneum. In other words, the underlying stromal layers of the two structures coalesce. The lysis of such an adhesive process is technically difficult and is associated with a very high percentage of recurrence.

Periadnexal adhesions usually coexist with other types of tubal disease. Thus, salpingo-ovariolysis is often an integral part of other reconstructive procedures. However, periadnexal adhesive disease may be the sole apparent lesion, in which case infertility depends on the severity and nature of these adhesions. Even in the presence of a patent tube, extensive adhesions may encapsulate the tube (especially the fimbriated end, the ovary, or both) and prevent ovum pickup (Fig. 21.9). By fixing the fimbriated end of the patent tube away from the ovary, adhesions could possibly distort the spatial relation and, hence, the functional relation that exists between these two organs. For example, the fimbriated end of a patent tube may be adherent to the anterior abdominal wall or the uterine fundus, whereas the ovary is fixed in the pouch of Douglas. Periovarian adhesions may also affect follicular development, as has been demonstrated in both animal and human studies. Human studies were usually performed on patients undergoing IVF treatment.

When salpingo-ovariolysis is performed with an open abdomen (laparotomy or minilaparotomy), adhesiolysis is usually commenced by defining the distal margins of the adhesions. The division of adhesions at their distal attachment frees the adnexa, making it possible to elevate and bring them closer to the abdominal wall. This move facilitates the remainder of the procedure. Elevation of the adnexa is achieved by the use of inert pads soaked in the irrigation fluid. Adhesiolysis is then completed by systematically excising the adhesions from the tubal serosa or ovarian surface (Fig. 21.14). With laparoscopic access, it is usually preferable to reverse this order and commence the adhesiolysis in the adnexa.

Adhesions are put on tension with a toothed forceps, and the site of incision is exposed. Division is effected electrosurgically or with appropriate microsurgical scissors. It is imperative to divide adhesions one layer at a time, slightly lateral to their attachments to the organ to avoid damaging the adjacent peritoneum. Adhesions are often composed of two layers, even though they may initially appear as a single layer. They tend to attach to an organ at two different levels. It is essential to enter between the two layers first, which permits exposure of the demarcation line between the adhesion and the mesothelium of the adjacent structure. Each layer of adhesion is then put on a stretch with toothed forceps, the demarcation line is identified,

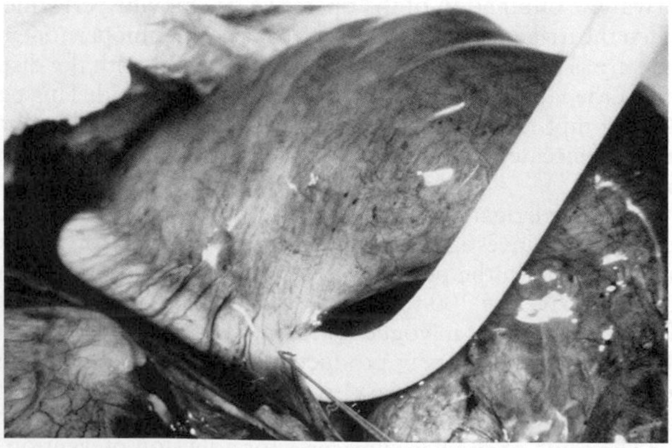

FIGURE 21.13. Salpingolysis. The space between the two involved structures facilitates division. See color version of figure.

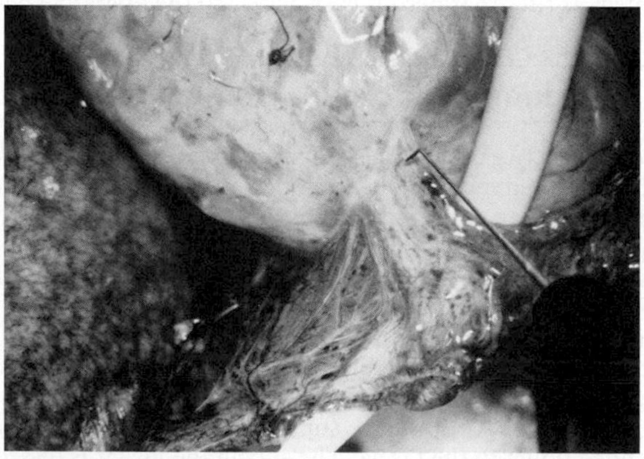

FIGURE 21.14. Ovariolysis. Broad adhesions that had already been divided at their distal margins are being excised from the ovary. See color version of figure.

and the adhesion is transected. With open access, placement of a Teflon rod under the incision line enhances exposure. Damage to the peritoneum or ovarian surface is avoided by keeping the transection line 1 mm away from these surfaces. Prominent vessels along the transection line are individually electrodesiccated.

When a microelectrode is used for this purpose, the electrosurgical unit is put on the blend setting, which on cut mode combines coagulating current with cutting current to provide concurrent hemostasis during the division of adhesions. Pure coagulating current (COAG mode) may be used to obtain hemostasis of individual bleeders, which are exposed under a jet of irrigation fluid. With open access, an elongating adaptor may be attached to the handle of the electrosurgical unit to facilitate adhesiolysis in the deeper parts of the pelvis.

All of the broad adhesions are excised and removed from the pelvis (Fig. 21.14). Shallow adhesions are simply divided. In this case, a small opening is made on the adhesion, through which a fine instrument or Teflon rod is introduced. This permits separation of the adjacent structures and better visualization of the adhesion, which is incised without damaging these structures. The procedure is completed with a thorough pelvic lavage with the irrigation solution mentioned earlier.

The technical principles are identical when laparoscopic access is used for the procedure. In this case, however, because there is no need to lift the adnexa close to the abdominal wall, the salpingo-ovariolysis is commenced with the tube and ovary. Once again, the performance of effective and safe salpingo-ovariolysis requires clear identification of each adhesive layer, which is grasped and retracted, permitting clear identification of the attachments to the organ of interest. The adhesions are incised parallel to the organ of interest and about 1 mm away to prevent damaging its mesothelial envelope (Figs. 21.15 and 21.16). Division is accomplished electrosurgically with a microelectrode or mechanically with the use of proper scissors. We use scissors for laparoscopic salpingo-ovariolysis and electrodesiccation to secure obvious vessels or bleeders encountered along the incision line. As described earlier, shallow adhesions are simply divided, whereas broad adhesions are excised (by dissecting them free at all points of attachment) and removed through one of the ancillary portals (Fig. 21.16).

Cohesive adhesions require identification of the dissection plane. This is achieved by making a small incision and developing a tissue plane either by spreading the jaws of the scissors, by blunt dissection, or by hydrodissection (injecting irrigation solution into the site under pressure). It is important to abstain from using thermal energy in such cases because of the inherent danger.

It should not be necessary to do a laparotomy solely for the purpose of salpingo-ovariolysis. Our primary approach in such cases has been to perform the procedure by way of laparoscopy, usually at the time of the diagnostic survey.

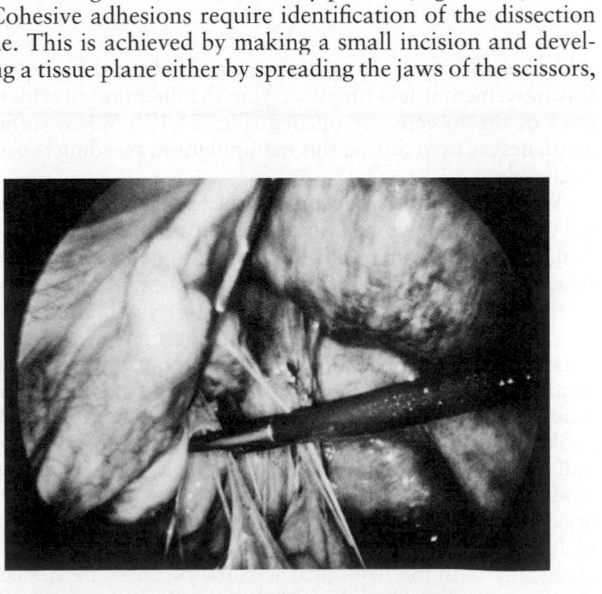

FIGURE 21.15. Salpingo-ovariolysis by laparoscopic access (same patient as in Figure 21.9). Division of adhesions parallel to the tube. See color version of figure.

Results of Salpingo-Ovariolysis

The reported intrauterine pregnancy rates resulting from open microsurgical salpingo-ovariolysis range from 41% to 57%. The rates for live births are 37% to 57%, and the rates for ectopic pregnancies are 5% to 8% of operated patients. In one of these studies, 33 of 63 (52.4%) patients who underwent microsurgical salpingo-ovariolysis achieved intrauterine pregnancies, and there were three (4.8%) ectopic pregnancies at 2-year follow-up. These 63 patients had been randomized to two cutting modalities: electrosurgery (n = 33) and CO_2 laser (n = 30). The results were identical in both subgroups. Indeed, there has been no demonstrable improvement in the outcome of such procedures with the use of lasers in both clinical and experimental studies.

The preexisting tubal patency and the uncontrolled nature of the salpingo-ovariolysis series reported in the literature may cast doubt on the value of this procedure. The Canadian Infertility Evaluation Study Group addressed this issue by studying treatment-dependent and treatment-independent pregnancies in patients with periadnexal disease whose fallopian tubes were not completely occluded. This was a multicenter, controlled, randomized study. The cumulative pregnancy rates were 59% among 69 patients in the group who underwent microsurgical salpingo-ovariolysis and only 16% among the 78 control patients who were not treated. This study confirms that pregnancies may occur in a small proportion of women with periadnexal adhesions and patent tubes and proves the therapeutic value of salpingo-ovariolysis in such cases.

In the early stages of development of operative laparoscopy, we demonstrated that laparoscopic salpingo-ovariolysis yields results similar to those obtained by microsurgery. We also stressed the importance of adhering to microsurgical principles in the performance of such procedures by laparoscopic access. We reported later a series of 92 patients who underwent salpingo-ovariolysis by laparoscopy. The duration of involuntary infertility was longer than 20 months for all patients. Periadnexal adhesions were severe in 79 patients and moderate in 13. Moreover, the series included only those patients in whom ovum pickup by the tube on the side with lesser disease was deemed impossible or greatly hampered. At the time of the survey, the patients had been monitored postoperatively for a period of 9 months or longer. Of the 92 patients, 57 (62%) achieved at least one intrauterine pregnancy, 54 (59%) had one or more live births, and five (5.4%) had ectopic pregnancies. Ten of the patients who did not get pregnant had a second-look laparoscopy that demonstrated no significant residual adhesive process.

Similar results were corroborated by other centers in Europe and North America. This demonstrates that the results of laparoscopic salpingo-ovariolysis, as expected, depend on the severity of the adhesions. The reported intrauterine pregnancy rates after laparoscopic salpingo-ovariolysis range from 51% to 62%, and ectopic pregnancy rates range from 5% to 8% of operated cases. Although no prospective, randomized trials exist, these results appear similar to those yielded by laparotomy.

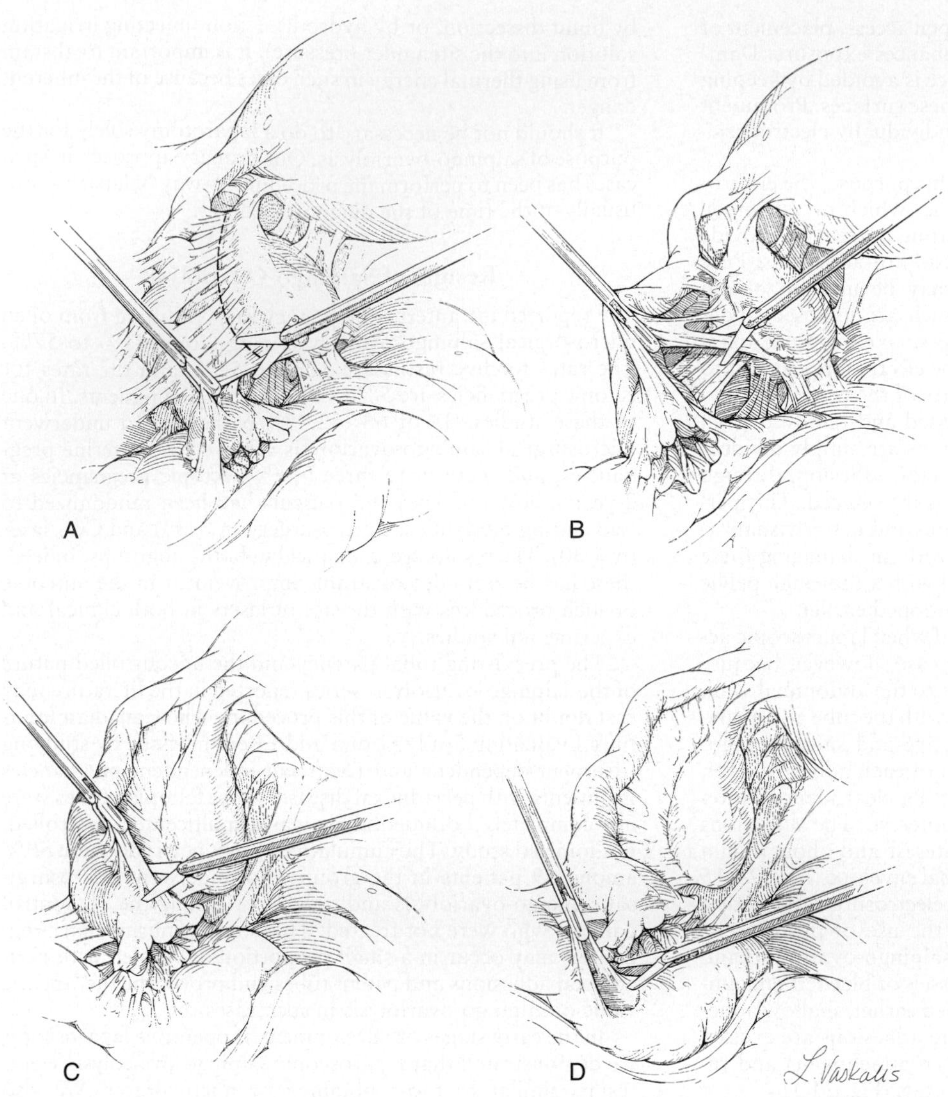

FIGURE 21.16. Salpingo-ovariolysis. A: Division of adhesions commences in a well-exposed area. B: Adhesions are stretched and are divided one layer at a time parallel to the organ of interest. C: Broad adhesions are freed at all points and removed from the peritoneal cavity. D: Salpingo-ovariolysis being completed. (From: Gomel V, Taylor PJ. *Diagnostic and operative gynecologic laparoscopy.* St Louis: Mosby; 1995:171, with permission.)

Fimbrioplasty

Fimbrioplasty is the reconstruction of the fimbriae or infundibulum in a tube that exhibits fimbrial agglutination or prefimbrial phimosis, and results in partial distal occlusion. Often, the tube and ovary are involved in adhesions, in which case salpingo-ovariolysis must precede the fimbrioplasty. The technique of fimbrioplasty, which will be described further, is the same irrespective of the access route used. Our approach is invariably by laparoscopic access.

Fimbrial phimosis results from the agglutination of the fimbriae. A small opening is usually present at the distal end of the tube unless this opening is covered by fibrous tissue. The latter usually becomes evident when the tube is distended by transcervical chromopertubation. When the opening is covered by fibrous tissue, this tissue must be incised or excised to gain access to the fimbriae. Agglutination of the fimbriae can be corrected simply by introducing a fine forceps (mosquito forceps by way of laparotomy or a 2-mm grasping or alligator forceps by way of laparoscopy) with jaws closed through the phimotic fimbrial opening. The jaws of the forceps are opened within the tubal lumen, and the forceps are gently withdrawn with the jaws open. Deagglutination is achieved by repeating this movement a few times, varying the direction in which the jaws of the forceps are opened (Fig. 21.17). When sufficient gentleness is used during this manipulation, bleeding is usually negligible.

When the stenosis is located at the level of the true abdominal tubal ostium, which is located at the apex of the infundibulum, the fimbriae may have a normal appearance. However, when chromopertubation is performed, the ampullary portion of the tube distends before any exit of dye solution. In this instance, it is necessary to place an incision on the antimesosalpingeal border of the tube, which commences at the infundibulum and continues past the stenotic area into the distal ampulla. The tube is stabilized by introducing a thin Teflon probe through the stenotic opening into the distal ampulla, and the incision is made electrosurgically by using a microelectrode. This is the approach we generally use. Alternatively, the area can be injected with 1 mL of dilute vasopressin solution (1 IU in 10 mL of normal saline), and the incision made mechanically with microsurgical scissors. Bleeders are desiccated electrosurgically. The edges of the two flaps thus created are folded back either by securing them to the adjacent ampullary serosa with no. 7-0 or 8-0 polyglactin 910 (Vicryl) sutures or by

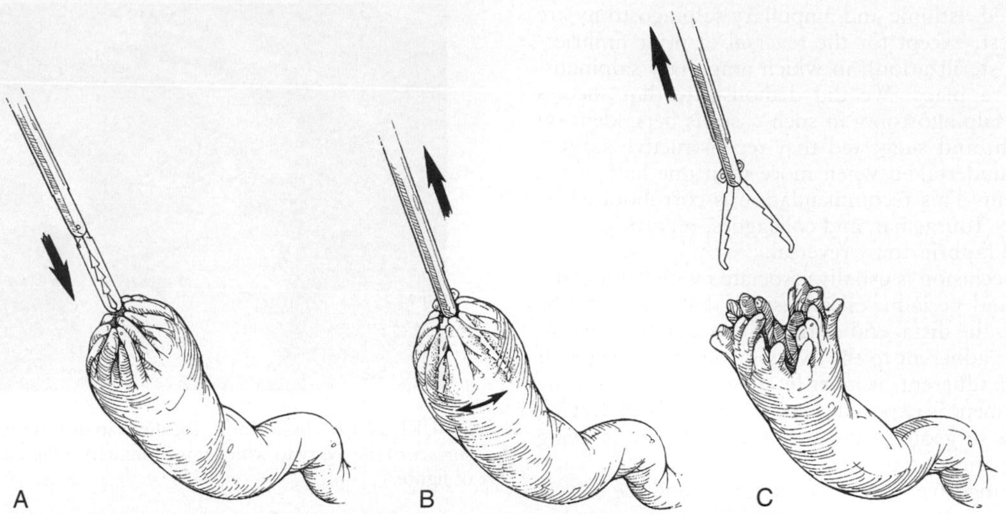

FIGURE 21.17. Fimbrioplasty: to free agglutinated fimbriae. A: The 3-mm alligator-jawed forceps is introduced through the stenosed opening. B: The jaws of the forceps are opened within the tube. C: The forceps is gently withdrawn while the jaws are kept open. (From: Gomel V, Taylor PJ. *Diagnostic and operative gynecologic laparoscopy.* St Louis: Mosby; 1995:173, with permission.)

electrosurgery (or a defocused CO_2 laser beam), which desiccates the serosal aspect of the flaps, causing them to fold backward (Fig. 21.18).

Results of Fimbrioplasty

Very few investigators have classified fimbrioplasty as an independent procedure. Most include such patients in their salpingostomy series. French and Belgian centers include fimbrioplasty (correction of partial distal tubal occlusion) as stage 1 in their salpingostomy series.

Patton and colleagues, in a series of microsurgical fimbrioplasty procedures in 40 patients, reported total intrauterine and ectopic pregnancy rates of 63% (25 patients) and 5% (2 patients), respectively, after 24 months of follow-up. The outcome of the intrauterine pregnancies and the live birth rates were not provided.

In 1983, Gomel reported 40 such patients, all treated by laparoscopic access. Live births occurred in 19 (48%), and two patients (5%) had tubal gestations. Mettler and associates reported a crude pregnancy rate of 31% among 51 women. The anatomic location and outcome of these pregnancies were not recorded. Dubuisson and colleagues reported 31 such patients. After 18 months of follow-up, eight patients (25.8%) had intrauterine pregnancies, and four (12.9%) had ectopic pregnancies. Donnez and colleagues (1986a), in a series of 100 patients, reported a total pregnancy rate of 61%. The location and outcome of these pregnancies were not provided. Canis and colleagues included 32 such patients with their salpingostomy patients; 16 (50%) of these achieved intrauterine pregnancies, but the outcome was not reported. Surprisingly, there were no tubal pregnancies.

Laparoscopic and open microsurgical fimbrioplasty appear to be comparable with regard to intrauterine pregnancy rates; however, with the former, the ectopic rate can be up to 14%.

Salpingostomy (Salpingoneostomy)

Salpingostomy, or salpingoneostomy, is the creation of a new stoma in a tube with a completely occluded distal end (hydrosalpinx). Salpingostomy can be terminal, ampullary, or isthmic, depending on the anatomic location at which the new

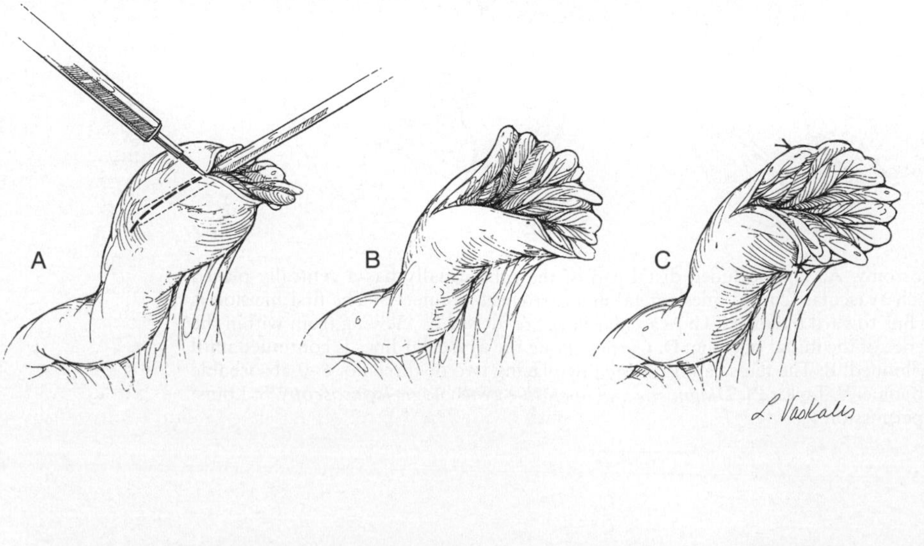

FIGURE 21.18. Fimbrioplasty: correction of prefimbrial phimosis. A and B: An incision is placed at the antimesosalpingeal border of the tube. C: Completed procedure with flaps everted. (From: Gomel V, Taylor PJ. *Diagnostic and operative gynecologic laparoscopy.* St Louis: Mosby; 1995:173, with permission.)

stoma is fashioned. Isthmic and ampullary salpingostomy are of historic interest, except for the reversal of prior fimbriectomy (Kroener's sterilization), in which ampullary salpingostomy may have a place. We did demonstrate that success with ampullary salpingostomy in such cases is dependent on ampullary length, and suggested that reconstructive surgery should only be undertaken when more than one half of the ampulla is present. This recommendation is corroborated by a recent study, by Tourgeman and colleagues, reporting on 41 women who had fimbriectomy reversal.

Distal tubal occlusion is usually associated with varying degrees of pelvic and periadnexal adhesions that must first be lysed. Thereafter, the distal end of the tube is examined to ensure that it is not adherent to the ovary or other structures. If the distal tube is adherent, it must be dissected free until the tuboovarian ligament is exposed (Fig. 21.19). Only by freeing the tube can the surgeon ensure that the neostomy is being performed at the appropriate site.

Once the salpingo-ovariolysis is completed and the tube is totally freed, it is distended by transcervical chromopertubation. The occluded terminal end of the tube is examined under magnification, which permits recognition of the relatively avascular zones that radiate from a central punctum. The tube is entered at this central point with use of the microelectrode or microsurgical scissors, and the incision is extended toward the ovary over an avascular line (Fig. 21.20). This incision fashions a new fimbria ovarica that maintains the tuboovarian relation. At this point in the procedure, it becomes possible to view the tube from within when placing additional incisions along its circumference to complete the creation of a new stoma. These additional incisions are made between endothelial folds, over avascular areas. In so doing, one avoids cutting through vascular mucosal folds, which will be shaped as fimbriae, and bleeding is minimized as a result. Any bleeding points that occur are exposed under a jet of irrigation fluid and desiccated individually with a microelectrode or microbipolar

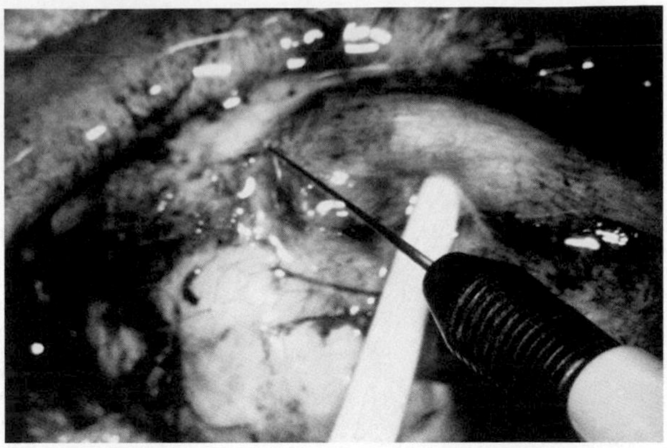

FIGURE 21.19. Dissection of the distal hydrosalpinx from the anterior surface of the ovary to which it is intimately adherent. See color version of figure.

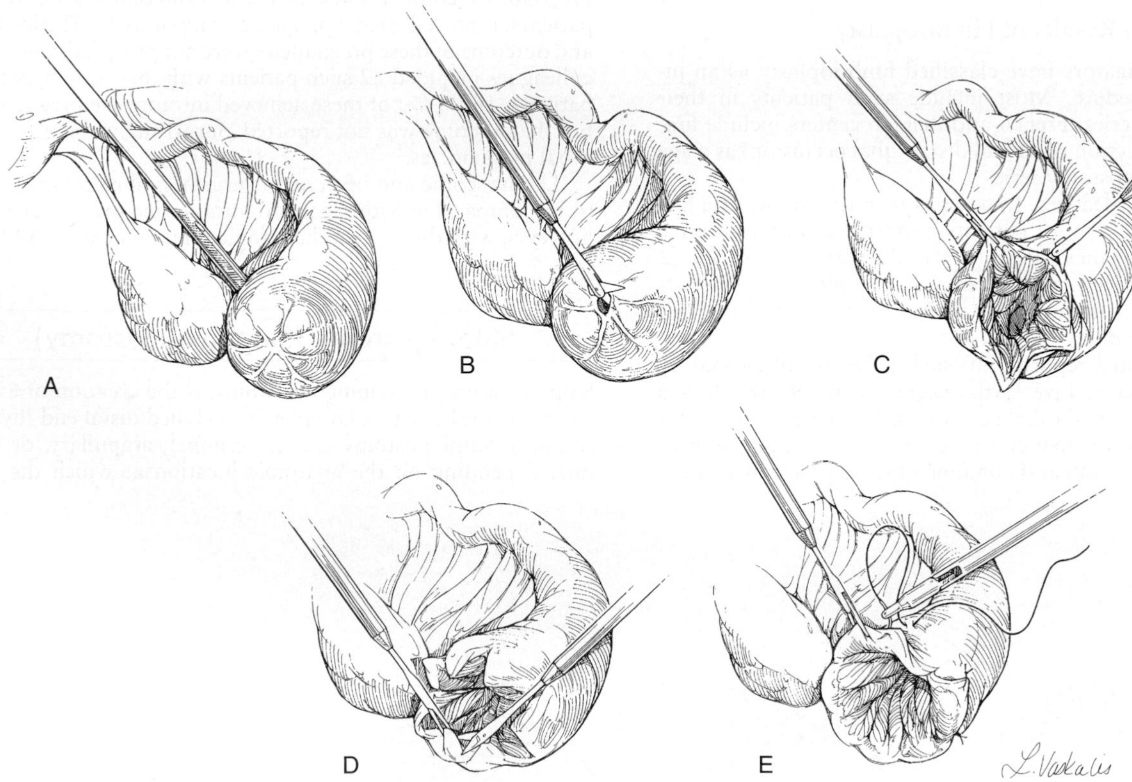

FIGURE 21.20. Salpingostomy. **A:** The occluded distal end of the tube usually has a centrally placed avascular area, from which avascular scarred lines extend in a cartwheel manner. **B:** The first incision is made along an avascular line toward the ovary. **C:** Avascular lines are incised by viewing from within the tube along the circumference of the initial opening. **D:** Cutting along the avascular lines is continued until a satisfactory stoma is fashioned. **E:** The flaps can be everted by placing two or three no. 6–0 absorbable synthetic sutures. (From: Gomel V, Taylor PJ. *Diagnostic and operative gynecologic laparoscopy.* St Louis: Mosby; 1995:174, with permission.)

forceps. Once a satisfactory stoma is achieved, the flaps created in the process are everted either by securing them without tension to the ampullary seromuscularis with interrupted no. 8-0 Vicryl sutures (Fig. 21.20) or by desiccating their serosal surface, which causes them to fold backward. Desiccation is achieved either electrosurgically with a ball-shaped electrode and a low power density or with CO_2 laser using a defocused beam. The procedure is concluded with a thorough pelvic lavage, as described earlier in this chapter.

Considering that the results of salpingostomy obtained by laparoscopy approach those obtained by open access, and considering further the significant improvement in IVF results, an open salpingostomy should be rarely indicated.

If during the initial diagnostic laparoscopy, the surgeon decides to perform the salpingostomy by open access and if the adnexa are found to be fixed by periadnexal adhesions, these adhesions can be lysed laparoscopically at their distal margins, thus mobilizing the adnexa. Such an undertaking permits the subsequent salpingostomy to be readily performed through a minilaparotomy incision. The same applies to cases of tubotubal anastomosis and more complex reconstructive procedures.

Results of Salpingostomy

In the major published series, the live birth rate after microsurgical salpingostomy ranges from 20% to 37%, and the ectopic pregnancy rate ranges from 5% to 18% (Table 21.3). The factors that affect the outcome of salpingostomy were reviewed earlier in this chapter. Work performed in the past 30 years has made it evident that the major determinants of the outcome of salpingostomy are the degree of preexisting tubal damage and the extent and nature of periadnexal adhesions (Figs. 21.21 and 21.22). As stated earlier in this chapter, the reported live birth rate after microsurgical salpingostomy in favorable cases (mild) ranges from 40% to 60%. This rate drops to less than 20% in unfavorable (severe damage) cases.

We reported a series of 90 patients who underwent microsurgical salpingostomy with a minilaparotomy incision. Nineteen (21.1%) were lost to follow-up and were considered failures. Twenty-seven (30%) patients achieved one or more intrauterine pregnancies, and eight (8.9%) had tubal pregnancies. Ectopic gestations occurred in two additional patients who also had intrauterine pregnancies. Twenty-three (25.6%) women were successful in having one or more live births. These 90 patients were assessed with the classification approved by

TABLE 21.3

RESULTS OF MICROSURGICAL SALPINGOSTOMY

Investigators	Year	Patients	Intrauterine pregnancies	Live births	Ectopic pregnancies
ACCESS BY LAPAROTOMY					
Swolin[a]	1975	33	9	8 (24.2%)	6
Gomel[b]	1978	41	12	11 (26.8%)	5
Gomel[b]	1980	72	22	21 (29.2%)	7
Larsson[c]	1982	54	21	17 (31.5%)	0
Verhoeven et al.[d]	1983	143	34	28 (19.6%)	3
Tulandi and Vilos[e]	1985	67	15	NS	3
Boer-Meisel et al.	1986	108	31	24 (22.2%)	19
Donnez and Casanas-Roux[a]	1986	83	26	NS	6
Kosasa and Hale	1988	93	37	34 (36.6%)	13
Schlaff et al.	1990	82	14	NS	6
Winston and Margara	1991	323	106	74 (22.9%)	32
ACCESS BY MINILAPAROTOMY					
Gomel	1990	90	27	23 (25.6%)	8
ACCESS BY LAPAROSCOPY					
Gomel[f]	1977	9	4	4	0
Daniell and Herbert[g]	1984	22	4	3 (13.6%)	1
Dubuisson et al.	1990	34	10	NS	1
Canis et al.	1991	55	13	NS	6
McComb and Paleologou	1991	22	5	5 (22.7%)	1
Dubuisson et al.	1994	90	29	26 (29.9%)	4
Oh	1996	82	29	NS	8
Millingos et al.	2000	61	14	NS	2
Taylor et al.	2001	139	44	25 (18%)	23

NS, not stated.
[a]Follow-up period more than 8 years.
[b]Follow-up period more than 1 year.
[c]Follow-up period more than 4 years.
[d]Twenty-three of these were iterative procedures; only three of these patients (13%) had live births.
[e]Thirty-seven of these procedures were performed with the carbon dioxide laser.
[f]Eight of the nine patients had prior salpingostomy by conventional techniques that resulted in reocclusion.
[g]Performed with the carbon dioxide laser.

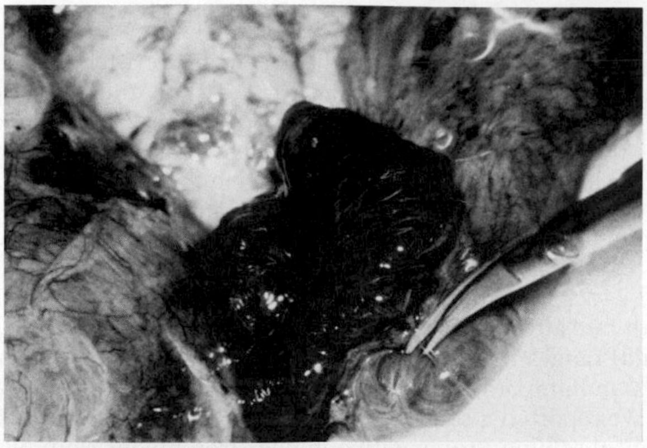

FIGURE 21.21. Microsurgical salpingostomy by open access. The tube is minimally dilated and has a well-preserved epithelium. See color version of figure.

the American Fertility Society. On the basis of this classification, 73 patients had extensive (severe) damage, and 17 had limited (mild) damage. In the group of 73 patients, 15 (20.5%) had one or more intrauterine pregnancies, and 13 (17.8%) had one or more live births. In the "mild" group of 17 patients, 12 (70.6%) had one or more intrauterine pregnancies, and 10 (58.8%) had one or more live births ($p < 0.05$) (Table 24.3). These observations emphasize the importance of a thorough preoperative investigation and proper patient selection.

On the surface, the results yielded by laparoscopic salpingostomy appear to be somewhat inferior to those obtained by open access. However, laparoscopic salpingostomy offers distinct advantages: It can be performed during the initial diagnostic laparoscopy, avoiding a second intervention and resulting in cost savings.

During the past decade, there have been many more reports about the deleterious effect of hydrosalpinx on the outcome of IVF treatment than reports on surgical reconstruction of the condition. This deleterious effect is more evident when hydrosalpinges are large enough to be visible at sonography. In such cases, salpingectomy, before IVF, clearly improves the outcome of this treatment. Several hypotheses have been put forward to explain the detrimental effect of a hydrosalpinx on fertility and specifically IVF outcome. A "wash-out effect" owing to the passage of the collected tubal fluid to the uterine cavity at the time when embryos are transferred is one such hypothesis. This wash out may also occur some time after transfer, as evidence suggests many embryos ascend to the tube after transfer and eventually return to the uterus when the tube assumes a prouterine transport. It is at this time that the fluid contained in the hydrosalpinx, by passing to the uterus, may wash the embryos out. Other hypotheses related to the hydrosalpinx fluid include an embryotoxic effect, bioactive factors in the fluid adversely effecting endometrial receptivity, and an inadequate glucose supply in this fluid. These hypotheses are controversial at present and the real mechanism remains to be elucidated.

The assumption that the deleterious effect of large hydrosalpinges may be owing to a washout of the transferred embryos is supported by a study of Van Voorhis and colleagues. They compared women with hydrosalpinges (n = 34) with women who had tubal disease but no hydrosalpinges (n = 124) undergoing IVF treatment. Women with hydrosalpinges were found to have a reduced clinical pregnancy rate (18% vs. 37%, $p = 0.053$), a reduced ongoing pregnancy rate (15% vs. 34%, $p = 0.051$), and reduced implantation rate (7% vs. 18%, $p = 0.003$) after IVF procedures. Among women who had hydrosalpinges, 16 had their hydrosalpinges aspirated at the time of oocyte retrieval, and 18 did not. Aspiration of hydrosalpinges was associated with a higher clinical pregnancy rate (31% vs. 5%, $p = 0.07$), a higher ongoing pregnancy rate (31% vs. 0%, $p = 0.015$), and a higher implantation rate (14 vs. 1%, $p = 0.015$) as reported by Van Voorhis and colleagues. However, others have indicated that aspiration of hydrosalpinx fluid is of little value before oocyte retrieval or embryo transfer.

A study from our department demonstrated that performing a salpingostomy in women with a unilateral hydrosalpinx and a contralateral patent tube improves embryo implantation. The salpingostomy in the study group yielded an intrauterine pregnancy rate that was significantly greater than that expected from the salpingostomy itself. It is hypothesized that the pregnancies occur through the preexiting patent tube, because the hydrosalpinx fluid no longer suppresses embryo implantation. We look forward to studies that would more precisely determine the value of salpingostomy for hydrosalpinx visible at ultrasound in patients undergoing IVF.

Tubotubal Anastomosis

The term *tubotubal anastomosis* refers to an anastomosis performed anywhere along the tube either to treat occlusions resulting from disease processes or to reverse a prior sterilization. The procedure used to repair proximal or cornual tubal disease is usually referred to as *tubocornual anastomosis* and will be discussed separately.

Microsurgery finds its ultimate application in tubotubal anastomosis. The precision afforded by this technique allows total excision of occluded or diseased portions, proper alignment, and excellent apposition of each layer of the proximal and distal tubal segments.

Tubotubal anastomosis is performed either to reverse a previous tubal sterilization or to reconstruct the tube after removal of a diseased portion that is often occluded and affects the tube at a site other than the fimbriated end. Depending on the tubal segments that are approximated, tubotubal anastomosis can be intramural–isthmic, intramural–ampullary, isthmic–isthmic, isthmic–ampullary, ampullary–ampullary, or ampullary–infundibular. This section first describes the fundamentals of tubotubal anastomosis and then the technical variations necessary to deal with each specific type of anastomosis.

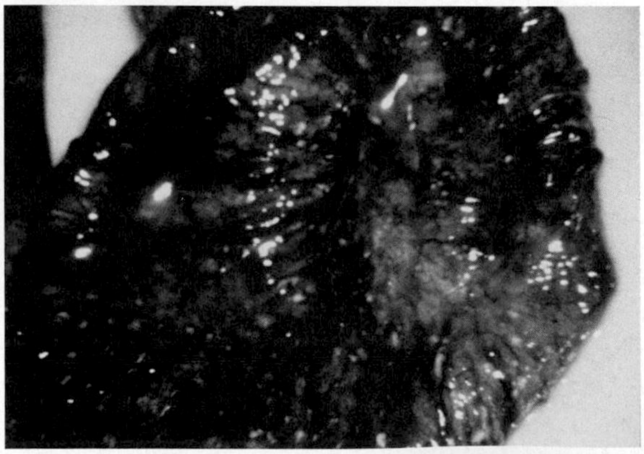

FIGURE 21.22. Microsurgical salpingostomy by open access. The tube is markedly dilated and exhibits a flat epithelium with poorly preserved folds. See color version of figure.

Basic Principles of Tubotubal Anastomosis

When periadnexal adhesions are present, salpingo-ovariolysis is first completed. When access is achieved through laparotomy or minilaparotomy, the side to be worked on is elevated with the use of pads soaked in irrigation solution. The contralateral adnexa is left in its natural position to prevent desiccation. When access occurs by way of laparoscopy, the mesosalpinx under the site of anastomosis may be injected with 1 to 2 mL of dilute vasopressin solution to reduce oozing and facilitate hemostasis.

The principles of tubotubal anastomosis are the same, irrespective of the mode of access used. The proximal tubal segment is distended by transcervical chromopertubation. This helps identification of the site of occlusion. The tube is transected, with appropriate scissors, adjacent to the site of occlusion or, in the case of a previous tubal sterilization, near the occluded end. The occluded end or occluded segment of the tube is grasped with a strong-toothed forceps to expose the site and facilitate the transection (Fig. 21.23A), which is effected with straight scissors or a sharp microblade. It is essential to halt the incision at the mesosalpinx, in the immediate periphery of the tubal muscularis, to avoid damaging the adjacent vascular arcade. Dye solution can now escape from the transected tubal lumen (Fig. 21.23B).

The occluded tubal segment is excised from the mesosalpinx electrosurgically or with scissors, the line of incision kept close to the tube to avoid damaging the vessels mentioned earlier (Fig. 21.23C). The cut surface is examined under high magnification to ensure that the tube is normal. Healthy tube is devoid of scarring and exhibits normal muscular and vascular architecture together with intact mucosal folds (Fig. 21.23D). Hemostasis is obtained by precise electrodesiccation of the more significant bleeders, which are located between the serosa and muscularis. Each is exposed by irrigation and desiccated with an insulated microelectrode. If open access is used, gentle compression of the tube between thumb and forefinger facilitates this process. Desiccation of minor bleeders is unnecessary because they stop spontaneously. Desiccation of the tubal epithelium must be avoided to prevent damaging it and adversely affecting future tubal function. Major tubal vessels (such as those composing the vascular arcade) may be divided inadvertently or by necessity. These can be electrodesiccated with monopolar or bipolar current. Overzealous electrodesiccation must be avoided to prevent devitalizing the anastomosis site.

When there is no significant luminal disparity between the two segments, the distal portion is prepared in a similar manner. Before transection, the distal segment is distended by descending hydropertubation, which consists of injecting a few milliliters of irrigation fluid or dilute dye solution through the fimbriated end to identify the distal limit of the occluded portion or, in the case of a prior sterilization, to identify the extremity of the stump. The tubal segments are approximated in two layers. The first of these joins the epithelium and muscularis, and the second joins the serosa. We generally use no. 8-0 Vicryl sutures swaged on a 130-micron-shaft, 4- or 5-mm-long, taper-cut needle for tubal anastomosis. The first suture of the inner musculoepithelial layer is always placed at the mesosalpingeal border (6-o'clock position) to ensure proper alignment of the two segments of tube. All of the sutures are placed in a way that positions the knots peripherally.

In exceptional circumstances when the distance between the two segments is great, the mesosalpinx adjacent to the cut ends of the two tubal segments can be approximated first, using a single interrupted no. 7-0 or 8-0 suture. This step brings the tubal segments into close proximity; thus, it facilitates placement of the sutures of the inner layer and reduces the tension that would have existed when tying these sutures.

Once the 6-o'clock suture is tied, the placement of three or more additional sutures (depending on the type of anastomosis) is required to appose the inner layer. These additional sutures can be placed by using a single strand of suture as a continuous series of loops, including the muscularis and the epithelium of the two segments (Figs. 21.23E and 21.24). The sutures are tied individually, after the division of the loop between each successive suture (Fig. 21.23F). This approach facilitates and speeds up suture placement. We advise against the use of a splint in the lumen of the tube because this does not facilitate the procedure and may traumatize the endothelium. Instead, if necessary, the cut surface may be stained with methylene blue or indigo carmine solution to accentuate the visibility of the individual layers.

After approximation of the inner layer, chromopertubation should demonstrate tubal patency and a watertight anastomotic site (Fig. 21.23G). The serosa is joined either with interrupted sutures or with two continuous sutures, one that runs anteriorly and the other posteriorly, starting at the antimesosalpingeal border (12 o'clock). Finally, the defect in the mesosalpinx is repaired (Fig. 21.23H).

Tubotubal Anastomosis to Repair Midtubal Disease

The most common reason to perform a tubotubal anastomosis is reversal of sterilization. Midtubal occlusions resulting from disease processes are rare. Such lesions usually affect the intramural or proximal isthmic segments and require a tubocornual type anastomosis.

The causes of midtubal occlusion include endometriosis and tubal pregnancy, usually undiagnosed or treated by observation. A tubal pregnancy treated medically with methotrexate administration or surgically by linear salpingotomy may result in tubal occlusion at the gestational site. Treatment of tubal pregnancy by segmental excision will leave the tube in two segments, as with tubal sterilization. Rare causes of occlusion include congenital absence of a midtubal segment and tuberculosis. In the latter instance, reconstruction is contraindicated.

In an intact tube, the site of occlusion may be apparent on inspection; palpation of the tube may identify an indurated segment that is the likely site of occlusion. As mentioned earlier, transcervical chromopertubation distends the proximal segment up to the site of occlusion and helps the surgeon define its proximal limit. The tube is transected either immediately proximal to the occluded segment or in the occluded zone itself. Successive transection of the tube at 1- to 2-mm intervals helps identify the normal segments proximal and distal to the occlusion site.

Irrespective of the type of anastomosis, the basic steps of the procedure are the same. The luminal diameter of the tube is not uniform and is significantly greater in the ampullary segment. The technical variations required largely depend on the disparity of the luminal calibers of the two segments to be joined.

Intramural–Isthmic Anastomosis

Anastomosis between the intramural and isthmic segments is the type of anastomosis most often required to treat cornual disease.

In most cases of reversal of sterilization, a short segment of isthmus is usually present. This short segment is frequently adherent to the side of the uterus as a result of retraction of the adjacent mesosalpinx, thus giving the appearance of total absence of the proximal tube. The presence of a portion of isthmus would have been evident from HSG. Transcervical

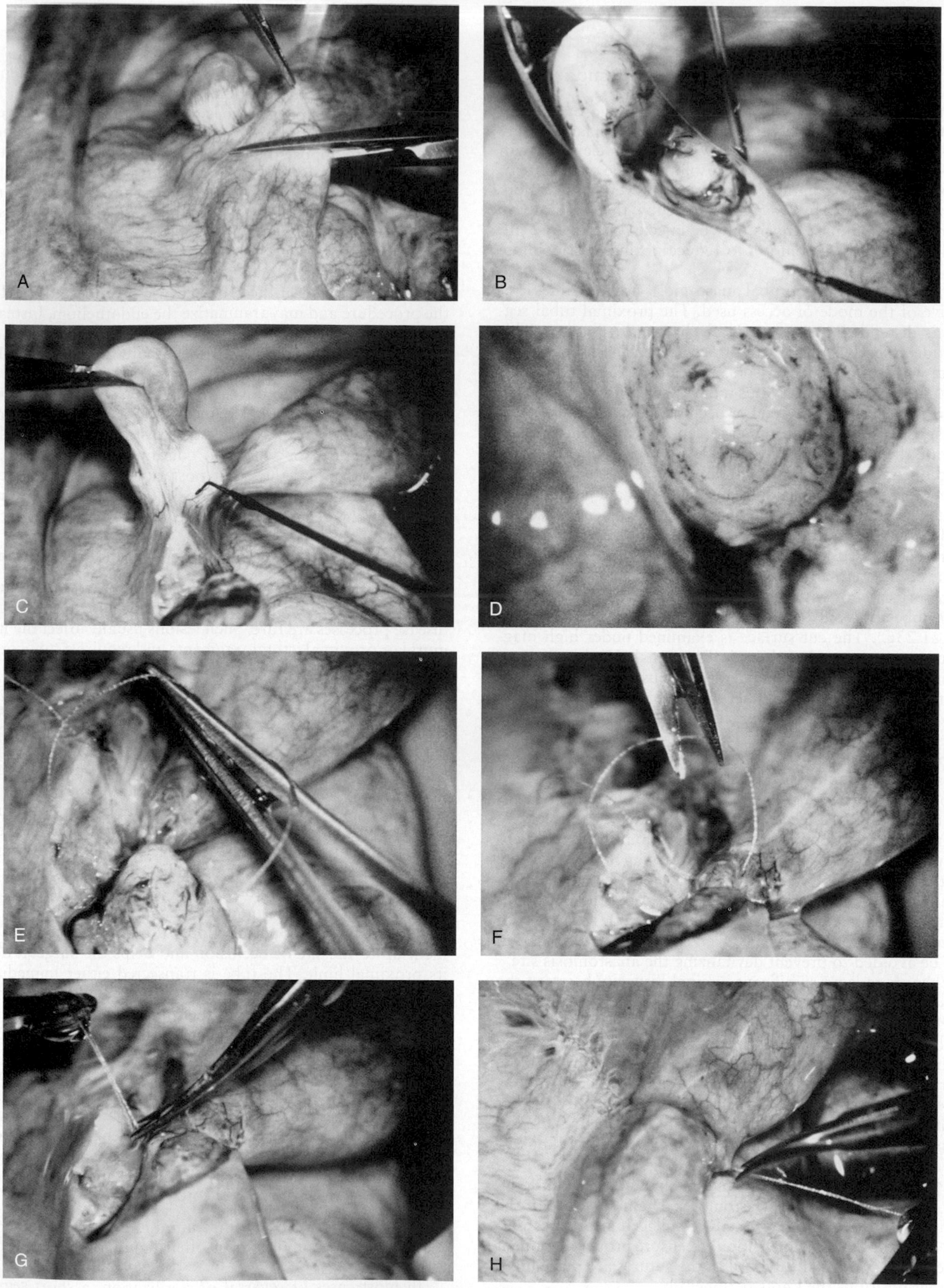

FIGURE 21.23. Microsurgical tubotubal anastomosis for reversal of Falope-ring sterilization. **A:** The occluded end of the isthmus is grasped, and the tube is transected with scissors. **B:** Dye solution escapes from the lumen. **C:** The occluded tubal segment is excised from the mesosalpinx electrosurgically by use of a microelectrode. **D:** The cut surface of the patent tube is assessed under high magnification. **E:** Once the 6-o'clock suture is tied, subsequent sutures can be placed with use of a single strand of suture as a continuous series of loops. **F:** Each suture is tied individually after the division of the loop between successive sutures. **G:** The apposition of the inner musculoepithelial layer is complete. **H:** The anastomosis is completed with approximation of the serosa. See color version of figure.

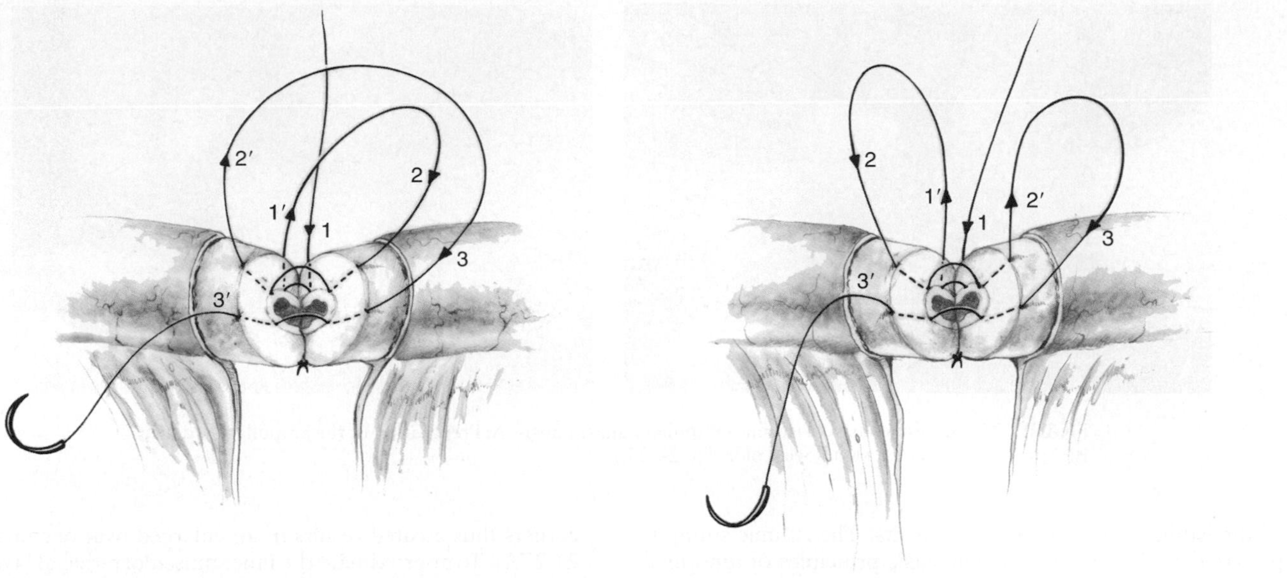

FIGURE 21.24. Microsurgical tubotubal anastomosis. Placement of sutures using a single strand of suture as a continuous series of loops.

chromopertubation distends this small segment of isthmus, facilitating identification of its distal margin and its dissection from the uterus. The dissection must be effected carefully to avoid damaging the tube itself and the vessels supplying it. The conservation and appropriate preparation of this segment, even when very small, convert the anastomosis to an isthmic–isthmic type and facilitate the procedure.

In the absence of any isthmus (as may be the case subsequent to either a tubal sterilization or excision of an isthmic pregnancy), maintenance of uterine distention by chromopertubation will indicate the site where the intramural segment should be sought, between the uterine insertion points of the round and ovarian ligaments. Excision of the serosa and underlying scar tissue over the distended area may permit the dye solution to stream out of the intramural segment. In some instances, it is also necessary to dissect the muscularis of this segment from the surrounding uterine muscle for 1 or 2 mm with microscissors or a microelectrode. After this, the tube is transected with microscissors. This process may have to be repeated until the patent tube is reached, at which point dye solution should stream out of the lumen (see Fig. 21.30).

Because of extensive vascularity, dissection in the cornua usually causes significant oozing that hinders visibility. When more than superficial dissection of this region is anticipated, initial infiltration with dilute vasopressin solution (1 U of vasopressin in 10 mL of normal saline) significantly decreases capillary oozing and facilitates the procedure. With use of a 30-gauge needle on a 3-mL syringe, the cornual region of the uterus is injected with 2 mL of this solution in a circular fashion under the serosa 1 cm medial to the uterotubal junction. The resulting vasoconstriction is recognized by serosal blanching.

In this type of anastomosis, there is no significant luminal disparity between the two segments of tube. Hence, the isthmus is simply transected near the occluded end and prepared, as described earlier. A two-layer anastomosis is then performed. Once the inner layer has been joined, the serosa and superficial muscle of the cornual region are approximated to the serosa of the isthmus. The defect under the tube is repaired by suturing the mesosalpinx to the serosa of the lateral edge of the uterus.

Intramural–Ampullary Anastomosis

The salient feature of intramural–ampullary anastomosis is the considerable luminal disparity that exists between the intramural and ampullary segments. The key technical issue lies in the preparation of the occluded proximal end of the ampulla, where an opening into the ampullary lumen, which is not much larger than that of the intramural segment, must be fashioned.

The intramural segment is first prepared as described under intramural–isthmic anastomosis. To identify the occluded end of the ampulla, which may be buried between the leaves of the mesosalpinx, the tube is distended with a few milliliters of dye or irrigation solution introduced through the fimbriated end. Alternatively, a malleable blunt probe can be introduced through the infundibulum and gently threaded toward the occluded end. With the use of microscissors, the serosa over the tip of the ampullary stump is incised in a circular manner. The serosa and any scar tissue under it are then excised to expose the muscularis of the occluded end. The center point of the exposed muscularis is grasped with toothed microforceps, and a small incision is made into the ampullary lumen with the microscissors. This opening is enlarged to correspond in size to the lumen of the proximal tubal segment by excising a tiny circular portion of muscularis and epithelium (Figs. 21.25A and 21.26). The resulting opening is slightly larger than the intramural lumen, but because of the absence of significant disparity, anastomosis of the two segments can be performed as described for isthmic–isthmic anastomosis.

Isthmic–Isthmic Anastomosis

Isthmic–isthmic anastomosis is the simplest type of anastomosis to perform. The lumina are comparable in size. The technique is the same as that described earlier under the basic principles of tubotubal anastomosis.

Isthmic–Ampullary Anastomosis

The salient feature of this type of anastomosis is also the considerable luminal disparity that usually exists between the lumina

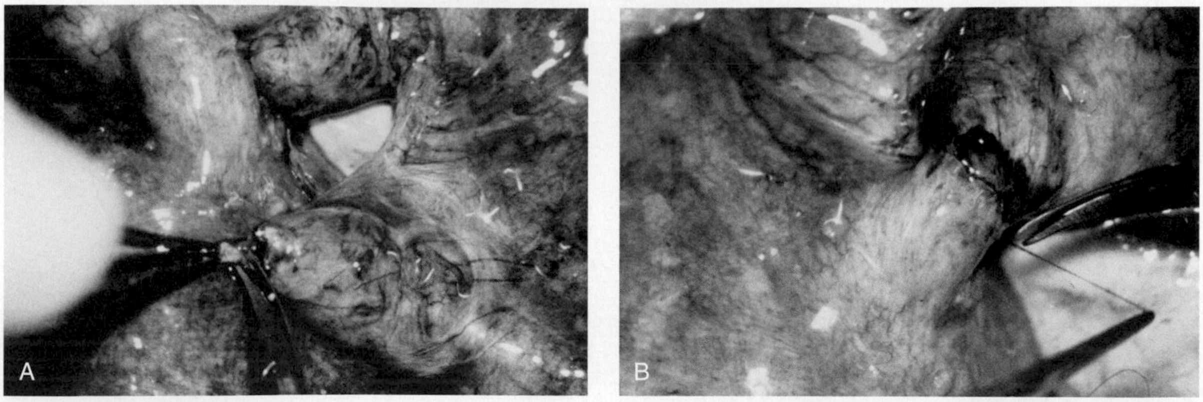

FIGURE 21.25. Microsurgical isthmic–ampullary anastomosis. A: Preparation of the ampullary segment. B: Approximation of serosa. (See Color Fig. 24.25.)

of the isthmic and ampullary segments. The isthmic stump is prepared as described under the basic principles of tubotubal anastomosis. In most instances, the occluded end of the ampullary stump will be free, enabling a lumen of appropriate diameter (comparable in size to that of the isthmic segment) to be fashioned, as described under intramural–ampullary anastomosis (Figs. 21.25A and 24.26). A two-layer anastomosis is then performed as described under the basic principles of tubotubal anastomosis (Fig. 21.25B). Although the muscularis of the ampulla is considerably thinner than that of the isthmus, this poses no problem in approximating the epithelium and muscularis of the two segments.

Occasionally, circumstances will not permit the use of the technique described earlier in the preparation of the occluded ampullary end. The ampullary stump may be occluded by a permanent suture or clip, and removal of this suture or clip may lead to the creation of an opening that is much larger than the isthmic lumen and through which lush epithelial folds will prolapse.

If the opening into the ampullary lumen is made significantly larger than that of the isthmic segment (either inadvertently or by necessity), it will be necessary to either enlarge the isthmic lumen or narrow the ampullary lumen. To enlarge the lumen of the isthmic segment, a 2- to 3-mm slit is made with scissors at its antimesosalpingeal border. Partial excision of the corners thus created results in an enlarged oval opening (Fig. 21.27A). To approximate the inner musculoepithelial layer, the 6-o'clock suture is placed first and tied. Five additional sutures are usually required, and these are placed as described earlier. The 12-o'clock suture must incorporate the muscularis and epithelium of the ampulla and the same tissues at the apex of the isthmic slit (Fig. 21.27B). Approximation of the serosa and closure of the defect in the mesosalpinx complete the anastomosis. An alternative approach is to reduce the size of the large ampullary opening. This is achieved by plicating the muscular layer surrounding the opening with interrupted sutures, after which the prolapsing epithelium is invaginated.

Ampullary–Ampullary Anastomosis

The proximal ampullary segment is transected near the occluded end, which is then excised from the mesosalpinx as previously described. An opening that corresponds in size to the lumen of the proximal segment is made in the occluded end of the distal ampullary segment, as described under isthmic–ampullary anastomosis.

In this type of anastomosis, the major difficulty to be overcome is the propensity of the ampullary epithelium to prolapse through the lumen. Although investigators such as Winston have advocated excision of these epithelial fronds, we advise against this approach because there could potentially be

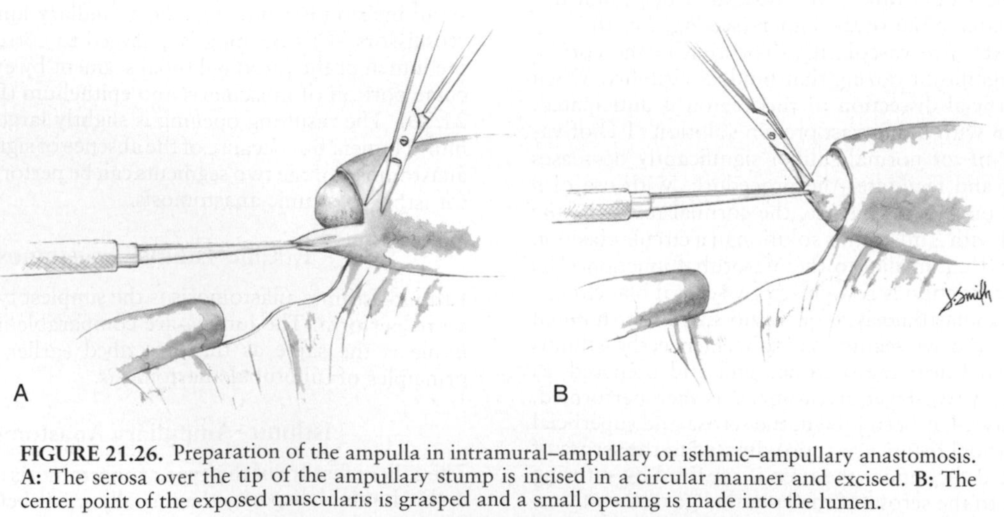

FIGURE 21.26. Preparation of the ampulla in intramural–ampullary or isthmic–ampullary anastomosis. A: The serosa over the tip of the ampullary stump is incised in a circular manner and excised. B: The center point of the exposed muscularis is grasped and a small opening is made into the lumen.

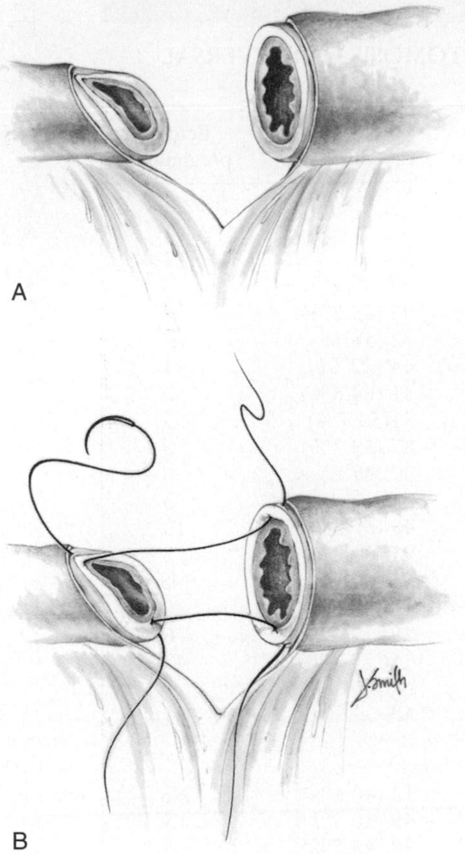

FIGURE 21.27. Isthmic–ampullary anastomosis in the presence of significant luminal disparity. A: Enlargement of the isthmic lumen. B: Placement of the 12-o'clock suture.

subsequent intratubal adhesion formation at this site. The epithelial fronds can be replaced with pressure from the irrigating solution or with the tip of the plain microforceps while the successive sutures of the inner layer are tied. One must be careful not to include these epithelial fronds within a suture or knot or between the segments that are being approximated. Because of the larger circumference of the ampulla, approximation of the two ampullary segments will require a greater number of interrupted sutures than in an isthmic–isthmic anastomosis.

Ampullary–Infundibular Anastomosis

An ampullary–infundibular anastomosis may be necessary when a distal ampullary portion of tube has been ablated or excised either during a prior sterilization or during removal of a tubal gestation, leaving distally the infundibular segment only. The occluded ampulla is prepared as described previously. To make anastomosis of the two segments possible, it is necessary to fashion an opening in the infundibular portion. To do so, a Teflon probe with a conical tip is introduced into the infundibulum from the fimbriated end, and a circular opening is fashioned with microscissors, from the medial side, corresponding in size to the lumen of the ampullary segment. A two-layer anastomosis is then performed.

Results of Tubotubal Anastomosis for Reversal of Sterilization

The major published series report live birth rates between 40% and 80% after microsurgical tubotubal anastomosis for reversal of sterilization (Table 21.4). The ectopic gestation rates are usually low.

The factors that affect the outcome of such procedures are multiple and include the following: the type of prior sterilization, the site of anastomosis, and the length of the reconstructed tube or tubes, which are interrelated factors; the presence of single versus double reconstructed oviducts; the status of the tubes (presence or absence of disease); the extent and nature of adhesions and the presence of other pelvic disease; the age of the patient; the status of other fertility parameters, especially that of the male partner; and last, but not least, the surgical technique used. Therefore, the outcome depends on the degree of rigor in selection criteria and the quality of the surgical technique. This is also corroborated by recent reports on sterilization reversal, which include two large series from Korea (Table 21.4). In our experience, in the absence of a male factor, the two most important parameters that predict outcome are the age of the female partner and the length of the reconstructed tube. A reconstructed tubal length of less than 4 cm adversely affects outcome; this likely reflects the loss of ampullary length and consequent loss of oviductal oocyte retention.

Tubotubal anastomosis by laparoscopic access to reconstruct a previous tubal sterilization or a prior segmental excision for tubal pregnancy is being performed in several centers. Whereas some investigators obtain satisfactory outcomes with this approach, others report significantly inferior results in comparison with open access. This is largely due to modification of the recognized microsurgical technique to make the laparoscopic procedure simpler to perform.

The first report on laparoscopic tubotubal anastomosis was a case report; instead of microsurgical suturing for the apposition of the tubal segments, they used a biologic glue over a stent. Pregnancy outcome was not reported. Early reports on tubotubal anastomosis were on small series, performed with simplified techniques, and although most of the cases were simpler forms of sterilization reversal, the results were relatively poor.

Most surgeons who attempted tubotubal anastomosis by laparoscopic access using the microsurgical technique described earlier found that operating times are prolonged. Many attempted to simplify the technique by using glue as described above or using only two sutures for the apposition of the prepared tubal segments, as first reported by Dubuisson and Swolin. In this technique, the first suture (4/0 Vicryl) approximates the mesosalpinx immediately beneath the two segments of tube, and the second (6/0 Vicryl) the tube at 12-o'clock position. The second suture incorporates the serosa and muscularis of the two segments of tube. There are several recent reports in the literature on this technique. There are also publications reporting on the laparoscopic use of a truly microsurgical, two-layer anastomosis technique. One of these is a large series by Yoon and colleagues, from Korea, which includes 202 cases. Fifteen of these were lost to follow-up, and one had no partner. The remaining 186 were monitored for a minimum of 12 months. One hundred fifty-four achieved intrauterine pregnancies, a rate of 77% if we consider, as most series do, the 15 cases lost to follow-up as failures. Ninety-eight were delivered of healthy infants, 25 pregnancies ended in abortion, and 31 patients had ongoing pregnancies at the time of the survey. If all 31 ongoing pregnancies would have resulted in a live birth, the live birth rate in this series would have been 64%. There

TABLE 21.4

RESULTS OF MICROSURGICAL TUBOTUBAL ANASTOMOSIS FOR REVERSAL OF STERILIZATION

Investigators	Year	Patients	Intrauterine pregnancies	Live births	Ectopic pregnancies
ACCESS BY LAPAROTOMY					
Gomel	1974	14	8	NS	1
Gomel	1980c	118	76	NS	1
Winston	1980	105	63	NS	3
Gomel[a]	1983b	118	96	93 (78.8%)	2
DeCherney et al.[b]	1983	124	84	72 (58.1%)	8
Schlosser et al.	1983	119	NS	44 (37%)	11
Silber and Cohen[c]	1984	48	33	31 (64.6%)	2
Henderson	1984	95	61	51(53.7%)	5
Paterson	1985	147	93	87 (59.2%)	5
Spivak et al.[d]	1986	83	48	39 (47%)	6
Boeckx et al.	1986	63	44	NS	3
Rock et al.	1987	80	58	49 (61.3%)	10
Xue and Fa[e]	1989	117	98	95 (81.2%)	2
Putman et al.	1990	86	64	55 (64%)	NS
teVelde et al.	1990	215	156	137 (63.7%)	8
Kim JD et al.[f]	1997	387	329	295 (76.2%)[f]	6
Kim SH et al.[g]	1997	1,118	505	366 (32.7%)[g]	42
Cha et al.	2001	44	31	NS	1
Wiegerinck et al.	2005	41	26	NS	1
ACCESS BY LAPAROSCOPY					
Dubuisson et al.[h]	1998	32	17	13 (40.6%)	NS
Bisonette et al.[h]	1999	102	64	49 (50.5%)i	5
Yoon et al.[j]	1999	202	154	98 (48.5%)[k]	5
Mettler et al.[h,l]	2001	28	15	15 (53.6%)	2
Cha et al.[j,m]	2001	37	28	NS	1
Ribeiro et al.	2003	26	13	NS	0
Wiegerinck et al.[m]	2005	41	15	NS	1

NS, not stated.
[a]Resurvey of 1980 series; follow-up period more than 18 months.
[b]Follow-up period more than 18 months.
[c]Follow-up period more than 4 years.
[d]Follow-up period more than 1 year.
[e]Follow-up period more than 3.5 years.
[f]Follow-up period more than 2 years. There were eight ongoing pregnancies in addition to the live births.
[g]Follow-up period more than 5 years. There were 31 ongoing pregnancies in addition to the live births.
[h]Tubal anastomosis performed with single-suture' technique.
[i]Tubal anastomosis performed by using two-layer microsurgical technique.
[k]There were 31 ongoing pregnancies in addition to the live births.
[l]A screening laparoscopy was performed, and only those having a distal tubal segment of 4 cm and a proximal segment of 3 cm were included.
[m]Comparative study with cases performed with open access.

were five cases of ectopic pregnancy. These results are not too dissimilar to those achieved by open access, which supports the premise that what is important is the technique used and not the mode of access. Cha and colleagues, also from Korea, further support this assumption. In their study, they compare the fertility outcome in 81 women who had microsurgical reversal of sterilization, 37 by laparoscopic and 44 by open access. The outcomes, as well as the intrauterine and tubal pregnancy rates, were similar in both groups (Table 21.4).

Attempts to develop simple techniques that would yield equivalent results by laparoscopic access continue to be made. A recent study reports the use of the following laparoscopic technique for tubal anastomosis: Once the tubal ends to be anastomosed were prepared, a splint was inserted into the proximal tube through a "guiding catheter" inserted vaginally. The splint was then introduced into the distal portion of the tube through the fimbriated end. The distal portion was aligned with the proximal segment over the splint. The seromuscularis of the two segments was fixed at the 3- and 9-o'clock positions using microclips of 3-mm size. Subsequently, fibrin glue was applied "on the anastomosis surface." The splint was taped externally to the Foley catheter and removed 4 hours after the end of the procedure. Although they report similar results for both the laparoscopic group and a control group (selected from patients whose procedure was performed through a Pfannenstiel incision), it is surprising that in the control group the cumulative rate of ongoing pregnancy at 3 years was only 52% and in the laparoscopic group only 45%. This is despite the fact that in the latter group, more than 90% of the sterilizations had been performed by clips or silastic rings, and their average age was only 34.9 years.

Robotically assisted tubal anastomosis has been explored by several groups. The largest series reported a similar pregnancy ratio for robotically assisted surgery as compared to mini laparotomy, however the cost and surgical time for robotically assisted tubal anastomosis was greater.

Using metaanalysis, Watson and colleagues examined the role of microsurgery versus macrosurgery in the reversal of sterilization. The available studies were limited by the lack of randomized controlled trials and the use of historical control groups. However, as expected, the use of magnification during sterilization reversal as well as during adhesiolysis and salpingostomy led to higher pregnancy and lower ectopic rates.

Microsurgical tubotubal anastomosis for reversal of sterilization produces excellent results that are principally dependent on the status and the length of the reconstructed tube. Live birth rates of 60% to 80% can be achieved, provided that the reconstructed tube is longer than 4 cm and the ampullary portion greater than 2 cm. The second most important factor is the woman's age. The tubal pregnancy rates are usually low.

The advantages of laparoscopic access are well recognized. These include a shorter hospital stay and recovery time and lower postoperative analgesic requirements. Our experience demonstrates that access by a minilaparotomy incision, as described earlier, provides the same advantages. We perform tubal anastomosis for reversal of sterilization, tubocornual anastomosis for pathologic tubal occlusion, and other more complex reconstructive microsurgical procedures via minilaparotomy using an operating microscope. Patients are admitted to hospital on the morning of surgery, and most are discharged a few hours postoperatively. Each surgeon must balance patient factors, his or her expertise, and the resources of the center in deciding how to approach such procedures.

Tubocornual Anastomosis for Proximal Tubal Disease

Various disease processes can affect the proximal tube and occlude the region of the uterotubal junction. On the basis of histologic studies on resected tubal segments, these occlusive lesions in order of frequency are as follows: obliterative fibrosis, chronic inflammation, salpingitis isthmica nodosa, intratubal endometriosis, and, rarely, ectopic gestation and tuberculosis. All of the published series report a varying but usually low percentage of cases with no demonstrable lesions. This may be related to tubal spasm (at the time of HSG or laparoscopy) or to the presence of tubal plugs or synechiae. Such conditions, as opposed to occlusive disease, are amenable to treatment with selective salpingography or tubal cannulation, which were discussed earlier in this chapter.

The management strategy in proximal tubal occlusion must take into account other variables, including the condition of the distal tube, the extent and nature of pelvic adhesions, the presence of associated pelvic disease, and the status of other fertility parameters, especially male factor infertility. This strategy must also respect the following principles: simplicity, reproducibility, and cost-effectiveness.

The selection of treatment must be individualized according to the investigative findings, the wishes of the couple, the expertise of the surgeon, and the results achieved by the center in which the couple will be managed. Fig. 21.28 diagrammatically summarizes the management of proximal tubal occlusion.

The traditional surgical treatment of occlusive proximal tubal disease was uterotubal implantation. The application of microsurgery has made it possible to perform an anastomosis instead, after removal of the affected tubal segment.

Central to this approach is the complete excision of the affected portion of tube, whether it is intramural or isthmic. In cases of pathologic occlusion, a portion of healthy intramural tube is usually spared, permitting the conservation of sometimes all but more often a part of this segment. In other instances, the whole intramural segment is involved in the disease process and must be excised. In such cases, microsurgery permits an anastomosis to be performed between the uterine tubal ostium and the healthy portion of isthmus. Depending on the extent of intramural tube that is excised and thus the site at which the anastomosis is performed, tubocornual anastomosis may be juxtamural, intramural, or juxtauterine (Fig. 21.29).

The cornual region of the uterus is infiltrated with dilute vasopressin solution. This is done by injecting 2 mL of this solution in a circular fashion under the serosa 1 cm medial to the uterotubal junction with use of a 30-gauge needle on a 3-mL syringe. Vasoconstriction is recognized by serosal blanching. The tube is then incised at the uterotubal junction, with care taken not to divide the arteriovenous arcade at its mesosalpingeal margin (Fig. 21.30). After transection of the tube, patency of the intramural segment is assessed by transcervical chromopertubation, and the normalcy of the cut surface is evaluated under high magnification.

If the intramural tube is found to be occluded or abnormal at this site, its musculature is dissected further from the surrounding uterine muscle, 1 to 2 mm at a time, toward the uterine cavity (Fig. 21.30A). The small portion of tube thus dissected is transected, and the cut surface is reassessed. If the intramural tube is still occluded or abnormal, the same procedure is repeated until normal patent tube is reached. Dye solution will spurt from the open lumen. It is essential that dissection of the intramural tube from the surrounding uterine muscle be effected at the level of the immediate periphery of the tubal muscularis (Fig. 21.30B). The preoperative HSG usually provides information about the length of the normal intramural segment and the extent of excision required. Transection of successive portions of the intramural tube can be achieved with either curved microscissors or especially designed cornual blade (Gomel cornual blade, Spingler-Tritt, Jestetten, Germany). By limiting the excised tissue to the intramural tube, there is little risk of creating a large defect at the cornu.

After the preparation of the cornual end, the occluded or abnormal isthmic segment is prepared by making serial cuts 1 to 2 mm apart, beginning at the initial transection site at the uterotubal junction and continuing until normal patent tube is identified (Fig. 21.30C, D). Patency of the distal segment is confirmed by descending hydropertubation, with injection of a few milliliters of dye or irrigation solution through the fimbriated end. Hemostasis of the cut end of the normal distal tube is obtained by precise electrocoagulation of bleeders located between the muscularis and serosa. The intervening abnormal tubal segments are excised from the mesosalpinx electrosurgically, avoiding the vascular arcade beneath the tube.

The intramural and isthmic segments are approximated in two layers as follows: The initial suture of the first layer, which incorporates the muscularis and epithelium of the two segments, is placed at the 6-o'clock position (Fig. 21.30E). If the anastomosis is superficial (juxtamural type), the suture is tied.

With anastomoses located deep in the cornua, as in intramural or juxtauterine types, the 6-o'clock suture is held with a clip until the remaining sutures have been placed, because

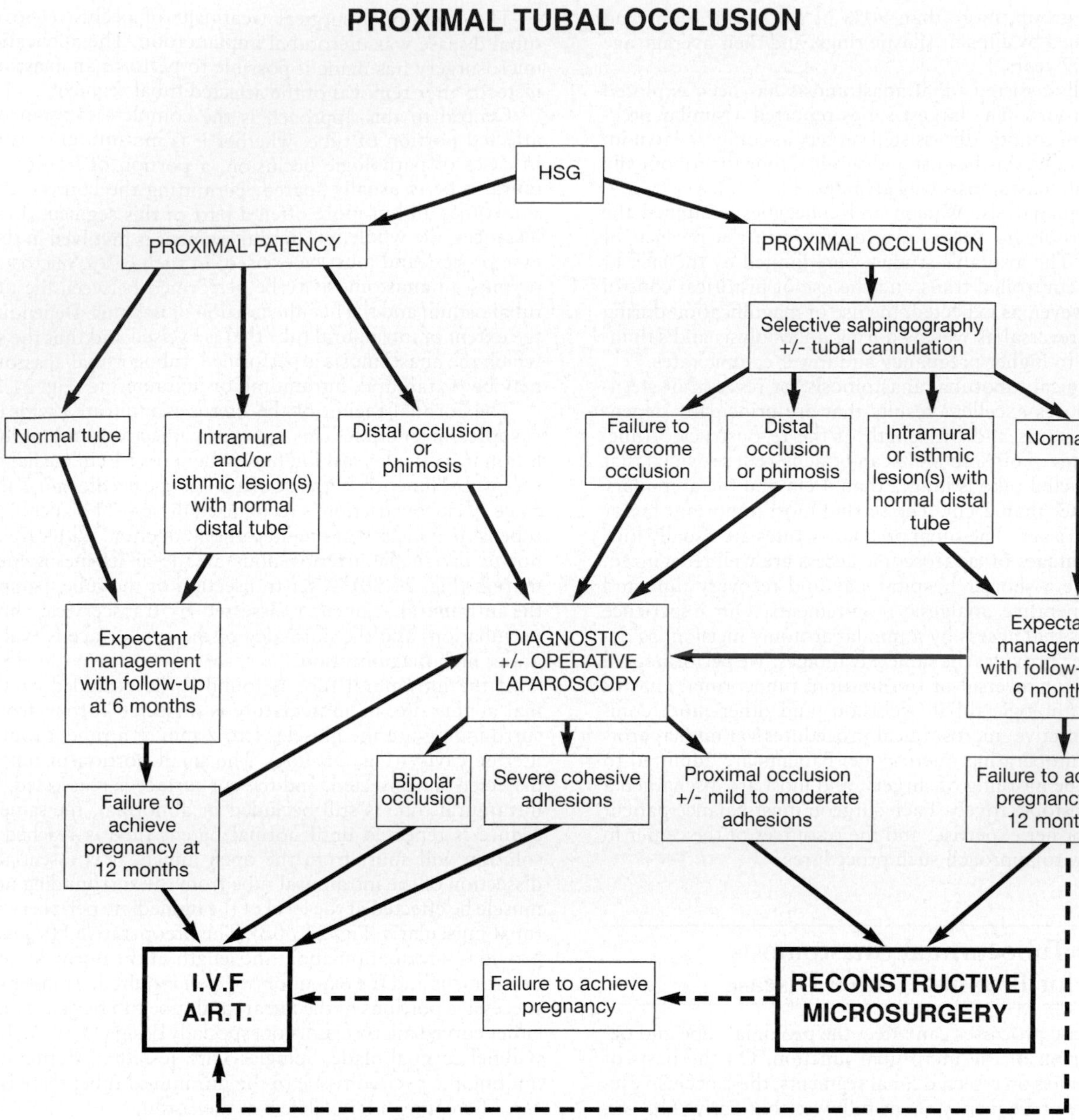

FIGURE 21.28. Management of proximal tubal occlusion. HSG, hysterosalpingogram; IVF, *in vitro* fertilization; ART, artificial reproductive technology. (Modified from: Gomel V, Dubuisson JB. *References en Gynecologie et Obstetrique*. September 1995:251, with permission.)

tying this initial suture would make placement of the subsequent sutures difficult if not impossible. In such cases, the subsequent sutures are placed with use of a continuous strand of suture, as described earlier (Fig. 21.30). This approach facilitates suture placement and prevents the individual sutures from becoming tangled. Three additional sutures, placed at cardinal points, are usually sufficient to join the inner layer. If the cornual crater is deep and the placement of sutures is difficult, this task can be facilitated by making a coronal incision on the uterus, above the cornual crater. The edges of this incision must be approximated at the end of the procedure.

If the distance between the two segments of tube is significant or if there is undue tension, it is necessary to hold the distal tubal segment close to the intramural segment while tying the sutures. Alternatively, a single no. 7-0 Vicryl suture is passed through the mesosalpinx below the cut end of the distal segment of tube and then through the border of the uterus immediately beneath the cornual crater. The suture is tied to bring the two segments into close proximity. The 6-o'clock suture is tied first. Then the loop between each succeeding suture is divided and tied in turn. After approximation of the first layer, the seromuscularis of the uterus is joined to the serosa of the tube with no. 8-0 sutures. The defect under the tube is closed by approximating the mesosalpinx to the lateral edge of the uterus (Fig. 21.30F, G).

Compared with tubouterine implantation, microsurgical tubocornual anastomosis offers several advantages: It largely maintains the integrity of the uterine cornua; preserves a longer tube; obviates the need for a cesarean section, except for obstetric reasons; and yields better results.

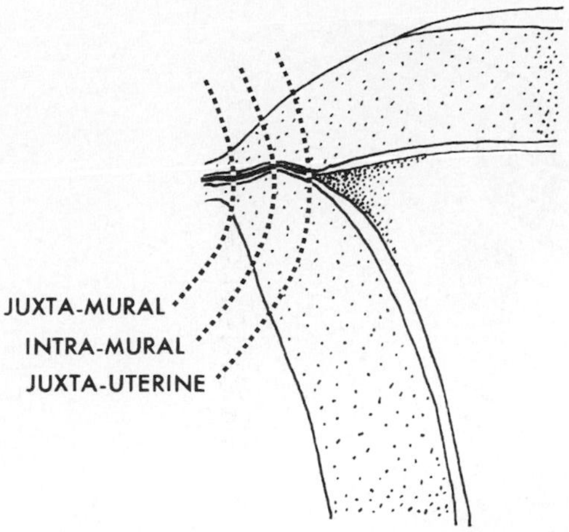

FIGURE 21.29. Types of tubocornual anastomosis.

Results of Tubocornual Anastomosis

Microsurgical tubocornual anastomosis for the treatment of occlusive cornual disease yields fairly good results in centers experienced with this procedure. The published series report live birth rates between 33% and 56% and ectopic pregnancy rates between 5% and 7% (Table 21.5). This table makes it clearly evident that there has been a paucity of reports regarding this procedure for more than a decade.

Rare Procedures and Technically Difficult Cases

Rare circumstances may be encountered that are amenable to microsurgical correction. Some of these circumstances are discussed in this section.

The technical difficulty of a procedure must be differentiated from the prognosis that the procedure offers. Furthermore, difficulty is a relative term because what is commonplace work for some may be difficult or even impossible for others to achieve. From the patient's standpoint, what is important is the prognosis—the yield associated with the surgical procedure. Furthermore, the prognosis is not necessarily inversely proportional to the difficulty of the procedure. For example, microsurgical tubocornual anastomosis to treat occlusive cornual lesions is one of the technically more difficult reconstructive tubal operations. However, centers experienced in this procedure achieve excellent results. An even more technically difficult operation is tuboovarian transposition.

Tuboovarian Transposition

In the case of a unicornuate uterus without an ipsilateral tube and ovary, the contralateral tube and ovary, if present, may be transposed while preserving their vascular pedicle. We performed such a procedure in a woman with a single left unicornuate uterus whose ipsilateral tube and ovary were removed subsequent to a left tubal pregnancy. On the right side, placed high on the pelvic sidewall, were an ovary and a short oviduct, composed of infundibulum and ampulla (Fig. 21.31A).

The uterus was mobilized centrally as follows: The left round ligament was divided near its inguinal insertion and dissected from the broad ligament with its vascular supply intact (Fig. 21.31A). The divided end of the round ligament was then affixed to the right inguinal region (Fig. 21.31B). Microsurgical transposition of the right ovary and tube with preservation of their vascular supply permitted anastomosis between the left intramural and right ampullary tubal segments (Fig. 21.31C). The ovary was mobilized further to achieve the proper spatial relation with the fimbrial extremity of the tube (Fig. 21.31D). In the third postoperative cycle, the patient was successful in achieving an intrauterine pregnancy, which resulted in a normal live birth. She has since had two more children. Since the publication of this report in May 1985, there have been at least five case reports of successful transposition of the fallopian tube without the ovary. These reports clearly illustrate the potential of surgery, even though technically difficult, in restoring fertility in the face of unusual pelvic anatomy.

Correction of Bipolar Tubal Disease

The results associated with surgical correction of bipolar (both proximal and distal) tubal occlusion are dismal. A report from the Mayo Clinic included 31 such patients: bipolar tubal occlusion of both tubes ($n = 13$) or their only remaining tube ($n = 5$); bilateral distal and unilateral proximal occlusion ($n = 7$); and bilateral proximal and unilateral distal occlusion ($n = 6$). Despite a mean follow-up period of more than 3 years, pregnancies occurred in only three patients. Furthermore, two of these were ectopic, and one was a spontaneous abortion.

Anastomosis of Contralateral Tubal Segments

A patient may have a healthy proximal segment of tube on one side, whereas on the opposite side, an ampullary–infundibular segment exists. In such a circumstance, microsurgical reconstruction of one functional tube can be achieved by anastomosis of the contralateral tubal segments behind the uterus, maintaining the physiologic relation between the tubal infundibulum and ovary. In the presence of both ovaries, the uteroovarian ligaments are first approximated with interrupted, nonabsorbable no. 4–0 or 5–0 nylon sutures. This brings the ovaries together and helps reduce tension in achieving the subsequent tubal anastomosis (Fig. 21.32). Successful delivery after such a procedure has been reported.

Approximation of the Fimbriated End of the Oviduct to the Contralateral Ovary

When a single ovary exists on the side opposite the patient's only tube, simple approximation of the fimbriated extremity of the tube to the ovary may be possible. The ovary is mobilized, and the mesovarium is fixed to the posterior surface of the uterus with nonabsorbable sutures. The contralateral oviduct is mobilized, and its mesosalpinx is sutured to the posterior aspect of the uterus. The nonabsorbable sutures are placed on the mesosalpinx about 1 cm from the tube. This will effectively place the infundibulum in close proximity to the ovary. Alternatively, the ovary can be transposed to the contralateral side with its vascular pedicle kept intact.

Iterative Reconstructive Surgery

Except in rare circumstances, there are no data to support the undertaking of an iterative surgical procedure when a prior reconstructive operation has failed.

Rare exceptions include cases of tubotubal anastomosis that failed for purely technical reasons, in which sufficient lengths of healthy tube is available for reconstruction. In such instances,

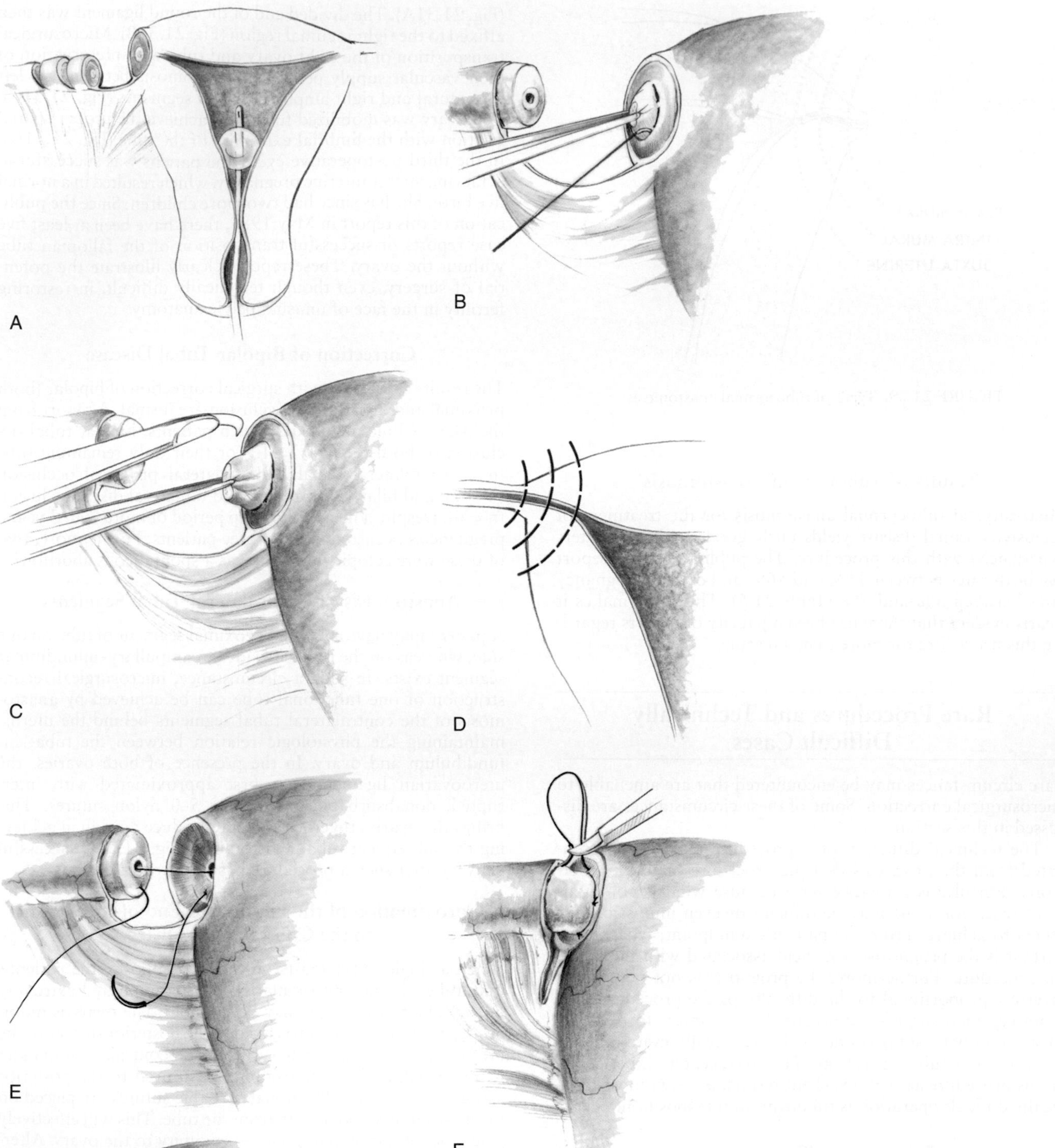

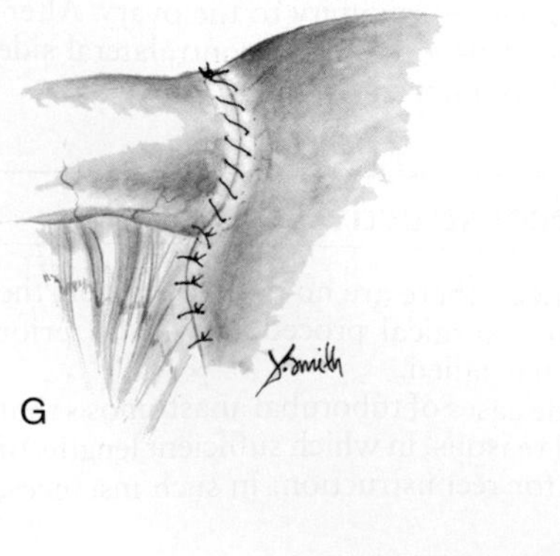

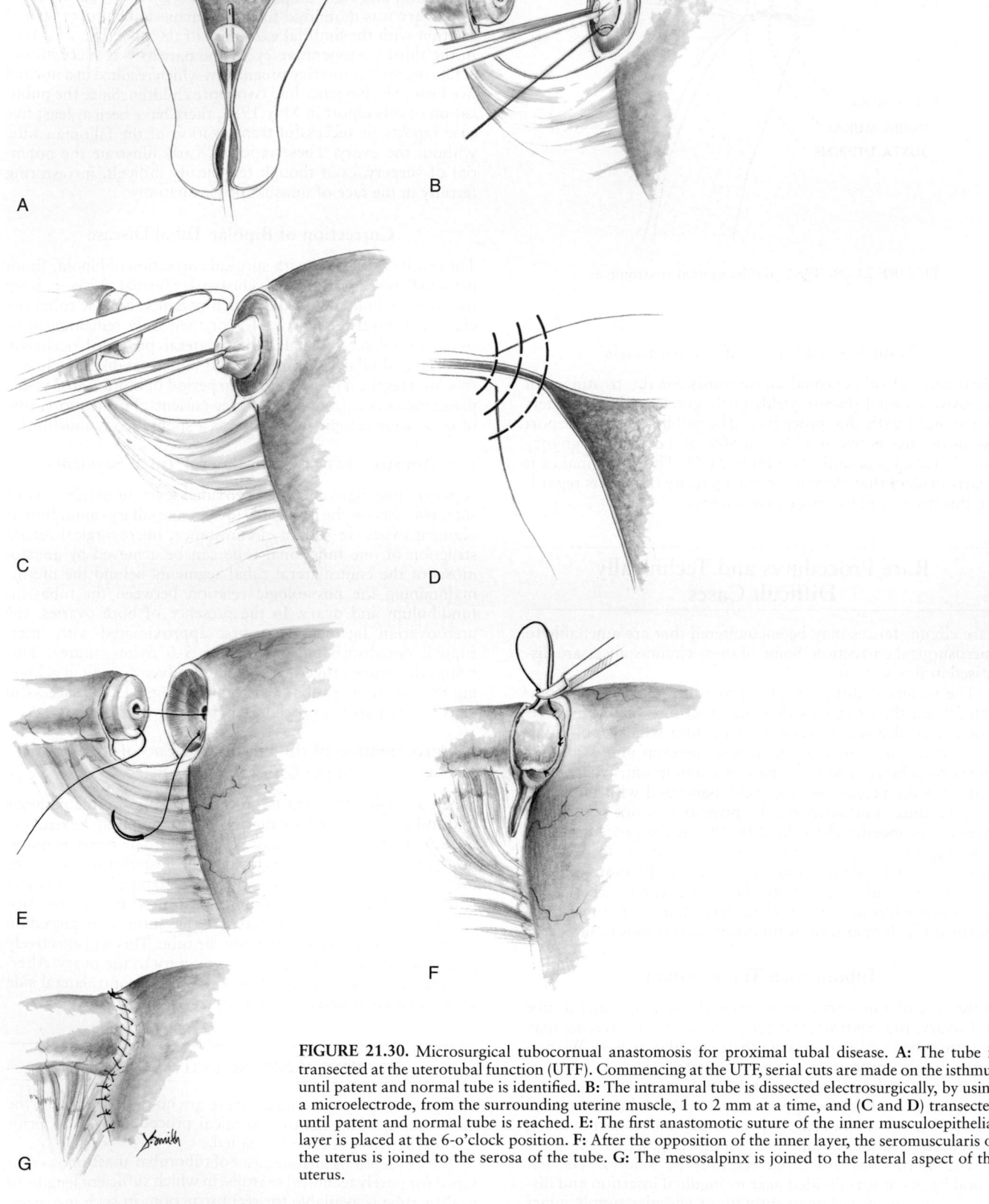

FIGURE 21.30. Microsurgical tubocornual anastomosis for proximal tubal disease. **A:** The tube is transected at the uterotubal function (UTF). Commencing at the UTF, serial cuts are made on the isthmus until patent and normal tube is identified. **B:** The intramural tube is dissected electrosurgically, by using a microelectrode, from the surrounding uterine muscle, 1 to 2 mm at a time, and (**C** and **D**) transected until patent and normal tube is reached. **E:** The first anastomotic suture of the inner musculoepithelial layer is placed at the 6-o'clock position. **F:** After the opposition of the inner layer, the seromuscularis of the uterus is joined to the serosa of the tube. **G:** The mesosalpinx is joined to the lateral aspect of the uterus.

TABLE 21.5

RESULTS OF MICROSURGICAL TUBOCORNUAL ANASTOMOSIS FOR OCCLUSIVE PROXIMAL TUBAL DISEASE

Investigators	Year	Patients	Intrauterine pregnancies	Live births	Ectopic pregnancies
Gomel	1977	13	NS	7 (53.8%)	1
Gomel	1980	38	21	20 (52.6%)	2
Winston	1980	49	NS	16 (32.7%)	2
McComb	1986	26	15	14 (53.8%)	2
Donnez and Casanas-Roux	1986	82	NS	36 (43.9%)	6
Gillett and Herbison	1989	32	19	18 (56.3%)	2
Tomazevic et al.[a]	1996	59	NS	27 (45.8%)	NS
Awartani and McComb	2003	26	12	NS	3

[a] Of the 32 operated patients who did not deliver within 2 years after surgery, 21 were treated with 66 cycles of *in vitro* fertilization, resulting in live births for 12.

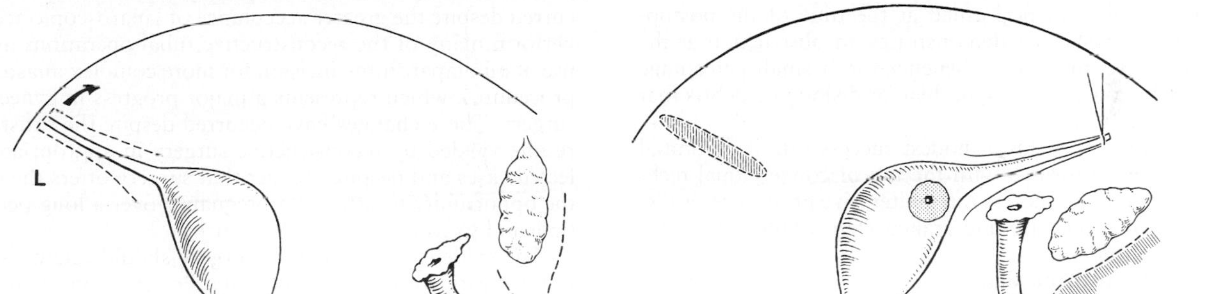

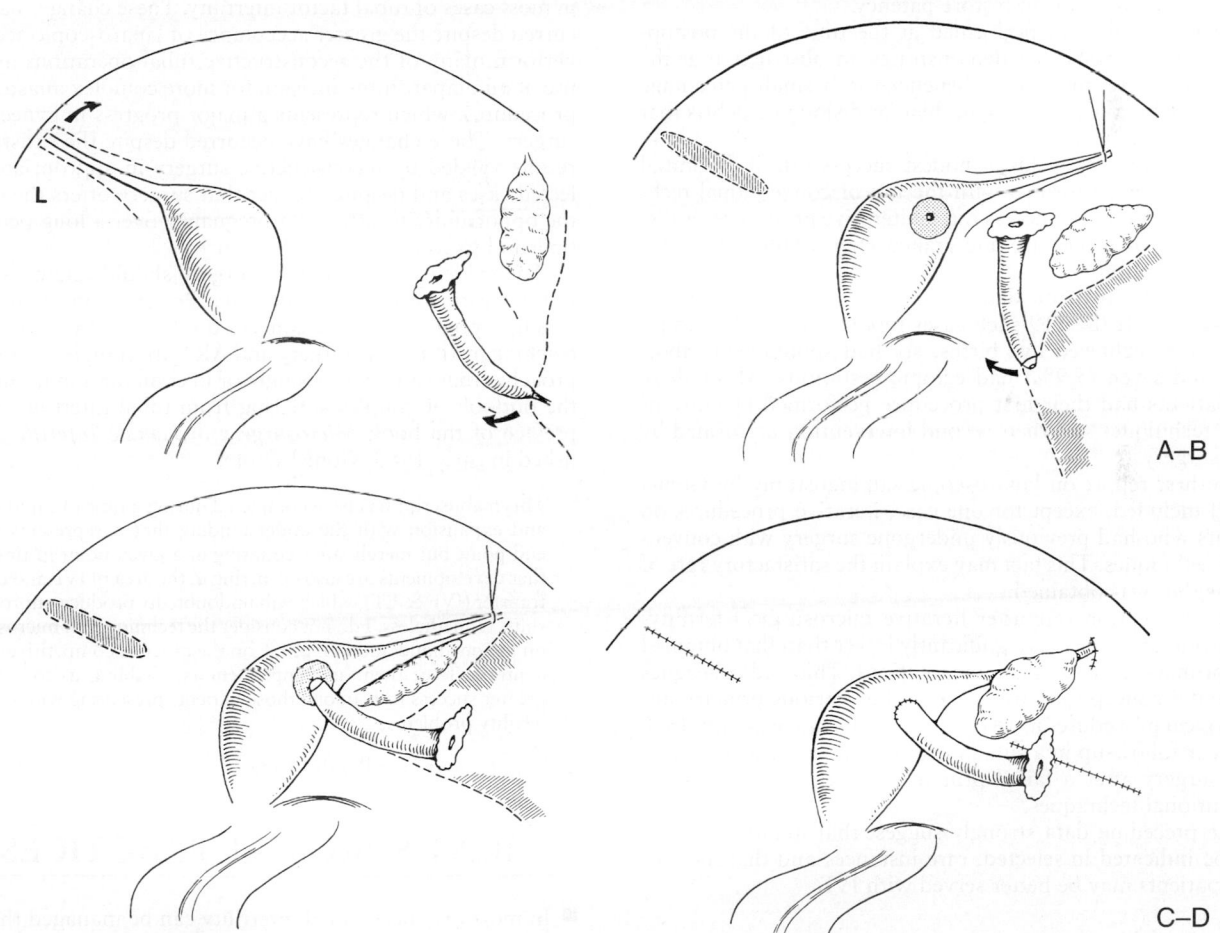

FIGURE 21.31. Microsurgical tuboovarian transposition. (From: Gomel V, McComb P. Microsurgical transposition of the human fallopian tube and ovary with subsequent pregnancy. *Fertil Steril* 1985;43:804, with permission.)

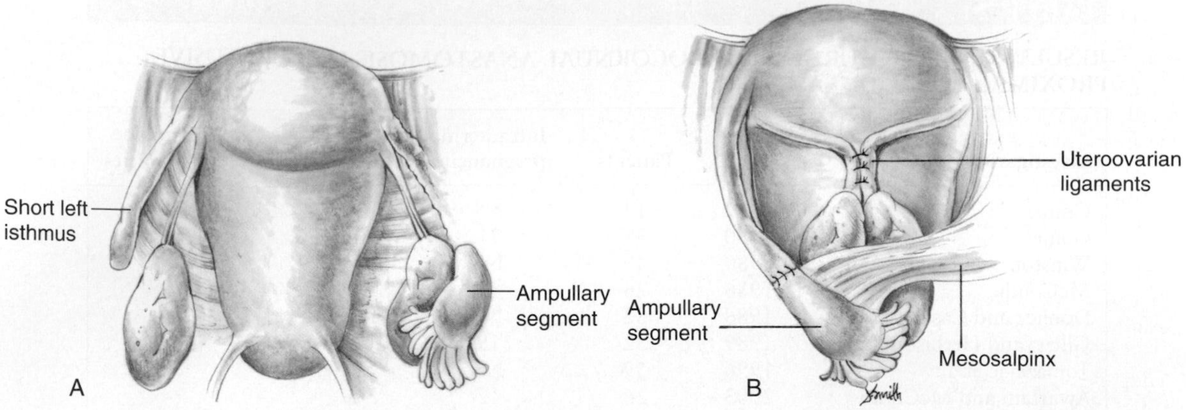

FIGURE 21.32. Microsurgical anastomosis of contralateral tubal segments. **A:** Isthmic segment of tube on left and ampullary–infundibular segment on right. **B:** The uteroovarian ligaments are approximated with nonabsorbable sutures behind the uterus; the left isthmic segment of tube is anastomosed to the right ampullary–infundibular segment.

an iterative microsurgical anastomosis may be undertaken if tubal cannulation fails to restore patency.

Tubal cannulation, performed at the time of the postoperative control HSG that demonstrates an obstruction at the anastomosis site, may prove beneficial in a small percentage of cases by breaking down synechiae or dislodging debris that may be present at this site.

Iterative surgery yields a modest success rate if the initial procedure was performed with the use of conventional techniques. However, the success rate of iterative procedures is disappointing when they are undertaken after a failed microsurgical intervention.

Most of the available data on iterative surgery concern salpingostomy. Of the 119 such cases reported in the literature, 18 (15.1%) achieved live births, six had spontaneous abortions, and seven (5.9%) had ectopic gestations. All of these 119 patients had their first procedure performed by conventional techniques and their second intervention performed by microsurgery.

The first report on laparoscopic salpingostomy by Gomel (1997) included, except for one case, iterative procedures on patients who had previously undergone surgery with conventional techniques. This fact may explain the satisfactory rate of success that was obtained.

The conception rate after iterative microsurgical fertility-promoting procedures is significantly lower than that obtained with primary microsurgical interventions. Thie and colleagues reported a conception rate of 51% after various primary microsurgical procedures in 161 patients. This rate was only 18% at 3-year follow-up in a similar group of 21 patients who had microsurgery after a failed primary operation performed by conventional techniques.

The preceding data strongly suggest that iterative surgery may be indicated in selected, rare instances and that most of these patients may be better served with IVF.

Observations on Current Practice

The enormous progress in IVF and ART in the past 20 years has been accompanied with the industrialization of this technology and its services all over the world. In parallel fashion, there has been a significant decline in the practice and teaching of reconstructive surgery. There is a paucity of publications on this subject. IVF is offered now, as a primary treatment option, in most cases of tubal factor infertility. These changes have occurred despite the greater acceptance of laparoscopic access to perform many of the reconstructive tubal operations and the use of minilaparotomy incision for more complex anastomotic procedures, which represents a major progress in gynecologic surgery. These changes have occurred despite the satisfactory results yielded by reconstructive surgery in appropriately selected cases and despite the fact that surgery offers the couple the opportunity to attempt a pregnancy over a long period of time and to conceive more than once.

The evidence suggests that surgery should retain its place in the treatment of tubal infertility. Preservation of the place of surgery will require a concerted effort on the part of the teaching institutions. Surgery and ART are complementary approaches that can be used singly or in combination to improve the outlook of couples suffering from tubal infertility. In the preface of the book *Microsurgery in Female Infertility,* published in early 1983, Gomel wrote:

> This manuscript has been completed during a time of rapid change and expansion with the understanding that it represents not an end point but merely an accounting at a given point in time. Further developments are also occurring in the area of IVF and embryo transfer (IVF & ET), which will undoubtedly produce improved results. Nonetheless, I do not consider the techniques of microsurgery on the one hand and IVF & ET on the other as competitive; on the contrary, I see them as complementary, enabling us to achieve a greater success rate among those patients presenting with complex fertility problems.

This statement is still valid today.

BEST SURGICAL PRACTICES

- In most instances, tubal infertility can be managed through surgery and/or ART. Each approach has unique advantages and disadvantages and can be used in isolation or in combination to improve the outlook of couples suffering from tubal infertility.
- Periadnexal adhesions, coexisting with other types of tubal disease or in isolation, can affect fertility by encapsulating the tube preventing ovum pickup or by distorting the spatial relation between the tube and ovary. Open or preferably

laparoscopic salpingoovariolysis is associated with intrauterine pregnancies rates of approximately 50% to 60% and a low incidence of ectopic pregnancy.

- In select cases of proximal tubal occlusion, selective salpingography or transcervical fallopian tube cannulation may be useful in overcoming obstruction. True pathologic tubal occlusion resulting from salpingitis isthmica nodosa, endometriosis, or extensive postinflammatory fibrosis, however, is best treated by microsurgical tubocornual anastomosis.
- Fimbrioplasty for fimbrial phimosis and salpingostomy for complete distal tubal obstruction involve the creation of an anatomically correct distal tubal ostia that will allow ovum pickup and restore tubal function. The success of these procedures depends on the degree of tubal disease.
- Distal tubal occlusion results in the accumulation of fluid within the tube, which is called *hydrosalpinx*. Hydrosalpinges that are visible with ultrasonography may adversely affect the results of VF treatment. They should be removed, proximally occluded, or drained surgically through the creation of a neosalpingostomy before IVF.
- Tubotubal anastomosis, for reversal of sterilization or a disease process that results in tubal occlusion, produces excellent results that are principally dependent on the status and the length of the reconstructed tube and the age of the female partner.
- Provided proper anastomotic technique is used, success of tubotubal anastomosis by laparoscopy approaches that of access by minilaparotomy; hence, each surgeon must balance patient factors, his or her expertise, and the resources of the center in deciding how to approach such procedures.
- Thoughtful surgical technique minimizing tissue damage is the hallmark of fertility-promoting tubal reconstructive surgery and is independent of the route of access but dependent on the skill and dedication of the surgeon.

Bibliography

Aboulghar MA, Mansour RT, Serour GI, et al. Transvaginal ultrasonic needle guided aspiration of pelvic inflammatory cystic masses before ovulation induction for in vitro fertilization. *Fertil Steril* 1990;53(2):311.

Ajonuma LC, Ng EH, Chan HC. New insights into the mechanisms underlying hydrosalpinx fluid formation and its adverse effect on IVF outcome. *Hum Reprod Update* 2002;8(3):255.

Alper MM, Garner PR, Spence JEH, et al. Pregnancy rates after hysterosalpingography with oil- and water-soluble contrast media. *Obstet Gynecol* 1986;68:6.

Awartani K, McComb PF. Microsurgical resection of nonocclusive salpingitis isthmica nodosa is beneficial. *Fertil Steril* 2003;79:1199.

Benadiva CA, Kligman I, Davis O, et al. In vitro fertilization versus tubal surgery: Is pelvic reconstructive surgery obsolete? *Fertil Steril* 1995;64:1051.

Bergh T, Ericson A, Hillensjo T, et al. Deliveries and children born after in-vitro fertilization in Sweden 1982–95: a retrospective cohort study. *Lancet* 1999;354:1579.

Bisonette F, Lapensee L, Bouzayen R. Outpatient laparoscopic tubal anastomosis and subsequent fertility. *Fertil Steril* 1999;72:549.

Boeckx W, Gordts S, Buysse K, et al. Reversibility after female sterilization. *BJOG* 1986;93:839.

Boer-Meisel ME, teVelde ER, Habbema JDF, et al. Predicting the pregnancy outcome in patients treated for hydrosalpinx: a prospective study. *Fertil Steril* 1986;45:23.

Bowman MC, Cooke ID. Comparison of fallopian tube intraluminal pathology as assessed by salpingoscopy with pelvic adhesions. *Fertil Steril* 1994;61:464.

Brosens IA, Puttemans PJ. Double-optic laparoscopy: salpingoscopy, ovarian cystoscopy and endo-ovarian surgery with the argon laser. *Baillieres Clin Obstet Gynaecol* 1989;3:595.

Bruhat MA, Mage G, Manhes H, et al. Laparoscopy procedures to promote fertility ovariolysis and salpingolysis: results of 93 selected cases. *Acta Eur Fertil* 1983;14:113.

Brundin A, Dahlborn M, Ahlberg-Ahre E, et al. Radionuclide hysterosalpingography for measurement of human oviduct function. *Int J Gynecol Obstet* 1989;28:53.

Canis M, Mage G, Pouly JL, et al. Laparoscopic distal tuboplasty: report of 87 cases and a 4 year experience. *Fertil Steril* 1991;56:616.

Caspi E, Halperin V, Bukovsky I. The importance of periadnexal adhesions in tubal reconstructive surgery for infertility. *Fertil Steril* 1979;31:296.

Centers for Disease Control and Prevention 2003 Assisted Reproductive Technology (ART) Report. Web site: www.cdc.gov/ART/ART2003

Centers for Disease Control and Prevention. CDC STD Surveillance Data 2004. Web site: www.cdc.gov/std/stats/

Cha SH, Lee MH, Kim JH, et al. Fertility outcome after tubal anastomosis by laparoscopy and laparotomy. *J Am Assoc Gynecol Laparosc* 2001;8:348.

Cohen J. The efficiency and efficacy of IVF and GIFT. *Hum Reprod* 1991;6:613.

Collins JA, Rowe TC. Age of the female partner is a prognostic factor in prolonged unexplained infertility: a multicenter study. *Fertil Steril* 1989;52:15.

Dan U, Oelsner G, Gruberg L, et al. Cerebral embolization and coma after hysterosalpingography with oil-soluble contrast medium. *Fertil Steril* 1990;53:939.

Daniell JF, Herbert CM. Laparoscopic salpingostomy using the CO_2 laser. *Fertil Steril* 1984;41:558.

Degueldre M, Vandromme J, Huong PT, et al. Robotically assisted laparoscopic microsurgical tubal reanastomosis: a feasibility study. *Fertil Steril* 2000;74(5):1020.

DeCherney AH, Mezer HC, Naftolin F. Analysis of failure of microsurgical anastomosis after mid-segment, non-coagulation tubal ligation. *Fertil Steril* 1983;39:618.

Dicker D, Ashkenazi J, Feldberg D, et al. Severe abdominal complications after transvaginal ultrasonographically guided retrieval of oocytes for in vitro fertilization and embryo transfer. *Fertil Steril* 1993;59:1313.

Donnez J, Casanas-Roux F. Prognostic factors of fimbrial microsurgery. *Fertil Steril* 1986a;46:200.

Donnez J, Casanas-Roux F. Prognostic factors influencing the pregnancy rate after microsurgical cornual anastomosis. *Fertil Steril* 1986;46:1089.

Donnez J, Nisolle M, Casanas-Roux F. CO_2 laser laparoscopy in infertile women with adnexal adhesions and women with tubal occlusion. *J Gynecol Surg* 1989;5:47.

Dubuisson JB, Bouquet de Jolıniere J, Aubriot FX, et al. Terminal tuboplasties by laparoscopy: 65 consecutive cases. *Fertil Steril* 1990;54:401.

Dubuisson JB, Chapron C. Single suture laparoscopic tubal re-anastomosis. *Curr Opin Obstet Gynecol* 1998;10:307.

Dubuisson JB, Chapron C, Morice P, et al. Laparoscopic salpingostomy: fertility results according to the tubal mucosal appearance. *Hum Reprod* 1994;9:334.

Erenus M, Zouves C, Rajamahendran DVM, et al. The effect of embryo quality on subsequent pregnancy rates after in vitro fertilization. *Fertil Steril* 1991;56:707.

Fayez JA. An assessment of the role of operative laparoscopy in tuboplasty. *Fertil Steril* 1983;39:476.

Filmar S, Gomel V, McComb P. The effectiveness of CO_2 laser and electromicrosurgery in adhesiolysis: a comparative study. *Fertil Steril* 1986;45:407.

FIVNAT 1989 et bilan general 1986–1989. *Contracept Fertil Sex* 1990;18:588.

Gillett WR, Herbison GP. Tubocornual anastomosis: surgical considerations and coexistent infertility factors in determining the prognosis. *Fertil Steril* 1989;51:241.

Glazener CMA, Loveden LM, Richardson SJ, et al. Tubo-cornual polyps: their relevance in subfertility. *Hum Reprod* 1987;2:59.

Gomel V. Laparoscopic tubal surgery in infertility. *Obstet Gynecol* 1975; 46:47.

Gomel V. Reconstructive surgery of the oviduct. *J Reprod Med* 1977a;18:181.

Gomel V. Salpingostomy by laparoscopy. *J Reprod Med* 1977b;18:265.

Gomel V. Tubal anastomosis by microsurgery. *Fertil Steril* 1977c;28:59.

Gomel V. Profile of women requesting reversal of sterilization. *Fertil Steril* 1978a;30:39.

Gomel V. Salpingostomy by microsurgery. *Fertil Steril* 1978b;29:380.

Gomel V. Causes of failure of reconstructive infertility microsurgery. *Clin Obstet Gynecol* 1980a;23:1269.

Gomel V. Clinical results of infertility microsurgery. In: Crosignani PG, Rubin BL, eds. *Microsurgery in female infertility.* London: Academic Press; 1980b:77.

Gomel V. Microsurgical reversal of sterilization: a reappraisal. *Fertil Steril* 1980c;33:587.

Gomel V. An odyssey through the oviduct. *Fertil Steril* 1983a;39:144.

Gomel V. *Microsurgery in female infertility.* Boston: Little, Brown; 1983b.

Gomel V. Salpingo-ovariolysis by laparoscopy in infertility. *Fertil Steril* 1983c;34:607.

Gomel V. Distal tubal occlusion. *Fertil Steril* 1988;49:946.

Gomel V. Operative laparoscopy: time for acceptance. *Fertil Steril* 1989;52:1.

Gomel V. From microsurgery to laparoscopic surgery: a progress. *Fertil Steril* 1995;63:464.

Gomel V, Erenus M. *The American Fertility Society, 46th Annual Meeting. Program Supplement* 1990:P-097–S106(abst).

Gomel V, Filmar S. Arrested tubal pregnancy. *Fertil Steril* 1987;48:1043.

Gomel V, McComb PF. Microsurgical transposition of the human fallopian tube and ovary with subsequent intrauterine pregnancy. *Fertil Steril* 1985; 43:804.

Gomel V, McComb PF. Microsurgery for tubal infertility. *J Reprod Med.* In press.

Gomel V, McComb PF. Unexpected pregnancies in women afflicted by occlusive tubal disease. *Fertil Steril* 1981;36:529.

Gomel V, Rowe TC. Microsurgical tubal reconstruction and reversal of sterilization. In: Wallach EE, Zacur HA, eds. *Reproductive medicine and surgery.* St Louis: Mosby; 1995:1074.

Gomel V, Swolin K. Salpingostomy: microsurgical technique and results. *Clin Obstet Gynecol* 1980;23:1243.

Gomel V, Taylor PJ. In vitro fertilization versus reconstructive tubal surgery. *J Assist Reprod Genet* 1992;9:306.

Gomel V, Taylor PJ. Reconstructive tubal surgery in the female. In: Insler V, Lunenfeld B, eds. *Infertility, male and female.* Edinburgh: Churchill Livingstone; 1993:481.

Gomel V, Taylor PJ. *Diagnostic and operative gynecologic laparoscopy.* St Louis: Mosby; 1995.

Gordts S, Boeckx W, Vasquez G, et al. Microsurgical resection of intramural tubal polyps. *Fertil Steril* 1983;40:258.

Gurgan T, Urman B, Yarali H, et al. Salpingoscopic findings in women with occlusive and nonocclusive salpingitis isthmica nodosa. *Fertil Steril* 1994;61: 461.

Henderson SR. The reversibility of female sterilization with the use of microsurgery: a report on 102 patients with more than one year of follow-up. *Am J Obstet Gynecol* 1984;149:57.

Henry-Suchet J, Loffredo V, Tesquier L, et al. Endoscopy of the tube (5 tuboscopy): its prognostic value for tuboplasties. *Acta Eur Fertil* 1985;16:139.

Hulka JF. Adnexal adhesions: a prognostic staging and classification system based on a five year survey of fertility surgery results at Chapel Hill, North Carolina. *Am J Obstet Gynecol* 1982;144:141.

Hull MGR, Glazener CMA, Kelly NJ, et al. Population study of causes, treatment, and outcome of infertility. *BMJ* 1985;291:1693.

Johnson NP, Mak W, Sowter MC. Surgical treatment for tubal disease in women due to undergo in vitro fertilisation. *Cochrane Database of Syst Rev* 2004;3:CD002125.

Jones HW Jr, Rock JA. On the reanastomosis of fallopian tubes after surgical sterilization. *Fertil Steril* 1978;29:702.

Kerin JF. Nonhysteroscopic falloposcopy: a proposed method for visual guidance and verification of tubal cannula placement for endotuboplasty, gamete and embryo transfer procedures. *Fertil Steril* 1992;57:1133.

Kerin JF, Williams DB, San Roman GA, et al. Falloposcopic classification and treatment of fallopian tube lumen disease. *Fertil Steril* 1992;57:731.

Kim JD, Kim KS, Doo JK, et al. A report on 387 cases of microsurgical tubal reversals. *Fertil Steril* 1997;68:875.

Kim SH, Shin CJ, Kim JG, et al. Microsurgical reversal of tubal sterilization: a report on 1118 cases. *Fertil Steril* 1997;68:865.

Kosasa TS, Hale RW. Treatment of hydrosalpinx using a single incision eversion procedure. *Int J Fertil* 1988;33:319.

Lang EK, Dunaway HH. Recanalization of obstructed fallopian tube by selective salpingography and transvaginal bougie dilatation: outcome and cost analysis. *Fertil Steril* 1996;66:210.

Larsson B. Late results of salpingostomy combined with salpingolysis and ovariolysis by electromicrosurgery in 54 women. *Fertil Steril* 1982;37:156.

Lauritsen JG, Pagel JD, Vangsted P, et al. Results of repeated tuboplasties. *Fertil Steril* 1982;37:68.

Letterie GS, Luetkehans T. Reproductive outcome after fallopian tube canalization and microsurgery for bipolar tubal occlusion. *J Gynecol Surg* 1992;8:11.

Luber K, Beeson CC, Kennedy JF, et al. Results of microsurgical treatment of tubal infertility and early second-look laparoscopy in the post-pelvic inflammatory disease patient: implications for in vitro fertilization. *Am J Obstet Gynecol* 1986;154:1264.

Lundberg S, Wramsby H, Bremmer S, et al. Radionuclide hysterosalpingography is not predictive in the diagnosis of infertility. *Fertil Steril* 1998;69(2):216.

Luttjeboer F, Harada T, Hughes E, et al. Tubal flushing for subfertility Cochrance Database Syst. Rev. 2007; July 18;(3):CD003718.

Madlenat P, DeBrux J, Palmer R. L'etiologie des obstructions tubaires proximales et son rle dans le prognostic des implantations. *Gynecologie* 1977;28:47.

Mahadevan MM, Wiseman D, Leader A, et al. The effects of ovarian adhesive disease upon follicular development in cycles of controlled stimulation for in vitro fertilization. *Fertil Steril* 1985;44:489.

Marana R, Muscatello P, Muzii L, et al. Perlaparoscopic salpingoscopy in the evaluation of the tubal factor in infertile women. *Int J Fertil* 1990;35:211.

Marchino GL, Gigante V, Gennarelli G, et al. Salpingoscopic and laparoscopic investigations in relation to fertility outcome. *J Am Assoc Gynecol Laparosc* 2001;8:218.

McComb P. Microsurgical tubocornual anastomosis for occlusive cornual disease: reproducible results without the need for tubouterine implantation. *Fertil Steril* 1986;46:571.

McComb P, Gomel V. Cornual occlusion and its microsurgical reconstruction. *Clin Obstet Gynecol* 1980;23:1229.

McComb PF, Lee NH, Stephenson MD. Reproductive outcome after microsurgery for proximal and distal occlusions in the same fallopian tube. *Fertil Steril* 1991;56:134.

McComb PF, Paleologou A. The intussusception salpingostomy technique for the therapy of distal oviductal occlusion at laparoscopy. *Obstet Gynecol* 1991;78:443.

McComb PF, Taylor RC. Pregnancy outcome after unilateral salpingostomy with a contralateral patent oviduct. *Fertil Steril* 2001;76:1278.

Medical Research International, Society for Assisted Reproductive Technology, The American Fertility Society. In vitro fertilization-embryo transfer (IVF-ET) in the United States: 1989 results from the IVF-ET Registry. *Fertil Steril* 1991;55:14.

Mettler L, Giesel H, Semm K. Treatment of female infertility due to tubal obstruction by operative laparoscopy. *Fertil Steril* 1979;32:384.

Mettler L, Ibrahim M, Lehmann-Willenbrock E, et al. Pelviscopic reversal of tubal sterilization with the one- to two-stitch technique. *J Am Assoc Gynecol Laparosc* 2001;8:353.

Millingos SD, Kallipolitis GK, Loutradis DC, et al. Laparoscopic treatment of hydrosalpinx: factors affecting pregnancy rate. *J Am Assoc Gynecol Laparosc* 2000;7:355.

Molloy D, Martin M, Speirs A, et al. Performance of patients with a "frozen pelvis" in an in vitro fertilization program. *Fertil Steril* 1987;47:450.

Munro MG, Gomel V. Fertility-promoting laparoscopically directed procedures. *Reprod Med Rev* 1994;3:29.

Musset R. *An atlas of hysterosalpingography.* Québec: Les Presses de l'Université Laval, 1979.

Navot D, Bergh PA, Williams MA, et al. Poor oocyte quality rather than implantation failure as a cause of age-related decline in female fertility. *Lancet* 1991;337:1375.

Novy MJ, Thurmond AS, Patton P, et al. Diagnosis of cornual obstruction by transcervical fallopian tube cannulation. *Fertil Steril* 1988;50:434.

Oh ST. Tubal patency and conception rates with three methods of laparoscopic terminal salpingostomy. *J Am Assoc Gynecol Laparosc* 1996;3:519.

Paavonen J, Eggert-Kruse W. Chlamydia trachomatis: impact on human reproduction. *Hum Reprod Update* 1999;5:433.

Pabuccu R, Ulgenalp I, Baser I, et al. Microsurgical transposition of the human fallopian tube. *Gynecol Obstet Invest* 1991;31:51.

Papaioannou S, Afnan M, Girling AJ, et al. Diagnostic and therapeutic value of selective salpingography and tubal catheterization in an unselected infertile population. *Fertil Steril* 2003;79:613.

Patton PE, Williams TJ, Coulam CB. Results of microsurgical reconstruction in patients with combined proximal and distal tubal occlusion: double obstruction. *Fertil Steril* 1987;48:670.

Patterson PJ. Factors influencing the success of microsurgical tuboplasty for sterilization reversal. *Clin Reprod Fertil* 1985;3(1):57–64.

Pauerstein CJ, Turner T, Eddy CA. A technique for evaluating functional patency of the oviduct. *Fertil Steril* 1977;28:777.

Putman JM, Holden AEC, Olive DL. Pregnancy rates following tubal anastomosis: Pomeroy partial salpingectomy versus electrocautery. *J Gynecol Surg* 1990;6:173.

Reich H, McGlynn F, Parents C, et al. Laparoscopic tubal anastomosis. *J Am Assoc Gynecol Laparosc* 1993;1:16.

Ribeiro SC, Tormena RA, Giribela CG, et al. Laparoscopic tubal anastomosis. *Int J Gynaecol Obstet* 2004;84(2):142.

Rock JA, Guzick DS, Katz E, et al. Tubal anastomosis: pregnancy success following the reversal of Falope ring or monopolar cautery sterilization. *Fertil Steril* 1987;48:13.

Rock JA, Katayama KP, Martin EJ, et al. Factors influencing the success of salpingostomy techniques for distal fimbrial obstruction. *Obstet Gynecol* 1978;52:591.

Rogers AK, Goldberg SM, Hammel JP, et al. Tubal anastomosis by robotic compared to outpatient minilaprotomy. *Obstet Gynecol* 2007;109(6):1375–1380.

Rowe TC, Gomel V, McComb P. Investigations of tuboperitoneal causes of female infertility. In: Insler V, Lunenfeld B, eds. *Infertility, male and female.* Edinburgh: Churchill Livingstone; 1993:253.

Rubin IC. Non-operative determination of patency of fallopian tubes in sterility: intrauterine inflation with oxygen and production of a subphrenic pneumoperitoneum. *JAMA* 1920;74:1017.

Rubin IC. Roentgendiagnostik der uterus tumorens mit hilfe von intrauterine collargol injectionen vorlaeufige mitteilung. *Zentralbl Gynakol* 1914;38: 658.

Rubin IC. Therapeutic aspects of uterotubal insufflation in sterility. *Am J Obstet Gynecol* 1945;50:621.

Rufat P, Olivennes F, deMouzon J, et al. Task force report on the outcome of pregnancies and children conceived by in vitro fertilization (France: 1987 to 1989). *Fertil Steril* 1994;61:324.

Russell JB, Rodriguez Z, Komins JI. The use of transvaginal ultrasound to aspirate bilateral hydrosalpinges prior to in vitro fertilization: a case report. *J In Vitro Fert Embryo Transfer* 1991;8(4):213.

Schlaff WD, Hassiakos DK, Damewood MD, et al. Neosalpingostomy and distal tubal obstruction: prognostic factors and impact of surgical technique. *Fertil Steril* 1990;54:984.

Schlösser HW, Frantzen C, Mansour N, et al. Sterilisation Refertilisierung. Erfahrungen und Ergebnisse bei 119 microchirurgisch refertilisierten Frauen. *Geburtshilfe Frauenheilkd* 1983;43:213.

Sedbon E, Bouquet de la Joliniere J, Boudouris O, et al. Tubal desterilization through exclusive laparoscopy. *Hum Reprod* 1989;4:158.

Silber SJ, Cohen R. Microsurgical reversal of tubal sterilization: factors affecting pregnancy rate, with long-term follow-up. *Obstet Gynecol* 1984;64:679.

Singhal V, Li TC, Cooke ID. An analysis of factors influencing the outcome of 232 consecutive tubal microsurgery cases. *BJOG* 1991;98:628.

Society for Assisted Reproductive Technology, American Society for Reproductive Medicine. Assisted reproductive technology in the United States and Canada: 1992 results generated from the American Fertility Society/Society for Assisted Reproductive Technology Registry. *Fertil Steril* 1994;62: 1121.

Society for Assisted Reproductive Technology, American Society for Reproductive Medicine. Assisted reproductive technology in the United States and Canada: 1993 results generated from the American Society for Reproductive Medicine/Society for Assisted Reproductive Technology Registry. *Fertil Steril* 1995;64:13.

Society for Assisted Reproductive Technology and American Society for Reproductive Medicine. Assisted reproductive technology in the United States: 1997 results generated from the American Society for Reproductive Medicine/Society for Assisted Reproductive Technology Registry. *Fertil Steril* 2000;74:641.

Spivak MM, Librach CL, Rosenthal DM. Microsurgical reversal of sterilization: a six-year study. *Am J Obstet Gynecol* 1986;154:355.

Strandell A, Lindhard A, Waldenstrom U, et al. Hydrosalpinx and IVF outcome: a prospective, randomized, multicentre trial in Scandinavia on salpingectomy before IVF. *Hum Reprod* 1999;14:2762.

Strandell A, Lindhard A, Waldenstrom U, et al. Hydrosalpinx and IVF outcome: cumulative results after salpingectomy in a randomized, controlled trial. *Hum Reprod* 2001;16:2403.

Strandell A, Waldenstrom U, Nilsson L, et al. Hydrosalpinx reduces in-vitro fertilization/embryo transfer pregnancy rates. *Hum Reprod* 1994;9:863.

Stumpf PG, March CM. Febrile morbidity following hysterosalpingography: identification of risk factors and recommendations for prophylaxis. *Fertil Steril* 1980;33:487.

Sweeney WJ III, Gepfert R. The fallopian tube. *Clin Obstet Gynecol* 1965;8:32.

Swolin K. Electro microsurgery and salpingostomy: long-term results. *Am J Obstet Gynecol* 1975;121:418.

Swolin K. Fertiltatsoperationen: Teil I and II. *Acta Obstet Gynecol Scand* 1967;46:204.

Tan SL, Royston P, Campbell S, et al. Cumulative conception and live birth rates after in-vitro fertilization. *Lancet* 1992;339:1390.

Taylor PJ, Collins JA. *Unexplained infertility.* New York: Oxford Medical Publications; 1992.

Taylor RC, Berkowitz J, McComb PF. Role of laparoscopic salpingostomy in the treatment of hydrosalpinx. *Fertil Steril* 2001;75:594.

Templeton AA, Mortimer D. The development of a clinical test of sperm migration to the site of fertilization. *Fertil Steril* 1982;37:410.

teVelde ER, Boer ME, Looman CWN, et al. Factors influencing success or failure after reversal of sterilization: a multivariate approach. *Fertil Steril* 1990;54:270.

Thie JL, Williams TJ, Coulam CB. Repeat tuboplasty compared with primary microsurgery for postinflammatory tubal disease. *Fertil Steril* 1986;45: 784.

Thurmond AS. Selective salpingography and fallopian tube recanalization. *AJR Am J Roentgenol* 1991;156:33.

Tomazevic T, Ribic-Pucelj M, Omahen A, et al. Microsurgery and in-vitro fertilization and embryo transfer for infertility resulting from pathological proximal tubal blockage. *Hum Reprod* 1996;11:2613.

Tourgeman DE, Bhaumik M, Cooke GC, et al. Pregnancy rates following fimbriectomy reversal via neosalpingostomy: a 10 years retrospective analysis. *Fertil Steril* 2001;76:1041.

Trimbos-Kemper TCM. Reversal of sterilization of women over 40 years of age: a multicenter survey in the Netherlands. *Fertil Steril* 1990;53:575.

Tulandi T. Salpingo-ovariolysis: a comparison between laser surgery and electrosurgery. *Fertil Steril* 1986;45:489.

Tulandi T, Collins JA, Burrows E, et al. Treatment-dependent and treatment-independent pregnancy among women with periadnexal adhesions. *Am J Obstet Gynecol* 1990;162:354.

Tulandi T, Vilos GA. A comparison between laser surgery and electrosurgery for bilateral hydrosalpinx: a two year followup. *Fertil Steril* 1985;44: 846.

Tureck RW, Garcia C-R, Blasco L, et al. Perioperative complications arising after transvaginal oocyte retrieval. *Obstet Gynecol* 1993;81:590.

Uher J, Rypacek F, Presl J. Transport of novel ovum surrogates in the human fallopian tube: a clinical study. *Fertil Steril* 1990;54:278.

Urman B, Gomel V, McComb P, et al. Midtubal occlusion: etiology, management, and outcome. *Fertil Steril* 1992;59:747.

Urman B, Zouves C, Gomel V. Fertility outcome following tubal pregnancy. *Acta Eur Fertil* 1991;22:205.

van Noord-Zaadstra BM, Looman CWN, Alsbach H, et al. Delayed childbearing: effect of age on fecundity and outcome of pregnancy. *BMJ* 1991;302: 1361.

Van Voorhis BJ, Sparks AE, Syrop CH, et al. Ultrasound guided aspiration of hydrosalpinges is associated with improved pregnancy and implantation rates after in-vitro fertilization cycles. *Hum Reprod* 1998;13:736.

Verhoeven HC, Berry H, Frantzen C, et al. Surgical treatment for distal tubal occlusion: a review of 167 cases. *J Reprod Med* 1983;28:293.

Watson A, Vandekerckhove P, Lilford R. Techniques for pelvic surgery in subfertility. *Cochrane Database Syst Rev* 2003;3:CD000221.

Westrom L. Effect of acute pelvic inflammatory disease on fertility. *Am J Obstet Gynecol* 1975;121:707.

Westrom L. Incidence, prevalence and trends of pelvic inflammatory disease and its consequences in industrialized countries. *Am J Obstet Gynecol* 1980;138:880.

Westrom L, Joesoef MR, Reynolds GH, et al. Pelvic inflammatory disease and infertility. *Sex Transm Dis* 1992;14:185.

Wiegerinck MA, Ronkema M, Van Kessel PH, et al. Sutureless re-anastomosis by laparoscopy versus microsurgical re-anastomosis by laparotomy for sterilization reversal: a matched colort study. *Hum Reprod* 2005;20(8):2355–2358.

Winston RML. Reversal of sterilization. *Clin Obstet Gynecol* 1980;23:1261.

Winston RML, Margara RA. Microsurgical salpingostomy is not an obsolete procedure. *BJOG* 1991;98:637.

Xue P, Fa Y-Y. Microsurgical reversal of female sterilization. *J Reprod Med* 1989;34:451.

Yoon TK, Sung HR, Kang HG, et al. Laparoscopic tubal anastomosis: fertility outcome in 202 cases. *Fertil Steril* 1999; 72:1121.

Zouves C, Erenus M, Gomel V. Tubal ectopic pregnancy after in vitro fertilization and embryo transfer: a role for proximal occlusion or salpingectomy after failed distal tubal surgery? *Fertil Steril* 1991;56:691.

Zouves C, Gomel V. Gamete intrafallopian transfer (GIFT): procedure-dependent and procedure-independent pregnancy. *Infertility* 1990;13:163.

CHAPTER 22 ■ ENDOMETRIOSIS

JOHN S. HESLA AND JOHN A. ROCK

DEFINITIONS

Adenomyoma—A manifestation of adenomyosis characterized as localized, encapsulated disease of the uterine wall, as compared with the more common diffuse pattern of extension of endometrial glands and stroma in the myometrium.

Adenomyosis—Heterotopic endometrial glands and stroma located deep within the myometrium, with glandular extension below the endometrial-myometrial interface of at least 2.5 mm.

American Society for Reproductive Medicine (ASRM) Classification of Endometriosis—A scoring system to quantify the location and extent of endometriosis with a scalar rather than numeric terminology. This documentation has been proposed to allow direct comparison of patient responses to medical and surgical treatments and to identify factors predictive of disease outcome.

Atypical peritoneal implants of endometriosis—Lesions of varying appearance, including vesicles, flat plaques, raised blebs, polypoid structures, areas of fibrosis and adhesion formation, and peritoneal defects. May be clear, yellow, brown, blue, or black in color, as compared with the readily recognized red or gray implants.

Cancer antigen-125 (CA-125)—A high-molecular-weight glycoprotein expressed on the cell surface of some derivatives of embryonic coelomic epithelium. CA-125 is often elevated in cases of mild-severe endometriosis, as well as other conditions, including acute pelvic inflammatory disease, adenomyosis, uterine leiomyoma, menstruation, pregnancy, epithelial ovarian cancer, pancreatitis, and chronic liver disease.

Endometrioma—A solitary, nonneoplastic mass containing endometrial tissue and blood.

Endometriosis—The presence and growth of functioning endometrial tissue containing glandular and stromal elements in places other than the uterus that often results in severe pain and infertility.

Hydrodissection—Forceful injection of physiologic irrigant through a small defect created in the surfaces to be separated, such as the peritoneum from the retroperitoneal tissue. This may aid in establishment of the plane of dissection.

Presacral neurectomy—Division of the superior hypogastric plexus; useful as an adjunctive procedure to eliminate the uterine component of dysmenorrhea that results from endometriosis.

Reflux menstruation—Reflux of menses through fallopian tube to ectopic site, especially the peritoneal cavity. Proposed by John Sampson as a mechanism for the origin of endometriosis in many women.

Uterine nerve ablation—Division of the uterosacral ligaments at a point approximately 1.5 cm distal to the cervix to interrupt many sensory nerve fibers of the cervix and uterine corpus. Has been proposed to alleviate severe dysmenorrhea.

Uterine suspension—Surgical technique of elevation of the adnexa to reduce adhesion formation at denuded peritoneal surfaces of the posterior cul-de-sac, uterine serosa, and broad ligament.

Endometriosis is a clinical and pathologic entity initially described by von Rokitansky in 1860 that is characterized by the presence of tissue resembling functioning endometrial glands and stroma outside the uterine cavity. These ectopic implants can be located throughout the pelvic cavity, including the ovaries, uterine ligaments, rectovaginal septum, parietal peritoneum, intestinal serosa, and appendix. Less common sites of involvement include the cervix, hernial sacs, the umbilicus, laparotomy and episiotomy scars, and the pleural and pericardial cavities (Fig. 22.1).

Although endometriosis has been extensively investigated over the past century, it remains an enigmatic disease process. The association between endometriosis and infertility is still undefined, and there are scant data to support the many hormonal and surgical therapies that have been proposed. In addition, the often subtle and varied appearances of endometriosis can make recognition and surgical staging difficult, thereby casting doubt on the utility of the classification systems that have been developed. Nevertheless, the findings of well-designed clinical trials and recent studies that have elucidated the pathogenesis of endometriosis have enabled a more rational approach to the medical and surgical management of this disease.

PREVALENCE

The estimated prevalence of endometriosis among population groups varies depending on the presenting symptoms. One to seven percent of asymptomatic women undergoing tubal ligation are diagnosed with the disease at laparoscopy; this range may approximate the prevalence in the general population. Among women with pelvic pain, the prevalence of endometriosis ranges from about 5% to 21%, and the disease has been diagnosed in 40% to 52% of women with severe dysmenorrhea. Cramer and colleagues, in a multicenter study, diagnosed endometriosis in 17% of women with primary infertility, and in other series the prevalence varied from about 9% to 50%. Verkauf prospectively identified endometriosis in 38.5% of infertile women and 5.2% of fertile women. Other studies have confirmed the odds that infertile women are seven to 10 times more likely to have endometriosis than their fertile counterparts. However, any postmenarchal woman is at risk, because endometriotic implants have been identified in postmenopausal women, in women with primary amenorrhea secondary to müllerian anomalies, and in 69.6% of teenagers who underwent diagnostic laparoscopy for chronic pelvic pain.

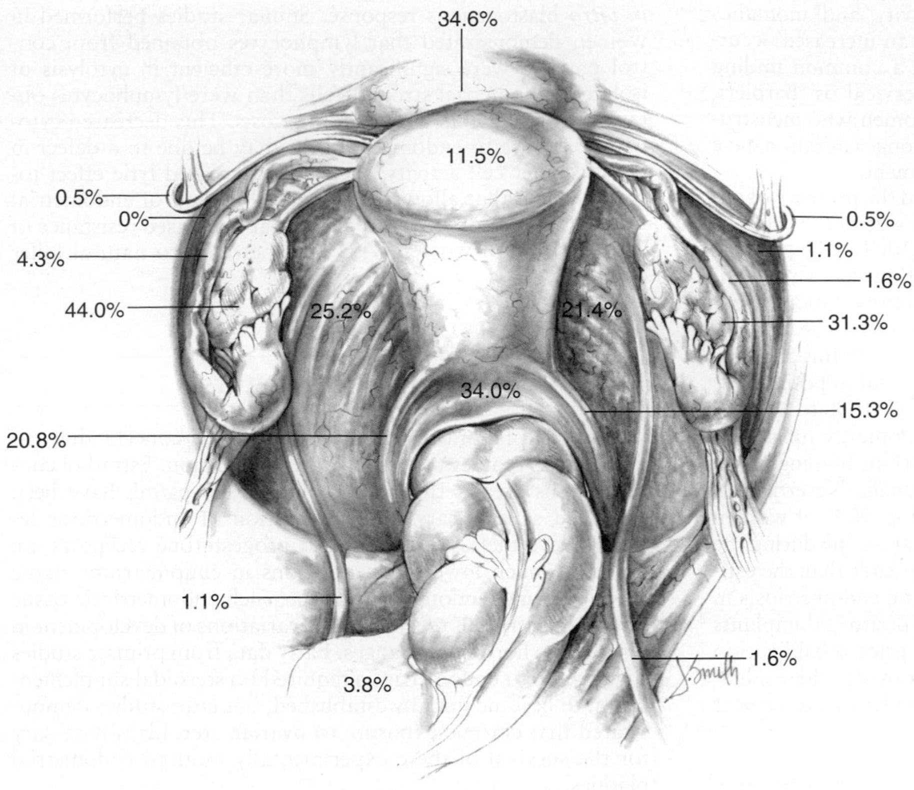

FIGURE 22.1. Anatomic locations of endometriosis implants in 182 consecutive infertility patients found to have endometriosis by laparoscopy. The rates shown indicate the percentage of all patients with implants in a given locale. (Redrawn from Jenkins S, Olive DL, Haney AF. Endometriosis: pathogenic implications of the anatomic distribution. *Obstet Gynecol* 1986;67:335.)

Several investigators have reported the possibility of a familial tendency to endometriosis. No studies have confirmed a human lymphocyte antigen linkage for the disease; a polygenic, multifactorial mode of inheritance has been suggested. Simpson and colleagues reported a 6.9% occurrence rate in first-degree female relatives, which compared with 1% for the non–blood-related control group.

HISTOGENESIS

The mechanism by which endometriosis develops is unknown, although there has been much discussion as to its origin (Table 22.1). A complete understanding of the histogenesis of the aberrant endometrial cells has been compromised because of the variations of disease presentation. Four major theories have been proposed:

1. The reflux and direct implantation theory suggests that viable endometrial cells reflux through the fallopian tubes during menstruation and implant on surrounding pelvic structures.
2. The coelomic metaplasia theory suggests that the multipotential cells of the coelomic epithelium may be stimulated to transform into endometrial-like cells.
3. The vascular dissemination theory suggests that endometrial cells enter the uterine vasculature or lymphatic system at menstruation and are transported to distant sites.
4. The autoimmune disease theory suggests that endometriosis is a disorder of immune surveillance that allows ectopic endometrial implants to grow.

TABLE 22.1

THEORIES FOR THE HISTOGENESIS OF ENDOMETRIOSIS

Transtubal regurgitation or retrograde menstruation
Direct implantation of endometrial cells
Metaplasia of coelomic epithelium
Lymphatic dissemination
Hematogenous spread
Activation of embryonic cell rests
Activation of wolffian rests
Metaplasia of urothelium
Hereditary factor
Immunologic factor

Reflux and Direct Implantation Theory

John Sampson first postulated that endometriosis arose from retrograde flow of fragments of endometrial tissue through the oviducts and into the peritoneal cavity. Much evidence validates this theory. The anatomic distribution of endometriosis as noted at laparoscopy is consistent with a reflux pattern of development; the most common sites of disease in the infertile woman are the ovary and uterosacral ligament, followed by the posterior uterus, posterior cul-de-sac, and posterior broad ligament. Endometriosis developed in monkeys when the uterus was surgically inverted to cause menstruation to occur intraperitoneally. Exposure of abraded peritoneum to endometrial cells has resulted in the growth of endometriotic implants in rabbits and rats. Endometriosis has developed in laparotomy, episiotomy, and cesarean section scars after surgical entrance into the endometrial cavity, and anomalies of the müllerian tract are associated with an increased occurrence of endometriosis. Endometriosis is a common finding in women with stenosis of the external cervical os (Barbieri, 1998). Epidemiologic data suggest that women who menstruate more frequently, more heavily, or for a longer duration have an increased likelihood of disease development.

Peritoneal implants of endometriosis and the presence of endometriomas are more common on the left side of the pelvis as compared with the right (Vercellini et al., 2004). The position of the sigmoid colon creates a sequestered microenvironment around the left adnexa, which facilitates implantation of endometrial cells regurgitated through the left tube. The large intestine does not provide the right hemipelvis with this anatomical shelter, because the cecum lies more cranial in position.

Focal endometriosis has been identified in 16% to 63% of proximal tubal segments after cautery or Pomeroy tubal sterilization, perhaps as a consequence of recurrent bathing of the healing terminal area with menstrual products. Nevertheless, bloody peritoneal fluid has been observed in 90% of women with patent fallopian tubes undergoing laparoscopy during the perimenstrual time period, a figure much greater than the estimated 2% to 5% prevalence of symptomatic endometriosis in women of reproductive age. Additionally, peritoneal implants have been identified in women who had a prior tubal ligation procedure and were undergoing laparoscopy for the evaluation of pelvic pain. Hence, other factors evidently are present to promote the ectopic implantation.

Coelomic Metaplasia Theory

The germinal epithelia of the ovary, endometrium, and peritoneum all originate from the same totipotential coelomic epithelium. The metaplasia theory postulates that these totipotential cells are transformed by repeated exposure to hormonal or infectious stimuli. This may explain the development of endometriotic lesions in unusual locations and in the odd cases of male patients in whom endometriosis develops after prostatectomy, orchiectomy, or prolonged treatment with estrogen. Reports of endometriosis in women with primary amenorrhea and an absence of functioning uterine endometrium and of endometriosis identified in mature teratomas also lend support to the metaplasia theory.

Vascular Dissemination Theory

Endometrial cells can be transported to extrauterine sites by blood vessels or the lymphatic system or by contamination of the pelvis or abdominal wall incision if the uterine cavity is surgically entered. Retroperitoneal endometriosis is hypothesized to arise from lymph vascular spread; 29% of patients with pelvic endometriosis documented on autopsy had pelvic lymph nodes that contained endometriosis. Theories of vascular dissemination help explain how endometriosis can develop in the lung or pericardium.

Autoimmune Disease Theory

Alterations in cellular immunity can facilitate the successful implantation of translocated endometrial cells. Compared with control subjects, monkeys with spontaneous endometriosis had both a lowered cell-mediated response to autologous endometrial tissue, as determined by skin testing, and a decreased *in vitro* blastogenesis response. Similar studies performed in women demonstrated that lymphocytes obtained from control patients were significantly more efficient in cytolysis of isolated endometrial stromal cells than were lymphocytes obtained from patients with endometriosis. This decreased cytotoxic response to endometrial cells may be due to a defect in natural killer cell activity, such as a decreased lytic effect toward stroma that allows ectopic development of endometrial fragments. In addition, there may be an increased resistance of endometrium in women with endometriosis to natural killer cytotoxicity.

Promoting Factors

Clinical and laboratory studies support the concept that endometriosis is an estrogen-dependent condition. Estradiol concentrations greater than approximately 60 pg/mL have been identified as necessary for proliferation of endometriotic lesions. Nevertheless, estrogen and progesterone receptors are found in much lower concentrations in endometriotic tissue than in normal endometrium tissue; such endometriotic tissue also frequently fails to show cyclic variations of development in response to hormonal changes. Early data from primate studies suggested that endometriosis required no steroidal supplementation to become initially established, but later studies demonstrated that chronic exposure to ovarian steroids is necessary for the survival of these experimentally induced endometrial plaques.

Growth factors can originate from the peritoneal environment to stimulate endometrial development. Platelet-derived growth factor, a macrophage secretory product, enhanced endometrial stromal cell proliferation in a dose-dependent manner. Similarly, macrophage-conditioned media promoted mouse endometrial stromal cell proliferation *in vitro,* and this activation was enhanced with the addition of estrogen. Increased concentrations of macrophage-derived growth factors, including vascular endothelial growth factor, have been identified in the peritoneal fluid of women with endometriosis. This suggests that changes in the vascular permeability and angiogenesis play an important role in the pathophysiology of this disease.

Molecular alterations in steroidogenic enzyme function have been implicated in the pathogenesis of endometriosis. Endometrial tissue from patients with endometriosis expresses aromatase P-450, whereas endometrium from control women without identifiable endometriosis does not. The presence of aromatase within endometriosis results in higher local production of estrogen necessary to support the growth and metabolic activity of the lesion.

Menstrual effluent contains factors that induce alterations in the peritoneal mesothelium, facilitating adhesion of endometrial cells. Attachment of endometrial cells is enhanced by induction of adhesion molecules and their receptors and the overexpression of matrix metalloproteinases and plasminogen activators. These factors ensure local destruction of the extracellular matrix. Suppression of matrix metalloproteinase production by progesterone decreased ectopic implantation of endometrium in the nude mouse, implicating these proteinases in the pathogenesis of endometriosis.

In summary, no single theory explains all cases of endometriosis, although the direct implantation mechanism seems the likely cause for most disease locations. Immunologic factors, inducing substances, or other mediators may explain the development of endometriosis in more distant sites.

NATURAL HISTORY

The natural history of endometriosis is not clearly understood. The disease appears to progress in most untreated patients, although spontaneous regression can occur in as many as 58% of milder cases. Surgical and medical therapies may promote a temporal regression but may not effectively eliminate microscopic, retroperitoneal, and hormonally resistant disease. Dmowski and Cohen described persistent disease in 15% of patients treated with danazol, and Henzl and associates noted a progression of disease during the course of treatment in 4% to 8% of patients receiving danazol or an analog of gonadotropin-releasing hormone (GnRH). When conservative surgery was combined with danazol or GnRH agonist therapy, the overall recurrence rate at 36 months was between 13.5% and 33%.

The effect of pregnancy on the clinical course of endometriosis is uncertain. Although Sampson proposed that pregnancy induces involution of implants, other authors recently described a variable response of endometriosis to pregnancy. It is possible that endometriosis becomes temporarily suppressed during pregnancy. McArthur and Ulfelder analyzed the clinical effect of pregnancy on endometriosis in 24 patients. They found that the behavior of endometriosis during the gravid state was extremely variable and that the regression of disease appeared to be due to decreased tissue responsiveness to hormonal stimulation rather than to actual necrosis of the lesions. More patients in their series experienced disease persistence than permanent regression. Monkey studies have confirmed these findings; the response of endometrial implants to pregnancy varied from total regression to significant progression.

Approximately 2% to 4% of early postmenopausal women suffer from endometriosis. These cases are usually associated with exogenous intake of estrogens or tamoxifen. Nevertheless, there are reports of symptomatic endometriosis in women older than 60 years of age who have not received steroid replacement therapy. Such cases presumably are secondary to the responsiveness of the residual lesions to low levels of estrogens that arise from peripheral conversion of ovarian and adrenal androgens.

PATHOPHYSIOLOGY

Gross Appearance

Signs of endometriosis may be evident on physical examination. Endometriosis can form tender nodules on the uterosacral ligaments that are readily palpable on rectovaginal examination. It may infiltrate the deepest portion of the pouch of Douglas and cause pain with defecation and, rarely, cyclic rectal bleeding. Lesions of endometriosis have been identified in the umbilicus, in the vulva, and in episiotomy scars. Complete ureteral obstruction has been reported. This can be temporarily reversed with the administration of GnRH agonists, progestogens, and danazol. Diaphragmatic involvement can lead to chronic, recurrent pneumothorax at the time of menstruation. Lesions have been identified in the upper and lower extremities, the pericardium, and the lung.

The gross appearance of endometriosis is extremely variable. On entering the abdomen, the surgeon may find a small, adherent nodule on one or both sides of the pelvis, usually attached to the posterior cul-de-sac and posterior surface of the uterus. Frequently, release of ovarian adhesions to mobilize the adnexa results in an egress of chocolate-colored or dark red fluid that is highly suggestive of endometriosis. Examination of the ovary may disclose a cyst that is rarely larger than 10 cm and has a dark, hemorrhagic lining. Endometriomas develop over a time span of a few months as a result of extensive intracystic hemorrhage. Reddish blue, fibrinous areas that represent small islands of endometriosis may be present on the ovarian cortex. Peritoneal implants vary in appearance from black, puckered lesions surrounded by a variable extent of fibrosis, to red polypoid material, to clear vesicles. Other appearances include yellow-brown peritoneal discoloration, white plaques, or scarring. The strong inflammatory stimulus of superficial lesions of endometriosis may promote fibrosis and invagination of adjacent peritoneal surfaces.

The fallopian tube is usually nonobstructed and free of gross disease, although peritubal adhesions can extend to adjacent structures, particularly in patients with extensive disease. Deeply infiltrating endometriotic nodules extend more than 5 mm beneath the peritoneum and may involve the uterosacral ligaments, bladder, ureters, or vagina. The depth of invasion has been correlated with pain symptomatology. Endometrial invasion of the rectal or sigmoidal wall can simulate malignancy or produce complete obstruction.

Microscopic Appearance

The essential diagnostic criterion is the presence of endometrial tissue, both stroma and glandular elements. This aberrant tissue resembles the uterine mucosa both histologically and physiologically. Secretory change and decidualization are seen in response to hormone influences in the luteal phase, and estrogen stimulates proliferation of the ectopic implants. Nevertheless, these functional changes are less uniform for implants than for the uterine mucosa.

The ultrastructural features of endometriosis are consistent with an incomplete response to the hormonal milieu. Endometriotic implants contain lower concentrations of progesterone and estrogen receptors than do corresponding normal endometrium, so the histologic response to progesterone is less profound. Gould and colleagues reported that the nucleus of endometriotic stromal cells had a marked degree of estrogen binding throughout the menstrual cycle, whereas stromal binding sites in the uterine endometrium were present only during the proliferative phase and not the secretory phase of the cycle. The differing responses of the two tissue types to steroid hormones were reflected by the modulation of estrogen binding and changes in glandular histology. Estrogen receptors did not undergo downregulation during the luteal phase of the cycle in endometriotic foci, despite an increase in endogenous progesterone concentration. Alterations in the quantity, activation, or function of the progesterone receptor may be responsible for this lack of change in estradiol receptors, the abnormal response of the ectopic endometrium to progesterone, and the failure of hormonal therapy in some patients.

Because of the pressure of retained blood in the cyst cavities of endometriomas, a large concentration of endothelial leukocytes heavily laden with hemosiderin (pseudoxanthoma cells) may be found, and the glandular lining may be nearly absent and replaced by reactive connective tissue elements. Biopsy may fail to yield histologic proof of the endometrial glands and stroma in about one third of all cases of typical clinical endometriosis, even if many tissue sections are analyzed.

The "chocolate cyst" description of the ovary is used synonymously with endometrial cyst or endometrioma. Nevertheless, other types of ovarian cysts may have a similar fluid content, including the hemorrhagic follicle, corpus luteum, or

TABLE 22.2

HISTOLOGY OF TUMORS ARISING IN ENDOMETRIOSIS

Histology	Numbers[a]	Incidence (%)
Endometrioid carcinoma		
Adenocarcinoma	96	46.4
Adenoacanthoma	43	20.8
Adenosquamous carcinoma	4	1.9
Clear cell carcinoma	28	13.5
Sarcoma, including mixed mesodermal tumor	24	11.6
Serous cystadenocarcinoma	6	2.9
Squamous cell carcinoma	3	1.4
Mucinous cystadenocarcinoma	2	1.0
Mixed germ cell tumor and adenocarcinoma	1	0.5
Totals	207	100

[a]Two patients had two different histologic patterns.
From Heaps JM, Nieberg RK, Berek JS. Malignant neoplasms arising in endometriosis. *Obstet Gynecol* 1990;75:1023, with permission.

cystadenoma. Pathologic confirmation of the diagnosis is always advised.

Approximately 0.7% to 1.0% of patients with endometriosis have lesions that undergo malignant transformation. Atypical glandular changes have been found in 3% to 6% of cases of ovarian endometriosis. Several histologic tumor types have been described (Table 22.2). Endometrioid adenocarcinomas account for 69% of reported lesions, with the ovary being the primary site in most cases. Rapidly enlarging endometriomas or those measuring greater than 10 cm should be sectioned carefully to search for malignant foci. Tumors arising in endometriosis are predominantly of low grade and confined to the site of origin. Progestogen therapy is recommended after surgical resection of these lesions.

Clinical Characteristics

The clinical features of endometriosis are varied, and the presentation depends on the site of growth and the severity of disease. The classic triad of dysmenorrhea, dyspareunia, and infertility has been described as characteristic of the disease (Table 22.3). Nevertheless, patients with extensive endometriosis may be clinically symptom free, and women with only minimal involvement may manifest disabling pelvic pain. Dysmenorrhea is a common symptom that most likely is associated with endometriosis if it develops after age 20 years, is progressive, and is not well relieved by nonsteroidal antiinflammatory agents or oral contraceptives. Spasmodic pain beginning before the onset of menstrual bleeding is another common symptom of patients with endometriosis. When the rectovaginal septum or uterosacral region is involved, the pain is often referred to the rectum or lower sacral and coccygeal regions because of premenstrual and menstrual swelling of ectopic implants. Dyschezia and constipation may be present. Dyspareunia is common, especially in cases of uterosacral or vaginal infiltration, fixed retroversion of the uterus, or ovarian fixation by adhesions. Again, there is no absolute correlation between the amount of visible endometriosis as seen at surgery and the extent of symptoms; minor disease involvement may result in severe pain, whereas massive areas of superficial endometriosis may cause no discomfort.

Other presenting symptoms can include signs of urinary tract involvement, such as hematuria or ureteral obstruction, unusual abdominal or adnexal masses, cyclic sciatica, catamenial pneumothorax or hemoptysis, and swollen and painful scars. Premenstrual spotting can occur for 3 to 7 days before the start of menses; this is a poorly recognized but relatively consistent sign of endometriosis. An endometrioma can leak, causing considerable pain, or it can rupture and produce a clinical picture much like that seen with a ruptured ectopic pregnancy or acute appendicitis. Nearly 10% of patients with

TABLE 22.3

SYMPTOMS ASSOCIATED WITH ENDOMETRIOSIS

Pelvic
Dysmenorrhea
Dyspareunia
Chronic pelvic pain
Sciatica
Premenstrual spotting
Gastrointestinal
Constipation
Diarrhea
Dyschezia
Tenesmus
Hematochezia
Urinary
Flank pain
Back pain
Abdominal pain
Urgency
Frequency
Hematuria
Pulmonary
Hemoptysis
Catamenial chest pain
Pneumothorax
Infertility

TABLE 22.4

POSSIBLE MECHANISMS BY WHICH ENDOMETRIOSIS CAUSES INFERTILITY

Mechanical interference
Pelvic adhesions
Chronic salpingitis
Altered tubal motility
Distortion of tuboovarian relations
Impaired oocyte pickup
Alterations in peritoneal fluid
Increased concentration of prostaglandins
Increased number of activated macrophages
Increased production of cytokines
Enhanced phagocytosis of sperm
Abnormal systemic immune system response
Increased cell-mediated gamete injury
Increased prevalence of autoantibodies
Antiendometrial antibody production
Hormonal or ovulatory dysfunction
Defective folliculogenesis
Luteinized unruptured follicle syndrome
Hyperprolactinemia
Luteal phase deficiency
Fertilization or implantation failure
Early spontaneous abortion

From Surrey ES, Halme J. Endometriosis as a cause of infertility. *Obstet Gynecol Clin North Am* 1989;16:79, with permission.

endometriosis present with acute symptoms that require exploration for diagnosis and treatment.

Approximately 20% to 40% of women with endometriosis are infertile. When extensive pelvic scarring or large endometriomas are present in the patient with endometriosis, the associated infertility can be clearly attributed to anatomic distortion. However, the pathophysiology of infertility in patients with less advanced disease is more controversial.

Endometriotic implants within the fallopian tube or ovary may promote a local inflammatory response that has a direct, deleterious effect on tubal function (Table 22.4). Oocyte pickup by the fallopian tube may be prevented despite the normal process of oocyte maturation and ovulation. Endometriosis and especially adenomyosis is associated with impeded hyperperistaltic and dysperistaltic uterotubal transport capacity. Chronic salpingitis was detected in 29 of 87 (33%) fallopian tubes of patients undergoing laparotomy for ovarian endometriosis; tubal obstruction was demonstrated in only one of these cases, although adhesions were present in 24%. Endometriosis has been identified in the resected segments of fallopian tubes in women undergoing tubal-cornual anastomosis for proximal tubal obstruction when there was no evidence of implants elsewhere in the pelvis. Others have reported a correlation between tubal endometriosis and chronic salpingitis in similar cases, although this finding has not been uniform.

Altered folliculogenesis or ovulation has been described in endometriotic patients who have undergone serial sonogram studies. An abnormal follicular growth rate and total growth period may disturb the normal synchronization of oocyte maturation, uterine receptivity, and ovulation. Tummon and coworkers reported that women with minimal endometriosis had more, yet smaller, follicles and lower preovulatory estradiol levels at the time of midcycle luteinizing hormone (LH) surge. Luteinized unruptured follicle (LUF) syndrome, a condition of normal ovulatory hormone secretion and luteinization of the follicle without the expected occurrence of ovulation, has been reported to be more common in patients with endometriosis. Mio and colleagues performed transvaginal ultrasound at least every other day from cycle day 8 through the third day after human chorionic gonadotropin (hCG) administration on 47 patients with endometriosis, predominantly minimal and mild, and 28 control patients with male factor infertility. LUF syndrome was diagnosed in 20 of 81 (24.7%) monitored cycles in endometriosis patients and in only 3 of 44 (6.8%) monitored cycles in control patients, a difference that achieved statistical significance. Schenken and associates also noted an increased rate of LUF and associated luteal phase deficiency in monkeys with surgically induced moderate to severe endometriosis. An absence of sonographic evidence of midcycle follicular collapse in patients with mild endometriosis has ranged from 4% to 35% in the literature.

Luteal phase function has been evaluated by endometrial biopsy and peripheral progesterone concentrations. There is insufficient evidence to conclusively link endometriosis with a deficiency of corpus luteum activity, although some studies have suggested the existence of a shortened luteal phase, delayed increase in progesterone secretion after ovulation, decreased progesterone secretion in the late luteal phase, and lowered serum estradiol levels during the early follicular phase.

The effect of endometriosis on fertilization and preimplantation development is widely debated. Peritoneal fluid from patients with endometriosis had a deleterious effect on sperm-oocyte interaction in homologous mouse and hamster fertilization assays. *In vitro* studies involving human zona pellucida confirmed an adverse effect of peritoneal fluid on sperm binding in this patient population, although others reported that peritoneal fluid from women with low-stage endometriosis had no detrimental effect on sperm motility characteristics. Peritoneal fluid from women with moderate and severe endometriosis caused declines in sperm motility and velocity. Exposure of two-cell mouse embryos to the peritoneal fluid or serum of patients with endometriosis has resulted in a decreased rate of cleavage and development to the blastocyst and hatching stages as compared with control nonendometriotic specimens. However, this association was not verified by similar studies of mouse embryo development and apoptosis.

Integrins are ubiquitous cell adhesion molecules that undergo dynamic alterations during the normal menstrual cycle in the human endometrium. The $\alpha v\beta 3$ vitronectin receptor integrin is normally expressed in endometrium during the periimplantation period; such expression may be lost in women with mild endometriosis, which may affect uterine receptivity.

A high frequency of spontaneous abortions in infertile women with endometriosis has been reported, although the relation was questioned because of potential control group bias. Naples and coworkers found that patients with endometriosis who refused treatment had the same abortion rate before and after diagnosis (26% and 25.5%). Studies of the last decade with appropriate control groups have demonstrated no substantial increase in the incidence of spontaneous abortion in women with endometriosis.

Mechanisms Influencing Symptoms

Because of the uncertain mechanisms causing infertility and pelvic pain in patients with minimal and mild endometriosis, many investigators have attempted to identify specific alterations in the peritoneal environment that would explain these symptoms. Significant increases or decreases in peritoneal fluid volume that are due to increased production by the ovaries, altered mesothelial permeability, or increases in the colloid osmotic pressure have been hypothesized to inhibit ovum capture by the fallopian tube or to adversely affect tubal transport. Koninckx and associates reported elevations in peritoneal fluid volume during cycle days 1 through 5 in patients with mild and moderate endometriosis. The quantity of fluid was comparable to that in control subjects during the remainder of the follicular phase. These authors described reduced volumes in the early luteal phase, which directly contrasts with findings reported by Oak and colleagues. Rock and associates evaluated patients during cycle days 8 through 12 and measured no difference in fluid volumes in patients with endometriosis compared with that in control subjects. Similar findings were noted by Rezai and associates. Hence, it appears unlikely that fluid volume alone plays a role in the establishment of infertility.

Peritoneal fluid from patients with minimal and mild endometriosis has been shown to increase macrophage proliferation *in vitro*. In addition, several studies have described increases in total macrophage number in the peritoneal fluid of patients with endometriosis. Hill and coworkers measured significant elevations in total leukocytes, macrophages, helper T cells, lymphocytes, and natural killer cells in women with stages I and II endometriosis. Activated macrophages may affect the reproductive process by altering sperm motility, fimbrial ovum capture, sperm-oocyte interaction, and early embryonic growth. Increased sperm phagocytosis by macrophages has been demonstrated by *in vivo* animal and *in vitro* human studies. Suginami and Yano have demonstrated the presence of an ovum capture inhibitor in peritoneal fluid from patients with endometriosis, which reduces fimbrial activity for ovum capture *in vitro*. This macromolecule may prevent contact between the fimbrial cells and cumulus oophorus.

Prostaglandins, interleukins, and other substances produced by macrophages may be harmful to reproduction. Fakih and colleagues demonstrated that interleukin-1 was present in the peritoneal fluid of almost all patients with endometriosis, but not in the fertile control group. Interleukins have been shown to adversely affect mouse embryo growth *in vitro*. In addition, interleukin-1 stimulated fibroblast proliferation, collagen deposition, and fibrinogen formation; hence, elevated concentrations of such lymphokines may account for the development of fibrosis and adhesions in advanced stages of endometriosis. Interleukin-6 secretion *in vitro* is upregulated in ectopic and eutopic endometrial stromal cells from women with endometriosis. Nevertheless, not all studies have confirmed the existence of a difference in interleukin activity between endometriosis patients and control groups. Decreased plasminogen activator activity in endometriotic implants may also be a cause for increased adhesion formation.

Bleeding from ectopic endometrial implants may promote the formation of free oxygen radicals. The iron in hemoglobin may be the catalyst of free radical reactions. Free radicals may damage proteins, carbohydrates, nucleotides, and lipids, resulting in tissue damage and *de novo* adhesions.

Chronic elevations in the level of peritoneal prostaglandins have been hypothesized to interfere with ovulation, to alter tubal mobility such that the embryo may arrive in the uterus at a suboptimal time for implantation, or to diminish corpus luteum function. Drake and associates measured the metabolites of prostacyclin and thromboxane A_2 in peritoneal fluid and noted a 10-fold increase in these levels in patients with endometriosis. Ylikorkla and colleagues confirmed these observations, although the increase in prostanoid metabolites in the patients with endometriosis was less than twice that of the controls. When cycle stage was experimentally controlled, Rock and coworkers, Rezai and associates, and others failed to demonstrate a significant change in prostaglandin levels in peritoneal fluid from patients with endometriosis as compared with control groups. In addition, prostaglandin concentrations did not vary between the follicular and luteal phase in either endometriosis patients or controls. Variations in collection of samples during the menstrual cycle, selection of control groups, and collection techniques have compromised the interpretation of data regarding the relative importance of prostanoid content in peritoneal fluid in the studies that have been published on this topic.

Alterations in the systemic immune response of endometriosis patients may influence fecundity. Cellular and humoral abnormalities have been reported in the peripheral blood and peritoneal fluid of women with endometriosis. Translocated endometrial cells may implant only in patients with an inherent defect in cell-mediated immunity. Functional changes in monocytes and macrophages, natural killer cells, cytotoxic T lymphocytes, and B cells suggest decreased surveillance, recognition, and destruction of misplaced endometrial cells and possible facilitation of their implantation. The endometrial proteins of menstrual fluid may be recognized as foreign by the host and trigger an autoimmune response. This host reaction can be variable, thus explaining why some women with a weak autoimmune response and varying extent of disease can conceive with no difficulty. Other investigators have confirmed a high prevalence of autoantibodies against endometrial and ovarian tissues in the sera and cervical and vaginal secretions of women with endometriosis.

Nonspecific polyclonal B-cell activation has been postulated to exist in endometriosis, but there is a lack of substantive data to demonstrate that this association contributes significantly to endometriosis-associated subfertility.

Dioxin, a pollutant that is known to decrease cell-mediated cytotoxicity by reducing the number of helper T cells, has been suggested as a causative factor in the high incidence of endometriosis in developed countries. Heilier and associates documented an increase in dioxinlike compounds in the serum of women with peritoneal endometriosis and deep endometriotic (adenomyotic) nodules. Moreover, a dose-dependent relation existed between dioxin exposure and the subsequent development and severity of endometriosis in the rhesus monkey after a latent period of more than 5 years.

Nevertheless, other studies have suggested that endometriosis may not promote immunologic alterations in the pelvis. In a retrospective analysis of the cell count and volume of peritoneal fluid in 135 infertile women with endometriosis, Haney and colleagues found a negative correlation between total cell numbers and extent of disease and no significant correlation between fluid volume and extent of disease. Similarly, in the rabbit model of endometriosis, there was no difference in peritoneal fluid volume, macrophage numbers, or macrophage activation in treated versus control animals.

Hence, the exact cause-and-effect relation between endometriosis and infertility in the absence of a distortion in pelvic anatomy remains unknown. In a recent study using an adhesion-free rabbit model of endometriosis, peritoneal implants did not adversely affect the number of corpora lutea, the oocyte recovery or fertilization rates, tubal transport, embryonic development and cleavage, or nidation index. Similarly, Mahmood and Templeton were unable to detect differences in hormonal patterns of the menstrual cycle, follicular growth, preovulatory peritoneal fluid volume and sex steroid concentration, rate of LUF, oocyte maturity, fertilization rate, or cleavage rate between patients with minimal and mild endometriosis and control women.

Little is known about the mechanisms by which endometriosis induces pain symptoms. Dyspareunia may be related to stimulation of pain fibers by stretching of scarred, inelastic tissue or by direct pressure on nodules of endometriosis embedded in fibrotic tissue. Endometriosis implants may secrete inflammatory substances such as prostaglandins, cytokines, and growth factors that initiate the sequence of events that result in the development of pain. Moreover, the extravasated debris and blood from endometriotic implants may stimulate an inflammatory reaction within the peritoneal cavity with production of the aforementioned substances.

DIAGNOSIS

Symptoms

Dysmenorrhea, dyspareunia, and pelvic, back, and rectal pain—the more common symptoms of endometriosis—have been assumed to be caused by endometrial implants. However, the development of such symptoms is not diagnostic of the disease state. In one random survey of women in the general population, more than 60% reported dyspareunia at some point in their lives, and 33% had persistent discomfort. The prevalence of laparoscopically diagnosed endometriosis in patients with chronic pelvic pain has ranged from 4% to 52% in published series. The age of peak diagnosis of endometriosis based on presenting symptom is pelvic pain, age 15 to 24 years; infertility, age 25 to 34 years; and dysfunctional uterine bleeding, age 35 to 44 years (Leibson et al.).

Some authorities have suggested that the symptoms may be dependent on the location of the implants, the presence of adhesions, distortion of ovarian anatomy by endometriosis, and involvement of other organs, such as the ureter or rectum. However, Fedele and colleagues found no significant association between the American Fertility Society (AFS; now known as the American Society for Reproductive Medicine) classification of disease stage and the presence and severity of dysmenorrhea, pelvic pain, and dyspareunia in a prospective study of 160 women. The pain profiles of the patients with ovarian lesions were similar to those of the patients with peritoneal or ovarian and peritoneal disease. Conversely, in a later study by the same group, ovarian endometriomas were the only lesions significantly associated with severe dysmenorrhea and pelvic pain in infertile women.

Koninckx and coworkers demonstrated that the presence of pelvic pain did not correlate with the total area of endometriosis, type of lesion, or volume of disease. The only significant discriminator proved to be the depth of infiltration; endometriotic lesions greater than 1 cm in depth were associated with severe discomfort (Fig. 22.2). This supports earlier data that strongly linked pain with deep infiltration of the fibromuscular tissue of the pelvis.

Pain symptoms generally correlate with fluctuations in steroid hormone concentrations. In response to cyclic stimulation by ovarian estradiol and progesterone, endometriotic lesions undergo epithelial and stromal proliferation, variable secretory changes, stromal pseudodecidual reaction, and periodic regression in a manner more disorganized than, yet similar to, that of normal endometrium. Surgical castration and ovarian hormonal suppressive therapy result in diminution of pain in most patients.

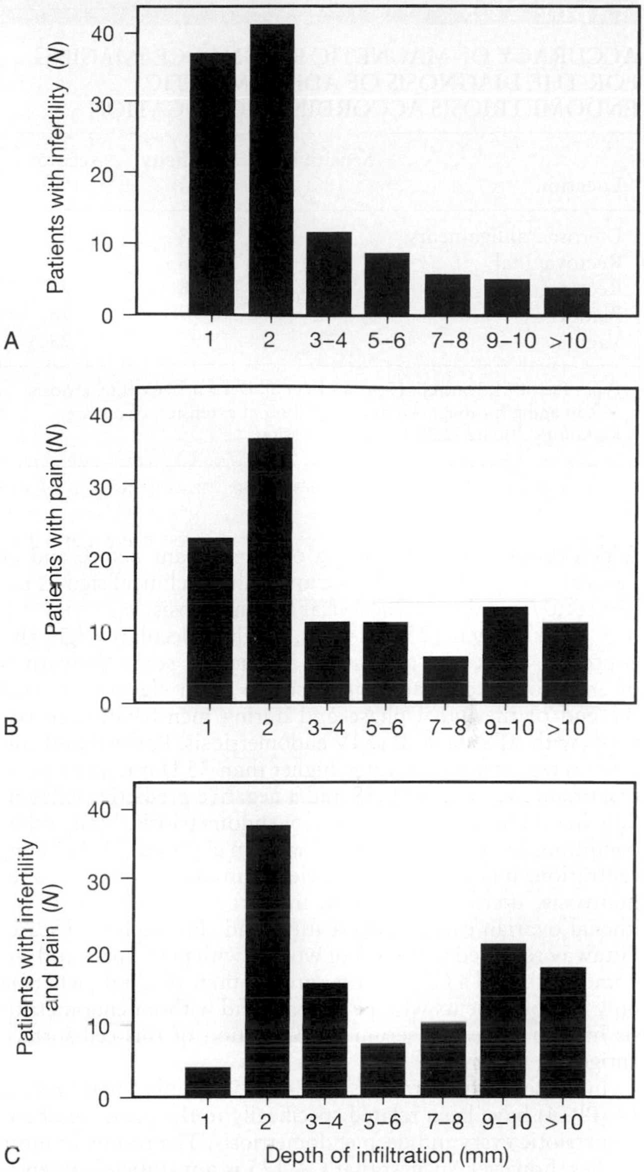

FIGURE 22.2. Frequency distributions of depth of infiltration of pelvic endometriosis in women with (A) infertility (N = 283), (B) pain (N = 119), or (C) infertility and pain (N = 48). (Redrawn from Koninckx PR, Mueleman C, Demeyere S, et al. Suggestive evidence that pelvic endometriosis is a progressive disease, whereas deeply infiltrating endometriosis is associated with pelvic pain. *Fertil Steril* 1991;55:759.)

Physical Findings

Bimanual pelvic examination may reveal tender uterosacral ligaments, cul-de-sac nodularity, induration of the rectovaginal septum, fixed retroversion of the uterus, adnexal masses, and generalized or localized pelvic tenderness. The adherent tube and ovary may constitute a tender, irregular mass that is similar in characteristics to the mass palpated in cases of chronic salpingo-oophoritis. Uterosacral nodules occasionally reach 1 cm or more in size. Lesions implanted in the retrocervical area or rectovaginal wall are frequently more easily felt than seen and can be missed if the physical examination is omitted.

TABLE 22.5

ACCURACY OF MAGNETIC RESONANCE IMAGING FOR THE DIAGNOSIS OF ADENOMYOTIC ENDOMETRIOSIS ACCORDING TO LOCATION

Location	Sensitivity (%)	Specificity (%)	Accuracy (%)
Uterosacral ligaments	76	83	80
Rectovaginal	80	98	97
Rectosigmoid	88	98	95
Bladder	88	99	98
Vagina	76	95	93

From Bazot M, Darai E, Hourani R, et al. Deep pelvic endometriosis: MR imaging for diagnosis and prediction of extension of disease. *Radiology* 2004;232:379, with permission.

A perceptible, painful swelling of the implant before and at menstruation remains a classic and reliable clinical sign of active rectovaginal or retrocervical endometriosis.

Cancer antigen-125 (CA-125), a high-molecular-weight glycoprotein expressed on the cell surface of some derivatives of embryonic coelomic epithelium, is often elevated toward the end of the luteal phase and during menstruation in patients with AFS stages II to IV endometriosis. Barbieri and colleagues reported that a value higher than 35 U/mL had a positive predictive value of 0.58 and a negative predictive value of 0.96 in establishing the presence of endometriosis. Many other conditions have been associated with an elevated CA-125 concentration, including acute pelvic inflammatory disease, adenomyosis, uterine leiomyoma, menstruation, pregnancy, epithelial ovarian cancer, pancreatitis, and chronic liver disease. Pittaway reported that 80% of women with pelvic pain and endometriosis had a CA-125 titer greater than 16 U/mL, whereas only 6% of patients with pelvic pain and without endometriosis had an increased serum concentration of this cell-surface antigen.

Increased concentrations of CA-125 and placental protein 14 (PP14) have been related specifically to the presence of endometriotic cysts and deep endometriosis. The results of most studies, however, suggest that CA-125 is not sufficiently sensitive to identify lesser stages of endometriosis and is therefore not reliable as a screening test. Doppler sonographic evaluation of resistance indices in the vessels of adnexal masses increases the sensitivity and negative predictive values of two-dimensional sonography and CA-125, but this yields many false-positive results because of the neovascularity of benign tumors. Magnetic resonance imaging (MRI) may be helpful in assessing deep pelvic and extrapelvic endometriosis (Table 22.5).

Visual Findings

The patient with unexplained lower abdominal pain or a presentation suggesting endometriosis requires laparoscopy for definitive diagnosis. Ultrasonography and other noninvasive procedures cannot provide the specific information needed to diagnose or classify the extent or severity of disease. For proper laparoscopic evaluation, a double puncture technique is essential. The ancillary probe or forceps placed through the lower abdominal sheath permits mobilization of the tubes and ovaries. A methodical regimented approach should be used to thoroughly inspect the lateral side walls, all ovarian surfaces, both sides of the broad ligaments, the bladder and bowel serosa, and the inferior aspects of the cul-de-sac. Uterine manipulation with a cannula fixed to the cervix facilitates evaluation of the uterosacral ligaments and rectal serosa. Photography and video recording are useful for documentation of findings.

Awareness of the wide range of visual appearances of endometriosis is necessary for accurate diagnosis and appropriate surgical therapy of the disease. Although darkly pigmented lesions are readily recognizable and are considered a classic presentation of endometriosis, less discernible yet common forms of implants were described as early as the 1920s, when Sampson noted "red raspberries, purple raspberries, blueberries, blebs, and peritoneal pockets." The black or blue puckered "powder-burn" implant is a late consequence of cyclic growth and regression of the lesion, to the point that bleeding and hemosiderin staining of the tissue have occurred. Biopsy of such areas reveals inactive endometrial glands and fibrous stroma.

Distinctive morphologic variations include vesicles, flat plaques, raised lesions, polypoid structures, areas of fibrosis and adhesion formation, and peritoneal defects (Table 22.6). Yellow, brown, blue, or black coloration is proportional to the amount of hemosiderin deposition. Red polypoid lesions share the closest histologic characteristics with native endometrium and are thought to have the greatest metabolic activity, as is suggested by their high concentrations of prostaglandin metabolites. Biopsy of nonpigmented implants (i.e., implants that are the same color as adjacent peritoneum) may reveal active endometriotic glands and stroma. White lesions are predominantly fibromuscular scarring with scattered glandular and stromal elements, and brown lesions are mainly hemosiderin deposits. Peritoneal defects and subovarian adhesions contain

TABLE 22.6

HISTOLOGIC CONFIRMATION OF LESIONS CATEGORIZED BY APPEARANCE

Investigators	Confirmation by appearance (%)						
	Black	White	Red	Glandular	Subovarian adhesions	Yellow-brown patches	Pockets
Jansen and Russell, 1986	—	81	81	67	50	47	47
Stripling et al., 1988	97	91	75	—	—	33	—
Martin et al., 1989	94	80	75	66	39	22	39

endometriosis in 40% to 70% of cases. Because other peritoneal lesions share morphologic features similar to those of endometriosis, the differential diagnosis is broad and includes old suture locations, epithelial malignancies, hemangioma, inflammatory reaction to infection or oil-based hysterosalpingogram dye, and carbon deposition from laser surgery. Rectovaginal endometriotic lesions consist of smooth muscle with active glandular epithelium and scanty stroma. They share similar characteristics to adenomyomas.

Small endometriotic lesions become more visible during the premenstrual and menstrual phases of the cycle, because during this time microfoci of peritoneal disease become congested with blood and debris. In addition, vascular dilatation, superficial hemorrhage, and ecchymosis formation cause accentuation of the more typical features of endometriosis. Performance of laparoscopy at a time when ovarian steroidogenesis is suppressed by medications such as GnRH analogs or progestogens can lead to inaccuracies in the assessment of extent of disease.

Jansen and Russell reported the presence of nonpigmented lesions in 38% of their 202 patients with biopsy-proven endometriosis; 15% had only nonpigmented implants. Most areas of pigmented endometriosis are surrounded by nonpigmented endometriosis. These subtle lesions may represent the first stage of development of peritoneal disease. Recognition of nonpigmented endometriosis may be enhanced by "painting" the peritoneum with the patient's blood or by filling the pelvis with irrigation fluid and submerging the laparoscope to appreciate the three-dimensional configuration of clear lesions. Subtle lesions are likely to originate from microscopic glands; they appear and disappear like blebs on the peritoneal surface. With progressive fibrosis, these implants become the classic pigmented, scarred lesions, and finally, when fibrosis replaces the stroma, they appear as white, inactive disease.

The ability to detect subtle lesions of endometriosis increases with the experience of the surgeon and is reinforced by histologic confirmation. Although depth perception is impaired when the monocular lens of the laparoscope is used to view the pelvic cavity, the magnification ability of this lens when closely approximated to the peritoneum may allow identification of subtle surface irregularities present in occult disease. Magnification up to 10× power can be obtained with the laparoscope, depending on the working distance. Microscopic implants of endometriosis not visible even with 10× magnification have been documented by scanning electron microscopy in peritoneal biopsies of patients with unexplained infertility who had no evidence of disease at the time of laparoscopy. A scanning electron microscopic study of samples of supposedly normal tissue from endometriosis patients has documented the presence of endometriotic foci in 25% of cases. Lesions as small as 200 μm have been identified through this technique. Hence, surgical treatment of all visible disease is more accurately described as cytoreductive rather than ablative.

An ovarian endometrial cyst is usually formed by an inversion of the ovarian cortex. The frontal surface of the ovary in proximity to the hilus is the most common site for the invagination process to occur. Adhesions are common from the ovary to the fossa ovarica or to the posterior leaf of the parametrium. Recognition of deep ovarian endometriosis is necessary for correct surgical staging. Small endometriomas were diagnosed in 48% of infertile women with mildly enlarged ovaries (3.5 to 5 cm in diameter) when the ovaries were punctured with a 16-gauge needle. The ovarian surfaces were without gross disease in this series of patients. Preoperative sonographic evaluation is a useful screening test for the presence of small endometrial cysts; their identification may affect the disease categorization to which the patient is assigned. Sonographic patterns may indicate purely cystic features, cystic features with few septations or minimal debris, complex combinations of cystic and solid elements, and largely solid features. More recently, fat-saturated MRI has been shown to be an acceptable tool for detecting endometriomas larger than 4 mm in diameter. Deep ovarian endometriosis is frequently associated with the presence of intestinal or more extensive pelvic disease.

Vercellini and colleagues studied the visual diagnostic parameters of ovarian endometriomas at laparotomy in 245 women with ovarian cysts. The gross characteristics that established the diagnosis included a size smaller than 12 cm in diameter; adhesions to the pelvic side wall, to the posterior broad ligament, or to both; the presence of powder-burn lesions; superficial endometriosis with adjacent puckering on the surface of the ovary; and tarry, thick, chocolate-colored fluid content. These criteria yielded a sensitivity of 97%, a specificity of 95%, and an accuracy of 96%.

An adnexal mass in a patient with known pelvic endometriosis cannot be assumed to be an endometrial cyst of the ovary. Ovarian malignancy must remain in the differential diagnosis; the size of the mass has been correlated with malignancy. In a study of 180 women, 1% of masses smaller than 5 cm, 11% of masses between 5 and 10 cm, and 72% of masses larger than 10 cm were malignant. Most of these malignant tumors were adenocarcinoma.

The rules that apply to the management of all women in whom an adnexal mass develops also apply to patients with endometriosis with an adnexal mass. Among women of reproductive age, unilateral adnexal masses that are cystic and unilocular with regular borders on ultrasound examination are likely to be benign, whereas masses with solid areas, septa, papillations, or irregular borders have a greater likelihood of being malignant. Endometriomas vary in their appearance but usually have regular borders and slightly thickened and diffuse internal echoes unless fresh hemorrhage is present. Sensitivity and specificity of transvaginal ultrasound have been reported by Eskenazi and colleagues to be 84% to 100% and 90% to 100%, respectively.

The depth of peritoneal infiltration by endometriosis cannot be evaluated by inspection alone. Deep endometriosis, which is almost exclusively localized to the posterior cul-de-sac and the uterosacral ligaments, is better detected by palpation and becomes even more apparent during excision. Deep endometriosis has been recognized to become smaller with increasing depth, although in some women, the largest volume is hidden under an adhesion involving the bowel or is buried in the rectovaginal septum. Diagnosis is enhanced if clinical examinations are performed during menstruation in women with chronic pelvic pain, severe dysmenorrhea, or deep dyspareunia. In most cases, a nodule is more palpable at this time.

Koninckx and Martin have described three types of infiltrating endometriosis. Type I is characterized by a large pelvic area of typical or subtle lesions surrounded by white sclerotic tissue. During excision, deep disease becomes obvious and grows progressively smaller with deeper sectioning of tissue (like a cone). Type II is formed by retraction of the bowel and is recognized clinically as a small classic lesion associated with retraction. In some women, no implant is visible, but induration is associated with the retraction. Excision usually reveals the presence of a nodule. Type III is nodular endometriosis of the rectovaginal septum. This category is clinically suspected at the time of rectovaginal examination when painful nodularities are noted. Occasionally, nodular endometriosis presents as small, typical lesions at laparoscopy or as dark blue cysts at the vaginal fornix during speculum examination. Type III disease is the most severe and often spreads laterally to involve the ureter.

CLASSIFICATIONS

Many endometriosis classification systems have been introduced to allow direct comparison of patient responses to medical and surgical treatments and to identify factors predictive of disease outcome. No system has yet been devised that is entirely satisfactory. AFS (renamed the American Society for Reproductive Medicine) organized a panel of experts in 1979 to develop a classification system that might serve as a basis for evaluating various therapies. The committee devised an innovative scheme based on the natural progression of the disease. Three anatomic areas—the peritoneum, ovary, and fallopian tube—were examined for the presence of endometriosis or adhesions, with allowances made for unilateral involvement. However, the system was not weighted for depth of infiltration of peritoneal implants. A point system instead assigned values to each area of disease involvement based on the presumption that implant area and adhesion characteristics were most often associated with disease prognosis. The stage of disease was determined by the cumulative score of the assigned points. This classification system was criticized for its arbitrary division of endometriosis into categories that did not necessarily reflect the true relative risk of disease sequelae, pain, and infertility.

The AFS classification was revised in 1985 to provide a more standard assessment of endometriosis for correlation of surgical treatment with distribution and severity of implants (Table 22.7). The point range of mild disease was expanded, and greater weight was given to deep endometriosis, dense adhesions, and cul-de-sac obliteration by adhesive disease. Although the revised staging system appropriately acknowledges the importance of adhesive disease and endometriomas, most women with extensive peritoneal disease in the absence of ovarian involvement, particularly deeply invasive implants, receive a very low score on laparoscopic inspection of the lesions.

This revised AFS classification has been widely used by investigators to categorize disease states. Nevertheless, direct comparison of treatment outcome is compromised by inconsistencies in the application of the staging criteria and by the great variations in medical and surgical therapeutic options being applied in the management of endometriosis. Evaluation of the extent of disease by laparoscopy may be limited by a lack of recognition of atypical implants, particularly if the patient is hypoestrogenic as a result of recent discontinuation of medical therapy for endometriosis. Furthermore, the divisions between stages of endometriosis remained arbitrary, the point score for ovarian involvement was weighted too heavily, and the classification scheme did not address disease involving the fallopian tubes, intestines, or urinary tract. Also, there were no parameters to indicate the present activity and state of evolution of the disease.

The Endometriosis Classification Subcommittee of the American Society for Reproductive Medicine (ASRM) released new recommendations in 1996 for the documentation of the extent and location of disease. One concern over the reproducibility of the scoring system was directed at the variability in assessing ovarian endometriosis and cul-de-sac obliteration. The subcommittee indicated that an endometriotic cyst should be confirmed by histology or by the presence of the following features: (i) cyst diameter less than 12 cm; (ii) adhesion to pelvic

TABLE 22.7

THE AMERICAN SOCIETY FOR REPRODUCTIVE MEDICINE REVISED CLASSIFICATION OF ENDOMETRIOSIS[a]

Endometriosis	<1 cm	1–3 cm	>3 cm
Peritoneum			
Superficial	1	2	4
Deep	2	4	6
Ovary			
Right superficial	1	2	4
Right deep	4	16	20
Left superficial	1	2	4
Left deep	4	16	20
Posterior			
Cul-de-Sac	Partial	Complete	
Obliteration	4	40	
Adhesions	<1/3 Enclosure	1/3–2/3 Enclosure	>2/3 Enclosure
Ovary			
Right filmy	1	2	4
Right dense	4	8	16
Left filmy	1	2	4
Left dense	4	8	16
Tube			
Right filmy	1	2	4
Right dense	4[b]	8[b]	16
Left filmy	1	2	4
Left dense	4[b]	8[b]	16

[a]Determination of the stage or degree of endometrial involvement is based on a weighted point system. The following categories have been established: stage I (minimal disease) 1–5 points; stage II (mild disease) 6–15 points; stage III (moderate disease) 16–40 points; stage IV (severe disease) >40 points.
[b]If the fimbriated end of the fallopian tube is completely enclosed, change the point assignment to 16.

side wall and/or broad ligament; (iii) endometriosis on surface of ovary; (iv) tarry, thick, chocolate-colored fluid content. Cul-de-sac obliteration should be considered partial if some normal peritoneum is visible below the uterosacral ligaments, but adhesions or endometriosis have obliterated part of the cul-de-sac. Complete obliteration exists when no peritoneum is visible below the uterosacral ligaments. Because information is accumulating to suggest that the morphologic appearance of the endometriotic implants may correlate with biologic activity and consequently fertility, the newly revised classification scheme requests the categorization of lesions as red, white, and black. The percentage of surface involvement of each implant type is to be documented.

This revised ASRM classification system is oriented toward the infertile population. Muzii and colleagues, using a pain questionnaire administered to women before surgery, found a significant correlation between the severity of dysmenorrhea and total revised ASRM score, partial score for deep disease, and partial score for adhesions. However, they found no correlation between the pain score for dysmenorrhea and the partial score for superficial disease, number of typical and atypical implants, or the total number of implants. Limited knowledge of the specific pathophysiologic alterations by which endometriosis can cause these symptoms has so far prevented any precise categorization of disease based on response to conventional therapies for these symptoms.

THERAPIES

Although women with endometriosis can present with a range of symptoms, therapy is usually initiated for the correction of pain, infertility, or a persistent pelvic mass. Pain and infertility can coexist in a patient; nevertheless, many women with endometriosis-associated infertility have relatively little or no discomfort. Treatment options vary depending on the clinical history and findings at the time of surgery.

Expectant Management

Treatment of mild and moderate endometriosis with hormonal preparations may not offer any advantage over expectant management in promoting conception. In studies by Seibel and colleagues, Hull and associates, and Telimaa, patients assigned to expectant management conceived earlier than the medically treated group, and the cumulative pregnancy rate was not higher for women receiving progestogens or danazol. This lack of enhancement of fecundity may be related to the lower number of estrogen, progesterone, and androgen receptors in endometriotic lesions as compared with normal endometrium. Nevertheless, patients who have pelvic pain or dysmenorrhea and minimal or mild disease do benefit from hormonal therapy.

The age of the patient and the duration of her infertility are important factors to consider in determining the appropriate therapy for the symptomatic individual. Laparoscopic laser ablation of milder stages of endometriosis appears to lessen the interval to conception, although the cumulative pregnancy rate may not be greater than that of women managed expectantly. Surgical therapy for more advanced disease results in a higher pregnancy rate than does expectant management or hormonal treatment, partly because of correction of mechanical factors that may be inhibiting ovulation or tubal function.

There is no direct evidence to support the contention that surgical treatment of minimal or mild endometriosis in the asymptomatic patient will hinder future disease progression and sequelae. The potential benefits of cytoreductive therapy must be weighed against the risk of adhesion formation through surgical devitalization of peritoneal surfaces.

Medical Treatment

Mild pain symptoms associated with endometriosis may be effectively treated with nonsteroidal antiinflammatory agents and oral contraceptives (Fig. 22.3). Additional endocrinologic therapies include progestogens, GnRH agonists, and danazol. These agents have similar degrees of efficacy in the relief of pain symptoms; side effects vary depending on their mechanism of action. At restoration of ovulation and of physiological levels of estrogen, both eutopic and ectopic endometrium resume metabolic activity. Therefore, medical therapy is symptomatic rather than curative, and most patients experience pain relapse at suspension of treatment.

Progestogens

By inhibiting the pituitary release of LH, progestogens suppress ovarian steroidogenesis and promote endometrial glandular atrophy, apoptosis, and extensive decidual transformation of the stroma. Progestogens oppose the growth-promoting effects of estrogens on the endometrial tissue by altering the clearance of the nuclear estrogen receptor and inducing 17β-hydroxysteroid dehydrogenase, which converts estradiol to the weaker estrone. Moreover, by eliminating cyclic bleeding and suppressing uterine contractility, progestogens prevent reflux menstruation, a potential stimulus for continued endometriosis development. Progestogens may prevent implantation and growth of regurgitated endometrium by inhibiting the expression of matrix mettalloproteinases and plasminogen activators. Moreover, progestogens have antiinflammatory properties.

Luciano and colleagues administered medroxyprogesterone acetate, 50 mg daily for 4 months, to symptomatic women with moderate to severe endometriosis. Improvement of pain, pelvic nodularity, and tenderness on examination occurred in 80% of patients. Twenty percent of women experienced breakthrough bleeding, and an additional 10% reported persistent cyclic bleeding. Minor weight gain, edema, and increased irritability were other described side effects, which were generally well tolerated. A lower daily dose of 30 mg may provide equivalent relief of symptoms. Bergqvist and Theorell administered this dose to patients for 6 months and found a similar improvement in quality-of-life scores as that achieved with the GnRH agonist nafarelin. Compared with the cost of GnRH agonists and danazol, which are the other commonly prescribed agents, the low cost of the medroxyprogesterone acetate is a notable advantage.

Norethindrone acetate has been shown to be effective in achieving amenorrhea and controlling disease symptoms. When used to treat moderate or severe pelvic pain after unsuccessful conservative surgery for symptomatic rectovaginal endometriosis, a dose of 3.5 mg per day for 12 months resulted in a 73% satisfaction rate (33/45). Vercellini and colleagues (2005) reported a substantial reduction in dysmenorrhea, deep dyspareunia, nonmenstrual pelvic pain, and dyschezia scores. Low-dose norethindrone acetate could be considered an effective, tolerable, and inexpensive first-choice medical alternative to repeat surgery in those with recurrent pain.

A similar response rate can be obtained with megestrol acetate. Doses of 40 mg per day for up to 24 months resulted in significant relief of dysmenorrhea, noncyclic pelvic pain, and dyspareunia in 86% of subjects.

Parenteral depot medroxyprogesterone acetate has also been used to produce long periods of amenorrhea and elicit

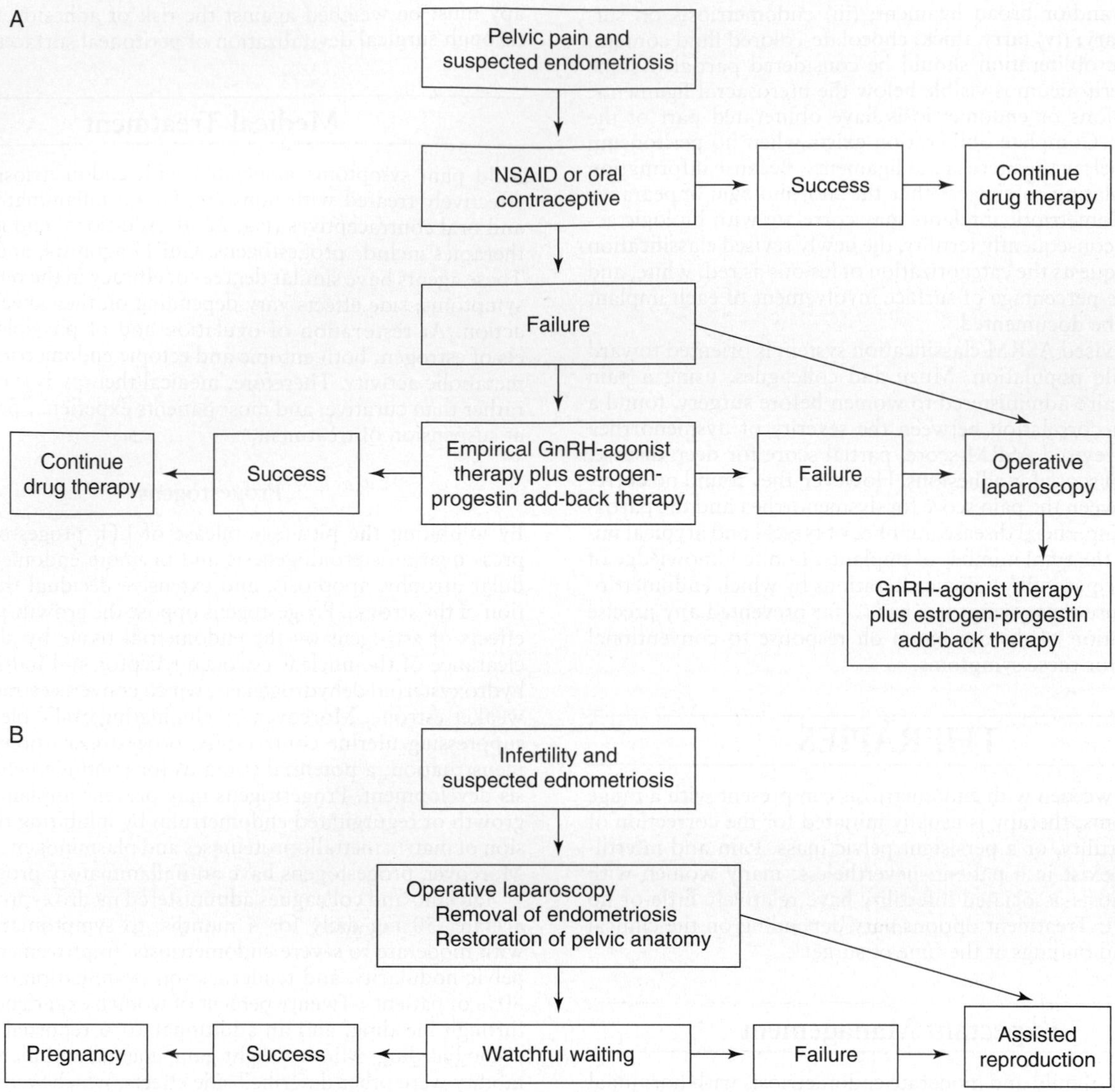

FIGURE 22.3. Algorithm for treatment of endometriosis-associated pain (A), and infertility (B). Where multiple pathways are shown, the path is guided by medical judgment and patient preference. In the infertility pathway, some practitioners dispense with the operative laparoscopy and recommend assisted reproductive technologies directly. (From Olive DL, Pritts EA. Treatment of endometriosis. *N Engl J Med* 2001;345:267, with permission.)

direct progestational changes of the endometrial tissue. A regimen of 150 mg intramuscularly every 3 months for 1 year has been used to manage endometriosis patients with moderate to severe pelvic pain. Twenty-nine of 40 subjects (72.5%) were satisfied with their pain relief after 1 year of therapy. An alternative regimen is 104 mg subcutaneously every 3 months. Frequent breakthrough bleeding can be troublesome to correct.

The rate of recurrence of symptomatic endometriosis after progestogen therapy appears to be related to the length of follow-up. Riva and colleagues reported an 18% rate after an average of 11 months, whereas Moghissi and Boyce described a 42% recurrence rate during a 2-year interval after discontinuation of medication.

Cyclic administration of low-dose oral contraceptive pills may result in relief of pelvic pain, particularly cramping associated with menstruation. This line of therapy should be considered for the woman with mild symptoms who is not attempting to conceive. Long-term continuous oral contraceptive use has been proposed for women with symptomatic endometriosis and menstruation-related pain who have failed a cyclic pill regimen. With such a regimen, the endometrium remains thin on sonogram studies, and endometriotic plaques subjected to a progestin-dominant pill are less active, usually less painful, and will undergo apoptosis. Low-dose (20 to 35 mg ethinyl estradiol) combination oral contraceptives may be given daily for 6 to 9 months without break to relieve pain or more severe dysmenorrhea. The dose may be increased to two or more tablets per day for several days to alleviate episodes of breakthrough bleeding. Eighty percent (40/50) were satisfied or very satisfied with continuous use of an oral contraceptive containing ethinyl estradiol (0.02 mg) and desogestrel (0.15 mg) for 2 years, and 96% experienced pain relief, although spotting and breakthrough bleeding were frequent side effects (Vercellini et al., 2003).

The levonorgestrel intrauterine device (IUD) has proven effective in relieving pelvic pain symptoms caused by peritoneal and rectovaginal endometriosis and in reducing the risk of recurrence of dysmenorrhea after conservative surgery. In a study by Lockhat and colleagues, an improvement in symptoms was observed in 96% throughout the 36 months of use, with only 11% experiencing pain symptoms at 18 months. The progestogen released by the IUD is rapidly absorbed by the subendometrial vascular network, which reduces menstrual flow by 70% to 90%.

Danazol

Danazol is a synthetic (2,3-isoxazole) derivative of 17α-ethinyl testosterone that was introduced into clinical practice by Greenblatt and colleagues in 1971 after good performance in uncontrolled trials. The drug gained rapid acceptance because of its effectiveness in relieving pain associated with endometriosis and in enhancing fertility. All of the progestational and the weak androgenic effects of the drug result from retention of the methyl group in the 19 position of the steroid nucleus, whereas the oral activity of danazol is ascribed to the ethinyl group at position 17.

The pharmacologic action of danazol is complex. By directly inhibiting GnRH secretion, the midcycle LH surge is ablated, although basal gonadotropin concentrations are maintained. The drug interacts with endometrial androgen and progesterone receptors, suppresses the activity of multiple enzymes necessary for ovarian and adrenal steroidogenesis, and displaces androgens from sex hormone–binding globulin, thereby augmenting androgen action on endometrial receptors. The decline in sex hormone–binding globulin induced by danazol lowers estradiol binding, increases estradiol clearance, and promotes a decline in the circulating level of this hormone. Hence, the derivative has direct androgenic and antiprogestational action on endometrial implants and creates a hypoestrogenic, hypoprogestational environment antagonistic to endometriosis. Moreover, by producing amenorrhea, danazol prevents peritoneal seeding of refluxed endometrial tissue. In addition, danazol is capable of suppressing elevated autoantibodies in several autoimmune diseases and has been shown to decrease immunoglobulin and autoantibody levels in women with endometriosis. In contrast to GnRH agonists, danazol use maintains a normal estrogenic state and increases bone mineral density over baseline.

The adverse effects of danazol reflect its anabolic, androgenic, and antiestrogenic properties and may be dose related. Weight gain, muscle cramps, decreased breast size, and vasomotor symptoms are noted in 50% or more of patients maintained on doses of 400 to 800 mg per day. In Buttram's 1985 series, 41% of patients treated with the standard dose of 800 mg per day gained more than 10 pounds during the course of therapy. The threefold increase in free testosterone can cause acne, oily skin, and deepening of the voice in a small percentage of recipients. High-density lipoprotein (HDL) cholesterol declines by 50% or more in response to the altered steroid concentrations; an 80% decrease in the HDL_2 subfraction has been reported. Most series have described a concomitant increase in low-density lipoprotein (LDL) cholesterol; the alteration in the ratio of HDL to LDL cholesterol may be an unacceptable risk to some patients. Because danazol is metabolized by the liver, modest elevations in serum glutamic oxaloacetic transaminase and serum glutamate pyruvate transaminase may arise. Reported idiopathic drug reactions include gastrointestinal disturbances, weakness, dizziness, skin rashes, headaches, and muscle cramps. Bothersome side effects occur in as many as 85% of patients, and at least 10% of women receiving danazol discontinue pharmacologic treatment because the adverse effects are intolerable. Combining danazol therapy with aerobic exercise appears to reduce the incidence of many of these androgenic side effects. Preliminary data from trials using danazol vaginal rings suggest that this route of administration may result in symptomatic improvement of pain while avoiding the androgenic side effects noted with oral administration.

Because of the potential androgenic action of this hormone on the developing fetus, the patient must not be pregnant when initiating therapy. Barrier contraception has been recommended for the entire course of treatment to eliminate the possibility of conception, although high doses of danazol usually cause anovulation.

The amenorrhea induced by danazol has been found to benefit patients with dysmenorrhea, dyspareunia, and cyclic pelvic pain associated with endometriosis. Young and Blackmore reviewed the effects of different dosages of danazol with respect to relief of symptoms in 452 patients. At a dose of 800 mg, 95% of patients noted relief of dysmenorrhea, and 89% reported relief of pelvic pain. At a dose of 400 mg, posttherapeutic relief was reduced by 10%. Moore and associates reported that pain associated with minimal and moderate pelvic endometriosis appeared to respond well to doses of danazol of 400 mg or less per day, whereas severe endometriosis was best treated with doses greater than 400 mg per day. A 6-year prospective study that evaluated the effectiveness of danazol at two doses (400 mg and 800 mg) in carefully classified patients concluded that there was no difference in side effects between the two doses and that gross resolutions of disease at second-look laparoscopy were similar. However, ovarian endometriosis greater than 1 cm did not respond as well to either dose of danazol as did peritoneal or ovarian disease less than 1 cm.

Recurrence of symptoms within 4 to 12 months of discontinuation of danazol therapy approached 50% in most studies. Puleo and Hammond found that pain recurred in 38% of patients after a mean of 6.9 months; active disease was found within 1 year in 51% of women. Lower daily doses of medication or courses of treatment less than 4 months in duration may result in a shorter symptom-free interval.

Clinical trials designed to assess the efficacy of medical therapy of minimal, mild, and moderate stages of disease refute the notion that danazol may enhance conception. Furthermore, conception is delayed while the patient is receiving danazol.

Gonadotropin-Releasing Hormone Agonists

GnRH agonists are available for use in the treatment of estrogen-dependent diseases such as endometriosis. Some of the more frequently studied analogs include leuprolide, nafarelin, buserelin, and goserelin. Alteration of the amino acid at position 6 and ethylamide replacement of the C-terminal amino acid of the native decapeptide hormone results in a GnRH agonist with increased resistance to lysosomal degradation. Pituitary receptor binding is enhanced, resulting in a decline in the number of receptors available for further occupancy. Continued administration of the GnRH agonist leads to a desensitization of the pituitary gonadotrope receptor and a reversible downregulation of the pituitary-ovarian axis. Ovarian estrogen secretion may reach castrate levels.

The initial response to GnRH agonist administration is a markedly increased secretion of pituitary stores of follicle-stimulating hormone (FSH) and LH. If therapy is begun in the follicular phase of the menstrual cycle, the developing follicle may respond to the flare in circulating gonadotropin levels with a rapid increase in estradiol production. Estradiol levels may remain elevated for 3 weeks before declining. GnRH agonist administration in the luteal phase leads to a more rapid decline in estrogen secretion, although FSH and LH levels remain elevated for 1 and 4 weeks, respectively.

GnRH agonist treatment results in improvement or resolution of pain symptoms in all stages of disease. Lemay and colleagues reported resolution of pain in 70% and improvement in discomfort in 15% of 24 subjects after 2 to 4 months of treatment with the agonist buserelin. Dyspareunia improved in 9% and disappeared in 91% of patients studied. The depot formulation of leuprolide acetate has also been shown to significantly reduce dysmenorrhea, pelvic pain, and pelvic tenderness in patients with endometriosis.

Henzl and associates, in a double-blind, multicenter study, treated 213 patients with either danazol or nafarelin. After 6 months of treatment, more than 80% of patients in all groups experienced a significant reduction in visible implants. A 43% reduction in AFS score was noted for each treatment group; there was no difference in response among patients receiving the 0.4- and 0.8-mg daily dose of nafarelin. Most patients continued to demonstrate some visible implants at the time of follow-up laparoscopy, and, as with danazol, there was some diminution in size of endometriomas but no effect on preexisting adhesions.

The optimal interval of GnRH analog administration has been widely debated. Six months of medication has been traditionally prescribed, although a significant reduction in implant volume occurs as early as 2 weeks after initiation of treatment in the rat model. A maximal effect was measured after 4 weeks of therapy in this animal study, suggesting that short courses of drug may be as efficacious as 6 months of continuous therapy. The regrowth of lesions after estrogen therapy has been reported years after the menopause; hence, hypoestrogenism results in inactivation rather than resolution of the disease.

Response to therapy may be dependent on route of administration. Donnez and colleagues reported that buserelin administration by a long-acting subcutaneous implant led to a greater reduction in endometriosis score, mitotic index, and endometrial cyst diameter than when given in an intranasal form. This may have been due to a greater consistency in hormonal release by the injected preparation.

As occurs with danazol and progestogen regimens, symptoms recur at variable periods after discontinuation of GnRH analog therapy. Subjective return of pain occurred in 57% of patients within 6 months of discontinuing leuprolide, although 37% with moderate or severe pelvic pain at baseline were still improved at 1 year. Franssen and colleagues noted a lasting and significant amelioration of dysmenorrhea and dyspareunia 6 months after completion of treatment; however, scores for chronic pelvic pain had nearly reached their pretreatment level once this time had elapsed. Patients with a higher disease stage at the onset are more likely to experience recurrence and to experience it earlier than patients with minimal disease. One treatment option for such patients may be a second 3-month course of GnRH analog. Henzl reported a significant decrease in mean pain scores and essentially no change in compact bone density in most patients when nafarelin was readministered for 3 months after a treatment-free interval of 6 months or more.

The effect of GnRH analog on endometriosis-associated infertility is difficult to assess because of a lack of an expectant management control group in most clinical studies. The preliminary pregnancy rates, which range from 0% to 60%, are derived from trials that do categorize response based on stage of disease.

Most of the side effects associated with GnRH analog therapy are related to hypoestrogenism. Hot flashes are common and can lead to sleep disturbances and chronic fatigue in extreme cases. Vaginal dryness, superficial dyspareunia, headaches, and depression have been reported. In general, these adverse effects are better tolerated than those experienced with danazol use. In addition, there are no undesirable changes in HDL, LDL, or total cholesterol throughout the prolonged period of hypoestrogenism induced by GnRH analog, unlike the changes accompanying danazol intake.

A decline in trabecular bone mineral content and an increase in urinary calcium excretion to menopausal levels occur during the course of GnRH analog therapy in about two thirds of patients. Quantitated computed tomographic studies consistently show significant loss of trabecular bone of the vertebrae and hip with GnRH analog exposure. Restoration of normal estrogen production after cessation of therapy appears to at least partially reverse these bone changes. In a study of the GnRH agonist goserelin, an 8.2% decline in density of the lumbar spine was measured after completion of 6 months of treatment; this improved to a mean loss of 5.4% at 6 months postcessation. Others found no significant change from baseline after a 6-month course of GnRH analog when bone density was assessed 6 months after treatment.

Concomitant administration of a progestogen during the course of GnRH analog therapy has been examined to ameliorate vasomotor symptoms and retard both urinary calcium excretion and radiologic evidence of loss of bone mineral density. Cedars and coworkers reported a diminution in the side effects mentioned earlier when medroxyprogesterone acetate was administered at a dose of 20 to 30 mg per day during the 6-month course of agonist therapy; however, laparoscopic evaluation after completion of therapy failed to reveal any improvement or suppression of active endometriosis with the combination regimen, and the regimen failed to significantly reduce symptoms of pelvic pain. Conversely, Makarainen and colleagues reported that medroxyprogesterone acetate, 100 mg per day, diminished hot flushes and the urinary excretion of calcium in women treated with goserelin acetate, 3.6 mg monthly, for 6 months. Second-look laparoscopy revealed equivalent diminution in extent of endometriosis when compared with the goserelin-progestin placebo group.

Norethindrone, the 19-nortestosterone progestin, has been shown to suppress both the painful symptoms of endometriosis and the extent of disease at laparoscopy when used in daily doses of 1.4 mg to 10 mg during GnRH agonist therapy. A randomized, double-blind study has demonstrated that GnRH agonist therapy may be safely and effectively extended for up to 1 year in the management of endometriosis-associated pelvic pain when prescribed in conjunction with low-dose sex steroid hormones. Hornstein et al. reported that norethindrone acetate, 5 mg, alone or in combination with conjugated equine estrogens, 0.625 mg daily, from the onset of depot leuprolide acetate therapy alleviated hypoestrogenic symptoms and preserved bone density while resulting in equivalent pain relief to that achieved by the placebo estrogen-progestin patient group. Others have treated a limited number of patients with a similar regimen for up to 10 years without detecting an adverse effect on bone mineral density. For women with relapse of endometriosis-associated pain, GnRH agonist with "add-back" progestin or progestin/estrogen therapy provides patients with a better quality of life than GnRH analog alone or oral contraceptive regimens.

The addition of calcium carbonate and alendronate or etidronate sodium, which are organic bisphosphonates, to the low-dose norethindrone acetate add-back therapy in patients with symptomatic endometriosis receiving prolonged GnRH agonist treatment may further minimize the adverse side effects of hypoestrogenism. Additional controlled studies will better establish the optimal medical management of this condition.

Conservative Surgery

Surgery is indicated for correction of pain, infertility, or other symptoms in patients with extensive pelvic endometriosis, or when hormonal manipulation fails to adequately diminish pain symptoms in women with lesser stages of disease. Surgery is successful in relieving pain in a very high percentage of cases and offers a better prognosis for pregnancy than does endocrine therapy in many cases of advanced disease.

The surgeon who has mastered the specialized techniques of operative laparoscopy can treat a wide range of pathologic findings at the time of diagnosis. Therapeutic planning depends on many factors, including the age of the patient, her desire for fertility or pain relief, the duration and intensity of her symptoms, the extent of disease, and previous treatments that have been undertaken. Preoperative rectoscopy-sigmoidoscopy and intravenous pyelography are recommended in patients with symptoms suggestive of deeply invasive endometriosis of the posterior cul-de-sac and rectovaginal septum. MRI may also be helpful in predicting the extension of disease (Table 22.5).

The decision of whether to perform surgical resection of endometriosis through the laparoscope or open abdomen is not entirely dependent on the stage of disease encountered. Laparoscopy can be considered for all cases unless there is difficulty in establishing the appropriate tissue planes of dissection or unless improved access is necessary for atraumatic manipulation of the involved organs. Specific endoscopic procedures include ablation of endometriotic implants, adhesiolysis, ovarian cystectomy, oophorectomy, and salpingectomy. Although the results and complications are similar, the cost savings with respect to decreased hospital expenses and loss of work time favor laparoscopy over laparotomy when other factors regarding risks and outcome are equal. Laparoscopy provides superior visualization of the posterior cul-de-sac and allows a high degree of magnification of peritoneal surfaces, which aids in the identification of subtle disease.

Conservative resection of disease by laparotomy is most valuable in cases of extensive, dense pelvic adhesions or endometriomas greater than 5 cm in diameter. In addition, deep involvement of the rectovaginal septum with fibrotic extension into the perirectal fossa, invasion of the bowel muscularis, and endometriotic infiltration in the region of the uterine vessels and ureter are generally best approached through the open abdomen for all but advanced endoscopic surgeons. The objective of the laparotomy procedure is complete excision of all endometriosis and associated adhesive disease to restore normal functional anatomy of the reproductive tract. The usual surgical approach is through a transverse suprapubic incision. A Maylard incision provides adequate exposure for presacral neurectomy and reconstructive surgery of ovarian endometriomas of almost any size.

Principles of Microsurgery

Microsurgical technique, or the philosophy of gentle manipulation of tissue in an attempt to avoid trauma, is the major tenet of pelvic reconstruction. The inflammation, trauma, coagulation, and foreign materials associated with conventional macrosurgical technique lead to tissue ischemia and adhesion formation because of local failure of the intrinsic peritoneal fibrinolytic system. Adhesion formation can be reduced by the application of loupe magnification or use of the operating microscope, reconstruction with fine, nonreactive sutures, precise hemostasis, and frequent irrigation of tissues with warmed lactated Ringer solution. Nevertheless, there are no definitive data to suggest that use of the particularly costly ancillary laser and the operating microscope has appreciably improved the reproductive prognosis in the surgical management of endometriosis through laparotomy. The magnification provided by laparoscopy in a closed surgical field matches these microsurgical principles.

Several basic techniques are available for the endoscopic ablation of endometriosis, including excision, coagulation, and vaporization. Coagulation can be achieved by monopolar or bipolar cautery, thermocoagulation, or, in some circumstances, laser, depending on the wavelength of energy applied. The extent of tissue penetration in electrocautery is related to the power and type of current, the duration of application, and the size of the electrode. Less tissue damage is achieved with bipolar than with monopolar cautery. The carbon dioxide (CO_2) laser is more precise than the fiber lasers, although CO_2 laser energy is strongly absorbed by water molecules and is rendered ineffective in the presence of blood. Meticulous technique that maintains serosal integrity may reduce the incidence of *de novo* adhesion formation.

Sites of Conservative Surgery

Peritoneum. Small lesions of superficial peritoneal endometriosis less than 5 mm in diameter are easily treated with laser or bipolar coagulation while under a constant stream of irrigation. Deep lesions or more extensive peritoneal disease must be excised with a tissue margin of at least 2 to 4 mm, because, as noted previously, microscopic lesions are commonly present in tissue adjacent to visible implants (Fig. 22.4). Ablation of deep disease by monopolar microdiathermy or CO_2 laser vaporization rather than excision of the disease may result in inadequate resection and a greater amount of ischemic damage to the tissue, heightening the propensity toward adhesion formation. Immobilizing adhesions can be merely divided during the preparatory phase of the procedure; precise excision is more easily accomplished after the involved organs are freed. Before dissection of the pelvic sidewall, the ureter must be identified and isolated; it frequently is displaced from its normal location by endometriotic adhesive disease. A Lucite, Teflon, or laparoscopic titanium probe can be used to isolate adhesions and protect adjacent structures during separation of the tissue planes. Suture placement can lead to foreign body reaction, tissue anoxia, and fibrosis and should therefore be avoided. Covering hemostatic, deperitonealized surfaces with an absorbable, oxidized, regenerated cellulose barrier (Interceed) significantly reduces the incidence, extent, and severity of postsurgical pelvic adhesions, even in patients with severe endometriosis. Alternatively, application of the Gore-Tex surgical membrane has been shown to result in a statistical reduction in adhesion score; this barrier can be removed at the time of a second-look laparoscopic procedure if its presence would impair tuboovarian function.

Estimations of the depth of endometrial implants at the time of laparoscopic resection relate well with histologic measurements. Superficial implants can be destroyed by bipolar cauterization; however, 25% of patients have lesions greater than 5 mm in depth. Deep (<5 mm) and very deep (<10 mm) lesions represent an active form of the disease and occur almost exclusively in patients who report pain. The superficial action of nonvaporizing modalities such as bipolar or thermal coagulation is

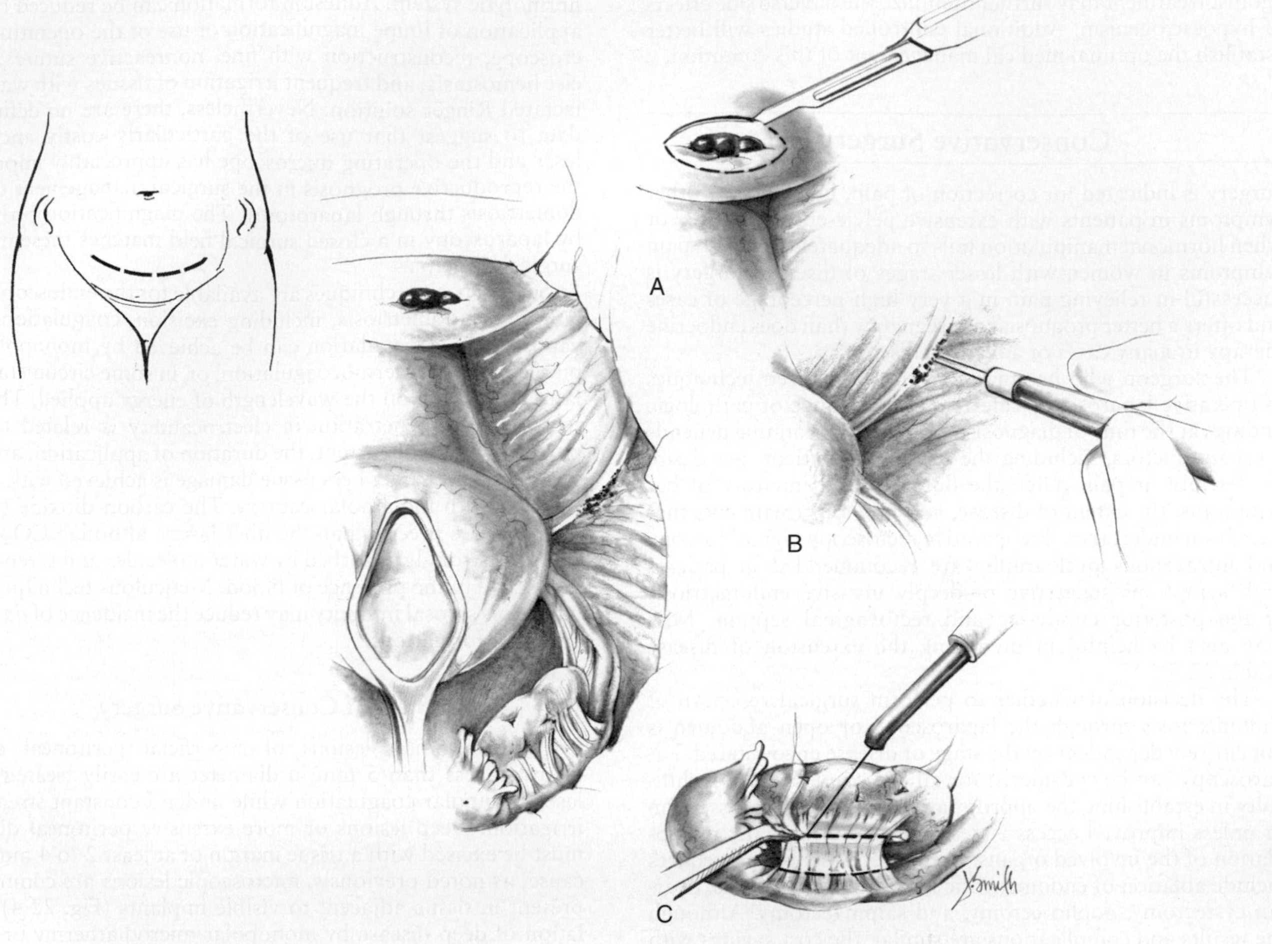

FIGURE 22.4. Excision or CO_2 laser vaporization of peritoneal implants. A: Superficial implants are vaporized by use of power densities between 1,000 and 3,000 W/cm^2, with a spot size of 0.8 to 1 mm, or they are cauterized with microbipolar forceps. More extensive peritoneal disease is excised. Very large defects can be closed with 5-0 or 6-0 polyglactin or polydioxanone sutures. Adhesion barriers can be placed. B: Endometriosis can be associated with extensive adnexal adhesions. C: Wide adhesion bands can be retracted with a glass rod or similar nonconductive probe and completely excised with a monopolar microelectrode.

not sufficient for deep disease. The diagnosis of retroperitoneal endometriosis is suggested by preoperative digital rectovaginal palpation and laparoscopic blunt probe palpation. The depth of infiltration of deep lesions appears to correlate poorly with the visible surface area of involvement. The laparoscopic treatment of deep disease is often complicated by the proximity of implants to vital structures such as the ureter, bladder, and vessels (Table 22.8).

Laparoscopic forceps are used to elevate and isolate the tissue to be excised. Instruments should be placed with care, because surgical manipulation of tissue that will not be resected may result in *de novo* adhesion formation. The diseased peritoneum may also be separated from underlying tissue by the technique of hydrodissection, which forcefully injects physiologic irrigant retroperitoneally through a small defect created in the peritoneum (Fig. 22.5). This retroperitoneal placement of fluid acts to dissipate CO_2 laser energy and, in so doing, promotes safer dissection or vaporization of the peritoneal surface. Coagulation or vaporization of disease in the ovarian fossa or near the uterosacral ligament should be undertaken only after clear identification of the ureter. Uterine manipulation with a Valtchev retractor may be used while treating lesions of the posterior cul-de-sac.

It is difficult to evaluate the depth of tissue damage with electrocauterization; however, laser vaporization allows visualization of the three-dimensional boundaries of every lesion. The laser beam should be applied until the bubbling of retroperitoneal areolar tissue is noted. The zone of thermal necrosis is minimal with the CO_2 laser, particularly when applied in the superpulse mode. In the region of the ureter, urinary bladder, colon, or large blood vessels, a single or repeat pulse mode of 0.05 to 0.1 second allows a depth of penetration of 100 to 200 μm. Irrigation of the pelvis washes off debris and carbon deposition and better exposes the base of the site of laser impact. A 2- to 4-mm clear margin is desired around each lesion treated. Excision of the involved peritoneum is superior to vaporization of implants when the extent of tissue penetration cannot be recognized.

Dissection of retroperitoneal disease can be facilitated by placing a bougie probe in the rectum and a sponge forceps in the vagina (Fig. 22.6). Traction in either direction opens the rectovaginal and perirectal spaces. Initial dissection of the

TABLE 22.8

SUGGESTED SURGICAL PROCEDURE ACCORDING TO CLASSIFICATION OF DEEPLY INFILTRATING ENDOMETRIOSIS (DIE)

DIE classification	Operative procedure
A: Anterior DIE	
Al: Bladder	Laparoscopic partial cystectomy
P: Posterior DIE	
PI: Uterosacral ligament	Laparoscopic resection of USL
P2: Vagina	Laparoscopically assisted vaginal resection of DIE infiltrating the posterior fornix
P3: Intestine	
Solely intestinal location	
Without vaginal infiltration (V−)	Intestinal resection by laparoscopy or by laparotomy
With vaginal infiltration (V+)	Laparoscopically assisted vaginal intestinal resection or exeresis by laparotomy
Multiple intestinal location	Intestinal resection by laparotomy

USL = uterosacral ligament.
From Chapron C, Fauconnier A, Vieira M et al. Anatomical distribution of deeply infiltrating endometriosis: surgical implications and proposition for a classification. *Hum Reprod* 2003;18:157, with permission.

anterior rectum provides a landmark of the retrovaginal space and permits posterior mobilization of the nodule. Subsequent lateral dissection is performed, followed by anterior dissection, which permits retrieval of the involved tissue.

Resection of deep posterior cul-de-sac nodules requires great endoscopic expertise. A combined laparoscopic-vaginal approach may be necessary to effectively remove these implants (Fig. 22.7). It is often helpful to have an assistant place his or her fingers deep in the vaginal fornices or a bougie probe in the rectum to indicate the sites of the nodules to ensure their complete removal. The direct palpation made possible through laparotomy may be required to recognize all indurated, deep lesions. A complete bowel preparation is mandatory in all cases of suspected deep endometriosis.

Electrosurgery should be avoided when extensive dissection is performed because it may be associated with widespread thermal damage and difficulty in recognizing tissue planes. Superficial invasion of the muscularis of bowel or bladder can be treated with laser vaporization or endocoagulation because of the precision and lack of penetration of these energy sources. Anterior cul-de-sac treatment should be accompanied by continuous bladder drainage.

Tubal endometriosis may distort the normal anatomic relationship of the distal tube to the ovary and in severe cases may cause complete fimbrial obstruction. Short pulses of CO_2 laser may be used to vaporize lesions while minimizing thermal damage. Endoscopic adhesiolysis of the distal tube may be accomplished with fine scissors or careful application of

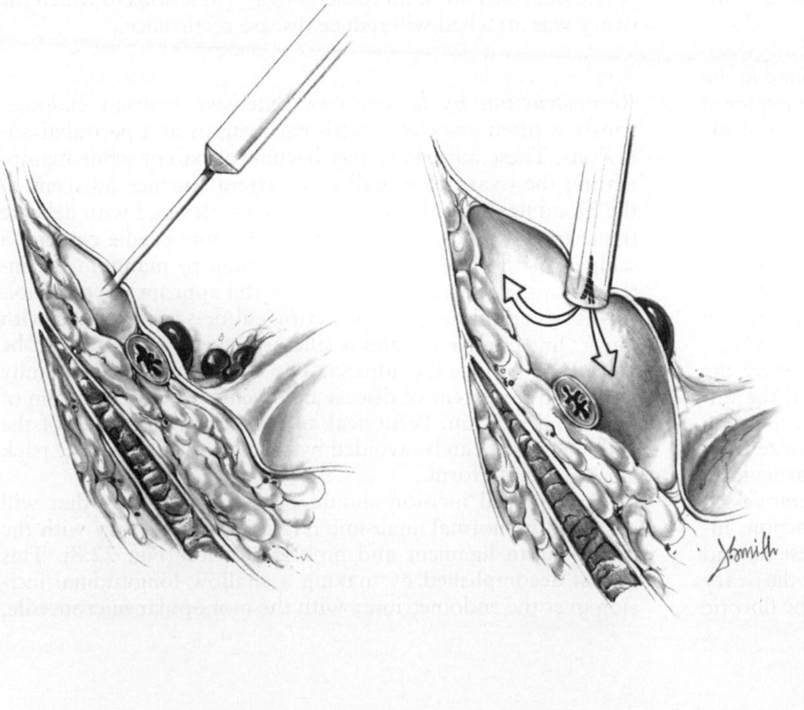

FIGURE 22.5. Hydrodissection.

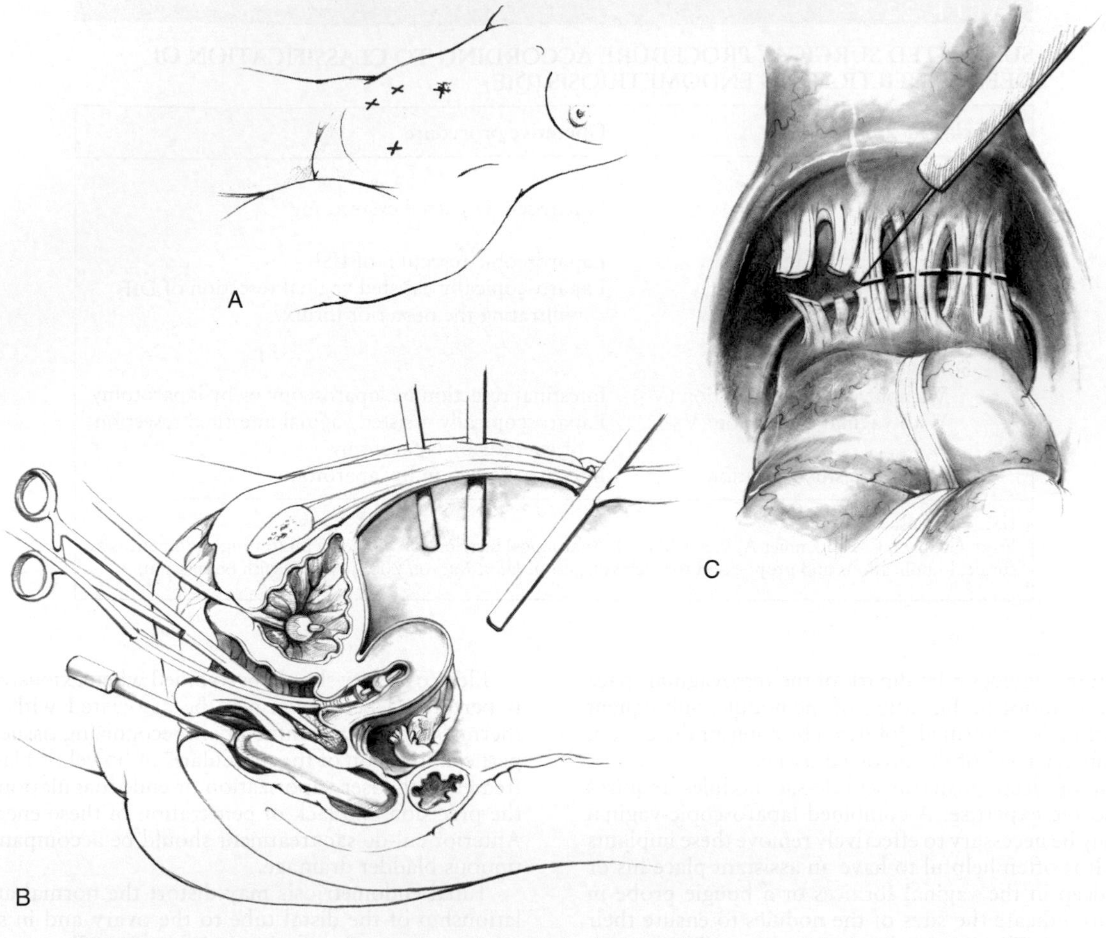

FIGURE 22.6. Laparoscopic therapy for endometriosis. **A:** Dorsal lithotomy positioning for surgery, with multiple puncture sites marked for placement of ancillary instruments. **B:** Traction on bougie in rectum and sponge forceps in vagina mobilize rectovaginal and perirectal spaces. Uterine manipulation cannula, bladder drainage, and multiple transabdominal instruments facilitate safe dissection. **C:** CO_2 laser division of endometriosis-associated adhesions extending from lower uterus to rectal serosa.

laser. Unipolar electrocautery should not be used on this tissue.

Defects in the parietal peritoneal surface are frequently associated with endometriosis and are most commonly found in the posterior cul-de-sac region. These defects should be explored and ablated even if they appear grossly normal because of the frequency of microscopic disease.

Ovary. Superficial endometriosis of the ovary usually presents as small, dark, punctate lesions located on and immediately beneath the cortical surface. This disease can be readily treated with laser or bipolar forceps under constant irrigation. Occasionally, however, the small, visible lesion may be merely the tip of a large endometrial cyst. If there is any doubt, the implant should be excised and the ovary explored to determine the extent of disease. Care should be taken to minimize thermal injury to surrounding ovarian tissue. This is particularly important near the fimbria ovarica, because postoperative adhesion formation could compromise distal tubal function. Inability to elevate the ovary is usually a sign of adhesions and endometriotic implants of the inferolateral surface of the ovary and the peritoneum of the ovarian fossa. Excising the fibrotic pelvic sidewall and/or uterosacral ligament lesions to which the ovary was attached will reduce disease recurrence.

Reconstruction by laparotomy. Extensive ovarian endometriosis is often associated with periovarian and peritubal adhesions. These adhesions may become apparent while manipulating the ovary to visualize the lateral surface adjacent to the broad ligament. Filmy adhesions are elevated with delicate tissue forceps and can be resected with fine-needle cautery, a scalpel, or the laser. Care must be taken to maintain the integrity of the ovarian capsule. After the appropriate adhesiolysis is accomplished, the posterior cul-de-sac is packed with moist, lint-free packs, and a silicon surgical platform can be placed to stabilize the adnexa. The ovary should be carefully examined for extent of disease involvement before creation of the initial incision. Peritoneal spillage of the contents of the endometrioma can be avoided by placement of a lint-free pack around the platform.

The cortical incision should be made in a way that will preserve the normal anatomic relations of the ovary with the uteroovarian ligament and fimbria ovarica (Fig. 22.8). This is best accomplished by making a shallow longitudinal incision over the endometrioma with the monopolar microneedle,

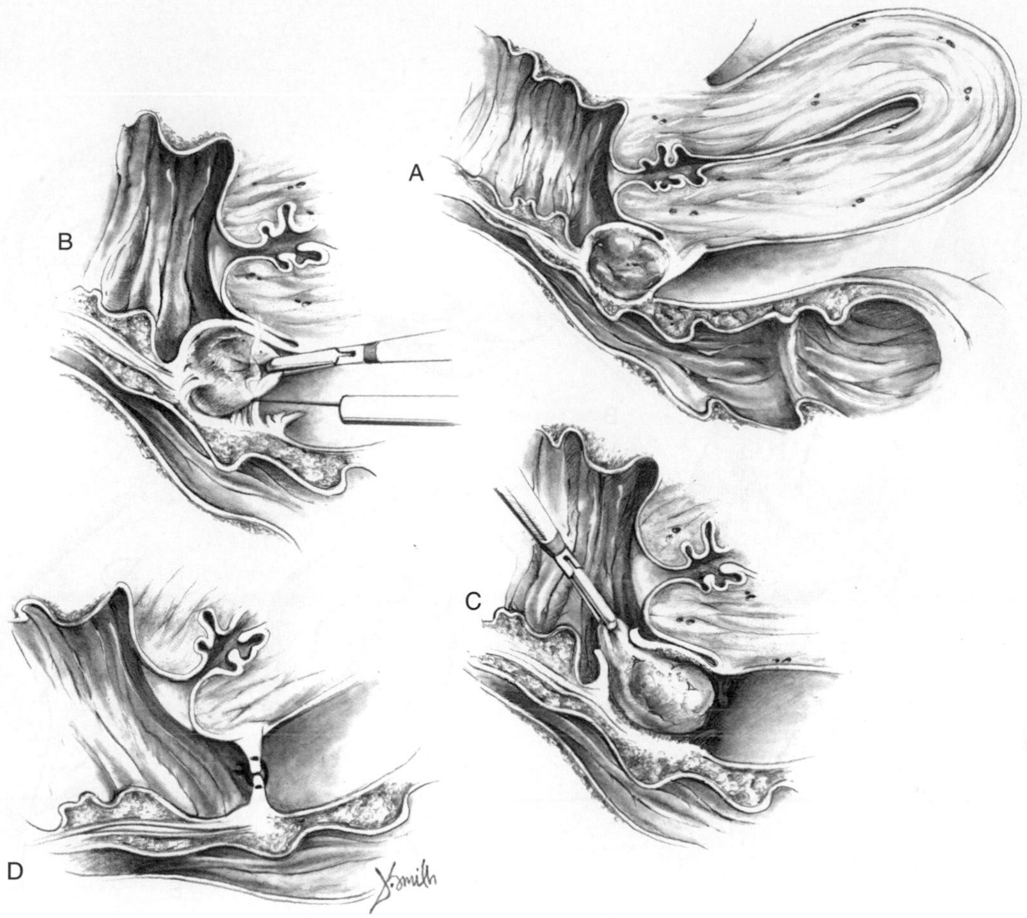

FIGURE 22.7. **A:** Deep laparoscopic dissection of the rectovaginal space, in combination with colpotomy, for the excision of a large endometriotic nodule of the rectovaginal septum. **B:** Initial laparoscopic dissection of nodule. **C:** Completion of dissection by way of colpotomy incision. **D:** Vaginal suture placement to reapproximate the rectovaginal septal defect.

scalpel, or laser. The surgeon should attempt to remove the endometrioma in an intact state; however, if the cyst cavity is inadvertently entered, an elliptical incision around the site of rupture is useful for exposure. The intact endometrioma can be transfixed with a traction suture of 2-0 nylon to facilitate creation of a cleavage plane between the cyst and normal ovarian tissue. Blunt, curved scissors or a flat probe or knife handle is used for dissection. Particular care must be taken when dissecting the hilar region to maintain hemostasis and preserve primordial follicles. An attempt should be made to preserve as much of the normal ovarian cortex as possible; pregnancies have been achieved with only a small fraction of remaining ovary.

The ovary is reconstructed by placing one or two pursestring sutures of 4-0 or 5-0 polyglactin, polyglycolic acid, or polydioxanone to eliminate the dead space and maximize hemostasis. This may be followed by placement of a running subcortical 5–0 suture of the same delayed-absorbable material (Fig. 22.8), if necessary. In some circumstances, less tissue distortion can be achieved by placing a deep layer of interrupted mattress sutures followed by additional layers of running sutures (Fig. 22.8). Suture on or extruding through the surface should be strictly avoided because of its adhesiogenic properties.

After the ovary has been carefully approximated, the posterior surfaces of the uterus and broad ligament are inspected for hemostasis wherever the ovary was previously adhered. Microbipolar cauterization may be necessary. Placement of an adhesion barrier is useful in separating raw peritoneal surfaces during the healing process.

Endoscopic therapy of ovarian endometriosis. Surgical treatment of endometriosis less than 4 to 5 cm in diameter can be accomplished with relative ease. However, endoscopic resection of larger lesions may be compromised by the presence of dense, cohesive adhesions and by difficulties removing the entire cyst wall because of the inability to find the plane of attachment of the fibrotic endometrioma to the ovarian cortex.

The endometrioma can be excised in an intact or ruptured state during the laparoscopic procedure. In either case, the technique is initiated by longitudinally incising the cortex overlying the cyst after achieving full mobilization of the ovary by adhesiolysis. The incision is generally made along the inferior pole on the opposite side to the hilus in such a manner as to preserve the apposition of healthy ovarian tissue to the fimbria. The cyst contents are immediately drained with the suction cannula, and the cavity is irrigated and inspected for papillary structures or other suspicious features. Often, the cyst ruptures during dissection of adhesions that bind the ovary to the pelvic sidewall. Under this circumstance, the plane of dissection between the cyst wall and the ovarian cortex can be established after identifying the site of rupture. The opening can be extended with the use of the needle electrode or laser.

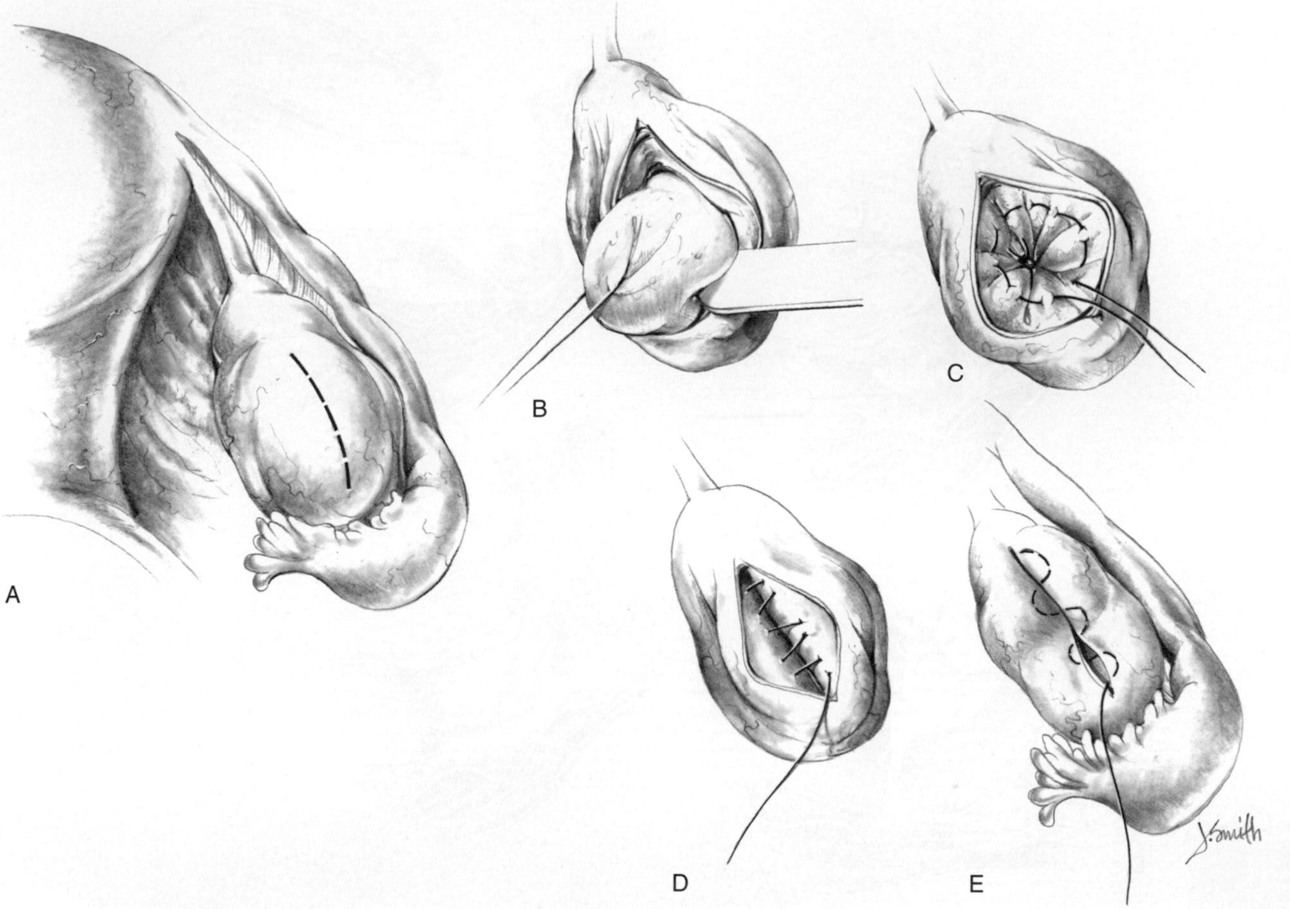

FIGURE 22.8. Excision of ovarian endometrioma through laparotomy. **A:** The ovarian cortex is gently incised so that the endometrial cyst is not entered. The incision is made along the longitudinal axis of the ovary. **B:** The endometrioma is then peeled out with the blunt knife handle. **C** and **D:** The ovarian defect is closed with two layers of pursestring sutures of 4-0 or 5-0 absorbable, nonreactive material. **E:** In the case of a deep defect, a more superficial running suture may be necessary before the cortical edges are approximated with 5-0 nonreactive, delayed-absorbable sutures.

With larger endometriomas, the normal ovarian cortex is stabilized with atraumatic forceps, and the cyst wall is grasped with biopsy forceps and stripped from the bed of normal ovarian tissue (Fig. 22.9). The dissection may be facilitated by removing a small circular rim of tissue around the adhesion site to begin the stripping procedure in a clearer field, where the endometrioma wall is less adhered to healthy ovarian tissue (Muzii et al., 2005). Judicious use of the needle electrode or hydrodissection may facilitate separation of the tissue planes. Remaining fragments of the cyst wall should be vaporized with laser or fulgurated by electrocautery. Hemostasis can be achieved with bipolar cautery.

An alternative technique involves sharp and blunt dissection to remove the cyst in an intact state. Hydrodissection is particularly useful with this approach. The cyst contents are carefully drained in a plastic laparoscopy pouch to facilitate clean removal from the peritoneal cavity.

Very small endometriomas less than 1 to 2 cm in size may be effectively treated by electrocoagulation of the mucosal lining. Because carbon dioxide laser is absorbed by fluid, complete ablation of the cyst wall with this energy source may be compromised in an environment rich in blood and hemosiderin.

The ovarian defect is usually left to heal spontaneously. Ischemia associated with suture placement can provoke adhesion formation after laparoscopic ovarian reconstruction. Low-power continuous carbon dioxide laser or bipolar coagulation can be applied to the inside wall of the redundant ovarian capsule to cause an inversion of the incised cortex. Most authors have reported excellent results with this no-suture technique.

Under the rare circumstances of persistent bleeding or poor apposition of ovarian tissue, the cortex may be reapproximated with sutures. If fine absorbable suture is used, the knot should be placed internally to minimize the possibility of it becoming a nidus for adhesion formation. The high incidence of adhesion formation after surgery for endometriosis, particularly at the site of the ovary or where dense adhesions were divided, underscores the importance of optimizing surgical techniques to potentially reduce adhesion formation.

Extensive cauterization of ovarian tissue can lead to a rise in FSH levels postoperatively and should be avoided. Post-surgical ovarian failure after laparoscopic excision of bilateral endometriomas is a rare but possible complication. There were three cases of premature ovarian failure among 126 patients who underwent laparoscopic excision of bilateral endometriomas in a recent series by Busaccca and colleagues,

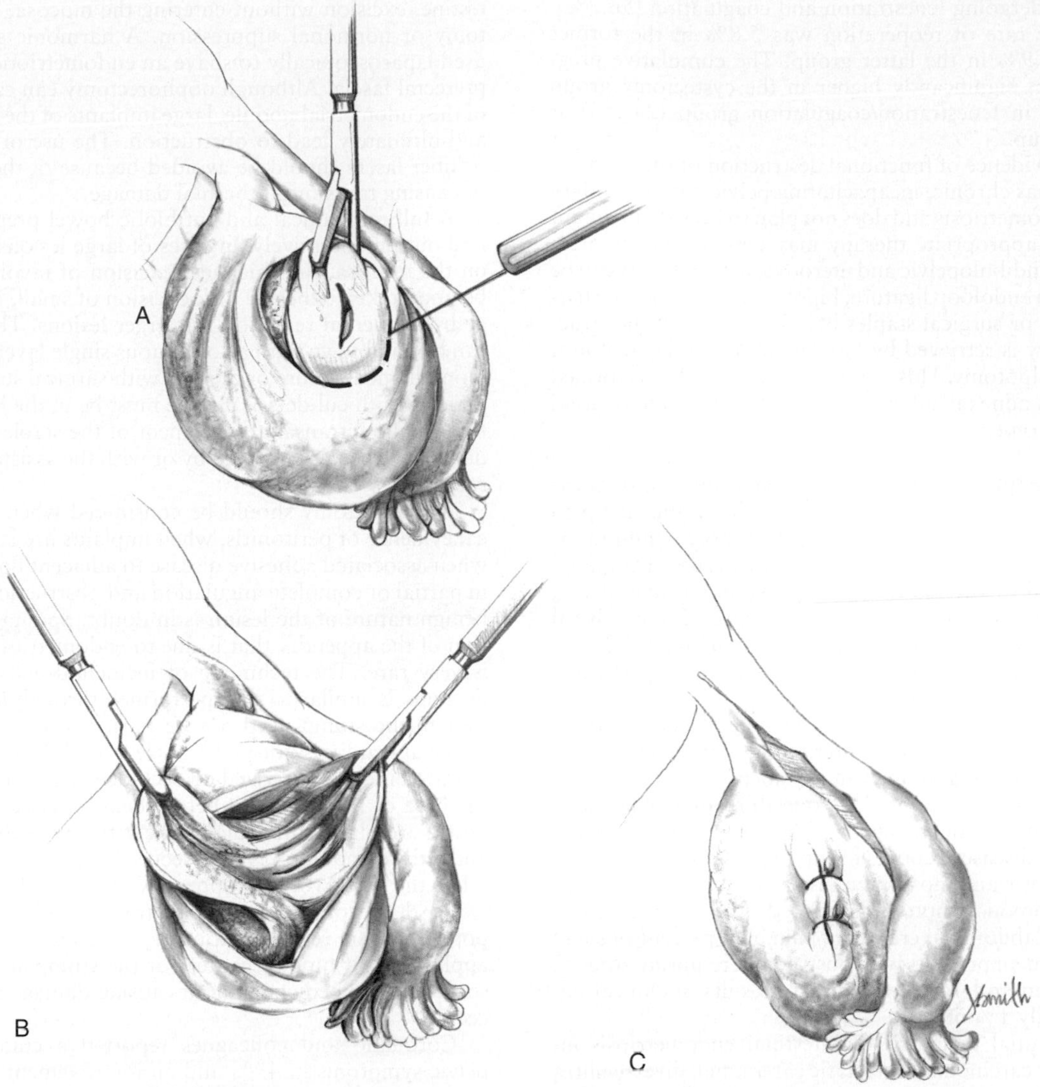

FIGURE 22.9. Laparoscopic ovarian cystectomy after fenestration of the cyst. A: The cut edges of the ovarian cortex and cyst wall are held and teased apart. B: The cyst wall can be stripped off by twisting it around the grasping forceps. Hydrodissection may be helpful. C: Large defects can be closed with laparoscopic suturing. Most incisions are left to heal by second intention.

corresponding to a rate of 2.4%. This may be caused by irreversible trauma to ovarian vasculature by electrocoagulation, excessive removal of ovarian tissue, and an autoimmune reaction caused by a severe, local inflammatory process.

Fayez and Vogel prospectively evaluated four laparoscopic methods for the treatment of endometriomas. Patients were treated postoperatively with danazol and underwent a second-look laparoscopy 8 weeks after their initial surgery. Complete excision with scissors successfully eliminated recurrence of the cysts, but adnexal adhesions had developed postoperatively in all cases. Mere incision and drainage of the cyst contents, followed by stripping or CO_2 laser vaporization of the lining, resulted in adhesion formation in only 25% to 37% of cases, but endometrioma cysts recurred in 21% to 22%. Other authors have used the potassium-titanyl-phosphate (KTP) laser to photocoagulate or remove the cyst lining of large endometriomas and have reported a very low rate of recurrence at 6 months after the procedure.

In a prospective study by Beretta and colleagues, patients were randomly allocated at the time of laparoscopy to undergo either cystectomy or drainage of the endometrioma and bipolar coagulation of the inner lining. No preoperative or postoperative adjunctive medical therapies were administered. The excision technique resulted in a lower 24-month cumulative recurrence rate of dysmenorrhea, deep dyspareunia, and nonmenstrual pelvic pain. The median interval between the operation and the recurrence of moderate to severe pelvic pain was longer in the cystectomy group (19 months) versus the drainage and coagulation group (9.5 months). In addition, the 24-month cumulative pregnancy rate was statistically significantly higher in the former group than in the latter group (66.7% versus 23.5%, respectively).

In a recent prospective, randomized clinical trial by Alborzi and associates, the rate of recurrence of pelvic pain and dysmenorrhea over a 2-year postoperative period was significantly less for those who underwent cystectomy (15.8%) as compared with those undergoing fenestration and coagulation (56.7%). Moreover, the rate of reoperation was 5.8% in the former group and 22.9% in the latter group. The cumulative pregnancy rate was significantly higher in the cystectomy group (59.4%) than in fenestration/coagulation group (23.3%) at 1-year follow-up.

If there is evidence of functional destruction of the ovary or if the patient has chronic, incapacitating pelvic pain secondary to ovarian endometriosis and does not plan to become pregnant in the future, appropriate therapy may consist of oophorectomy. The infundibulopelvic and uteroovarian ligaments can be ligated with an endoloop ligature, bipolar coagulation, the harmonic scalpel, or surgical staples before excision of the structure. The ovary is retrieved by morcellation, minilaparotomy, or posterior colpotomy. This type of surgery must be performed carefully when adnexal adhesions are present to avoid ovarian remnant syndrome.

Intestines. Intestinal involvement has been estimated to occur in 3% to 15% of women with endometriosis and in up to 50% of patients with severe disease. The most common areas of intestinal involvement are the rectum and rectosigmoid colon, followed by the sigmoid colon, cecum, terminal ileum, proximal colon, and appendix. The incidence of appendiceal endometriosis has been estimated at approximately 0.8% of all appendectomies; 3% to 5% of patients with endometriosis have appendiceal involvement.

Symptoms that should arouse suspicion of colorectal involvement include constipation alternating with diarrhea, rectal pain, tenesmus, dyspareunia, and dysmenorrhea. Cyclic rectal bleeding is seen in as many as one third of women with rectosigmoid involvement, but the mucosa is rarely invaded. Small intestine disease accounts for up to 16% of gastrointestinal endometriosis and most often involves the terminal ileum. The most common symptom associated with disease in this location is midabdominal cramping pain. Ten percent of small bowel involvement presents with obstruction requiring surgery. The more common large bowel disease results in clinical obstruction in only 1% of cases.

The differential diagnosis of intestinal endometriosis includes primary carcinoma, metastatic carcinoma, diverticulitis, inflammatory bowel disease, irritable bowel syndrome, pelvic inflammatory disease, radiation colitis, and ischemic stricture. Endometrial adenocarcinomas have been reported in the colon and rectum but are exceedingly rare in comparison with the relatively large numbers of patients with colorectal endometriosis.

Preoperative or intraoperative rigid sigmoidoscopy may be helpful in ruling out primary colorectal malignancy. An intact mucosa effectively rules out primary colorectal malignancy. The greatest chance of diagnosing colorectal endometriosis occurs when the examination is performed at the time of menstruation. Although endometriosis rarely invades the intestinal mucosa, mucosal distortion is possible secondary to infiltration of the submucosa.

Pelvic and rectal pain is the major symptom that leads to colorectal resection in patients with advanced endometriosis. Bowel resection should be undertaken in the symptomatic patient or when there is a suspicion of malignancy; however, the frequency of such indications is small. In a series authored by Prystowsky and colleagues of 1,573 consecutive patients with endometriosis, only 11 women (0.7%) required bowel resection. Resection is usually undertaken for lesions producing partial obstruction because most of these lesions are fibrotic and unresponsive to hormonal manipulation. Recommended approaches for less extensive lesions include CO_2 laser vaporization of superficial serosal disease of the rectum or large intestine, excision without entering the mucosa, and oophorectomy or hormonal suppression. A harmonic scalpel may be used laparoscopically to shave an endometriotic nodule in the prerectal fascia. Although oophorectomy can cause regression of the endometrial nodule, large implants of the bowel can scar and ultimately lead to obstruction. The use of electrocautery or fiber lasers should be avoided because of their greater risk of causing transmural thermal damage.

A full mechanical and antibiotic bowel preparation is carried out preoperatively. In cases of large lesions that encroach on the mucosa, full-thickness excision of involved bowel can be undertaken either by disk excision of small, isolated lesions or by segmental resection for larger lesions. The anastomosis can be hand sewn with a continuous single layer of absorbable monofilament suture or created with surgical staples; however, patients with cul-de-sac disease must be in the lithotomy position to allow transanal placement of the stapler. These procedures have been performed by or with the assistance of general surgeons.

Appendectomy should be considered when there is physical evidence of peritonitis, when implants are large and active, when associated adhesive disease to adjacent bowel may result in partial or complete angulation and obstruction, or when the benign nature of the lesion is in doubt. Spontaneous perforation of the appendix that is due to endometriotic involvement is very rare. The technique of incidental endoscopic appendectomy is similar to that performed through laparotomy, although the stump need not be buried in the cecum. The tip of the appendix is grasped and elevated. The appendiceal vessels are bipolar cauterized or occluded with surgical clips near the base of the appendix before being excised. Two loop ligatures are placed immediately next to each other at the base, and a third endoloop is then secured approximately 5 mm distal to the first two. The appendix may then be transected between the second and third ligature and placed in a surgical pouch for safe retrieval from the abdominal cavity. Judicious application of bipolar cautery at the stump sterilizes the raw surface of the pedicle without causing damage to the adjacent cecum.

Coronado and colleagues reported a complete relief of pelvic symptoms in 49% and an improvement in 39% of patients who underwent full-thickness resection of the colon; 39% of patients in the series achieved a term pregnancy. In a later series by the same colorectal surgeons of 130 patients who underwent aggressive, conservative surgical management for advanced disease, the operative procedures performed included low anterior resection with anastomosis to the extraperitoneal rectum (n = 109), sigmoid resection (n = 10), disk excision of the rectum (n = 7), ileocecal resection (n = 2), and small bowel resection (n = 2). Twenty-four of 49 patients (49%) who attempted to conceive delivered a viable child.

The sequelae of intestinal endometriosis may not appear until the patient is postmenopausal. Although the endometriosis can become inactive, the resulting cicatrization can lead to a decrease in the bowel lumen and to symptoms of obstruction.

Urinary Tract. Endometriosis involving the urinary tract is relatively rare. The spectrum of disease severity varies from incidental findings at laparoscopy, laparotomy, or cystoscopy to more significantly associated hematuria, flank pain, hypertension, and ureteral obstruction. Bladder and ureteral involvement represent 85% and 15% of cases, respectively. Cystoscopy and intravenous pyelography are helpful studies in documenting the extent of disease. Vesical endometriosis can be treated by hormonal suppressive therapy or partial cystectomy. These nodular lesions develop within the muscularis and are typically seen with partial or complete obliteration of the anterior cul-de-sac. Conservative surgical treatment of bladder endometriosis is effective in ensuring long-term relief in most cases of endometriosis affecting the vesical dome, whereas success rates for deeper lesions involving the vesical base and the vesicouterine septum are lower, depending on the degree of surgical radicalness (Fedele et al., 2005).

Extrinsic ureteral compression by endometriosis presents four times more frequently than intrinsic involvement and is most likely to occur in the region of the ovarian fossa. Patients with paracervical and extensive uterosacral ligament disease are also at risk. The preferred treatment for ureteral obstruction is ureterolysis or resection of the involved segment followed by ureteroneocystostomy or ureteroureterostomy.

Involvement of peritoneum overlying the ureter is amenable to resection by laparotomy or laparoscopy. An incision is made in normal peritoneum adjacent to the involved area. The inferior margin of the incision is grasped and deviated medially, and the ureter is separated from the peritoneum bluntly or by hydrodissection. The peritoneal lesion can be excised or vaporized. Periureteral vessels must remain intact to prevent ischemia and resultant fistula formation. If the peritoneum is adhered and the lesion cannot be dissected, the ureter is likely involved in the disease process. Ureteroneocystostomy should be considered.

Incisional Scars. Surgical scars are occasionally the sites of endometriotic implantation. Perineal, vaginal, and vulvar scars, particularly episiotomies, colporrhaphies, and Bartholin gland excisions, are likely areas for involvement by endometriosis. There is often a history of delayed wound healing of the incisional scar infiltrated with endometriosis. These implants typically appear as either deep-lying or subcutaneous nodules infiltrating the fascia and muscle. Bleeding into the tissues at the time of menstruation can cause cyclic local pain, tenderness, and discoloration; however, the nodule may lie too deep for detection of any color change through the skin. If the nodule is superficial, cyclic bleeding or ulceration may be apparent.

In most instances, incisional endometriomas have followed surgical procedures that violated the uterine cavity and allowed the endometrium to be transplanted. Wespi and Kletzhändler suggested that the frequency might approach 5% among patients having cesarean section or hysterectomy. Metroplasty and myomectomy also increase the risk of incisional endometriosis. Indeed, endometriosis has been reported along the needle tracts after amniocentesis or saline injection for abortion. Careful flushing and irrigation of the abdomen and of the incision during closure should minimize the chance of contamination when incision into the uterine cavity is required.

Episiotomy scars and cervical and vaginal lacerations also serve as implantation sites after delivery. The chance is significantly increased when postpartum curettage is performed. Paull and Tedeschi reported 15 instances in 2,208 deliveries when curettage was carried out and no instances in 13,800 deliveries without curettage.

Management, usually best accomplished by local excision, is both diagnostic and curative. Various hormonal regimens may be appropriate if it is imperative to avoid surgery. However, malignancy can occur in each area of ectopic endometriosis, and histologic confirmation of the tentative diagnosis is recommended.

Thorax. Thoracic endometriosis is an uncommon disease with varying clinical presentations. The diagnosis is almost always established on clinical grounds. In a report of 65 cases of thoracic endometriosis (Foster et al.), pleural and lung parenchymal disease presented with different clinical features. Ninety-three percent of women with pleural disease developed pain with right-sided pneumothorax or pleural effusion. Because numerous right diaphragmatic defects were noted in patients with pleural involvement, pleural implants are believed to be secondary to tubal regurgitation and transport of endometrial tissue through the diaphragmatic defects. Other symptoms may include upper quadrant abdominal pain or referred pain to the shoulder. Disease involving the lung parenchyma produced hemoptysis rather than the pleuritic symptoms. Previous pelvic surgery was more common among women who had parenchymal endometriosis; however, pelvic endometriosis was found more often in those with pleural disease.

Catamenial pneumothorax or hemoptysis should alert the physician to the possibility of thoracic endometriosis. The chest roentgenogram is usually of little value in diagnosing this disease; however, cytology, aspiration biopsy, and pleuroscopy may be useful. Massive effusion and bleeding can occur, but this presentation is more commonly associated with a malignancy. GnRH agonist or surgical treatment may be effective in the symptomatic patient. Surgical pleural abrasion may be superior to hormonal treatment in the long-term management of pneumothorax.

Adjunctive Procedures of Conservative Surgery

Uterine Suspension. Uterine suspension techniques have been devised to reduce adhesion formation at denuded peritoneal surfaces of the posterior cul-de-sac, uterine serosa, and broad ligament. Elevation of the adnexa may prevent adhesion reformation of the ovary or fallopian tube at a site where existing adhesions have been excised. This procedure may be particularly useful in the case of a posterior or retroflexed uterus. It is indicated in selected cases of dyspareunia after resection of posterior cul-de-sac endometriosis. There is no evidence to suggest that uterine suspension is detrimental to subsequent pregnancies, although it is of unproven efficacy in enhancing fertility or as an adjunct in the treatment of endometriosis-associated pelvic pain. The modified Gilliam procedure offers certain advantages over other uterine suspensions because of its maintenance of normal anatomic relations. Shortening the round ligament through the internal inguinal ring eliminates the opening that is made lateral to the point of the ligament's attachment to the abdominal wall in the Olshausen suspension procedure.

When a modified Gilliam suspension is performed via laparotomy, the uterus is elevated, and a 2-0 absorbable suture is placed around each round ligament about 3 to 4 cm from its insertion into the uterus (Fig. 22.10). The edge of the rectus fascia is grasped by a Kocher clamp at the level of the anterosuperior spine of the ileum. The adjacent peritoneal edge is grasped with a Kelly clamp. The rectus fascia is separated from the underlying musculature with blunt dissection. A long Kelly clamp is inserted between the fascia and muscle to the level of the inguinal ring while displacing the peritoneum superiorly. This clamp is inserted through the ring and along the round ligament by gently opening and closing the instrument. The insertion is facilitated by placing traction on the suture to stabilize the round ligament. The peritoneum overlying the ligament is then incised at a point adjacent to the suture, and the suture is grasped by the Kelly clamp. By withdrawing the clamp, the round ligament is brought through the internal ring and outside of the peritoneal cavity; it can then be sutured to the rectus sheath with 2-0 interrupted delayed-absorbable sutures. These sutures must be placed through the round ligament without

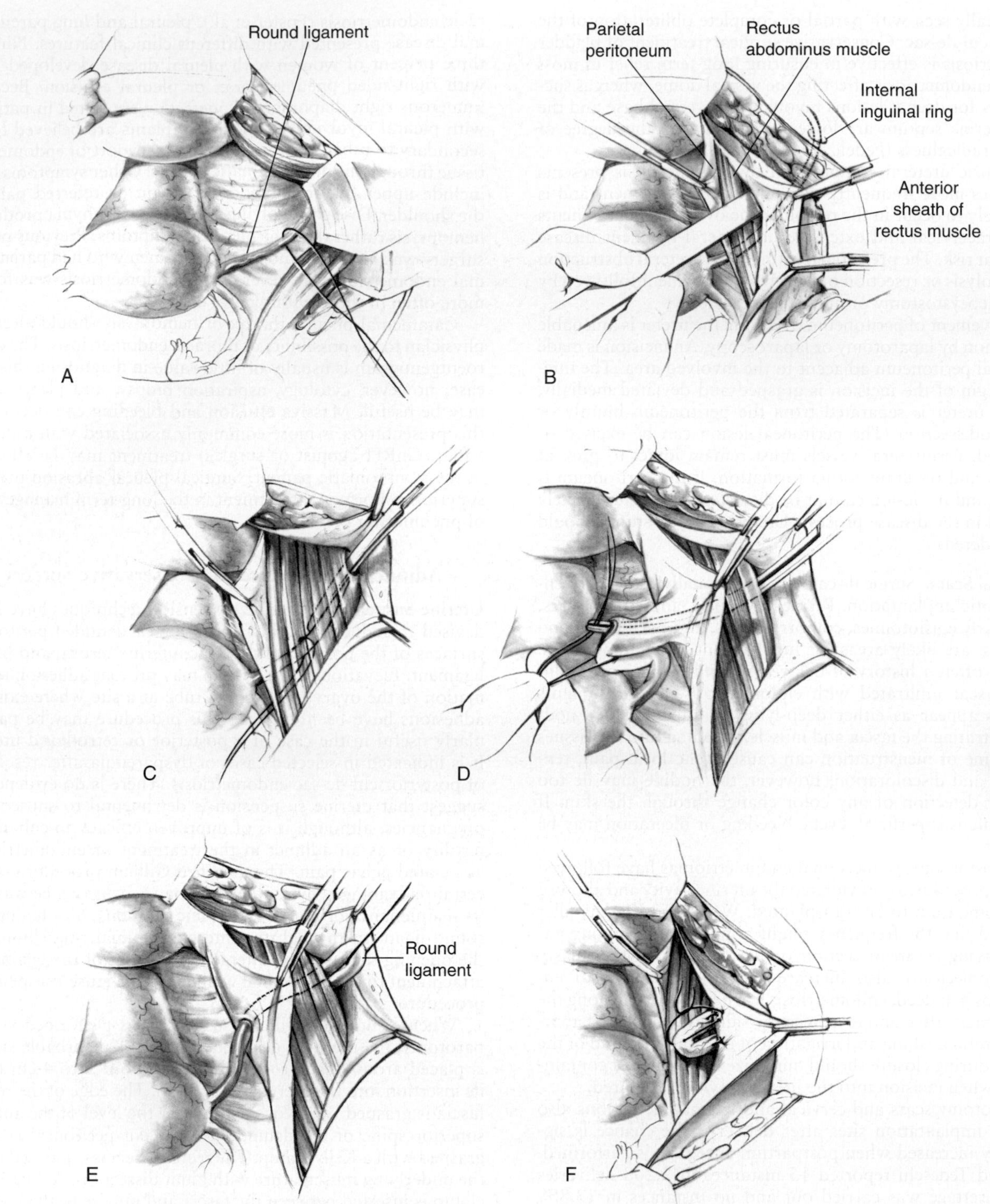

FIGURE 22.10. Modified Gilliam suspension. A: A chromic suture is placed around the round ligament about 3 to 4 cm from the uterine cornu. B: The rectus fascia is grasped with Kocher clamps and separated from the belly of the rectus muscle bluntly with the index finger or knife handle. C: The parietal peritoneum is grasped with Kelly forceps. A long Kelly forceps is introduced through the internal inguinal ring as it passes over the belly of the rectus. D: The Kelly clamp is brought through the internal inguinal ring and along the round ligament to a point adjacent to the chromic stay suture. A knife is used to open the peritoneum. The ends of the chromic suture are grasped by the Kelly clamp. E: As traction is applied to the suture, a knuckle of the round ligament passes through the internal ring. F: Three sutures of 2-0 delayed-absorbable or silk suture are placed, fixing the ligament to the rectus fascia in a manner that will not interrupt the blood supply.

encircling the ligament and thus occluding its blood supply. This procedure is repeated on the opposite side.

At the end of the suspension, the surgeon's hands should be introduced into the abdomen to ascertain whether there is a loop of round ligament lateral to the point where the ligament has been withdrawn from the peritoneal cavity. If so, this should be corrected to prevent strangulation of the involved segment lying between the ligament and abdominal wall. In addition, the fallopian tube should be inspected to ensure that its course has not been disturbed. This can occur if the traction suture has been placed through a segment of round ligament too close to the uterus.

Laparoscopic suspension is possible after placement of a trocar and sheath approximately 5 cm lateral to the midline and 3 cm above the inguinal ligament. The anterior rectus fascia in this site is tagged with suture. The round ligament is grasped at the usual site with laparoscopic forceps to elevate the ligament to the tagged anterior fascia, where it is sutured in place with nonabsorbable suture. The desired positioning of the uterus is confirmed laparoscopically.

Presacral Neurectomy. Presacral neurectomy, or division of the superior hypogastric plexus, is useful as an adjunctive procedure to eliminate the uterine component of dysmenorrhea that results from endometriosis. Sixty percent to 85% of patients with secondary dysmenorrhea experience complete relief of symptoms. There is no evidence that presacral neurectomy enhances fertility.

A significantly greater relief of midline pelvic pain is achieved when endometriosis resection is combined with presacral neurectomy compared with conservative resection alone. In a series by Tjaden and colleagues, all 17 patients undergoing presacral neurectomy noted a complete resolution of midline pelvic pain, and only two of these had a recurrence of pain within the 42-month follow-up period. Endometriosis rarely provokes exclusively midline pelvic pain, however, and lateralizing adnexal pain and deep dyspareunia are not affected by this procedure. Careful patient selection is necessary if the desired outcome is to be achieved.

The hypogastric plexus consists of fine strands of nerves embedded in a delicate areolar tissue. The plexus is formed as a continuation of the aortic and inferior mesenteric plexuses and passes over the bifurcation of the aorta. It then continues below the promontory of the sacrum before dividing into the right and left inferior hypogastric nerves. The presacral neurectomy procedure can be performed through a transverse Maylard incision or longitudinal incision that adequately exposes the region of the bifurcation of the aorta (Fig. 22.11). At the time of laparotomy, the descending colon is packed superiorly and to the left to expose the left margin of the hypogastric plexus. The posterior peritoneum overlying the sacrum is elevated and incised with the scalpel. The incision is extended caudally with scissors for about 5 cm to the third or fourth sacral vertebra and cranially to just below the bifurcation of the aorta. The margin of the posterior peritoneum can be drawn upward and outward by a stay suture or an Allis clamp. A Kitner sponge is then used to dissect the areolar tissue and associated nerve fibers off the posterior aspect of the peritoneal flap. The right ureter is readily visible and can be retracted laterally, and the areolar tissue is dissected from it without disturbing its blood supply. The common iliac artery, which lies just below the ureter, is freed superiorly from the adjacent tissue. A right-angle clamp or probe can be introduced medially next to the promontory to elevate the sheath and allow blunt dissection underneath it. Care must be taken to avoid the middle sacral vessels that may be left intact on the surface of the promontory. Injury to the middle sacral vein can result in significant blood loss. Hemorrhage is controlled with cautery, suture ligation, hot packs, hypogastric vessel ligation, use of an absorbable gelatin sponge (Gelfoam) or microfibular collagen (Avitene), or packing with bone wax.

The areolar tissue is taken off the left flap of peritoneum until the superior hemorrhoidal vessels are exposed. These vessels should remain on the peritoneum but are bluntly freed from the overlying tissue. By elevating the sheath, several vessels that feed into the left common iliac vein can be identified. These branches are isolated, clamped, and tied as they are visualized. When the plexus has been isolated, a Babcock clamp can be used to elevate the sheath. Two 2-0 absorbable or silk sutures are placed around the proximal and distal aspects of a 5-cm segment of the plexus and are loosely tied. The tonsil clamp is applied to each end of the nerve bundle. As the clamps are removed, the sutures are slipped down over the crushed areas and tied securely. The intervening portion of the plexus is then excised. The peritoneum may then be approximated with absorbable suture.

In less than 10% of cases, the pelvic mesocolon is inserted in front of the interiliac trigone and the nerve bundle cannot be reached by simple incision of the peritoneum. In these cases, the chief branches of the inferior mesenteric artery must be moved to the left to expose the triangular space between the two common iliac arteries. Unless there is adequate exposure and meticulous dissection, incomplete resection of the superior hypogastric plexus can occur, resulting in suboptimal denervation.

A laparoscopic approach to presacral neurectomy has also been described. This technique involves insertion of a 10-mm trocar sheath 3 cm above the symphysis pubis and placement of two accessory ports in each iliac fossa. Steep Trendelenburg position with a left lateral tilt is required to allow displacement of the intestines cephalad to expose the bifurcation of the aorta and sacral promontory. After retraction of the sigmoid colon and vasopressin infiltration of the sacral promontory area, the parietal peritoneum is grasped and elevated, and a transverse incision is performed from the major vessels or ureter on the right to the mesentery of the sigmoid on the left. The presacral nerve is isolated by developing the avascular space between the nerve and right internal iliac artery down to the periosteum via blunt dissection. Segments of the superior hypogastric plexus are removed by sharp dissection after thorough diathermy. The entire length of removed nerve plexus should not exceed 3 to 4 cm. Venous bleeding is controlled with bipolar cautery. Meticulous hemostasis must be ensured at the completion of the operation. This technique should only be performed by experienced laparoscopic surgeons because the vascular complications can be serious.

In a review of 655 laparoscopic presacral neurectomy procedures, Chen and Soong reported a 0.6% rate of major complications, including one case of injury of the right internal iliac artery and three cases of chylous ascites.

Polan and DeCherney reported that the combination of presacral neurectomy and conservative surgery in women with chronic pelvic pain, endometriosis, and pelvic inflammatory disease increased total postoperative pain relief from 26% to 75%, although only a small number of patients were included in this laparotomy series. Lee and coworkers performed presacral neurectomy via laparotomy in 50 women with chronic pelvic pain. Dysmenorrhea resolved in 73% of the cases, dyspareunia lessened in 77%, and acyclic pain improved in 63%. The uterosacral ligaments were resected in half of the subjects in this study, but this did not seem to affect the overall rate of pain relief. In a randomized clinical trial of women with

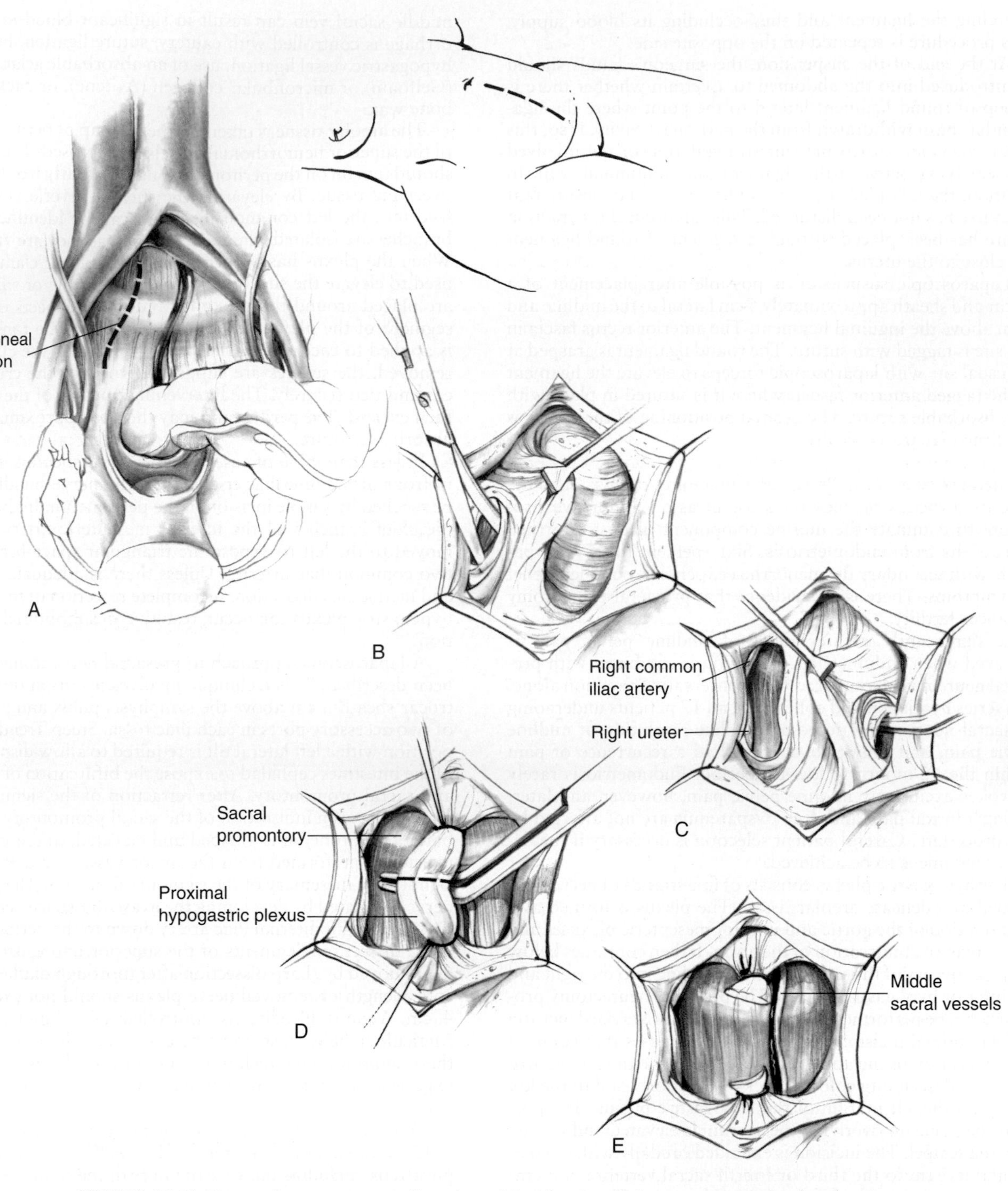

FIGURE 22.11. Presacral neurectomy. **A:** Location of incision in relation to anatomic landmarks. A Maylard incision can also be used in some cases. The descending colon is displaced superiorly and to the left for good exposure of the left margin of the hypogastric plexus. **B:** A Kitner sponge is used to dissect the areolar tissue medially and off the posterior aspect of the peritoneal flap. The right ureter can be identified easily. **C:** The areolar nerve-bearing tissue is dissected from the peritoneum on the left side, exposing the left internal iliac vessels and superior hemorrhoidal vessels. **D:** The plexus is isolated and elevated off the sacral promontory. A segment of plexus about 5 cm in length is isolated with 2-0 silk sutures. **E:** The plexus is excised. Note relation between pedicles of the nerve bundle and adjacent structures.

moderate to severe endometriosis and pelvic pain undergoing conservative surgical therapy, Candiani and colleagues reported a recurrence of midline menstrual pain in 23% of women who underwent presacral neurectomy versus a 42% recurrence in those who did not. This difference reached the limit of statistical significance ($p = 0.06$).

In an uncontrolled laparoscopic study by Nezhat and associates of 100 women subjected to vaporization of endometriosis and presacral neurectomy, the symptoms of pelvic pain, dysmenorrhea, and dyspareunia were reduced by more than 50% in 74, 61, and 55 patients, respectively, over the 1-year follow-up period. The stage of endometriosis did not correlate with the degree of pain improvement achieved. More recently, in a prospective, randomized, double-blind, controlled trial, Zullo and colleagues reported that the performance of laparoscopic presacral neurectomy improved the cure rate in women treated with conservative laparoscopic surgery for severe dysmenorrhea caused by endometriosis as compared with those who underwent mere ablation of endometriosis (85.7% vs. 57.1% at 12 months, $p < 0.05$).

Two common side effects of the presacral neurectomy procedure have been observed. Constipation may require laxatives or stool softeners for a period of 3 to 4 months. The vaginal dryness that develops in as many as 10% to 15% of patients is transient and usually resolves within 6 months. Difficulty with micturition is an infrequent complication that rarely lasts for more than 1 or 2 months. A painless first stage of labor has been reported in women who have undergone presacral neurectomy.

Uterine Nerve Ablation. The technique of uterosacral neurectomy was initially described by Ruggi in 1899. Later popularized by Doyle, it has since been adapted for performance during laparoscopic procedures for the alleviation of dysmenorrhea. Sympathetic fibers T10 to L1 are contained within the inferior hypogastric plexus and course along the inferior vena cava and sacrum to enter the uterus through the nerves of the uterosacral ligaments and accompanying uterine arteries. The parasympathetic components of the paracervical nerves originate from S1 through S3 or S4, travel within the nervi erigentes, and emerge in the lateral pelvis to form the Frankenhäuser ganglia lateral to the cervix. Division of the uterosacral ligaments at a point approximately 1.5 cm distal to the cervix should interrupt many sensory nerve fibers of the cervix and uterine corpus.

In general, uterine nerve ablation by laser is preferable to electrocautery because it is less likely to cause undesirable thermal damage. The course of the ureters and adjacent vasculature should be noted before commencement of dissection. The uterosacral ligaments are exposed by manipulating the uterine cannula to anteflex the corpus and by applying pressure to the posterior cervix with an ancillary laparoscopic probe.

The initial incision is made on the medial aspect of the ligament at its junction with the uterus. A second incision is made just lateral to the uterosacral ligament and medial to the ureter. The ligament is then grasped with forceps and stretched toward the sidewall. The CO_2 laser is used to vaporize a 2- to 5-cm area of each ligament to a depth of approximately 1 cm. This division should be centered approximately 1.5 cm distal to the cervix. The posterior aspect of the cervix between the insertions of the uterosacral ligaments may be superficially vaporized to interrupt the sensory fibers crossing to the contralateral side. Because extension of the beam too far lateral or posterior from the ligament can result in considerable bleeding, the surgeon should have immediate access to bipolar cautery, endocoagulation, or hemostatic clips. Fiber lasers such as the KTP/532 offer the advantages of increased hemostasis and lack of carbon plume, compared with the CO_2 instrument. If bipolar diathermy is used to fulgurate the uterosacral ligament, laparoscopic scissors are used to excise the segment of ligament in question.

Early retrospective and often uncontrolled clinical trials suggested that the laparoscopic uterosacral neurectomy technique might be efficacious. Feste reported significant improvement in the symptoms of primary dysmenorrhea or dysmenorrhea associated with endometriosis in 71% of a series of 42 patients. In a similar series of 100 patients by Donnez and Nisolle, 50% experienced complete relief, 41% had mild to moderate relief, and 9% described no relief. Using the carbon dioxide laser, Davis observed a considerable improvement in dysmenorrhea in 135 of 146 women (92%) with endometriosis and an improvement in dyspareunia in 103 of 109 women (94%) with endometriosis who underwent uterine nerve ablation and vaporization of endometriosis. This therapeutic benefit did not seem to differ among revised ASRM classification stages of endometriosis. Lichten and Bombard published a randomized, prospective, double-blind study of laparoscopic uterosacral nerve ablation for the treatment of severe or incapacitating dysmenorrhea unresponsive to oral contraceptives and nonsteroidal antiinflammatory agents. None of the control patients noted improvement, whereas 9 of 11 in the treated group had almost complete relief at 3 months, and 5 of 11 described complete relief from dysmenorrhea 1 year after surgery. Patients with endometriosis were not included in this small series.

Surgical resection of pelvic endometrial implants may be all that is necessary to alleviate discomfort in most endometriosis patients. In a double-blind, randomized controlled laparoscopic trial, Johnson and colleagues found that uterine nerve ablation was effective in reducing dysmenorrhea in the absence of endometriosis, but the addition of this procedure to the surgical treatment of endometriosis was not associated with a significant difference in any pain outcomes. Similarly, Vercellini and colleagues could not demonstrate the efficacy of this procedure.

Uterine nerve ablation by laparotomy fell from favor before it was revived as an endoscopic technique. The potential neurological, intestinal, orthopedic, and psychological components of pain should be considered before subjecting the patient to a procedure that, although now performed endoscopically, carries some surgical risk, and whose effectiveness has been questioned because of the small number of cases evaluated. Complications associated with transection of the uterosacral ligaments include ureteral damage, bowel damage, and postoperative hemorrhage, which, if undetected, may result in death. Uterine prolapse has recently been described as a potential long-term side effect of the procedure.

Second-Look Laparoscopy

Second-look laparoscopy has been suggested as an appropriate procedure for additional lysis of pelvic adhesions in patients who have undergone a laparotomy or a laparoscopy for the resection of endometriosis. If scheduled 8 days to 6 weeks after the initial dissection, second-look laparoscopy allows separation of *de novo* adhesions that are still relatively filmy in consistency. In addition, laparoscopy after pelvic reconstructive surgery provides an opportunity to assess future prognosis for fertility.

Early second-look laparoscopy after endoscopic treatment of endometriomas has revealed a recurrence rate of endometriomas of 15% to 20%. Equally significant are the nearly 20% incidence of *de novo* adhesion formation and the 40% to 82% recurrence rate of dense adhesions. Second-look laparoscopy allows treatment of these findings; however, there is little direct evidence that this secondary surgical procedure will increase the cumulative pregnancy rate.

Surgical Outcomes

No classification schedule for endometriosis provides an accurate correlation between extent of disease and pregnancy rate. Nevertheless, point categorization through the revised ASRM classification does provide a framework in which to report outcomes of therapy.

Fertility. In a review of the surgical outcome expected through laparoscopic therapy for minimal and mild endometriosis, the crude pregnancy rate following cautery or laser ablation of implants was 54% to 58% (Cook and Rock). Life-table analysis showed similar conception rates following laparoscopy and laparotomy to excise minimal or mild stages of endometriosis. Hence the performance of a laparotomy is not warranted for lesser stages of disease.

Treatment of mild endometriosis via laparoscopic excision or electocoagulation resulted in similar reproductive outcomes in a retrospective study by Tulandi and Al-Took. The total pregnancy rate was 53.5% in the excision group and 57.1% in the electrosurgery group. The mean interval between surgery and conception was 10.7 months in the electrosurgery group and 13.3 months in the excision group. Excision of tissue may result in more complete removal of infiltrating endometriosis, which should be of particular benefit to patients with deep nodules.

The stage of disease as categorized by the modified ASRM classification of endometriosis did not predict subsequent reproductive performance in a 2006 study by Vercellini and colleagues. Five hundred and thirty-seven infertile women with endometriosis undergoing first-line conservative laparoscopic surgery were followed for a mean of 32 months postoperatively. The cumulative probability of pregnancy at 3 years following laparoscopy was 47% (51% at stage I, 45% at stage II, 46% at stage III, and 44% at stage IV; log-rank test, $[chi]^2 = 1.50$, $P = 0.68$).

Expectant management of mild to moderate endometriosis after diagnosis by laparoscopy yields a crude pregnancy rate of about 50%, which has brought into question whether surgical therapy of lesser stages of disease actually enhances fertility. In a retrospective study comparing the efficacy of electrosurgical treatment of endometriosis with the efficacy of expectant management in minimal and mild endometriosis-associated infertility, Tulandi and Mouchawar reported that the cumulative probability of conception was significantly higher among patients treated surgically. Moreover, metaanalysis of the two randomized prospective trials showed that laparoscopic electrosurgery or laser to resect or ablate stage I–II endometriosis implants and adhesions resulted in a significantly higher fecundity rate as compared with the control group undergoing diagnostic laparoscopy only. The largest trial (Marcoux et al., 1997) clearly supported this outcome, with an increased chance of pregnancy (odds ratio [OR] 2.03, 95% confidence interval [CI] 1.28–3.24) and ongoing pregnancy rate after 20 weeks (OR 1.95, 95% CI 1.18–3.22) (Fig. 22.12), but the smaller trial (Parazzini, 1999) did not show benefit (pregnancy OR 0.76, 95% CI 0.31–1.88; live birth OR 0.85, 95% CI 0.32–2.28). When the ongoing pregnancy and live birth rates from these two studies were combined, there was a statistically significant increase with surgery (OR 1.64, 95% CI 1.05–2.57) (Jacobson et al). The findings suggest that for every 12 patients having stage I or II endometriosis diagnosed at laparoscopy, there will be one additional successful pregnancy if ablation or

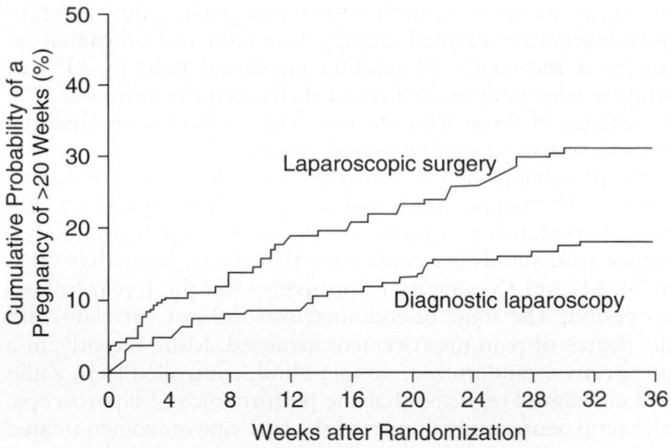

FIGURE 22.12. Cumulative probability of a pregnancy carried beyond 20 weeks in the 36 weeks after laparoscopy in women with endometriosis, according to study group. (From Marcoux S, Maheux R, Béribé S. Laparoscopic surgery in infertile women with minimal or mild endometriosis. *N Engl J Med* 1997;337:217.)

resection of visible endometriosis is performed, compared with no treatment.

Operative treatment of moderate or severe disease does offer a greater likelihood of conception than does expectant management, in part because of correction of mechanical factors such as adhesions. The overall crude pregnancy rate reported by various studies of conservative laparotomy for endometriosis that stratified reproductive results by disease severity was 38%, with a monthly fecundity rate averaging 1.4% to 1.5% (Cook and Rock). Laparoscopic treatment of severe endometriosis offered a mean crude pregnancy rate of 47.6% in a small compilation of series. Hence, expert laser laparoscopists have reported results that appear to be as good as those obtained through the open abdomen, although there are inadequate data for direct comparison of outcomes of the two surgical modalities, and the correct identification and classification of disease may vary between laparotomy and laparoscopy groups. Life-table analysis demonstrated that pregnancy is most likely to occur during the first 36 months after surgery. Furthermore, the duration of infertility and, perhaps, patient age may have a greater impact on cumulative pregnancy rates than the actual stage (revised ASRM stages I through IV) of the disease.

Pain. In a prospective, randomized double-blind, controlled trial of laser laparoscopy in the treatment of pelvic pain associated with minimal to moderate endometriosis, Sutton and associates found that 62.5% of the laser-treated women reported symptom improvement at 6 months as compared with 22.6% of those treated expectantly. Symptom relief continued at 1 year in 90% of those who initially responded. Moreover, in a more recent randomized, blinded, crossover study, 80% percent of patients who underwent excisional surgery had symptomatic improvement as compared with 30% of the placebo group (Abbott et al., 2004).

The technique of surgically treating lesser stages of endometriosis may not significantly influence pain relief, as long as the surgeon is aware of the depth of extension of the lesions. In a recent randomized study by Wright and colleagues, both excision and ablation of mild endometriosis produced good symptomatic relief and reduction of pelvic tenderness (67%).

Long-term improvement in quality of life can be achieved with laparoscopic excision of endometriosis. In a prospective, observational cohort study of 176 women with chronic pelvic pain with surgically diagnosed endometriosis, pain scores were highly significantly reduced at 2 to 5 years following resection in the categories of dysmenorrhea, dyspareunia, nonmenstrual pain, and dyschezia. The chance of requiring further surgery was 36%. Of note, almost one third who had further surgery had no evidence of endometriosis, either macroscopically or histologically, at the time of reoperation (Abbott et al., 2003).

Aggressive and complete excision of deep endometriosis is justified. Resection of deep endometriosis relieved dyspareunia in 40% and dysmenorrhea in 60% of cases. Nezhat and associates noted moderate to complete relief of pain in 162 of 175 women; however, some patients in this series had several surgical interventions. Preliminary analysis of the surgical results in 250 women in whom deep endometriosis had been excised with CO_2 laser showed a cure rate of pelvic pain in 70% and a recurrence rate of less than 5% over a 5-year follow-up period. Vercellini and colleagues (2006) reported that conservative surgery for rectovaginal endometriosis in infertile women did increase the pain-free survival time, although it did not modify the reproductive prognosis over expectant management. The recurrence rate of clinically detectable endometriosis is higher when the depth of infiltration is greater than 5 mm at the time of initial surgery, no matter the site of the lesion.

Persistence of dysmenorrhea and nonmenstrual pain after optimal endometriosis surgery may indicate adenomyosis. In a recent study by Parker and colleagues, chronic pelvic pain was significantly more likely to persist with uterine junctional zone thickness greater than 11 mm on preoperative MRI.

Recurrent Surgery

Rock and colleagues have shown that 13.5% of patients initially treated with conservative surgery required subsequent operative procedures. Wheeler and Malinak noted a cumulative recurrence rate at 3 and 5 years after conservative surgery of 13.5% and 40.3%, respectively. Neither the initial staging nor the ability to conceive after the initial surgery greatly affected the recurrence rates. Redwine reported a cumulative recurrence rate of 19% at 5 years after conservative laparoscopic excision of endometriosis by sharp dissection.

Laparoscopic excision of ovarian endometriomas by the stripping technique is associated with a lower reoperation rate than that of fenestration. In a study of patients who underwent laparoscopic cystectomy of ovarian endometriomas of greater than 3 cm in diameter, Busacca and colleagues reported a cumulative rate of ultrasonographic recurrence of 11.7% over 48 months.

A second cytoreductive procedure may benefit some infertile women who have undergone surgery in the past if assisted reproductive technologies are not pursued. A cumulative pregnancy rate of 32.4% at 35.4 months was achieved by Fedele and colleagues (2006) after a second conservative laparoscopic stripping procedure for recurrent endometriomas. The recurrence of pain (17.4%) was similar to that experienced after the primary laparoscopic stripping procedure. However, if the initial surgery fails to restore fertility in patients with stage III or stage IV endometriosis, *in vitro* fertilization (IVF) may be more beneficial than reoperation for those who are otherwise aysmptomatic. Pagidas and colleagues compared the outcome of a second operation for stage III or IV endometriosis-related infertility versus proceeding directly to IVF. The cumulative pregnancy rate 9 months after surgery was 24.4%, compared with a pregnancy rate of 33.4% after one trial of IVF and a cumulative pregnancy rate of 69.6% after two trials of IVF.

Combination Medical and Surgical Treatment

Preoperative and postoperative medical therapies have been proposed as treatment adjuncts to conservative resection of endometriosis to enhance fertility. Preoperative suppression of disease with hormonal agents may facilitate the surgical procedure by reducing tissue vascularity, and the greater ease in tissue dissection may decrease adhesion formation during the postoperative period. The preoperative hormonal agents also eliminate the corpus luteum that might otherwise be mistaken for an endometrioma. However, they may also reduce the size of endometriosis implants, making them less recognizable after short-term drug therapy. In a controlled clinical trial by Muzii et al, a 3-month course of GnRH agonist treatment before laparoscopy for endometrioma excision failed to result in a reduction in operative time or recurrence rate of disease during a 1-year follow-up period. There are no substantive data to justify hormonal treatments before surgery to improve the success of surgery.

Initiation of postoperative medical therapy may inhibit the activity of any residual disease, suppress ovulation, and decrease the possibility of adverse effects of peritoneal spillage of disease at the time of resection. Postoperative medical therapy has a serious drawback, however; the patient is unable to attempt conception for several months. Andrews and Larsen have noted that the best chance for postsurgical conception occurs during the first 6 months after conservative surgery by laparotomy. Thus, suppressing ovulation during that critical period may be counterproductive. Treatment with a GnRH agonist after surgery does not improve fertility as compared with expectant management (Busacca et al.).

Contemporary management of women with endometriosis-associated pelvic pain involves both surgical and long-term medical therapy. When cytoreductive laparoscopy is followed by a 6-month course of GnRH analog, there is a significant delay in the return of endometriosis symptoms requiring further treatment. In a randomized, prospective study, Hornstein and colleagues found that this interval was more than 24 months in those receiving nafarelin versus 11.7 months in the placebo group. A shorter duration of hormonal therapy during the postoperative period may be inadequate in reducing recurrence risk. A 3-month course of nafarelin following surgical therapy of stage III and IV endometriosis was ineffective in reducing pain scores as compared with placebo. Postoperative administration of low-dose, cyclic oral contraceptives for 6 months delayed the recurrence of pain symptoms and endometriomas at 12 months, but no significant differences were detected at 24 months or 36 months following laparoscopic excision.

Hysterectomy

The number and rate of hysterectomies performed for endometriosis increased steadily from the 1960s to the 1980s, more so than for other diagnoses. The reported rate for 1982 to 1984 was more than double the rate for 1965 to 1967, although the exact reasons for the increase remain uncertain. Although statistically significant increases for hysterectomy rates were observed from 1994 through 1998, the increase was limited, and the curve remained nearly flat. Endometriosis was the primary indication for 20.8% of white women and 9.7% of black women undergoing hysterectomy in the United States from 1994 to 1999. Because of concern over the risk of recurrence even after definitive surgical therapy, bilateral oophorectomy was performed at the time of hysterectomy in 52% of women 44 years of age or younger and in 81% of women 45 years of age or older.

Definitive surgery offers prompt, complete, and long-term relief of pain from endometriosis more often than do the various available medical regimens. Most hysterectomies for endometriosis are performed by the abdominal route; in selected cases, laparoscopy may allow lysis of complicating adhesions or large implants, thus allowing safe vaginal hysterectomy. When the posterior cul-de-sac is obliterated and extensive fibrosis is present deep in the pelvis, subtotal hysterectomy may be indicated.

The recurrence of cyclic pain associated with endometriosis after hysterectomy with preservation of normal ovaries has been estimated at 3% to 7%. Nevertheless, in a study of 138 women who underwent hysterectomy with the diagnosis of endometriosis at the Johns Hopkins Hospital, ovarian conservation was associated with a 6.1 times greater risk of development of recurrent pain and an 8.1 times greater risk of reoperation as compared with oophorectomy at the time of hysterectomy. Laparoscopic resection of invasive peritoneal and intestinal disease that persists after castration may result in an improvement in pain symptoms. Hysterectomy does not improve symptoms in 25% of cases of chronic pelvic pain when the uterus is believed to be the source of the pain.

Minute, hormonally active ovarian fragments may be detected in women with symptomatic endometriosis, even after total abdominal hysterectomy and bilateral salpingo-oophorectomy. This ovarian remnant syndrome is the result of incomplete excision of cortical tissue at the time of extirpative surgery for endometriosis or pelvic inflammatory disease. Most ovarian remnants are retroperitoneal in location, and they are often densely adhered to pelvic sidewall structures, including the ureter, hypogastric vessels, and bladder base. Complete surgical removal may be difficult.

Estrogen replacement therapy after total hysterectomy and bilateral oophorectomy is associated with less than a 10% rate of recurrence of endometriosis. A cause-and-effect relation between estrogen replacement and malignancy in endometriosis has not been established, suggesting that progestational agents need not be prescribed together with estrogens after hysterectomy for a diagnosis of endometriosis. However, administering both progestin and estrogen may be theoretically beneficial if the disease was incompletely resected or deeply invasive, contained atypical epithelial changes, or is recurrent. Women who begin estrogen replacement therapy immediately after total abdominal hysterectomy and bilateral salpingo-oophorectomy are at no greater risk of recurrent pain than those who delay estrogen therapy for more than 6 weeks postoperatively.

Women with endometriosis were shown by Modugno and colleagues to be at increased risk of developing ovarian cancer (OR 1.32; 95% CI 1.06–1.65). Hysterectomy and the use of oral contraceptives for greater than 10 years substantially reduce this risk.

ENDOMETRIOSIS AND ASSISTED REPRODUCTIVE TECHNOLOGIES

If spontaneous conception is not achieved within 3 years of surgical resection of endometriosis or within 1 year of repair of tubal obstruction associated with endometriosis, the odds are poor that it ever will occur. Techniques in assisted reproduction have been widely used during the past two decades for the management of endometriosis-associated infertility unresponsive to cytoreductive surgical or hormonal therapy. IVF removes gametes and zygotes from a potentially harmful environment and may bypass pelvic adhesions associated with endometriosis. Endometriosis is the sole identifiable cause of infertility in 25% to 35% of women undergoing IVF/embryo transfer.

The impact of endometriosis on the outcome of IVF has been controversial. Several studies have noted that the responses to gonadotropic stimulation, the numbers of preovulatory oocytes, the fertilization and cleavage rates, and the clinical pregnancy rates associated with stage I and stage II endometriosis have been equivalent to rates associated with tubal disease and unexplained infertility. Kuivasaari et al. reported that there was a significantly lower pregnancy rate and embryo implantation rate per fresh embryo transfer after pooled cycles (1–4) among women with stage III/IV endometriosis (22.6%) compared with stage I/II (40%) or tubal infertility (36.6%). However, when adjusted for confounding variables, Barnhart and colleagues in 2002 found that there was a significantly negative association between endometriosis of all stages and IVF outcome. This metaanalysis pooled data from 22 nonrandomized studies regarding IVF success rates in patients with endometriosis versus control patients without endometriosis and with tubal infertility. Most of these series included small numbers of subjects. The authors concluded that there was a 54% reduction in pregnancy rate after IVF in patients with endometriosis and that the success was even poorer when the staging of endometriosis was higher. Subsequent studies have disputed these findings.

Poor IVF outcome in severe endometriosis may be related to oocyte or embryo factors rather than decreased uterine receptivity. Diaz and colleagues found that a history of severe endometriosis in recipients of donor oocytes had no effect on embryo implantation rates or clinical pregnancy rates as compared with recipients who did not have a history of endometriosis.

In general, women with endometriosis have a lower ovarian response to gonadotropin stimulation. One reason for this response may be previous ovarian resection. Studies recruiting women with a history of surgical excision of a unilateral endometrioma and comparing subsequent ovarian responsiveness to gonadotropin stimulation in the affected and contralateral intact gonad indicate that excision of endometriomas is associated with a quantitative damage to ovarian follicular reserve. However, this lower oocyte yield following surgery has not necessarily led to decreased pregnancy rates.

Recent retrospective studies have suggested that routine laparoscopic cystectomy for endometriomas before commencing an IVF cycle does not improve IVF outcomes. Aside from a lower peak estradiol level on the day of hCG administration and a higher total gonadotropin dose administered to women previously operated on for an endometrioma, no significant differences were found between the resected endometrioma group and the intact endometrioma group among the different variables analyzed (Garcia-Velasco et al.). Pre-IVF excision of ovarian endometriomas in symptomatic women did not impair nor enhance IVF or intracytoplasmic sperm injection success rates.

Another recent retrospective study indicated that women with a history of past or current endometriomas had fewer oocytes retrieved during IVF than tubal factor controls, but the fertilization rate, embryo quality, or pregnancy outcome was not affected (Suzuki et al.).

Tinkanen and Kujansuu studied the effects of operative treatment of recurrent ovarian endometriosis on the pregnancy rate with IVF. They compared 45 patients with ultrasound-diagnosed ovarian endometriosis during IVF treatment, 36 of the cases being recurrences after previous operation, with 55 patients who had undergone past endometrioma resection and had no evidence of recurrence before IVF. Patients with endometriomas had significantly more embryos for transfer compared with women without endometriomas. The clinical pregnancy rate was 38% in the endometrioma group compared with 22% in the no-endometrioma group. The women who had surgery with no recurrent endometriosis may have had a more extensive resection as compared with those with recurrent endometriomas following initial surgery. Radical surgery could result in diminished ovarian reserve.

Hence, the hypothesis that surgical therapy of endometriosis increases IVF pregnancy rates is not clearly validated by the available evidence. Endometrioma resection may compromise or destroy adjacent normal ovarian tissue by removing part of the ovarian cortex and thus reducing ovarian reserve. Moreover, elective aspiration of endometriomas is associated with an increased risk of infection, even with the prophylactic use of antibiotics. On the other hand, larger endometriomas may interfere with follicular recruitment, may impose difficulties during oocyte retrieval, and may theoretically produce substances that are toxic to maturing oocytes and affect cell cleavage after fertilization.

The presence of significant pelvic pain symptoms, number of previous surgical interventions for endometriosis, and the patient's age and ovarian reserve must be taken into consideration in establishing an individualized treatment plan (Fig. 22.3). Further randomized clinical trials are needed to elucidate the relative effects of mild peritoneal endometriosis and advanced stages of disease associated with endometriomas and pelvic adhesions on the outcome of IVF.

The relative value of initial medical therapy before use of assisted reproductive technologies remains controversial. Dicker and associates noted that 35 women with severe endometriosis who underwent 6 months of ovarian suppression with a GnRH analog had a higher clinical pregnancy rate per cycle and per transfer than did 32 women who received ovarian stimulation for IVF without prior GnRH treatment (per cycle, 25% versus 3.9%; per transfer, 33% versus 5.3%). The majority of retrospective studies and one small randomized controlled trial suggested that the reproductive outcome in women with endometriosis undergoing IVF is improved in all stages of disease, and particularly in patients with moderate-severe endometriosis, after prolonged (e.g., 3 month) down-regulation with GnRH agonist before starting ovarian stimulation.

Gamete intrafallopian transfer (GIFT) may overcome impairment of sperm transport to the fallopian tube, failed ovum capture, or abnormalities in the peritoneal environment associated with endometriosis, although the presence of any anatomic disorders of the fallopian tubes has negative prognostic significance for a successful outcome for this procedure. Hulme and colleagues performed GIFT on 46 infertile patients with minimal to moderately active endometriosis not previously treated by medical or surgical methods. The only prerequisite was patency of at least one fallopian tube. The pregnancy rate per GIFT cycle was 30.5% (18/59), which compared with a clinical pregnancy rate of 25.8% for all patients undergoing the procedure at their unit. One or more endometriomas were aspirated from the ovaries at the time of follicle aspiration in 11 patients; 4 of the 11 achieved live births with GIFT. Nevertheless, Guzick and associates, in a case-control study, found that pelvic endometriosis significantly impaired the efficacy of GIFT. Of 114 laparoscopic oocyte retrievals performed in the endometriosis group, there were 37 pregnancies (32.5%) and 25 deliveries (23.7%); of the 214 retrievals in the control group, there were 101 pregnancies (47.2%) and 76 deliveries (35.5%).

Controlled ovarian hyperstimulation (COH) with human menopausal gonadotropins or pure FSH together with intrauterine insemination (IUI) has been proposed as a method to increase cycle fecundity of patients with endometriosis, although few series have been published to date (Table 22.9). By increasing the number of oocytes released at the time of ovulation and introducing a high concentration of spermatozoa into the female reproductive tract, the chance for conception is improved, merely because of the larger number of gametes available for fertilization. In addition, subtle abnormalities of folliculogenesis, corpus luteum function, tubal motility, or sperm function may be corrected with this therapy. Cycle fecundity rates associated with COH/IUI therapy in patients with endometriosis-associated infertility have ranged from 9% to 13%, although these series did not include a nontreatment control group. One recent prospective randomized study found

TABLE 22.9

CYCLE FECUNDITY IN WOMEN WITH STAGE I OR II ENDOMETRIOSIS, ACCORDING TO TREATMENT

	Unexplained infertility	Endometriosis-associated infertility			
Group treatment	Guzick et al.	Deaton et al.,	Chaffkin et al.	Fedele et al.	Kemmann et al.
No treatment or intracervical					
Insemination	0.02	0.033	–	0.045	0.028
IUI	0.05[a]	–	–	–	–
Clomiphene	–	–	–	–	0.066
Clomiphene/IUI	–	0.095[a]	–	–	–
Gonadotropins	0.04[a]	–	0.066	–	0.073[a]
Gonadotropins/IUI	0.09[a]	–	0.129[a]	0.15[a]	–
IVF	–	–	–	–	0.222[a]

[a] $P<.05$ for treatment vs. no treatments.
IUI, intrauterine insemination; IVF, *in vitro* fertilization.
From the Practice Committee of the American Society for Reproductive Medicine. *Fertil Steril* 2004;82 (suppl1):S40, with permission.

a higher pregnancy rate with COH/IUI following at least 6 weeks of GnRH agonist suppression in patients with advanced stages of endometriosis.

Fedele and associates reported that superovulation with timed intercourse was not associated with a better cumulative, crude pregnancy rate than expectant management in infertile women with endometriosis stages I and II, although the cycle fecundity rate was improved. However, a more recent randomized, controlled trial of COH and IUI for infertility associated with stage I and II endometriosis demonstrated a live birth rate of 11% per cycle in the treatment group and 2% in the control group. Others reported that ovarian stimulation or induction using gonadotropins results in higher fecundity rates than no treatment, but the clinical pregnancy rate after treatment was still significantly lower in the endometriosis group (6.5%) than in women with unexplained infertility (15%) (Nuoja-Huttunen et al.). There was no surgical treatment of endometriosis before therapy with COH and IUI in these latter studies.

In a 2006 retrospective study by Webrouck and colleauges, the clinical pregnancy rate per cycle of COH and IUI in women with minimal and a mild endometriosis who underwent laparoscopic excision of lesions within 7 months of onset of treatment was 21% or 18.9%, respectively, which was comparable to that achieved in patients with unexplained infertility, 20.5%. The mean age of the patients with endometriosis in this study was 31 years. The cumulative live birth rate of nearly 70% within four cycles suggest that COH and IUI may be appropriate first-line therapy in patients younger than 35 who have not become pregnant within 6 to 12 months after surgical treatment of minimal to mild endometriosis and who have no other infertility risk factors. The clinical history must be carefully weighed when planning a sequence of therapy for the infertile patient with endometriosis.

Temporary exposure to very high estradiol levels in women during COH for IVF or intrauterine insemination is not a major risk factor for endometriosis recurrence in women treated with assisted reproductive technology.

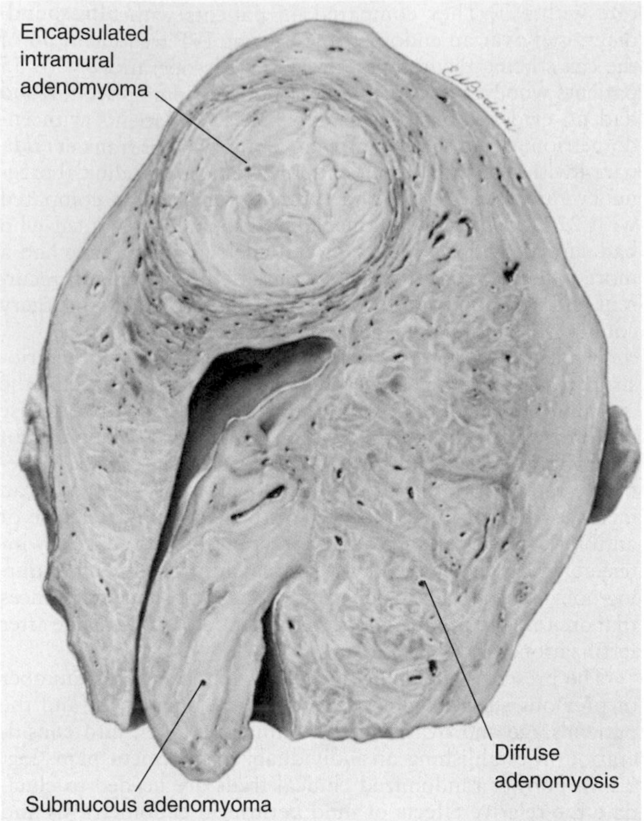

FIGURE 22.13. Uterus showing three types of adenomyomatous growth: encapsulated intramural adenomyoma, submucous adenomyoma, and diffuse adenomyosis of walls.

ADENOMYOSIS

Adenomyosis is defined as heterotopic endometrial glands and stroma located deep within the myometrium. This disease can be categorized as diffuse or local in its distribution. Diffuse adenomyosis can be relatively localized but is never encapsulated (Fig. 22.13). The uterus itself is usually mildly enlarged, rarely to more than twice-normal size, and is generally symmetric. Cut sections of the myometrium reveal a coarse trabecular pattern of interlacing musculature and fibrous tissue with small islands of endometrium that are often dark and hemorrhagic. Localized, encapsulated disease of the uterine wall is termed *adenomyoma,* to distinguish this manifestation of adenomyosis from the more usual diffuse pattern. An adenomyoma is always located mainly within the wall of the uterus but may project into the uterine cavity to become further known as a *submucous adenomyoma.* This encapsulated, submucous form of adenomyosis disease resembles the leiomyoma.

The most widely accepted theory of the origin of adenomyosis is that endometrial tissue within the myometrium is of müllerian origin. Its presence in this location is the result of a direct, downward extension of the endometrium of the uterine cavity. Serial sectioning of tissue has revealed a direct continuity between the basalis portion of the endometrium and the endometrial islands within the areas of adenomyosis. Endometrial extensions sometimes are present through the full thickness of the myometrium to the serosal surface of the uterus. Occasionally, only subserosal adenomyosis is seen. Subserosal adenomyosis is often associated with pelvic endometriosis and may cause the lymphatic spread of endometrial fragments.

The intramural islands generally have the same histologic appearance as the basalis of the endometrium (Fig. 22.14) and often respond to estrogen stimulation by demonstrating a proliferative or, occasionally, cystic hyperplastic pattern. Cellular atypia is rare. The effect of progestational agents on the ectopic endometrium is less predictable. Secretory changes in the glands are uncommon except in pregnancy, when a decidual reaction of the stroma is anticipated. Unlike endometriosis, adenomyotic lesions are not characterized by a pronounced hemorrhagic tendency or inflammatory response. In the absence of hormonal stimulation, adenomyosis becomes atrophic. Adenocarcinomas involving adenomyosis are characterized by a history of prior exogenous estrogen use, by low histologic grades, and by an excellent prognosis.

Adenomyosis can be definitively diagnosed only through histologic sections of myometrium. The reported incidence of the disease varies widely among institutions, from 8% to 62%, depending on the criteria used for diagnosis and on the thoroughness with which the excised uterine tissue is studied. The usual criterion for diagnosis is glandular extension below the endometrial-myometrial interface of greater than 2.5 mm, whereas adenomyosis subbasalis can be defined as minimally

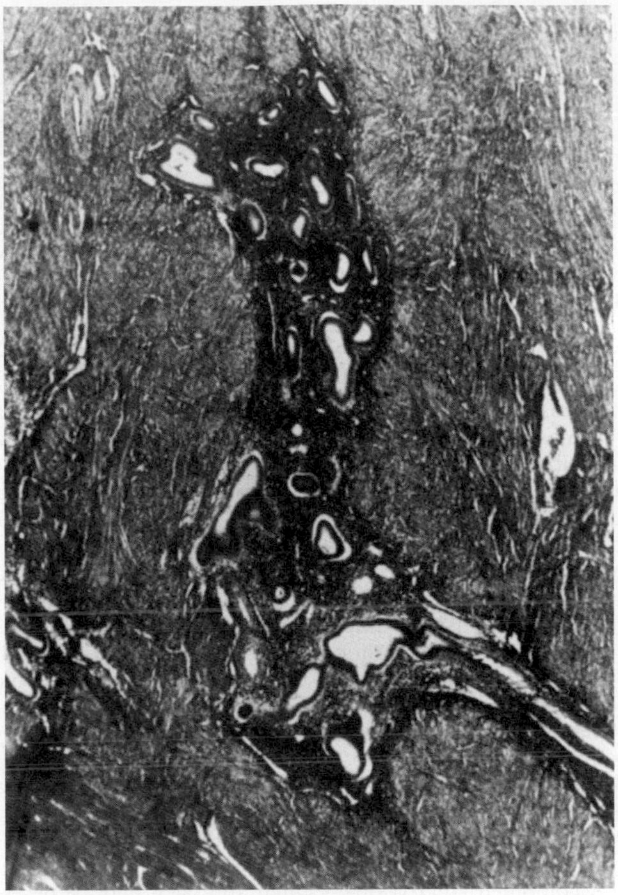

FIGURE 22.14. Area of adenomyosis. Compact stroma and proliferative, slightly hyperplastic glands surrounded by hypertrophied myometrium.

invasive adenomyosis extending less than 2 mm beneath the basal endometrium. The incidence of adenomyosis begins to rise in the mid-30s and peaks in the fifth decade. Infertility is not common, although most patients are multiparous. About 12% have coexisting external endometriosis. Adenomyosis is often discovered incidentally in patients undergoing surgery for uterine leiomyomas.

Symptoms

Adenomyosis is often an incidental pathologic finding, and approximately 35% of cases are asymptomatic. Dysmenorrhea is more likely to be reported when glandular invasion exceeds 80% or more of the myometrium. Pain can be severe, cramping, or knifelike, and may occur up to 1 week before the onset of menstrual flow. The pattern of dysmenorrhea is likely associated with bleeding episodes within the deep-lying islands of endometrium. Menorrhagia can be a consequence of the increased surface area of the enlarged uterine cavity. In addition, extensive involvement of the myometrium can interfere with the normal contractility of the uterine musculature and can lead to excessive bleeding. Nevertheless, data collected from 1,851 hysterectomies for the prospective, multicenter Collaborative Review of Sterilization study indicate that adenomyosis occurs as often in asymptomatic uteri removed for prolapse (19%) as in uteri removed for excessive bleeding (22%) or pain symptoms (15%). Uterine adenomyosis is significantly associated with pelvic endometriosis, with a prevalence of up to 90%. By impairing uterine sperm transport, adenomyosis may be a leading factor of infertility in women with endometriosis.

Pelvic Findings

The uterus may be very firm to palpation and is usually enlarged to not more than twice its normal size. As it is classically described, the adenomyotic enlargement occurs in the anteroposterior dimension, a reflection of the more prominent involvement of the posterior uterine wall. In the more common diffuse type of adenomyosis, the uterus is a symmetrically enlarged, globular structure. Encapsulated adenomyomata may cause the uterus to be irregular or asymmetric, much as it is when leiomyomata are present. At times, particularly during menstruation, the enlarged uterus is tender on examination.

Diagnosis

Adenomyosis should always be suspected in a woman with dysmenorrhea and menorrhagia of increasing severity her fourth or fifth decade, particularly if the uterus is symmetrically enlarged, firm, and tender. An exact preoperative diagnosis is often difficult to establish because dysfunctional uterine bleeding and multiple small leiomyomas can present in a similar fashion. Gambone and colleagues reported that a presumptive diagnosis of adenomyosis was verified in only 38% of hysterectomy specimens. The diagnosis can be histologically established before hysterectomy only in the rare case in which excessive myometrium is removed during curettage or a polypoid submucous adenomyoma is excised. However, hysteroscopic myometrial biopsy of the posterior uterine wall with use of a 5-mm loop electrode has been shown to effectively establish the diagnosis in women with menorrhagia.

Hysterosalpingography of the adenomyomatous uterus with water-based media can occasionally demonstrate multiple spiculations or tuft defects leading from the uterine cavity to the myometrial wall; however, similar findings can occur in cases of vascular or lymphatic extravasation. MRI has proved to be highly accurate for distinguishing adenomyosis from leiomyomata; on T2-weighted images, adenomyosis appears as an ill-defined, relatively homogeneous, low-signal-intensity area embedded with sparse, high-intensity spots. The optimal junctional zone thickness value for establishing the diagnosis of adenomyosis is 12 mm or more. Several studies have shown that the sensitivity and specificity of MRI to diagnose adenomyosis ranges from 86% to 100% in a symptomatic patient population.

Recent studies have also suggested an important role for transvaginal ultrasound in distinguishing adenomyosis from leiomyomata. By using the diagnostic criterion of the presence of unencapsulated, heterogeneous, myometrial areas within round anechoic areas 1 to 3 mm in diameter, Fedele and colleagues noted a sensitivity of 80%, a specificity of 74%, a negative predictive value of 81%, and a positive predictive value of 73%. Nevertheless, when transvaginal sonography and MRI have been prospectively compared, the latter has been significantly more accurate in correctly establishing the diagnosis.

Hormone receptor studies have documented the presence of steroid receptors in adenomyotic foci. Estrogen receptors are more consistently present than are progesterone receptors, which are completely absent in 40% of cases evaluated. Progestins or cyclic estrogen-progestin combination preparations offer little aid in treatment, although recent reports indicated that adenomyosis-associated menorrhagia can be controlled with the insertion of a levonorgestrel-releasing intrauterine device or a danazol-loaded intrauterine device. GnRH agonist therapy for 6 months resulted in the disappearance of pain symptoms and a decline in uterine volume in 65% of cases of biopsy-proven adenomyosis, but the dysmenorrhea and menorrhagia recurred at the end of treatment. Nevertheless, extended intermittent use of these agonists can effectively relieve pain symptoms while having the significant advantage of preserving fertility between treatments.

Curettage does not aid in establishing the diagnosis of adenomyosis and is ineffective as treatment, although it may be required because of abnormal bleeding. The need for surgery, therefore, is based on continued menorrhagia and dysmenorrhea rather than on an estimation of uterine size or even the known presence of adenomyosis or leiomyomata. The definitive treatment for abnormal bleeding caused by adenomyosis is hysterectomy. The vaginal route is preferred if the size of the uterus is appropriate and no other pelvic abnormalities are present. Under certain circumstances, as with a younger patient who wishes to retain her reproductive capability, excision of an encapsulated adenomyoma should be considered instead of hysterectomy. Such situations arise infrequently because adenomyosis is generally diffuse and usually occurs in multiparous women who are no longer interested in childbearing. The precise efficacy of hysteroscopic endometrial resection, laparoscopic myometrial reduction, and myometrial excision as conservative surgical procedures for adenomyosis has yet to be proved. Endometrial ablation is ineffective as treatment for deep, subserosal adenomyosis.

Interventional radiological techniques have been described to selectively embolize the uterine vessels in women with adenomyosis. Although short-term results of uterine artery embolization to treat adenomyosis appeared encouraging, midterm results were disappointing, with only 55% of treated patients showing clinical improvement after 2 years (Pelage et al). Preliminary trials have suggested that magnetic resonance-guided focused ultrasound surgery may be used in the future to destroy focal adenomyosis.

Hysterectomy should be considered in the severely symptomatic patient when ultrasonography, MRI, or myometrial biopsy demonstrates deep adenomyosis.

BEST SURGICAL PRACTICES

- Surgery is indicated for correction of pain, infertility, or other symptoms in patients with extensive pelvic endometriosis, or when hormonal manipulation fails to adequately diminish pain symptoms in women with lesser stages of disease.
- Preoperative rectoscopy-sigmoidoscopy and intravenous pyelography are recommended in patients with symptoms suggestive of deeply invasive endometriosis of the posterior cul-de-sac and rectovaginal septum. Preoperative ultrasound and MRI may help to categorize the extent of ovarian involvement and location of deeply infiltrating disease. A bowel prep before surgery may facilitate optimal performance and safety of the surgical procedure, particularly when deep disease is anticipated.
- Laparoscopy can be considered for all cases unless there is difficulty in establishing the appropriate tissue planes of dissection or unless improved access is necessary for atraumatic manipulation of the involved organs. Conservative resection of disease by laparotomy is most valuable in cases of extensive, dense pelvic adhesions or endometriomas greater than 5 cm in diameter. In addition, deep involvement of the rectovaginal septum with fibrotic extension into the perirectal fossa, invasion of the bowel muscularis, and endometriotic infiltration in the region of the uterine vessels and ureter are generally best approached through the open abdomen for all but advanced endoscopic surgeons.
- The philosophy of gentle manipulation of tissue in an attempt to avoid trauma is the major tenet of pelvic reconstruction. Adhesion formation can be reduced by magnification of the surgical site, avoidance of suture unless clearly indicated, reconstruction with fine nonreactive suture, precise hemostasis, and frequent irrigation of tissues with warmed solution.
- Less tissue damage is achieved with bipolar than with monopolar cautery. Ablation of deep disease by monopolar microdiathermy or CO_2 laser vaporization rather than excision of the disease may result in inadequate resection and a greater amount of ischemic damage to the tissue, heightening the propensity toward adhesion formation. Deep lesions or more extensive peritoneal disease must be excised with a tissue margin of at least 2 to 4 mm, because microscopic lesions are commonly present in tissue adjacent to visible implants. Twenty-five percent of patients have lesions greater than 5 mm in depth.
- Coagulation or vaporization of disease in the ovarian fossa or near the uterosacral ligament should be undertaken only after clear identification of the ureter. Resection of deep posterior cul-de-sac nodules requires great endoscopic expertise. A combined laparoscopic-vaginal approach may be necessary.
- Inability to elevate the ovary is usually a sign of adhesions and endometriotic implants of the inferolateral surface of the ovary and the peritoneum of the ovarian fossa. When removing an endometrioma, the cortical incision should be made in a way that will preserve the normal anatomic relations of the ovary with the uteroovarian ligament and fimbria ovarica. Suture on or extruding through the surface should be avoided when possible because of its adhesiogenic properties. With larger endometriomas, the normal ovarian cortex is stabilized with atraumatic forceps, and the cyst wall is grasped with biopsy forceps and stripped from the bed of normal ovarian tissue. The dissection may be facilitated by removing a small circular rim of tissue around the adhesion site to begin the stripping procedure in a clearer field, where the endometrioma wall is less adhered to healthy ovarian tissue. The rate of recurrence of pelvic pain and dysmenorrhea over a 2-year postoperative period is significantly less for those patients who are managed by cystectomy as compared with those undergoing fenestration and coagulation. Moreover, the rate of reoperation is less and the cumulative pregnancy rate is higher in the cystectomy group. Extensive cauterization or resection of ovarian tissue can lead to a rise in FSH levels postoperatively and should be avoided.
- Aggressive and complete excision of deep endometriosis is justified. The recurrence rate of clinically detectable endometriosis is higher when the depth of infiltration is greater than 5 mm at the time of initial surgery, no matter the site of the lesion. A second cytoreductive procedure may benefit some infertile women who have undergone surgery in the past, although assisted reproductive

technologies would lead to a higher chance of conceiving for most patients who failed primary surgery. The hypothesis that surgical therapy of endometriosis increases IVF pregnancy rates is not clearly validated by the available evidence.

- Uterine suspension is of unproven efficacy in enhancing fertility or as an adjunct in the treatment of endometriosis-associated pelvic pain.
- Presacral neurectomy, or division of the superior hypogastric plexus, is useful as an adjunctive procedure to eliminate the uterine component of dysmenorrhea that results from endometriosis. Uterine nerve ablation may be effective in reducing dysmenorrhea in the absence of endometriosis, but the addition of this procedure to the surgical treatment of endometriosis has not been associated with a significant difference in any pain outcomes.

Bibliography

Abbott JA, Howe J, Clayton RD, et al. The effects and effectiveness of laparoscopic excision of endometriosis: a prospective study with 2-5 year follow-up. *Hum Reprod* 2003;18:1922.

Abbott J, Howe J, Hunter D, et al. Laparoscopic excision of endometriosis: a randomized, placebo-controlled trial. *Fertil Steril* 2004;82:878.

Aboulghar MA, Mansour RT, Serour G, et al. The outcome of *in vitro* fertilization in advanced endometriosis with previous surgery: a case-controlled study. *Am J Obstet Gynecol* 2003;188:371.

Adamson GD, Hurd SJ, Pasta DJ, et al. Laparoscopic endometriosis treatment: is it better? *Fertil Steril* 1993;59:35.

Adamson GD, Subak LL, Pasta DJ, et al. Comparison of CO_2 laser laparoscopy with laparotomy for the treatment of endometriomata. *Fertil Steril* 1992;57:965.

Albourzi S, Momtahan M, Parsanezhad M, et al. A prospective, randomized study comparing laparoscopic ovarian cystectomy versus fenestration and coagulation in patients with endometriomas. *Fertil Steril* 2004;82:1633.

American Fertility Society. The classification of endometriosis. *Fertil Steril* 1979;32:633.

American Fertility Society. Revised American Fertility Society classification of endometriosis: 1985. *Fertil Steril* 1985;43:351.

American Society for Reproductive Medicine. Revised American Society for Reproductive Medicine classification of endometriosis: 1996. *Fertil Steril* 1997;67:817.

Andrews WE, Larsen GD. Endometriosis: treatment with hormonal pseudopregnancy and/or operation. *Am J Obstet Gynecol* 1974;118:643.

Ascher SM, Arnold LL, Patt RH, et al. Adenomyosis: prospective comparison of MR imaging and transvaginal sonography. *Radiology* 1994;190:803.

Awadalla SG, Friedman CI, Haq AU, et al. Local peritoneal factors: their role in infertility associated with endometriosis. *Am J Obstet Gynecol* 1987;157:1207.

Ayers JW, Birenbaum DL, Menon KM. Luteal phase dysfunction in endometriosis: elevated progesterone levels in peripheral and ovarian veins during the follicular phase. *Fertil Steril* 1987;47:925.

Badawy SZA, Cuenca V, Kaufman L, et al. The regulation of immunoglobulin production by B cells in patients with endometriosis. *Fertil Steril* 1989;51:770.

Bailey HR, Ott MT, Hartendorp P. Aggressive surgical management for advanced colorectal endometriosis. *Dis Colon Rectum* 1994;37:747.

Barbieri RL. Etiology and epidemiology of endometriosis. *Am J Obstet Gynecol* 1990;162:565.

Barbieri RL. Hormone treatment of endometriosis: the estrogen threshold hypothesis. *Am J Obstet Gynecol* 1992;166:740.

Barbieri RL. Stenosis of the external os: an association with endometriosis in women with chronic pelvic pain. *Fertil Steril* 1998;70:571.

Barbieri RL, Niloff JM, Bast RC Jr, et al. Elevated serum concentrations of CA-125 in patients with advanced endometriosis. *Fertil Steril* 1986;45:630.

Barbieri RL, Ryan KJ. Danazol: endocrine pharmacology and therapeutic applications. *Am J Obstet Gynecol* 1981;141:453.

Barnhart K, Dunsmoor-Su R, Coutifaris C. Effect of endometriosis on *in vitro* fertilization. *Fertil Steril* 2002;77:1148.

Beretta P, Franchi M, Ghezzi F, et al. Randomized clinical trial of two laparoscopic treatments of endometriomas: cystectomy versus drainage and coagulation. *Fertil Steril* 1998;70:1176.

Bergqvist A, Theorell T. Changes in quality of life after hormonal treatment of endometriosis. *Acta Obstet Gynecol Scand* 2001;80:628.

Biberoglu KO, Behrman SJ. Dosage aspects of danazol therapy in endometriosis: short term and long term effectiveness. *Am J Obstet Gynecol* 1981;138:645.

Brosens IA, Koninckx PR, Corveleyn PA. A study of plasma progesterone, oestradiol-17β, prolactin and LH levels and of the luteal phase appearance of the ovaries in patients with endometriosis and infertility. *BJOG* 1978;85:246.

Brosens I, Vasquez G, Gordts S. Scanning electron microscopy study of the pelvic peritoneum in unexplained infertility and endometriosis. *Fertil Steril* 1984;41:215.

Bruner KL, Mastrisian LM, Rodgers WH, et al. Suppression of matrix metalloproteinases inhibits establishment of ectopic lesions by human endometrium in nude mice. *J Clin Invest* 1997;99:2851.

Busacca M, Marana R, Caruana P, et al. Recurrence of ovarian endometriomas after laparoscopic excision. *Am J Obstet Gynecol* 1999;180:519.

Busacca M, Riparini J, Somigliana E, et al. Postsurgical ovarian failure after laparoscopic excision of bilateral endometriomas. *Am J Obstet Gynecol* 2006;195:421.

Buttram VC Jr, Reiter RC, Ward S. Treatment of endometriosis with danazol: report of a 6 year prospective study. *Fertil Steril* 1985;43:353.

Candiani GB, Fedele L, Vercellini P, et al. Presacral neurectomy for the treatment of pelvic pain associated with endometriosis: a controlled study. *Am J Obstet Gynecol* 1992;167:100.

Candiani GB, Fedele L, Vercellini P, et al. Repetitive conservative surgery for recurrence of endometriosis. *Obstet Gynecol* 1991;77:421.

Candiani GB, Vercellini P, Fedele L, et al. Conservative surgical treatment for severe endometriosis in infertile women: are we making progress? *Obstet Gynecol Surv* 1991;48[Suppl 7]:490.

Candiani GB, Vercellini P, Fedele L, et al. Conservative surgical treatment of rectovaginal septum endometriosis. *J Gynecol Surg* 1992;8:177.

Candiani GB, Vercellini P, Fedele L. Laparoscopic ovarian puncture for correct staging of endometriosis. *Fertil Steril* 1990;53:994.

Canis M, Mage G, Wattiex A, et al. Second-look laparoscopy after laparoscopic cystectomy of large ovarian endometriomas. *Fertil Steril* 1992;58:617.

Carpenter SE, Markham SM, Rock JA. Exercise may reduce side effects of danazol. *Infertility* 1988;2:259.

Cedars MI, Lu JK, Meldrum DR, et al. Treatment of endometriosis with a long-acting gonadotropin releasing hormone agonist plus medroxyprogesterone acetate. *Obstet Gynecol* 1990;75:641.

Chaffkin LM, Nulsen JC, Luciano AA, et al. A comparative analysis of the cycle fecundity rates associated with combined human menopausal gonadotropin (hMG) and intrauterine insemination (IUI) versus either hMG or IUI alone. *Fertil Steril* 1991;55:252.

Cheesman KL, Ben-Nun I, Chatterton RT Jr, et al. Relationship of luteinizing hormone, pregnanediol-3-glucuronide and estriol-16-glucuronide in urine of infertile women with endometriosis. *Fertil Steril* 1982;38:542.

Cheesman KL, Cheesman SD, Chatterton RT, et al. Alterations in progesterone metabolism and luteal function in infertile women with endometriosis. *Fertil Steril* 1983;40:590.

Chen FP, Soong YK. The efficacy and complications of laparoscopic presacral neurectomy in pelvic pain. *Obstet Gynecol* 1997;90:974.

Chong AP, Luciano AA, O'Shaughnessy AM. Laser laparoscopy versus laparotomy in the treatment of infertility patients with severe endometriosis. *J Gynecol Surg* 1990;6:179.

Coddington CC, Oehninger S, Cunningham DS, et al. Peritoneal fluid from patients with endometriosis decreases sperm binding to the zona pellucida in the hemizona assay: a preliminary report. *Fertil Steril* 1992;57:783.

Confino E, Harlow L, Gleicher N. Peritoneal fluid and serum autoantibody levels in patients with endometriosis. *Fertil Steril* 1990;53:242.

Cook AS, Rock JA. The role of laparoscopy in the treatment of endometriosis. *Fertil Steril* 1991;55:663.

Cornillie FJ, Oosterlynck D, Lauweryns JM, et al. Deeply infiltrating pelvic endometriosis: histology and clinical significance. *Fertil Steril* 1989;53:978.

Coronado C, Franklin RR, Lotze EC, et al. Surgical treatment of symptomatic colorectal endometriosis. *Fertil Steril* 1990;53:411.

Cramer DW, Missmer SA. The epidemiology of endometriosis. *Ann N Y Acad Sci* 2002;955:11.

Cramer DW, Wilson E, Stillman RJ, et al. The relation of endometriosis to menstrual characteristics, smoking, and exercise. *JAMA* 1986;255:1904.

Cullen TS. The distribution of adenomyomata containing uterine mucosa. *Arch Surg* 1919;80:130.

Czernobilsky B, Morris W. A histologic study of ovarian endometriosis with emphasis on hyperplastic and atypical changes. *Obstet Gynecol* 1979;53:318.

Czernobilsky B, Silverstein A. Salpingitis in ovarian endometriosis. *Fertil Steril* 1978;30:45.

Damewood MD, Hesla JS, Schlaff WD, et al. Effect of serum from patients with minimal to mild endometriosis on mouse embryo development in vitro. *Fertil Steril* 1990;54:917.

Daniell JF. Fiberoptic laser laparoscopy. *Baillieres Clin Obstet Gynaecol* 1989;3:545.

Davis GD. Management of endometriosis and its associated adhesions with the CO_2 laser laparoscope. *Obstet Gynecol* 1986;68:422.

Davis GD, Brooks RA. Excision of pelvic endometriosis with the carbon dioxide laser laparoscope. *Obstet Gynecol* 1988;72:816.

Dawood MY. Impact of medical treatment of endometriosis on bone mass. *Am J Obstet Gynecol* 1993;168:674.

Dawood MY, Kahn-Dawood FS, Wilson L Jr. Peritoneal fluid prostaglandins and prostanoids in women with endometriosis, chronic pelvic inflammatory disease, and pelvic pain. *Am J Obstet Gynecol* 1984;148:391.

DeLeon FD, Vijayakumar R, Brown M, et al. Peritoneal fluid volume, estrogen, progesterone, prostaglandin, and epidermal growth factor concentrations in patients with and without endometriosis. *Obstet Gynecol* 1986;68:189.

Diaz I, Navarro J, Blasco L, et al. Impact of stage III–IV endometriosis on recipients of sibling oocytes: matched case-control study. *Fertil Steril* 2000;74:31.

Dicker D, Feldberg D, Goldman JA, et al. The impact of long-term gonadotropin-releasing hormone analogue treatment on preclinical abortions in patients with severe endometriosis undergoing in vitro fertilization-embryo transfer. *Fertil Steril* 1992;57:597.

Dickey RP, Olar TT, Taylor SN, et al. Relationship of follicle number, serum estradiol, and other factors to birth rate and multiparity in human menopausal gonadotropin-induced intrauterine insemination cycles. *Fertil Steril* 1991;56:89.

diZerega G, Hodgen G. Endometriosis: role of ovarian steroids in initiation, maintenance, and suppression. *Fertil Steril* 1980;33:649.

Dlugi AM, Miller JD, Knittle J, et al. Lupron depot (leuprolide acetate for depot suspension) in the treatment of endometriosis: a randomized, placebo-controlled, double-blind study. *Fertil Steril* 1990;54:419.

Dmowski WP, Cohen MR. Treatment of endometriosis with an antigonadotropin, danazol: a laparoscopic and histologic evaluation. *Obstet Gynecol* 1975;46:147.

Dmowski WP, Radwanska E, Binor Z, et al. Mild endometriosis and ovulatory dysfunction: effect of danazol treatment on success of ovulation induction. *Fertil Steril* 1986;46:784.

Dmowski WP, Steele RW, Baker GF. Deficient cellular immunity in endometriosis. *Am J Obstet Gynecol* 1981;141:377.

Döberl A, Berquist A, Jeppson S, et al. Regression of endometriosis following the shorter treatment with, or lower dose of, danazol. *Acta Obstet Gynecol Scand Suppl* 1984;123:51.

Dodin S, Lemay A, Maheux R, et al. Bone mass in endometriosis patients treated with GnRH agonist implant or danazol. *Obstet Gynecol* 1991;77: 410.

Dodson WC, Haney AF. Controlled ovarian hyperstimulation and intrauterine insemination for treatment of infertility. *Fertil Steril* 1991;55:457.

Donnez J, Nisolle M. CO_2 laser laparoscopic surgery: adhesiolysis, salpingostomy, laser uterine nerve ablation and tubal pregnancy. *Baillieres Clin Obstet Gynaecol* 1989;3:525.

Donnez J, Casanas-Roux F, Ferin J, et al. Tubal polyps, epithelial inclusions, and endometriosis after tubal sterilization. *Fertil Steril* 1984;41:56.

Donnez J, Nisolle-Pochet M, Clerckx-Braun F, et al. Administration of nasal buserelin as compared with subcutaneous buserelin implant for endometriosis. *Fertil Steril* 1989;52:25.

Doyle JB. Paracervical uterine denervation by transection of the cervical plexus for the relief of dysmenorrhea. *Am J Obstet Gynecol* 1955;70:11.

Drake TS, O'Brien WF, Ramwell PW, et al. Peritoneal fluid thromboxane B_2 6-keto-prostaglandin F_{1a} in endometriosis. *Am J Obstet Gynecol* 1981;140:401.

Dunselman GA, Dumoulin JC, Land JA, et al. Lack of effect of peritoneal endometriosis on fertility in the rabbit model. *Fertil Steril* 1991;56:340.

Eskenazi B, Warner M, Bonsignore L, et al. Validation study of nonsurgical diagnosis of endometriosis. *Fertil Steril* 2001:76,929.

Evers JL. The second look laparoscopy for evaluation of the results of medical treatment of endometriosis should not be performed during ovarian suppression. *Fertil Steril* 1987;47:502.

Fahaeus L, Larsson-Cohn U, Ljungberg S, et al. Profound alterations of the lipoprotein metabolism during danazol treatment in premenopausal women. *Fertil Steril* 1984;42:52.

Fakih H, Baggett B, Holtz G, et al. Interleukin-1: a possible role in the infertility associated with endometriosis. *Fertil Steril* 1987;47:218.

Fakih HN, Tamura R, Kesselman A, et al. Endometriosis after tubal ligation. *J Reprod Med* 1985;30:939.

Fayez JA, Collazo LM. Comparison between laparotomy and operative laparoscopy in the treatment of moderate and severe endometriosis. *Int J Fertil* 1990;35:252.

Fayez JA, Vogel MF. Comparison of different treatment methods of endometriomas by laparoscopy. *Obstet Gynecol* 1991;78:660.

Fedele L, Bianchi S, Bocciolone L, et al. Pain symptoms associated with endometriosis. *Obstet Gynecol* 1992;79:767.

Fedele L, Bianchi S, Dorta M, et al. Transvaginal ultrasonography in the differential diagnosis of adenomyoma versus leiomyoma. *Am J Obstet Gynecol* 1992;167:603.

Fedele L, Bianchi S, Marchini M, et al. Superovulation with human menopausal gonadotropins in the treatment of infertility associated with minimal or mild endometriosis: a controlled randomized study. *Fertil Steril* 1992;58: 28.

Fedele L, Bianchi S, Zanconato G, et al. Laparoscopic excision of recurrent endometriomas: long-term outcome and comparison with primary surgery. *Fertil Steril* 2006: 85:694.

Fedele L, Bianchi S, Zanconato G, et al. Long-term follow-up after conservative surgery for bladder endometriosis. *Fertil Steril* 2005;83:1729.

Fedele L, Parazzini F, Bianchi S, et al. Stage and localization of pelvic endometriosis and pain. *Fertil Steril* 1990;53:155.

Feste JR. Laser laparoscopy: a new modality. *J Reprod Med* 1985;30:413.

Foster DC, Stern JL, Buscema J, et al. Pleural and parenchymal pulmonary endometriosis. *Obstet Gynecol* 1981;58:552.

Franssen AM, Kaver FM, Chadha DR, et al. Endometriosis: treatment with gonadotropin-releasing hormone agonist buserelin. *Fertil Steril* 1989; 51:401.

Gambone JC, Reiter RC, Lerich JB, et al. The impact of a quality assurance process in the frequency and confirmation rate of hysterectomy. *Am J Obstet Gynecol* 1990;163:545.

Gant NF. Infertility and endometriosis: comparison of pregnancy outcomes with laparotomy versus laparoscopic techniques. *Am J Obstet Gynecol* 1992;166:1072.

Garcia-Velasco JA, Mahutte NG, Corona J, et al. Removal of endometriomas before in vitro fertilization does not improve fertility outcomes: a matched, case-control study. *Fertil Steril* 2004;81:1194.

Glatt AE, Zinner SH, McCormack WM. The prevalence of dyspareunia. *Obstet Gynecol* 1990;75:433.

Gould SF, Shannon JM, Cunha GR. Nuclear estrogen binding sites in human endometriosis. *Fertil Steril* 1983;39:520.

Granberg S, Wikland M, Jansson I. Macroscopic characterization of ovarian tumors and the relation to the histologic diagnosis: criteria to be used for ultrasound evaluation. *Gynecol Oncol* 1989;35:139.

Greenblatt RB, Dmowski WP, Mahesh VB, et al. Clinical studies with an antigonadotropin danazol. *Fertil Steril* 1971;22:102.

Grow DR, Filer RB. Treatment of adenomyosis with long-term GnRH analogues: a case report. *Obstet Gynecol* 1991;78:538.

Gruenwald P. Origin of endometriosis from the mesenchyme of the coelomic walls. *Am J Obstet Gynecol* 1942;44:470.

Guzick DS. Clinical epidemiology of endometriosis and infertility. *Obstet Gynecol Clin North Am* 1989;16:43.

Guzick DS, Yao YA, Berga SL, et al. Endometriosis impairs the efficacy of gamete intrafallopian transfer: results of a case-control study. *Fertil Steril* 1994;62:1186.

Habuchi T, Okagaki T, Miyakawa M. Endometriosis of bladder after meno pause. *J Urol* 1991;145:361.

Halme J, Hammond MG, Hulka JK, et al. Retrograde menstruation in healthy women and in patients with endometriosis. *Obstet Gynecol* 1984;64: 151.

Halme J, White C, Kauma S, et al. Peritoneal macrophages from patients with endometriosis release growth factor activity in vitro. *J Clin Endocrinol Metab* 1988;66:1044.

Haney AF, Jenkins S, Weinberg JB. The stimulus responsible for the peritoneal fluid inflammation observed in infertile women with endometriosis. *Fertil Steril* 1991;56:408.

Heaps JM, Nieberg RK, Berek JS. Malignant neoplasms arising in endometriosis. *Obstet Gynecol* 1990;75:1023.

Heilier JF, Nackers F, Verougstraete V, et al. Increased dioxin-like compounds in the serum of women with peritoneal endometriosis and deep endometriotic (adenomyotic) nodules. *Fertil Steril* 2005;84:305.

Henzl MR. Gonadotropin-releasing hormone analogs: update on new findings. *Am J Obstet Gynecol* 1992;166:757.

Henzl MR, Corson SL, Moghissi K, et al. Administration of nasal nafarelin as compared with oral danazol for endometriosis. *N Engl J Med* 1988;318:485.

Hickman TN, Namnoum AB, Hinton EL, et al. Timing of estrogen replacement therapy following hysterectomy with oophorectomy for endometriosis. *Obstet Gynecol* 1998;91:673.

Hill JA, Faris HM, Schiff I, et al. Characterization of leukocyte subpopulations in the peritoneal fluid of women with endometriosis. *Fertil Steril* 1988;50:216.

Hornstein MD, Hemmings R, Yuzpe AA, et al. Use of nafarelin versus placebo after reductive laparoscopic surgery for endometriosis. *Fertil Steril* 1997;68:860.

Hornstein MD, Surrey ES, Weisberg GW, et al. Leuprolide acetate depot and hormonal add-back in endometriosis: a 12-month study. *Obstet Gynecol* 1998;91:16.

Houston DE, Noller RL, Melton LJ III, et al. Incidence of pelvic endometriosis in Rochester, Minnesota 1970–1979. *Am J Epidemiol* 1987;125:959.

Hull ME, Moghissi KS, Magyar DF, et al. Comparison of different treatment modalities of endometriosis in infertile women. *Fertil Steril* 1987;47:40.

Hulme VA, van der Merwe JP, Kruger TF. Gamete intrafallopian transfer as treatment for infertility associated with endometriosis. *Fertil Steril* 1990;53:1095.

Igarashi M, Abe Y, Fukuda M, et al. Novel conservative medical therapy for uterine adenomyosis with a danazol-loaded intrauterine device. *Fertil Steril* 2000;74:412.

Ishimaru T, Masuzaki H. Peritoneal endometriosis: endometrial tissue implantation as its primary etiologic mechanism. *Am J Obstet Gynecol* 1991;165:210.

Jacobson TZ, Barlow DH, Koninckx PR, et al. Laparoscopic surgery for subfertility associated with endometriosis. *Cochrane Database Syst Rev* 2002;4:CD001398.

Jänne O, Kauppila A, Kukko E, et al. Estrogen and progestin receptors in endometriosis lesions: comparison with endometrial tissue. *Am J Obstet Gynecol* 1981;141:562.

Jansen RP, Russell P. Nonpigmented endometriosis: clinical, laparoscopic, and pathologic definition. *Am J Obstet Gynecol* 1986;155:1154.

Javert CT. Pathogenesis of endometriosis based on endometrial homeoplasia direct extension, exfoliation and implantation, lymphatic and hematogenous metastasis. *Cancer* 1949;2:399.

Jenkins S, Olive DL, Haney AF. Endometriosis: pathogenetic implications of the anatomic distribution. *Obstet Gynecol* 1986;67:335.

Johnson JV, Roxek MM, Moreno AC, et al. Surgically induced endometriosis does not alter peritoneal factors in the rabbit model. *Fertil Steril* 1991;56:343.

Johnson NP, Farquhar CM, Crossley S, et al. A double-blinded randomized controlled trial of laparoscopic uterine nerve ablation for women with chronic pelvic pain. *BJOG* 2004;111:950.

Killick S, Elstein M. Pharmacologic production of luteinized unruptured follicles by prostaglandin synthetase inhibitors. *Fertil Steril* 1987;47:773.

Kim CH, Cho YK, Mok JE. Simplified ultralong protocol of gonadotrophin-releasing hormone agonist for ovulation induction with intrauterine insemination in patients with endometriosis. *Hum Reprod* 1996;11:398.

Koninckx PR, Braet P, Kennedy SH, et al. Dioxin pollution and endometriosis in Belgium. *Hum Reprod* 1994;9:1001.

Koninckx P, Ide P, Vandenbroucke W, et al. New aspects of the pathophysiology of endometriosis and associated infertility. *J Reprod Med* 1980;24:257.

Koninckx PR, Martin DC. Deep endometriosis: a consequence of infiltration or retraction or possibly adenomyosis externa? *Fertil Steril* 1992;58:924.

Koninckx PR, Mueleman C, Demeyere S, et al. Suggestive evidence that pelvic endometriosis is a progressive disease, whereas deeply infiltrating endometriosis is associated with pelvic pain. *Fertil Steril* 1991;55:759.

Koninckx PR, Rittinen L, Seppälä M, et al. CA-125 and placental protein 14 concentrations in plasma and peritoneal fluid of women with deeply infiltrating pelvic endometriosis. *Fertil Steril* 1992;57:523.

Kuivasaari P, Hippeläinen M, Anttila M, et al. Effect of endometriosis on IVF/ICSI outcome: stage III/IV endometriosis worsens cumulative pregnancy and live-born rates. *Hum Reprod* 2005;20:3130.

Lamb K, Hoffman RG, Nichols TR. Family trait analysis: a case-control study of 43 women with endometriosis and their best friends. *Am J Obstet Gynecol* 1986;154:596.

Laufer MR. Identification of clear vesicular lesions of atypical endometriosis: a new technique. *Fertil Steril* 1997;68:739.

Laufer MR, Goitein L, Bush M, et al. Prevalence of endometriosis in adolescent girls with chronic pelvic pain not responding to conventional therapy. *J Pediatr Adolesc Gynecol* 1997;10:199.

Leach RE, Arneson BW, Ball GD, et al. Absence of antisperm antibodies and factors influencing sperm motility in the cul-del-sac fluid of women with endometriosis. *Fertil Steril* 1990;53:351.

Lee NC, Dicker RC, Rubin GL, et al. Confirmation of the preoperative diagnoses for hysterectomy. *Am J Obstet Gynecol* 1984;150:283.

Lee RB, Stone K, Magelssen D, et al. Presacral neurectomy for chronic pelvic pain. *Obstet Gynecol* 1986;69:517.

Leibson CL, Good AE, Hass SL, et al. Incidence and characterization of diagnosed endometriosis in a geographically defined population. *Fertil Steril* 2004:82:314.

Lemay A, Maheux R, Faure N, et al. Reversible hypogonadism induced by a luteinizing hormone-releasing hormone (LH-RH) agonist (buserelin) as a new therapeutic approach for endometriosis. *Fertil Steril* 1984;41:863.

Lessey BA, Castelbaum AJ, Sawin SW, et al. Aberrant integrin expression in the endometrium of women with endometriosis. *J Clin Endocrinol Metab* 1994;79:643.

Lichten EM, Bombard J. Surgical treatment of primary dysmenorrhea with laparoscopic uterine nerve ablation. *J Reprod Med* 1987;32:37.

Lockhat FB, Emembolu JO, Konje JC. The efficacy, side-effects and continuation rates in women with symptomatic endometriosis undergoing treatment with an intra-uterine administered progestogen (levonorgestrel): a 3 year follow-up. *Hum Reprod* 2005;20:789.

Loh FH, Tan AT, Kumar J, et al. Ovarian response after laparoscopic ovarian cystectomy for endometriotic cysts in 132 monitored cycles. *Fertil Steril* 1999;72:316.

Luciano AA, Hauser KS, Chapler FK, et al. Effects of danazol on plasma lipids and lipoprotein levels in healthy woman and in women with endometriosis. *Am J Obstet Gynecol* 1983;145:422.

Luciano AA, Turksoy RN, Carleo J. Evaluation of oral medroxyprogesterone acetate in the treatment of endometriosis. *Obstet Gynecol* 1988;72:323.

Mahmood TA, Templeton A. Folliculogenesis and ovulation in infertile women with mild endometriosis. *Hum Reprod* 1991;6:225.

Mahmood TA, Templeton A. Pathophysiology of mild endometriosis: review of literature. *Hum Reprod* 1990;5:765.

Mahmood TA, Templeton A. Peritoneal fluid volume and sex steroids in the preovulatory period in mild endometriosis. *BJOG* 1991;98:179.

Mahmood TA, Arumugam K, Templeton AA. Oocyte and follicular fluid characteristics in women with mild endometriosis. *BJOG* 1991;98:573.

Makarainen L, Ronnberg L, Kauppila A. Medroxyprogesterone acetate supplementation diminishes the hypoestrogenic side effects of gonadotropin-releasing hormone agonist without changing its efficacy in endometriosis. *Fertil Steril* 1996;65:29.

Marcoux S, Maheux, Bérubé S, et al. Laparoscopic surgery in infertile women with minimal or mild endometriosis. *N Engl J Med* 1997;337:217.

Marrs RP. The use of potassium-titanyl-phosphate laser for laparoscopic removal of ovarian endometriomas. *Am J Obstet Gynecol* 1991;164:1622.

Martin D. Laparoscopic treatment of ovarian endometriomas. *Clin Obstet Gynecol* 1991;34:452.

Martin DC, Hubert GD, Levy BS. Depth of infiltration of endometriosis. *J Gynecol Surg* 1989;5:55.

Martin DC, Hubert GD, Vander Zwaag R, et al. Laparoscopic appearances of peritoneal endometriosis. *Fertil Steril* 1989;51:63.

Max E, Sweeney WB, Bailey HR, et al. Results of 1,000 single-layer continuous polypropylene intestinal anastomoses. *Am J Surg* 1991;162:461.

McArthur JW, Ulfelder H. The effect of pregnancy upon endometriosis. *Obstet Gynecol Surv* 1965;20:709.

McCausland AM. Hysteroscopic myometrial biopsy: its use in diagnosing adenomyosis and its clinical application. *Am J Obstet Gynecol* 1992;166:1619.

Meldrum DR, Chang RJ, Lu J, et al. "Medical oophorectomy" using a long-acting GnRH agonist: a possible new approach to the treatment of endometriosis. *J Clin Endocrinol Metab* 1982;54:1081.

Meresman GF, Auge L, Baranao RI, et al. Oral contraceptives suppress cell proliferation and enhance apoptosis of eutopic endometrial tissue from patients with endometriosis. *Fertil Steril* 2002;77:1141.

Metzger DA, Olive DL, Stohs GF, et al. Association of endometriosis and spontaneous abortion: effect of control group selection. *Fertil Steril* 1986;45:18.

Meyer R. Über Stand der Frage der Adenomyositis und Adenomyome im Allgemeinen und ins Besondere über Adenomyositis seroepithelialis und Adenomyometritis sarcomatosa. *Zentralbl Gynakol* 1919;36:745.

Mio Y, Toda T, Harada T, et al. Pathophysiology of infertility associated with endometriosis: luteinized unruptured follicle in the early stages of endometriosis as a cause of unexplained infertility. *Am J Obstet Gynecol* 1992;167:251.

Missmer SA, Hankinson SE, Spiegelman D, et al. Reproductive history and endometriosis among premenopausal women. *Obstet Gynecol* 2004;104:965.

Mittal KR, Barwick KW. Endometrial adenocarcinoma involving adenomyosis without true myometrial invasion is characterized by frequent preceding estrogen therapy, low histologic grades, and excellent prognosis. *Gynecol Oncol* 1993;49:197.

Modugno F, Ness RB, Allen GO, et al. Oral contraceptive use, reproductive history, and risk of epithelial ovarian cancer in women with and without endometriosis. *Am J Obstet Gynecol* 2004: 191:733.

Moen M, Bratlie A, Moen T. Distribution of HLA antigens among patients with endometriosis. *Acta Obstet Gynecol Scand Suppl* 1984;123:25.

Moghissi KS, Boyce CR. Management of endometriosis with oral medroxyprogesterone acetate. *Obstet Gynecol* 1976;47:265.

Moore EE, Harger JH, Rock JA, et al. Management of pelvic endometriosis with low-dose danazol. *Fertil Steril* 1981;36:15.

Moore JG, Binstock MA, Growdon WA. The clinical implications of retroperitoneal endometriosis. *Am J Obstet Gynecol* 1988;158:1291.

Moore JG, Hibbard LT, Growdon WA, et al. Urinary tract endometriosis: enigmas in diagnosis and management. *Am J Obstet Gynecol* 1979;134:162.

Morcos RN, Gibbons WE, Findlay WE. Effect of peritoneal fluid on in vitro cleavage of 2-cell mouse embryos: possible role in infertility associated with endometriosis. *Fertil Steril* 1985;44:678.

Murphy AA, Green WR, Bobbie D, et al. Unsuspected endometriosis documented by scanning electron microscopy in visually normal peritoneum. *Fertil Steril* 1986;46:522.

Murphy AA, Schlaff WD, Hassiakos D, et al. Laparoscopic cautery in the treatment of endometriosis-related infertility. *Fertil Steril* 1991;55:246.

Muscato JJ, Haney AF, Weinberg JB. Sperm phagocytosis by human peritoneal macrophages: a possible cause of infertility in endometriosis. *Am J Obstet Gynecol* 1982;144:503.

Muzii L, Bellati F, Palaia I, et al. Laparoscopic stripping of endometriomas: a randomized trial on different surgical techniques. Part I: Clinical results. *Hum Reprod* 2005:20:1981.
Muzii L, Marana R, Caruana P, et al. The impact of preoperative gonadotropin-releasing hormone agonist treatment on laparoscopic excision of ovarian endometriotic cysts. *Fertil Steril* 1996;65:1235.
Muzii L, Marana R, Caruana P, et al. Postoperative administration of monophasic combined oral contraceptives after laparoscopic treatment of ovarian endometriomas: a prospective, randomized trial. *Am J Obstet Gynecol* 2000;183;588.
Muzii L, Marana R, Pedulla S, et al. Correlation between endometriosis-associated dysmenorrhea and the presence of typical and atypical lesions. *Fertil Steril* 1997;68:19.
Namnoum AB, Hickman TN, Goodman SB, et al. Incidence of symptom recurrence after hysterectomy for endometriosis. *Fertil Steril* 1995;64:898.
Naples JD, Batt RE, Sadigh A. Spontaneous abortion rate in patients with endometriosis. *Obstet Gynecol* 1981;57:509.
Nezhat C, Nezhat F, Pennington E. Laparoscopic treatment of infiltrative rectosigmoid colon and rectovaginal septum endometriosis by the technique of video laparoscopy and the CO_2 laser. *BJOG* 1992;99:664.
Nezhat C, Seidman DS, Nezhat F, et al. Laparoscopic surgical management of diaphragmatic endometriosis. *Fertil Steril* 1998;69:1048.
Nezhat CH, Seidman DS, Nezhat FR, et al. Long-term outcome of laparoscopic presacral neurectomy for the treatment of central pelvic pain attributed to endometriosis. *Obstet Gynecol* 1998;91:701.
Nishida M. Relationship between the onset of dysmenorrhea and histologic findings in adenomyosis. *Am J Obstet Gynecol* 1991;165:229.
Noble LS, Simpson ER, John A, et al. Aromatase expression in endometriosis. *J Clin Endocrinol Metab* 1996;81:174.
Nuoja-Huttunen S, Tomas C, Bloigu R, et al. Intrauterine insemination treatment in subfertility: an analysis of factors affecting outcome. *Hum Reprod* 1999;14:698.
Oak MK, Chantler EN, Williams CA, et al. Sperm survival studies in peritoneal fluid from infertile women with endometriosis and unexplained infertility. *Clin Reprod Fertil* 1985;3:297.
Olive DL, Henderson DY. Endometriosis and müllerian anomalies. *Obstet Gynecol* 1987;69:412.
Olive DL, Lee KL. Analysis of sequential treatment protocols for endometriosis-associated infertility. *Am J Obstet Gynecol* 1986;154:613.
Olive DL, Martin DC. Treatment of endometriosis-associated infertility with CO_2 laser laparoscopy: the use of one- and two-parameter exponential models. *Fertil Steril* 1987;48:18.
Olive DL, Montoya I, Riehl RM, et al. Macrophage-conditioned media enhance endometrial stromal cell proliferation in vitro. *Am J Obstet Gynecol* 1991;164:953.
Oosterlynck DJ, Cornillie FJ, Waer M, et al. Women with endometriosis show a defect in natural killer cell activity resulting in a decreased cytotoxicity to autologous endometrium. *Fertil Steril* 1991;56:45.
Pagidas K, Falcone T, Hemmings R, et al. Comparison of reoperation for moderate (stage III) and severe (stage IV) endometriosis-related infertility with in vitro fertilization-embryo transfer. *Fertil Steril* 1996;65:791.
Parazzini F. Ablation of lesions or no treatment in minimal-mild endometriosis in infertile women: a randomized trial. *Gruppo Italiano per lo Studio dell'Endometriosi. Hum Reprod* 1999;14:1332.
Parazzini F, Fedele L, Busacca M, et al. Postsurgical medical treatment of advanced endometriosis: results of a randomized clinical trial. *Am J Obstet Gynecol* 1994;171:1205.
Parker JD, Leondires M, Sinaii N. Persistence of dysmenorrhea and nonmenstrual pain after optimal endometriosis surgery may indicate adenomyosis. *Fertil Steril* 2006;86:711.
Paull T, Tedeschi LG. Perineal endometriosis at the site of episiotomy scar. *Obstet Gynecol* 1972;40:28.
Pelage JP, Jacob D, Fazel A, et al. Midterm results of uterine artery embolization for symptomatic adenomyosis: initial experience. *Radiology* 2005;234: 948.
Pinkert T, Catlow C, Straus R. Endometriosis of the urinary bladder in a man with prostatic carcinoma. *Cancer* 1979;43:1562.
Pittaway DE, Daniell JF, Maxson WS. Ovarian surgery in an infertility patient as an indication for a short-interval second-look laparoscopy: a preliminary study. *Fertil Steril* 1985;44:611.
Pittaway DE, Douglas JW. Serum CA-125 in women with endometriosis and chronic pelvic pain. *Fertil Steril* 1989;51:68.
Pittaway DE, Vernon C, Fayez JA. Spontaneous abortions in women with endometriosis. *Fertil Steril* 1988;50:711.
Pokras R, Hufnagel VG. Hysterectomy in the United States, 1965–84. *Am J Public Health* 1988;78:852.
Polan ML, DeCherney A. Presacral neurectomy for pelvic pain in infertility. *Fertil Steril* 1980;34:557.
Prystowsky JB, Stryker SJ, Ujiki GT, et al. Gastrointestinal endometriosis: incidence and indications for resection. *Arch Surg* 1988;123:855.
Puleo JG, Hammond CB. Conservative treatment of endometriosis externa: the effects of danazol therapy. *Fertil Steril* 1983;40:164.
Punnonen R, Soderstrom P, Alanen A. Isthmic tubal occlusion: etiology and histology. *Acta Eur Fertil* 1984;15:39.
Ranney B. Endometriosis IV: hereditary tendency. *Obstet Gynecol* 1971;37:734.
Redwine DB. Conservative laparoscopic excision of endometriosis by sharp dissection: life table analysis of reoperation and persistent or recurrent disease. *Fertil Steril* 1991;56:28.
Redwine DB. The distribution of endometriosis in the pelvis by age groups and fertility. *Fertil Steril* 1987;47:173.
Redwine DB. Endometriosis persisting after castration: clinical characteristics and results of surgical management. *Obstet Gynecol* 1994;83:405.
Redwine DB. Peritoneal blood painting: an aid in the diagnosis of endometriosis. *Am J Obstet Gynecol* 1989;161:865.
Redwine DB. Ovarian endometriosis: a marker for more extensive pelvic and intestinal disease. *Fertil Steril* 1999;72:310.
Rezai N, Ghodgaonkar RB, Zacur HA, et al. Cul-de-sac fluid in women with endometriosis: fluid volume, protein and prostanoid concentration during the periovulatory period—days 13 to 18. *Fertil Steril* 1987;48:29.
Rier SE, Martin DC, Bowman RE, et al. Endometriosis in rhesus monkeys (Macaca mulatta) following chronic exposure to 2,3,7,8-tetrachlorodibenzo-p-dioxin. *Fundam Appl Toxicol* 1993;21:433.
Riva HL, Kawasaki DM, Messinger AJ. Further experience with norethynodrel in treatment of endometriosis. *Obstet Gynecol* 1962;19:111.
Rivlin ME, Miller JD, Krueger RP, et al. Leuprolide acetate in the management of ureteral obstruction caused by endometriosis. *Obstet Gynecol* 1990;75:532.
Rock JA, Dubin NH, Ghodgaonkar RB, et al. Cul-de-sac fluid in women with endometriosis: fluid volume and prostanoid concentration during the proliferative phase of the cycle—days 8–12. *Fertil Steril* 1982;37:747.
Rock JA, Guzick DS, Jones HW Jr. The efficacy of accessory surgical intervention in conjunction with resection and fulguration of endometriosis. *Infertility* 1981;4:193.
Rock JA, Guzick DS, Sengos C, et al. Evaluation of pregnancy success with respect to extent of disease as categorized using contemporary classification systems. *Fertil Steril* 1981;35:131.
Rock JA, Parmley TH, King TM, et al. Endometriosis and the development of tuboperitoneal fistulas after tubal ligation. *Fertil Steril* 1981;35:16.
Ruggi G. Della sympatectamia al collo ed ale ad ome. *Policlinico* 1899;193.
Sakamoto A. Subserosal adenomyosis: a possible variant of pelvic endometriosis. *Am J Obstet Gynecol* 1991;165:198.
Saleh A, Tulandi T. Reoperation after laparoscopic treatment of ovarian endometriomas by excision and by fenestration. *Fertil Steril* 1999;72:322.
Sangi-Haghpeykar H, Poindexter AN. Epidemiology of endometriosis among parous women. *Obstet Gynecol* 1995;85:983.
Sampson JA. Benign and malignant endometrial implants in peritoneal cavity, and their relation to certain ovarian tumors. *Surg Gynecol Obstet* 1924;38: 287.
Sampson JA. Peritoneal endometriosis due to menstrual dissemination of endometrial tissue into the peritoneal cavity. *Am J Obstet Gynecol* 1925;14:422.
Schenken RS, Asch RH, Williams RF, et al. Etiology of infertility in monkeys with endometriosis: luteinized unruptured follicles, luteal phase defects, pelvic adhesions and spontaneous abortions. *Fertil Steril* 1984;41:122.
Schenken RS, Williams RF, Hodgen GD. Effect of pregnancy on surgically induced endometriosis in cynomolgus monkeys. *Am J Obstet Gynecol* 1987;157:1392.
Schlaff WD, Dugoff L, Damewood MD, et al. Megestrol acetate for treatment of endometriosis. *Obstet Gynecol* 1990;75:646.
Schmidt CL. Endometriosis: a reappraisal of pathogenesis and treatment. *Fertil Steril* 1985;44:157.
Schneider VL, Schneider A, Reed KL, et al. Comparison of Doppler with two-dimensional sonography and CA-125 for prediction of malignancy of pelvic masses. *Obstet Gynecol* 1993;81:983.
Schweppe KW, Wynn RM. Ultrastructural changes in endometriotic implants during the menstrual cycle. *Obstet Gynecol* 1981;58:465.
Schweppe KW, Wynn RM, Beller FK. Ultrastructural comparison of endometriotic implants and eutopic endometrium. *Am J Obstet Gynecol* 1984;148:1024.
Seibel MM, Berger MJ, Weinstein FG, et al. The effectiveness of danazol on subsequent fertility in minimal endometriosis. *Fertil Steril* 1982;38:534.
Sekiba K, Obstetrics and Gynecology Adhesion Prevention Committee. Use of Interceed (TC7) absorbable adhesion barrier to reduce postoperative adhesion reformation in infertility and endometriosis surgery. *Obstet Gynecol* 1992;79:518.
Serta RT, Rufo S, Seibel MM. Minimal endometriosis and intrauterine insemination: does controlled ovarian hyperstimulation improve pregnancy rates? *Obstet Gynecol* 1992;80:37.
Shook TE, Nyberg LM. Endometriosis of the urinary tract. *Urology* 1988;31:1.
Simpson JL, Elias S, Malinak LR, et al. Heritable aspects of endometriosis. I. Genetic studies. *Am J Obstet Gynecol* 1980;137:325.
Simpson JL, Malinak LR, Elias S, et al. HLA associations in endometriosis. *Am J Obstet Gynecol* 1984;148:395.
Somigliana E, Vercellini P, Viganc P, et al. Should endometriomas be treated before IVF-ICSI cycles?. *Hum Reprod Update* 2006: 12:57.

Steele RW, Dmowski WP, Marmer DJ. Immunologic aspects of human endometriosis. *Am J Reprod Immunol* 1984;6:33.

Stock RJ. Postsalpingectomy endometriosis: a reassessment. *Obstet Gynecol* 1982;60:560.

Stovall TG, Ling FW, Crawford DA. Hysterectomy for chronic pelvic pain of presumed uterine etiology. *Obstet Gynecol* 1990;75:676.

Strathy JH, Molgaard CA, Coulam CB, et al. Endometriosis and infertility: a laparoscopic study of endometriosis among fertile and infertile women. *Fertil Steril* 1982;38:667.

Stripling MC, Martin DC, Chatman DL, et al. Subtle appearance of pelvic endometriosis. *Fertil Steril* 1988;49:425.

Sueldo CE, Lambert H, Steinleitner A, et al. The effect of peritoneal fluid from patients with endometriosis on murine sperm–oocyte interaction. *Fertil Steril* 1987;48:697.

Suginami H, Yano K. An ovum capture inhibitor (OCI) in endometriosis peritoneal fluid: an OCI-related membrane responsible for fimbrial failure of ovum capture. *Fertil Steril* 1988;50:648.

Surgical Membrane Study Group. Prophylaxis of pelvic sidewall adhesions with Gore-Tex surgical membrane: a multicenter clinical investigation. *Fertil Steril* 1992;57:921.

Surrey ES, Halme J. Effect of platelet-derived growth factor on endometrial stromal cell proliferation in vitro: a model for endometriosis? *Fertil Steril* 1991;56:672.

Surrey ES, Gambone JC, Lu JK, et al. The effects of combining norethindrone with a gonadotropin-releasing hormone agonist in the treatment of symptomatic endometriosis. *Fertil Steril* 1990;53:620.

Surrey ES, Voigt B, Fournet N, et al. Prolonged gonadotropin-releasing hormone agonist treatment of symptomatic endometriosis: the role of cyclic sodium etidronate and low-dose norethindrone "add-back" therapy. *Fertil Steril* 1995;63:747.

Sutton CJ, Ewen SP, Whitelaw N, et al. Prospective, randomized, double-blind, controlled trial of laser laparoscopy in the treatment of pelvic pain associated with minimal, mild, and moderate endometriosis. *Fertil Steril* 1994;62:696.

Suzuki T, Ixumi S, Matsubayashi H, et al. Impact of ovarian endometrioma on oocytes and pregnancy outcome in in vitro fertilization. *Fertil Steril* 2005;83:908.

Takahashi K, Okada S, Ozaki T, et al. Diagnosis of pelvic endometriosis by "fat-saturation" technique. *Fertil Steril* 1994;62;973.

Tamaya T, Motoyama T, Ohono Y, et al. Steroid receptor levels and histology of endometriosis and adenomyosis. *Fertil Steril* 1979;31:396.

Telimaa S. Danazol and medroxyprogesterone acetate inefficacious in the treatment of infertility in endometriosis. *Fertil Steril* 1988;50:872.

Te Linde RW, Scott RB. Experimental endometriosis. *Obstet Gynecol* 1978;130:569.

Thomas EJ, Lenton EA, Cooke ID. Follicle growth patterns and endocrinological abnormalities in infertile women with minor degrees of endometriosis. *BJOG* 1986;93:852.

Tinkanen H, Kujansuu E. In vitro fertilization in patients with ovarian endometriomas. *Acta Obstet Gynecol Scand* 2000;79:119.

Tjaden B, Schlaff WD, Kimball A, et al. The efficacy of presacral neurectomy for the relief of midline dysmenorrhea. *Obstet Gynecol* 1990;76:89.

Togashi K, Ozasa H, Konishi I, et al. Enlarged uterus: differentiation between adenomyosis and leiomyoma with MR imaging. *Radiology* 1989;171:531.

Tseng JF, Ryan IP, Milam TD, et al. Interleukin-6 secretion in vitro is upregulated in ectopic and eutopic endometrial stromal cells from women with endometriosis. *J Clin Endocrinol Metab* 1996;81:1118.

Tulandi T, Al-Took S. Reproductive outcome after treatment of mild endometriosis with laparoscopic excision and electrocoagulation. *Fertil Steril* 1998;69:229.

Tulandi T, Mouchawar M. Treatment-dependent and treatment-independent pregnancy in women with minimal and mild endometriosis. *Fertil Steril* 1991;56:790.

Tummon IS, Asher LJ, Martin JS, et al. Randomized controlled trial of superovulation and insemination for infertility associated with minimal or mild endometriosis. *Fertil Steril* 1997;68:8.

Tummon IS, Colwell KA, MacKinnoa CJ, et al. Abbreviated endometriosis-associated infertility correlates with in vitro fertilization success. *J In Vitro Fert Embryo Transfer* 1991;8:149.

Tummon IS, Maclin VM, Radwanska E, et al. Occult ovulatory dysfunction in women with minimal endometriosis and unexplained infertility. *Fertil Steril* 1988;50:716.

Uchima FDA, Edery M, Iguchi T, et al. Growth of mouse endometrial luminal epithelial cells in vitro: functional integrity of the oestrogen receptor system and failure of oestrogen to induce proliferation. *J Endocrinol* 1991;128:115.

Uohara JK, Kovara TY. Endometriosis of the appendix: report of 12 cases and review of the literature. *Am J Obstet Gynecol* 1975;121:423.

Vaughan Williams CA, Oak MK, Elstein M. Cyclical gonadotrophin and progesterone secretion in women with minimal endometriosis. *Clin Reprod Fertil* 1986;4:259.

Vercellini P, De Giorgi O, Oldani S, et al. Depot medroxyprogesterone acetate versus an oral contraceptive combined with very-low-dose danazol for long-term treatment of pelvic pain associated with endometriosis. *Am J Obstet Gynecol* 1996;175:396.

Vercellini P, Fedele L, Aimi G, et al. Reproductive performance, pain recurrence and disease relapse after conservative surgical treatment for endometriosis: the predictive value of the current classification system. *Hum Reprod* 2006;21:2679.

Vercellini P, Fedele L, Bianchi S, et al. Pelvic denervation for chronic pain associated with endometriosis: fact or fancy? *Am J Obstet Gynecol* 1991; 165:745.

Vercellini P, Frontino G, De Giorgi O. Continuous use of an oral contraceptive for endometriosis-associated recurrent dysmenorrhea that does not respond to a cyclic pill regimen. *Fertil Steril* 2003;80(3):560.

Vercellini P, Pietropaolo G, De Giorgi O, et al. Reproductive performance in infertile women with rectovaginal endometriosis: is surgery worthwhile? *Am J Obstet Gynecol* 2006;195:1303.

Vercellini P, Pietropaolo G, De Giorgi O, et al. Treatment of symptomatic rectovaginal endometriosis with an estrogen-progestogen combination versus low-dose norethindrone acetate. *Fertil Steril* 2005;84:1375.

Vercellini P, Vendola N, Bocciolone L, et al. Reliability of visual diagnosis of ovarian endometriosis. *Fertil Steril* 1991;56:1198.

Verkauf BS. The incidence, symptoms, and signs of endometriosis in fertile and infertile women. *J Fla Med Assoc* 1987;74:671.

Vernon MW, Beard JS, Graves K, et al. Classification of endometriotic implants by morphologic appearance and capacity to synthesize prostaglandin F. *Fertil Steril* 1986;46:801.

Vigano P, Vercellini P, Di Blasio AM, et al. Deficient antiendometrium lymphocyte-mediated cytotoxicity in patient with endometriosis. *Fertil Steril* 1991;56:894.

von Rokitansky C. Ueber Uterusdrusen-Neubildung im Uterus und Varialsarcomen. *Zkk Gesellsch d Aerzte zu Wien* 1860;37:577.

Wardle PG, Hull MG. Is endometriosis a disease? *Baillieres Clin Obstet Gynaecol* 1993;7:673.

Weed JC, Arquembourg PC. Endometriosis: can it produce an automimmune response resulting in infertility? *Clin Obstet Gynecol* 1980;23:885.

Wentz AC. Premenstrual spotting: its association with endometriosis but not luteal phase inadequacy. *Fertil Steril* 1980;33:605.

Werbrouck E, Spiessens C, Meuleman C, et al. No difference in cycle pregnancy rate and in cumulative live-birth rate between women with surgically treated minimal to mild endometriosis and women with unexplained infertility after controlled ovarian hyperstimulation and intrauterine insemination. *Fertil Steril* 2006;86:566.

Wespi HJ, Kletzhändler M. Uber Narbenendometriosen. *Mschr Geburtsh Gynakol* 1940;111:169.

Wheeler JM, Malinak LR. Recurrent endometriosis: incidence, management, and prognosis. *Am J Obstet Gynecol* 1983;146:247.

Wheeler JM, Johnston BM, Malinak LR. The relationship of endometriosis to spontaneous abortion. *Fertil Steril* 1983;39:656.

Wilcox LS, Koonin LM, Pokras R, et al. Hysterectomy in the United States, 1988-1990. *Obstet Gynecol* 1994;83:549.

Wihemsson L, Lindblom B, Wiqvist N. The human uterotubal junction: contractile patterns of different smooth muscle layers and the influence of prostaglandin F_2, prostaglandin $F_{2\alpha}$ and prostaglandin I_2 *in vitro*. *Fertil Steril* 1979;32:303.

Wood C, Maher P, Hill D. Biopsy diagnosis and conservative surgical treatment of adenomyosis. *Aust N Z J Obstet Gynaecol* 1993;33:319.

Wright J, Lotfallah H, Jones K, et al. A randomized trial of excision versus ablation for mild endometriosis. *Fertil Steril* 2005;83:1830.

Yaron Y, Peyser MR, Samuel D, et al. Infected endometriotic cysts secondary to oocyte aspiration for in-vitro fertilization. *Hum Reprod* 1994;9:1759.

Yanushpolsky EH, Best CL, Jackson KV, et al. Effects of endometriomas on oocyte quality, embryo quality, and pregnancy rates in *in vitro* fertilization cycles: a prospective, case-controlled study. *J Assist Reprod Genet* 1998;15:193.

Vercellini P, Chapron C, Fedele L, et al. Evidence for asymmetric distribution of lower intestinal endometriosis. BJOG. 2004;111:1213.

Ylikorkla O, Koskimies A, Laathainen T, et al. Peritoneal fluid prostaglandins in endometriosis, tubal disorders, and unexplained infertility. *Obstet Gynecol* 1984;63:616.

Young MD, Blackmore WP. The use of danazol in the management of endometriosis. *J Int Med Res* 1977;5[Suppl 3]:86.

Zanagnolo VL, Beck R, Schlaff WD, et al. Time-related effects of gonadotropin-releasing hormone analog treatment in experimentally induced endometriosis in the rat. *Fertil Steril* 1991;55:411.

Zullo F, Palomba S, Zupi E, et al. Effectiveness of presacral neurectomy in women with severe dysmenorrhea caused by endometriosis who were treated with laparoscopic conservative surgery: a 1-year prospective randomized double-blind controlled trial. *Am J Obstet Gynecol* 2003;189:5.

Vercellini P, [illegible] G, [illegible] S, et al. Severe [illegible] [illegible] and [illegible] [illegible] combined with [illegible] for [illegible] pain associated with endometriosis. [illegible] 2003;[illegible].

Vercellini P, Pasinetti E, Aimi G, et al. [illegible] performance [illegible] [illegible] [illegible] for [illegible] [illegible] [illegible]. [illegible] 2002;[illegible].

[illegible] [illegible] [illegible] for chronic pelvic pain [illegible]. [illegible] 1995;[illegible].

[illegible] [illegible] [illegible] [illegible] [illegible] [illegible] chronic pelvic pain [illegible]. [illegible] 2003;[illegible].

[illegible] [illegible] [illegible] of chronic pelvic pain [illegible] [illegible] [illegible] 2004;[illegible].

[illegible] P, [illegible] G, [illegible] C, et al. [illegible] [illegible] [illegible] [illegible] [illegible]. [illegible] 2002;[illegible].

[illegible] P, [illegible] [illegible], [illegible] J, et al. [illegible] [illegible] [illegible]

[redacted]

[illegible] [illegible] [illegible] [illegible] [illegible]. 1999;[illegible].

[illegible] [illegible] [illegible] [illegible]. [illegible] 1991;[illegible].

[illegible] [illegible] [illegible] [illegible] [illegible] [illegible]. [illegible] 1994;[illegible].

[illegible] [illegible] [illegible] [illegible] [illegible] [illegible]. [illegible] 1990;[illegible].

[illegible] [illegible] [illegible] [illegible] [illegible] [illegible] [illegible] [illegible] [illegible] 2000;[illegible].

[illegible] [illegible] [illegible] [illegible] [illegible]. [illegible] 1994;[illegible].

[illegible] [illegible] [illegible] [illegible] [illegible]. [illegible] 1991;[illegible].

[illegible] [illegible] [illegible] [illegible] [illegible]. [illegible] 1999;[illegible].

[illegible] [illegible] [illegible] [illegible] [illegible]. [illegible] 1991;[illegible].

[illegible] [illegible] [illegible] [illegible] [illegible] [illegible]. [illegible] 2004;[illegible].

[illegible] [illegible] [illegible] [illegible] [illegible] [illegible]. [illegible] 1991;[illegible].

[illegible] [illegible] [illegible] [illegible] [illegible] [illegible]. [illegible] 2004;[illegible].

[illegible] [illegible] [illegible] [illegible] [illegible] [illegible]. [illegible] 1998;[illegible].

[illegible] [illegible] [illegible] [illegible]. [illegible] 1989;[illegible].

[illegible] [illegible] [illegible] [illegible] [illegible]. [illegible] 1998;[illegible].

[illegible] [illegible] [illegible] [illegible] [illegible] [illegible]

Steele RW, [illegible] WR, [illegible] CL, [illegible] aspects of [illegible] [illegible]. [illegible] 1985;[illegible].

[illegible] [illegible] [illegible] [illegible]. [illegible] 1987;[illegible].

[illegible] [illegible] [illegible] [illegible] [illegible] [illegible]. [illegible] 1990;[illegible].

[illegible] [illegible] [illegible] [illegible] [illegible] [illegible] [illegible]. [illegible] 1993;[illegible].

[illegible] [illegible] [illegible] [illegible] [illegible]. [illegible] 1990;[illegible].

[illegible] [illegible] [illegible] [illegible] [illegible] [illegible]. [illegible] 1998;[illegible].

[illegible] [illegible] [illegible] [illegible] [illegible] [illegible]. [illegible] 1990;[illegible].

[illegible] [illegible] [illegible] [illegible] [illegible] [illegible]. [illegible] 1993;[illegible].

[illegible] [illegible] [illegible] [illegible]

[redacted]

[illegible] [illegible] [illegible] [illegible]. 1993;[illegible].

[illegible] [illegible] [illegible] [illegible] [illegible] [illegible] [illegible]. [illegible] 1999;[illegible].

[illegible] [illegible] [illegible] [illegible] [illegible] [illegible]. [illegible] 2002;[illegible].

[illegible] [illegible] [illegible] [illegible] [illegible]. [illegible] 1994;[illegible].

[illegible] [illegible] [illegible] [illegible] [illegible] [illegible]. [illegible] 1994;[illegible].

[illegible] [illegible] [illegible] [illegible] [illegible]. [illegible] 1990;[illegible].

[illegible] [illegible] [illegible] [illegible] [illegible] [illegible]. [illegible] 1998;[illegible].

[illegible] [illegible] [illegible] [illegible] [illegible] [illegible]. [illegible] 1991;[illegible].

[illegible] [illegible] [illegible] [illegible] [illegible] [illegible]. [illegible] 2000;[illegible].

[illegible] [illegible] [illegible] [illegible] [illegible] [illegible]. [illegible] 1997;[illegible].

[illegible] [illegible] [illegible] [illegible] [illegible] [illegible]. [illegible] 1998;[illegible].

[illegible] [illegible] [illegible] [illegible] [illegible] [illegible]. [illegible] 2004;[illegible].

[illegible] [illegible] [illegible] [illegible] [illegible] [illegible]. [illegible] 1999;[illegible].

SECTION V SURGERY FOR BENIGN GYNECOLOGIC CONDITIONS

CHAPTER 23 ■ SURGICAL CONDITIONS OF THE VULVA

IRA R. HOROWITZ, JOSEPH BUSCEMA, AND BHAGIRATH MAJMUDAR

DEFINITIONS

Bubo—Enlarged, suppurative inguinal lymph node characteristic of chancroid.

Burow's solution—A soothing aluminum sulfate solute that can be used as a soak or wet compress for inflamed or irritated skin or mucous membrane.

Cavitron Ultrasonic Surgical Aspirator (CUSA)—An electromechanical surgical instrument that is useful in soft tissue dissection. Using focused ultrasound, superficial tissue is sheared off and aspirated through the wand tip. It has been used to treat condyloma and vulvar intraepithelial neoplasia.

Donovan body—An intracytoplasmic Gram-negative, rod-shaped bacteria characteristically identified in histocytes associated with granuloma inguinale.

Fournier's gangrene—An older term for necrotizing fasciitis.

Keyes biopsy instrument—A pencil-like biopsy instrument with a sharp, hollow, cylindrical tip that is rotated while pressed against the skin. It cuts a small, cylindrical biopsy, which is then elevated with tissue forceps and cut off at the base with scissors or a knife.

Necrotizing fasciitis—A severe, rapidly progressive, life-threatening infection of the subcutaneous tissue and fascia that may involve the vulva. Synergistic bacterial infection with multiple organisms, it is associated with vascular thrombosis leading to necrosis of the skin and subcutaneous tissue of fascia. It is treated with aggressive broad-spectrum antibiotic coverage and wide surgical debridement.

Silvadene cream—A 1% silver sulfadiazine cream, which is commonly used on the vulva following laser therapy or surgery to minimize the risk of cellulitis or wound infection and to sooth the postoperative wound site.

Vulvar intraepithelial neoplasia (VIN)—A preinvasive neoplastic condition of the vulva.

Vulvar vestibulitis—A painful condition of the vulva of uncertain etiology. It is characterized by (i) severe pain on vestibular touch or attempted vaginal entry, (ii) tenderness to pressure localized within the vulvar vestibule, and (iii) minimal physical findings consisting of slight erythema within the vestibule.

Word catheter—A small latex catheter with an inflatable balloon to hold it in place. It is inserted to drain a Bartholin's duct abscess.

The vulva and the adjacent perianal skin are designated the anogenital area. These tissues are derived from ectoderm and are considered separately from the vagina and cervix, which are of mesodermal origin. Multifocal diseases, particularly human papillomavirus (HPV), can affect all of the aforementioned epithelia. A complete vulvar examination should, therefore, include the vulva, perineum, anal area, urethral meatus, buttocks, and thighs. It is difficult to appreciate subtle skin changes in patients with dark skin; therefore, an adequate light source is necessary.

VULVAR DERMATOSES

In 1987, the International Society for the Study of Vulvovaginal Diseases (ISSVD) revised the terminology to describe the nonneoplastic epithelial disorders of the vulva, which include psoriasis, lichen planus, lichen simplex chronicus, candidiasis, and condyloma acuminata. In their 1976 classification, the ISSVD categorized hyperplastic dystrophy with and without atypia. In the classification of 1987, squamous cell hyperplasia is without atypia, and lesions with atypia are considered vulvar intraepithelial neoplasia (VIN).

The terms *kraurosis* and *leukoplakia* have been overused in the past. In 1877, Schwimmer reported that leukoplakia on the buccal surfaces of the mouth was a premalignant lesion, and Beisky later described kraurosis as an atrophic lesion similar to lichen sclerosus. Because of these early reports, every lesion on the vulva that appeared white and constricted the vaginal outlet was called kraurosis. Moreover, conditions as varied as leukoderma and invasive cancer have been called leukoplakia. Other terms, such as *primary senile atrophy* and *atrophic leukoplakia,* have been used interchangeably. They are nonspecific and should be eliminated. The epidermis may be thickened and the skin markings accentuated (lichenification), but the extent of the epithelial proliferation cannot be assessed without biopsy. Usually a 3- or 4-mm Keyes punch biopsy is used to obtain a small biopsy in the office under local anesthesia (Fig. 23.1). The specimen is oriented with the epithelial surface up on a square of filter paper or Telfa before being placed in fixative. This allows correct orientation of the tissue so that a full-thickness, nontangential, microscopic section can be prepared. Occasionally, experienced clinicians make a tentative diagnosis based on history and physical examination. A trial of topical therapy may be used for 6 to 8 weeks to evaluate the response; if the response is less than satisfactory or if there is any suspicion of invasive cancer, a biopsy must be done.

Although some physicians have suggested that lichen sclerosus and kraurosis have different histopathologies, their microscopic appearance is similar. A safe approach would be for surgeons to describe the anatomic appearance (i.e., whether the vulva is shrunken and constricted or thickened and leathery), leaving it up to the pathologist, who is familiar with both histology and anatomy, to define the cellular and histologic abnormalities.

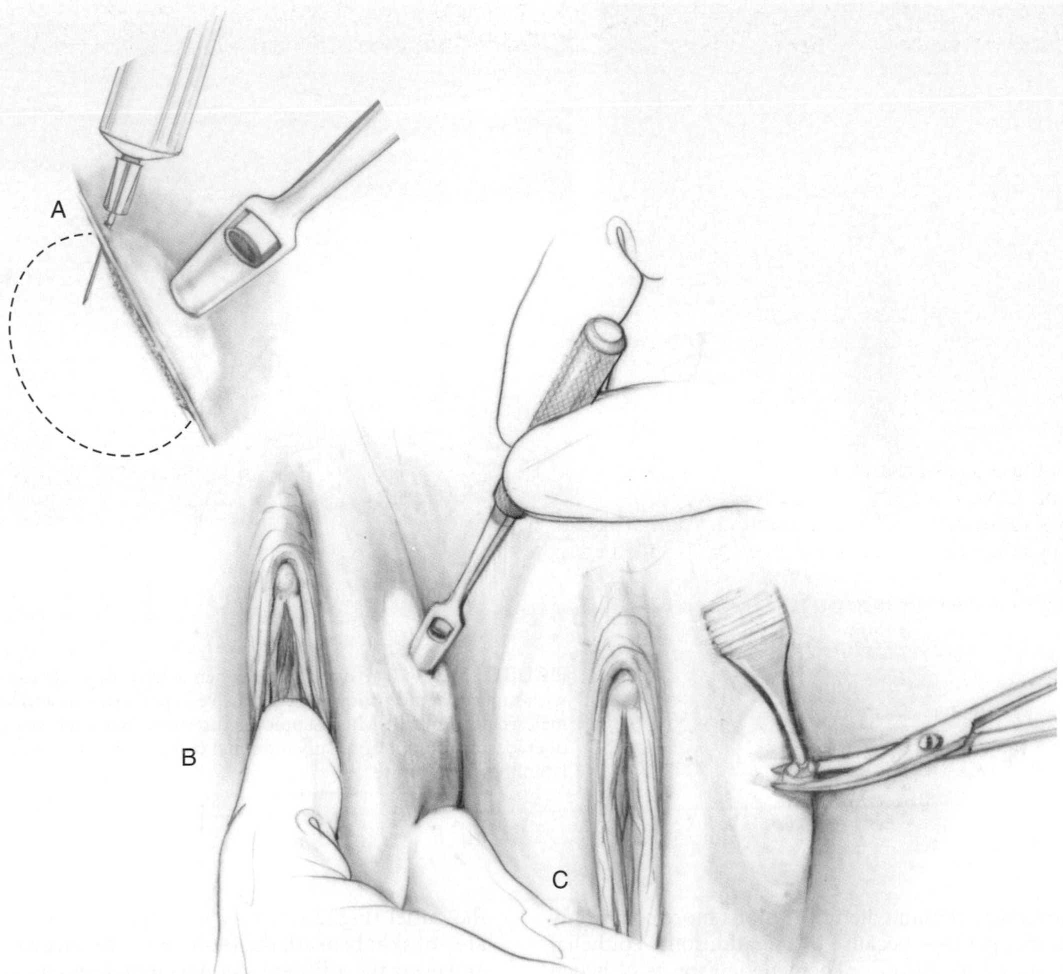

FIGURE 23.1. Biopsy of the vulva. **A:** The skin and subcutaneous tissue is infiltrated with local anesthetic using a small needle. **B:** A 3- or 4-mm Keyes punch biopsy instrument is firmly pressed against the skin to be biopsied and gently rotated. **C:** The small core of skin and subcutaneous tissue separated by the Keyes punch is elevated by small toothed tissue forceps and trimmed off at the base with curved iris scissors. Pressure is applied to the biopsy site, and the base is cauterized with silver nitrate sticks.

Hyperkeratosis

Both chronic infections and benign tumors, most commonly condylomata acuminata, appear white because keratin absorbs moisture, which reflects light back to the observer.

To avoid the ambiguous term *leukoplakia,* Jeffcoate, in 1966, introduced the term *dystrophy* into the nomenclature of benign epithelial lesions of the vulva. Predictions about the malignant potential of vulvar dystrophy vary; of all the types of dystrophy, the one most often benign is lichen sclerosus. As noted earlier, the terminology for vulvar dystrophies has been altered. Vulvar dystrophy has been classified in three categories: squamous hyperplasia, lichen sclerosus, and VIN. Typical squamous cell hyperplasia is characterized by a thickened, hyperkeratotic squamous epithelium, elongated rete pegs, and often an infiltration of the underlying tissue with chronic inflammatory cells. Typical hyperplasia is a benign form of chronic dermatitis with hyperkeratosis and acanthosis; thus, the designation "dystrophy" should be eliminated.

Depigmentation Lesions

Leukoderma and *vitiligo* are terms that are used interchangeably. Treatment is not required unless the symptoms of the commonly associated chronic dermatitis cannot be controlled by local medications. The hyperkeratotic lesions comprise a number of diverse entities that share a white to grayish white epithelial appearance in a moist environment. Biopsy is the only reliable criterion for accurate assessment.

Lichen Sclerosus

Lichen sclerosus is characterized by hyperkeratosis, thinning of the epidermis, loss of rete peg architecture, collagenization of the underlying tissue, and associated middermal inflammatory infiltrate (Fig. 23.2). It can occur at any age. The disease has been noted in the prepubertal child, and it occurs during the menstrual years. Nevertheless, it is seen most often in

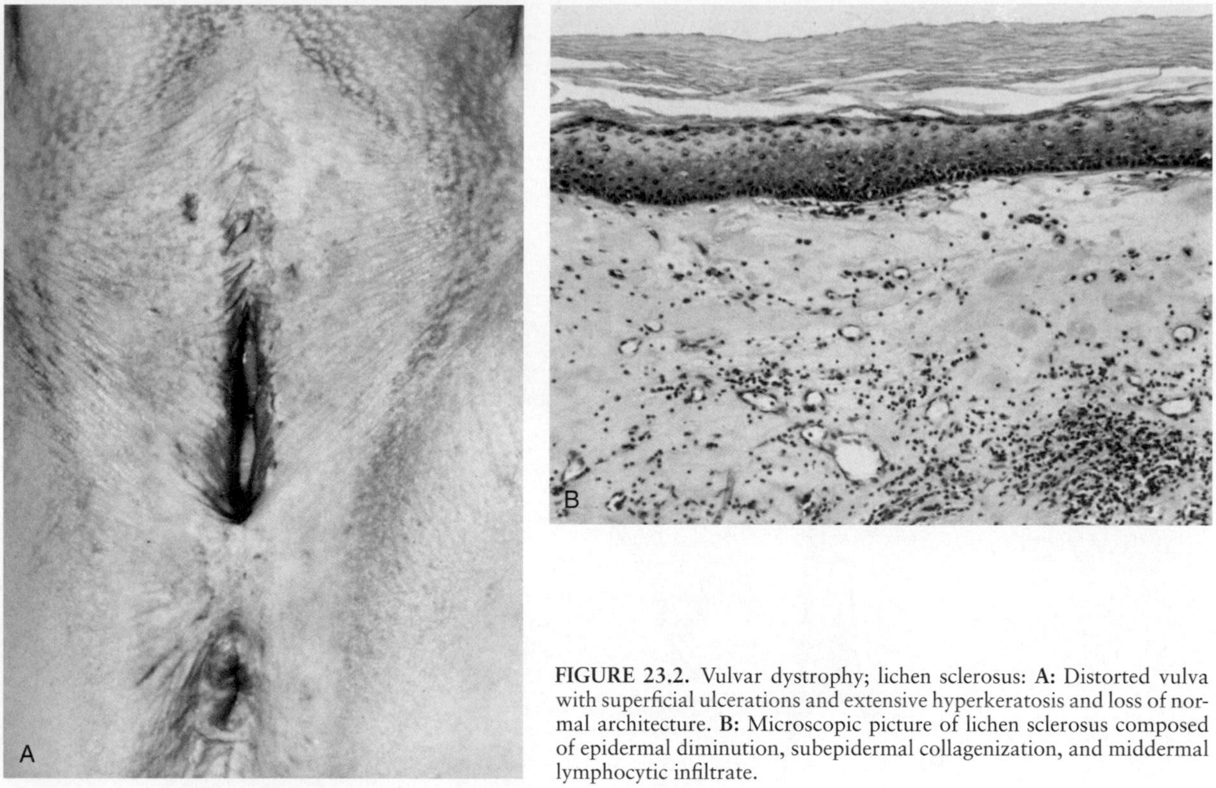

FIGURE 23.2. Vulvar dystrophy; lichen sclerosus: **A:** Distorted vulva with superficial ulcerations and extensive hyperkeratosis and loss of normal architecture. **B:** Microscopic picture of lichen sclerosus composed of epidermal diminution, subepidermal collagenization, and middermal lymphocytic infiltrate.

the postmenopausal woman when the lesions more commonly are symptomatic, perhaps because of the additional epithelial compromise caused by atrophy. The genetic aspects of lichen sclerosus have not been clearly identified, but the finding of lesions in both mother and child has been documented.

If biopsy specimens reveal lichen sclerosus, the patient should be treated with ultrapotent corticosteroids. Many series over the past few years have shown an excellent clinical response to 0.05% clobetasol proportionate topical ointment or cream. In a series of 81 women with biopsy-proven lichen sclerosus, Lorenz and coworkers reported that 77% had complete remission of symptoms and another 18% experienced significant improvement. Patients were treated with topical application of clobetasol cream twice daily for 1 month, at bedtime for another month, and, finally, twice a week for 3 months. They continued to use the cream on an "as needed" basis once or twice a week. Many patients continue to require occasional episodic therapy for symptomatic flare-ups, but the long-term effects of these ultrapotent steroids on the vulva have not been well studied. Some experts recommend maintenance therapy with lower potency corticosteroids, such as triamcinolone or 0.1% betamethasone. Topical testosterone has been recommended in the past, but Bornstein and associates compared the results of 2% testosterone propionate with 0.05% clobetasol dipropionate; at 1 year follow-up, 80% of the clobetasol treated patients reported symptomatic improvement compared with 40% of those treated with testosterone.

Many patients with chronic vulvar dermatitis, stenosis of the outlet specifically related to lichen sclerosus, and vestibulitis have an associated constriction of the vaginal outlet with resultant dyspareunia. Local intravaginal or vulvar applications of estrogen do not improve this condition. Plastic surgery to the outlet (Fig. 23.3) may be helpful. By excising a triangular area of skin beneath the fourchette, the surgeon can undermine and evert the adjacent vaginal epithelium, incise the transverse perineal muscle and fascia, and cover the denuded area with a flap of vaginal mucosa. The procedure is simple, and the use of delayed-absorbable suture material lessens the incidence of wound breakdown, which commonly occurs when absorbable suture is used. The results of this procedure have been most satisfactory; about 95% of patients are greatly relieved of dyspareunia. Breech and Laufer have reported good results in a few patients by suturing a protective covering of oxidized regenerated cellulose gauze (Surgicel, Johnson & Johnson, Arlington, TX) to the raw surfaces of the inner labia and clitoris after division of intracoital adhesions to prevent recurrence.

VULVAR INTRAEPITHELIAL NEOPLASIA

The first two cases of carcinoma *in situ* (CIS) of the skin were described by Bowen in 1912. Bowen also stated that although stromal invasion had not developed in patients observed over periods of 12 to 16 years, curettage and cauterization did not eliminate recurrence of the lesions.

In 1958, Woodruff and Hildebrandt reported 13 cases of VIN. They suggested that because the histology varied from one area to another in the same section, the general term *carcinoma in situ* should be used to designate the lesion. Today, the term *vulvar intraepithelial neoplasia* is commonly used, and vulvar intraepithelial lesions were originally subdivided into VIN I, corresponding to mild dysplasia; VIN II, similar to moderate

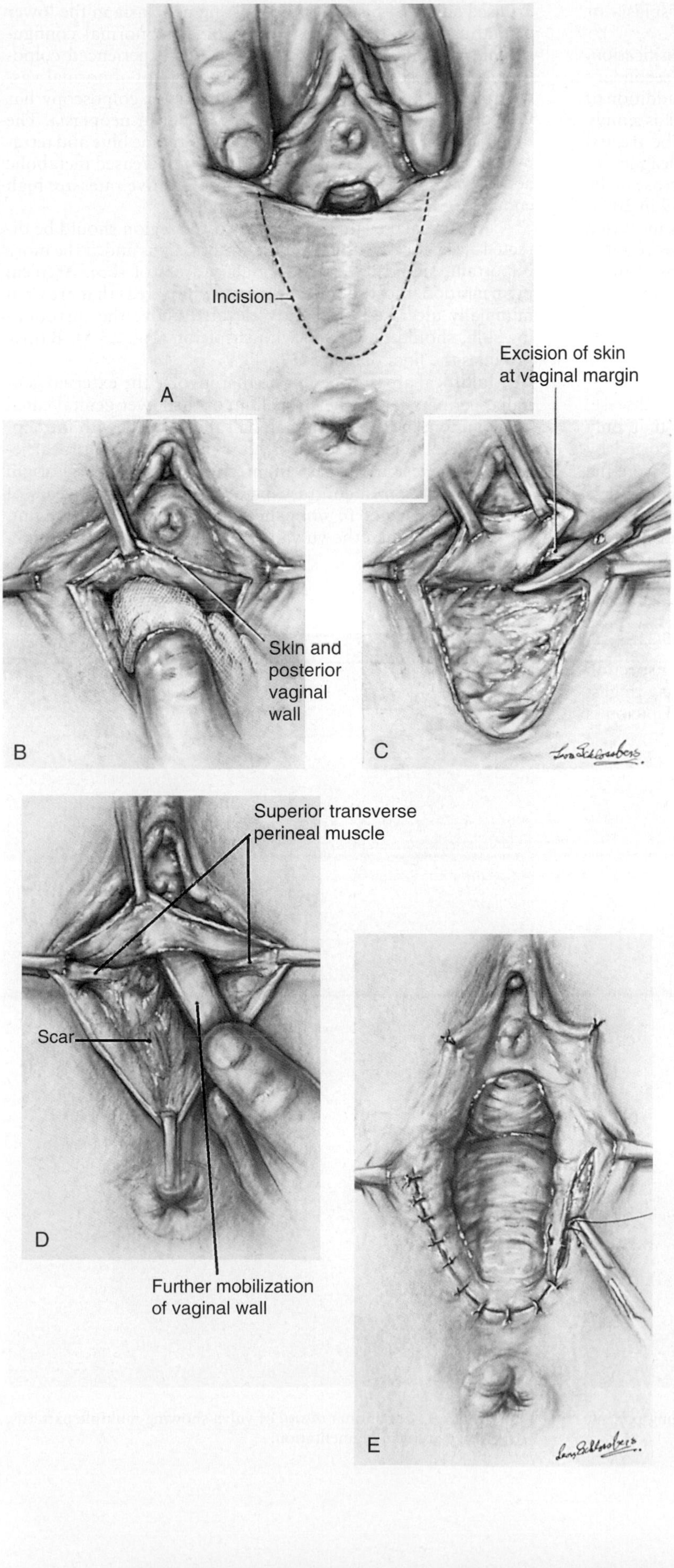

FIGURE 23.3. Perineoplasty. **A:** The incisional line is identified. The incision must be sufficiently extensive to allow for postoperative retraction and subsequent constriction of the outlet. **B:** The vagina is undermined to allow for exteriorization without tension. **C:** The scarred skin of the fourchette is excised. The vaginal epithelium is preserved for exteriorization. The vaginal epithelium is sufficiently undermined for the margins to be approximated to the skin (**D**) without tension (**E**). Occasionally, a small incision is made into the midline of the exteriorized mucosa to allow for an adequate outlet without tension.

dysplasia; and VIN III, corresponding to severe dysplasia or CIS, similar to the classification of cervical disease.

However, in 2004, the ISSVD changed the classification, eliminating the term *VIN I*. VIN I is thought to be secondary to viral changes and not a reproducible diagnosis. In addition to eliminating VIN I, they combined VIN II and VIN III as simply VIN, the expectation being that these lesions will be treated as high-grade preinvasive neoplasms. Jones and colleagues, in their review of 405 women with VIN, reported a decrease in the mean age of patients with VIN from 50 in 1980 to 39 in 2003. The increased prevalence of HPV infection as well as increased awareness by patients, clinicians, and pathologists has resulted in an increase in the diagnosis of VIN and, perhaps, a more common identification of these lesions in younger women.

Symptoms

Pruritus is the predominant symptom of most vulvar disease, including cancer, yet itching was the primary symptom in only 50% of patients with *in situ* cancer in a series reported by Buscema and associates. Other presenting symptoms were the presence of a lump, bleeding, and pain. In a small percentage of the cases, the lesion was discovered on routine examination; but in others, the diagnosis commonly was made in patients seen during follow-up of cervical neoplasia.

Diagnosis

The best technique for early diagnosis is careful inspection of the external genitalia—including perianal areas, thighs, and buttocks—under a bright light (Fig. 23.4). If suspicion is aroused either by history or preexisting neoplasia in the lower genital canal or by the suggestion of an abnormal configuration, magnification should be used. An experienced colposcopist can describe white lesions and areas of abnormal vasculature. As a screening procedure, however, colposcopy has not contributed to the early detection of vulvar neoplasia. The use of nuclear staining, specifically 1% toluidine blue and tetracycline fluorescence, has delineated foci of increased metabolic activity, but the false-negative and false-positive rates are high enough to make the results unpredictable.

Careful visual evaluation of the vulvar region should be directed at the focally white, hyperkeratotic areas and at the more important, slightly elevated, papillary areas of skin. Atypical pigmentation, most significantly gray-white areas that are even minimally ulcerated or slightly elevated above the surrounding skin, should be viewed with suspicion (Fig. 23.5). Biopsy provides the final diagnosis.

Multifocal areas of neoplasia that involve the external genitalia, perineum, and the epithelium of the lower genital canal are common; in fact, more than half the patients with intraepithelial disease in the lower genital tract have multifocal lesions. These lesions suggest an infectious, possibly viral origin for the neoplasia. In contrast, patients older than 60 years of age with invasive or *in situ* cancer more commonly have unifocal disease. When the vulva is the primary site of the lesion,

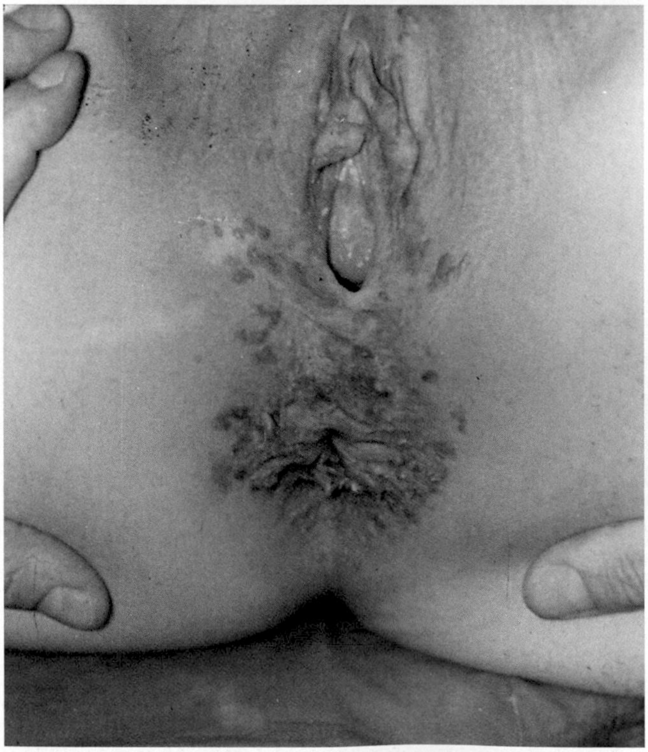

FIGURE 23.4. Multiple foci of carcinoma *in situ* in a young patient. Note the vulvar and perianal involvement.

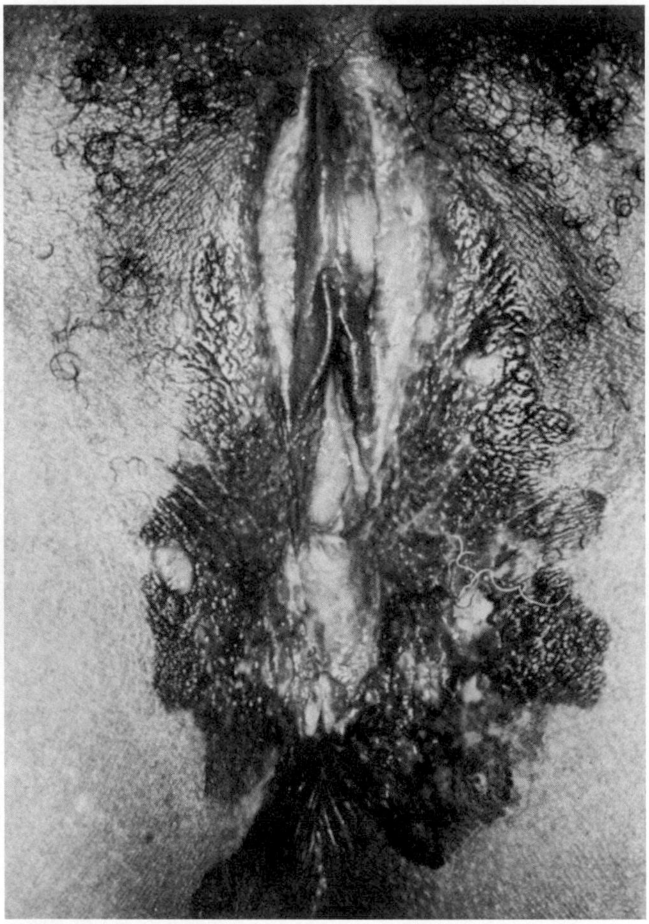

FIGURE 23.5. Carcinoma *in situ* of vulva showing multiple patterns, particularly atypical pigmentation.

the cervix, vagina, and perianal areas are frequent sites for associated neoplastic alterations. The combination of vulvar and cervical cancer makes up about 20% of all multicentric neoplasia in the lower genital tract.

The most pressing question about multifocal disease is whether invasive disease that develops from *in situ* lesions will arise in many foci or in only one focus. Only two of our patients with *in situ* neoplasia younger than 40 years of age have developed invasive cancer, and both cases appeared as solitary perianal lesions. Because the vulva and the cervix are of different embryologic origins, the tendency to correlate the histopathology of one area with that of the other may be unrewarding. For example, the full-thickness changes that signal cervical intraepithelial neoplasia are not as comparable when they occur on the vulva. Keratinization at the rete tips with intraepithelial pearl formation may indicate, on the other hand, a preinvasive disease in the anogenital area anywhere.

Pathologic Diagnosis

Biopsy with a Keyes punch can be performed in the office with the use of local anesthesia. Knife biopsies often are tangential and contain only the superficial layers, which results in a less than accurate histologic interpretation. Correct orientation of the tissue in the fixative is mandatory if accurate evaluation of the specimen is to be rendered. Such orientation can be obtained by placing the biopsy specimen on filter paper or Telfa with the epithelial surface exposed, so that the pathologist can embed the specimen accurately. Tangential cutting may result in the erroneous diagnosis of invasive disease. Cytology has not proved to be a satisfactory screening technique in the evaluation of the precursory cellular atypias in vulvar neoplasia.

The classic bowenoid changes vary from one microscopic section to another, but typical sections show loss of polarity, hyperchromasia, anaplasia, individual cell keratinization, corps ronds, and mitotic activity on the surface (Fig. 23.6). Abnormal mitosis may abound. Other gross variations include the

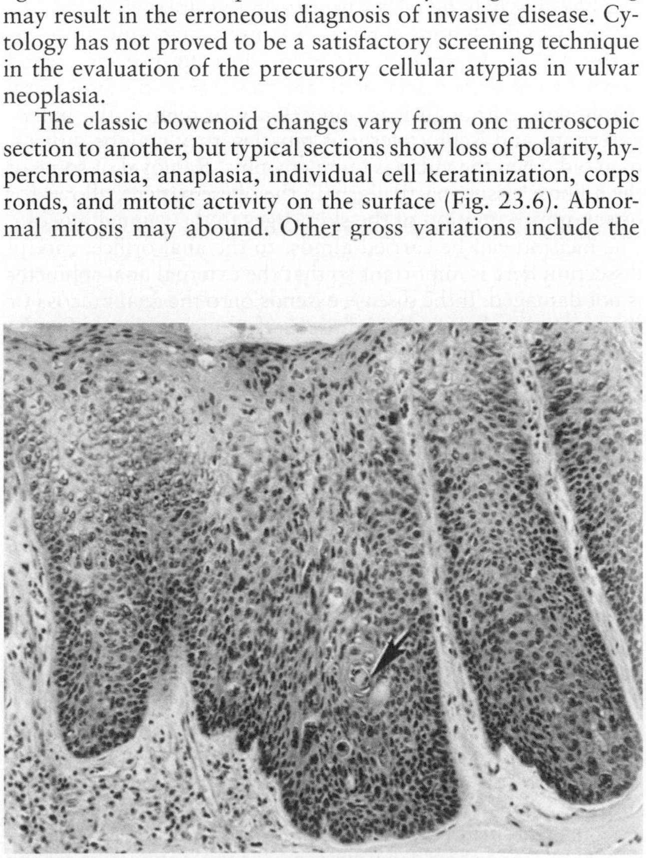

FIGURE 23.6. Carcinoma *in situ* of the vulva. There is full-thickness alteration in the architecture with elongation and distortion of the rete pegs. At arrow, there is intraepithelial pearl formation (×160).

erythroplastic lesion (erythroplasia of Queyrat) with immature cells extending from base to surface, and lesions that appear almost normal, being marked only by intraepithelial pearl formation at the rete tips in a background of marked dysplasia. Papillary lesions showing changes of high-grade dysplasia were previously designated as *bowenoid papulosis,* a term discontinued by ISSVD.

Treatment and Results

Although **surgical excision** of vulvar intraepithelial neoplasia is favored, patients typically do not require total vulvectomy. Modesitt and colleagues found invasive cancer in 22% of patients with biopsies consistent with VIN III. Vulvectomy may be appropriate for selected patients who are elderly, particularly if they have extensive disease, or for patients with Paget disease. Wide local excision usually is successful, but an attempt should be made to obtain clear margins. The adjacent loose skin of the vulva provides sufficient extra skin to cover minor defects without a skin graft and without significant deformity. The incidence of recurrence is no greater with local excision than with total vulvectomy, but it still approaches 30% to 40%. Positive margins have been indicative of an increased risk of recurrence in some series. Unless invasive cancer is suspected in the area of the positive margins, immediate reexcision is usually not indicated, but careful follow-up is necessary because recurrence is common. Brown has suggested CO_2 laser vaporization around the surgical margins will decrease the risk of recurrence.

A **skinning vulvectomy**, in which the epidermis and underlying dermis of the vulva and often the perineal area are removed and replaced by a skin graft, has been used for the treatment of extensive or multifocal vulvar *in situ* disease. This procedure is usually recommended in younger women with extensive lesions in an attempt to restore normal anatomy and sexual function. However, the technique requires surgery at a donor site, which produces an additional scar in a patient who usually is young. Furthermore, it imposes prolonged bed rest, near complete immobilization of the lower extremities, and indwelling bladder catheterization for 5 to 6 days while the skin graft heals.

The **carbon dioxide laser** has been successfully used in the treatment of *in situ* vulvar neoplasia. This approach is of particular appeal for the younger patient with multifocal, viral proliferative disease. This subset of patients with VIN is undoubtedly at lower risk for occult invasion. Emphasis in therapy should be directed toward preservation of maximum tissue and vulvar function. Given these considerations and the reality of recurrences, laser ablation provides an effective medium. Pretreatment requirements include careful examination of the lower genital tract and the liberal use of biopsies to identify areas of possible invasion and multicentric disease. The risk of invasive cancer is greater in the older patient. The desire for cosmetic results is less, so the use of surgical excision is favored in older women.

The laser itself is directed colposcopically after examination of tissues prepared by the application of dilute acetic acid. The latter may enhance detection of minimal viral changes not readily seen with the naked eye. Although benign condylomata can be adequately treated by superficial vaporization (so-called first and second plane), laser treatment of VIN must address the extension of disease into the hair follicles (pilosebaceous ducts). This mandates deeper laser vaporization beyond the papillary dermis and into the upper reticular dermis (third plane). The colposcope permits recognition of landmarks that characterize these levels. Baggish and coworkers identified skin appendage involvement in 36% of cases of vulvar *in situ* carcinoma and predicted that laser vaporization to a depth of 2.5 mm would effectively treat involved appendages in 95% of cases. Shatz and associates advocated ablation of VIN to a depth of 1 to 2 mm in nonhairy and hairy skin to achieve similar success. In laser treatment of VIN, the use of appropriate power densities should be emphasized. Low-power densities lead to thermal conduction injury in adjacent and underlying normal tissue. The latter increases the risk of scarring. Power densities of greater than 750 W/cm^2 are recommended. However, the deeper extent of vaporization required for VIN III, particularly in hair-bearing areas of the vulva, results in considerably greater postoperative pain, a longer period of healing, and an increased risk of scarring and subsequent chronic pain and dyspareunia; therefore many experts have abandoned the use of the laser in favor of surgical excision for VIN III. Bornstein and Kaufman have proposed combining laser ablation with surgical excision in the treatment of selected patients with VIN. Laser is used particularly in areas where excision hampers preservation of anatomy, such as in the clitoral region. Laser therapy for VIN should probably be reserved for experienced laser surgeons and colposcopists.

The **Ultrasonic Surgical Aspirator** can assist the surgeon in ablating to depths comparable to those achieved with the CO_2 laser. The advantage of this instrument is its ability to obtain additional tissue that might identify an occult cancer. Ultrasonic Surgical Aspirator and laser ablation also may be used to treat perianal intraepithelial neoplasia. In this setting, two concerns should be kept in mind. This location appears to be associated with a greater risk for the development of invasive squamous cancer, and the likelihood of fibrosis, scarring, and stricture is heightened. As with all treatments for VIN, the potential for recurrence and the need for further follow-up must be appreciated. With ablative approaches such as laser, diligence must be exercised to exclude invasion.

Topical agents have been used in the treatment of VIN with inconsistent results. Most notable among these topical treatments has been 5-fluorouracil (5-FU, Efudex 5%). Efudex is not recommended by the manufacturer for this use, and they specifically recommend against its use in the vagina. The mechanism of action appears to be related to the inhibition of DNA and RNA synthesis; the latter is not specific to dysplastic or HPV-infected cells. Normal epithelium is susceptible to the agent, and a component of hypersensitivity reaction appears operative in its mode of action. For cases in which treatment is effective, denudation of the epithelium is a requisite for success. This understandably leads to localized discomfort and pain, often reported as intense burning. Treatment regimens with topical 5-FU are diverse, and no standardized administration protocol has been widely adopted. One technique is topical application on an alternate-night basis for as long as 6 weeks; patient compliance problems typically lead to earlier curtailment. Among young patients with erythroplastic VIN, a 50% to 60% complete response rate has been reported. The hyperkeratotic VIN lesion has not proved to be as responsive to 5-FU.

In a 41-year review of 405 women, Jones and colleagues observed that more than 50% of women treated with laser ablation or surgical resection required an additional procedure within 14 years. Fifty percent of patients with positive surgical margins required additional treatment within 5 years. In comparison with positive margins, women with negative margins had a 15% chance of requiring additional therapy. Brown and colleagues, in a small series of 33 patients, noted a decrease in recurrence with a combination of surgical excision and laser vaporization at the margins.

TECHNIQUE OF CONSERVATIVE (SIMPLE) VULVECTOMY

Conservative (simple) vulvectomy is recommended in many patients with widespread VIN when it may be difficult to rule out invasive cancer or Paget disease of the vulva. It may also be appropriate when premalignant lesions, such as granulomatous diseases, do not respond to medical therapy or wide local excision.

An outline of the surgical margins is made with a surgical marking pen (Fig. 23.7). The initial incision should be made at the vaginal outlet so that the urethral borders can be well demarcated and the vaginal epithelium undermined for a short distance. If the incision is begun at the lateral skin margins, bleeding can mask the area, making the incision at the outlet more difficult to define. When the first incision is made at the outlet, a small pack can be placed into the vagina to control the bleeding while the elliptic incision at the outer skin margins of the lesion is made. The skin incision usually encompasses most of the labia majora, depending on the extent of the lesion. The incision through the skin is made with a knife to avoid tissue necrosis that occurs at the skin margins when an electrosurgical instrument is used. Minor vessels can be coagulated.

Major bleeding concerns may arise at the clitoris, particularly from the dorsal vein. Hemostatic sutures must be used to control the bleeding. A second point of concern is the pudendal vessels, which enter at the lower one third of the vulva close to the opening of the Bartholin duct. Branches of the pudendal vessels extend down to the anus as the inferior hemorrhoidals, and bleeding may be rather profuse in this area.

Because the lesions for which conservative vulvectomy is performed are superficial, dissection does not need to extend down to the deep fascia or to the muscles of the urogenital diaphragm. Although it is unnecessary to remove the bulbocavernous and ischiocavernous muscles, they may be difficult to avoid when the vulva is quite atrophic. Removal of some of the adipose tissue, particularly in the obese patient, allows for better approximation of the skin edges to the vaginal mucosa. The incision can be carried almost to the anal orifice; careful dissection here is important so that the external anal sphincter is not damaged. If the disease extends onto the anal mucosa or the protruding hemorrhoidal tissue, the mucosa should first be carefully dissected from the underlying external sphincter, excised with the tumor-free margins, and sutured to the perianal skin with 3–0 delayed-absorbable material. In the remaining vulva, the underlying tissues are approximated in layers with absorbable sutures, and the skin edges are approximated with interrupted absorbable sutures (Fig. 23.7). If bleeding is a problem, a small suction drain can be placed at the lower end of the incision, but it is much better to achieve meticulous hemostasis and use a firm pack against the area for 24 hours.

During closure of the perineal defect above the anal orifice and posterior vaginal introitus, the surgeon should evert the vaginal epithelium over the perineum in approximation to the anal orifice rather than suture the lateral skin edges snugly across the perineum and fourchette. Everting the vaginal mucosa allows for satisfactory coitus, whereas tightly approximated skin across the posterior fourchette may constrict the vaginal introitus and predispose to pain, dyspareunia, and fissuring.

When the firm packing has been removed after 24 hours, the entire area should be exposed. Initial application of ice packs to the operative site for 24 to 48 hours seems to provide more comfort to the patient than heat. Later, warm air blown across the perineum is both comforting and therapeutic

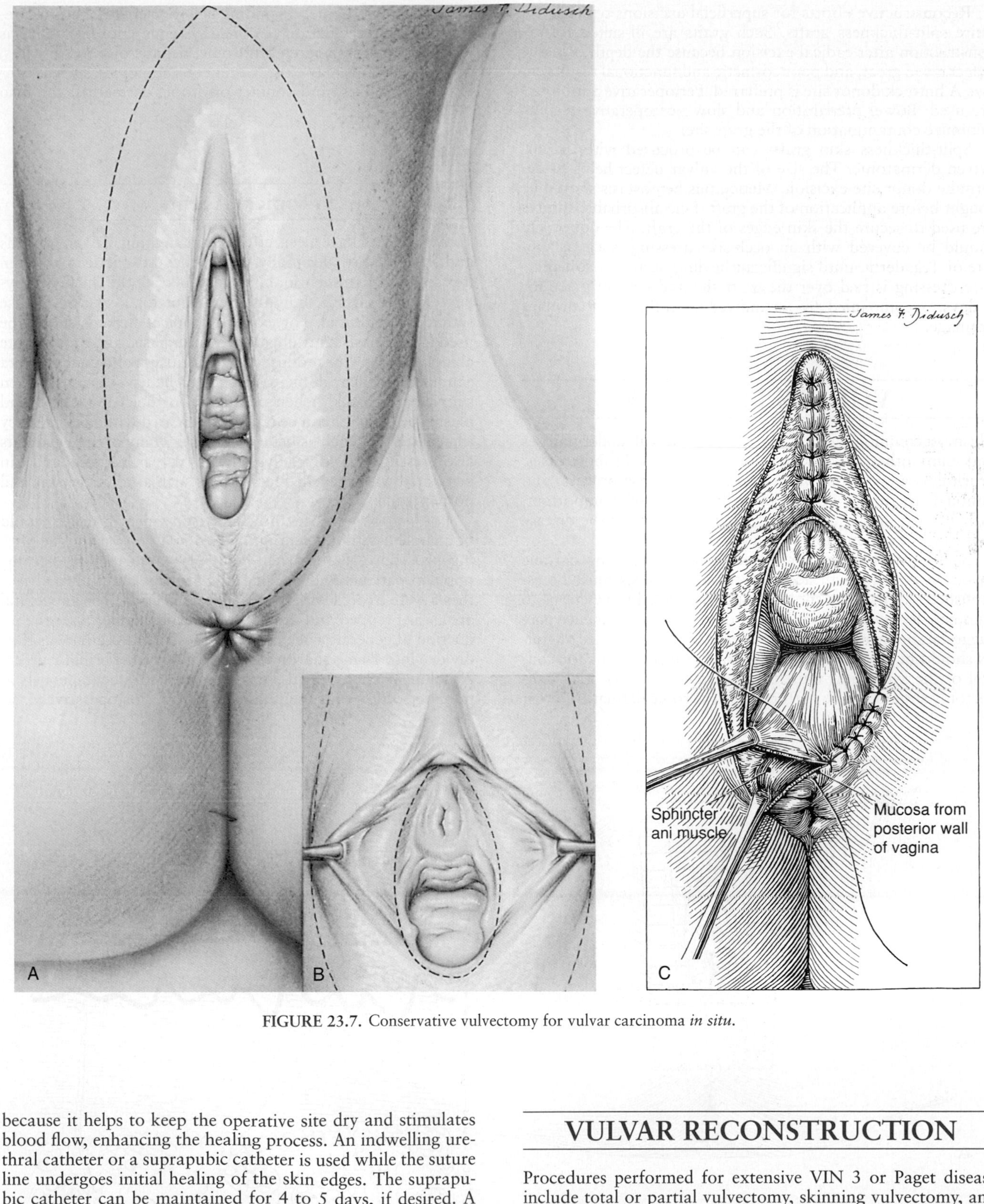

FIGURE 23.7. Conservative vulvectomy for vulvar carcinoma *in situ.*

because it helps to keep the operative site dry and stimulates blood flow, enhancing the healing process. An indwelling urethral catheter or a suprapubic catheter is used while the suture line undergoes initial healing of the skin edges. The suprapubic catheter can be maintained for 4 to 5 days, if desired. A single dose of a cephalosporin such as Cefazolin (1g) intravenously is recommended immediately before surgery. Infrequently, a local cellulitis may develop, necessitating antibiotic therapy; extended-spectrum cephalosporins and semisynthetic penicillins have proved effective.

VULVAR RECONSTRUCTION

Procedures performed for extensive VIN 3 or Paget disease include total or partial vulvectomy, skinning vulvectomy, and multiple wide excisions. These may occasionally result in large denuded areas, creating challenges for reconstruction. With the advent of laser ablation and the Ultrasonic Surgical Aspirator, fewer procedures such as skinning vulvectomy are performed for VIN.

Reconstructive efforts for superficial excisions typically require split-thickness grafts. Such grafts are ill-suited for reconstruction after radical excision because the depth of tissue defect is too great, and poor cosmetic and functional results ensue. A buttock donor site is preferred. Perioperative antibiotics are used. Bowel preparation and slow postoperative feeding minimize contamination of the graft site.

Split-thickness skin grafts can be procured with an air-driven dermatome. The size of the vulvar defect helps to determine donor site excision. Meticulous hemostasis should be sought before application of the graft. Fine absorbable sutures are used to secure the skin edges of the graft. The donor site should be covered with an occlusive dressing, such as Op-Site or Tegaderm, until significant healing occurs. A soft pressure dressing is tied over the graft site and kept in place for 5 days, accompanied by an indwelling catheter for urinary drainage.

VUVLAR PRURITUS

The most common symptom associated with vulvar dermatoses and many other vulvar conditions is pruritus. In most cases, pruritus is a symptom of an underlying disease process, and although treatment of this annoying symptom is important, the clinician should attempt to diagnose and treat the disease that causes the symptom of pruritus.

Before any therapy for vulvar lesions caused by chronic irritation is begun, an accurate tissue diagnosis must be established. All patients should be given detailed instructions to eliminate local irritants. A history of urinary incontinence may suggest a source of chronic vulvar irritation. Associated vaginitis should be treated vigorously. Topical medications for control of the symptoms must be given a satisfactory trial. Vulvectomy should not be performed for chronic dermatitis or for the benign dystrophies, including lichen sclerosus, before careful histologic evaluation is done. Systemic etiologies such as diabetes, anxiety, Sjögren syndrome, hepatic or renal diseases, or drug reactions may exist. Cutaneous etiologies, such as candidiasis, vaginitis, and contact or atopic dermatitis, can also occur.

Topical Agents

Topical agents have been effective in treating vulvar pruritus and should be tried initially. When they are ineffective, often it is secondary to their inability to penetrate the thickened hyperkeratotic surface. Initially, treatment for a specific disease should be instituted. For example, topical steroids should be used for psoriasis, antifungals for candidiasis, and appropriate ablative therapy for molluscum contagiosum and condylomata acuminata. Vulvar dermatoses such as lichen sclerosus, lichen simplex chronicus, lichen planus, seborrheic dermatitis, and plasma cell vulvitis can be effectively treated with high-potency topical steroids such as betamethasone. Many of these patients also present with vulvar dysesthesia (vulvar burning) and can be treated with tricyclic medications such as amitriptyline and nortriptyline.

For historic purposes, no chapter on vulvar pruritus would be complete without mentioning alcohol injection and the Mering procedure. Before treatment with amitriptyline became popular, patients with recalcitrant pruritus and vulvar dysesthesia were treated with local alcohol injection. The anogenital area was prepped and draped in a sterile manner after the induction of general or regional anesthesia. The region was then divided into 1-cm squares with a marking pen of brilliant green. Absolute alcohol, 0.2 mL, was then injected subcutaneously at the intersection of these lines (Fig. 23.8). Postoperatively, the

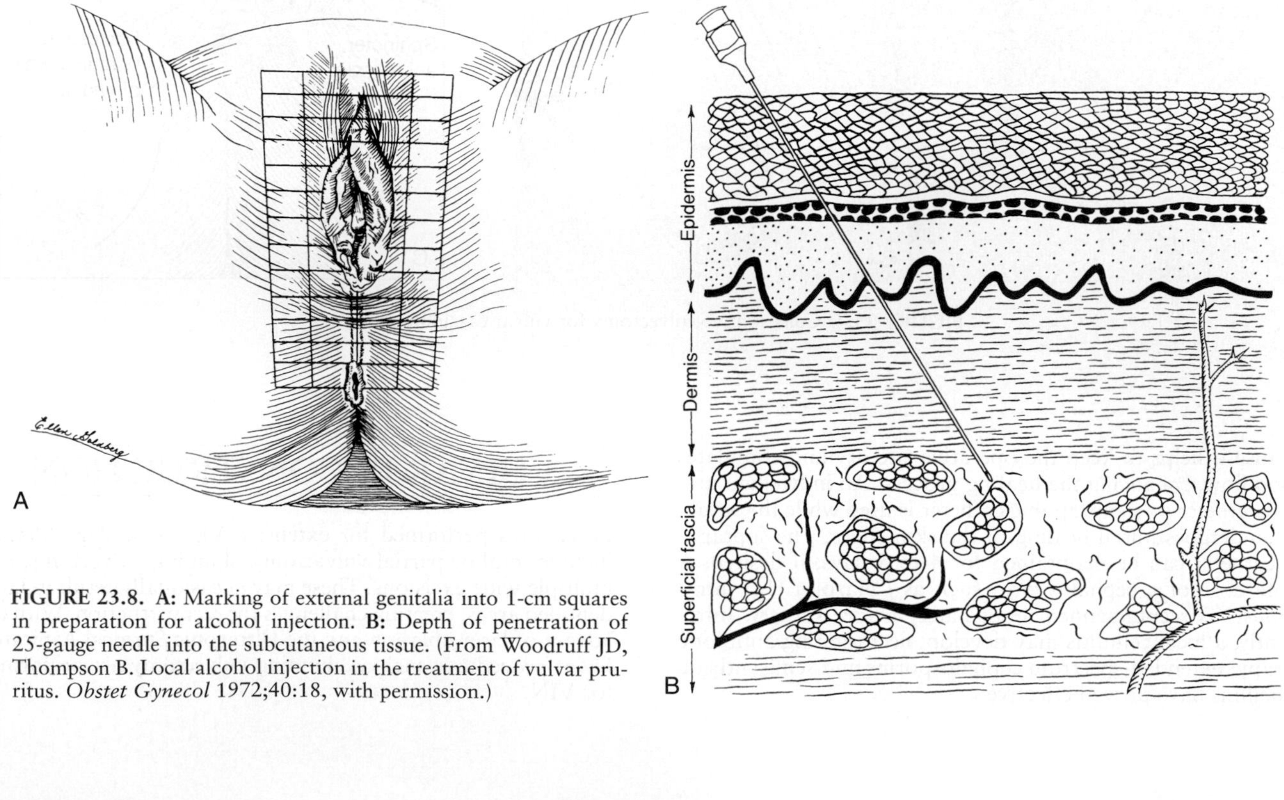

FIGURE 23.8. A: Marking of external genitalia into 1-cm squares in preparation for alcohol injection. **B:** Depth of penetration of 25-gauge needle into the subcutaneous tissue. (From Woodruff JD, Thompson B. Local alcohol injection in the treatment of vulvar pruritus. *Obstet Gynecol* 1972;40:18, with permission.)

patients were treated with cold packs and cool sitz baths for 1 week.

Mering Procedure

Because of the effectiveness of topical high-potency steroid creams, the Mering procedure is rarely used to treat vulvar pruritus in the United States today. It requires hospitalization and careful surgical technique (Fig. 23.9). The skin is shaved and thoroughly cleaned, and the incision is outlined with a marking pencil. The incision is made on the outer surface of the labium majus. It extends to the fascia of the urogenital diaphragm from the level of the clitoris to slightly beyond the fourchette and may continue inferiorly to the level of the anal orifice, depending on the extent of the pruritus. The nerves in the adjacent tissue are severed with a finger placed on each side, moving from the lateral aspect of the clitoris toward the midline, over the clitoris, where the fingers meet. The procedure interrupts branches of the ilioinguinal and genitofemoral nerves (Fig. 23.10). Blunt dissection extends posteriorly to the lateral side of the rectum, outside the external anal sphincter. If the perianal area is involved, blunt dissection may extend to the posterior limit of the anal orifice, where the two fingers meet behind the anus in the midline breaking up the branches of the pudendal nerve.

It is important that hemostasis be meticulously maintained. A small, flat Jackson-Pratt drain should be placed under the flap on each side. The subcutaneous tissue is approximated with absorbable sutures, and the skin is sutured with polyglycolic acid or polyglactin 910 material. The area must be packed tightly for 24 hours, and the patient should use ice packs or cool tub baths. Domeboro sitz baths (Burow's solution) may help to relieve edema.

VULVAR PAIN AND VULVODYNIA

Vulvar pain is another common symptom of vulvar disease. It may be produced by a wide variety of vulvar conditions or, occasionally, primary vulvodynia without any identifiable underlying diagnosis may be encountered. The ISSVD has defined vulvodynia as "vulvar discomfort, most often described as burning pain, occurring in the absence of relevant visible findings or a specific, clinically identifiable, neurologic disorder." The classification of vulvar pain is presented in Table 23.1.

There are many types of vulvar conditions that cause vulvar pain, including infections (candidiasis, herpes, etc.), inflammatory conditions (contact dermatitis), neoplasia (vulvar intraepithelial neoplasia, Paget disease, etc.) and neurologic conditions (herpetic neuralgia, neuroma, etc.). A careful diagnostic evaluation, usually including a biopsy of the vulva, is indicated to identify any of these lesions so that the correct therapy can be instituted. However, despite a careful and thorough workup, some patients will have vulvar pain for which an underlying diagnosis cannot be found. These patients are thus diagnosed with vulvodynia as defined above. The syndrome may be either localized to one area of the vulva or generalized, and the pain may be present all the time (unprovoked) or only when the vulva is touched or pressed (provoked). Vulvodynia involving the vulvar vestibule has been called *vulvar vestibulitis* or *vestibulodynia*. It is a clinical syndrome

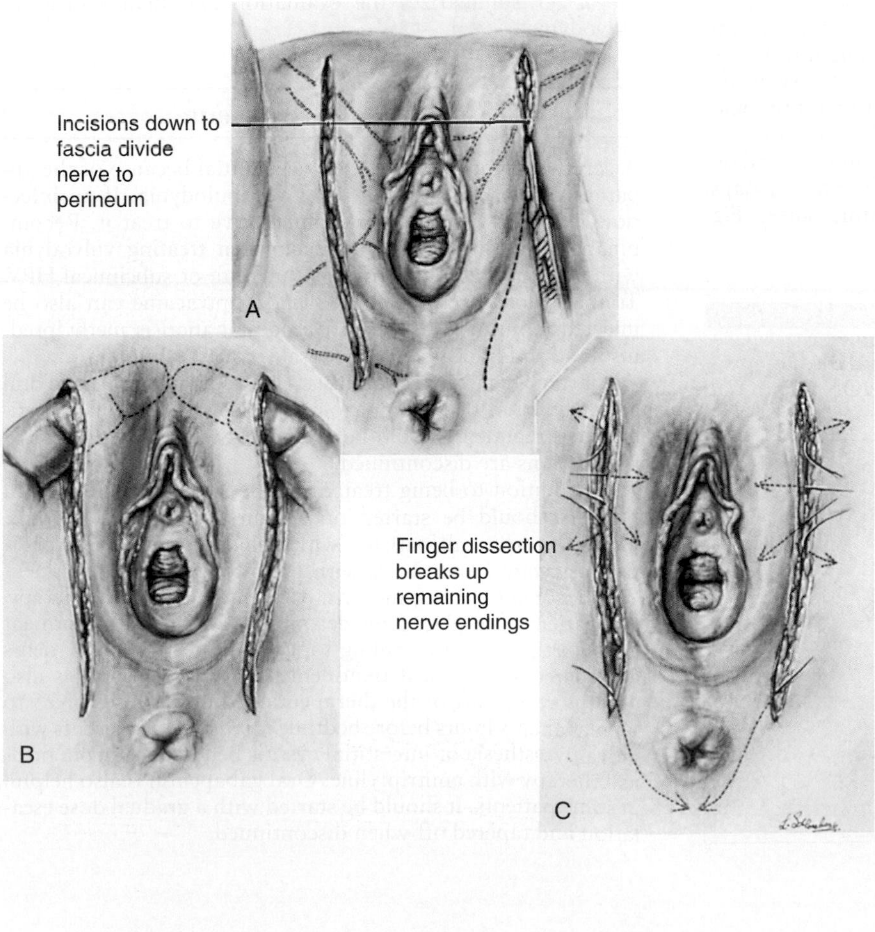
Incisions down to fascia divide nerve to perineum
A
B
Finger dissection breaks up remaining nerve endings
C

FIGURE 23.9. The Mering procedure. **A:** The incisions are made at the lateral margins of the labia majora, extending to the level of the clitoris superiorly and the anal orifice inferiorly. The depth of dissection is the deep fascia, to incise the adipose tissue and the nerves. **B:** The finger dissects the underlying tissue, breaking up the fibers of the pudendal, ilioinguinal, and genitofemoral nerves. **C:** The underlying tissues are carefully approximated to attain good hemostasis. A small drain should be inserted at the most dependent aspect of the incision to avoid the accumulation of blood in the operative sites.

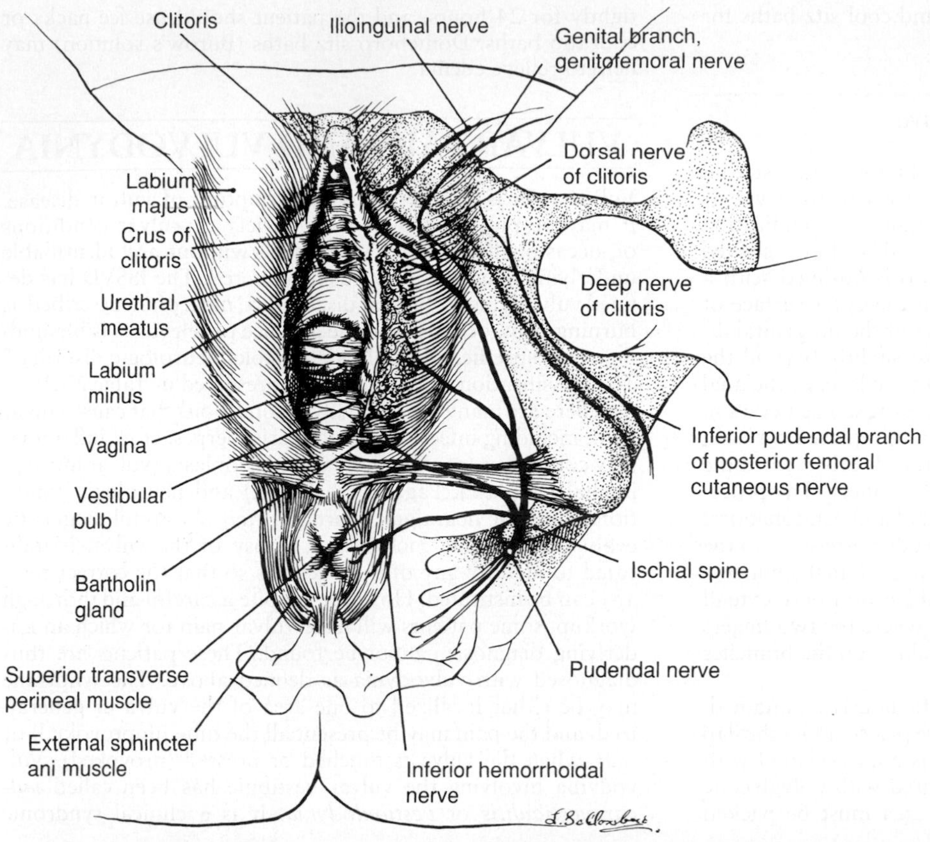

FIGURE 23.10. Nerve supply to anogenital region. (From Woodruff JD, Julian CG. In: Ridley JH, ed. *Gynecologic surgery: errors, safeguards and salvage.* Baltimore: Williams & Wilkins, 1974, with permission.)

consisting of the following characteristics: (i) severe pain on vestibular touch or attempted vaginal entry, (ii) tenderness to pressure localized within the vulvar vestibule, and/or (iii) physical findings confined to vestibular erythema of varying degrees. This syndrome is chronic and multifactorial. Etiologies include chronic or recurrent candidiasis, HPV infections, recurrent bacterial vaginosis, trauma, chemical and surgical destructive techniques, alterations of vaginal pH, irritants (soaps, detergents, douches, deodorants), and idiopathic causes. Figure 23.11 summarizes the evaluation and management of vulvodynia.

TABLE 23.1

INTERNATIONAL SOCIETY FOR THE STUDY OF VULVOVAGINAL DISEASES CLASSIFICATION OF VULVAR PAIN

A. Vulvar pain related to a specific disorder
- Infectious
- Inflammatory
- Neoplastic
- Neurologic

B. Vulvodynia
1. Generalized
   a. Provoked (sexual or nonsexual)
   b. Unprovoked (spontaneous)
   c. Mixed (provoked and nonprovoked)
2. Localized (i.e., Vestibule, clitoris, vulva)
   a. Provoked (sexual or nonsexual)
   b. Unprovoked (spontaneous)
   c. Mixed (provoked and nonprovoked)

Medical Treatment

A careful diagnostic evaluation is essential because of the apparent multifactorial etiology of vestibulodynia. If an infectious etiology is present, it is imperative to treat it. Recombinant alpha-interferon is efficacious in treating vulvodynia with a history of condylomata acuminata or subclinical HPV. Triamcinolone acetonide 0.1% and bupivacaine can also be injected monthly. An alternative combination is methylprednisolone and lidocaine submucosal.

Chronic recurrent candidiasis is treated with prolonged oral administration of ketoconazole or fluconazole. Topical anticandidal regimens should be prescribed when oral antifungal medications are discontinued.

In addition to being treated for the infectious etiology, all patients should be started on a course of topical steroids. Horowitz treats all patients with vulvodynia with hydrocortisone acetate 1% or 2.5% with 1% pramoxine HCl ointment (Pramosone) for 2 to 3 months. After 3 months of this therapy, the patients are placed on desoximetasone 0.25% ointment (Topicort). Only after failing topical steroids are the patients considered for surgical treatment. Oral amitriptyline is also an important part of the therapeutic regimen. Doses of 25 to 75 mg taken 3 hours before bedtime is prescribed. Patients with vulva dysesthesia or interstitial cystitis benefit most from medical therapy with amitriptyline. Oral gabapentin is also helpful in some patients. It should be started with a gradual dose escalation and tapered off when discontinued.

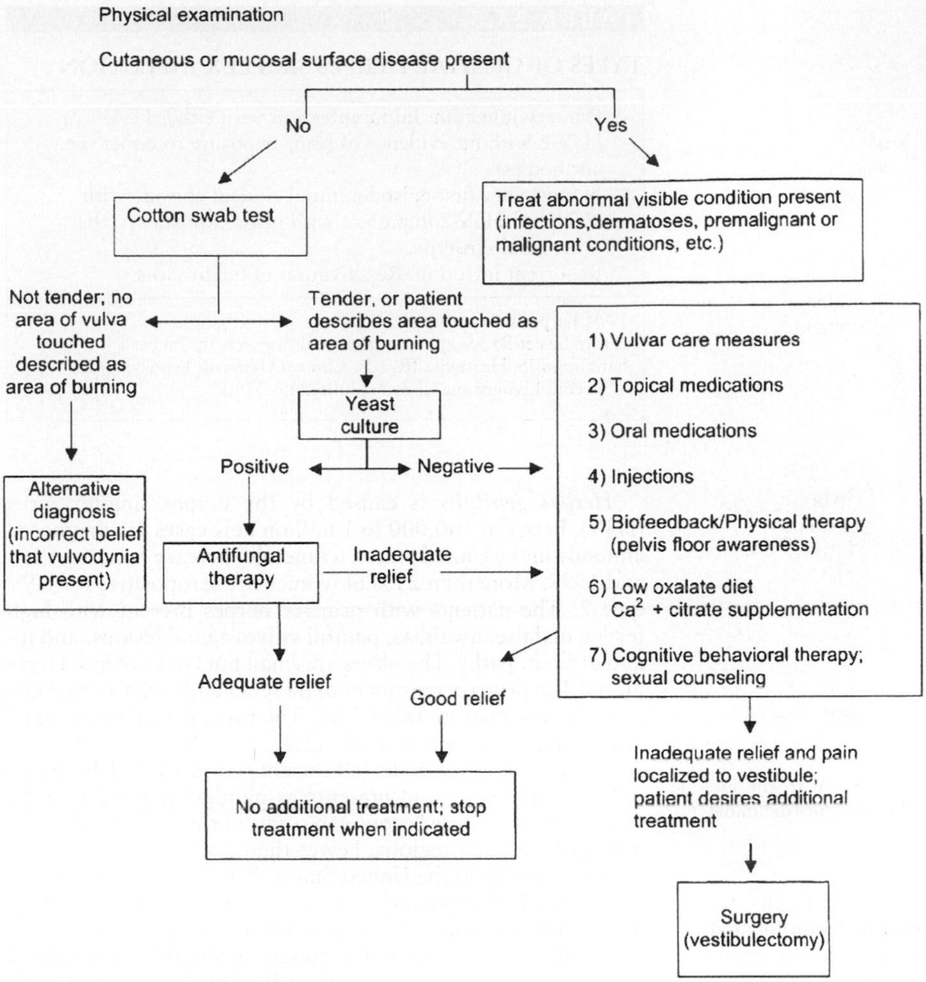

FIGURE 23.11. Vulvodynia algorithm. (From Haefner HK, Collins ME, Davis GD, et al. The vulvodynia guideline. *J Low Genit Tract Dis* 2005;9[1]:42.)

Surgical Treatment

Carbon dioxide laser ablation of the vestibular glands has not been shown to be optimal and has resulted in scarring and increased dyspareunia in some patients. In 1995, Reid and associates reported long-term results with the flashlamp-excited dye laser in nonresponders to medical therapy. Those with poor responses to laser vaporization were then treated with gland resection. Overall response rates were 62% to 80%, depending on the distribution of tenderness. However, long-term follow-up has been disappointing, and this approach remains controversial.

Primary surgical therapy has produced relief of symptoms in 75% to 90% of patients. This technique was initially described by Woodruff and associates in 1981 and Friedrich in 1987, and was modified by Marinoff and Turner in 1991 to include the periurethral Skene gland openings. The outer incision extends circumferentially from the periurethral glands along Hart's line to the contralateral glands. The proximal vaginal margin is just inside the hymenal ring. This horseshoe-shaped epithelium is superficially excised and sent for histologic diagnosis. In almost all cases, the histology consists of nonspecific periglandular chronic inflammation, much less impressive than might be expected based on the severe symptoms reported. As in a perineoplasty, the vaginal mucosa is undermined and the vagina advanced to approximate edges. The wound is closed in two interrupted layers of 3-0 polyglactin 910 (Vicryl) or polyglycolic acid (Dexon) sutures (Fig. 23.12). Postoperative treatment is the same as for perineoplasty. Coitus should be avoided for 2 to 3 months after surgery.

Several of Horowitz's patients (unpublished report) had severe levator spasm secondary to anticipation of activities associated with vulvar pain. This learned response has been treated successfully with biofeedback in several patients. Glazer and colleagues were the first to report the treatment of vulvar vestibulitis syndrome with electromyographic biofeedback of pelvic floor musculature. Seventy-eight percent (22 of 28) resumed coitus by the end of the treatment period.

VULVAR INFECTIONS

Although infections involving the vulva are treated with antibiotics rather than surgery, their appearance may resemble carcinoma *in situ* or even invasive cancer of the vulva. An accurate diagnosis may require cultures, viral testing, or even biopsy. Appropriate therapy is based on a correct diagnosis. Treatment of vulvitis secondary to an infectious process varies depending on the infection present. Viral infections such as HPV are strongly associated with intraepithelial neoplasia and carcinoma. These lesions are discussed later in this chapter.

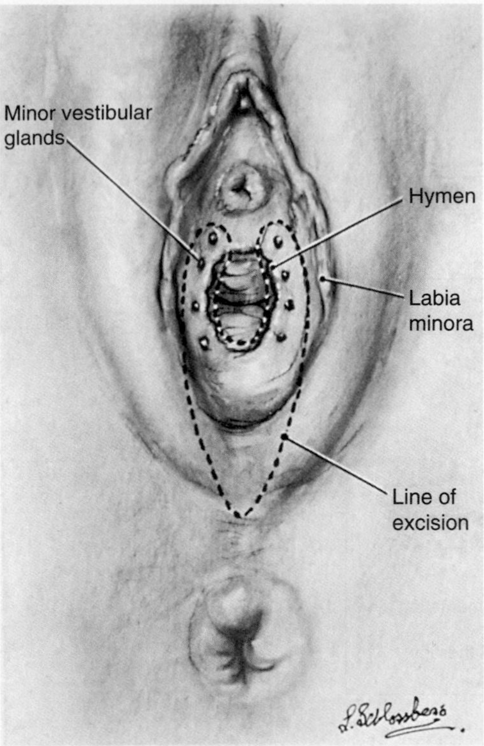

FIGURE 23.12. The minor vestibular glands exit lateral to the hymenal ring. They are very superficial and thus seldom produce definable "nodules," even when chronically infected.

Molluscum contagiosum, a member of the pox family, requires accurate identification and resection of the umbilicated lesions with a dermal curette. These lesions are usually circular and umbilicated. *Molluscum contagiosum* in an adult may be an indicator of underlying human immunodeficiency virus (HIV) infection. Therefore, the patient's background should be appropriately discussed.

TABLE 23.3

TYPES OF GENITAL HERPES SIMPLEX INFECTION

- Primary infection: Initial infection with either HSV-1 or HSV-2 without evidence of prior exposure to either (i.e., antibodies).
- Nonprimary first episode: Initial clinical episode with HSV-1 or HSV-2 in patient with prior exposure to the other viral serotype.
- Recurrent infection: Reactivation of latent virus.

HSV, herpes simplex virus.
(From Sweet RL. Sexually transmitted diseases. In: Bieber EJ, Sanfilippo JS, Horowitz IR, eds. *Clinical Gynecol*; Pennsylvania: Churchill Livingstone Elsevier, 2006;249–258.)

Herpes genitalis is caused by the herpes simplex virus (HSV). Between 500,000 to 1 million new cases are diagnosed annually in the United States, a ninefold increase between 1966 and 1997. More than 25% of women are seropositive for HSV type 2. The patients with primary herpes present with high fevers, malaise, myalgias, painful vulvovaginal lesions, and inguinal adenopathy. The ulcers are small but coalesce into larger ulcers. The primary treatment of these sexually transmitted diseases is presented in Table 23.2. The three categories of HSV infection are outlined in Table 23.3.

Granuloma inguinale (Donovanosis) is caused by *Klebsiella granulomatis* and presents as painless papular nodules or ulcerations. These lesions can occur in the genital, perianal, oral, and inguinal regions. Fewer than 100 new cases are reported annually in the United States. When large and destructive, *Granuloma inguinale* can simulate malignancy. Cytology and biopsy accompanied with Warthin Starry stains may establish the true diagnosis. The condition should be considered in all cases in which clinically malignant lesions are repetitively negative by biopsies. No U.S. Food and Drug Administration (FDA)-approved polymerase chain reaction (PCR) tests are available to date. The 2006 Centers for Disease Control and

TABLE 23.2

CDC-RECOMMENDED TREATMENT OF SEXUALLY TRANSMITTED DISEASES

Disease	Primary treatment	Alternate treatment
Herpes		
First episode	Acyclovir 400 mg PO TID × 7–10 days Famciclovir 200 mg PO TID 7–10 days Valacyclovir 1 g PO BID 7–10 days	Acyclovir 200 mg PO 5 × day × 7–10 days
Suppressive	Acyclovir 400 mg PO BID Valacyclovir 500 mg PO daily Valacyclovir 1 g PO daily	Famciclovir 250 mg PO BID
Episodic	Acyclovir 400 mg PO TID × 5 days Acyclovir 800 mg PO BID × 2 days Famciclovir 125 mg PO BID × 5 days Famciclovir 1,000 mg PO BID × 1 day Valacyclovir 500 mg PO BID × 3 days Valacyclovir 1.0 g daily × 5 days	Acyclovir 800 mg PO BID × 5 days

BID, twice a day; PO, by mouth; TID, three times a day.
Available at: www.cdc.gov/std/treatment/2006/genital-ulcers.html.

Prevention (CDC)-recommended treatment regimen is doxycycline 100 mg orally twice daily for 3 weeks or until lesions have completely healed. Alternative treatment regimens include:

Azithromycin 1 g orally once per week for at least 3 weeks and until all lesions have completely healed
OR
Ciprofloxacin 750 mg orally twice a day for at least 3 weeks and until all lesions have completely healed
OR
Erythromycin base 500 mg orally four times a day for at least 3 weeks and until all lesions have completely healed
OR
Trimethoprim-sulfamethoxazole one double-strength (160 mg/800 mg) tablet orally twice a day for at least 3 weeks and until all lesions have completely healed

Lymphogranuloma venereum (LGV) is caused by *Chlamydia trachomatis* types L1, L2, and L3. LGV presents with papular or vesicular lesions on the vulva that can also ulcerate. LGV lesions are usually painless and heal spontaneously. As with herpes, these patients present with headaches, myalgias, arthralgias, and inguinal adenopathy. The 2006 CDC treatment guidelines recommend doxycycline 100 mg orally twice daily for 21 days. Alternatively, the patient can be treated with erythromycin base 500 mg orally four times daily for 21 days.

Chancroid is caused by *Haemophilus ducreyi*. The chancroid lesions present as multiple papules that become pustular and ulcerate. These lesions are very tender and have a ragged edge sitting on an erythematous base (halo). More than 50% of these patients present with large inguinal lymph nodes called buboes. These lymph nodes may become suppurative. Lymph nodes and soft tissue in the inguinal area can also be involved secondary to LGV and granuloma inguinale. The 2006 CDC treatment guidelines are as follows:

Recommended Regimens
Azithromycin 1 g orally in a single dose
OR
Ceftriaxone 250 mg intramuscularly in a single dose
OR
Ciprofloxacin 500 mg orally twice a day for 3 days (ciprofloxacin is contraindicated for pregnant and lactating women)
OR
Erythromycin base 500 mg orally three times a day for 7 days

Syphilis is caused by the spirochete *Treponema pallidum*. The primary lesions usually have a painless, coin-shaped ulcer with a raised border and an indurated base. They can present 10 to 90 days after exposure and resolve in 2 to 6 weeks. Untreated syphilis results in a secondary phase characterized by skin rash, generalized adenopathy, and moist, papular anogenital lesions called condyloma latum. This is followed by a latent phase leading to tertiary syphilis. The latter can involve the cardiovascular, musculoskeletal, or central nervous system. *T. pallidum* can also cross the placenta and result in syphilis in the newborn infant. More than one sexually transmitted disease can be seen in the same patient and can combine with acquired immunodeficiency syndrome (AIDS). See Table 23.4 for CDC 2006 guidelines.

Necrotizing Fasciitis

Necrotizing fasciitis of the vulva is a very serious destructive infection characterized by rapid progression and a high mortality rate ranging from 12% to 60%. It represents a surgical emergency. Multiple bacterial pathogens are implicated, including staphylococci, A. streptococci, *Escherichia coli, Peptostreptococcus*, *Provotella* and *Porphyromonas* spp, *Bacteroides fragilis,* and *Clostridium* spp. Associated vascular thrombosis leads to skin and subcutaneous tissue necrosis. Fisher's criteria have been emphasized in the diagnosis and help to exclude clostridial infections. Brook and Frazier isolated mixed aerobic-anaerobic flora in 68% of specimens, 10% facultative or aerobic bacteria, and 22% exclusively anaerobic organisms. Diabetes mellitus is the most common predisposing condition, although other factors, such as radiation, have been identified. The most common clinical findings are necrosis, fever tachycardia, leukocytes, edema and foul odor.

Devascularization of the skin proceeds with sparing of underlying muscle and bone. Early skin changes include hemorrhagic bullous formation. Typically, the underlying fascial necrosis exceeds the boundaries of visible skin involvement. Inflammatory alterations and edema usually are present. Most patients present with fever, tachycardia, and signs of systemic toxic reaction. Prompt diagnosis is important because this disorder progresses rapidly.

Treatment combines expeditious surgery, antibiotics, and maintenance of circulation and tissue oxygenation. Surgical treatment should include aggressive excision of nonviable skin, subcutaneous tissue, and avascular fascia. Extensive debridement down to and including the fascia must be performed until viable, well-vascularized tissue margins are identified. Wounds are packed, not primarily closed. High-dose broad-spectrum antibiotic coverage is administered, and associated medical conditions such as dictates are managed aggressively. These patients are frequently very sick, and renal failure and acute adult respiratory distress syndrome commonly complicate their management. The operation for additional debridement or subsequent skin grafting is also common. ***Fournier's gangrene*** presents in a manner similar to that of necrotizing fasciitis and nonclostridial myonecrosis. Infections develop in the labia and spread to the perineum, buttocks, and abdominal wall. Treatment consists of a combination of surgery, broad-spectrum antibiotics, and hyperbaric oxygen.

Hidradenitis Suppurativa

An infectious process commonly demanding extensive local surgery is suppurative hidradenitis. This pustular disease begins as an infection in the apocrine sweat glands. The early manifestations often are cyclic, because the secretory activity of the apocrine glands corresponds to the progestational phase of the menstrual cycle. Consequently, in the early stages of the disease or in the chronic pruritic phase (Fox-Fordyce disease), the use of hormonal therapy, such as oral contraceptives, may help to modify the secretory activity of the glands. Once the disease extensively involves the deeper tissues, local and systemic agents usually are ineffective. Isotretinoin (Accutane) has been effective in some cases, but care must be taken in prescribing this agent because it is a powerful teratogen. Culturing exudates and treating with appropriate antibiotics may provide palliation and further delay surgery. The pustules often infect the entire area, so that pressure at one point may produce exudation of purulent material from sinus tracts (Fig. 23.13A). Multiple bacteria have been isolated from patients with hidradenitis suppurativa (Table 23.5). Because the entire anogenital area is honeycombed by the underlying infection, simple incision into a few of the pustules is useless. Extensive debridement must be performed to allow healing from the base.

TABLE 23.4

CDC-RECOMMENDED TREATMENT OF SYPHILIS IN ADULTS, 2006

Primary and secondary syphilis
Recommended regimen
Benzathine penicillin G, 2.4 million units IM in a single dose
Penicillin allergy (nonpregnant)
Doxycycline 100 mg orally twice a day for 2 weeks
OR
Tetracycline 500 mg orally four times a day for 2 weeks

Latent syphilis
Early latent syphilis (<1 year)—recommended regimens
Benzathine penicillin G, 2.4 milling units IM in a single dose
Late latent syphilis (>1 year)—recommended regimens
Benzathine penicillin G, 7.2 million units total, administered as three doses of 2.4 million units IM each, at 1-week intervals
Penicillin allergy (nonpregnant)
Doxycycline 100 mg orally twice a day
OR
Tetracycline 500 mg orally four times a day
Both drugs administered for 2 weeks if duration of infection known to have been <1 year; otherwise, administer for 4 weeks.

Tertiary syphilis
Recommended regimen
Benzathine penicillin G, 7.2 million units total, administered as three doses of 2.4 million units IM, at 1-week intervals
Penicillin allergy (nonpregnant)
Doxycycline 100 mg orally twice a day
OR
Tetracycline 500 mg orally four times a day
Both drugs administered for 2 weeks if duration of infection known to have been <1 year; otherwise, administer for 4 weeks.

Neurosyphilis
Recommended regimen
Aqueous crystalline penicillin G 18 million to 24 million units per day, administered in 3 million to 4 million units IV every 4 hours, for 10–14 days
Alternative regimen (if compliance assured)
Procaine penicillin 2.4 million units IM daily
PLUS
Probenecid 500 mg orally four times a day, both for 10–14 days
Penicillin allergy (nonpregnant)
Ceftriaxone 2 G daily either IM or IV for 10–14 days

Syphilis during pregnancy
Recommended regimens
Penicillin regimen appropriate for the pregnant woman's stage of syphilis. Some experts recommend additional therapy (e.g., a second dose of benzathine penicillin 2.4 million units IM) 1 week after the initial dose, particularly for women in the third trimester and for those who have secondary syphilis during pregnancy.
Penicillin allergy
A pregnant woman with a history of penicillin allergy should be treated with penicillin after desensitization.

IM, intramuscularly; IV, intravenously.
Available at www.cdc.gov/std/treatment/2006/genital-ulcers.html.

The incision extends into the underlying fat, and the involved skin is removed in segments, leaving bridges of normal skin between the excised pustules. Loose approximation of the skin edges can be performed with polyglycolic acid or polyglactin 910 suture material; more commonly, the entire area is left open and treated locally to promote granulation (Fig. 23.13B). Results of therapy are rewarding in most cases, and skin grafting usually is unnecessary. The patient must be treated with antibiotics based on cultures obtained from the draining sinuses both before and after surgery. Radical vulvectomy is occasionally indicated for extensive disease of the vulvar, inguinal, and perineal areas, but generally simple vulvectomy is usually effective. It is imperative that a thorough histologic evaluation be performed by the pathologist. Squamous cell carcinoma has been reported to arise in diffuse perineal suppurative hidradenitis. Myocutaneous flaps or

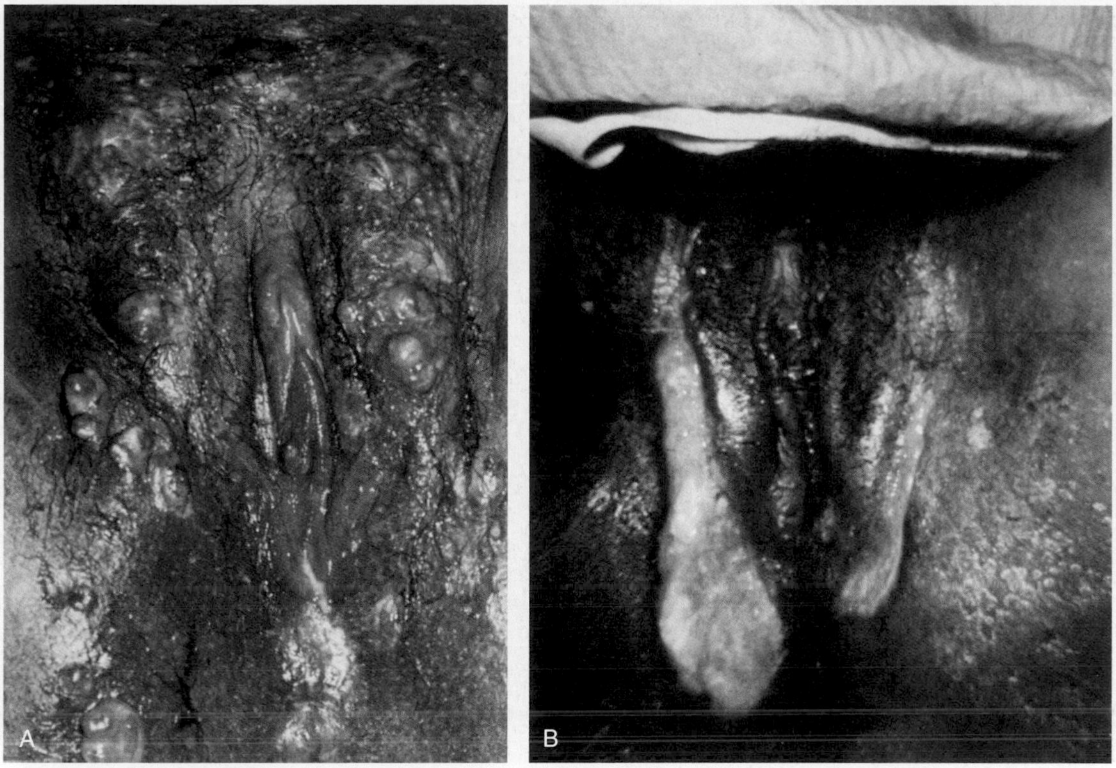

FIGURE 23.13. A: Extensive suppurative hidradenitis with numerous communicating sinuses. B: Same vulva 4 weeks after debridement with exuberant granulations (complete healing in 2 months).

split-thickness skin grafts can be placed in a two-stage procedure. This will allow the infections to clear before the raw vulvar surface is grafted. Wet to dry dressings are used 48 hours to 2 weeks before grafting.

Harrison and colleagues have reported a 37% recurrence rate in patients with inguinal or perineal lesions. In their series of 106 patients, Rompel and Petres experienced 17.8% complication rate with surgery and only a 2.5% recurrence in the operative field.

TABLE 23.5

BACTERIA INVOLVED IN HIDRADENITIS SUPPURATIVA

Gram-positive organisms	Gram-negative organisms
Staphylococcus aureus	*Acinetobacter*
Staphylococcus epidermidis	*Pseudomonas aeruginosa*
Staphylococcus hominis	*Bacteroides*
Streptococcus milleri	*Fusobacterium*
Streptococcus pyogenes	*Prevotella*
Propionibacterium acnes	
Peptostreptococcus	
Corynebacterium	
Lactobacillus	

(From Faro S. Vulvovaginal infections. In: Bieber EJ, Sanfilippo JS, Horowitz IR, eds. *Clinical Gynecol*; Pennsylvania: Churchill Livingstone Elsevier, 2006;249–258.

CROHN DISEASE

Crohn disease, a chronic granulomatous inflammatory disease of the bowel, affects the vulva and perianal area in about 25% to 30% of the cases in which there is classic intestinal involvement. The draining sinuses often communicate with the vagina or the rectum, thus resulting in the formation of fistulous tracts (Fig. 23.14A). On rare occasions, the vulva may be primarily involved, even though the small and large bowel apparently are not affected or affected subsequently. Crohn disease can also present as unilateral labial hypertrophy.

Before any surgical therapy is begun, the diagnosis can be confirmed by studying the bowel or by obtaining a biopsy specimen of the affected tissues in the perineum. The presence of noncaseating granuloma without demonstrable organisms is characteristic of Crohn disease (Fig. 23.14B). Further deterioration of the tissue may result from attempts to excise a draining sinus produced by Crohn disease. Rectal incontinence can result from destruction of the anal sphincter or the development of a rectovaginal fistula. Approximately 9% of rectovaginal fistulas are secondary to Crohn disease.

Immunocytochemistry of Crohn's lesions has documented *Escherichia coli* and streptococcal antigens. In addition to short-term metronidazole, patients have responded to prolonged treatment (3–6 months) with broad-spectrum antibiotics such as ciprofloxacin. Methotrexate therapy is effective in reducing the requirement for prednisone in patients with chronically active Crohn disease. Other drugs used in the medical management of Crohn disease include 5-aminosalicylic acid, cyclosporine, azathioprine, 6-mercaptopurine, mesalamine, and infliximab (Remicade®).

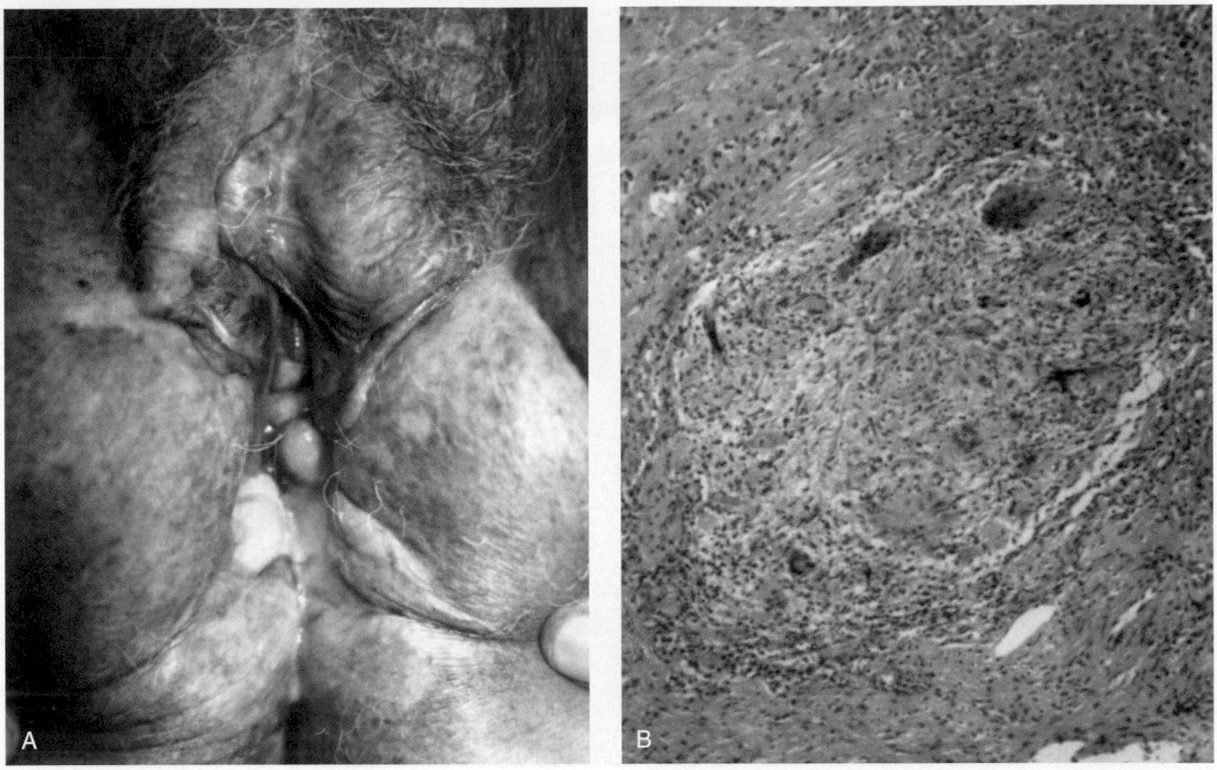

FIGURE 23.14. Crohn disease. **A:** Vulva showing multiple fistulae and fibrosis causing tissue contraction and distortion. **B:** Microscopic section to show noncaseating granuloma. No microorganisms were seen by special stains.

In addition to pharmacotherapy, a submucosal anal pull-through procedure may bring relief. Layered surgical repair of a fistula caused by Crohn disease usually is unsuccessful, particularly without appropriate medical management. However, after appropriate medical therapy, surgical excision of the tract is usually effective (see Chapter 39). Results are difficult to predict because multiple areas of the terminal colon and small intestine may be affected, and any affected area may involve the vagina or perineum. Medical therapy should always be given during this type of surgical procedure and should be continued postoperatively for at least 2 months.

TRAUMA

Major trauma to the vulva most often occurs when young girls experience injuries as a result of sledding or bicycling accidents. Hematomas and occasionally lacerations can develop when the vaginal area forcefully comes in contact with the crossbar of a bicycle (as during a fall from a bicycle seat), or when the girl is thrown from a sled against an obstacle such as a tree or fence. Trauma also can result from sexual assault, and the gynecologist must be sensitive to this possibility even when the initial history suggests another etiology. Women or girls who are victims of sexual assault should receive testing for pregnancy and sexually transmitted diseases. These patients should be referred to counseling and encouraged to report the abuse to state officials. All minors should be reported to the state by the examining physician.

Most traumatic injuries do not require surgical attention. An examination under anesthesia may be useful to adequately evaluate the extent of the injury. If surgical repair is not required, patients should be treated conservatively with activity restriction and with the immediate and continued use of Burow's solution (aluminum sulfate, calcium acetate; available as Domeboro tablets or powder) added to the sitz bath to reduce edema. Antibiotics may be used as prophylaxis against superinfection in damaged tissues. If a hematoma increases in size and extends well into the perineum or over the lower abdominal wall, incising the vulvar skin, evacuating the hematoma and ligating the bleeding vessels may reduce the period of convalescence. An alternative would be to use selective arterial embolization. Goldman and coworkers reported 30% of patients with genital trauma not associated with parturition have a urologic injury. When a hematoma produces urethral obstruction, evacuation may reduce the time an indwelling urethral catheter is needed. If the hematoma is not expanding, it should be followed conservatively. Most vulvar hematomas resolve spontaneously; surgical intervention, on the other hand, can result in significant morbidity, including infection. Frequently, a distinct bleeding site is not identified. If, however, the clot becomes secondarily infected, it requires prompt evacuation and drainage. Lacerations into the rectum or urethra should be repaired expeditiously.

CYSTS OF THE VULVA

Bartholin Duct Cysts

Obstruction of the Bartholin duct, usually near the orifice, is common. Although such obstructions can result from

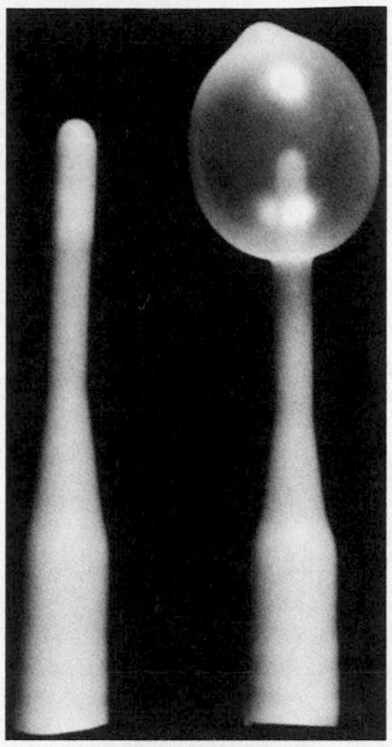

FIGURE 23.15. The Word catheter (*left*) is inserted into the Bartholin duct cyst through a vaginal incision. The bulb is inflated with saline solution (*right*), and the end of the catheter is placed in the vagina.

gonococcal infection, other infections and trauma more commonly explain the occlusion. During a mediolateral episiotomy or a posterior colporrhaphy, for example, sutures can easily injure or even ligate the duct. The lining of the main cyst is transitional epithelium. The mucus-secreting glands are not affected by the obstruction but may be distorted by the infectious process. During the acute infection, which may precede the actual cyst formation, an abscess often develops with symptoms of tenderness, swelling, and erythema. Depending on the cause, secretion from the cyst may be mucoid or cloudy.

Incision and drainage bring almost immediate relief to the patient and can be accomplished under local anesthesia. A small wick can be left in the cavity to maintain adequate drainage. A small incision (2 cm) is made in the cyst wall in the area of the normal duct orifice, and a culture is obtained for *Neisseria gonorrhoeae,* Chlamydia, and aerobic and anaerobic bacteria. A Word catheter (Fig. 23.15) is inserted and the catheter bulb inflated with 2 to 3 mL of saline. If the catheter remains in place for 3 to 4 weeks, the tract becomes epithelialized, and the catheter can be removed. Broad-spectrum antibiotics are given before surgery.

Marsupialization seldom can be accomplished during the acute stage, but the procedure is useful for chronic or recurrent abscesses. Injection of an antibiotic into the abscess has been tried as treatment for the acute infection but has proved to be less effective than systemic antibiotic therapy.

Most Bartholin duct cysts are uninfected and asymptomatic. They are usually found during routine pelvic examinations. Patients may even be unaware of large cysts. When symptoms do occur, most patients report discomfort during coitus or pain while sitting or walking. These require marsupialization only if they are symptomatic. Table 23.6 differentiates between a Bartholin cyst and abscess.

Technique of Marsupialization

Drainage of a Bartholin duct cyst by marsupialization is not as technically involved as excision and eliminates many complications. The procedure makes it possible to avoid excising the gland with the cyst and to preserve the secretory function of the gland for lubrication.

Marsupialization has had limited use since the Word catheter was introduced. The catheter accomplishes the same result as surgery with minimal or no trauma. The nipple of the catheter can be inserted into the vagina. There is essentially no discomfort with the procedure, and coitus can be resumed normally. Because this procedure can be performed with local analgesia in the office setting and yields results comparable to those of marsupialization, its use should be encouraged.

The marsupialization can be performed under local, regional, or general anesthesia. A wedged-shaped, vertical incision is made in the vaginal mucosa over the center of the cyst, just outside the hymenal ring, with a 15 blade (Fig. 23.16A). The incision should be as wide as possible to enhance the postoperative patency of the stoma. After the cyst wall is opened and the cyst is drained of its contents, the lining of the cyst is everted and approximated to the vaginal mucosa with interrupted sutures of 3-0 delayed-absorbable material (Fig. 23.16B). Drains and packs are not necessary, but the patient's postoperative care should include daily sitz baths beginning on the third or fourth postoperative day.

As a result of closure and secondary fibrosis of the orifice after marsupialization, 10% to 15% of cysts recur. Abscess formation is another occasional sequela of marsupialization.

TABLE 23.6

DIFFERENTIATION BETWEEN BARTHOLIN ABSCESS AND BARTHOLIN CYST

Bartholin abscess	Bartholin cyst
Enlarged gland	Enlarged gland
Erythema present in skin overlying and surrounding the gland	Erythema absent
Skin overlying the gland typically warm to the touch	No increase in temperature
Fever present, especially with tachycardia	Fever absent
Advancing cellulitis can be present	Cellulitis absent
WBC count elevated	WBC count not elevated
Bacteria and WBCs are present in fluid (pus) contained within Bartholin gland	No bacteria or WBCs present in (serous) fluid contained within the cyst

WBC, white blood cell.
(From Faro S. Vulvovaginal infections. In: Bieber EJ, Sanfilippo JS, Horowitz IR, eds. *Clinical Gynecol*; Pennsylvania: Churchill Livingstone Elsevier, 2006;249–258.)

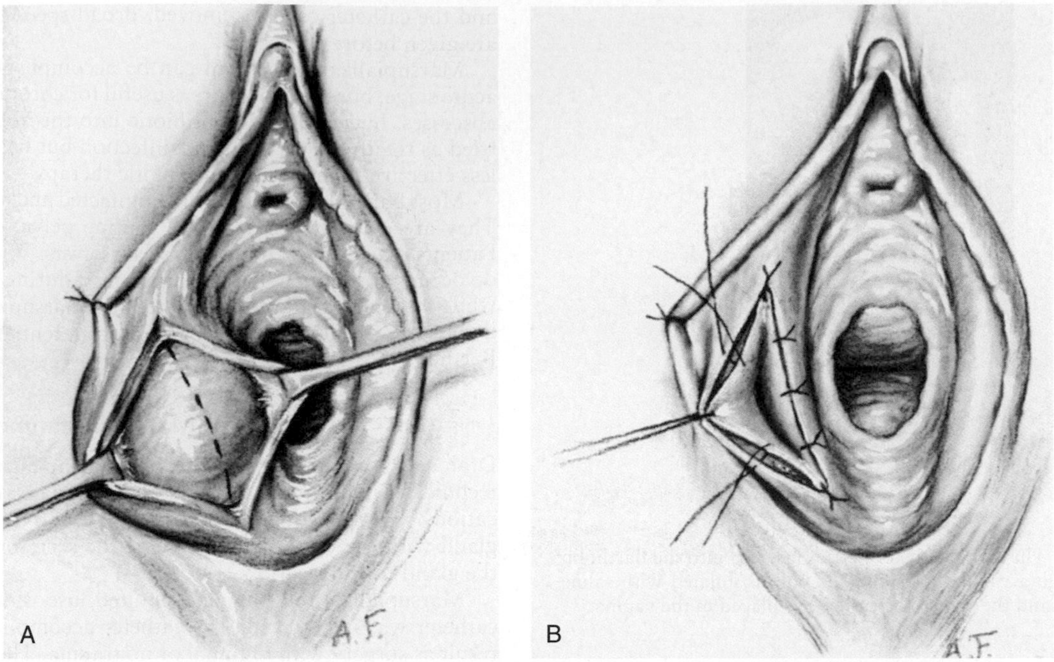

FIGURE 23.16. **A:** Incision for marsupialization. **B:** Marsupialization. (From Tancer ML, Rosenberg M, Fernandez D. Cysts of the vulvovaginal [Bartholin's] gland. *Obstet Gynecol* 1956;7:609.)

Technique of Excision

It is seldom necessary to excise a Bartholin duct cyst, particularly in the younger patient, unless there is induration at the base. The latter may signify deep-seated infection that is inaccessible by marsupialization. Conversely, this may represent neoplasm in the base of the gland, an issue of greater concern in the patient older than 40 years of age or in patients with coexisting Paget disease. An elliptical incision in the vaginal mucosa is made as close as possible to the site of the gland orifice with a 15 blade (Fig. 23.17). An incision on the mucosal side is preferable because an incision through the vulvar skin makes it difficult to dissect the cyst wall from the skin without incising or tearing the skin. If an opening is accidentally made through the skin, a permanent fenestration may result. Difficulty is not usually encountered during dissection of the cyst from the inner surface of the vulvar skin when the incision is made on the mucosal side. Excising a small ellipse of mucosa with the cyst allows the surgeon to have a site for traction and reduces the risk of rupturing the cyst. Because cyst formation usually is preceded by inflammation, the wall is adherent and cannot be easily enucleated with blunt dissection only. The blunt-pointed Mayo scissors serve admirably for sharp dissection of the cyst from its bed (Fig. 23.17C). The cyst can be mobilized further with the handle of the scalpel. A large cyst may develop posteriorly and may approximate the rectum. The rectal wall can easily be distinguished from the cyst by inserting a finger into the rectum during dissection.

Complete removal of the gland tissue adherent to the cyst wall is essential because residual glandular tissue may result in the formation of a tender nodule or recurrent cyst. If the margins of the cyst have become obscured, the cyst can be opened and the wall dissected from the surrounding tissue.

Directly beneath the Bartholin duct is the vestibular bulb, which is composed of anastomosing venous channels. In the dissection of the gland from the vestibular bulb, additional care must be taken to avoid troublesome bleeding. To ensure permanent hemostasis, the entire cavity must be obliterated by approximating the walls with fine delayed-absorbable suture material after excision of the cyst.

Approximation of the vaginal mucosa is best accomplished with a continuous or interrupted mucosal suture of 3–0 delayed-absorbable material. Persistent bleeding from the labia or vestibular bulb may cause a postoperative hematoma of the labia, which can progress to include the mons pubis and the abdominal wall beneath the Scarpa fascia. Bed rest, ice packs, and a pressure dressing on the vulva are the methods of treatment for a hematoma; attempts to ligate the venous bleeding points are futile. Although the blood usually reabsorbs with time, sometimes evacuation and drainage are necessary. If the bleeding deep in the bed of the gland seems uncontrollable, deep mattress sutures can be placed from the skin through the bleeding bed into the vagina. The sutures should not be tied too tightly because necrosis may result, with fenestration of the vaginal outlet. A small drain should be stitched into the bed with fine absorbable sutures to avoid the accumulation of blood and serous fluid.

Hydrocele or Cyst of the Canal of Nuck

Hydrocele is an uncommon vulvar cyst. The cyst appears as a dilatation in the labium majus and adjacent labium minus and must be differentiated from a Bartholin duct cyst. Figure 23.18 shows a hydrocele. The patient underwent two procedures for drainage of a Bartholin duct cyst, but the mass recurred after each procedure.

A **hydrocele** is a cystic, fluid-filled hernia of the peritoneum that accompanies the round ligament and extends from the inguinal canal into the vulva. When this sac extends into the

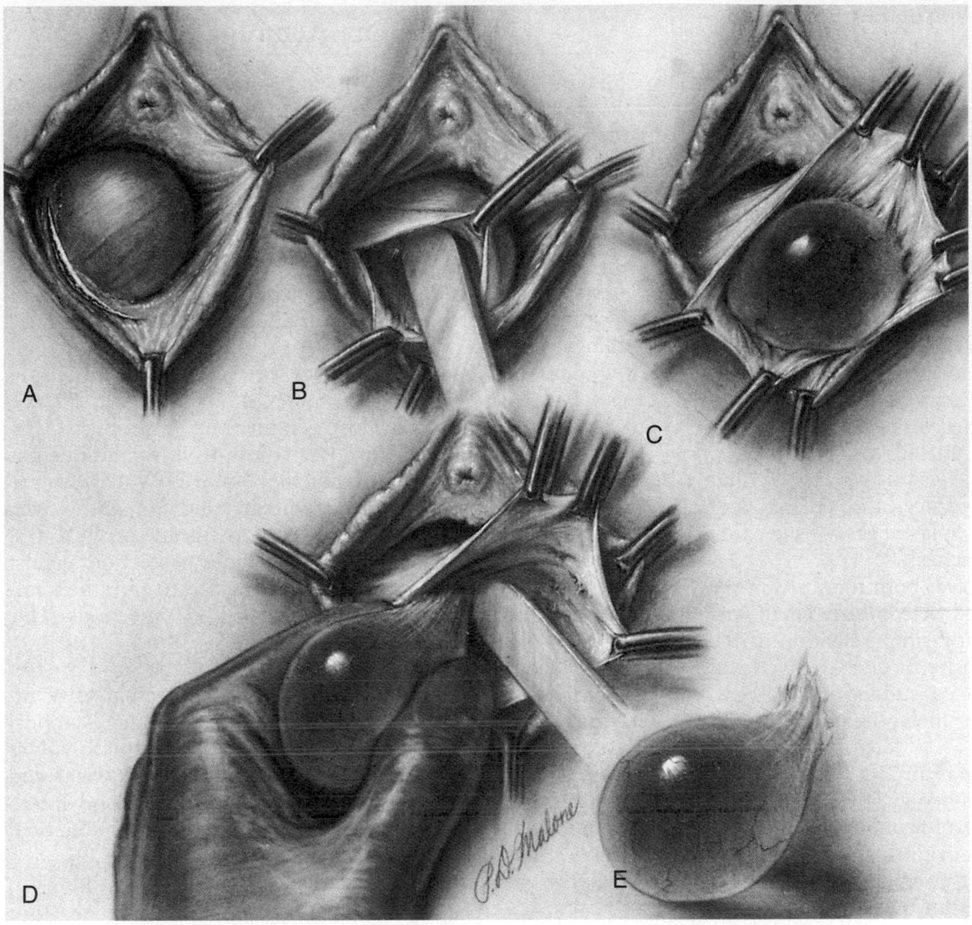

FIGURE 23.17. Excision of a Bartholin gland cyst. A: An incision is made in the mucosa over the cyst. B: Dissection is begun, using the handle of the scalpel. C: Dissection has been continued by sharp and blunt dissection. D: Dissection is almost complete. E: Intact cyst after removal.

inguinal canal, it is known as a cyst of the canal of Nuck. On rare occasions, a loop of intestine may follow the pathway of the round ligament, forming a hernia in the vulva. When a hydrocele is treated as a Bartholin duct cyst by incision and drainage, peritoneal fluid may reaccumulate above the drainage site, and the hydrocele recurs.

Surgical treatment for a hydrocele begins with an incision into the cystic mass. The external inguinal ring is identified by inserting a finger in the cyst anteriorly to the inguinal canal. The peritoneal lining is excised from the cavity, and the external inguinal ring is closed along with the subjacent tissue in the anterior vulva. If a hernia is present, inguinal herniorrhaphy

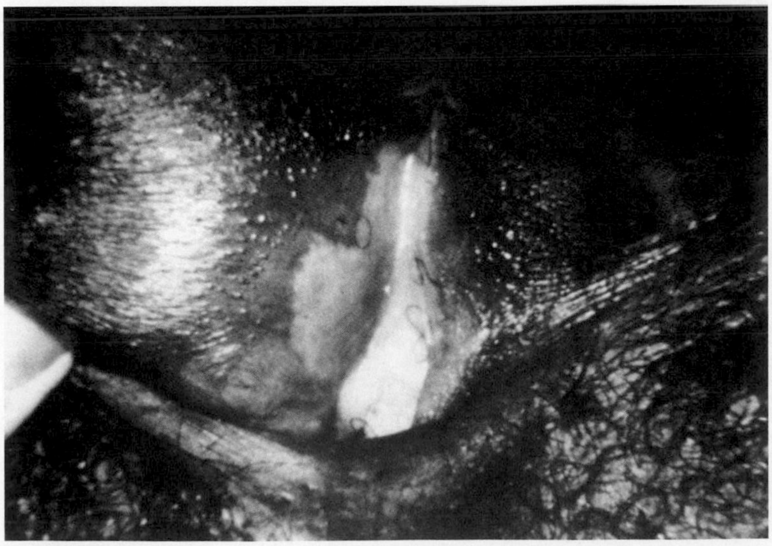

FIGURE 23.18. A hydrocele is caused by the extension of a peritoneal sac with the round ligament from the inguinal canal into the vulva.

should be performed along with excision of the peritoneal covering of the round ligament.

SOLID TUMORS OF THE VULVA

The incidence of solid, benign tumors in the vulva is low; but a variety of benign tumors, including fibromas, fibromyomas, lipomas, hemangiomas, neurofibromas, and endometriomas have all been reported. These tumors can originate from any of the three germinal layers that constitute the anogenital area. One occasionally sees a solid vulvar tumor composed of benign breast tissue or a benign fibroadenoma (Fig. 23.19). Lactational changes can be seen in this tissue. Such an event is accounted for by the embryologic milk line caudally ending in the vulvar area. Degenerative changes and necrosis often occur in the larger tumors and should not be confused with malignancy. Lipomas often are mistaken for cystic lesions because of their consistency, whereas hernias and hydroceles of the canal of Nuck must be differentiated from neoplastic growths because they require different surgical approaches.

Most solid tumors should be excised, both to ascertain the diagnosis and to relieve the patient's discomfort. Small, pedunculated tumors can be removed by simple ligation of the stalk; the deeply situated lesions require more extensive local dissection. All nevi showing hemorrhage, sudden enlargement, and pruritus should be suspected to be melanomas and excised widely.

The boundaries of such mesodermal tumors are difficult to delineate, but most of the tumors are benign. Even recurrence does not signify malignant alteration; a fibromyoma may recur if incompletely excised, even when the original specimen had no histologic evidence of malignancy. Although a sarcoma rarely arises in the vulva, histologic studies must be carefully made because degenerating atypical multinucleated cells of a benign or reactive tissue can be mistakenly diagnosed as malignant.

As in any vulvar surgery, hemostasis is important because compression is difficult to obtain in these soft tissues. Extravasation of blood can dissect the fascial planes well out to the vulva, thigh, flanks, and abdominal wall. Closed suction drains should be used in the wounds if hemostasis is not complete.

Condyloma Acuminatum

Condyloma acuminatum is one morphologic manifestation of HPV infection in the lower genital tract. These polypoid lesions have an incubation period ranging from several weeks to 8 months; however, clinical infection usually is apparent 6 to 8 weeks after exposure. Transmission of the virus is attributed to coitus, and the process is efficient, because most sexual partners are affected subclinically if not clinically. The disease process continues increasing in prevalence. Interestingly, clinically apparent condyloma constitute only a fraction of HPV infections. Most are undetected in asymptomatic patients with no clinical findings.

Numerous HPV subtypes have been identified. HPV subtypes 6, 11, 16, 18, 31, 33, 35, 39, 45, 51, 52, 56, 58, 59, 68, and 69 account for most genital tract infections. Careful histopathologic and virologic study of vulvar lesions has demonstrated an association of HPV 6 and HPV 11 with approximately 90% of exophytic vulvar condylomata, as well as flat cervical condylomas and some low-grade cervical dysplasias. The quadrivalent vaccine provides protection against HPV subtypes 6, 11, 16, and 18. It is not effective for the treatment of already existing condyloma or HPV infections. This vaccine is further discussed in Chapter 46.

Condylomata acuminata that manifest on the vulva are frequently associated with cervical, vaginal, and anal HPV infection. Careful clinical evaluation mandates vaginal/cervical cytology and colposcopy in patients who present with vulvar warts. This is appropriate not only to exclude cervical and vaginal dysplasia but also to define the extent of condylomatous involvement and permit appropriate tailoring of regional therapy.

Condylomata acuminata are small and usually multifocal lesions. They may be accompanied by pruritic discomfort or irritation. Warts initially may be reddish brown because of parakeratosis; however, with time and exposure to local trauma, they become gray or white. The latter appears to be associated with hyperkeratosis and the generalized keratin disturbance associated with viral infection (Fig. 23.20). Unless they are traumatized, bleeding is not a typical feature. In pregnancy, however, because of marked vascular alterations,

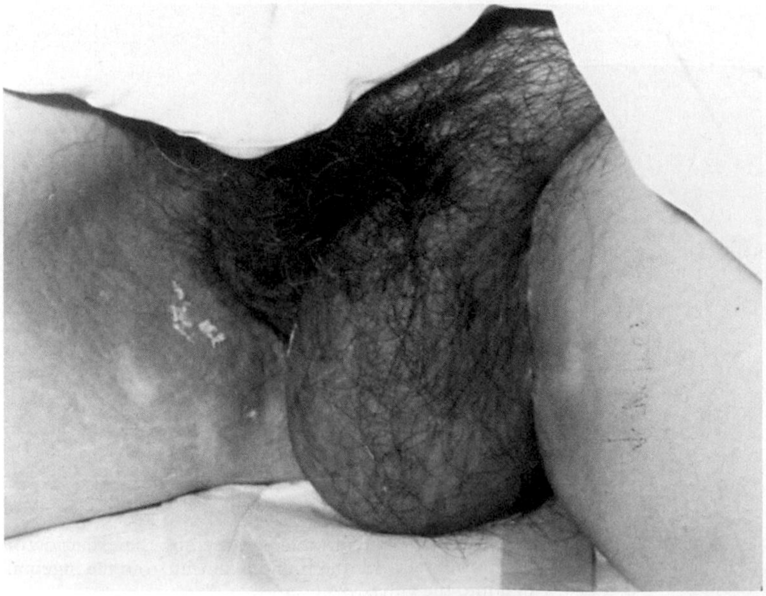

FIGURE 23.19. Fibroadenoma of the vulva arising from the embryonic breast tissue, the caudal end of the milk line.

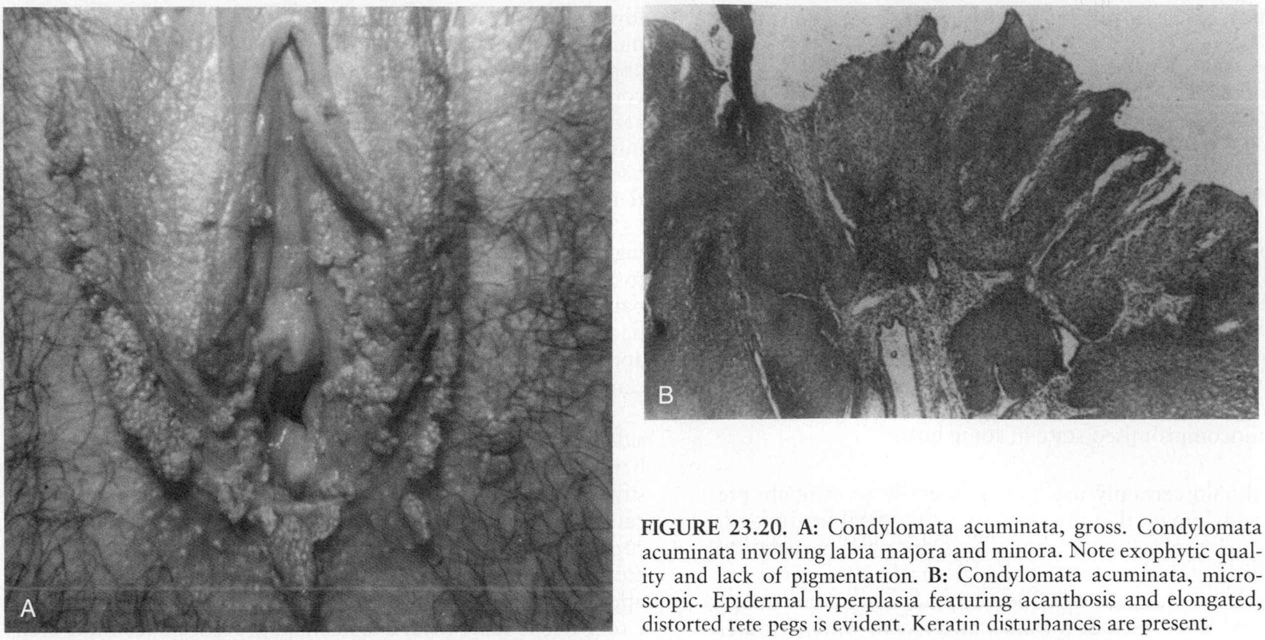

FIGURE 23.20. **A:** Condylomata acuminata, gross. Condylomata acuminata involving labia majora and minora. Note exophytic quality and lack of pigmentation. **B:** Condylomata acuminata, microscopic. Epidermal hyperplasia featuring acanthosis and elongated, distorted rete pegs is evident. Keratin disturbances are present.

condyloma of the vagina and perineum can be a source of abundant bleeding if laceration occurs. Massive vulvar and perianal condylomata may occur in certain circumstances, preventing identification of the introitus and anal orifice; conditions that foster this growth potential include immunosuppression and, less frequently, pregnancy (Fig. 23.21). Those lesions that were previously called *giant condyloma* are now regarded as *verrucous carcinoma*. In the spectrum of condylomatous growths, the dividing line between condyloma and verrucous carcinoma is indistinct because of the structural benignancy of both.

Various treatment approaches are available and are characterized by their inability to eliminate the offending agent: the virus. Interferon offers a nonspecific antiviral therapy. Flulike effects should be anticipated for at least several weeks. Efficacy has been demonstrated with this technique, although treatment is cumbersome, can be costly, and remains investigational. Its primary role has not been defined.

Topical Therapy

At the present time, only a variety of ablative approaches are available for management of condyloma. These should be individualized with consideration of prior treatment, volume and location of disease, the presence or absence of associated dysplasia, and other idiosyncratic patient factors. The most common approach to vulvar condylomata is the local application of 25% podophyllum resin, often prepared in benzoin. This method, although reasonably well tolerated in the office setting, often requires numerous applications. Burning discomfort ensues after sustained contact, which is necessary for efficacy. Most recommend that the agent be left in place for 6 hours before tub baths, so compliance may be problematic. Podophyllum appears to be more effective on exophytic, rather than flat, condylomata. Use is restricted to the vulva in nonpregnant patients; vaginal application may lead to undesirable absorption and neurotoxicity. An alternative is halogenated acetic acid, either bichloracetic or trichloroacetic (TCA). Our preference is 90% TCA. This agent quickly interacts with cellular proteins, inducing a coagulative effect, and rapidly turns lesions a brilliant white. Advantages include its ability to sustain a prompt chemical effect on the condyloma, its availability for intravaginal use and use during pregnancy, and the fact that is can be rapidly neutralized with sodium bicarbonate,

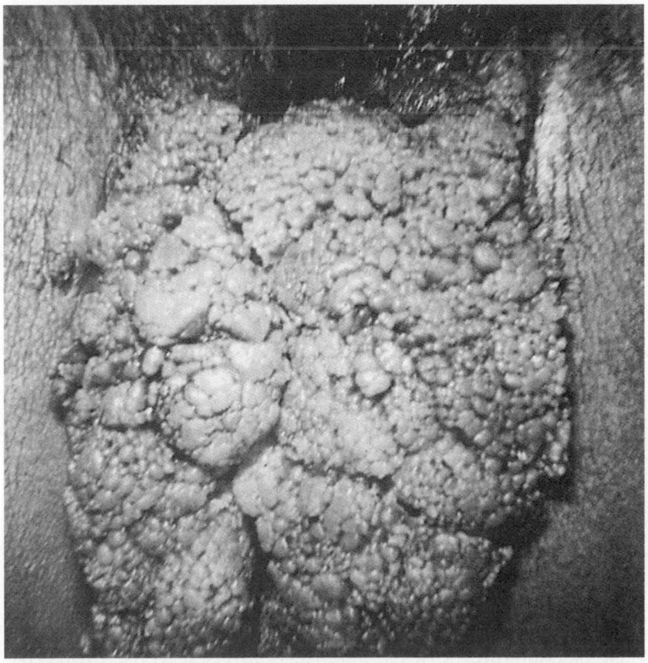

FIGURE 23.21. Massive condylomata acuminata now considered as verrucous carcinoma. Note abundant exophytic lesions producing confluent, cauliflowerlike growth. Lesion is present on perineum and totally obscures anal orifice. Patient is 23 years old and is maintained on prednisone because of neurosarcoidosis.

which may be dissolved in water and applied as a cooling paste.

Excision or Ablation

Surgical excision, electrosurgical, destruction, and laser ablation are reserved for certain patients.

Criteria for selection may include the following:

- Extensive volume of condylomata exceeding what may be resolved with chemical agents
- Multicentric HPV infections, particularly with involvement of the vagina, urethra, or anus
- Failure of concerted office therapy with topical chemical agents
- Additional presence of significant intraepithelial neoplasia
- Immunocompromised state in some hosts

One should certainly use biopsy liberally to evaluate presumed condylomata that are refractory to topical treatment or that have an atypical appearance. This helps prevent sustained, ineffective chemical treatment of high-grade VIN, often presenting as a flat and pigmented verrucous lesion in the younger patient, and helps exclude a frank cancer with warty features. Large, sessile condylomata or those that grow rapidly, bleed abnormally, or become necrotic or invasive should arouse the suspicion of malignancy.

Cryotherapy has been used on the vulva to eradicate warts. The freezing induces localized tissue necrosis. Although healing usually is satisfactory, and numbing effects induce analgesia, application is limited by delivery systems and probe-tip sizes. Larger condylomatous masses are more difficult to treat, as are vaginal lesions. Depth of apparent tissue destruction can be difficult to assess.

Electrocautery with a loop has been used effectively, particularly with massive lesions. Analgesic needs are definitely a factor in this approach. Smaller lesions may be fulgurated. Buildup of charred tissue can be removed by abrasion to identify residual warty tissue. The precision and depth of tissue injury can be problematic.

Colposcopically directed laser ablation performed by trained personnel in appropriately selected cases may afford effective treatment. Condylomatous lesions may be vaporized; starting at the center of the lesion causes the wart to collapse inward toward the beam. The level of the adjacent normal skin should be selected as a landmark. In treating condylomata, there is no need for deep laser vaporization into the dermis, exceeding the so-called first laser surgical plane. Issues of appropriate power density may be debated; however, the inexperienced laser surgeon should use lower-power densities (larger spot size or lower laser output) to protect against unnecessarily deep laser injury. In experienced hands, higher laser output may be feasible, which speeds the procedure. Power densities of 500 to 800 W/cm^2 normally are used for vaporization. Lower power densities are associated with undesirable thermal injury to adjacent tissues. Sites of laser vaporization should be wiped with moistened gauze sponges to remove carbon and thermally coagulated tissue and to permit accurate assessment of depth and remaining disease. Large lesions can be dealt with by laser excision followed by vaporization at the base (see Chapter 15). Clinicians are advised to use protective eyewear during vaporization to prevent possible conjunctival condyloma.

Brush laser vaporization of the normal epithelium surrounding warty lesions is commonly done to destroy subclinical HPV and reduce the risk of clinical recurrence. This technique uses lower power densities (200 to 300 W/cm^2) to superficially denude 1 to 2 cm of adjacent epidermis. The rationale for this approach is the presence of HPV in tissue proximal to the condyloma, as demonstrated by Ferenczy and colleagues. Brush vaporization and laser treatment of so-called subclinical HPV infection that may be appreciated with the colposcope have been proposed to lessen the viral reservoir and reduce recurrence rates.

Even with vaporization of grossly normal tissue surrounding the visible lesions, recurrences must be anticipated in 25% to 50% of patients with extensive disease treated with the laser, particularly if the patient is immunocompromised. These patients require further treatment with either laser or chemical approaches, such as 5-FU topically. If disease is minimal, they can be observed.

Patients subjected to extensive laser treatment require considerable local care while healing proceeds. Cool tub or sitz baths with Burow's solution followed by the application of silver sulfadiazine (Silvadene) cream and 5% lidocaine (Xylocaine) ointment often afford relief and protect against bacterial superinfection. Narcotics for pain management are appropriate short-term drugs. Prophylactic systemic antibiotics do not appear to be indicated. Weekly office follow-up is advised for 2 to 3 weeks to assess tissue healing, prevent undesirable areas of tissue agglutination, and allow potential early identification of recurrences, which can be managed with chemical ablation. Patients should be followed up carefully for several months after treatment to monitor for recurrences.

The Cavitron Ultrasonic Surgical Aspirator (CUSA) has also been efficacious in treating condyloma. Tissue cell damage is 25 to 30 mm, which is similar to that caused by a cold scalpel. This contrasts with electrocautery at 75 to 100 mm. The tip vibrates at 23,000 cycles per second. Tissue is fragmented and aspirated, providing a specimen for histologic evaluation. Regardless of the selected approach to therapy, all patients should be advised to have their consorts examined to lessen the risk of reexposure to lesions with a large viral burden. This theoretically helps diminish treatment failures. Patients with HIV or other types of immunosuppression need to be more closely followed up.

Hidradenoma (Sweat Gland Tumor) of the Vulva

A rare benign tumor of the vulva, hidradenoma, was first described by Schickele in 1902. The tumor is characterized by its intricate papillary adenomatous pattern, which may be readily mistaken for cancer.

Clinically, a hidradenoma is small, rarely more than 1 cm in diameter (Fig. 23.22A). Its consistency can range from firm to as soft as a sebaceous cyst, with which it is often confused. Most of these lesions are found in the interlabial folds, in the labia majora, or in the perineum. Because these tumors are apocrine in origin, the labia minora location is unusual. The occasional occurrence of reddish brown pulpy material on the surface results when the tumor is evulsed through the duct of the sweat gland.

These lesions have been carefully studied in numerous laboratories, and the complex microscopic patterns have been repeatedly stressed (Fig. 23.22B). The superficial papillary adenomatous pattern appears aggressive, but careful inspection shows that the glandular structures are lined by a single layer of well-organized cuboidal cells. In some parts of the tumor, the pink-staining secretory elements can be identified superficial to

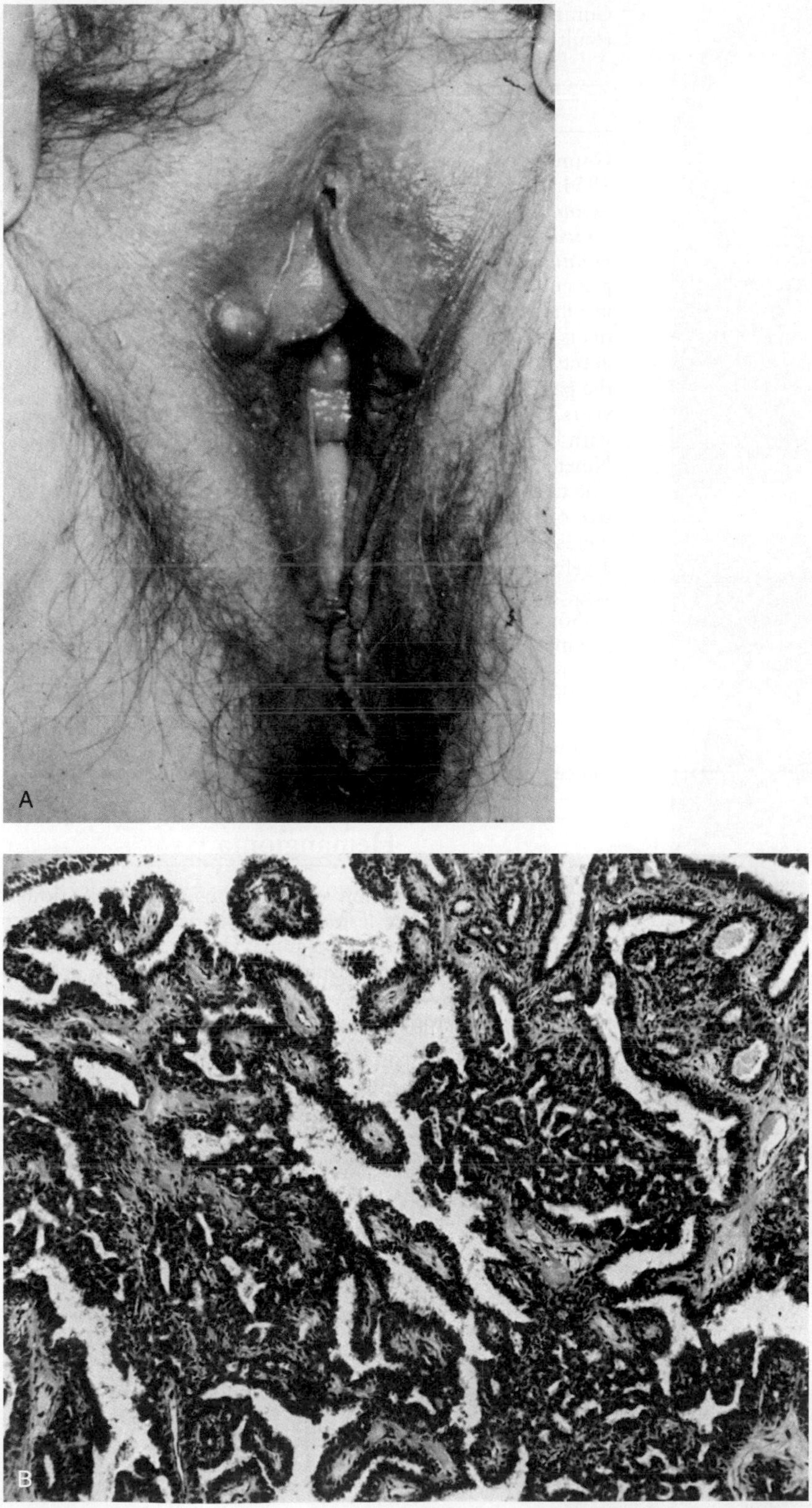

FIGURE 23.22. **A:** Hidradenoma of the vulva. **B:** Low-power magnification section of hidradenoma of the vulva. (**A:** From Novak E, Woodruff JD. *Obstetric and gynecologic pathology.* 7th ed. Philadelphia: WB Saunders; 1974.)

the basal layer. Beneath the epithelium is an indefinite layer of flattened myoepithelial cells. When the clear cell variant of the myoepithelium proliferates, an ominous picture is created, yet this clear cell hidradenoma also behaves in a benign manner. Although hidradenocarcinoma occasionally does occur, a finding of distinct adenocarcinoma in the vulva should initiate a search to rule out a metastatic lesion from another primary site.

Hidradenomas are classically asymptomatic, and most lesions are discovered during a routine pelvic examination.

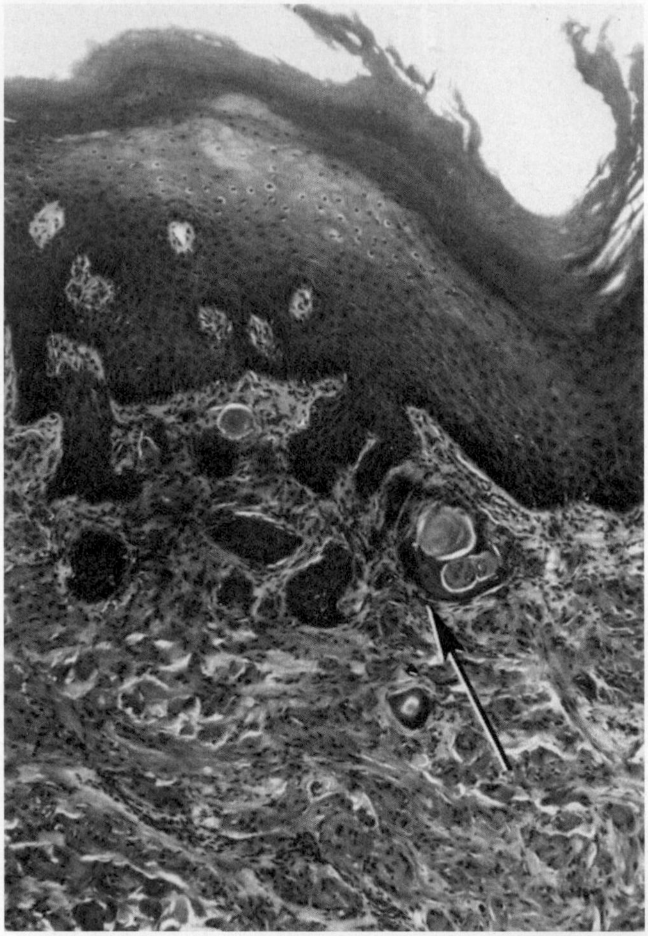

FIGURE 23.23. Granular cell tumor. Note the pseudoepitheliomatous hyperplasia, nests of large, pale "granular cells" beneath the epithelium.

Curative treatment consists of local excision; recurrences result only from incomplete excision.

Granular Cell Tumors

Granular cell tumors (GCTs) were first described by Weber in 1854. It wasn't until 1926 that Abrikossoff coined the term *myoblastoma*. Later, the tumor was termed *granular cell schwannoma*. The current nomenclature recognizes the term *granular cell tumor*. Although frequently benign, GCTs can present as a malignant form that is multicentric and metastatic in vital organs. Horowitz and associates reported on 20 patients presenting with GCTs of the vulva over a 31-year period at the Emory University Teaching Hospitals. Seventy percent of the patients were African American, and the mean age was 50 years. Ninety percent of the lesions were on the labia majora, with lesion size ranging from 0.4 × 0.4 cm to 7 × 8 × 12 cm. Nineteen of 20 patients were treated with a wide local excision. The twentieth patient required radical excision because of the size of the lesion. This patient eventually died of pulmonary metastasis. Only two patients presented with multiple lesions. Twelve lesions were stained for S-100. All were positive, which suggests a neural Schwann cell origin.

Sometimes the overlying pseudoepitheliomatous changes are misinterpreted as invasive cancer (Fig. 23.23). Identification is possible with recognition of the granular cells dispersed within the underlying stroma or within the tumor. In a few patients, GCT has behaved in a malignant fashion, but an appearance of a second lesion at a site outside the vulva usually indicates multiple primary lesions rather than metastasis.

Hemangioma

Hemangiomas are common vulvar lesions that usually do not require treatment. The lesions normally are small, are often multiple, and may bleed with trauma. On occasion, keratinization causes the superficial surface to appear white or gray-white (angiokeratoma). Hemangiomas should be differentiated from small varicosities, which commonly are seen in the postmenopausal patient.

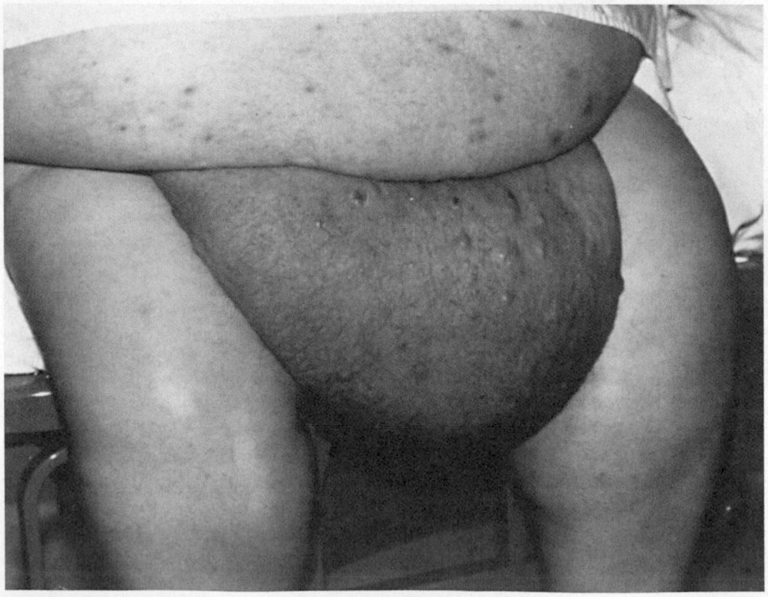

FIGURE 23.24. A benign angiolipoma noted for its massive size.

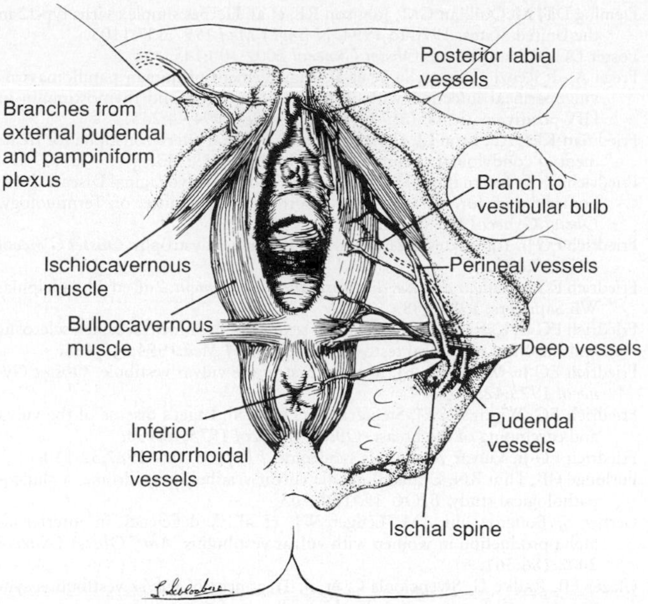

FIGURE 23.25. Vascular supply of the vulva.

An accurate diagnosis is imperative because a malignant melanoma can be misinterpreted as a hemangioma. The abrupt appearance of any pigmented lesion demands biopsy. In 2 of 11 melanomas seen in our clinic, the lesions were diagnosed as hematoma or angioma, and a correct diagnosis was provided only by histologic study. Angiokeratoma, a benign tumor, is a distinct clinicopathologic entity. Aggressive angiomyxoma, although structurally benign, is known for its large size and local recurrences. Some tumors, although benign, can be massive in size and thereby pose operative problems (Fig. 23.24).

The best treatment for congenital hemangioma is careful observation. The lesions regress spontaneously in almost all cases, and attempts at excision may be mutilating. If bleeding is a problem, the troublesome vascular channels can be treated by surgical ligation or embolization.

Varicocele and Varices

Varices are common on the vulva, and the larger lesions are almost routinely unilateral. As with most varicosities, treatment depends on size and symptoms. Whereas varicoceles in the scrotum arise from dilatation of the veins in the pampiniform plexus of the inguinal canal, the lesions on the vulva arise from the pudendal veins (Fig. 23.25). Careful evaluation usually demonstrates more extensive involvement of the tributaries of the hypogastric vein with varicosities of the gluteal vessels over the buttock.

If the patient experiences discomfort from the engorgement that follows exercise or standing for long periods, ligation is indicated with excision of the segment of vulvar skin that contains the varices. Knowledge of the intricate vascular system that supplies the external genitalia is necessary to ensure that surgery will result in long-term success and will prevent recurrences. Horowitz has treated several patients using selective embolization with success.

BEST SURGICAL PRACTICES

- Vulvar diseases are multiple and may be difficult to diagnose. Many inflammatory conditions clinically resemble cancer.
- Bartholin gland abscesses are usually treated with antibiotics and insertion of a Word catheter. Marsupialization or excision is rarely used today. The possibility of cancer of Bartholin gland should be considered in the postmenopausal women with a new mass involving Bartholin gland.
- Vulvodynia can be caused by infectious, inflammatory, neurologic, or neoplastic conditions of the vulva. When no underlying cause of vulvar pain can be demonstrated, oral amitriptyline and gabapentin as well as topical steroid creams should be tried. Local injection with triamcinolone and bupivacaine can also be used. If vulvar vestibulodynia is diagnosed, an extended perineoplasty has been effective in many patients.
- Vulvar condyloma are caused by some types of HPV (90% are due to type 6 and 11). These lesions may be self-limiting and resolve spontaneously. They do not undergo malignant transformation. If numerous, large, or symptomatic, they can be successfully treated with topical podophyllin, podofilox, or trichloroacetic acid. These lesions may also be destroyed or removed with electrosurgical desiccation, CUSA, CO_2 laser, or simple excision. These lesions may be difficult or impossible to eradicate in immunocompromised patients.
- VIN should be diagnosed by biopsy. It may be caused by certain types of HPV, especially in younger women. If untreated, it may progress to invasive cancer. It can be treated by laser ablation, but surgical excision is usually recommended. A variety of techniques have been used, depending on the size and location of the lesion or lesions.

ACKNOWLEDGMENTS

The authors want to recognize the late Dr. J. Donald Woodruff, who has been a coauthor of this chapter for several editions and who has served as a mentor to the current authors.

Bibliography

Abramov Y, Elchalal U, Abramov D, et al. Surgical treatment of vulvar lichen sclerosus: a review. CME review article. *Obstet Gynecol* 1996;51:3.

Abrikossoff AI. Über myome, ausgehend von der guer gestreiften willkürlichen muskulatur. Virchows Archiv für pathologische Anatomie and Physiologie und für Klinische Medizin, 1926;260:215–223.

Adelson MD. Ultrasonic surgical aspiration in the treatment of vulvar disease [Letter, Comment]. *Obstet Gynecol* 1991;78(3 Pt 1):477.

Aranda FI, Laforga JB. Nodular fasciitis of the vulva: report of a case with immunohistochemical study. *Pathol Res Pract* 1998;194:805.

Ault KA, Giuliano AR, Edwards RP, et al. A phase I study to evaluate a human papillomavirus (HPV) type 18 L1 VLP vaccine. *Vaccine* 2004;22:3004.

Bachmann GA, Raymond R, Arnold LD, et al. Chronic vulvar and other gynecologic pain: prevalence and characteristics in a self-reported survey. *J Reprod Med* 2006;1:3.

Baggish MS, Miklos JR. Vulva pain syndrome: a review. *Obstet Gynecol Surv* 1995;50:618.

Baggish MS, Sze EH, Adelson MD, et al. Quantitative evaluation of the skin and accessory appendages in vulvar carcinoma in situ. *Obstet Gynecol* 1989;74:169.

Barbero M, Micheletti L, Preti M, et al. Biologic behavior of vulvar intraepithelial neoplasia: source, logic and clinical parameters. *J Reprod Med* 1993;38:108.

Beisky A. Über Kraurosis Vulvae. Z *Heik* (Prague) 1885;6:69.

Bloss JD. The use of electrosurgical techniques in the management of premalignant diseases of the vulva, vagina, and cervix: an excisional rather than an ablative approach. *Am J Obstet Gynecol* 1993;169:1081.

Bronstein J, Abramovici H. Combination of subtotal perineoplasty and interferon for the treatment of vulvar vestibulitis. *Gynecol Obstet Invest* 1997;44:53.

Bronstein J, Heifetz S, Kellner Y, et al. Clobetasol dipropionate 0.05% versus testosterone propionate 2% topical application for severe vulvar lichen sclerosus. *Am J Obstet Gynecol* 1998;178:80.

Bornstein J, Kaufman RH. Combination of surgical excision and carbon dioxide laser vaporization for multifocal vulvar intraepithelial neoplasia. *Am J Obstet Gynecol* 1988;158:459.

Bornstein J, Lahat N, Sharon A, et al. Telomerase activity in HPV-associated vulvar vestibulitis. *J Reprod Med* 2000;45(8):643.

Bornstein J, Pascal B, Abramovici H. Intramuscular beta-interferon treatment for severe vulvar vestibulitis. *J Reprod Med* 1993;38:117.

Bornstein J, Sova Y, Atad J, et al. Development of vaginal adenosis following combined 5-fluorouracil and carbon dioxide laser treatments for diffuse vaginal condylomatosis. *Obstet Gynecol* 1993;81:896.

Bornstein J, Zarfati D, Fruchter O, et al. A repetitive DNA sequence that characterizes human papillomavirus integration site into the human genome is present in vulvar vestibulitis. *Eur J Obstet Gynaecol Reprod Biol* 2000;89:173.

Bouchard S, Yazbech S, Lallier M. Perineal hemangioma, anorectal malformation, and genital anomaly: a new association? *J Pediatr Surg* 1999;34:1133.

Bowen JD. Precancerous dermatoses. *J Cutan Dis* 1912;30:241.

Breech LL, Laufer MR. Surgicel in the management of labial and clitoral hood adhesions in adolescents with lichen sclerosus. *J Pediatr Adolesc Gynecol* 2000;13:21.

Bresci G, Parisi G, Banti S. Long term therapy with 5-aminosalicylic acid in Crohn's disease: is it useful? Our four years' experience. *Int J Clin Pharmacol Res* 1994;14:133.

Brook I, Frazier EH. Clinical and microbiological features of necrotizing fasciitis. *J Clin Microbiol* 1995;33:2382.

Brown JV III, Goldstein BH, Rettenmaier MA, et al. Laser ablation of surgical margins after excisional partial vulvectomy for VIN: effect on recurrence. *J Reprod Med* 2005;50:345.

Buscema J, Naghashfar Z, Sawada E, et al. The predominance of human papillomavirus type 16 in vulvar neoplasia. *Obstet Gynecol* 1988;71:601.

Buscema J, Stern J, Woodruff JD. The significance of histologic alterations adjacent to invasive vulvar carcinoma. *Am J Obstet Gynecol* 1980;137:902.

Buscema J, Woodruff JD, Parmley TH, et al. Carcinoma in situ of the vulva. *Obstet Gynecol* 1980;55:225.

Calvillo O, Skaribas IM, Rockett C. Computed tomography-guided pudendal nerve block: a new diagnostic approach to long-term anoperineal pain: a report of two cases. *Reg Anesth Pain Med* 2000;25:420.

Centers for Disease Control and Prevention. National Disease and Therapeutic Index (IMS American Ltd.). Available at www.cdc.gov.

Collins CG, Hansen LH, Theriot EA. Clinical stain for use in selecting biopsy sites in patients with vulvar disease. *Obstet Gynecol* 1966;28:158.

Coppelson M. Colposcopic features of papillomaviral infection and premalignancy in the female lower genital tract. *Dermatol Clin* 1991;9:251.

Crum CP, McLachlin CM, Tate JE, et al. Pathobiology of vulvar squamous neoplasia. *Curr Opin Obstet Gynecol* 1997;9:63.

Dalziel KL, Millard R, Wojnarowska F. The treatment of vulval lichen-sclerosus with a very potent topical steroid (clobetasol propionate 0.05%) cream. *Br J Dermatol* 1991;124:461.

Davis BL, Robinson DG. Diverticula of the female urethra: assay of 120 cases. *J Urol* 1970;104:850.

DeSimone CP, Crisp MP, Ueland FR. Concordance of gross surgical and final fixed margins in vulvar intraepithelial neoplasia 3 and vulvar cancer. *J Reprod Med* 2006;6:1285.

DiBonito L, Falconieri G, Bonifacio-Gori D. Multicentric papillomavirus infection of the female genital tract: a study of morphologic pattern, possible risk and viral prevalence. *Pathol Res Pract* 1993;189:1023.

DiPaola GR, Gomez-Rueda N, Arrighi L. Relevance of microinvasion in carcinoma of the vulva. *Obstet Gynecol* 1975;45:647.

Edwards L. New concepts in vulvodynia. *Am J Obstet Gynecol* 2003;189(Suppl):S24.

Ersan Y, Ozgultelxin R, Cetinkale O, et al. Fournier-gangran. *Langenbecks Arch Chir* 1995;380:139.

Farley DE, Katz VL, Dotters DT. Toxic shock syndrome associated with vulvar necrotizing fasciitis. *Obstet Gynecol* 1993;82:4:660.

Feagan BG, Rochon J, Fedorak RN, et al. Methotrexate for the treatment of Crohn's disease: the North American Crohn's Study Group Investigators. *N Engl J Med* 1995;332:292.

Feller ER, Ribaudo S, Jackson ND. Gynecologic aspects of Crohn's disease. *Am Fam Physician* 2001;64:1725.

Ferenczy A, Mitao M, Nagai N, et al. Latent papillomavirus and recurring genital warts. *N Engl J Med* 1985;313:784.

Fischer GO. The commonest causes of symptomatic vulvar disease: a dermatologist's perspectives. *Australas J Dermatol* 1996;1:12.

Fisher JR, Conway MJ, Takeshita RT, et al. Necrotizing fasciitis: importance of roentgenographic studies for soft-tissue gas. *JAMA* 1979;241:803.

Fleming DT, McQuillian GM, Johnson RE, et al. Herpes simplex virus type 2 in the United States, 1976 to 1994. *N Engl J Med* 1997;337:1105.

Foster DC. Vulvar disease. *Obstet Gynecol* 2002;100:145.

Frega A, di Renzi F, Stentella P, et al. Management of human papillomavirus vulvoperineal infection with systemic *b*-interferon and thymostimulin in HIV-positive patients. *Int J Gynaecol Obstet* 1994;44:255.

Friedman-Kien AE, Eron LJ, Conaut M, et al. Natural interferon alpha for treatment of condylomata acuminata. *JAMA* 1988;259:533.

Friedrich EG Jr. International Society for the Study of Vulvovaginal Disease. New nomenclature for vulvar disease: report of the Committee on Terminology. *Obstet Gynecol* 1976;47:122.

Friedrich EG Jr. Topical testosterone for benign vulvar dystrophy. *Obstet Gynecol* 1971;37:677.

Friedrich EG Jr. *Vulvar disease: diagnosis and management*. 2nd ed. Philadelphia: WB Saunders; 1983:488.

Friedrich EG Jr, Kalra PS. Serum levels of sex hormones in vulvar lichen sclerosus and the effect of topical testosterone. *N Engl J Med* 1984;310:488.

Friedrich EG Jr, Wilkinson EJ. Mucous cyst of the vulvar vestibule. *Obstet Gynecol* 1973;42:407.

Friedrich EG, Wilkinson EJ, Steingraeber PH, et al. Paget's disease of the vulva and carcinoma of the breast. *Obstet Gynecol* 1975;46:130.

Friedrich EG Jr. Vulvar vestibulitis syndrome. *J Reprod Med* 1987;32:110.

Furlonge CB, Thin RN, Evans BE, et al. Vulvar vestibulitis syndrome: a clinicopathological study. *BJOG* 1991;98:703.

Gerber S, Bongiovanni AM, Ledger WJ, et al. A deficiency in interferon-alpha production in women with vulvar vestibulitis. *Am J Obstet Gynecol* 2002;186:361.

Glazer HI, Radke G, Swencionis C, et al. Treatment of vulvar vestibulitis syndrome with electromyographic biofeedback of pelvic floor musculature. *J Reprod Med* 1995;40:283.

Goldman HB, Idom CB, Dmochowski RR. Traumatic injuries of the female external genitalia and their association with urological injuries. *J Urol* 1998;159:956.

Haefner HK. Critique of new gynecologic surgical procedures: surgery for vulvar vestibulitis. *Clin Obstet Gynecol* 2000;43:689.

Haefner HK, Collins ME, Davis GD, et al. The vulvodynia guideline. *J Low Genit Tract Dis* 2005;9:40.

Haefner HK, Tate JE, McLachlin CM, et al. Vulvar intraepithelial neoplasia: age, morphological phenotype, papillomavirus DNA, and coexisting invasive carcinoma. *Hum Pathol* 1995;26:147.

Haley JC, Mirowski GW, Hood AF. Benign vulvar tumors. *Semin Cutan Med Surg* 1998;17:196.

Harrison BJ, Mudge M, Hughes LE. Recurrence after surgical treatment of hidradenitis suppurativa. *BMJ* 1987;294:487.

Hatch K. Colposcopy of vaginal and vulvar human papillomavirus and adjacent sites. *Obstet Gynecol Clin North Am* 1993;20:203.

Hatch KD. Vulvovaginal human papillomavirus infections: clinical implications and management. *Am J Obstet Gynecol* 1991;165:1183.

Herzog TJ, Rader JS. The Ultrasonic Surgical Aspirator in the gynecologic oncology patient. *Adv Obstet Gynecol* 1994;1:325.

Hoffman MS, Pinelli DM, Finan M, et al. Laser vaporization for vulvar intraepithelial neoplasia III. *J Reprod Med* 1992;37:135.

Hoffman MS, Roberts WS, LaPolla JP, et al. Laser vaporization of grade 3 vaginal intraepithelial neoplasia. *Am J Obstet Gynecol* 1991;165:1342.

Horowitz BJ. Interferon therapy for condylomatous vulvitis. *Obstet Gynecol* 1989;73:446.

Horowitz IR, Copas P, Majmudar B. Granular cell tumors of the vulva. *Am J Obstet Gynecol* 1995;173:1710.

Horowitz IR, Gomella LG, eds. *Obstetrics and gynecology on call*. 1st ed. East Norwalk, CT: Appleton & Lange; 1992:167.

International Society for the Study of Vulvar Disease, Committee on Terminology. New nomenclature for vulvar disease. *Obstet Gynecol* 1989;160:769.

Japaze H, Dinh T, Woodruff JD. Verrucous carcinoma of the vulva: study of 24 cases. *Obstet Gynecol* 1982;60:462.

Jeffcoate TNA. Chronic vulvar dystrophies. *Am J Obstet Gynecol* 1966;95:61.

Jeffries DJ. Acyclovir update. *BMJ* 1986;293:1523.

Jones RW, Rowan DM, Stewart AW. Vulvar intraepithelial neoplasia: aspects of the natural history and outcome of 405 women. *Obstet Gynecol* 2005;106:1319.

Julian CG, Callison J, Woodruff JD. Plastic management of extensive vulvar defects. *Obstet Gynecol* 1971;38:193.

Kehoe S, Luesley D. Pathology and management of vulval pain and pruritus. *Curr Opin Obstet Gynecol* 1995;1:16.

Kent HL, Wisniewski PM. Interferon for vulvar vestibulitis. *J Reprod Med* 1990;35:1138.

Kizer JR, Bellah RD, Schnaufer L, et al. Meconium hydrocele in a female newborn: an unusual case of a labial mass. *J Urol* 1995;153:188.

Kornbluth A, Marion JF, Solomon P, et al. How effective is current medical therapy for severe ulcerative and Crohn's colitis? An analytic review of selected trials. *J Clin Gastroenterol* 1995;20:280.

Koutsky LA, Ault KA, Wheeler CM. A controlled trial of a human papillomavirus type 16 vaccine. *N Engl J Med* 2002;347:1645.

Larsen J, Peters K, Petersen CS, et al. Interferon alpha-2*b* treatment of symptomatic chronic vulvodynia associated with koilocytosis. *Acta Derm Venereol* 1993;73:385.

Le T, Hicks W, Menard C, et al. Preliminary results of 5% imiquimod cream in the primary treatment of vulva intraepithelial neoplasia grade 2/3. *Am J Obstet Gynecol* 2006;194:377.

Lijnen RL, Blindeman LA. VIN III (bowenoid type) and HPV infection. *Br J Dermatol* 1994;131:728.

Lorenz B, Kaufman RH, Kutzner S. Lichen sclerosus–therapy with clobetasol propionate. *J Reprod Med* 1998;43:790.

Majmudar B. Tumors of the vulva, Section 15. In: *Conn's current therapy 2000*. Philadelphia: WB Saunders, 2000.

Majmudar B, Castellano PZ, Wilson RW, et al. Granular cell tumors of the vulva. *J Reprod Med* 1990;35:1008.

Mann MS, Kaufman RH, Brown D Jr, et al. Vulvar vestibulitis: significant clinical variables and treatment outcome. *Obstet Gynecol* 1992;79:122.

Mao C, Koutsky LA, Ault KA, et al. Efficacy of human papillomavirus-16 vaccine to prevent cervical intraepithelial neoplasia: a randomized controlled trial. *Obstet Gynecol* 2006;107(1):18.

Marinoff SC, Turner ML. Vulvar vestibulitis syndrome: an overview. *Am J Obstet Gynecol* 1991;165:2:1228.

Marinoff SC, Turner ML, Hirsch RP, et al. Intralesional alpha interferon: cost-effective therapy for vulvar vestibulitis syndrome. *J Reprod Med* 1993;38:19.

Massad LS. Applying the new ISSVD terminology on precursors of vulvar squamous cell carcinoma to management. *J Low Genit Tract Dis* 2006;10:135.

Matthews D. Marsupialization in the treatment of Bartholin's cyst and abscesses. *Obstet Gynaecol Br Commonw* 1966;73:1010.

McKay M. Dysesthetic (essential) vulvodynia treatment with amitriptyline. *J Reprod Med* 1993;38:9.

McKay M. Subsets of vulvodynia. *J Reprod Med* 1988;3308:695.

McKay M. Vulvodynia: diagnostic patterns. *Dermatol Clin* 1992;10:423.

McKay M, Frankman O, Horowitz BJ, et al. Vulvar vestibulitis and vestibular papillomatosis: report of the ISSVD Committee on Vulvodynia. *J Reprod Med* 1991;36:413.

Mering JH. A surgical approach to intractable pruritus vulvae. *Am J Obstet Gynecol* 1952;64:619.

Modesitt SC, Waters AB, Walton L, et al. Vulvar intraepithelial neoplasia III: occult cancer and the impact of margin status on recurrence. *Obstet Gynecol* 1998;92(6):962.

Morin C, Bouchard C, Brisson J, et al. Human papilloma-viruses and vulvar vestibulitis. *Obstet Gynecol* 2000;95(5):683.

Moscicki A, Palefsky JM, Gonzales J, et al. Colposcopic and histologic findings and human papillomavirus (HPV) DNA test variability in young women positive for HPV DNA. *J Infect Dis* 1992;166:951.

Moyal-Barracco M, Lynch P. 2003 ISSVD terminology and classification of vulvodynia. *J Reprod Med* 2004;49:772.

Murina F, Tassan P, Roberti P, et al. Treatment of vulvar vestibulitis with submucous infiltrations of methylprednisolone and lidocaine: an alternative approach. *J Reprod Med* 2001;46:713.

Novak ER, Woodruff JD. *Gynecologic and obstetric pathology*. 8th ed. Philadelphia: WB Saunders; 1979.

O'Connell JX, Young RH, Nielsen GP, et al. Nodular fasciitis of the vulva: a study of six cases and literature review. *Int J Gynecol Pathol* 1997;16:117.

O'Farrell N. Donovanosis. In: Holmes KK, Sparling PF, Mardh P-A, et al. (eds). *Sexually transmitted diseases*. New York: McGraw-Hill; 1999:525.

Paavonen J. Vulvodynia: a complex syndrome of vulvar pain. *Acta Obstet Gynecol Scand* 1995;74:2343.

Parks JS, Jones RW, McLean MR, et al. Possible etiologic heterogeneity of vulvar intraepithelial neoplasia: a correlation of pathologic characteristics with human papillomavirus detection by in situ hybridization and polymerase chain reaction. *Cancer* 1991;67:1599.

Patsner B. Treatment of vaginal dysplasia with loop excision: report of five cases. *Am J Obstet Gynecol* 1993;169:179.

Pincus SH. Vulvar dermatoses and pruritus vulvae. *Dermatol Clin* 1992;10:297.

Price LM, Mendolsohn SS, Youngs GR, et al. Unilateral vulvar hypertrophy and Crohn's disease. *Int J STD AIDS* 1995;6:146.

Rader JS, Leake JF, Dillon MB, et al. Ultrasonic surgical aspiration in the treatment of vulvar disease. *Obstet Gynecol* 1991;77:573.

Raley JC, Followwill KA, Zimet GD, et al. Gynecologists' attitudes regarding human papilloma virus vaccination: a survey of Fellows of American College of Obstetricians and Gynecologists. *Infect Dis Obstet Gynecol* 2004;12(3–4):127.

Reed BD, Caron AM, Gorenflo DW, et al. Treatment of vulvodynia with tricyclic antidepressants: efficacy and associated factors. *J Low Genit Tract Dis* 2006;4:245.

Reid R, Greenberg M, Jenson AB, et al. Sexually transmitted papillomaviral infections. I. The anatomic distribution and pathologic grade of neoplastic lesions associated with different viral types. *Am J Obstet Gynecol* 1987;156:212.

Reid R, Greenberg MD, Lorincz AT, et al. Superficial laser vulvectomy. IV. Extended laser vaporization and adjunctive 5-fluorouracil therapy of human papillomavirus–associated vulvar disease. *Obstet Gynecol* 1990;76:439.

Reid R, Greenberg MD, Pizzuti DJ, et al. Superficial laser vulvectomy. *Am J Obstet Gynecol* 1992;166:815.

Reid R, Omoto KH, Precop SL, et al. Flashlamp-excited dye laser therapy of idiopathic vulvodynia is safe and efficacious. *Am J Obstet Gynecol* 1995;172:1684.

Rompel R, Petres J. Long-term results of wide surgical excision in 106 patients with hidradenitis suppurativa. *Dermatol Surg* 2000;26:638.

Santos JV, Baudet JA, Lasellas FJ, et al. Intravenous cyclosporine for steroid-refractory attacks of Crohn's disease: short and long term results. *J Clin Gastroenterol* 1995;20:207.

Schickele G. Weitere Beiträge zur Lehre der mesonephris chen Tumoren. Hegars Beitr. zur Geburtshilfe und gynäkologic, Bd. 6, H.3, 1902.

Schover L, Youngs DD, Cannata NW. Psychosexual aspects of the evaluation and management of vulvar vestibulitis. *Am J Obstet Gynecol* 1992;167:630.

Schwimmer E. Die idiopathischen Schleimhautplaugues der mundhohle (Leukoplakia buccalis). *Arch Dermat Syph* 1877;9:611–570.

Scurry J, Campion M, Scurry B, et al. Pathologic audit of 164 consecutive cases of vulvar intraepithelial neoplasia. *Int J Gynecol Pathol* 2006;25:176.

Scurry J, Wilkinson EJ. Review of terminology of precursors of vulvar squamous cell carcinoma. *J Low Genit Tract Dis* 2006;10:161.

Shakla VK, Hughes LE. A case of squamous cell carcinoma complicating hidradenitis suppurativa. *Eur J Surg Oncol* 1995;21:106.

Shatz P, Bergeron C, Wilkinson EJ, et al. Vulvar intraepithelial neoplasia and skin appendage involvement. *Obstet Gynecol* 1989;74:769.

Sherman KJ, Daling JR, Chu J, et al. Genital warts, other sexually transmitted diseases, and vulvar cancer. *Epidemiology* 1991;2:257.

Sideri M, Jones RW, Wilkinson EJ, et al. Squamous vulvar intraepithelial neoplasia: 2004 modified terminology, ISSVD Vulvar Oncology Subcommittee. *J Reprod Med* 2005;50:807.

Sobel JD. Management of recurrent vulvovaginal candidiasis with intermittent ketoconazole prophylaxis. *Obstet Gynecol* 1985;65:435.

Sonnendecker EW, Sonnendecker HE, Wright CA, et al. Recalcitrant vulvodynia: a clinicopathological study. *S Afr Med J* 1993;83:730.

Taussig FJ. *Diseases of the vulva*. New York: Appleton Century-Crofts; 1931.

Theusen B, Andreasson B, Bock JE. Sexual function and somatopsychic reactions after local excision of vulvar intra-epithelial neoplasia. *Acta Obstet Gynecol Scand* 1992;71:126.

Turner ML, Marinoff SC. General principles in the diagnosis and treatment of vulvar diseases. *Dermatol Clin* 1992;10:275.

Umpierre SA, Kaufman RH, Adam E, et al. Human papillomavirus DNA in tissue biopsy specimens of vulvar vestibulitis patients treated with interferon. *Obstet Gynecol* 1991;78:693.

van Beurden M, ten Kale FJ, Smits HL, et al. Multifocal vulvar intraepithelial neoplasia grade III and multicentric lower genital tract neoplasia associated with transcriptionally active human papillomavirus. *Cancer* 1995;75:2879.

Villa LL, Costa RLR, Petta CA, et al. Prophylactic quadrivalent human papillomavirus (types 6, 11, 16, and 18) L1 virus-like particle vaccine in young women: a randomised double-blind placebo-controlled multicentre phase II efficacy trial. *Lancet Oncol* 2005;6(5):271.

Vuopala S, Pollanen R, Kaappila A, et al. Detection and typing of human papillomavirus infection affecting the cervix, vagina, and vulva: comparison of DNA hybridization with cytological, colposcopic and histological examination. *Arch Gynecol Obstet* 1993;253:75.

Weber CO. Anatomische Untersuchang einer hypertropphischen Zunge nebst Bemrkungen uber die nenbildung guergestreifter muskel fasern. Virchows Arch A Pathol Anat Histopathl, 1854;7:115–125.

Welsh DA, Powers JS. Elevated parathyroid hormone-related protein and hypercalcemia in a patient with cutaneous squamous cell carcinoma complicating hidradenitis suppurativa. *South Med J* 1993;86:1403.

Wharton LR Jr, Everett HS. Primary malignant Bartholin gland tumors. *Obstet Gynecol Surv* 1951;6:1.

Wilkinson EJ, Guerrero E, Daniel R, et al. Vulvar vestibulitis is rarely associated with human papillomavirus infection types 6, 11, 16, or 18. *Int J Gynecol Pathol* 1993;12:344.

Woodruff JD, Genadry R, Poliakoff S. Treatment of dyspareunia and vaginal outlet distortions by perineoplasty. *Obstet Gynecol* 1981;57:750.

Woodruff JD, Hildebrandt EE. Carcinoma in situ of the vulva. *Obstet Gynecol* 1958;12:414.

Woodruff JD, Julian C, Paray T, et al. The contemporary challenge of carcinoma in situ of the vulva. *Am J Obstet Gynecol* 1973;115:677.

Woodruff JD, Richardson EH Jr. Malignant vulvar Paget's disease. *Obstet Gynecol* 1957;10:10.

Woodruff JD, Sussman J, Shakfeh S. Vulvitis circumscripta plasmacellularis. *J Reprod Med* 1989;34:369.

Woodruff JD, Thompson B. Local alcohol injection in the treatment of vulvar pruritus. *Obstet Gynecol* 1972;40:18.

Woodruff JD, Genadry R, Poliakoff S. Treatment of dyspareunia and vaginal outlet distortions by perineoplasty. *Obstet Gynecol* 1981;57:750.

Wu AY, Sherman ME, Rosenshein NB, et al. Pathologic evaluation of gynecologic specimens obtained with the Cavitron ultrasonic surgical aspirator (CUSA). *Gynecol Oncol* 1992;44:28.

Wysoki RS, Majmudar B, Willis D. Granuloma inguinale (donovanosis) in women. *J Repro Med* 1988;33:709.

CHAPTER 24 ■ SURGICAL CONDITIONS OF THE VAGINA AND URETHRA

CELIA E. DOMINGUEZ, JOHN A. ROCK, AND IRA R. HOROWITZ

DEFINITIONS

Genitoplasty—Surgical reconstruction of external genitals.

Hematocolpos—A condition in which menstrual blood accumulates inside the vagina and distends it; most commonly associated with obstructing vaginal anomalies.

Hermaphroditism—A condition in which there is a combination of disparate or contradictory elements; most commonly used to describe an individual who has both male and female sexual characteristics and organs (synonyms: intersex, androgyne).

Imperforate hymen—The hymen usually is perforated during embryonic life to establish a connection between the lumen of the vaginal canal and the vaginal vestibule, and it usually is torn early in the prepubertal years. If canalization fails and there are no perforations, the hymen is called imperforate.

Pseudohermaphrodism—A condition in which the gonads are of one sex (genetically XX or XY), but in which the physical/phenotypical appearance is of the opposite sex. Genetically female individuals (chromosomes XX, thus with female gonads/ovaries) presenting with significant male secondary sex characteristics and genetically male individuals (chromosome XY thus with male gonads/testes) presenting with significant female secondary sex characteristis.

THE VAGINA

The Imperforate Hymen and Its Complications

The hymen, the junction of the sinovaginal bulbs with the urogenital sinus (UGS), is a thin mucous membrane, sometimes cribriform in appearance, which is composed of endoderm from the UGS epithelium. The müllerian ducts meet the sinovaginal bulbs at the most cephalad tip of the invaginating UGS. The vaginal plate elongates and canalizes to form the vagina. If the vaginal plate does not canalize, a transverse vaginal septum is the result. Canalization of the most caudal portion of the vaginal plate at the UGS establishes a patent hymen. The hymen usually is perforated during embryonic life to establish a connection between the lumen of the vaginal canal and the vaginal vestibule, and it usually is torn early in the prepubertal years. If canalization fails and there are no perforations, the hymen is called *imperforate*.

Although variations in hymen development occur, complete blockage by the hymen of the vaginal orifice is rare, occurring in approximately 0.05% to 0.1% of newborn girls. In 1986, Mor and colleagues described the types of hymenal shape in the newborn infant from examination performed within the first 24 hours of life. In 53.5%, a smooth hymen with a central orifice was observed; a folded hymen with a central orifice was seen in 27%; a folded hymen with an eccentric orifice occurred in 4.5%; an anterior opening of the hymen was in 10.8%; a posterior opening was found in 0.6%. The researchers found that 3% had hymenal bands and 0.3% of the newborns had an almost imperforate hymen. Pokorny and Kozinetz described the various configurations and anatomic details of the prepubertal hymen. In a case series of 265 children with known genital problems, three main hymenal configurations were observed: fimbriated, circumferential, and posterior rim. Interestingly, bleeding without a history of trauma was associated with hymenal bumps or breaks suggestive of trauma (31%) or with other hemorrhagic vulvar lesions (40%).

Stelling and colleagues have recently evaluated the genetic transmission of imperforate hymen and reported that the occurrence of imperforate hymen in two consecutive generations of a family is consistent with a dominant mode of transmission, either sex-linked or autosomal. It has also been reported that transmission may be recessively inherited. Taken together, they concluded that imperforate hymen is caused by mutations of several genes and emphasized the importance of evaluation of all family members of affected patients.

Symptoms

If an imperforate hymen is noticed before puberty, the condition can be treated when it is entirely asymptomatic. Cases that are recognized at birth present with a thin bulging membrane between the labia, which represents a mucocolpos. When the hymen is incised, the vagina is found to contain mucoid fluid that is the result of accumulated cervical secretion. This is caused by the stimulation of the infant's cervical mucous glands by maternal estrogen in the presence of an intact hymen. Prenatal diagnosis of imperforate hymen and mucocolpos has been described with second-trimester antenatal sonography demonstrating a thin membrane that distended the vagina and spread the labia majora.

Although by performing a careful inspection of the external genitalia, an imperforate hymen may be diagnosed at any age, most commonly imperforate hymen is not detected until puberty, with girls presenting at age 13 to 15 years, when symptoms begin to appear but menstruation appears not to have begun. In 2005, Posner and Spandorfer hypothesized that children with late diagnoses would be more likely to be symptomatic, undergo more diagnostic testing, and lack appropriate documentation in their medical records of adequate examinations compared with children with the diagnoses of imperforate hymen made at an earlier age. They reported a bimodal distribution of age at diagnosis with 43% (n = 10) of girls

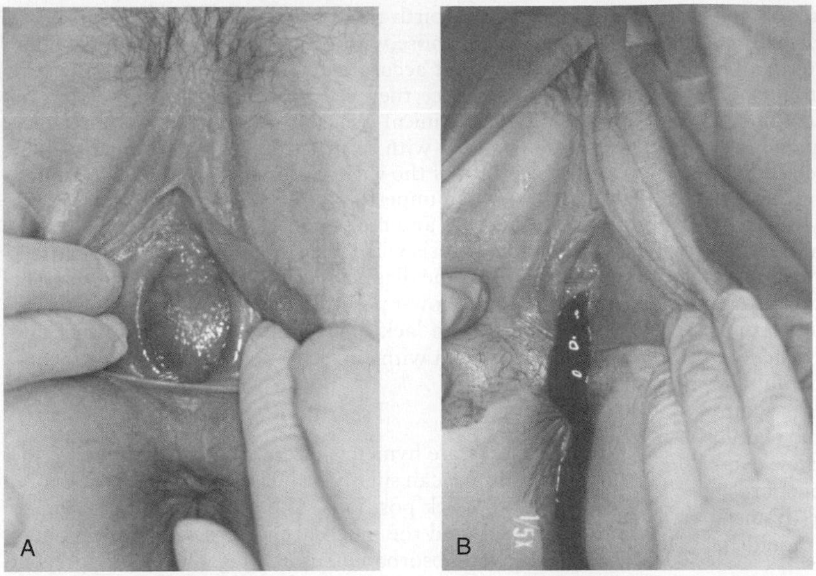

FIGURE 24.1. **A:** An imperforate hymen, membrane protrusion with a dark tinge posterior representing a hematocolpos. **B:** Extrusion of accumulated blood at time of incision into membrane. See color version of figure.

diagnosed younger than age 8 and 57% (n = 13) at or older than age 8. Among older girls, 100% were symptomatic with abdominal pain and/or urinary symptoms. They found that in the young girls, in 90% of cases, the diagnosis was incidental. On review of the older girls' medical records, they found that the majority lacked description of breast and pubic hair development, and almost half did not have menstrual history documented. The older group was more likely to present symptomatically and to undergo ancillary testing. They conclude that incorporating an examination of the external genitalia into routine practice of clinicians caring for children can prevent the significant delays in diagnosis of imperforate hymen, misdiagnosis, and potential morbidity associated with the latter group.

The symptoms girls present with after the onset of puberty are due to the accumulation of menstrual blood within the vaginal outlet tract. The blood of the first cycle period or two is collected in the vagina, which can hold a large volume of blood without undue stretching and with no other symptoms. This accumulated menstrual blood in the vagina is called *hematocolpos.* The patient may feel a slight fatigue and have cramping discomfort suggesting menstruation, but she has no history of any passage of menstrual blood through the vaginal outlet. Figure 24.1A shows bulging of the imperforate hymen, which may be dark in color because of occult blood showing through the stretched mucous membrane; Figure 24.1B shows extrusion of accumulated blood after the hymen is incised.

As menstruation continues to occur, however, the vagina becomes greatly overdistended, and the cervical canal also begins to dilate. Accumulation of menstrual blood in the uterine cavity, with subsequent hematometra, may occur. When the intrauterine pressure reaches a certain point, retrograde passage of blood into the tubes causes hematosalpinx. Associated or other adhesion formation within or at the fimbriated ends of the tubes may seal them, so that little or no blood enters the peritoneal cavity. In some cases, however, blood passes freely into the peritoneal cavity, forming hematoperitoneum (Fig. 24.2). A

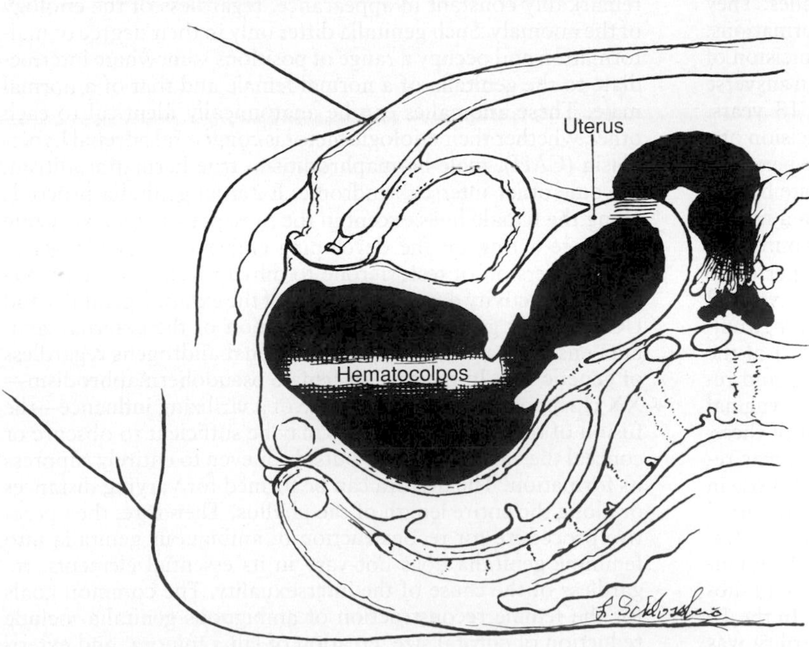

FIGURE 24.2. Hematocolpos, hematometra, hematosalpinx, and hematoperitoneum consequent to an imperforate hymen.

tender mass often is palpable suprapubically, the result of uterine enlargement and upward displacement, bladder distention, or both. If hematoperitoneum occurs, the irritation of the free blood may cause all the symptoms and signs of peritonitis.

The most common symptoms of vaginal overdistention are lower abdominal pain, discomfort in the pelvis, and pain in the lower back. Hematocolpos should be included in the differential diagnosis of amenorrheic girls presenting with persistent lower back pain. Irritation of the sacral plexus is believed to be the etiology of this referred pain pattern. The lower abdominal discomfort often is aggravated on defecation, and if extensive blood accumulation occurs in the vagina, constipation may result from pressure and obstruction of the underlying rectum. Urination can be difficult as a result of pressure of the distended vagina, which can compress the urethra and prevent emptying of the bladder; urinary obstruction can ensue. Bladder symptoms can present as cramplike pains in the suprapubic region, along with symptoms of dysuria, frequency, and urgency; overflow incontinence may eventually develop, and hydronephrosis is a rare complication. Girls presenting with severe dysmenorrhea and duplicate vagina and didelphic uterus should be evaluated for unilateral imperforate hymen.

Rock and colleagues followed pregnancy success subsequent to the surgical correction of imperforate hymen between 1945 and 1981 at the Johns Hopkins Hospital. Twenty-two patients of mean age 14.7 years were admitted for surgical correction of imperforate hymens. Associated anomalies, including urinary tract anomalies, were rare. Thirteen patients subsequently conceived, and 10 patients were observed to have living children. Liang and colleagues in 2003 reported on the long-term postoperative evaluation of 15 patients with imperforate hymen. They conducted questionnaires and telephone interviews regarding sexuality, fertility, menstrual problems, micturition, and defecation. The mean postoperative follow-up was 8.5 years, with the mean age at diagnosis being 13.2 years. The women reported being markedly relieved of their presenting symptoms after hymenectomy. There were some who reported having irregular menstruation, and 6/15 reported dysmenorrhea. The authors reported that most patients fared well in terms of fertility and sexual function. Joki-Erkkila and colleagues in 2003 also reported on presenting and long-term fecundity in women with obstructing vaginal anomalies. They identified 26 women with obstructive vaginal malformations. Sixteen had transverse obstructions: 13 underwent incision of an imperforate hymen and 3 excision of a complete transverse vaginal septum, with a mean follow-up period of 13 years. The remaining 10 had obstructive hemivagina and incision of a "longitudinal" vaginal septum with a mean follow-up period of 16 years. The transverse obstruction girls (imperforate hymen or transverse vaginal septum) were diagnosed within a month from their primary symptoms compared with 27 months for those with longitudinal obstruction. None with imperforate hymen required reoperation, but 2/3 with transverse vaginal septum did for vaginal constriction, and 3/10 with longitudinal vaginal septum had reexcision of their septum. All of the 10 women with longitudinal obstruction had uterine and renal malformations, whereas in those with a transverse vaginal obstruction, only 6 underwent renal evaluation, and of these, 2 had double ureters. Dysfunctional uterine bleeding was reported by 19% of those in the transverse and 40% of those in the longitudinal obstruction group; dyspareunia was reported in 30% of the transverse and none in the longitudinal; and dysmenorrhea was reported in 19% of transverse and 20% of longitudinal. No endometriosis was found in women who had subsequently had a laparotomy or laparoscopy (18/26). In the 14 who were attempting to conceive, difficulty with fertility was not diagnosed. Twenty-five (89%) out of 28 pregnancies ended in delivery, the live birth rate of the longitudinal group being 82%, and 94% in those with transverse obstruction. The authors concluded that accurate diagnosis, along with adequate treatment, can reduce the need for reoperations and that no specific long-term clinical gynecologic symptoms were identified in these women with obstructing vaginal anomalies. The great distensibility of the vagina probably protects the adolescent patient with an imperforate hymen from abnormal retrograde menstruation, and the possible subsequent development of pelvic endometriosis with imperforate hymen as the cause is unlikely as long as the diagnosis is made reasonably early. The recent long-term follow-up studies are helpful in counseling patients with respect to lack of a negative effect on fertility and pregnancy in women with correction of imperforate hymen.

Treatment

When an imperforate hymen is discovered before puberty, the hymenal membrane can simply be incised, preferably at the 2-, 4-, 8-, and 10-o'clock positions. The quadrants of the hymen are then excised, and the mucosal margins are approximated with fine delayed-absorbable suture (Fig. 24.3). To prevent scarring and stenosis, which could result in dyspareunia, the hymenal tissue should not be excised too close to the vaginal mucosa. All unnecessary intrauterine instrumentation should be avoided because if hematocolpos has already developed (Fig. 24.2), there is the risk of perforating the thin, overstretched uterine wall.

No further surgical intervention is generally needed. If the uterine mass does not regress within 2 to 3 weeks, however, inspection and dilatation of the cervix should be performed to make certain that drainage from the uterus is satisfactory.

Anomalies of the External Genitalia and Vagina

Construction of Female External Genitalia

Sexually ambiguous external genitalia defects of the UGS are remarkably constant in appearance, regardless of the etiology of the anomaly. Such genitalia differ only in their degree of malformation and occupy a range of positions somewhere intermediate to the genitalia of a normal female and that of a normal male. These anomalies can be anatomically identical to each other, whether their etiologic factor is congenital adrenal hyperplasia (CAH), male hermaphroditism, true hermaphroditism, or some other intersex syndrome. External genitalia proceeds along the female lines except in the presence of some virilizing influence acting on the developing embryo (i.e., androgens). The conversion of testosterone to dihydrotestosterone by 5α-reductase activity occurs in the skin of the external genitalia and UGS in early gestation. Masculinization of the external genitalia ensues in the presence of functional androgens regardless of genetic sex. In the case of female pseudohermaphrodism—XX chromosomes in the presence of a virilizing influence—the fusion of the scrotolabial folds may be sufficient to obscure or conceal the vagina from the outside or even to entirely suppress its formation. The urethra can be formed for varying distances or along the entire length of the phallus. Therefore, the operative procedure for reconstruction of ambiguous genitalia into feminine genitalia does not vary in its essential elements, regardless of the cause of the intersexuality. The common goals for the female reconstruction of ambiguous genitalia include reduction of clitoral size, creation of labia minora, and exteriorization of the vagina.

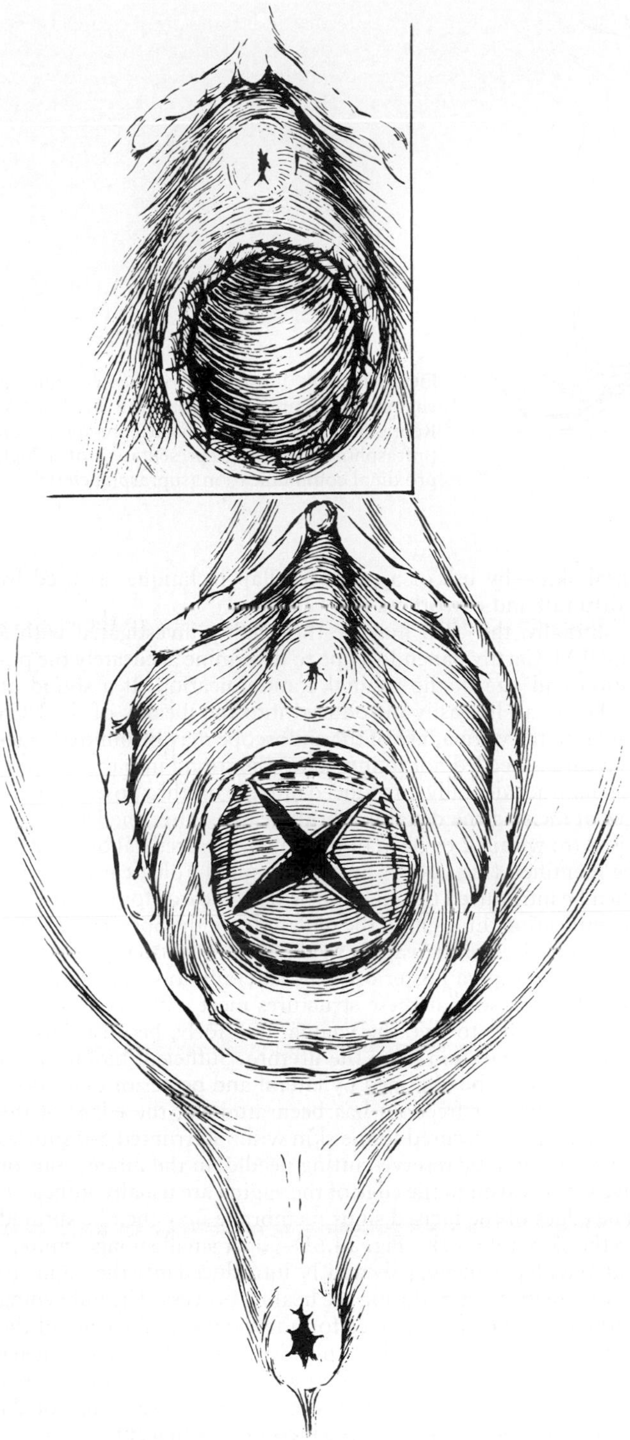

FIGURE 24.3. Excision of imperforate hymen. Stellate incisions are made through the hymenal membrane at the 2-, 4-, 8-, and 10-o'clock positions. The individual quadrants are excised along the lateral wall of the vagina, avoiding excision of the vagina. (*Inset*) Margins of vaginal mucosa are approximated with fine delayed-absorbable suture.

Any reconstruction of the external genitalia with the objective of producing normal female appearance and function requires a full understanding of the surgical anatomy. It is essential to accurately identify the site of communication of the vagina with the UGS. In their classic paper in 1969, Hendren and Crawford recognized the variability of the communication of the vaginal insertion into the UGS. Figure 24.4 illustrates the spectrum of vaginal communication with the urethra, with Figure 24.4A representative of a low distal communication (infrasphincteric) and Figure 24.4B representative of a high proximal communication (suprasphincteric). In 95% of cases, the vaginal communication is in relation to the caudal UGS derivatives (infrasphincteric) with the vagina communicating with that portion of the UGS that in a man gives rise to the membranous portion of the male urethra and that in the woman becomes the vaginal vestibule. If this usual relation is confirmed at surgery, the persistent, anomalous UGS may be incised to the vaginal communication without fear of disturbing the urinary sphincter. In less than 5% of cases, the vagina communicates high, with the portion of the UGS that becomes the prostatic urethra in the man or the entire urethra in the woman (suprasphincteric). Knowledge of the possible variants in communication of the vagina with the UGS is critical before entertaining surgical correction. Preoperatively genitography showing the relationship of the UGS, urethra, vagina, and bladder may be helpful. Contrast is injected retrogradely through the perineal meatus of the UGS. Delineation of this anatomy can be elucidated at the time of surgery with the use of endoscopy to evaluate where the vagina communicates with the UGS. In 1989, Bargy and colleagues described the anatomic lesions in the intersexual states based on clinical and anatomic observations.

One objective of the reconstruction procedure for external genitalia is to delay the procedure until the anomalous structures are of a size to permit easy identification of all structures. As observed by Azziz and coworkers, vaginal repair may be delayed until menarche, when maturity and the desire for sexual activity are usually well established. There is present debate in the need for early reconstruction for the sole purpose of cosmesis to prevent embarrassment or anxiety to the patient's family. Crouch and Creighton have recently revisited the long-standing dictum of early surgical correction of ambiguous genitalia for intersex conditions. They report that some advocate the "one-stage" procedure in infancy, but that others advocate deferral of vaginal surgery until after puberty, especially given that many patients require further surgery at adolescence. It has been believed that the intersex child may be psychologically damaged by the "appearance" of uncorrected external genitalia if not performed at infancy, but unfortunately to date little research on this exists.

Most hermaphrodites reared as girls have a vagina or vaginal pouch, although in some instances, it is rudimentary. Only rarely is there no vagina, despite ambiguity of the external genitalia. The choice of operative procedure must conform to the observed anatomy. Thus, these choices are considered in the context of several categories based on anatomic structure of the anomaly.

When the Vagina is Present and the Vaginosinus Communication is Low. The basic operation is, in essence, a modification of one described at length by Young that was previously performed successfully by various surgeons, notably in Europe. Patients with adrenal hyperplasia usually require only reconstruction of the external genitalia. However, when exploratory laparotomy is necessary to remove contradictory sex structures in other types of intersexuality or to establish the diagnosis, reconstruction of the genitalia may be considered at the same operation.

If an operation is deemed necessary at a very young age, the structures can be so small that it is impossible to introduce a finger into the UGS, and all tissues must be grasped throughout the operation with fine delicate tissue forceps. Operating loupes

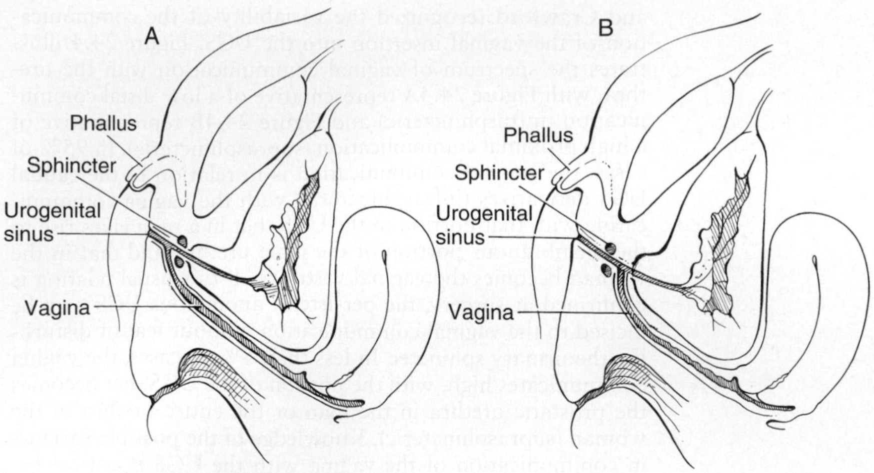

FIGURE 24.4. Illustration of the spectrum of vaginal communication with the urethra. **A:** Representative of a low distal communication (infrasphincteric). **B:** Representative of a high proximal communication (suprasphincteric).

(2.5–3) are of great benefit to the surgeon. Small bipolar forceps and microscissors are also useful. Fine 5-0 or 6-0 synthetic absorbable sutures on an atraumatic needle is used throughout the procedure.

In cases of simple labial fusion, a cutback vaginoplasty (Fig. 24.5) would be sufficient to restore "normal" female genital anatomy. In cases of low vaginal confluence with the UGS (Fig. 24.4A), reconstruction may be done either by freeing the posterior vaginal wall and suturing up to the perineal external opening (Fig. 24.6) or—if a patient has copious subcutaneous fat and difficulty exists in approximating the vagina to the perineal skin—by use of a posterior flap technique, as used by Fortunoff and coworkers (Fig. 24.7).

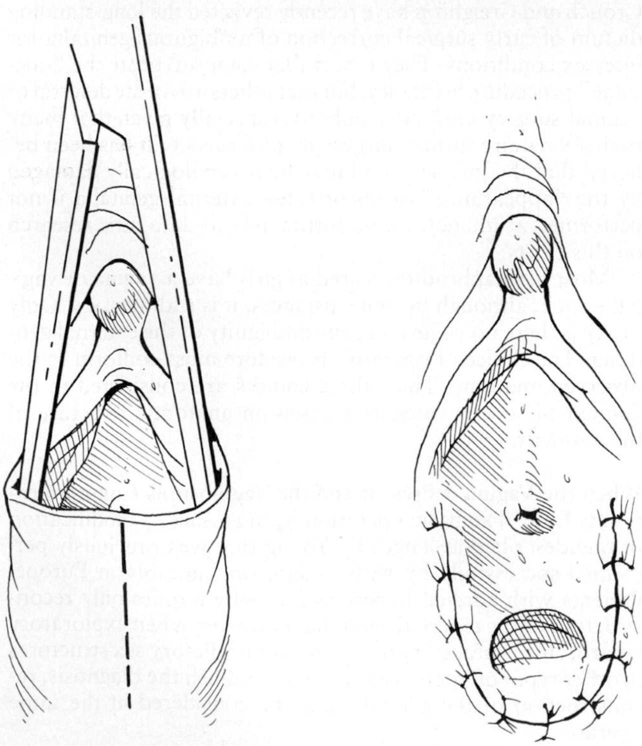

FIGURE 24.5. In cases of simple labial fusion, a cutback vaginoplasty is sufficient to restore "normal" female genital anatomy.

Initially, the UGS may be thoroughly investigated with a small McCarthy panendoscope to determine accurately the position and size of the vaginal communication. If a sound or catheter can be easily introduced into the meatus of the UGS and into the vagina, use of the endoscope may be omitted. Special care is needed not to introduce the sound into the urethra. A sound accidentally introduced into the urethra poses the danger of incising the distal urethral meatus. After the UGS is incised (to within 2 or 3 cm of the anus), the urethral orifice may be identified (Fig. 24.6A and B). A small Foley catheter may then be introduced through the urinary meatus for purposes of identification throughout the remainder of the operation. To attach the edges of the vagina to the skin, it is usually necessary to free the vagina posteriorly and laterally to secure sufficient mobilization so that these structures meet with no tension. It is unnecessary to free the vagina anteriorly, because this requires its separation from the urethra. Sufficient mobilization can ordinarily be obtained by lateral and posterior dissection. When sufficient freedom has been attained, the edges of the vagina may be secured to the skin with interrupted 5-0 sutures on an atraumatic reserve-cutting needle. In the infant, four or five sutures around the edge of the vagina are usually sufficient. The edges of the incised sinus membrane may then be sutured to the skin anteriorly (Fig. 24.6D–G). A small sponge impregnated with petroleum jelly may be introduced into the vagina to maintain its patency during the healing process. The indwelling catheter may be left in place for a few days until edema of the surrounding structures has subsided. An indwelling catheter is particularly useful in children with metabolic disorders that require accurate urine collection. A pressure dressing for 24 hours reduces the incidence of incisional hematoma.

Figure 24.7 illustrates vaginoplasty with a posterior flap as advocated by Fortunoff and is useful in cases with anticipated difficulty in bringing the vaginal orifice to the outside. Briefly, a posterior-based U-flap is drawn, with corners on either side of the perineal body near the rectum (Fig. 24.7A–C). This flap must be wide enough for tension-free anastomosis. This posterior flap is dissected in the midline and is carried out between the rectum and UGS.

Sutures are individually placed through the posterior-based flap and into the split posterior vagina. Sutures are tied after all have been placed. Because the anterior wall is not disturbed, no anterior flap is required. Finally, the phallic skin is

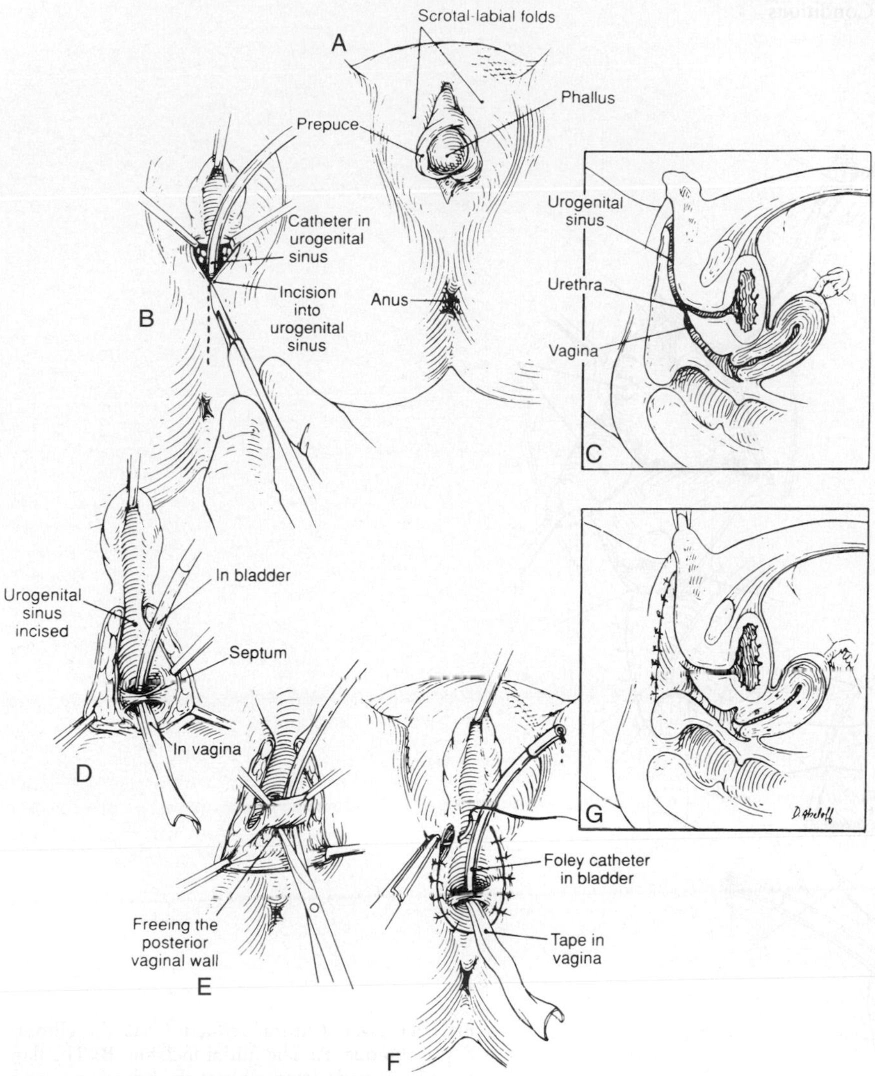

FIGURE 24.6. A: The external genitalia of an 18-month-old girl with congenital adrenal hyperplasia. The operation is the same, regardless of the etiology of the "virilizing" deformity. **B:** Beginning of the operation. Incision into the urogenital sinus. If the external meatus is large enough and the urogenital sinus will accommodate it, it is sometimes possible to introduce a catheter into the bladder through the urethra and introduce a sound into the vagina beside this. When the structures are large enough, this maneuver greatly facilitates the operative procedure by ensuring their identification. **C:** Lateral view showing the relations among the various structures. **D:** Situation after incision of the urogenital sinus. **E:** With the glass catheter in the bladder, the posterior vaginal wall is freed to make it possible to bring it to the skin edge without undue tension. **F:** The operative situation after the edges of the vagina are sutured to the skin and after the edges of the mucous membrane of the urogenital sinus are also sutured to the skin along the line of incision. **G:** Lateral view at the completion of the operation.

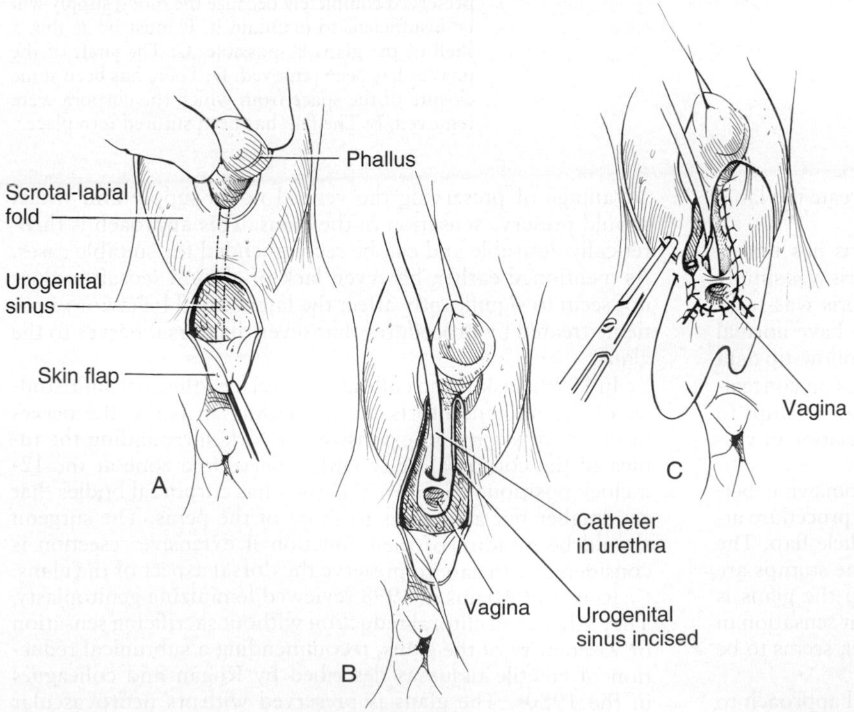

FIGURE 24.7. A posterior flap technique for when there is difficulty bringing the vaginal orifice to the outside.

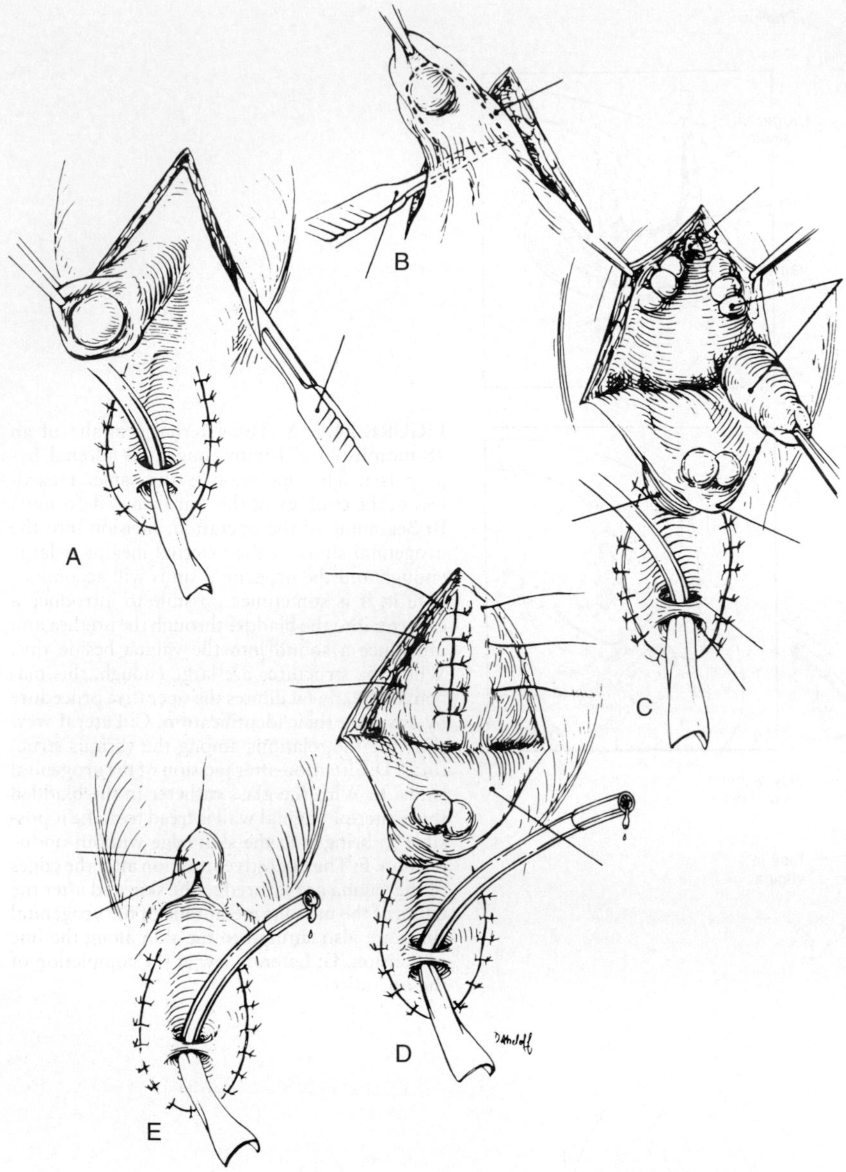

FIGURE 24.8. Clitoral reduction via the clitoral flap technique. **A:** The initial incision. **B:** The flap must be as wide as possible at the base to preserve the circulation for the glans. The glans cannot be preserved completely because the blood supply will be insufficient to maintain it. It must be as thin a shell of the glans as possible. **C:** The shaft of the phallus has been removed. **D:** There has been some closure of the space from which the corpora were removed. **E:** The flap has been sutured into place.

divided in the midline and moved inferiorly to create the labia minora.

Surgical reconstruction of an enlarged clitoris has undergone significant evolution. Traditionally, the clitoris was simply amputated, and a nonfunctioning cosmetic clitoris was fashioned. Although several children so treated now have normal adult sexual function, the literature is lacking in follow-up data on large patient groups. Surgical efforts now focus on concealment, plication, resection, and reduction, with an attempt to provide a normal cosmesis without sacrificing sensation or vascularity of the glans.

The clitoral flap technique has provided a somewhat better cosmetic result than simple amputation. This procedure attempts to preserve a shell of the glans on a pedicle flap. The shaft of the clitoris is subtotally resected, and the stumps are reanastomosed (Fig. 24.8). The nerve supply to the glans is severed during this procedure, with the result that sensation in the glans is diminished. Sexual function, however, seems to be satisfactory.

Rajfer and colleagues have suggested a dorsal approach to the subtotal resection of the corpora (Fig. 24.9), which has the advantage of preserving the ventral nerve supply and which should preserve sensation in the glans. This approach is theoretically desirable and can be recommended for suitable cases. As mentioned earlier, however, lack of clitoral sensation does not seem to significantly affect the later sexual behavior of patients treated by procedures that sever the dorsal nerves to the glans.

In 1999, Baskin and colleagues described the anatomic studies of the human clitoris. As in the human penis, the nerves in the clitoris form an extensive network surrounding the tunica of the corporeal body with a nerve-free zone at the 12-o'clock position. The normal clitoris has corporeal bodies that are smaller but analogous to those of the penis. The surgeon should be mindful of their function if extensive resection is considered with care to preserve the dorsal aspect of the glans.

Rink and Adams in 1998 reviewed feminizing genitoplasty. They advocated clitoral reduction without sacrificing sensation or vascularity of the glans, recommending a subtunical reduction of erectile tissue as described by Kogan and colleagues in the 1980s. The glans is preserved with its neurovascular supply intact along Buck's fascia and the dorsal tunic of the

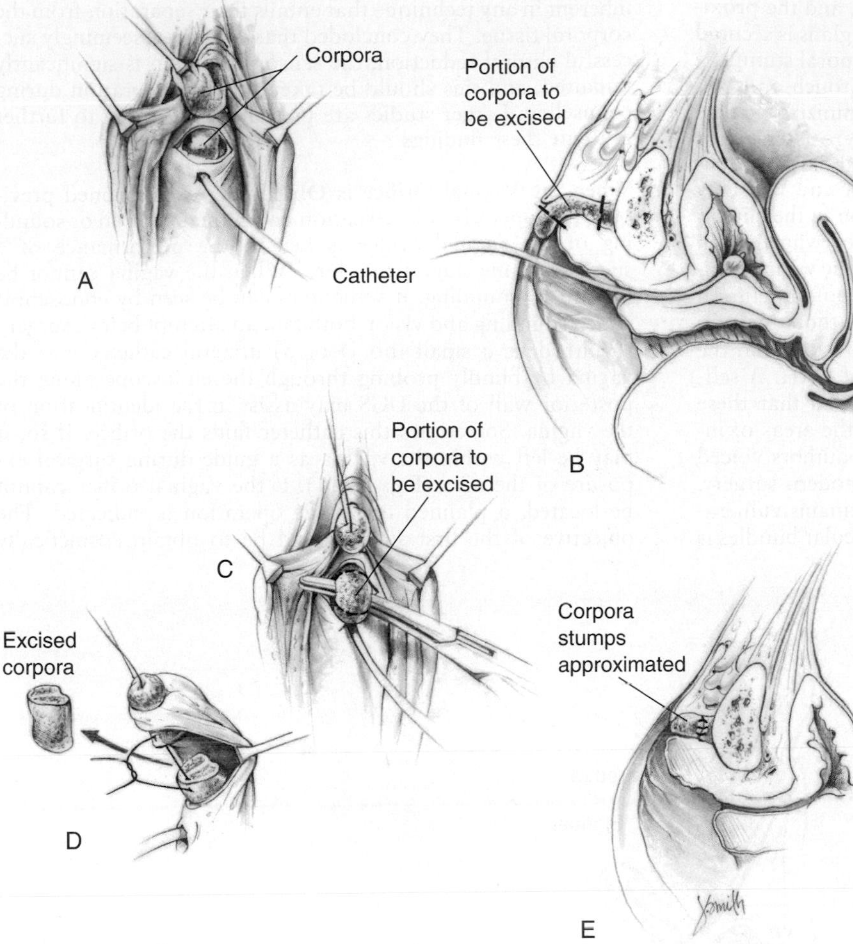

FIGURE 24.9. Clitoral reduction with the corpora exposed through a dorsal incision (operation of Rajfer and colleagues). A through C: Corpora are approached and removed through a posterior incision in the phallus. D: Diagram of the excised portion of the corpora. E: The corpora are removed and stumps approximated.

corpora, yet the cavernous erectile tissue is excised. Figure 24.10 illustrates this surgical management; additionally, the phallus is degloved, and this skin is used to create the labia minora. An incision is made around the corona of the phallus and continued inferiorly around the urethral meatus. Preservation of this meatal plate improves cosmesis and increases blood supply to the glans. The neurovascular bundle is identified, with lateral incisions into the tunica of the corpora along the phallus from the glans backward proximal to the corporal bifurcation. The cavernous erectile tissue is dissected from the

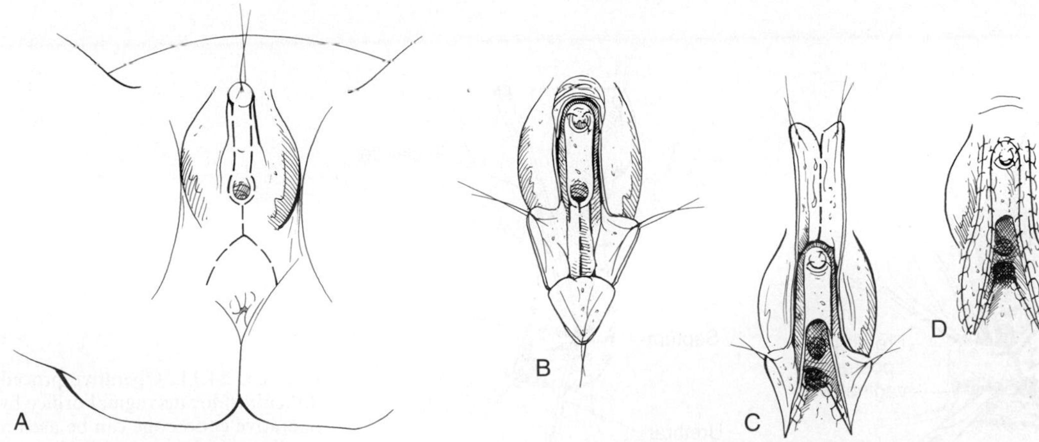

FIGURE 24.10. Surgical management of the clitoris with creation of labia minora and a posterior flap technique for vaginoplasty. A: Incision around the corona of the phallus continued inferiorly around the urethral meatus. B: Proposed incision into the posterior wall of the urogenital sinus. C: Degloving of the phallus. Sutures are individually placed through the posterior based flap and into the split posterior vagina. D: The phallic skin is divided in the midline and moved inferiorly to create the labia minora. (From Rink RC, Adams MC. Feminizing genitoplasty: state of the art. *World J Urol* 1998;16:212, with permission.)

inferior aspect of the dorsal tunic and excised, and the proximal and dorsal corpora are suture ligated. The glans is secured to the inferior aspect of the pubis or to the corporal stumps.

In a pilot study of six women in 2003, Crouch and colleagues reported on genital sensation after feminizing genitoplasty for women with CAH. These women were assessed for thermal, vibratory, and light-touch sensory thresholds in the clitoris and vagina using a genitosensory analyzer and Von Frey filaments. Highly abnormal results for sensation in the clitoris were found in the six women studied. In three who had an introitus capable of admitting a vaginal probe, the vaginal sensory data was considered normal. Given an abnormal clitoral sensation and normal vaginal sensation, the authors hypothesize that the abnormal clitoral findings may result from the surgical reconstruction rather than an effect of CAH. A self-administered sexual function assessment revealed that these women had sexual difficulties, particularly in the areas of infrequency of intercourse and anorgasmia. The authors voiced their concerns with the stated superiority of modern surgery. They stated that the vascularity of the glans remains vulnerable and that the risk of damage to the neurovascular bundles is inherent in any technique that entails their separation from the corporal tissue. They concluded that even after seemingly successful clitoral reduction, the sensory function is significantly impaired, and this should be taken into consideration during counseling. Larger studies are presently under way to further evaluate these findings.

When the Vaginal Orifice is Obscured. As mentioned previously, preoperative identification and catheterization or sounding of the vaginal orifice is key to the performance of a successful, one-stage procedure. When the vagina cannot be located by sounding, it sometimes can be seen by endoscopy. When sounding and vision both fail, an attempt before surgery to introduce a small (no. 4 or 5) ureteral catheter into the vagina by blindly probing through the endoscope along the posterior wall of the UGS may assist in the identification of the vagina. Sometimes this catheter finds the orifice. If so, it may be left within the vagina as a guide during surgical exposure of the area (Fig. 24.11). If the vaginal orifice cannot be located, a planned two-stage operation is indicated. The objective of the first stage would be to obtain cosmetically

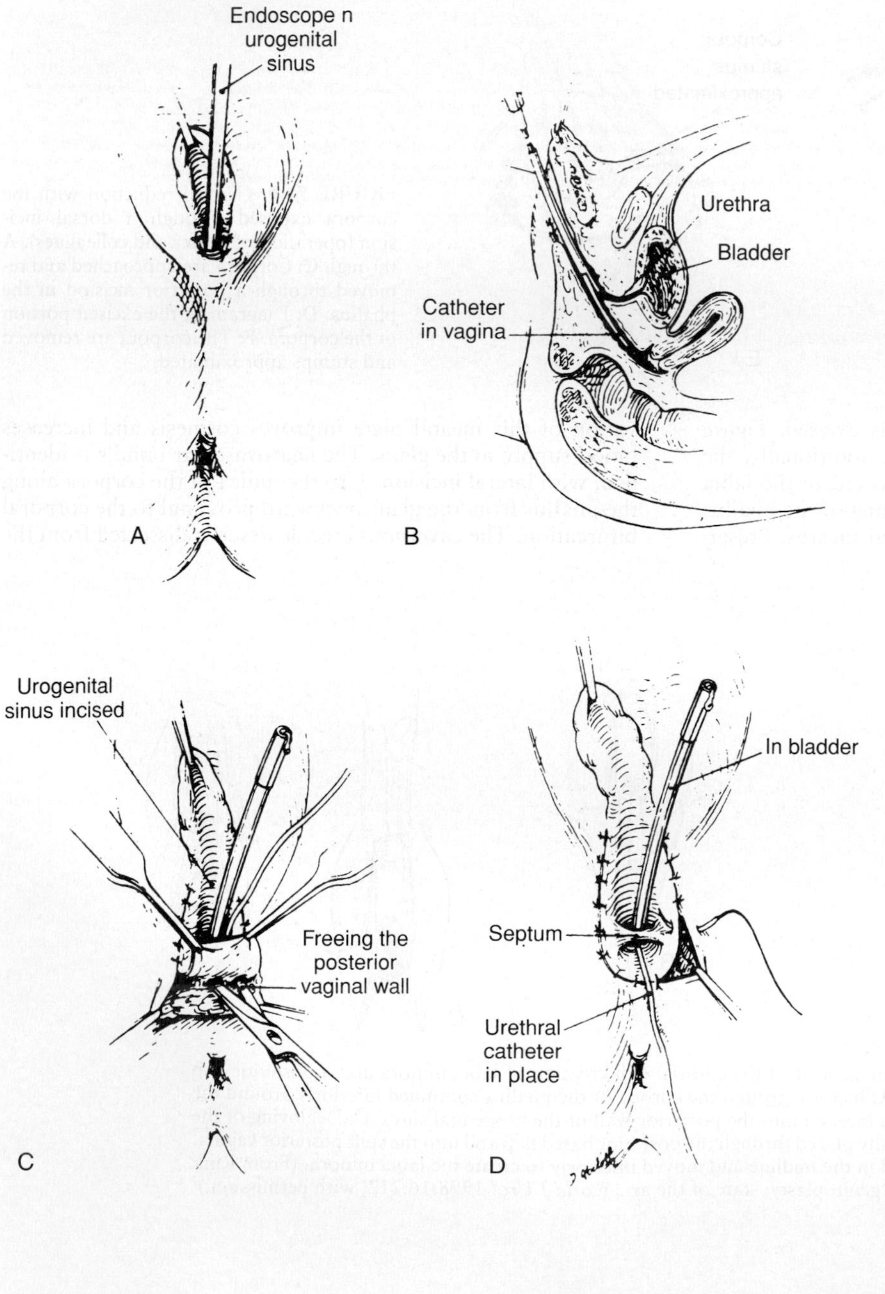

FIGURE 24.11. Operative procedure when it is difficult to locate vaginal orifice by sounding. An operative endoscope can be used to probe with a small ureteral catheter. **A:** The orifice is enlarged to accommodate the endoscope. **B:** The tip of the catheter has found the vaginal opening and entered the vagina. **C:** Freeing the posterior vaginal wall with the ureteral catheter in the vagina and a stiff catheter in the urethra. **D:** The vaginal portion of the operation is complete.

satisfactory female genitalia by reducing the clitoris and partially excising the UGS without exteriorizing the vagina. During the planned second stage, exteriorization of the vagina can be performed. The second stage should be postponed until identification of the vaginal orifice by sounding becomes possible. This may require waiting for puberty for estrogenization of the area. If dilators are needed for patency postoperatively, this surgery should be delayed until the girl is sufficiently mature for their appropriate use. This will maximize the success of the reoperation.

When the Vaginosinus Communication is Blocked. Rarely does the vagina not communicate with the UGS. The vagina with the UGS is homologous with the hymenal area, and the hymen rarely is imperforate in an otherwise normal woman. For such a circumstance, we have found it helpful to pass a uterine sound downward through the fundus via hysterotomy into the vagina, thus forming a protrusion on the perineum. With such a guide, the edges of the vaginal epithelium can be located and sutured to the skin (Fig. 24.12). Until the uterus enlarges somewhat from its infantile state, the cavity is not large enough to accommodate even a uterine sound. Therefore, if such an operation is contemplated, it should not be done until there is a palpable enlargement of the uterus at the onset of puberty. Evaluation of uterine volume sonographically as a predictor of uterine size adequacy may be helpful.

When the Vaginosinus Communication is High. Hendren has been especially interested in patients whose vaginosinus communication involves the proximal urethra (suprasphincteric). He has advocated an operation that disconnects the vagina from the urethra and repositions the vaginal orifice in the perineum, the "pull-through" vaginoplasty. In his hands, this procedure seems to have been satisfactory for some patients. The procedure requires positioning the new vaginal orifice in the perineum (Fig. 24.13). The vast majority of patients with ambiguous external genitalia and a vagina have a vaginosinus communication well distal to the proximal urethra (infrasphincteric), and consideration of the procedure advocated by Hendren is not necessary. In patients in whom the vagina enters the UGS proximal to the external sphincter, the pull-through vaginoplasty of Hendren and Crawford or the method described by Passerini-Glazel can be used to prevent incontinence. Hendren and Crawford's vaginal pull-through remains the basis for reconstruction today. Modification to this procedure has evolved in an attempt to decrease the complexity and decrease the tendency of an isolated vagina toward stenosis. Rink and coworkers have favored a one-stage procedure using a perineal prone approach with no division of the rectum.

Results of Revision of External Genitalia. Among 28 patients with adrenogenital syndrome and good follow-up treated at the Johns Hopkins Hospital, 22 (87.6%) needed further vaginal reconstructive surgery to achieve an adequate vaginal size

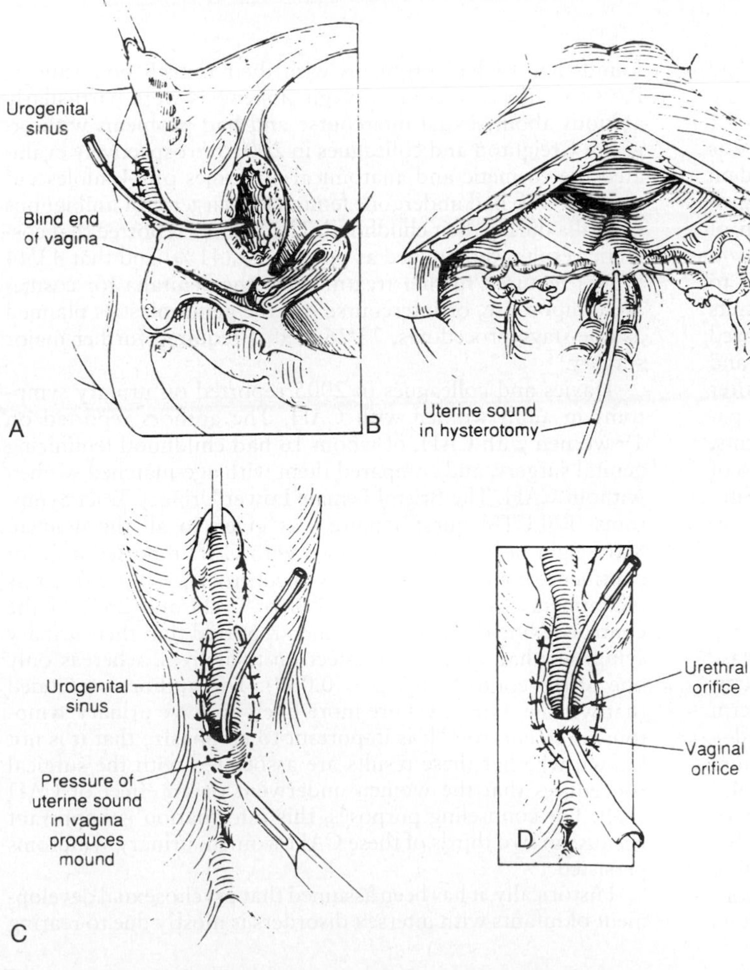

FIGURE 24.12. A: A situation in which the vaginal orifice is imperforate. B: A uterine sound has been passed through the fundus into the vagina. C: The tip of the sound can be palpated in the perineum. D: The completed procedure.

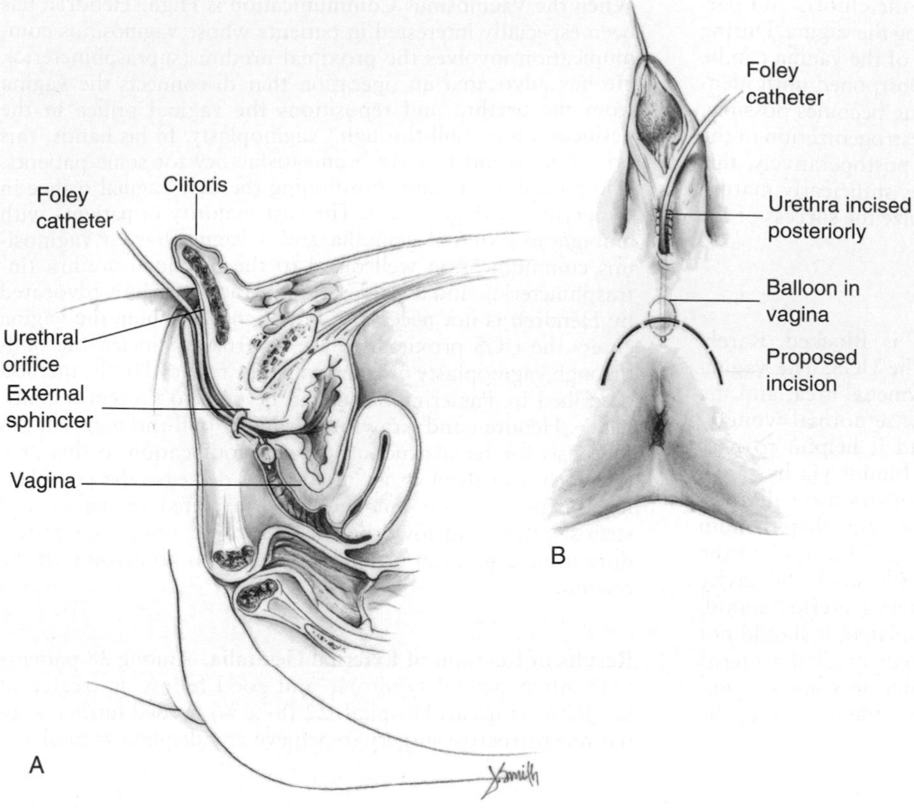

FIGURE 24.13. A perineal pull-through vaginoplasty according to Hendren. **A:** Sagittal view in diagram of high suprasphincteric vaginal communication to the urogenital sinus. A small Foley catheter is placed in the vagina to aid in its manipulation and localization. **B:** The location of the initial incision in relation to the balloon in the vagina.

to allow comfortable intercourse. Of the 22 patients, five had undergone more than one surgical attempt at reconstruction. The mean age of patients undergoing repeat procedures was 7.1 years. The mean age at first surgery for the whole group was 23.6 months. Vaginal reconstructive surgery was performed on 18 of these patients and was successful in 13 (72%) of the procedures. It generally is recommended that exteriorization of the vagina be postponed until near puberty, when feminization occurs and the young woman is sufficiently mature to comply with a postoperative dilatation program. The results of exteriorization performed during infancy must be followed up carefully for evidence of narrowing. In 1997, Costa and colleagues evaluated the vaginal size and sexual activity after different techniques of feminization of external genitalia in patients with pseudohermaphrodism. In their series of patients, all who underwent clitoroplasty reported orgasms, and 29% of the patients who had clitoridectomy reported no orgasms. Fifty percent of the patients who submitted to neovaginoplasty reported pain or bleeding during sexual intercourse. Satisfactory sexual intercourse was reported by 87% after vaginal dilation with acrylic molds.

In 2000, Krege and colleagues reported on the long-term follow-up of female patients with CAH from 21-hydroxylase deficiency, with special emphasis on the results of vaginoplasty. They reported that the main problem during the long-term follow-up was intravaginal stenosis, with all those affected—9 of 25 (36%)—having undergone a single-stage procedure early in life to correct ambiguous genitalia (mean age, 4.7 years; range, 2 to 9 years). The authors suggested that vaginoplasty should be undertaken at the beginning of puberty, because higher estrogen levels may prevent stenosis and dilatation may be performed. In addition, 16 patients answered questionnaires that included psychological profile, and the researchers found that 14 had problems with their overall body image. Patients with correction of vaginal stenosis were particularly anxious about sexual intercourse and had problems with orgasm. Creighton and colleagues in 2001 retrospectively evaluated the cosmetic and anatomical outcomes of 44 adolescent patients who had undergone feminizing surgery for ambiguous genitalia during their childhood. The authors reported that cosmetic results were judged as poor in 18 (41%) and that 43/44 (98%) required further treatment to the genitalia for cosmesis, tampon use, or intercourse. Of the genitoplasties planned as one-stage procedures, 23/26 (89%) required further major surgery.

Davies and colleagues in 2005 reported on urinary symptoms in adult women with CAH. The authors reported on 19 women with CAH, of whom 16 had childhood feminizing genital surgery, and compared them with age-matched women without CAH. The Bristol Female Lower Urinary Tract Symptoms (BFLUTS) questionnaire was given to all the women. Sixty-eight percent of the women with CAH reported urge incontinence compared with 16% of controls ($p = 0.003$). Stress incontinence was present in 47% of CAH and 26% of the controls. Nine of the CAH women reported that their urinary symptoms had an adverse effect on their lives, whereas only one of the controls did ($p = 0.008$). The authors concluded that women with CAH are more likely to have urinary symptoms than controls. It is important to emphasize that it is not known whether these results are associated with the surgical procedures that the women underwent or an effect of CAH itself. For counseling purposes, this information is important because in two thirds of these CAH women, urinary symptoms persisted.

Historically, it has been assumed that psychosexual development of infants with intersex disorders is mostly due to rearing

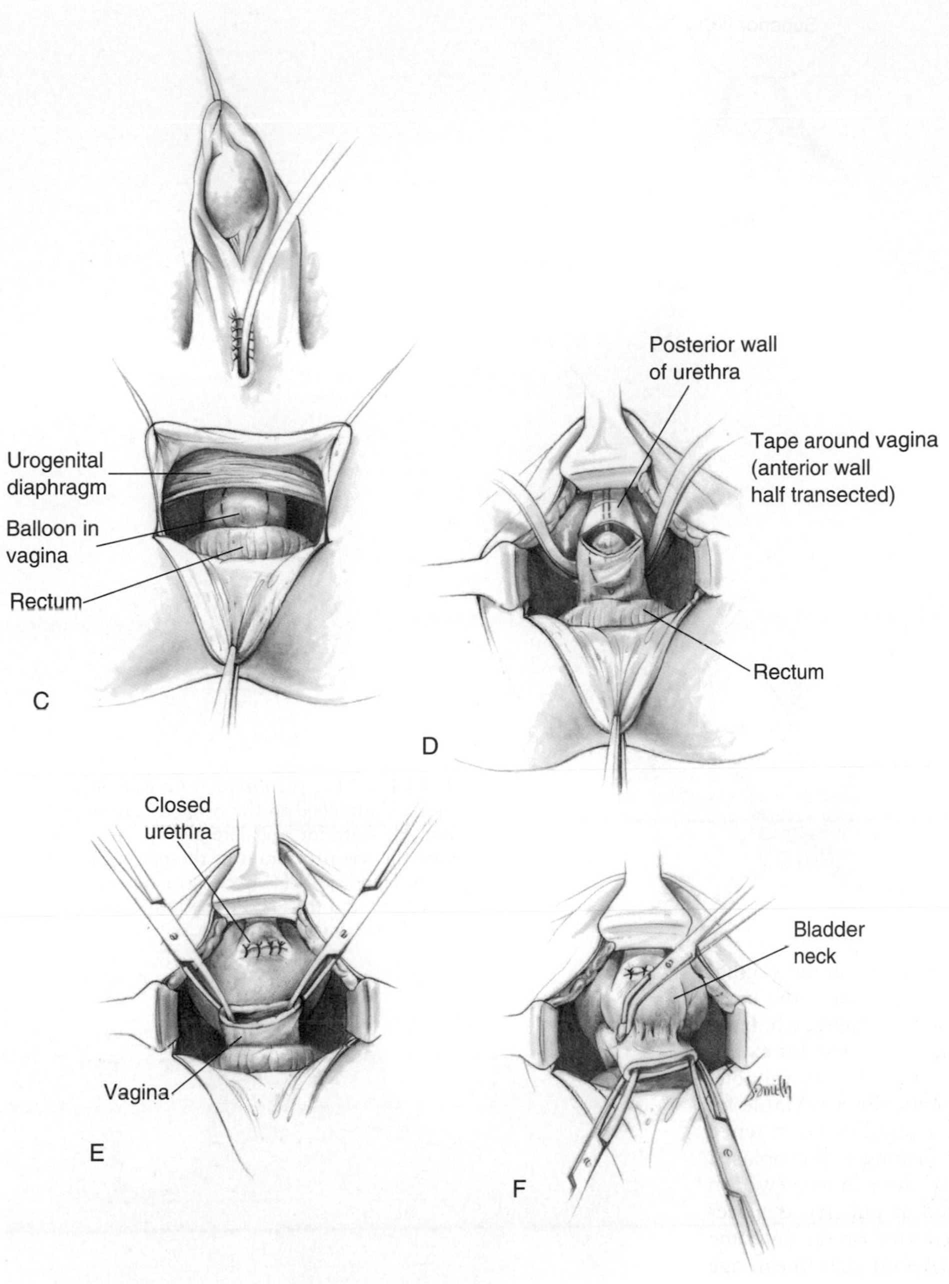

FIGURE 24.13. (*Continued*) **C:** The flap is retracted posteriorly, and the dissection is carried along the anterior wall of the rectum until the vagina (as identified by the balloon) is approached. **D:** The vagina is identified by the Foley balloon catheter. The vagina is open. Care should be taken to pull a flap of vagina distal so that there will be no problem in closing the urethra. **E:** The urethra is closed. Clips are placed on the vagina to bring it down to the perineum. **F:** The vagina is further mobilized.

rather than being intrinsic. Over the past decade, the role of testosterone imprinting of the fetal brain has been studied to evaluate the role of this hormone in determining male sexual orientation. Studies in the 1990s of girls with CAH have confirmed that such children engage in more rough-and-tumble play than their affected peers and that difficulties with adjustment to their assigned sex may exist. Nonetheless, few studies have been conducted to address the social, psychological, and sexual outcomes for affected adolescents and adults, although it appears that most function in the normal range and are well adjusted. The majority of girls appear not to overtly demonstrate sexual identity problems.

Ozbey and coauthors reported on the experience of sex (re)assignment in genotypic female (46XX) patients with CAH when complicated by delayed presentation and inadvertent assignment. They reported on 70 patients with CAH who between 1983 and 2002 were counseled for sex assignment. They evaluated age at diagnosis and operation, the degree of virilization, parental consanguinity, and the sex preference of the families as factors determining sex (re)assignment decision-making. Forty-one of seventy (59%) presented after the neonatal period, and in these cases, all of the parents had assumed or were advised of a sex based on external genitalia appearance. Forty-nine of seventy were reared as girls and 21 were reared as "boys." Of these 21 "boys," only nine could be reassigned as girls (mean age 7.9 months), and the other 12, with mean age at presentation of 55.8 months, were reared as "boys" in compliance with the parents' and the study group's decision. These "boys" underwent appropriate masculinizing reconstructive surgery. They concluded that age of presentation was critical for the ability to correctly assign the sex of patients with CAH.

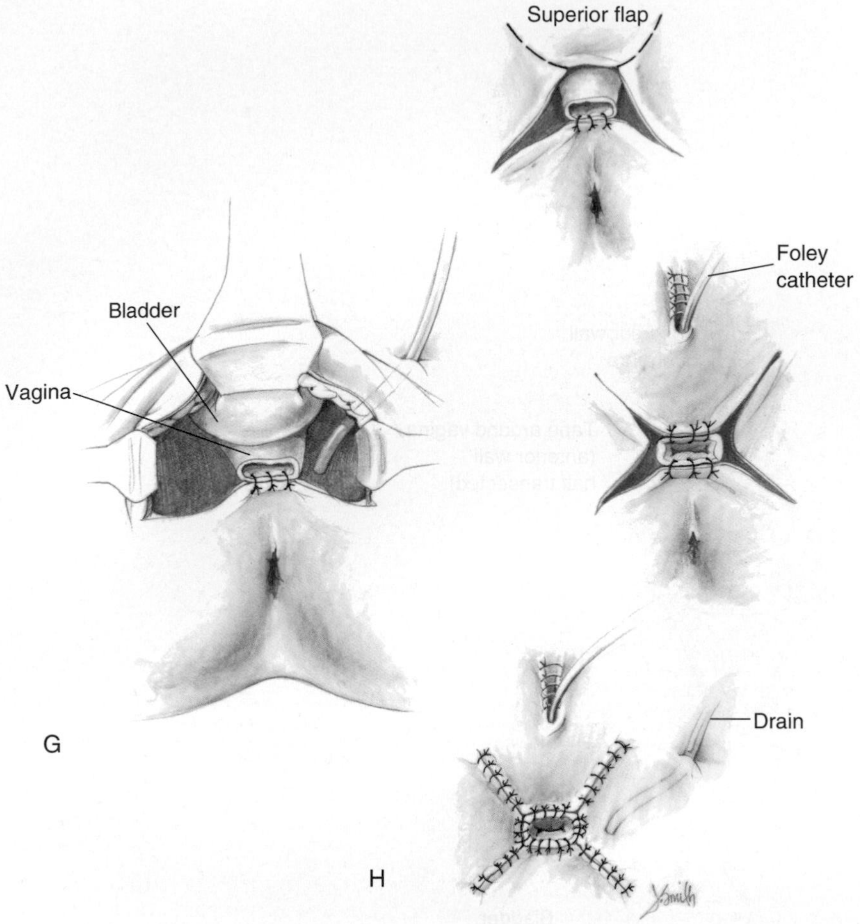

FIGURE 24.13. (*Continued*) **G:** The edge of the vagina is attached to the original flap of perineal skin. **H:** Anterior and lateral flaps are attached. Note the use of a drain in the perivaginal space. (From Hendren WH. Reconstructive problems of the vagina and the female urethra. *Clin Plast Surg* 1980;7:207, with permission.)

Secondary Operations. A secondary operation on the vaginal outlet may be required. This is generally the case if the basic operation is deliberately accomplished in two stages, whatever the reason. A secondary operation may be indicated, for example, when an infant's vaginal orifice is not readily identifiable, yet it seems desirable to construct cosmetically acceptable female genitalia at a very early age. Care should be taken when considering the appropriate age for performing a clitoroplasty. Some have recommended that this can be done in the newborn and that the vagina may be exteriorized at puberty as a second operation. Alizai and colleagues reported on the outcome of feminizing genitoplasty in 14 postpubertal girls (mean age 13.1 years) with CAH. These girls were assessed under anesthesia by a pediatric urologist, plastic/reconstructive surgeon, and gynecologist. Thirteen of fourteen had previously undergone feminizing genitoplasty in early childhood. The authors reported that the outcome of clitoral surgery was unsatisfactory (clitoral atrophy or prominent glans) in six of the girls. Additional vaginal surgery was necessary for normal comfortable intercourse in 13 of the girls. In the girls with a history of vaginal reconstruction in infancy, fibrosis and scarring were prominent. The authors concluded that these results were disappointing, even in the girls who had their surgery performed by specialist surgeons. The authors highlighted the importance of late follow-up and the challenges in the prevailing assumption that total correction can be achieved with a single-stage operation in infancy. When the complete operation is attempted at an early age, the vagina is sometimes not satisfactorily exteriorized. Vaginal stenosis may require reconstruction at the time of puberty (Fig. 24.14). In this circumstance, there usually has

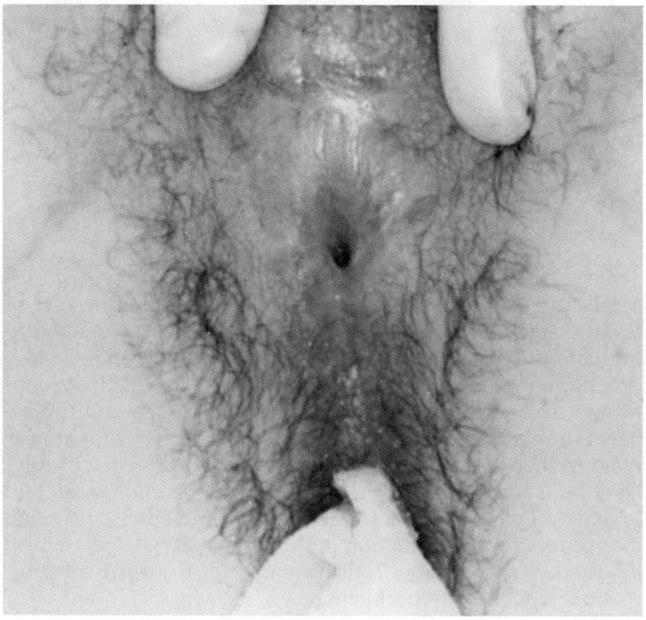

FIGURE 24.14. External genitalia of a 15-year-old patient with vaginal stenosis. Revision of the external genitalia, including an exteriorization of the vagina, had been performed in infancy.

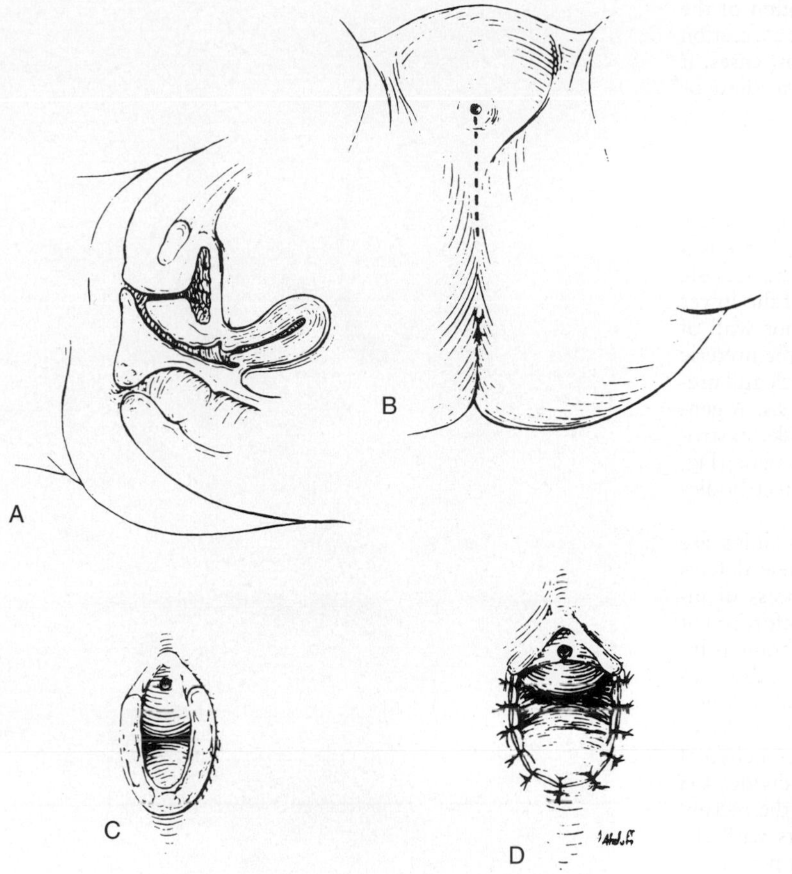

FIGURE 24.15. A: Repeated operation on the vaginal outlet when the operation was not completed at the first procedure. B: The posterior incision. C: The vagina is exposed. D: The closure.

been a failure to carry the midline incision far enough posteriorly, and a second procedure is required to complete the first one by continuing the midline incision far enough posteriorly.

In other cases, contraction at the vaginal outlet may occur even if the operation is adequately performed. A minor revision of the vaginal orifice is required to enlarge the vaginal orifice by making an incision in the midline and closing it at 90 degrees to the original axis of the incision (Fig. 24.15). In some instances, it may be necessary to create flaps to enlarge the vaginal orifice (Fig. 24.16).

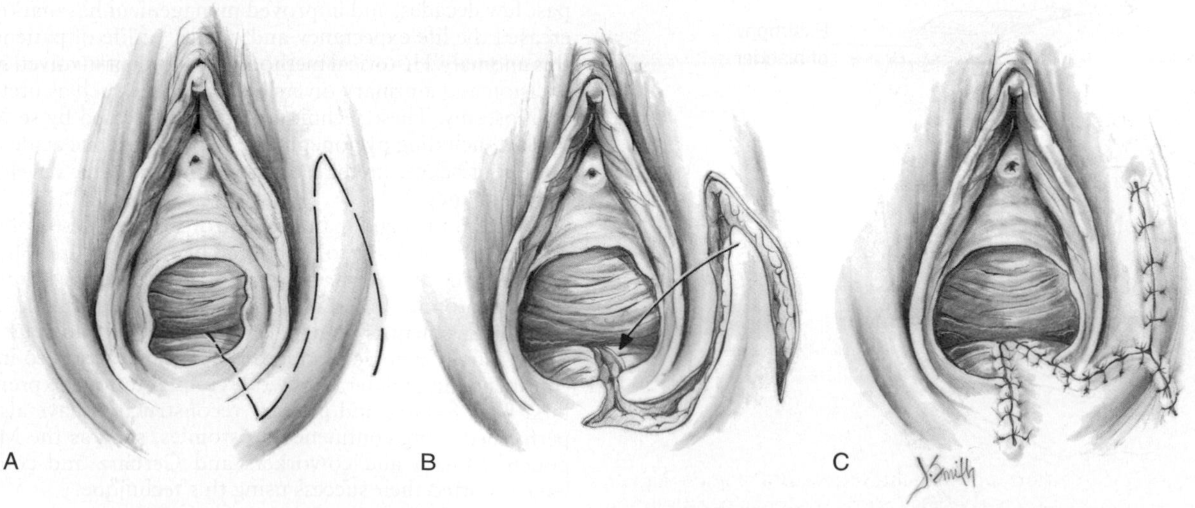

FIGURE 24.16. Labial cutaneous flap. A: An incision is made through the labia skin and subcutaneous fat. B: The flap is rotated into the perineotomy incision. C: The flap is sutured in place by interrupted 3–0 delayed-absorbable sutures. This may be repeated on the other side if required.

It should be emphasized that simple exteriorization of the lower vaginal tract can be combined with cosmetic correction of virilized external genitalia in infancy, but in most cases, it is best to defer definitive reconstruction of the intermediate or high vagina until after puberty.

Bladder Exstrophy

Exstrophy of the bladder is a rare congenital anomaly occurring in live births in a 1:25,000 to 1:40,000 ratio. There is a male predominance over females in a ratio of about 2:1. Classic bladder exstrophy is characterized by (i) absence of the lower anterior abdominal wall, (ii) absence of the anterior wall of the bladder so that the posterior bladder wall and the ureteric orifices are exposed, (iii) a poorly defined bladder neck and urethra, and (iv) wide separation of the pubic symphysis. A genital abnormality typically present in girls with bladder exstrophy is anterior displacement and narrowing of the vagina (Fig. 24.17) and separation of the clitoris into two distinct bodies (Fig. 24.18).

Bladder exstrophy, cloacal exstrophy, and epispadias are variants of the exstrophy epispadias complex. These defects have been attributed to failure of the normal process of ingrowth of mesoderm and the consequent lack of reinforcement of the cloacal membrane. The normal cloacal membrane is bilaminar and occupies the caudal end of the germinal disc. An ingrowth of mesenchyme between the ectodermal and endodermal layers of the cloacal membrane forms the lower abdominal wall musculature and the pelvic bones. After mesenchymal ingrowth occurs, descent of the urorectal septum divides the cloacal membrane into the bladder anteriorly and the rectum posteriorly. The urorectal septum eventually meets with the posterior remnant of the cloacal membrane, which perforates to form the anal and UGS openings. The paired genital tubercles migrate medially and fuse in the midline anterior to the cloacal membrane before perforation. Without its normal support from mesenchymal derivatives, the cloacal membrane is subject to premature rupture. Depending on the extent of the infraumbilical defect and the stage of development when rupture occurs, bladder exstrophy, cloacal exstrophy, or epispadias develops (Fig. 24.19).

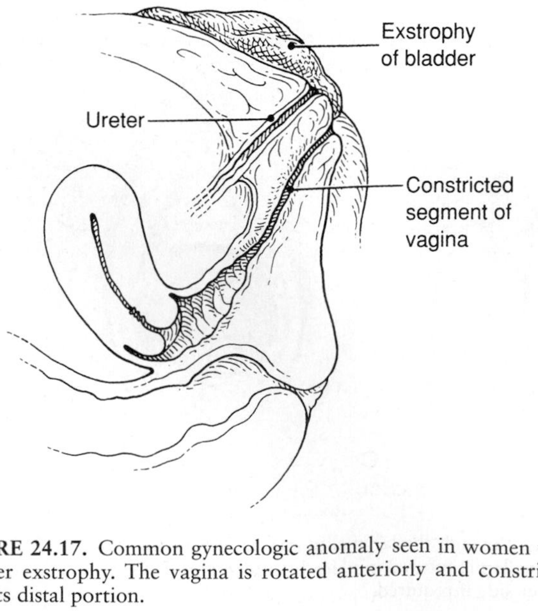

FIGURE 24.17. Common gynecologic anomaly seen in women with bladder exstrophy. The vagina is rotated anteriorly and constricted over its distal portion.

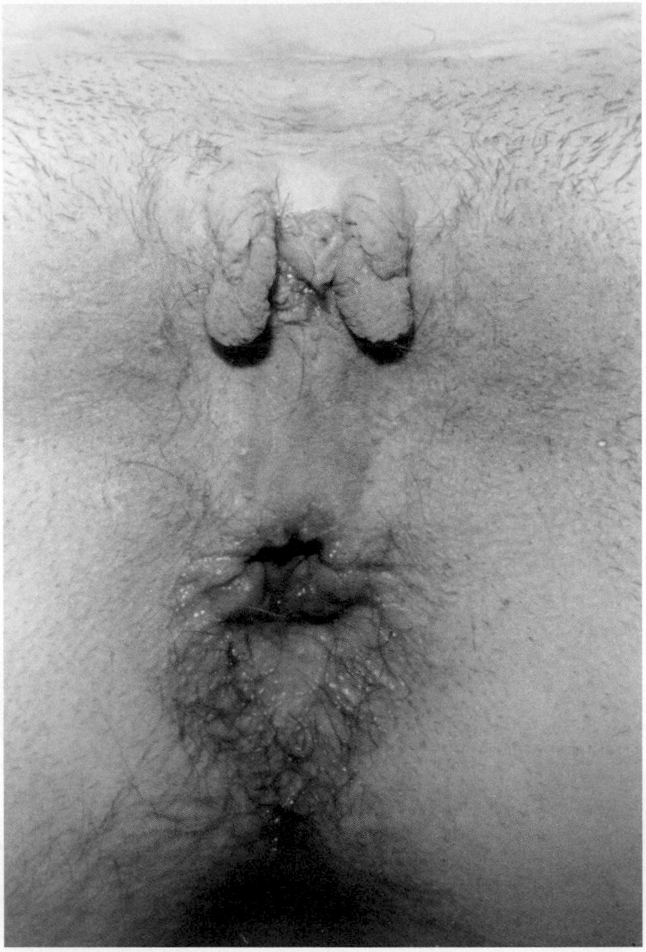

FIGURE 24.18. Preoperative photograph of a patient undergoing reconstruction of the external genitalia. Note the bifid clitoris and small anterior vaginal orifice.

Treatment. Our understanding of appropriate urologic management of bladder exstrophy has evolved greatly over the past few decades, and improved management has markedly increased the life expectancy and quality of life of patients with this anomaly. Historical methods of treatment involved bladder excision and a urinary diversion procedure such as ureterosigmoidostomy. These techniques are complicated by serious sequelae, including pyelonephritis, hyperchloremic acidosis, rectal incontinence, ureteral obstruction, and later development of malignancy.

Modern urologic management of bladder exstrophy relies on a staged approach to functional bladder closure. The initial procedure consists of primary bladder closure with or without iliac osteotomies to aid closure of the pelvic ring and growth and improvement of bladder capacity. The second-stage procedures usually involve bladder neck reconstruction to improve continence and bilateral ureteral reimplantations to prevent reflux. Both failures and primary reconstruction have also been performed using continence urostomies, such as the Mainz II pouch. Mingin and coworkers and Gerharz and colleagues have reported their success using this technique.

The prognosis using modern-day procedures is good. Although deficiency of the pelvic floor and a predisposition for pelvic organ prolapse are not unusual with bladder exstrophy, the condition of bladder exstrophy itself can often be corrected,

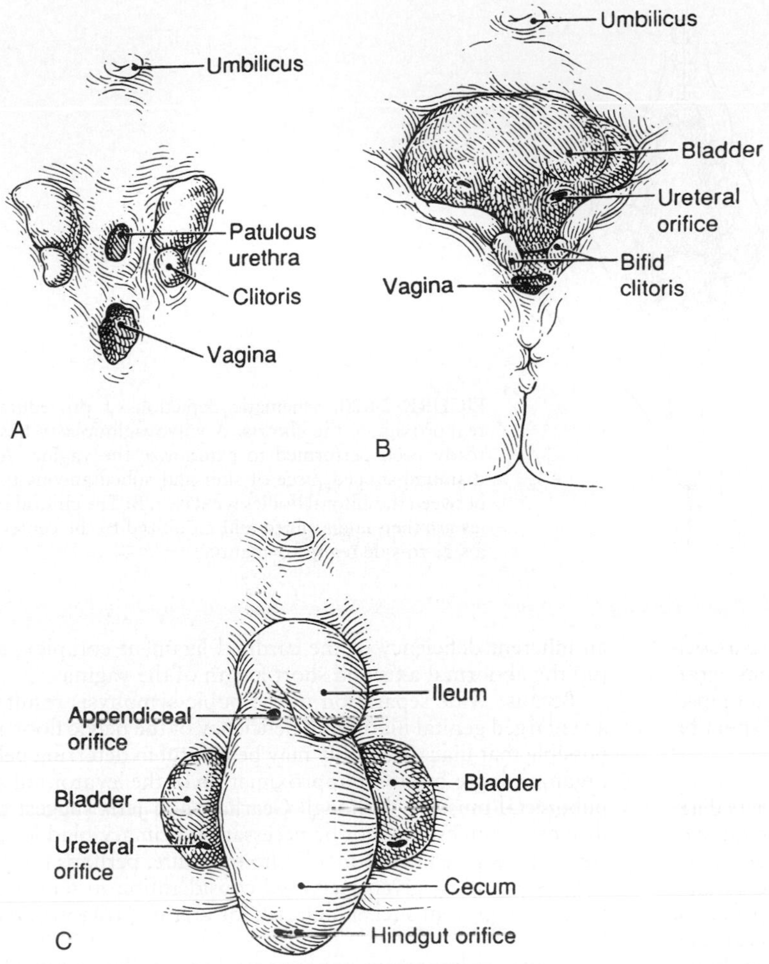

FIGURE 24.19. Anatomic features of (A) epispadias, (B) classic bladder exstrophy, and (C) cloacal exstrophy in females.

and associated genital anomalies can be managed to allow comfortable sexual activity and possibly even pregnancy.

The adjunctive procedures that may be important with surgical correction of bladder exstrophy are those that address the correction of anterior displacement and narrowing of the vagina, and separation of the clitoris into two distinct bodies that are so typically associated with bladder exstrophy.

The procedure for correcting the external genitalia has evolved from one that was first described by Howard Jones Jr. in 1973. Particular emphasis is placed on attainment of an adequate vaginal diameter without further predisposing to subsequent prolapse. The first step is vertical incision into the posterior raphe of what resembles fused scrotolabial folds; next, Allis clamps are placed laterally for traction. Fine-needle point electrocautery is then used to further open the incision, with special care taken not to take this incision too far posteriorly. The lateral portions of the incision are secured with 3-0 nonreactive absorbable sutures for further traction. The posterior vaginal edges are undermined to allow their mobilization to the exterior. The vaginal mucosa is then approximated to the perineal surface with interrupted and figure-of-eight sutures, incorporating the superficial perineal muscles into the closure. In the more posterior portion of the closure, 2–0 nonreactive absorbable suture is used, because this is the area of greatest tension. At completion, there is a significant increase in the diameter of the vagina, and the vaginal orifice usually accommodates two fingers.

Postoperative active dilatation therapy has recently been advocated. Experience with management of ambiguous genitalia has shown a decrease in the incidence of postoperative vaginal stenosis if dilatation therapy is employed during the constrictive phase (the first 6 weeks) of healing. For this reason, following reconstruction of the external genitalia and exteriorization of the vagina, appropriately sized Lucite dilators are used once or twice a day for this 6-week period or until healing is complete.

Reapproximation of the bifid clitoris (Fig. 24.20) is primarily cosmetic and is not always performed. The technique involves excising a diamond-shaped area of skin and subcutaneous tissue between the clitoral bodies. The medial aspect of each side of the clitoris is then denuded and undermined to allow a central reapproximation with a side-to-side closure.

Adjunctive Treatments. Stanton mentioned that perineotomy was performed in six patients with bladder exstrophy in which the labia and clitoris were reapproximated by a Z-plasty technique. Still others have described rather extraordinary efforts to restore the mons pubis and female escutcheon with skin flaps of hair-bearing areas. These latter reports, however, fail to mention correction of the vaginal anomaly.

Other series have described a wide range of both genital and extragenital abnormalities in association with bladder exstrophy. Stanton reviewed 70 patients with bladder exstrophy and observed an increased incidence of various müllerian

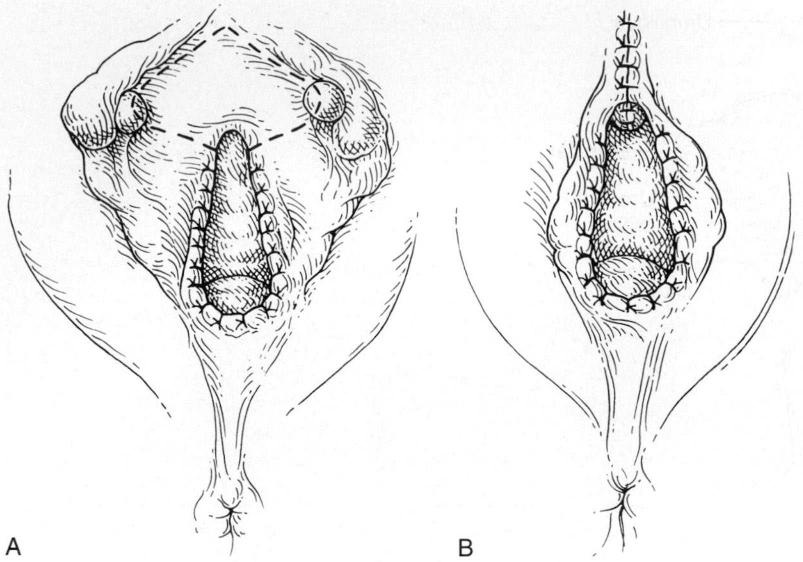

FIGURE 24.20. Schematic depiction of procedure to reapproximate the clitoris. A vulvovaginoplasty has already been performed to exteriorize the vagina. **A:** A diamond-shaped piece of skin and subcutaneous tissue between the clitoral bodies is excised. **B:** The clitoral bodies are then undermined and mobilized to the center for a side-to-side reapproximation.

anomalies. Eleven patients were also observed to have associated rectal prolapse. Blakely and Mills observed various extragenital abnormalities in their series, including rectal prolapse, imperforate anus, exophthalmos, renal agenesis, and spina bifida.

Results. Jones reviewed the records of all female patients diagnosed with bladder exstrophy at Johns Hopkins Hospital over a 20-year time span. Of 18 patients with adequately described external genitalia, 13 had small, anteriorly displaced vaginal orifices, and the remaining five patients had vaginal orifices of normal size and location. Therefore, although demonstrating phenomena very typical of bladder exstrophy, all female patients do not demonstrate the defect of narrowing of the vagina. Damario and colleagues have recently updated the Hopkins series, documenting continuing excellent long-term results.

Several series have reviewed subsequent pregnancy outcomes in patients with bladder exstrophy. Clemetson extensively reviewed the literature in 1958 and found 45 patients who underwent 64 pregnancies. A very high incidence of uterine prolapse was observed both before and after pregnancy. In addition, there was a higher incidence of premature labor and malpresentations (24%). Krisiloff and colleagues also reported a high incidence of uterine prolapse related to pregnancy, which occurred in 6 of 7 women. Burbige and coworkers reported on 14 pregnancies in patients with a history of bladder exstrophy. Uterine prolapse occurred in 7 of 11 patients, all of whom had undergone a previous urinary diversion procedure.

The mode of delivery in patients with prior urinary diversion procedures has primarily been spontaneous vaginal delivery. The increased incidence of premature labor and malpresentation, however, has warranted an increased rate of cesarean sections for obstetric indications. In patients with a prior bladder reconstruction, most surgeons advocate an elective cesarean section to eliminate stress on the pelvic floor and to avoid trauma to the delicate urinary sphincter mechanism.

Management of Uterine Prolapse with Bladder Exstrophy. Several mechanisms have been proposed to explain the high incidence of uterine prolapse in patients with bladder exstrophy. These mechanisms include (i) a deficiency of the pelvic floor that is due to the wide separation of the pubic symphysis, (ii) an inherent deficiency of the cardinal ligament complex, and (iii) the abnormal axis and short length of the vagina.

Because wide separation of the pubic symphysis results in an enlarged genital hiatus and deficiency of the pelvic floor, it is possible that iliac osteotomy may be helpful in deterring pelvic organ prolapse by closer approximation of the levator ani and puborectal muscles. Although Gearhart and Jeffs suggest that iliac osteotomies may not be necessary if primary bladder closure is performed in the first 72 hours of life, perhaps the procedure should be given increased consideration in female patients who present such a high risk for uterine prolapse later in life.

It appears important not to extend the midline perineal incision too far posteriorly in revision of the genitalia in these patients. As the incision proceeds posteriorly, the midline septum thickens to approximately 2 cm. At this point, the levator ani muscles may be severed, further enlarging the genital hiatus. It is prudent, therefore, to be more conservative; postoperative dilator therapy may aid in achieving further vaginal diameter if needed.

A case referred to us illustrated this point. A 16-year-old nulliparous patient with bladder exstrophy and a history of staged bladder reconstruction underwent revision of the external genitalia. A large posterior incision into the perineal body had left a gaping introitus, and uterine prolapse had occurred several months after this procedure. Our initial approach was to reconstruct the perineal body to help contain the uterus and improve support to the pelvic floor. This reconstruction has been successful, without further prolapse 5 years after the procedure. Blakely and Mills, who observed uterine prolapse occurring very soon after enlargement of the vaginal introitus, reported a similar case.

Management of uterine prolapse associated with bladder exstrophy may be difficult. The patient frequently desires preservation of her childbearing capacity. Sacrospinous fixation of the cervix may be considered, although an abnormally short vagina may produce difficulty in obtaining the suspension without significant suture bridges. An abdominal sacrocervicopexy may also be considered. Dewhurst and coworkers described this approach in 1980. They suspended the uterus to the sacrum using Ivalon sponge in a patient with procidentia following repair of bladder exstrophy.

The high historical incidence of uterine prolapse and the potential difficulties managing this problem highlight the need for the reconstructive surgeon to give extra thought and care to revision of the external genitalia in women with bladder exstrophy. Inappropriate reconstruction may actually accelerate genital prolapse. In addition, elective cesarean section may be the most judicious mode of delivery for limiting traumatic insults to the pelvic floor that could further increase the propensity for prolapse. Ricci and coworkers evaluated 17 patients (15 children, 2 young adults) with bladder exstrophy for latex allergy. Twelve shared latex sensitization, with five demonstrating symptoms. The multiple operative and cystoscope procedures performed on this group of patients has resulted in significant latex exposure and sensitization similar to that seen in health care workers.

Carcinoma of the Vagina

Carcinoma of the vagina is uncommon, occurring in less than 2% of patients with gynecologic malignancies. The average age at presentation is 60 years. Vaginal carcinoma is most frequently secondary to metastases from tumors of the cervix and vulva rather than originating in the vagina. Lesions that encroach on the outer vagina from the vulva must be separated from lesions that originate in the vaginal canal to be considered a vaginal primary.

The International Federation of Obstetrics and Gynecology (FIGO) has agreed on the following exclusionary criteria for the classification of vaginal cancer:

1. A vaginal growth extending to the portio of the cervix and reaching the area of the external os should always be considered a carcinoma of the cervix.
2. A vulvar growth that has extended to the vagina should be classified as carcinoma of the vulva.
3. A vaginal growth that is limited to the urethra should be classified separately as carcinoma of the urethra.

Clinicians now satisfy the staging criteria for the diagnosis of primary carcinoma of the vagina by showing a histologically negative cervix, urethra, vulva, and endometrium.

The criteria for the definition of primary carcinoma of the vagina were established after many clinicians reported the recurrence of vaginal lesions after treatment of carcinoma in situ of the cervix. Tumors recurred in 1% to 6% of cases. Today, extension of carcinoma in situ and invasive carcinoma of the cervix to the vaginal fornices or upper vagina can be easily identified with the use of colposcopy.

The clinical stages of carcinoma of the vagina agreed on by FIGO are listed in Table 24.1. In 1973, Perez and coworkers proposed that stage II be divided into stage IIa and IIb to provide a more accurate definition of the extent of the lesion. In the proposed modified FIGO classification, stage IIa includes subvaginal infiltration not extending into the parametrial regions, whereas stage IIb includes parametrial or paravaginal infiltration not extending to the pelvic wall. This classification has not been accepted by FIGO. Creasman and colleagues queried the National Cancer Data Base (NCDB), a central registry of hospital case data, for 1985 through 1994. Of the 4,885 cases, 75% were invasive and 90% epithelial. Survival at 5 years was as follows: stage 0, 96%; stage I, 73%; stage II, 58%; stage III-IV, 36%. The overall 5-year survival rate with melanoma was 14%.

TABLE 24.1

INTERNATIONAL FEDERATION OF OBSTETRICS AND GYNECOLOGY CLASSIFICATION OF VAGINAL CARCINOMA

Preinvasive Carcinoma	
Stage 0	Carcinoma in situ, intraepithelial carcinoma.
Invasive Carcinoma	
Stage I	Carcinoma limited to the vaginal wall.
Stage II	Carcinoma involving the subvaginal tissue, but not extending onto the pelvic wall.
Stage III	Carcinoma extending onto the pelvic wall.
Stage IV	Carcinoma extending beyond the true pelvis or involving the mucosa of the bladder or rectum. Bullous edema that does not permit a case to be allotted to stage IV.
Stage IVa	Spread of the growth to adjacent organs.
Stage IVb	Spread to distant organs.

From Pettersson F, ed. *Annual report on the results of treatment in gynecologic cancer.* Stockholm: FIGO; 1988:174.

Symptoms

The diagnosis of vaginal tumors frequently is delayed because of the lack of early symptoms. Progressive vaginal discharge and postmenopausal bleeding are the most frequent symptoms. Postcoital bleeding can also herald the presence of a vaginal or cervical carcinoma. More than 10% of patients are asymptomatic at the time of diagnosis.

Women with a history of vaginal, vulvar, and cervical intraepithelial neoplasia have an increased risk of vaginal carcinoma. These patients should receive annual Papanicolaou smears even if they have undergone a hysterectomy. Having a hysterectomy for other than preneoplastic or neoplastic conditions does not increase the risk for developing vaginal carcinoma.

The symptoms of vaginal carcinoma resemble those of cervical carcinoma, except that obvious bleeding occurs later than with neoplasms on the cervix. The overt bleeding eventually forces the patient to see her physician for diagnosis. The type of pelvic pain is frequently indicative of lesion location. The posterior vagina, the most common location of vaginal carcinomas, presents with tenesmus and other bowel symptoms. Anterior tumors, on the other hand, result in urethral and bladder symptoms.

Histopathology

The most common histologic type of primary vaginal tumor is squamous carcinoma, which accounts for 84% to 90% of all vaginal cancers (Table 24.2). Adenocarcinoma, including diethylstilbestrol (DES)-related cases, represents about 4% to 9% of vaginal cancers. Sarcomas, including leiomyosarcoma and sarcoma botryoides, account for 2% to 3% of vaginal lesions, and melanomas account for 1% to 2% of malignant neoplasms of the vagina. Rare tumors, such as endodermal sinus tumors or neoplasms originating in embryologic cloacal remnants, may form a transitional cell neoplasm that involves the vagina.

Squamous carcinoma of the vagina is discovered in 10% to 15% of cases after the finding of squamous cancer in other parts of the lower genital tract, such as the vulva or cervix. This has led to the theory of multicentric origin of squamous cancer

TABLE 24.2

HISTOLOGIC TYPES OF VAGINAL CANCER AND FREQUENCY OF OCCURRENCE

Type	Frequency (%)
Squamous carcinoma	85–90
Adenocarcinoma (including DES-related)	4–9
Sarcoma	2–3
Melanoma	2–3
Other	1–2

DES, diethylstilbestrol.

in the lower genital tract. Woodruff and Parmley and others emphasize this correlation and have recommended that patients with squamous cancer in one area be categorized as high risk for the development of squamous carcinoma in other sites of the lower genital tract. A viral etiology, such as the human papillomavirus, is most likely responsible for these findings.

Carcinoma may arise in the neovagina lined with a split-thickness skin graft from the buttock or lateral thigh. Carcinoma of the neovagina is a rare cancer; only nine cases have been reported. The primary carcinoma seems to be related to the transplanted tissue. In three cases, adenocarcinoma was associated with the use of a large or small bowel intestinal graft for vaginal reconstruction. Five cases of squamous cell cancer arising from the graft have been documented. The transplanted epithelium in the vagina may be exposed to an unidentified carcinogen or mutagen, as has been documented with the vulva, and can undergo malignant transformation in this environment. These observations underscore the need for regular pelvic examinations after operative vaginoplasty with either a bowel graft or a split-thickness skin graft.

DES, a nonsteroidal estrogenic hormone thought to enhance embryo implantation and placental development, was introduced into clinical obstetrics in 1944 in Boston and became popular and widely used during the next two decades. Women with a history of previous spontaneous abortions or other risk factors for early pregnancy loss of multiple gestations were given DES. It is known now that DES use during the first trimester of pregnancy may cause vaginal neoplasia. It was not until the late 1960s, however—when a cluster of cases of adenocarcinoma appeared in young women younger than age 25 years (all offspring of DES-treated women)—that Herbst and colleagues connected the result with the unusual cause.

From 1944 to 1970, about 1.5 to 2 million female offspring were exposed to DES. Fortunately, the incidence of vaginal adenocarcinoma in these young women has been quite low, ranging from 0.14 to 1.4 in 1,000 exposed women. More than 500 documented cases have been reported to the DES registry to date.

Observations of the development of vaginal adenosis and adenocarcinoma in teenage girls whose mothers were given DES before the 18th week of pregnancy brought new insights to the study of squamous tumor cells in the lower genital tract and greatly increased our understanding of the embryologic development of the vagina. The effect of the DES drug provided an indisputable histologic foundation for the development of an uncommon vaginal adenocarcinoma in women younger than 29 years of age. Twenty-five percent of women exposed in utero have anatomic cervical, vaginal, and urinary tract abnormalities.

The DES-associated adenocarcinoma originally was thought to arise from mesonephric remnants in the vagina, and the disease consequently was mislabeled as a clear cell carcinoma. However, electron microscopic analysis of the ultrastructure of both the adenocarcinoma and the vaginal adenosis allowed Fenoglio and colleagues to clearly define these lesions as composed of columnar epithelium, similar in all respects to endocervical epithelium, and of paramesonephric (müllerian) origin. The colposcopic studies of Stafl and Mattingly and of others confirm these observations.

Vaginal adenosis has been found by colposcopic examination to occur in 34% to 90% of exposed offspring and vaginal adenocarcinoma in 50%. Although the hypothesis is still unproven, there is a strong possibility that the benign vaginal lesion is the cell of origin for vaginal adenocarcinoma. The risk of development of clear cell adenocarcinoma in an exposed woman between birth and age 34 is 1 in 1,000.

Etiology

During embryologic development, the vagina is formed from the columnar epithelium of the müllerian ducts and UGS. The tissue then transforms into squamous epithelium, so that the vaginal and cervical epithelium have a common embryologic origin. Squamous metaplasia within the vaginal adenosis has been observed with a colposcope, and transformation of the metaplastic tissue also has been demonstrated in the development of intraepithelial neoplasia. Although many agents have been postulated as carcinogenic factors, none have been positively demonstrated. It is quite possible that squamous carcinoma arises from the effects of an oncogenic agent on the transformation zone within the foci of vaginal adenosis. The studies now being done on the effects of DES may find some interesting causative factors that influence vaginal carcinoma.

Carcinoma of the vagina also may share a common causative denominator with cervical carcinoma. Because slightly more than 50% of the cases occur in the posterior wall of the upper third of the vagina, which is the end point of vaginal coitus, vaginal carcinoma could be venereally induced. As with cervical carcinoma, primary carcinoma of the vagina usually occurs in sexually active women. Except for the cases of adenocarcinoma in young women exposed to DES, squamous carcinoma of the vagina is unquestionably associated with sexual activity. As with cervical intraepithelial neoplasia and carcinoma, the human papillomavirus is probably responsible for the majority of vaginal carcinomas.

Site of Lesion

Plentl and Friedman found that 51% of vaginal carcinoma lesions occur in the upper third of the vagina, 30% in the lower third, and 19% in the middle third. In the lower third, lesions most often occur in the anterior wall, whereas in the upper third, lesions most often appear in the posterior vaginal wall. Although the location is observed on diagnosis, the precise site of origin is difficult to pinpoint because the tumors usually have spread to various parts of the vagina by that time.

Pathways of Spread

The lymphatic drainage of the vagina takes place through different pathways. The upper third drains by way of the cervical lymphatics, the lower third passes by way of the vulvar lymphatics, and the middle third communicates with both the upper and the lower lymphatic channels. The vaginal vault and the anterior wall of the upper vagina drain to the interiliac pelvic lymph nodes, where they communicate with the external iliac, the hypogastric, and the common iliac nodes. The lymphatic drainage of the posterior vagina communicates directly with the deep pelvic nodes, including the inferior gluteal, sacral, and rectal nodes.

Because the major pathways of lymphatic drainage are to the superior and inferior gluteal muscles and the common iliac lymph nodes, the potential for extrapelvic spread of vaginal carcinoma is great. When extrapelvic spread occurs, prognosis usually is poor. The primary site of origin of the tumor is an important indicator of lymph node metastases, whether the tumor will metastasize to the inguinal-femoral chain or to the deep pelvic lymph nodes. When the disease involves the lower third of the vagina, 6% to 7% of patients have metastases to the inguinal-femoral lymph nodes.

Diagnosis

In general, invasive carcinoma of the vagina appears as either a raised exophytic lesion or an ulcerative, depressed lesion in the vaginal wall. Biopsy can be performed on both types of lesions easily, and diagnosis can be established without difficulty. Vaginal cytology usually is positive if an adequate cell sample is obtained from the exfoliated lesion, although, as often happens with cervical carcinoma, many cases of false-negative cytology occur even when an invasive lesion is present. Colposcopy, Lugol solution, or both can be used to demarcate the areas for biopsy, although iodine staining usually is unnecessary if the lesion is clearly visible.

Identifying vaginal carcinoma at an early stage can be a major problem because the first lesions appear within the epithelial cells, frequently indistinguishable from the remainder of the vaginal epithelium. Only by colposcopic examination or with iodine staining can alterations in the surface epithelium of the vagina be identified. Ng and associates have achieved an accuracy of 88% to 90% in detecting dysplastic lesions in DES-exposed patients with adenosis, but their technique requires separate, four-quadrant vaginal smears from the walls of the vagina to increase the sensitivity of the Papanicolaou smear. Herbst and coworkers emphasize the advantage of iodine staining of the vagina to reveal occult lesions that may be associated with adenosis. Stafl and Mattingly reported an accuracy of 96% in detecting abnormal epithelial lesions of the vagina in DES-exposed women by careful examination and colposcopy.

Because the vaginal speculum can obscure surface lesions and delay early diagnosis, the instrument should be rotated during the examination so that the entire canal can be inspected. With iodine staining, the clinician can detect multifocal lesions, but the entire vagina also should be cytologically tested. A thorough colposcopic examination can be used to detect vaginal carcinoma if the clinician has that expertise.

Treatment

Primary vaginal carcinoma is treated either with surgery or with radiotherapy. The choice of treatment depends on three factors: the size of the lesion, the location of the tumor in the vagina, and the clinical stage of the disease.

Stage 0 Lesions. Easiest to treat by far is vaginal intraepithelial neoplasia III (VAIN III), and it offers the most hopeful prognosis. Either surgery or radiotherapy can be used, depending on the location of the lesion. If the disease is located in the upper vagina and the margins of the disease are distinct, a partial vaginectomy, with or without hysterectomy, is a practical and successful method of treatment.

The carbon dioxide laser has proved to be a simple, effective means of treating noninvasive vaginal carcinoma. Laser therapy offers conservative treatment for both focal and multicentric lesions without impairment of normal coital function. Because there is a risk of residual disease in 10% of laser-treated patients, careful colposcopic and cytologic follow-up are critical. Histologic study is difficult after the carbon dioxide laser vaporizes the treated lesions. An alternative ablative technique is the ultrasonic surgical aspirator, the tip of which vibrates 23,000 times per second, fragmenting and aspirating the tissue in contact with it. This technique permits histologic evaluation of the collected tissue fragments. The operative site also heals faster secondary to decreased thermal damage. Robinson and colleagues reported their experience in treating 46 patients with VAIN. Sixty-six percent (29) of those initially treated with ultrasonic surgical aspiration did not have recurrence. Fifty-two percent of patients treated for recurrent disease (17) did not experience a recurrence. The mean duration of follow-up was 21 months.

Nonsurgical methods such as administration of 5-fluorouracil vaginal cream have also proved efficacious in treating VAIN.

Radiation therapy is rarely used to treat VAIN. However, radiation is an excellent modality for suspected invasion when the medical risk for further evaluation by surgery is too great.

A vaginal cylinder, such as the Bloedorn applicator, can be used for radiotherapeutic treatment to deliver 70 Gy to the vaginal surface over a period of about 72 hours. If the lesion is confined to the vaginal fornices, vaginal colpostats can be used to deliver a similar dosage. Lesions in the lower third of the vagina may be treated by partial vaginectomy or by intravaginal irradiation using a variety of brachytherapy techniques.

Stage I Lesions. Surgery, radiation, or both are the primary modalities for treating vaginal carcinomas. Lesions in the vaginal fornix can be treated with a radical Wertheim hysterectomy, partial vaginectomy, and bilateral pelvic lymphadenectomy. Treatment for this lesion is similar to that for stage Ib cervical carcinoma. If pelvic lymph nodes are histologically positive or if paraaortic lymph nodes look suspicious, a paraaortic lymphadenectomy should be performed. If the lymph nodes are histologically positive for carcinoma, pelvic radiation with or without paraaortic radiation should be administered. As with cervical carcinoma, the size of the lesion is prognostic of our ability to adequately treat these patients with primary surgery. Large lesions not permitting clear surgical margins (e.g., proximity to the bladder or rectum) should be treated with primary radiation therapy. Radical surgery also may require the replacement of the upper vagina with a split-thickness skin graft to reestablish normal vaginal length for a sexually active woman. Irradiation therapy is an alternative treatment for this stage of disease.

The radical Wertheim hysterectomy has been quite successful in treating stage I adenocarcinoma in young women who were exposed to DES in utero. More than 75% of patients are cured. Magrina and associates treated a patient with stage I disease at their institution with laparoscopic radical parametrectomy and pelvic and aortic lymphadenectomy. The role of laparoscopy in the treatment of vaginal carcinoma will continue to expand. Although its role in parametrectomy may be debated, laparoscopy to excise the pelvic and periaortic nodes before radiation may be beneficial to patients with advanced disease.

Sentinel Node Detection. Sentinel node detection in vaginal carcinoma has not gained universal acceptance. Gynecologic tumor—such as cervical and vulvar—have been much more amicable to sentinel node detection and biopsy. Van Dam and colleagues used ^{99m}TC-labeled nanocolloids in primary and recurrent vaginal carcinomas. Nodes were identified laparoscopically and resected. Three of four patients had nodes identified through sentinel node detection.

Radiation therapy is the preferable treatment for large proximal lesions or middle or distal vaginal tumors. A combination of teletherapy (external beam) and interstitial or intracavity therapy is used.

Stage II and Stage III Lesions. More extensive lesions of the vagina pose an extremely difficult therapeutic problem for the gynecologist. Because the levator ani muscles of the pelvic diaphragm surround the vagina, penetration of the lateral wall of the vagina by the invasive tumor frequently is associated with fixation of the disease to the adjacent pelvic musculature. Even radical surgery cannot effectively control the disease when it extends beyond the confines of the vagina into the paravaginal tissues. Instead, the major method of treatment for stage II and stage III lesions is radiotherapy.

When stage II lesions involve the anterior or posterior wall of the vaginal septum, an anterior or posterior exenteration with pelvic node dissection may be required. When the disease includes the lower third of the vagina, a groin dissection is necessary also. Because surgery must be so extensive, its usefulness is limited when the disease affects the paravaginal region (stage IIb) or the lateral vaginal wall (stage III).

Stage IV Lesions. When advanced lesions involve only the bladder or the rectum, exenteration may be required to control the disease effectively. Unfortunately, pelvic exenteration, either anterior or posterior, can be used only when there is no other extension of the disease, and it is rare for the bladder and rectum to be involved without involvement of the adjacent paravaginal tissues. If the patient is not an acceptable surgical risk for exenteration, external beam megavoltage irradiation therapy followed by intravaginal or interstitial irradiation can be used to control the local disease and to offer palliation. If the tumor does not respond after 5,000 cGY of irradiation treatment to the whole pelvis, an exenteration may be required to control the disease in properly selected patients. Exenteration is also recommended for central recurrences without lymph node metastasis.

Advanced/Recurrent Disease. Pelvic exenteration is the best treatment for patients who have failed primary irradiation therapy of vaginal carcinoma. As with cervical carcinoma, it is imperative that the recurrences be central and nodes radiographically negative. Before performing the exenteration, pelvic and periaortic nodes are sent for frozen section. Depending on the age of the patient, continent urinary diversions, neovaginal, and primary end-to-end colon anastomosis are performed when possible. Berek and colleagues reported on their 45-year pelvic exoneration experience at UCLA. Survival for cervical/vaginal cancers was 73% at 1 year, 57% at 3 years, and 54% at 5 years (Fig. 24.21). Positive margins had a deleterious effect on survival (Fig. 24.22).

Irradiation Therapy

Irradiation treatment of vaginal carcinoma is easily divided between lesions in the upper and middle thirds and the lower third of the vagina.

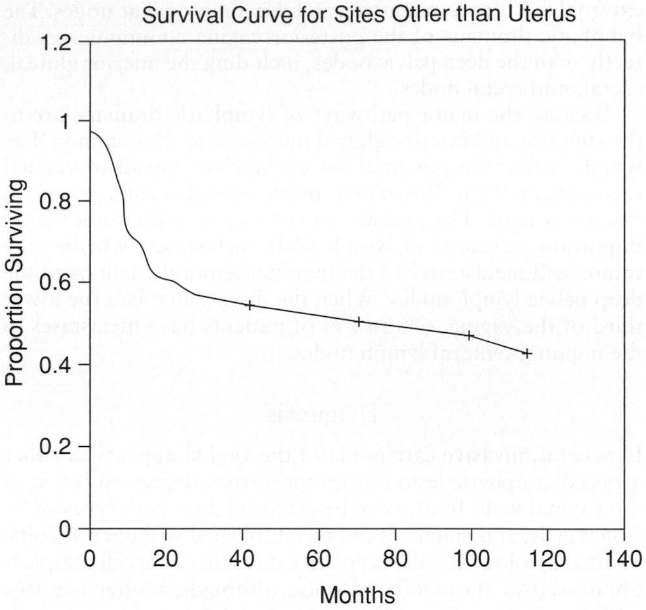

FIGURE 24.21. Survival of patients with recurrent cervical and vaginal cancers following pelvic exenteration. (From Berek JS, Howe C, Lagasse LD, et al. Pelvic exenteration for recurrent gynecologic malignancy: survival and morbidity analysis of the 45-year experience at UCLA. *Gynecol Oncol* 2005;99:157.)

Upper and Middle Thirds of the Vagina. Because the lymphatic drainage of the upper and middle vagina extends through the hypogastric and pelvic nodes, full pelvic irradiation is necessary. Treatment usually includes a combination of techniques.

External beam megavoltage therapy using 4,500 to 5,000 cGY focused on the midplane of the pelvis is used to treat the full pelvis and to encompass the vagina. A vaginal implant of

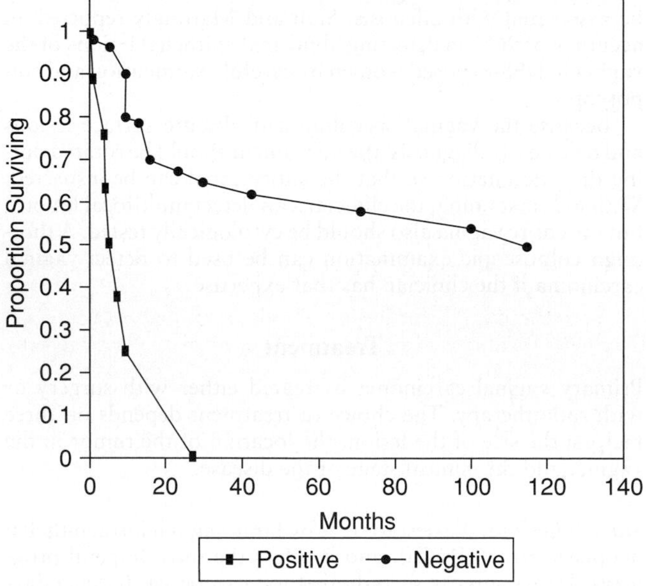

FIGURE 24.22. Survival based on status of surgical margins. (From Berek JS, Howe C, Lagasse LD, et al. Pelvic exenteration for recurrent gynecologic malignancy: survival and morbidity analysis of the 45-year experience at UCLA. *Gynecol Oncol* 2005;99:158.)

TABLE 24.3

ABSOLUTE 5-YEAR SURVIVAL AFTER IRRADIATION THERAPY FOR CARCINOMA OF THE VAGINA

	Proportion Surviving				
FIGO Stage	M. D. Anderson Hospital[a] 1948–1967	University of Maryland[e] 1970–2000	Washington University[b] 1957–1970	Vienna University[c] 1950–1977	1950–1977
I	/16 (69%)	/50 (85%)	/6 (83%)	/39 (85%)	/60 (75%)
II	/19 (68%)	/97 (78%)	/31 (64%)	/60 (47%)	/95 (45%)
IIa		/20 (65%)	/39 (51%)		
IIb		/11 (63%)	/21 (33%)		
III	/15 (27%)	/39 (58%)	/20 (40%)	/12 (33%)	/145 (30%)
IV	/11 (0%)	/7	/7 (0%)	/8 (19%)	/62 (19%)
I–IV	/61 (46%)		/64 (52%)	/119[d] (53%)	/362 (40%)

[a]Data from Hilgers RD. Squamous cell carcinoma of the vagina. *Surg Clin North Am* 1978;58:25.
[b]Data from Perez CA, Camel HM. Long-term follow-up in radiation therapy of carcinoma of the vagina. *Cancer* 1982;49:1308.
[c]Data from Kucera H, Langer M, Smekal G, et al. Radiotherapy of primary carcinoma of the vagina: management and results of different therapy schemes. *Gynecik Ibcik* 1985;21:87.
[d]Not included in the figure 119 are 15 patients of the total patient group of 134 who were stage 0.
[e]Data from Pecorelli S, ed. FIGO annual report on the results of treatment in gynecological cancer. *Int J Gynecol Obstet* 2003;83:27.

radium, cesium, or iridium follows, delivering an additional 3,000 to 4,000 cGY to a depth of 0.5 to 1.0 cm or more, depending on the thickness of the lesion.

At the M.D. Anderson Hospital, Brown and coworkers demonstrated the efficacy of using a radium needle implant for localized lesions. When the implant is used, high doses of radiation to the entire vagina, bladder, and rectum are avoided. Interstitial needles and iridium wires have been used as a primary treatment for localized vaginal lesions, and they can be used for persistent disease.

Lower Third of the Vagina. Lesions in the lower third of the vagina frequently metastasize to the inguinal-femoral lymphatics and must be treated with full external and intravaginal irradiation followed by external beam irradiation treatment to the inguinal-femoral lymph nodes. The inguinal-femoral regions require either a surgical groin dissection or the application of 5,000 to 6,000 cGY of electron beam teletherapy in addition to full pelvic irradiation. When vaginal lesions have metastasized to the groin lymph nodes, the cure rate is equally poor for both methods. In general, the presence of tumor in the groin nodes is a poor prognostic sign, suggesting that the deep pelvic nodes also may be involved in about 6% to 7% of cases. Because the incidence of vaginal cancer is so low, the exact frequency with which the deep pelvic nodes are involved has not been documented.

Chemoradiation for large bulky lesions may play a role in vaginal carcinoma, just as it does in cervical or vulvar lesions. Agents such as cisplatin, 5-fluorouracil, and hydroxyurea have been successfully used.

The number of patients with vaginal carcinoma reported to the FIGO registry by international clinics between 1979 and 1981 totals 547. Seventy-eight percent of these patients were treated by radiation. Only 38.6% of these patients were alive at 5 years. Results from other institutions that primarily have followed radiation therapy show that only stage I lesions have an adequate 5-year survival rate (Table 24.3).

In a retrospective analysis of 134 patients with carcinoma of the vagina treated at Washington University, Perez and Camel report an actuarial disease-free, 5-year survival rate of 85% for stage I lesions, 51% for stage IIa lesions, 33% for stage IIb lesions, 33% for stage III lesions, and 19% for stage IV lesions. The actuarial study demonstrated that beyond stage I of the disease, control is poor. For stage IIa lesions, local control of the disease was achieved in only 65% of cases at the University of Maryland because external irradiation was not used in all cases. Pelvic control was achieved in 48% of stage IIb and stage III lesions, but in none of the seven patients (0%) with stage IV disease.

Overall survival rates for stages I through IV from published reports are outlined in Table 24.4. The highest survival rates are observed in stage I disease, whereas few patients survive for 5 years after the diagnosis of stage IV disease.

THE URETHRA

The female urethra develops from the caudal end of the UGS after it separates from the vaginal canal between the 8th and 12th week of embryologic life. Because the vagina and urethra are so closely integrated, the urethra shares many common disease processes and anatomic defects with the vagina. Bacteria in the lower genital tract frequently colonize in the outer urethra, harbor in the paraurethral glands, and enter the bladder to produce acute infections. A bacterial infection in the lower genital tract may not become clinically manifest for several years, until a Skene duct cyst or a urethral diverticulum develops.

Estrogen deficiency causes atrophic changes of the vaginal mucosa and can have a similar effect on the urethral mucosa. Thinning of the epithelium and irritation of the sensory nerve fibers can cause urinary frequency and dysuria. Prolapse at the external meatus also may result from atrophic changes of the urethra.

Diverticulum of the Urethra

Despite the many documented cases of urethral diverticula, the condition has not been well recognized by the medical profession. Anderson observed a urethral diverticulum in 3% of 300 cases undergoing treatment for cervical carcinoma. The condition probably occurs more frequently than it is diagnosed;

TABLE 24.4

CARCINOMA OF THE VAGINA: COMPARISON OF SURVIVAL (%)

		Stage				
Investigators	Years Studied	I	II	III	IV	Total
Puthawala et al., 1983[a]	1976–1979	100	75	22	0	56
Gallup et al., 1987[a]	1971–1984	100	50	0	25	43
Brown et al., 1971[a]	1948–1967	69	68	27	0	46
Nori et al., 1983[a]	1950–1974	71	61	33	0	42
Perez, 1981[a]	1965–1981	81	42	30	9	50
Prempree, 1982[a]	1957–1975	78	57	39	0	48
Benedet et al., 1983[a]	1950–1980	71	50	15	0	45
Manetta et al., 1988[a]	1976–1986	71	47	33	33	48
Eddy et al., 1991[b]	1970–1989	84	70	45	35	28
Stock et al., 1995[b]	1962–1992	100	67	53	0	15
Creasman et al., 1998[b]	1985–1994	792	73	58	58	58
Frank et al., 2003[b]	1970–2000	165	78	56	37	46
Viswanathan et al., 2003[b]		58	70	64	32	0
Tabata et al., 2002[b]	1957–1995	51	82	70	0	0
Mock et al., 2003[b]		86	41	43	37	0
Otton et al., 2004[b]	1982–1998	70	71	48		

[a]Adapted from Manetta A, Perito JL, Larson JE, et al. Primary invasive carcinoma of the vagina. *Obstet Gynecol* 1988;72:77.
[b]Adapted from Creasman WT. Vaginal cancers. *Curr Opin Obstet Gynecol* 2005;17:71.

whenever an article reporting on urethral diverticulum appears in the literature, there is a coincident upsurge in the number of cases diagnosed. According to the National Hospital Discharge Survey Data Base (1979–1998), 27,000 inpatient procedures were performed for the repair of urethral diverticula in the United States over a 19-year period. The surgical treatment is three times as high in African American women. Moreover, the rate of inpatient surgery is decreasing.

Etiology

In 1941, Parmenter suggested several congenital factors that could develop into a urethral diverticulum, including Gartner duct, a faulty union of primal folds, cell nets, and wolffian ducts or vaginal cysts that rupture into the urethra. Additional possible causes include trauma at childbirth, surgical trauma, urethral stone, urethral stricture, and infection of the urethral glands.

Of the many possible causes of urethral diverticula that have been considered, none have been proved. Two of the most probable causes are *Gonococcus neisseria* infection (although gonococci are seldom cultured) and infection of the suburethral tissue by vaginal flora. Huffman's experiments support the notion that a suburethral infection can develop into an abscess that becomes lined with epithelium. Huffman demonstrated periurethral openings by constructing wax models of infected urethras. The usual organisms cultured are *Escherichia coli, Aerobacter aerogenes,* and other gram-negative bacilli; *Staphylococcus aureus;* and *Streptococcus faecalis.*

Symptoms

Dysuria, urgency, frequency, and hematuria occurred together in 85% to 90% of 32 cases reviewed by Peters and Vaughn. Other frequently occurring symptoms are a lump in the vagina caused by protrusion of the diverticulum sac into the vagina, dyspareunia (intermittent discharge from the urethra), and pain on walking. Pyuria and cystitis also occur, depending on the location of the diverticular orifice. If the opening is sufficiently close to the outer end of the urethra, there may be no leakage of purulent exudate back into the bladder, which may explain the absence of symptoms of cystitis in 5% of cases. If the diverticulum is located in the posterior urethra near the urethrovesical junction, stress urinary incontinence may be a significant symptom. In a review of 70 cases from the Johns Hopkins Hospital, Ginsberg and Genadry found that 17% of the diverticula were located in the proximal (outer) urethra, 43% in the midurethra, and 31% in the distal (posterior) urethra; in the remaining cases, the site was not specifically identified.

Not only are urinary tract symptoms the most common clinical expression of the urethral lesion, but a history of recurrent refractory cystitis is a clue that a diverticulum is the source of the infection.

Diagnosis

Urethral diverticula usually are small, varying from 3 mm to 3 cm in diameter. Some of the larger sacs cover the entire length of the urethra. On palpation of a suburethral mass, tenderness commonly is found. Pressure on the mass may cause the escape of urine or exudate from the urethral meatus.

An examination of the floor of the urethra through the water cystoscope while suburethral pressure is being applied reveals an opening in 50% to 70% of cases. The pressure may force contents of the diverticulum into the urethra while it is being viewed. Some of the openings are extremely small and may be missed. Inflammatory swelling can result in edema of the orifice, which makes visualization difficult or impossible.

The diagnosis of urethral diverticulum is firmly established by means of positive-pressure urethrography (PPUG). A special catheter is used to block the urethra at both ends and to fill it and the diverticulum under pressure with water-soluble contrast medium (Figs. 24.23–24.25). If the urethral orifice to the diverticulum is quite large, a voiding cystourethrogram

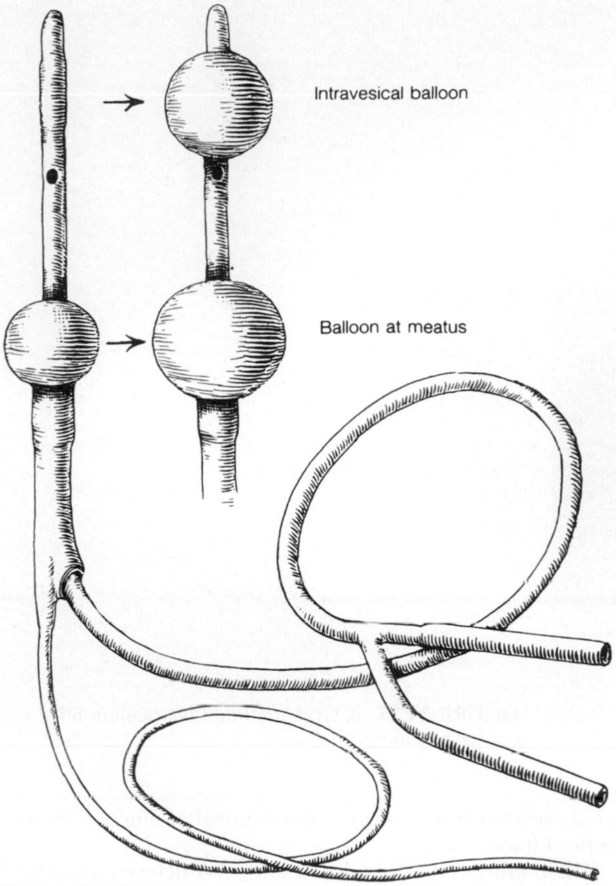

FIGURE 24.23. Double-ballooned catheter for positive-pressure urethrography. (From Davis JH, Cian L. Positive-pressure urethrography: a new diagnostic method. *J Urol* 1958;80:34, with permission.)

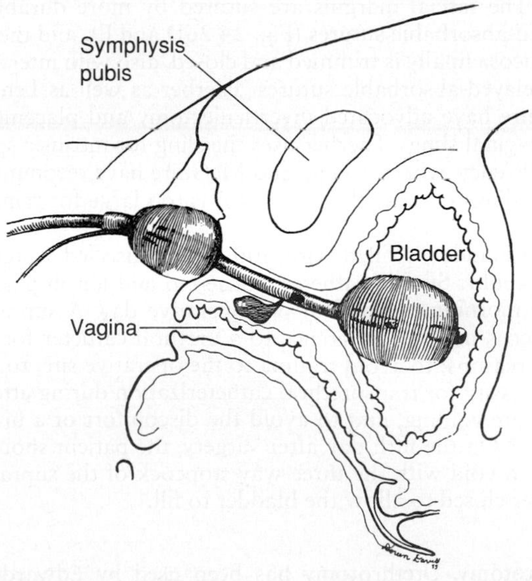

FIGURE 24.24. Double-ballooned catheter inserted for positive-pressure urethrography. (From Davis JH, Cian L. Positive-pressure urethrography: a new diagnostic method. *J Urol* 1958;80:34, with permission.)

together with a positive pelvic film may demonstrate the diverticulum. Although not as sensitive as PPUG, VCUG (voiding cystourethrography) may assist in identifying a urethral diverticulum. Wang and Wang compared VCUG and PPUG in evaluating 120 women. Twenty of 120 women demonstrated diverticulum. Thirteen were positive on PPUG and 10 with VCUG. If the surgeon's suspicion is high for urethral diverticulum, magnetic resonance imaging (MRI) should be considered if both the PPUG and VCUG studies are negative.

More recently, Chou and associates have suggested that a new method, virtual computerized tomography urethroscopy, increases the accuracy of diagnoses. The diverticulum orifice is less likely to be missed, especially when an inflammatory process or obstructed orifice exists. Gerrard and colleagues have suggested that transvaginal ultrasound is effective for evaluating patients with suspected urethral diverticulum. The technique is accurate, low cost, and readily available and should be considered as an initial screening technique for women when one suspects a urethral diverticulum. Computerized tomography and MRI have better defined diverticular anatomy. Neitlich and colleagues have suggested MRI to be more sensitive than double balloon urethrography. These techniques should be considered after other conventional methods have not defined the diverticulum.

Occasionally a diverticulum occurs with no clinical evidence of inflammation. If the diverticulum is diagnosed during a careful pelvic examination, and if the patient is completely asymptomatic except for a previous history of urinary tract problems, surgery is not necessary. With a complication rate of 15% to 20%, diverticulectomy should not be considered a quick and easy procedure. Removal of an asymptomatic urethral diverticulum may create more problems than it prevents, particularly if the sac is small or located in the floor of the posterior urethra. Only if a patient experiences acute or recurrent symptoms should urethral surgery be performed. Leng and McGuire classify urethral diverticulum as true versus pseudodiverticulum (Table 24.5).

Treatment

A diverticulum that requires treatment must be completely excised before the defect in the urethra can be closed. Failure to remove the entire diverticulum results only in recurrence of the problem. Many techniques have been used to identify the anatomic boundaries of the diverticulum. One popular method is to pass a sound into the diverticulum through the urethral orifice. Another method is to distend the diverticulum by injecting it with fibrinogen and thrombin mixed in a syringe to form a firm fibrin clot. However, direct anatomic dissection of the diverticulum from the paraurethral fascia and vaginal wall without visual enhancement of the anatomic boundaries offers a better success rate. The smooth covering of a diverticulum protruding into the vagina can be easily distinguished from the rugal folds of the vaginal mucosa.

If the wall of the diverticulum is left unopened until the dissection has reached the base of the diverticulum sac, its neck can be visualized directly while it is removed. Inadvertent removal of a portion of the urethral floor along the base of the diverticulum is too common an error; if the mucosa is closed with too much tension, a urethral stricture or a postoperative fistula may result.

Excision and Layered Closure. A midline incision is made through the vaginal mucosa, which is then separated from the wall of the diverticulum (Fig. 24.26A). The wall of the

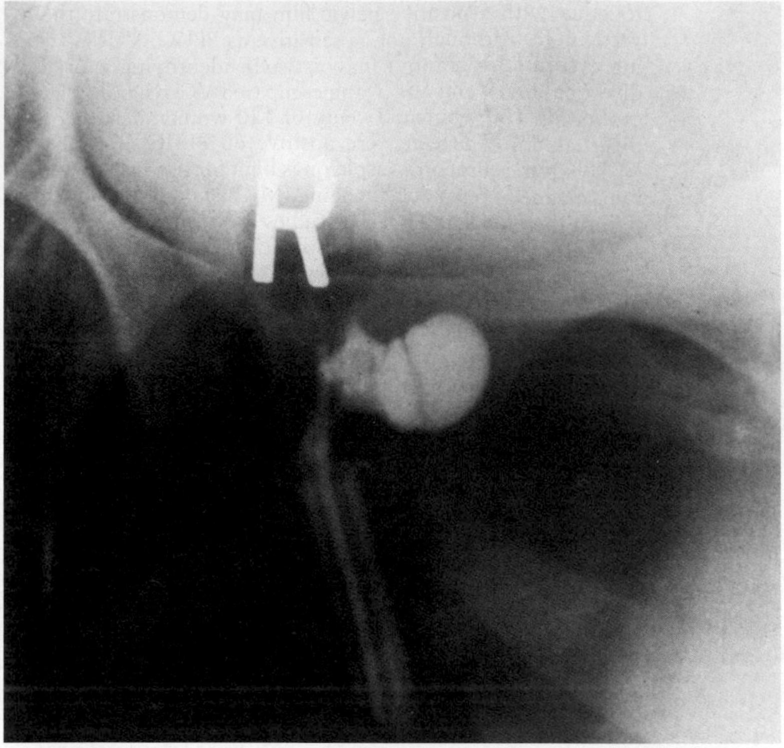

FIGURE 24.25. A large urethral diverticulum filled with contrast medium.

diverticulum also is dissected from the paraurethral fascia in as wide a circumference as can be developed.

The diverticulum is opened and the interior of the cavity is inspected. If the orifice of the diverticulum is large, the opening of the urethra can easily be seen, especially if a catheter has been placed in the urethra and bladder (Fig. 24.26B). The rest of the thin, friable mucosa of the diverticulum is separated from the vaginal mucosa and fascia before the neck of the diverticulum is trimmed near the urethral orifice. The lining of the diverticulum is friable because of inflammatory changes and the thin layer fragments during the dissection. Meticulous sharp dissection is required to separate the lining completely from the vagina and from the floor of the urethra. We repeat, in caution, that the neck of the diverticulum should be carefully resected to avoid eversion and to prevent the removal of mucosa from the urethral floor.

The urethral defect is closed with 3-0 delayed-absorbable sutures interrupted so that the edges can be inverted (Fig. 24.26C). After the interrupted sutures are tied, the paraurethral fascia is closed in a double-layer "vest-over-pants" technique in which the layer of fascia from one side of the urethra is sutured beneath the opposite and overlapping fascia and fastened to the urethral wall on that opposite side. The top layer of fascia is then sutured at its edge to the underlying fascial layer. The fascial margins are sutured by more durable 2-0 delayed-absorbable sutures (Fig. 24.26D and E), and the vaginal mucosa finally is trimmed and closed, also with interrupted 2–0 delayed-absorbable sutures. Faerber as well as Leng and McGuire have advocated diverticulectomy and placement of pubovaginal slings. Faerber uses the sling for intrinsic sphincter deficiency, whereas Leng and McGuire have recommended fascial slings to close the defect if it is too large for reinforcement.

The bladder is filled with 300 mL of distilled water, and a suprapubic Silastic catheter is inserted and left in place until the morning of the fifth postoperative day. A suprapubic catheter is used in preference to a urethral catheter for three major reasons: to avoid trauma to the operative site, to avoid the necessity for transurethral catheterization during attempts to initiate voiding, and to avoid the discomfort of a urethral catheter. On the fifth day after surgery, the patient should attempt to void with the three-way stopcock of the suprapubic catheter closed to allow the bladder to fill.

TABLE 24.5

URETHRAL DIVERTICULUM

True Diverticulum	Pseudodiverticulum
No prior urethral surgery	History of urethral surgery
Chronic recurring symptoms of urgency, dysuria, dyspareunia, dribbling	Relatively few voiding symptoms
Chronic lower urinary tract infections	Cystoscopy demonstrates broad-mouthed ostium to diverticulum
Narrow-necked ostium not readily apparent on radiography or cystoscopy	More likely to have stress incontinence

From Leng WW, McGuire EJ. Management of female urethral diverticula: a new classification. *J Urol* 1998;160(4)1297.

Urethrotomy. Urethrotomy has been used by Edwards and Beebe and by Kropp to treat diverticula. Splitting the floor of the urethra from the meatus down its full length to the site of the orifice of the diverticulum allows the sac to be well visualized during excision. As a rule, however, cases of urethral

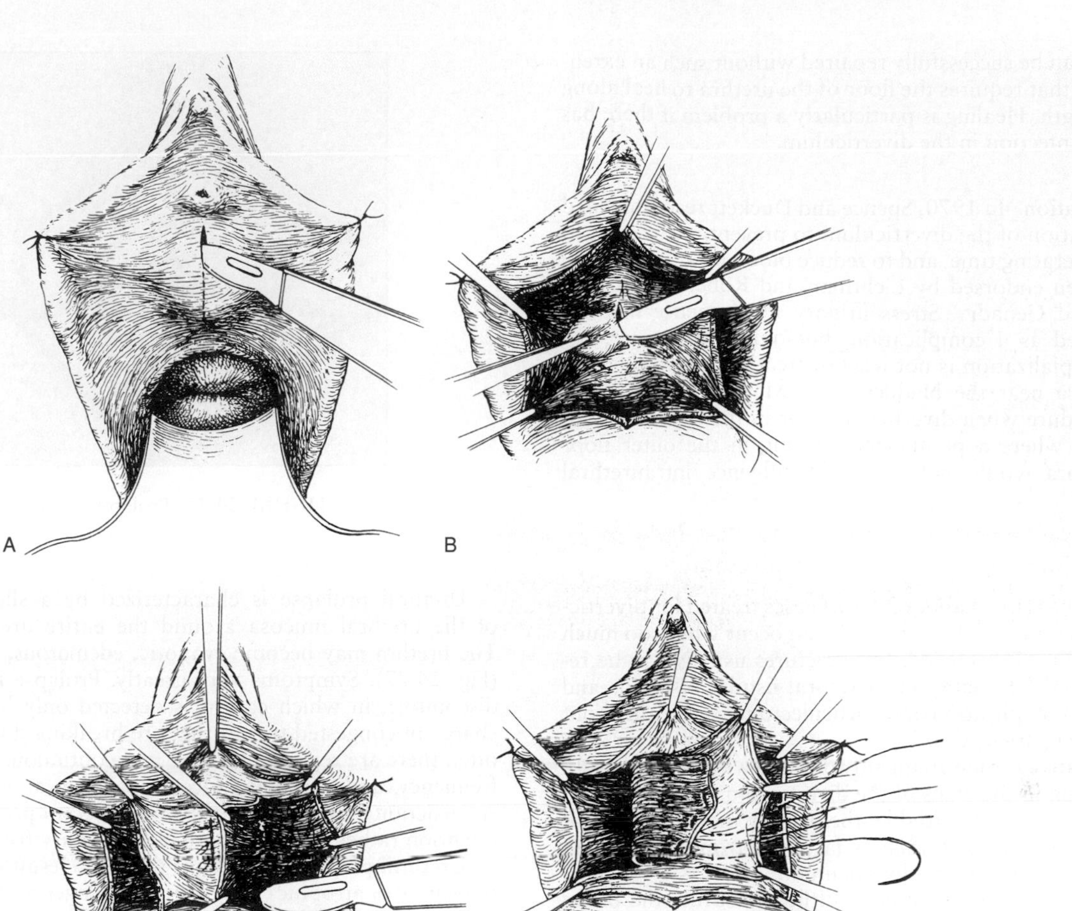

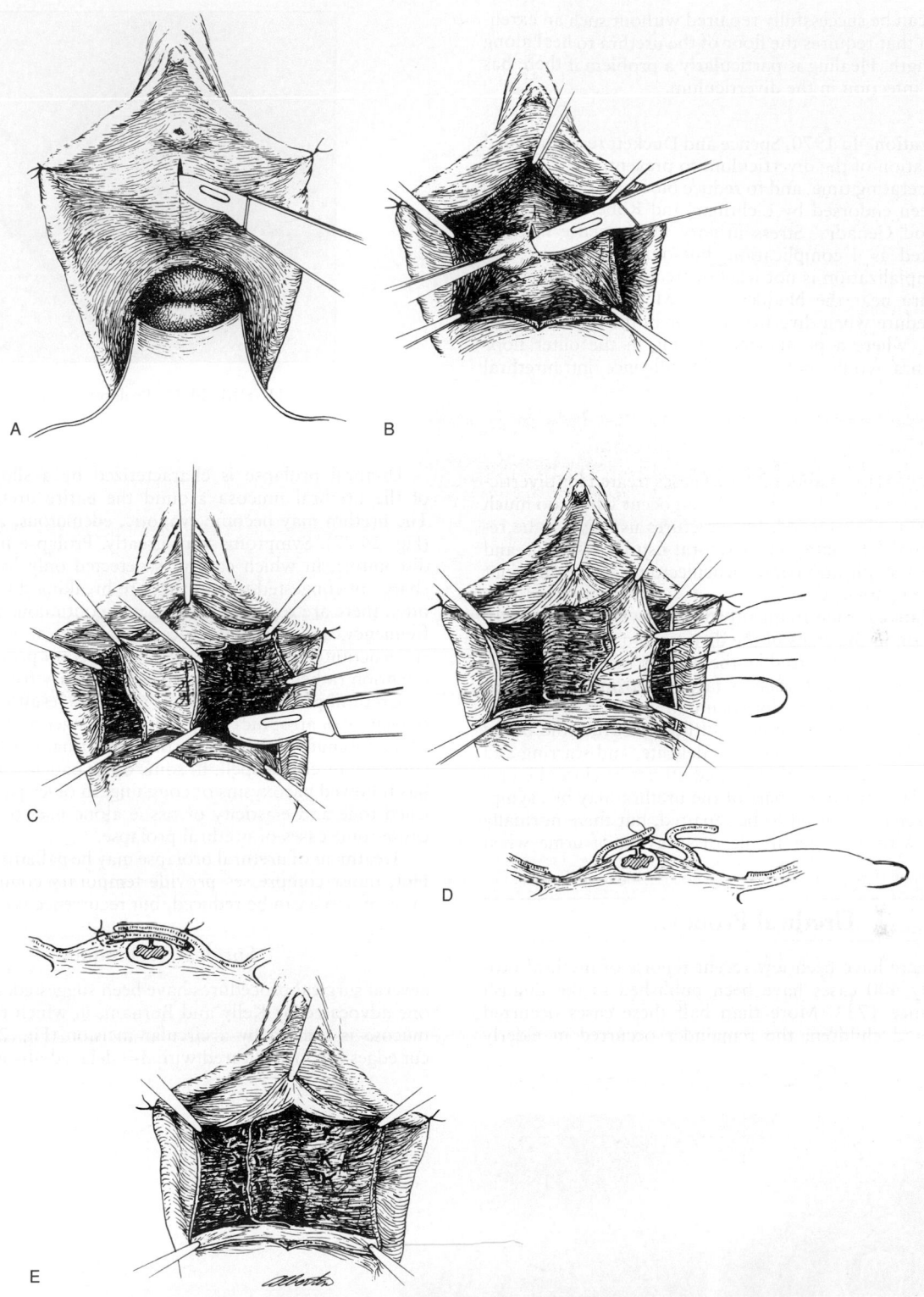

FIGURE 24.26. Suburethral diverticulum. **A:** A midline vaginal incision is made over the diverticulum. **B:** The diverticulum is dissected from the vaginal mucosa and surrounding fascia. Freed diverticulum is excised from the floor of the urethra, avoiding removal of an excessive amount of the urethral wall. **C:** The urethra is closed with interrupted 3-0 delayed-absorbable sutures placed through the muscularis and mucosa to ensure mucosa-to-mucosa approximation. The paraurethral fascia is mobilized with sharp dissection from the vaginal mucosa. **D:** The paraurethral fascia is plicated beneath the urethral incision, using the vest-over-pants technique. The inner layer of fascia is sutured to the undersurface of the outer layer using horizontal mattress sutures of 2-0 delayed-absorbable material. The inset is a cross-sectional view of suture placement. **E:** Completion of vest-over-pants plication of paraurethral fascia over the floor of the urethra. The free margin of the outer fascia is sutured to the inner fascial layer. The inset is a cross-sectional view of suture placement.

diverticula can be successfully repaired without such an extensive incision that requires the floor of the urethra to heal along its entire length. Healing is particularly a problem if there has been recent infection in the diverticulum.

Marsupialization. In 1970, Spence and Duckett recommended marsupialization of the diverticulum to prevent recurrence, to minimize operating time, and to reduce blood loss. This procedure has been endorsed by Lichtman and Robertson and by Ginsberg and Genadry. Stress urinary incontinence has not been reported as a complication, but only, we suspect, because marsupialization is not used to treat lesions in the posterior urethra near the bladder base. Marsupialization is a useful procedure when diverticula occur in the outer third of the urethra, where a permanent opening in the outer floor of the urethra would not adversely influence intraurethral pressure.

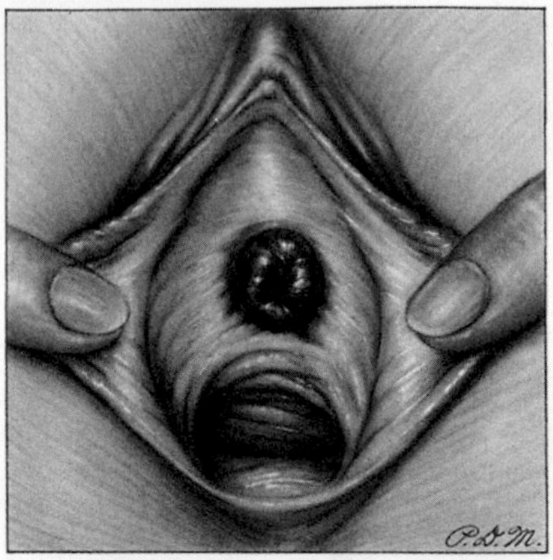

FIGURE 24.27. Prolapsed urethra.

Complications of Diverticulectomy

Complications arise in about 20% of cases treated for diverticula of the urethra. Urethral stricture can occur when too much urethral mucosa is removed, but strictures usually can be resolved by urethral dilatations. Urethral fistula, a serious and troublesome complication of diverticulectomy, occurs in about 5% of treated patients.

Postoperative fistulas frequently develop when acute or subacute infection in the walls of the diverticulum causes the urethral mucosa to become friable; the urinary incontinence that develops from urethral fistulas is far more troublesome than the initial symptoms of the diverticulum.

Closure of a urethral fistula is difficult because the blood supply to the floor of the urethra is delicate, and scarring and infection often develop with repeated efforts to close the urethra. A fistula in the outer part of the urethra may be asymptomatic and may not need to be repaired, but there normally are reports with an outer fistula of spraying of urine when voiding.

Urethral Prolapse

Although there have been few recent reports of urethral prolapse, nearly 400 cases have been published in the English literature since 1732. More than half these cases occurred in infants and children; the remainder occurred in elderly patients.

Urethral prolapse is characterized by a sliding outward of the urethral mucosa around the entire urethral meatus. The urethra may become cyanotic, edematous, and infarcted (Fig. 24.27). Symptoms vary greatly. Prolapse may cause no discomfort, in which case it is detected only by bloody discharge of congested tissues that are breaking down, but more often there are reports of severe and continuous pain, urinary frequency, and tenesmus. Occasionally, in a small child, tissue reaction and edema of the outer urethra produces urinary retention rather than the more usual urinary frequency.

Urethral prolapse is thought to be the result of poor development of or atrophic changes in the collagen and elastic tissues of the submucosa. In infants, prolapse usually follows a severe coughing or crying spell. In some older patients, too, prolapse has followed paroxysms of coughing. In older patients, diminished tone and elasticity of tissue alone may be sufficient to cause some cases of urethral prolapse.

Treatment of urethral prolapse may be palliative or surgical. Hot, moist compresses provide temporary comfort. A small mass of tissue can be reduced, but recurrence is common.

Surgical Techniques

Several surgical procedures have been suggested, including the one advocated by Kelly and Burnam, in which the prolapsed mucosa is excised by a circular incision (Fig. 24.28A). The cut edges are then sutured with 3-0 delayed-absorbable suture

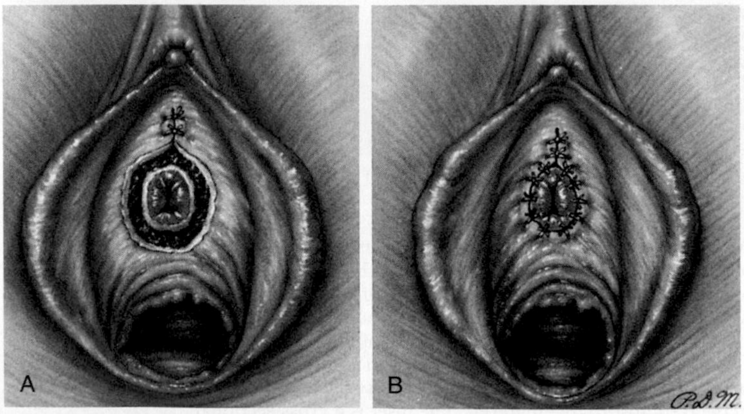

FIGURE 24.28. Operation for urethral prolapse. **A:** The prolapsed mucosa has been excised. **B:** Completed operation. Cut edges of urethral and vaginal mucosa are sutured with 3–0 delayed-absorbable sutures.

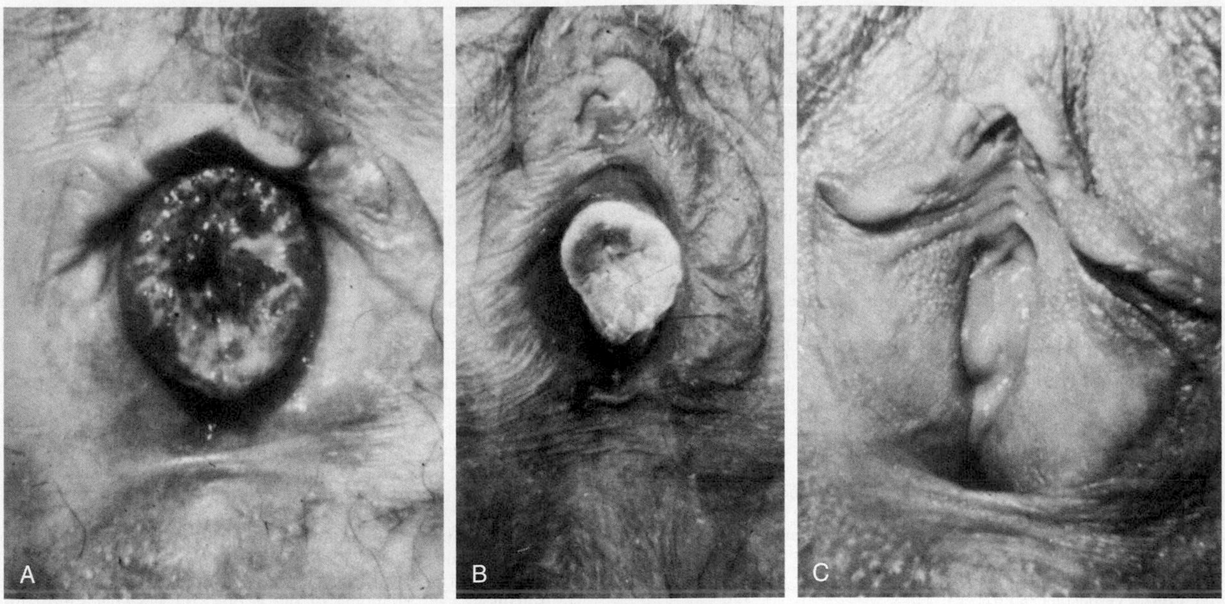

FIGURE 24.29. Cryosurgery in the treatment of urethral prolapse. A: Urethral prolapse in an elderly woman. B: Regression of urethral prolapse after cryosurgery. C: Repeated cryosurgery of urethral prolapse resulted in complete regression and healing of the urethral meatus within 8 weeks.

material, avoiding an excessive number of stitches, which can result in stricture of the urethral meatus (Fig. 24.28B). In most cases, this circumcision technique has proved to be the preferred method of correction.

Cryosurgery also has been used to treat urethral prolapse. The method is extremely effective in producing complete annular necrosis and healing of the prolapsed tissue (Fig. 24.29). The cryosurgery procedure can be performed without anesthesia, although for a young child, a local anesthetic is advisable. A suprapubic Silastic catheter is inserted and is left in postoperatively to permit bladder drainage until complete, spontaneous voiding can occur. The catheter also helps to prevent postoperative trauma at the suture line around the meatus.

BEST SURGICAL PRACTICES

- Incorporating an exam of the external genitalia into routine practice of clinicians caring for children can prevent delays in diagnosing imperforate hymen, misdiagnosis, and potential morbidity. To prevent scarring, stenosis, and subsequent dyspareunia in women with imperforate hymen, the hymenal tissue should not be excised too close to the vaginal mucosa.
- Sexually ambiguous external genitalia defects of the UGS are remarkably constant in appearance regardless of the etiology and differ only in degree of malformation, ranging somewhere intermediate to that of a normal girl and that of a normal boy. Thus, operative procedure for reconstruction of ambiguous genitalia into feminine genitalia does not vary in its essential elements.
- The common goals for the female reconstruction of ambiguous genitalia include reduction of clitoral size, creation of labia minora, and exteriorization of the vagina. Any reconstruction of the external genitalia with the objective of producing normal female appearance and function requires a full understanding of the surgical anatomy.
- It is essential to accurately identify the site of communication of the vagina with the UGS in female reconstruction of ambiguous genitalia. Knowledge of the possible variants in communication of the vagina with the UGS is critical before entertaining surgical correction.
- One objective of the reconstruction procedure for external genitalia is to delay the procedure until the anomalous structures are of a size to permit easy identification of all structures. Repair may be delayed until menarche, when maturity and the desire for sexual activity are usually well established.
- Surgical efforts of clitoral reduction focus on concealment, plication, resection, and reduction, with an attempt to provide a normal cosmesis without sacrificing sensation or vascularity of the glans. Even after seemingly successful clitoral reduction, the sensory function is significantly impaired, and this should be taken into consideration during counseling.
- Preoperative identification and catheterization or sounding of the vaginal orifice is key to the performance of a successful, one-stage procedure.
- It generally is recommended that exteriorization of the vagina be postponed until near puberty because higher estrogen levels may prevent stenosis, and sufficiently maturity in the patient is needed to comply with a postoperative dilatation program.
- When the complete operation is attempted at an early age, the vagina is sometimes not satisfactorily exteriorized. It should be emphasized that simple exteriorization of the lower vaginal tract can be combined with cosmetic correction of virilized external genitalia in infancy, but in most cases, it is best to defer definitive reconstruction of the intermediate or high vagina until after puberty.

Bibliography

Abramova L, Parekh J, Irvin WP, et al. Sentinel node biopsy in vulvar and vaginal melanoma; presentation of six cases and literature review. *Ann Surg Oncol* 2002;9:840.

Agrawal PP, Singhal SS, Neema JP, et al. The role of interstitial brachytherapy using template in locally advanced gynecological malignancies. *Gynecol Oncol* 2005;99:169.

Al-Kurdi M, Monaghan JM. Thirty two years experience in management of primary tumors of the vagina. *BJOG* 1981;88:1145.

Alizai NK, Thomas DFM, Lilford RJ, et al. Feminizing genitoplasty for congenital adrenal hyperplasia: what happens at puberty? *J Urol* 1999;161:1588.

Anderson MJ. The incidence of diverticula of the female urethra. *J Urol* 1967;98:96.

Azziz R, Mulaikal RM, Migeon CJ, et al. Congenital adrenal hyperplasia: long-term results following vaginal reconstruction. *Fertil Steril* 1986;46:1011.

Bailez MM, Gearhart JP, Migeon C, et al. Vaginal reconstruction after initial construction of the external genitalia in girls with salt-wasting adrenal hyperplasia. *J Urol* 1992;148:680.

Ball HG, Berman ML. Management of primary vaginal carcinoma. *Gynecol Oncol* 1982;14:154.

Bargy F, Laude F, Barbet JP, et al. The anatomy of intersexuality. *Surg Radiol Anat* 1989;11:103.

Baskin LS, Erol A, Li YW, et al. Anatomical studies of the human clitoris. *J Urol* 1999;162:1015.

Benedet JL, Murphy KJ, Fairey RN, et al. Primary invasive carcinoma of the vagina. *Obstet Gynecol* 1983;62:715.

Benjamin J, Elliott L, Cooper JF, et al. Urethral diverticulum in the adult female: clinical aspects, operative procedure, and pathology. *Urology* 1974;3:1.

Berek JS, Howe C, Legasse LD, et al. Pelvic exenteration for recurrent gynecologic malignancy: survival and morbidity analysis of the 45-year experience at UCLA. *Gynecol Oncol* 2005;99(1):153–9.

Blaikley JB, Dewhurst CJ, Ferreira HP, et al. Vaginal adenosis: clinical and pathological features with special reference to malignant change. *J Obstet Gynaecol Br Commonw* 1971;78:1115.

Blakely CR, Mills WG. The obstetric and gynaecological complications of bladder exstrophy and epispadias. *BJOG* 1981;88:167.

Breslow A. Thickness, cross-sectional areas, and depths of invasion in the prognosis of cutaneous melanoma. *Ann Surg* 1970;172:902.

Brown GR, Fletcher GH, Rutledge FN. Irradiation of in situ and invasive squamous cell carcinoma of the vagina. *Cancer* 1971;28:1278.

Burbige KA, Hensle TW, Chambers WJ, et al. Pregnancy and sexual function in women with bladder exstrophy. *Urology* 1986;28:120.

Burrows LJ. Surgical procedures for urethral diverticula in women in the United States, 1979-97. *Int Urogynecol J Pelvic Floor Dysfunct* 2005;16(2):158.

Choo YC, Anderson DG. Neoplasms of the vagina following cervical carcinoma. *Gynecol Oncol* 1982;14:125.

Chou CP, Huang JS, Yu CC, et al. Urethral diverticulum: diagnosis with virtual CT urethroscopy. *AJR Am J Roentgenol* 2005;184(6):1889.

Chung AF, Casey MJ, Flanner JT, et al. Malignant melanoma of the vagina: report of 19 cases. *Obstet Gynecol* 1980;55:720.

Clemetson CA. Ectopia vesicae and split pelvis: an account of pregnancy in a woman with treated ectopia vesicae and split pelvis, including a review of the literature. *J Obstet Gynaecol Br Emp* 1958;65:973.

Committee on Genetics, 1999-2000, Kaye CI, Cunniff C, et al. Evaluation of the newborn with developmental anomalies of the external genitalia. *Pediatrics* 2000;106:138.

Costa EM, Mendonca BB, Inacio M, et al. Management of ambiguous genitalia in pseudohermaphrodites: new perspectives on vaginal dilation. *Fertil Steril* 1997;67:229.

Creasman WT. Vaginal cancers. *Curr Opin Ob Gyn.* 2005;17(1):71–76.

Creasman WT, Phillips JL, Menck HR. The National Cancer Data Base report on cancer of the vagina. *Cancer* 1998;83(5):1033–1040.

Creighton SM, Minto CL, Steele SJ. Objective cosmetic and anatomical outcomes at adolescence of feminizing surgery for ambiguous genitalia done in childhood. *Lancet* 2001;358:124.

Crouch NS, Creighton SM. Minimal surgical intervention in the management of intersex conditions. *J Pediatr Endocrinol* 2004;17(12):1591.

Crouch NS, Minto CL, Laio KLM, et al. Genital sensation after feminizing genitoplasty for congenital adrenal hyperplasia: a pilot study. *BJU Int* 2003;91: 5.

Curra QJ, Rendtorff RC, Chandler RW, et al. Female gonorrhea: its relationship to abnormal uterine bleeding, urinary tract symptoms and cervicitis. *Obstet Gynecol* 1975;45:195.

Dalrymple JL, Russell AH, Lee SW, et al. Chemoradiation for primary invasive squamous carcinoma of the vagina. *Int J Gynecol Cancer* 2004;14: 110.

Damario MA, Carpenter SE, Jones HW Jr, et al. Reconstruction of the external genitalia in females with bladder exstrophy. *Int J Gynaecol Obstet* 1994;44:245.

Davis BL, Robinson DG. Diverticula of the female urethra: assay of 120 cases. *J Urol* 1970;104:850.

Davis HJ, Cian LG. Positive pressure urethrography: a new diagnostic method. *J Urol* 1958;80:34.

Davis HJ, Te Linde RW. Urethral diverticula: an assay of 121 cases. *J Urol* 1956;75:753.

Dewhurst J, Topliss PH, Shepherd JH. Ivalon sponge hysterosacropexy for genital prolapse in patients with bladder exstrophy. *BJOG* 1980;87:67.

DiSaia PJ, Morrow CP, Townsend DE. Synopsis of gynecologic oncology. New York: John Wiley & Sons, 1975.

Eddy GL, Marks RD, Miler MC III, et al. Primary invasive vaginal carcinoma. *Am J Obstet Gynecol* 1991;165:282.

Edwards E, Beebe RA. Diverticula of female urethra. Review: new procedure for treatment: report of 5 cases. *Obstet Gynecol* 1955;5:729.

Faerber GJ. Urethral diverticulectomy and pubovaginal sling for simultaneous treatment of urethral diverticulum and intrinsic sphincter deficiency. *Techniques in Urology* 1998;4:192.

Fenoglio C, Ferenczy A, Richard RM, et al. Scanning and transmission electron microscopic studies of vaginal adenosis and the cervical transformation zone in progeny exposed in utero to diethyl-stilbestrol. *Am J Obstet Gynecol* 1976;126:170.

Fortunoff FS, Latimer JK, Edson M. Vaginoplasty technique for female pseudohermaphrodites. *Surg Gynecol Obstet* 1964;118:545.

Frank SJ, Jhingran A, Levenback C, et al. Definitive radiation therapy for squamous cell carcinoma of the vagina. *Int J Radiat Oncol Biol Phys* 2005;62:138.

Frank SJ, Jhingran A, Levenback C, et al. Definitive treatment of vaginal cancer with radiation therapy. [Abstract 116] *Int J Radiat Oncol Biol Phys* 2003;57(Suppl.):S194.

Frick HC. Primary carcinoma of the vagina. *Am J Obstet Gynecol* 1968;101:695.

Frick HC, Jacox HW, Taylor HC. Primary carcinoma of the vagina. *Am J Obstet Gynecol* 1968;101:695.

Gallup DG, Morley GW. Carcinoma in situ of the vagina: a study and review. *Obstet Gynecol* 1975;46:334.

Gallup DG, Talledo OE, Shah KJ, et al. Invasive squamous cell carcinoma of the vagina: a 14-year-old study. *Obstet Gynecol* 1987;69:782.

Gearhart JP, Jeffs RD. State-of-the-art reconstructive surgery for bladder exstrophy at the Johns Hopkins Hospital. *Am J Dis Child* 1989: 143:1475.

Gerharz EW, Hohl UN, Weingartner K, et al. Experience with the Mainz modification of ureterosigmoidostomy. *Br J Surg* 1998;86:427.

Gerrard ER Jr., Lloyd LK, Kubricht WS, et al. Transvaginal ultrasound for the diagnosis of urethral diverticulum. *J Urol* 2003;169(4):1395.

Ginsberg DS, Genadry R. Suburethral diverticulum: classification and therapeutic considerations. *Obstet Gynecol* 1983;61:685.

Hamilton W, Boyd JD, Mossman HW. *Human embryology.* 3rd ed. Cambridge: W Heffer & Sons, 1962.

Hellman K, Silfversward C, Nilsson B, et al. Primary carcinoma of the vagina: factors influencing the age at diagnosis. The Radiumhemmet series 1956-96. *Int J Gynecol Cancer* 2004;14:491.

Hendren WH. Reconstructive problems of the vagina and the female urethra. *Clin Plast Surg* 1980;7:207.

Hendren WH. Surgical management of urogenital sinus abnormalities. *J Pediatr Surg* 1977;12:339.

Hendren WH, Crawford JD. Adrenogenital syndrome: the anatomy of the anomaly and its repair. *J Pediatr Surg* 1969;4:49.

Herbst AL, Cole P, Norusis MJ, et al. Epidemiologic aspects and factors related to survival in 384 registry cases of clear cell adenocarcinoma of the vagina and cervix. *Am J Obstet Gynecol* 1979;153:876.

Herbst AL, Scully RE, Robbo SJ. The significance of adenosis and clear-cell adenocarcinoma of the genital tract in young females. *J Reprod Med* 1975;14:5.

Herbst AL, Ulfelder H, Poskanzer EC. Adenocarcinoma of the vagina: association of maternal stilbestrol therapy with tumor appearing in young women. *N Engl J Med* 1971;284:878.

Herman JM, Homesley HD, Dignan MB. Is hysterectomy a risk factor for vaginal cancer?. *JAMA* 1986;256:601.

Herzog TJ, Rader JS. The ultrasonic surgical aspirator in the gynecologic oncology patient. In: Rock JA, Faro S, Gant NF Jr, et al., eds. *Advances in obstetrics and gynecology.* Vol. 1. St Louis: Mosby-Year Book, 1994:325.

Hilgers RD. Pelvic exenteration for vaginal embryonal rhabdomyosarcoma: a review. *Obstet Gynecol* 1975;45:175.

Hilgers RD. Squamous cell carcinoma of the vagina. *Surg Clin North Am* 1978;58:25.

Hines M. Abnormal sexual development and psychosexual issues. *Baillieres Clin Endocrinol Metab* 1998;12:173.

Hines M, Kaufman FR. Androgen and the development of human sex-typical behavior: rough-and-tumble play and sex preferred playmates in children with congenital adrenal hyperplasia (CAH). *Child Dev* 1994;65:1042.

Hoffman MJ, Adams WE. Recognition and repair of urethral diverticula. *Am J Obstet Gynecol* 1965;92:106.

Honig A, Rieger L, Kristen P, et al. A case review of metastasizing invasive hydatidiform mole. Is less-less good? Review of the literature with regard to adequate treatment. *Eur J Gynaecol Oncol* 2005;26:158.

Hopkins MP, Morley GW. Squamous cell carcinoma of the neovagina. *Obstet Gynecol* 1987;69:525.

Houghton CRS, Iversen T. Squamous cell carcinoma of the vagina: a clinical study of the location of the tumor. *Gynecol Oncol* 1982;13:365.

Huffman JW. The detailed anatomy of the paraurethral ducts in the adult human female. *Am J Obstet Gynecol* 1948;55:86.

Hutch JA. *Anatomy and physiology of the bladder, trigone and urethra.* New York: Appleton-Century-Crofts, 1972.

International Federation of Obstetrics and Gynecology. *Annual report on the results of treatment of carcinoma of the uterus, vagina and ovary.* Vol. 18. Stockholm: Norestedt, 1982.

Jahnke A, Domke R, Makovitzky J, et al. Vaginal metastasis of lung cancer: a case report. *Anticancer Res* 2005;25:1645.

Joki-Erkkila MM, Heinonen PK. Presenting and long-term clinical implications and fecundity in females with obstructing vaginal malformations. *J Pediatr Adolesc Gynecol* 2003;16(5):307.

Jones HW Jr. An anomaly of the external genitalia in female patients with exstrophy of the bladder. *Am J Obstet Gynecol* 1973;117(6):748.

Jones HW Jr, Verkauf BS. Surgical treatment in congenital adrenal hyperplasia: age at operation and other prognostic factors. *Obstet Gynecol* 1970;36:1.

Kamat MH, DelGaiso A, Seebode D. Urethral prolapse in female children. *Am J Dis Child* 1969;118:691.

Kanbour AE, Klionsky BK, Murphy AL. Carcinoma of the vagina following cervical cancer. *Cancer* 1974;34:1838.

Kelly HA, Burnam CF. Malfunctions of the urethra. In: Kelly HA, ed. *Diseases of the kidneys, ureters, and bladder.* New York: D Appleton, 1922: 564.

Klaus H, Stein RT. Urethral prolapse in young girls. *Pediatrics* 1973;52:645.

Klobe JM. *Pathologische Anatomieder weiblichen sexual Organe.* Vien 1864.

Kogan SJ, Smey P, Levitt SB. Subtunical total reduction clitoroplasty: a safe modification of existing techniques. *J Urol* 1983;130(4):746.

Krege S, Walz KH, Hauffa BP, et al. Long term follow-up of female patients with congenital adrenal hyperplasia from 21-hydroxylase deficiency, with special emphasis on the results of vaginoplasty. *BJU Int* 2000;86:253.

Krisiloff M, Puchner PJ, Tretter W, et al. Pregnancy in women with bladder exstrophy. *J Urol* 1978;119:478.

Kropp KA. The female urethra. In: Glenn JF, ed. *Urologic surgery.* Hagerstown, MD: Harper & Row, 1975.

Kucera H, Langer M, Smekal G, et al. Radiotherapy of primary carcinoma of the vagina: management and results of different therapy schemes. *Gynecik Ibcik* 1985;21:87.

Lamoreaux WT, Grigsby PW, Dehdashti F. FDG-PET evaluation of vaginal carcinoma. *Int J Radiat Oncol Biol Phys* 2005;62:733.

Latourette HB. End results of treatment of cancer of vagina. *Ann N Y Acad Sci* 1964;114:1020.

Lee RA. Diverticulum of the urethra: clinical presentation, diagnosis and management. *Clin Obstet Gynecol* 1984;27:490.

Lee RA, Symmonds RE. Recurrent carcinoma in situ of the vagina in patients previously treated for in situ carcinoma of the cervix. *Obstet Gynecol* 1976;48:61.

Leng WW, McGuire EJ. Management of female urethral diverticula: a new classification. *J Urol* 1998;160:1297.

Lialios G, Plantaniotis G, Kallitsaris A, et al. Vaginal metastasis from renal adenocarcinoma. *Gynecol Oncol* 2005;98:172.

Liang C-C, Chang S-D, Soong Y-K. Long-term follow-up of women who underwent surgical correction for imperforate hymen. *Arch Gynecol Obstet* 2003;269(1):5.

Lichtman A, Robertson J. Suburethral diverticula treated by marsupialization. *Obstet Gynecol* 1976;47:203.

Lintgen C, Herbert P. Clinical-pathological study of 100 female urethras. *J Urol* 1946;55:298.

Livermore GR. Treatment of prolapse of the urethra. *Surg Gynecol Obstet* 1921;32:557.

Magrina JF, Walter AJ, Schild SE. Laparoscopic radical parametrectomy and pelvic and aortic lymphadenectomy for vaginal carcinoma: a case report. *Gynecol Oncol* 1999;75:514.

Manetta A, Gutrecht EL, Berman ML, et al. Primary invasive carcinoma of the vagina. *Obstet Gynecol* 1990;76:639.

Manetta A, Perito JL, Larson JE, et al. Primary invasive carcinoma of the vagina. *Obstet Gynecol* 1988;72:77.

Marcus R Jr, Million RR, Daly JW. Carcinoma of the vagina. *Cancer* 1978;42:2507.

Marcus SL. Multiple squamous cell carcinoma involving the cervix, vagina and vulva: the theory of multicentric origin. *Am J Obstet Gynecol* 1960;80:802.

Melneck S, Cole P, Anderson D, et al. Rates and risks of DES-related clear cell adenocarcinoma of the vagina and cervix. *N Engl J Med* 1987;316:514.

Merino MJ. Vaginal cancer: the role of infectious and environmental factors [Review]. *Am J Obstet Gynecol* 1991;165:1255.

Mingin GC, Stock JA, Hanna MK. The Mainz II pouch: experience in 5 patients with bladder exstrophy. *J Urol* 1999;162:846.

Mock U, Kucera H, Fellner C, et al. High dose-rate (HDR) brachytherapy with or without external beam radiotherapy in the treatment of primary vaginal carcinoma: long-term results and side effects. *Int J Radiat Oncol Biol Phys* 2003;56:950–957.

Mor N, Merlob P, Reisner SH. Types of hymen in the newborn infant. *Eur J Obstet Gynecol Reprod Biol* 1986;22:225.

Murad TM, Durant JR, Maddox WA, et al. The pathologic behavior of primary vaginal carcinoma and its relationship to cervical cancer. *Cancer* 1975;35:787.

Nakagawa S, Koga K, Kuga K, et al. The evaluation of the sentinel node successfully conducted in a case of malignant melanoma of the vagina. *Gynecol Oncol* 2002;86:387.

Neitlich JD, Foster HE Jr,Glickman MG, et al. Detection of urethral diverticula in women: comparison of a high-resolution fast spin echo technique with double balloon urethrography. *J Urol* 1998;159(2):408.

Ng AB, Reagan JW, Hawliczek S, et al. Cellular detection of vaginal adenosis. *Obstet Gynecol* 1975;46:323.

Nomura Y, Yamakado K, Tanaka H, et al. Letters to the editor: radiofrequency ablation for the treatment of hemorrhagic vaginal cancer. *JVIR* 2005:1557.

Nori D, Hilaris BS, Shu F. Radiation therapy of primary vaginal carcinoma. *Int J Radiat Oncol Biol Phys* 1981;70:20.

Nori D, Hilaris B, Stanimir G, et al. Radiation therapy of primary vaginal carcinoma. *Int J Radiat Oncol Biol Phys* 1983;8:1471.

Orr JW, Dosoretz DD, Mahoney D. Surgically (laparotomy/laparoscopy) guided placement of high dose rate interstitial irradiation catheters (LG-HDRT): technique and outcome. *Gynecol Oncol* 2006;100:145.

Otton GR, Nicklin JL, Dickie GJ, et al. Early stage vaginal carcinoma – an analysis of 70 patients. *Int J Gynecol Cancer* 2004;14:304–310.

Oudoux A, Rousseau T, Bridji B. Interest of F-18 fluorodeoxyglucose positron emission tomography in the evaluation of vaginal malignant melanoma. *Gynecol Oncol* 2004;95:765.

Ozbey H, Darendeliler F, Kayserili H, et al. Gender assignment in female congenital adrenal hyperplasia: a difficult experience. *BJU Int* 2004;94(3): 388.

Parmenter FJ. Diverticulum of the urethra. *J Urol* 1941;45:749.

Passerini-Glazel G. A new 1-stage procedure for clitorovaginoplasty in severely masculinized female pseudohermaphrodites. *J Urol* 1989;142:565.

Pathak UN, House MJ. Diverticulum of the female urethra. *Obstet Gynecol* 1970;36:789.

Perez CA. Definitive radiotherapy for carcinoma of the vagina. *Int J Radiat Oncol Biol Phys* 1981;7:20.

Perez CA, Arneson AN, Dehner LP, et al. Radiation therapy in carcinoma of the vagina. *Obstet Gynecol* 1974;44:862.

Perez CA, Arneson AN, Galakatos A, et al. Malignant tumors of the vagina. *Cancer* 1973;31:36.

Perez CA, Camel HM. Long-term follow-up in radiation therapy of carcinoma of the vagina. *Cancer* 1982;49:1308.

Peters WA III, Kumar NB, Morley GW. Carcinoma of the vagina. *Cancer* 1985;55:892.

Peters WA, Vaughn EJ Jr. Urethral diverticula in the female: etiologic factors and postoperative results. *Obstet Gynecol* 1976;47:549.

Pettersson F. *Annual report on the results of treatment in gynecological cancer.* Stockholm: FIGO; 1988: 174.

Pirtoli L, Santoni R. Radiation therapy of the primary vaginal carcinoma. *Acta Radiol Oncol Radiat Phys Biol* 1980;19:353.

Plentl AA, Friedman EA. *Lymphatic system of the female genital tract.* Philadel phia: WB Saunders, 1971.

Pokorny SF, Kozinetz CA. Configuration and other anatomic details of the prepubertal hymen. *Adolesc Pediatr Gynecol* 1988;1:97.

Posner JC, Spandorfer PR. Early detection of imperforate hymen prevents morbidity from delays in diagnosis. *Pediatrics* 2005;115(4):1008.

Prempree T. Role of radiation therapy in the management of primary carcinoma of the vagina. *Acta Radiol [Oncol]* 1982;21:195.

Prempree T, Vlravathana T, Slawson RG, et al. Radiation management of primary carcinoma of the vagina. *Cancer* 1977;40:101.

Pride GL, Bucher DA. Carcinoma of vagina 10 or more years following pelvic irradiation therapy. *Am J Obstet Gynecol* 1977;127:513.

Pride GL, Schultz AE, Chuprevich TW, et al. Primary invasive carcinoma of the vagina. *Obstet Gynecol* 1979;53:218.

Puthawala A, Sved AM, Nalick R, et al. Integrated external and interstitial radiation therapy for primary carcinoma of the vagina. *Obstet Gynecol* 1983;62:367.

Rajfer J, Ehrlich RM, Goodwin WE. Reduction clitoroplasty via ventral approach. *J Urol* 1982;128:341.

Rastogi BL, Bergman B, Angawall L. Primary leiomyosarcoma of the vagina: a study of five cases. *Gynecol Oncol* 1984;18:77.

Reddy S, Lee MS, Graham JE, et al. Radiation therapy in primary carcinoma of the vagina. *Gynecol Oncol* 1987;26:19.

Reid GC, Schmidt RW, Roberts JA, et al. Primary melanoma of the vagina: a clinicopathologic analysis. *Obstet Gynecol* 1989;764:190.

Reiner WG. Sex assignment in the neonate with intersex or inadequate genitalia. *Arch Pediatr Adolesc Med* 1997;151:1044.
Reuben SC, Young J, Mikuta JJ. Squamous carcinoma of the vagina: treatment, complications, and long-term follow-up. *Gynecol Oncol* 1985;20:346.
Ricci G, Gentili A, Di Lorenzo F, et al. Latex allergy in subjects who had undergone multiple surgical procedures for bladder exstrophy: relationship with clinical intervention and atopic diseases. *BJU Int* 1999;84:1058.
Ries J, Ludwig H. Zur therapie des primaren karzinoms der vagina. *Strahlentherapie* 1962;118:92.
Rink RC, Adams MC. Feminizing genitoplasty: state of the art. *World J Urol* 1998;16:212.
Rink RC, Pope JC, Kropp BP, et al. Reconstruction of the high urogenital sinus: early perineal prone approach without division of the rectum. *J Urol* 1997;158:1293.
Robinson JB, Sun CC, Bodurka-Bevers D, et al. Cavitational ultrasonic surgical aspiration for the treatment of vaginal intraepithelial neoplasia. *Gynecol Oncol* 2000;78:235.
Rock JA, Katz E. Ambiguous genitalia. *Semin Reprod Endocrinol* 1987;5:327.
Rock JA, Schlaff WD. Congenital adrenal hyperplasia: the surgical treatment of vaginal stenosis. *Int J Gynaecol Obstet* 1986;24:417.
Rock JA, Zacur HA, Dlugi AM, et al. Pregnancy success following the surgical correction of imperforate hymen as compared to the complete transverse vaginal septum. *Obstet Gynecol* 1982;59:448.
Rubin SC, Young J, Mikuta JJ. Squamous carcinoma of the vagina: treatment, complications, and long-term follow-up. *Gynecol Oncol* 1985;20:346.
Rutledge FN. Cancer of the vagina. *Am J Obstet Gynecol* 1967;97:635.
Rutledge FN, Boronow RC, Wharton JT. *Gynecologic oncology.* New York: John Wiley & Sons, 1976.
Samant R, Tam T, Dahrouge S, et al. Radiotherapy for the treatment of primary vaginal cancer. *Radiother Oncol* 2005;77:133.
Sander R, Nuss RC, Rhadgan RM. DES-associated vaginal adenosis followed by clear-cell adenocarcinoma. *Int J Gynecol Pathol* 1986;5:362.
Schubert G. Uber scheidenbildung bei angeborenem vaginaldefekt. *Zbl Gynak* 1911;45:1017.
Sholem SL, Wechsler M, Roberts M. Management of the urethral diverticulum in women: a modified operative technique. *J Urol* 1974;112:485.
Smith FR. Clinical management of cancer of the vagina. *Ann N Y Acad Sci* 1964;114:1012.
Smith WG. Invasive carcinoma of the vagina. *Clin Obstet Gynecol* 1981;24:503.
Spence H, Duckett J. Diverticulum of the female urethra: clinical aspects and presentation of simple operative technique for cure. *J Urol* 1970;104:432.
Spirtos IM, Doshi BP, Kapp DS, et al. Radiation therapy for primary squamous cell carcinoma of the vagina: the Stanford University experience. *Gynecol Oncol* 1989;35:20.
Stafl A, Mattingly RF. Vaginal adenosis: a precancerous lesion? *Am J Obstet Gynecol* 1974;120:666.
Stanton SL. Gynecologic complications of epispadias and bladder exstrophy. *Am J Obstet Gynecol* 1974;119:749.
Stelling JR, Gray MR, Davis AJ, et al. Dominant transmission of imperforate hymen. *Fertil Steril* 2000;74:1241.
Stern A, Patel S. Diverticulum of the female urethra: value of the postvoid bladder film during excretory urography. *Radiology* 1976;121:22.
Stock RG, Chen AS, Seski J. A 30-year experience in the management of primary carcinoma of the vagina: analysis of prognostic factors and treatment modalities. *Gynecol Oncol* 1995;56:45.
Stuart GC, Allen HH, Anderson RJ. Squamous cell carcinoma of the vagina following hysterectomy. *Am J Obstet Gynecol* 1981;139:311.
Tabata T, Taheshirma N, Nishida H, et al. Treatment failure in vaginal cancer. *Gynecol Oncol* 2002;84:309–314.
Tait L. Sacular dilatation of the urethra: removal, cure. *Lancet* 1875;2:625.
Thigpen JT, Blessing JA, Homesley HD, et al. A phase II trial of cisplatin in advanced recurrent cancer of the vagina: a GOG study. *Gynecol Oncol* 1986;23:101.
Underwood PB, Smith RT. Carcinoma of the vagina. *JAMA* 1971;217:46.
Usherwood MM. Management of vaginal carcinoma after hysterectomy. *Am J Obstet Gynecol* 1975;122:352.
van Dam P, Sonnemans H, van Dam P-J, et al. Sentinel node detection in patients with vaginal carcinoma. *Gynecol Oncol* 2004;92:89.
Viswanathan A, Bishop K, Lee H, et al. The impact of brachytherapy dose in vaginal cancer [Abstract 1135]. *Int J Radiat Oncol Biol Phys* 2003;57(Suppl.):343.
Wang AC, Wang CR. Radiologic diagnosis and surgical treatment of urethral diverticulum in women: a reappraisal of voiding cystourethrography and positive pressure urethrography. *J Reprod Med* 2000;45:377.
Weed JC, Lozier C, Daniel SJ. Human papilloma virus in multifocal, invasive female tract malignancy. *Obstet Gynecol* 1983;62:832.
Wharton JT. Carcinoma of the vagina. In: Rutledge F, Boronow RC, Wharton JT, eds. *Gynecologic oncology.* New York: John Wiley & Sons; 1976:259.
Wharton JT. Carcinoma of the vagina and urethra. In: Rovinsky D, ed. *Obstetrics and gynecology.* Hagerstown, MD: Harper & Row, 1972.
Wharton JT, Kearns W. Diverticulum of the female urethra. *J Urol* 1950;63:1063.
Wheeless CR Jr, McGibbon B, Dorsey JH, et al. Gracilis myocutaneous flap in reconstruction of the vulva and female perineum. *Obstet Gynecol* 1979;54:97.
Whelton JA, Kottmeier HL. Primary carcinoma of the vagina. *Acta Obstet Gynecol Scand* 1962;41:22.
Winderl LM, Silverman RK. Prenatal diagnosis of congenital imperforate hymen. *Obstet Gynecol* 1995;85(5 pt 2):857.
Woodruff JD, Parmley TH. Epidermoid carcinoma of the vagina. In: Hafez EC, Evans TN, eds. *The human vagina.* New York: Elsevier North Holland, 1979.
Young HH. *Genital abnormalities, hermaphroditism and related adrenal diseases.* Baltimore: Williams & Wilkins, 1937.
Young RH, Scully RE. Endodermal sinus tumor of the vagina: a report of nine cases and review of the literature. *Gynecol Oncol* 1984;18:380.
Zambo K, Koppan M, Paal A. Sentinel lymph nodes in gynaecological malignancies: frontline between TNM and clinical staging systems? *Eur J Nucl Med Mol Imaging* 2003;30:1684.

CHAPTER 25 ■ SURGERY FOR ANOMALIES OF THE MÜLLERIAN DUCTS

JOHN A. ROCK AND LESLEY L. BREECH

DEFINITIONS

Hematometra—The distension of the uterus with blood or menstrual fluid.

Hematometrocolpos—The distension of the uterus and vagina with blood or menstrual fluid; because the vaginal wall is more distensible, the vagina will preferentially fill before the uterus.

Hydrocolpos—The distension of the vagina with fluid; often seen in infants with complex reproductive anomalies.

Metroplasty—Uterine reconstructive procedure.

Uterine anlagen—An underdeveloped uterine structure that is a remnant of a single embryologic müllerian duct.

Maldevelopment of the müllerian ducts occurs in a variety of forms, and each anomaly is distinctive. Nevertheless, some generalizations can be made. Classifications of vaginal anomalies based on certain anatomic findings are useful in organizing the type of malformation, but there usually are exceptions to each rule. Thus, what appears, after a preliminary diagnostic evaluation, to be an apparently isolated vaginal malformation may be found later to be associated with a uterine or renal anomaly. A comprehensive preoperative evaluation of patients with suspected malformations of the müllerian ducts is essential, but a clear understanding of the particular anomaly may not be established until the time of surgical correction. Reproductive surgeons must therefore be equally skilled in both uterine and vaginal reconstruction.

The patient with a uterovaginal anomaly often relies entirely on her physician to clarify the reproductive consequences associated with her diagnosis. The physician can help to allay her anxieties by making a prompt evaluation and giving a full and accurate description of the reproductive implications or the obstetric consequences of her particular uterovaginal anomaly.

CLASSIFICATION OF UTEROVAGINAL ANOMALIES

Classifications of uterovaginal anomalies originally were organized on the basis of clinical findings. Our improved understanding of the embryologic development of most uterovaginal anomalies has enabled categorization on this basis. The 1988 American Fertility Society (AFS) classification of müllerian anomalies (Table 25.1) offers an alternative based on the degree of failure of normal uterine development. Anomalies are grouped according to similarities of clinical manifestations, treatment, and prognosis for fetal salvage. The AFS classification system is weighted primarily toward disorders of lateral fusion and does not include associated vaginal anomalies, although the scheme does allow the user to describe anomalies involving the vagina, tubes, and urinary tract as associated malformations.

No classification of müllerian maldevelopment can focus entirely on the uterus, however. The vagina is often involved, and sometimes the tubes are involved as well. This discussion follows a suggested modification of the AFS classification of uterovaginal anomalies (Table 25.2) that comprises four groups based on embryologic considerations.

Class I: Dysgenesis of the Müllerian Ducts

Dysgenesis of the müllerian ducts, which includes agenesis of the uterus and vagina (the Mayer-Rokitansky-Küster-Hauser syndrome), is an impairment of the reproductive system characterized by no reproductive potential other than that achieved by *in vitro* fertilization in a host uterus.

Class II: Disorders of Vertical Fusion of the Müllerian Ducts

Disorders of vertical fusion can be considered to represent faults in the junction between the down-growing müllerian ducts (müllerian tubercle) and the up-growing derivative of the urogenital sinus. Typically, these disorders are characterized by an atretic portion of vagina that can be quite thick, extending through more than half the distance of the vagina, or it can be quite thin and limited to a small obstructing membrane.

Regardless of the length of the septum, a disorder of vertical fusion should be regarded as a transverse vaginal septum and classified as either obstructed or unobstructed. The so-called partial vaginal agenesis with uterus and cervix present is probably a misnomer for a large segment of atretic vagina. Cervical agenesis or dysgenesis is also included in the group of disorders of vertical fusion.

Class III: Disorders of Lateral Fusion of the Müllerian Ducts

Disorders of lateral fusion of the two müllerian ducts can be symmetric-unobstructed, as with the double vagina, or asymmetric-obstructed, as with unilateral vaginal obstruction. Obstructions associated with disorders of lateral fusion are particularly noteworthy in that they are observed clinically only as unilateral obstructions that almost invariably are associated with absence of the ipsilateral kidney. Bilateral obstruction is

TABLE 25.1

AMERICAN FERTILITY SOCIETY CLASSIFICATION OF MÜLLERIAN ANOMALIES[a]

Classification Anomaly
Class I. Segmental, müllerian agenesis–hypoplasia
A. Vaginal
B. Cervical
C. Fundal
D. Tubal
E. Combined anomalies
Class II. Unicornuate
A. Communicating
B. Noncommunicating
C. No cavity
D. No horn
Class III. Didelphys
Class IV. Bicornuate
A. Complete (division down to internal os)
B. Partial
Class V. Septate
A. Complete (septum to internal os)
B. Partial
Class VI. Arcuate
Class VII. Diethylstilbestrol related

[a]This classification allows the user to indicate the malformation type and provides additional findings to describe associated variations involving the vagina, cervix, tubes (right, left), and kidneys (right, left). Adapted from the American Fertility Society. Classification of müllerian anomalies. *Fertil Steril* 1988;49:944.

thought to be associated with bilateral kidney agenesis and subsequent nonviability of the developing embryo.

The three varieties of asymmetric obstruction with ipsilateral renal agenesis are as follows:

1. Unicornuate uterus with a noncommunicating horn that contains menstruating endometrium
2. Unilateral obstruction of a cavity of a double uterus
3. Unilateral vaginal obstruction

The five groups of symmetric-unobstructed disorders of lateral fusion are as follows:

1. The didelphic uterus
2. The septate uterus
3. The bicornuate uterus
4. The T-shaped uterine cavity, which may be hypoplastic and irregular, and which is associated with diethylstilbestrol (DES) exposure *in utero*
5. The unicornuate uterus with or without a rudimentary horn

The first three groups are types of double uteri; differentiation between a septate uterus (second group) and a bicornuate uterus (third group) requires visualization of the fundus. The septum within the septate uterus is complete or partial. When the septum is complete, there inevitably are two cervices with a longitudinal vaginal septum that can extend to the introitus or partially down the vagina. The bicornuate uterus also can have a partial or almost complete separation of the uterine cavities. The term *arcuate uterus* is used primarily by radiologists to refer to a slight septum in the uterine fundus that forms no clear separation of the uterine cavities. This type of uterus is usually included in the category of partial septate uterus.

TABLE 25.2

AMERICAN FERTILITY SOCIETY CLASSIFICATION OF UTEROVAGINAL ANOMALIES

Class I. Dysgenesis of the müllerian ducts
Class II. Disorders of vertical fusion of the müllerian ducts
A. Transverse vaginal septum
1. Obstructed
2. Unobstructed
B. Cervical agenesis or dysgenesis
Class III. Disorders of lateral fusion of the müllerian ducts
A. Asymmetric-obstructed disorder of uterus or vagina usually associated with ipsilateral renal agenesis
1. Unicornuate uterus with a noncommunicating rudimentary anlage or horn
2. Unilateral obstruction of a cavity of a double uterus
3. Unilateral vaginal obstruction associated with double uterus
B. Symmetric-unobstructed
1. Didelphic uterus
a. Complete longitudinal vaginal septum
b. Partial longitudinal vaginal septum
c. No longitudinal vaginal septum
2. Septate uterus
a. Complete
1) Complete longitudinal vaginal septum
2) Partial longitudinal vaginal septum
3) No longitudinal vaginal septum
b. Partial
1) Complete longitudinal vaginal septum
2) Partial longitudinal vaginal septum
3) No longitudinal vaginal septum
3. Bicornuate uterus
a. Complete
1) Complete longitudinal vaginal septum
2) Partial longitudinal vaginal septum
3) No longitudinal vaginal septum
b. Partial
1) Complete longitudinal vaginal septum
2) Partial longitudinal vaginal septum
3) No longitudinal vaginal septum
4. T-shaped uterine cavity (diethylstilbestrol related)
5. Unicornuate uterus
a. With a rudimentary horn
1) With endometrial cavity
a) Communicating
b) Noncommunicating
2) Without endometrial cavity
b. Without a rudimentary horn
Class IV. Unusual configurations of vertical-lateral fusion defects

Modified from the American Fertility Society. Classification of müllerian anomalies. *Fertil Steril* 1988;49:944.

The unicornuate uterus may have an attached horn with a cavity that communicates with the unicornuate uterus, or there may be no uterine horn or a uterine horn with no cavity. Some debate has focused on whether the unicornuate uterus with a communicating horn can represent a hypoplastic side of a bicornuate uterus.

Class IV: Unusual Configurations of Vertical-Lateral Fusion Defects

This final category includes combinations of uterovaginal anomalies and other disorders. Unusual uterovaginal configurations have been described that do not fit a particular category, and vertical and lateral fusion disorders can coexist.

Unusual configurations of vertical-lateral fusion defects can be seen with abnormalities of the lower urinary tract. Singh and coworkers have described a patient who was noted to have a persistent hymen and a longitudinal vaginal septum with a didelphic uterus. The patient was noted also to have a double urethra and bladder and left renal agenesis.

Obstructive lesions require immediate attention to relieve retrograde flow of trapped mucus and menstrual blood and increasing pressure on surrounding organs and structures. When no obstruction is present, attention may not be required immediately, but it will always be required eventually to establish or improve reproductive or coital function.

EMBRYOLOGY

The reproductive organs in the female (and in the male) consist of external genitalia, gonads, and an internal duct system between the two. These three components originate embryologically from different primordia and in close association with the urinary system and hindgut. Thus, the developmental history is complex (Figs. 25.1 and 25.2). Even in the 3.5- to 4-mm embryo, it is possible to recognize the bilateral thickenings of the coelomic epithelium known as the gonadal ridges medial to the mesonephros (primitive kidney) in the dorsum of the coelomic cavity. At about the sixth week of gestation, in the 17- to 20-mm embryo, the gonad can be distinguished as either a testis or an ovary.

In the female, the labia minora and majora develop from the labioscrotal folds, which are ectodermal in origin. The phallic portion of the urogenital sinus gives rise to the urethra. The müllerian (paramesonephric) duct system is stimulated to develop preferentially over the wolffian (mesonephric) duct system, which regresses in early female fetal life. The cranial parts of the wolffian ducts can persist as the epoöphoron of the ovarian hilum; the caudal parts can persist as Gartner's ducts. The müllerian ducts persist and attain complete development to form the fallopian tubes, the uterine corpus and cervix, and a portion of the vagina.

Origin of the Müllerian Ducts

About 37 days after fertilization, the müllerian ducts first appear lateral to each wolffian duct as invaginations of the dorsal coelomic epithelium. The site of origin of the invaginations remains open and ultimately forms the fimbriated ends of the fallopian tubes. At their point of origin, each of the müllerian ducts forms a solid bud. Each bud penetrates the mesenchyme lateral and parallel to each wolffian duct. As the solid buds elongate, a lumen appears in the cranial part, beginning at each coelomic opening. The lumina extend gradually to the caudal growing tips of the ducts.

Eventually, the caudal end of each müllerian duct crosses the ventral aspect of the wolffian duct. The paired müllerian ducts continue to grow in a medial and caudal direction until they eventually meet in the midline and become fused together in the urogenital septum. A septum between the two müllerian ducts gradually disappears, leaving a single uterovaginal canal lined with cuboidal epithelium. Failure of reabsorption of this septum can result in a septate uterus. The most cranial parts of the müllerian ducts remain separate and form the fallopian tubes. The caudal segments of the müllerian ducts fuse to form the uterus and part of the vagina. The cranial point of fusion is the site of the future fundus of the uterus. Variations in this site of fusion can result in an arcuate or bicornuate uterus. Complete failure of fusion can result in a didelphic uterus.

Isolated case reports continue to challenge established embryologic mechanisms of müllerian development. Dunn and Hantes reported a case of a double cervix and vagina with a blind cervical pouch challenging the theory of unidirectional fusion. Engmann and colleagues reported a unicornuate uterus with normal external uterine morphology, with bilateral fallopian tubes; however, only the right fallopian tube communicated with the uterine cavity. The patient suffered from pain because of the obstruction egress of the stimulated endometrial tissue. The patient was treated with removal of the obstructed cavity. The authors propose that this may represent failure of canalization of one of the müllerian ducts. Additional reports are necessary to fully evaluate potential variations in embryological development.

Development of the Vagina

The vagina is formed from the lower end of the uterovaginal canal, which developed from the müllerian ducts and the urogenital sinus (Fig. 25.2). The point of contact between the two is the müllerian tubercle. A solid vaginal cord results from proliferation of the cells at the caudal tip of the fused müllerian ducts. The cord gradually elongates to meet the bilateral endodermal evaginations (sinovaginal bulbs) from the posterior aspect of the urogenital sinus below. These sinovaginal bulbs extend cranially to fuse with the caudal end of the vaginal cord, forming the vaginal plate. Subsequent canalization of the vaginal cord occurs, followed by epithelialization with cells derived mostly from endoderm of the urogenital sinus. Recent proposals hold that only the upper one third of the vagina is formed from the müllerian ducts and that the lower vagina develops from the vaginal plate of the urogenital sinus. Recent studies also suggest that the vaginal canal is actually open and connected to a patent uterus and tubes, even in early embryonic life, and that the vagina does not form and later become canalized from an epithelial cord of squamous cells growing upward from the urogenital sinus. Most investigators now suggest that the vagina develops under the influence of the müllerian ducts and estrogenic stimulation. There is general agreement that the vagina is a composite formed partly from the müllerian ducts and partly from the urogenital sinus.

At about the 20th week, the cervix takes form as a result of condensation of stromal cells at a specific site around the fused müllerian ducts. The mesenchyme surrounding the müllerian ducts becomes condensed early in embryonic development and eventually forms the musculature of the female genital tract. The hymen is the embryologic septum between the sinovaginal bulbs above and the urogenital sinus proper below. It is lined by an internal layer of vaginal epithelium and an external layer of epithelium derived from the urogenital sinus (both of endodermal origin), with mesoderm between the two. It is not derived from the müllerian ducts.

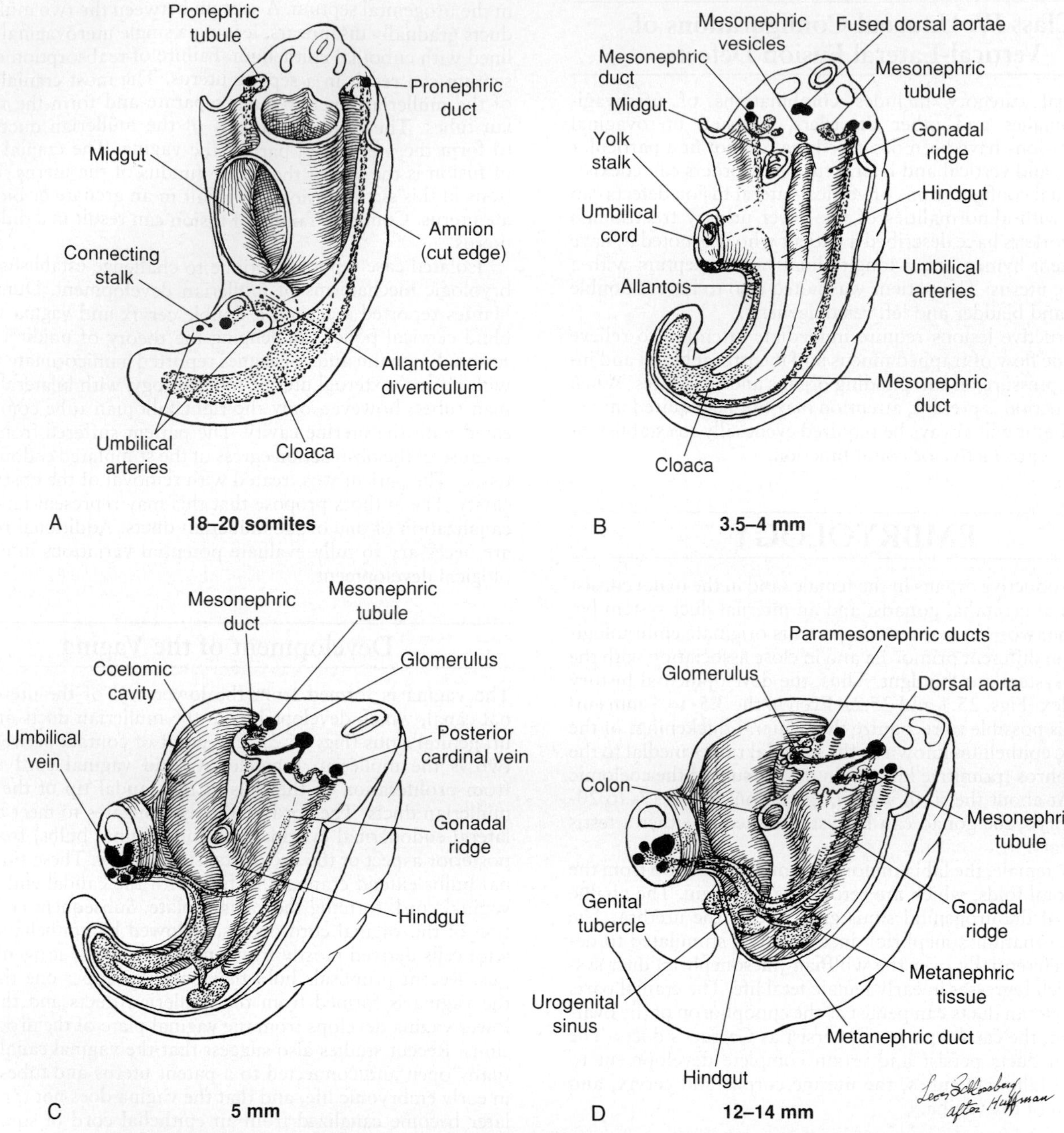

FIGURE 25.1. Diagrammatic representation of the development of the female reproductive organs and structures in early embryogenesis. **A:** At the 18- to 20-somite stage (fourth week), the gonadal ridges have not yet begun to form. **B:** In the 3.5- to 4-mm embryo (fifth week), the gonadal ridges can be recognized as thickenings of the coelomic cavity just medial to the mesonephric tubules. (Gonadal differentiation into either testis or ovary does not occur until the sixth week of development.) The allantoenteric diverticulum is joined caudally to the dilated cloaca. **C** and **D:** The genital tubercle and labial folds form in the region just anterior to the cloaca. The cloaca later divides into the ventral urogenital sinus and the dorsal rectum. The development of the urinary system closely parallels that of the reproductive system. The nonfunctioning pronephric tubules shown in (**A**) develop to form the mesonephric ducts shown in (**B**) and (**C**). The permanent kidneys eventually develop from the metanephric tissue, and the urinary collecting system develops from the metanephric ducts. The paramesonephric (müllerian) ducts are apparent by the 12- to 14-mm stage (**D**). (Their subsequent development is illustrated in Figure 25.2.)

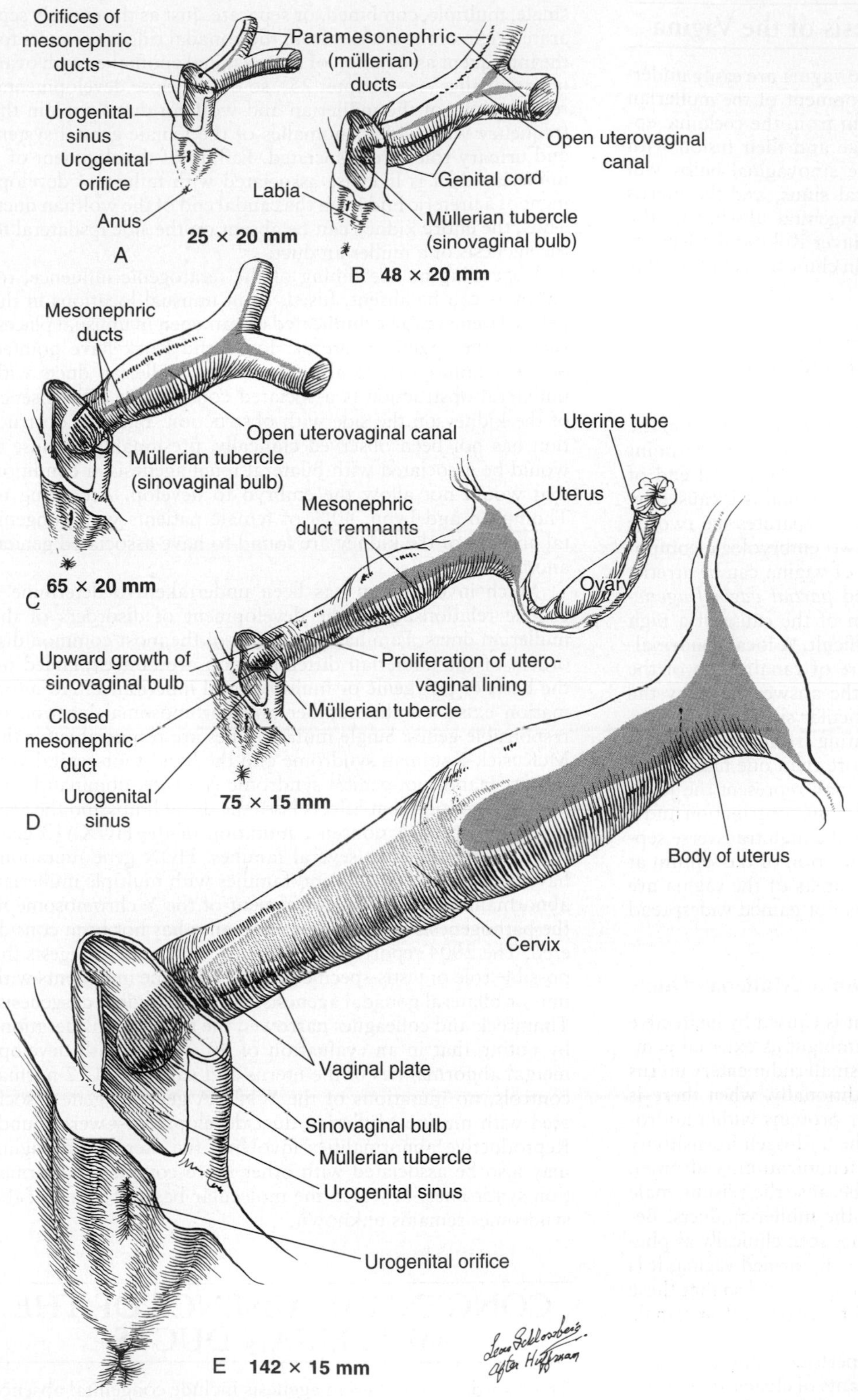

FIGURE 25.2. Further development of the paramesonephric (müllerian) ducts and the urogenital sinus. **A:** Early development of the paramesonephric ducts. The cranial ends of the paramesonephric ducts develop first. These ends remain open to form the fimbriated ends of the fallopian tubes. The paramesonephric ducts grow caudally and cross the mesonephric ducts ventrally. **B:** Eventually, they fuse together to form the uterovaginal canal. **C:** Further caudal development brings this structure into contact with the wall of the urogenital sinus, producing the müllerian tubercle. The caudal ends of the fused paramesonephric ducts form the uterine corpus and cervix. Together with the urogenital sinus, they also form the vagina. The cranial point of fusion of the paramesonephric ducts marks the location of the future uterine fundus. The fallopian tubes form from the unfused cranial parts of the paramesonephric (müllerian) ducts. The proliferation of the lining of the uterovaginal canal above the upward growth of the sinovaginal bulb from below (**D**) forms the vaginal plate (**E**), which later becomes canalized to leave an open vaginal canal. Thus, the vagina is of composite origin. The mesonephric ducts in the female degenerate but can persist into adult life as Gartner's ducts.

Anomalies in Organogenesis of the Vagina

Anomalies in the organogenesis of the vagina are easily understood. If there is failure in the development of the müllerian ducts at any time between their origin from the coelomic epithelium at 5 weeks of embryonic age and their fusion with the urogenital sinus at 8 weeks, the sinovaginal bulbs will fail to proliferate from the urogenital sinus, and the uterus and vagina will fail to develop. Congenital absence of the uterus and the vagina, known as the Mayer-Rokitansky-Küster-Hauser syndrome, is the most common clinical example of this anomaly.

Transverse Vaginal Septum

A transverse vaginal septum can develop at any location in the vagina but is more common in the upper vagina at the point of junction between the vaginal plate and the caudal end of the fused müllerian ducts. This defect presumably is caused by failure of absorption of the tissue that separates the two or by failure of complete fusion of the two embryologic components of the vagina. A large segment of vagina can be atretic. In past reviews, this has been termed *partial vaginal agenesis with a uterus present.* Elucidation of the cause of a high transverse vaginal septum is more difficult. A local abnormality of the vaginal mesoderm or failure of canalization of the epithelial vaginal plate can provide the answer, but why the abnormality should occur at this particular site is not evident. The proportion of the vagina originating from the urogenital sinus can at times be considerably more than one fifth, and a high transverse vaginal septum thus may represent the junction of an abnormally long urogenital sinus contribution and a short müllerian portion. Alternatively, the high transverse septum could be the sequela of a local infection of the septum at the end of the vagina. Septa in other areas of the vagina are unexplained by this theory, which has not gained widespread acceptance.

Disorders of Ineffective Suppression of Müllerian Ducts

When abnormal gonadal development is caused by ineffective suppression of the müllerian ducts, ambiguous external genitalia frequently are accompanied by a small rudimentary uterus or a partially developed vagina. Additionally, when there is a genetic loss of cytoplasmic receptor proteins within androgenic target cells, such as occurs in the androgen insensitivity syndrome (formerly called testicular feminization syndrome), the vagina is incompletely developed because the existing male gonads suppress the development of the müllerian ducts. Because these genetically male patients are seen clinically as phenotypic XY females without a completely formed vagina, it is important that a vagina be surgically constructed so that these patients may have satisfactory sexual function in their female gender role.

Congenital rectovaginal fistula, imperforate (covered) anus, hypospadias, and other anatomic variants of cloacal dysgenesis also can occur. These anomalies can be associated with maldevelopment of the müllerian and mesonephric duct derivatives.

Müllerian Duct Abnormalities

Abnormalities in the formation or fusion of the müllerian ducts can result in a variety of anomalies of the uterus and vagina: single, multiple, combined, or separate. Just as the entirely separate origin of the ovaries from the gonadal ridges accounts for the infrequent association of uterovaginal anomalies with ovarian anomalies (see Chapter 25), so do the close developmental relationships of the müllerian and wolffian ducts explain the frequency with which anomalies of the female genital system and urinary tract are associated. Failure of development of a müllerian duct is likewise associated with failure of development of a ureteric bud from the caudal end of the wolffian duct. Thus, the entire kidney can be absent on the side ipsilateral to the agenesis of a müllerian duct.

Depending on the timing of the teratogenic influence, renal units can be absent, fused, or in unusual locations in the pelvis. Ureters can be duplicated or can open in unusual places, such as the vagina or uterus. Jones and Rock have pointed out that failure of lateral fusion of the müllerian ducts with unilateral obstruction is associated consistently with absence of the kidney on the side with obstruction. Bilateral obstruction has not been observed clinically, presumably because it would be associated with bilateral renal agenesis, a condition that would not allow the embryo to develop. According to Thompson and Lynn, 40% of female patients with congenital absence of the kidney are found to have associated genital anomalies.

Much investigation has been undertaken to determine a genetic relationship in the development of disorders of the müllerian ducts. Familial aggregates of the most common disorders of the müllerian differentiation are best explained on the basis of polygenic or multifactorial inheritance. No information exists on the number and chromosomal location of responsible genes. Single mutant genes are responsible for the McKusick-Kaufman syndrome and the hand-foot-genital syndrome. Hand-foot-genital syndrome is a rare, dominantly inherited condition that affects both the distal limbs and the genitourinary tract. A nonsense mutation of the HOXA13 gene has been identified in several families. HOX gene mutations have been reported in several families with multiple müllerian abnormalities. To date, involvement of the Y chromosome in the pathogenesis of müllerian anomalies has not been considered. The 2004 report by Plevraki and colleagues suggests the possible role of testis-specific protein 1-Y gene in patients with uni- or bilateral gonadal agenesis and uterovaginal dysgenesis. Timmreck and colleagues narrowed the genetic considerations by noting that in an evaluation of 40 women with developmental abnormalities of the uterus and vagina and 12 normal controls, no mutations of the WNT7A gene—a gene associated with murine Müllerian duct development—were found. Reproductive abnormalities involving the uterus and vagina may also be associated with other more complex malformation syndromes, in which the molecular basis of many of the syndromes remains unknown.

CONGENITAL ABSENCE OF THE MÜLLERIAN DUCTS

The disorders of müllerian agenesis include congenital absence of the vagina and uterus. Often referred to in the literature simply as congenital absence of the vagina (vaginal agenesis), this condition is more accurately labeled aplasia (or dysplasia) of the müllerian ducts because the lower vagina generally is normal, but the middle and upper two thirds are missing. Despite the absence of the uterus, rudimentary uterine primordia are found that are comparable to each other in size and appearance. Tubes and ovaries in patients with congenital absence of the müllerian ducts generally are normal. The syndrome, usually referred to as the Mayer-Rokitansky-Küster-Hauser (MRKH) syndrome, is associated with a heterogeneous group of disorders that have a variety of genetic, endocrine, and metabolic manifestations and associated anomalies of other body systems.

Characteristics of Women with Müllerian Agenesis

- Congenital absence of the uterus and vagina (small rudimentary uterine bulbs are usually present with rudimentary fallopian tubes)
- Normal ovarian function, including ovulation
- Sex of rearing: female
- Phenotypic sex: female (normal development of breasts, body proportions, hair distribution, and external genitalia)
- Genetic sex: female (46,XX karyotype)
- Frequent association of other congenital anomalies (skeletal, urologic, and especially renal)

Partial agenesis of the vagina with the uterus present and a transverse vaginal septum both are categorized as disorders of vertical fusion. These two disorders have a low incidence of associated urinary tract anomalies, another circumstance that sets them apart from the MRKH syndrome.

Realdus Columbus first described congenital absence of the vagina in 1559. In 1829, Mayer described congenital absence of the vagina as one of the abnormalities found in stillborn infants with multiple birth defects. Rokitansky in 1838 and Küster in 1910 described an entity in which the vagina was absent, a small bipartite uterus was present, the ovaries were normal, and anomalies of other organ systems (renal and skeletal) were frequently observed. Hauser and associates emphasized the spectrum of associated anomalies. Pinsky suggested that congenital absence of the vagina is part of a symptom complex and not a true syndrome. Over the years, the disorder has come to be known as the Mayer-Rokitansky-Küster-Hauser syndrome, the Rokitansky-Küster-Hauser syndrome, or simply the Rokitansky syndrome (Fig. 25.3). Counseller found that the condition occurred once in 4,000 female admissions to the Mayo Clinic. Evans estimated that vaginal agenesis occurred once in 10,588 female births in Michigan from 1953 to 1957.

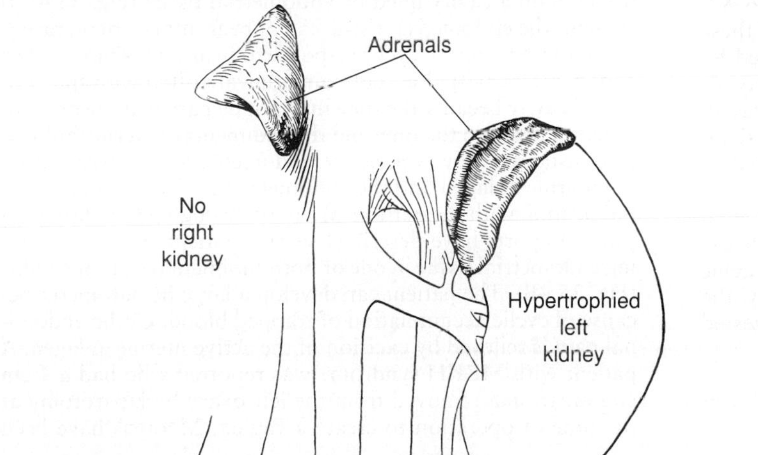

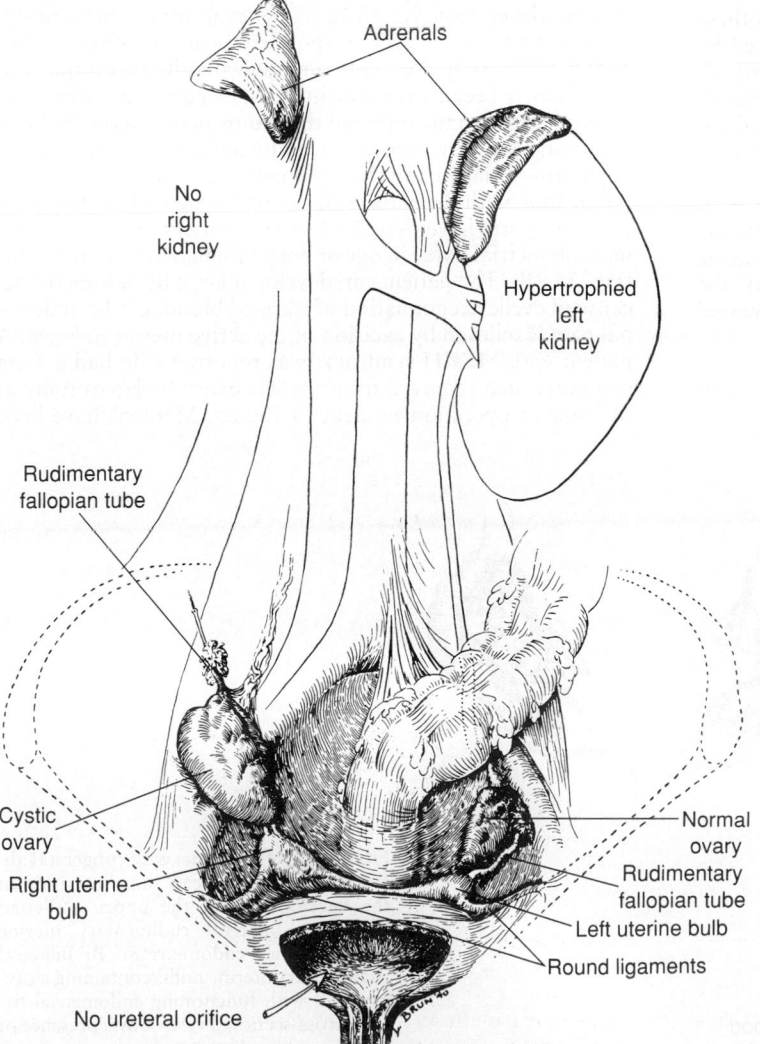

FIGURE 25.3. Typical findings in a patient with Mayer-Rokitansky-Küster-Hauser syndrome. Note the absence of the right kidney and right ureteral orifice. The uterus is represented by bilateral rudimentary uterine bulbs joined by a band behind the bladder. The ovaries appear normal although there is malposition of the right ovary.

Individuals with an absent vagina and the classic MRKH syndrome usually are first seen by a gynecologist at age 14 to 15 years, when the absence of menses causes concern. Such young women have a normal complement of chromosomes (46,XX) and usually have normal ovaries and secondary sex characteristics, including external genitalia. Menstruation does not appear at the usual age because the uterus is absent, but ovulation occurs regularly. There are some exceptions to the rule of normal ovaries. For example, polycystic ovaries and gonadal dysgenesis have been reported in patients with congenital absence of the vagina. Plevraki and colleagues reinforced the importance of consideration of such conditions, as one of the six women with MRKH evaluated over a 12-month period demonstrated hypergonadotropic hypogonadism that was due to the bilateral absence of gonadal tissue. Additionally, nested polymerase chain reaction demonstrated the presence of testis-specific protein 1-Y-linked (TSPY) gene in two women.

Etiologic Factors

An exclusively genetic etiology cannot be ascribed to vaginal agenesis because almost all patients have a normal karyotype (46,XX) and because the discordance of vaginal agenesis in three sets of monozygotic twins has been reported. The occurrence of complete vaginal agenesis in sisters with a 46,XX karyotype suggests an autosomal mode of inheritance for these patients. Shokeir investigated the families of 13 unrelated females with aplasia of müllerian duct derivatives. Similarly affected females were found in 10 families. Usually there was an affected female paternal relative, suggesting female-limited autosomal dominant inheritance of a mutant gene transmitted by male relatives.

Other investigators point to the variety of associated anomalies as support for the etiologic concept of variable expression of a genetic defect possibly precipitated by teratogenic exposure between the 37th and the 41st gestational day, the time during which the vagina is formed. Knab has suggested five possible etiologic factors of the MRKH syndrome:

1. Inappropriate production of müllerian regressive factor in the female embryonic gonad
2. Regional absence or deficiency of estrogen receptors limited to the lower müllerian duct
3. Arrest of müllerian duct development by a teratogenic agent
4. Mesenchymal inductive defect
5. Sporadic gene mutation

Knab believes that the teratogenic and the mutant gene etiologies are the most probable.

Anomalies Associated with Müllerian Agenesis

Many patients with müllerian agenesis have associated anomalies of the upper müllerian duct system together with associated anomalies of other organ systems. By gentle rectal examination, the physician can feel an absence of the midline müllerian structure that should represent the uterus. The physician instead feels a smooth band (possibly a remnant of the uterosacral ligaments) that extends from one side of the pelvis to the other. In MRKH syndrome, the uterus is represented by bilateral rudimentary uterine bulbs that vary in size, are not usually palpable, are connected to small fallopian tubes, and are located on the lateral pelvic side wall adjacent to normal ovaries. Depending on their size, these rudimentary uterine bulbs may or may not contain a cavity lined by endometrial tissue (Fig. 25.4). If present, the endometrial tissue can appear immature or, rarely, can show evidence of cyclic response to ovarian hormones. The endometrial cavity does not communicate often with the peritoneal cavity because the tube may not be patent at the point of junction between the tube and the rudimentary uterine bulb. In rare instances, however, active endometrium can exist within the uterine anlagen and the endometrial cavity, enabling communication with the peritoneal cavity through patent fallopian tubes. Reports have described several patients with functioning endometrial tissue in one or both rudimentary uterine bulbs (Fig. 25.4B). The patient can develop a large hematometra because of cyclic accumulation of trapped blood. Cyclic abdominal pain is relieved by excision of the active uterine anlagen. A patient with MRKH syndrome was reported who had a 4-cm endometrioma removed from the left ovary by laparotomy at the time of operation to create a vagina. Myomas have been

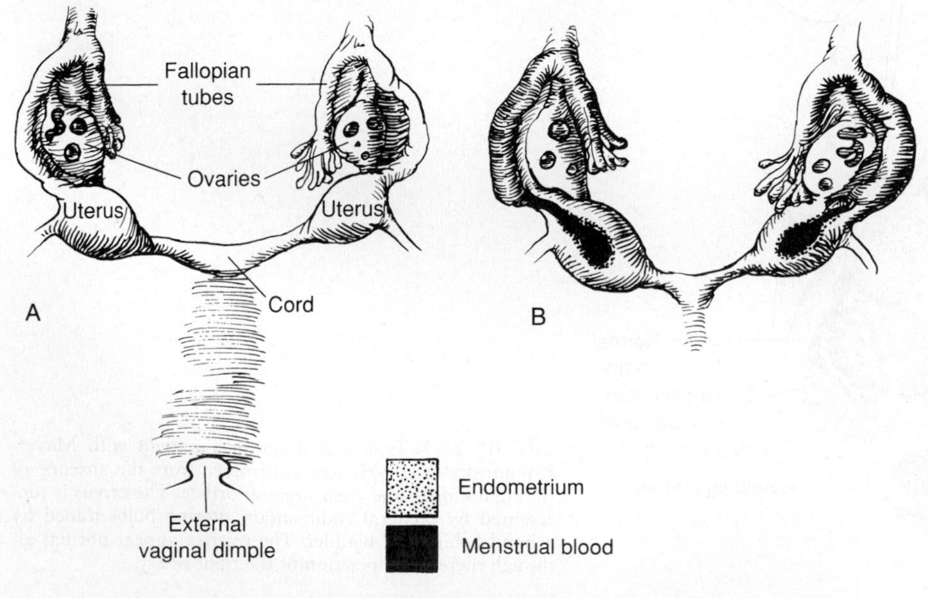

FIGURE 25.4. Patients with congenital absence of the vagina can show variation in the development of the upper müllerian ducts. **A:** Bilateral rudimentary uterine bulbs without endometrium. **B:** Bilateral rudimentary uterine bulbs containing a cavity lined with functioning endometrial tissue. Cross-sectional view shows presence of menstrual blood.

known to form in the muscular wall, and mild dysmenorrhea has been attributed to their presence. A small myoma has been found, in addition to the tube and ovary, in the inguinal canal and in the inguinal hernia sac.

Chakravarty and colleagues and Singh and Devi have demonstrated that the rudimentary bulbs have the potential for function. These authors used these rudimentary uterine bulbs to reconstruct a midline uterus. The reconstructed uterus was then connected to a newly constructed vagina. A surprising number of patients who have undergone this procedure have experienced cyclic menstruation, although recurrent stenosis and obstruction of the rudimentary horns are the most common results of such efforts. The authors of this chapter have had no experience with this technique and question its usefulness. However, these rudimentary uterine bulbs usually are insignificant structures that cause no problems.

Associated Urologic and Renal Anomalies

Fore and associates reported that 47% of patients in whom evaluation of the urinary tract was performed had associated urologic anomalies. In other studies, approximately one third of patients with complete vaginal agenesis were found to have significant urinary anomalies, including unilateral renal agenesis, unilateral or bilateral pelvic kidney, horseshoe kidney, hydronephrosis, hydroureter, and a variety of patterns of ureteral duplication. A significant number of patients with partial vaginal agenesis also have associated urinary tract anomalies.

Associated Skeletal and Other Anomalies

Associated skeletal anomalies have been recognized since congenital absence of the vagina was first described. In a review of 574 reported cases, Griffin and associates found a 12% incidence of skeletal abnormalities. Most of these abnormalities involve the spine (wedge vertebrae, fusions, rudimentary vertebral bodies, and supernumerary vertebrae), but the limbs and ribs also can be involved. Other anomalies include syndactyly, absence of a digit, congenital heart disease, and inguinal hernias, although the latter are more often present in patients with androgen insensitivity syndrome than in patients with MRKH syndrome (Fig. 25.3). Consideration of cardiac anomalies is also important, as Pittock and colleagues reported a substantial incidence of cardiac defects (16%) when reviewing a group of 25 patients with MRKH at the Mayo Clinic.

Treatment for Disorders of Müllerian Agenesis Preoperative Considerations

If functioning endometrial tissue is present with the anlagen, then symptoms from cryptomenorrhea will begin shortly after female secondary sex characteristics develop. Prompt removal of the active uterine bulbs affords complete relief of symptoms.

Occasionally, older patients with the classic MRKH syndrome consult a gynecologist because of difficult or painful intercourse. The indication for operation in these patients is obvious. Of all patients, they are the most satisfied with the operative results.

Most commonly, patients age 14 to 16 years are seen by a gynecologist because of primary amenorrhea. An examination may not have been done by a previous physician because the patient was "too young," but various hormonal medications may have been given with hope that menstruation would begin. An inaccurate examination may have led to the mistaken diagnosis of imperforate hymen. Futile attempts to incise the hymen may have resulted in scarring of the apex of the vaginal dimple before a correct diagnosis of congenital absence of the vagina was finally made. In the past, it was customary to advise delaying surgery to create a vagina for these young patients until just before their marriage. This led to difficulties, particularly when complications developed that required a delay in marriage until the vagina healed completely. More recently, it has become usual to perform the procedure when patients are 17 to 20 years old and are emotionally mature and intellectually reliable enough to manage the potential postoperative requirements for care, including manipulation of the vaginal form or the potential use of dilators.

Psychological Preparation of the Patient

Insufficient attention has been given to the psychological aspects of this problem. The patient with congenital absence of the vagina cannot be made into a whole person simply by creating a perineal pouch for intercourse. Establishment of sexual function is only one concern and may be the easiest problem to correct. Evans reported that 15% of his patients have real psychiatric difficulty. He and David and associates suggest that psychiatric help should be initiated before the operation. Weijenborg and ter Kuile described the effect of a group program on women with Rokitansky syndrome. The authors held group sessions conducted by a gynecologist, a female social worker, and a woman with Rokitansky syndrome. Seventeen patients participated. Three women had elected not to create a vagina, six women created a vagina by dilatation or sexual activity, and eight women had undergone a vaginoplasty. Indices of psychological distress were measured before the program, at initiation of the program, and at the last group session. The results demonstrated that women with Rokitansky syndrome felt less anxious, less depressed, and less sensitive to interpersonal contact after participation in the semistructured program. These data support the value of group interaction in patients with Rokitansky syndrome.

Learning about this anomaly, especially at a young age, is a shock and is accompanied by diminished self-esteem. Such patients can be encouraged by having their gynecologist offer appropriate surgery to establish coital function. The gynecologist can point out that, functionally, the patient will be like thousands of young women who have had a hysterectomy because of serious pelvic disease and who have satisfied their desire to be a parent through adoption or gestational surrogacy.

When counseling patients at the time of diagnosis, gestational surrogacy should definitely be included in the discussion. Until recently, the literature had provided only sparse evidence regarding the use of this modality in this population. Beski and colleagues confirmed the use of gestational surrogacy in a small population. The treatment cycles resulted in six clinical pregnancies (42.9% pregnancy rate per embryo transfer and 54.5% per oocyte retrieval) and three live births (21.4% per embryo transfer, 27.3% per retrieval, and 50% per patient). Several authors have reported on the genetic offspring of patients with vaginal agenesis. Petrozza and colleagues reported a retrospective study in 1997, describing a large number of treatment cycles for patients with Rokitansky syndrome. The authors attempted to determine an inheritance pattern of the syndrome through a questionnaire sent to all centers performing surrogacy treatment in the United States. A total of 162 *in vitro* fertilization/surrogacy treatment cycles were reviewed for 58 patients with congenital agenesis of the uterus and vagina. The treatment resulted in 34 live births (17 girls, 17 boys). One child had a nonspecific middle ear defect and hearing loss. The authors concluded that congenital absence of the uterus and vagina was not commonly inherited in a dominant fashion. These findings suggest inheritance of this disorder in children of affected mothers is likely via a polygenic mechanism.

Patient Cooperation

Regardless of which operative technique is chosen, the patient must cooperate if the operation is to be successful. When a McIndoe operation is performed, patients must understand the need to wear a form continuously for several months and intermittently for several years until the vagina is no longer subject to constriction and until regular intercourse is taking place. The operation should not be performed until preoperative interviews determine that the patient understands her essential role in its success. This is especially important when the patient is a young teenager. The single most important factor in determining the success of vaginoplasty is the psychosocial adjustment of the patient to her congenital vaginal anomaly.

Laboratory and Diagnostic Testing

A complete chromosomal analysis should be performed in all patients. If there is a suspicion of ovarian dysgenesis, androgen insensitivity syndrome, or some aberration of the classic MRKH syndrome, then a consideration of additional SRY analysis should be entertained to assess the possible presence of any Y chromosome. An intravenous pyelogram should be done preoperatively. This also provides an adequate survey for anomalies of the spine. If a pelvic mass is present, then additional special studies, including ultrasonography, should be performed to differentiate between hematometra, hematocolpos, endometrial and other ovarian cysts, and pelvic kidney. In some centers, magnetic resonance imaging (MRI), combined with an magnetic resonance urogram, may facilitate the evaluation of the reproductive, urologic, and skeletal systems with one radiographic study.

Evaluation of Cyclic Pain

Some patients without a pelvic mass report cyclic pain. This pain can be ovulatory or possibly a result of dysmenorrhea originating in well-developed rudimentary uterine bulbs. The physician can differentiate between the two by asking the patient to keep a basal body temperature chart and to mark the days when pelvic pain is present. Occasionally there is a question about whether a patient has congenital absence of the vagina or an imperforate hymen with cryptomenorrhea. The diagnosis is clarified before operative intervention by using radiographic imaging. Pelvic ultrasonography can often detect hematocolpos or an obstructed uterine anlagen distended with menstrual blood. An MRI can differentiate the two diagnoses, if necessary.

TABLE 25.3

CLASSIFICATION OF METHODS TO FORM A NEW VAGINA

Nonsurgical (intermittent pressure on the perineum)
Active dilatation
Passive dilatation
Surgical
Without use of abdominal contents
Without cavity dissection
Vulvovaginoplasty
Constant pressure (Vecchietti)
No attempt to line cavity (now unacceptable)
Lining cavity with grafts
Split-thickness skin grafts (McIndoe operation)
Dermis grafts
Amnion homografts
Lining cavity with flaps
Musculocutaneous flaps
Fasciocutaneous flaps
Subcutaneous pedicled skin flaps
Labial skin flaps (can be created with tissue expander)
Penoplasty (transsexualism)
With use of abdominal contents (cavity lining with)
Peritoneum
Free intestinal graft
Pedicled intestine

METHODS OF CREATING A VAGINA

There is no unanimity of opinion regarding the correct approach to the problem of vaginal agenesis (Table 25.3). With the development of the Ingram method for vaginal dilatation, fewer patients require surgical vaginoplasty. The role of tissue expanders in vaginoplasty has been reviewed by Patil and Hixon. Labial expansion with an expander having a capacity of 250 mL provides a flap 10 cm long and 8 cm wide with a 4-cm projection. Thus, well-vascularized flaps can be available to provide an outlet for stenosis-free vaginoplasty. This approach has been suggested to maximize the success of surgical vaginoplasty. A review of the methods devised for the formation of a vagina follows. The editors of this book have found the modified McIndoe technique to give the most consistently satisfactory results.

Nonsurgical Methods

In 1938, Frank described a method of creating an artificial vagina without operation. In 1940, he reported remarkably satisfactory results in eight patients treated with this method. His follow-up study showed that a vagina formed in this manner remained permanent in depth and caliber, even in patients who neglected dilatation for more than 1 year. It has been emphasized that the pelvic floor itself is embryologically deficient in some patients. Indeed, the ease with which some patients are able to create a vagina with intercourse alone or with other intermittent pressure techniques can be explained on this basis. Five patients were reported to have developed enteroceles, one after coitus alone, three after a Williams vulvovaginoplasty, and three after a McIndoe operation. This complication can

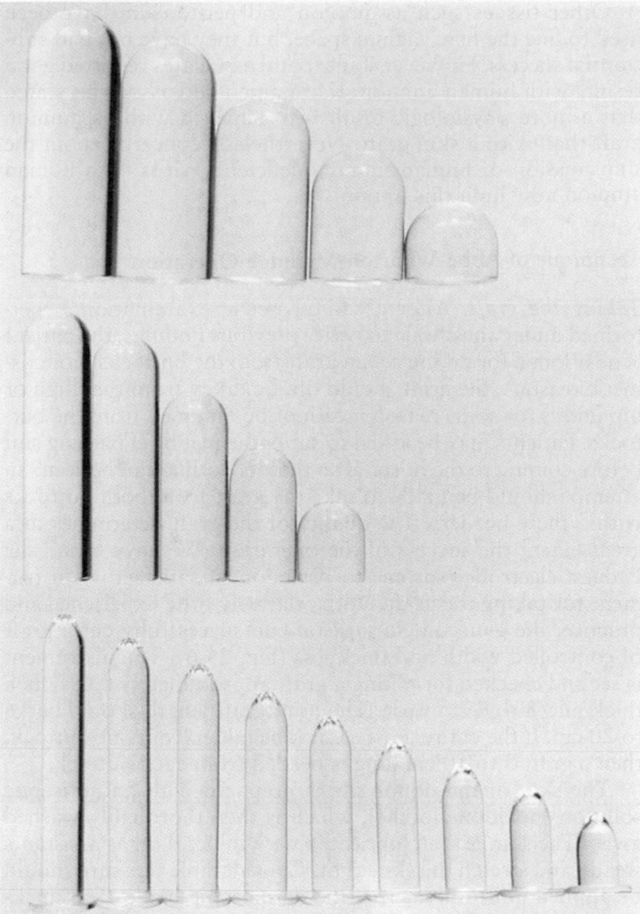

FIGURE 25.5. Vaginal dilators for use in Ingram passive dilatation technique to create a new vagina. The set consists of 19 dilators of increasing length and width. (Courtesy of Faulkner Plastics, Tampa, FL.)

develop when the vaginal mucosa is brought in close proximity to the pelvic peritoneum, but a relative embryologic weakness or an absence of endopelvic fascia can also contribute to this complication. Rock, Reeves, and associates at the Johns Hopkins Hospital reported that an initial trial of vaginal dilatation was successful in 9 of 21 patients.

Prompted by the rewarding results of Broadbent and Woolf, Ingram has described a passive dilatation technique of creating a new vagina. Instructing his patients in the insertion of dilators (Fig. 25.5) specially designed for use with a bicycle seat stool, Ingram was able to produce satisfactory vaginal depth and coital function in 10 of 12 cases of vaginal agenesis and 32 of 40 cases of various types of stenosis.

The Ingram technique for passive dilatation has several advantages. The patient is not required to press the dilator against the vaginal pouch. A series of graduated Lucite dilators slowly and evenly dilate the neovaginal space. The patient should be carefully instructed in the use of dilators, as recommended by Ingram, beginning with the smallest dilator. The patient is shown and instructed with the use of a mirror how to place a dilator against the introital dimple. The dilator may be held in place with a supportive undergarment and regular clothing worn over this.

TABLE 25.4

OUTCOMES OF PATIENTS WITH VAGINAL AGENESIS WHO ATTEMPTED DILATATION

Patients	Totals	Percent
Successful dilatation	34/37	91.9%[a]
Failed dilatation	3/37	8.1%

[a] $p < 0.001$.
Modified from Roberts CP, Haber MJ, Rock JA. Vaginal creation for muüllerian agenesis. *Am J Obstet Gynecol* 2001;185:1349.

The patient is shown how to sit on a racing type bicycle seat that is placed on a stool 24 inches above the floor. She is instructed to sit leaning slightly forward with the dilator in place for at least 2 hours per day at intervals of 15 to 30 minutes. Follow-up is usually at monthly intervals, and the patient can expect to graduate to the next size larger dilator about every month. An attempt at sexual intercourse may be suggested after the use of the largest dilator for 1 or 2 months. Continued dilatation is recommended if intercourse is infrequent. In our experience, functional success rates are outstanding. Rock and Roberts reported the largest series of vaginal agenesis patients who used the Ingram method of dilatation to create a neovagina. The records of 51 patients with müllerian agenesis were reviewed: 37 patients attempted vaginal dilatation and 14 young women underwent a surgical intervention. Functional success was defined as satisfactorily achieving intercourse or accepting the largest dilator without discomfort in the clinic visit. All patients were followed up for at least 2 years and for an average of 9.25 years. Functional success was achieved in 91.9% of those who attempted dilatation (Table 25.4). Thus, passive dilatation should be suggested as an initial therapy for vaginal creation. If dilatation is unsuccessful, operative vaginoplasty is indicated.

Surgical Methods

During the past 3 decades, experience has proved the Abbe-Wharton-McIndoe procedure (more popularly called the McIndoe operation) for dealing with complete absence of a vagina to be generally superior to others in most cases. In special circumstances, alternative methods of creation of a neovagina may be indicated.

Historical Development of Surgical Procedures

In 1907, Baldwin used a double loop of ileum to line a space dissected between the rectum and bladder, leaving the mesentery connected to the bowel. The continuity of the intestinal tract was reestablished by an end-to-end anastomosis. He reported that the new vagina was absolutely normal in every way. In 1910, Popaw constructed a vagina using a portion of the rectum that was moved anteriorly. This operation was modified by Schubert in 1911. The rectum was severed above the anal sphincter and moved anteriorly to serve as the vagina. The sigmoid was sutured to the anus to reestablish the continuity of the intestinal tract. Both operations had soberingly high morbidity and mortality rates, and their popularity declined. Today, segments of sigmoid are used most often to create a vaginal pouch or extend vaginal length in patients who have lost vaginal function as a result of extensive surgery or irradiation for pelvic malignancy. Some patients who are treated for multiple genitourinary or gastrointestinal abnormalities may be treated with a bowel vaginoplasty during a combined procedure.

Less formidable procedures involving dissection of a space between the bladder and rectum and lining of this space with flaps of skin from the labia or inner thighs also were tried. Marked scarring resulted, and hair usually grew in the vagina. Extensive plastic procedures to construct a vagina are no longer necessary or desirable and have been discarded in favor of safer procedures unless there is the problem of maintaining a vaginal canal after an extensive exenterative operation for pelvic malignancy. In this case, the physician may want to consider using the gracilis myocutaneous flap technique described by McCraw and associates in 1976.

The Abbe-Wharton-McIndoe Operation

The operation most popular today for creating a new vagina began with simple surgical attempts to create a space between the bladder and the rectum. These early attempts were often made in patients with cryptomenorrhea. However, such a space usually would constrict because the surgeon would fail to recognize the importance of prolonged continuous dilatation until the constrictive phase of healing was complete.

At the Johns Hopkins Hospital in 1938, Wharton combined an adequate dissection of the vaginal space with continuous dilatation by a balsa form that was covered with a thin rubber sheath and was left in the space. He did not use a split-thickness skin graft. Instead, he based his operation on the principle that the vaginal epithelium has remarkable powers of proliferation and in a relatively short time will cover the raw surface. Recalling that a similar process occurs in the fetus when the epithelium of the sinovaginal bulbs and the urogenital sinus form the vaginal canal, Wharton merely applied this same principle in the adult. This simple procedure is entirely satisfactory as long as the space is kept dilated long enough to allow the epithelium to grow in. Occasionally, however, even after several years, the vault of the vagina remains without epithelial covering. Coital bleeding and leukorrhea result from the persistent granulation tissue, and there is a tendency for vaginas constructed by this method to be constricted by scarring in the upper portion. In Counseller's 1948 report from the Mayo Clinic of 100 operations to construct a new vagina, 14 were performed by Wharton's method, with excellent results in all 14 patients. It was stated that the disadvantages of persistent granulation tissue with bleeding and leukorrhea were of no consequence. This has not been the experience of the editors of this book.

When inlay skin grafts were first used to construct a new vagina, the results were poor because the necessity for dilatation of the new vagina again was not recognized. Severe contraction, uncontrolled by continuous or intermittent dilatation, almost invariably spoiled the results. Although Heppner, Abbe, and others preceded him by many years in using a skin-covered prosthesis in neovaginal construction, it was Sir Archibald McIndoe, at the Queen Victoria Hospital in England, who popularized the method and gave it substantial clinical trial. He emphasized the three important principles used today in successful operations for vaginal agenesis:

1. Dissection of an adequate space between the rectum and the bladder
2. Inlay split-thickness skin grafting
3. The cardinal principle of continuous and prolonged dilatation during the contractile phase of healing

Other tissues such as amnion and peritoneum have been used to line the new vaginal space, but they have not had substantial success. However, Tancer and associates reported good results with human amnion. Karjalainen and associates stated that a more physiologic result was achieved with an amnion graft than with a skin graft. Nevertheless, concerns about the transmission of human immunodeficiency virus with human amnion now limit this option.

Technique of Abbe-Wharton-Mcindoe Operation

Taking the graft. After a careful pelvic examination is performed under anesthesia to verify previous findings, the patient is positioned for taking a skin graft from the buttocks. For cosmetic reasons, the graft should not be taken from the thigh or hip unless for some reason it cannot be obtained from the buttocks. Patients may be asked to sunbathe in a brief bathing suit before coming to the hospital so that its outline can be seen; an attempt should be made to take the graft from both buttocks within these borders. The quality of the graft determines to a great extent the success of the operation. We have found the Padgett electrodermatome to be the most satisfactory instrument for taking the graft. With relatively little experience and practice, the gynecologic surgeon can successfully cut a graft of controlled width and thickness (Fig. 25.6). The instrument is set and checked for taking a graft approximately 0.018 inch thick and 8 to 9 cm wide. The total graft length should be 16 to 20 cm. If the entire graft cannot be taken from one buttock, then a graft 8 to 10 cm long is needed from each buttock.

The skin of the donor site is prepared with an antiseptic solution (povidone-iodine), which is then thoroughly washed away. The skin is then lubricated with mineral oil as assistants steady and stretch the skin tight. Considerable pressure should be applied uniformly across the dermatome blade. The thickness of the graft must have minimal variation. A graft that is a little too thick is better than one that is a little too thin. There should be no breaks in the continuity of the graft. The graft is placed between two layers of moist gauze and the donor sites are dressed. The donor site is soaked with a dilute solution of epinephrine for hemostasis, and a sterile dressing is applied. A pressure dressing is then placed over the site; this dressing can be removed on the seventh postoperative day. The sterile dressing dries in place over the donor site and ultimately will fall off by itself. Moistened areas on the dressing can be dried with cool air. If there is separation and evidence of some superficial infection, then merbromin can be applied to these areas.

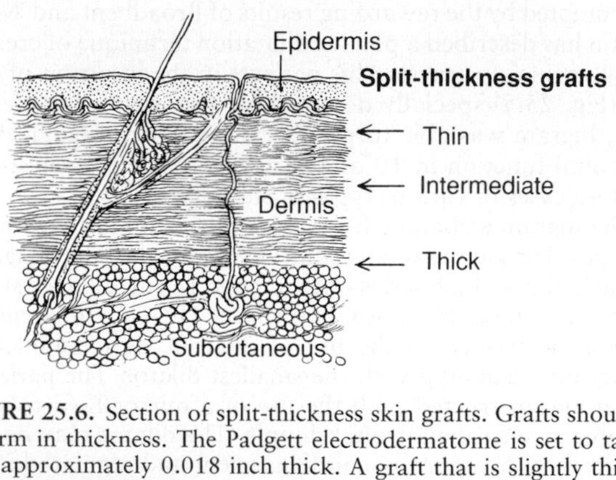

FIGURE 25.6. Section of split-thickness skin grafts. Grafts should be uniform in thickness. The Padgett electrodermatome is set to take a graft approximately 0.018 inch thick. A graft that is slightly thick is better than a thin graft.

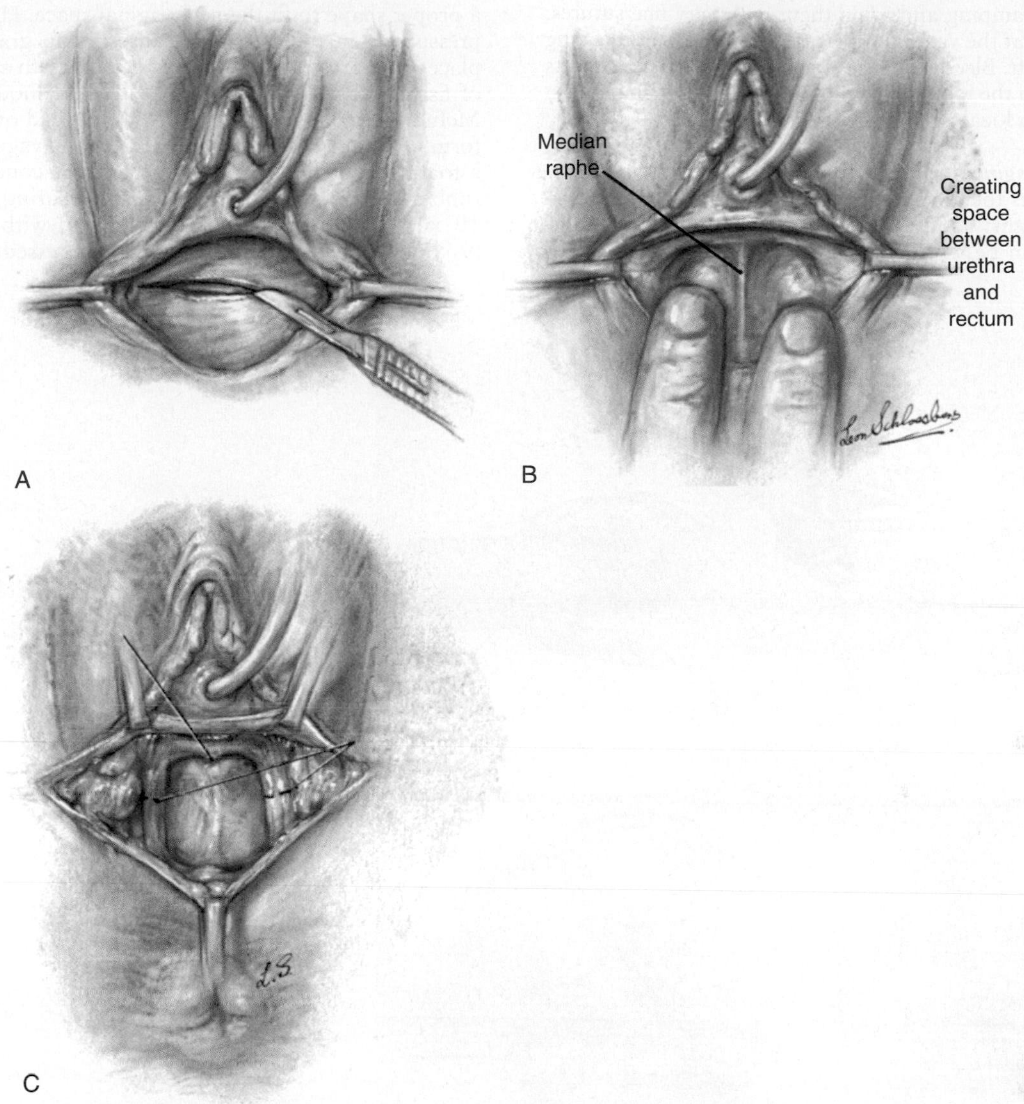

FIGURE 25.7. The McIndoe procedure. **A:** A transverse incision is made in the apex of the vaginal dimple. **B:** A channel can usually be dissected on each side of the median raphe. The median raphe is then divided. Careful dissection prevents injury to the bladder and rectum. **C:** A space between the urethra and bladder anteriorly and the rectum posteriorly is dissected until the undersurface of the peritoneum is reached. Incision of the medial margin of the puborectalis muscles will enlarge the vagina laterally.

Creating the neovaginal space. The patient is placed in the lithotomy position, and a transverse incision is made through the mucosa of the vaginal vestibule (Fig. 25.7A). The space between the urethra and bladder anteriorly and the rectum posteriorly is dissected until the undersurface of the peritoneum is reached. This step may be safer with a catheter in the urethra and sometimes a finger in the rectum to guide the dissection in the proper plane. After incising the mucosa of the vaginal vestibule transversely, the physician often is able to create a channel on each side of a median raphe (Fig. 25.7B), starting with blunt dissection and then dilating each channel with Hegar dilators or with finger dissection. In some instances, it may be necessary to develop the neovaginal space by dissecting laterally and bringing the fingers toward the midline. The median raphe is then divided, thus joining the two channels. This maneuver is helpful in dissecting an adequate space without causing injury to surrounding structures.

To avoid subsequent narrowing of the vagina at the level of the urogenital diaphragm, it may be helpful to incise the margin of the puborectalis muscles bilaterally along the midportion of the medial margin (Fig. 25.7C). Although useful in all circumstances, incision of the puborectalis muscle is more important in cases of androgen insensitivity syndrome with android pelvis, in which the levator muscles are more taut against the pelvic diaphragm, than in cases of gynecoid pelvis. Incision of the puborectalis muscle causes no difficulty with fecal incontinence, significantly improves the ease with which the vaginal form can be inserted into the canal in the postoperative period, and has eliminated the problem of contracture of the upper vagina caused by a poorly applied form. The dissection should be carried as high as possible without entering the peritoneal cavity and without cleaning away all tissue beneath the peritoneum. A split-thickness skin graft will not take well when applied against a base of thin peritoneum. All bleeders should be ligated by clamping and tying them with very fine sutures. It is essential that the vaginal cavity be dry to prevent bleeding beneath the graft. Bleeding causes the graft to separate from its bed, resulting in the inevitable failure of the graft to implant in that area and in local graft necrosis.

Preparing the vaginal form. Early skin grafts were formed over balsa, which has the advantages of being an inexpensive, easily available, light wood that can be sterilized without difficulty. It also can be whittled easily in the operating room to a proper shape to fit the new vaginal space. However, uneven pressure from the form can cause a skin graft to slough in places, and pressure spots are associated with an increased risk of fistula formation. The Counseller-Flor modification of the McIndoe technique (Fig. 25.8) uses, instead of the rigid balsa form, a foam rubber mold shaped for the vaginal cavity from a foam rubber block and covered with a condom. The foam rubber is gas sterilized in blocks measuring approximately 10 × 10 × 20 cm. The block is shaped with scissors to approximately twice the desired size, compressed into a condom,

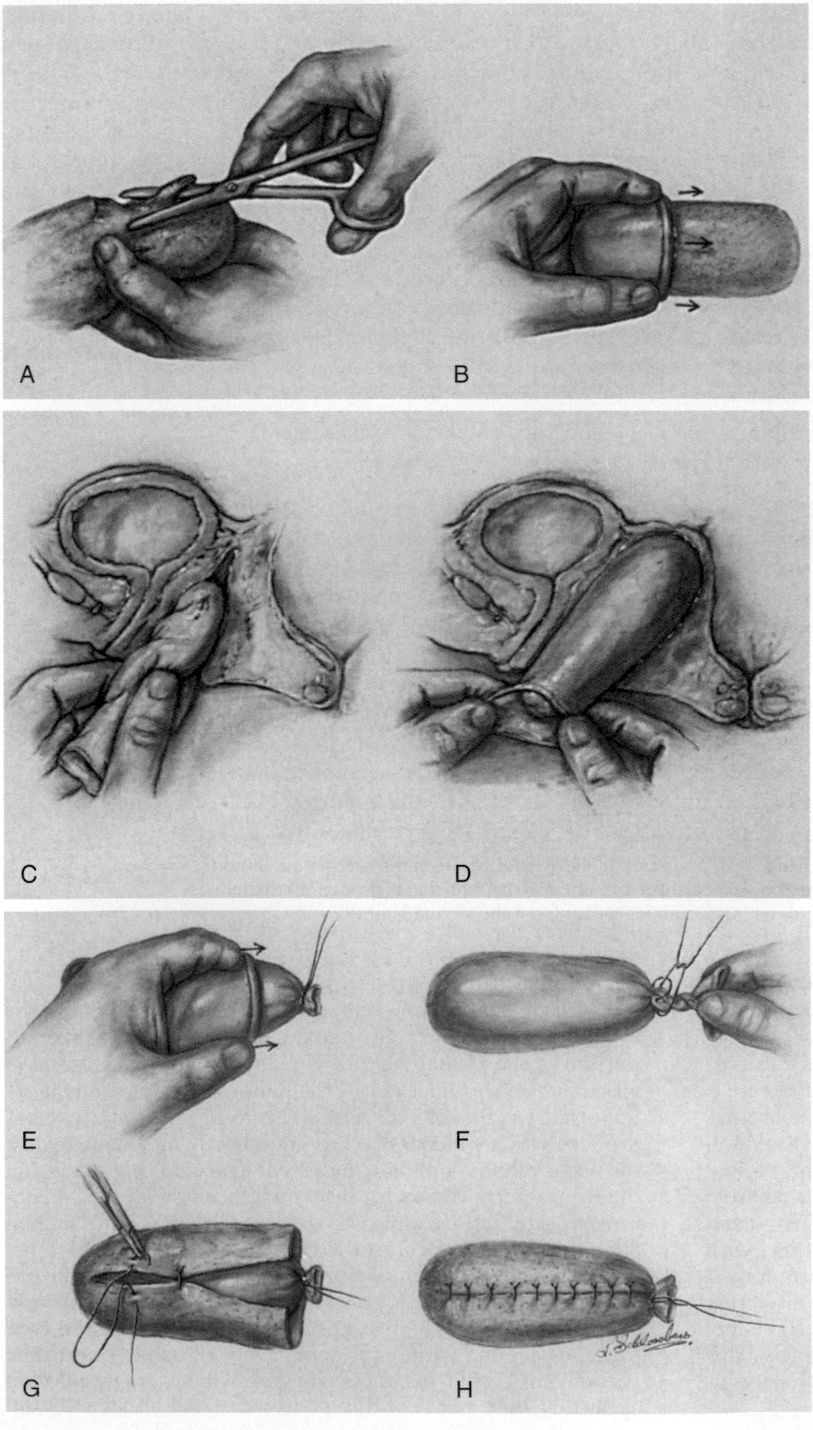

FIGURE 25.8. Counseller-Flor modification of the McIndoe technique. **A:** A form is cut from a foam rubber block. **B:** A condom is placed over the form. **C:** The form is compressed and placed into the vagina. **D:** Air is allowed to expand the foam rubber, which accommodates to the neovaginal space. The condom is closed and the form removed. A second condom is placed over the form (**E**) and tied securely (**F**). **G:** The graft is then sewn over the form with interrupted 5–0 nonreactive sutures. **H:** The undersurfaces of the sutured edges of the graft are exteriorized. The vaginal form is ready for insertion into the neovagina.

and placed into the neovagina (Fig. 25.8A through C). The form is left in place for 20 to 30 seconds with the condom open to allow the foam rubber to expand and conform to the neovaginal space (Fig. 25.8D). The condom is then closed, and the form is withdrawn. The external end is tied with 2-0 silk, and an additional condom is placed over the form and tied securely (Fig. 25.8E and F).

Sewing the graft over the vaginal form. The skin graft is then placed over the form and its undersurface exteriorized and sewn over the form with interrupted vertical mattress 5-0 nonreactive sutures (Fig. 25.8G and H). Where the graft is approximated, the undersurfaces of the sutured edges are also exteriorized.

The graft should not be "meshed" to make it stretch farther, and the edges of the graft should be approximated meticulously around the form without gaps. Granulation tissue develops at any place where the form is not covered with skin. Contraction usually occurs where granulation tissue forms. After the form has been placed in the neovaginal space, the edges of the graft are sutured to the skin edge with 5-0 nonreactive absorbable sutures, with sufficient space left between sutures for drainage to occur. The physician must be careful not to have the form so large that it causes undue pressure on the urethra or rectum. A balsa form should have a groove to accommodate the urethra. With a foam rubber form, this is unnecessary. A suprapubic silicone catheter is placed in the bladder for drainage. If the labia are of sufficient length, then the form can be held in place by suturing the labia together with two or three nonreactive sutures.

Replacing with a new form. After 7 to 10 days, the form is removed and the vaginal cavity is irrigated with warm saline solution and inspected. This is usually performed with mild sedation and without an anesthetic. The cavity should be inspected carefully to determine whether the graft has taken satisfactorily in all areas of the new vagina. Any undue pressure by the form should be noted and corrected. It is especially important that there not be too much pressure superiorly against the peritoneum of the cul-de-sac. Such a constant upward pressure could result in weakness with subsequent enterocele formation. The new vaginal cavity must be inspected frequently to detect and to prevent pressure necrosis of the skin graft.

The patient is given instructions on daily removal and reinsertion of the form and is taught how to administer a low-pressure douche of clear warm water. She is advised to remove the form at the time of urination and defecation, but otherwise to wear it continuously for 6 weeks. A neoprene form, which is much easier to remove and keep clean than a foam rubber form, is substituted for the original form in 6 weeks. A new form is molded with a sterile sheath cover (condom) to fit the size of the vaginal canal. The patient is instructed to use the form during the night for the following 12 months. If there has been no change in the caliber of the vagina by that time, then it is unlikely to occur later, and insertion of the form at night can be done intermittently until coitus is a frequent occurrence. However, if there is the slightest difficulty in inserting the form, then the patient should be advised to use the form continuously again. Most patients are able to maintain the form in place simply by wearing tighter underclothes and a perineal pad. Douches are advisable during residual vaginal healing and discharge.

Results and Complications. Results with the McIndoe operation have improved over the years. Recently reported percentages of satisfactory results have ranged from 80% to 100%. The serious complications formerly associated with the McIndoe operation have been significantly reduced by improvements in technique and greater experience. Serious complications do still occur, however, including a 4% postoperative fistula rate (urethrovaginal, vesicovaginal, and rectovaginal), postoperative infection, and intraoperative and postoperative hemorrhage. Failure of graft take is also still reported as an occasional complication. Failure of graft take often leads to the development of granulation tissue, which might require reoperation, curettage of the granulation tissue down to a healthy base, and even regrafting. Minor granulation can be treated with silver nitrate application. The functional result is more important than the anatomic result in evaluating the success of this operation. Although a vagina of only 4 cm is adequate for some couples, in most instances a vagina smaller than 4 cm causes major problems.

The postoperative results have improved significantly since the balsa vaginal form was replaced by the foam rubber form. Between 1950 and 1989, the McIndoe operation was performed on 94 patients at the Johns Hopkins Hospital. During these 39 years, 83% of the 94 patients had a 100% take of the graft; in only three cases was there a significant area over which the graft failed.

Urethrovaginal fistula has become even more infrequent since the introduction of the suprapubic catheter and the foam rubber form. The catheter is removed when the patient is voiding well and has no residual urine. In general, the patient is able to void without difficulty within the first few days of the procedure. Prophylactic broad-spectrum antibiotics started within 12 hours of surgery and continued for 7 days are of definite value in reducing the incidence of graft failures from infection in the operative site.

Because of the excellent results obtained after a modified McIndoe vaginoplasty, this operation is recommended as the procedure of choice for women unable or unwilling to obtain a neovagina with dilatation methods. Women with a flat perineum with no dimple or pouch have no alternative other than the McIndoe vaginoplasty to obtain a neovagina for comfortable sexual relations.

Desirability of the modified McIndoe procedure may be increased by the use of alternative graft harvest sites to conceal possible aesthetic concerns of the buttock site, as proposed by Höckel and colleagues. The authors proposed the use of split skin harvesting from the scalp because thin (0.25-mm) split skin grafts do not seem to hamper hair growth at the donor site nor lead to hair growth at the recipient site. Because alopecia has been reported as a complication associated with technical errors, more experience is necessary before advocating the scalp as a potential graft harvest site.

It is important that a McIndoe operation be performed correctly the first time. If the vagina becomes constricted because of granulation tissue formation, injury to adjacent structures, or failure to use the form properly, then subsequent attempts to create a satisfactory vagina are more difficult. The first operation has the best chance of success.

Ozek, like many other surgeons, modified the McIndoe procedure by describing an X-type perineal incision and the use of a perforated vaginal mold during the postoperative period. He postulated that this incision minimized stricture at the vaginal introitus and provided greater ease of dissection of the vaginal cavity. He reinforced that the overall procedure is simple with a generally uneventful postoperative course. Complications included infection, failure of skin graft take, stress urinary incontinence, partial graft loss, and vaginal stricture. All were treated satisfactorily except the patient with stress urinary incontinence.

Despite any minor modifications of the McIndoe vaginoplasty, the essential components of dissection of an adequate space, split-thickness skin grafting, and continuous dilatation during the contractile phase of healing remain unchanged. Recent reviews continue to support the safety and efficacy of the procedure. Hojsgaard and Villadsen reported 26 patients who underwent vaginoplasty, 18 of whom had Rokitansky syndrome. All patients were recorded as having a satisfactory result with complete graft take, adequate vaginal dimensions, and no strictures or fistulas giving symptoms. Complete take was achieved in 33% of patients within a week postoperatively, and after one further grafting procedure, an additional 38% had complete take. The intraoperative and early postoperative complications were perforation of the rectum in one patient (3.8%) and postoperative bleeding in three patients (11.5%). The late complications were vaginal stricture in three patients (11.5%), urethrovaginal fistula in two patients (7.7%), and rectovaginal fistula in one patient (3.8%). Alessandrescu and colleagues described the surgical management of 201 cases of Rokitansky syndrome. The surgeon substituted a modified transverse perineal incision and a perforated, rigid plastic mold. Intraoperative and postoperative complications consisted of two rectal perforations (1%), eight graft infections (4%), and 11 infections of graft site origin (5.5%). Sexual satisfaction was investigated with both objective and subjective criteria. Among the 201 cases, 83.6% had anatomic results evaluated as "good," 10% as "satisfactory," and 6.5% as "unsatisfactory." More than 71% of patients rated their sexual life as "good" or "satisfactory" and reported that they had been able to experience orgasms related to vaginal intercourse. Twenty-three percent reported the ability to have sexual intercourse but had no ability to achieve orgasm, and only 5% percent expressed dissatisfaction with their sexual performance. Strickland and colleagues reported on the coital satisfaction, perception of vaginal competence, and impact on lifestyle of adult women undergoing vaginoplasty as adolescents. Ten of 22 women responded to a questionnaire at a median of 18 years (range = 5–13 years) following surgical intervention with a McIndoe vaginoplasty. All of the women had sexual experience, and 80% were sexually active at the time of evaluation. The most frequent difficulty reported was vaginal dryness and lack of lubrication with sexual intercourse. Ninety percent of the subjects expressed satisfaction that sexual ability was acceptable. This experience also supports the role of the McIndoe vaginoplasty in providing young women with vaginal agenesis long-term coital ability and minimal disabilities.

Development of malignancies. Several case reports exist of malignant disease developing in a vagina created by various techniques; these reports were reviewed by Gallup and colleagues, as well as others. The authors reported a patient who was initially treated for intraepithelial malignancy by total vaginectomy combined with a split-thickness skin graft vaginoplasty to reconstruct a functional vagina. The authors noted a lesion in her vaginal apex 7 years later. These findings suggest that epithelium transplanted to the vagina can assume the oncogenic potential of the lower reproductive tract. The evidence supports a risk of neoplastic change in both skin and bowel grafts, with a reported average interval from vaginoplasty to diagnosis on the order of 19 years. Epithelium transplanted to the vagina will assume the oncogenic potential of the lower reproductive tract. Consideration of a plan for surveillance and counseling regarding transmission risk for virally related dysplastic change in the lower genital tract is also extremely important for any patients undergoing neovaginoplasty.

The Williams Vulvovaginoplasty

Construction of a perineal bridge to help contain the vaginal mold was a routine part of the operation described by McIndoe, but it was not adopted subsequently by others. However, Williams described a similar vulvovaginoplasty procedure in 1964 and advised that it could be used to create a vaginal canal. In 1976, he reported that the procedure was unsuccessful in only 1 of 52 patients. Feroze and coworkers reported that the anatomic results were good in 22 of 26 patients. According to these authors, the advantages of the Williams operation are its technical simplicity, its absence of serious local complications even when performed as a repeat procedure, the ease of postoperative care, the absence of postoperative pain, the speed of recovery, the possible elimination of dilators and consequent applicability to patients who do not intend to have regular intercourse in the near future, and the higher success rates of primary and repeat procedures. The technique is not applicable to patients with poorly developed labia. It does result in an unusual angle of the vaginal canal, which is reported to straighten to a more normal direction with intercourse. If a very high perineum is created, urine can momentarily collect in the pouch after urination, giving the impression of postvoid incontinence. Failure of the suture line to heal by primary intention results in a large area of granulation tissue and most likely an unsatisfactory result.

Williams believes that if the urethral meatus is patulous, a vulvovaginoplasty should not be performed because the urethra might be stretched further by coitus. He suggests that varying deficiencies in muscular and fascial tissue can explain why some patients with uterovaginal agenesis are able to develop a satisfactory vaginal canal with simple intermittent pressure with coitus, whereas others are prone to develop enteroceles.

The technique of vulvovaginoplasty described by Williams is as follows (Fig. 25.9). A horseshoe-shaped incision is made in the vulva to extend across the perineum and up the medial side of the labia to the level of the external urethral meatus. The success of the operation depends on the appropriation of sufficient skin to line the new vagina. For this reason, the initial mucosal incisions are made as close to the hairline as possible and approximately 4 cm from the midline. After complete mobilization, the inner skin margins are sutured together with knots tied inside the vaginal lumen. A second layer of sutures approximates subcutaneous fat and perineal muscles for support. Finally, the external skin margins are approximated with interrupted sutures. If the procedure is performed properly, it should be possible to insert two fingers into the pouch to a depth of 3 cm. An indwelling bladder catheter is used. The patient is confined to bed for 1 week to avoid tension on the suture line. Examinations are avoided for 6 weeks, at which time the patient is instructed in the use of dilators.

Capraro and Gallego have advised a modification of the Williams technique. They make the U-shaped incision in the skin of the labia majora at the level of the urethra or even lower, claiming that this modification results in a vulva more normal to sight and touch and still satisfactory for intercourse, and that it avoids trapping stagnant urine in the vaginal pouch. Other modifications have been made by Feroze and associates and by Creatsas. Creatsas's modification of Williams procedure involves incisions at the hymenal ring and the use of delayed absorbable suture. The outcomes of adolescent women who underwent either the Williams vaginoplasty or the modification were summarized by Creatsas. One hundred and one women were treated for MRKH with the modified procedure. Ninety-seven percent of patients had a neovaginal length of 10 to 12 cm with a width of 5 centimeters. No wound

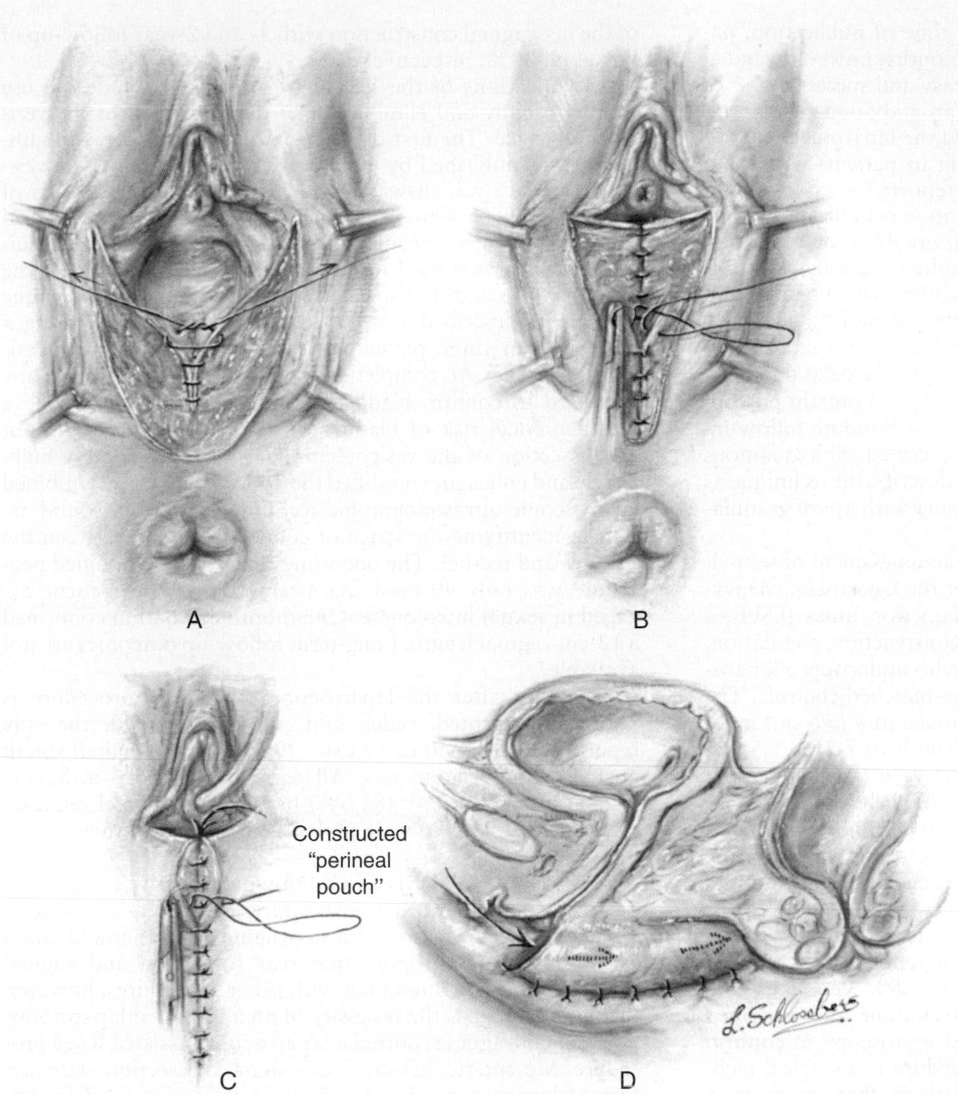

FIGURE 25.9. The Williams vulvovaginoplasty. A through C: No. 3–0 polyglycolic acid sutures can be used throughout to close both inner and outer skin margins and the tissue between. D: The entrance to the pouch should not cover the external urethral meatus.

separations or bleeding with intercourse were reported; however, these complications did occur in 20% of the patients who underwent the Williams vaginoplasty (10 young women). An assessment of sexual satisfaction was performed on the entire population; 94.4% of patients described her sexual life as satisfactory. Deligeoroglou and colleagues in Greece published supportive data regarding the Creatsas modification by describing both anatomic and functional success of 116 adolescents who underwent the procedure over a 15-year period. The physical exam findings were documented; however, the follow-up period was not clearly addressed.

The Williams vulvovaginoplasty is a useful operation and should certainly be considered the operation of choice for patients needing a follow-up to an unsatisfactory McIndoe operation or a supplement to a small vagina resulting from extensive surgery or radiation therapy. It remains an option for the rare patient with a solitary kidney low in the pelvis who does not have room for dissection of an adequate vaginal space.

Alternative Techniques

Schätz and colleagues reported three patients who underwent the George modification of the Wharton-Sheares neovaginoplasty technique. Wharton combined an adequate dissection of the vaginal space with continuous dilatation by a balsa form that was covered with a thin rubber sheath and was left in the space. His operation was based on the principle that the vaginal epithelium will proliferate and, in a relatively short time, will cover the raw surface. This modification of an already simple procedure may provide an alternative in areas where multidisciplinary, reconstructive pelvic surgery teams are not available. Because the procedure includes the mere dilatation of the bilateral müllerian ducts and lining of the superior aspect with peritoneum, it eliminates some of the more complex aspects of the other surgical options. However, with a mean follow-up period reported as only 12 months (range of 2–23 months), reported long-term complications associated with the Wharton method (persistent granulation tissue, coital bleeding, leukorrhea, and scarring of the upper portion) cannot be fully evaluated. Longer follow-up and a larger patient experience are both necessary to consider if this procedure should an option for patients with MRKH.

Moyotoma and colleagues described 10 patients who were diagnosed with vaginal agenesis and were treated with oxidative regenerated cellulose fabric (Interceed). Operative time (<30 minutes) and postoperative hospitalization (2 days) were significantly shorter than that for a traditional skin graft. Vaginal depth was 8 to 10 cm, and no significant operative complications were reported. At the time of publication, patients had only been followed for 6 months; however, vaginal intercourse was already reported as easy and successful.

Several authors, including Adamyan and Soong, and Templeman and colleagues, have described the laparoscopic use of the peritoneum to create a neovagina in patients with vaginal agenesis. Adamyan and Soong reported a group of 45 patients without significant postoperative complications. The most common postoperative problem involved the formation of granulation tissue at the vaginal vault. Templeman and colleagues described the laparoscopic mobilization of peritoneum for the creation of a neovagina in only one patient. The peritoneum was grasped through a perineal dissection and sutured to the introitus. A pursestring closure was placed at the apex. Stenting of the neovagina was continued for 3 months postoperatively followed by rigid dilator use. At 9-month follow-up evaluation, an 8- by 2-cm vagina was described, with squamous epithelialization present. Both groups describe the technique as safe and efficient, producing a neovagina with apical granulation tissue as the only complication.

Giannesi and colleagues reported an assessment of sexuality via a self-report questionnaire after the laparoscopic Davydov procedure. The Female Sexual Function Index (FSFI), a validated measure in the vaginal reconstruction population, was administered to both 28 women who underwent a laparoscopic Davydov procedure and 28 age-matched controls. The anatomical result was judged to be satisfactory (>6 cm) in 26 of 28 patients with a mean vaginal length of 7.2 ± 1.5 cm. No statistical difference was found between the subjects and the controls in all six domains of the FSFI; however, the authors note that 6 of the 25 (24%) operative subjects who completed the entire FSFI had a poor FSFI result. Of note, the areas of greatest concern were in the areas of lubrication and pain.

The Vecchietti operation was first described in 1965 by Giuseppe Vecchietti. He subsequently reported his cumulative 14-year experience in 1979 and 1980. Veronikus and colleagues reviewed the use of the technique and described a laparoscopic modification that uses cystoscopy to confirm bladder integrity. The Vecchietti procedure is a surgical technique for the treatment of vaginal agenesis that constructs a dilatation-type neovagina in 7 to 9 days. The procedure uses specialized equipment including a traction device, a ligature carrier, and an acrylic shaped olive. The process is in two steps, with essential operative and postoperative components. The operative phase involves positioning the olive at the perineum and the traction sutures extraperitoneally. Classically performed through a Pfannenstiel incision, the ligature carrier introduces the suture into a newly dissected vesicorectal space. The olive is threaded with suture at the perineum, and the suture is reintroduced at the abdomen. The suture is then guided lateral to the rectus muscles bilaterally in a subperitoneal fashion and advanced along the sidewall. The traction device, which provides constant traction on the olive, is positioned on the abdomen. During the postoperative invagination phase, the neovagina is created by applying constant traction to the olive. The process reportedly occurs at a rate of 1.0 to 1.5 cm per day, developing a 10- to 12-cm vagina in 7 to 9 days. Patients are instructed on the use of a vaginal obturator to be used as an outpatient. Borruto reported on Vecchietti's personal series of vaginal agenesis patients, comprising 522 consecutive patients. The surgical complications included one bladder and one rectal puncture with the ligature carrier and three cases of vaginal vault bleeding. At 100% follow-up at 1 month, dyspareunia was initially reported to be 12%, but resolved in all cases by 3 months. There were no reported failures of the neovaginal construction with 1- and 2-year follow-up of 70% and 30%, respectively.

Modifications of the Vecchietti approach include the use of laparoscopy and elimination of the dissection of the vesicorectal space. The first description of a laparoscopic modification was published by Gauwerky and colleagues. The vesicorectal space was dissected laparoscopically. The threads of the olive device were positioned using a probe introduced into the abdomen through the perineum. Six small abdominal incisions were used for laparoscopic instruments and the traction springs of the specialized device. In 1995, Laffarque and others described a laparoscopic intervention, creating a neovagina in three patients without dissection of the vesicorectal space. At completion of the procedure, cystoscopy was used to confirm bladder integrity. Some experts believe the theoretical risk of bladder or rectal perforation without the dissection of the vesicorectal space is unacceptably high. Fedele and colleagues modified the approach to use a combined laparoscopic-ultrasonographic technique. The ultrasound assists in identifying the space of connective tissue between the bladder and rectum. The operating time for this modified procedure was only 40 minutes. After 10 days, the patient engaged in sexual intercourse. One-month evaluation confirmed a 12-cm vaginal length. Long-term follow-up outcomes are not available.

Sexuality after the laparoscopic Vecchietti procedure is poorly documented. Fedele and colleagues provide the only report, describing 50 of 52 cases (96%) with a vaginal length greater than 7 centimeters. All patients succeeded in having vaginal intercourse, 49 (82.6%) had a stable sexual relationship, and 49 (94.2%) were globally satisfied with their sexual life.

Bowel vaginoplasty is a well-known alternative for creation of a neovagina. The Ruge procedure and others are characterized by the formation of a neovagina using sigmoid colon grafts. Advocates propose that scar formation and vaginal stenosis occur less often than with other procedures; however, the disadvantage is the necessity of an abdominal laparotomy. Ota and colleagues reported a laparoscopic-assisted Ruge procedure. Mesenteric dissection and sigmoid resection were performed laparoscopically. A 3.5-cm incision was used for appropriate bowel suturing. The segment of sigmoid colon was mobilized and brought to the introitus. The serosal layer of the pediculate end was stabilized to pelvic peritoneum. The patient remained hospitalized for 14 days. The benefit of this modification is certainly the accomplishment of a difficult surgical procedure endoscopically. Other advantages include the functional, ample vaginal length (12 cm) without postoperative dilatation. Disadvantages include the extended postoperative hospitalization period and the small number of patients evaluated.

Reported surgical outcomes by authors such as Hensle and colleagues and Communal and associates support the role of sigmoid neovaginoplasty, especially in patients with MRKH. Until recently, long-term data regarding sexual function had not been available. Parsons and colleagues retrospectively reviewed 28 cases at a mean of 6.2 years after sigmoid vaginoplasty. Seventy-nine percent of patients were reportedly "very satisfied" with sexual function, and 21% were "comfortable" with the outcome. Communal and colleagues administered the FSFI to 11 patients after creation of a sigmoid neovagina. The mean score of the 8 women who were attempting intercourse was reported to be equivalent to that of "normal" patients without vaginal agenesis. Hensle and colleagues provided additional information by reporting the sexual function of 57 patients who underwent creation of a bowel neovagina.

Forty-two of the patients were reported to have MRKH. Eight patients underwent ileovaginoplasty; two patients were then subsequently treated with a colonic neovagina. The follow-up period varied from 18 months to 24 years with a mean of 8.8 years. Outcomes were evaluated both by a retrospective chart review and the female sexual dysfunction questionnaire (FSDQ) described as an Institutional Review Board–approved, validated instrument. Of the 36 patients who responded, 31 were sexually active. Seventy-eight percent of the entire group of patients, including additional diagnoses precipitating neovaginoplasty, reported sexual desire, 33% sexual arousal, 33% sexual confidence, and 78% sexual satisfaction. Also, 56% reported frequent orgasms, 22% occasional orgasms, and 22% no orgasms. Thirty-two patients (89%) reported adequate lubrication for sexual activity; 34 patients used home douching, and 20 required pads for mucus production.

Makinoda and colleagues reported a nongrafting method of vaginal creation. This group reported 18 women who underwent a two-step protocol. The initial step used noninvasive dilatation using a vaginal mold based on the technique of Frank. The second step was a surgical procedure via a perineal approach. The apex of the dilated vaginal space was incised, and further dissection between the bladder and rectum was carried to the peritoneal cavity. After peritoneal perforation, the uterine structures, when present, were pulled down and sutured to the newly created vaginal space. A firm vaginal mold was inserted and recommended for use for 6 months postoperatively. The authors propose a benefit of avoidance of grafting. The time course for success with the initial dilatation step may be unacceptably long in many patients (mean $= 10.90 \pm 9.8$ months). No significant surgical complications were reported despite the theoretical risk of ureteral contortion and kinking when pulling the rudimentary uterine structures inferiorly. During the follow-up period, shrinkage of the vaginal length and diameter was noted in some patients who had been noncompliant with the mold or without coitus. The authors noted a minimal vaginal length of 5 cm in a patient who was noncompliant with the mold and not sexually active. The authors dispute the necessity of any lining of the neovaginal space. In their experience, significant narrowing or contraction of the margins did not occur. They maintain that the vaginal space is maintained by suturing the muscular buds of the uterus to the pressure-created neovaginal space.

A spatial W-plasty technique using a full-thickness unilateral groin graft has been described in a limited number of patients by Chen and others. The authors advocate an earlier intervention with the premise that a full-thickness graft may grow as the patient grows. This is recommended to eliminate psychological issues in patients who would be treated during the late teens, when sexual identity may be forming.

Acquired Vaginal Insufficiency

Unusual types of infection and atrophy can rarely cause closure of part of the vagina, but acquired vaginal inadequacy most often is the result of treatment of various gynecologic malignancies with surgery or radiation, or a combination of both. Restoration and maintenance of vaginal function are important elements of the treatment plan for such malignancies, especially when the patient is young and otherwise healthy. The unique surgical challenges associated with creation of a neovagina in patients treated with radiation therapy require the experience and expertise of surgeons familiar with this population. The techniques of vaginal reconstruction in gynecologic oncology have been reviewed by Magrina and Masterson, by Pratt, and by McCraw and associates.

DISORDERS OF VERTICAL FUSION

The problems associated with vertical fusion include transverse vaginal septum with or without obstruction. Although imperforate hymen is a vertical fusion problem, the hymen is not a derivative of the müllerian ducts; therefore, this condition is discussed elsewhere (see Chapter 24).

Transverse Vaginal Septum

No reliable epidemiologic data exist regarding the incidence of transverse vaginal septum. Reported incidences vary from 1 in 2,100 to 1 in 72,000. It is probably less common than congenital absence of the vagina and uterus. It has been diagnosed in newborns, infants, and older adolescent girls. Its etiology is unknown, although McKusick has suggested that some and perhaps most cases are the result of a female sex-limited autosomal recessive transmission. There is a developmental defect in vaginal embryogenesis that leads to an incomplete fusion between the müllerian duct component and the urogenital sinus component of the vagina. The incomplete vertical fusion results in a transverse vaginal septum (AFS class IIA) that varies in thickness and can be located at almost any level in the vagina (Fig. 25.10). Lodi has reported that 46% occur in the upper vagina, 40% in the midvagina, and 14% in the lower vagina. Rock, Zacur, and associates have noted septa in the upper, middle, and lower thirds of the vagina in 46%, 35%, and 19% of patients, respectively. In general, the thicker septum is noted to be more common closer to the uterine cervix. In contrast to congenital absence of the müllerian ducts, the transverse vaginal septum is associated with few urologic or other anomalies. Imperforate anus and bicornuate uterus can be found, as reported by Mandell and colleagues. The lower surface of the transverse septum is always covered by squamous epithelium. The upper surface can be covered by glandular epithelium, which is likely to be transformed into squamous epithelium by a metaplastic process after correction of the obstruction.

In neonates and young infants, imperforate transverse vaginal septum with obstruction can lead to serious and life-threatening problems caused by the compression of surrounding organs by fluid that has collected above the septum. The fluid undoubtedly comes from endocervical glands and müllerian glandular epithelium in the upper vagina that have been stimulated by the placental transfer of maternal estrogen. Continued fluid collection in infants, even after the first year, has been reported; thus, the possibility of a fistula between the upper vagina and the urinary tract should be considered. The distended upper vagina creates a large pelvic and lower abdominal mass that can displace the bladder anteriorly, displace the ureters laterally with hydroureters and hydronephrosis, compress the rectum with associated obstipation and even intestinal obstruction, and limit diaphragmatic excursion to indirectly compress the vena cava and produce cardiorespiratory failure. Fatalities have been reported. The hydrocolpos develops along the axis of the upper vagina and therefore may not necessarily cause the outlet or perineum to bulge when there is compression of the mass from above. After careful preoperative radiologic and endoscopic investigations of the infant, the septum should be removed through a perineal approach. Bilateral Schuchardt incisions may be required to ensure that the septum has been removed. Because of the subsequent tendency for vaginal stenosis and reaccumulation of the fluid in the upper vagina, follow-up studies to assess the recurrence of urinary obstruction are important. Vaginal reconstruction may be

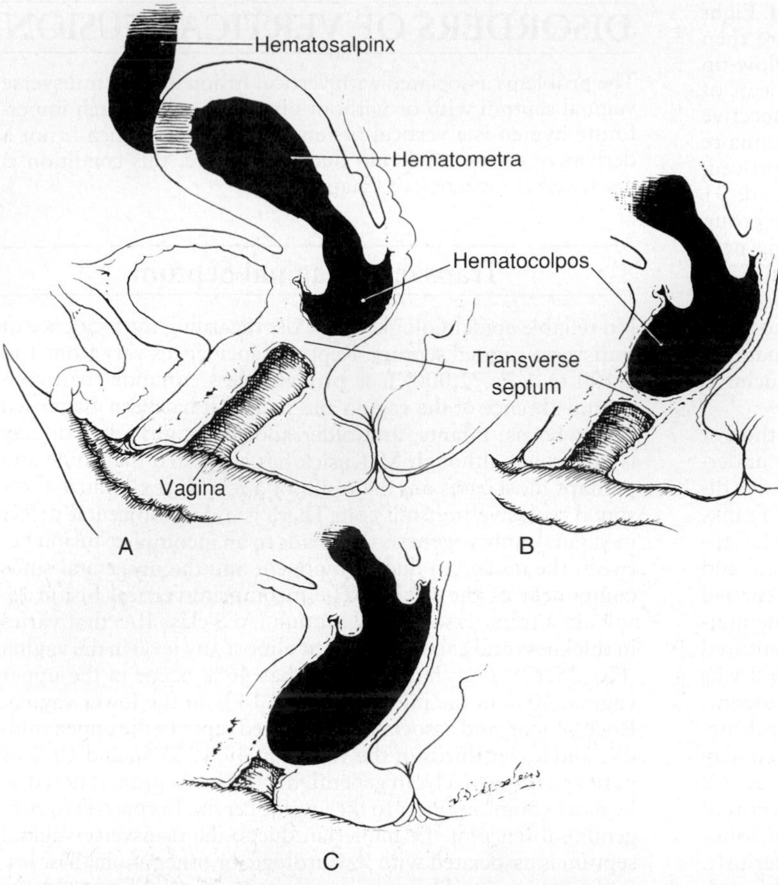

FIGURE 25.10. Positions of septum responsible for complete vaginal obstruction. High (A), mid (B), and low (C) transverse vaginal septa. Note the position of the hematocolpos. Lower vaginal septa allow more blood to accumulate in the upper vagina. The vaginal mass shown in (C) is more accessible through rectovaginal examination.

required in later years to allow satisfactory menstruation and coitus.

A hematocolpos may not develop until puberty. Symptoms include cyclic lower abdominal pain, no visible menstrual discharge, and gradual development of a central lower abdominal and pelvic mass. Sometimes a small tract opens in the septum, some menstrual blood escapes periodically, and symptoms are variable. A septum large enough to allow pregnancy to occur can still cause dystocia during labor. Cyclic hematuria may be present if a communication between the bladder and upper vagina exists. The pelvic organs of a woman with a transverse vaginal septum are shown in Figure 25.11. The woman developed severe cyclic pain at the time of onset of menstruation, but there was no external bleeding until menstrual blood finally began to flow through the small sinus. Pelvic examination per rectum revealed a cervix and a normal-sized corpus. The ovaries were palpable but adherent, probably because of organized blood from hematosalpinx and hematoperitoneum. Remarkably, the woman had little dysmenorrhea after beginning to menstruate externally. Coitus was fairly satisfactory before surgical correction, but the shortness of the vagina was something of a handicap. The obstructing membrane was excised, and an anastomosis of the upper and lower vagina was performed.

The findings of 26 patients with complete transverse vaginal septum reported from the Johns Hopkins Hospital by Rock, Zacur, and colleagues have shown that associated congenital anomalies include urinary tract anomalies, coarctation of the aorta, atrial septal defect, and malformations of the lumbar spine. Vaginal patency and coital function were successfully established in all patients, and 7 of 19 patients attempting pregnancy eventually had children. The incidence of endometriosis and spontaneous abortion was high. A lower pregnancy rate and more extensive endometriosis were present when the transverse septum was located high in the vagina, suggesting that retrograde flow through the uterus and fallopian tubes occurs earlier in these patients. More extensive dissection between the bladder and rectum was required to identify the upper vagina when the septum was thick and high. Exploratory laparotomy was necessary in five patients to guide a probe through the uterine fundus and cervix and to assist in locating a high hematocolpos.

Surgical Technique for a Transverse Vaginal Septum

A transverse incision is made through the vault of the short vagina (Fig. 25.11A). A probe is introduced through the septum after a portion of the barrier has been separated by sharp and blunt dissection. The physician usually finds some areolar tissue in dissecting the space between the vagina and the rectum. Palpation of a urethral catheter anteriorly and insertion of a double-gloved finger along the anterior wall of the rectum posteriorly provides the proper surgical guidelines so that the bladder and rectum can be avoided during this blind procedure. After the dissection is continued for a short distance, the cervix can usually be palpated, and continuity can be established with the upper segment of the vagina (Fig. 25.11B and C). The lateral margins of the excised septum are extended widely by sharp knife dissection to avoid postoperative stricture formation. The edges of the upper and the lower vaginal

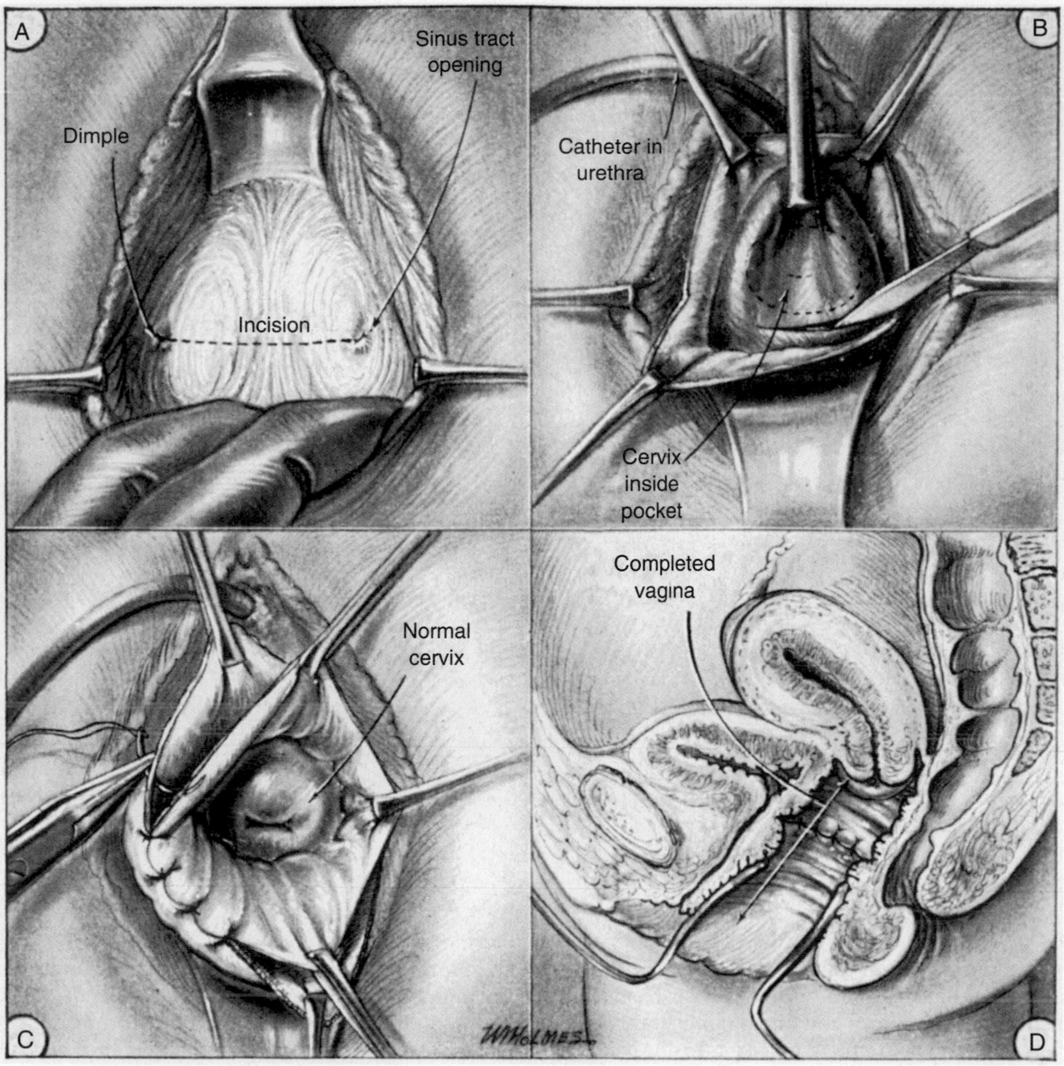

FIGURE 25.11. Surgical correction of transverse vaginal septum. **A:** The upper end of a short vagina. The small sinus tract opening, through which the patient menstruated, is shown. The line of incision is drawn through the mucous membrane between the vaginal dimple and the sinus. **B:** Areolar tissue is dissected through to the pocket of mucosa that covered the cervix. The mucosa is incised. **C:** An anastomosis is made between the lower vagina and the upper vagina. **D:** Completed vagina. It is slightly shorter than normal but of normal caliber.

mucosa are undermined and mobilized enough to permit anastomosis with the use of interrupted delayed-absorbable sutures (Fig. 25.11C). Figure 25.11D shows the completed anastomosis with a vagina that is of normal caliber but has a length slightly shorter than average. A soft foam rubber vaginal form covered with a sterile latex sheath can be placed in the vagina and removed in 10 days for evaluation of the healing process. The form can be worn for 4 to 6 weeks until complete healing has occurred. After this, coitus is permitted. If the patient is not sexually active, then vaginal dilatation may be necessary to maintain established patency. Alternatively, a silicone elastomer (Silastic) vaginal form can be inserted at night until the constrictive phase of healing is complete.

High Transverse Vaginal Septum. If the length of the obstructing transverse vaginal septum is such that reanastomosis of the upper and lower vagina is impossible, as is the case with a high transverse vaginal septum, in which a significant portion of vagina is atretic, then a space is created between the rectum and bladder to permit identification of the obstructed vagina (Fig. 25.12). The mass that has resulted from accumulated menstrual blood must be distinguished from the bladder anteriorly and the rectum posteriorly, a process that is facilitated by the mass itself. When differentiation is impossible, however, exploratory laparotomy can be performed. During this procedure, a probe is passed through the fundus of the uterus to tent out the vaginal septum and enable the surgeon to excise it from below and resect it safely.

In most surgical procedures to remove the high transverse vaginal septum, the obstructing membrane can be readily identified (Fig. 25.13), after which the operator can probe the mass with an aspirating needle to identify old menstrual blood. The upper vagina is then opened and the septum excised. Because

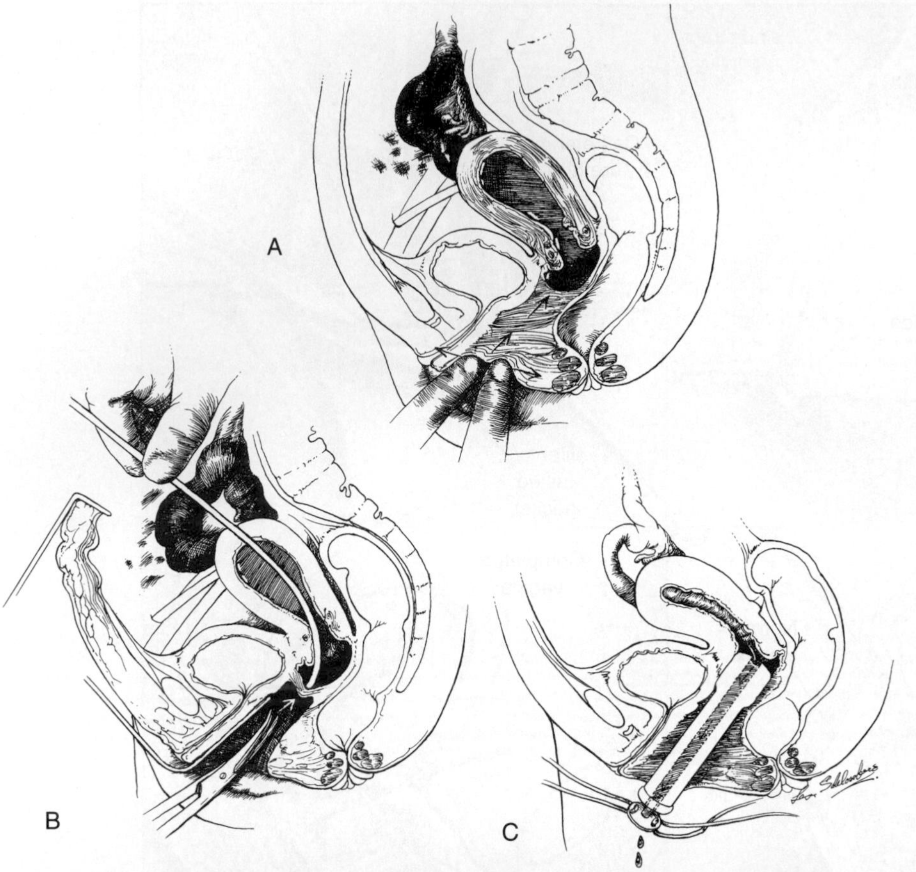

FIGURE 25.12. Correction of an atretic vagina. **A:** A large portion of atretic vagina is palpated with two fingers. Once the vaginal space is developed, it may be necessary to open the abdomen via laparotomy and pass a probe through to the uterine fundus (**B**) to tent out the septum, which may then be safely excised. **C:** An acrylic resin (Lucite) form is then placed into the vagina and secured with rubber straps.

the distance between the septum and the upper vagina is too great to permit an anastomosis, an indwelling acrylic resin (Lucite) form, consisting of a bulbous end and a channel through which menstrual blood can drain, is placed into the vagina and anchored with a retaining harness. The bulbous end of the form, in most instances, is retained in the upper vagina and should be left in place for 4 to 6 months while epithelialization is accomplished. After its removal, vaginal dilatation should be practiced on a daily basis for 2 to 4 months to prevent contracture of the space. It is essential to the success of the operation that the new space not become constricted; to avoid constriction, the form must be worn for many months during the constrictive phase of healing. As an alternative to the Lucite form, the physician can consider using a split-thickness graft to bridge the gap. The graft is usually sutured *in situ* in the vagina rather than sutured to a form. An ingenious but rather complicated Z-plasty method of bridging the gap has been described by Garcia and by Musset. A simpler flap method was described by Brenner and associates.

A transverse vaginal septum diagnosed after the onset of puberty presents numerous problems. Often, a large segment of the vagina is absent, making anastomosis of the upper and lower segments difficult. Furthermore, postoperative vaginal dilatation is necessary to prevent stenosis at the anastomosis site. Poor compliance with dilatation in a poorly motivated pubertal patient is always a concern. However, rarely is the surgeon able to delay vaginoplasty until the patient is more mature because of increasingly severe cyclic abdominal pain caused by the hematocolpos. Thus, a difficult vaginoplasty can have less than optimal results.

Hurst and Rock have described an alternative approach to maximize surgical resection and anastomosis in women with a high transverse vaginal septum. Aspiration of the hematocolpos under ultrasound guidance was necessary to relieve the acute pain and delay surgery. Continuous oral contraceptives were used to delay recurrence of hematocolpos. Most important, vaginal dilatation was used to lengthen the lower vaginal segment to facilitate resection and reanastomosis (Fig. 25.14). In all three patients, the approach was successful.

Congenital Absence or Dysgenesis of the Cervix

Agenesis or atresia of the cervix (AFS class IIB) is a relatively infrequent müllerian anomaly. When this anomaly does occur, it is often in association with absence of a portion or all of the vagina. In many cases of cervical agenesis or atresia, retention of menstrual blood initiates symptoms of cyclic lower abdominal pain without menstrual flow, causing the patient to seek gynecologic evaluation and care. In past times, diagnosis was suspected on the basis of a history and physical findings but was not proved until the time of surgery. Today, diagnosis of cervical agenesis or atresia is still usually difficult before operation, but the possibility of making a correct diagnosis before surgery does exist, with the help of modern diagnostic tools. Early diagnosis offers significant advantages in patient care, the most important of which is effective presurgical planning and preparation.

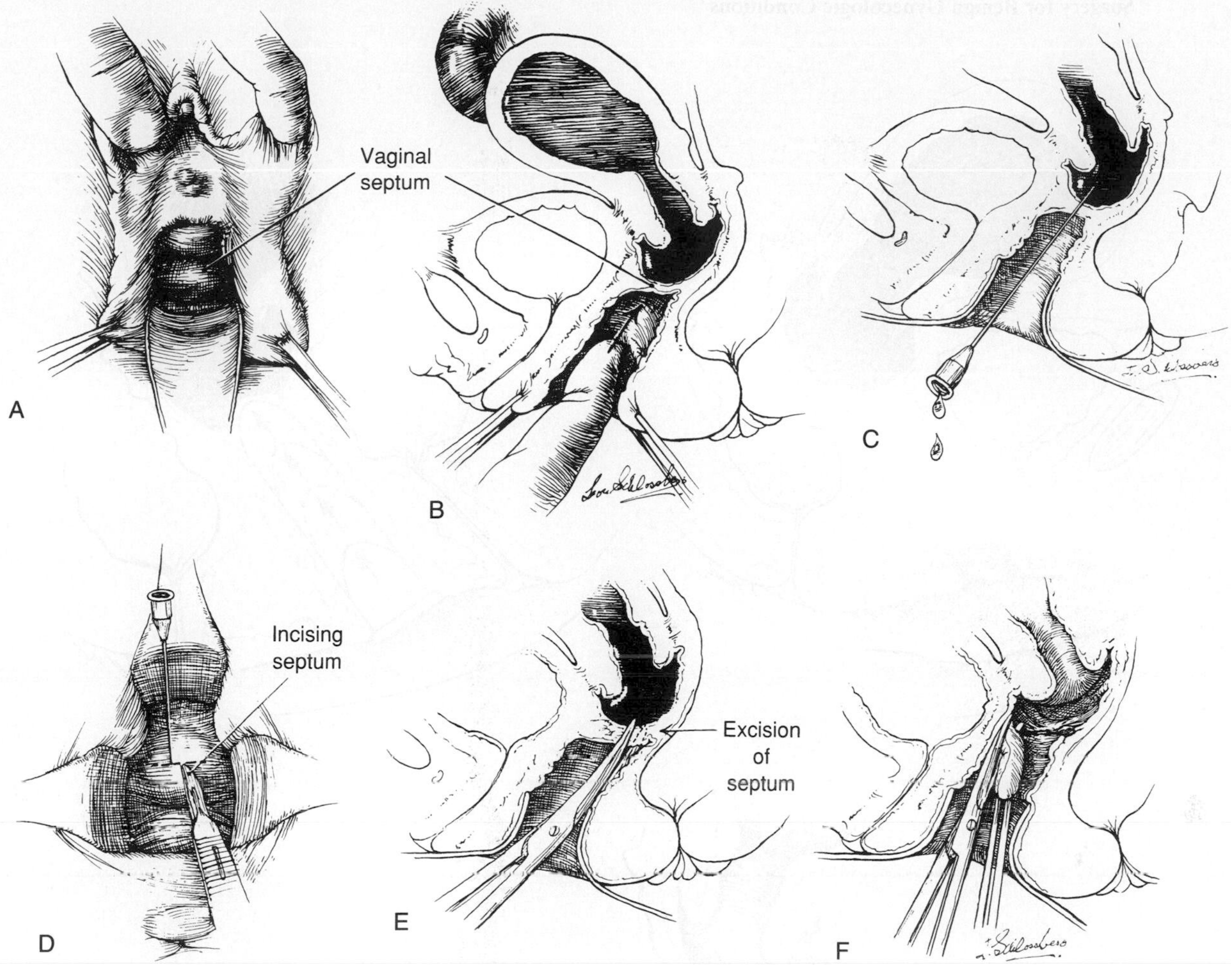

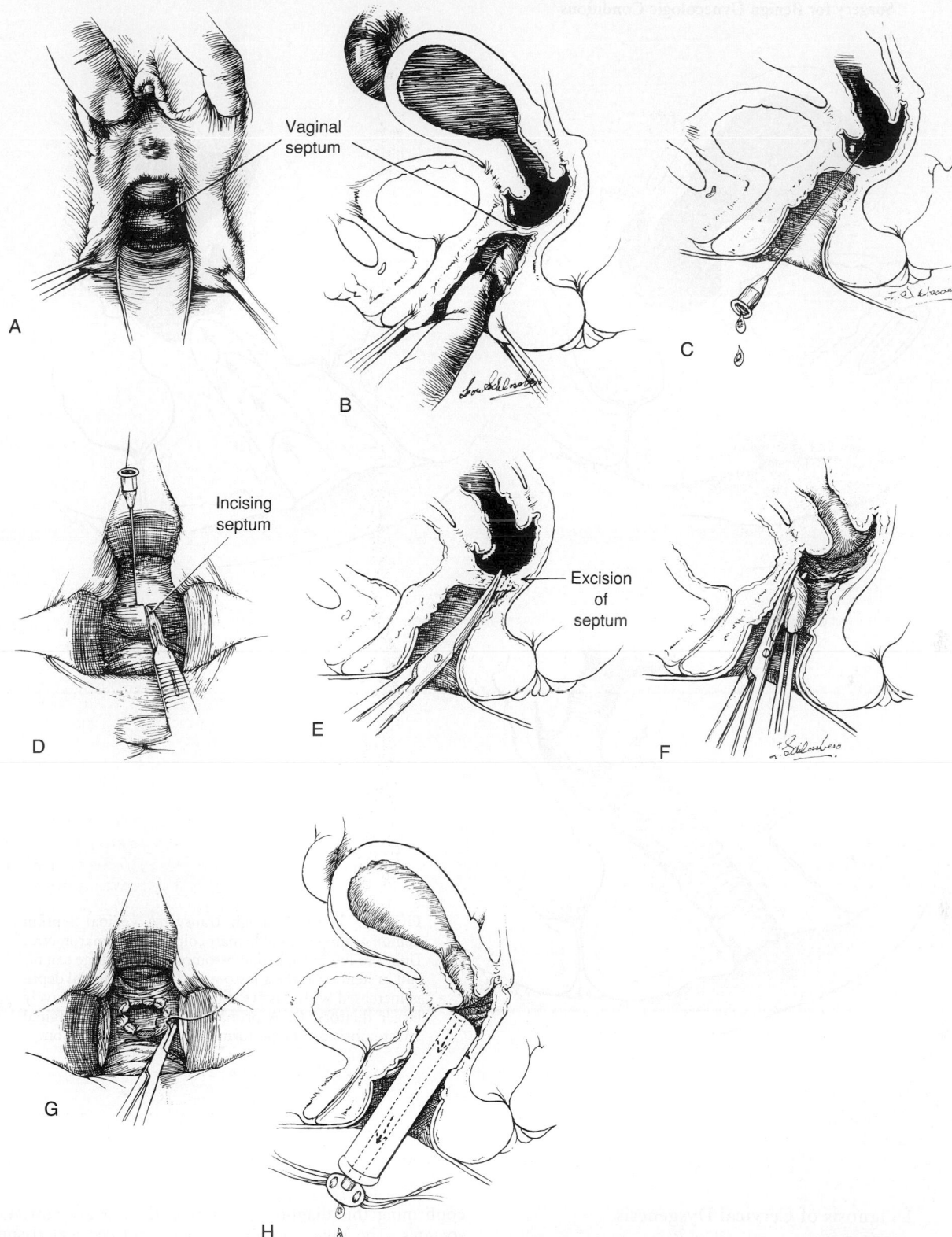

FIGURE 25.13. A high transverse vaginal septum. **A:** The neovaginal space is dissected, revealing a high obstructing vaginal membrane. **B:** This can be palpated with the middle finger. **C:** A needle is then placed into the mass. **D:** The incision is made with a sharp knife, and considerable bleeding can occur. **E:** The septum is excised. **F:** The septum is removed. **G:** After the septum is removed, the wall of the septum is oversewn with interrupted sutures of 2–0 chromic catgut. **H:** Because the distance between the septum and the upper vagina is too great to allow anastomosis, an acrylic resin (Lucite) form is placed in the vagina so that epithelialization can occur over the form while vaginal patency is maintained. The form, in place, is fitted with a plastic retainer. Rubber straps can be placed through the retainer and attached to a waist belt to allow constant upper pressure so that the form is retained in the upper vagina. Modification of this method includes a small adapter to allow drainage through the acrylic resin (Lucite) form, preventing the accumulation of old blood and mucus in the upper vagina. (From Rock J. Anomalous development of the vagina. *Semin Reprod Endocrinol* 1986;4:24, with permission.)

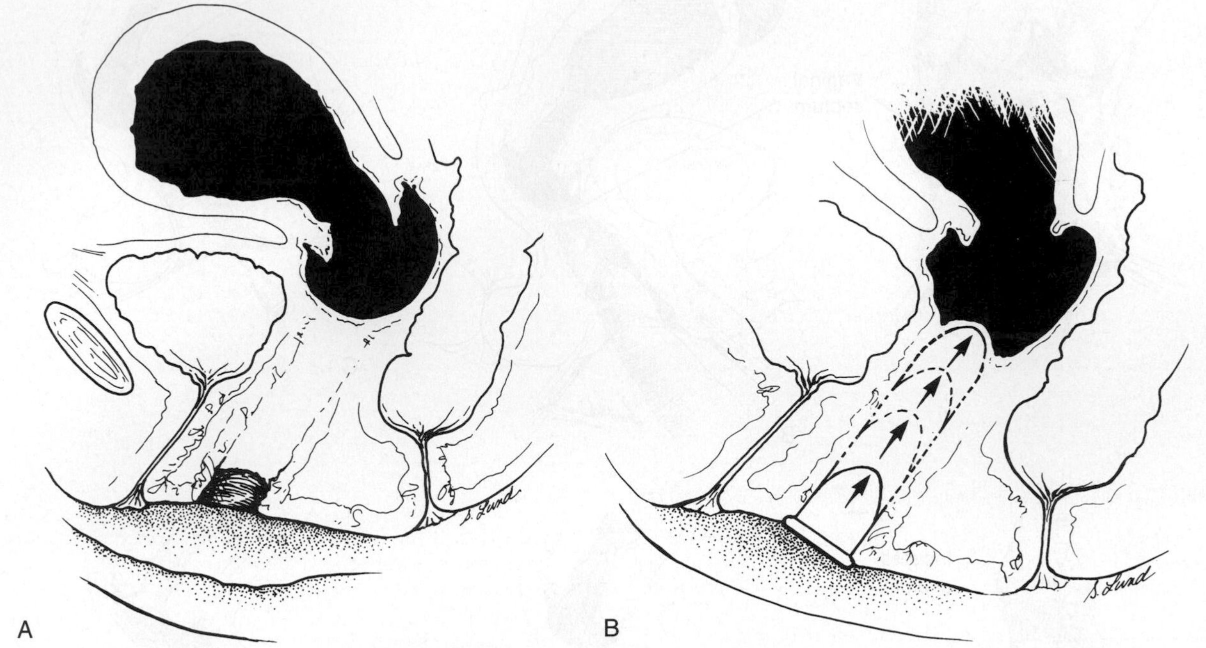

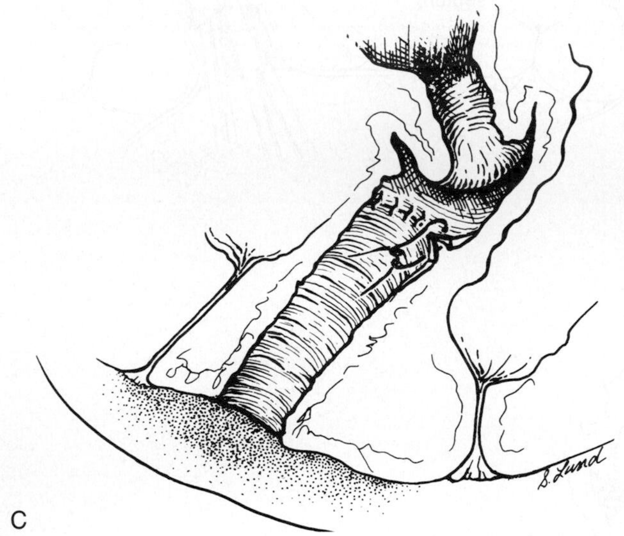

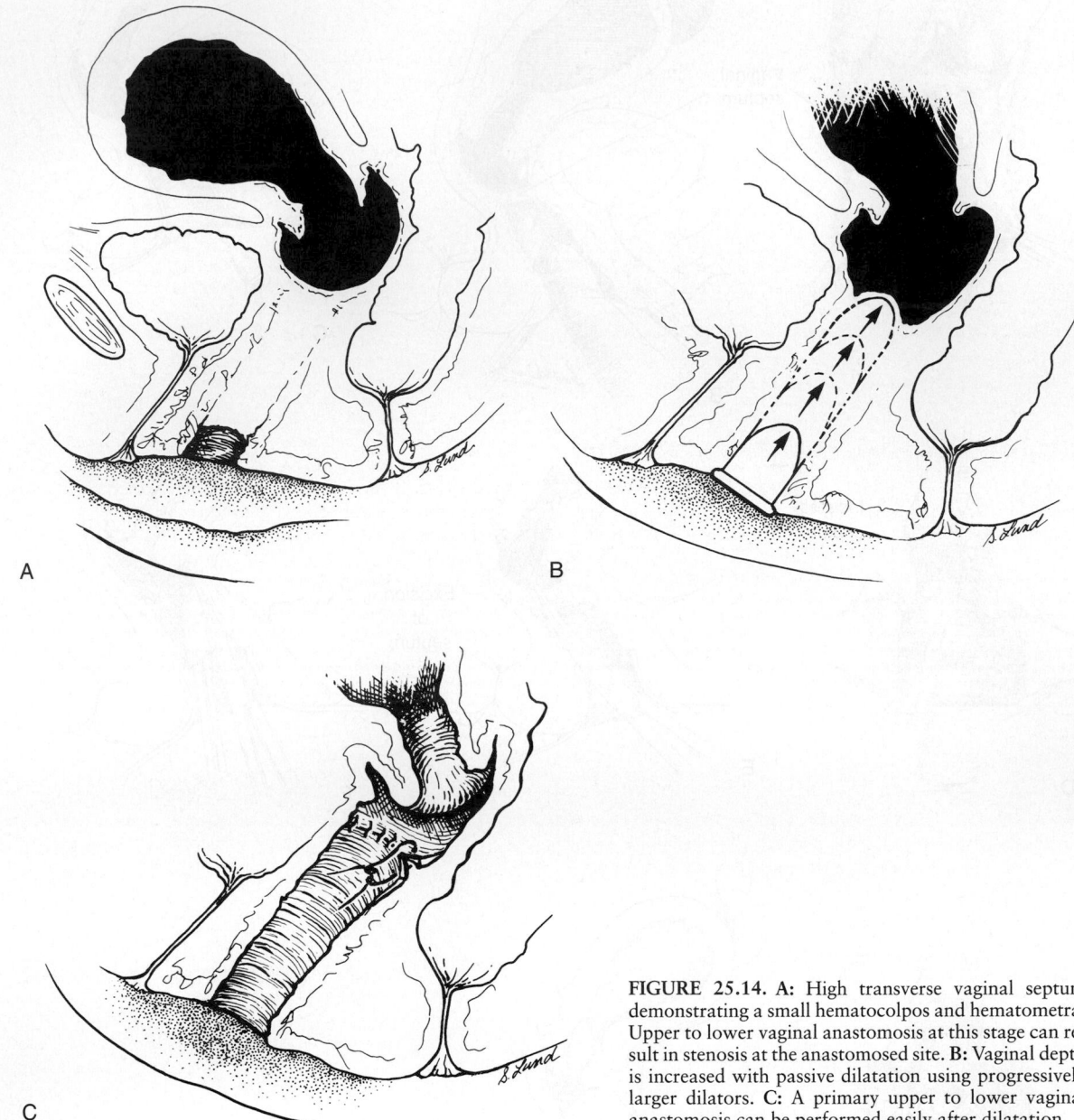

FIGURE 25.14. A: High transverse vaginal septum demonstrating a small hematocolpos and hematometra. Upper to lower vaginal anastomosis at this stage can result in stenosis at the anastomosed site. **B:** Vaginal depth is increased with passive dilatation using progressively larger dilators. **C:** A primary upper to lower vaginal anastomosis can be performed easily after dilatation.

Diagnosis of Cervical Dysgenesis

Patients with congenital absence of the cervix present a diagnostic challenge. Patients with cervical aplasia with a functioning midline uterine corpus have aplasia of the lower two thirds of the vagina with an upper vaginal pouch. Similarly, some patients have a considerable atretic segment of vagina and an upper vaginal pouch with a properly developed uterine cervix and corpus above. Differentiation of these two müllerian anomalies is essential. Ultrasonography may be helpful. Valdes and associates have reported the use of preoperative ultrasonography in the evaluation of two patients with atresia of the vagina and cervix. MRI has been found to be helpful in confirming this diagnosis, as reported by Markham and associates. The lower uterine segment and cervical tissue can be carefully examined (Fig. 25.15). With cervical dysgenesis, there is no vaginal dilatation with the accumulation of blood, as seen with a high transverse vaginal septum. Both ultrasonography and MRI are most helpful when they are correlated with the findings of a careful pelvic examination under anesthesia.

Anatomic Variations of Congenital Cervical Anomalies

Two basic categories of cervical anomalies have been observed in several configurations. Patients exhibiting the first type,

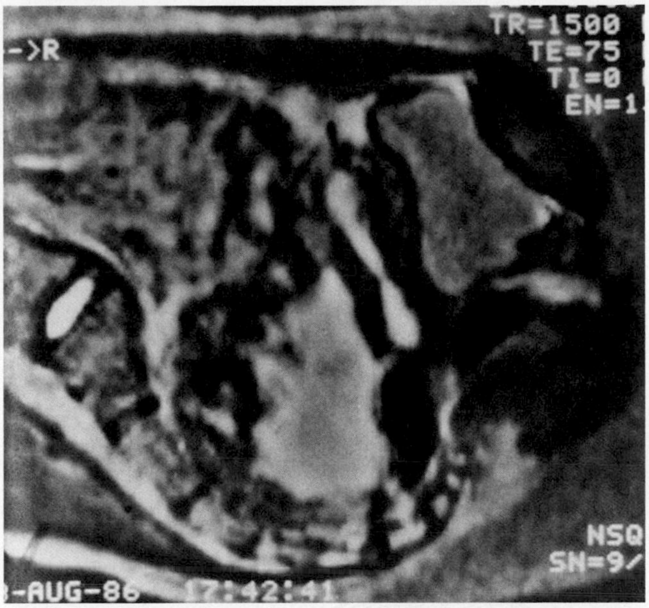

FIGURE 25.15. Magnetic resonance T1-weighted image showing atretic segment of distal cervix. The tip of an atretic cervix is shown. No vagina is noted.

cervical aplasia, lack a uterine cervix (Fig. 25.16A), and the lower uterine segment narrows to terminate in a peritoneal sleeve at a point well above the normal communication with the vaginal apex. The second type, cervical dysgenesis, can be described as four subtypes:

1. Cervical body consisting of a fibrous band of variable length and diameter (endocervical glands may be noted on pathologic examination) (Fig. 25.16B)
2. Intact cervical body with obstruction of the cervical os (the cervix is usually well formed, but a portion of the endocervical lumen is obliterated) (Fig. 25.16C)
3. Stricture of the midportion of the cervix (which is hypoplastic with a bulbous tip and no identifiable cervical lumen) (Fig. 25.16D)
4. Fragmentation of the cervix (with portions that can be palpated below the fundus and that are not connected to the lower uterine segment) (Fig. 25.16E)

Associated anomalies of the urinary tract are rare, but they do occur. Variable portions of the vagina can be atretic. Cervical obstruction is most often associated with a vagina of normal length.

Treatment

When both the vagina and cervix are absent and a functioning uterine corpus is present, it is difficult to obtain a satisfactory fistulous tract through which menstruation can occur. Many methods have been tried, most of them involving creation of a passage through the dense fibrous tissue between the uterine cavity and the vagina and placement of a stent to keep the tract open. Occasional successes in maintaining an open passageway and normal cyclic menstruation have been reported, but endocervical glands do not develop, and there is no way to compensate for the absence of the cervical mucus, which plays an important role in sperm transport. Even though cyclic ovulatory periods can be achieved in a few patients, pregnancy is unlikely. Eventually the uterovaginal tract closes from constriction by fibrous tissue. Endometriosis can develop along the tract. Endometriosis also can develop in ovaries and other pelvic sites because of retrograde menstruation. Recurrent and severe pelvic infection is a common problem and may require total hysterectomy and removal of both ovaries. As *in vitro* fertilization procedures began to offer the possibility for a host uterus to carry a pregnancy to term, procedures to establish a fistulous tract were abandoned. Nevertheless, Cukier and associates in 1986 reported treating a patient with congenital absence of the cervix by construction of a splint that extended into the neocervical canal such that a split-thickness skin graft could actually be placed within the endocervical canal. This patient has continued to menstruate without difficulty, although pregnancy has not been accomplished.

Many authors have recommended hysterectomy as an initial procedure for a patient with a functioning uterine corpus and congenital absence of the cervix and vagina. A hysterectomy eliminates much needless suffering from associated problems such as cryptomenorrhea, sepsis, endometriosis, and multiple operations. If the hysterectomy is performed soon enough, before the problems become great, it may be possible to conserve the ovaries and their useful functions. The reconstructive surgeon should be prepared to perform a vaginoplasty with use of a split-thickness graft if hysterectomy is performed, particularly if there has been a vaginal dissection. If the neovaginal space is allowed to close and scar, then future operations to develop an adequate neovagina are associated with increased risks of graft failure and fistula formation.

Despite the overall poor results from reconstruction for congenital absence of both the cervix and the vagina, clinical experience suggests that cannulization procedures can be worthwhile for a few carefully selected cases with adequate stroma to allow a cervicovaginal anastomosis. If a long segment of cervix is fibrous cord, a cervical grafting technique may be required. If a fragmented cervix is noted, then hysterectomy is usually warranted. Those few patients who have achieved a pregnancy after cervical reconstruction have had a well-formed cervical body.

Anecdotal case reports occasionally appear in the literature confirming the necessity of palpable cervical tissue. Letterie described the development of a cervicovaginal tract in an adolescent patient with a core of cervical tissue. The tract remained patent for menstrual flow for 2 years; however, pregnancy had not yet been attempted. Data published by the senior author regarding the long-term follow-up of 21 patients with abnormal cervical development support the success of cannulization in only selected patients with sufficient rudimentary cervical tissue. All of the patients with fragmentation of the cervix ($n = 4$) eventually underwent hysterectomy. Only those patients with a well-formed cervical body, with at least a palpable cord or only distal obstruction, achieved successful surgical outcomes (4/7 patients). Only one patient, with distal obstruction, treated with cannulization using a full-thickness skin graft, achieved pregnancy.

Others have reported the anastomosis of a well-developed distal vagina to a substantial midline uterine body. Creighton and colleagues described the use of the laparoscope for this procedure; however, Deffarges and associates examined the outcomes of 18 patients after open uterovaginal anastomosis. Twenty-two percent of patients required additional surgery. Eighty-three percent of the cases were associated with upper genital tract complications. Six spontaneous pregnancies were also reported in four of the patients. Despite the small potential for pregnancy, it is imperative to realize the potential for complications, including sepsis and even death as a result of ascending infection.

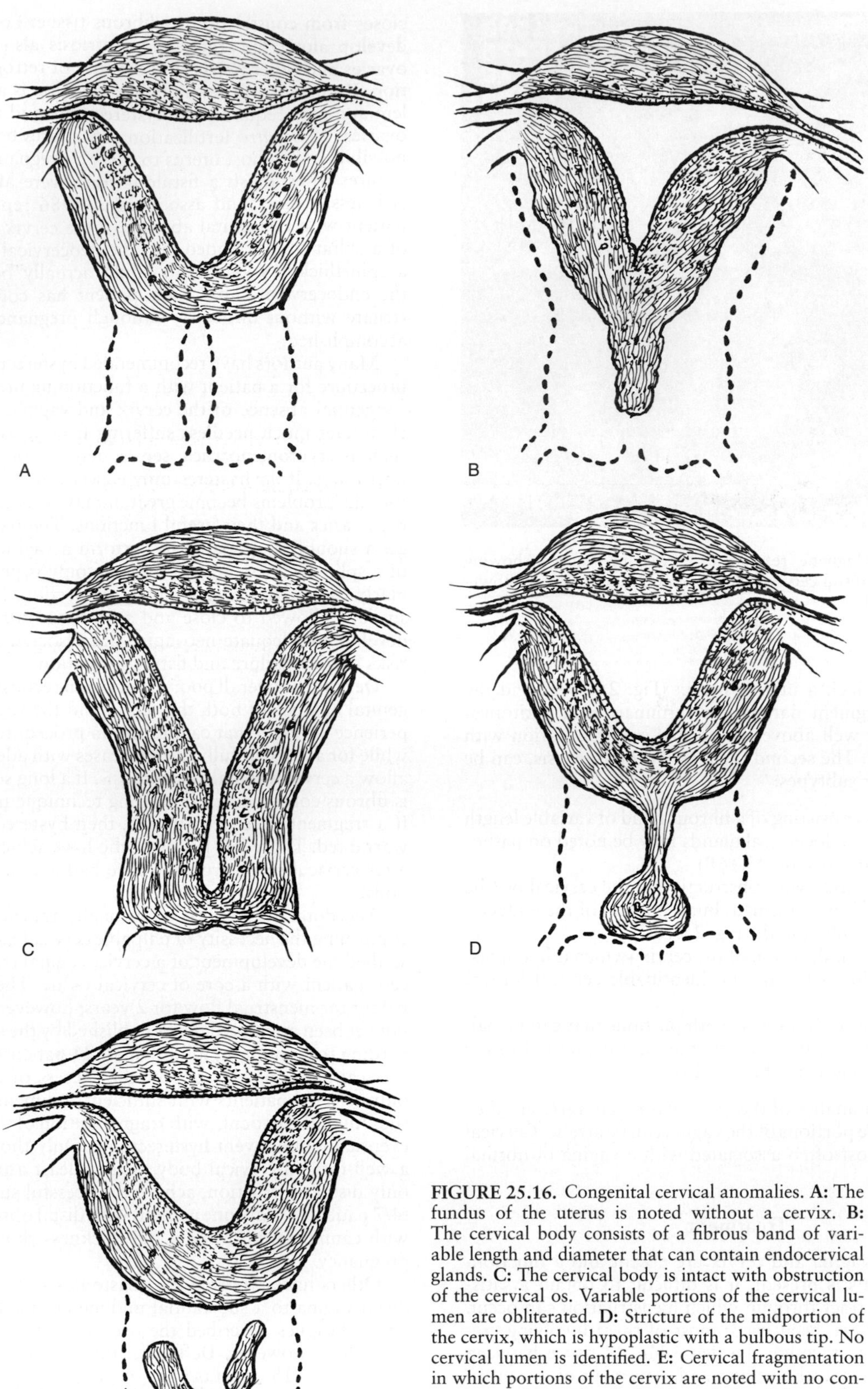

FIGURE 25.16. Congenital cervical anomalies. **A:** The fundus of the uterus is noted without a cervix. **B:** The cervical body consists of a fibrous band of variable length and diameter that can contain endocervical glands. **C:** The cervical body is intact with obstruction of the cervical os. Variable portions of the cervical lumen are obliterated. **D:** Stricture of the midportion of the cervix, which is hypoplastic with a bulbous tip. No cervical lumen is identified. **E:** Cervical fragmentation in which portions of the cervix are noted with no connection to the uterine body. Hypoplasia of the uterine cavity can be associated with cervical cord fragmentation.

The surgical approach for the rare opportunity for cervical cannulation remains a challenge. Several additional factors may also influence the surgical outcome: the size of the created channel, the duration of stenting of the channel, the presence of rudimentary endocervical glands in the region of the created channel, the presence of a native vagina adjacent to the created channel, or the number of menses allowed to flow through the stented channel. Because the surgical approach for cervical cannulation is based only on several case reports, there is truly limited data regarding safety and efficacy to share with patients and families. A frank discussion with both the patient and her family regarding the potential risks and morbidity is imperative. Even reportedly successful attempts have involved multiple surgical interventions, such as a reported cervicoplasty with bladder mucosa described by Bugamann and colleagues; the 12-year-old patient had to undergo at least one previously failed attempt at reconstruction before the reported successful procedure. Very young adolescents may be subjected to multiple surgical procedures without good evidence of success.

DISORDERS OF LATERAL FUSION

Failures of lateral fusion of the two müllerian ducts cause vaginal anomalies that are grouped as obstructed or unobstructed.

The Unobstructed Double Uterus (Bicornuate, Septate, or Didelphic Uterus)

Complete failure of medial fusion of the two müllerian ducts can result in complete duplication of the vagina, cervix, and uterus. Partial failure of fusion can result in a single vagina with a single or duplicate cervix and complete or partial duplication of the uterine corpus. A failure of absorption of the uterine septum between the two fused müllerian ducts causes the septum to persist inside the uterus to a variable extent while the external appearance remains that of a single uterus. The septum can be so complete that it divides both the uterine cavity and endocervical canal into two equal or unequal components. More often, incomplete disappearance of the septum leaves only the upper uterine cavities divided. Each of these and a variety of other forms of double uteri have their own individual features of clinical significance. When no obstruction is present, surgical reconstruction is performed primarily because of difficulties with reproduction.

Some aspects of lateral fusion disorders remain controversial because information is still inaccurate or incomplete. Many reports are based on small samples of selected patients, patients who have been diagnosed as having one anomaly or another based on incomplete data, and patients who have received unification operations without preliminary studies to rule out other causes of reproductive difficulty. A comparison of results from one series to the next is difficult because authors have used different classifications based on a variety of embryologic, anatomic, physiologic, functional, and radiologic considerations. Unknown numbers of uterine anomalies may have escaped detection because reproductive performance is generally acceptable and gynecologic difficulties do not necessarily occur.

The müllerian ducts undergo multiple steps in development, including caudal, medial growth followed by fusion and later resorption of the remaining septum. Apoptosis has been proposed as a mechanism by which the septum regresses. Bcl-2, a protein involved in regulating apoptosis, was found to be absent from the septa of several uteri. The absence of this critical protein may play a pivotal role in the persistence of the septum and lateral fusion disorders.

Historical Development of Surgical Procedures

Ruge, in 1882, first reported excision of a uterine septum in a woman who had suffered two pregnancy losses. The woman subsequently carried a pregnancy to term. Paul Strassmann of Berlin and later Erwin Strassmann, his son, were strong advocates of uterine unification operations. The studies of Jones and Jones have contributed greatly to modern understanding of the management of uterine anomalies. Their studies began with a report in 1953 of a series that was started in 1936. Updates have been published from time to time. Wheeless, Rock, Andrews, and others have joined in these reports.

Diagnosis of Uterine Anomalies

If a uterine anomaly is associated with obstruction of menstrual flow, then it causes symptoms that will come to the attention of the gynecologist shortly after menarche. Unobstructed uterine anomalies are diagnosed later in a variety of circumstances. Young girls may notice difficulty in using tampons or later difficulty in coitus if a longitudinal vaginal septum is present. This can lead to the diagnosis of an associated uterine anomaly. A patient with an anomalous upper urinary tract on intravenous pyelogram may be found to have a uterine anomaly on gynecologic evaluation. A uterine anomaly is occasionally found when a patient reports dysmenorrhea or menorrhagia or when a dilatation and curettage (D&C) is performed for abortion or some other indication. A palpable mass may be a uterine anomaly but should be confirmed as such by ultrasonography, hysterography, or laparoscopy. Woelfer and colleagues recently described the use of three-dimensional ultrasonography in screening for congenital uterine anomalies. During an investigation of the correlation of uterine anomalies with obstetric complications, the authors assessed the potential value of three-dimensional ultrasound for screening. More than 100 women with uterine anomalies were identified. Seventy-two arcuate uteri, 29 septate, and five bicornuate uteri were described. The authors emphasized how the three-dimensional ultrasound may overcome the limitations of conventional two-dimensional ultrasonography in providing a coronal view of the uterus, thus differentiating between arcuate, bicornuate, and subseptate uteri. This technique remains investigational. Semmens has pointed out that the diagnosis of a uterine anomaly can also be made from astute observation of an abnormal uterine contour during pregnancy, either in the antepartum period or at the time of abdominal or vaginal delivery. The abnormal contour is caused by a combination of fetal malpresentation and an anomalous uterus. An anomalous uterus can also be diagnosed when a pregnancy occurs despite the presence of an intrauterine contraceptive device. Persistent postmenopausal bleeding despite recent D&C can lead to a diagnosis of an anomalous uterus. Sometimes the diagnosis is made as an incidental finding at laparotomy. However, most uterine anomalies are diagnosed after hysterosalpingography to evaluate infertility or reproductive loss, usually from repeated spontaneous abortion.

Uterine Anomalies and Reproductive History

Although some uterine anomalies can cause infertility, most patients with uterine anomalies are able to conceive without difficulty. There is no question that uterine anomalies can be associated with perfectly normal reproductive performance. Overall, however, the incidences of spontaneous abortion, premature birth, fetal loss, malpresentation, and cesarean section are clearly increased when a uterine anomaly is present. It is impossible to predict which patients with uterine anomalies will have these problems.

Etiology of Reproductive Failure

The etiology of reproductive failure in patients with uterine anomalies remains unclear. Mahgoub believes that the presence of a uterine septum can lead to abortion because of diminished intrauterine space for fetal growth or because of implantation of the placenta on a poorly vascularized septum. Mizuno and associates have attached importance to the inadequacy of vascularization of the uterine septum. Associated cervical incompetence, luteal phase insufficiency, and distortion of the uterine milieu have all been implicated in the etiology of increased reproductive loss. However, it is as yet unexplained why some patients with a uterine anomaly have normal reproductive function, whereas others abort early in pregnancy. Interestingly, it has been reported that the chance for a liveborn child increases with each pregnancy loss. It is unknown whether this apparent "conditioning" of the uterus is due to better vascularization, better myometrial stretching and accommodation, or some other factor.

A medical history of three or more episodes of spontaneous abortion or premature labor merits hysterosalpingography to determine whether structural abnormalities of the uterus are present. An abnormality is found in about 10% of such cases. Among chronic early second-trimester aborters, the incidence may be higher. The etiology of spontaneous abortion is complex, and a complete workup should be done even when an anomalous uterus has been found. A careful history should include a detailed discussion of each previous pregnancy loss and inquiry into DES exposure or other drug or chemical toxicity, specific medical illnesses, and exposure to contagious diseases. A family history should emphasize reproductive failures among family members of both the patient and the husband. Specific medical diseases such as thyroid disease, diabetes mellitus, renal disease, and systemic lupus erythematosus should be ruled out. The possibility of infection by such agents as *Neisseria gonorrhoeae, Chlamydia, Mycoplasma, Toxoplasma,* and *Listeria* should be considered. Chromosome analyses should be done. Abnormalities in aborted tissue are found in more than 50% of spontaneous abortions, and abnormalities appear in up to one fourth of couples with a history of habitual abortion. Identifying such couples makes it possible to offer genetic counseling for subsequent pregnancies. Uterine leiomyomas, especially lower uterine segment and submucous leiomyomas, can cause spontaneous abortion. Basal body temperature charts, serum progesterone determinations, and endometrial biopsies timed in the luteal phase help determine the presence of luteal phase deficiency. The cervix should be studied for incompetence.

Couples with multiple etiologies for reproductive loss should have all other problems corrected before metroplasty is considered. Indeed, correcting other factors first may correct the problem of reproductive loss without metroplasty. In 1977, Rock and Jones reported on seven patients who had anomalous uterine development and extrauterine factors in the etiology of their reproductive loss. These patients had already had 16 pregnancies, 5 (29%) of which resulted in a liveborn child. After therapy to correct the extrauterine factor, the success rate increased to 71%. Stoot and Mastboom reported an impressive increase in reproductive performance among uterine anomaly patients by simple improvement of abnormal carbohydrate metabolism.

Hysterographic Studies

Proper technique during the performance of hysterosalpingography to diagnose uterine anomalies is important. The hysterogram must be taken at right angles to the axis of the uterus for a true assessment of the deformity to be made. The study is best done under fluoroscopy. A septate uterus cannot be distinguished from a bicornuate uterus by hysterogram alone (Fig. 25.17). The external uterine configuration also cannot usually be determined by pelvic examination alone, but some idea of the configuration can be obtained by ultrasonography. McDonough and Tho have suggested the use of double-contour pelvic pneumoperitoneum-hysterographic studies for precise identification of müllerian malformations. Of course, laparoscopy is even more certain. If the uterine corpus has not been previously visualized, the physician must be prepared to correct either anomaly (i.e., obstructed or unobstructed), depending on the findings at laparotomy.

Additional Testing

A complete investigation should also include an assessment of tubal patency and an intravenous pyelogram. A variety of upper urinary tract anomalies are seen, including absence of one kidney, horseshoe kidney, pelvic kidney, duplication of the collecting system, and ectopically located ureteral orifices. The lower urinary tract (bladder and urethra) is much less often anomalous.

The Double Uterus and Obstetric Outcome

The percentage of full-term pregnancies with various types of double uteri in an unselected series of women who have not been operated on is unknown. For all types combined, it is probably approximately 25%. In patients selected for operation, it probably increases from approximately 5% to 10% to approximately 80% to 90%. Because patients with uterine anomalies who have relatively normal obstetric histories cannot be identified, there is confusion in the literature about which anomalies are more often associated with obstetric difficulties and which are relatively benign in their effect. Special diagnostic procedures to detect uterine anomalies are not usually performed before reproductive performance is tested. A didelphic uterus is the exception. This anomaly can be diagnosed easily on routine pelvic examination by identification of two complete cervices and perhaps also a longitudinal vaginal septum. A study by Heinonen in Finland of 182 women with uterine anomalies indicated that pregnancies in the septate uterus had a better fetal survival rate (86%) than they did in the complete bicornuate uterus (50%) or in the unicornuate uterus (40%). These findings differ from prevailing opinions that the septate uterus is associated with the highest reproductive loss, as proposed by Jones and Jones. A recent report by Woefler and associates supports Jones and Jones's opinions by noting that women with a septate uterus had a significantly higher proportion of first trimester loss than women with a normal uterus.

In 1968, Capraro and colleagues reported on 85 patients with uterine anomalies seen between 1962 and 1966. One uterine anomaly was seen for every 645 admissions (0.145%). Metroplasty was considered necessary in only 14 (16%) of these 85 cases. According to Jones and Jones, only one third of patients with a double uterus have important reproductive problems. In most instances, the presence of a double uterus is not in itself an indication for metroplasty.

In 1980, Jewelewicz and coworkers estimated the spontaneous abortion rate to be 33.8% in women with a bicornuate

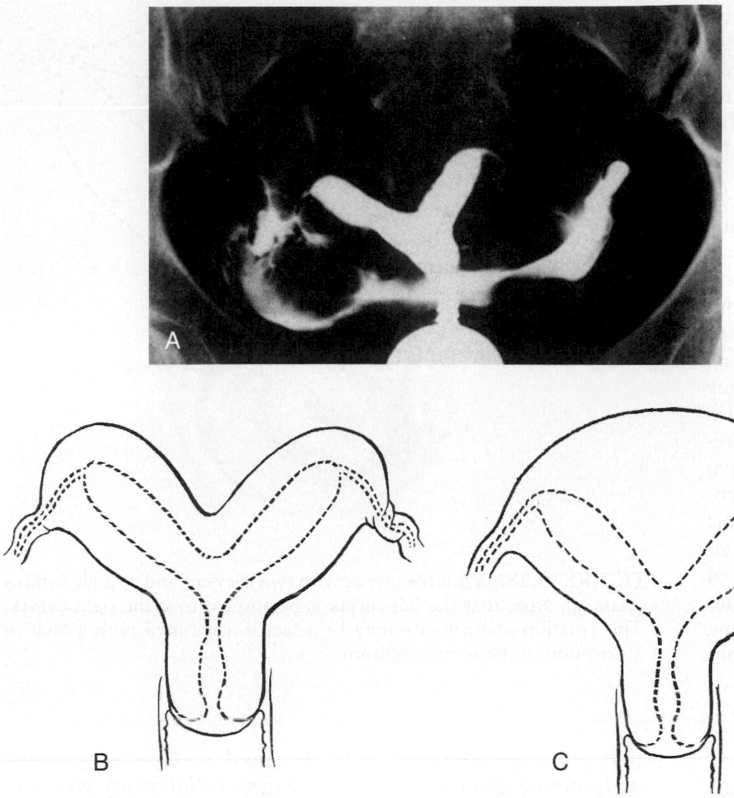

FIGURE 25.17. A: A hysterogram of a double uterus. A bicornuate uterus (B) and a septate uterus (C) are types of double uteri. Visualization of the fundus is required to determine the type of uterus.

uterus, 22.2% in those with a septate uterus, and 34.6% in those with a unicornuate uterus. More recently, Ludmir and associates reported that high-risk obstetric intervention did not significantly increase the fetal survival rate for uncorrected uterine anomalies. Capraro and associates found a preoperative fetal salvage rate of 33.3% for the septate uterus, 10% for the bicornuate uterus, and 0% for the didelphic uterus. Postoperatively, the fetal salvage rate was 100% for the bicornuate uterus, 80% for the septate uterus, and 66% for the didelphic uterus. The report gives the improved salvage figures, compared with several previous studies, after abdominal metroplasty.

Ravasia and colleagues described the incidence of uterine rupture in a cohort of women with müllerian duct anomalies who attempted vaginal birth after cesarean delivery (VBAC). Of the 1,813 patients who attempted VBAC between 1992 and 1997, only 25 patients with known müllerian duct anomalies attempted a trial of labor. This included 14 patients with a bicornuate uterus, five with a septate uterus, four with a unicornuate uterus, and two with uterine didelphys. Uterine rupture was diagnosed in two patients with müllerian anomalies. The authors proposed several mechanisms for the greater incidence of uterine rupture in this population: abnormal development of the lower uterine segment, previous scar similar to a vertical or classic incision, and the possibility of abnormal traction on the uterine scar during labor.

The Didelphic Uterus. A didelphic uterus with two hemicorpora is easily diagnosed because all patients have two hemicervices visible on speculum examination, and most, if not all, have a longitudinal sagittal vaginal septum. In the series reported by Heinonen and associates, all 21 patients with a didelphic uterus had a vaginal septum. Conversely, a patient with a longitudinal vaginal septum usually has a didelphic uterus. The indication for uterine unification is related to the role of this anomaly as an etiologic factor in reproductive loss. Of all the uterine anomalies (except arcuate uterus), the didelphic uterus is associated with the best possibility of a successful pregnancy. However, there is still some increase in perinatal mortality, premature birth, breech presentation, and cesarean section for delivery. Heinonen and associates reported a fetal survival rate of 64% without metroplasty. Musich and Behrman stated that the didelphic uterus offers the best chance for a successful pregnancy (57%) and should not be considered an appropriate indication for metroplasty. However, W. S. Jones considered the didelphic uterus to give the worst obstetric outcome. In the opinion of the editors of this book, a unification operation for a didelphic uterus is not often indicated, and the results may be disappointing, especially when an attempt is made to unify the cervix. Not only is this procedure technically difficult in a complete didelphic anomaly, but it can also result in cervical incompetence or cervical stenosis.

The Septate Uterus. Most patients who are evaluated for repeated abortion and who are found to have a uterine anomaly have a septate uterus. A few have other anomalies, mostly the bicornuate uterus. Proctor and Haney's review of women with recurrent first-trimester pregnancy loss reinforce the role of the septate uterus in repeated pregnancy loss. Of 35 women reviewed with a divided uterine cavity on hysterosalpingogram, all women were found through diagnostic hysteroscopy and laparoscopy to have a septate uterus. In our experience, fetal survival rates are higher after septate uterus repair than after other repairs. In 1977, Rock and Jones reported on 43 patients with septate uteri selected for Jones metroplasty at the Johns Hopkins Hospital. Of these 43 patients, 95% became pregnant postoperatively, 73% carried to term, and 77% delivered a liveborn child. Similarly, hysteroscopic metroplasty for the septate uterus provides a substantial improvement in obstetric outcome. Data obtained from retrospective studies suggest that hysteroscopic metroplasty is associated with favorable outcomes, with a pregnancy rate of approximately 80% and a miscarriage rate of only approximately 15%. Recent prospective observational studies reported similar findings. Pabuccu and Gomel reported the reproductive outcome of 61 patients; however, the patients had unexplained infertility and nearly 15% were also treated with cervical cerclage. Litta and colleagues also reported an 83.3% term delivery rate in their population of women with a septate uterus who underwent hysteroscopic metroplasty. Patton and colleagues described 16 women with a complete uterine septum. The preoperative pregnancy loss rate was 81%. Eleven of the fourteen septa treated with a hysteroscopic approach were successfully removed. The remaining three unsuccessful hysteroscopic procedures and two additional patients were treated using the Tompkins metroplasty. Postoperatively, 9 women conceived after hysteroscopic surgery, and term live births occurred in 9 of 12 (75%) conceptions. The most controversial area remains the resection of the cervical portion of the septum. Parsanezhad and colleagues reported a multicenter, randomized controlled trial regarding the management of the cervical septum. Surgical issues, complications, and pregnancy outcomes were compared. Operating times, distending media deficits, and perioperative complications were all substantially better in the cervical septum resection group. The reproductive outcomes were similar; however, the cesarean section rate was higher in the group in which the cervical septum was spared. The histologic features of the septum in this abnormal uterus have been described. Dabirashrafi and colleagues noted less connective tissue in uterine septa. Poor decidualization and placentation were suggested as a cause.

Finally, the AFS class VA uterus (a double cervix and uterine cavity with a single fundus) can result from a rotation abnormality during the descent of the müllerian ducts. Among the reported cases of the septate uterus, the incidence of the complete septum involving the cervix varies from 4% to 29%. If the dextrorotating müllerian ducts overrotate, the senior author theorizes that the septum fails to absorb after fusion of the ducts (J. A. Rock, personal observations, 1991). In virtually every patient with a complete septate uterus, the left cervix is higher than the right. In one patient, one cervix has been noted above the other (Fig. 25.18). This rotation abnormality may be a factor associated with lack of absorption of the uterine septum in these patients.

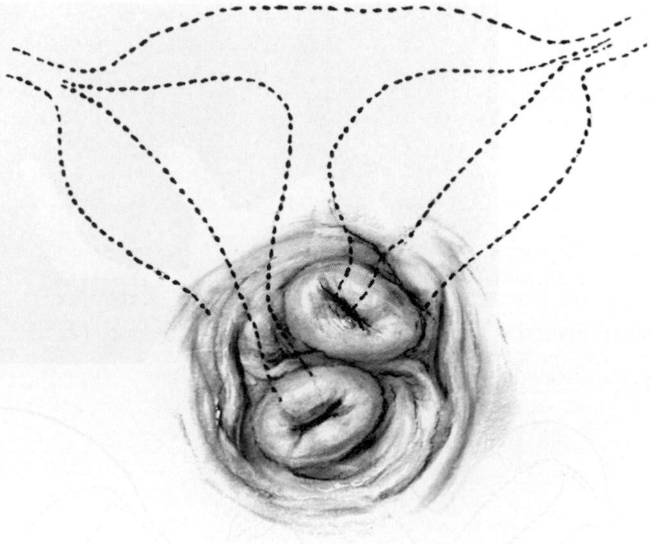

FIGURE 25.18. A double uterus with two cervices and a single fundus (class V). Note that the left cervix is positioned over the right cervix. This rotation abnormality may be a factor associated with a lack of absorption of the uterine septum.

Uterine Anomalies and Menstrual Difficulties

Dysmenorrhea and abnormal and heavy menstrual bleeding have been reported to occur more frequently with any form of double uterus and to be relieved after unification operations. Capraro and associates reported several cases in which dysmenorrhea was cured by metroplasty. Erwin Strassmann also believed that all cases of dysmenorrhea and menorrhagia associated with uterine anomalies were relieved by unification of the two uterine cavities. Generally, however, dysmenorrhea and menorrhagia are inappropriate indications for uterine unification, and the operation should not be performed solely for these reasons.

Uterine Anomalies and Infertility

Opinions differ considerably in terms of whether infertility is a proper indication for metroplasty. Erwin Strassmann stated that primary infertility could be cured in 60% of patients with uterine anomaly if all other causes of infertility were excluded. Strassmann reported eight metroplasties for primary sterility that yielded nine pregnancies and seven liveborn children, although the number of patients who conceived was not given. Similar reports of small numbers of patients can be found throughout the literature. Heinonen and Pystynen indicated that uterine anomalies are rarely the reason for infertility. Nonuterine causes of infertility must be ruled out before metroplasty, as a last resort, is considered.

Certainly, a full infertility investigation to rule out other causes should be completed before the anomalous uterus is blamed. Even when no other cause for infertility is found, if the uterus is septate or bicornuate, then there may not be any proper indication for metroplasty. This question of when to perform metroplasty simply has not yet been answered. The decision is difficult and becomes even more difficult when the opportunity for metroplasty presents itself because a septate or bicornuate uterus requires laparotomy for some other reason, such as endometriosis or tubal occlusion.

Surgical Technique for Uterine Unification

Traditionally, the septate uterus has been unified with either the Jones or the Tompkins procedure. Clinical reports by Chervenak and Neuwirth; by Daly, Walters, and colleagues; by DeCherney and associates; and and Israel and March have favorably compared hysteroscopic or resectoscopic incision of a uterine septum with the more traditional transabdominal approach. Term pregnancy rates after these procedures have approached 80% to 85%. Several attempts may be necessary to incise a wide septum, although the septum usually can be incised completely at the first operation.

Transcervical Lysis of the Uterine Septum. Abdominal metroplasty for transfundal incision or for excision of the septum associated with the septate uterus generally has been abandoned. With hysteroscopic scissors, the procedure can be tedious, especially with a large, broad septum. Although the hysteroscope and scissors are still used for cutting the septum, the resectoscope has been found to be comparable. The optics are excellent, and the septum can be electrosurgically incised with little difficulty. Laser-assisted procedures have also been described.

Before transcervical lysis of a uterine septum, a gonadotropin-releasing hormone agonist may be given for 2 months to reduce the amount of endometrium that can obscure the surgeon's view during the procedure. Many authors do not consider routine preoperative preparation of the endometrium essential and may only use medications in procedures involving exceptionally wide septa or complete septa that involve the lower one third of the uterine cavity or the cervical canal. If medical preparation is not used, surgical intervention should be scheduled during the early proliferative phase of the cycle to avoid bleeding and impaired visualization from a vascular endometrium associated with the secretory phase. Transcervical lysis is usually performed in conjunction with laparoscopy under general endotracheal anesthesia. The uterine cavity is distended with dextran 70 (Hyskon) by way of the resectoscope, which is inserted into the cervix. The septum is then electrosurgically incised by advancing the cutting loupe, using the trigger mechanism of the resectoscope. The uterine septum is incised until the tubal ostia are visualized and there is no appreciable evidence of the septum. The procedure is performed under simultaneous laparoscopy to limit the risks of uterine perforation. The laparoscopic light can be turned off so that the light from the hysteroscope can be clearly visualized through the fundus. Most patients can be discharged within 4 hours of the procedure. There is no role for placement of a postoperative intrauterine device. The benefit of routine procedure-related antibiotic therapy has not been well supported with evidence; however, it is recommended to administer antibiotics before the procedure and to continue for 5 days after surgery to limit the risks of infection. If excessive bleeding occurs after the procedure, a Foley catheter should be placed in the uterine cavity for tamponade and removed in 4 to 6 hours. Hormonal therapy is the most commonly used postoperative treatment regimen. The aim of the treatment is the promotion of rapid epithelialization. Dabirashrafi and colleagues reported that estrogen therapy did not appear to demonstrate a benefit. Further evidence is necessary before dismissing the current trend of postoperative estrogen therapy.

Transcervical lysis also can be performed to repair a complete septate uterus (i.e., a single fundus with two cavities and two cervices). In this instance, a no. 8 Foley catheter is inserted into one cervix and indigo carmine is injected into the cavity. The other cavity is distended with dextran 70 (Hyskon) by way of the resectoscope. The septum is electrosurgically incised at a point above the internal cervical os until the Foley catheter is visualized. The septum is then incised in a superior direction until the tubal ostium is visualized and there is no appreciable septum (Fig. 25.19).

After transcervical lysis of a uterine septum, a 2-month delay before attempting pregnancy is suggested to allow complete resorption of the septum. Delivery may be vaginal. The Jones procedure is used to repair a septate uterus when a particularly broad septum cannot be easily incised with the resectoscope. The Strassmann procedure is used for unification of a bicornuate uterus. The safety and efficacy of hysteroscopic resection of the uterine septum in patients with a class VA septate uterus has been demonstrated by the senior author. Historically, case reports, such as that of Hundley and colleagues, were the only source of information about this interesting variant; however, one of the largest populations of patients with a complete septum was reported in 1999 by Roberts and Rock. The patients underwent hysteroscopic metroplasty with preservation of the cervical portion of the septum. With the exception of one case

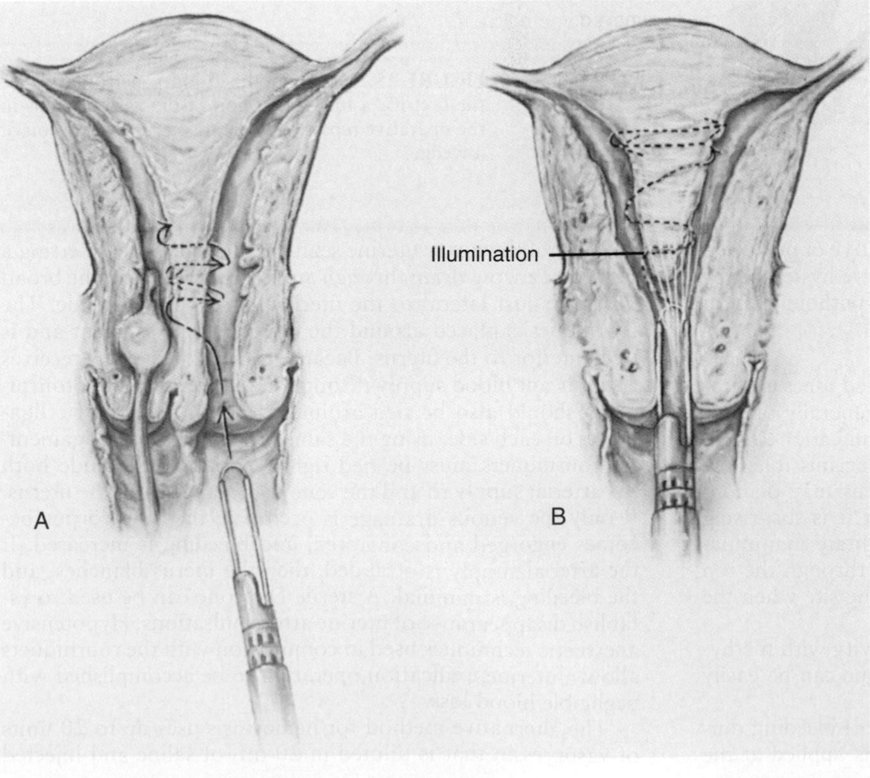

FIGURE 25.19. Resectoscopic metroplasty. **A:** A Foley catheter is placed in one cavity of a complete septate uterus (American Fertility Society class VA uterus). The resectoscope is inserted in the opposite cavity, and the septum is incised until the Foley is visualized. The septum can be easily incised with the resectoscope until both internal os are visible. **B:** A septate uterus with a single cervix. The septum can be incised with the straight loupe of the resectoscope.

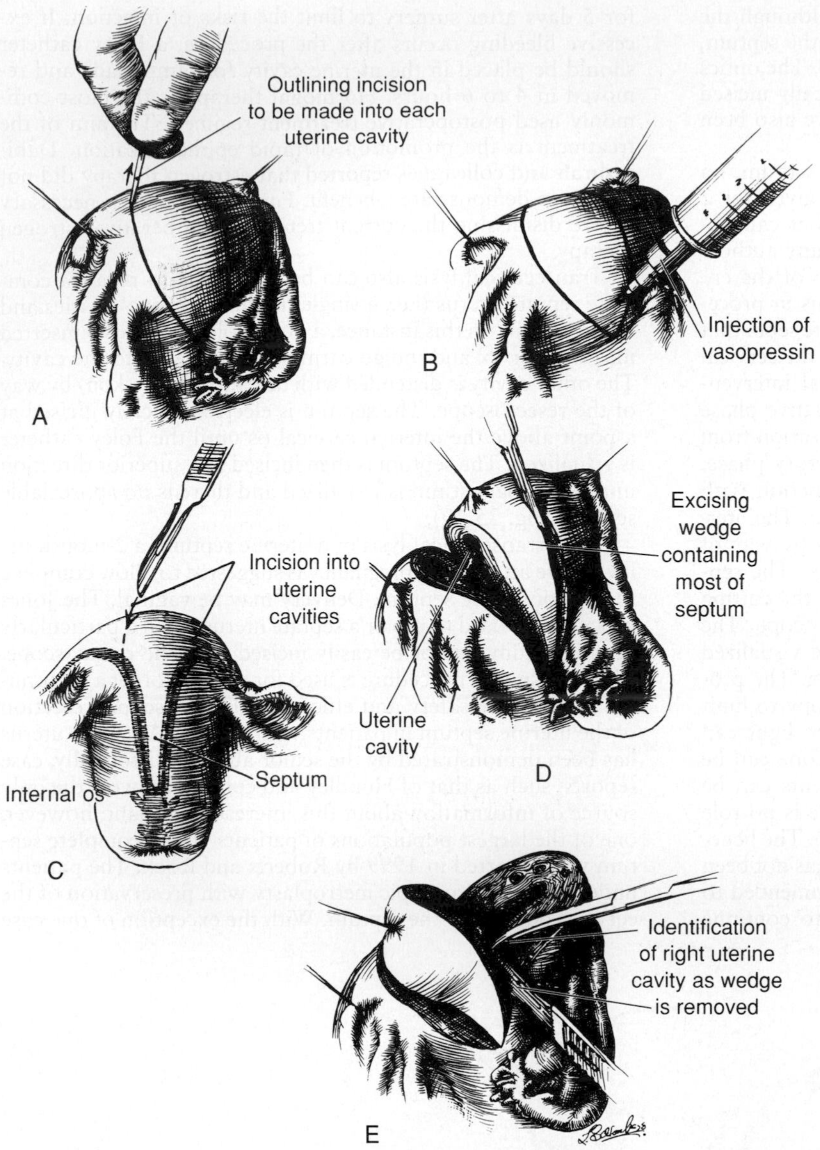

FIGURE 25.20. The modified Jones metroplasty. See the text for a full description of the various steps in the operative repair of a septate uterus by excision of a wedge.

of pulmonary edema, no significant intraoperative or postoperative complications were reported. Postoperative hysteroscopy revealed only minor fundal septal remnants without clinical significance.

The Modified Jones Metroplasty. In the modified Jones unification operation (Fig. 25.20), the abdomen is generally opened through a transverse incision. If only the unification operation is planned, then a Pfannenstiel incision is permissible. The pelvic viscera are inspected. The septate uterus may demonstrate a median raphe across the fundus, but it is surprising how often the corpus looks normal. To facilitate manipulation, a traction suture of heavy silk is placed through the top of the septum. This suture is removed from the site when the septum is excised.

No attempt is made to stain the uterine cavity with methylene blue. Normal unstained endometrial tissue can be easily differentiated from the myometrium.

There are essentially two methods to control bleeding during this procedure. In the first, a tourniquet is applied at the junction of the lower uterine segment and cervix by inserting a 0.5-inch Penrose drain through an avascular space in the broad ligaments just lateral to the uterine vessels on each side. The tourniquet is placed around the lower uterine segment and is tied anterior to the uterus. Because the uterine corpus receives a significant blood supply through the ovarian arteries, tourniquets should also be tied around the infundibulopelvic ligaments on each side, using the same hole in the broad ligament. All tourniquets must be tied tightly enough to occlude both the arterial supply to and the venous drainage from the uterus. If only the venous drainage is occluded, then the corpus becomes engorged and congested, and bleeding is increased. If the arterial supply is occluded, then the uterus blanches, and the bleeding is minimal. A sterile Doptone can be used to establish disappearance of uterine artery pulsations. Hypotensive anesthetic techniques used in conjunction with the tourniquets allow a uterine unification operation to be accomplished with negligible blood loss.

The alternative method for hemostasis uses up to 20 units of vasopressin that is diluted in 20 mL of saline and injected

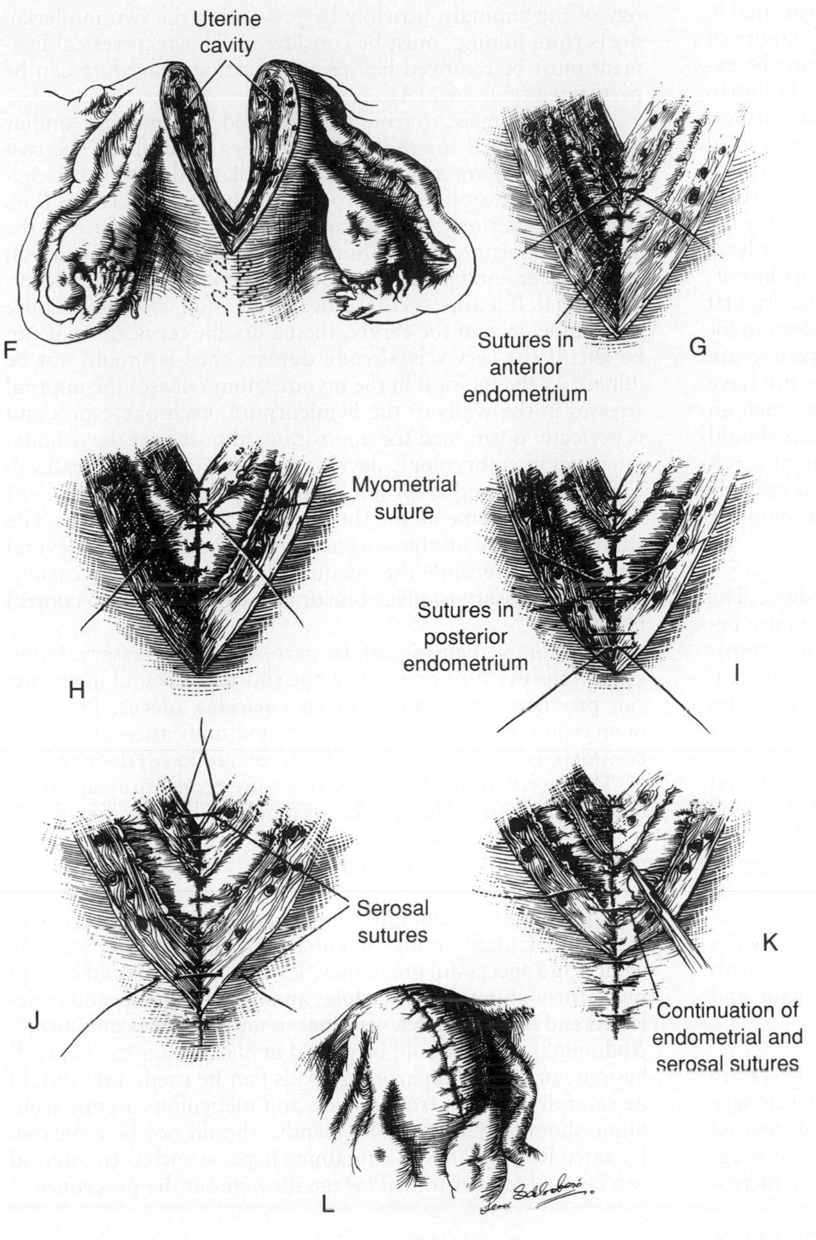

FIGURE 25.20. (*Continued*)

into the anterior and posterior walls of the uterus before the incision is made.

The uterine septum should be surgically excised as a wedge (Fig. 25.20D). The incisions begin at the fundus of the uterus. The approach to the endometrial cavity should be handled carefully so that it is not transected (Fig. 25.20E). The original incisions at the top of the fundus are usually within 1 cm—and sometimes even less—of the insertion of the fallopian tubes. If the incision is directed toward the apex of the wedge, however, there seems to be little danger of transecting the tube across its interstitial transit in the myometrium.

After the wedge has been removed, the uterus is closed in three layers with interrupted stitches; 2–0 nonreactive suture on an atraumatic tapered needle is convenient. Two sizes of needles are needed: a half-inch needle for the inner and intermediate layers and a large needle (three fourths half-round) for the outer muscular layer. The inner layer of stitches must include about one third of the thickness of the myometrium, because the endometrium alone is too delicate to hold a suture and will be cut through. The inner sutures should be placed through the endometrium and the myometrium in such a way that the knot is tied within the endometrial cavity (Fig. 25.20G–H). While the suture is being tied, the two lateral halves of the uterus should be pressed together both manually and with the guy sutures to relieve tension on the suture line and to reduce the possibility of cutting through. These sutures are placed alternately, first anterior and then posterior. After the first few stitches are placed and before the first layer is completed, the second layer can be started to reduce tension.

As the operation proceeds, the third layer of stitches is begun in the serosa both anteriorly and posteriorly (Fig. 25.20I–K). Finer, nonreactive suture material can be used to approximate the serosal edges of the uterus more precisely to prevent adhesion formation to the suture line (Fig. 25.20K–L). By the conclusion of the operation, the uterus appears near normal in configuration. The striking feature is usually the proximity of the insertions of the fallopian tubes. Special care must be exercised not to obstruct the interstitial portions of the fallopian tubes while placing the fundal myometrial and serosal sutures.

The final size of the uterine cavity seems to be relatively unimportant to reproductive capability; uterine symmetry appears to be a more important factor. Often the constructed cavity is quite small compared with the normal uterus. Whether the surgeon removes the septum with the Jones procedure or lyses the septum transcervically, postoperative hysterogram films often show small dog-ears that are leftover tags from the original bifid condition of the uterus. Such dog-ears do not seem to interfere with function, although a postoperative roentgenogram cannot be considered normal in the sense that it does not have the appearance of a normal endometrial cavity after such an operation. If a double cervix is present, the physician should not attempt to unify the cervix because an incompetent cervical os will result. To allow the uterine incision the best possible opportunity to heal, a delay of 4 to 6 months in attempting pregnancy is advised after abdominal metroplasty.

The Jones Metroplasty Versus The Tompkins Procedure. The technique of modified Jones metroplasty is a compromise between the classic Jones metroplasty and the Tompkins metroplasty. In the Jones operation, the entire septum is removed. In the Tompkins operation, a single median incision divides the uterine corpus and septum in half. The incision is carried inferiorly until the endometrial cavity is reached. Each lateral septal half is then incised to within 1 cm of the tubes. No septal tissue is removed. The myometrium is reapproximated, taking care not to place sutures too close to the interstitial portion of the tubes. Proponents of the Tompkins technique suggest that it is simpler than the classic Jones procedure, that it conserves all myometrial tissue and leaves the uterotubal junction in a more normal and lateral position, and that it provides better results than the Jones metroplasty. Good results with the Tompkins technique have been reported by McShane and colleagues.

The Wedge Metroplasty Versus Transcervical Lysis. There are obvious advantages to a transcervical incision of a uterine septum for patients with a septate uterus. Morbidity is decreased after the procedure, and delivery can be vaginal. Term pregnancy rates are comparable with those after abdominal metroplasty for repeated pregnancy wastage.

Most of the septa associated with a septate uterus can be cut through the cervix by way of the hysteroscope or the resectoscope. Nevertheless, cases of broad uterine septum can benefit from the wedge metroplasty, and reconstructive surgeons should be knowledgeable in its performance.

The Strassmann Metroplasty The Strassmann procedure is not easily adapted to the septate uterus, but it is the procedure of choice for unification of the two endometrial cavities of an externally divided uterus, both bicornuate and didelphic (Fig. 25.21). A bicornuate uterus cannot be repaired through transcervical lysis because perforation will result. When there has been failure of fusion of the two müllerian ducts, inspection of the pelvic cavity often reveals a broad peritoneal band that lies in the middle between the two lateral hemicorpora. This rectovesical ligament is attached anteriorly to the bladder, folds over and is attached between the uterine cornua, continues posteriorly in the cul-de-sac, and ends with its attachment to the anterior wall of the sigmoid and rectum. It is not invariably present, but when it is, its potential significance in the etiology of the anomaly, possibly by preventing the two müllerian ducts from joining, must be considered. This rectovesical ligament must be removed before a unification procedure can be performed (Fig. 25.21A).

For hemostasis, tourniquets are used in a manner similar to that described for the modified Jones procedure. The two uterine cornua are incised on their median sides in their longitudinal axes, deeply enough to expose the uterine cavities (Fig. 25.21B). Superiorly, the incision must not be too close to the interstitial portion of the fallopian tubes. Inferiorly, the incision is carried far enough to join the two sides into a single endocervical canal. If it appears that a deeper incision will compromise the competence of the cervix, then a double cervical canal can be left. If the cervix is already duplex, then it should not be joined. As the incision in the myometrium releases the internal stresses in the walls of the hemicorpora, each one everts and is perfectly positioned for apposition, almost as if the original intention in embryologic development is finally to be realized. The suture technique for joining the two sides (Fig. 25.21C–E) is exactly the same as for the modified Jones procedure. The suture line in the uterine corpus should be observed for several minutes to determine the adequacy of hemostasis. Occasionally it is necessary to place one or two extra sutures to control bleeding.

A uterine suspension can be performed as necessary. However, in the event of pregnancy, the shortened round ligaments can produce symptoms from an enlarging uterus. Presacral neurectomy in association with uterine unification should be considered only in patients with severe midline dysmenorrhea.

The cervix should be dilated to ensure proper drainage from the uterine cavity. This can be accomplished transvaginally after the abdominal procedure or from above by inserting a dilator through the cervical canal into the vagina to be removed later.

The operative technique should always be consistent with the goal of maintaining or enhancing fertility and possibly achieving a successful pregnancy. Tissue surfaces should be kept moist throughout the procedure, and instruments should be selected and used in such a way that tissue damage is minimized. Abdominal packs should be placed in plastic bags to avoid adhesions, or no-lint laparotomy pads can be used. Talc should be carefully washed from gloves, and meticulous aseptic technique should be used. The appendix should not be removed. Lactated Ringer solution containing heparin and corticosteroid can be used for peritoneal lavage throughout the procedure.

Cervical Incompetence Associated with a Double Uterus

When a patient with an anomalous uterus, with or without unification, becomes pregnant, she must be watched closely for evidence of cervical incompetence, especially if a history of previous reproductive loss suggests cervical incompetence. Heinonen and associates improved fetal survival rate from 57% to 92% by cervical cerclage. Cerclage was used mostly in patients with a partial bicornuate uterus. In these patients, the fetal salvage rate was improved from 53% before cerclage to 100% afterward. Prematurity also was decreased, from 53% to 3%. The authors stress that cervical incompetence, not the uterine anomaly, is the proper indication for cerclage in these patients. However, the frequency with which these problems are found together suggests the importance of doing a careful evaluation for both problems. Some reproductive losses from a uterine anomaly might be prevented by cerclage of an incompetent cervix during metroplasty. However, routine cerclage at the time of metroplasty is not recommended.

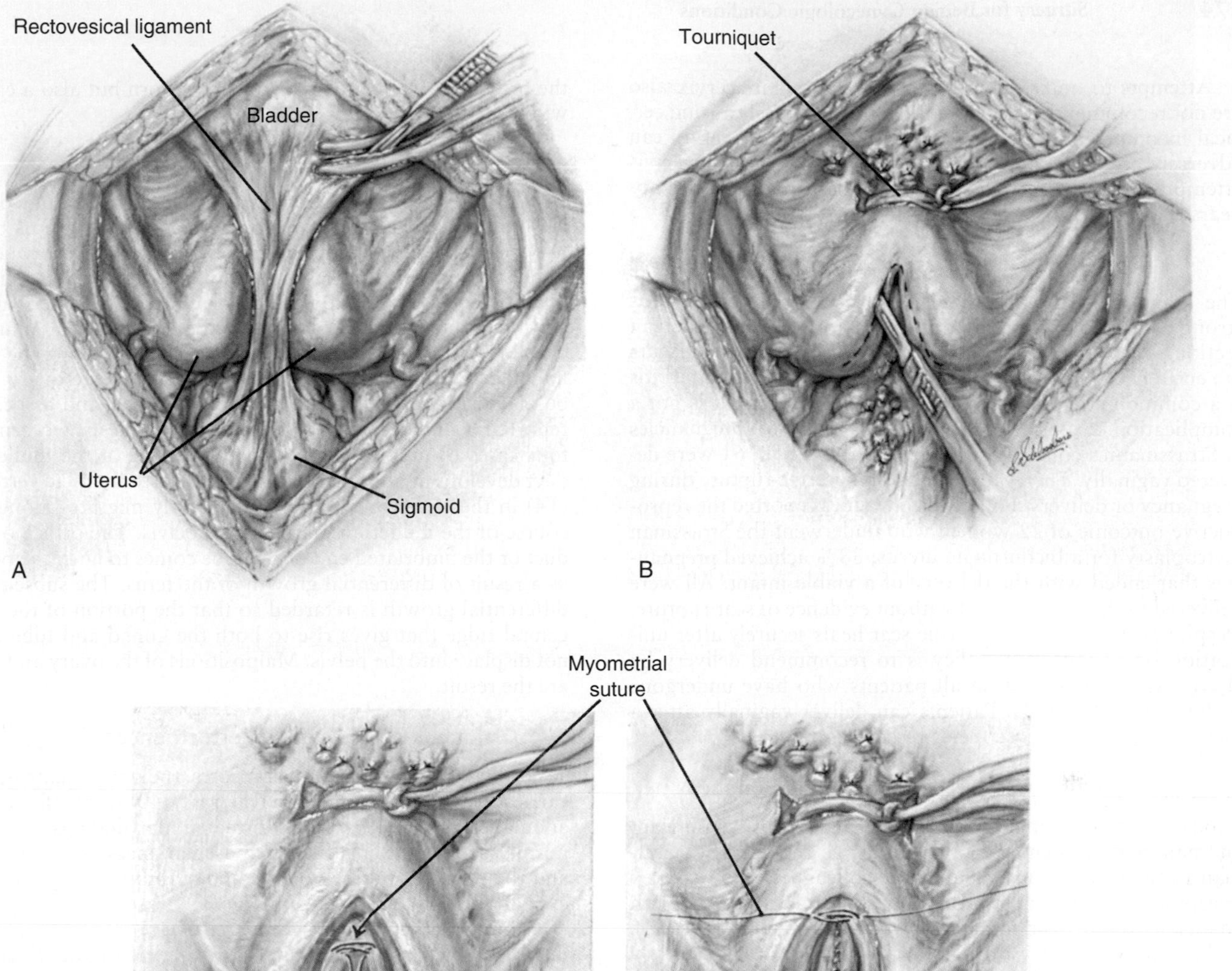

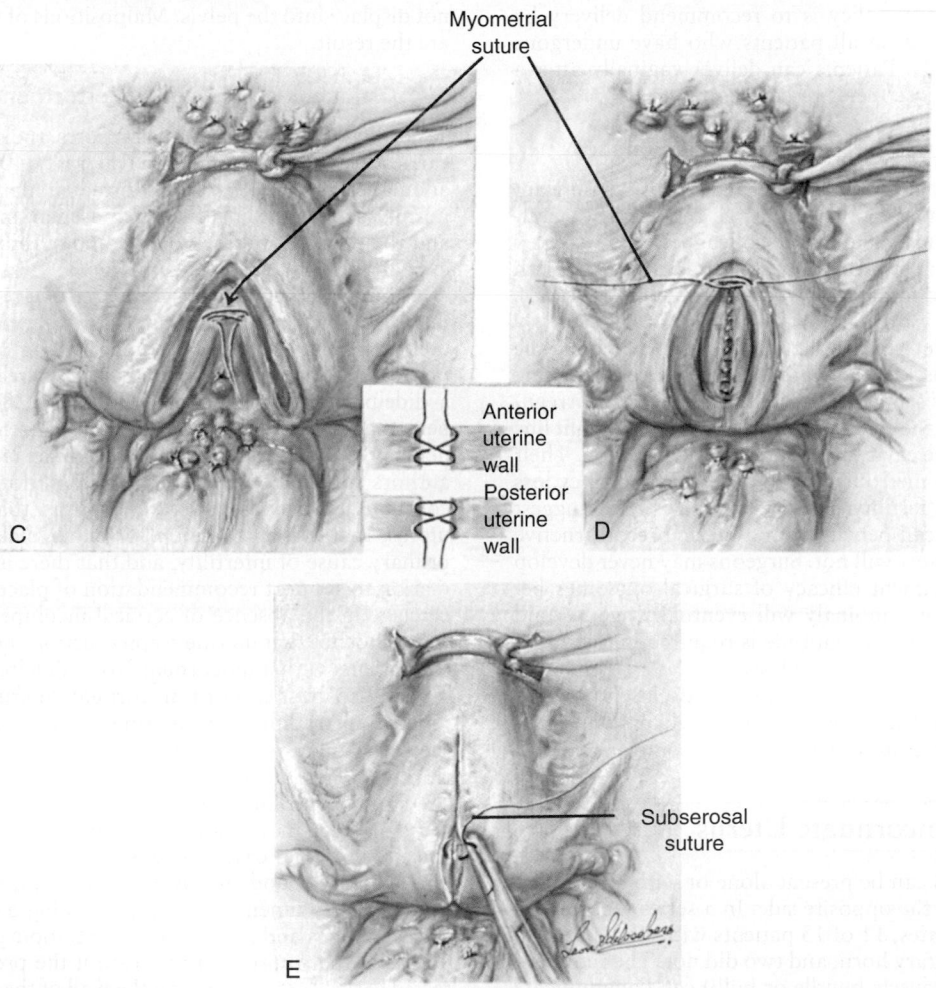

FIGURE 25.21. The Strassmann metroplasty with modification. **A:** If a rectovesical ligament is found, it should be removed. **B:** An incision is made on the medial side of each hemicorpus and carried deep enough to enter the uterine cavity. The edges of the myometrium will evert to face the opposite side. **C** and **D:** The myometrium is approximated by use of interrupted vertical figure-of-eight 3–0 polyglycolic acid sutures. One should avoid placing sutures too close to the interstitial portion of the fallopian tubes. **E:** A continuous 5–0 polyglycolic acid subserosal suture is used as a final layer. Tourniquets are removed, and defects in the broad ligament are closed.

Attempts to unify a double cervix or a septate cervix also are not recommended because of the possibility of causing cervical incompetence. However, a double or septate cervix can adversely affect the outcome of delivery if vaginal delivery is attempted, and delivery should be by cesarean section if it appears that the cervix will cause dystocia.

Mode of Delivery after Metroplasty

The scar formed in the myometrium after unification is as strong as, if not stronger than, the scar formed after cesarean section. The biologic conditions under which healing occurs are entirely different in these two situations. Endomyometritis is a common complication after cesarean section but is not a complication of uterine unification. Of 71 known pregnancies in Strassmann's collected series reported in 1952, 61 were delivered vaginally. There were no cases of uterine rupture during pregnancy or delivery. Lolis and colleagues reported the reproductive outcome of 22 women who underwent the Strassman metroplasty for a bicournuate uterus; 88% achieved pregnancies that ended with the delivery of a viable infant. All were delivered by cesarean section without evidence of scar rupture. Despite evidence that the uterine scar heals securely after unification operations, our policy is to recommend delivery by elective cesarean section in all patients who have undergone abdominal metroplasty. Patients can deliver vaginally after a metroplasty by hysteroscope or resectoscope.

Diethylstilbestrol-Related Uterine Anomalies

Exposure of the female fetus to DES can cause significant anomalous development of the uterus, as reported by Kaufman and associates and by Haney and colleagues. The T-shaped uterus is the variant most commonly seen. It is associated with an increased rate of spontaneous abortions, preterm deliveries, and ectopic pregnancies.

Nagel and Malo determined the feasibility of correcting the uterine malformations seen in DES-exposed women by incising constriction rings and septa. Their goal was to incise the irregular uterine walls until the cavity assumed a smooth, straight line from the lower uterine cavity to the uterine tubal ostium. Their results suggested that metroplasty can decrease pregnancy loss but does not enhance fertility. The editors of this book suggest that the rare patient can benefit from a uterine reconstructive procedure, but that most will not. Surgeons may never develop a large series to document efficacy of surgical outcomes because patients with this anomaly will eventually age beyond reproductive years, and some latitude is required in cases that might possibly benefit from metroplasty.

DES-exposed patients must be monitored closely for evidence of dilatation and effacement of the cervix early in pregnancy. Cervical cerclage may be indicated in some patients.

Unicornuate Uterus

A unicornuate uterus can be present alone or with a rudimentary horn or bulb on the opposite side. In a series reported by Heinonen and associates, 11 of 13 patients with a unicornuate uterus had a rudimentary horn, and two did not. The rudimentary anlage (uterine muscle bundle or bulb) can communicate directly with the unicornuate uterus. In some instances, there is no cavity within the anlage, or there is no rudimentary horn. Most rudimentary horns are noncommunicating (90% according to O'Leary and O'Leary). The two sides may be connected by a fibromuscular band, or there may be no connection and no communication between the two uterine cavities. Fedele and associates have found sonography useful in determining the presence of not only a rudimentary horn but also a cavity within.

Associated Anomalies

Urinary tract anomalies are often associated with a unicornuate uterus. On the side opposite the unicornuate uterus there may be a horseshoe or a pelvic kidney, or the kidney may be hypoplastic or absent. This is especially true if there is associated müllerian duct obstruction. When all müllerian duct derivatives and the kidney are absent on one side, this implies failure of development of the entire urogenital ridge, including the genital ridge where the ovary forms. In addition, the ovary may be malpositioned (Fig. 25.22). Rock, Parmley, and associates reported a unilateral ovary located above the pelvic brim in four cases of uterine anomalies. The orifice of the müllerian duct develops at about the level of the fourth thoracic vertebra (T4) in the embryo. The tip subsequently migrates along the course of the müllerian duct into the pelvis. The orifice of the duct or the fimbriated end of the tube comes to lie in the pelvis as a result of differential growth of the fetus. The subsequent differential growth is retarded so that the portion of the urogenital ridge that gives rise to both the gonad and tube does not displace into the pelvis. Malpositions of the ovary and tube are the result.

Reproductive Performance

According to Heinonen and associates, the unicornuate uterus carries the poorest fetal survival rate (40%) of all uterine anomalies. In 1957, Jones reported similar findings. The abnormal shape, the insufficient muscular mass of the uterus, and the reduced uterine volume and inability to expand may explain the poor obstetric outcome.

Moutos and colleagues compared the reproductive performance of the unicornuate uterus with that of the didelphic uterus. Twenty of the 29 women with a unicornuate uterus produced a total of 40 pregnancies, whereas 13 women with a didelphic uterus produced a total of 28 pregnancies. The percentages of pregnancies resulting in preterm delivery, term delivery, and living children were similar in both groups. The authors concluded that reproductive performance of the unicornuate uterus was not different from that of the didelphic uterus, that it is uncommon for either malformation to be a primary cause of infertility, and that there is insufficient information to support recommendation of placement of a cervical cerclage in the absence of cervical incompetence. Thus, there is no evidence that uterine reconstruction should be performed for patients with a unicornuate (or a didelphic) uterus.

Because most cases of unicornuate uterus have a noncommunicating rudimentary uterine horn on the opposite side, there is danger of pregnancy in the rudimentary horn from transperitoneal migration of sperm or ovum from the opposite side. According to Holden and Hart, approximately 350 cases of pregnancy in a rudimentary horn have been reported since the original case report by Mauriceau in 1669. O'Leary and O'Leary found the corpus luteum on the side contralateral to the rudimentary horn containing a pregnancy in 8% of cases. Signs and symptoms of an ectopic pregnancy develop with eventual rupture of the horn if the pregnancy is not detected early. Rupture through the wall of the vascular rudimentary horn is associated with sudden and severe intraperitoneal hemorrhage and shock. Death can occur in a few minutes. It is surprising that the current mortality rate has decreased to 5%.

Very little, if anything, can be done to improve the reproductive performance of patients with a unicornuate uterus. The physician should observe closely for cervical incompetence and

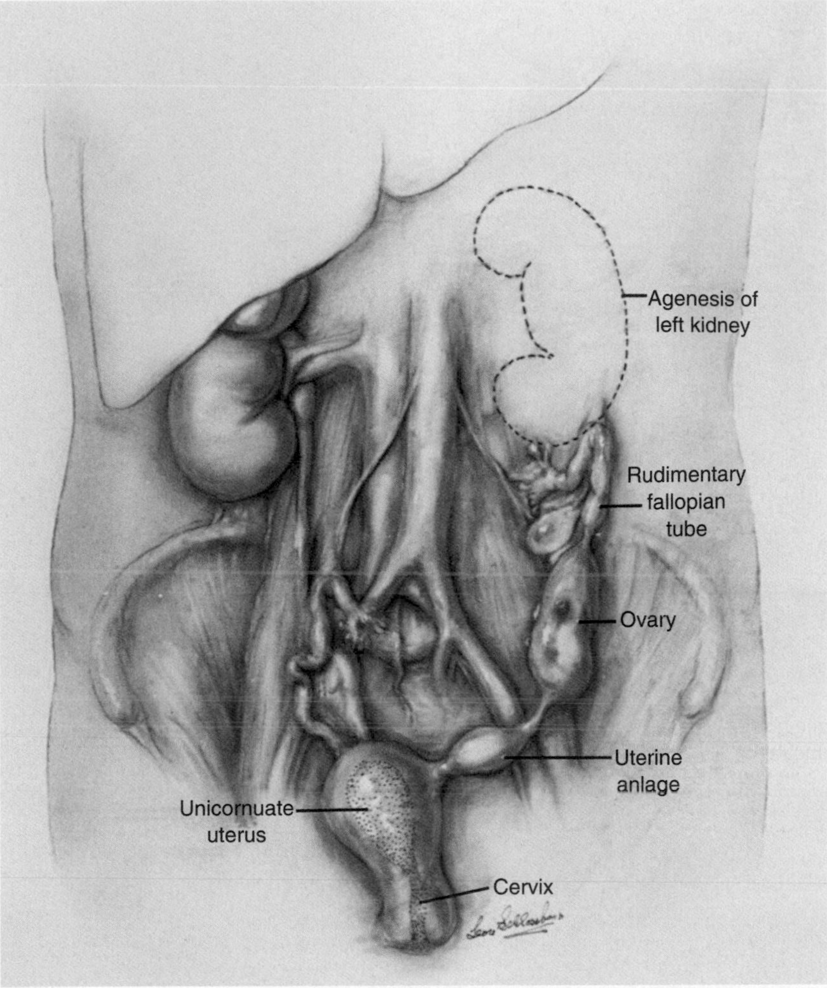

FIGURE 25.22. A unicornuate uterus associated with ovarian malposition on the left. Note that the ovary and the tube are slightly above the pelvic brim. In this instance, the ovary measured 6 inches long.

perform cerclage as indicated. Andrews and Jones have suggested that removal of the rudimentary uterine horn may improve the chances of a successful pregnancy, but the experience is too small to support a definite recommendation. Cases of asymmetric development of the unicornuate uterus with an opposing rudimentary uterine horn are not amenable to unification.

Longitudinal Vaginal Septum

Failure of fusion of the lower müllerian ducts that form the vagina can result in a vagina with a longitudinal septum. The septum can be partial or complete. Young patients have difficulty using tampons. In cases of didelphic uterus with a longitudinal vaginal septum, one uterine hemicorpus is usually better developed than the other. If intercourse consistently occurs on the vaginal side connected to the uterine hemicorpus that is less well developed, then infertility or repeated abortion could result. For these reasons, the septum should be removed (when the patient is not pregnant) unless there is a contraindication. This can usually be accomplished easily with reasonable precautions against injury to the urethra, bladder, and rectum.

Haddad and colleagues reported their experience over a 24-year period with management of the longitudinal vaginal septum. The retrospective review of 202 patient charts described a complete septum (extending from cervix to introitus) in 45.6% of patients, high partial in 36.1%, and a medium or low partial, involving only the distal vagina, in 18.3%. Uterine malformations were noted in 87.8% of cases. The frequency of uterine malformations was 99.4% in cases of complete or partial high septum and 30.3% in cases of partial medium or low septum. The most common malformation was class VA complete septate uterus in 59.5% of malformations, followed by class III didelphys uterus (24.3%) and class VB partial septate uterus (15%). Section or resection was performed in 201 cases. Bladder injury in one patient was the only reported complication. As highlighted by the high prevalence of associated uterine malformations in this review, management should always include an assessment of uterine anatomy.

Asymmetric Obstruction of the Uterus or Vagina

Unicornuate Uterus and Noncommunicating Uterine Anlagen Containing Functional Endometrium

If one müllerian duct develops normally while the opposite müllerian duct fails to develop or develops incompletely, then a relatively normal unicornuate uterus is found on one side and the cervix, musculature, uterine cavity, endometrium, fallopian tube, blood supply, and ligamentous attachments are

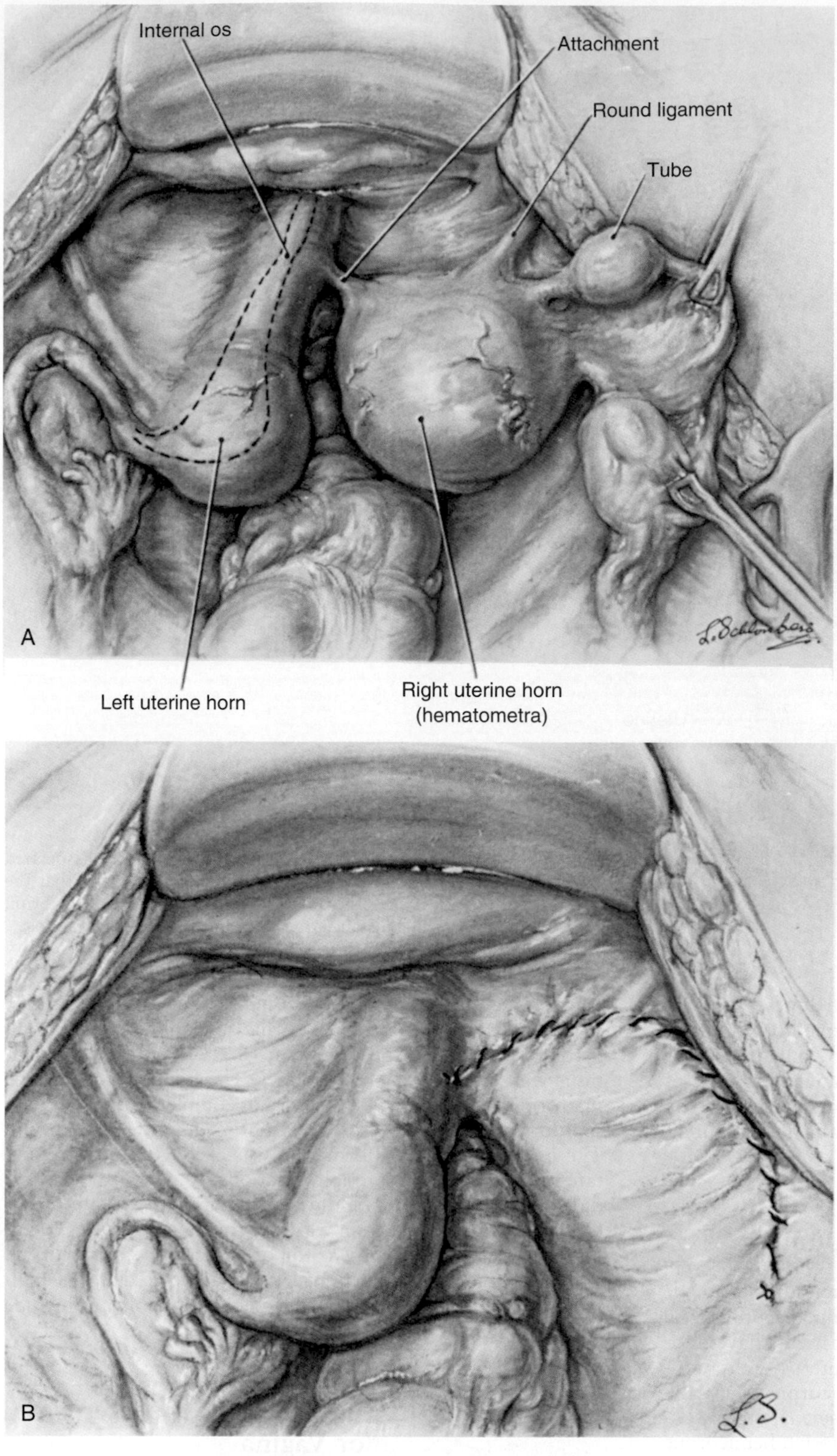

FIGURE 25.23. **A:** A noncommunicating rudimentary horn with functional endometrium that contains menstrual blood under pressure. Note the congenital abnormality of the fallopian tube, which prevented retrograde menstruation. **B:** The same patient after excision of the rudimentary horn.

absent or hypoplastic to a varying degree on the other side. Obstruction to menstruation can also occur to varying degrees on the improperly developed side. For example, if a rudimentary uterine horn does not communicate externally but does have an endometrium-lined uterine cavity, then clear symptoms of obstructed menstruation may begin soon after menarche, and severe dysmenorrhea will be present. Cryptomenorrhea can be overlooked as the diagnosis because there is cyclic menstruation from the opposite side. It is important to make the diagnosis as soon as possible, because if the lumen of the tube communicates with the endometrial cavity of the rudimentary uterus, then retrograde menstruation and pelvic endometriosis will develop, and reproductive potential can be destroyed. During the operation illustrated in Figure 25.23, which was performed to remove an obstructed rudimentary uterine horn, the fallopian tube was obstructed, and retrograde menstruation was impossible. Occasionally, the fallopian tube connected to the rudimentary uterine horn may not be patent because of incomplete development. Multiple case reports regarding the laparoscopic resection of obstructed uterine anlagen have supported the use of multiple techniques (stapling, bipolar or monopolar cautery, and the harmonic scalpel). Fedele and colleagues reported a series of 10 patients who have done well; however, the follow-up was only reported out to 6 months postprocedure. The authors strongly recommend the removal of the associated fallopian tube to minimize the risk of an ectopic pregnancy.

Unilateral Obstruction of a Cavity of a Double Uterus

Another example of a rare obstructed lateral fusion problem is the complete septum between two uterine cavities illustrated in Figure 25.24. One cavity communicated with a cervix and the other did not. This could represent an example of unilateral failure of cervical development. The patient reported incapacitating dysmenorrhea that appeared shortly after the menarche and lasted 5 days. A tense, cystic mass was palpable in the right half of the pelvis. The operation, described originally by Jones in the second edition of this book, consisted of making an incision through the anterior wall of the cystic right portion of the uterus. It was found to contain old menstrual blood. The entire septum was excised, and the uterus was reconstructed by anastomosis of the two cavities. A continuous lockstitch was reinforced by interrupted myometrial sutures, and the plastic reconstruction of the uterus was completed by a third layer of interrupted sutures uniting myometrium and serosa. Steinkampf and colleagues reported a similar case in a 17-year-old girl with progressive pelvic pain. The authors described an accessory noncommunicating uterine cavity, which they treated by excision at laparotomy.

Sanders and colleagues described several cases in which the role of interventional radiology was crucial in the management of obstructive anomalies. The report described the drainage of a noncommunicating right uterine cavity distended with blood in a unicornuate uterus in a 14-year-old patient. Adequate access was established by using ultrasound-guided

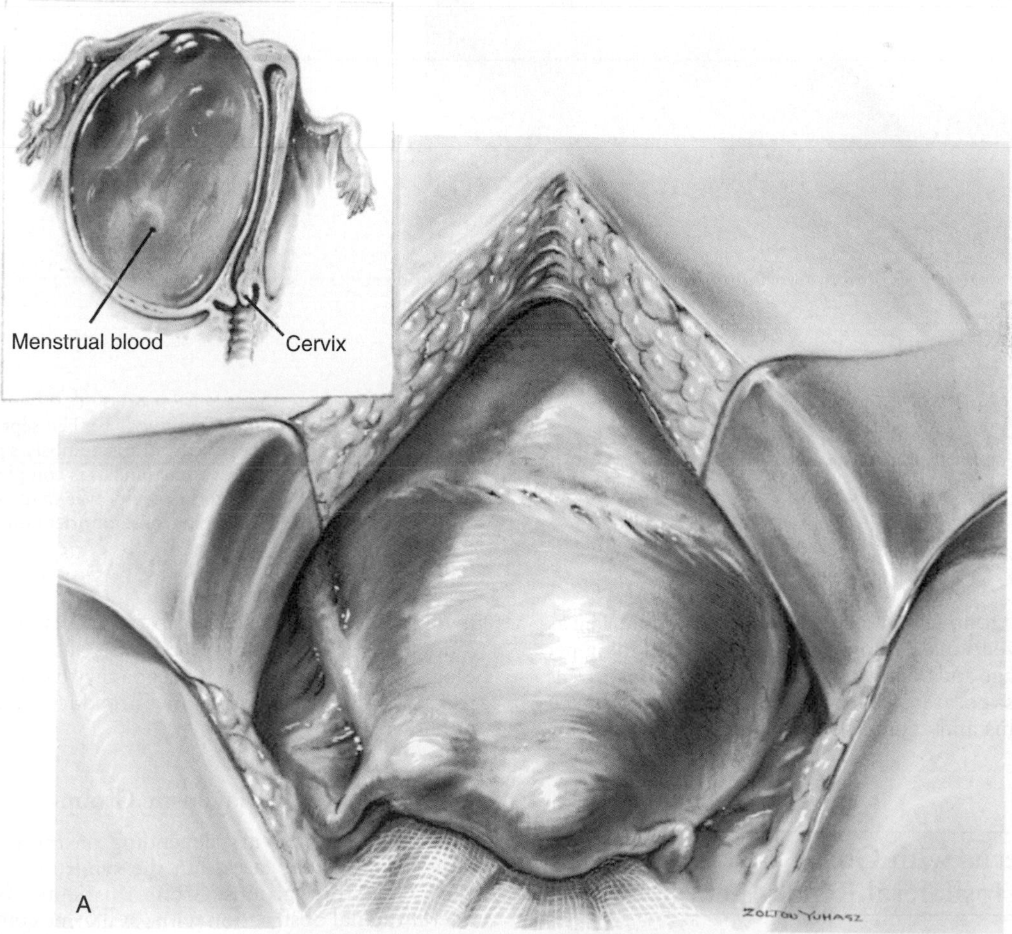

FIGURE 25.24. A: A double uterus seen at operation. Hematometra in the right uterine cavity (*inset*), which does not communicate with the other cavity or the cervical canal.

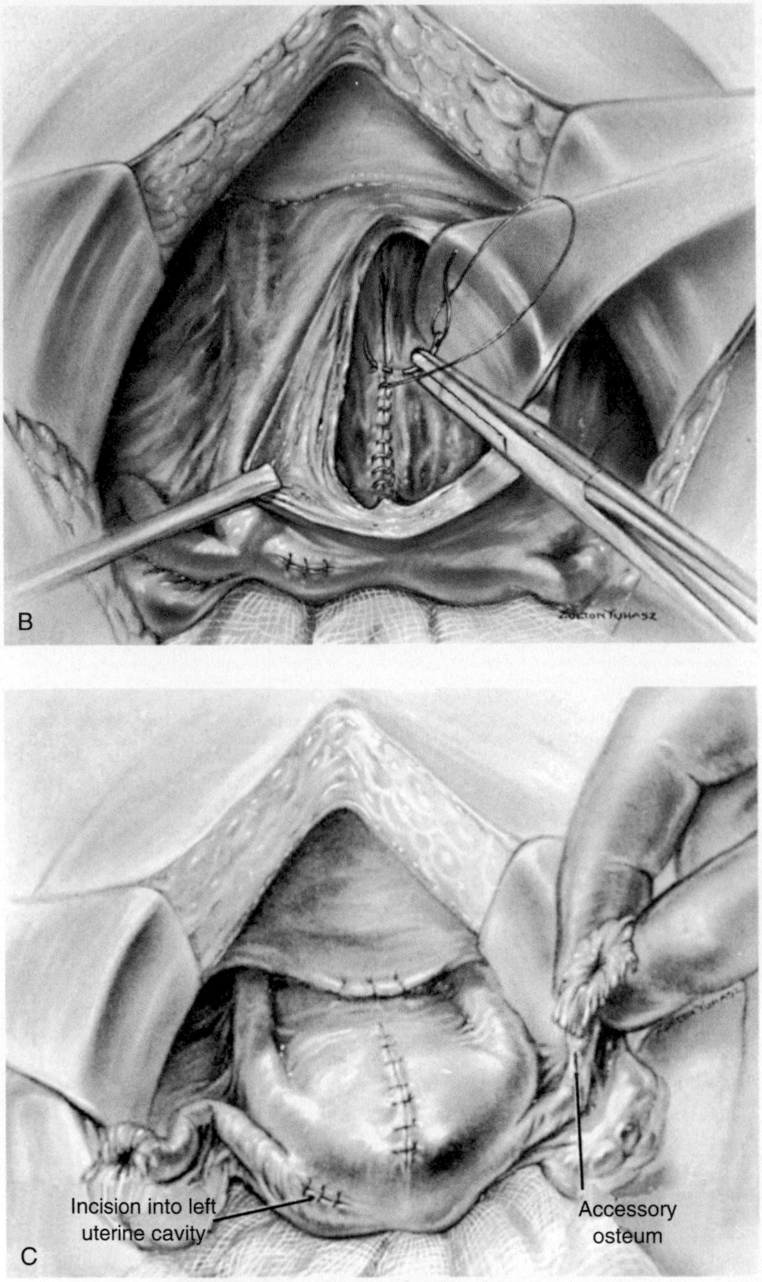

FIGURE 25.24. (*Continued*) **B:** The septum of the double uterus has been excised and anastomosis is performed to unite the two cavities. **C:** Anastomosis is completed. The small incision in the left uterine cavity was made before the septum was removed for the purpose of orientation.

needle aspiration followed by a hysteroscopic excision. The assistance of interventional radiologic procedures, including percutaneous drainage and dilatation of small maldeveloped areas, may allow access to areas otherwise inaccessible by conventional mechanisms and assist in preserving reproductive function.

Double Uterus with Obstructed Hemivagina and Ipsilateral Renal Agenesis

The unique clinical syndrome consisting of a double uterus, obstruction of the vagina (unilateral, partial, or complete), and ipsilateral renal agenesis is rare. The renal agenesis (mesonephric involution) on the side of the obstructed vagina associated with a double uterus and double cervix is suggestive of an embryologic arrest at 8 weeks of pregnancy that simultaneously affects the müllerian and metanephric ducts. The exact cause is unknown.

Diagnostic Groups

Clinical symptoms vary depending on the uterovaginal relations in individual cases, but the syndrome can be described generally in three groups. Group 1 patients have complete unilateral vaginal obstruction without uterine communication, resulting in a paravaginal mass and symptoms of severe dysmenorrhea and lower abdominal pain. Menses are regular. Group 2 patients have an incomplete unilateral vaginal obstruction

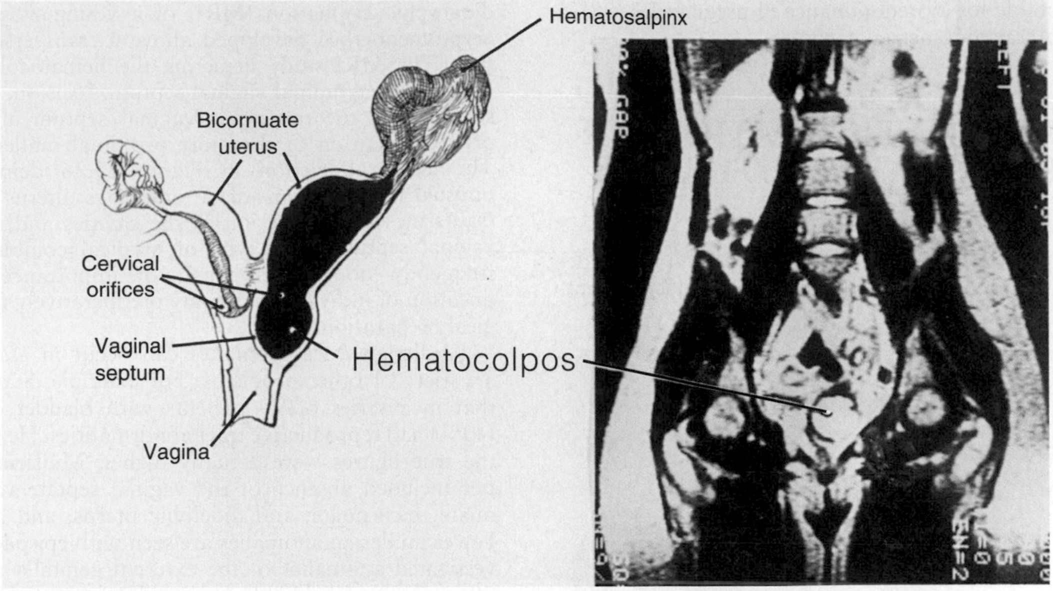

FIGURE 25.25. A double uterus with unilateral complete vaginal obstruction and ipsilateral renal agenesis. Magnetic resonance imaging reveals the left hematocolpos, both uteri, and absence of the left kidney on the side of the vaginal obstruction.

without uterine communication. The presenting symptoms are lower abdominal pain, severe dysmenorrhea, excessive foul mucopurulent discharge, and, in some instances, intermenstrual bleeding. Group 3 patients have complete vaginal obstruction with a laterally communicating double uterus. They have a paravaginal mass, lower abdominal pain, and dysmenorrhea. Menses are regular. A 10-year review of patients with this anomaly was published by Phupong and colleagues. Most patients presented with dysmenorrhea (73%) or a pelvic or paravaginal mass (71%). The right uterus and vagina were affected in 63.5% of patients.

Because menses in patients with this syndrome are rarely irregular, the possibility of this syndrome as a diagnosis can easily be overlooked. A careful pelvic examination is necessary to make the correct diagnosis. MRI can identify the obstructed vagina, double uterus, and absence of a kidney on the side of the obstruction (Fig. 25.25), but it may not be helpful if there is incomplete vaginal obstruction or a uterine communication.

Complete unilateral vaginal obstruction (group 1) can go unrecognized for a number of years after the onset of menses. The vagina is quite distensible and can accommodate a large amount of accumulated blood in the obstructed side. There is sufficient absorption of menstrual blood between periods so that each subsequent flow can add to the increments of accumulated blood without pain. Nevertheless, once retrograde menstruation occurs, endometriosis invariably is the result.

Surgical Treatment

Careful excision of the vaginal septum is the treatment of choice for a unilateral vaginal obstruction. Prophylactic antibiotics should be administered before surgery. After opening the vaginal pouch, the surgeon should use suction and lavage to remove the pooled blood and mucus. Phupong and colleagues' review also confirms the successful use of this primary therapy in 84.3% of patients. Haddad and colleagues reported a similar experience in a report describing patient management over a 27-year period. Excision of the vaginal septum was successful in 88% of patients, with complete excision in one procedure in 92% of those patients. In cases of pyocolpos or hematocolpos, distention and stretching of the septal tissue may increase the risk of inadequate resection and possible postoperative stenosis; the authors found the use of a two-step graduated resection advantageous to ensure adequate resection. A limited resection (3 cm) was performed to allow adequate drainage, followed by a return to the operating room in approximately 1 month to remove any remaining septum.

Because the obstructing septum is usually thick, removal can be difficult. Clamps should be used to isolate a generous vaginal pedicle while the suture is being tied in place to prevent slippage of tissue. Such pedicles generally retract during healing, and formation of a vaginal stenosis is avoided. In most instances, surgery is restricted to excision of the septum, and abdominal exploration is unnecessary. Uterine reconstruction is not indicated for cases of lateral communication of the uterine horns. Some authors have reported the use of hemihysterectomy in patients with a high, thick-walled obstruction, massive ovarian involvement, endometriosis, or adenomyosis; however, this is generally not recommended in young patients.

Reproductive Performance

Reproductive performance for patients with this disorder is usually consistent with that of patients with a double uterus unless the delay in diagnosis and resection of the obstructing septum has been sufficient to destroy tubal function or to cause the development of endometriosis. Haddad and colleagues' review was notable for a predominance of pregnancies (80%) in the contralateral endometrial cavity.

UNUSUAL CONFIGURATIONS OF VERTICAL-LATERAL FUSION DEFECTS

Unusual configurations of both vertical and lateral fusion defects may occur simultaneously. Figure 25.26 depicts the radiographic evaluation (MRI) of a young woman in whom cryptomenorrhea developed above a transverse vaginal septum. The MRI study depicting the hematocolpos also suggests the longitudinal vaginal septum. Incision, drainage, and resection of the transverse vaginal septum allowed appropriate evaluation of the more proximal müllerian anatomy. The artist's depiction in Figure 25.26 demonstrates the unusual constellation of a didelphys uterus with an intrauterine communication of the cavities and a longitudinal vaginal septum. This type of atypical combination occurs frequently enough to emphasize the importance of proper delineation of individual anatomy preoperatively for proper surgical preparation.

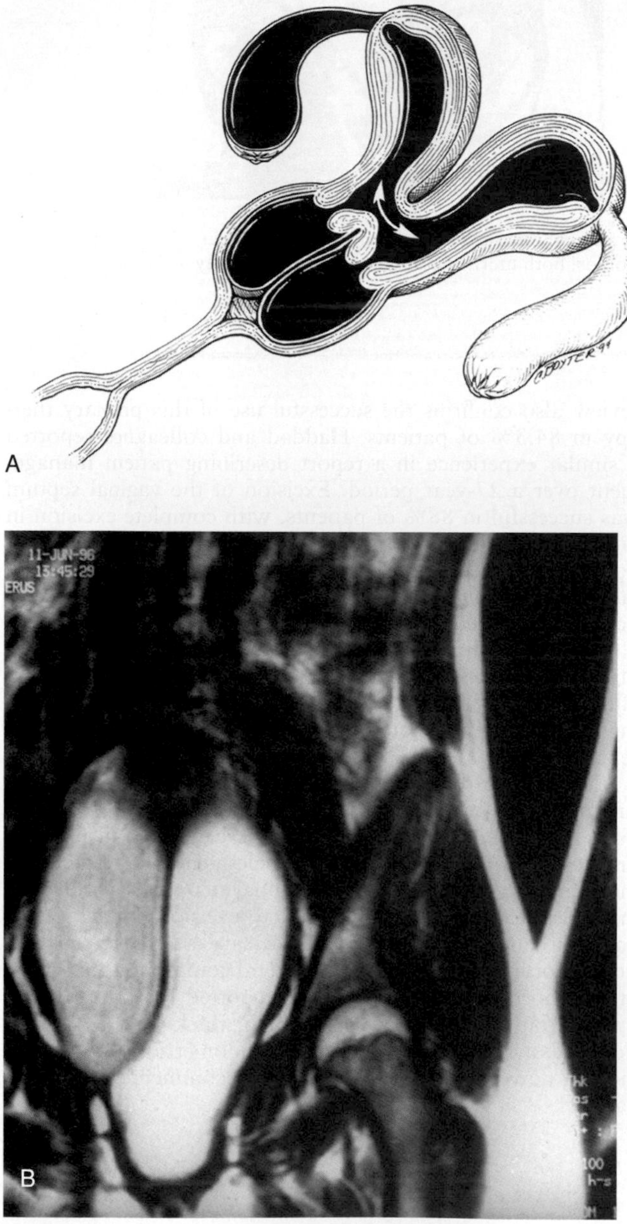

FIGURE 25.26. An unusual combination of both vertical and lateral fusion defects. A: A didelphys uterus with an intrauterine communication and a longitudinal vaginal septum are present proximal to a transverse vaginal septum. B: The magnetic resonance image demonstrates the presence of both septa.

Müllerian duct anomalies can occur in association with a variety of other problems. For example, Stanton reported that in a series of 70 patients with bladder exstrophy, 30 (43%) had reproductive tract abnormalities. He suggested that the true figures were actually higher. Müllerian abnormalities included absence of the vagina; septate vagina; unicornuate, bicornuate, and didelphic uterus; and absent uterus. Fewer müllerian anomalies are seen with epispadias. Jones investigated anomalies of the external genitalia and vagina in 30 patients with bladder exstrophy seen at the Johns Hopkins Hospital and suggested operative techniques for correction of these anomalies. Techniques for the management of other gynecologic and obstetric problems (especially uterine prolapse) also have been discussed by Weed and McKee and by Blakeley and Mills. A number of other rare combinations of congenital malformations of the vagina and perineum have been found in association with uterine anomalies. Their surgical correction, especially in children, is reported by Hendren and Donahoe and by others. Several authors have considered the uterovaginal anomalies that occur in association with multiple other gastrointestinal and genitourinary abnormalities. Goh and colleagues described an infant girl with complete duplication of the bladder, urethra, uterus, and vagina associated with a urogenital sinus and an anterior ectopic anus. Gastol and colleagues and Magalhaes and associates also described children with complete duplication of the bladder, urethra, vagina, and uterus. These complex anomalies include significantly more defects than lateral fusion concerns in the müllerian ducts. These cases emphasize the variable anatomy in this rare group of anomalies and that a substantial effort should be placed on defining anatomy before surgical exploration and management. Sheldon and colleagues reviewed 13 consecutive cases of vaginal reconstruction in pediatric patients with multisystem anomalies. The review emphasized several important principles involved in the surgical management: (i) all anticipated perineal reconstruction should be performed in a single stage, (ii) urethral catheterization has an important role, (iii) urinary reconstruction is often intimately involved in the vaginal reconstruction, (iv) avoidance of overlapping suture lines is essential for optimal healing, (v) maximum growth potential of the neovagina should be considered, and (vi) meticulous follow-up of proper routine dilatation of the neovagina should be expected. Coordinated reconstruction of all organ systems is especially important in these complex cases.

Müllerian duct anomalies are seen with the McKusick-Kaufman syndrome, an autosomal recessive disorder. Other clinical findings reported with this syndrome include hydrometrocolpos, postaxial polydactyly, syndactyly, congenital heart disease, intravaginal displacement of the urethral meatus, and anorectal anomalies. In 1982, Jabs and colleagues added an unusual case to the few cases previously reported in the literature.

Müllerian duct anomalies may also affect the development of the fallopian tube. Although extremely rare, episodes of unilateral or bilateral absence of the fallopian tube have been reported. Of the less than 10 cases in the literature, Eustace reported two of the described cases. He hypothesized that compromise of the local blood supply to the caudal aspect of the müllerian duct was a more likely cause than a fusion disorder. This situation could affect fallopian tube development to a variable extent with even some effect on ovarian development.

BEST SURGICAL PRACTICES

- Vaginal dilatation should be the first line of treatment for creation of a neovagina in patients with müllerian agenesis.
- The gynecologic literature continues to support the role of the McIndoe vaginolasty as a safe and effective procedure for surgical creation of a neovagina, when necessary.
- Appropriate preoperative evaluation of reproductive and pelvic anatomy remains a critical step before a patient is taken to the operating room for treatment of any müllerian anomaly.
- In patients with müllerian agenesis, removal of uterine anlagen that contain endometrium and have the potential to cause obstruction and subsequent pelvic pain should be strongly considered.
- Hysteroscopic metroplasty is a successful, minimally invasive technique for removal of a uterine septum.
- Resection of a uterine septum has been shown to improve pregnancy success in patients with a history of recurrent pregnancy loss.
- Strassman metroplasty should be considered in select women with a bicornate uterus who have experienced recurrent pregnancy loss or preterm delivery.

Bibliography

Abbe R. New method of creating a vagina in a case of congenital absence. *Med Rec* 1898;54:836.

Adamyan LV. Laparoscopic management of vaginal aplasia with or without functional noncommunicating rudimentary uterus. In: Arrequi ME, Fitzgibbons RJ, Katkhouda N, et al., eds. *Principles of laparoscopic surgery*. New York: Springer-Verlag; 1995: 646.

Adamyan LV, Maurvatov KD, Sorour YA, et al. Medicogenetic features and surgical treatment of patients with congenital malformations of the uterus and vagina. *Int J Fertil* 1996;41:293.

Alessandrescu D, Peltecu GC, Buhimschi CS, et al. Neocolpopoiesis with split-thickness skin graft as a surgical treatment of vaginal agenesis: retrospective review of 201 cases. *Am J Obstet Gynecol* 1996;175:131.

American Fertility Society classification of müllerian anomalies. *Fertil Steril* 1988;49:952.

Andrews MC, Jones HW. Impaired reproductive performance of the unicornuate uterus: intrauterine growth retardation, infertility, and recurrent abortion in five cases. *Am J Obstet Gynecol* 1982;144:173.

Baldwin A. Formation of an artificial vagina by intestinal transplantation. *Am J Obstet Gynecol* 1907;56:636.

Baldwin JF. The formation of an artificial vagina by intestinal transplantation. *Ann Surg* 1984;40:398.

Beski S, Gorgy A, Venkat G, et al. Gestational surrogacy: a feasible option for patients with Rokitansky syndrome. *Hum Reprod* 2000;15:2326.

Blakeley CR, Mills WG. The obstetric and gynaecological complications of bladder exstrophy and epispadias. *BJOG* 1981;88:167.

Borruto F. Mayer-Rokitansky-Küster syndrome: Vecchietti's personal series. *Clin Exp Obstet Gynecol* 1992;19:273.

Brenner P, Sedlis A, Cooperman H. Complete imperforate transverse vaginal septum. *Obstet Gynecol* 1965;25:135.

Broadbent TR, Woolf RM. Congenital absence of the vagina: reconstruction without operation. *Br J Plast Surg* 1977;30:118.

Bugamann P, Amaudruz M, Hanquinet S, et al. Uterocervicoplasty with a bladder mucosa layer for treatment of complete cervical agenesis. *Fertil Steril* 2002;77;831.

Busacca M, Perino A, Venezia R. Laparoscopic-ultrasonographic combined technique for the creation of a neovagina in Mayer-Rokitansky-Küster-Hauser syndrome. *Fertil Steril* 1996;66:1039.

Buttram VC Jr. Müllerian anomalies and their management. *Fertil Steril* 1983;40:159.

Buttram VC Jr, Gibbons WE. Müllerian anomalies: a proposed classification (an analysis of 144 cases). *Fertil Steril* 1979;32:40.

Capraro VJ, Chuang JT, Randall CL. Improved fetal salvage after metroplasty. *Obstet Gynecol* 1968;29:97.

Capraro VJ, Gallego MB. Vaginal agenesis. *Am J Obstet Gynecol* 1976;124:98.

Chakravarty BN. Congenital absence of the vagina and uterus—simultaneous vaginoplasty and hysteroplasty. *J Obstet Gynecol India* 1977;27: 627.

Chakravarty BN, Gun KM, Sarkar K. Congenital absence of vagina: anatomico-physiological consideration. *J Obstet Gynecol India* 1977;27:621.

Chen YT, Cheng T, Lin H, et al. Spatial W-plasty full thickness skin graft for neovaginal reconstruction. *Plast Reconstr Surg* 1994;94:727.

Chervenak FA, Neuwirth RS. Hysteroscopic resection of the uterine septum. *Am J Obstet Gynecol* 1981;141:351.

Communal PH, Chevret-Measson M, Golfier F, et al. Sexuality after sigmoid colpopoiesis in patients with Mayer-Rokitansky-Kuster-Hauser syndrome. *Fertil Steril* 2003;80:600.

Counseller VS. Congenital absence of the vagina. *JAMA* 1948;136:861.

Counseller VS, Davis CE. Atresia of the vagina. *Obstet Gynecol* 1968;32:528.

Counseller VS, Flor FS. Congenital absence of the vagina. *Surg Clin North Am* 1957;37:1107.

Creatsas GC. Creatsas modification of Williams vaginoplasty. *J Gynecol Surg* 1991;7:219.

Creatsas G, Deligeoroglou E, Makrakis E, et al. Creation of a neovagina following vaginoplasty and the Creatsas modification in 111 patients with Mayer-Rokitansky-Küster-Hauser syndrome. *Fertil Steril* 2001;76:1036.

Creighton SM, Davies MC, Cutner A. Laparoscopic management of cervical agenesis. *Fertil Steril* 2006;85:1510.

Cukier J, Batzofin JH, Conners JS, et al. Genital tract reconstruction in a patient with congenital absence of a vagina and hypoplasia of the cervix. *Obstet Gynecol* 1986;68:325.

Dabirashrafi H, Bahadori M, Mohammad K, et al. Septate uterus: new idea on the histologic features of the septum in the abnormal uterus. *Am J Obstet Gynecol* 1995;172:105.

Daly DC, Tohan N, Walters C, et al. Hysteroscopic resection of the uterine septum in the presence of a septate cervix. *Fertil Steril* 1983;39:560.

Daly DC, Walters CA, Soto-Albors CE, et al. Hysteroscopic metroplasty: surgical technique and obstetrical outcome. *Fertil Steril* 1983;39:623.

David A, Carvil D, Bar-David E, et al. Congenital absence of the vagina: clinical and psychological aspects. *Obstet Gynecol* 1975;46:407.

Davydov SN. Colpopoiesis from the peritoneum of the uterorectal space. In: *Proceedings of the Ninth World Congress of Obstetrics and Gynecology, Tokyo, 1979*. Amsterdam: Excerpta Medica, 1980: 793.

DeCherney A, Polan ML. Hysteroscopic management of intrauterine lesions and intractable uterine bleeding. *Obstet Gynecol* 1983;61:392.

DeCherney AH, Russell JB, Graebe RA, et al. Resectoscopic management of müllerian fusion defects. *Fertil Steril* 1986;45:726.

Deffarges JV, Haddad B, Musset R, et al. Utero-vaginal anastomosis in women with uterine cervix atresia: long term follow-up and reproductive performance. A study of 18 cases. *Hum Reprod* 2001;16:1722.

Deligeoroglou E, Makrakis E, Papagianni V. The Creatsas modification of Williams vaginoplasty. *J Gynecol Surg* 2003;19:121.

Dietrich JE, Young AE, Young RL. Resection of a non-communicating uterine horn with the use of the harmoni scalpel. *J Pediatr Adolesc Gynecol* 2004;17:407.

Dillon WP, Mudaliar NA, Wingate NB. Congenital atresia of the cervix. *Obstet Gynecol* 1979;54:126.

Dunn R, Hantes J. Double cervix and vagina with a normal uterus and blind cervical pouch: a rare mullerian anomaly. *Fertil Steril* 2004;82:458.

Engmann L, Schmidt D, Nulsen J, et al. An usual anatomic variation of a unicornuate uterus with normal external uterine morphology. *Fertil Steril* 2004;82:950.

Eustace DL. Congenital absence of fallopian tube and ovary. *Eur J Obstet Gynecol Reprod Biol* 1992;46:157.

Evans TN. The artificial vagina. *Am J Obstet Gynecol* 1967;99:944.

Evans TN, Poland ML, Boving RL. Vaginal malformations. *Am J Obstet Gynecol* 1981;141:910.

Farber M, Marchant DJ. Reconstructive surgery for congenital atresia of the uterine cervix. *Fertil Steril* 1976;27:1277.
Farber M, Mitchell GW. Bicornuate uterus and partial atresia of the fallopian tube. *Am J Obstet Gynecol* 1979;134:881.
Farber M, Mitchell GW. Surgery for congenital anomalies of müllerian ducts. *Contemp Obstet Gynecol* 1977;9:63.
Farber M, Mitchell GW. Surgery for congenital absence of the vagina. *Obstet Gynecol* 1978;51:364.
Fayez JA. Comparison between abdominal and hysteroscopic metroplasty. *Obstet Gynecol* 1986;68:399.
Fedele L, Bianchi S, Zanconato G, et al. Laparoscopic creation of a neovagina in patients with Rokitansky syndrome: analysis of 52 cases. *Fertil Steril* 2000;74:384.
Fedele L, Bianchi S, Zanconato G, et al. Laparoscopic removal of the cavitated noncommunicating rudimentary uterine horn: surgical aspects in 10 cases. *Fertil Steril* 2005;83:432.
Fedele L, Borruto F, Bianchi S, et al. A new laparoscopic procedure for creation of a neovagina in Mayer-Rokitansky-Küster-Hauser syndrome. *Fertil Steril* 1996;66:854.
Fedele L, Doeta M, Vercellini P, et al. Ultrasound in the diagnosis of subclasses of unicornuate uterus. *Obstet Gynecol* 1988;71:274.
Feroze RM, Dewhurst CJ, Welply G. Vaginoplasty at the Chelsea Hospital for women: a comparison of two techniques. *BJOG* 1975;82:536.
Fore SR, Hammond CB, Parker RT, et al. Urologic and genital anomalies in patients with congenital absence of the vagina. *Obstet Gynecol* 1975;46:410.
Frank RT. The formation of an artificial vagina without operation. *Am J Obstet Gynecol* 1938;35:1053.
Frank RT. The formation of an artificial vagina without operation. *N Y State J Med* 1940;40:1669.
Frank RT, Geist SH. The formation of an artificial vagina by a new plastic technic. *Am J Obstet Gynecol* 1927;14:712.
Gallup DG, Castle CA, Stock RJ. Recurrent carcinoma in situ of the vagina following split thickness skin graft vaginoplasty. *Gynecol Oncol* 1987;26:98.
Garcia J, Jones HW. The split thickness graft technic for vaginal agenesis. *Obstet Gynecol* 1977;49:328.
Garcia RF. Z-plasty for correction of congenital transverse vaginal septum. *Am J Obstet Gynecol* 1967;99:1164.
Gastol P, Baka-Jakubiak L, Skobejko-Wlodarska L, et al. Complete duplication of the bladder, urethra, vagina, and uterus in girls. *Urology* 2000;55:578.
Gauwerky JFH, Wallwiener D, Bastert G. An endoscopically assisted technique for reconstruction of a neovagina. *Arch Gynecol Obstet* 1992;252:59.
Geary WL, Weed JC. Congenital atresia of the uterine cervix. *Obstet Gynecol* 1973;42:213.
Genest D, Farber M, Mitchell GW, et al. Partial vaginal agenesis with a urinary-vaginal fistula. *Obstet Gynecol* 1981;58:130.
Giannesi A, Marchiole P, Benchaib M, et al. Sexuality after laparoscopic Davydov in patients affected by congenital vaginal agenesis associated with uterine agenesis or hypoplasia. *Hum Reprod* 2005;20:2954.
Goh DW, Davey RB, Dewan PA. Bladder, urethral, and vaginal duplication. *J Pediatr Surg* 1995;30:125.
Goodman FR, Bacchelli C, Brady AF, et al. Novel HOXA13 mutations and the phenotypic spectrum of hand-foot-genital syndrome. *Am J Hum Genet* 2000;67:197.
Goodman FR, Scambler PJ. Human HOX gene mutations. *Clin Genet* 2001;59:1.
Graves WP. Method of constructing an artificial vagina. *Surg Clin North Am* 1921;1:611.
Griffin JE, Edwards C, Madden JD, et al. Congenital absence of the vagina. *Ann Intern Med* 1976;85:224.
Haddad B, Barranger E, Paniel BJ. Blind hemivagina: long-term follow-up and reproductive performance in 42 cases. *Hum Reprod* 1999;14:1962.
Haddad B, Louis-Sylvestre C, Poitout P, et al. Longitudinal vaginal septum: a retrospective study of 202 cases. *Eur J Obstet Gynecol Reprod Biol* 1997;74:197.
Haney AF, Hammond CB, Soules MR, et al. Diethylstilbestrol-induced upper genital tract abnormalities. *Fertil Steril* 1979;29:142.
Hauser GA, Keller M, Koller T. Das Rokitansky-Küster Syndrom. Uterus bipartitus solidus rudimentarius cum vagina solida. *Gynecologia* 1961;151:111.
Hauser GA, Schreiner WE. Das Mayer-Rokitansky-Küster Syndrom. *Schweiz Med Wochenschr* 1961;91:381.
Heinonen PK. Longitudinal vaginal septum. *Eur J Obstet Gynecol Reprod Biol* 1982;13:253.
Heinonen PK, Pystynen PP. Primary infertility and uterine anomalies. *Fertil Steril* 1983;40:291.
Heinonen PK, Saarikoski S, Pystynen P. Reproductive performance of women with uterine anomalies. *Acta Obstet Gynecol Scand* 1982;61:157.
Hendren WH, Donahoe PK. Correction of congenital abnormalities of the vagina and perineum. *J Pediatr Surg* 1980;15:751.
Hensle TW, Shabsigh A, Shabsigh R, et al. Sexual function following bowel vaginoplasty. *J Urol* 2006;175:2283.
Hickok LR. Hysteroscopic treatment of the uterine septum: a clinician's experience. *Am J Obstet Gynecol* 2000;182:1414.
Höckel M, Menke H, Germann G. Vaginolasty with split skin grafts from the scalp: optimization of the surgical treatment for vaginal agenesis. *Am J Obstet Gynecol* 2003;188:1100.
Hojsgaard A, Villadsen I. McIndoe procedure for congenital vaginal agenesis: complications and results. *Br J Plast Surg* 1995;48:97.
Holden R, Hart P. First-trimester rudimentary horn pregnancy: prerupture ultrasound diagnosis. *Obstet Gynecol* 1983;61[Suppl]:56.
Homer HA, Li T, Cooke ID. The septate uterus: a review of management and reproductive outcome. *Fertil Steril* 2000;73:1.
Hucke J, Pelzer V, Bruyne FD, et al. Laparoscopic modification of the Vecchietti-operation for creation of a neovagina. *J Pelvic Surg* 1995;1:191.
Hundley AF, Fielding JR, Hoyte L. Double cervix and vagina with septate uterus: an uncommon müllerian malformation. *Obstet Gynecol* 2001;98:982.
Hurst BS, Rock JA. Preoperative dilatation to facilitate repair of high transverse vaginal septum. *Fertil Steril* 1992;57:1351.
Ingram JM. The bicycle seat stool in the treatment of vaginal agenesis and stenosis: a preliminary report. *Am J Obstet Gynecol* 1981;140:867.
Israel R, March CM. Hysteroscopic incision of the septate uterus. *Am J Obstet Gynecol* 1984;149:66.
Jabs EW, Leonard CO, Phillips JA. New features of the McKusick-Kaufman syndrome. *Birth Defects* 1982;18:161.
Jacob JH, Griffin WT. Surgical reconstruction of congenital atresia of the cervix. *Am J Obstet Gynecol* 1961;82:923.
Jacobsen LJ, DeCherney A. Shall we operate on Müllerian defects? Results of conventional and hysteroscopic surgery. *Fertil Steril* 2000;73:1376.
Jeffcoate TNA. Advancement of the upper vagina in the treatment of haematocolpos and haematometra caused by vaginal aplasia: pregnancy following the construction of an artificial vagina. *J Obstet Gynaecol Br Comm* 1969;76:961.
Jewelewicz R, Husami N, Wallach EE. When uterine factors cause infertility. *Contemp Obstet Gynecol* 1980;16:95.
Jones HW. An anomaly of the external genitalia in female patients with exstrophy of the bladder. *Am J Obstet Gynecol* 1973;117:748.
Jones HW. Reproductive impairment and the malformed uterus. *Fertil Steril* 1981;36:137.
Jones HW, Delfs E, Jones GE. Reproductive difficulties in double uterus: the place of plastic reconstruction. *Am J Obstet Gynecol* 1956;72:865.
Jones HW, Jones GE. Double uterus as an etiological factor in repeated abortion: indications for surgical repair. *Am J Obstet Gynecol* 1953;65:325.
Jones HW, Mermut S. Familial occurrence of congenital absence of the vagina. *Am J Obstet Gynecol* 1972;114:1100.
Jones HW, Rock JA. *Reparative and constructive surgery of the female generative tract*. Baltimore: Williams & Wilkins, 1983.
Jones HW, Wheeless CR. Salvage of the reproductive potential of women with anomalous development of the müllerian ducts: 1868–1968–2068. *Am J Obstet Gynecol* 1969;104:348.
Jones TB, Fleischer AC, Daniell JF, et al. Sonographic characteristics of congenital uterine abnormalities and associated pregnancy. *J Clin Ultrasound* 1980;8:435.
Jones WS. Obstetric significance of female genital anomalies. *Obstet Gynecol* 1957;10:113.
Karjalainen O, Myllynenl O, Kajanoja P, et al. Management of vaginal agenesis. *Ann Chir Gynaecol* 1980;69:37.
Kaufman RH, Binder GL, Gray PM, et al. Upper genital tract changes associated with exposure in utero to diethylstilbestrol. *Am J Obstet Gynecol* 1977;128:51.
Knab DR. *Müllerian agenesis: a review*. Bethesda, MD: Department of Gynecology/Obstetrics, Uniformed Services University School of Medicine and Naval Hospital, 1983.
Kuster H. Uterus bipartitus solidus rudimentarius cum vagina solida. *Z Geb Gyn* 1910;67:692.
Kusuda M. Infertility and metroplasty. *Acta Obstet Gynecol Scand* 1982;61:407.
Laffarque F, Giacalone PL, Boulot P, et al. A laparoscopic procedure for the treatment of vaginal aplasia. *BJOG* 1995;102:565.
Lawrence A. Vaginal neoplasia in a male-to-female transsexual: Case report, review of the literature, and recommendations for cytological screening. *The International Journal of Transgenderism* 2001;5(1):1721.
Lees DH, Singer A. Vaginal surgery for congenital abnormalities and acquired constructions. *Clin Obstet Gynecol* 1982;25:883.
Letterie GS. Combined congenital absence of the vagina and cervix. *Gynecol Obstet Invest* 1998;46:65.
Litta P, Pozzan C, Merlin F, et al. Hysreoscopic metroplasty under laparoscopic guidance in infertile women with septate uteri. *J Reprod Med* 2004;49:274.
Lodi A. Contributo clinico statistico sulle malformazion della vagina osservate nella clinica Obstetrica e Ginecologica di Milano dal 1906 al 1950. *Ann Ostet Ginecol Med Perinat* 1951;73:1246.
Lolis DE, Paschopoulos M, Makrydimas G, et al. Reproductive outcome after Strassman metroplasty in women with a bicornuate uterus. *J Reprod Med* 2005;50:297.

Ludmir J, Samuels P, Brooks S, et al. Pregnancy outcome of patients with uncorrected uterine anomalies managed in a high risk obstetric setting. *Obstet Gynecol* 1990;75:907.

Maciulla GJ, Heine MW, Christian CD. Functional endometrial tissue with vaginal agenesis. *J Reprod Med* 1978;21:373.

Magalhaes ML, Campos LA, Souza LC, et al. A case of association of duplication of the urogenital and intestinal tracts. *J Pediatr Adolesc Gynecol* 1999;12:165.

Magrina JF, Masterson BJ. Vaginal reconstruction in gynecological oncology: a review of techniques. *Obstet Gynecol Surv* 1981;36:1.

Mahgoub SE. Unification of a septate uterus: Mahgoub's operation. *Int J Gynecol Obstet* 1978;15:400.

Makinoda S, Nishiya M, Sogame M, et al. Non-grafting method of vaginal construction for patients of vaginal agenesis without functioning uterus (Mayer-Rokitansky-Küster Syndrome). *Int Surg* 1996;81:385.

Mandell J, Stevens PS, Lucey DT. Diagnosis and management of hydrometrocolpos in infancy. *J Urol* 1978;120:262.

Markham SM, Parmley TH, Murphy AA, et al. Cervical agenesis combined with vaginal agenesis diagnosed by magnetic resonance imaging. *Fertil Steril* 1987;48:143.

Matsui H, Seki K, Sekiya S. Prolapse of the neovagina in Mayer-Rokitansky-Küster-Hauser syndrome. *J Reprod Med* 1999;44:548.

McCraw JB, Massey FM, Shanklin KD, et al. Vaginal reconstruction with gracilis myocutaneous flaps. *Plast Reconstr Surg* 1976;58:176.

McDonough PG, Tho PT. Use of pelvic pneumoperitoneum: a critical assessment of 12 years experience. *South Med J* 1974;67:517.

McIndoe AH. The treatment of congenital absence and obliterative conditions of the vagina. *Br J Plast Surg* 1950;2:254.

McIndoe AH, Banister JB. An operation for the cure of congenital absence of the vagina. *J Obstet Gynaecol Br Emp* 1938;45:490.

McKusick VA. Transverse vaginal septum (hydrometrocolpos). *Birth Defects* 1971;7:326.

McKusick VA, Bauer RL, Koop CE, et al. Hydrometrocolpos as a simply inherited malformation. *JAMA* 1964;189:119.

McKusick VA, Weilbaccher RG, Gragg GW. Recessive inheritance of a congenital malformation syndrome. *JAMA* 1968;204:111.

McShane PM, Reilly RJ, Schiff I. Pregnancy outcomes following Tompkins metroplasty. *Fertil Steril* 1983;40:190.

Mizuno K, Koike K, Ando K, et al. Significance of Jones-Jones operation on double uterus: vascularity and dating of endometrium in uterine septum. *Jpn J Fertil Steril* 1978;23:9.

Motoyama S, Laoag-Fernandez JB, Mochizuki S, et al. Vaginoplasty with Interceed absorbable adhesion barrier for complete squamous epithelialization in vaginal agenesis. *Am J Obstet Gynecol* 2003;188:1260.

Moutos DM, Damewood MD, Schlaff WD, et al. A comparison of the reproductive outcome between women with a unicornuate uterus and women with a didelphic uterus. *Fertil Steril* 1992;58:88.

Murphy AA, Krall A, Rock JA. Bilateral functioning uterine anlagen with the Rokitansky-Mayer-Küster-Hauser syndrome. *Int J Fertil* 1987;32:296.

Musich JR, Behrman SJ. Obstetric outcome before and after metroplasty in women with uterine anomalies. *Obstet Gynecol* 1978;52:63.

Musset R. Traitement chirurgical des cloisans transversales due vagin d'origine congenitale par la plastie en "Z" a l'Hopital Lariboisiere. *Gynec et Obstet* 1956;55:382.

Nagel TC, Malo JW. Hysteroscopic metroplasty in diethylstilbestrol-exposed uterus and similar fusion anomalies. *Fertil Steril* 1993;59:502.

Niver DH, Barrette G, Jewelewicz R. Congenital atresia of the uterine cervix and vagina: three cases. *Fertil Steril* 1980;33:25.

Nunley WC, Kitchin JD. Congenital atresia of the uterine cervix with pelvic endometriosis. *Arch Surg* 1980;115:757.

O'Leary JL, O'Leary JA. Rudimentary horn pregnancy. *Obstet Gynecol* 1963;22:371.

Ota H, Tanaka J, Murakami M, et al. Laparoscopy-assisted Ruge procedure for the creation of a neovagina in a patient with Mayer-Rokitansky-Küster-Hauser syndrome. *Fertil Steril* 2000;73:641.

Ozek C, Gurler T, Alper M, et al. Modified McIndoe procedure for vaginal agenesis. *Ann Plast Surg* 1999;43:393.

Pabuccu R, Gomel V. Reproductive outcome after hysteroscopic metroplasty in women with septate uterus and otherwise unexplained infertility. *Fertil Steril* 2004;28:1675.

Parsanezhad ME, Alborzi S, Zarei A, et al. Hysteroscopic metroplasty of the complete uterine septum, duplicate cervix, and vaginal septum. *Fertil Steril* 2006;85:1473.

Parsons JK, Gearhart SL, Gearhart, JP. Vaginal reconstruction utilizing sigmoid colon: complications and long term results. *J Pediatr Surg* 2002;37:629.

Patton PE, Novy MJ, Lee DM, et al. The diagnosis and reproductive outcome after surgical treatment of the complete septate uterus, duplicated cervix, and vaginal septum. *Am J Obstet Gynecol* 2004;190:1669.

Patil V, Hixon FP. The role of tissue expanders in vaginoplasty for congenital malformations of the vagina. *Br J Urol* 1992;70:554.

Petrozza JC, Gray MR, Davis AJ, et al. Congenital absence of the uterus and vagina is not commonly transmitted as a dominant genetic trait: outcomes of surrogate pregnancies. *Fertil Steril* 1997;67;387.

Phupong V, Pruksananonda K, Taneepanichskul S, et al. Double uterus with unilaterally obstructed hemivagina and ipsilateral renal agenesis: a variety presentation and a ten-year review of the literature. *J Med Assoc Thai* 2000;83:569.

Pinsky L. A community of human malformation syndromes involving the müllerian ducts, distal extremities, urinary tract, and ears. *Teratology* 1974;9:65.

Pittock ST, Babovic-Vuksanovic D, Lteif A. Mayer-Rokitansky-Kuster-Hauser anomaly and its associated malformations. *Am J Med Genet* 2005;135A:314.

Plevraki E, Kita M, Goulis DG, et al. Bilateral ovarian agenesis and the presence of the testis specific protein 1-Y-linked gene: two new features of Mayer-Rokitansky-Küster-Hauser syndrome. *Fertil Steril* 2004;81:689.

Popaw DD. Utilization of the rectum in construction of a functional vagina. *Russk Virach St Peter* 1910;43:1512.

Pratt JH. Vaginal atresia corrected by use of small and large bowel. *Clin Obstet Gynecol* 1972;15:639.

Proctor JA, Haney AF. Recurrent first trimester pregnancy loss is associated with uterine septum but not with bicornuate uterus. *Fertil Steril* 2003;80:1212.

Ravasia DJ, Brain PH, Pollard JK. Incidence of uterine rupture among women with mullerian duct anomalies who attempt vaginal birth after cesarean delivery. *Am J Obstet Gynecol* 1999;181:877.

Roberts CP, Haber MJ, Rock JA. Vaginal creation for müllerian agenesis. *Am J Obstet Gynecol* 2001;185:1349.

Rock JA, Baramki TA, Parmley TH, et al. A unilateral functioning uterine anlage with müllerian duct agenesis. *Int J Gynecol Obstet* 1980;18:99.

Rock JA, Carpenter SE, Wheeless CR, et al. The clinical management of maldevelopment of the uterine cervix. *J Pelvic Surg* 1995;1:129.

Rock JA, Jones HW. The clinical management of the double uterus. *Fertil Steril* 1977;28:798.

Rock JA, Jones HW. The double uterus associated with an obstructed hemivagina and ipsilateral renal agenesis. *Am J Obstet Gynecol* 1980;138:339.

Rock JA, Jones HW Jr. Vaginal forms for dilatation and/or to maintain vaginal patency. *Fertil Steril* 1984;42:187.

Rock JA, Parmley T, Murphy AA, et al. Malposition of the ovary associated with uterine anomalies. *Fertil Steril* 1986;45:561.

Rock JA, Reeves LA, Retto H, et al. Success following vaginal creation for müllerian agenesis. *Fertil Steril* 1983;39:809.

Rock JA, Roberts CP, Hesla JS. Hysteroscopic metroplasty of the class Va uterus with preservation of the cervical septum. *Fertil Steril* 1999;72:942.

Rock JA, Schlaff WD. The obstetrical consequences of uterovaginal anomalies. *Fertil Steril* 1985;43:681.

Rock JA, Schlaff WD, Zacur HA, et al. The clinical management of congenital absence of the uterine cervix. *Int J Gynecol Obstet* 1984;22:229.

Rock JA, Zacur HA. The clinical management of repeated early pregnancy wastage. *Fertil Steril* 1983;39:123.

Rock JA, Zacur HA, Dlugi AM, et al. Pregnancy success following surgical correction of imperforate hymen and complete transverse vaginal septum. *Obstet Gynecol* 1982;59:448.

Rotmensch J, Rosensheim N, Dillon M, et al. Carcinoma arising in the neovagina: case report and review of the literature. *Obstet Gynecol* 1983;61:534.

Ruge E. Ersatz der durch die flexur mittels laparotomie. *Dtsch Med Wochenschr* 1914;40:120.

Sanders BH, Machan LS, Gomel V. Complex uterine surgery: a cooperative role for interventional radiology with hysteroscopic surgery. *Fertil Steril* 1998;70:952.

Schätz T, Huber J, Wenzl R. Creation of a neovagina according to Whartion-Sheares-George in patients with Mayer-Rokitansky-Küster-Hauser syndrome. *Fertil Steril* 2005;83:437.

Schubert G. Uber Scheidenbildung bei angeborenem Vaginaldefekt. *Zentralbl Gynaekol* 1911;45:1017.

Semmens JP. Abdominal contour in the third trimester: an aid to diagnosis of uterine anomalies. *Obstet Gynecol* 1965;25:779.

Sheldon CA, Gilbert A, Lewis AG. Vaginal reconstruction: critical technical principles. *J Urol* 1994;152:190.

Shokeir MHK. Aplasia of the müllerian system: evidence for probably sex-limited autosomal dominant inheritance. *Birth Defects* 1978;14:147.

Simpson JL. Genetics of the female reproductive ducts. *Am J Med Genet* 1999;89:224.

Singh KJ, Devi L. Hysteroplasty and vaginoplasty for reconstruction of the uterus. *Int J Gynaecol Obstet* 1980;17:457.

Singh M, Gearheart JP, Rock JA. Double urethra, double bladder, left renal agenesis, persistent hymen, double vagina and uterus didelphys. *Adolesc Pediatr Gynecol* 1993;6:99.

Soong YK, Chang FH, Lai YM, et al. Results of modified laparoscopically assisted neovaginoplasty in 18 patients with congenital absence of the vagina. *Hum Reprod* 1996;11:200.

Stanton SL. Gynecologic complications of epispadias and bladder exstrophy. *Am J Obstet Gynecol* 1974;119:749.

Steinkampf MP, Manning MT, Dharia S, et al. An accessory uterine cavity as a cause of pelvic pain. *Obstet Gynecol* 2004;103:1058.

Stoot JE, Mastboom JL. Restriction on the indications for metroplasty. *Acta Eur Fertil* 1977;8:79.

Strassmann EO. Operations for double uterus and endometrial atresia. *Clin Obstet Gynecol* 1961;4:240.

Strassmann EO. Plastic unification of double uterus. *Am J Obstet Gynecol* 1952;64:25.

Strassmann P. Die operative vereinigung eines doppelten uterus. *Zentralbl Gynakol* 1907;29:1322.

Strickland JL, Cameron WJ, Krantz KE. Long-term satisfaction of adults undergoing McIndoe vaginoplasty as adolescents. *Adolesc Pediatr Gynecol* 1993;6:135.

Tancer ML, Katz M, Veridiano NP. Vaginal epithelialization with human amnion. *Obstet Gynecol* 1979;54:345.

Templeman CL, Hertweck SP, Levine RL, et al. Use of laparoscopically mobilized peritoneum in the creation of a neovagina. *Fertil Steril* 2000;74:589.

Thompson DP, Lynn HB. Genital anomalies associated with solitary kidney. *Mayo Clin Proc* 1966;41:538.

Thompson JD, Wharton LR, Te Linde RW. Congenital absence of the vagina. *Am J Obstet Gynecol* 1957;74:397.

Timmreck LS, Pan HA, Reindollar RH, et al. WNT7A mutations in patients with müllerian duct abnormalities. *J Pediatr Gynecol* 2003;16:217.

Tompkins P. Comments on the bicornuate uterus and twinning. *Surg Clin North Am* 1962;42:1049.

Ulfelder H, Robboy SJ. The embryologic development of the human vagina. *Am J Obstet Gynecol* 1976;126:769.

Valdes C, Malini S, Malinak L. Sonography in the surgical management of vaginal and cervical atresia. *Fertil Steril* 1983;40:263.

Vecchietti G. Neovagina nella sindrome di Rokitansky-Küster-Hauser. *Attual Ostet Ginecol* 1965;11:129.

Vecchietti G. Le neo-vagin dans le syndrome de Rokitansky-Küster-Hauser. *Rev Med Suisse Romane* 1979;99:593.

Vecchietti G. Die neovagina beim Rokitansky-Küster-Hauser-Syndrom. *Gynäkologe* 1980;13:112.

Vecchietti G, Ardillo L. *La sindrome di Rokitansky-Küster-Hauser: fisiopatologia e clinica dell aplasia vaginale con corni uterini rudimentali*. Roma: Societa Editrice Universo, 1970.

Veronikus DK, McClure GB, Nichols DH. The Vecchietti operation for constructing a neovagina: indications, instrumentation, and techniques. *Obstet Gynecol* 1997;90:301.

von Rokitansky KE. Ober die sogenannten Verdoppelungen des uterus. *Med Jb Ost Stoat* 1938;76:39.

Weed JC, McKee DM. Vulvoplasty in cases of exstrophy of the bladder. *Obstet Gynecol* 1974;43:512.

Weijenborg PT, ter Kuile MM. The effect of a group programme on women with the Mayer-Rokitansky-Küster-Hauser-Syndrome. *BJOG* 2000;107: 365.

Wharton LR. Congenital malformations associated with developmental defects of the female reproductive organs. *Am J Obstet Gynecol* 1947;53:37.

Wharton LR. Further experiences in construction of the vagina. *Ann Surg* 1940;111:1010.

Wharton LR. A simple method of constructing a vagina. *Ann Surg* 1938;107:842.

Williams EA. Congenital absence of the vagina, a simple operation for its relief. *J Obstet Gynaecol Br Comm* 1964;71:511.

Williams EA. Uterovaginal agenesis. *Ann R Coll Surg Engl* 1976;58:266.

Williams EA. Vulvo-vaginoplasty. *Proc R Soc Med* 1970;63:40.

Woelfer B, Salim R, Banerjee S. Reproductive outcomes in women with congenital uterine anomalies detected by three-dimensional ultrasound screening. *Obstet Gynecol* 2001:98;1099.

CHAPTER 26 ■ NORMAL AND ABNORMAL UTERINE BLEEDING

WILLIAM J. BUTLER AND DAVID E. CARNOVALE

DEFINITIONS

Amenorrhea—The absence of menstrual bleeding for more than 6 months.

Breakthrough bleeding—Intermenstrual bleeding that occurs despite the use of exogenous hormones.

Dysfunctional uterine bleeding (DUB)—Abnormal uterine bleeding occurring in the absence of identifiable pathology. It is often subdivided into ovulatory DUB and anovulatory DUB. DUB is a diagnosis of exclusion.

Dysmenorrhea—Painful menstruation.

Interval bleeding—Bleeding between menstrual cycles.

Menorrhagia—Prolonged menstrual bleeding that is excessive in amount, duration, or both that occurs at regular intervals.

Metrorrhagia—Menstrual bleeding occurring at irregular intervals that is normal in amount and may or may not be prolonged.

Oligomenorrhea—A menstrual cycle interval of more than 37 days.

Polymenorrhea—A menstrual cycle interval of less than 21 days.

Postmenopausal bleeding—Uterine bleeding occurring more than 12 months after the last menstrual period of a menopausal woman.

Reproductive capability in a young woman begins at the point of menarche, which is the beginning of cyclic uterine bleeding in the anatomically and physiologically normal female. Menarche marks the beginning of an important stage in a young woman's physical reproductive maturation and development. Even before the onset of this entirely natural but potentially disturbing function, a young woman's early psychological reactions to menstruation, and probably also her lifelong view, can be influenced by the accuracy of her information and the degree of empathy with which this knowledge has been conveyed to her.

Many women, perhaps appropriately, conclude that any departure from their personal menstrual experience is abnormal, and they will seek treatment for these departures. Conversely, some women accept or perhaps ignore even significant variations in their menstrual function, sometimes to the extent that serious health impairment occurs (e.g., severe iron-deficiency anemia).

Clinical experience has led to empiric definitions of variations in menstrual pattern that constitute abnormal uterine bleeding. Various terms are in general use to facilitate description and record keeping regarding patterns of uterine bleeding. We defined above some of the terms used in this discussion.

Current medical therapies are quite effective in the management of most of the disturbances of menstrual function that occur in the absence of infection, gestation, or uterine tumor. The success of these therapies depends on a complete understanding of normal menstrual physiology and of the effects of the various agents available for treatment. New surgical diagnostic and therapeutic technologies are becoming available to aid in the management of patients who fail to respond to conventional endocrine manipulation by medical therapies.

NORMAL MENSTRUAL PHYSIOLOGY

Menstruation is the physiologic shedding of the endometrium associated with uterine bleeding that occurs at monthly intervals from menarche to menopause. In the years between these two physiologic landmarks, menstruation will occur 400 to 500 times in the average woman. According to the classical theory of the physiology of menstruation, it is the superficial functional layer of the endometrium that is shed during menstruation, and regeneration proceeds from the remaining intact basalis.

Recent work in humans has confirmed the presence of endometrial stem cells, which most likely are located in niches within the basalis layer. Additionally, it appears that these progenitor cells are hormonally independent. The proliferative potential of these cells is maintained in the noncycling state as demonstrated by their ability to regenerate endometrium in postmenopausal women given hormone replacement therapy.

The amazing regenerating properties of the endometrium and its ability to support and nourish a fertilized ovum is an extremely complex system that appears to involve numerous endocrine, paracrine, and autocrine interactions. At the endometrial level, all three inhibin subunits are expressed in the human. It is believed that these dimeric glycoproteins may be involved in endometrial maturation, such as angiogenesis, decidualization, and tissue remodeling. Epidermal growth factors (EGF) are extremely important in human embryogenesis, development, and proliferation differentiation. Human endometrial cells have been shown to express all four EGF receptors and two ligands amphiregulin (AF) and transforming growth factor alpha (TGF-α). Other substances with known angiogenic properties, such as leptin and erythropoietin, have also been shown to be expressed along with their receptors by human endometrium.

This process of monthly shedding and regeneration can occur as often as it does without producing permanent tissue damage possibly because most of the functional endometrium is conserved during menses and because the metamorphosis from proliferative to secretory endometria is controlled not only by processes of cell desquamation and reproliferation but also by dynamic and interactive processes of the endocrinologic and reproductive systems involving many organs. Any interruption of these normal but quite complex cyclic processes can lead to irregularities in endometrial breakdown and to dysfunctional uterine bleeding (DUB).

ENDOCRINOLOGY

The endometrium is an endocrine organ that responds to circulating blood levels of estrogen and progesterone. These two steroids alone are sufficient to induce growth and maturation of an endometrium that can support blastocyst implantation, as has been demonstrated by their sequential administration to patients with ovarian failure to prepare for the transfer of donated embryos. Estradiol (E_2) production by the developing follicle stimulates metabolic activity in the endometrium. E_2 has multiple effects that are mediated through binding to estrogen receptors. There are two estrogen receptors: alpha and beta. The estrogen receptors are members of a hormone receptor family that includes not only the other steroid receptors but also receptors for vitamin D and thyroid hormone. All receptors in this family have three domains. The regulatory domain at the amino acid terminal binds regulatory protein factors. The hormone-binding domain on the carboxy terminal, with its contiguous hinge region, undergoes conformational changes when a steroid hormone binds to it, allowing DNA binding. The DNA-binding domain binds to the hormone-responsive elements in the target gene. The conformation of the DNA-binding domain consists of the highly conserved zinc finger structures that interact with complementary patterns in the DNA.

Steroid hormones have relatively low molecular weights and are rapidly transported into cells by passive diffusion. Binding of a steroid hormone to the intranuclear receptors transforms and activates the hormone receptor complex to allow DNA binding to specific hormone response elements and initiates subsequent transcription. Both estrogen and progesterone receptors bind to their response elements as dimers. After gene activation, the hormone receptor complex undergoes processing with dissociation and loss of activity.

Transcription of target genes with mRNA synthesis leads to translation with synthesis of proteins on ribosomes in the cytoplasm. The biologic effects of E_2 are mediated through this protein synthesis.

Estrogen and Progesterone Receptor Induction

One important function of estrogen is the induction of synthesis of its own and other steroid hormone receptors, called replenishment. Estrogen receptors reach a maximum concentration in the middle-to-late proliferative phase of the menstrual cycle. Progesterone receptors are also induced, and their concentration peaks in the late proliferative phase. Progesterone then blocks the estrogen replenishment mechanism, possibly by accelerating receptor turnover and inhibiting E_2-induced gene transcription. Enough progesterone receptors persist throughout the luteal phase, however, to maintain endometrial responsiveness and induction of deciduation.

Estrogen and Progesterone Target Genes

Target genes of the E_2 receptor complex code for the synthesis of numerous proteins, including structural proteins, enzymes, and growth factors. The relative roles played by the alpha and beta estrogen receptors in the endometrium have yet to be completely elucidated. The net effect of estrogenic stimulation is to induce DNA synthesis and mitotic activity with proliferation of the endometrial glands and stroma. The results are cessation of menstrual flow and an increase in the thickness of the endometrium.

Progesterone also has multiple biologic effects mediated through its receptors. It actively inhibits synthesis of both its own receptors and estrogen receptors, although sufficient progesterone receptors remain throughout the luteal phase of the cycle to mediate maturation and secretory differentiation of the endometrium. The net effect is to antagonize estrogenic metabolic activity with suppression of DNA synthesis in endometrial cells, which results in dynamic inhibition of cell mitosis. Progesterone is also responsible for the active induction of synthesis of various cytoplasmic enzymes, the secretion of proteins such as prolactin-dependent and progesterone-dependent endometrial peptide from decidualized stromal cells, and the stabilization of lysosomes, all of which may play an important role in the onset of menstruation.

Histology and Physiology

The postmenstrual endometrium that remains after collapse and partial shedding during menstruation consists of a thin but stable layer of basalis cells and the dense irregular remnants of the stromal cell–derived stratum spongiosum. The glands are narrow and lined by low cuboidal epithelial cells with few mitoses. The glandular stromal cells are small and spindly with little cytoplasm or mitotic activity. Protein synthesis and secretory activity are minimal. It is on this substrate of basal and stromal cells that estrogen induces a proliferative response.

Early Proliferative Phase

Mitotic activity results in growth and pseudostratification of the glandular epithelial cells. With development and elongation of the glands, the epithelial cells assume a more columnar shape, with secretory granules in the cytoplasm, and glycogen begins to collect in the basal vacuoles. Arteriolar vessels grow up into the endometrium as part of the general proliferative response. The stromal cells also proliferate and expand from a dense compact state to an expanded matrix by transient edema. The combined effects of proliferation and expansion cause the endometrium to grow in this phase to a thickness of 3 to 5 mm.

The increased mitotic activity that results in proliferation is mediated by way of estrogen induction of various peptide growth factors. Epidermal growth factor and insulinlike growth factor I (IGF-I) are two potent mitogens with synthesis that is stimulated by estrogen in endometrial epithelial and stromal cells. Endothelin-1 is a vasoactive peptide with mitogenic activity; its synthesis is induced by both estrogen and growth factors, and its metabolism is enhanced by progesterone. Endothelin-1 may play a role in proliferation and in menstruation. The various peptides that are secreted from stromal and epithelial cells to form the extracellular matrix of the endometrium can be either induced or suppressed by both estrogen and progesterone. Fibronectin, for example, is suppressed by progesterone, whereas several integrin subtypes are stimulated by progesterone. These peptides may have a functional role in proliferation, differentiation, and embryo implantation.

Angiogenesis allows both repair of the endometrium after menstruation and supports cellular proliferation for regrowth during the follicular phase. It is supported and promoted by multiple growth factors. An important role is played by vascular endothelial growth factor (VEGF). VEGF mRNA expression is induced by E_2 and increases from the early proliferative phase through the secretory phase (Torry and Torry). VEGF is produced by the glandular epithelial cells, although some stromal expression is evident in the secretory phase. The increased expression throughout the cycle supports a possible role of VEGF in expansion and coiling of the spiral arterials. Changes in VEGF expression have been detected in women with abnormal uterine bleeding, supporting a possible role in the pathogenesis of menorrhagia (Kooy et al.).

E_2 induces several enzymes (alkaline phosphatase, 5α-reductase, and possibly phospholipase A_2). Phospholipase A_2, which releases arachidonic acid from phospholipid esters, controls the rate-limiting step in prostaglandin synthesis. E_2 also stimulates cyclooxygenase synthesis of prostaglandin $F_{2\alpha}$ ($PGF_{2\alpha}$) and prostaglandin E_2 (PGE_2), both of which have a role in menstrual function. $PGF_{2\alpha}$ has vasoconstrictive and muscle contraction effects. PGE_2 is generally a vasodilator but can also cause contractions in uterine smooth muscle. Alterations in the relative levels of $PGF_{2\alpha}$ and PGE_2 are known to change menstrual bleeding patterns.

Late Proliferative Phase

Ovulation with corpus luteum formation and significant progesterone secretion leads to secretory transformation in the late proliferative–phase endometrium. Progesterone inhibits both estrogen and progesterone receptor synthesis and inhibits DNA synthesis and mitosis. This inhibition process is accompanied by the development of RNA-filled channels between the nucleoli and nuclear membranes that are responsible for the progesterone-induced active synthesis of cytoplasmic enzymes during the secretory phase of the cycle.

The Secretory Phase

The cytoplasmic enzymes 17β- and 20α-hydroxysteroid dehydrogenase (HSD) are induced by progesterone and modulate steroid activity. The enzyme 17β-HSD catalyzes the conversion of E_2 to the relatively weaker estrogen estrone, which, when sulfated by estrogen sulfotransferase, can no longer bind to estrogen receptors. The enzyme 20α-HSD alters progesterone receptor binding and activity. Cytoplasmic lytic enzymes such as acid phosphatase are also induced by progesterone but are kept inactive within Golgi-derived lysosomes, the membranes of which are stabilized by progesterone. IGF II is synthesized locally by middle-to-late secretory-phase endometrium and appears to be involved in the differentiation response of the endometrium to progesterone. IGF binding protein I also appears at this time and is regulated by the IGFs and by relaxin. Other autocrine or paracrine agents secreted locally by decidual cells are relaxin, progesterone-dependent endometrial peptide, and prolactin.

Progesterone has also been shown to induce the activity of metalloendopeptidase, which degrades the endothelin-1 peptide. Withdrawal of progesterone can lead to increased endothelin-1 activity with vasospasm and initiation of menstrual bleeding. Several investigators have described increased levels of protease inhibitors, such as α_1-antitrypsin and antithrombin III, in secretory-phase uterine fluid, which may also be involved in the mechanism of menstrual bleeding.

The Luteal Phase

Morphologically, secretory transformation of the endometrium results in coiling of the spiral arterioles and endometrial glands. The endometrium reaches its maximum thickness of 5 to 6 mm and maintains this thickness throughout the luteal phase. The subnuclear intracytoplasmic glycogen vacuoles in the basal glandular cells transpose to the apex and are expelled into the glandular lumen. The stromal cells subsequently flatten into a low cuboidal form. Stromal cell differentiation from reticular spindle-shaped cells into plump predecidual cells and phagocytic granulated cells defines two layers in the functional endometrium known as the superficial compactum and the deeper spongiosum. The spongiosum has a loose edematous matrix that is the consequence of increased capillary permeability, mediated possibly by prostaglandins. The predecidual, late secretory–phase stromal cells produce several metabolically active substances, as previously described, and are infiltrated by migratory leukocytes. The release of lysosomal enzymes from endometrial cells and possibly also from leukocytes may be involved in the initiation of menstruation.

Menstruation

Menstruation is controlled by many complex, interrelated, and incompletely understood factors. Normal menstruation results from progesterone withdrawal from the estrogen-primed endometrium. Changes that occur in the endometrium during menstruation were described by Markee by observation of endometrial tissue transplanted to the anterior chamber of the eyes of rhesus monkeys. Markee described cyclic changes in endometrial vascularity and the development of coiled vessels supplying the superficial two thirds of the endometrium. The estrogen-primed endometrium of the follicular phase is compact, with relatively underdeveloped vasculature. Progesterone converts this endometrium into a thick, edematous, secretory lining that is glycogen enriched and prepares the metabolically active stroma and glands with an increased vasculature to receive and nourish a fertilized ovum. If implantation does not occur, estrogen and progesterone levels fall, prostaglandin synthesis occurs, and lysosomal membranes rupture, causing constriction of the spiral arterioles, ischemic necrosis, and sloughing of the endometrium superficial to the basalis layer.

Lysosomal release and ischemic necrosis has been believed to be the main mechanism for normal menstrual bleeding for many years. However, the difficulty in detecting cell necrosis during menstruation and viability of menstrual fragments has raised a number of questions about this theory. Current data support the "metalloproteinase theory" as the mechanism leading to menstrual tissue breakdown and shedding. Matrix metalloproteinases (MMPs), lytic enzymes in conjunction with activated endometrial stromal granulocytes, macrophages, and mast cells together are now thought by most investigators to cause menstruation. It is believed that tissue inhibitors of metalloproteinases (TIMPs) remain constant throughout the menstrual cycle. Before menstruation, production and activation of MMPs increases in an environment of stable amounts of TIMPs, leading to an altered MMPs/TIMPS ratio, resulting in tissue breakdown. Estrogen and progesterone, along with cytokines, appear to play a significant role in the regulation and expressions of the MMPs. High levels of progesterone are believed to inhibit MMP production and activity. This would explain endometrial tissue breakdown that occurs coincident with dropping progesterone levels from an involuting corpus luteum.

In the second part of the menstrual phase, mitotic activity resumes, and epithelial regeneration begins. This process occurs even while menstrual bleeding continues. Horizontal growth from the stem cells of the glands present in niches within the basalis layer continues the regenerative process. New blood capillaries are formed by the stimulating effect vascular endothelial growth factor (VEGF) and thymidine phosphorylase (TP) secreted by both epithelial and stromal cells. Continuous proliferation of stem cells is ensured by high telomerase activity.

This process begins in the premenstrual phase of the cycle with cessation of synthesis and inspissation of ground substance and supporting tissues by lytic enzymes released from lysosomes, which causes loss of fluids and compression of the endometrium, tonic contractions of spiral arterioles with reduction of blood flow to the tissues, loss of stromal edema, and kinking of the coiled spiral arterioles caused by the reduction in endometrial thickness.

A generalized state of ischemia develops in the superficial layers of endometrium, and bleeding into the stroma begins. Acid phosphatase and prostaglandin substances released from autolyzed cells, together with increased endothelin-1 activity, cause more intense vasoconstriction of spiral arterioles, and devitalized tissues finally slough as small hemorrhages in the stroma coalesce. According to Beller, coagulation factors are decreased in normal menstrual discharge. Fibrinogen is absent, plasminogen is converted to plasmin by released peptidases, and the amount of plasmin inhibitor is decreased. Menstrual blood generally does not clot, but it can form red blood cell aggregates with mucoid substances, mucoproteins, and glycogen as it collects in the vagina. These red cell aggregates may appear to be blood clots, but they contain no fibrin. In the presence of very heavy flow, however, clotting can occur.

According to classical theory, during menstruation the superficial compacta and the intermediate stratum spongiosum layers of the endometrium are shed, leaving only the basalis layer intact. New endometrium is regenerated from the basalis. Regeneration of new capillaries from the basalis has been observed by Markee, and restoration of the endometrial circulation has been correlated with the cessation of menstrual bleeding. Blood loss from the process of normal menstruation is limited by recovery of tone in the myometrium and endometrial vasculature, cessation of cellular autolysis, eventual clotting over the endometrial surface, and eventual active regeneration of glands, stroma, and vessels in the basalis layer in response to rising estrogen levels in the new cycle. The retained basalis endometrium is protected from destruction by lysosomal enzymes by a mucinous carbohydrate coat that covers the free surfaces of endometrial cells. This mechanism for retention of some endometrium during menstruation may explain the lack of permanent damage during the years of menstruation.

Endometrial regression during menstruation is described by classical theory as the result of four processes: autophagia, heterophagia, extrusion of secretory products, and elimination of fluids with some, but not complete, shedding of tissue. Autophagia and heterophagia are the kindred processes of intracellular lytic digestion of debris in vacuoles and of extracellular lytic digestion of debris taken up by phagosomes. Both processes eliminate damaged tissue to allow regeneration of normal endometrial cells. With fluid loss and secretion, the functionalis (the remaining functional basalis) regresses to a resting state, ready to regenerate in the next cycle. These two processes can only partially explain the observation that initial endometrial regeneration occurs in the absence of estrogen. This initial lack of estrogen dependence can also be secondary to the lesser proliferative response required after regression, compared with complete endometrial shedding. Much work remains to be done to define the complex processes involved in menstruation.

ABNORMALITIES OF THE MENSTRUAL CYCLE

Given the complexities and varieties of possible alterations of the systems that control menstruation, it is not surprising that abnormal uterine bleeding should occur even in the absence of obvious disease. Prolonged estrogen stimulation can result in endometrium that outgrows its blood supply and has asynchronous development of endometrial glands, stroma, and blood vessels. Any failure of progesterone production can also profoundly affect endometrial glands, stroma, and blood vessels. Abnormal synthesis of acid mucopolysaccharides can result in the release of excessive amounts of hydrolytic enzymes into the stroma. Lysosome release from endometrial glands, influenced by plasma progesterone levels, can affect menstrual flow. The endometrium and myometrium of patients with menorrhagia produce altered types of prostaglandins. Smith and associates have shown that the amount of menstrual flow is influenced by a change in the endometrial conversion of prostaglandin endoperoxide from PGF_2 to PGE_2 and that women with menorrhagia synthesize mainly the vasodilator PGE_2 in the endometrium.

Menstruation has three clinical characteristics: the menstrual interval or cycle length, the duration of flow, and the amount of flow. The mean cycle length is 28 to 29 days, although a menstrual interval of 21 to 37 days can be considered normal. A menstrual interval shorter than 21 days is defined as polymenorrhea. A menstrual interval longer than 37 days is defined as oligomenorrhea. Amenorrhea is the absence of menses for 6 months or longer. The menstrual interval can vary from month to month by several days. Regularity of the menstrual cycle is more important than exact approximation to the 28-day mean menstrual interval. Variation in the length of the menstrual interval in regular ovulatory cycles usually occurs in the preovulatory (proliferative) phase of the cycle and is more frequent among postmenarchal teenagers and in women approaching menopause.

A duration of flow of 7 days or less is considered normal. A patient bleeding beyond 7 days enters the intermenstrual phase of the cycle, which is defined as metrorrhagia. Regardless of the length of the menstrual flow, 70% of the blood loss usually occurs by the second day and 90% by the third day. The mean menstrual blood loss for a normal period is about 40 mL. A total blood loss of 20 to 80 mL, representing 10 to 35 mg iron, has long been accepted as within the normal range. Menstrual blood loss of 80 mL or less was established as the upper limit of normal, as this is the 95th percentile in healthy women with normal iron stores measured in a population of Swedish women in the 1960s. Clinically, the use of such a statistical cutoff for a value that is not likely to be measured and is likely to vary among populations depending on diet, health, and genetics is very limited. Additionally, it has recently been shown that the 80 mL value has neither the sensitivity or specificity for disease, compromised iron status, or adverse impact of periods. The determination of the normalcy of menstrual bleeding amount is better addressed in the context of the particular woman's circumstances. Concerns about anemia in a particular patient should be investigated with appropriate laboratory tests for iron stores. A thorough menstrual history should establish the patient's perception of the heaviness of her flow, impact on her life, difficulty with containment of flow, and associated symptoms. For some patients, their problem may be acute unmanageable menstrual bleeding in the first few days rather than the overall volume leading to anemia. Other patients may have noticed a significant increase in menstrual bleeding that may be due to uterine myomas.

Iron-deficiency anemia is a late manifestation of excessive menstruation. Serum iron (ferritin) levels are more sensitive than hematocrit and hemoglobin levels for detection of iron depletion before anemia develops, as shown by Guillebaud and colleagues. We believe that development and routine use of a convenient, standardized, objective method for measuring menstrual blood loss would significantly improve the clinical practice of gynecology. One fifth of women have a problem with excessive menstrual blood loss sometime during their reproductive years. The method of Hallberg and Nilsson for quantification of iron and blood loss is based on the simultaneous use of tampons and pads for the collection of menstrual blood. Menstrual blood is extracted with 5% sodium hydroxide, which converts hemoglobin to alkaline hematin. The concentration is then determined spectrophotometrically. The method is simple and gives accurate results but is not widely used.

DYSFUNCTIONAL UTERINE BLEEDING

DUB is a symptom complex that includes any condition of abnormal uterine bleeding in the absence of pregnancy, neoplasm, infection, or other intrauterine lesion. Such bleeding is most often the result of endocrinologic dysfunction that inhibits normal ovulation.

Chronic Anovulation and Dysfunctional Uterine Bleeding

The state of chronic anovulation is the result of unopposed estrogen stimulation of the endometrium with consequent irregular breakdown and bleeding. Chronic anovulation syndrome is a "wastebasket" diagnosis for multiple endocrine etiologies. Hyperthyroidism and hypothyroidism, hyperprolactinemia, hormone-producing ovarian tumors, and Cushing disease are all endocrine syndromes that can induce anovulation, but the primary etiology of DUB is chronic anovulation syndrome, often commonly described as the polycystic ovary or Stein-Leventhal's syndrome. Any imbalance in hypothalamic pulsatile release of gonadotropin-releasing hormone (GnRH), in pituitary synthesis or release of follicle-stimulating hormone (FSH) or luteinizing hormone (LH), or in ovarian follicular production of E_2, androgens, or progesterone can upset the delicate balances that induce cyclic ovulation and normal menstrual function. Exogenous androgen production in the adrenal glands and estrone production in adipose tissue produce identical clinical pictures.

Abnormal bleeding associated with ovulatory cycles thus requires careful differential diagnosis. Patients at the extremes of reproductive function, both perimenarchal and perimenopausal, require evaluations modified to recognize their unique clinical situations. A clear understanding of the diverse etiologies of DUB will lead to easier and more practical diagnostic schemes and more effective therapeutic interventions.

Abnormal Ovulation and Dysfunctional Uterine Bleeding

Although the most frequent cause of DUB is anovulation, histologic studies consistently show that 15% to 20% of DUB patients have secretory endometrium, indicative of at least intermittent, if not regular, ovulation. The differential diagnosis of abnormal bleeding with ovulation differs from that of anovulation. Ovulatory patients with abnormal bleeding are more likely to have an underlying organic pathology and are not, therefore, true DUB patients by strict definition.

Aksel and Jones studied endometria of patients with dysfunctional bleeding and found hyperplasia in 63% of cases; secretory endometrium was observed in 17%, and nonsecretory endometrium of the interval, postmenstrual, or atrophic type made up the remaining 20%. Thus, at least 17% of patients in this series had normal cyclic hormonal function and ovulation before the endometrium was examined, and it is possible that many patients with the postmenstrual type of endometria would have shown secretory changes if curettage had been performed somewhat later. In addition to histologic confirmation of ovulation by the presence of secretory endometrium, ovulation can be documented by basal body temperature charting, urinary LH surge detection, or prospective hormonal evaluation. In some cases, the prospective hormonal studies using daily serum estrogen and progesterone levels are more accurate for defining ovulatory status than are the historically accepted studies of endometrial histology, which can be misleading because of previous hormonal therapy. A serum progesterone concentration exceeding 3 ng/mL in the luteal phase of the cycle indicates ovulation.

Diagnostic Imaging Techniques

Diagnostic vaginal ultrasound can be particularly useful in cases of ovulatory abnormal uterine bleeding. A nonrandomized study of 45 otherwise unselected patients with abnormal uterine bleeding demonstrated anatomic pathology in 31% by vaginal ultrasound compared with 9% by clinical examination. Pathologic findings included leiomyoma uteri, polyps, and abnormal endometrial architecture. If these data are confirmed by later studies, the implication is that true DUB in ovulatory patients may be even more rare than the currently accepted figure of 15% to 20%. Endovaginal ultrasound is also of particular value in cases of perimenopausal and postmenopausal abnormal bleeding, which will be discussed later (Fig. 26.1).

Saline infusion sonography (SIS) is a technique to improve visualization of the endometrial cavity during transvaginal ultrasonography. The technique involves a pelvic examination with placement of an open-sided bivalve speculum. The cervix is prepared with antiseptic solution, and a small catheter is inserted through the cervical os for instillation of sterile saline. A number of catheters are available both with and without small balloons, which are useful in the case of a parous cervix. The speculum is then removed, and the endometrial cavity is distended with sterile saline during transvaginal ultrasonography. Dueholm and colleagues compared the accuracy of saline infusion sonography with transvaginal sonography, hysteroscopy, and magnetic resonance imaging (MRI). In 108 patients with abnormal uterine bleeding, pain, endometriosis, or myomas,

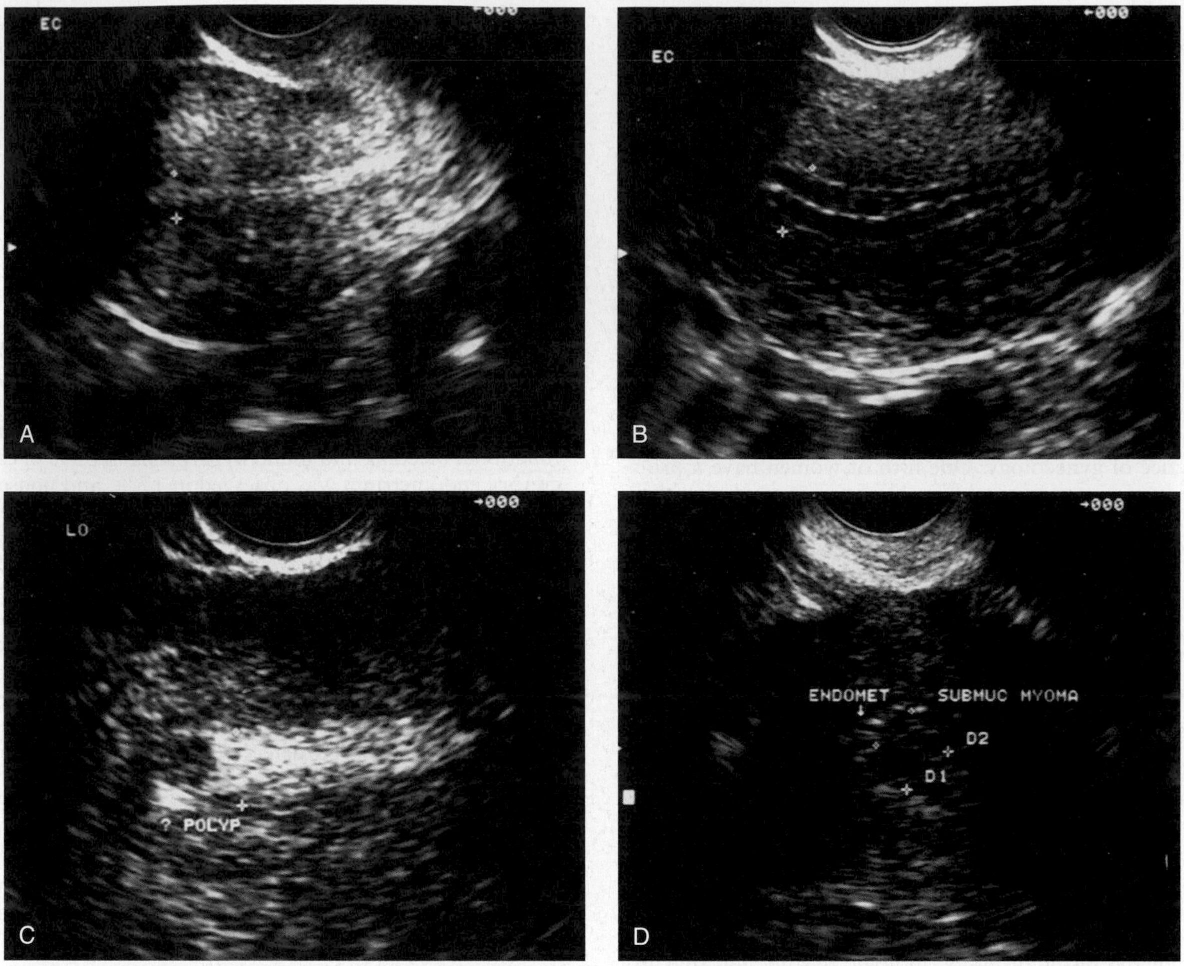

FIGURE 26.1. **A:** Single-line endometrium consistent with postmenstruation, early proliferation, and postmenopause. **B:** Three-line endometrium from estrogen stimulation, late follicular phase. **C:** Endometrial polyp in hyperechoic thickened endometrium consistent with luteal phase or hyperplasia–neoplasia. **D:** Submucous myoma with distortion of endometrial cavity marked by single-line endometrium.

SIS had an overall sensitivity comparable to the gold standard of hysteroscopy and better than either MRI or transvaginal sonography. MRI had the highest sensitivity for submucous myomas, but a relatively low sensitivity for other intrauterine pathology, such as polyps. As SIS is a less invasive procedure than a surgical technique, such as hysteroscopy, and is much less expensive than MRI, it should be the procedure of choice for imaging of the endometrial cavity in patients with abnormal uterine bleeding.

Proper evaluation of abnormal bleeding in the ovulatory patient demands assessment for other less common causes of bleeding. According to Claessens and Cowell, bleeding dyscrasias are particularly common in perimenarchal patients, up to 19% of whom have a primary coagulation disorder, such as idiopathic thrombocytopenic purpura or von Willebrand disease. An ad hoc consensus conference that met in May 2004 concluded that underlying hemostatic disorders were a more common cause of menorrhagia in adult women than has been currently recognized (Munrow and Lukes). The most common of these coagulopathies is von Willebrand disease. The incidence of von Willebrand disease in the general population has been estimated at 0.8% to 1.3%. The consensus conference calculated, by review of the literature, an incidence of 13.2% (range 11.2%–15.5%) in healthy women with menorrhagia. Conversely, women with von Willebrand disease report menorrhagia in 78% to 93% of patients. Other inherited disorders of hemostasis are relatively rare. Other disorders of platelet number and function have variable effects on menstrual bleeding, depending on their severity. Treatment of abnormal uterine bleeding secondary to coagulopathy may involve medical management with tranexamic acid, desmopressin acetate (DDAVP), hormonal therapy, or a progestin-containing intrauterine device (IUD). Endometrial ablation is also appropriate in these patients.

Hemorrhagic diatheses can occur with leukemia, with chemotherapy treatment, or as secondary to oral anticoagulant therapy or ingestion of foods or drugs that inhibit platelet aggregation. Infection has been shown to cause abnormal uterine bleeding. Mobiluncus species identified in cases of abnormal bleeding respond to oral metronidazole therapy. Chlamydia has been implicated in abnormal bleeding, particularly with concurrent use of oral contraceptives. Menorrhagia has been described as an early symptom in patients with subclinical hypothyroidism before diagnosis of overt disease. Thyroid replacement in a normal physiologic dosage will resolve the abnormal bleeding.

Arteriovenous malformation is a very rare cause of ovulatory bleeding. In a report by Fleming and colleagues, only two cases were diagnosed before definitive surgery; the diagnosis was by pelvic angiography.

The reported association between tubal ligation and new onset of abnormal uterine bleeding should also be noted. Although numerous anecdotal reports exist, no underlying pathologic changes in anatomy or hormone production have ever been documented. Long-term follow-up studies do not confirm an increased incidence of abnormal bleeding in these patients but do implicate biased patient perception. Patients who discontinue oral contraceptive use after tubal ligation have heavier and more painful bleeding, whereas patients who have intrauterine devices removed after sterilization have improved menstrual symptomatology.

Pathophysiology

As stated earlier, the most common etiology for DUB is estrogen withdrawal or estrogen breakthrough bleeding in an anovulatory patient. In the absence of progesterone exposure to cause inhibition of DNA synthesis and mitosis, the estrogenic proliferative response causes stromal cell growth to exceed the structural integrity of its stromal matrix, and the endometrium breaks down with irregular bleeding. Unopposed estrogen results in vascular endometrial tissue with relatively scant stroma, giving glands a back-to-back appearance. The endometrium is fragile and undergoes repetitive spontaneous breakdown. In the absence of normal control mechanisms to limit menstrual blood loss, bleeding can be prolonged and excessive.

Other contributing factors are the lack of coordinated vasoconstriction and the release of lytic enzymes, which occurs in a normal progesterone-stimulated endometrium. The absence of progesterone stimulation of metalloendopeptidase increases endothelin-1 activity, which contributes to vasospasm. Lysosomal enzymes inappropriately released in the absence of progesterone stabilization of the lysosomal membrane further contribute to structural breakdown.

Many questions still remain about the mechanisms responsible for all cases of DUB. Although the above makes sense in certain circumstances, it does not explain clinical scenarios such as bleeding unresponsive to hormonal manipulation after structural lesions have been ruled out. The same lytic enzymes, MMPs, and their inhibitors involved in normal menstrual bleeding have been found to have aberrant locally restricted expression, activation, and uncontrolled activity in the endometrial tissue biopsy specimens from women with metrorrhagia.

Hemostasis in a bleeding endometrium depends both on coagulation, with thrombus formation forming plugs in superficial blood vessels, and on vasoconstriction of spiral arterioles; generalized endometrial collapse with compression of bleeding vessels can also contribute. The lack of coordinated vasoconstriction and the irregular structural collapse lead to irregular and often heavy bleeding. The amount of bleeding correlates directly with the level of estrogen stimulation. The chronic high estrogen milieus seen in cases of obesity and chronic anovulation, and in perimenarchal and perimenopausal patients, cause the greatest amount of DUB blood loss.

Unopposed estrogen stimulation can, over time, induce a hyperplastic response in the proliferating endometrium (Fig. 26.2A). Such hyperplasia can eventually develop the cytologic changes associated with neoplasia: atypical adenomatous hyperplasia or even low-grade adenocarcinoma. Such cellular transformation takes time, as much as 10 to 20 years; a young patient with DUB has a low risk of hyperplasia or neoplasia and generally does not require endometrial sampling. The perimenopausal patient has a substantially higher risk, however, and sampling is mandated.

Making the Differential Diagnosis

DUB occurs most frequently at the extremes of menstrual life, but it can develop at any intervening time. The characteristics of DUB are variable, from infrequent heavy flow (oligomenorrhea) to almost continuous spotting or bleeding. The age at onset and duration of irregularity can provide important

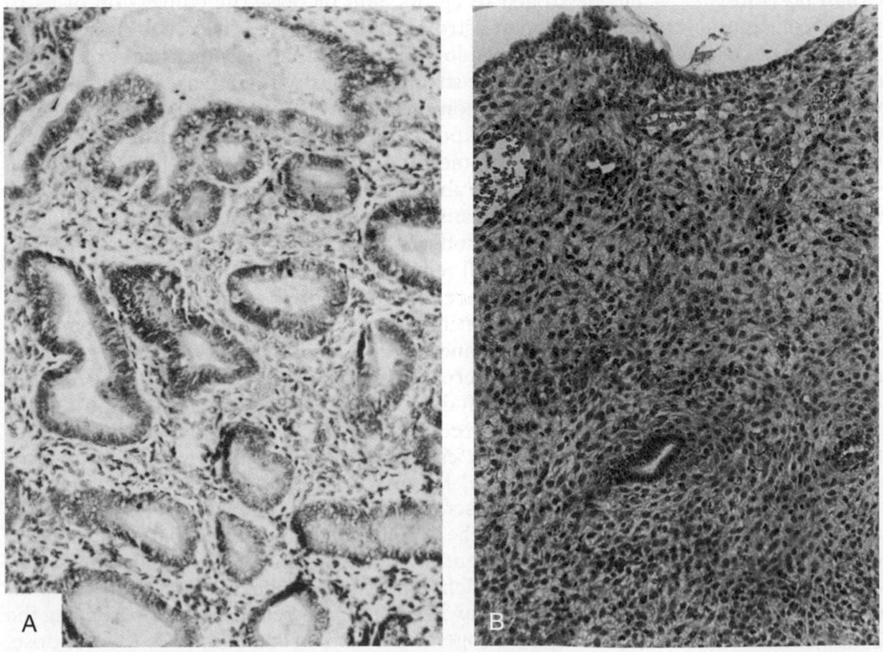

FIGURE 26.2. A: Endometrial hyperplasia before treatment showing hyperplastic cellular changes of glands. B: Hyperplastic endometrium after continuous progestin treatment.

clues to etiology. Anovulation is common in the perimenarchal girl. More than 50% of cycles are anovulatory in the first 2 years after menarche. Complications of pregnancy are also common in this age group and must be ruled out before initiation of treatment for DUB. New sensitive radioimmunoassays for the beta subunit of human chorionic gonadotropin are accurate for evaluating the possibility of pregnancy without invasive tissue sampling. Although relatively rare, endocrinologically active ovarian neoplasms do occur and should be particularly excluded in prepubertal vaginal bleeding. Other causes of irregular bleeding in the adolescent include genital trauma and coagulopathies such as idiopathic thrombocytopenic purpura and von Willebrand disease. As previously mentioned, the Claessens and Cowell review of children's hospital admissions for menorrhagia reports an overall 19% incidence of primary coagulation disorders and a 50% incidence in patients presenting at the time of menarche. Some more recent studies have disputed this high figure and cited a lower risk of 5%. Given the new data on von Willebrand disease in adult female menorrhagia, this newer figure is questionable, and coagulopathies should still be considered a significant cause of abnormal uterine bleeding in adolescents. The most common diagnosis is idiopathic thrombocytopenic purpura, but platelet disorders such as von Willebrand and Glanzmann diseases, thalassemia, and leukemia are also found.

The adult patient with DUB can have either an acute or a chronic history of menstrual irregularity. Onset at menarche and persistence into adulthood is a classic history for chronic anovulation syndrome, but nonclassical adrenal hyperplasia must be differentiated when there is coexistent androgen excess. The differential diagnosis can be made by obtaining a baseline 17α-hydroxyprogesterone level. A level less than 200 ng/dL rules out partial adrenal 21-hydroxylase enzyme deficiency. An elevated baseline 17α-hydroxyprogesterone requires a cosyntropin stimulation test to confirm the nonclassical adrenal hyperplasia diagnosis. A more acute history requires a differential diagnosis of other endocrinologic causes of anovulation, for example, thyroid and prolactin disorders, complications of pregnancy, neoplastic processes such as fibroids or hormone-producing ovarian tumors, intrauterine lesions such as polyps and synechiae, and coagulopathies. Adult patients with menorrhagia are at higher risk than previously thought to have a bleeding diathesis. Dilley and colleagues identified coagulopathies in 10.7% of 121 patients in a case control study. The majority of cases were von Willebrand disease. Women older than the age of 30 years with a history consistent with chronic anovulation should undergo endometrial sampling because of their greater risk of hyperplasia and neoplasia. Perimenopausal women with DUB have an even higher risk of hyperplasia and neoplasia and should always undergo extensive endometrial sampling, in most cases by dilatation and curettage (D&C).

Several years before menopause, menstrual cycles usually shorten secondary to a decreased proliferative phase, with resultant moderate elevation of FSH and subsequent frequent anovulatory cycles. This unopposed estrogen environment is conducive to the development of both DUB and hyperplasia. Appropriate evaluation of the perimenopausal and postmenopausal patient will be thoroughly discussed later in this chapter.

A diagnosis of DUB is often a diagnosis of exclusion. Problems of pregnancy such as incomplete or missed abortion, subinvolution of the placental site, placental polyp, trophoblastic disease, and extrauterine pregnancy must be ruled out. All gynecologic malignancies can cause abnormal bleeding. Common epithelial tumors of the ovary can produce estrogen and cause uterine bleeding. Submucous leiomyomata and endometrial polyps can be present in older women but are not a problem in the differential diagnosis of adolescents. Excessive anovulatory bleeding is common with polycystic ovarian disease, with functional cysts of the ovary, and perhaps in some cases of luteal phase deficiency.

The patient workup for abnormal uterine bleeding should include a complete history and physical examination. Pelvic examination may disclose an adnexal mass, evidence of genital trauma or laceration, or a fibroid uterus. Laboratory studies should include thyroid function tests and the evaluation of levels of human chorionic gonadotropin, FSH, LH, prolactin, and serum androgens, if indicated. A significant increase in dehydroepiandrosterone sulfate indicates a need to screen for nonclassical adrenal hyperplasia. A serum progesterone level measurement is useful for assessment of ovulatory status. A complete blood count with platelet and coagulation studies is appropriate, and a bleeding time may be indicated to assess platelet function. As mentioned earlier, endovaginal ultrasound and SIS are valuable adjuncts to pelvic examination. They are particularly informative for assessment of intrauterine or extrauterine pregnancies and pelvic masses detected on examination. Occasionally, they may also reveal anatomic pathology not detected by other means (Fig. 26.1). Invasive tissue-sampling procedures include endometrial sampling and D&C. A D&C is preferable in the perimenopausal or postmenopausal patient and may also be indicated when there is clinical suspicion of an abnormal pregnancy. A D&C is relatively contraindicated in the adolescent. Hysterosalpingography and hysteroscopy also have potential benefit and will be reviewed later in this chapter.

Treatment

Because most patients with DUB have an underlying etiology of chronic anovulation with unopposed estrogen stimulation of the endometrium, medical treatment with progestational compounds is the mainstay of therapy. Precise amounts can differ depending on the patient's age, but adequate progestin stimulation will decrease DNA synthesis and cell proliferation, deplete estrogen receptors, and increase the conversion of E_2 to the less potent estrone sulfate. These effects will induce maturation of the endometrium, healing of superficial breaks, enhancement of the stromal matrix with increased structural stability, and cessation of bleeding. Withdrawal of the progestin after adequate exposure results in orderly and uniform shedding of the endometrium with a finite self-limited bleed. The progestin dosage and duration of therapy must induce a complete secretory transformation; otherwise, complete inhibition of all estrogenic effects will fail, and islands of proliferative endometrium will remain.

Whitehead and colleagues have shown that postmenopausal estrogen replacement mimics the unopposed estrogen environment of chronic anovulation, and that 4% of patients develop endometrial hyperplasia with only 7 days of progestin exposure, 2% with 10 days of exposure, and 0% with 12 days of exposure. They recommend 12 days of progestin every month to counteract the estrogen proliferative effects. Medroxyprogesterone acetate, 10 mg, or norethindrone acetate, 5 mg per day, may be prescribed. After initial control of the dysfunctional bleeding, the 12-day course can be repeated at monthly intervals to prevent the development of hyperplasia. It is convenient to start each new course on the first day of each month. A regular withdrawal can be expected to start either during the last 2 days of progestin or within several days of the last dose.

Failure to withdraw could signify pregnancy, development of a hypoestrogenic state, or, rarely, induction of ovulation by progestin stimulation of the estrogen-primed patient. In such a case of endogenous progesterone production, the menses can be delayed 2 weeks. A word of caution: This regimen is not contraceptive.

An alternative method for delivery of a progestin to control dysfunctional bleeding and menorrhagia is local administration with a progestin-impregnated IUD. Numerous studies have demonstrated significant reductions in menstrual blood loss in patients using the progestin-impregnated IUD. Xiao and colleagues showed reductions of more than 80% at up to 36 months. Irvine and associates performed a randomized trial of 44 women with menorrhagia, comparing a levonorgestrel IUD with cyclic progestin therapy. The IUD group had blood loss reduced by 90%, along with higher patient satisfaction, compliance, and continuation. A comparison of endometrial resection with the levonorgestrel IUD showed highly significant decreases in menstrual blood loss with both treatment arms (Rauramo et al.). The incidence of complications was similar in both groups, and 3-year follow-up rates were similar. Seventeen percent of the resection group required follow-up surgery. Other studies have shown a significant cost benefit to use of the levonorgestrel IUD compared with surgical management of abnormal uterine bleeding, including hysterectomy. As noted earlier, the levonorgestrel IUD has also shown to be effective in controlling menorrhagia in patients with hemostatic disorders such as von Willebrand disease.

Chronic unopposed estrogen can produce a very lush endometrium that can bleed heavily during progestin withdrawal. Speroff and colleagues recommend treatment using combination oral contraceptives in a step-down regimen. Two to four pills are given daily, one every 6 to 12 hours, for 5 to 7 days for acute control of bleeding. This will usually control acute bleeding within 24 to 48 hours, allowing time to complete the diagnostic evaluation. Withdrawal of medication will result in a heavy bleed. On the fifth day of this bleed, a low-dose cyclic oral contraceptive is started and repeated for three cycles to allow orderly regression of the excessive proliferative endometrium. Alternatively, the dosage of combination pills can be tapered (four times a day, then three times a day, then two times a day) over 3 to 6 days and then continued at one pill every day. Combination oral contraceptives induce atrophy of the endometrium because the chronic estrogen–progestin exposure suppresses pituitary gonadotropins and inhibits endogenous steroidogenesis. They are useful for long-term management of DUB in patients without contraindications and have the added benefit of pregnancy prevention. Particularly in perimenarchal patients, heavy prolonged bleeding can denude the basal endometrium and make it unresponsive to progestins. Curettage for control of hemorrhage is contraindicated because of a high risk of development of intrauterine synechiae (Asherman syndrome) if the basalis is curetted. High-dose intravenous estrogen (conjugated estrogens 25 mg every 4 hours until bleeding abates) will give acute control by proliferative repair of the endometrium and by direct effects on coagulation, including increased fibrinogen and platelet aggregation. Megestrol 20 mg twice daily is also an excellent method for obtaining acute control of abnormal uterine bleeding without the side effects of intravenous estrogen treatment. It will be effective in any situation other than one in which the entire endometrium has sloughed, leaving only basalis. A progestin alone or oral conjugated estrogens in combination with a progestin can then be used to induce orderly withdrawal bleeding.

Hysteroscopy of patients who fail to respond to hormonal therapy may reveal previously missed pathology, such as a submucous myoma or polyp. These diagnoses are particularly common in patients with ovulatory dysfunctional bleeding. If a diagnostic curettage has not been previously performed, one can be performed in conjunction with the hysteroscopy, both for diagnosis and for temporary therapy. If atypical hyperplasia has been identified and preservation of fertility is desired, more aggressive progestin therapy is recommended. Medroxyprogesterone acetate, 30 mg, or megestrol, 20 to 40 mg, daily for 3 months should be monitored by repeat endometrial sampling to assess the efficiency of the medical treatment (Fig. 26.2B). If atypical hyperplasia persists, very high-dose progestin protocols can be tried, but hysterectomy must be considered.

Menorrhagia can be reduced when prostaglandin E_2 and prostacyclin synthesis are decreased by nonsteroidal antiinflammatory medications. These drugs inhibit the cyclooxygenase enzyme necessary for endometrial production of prostaglandin under estrogen stimulation and thus alter the relative production of the proaggregation vasoconstrictor thromboxane A_2 and the antiaggregation vasodilator prostacyclin. Pathology studies have confirmed that this improves both platelet aggregation and vasoconstriction. Fraser and colleagues (1981) demonstrated these compounds to be most effective when given in therapeutic dosages for 7 to 10 days before the expected onset of the next menstrual period in ovulatory DUB patients, but they are commonly started with the onset of menses and continued throughout the bleeding episode with good success.

For coagulation disorders, 1-desamino-8-D-arginine vasopressin (also known as desmopressin, or simply DDAVP) increases coagulation factor VIII with a therapeutic effect lasting about 6 hours. It is best administered intravenously, 0.3 μg/kg in 50 mL saline over 15 to 30 minutes, but can be used intranasally. Antifibrinolytic agents such as ϵ-aminocaproic acid and tranexamic acid can decrease blood loss up to 50%, but their significant central nervous system and gastrointestinal side effects and the purported risk of intracranial arterial thrombosis have traditionally limited their applicability. New data do not support a significant thrombotic risk, and traxenamic acid is widely available in Europe for use in menorrhagia. Ergot derivatives are ineffective for treatment of menorrhagia. Local delivery of progestational agents by way of an intrauterine device has been demonstrated by Milsom and colleagues to be extremely effective, with more than a 90% reduction in bleeding in some patients. This has the potential to provide long-term therapy for patients with chronic bleeding unresponsive to other therapies.

Long-acting derivatives of GnRH agonists down-regulate pituitary synthesis of FSH and LH and induce "medical castration." Withdrawal of endogenous steroid stimulation will result in endometrial atrophy. Various delivery options are available, including intranasal delivery, daily subcutaneous delivery, monthly intramuscular depot, and subcutaneously implanted pellet analog. GnRH agonists are not effective in acute control of abnormal bleeding. At least 2 to 4 weeks are required for adequate suppression of gonadotropin production and inhibition of steroidogenesis. Long-term therapy can effectively control blood loss with chronic DUB secondary to chronic systemic illness, thrombocytopenia, or other coagulopathies. Because of the profoundly hypoestrogenic state induced by these drugs, there is accelerated bone resorption and the risk of development of significant osteoporosis. Therefore, long-term therapy requires "add-back" treatment with an estrogen-progestin combination to prevent bone loss. GnRH agonists can also be used as adjuncts for endometrial preparation before endometrial ablation.

Ablation or destruction of the endometrium has been advocated for treatment of chronic abnormal bleeding unresponsive to medical management in the presence of a normal endometrial cavity and the absence of submucous leiomyomata, endometrial hyperplasia, or neoplasia. Although there has been significant disagreement regarding the appropriate indications for this procedure, it has been widely applied with varying success. The original methods included use of hysteroscopy with the Nd:YAG laser, electrosurgical roller-ball cauterization, or endomyometrial resection using a loop electrode. These hysteroscopic surgical techniques require special training. More recently, new techniques have been described to ablate the endometrial cavity without the requirement for hysteroscopy. These include thermal balloon ablation, direct instillation of heated saline, cryoablation with a cryoprobe, microwave endometrial ablation, and use of radiofrequency electromagnetic energy (Corson et al.; O'Connor and Magos; Rutherford et al.; Sharp et al.; Singer et al.; Weisberg et al.). Success rates reported with the various techniques have ranged from 60% to 95% of patients achieving either hypomenorrhea or amenorrhea. Pretreatment with danazol, GnRH analogs, or suction curettage to thin the endometrium appears to improve long-term success rates (Brooks; Donnez et al.). Seeras and Gilliland reported resumption of menstruation in 44% of women after ablation if they had not received preoperative endometrial suppression.

A number of comparison studies have looked at success rates of the various techniques to determine relative efficacy, complication rates, and relative cost. Meyer and colleagues compared roller-ball ablation with thermal balloon ablation in a prospective, randomized trial. A greater percentage of women in the roller-ball group (27.2%) were amenorrheic at their 12-month follow-up than were women in the uterine balloon group (15.2%). The rates of hypomenorrhea plus amenorrhea were not significantly different (balloon, 80.2%; roller ball, 84.3%). Overall patient satisfaction was equivalent. The complication rate was 3.2% in the hysteroscopic roller-ball group with no significant intraoperative complications in the thermal balloon group. A comparison of thermal balloon ablation with the progestin-containing IUD showed similar results as far as overall satisfaction; however, bleeding scores were lower and amenorrhea rates higher in the IUD group (Busfield et al.). Corson, with follow-up by Goldrath, performed a prospective randomized trial of endometrial ablation using the Hydro ThermAblator (HTA; Boston Scientific Corporation, Natick, MA, USA) versus roller ball (Figs. 26.3 and 26.4). This system uses heated saline flowing free under low pressure to ablate the endometrium under hysteroscopic guidance. Success rates for both groups were comparable at 3 years with amenorrhea rates of 53% for HTA and 46% for roller ball, and overall satisfaction rates of 98% and 97%, respectively. There were no significant differences in complication rates or repeat surgical procedures.

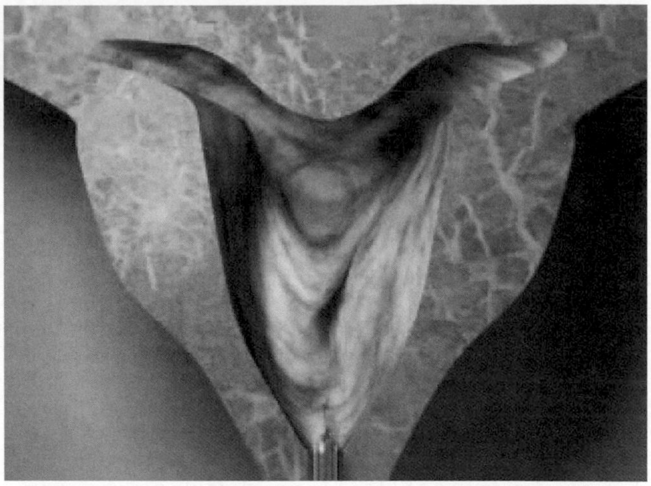

FIGURE 26.3. Hydro ThermAblator (HTA; Boston Scientific Corporation, Natick, MA, USA).

The Novasure system (Cytyc Corporation, Palo Alto, CA, USA) uses radiofrequency current through a mesh electrode that conforms to the endometrial cavity to ablate the endometrium. Tissue desiccation is rapid compared with thermal devices and requires no pretreatment of the endometrium. The overall success rate of 88.3% and amenorrhea rate of

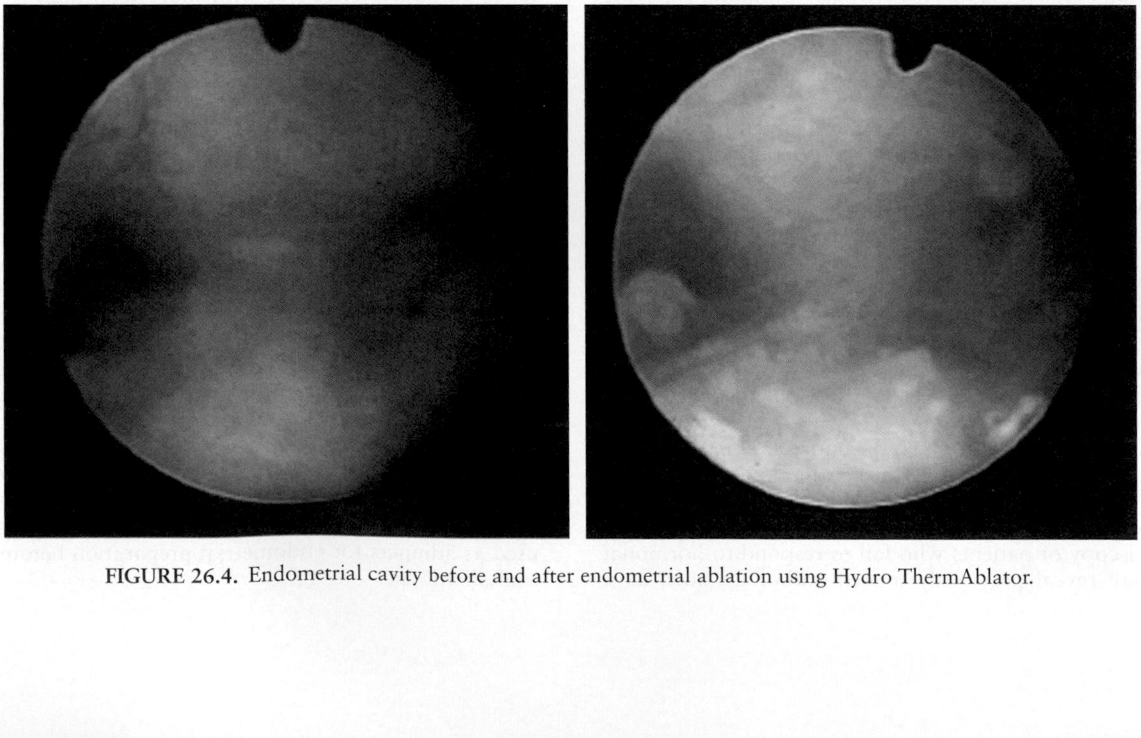

FIGURE 26.4. Endometrial cavity before and after endometrial ablation using Hydro ThermAblator.

41% for Novasure-treated patients were higher than 81.7% and 35% rates, respectively, for endometrial resection in a randomized trial (Cooper et al.). A randomized trial versus Hydro ThermAblation also demonstrated higher amenorrhea rates (Bongers et al.). Microwave energy can also be used to ablate endometrium. The MEA (Microsulis Americas, Pampano Beach, FL, USA) device was tested in a prospective randomized trial comparing it with roller-ball ablation (Cooper et al.). Success rates were 87% and 83.2%, respectively, for MEA and roller ball. Amenorrhea rates were 61.3% for MEA and 51% for the roller-ball group. This trial also included patients with up to 3-cm submucous myomas. Subgroup analysis did not show any difference in the success rate in this group.

Endomyometrial resection has been reported to have higher amenorrhea rates compared with rates for other techniques (Kooy et al.). Vercellini and colleagues compared myometrial resection with endometrial ablation using a vaporizing electrode similar to a roller ball. Amenorrhea rates were 48% for the endomyometrial resection group and 36% for the ablation group, although overall patient satisfaction rates were equivalent. Difficulty of surgery and mean fluid deficit were both described as greater in the resection group. Comparison of endometrial ablation with laser versus endomyometrial resection showed equivalent amenorrhea rates of approximately 45%, with overall patient satisfaction rates of 90% (Battacharya et al.).

Operative hysteroscopic techniques require specialized training, and complications, although relatively infrequent, can be significant. A multihospital survey in The Netherlands reported an overall complication rate for hysteroscopy of 0.28% (Jansen et al.). Diagnostic hysteroscopy had a significantly lower complication rate than that of operative hysteroscopy (0.13% vs. 0.95%). The most frequent surgical complication was uterine perforation (0.76%). Reported complication rates for hysteroscopic ablation procedures are significantly higher. O'Connor and Magos followed 525 women for up to 5 years after endometrial resection. They reported a 6% incidence of intraoperative complications and a 3% incidence of postoperative complications. They also reported a 15% complication rate in patients who required a repeat ablative procedure. The "Mistletoe" survey from the Royal College of Obstetricians and Gynaecologists recorded endomyometrial resection complication rates of 7.2% but only 4% for roller-ball and laser ablations (Overton et al.). A prospective trial of thermal balloon versus rollerball ablation reported intraoperative complications in 3.2% of the roller-ball patients but no significant intraoperative complications in the thermal balloon patients (Meyer et al.). Reported complications include uterine perforation with hemorrhage, laser or electrosurgical damage to the bowel, excessive absorption of distending medium with fluid overload, hyponatremia and pulmonary edema, and persistence of bleeding requiring repeat ablation or hysterectomy. The reported complication rates do compare favorably with reported morbidity rates for women undergoing hysterectomy, which range from 7% to 15% (Summitt et al.).

There is concern regarding the potential outcome of pregnancies conceived after endometrial ablation. A literature review (Cook and Seman) reports a miscarriage rate of 21.7%, a preterm rate of 26.1%, and a perinatal mortality rate of 11.8%. Of those pregnancies that continued beyond 20 weeks, 35.3% were described as having abnormal placental adherence, including placenta accreta and increta. The hysterectomy rate for this series of patients was 8.9%. These outcomes were attributed to the possible presence of intrauterine synechiae, although in most cases, no direct endometrial cavity assessment was done.

Another concern has been possible obliteration of warning signs heralding the development of endometrial carcinoma, with subsequent delay in diagnosis. Endometrial ablation procedures usually result in a narrowed tubular uterine cavity without the obliteration seen in Asherman syndrome, but are rarely expected to result in total ablation of all endometrial tissue. Several cases of postablation endometrial carcinoma have now been reported (Brooks-Carter et al., Copperman et al.). The cost of endometrial ablation does compare favorably with that of hysterectomy, with hysterectomy reported as 58% more expensive when all costs, including lost work time, are considered (Vilos et al.).

D&C is both diagnostic and therapeutic. Removal of the structurally fragile bleeding endometrium allows restoration of normal hemostatic events, with regeneration of the integrity of the endometrium and restoration of the normal proliferative response. If the patient fails to respond to medical therapy, repeated curettage, or even endometrial ablation, then more definitive therapy, such as hysterectomy, should be considered, taking into account the age of the patient and her desire for future childbearing. It has been estimated that 2 million women in the United States are seen annually with reports of excessive uterine bleeding, and about 150,000 undergo hysterectomy, which accounts for 20% to 30% of all hysterectomies performed.

In general, the ovulatory type of bleeding has the poorest response to replacement hormonal therapy and the highest incidence of recurrence. Although a hysterectomy can be considered an admission of therapeutic defeat, it is frequently an expeditious method of resolving this refractory and recurrent type of DUB. When bleeding persists after repeated curettage and cyclic hormonal therapy, hysterectomy may be required. If other conditions are present that should be corrected surgically, such as a relaxed vaginal outlet, rectocele, cystocele, or uterine descensus, we recommend vaginal hysterectomy with support of the vaginal vault and repair of the vaginal wall relaxation. When hysterectomy is indicated in premenopausal women younger than 50 years of age, normal ovarian tissue is conserved. In a patient younger than 30 years of age, radical surgical treatment should be strongly avoided; one can almost always control uterine bleeding by repeated curettage or by increasing amounts of cyclic hormone therapy. Today, the availability and use of estrogen and progesterone have changed the need for hysterectomy to treat DUB. Hysterectomy is not indicated in young women but may be indicated in older women when hormonal therapy and repeated curettage have failed.

Blood transfusions are seldom required when DUB is associated with anemia, but they may be given if the anemia is so severe that symptoms are present. Oral iron therapy should be started at the first sign of heavy menstruation to prevent depletion of iron stores, and it should be given for 3 to 6 months after normal hemoglobin and hematocrit levels have been restored in patients with iron-deficiency anemia.

PERIMENOPAUSAL AND POSTMENOPAUSAL BLEEDING

When uterine bleeding occurs more than 12 months after the last regular menstrual period, it is defined as postmenopausal bleeding. For a period varying from months to years before menopause, the individual patient may experience irregular patterns of bleeding. Often the first sign is a shortening of the menstrual interval secondary to premature elevation in FSH, followed by intermittent periods of amenorrhea

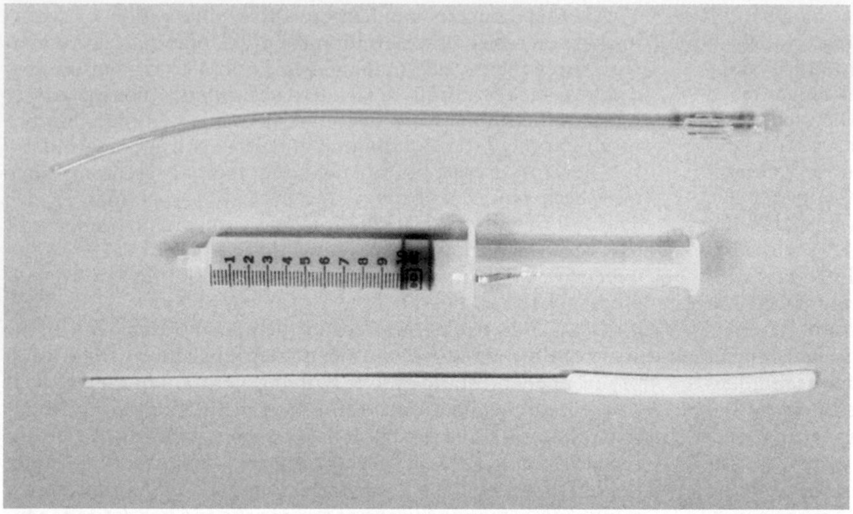

FIGURE 26.5. An endometrial suction sampling (UTER CYTE) instrument with syringe vacuum.

alternating with heavy bleeding consistent with oligoovulation or anovulation. With this clinical picture, special consideration must be given to ruling out a neoplastic process as the source of the bleeding. The first diagnostic consideration is to ensure that the bleeding originates from the uterus. In elderly women especially, bleeding from the urethra or rectum may be reported as vaginal bleeding. Vaginal or cervical lesions causing the bleeding should be diagnosed readily with careful inspection or biopsy. Cancers of the vagina or cervix or cervical polyps can also be readily diagnosed and appropriate treatment rendered.

When the source of the bleeding is determined to be the uterine cavity, sampling of the endometrium for pathology examination is usually considered to be mandatory. Although D&C continues to be a commonly performed procedure for both its diagnostic and therapeutic benefits, office endometrial biopsy can often expedite appropriate evaluation and therapy. Many instruments have been devised for the sampling of endometrial tissue and evaluation of the endometrial cavity. The standard instrument used for many years has been the Novak curet. Although this curet was initially devised to obtain a sample of the endometrium by suction and aspiration, it is most commonly used as a miniature curet that contains a serrated edge surrounding its biopsy aperture. The curet is about 5 mm in diameter and can usually be passed without dilatation through a small cervical canal, even in nulliparous women. Occasionally, the postmenopausal cervical canal is stenotic and difficult to penetrate. Because of the discomfort associated with passage of the Novak curet, newer Silastic curets have been developed. These have a smaller diameter (3 mm), are flexible, and are often better tolerated by patients. They can be difficult to pass through a truly stenotic cervix because of their pliability. Often there is an accompanying syringe that attaches and develops effective vacuum pressure to improve the size of the sample obtained (Fig. 26.5). A four-quadrant endometrial biopsy with passes along the anterior and posterior and both lateral walls of the endometrial cavity is recommended for diagnosis of abnormal bleeding. Another potentially useful device not requiring a syringe to develop negative pressure is a disposable plastic tube with a 3.1-mm outer diameter, an aspiration port, and solid plastic obturator at its tip. The obturator fits so closely that its slow withdrawal from the uterine cavity causes sufficient suction to obtain an adequate endometrial specimen in most cases (Fig. 26.6). However, the endometrial surface area sampled is small (5%) and can easily miss polyps, submucous myomas, and endometrial carcinoma that occupies only a small portion of the endometrial cavity (Guido et al.). Because of the small aperture of this device and its almost total reliance on suction to obtain a specimen, the architecture of the obtained biopsy may be somewhat distorted.

Vacuum suction curettage has gained some popularity as an office procedure for endometrial sampling that does not require general anesthesia. A small metal or plastic cannula with an outside diameter of 3 mm that has a slightly curved tip and an opening on the concave surface for easier insertion through a small endocervical canal is connected to a plastic collection chamber, which in newer models is a large syringe rather than the old pumps or faucets. Several studies have compared the results of suction curettage with those of regular curettage under anesthesia in the same patient. Cohen and colleagues

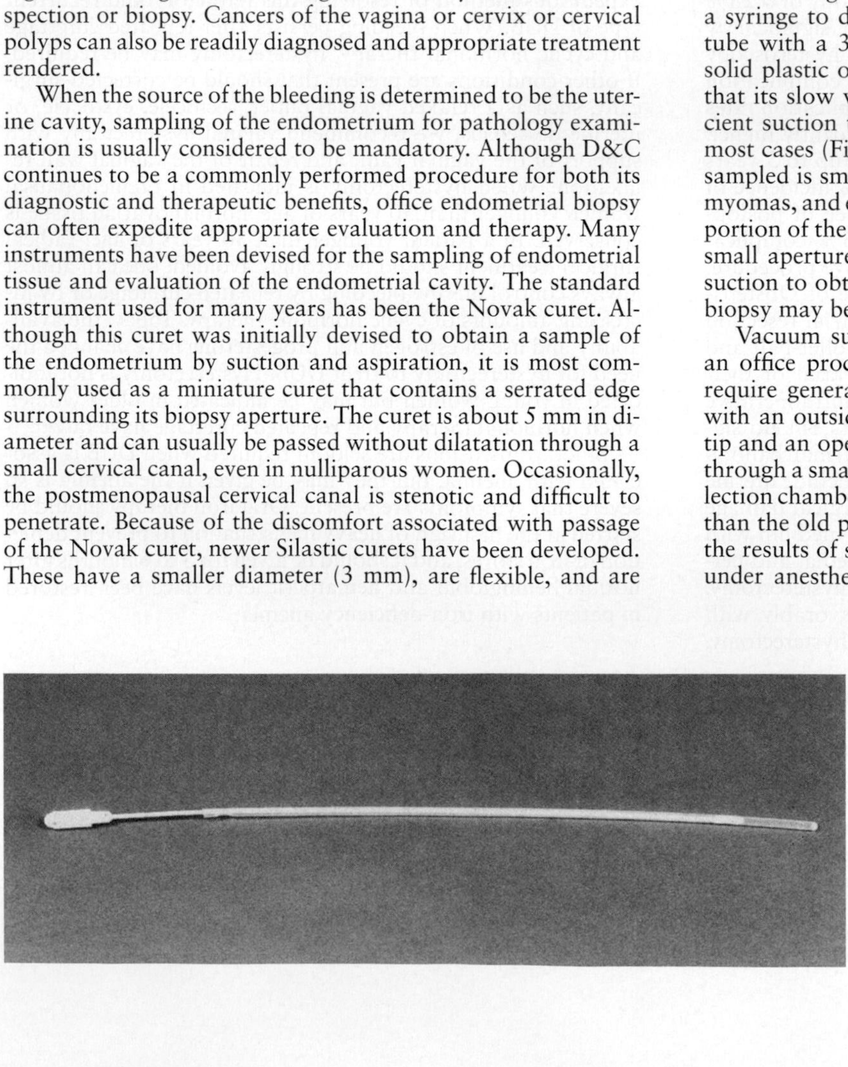

FIGURE 26.6. A useful suction endometrial sampling Pipelle instrument, with 3.1 mm in outside diameter and no pump or syringe required.

studied 98 patients; in 93, they found identical histologic patterns with both methods. In five patients, there was no correlation between the results of the two techniques, and none of these had cancer. At the Medical University of South Carolina, Lutz and colleagues found suction curettage to be 98% accurate in evaluating high-risk women with abnormal bleeding for endometrial malignant disease.

These new tools require little or no cervical dilatation and permit almost painless endometrial sampling. A quick-acting, nonsteroidal antiinflammatory drug (e.g., 550 mg naproxen sodium) administered 15 to 30 minutes before curetting provides satisfactory analgesia for most patients. If dilatation of the cervix is required, paracervical block anesthesia can be initiated by injecting 4 to 5 mL of 1% lidocaine at the 3-o'clock and 9-o'clock positions in the paracervical tissues, exercising care to avoid intravascular injection.

The principal value of an endometrial biopsy is that a formal D&C under anesthesia has been avoided if the removed tissue contains adenocarcinoma. If the cause of postmenopausal bleeding is not identified in a screening endometrial biopsy, however, then a standard curettage is obligatory. In office biopsies of the endometria of more than 20,000 patients of all ages, Hofmeister detected 273 cases of endometrial carcinoma, 32 of which (14.28%) were totally asymptomatic. The endometrial carcinoma detection rate was 1.76% of the total group of 23,202 patients. Hofmeister's routine office endometrial biopsies using a modification of the Novak and Randall curet provide one of the largest clinical experiences of this instrument to date. Unfortunately, only patients who had continued uterine bleeding or who demonstrated an atypical pattern in the office biopsy were subjected to a complete curettage. Therefore, the true-negative and false-negative rate for the Novak type of curet in the detection of endometrial cancer has not been determined accurately. In other studies, summarized by Cohen and colleagues, the accuracy of detection of endometrial cancer by endometrial curettage varied from 76% to 92%. However, a thorough endometrial curettage under anesthesia is also not infallible in the detection of endometrial cancer. Bettocchi and colleagues evaluated the diagnostic accuracy of endometrial curettage in 397 patients. D&C failed to detect intrauterine pathology in 62.5% of patients, including four cases of complex hyperplasia and five cases of endometrial adenocarcinoma as well as many endometrial polyps and submucous myomas.

Vaginal ultrasound has been investigated as a screening tool in patients with postmenopausal bleeding. The average thickness of the postmenopausal endometrial stripe has been reported as 2.3 + 1.8 mm, with a range of 0 to 10 mm, in a series of 300 asymptomatic women. Twenty-two had endometrial stripes of 5 mm or larger, and all had benign pathology. In a series of 51 cases of postmenopausal bleeding, Nasri and colleagues reported that if the endometrial thickness was less than 5 mm, the pathology would show either inactive or no endometrial tissue. Karlsson and associates reported on 1,168 women with postmenopausal bleeding. Patients with an endometrial echo of less than 4 mm had a sensitivity of 96% and a specificity of 68% for detecting endometrial pathology. If a 5-mm cutoff was used, two endometrial carcinomas would have been missed. In another study by Gull and colleagues, 198 women screened for postmenopausal bleeding had an endometrial thickness of 5 mm or greater. Endometrial sampling diagnosed 36 primary endometrial cancers, one metastatic breast cancer, and three cases of atypical endometrial hyperplasia. Of 163 women with an endometrial stripe of 4 mm or less, only one was found to have endometrial cancer. Other series have shown that an endometrial thickness of greater than 8 mm is an indication for endometrial sampling, regardless of whether there is a report of bleeding. This will detect most, if not all, endometrial cancers. A metaanalysis reviewing the accuracy of transvaginal sonography reported that 96% of women with endometrial cancer and 92% of women with other endometrial diseases had an endometrial echo of greater than 5 mm (Smith-Bindman et al.). The false-positive rate was dependent on the use of hormone replacement therapy, with nonusers having a false-positive risk of 8%, whereas those on hormones had a 23% false-positive rate. SIS can be used to further evaluate patients with thickened endometrial stripes to detect structural problems such as polyps as an adjunct to endometrial sampling. Although the exact indications for patient screening and parameters for follow-up need to be more precisely defined, vaginal ultrasound appears to have promise as a noninvasive method for evaluating the postmenopausal patient.

Office hysteroscopy using new smaller-diameter flexible or rigid hysteroscopes is growing in popularity because it enables selective biopsy of the areas of visualized endometrium that appear most likely to contain a neoplastic process. A blind endometrial biopsy that reveals benign endometrial histology does not absolutely preclude the presence of a malignant process elsewhere within the endometrium. A neoplastic transformation in the endometrium is often a focal abnormality. Another major advantage of hysteroscopy is the diagnosis of endometrial polyps, submucous myomas, or other sources of bleeding that may not always be identified by endometrial biopsy or conventional curettage. In a series of 110 cases of postmenopausal bleeding, the causes of 95 were identified as endometrial polyps or submucous myomas. Only two cases of early adenocarcinoma were identified. Operative hysteroscopy, endometrial ablation, or both successfully controlled bleeding in most cases of benign disease. In cases of postmenopausal uterine bleeding, the recommended diagnostic procedures may or may not produce a tissue sample of endometrium. It is not uncommon to obtain no tissue from patients with marked hypertension or from patients undergoing chronic anticoagulant therapy. This lack of tissue is also consistent with bleeding from an atrophic endometrium, which is a benign condition. When endometrium is present, a wide range of histology can be observed. Occasionally, simple proliferative endometrium is found. The endometrium can exhibit simple hyperplasia, more marked adenomatous hyperplasia, or hyperplasia with atypical cells, resulting in a diagnosis of atypical endometrial hyperplasia. Later in the menopausal years, it is not uncommon for the endometrium to have the characteristics of cystic hyperplasia, often referred to in the older literature as "Swiss cheese hyperplasia."

Hormone-induced postmenopausal uterine bleeding can be the result of endogenous or exogenous hormonal effects. The proliferation of endometrium in a patient who is not receiving exogenous hormonal therapy is generally attributed to endogenous production of estrone. Estrone is the peripheral conversion product of the weak androgenic precursor androstenedione (85% from adrenal, 15% from ovary), and its synthesis occurs primarily in adipose tissue. In the absence of exogenous hormonal therapy, one must also exclude the possibility of an estrogen-producing ovarian tumor (granulosis cell tumor).

Management of perimenopausal bleeding in the absence of significant hyperplasia or neoplasia is essentially the same as for DUB in a younger patient. One recently accepted method that in the past was proscribed is the use of low-dose oral contraceptives. The Food and Drug Administration has approved them for patients older than 40 years of age in the absence of specific contraindications, such as hypertension, hyperlipidemia, and smoking. They provide excellent cycle control with a monthly withdrawal bleed and suppression of the endometrium. Oral contraceptives can be continued until an FSH level greater than 40 IU/L during the week of placebo pills confirms ovarian failure. Standard postmenopausal hormone replacement can then be used. A sequential program of 12 days of progestin, 5 to 10 mg medroxyprogesterone acetate, or 5 mg norethindrone acetate on a monthly basis is an alternative and is continued until failure of withdrawal bleeding occurs, indicating the need for estrogen replacement. Because recent studies indicate that perimenopausal patients are relatively hypoestrogenic and can be at risk for accelerated bone loss before the actual onset of menopause, some clinicians recommend concurrent estrogen replacement even in the perimenopausal patient.

Endometrial hyperplasia requires a more aggressive progestational regimen. Atypical adenomatous endometrial hyperplasia is considered by most to be the equivalent of an intraepithelial malignancy, and hysterectomy is often advised. Management of several types of endometrial hyperplasia other than atypical adenomatous hyperplasia can generally be accomplished by monthly administration of a progestin such as medroxyprogesterone acetate, 10 mg per day for 12 days, or norethindrone acetate, 5 mg per day for 12 days. Another endometrial biopsy should be obtained within 3 to 6 months to assess for resolution of the hyperplasia. A more aggressive hormonal regimen uses continuous high-dose progestin for 3 to 6 months (i.e., megestrol, 20 to 160 mg per day).

Any of the regimens currently in use for postmenopausal hormonal replacement therapy can cause uterine bleeding. Unopposed estrogen is no longer recommended for postmenopausal hormone replacement in the case of an intact uterus because hyperplasia develops in 18% to 32% of cases and because unopposed estrogen has an up to sevenfold increased risk of endometrial carcinoma. Cyclic estrogen-progestin regimens significantly decrease this risk to less than 1% with 12 days of progestin. There are numerous dosage regimens for the use of conjugated estrogens, 0.625 to 1.25 mg; micronized E_2, 1 to 2 mg; esterified estrogens, 0.625 to 1.25 mg; and E_2 patches. Although estrogen replacement therapy performs well if used for only 21 to 25 days of the month, there is no clinical reason for its discontinuance, and recent recommendations are to continue it throughout the entire cycle. The progestin regimens are those that have already been outlined. The bleeding that accompanies these commonly used continuous-estrogen and cyclic-progestin regimens should occur predictably, at the conclusion of the progestin phase of the cyclic administration. Most investigators of the subject now agree that the predictable and appropriately timed withdrawal bleeding that occurs with these regimens does not require sampling for endometrial histology. Continuous daily regimens of estrogen and low-dose progestin replacement therapy (i.e., conjugated estrogen, 0.625 mg, and medroxyprogesterone acetate, 2.5 mg) are commonly accompanied by irregular bleeding patterns for at least 4 to 8 months after initiation of the regimen. They are used with the anticipation that over months of use, the proportion of women becoming completely amenorrheic will increase, and for most women, the long-term benefits with these regimens will outweigh those of the conventional cyclic regimen, in which most women bleed regularly at the conclusion of the progestin phase of the cycle for at least 6 to 24 months. As a general rule, just as intermenstrual bleeding during the regular menstruating years dictates investigation and management, so do patterns of postmenopausal bleeding not following an anticipated schedule require investigation and management.

The most important point about the significance of postmenopausal bleeding is its frequent association with gynecologic malignancy, particularly endometrial carcinoma. Although the incidence of malignancy to explain postmenopausal bleeding has decreased in recent decades, diagnostic efforts must carefully consider and rule out possible malignancy by use of appropriate diagnostic procedures, especially careful pelvic examination and uterine curettage. An endometrial biopsy is helpful for the diagnosis of suspected endometrial carcinoma only if the biopsy is positive. The definitive method for obtaining adequate histology for diagnosis is D&C.

DILATATION OF THE CERVIX

Recamier invented the curet in 1943. Since then, dilatation of the cervix with curettage of the endometrial cavity has become the second most frequently performed gynecologic procedure in the United States. Curettage is used to diagnose uterine malignancy, to complete an incomplete or missed abortion, to evaluate the causes of infertility, to relieve dysmenorrhea, and to control DUB. Improved medical therapies for DUB and dysmenorrhea have made dilatation of the cervix and curettage of the uterus less necessary for these two problems, especially in young women.

Dilatation of the cervix is performed as a preliminary step to curettage of the uterine cavity. As a therapeutic measure, it is used for acquired or congenital cervical stenosis, for dysmenorrhea, for introduction of intracervical and intrauterine radium or cesium, occasionally for insertion of an intrauterine contraceptive device, or for allowing drainage of the uterine cavity in the presence of pyometra, as well as a part of other operations on the cervix.

Most indications for cervical dilatation are obvious. In connection with primary dysmenorrhea, however, there is room for controversy. It is a recognized fact that many cases of primary dysmenorrhea are not cured by cervical dilatation. Because of frequent failures, some gynecologists have almost abandoned it as a therapeutic technique. We do not subscribe totally to this pessimistic point of view. Unfortunately, in most instances, it is impossible to detect those cases of dysmenorrhea that will be relieved by cervical dilatation. Often the operation must be performed as a therapeutic test, but it is fortunately such a minor procedure that its performance is justified on that basis. In nulliparous women in whom pain is greatest just before or during the early part of the menstrual flow, there is a possibility of relief from the pain by cervical dilatation. The result is unpredictable, however, and we advise permitting the patient to decide whether menstrual pain is sufficiently severe to justify an operation that is of limited or possibly no benefit.

Ibuprofen, naproxen sodium, and mefenamic acid have proved to be so effective in the management of dysmenorrhea that a thorough trial of these agents is indicated. It is now evident that endometriosis can occur much earlier than was once believed; dysmenorrhea unrelieved by these nonsteroidal antiinflammatory drugs or oral contraceptives should be considered an indication for laparoscopy.

Postmenopausal Cervical Stenosis

In cases of postmenopausal cervical stenosis, pyometra may be discovered by uterus sounding. The pus should be cultured for anaerobic and aerobic organisms, and the cervix should be dilated. A short, soft, rubber or plastic tube can be sutured in place to keep the cervical canal open while the uterine cavity is draining. Although antibiotics may not be strictly necessary in all cases, fever and pelvic pain and tenderness herald the onset of spreading pelvic infection.

Curetting a pyometra can produce parametritis or wider pelvic cellulitis. Because the risk of perforation, with the potential for development of serious peritonitis, is increased during curettage, it should be delayed until adequate drainage has occurred (3 to 10 days, depending on the magnitude of the pyometra), and antibiotic therapy should be used. Curettage is mandatory to exclude the endocervical or endometrial malignancies frequently associated with pyometra.

Technique of Cervical Dilatation

The patient is placed on the table in the lithotomy position. A careful pelvic examination locates the position of the uterine corpus, and the vagina and the perineum are cleaned with the usual vaginal preparation of povidone-iodine (Betadine). The cervix is grasped with a four-pronged tenaculum (Fig. 26.7A) and gently drawn toward the vaginal outlet. I favor the straight Jacobs clamp, especially when difficult dilatation is either anticipated or encountered. It is much less likely to cause cervical laceration than is the single-tooth tenaculum. A sound (Fig. 26.7B) is passed carefully through the cervical canal into the uterine cavity to avoid creating a false passage. Resistance is greatest at the internal cervical os. Occasionally, a fine silver probe is needed for finding the proper passage if the canal is stenotic. Passing the uterine sound provides confirmatory information about the position of the uterus, the length of the uterine cavity, and the angulation between the cervical canal and the uterine cavity. The degree of stenosis of the cervical canal can be detected in this manner. Sounding the uterus is contraindicated in the presence of a pregnancy because of the increased risk of perforating the soft myometrium.

The cervical canal is dilated with a small Hegar dilator (Fig. 26.8). The uterine wall can be perforated by improper passage of the dilator; the cause usually is lack of knowledge or disregard of the position of the uterus. When acute anteflexion is present, the dilator can perforate posteriorly (Fig. 26.9). When retrodisplacement exists, the perforation usually occurs anteriorly (Fig. 26.10). These two complications can be avoided by sounding the uterine cavity before dilating the cervix and by following the direction of the endocervical canal and uterine cavity indicated by the sound. The dilator rarely perforates the fundus except when there is an atrophic postmenopausal uterus or when an invasive tumor or pregnancy has softened the uterine wall. After either the 3- or 4-mm Hegar dilator is passed, successively larger ones are used. For ordinary curettage, dilatation to 8 or 9 mm suffices. When the dilatation is for dysmenorrhea, we prefer to carry the dilatation up to 10 mm. Be aware of concerns that excessive dilatation can be associated with an incompetent cervix in a subsequent pregnancy. If cervical dilatation is difficult, half-size Hegar dilators with incremental diameters of 0.5 mm are useful (Fig. 26.8).

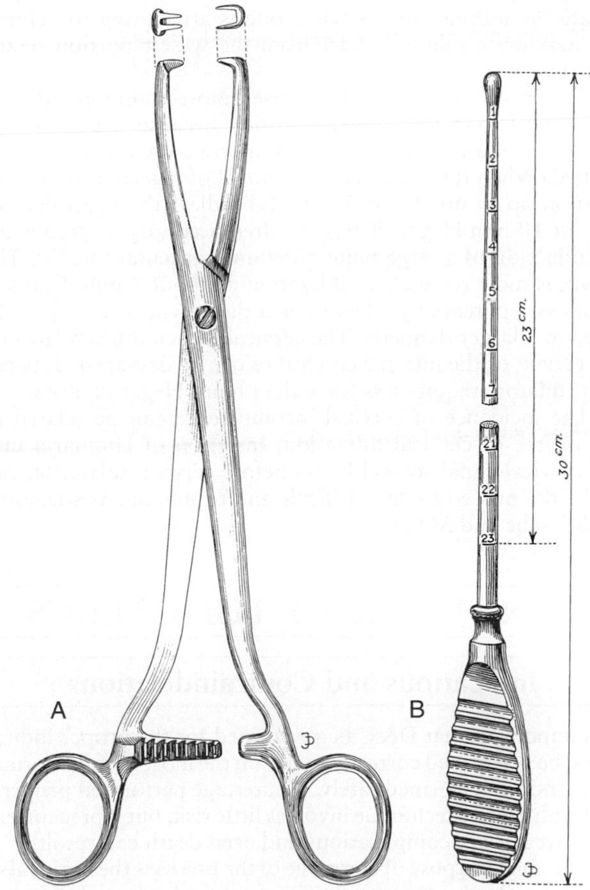

FIGURE 26.7. A: Straight Jacobs clamp, used for pulling down cervix when performing curettage. B: Uterine sound.

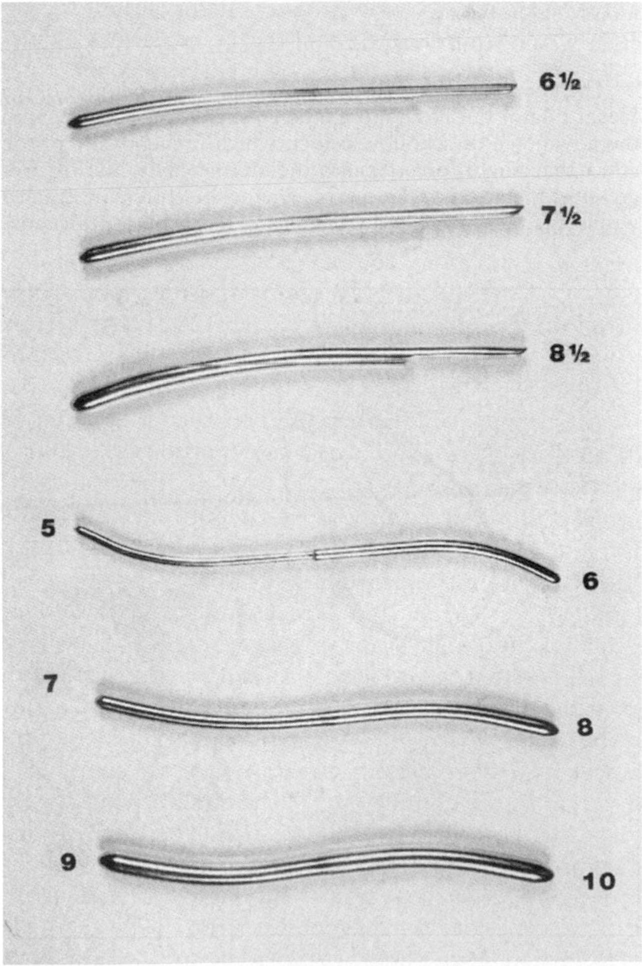

FIGURE 26.8. Graduated Hegar dilators and "half-size" Hegar dilators.

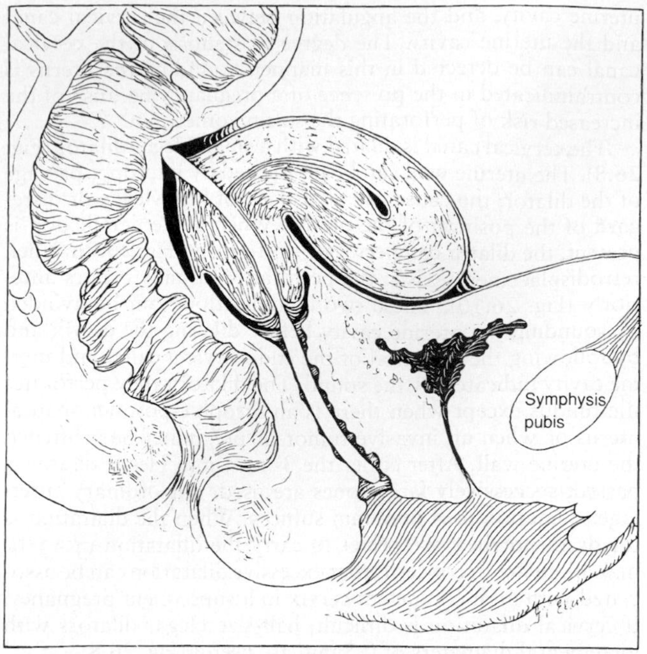

FIGURE 26.9. Perforation of the acutely anteflexed uterus. The uterus was thought to be in retroposition, and the Hegar dilator was erroneously directed posteriorly.

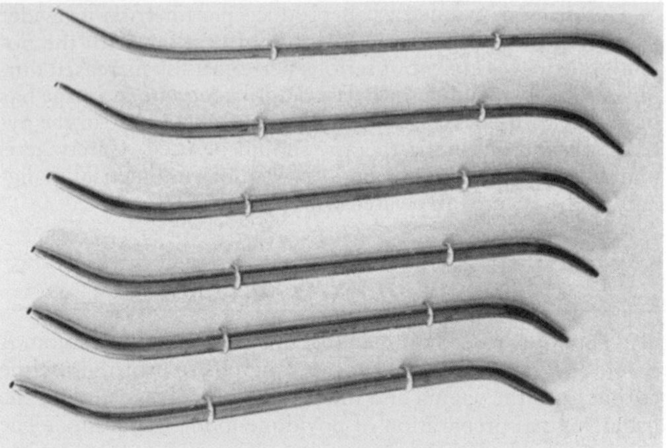

FIGURE 26.11. Hank-Bradley dilators in graduated sizes. Note central canal that extends through length of dilator.

The Hank-Bradley dilator has the shape and contour of the Hegar dilator but has a more tapered shank (Fig. 26.11), with the advantage of a hollow center, which prevents any piston effect that might force air into the uterine cavity during progressive dilatation of the cervix. The positive pressure created within the uterine cavity by passing a Hegar dilator can cause blood, endometrium, fragments of neoplastic tissue, or infected material to be forced into the fallopian tubes or peritoneal cavity. Beyth and colleagues have demonstrated that significant numbers of patients have endometrial tissue in their peritoneal fluid after curettage, and there is a possibility of reflux of endometrial carcinoma cells into the peritoneal cavity with forceful dilatation of a postmenopausal cervix harboring endometrial carcinoma. In the small postmenopausal uterus, however, it is quite easy for the tip of the Hank-Bradley dilator to perforate the uterine fundus when one is attempting to achieve the maximum dilating effect from the widest portion of the instrument.

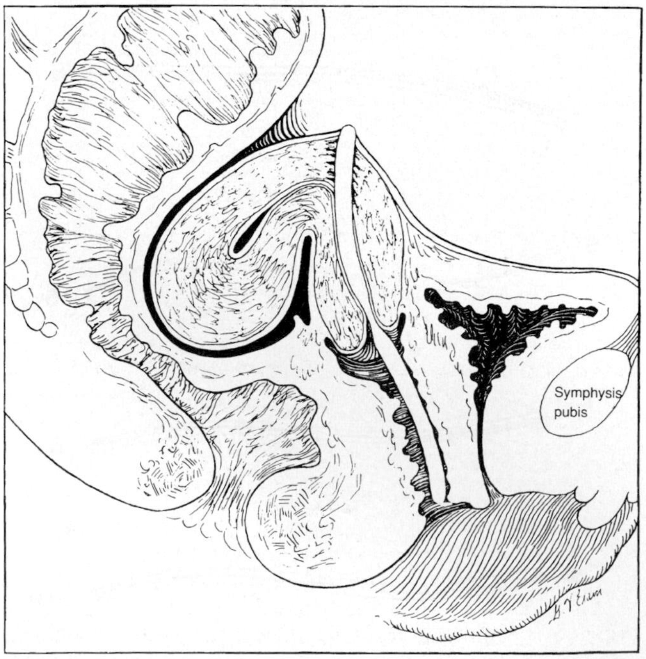

FIGURE 26.10. Perforation of the retroflexed uterus. The uterus was thought to be in anteposition, and the Hegar dilator was erroneously directed anteriorly.

The Hank-Bradley dilator is used more commonly during curettage for an incomplete abortion because it permits the release of blood through the dilator while the cervix is being dilated. When dilatation is for removal of placental tissue, dilatation up to no. 19 or 20 Hank-Bradley (the equivalent of a 9- or 10-mm Hegar dilator) is often necessary to permit the introduction of a large blunt curet and placental forceps. The cervix is most resistant to dilatation at about 8 mm. Cervical injury is a potential problem when the cervix is forcefully dilated to a larger diameter. The cervical tenaculum can lacerate the cervix, or the internal cervical os can be damaged. Tapered Pratt dilators require less force than blunt Hegar dilators.

The incidence of cervical incompetence can be related to the degree of cervical dilatation. Insertion of laminaria into the cervical canal several hours before cervical dilatation can make the procedure less difficult and traumatic, as suggested by Manabe and Manabe.

CURETTAGE OF THE UTERUS

Indications and Contraindications

It is important that D&C be performed for the proper indications, be performed correctly to obtain the most useful information, and be performed safely. A curettage performed properly and with aseptic technique involves little risk, but if precautions are disregarded, complications and even death can result.

The chief purpose of curettage of the uterus is the removal of endometrial or endocervical tissue for histologic study of cases of abnormal uterine bleeding. Although classical curettage of the uterus continues to be a useful procedure, new practices and instrumentation permit the procurement of endometrium as a screening diagnostic test under many circumstances. Appropriate use of such procedures can reduce significantly the need for operating room curettage. Careful pelvic examination under relaxation anesthesia has been an important adjunctive diagnostic aid to conventional D&C, but the precision and availability of ultrasound and other imaging techniques have brought them to the forefront of importance in diagnosis.

Outpatient Curettage

Over the years, there have been efforts to lower the cost of D&C by making it an outpatient procedure. In 1957, Vermeeren and associates presented a series of 10,000 minor gynecologic operations performed on an outpatient basis on the gynecology service at the Johns Hopkins Hospital. The results were more than satisfactory. These women were usually operated on under general anesthesia and were discharged after recovery from anesthesia. D&C was the operation most frequently performed. The success and safety of such a program depend, of course, on the careful selection of patients and the willingness of the practitioner to admit a patient for observation should complications occur. Today, D&C is often performed satisfactorily on an outpatient basis or in an ambulatory surgery center. Reports by Sandmire and Austin and by Martin and Rust are among many that record favorable experiences with this procedure.

As mentioned earlier, endometrial sampling today is often performed by biopsy, suction, or D&C as an office procedure. Although these relatively easy outpatient techniques for evaluating endometrium histology can often provide a correct diagnosis, they do not fulfill the requirement of a thorough curettage for absolute determination of the etiology of uterine bleeding. One can have total confidence in the biopsy or office curettage findings only if they show frank adenocarcinoma. If the histology of the office procedures is negative, one cannot rule out this serious condition. Even in the most experienced hands, endometrial carcinoma can be quite elusive. A further note of caution is that none of the office endometrial sampling methods can ensure the removal of an endometrial polyp. Therefore, endometrial carcinoma in a polyp could be missed, as could a polyp that is a source of benign bleeding. Office sampling techniques are used only as screening procedures; if the results are negative, a more thorough D&C under anesthesia is indicated. Office hysteroscopy can sometimes be an alternative to D&C to identify missed pathologies, such as a polyp or a submucous myoma, or to allow directed biopsy of a suspicious endometrium.

Indications for obtaining endometrial histology by one or more of the aforementioned methods include the following:

- Abnormal bleeding at any premenopausal age, especially when not corrected promptly by medical management, in women older than 35 years of age, or if a submucous myoma is suspected (include hysteroscopy or hysterosalpingography)
- Postmenopausal bleeding of any amount, regardless of a finding of atrophic vaginitis, polyp, or urethral caruncle
- Prehysterectomy in the postmenopausal woman to exclude endocervical or endometrial carcinoma
- Postmenopausal vaginal surgery without hysterectomy

When office procedures fail to establish the diagnosis, it is preferable to use a general anesthetic during D&C. The procedure is more comfortable for the patient and easier to perform with the patient fully relaxed, and most patients will opt for a general anesthetic for this procedure. A D&C under general anesthesia also provides an ideal opportunity for thorough examination of the pelvic organs. Before the examination, the bladder should be empty and an enema should have been given and expelled. The pelvic examination should be performed after the anterior abdominal wall is relaxed from the anesthesia and before the patient is draped. Occasionally, new and important pelvic findings will be discovered. In a study of 2,666 women requiring curettage, McElin and colleagues found unanticipated adnexal masses in 30 women during pelvic examination under anesthesia before D&C. Twenty-eight masses were benign, and two were malignant. When women who are serious medical risks require curettage for postmenopausal bleeding, the operation is performed without anesthetic other than hypodermic or intravenous administration of a sedative combined with paracervical nerve block.

A single curettage will not remove all of the surface endometrium completely from the uterine cavity. Repeated studies have demonstrated the inability of a thorough curettage to remove more than 50% to 60% of the endometrium when the procedure has been performed by experienced gynecologists immediately before a planned hysterectomy. Stock and Kanbour, from McGee Hospital in Pittsburgh, observed that in 60% of hysterectomy specimens studied, less than 50% of the endometrial surface had been removed by a prehysterectomy curettage. They also found 26 cases of endometrial carcinoma that had been classified as clinically normal-appearing tissue on prehysterectomy curettage; six of these carcinomas were reported as benign on frozen section. These facts and other similar experiences indicate that it is difficult to be certain of the histology of the endometrium by gross examination of the curetting. If the symptoms warrant a curettage, then the endometrium deserves a full histologic diagnosis.

Curettage is also performed for bleeding from a cervical stump and is frequently performed as part of a cervical conization to rule out extension of cervical carcinoma into the endometrium. Helmkamp and associates found no evidence of endometrial abnormality in any of 114 curettage specimens removed at the time of 114 cervical conizations. These investigators recommend that curettage at the time of cervical conization should not be performed routinely but should be performed selectively in postmenopausal and perimenopausal patients when the cytology smear shows abnormal glandular cells or when an intrauterine abnormality is suspected.

The chief contraindication to curettage is infection. Acute endometritis and salpingitis are conditions under which curettage should be avoided. If curettage is necessary for removal of infected placental tissue, it should be preceded by a period of parenteral antibiotic therapy adequate to achieve therapeutic tissue levels of antibiotics. Endometritis associated with retained products of conception will remain unresolved until the infected necrotic material is cast off spontaneously or until it is removed by the curet. Curettage is also contraindicated when pyometra is present.

Technique of Curettage of the Uterus

After the patient is anesthetized and placed in the lithotomy position, the bladder is emptied with a catheter. The pelvic organs are examined thoroughly before the patient is prepped and draped. The procedure includes a bimanual rectovaginal–abdominal examination. The examination under anesthesia is one of the most informative features of this operation because it can provide anatomic details of the reproductive tract that are unrecognizable without anesthesia. The vagina and perineum are cleaned with the usual technique.

Fractional curettage is an attempt to remove tissue samples from the endocervical canal apart from tissue removed from the endometrial cavity. The cervical canal should be curetted before dilatation of the cervical canal and curettage of the endometrial cavity. The special shape of the small Gusberg curet makes it particularly useful for curetting the endocervix. Differential curettage of the endocervix, separate from the endometrium, is important for diagnosis of endometrial carcinoma that may have extended to the endocervix. All cases of perimenopausal bleeding should be fractionally curetted; this procedure is too often neglected. If the endocervical curettage is not performed, a second fractional curettage is required to determine the anatomic boundaries of endometrial carcinoma. The value of fractional curettage has been questioned, but Chen and Lee and others have emphasized the importance of cervical stromal invasion, rather than the finding of tumor tissue, as the crucial criterion in endocervical curetting affecting staging and prognosis.

The uterine cavity is then sounded to determine its size and to confirm the position determined from examination under anesthesia. The cervical canal is dilated with the Hegar or Hank-Bradley dilator. A dilatation to 8 or 9 mm by a Hegar dilator is sufficient for the usual diagnostic curettage. A gauze is placed in the posterior vaginal fornix along the posterior retractor so that the blood and the endometrium removed from the uterus can fall on it (Fig. 26.12). Before the curettage is performed, the uterine cavity is explored for endometrial polyps

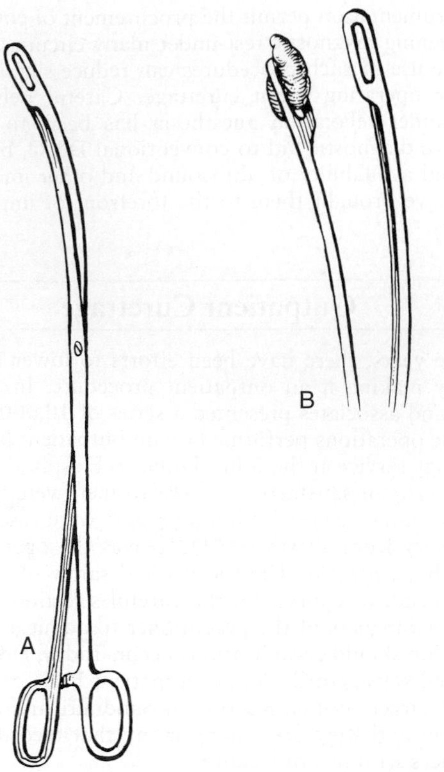

FIGURE 26.13. A: Ureteral stone forceps, an excellent instrument for removing endometrial polyps. **B:** A polyp, grasped in forceps, that was missed at curettage.

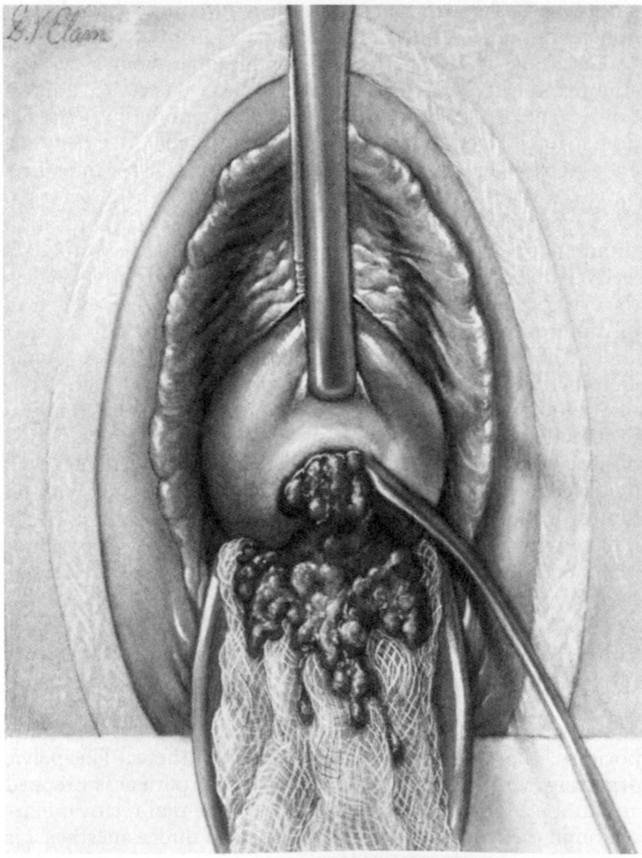

FIGURE 26.12. Method of collecting curettings and blood on gauze.

by use of a narrow stone forceps (Fig. 26.13). This forceps can be opened and closed as the tip of the forceps is moved systematically across the dome of the uterus and the anterior and posterior walls. An endometrial polyp can be easily missed with an ordinary curet, and unnecessary hysterectomies have been performed because of supposed persistent or recurrent dysfunctional bleeding after a curettage (Fig. 26.14). If polyp forceps are routinely used, such operations can be avoided. It is easier to identify and remove an endometrial polyp if the uterine cavity is explored with the stone forceps before the uterus is curetted. In a 28-month period during which forceps were used routinely at the Johns Hopkins Hospital, Josey found that endometrial polyp was diagnosed 130 times. In 83 of these cases, the polyp was removed by forceps. Although the sessile form of a submucous myoma is diagnosed easily by noting an irregularity of the uterine wall with the curet, the pedunculated variety, like the endometrial polyp, can escape detection because of its narrow stalk. Often, such a leiomyoma can be grasped with the polyp forceps. A uterine septum can also be detected with the forceps. Alternatively, hysteroscopy can be used to evaluate the cavity before curettage.

A small-sized or medium-sized, malleable, bluntly serrated curet (Fig. 26.15) is then introduced into the uterus, and the entire uterine cavity is systematically curetted. The anterior, lateral, and posterior walls are scraped gently but firmly, and finally, the top of the cavity is scraped with a side-to-side movement (Fig. 26.16). The handle of the curet should never be held against the palm of the hand. Instead, it should be held gently, as one would hold a pencil. The instrument is held loosely as it is inserted for the full distance. Pressure is then exerted

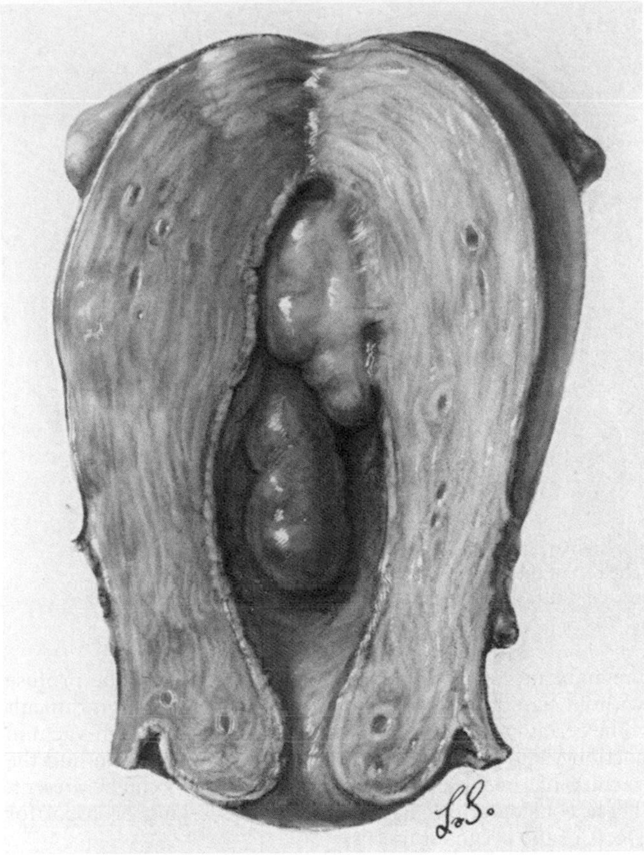

FIGURE 26.14. Opened uterus, showing two separate endometrial polyps.

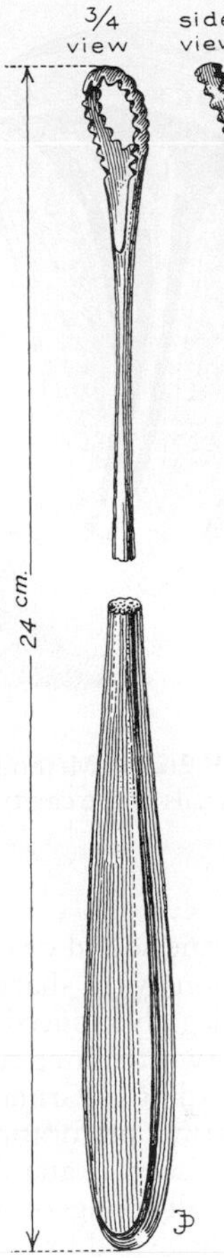

FIGURE 26.15. Small serrated curet for routine curettage.

against the uterine wall as the curet is drawn in an outward direction. Because the instrument is malleable, its curvature can be changed to conform to the contour of the uterine cavity. A uterine "cry," vibrations felt in the hand holding the curet, is often used as a sign that adequate tissue has been removed.

The unclotted blood is absorbed quickly by the gauze sponge, leaving the relatively clean endometrium to be placed in a prepared container with appropriate fixative. Again, the curettings should never be mashed or scraped but should be picked carefully from the sponge with a smooth-tip forceps and placed immediately in the fixative. The curettings should be examined carefully at this time for fatty tissue or other unusual tissue. Fragments of hyperplastic endometrium sometimes appear tan or yellow.

When curettage is performed as a curative measure for removal of placental tissue, a large, blunt, smooth curet is used to lessen the possibilities of perforation and endometrial sclerosis. The larger and softer the uterus, the larger the curet should be and the more care one should exercise to avoid these complications. When large masses of placental tissue are present, ovum forceps are most useful when used in conjunction with the curet. High vacuum suction is now used almost routinely for placental tissue removal.

Routine blind biopsy of the cervix is usually unrewarding if a negative cytologic smear has been obtained and there is no suspicious cervical lesion. We no longer do a blind biopsy of the cervix at the time of curettage unless an abnormal lesion is present. If a patient's recent cytologic results are normal and she has a profuse, recurrent, mucous discharge associated with cervicitis and nabothian cysts, cervical cauterization or laser vaporization can be done at the time of curettage, but biopsy confirmation to exclude occult malignancy should be obtained.

Complications of Cervical Dilatation and Uterine Curettage

If the position and the consistency of the uterus are carefully observed on bimanual examination under anesthesia before curettage is begun, perforation will rarely occur. When the position of the uterus is not known to the operator, perforation occurs with remarkable ease. Special care should be exercised with a uterus that is acutely anteflexed or retroflexed. With cervical stenosis, pregnancy, or intrauterine malignancy, perforation is more likely. The postmenopausal atrophic uterus can be perforated with only slight force applied to the uterine sound or the curet. Perforation is discovered when the sound or the curet fails to encounter resistance where it normally should, as judged by the palpated size of the uterus. Abdominal ultrasound visualization of the uterus, cervix, and endocervical canal, which may require a distended bladder, can be useful in guiding the passage of either a dilator or a curette through the endocervical canal into the endometrial cavity.

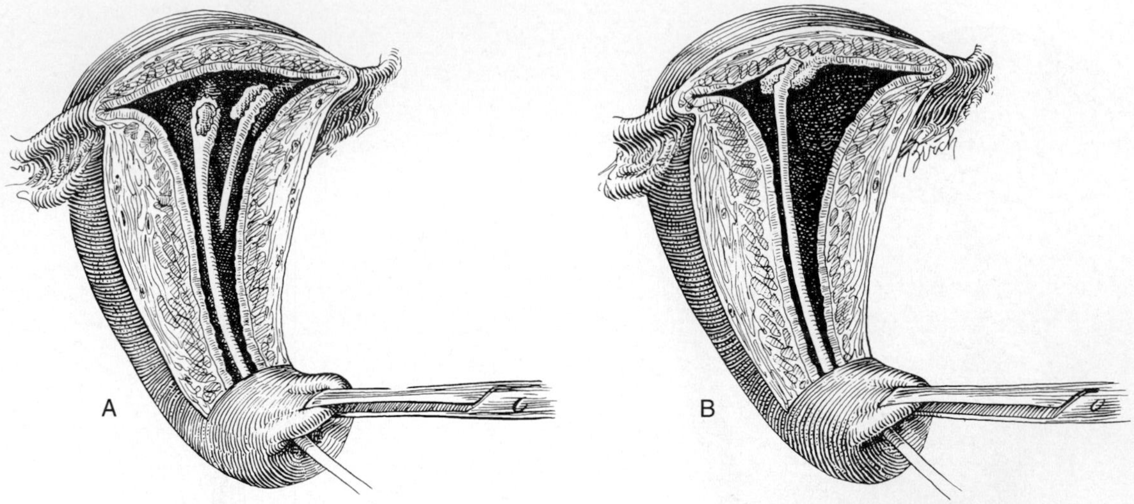

FIGURE 26.16. Method of curetting the uterine cavity systematically. **A:** The anterior, posterior, and lateral walls of the cavity are curetted systematically. **B:** The top of the cavity is then curetted thoroughly.

Perforation by the uterine sound or cervical dilator causes less damage than perforation by the sharp curet or suction cannula. Sharp curettage for legally induced abortion has a major complication rate that is two to three times higher than that for suction curettage, according to Grimes and Cates. The two principal dangers of uterine perforation are bleeding and trauma to the abdominal viscera. Lateral perforation through the uterine vessels is especially dangerous from the standpoint of intraperitoneal hemorrhage and broad ligament hematoma formation. Damage can occur to the bowel, omentum, mesentery, ureter, and fallopian tube. Perforation of the anterior or posterior wall of the uterus by a small curet in performing a diagnostic curettage is usually not a serious accident. However, it is usually necessary to discontinue curettage. One must watch carefully for signs of hemorrhage or infection. If signs of hemorrhage develop, the abdomen should be opened and the uterine wound sutured. If signs of infection occur, broad-spectrum antibiotics should be given. If a pelvic abscess develops, the abscess should be drained if possible. Serious hemorrhage or infection occurs only rarely. When serious damage from perforation is suspected, laparoscopy can be performed to assess the extent of the damage and the needed repair. According to MacKenzie and Bibby, complications occurred in 1.7% of cases of D&C. McElin and colleagues reported that 0.5% of cases had postoperative febrile morbidity after D&C. Uterine perforation occurred in 0.63% of cases.

One should be absolutely certain that the endometrial cavity has been entered when D&C is performed for postmenopausal bleeding. A relatively stenotic internal cervical os and a fear of uterine perforation can prevent entry into the uterine cavity above the internal cervical os, resulting in failure to curet the uterine cavity and consequent failure to diagnose the cause of the bleeding. Again, ultrasound can be a valuable tool for confirming placement of the curette tip in the endometrial cavity.

Perforation of a pregnant uterus is a more serious complication than is perforation of the nonpregnant uterus. First, there is the requirement that all remaining pregnancy tissue be completely removed to prevent sepsis. To accomplish this blindly when there is a defect in the uterine wall is unsafe. Second, the pregnant uterus is a much more vascular organ than is the nonpregnant uterus, and intraperitoneal bleeding can be profuse without significant external bleeding. Third, it often is difficult to be certain when the perforation occurred. If a high-vacuum suction vacuret has passed through the myometrium and the vacuum has been activated, major bowel injury can be present. These considerations have led to the following protocol for D&C of the pregnant uterus:

1. Never activate the vacuum suction if there is any question about the safe location of the vacuret within the uterine cavity.
2. Laparoscope any pregnant uterus that is possibly perforated. With the laparoscope in place, a second operator can evacuate remaining placental tissue while the laparoscopist monitors safety. Many perforations in which no other visceral damage has occurred are fundal. If laparoscopic observation confirms that bleeding is minimal, the perforation can be managed conservatively with antibiotics and serial hematocrit determination for 24 to 48 hours. If there is no evidence of continued bleeding or developing infection, the patient can be discharged.
3. During laparoscopy, if there is any evidence of intestinal injury or any suspicion of such injury, or if bleeding is significant, then laparotomy is mandatory. Unfortunately, bowel injury by high-vacuum suction may require bowel resection and anastomosis.

Figure 26.17 shows a uterus removed immediately after a perforation because of intraperitoneal bleeding. Word analyzed 70 accidental uterine perforations. Among these, an unplanned hysterectomy was performed on seven unprepared patients. In none of these cases did the intraperitoneal findings indicate the need for hysterectomy. In fact, hysterectomy compounded the surgical error. Fifty-five patients were treated conservatively, and only one developed a complication, in the form of a pelvic abscess that was drained by colpotomy. Forty-one of the 70 perforations occurred in postmenopausal women.

When a large, boggy, postabortion or puerperal uterus is perforated by a large curet or placental forceps in removing placental tissue, there is more danger of hemorrhage, infection, or injury to bowel. The treatment protocols and the procedures

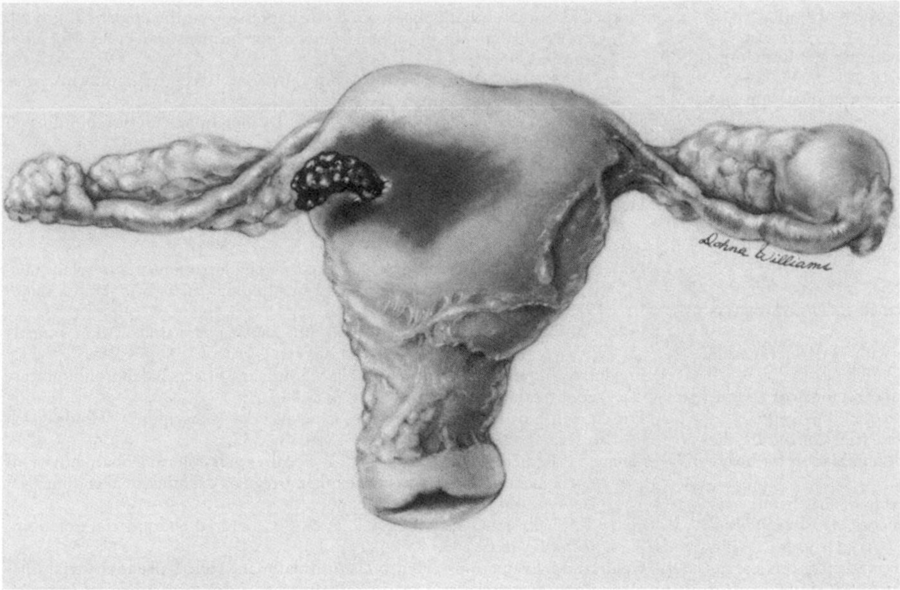

FIGURE 26.17. Result of uterine perforation. Specimen removed directly after perforation.

for these serious complications are discussed elsewhere in this textbook.

Asherman syndrome is a pathologic condition of intrauterine adhesions that can cause secondary amenorrhea, other menstrual irregularities, infertility, or recurrent abortion. Numerous investigators have shown a strong association between puerperal D&C and the formation of synechiae that can partially or completely obliterate the endometrial cavity. No incidence figures are available because no prospective studies have been performed, but factors other than pregnancy that increase the risk of endometrial sclerosis after D&C are infection, scant endometrium that exposes the basalis to trauma, and a hypoestrogenic state. Rarely, significant synechiae are seen in the absence of an antecedent curettage. Cases have been reported after severe endometritis, tuberculosis, myomectomy, and cesarean section. Diagnosis is made by clinical history, hysterosalpingography, or hysteroscopy. Therapy requires lysis of adhesions by repeat curettage or, preferably, by hysteroscopic scissors or KTP laser.

Patency of the uterine cavity is maintained with an intrauterine device or balloon catheter, and endometrial regeneration is stimulated by oral estrogen therapy. The prognosis with significant adhesions is poor. Only 40% of patients will become pregnant, and about half of these will undergo spontaneous abortion or premature delivery. Consideration should be given to the risks of adhesion formation before the curettage of a pregnant or infected uterus, and possibly a less vigorous scraping should be performed in an attempt to minimize endometrial trauma.

BEST SURGICAL PRACTICES

- Although hysteroscopy is the gold standard for evaluating endometrial cavity pathology, saline infusion sonography (SIS) has comparable sensitivity and is less invasive and less expensive.
- Historic data showed higher amenorrhea rates with endometrial ablation using endomyometrial resection. However, newer techniques of hydrothermablation, radiofrequency current, and microwaves have comparable amenorrhea rates. Hydrothermablation has the advantage of visualization of the endometrial cavity, radiofrequency ablation does not require endometrial pretreatment, and microwave endometrial ablation has been reported to be successful in the presence of small submucous myomas.
- Endometrial sampling can be done by Pipelle, four quadrant endometrial biopsy, or formal dilatation and curettage (D&C). All of these techniques can miss significant lesions, and the concurrent use of vaginal ultrasonography or SIS will improve sensitivity.
- Hysteroscopy is a valuable adjunct to D&C, particularly in the patient at higher risk for focal endometrial pathology that might be missed on endometrial sampling.
- Abdominal ultrasound guidance may reduce the risk of complications such as perforation during difficult cervical D&C, such as in the stenotic postmenopausal patient or in the case of a large uterus.

Bibliography

Aksel S, Jones GS. Etiology and treatment of dysfunctional uterine bleeding. *Obstet Gynecol* 1974;44:1.

Anderson ABM, Haynes PJ, Guillebaud J, et al. Reduction of menstrual blood loss by prostaglandin synthesis inhibition. *Lancet* 1976;1:774.

Andolf E, Dahlander K, Aspenberg P. Ultrasonic thickness of the endometrium correlated to body weight in asymptomatic postmenopausal women. *Obstet Gynecol* 1993;82:936.

Asherman J. Amenorrhea traumatica (atretica). *J Obstet Gynaecol Br Emp* 1948;55:23.

Atwood JT, Toth TL, Schiff I. Abnormal uterine bleeding in the perimenopause. *Int J Fertil* 1993;38:261.

Azziz R, Zacur HA. 21-Hydroxylase deficiency in female hyperandrogenemia. *J Clin Endocrinol Metab* 1989;69:577.

Barnett JM. Suction curettage on unanesthetized outpatients. *Obstet Gynecol* 1973;42:672.

Battacharya S, Cameron IM, Parkin DE, et al. A pragmatic randomized comparison of transcervical resection of the endometrium with endometrial laser ablation for the treatment of menorrhagia. *BJOG* 1999;106:360.

Bayer SR, DeCherney AH. Clinical manifestations and treatment of dysfunctional uterine bleeding. *JAMA* 1993;269:1823.

Beller FK. Observations on the clotting of menstrual blood and clot formation. *Am J Obstet Gynecol* 1971;3:535.

Bettocchi S, Ceci O, Vicino M, et al. Diagnostic inadequacy of dilatation and curettage. *Fertil Steril* 2001;75:803.

Beyth Y, Yaffe H, Levii I, et al. Retrograde seeding of endometrium: a sequela of tubal flushing. *Fertil Steril* 1975;26:1094.

Bongers M, Bourdrez P, Mol B, et al. Randomised controlled trial of bipolar radio-frequency endometrial ablation and balloon endometrial ablation. *BJOG* 2004;111:1095.

Brooks PG. Complications of operative hysteroscopy: how safe is it?. *Clin Obstet Gynecol* 1993;35:256.

Brooks PG. Hysteroscopic surgery using the resectoscope: myomas, ablation, septae and synechiae: does pre-operative medication help?. *Clin Obstet Gynecol* 1993;35:249.

Brooks PG, Serden SP. Endometrial ablation in women with abnormal uterine bleeding aged fifty and over. *J Reprod Med* 1992;37:682.

Brooks-Carter GN, Killackey MA, Neuwirth RS. Adenocarcinoma of the endometrium after endometrial ablation. *Obstet Gynecol* 2000;96:836.

Busfield R, Farquhar C, Sowter M, et al. A randomized trial comparing the levonorgestrel intrauterine system and thermal balloon ablation for heavy menstrual bleeding. *BJOG* 2006;113:257.

Cameron IT, Haining R, Lumsden M-A, et al. The effects of mefenamic acid and norethisterone on measured menstrual blood loss. *Obstet Gynecol* 1990;76:85.

Chen SS, Lee L. Reappraisal of endocervical curettage in predicting cervical involvement by endometrial carcinoma. *Obstet Gynecol* 1986;31:50.

Chiazze L Jr, Brayer FT, Macisco JJ Jr, et al. The length and variability of the human menstrual cycle. *JAMA* 1968;203:377.

Claessens EA, Cowell CA. Acute adolescent menorrhagia. *Am J Obstet Gynecol* 1981;139:227.

Cohen CJ, Gusberg SB, Koffier D. Histologic screening for endometrial cancer. *Gynecol Oncol* 1974;2:279.

Cook J, Seman E. Pregnancy following endometrial ablation: case history and literature review. *Obstet Gynecol Surv* 2003;58:551.

Cooper J, Anderson T, Fortin C, et al. Microwave endometrial ablation vs. rollerball electroablation for menorrhagia: a multicenter randomized trial. *J Am Assoc Gynecol Laparosc* 2004;11:394.

Cooper J, Gimpelson R, Laberge P, et al. A randomized multicenter trial of safety and efficacy of the Novasure system in treatment of menorrhagia. *J Am Assoc Gynecol Laparosc* 2002;9:418.

Copperman AB, DeCherney AH, Olive DL. A case of endometrial cancer following endometrial ablation for dysfunctional uterine bleeding. *Obstet Gynecol* 1993;82:640.

Corson S. A multicenter evaluation of endometrial ablation by Hydro ThermAblator and rollerball for treatment of menorrhagia. *J Am Assoc Gynecol Laparosc* 2001;8:359.

Corson SL, Brill AI, Brooks PG, et al. Interim results of the American VESTA trial of endometrial ablation. *J Am Assoc Gynecol Laparosc* 1999;6:45.

Coulam CB, Annegers JF, Kranz JS. Chronic anovulation syndrome and associated neoplasia. *Obstet Gynecol* 1983;61:403.

Crosignani PG, Vercellini P, Mosconi P, et al. Levonorgestrel-releasing intrauterine device versus hysteroscopic endometrial resection in the treatment of dysfunctional uterine bleeding. *Obstet Gynecol* 1997;90:257.

Davies AJ, Anderson ABM, Turnbull AC. Reduction by naproxen of excessive menstrual bleeding in women using intrauterine devices. *Obstet Gynecol* 1981;57:74.

Denis R Jr, Barnett JM, Forbes SE. Diagnostic suction curettage. *Obstet Gynecol* 1973;42:301.

DeVore G, Owens O, Case NL. Use of intravenous Premarin in the treatment of dysfunctional uterine bleeding: a double-blind randomized control study. *Obstet Gynecol* 1982;59:285.

Dickson RB, Johnson MD, el-Ashry D, et al. Breast cancer: influence of endocrine hormones, growth factors and genetic alterations. *Adv Exp Med Biol* 1993;330:119.

Dickson RB, Lippman ME. Estrogenic regulation of growth and polypeptide growth factor secretion in human breast carcinoma. *Endocr Rev* 1987;8:39.

Dilley A, Drews C, Miller C, et al. Von Willebrand disease and other inherited bleeding disorders in women with diagnosed menorrhagia. *Obstet Gynecol* 2001;97:630.

Dodson MG. Use of transvaginal ultrasound in diagnosing the etiology of menometrorrhagia. *J Reprod Med* 1994;39:362.

Donnez J, Vilos G, Gannon MJ, et al. Goserelin acetate (Zoladex) plus endometrial ablation for dysfunctional uterine bleeding: a large randomized double-blind study. *Fertil Steril* 1997;68:29.

Dueholm M, Lundorf E, Hansen ES, et al. Evaluation of the uterine cavity with magnetic resonance imaging, transvaginal sonography, hysterosonographic examination, and diagnostic hysteroscopy. *Fertil Steril* 2001;76:350.

Economos K, MacDonald PC, Casey ML. Endothelin-1 gene expression and protein biosynthesis in human endometrium: potential modulator of endometrial blood flow. *J Clin Endocrinol Metab* 1992;74:14.

Ejskjær K, Sørensen BS, Poulsen SS, et al. Expression of the epidermal growth factor system in human endometrium during the menstrual cycle. *Mol Hum Reprod* 2005;11:543.

Evans RM. The steroid and thyroid hormone receptor family. *Science* 1988;240:889.

Falcone T, Desjardins C, Bourgue J, et al. Dysfunctional uterine bleeding in adolescents. *J Reprod Med* 1994;39:761.

Fleming H, Oster AG, Pickel H, et al. Arteriovenous malformations of the uterus. *Obstet Gynecol* 1989;73:209.

Fraser IS, Baird DT. Blood production and ovarian secretion rates of estradiol-17, 3 and estrone in women and dysfunctional uterine bleeding. *J Clin Endocrinol Metab* 1974;38:727.

Fraser IS, Michie EA, Wide L, et al. Pituitary gonadotropins and ovarian function in adolescent dysfunctional uterine bleeding. *J Clin Endocrinol Metab* 1973;37:407.

Fraser IS, Pearse C, Shearman RP, et al. Efficacy of mefenamic acid in patients with a complaint of menorrhagia. *Obstet Gynecol* 1981;58:543.

Friedman AJ, Juneau-Norcross M, Rein MS. Adverse effects of leuprolide acetate depot treatment. *Fertil Steril* 1993;59:448.

Fritsch N. Ein Fall von volligen Schwund der gebarmutter Hohle nach Auskratzung. *Zentralbl Gumsrl* 1894;18:1337.

Galant C, Berlière M, Dubois D, et al. Focal expression and final activity of matrix metalloproteinases may explain irregular dysfunctional endometrial bleeding. *Am J Path* 2004;165:83.

Garry R, Shelly-Jones D, Mooney P, et al. Six hundred endometrial ablations. *Obstet Gynecol* 1995;85:24.

Goldrath M. Evaluation of Hydro ThermAblator and rollerball endometrial ablation for menorrhagia 3 years after treatment. *J Am Assoc Gynecol Laparosc* 2003;10:505.

Gregg RH. The praxiology of the office dilatation and curettage. *Am J Obstet Gynecol* 1981;140:179.

Grimes D. Estimating vaginal blood loss. *J Reprod Med* 1979;22:190.

Grimes D, Cates W Jr. Complications from legally induced abortion: a review. *Obstet Gynecol Surv* 1979;34:177.

Guidice LC, Dsupin BA, Jin IH, et al. Differential expression of messenger ribonucleic acids encoding insulin-like growth factors and their receptors in human uterine endometrium and decidua. *J Clin Endocrinol Metab* 1993;76:1115.

Guido R, Kanbour-Shakir A, Rulin M, et al. Pipelle endometrial sampling: sensitivity in the detection of endometrial lesions. *J Reprod Med* 1995;40:553.

Guillebaud J, Barnett MD, Gordon YB. Plasma ferritin levels as an index of iron deficiency in women using intrauterine devices. *BJOG* 1979;86:51.

Gull B, Carlsson SA, Karlsson B, et al. Transvaginal ultrasonography of the endometrium in women with postmenopausal bleeding: Is it always necessary to perform an endometrial biopsy?. *Am J Obstet Gynecol* 2000;182:509.

Hallberg L, Hogdahl A, Nilsson L, et al. Menstrual blood and iron deficiency. *Acta Med Scand* 1966;180:639.

Hallberg L, Nilsson L. Constancy of individual menstrual blood loss. *Acta Obstet Gynecol Scand* 1964;43:352.

Hallberg L, Nilsson L. Determination of menstrual blood loss. *Scand J Clin Lab Invest* 1964;16:244.

Handwerger S, Richards RG, Markoff E. The physiology of decidual prolactin and other decidual protein hormones. *Trends Endocrinol Metab* 1992;3:91.

Haynes PJ, Hodgson H, Anderson ABM, et al. Measurement of menstrual blood loss in patients complaining of menorrhagia. *BJOG* 1997;84:763.

Healy DL, Hogden GD. The endocrinology of human endometrium. *Obstet Gynecol Surv* 1983;38:509.

Helmkamp BF, Denslow BL, Boufiglio TA, et al. Cervical conization: when is dilatation and curettage indicated? *Am J Obstet Gynecol* 1983;146:893.

Hofmeister FJ. Endometrial biopsy: another look. *Am J Obstet Gynecol* 1974;118:773.

Hofmeister FJ. Endometrial curettage. In: Symmonds CM, Zuspan FT, eds. *Clinical and diagnostic procedures in obstetrics and gynecology*. New York: Marcel Dekker, 1984.

Hunt JS, Chen H-L, Hu X-L, et al. Tumor necrosis factor-a messenger ribonucleic acid and protein in human endometrium. *Biol Reprod* 1992;47:141.

Irvine G, Campbell-Brown M, Lumsden M, et al. Randomized comparative trial of the levonorgestrel intrauterine system and norethisterone for treatment of idiopathic menorrhagia. *BJOG* 1998;105:592.

Jansen FW, Vredevoogd CB, Van Ulzen K, et al. Complications of hysteroscopy: a prospective multicenter study. *Obstet Gynecol* 2000;96:266.

Jensen J. Contraceptive and therapeutic effects of the levonorgestrel intrauterine system: an overview. *Obstet Gynecol Surv* 2005;60:604.

Jensen JA, Jensen JG. Abragio mucosae uteri e aspiratione. *Ugeskr Laeger* 1968;130:2121.

Jensen JG. Vacuum curettage. Outpatient curettage without anesthesia: a report of 350 cases. *Dan Med Bull* 1970;17:199.

Josey WE. Routine intrauterine forceps exploration at curettage. *Obstet Gynecol* 1958;11:108.

Joshi SG. Progestin-regulated proteins of the human endometrium. *Semin Reprod Endocrinol* 1983;1:221.

Kadir R, Lukes A, Kouides P, et al. Management of excessive menstrual bleeding in women with hemostatic disorders. *Fertil Steril* 2005;84:1352.

Karlsson B, Granberg S, Wikland M, et al. Transvaginal ultrasonography of the endometrium in women with postmenopausal bleeding: a Nordic multicenter study. *Am J Obstet Gynecol* 1995;172:1488.

Kelly HA. Curettage without anesthesia on the office table. *Am J Obstet Gynecol* 1925;9:78.

King RJB. Structure and function of steroid receptors. *J Endocrinol* 1987; 114:341.

Klein SM, Garcia CR. Asherman's syndrome: a critique and current review. *Fertil Steril* 1973;24:722.

Kooy J, Taylor NH, Healy DL, et al. Endothelial cell proliferation in the endometrium of women with menorrhagia and in women following endometrial ablation. *Hum Reprod* 1996;11:1067.

Krettek JE, Arkin SI, Chaisilwattana P, et al. Chlamydia trachomatis in patients who used oral contraceptives and had intermenstrual spotting. *Obstet Gynecol* 1993;81:728.

Kubrinsky NL, Tulloch H. Treatment of refractory thrombocytopenic bleeding with desamino-8-D-arginine vasopressin (desmopressin). *J Pediatr* 1988;112:993.

Larsson PG, Bergman BB. Is there a causal connection between motile curved rods, *Mobiluncus* species and bleeding complications?. *Am J Obstet Gynecol* 1986;154:107.

Laufer MR, Mitchell SR. Treatment of abnormal uterine bleeding with gonadotropin-releasing hormone analogues. *Clin Obstet Gynecol* 1993;36:668.

Leather A, Studd J, Watson N, et al. The prevention of bone loss in young women treated with GnRH analogues with "add-back" estrogen therapy. *Obstet Gynecol* 1993;81:104.

Lessey BA, Castelbaum AJ, Sawin SW, et al. Further characterization of endometrial integrins during the menstrual cycle and in pregnancy. *Fertil Steril* 1994;62:497.

Lessey BA, Damjanovich L, Cautifaris C, et al. Integrin adhesion molecules in the human endometrium: correlation with normal and abnormal menstrual cycle. *J Clin Invest* 1992;90:188.

Lomano JM. Photocoagulation of the endometrium with the Nd:YAG laser for the treatment of menorrhagia: a report of 10 cases. *J Reprod Med* 1986: 31:149.

Lukes A, Kadir R, Peyvandi F, et al. Disorders of hemostasis and excessive menstrual bleeding: prevalevie and clinical impact. *Fertil Steril* 2005;84: 1338.

Lutz MH, Underwood PB Jr, Kreutner A, et al. Vacuum aspiration: an efficient outpatient screening technique for endometrial disease. *South Med J* 1977;70:393.

MacKenzie IZ, Bibby JG. Critical assessment of dilatation and curettage in 1,029 women. *Lancet* 1978;2:566.

Manabe Y, Manabe A. Nelaton catheter for gradual and safe cervical dilatation: an ideal substitute for laminaria. *Am J Obstet Gynecol* 1981;140:465.

March CM. Hysteroscopy. *J Reprod Med* 1992;37:293.

Markee JE. Menstruation in intraocular endometrial transplants in the rhesus monkey. *Contr Embryol Carneg Justn* 1940;28:219.

Martin PL, Rust JA. Surgical gynecology for the ambulatory patient. *Clin Obstet Gynecol* 1974;17:205.

McElin TW, Burd CC, Reeves BD, et al. Diagnostic dilatation and curettage. *Obstet Gynecol* 1969;33:807.

Mengert WF, Slate WG. Diagnostic dilatation and curettage as an outpatient procedure. *Am J Obstet Gynecol* 1960;79:727.

Meyer WR, Walsh BW, Grainger DA, et al. Thermal balloon and roller ball ablation to treat menorrhagia: a multicenter comparison. *Obstet Gynecol* 1998;92:98.

Milsom I, Andersson K, Andersch B, et al. A comparison of flurbiprofen, tranexamic acid and a levonorgestrel-releasing intrauterine contraceptive device in the treatment of idiopathic menorrhagia. *Am J Obstet Gynecol* 1991;164:879.

Mishell DR Jr, Connel E, Haney A, et al. Oral contraception for women in their 40s. *J Reprod Med* 1990;35:447.

Mularoni A, Mahfoudi A, Beck L, et al. Progesterone control of fibronectin secretion in guinea pig endometrium. *Endocrinology* 1992;131:2127.

Munrow, Lukes A. Abnormal uterine bleeding and underlying hemostatic disorders: report of a consensus process. *Fertil Steril* 2005;84:1335.

Mylonas I, Jeschke U, Wiest I, et al. Inhibin/activin subunits alpha, beta-A and beta-B are differentially expressed in normal human endometrium throughout the menstrual cycle. *Histochem Cell Biol* 2004;122:461.

Narula RK. Endometrial histopathology in dysfunctional uterine bleeding. *J Obstet Gynaecol India* 1967;17:614.

Nasri MN, Shepherd JH, Setchell ME, et al. The role of vaginal scan in measurement of endometrial thickness in postmenopausal women. *BJOG* 1991;98:470.

Nilsson L, Rybo G. Treatment of menorrhagia. *Am J Obstet Gynecol* 1971; 110:713.

Novak E. Relation of hyperplasia of endometrium to so-called functional uterine hemorrhage. *JAMA* 1920;75:292.

Novak E. A suction curette apparatus and endometrial biopsy. *JAMA* 1935; 104:1497.

O'Connor H, Magos A. Endometrial resection for the treatment of menorrhagia. *N Engl J Med* 1996;335:151.

Osmers R. Transvaginal sonography in endometrial cancer. *Ultrasound Obstet Gynecol* 1991;2:2.

Overton C, Hargreaves J, Maresh M. A national survey of the complications of endometrial destruction for menstrual disorders: the "the Mistletoe" study. *BJOG* 1997;102:1351.

Pacheco JC, Kempers RD. Etiology of postmenopausal bleeding. *Obstet Gynecol* 1968;32:40.

Rauramo I, Elo I, Istre O. Long-term treatment of menorrhagia with levonorgestrel intrauterine system versus endometrial resection. *Obstet Gynecol* 2004;104:1314.

Reyniak JV. Dysfunctional uterine bleeding. *J Reprod Med* 1976;17:293.

Rodgers WH, Osteen KG, Matrisian LM, et al. Expression and localization of matrilysin, a matrix metalloproteinase, in human endometrium during the reproductive cycle. *Am J Obstet Gynecol* 1993;168:253.

Rubin MC, Davidson AR, Philliber SG, et al. Long-term effect of tubal sterilization on menstrual indices and pelvic pain. *Obstet Gynecol* 1993;82:118.

Rutherford TJ, Zreik TG, Troiano RN, et al. Endometrial cryo ablation, a minimally invasive procedure for abnormal uterine bleeding. *J Am Assoc Gynecol Laparosc* 1998;5:23.

Sandmire HF, Austin SD. Curettage as an office procedure. *Am J Obstet Gynecol* 1974;119:82.

Schaedel Z, Dolan G, Powell M. The use of the levonorgestrel-releasing intrauterine system in the management of menorrhagia in women with hemostatic disorders. *Obstet Gynecol* 2005;193:1361.

Schwab K, Chan R, Gargett C. Putative stem cell activity of human endometrial epithelial and stromal cells during the menstrual cycle. *Fertil Steril* 2005;84:1124.

Seeras RC, Gilliland GB. Resumption of menstruation after amenorrhea in women treated by endometrial ablation and myometrial resection. *J Am Assoc Gynecol Laparosc* 1997;4:305.

Sharp NC, Cronin N, Feldberg I, et al. Microwaves for menorrhagia: a new fast technique for endometrial ablation. *Lancet* 1995;346:1003.

Singer A, Almanza R, Rutierrez A, et al. Preliminary clinical experience with a thermal balloon ablation method to treat menorrhagia. *Obstet Gynecol* 1994;83:732.

Sivridis E, Giatromanolaki A. New insights into the normal menstrual cycle—regulatory molecules. *Histol Histopathol* 2004;19:511.

Smith SK, Abel MH, Kelly RW, et al. Prostaglandin synthesis in the endometrium of women with ovular dysfunctional uterine bleeding. *BJOG* 1981;88:434.

Smith SK, Abel MH, Kelly RW, et al. A role for prostacyclin (PGI_2) in excessive menstrual bleeding. *Lancet* 1981;1:522.

Smith-Bindman R, Kerlikowske K, Feldstein V, et al. Endovaginal ultrasound to exclude endometrial cancer and other endometrial abnormalities. *JAMA* 1998;280:1510.

Southam AI, Richard RM. The prognosis for adolescents with menstrual abnormalities. *Am J Obstet Gynecol* 1966;94:637.

Speroff L, Glass RH, Kase NG. Dysfunctional uterine bleeding. In: *Clinical gynecologic endocrinology and infertility*. 6th ed. Baltimore: Lippincott Williams & Wilkins; 1999:575.

Stefos T, Sotiriadis A, Tsanadis G, et al. Serum leptin and erythropoietin during menstruation. *Clin Exp Obstet Gynecol* 2005;32:41.

Stock RJ, Kanbour A. Pre-hysterectomy curettage: an evaluation. *Obstet Gynecol* 1975;45:537.

Summitt RJ Jr, Stovall TG, Steege JF, et al. A multicenter randomized comparison of laparoscopically assisted vaginal hysterectomy and abdominal hysterectomy candidates. *Obstet Gynecol* 1998;92:321.

Swartz DP, Jones GES. Progesterone in anovulatory uterine bleeding: clinical observations. *Fertil Steril* 1957;8:103.

Taylor PJ, Graham G. Is diagnostic curettage harmful in women with unexplained infertility? *BJOG* 1982;89:296.

Teare AJ, Rippey JJ. Dilatation and curettage. *S Afr Med J* 1979;55:535.

Torry DS, Torry RJ. Angiogenesis and the expression of vascular endothelial growth factor in endometrium and placenta. *Am J Reprod Immunol* 1997;37:21.

Townsend DE, Fields G, McCausland A, et al. Diagnostic and operative hysteroscopy in the management of persistent postmenopausal bleeding. *Obstet Gynecol* 1993;82:419.

Tseng L, Gusberg SB, Gurpide E. Estradiol receptor and 17β-dehydrogenase in normal and abnormal human endometrium. *Ann N Y Acad Sci* 1977; 286:190.

Van Eijkeren MA, Christiaens GC, Geuze JH, et al. Effects of mefenamic acid on menstrual hemostasis in essential menorrhagia. *Am J Obstet Gynecol* 1992;166:1419.

Van Eijkeren MA, Christiaens GC, Haspels AA, et al. Measured menstrual blood loss in women with a bleeding disorder or using oral anticoagulant therapy. *Am J Obstet Gynecol* 1990;162:1261.

Van Eijkeren MA, Christiaens GC, Sixma JJ, et al. Menorrhagia: a review. *Obstet Gynecol Surv* 1989;4:421.

Vercellini P, Oldani S, Yaylayan L, et al. Randomized comparison of vaporizing electrode and cutting loop for endometrial ablation. *Obstet Gynecol* 1999;94:521.

Vermeeren J, Chamberlain RR, Te Linde RW. Ten thousand minor gynecologic operations on an outpatient basis. *Obstet Gynecol* 1957;9:139.

Vilos GA, Pispidkis JT, Botz CK. Economic evaluation of hysteroscopic endometrial ablation versus vaginal hysterectomy for menorrhagia. *Obstet Gynecol* 1996;88:241.

Warner P, Critchley H, Lumsden M, et al. Menorrhagia II: Is the 80-mL blood loss criterion useful in management of complaint of menorrhagia?. *Am J Obstet Gynecol* 2004;190:1224.

Weisberg M, Goldrath MH, Berman J, et al. Hysteroscopic endometrial ablation using free heated saline for the treatment of menorrhagia. *J Am Assoc Gynecol Laparosc* 2000;7:311.

Whitehead MI, Frazier D. The effects of estrogens and progestogens on the endometrium. *Obstet Gynecol Clin North Am* 1987;14:299.

Whitehead MI, King RJ, McQueen J, et al. Endometrial histology and biochemistry in climacteric women during estrogen and estrogen/progestogen therapy. *J R Soc Med* 1979;72:322.

Wilansky DL, Greisman B. Early hypothyroidism in patients with menorrhagia. *Am J Obstet Gynecol* 1989;160:673.

Wilborn WH, Flowers CE Jr. Cellular mechanisms for endometrial conservation during menstrual bleeding. *Semin Reprod Endocrinol* 1984;2:307.

Word B. Current concepts of uterine curettage. *Postgrad Med* 1960;28:450.

Word B, Gravlee LC, Wideman GL. The fallacy of simple uterine curettage. *Obstet Gynecol* 1958;12:642.

Xiao B, Wus-C, Chong J, et al. Therapeutic effects of the levonorgestrel-releasing intrauterine system in the treatment of idiopathic menorrhagia. *Fertil Steril* 2003;79:963.

CHAPTER 27 ■ TUBAL STERILIZATION

HERBERT B. PETERSON, AMY E. POLLACK, AND JEFFREY S. WARSHAW

DEFINITIONS

Air embolism—Potential complication of laparoscopic abdominal insufflation with the Veress needle, associated with "vapor lock" of the right ventricle, which occludes blood flow and results in cardiovascular collapse. A "cog wheel" murmur can sometimes be heard.

Bipolar coagulation—Method of tubal occlusion usually performed via laparoscopy that causes electrocoagulation of the tube when current is applied by grasping forceps; one jaw of the forceps is an active electrode, and the other is a return electrode. There is less chance for unintended thermal injuries than with unipolar coagulation, and the chance of unintended thermal injury by capacitive coupling is virtually eliminated. However, less widespread thermal destruction of the tube increases the chance for sterilization failure relative to unipolar coagulation unless the surgeon uses techniques that maximize the likelihood of adequate tubal coagulation.

Capacitive coupling—Unintended consequence of laparoscopic use of unipolar coagulation, which under certain conditions can result in a charge being transferred to the operative laparoscope or conductive laparoscopic sheath. Subsequent occult transference of this charge to intestines can lead to thermal injury and subsequent infectious morbidity or mortality.

Cumulative failure rates—Contrary to previous beliefs, tubal sterilization failures are not isolated to a narrow window of time after the procedure, but rather increase cumulatively with each passing year following sterilization. Younger women, who are more fecund at sterilization and for years after, have higher failure rates initially and over time.

Irving method—Method of partial salpingectomy that buries the end of the proximal tubal stump in the myometrium of the uterus, in an attempt to reduce the rate of tuboperitoneal fistula.

Luteal phase pregnancy—Refers to pregnancies that occurred before sterilization but were detected after sterilization. Such pregnancies may be erroneously attributed to sterilization "failure."

Open laparoscopy—Laparoscopic procedure begun without prior insufflation by directly visualizing, elevating, and incising the layers of the abdominal wall near the umbilicus. Has the benefit of reducing vascular injuries and, potentially, bowel injuries associated with blind direct Veress needle and trocar insertion.

Parkland method—Method of partial salpingectomy that involves ligation of the tube in two places, followed by excision of the intervening segment of tube. Achieves immediate separation of severed tubal ends.

Pomeroy method—Method of partial salpingectomy that involves ligation, followed by excision, of a loop of tube. No attempt to bury the severed ends of tube.

Poststerilization regret—Regret after the decision to undergo surgical sterilization can be related to several factors, including preexisting patient characteristics, subsequent changes in the patient's situations or attitudes, and dissatisfaction resulting from adverse side effects caused or perceived to be caused by the procedure. Studies have identified young age at tubal sterilization as a risk factor for later regret.

Posttubal ligation syndrome—Refers to the historic perception that menstrual disturbances could result from tubal sterilization. This term is outdated, as substantial evidence against such a syndrome now exists. Women who undergo sterilization are no more likely than their nonsterilized counterparts to experience a syndrome of menstrual abnormalities.

Silicone rubber banding—Method of tubal occlusion usually performed via laparoscopy in which a silicone rubber band is applied to the isthmic portion of the tube. The technique is most effective when the tube has normal anatomy and the operator is experienced with the technique of application. The possibility of tubal transection, and resultant hemorrhage, appears to be highest with this technique.

Sterilization timing—Sterilization can be performed in relation to pregnancy (following vaginal delivery, cesarean section, or abortion) or remote from pregnancy (interval sterilization).

Tubal clips—Methods of tubal occlusion usually performed via laparoscopy in which a Filshie or Hulka clip is applied to the isthmic portion of the tube. The technique is most effective when the tube has normal anatomy and the operator is experienced with the technique of application. These methods inflict the narrowest zone of tubal damage (3–5 mm), affording a greater chance of sterilization reversal when compared with other methods.

Tuboperitoneal fistula—Poststerilization communication of the proximal tubal stump with the peritoneal cavity, which can result in sterilization failure, including ectopic gestation. Theoretically may be reduced by leaving a proximal tubal stump of 2 cm and by minimizing ligature-induced necrosis at the site of tubal interruption.

Uchida method—Method of partial salpingectomy that buries the end of the proximal tubal stump within the leaves of the mesosalpinx in an attempt to reduce the rate of tuboperitoneal fistula.

Unipolar coagulation—Method of tubal occlusion usually performed via laparoscopy that causes electrocoagulation of the tube when current is applied by grasping forceps; both jaws of the forceps serve as an active electrode. The high effectiveness rates observed with this method are a property of the wide zone of thermal destruction of the tube that results, but this same property increases morbidity from unintended thermal injuries. Surgeon must be vigilant regarding possibility of capacitive coupling.

In proposing the concept of tubal sterilization in 1842, James Blundell suggested the following:

> ... the operator ... ought to remove a portion, say one line, of the Fallopian tube, right and left, so as to intercept its caliber—the larger blood vessels being avoided. Mere divisions of the tube might be sufficient to produce sterility, but the further removal of a portion of the tube appears to be surer practice. I recommend this precaution, therefore, as an improvement of the operation.

Samuel Smith Lungren of Toledo, Ohio, is credited with having performed the first tubal sterilization in 1880, after having performed a cesarean section for a woman whose previous child was also born by cesarean section because of a contracted pelvis. During the second cesarean section, Lungren intended to remove the woman's ovaries to prevent future pregnancy, but instead decided that "the risk would be lessened and the same result would be accomplished by tying both Fallopian tubes with strong silk ligatures about one inch from the uterus." At the time of Lungren's successful tubal sterilization, laparotomy was a life-threatening procedure; thus, the performance of tubal sterilization at the time of cesarean section to prevent future pregnancy was potentially lifesaving. In 1919, Madlener reported on 85 tubal sterilizations performed at the time of laparotomy for other reasons, including cesarean section; three of the 85 women died postoperatively from infection. Because of the extreme risks, performing a laparotomy for the sole purpose of tubal sterilization remained an unpopular idea until the mid-20th century. Indeed, when three deaths occurred from 1936 to 1950 among 1,022 women who had postpartum Pomeroy sterilization, the investigators concluded that the risk for sterilization was comparable to that for multiparity and that "sterilization because of great multiparity alone cannot be justified on medical grounds" (Prystowsky and Eastman).

In addition to concerns about safety, the early history of tubal sterilization included debate about the appropriateness of tubal sterilization for fertility control. At the 21st Annual Meeting of the American Gynecological Society in 1886, participants debated a woman's right to undergo surgical sterilization. During this debate, Edward P. Davis said, "I hold it [sterilization] to be the right of a woman who is in a condition to which natural delivery is impossible. . . ." H.J. Garrigues objected by saying,

> We must leave that to Nature or to God. . . . I do not think that the woman has a right of that kind. . . . The mere fact that she does not want to have more children should not decide the question. (Speert)

The availability and acceptability of tubal sterilization as a method of fertility control remained limited until the mid-20th century, and, accordingly, tubal sterilization remained uncommon in the United States and around the world until the 1960s. In the 1970s, the worldwide popularity of tubal sterilization increased dramatically. Between 1970 and 1980, the estimated number of tubal sterilizations increased markedly in Europe, China, India, other parts of Asia, and Latin America. In the United States, the number of tubal sterilizations increased nearly fourfold—from about 200,000 in 1970 to about 700,000 in 1977. Among the factors affecting this increase were the availability and acceptability of two new surgical approaches—minilaparotomy and laparoscopy. In contrast to laparotomy for sterilization, these approaches were safer, allowed for surgery without hospitalization, reduced recovery time, and gave a better cosmetic result. Minilaparotomy has been used in many developing countries, and laparoscopy has been used in many developed countries, as well as in the United States.

Minilaparotomy for interval sterilization (i.e., sterilization at a time unrelated to pregnancy) requires a 2.5- to 3.0-cm suprapubic incision. The technique was first described by Uchida and colleagues in Japan in 1961. It was used in the early 1970s in Thailand by Vitoon and associates and then rapidly gained acceptance worldwide. Laparoscopy for tubal sterilization was first proposed by Anderson (1937) and later described by Power and Barnes (1941). The use of laparoscopy in Europe was encouraged by the work of Palmer (France), Steptoe (Britain), and Frangenheim (Germany), and use of the technique rapidly gained popularity in the 1970s, particularly in Europe and the United States.

In the United States, the increased use of tubal sterilization in the 1970s occurred concurrently with the widespread availability and acceptability of laparoscopy. In 1970, less than 1% of sterilizations were performed with a laparoscope, but by 1975, more than one third of the 550,000 women who had tubal sterilization had the procedure performed laparoscopically. This transition was associated with a marked reduction in length of hospital stay for tubal sterilization—from 6.5 nights in 1970 to 4 nights in the years 1975 to 1978. By 1987, one third of tubal sterilizations in the United States required no overnight hospital stay, and 79% of these were performed by way of laparoscopy.

Sterilization is now the method of family planning most commonly used in the world. In 1995, about 223 million couples used sterilization (of themselves or their spouses) for contraception; 180 million were women using tubal sterilization and 43 million were men using vasectomy.

Thus, the developing world accounts for most of the use of sterilization. Nearly half of all users are in China, and more than one fourth are in India. Vasectomy accounts for only a small percentage of sterilization procedures in developing countries except for China, India, and South Korea. In nearly all countries, the prevalence of tubal sterilization exceeds that of vasectomy. Worldwide, the ratio of female-to-male sterilization is 4 to 1.

In the United States, more than 3 million tubal sterilizations were performed in 1994–1996. Approximately one-half were postpartum procedures; of these, 58% were performed after vaginal delivery and 42% were concurrent with cesarean section. Of the approximately one-half of tubal sterilizations performed as interval procedures, 96% were performed on an outpatient basis. Among interval sterilizations, laparoscopy was used as the surgical approach in 89% of procedures performed in outpatient settings and 53% of those performed in inpatient settings.

In the United States, sterilization has also become the most commonly used method of contraception among married couples. The proportion of couples who used contraception that chose sterilization more than doubled from 1973 (16%) to 2002 (36%). Most of this increase was in female sterilization—from 9% in 1973 to 27% in 2002; there was little to no increase in male sterilization over this period (8% in 1973 and 9% in 2002). Among U.S. women using contraception in 2002, 10% 25 to 29 years old, 19% 30 to 34 years old, 29% 35 to 40 years old, and 35% 40 to 44 years old had undergone tubal sterilization.

TIMING OF STERILIZATION

Tubal sterilization can be performed at the time of cesarean section, shortly after delivery or induced abortion, or at a time unrelated to pregnancy. About one half of tubal sterilizations in the United States are performed at a time unrelated to pregnancy. The timing of tubal sterilization can influence the choice of anesthetic, surgical approach, and method of tubal occlusion. For example, most sterilizations performed concurrently with cesarean section require no separate anesthesia and involve partial salpingectomy as the method of tubal occlusion. Most tubal sterilizations performed after vaginal delivery are done by minilaparotomy with subumbilical incisions and partial salpingectomy. Tubal sterilization not associated with birth usually is performed by laparoscopy (with use of coagulation, silicone rubber band application, or clip application) or minilaparotomy (with use of partial salpingectomy).

PREOPERATIVE EVALUATION

The candidate for sterilization should be extensively counseled. The intended permanence of the procedure, alternatives to sterilization, and risks of surgery should be discussed. For couples desiring sterilization, no such discussion is complete without consideration of vasectomy as an alternative. Women also should be made aware that sterilization failure can occur and that the relative likelihood of ectopic pregnancy is increased when sterilization failure does occur.

The workup of women who are to undergo tubal sterilization includes a history and physical examination and a laboratory evaluation, as indicated. Consideration should be given to whether the woman might be pregnant at the time of sterilization, and pregnancy testing should be ordered as necessary.

A careful gynecologic history and examination also are necessary before sterilization. Women with gynecologic disease or symptoms may require additional diagnostic or therapeutic measures. Some ultimately may be better served by other surgical procedures, either instead of or in addition to sterilization. For example, some women with enlarged and symptomatic uterine leiomyomata and women with symptomatic pelvic relaxation may benefit more from hysterectomy than from tubal sterilization. Others, such as women with abnormal cervical cytology, need careful evaluation before a decision can be made about preventing or treating invasive cervical cancer.

ANESTHESIA

Complications of general anesthesia are the leading cause of death attributed to sterilization in the United States. The risks inherent in general anesthesia are exacerbated by its use postpartum and during laparoscopy. The special requirements of general anesthesia for laparoscopy have been well described.

Except for the use of conduction anesthesia postpartum, general anesthesia is the technique most often used for female sterilization in the United States. A 1988 survey of members of the American Association of Gynecologic Laparoscopists revealed that the number of providers of tubal sterilization who used local anesthesia for laparoscopic sterilization had increased from 4% (in the 1982 survey) to 8%. Worldwide, more than 75% of tubal sterilization procedures are performed under local anesthesia. A discussion of the technology and regimen for administering general or conduction anesthesia is beyond the scope of this chapter. Instead, we focus on local anesthesia because of its increasing use in outpatient settings for many types of surgery.

Sterilization by laparoscopy or minilaparotomy can be performed safely under local anesthesia. The patient avoids the risks associated with general anesthesia, spends less time sedated or anesthetized, and has a more rapid recovery. Nausea and vomiting are less likely to occur, and the patient is awake to report symptoms that can indicate the occurrence of a complication. Television technology has made it possible for the patient to observe the procedure if she desires. Furthermore, the overall expense often is reduced compared with procedures done under general anesthesia.

In the United States, the overall morbidity rate for female sterilization is so low that it is difficult to obtain a sample large enough to demonstrate a comparative safety advantage for local versus general anesthesia. One U.S. study randomly assigned 100 women to either local or general anesthesia for laparoscopic sterilization. Serious or life-threatening events did not occur in either group. However, women who had general anesthesia were more likely to have intraoperative hypotension, hypertension, or tachycardia, which suggests that these women were hemodynamically less stable and may have been at increased risk for cardiovascular complications. In another study, 125 women were randomly allocated to the use of local or general anesthesia for laparoscopic sterilization. Women who had general anesthesia were more likely to develop hypotension; hypertension was more common in the local anesthesia group. No women in either group had tachycardia.

Operating under local anesthesia incurs several possible disadvantages. The patient's anxiety may be increased; therefore, the surgeon must use a decisive and gentle surgical technique while talking with the patient. The patient may feel discomfort; thus, the physician must have a thorough understanding of the use of sedative and analgesic drugs. Although obesity can complicate the use of local anesthesia, several studies indicate that local anesthesia can be used successfully for obese women. Women with a history of multiple abdominal or pelvic surgical procedures or peritonitis may need additional anesthesia if the procedure is difficult or prolonged. Additional anesthesia also may be required during minilaparotomy if the abdominal incision needs to be extended. One U.S.-based retrospective study reviewed 2,827 outpatient laparoscopic sterilizations performed under local anesthesia and mild sedation from 1980 to 1988. The mean operating time was 10.0 (±5.1) minutes, and the mean anesthesia time was 23.3 (±6.9) minutes. The hospital cost to the patient was reduced 65% to 85%. Another U.S. study reported on 358 minilaparotomies for interval sterilization performed under local anesthesia. The average operating time was 21 minutes, and no complications were reported. In both series, the local anesthetic was 0.5% bupivacaine hydrochloride used alone or in combination with lidocaine. In one series, midazolam hydrochloride and fentanyl citrate were used for mild intravenous sedation; in the other series, meperidine hydrochloride and diazepam were used.

For local infiltration and paracervical block, agents of intermediate intrinsic potency (defined as the minimum concentration required to produce a block within 5 to 10 minutes), such as lidocaine or mepivacaine, have been found suitable. Both are amides with good stability and low toxicity. Onset of analgesic effects is rapid, even when a low concentration of medication is used, and the duration of the effect is sufficient for the procedure but not prolonged (about 1.5 hours when the medication is given in plain solution). Bupivacaine, a more potent and a longer-acting amide, is frequently used in the United States. However, the short duration of action provided by lidocaine or mepivacaine is preferred by some because it allows for awareness of any abnormal degree of persistent pain and early diagnosis of complications, such as hematoma formation.

SURGICAL APPROACH

Minilaparotomy

The minilaparotomy approach to tubal occlusion can be used in the interval or postpartum period. Although interval sterilization by minilaparotomy is the sterilization procedure most frequently performed in many countries, it is not a common procedure in the United States. Minilaparotomy in the United States often is used preferentially among women considered to be at increased risk for laparoscopy.

Interval minilaparotomy is performed with use of a 2- to 3-cm midline vertical or transverse suprapubic incision. In patients with an enlarged uterus resulting from uterine leiomyomata or other benign conditions, the minilaparotomy incision should be made at the level of the uterine fundus to ensure access to the fallopian tubes. A uterine manipulator is placed through the cervix just before surgery and is used to bring the uterus toward the incision. Placement of a paracervical block before insertion of the uterine manipulator reduces discomfort for patients having surgery under local anesthesia. The abdomen is then entered with the approach that is used for laparotomy; small handheld retractors and the Trendelenburg position are used to enhance exposure. Once the uterus is identified, a tubal hook or a finger is placed posteriorly at the top of the fundus and moved along the uterus. The fallopian tube is identified first by the fimbriated end, and then the midportion of the fallopian tube is grasped with a small Babcock clamp and elevated through the abdominal incision. Tubal occlusion most often is performed by use of the modified Pomeroy or Parkland technique. However, clips or rings can be applied through the minilaparotomy incision with modified instruments originally developed for use through the operating laparoscope.

Postpartum minilaparotomy is performed in a manner similar to that of interval minilaparotomy. It is ideally performed before the onset of postpartum uterine involution while the uterine fundus is high in the abdomen (within 48 hours of delivery). A 2- to 3-cm subumbilical vertical or semicircular incision is made in the midline where the abdominal wall is thin. Because of the proximity of the enlarged uterus to the incision, access to the fallopian tubes is easier than it is with an interval approach. A uterine manipulator is unnecessary when minilaparotomy is performed in the postpartum period.

Laparoscopy

> The magic is in the magician, not in the wand. . . . Entering the abdomen is the most dangerous part of the laparoscopic procedure. (Hulka and Reich)

The laparoscopic instrumentation, including laparoscope, light cables and light source, insufflator and tubing, and video camera and television, if used, should be set up and tested for proper functioning before any incisions are made. If a Veress needle is to be used, it is good practice to attach it to the insufflation tubing and test that gas flows freely through it. High line pressures (3 mm Hg or higher) during low-flow insufflation (1 L/min) through a Veress needle that has yet to be inserted into the abdominal cavity suggest that the needle has some occlusion. Checking for occlusion before inserting the needle can avoid the multiple attempts at needle placement that might occur in the belief that incorrect placement, rather than needle occlusion, is the cause of resistance to flow. It is convenient, while waiting for surgery, to have the end of the laparoscope bathing in warm sterile fluid to prevent it from fogging when it is inserted into the abdominal cavity.

A no. 11 scalpel blade is used to make a single vertical incision in the lower rim of the umbilicus. This must be done carefully because the aorta can lie just a few centimeters beneath the abdominal wall, particularly in a thin patient. The abdominal wall is lifted away from the aorta by pinching the skin beneath the umbilicus between thumb and index finger. The umbilicus is elevated with one hand while the surgeon's other hand makes the controlled incision.

The Veress needle is disconnected from the insufflation tubing before insertion. The stopcock on the needle then is placed in the open position, and the spring action of the needle is tested for smooth operation. Elevating the abdominal wall and using the Veress needle with the stopcock open allows air to rush into the previously gas-free abdominal cavity when the end of the needle penetrates the peritoneal layer. The in-rushing air, if heard, is one of the first indicators that successful abdominal entry has occurred. Outflow of blood likewise can serve as an immediate indicator of vessel injury. Allowing air to rush in also can cause the bowel to fall away from the abdominal wall.

The terminal aorta is palpated, even in a moderately obese patient, through the abdominal wall in the midline, just above or at the umbilicus. The pulsations of the aorta are lost in the midline just beneath the umbilicus, corresponding to the sacral hollow. The aorta bifurcates at the level of L4, which corresponds to the summits of the iliac crests. This is a more reliable landmark for bifurcation of the aorta than the umbilicus. The Veress needle is placed through the umbilical incision and is directed at an angle toward the sacral hollow or uterine fundus (to avoid the aorta) and in the midline (to avoid the iliac vessels). Elevating the abdominal wall during this placement increases the distance between the Veress needle and major vessels. While placing the Veress needle, the surgeon should hold the needle like a dart, being careful not to impede the action of the spring mechanism. Resistance at the tip of the needle causes the blunt cannula inside the needle to be pushed back, and the spring mechanism at the hub of the needle extends. When resistance at the tip of the advancing needle is lost, as occurs with successful penetration of the peritoneal cavity, the blunt cannula inside the needle advances back out to the tip, and the spring mechanism at the hub of the needle snaps back in. Observing the spring mechanism for this snap can serve as a sign to test for successful placement. Often there are two snaps—the first when the fascia is penetrated and the second with peritoneal penetration. Continuing to advance the needle tip much beyond the point of penetration of the parietal peritoneum risks placing the needle tip between loops of bowel or under the omental apron, both of which can cause resistance to flow and can result in reinsertion of the needle. Continued advancement of the Veress needle also risks vascular injury. The needle tip should not be moved laterally once the tip is inserted in the abdomen; any simple vascular puncture could be transformed into a major laceration if the needle tip is moved from side to side. Once abdominal penetration is made with the Veress needle, the needle should be stabilized carefully until the safety checks have been completed. The needle should not be moved, and a laparotomy should be performed immediately if major vascular injury is suspected.

The distance between skin and fascia can increase with increasing patient obesity. A given angle of entry of the Veress needle that successfully penetrates the peritoneal cavity in a thin patient might fall far short of the peritoneum in an obese patient. To bring the peritoneal cavity within the physical length of the Veress needle, it is often necessary to pursue entry with a trajectory closer to the vertical. However, this also directs the Veress needle toward the aorta and therefore should be attempted only by experienced surgeons, and with extreme care. Alternatively, open laparoscopy can be performed.

Several safety checks for correct intraabdominal placement can be performed while the Veress needle is held steady. The instillation of 5 to 10 mL of sterile saline through the needle, followed immediately by aspiration, can be helpful. The fluid should meet little resistance, and, more important, scant fluid should return on reaspiration. Reaspiration of fluid suggests that the needle tip is in a small enclosed space that does not allow immediate dispersion of the instilled fluid. Reaspiration of feculent fluid or bloody fluid suggests bowel or vascular penetration, respectively. Simple penetration of the bowel with a Veress needle does not mandate immediate exploratory laparotomy. Depending on the setting and the skill level of the surgeon, reinsertion of the needle or open laparoscopy, followed by laparoscopic visualization of the intestine, can be pursued.

A second safety check consists of attaching a filled 10-mL syringe to the hub of the Veress needle and then removing the plunger. Elevation of the abdominal wall at this point should cause an increased negative intraperitoneal pressure, which allows the fluid in the syringe to drain passively into the abdominal cavity through an open stopcock. Alternatively, a drop of saline (drip test) can be placed on the hub of the Veress needle, and, with the stopcock open, elevation of the abdominal wall should result in the drop flowing downward freely.

Once these safety checks are performed, insufflation is begun at 1 L/min or less. Initial insufflation pressures often are 5 mm Hg or less in thin patients and, even with correct needle placement, can be 10 mm Hg or more in obese patients. An intraabdominal pressure greater than 15 mm Hg during insufflation generally is avoided to prevent respiratory compromise and decreased venous return secondary to vena caval compression. Abdominal distention increases the distance between the abdominal wall and major pelvic vessels, and this increases the safety buffer when the trocar is inserted. However, the abdomen should not be distended so taut that it is difficult to manually elevate it for trocar insertion.

During insufflation, a shift from dullness to tympany with percussion over the liver is indicative of pneumoperitoneum formation. It also is prudent for the surgeon to pay attention to the electrocardiogram rhythm during insufflation, because the sudden appearance of premature ventricular contractions can be an indicator of intravascular insufflation. Sudden vascular collapse during insufflation can be caused by a gas embolism into the right side of the heart, and at times this life-threatening event can be signaled by a new "cog wheel" or "mill wheel" murmur. Rapidly tilting the patient into Trendelenberg position and onto her left side and advancing a Swan-Ganz catheter into the right heart for aspiration can be life-saving.

Once insufflation is complete, the Veress needle is removed, and the umbilical incision is widened to accommodate the trocar and sleeve. An incision that is too large can result in leakage of gas around the sleeve. An incision that is too small can restrict access. The trocar should be checked before insertion to ensure that it is sharp; a dull trocar potentially is dangerous because it requires increased force for abdominal entry.

The trocar is grasped as shown in Figure 27.1. The middle finger serves as a stopper, preventing the forward momentum following fascial puncture from carrying the trocar deep into the pelvis. The precautions for insertion of the Veress needle pertain even more to insertion of the trocar; the abdominal wall is elevated, and the trocar is directed toward the hollow of the sacrum or the uterine fundus, and a midline trajectory is followed.

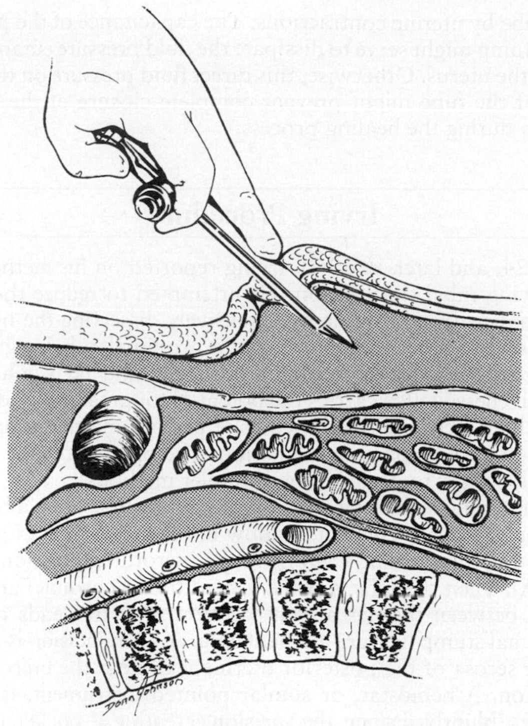

FIGURE 27.1. Trocar entry. When inserting the trocar through the abdominal wall, the trocar is "palmed" in the surgeon's dominant hand, with the extended middle finger serving as a stopper to deep abdominal penetration. If the surgeon's hand is too small to accomplish this, open laparoscopy should be considered.

Open laparoscopy is performed without previous creation of a pneumoperitoneum. The skin beneath the umbilicus is incised sufficiently with a scalpel in either a vertical or transverse direction to adequately visualize the underlying fascia. The skin is released, and the fascia is grasped and elevated. The fascia is then incised in the midline, and the opening is stretched with a hemostat or incised to a length just sufficient to visualize the underlying peritoneum, which in turn is elevated and incised. Each angle of the fascial incision is sutured with a no. 0 absorbable stitch but not tied. The Hasson blunt cannula and sleeve are then placed through the opening of the peritoneum. The blunt cannula then is removed, and the abdomen is insufflated through the port found on the sleeve.

METHOD OF TUBAL OCCLUSION

All tubal sterilization methods rely on correct identification of the fallopian tube for success. With any of the methods, the tube should be followed out to its fimbriated end to confirm that the correct structure has been identified.

Theoretically, the risk of tuboperitoneal fistula formation can be reduced by preserving a proximal tubal segment 1 to 2 cm in length. It is possible that the proximal tubal stump serves as a distensible reservoir for the small amount of uterine fluid that is normally forced through the interstitial portion of the tube by uterine contractions. The capacitance of the proximal stump might serve to dissipate the fluid pressure emanating from the uterus. Otherwise, this direct fluid pressure on the cut end of the tube might prevent complete closure of the tubal lumen during the healing process.

Irving Procedure

In 1924, and later, in 1950, Irving reported on his method of achieving tubal sterilization. He attempted to reduce the risk of tuboperitoneal fistulae by extensively dissecting the ligated ends of the tubes and burying the proximal tubal segment. Although the extra dissection in this technique likely enhances effectiveness, it also carries the potential for greater blood loss, as well as increases the difficulty of performing the technique through a minilaparotomy incision. The procedure also takes slightly longer to perform than simpler methods.

The Irving technique is accomplished by first using a hemostat or scissors to create a window in the mesosalpinx just beneath the tube, about 4 cm from the uterotubal junction (Fig. 27.2A). Then the tube is twice ligated (no. 1 chromic) and divided between the ties at this location. The free ends of the proximal stump ligature are held long. A 1-cm incision is made in the serosa of the posterior uterine wall near the uterotubal junction. A hemostat, or similar pointed instrument, is then used to bluntly deepen the incision, creating a pocket in the uterine musculature about 1 to 2 cm deep (Fig. 27.2B). The two free ends of the proximal stump ligature, previously held long, are then individually threaded onto a curved needle and brought deep into the myometrial tunnel and out through the uterine serosa (Fig. 27.2C). Traction on the sutures then draw the ligated proximal stump deep into the myometrial tunnel, and tying the free sutures fix the tube in this buried location (Fig. 27.2D). Often this can be accomplished without incising the mesosalpinx, but if extra mobilization of the proximal stump is needed, or if the proximal stump mesosalpinx appears in danger of being torn when traction is applied, then the mesosalpinx under the proximal tubal segment can be incised partly back toward the uterus. The serosal opening of the myometrial tunnel is then plicated closed around the tube with use of a fine absorbable suture, but great care should be exercised to avoid compromising the tube as it enters the tunnel. Strangulation or damage to the tube with this stitch could cause necrosis and fistula formation in the extramyometrial portion of the proximal tube. No treatment of the distal tubal stump is necessary, but some surgeons choose to bury that segment in the mesosalpinx.

Modified Pomeroy Procedure

Bishop and Nelms, colleagues of Pomeroy, reported on the Pomeroy technique for tubal occlusion in 1930. They were

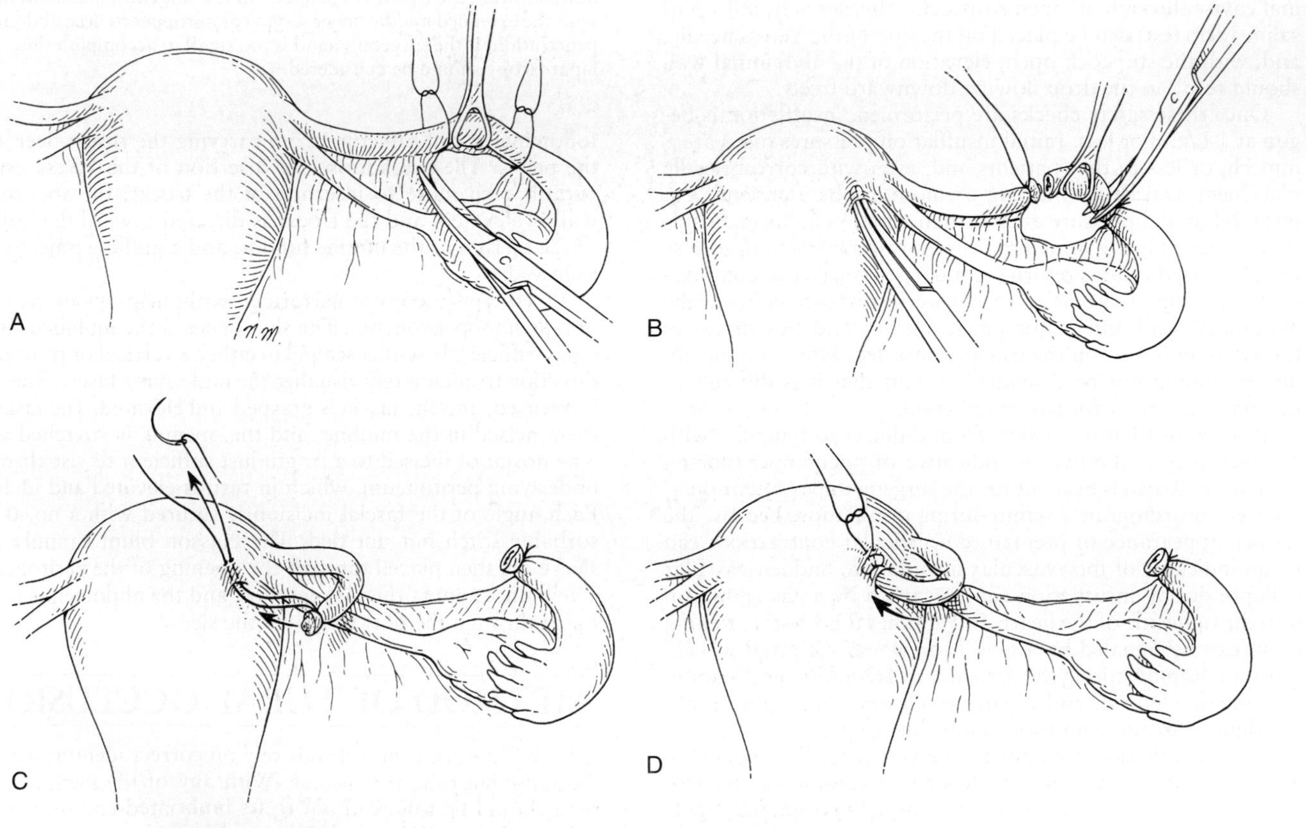

FIGURE 27.2. Irving method. **A:** A fenestration is made beneath the tube about 4 cm from the uterotubal junction using scissors or a hemostat. **B:** The tube is then twice ligated and a portion resected. A deep pocket is created in the myometrium on the posterior uterus. The dashed line shows the line of incision if added mobilization of the proximal tube is necessary to bury the end of the tube in the myometrium. **C:** The tagged ends of the tube are sutured deep into the myometrial tunnel and out through the uterine serosa. **D:** Tying these sutures secures the cut end of the proximal tube deep in the myometrial pocket.

careful to point out the importance of using absorbable suture as opposed to permanent suture.

In this method, the tube is grasped in its midportion, usually with a small atraumatic clamp such as the Babcock, and a loop of tube is elevated (Fig. 27.3A). The base of the loop is ligated with no. 1 plain catgut, leaving a 2-cm proximal stump of isthmus, and the sutures are held long. A 2- to 3-cm portion of tube in the ligated loop is transected and removed with scissors (Fig. 27.3B). Bishop and Nelms, in the original report on this method, pointed out that ligation was performed with a double strand of absorbable chromic catgut suture to allow the cut tubal ends to quickly separate after surgery. It was their belief that this would allow the ends to naturally fibrose and peritonealize without fistulization or communication. This also is the rationale for the common modification of the Pomeroy technique, in which the original chromic suture is replaced by plain catgut because of the more rapid degradation of the latter. Surgeons have a tendency to strenuously tighten the catgut ligature around the tube (as though the tighter the ligature, the better the occlusion), but this appears to go against the very principles of the procedure. This tightening can result in greater strangulation and necrosis of the adjoining tubal segments, potentially increasing the risk of fistula formation and failure. Taking time to identify the muscular tube, which is often seen pouting from each of the severed limbs of the ligated tube, is a good habit to develop, as is checking the tubal stumps for hemostasis. Resection of a limited amount of tube, restricted to the isthmic section, is ideal should unexpected future reanastomosis be requested. Making the knuckle of tube in the loop too small, however, can result in only a shave excision of the side of the tube, with incomplete transection of the lumen. To avoid incomplete resection, the mesosalpinx within the ligated loop should be perforated with scissors before the tubal limb on each side of this window is individually cut. It is important not to cut the loop so close to the suture that only short distal segments of tube remain beyond the tie. These short limbs can easily slip out of the ligature and cause delayed bleeding.

The Pomeroy method minimizes bleeding by compressing and sealing the vascular mesosalpinx before tubal transection. It is not unusual when performing tubal sterilization at the time of cesarean section to find the mesosalpinx greatly engorged with distended veins. Elevation of the uterus through the abdominal incision often facilitates tubal occlusion by allowing the vessels to drain and decompress. It is important when replacing the uterus into the peritoneal cavity to lead with one adnexa at a time while protecting the tubal ligation site on that side. Otherwise, when the uterus is replaced, a tight fit can cause the adnexa to be squeezed against the incision, with resultant avulsion of the ligature and postoperative bleeding. When a Pomeroy ligation is performed through a minilaparotomy incision, the ligation sutures are held while the tube is cut. This prevents retraction of the cut tubal stumps into the peritoneal cavity before they can be adequately examined and before hemostasis can be ensured. After examination is complete, the sutures are cut, and the tubal stumps are allowed to retract into the abdomen.

It is also possible to perform a modified Pomeroy tubal ligation as a laparoscopic interval procedure. In this technique, a laparoscope with an operating channel is placed through the umbilical port, and a 5-mm midline suprapubic cannula is introduced under direct vision. A plain gut Roeder loop (endoscopic slip knot) is introduced through the 5-mm port. A grasper is introduced through the operative channel of the laparoscope, advanced through the suture loop, and the appropriate portion of tube is grasped and retracted back through the loop. The slip knot of the loop is then tightened, ligating a knuckle of the tube. Scissors are then introduced through the operative scope, and the suture is cut. With use of a grasper through the 5-mm port, the loop of tube is held on tension while the scissors are used through the operative channel to transect the tube above the ligature. When the procedure is complete and the tubal segment has been resected, the grasper is used through the operative channel to hold the specimen while the operative scope and grasper are removed together through the

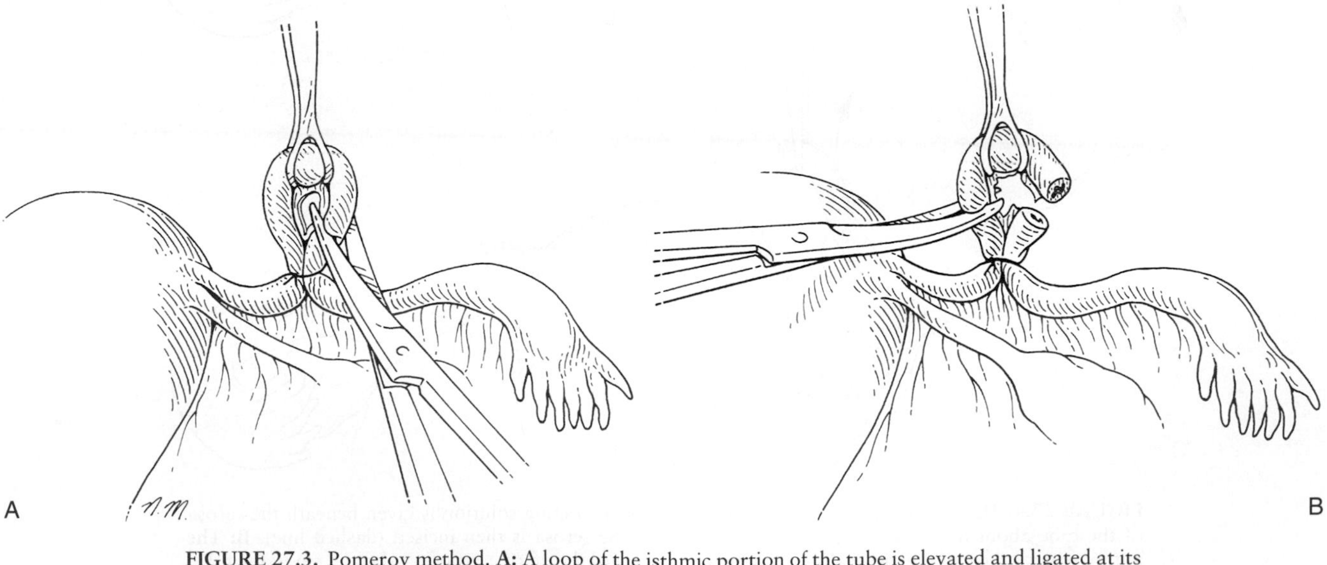

FIGURE 27.3. Pomeroy method. A: A loop of the isthmic portion of the tube is elevated and ligated at its base with one or two ties of no. 1 plain catgut suture. If performed through a minilaparotomy incision, these ties should be held long to prevent premature retraction of the tubal stumps into the abdomen when the loop of tube is transected. B: A fenestration is bluntly created through the mesentery within the tubal loop, and each limb of the tube on either side of this fenestration is individually cut. The cut ends of the tube are inspected for hemostasis and allowed to retract into the abdomen.

umbilical sleeve. In contrast to most other methods of laparoscopic sterilization, this technique has the advantage of producing a surgical specimen for evaluation.

Uchida Method

Originally reported on in 1961, and reported on in revised form in 1975, the Uchida method, like the Irving procedure before it, recognized the role of fistula formation in tubal sterilization failures and included steps to prevent this complication.

This method begins by having the surgeon grasp the tube in its midportion, about 6 to 7 cm from the uterotubal junction. A 1:1,000 epinephrine in saline solution is injected subserosally, creating a bleb over the tube that is then incised (Fig. 27.4A). The muscular tube, which often can be seen springing up through the serosal incision, then is divided between two hemostats. The serosa over the proximal tubal segment is dissected bluntly toward the uterus, exposing about 5 cm of the proximal tubal segment (Fig. 27.4B). The tube then is ligated with no. 0 chromic suture near the uterotubal junction, and this 5-cm segment of exposed tube is resected. The shortened proximal stump is allowed to retract into the mesosalpinx (Fig. 27.4C). The serosa around the opening in the mesosalpinx is sutured in a pursestring fashion with a fine absorbable stitch. Simultaneous ligation of the distal tube and gathering of the mesosalpinx around the distal stump are accomplished when the pursestring suture is tied (Fig. 27.4D). This step also fixes the distal stump in a position open to the peritoneal cavity while burying the proximal stump within the leaves of the mesosalpinx.

Uchida added fimbriectomy to the procedure in 1975 to enhance effectiveness. Some surgeons omit this step, and in addition excise only 1 to 2 cm of tube (rather than the recommended 5 cm) to permit future tubal anastomosis.

Parkland Method

In this method, made popular during the 1960s at Parkland Memorial Hospital, the tube is grasped in its midportion with a Babcock clamp, and a hemostat or scissors is used to create

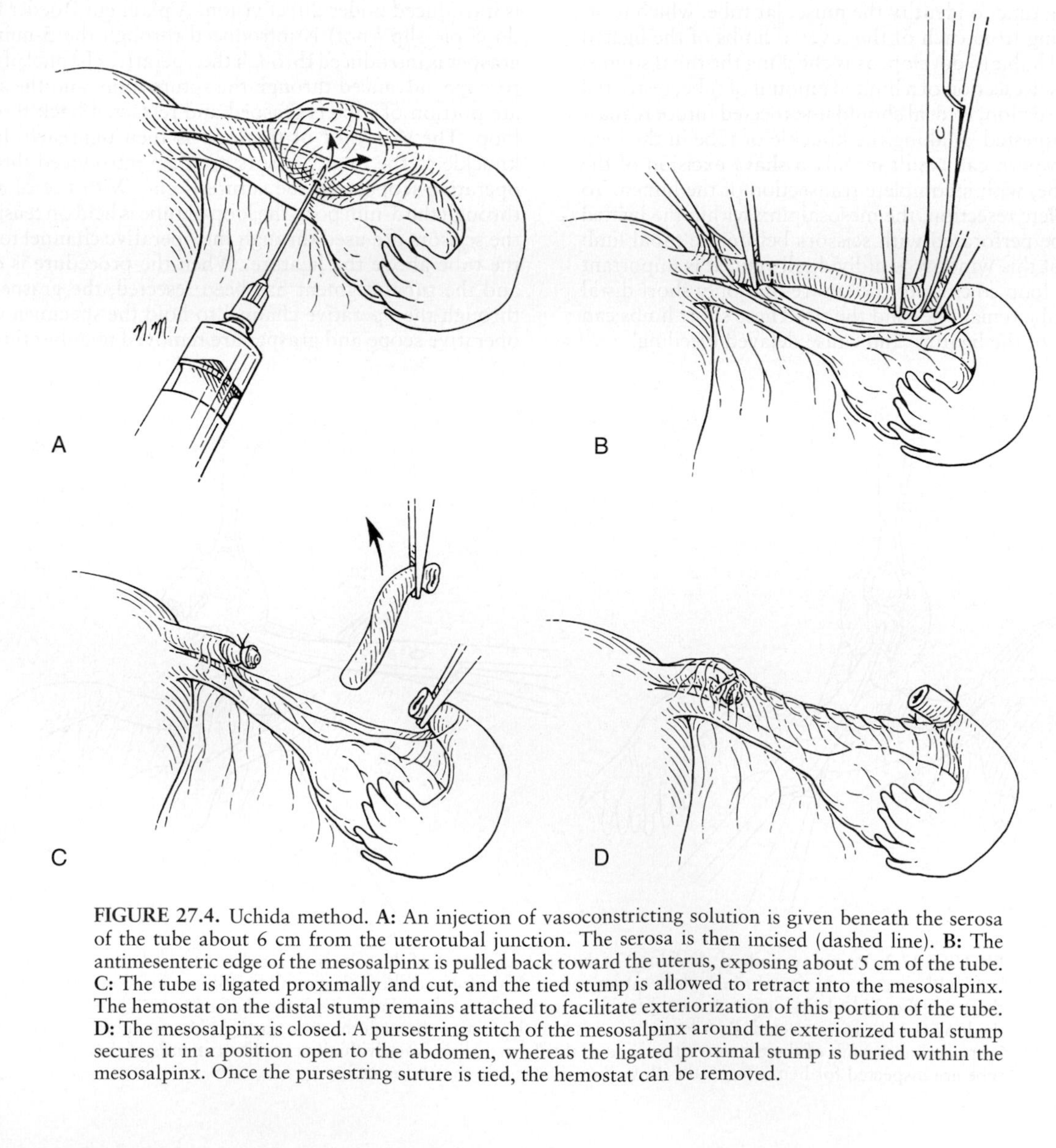

FIGURE 27.4. Uchida method. **A:** An injection of vasoconstricting solution is given beneath the serosa of the tube about 6 cm from the uterotubal junction. The serosa is then incised (dashed line). **B:** The antimesenteric edge of the mesosalpinx is pulled back toward the uterus, exposing about 5 cm of the tube. **C:** The tube is ligated proximally and cut, and the tied stump is allowed to retract into the mesosalpinx. The hemostat on the distal stump remains attached to facilitate exteriorization of this portion of the tube. **D:** The mesosalpinx is closed. A pursestring stitch of the mesosalpinx around the exteriorized tubal stump secures it in a position open to the abdomen, whereas the ligated proximal stump is buried within the mesosalpinx. Once the pursestring suture is tied, the hemostat can be removed.

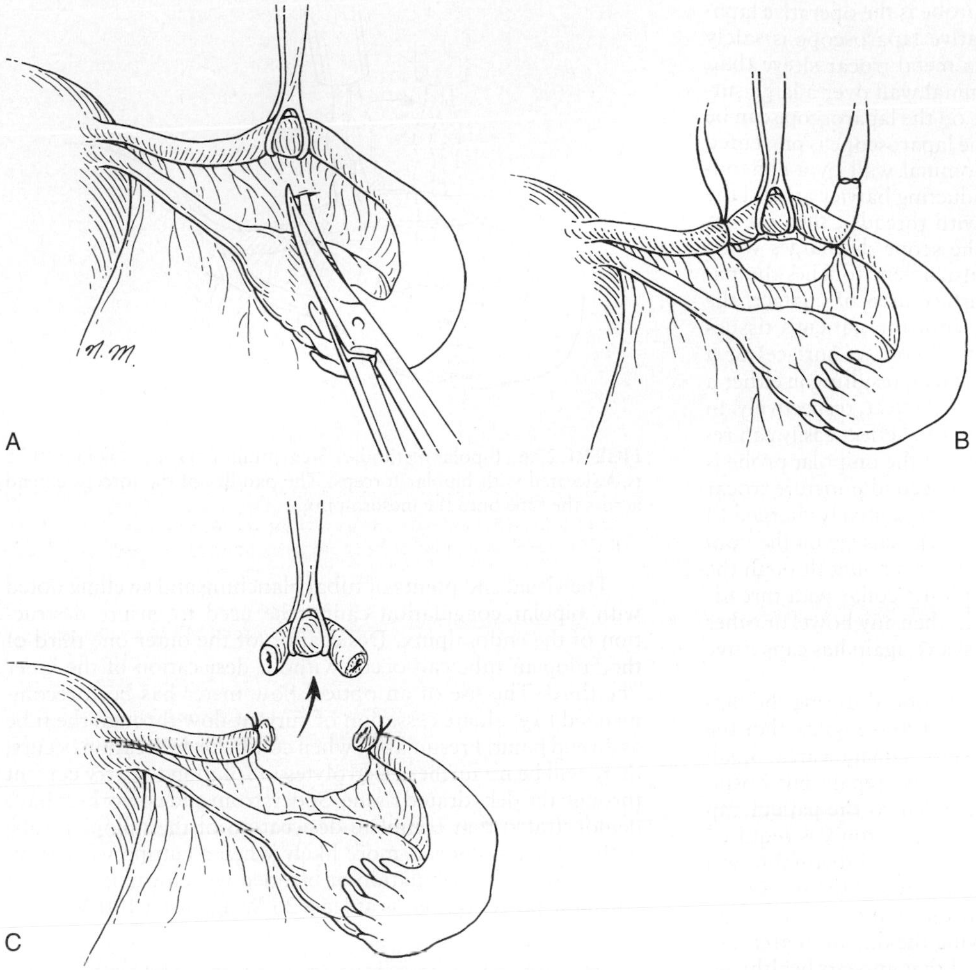

FIGURE 27.5. Parkland method. **A:** A 2- to 3-cm fenestration is made beneath the isthmic portion of tube either with scissors or bluntly with a hemostat. **B:** Ligation of the tube. Pulling up on the suture during ligation or during transection of the tube can shear the tube off the underlying mesentery, resulting in troublesome bleeding. **C:** Portion of tube removed.

a window in an avascular area of the mesosalpinx just beneath the isthmic portion of the tube (Fig. 27.5A). The window is stretched to about 2.5 cm in length by opening the hemostat. Two ligatures of no. 0 chromic material are passed through the window, and the tube is ligated proximally and distally, leaving a 2-cm proximal stump of isthmic tube (Fig. 27.5B). The intervening segment of tube between the ties then is resected (Fig. 27.5C). In contrast to the Pomeroy method, in which the resected portions of the tubes are ligated together and later separate when the suture weakens, immediate separation of the tubal ends is accomplished with the Parkland method. Care should be taken to avoid undue traction on the ligatures while resecting the tubal segments, because this could result in tearing of the mesosalpinx and excessive bleeding.

Unipolar Coagulation

Unipolar coagulation was the first method of laparoscopic tubal occlusion to achieve widespread use. However, reports of electrical complications, particularly thermal bowel injury, resulted in a significant decline in this method's popularity as soon as alternative methods of laparoscopic tubal occlusion became available in the mid-1970s. In unipolar coagulation, a specially designed insulated grasping forceps is introduced through the operating channel of the laparoscope or independently through a 5-mm second puncture port. As a safety precaution, attachment of the electric cable to the grasping forceps should be delayed until the surgeon is ready to coagulate the fallopian tube.

With unipolar coagulation, as much as 3 to 5 cm of tube can be destroyed with a single burn, with occult damage occurring beyond the visual zone of desiccation. For this reason, the isthmic–ampullary portion of the tube should be carefully identified and grasped about 5 cm from the uterus to preserve some length of proximal tube. The jaws of the grasping forceps should completely encircle the fallopian tube and include a portion of the mesosalpinx as well. The tube should be elevated away from adjacent structures, such as bowel and bladder, before current is applied for about 5 seconds. If a second burn is required, it should be applied to the proximal rather than the distal portion of the tube. The current should be turned off before the tube is released and the grasping forceps are retracted into the laparoscope. Both jaws of the grasping forceps serve as active electrodes and will burn any structure they touch while current is applied.

The thermal injuries to abdominal viscera that are seen with unipolar coagulation are, in some cases, likely attributable to the phenomenon of capacitive coupling. The current flowing down the unipolar probe creates an electromagnetic field that can transfer an electric charge to any conductor surrounding the probe. The greater the voltage being used with the probe, the greater this capacitive effect. In the case of laparoscopic unipolar coagulation for sterilization, the conductor surrounding the insulated unipolar probe is the operative laparoscope itself. As long as the operative laparoscope is safely grounded (usually by contact with a metal trocar sleeve that, in turn, is in contact with the abdominal wall over a large surface area), then the capacitive charge on the laparoscope can be harmlessly dissipated. If, however, the laparoscope is prevented from safely grounding into the abdominal wall by a nonconducting trocar sleeve or by a nonconducting barrier around the trocar sleeve (e.g., a plastic collar with threads), then the capacitive charge that builds up on the scope discharges when and wherever any portion of that instrument touches the patient's tissues. Depending on the surface area of contact, the discharging current from the scope into the patient's tissues has either a high current density (small contact surface) or a low current density (large contact surface), resulting in either a large thermal effect or a minimal thermal effect, respectively. In the case of contact with bowel, this thermal effect easily can result in delayed necrosis and peritonitis. If the unipolar probe is brought into the abdomen by way of a second puncture trocar sheath, then it is the sheath itself that is capacitively charged (if it is made of a conducting material). If the charge on the conducting trocar sleeve is prevented from grounding through the abdominal wall (as could occur if a plastic collar with threads is being used around the trocar sleeve), then any bowel or other grounded tissue touching the trocar sleeve again has capacitive current flowing into it.

If thermal injury to the intestine is noticed during the laparoscopic procedure, then it is important to recognize that the injury can extend well beyond the visibly damaged area. Small burns of the bowel serosa may not require repair, but hospitalization for 5 to 7 days is recommended so the patient can be observed for delayed peritonitis. A laparotomy is required if peritonitis occurs. A large area of superficial thermal bowel injury, or one that is thought to extend beyond the serosa, requires resection of that portion of intestine with a 5-cm margin on either side of the lesion. Oversewing the damaged area can result in stitches being placed in bowel that appears healthy visually but in reality is destined to necrose from occult thermal or electrical injury.

Bipolar Coagulation

The use of bipolar coagulation for tubal sterilization was reported by Rioux and Cloutier in 1974. With bipolar coagulation, current flows from one jaw of the grasper to the other, requiring only the intervening tissue of the patient within the jaws of the instrument to complete the circuit. This eliminates the need for a distant ground plate. Compared with unipolar coagulation, which uses the patient's body to complete the circuit, bipolar coagulation applies current in a more discrete manner (a 1.5- to 3-cm zone of thermal injury) and with an increased element of safety. Capacitive coupling does not occur with bipolar forceps because the field effects from the equal but opposite currents that flow in both directions along the shaft of the instrument cancel out one another.

Once the fallopian tube is carefully identified, it is grasped in the distal isthmic section with the bipolar forceps in such a way that the tube is completely encircled, including a portion of the mesosalpinx (Fig. 27.6). The tube then is elevated away from any adjacent structures, and current is applied. Two additional contiguous areas similarly are coagulated to ensure at least a 3-cm area of desiccation. As with unipolar coagulation, an effort should be made to leave the proximal 2 cm of tube undisturbed to reduce the risk of tuboperitoneal fistula formation.

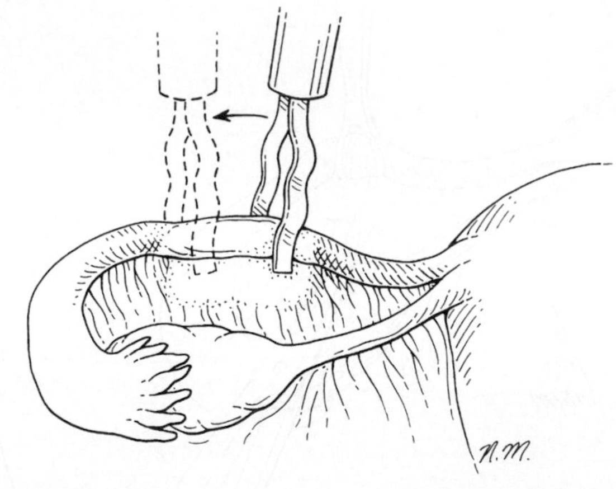

FIGURE 27.6. Bipolar method. A 3-cm minimum zone of isthmic tube is desiccated with bipolar forceps. The paddles of the forceps extend across the tube onto the mesosalpinx.

The visual end points of tubal blanching and swelling noted with bipolar coagulation cannot be used to ensure destruction of the endosalpinx. Desiccation of the outer one third of the fallopian tube can occur without desiccation of the inner one third. The use of an optical flow meter has been recommended to evaluate cessation of current flow through the tube as an end point. Presumably, when complete desiccation occurs, there will be no further electrolytes in solution to carry current through the dehydrated tissue. Soderstrom and coworkers have demonstrated that complete desiccation of the fallopian tube with bipolar systems is more likely when a cutting waveform, as opposed to a coagulation or blended waveform, is used and when the power output is at least 25 W against a 100-V load.

Silicone Rubber Bands

High complication rates with the use of unipolar coagulation led to the pursuit of safer, nonthermal methods that could be applied laparoscopically. The first of these methods to gain popularity was the silicone rubber band, developed by Yoon and coworkers in the early 1970s.

The band is introduced with a specially designed endoscopic applicator that can be delivered either through the operating channel of a laparoscope or a separate second puncture port. The band is first stretched over the distal end of the applicator barrel (immediately before use to avoid extended deformation of the band). A transcervical uterine manipulator can be used to help achieve proper exposure. After the device is introduced into the abdominal cavity, grasping tongs are extended from within the applicator barrel. One of the tongs is used to gently hook and elevate the isthmic portion of the tube about 3 cm from the uterus. The tongs then are retracted into the applicator, which closes both arms of the tongs around the grasped tube while pulling the loop of tube up into the barrel (Fig. 27.7). The surgeon must take care in ensuring that the tube is completely encircled by the tongs as they are retracted into the applicator. Failure to do this can result in a band that is only tangentially applied to the tube (failing to occlude its lumen) or applied only to the mesosalpinx.

It is important to avoid excessive traction on the tube during retraction of the tongs. The surgeon should slowly advance the entire applicator toward the tube while gradually retracting the tongs and tube up into the applicator. Failure to do this

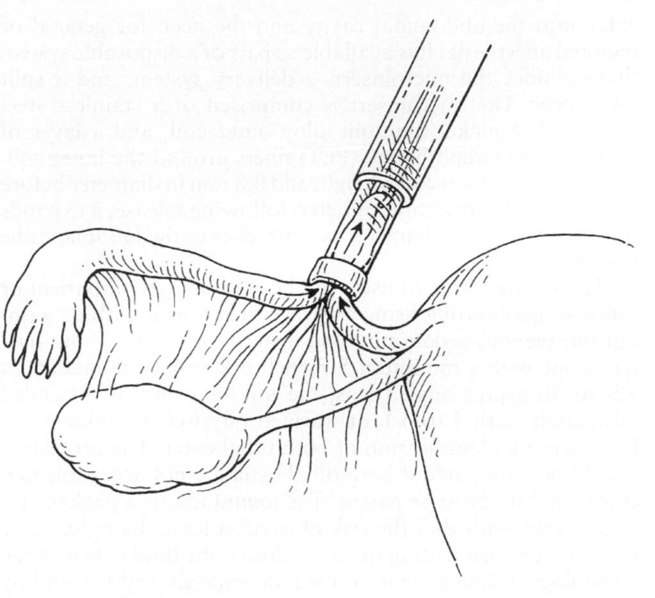

FIGURE 27.7. Silicone band method. The isthmic portion of the tube is retracted into the applicator barrel using grasping tongs, which should completely surround the tube. The applicator barrel is advanced toward the tube during this retraction process to avoid excessive traction on the tube and its mesentery.

can result in mesosalpingeal hemorrhage and tubal laceration. Once the loop is fully retracted into the device, the band is slid off the applicator barrel and onto the base of the loop.

About 1.5 to 2 cm of tube is contained in the constricted loop. After devascularization, this portion of tube becomes anoxic and resorbs over time. Eventually, the band no longer encircles any tube, and later it is often found in the mesosalpinx. Apart from the 2-cm loop of encircled tube, very little destruction is caused by the band, and 2 mm lateral to the area of constriction of the tube is relatively undisturbed.

It is difficult to apply a band to edematous or thickened fallopian tubes successfully. Tubal adhesions can reduce the mobility of the tube and preclude pulling an adequate loop of tube into the applicator. Additional rings can be applied to the cut edges if transection of the mesosalpinx or tube with accompanying hemorrhage occurs. Bipolar or unipolar coagulation can be used if this is unsuccessful.

Spring Clip

The use of a spring clip for tubal sterilization was reported by Hulka and colleagues in 1973. The introducer for the clip can be delivered into the abdomen through the operative channel of the laparoscope or a second puncture cannula (Fig. 27.8). Because the clip must be applied exactly perpendicular to the long axis of the fallopian tube, it is helpful at times to use the two-puncture method—placing the tube on stretch by use of a transcervical uterine manipulator and a grasping forceps inserted through the operating channel of the laparoscope, and introducing the applicator through the second puncture port.

The clip is held in a cradle by the applicator and can be closed and opened on the tube multiple times until an acceptable application is achieved. At this point, further pressure on the thumb device of the applicator drives the spring mechanism over the jaws of the clip, locking it closed. If improper application is determined at this point, the clip cannot be removed,

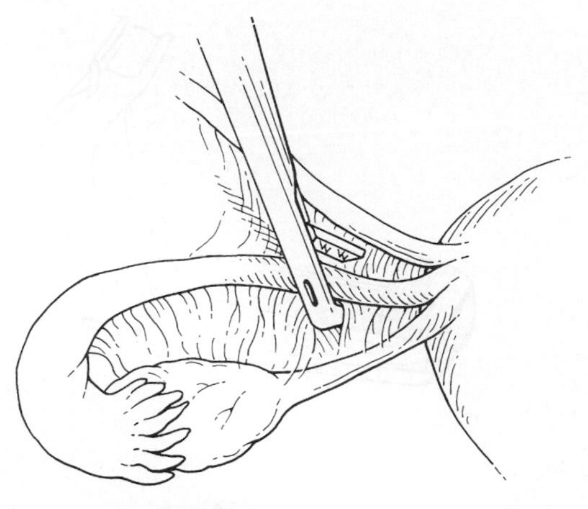

FIGURE 27.8. Spring clip method. The clip is applied to the midisthmus (about 2 cm from the cornua) at a 90-degree angle to the long axis of the tube. The hinge of the clip should be pressed against the tube, and the tips of the clip should extend onto the mesosalpinx.

and another clip has to be placed. To be effective, the clip must be applied to the isthmic portion of the tube, about 2 cm from the uterus and exactly at right angles to the long axis of the tube. It must be applied fully advanced over the tube, with the hinge of the clip pressing against the tube and with the tips of the jaws of the clip extending beyond the tube onto the mesosalpinx, creating a characteristic fold in the mesosalpinx when the clip is closed. The tube is not elevated when applying the clip, in contrast to the techniques used in coagulation and band application.

The clip, like the silicone rubber band, is most likely to be successful when applied to a normal tube. Tubal distortion, thickening, and adhesions make correct application difficult and often impossible.

A considerable advantage to the clip method of sterilization is that only 3 mm of tube is compressed by the clip, and minimal collateral damage occurs in the adjacent tissue. As a result, anastomosis procedures after clip sterilization often are highly successful.

Filshie Clip

The Filshie clip was first introduced in Europe in 1975, and the hinged Mark VI model was approved for use in the United States by the U.S. Food and Drug Administration (FDA) in 1996. The device has titanium jaws lined with silicone rubber and is used with specially designed applicators that are available in both single- and double-puncture versions for use with laparoscopy or minilaparotomy. The Filshie clip has a hinge on one end and a small curve on the other and is designed to be placed on the isthmic portion of the fallopian tube approximately 1 to 2 cm from the cornua (Fig. 27.9).

To be effective, the jaws of this clip, as with the spring clip, must include the entire circumference of the tube. Only one properly applied clip needs to be applied to each fallopian tube. Once the tube is occluded, both the tube and the silicone rubber lining of the clip are compressed. Over time, about 3 to 5 mm of the compressed tissue undergoes avascular necrosis, and the compressed silicone rubber expands. Eventually, plical attenuation and fibrosis of the adjacent tubal segments occurs, and the clips are peritonealized.

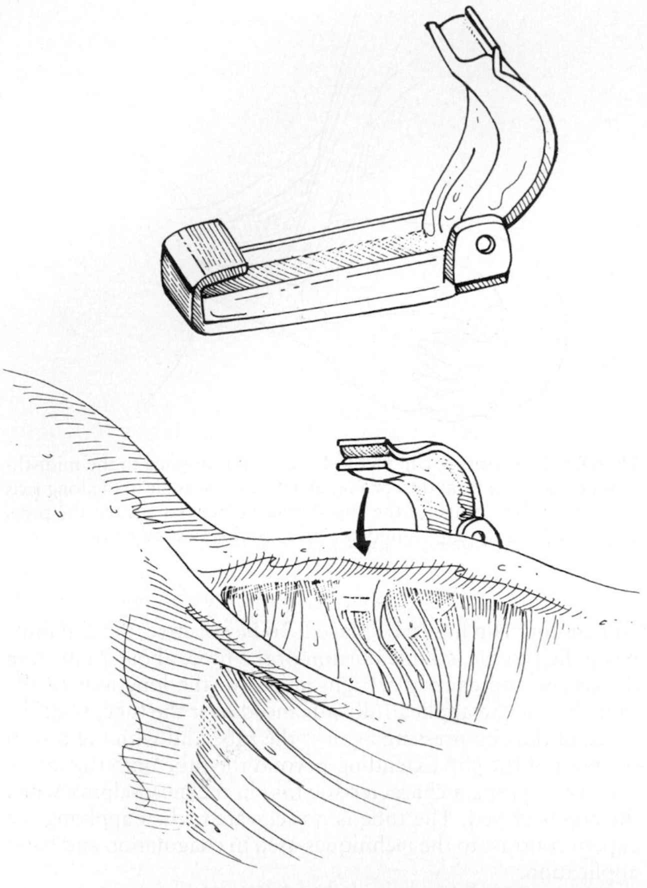

FIGURE 27.9. Filshie clip method. The clip is applied to the midisthmus (about 1 to 2 cm from the cornua) with the lower jaw of the clip being visible in the mesosalpinx to assure that the entire circumference of the tube is included.

The clip is placed into the applicator, and the applicator and clip then are introduced through the cannula with the jaws of the clip in a partially closed position so that the instrument with the clip in place can be used to manipulate the fallopian tube into proper position. The clip may close prematurely if too much pressure is placed on the handle of the applicator. The lower jaw of the clip, with its small curve at the tip, should be seen through the mesosalpinx to assure that the clip includes the entire circumference of the isthmic portion of the tube before the clip is applied. Because of the clip's hinge and the silicone lining of the jaws, the tubes can be manipulated and released several times for better positioning of the clip. Gentle pressure is placed on the applicator handle once desired placement is obtained, which causes the upper jaw of the clip to flatten and lock under the curved tip of the lower jaw. The clip should be closed slowly to avoid transection of the fallopian tube, which is more likely with edematous tubes. A clip can be placed on each transected end if transection occurs. Many surgeons recommend the use of a double-puncture technique to assure proper placement.

Essure™

The Essure™ microinsert was approved by the FDA for use as an interval tubal sterilization device in late 2002. The device is inserted transcervically via hysteroscopy and thus avoids both entry into the abdominal cavity and the need for general or regional anesthesia. It is available as part of a disposable system that includes the microinsert, a delivery system, and a split introducer. The microinsert is comprised of a stainless steel inner coil, a nickel titanium alloy outer coil, and a layer of polyethylene terephthalate (PET) fibers around the inner coil. The microinsert is 4 cm in length and 0.8 mm in diameter before release from the insertion catheter; following release, it expands to 1.5 to 2.0 mm in diameter as it attaches to the fallopian tube (Fig. 27.10).

The Essure™ microinsert can be placed in an outpatient or office surgery setting using a paracervical block with or without intravenous sedation. Using a sterile standard 5-mm hysteroscope with a minimum 5 French operating channel and a 12- to 30-degree angled lens, the uterine cavity is distended adequately with 2 to 3 L of warmed physiologic saline to allow accurate identification of both tubal ostia. The procedure should be terminated if both tubal ostia are not accessible and considered likely to be patent. The manufacturer's package insert recommends that the risk of hypervolemia be reduced by immediately terminating the procedure if the fluid deficit of the physiologic saline distension medium exceeds 1500 cc and by limiting the time of the hysteroscopic procedure to a maximum of 20 minutes.

The Essure™ microinsert is designed to be placed in the fallopian tube across the uterotubal junction where the tube exits the uterine wall but with 5 to 10 mm (the equivalent of 3–8 coils) still trailing into the uterus. This is achieved by inserting the delivery catheter with the microinsert into the proximal tubal lumen to the level indicated by the black position marker on the catheter. When the device is correctly placed, the delivery catheter is withdrawn, and the delivery wire is separated from the microinsert. The trailing end of the coils aids in anchoring the device to decrease the risk of expulsion. The device is also anchored as it expands in the tube at placement, but occlusion is not considered adequate without tissue ingrowth from the tubal wall into the coils that occurs as a result of an inflammatory and fibrotic response to the PET fibers in the inner coil. A hysterosalpingogram (HSG) must be performed 3 months postinsertion to assure complete bilateral tubal occlusion. Alternate contraception should be used until occlusion is documented.

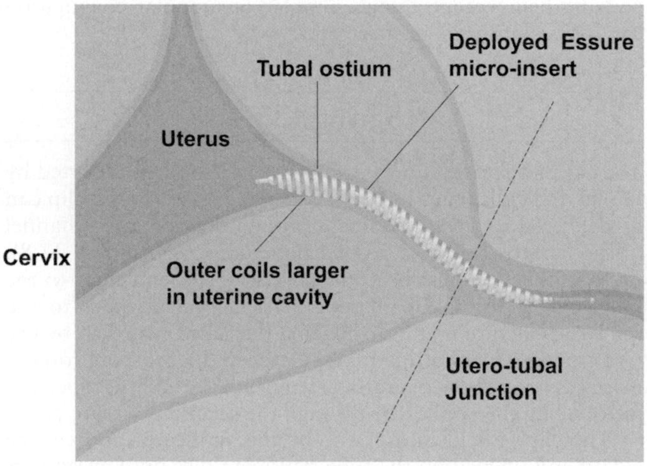

FIGURE 27.10. Essure method. The Essure microinsert is designed to be placed in the fallopian tube across the uterotubal junction where the tube exits the uterine wall but with 5 to 10 mm (the equivalent of 3–8 coils) still trailing into the uterus.

In early studies, 14% of microinsert attempts failed on one or both sides, with the first attempt using the braided catheter. Although the rate of failed attempts was reduced as training improved, the insertion failure rate remained considerable at 10%. A newly designed coil catheter system has replaced the original one; initial tests suggest an improved rate of successful single-attempt bilateral placements, but these encouraging findings require confirmation in the general population.

The Essure™ microinsert is indicated, as for other methods of sterilization, only for women who are certain about their desire to terminate future fertility. The microinserts are not removable, and several coils project into the uterine cavity, making *in vitro* fertilization less feasible. Thus, this method has less potential for a desired subsequent pregnancy than laparoscopic or minilaparotomy tubal sterilization should regret occur.

Women with a known hypersensitivity to nickel should not have the Essure™ microinsert inserted because the outer coil is made of nickel-titanium alloy.

IMMEDIATE COMPLICATIONS

Mortality

In an international study of 41,834 sterilizations performed from 1971 to 1979 in 28 countries, the estimated case-fatality rate was 13.4 per 100,000 interval tubal sterilization procedures, 53.3 per 100,000 postabortion sterilization procedures, and 43.4 per 100,000 sterilizations after vaginal delivery. At least some of the differences in case-fatality rates between interval tubal sterilization and sterilization associated with pregnancy were likely attributable to complications of pregnancy termination or delivery rather than tubal sterilization per se.

The potential health impact of tubal sterilization in countries that have a high rate of maternal mortality can be assessed by analyzing sterilization-attributable deaths in Bangladesh. In the first of two epidemiologic investigations, 28 deaths were attributed to tubal sterilization in two geographic areas; the case-fatality rate was 19 deaths per 100,000 tubal sterilizations. In the second investigation, 19 deaths were identified nationwide, for a case-fatality rate of 12.4 deaths per 100,000 procedures. Anesthesia overdosage, tetanus, and hemorrhage were the leading causes of death in both investigations. On the basis of an estimated maternal mortality rate of 570 per 100,000 live births, more than 1,000 maternal deaths for each 100,000 tubal sterilizations performed would have been averted during the reproductive years of the cohort.

In the United States, deaths attributable to tubal sterilization are rare. Based on an assessment of tubal sterilizations performed in U.S. hospitals in 1979 and 1980, the estimated case-fatality rate for tubal sterilization is one to two per 100,000 procedures. Complications of general anesthesia are the leading cause of sterilization-attributable death. In a survey of deaths attributable to tubal sterilization in the United States from 1977 to 1981, 29 deaths were identified: 11 followed complications of general anesthesia, seven were caused by sepsis, four were caused by hemorrhage, three were caused by myocardial infarction, and four were related to other causes.

At least some of these deaths are preventable. Safer use of general anesthesia or use of local anesthesia, particularly for interval laparoscopic and minilaparotomy procedures, should reduce the risk of death from anesthesia. Of the seven identified deaths caused by sepsis from 1977 to 1981, three were associated with the use of unipolar electrocoagulation. Safer use of unipolar coagulation or alternative methods of tubal occlusion reduces the risk of thermal bowel injury. Three of the four deaths attributable to hemorrhage occurred after major vessel laceration during abdominal entry for laparoscopy. Safer insertion of the Veress needle and trocar or use of alternative techniques, such as open laparoscopy or minilaparotomy, should reduce the risk of such laceration.

Morbidity

Morbidity attributable to tubal sterilization is uncommon but not rare. The risks for and types of morbidity vary somewhat by surgical approach and method of tubal occlusion. Direct comparisons of minilaparotomy and laparoscopy for tubal sterilization are limited, but studies suggest several differences. In a nonrandomized study in 23 countries, 7,053 women who had silicone rubber band application by way of laparoscopy were compared with 3,033 women who had silicone rubber band application by minilaparotomy and 5,081 women who had modified Pomeroy ligation by minilaparotomy. The surgical complication rates were 2.04%, 1.45%, and 0.79% for the three groups, respectively. In a smaller but randomized study in eight centers, 791 women who had modified Pomeroy occlusion by minilaparotomy were compared with 819 women who had occlusion from electrocoagulation (technique not specified) by way of laparoscopy. Major complications occurred in 1.5% of the women in the minilaparotomy group and 0.9% of the women in the laparoscopy group. Minor complications, which are more common, occurred in 11.6% of women in the former group and 6.0% in the latter group.

In a U.S. multicenter, collaborative study, major complications were more common among women who had minilaparotomy (3.5%) than among those who had interval laparoscopic sterilization (1.6%). However, women in the study were not randomly assigned to groups, and the sterilization procedures were performed in institutions where most interval tubal sterilizations were done by way of laparoscopy. Thus, minilaparotomy sterilizations may have been performed selectively for women at increased risk for complications.

Although the overall complication rates are similar for minilaparotomy and laparoscopy, the types of complications appear to vary. Complications of minilaparotomy usually are not serious and typically include minor wound infection, longer operating time, slightly longer postoperative convalescence, and greater postoperative pain. Laparoscopic complications are more likely to include rare but life-threatening hemorrhage and viscus perforations during abdominal entry, and thermal bowel injury during electrocoagulation. A study of 100,000 laparoscopies in France suggests that major vessel laceration occurs in three of 10,000 procedures. In a study conducted in the United Kingdom, major vessel laceration occurred in nine of 10,000 laparoscopies.

Some of the most serious complications of both interval minilaparotomy and laparoscopy occur during abdominal entry. Bladder laceration during suprapubic minilaparotomy can occur, but usually it is recognized during surgery and is repaired easily. Major vessel and bowel laceration during needle or trocar insertion for laparoscopy are more difficult to recognize or repair, and delayed treatment of these injuries can be fatal. Meticulousness is required to reduce the risks of abdominal entry. Comparative studies of open versus conventional laparoscopy are limited and have insufficient power to assess the risk of life-threatening complications, but use of open laparoscopy should markedly reduce the risk of major vessel laceration and should reduce, to a lesser extent, the risk of bowel laceration. The use of open laparoscopy can be particularly advantageous for women known or strongly suspected to have multiple abdominal or pelvic adhesions. However, even open laparoscopy can result in bowel injury if the bowel is adherent to the anterior abdominal wall.

The method of tubal occlusion chosen influences the risk for and type of complications during laparoscopy. Thermal bowel injury is more common with unipolar than bipolar coagulation, but it can occur during the latter if the bowel is grasped and coagulated. Transection of the fallopian tube can occur with any technique, particularly when an attempt is made to mobilize the fallopian tube in the presence of thick peritubal adhesions. Tubal transection is most likely to occur when silicone rubber bands are used, but any resultant bleeding usually can be managed by the application of a second ring or by the use of coagulation.

DELAYED COMPLICATIONS

Pregnancy

Tubal sterilization is highly effective in preventing pregnancy. A frequently cited failure rate is four pregnancies per 1,000 sterilization procedures. However, a range of failure rates is more likely to portray the risk of pregnancy after sterilization. The determinants of that range are likely to include the method of tubal occlusion, surgical technique, and the age of the woman at sterilization. In the U.S. Collaborative Review of Sterilization, a multicenter, prospective, cohort study, 10,685 women undergoing tubal sterilization in medical centers in nine U.S. cities from 1978 to 1987 were followed for up to 8 to 14 years. A total of 143 sterilization failures were identified with the 10-year cumulative probability of failure, ranging from 7.5 per 1,000 procedures (for unipolar coagulating procedures and postpartum partial salpingectomy procedures) to 36.5 per 1,000 (for spring clip application procedures). The failure rates for most methods of tubal occlusion were higher for women aged 18 to 27 years at sterilization (as high as 54.3 and 52.1 per 1,000 bipolar coagulation and spring clip applications, respectively) than for women aged 34 to 44 years at sterilization (as low as 1.8 and 3.8 per 1,000 unipolar coagulation and postpartum partial salpingectomy procedures, respectively).

This large U.S. multicenter study, along with two smaller studies in Thailand and Belgium, have dispelled the widely held belief that nearly all pregnancies after sterilization occur in the first year or two after the procedure. In the Thai study, 418 women were followed for 6 to 10 years after sterilization, and only one of four pregnancies identified occurred within 2 years of the procedure. In the Belgian study, of 17 pregnancies after 1,437 sterilizations by bipolar coagulation, none occurred within 12 months of electrocoagulation, and eight occurred more than 24 months after the procedure. In the U.S. study, the 10-year cumulative probability of pregnancy after bipolar coagulation (24.8 per 1,000 procedures) was about 10 times the probability (2.3 per 1,000) at 1 year. Further, pregnancies occurred in the tenth year after all four methods of laparoscopic sterilization studied (bipolar and unipolar coagulation, silicone rubber band application, and spring clip application).

The fact that the risk of pregnancy after sterilization only can be determined after long-term follow-up creates a dilemma in interpreting published failure rates. For example, the failure rates in the U.S. Collaborative Review of Sterilization for six methods of tubal occlusion were based on procedures performed in the late 1970s and 1980s when laparoscopic sterilization was fairly new. Whether failure rates for procedures performed in the past reflect the risk for current procedures is unclear. In an analysis of bipolar coagulation procedures in the U.S. Collaborative Review of Sterilization, the 5-year cumulative probability of pregnancy for women sterilized in 1978 to 1982 (19.5 per 1,000 procedures) was significantly greater than that for women sterilized in 1985 to 1987 (6.3 per 1,000 procedures). Further, most of the procedures evaluated in that study were performed in teaching institutions; it is unclear whether procedures performed in teaching institutions can be generalized outside such settings.

Luteal phase pregnancy, or pregnancy diagnosed after sterilization but conceived before sterilization, is estimated to occur in two to three per 1,000 sterilization procedures. The most effective strategy for reducing the risk for luteal phase pregnancy is to time the sterilization procedure to occur during the follicular phase of the menstrual cycle. Reliance on dilatation and curettage at the time of sterilization is substantially less effective. The likelihood of luteal phase pregnancy occurring also depends on the method of contraception used before tubal sterilization. Women who use steroid hormonal contraceptives or intrauterine devices are at substantially lower risk for luteal phase pregnancy than are women who use barrier methods or no method of contraception. Testing for pregnancy by using an enzyme-linked immunosorbent assay pregnancy test as indicated before sterilization also reduces the risk for luteal phase pregnancy.

The likelihood of ectopic pregnancy occurring is increased when pregnancy occurs after sterilization. In the U.S. Collaborative Review of Sterilization, the highest proportion of ectopic pregnancies among all pregnancies after sterilization was among women who underwent bipolar coagulation (65%), followed by interval partial salpingectomy (43%), silicone rubber band application (29%), postpartum partial salpingectomy (20%), unipolar coagulation (17%), and spring clip application (15%). The proportion of pregnancies that were ectopic increased over time; for all methods combined, the proportion of ectopic pregnancies was three times greater in the fourth through tenth years after sterilization (61%) than in the first 3 years (20%). The pregnancies that occurred in the tenth year after unipolar and bipolar coagulation, silicone rubber band application, and spring clip application were all ectopic. All but one (an ovarian pregnancy after bipolar coagulation) of the 47 ectopic pregnancies identified in the study were tubal pregnancies. The index of suspicion for ectopic pregnancy should be high when pregnancy is suspected after tubal sterilization. Pregnancy should be confirmed by use of a highly sensitive pregnancy test as soon as feasible.

A woman's individual risk for ectopic pregnancy can be considered in both absolute and relative terms. Her absolute risk is determined by the likelihood that the sterilization procedure can fail to prevent pregnancy and the likelihood that a resulting pregnancy will be ectopic. This risk is also relative to the risk for ectopic pregnancy that a woman had before tubal sterilization. Depending on the method of contraception used before sterilization, some women may be at greater risk for ectopic pregnancy after tubal sterilization. In a report from a case-control study in Seattle, both postpartum sterilization and interval sterilization were associated with a lower risk of ectopic pregnancy than was use of no contraception. However, women who had interval tubal sterilization had a higher risk of ectopic pregnancy than did women who were using oral contraceptives or barrier methods of contraception. In contrast, the risk for ectopic pregnancy was similar between women who had postpartum tubal sterilization and those who used oral contraceptives or barrier contraception.

Careful attention to surgical technique is required to maximize sterilization effectiveness. To reduce the risk of pregnancy after bipolar coagulation, Soderstrom and colleagues identified determinants of complete electrocoagulation. In the U.S. Collaborative Review of Sterilization, women undergoing bipolar coagulation later in the study who had three or more sites of coagulation had a 5-year cumulative probability of failure of 3.2 per 1,000 procedures. This is similar to the 5-year probability for unipolar coagulation (2.3 per 1,000) and substantially lower than that for women undergoing bipolar coagulation with fewer than three sites of coagulation (12.9 per 1,000). Stovall and coworkers reported on the use of silicone rubber bands and spring clips in a residency training program; all of 20 sterilization failures were associated with improper application of the occlusive device on gross and microscopic evaluation after subsequent bilateral salpingectomy. In the U.S. Collaborative Review of Sterilization, the risks of pregnancy were significantly increased among women who had a silicone rubber band applied solely to the distal one third of at least one fallopian tube and among women who had a spring clip applied to a site other than the proximal one third of at least one tube.

The likelihood of sterilization failure depends not only on the sterilization technique but also on patient and physician factors. For example, proper application of silicone rubber bands and spring clips generally is difficult in the presence of thickened tubes or dense pelvic adhesions; under such circumstances, alternative techniques usually are preferred. As noted, failure rates generally are higher for women sterilized at younger ages, not only because they are more fecund at the time of sterilization than older women, but also because they have a longer period after sterilization during which it would be feasible for pregnancy to occur. The latter consideration, which is an issue because it is now clear that pregnancy can occur for many years after sterilization, also applies to any temporary method of contraception that a woman chooses to use. For example, based on data from the U.S. Collaborative Review of Sterilization, a woman sterilized at 28 to 33 years old has a 10-year chance of pregnancy of less than 1% to about 3%, depending on the method of tubal occlusion. The comparable risk for 10 years of use of the Copper T 380 intrauterine device is about 2%, but the typical failure rate for oral contraceptive use is about 6% to 8% in just the first 12 months of use. Data regarding the long-term failure rates of the Filshie clip and the Essure™ microinsert are less complete than those for the other commonly used techniques. However, based on data to date, both appear highly effective with proper placement.

Menstrual Changes

After nearly a half century of debate, questions regarding the existence of a posttubal ligation syndrome of menstrual abnormalities appear to be largely resolved. Questions arose initially when Williams and colleagues reported in 1951 that sterilized women had a higher-than-expected occurrence of menorrhagia and metrorrhagia. Studies in the 1970s appeared to support the existence of a poststerilization syndrome, but most of those studies had major methodologic shortcomings, including failure to account for factors other than sterilization per se that might have influenced poststerilization menstrual changes. One such factor was the use of oral contraceptives; in the United States, as many as 30% of women may use oral contraceptives immediately before tubal sterilization, and many of these women have menstrual changes after sterilization attributable solely to cessation of oral contraceptive use. Although one well-controlled study (Shain et al., 1989) in the 1980s identified poststerilization menstrual changes, nearly all other studies reported in the 1980s that controlled for factors such as cessation of oral contraceptive use found little or no evidence of a poststerilization syndrome at 1 to 2 years after sterilization.

Until the 1990s, questions remained about whether menstrual changes attributable to sterilization may occur several years after the procedure. Two U.S. multicenter, prospective, cohort studies argue strongly against such an occurrence. In the first, reported in 1993, 500 women were evaluated at 6 to 10 months and 3 to 4.5 years after sterilization. When women who were taking oral contraceptives were excluded, no significant differences in seven menstrual parameters were found between sterilized women and two groups of nonsterilized women.

In the second, reported in 2000, 9,514 sterilized women enrolled in the U.S. Collaborative Review of Sterilization were compared with 573 women whose husbands underwent vasectomy. All women were asked the same questions about six menstrual parameters before tubal sterilization or the husband's vasectomy and again at annual follow-up interviews for up to 5 years. The sterilized women were no more likely than the nonsterilized women to report changes in intermenstrual bleeding or cycle length. The sterilized women were more likely than the nonsterilized women to have decreases in the number of days of bleeding and the amount of bleeding and menstrual pain; they were also more likely to have an increase in cycle irregularity. When the risk of menstrual abnormalities was evaluated by method of tubal occlusion, there were no significant differences between the women sterilized by any of six methods and the women whose husbands underwent vasectomy in amount or duration of menstrual bleeding, intermenstrual bleeding, or menstrual pain. Women undergoing three methods of sterilization (silicone rubber band application, interval partial salpingectomy, and thermocoagulation) were more likely than nonsterilized women to have an increase in cycle irregularity, whereas women undergoing two other methods (unipolar and bipolar coagulation) were more likely to have decreases in cycle irregularity. This latter observation suggests strongly that the differences between sterilized and nonsterilized women in the likelihood of cycle irregularity and other menstrual features were attributable to chance or unmeasured differences between the study groups. Finally, sterilized women were compared with nonsterilized women for risk of a syndrome consisting of persistent increases in either amount of bleeding, days of bleeding, or intermenstrual bleeding; no significant differences were identified.

Although sterilization procedures have been hypothesized to adversely affect ovarian function, laboratory studies have identified no consistent abnormalities that reflect ovarian dysfunction. Further, the biological plausibility of such an occurrence is uncertain. The tubal branch of the uterine artery, which often is occluded during sterilization, connects with the ovarian branch of the uterine artery; thus, interrupting the tubal branch could affect the blood supply to the ovary. However, blood also is supplied to the ovary by the ovarian artery, which branches directly off the aorta and is remote from the site of tubal occlusion. The possibility has been raised that tubal occlusion could damage the ovary by acutely increasing pressure in the uteroovarian arterial loop. However, as noted, neither laboratory nor epidemiologic studies find changes consistent with acute injury to the ovary, and there is now strong evidence against the occurrence of sterilization-attributable menstrual abnormalities within 5 years of the procedure.

Some women who have no menstrual abnormalities before sterilization have them later, and for other women, menstrual abnormalities before sterilization resolve. To consider the former group as having a syndrome is inappropriate unless the latter group is considered to have an opposing syndrome. Although menstrual abnormalities are common among sterilized women, they also are common among nonsterilized women of similar ages. The balance of the evidence to date suggests strongly that sterilized women are no more likely than comparable nonsterilized women to have menstrual abnormalities.

Hysterectomy

Tubal sterilization and hysterectomy are common procedures in the United States, and any relation between the two has important consequences. Tubal sterilization could increase the risk for hysterectomy by increasing either the reality or the perception that a poststerilization syndrome occurs. As noted, the evidence against such a syndrome is now strong; thus, it should not be an indication for hysterectomy. Alternatively, the fact that a woman has had tubal sterilization could affect decision making about further surgery. At least three studies suggest that this effect can occur. Cohen studied 4,374 women 25 to 44 years old who had tubal sterilization in 1974 while enrolled in a universal health insurance plan in Canada. Women 25 to 29 years old at the time of sterilization were 1.6 times more likely than nonsterilized women to have a hysterectomy at a later time. However, women 30 years or older at the time of sterilization were no more likely than nonsterilized women to have a hysterectomy subsequently. Goldhaber and colleagues, who studied 39,502 women sterilized from 1971 to 1984, found that women sterilized at 20 to 24 years old were 2.4 times more likely than nonsterilized women to have a hysterectomy subsequently. For other sterilized women, the risk for hysterectomy steadily decreased with increasing age; women sterilized at 40 to 49 years old had no increased risk. Stergachis and associates studied 7,414 women sterilized from 1968 to 1983 and found that women sterilized at 20 to 29 years old were 3.4 times more likely than nonsterilized women to subsequently have a hysterectomy. Women sterilized at 30 years old or older had no increased risk for hysterectomy.

The fact that the increased risk for hysterectomy was concentrated among women sterilized at a young age in the noted studies suggests that any increased risk for hysterectomy after tubal sterilization is not biologic in etiology but attributable to other factors, such as removal of fertility preservation as a factor in decision making. In the U.S. Collaborative Review of Sterilization, women sterilized at 34 years old and younger were four to five times more likely to undergo hysterectomy than women the same age whose husbands underwent vasectomy. However, women sterilized at 35 years old and older were also four to five times more likely to undergo hysterectomy than women whose husbands underwent vasectomy, suggesting that fertility preservation does not explain all differences in decision making between sterilized and nonsterilized women.

In the U.S. Collaborative Review of Sterilization, the cumulative probability of undergoing hysterectomy within 14 years after sterilization was 17%. Although women with gynecologic disorders at the time of sterilization were at greater risk of hysterectomy, most women who reported gynecologic disorders at sterilization did not undergo hysterectomy within the follow-up period. For example, women who reported having a history of endometriosis at sterilization were more likely to undergo hysterectomy than women without a history of endometriosis; the probability of women reporting endometriosis undergoing hysterectomy within 14 years was 35%, versus 15% for women without endometriosis. Similarly, women who reported having a history of uterine leiomyomata at sterilization were more likely to undergo hysterectomy than women without a history of leiomyomata; the 14-year cumulative probability of hysterectomy among women reporting leiomyomata was 27% versus 14% for women without leiomyomata.

Regret

The decision to undergo sterilization is serious to both men and women because the intent is to permanently terminate fertility. Although microsurgical methods of reversal are available, these methods require special skill, the procedures are complicated and lengthy, the costs are high, and none of the methods guarantees success.

Findings from studies of poststerilization regret provide useful information for presterilization counseling. Sterilization regret is a complex condition that is often causally linked to unpredictable life events. The risk factors for regret described here should not be used as reasons for restricting access to sterilization. Instead, they should be used to identify persons who may need extensive counseling. Presterilization counseling has been shown to correlate with poststerilization satisfaction.

Poststerilization regret can arise from several factors, including preexisting patient characteristics, subsequent changes in the patient's social situations or attitudes, and dissatisfaction resulting from adverse side effects caused or perceived to be caused by the procedure. Estimates of the prevalence of sterilization regret vary widely by measure of indication of regret and geographic region. During the last two decades, U.S.-based studies have reported rates of poststerilization regret ranging from 0.9% to 26.0%. The wide range reflects, in part, differences in study design and questions asked of respondents. In general, the likelihood of a woman expressing regret after sterilization appears to increase over time. In the U.S. Collaborative Review of Sterilization, the cumulative probability of regret increased from 4% at 3 years after sterilization to 8% at 7 years and 13% at 14 years. The 5-year cumulative probability of regret after tubal sterilization (7%) was similar to that for women whose husbands underwent vasectomy (6%).

In the 1982 National Survey of Family Growth, about 10% of women who had been sterilized reported that they would have the sterilization reversed if it were safe to do so. In the U.S. Collaborative Review of Sterilization, 14% of sterilized women reported that they had sought information about tubal reanastomosis at least once within 14 years of sterilization; only 1% actually obtained a reversal.

At least five studies have identified young age at sterilization as the strongest predictor of later regret of sterilization. In the U.S. Collaborative Review of Sterilization, young age at sterilization also was a strong predictor of regret, regardless of parity or marital status. After adjusting for other risk factors, women 30 years of age or younger at sterilization were about twice as likely as older women to express regret within 14 years of sterilization. Similarly, the cumulative probability of expressing regret within 14 years was 20% for women 30 years old or younger versus 6% for women older than 30 years at sterilization. Likewise, the 14-year cumulative probability of requesting information about reversal was 40% among women sterilized at 18 to 24 years old and, after adjustment for other risk factors, women 18 to 24 years old were almost four times as likely as women 30 years old or older to request information about reversal. Although low parity has been identified as a risk factor for regret in some studies, it was not an independent risk factor in other studies after control for factors such as young age at the time of sterilization. The U.S. Collaborative

Review of Sterilization also found that women identifying tubal substantial conflict with their husbands or partners before sterilization were more than three times as likely to regret their decision and more that five times as likely to request sterilization reversal.

Timing of the procedure in relation to pregnancy has been reported as a risk factor for regret. Several studies found that women who had tubal sterilization concurrent with cesarean section or following vaginal delivery or abortion were more likely to regret sterilization, but studies have been inconsistent in this regard. In the U.S. Collaborative Review of Sterilization, the 14-year cumulative probability of regret was nearly identical for women whose sterilizations were concurrent with cesarean section (16%), after vaginal delivery (18%), and within 1 year of pregnancy (18%). The probability of regret decreased with time since the birth of the youngest child; women with 8 or more years since the birth of the youngest child had a probability of only 5%, a rate similar to that for women with no previous births (6%).

In summary, indicators of regret can vary significantly by cultural and individual circumstances. Most studies have found that age younger than 30 years is an independent risk factor for regret. The presterilization counseling for women in this age group should place special emphasis on the risk for regret. Other risk factors, such as time in relation to an obstetric event, ambivalence, or unstable life circumstances, should be assessed with each patient on an individual basis.

Sexual Function

In the U.S. Collaborative Review of Sterilization, approximately 80% of women undergoing interval sterilization reported no consistent change in either sexual interest or pleasure in the first 2 years after the procedure. Of women reporting a consistent change, women were 10 and 15 times more likely to report positive changes in sexual interest or pleasure than negative ones.

Cancer

Although there is no evidence that tubal sterilization increases the risk for cancer at any site, studies are inconsistent regarding a possible reduction in risk of breast cancer after sterilization. One large prospective study by the American Cancer Society found that tubal sterilization reduced the risk of breast cancer mortality but only among women sterilized before 1975. It is unclear whether women who were sterilized had rates of screening mammography similar to those of nonsterilized women; thus, women who underwent tubal sterilization may have had greater access to screening services. A retrospective cohort study using data from the Ontario Cancer Registry found a reduced risk of breast cancer incidence among sterilized women, but that study was unable to control for potentially confounding variables. Two population-based case-control studies supported by NIH that did control for confounding found no effect of sterilization on breast cancer risk. Thus, at this point, it is unclear whether there is any biologic relationship between tubal sterilization and reduction in risk of subsequent breast cancer.

Several studies have identified a reduced risk of ovarian cancer after tubal sterilization. Hankinson and colleagues reported on the first large prospective cohort study of this relation; the risk of ovarian cancer for women who had tubal sterilization was one third that of nonsterilized women. In a pooled analysis of case-control studies, Whittemore and coworkers found a reduced risk of ovarian cancer after tubal sterilization. Whether the observed reduction in risk of ovarian cancer is a real protective effect or is attributable to some other factor remains unclear. However, there is reason for optimism that reduction in risk of ovarian cancer may be an important noncontraceptive health benefit of tubal sterilization.

VASECTOMY AS A SURGICAL ALTERNATIVE

Some couples who have chosen surgical sterilization for permanent contraception have difficulty in deciding whether vasectomy or tubal sterilization is most appropriate. Although numerous individual- or couple-related concerns can influence the decision, many couples include considerations about safety and effectiveness in their decision making. To assist such couples, we provide a brief overview of the health effects of vasectomy.

In regard to immediate surgical complications, vasectomy is a remarkably safe procedure. Serious morbidity and death are extremely rare. Fairly minor complications, such as scrotal swelling, ecchymosis, and pain, occur in up to 50% of men who have a vasectomy, but these symptoms usually resolve spontaneously within 1 to 2 weeks. Vasectomy generally has been performed through two incisions in the scrotum, one overlying each vas. Hematoma formation usually occurs in about 2% of such procedures; infections usually occur in less than 2%. In 1985, a new vasectomy technique was introduced, referred to as no-scalpel vasectomy. It reduced the already-low rate of minor complications. In most reports, pregnancy rates after vasectomy are less than 1%. Unlike tubal sterilization, vasectomy is not immediately effective. Three months are required to flush the vasa of viable sperm. This should be confirmed by a postvasectomy semen analysis at 3 months or more after the procedure.

In 1978, questions about the long-term health effects of vasectomy were raised when an increased risk for atherosclerosis was found among monkeys that had had a vasectomy. At least nine subsequent epidemiologic studies in men found no such increased risk, and later findings in monkeys did not support an increased risk. Thus, vasectomy does not affect the risk for subsequent cardiovascular disease. These studies also provided strong evidence that vasectomy does not increase overall mortality. More recently, questions were raised about the risk of prostate cancer after vasectomy. A 1998 metaanalysis of 14 observational studies concluded that the evidence for an association between vasectomy and prostate cancer was of low quality because of biases that overestimate the effect of vasectomy, and that any association is likely not a causal one. Subsequently, a large population-based study in New Zealand found no relation between vasectomy and risk of prostate cancer. Thus, the evidence to date argues strongly against any causal relationship.

Questions remain regarding a potential syndrome of postvasectomy pain. The purported syndrome has been varyingly defined as chronic testicular, epididymal, or scrotal pain, and the proposed causes include epididymal congestion, nerve entrapment, and sperm granulomas. Although a few small, uncontrolled surveys found rates of such pain as high as 2% to 15%, the largest and best study found the incidence of epididymitis-orchitis more than 12 months after vasectomy to be 24.7 per 10,000 person-years versus 13.6 per 10,000 person-years among men who did not undergo vasectomy. Although uncertainties remain, it is likely that a small percentage of men will indeed experience chronic pain after vasectomy. It appears, based on limited information, that many such men will respond to conservative measures and that surgical management, including vasectomy reversal, may help others.

BEST SURGICAL PRACTICES

- Preprocedure assessment and counseling are essential elements in a successful sterilization procedure. Counseling regarding failure rates, risks, and risk factors for later regret should be performed. Preprocedure cytologic screening and day-of-surgery pregnancy testing are encouraged if indicated.
- General anesthesia is the leading cause of death of tubal sterilizations in the United States. Although tubal sterilizations can usually be performed safely under local anesthesia, general anesthesia is used more often in the United States. One of the reasons that vasectomy is safer than tubal sterilization is that general anesthesia is rarely required.
- A major portion of morbidity and mortality associated with laparoscopic methods of sterilization is related to entry into the abdominal cavity. Open laparoscopy can reduce the incidence of major vascular injury at entry. In closed laparoscopy technique, meticulous attention to details of entry can help reduce injury.
- Safety measures with insertion of the Veress needle include directing it in the midline, toward the hollow of the sacrum or uterine fundus, and not laterally toward the major vessels, while simultaneously elevating the abdominal wall away from the dorsal vascular structures. The aortic bifurcation occurs at the level of the summits of the iliac crests and should be avoided. The Veress needle should be inserted with the port open and held in a manner to avoid occluding the spring mechanism of the inner safety obturator. Infiltration followed by aspiration of 5 to 10 cc of sterile fluid through the Veress needle can help identify malposition of the tip of the needle. Negative intraperitoneal pressure induced by elevation of the abdominal wall can be used in a variety of fluid tests at the hub of the Veress needle to confirm proper needle placement (e.g., drip test). Return of blood through the Veress needle should prompt immediate laparotomy, and the Veress needle should be left in place until the site of injury is identified, as is also the case with trocar/sleeve insertion. Insufflation should proceed at a rate no greater than 1 L/min, and the starting insufflation pressure should be less than 10 mm Hg. Intravascular insufflation can first manifest as an irregular heart rhythm, "cog wheel" heart murmur, and then result in vascular collapse. Immediate Trendelenberg and left lateral positioning can be lifesaving. Insufflation to greater than 15 mm Hg pressure should be attempted with only the greatest of care and with close monitoring of possible compromise of cardiac venous return and respiratory function. When inserting the umbilical or accessory trocar, "palming" the trocar with the surgeon's middle finger along the shaft of the instrument can serve as a safety stopper to sudden uncontrolled deep advancement of the sharp trocar tip when fascial bursting pressure is finally exceeded. Accessory trocars, if used, should be advanced under direct visualization.
- With all the techniques of tubal sterilization, success is dependent on correct identification of the tube, and hasty tubal identification, without taking the time to follow the tubes out to their fimbriated ends (if not distorted by adhesions), can result in procedural failure.
- Nearly all the techniques of tubal sterilization involve the isthmic portion of the fallopian tube, which is the narrowest and most uniform caliber portion of the extramural tube. However, it is suggested that 2 cm of the isthmic portion of the tube be left at the cornu, proximal to the site of tubal interruption, to theoretically reduce the incidence of tuboperitoneal fistula. Aggressive overtightening of ligatures, just as avoided in surgical technique elsewhere in the body, should likewise be avoided at time of tubal interruption, as strangulation and necrosis of the tube can lead to fistulization and failure rather than success. Ligatures applied during partial salpingectomy methods of sterilization (e.g., Pomeroy, Parkland) at the time of cesarean delivery are at risk of dislodgement by shearing forces when the uterus is restituted into the abdominal cavity at the end of the procedure. Care should be exerted to protect the ligated areas as one and then the other adnexa is replaced into the abdomen.
- Laparoscopic unipolar coagulation of the fallopian tube is one of the most successful methods of sterilization, likely attributed to the approximately 5-cm zone of thermal destruction that results. However, the risk for thermal injuries is also highest with this method, unless the safe application of unipolar energy at laparoscopy and the concept of capacitive coupling is understood by the surgeon. Greater tubal destruction and sterilization success with this method go hand in hand with least likelihood that reversal could ever be achieved.
- Laparoscopic bipolar coagulation creates a smaller zone of thermal injury (approximately 3 cm) than unipolar and is also not likely to result in indirect thermal injury by capacitive coupling. Three contiguous burns over a 3-cm length of tube, beginning approximately 3 cm from the cornu and moving toward the fimbriated end, is recommended. Also recommended is use of the cutting waveform, delivering at least 25 W of bipolar energy (continuous waveform by default) and the use of an optical flow meter to estimate when coagulation (and flow of current) is complete.
- Silastic band application requires familiarity with the applicator and the tendency of its grasping tongs to transect the fallopian tube when trying to retract a knuckle of tube into the hollow applicator cannula. Tethered or thickened tubes are at greatest risk of transection and should be avoided. A complete encirclement of the tube by the grasping tongs is necessary if a partial or tangential application of the ligating band is to be avoided.
- Hulka and Filshie clips are reliable methods of tubal interruption but require strict adherence to surgical technique to be successful. Application at right angles to the tube, 2 cm from the uterus, without excessive tubal elevation, and with the tips of the clips advanced onto the mesosalpinx are the key points of the application. Clips are associated with minimal tubal destruction (3 mm) and are therefore the most amenable to tubal reversal.
- Essure microinserts are placed transcervially via hysteroscopy. Care should be taken to identify both tubal ostia and to insert the device into the proximal lumen to the level marked on the catheter. Hypervolemia should be avoided, and a follow-up HSG must be performed at 3 months postinsertion. Alternate contraception should be used until occlusion is documented.

Bibliography

Allyn DP, Leton DA, Westcott NA, et al. Presterilization counseling and women's regret about having been sterilized. *J Reprod Med* 1986;31:1027.

Anderson ET. Peritoneoscopy. *Am J Surg* 1937;35:36.

Bernal-Delgado E, Latour-Perez J, Pradas-Arnal F, et al. The association between vasectomy and prostate cancer: a systematic review of the literature. *Fertil Steril* 1998;70:191.

Bhiwandiwala PP, Mumford SD, Feldblum PJ. A comparison of different laparoscopic sterilization occlusion techniques in 24,439 procedures. *Am J Obstet Gynecol* 1982;144:319.

Bhiwandiwala PP, Mumford SD, Kennedy KI. Comparison of the safety of open and conventional laparoscopic sterilization. *Obstet Gynecol* 1985;66:391.

Bishop E, Nelms WF. A simple method of tubal sterilization. *N Y State Med J* 1930;30:214.

Bordahl PE, Raeder JC, Nordentoft J, et al. Laparoscopic sterilization under local or general anesthesia? A randomized study. *Obstet Gynecol* 1993;81:137.

Boring CC, Rochat RW, Becerra J. Sterilization regret among Puerto Rican women. *Fertil Steril* 1988;49:973.

Brinton LA, Gammon MD, Coates RJ, et al. Tubal ligation and risk of breast cancer. *Br J Cancer* 2000;82:1600.

Calle EE, Rodriguez C, Walker KA, et al. Tubal sterilization and risk of breast cancer mortality in U.S. women. *Cancer Causes Control* 2001;12:127.

Chamberlain G, Brown JC, eds. *Gynaecological laparoscopy: the report of the confidential inquiry into gynaecological laparoscopy*. London: The Royal College of Obstetricians and Gynaecologists, 1978.

Cheng MCE, Cheong J, Ratnam SS, et al. Psychosocial sequelae of abortion and sterilization: a controlled study of 200 women randomly allocated to either a concurrent or interval abortion and sterilization. *Asia Oceania J Obstet Gynaecol* 1986;12:193.

Chi I-C, Feldblum PJ. Luteal phase pregnancies in female sterilization patients. *Contraception* 1981;23:579.

Choe JM, Kirkemo AK. Questionnaire-based outcomes study of nononcological post-vasectomy complications. *J Urol* 1996;155:1284.

Cohen MM. Long-term risk of hysterectomy after tubal sterilization. *Am J Epidemiol* 1987;125:410.

Costello C, Hillis SD, Marchbanks PA, et al. The effect of interval tubal sterilization on sexual interest and pleasure. *Obstet Gynecol* 2002;100:511.

Cox B, Sneyd MJ, Paul C, et al. Vasectomy and risk of prostate cancer. *JAMA* 2002; 287:3110.

DeStefano F, Greenspan JR, Ory HW, et al. Demographic trends in tubal sterilization: United States, 1970–1978. *Am J Public Health* 1982;72:480.

DeStefano F, Perlman JA, Peterson HB, et al. Long-term risks of menstrual disturbances after tubal sterilization. *Am J Obstet Gynecol* 1985;152:835.

Dueholm S, Zingenburg HJ, Sandgren G. Late sequelae after laparoscopic sterilization in the pregnant and nonpregnant woman. *Acta Obstet Gynecol Scand* 1987;66:227.

Emens JM, Olive JE. Timing of female sterilization. *BMJ* 1978;2:1126.

Engender Health. Contraceptive Sterilization: *global issues and trends*. New York: Engender Health; 2002:xii.

Escobedo LG, Peterson HB, Grubb GS, et al. Case-fatality rates for tubal sterilization in U.S. hospitals, 1979 to 1980. *Am J Obstet Gynecol* 1989;160: 147.

Essure^{TM} Permanent Birth Control System. Instructions.2002. Conceptus, Inc.

Filshie GM, Casey D, Pogmore JR, et al. The titanium/silicone rubber clip for female sterilization. *BJOG* 1981: 88:655.

Fishburne JI. Anesthesia for laparoscopy: considerations, complications, and techniques. *J Reprod Med* 1978;21:37.

Gentile GP, Kaufman SC, Helbig DW. Is there any evidence for a post-tubal sterilization syndrome?. *Fertil Steril* 1998;69:179.

Goldhaber MK, Armstrong MA, Golditch IM, et al. Long-term risk of hysterectomy among 80,007 sterilized and comparison women at Kaiser Permanente, 1971–1987. *Am J Epidemiol* 1993;138:508.

Grimes DA. Primary prevention of ovarian cancer. *JAMA* 1993;270:2855.

Grimes DA, Peterson HB, Rosenberg MJ, et al. Sterilization-attributable deaths in Bangladesh. *Int J Gynaecol Obstet* 1982;20:149.

Grimes DA, Satterthwaite AP, Rochat RW, et al. Deaths from contraceptive sterilization in Bangladesh: rates, causes, and prevention. *Obstet Gynecol* 1982;60:635.

Grubb GS, Peterson HB. Luteal phase pregnancy and tubal sterilization. *Obstet Gynecol* 1985;66:784.

Handa VL, Berlin M, Washington AE. A comparison of local and general anesthesia for laparoscopic tubal sterilization. *J Womens Health* 1994;3: 135.

Hankinson SE, Hunter DJ, Colditz GA, et al. Tubal ligation, hysterectomy, and risk of ovarian cancer: a prospective study. *JAMA* 1993;270:2813.

Healy B. From the National Institutes of Health: Does vasectomy cause prostate cancer? *JAMA* 1993;269:2620.

Henshaw SK, Singh S. Sterilization regret among U.S. couples. *Fam Plann Perspect* 1986;18:238.

Hillis SD, Marchbanks PA, Tylor LR, et al. Higher hysterectomy risk for sterilized than nonsterilized women: findings from the U.S. Collaborative Review of Sterilization. *Obstet Gynecol* 1998;91:241.

Hillis SD, Marchbanks PA, Tylor LR, et al. Poststerilization regret: findings from the United States Collaborative Review of Sterilization. *Obstet Gynecol* 1999;93:889.

Hillis SD, Marchbanks PA, Tylor LR, et al. Tubal sterilization and the long-term risk of hysterectomy: findings from the United States Collaborative Review of Sterilization. *Obstet Gynecol* 1997;89:609.

Holt VL, Chu J, Daling JR, et al. Tubal sterilization and subsequent ectopic pregnancy: a case-control study. *JAMA* 1991;226:242.

Hulka JF, Fishburne JI, Mercer JP, et al. Laparoscopic sterilization with a spring clip: a report of the first fifty cases. *Am J Obstet Gynecol* 1973;116: 715.

Hulka JF, Peterson HB, Phillips JM. American Association of Gynecologic Laparoscopists' 1988 membership survey on laparoscopic sterilization. *J Reprod Med* 1990;35:584.

Hulka JF, Reich H. *Textbook of laparoscopy*. 2nd ed. Philadelphia: WB Saunders; 1994:85.

Irving FC. Tubal sterilization. *Am J Obstet Gynecol* 1950;60:1101.

Irwin KL, Lee NC, Peterson HB, et al. Hysterectomy, tubal sterilization and the risk of breast cancer. *Am J Epidemiol* 1988;127:1192.

Jamieson DJ, Costello C, Trussell J, et al. The risk of pregnancy after vasectomy. *Obstet Gynecol* 2004;103:848.

Jamieson DJ, Hillis SD, Duerr A, et al. Complications of interval laparoscopic sterilization: findings from the United States Collaborative Review of Sterilization. *Obstet Gynecol* 2000;96:997.

Jamieson DJ, Kaufman SC, Costello C, et al. A comparison of women's regret after vasectomy versus tubal sterilization. *Obstet Gynecol* 2002;99:1073.

Kerin J, Munday D, Ritossa M, et al. Essure hysteroscopic sterilization: results based on utilizing a new coil catheter delivery system. *J Am Assoc Gynecol Laparosc* 2004;11:388.

Kjer JJ, Knudsen LB. Ectopic pregnancy subsequent to laparoscopic sterilization. *Am J Obstet Gynecol* 1989;160:1202.

Koetsawang S, Gates DS, Suwanichati S, et al. Long-term follow-up of laparoscopic sterilizations by electrocoagulation, the Hulka clip, and the tubal ring. *Contraception* 1990;41:9.

Kreiger N, Sloan M, Cotterchio M, et al. The risk of breast cancer following reproductive surgery. *Eur J Cancer* 1999;35:97.

Layde PM, Peterson HB, Dicker RC, et al. Risk factors for complications of interval tubal sterilization by laparotomy. *Obstet Gynecol* 1983;62:180.

Leader A, Galan N, George R, et al. A comparison of definable traits in women requesting reversal of sterilization and women satisfied with sterilization. *Am J Obstet Gynecol* 1983;145:198.

Levinson CJ, Daily HJ, Skinner SJ. Pathologic changes in the fallopian tube after Silastic ring occlusion. In: Phillips JM, ed. *Endoscopy in gynecology*. Downey, CA: American Association of Gynecologic Laparoscopists; 1978: 180.

Lichter ED, Laff SP, Friedman EA. Value of routine dilation and curettage at the time of interval sterilization. *Obstet Gynecol* 1986;67:763.

Lipscomb GH, Spellman JR, Ling FW. The effect of same-day pregnancy testing on the incidence of luteal phase pregnancy. *Obstet Gynecol* 1993;82: 411.

Liskin L, Pile JM, Quillin WF. Vasectomy—safe and simple. *Popul Rep D* 1983;4:D61.

Liskin L, Rinehart W. Minilaparotomy and laparoscopy: safe, effective, and widely used. *Popul Rep C* 1985;9:c-127.

Mackay AP, Kicke BA, Jr., Koonin LM, et al. Tubal sterilization in the United States, 1994–1996. *Fam Plan Perspect* 2001;33:161.

Madlener M. γber sterilisierende operationen an den tuben. *Zentralbl Gynakol* 1919;20:380.

Makar AP, Vanderheyden JS, Schatteman EA, et al. Female sterilization failure after bipolar electrocoagulation: a six-year retrospective study. *Eur J Obstet Gynecol Reprod Biol* 1990;37:237.

Marcil-Gratton N. Sterilization regret among women in metropolitan Montreal. *Fam Plann Perspect* 1988;20:222.

Marquette CM, Koonin LM, Antarsh L, et al. Vasectomy in the United States 1991. *Am J Public Health* 1995;85:644.

Massey FJ Jr, Bernstein GS, O'Fallon WM, et al. Vasectomy and health: results from a large cohort study. *JAMA* 1984;252:1023.

McMahon AJ, Buckley J, Taylor A, et al. Chronic testicular pain following vasectomy. *Br J Urol* 1992;69:188.

Mintz M. Risks and prophylaxis in laparoscopy: a survey of 100,000 cases. *J Reprod Med* 1977;18:269.

Mosher WD, Martinez GM, Chandra A, et al. *Use of contraception and use of family planning services in the United States: 1982–2002. Advance data from vital and health statistics*. No 350. Hyattsville, MD: National Center for Health Statistics, 2004.

Mumford SD, Bhiwandiwala PP, Chi I-C. Laparoscopic and minilaparotomy female sterilisation compared in 15,167 cases. *Lancet* 1980;2:1066.
Nirapathpongporn A, Huber DH, Krieger JN. No-scalpel vasectomy at the King's birthday vasectomy festival. *Lancet* 1990;335:894.
Nisanian A. Outpatient minilaparotomy sterilization with local anesthesia. *J Reprod Med* 1990;35:380.
Penfield AJ. The Filshie clip for female sterilization: a review of world experience. *Am J Obstet Gynecol* 2000;182:485.
Peterson HB, Curtis KM. Long-acting methods of contraception. *N Engl J Med* 2005;353:2169.
Peterson HB, DeStefano F, Rubin GL, et al. Deaths attributable to tubal sterilization in the United States, 1977 to 1981. *Am J Obstet Gynecol* 1983;146:131.
Peterson HB, Greenspan JR, DeStefano F, et al. The impact of laparoscopy on tubal sterilization in United States hospitals, 1970 and 1975 to 1978. *Am J Obstet Gynecol* 1981;140:811.
Peterson HB, Howards SS. Vasectomy and prostate cancer: the evidence to date. *Fertil Steril* 1998;70:201.
Peterson HB, Huber DH, Belker AM. Vasectomy: an appraisal for the obstetrician-gynecologist. *Obstet Gynecol* 1990;76:568.
Peterson HB, Hulka JF, Spielman FJ, et al. Local versus general anesthesia for laparoscopic sterilization: a randomized study. *Obstet Gynecol* 1987;70:903.
Peterson HB, Jeng G, Folger SG, et al. The risk of menstrual abnormalities after tubal sterilization. *N Engl J Med* 2000;343:1681.
Peterson HB, Xia Z, Hughes JM, et al. The risk of ectopic pregnancy after tubal sterilization. *N Engl J Med* 1997;336:762.
Peterson HB, Xia Z, Hughes JM, et al. The risk of pregnancy after tubal sterilization: findings from the U.S. Collaborative Review of Sterilization. *Am J Obstet Gynecol* 1996;174:1161.
Peterson HB, Xia Z, Wilcox LS, et al. Pregnancy after sterilization with bipolar electrocoagulation. *Obstet Gynecol* 1999;94:163.
Peterson HB, Xia Z, Wilcox LS, et al. Pregnancy after tubal sterilization with silicone rubber band and spring clip application. *Obstet Gynecol* 2001;97:205.
Piccinino LJ, Mosher WD. Trends in contraceptive use in the United States: 1982–1995. *Fam Plann Perspect* 1998;30:4.
Pitaktepsombati P, Janowitz B. Sterilization acceptance and regret in Thailand. *Contraception* 1991;44:623.
Poindexter AN, Abdul-Malak M, Fast J. Laparoscopic tubal sterilization under local anesthesia. *Obstet Gynecol* 1990;75:5.
Power FH, Barnes AC. Sterilization by means of peritoneoscopic tubal fulguration. *Am J Obstet Gynecol* 1941;41:1038.
Prystowsky H, Eastman NJ. Puerperal tubal sterilization: report of 1,830 cases. *JAMA* 1955;158:463.
Rennie AL, Richard JA, Milne MK, et al. Post-partum sterilisation—an anaesthetic hazard?. *Anaesthesia* 1979;34:267.
Rioux JE, Cloutier D. A new bipolar instrument for tubal sterilization. *Am J Obstet Gynecol* 1974;119:737.
Rochat RW, Bhiwandiwala PP, Feldblum PJ, et al. Mortality associated with sterilization: preliminary results of an international collaborative observational study. *Int J Gynaecol Obstet* 1986;24:275.
Ross JA, Frankenberg E. Sterilization. In: Ross JA, Frankenberg E, eds. *Findings from two decades of family planning research*. New York: Population Council; 1993:57.
Rulin MC, Davidson AR, Philliber SG, et al. Long-term effect of tubal sterilization on menstrual indices and pelvic pain. *Obstet Gynecol* 1993;82:118.
Rulin MC, Turner JH, Dunworth R, et al. Post-tubal sterilization syndrome—a misnomer. *Am J Obstet Gynecol* 1985;151:13.
Schmidt JE, Hillis SD, Marchbanks PA, et al. Requesting information about and obtaining reversal after tubal sterilization: findings from the U.S. Collaborative Review of Sterilization. *Fertil Steril* 2000;74:892.
Schwartz D, Wingo PA, Antarsh L, et al. Female sterilizations in the United States, 1987. *Fam Plann Perspect* 1989;21:209.
Shain RN, Miller WB, Holden AEC. Married women's dissatisfaction with tubal sterilization and vasectomy at first-year follow-up: effects of perceived spousal dominance. *Fertil Steril* 1986;45:808.
Shain RN, Miller WB, Mitchell GW, et al. Menstrual pattern change one year after sterilization: results of a controlled, prospective study. *Fertil Steril* 1989;52:192.
Shy KK, Stergachis A, Grothaus LG, et al. Tubal sterilization and risk of subsequent hospital admission for menstrual disorders. *Am J Obstet Gynecol* 1992;166:1698.
Siegler AM, Grunebaum A. A short history of tubal sterilization. In: Phillips JM, ed. *Endoscopic female sterilization: a comparison of methods*. Downey, CA: American Association of Gynecologic Laparoscopists; 1983:3.
Soderstrom R. Electrical safety in laparoscopy. In: Phillips JM, ed. *Endoscopy in gynecology*. Downey, CA: American Association of Gynecologic Laparoscopists; 1978:306.
Soderstrom RM, Levy BS, Engel T. Reducing bipolar sterilization failures. *Obstet Gynecol* 1989;74:60.
Speert H. *Obstetrics and gynecology in America: a history*. Chicago: American College of Obstetricians and Gynecologists; 1980:68.
Stergachis A, Shy KK, Grothaus LC, et al. Tubal sterilization and the long-term risk of hysterectomy. *JAMA* 1990;264:2893.
Stovall TG, Ling FW, O'Kelley KR, et al. Gross and histologic examination of tubal ligation failures in a residency training program. *Obstet Gynecol* 1990;76:461.
Trussell J, Hatcher RA, Cates W, et al. A guide to interpreting contraceptive efficacy studies. *Obstet Gynecol* 1990;76:558.
Trussell J, Kost K. Contraceptive failure in the United States: a critical review of the literature. *Stud Fam Plann* 1987;18:237.
Uchida H. Uchida tubal sterilization. *Am J Obstet Gynecol* 1975;121:153.
Whittemore AS, Harris R, Itnyre J, et al. Characteristics relating to ovarian cancer risk: collaborative analysis of 12 U.S. case-control studies. II. Invasive epithelial ovarian cancers in white women. *Am J Epidemiol* 1992;136:1184.
Williams EL, Jones HE, Merrill RE. The subsequent course of patients sterilized by tubal ligation: a consideration of hysterectomy for sterilization. *Am J Obstet Gynecol* 1951;61:423.
World Health Organization Task Force on Female Sterilization, Special Programme of Research, Development and Research Training in Human Reproduction. Minilaparotomy or laparoscopy for sterilization: a multicenter, multinational, randomized study. *Am J Obstet Gynecol* 1982;143:645.
Wortman J. Female sterilization by minilaparotomy. *Popul Rep C* 1974;5:c-53.
Wortman J, Piotrow P. Laparoscopic sterilization—a new technique. *Popul Rep C* 1973;1:c-1.
Yoon IB, Wheeless CR, King TM. A preliminary report on a new laparoscopic sterilization approach: the silicone rubber band technique. *Am J Obstet Gynecol* 1974;120:132.

CHAPTER 28 ■ SURGERY FOR BENIGN DISEASE OF THE OVARY

JOSEPH S. SANFILIPPO AND JOHN A. ROCK

DEFINITIONS

Accessory ovary—An additional ovarian mass close to the normally placed ovary and connected to it by the uteroovarian or infundibulopelvic ligament.

Fimbria ovarica—The structure attaching the infundibulum of the fallopian tube to the distal pole of the ovary. It is vitally important to the fimbrial ovum capture mechanism.

Gore-Tex surgical membrane—A permanent, nonporous material of expanded polytetrafluoroethylene. It may be used as a peritoneal substitute to prevent adhesions.

Interceed—An absorbable material consisting of oxidized regenerated cellulose. It functions as a temporary barrier to prevent adherence of serosal surfaces and has demonstrated efficacy in the peritoneal cavity.

Malpositioned ovary—An ovary located above the pelvic brim because of a lack of normal descent into the pelvis. It may be elongated, but it remains attached to the uterus by the uteroovarian ligament and to the fallopian tube by the fimbria ovarica.

Ovarian cortex—The outer layer of the ovary consisting of an outer zone, which is mainly collagenous (tunic albuginea), and an inner zone, which is less fibrous and more cellular and contains the germ cells (primordial follicles).

Ovarian medulla—The inner region surrounding the helium of the ovary. It contains no follicles, only blood vessels and the remnants of the tubular structures that are homologous to the male testis (rete testis).

Ovarian remnant—Persistent ovarian tissue unintentionally left behind following oophorectomy.

Paradoxic oophorectomy—A concept suggesting that removing an ovary on the side of unilateral obstruction or absence of a fallopian tube may improve fertility. Removal of one ovary supposedly promotes repeated ovulations from the ovary opposite the remaining patent fallopian tube.

Residual ovary—Symptomatic ovarian tissue following removal of the ovary.

Supernumerary ovary—An additional ovary that has no direct or ligamentous connection with a normally placed ovary. It is located at some distance from the normally placed ovaries.

Tumor markers—Substances identified in higher than normal amounts in blood, urine, or body tissues of patients with specific malignancies. They are produced directly by the tumor or as a response to the presence of cancer, i.e., indirect marker.

Tunica albuginea—Condensed ovarian stroma that forms a fibrous capsule.

Management of benign disease of the ovary continues to unfold with new and challenging clinical alternatives. Progress has occurred with regard to ovarian reconstruction. The population is living longer, and cancer survivors are increasing exponentially. All of this leads us to focus on enhancing our understanding of preservation of ovarian function, determining treatment related to decreased adhesion formation, and addressing a host of other aspects related to ovarian activity.

It has been established that the ovaries and fallopian tubes are sensitive to ischemia from surgical trauma; adhesions may develop as a result; and the normal anatomic relationship between fallopian tubes, ovaries, and uterus may be altered. Knowledge regarding anatomy and embryology of the ovaries and other reproductive organs complemented by mastery of the principles and skills of microsurgery are the prerequisites for excellent results following ovarian reconstructive surgery. Embryology and anatomy are addressed in this chapter with emphasis on the importance of the anatomic relations of the ovary to other pelvic organs in the section on the evaluation and management of an adnexal mass. State-of-the-art surgical procedures—both via minimally invasive as well as laparotomic approaches and techniques devised for the reconstruction of the ovary—for restoration of normal pelvic anatomy are presented in the context of specific pathology or other abnormal conditions that require surgical intervention. This chapter also focuses on pediatric and adolescent surgical procedures that are performed when ovarian pathology is identified.

EMBRYOLOGY

The reproductive system is derived from mesoderm. The primordium of the urogenital ridge, it is divided into two segments. One is the nephrogenic ridge, i.e., metanephros derivatives, the renal system; the other is the gonadal ridge for development of the reproductive tract. Gonads are a reflection of three origins: mesothelium, mesenchyme, and primordial germ cells. The paramesonephros gives rise to the fallopian tubes and the uterus. Two gonadal ridges arise early in gestation (4 to 5 weeks) in the developing embryo as thickening on the medial aspect of the coelomic cavity adjacent to the mesonephros. These gonadal outgrowths are composed of coelomic epithelium and underlying mesenchyme projecting into the future peritoneal cavity. The epithelial and mesenchymal cells of the gonadal primordia are of mesodermal origin (large, spherical ovoid germ cells that originate extragonadally in the wall of the yolk sac and migrate to the developing gonads). Until the 6th week of gestation, the gonads of the two sexes remain morphologically indistinguishable. The presumptive ovaries remain undifferentiated until the onset of meiosis at the end of the first trimester. The ovarian cortex is a single germinal epithelium.

The tunica albuginea lies beneath the cortex and is composed of connective tissue. The stroma is composed of fibroblasts, smooth muscle, endothelium, and interstitial cells, including undifferentiated theca cells and corpora albicans.

Sexual differentiation requires initiation by various genes, along with a single gene determinant on the Y chromosome (TDF, testis-determining factor), which is necessary for testicular differentiation. In XX individuals (in the absence of a Y chromosome), the bipotential gonad develops into an ovary.

The mechanisms responsible for gonadal sex differentiation are largely unknown. Investigators have theorized the presence of a testicular determining factory (H-Y cell-surface antigen on the short arm of the Y chromosome) that is elaborated by a specific gene. Meiosis-inducing and -preventing substances, both of which are produced by cells derived from mesonephric structures adjacent to the gonad, are the agents of regulation of ovarian and testicular germ cell differentiation. The balance between these two substances varies between the two sexes and at different stages of development. The meiosis-inducing substance predominates in the fetal ovary. Maternal ovarian hormone production is not required for differentiation of the germ cells or, apparently, for later development of the fetal reproductive tract. Various ultrastructural studies have shown no specific changes in fetal granulosa cells that can be definitely associated with steroid hormone secretion such as is identified in the fetal Leydig cells. Thecal cells play an essential role in steroid synthesis in the adult ovary, but they do not appear until later in gestation and even then retain a relatively undifferentiated appearance. Fetal pituitary gonadotropin production begins as early as 10 weeks' gestation and reaches peak levels at midgestation. Gonadotropins have a major influence on follicular development in the adult ovary, but evidence for a similar function in the fetus is lacking.

GENE EXPRESSION

Specific follicular cell receptors bind growth factors, which are locally synthesized with the ultimate effect of intracellular signaling and protein kinase activation. This activity affects transcription of targeted genes. Gene expression is involved in follicle development, ovulation, and corpus luteum and corpus albicans formation. Transcription factors include protooncogenes, C-myc, and CCAAT/enhancer binding protein.

FEMALE FETAL DEVELOPMENT

The ovarian surface cortex, during the early prefollicular stage, is characterized by germ cells and granulosa cells organized in cords and sheets, but the cortex lacks specific conformation. The final distinctive change to occur in the fetal ovary is the onset of meiosis at the 11th or 12th week of gestation. Meiosis is preceded by differentiation of primitive germ cells into actively dividing mitotic cells called *oogonia*. The mitotic divisions of the oogonia are associated with complete separation at telophase, leaving the daughter cells connected by intracellular bridges. After a series of mitotic divisions, there is progressive entry of cells into meiosis, beginning in the innermost cortex and gradually extending to the periphery. These cells passing through the various stages of the first meiotic prophase are then designated *oocytes*. By late gestation, all surviving oocytes have advanced to the diplotene stage. Further differentiation of the oocytes is arrested at this stage and does not resume until ovulation begins at menarche, about 12 years later.

Follicular formation begins at 18 to 20 weeks' gestation and continues throughout the remaining weeks of fetal development. All the surviving oocytes are surrounded by adjacent granulosa cells; oocyte and follicular growth are well established by the late fetal and early neonatal period. The constant degeneration and loss of oocytes before their incorporation into the follicles reduces their numbers to only 1 to 2 million (follicles) in the newborn ovary.

ANATOMY

The dimensions of the adult ovary vary from individual to individual but average 3 to 5 cm in length, 2 to 3 cm in width, and 1 to 2 cm in diameter, with a weight of 3 to 8g. The ovarian capsule is smooth in childhood, but its surface becomes pitted from follicular maturation and atresia.

The size, shape, and position of the ovary in the pelvis are somewhat variable, and both the consistency and the follicular changes taking place within the ovary vary with stage of the menstrual cycle. The ovary typically is anchored to the side wall of the pelvis in the shallow peritoneal fossa of Waldeyer formed between the angle of proximity of the ovary to the ureter. This knowledge is important before dissecting the ovary off the pelvic side wall.

The ovary is connected to the uterus by the uteroovarian ligament, to the posterior aspect of the broad ligament by the mesovarium ligament, and to the lateral pelvic sidewall by the infundibulopelvic ligament (Fig. 28.1). The mesovarium ligament attaches to the mesentery of the ovary. The other two ligaments are attached at the hilum of the ovary.

The ovary migrates downward from high in the abdomen during embryonic life. The infundibulum of the fallopian tube extends onto the ovary and is attached to it at its most distal pole by the fimbria ovarica. The relation of the ovary to the fimbria ovarica and to the uteroovarian ligament is crucial, and they should be carefully maintained during ovarian reconstruction.

During embryogenesis, the ovary may assume an unusual appearance (i.e., it may be septate) or assume an unusual position (Fig. 28.2). An accessory ovary (Fig. 28.2A) usually is close to or is connected to a normally placed ovary. An accessory ovary also may be attached to the broad, uteroovarian or infundibulopelvic ligaments. Unlike the accessory ovary, a supernumerary ovary (Fig. 28.2B) must have an independent embryologic origin. It may develop from a primordium such as arrested migrating gonadocytes. A supernumerary ovary consists of typical ovarian tissue but has no direct or ligamentous connection with a normally placed ovary. A supernumerary ovary is thus a true third ovary that has independent function and is located at a point that is distant to a normally placed ovary. Ovarian malposition (Fig. 28.2C) also may occur when the ovary fails to descend into the pelvis to assume its normal location. In ovarian malposition, the ovary is attached as it should be to the uterus by the uteroovarian ligament and to the fallopian tube by the fimbria ovarica, but it may lie adjacent to the liver or spleen. The ovary is elongated and may measure up to 15 cm in length. The fallopian tube attaching to such a malpositioned ovary may be 20 to 26 cm in length, almost twice its normal length.

The normal ovary has a surface covering composed of a single layer of flattened, germinal epithelial cells. This layer is contiguous at the ovarian hilum, with the peritoneal epithelium

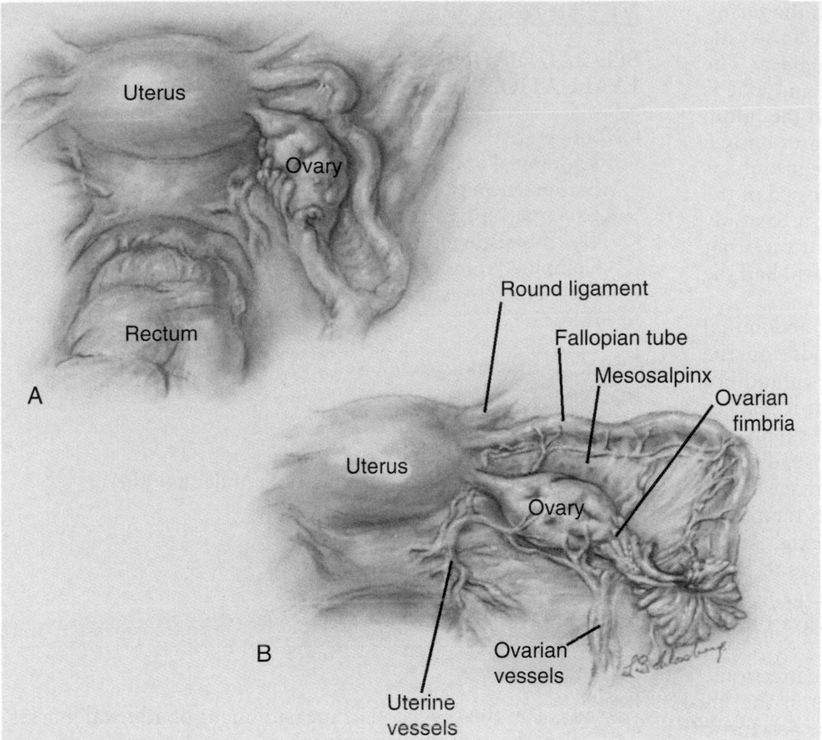

FIGURE 28.1. Normal anatomy of the ovary. **A:** Anatomic relations of the uterus, tube, and ovary. **B:** The infundibulum of the oviduct extends onto the ovary and is attached at its most distal pole (ovarian fimbria). The mesovarian is the mesentery of the ovary. Each ovary is attached at the hilum.

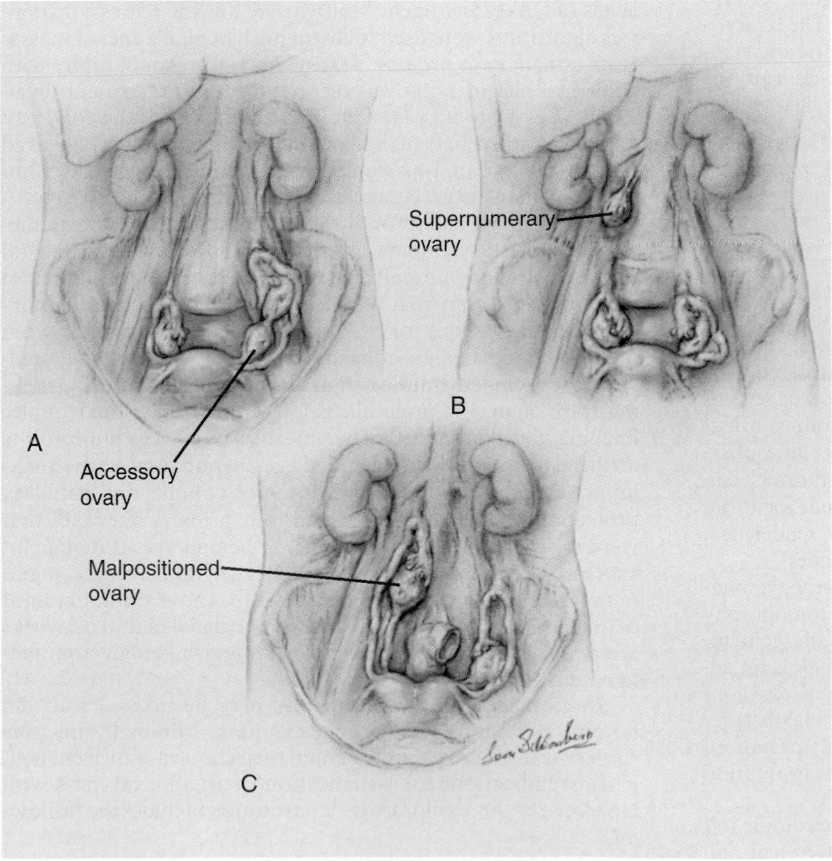

FIGURE 28.2. Ovarian anomalies. **A:** Accessory. **B:** Supernumerary. **C:** Malpositioned.

of the posterior leaf of the broad ligament. Beneath the germinal epithelium is a second layer of condensed ovarian stroma that forms a fibrous capsule, i.e., the tunica albuginea. The area through which the vessels and nerves enter and exit is called the hilum of the ovary. Immediately around the hilum and extending into the substance of the ovary is an area known as the medulla, which is covered by the cortex. The medulla is composed of fibrous tissue unlike the condensed stroma of the ovarian cortex. The medulla contains no follicles; it has only blood vessels and the remnants of the tubular structure that would have developed into a testis (i.e., the rete ovarii) had the fetus been male.

The ovarian artery arises on each side of the abdominal aorta just below the renal arteries. The artery descends from the aorta and crosses the ureter obliquely to enter the infundibulopelvic ligament on its course to the ovary. When it reaches the broad ligament, the ovarian artery branches to supply the fallopian tube and ovary before it finally anastomoses directly with the uterine artery to form a continuous arcade in the broad ligament. The ovarian veins are situated mainly in the mesosalpinx, where they give rise to the pampiniform plexus. At the outer end of the broad ligament, this plexus coalesces to form a single, large ovarian vein. The ovarian vein accompanies the ovarian artery to terminate in the inferior vena cava on the right and the renal vein on the left.

The lymphatic vessels of the ovary drain in three directions. The main group accompanies the ovarian vessels in the infundibulopelvic ligament and eventually reaches the periaortic nodes in the vicinity of the kidney. Other lymphatic channels communicate with channels of the opposite ovary by crossing the fundus of the uterus through the ovarian ligament. Some channels drain through the ovarian and round ligaments into the superficial inguinal lymph nodes in the groin. The ovary is supplied by both motor and sensory parasympathetic and sympathetic nerves, which accompany the ovarian vessels from the abdomen as they pass into the infundibulopelvic ligament to reach the hilum of the ovary. The segmented nerves supply the ovary from T10 and T11.

ADNEXAL MASS

The uterine adnexa (gynecologic origin) consist of the ovaries, the fallopian tubes, and the uterine ligaments. Although adnexal pathology often involves one of these structures, contiguous tissue of nongynecologic origin also may be involved. The bimanual examination is the most practical method of screening for an adnexal mass. When such a mass is found, its initial characteristics should be carefully described so that any subsequent change can be appreciated and the nature of the mass can be better ascertained. The description should include location, size (in centimeters), consistency, shape, mobility, tenderness, bilaterality, and associated findings (e.g., fever, ascites).

Adjunctive diagnostic techniques such as sonography, magnetic resonance imaging (MRI), and computed tomography (CT) may help delineate the nature of adnexal enlargement. Pelvic ultrasonography, especially three dimensional, is an accurate means of determining the location, size, extent, and consistency of pelvic masses and is also useful for detecting obstructive uropathy, ascites, and metastasis. Other more specialized diagnostic procedures also may be necessary for the evaluation of an adnexal mass (Table 28.1).

CT scanning has been particularly useful in gynecologic oncology because it helps define the extent of paracervical and parametrial involvement and allows a reasonable determination of the resectability of malignant neoplasms. MRI has surpassed CT in the precision of measurement of adnexal masses. MRI also allows a clear definition of the relationship of adjacent organs.

TABLE 28.1

SPECIAL DIAGNOSTIC PROCEDURES FOR THE EVALUATION OF AN ADNEXAL MASS

Nonoperative Noninvasive
Abdominal and pelvic radiography
Barium enema
Excretory urography
Gastrointestinal series with small bowel follow-through
Computed tomography scan
Magnetic resonance imaging
β-hCG
CA-125
Nonoperative Invasive
Culdocentesis
Pelvic arteriography
Operative Noninvasive
Abdominal and pelvic examination under anesthesia
Operative Invasive
Culdoscopy
Laparoscopy
Exploratory posterior colpotomy
Exploratory laparotomy

In a study conducted by Timmerman and coworkers, assessment was made of the use of both ultrasound and circulating levels of CA-125 antigen. Multivariate logistic regression analysis algorithms were used to distinguish benign adnexal masses from a malignant process. Transvaginal ultrasonography with color Doppler imaging was recorded in the 191 patients evaluated, ages 18 to 93 years. Of interest, 26.7% of the cohort of patients studied had malignant tumors. The authors believed that regression analysis could be used to accurately discriminate malignant from benign adnexal masses preoperatively.

An intriguing aspect of ultrasound assessment is the prediction of malignancy in adnexal masses using an artificial neural network. Taylor and colleagues reported generating a neural network algorithm that enabled computing of a probability of malignancy score for preoperative discrimination between malignant and benign adnexal masses. A retrospective analysis that included training in artificial neural network assessing transvaginal B-mode ultrasonography and color Doppler imaging was determined. The variables that were put into the artificial neural network included age, menopausal status, maximum diameter of the neoplasm, tumor volume, and papillary projections. The results identified four primary variables that were most effective in distinguishing benign versus malignant processes. These variables included age, time-average maximum velocity, papillary projection score, and maximum tumor diameter. The authors concluded that artificial neural networks are a useful clinical parameter to distinguish benign from malignant ovarian masses.

Surgical intervention ultimately may be necessary to determine the nature of the adnexal mass. Minimally invasive surgery is useful to exclude benign ovarian or nonovarian neoplasms. Indications for visualization of an adnexal mass with laparoscopy or exploratory laparotomy include the following:

- Ovarian mass >6 cm in diameter
- Adnexal mass >10 cm in diameter

- Any solid mass first developing after menopause
- Failure to discover the nature of the mass (e.g., leiomyoma) with radiologic or sonographic imaging techniques

One of the major goals of the evaluation of the adnexal mass is to rule out malignancy. There is an age-dependent risk for a malignant adnexal mass. The incidence of malignant neoplasm increases significantly after age 50 years. Increased size of the adnexal mass is associated with an increased risk of malignancy.

Granberg and colleagues found that less than 1% of masses smaller than 5 cm were malignant, less than 11% of masses 5 to 10 cm were malignant, and 72% of masses larger than 10 cm were malignant. Sassone and associates, in an evaluation of women of all ages (mean age, 41 years) by transvaginal sonography, found that 3% of masses smaller than 5 cm and 7% of masses 5 to 10 cm were malignant; the incidence of malignancy for masses larger than 10 cm was 13%.

Endometriosis is a common cause of an adnexal mass. An endometrial cyst of the ovary may develop into an endometrioma. Leakage of blood from the cyst may cause peritoneal irritation, pelvic adhesions, and pelvic organ fixation.

Tuboovarian inflammatory complex usually is the result of incompletely treated or unresolved subacute, chronic pelvic inflammatory disease (PID) in the walled-off area surrounding the pelvic structure.

Uterine leiomyomata cause nodularity and consequent irregular conformation of the uterus. The uterus may become enlarged and may present as an abdominal mass. The inability to distinguish a leiomyoma from an ovarian tumor on pelvic examination is an indication for further diagnostic evaluation.

Adnexal enlargement may be the result of carcinoma of the rectum, appendix, or bladder. Patients present with a variety of symptoms according to the organ involved. A complete and thorough evaluation is necessary to delineate the etiology of a neoplasm.

An adnexal mass may be noted in cases of acute abdomen. The differential diagnosis should include adnexal torsion, ruptured hemorrhagic cyst, degenerating leiomyomata, ectopic pregnancy, unruptured tuboovarian abscess, acute appendicitis with or without abscess formation, and diverticular disease of the sigmoid colon. A careful history, pelvic examination, and appropriate imaging studies often allow a prompt diagnosis.

Although every adnexal mass requires individual evaluation and management, it is possible to make a number of useful general recommendations. Expectant management is justified only when an asymptomatic physiologic cyst is suspected. Most cysts greater than 6 cm in diameter require a thorough evaluation. Imaging techniques are invaluable for characterizing the nature of the adnexal enlargement, but these procedures do not replace a careful medical history and thorough physical and pelvic examination.

ADNEXAL MASS DURING PREGNANCY

The incidence of adnexal mass in pregnancy requiring surgical intervention has been reported to occur in 1 in 81 to 2,500 pregnancies. When an adnexal mass is noted incidentally on ultrasound during pregnancy, the majority of small, simple cysts do not pose a risk to the pregnancy. Furthermore, most large or sonographically complex masses spontaneously resolve, as reported by Bernhard and colleagues. This study evaluated 18,391 ultrasound studies done in an obstetric population for which 432 women were identified with an adnexal mass. The incidence of adnexal masses was 2.3% in the pregnant population evaluated. In addition, the rate of torsion of the adnexal mass was 1%, and the rate of malignancy was also reported as 1%.

Before operative intervention, a complete assessment of the fetus—including ultrasound to rule out a lethal anomaly and to document cardiac activity—is in order. The optimal time for elective surgery is during the second trimester. The patient should be informed of the increased risk of preterm labor and delivery. The patient should be placed in the left lateral tilt position to avoid inferior vena cava compression and associated uteroplacental insufficiency. Postoperatively, the fetus should be placed on continuous fetal heart rate monitoring.

The most effective approach in management of adnexal masses during pregnancy remains a point of controversy (i.e., laparoscopy versus laparotomy). In a series of 88 pregnant women who underwent 93 surgical procedures for suspected adnexal pathology, laparoscopy was performed during the first trimester in 39 patients. The remaining 54 patients underwent laparotomy, 25 during the first trimester and 29 during the second trimester. Neither intraoperative nor postoperative internal complications were reported in the series. Five of 39 women undergoing the first-trimester surgery had a spontaneous abortion. During the first trimester, a Veress needle was used for insufflation, and the procedure was in essence conducted in a manner virtually identical to that in the nonpregnant state (i.e., closed laparoscopy). It was concluded that laparoscopic gynecologic surgery is safe during pregnancy when conducted in the first trimester.

ULTRASOUND

Ultrasound is useful in predicting malignancy (Table 28.2). Characteristic features of benign versus malignant neoplasms have been reported. Collated data from studies of ultrasound accuracy in the prediction of malignancy have an average positive predictive value of 74% and an average sensitivity of 88% (Table 28.3).

Weiner and coworkers have used transvaginal color flow imaging before exploratory surgery to study the impedance to blood flow in women with an adnexal mass. Intramural blood vessels consistently demonstrated low impedance to flow with

TABLE 28.2

ULTRASOUND CHARACTERISTICS OF THE OVARY

Benign Pattern
Simple cyst without internal echoes
Simple cyst with scattered echoes
Polycystic echoes
Polycystic echoes with thick septum
Sessile or polypoid smooth mural echoes
Central dense round echoes
Thin or thick multiple linear echoes
Thin or thick multiple linear echoes with dense part
Malignant Pattern
Cystic echoes with papillary or indented mural part
Polycystic echoes with irregular thick septum and solid part
Solid pattern (.50%) heterogeneous component with irregular cystic part
Completely solid with homogeneous component
Low impedance to flow (color Doppler)

TABLE 28.3

ULTRASOUND ACCURACY IN PREDICTION OF MALIGNANCY

Author	Patients (*n*)	Malignancy prevalence	Positive predictive value (%)	Negative predictive value (%)	Sensitivity	Specificity
Kobayashi 1976	406	15	31	93	71	73
Meire et al. 1978	51	35	83	91	83	91
Pussell 1980	25	48	83	91	83	84
Herrmann et al. 1987	241	21	75	95	82	93
Finkler et al. 1988	102	36	88	81	62	95
Benacerraf et al. 1990	100	30	72	91	80	87
Granberg et al. 1989	180	21.5	74	95	82	92
Sassone et al. 1991	143	10	87	100	100	83

a pulsatility index less than 1:16 in women with malignant tumors. The sensitivity and specificity of the preoperative pulsatility index in detecting malignant ovarian tumors were 94% and 97%, respectively. Kurjak and colleagues found that vessels with a low-resistance index near the center of the mass or within papules or septa were highly correlated with malignancy. Therefore, transvaginal color flow imaging may be a useful clinical tool in the preoperative evaluation of ovarian masses.

Doppler resistance index has been used as a "vascular" scoring system. Color Doppler ultrasonography appears to be a reliable method in presurgically evaluating ovarian neoplasms.

Transvaginal color Doppler sonography has identified the following parameters as useful in determining malignant versus benign ovarian masses: number of vessels detected in each tumor, tumor vessel location (central versus peripheral), peak systolic velocity, lowest resistance index, mean resistance index, lower pulsatility index, and mean pulsatility index. Color Doppler signals were detected in 100% of malignant masses and 75% of benign masses, with the difference being statistically significant as reported by Alcazar and associates. Tumor vessel location appears to be central in virtually all malignant masses. Overall, the receiver operating characteristic curves generated can be used to predict malignant processes. The lowest resistance index was associated with the majority of malignant tumors.

Three-dimensional ultrasonographic technology has been used to evaluate adnexal masses. Images are dissected in XYZ planes and can be focused especially on areas suggestive of malignancy. Three-dimensional ultrasonography facilitates real-time analysis of acquired image data and allows reassessment of the findings at the time of the original ultrasound. Three-dimensional transvaginal ultrasonographic technology appears to enhance and facilitate morphologic assessment of benign as well as malignant ovarian masses.

TUMOR MARKERS

Tumor markers are substances that are identified in higher than normal amounts in blood, urine, or body tissues of patients with specific malignancies. The tumor marker is produced by the tumor per se or as a response to the presence of cancer. They are not unique to malignant processes and can be elevated with benign conditions. Tumor markers are not elevated in every patient with malignancy, especially in the early stages of the disease. Many (tumor markers) are not specific for a particular type of cancer; therefore, there are limitations to the use of tumor markers.

CA-125 is a tumor-associated antigen to an antibody expressed by about 80% of patients with epithelial ovarian cancer. It can be increased by nongynecologic malignancies with involvement of the pleura or peritoneum and by benign conditions that result in ascites. Because of the many medical diagnoses that give false-positive CA-125 results, CA-125 cannot be used for general population screening for ovarian cancer in either premenopausal or postmenopausal women. However, in menopausal women who present with a pelvic mass, CA-125 can help differentiate benign from malignant masses.

Because menopausal women have fewer gynecologic diseases that give false elevation of CA-125, the test is more sensitive and specific in this age group. Several authors have demonstrated that a panel of assays can improve both sensitivity and specificity in the detection of ovarian malignancies. For example, Soper and associates demonstrated 100% specificity and predictive value for CA-125 with TAG 72 or CA-15–3. Table 28.4 provides specific markers and their clinical application.

The clinical findings listed in Tables 28.3 through 28.6 are often helpful in differentiating a malignant from a benign neoplasm. All ovarian neoplasms larger than 6 cm in diameter with a solid component should undergo investigation. The postmenopausal ovary is usually small and nonpalpable. Enlargement of the postmenopausal ovary requires immediate investigation. Symptoms of ovarian neoplasms usually depend on their size, rate of growth, and position in the pelvis or abdomen. Symptoms may include vague lower abdominal fullness or pressure discomfort. Larger masses rise out of the true pelvis and may cause abdominal enlargement with varicosities and edema of the lower extremities. Most ovarian neoplasms are asymptomatic until they enlarge or involve adjacent organs and structures.

LAPAROSCOPIC MANAGEMENT OF AN OVARIAN MASS

The pelvic (adnexal) mass may be of gynecologic or nongynecologic origin (Table 28.5). Specific clinical findings are helpful to differentiate a malignant from a benign neoplasm (Table 28.6). It is important to establish whether the mass is of ovarian origin and to understand that a mass causing an ovary to enlarge to >6 cm in diameter should be considered potentially malignant until proven otherwise. The most common ovarian mass is the physiologic ovarian cyst, which is caused by failure

TABLE 28.4

TUMOR MARKERS-ADNEXAL MASSES

Marker	Comments
CA-125	80% nonmucinous ovarian carcinomas have elevation of CA-125. Decreasing levels generally indicate response to therapy. Used to identify recurrences.
CEA	Primary use is to monitor recurrence of colon cancer. Oncofetal antigen-Ag complex glycoprotein, 20,000 d associated with plasma membrane of tumor cells. Increased with ovarian cancer and with melanoma, breast, pancreatic, stomach, cervical, bladder, kidney, thyroid, and liver cancer. Inflammatory bowel disease and smoking elevates CEA.
cMyc	Amplified in 30%–50% of ovarian tumors. The protein is simultaneously overexpressed.
CMycRA	Associated with aneuploidy in ovarian malignant cell progression.
BRCA-1	Associated with mutations of breast tumor–related antigen. BRCA-1 tumor suppressor gene has been identified; 63% risk of developing ovarian cancer with positive BRCA-1 gene.

of a follicle to rupture or to regress. Physiologic ovarian cysts normally are <6 cm in diameter, smooth, mobile, and slightly tender to palpation. They usually contain straw-colored fluid and may be associated with menstrual irregularity. Physiologic ovarian cysts smaller than 6 cm usually regress by absorption of the fluid or spontaneous rupture. The premenopausal patient may be managed conservatively over two menstrual cycles. If regression fails to occur over two periods of observation or if enlargement is noted, reassessment is indicated.

Oral contraceptives have been suggested as an alternative treatment for functional cysts. The combination-type oral contraceptives send negative feedback to the pituitary gland to decrease gonadotropin stimulation of the ovary, which causes regression of the cyst. Steinkampf and colleagues noted that the rate of disappearance of functional ovarian cysts was not affected by estrogen-progestin treatment; nevertheless, a patient taking oral contraceptives with an adnexal mass should be thoroughly investigated.

Failure of the corpus luteum to regress (in the nonpregnant patient) may cause development of a corpus luteum cyst. The size of the corpus luteum cyst varies according to the amount of blood contained within the cyst. A large corpus luteum may rupture and cause intraperitoneal hemorrhage. Amenorrhea or irregular uterine bleeding may accompany the development of a corpus luteum cyst. A sensitive pregnancy test, ultrasonography, and laparoscopy can be used to differentiate an ectopic pregnancy from a persistent corpus luteum.

A theca-lutein cyst, which may be associated with gestational trophoblastic disease or pregnancy, is the result of luteinization of the ovary by human chorionic gonadotropin (hCG). Many of these cysts are bilateral and multicystic. A reduction in hCG levels usually leads to their spontaneous regression.

TABLE 28.5

CLASSIFICATION OF THE ADNEXAL MASS

Gynecologic origin	Nongynecologic origin
Nonneoplastic	Nonneoplastic
Ovarian	Appendiceal abscess
Physiologic cysts	Diverticulosis
Follicular	Adhesions of bowel and omentum
Corpus luteum	
Theca-lutein cyst	Peritoneal cyst
Luteoma of pregnancy	Feces in rectosigmoid
Polycystic ovaries	Urine in bladder
Inflammatory cysts	Pelvic kidney
Urachal cyst	
Nonovarian	Anterior sacral meningocele
Ectopic pregnancy	Neoplastic
Congenital anomalies	Carcinoma
Embryologic remnants	Sigmoid
Tubal	Cecum
Pyosalpinx	Appendix
Hydrosalpinx	Retroperitoneal neoplasm
Bladder	Presacral teratoma
Neoplastic	
Ovarian	
Nonovarian	
Leiomyomata	
Paraovarian cyst	
Endometrial carcinoma	
Tubal carcinoma	

Adapted from Hall DJ, Hurt WG. The adnexal mass. *J Fam Pract* 1982;14:135, with permission.

TABLE 28.6

CLINICAL FINDINGS SUGGESTING BENIGN OR MALIGNANT ADNEXAL MASS

Benign	Malignant
Unilateral	Bilateral
Cystic	Solid
Mobile	Fixed
Smooth	Irregular
No ascites	Ascites
Slow growth	Rapid growth
Young patient	Older patient

Polycystic ovarian disease (PCOD) is associated with bilaterally enlarged ovaries with a smooth surface. The ovaries contain multiple follicular cysts; many patients are obese and hirsute and have accompanying anovulation (see Ovarian Surgery for Polycystic Ovarian Disease).

Congenital anomalies of the müllerian system and vestigial remnants of the wolffian system are of gynecologic, if not strictly ovarian, origin. Müllerian anomalies should be considered in the differential diagnosis of an adnexal mass. Uterine anomalies ofentimes are associated with cyclic pain from development of hematometra, whereas an enlarged paraovarian cyst may be asymptomatic.

OVARIAN REMNANT SYNDROME

The ovarian remnant occurs in patients who have had previous oophorectomy with or without hysterectomy. The symptomatic patient may present with or without a palpable mass or with a palpable pelvic mass but no symptoms. Pathologic investigation confirms the presence of ovarian tissue when there should be none.

The ovarian remnant syndrome differs from the residual ovarian syndrome in that with the latter, the ovary is purposely saved, and a pathologic process subsequently develops in the ovary. The ovarian remnant syndrome follows attempted oophorectomy.

Minke and associates demonstrated that devascularization of ovarian tissue can occur with reimplanting on intact or abraded peritoneal surfaces, where it may resume endocrine function. Thus, the authors suggest that great care should be exercised to remove all ovarian tissue, particularly when oophorectomy is performed through the laparoscope.

Ultrasonography remains a valuable tool in establishing the diagnosis of ovarian remnant syndrome. The use of both transabdominal sonography and transvaginal sonography with use of color Doppler identification of the mass acquires information with respect to both arterial and venous flow. This facilitates identification of ovarian tissue. With respect to diagnosis, use of gonadotropin-releasing hormone (GnRH) agonist stimulation test has specific utility. The patient often presents with chronic pelvic pain with or without a pelvic mass. Use of GnRH agonist stimulation test allows identification of the presence of functioning ovarian tissue in association with ovarian remnant syndrome. Associated chronic pelvic pain frequently responds to suppressive therapy. Initially, the gonadotropin flare results in increased production of estradiol and allows confirmation of the diagnosis. As treatment is continued, the GnRH agonist often proves efficacious in relief of pelvic pain.

Symmonds and Petit identified three major factors that may complicate the initial surgery and make it difficult or impossible for the surgeon to ascertain whether all ovarian tissue has been removed: increased pelvic vascularity, which renders hemostasis difficult; adhesions, which distort the anatomy and make dissection difficult; and neoplasms, which also distort the anatomy. The most common preexisting disease is endometriosis, followed in frequency by pelvic inflammatory disease. Patients with ovarian remnant syndrome often present with both pelvic pain and a mass. The quality of the pain varies, often cyclically, and ranges from a sensation of pressure or dull aching to a severe stabbing pain.

The clinical diagnosis of ovarian remnant syndrome can be difficult. A finding of premenopausal levels of follicle-stimulating hormone (FSH) may facilitate the diagnosis. Sonography (especially vaginal) may be of some value, and a CT scan or MRI may be useful for defining the physical relation of the ovarian remnant to surrounding structures.

The treatment of choice is adequate excision of the ovarian remnant with removal of contiguous adherent tissue such as pelvic peritoneum, bowel serosa, the underlying involved ligament, and alveolar and vascular tissues (Fig. 28.3). Excision of ovarian tissue may require a retroperitoneal dissection to define the relation of the ureter to the bowel and ovary. Special care should be taken to carefully define all anatomic relations before extirpation of the remnant.

Magtibay and colleagues addressed the surgical management of patients with ovarian remnant syndrome at the Mayo Clinic. All operations for residual ovary syndrome were performed by laparotomy. Of 186 patients who underwent a wide dissection and removal of the remnant, a moderate risk of bowel, bladder, or ureteral injury was noted; however, 90% of patients had complete resolution or marked improvement of symptoms after surgery.

Laparoscopic excision of ovarian remnant ovaries is feasible. A laparoscopic retroperitoneal approach that allows dissection of the course of the ureters with coagulation and dissection of the infundibulopelvic ligament and the uterine vessels can be accomplished. Surgeons with appropriate laparoscopic skills can consider this surgical approach. There is potential for ureteral injury as well as cystotomy and bowel injury.

RESIDUAL OVARY

Based on the clinical circumstance, the gynecologic surgeon should consider the value of ovarian conservation at the time of hysterectomy for benign disease. Some authors have noted the incidence of malignant neoplasm in retained ovaries as a reason for prophylactic oophorectomy, and others have noted the presence of "residual ovary syndrome," characterized by either recurrent pelvic pain or a persistent pelvic mass (Fig. 28.4). However, Funt followed up 992 patients after conservation of one or both ovaries at the time of hysterectomy and reported that none developed ovarian malignancy, and only 1.4% required subsequent surgical intervention for adnexal pathology. The benefits of preserved ovarian function thus appear to substantially outweigh the risk of subsequent ovarian pathology requiring further surgery. Before surgery, the gynecologic surgeon should discuss the various risks and benefits of castration and should encourage the patient to participate in any decision concerning the fate of her ovaries.

GnRH agonists have been used to assess response of residual ovaries with chronic pelvic pain followed by surgical intervention to remove the residual ovarian tissue. Resolution of pelvic pain in six treated patients occurred with the analog (GnRH agonist) and persisted with surgical extirpation of the ovarian tissue. Suppression of ovarian function by GnRH agonists allows differentiation of pelvic pain caused by residual ovary from other sources and thus should be a prerequisite to surgical intervention.

In a retrospective report of 20 years' experience with residual ovary syndrome in which 2,561 hysterectomies were performed, the incidence of residual ovary syndrome was 2.85%. Thus, 1 in 35 women who undergo hysterectomy with ovarian preservation become symptomatic—that is, they experience pelvic pain often with the presence of a benign cyst. Patients should be counseled preoperatively with respect to the potential for residual ovary syndrome when the initial surgical intervention is anticipated. In addition to chronic pelvic pain, a pelvic mass and dyspareunia include the "cluster of symptoms" that can occur in patients who have undergone previous hysterectomy.

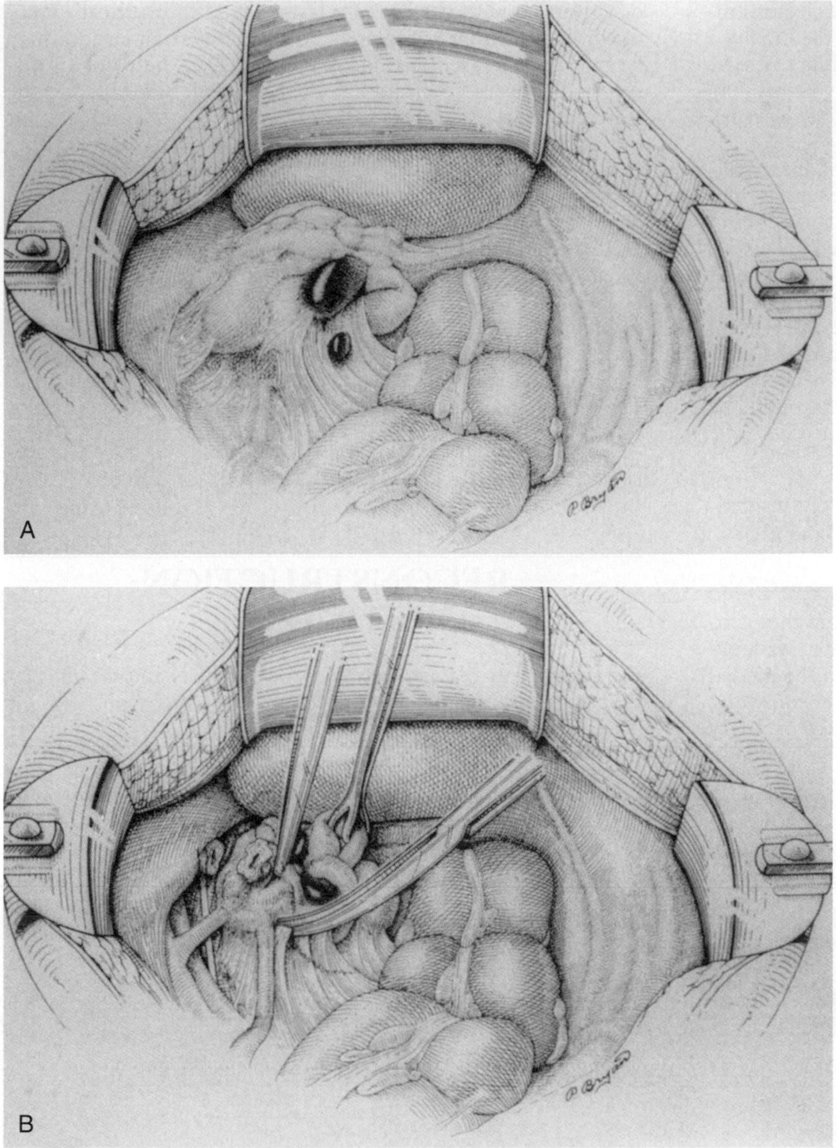

FIGURE 28.3. A: Not infrequently, the ovarian remnant may adhere to the bowel and the pelvic sidewall peritoneum. B: The ureter must be visualized and its relation to the bowel and ovarian remnant established. This may require development of the pararectal and rectovaginal spaces.

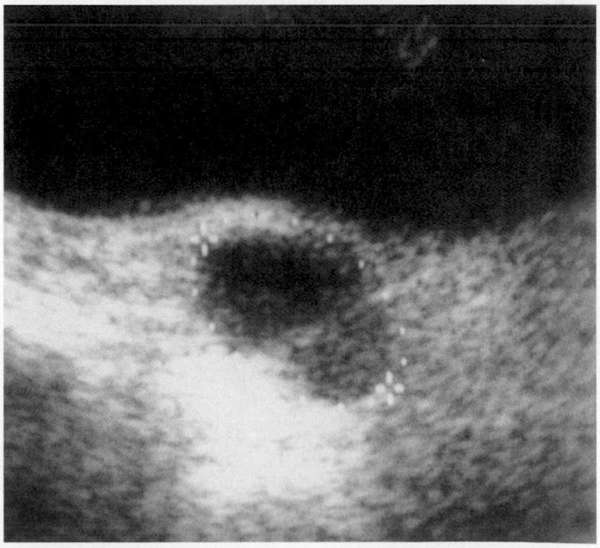

FIGURE 28.4. Abdominal sonogram showing a residual ovary with presumed follicular activity.

ADNEXAL TORSION

Torsion of the adnexa is an infrequent cause of pain in the lower abdomen. However, torsion is a common gynecologic surgical emergency, with a prevalence of 2.7%. Treatment of adnexal torsion is considered an emergency because peritonitis and death can result. Any portion of the adnexa (tube or ovary) may undergo torsion. It may occur in neoplastic ovaries or as a consequence of hyperstimulation.

The clinical findings of torsion are nonspecific. For this reason, delay in diagnosis and surgical intervention is common. The classic presentation is the acute onset of abdominal pain with clinical evidence of peritonitis and an adnexal mass. However, according to Bayer and Wiskind, the presenting findings in most patients are nonspecific and unimpressive. Torsion is more likely to occur during ovulation or as a premenstrual event associated with increased pelvic congestion; the authors found no correlation between the phase of the cycle and the onset of the symptoms.

Historically, the adnexa usually were removed because some authors suggested that untwisting the adnexa could increase the risk of thromboembolism. This has not been well substantiated. There is growing evidence that unwinding the involved adnexa to observe for tissue reperfusion and viability is safe. Nevertheless, a significant delay in surgical intervention may result in irreversible necrosis, requiring removal of the tube, ovary, or both.

The minimally invasive surgical management of adnexal torsion has been increasing in efficacy. Mage and colleagues found that unwinding the adnexa was possible in most patients in their series, and no further intervention was required. Likewise, Shalev and Peleg demonstrated that laparoscopic detorsion of the adnexa is safe and reliable as a primary treatment of this condition. Thus, the weight of evidence warrants conservation of the adnexa, if there is evidence of reperfusion and if significant delay has not resulted in irreversible tissue necrosis. In most instances, detorsion may be accomplished through the laparoscope.

SURGERY OF THE OVARIAN SURFACE

Surgery to remove adhesions or endometriosis from the ovarian surface is not unusual and primarily accomplished via laparoscopy. *De novo* adhesions or adhesions between the medial surface of the ovary and the broad ligament may be filmy and vascular (Fig. 28.5A), and may be excised by fine electrocautery or vaporized with the use of a laser (Fig. 28.5B). More extensive adhesions that completely cover the ovarian surface may be thick and avascular (Fig. 28.5C and D). The plane of dissection between the broad ligament or pelvic sidewall and the adherent ovarian surface must be developed with care so as not to remove or damage the peritoneum while excising the adhesion (Fig. 28.5D). Multiple, small adhesions distributed over the ovarian surface, once coagulated, can be gently removed from the ovary without trauma to the ovarian cortex.

If the lateral aspect of the ovary is densely adherent to the broad ligament, it may be necessary to dissect the ovary free. Some cases require that a large area of the sidewall or the broad ligament be denuded; reperitonealization can be accomplished with 7–0 fine, nonreactive suture material.

Small endometrial implants can be fulgurated or vaporized. The resulting small ovarian defect usually does not require closure. Care should be taken to ensure that the endometriosis is superficial and that the implant is not actually the tip of a large endometrioma within the substance of the ovary.

RECONSTRUCTION OF THE OVARY

Before ovarian reconstruction is begun, it is important that proper mobilization of the ovary be accomplished for reestablishment of normal anatomic relations. Once complete

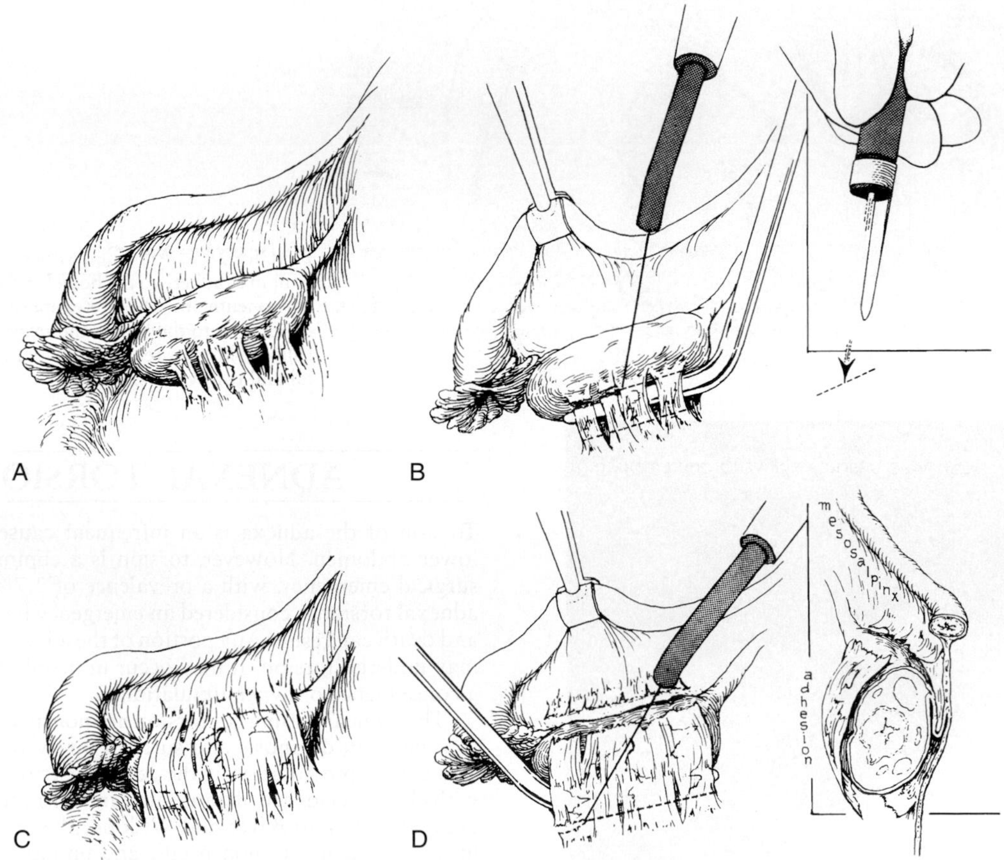

FIGURE 28.5. Ovarian adhesions. **A:** Filmy adhesions between the medial aspect of the ovary and the pelvic sidewall. **B:** These may be removed with laser or fine electrocautery with use of a quartz or glass rod, respectively, as a backstop. **C:** The ovary may be enveloped by adhesions. **D:** Care should be taken to tent up the adhesions so that the peritoneum is not damaged or incised.

excision of the involved ovarian pathology has been accomplished, the main objectives of ovarian reconstruction are atraumatic closure of the stroma and cortex and prevention of adhesion formation. The principles for accomplishing this goal include gentle tissue handling, hemostasis, the use of fine (and ideally minimally reactive) suture material, and an effort to "bury knots" for the prevention of adhesions.

The restoration of normal-appearing anatomy is the most logical approach for creating maximal ovarian surface, which facilitates ovum pickup by the fallopian tube. Controversy continues as to whether it is more appropriate to completely excise or lyse paraovarian and peritubal adhesions.

The most important aspect of ovarian reconstruction is reapproximation of the cortex with the use of atraumatic techniques, including fine absorbable suture material. On completion of the procedure, intraabdominal lavage should be used, ideally with a physiologic substance such as lactated Ringer solution. Every effort should be made to remove all blood from the peritoneal cavity, preferably with the patient taken out of the Trendelenburg position.

The approach to resection of an ovarian cyst should be planned so as to minimize adhesion formation. The incidence of *de novo* adhesion formation appears to be decreased when the initial approach is through laparoscopy. The Operative Laparoscopy Study Group assessed the issue of frequency and severity of adhesion reformation and of *de novo* adhesions after operative laparoscopy. In a multicenter collaborative approach that included early second-look intervention, 68 patients underwent operative laparoscopic procedures, including adhesiolysis as well as ovarian cystectomy. The scoring of adhesions noted during the second-look laparoscopy occurred at nine sites (each ovary, each fallopian tube, omentum, cul-de-sac, pelvic sidewall, and large and small bowel). The study concluded that adhesion reformation is a frequent occurrence and that *de novo* adhesion formation occurred less frequently after initial operative laparoscopy.

A number of agents have been advocated for preventing adhesions, including oxidized regenerated cellulose [Interceed (TC7), Johnson & Johnson Medical, Arlington, TX], which is an absorbable barrier that promotes reepithelialization of the affected area. Pagidas and Tulandi compared Interceed with Ringer lactate solution for adhesion prevention. Ringer lactate solution was as effective as Interceed in decreasing adhesion formation. Haney and colleagues compared oxidized regenerated cellulose with expanded polytetrafluoroethylene (Gore-Tex surgical membrane). The results indicated that expanded polytetrafluoroethylene was associated with fewer postsurgical adhesions. Other agents include sodium hyaluronate carboxymethyl cellulose (Seprafilm).

Functional Ovarian Cysts

Physiologic cyst enlargement of the ovary may occur as a sequela of failure of either follicular rupture or corpus luteum regression. The latter is termed Halban syndrome. The former has been associated with luteinized unruptured follicle syndrome, in which "intraovarian ovulation" is thought to occur; this is a diagnosis usually established with ultrasound. In general, functional ovarian cysts regress spontaneously; however, they may persist and become symptomatic, reaching dimensions as large as 10 cm in diameter. The obvious and most feasible approach is observation, because most such cysts are self-limited. The cyst, however, may prove to be a source of continued pelvic pain or may adhere to the posterior broad ligament, producing persistent symptoms. The potential for adnexal torsion always exists with an ovarian cyst.

RESECTION OF BENIGN CYSTS

Surgical intervention often is initiated with a laparoscopic approach, which permits completion of fenestration of the nonneoplastic ovarian cyst. The cyst lining is stripped from the remaining "normal ovary," and ovarian reconstruction takes place. In several series of laparoscopic management of ovarian cysts, a simple follicular or luteal cyst was identified in most patients evaluated for pelvic pain. In a series by Kleppinger, 31 of 64 ovarian cysts were noted to fall into this category.

Surgical Techniques

Laparotomy

An elliptic incision is made through the thin ovarian cortex of a benign cyst (Fig. 28.6). The end of the knife handle is then inserted and a plane developed over the cyst wall. Alternatively, fine-needle electrocautery can be used to develop a plane, and microsurgical scissors can be used to separate the cyst wall from the ovarian cortex. Low-power magnification (i.e., surgical loupes) often assists the surgeon in identifying the correct plane between the cyst wall and the ovarian parenchyma. After the cyst wall has been completely separated from its adherent attachments to the thin ovarian cortex, it can be shelled out without rupture. However, even with the gentlest technique, rupture can occur because of the friability of the cyst wall. Before the cyst is shelled out, it is important to pack the cul-de-sac with moist, lint-free pads so that, if rupture does occur, spillage does not contaminate the pelvic cavity. After the cyst has been removed, the dead space can be obliterated with a pursestring suture of fine gauge 7–0 nonreactive material. Alternatively, 5–0 nonreactive vertical mattress sutures or figure-of-eight, or both, can be placed to approximate the lateral walls of the ovary. The ovarian surface is then neatly reapproximated with a subcortical running suture of 7–0 fine-gauge nonreactive material (Fig. 28.6D). If the cortex is quite friable, it may be necessary to place interrupted 7–0 sutures to achieve adequate approximation. Some authors advocate leaving the ovary open after cystectomy. To date, there have been no controlled trials evaluating postoperative adhesion formation when the incised ovarian surface is or is not reapproximated.

In some instances, there is excessive redundant thin cortex, which may present a special problem in ovarian reconstruction. The amount of cortex removed depends on the position of the cyst as well as its overall size. Careful assessment of the ovary is necessary before the initial incision is made. The incision in the ovarian cortex facilitates symmetric reconstruction. The redundant cortex can be removed and the dead space obliterated with an internal closure, with care taken that suture material does not penetrate the ovarian cortex. This prevents ischemia and adhesion formation. The infolding technique recommended by Kistner and Patton may result in anatomic distortion and puckering of the ovarian cortex. The "baseball" closure allows careful approximation of cortical edges when redundancy is noted (Fig. 28.7).

Concern over ovarian surgery via laparotomy has been reported. In an older reference of 36 young women operated on for an ovarian cyst, 45% were noted subsequently to be infertile. The author, Van der Watt, conveyed the importance of not interfering with functional cysts in "normal ovaries,"

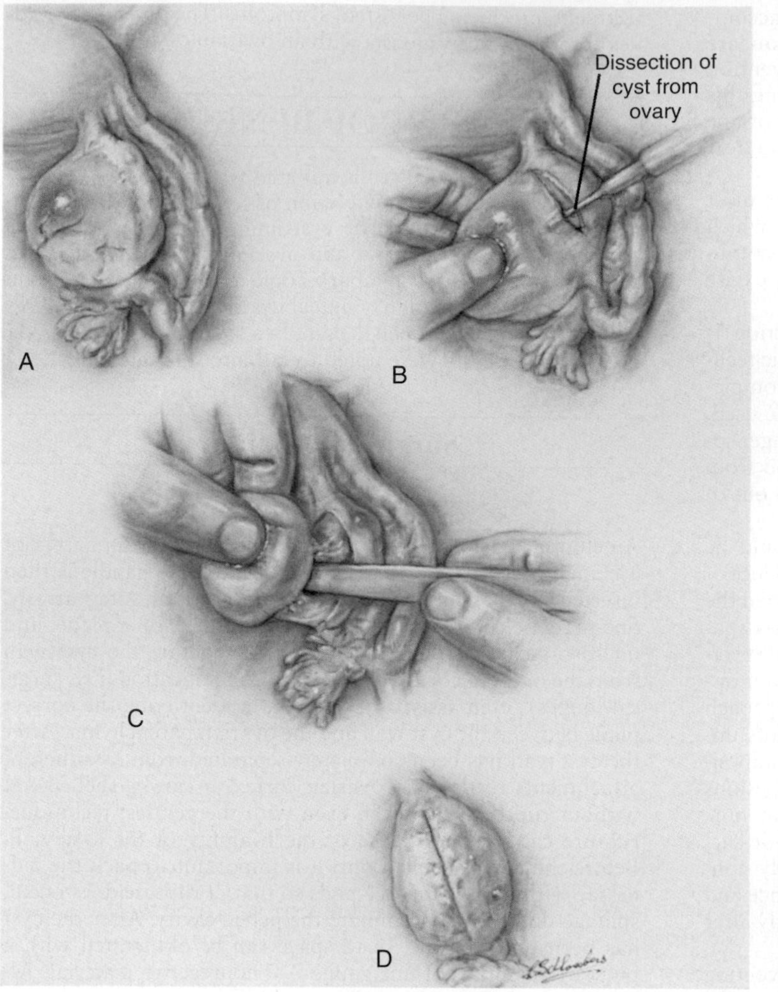

FIGURE 28.6. Resection of benign cyst. **A:** Thin-walled ovarian cyst. **B:** An incision is made through the cortex. **C:** A plane is developed by the use of blunt dissection. The inner ovarian stroma may be approximated with a pursestring suture of 5–0 nonreactive material. **D:** The ovarian cortex is approximated with 7–0 nonreactive suture material.

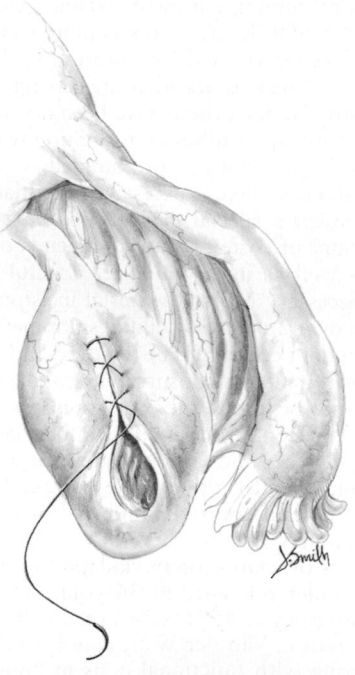

FIGURE 28.7. Closure of the ovary with a baseball stitch.

because resulting adhesion formation could compromise fertility. It was advocated that benign ovarian cysts should not be removed at the time of surgery for other indications unless they are sufficiently large to interfere with tubal function or cause discomfort to the patient.

Minimally Invasive Surgery

Specific skill levels reflecting both the degree of operator expertise and appropriate instrumentation provide clinicians with four levels of training. Level I stands for equipment needs and potential surgical procedures for basic operative laparoscopy, including such entities as diagnostic laparoscopy, tubal sterilization, lysis of filmy adhesions, and biopsy. Level II reflects the clinician's ability to perform linear salpingostomy for ectopic pregnancy, salpingectomy, lysis of vascular adhesions, and elimination of endometriotic implants. Level III includes the ability to perform salpingo-oophorectomy, lysis of extensive adhesions (including bowel adhesions), ovarian cystectomy, appendectomy, myomectomy, laparoscopic-assisted hysterectomy, and neosalpingostomy, as well as the ability to treat tuboovarian abscess and uterine suspension. Level IV includes bowel resection, anastomosis, pelvic lymphadenectomy, presacral neurectomy, tubal reanastomosis, and excision of deep, infiltrating vaginal, paravaginal, and rectal endometriosis.

A number of principles should be followed as surgeons proceed with the correction of pelvic abnormalities that are amenable to a laparoscopic approach. The first is to restore normal anatomy. Once the ovary is stabilized, ideally with an atraumatic forceps, an appropriately planned ovarian incision can be made to correct the pathology encountered. Every effort should be made not to spill the contents.

Large amounts of irrigation solution should be used. In some instances, the cyst wall can be stripped (Fig. 28.8), electrocoagulated, or vaporized. The ovarian incision can then be either left open to heal by primary intention or reapproximated with sutures with either extracorporal or intracorporal suture-tying techniques. When this procedure is completed, the pelvis is irrigated with large amounts of irrigation solution (Ringer lactate), and the patient is taken out of the Trendelenburg position to facilitate removal of any blood products that remain in the peritoneal cavity.

One alternative to suturing is to reapproximate incised segments of ovarian cortex with the use of bipolar coagulation to provide coaptation of the incised segment of the ovary. There is continued debate regarding the use of adhesion prevention materials.

A number of potential pitfalls continue to be of concern in the laparoscopic approach to ovarian lesions. These have been addressed by Seltzer and colleagues and include the following:

- The potential for disruption of an ovarian malignancy
- Whether observation-recommended surgical intervention would be the most feasible alternative
- Potential for increased duration of the surgical procedure if done endoscopically
- Total cost
- Potential for incomplete resection of an ovarian lesion laparoscopically

One can view laparoscopic approach to the adnexal mass based on age. Specifically, in the pediatric patient, problems such as torsion, hemorrhagic cysts, benign neoplasm (e.g., teratoma), as well as oophorectomy have been reportedly addressed via the laparoscope. One advantage over laparotomy is the ability to better visualize the entire lower abdomen and pelvis, including the opposite ovary. In the adult, depending on the clinical circumstance, cyst aspiration, cystectomy, or oophorectomy can be accomplished laparoscopically.

Predictors of clinical outcomes in the laparoscopic management of adnexal mass has been addressed by Havrilesky and coauthors. The authors noted that adnexal mass thought to be benign preoperatively were successfully managed laparoscopically in three fourths of the patients. Adverse events were attributable to concurrent hysterectomy rather than removal of the adnexal mass. Malignancy occurred in 2%, and laparoscopic management was not associated with adverse outcomes.

Concern is expressed for an ovarian neoplasm subsequently noted to be malignant. In a countrywide survey in Austria, Wenzl and colleagues reported on 54,198 laparoscopies; 16,601 were performed for adnexal masses, and 108 cases of ovarian tumors were subsequently found to be malignant. Of the 108 cases, 20 were managed laparoscopically, 22 by immediate laparotomy, and the rest by delayed laparotomy (3 to 1,415 days). The authors concluded that laparoscopic surgery with the finding of an ovarian malignancy is rare: 0.65% of all endoscopic surgical procedures. If a malignancy is identified, laparotomy is recommended for optimal staging and treatment.

The extent of damage to ovarian reserve associated with laparoscopic excision of endometriomas was studied by Ragni and coauthors. A reduced number of dominate follicles, oocytes, embryos, and high-quality embryos was observed in the operated gonad. Fertilization rate and rate of good-quality

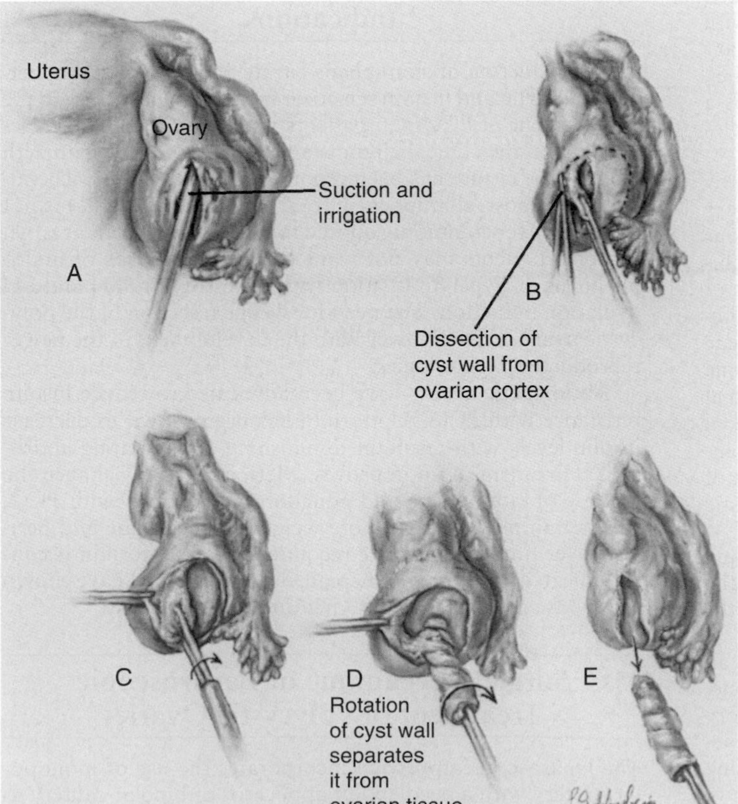

FIGURE 28.8. Removal of a small ovarian endometrial cyst through the laparoscope. **A:** After incision of the ovarian cortex, the contents of the endometrioma are removed with suction and irrigation. **B:** The plane between the ovary and the cyst wall is developed by using traction and twisting the forceps clockwise. **C:** The endometrial cyst wall is grasped with forceps. **D:** The cyst wall separates from the ovarian tissue by use of a twisting motion. The ovarian defect may be left open to heal by secondary intention or may be closed with vertical mattress sutures. **E:** The cyst wall is removed.

embryos were similar in operated and control groups. Laparoscopic excision of endometriomas is associated with a quantitative but not a qualitative damage to ovarian reserve.

OVARIAN SURGERY FOR POLYCYSTIC OVARIAN DISEASE

Signs and symptoms of polycystic ovarian (PCO) syndrome begin at puberty. PCO is a sign, not a diagnosis. In a consensus meeting held in Rotterdam, the American Society for Reproductive Medicine and the European Society for Human Reproduction and Embryology agreed that two of the following criteria must be met once other endocrinopathies have been ruled out (i.e., Cushing, adrenal hyperplasia):

- Oligoamenorrhea
- Clinical and or biochemical evidence for hyperandrogenemia
- Polycystic-appearing ovaries on ultrasound

The polycystic ovary may result from a virilizing ovarian or adrenal neoplasm or from congenital adrenal hyperplasia, or it may result from suboptimal hypothalamic-pituitary function at puberty. The exact mechanism for the development of ovulatory failure has been attributed to androgen overproduction and its effect on the hypothalamic-pituitary ovarian axis.

Stein and Leventhal, during the period 1902 to 1935, noted that a group of women had evidence for what is currently called polycystic ovaries at the time of laparotomy. Specifically, in 1935, Stein and Leventhal reported seven patients with the hallmarks of PCO.

The histologic findings in a polycystic ovary cover a broad spectrum, ranging from the originally described typical "Stein-Leventhal" type of polycystic ovary with a large number of follicular cysts and few atretic cysts in which there is marked stromal hyperplasia and hyperthecosis, to a smaller ovary with a few follicular cysts and atretic follicles. The polycystic ovary may exhibit microscopic islands of luteinized thecal cells, i.e., hyperthecosis, scattered in the stroma, but usually there is a thickened, fibrosed tunica with a large number of cystic follicles beneath this thickened capsule.

There are several hypotheses regarding the mechanism by which ovarian drilling (wedge resection) of the polycystic ovary resolves ovulatory failure. The theory stating that the fibrous capsule acts as a mechanical barrier to the ovulatory follicle has been refuted. Evidence against this theory consists of the observation that if one ovary is removed, ovulation occurs from the other ovary. In addition, the use of clomiphene citrate results in ovulation through an intact capsule. Some have stated that neonatal androgens may cause an abnormal hypothalamic-pituitary axis, resulting in abnormal gonadal patterns. This theory is not widely accepted. Neonatal androgen treatment in rats is associated with masculinization of the hypothalamus and with ovulatory failure with polycystic ovaries.

The most popular theory explaining how ovarian drilling results in the resumption of ovulatory cycles notes that the removal of androgen-secreting stroma and theca reduces the amount of abnormal steroid production in the ovary. After wedge resection, there is usually a decrease in the mean level of 17*a*-hydroxyprogesterone, dehydroepiandrosterone, androstenedione, and testosterone, as well as a transitory decrease in estradiol. This reduction in the steroidogenesis of androgens, allowing normalization of the luteinizing hormone (LH): follicle stimulating hormone (LH:FSH) ratio, results in the resumption of ovulatory cycles. Ovarian renin-angiotensin activity is enhanced with PCO. This system—renin-angiotensin—remains unaltered following ovarian electrocautery (i.e., ovarian drilling), even though serum levels of LH, testosterone, and androstenedione decline.

Sex hormone–binding globulin (SHBG) concentrations following electrocautery with PCO have been evaluated. Whereas there were significant decreases in serum androgens and gonadotropins, the concentration of SHBG increased in the serum. Gjonnaess has reported that there is no change with respect to dehydroepiandrosterone sulfate (DHEAS) with ovarian drilling. This is indicative of neural alteration in the pituitary-adrenal axis in comparison to the pituitary-ovarian axis.

A more recent consensus (2007) regarding PCOS focused on treatment. The results noted better pregnancy rates with use of clomiphene citrate or clomiphene citrate plus the insulin sensitizer metformin in comparison to metformin alone. They also felt that there is a role for ovarian drilling.

There is some debate as to the amount of ovarian mass that should be removed at the time of wedge resection. Halbe and coworkers attempted to clarify this question by removing different amounts of ovarian cortex and medulla from a random selection of patients with polycystic ovarian disease. Thirty-eight of 62 patients were interested in conception. The 38 patients were divided into three groups, the first of which underwent removal of not more than one fifth of the original ovarian size. The second group had one third of the ovarian mass removed, and the third group had one half to three fourths of the original ovarian size reduced. The resumption of ovulatory cycles was recorded at 53%, 71%, and 91%, respectively. The authors concluded that the best ovulatory rate and the best pregnancy rate resulted after removal of at least half of the ovarian medulla.

Indications

The introduction of clomiphene citrate and the oral antihyperglycemic drug and insulin sensitizer metformin has changed the management of PCOD in patients who desire pregnancy. Depending on the clinical circumstance, the conception rate with clomiphene citrate has been reported at 50% to 60%. The incidence of post–clomiphene citrate birth defects (3.1%) is not increased over commonly quoted rates for populations at large.

Some patients may not want to accept the risks of multiple births or hyperstimulation with pure FSH or FSH and LH ovulation induction. The need for wedge resection of the polycystic ovary is much lower with the development of the newer reproductive technologies.

Antidiabetic agents have been advocated to reduce insulin resistance with PCO. Metformin has been shown to decrease insulin levels with resultant diminishing of circulating androgens. Hirsutism often improves. Metformin may enhance the efficacy of clomiphene and gonadotropin therapy with PCO. Metformin may also promote weight loss. Baseline and periodic liver function tests are recommended. Metformin is contraindicated with renal or hepatic disease. Patients have shown a response at dosages of 500 mg three times per day.

Surgical Technique of Laparoscopic Treatment of Polycystic Ovaries

The laparoscopic approach incorporates the use of monopolar cautery with a needlepoint applicator or bipolar cautery to drill holes several millimeters apart through the ovarian cortex (Fig. 28.9). Care should be exercised to avoid the hilum because bleeding could result if it is penetrated. It is important to achieve hemostasis over the drilled areas.

The ovarian drilling technique includes a 5-mm second puncture placed suprapubically, through which suction irrigation or grasping of tissues can be performed. All visible subcapsular follicles are vaporized, and a 2- to 4-mm–diameter crater is made randomly in the ovarian stroma. Hemostasis is accomplished with bipolar forceps.

Ovarian coagulation can be accomplished with unipolar punch biopsy forceps or a needle electrode. The power setting is 20 to 30 W in a cutting mode. The cortex is usually penetrated at 10 to 15 sites for a depth of 3 to 5 mm. Caution is exercised to minimize thermal damage. Smaller ovaries may require fewer cauterization sites.

There are no randomized controlled studies addressing the efficacy of the laparoscopic approach to ovarian drilling. Twenty-seven studies were evaluated by Donesky and Adashi and involved a total of 729 patients. The ovulation rate was 84.2%, and the pregnancy rate was 55.7%. These authors emphasized that well-designed studies are needed in this area, which would encompass the PCO population proposed for laparoscopic drilling. This cohort of patients would require a well-documented clinical and biochemical finding of PCO, documented long-standing infertility (2 years or more), evidence for failure of clomiphene citrate, absence of correction of other infertility factors, randomization into a treatment group, and standardized documented follow-up, with particular attention to postovulatory patterns.

Complications

The major concern is that of adhesion formation after either wedge resection or laparoscopic drilling. Toaff and associates noted extensive peritubular and periovarian adhesions in a small series (seven) of patients who did not conceive after bilateral wedge resection. One other concern is that of bilateral ovarian atrophy as a reflection of aggressive ovarian resection. This is a rare complication of the procedure. Thus, iatrogenic consequences of the surgical approaches must be discussed with the patient preoperatively. There is continued controversy as to whether a bilateral wedge resection approach results in suboptimal pregnancy rates because of postoperative adhesion formation. The principles of microsurgery must be reemphasized (e.g., gentle tissue handling, precise hemostasis, keeping tissues moist).

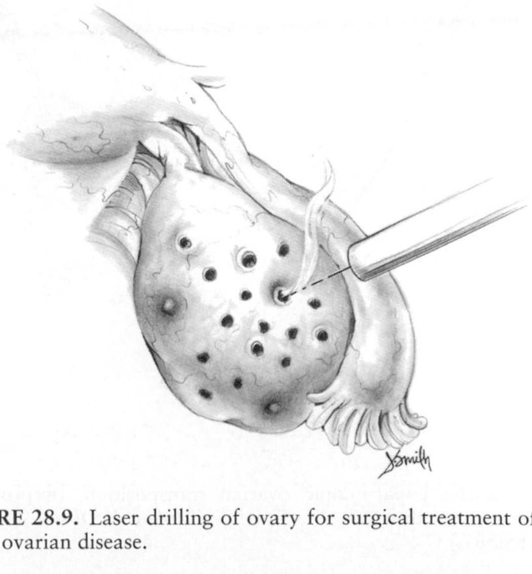

FIGURE 28.9. Laser drilling of ovary for surgical treatment of polycystic ovarian disease.

PARADOXICAL OOPHORECTOMY

Paradoxical oophorectomy is the removal of severely pathologic adnexa to improve fertility in patients with strictly unilateral tubal disease. Consideration of removal of the contralateral ovary when there is single tubal patency (i.e., paradoxical oophorectomy) has perhaps taken on a new perspective with the advent of assisted reproductive technology (ART). From a historical point of view, it has been advocated that a patient with one functional tube would benefit from paradoxical oophorectomy, thus ensuring that ovulation would occur repeatedly on the appropriate side. Scott and coworkers reported a series of 24 patients with unilateral tubal patency diagnosed by retrograde injection at laparotomy. Contralateral oophorectomy or salpingo-oophorectomy was performed on all patients, and 16 women subsequently had 21 pregnancies, for a pregnancy rate of 67%. The authors suggested that the frequency with which transperitoneal migration occurs may be a factor. Hallet noted that one in five tubal ectopic pregnancies has a corpus luteum. On the contralateral side, Jansen noted an intrauterine pregnancy rate of 18.7% ($n = 91$), contrasted with bilateral salpingostomy for hydrosalpinges in the presence of only one ovary wherein the pregnancy rate was 43.8% ($n = 16$). With unilateral salpingostomy or bilateral division of adhesions, pregnancy rates were comparable to those after bilateral salpingolysis. The mean surgery-pregnancy interval was longer after unilateral salpingostomy (104 weeks) than after bilateral salpingolysis (45 weeks). The author suggested that salpingo-oophorectomy may be preferable to salpingoneostomy for unilateral hydrosalpinx.

Perhaps the major concern is for the patient who presents with tubal ectopic gestation in which the opposite (i.e., normal-appearing) adnexa appears to be unaffected. The paradoxical salpingo-oophorectomy approach has been advocated with this circumstance by Scott and coworkers. It has been advocated to wait at least 2 years after diagnostic laparoscopy reveals extensive unilateral disease before proceeding with paradoxical oophorectomy.

Randomized, carefully controlled clinical trials are necessary to further evaluate the efficacy of paradoxical oophorectomy. The risks and benefits must be carefully considered both preoperatively and intraoperatively, especially if the patient is a candidate for ART. There is clear evidence that increased numbers of ova can be recovered when both ovaries are *in situ*. Increased pregnancy success after superovulation is a reflection of the number of ovaries (one versus two)—the total number of follicles available for stimulation.

Laparoscopic Oophorectomy

The general principles of laparoscopic oophorectomy include placing the patient in the Trendelenburg position, with appropriate planning of ports for the proposed procedure, and planning for removal of the affected adnexa. Pelvic washings and the use of frozen section may be germane to the task at hand. After restoration of normal anatomy and adhesiolysis as indicated, the adnexa are gently placed on stretch. They are approached from either the infundibulopelvic ligament or the insertion of the round ligament. Regardless of the approach chosen, identification of the ureter is of paramount importance. The infundibulopelvic ligament is identified and coagulated. The broad ligament is incised, beginning at the round ligament, and further dissection is performed with an irrigation dissection probe into the retroperitoneal space. Every effort must be made to completely remove all ovarian tissue to prevent ovarian remnant syndrome.

Tissue Removal

Once the adnexa have been completely freed, if benign disease is extremely likely, desiccation of the tissue and thus segmental removal is appropriate. However, if there is concern for the pathology, use of an endoscopic pouch is appropriate. In this circumstance, every effort is made to remove the ovary intact. Careful inspection of the operative site and a check for any bleeding are recommended. In addition, the end-point pressure of CO_2 insufflation should be reduced with suctioning of some of the CO_2 to check for any tamponade effect. As with all laparoscopic procedures, the patient should be monitored carefully after surgery for any signs of intraperitoneal bleeding.

FERTILITY PRESERVATION WITH CANCER

As response to both medical and surgical therapies continue to result in increasing numbers of survivors, gynecologic surgeons must be kept abreast of current thinking in this field. Cryopreservation of ovarian-tissue, nonfertilized, immature germ cells is receiving increased attention including in prepubertal girls. Medical agents, including letrozole and tamoxifen, have been used as ovarian stimulants for cryopreservation in women with breast cancer. Tamoxifen resulted in two to five times higher embryo yield than natural cycle *in vitro* fertilization (IVF). The best prognosis for fertility appears to preserve gametes before initiation of chemotherapy for cancer. Ovarian transplantation with subsequent embryo generation has been reported after restoration of ovarian function by heterotopic transplantation. Ovarian transplantation remains an experimental technique at this point in time. Ovarian cortical tissue strip retrieval is amenable to a laparoscopic approach. Autologous, orthotopic transplantation after cryopreservation has been successfully used to restore fertility. Ovarian tissue banking and autografting of ovarian cortex are promising therapies for patients with ovarian failure. Kim and coauthors have verified the correlation between ischemic tissue damage and the duration of ischemia. The authors noted the ovarian cortex could tolerate ischemia for at least 3 hours. Thus, it appears that the future of ovarian transplantation depends on the postgrafting ischemia time by effective revascularization techniques.

OVARIAN TRANSPOSITION BEFORE RADIOTHERAPY

Lemevel and coworkers reported laparoscopic transposition in a patient being treated for Hodgkin disease before receiving radiotherapy. The ovaries were laparoscopically suspended out of the field of radiation. Iatrogenic menopause did not occur in the four patients for which this was reported. Other authors have reported similar recommendations. Bisharah and Tulandi have recommended transection of the ovarian ligament and transposition of the ovaries without affecting the fallopian tubes. This is associated with positioning of the ovaries laterally and anteriorly at the level of the anterosuperior iliac spines (Fig. 28.10).

Gonads are sensitive to irradiation. Whole-body, abdominal, or pelvic irradiation can cause ovarian damage and adversely affect uterine function. It is estimated that the sensitivity of oocytes to radiation is an LD50 of 2 Gy (the lethal dose required to eliminate 50% of the oocytes).

Cytotoxic drugs are classified as follows:

High risk: Cyclophosphamide, ifosfamide, chlormethine, busulfan, melphalan, procarbazine, and chlorambucil

Moderate risk: Cisplatin, carboplatin, and doxorubicin

Low risk: Vincristine, methotrexate, Dactinomycin, bleomycin, mercaptopurine, and vinblastine

Attempts have been made to assess ovarian function and "ovarian reserve." This has included evaluation of ovarian volume; serum inhibin B, secreted by antral developing follicles; and antimüllerian hormone, a glycoprotein expressed in fetal tissue and preantral and small antral follicles, but in the adult, when levels are lowered (i.e., in cancer survivors), the ovarian reserve is decreased.

One alternative to oophoropexy is ooctye retrieval, fertilization, and cryopreservation—i.e,. ART/IVF. Preserving unfertilized oocytes remains an area of research as prognosis for fertility overall is poor.

Fertility outcome following ovarian transposition and pelvic irradiation for pelvic cancer has been addressed in a total of 37 consecutive cases by Morice and colleagues. Patients were treated for clear cell adenocarcinoma of the vagina or cervix, ovarian dysgerminoma, and sarcoma. The pregnancy rate was 15% (4/27) in patients attempting pregnancy with clear cell

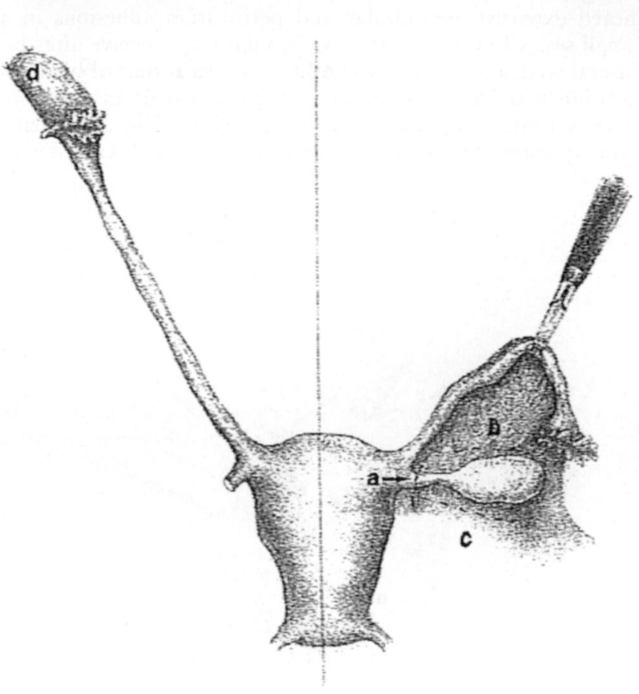

FIGURE 28.10. Laparoscopic ovarian transposition. (Reproduced with permission Bisharah M, Tulandi T, *Am J Obstet Gynecol* 2003;188:367.)

adenocarcinoma of the vagina or cervix. In the dysgerminoma and sarcoma group, 80% pregnancy occurred (8/10). Thus, the prognosis for future fertility following ovarian transposition and irradiation should be considered for discussion in selected patients before radiotherapy. The subject of fertility preservation in cancer survivors has been addressed by the Ethics Committee of the American Society for Reproductive Medicine, the main focus of which is that physicians should inform cancer survivors of their alternatives and include them in pretherapy discussion of alternatives before initiation of treatment.

OVARIAN CYSTS IN NEONATE AND PREPUBERTAL CHILD

In a retrospective study of 65 fetal ovarian cysts noted by ultrasound, 57% were located on the left, 36% were on the right, and 7% were bilateral. In 17 patients, intervention was required after delivery because of persistence and/or enlargement. The histologic results included follicular cysts in 12 cases, a lymphangioma, and one teratoma; the remaining were amenable to aspiration. The authors, Mittermayer and colleagues, conclude that lack of regression requires intervention in the neonatal period. Ovarian cysts in the neonate >5 cm in diameter have an increased chance of torsion.

Ovarian surgery in the premenarchal girl has been evaluated in a study from the University of Michigan in 52 patients, 50% of whom were less than 1 year and 31% between 1 and 8 years old. The most common presentation was abdominal/pelvic mass ($n = 24$), and the postoperative diagnoses included torsion in 18 and malignancy in 5 patients. Histopathologic evaluation included hemorrhagic infarction, dysgenetic gonads, simple cysts, teratoma, theca lutein cyst, fibroma, neuroblastoma, germ cell tumor, gonadoblastoma, and metastatic Wilms tumor.

LAPAROSCOPIC OVARIAN SURGERY IN THE PEDIATRIC OR ADOLESCENT PATIENT

A number of gynecologic problems from the neonatal period through adolescence can be addressed laparoscopically. Entities such as ovarian torsion, acute PID (diagnosis and treatment complementing antimicrobial therapy), torsion, and benign neoplasms must be considered in this age group. In addition, gonadectomy for problems such as male pseudohermaphroditism is amenable to the laparoscopic approach.

Follicular cysts appear to be of particular concern in both the pediatric and adolescent patient because they present with abdominal pain. An abdominal or pelvic mass can be identified on physical examination. The clinician must always keep in mind the importance of appropriate preoperative assessment (with the use of ultrasound and other clinical parameters) in deciding which patients are candidates for operative intervention. Depending on the clinical circumstance, a conservative approach in this age group is advocated; appropriate concern must be given (especially in the pediatric patient) to the potential for malignancy with ovarian masses, particularly if a solid component is identified.

The literature attests to operative intervention of ovarian cysts that appear to be nonfunctional. One of these was reported in a 1.5-month-old infant in whom ultrasound showed evidence of an ovarian mass. At laparotomy, the mass proved to be consistent with right ovarian torsion and necrosis, and it required adnexectomy. In one other reported case, a follicular-appearing cyst seen on ultrasound was associated with rapidly progressive virilization and a markedly elevated plasma testosterone level (289 ng/dL); histologic evaluation identified a granulosa cell tumor with mild luteinization.

The feasibility of aspirating an ovarian cyst continues to be controversial. In two case reports, laparoscopic puncture and aspiration of a malignant ovarian cyst was performed. Preoperative ultrasound indicated that the involved adnexal mass had a benign nature. Cytologically negative fluid was obtained from the aspirate. Eight weeks after operation, extensive disseminated ovarian carcinoma was noted at laparotomy.

Endoscopic surgery continues to broaden its horizon with expansion into laparoscopic surgical care beginning with the neonate. The use of 2-mm laparoscopes with the addition of 2- to 3-mm instrumentation has facilitated the diagnostic and therapeutic aspects of laparoscopy in this age group. Miniaturized video camera systems are necessary when one uses the 2-mm laparoscope telescope. When a decision is made to proceed with laparoscopy in a neonate or infant, general endotracheal anesthesia is used. Ideally, prophylactic antibiotics are administered preoperatively. The stomach is emptied with a suction catheter when the patient is asleep, and the bladder is emptied by use of the Crede maneuver. The abdominal wall is thinner and more elastic in the child than in the adolescent or adult. One must take this into consideration when introducing instrumentation, because it may be easier to insufflate in the subcutaneous space of the child than in the subcutaneous space of an adult. A Veress needle can be used with insufflation of carbon dioxide at 0.5 L/min. In infants, the end point of peritoneal distending pressure should be set at 6 to 8 mm Hg; in the pediatric patient, 8 to 10 mm Hg; in the older child or adolescent, 10 to 12 mm Hg.

After surgery, the trocar sites can be sutured in children, whereas in neonates and infants, the use of Steri-Strips (3M, St. Paul, MN) or other wound-closure bandages is usually adequate for reapproximation of the incised skin edges. Waldschmidt and Schier reported a series of 136 laparoscopic surgical procedures in neonates and infants. The most frequent indications were lysis of adhesions, abdominal cysts and neoplasms, gonadectomy, appendectomy, and cholecystectomy. A 1,400-g preterm infant was the only one in the series who suffered a complication (hernia at the incision site). Thus, adnexal pathology in this age group appears to be amenable to a laparoscopic approach.

Procedures such as transposition of an ovary before radiotherapy, bilateral gonadal excision in a male pseudohermaphrodite (i.e., Y-bearing chromosomal analysis), adnexal torsion, suspected salpingitis, and endometriosis all have been identified in this age group. The authors concluded that because the morbidity is low and recovery is likely, the laparoscopic approach should be considered.

Although certain procedures in the child do not differ significantly from those in the adult, the early diagnosis of ovarian pathology (e.g., adnexal torsion) can result in a significant advantage in terms of managing the patient and preserving ovarian tissue.

BEST SURGICAL PRACTICES

- Minimally invasive surgery can be used to evaluate and manage ovarian masses ≥6 cm and adnexal masses ≥10 cm.

- Before operative intervention in a pregnant patient with a symptomatic adnexal mass, complete assessment of the fetus—including ultrasound to rule out any fetal anomalies—is recommended. The optimal time for elective intervention is during the second trimester. The patient should be informed regarding preterm labor and delivery. The surgical procedure ideally is performed in the left lateral decubitus position.
- Transvaginal color Doppler sonographic assessment of ovarian malignant masses includes number of vessels detected, location of tumor vessels (central vs. peripheral), determination of peak systolic velocity, low-resistance index, mean-resistance index, and lower-pulsatility index.
- The major goal of the evaluation of a pelvic mass is to rule out malignancy. All ovarian neoplasms >6 cm with a solid component should undergo a thorough evaluation to try to rule out cancer.
- In management of ovarian remnant syndrome, treatment of choice is adequate excision of the remnant ovarian tissue and contiguous adherent tissues, i.e., pelvic peritoneum, bowel serosa, and underlying involved alveolar and/or vascular tissues. Retroperitoneal dissection may be required.

Bibliography

Abbott D, Dumesic D, Franks S. Developmental origin of polycystic ovary syndrome—a hypothesis. *J Endocrinol* 2002;174:1.

Adashi EY, Rock JA, Guzick D, et al. Fertility following bilateral ovarian wedge resection: a critical analysis of 90 consecutive cases of the polycystic ovary syndrome. *Fertil Steril* 1981;35:320.

Adhesion Barrier Study Group. Interceed (TC-7). Prevention of post surgical adhesions by Interceed (TC-7). *Fertil Steril* 1989;51:933.

Alborzi S, Momtahan M, Parsanezhad ME, et al. A prospective, randomized study comparing laparoscopic ovarian cystectomy versus fenestration and coagulation in patients with endometriomas. *Fertil Steril* 2004;82(6):1633.

Alcazar J, Ruiz-Perez M, Errasti T. Transvaginal color-Doppler sonography in adnexal masses: Which parameter performs best?. *Ultrasound Obstet Gynecol* 1996;8:114.

American Society for Reproductive Medicine. Fertility preservation and reproduction in cancer patients. *Fertil Steril* 2005;83(6):1622.

Andolf E, Jorgensen C, Astedt B. Ultrasound examination for detection of ovarian carcinoma in risk groups. *Obstet Gynecol* 1990;75:106.

Anttila L, Tenttila T, Matinlauri I, et al. Serum total renin levels after ovarian electrocautery in women with polycystic ovary syndrome. *Gynecol Endocrinol* 1998;12:327.

Babaknia A, Calfopoulos P, Jones HW Jr. The Stein-Leventhal syndrome and coincidental ovarian tumors. *Obstet Gynecol* 1976;47:223.

Bayer AI, Wiskind AK. Adnexal torsion: Can the adnexa be saved?. *Am J Obstet Gynecol* 1994;171:1506.

Bernhard LM, Klebba PK, Gray DL, et al. Predictors of persistence of adnexal masses in pregnancy. *Obstet Gynecol* 1999;93:585.

Bisharah M, Tulandi T. Laparoscopic preservation of ovarian function: an underused procedure. *Am J Obstet Gynecol* 2003;188:367.

Carey M, Slack M. GnRH analogue in assessing chronic pelvic pain in women with residual ovaries. *BJOG* 1996;103:150.

Caruso A, Caforio L, Testa A, et al. Transvaginal color Doppler ultrasonography in the presurgical characterization of adnexal masses. *Gynecol Oncol* 1996;63:184.

Casper RF, Greenblatt EM. Laparoscopic ovarian cautery for induction of ovulation in women with polycystic ovary disease. *Semin Reprod Endocrinol* 1990;8:209.

Chan L, Lin W, Uerpairojkit B, et al. Evaluation of adnexal masses using three-dimensional ultrasonographic technology: preliminary report. *J Ultrasound Med* 1997;16:349.

Damewood M, Hesla H, Lowen M, et al. Induction of ovulation and pregnancy following lateral oophoropexy for Hodgkin's disease. *Int J Gynecol Obstet* 1990;33:369.

Davidoff AM, Hebra A, Kerr J, et al. Laparoscopic oophorectomy in children. *J Laparoendosc Surg* 1996;6(Suppl 1):SIIS.

Dexel A, Efrat Z, Orvito R, et al. The residual ovary syndrome: a 20 year experience. *Eur J Obstet Gynecol Reprod Biol* 1996;68:159.

Diamond MP, Daniell JF, Feste J, et al. Adhesion reformation and de novo adhesion formation after reproductive pelvic surgery. *Fertil Steril* 1987;47:864.

Dolgin S. Ovarian masses in the newborn. *Semin Pediatr Surg* 2000;9:121.

Donesky BW, Adashi EY. Surgically induced ovulation in the polycystic ovary syndrome: wedge resection revisited in the age of laparoscopy. *Fertil Steril* 1995;63:439.

Ehrman DA. Medical progress: polycystic ovary syndrome. *N Engl J Med* 2005;352:1223.

Einhorn N, Bast RC Jr, Knapp RC, et al. Preoperative evaluation of serum CA 125 levels in patients with primary epithelial ovarian carcinoma. *Obstet Gynecol* 1986;67:414.

Farquhar C, Vandekerckhove P, Lilford R. Laparoscopic drilling by diathermy or laser for ovulation induction in anovulatory polycystic ovary syndrome. *Cochrane Database Syst Rev* 2001;4:1.

Finkler NJ, Benacerraf B, Lavin PT, et al. Comparison of serum CA-125, clinical impression, and ultrasound in the postoperative evaluation of ovarian masses. *Obstet Gynecol* 1988;72:659.

Funt M. The residual adnexa: asset or liability? *Am J Obstet Gynecol* 1977;129:251.

Gillman J. The development of the gonads in man with a consideration of the role of fetal endocrine and the histogenesis of ovarian tumors. *Contrib Embryol* 1948;32:81.

Gjonnaess II. Late endocrine effects of electrocautery in women with polytcystic ovary syndrome. *Fertil Steril* 1998;69:697–701.

Granberg S, Wickland M. A comparison between ultrasound and gynecologic examination for detection of enlarged ovaries in a group of women at risk for ovarian carcinoma. *J Ultrasound Med* 1988;7:59.

Granberg S, Wikland M, Jansson I. Macroscopic characterization of ovarian tumors and the relation to the histologic diagnosis: criteria to be used for ultrasound evaluation. *Gynecol Oncol* 1989;35:139.

Grogan RH. Reappraisal of the residual ovary. *Am J Obstet Gynecol* 1967;97:124.

Gurgan T, Yarali H, Urman B. Laparoscopic treatment of polycystic ovarian disease. *Hum Reprod* 1994;9:573.

Halbe HW, da Fonseca AM, Silva P deP, et al. Stein-Leventhal syndrome. *Am J Obstet Gynecol* 1972;114:280.

Hallet JC. Repeat octopic pregnancy: a study of 123 consecutive cases. *Am J Obstet Gynecol* 1975;122:520.

Haney AF, Doty E. Murine peritoneal injury and de novo adhesion formation caused by oxidized-regenerated cellulose (Interceed [TC7]) but not expanded to polytetrafluoroethylene (Gore-Tex surgical membrane). *Fertil Steril* 1992;57:202.

Haney AF, Hesla J, Hurst BS, et al. Expanded polytetrafluoroethylene (Gore-Tex surgical membrane) is superior to oxidized regenerated cellulose (Interceed TC7) in preventing adhesions. *Fertil Steril* 1995;63:1021.

Havrilesky LJ, Peterson BL, Dryden DK, et al. Predictors of clinical outcomes in the laparoscopic management of adnexal masses. *Obstet Gynecol* 2003;102(2):243.

Heinrich U, Eberlein-Gonska M, Benz G, et al. Late-onset 30-hydroxysteroid dehydrogenase deficiency with virilization induced by a large ovarian cyst. *Horm Res* 1993;40:227.

Heloury Y, Guiberteau V, Sagot P, et al. Laparoscopy in adnexal pathology in the child: a study of 28 cases. *Eur J Pediatr Surg* 1993;3:75.

Hernandez E, Miyazawa K. The pelvic mass: patients' ages and pathologic findings. *J Reprod Med* 1988;33:361.

Jansen RP. Surgery pregnancy time intervals after salpingolysis, unilateral salpingostomy and bilateral salpingostomy. *Fertil Steril* 1980;34:222.

Jawad A, Al-Meshari A. Laparoscopy for ovarian pathology in infancy and childhood. *Pediatr Surg Int* 1998;14:62.

Jeffcoate TA. *Principles of gynecology*. London: Butterworths; 1975.

Jeremias E, Bedaiwy MA, Nelson D, et al. Assessment of tissue injury in cryopreserved ovarian tissue. *Fertil Steril* 2003;79(3):651.

Kamprath S, Possover M, Schneider A. Description of a laparoscopic technique for treating patients with ovarian remnant syndrome. *Fertil Steril* 1997;68:663.

Kim SS, Yang HW, Kang HG, et al. Quantitative assessment of ischemic tissue damage in ovarian cortical tissue with or without antioxidant (ascorbic acid) treatment. *Fertil Steril* 2004;82(3):679.

Kiran G, Kiran H, Coban YK, et al. Fresh autologous transplantation of ovarian cortical strips to the anterior abdominal wall at the Pfannenstiel incision site. *Fertil Steril* 2004;82(4):954.

Kistner RW, Patton GW. Surgery of the ovary. In: *Atlas of infertility surgery.* Boston: Little, Brown; 1975;105:177.

Kleppinger RK. Ovarian cyst fenestration via laparoscopy. *J Reprod Med.* 1978;21:16.

Kobayashi M. Use of diagnostic ultrasound in trophoblastic neoplasms and ovarian tumors. *Cancer* 1976;38:441.

Kojima E. Ovarian wedge resection with contract Nd:YAG laser irradiation used laparoscopically. *J Reprod Med* 1989;34:444.

Kurjak A, Predanic M, Kupesic-Urek S, et al. Transvaginal color and pulsed Doppler assessment of adnexal tumor vascularity. *Gynecol Oncol* 1993;50:3.

Larsen JF, Pedersen OD, Gregersen E. Ovarian cyst fenestration via the laparoscope. *Acta Obstet Gynecol Scand* 1986;65:539.

Laxman D, Burgman A, Sagi J, et al. The postmenopausal adnexal mass: correlation between ultrasonic and pathologic findings. *Obstet Gynecol* 1991;77:726.

Lemevel A, Bourdin S, Harousseau J, et al. Ovarian transposition by laparoscopy before radiotherapy in the treatment of Hodgkin's disease. *Cancer* 1998;83:1420.

Litos M, Furara S, Chin K. Supernumerary ovary: a case report and literature review. *J Obstet Gynaecol* 2003;23:325.

Mage G, Canis M, Mandes II, et al. Laparoscopic management of adnexal torsion: a review of 35 cases. *J Reprod Med* 1989 Aug;34:520–4.

Magtibay PM, Nyholm JL, Hemandez JL, Podratz KC. Ovarian Remnant Syndrome. *Am J Obstet Gynecol* 2005 Dec;193(6):2062–6.

Maiman M, Seltzer V, Boyce J. Laparoscopic excision of ovarian neoplasms subsequently found to be malignant. *Obstet Gynecol* 1991;77:563.

Malkasian G Jr, Knapp R, Lavin PT, et al. Preoperative evaluation of serum CA125 levels in premenopausal and postmenopausal patients with pelvic masses: discrimination of benign from malignant disease. *Am J Obstet Gynecol* 1988;159:341.

Merritt DR. Torsion of the uterine adnexa: a review. *Adolesc Pediatr Gynecol* 1991;4:3.

Minke T, Depond W, Winkelmann T, et al. Ovarian remnant syndrome: study in laboratory rats. *Am J Obstet Gynecol* 1994: 171:1440.

Mittermayer C, Blaicher W, Grassauer D, et al. Fetal ovarian cysts: developmental and neonatal outcome. *Ultraschall Med* 2003;24:21.

Morice P, Thiam-Ba R, Castaige D, et al. Fertility results after ovarian transposition for pelvic malignancies treated by external irradiation or brachytherapy. *Hum Reprod* 1998;13:660.

Oehler M, Wain G, Brand A. Gynaecological malignancies in pregnancy: a review. *Aust N Z Obstet Gynaecol* 2003;43:414.

Oktay K. Fertility preservation: an emerging discipline in the care of young paients with cancer. *Lancet Oncol* 2005;6:192.

Oktay K, Alp Aydin B, Karlikaya G. A technique for laparoscopic transplantation of frozen-banked ovarian tissue. *Fertil Steril* 2001;75(6):1212.

Oktay K, Buyuk E, Rosenwaks Z, et al. A technique for transplantation of ovarian cortical strips to the forearm. *Fertil Steril* 2003;80(1):193.

Operative Laparoscopy Study Group. Postoperative adhesion development after operative laparoscopy: evaluation at early second-look procedures. *Fertil Steril* 1992;55:700.

Pabuccu R, Onalan G, Goktolga U, et al. Aspiration of ovarian endometriomas before intracytoplasmic sperm injection. *Fertil Steril* 2004;82(3):705.

Pagidas K, Tulandi T. Effects of Ringer's lactate, Interceed (TC7) and Gore-Tex surgical membrane on post-surgical adhesion formation. *Fertil Steril* 1992;57:199.

Quint EH, Smith YR. Ovarian surgery in premenarchal girls. *J Pediatr Adolesc Gynecol* 1999;12:27–30.

Ragni G, Somigliana MD. Damage to ovarian reserve with laparoscopic excision. *Am J Obstet Gynecol* 2005;193:1908.

Ragni G, Somigliana E, Benedotti F, Paffoni A, Vegetti W, Restelli L, Crosignant PG. Damage to ovarian reserve associated with laparoscopic excision of endometriomas: a quantitative rather than a qualitative injury. *Am J Obstet Gynecol* 2005 Dec;193(6):1908–14.

Rane A, Ohizua O. "Acute" residual ovary syndrome. *Aust N Z J Obstet Gynaecol* 1998;38:447.

Rotterdam ESHRE/ASRM PCOS Consensus Workshop Group. Revised 2003 consensus on diagnostic criteria and long-term health risks related to polycystic ovary syndrome. *Fertil Steril* 2004;81:19.

Sassone AM, Timor-Tritsch IE, Artner A, et al. Transvaginal sonographic characterization of ovarian disease: evaluation of a new scoring system to predict ovarian malignancy. *Obstet Gynecol* 1991;78:70.

Schmeler K, Mayo-Smith W, Peipert J, et al. Adnexal masses in pregnancy: surgery compared with observation. *Obstet Gynecol* 2005;105:1098.

Schwobel MG, Stauffer UG. Surgery of the female gonads. *Zeitschrift fur kinderchirurgie* 1988;43:289.

Scott JS, Lynch EM, Anderson JA. Surgical treatment of female infertility; value of paradoxical oophorectomy. *BMJ* 1976;1:631.

Scott RT, Beatse SN, Illions EH, et al. Use of the GnRH agonist stimulation test in the diagnosis of ovarian remnant syndrome: a report of three cases. *J Reprod Med* 1995;40:143.

Seltzer V, Maiman M, Boyce J. Laparoscopic survey in the management of ovarian cysts. *Female Patient* 1992;17:19.

Shalev E, Mann S, Romano S, et al. Laparoscopic detorsion of adnexa in childhood: a case report. *J Pediatr Surg* 1991;26:1145.

Shalev E, Peleg D. Laparoscopic treatment of adnexal torsion. *Surg Obstet Gynecol* 1993;176:448.

Sherard G, Hodson C, Williams HJ, et al. Adnexal masses and pregnancy: a 12 year experience *Am J Obstet Gynecol* 2003;189:358.

Soper JT, Hunter VJ, Daly L, et al. Preoperative serum tumor-associated antigen levels in women with pelvic masses. *Obstet Gynecol* 1990;75:249.

Soriano D, Wefet Y, Seidman D, et al. Laparoscopy versus laparotomy in the management of adnexal masses during pregnancy. *Fertil Steril* 1999;71:955.

Stein I, Leventhal ML. Amenorrhea associated with bilateral polycystic ovaries. *Am J Obstet Gynecol* 1935;29:181.

Steinkampf MP, Hammond KR, Blackwell RE. Hormonal treatment of functional ovarian cysts: a randomized prospective study. *Fertil Steril* 1990;54:775.

Symmonds RE, Petit P. Ovarian remnant syndrome. *Obstet Gynecol* 1979;54:175.

Tawa K. Ovarian tumors in pregnancy. *Am J Obstet Gynecol* 1964;90:5111.

Taylor A, Jurkovic D, Bourne T, et al. Sonographic prediction of malignancy in adnexal masses using an artificial neural network. *BJOG* 1999;106:21.

Terz J, Barber H, Bronschwig A. Incidence of carcinoma in the retained ovary. *Am J Surg* 1967;113:511.

Timmerman D, Bourne T, Tailor A, et al. A comparison of methods for preoperative discrimination between malignant and benign adnexal masses: the development of a new logistic regression model. *Am J Obstet Gynecol* 1999;181:57.

Toaff R, Toaff ME, Peyser MR. Infertility following wedge resection of the ovaries. *Am J Obstet Gynecol* 1976;124:92.

Trimbos-Kemper TC, Trimbos JB, van Hall EV. Management of infertile patients with unilateral tubal pathology by paradoxical oophorectomy. *Fertil Steril* 1982;37:623.

Tulandi T, Al Took S. Laparoscopic ovarian suspension before a radiation therapy. *Fertil Steril* 1998;70:381.

Van der Watt J. The mutilated ovary syndrome. *S Afr Med J* 1970;44:687.

Waldschmidt J, Schier F. Laparoscopic surgery in neonates and infants. *Eur J Pediatr Surg* 1991;1:145.

Wallace WH, Anderson R, Irvine DS. Fertility preservation for young patients with cancer: who is at risk and what can be offered? *Lancet Oncol* 2005;6:209.

Weiner Z, Thaler I, Beck D, et al. Differentiating malignant from benign ovarian tumors with transvaginal color flow imaging. *Obstet Gynecol* 1992;79:159.

Wenzl R, Lehner R, Husslein P, et al. Laparoscopic surgery in cases of ovarian malignancy: an Austria-wide survey. *Gynecol Oncol* 1996;63:57.

White M, Stella J. Ovarian torsion: 10 year perspective. *Emerg Med Australas* 2005;17:231.

Williams RS, Mendenhall N. Laparoscopic oophoropexy for preservation of ovarian function before pelvic node irradiation. *Obstet Gynecol* 1992;80:541.

Witschi E. Embryology of the ovary. In: *The ovary.* Baltimore: Williams & Wilkins;1963;1.

Witschi E. Migration of the germ cells of human embryos from the yolk sac to the primitive gonadal folds. *Contrib Embryol* 1948;32:69.

CHAPTER 29 ■ PERSISTENT OR CHRONIC PELVIC PAIN

JOHN F. STEEGE

DEFINITIONS

Allodynia—Pain resulting from a nonnoxious stimulus.

Hyperalgesia—Painful sensation of abnormal severity following noxious stimulation.

Neuropathic pain—Pain persisting after healing of disease or trauma-induced tissue damage.

Neuroplasticity—The malleability of central pain perception mechanisms in response to chronic pain states.

Nociceptor—A nerve receptor for pain.

Chronic pelvic pain (CPP) is defined as pain present either intermittently or continuously for 6 months or more. Although much work remains to be done concerning the epidemiology of the disorder, preliminary surveys suggest that it may affect 5% to 15% of women at some time in their lives, predominantly during their reproductive years. The gynecologist confronts this problem on a regular basis. Many organic and functional disorders of the reproductive, gastrointestinal, urinary tract, and musculoskeletal systems may contribute nociceptive stimuli to the problem. Dysfunction or organic disease in one organ system may induce nociception in an adjacent system in the manner of "cross-talk." In addition, by dysregulation of neurologic pathways, pain can become an illness in itself when it lasts longer than 4 to 6 months. This chapter reviews the common structural and functional components of CPP, describes the criteria for a chronic pain syndrome (CPS), and offers a theoretical model to explain the evolution of chronic pain over time.

Many pain disorders are deemed "chronic" by virtue of their duration—that is, 6 months or longer. In practice, this usually connotes decreased function (perhaps even disability) as well as progressive behavioral and affective changes. Although this definition is useful as a benchmark, some victims of chronic pain may develop these characteristics sooner than 6 months into the problem, and others may endure severe pain for years while remaining surprisingly functional and well adjusted. As suggested later, it is therefore perhaps useful to use additional behavioral and psychometric criteria to the chronologic definition of "chronic" to focus diagnostic and treatment efforts.

HISTORY

Over the past 50 years, the study of CPP has gone through significant changes in approach. Investigations undertaken before the development of laparoscopy focused on correlations between pelvic pain and psychologic distress. This approach was prompted by the fact that the two most common organic contributors to CPP—endometriosis and adhesions—can be difficult to diagnose by history and physical examination alone. In the absence of palpable pathology, the gynecologist of the 1950s and 1960s was understandably reluctant to subject a patient to laparotomy to investigate pain. During this era, the prevailing cartesian theory of pain perception suggested that pain should be somewhat proportional to the degree of tissue damage found. (If the pathology was not big enough to palpate, it was seldom operated on.) Although this was sufficient to explain most acute pain, the cartesian model fails to explain the majority of chronic pain disorders, in gynecology as well as other areas of medicine. The gate control theory, promulgated by Melzack and Wall in 1965, allowed integration of physical and psychologic parameters, and explained how chronic pain can be quite different from acute pain. The model also suggests that information flows in two directions regarding pain: (i) nociceptive signals from peripheral tissue ascend through the spinal cord to higher centers, and (ii) central centers can modulate, via descending signals altering spinal cord neurotransmitter and interneuron activity, the transmission of these nociceptive signals from the periphery. Deterioration of these regulatory processes were thought to potentially account for development of chronic pain states by allowing too many peripheral signals through the spinal cord "gates."

While these changes in pain theory were stimulating the field of pain research, gynecologists were busy developing laparoscopy. Previously cherished myths soon fell by the wayside: for example, endometriosis is seldom found in adolescents or African Americans. With these observations came the hope that laparoscopic and medical treatment of this pathology would fix CPP. Reports of CPP from that era focused on "laparoscopy-negative" patients; indeed, some pelvic pain clinics required a negative laparoscopy as an entry criterion, implying that if some pathology were found, it must be a "real" cause for pain. Subsequent experience has shown that even though treatment of laparoscopically diagnosed pathology is often helpful, the clinical reality is more complex:

1. In many instances, the organic pathology found at laparoscopy may be incidental and not related to the pain.
2. In those with pathology that does contribute to nociception, the pain experienced by the patient may be the sum of this contribution plus signals from some or all of the disorders listed in Table 29.1.

Consider the research of the 1980s that documented a distressingly high prevalence of physical and sexual abuse. Epidemiologic surveys of community samples revealed that as many as 25% to 30% of adult women reported having experienced sexual abuse during childhood. Studies of women attending pelvic pain clinics, especially those based in psychiatric settings, showed that up to 60% of these women had been abused. These observations led to the speculation that the experience of abuse may make a person more vulnerable to the

TABLE 29.1

POSSIBLE CAUSES OF PELVIC PAIN IN LAPAROSCOPY-NEGATIVE PATIENTS

Gastrointestinal
Constipation
Irritable bowel syndrome
Inflammatory bowel disease
Diverticulitis
Urinary
Urethral syndrome
Interstitial cystitis
Musculoskeletal or Neurologic
Pelvic floor tension myalgia
Piriformis syndrome
Nerve entrapment
Ventral hernia
Rectus tendon strain
Myofascial pain
Back or pelvic postural changes
Gynecologic
Pelvic vascular congestion
Cervical stenosis

From Steege JF, Stout AL, Somkuti SG. Chronic pelvic pain: toward an integrative model. *Obstet Gynecol Surv* 1993;48:95, with permission.

development of CPP or perhaps be a specific cause for pain. Currently, preliminary studies using positron-emission tomography and functional magnetic resonance imaging (MRI) methods suggest that the experience of abuse may indeed leave its neurophysiologic footprints: Stressful stimuli produce different central response patterns in abused versus nonabused subjects. However, detection of abuse in a patient's history seems to prompt referral for tertiary care, whereas symptom levels in various pain disorders [e.g., irritable bowel syndrome (IBS)] are similar in referred and nonreferred patients. The presence of an abuse history means that the evaluating health professionals need to take this into account, but it does not necessarily imply that the abuse is causally involved in the development of the pain. The impact of a history of abuse on the outcome of treatment of organic pathology should be the subject of further research.

Finally, even the gate control theory is held to be inadequate to explain clinical manifestations of pain. The neuromatrix theory, described by Melzack, is an expansion that includes the notion of neuroplasticity, among other elements. The concept of neuroplasticity suggests that experience can change the neurophysiologic behavior of the central nervous system in a manner that influences the subsequent processing of nociceptive stimuli. It may explain the apparent development of pain responses to stimuli usually thought of as nonpainful (allodynia), as well as exaggerated responses to painful stimuli (hyperalgesia). Every practicing gynecologist has seen patients whose pain responses seem out of proportion to the pathology found. This may reflect the emotional meaning of the problem for the patient, as well as past or present emotional trauma, but it may also be the result of nociceptive mechanisms not yet understood (e.g., the mechanism of pain from endometriosis) or the result of sensitization of spinal cord interneurons that have become pain generators as a result of being on the receiving end of peripheral nociceptive stimuli for prolonged periods. When nociception has been emanating from one organ system for a period of time, adjacent organs may join the chorus. A common example is the finding that pain from endometriosis and bladder symptoms coexist more than one might expect. Vulvar vestibulitis overlaps with interstitial cystitis in a similar manner. On occasion, one is confronted with the unfortunate patient with multiple somatosensory disorders—e.g., she might have IBS, endometriosis, interstitial cystitis, fibromyalgia, chronic fatigue syndrome, etc., all at the same time. Such observations have led some investigators to pursue potential genetic variations in central neurotransmitter networks that might predispose to the development of multiple such disorders.

The above is the negative side of neuroplasticity. The positive side of the neuroplasticity concept is that, perhaps, given enough time and the right treatment, even seemingly intractable chronic pain problems may ameliorate to the point of allowing substantially improved function. This chapter reviews the various organic, psychologic, and physiologic factors that contribute to CPP, outlines methods of evaluation, gives suggestions for treatment, and finishes with a discussion of an integrated model of the development of CPP.

CONTRIBUTIONS OF TISSUE DAMAGE TO PAIN

Endometriosis

A recent review summarized laparoscopic findings from 2,615 patients in 15 studies (nine retrospective, six prospective). Endometriosis was found in 2% to 51% of patients, suggesting that referral biases lead to very skewed samples. Clearly, not every woman with pain has endometriosis, nor does every woman with endometriosis have pain, although women with the disease had pain more often than those without it. A number of previous studies of CPP either described only patients without organic laparoscopic findings or stratified patients according to the presence or absence of physical pathology. The description of atypical (nonpigmented) endometriosis by Jansen and Russell in 1986 calls these classifications into question. Laparoscopy studies published before that time reported that 11% of women with CPP had endometriosis, whereas three similarly conducted studies published since 1986 reported a 41% prevalence of endometriosis in women undergoing laparoscopy for CPP. The pre-1986 literature on pelvic pain must be reevaluated with this information in mind. Many studies may have included women with endometriosis in the anatomically normal group, thus generating erroneous conclusions about the entirely psychogenic nature of their pain.

The first symptom of significant endometriosis is often increased dysmenorrhea alone, but other pain often develops, and its duration and severity often progress as the disease advances, to the point that it can be present almost constantly. Again, the severity of the pain correlates poorly with the amount of diffuse peritoneal disease, but may vary more directly with deeply infiltrative cul-de-sac disease. Fear of worsened pain, impaired fertility, or recurrent disease after treatment can increase pain levels. Of the many women on whom we have performed laparoscopy for recurrent pain following complete hysterectomy and adnexectomy for endometriosis, only a small minority (3% to 5%) proved to have recurrent disease. Most cases of postoperative pain have been attributable to a combination of postoperative adhesions, fear of recurrent disease, and functional problems such as levator spasm and IBS.

When endometriosis is strongly suspected, and initial treatment with oral contraceptives has failed, diagnostic laparoscopy should be the next step. One widely discussed study (Ling et al. 1999) concluded that a careful clinical history and physical examination can predict the presence of endometriosis in about 80% of cases. However, this was done in the setting of a strict research protocol; the diagnostic sensitivity of this approach in general clinical practice is likely much lower. Unfortunately, the study is often misinterpreted as implying that relief of pain following GnRH treatment is also *specific*—i.e., makes the diagnosis of endometriosis. Careful reading of the data reveals that this is not the case: the frequency of relief following GnRH treatment was the same in women with and without endometriosis. In addition, pain sensitivity is known to increase perimenstrually even in women without gynecologic pain problems. This may mean that nociceptive from pain disorders outside the reproductive tract may also improve when menstrual cyclicity is eliminated. For example, symptoms from IBS have been shown to be reduced in women taking GnRH agonists. Hence, although *failure* to relieve pain with a GnRH agonist would appear to strongly support the notion that the reproductive organs are not involved, relief of pain with these medications does not prove that they are to blame.

Hysterectomy and bilateral salpingo-oophorectomy relieve endometriosis-related pain in more than 90% of cases. When one or both ovaries are preserved, the recurrence rate is estimated to be 30% or higher, but this figure includes endometriosis of all stages. Some practitioners believe that if disease does not involve the ovaries, surgical excision of the disease, with ovarian conservation, results in an acceptable 5% to 10% recurrence rate over the subsequent 5 years. Further investigation of this unorthodox approach is warranted.

Pelvic Adhesions

In a review by Steege and colleagues, 6% to 55% of the 2,615 patients who underwent laparoscopy for pelvic pain had pelvic adhesions. As is the case for endometriosis, the site of adhesive disease correlated well with the site of pain, but the intensity of pain was unrelated to the extent of adhesions present. Nociceptive signals from the damaged tissue seem subject to modulation at the spinal cord level and interpretation in higher centers. Adhesions are most likely stable anatomically a few months after injury (e.g., surgery, infection), but the intensity of associated pain can progress. After about 6 months of pain experience, complex relationships among physical, emotional, and cognitive factors can exist that require comprehensive treatment.

Pelvic Support

Although problems with pelvic relaxation are common in women in their sixth or seventh decade of life, most patients at pain clinics are in their third or fourth decade. The implication is that cases of pain associated with pelvic support problems constitute the minority of pelvic pain problems.

Pelvic relaxation usually leads to reports of heaviness, pressure, dropping sensations, or aching. In attempting to hold in prolapsing organs, the patient may be tensing the levator plate and contributing to tenderness during daily activities and intercourse. Fear of (or actual) loss of urinary control during coitus can add to the discomfort by impairing physiologic sexual response.

Excess mobility of the pelvic organs (universal joint or Allen-Masters syndrome) attributed to childbirth or other traumatic causes of ligament (especially broad ligament) tears in uterine supports has been implicated in CPP. Such highly subjective physical examination findings are difficult to document rigorously, and because surgery has been the traditional primary treatment, controlled studies of the association of pain with ligamentous tears have not been possible.

Uterine retroversion is another controversial potential etiology for CPP, particularly in the form of deep dyspareunia. Uncontrolled clinical series of uterine suspension procedures for pelvic pain suggest that the most frequent scenario involves a combination of uterine retroversion (most often innocent by itself) with new intrinsic uterine pathology (e.g., adenomyosis, myomas) or nearby cul-de-sac or adnexal pathology (e.g., endometriosis, adhesions, ovary prolapsed into the cul-de-sac). On occasion, these anatomic circumstances, combined with a new partner of more generous penile dimensions, produce new deep dyspareunia.

Generally speaking, uterine suspension procedures have earned a mixed reputation at best, as many versions yield short-term benefit at best. A recently developed laparoscopic procedure uses permanent suture that is woven through almost the entire length of the round ligament on each side. As support is dependent on the suture and less on shortening an intrinsically weak round ligament, maintenance of anteversion appears to be better and may even persist following pregnancy in some cases.

Pelvic Congestion

Overfilling (congestion) of the pelvic venous system has been implicated as a cause of dull chronic aching pain that usually is worse at the end of the day after prolonged standing, premenstrually, and after coitus not accompanied by orgasm. The pain is occasionally unilateral, is usually present in multiparous women, and is likely due to anatomic causes, at least in part. The high comorbidity with psychologic distress indicates that psychophysiologic factors may also contribute. Medroxyprogesterone can help (by eliminating the menstrual cycle), but the best long-term results have followed psychotherapy in conjunction with this medication. In any case, good radiologic studies in women who are awake during the procedure have documented increased pelvic venous diameter in those affected. Veins cannot be reliably evaluated during laparoscopy because of confounding effects such as position and fluid load.

Residual Ovary

When the uterus has been removed, with or without removal of one ovary, the remaining ovary or ovaries can become symptomatic in 1% to 4% of women. In many instances, benign functional ovarian cysts can form and can be transiently symptomatic. Pain from the ovary can be increased by confinement of the ovary within postoperative adhesions, rupture or leakage of a cyst prompting additional adhesion formation, or attachment of the ovary to the sigmoid colon or vaginal apex by postoperative adhesions. In the case of attachment to the vaginal apex, deep dyspareunia can result when the vaginal apex is struck. When this pain causes diminished sexual response, loss of the normal vaginal apex expansion and elongation that is part of sexual response can leave the ovary or ovaries closer to the introitus, thus aggravating the deep dyspareunia.

Ovarian Remnant

A more difficult situation can develop if a small fragment of ovarian tissue is left behind during attempted oophorectomy. In most instances, this happens when extensive pelvic adhesive disease or endometriosis made the dissection difficult. Within 1 to 3 years of the attempted oophorectomy, continued follicle-stimulating hormone (FSH) stimulation will result in growth of the ovarian fragment, often producing an intermittently symptomatic pelvic mass located along the course of the ovarian vascular supply. This problem is uncommon, but not rare, as implied by early case series. The prevalence of asymptomatic ovarian remnants is unknown. As in the case of the residual ovary, the remnant can produce dyspareunia if it is located close to the vaginal apex.

Vaginal Apex Pain

Following hysterectomy, pain may persist or recur because of intrinsic sensitivity of the vaginal apex. Although the cuff may appear to have healed perfectly well, gentle examination with a cotton-tipped applicator may reveal focal sensitivity of moderate to severe degree, often located in one lateral fornix or the other, and often replicating the reported pain of dyspareunia. When this is not done, the unaware examiner may then, noting pain upon traditional bimanual examination, mistakenly conclude that the source of nociception lies cephalad, for example, in a remaining ovary, pelvic scarring, or bowel adhesions.

The diagnosis may be confirmed by noting elimination of the pain following injection of local anesthetic. The pain appears to be neuropathic in nature, by virtue of the typical descriptors used (burning, stinging, sharp), and by virtue of the treatments that seem to benefit some patients (overnight applications of 5% lidocaine ointment, low doses of nortriptyline, and medications such as gabapentin, lamotrigene, and Lamictal). Surgical revision of the vaginal apex, often done laparoscopically, may give good initial relief in about two thirds of patients, but pain tends to recur to a degree over the subsequent 2 to 3 years.

Musculoskeletal Problems

Musculoskeletal changes can become involved with CPP, either as the primary problem or as a secondary reaction to the pelvic pain. Dysmenorrhea can be referred to the midline of the low back, especially when the uterus is retroverted. Pain can also be referred to the midline of the low back in the presence of cul-de-sac endometriosis. An ovary fixed to the pelvic sidewall can refer pain to the ipsilateral low back and lower quadrant.

The muscular problem that most often produces pelvic pain is pelvic floor tension myalgia. Intermittent or constant painful contraction of the levator plate can be present as a primary psychophysiologic problem, but contraction is more often a reaction to some other source of pain. Even when the primary source of pain is successfully treated, the reactive muscle contraction can persist as a learned response, in much the same way that vaginal introital muscle spasm (vaginismus) can persist after transient but repeated painful vaginal events.

Lumbar musculature can become tender as a primary problem or in reaction to subtle changes in posture and motion. Trigger points can be present in the low back and gluteal areas in the muscles best inspected by pelvic examination (e.g., levator plate, piriformis, obturator internus).

The piriformis and obturator muscles warrant additional mention because they are seldom appreciated as possible sources of pain. These muscles are external rotators of the leg, and rotation against resistance can allow detection of tender spasm of the muscles during the pelvic examination. The sciatic nerve can traverse the belly of the piriformis as a normal anatomic variant, producing symptoms similar to sciatica when the muscle is in spasm.

Myofascial Pain

Focal lower quadrant abdominal wall pain can be produced by entrapment of the genitofemoral and ilioinguinal nerves, as described by Applegate. Such entrapment appears most often after Pfannenstiel abdominal incisions. Slocumb has advanced the theory that myofascial trigger points account for a large fraction of CPP. In my experience, abdominal wall components may be the primary cause for pain in some cases, but are more often a later reaction to the long duration of pain from some other source. Reiter and Gambone reported that 14% of 122 laparoscopy-negative women had myofascial pain probably related to a previous surgical incision.

Medical Comorbidity

The cause of chronic lower abdominal or pelvic pain often involves nongynecologic systems (Table 29.1). A careful history and close physical examination of gastrointestinal, urologic, musculoskeletal, and neurologic systems are needed to evaluate the contributions of nongynecologic systems to CPP. Most of the available literature examines these problems of other systems independently of each other and without reference to their relevance to CPP or to the overall prevalence of these disorders in CPP.

The gastrointestinal system is perhaps the most common nongynecologic source of pelvic pain. Constipation and IBS occur most frequently, although inflammatory bowel disease and diverticulitis can at times present with pain alone. Women with IBS may have increased relaxin levels (produced by a dysfunctional corpus luteum) as one of many possible contributing factors. As previously mentioned, treatment with a gonadotropin-releasing hormone (GnRH) agonist may reduce symptoms of IBS.

Urologic problems, which are less easily confused with gynecologic disorders, are perhaps second in terms of prevalence. The urethral syndrome (frequency, urgency, and dysuria in the absence of bacteriuria), interstitial cystitis, and bladder spasms are all accompanied by significant anxiety and depression symptoms. The symptoms of these three disorders are very similar to those in a population of gynecologic CPP patients. Structured questionnaires [e.g., the Pain, Urgency, Frequency (PUF) scale] help detect symptoms possibly emanating from the bladder, but in some patients, a "positive" score can be achieved on the basis of other components of pelvic pain alone, without specific bladder symptoms, hence making this measure perhaps too *sensitive*, and hence insufficiently *specific*. A history (whether pain occurs during micturition, daily activities, or coitus) does not always reveal the involved system, but careful pelvic examination with stepwise gentle palpation of the urethra, bladder base, and bladder may help the physician identify from the patient's response the site of the pain she is experiencing.

Many patients do not experience the problems described here in pure form, but rather in varying degrees of intensity, with varying contributions to an individual's total discomfort. Indeed, we suspect that shared innervation of pelvic organs may often lead to subsyndromal symptoms in an organ system that neighbors one with organic pathology. Such patients may have a multifaceted somatosensory disorder, as opposed to being the unfortunate victim of multiple unrelated organ-specific disease processes. Close attention to such nuances of detail is warranted both in clinical management and in published reports.

PSYCHOLOGIC FACTORS

Personality

The links between chronic pain and individual psychology and personality style have been sought after and discussed in the psychiatric literature for many years. Some early reports implied that women who reported CPP had a high prevalence of feminine identity problems related to conflicts about adult sexuality, psychiatric disturbance characterized by mixed character disorder with predominant schizoid features, high neuroticism, and unsatisfactory relationships. Although these initial studies were an important beginning, the high prevalence of psychopathology in some reported samples did not seem applicable to significant numbers of CPP patients seen in practice. The findings are difficult to interpret, partly because there is a lack of clarity concerning the operational definition of CPP that was used. Biases in patient selection and interviewer information, inadequate control groups, and the absence of diagnostic laparoscopy also contribute to the confusion. Despite these shortcomings, it seems apparent that disorders of personality, especially borderline personality, are overrepresented both in the general population of severe chronic pain patients and in the population of pelvic pain patients. In primary care, such patients usually are seen less often. In any case, a label of personality disorder should not be applied indiscriminately to every angry patient by her frustrated physician. People who have difficulties maintaining satisfactory relationships and function in life, even when these difficulties are caused in part by subsyndromal personality problems, can be more vulnerable to nociceptive signals from tissue damaged by endometriosis, infection, or surgery. Unmet dependency needs may lead them to seek external solutions such as medications and further surgery, rather than to rely on their own impaired coping skills.

Depression

Focusing specifically on a CPP sample that had been evaluated by diagnostic laparoscopy, Walker and associates found that women with CPP (with and without positive laparoscopic findings) met criteria for lifetime major depression, current major depression, lifetime substance abuse, adult sexual dysfunction, and somatization more often than did control subjects. Stout and Steege found that 59% of 294 women seeking evaluation at a pelvic pain clinic scored in the depressed range (greater than 16) on the Center for Epidemiologic Studies Depression Scale at the time of their initial visit. Slocumb and colleagues reported that patients with an abdominal pelvic pain syndrome scored higher as a group on scales of anxiety, depression, anger-hostility, and somatization on the Hopkins Symptom Checklist; however, 56% of the total sample scored within the normal range on all scales.

Because no study of CPP has assessed its association with depression over time, no statement can be made as to whether depressive symptoms are a predisposing factor leading to, or a reaction to, the pain condition. There seem to be two distinct groups of CPP patients: one in which pain and depression are common final presentations reached by a number of pathways and another in which depression develops in reaction to pain, as is the case with many other acute and chronic medical diseases.

History of Sexual Abuse

Women seeking treatment for CPP have a high prevalence of sexual trauma in their personal histories. In Reiter's study of 106 women with CPP, 48% had a history of major psychosexual trauma (molestation, incest, or rape) compared with 6.5% of 92 pain-free control subjects presenting for annual routine gynecologic examination ($p < 0.001$). The high prevalence of reports of psychosexual trauma elicited from pelvic pain patients supports the hypothesis that pelvic pain is specifically and psychodynamically related to sexual abuse. However, Rapkin and colleagues did not find a higher prevalence of childhood or adult sexual abuse in a group of women with CPP compared with women with chronic pain in other locations, although women with CPP reported a higher incidence of childhood sexual abuse. These findings argue against a unique relation between sexual abuse and CPP and suggest that abusive experiences promote the chronicity of many different painful conditions. Morrison also reported an association between sexual abuse and a wide variety of pathologic conditions. Jamieson and Steege, in a survey of 581 women seen in primary care practices, found that 28% of women reported having been sexually abused as children and 26% as adults. In this study, those abused only in childhood did not have an increased prevalence of CPP or other pain disorders, whereas those who had suffered abuse both as children and adults did.

When such a history is documented, the clinician and patient together must judge whether the feelings surrounding these events are intense enough to intrude upon the present. If so, psychotherapeutic help may be indicated. If not, although the memories may be painful, further emotional work on this area may not be beneficial. The treatment literature on the sequelae of abuse (and their treatment) is disappointing, especially when the abuse occurred in the distant past. In either case, it is difficult to judge whether these events are directly relevant to the present pain and hence demand attention, or whether they contribute to a psychologically vulnerable substrate acted upon by subsequent physical and emotional events. In these circumstances, it may be worthwhile to suggest further mental health evaluation as an exploratory measure, being careful not to imply that the patient is being referred because the physician is certain that the abuse is related to the development of the pain.

Sexual Dysfunction

In clinical practice, women presenting with CPP often report a high incidence of marital distress and sexual dysfunction, particularly dyspareunia. Stout and Steege found that 56% of 220 married women scored in the maritally distressed range (less than 100) on the Locke-Wallace Marital Adjustment Scale at the time of initial visit. A high level of marital distress has also been reported in other chronic pain patients and their spouses. Although some women report satisfactory sexual functioning before the onset of pain symptoms, others appear to have long-standing impairments in sexual response. In our experience, sexual difficulties are often the problem that makes a person seek help for her pain.

DIAGNOSTIC STRATEGIES

Recognizing a Chronic Pain Syndrome

Many women can experience pain for longer than 6 months without becoming debilitated; although their pain is chronic, such women are not described as having a CPS. The following are the common clinical hallmarks of true CPS:

1. Duration of 6 months or longer
2. Incomplete relief by most previous treatments
3. Significantly impaired physical function at home or at work
4. Signs of depression (sleep disturbance, weight loss, loss of appetite)
5. Pain out of proportion to pathology
6. Altered family roles

Of the signs of depression, sleep disturbance is usually the first to appear. Careful questioning is needed to distinguish awakening caused by pain from awakening that just happens. In the true vegetative sign, the person usually cannot get back to sleep even if pain is relieved (by medication or other means).

The alteration of family roles is perhaps the most important of those mentioned. This includes changed responsibilities for household, children, finances, and so forth. Initially intended as helpful, such changes may in the long run diminish the patient's self-esteem and progressively reduce her family's interactions with her to little more than checking on her pain. Over time, this covertly reinforces the symptom of pain and imparts to it unintended value as a major means of maintaining communication within the family.

Simultaneous Medical and Psychosocial Evaluation

When the aforementioned markers of CPS are present, one should surrender the need to immediately discover how much of the pain problem is physical and how much is psychologic. Rather than guess, it is useful to ask two separate questions: Is there physical disease that requires medical or surgical treatment? Is there emotional or psychological distress that requires treatment?

It is useful to directly state that the precise connection between these two cannot be measured; this can help diminish the patient's fear that she will be told "it's all in her head." The patient can then be more open to sharing her personal and emotional concerns. If this statement is made early in the evaluation, before all physical evaluations have been carried out, the patient is likely to be less defensive. At this stage, a mental health consultant has a better chance of developing rapport with the patient and will be a more helpful collaborator when needed.

History Taking

The site, duration, pattern during activities, relation to position changes, and association with bodily functions are all important elements of pain. For example, pain that is focal and positional is more often associated with adhesive disease; pain that is absent in the morning but worsens progressively during the day may be associated with pelvic congestion or pelvic floor muscle dysfunction. The patterns of pain associated with endometriosis are discussed earlier.

The chronology of the pain is critical. As CPS develops, pain can be present over a progressively larger area despite stable organic pathology. Interpreting this as the breakdown or wearing out of physiologic systems that deal with pain signals has some biologic validity and may make sense to the patient.

From a cognitive perspective, it is invaluable to discern the patient's and her family's ideas about the causes of and future for her pain. Fears of cancer can be discovered even if this diagnosis was never even remotely considered by the clinician. Less dramatic, but equally powerful, attributions of cause can emerge, such as pelvic infection that is due to sexual acts remote in time, arguments with a spouse, divine retribution, and so forth.

Physical Examination

The exam begins with single finger palpation of the abdominal wall, with and without having the patient flex the rectus muscles. A positive Carnett sign (persistent or increase tenderness when palpation is done in the presence of abdominal wall flexion) implies at least a contribution to the pain from abdominal wall myofascial sources. On occasion, gentle fingertip palpation of the abdominal wall can detect such trigger points in the musculature.

Pelvic exam then begins with external review of the vulva and vestibule. Gentle palpation with a cotton swab can detect areas of sensitivity compatible with vestibulitis in the introitus or trigger points higher in the vagina.

Guiding a patient through contraction-relaxation sequences of the abdominal, thigh, and vaginal introital muscles can reduce the discomfort of the examination and can indicate the patient's degree of control over muscle tension. Single-digit palpation of the levator plate, piriformis, and obturator muscles can elicit tenderness compatible with the label of pelvic floor tension myalgia. This condition is often present as a sequel to some other pelvic pain, but it can become a problem in itself. Discomfort is usually felt as pelvic pressure and radiation pain to the sacrum, near the insertions of the levator plate muscles.

Single-digit palpation should also be used to discover areas of tenderness in the cervix, uterus, and adnexa as well. Premature addition of the abdominal hand to the exam adds in nociceptive signals from abdominal wall myofascial components that may lead the examiner to overattribute pain to the viscera. Finally, the abdominal hand is added to assess size, shape, and mobility of pelvic structures. Adnexal thickening and mobility, pelvic relaxation, coccygeal tenderness, and foci of pain that reproduce dyspareunia should be noted.

Laboratory Tests

Imaging Studies

In the case of CPS, it has already been established that intensity of pain does not correlate well with extent of organic pathology. It follows that if the physical examination is relatively benign and is not severely limited by body habitus, extensive imaging usually adds little to the database needed before laparoscopy is performed. This is especially true in the case of organ-specific studies (intravenous pyelography, barium enema, colonoscopy) in the absence of symptoms or signs pointing to a specific organ system (e.g., blood in the stools). If the patient has had multiple previous surgeries, high-resolution studies such as MRI and computed tomography scans are often misleading because of postoperative artifact. "Cystic masses" seen on such studies often prove to be nothing more than pockets of adhesions or peritoneal inclusion cysts.

Blood Studies

Relatively few hematologic or chemical measures are of use in diagnosing CPP. An elevated leukocyte count and erythrocyte sedimentation rate may make the clinician suspect chronic pelvic inflammatory disease even when cervical cultures are negative for the most common sexually transmitted diseases. The cancer antigen-125 test is positive in advanced endometriosis but is not sufficiently sensitive to detect early-stage disease or reliably monitor its response to treatment. If any remnant ovarian tissue is present, FSH and estradiol levels remain in premenopausal ranges in almost all instances. Replacement estrogen therapy should be withdrawn 3 weeks before these levels are measured.

Anesthetic Blocks

Injection of small volumes of a local anesthetic, 1 to 5 mL of 1% lidocaine or 0.5% bupivacaine, blocks pain from either an entrapped segmental nerve (e.g., ilioinguinal) or an abdominal wall trigger point. In the latter case, such blocks can be therapeutic as well as diagnostic. Many anesthesia pain clinics administer epidural or spinal anesthetics to distinguish pain arising from peripheral organs from pain that has become completely central in origin.

In some instances, it is useful to attempt transvaginal blocks with the same local anesthetics for vaginal apex pain, as discussed above. Local blocks can be therapeutic as well as diagnostic. A series of three or four blocks administered 1 to 2 weeks apart may give relief for months to years in some instances.

In most cases, a history and careful routine physical examination distinguishes central from lateral sources of pelvic pain. When this discrimination is difficult, it may be useful to administer a transvaginal uterosacral block (blocking most uterine innervation) and then repeat the pelvic examination. When this relieves the pain, the pain can be assumed to arise from the uterus, but if the pain is not relieved, one cannot distinguish a failed block from pain of nonuterine origin.

Psychologic Tests and Interviews

To distinguish physical from psychologic causes for pain, many studies of CPP have used traditional psychologic instruments that were developed to measure general psychopathology or personality factors. In some studies, more abnormalities are detected in women without physical pathology at laparoscopy. In other papers, women with organic disease who have had pain for a long time appear equally distressed in their questionnaire responses. These psychometric instruments generally have little face value for chronic pain patients, and their use often confirms the patient's fears that the health care provider thinks she is "crazy" or that the pain is "all in her head." Once again, the question of whether the emotional distress identified by these instruments is an antecedent to or a consequence of persistent pain remains unanswered. A more complete review of the psychometric instruments that have been used to study CPP is presented elsewhere.

Psychometric tests are most useful when they are interpreted by a psychologist who has interviewed the patient, and they serve best as a means to better understand the patient's strengths and weaknesses, rather than as a means to decide who needs surgery.

Laparoscopy

Great strides have been made in operative laparoscopy in the past two decades. New techniques and new terminology (e.g., pelviscopy) imply new "magic" to the physician and public alike. Laparoscopy should be liberally performed for diagnostic purposes, and ablation/excision of endometriosis and lysis of adhesions are no doubt useful procedures. However, the premature surgical procedure errs in the notion that pain is "hardwired" to pelvic pathology. The available evidence clearly argues against this. When a CPS is clinically evident, results of laparoscopic treatment alone, despite comparable pathology, are much less impressive. For a patient with the clinical markers of CPS listed earlier, the complete workup as described should be performed before laparoscopy.

In some puzzling cases, we have performed laparoscopy under local anesthesia to "pain map" the pelvis. A 2-mm laparoscope and a small suprapubic probe are placed with the use of short-acting intravenous analgesia (remifentanyl) and local lidocaine 1%. Having been oriented to the procedure beforehand, as each organ is touched, she is asked (i) "Does this give you the pain you get?" and (ii) "Please rate the pain." She responds with a number picked from a scale of 1 to 10, with 10 signifying the "worst pain you could imagine." This technique may make it possible to determine whether visualized pathology is causing nociceptive signals or to discriminate visceral from somatic pain.

It is possible in some cases to block the superior hypogastric plexus during pain mapping to better predict benefit from presacral neurectomy. In this approach, mapping is done before and after injecting 10 mL of 1% lidocaine just underneath the peritoneum over the sacrum, using a 7-inch, 22-gauge spinal needle.

MANAGEMENT

Physicians use specific treatments in chronic pain depending on the model of pain perception that they follow. The surgically oriented gynecologist often tacitly follows the cartesian model, attempting to eliminate organic tissue damage to diminish pain proportionately. The behaviorist, cognitive therapist, and insight-oriented psychotherapist use approaches consistent with each one's basic therapeutic orientation, whereas advocates of the gate control theory use medications and other treatments that make sense based on that theory. The following represents an eclectic treatment approach. The treatment literature is considerably sparser than is the literature exploring the etiology of CPP.

General Principles

A complete evaluation of CPS often reveals a number of contributing factors, such as bladder irritability, irregular bowel function, poor posture, and emotional and relationship stresses, in addition to laparoscopically visualized pathology. Treating each component sequentially is common practice but often ends in frustration because each treatment addresses only a part of the problem. Simultaneous treatments often begin with disquieting multiple drug therapy but allow better relief. Close follow-up at regularly scheduled visits allows gradual tapering of medications over time. Planned visits also provide support and a coping mechanism for the patient. When the patient is essentially required to feel worse to be seen again, the pain may be tacitly reinforced.

Medication Use

Analgesics

Advocates of the operant conditioning model suggest that analgesics be taken continuously, in a non–pain-contingent fashion. This eliminates the need to demonstrate pain behaviors or voice pain symptoms to justify the use of medication, thus eliminating the tendency of medication to act as a reinforcer of pain behaviors. This approach is benign enough when relatively nontoxic and nonaddicting medications such as acetaminophen are used, but it presents potential hazards when drugs such as the following are used: nonsteroidal antiinflammatory drugs (NSAIDs; gastric irritation, renal damage); aspirin or NSAIDs in combination with the milder narcotics, such as codeine, oxycodone, and pentazocine (constipation, sedation, habituation); and pure narcotics (addiction, diminished analgesic potency over time). When well tolerated, all three types of drugs can serve well in appropriate patients (without histories of substance abuse). Indeed, contrary to common perception, there is support for the notion that chronic low-dose opiate therapy may allow good return of function without adverse side effects in those who have failed intensive pain clinic treatments.

Antidepressants

This class of drugs, particularly the tricyclic antidepressants, can potentiate the effects of analgesics in CPS, even when given at doses less than those usually used in the treatment of depression. Agents such as fluoxetine (Prozac) show promise and have a low level of side effects. Few controlled trials of antidepressants have been carried out in CPP patients.

Anxiolytics

Anxiolytic drugs are certainly widely prescribed by gynecologists, although it is uncertain how often they are given for pain. In one study, alprazolam, a triazolobenzodiazepine with mixed anxiolytic and antidepressant effects, had a surprising degree of analgesic effect in moderate to high doses in patients with chronic pain of malignant origin and concomitant mood changes or anxiety. These patients were already receiving narcotics, which may suggest that alprazolam potentiates the analgesic effect of narcotics. Their role in conjunction with nonnarcotic analgesics is uncertain, and the addiction potential is obvious.

Other Medications

Nonanalgesic and nonpsychotropic drugs also have potential roles in the treatment of specific pelvic conditions. For example, medroxyprogesterone acetate treatment sufficient to suppress ovarian function may reduce the diameter of engorged pelvic veins and thus reduce the discomfort of pelvic congestion. However, the longest-lasting relief was observed when psychotherapy was used as well.

The use of GnRH agonists has been recommended to distinguish gynecologic from nongynecologic sources of pain; however, these agents also relieve the symptoms of IBS, probably by reducing serum relaxin levels. When the differential diagnosis includes ovarian remnant syndrome, residual ovary syndrome, or any other disorder influenced by the menstrual cycle, the impact of GnRH agonists on pelvic pain must be interpreted with caution in anyone with symptoms at all compatible with bowel dysfunction. In addition, pain threshold has been shown to be lower premenstrually, even in asymptomatic women. The impact of the menstrual cycle itself in chronic pain patients has not been well explored, but it seems likely that it may impart some cyclicity even to conditions unrelated to the reproductive tract. Cyclicity of symptoms must therefore be interpreted with caution, and the obliteration of symptoms or of their cyclicity by pharmacologically obliterating the menstrual cycle does not demonstrate a gynecologic cause. To address the most common clinical circumstance: relieving pain with a GnRH agonist does not prove that the pain is due to endometriosis, nor does it prove that pain comes from the reproductive tract, as discussed above.

Surgery

Two basic surgical approaches have been used to treat CPP: removing pelvic organs and treating visible disease while leaving the pelvic organs in place. Only the former approach has been evaluated for efficacy to any degree.

In the United States, about 12% of hysterectomies are performed with pelvic pain as the primary indication. An additional 6.1% are performed for endometriosis or adenomyosis, and 5.1% are performed for pelvic inflammatory disease; no doubt many in these two categories also involve symptoms of pain. In about one third of hysterectomies performed for pain, no pathology is found. Despite the frequency of pain as an indication for this procedure, data regarding efficacy are surprisingly sparse. One report notes relief in 78% of women after hysterectomy for pelvic pain of uterine etiology (women with adnexal or other pelvic disease were excluded). However, the presence or absence of uterine pathology (adenomyosis or leiomyomata) had no bearing on whether pain was relieved. It cannot be determined from the report (Table 29.1) whether failure to obtain relief was due to the presence of other pelvic conditions, postoperative adhesion formation, or psychologic reasons. Symptom substitution was not evaluated in the report. Relief of pain by removal of the normal uterus is even more puzzling; apparently this was not accounted for by concomitant procedures performed for deficient pelvic support. Some of these cases may have involved pelvic congestion or perhaps other mechanisms even less well understood. A 22% failure rate emphasizes the need for careful preoperative evaluation of all potentially contributing factors, both physical and emotional.

According to two recent reports, hysterectomy performed in primary care settings was very effective for the treatment of CPP. In a prospective observational study of private practices in Maine, Carlson and associates reported that at a 1-year follow-up, satisfaction with the outcome of surgical treatment was much higher than satisfaction with the outcome of medical therapy. However, about one third of women improved substantially on medical therapy, and perhaps women were more likely to undergo operation when organic pathology was demonstrable. In the Maryland Women's Health Study, 1,299 women were interviewed at length before hysterectomy for benign disease and at 3, 6, 12, and 24 months after surgery. In more than 90% of cases, the procedure was well tolerated and did not result in postoperative depression or a decline in sexual functioning. In the subset of women with pain as the primary indication for surgery, relief of pain occurred in more than 80%, indicating that the clinicians involved generally used good judgment and technique. In general, women with preoperative depression or sexual dysfunction did not fare as well as their less symptomatic counterparts, although even when hysterectomy is performed in women with both depression and chronic pelvic pain, slightly more than 80% are improved emotionally and in terms of pain at 2-year follow-up.

Adnexal and other intrapelvic diseases, usually endometriosis or adhesions that are due to either postoperative changes or chronic pelvic inflammatory disease, have been treated by both laparotomy and laparoscopy. Use of the CO_2 laser during laparotomy does not improve the results of standard infertility surgical techniques as evaluated by second-look laparoscopy and by pregnancy rate.

Laparoscopy is probably superior to laparotomy for treating adhesive disease. In the rabbit model, infliction of injuries with the laser by way of laparotomy resulted in adhesion formation, but no adhesions formed when identical damage was caused by laparoscopy. In the rabbit and the human, adhesiolysis is more effective with laparoscopy than with laparotomy. However, none of the large clinical trials of laparoscopic adhesiolysis evaluate the effects of the procedures on pain.

Although second-look verification of effective adhesiolysis is lacking, results of several studies on the treatment of pelvic adhesions for the relief of pain are encouraging. Even when treated by laparotomy, with the use of infertility techniques, 28 of 42 (65%) patients reported cure or improvement of pain. In a sample of mostly primary care patients, 84% of 65 patients had relief of pain after laser laparoscopic adhesiolysis with follow-up intervals of 1 to 5 years. In Sutton's large series, 85% had pain relief at 1 year. Steege and Stout reported that 15 of 20 (75%) patients without a CPS who were undergoing laser laparoscopic adhesiolysis had good relief of pain at a follow-up 6 to 12 months after surgery. However, if a CPS was present, only 4 of 10 (40%) patients with equivalent adhesive disease obtained relief. The greater the emotional and behavioral disability, the greater the need for combined medical, surgical, and mental health management.

Several studies support an association between pelvic pain and endometriosis, although a strict quantitative relationship is lacking. In terms of surgical treatment of pain from endometriosis, laser ablation results in relief of pain in about 60% of women at 1 year follow-up, compared with 96% treated by laparoscopic excision of the disease. A randomized trial comparing these two methods has not been done. The benefits of surgical excision may be prolonged by subsequent medical therapy. Numerous studies have been done of postsurgical treatment with hormonal medications. Oral contraceptives, Danocrine, progestins, and GnRH agonists (with and without add-back estrogen/progestin) have all been shown to be effective. Although the GnRH agonists have become perhaps the most widely used of these, definitive evidence for their superiority is lacking. The more economical and less physiologically intrusive approach would seem to favor sex steroids over GnRH agonists. Most troublesome in reviewing all of these studies is the observation that dyspareunia is the symptom that is most refractory to treatment, testifying to its multifactorial nature.

Presacral neurectomy, as an adjunct to surgical excision of endometriosis, has been evaluated for its effect on pelvic pain. In a retrospective sample of 71 women undergoing conservative resection of endometriosis by way of laparotomy, 35 (50%) who also had presacral neurectomy enjoyed significantly greater improvement in both dysmenorrhea and dyspareunia, with 75% to 95% obtaining improvement. Two subsequent retrospective reports noted that similar percentages (about 75%) of women obtained pain relief after endometriosis surgery that included presacral neurectomy, compared with about 25% who obtained relief without neurectomy.

Two studies on the treatment of presacral neurectomy as adjunctive therapy along with conservative resection for stage III–IV endometriosis reached different conclusions about the additive value of presacral neurectomy. Tjaden and associates performed conservative resection by way of laparotomy and randomized eight women to receive or not receive presacral neurectomy. All the neurectomized women improved dramatically, whereas the others did not. The institutional review board mandated stopping the study because statistical significance had been reached. The authors then reported an open clinical series in which 15 of 17 women improved substantially after conservative resection with presacral neurectomy. Candiani and colleagues reached a different conclusion after randomizing 71 women to receive or not receive presacral neurectomy along with conservative resection of advanced endometriosis. They found that central dysmenorrhea improved slightly more in neurectomized women, but daily pain and dyspareunia were not improved by adding presacral neurectomy to the procedure. The literature is therefore inconclusive regarding the value of the neurectomy procedure.

Laparoscopic treatment of even severe endometriosis has a growing number of advocates. Again, the focus has been on fertility rates, but one prospective report notes prolonged pain relief in two thirds of patients. The ability to perform presacral neurectomy by way of laparoscopy should not provoke wide adoption of the procedure without careful consideration of these data.

An ovarian remnant should be removed if it is persistently symptomatic despite all reasonable attempts at medical suppression and if menopause cannot be expected in the patient's near future. Whether performed by laparoscopy or laparotomy, the dissection should be detailed and should include all the peritoneum surrounding the mass. The ureter and pelvic sidewall vessels should be exposed and carefully freed from the specimen. When a GnRH agonist has been used preoperatively for symptom control or to distinguish the relative contributions made by the remnant and other pelvic pathology, such as adhesions, the remnant tissue may become so small as to make it difficult to identify. Hence, if a palpable (or ultrasonically visible) mass disappears after GnRH agonist treatment, it may be wise to allow time for it to regrow before pursuing surgical excision. When the remnant is small, some surgeons have stimulated the remnant with clomiphene citrate to make it easier to find.

Finally, the peritoneal windows syndrome must be mentioned. Openings in the peritoneum covering the posterior broad ligament and the cul-de-sac of Douglas, or peritoneal "windows," have been noted since the 1950s and were associated with endometriosis by Chatman. Excision and closure of the windows have been anecdotally reported, but the value of these operations in treating pain associated with the disease remains to be demonstrated. It is my practice to excise the peritoneum involved with the window, but not to stitch the area closed. Microscopic endometriosis is found in many cases.

Alternative Treatments

Biofeedback, transcutaneous electric nerve stimulation units, relaxation training, and individual and couples counseling all have their appropriate roles in individual cases, but none is so clearly applicable or effective that its automatic use is supported in cases of CPP. In keeping with the approach outlined in the earlier discussion of medications, problems requiring counseling should be addressed but should be treated as issues separate from the discussion of appropriate surgical approaches. Cause-and-effect relations are difficult to demonstrate even in retrospect when psychologic assistance works.

Management Overview

The most effective clinical approach requires simultaneous treatment of as many factors as possible: anatomic, musculoskeletal, functional bowel and bladder, psychologic, and so forth. Patient and physician must contract for the long term and work from a rehabilitation perspective, rather than hope that the latest single addition to the treatment will prove to be the answer. The physician, to prevent frustration and feelings of defeat, must often play the role of helping to manage and relieve the pain while helping to maximize function, even when pain persists. To the surgically trained gynecologist who prefers a clear-cut single answer to a clinical problem, this can be the most difficult part of dealing with the problem of CPP.

THE EVOLUTION OF A CHRONIC PAIN SYNDROME

As is apparent from this discussion, CPP is a heterogeneous problem, not a single diagnosis, and no single etiologic hypothesis is clearly supported. Most of the hypotheses reviewed here have some credible evidence supporting them; none have been sufficiently validated.

Some patients appear to have a pure version of one or the other of the syndromes described, whereas many others present with several or many simultaneously. Psychologic and neurologic mechanisms are proposed here to explain how the evolution of chronic pain may occur, regardless of the particular tissue damage or functional disorder that may first have provided nociceptive stimuli. We suggest the following elements (Fig. 29.1): biologic events sufficient to initiate nociception, alterations of lifestyles and relations over time, recruitment of neighboring organ systems, anxiety and affective disorders, and a circular interaction (vicious cycle) among these elements.

Biologic Events Sufficient to Initiate Nociception

Sexually transmitted diseases, endometriosis, recurrent bladder and vaginal infections, primary or secondary functional dyspareunia, alterations of bowel habit, muscular dysfunction, pelvic congestion, and gynecologic or other abdominal surgeries (Table 29.1) may contribute individually or in combination.

Alteration of Lifestyle and Relations

Physical activities at home and recreational pursuits can suffer. Believing that rest usually helps in the treatment of most causes of acute pain, the patient may assume that the same applies to chronic pain and may thus restrict herself more than actual discomfort dictates. Family members start to regard the patient as sick and leave her out of many activities, thus reducing her roles within the family structure. With time, concern for and discussion of her pain can become the family's major pattern of communication with the pain victim. If sexual intimacy has been the major means of emotional sharing and smoothing over of differences, and if this intimacy is reduced, then the altered pattern of interactions may take hold more quickly.

Anxiety and Affective Disorders

Depression can occur as a cumulative result of the disability suffered, or the pain can bring on an episode of depression in a patient already biologically vulnerable. The observation most relevant here is that pain patients with a family history of depression can derive the most benefit from tricyclic antidepressants.

The Vicious Cycle

Diminished activity, altered family roles and social supports, anxiety, and affective disturbances can influence nociception by a variety of central pathways, ultimately altering spinal cord "gating" of nociceptive signals. Cognitions about the pain can play an additional role.

Several important modifying influences can be present in addition to these major pathways (Fig. 29.2). Incest and other forms of sexual abuse have attracted the most attention as possible forerunners of CPP. However, CPP is clearly not a unique or specific sequel to sexual abuse, and a large proportion of CPP patients have not been abused in this manner. Victims of sexual abuse have many negative emotional sequelae; pain problems often occur after abuse, but they are not necessarily directly caused by the abuse.

Sexual abuse perpetrated by a family member is a clear indication of a psychologically detrimental environment of rearing that might have led to disturbances in character and personality

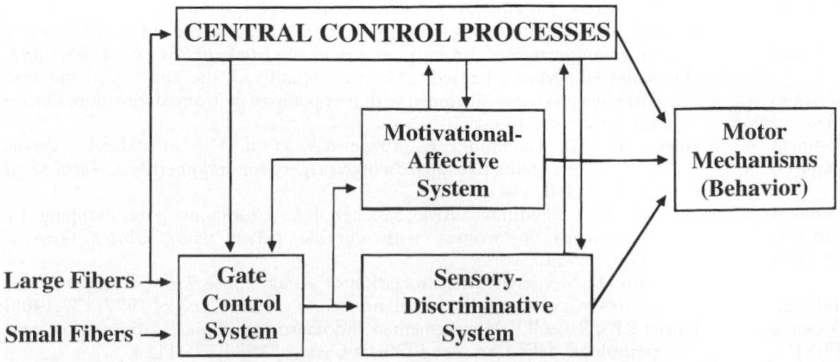

FIGURE 29.1. The gate control theory of pain perception.

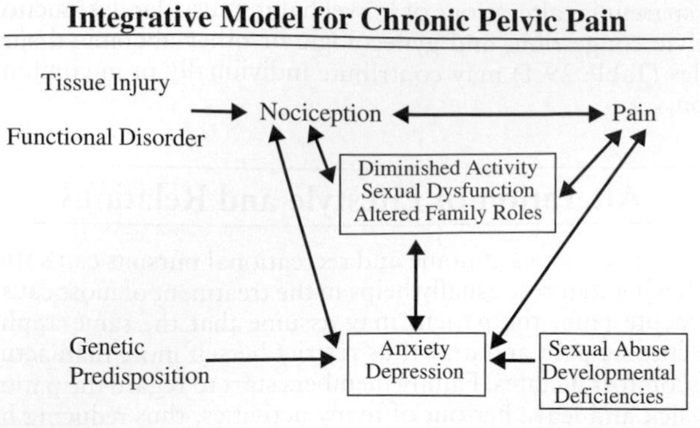

FIGURE 29.2. An integrative model for chronic pelvic pain, including elements of gate control theory, cognitive-behavioral theory, and the operant conditioning model.

development perhaps equal in importance to the terrible trauma of the abuse itself. Learning more about the factors that can mitigate the impact of sexual abuse in general will facilitate our understanding of the psychologic vulnerabilities that can make a particular person more susceptible to development of CPP or other chronic pain disorders.

A genetic predisposition to depression also allows the vicious cycle to become easily established and strengthened over time. Antidepressant medications play an important role in the overall therapeutic plan in such cases. A relatively new area of research in pain is dealing with possible genetically determined variations in central neurotransmitter processes that may predispose to the development of pain syndromes.

Several authors have suggested that the concept of perceived control best explains the development of affective changes accompanying chronic pain, regardless of the location of the pain. The individual who sees herself as having little control over the physical and emotional events affecting her may be most vulnerable to development of a CPS. It may be reasonable to consider this variable as a culmination of the effects of affective change, activity, family roles, sexual dysfunction, and previous victimization experiences.

The longer that pain has been a part of the person's life, and the more psychologic vulnerabilities she carries forward to the present, the less likely it is that any treatment of the tissue damage itself will be effective in relieving pain and restoring physical and emotional function. However, as treatment studies show, the organic contribution to chronic pain can seldom be dismissed entirely. The more difficult task is the selection of an efficient and cost-effective combination of treatment approaches aimed at the most important factors acting in the present.

BEST SURGICAL PRACTICES

- A complete medical and psychosocial history, as well as a pain-oriented physical and pelvic examination, should be completed before diagnostic laparoscopy is performed.
- Laparoscopic pain mapping under conscious sedation is sometimes useful for evaluating the contributions to pain made by the various pelvic organs.
- For endometriosis that extends beyond the superficial peritoneum, excision may be more effective than ablation by various energy sources.
- Neuropathic and musculoskeletal components of chronic pelvic pain often require treatment both before and after appropriate pelvic surgery.
- Whenever possible, a minimally invasive (laparoscopic) approach is especially appropriate for chronic pain patients.

Bibliography

Applegate WV. Abdominal cutaneous nerve entrapment syndrome. *Surgery* 1972;71:188.

Barbot J, Parent B, Dubuisson JB, et al. A clinical study of the CO_2 laser and electrosurgery for adhesiolysis in 172 cases followed by early second-look laparoscopy. *Fertil Steril* 1987;48:140.

Beard RW, Belsey EM, Lieberman BA, et al. Pelvic pain in women. *Am J Obstet Gynecol* 1977;128:566.

Beard RW, Highman JH, Pearce S, et al. Diagnosis of pelvic varicosities in women with chronic pelvic pain. *Lancet* 1984;2:946.

Candiani GB, Fedele L, Vercellini P, et al. Presacral neurectomy for the treatment of pelvic pain associated with endometriosis: a controlled study. *Am J Obstet Gynecol* 1992;167:100.

Carlson KJ, Miller BA, Fowler FJ. The Maine Women's Health Study: II. Outcomes of nonsurgical management of leiomyomas, abnormal bleeding, and chronic pelvic pain. *Obstet Gynecol* 1994;83:566.

Castelnuovo-Tedesco P, Krout BM. Psychosomatic aspects of chronic pelvic pain. *Int J Psychiatry Med* 1970;1:109.

Chan CLK, Wood C. Pelvic adhesiolysis: the assessment of symptom relief by 100 patients. *Aust N Z J Obstet Gynaecol* 1985;25:295.

Chatman DL, Zbella EA. Pelvic peritoneal defects and endometriosis: further observations. *Fertil Steril* 1986;46:711.

Crisson JE, Keefe FJ. The relationship of locus of control to pain coping strategies and psychological distress in chronic pain patients. *Pain* 1988;35:147.

Diamond MP, Daniell JF, Johns DA, et al. Postoperative adhesion development after operative laparoscopy: evaluation at early second-look procedures. *Fertil Steril* 1991;55:700.

Diamond MP, Daniell JF, Martin DC, et al. Tubal patency and pelvic adhesions at early second-look laparoscopy following intra-abdominal use of the carbon dioxide laser: initial report of the Intra-abdominal Laser Study Group. *Fertil Steril* 1984;42:717.

Dicker RC, Greenspan JR, Straus LT, et al. Complications of abdominal and vaginal hysterectomy among women of reproductive age in the United States: the collaborative review of sterilization. *Am J Obstet Gynecol* 1982;144:841.

Duncan CH, Taylor HC. A psychosomatic study of pelvic congestion. *Am J Obstet Gynecol* 1952;64:1.

Farquhar CM, Rogers V, Franks S, et al. A randomized controlled trial of medroxyprogesterone acetate and psychotherapy for the treatment of pelvic congestion. *BJOG* 1989;96:1153.

Fedele L, Parazzini F, Bianchi S, et al. Stage and localization of pelvic endometriosis and pain. *Fertil Steril* 1990;53:155.

Fernandez F, Adams F, Holmes VF. Analgesic effect of alprazolam in patients with chronic, organic pain of malignant origin. *J Clin Psychopharmacol* 1987;7:167.

Fordyce WE. *Behavioral methods of control of chronic pain and illness*. St. Louis: CV Mosby, 1976.

Garcia C-R, David SS. Pelvic endometriosis: infertility and pelvic pain. *Am J Obstet Gynecol* 1977;129:740.

Gidro-Frank L, Gordon I, Taylor HC. Pelvic pain and female identity: a survey of emotional factors in 40 patients. *Am J Obstet Gynecol* 1960;79:1184.

Gross R, Doerr H, Caldirola D, et al. Borderline syndrome and incest in chronic pelvic pain patients. *Int J Psychiatry Med* 1980/81;10:79.

Haber J, Roos C. Effects of spouse abuse and/or sexual abuse in the development and maintenance of chronic pain in women. *Adv Pain Res Ther* 1985;9:889.

Hartmann KE, Ma C, Lamvu GM, et al. Quality of life and sexual function after hysterectomy in women with preoperative pain and depression. *Obstet Gynecol* 2004;104(4):701.

Hornstein MD, Hemmings R, Yuzpe AA, et al. Use of nafarelin versus placebo after reductive laparoscopic surgery for endometriosis. *Fertil Steril* 1997;68:860.

Howard FM, El-Minawi AM, Sanchez RA. Conscious pain mapping by laparoscopy in women with chronic pelvic pain. *Obstet Gynecol* 2000;96:934.

Jamieson DJ, Steege JF. The association of sexual abuse with pelvic pain complaints in a primary care population. *Am J Obstet Gynecol* 1997; 177:1408.

Jansen RPS, Russell P. Nonpigmented endometriosis: clinical, laparoscopic, and pathologic definition. *Am J Obstet Gynecol* 1986;155:1154.

Keye WR, Hansen LW, Astin M, et al. Argon laser therapy of endometriosis: a review of 92 consecutive patients. *Fertil Steril* 1987;47:208.

Kjerulff KH, Langenberg PW, Rhodes JC, et al. Effectiveness of hysterectomy. *Obstet Gynecol* 2000;95:319.

Kresch AJ, Seifer DB, Sachs LB, et al. Laparoscopy in 100 women with chronic pelvic pain. *Obstet Gynecol* 1984;64:672.

Lamvu G, Robinson B, Zolnoun D, et al. Vaginal apex revision: a treatment option for vaginal apex pain. *Obstet Gynecol* 2004;104(6):1340.

Lee RB, Stone K, Magelssen D, et al. Presacral neurectomy for chronic pelvic pain. *Obstet Gynecol* 1986;68:517.

Ling FW, for the Pelvic Pain Study Group. Randomized controlled trial of depot leuprolide in patients with chronic pelvic pain and clinically suspected endometriosis. *Obstet Gynecol* 1999;93:51.

Luciano AA, Maier DB, Koch EL, et al. A comparative study of postoperative adhesions following laser surgery by laparoscopy versus laparotomy in the rabbit model. *Obstet Gynecol* 1989;75:220.

Mathias JR, Clench MH, Roberts PH, et al. Serum relaxin levels detected in women with functional bowel disease and reduced by leuprolide acetate (LA) therapy. *Gastroenterology* 1993;104[Suppl 4]:A549.

Mattingly RF, Thompson JD. Leiomyomata uteri and abdominal hysterectomy for benign disease. In: *Te Linde's operative gynecology*. 6th ed. Philadelphia: JB Lippincott; 1985:227.

Melzack R. From the gate to the neuromatrix. *Pain* 1999;82[Suppl 6]:121.

Melzack R. Neurophysiologic foundations of pain. In: Sternbach RA, ed. *The psychology of pain*. New York: Raven Press, 1986:1.

Melzack R, Wall PD. Pain mechanisms: a new theory. *Science* 1965;150:971.

Morrison J. Childhood sexual histories of women with somatization disorder. *Am J Psychiatry* 1989;146:239.

Nezhat CR, Nezhat FR, Metzger DA, et al. Adhesion reformation after reproductive surgery by videolaseroscopy. *Fertil Steril* 1990;53:1008.

Olive DL. Endometriosis. *N Engl J Med* 1993;328:1759.

O'Shaughnessy A, Check JH, Nowroozi K, et al. CA-125 levels measured in different phases of the menstrual cycle in screening for endometriosis. *Obstet Gynecol* 1993;81:99.

Portenoy RK, Foley KM. Chronic use of opioid analgesics in non-malignant pain: report of 38 cases. *Pain* 1986;25:171.

Prentice A, Deary AJ, Bland E. Progestins and anti-progestagens for pain associated with endometriosis (Cochrane Review). In: *The Cochrane Library, Issue 2*. Oxford: Update Software, 2001.

Prentice A, Deary AJ, Goldbeck-Wood S, et al. Gonadotropin-releasing hormone analogues for pain associated with endometriosis (Cochrane Review). In: *The Cochrane Library, Issue 2*. Oxford: Update Software, 2001.

Rapkin AJ, Kames LD, Darke LL, et al. History of physical and sexual abuse in women with chronic pain. *Obstet Gynecol* 1990;76:92.

Raskin DE. Diagnosis in patients with chronic pelvic pain [Letter]. *Am J Psychiatry* 1984;141:824.

Redwine DB. Conservative laparoscopic excision of endometriosis by sharp dissection: life table analysis of reoperation and persistent or recurrent disease. *Fertil Steril* 1991;56:628.

Reiter RC. Occult somatic pathology in women with chronic pelvic pain. *Clin Obstet Gynecol* 1990;33:154.

Reiter RC, Gambone JC. Demographic and historic variables in women with idiopathic chronic pelvic pain. *Obstet Gynecol* 1990;75:428.

Rudy TE, Kerns RD, Turk DC. Chronic pain and depression: toward a cognitive-behavioral mediation model. *Pain* 1988;35:129.

Selak V, Farquhar C, Prentice A, et al. Danazol for pelvic pain associated with endometriosis (Cochrane Review). In: *The Cochrane Library, Issue 2*. Oxford: Update Software, 2001.

Simons DG, Travell J. Myofascial trigger points: a possible explanation. *Pain* 1981;10:100.

Sinaki M, Merritt JL, Stillwell GK. Tension myalgia of the pelvic floor. *Mayo Clin Proc* 1977;52:717.

Slocumb J. Neurological factors in chronic pelvic pain: trigger points and the abdominal pelvic pain syndrome. *Am J Obstet Gynecol* 1984;149:536.

Slocumb JC, Kellner R, Rosenfeld RC, et al. Anxiety and depression in patients with the abdominal pelvic pain syndrome. *Gen Hosp Psychiatry* 1989;11:48.

Steege JF. Dyspareunia and vaginismus. *Clin Obstet Gynecol* 1984;27:750.

Steege JF. Ovarian remnant syndrome. *Obstet Gynecol* 1987;70:64.

Steege JF, Metzger DA, Levy BS. *Chronic pelvic pain: an integrated approach*. Philadelphia: WB Saunders, 1998.

Steege JF, Stout AL. Resolution of chronic pelvic pain following laparoscopic adhesiolysis. *Am J Obstet Gynecol* 1991;165:278.

Steege JF, Stout AL, Somkuti SG. Chronic pelvic pain: toward an integrative model. *Obstet Gynecol Surv* 1993;48:95.

Stout AL, Steege JF. *Psychosocial and behavioral self-reports of chronic pelvic pain patients*. Presented at the meeting of the American Society for Psychosomatic Obstetrics and Gynecology, Houston, TX, March 1991.

Stout AL, Steege JF, Dodson WC, et al. Relationship of laparoscopic findings to self-report of pelvic pain. *Am J Obstet Gynecol* 1991;164:73.

Stovall TG, Ling FW, Crawford DA. Hysterectomy for chronic pelvic pain of presumed uterine etiology. *Obstet Gynecol* 1990;75:676.

Summitt RL, Ling FW. Urethral syndrome presenting as chronic pelvic pain. *J Psychosom Obstet Gynaecol* 1991;12(Suppl):77.

Sutton CJ, Ewen SP, Whitelaw N, et al. Prospective, randomized, double blind controlled trial of laser laparoscopy in the treatment of pelvic pain associated with minimal, mild, and moderate endometriosis. *Fertil Steril* 1994;62:696.

Sutton C, MacDonald R. Laser laparoscopic adhesiolysis. *J Gynecol Surg* 1990;6:155.

Sutton CJ, Pooley AS, Ewen SP, et al. Follow-up report on a randomized, controlled trial of laser laparoscopy in the treatment of pelvic pain associated with minimal to moderate endometriosis. *Fertil Steril* 1997;68:1070.

Tjaden B, Schlaff WD, Kimball A, et al. The efficacy of presacral neurectomy for the relief of midline dysmenorrhea. *Obstet Gynecol* 1990;76:89.

Tulandi T. Adhesion reformation after reproductive surgery with and without the carbon dioxide laser. *Fertil Steril* 1987;47:704.

Tulandi T. Salpingo-ovariolysis: a comparison between laser surgery and electrosurgery. *Fertil Steril* 1986;45:489.

Vercellini P, Trespidi L, Colombo A, et al. A gonadotropin-releasing hormone agonist versus a low-dose oral contraceptive for pelvic pain with endometriosis. *Fertil Steril* 1993;60:75.

Walker EW, Katon W, Harrop-Griffiths J, et al. Relationship of chronic pelvic pain to psychiatric diagnoses and childhood sexual abuse. *Am J Psychiatry* 1988;145:75.

Walters MD. Definitive surgery. In: Schenken RS, ed. *Endometriosis: contemporary concepts in clinical management*. Philadelphia: JB Lippincott, 1989: 267.

Winkel CA, Bray M. Treatment of women with endometriosis using excision alone, ablation alone, or ablation in combination with leuprolide acetate. Proceedings of the 5th World Congress on Endometriosis, Yokahama, Japan, 1996:55.

CHAPTER 30 ■ PELVIC INFLAMMATORY DISEASE

MARK G. MARTENS

DEFINITIONS

Bacterial vaginosis (BV)—A vaginal condition demonstrated by a replacement of the normal lactobacillus predominant vaginal flora with a mixture of facultative and obligate anaerobes, mycoplasma, and other species, resulting in a malodorous discharge. The presence of *Gardnerella vaginalis* without symptoms is not synonymous with BV.

Colpotomy—Incision into and through the vaginal epithelium into a cavity (often abscess or pelvic/abdominal cavity).

Febrile morbidity—Temperature equal to or greater than 100.4°F or 38°C on two separate occasions (greater than 4 hours apart), starting 24 hours after the initiating event.

Fever—Temperature equal to or greater than 99.6°F or 37.5°C.

Lower genital tract infection (LGTI)—An alternative term used to describe infection limited to the cervix and/or vulva and vagina.

Mollicutes—Class of organisms that includes *Chlamydia, Mycoplasma, Ureaplasma,* and other species.

Outpatient therapy—Previously synonymous with oral therapy; however, the term now includes oral, ambulatory intravenous, or intermittent injectable therapies.

Parenteral therapy—Usually denotes intravenous (antibiotic) therapy, but not necessarily given while hospitalized.

Pelvic inflammatory disease (PID)—A general term used to refer to infection and inflammation of the upper genital tract in women.

Phlegmon—A massive infiltration of inflammatory cells into infected soft tissue resulting not in an abscess, but a "woody induration" sensation upon examination/palpation.

Prevotella—Newly named genus that now includes several species formerly called Bacteroides (e.g., *Bacteroides bivia*).

Salpingitis—Infection/inflammation of one or both of the fallopian tubes (often incorrectly used as an equivalent to all PID).

Tuboovarian abscess (TOA)—A term used to describe an abscess incorporating the fallopian tube and ovary.

Upper genital tract infection (UGTI)—A more descriptive term used alternatively to PID.

Pelvic inflammatory disease (PID) is one of the most serious infections facing women today. According to Velebil and colleagues, it is the most common gynecologic reason for hospitalization and emergency department visits in the United States each year. Untreated or unsuccessfully treated women may suffer life-threatening consequences, and even adequately treated women are at much higher risk for potentially serious sequelae. PID is a spectrum of diseases initially involving the cervix, uterus, and fallopian tubes. Acute PID, the acute clinical syndrome, is most often attributed to an ascending spread of microorganisms from the vagina and endocervix to the endometrium, fallopian tubes, and contiguous structures. The terms *acute PID* and *acute salpingitis* are often used interchangeably, but PID is not limited to tubal infection only. A more descriptive term to differentiate the severity and extent of various forms of PID was introduced by Hemsell and colleagues: *upper genital tract infection (UGTI)*. This is differentiated from *lower genital tract infection (LGTI)* because response to treatment appears to be different in these two entities. PID was previously categorized as inpatient or outpatient treatment groups, which sometimes did not accurately reflect the severity of illness.

Sexually transmitted diseases (STDs) have been reported at epidemic proportions in the United States, with the Centers for Disease Control and Prevention (CDC) estimating 19 million new infections each year. The incidence of chlamydia infections increased almost 6%, with 929,000 cases reported and 2.8 million new cases suspected annually. Gonorrhea incidence has decreased 70% since 1975, but is still estimated to occur in more than 60,000 women each year in the United States. For women, acute PID is the most common and important complication of STDs. Bell and Holmes in the 1980s estimated that 1 million women a year were treated for acute salpingitis in the United States, but recent estimates by Sutton and colleagues estimated a decrease in cases of PID to less than 800,000 per year and a 68% decrease in hospitalized PID from 1995 to 2001. About 250,000 to 300,000 women are hospitalized each year with a diagnosis of salpingitis or PID. The disease generates nearly 2.5 million visits to physicians, and an estimated 150,000 surgical procedures are performed for complications every year. According to Sutton and colleagues, the direct and indirect costs of PID and its sequelae now total $2 billion and $10 billion in the United States, respectively. In terms of overall incidence, acute PID occurs in about 1% to 2% of young, sexually active women each year. PID is the most common serious bacterial infection in women age 16 to 25 years, and the resultant morbidity exceeds that produced by all other infections combined for this age group.

ETIOLOGY

Within certain geographic areas or populations, *Neisseria gonorrhoeae* is a common cause of PID; however, most cases of acute PID are the result of a polymicrobial infection caused by organisms ascending from the vagina and cervix to infect the lining of the endometrium and fallopian tube. Approximately 85% of cases are natural, noniatrogenic occurring infections in sexually active women of reproductive age. The remaining 15% of infections occur after procedures that break the cervical mucous barrier, such as placement of an intrauterine device (IUD), endometrial biopsy, or uterine curettage, which allow vaginal flora to infect the upper genital tract.

In the United States, nontuberculous acute PID was traditionally separated into gonococcal and nongonococcal disease, depending on the isolation of *N. gonorrhoeae* from the endocervix. A variety of organisms can be isolated from the endocervix; therefore, it is difficult to determine which of these organisms cause PID and which are normal cervicovaginal flora and only present as colonizers in the upper genital tract at time of diagnosis. While upper genital tract organisms are probably more indicative of the causative organisms, they are often difficult to obtain without suspecting endocervical contamination during the diagnostic procedure. Bacterial organisms cultured directly from tubal fluid may commonly include *N. gonorrhoeae, Chlamydia trachomatis,* endogenous aerobic and anaerobic bacteria, and genital *Mycoplasma* species. Laparoscopic studies have demonstrated a correlation of no more than 50% between endocervical and tubal cultures, but the presence of *N. gonorrhoeae* is usually considered an important causative factor. However, endocervical gonorrhea does not necessarily indicate its sole pathogenic nature in all cases. Direct fallopian tube cultures have demonstrated that tubal infections are often polymicrobial. The type and number of species vary depending on the stage of the disease. Gonorrhea, for example, is often cultured from the cervix during the first 24 to 48 hours of the disease but is often absent later. Similarly, fewer organisms are cultured late in the disease, and anaerobic bacteria such as *Prevotella, Bacteroides, Peptococcus,* and *Peptostreptococcus* species tend to predominate. Whether these anaerobes play a causative role or increase in number and frequency as a result of the inflammatory response is uncertain. Sweet has summarized the literature by stating that in approximately one third of women with PID, *N. gonorrhoeae* is the only organism recovered by direct tubal or cul-de-sac culture. One third have a culture positive for *N. gonorrhoeae* plus a mixture of endogenous aerobic and anaerobic flora, and the remaining one third have only aerobic and anaerobic organisms. Chow and colleagues and Monif and colleagues have postulated that the gonococcus may initiate acute PID and produce tissue damage. This damage changes the local environment, which in turn allows anaerobic and aerobic organisms from the vaginal and cervical flora to invade the upper genital tract. Both Eschenbach and Sweet have suggested that not all PID follows gonococcal infection and that acute PID initially may also have a polymicrobial etiology.

According to Sweet and Gibbs, about 20% of all women with salpingitis have tubal cultures positive for *C. trachomatis. N. gonorrhoeae* and *C. trachomatis* are found in the same individual 25% to 40% of the time. Scandinavian studies by Eilard and coworkers have reported the recovery of *C. trachomatis* from the cervix in 22% to 47% of women with acute PID. *C. trachomatis* by itself produces a mild form of salpingitis with an insidious onset. In contrast to gonorrhea, *Chlamydia* can remain in the fallopian tubes for months or years after initial colonization of the upper genital tract. Svensson and colleagues found that women with *C. trachomatis* infection at laparoscopy had the most severe fallopian tube involvement, probably because of its clinically silent or minimally symptomatic nature, which results in difficult or delayed diagnosis and therefore delayed or absent treatment. The two major sequelae of acute PID are tubal infertility and ectopic pregnancy. These have been strongly associated with prior chlamydial infection as a consequence of intratubal and peritubal adhesions.

Although *C. trachomatis* is generally believed to be one of the most common causes of PID, along with *N. gonorrhoeae,* its etiologic role is very different. *N. gonorrhoeae* is a Gram-negative diplococcus with rapid growth that is due to a rapid cycle of about 20 to 40 minutes to divide. This results in a logarithmic increase in the number of organisms once *N. gonorrhoeae* reaches an area such as the endometrium or fallopian tube, where growth is relatively unimpeded. This rapid increase in the number of Gram-negative bacteria usually results in a rapid and intense inflammatory response by the woman's host defenses. The response to this rapid bacterial growth is proliferation and aggregation of white blood cells and their inflammatory products. Migration of this bacterial and leukocytic mixture through the fallopian tube to the ovary and peritoneal cavity, and back to the cervix and vagina, causes the symptoms that are pathognomonic of acute PID.

C. trachomatis, however, is a slow-growing intracellular organism. Its lack of mitochondria results in its obligatory intracellular existence and also causes its growth cycle to be extremely slow compared with *N. gonorrhoeae* and nonintracellular microorganisms. The growth cycle of *Chlamydia* is 48 to 72 hours; therefore, several weeks to months are required for the growth to reach numbers sufficient to cause clinical symptoms, if at all. Its slow growth does not induce a rapid or violent inflammatory response. This explains the slow and insidious nature of the symptoms of acute *C. trachomatis* infections. However, because of its intracellular growth cycle, the release of the elementary bodies (its infectious vehicle) occurs by rupture of the cell that it has invaded. The repeated occurrence of elementary body infection of susceptible cells—and their subsequent destruction by rupture—is the major mechanism by which *C. trachomatis* causes disease in acute pelvic infections. Also, because of its slow growth and lack of acute inflammatory response and clinical symptoms, treatment is often delayed or not started at all, adding to the extended tissue destruction and PID sequelae.

The lack of acute symptoms does not lessen the importance of *Chlamydia* as a PID pathogen. Not only does the tissue destruction result in severe complications such as ectopic pregnancy and infertility, but also the tissue damage provides fertile ground for the growth of secondarily infecting aerobic and anaerobic bacteria. This necrotic tissue is an excellent growth medium, and the epithelial damage enhances the breakdown of the surface defense mechanisms. The importance of *Chlamydia* was documented during the 1980s when treatment of acute PID was initially believed to be successfully accomplished with regimens not active against *C. trachomatis.* However, although success was evident with short-term follow-up, long-term follow-up demonstrated that treatment of *C. trachomatis* was necessary. PID regimens without *Chlamydia* coverage resulted in an increased incidence of long-term complications such as abscesses and chronic pelvic pain, with resultant increased surgical intervention. Therefore, modern treatment of PID includes *C. trachomatis* coverage, even though this organism may not be the cause of the acute symptoms.

Nongonococcal infections are believed to be the result of acute bacterial infections or possibly a preceding or previously treated *C. trachomatis* UGTI. This is confirmed by the high incidence of *Chlamydia* antibodies in patients with acute PID, ectopic pregnancy, and infertility.

In addition to *N. gonorrhoeae, Chlamydia,* and aerobic and anaerobic bacteria, other microorganisms have been implicated as etiologic agents in acute salpingitis. Bacterial vaginosis–related organisms such as *Gardnerella, Mycoplasma hominis,* and *Ureaplasma urealyticum* have also been suggested as causal agents in acute salpingitis by Ness and colleagues (2005). However, their role remains controversial, and this study contradicts a study from the previous year by a similar group of investigators. Cervical cultures positive for both *M. hominis* and *U. urealyticum* have been recovered from women with PID. However, the rate of isolation can be as high as 75%, which is not statistically different from that of women who are sexually active but without PID (baseline rate of about 50%), as found by Lemeke and Lsonka. However, evidence is recently accumulating that *Mycoplasma genitalium* may play a role in PID, with Ross of Great Britain calling for the development of reliable tests for its identification and susceptibility.

RISK FACTORS

Several factors that predispose to the development of acute PID have been identified. Risk factors are important considerations in both the clinical management and prevention of UGTIs. There is a strong correlation between exposure to STDs and PID. In the United States, recent studies have confirmed this association with the recovery of *N. gonorrhoeae* or *C. trachomatis* in about 50% of patients hospitalized with acute PID. Age at first intercourse, frequency of intercourse, number of sexual partners, and marital status are all associated with the frequency of exposure to STDs and thus are associated with PID. Women with multiple partners have an increased risk (four to six times normal) for development of acute salpingitis, compared with women who have monogamous sexual relations. Recently, Ness and colleagues have demonstrated the validity of a *Chlamydia* risk factor scoring system for the prediction of 74% of PID. Significant factors included age at first sex, cervicitis, history of PID, family income, smoking, medroxyprogesterone use, and sex with menses.

The incidence of acute PID decreases with advancing age. Adolescent girls are at significant risk for development of acute salpingitis. Westrom reported that nearly 70% of women with PID were younger than 25 years of age, 33% experienced their first infection before the age of 19, and 75% were nulliparous. The risk for development of acute PID in a sexually active adolescent female patient was 1:8, whereas the risk was 1:80 for a sexually active woman 24 years of age or older. Several reasons have been suggested for this increased risk. The two microorganisms most commonly considered to be the inciting agents in cases of PID, *N. gonorrhoeae* and *C. trachomatis,* have a predilection for columnar epithelium. As suggested by Schaefer and by Sweet and colleagues, cervical columnar epithelium is exposed to a greater extent in younger individuals and recedes into the cervical canal with increasing age.

Clinical and laboratory studies have documented that the use of contraceptives changes the relative risk for development of PID. Multiple case-controlled studies have shown an increased risk of acute PID in women who wear an IUD. It has been estimated that IUD users have a threefold to fivefold increased risk for development of acute PID. In a report by Tatum and colleagues of animal model investigations, it was suggested that multifilament strings may be a major contributing factor in the increased risk of PID. Barrier methods of contraception (condoms, diaphragms, and spermicidal preparations) are effective both as mechanical obstructive devices and as chemical barriers. A nearly 60% decrease in the risk of PID has been demonstrated among women using a barrier method of contraception. Recently, Ness and colleagues found a 30% to 60% decrease in recurrent PID in women using condoms consistently.

Oral contraceptives have also been shown to reduce the risk of acute PID. The mechanism for such protection remains speculative. The thicker cervical mucus produced by the progestin component of oral contraceptives is believed to inhibit sperm and accompanying bacteria penetration into the upper genital tract. The decrease in duration of menstrual flow accompanying oral contraceptive use theoretically creates a shorter interval for bacterial colonization. Svensson and coworkers reported that in addition to protecting against PID, the use of oral contraceptive pills was associated with a better prognosis for future fertility than was seen in women with acute PID using other contraceptive methods or no contraceptive methods. The pill's ability to inhibit ovulation presumably helps from providing a nidus for tuboovarian abscess formation.

Surgical procedures of the female genital tract also place the patient at risk for PID. About 15% of pelvic infections occur after procedures that break the cervical mucous barrier, allowing for colonization of the upper genital tract. Eschenbach and Holmes reported that these procedures include endometrial biopsy, curettage, IUD insertion, hysteroscopy, and hysterosalpingography. The incidence of UGTI associated with first-trimester abortions is about 1 in 200 cases. Recent practice has emphasized the use of prophylactic antibiotics in high-risk cases to attempt to decrease the incidence of iatrogenic acute PID. Two randomized trials have indicated that the treatment of bacterial vaginosis (BV) with metronidazole substantially reduced postabortion PID (Jackson and Luton and Dunstable Hospital).

Acute salpingitis occurring in a woman with a previous tubal ligation was once believed to be rare. Phillips and D'Abling reported that acute PID developed in the proximal stump of previously ligated fallopian tubes in 1 of 450 women hospitalized for acute salpingitis. However, many cases may be undiagnosed because of the absence of peritoneal signs.

Previous acute PID is also a risk factor for future episodes of the disease. Another acute tubal infection develops in about 25% of women who have had acute PID. The exact mechanism for this increased susceptibility has not been determined, but it may be loss of the natural protective mechanisms of the fallopian tube lining against microorganisms. This increased risk may be related to the sexual habits of the woman involved, such as reinfection from an untreated male partner or genital tract damage from the initial infection. Eschenbach has documented that more than 80% of male contacts are not treated.

DIAGNOSIS

Acute PID presents with a broad spectrum of clinical symptoms. The differential diagnosis of acute PID includes acute appendicitis, endometriosis, torsion or rupture of an adnexal mass, ectopic pregnancy, and LGTI.

Common clinical manifestations include lower abdominal pain, cervical motion tenderness, and adnexal tenderness and may include fever, cervical discharge, and leukocytosis. Historically, the diagnosis of acute PID was not established unless the patient had the triad of lower abdominal and pelvic pain, fever, and leukocytosis.

Jacobson and Westrom have shown that all three are present in only 15% to 30% of actual PID cases. In addition, about 50% of patients initially present with a normal temperature and white blood cell (WBC) count. Pain in the lower abdomen and pelvis is by far the most common symptom of acute PID. It occurs in more than 90% of patients at initial presentation. The pain is usually described as constant and dull and is accentuated by motion and sexual activity. Generally, the pain is of recent onset, usually less than 7 days. About 75% of patients with PID have an associated endocervical infection and coexistent purulent vaginal discharge. Nausea and vomiting are comparably late symptoms in the course of the disease. Abnormal vaginal bleeding, especially menorrhagia, or spotting, is noted in about 40% of patients. The CDC has established the criteria for making the diagnosis of salpingitis based on clinical grounds. The most recent update includes that only signs

TABLE 30.1

CRITERIA FOR THE DIAGNOSIS OF ACUTE SALPINGITIS

Empirical treatment of PID should be initiated in sexually active young women and other women at risk for STDs if they are experiencing pelvic or lower abdominal pain, if no cause for the illness other than PID can be identified, and if one or more of the following minimum criteria are present on pelvic examination:

- Cervical motion tenderness *or* uterine tenderness *or* adnexal tenderness

The requirement that all three minimum criteria be present before the initiation of empiric treatment could result in insufficient sensitivity for the diagnosis of PID. The presence of signs of lower genital tract inflammation, in addition to one of the three minimum criteria, increases the specificity of diagnosis. In deciding on the initiation of empiric treatment, clinicians should also consider the risk profile of the patient for STDs.

More elaborate diagnostic evaluation frequently is needed because incorrect diagnosis and management might cause unnecessary morbidity. These additional criteria may be used to enhance the specificity of the minimum criteria. The following additional criteria can be used to enhance the specificity of the minimum criteria and support a diagnosis of PID:

- Oral temperature >101°F (>38.3°C)
- Abnormal cervical or vaginal mucopurulent discharge
- Presence of abundant numbers of WBC on saline microscopy of vaginal secretions
- Elevated ESR
- Elevated C-reactive protein
- Laboratory documentation of cervical infection with *N. gonorrhoeae* or *C. trachomatis*

The majority of women with PID have either mucopurulent cervical discharge or evidence of WBC on a microscopic evaluation of a saline preparation of vaginal fluid. If the cervical discharge appears normal and no WBCs are observed on the wet prep of vaginal fluid, the diagnosis of PID is unlikely, and alternative causes of pain should be investigated. A wet prep of vaginal fluid offers the ability to detect the presence of concomitant infections (e.g., bacterial vaginosis and trichomoniasis).

The most specific criteria for diagnosing PID include the following:

- Endometrial biopsy with histopathologic evidence of endometritis
- Transvaginal sonography or magnetic resonance imaging techniques showing thickened, fluid-filled tubes with or without free pelvic fluid or tuboovarian complex, or Doppler studies suggesting pelvic infection (e.g., tubal hyperemia)
- Laparoscopic abnormalities consistent with PID

A diagnostic evaluation that includes some of these more extensive studies might be warranted in certain cases. Endometrial biopsy is warranted in women undergoing laparoscopy who do not have visual evidence of salpingitis, as some women with PID have endometritis alone.

ESR, erythrocyte sedimentation rate; PID, pelvic inflammatory disease; STD, sexually transmitted disease; WBC, white blood cell.

of pelvic and abdominal pain are required for a diagnosis of PID and eliminates leukocytosis and fever as essential criteria (Table 30.1).

Perihepatic inflammation and adhesions, more commonly known as the Fitz-Hugh-Curtis syndrome, develop in 1% to 10% of patients with acute PID. Signs and symptoms include right upper quadrant pain, pleuritic pain, and tenderness in the right upper quadrant when the liver is palpated. Usually the symptoms and signs of this syndrome are preceded by the clinical onset of acute PID. The condition is often mistakenly diagnosed as either acute cholecystitis or pneumonia. Fitz-Hugh-Curtis syndrome is believed to develop from vascular or transperitoneal dissemination of either *N. gonorrhoeae* or *C. trachomatis* to produce the perihepatic inflammation. Other organisms may be involved, but limited data exist on their causality.

Jacobson and Westrom attempted to correlate the clinical diagnosis of acute salpingitis with laparoscopic pelvic findings. Of 814 women in whom laparoscopy was performed for presumed acute PID, 512 (65%) had visual evidence of salpingitis; 184 (23%) had normal visual findings; and 98 (12%) had other pelvic pathology. Because of the positive clinical findings, many of the patients with normal findings were suspected to have early PID with endometritis and endosalpingitis without visual evidence of tubal or pelvic damage. Thus, **laparoscopy** is limited as a method of diagnosing the early stages of PID, but it is important to rule out non-PID surgical emergencies, such as appendicitis, and other entities requiring different treatment modalities, such as endometriosis.

Despite these shortcomings of early diagnosis, laparoscopic visualization of the pelvis is still the most accurate method of confirming the diagnosis of acute PID. However, it is logistically and economically impractical for all patients suspected of having acute PID to undergo diagnostic laparoscopy in the United States. Therefore, the diagnosis of most episodes of acute PID is often made on the basis of clinical history and physical examination. Although it is suggested that laparoscopy be offered to all patients with an uncertain diagnosis, it is strongly indicated for patients who are not responding to therapy in an effort to confirm the diagnosis, obtain cultures from the cul-de-sac or fallopian tubes, and drain pus if necessary. In summary, laparoscopic studies have shown the following:

1. The clinical diagnosis of acute PID may be inaccurate.
2. Acute PID is sometimes found in patients undergoing laparoscopy for other causes of pelvic pain.
3. Laparoscopy is a relatively safe method for making the visual diagnosis of the latter stages of PID, and thus assessing future fertility prognosis and planning.
4. Laparoscopy is an excellent means of obtaining cultures directly from the tube.

The appearance of the pelvic organs can vary from erythematous, indurated, edematous oviducts, to pockets of purulent material, to a large pyosalpinx or tuboovarian abscess. However, although no disease may be evident in early stages, it is imperative to render treatment to all stages to avoid long-term sequelae.

Other less invasive methods of diagnosis have been suggested for verifying a clinical diagnosis of acute PID. **Endometrial biopsy** is one alternative to laparoscopy. Paavonen and associates reported a 90% correlation between histologic endometritis and laparoscopically confirmed salpingitis. However, results may be delayed up to 2 to 3 days, making its clinical applicability limited. **Ultrasonography** is of limited value for patients with mild or moderate pelvic PID. Thus, the routine use of sonography in patients with acute salpingitis does not appear to be indicated. Ultrasound is helpful in distinguishing an adnexal mass, especially in patients who demonstrate a lack of response to antimicrobial therapy in the initial 48 to 72 hours of therapy. Sonohysterography, an ultrasound examination using the instillation of saline to better define pelvic structures, is not indicated at this time for patients suspected of having PID because no studies have been performed to demonstrate its safety in the event that pathogens are dispersed into the upper genital tract in the process of instilling the saline. **Culdocentesis,** with evidence of purulent peritoneal fluid, is helpful in the diagnosis of acute PID. With acute PID, the WBC count of peritoneal fluid is greater than 30,000 cells/mL, compared with a WBC count of 1,000 cells/mL in women without peritoneal inflammation. However, other infections, such as appendicitis and diverticulitis, among others, can also cause purulent pelvic fluid and a false diagnosis of PID.

Laboratory tests can be obtained, but their results lack sufficient sensitivity and specificity to make them an important factor in establishing the diagnosis. Leukocytosis is not a reliable indicator of acute PID, nor does it accurately correlate with the severity of tubal inflammation or need for hospitalization. Less than 50% of women with acute PID have a WBC count greater than 10,000 cells/mL. Similarly, the erythrocyte sedimentation rate (ESR), which for years was a routine laboratory test for women with acute PID, is nonspecific and is a crude indicator of severity of disease. The ESR is elevated higher than 15 mm/hr in about 75% of women with laparoscopically confirmed acute salpingitis. However, 53% of women with pelvic pain and normal-appearing pelvic organs also have an elevated ESR. Plasma proteins, such as C-reactive protein and antichymotrypsin, have been studied to determine whether they help in the diagnosis of acute PID. They have been found to be more sensitive than the ESR. Other investigators have found that **decreased or absent isoamylase in peritoneal fluid** in cases of acute PID is the best nonculture laboratory test for the disease. The major disadvantages of this test are that it requires several hours to complete and that peritoneal fluid must be obtained.

Other evaluation has revealed various inflammatory cytokines to be associated with pelvic infections; however, these tests are not commercially available to a useful extent. Because most cases of UGTI are associated with, and preceded by, lower genital tract infection, examination of the endocervix for inflammation, Gram stain, and culture for both *N. gonorrhoeae* and *C. trachomatis* are important for proper evaluation. A negative Gram-stained smear of the endocervix does not rule out upper tract infection. However, most studies have found that acute PID is rare without a concomitant increase in inflammatory cells in the vagina and the cervix.

SEQUELAE

Infertility

One fourth of all women who have had acute salpingitis experience one or more long-term sequelae. The most common is involuntary infertility, which occurs in about 20% of patients. PID ranks as one of the major causes of infertility. Before antibiotic therapy, 50% to 70% of women who had experienced UGTIs became sterile. The sequelae of infections vary from a patent oviduct, to peritubular and periovarian adhesions that may interfere with ovum pickup, to complete tubal obstruction. The infertility rate increases directly with the number of episodes of acute pelvic infection. Also, women with mild disease are seven times less likely to suffer tubal obstruction than women with severe PID.

Ectopic Pregnancy

The chance of ectopic pregnancy is increased 6- to 10-fold in patients with a previous episode of acute salpingitis. Pathologic studies estimate that at least 50% of ectopic pregnancies occur in fallopian tubes damaged by previous salpingitis. The mechanism for the increased rate is believed to be interference of ovum transport through the tube or entrapment of the ovum secondary to microscopic tubal damage.

Chronic Pelvic Pain

The chance that chronic pelvic pain will develop in a woman after acute salpingitis is four times that of control subjects without pelvic infection (20% vs. 5%). Chronic pelvic pain can be caused by a hydrosalpinx. A hydrosalpinx is presumably the end-stage development of a pyosalpinx. The pain can also be related to adhesions surrounding the ovary. All patients with chronic pelvic pain believed to be caused by acute PID should undergo laparoscopy or laparotomy to establish the cause of the chronic pain and rule out other diseases such as endometriosis, which require different treatment, or the presence of pelvic adhesions, which can often be directly resolved.

A tuboovarian complex is a collection of pus within an anatomic space created by adherence to adjacent organs. The incidence of true adnexal abscess is about 10% in women with acute PID. Landers and Sweet noted a 20% rate of early treatment failure (after 48 to 72 hours) of antibiotic therapy as a result of persistent pain or enlargement of a tuboovarian abscess or complex. In addition, according to Landers and Sweet, 31% required an operation several weeks to months after their acute infections for persistent disease or pain.

MORTALITY

Before antibiotic therapy, the mortality rate associated with acute PID was 1%. Most of these deaths resulted from rupture of tuboovarian abscesses. Today, death associated with PID is rare, but the mortality rate can still be as high as 5% to 10% for ruptured tuboovarian abscesses, even with modern medical and operative therapy. This is mostly the result of subsequent development of adult respiratory distress syndrome (ARDS), a condition often associated with serious infection or delayed treatment.

TREATMENT

The therapeutic goals in the management of acute PID include both elimination of the acute infection and symptoms and prevention of long-term sequelae such as infertility, ectopic pregnancy, chronic pelvic pain, and the residue of infection. Antibiotic treatment should be started as soon as cultures have been obtained and diagnosis is confirmed or strongly suspected. Treatment is based on the consensus that PID is polymicrobial in cause. Empirical antibiotic protocols should cover a wide range of bacteria, including *N. gonorrhoeae, C. trachomatis,* anaerobic rods and cocci, Gram-negative aerobic rods, Gram-positive aerobes, and *Mycoplasma* species. Despite general agreement that broad-spectrum therapy is appropriate, questions persist regarding optimal therapeutic regimens.

Controversy has arisen over the issue of outpatient treatment with oral antibiotics versus inpatient treatment with parenteral antibiotics. There are no data available to evaluate the efficacy of hospital versus ambulatory management of acute PID. In the United States, three of four women with acute pelvic infection are treated as outpatients for their disease. In Scandinavia, which has a different health care system, most women are treated as inpatients. In 2006, the CDC published recommended treatment guidelines for outpatient management of acute PID (Table 30.2). Some of the treatment regimens are

TABLE 30.2

CDC-RECOMMENDED TREATMENT REGIMENS FOR ORAL THERAPY OF ACUTE PELVIC INFLAMMATORY DISEASE

Oral therapy can be considered for women with mild to moderately severe acute PID, as the clinical outcomes among these women are similar to those treated with inpatient therapy. The following regimens provide coverage against the frequent etiologic agents of PID. Patients who do not respond to oral therapy within 72 hours should be reevaluated to confirm the diagnosis and should be administered parenteral therapy on either an outpatient or inpatient basis.

Regimen A

Levofloxacin 500 mg orally once daily for 14 days[a]

OR

Ofloxacin 400 mg orally once daily for 14 days[a]

WITH OR WITHOUT

Metronidazole 500 mg orally twice a day for 14 days

Oral ofloxacin has been investigated as a single agent in two well-designed clinical trials, and it is effective against both *N. gonorrhoeae* and *C. trachomatis*. Despite the results of these trials, lack of anaerobic coverage with ofloxacin is a concern; the addition of metronidazole to the treatment regimen provides this coverage. Levofloxacin is as effective as ofloxacin and may be substituted. Azithromycin has been demonstrated in one randomized trial to be an effective regimen for acute PID. The addition of metronidazole should be considered, as anaerobic organisms are suspected to be involved in the etiology of most cases of PID. Metronidazole will also treat bacterial vaginosis, which often is associated with PID.

Regimen B

Ceftriaxone 250 mg IM in a single dose

PLUS

Doxycycline 100 mg orally twice a day for 14 days

WITH OR WITHOUT

Metronidazole 500 mg orally twice a day for 14 days

OR

Cefoxitin 2 g IM in a single dose and probenecid, 1 g orally administered concurrently in a single dose

PLUS

Doxycycline 100 mg orally twice a day for 14 days

WITH OR WITHOUT

Metronidazole 500 mg orally twice a day for 14 days

OR

Other parenteral third-generation cephalosporin (e.g., ceftizoxime or cefotaxime),

PLUS

Doxycycline 100 mg orally twice a day for 14 days

WITH OR WITHOUT

Metronidazole 500 mg orally twice a day for 14 days

The optimal choice of a cephalosporin for Regimen B is unclear; although cefoxitin has better anaerobic coverage, ceftriaxone has better coverage against *N. gonorrhoeae*. Clinical trials have demonstrated that a single dose of cefoxitin is effective in obtaining short-term clinical response in women who have PID. However, the theoretical limitations in its coverage of anaerobes may require the addition of metronidazole to the treatment regimen. Metronidazole also will effectively treat BV, which is frequently associated with PID. No data have been published regarding the use of oral cephalosporins for the treatment of PID. Limited data suggest that the combination of oral metronidazole plus doxycycline after primary parenteral therapy is safe and effective.

Alternative Oral Regimens

Although information regarding other outpatient regimens is limited, one other regimen has undergone at least one clinical trial and has broad-spectrum coverage. Amoxicillin/clavulanic acid plus doxycycline was effective in obtaining short-term clinical response in a single clinical trial; however, gastrointestinal symptoms might limit compliance with this regimen.

BV, bacterial vaginosis; CDC, Centers for Disease Control and Prevention; IM, intramuscularly; PID, pelvic inflammatory disease.

[a]Quinolones should not be used in persons with a history of recent foreign travel or partners' travel, infections acquired in California or Hawaii, or in other areas with increased QRNG (quinolone-resistant *Neisseria gonorrhoeae)* prevalence.

based on the controversial premise that it may be adequate to cover just a few of the major etiologic agents (*N. gonorrhoeae* and *C. trachomatis*) involved in acute salpingitis. As a result, studies have documented a 10% to 20% treatment failure rate for women receiving oral antibiotics as outpatients compared with a 5% to 10% failure rate for women without an abscess receiving intravenous antibiotics as inpatients, where broader coverage is used. The inclusion of the quinolone arm, ofloxacin, and levofloxacin in the outpatient treatment regimen does permit broader oral coverage of probable pathogens, but this still may not be adequate for serious disease. It is important to reevaluate patients within 48 to 72 hours of initiating outpatient therapy to determine the response of the disease. If a poor response has been obtained, the patient should be hospitalized with parenteral antibiotics and possible laparoscopic evaluation in the hope of preventing or limiting the sequelae of PID.

Ideally, every woman with acute PID should be hospitalized for the first few days for parenteral antibiotic treatment. Because this may not be practical because of limited economic or physical facility resources, the clinician who diagnoses acute salpingitis in the office or emergency department is faced with the question of which patient to hospitalize. Indications for the hospitalization of patients with acute salpingitis are also defined by the CDC in the 2006 guidelines (Table 30.3). In the past, the CDC has suggested that all adolescents with salpingitis be hospitalized because of their high noncompliance rate and to optimize treatment to prevent damage to the reproductive tract, which could affect future fertility and result in chronic pelvic pain. Recently, Kelly and colleagues found a high incidence and recurrence in adolescents, perhaps related to poor compliance. However, the CDC's new policy is to use the same criteria for hospitalization as for older women. This recommendation is not agreed upon by all infectious disease groups because of the seriousness of inadequately treated PID in the younger, often noncompliant population.

Another indication for hospitalization is the presence of an adnexal or pelvic abscess. Outpatient therapy may not provide antibiotic levels high enough to penetrate an abscess, and rupture of the abscess may have serious consequences. Women in whom the definitive diagnosis of acute PID is in question should also be hospitalized, and additional diagnostic measures should be instituted. As previously stated, at least 10% of all patients have other serious diagnoses, such as acute appendicitis, ectopic pregnancy, or adnexal torsion, and these should be ruled out. Patients with serious illness, patients with nausea and vomiting, patients who are unable to follow or tolerate outpatient therapy, and patients with a previously failed outpatient oral regimen also should be hospitalized and given parenteral antibiotics. A recent trial by Ness and colleagues investigating the outcomes in patients randomized to inpatient or outpatient did not find differences in short-term outcomes, but difficulties in patient selection and randomization may not permit these results to be applicable to all PID patients.

TABLE 30.3

CRITERIA FOR HOSPITALIZATION OF PATIENTS WITH ACUTE PELVIC INFLAMMATORY DISEASE

The following criteria for hospitalization are suggested:

- Surgical emergencies (such as appendicitis) cannot be excluded.
- The patient is pregnant.
- The patient does not respond clinically to oral antimicrobial therapy.
- The patient is unable to follow or tolerate an outpatient oral regimen.
- The patient has severe illness, nausea and vomiting, or high fever.
- The patient has a tuboovarian abscess.

The 2006 CDC guidelines for inpatient treatment of acute PID describe two regimens (Table 30.4). Regimen A is a combination of oral or parenteral doxycycline plus intravenous cefoxitin or cefotetan. Other third-generation cephalosporins can be substituted, such as ceftizoxime (Cefizox) or cefotaxime (Claforan). All of these agents are effective against penicillinase-producing *N. gonorrhoeae, Peptostreptococcus,* and other anaerobic species, as well as *Escherichia coli* and other aerobic (facultative) species. Ceftriaxone is recommended by the CDC; however, its poor anaerobic activity and lack of trials do not make it an acceptable alternative for several investigators. Doxycycline can be given intravenously if the patient is unable to tolerate oral therapy, but it must be infused very slowly to prevent pain and sclerosis of the vein. Oral doxycycline has been demonstrated to be equally effective because of the slow growth cycle of *Chlamydia* and the requirement of prolonged treatment. A recent study by Viberga and colleagues investigating the microbiology of IUD-related infection found an increased recovery of *Fusobacterium* and *Peptostreptococcus* species, which generally are covered by both cephalosporin and clindamycin. A possible disadvantage of the cephalosporin-doxycycline combination is that these two antibiotics may be less than ideal for anaerobic infections or for a pelvic abscess.

Regimen B is a combination of clindamycin and an aminoglycoside (gentamicin). This combination provides excellent activity against anaerobes, Gram-negative aerobes, and Gram-positive aerobes. Historically, it has been the preferred regimen for patients with an abscess, IUD-related infections, or pelvic infections after a diagnostic or operative procedure. However, there are few data to prove that it is significantly more effective than the cephalosporin regimens. A possible disadvantage of regimen B is that it may not provide optimal activity against *C. trachomatis* and *N. gonorrhoeae*. Clindamycin in high doses (900 mg in 8 hours) has good activity against *Chlamydia,* and *in vitro* studies by Martens and colleagues have demonstrated effectiveness against 90% of *C. trachomatis* strains. Doxycycline is believed to be the most effective chlamydial agent according to *in vitro* testing and is often used for at least 7 days to complete treatment when the patient is switched from parenteral to posthospitalization therapy. Also, the CDC recommendation of once-daily dosing for gentamicin is not based on any data on PID patients and should be used only if indicated for renal considerations.

Each regimen stresses two concepts: the polymicrobial etiology of acute pelvic infection and the necessity of protecting against *C. trachomatis* and *N. gonorrhoeae*. With both protocols, the CDC recommends a minimum of at least 24 hours of intravenous treatment after clinical improvement. Both protocols also require completion of a 14-day course of oral antibiotics (doxycycline or clindamycin) to eradicate slow-growing organisms such as *C. trachomatis*.

Alternative inpatient parenteral regimens are included in the 2006 CDC PID guidelines (Table 30.4). The CDC lists only the β-lactamase inhibitor combination ampicillin-sulbactam (Unasyn), but piperacillin-tazobactam has been demonstrated by Hemsell and colleagues, Sweet and colleagues, and others

TABLE 30.4

CDC-RECOMMENDED TREATMENT REGIMENS FOR PARENTERAL THERAPY OF ACUTE PELVIC INFLAMMATORY DISEASE

Regimen A
Cefotetan 2 g IV every 12 hours
OR
Cefoxitin 2 g IV every 6 hours
PLUS
Doxycycline 100 mg orally or IV every 12 hours
Because of pain associated with infusion, doxycycline should be administered orally when possible, even when the patient is hospitalized. Both oral and IV administration of doxycycline provide similar bioavailability.
Parenteral therapy may be discontinued 24 hours after a patient improves clinically, and oral therapy with doxycycline (100 mg twice a day) should continue to complete 14 days of therapy. When tuboovarian abscess is present, many health care providers use clindamycin or metronidazole with doxycycline for continued therapy rather than doxycycline alone, because it provides more effective anaerobic coverage.
Clinical data are limited regarding the use of other second- or third-generation cephalosporins (e.g., ceftizoxime, cefotaxime, and ceftriaxone), which also may be effective therapy for PID and may replace cefotetan or cefoxitin. However, these cephalosporins are less active than cefotetan or cefoxitin against anaerobic bacteria.
Regimen B
Clindamycin 900 mg IV every 8 hours
PLUS
Gentamicin loading dose IV or IM (2 mg/kg of body weight) followed by a maintenance dose (1.5 mg/kg) every 8 hours. Single daily dosing may be substituted.
Although use of a single daily dose of gentamicin has not been evaluated for the treatment of PID, it is efficacious in other analogous situations. Parenteral therapy can be discontinued 24 hours after a patient improves clinically; continuing oral therapy should consist of doxycycline 100 mg orally twice a day or clindamycin 450 mg orally four times a day to complete a total of 14 days of therapy. When tuboovarian abscess is present, many health care providers use clindamycin for continued therapy rather than doxycycline, because clindamycin provides more effective anaerobic coverage.
Alternative Parenteral Regimens
Limited data support the use of other parenteral regimens, but the following three regimens have been investigated in at least one clinical trial, and they have broad-spectrum coverage.
Levofloxacin 500 mg IV once daily[a]
WITH OR WITHOUT
Metronidazole 500 mg IV every 8 hours
OR
Ofloxacin 400 mg IV every 12 hours[a]
WITH OR WITHOUT
Metronidazole 500 mg IV every 8 hours
OR
Ampicillin/sulbactam 3 g IV every 6 hours
PLUS
Doxycycline 100 mg orally or IV every 12 hours
IV ofloxacin has been investigated as a single agent; however, because of concerns regarding its spectrum, metronidazole may be included in the regimen. Levofloxacin is as effective as ofloxacin and may be substituted; its single daily dosing makes it advantageous from a compliance perspective. One trial demonstrated high short term clinical cure rates with azithromycin, either alone for 1 week (at least one IV dose, followed by oral therapy) or with a 12-day course or metronidazole. Ampicillin/sulbactam plus doxycycline is effective coverage against *C. trachomatis*, *N. gonorrhoeae*, and anaerobes and for patients who have tuboovarian abscess.

CDC, Centers for Disease Control and Prevention; IM, intramuscularly; IV, intravenously; PID, pelvic inflammatory disease.
[a]Quinolones should not be used in persons with a history of recent foreign travel or partners' travel, infections acquired in California or Hawaii, or in other areas with increased QRNG (quinolone-resistant *Neisseria gonorrhoeae)* prevalence.

to have excellent *in vitro* and *in vivo* activity against PID and its pathogens.

MANAGEMENT OF SEX PARTNERS

Male sex partners of women with PID should be examined and treated if they had sexual contact with the patient during the 60 days preceding the patient's onset of symptoms. Evaluation and treatment is imperative because of the risk for reinfection of the patient and the strong likelihood of urethral gonococcal or chlamydial infection in the sex partner. Male partners of women who have PID caused by *C. trachomatis* and/or *N. gonorrhoeae* often are asymptomatic.

Management of acute PID should include treatment of the male partner and education for the prevention of reinfection, including the use of proper contraception. The importance of treating sexual partners cannot be overstressed. Eschenbach reported that 25% of gonococcal PID patients were readmitted to the hospital within 10 weeks of the initial treatment. A study of gonococcal PID noted that 13% of male partners screened were asymptomatic urethral carriers and that even higher rates for *C. trachomatis* were present. These partners should be treated with one of the regimens for uncomplicated gonorrhoeae and chlamydial infection (i.e., ceftriaxone, 125 mg intramuscularly, followed by oral doxycycline, 100 mg twice a day for 7 days, oral azithromycin in 1 g or ofloxacin 300 mg b.i.d. for 7 days orally). Women with acute PID often return to the same social situations they were in before treatment. It is hoped that treating sexual partners and educating patients with regard to contraception would decrease the incidence of recurrent infections and affect the often poor prognosis for future fertility.

HIV INFECTION

Differences in the clinical manifestations of PID between human immunodeficiency virus (HIV)-infected women and HIV-negative women have not been well delineated. In early observational studies, HIV-infected women with PID were more likely to require surgical intervention. In recent, more comprehensive observational and controlled studies, HIV-infected women with PID had similar symptoms when compared with uninfected controls. They were more likely to have a tuboovarian abscess, but responded equally to standard parenteral and oral antibiotic regimens when compared with HIV-negative women. The microbiologic findings for HIV-positive and HIV-negative women were similar, except for (a) higher rates of concomitant *M. hominis*, candida, streptococcal, and HPV infections and (b) HPV-related cytologic abnormalities among those with HIV infection. Whether the management of immunodeficient HIV-infected women with PID requires more aggressive interventions (e.g., hospitalization or parenteral antimicrobial regimens) had not been determined.

SURGICAL MANAGEMENT

Laparotomy should generally be reserved for patients with surgical emergencies such as ruptured abscesses or definitive treatment of failed medical management. Laparoscopy, however, is an underused but usually helpful procedure for diagnosis, prognosis, and possibly treatment of PID. Laparoscopic evaluation should be considered in all patients with a differential diagnosis of PID and without laparoscopic surgery contraindications.

Laparoscopy is important not only to diagnose PID but also to rule out surgical emergencies, such as appendicitis and ruptured abscesses. It also prevents inappropriate management of patients with noninfectious problems, such as endometriosis. These patients need additional surgical and medical management, not antibiotic therapy and delayed diagnosis. In addition, evaluation of the extent of the inflammatory process in confirmed PID is helpful in establishing a prognosis and further management plan if initial treatment fails. Patients with evidence of current or previous abscesses have a higher failure rate with antibiotic therapy. Also, treatment of unilateral abscesses may necessitate surgical management to avoid the spread of the infection to the other tube and ovary.

Cultures obtained from the peritubal region or from the peritoneal cavity can also be helpful for identifying organisms resistant to initial management. This has become increasingly important in light of the increasing rate of clindamycin-resistant anaerobes and the elimination of metronidazole from the CDC-recommended inpatient guidelines. Laparoscopic management of PID that appears helpful includes copious drainage of the pelvis with normal saline or preferably Ringer solution. Antibiotic inclusion in the lavage fluid has not been demonstrated to be helpful to date. Laparoscopic manipulation or drainage of documented pelvic abscesses has been attempted by several investigators.

Henry-Suchet and associates reported the successful use of laparoscopy to diagnose and drain tuboovarian abscesses in 50 women. Adhesions were lysed, and the abscesses were drained through the laparoscope. All patients received intravenous antibiotics. Forty-five of the 50 (90%) patients were cured. Reich and McGlynn had a similar experience in 25 women with pelvic abscesses treated laparoscopically. Four of seven women desiring pregnancy conceived, and two women had unplanned pregnancies. However, the diagnosis of abscesses is not uniform in these studies. Also, it is of concern that similar results will not necessarily be demonstrated in less experienced hands. Anatomically, drainage of abscesses within the pelvic cavity by laparoscope will not drain the entire abscess contents out of the pelvic cavity, and despite how extensive the lavage or laparoscopic removal is, pus and bacteria will be spilled and exposed to the pelvic cavity. This is contrary to the natural defense mechanism of the body of isolating and containing the inflammation-causing organisms within an abscess. Therefore, laparoscopic drainage of pelvic abscesses should be undertaken only by experienced laparoscopic surgeons and with the patient's full understanding of all other options.

Laparotomy with extensive pelvic surgery was often recommended in the past, before the development of broad-spectrum antibiotics.

If a patient has been hospitalized on several occasions for acute exacerbation of PID with bilateral tuboovarian abscesses to the point where the future surgical risk increases significantly, definitive surgical intervention may be indicated. The operation should be done when the infection is quiescent, if possible. The surgery may still be difficult, but there will be fewer complications than when patients are operated on in the acute phase of the infection. The timing of the operative intervention is important. There should be complete absorption of the inflammatory exudate surrounding the focus of the infection, as seen radiologically. Bimanual pelvic examination should be possible without producing a marked or persistent febrile response. It has been suggested that definitive surgery be delayed for 2 to 3 months after the recent exacerbation for more complete resolution of the infection. Ideally, the patient should have a normal ESR, WBC, and hematocrit, and relatively nontender pelvic organs, except possibly with motion.

Kaplan and associates recommended more aggressive management in patients who exhibit either no clinical response or only partial response after 24 to 72 hours. Their approach included a total abdominal hysterectomy and bilateral salpingo-oophorectomy and was thought to reduce the protracted period of intensive medical therapy in a group of patients who would eventually require surgery. They noted that conservative management of their cases usually resulted in protracted periods of intensive care and repeated hospital admissions, and rarely in subsequent pregnancies. However, the early surgical intervention described above was associated with six incidences of injury to the bowel and additional postoperative complications. Unfortunately, patients with acute pelvic abscess are frequently young, and future childbearing is often desired, even though it may be impossible without intervention such as *in vitro* fertilization for most patients. Conservation of ovarian function for these young women is an important benefit of medical management. Some differences in the percentage of patients responding to conservative management in different studies and different geographic locations might be explained by differences in the predominant microorganisms causing the infection at these locations and their sensitivity to the antibiotics used.

Older studies of the management of patients with pelvic abscess, which emphasized the early use of surgery, are no longer pertinent, because modern antibiotic drugs were not available then. Collins and Jansen in 1959 had an early failure rate of 10% for conservative medical therapy. However, 113 of their 174 patients required later surgery, which corresponds to a late failure rate of 65%. Ginsburg and associates reviewed cases of 160 patients treated for tuboovarian abscess during the years 1969 to 1979. The early failure rate with broad-spectrum antibiotics was 31%, whereas the late failure rate was an additional 21%. Thus, with an average follow-up period of 25.5 months, 48% did not require later surgery. Subsequent reports by Hager and colleagues and by Landers and Sweet support conservative management.

When conservative management fails and a pelvic abscess is noted dissecting the rectovaginal septum, drainage by way of colpotomy may be possible.

POSTERIOR COLPOTOMY

In a classic article, Wharton described various techniques of vaginal drainage of pelvic abscess. Today, posterior colpotomy is done to evacuate pus and to establish drainage from a pelvic abscess that presents in the cul-de-sac.

There are three requirements for colpotomy drainage of a pelvic abscess.

1. The abscess must be midline or nearly so.
2. The abscess should be adherent to the cul-de-sac peritoneum and should dissect the rectovaginal septum to assure the surgeon that the drainage will be extraperitoneal and that pus will not be disseminated transperitoneally.
3. The abscess should be cystic or fluctuant to ensure adequate drainage.

Occasionally, a cul-de-sac abscess can be successfully drained without dissecting the septum. However, the serosal surface of the abscess should be adherent to the cul-de-sac peritoneum. Ultrasonography may be helpful in locating the pockets of pus.

After adequate anesthesia, the patient is placed in the lithotomy position. It is essential that a thorough examination of the pelvis be performed under anesthesia so that the operator knows the size and position of the mass that is to be drained.

After preparation and draping in the dorsal lithotomy position, the posterior lip of the cervix is grasped with a tenaculum and drawn down and forward. The vaginal mucosa of the posterior vaginal fornix is incised just below the reflection of the vaginal mucosa onto the cervix, and the transverse incision is widened with a pair of long scissors (Fig. 30.1A). The incision must be large enough to allow adequate exploration and drainage of the abscess cavity with the index finger. The cul-de-sac peritoneum and abscess wall are punctured with a long Kelly clamp (Fig. 30.1B). As the abscess wall is perforated, there is a definite sensation of puncturing a cystic cavity. If blood or pus is present, this is soon seen in the upper vagina. The jaws of the clamp are spread, and the flow of liquid from the cul-de-sac is increased. A sample of the purulent exudate is sent to the microbiology laboratory for appropriate culture and sensitivity. Collection of the specimen anaerobically with a capped syringe with rapid transport to the laboratory allows the more fastidious flora to be defined. A direct smear for Gram stain is also made from the pus and examined for predominating organisms.

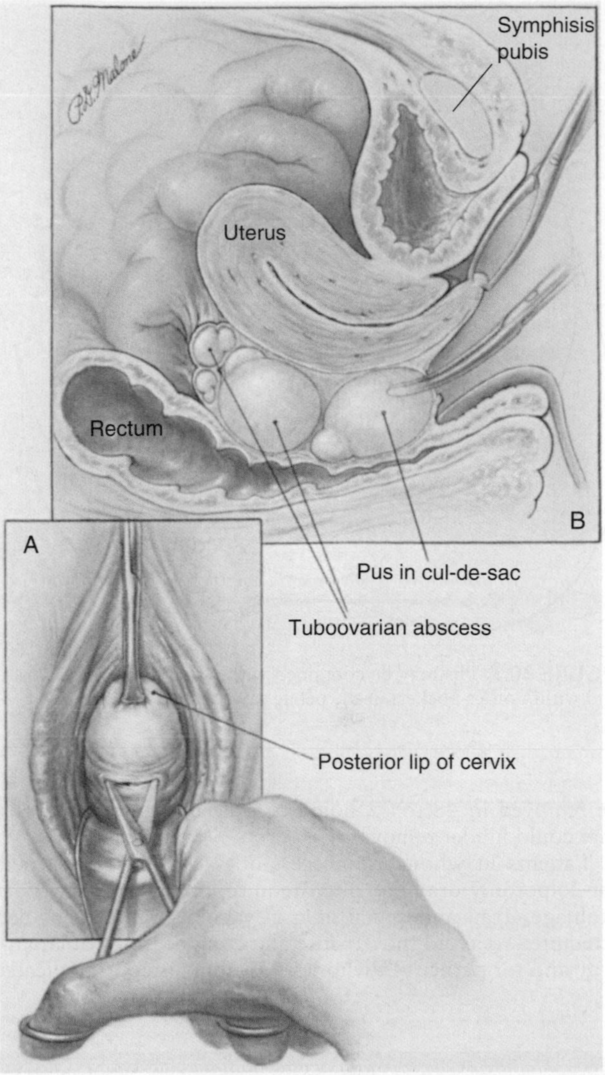

FIGURE 30.1. Posterior colpotomy. **A:** A transverse incision is made through the vaginal mucosa at the junction of the posterior vaginal fornix with the cervix. **B:** A Kelly clamp is thrust through the abscess wall.

There may be more than one compartment in an abscess cavity (Fig. 30.2). It is desirable to insert an index finger in the cavity and explore. Fibrous adhesions within the cavity can be gently broken. If another abscess wall is felt, it can often be cautiously and safely punctured under the guidance of a finger. Exploration and manipulation should be done carefully to avoid intraperitoneal rupture of the abscess or perforation of the bowel. To allow adequate drainage, the vaginal incision should be at least 2 cm wide. If pus has been obtained, one or two drains are inserted into the abscess cavity and anchored with fine absorbable suture to permit easy removal. Penrose or closed suction drainage systems can be used. These are left for several days or longer. Wharton has emphasized the importance of prolonged drainage. A suture or two may be required to control bleeding from the vaginal mucosa. However, if a mushroom (Malecot) catheter is used for drainage, it should

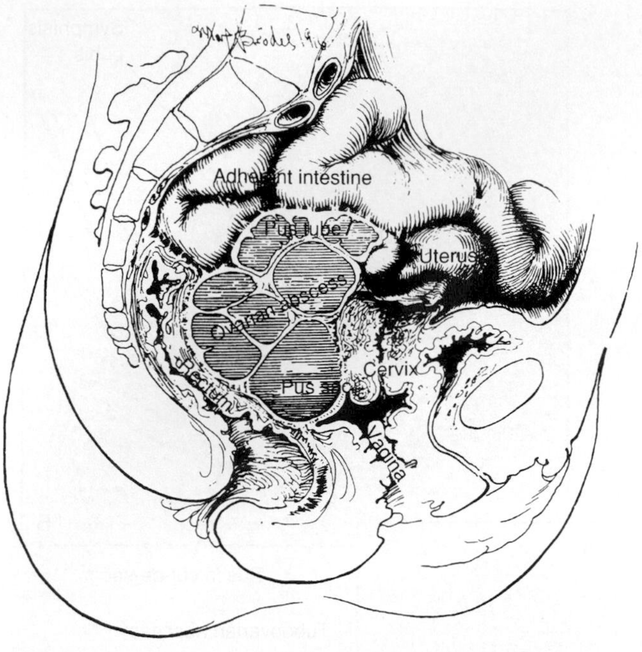

FIGURE 30.2. Pus may be contained within the tuboovarian abscess and within other pockets in the pelvic cavity.

be removed in 48 to 72 hours to prevent significant fibrosis that could hinder removal.

Patients in whom the abscess does not meet the criteria for colpotomy drainage often require laparotomy and direct drainage. Transabdominal or transvaginal drainage has been attempted to avoid the expense and complications of laparotomy and for patients in whom laparotomy is contraindicated.

Experience with **percutaneous drainage** of intraabdominal and pelvic abscesses under ultrasonographic or computed tomographic (CT) guidance has been reported by Olak and associates, and by others. Worthen and Gunning used percutaneous catheter drainage of 11 abscesses in nine patients and achieved a cure rate of 77%. Two patients required surgical intervention subsequently. In 19 patients, simple percutaneous aspiration of 23 abscesses was successful, with a 94% cure rate. The attempt at aspiration failed in seven patients (Fig. 30.3). The Grady Memorial Hospital experience, as reported by Tyrrel and associates, is similar. CT-guided percutaneous drainage in eight patients with tuboovarian abscess resulted in recovery without surgery in seven. One patient had marked clinical improvement but still required a posterior colpotomy. No complications occurred. Loy and associates have reported that the simultaneous use of real-time pelvic ultrasonography can facilitate transvaginal drainage of a pelvic abscess. If patients do not respond to intravenous antibiotics and percutaneous drainage or aspiration, surgical intervention is required.

The long-term effects of pus and organisms released into the pelvis from the puncture site are unknown. However, short-term success rates are good, and surgical drainage of acute abscess is a basic principle. Therefore, needle drainage can be considered with proper patient selection and appropriate informed consent, which includes other management options.

If **exploratory laparotomy** is necessary, the patient can be positioned in Allen universal stirrups. A lower abdominal transverse Maylard incision is ideal because it affords good exposure to the lateral adnexal pelvic organs and pelvic side walls. Pelvic adhesions should be released, and the bowel should be packed off before the pelvic dissection commences. During the dissection, free pus is often spilled, and the upper abdomen should be isolated from this, if possible. When a ruptured abscess is encountered, the exudate is collected and sent immediately to the laboratory for Gram stain, anaerobic and aerobic cultures, and antimicrobial sensitivity studies. The easiest way to obtain the material for anaerobic culture is simply to collect

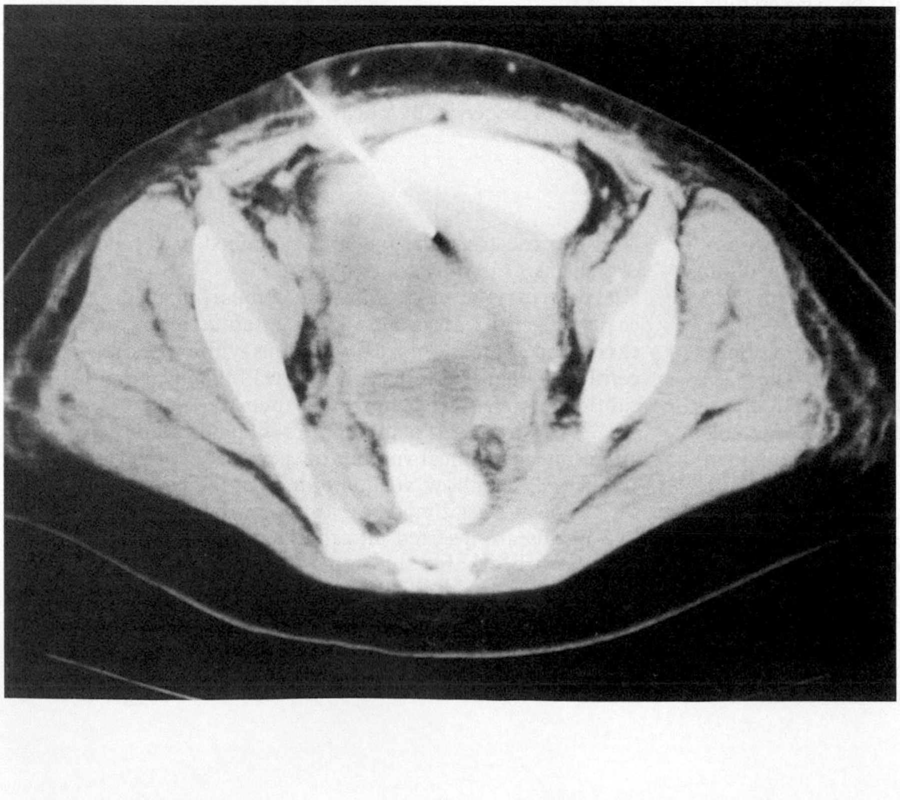

FIGURE 30.3. Transabdominal needle aspiration of a pelvic abscess under guidance of computed tomography. Drainage tube is also placed.

it in an airtight syringe and to submit a small piece of the abscess wall in an airtight container. The easiest place to begin the dissection is in the round ligament, which is the most consistently available and identifiable landmark. Following the round ligament medially always leads to the uterine corpus. Variations in the usual technique for the operation may be required because of extensive disease, dense adhesions, indurated and edematous tissue, and distorted anatomy. For example, it is sometimes convenient to perform the central dissection first (i.e., a subtotal hysterectomy). This allows more space and adequate exposure to perform the required adnexal surgery. Tuboovarian inflammatory masses may be found densely adherent in the cul-de-sac to the uterus, to the posterior surface of the broad ligament, and to the lateral pelvic sidewall. There is risk of injury to the ureters, sigmoid, rectum, and small intestines. The method of dissection used depends on the nature of the adhesions. Soft, fresh adhesions can be broken gently and easily with finger dissection. Dense fibrotic adhesions must be carefully dissected and cut with scissors. The dissection can be especially difficult and risky if pelvic tissues are intensely indurated, as in ligneous pelvic cellulitis. If the infundibulopelvic ligament can be clamped, cut, and securely ligated, one can gain access to the lateral retroperitoneal space and identify the ureter. This facilitates a safe dissection of the abscess wall away from the ureter. In cases with extensive disease involving one or both adnexa, the use of preoperative ureteral catheterization may be helpful in identifying the location of the pelvic ureters. With tuboovarian abscess, the anatomic limits of the ovary may be difficult to define. If the ovary is to be removed, it should be removed completely to prevent subsequent development of ovarian remnant syndrome.

When both adnexa must be removed, a hysterectomy should be entertained if extensive uterine involvement is suspected. In some cases, only a subtotal hysterectomy is feasible. However, if the lower uterine segment can be visualized, the cervix can usually be excised after removal of the adnexa and the uterine corpus. The operative field should be copiously irrigated. The vaginal vault should be left open for drainage. A Penrose drain can be inserted and then removed several days later. Suspension of the vaginal vault and reperitonization of the pelvis are accomplished in the usual manner, if possible. A routine closure of the abdominal incision is performed. Jackson-Pratt suction drains are often placed above the fascia and brought out through a separate incision.

Because the patient has been placed in the Allen universal stirrups for laparotomy, ureteral integrity can be confirmed as discussed elsewhere. Five milliliters of indigo carmine is given intravenously, and a cystoscope is placed in the bladder. Blue dye can then be seen flowing from each ureteral orifice.

In the past, it was standard practice to do a bilateral salpingo-oophorectomy in almost all patients who had a laparotomy for acute pelvic abscess. This practice was based on the belief that the disease is almost always severe in both adnexa. Recent studies have suggested that as many as 25% to 50% of patients will have a relatively normal tube and ovary on one side. This may be especially true of patients whose infection is associated with IUD use. Golde and associates reported that 37 of 85 patients (44%) with tuboovarian abscesses confirmed at operation had unilateral abscesses; 20 were using an IUD. The studies of Landers and Sweet, Hager and Majmudar, and Ginsburg and coworkers also found a higher percentage of unilateral adnexal disease than was previously reported. In light of these findings, conservative adnexal surgery may be possible in some patients. We have no hesitation in leaving a relatively normal tube and ovary at the time of hysterectomy with removal of the opposite adnexa for acute pelvic abscess. When the uterus is removed and the continuity between the conserved tube and the lower genital tract is interrupted, there is little risk of a new infection. If a strictly unilateral pelvic abscess is found at laparotomy, removal of the affected tube and ovary only, leaving in the uterus and the opposite adnexa, is acceptable in a patient who wishes to preserve fertility. However, *in vitro* fertilization techniques may be required to accomplish pregnancy. Such a patient does have a risk of recurrent tuboovarian abscess. It is especially important that her sexual partner be examined and receive treatment when indicated.

In recent years there have been advances in reproductive technology that allow infertile patients to conceive and carry pregnancies to term under the most extraordinary circumstances. It has been possible, for example, to accomplish a successful pregnancy in a woman who has a uterus but no ovaries by instillation of a donated fertilized ovum into a suitably prepared uterus. Such a sophisticated procedure is not available to a large number of patients. However, in light of the recent findings of the risk of estrogen plus progesterone treatment from the Women's Health Initiative Study, the option of leaving in the uterus when bilateral salpingo-oophorectomy is to be performed should be discussed with the patient, especially if she is young and nulliparous.

In summary, patients with an acute pelvic abscess should be hospitalized for treatment with parenteral broad-spectrum antibiotics. Surgery is indicated if the diagnosis is uncertain, if intraperitoneal rupture is diagnosed or suspected, or if the patient fails to respond to medical management.

RUPTURED PELVIC ABSCESS

A tuboovarian or pelvic abscess can rupture spontaneously into the rectum or sigmoid colon, into the bladder, or into the free peritoneal cavity. A pelvic abscess almost never ruptures spontaneously into the vagina unless the patient had a previous posterior colpotomy for drainage of an abscess. Under these circumstances, a recurrent pelvic abscess can dissect along the tract of the previous posterior colpotomy incision and drain spontaneously through the vagina.

Spontaneous drainage through the rectum or sigmoid colon usually occurs in a patient whose abscess is too high to drain with a posterior colpotomy. In other words, although the abscess is fluctuant and midline, it is not yet dissecting the rectovaginal septum. While waiting for the abscess to come down, a sudden unexpected improvement in the patient's condition is noted, and she will confirm that pus has begun to drain through the anus. Further improvement in her condition usually occurs. A posterior colpotomy is not needed and, indeed, is contraindicated because doing so could cause a rectovaginal fistula to form.

Spontaneous drainage through the bladder is rare. It occurs most commonly in elderly women with chronic abscesses developing from ruptured sigmoid diverticula. Only rarely does a chronic tuboovarian or pelvic abscess rupture and drain through the bladder, causing secondary infection of the bladder. When the abscess is removed with laparotomy, a defect in the bladder wall is noted. The indurated tissue around the defect should be removed and the defect closed with 3–0 delayed-absorbable suture in two layers. A Foley catheter can be left in place for 10 to 14 days while healing of the bladder wall takes place.

Of all the complications that can result from PID, intraabdominal rupture of a tuboovarian abscess is the most life-threatening. Mortality from this complication is due to septic shock and the complications of generalized peritonitis, and the mortality rate can approach up to 10% in patients with warm shock.

Abscesses can rupture spontaneously, after bimanual examination or accidental trauma. Bacteriologic study of the contents of the abscess has historically been unrewarding; a specific organism has been isolated in less than 50% of cases. The gonococcus is rarely identified in a pelvic abscess. Careful aerobic and anaerobic cultures often demonstrate the presence of a mixed infection that includes anaerobic organisms. McNamara and Mead reviewed the results of three separate studies that demonstrated 31 positive isolates of anaerobes in 30 patients with a pelvic abscess. Landers and Sweet have also confirmed similar findings in their series.

Diagnosis of Ruptured Tuboovarian Abscess

The major clinical symptom of ruptured tuboovarian abscess is acute, progressive pelvic pain that is usually so severe that the patient can accurately identify the time and place of its occurrence. In a classic series from the Johns Hopkins Hospital reported by Vermeeren and Te Linde, the average age of patients with a ruptured tuboovarian abscess was 33 years, which is at least 10 years older than the average age of patients with acute PID. About 2% of these patients are postmenopausal. To our knowledge, only two cases of ruptured tuboovarian abscess in a pregnant patient have been reported. Often, there is a history of recurrent attacks of PID, with a sudden increase in the severity and extent of abdominal pain during a recent exacerbation of infection. On examination, the patient appears seriously ill and dehydrated, with rapid, shallow respirations. The abdomen is distended and quiet, with diminished or absent bowel sounds. Signs of generalized peritonitis, direct and rebound tenderness, muscle rigidity, and shifting dullness may be noted. A pelvic mass is palpable in more than 50% of cases. Tachycardia is common. Shock can be present or can develop while the patient is under observation. It is due to accumulation of fluids in peripheral tissues and later failure of compensatory vasoconstrictor mechanisms. The patient's temperature is usually greater than 101°F, but it can also be normal and even subnormal late in the course. The leukocyte count is likely to be more than 15,000, but it also can be normal. Severe leukopenia is an ominous sign. A culdocentesis is a valuable diagnostic aid and was positive for purulent material in 70% of the cases in the Mickal and Sellmann series. An abdominal radiograph usually shows a paralytic ileus, sometimes evidence of free fluid in the peritoneal cavity, and atelectasis in the lung bases. A CT scan of the pelvis and abdomen is most helpful and will usually confirm the pelvic abscess with free purulent fluid in the upper abdomen. It may also suggest an alternative diagnosis such as a ruptured appendix or acute cholecystitis. Drainage of a pelvic abscess can also be done percutaneously under CT scan or ultrasound guidance.

Treatment of Ruptured Tuboovarian Abscess

The longer the delay in the operative treatment of ruptured tuboovarian abscess, the greater the primary mortality rate. In the series by Vermeeren and Te Linde from the Johns Hopkins Hospital, death occurred less than 90 hours after the time of rupture in 88% of fatal cases, both operative and nonoperative.

As time passes after rupture of a tuboovarian abscess, septic peritonitis becomes more severe and generalized. The passage of time allows the development of septic shock from greater absorption of bacteria and bacterial endotoxins, and secretion of great quantities of fluid into the peritoneal cavity across inflamed peritoneal surfaces. Fluid shifts from the intravascular compartment to interstitial spaces as a result of the increased vascular permeability of the inflamed peritoneal membrane. This leads to hypovolemia, decreased cardiac output, decreased central venous pressure, hypotension, vasoconstriction, increased peripheral resistance, decreased tissue perfusion, metabolic acidosis, ARDS, decreased renal glomerular perfusion and filtration with decreased urine flow, severe hypoxemia, multiple organ system failure, and death. The prompt diagnosis and treatment of intraperitoneal rupture of a tuboovarian abscess is essential to minimize the risk of mortality of generalized peritonitis.

The treatment of patients with ruptured tuboovarian abscess can be divided into three phases: preoperative, operative, and postoperative.

Preoperative Phase

Surgery should be undertaken after rapid but adequate preoperative preparation. The patient should be typed and crossmatched with 2 to 4 units of packed red blood cells. Monitoring of central venous pressure is essential for proper evaluation of the hemodynamics of this condition because many patients are dehydrated, in shock, and anemic. Swan-Ganz catheter placement may be preferable because it allows pulmonary capillary wedge pressure and pulmonary artery pressure determinations that are helpful in assessing the adequacy of fluid replacement and in detecting fluid overload. Variable amounts of fluid, sometimes tremendous amounts, are lost into the peritoneal cavity and intestinal tract because of peritonitis. Emergency blood chemistry determinations (e.g., serum electrolytes, creatinine, glucose, bilirubin, and alkaline phosphatase) are obtained, and intravenous fluids, preferably Ringer lactate, are started immediately. Crystalloid solutions for fluid volume resuscitation are preferred for most patients with septic peritonitis. It may be advantageous to use partial colloid resuscitation in some patients with evidence of cardiopulmonary dysfunction because a smaller total volume is required. An excess of intravenous crystalloid solution may result in fluid overload.

Vigorous broad-spectrum intravenous antibiotic therapy should be instituted. An indwelling urethral catheter is used to monitor fluid intake with hourly urine output. Combating shock is a primary concern throughout treatment. Clinical assessment of respiratory function should be made. A distended tender abdomen may cause rapid, shallow respirations and use of accessory muscles for ventilation. Arterial blood gases may indicate mild hypoxemia, in which case oxygen should be administered. If anemia is severe, blood transfusion should be started before surgery. When the patient has been properly prepared, immediate surgery should be undertaken. The results of treatment are better if major metabolic and hemodynamic problems are corrected before operation, but one cannot waste time in treating a critically ill patient with septic peritonitis.

Operative Phase

The anesthetic of choice depends on the preference and experience of the anesthesiologist and the medical condition of the patient.

The operation should be performed as rapidly as possible. Because speed as well as access to the upper abdomen may be required, a lower midline incision should be used. It can be quickly extended above the umbilicus if necessary.

The patient should not be put in the Trendelenburg position until the abdomen is packed off, and no more of a dependent position should be used than is needed to prevent further dissemination of pus into the upper abdomen. When the abdomen is opened, any odor that is present should be noted. An unpleasant, putrid odor is indicative of infection with anaerobic organisms. Pus from the abdomen should be collected correctly for both aerobic and anaerobic culture and for Gram stain, and be promptly transported to the laboratory. Organisms grown should be tested for sensitivity to various antibiotics.

The operation of choice is removal of the free pus, together with the abscess, the uterus, the tubes, and usually the ovaries. Only occasionally is it possible to leave an ovary in a patient with a ruptured pelvic abscess. If rupture has occurred from a strictly unilateral tuboovarian abscess, with a relatively normal tube and ovary on the opposite side, a unilateral salpingo-oophorectomy can be performed, especially if the patient is young. However, the risk of a recurrent abscess in the opposite tube and ovary is high if the uterus is also left in place. When the uterus is removed along with the tuboovarian abscess, the risk of recurrent abscess in the opposite adnexa is reduced. When hysterectomy is performed, usually a total hysterectomy can be done. However, even in the best surgical hands, a subtotal hysterectomy is faster than a total one and is sometimes justified. It is probable that the mortality rate would be increased if total hysterectomies were always performed. Although we believe firmly in total hysterectomy, we do not believe in performing it when the danger of total hysterectomy exceeds the danger from a retained cervix. Except in the young patient, it is often better to remove the corpus than to perform a unilateral adnexectomy alone. Furthermore, the opposite adnexa is significantly involved in most patients, and subsequent operation may be necessary if conservation of one side is practiced, as was required in 35% of Pedowitz and Bloomfield's cases. This is contrary to what has been described earlier in the surgical treatment of an unruptured abscess, because the risk of incomplete eradication of the immediate infection in an acutely ill patient with rupture, peritonitis, and possibly septic shock is much higher. Therefore, definitive surgical treatment is usually recommended in severely ill patients with ruptured abscess.

The technical performance of the procedure may be difficult, but is similar to that described earlier for laparotomy followed by failed colpotomy drainage or suspected rupture. Anatomy is distorted, dependable landmarks are obscured, and tissues are thick, edematous, friable, and inflamed. Loops of densely adherent intestine must be separated carefully to avoid injury. Injury to the serosa of distended bowel occurs commonly and often requires repair. Any entry into the lumen of the bowel must be recognized and repaired. Retroperitoneal planes of dissection can be used to advantage in identifying the ureters and removing inflammatory adnexal masses. Otherwise, it is likely that fragments of ovary will be left behind, which can subsequently cause signs and symptoms of the ovarian remnant syndrome. As much of the remaining abscess wall as possible should be removed without causing unnecessary additional bleeding. Pieces of the abscess wall can be left adherent to the pelvic sidewall and cul-de-sac. Oozing of blood from all dissected tissue has been likened to "cinder bed bleeding" and is difficult to control.

The upper abdomen should be carefully explored for collections of pus in the subdiaphragmatic and subhepatic regions. If an upper abdominal abscess is found, it may be necessary to place a closed suction drain into the abscess cavity through the upper abdominal wall.

Before the incision is closed, the abdominal cavity should be irrigated with copious quantities of warm sterile saline to remove remaining bacteria and debris. There is always some fear of dissemination of the infection by copious irrigation. However, this disadvantage is far outweighed by the benefit of diluting and removing bacteria and necrotic debris. We do not add antiseptics or antibiotics to the irrigating solution. If hemostasis is poor or if considerable necrotic material is left behind, there may be some benefit from peritoneal drainage with closed suction catheters. Closed suction drains can be placed through a separate stab wound in the abdominal wall, through the cul-de-sac, or through the vaginal vault when a total hysterectomy has been done, but the drainage of free peritoneal exudate in the upper abdomen is of no therapeutic value.

The abdominal incision is closed with a Smead-Jones technique or with a continuous suture taking large bites of tissue. A monofilament suture of polypropylene or nylon should be used. Retention sutures can be placed but are not usually necessary. The incision should be irrigated with warm saline. When there has been gross contamination of the incision, the subcutaneous fat and skin should be left open and packed lightly with gauze soaked in an antibiotic or dilute acetic acid solution. The wound is repacked daily and inspected. In 4 to 5 days, if the tissues are healthy, the incision is closed secondarily with sutures. Alternatively, the edges can be drawn together with sterile adhesive strips.

Postoperative Phase

Postoperative care should consider shock, infection, ileus, and fluid imbalances. Complications of the late postoperative period include pelvic and abdominal abscesses, intestinal obstruction, intestinal fistulas, incisional breakdown with or without evisceration, pulmonary embolus, continued sepsis, and disseminated intravascular coagulation. Serious medical diseases such as uncontrolled diabetes or renal or pulmonary failure (ARDS) further complicate recovery from this potentially lethal disease.

Septic shock should be combated with blood (when indicated for a hemoglobin less than 7.0 g), Ringer lactate, respiratory support, and, if necessary, vasoactive substances. Infection is controlled by the continued aggressive use of broad-spectrum intravenous antibiotics until the patient can take antibiotics orally. When the results of the antibiotic sensitivity studies on the operative specimen are available, a change to more effective agents should be considered, but only if the patient shows evidence of continued sepsis. Antibiotics should not necessarily be changed on the basis of sensitivity studies if the patient is improving clinically. Sometimes the patient's condition improves initially, only to show signs of recurring intraabdominal infection the second week after operation. Under these circumstances, it is appropriate to change antibiotics. Antibiotics should be continued until the patient is afebrile with only a mild leukocytosis or mildly elevated C-reactive protein and is able to eat a regular diet. A long period of treatment with antibiotics may result in complications such as pseudomembranous enterocolitis.

The semi-Fowler position may help prevent subphrenic and subdiaphragmatic abscess formation. Patients with signs of continued intraabdominal sepsis should have CT scans to identify collections of pus. If found, CT-directed drainage may be possible.

Constant intestinal suction by means of a long intestinal tube is a very important feature of postoperative care. A dynamic ileus persists postoperatively for a variable period and is best treated with the long intestinal tube until there is evidence of peristalsis and the patient is passing flatus.

Close attention to fluid balance and blood chemistry determinations is mandatory. Frequently, patients with ruptured tuboovarian abscess may have poor kidney function. The fluid output and serum creatinine should be followed closely.

PRIMARY OVARIAN ABSCESS

A primary ovarian abscess is an entity distinctly different from tuboovarian abscess. A tuboovarian abscess is one in which the abscess wall is composed of fallopian tube and ovarian parenchyma. A primary ovarian abscess, on the other hand, is one in which the infection occurs in the parenchyma of the ovary. Unlike tuboovarian abscess, it is an unusual condition. Interest in primary ovarian abscess was stimulated by the 1964 report of Willson and Black. According to a review by Wetchler and Dunn, 120 cases had been reported by 1985.

Although bacteria can gain access to the ovarian parenchyma by hematogenous or lymphatic spread, it is probable that most primary ovarian abscesses occur because bacteria present around the ovary gain access to the parenchyma through a break in the ovarian capsule. This can occur naturally by ovulation or it can be broken by a surgical procedure. Bacteria come from the fallopian tube, from the vagina during or after hysterectomy, from intrauterine infection associated with an IUD, or from appendicitis, diverticulitis, or any other condition that is associated with peritonitis. A primary ovarian abscess is usually unilateral. However, its occurrence simultaneously in both ovaries and during pregnancy seems to support the occasional hematogenous or lymphatic spread, or both. Primary ovarian abscess has been reported secondary to infections at distant sites (tonsillitis, typhoid, parotitis, and tuberculosis).

Diagnosis of an unruptured primary ovarian abscess can be difficult because of the variable clinical presentation. Lower abdominal pain and fever are usually present. Lower abdominal and pelvic tenderness and an adnexal mass may be present, but the pelvic examination is sometimes not helpful. Although an event predisposing to primary ovarian abscess (e.g., surgery, IUD use, appendicitis, or systemic infection) may be uncovered in the history, the event is sometimes remote. Ultrasonography and CT can be helpful in identifying an abscess cavity. If an ovarian abscess ruptures, the clinical picture is much the same as in ruptured tuboovarian abscess, with abdominal distention, direct and rebound tenderness, ileus, and sometimes shock. The patient appears gravely ill, and the need for immediate surgery is usually obvious.

The management of patients with primary ovarian abscess is similar to the management of patients with acute tuboovarian abscess. If the abscess is not ruptured, medical management with antibiotics for both anaerobic and aerobic organisms plus supportive care is indicated. A failure to respond or deterioration in the patient's condition suggests alteration in antibiotic coverage or possible exploratory surgery, or both, to remove the abscess. Ruptured ovarian abscess requires immediate laparotomy after a brief but intense effort to stabilize the patient and start antibiotic therapy. At operation, only the affected ovary need be removed. The tubes and the uterus can be conserved. If both ovaries are involved, they should be removed. For a patient who is not interested in conception in the future, the uterus and both tubes can also be removed. If the patient is interested in pregnancy, the uterus and fallopian tubes can be left in place for possible implantation of a donated egg in the future.

SURGERY FOR CHRONIC PELVIC INFLAMMATORY DISEASE

Although the gonococcus may be responsible for initiating acute salpingitis, which is short-lived, the residual chronic salpingitis is usually due to secondary invaders, both aerobic and anaerobic, or perhaps to an initial infection with *C. trachomatis*. As a result of the initial infection or from subsequent secondary exacerbations, the fimbria can become occluded and the tubes bound to the ovaries with adhesions. In addition, the bowel can become adherent to the broad ligament and the adnexal structures, and the fascia and loose connective tissue of the broad ligament can be converted into an indurated, brawny structure typical of ligneous induration. This can extend to include tissues beneath the peritoneum on the lateral pelvic sidewall, where ligneous pelvic cellulitis can cause ureteral obstruction. If the chronic infection persists, serious effusion from the inflammatory process within the endosalpinx produces a hydrosalpinx that can ignite periodically with secondary subacute pelvic infection or can progress to produce a pyosalpinx and tuboovarian abscess. If the subacute infection is left untreated or is treated inadequately, spontaneous intraabdominal rupture or leakage of an old tuboovarian abscess can occur. In a review of this subject, Heaton and Ledger identified this problem principally in premenopausal women, with only 1.7% of patients with a tuboovarian abscess being postmenopausal.

The signs and symptoms of chronic PID that most often require surgical treatment include severe, persistent, progressive pelvic pain, usually bilateral, although occasionally localized in one of the lower abdominal quadrants; repeated exacerbations of PID requiring multiple hospitalizations and recurrent medical treatment; progressive enlargement of a tuboovarian inflammatory mass, especially if it cannot be distinguished from a neoplastic tumor of the ovary; severe dyspareunia related to the chronic pelvic infection; and bilateral ureteral obstruction from ligneous cellulitis. It was formerly accepted that a history of previous colpotomy for drainage of a pelvic abscess was sufficient reason in itself to justify definitive abdominal surgery later for removal of the uterus and adnexa. We have seen several patients who have become pregnant after posterior colpotomy for drainage of a cul-de-sac abscess and who have remained relatively free of symptoms for long periods. Today, previous posterior colpotomy for pelvic abscess drainage is not a sufficient indication by itself for definitive abdominal surgery.

Selection of Operation

The final decision regarding the proper operation for the surgical management of chronic PID is usually made with the abdomen open. Consideration must be given not only to the pathologic lesions found at operation but also to the patient's age, parity, desire for children, previous history of pelvic disease, and other associated pelvic disease and symptoms. Because a knowledge of all these is essential to the best surgical judgment, the operator should be thoroughly familiar with the patient, her history, and her desires.

In the surgical management of chronic PID, the question of removal or retention of the ovary at the time of hysterectomy and salpingectomy has been left open to conjecture and individual surgical opinion in most instances. This question

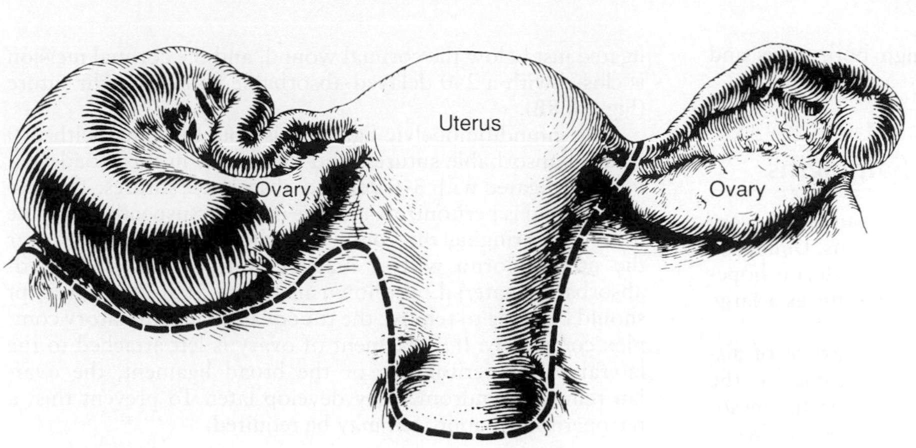

FIGURE 30.4. Total abdominal hysterectomy and unilateral salpingo–oophorectomy from extensive chronic salpingo–oophoritis. A small hydrosalpinx on the opposite side can be left in to preserve blood supply to the ovary.

was the subject of a study by Weiner and Wallach of the ovarian histology in ovaries removed from patients with PID. In 40 consecutive women who underwent oophorectomy during surgical treatment of PID, nearly 50% of the removed ovaries were free of inflammatory disease and demonstrated normal follicular activity. The study concluded that ovarian histology was usually normal among patients who gave no history of dysfunctional uterine bleeding. Therefore, the menstrual history of such patients should be helpful in the decision regarding ovarian conservation or ablation. Kirtley and Benigno have reviewed our experience with ovarian conservation at the time of surgery for PID. In this series, 98 (82%) patients who required surgery had a total abdominal hysterectomy and bilateral salpingo-oophorectomy. In 22 patients (18%), either part or all of an ovary was retained. Of the 22 patients, 15 were available for follow-up hormonal assays. The mean follow-up time was 58 months. Cyclic ovarian function was confirmed in all but two patients. In the two patients with ovarian failure, other significant disease processes were also present. No patient suffered a complication as a result of adnexal conservation. We believe that normal ovarian tissue should be conserved at the time of definitive surgery for PID. The release of peritubal adhesions in mild chronic PID is indicated occasionally in women in whom future childbearing is desired, as long as the tubes can be shown to be patent, usually by transfundal chromotubation after the lower uterine isthmus is occluded by a Ziegler clamp. This type of procedure provides the most rewarding pregnancy rate of all types of tubal reconstructive surgery. More often, one tube is hopelessly closed and the opposite tube is patent after release of adhesions. In such a case, unilateral salpingectomy may be required if reconstructive surgery is not possible. Many other procedures are available in the treatment of this disease, including salpingo-oophorectomy with or without hysterectomy (Figs. 30.4 and 30.5).

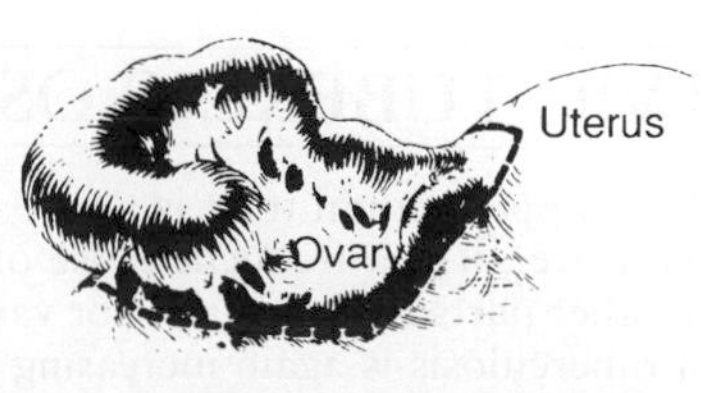

FIGURE 30.5. When significant chronic pelvic inflammatory disease involves only one adnexa and preservation of uterine function is indicated, a unilateral salpingo-oophorectomy can be performed.

In most instances of surgery for chronic PID, total abdominal hysterectomy and bilateral salpingo-oophorectomy are necessary to remove the primary tubal pathology because of inflammatory damage of both tubes and ovaries. Total abdominal hysterectomy and bilateral salpingo oophorectomy (Fig. 30.6) have been performed for severe actinomycosis infection.

If the uterus is removed and an ovary is preserved, it may be preferable to leave the entire adnexa in place in the absence of active tubal infection rather than compromise the venous drainage or the arterial blood supply to the ovary with subsequent cystic changes that may require an additional operative procedure later. Once the continuity of the tubal lumen from the uterine cavity is broken, the chronically inflamed tube does not usually produce subsequent symptoms, as shown by Falk in his series of cases with interstitial tubal resection. A small hydrosalpinx on the same side as the normal ovary can also be left in place so that ovarian blood supply is not disturbed during an attempt to remove the tube. When it is considered advisable to remove both adnexa because of the extent of the tuboovarian disease, a total hysterectomy may also be considered unless the uterus is hopelessly encased in pelvic scar tissue and densely adherent to the pelvic viscera.

In the optimum case, especially in a young woman who wishes to establish or maintain the possibility of future fertility, conservative surgery may be desirable, with the hope that pregnancy can be accomplished through *in vitro* fertilization techniques. In this situation, the uterus and one adnexa should be conserved, and the ovary should be positioned in the pelvis so an ovum can be harvested later through the laparoscope or through the vagina. As mentioned earlier, if the patient wishes,

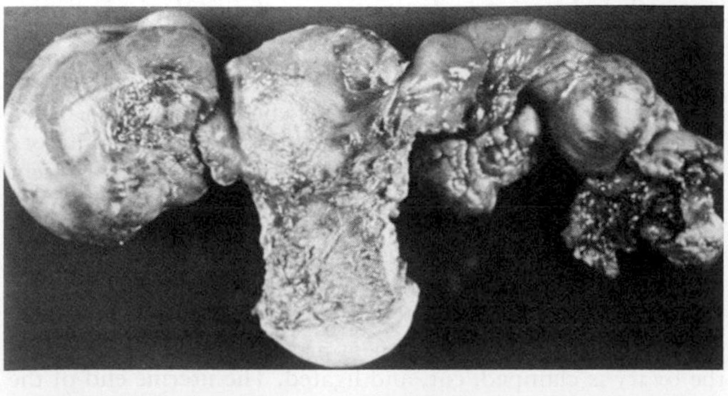

FIGURE 30.6. Total abdominal hysterectomy and bilateral salpingo-oophorectomy for severe pelvic actinomycosis.

the uterus can be left in place even though both tubes and ovaries have been removed.

Salpingectomy for Chronic Salpingitis

At the time of surgery for the treatment of chronic PID, every effort should be made to retain uninvolved organs. Unilateral salpingectomy should be considered when the oviduct is hopelessly destroyed by the disease process and presents as a large hydrosalpinx.

Once the abdomen has been opened and the extent of disease evaluated, the adhesions binding the tube are cut, and the tube is freed. It is held by a Kelly clamp placed on the mesosalpinx just beneath the fimbriated end. The mesosalpinx is then clamped and cut, with a succession of small bites taken as close to the tube as possible (Fig. 30.7A). Removal of a chronic hydrosalpinx can also be done laparoscopically.

Keeping the operative trauma as far as possible from the ovary that is to be retained lessens the danger of imperiling its blood supply. Experience has shown that the ovary whose tube has been removed is more apt to become cystic than the ovary whose tube has been left undisturbed. Therefore, it seems logical to interfere as little as possible with the blood supply of the ovary by hugging the tube closely when excising it.

The tube is excised at the uterine cornu in a wedge-shaped manner, as indicated in Figure 30.7B. A wide, figure-of-eight 2–0 delayed-absorbable suture is placed in the cornu before the wedge is excised and is tightened as the interstitial portion of the tube is removed. If there is palpable extension of the inflammation at the uterine cornu (so-called salpingitis isthmica nodosa), the wedge may be large.

The wound in the uterus is closed with one or more 2–0 delayed-absorbable figure-of-eight sutures (Fig. 30.7B). The vessels in the mesosalpinx are ligated with transfixion 3–0 delayed-absorbable sutures. The advantage of the transfixion suture is that it does not slip off the tissue when tied as the clamp is withdrawn (Fig. 30.7C).

A mattress suture of 3–0 delayed-absorbable material is used to bring the broad and round ligaments over the cornual wound (Fig. 30.7D). This suture passes just beneath the round ligament, so that the ligament is not strangulated when the suture is drawn tight. When this suture is tied, the cornual wound is covered with the broad ligament, and the uterus is suspended to some extent in a manner similar to that used in the Coffey suspension. Usually, a second mattress or interrupted suture is necessary to cover the mesosalpinx completely, as shown in Figure 30.7E.

Salpingo-oophorectomy for Chronic Salpingitis

As in salpingectomy, the abdomen is entered through a transverse Maylard incision. The chronic tuboovarian inflammatory mass is first dissected free, and the infundibulopelvic ligament is identified. It is doubly clamped with Ochsner clamps, and a third clamp is applied to control back-bleeding (Fig. 30.8A). The ureter must be identified before the infundibulopelvic ligament is clamped, cut, and ligated.

After the infundibulopelvic ligament is cut and ligated, the remainder of the broad ligament attachment of the tube and the ovary is clamped, cut, and ligated. The uterine end of the tube and the ovarian ligament are excised from the uterus in a wedge-shaped manner. The ascending uterine vessels are ligated just below the cornual wound, and the cornual incision is closed with a 2–0 delayed-absorbable figure-of-eight suture (Fig. 30.8B).

The infundibulopelvic ligament is doubly ligated with 2–0 delayed-absorbable sutures, and the vessels in the broad ligament are ligated with 3–0 delayed-absorbable sutures. The cornual wound is peritonized, and the uterus is suspended to some degree by bringing the round and the broad ligaments over the uterine cornu with a mattress suture of 2–0 delayed-absorbable material, as shown in Figure 30.8C. An attempt should be made to remove the tuboovarian inflammatory complex completely. If a fragment of ovary is left attached to the lateral pelvic peritoneum or the broad ligament, the ovarian remnant syndrome may develop later. To prevent this, a retroperitoneal approach may be required.

Identification of the Ureter

Identification of the course of the ureter in a pelvis in which the anatomy has become obliterated as a result of PID is one of the most important techniques for the gynecologic surgeon. In the surgical treatment of this disease, one may find a tuboovarian inflammatory mass that is located between the leaves of the broad ligament and extends to the lateral pelvic wall. It is not uncommon for the ligneous induration of the thickened parietal peritoneum to obscure completely the location and course of the pelvic ureter so that dissection of the diseased adnexa produces a surgical risk to the urinary tract, requiring great technical skill to avoid ureteral injury. Knowledge of the normal anatomic location of the pelvic ureters is essential so that these vital structures can be identified before an attempt is made to remove the adnexal masses. Division of the round ligament allows access to the lateral pelvic wall beneath the peritoneum. After the round ligament is divided, the peritoneum is incised inferiorly toward the internal cervical os and superiorly just lateral to the infundibulopelvic ligament. The peritoneum is easily reflected medially away from the pelvic sidewall with finger dissection, and the ureter is identified. It remains attached to the peritoneum. If there is difficulty with this procedure, the ureter can usually be identified as it crosses over the common iliac artery just above its bifurcation, and it can be traced downward.

Such patients may have a preoperative ureteral catheterization when there is clinical evidence of large, adherent adnexal masses. However, if such an anatomic problem is encountered at the time of laparotomy, an incision can be made in the dome of the bladder that allows the passage of ureteral catheters. If the patient has been positioned in the Allen universal stirrups for operation, intraoperative cystoscopy with passage of ureteral stents is easily accomplished. At the end of the operation, 5 mL of indigo carmine is given intravenously. With a cystoscope in the bladder, the dye can be seen effusing from both ureteral orifices, confirming that the ureters have not been injured or compromised.

PELVIC TUBERCULOSIS

Tuberculosis of the upper genital tract is a rare disease in the United States. However, it is a frequent cause of chronic PID and infertility in other parts of the world. For various reasons, the incidence of tuberculosis is again increasing in the United States. Therefore, cases of tuberculosis-associated PID may also become more evident. It should always be considered in the differential diagnosis of pelvic pain in immigrants, especially those

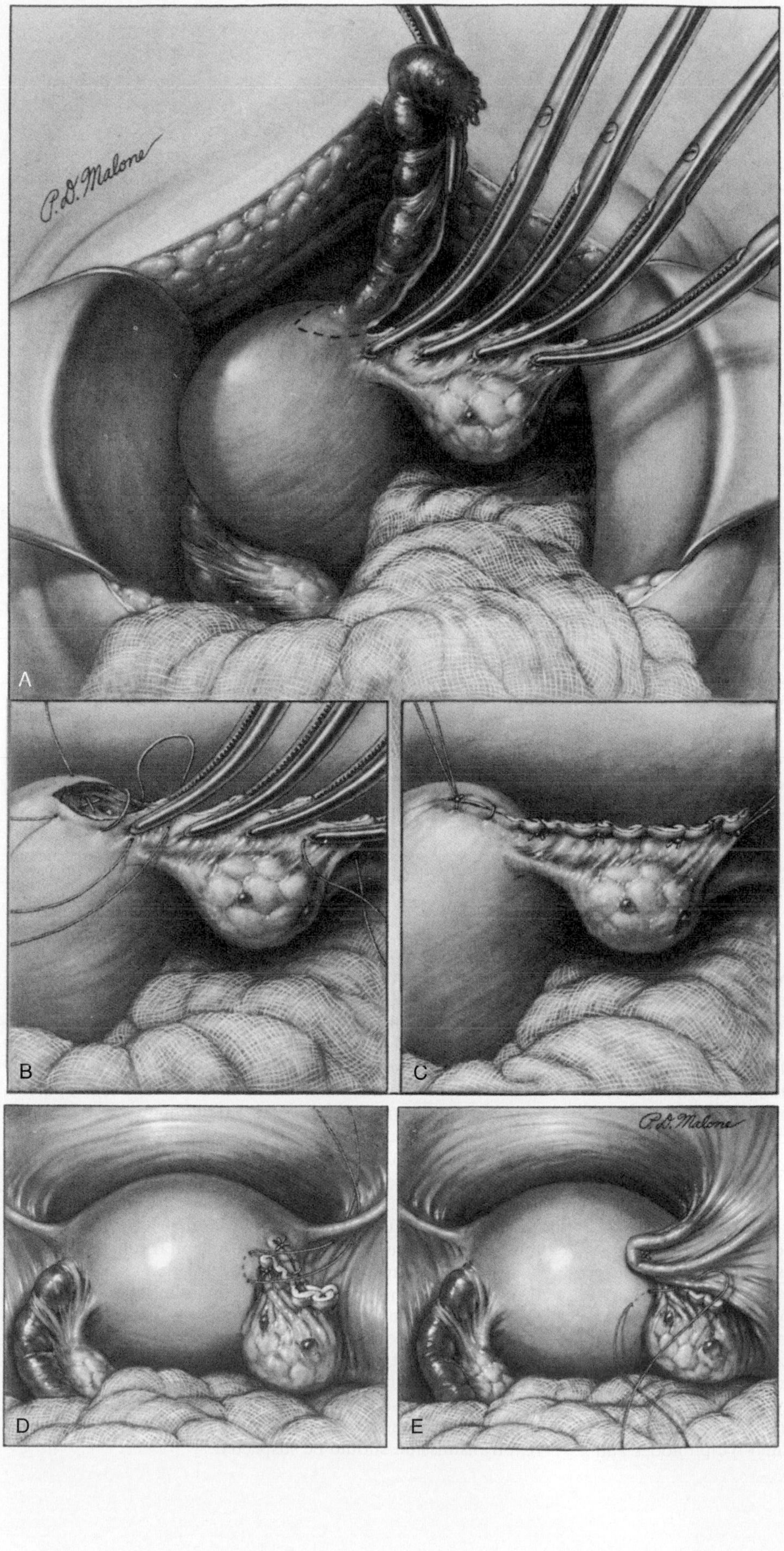

FIGURE 30.7. Salpingectomy. **A:** Mesosalpinx is clamped with multiple Kelly clamps and cut. Dotted lines indicate cornual excision, which is elective. **B:** Cornual wound is closed with 2–0 delayed-absorbable suture. **C:** Mesosalpinx vessels are transfixed. **D:** Mattress suture is placed to cover operative area. **E:** Round ligament and broad ligament cover operative area.

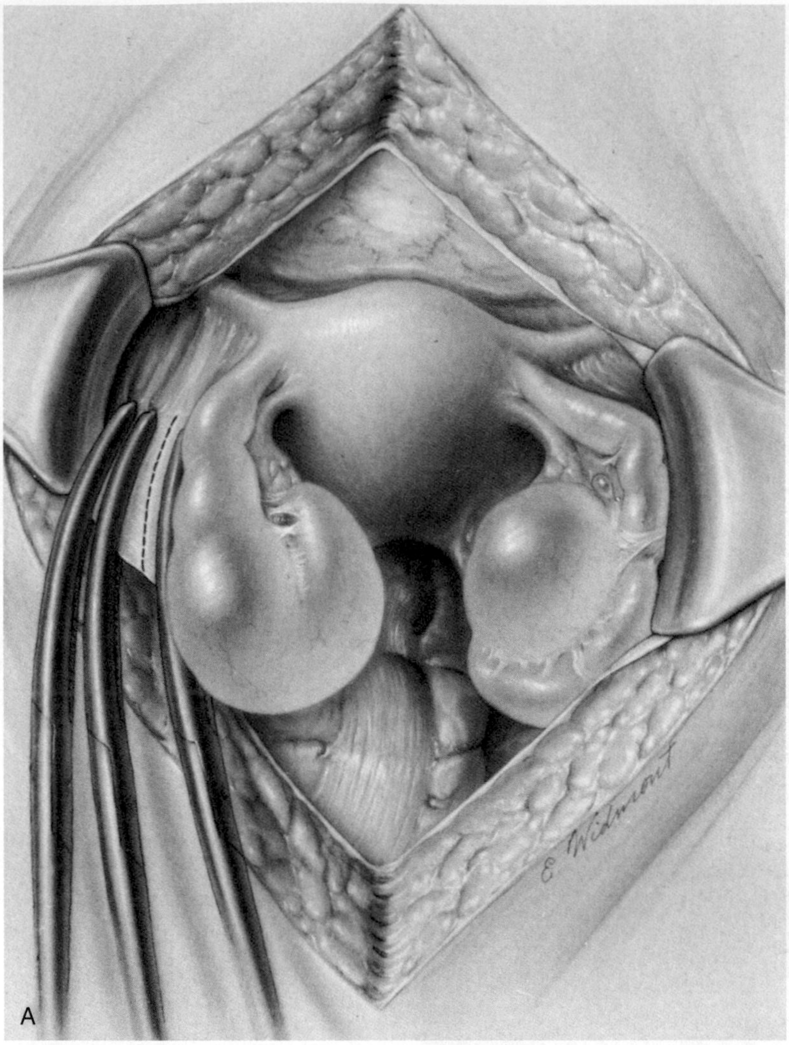

FIGURE 30.8. Salpingo-oophorectomy. **A:** The infundibulopelvic ligament is doubly clamped. Another clamp is placed to control back-bleeding. Dotted line indicates incision.

from Asia, the Middle East, and Latin America, and in patients with HIV. Pelvic tuberculosis is produced primarily by either *Mycobacterium tuberculosis* or *Mycobacterium bovis*. The primary site of infection for tuberculosis is usually the lung, with lymphatic spread from the Ghon complex to regional lymph nodes at the hilum usually occurring within 1 to 2 years. More rapid dissemination is due to hematogenous spread, which results in miliary disease often within the first year. The fallopian tubes are the predominant site of pelvic tuberculosis, but the bacilli also spread to the endometrium and occasionally the ovaries.

No location in the body is immune to the development of metastatic foci of infection. Tuberculosis of the bone, meninges, kidney, epididymis, fallopian tubes, and other sites can develop. At some sites of miliary spread, the lesions can remain quiescent for long periods before reactivation and further spread of the disease. Direct extension from one organ or system to an adjacent organ or system can also occur. Organs of the female reproductive tract are usually infected by hematogenous miliary spread from a primary pulmonary lesion, by hematogenous spread from a secondary miliary site, by lymphatic spread from a primary pulmonary site to intestinal lymph nodes and then to the pelvis, or by direct extension from adjacent abdominal organs (small intestines, appendix, rectum, bladder) that are the site of tuberculous infection. Fistulas between the intestinal tract and the fallopian tubes have been reported with pelvic tuberculosis.

A venereal transmission of the disease has been reported, with primary genital infection in the woman occurring after coitus with a sexual partner who had tuberculosis of the genitourinary tract. According to Sutherland and MacFarlane, it is not possible to prove conclusively that genitourinary tuberculosis in the man can be transmitted to the woman through sexual intercourse. Because it has been shown that *M. tuberculosis* is present in the sperm of men with urogenital tuberculosis, the possibility of transmission to the pelvic organs of the woman through intercourse must be accepted. Sutherland presents five cases in which sexual transmission of genitourinary tuberculosis from man to woman presumably occurred. However, of 128 husbands of women with genital tuberculosis, only five (3.9%) were found to have active genitourinary tuberculosis. When tuberculosis of the vulva, vagina, and cervix is present without evidence of tuberculosis elsewhere in the body, venereal transmission should be suspected.

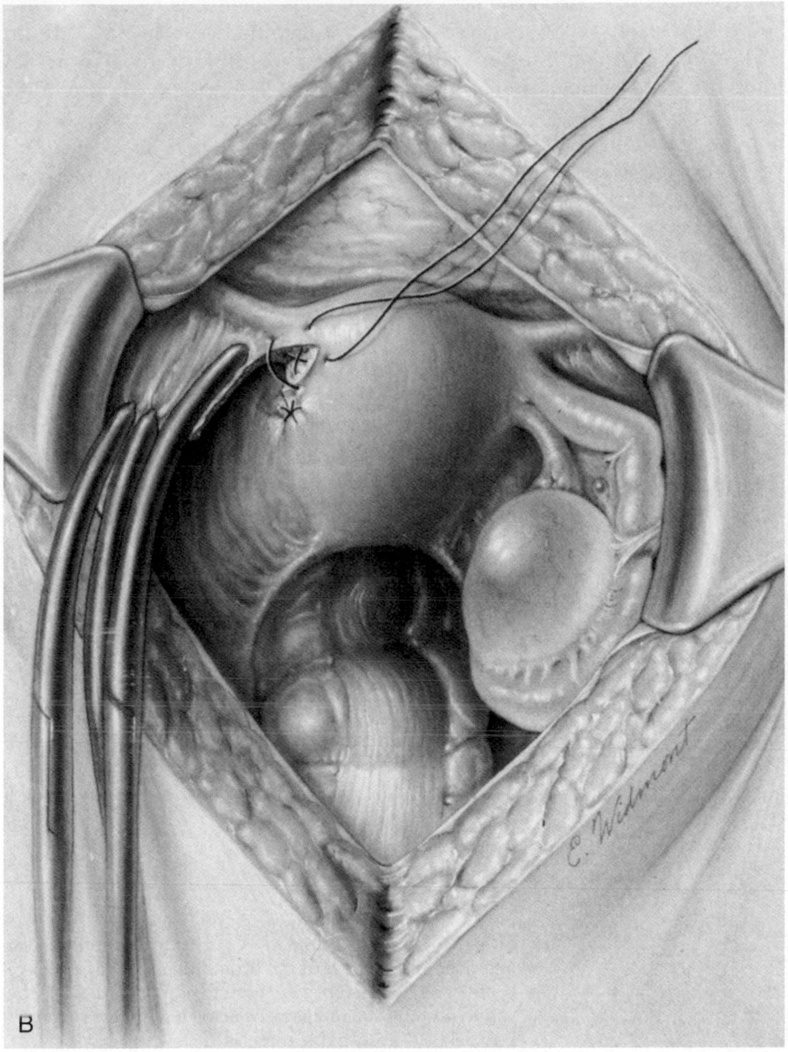

FIGURE 30.8. (*Continued*) **B:** A suture has been placed to ligate the ascending uterine vessels just below the cornual incision. The cornual incision is closed with a figure-of-eight suture of 2–0 delayed-absorbable material.

Pathology of Pelvic Tuberculosis

Both fallopian tubes are involved in almost all patients with pelvic tuberculosis. About one half of patients with tuberculous salpingitis have tuberculous endometritis. Tuberculosis of the cervix is present in 5% of cases. The vagina and vulva are rarely involved. At operation, one may find evidence of generalized tuberculous peritonitis with small, grayish white tubercles covering all peritoneal surfaces of the abdominal and pelvic organs. The mucosa of the fallopian tubes may not be involved in generalized serosal tuberculous infection. At a later stage of infection, tuberculous salpingitis may grossly resemble other forms of PID involving the adnexa. Unless tubercles are seen, the diagnosis may not be apparent until microscopic sections are examined by the pathologist. A large pyosalpinx may contain the caseous material of a tuberculous infection but may also contain the purulent exudate of a secondary infection with other common organisms. Tubercles form in the lining of the tube. Some have caseation at the center, with giant cells and epithelioid cells. A proliferation of the mucosal lining of the fallopian tube may resemble a primary tubal carcinoma microscopically and may be confusing to the pathologist.

Tuberculous peritonitis is commonly associated with tuberculosis of the pelvis. Clinically, tuberculous peritonitis can be divided into two groups. In "wet" peritonitis there is an outpouring of straw-colored fluid into the peritoneal cavity, producing ascites. The peritoneum of the parietal wall and viscera is covered with innumerable small tubercles (Fig. 30.9). The tubes, in addition to being covered with miliary tubercles on the serosal surface, are usually slightly enlarged and distended. In contrast to other forms of salpingitis, the fimbriae may be patent. Within the tubal wall and tubal mucosa, the histology is typical of tuberculosis, with tubercle formation, multinucleated giant cells, and epithelioid reaction (Fig. 30.10). In advanced cases, frank caseation is present. This pattern is usually associated with hematogenous spread of the tuberculous organism to the peritoneal surfaces and the pelvic organs.

Another type of tuberculous peritonitis encountered in women is the "dry" or adhesive type. Bowel adheres to bowel by innumerable dense adhesions that blend with the musculature. The muscle of the bowel is often invaded to some degree by the tuberculous process. Separation of these adhesions is extremely difficult surgically, and accidental injury to the bowel is common. The pelvic organs show evidence of tuberculous

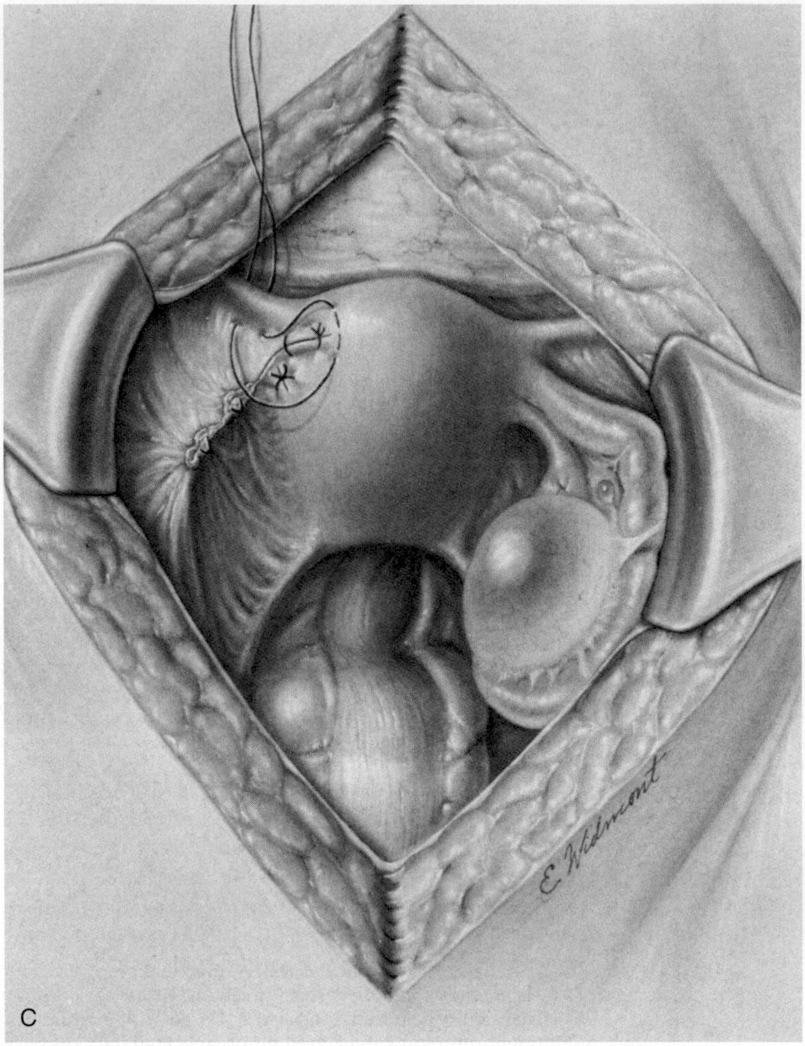

FIGURE 30.8. (*Continued*) **C:** The infundibulopelvic ligament and the rest of the broad ligament vessels have been ligated. The cornual wound is covered with the round and the broad ligament using a mattress suture of 2–0 delayed-absorbable material.

salpingitis with enlargement of the tubes and occasionally pyosalpinges and even tuboovarian abscess formation.

Tuberculous involvement of the myometrium is rare. Tuberculous endometritis, however, is common, occurring in 60% to 70% of women with pelvic tuberculosis. Microscopically, tubercles are seen scattered throughout the endometrium, but they may be scanty. Tubercles are often seen in the endometrium removed by curettage in the premenstrual phase and are usually located in the endometrium adjacent to the tubal ostia. Apparently, the uterine cavity is protected from advanced tuberculous infection by the cyclic shedding of endometrial tissue in the reproductive years. Even in advanced pelvic tuberculous infections, evidence of caseation, fibrosis, and calcification are rarely seen in the uterine cavity. Occasionally, the endometrial cavity is obliterated by extensive adhesions. Total destruction of the endometrium can result in amenorrhea. Tuberculous pyometra can also develop, especially in postmenopausal women with an occluded internal cervical os.

Tuberculous lesions of the cervix are rare. They can be either ulcerative or exophytic and can resemble a primary cervical malignancy or granuloma inguinale of the cervix. When there is a tuberculous lesion of the cervix, the cervical biopsy often reveals tubercles.

A tuberculous infection of the ovary usually involves only the surface of the ovary and represents simply an extension of infection from the peritoneal cavity and the adjacent fallopian tubes. The infection is usually limited to a perioophoritis. Tuberculous caseation can be found within the ovarian parenchyma, although this is uncommon. Presumably, it occurs as a result of hematogenous spread to the ovarian parenchyma rather than by direct extension through the ovarian capsule. However, a break in the ovary caused by ovulation may also allow the tubercular bacilli to gain access to the ovarian parenchyma. The ovaries are involved in about 25% of cases of pelvic tuberculosis.

It is uncommon for tuberculosis to involve the vulva and vagina. It is seen in only 2% of patients with pelvic tuberculosis. The gross appearance may be ulcerative with multiple sinuses, it may be hypertrophic with elephantiasis, or it may be similar to that of carcinoma.

Throughout the pelvic organs, the microscopic picture is similar, with tubercles of granulomatous inflammation, Langhans' giant cells, epithelioid cells, and central caseation associated with chronic inflammation. With special stains, acid-fast bacilli can be demonstrated on careful microscopic examination of the tubercles.

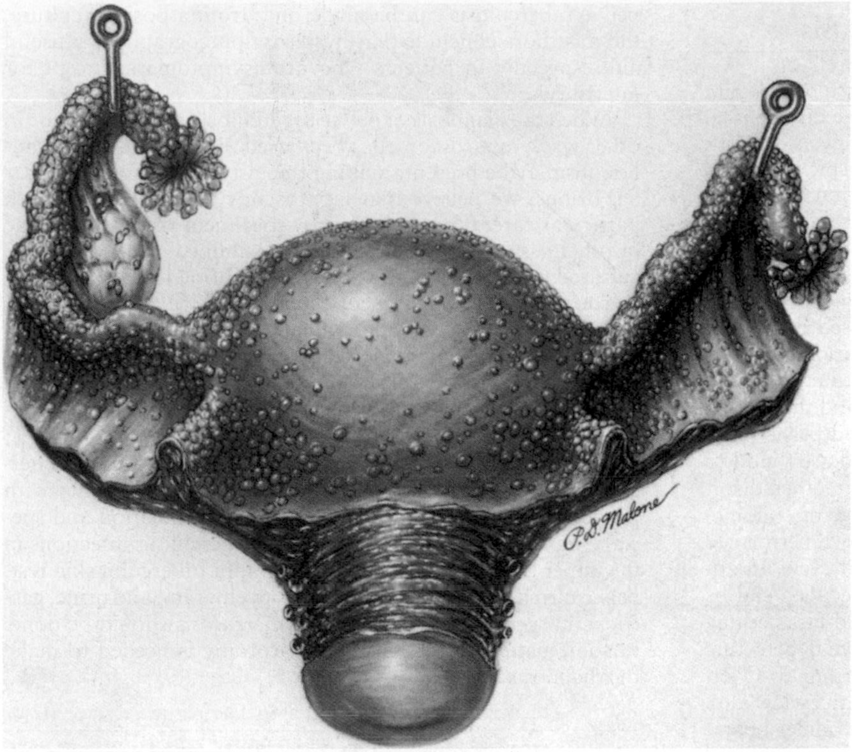

FIGURE 30.9. Typical specimen of tuberculosis of the reproductive organs as part of generalized tuberculous peritonitis.

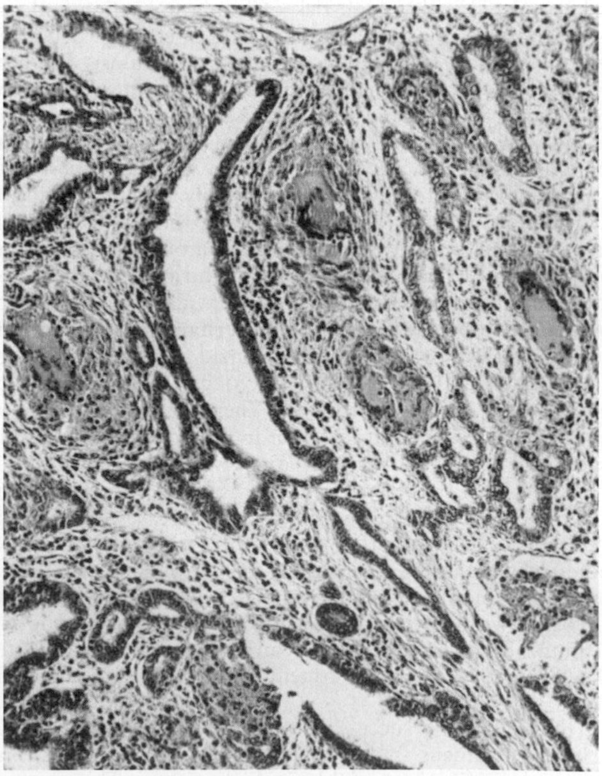

FIGURE 30.10. Tuberculosis of the fallopian tube. Note the multinucleated giant cells.

Clinical Features of Pelvic Tuberculosis

Pelvic tuberculosis occurs most often in patients between the ages of 20 and 40 years. The age of patients with gynecologic tuberculosis has changed in recent years; the proportion of patients older than 40 years of age is now much higher than it was in the past. Falk and associates found that the incidence of pelvic tuberculosis in postmenopausal Swedish women is increasing. This was also the opinion of Sutherland, who reported an investigation from Glasgow in which 26 of 701 patients (3.7%) with proven gynecologic tuberculosis were postmenopausal.

The most common clinical symptoms of pelvic tuberculosis include pelvic pain, general malaise, menstrual irregularity, and infertility. Brown and associates found that menstrual irregularity occurred in nearly 50% of patients, whereas amenorrhea or oligomenorrhea was present in 27%. A low-grade fever that on occasion can produce a fulminating septic course is noted in most cases of active or subacute disease. The failure of fever to subside with high doses of broad-spectrum antibiotics is a classic feature of pelvic tuberculosis. A clinical course that is refractory to antibiotic therapy for the usual PID should alert the clinician to the possibility of tuberculosis.

Among patients with pulmonary tuberculosis, the incidence of pelvic tuberculosis generally varies between 10% and 20%. Falk and associates noted that 38% of women with genital tuberculosis had previously had tuberculosis in other organs, usually the lungs. Often, the patient's clinical course is that of a chronic indolent illness.

Diagnosis of Pelvic Tuberculosis

The clinical symptoms and signs of pelvic tuberculosis should direct the clinician to the diagnosis. However, the disease is so uncommon that it is seldom encountered in the gynecologist's usual practice; therefore, the clinical index of suspicion is generally low. In many cases, the clinical presentation is obscure and the diagnosis is delayed. Howard Kelly once said that when competent gynecologists disagree about the diagnosis of an obscure pelvic condition, it usually is diagnosed as either an "old ectopic pregnancy or pelvic tuberculosis."

More than two thirds of the cases are diagnosed at the time of laparotomy performed for some other indication or at the time of investigation for infertility or abnormal uterine bleeding. The most common symptom is infertility, and the second most common symptom is lower abdominal and pelvic pain. Some patients are completely asymptomatic and are found to have pelvic tuberculosis during examination for other disorders such as infertility. A dilatation and curettage or endometrial biopsy is diagnostic in some cases, especially if performed in the late premenstrual phase of the menstrual cycle. In addition to standard microscopic sections, the specimen can be examined by fluorescent antibody technique. Acid-fast staining of tissue or culture of menstrual blood is effective in detecting the organism in only about 10% of cases, according to Overbeck. The menstrual blood can be collected in a cervical cap. The culture or inoculation can be repeated many times before a positive result is obtained. Acid-fast stains of tissue suspected of tuberculous infection are important to confirm the diagnosis. Because some acid-fast bacilli are not tuberculous bacilli, it is important to obtain a positive culture whenever possible. A negative evaluation of the endometrium does not rule out pelvic tuberculosis, because the disease can be present in the fallopian tubes without tuberculous endometritis in 30% to 40% of cases.

On pelvic examination, bilateral adnexal tenderness is the rule. The tenderness is usually less marked than with acute gonococcal or streptococcal infections. Occasionally, a large tuberculous tuboovarian abscess is palpated on pelvic examination and even felt through the abdominal wall. The classic doughy feel of the broad ligament suggests a tuberculous inflammatory disease that is produced by a combination of thickening of the broad ligament, adherent bowel, and some ascitic fluid. On occasion, cul-de-sac nodules representing tubercles on the serosal surfaces of pelvic organs can be felt. The clinical detection of ascites is the strongest evidence obtainable in favor of pelvic tuberculosis. It was present in one fifth of the cases reported by Brown and associates. However, other causes of ascites must be considered, including ovarian carcinoma and cirrhosis of the liver. In differentiating tuberculous salpingitis from neisserial infections, the finding of a virginal outlet in the presence of obvious tubal inflammation should lend strength to the diagnosis of pelvic tuberculosis.

The diagnosis of tuberculosis cannot be made with certainty from a hysterosalpingogram, but it may be helpful. The radiographic criteria for a suspicion of pelvic tuberculosis by hysterosalpingogram have been described by Klein and associates as follows: calcified lymph nodes or smaller, irregular calcifications in the adnexal areas; obstruction of the fallopian tube in the zone of transition between the isthmus and the ampulla; multiple constrictions along the course of the fallopian tube; endometrial adhesions or deformity or obliteration of the endometrial cavity in the absence of a history of curettage or abortion; and vascular or lymphatic extravasation of contrast material. Although a conclusive diagnosis of pelvic tuberculosis can be made only from a positive culture, these authors conclude that hysterosalpingography is a useful aid, especially in patients who are asymptomatic except for infertility.

When the diagnosis of pelvic tuberculosis cannot be made in other ways, laparoscopy has been used. Because numerous adhesions may be present, making the introduction of the trocar hazardous, we believe that laparoscopy should be used with particular care. If possible, biopsy specimens of tubal fimbriae or other suspicious areas should be examined histologically or cultured to confirm the diagnosis. In addition to disclosing numerous adhesions, laparoscopy may reveal widespread miliary tubercles involving the omentum and peritoneal surfaces. Matted adnexal masses may be seen. Microscopic examination of peritoneal fluid shows a predominance of lymphocytes.

Vaginal cytology is of limited value in diagnosing tuberculosis. The cytologist must be familiar with the morphology of epithelioid cells in the vaginal smear. Only in cases of tuberculosis of the cervix may cytology be helpful. Patients with pelvic tuberculosis should also have an examination and special diagnostic procedures to rule out tuberculous infections in the upper genital tract. Chest radiograph, tuberculin skin test, pelvic ultrasonography, intravenous pyelogram, and urine, gastric, and sputum cultures for *M. tuberculosis* should be done. In some patients, exploratory laparotomy is needed to make the diagnosis.

Treatment of Pelvic Tuberculosis

Before the advent of antituberculous drug therapy, surgery was often used in the treatment of pelvic tuberculosis. Primary surgical treatment was technically difficult, sometimes ineffective, and associated with a high risk of fistula formation and persistent draining sinuses. With the advent of effective drug therapy, the surgical treatment for genital tuberculosis has been restricted to specific indications. Beginning with streptomycin more than 30 years ago, and later isoniazid and paraaminosalicylic acid, it became evident that many cases of pelvic tuberculosis could be cured or controlled with antituberculous drug therapy. There have been major advances in the antibiotic treatment of this disease, including the use of isoniazid with rifampin, with or without ethambutol, given sometimes for a period of 2 years or longer. Sutherland analyzed the results obtained with various drug schedules. The drugs that have been used to treat tuberculosis are isoniazid, rifampin, streptomycin, ethambutol, and pyrazinamide. Isoniazid and rifampin are the most effective and have the lowest toxicity. They should be the foundation of most drug regimens. The addition of ethambutol may not be of benefit, at least not in pulmonary tuberculosis. Severe and sometimes fatal hepatitis, which can develop even after months of treatment, has been associated with isoniazid therapy. The risk of developing hepatitis increases with age and with the daily consumption of alcohol. Liver function studies should be done before treatment is started, and patients should be carefully monitored with liver function studies throughout the course of therapy and later. The regimen options and dosage recommendations of the American Thoracic Society and the CDC from 1993 for the treatment of tuberculosis are given in Tables 30.5 and 30.6.

The therapeutic success of modern antituberculous drug treatment regimens is difficult to assess in view of the limited number of cases available in the literature. The cure rate varies in the literature from 65% to 95%. Kardos removed the fallopian tubes from 168 patients after medical treatment for 10 months and found active tuberculosis in 35% of the

TABLE 30.5

REGIMEN OPTIONS FOR THE INITIAL TREATMENT OF TUBERCULOSIS

Option 1	Option 2	Option 3
Administer daily INH, RIF, and PZA for 8 wk, followed by 16 wk of INH and RIF daily or 2–3 times/wk.[a] In areas where the INH resistance rate is not documented as less than 4%, EMB or SM should be added to the initial regimen until susceptibility to INH and RIF is demonstrated. Continue treatment for at least 6 mo, and 3 mo beyond culture conversion. Consult a tuberculosis medical expert if the patient is symptomatic or smear or culture positive after 3 mo.	Administer daily INH, RIF, PZA, and SM or EMB for 2 wk, then administer the same drugs 2 times/wk[a] for 6 wk (by DOT). Next, administer INH and RIF 2 times/wk for 16 wk (by DOT). Consult a tuberculosis medical expert if the patient is symptomatic or smear or culture positive after 3 mo.	Treat by DOT, 3 times/wk[a] with RIF, PZA, and EMB or SM for 6 mo.[b] Consult a tuberculosis medical expert if the patient is symptomatic or smear or culture positive after 3 mo.

INH, isomazid; RIF, rifampin; PZA, pyrazinamide; EMB, ethambutol hydrochoride; SM, streptomycin sulfate; DOT, directly observed therapy.
[a]All regimens administered two times a week or three times a week should be monitored by DOT for the duration of therapy.
[b]The strongest evidence from clinical trials is the effectiveness of all four drugs administered for the full 6 months. There is weaker evidence that SM can be discontinued after 4 months if the isolate is susceptible to all drugs. The evidence for stopping PZA before the end of 6 months is equivocal for the three-times-a-week regimen, and there is no evidence on the effectiveness of this regimen with EMB for less than full 6 months.

surgical specimens. The experience of Sutherland suggests, however, that the results of treatment may be improved with newer drugs. The patients under treatment must be followed up closely for evidence of regression or remission of the pelvic tuberculosis. Only about 50% of patients with genital tuberculosis have the disease in the endometrial cavity; therefore, repeat endometrial biopsies and culture of menstrual egress provides only limited diagnostic information. The progress of the disease can be monitored closely by evaluating the size of adnexal masses with pelvic examinations and ultrasonography, as well as tracking the ESR, WBC count, and temperature response. Prolonged follow-up is probably indicated in all cases, because recurrence of the tuberculous pelvic lesion 5 years and even later after the end of drug treatment has occasionally been found.

Surgery in the management of patients with pelvic tuberculosis should be reserved for specific indications, as outlined by Schaefer and by Sutherland. In general, surgery is reserved for those patients who have failed to respond to an adequate trial of medical therapy. Our indications for the surgical treatment of pelvic tuberculosis include the following:

1. Persistence or enlargement of an adnexal mass after 4 to 6 months of antituberculous antibiotic therapy. The rare possibility of an ovarian tumor must always be considered, even though pelvic tuberculosis is also present. In a 1980 report by Sutherland, the persistence or development of substantial pelvic masses was the indication for surgery in 36 of 91 women with proven tuberculosis of the genital tract treated by surgery. Pelvic ultrasonography should be useful in following the response of adnexal masses to treatment.
2. Persistence of pelvic pain or recurrence of pelvic pain while on medical therapy. In Sutherland's report, 40 of 91 patients were operated on because of pain.

TABLE 30.6

DOSAGE RECOMMENDATIONS FOR THE INITIAL TREATMENT OF TUBERCULOSIS

Drug	Dosage: Daily	Dosage: Two times a week	Dosage: Three times a week
Isoniazid	5 mg/kg Max 300 mg	15 mg/kg Max 900 mg	15 mg/kg Max 900 mg
Rifampin	10 mg/kg Max 600 mg	10 mg/kg Max 600 mg	10 mg/kg Max 600 mg
Pyrazinamide	15–30 mg/kg Max 2 g	50–70 mg/kg Max 4 g	50–70 mg/kg Max 3 g
Ethambutol hydrochloride	5–25 mg/kg Max 2.5 g	50 mg/kg Max 2.5 g	25–30 mg/kg Max 2.5 g
Streptomycin sulfate	15 mg/kg Max 1 g	25–30 mg/kg Max 1.5 g	25–30 mg/kg Max 1 g

3. Primary unresponsiveness of the tuberculous infection to antibiotic therapy, as shown by persistent spiking temperature, leukocytosis, elevated ESR, and evidence on biopsy specimens of continued endometrial infection. Of the 91 women in Sutherland's report, 10 were operated on because of persistence of endometrial tuberculosis.
4. Difficulty in obtaining patient cooperation for continued long-term therapy. In these cases, we are accustomed to giving a brief course of streptomycin, 0.5 g every 12 hours intramuscularly for 1 week before surgery, to perform definitive surgery, and then we give 0.5 g every 24 hours in the postoperative period for 2 weeks. A persistent effort should be made to obtain the patient's cooperation for continued antituberculous therapy postoperatively. It is advisable to continue treatment for a year or longer. Isoniazid and rifampin should be used if possible. A common reason for failure of treatment is a tendency for the physician to discontinue drugs after only a few months because the patient appears well.

The preferred surgical treatment includes total abdominal hysterectomy and bilateral salpingo-oophorectomy. The nature of this inflammatory disease may make this operative procedure technically difficult, with an increased risk of injury to bowel and bladder. Consequently, in the event of a frozen pelvis from pelvic tuberculosis, it is occasionally necessary to perform only a subtotal abdominal hysterectomy and adnexectomy.

Adhesions, which are invariably present and usually widespread, may make the dissection more difficult and injury more likely. However, it is usually possible to do this operation without a high incidence of bowel fistulas and other significant complications. Sutherland reported the results of surgery in 77 patients operated on while antituberculous therapy was administered. There were no deaths, no fistulas, and few late complications.

For young patients who are eager to attempt future childbearing, conservative adnexectomy should be carried out only if it is possible to do so after the extent of the adnexal disease is carefully evaluated and is found to be minimal. It is unwise for the surgeon to be committed to a specific operative procedure before the time of surgery, because conservative pelvic surgery for tuberculosis may constitute poor surgical judgment once the operative findings are known. The patient should be forewarned that conservative surgery will be performed only if the disease is minimal and such surgery is considered medically advisable.

Conservation of an ovary at the time of operation for pelvic tuberculosis is occasionally possible if the ovary is involved only on its surface. However, if one finds gross evidence of ovarian enlargement or other gross evidence of infection deep in the ovarian parenchyma, the ovary should be removed. Bisection of ovaries to assess the presence of disease deep in the ovarian parenchyma is not advisable.

Reactivation of silent pelvic tuberculosis after tubal reconstructive surgery has been reported by Ballon and associates and by others. We believe that reconstructive tubal surgery has no place in the management of patients whose infertility is the result of bilateral tubal obstruction from tuberculous salpingitis.

Pregnancy after Pelvic Tuberculosis

It is evident from the literature, including the studies of both Schaefer and Sutherland, that only about 5% of patients with genital tuberculosis are capable of becoming pregnant, and only 2% carry a pregnancy to term. It is also evident that in the presence of tuberculous tuboovarian abscesses, pregnancy is extremely rare, and conservative surgery for the purpose of preserving fertility is unwarranted. Only when there is minimal pelvic disease without adnexal masses should conservative surgery be considered.

BEST SURGICAL PRACTICES

- Laparoscopy should be discussed with all patients suspected of pelvic inflammatory disease to confirm the diagnosis and to rule out other surgical emergencies such as appendicitis, ectopic pregnancy, or ruptured abscess. However, patients at high risk for complications or with contraindications to laparoscopy can be started on antimicrobial therapy and followed for 24 to 48 hours for a response. With the advent of very effective antimicrobial therapy, strong consideration should be given for surgical expiration if the patient fails initial therapy or symptomatology changes suggesting an alternative diagnosis. If laparoscopy is not selected as initial management, an endometrial sampling for detection of inflammatory cells and bacterial culture is usually helpful.
- Sonohysterography is contraindicated in patients suspected of having PID. Culdocentesis with the finding of purulent peritoneal fluid may indicate PID, but does not rule out appendicitis or diverticulitis.
- Posterior colpotomy requires midline abscess, an abscess that is adherent to cul-de-sac peritoneum and dissects the rectovaginal septum, and a cystic or fluctuant abscess.
- Hysterectomy is no longer absolutely necessary if salpingo-oophrectomy is needed for treatment of tuboovarian abscesses. Copious irrigation with lactated Ringer is essential if an abscess has ruptured or pus is present in the abdomen. Antibiotic irrigation has not demonstrated additional benefit or risk. If hysterectomy is necessary after bilateral salpingo-oophrectomy, the vaginal vault should be left open for drainage (with or without a Penrose drain).
- Swam-Ganz catheter placement is helpful in monitoring central venous pressure in patients undergoing surgery for ruptured tuboovarian abscess.

Bibliography

Ballon SC, Clewell WH, Lamb EJ. Reactivation of silent pelvic tuberculosis by reconstructive tubal surgery. *Am J Obstet Gynecol* 1975;122: 991.

Bell TA, Holmes KK. Age-specific risks of syphilis, gonorrhea, and hospitalized pelvic inflammatory disease in sexually experienced U.S. women. *Sex Transm Dis* 1989;11:291.

Brown AB, Gilbert RA, Te Linde RW. Pelvic tuberculosis. *Obstet Gynecol* 1953;2:476.

Centers for Disease Control and Prevention. Initial therapy for tuberculosis in the era of multidrug resistance. *JAMA* 1993;270:694.

Centers for Disease Control and Prevention. Sexually transmitted diseases: treatment guidelines. *MMWR Morb Mortal Wkly Rep* 2006;55(RR-11): 56.

Centers for Disease Control and Prevention. Trends in reportable sexually transmitted diseases in the United States, 2004. November 2005. Available at: http://www.cdc.gov/std/stats/trends2004.htm.

Chow AW, Pattern V, Marshall JR. The bacteriology of acute pelvic inflammatory disease. *Am J Obstet Gynecol* 1975;122:876.

Collins CG, Jansen FW. Management of tubo-ovarian abscess. *Clin Obstet Gynecol* 1959;2:512.

Eilard ET, Brorsson JE, Hanmark B, et al. Isolation of *Chlamydia* in acute salpingitis. *Scand J Infect Dis* 1976;9:82.

Eschenbach DA. Epidemiology and diagnosis of acute pelvic inflammatory disease. *Obstet Gynecol* 1980;55:142.

Eschenbach DA, Holmes KK. Acute PID: current concepts of pathogenesis, etiology and management. *Clin Obstet Gynecol* 1975;18:35.

Falk HC. Cornual resection for the treatment of recurrent salpingitis. *Am J Surg* 1951;81:595.

Falk V, Ludviksson K, Argen G. Genital tuberculosis in women. Analysis of 187 newly diagnosed cases from 47 Swedish hospitals during the ten-year period 1968 to 1977. *Am J Obstet Gynecol* 1980;138:974–7.

Fitz-Hugh T. Acute gonococcic peritonitis of the right upper quadrant in women. *JAMA* 1934;102:2084.

Franklin EW 3rd, Hevron JE Jr, Thompson JD. Management of pelvic abscess. *Clin Obstet Gynecol* 1973;16:66.

Ginsburg DS, Stern JL, Hamod KA, et al. Tubo-ovarian abscess: a retrospective review. *Am J Obstet Gynecol* 1980;138:1055.

Golde SH, Israel R, Ledger WJ. Unilateral tubo-ovarian abscess: a distinct entity. *Am J Obstet Gynecol* 1977;17:807.

Hager WD, Eschenbach DA, Spence MR, et al. Criteria for diagnosis and grading of salpingitis. *Obstet Gynecol* 1983;61:113.

Hager WD, Majmudar B. Pelvic actinomycosis in women using intrauterine contraceptive devices. *Am J Obstet Gynecol* 1979;133:60.

Hager WD, McDaniel PS. Treatment of serious obstetric and gynecologic infections with cefoxitin. *J Reprod Med* 1983;28:337–40.

Heaton FC, Ledger WJ. Postmenopausal tubal ovarian abscess. *Obstet Gynecol* 1976;47:90.

Hemsell DL, Ledger WJ, Martens M, et al. Concerns regarding the Centers for Disease Control's published guidelines for pelvic inflammatory disease. *Clin Infect Dis* 2001;32:103.

Hemsell DL, Wendel GD, Hemsell PG, et al. Inpatient treatment for uncomplicated and complicated acute pelvic inflammatory disease: ampicillin/sulbactam vs. cefoxitin. *Infect Dis Obstet Gynecol* 1993;1:123.

Henry-Suchet, Soler A, Loffredo V. Laparoscopic treatment of tubo-ovarian abscesses. *J Reprod Med* 1984;29:579.

Jackson P, Ridley WJ, Pattison NS. Single dose metronidazole prophylaxis in gynaecological surgery. *N Z Med J* 1979;89:243–5.

Jacobson L, Westrom L. Objectivized diagnosis of acute pelvic inflammatory disease. *Am J Obstet Gynecol* 1969;105:1088.

Kaplan AL, Jacobs WM, Ehresman JR. Aggressive management of pelvic abscess. *Am J Obstet Gynecol* 1967;98:982.

Kaplan RL, Sahn SA, Petty TL. Incidence and outcome of the respiratory distress syndrome in gram-negative sepsis. *Arch Intern Med* 1979;1939: 867.

Kardos F. Late results in women with genital tuberculosis. *Obstet Gynecol* 1967;29:247.

Kelly AM, Ireland M, Aughey D. Pelvic inflammatory disease in adolescents: high incidence and recurrence rates in an urban teen clinic. *J Pediatr Adolesc Gynecol* 2004;17:383.

Kelly H. *Operative gynecology, vol. II*. New York: Appleton, 1898:199, 212, 374, 412, 432, 433.

Kirtley L, Benigno BB. *The residual adnexa following surgery for pelvic inflammatory disease*. Resident Research Day. Atlanta: Emory University School of Medicine, Gynecology and Obstetrics Department, 1979. Unpublished data.

Klein TA, Richmond JA, Mishell DR Jr. Pelvic tuberculosis. *Obstet Gynecol* 1976;48:99.

Landers DV, Sweet RL. Tubo-ovarian abscess: contemporary approach to management. *Rev Infect Dis* 1983;5:876.

Larsen B. Pelvic inflammatory disease in teenagers. *Clinical Advances in the Treatment of Infections* 1991;5:1–8.

Lemeke R, Lsonka GW. Antibodies against pleuropneumonia-like organisms in patients with salpingitis. *Br J Vener Dis* 1962;38:212.

Loy RA, Gallup DG, Hill JA, et al. Pelvic abscess: examination and transvaginal drainage guided by real-time ultrasonography. *South Med J* 1989;82: 788.

Luton and Dunstable Hospital Study Group. Metronidazole in the prevention and treatment of bacteroides infections in gynaecological patients. *Lancet* 1974;304:1543.

Martens MG, Faro S, Maccato M, et al. In-vitro susceptibility testing of clinical isolates of *Chlamydia trachomatis*. *Infect Dis Obstet Gynecol* 1993;1: 40.

McNamara MT, Mead PB. Diagnosis and management of the pelvic abscess. *J Reprod Med* 1976;17:299.

Mickal A, Sellmann AH. Management of tubo-ovarian abscess. *Clin Obstet Gynecol* 1969;12:252.

Mickal A, Sellmann AH, Beebe JL. Ruptured tubo-ovarian abscesses. *Am J Obstet Gynecol* 1968;100:432.

Monif GR. Clinical staging of acute bacterial salpingitis and its therapeutic ramifications. *Am J Obstet Gynecol* 1982;143:489.

Monif GR. Significance of polymicrobial bacterial superinfection in the therapy of gonococcal endometritis-salpingitis-peritonitis. *Obstet Gynecol* 1980;55:1545.

Monif GR, Welkos SL, Baer H, et al. Cul-de-sac isolates from patients with endometritis-salpingitis-peritonitis and gonococcal endocervicitis. *Am J Obstet Gynecol* 1976;126:158.

Ness RB, Hillier SL, Kip KE, et al. Bacterial vaginosis and risk of pelvic inflammatory disease. *Am J Obstet Gynecol* 2004;104:761.

Ness RB, Kip KE, Hillier SL, et al. A cluster analysis of bacterial vaginosis-associated microflora and pelvic inflammatory disease. *Am J Epidemiol* 2005;162:585.

Ness RB, Randall H, Richter HE, et al. Condom use and the risk of recurrent pelvic inflammatory disease, chronic pelvic pain, or infertility following an episode of pelvic inflammatory disease. *Am J Public Health* 2004;94:1327.

Ness RB, Trautmann G, Soper DE. Effectiveness of treatment strategies of some women with pelvic inflammatory disease: a randomized trial. *Obstet Gynecol* 2005;106:573.

Ness RB, Smith KJ, Chang CC, et al. Prediction of pelvic inflammatory disease among young, single, sexually active women. *Sex Transm Dis* 2006;33: 137.

Olak J, Christon NV, Stein LA, et al. Operative vs. percutaneous drainage of intra-abdominal abscesses. *Arch Surg* 1986;121:141.

Overbeck L. Is tuberculosis of the female urogenital tract an entity? *J Obstet Gynaecol Br Commonw* 1966;73:624.

Paavonen J, Kiviat N, Brunham RC, et al. Prevalence and manifestations of endometritis among women with cervicitis. *Am J Obstet Gynecol* 1985;152:280.

Pedowitz P, Bloomfield R. Ruptured adnexal abscess (tubo-ovarian) with generalized peritonitis. *Am J Obstet Gynecol* 1964;88:721.

Peterson HB, Walker CK, Kahn JG, et al. Pelvic inflammatory disease: key treatment issues and options. *JAMA* 1991;266:2605.

Phillips AJ, D'Abling G. Acute salpingitis subsequent to tubal ligation. *Obstet Gynecol* 1986;67:55.

Reich H, McGlynn F. Laproscopic treatment of tuboovarian and pelvic abscess. *J Reprod Med* 1987;32:747–752.

Rivlin MR, Hunt JA. Ruptured tubo-ovarian abscess: is hysterectomy necessary?. *Obstet Gynecol* 1983;61:169.

Ross JD. Is mycoplasma genitalium cause of pelvic inflammatory disease? *Infect Dis Clin North Am* 2005;19:407.

Rossouw JE, Anderson GL, Prentice RL, LaCroix AZ, Kooperberg C, Stefanick ML, Jackson RD, Beresford SA, Howard BV, Johnson KC, Kotchen JM, Ockene J. Writing Group for the Women's Health Initiative Investigators. Risks and benefits of estrogen plus progestin in healthy postmenopausal women: principal results From the Women's Health Initiative randomized controlled trial. *JAMA* 2002;288:321–33.

Schaefer G. Female genital tuberculosis. *Clin Obstet Gynecol* 1976;19:223.

Sutherland AM. Laparoscopy in diagnosis of pelvic tuberculosis. *Lancet* 1979;2:95.

Sutherland AM. The management of genital tuberculosis in women. *Gazzet San* 1970;19:180.

Sutherland AM. Postmenopausal tuberculosis of the female genital tract. *Obstet Gynecol* 1982;59:545.

Sutherland AM. Surgical treatment of tuberculosis of the female genital tract. *BJOG* 1980;87:610.

Sutherland AM. Twenty-five years' experience of the drug treatment of tuberculosis of the female genital tract. *BJOG* 1977;84:881.

Sutherland AM. The treatment of tuberculosis of the female genital tract with rifampicin, ethambutol, and isoniazid. *Arch Gynecol* 1981;230:315.

Sutherland AM. The changing pattern of tuberculosis of the female genital tract. A thirty year survey. *Arch Gynecol* 1983;234:95–101.

Sutherland AM, MacFarlane JR. Transmission of genitourinary tuberculosis. *Health Bull (Edinb)* 1982;40:87.

Sutton MY, Strenberg M, Zaida A, et al. Trends in pelvic inflammatory disease hospital discharges and ambulatory visits, United States, 1985–2001. *Sex Transm Dis* 2005;32:778.

Svensson L, Westrom L, Ripa KT, et al. Differences in some clinical laboratory parameters in acute salpingitis related to culture and serologic findings. *Am J Obstet Gynecol* 1980;138:1017.

Svensson L, Westrom L, Mardh PA. Contraceptives and acute salpingitis. *JAMA* 1987;251:2553.

Sweet RL. PID and infertility in women. *Infect Dis Clin North Am* 1987;1: 199.

Sweet RL, Draper DL, Schacter J, et al. Microbiology and pathogenesis of acute salpingitis as determined by laparoscopy: What is the appropriate site to sample? *Am J Obstet Gynecol* 1980;138:985.

Sweet RL, Gibbs RS. *Infectious diseases of the female genital tract*. Baltimore: Williams & Wilkins, 1990:241.

Sweet RL, Roy S, Faro S, et al. Piperacillin-tazobactam versus clindamycin and gentamicin in the treatment of hospitalized women with pelvic infection. *Obstet Gynecol* 1994;83:280.

Sweet RL, Schacter J, Robbie M. Failure of beta-lactam antibiotics to eradicate *Chlamydia trachomatis* in the endometrium despite clinical care of acute salpingitis. *JAMA* 1983;250:2641.

Tatum HJ, Schmidt FH, Phillips D, et al. The Dalkon shield controversy: structural and bacteriological studies of IUD trials. *JAMA* 1975;231: 711.

Tyrrel RT, Murphy FB, Bernardino ME. Tubo-ovarian abscesses: CT-guided percutaneous drainage. *Radiology* 1990;175:87.

Velebil P, Wingo PA, Xia Z, et al. Rate of hospitalization for gynecologic disorders among reproductive-age women in the United States. *Obstet Gynecol* 1995;86:764.

Vermeeren J, Te Linde RW. Intraabdominal rupture of pelvic abscesses. *Am J Obstet Gynecol* 1954;68:402.

Viberga I, Odlind V, Lazdane G, Kroica J, Berglund L, Olofsson S. Microbiology profile in women with pelvic inflammatory disease in relation to IUD use. *Infect Dis Obstet Gynecol* 2005;13:183–90.

Washington AE, Cates W Jr, Zaidi AA. Hospitalization for PID: epidemiology and trends in the U.S., 1975 to 1981. *JAMA* 1984;251:2529.

Weiner S, Wallach EE. Ovarian histology in pelvic inflammatory disease. *Obstet Gynecol* 1974;43:431.

Westrom L. Incidence, prevalence and trends of acute pelvic inflammatory disease and its consequences in industrialized countries. *Am J Obstet Gynecol* 1980;138:880.

Westrom L. Introductory address: treatment of pelvic inflammatory disease in view of etiology and risk factors. *Sex Transm Dis* 1984;11:437.

Wetchler SJ, Dunn LJ. Ovarian abscess: report of a case and a review of the literature. *Obstet Gynecol Surv* 1985;40:476.

Wharton LR. Pelvic abscess: a study based on a series of 716. *Arch Surg* 1921;2:246.

Willson JR, Black JR. Ovarian abscess. *Am J Obstet Gynecol* 1964;90:34.

Worthen NJ, Gunning JE. Percutaneous drainage of pelvic abscesses: management of the tubo-ovarian abscess. *J Ultrasound Med* 1986;5:551.

CHAPTER 31 ■ LEIOMYOMATA UTERI AND MYOMECTOMY

LESLEY L. BREECH AND JOHN A. ROCK

DEFINITIONS

Intravenous leiomyomatosis—Smooth muscle tumor that consists of polypoid intravascular projections into the veins of the parametrium and broad ligaments.

Leiomyomatosis peritonealis disseminata—A benign reparative process in which fibroblasts replace soft peritoneal decidua on subperitoneal surfaces of the uterus and other pelvic and abdominal viscera resulting in nodules with a pseudoleiomyomatous pattern.

Menorrhagia—Prolonged (>7 days) or heavy (>80 mL) menstrual bleeding occurring at regular intervals.

Metrorrhagia—Prolonged (>7 days) episodes of menstrual bleeding occurring at irregular intervals.

Menometrorrhagia—Heavy, prolonged bleeding occurring at irregular intervals.

Submucosal—Present within the uterine myometrium just below the basal layer of the endometrial lining.

Subserosal—Present within the uterine myometrium just below the serosal or peritoneal covering of the uterus.

Leiomyomata are the most common tumors of the uterus and the female pelvis. This chapter discusses the pathologic and clinical features of uterine leiomyomata, the choice of treatment, and the indications and techniques for myomectomy.

Hysterectomy is sometimes required for the management of leiomyomata. It is also performed for many other indications, but leiomyomata uteri is the most common indication for hysterectomy. Refer to Chapter 32 for a complete discussion of hysterectomy.

Advances in gynecologic surgery just 100 years ago finally brought this common and sometimes fatal disease of women under reasonable control. Before the 20th century, no effective treatment was available. Uterine leiomyomata often grew to enormous size and caused great suffering from bleeding, pain, and emaciation (Fig. 31.1). Death from this benign disease was not uncommon. Progress in gynecologic surgery and anesthesia finally allowed the safe removal of these tumors by skilled gynecologic surgeons.

No one played a more important role in this endeavor than Drs. Kelly and Cullen. Working together at the Johns Hopkins Hospital, they gradually developed surgical techniques that were successful in preventing and controlling intraoperative hemorrhage. Several illustrations from their magnificent treatise, *Myomata of the Uterus,* published in 1907, are included in this chapter. In the preface, Cullen wrote:

> It was my good fortune to come to Baltimore in 1891, shortly after the hospital opened. At that time many cases of myoma were considered inoperable, and even when hysterectomy was undertaken it was only in the cases in which a stout rubber ligature could be temporarily tied around the cervix and when, as happened in some cases, this ligature slipped, alarming hemorrhage followed. Then came the systematic controlling of each of the cardinal vessels; later the bisection, and finally the transverse severance of the cervix as a preliminary feature of the operation in exceptionally difficult cases, until at present a myomatous uterus that cannot be removed is almost unheard of. I have watched the gradual simplication of the surgical procedures with the greatest interest. Many American surgeons have had much to do with the wonderful advance in this direction, but I know of no other man, either here or abroad, who has done as much toward this advancement as Howard A. Kelly.

The mortality rate for 1,373 operations performed for uterine leiomyomata at the Johns Hopkins Hospital between 1889 and 1906 was 5.75%; it was less than 1% for 238 operations performed between 1906 and 1909. In 55 patients, no operation was attempted because of refusal or the patient's weakened condition. Among these patients, 21 deaths occurred in the hospital. Death from uterine leiomyomata is a rare occurrence today. The almost total elimination of mortality caused by this tumor represents a major milestone in the health care of women.

During the past century, hysterectomy and myomectomy by the traditional and classic techniques have been the main treatment for women with uterine leiomyomata and significant symptoms, and they continue to be so today. Each year in the United States, more than 200,000 hysterectomies are performed with uterine leiomyomata as the primary indication. However, this traditional management will change in the future, for several reasons:

1. Concern regarding the increasing costs of health care has focused on the need to use effective but less expensive methods of management of uterine leiomyomata.
2. Advances in surgical technology now allow certain patients to be treated with new, minimally invasive techniques, including laparoscopic hysterectomy, laparoscopic-assisted vaginal hysterectomy, laparoscopic myomectomy, laparoscopic myoma coagulation (myolysis), and hysteroscopic resection of submucous myomata. Under proper circumstances, these procedures can be safe, effective, and less costly, but more time is needed before they will be available to a greater number of patients in need.
3. Interest in nonsurgical management also appears to be increasing with more data available regarding minimally invasive procedures, including uterine artery embolization. This procedure has emerged from an investigational realm to common clinical practice. As more long-term data become available, outcomes and prognosis are becoming more clearly delineated.
4. A medical approach to the management of patients with leiomyomata is now available. Gonadotropin-releasing hormone (GnRH) analogs, administered for 3 to 6 months, cause most uterine leiomyomata to shrink. However, the

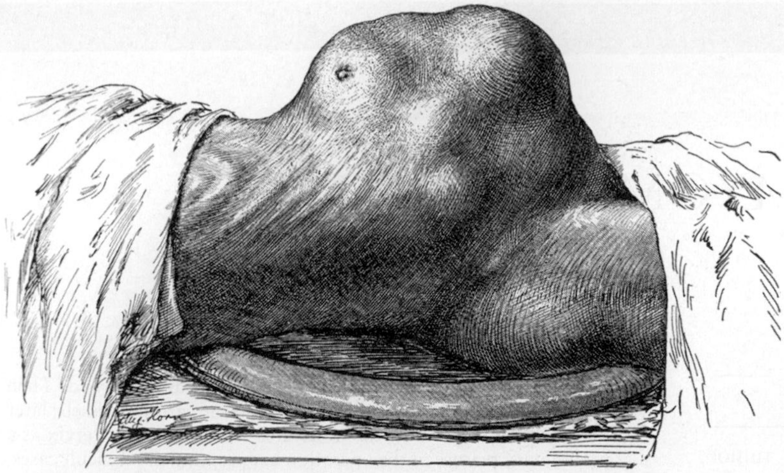

FIGURE 31.1. The patient is thin and emaciated, the outline of the ribs being prominent. Such advanced and neglected cases of multiple uterine leiomyomata are rarely seen today.

myomata regain their original size several months after the GnRH analog is discontinued. This medical regimen has been useful as an adjunct to surgical management. Women who become symptomatic with leiomyomata just before menopause can be treated temporarily with GnRH analogs and can possibly avoid surgical therapy.

5. Uterine leiomyoma are a major public health and women's health care problem. Society has a legitimate reason for interest and concern and has questioned the advisability of hysterectomy for the management of most cases of uterine leiomyomata. Many women insist on the preservation of uterine function for future childbearing, and sometimes even when future childbearing is not desired or not likely to occur. There will probably be a greater emphasis on expectant management, medical management, minimally invasive surgical procedures, and conservational management of uterine leiomyomata in the future.

In the future, the traditional and classic techniques of hysterectomy and myomectomy will be required less often for patients with symptomatic leiomyomata. At present, however, these operations are still appropriate in many situations.

ETIOLOGY, PATHOLOGY, AND GROWTH CHARACTERISTICS OF UTERINE LEIOMYOMATA

A leiomyoma is a benign tumor composed mainly of smooth muscle cells but containing varying amounts of fibrous connective tissue. The tumor is well circumscribed but not encapsulated. Various terms are used to refer to the tumor, such as *fibromyoma, myofibroma, leiomyofibroma, fibroleiomyoma, myoma, fibroma,* and *fibroid*. The latter designation is the one most commonly used, but it is the least accurate and acceptable. The term *leiomyoma* is a reasonably accurate one that emphasizes the origin of this tumor from smooth muscle cells and the predominance of the smooth muscle component. The tissue culture work of Miller and Ludovici suggested an origin from smooth muscle cells. The studies of Townsend and associates suggest a unicellular origin for leiomyomata.

Leiomyomata are the most common tumors of the uterus and female pelvis. It is impossible to determine their true incidence accurately, although the frequently quoted incidence of 50% found at postmortem examinations seems reasonable. Leiomyomata are responsible for about one third of all hospital admissions to gynecology services. It is well recognized that the incidence is much higher in black women than in white. In a careful study of leiomyomata among women in Augusta, Georgia, Torpin and associates found the incidence among black women to be three and one third times that among white women. There is no explanation for this racial difference. Leiomyomata also are larger and occur at a younger age in black women. In our experience, a large degenerating intramural leiomyoma was removed from a 1-year-old black girl; the tumor had enlarged the uterus to the level of the umbilicus. In black women, leiomyomata are not uncommon before 30 years of age. However, they are uncommon in any women before 20 years of age. Patients with uterine leiomyomata often have a positive family history of uterine leiomyomata. This suggests the presence of a gene encoding for their development.

About 40% to 50% of leiomyomas show karyotypically detectable chromosomal abnormalities that are both nonrandom and tumor specific. Identified chromosomal abnormalities include t(12;14)(q15;q23–24), del(7)(q22q32), rearrangements involving 6p21, 10q, trisomy 12, and deletions of 3q. Interestingly, a recent study of 217 myomas found a positive correlation between the presence of a cytogenetic abnormality and the anatomic location of the myoma. In this study by Brosens and colleagues, submucous myomas were consistently shown to have fewer cytogenetic abnormalities when compared with intramural and subserous lesions (12% vs. 35% and 29%, respectively). An increased prevalence in certain races, twin studies indicating higher correlation with hysterectomy in monozygotic twins, and increased incidence in first-degree relatives all seem to support an inherited predisposition. The true genetic contribution to the development of uterine leiomyoma remains to be defined.

Most of the data concerning the incidence of uterine leiomyomata are based on gross examination of the uterus, routine pathology reports, or the clinical diagnosis of uterine leiomyomata. Cramer and Patel subjected 100 uteri to gross serial sectioning at 2-mm intervals. They found 649 leiomyomata, roughly threefold the number identified by routine pathologic examination. Admittedly, some were only a few millimeters in diameter, but all were grossly visible. In 48 uteri with no mention of leiomyomata in the routine report, 27 were found to have small tumors. The incidence of leiomyomata was the same in premenopausal and postmenopausal uteri, although the average number of leiomyomata and the average size of the largest leiomyoma were greater in the premenopausal women. This work has important implications for future epidemiologic studies. It also suggests that it is almost never possible to surgically remove all leiomyomata when a myomectomy is performed.

The growth of leiomyomata is dependent on estrogen production. The tumors thrive during the years of greatest ovarian activity. Continuous estrogen secretion, especially when uninterrupted by pregnancy and lactation, is thought to be the most important underlying risk factor in the development of myomata. After menopause, with regression of ovarian estrogen secretion, growth of leiomyomata usually ceases. Actual regression in the tumor size may occur. There are rare instances, however, of postmenopausal growth of benign leiomyomata, suggesting the possibility of postmenopausal estrogen production either in the ovary or elsewhere. Postmenopausal ovarian cortical stromal hyperplasia may be associated with an increase in estrogen secretion by the ovary. The postmenopausal ovarian stroma in a variety of presumably inactive ovarian tumors, including mucinous cysts and Brenner tumors, can also produce estrogen. When a central pelvic tumor presumed to be uterine leiomyomata enlarges after menopause, one should think of the possibility of malignant change in the leiomyoma itself or in the adjacent myometrium, or of the growth of a new pelvic tumor of extrauterine origin.

Older nulliparous women have an increased risk of developing leiomyomata. However, in multiparous women, the relative risk decreases with each pregnancy. A woman who has had five term pregnancies has only one fifth the risk of a nulliparous woman of developing myomata. The risk is reduced in women who smoke and is increased in obese women; this is possibly related to the conversion of androgens to estrogen by fat aromatase.

The observation that leiomyomata may show significant enlargement during pregnancy provides further clinical evidence of the relation of estrogen and progesterone to the growth of these tumors. However, a better blood supply during pregnancy might also encourage their growth. In a prospective ultrasonographic study of 29 pregnant patients with uterine leiomyomata, Aharoni and associates found no evidence of enlargement of the myomata in 78%. Lev-Toaff and colleagues also confirmed that some leiomyomata do enlarge during pregnancy in response to estrogen and progesterone.

In the initial two decades following the introduction of oral contraceptives containing high-dose estrogen, there was a striking increase in the occurrence of large leiomyomata among young women of all racial backgrounds who took these pills. Although the growth of uterine leiomyomata is not invariably stimulated, oral contraceptives containing high-dose estrogen should not be prescribed for women with these tumors. Oral contraceptives with low-dose estrogen are less likely to stimulate growth. According to Parazzini and associates, there is no significant relation between the occurrence or growth of leiomyomata and the newer oral contraceptives that contain much smaller amounts of estrogens and progestins, and some believe that the risk of developing myomata is reduced with these low-dose pills.

Scientific investigators have been intrigued by the observation that leiomyomata develop during the reproductive years, sometimes grow during pregnancy, and regress after menopause. Nelson, Lipschutz, and others have produced multiple leiomyomata artificially on the serosal surface of the uterus and other peritoneal surfaces in guinea pigs given prolonged estrogen injections. Spellacy and coworkers found that levels of plasma estradiol were the same in patients with and without leiomyomata. However, Wilson and associates found a significantly higher concentration of estrogen receptors in leiomyomata than in myometrium. Farber and colleagues reported that these tumors bind about 20% more estradiol per milligram of cytoplasmic protein than does the normal myometrium of the same organ. This observation was not uniformly true for all leiomyomata, suggesting that different cellular components with a leiomyoma may be associated with different biologic activity. Otubu and coworkers found the concentration of estradiol to be significantly higher in leiomyomata than in normal myometrium, especially in the proliferative phase of the menstrual cycle. Soules and McCarty reported that leiomyomata had more estrogen receptors than did normal uterine tissues in the first phase (days 1 through 9) and in the second phase (days 10 through 18) of the menstrual cycle. Gabb and Stone found that the ability to convert estradiol to estrone was similar in leiomyomata and myometrium. However, Pollow and associates found the conversion of estradiol into estrone to be significantly lower in leiomyomata than in myometrium. This difference in conversion rate could result in a relative accumulation of estrogen in a leiomyoma, causing a hyperestrogenic state within the tumor and surrounding tissues. The enzyme 17β-hydroxy dehydrogenase accelerates the conversion of estradiol to estrone. Leiomyomata have a low concentration of 17β hydroxy dehydrogenase, which results in a relative accumulation of estradiol in leiomyomatous tissue. These findings may explain the myometrial hypertrophy that is invariably present with leiomyomata.

Other abnormalities in endocrine function have also been suggested. Ylikorkala and colleagues found that pituitary function may be abnormal in women with leiomyomata. Patients with leiomyomata had a low follicle-stimulating hormone level and a diminished follicle-stimulating hormone response to pituitary GnRH. There was an excessive prolactin response to thyrotropin-releasing hormone. Spellacy and colleagues found that the peak levels of human growth hormone reached during a hypoglycemic test were twice as high in patients with leiomyomata as in the control group. Reddy and Rose suggested the possibility that 5α-reduced androgens may play a role in the pathophysiology of uterine leiomyomata, because a significant increase in 5α-reductase has been found in leiomyoma tissue as compared with myometrium and endometrium. Influenced by the experimental investigations of Lipschutz and associates, Goodman in 1946 treated patients with uterine leiomyomata with progesterone and noted a decrease in tumor size in all patients. However, Segaloff and colleagues reported no effect in their study. Goldzieher and coworkers produced histologic evidence of extensive degenerative changes in leiomyomata by administering high-dose progestin therapy (medrogestone in high doses for 21 days). Filiceri and associates have reported the regression of a uterine leiomyoma after long-term administration of a long-acting luteinizing hormone-releasing hormone agonist given to suppress ovarian estrogen secretion. Coutinho successfully used a potent 19-norsteroid antiestrogen–antiprogesterone to treat excessive uterine bleeding in 16 patients with uterine leiomyomata. A reduction in the size of the tumors was noted.

Although the exact etiology of uterine leiomyomata is not known, the puzzle may be solved bit by bit by the research of Kornyei and colleagues, Wilson and coworkers, Tamaya and associates, Buchi and Keller, Sadan and colleagues, and others who continue to investigate estrogen and progesterone as possible growth factors. Although some data are conflicting, evidence suggests that both estrogen and progesterone are involved in the growth of uterine leiomyomata. The possibility that progesterone may play a role in the growth of leiomyomata is suggested by the work of Kawaguchi and coworkers, who found a higher mitotic count in leiomyomata obtained in the proliferative phase of the menstrual cycle.

Anderson and associates have shown that medroxyprogesterone acetate, a progestin, causes a decrease in connexin-43 messenger ribonucleic acid levels in primary cultures of human myometrium and leiomyoma. Connexin-43 is a gap junction protein whose formation is stimulated by 17β-estradiol.

According to the research data of Brandon and colleagues, progesterone receptor messenger ribonucleic acid is overexpressed in uterine leiomyomata, compared with normal adjacent myometrium, suggesting that amplified progesterone-mediated signaling is instrumental in the abnormal growth of these tumors. It is possible that the increased amount of progesterone receptor is caused by an alteration of estrogen or estrogen receptors in leiomyomata. The work of Kastner and coworkers and Nardulli and associates has demonstrated that progesterone receptor expression is regulated by estrogen.

Research in recent years has also focused on polypeptide growth factors in the stimulation of growth of leiomyomata. Polypeptide growth factors that have been investigated include epidermal growth factor, transforming growth factor-alpha and beta, insulinlike growth factor (IGF), platelet-derived growth factor, vascular endothelial growth factor, and basic fibroblast growth factor. Other growth factors may also be involved. Polypeptide growth factor research has been performed by Goustin and colleagues, by Hoffmann and coworkers, by Lumsden and associates, and by others. A brief review of this research has been written by Vollenhoven and associates, who have been involved in the study of IGFs in uterine leiomyomata.

Results from a study by Strawn and colleagues demonstrate that IGF-I stimulates leiomyoma growth in a dose-related manner over that of normal myometrial tissue in monolayer culture. This stimulatory effect, in the absence of sex steroid hormones or other growth factors, provides additional support that IGF-I may play an important direct role in the pathogenesis of these tumors, possibly by modulating the response of these tumors to various levels of sex steroids. Dawood and Kahn-Dawood were unable to find any significant elevation in peripheral levels of serum IGF-I in nonpregnant premenopausal women with uterine leiomyomata of 14 weeks' gestational size. The authors state, "Nevertheless, the finding does not detract from the potential paracrine or autocrine role that IGF-I produced by leiomyoma cells may have either on the growth of its own or adjacent myomas or on the vascular supply and blood flow of the uterus and myomas."

Rein and coworkers have proposed a hypothesis to explain the pathogenesis of myomata. This hypothesis suggests a critical role for progesterone in their growth. They state:

> The initiation and growth of myomas likely involves a multistep cascade of separate tumor initiators and promotors. The initial neoplastic transformation of the normal myocyte involves somatic mutations. Although the initiators of the somatic mutations remain unclear, the mitogenic effect of progesterone may enhance the propagation of somatic mutations. Myoma proliferation is the result of clonal expansion and likely involves the complex interactions of estrogen, progesterone, and local growth factors. Estrogen and progesterone appear equally important as promotors of myoma growth.

To treat patients with uterine leiomyomata properly, the gynecologic surgeon must be familiar with their pathology, growth characteristics, and clinical features. Leiomyomata may be single, but most are multiple. They develop most commonly in the uterine corpus and much less often in the cervix. They may develop in the round ligaments, but this is rare. Because they arise in the myometrium, they are all interstitial or intramural in the beginning. As they enlarge, they can remain intramural, but growth often extends in an internal or external direction. Thus, the tumor can eventually become subserous or submucous in location. A subserous tumor can become pedunculated and occasionally parasitic, receiving its blood supply from another source, usually the omentum. A submucous tumor can also become pedunculated and may gradually dilate the endocervical canal and protrude through the cervical os. Indeed, a submucous myoma may descend through the vagina. Rarely, chronic uterine inversion results if the prolapsing submucous leiomyoma is attached to the top of the endometrial cavity and pulls the uterine fundus downward through the cervix.

In general, subserous leiomyomata contain more fibrous tissue than submucous leiomyomata. However, submucous leiomyomata contain more smooth muscle tissue than subserous leiomyomata. Sarcomatous change is more common in submucous tumors.

The typical uterine leiomyoma is a firm multinodular structure of variable size. The largest tumor, reported by Hunt in 1888, weighed more than 65 kg. Tumors of 4 to 5 kg are not rare, but most are smaller. In the operating room, leiomyomata appear as nodular tumors of different sizes that distort the uterus in various ways, depending on their size, location, and direction of growth. Growth between the leaves of the broad ligament and origin from the cervix may make surgical removal difficult. Subserous and subserous pedunculated tumors, as well as intraligamentous tumors, may create problems in diagnosis because they are difficult to distinguish from tumors arising from the adnexal organs (Fig. 31.2). When tumors cause symmetric enlargement of the uterus, they may be mistaken for a pregnant uterus on bimanual examination.

The "normal" intramural leiomyoma on section protrudes from the surrounding compressed myometrium. Ordinarily there is a clear distinction between the myoma and the myometrium so that dissection between the two is easy to accomplish. Myomata usually can be removed from surrounding myometrium with ease. Although these tumors are not encapsulated, a clear distinction can usually be made between a myoma and the myometrium that surrounds it. The cut surface appears as glistening pinkish white and gray. It is firm, and there is a whorllike arrangement of the muscle and the fibrous tissue. In contrast to this typical appearance, the myometrium may be thickened by a diffuse, ill-defined nodularity of smooth muscle. This so-called diffuse leiomyomatosis usually involves all parts of the myometrium and causes symmetric enlargement of the uterine corpus. The nodules of smooth muscle are not distinct, contain little collagen, and merge with one another and the surrounding hypertrophied myometrium.

The extracellular matrix of leiomyomata is composed mostly of collagen but also contains proteoglycans and fibronectin. According to Fujita, myomata contain 50% more collagen than does normal myometrium, and the ratio of collagen type I to collagen type III is increased in myomata. Proteoglycans provide hydrated spaces between myoma cells. Fibronectin is a glycoprotein that mediates adhesion between myoma cells and extracellular matrix.

The most common change in leiomyomata is hyaline degeneration. The cut surface of a hyalinized area is smooth and

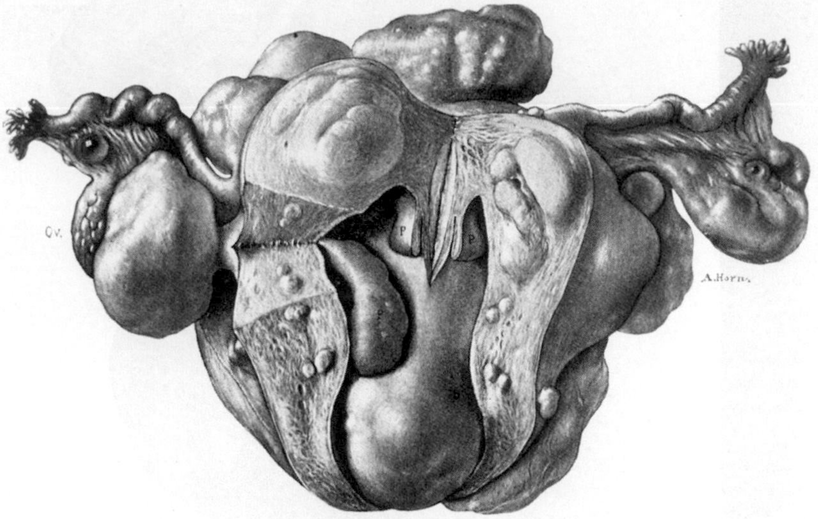

FIGURE 31.2. The uterine corpus is almost completely replaced by small and large myomas in intramural, subserous, and submucous positions. Some are pedunculated. A pedunculated submucous myoma is dilating the endocervical canal. A pedunculated subserous myoma is adjacent to the left ovary and will interfere with its palpation.

homogeneous and does not show the whorllike arrangement of the rest of the leiomyoma. Almost all leiomyomata, except the smallest, have scattered areas of hyaline degeneration. Eventually these may become liquefied and form cystic cavities filled with clear liquid or gelatinous material (Fig. 31.3). Sometimes the cystic change is so great that the leiomyoma becomes a mere shell and is truly a cystic tumor. Softness of a tumor does not necessarily indicate cystic degeneration. Fleshy leiomyomata may be equally soft.

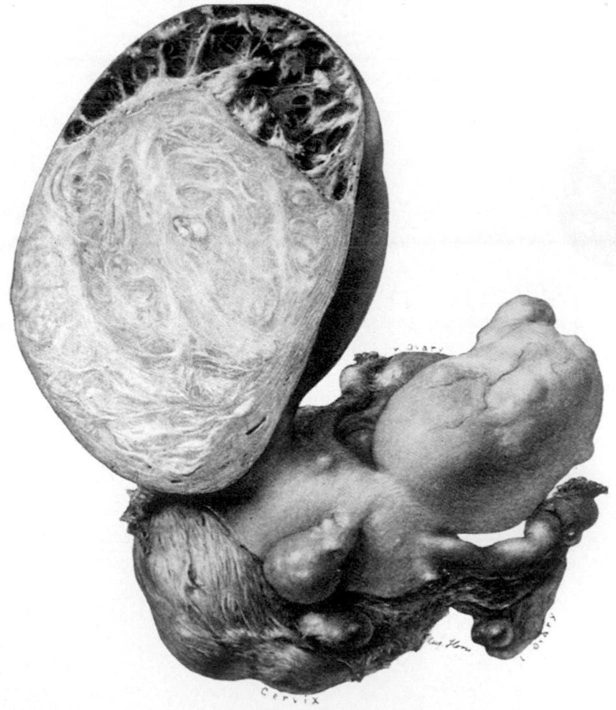

FIGURE 31.3. Multiple leiomyomata are present. A large subserous myoma has undergone partial cystic degeneration.

Over time, with continued diminished blood supply and ischemic necrosis of tissue, calcium phosphates and carbonates are deposited in myomata. Their presence is evidence of a continuum of degenerative changes. The calcium may be deposited in varying amounts. If it is deposited at the periphery of the tumor, the leiomyoma may resemble a calcified cyst. Other calcified leiomyomata may show an irregular or diffuse distribution throughout with a honeycomb or mulberry appearance. When the degenerative change is advanced, the leiomyoma may become solidly calcified. Such calcified tumors have been called "wombstones." Calcified leiomyomata are seen most often in elderly women, in black women, and in women who have pedunculated subserous tumors. They are easily seen radiographically (Fig. 31.4).

Leiomyomata may undergo changes as a result of infection. Submucous leiomyomata are most commonly infected when they protrude into the uterine cavity, or especially into the vagina (Fig. 31.5). The pedunculated submucous leiomyoma thins out the endometrium as it grows inward, and eventually the surface becomes ulcerated and infected (Fig. 31.6). An intramural leiomyoma in an involuting puerperal uterus can also become infected when endometritis is present. Microscopic abscesses can be found, and gross abscesses occasionally occur, particularly if the leiomyoma descends as low as the cervical canal. Such infections are usually streptococcal and may be virulent. *Bacteroides fragilis* infections also occur. Parametritis, peritonitis, and even septicemia may result.

Necrosis of a leiomyoma is caused by interference with its blood supply. Occasionally a pedunculated subserous leiomyoma twists, and if an operation is not done immediately, infarction results. Necrosis sometimes occurs in the center of a large tumor simply as a result of poor circulation. Necrotic leiomyomata are dark and hemorrhagic in the interior. Eventually the tissue breaks down completely. So-called red or carneous degeneration is seen occasionally, especially in association with pregnancy. This condition is thought to result from poor circulation of blood through a rapidly growing tumor. Thrombosis and extravasation of blood into the myoma tissue are responsible for the reddish discoloration (Fig. 31.7).

A subserous and especially a subserous pedunculated myoma may gradually outgrow its blood supply (Fig. 31.8). To keep the myoma tissue from undergoing complete ischemic

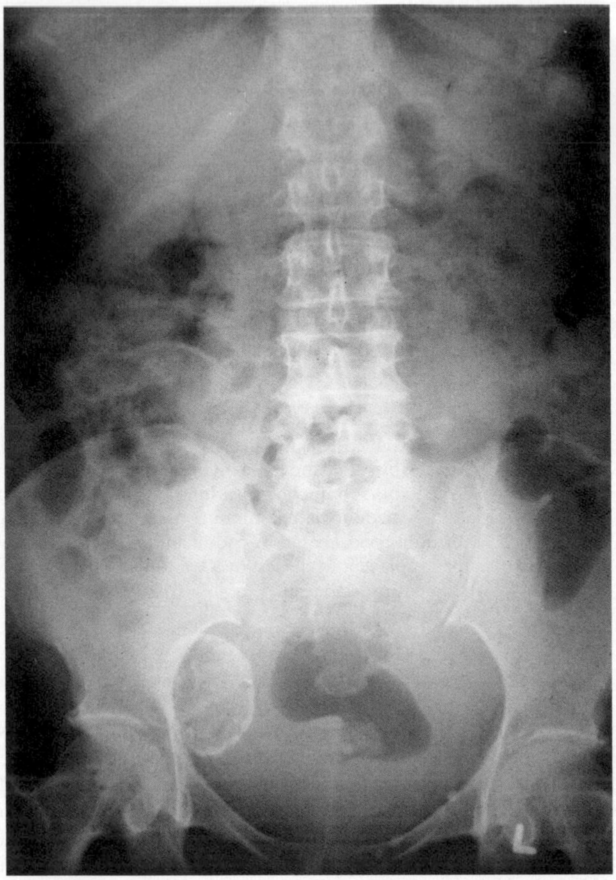

FIGURE 31.4. An abdominal radiograph shows typical calcification in a leiomyoma.

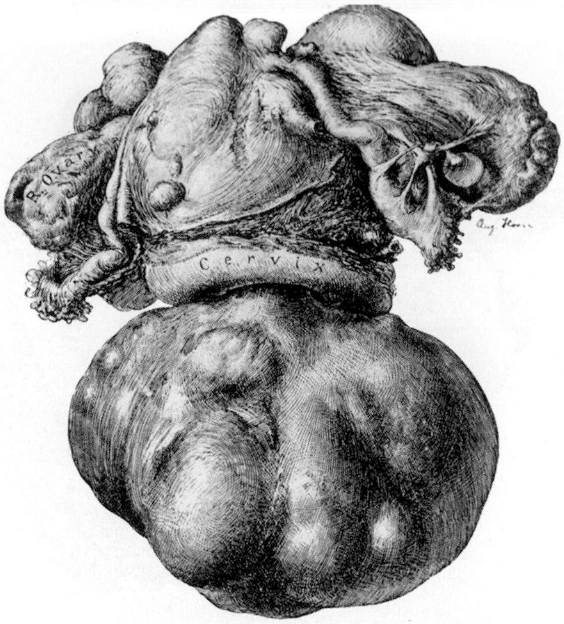

FIGURE 31.5. A large submucous pedunculated myoma has dilated the cervix and is now located in the vagina. Its pedicle is attached inside the uterine cavity. Morcellation of the myoma performed transvaginally allows clamping and ligation of the pedicle.

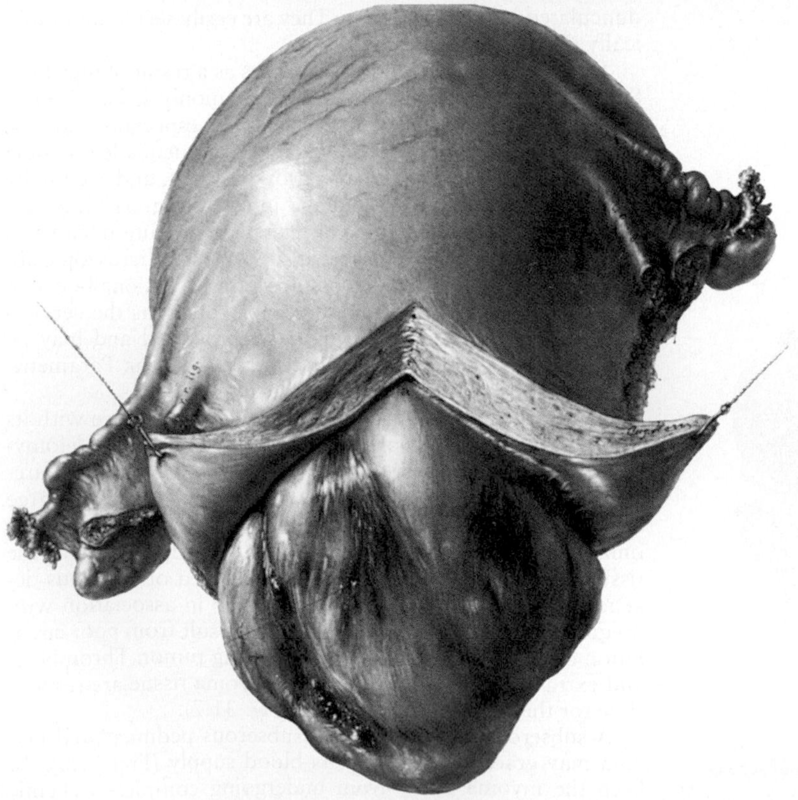

FIGURE 31.6. Pedunculated submucous myoma showing necrosis and ulceration.

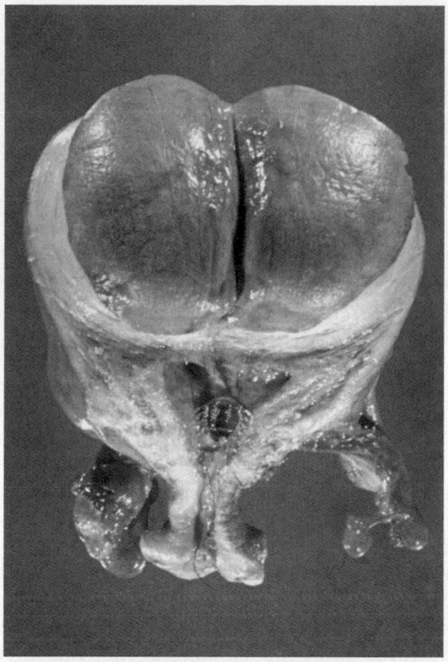

FIGURE 31.7. Degenerating leiomyoma showing carneous discoloration caused by thrombosis and extravasation of blood into the myoma tissue. A Dalkon shield can be seen in the endometrial cavity. See color version of figure.

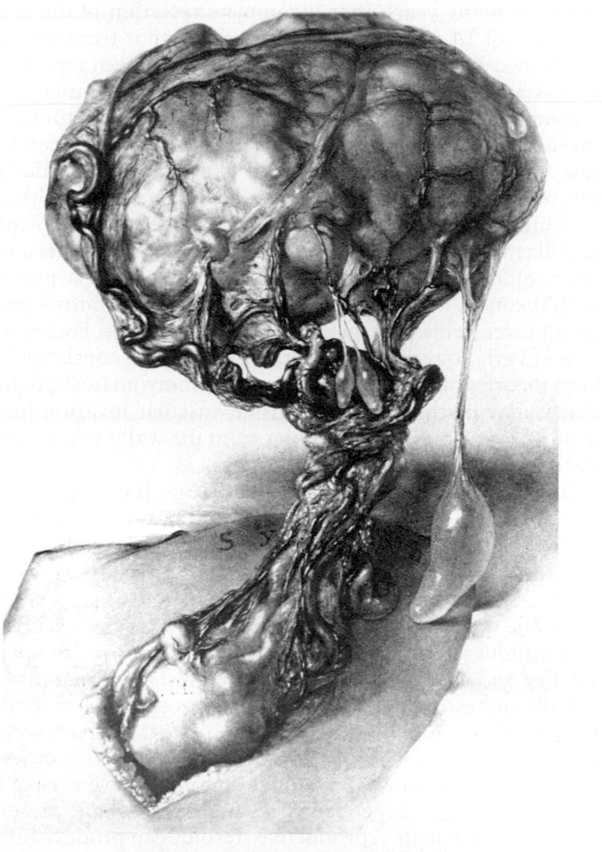

FIGURE 31.8. A subserous pedunculated myoma receives tenuous blood supply through its uterine pedicle. Such a myoma may wander in the upper abdomen and eventually receive its blood supply from other sources. It may also twist on its pedicle and undergo infarction.

necrosis, the omentum becomes adherent to the peritoneal surface of a pedunculated subserous myoma and provides whatever blood supply is needed. Eventually, the pedicle may disappear or twist, and the myoma will become completely free from the uterus, wander in the upper abdomen, and receive its "parasitic" blood supply from the omentum and other sources.

On occasion, fat occurs in leiomyomata as true fatty degeneration. The cut surface may have a yellowish discoloration. Infrequently, a deposit of true fat may form a fibrolipoma; however, the presence of fat in a leiomyoma is rare. Indeed, if fat is seen grossly or microscopically in a curettage specimen, one should not assume that it represents fatty degeneration of a leiomyoma. One should assume that the uterus has been perforated and that fragments of fat have been curetted from the mesentery or omentum.

The most important, but rare, change in a leiomyoma is sarcomatous degeneration. There is much variation in the reported incidence of sarcoma in leiomyomata. The incidence given by Novak is 0.7%. However, a review of 13,000 myomata by Montague and associates at the Johns Hopkins Hospital revealed 38 cases of malignant change, the incidence of sarcoma thus being 0.29%. Corscaden and Singh indicated by their study that the true incidence of sarcoma developing within uterine leiomyomata is no higher than 0.13% and is probably as low as 0.04%. It should be remembered that because most women with uterine leiomyomata do not undergo surgical removal, the true incidence of sarcoma in leiomyomata is probably much lower than 1 per 1,000 (0.1%).

After hysterectomy in 1,429 patients with presumed benign leiomyomata, the histologic diagnosis of leiomyosarcoma was made in seven (0.49%), according to a study by Leibsohn and coworkers. There was no evidence of malignancy in the endometrial sampling of any of these seven patients, and the diagnosis was suspected intraoperatively in only three. Uterine weights ranged from 120 to 1,100 g. In a woman between 41 and 50 years of age with presumed symptomatic leiomyomata, there is a 1 in 112 chance of a leiomyosarcoma being present, according to these authors. This information has important implications in the consideration of conservative or delayed treatment for these women. Parker and associates found that the total incidence of uterine sarcomas (leiomyosarcoma, endometrial stromal sarcoma, and mixed mesodermal tumor) among patients operated on for presumed benign uterine leiomyoma is lower (0.23%) than the 0.49% reported by Leibsohn and coworkers.

The difficulty in defining the true incidence of sarcomatous change is understandable if one is familiar with the histology of leiomyomata. Abundantly cellular leiomyomata are relatively common, and at first glance they suggest sarcoma; however, they lack a significant number of mitotic figures, and patients from whom such tumors are removed all remain well. Misinterpretation of the histologic picture of this type of cellular leiomyoma undoubtedly accounts for the increased incidence of leiomyosarcoma reported by some. When cutting into leiomyomata in the operating room, the surgeon finds that sarcomatous areas have a somewhat characteristic appearance, although the histologic diagnosis certainly cannot be made by gross examination. A sarcoma is likely to occur in a rather large leiomyoma and toward the center of the tumor, where the blood supply is poorest. Instead of being firm fibrous tissue that grates when scraped with a knife blade, the tissue is soft and homogeneous, and is described as resembling raw pork. Later, as necrosis of the malignant tissue occurs, it becomes more friable and hemorrhagic.

It has been difficult to understand uterine leiomyosarcoma because pathologists do not agree on the criteria necessary for diagnosis. Some pathologists rely on the mitotic count. All tumors with less than five mitotic figures per 10 high-power fields are considered benign. All tumors with more than 10 mitotic figures per 10 high-power fields are called malignant. Those in between can be called smooth muscle tumors of uncertain malignant potential.

Other pathologists believe the mitotic count may have some significance but choose to rely instead on the presence of nuclear hyperchromatism, nuclear pleomorphism, or giant cells and other bizarre cell forms to make the diagnosis. Corscaden and Singh believe that no combination of histologic features is reliable and that only smooth muscle tumors that metastasize or recur are definitely malignant. We believe that all of these features should be taken into consideration for diagnosis and prognosis. When the tumor is confined to the uterus, both mitotic grade and histologic grade are important in the diagnosis and prognosis. A poor prognosis is associated with high mitotic counts and extremely atypical and anaplastic cytologic features. Bell and colleagues at Stanford University Medical Center assessed a variety of histopathologic features of 213 problematic smooth muscle neoplasms for which there were at least 2 years of clinical follow-up data. From the wide variety of light-microscopic features assessed, the important predictors that emerged were mitotic index, the degree of cytologic atypia, and the presence or absence of coagulative tumor cell necrosis. Previously, the mitotic index was relied on exclusively to determine whether a uterine smooth muscle tumor was benign or malignant, but currently an approach is used that incorporates additional histopathologic features.

A normal chromosome complement (46,XX) was observed by Meloni and coworkers in about 50% of leiomyoma cases. About 50% showed clonal abnormalities, such as those of chromosomes 1, 7, and 13, and t(12;14). Interstitial deletions of chromosome 7 were the ones most often involved, suggesting that this abnormality may be of primary importance in the cellular proliferation of leiomyomata. A relation between more aggressive histology and chromosomal abnormalities was also suggested.

Tumors that show obvious evidence of blood vessel invasion or spread to contiguous organs are rarely cured. The extent of the disease at the time of initial diagnosis is of even greater significance. In other words, when the diagnosis is suspected for the first time by the pathologist when he examines routine sections from a uterine leiomyoma, the patient almost always survives. However, if the diagnosis is made preoperatively by the gynecologist or is suspected during the operative procedure because of invasion of surrounding organs, the prognosis is grave.

An unusual atypical smooth muscle tumor was first described in the stomach by Martin and associates in 1960. Variously called *bizarre leiomyoma, leiomyoblastoma, clear-cell leiomyoma,* and *plexiform tumorlet,* these atypical smooth tumors probably all belong together. The term *epithelioid leiomyoma* was adopted by the World Health Organization. Kurman and Norris have proposed that this term be used for all atypical leiomyomata. Histologically, the characteristic feature is the mixture of rounded polygonal cells and multinucleated giant cells present in epithelioid clear-cell and plexiform patterns. Clinically, in the uterus most of these tumors are benign. They may rarely exhibit malignant potential. Malignancy is difficult to predict from histologic criteria because some metastases occurred from tumors that demonstrated very few mitoses. Kurman and Norris have suggested, however, that epithelioid neoplasms having more than five mitotic figures per 10 high-power fields should be called *epithelioid leiomyosarcomas* and that the term *epithelioid leiomyoma* should be applied when there is a lower level of mitotic activity. Although combination therapy (surgery plus radiation therapy or chemotherapy) may not be indicated for a patient with an epithelioid leiomyoma, follow-up should be considered essential, as emphasized by Klunder and colleagues.

An unusual benign form of leiomyomata uteri, *intravenous leiomyomatosis,* was first recognized at the turn of the 20th century and has been reported sporadically since then. Before 1982, about 50 cases had been reported, according to Bahary and coworkers. Probably at least that many have been reported since. Marshall and Morris presented the first detailed report of this entity in the American literature in 1959. The characteristic feature of this peculiar smooth muscle tumor is the extension of the polypoid intravascular projections into the veins of the parametrium and broad ligaments. Although there may be some difficulty in distinguishing such lesions from low-grade sarcoma, they are distinctly different histologically from stromatosis uteri because the intravenous plugs are mainly smooth muscle in origin. In 1966, Edwards and Peacock collected 32 cases of intravenous leiomyomatosis, including two cases of their own, and reviewed the clinical experience with this condition. In approximately 50% of the cases, the intravenous tumor was confined to the parametrium; in 75%, it extended no further than the veins of the broad ligament. The observations of Edwards and Peacock suggest that the severed intravenous extensions are probably incapable of independent parasitic existence and remain dormant after removal of the uterus. However, the cases presented by Bahary and associates tend to refute this idea. Total surgical excision of the tumor should be attempted for successful therapy. Some patients have survived for many years after incomplete resection of the tumor. A review of 14 cases of this rare uterine tumor from the file of the Armed Forces Institute of Pathology has been reported by Norris and Parmley. In this series, two of three patients with incomplete resection had a recurrence; the recurrent tumor was excised surgically, and the patients were alive and free of disease 5 and 11 years after operation. The authors concluded that this tumor behaves clinically like a benign neoplasm, although its wormlike extensions may involve uterine, vaginal, ovarian, and iliac veins. The uterine veins in the broad ligaments are the most common sites of extension. The mitotic index is quite low, with the most active lesions showing only one mitosis per 15 high-power fields. The material from the Armed Forces Institute of Pathology provides histologic evidence consistent with both theories of origin of intravenous leiomyomatosis, namely, that it may be the result of unusual vascular invasion from a leiomyoma or may arise *de novo* from the wall of veins within the myometrium.

Extension of benign leiomyomatosis up the vena cava and into the right atrium has been reported in several cases, with a fatal outcome in some. Before 1994, approximately 27 cases of intravenous leiomyomatosis extending to the heart were reported. Several recent cases requiring open-heart surgery to remove the intracardiac tumor thrombosis have been successful and without recurrence. All reported cases occurred in women. Tierney and colleagues reported that substantial quantities of cytoplasmic estradiol and progesterone receptors were found in the right atrial tumor removed from a patient with intravenous leiomyomatosis. Their patient was treated with the antiestrogen tamoxifen because of residual tumor in the vena cava that could be estrogen dependent. Irey and Norris have presented evidence that female reproductive steroids can produce intimal proliferation of veins in predisposed persons. Interestingly, of the 30 patients with leiomyomata and leiomyosarcomas of the vena cava reviewed by Wray and Dawkins, 80% were female. Both intravenous leiomyomatosis and benign metastasizing leiomyoma have been reported to metastasize to the lung. As suggested by Banner and coworkers, by Horstmann and associates, and by Evans and colleagues, oophorectomy may be indicated in patients with these conditions, again because of the possibility that these tumors may be estrogen dependent or that estrogens may have the ability to stimulate their development, whether in a uterine or extrauterine location and whether they appear to be endothelial or mesenchymal in origin.

The possibility of metastases from a histologically benign uterine leiomyoma has been discussed by Idelson and Davids and by Clark and Weed. When such a case occurs, it is usually settled by finding a sarcomatous component in the leiomyoma or by finding evidence of intravenous leiomyomatosis. However, multiple cases have now been reported in which a benign uterine leiomyoma metastasized. Idelson and Davids' case showed metastases to the aortic lymph nodes. The patient reported by Cramer and associates had metastatic tumor to the omentum, ovary, periaortic lymph node, and lung. In each location, the histology and estrogen receptor content of the tumor resembled those of a benign leiomyoma. The recommended treatment consists of surgical removal with castration and little or no estrogen replacement.

Leiomyomatosis peritonealis disseminata is sometimes confused with intravenous leiomyomatosis. However, only subperitoneal surfaces of the uterus and other pelvic and abdominal viscera are involved with leiomyomatosis peritonealis disseminata, and invasion of the lumen of blood vessels does not occur. Only about 15 cases have been reported, according to Pearce. All occurred in patients in the reproductive years who often had large uterine leiomyomata and were usually pregnant or taking oral contraceptives. The condition is likely to be confused with a disseminated intraabdominal malignancy, but it is entirely benign histologically and clinically. Parmley and colleagues have demonstrated the histologic similarities between this peritoneal lesion and the decidual change of the mesothelium in the pelvis, and they propose that the condition represents a benign reparative process in which fibroblasts replace soft peritoneal decidua. They suggest that this fibrocytic reaction occurs during pregnancy and especially in the postpartum period, resulting in nodules with a pseudoleiomyomatous pattern. Similar findings have been noted in patients with endometriosis treated with prolonged Enovid therapy. These findings indicate that prolonged and continuous stimulation of subperitoneal decidua by either endogenous or exogenous estrogen and progesterone is important in the pathogenesis of this condition. Parmley and coworkers suggest that the condition is more appropriately called *disseminated fibrosing deciduosis*. Goldberg and associates, on the other hand, on the basis of electron microscopy studies, believe that the tumors arise from smooth muscles of small blood vessels. This has been confirmed by Ceccacci and colleagues. It has been possible to show a continuum from fibroblastic cells through myofibroblasts to leiomyocytes. Although the cell of origin of this tumor is still controversial, the tumor is benign, and the acceptable treatment to date is total abdominal hysterectomy and bilateral salpingo-oophorectomy. If this tumor occurs in the omentum, an omentectomy should also be performed to define more clearly the histologic nature of the lesion.

In attempting to distinguish between benign and malignant disease in a patient with uterine leiomyomata who also has unusual clinical findings, it is appropriate to keep the entities mentioned earlier (intravenous leiomyomatosis, atypical bizarre leiomyoma, benign metastasizing leiomyoma, and disseminated intraperitoneal leiomyomatosis) in mind. Although they all have features similar to those of malignant disease, they are almost always benign and amenable to treatment. One should also remember that benign uterine leiomyomata have been associated with pseudo-Meigs syndrome in a few cases. Meigs reported five cases in 1954. In these cases, the ascites did not reappear after removal of the uterine leiomyomata.

There is a high frequency of endometrial hyperplasia when the uterus contains leiomyomata. Degligdish and Loewenthal reported that cystic glandular hyperplasia is often found in the endometrium at the margin of the leiomyoma. Yamamoto and coworkers have reported high concentrations of estrone and estrone sulfatase activity in the endometrium overlying a myoma. They suggest that the local hyperestrogenism in the endometrium overlying a leiomyoma may assist in the genesis or enlargement of these tumors.

Gynecologic surgeons are especially concerned about the vascularity of individual leiomyomata and about the blood flow to the uterus in the presence of multiple and sometimes very large leiomyomata. These considerations are pertinent when surgery, especially myomectomy, is contemplated.

According to Vollenhoven and associates, the vascularization of leiomyomata was studied by Vasserman and colleagues, and the findings were presented to the World Congress of Gynecology and Obstetrics in 1988. Using femoral arteriography, selective intraoperative angiography, radiography, and injection of surgical specimens, these investigators showed that leiomyomata have a rich vascular supply, including blood lakes within tumors. They found more than one nutrient vessel per myoma. Venous channels were predominantly peripheral, whereas the arterial supply was both internal and peripheral. Farrer-Brown and coworkers, using radiologic methods, demonstrated that myomata in various locations within the myometrium can cause congestion and dilatation of endometrial venous plexuses by obstructing venous return. These obstructions can result in ectasia of endometrial and myometrial venules (Fig. 31.9). The degree of vascularity of leiomyomata was also studied by Karlsson and Persson. Vascularity varied from many, to few, to no intrinsic vessels demonstrable. Generally, the sum of the width of the uterine arteries increases with the size of the uterus, but the diameter of the two sides sometimes differs markedly. A rich vascularity was found in 22 of 34 uteri with leiomyomata, but with increasing size there is a tendency to less vascularity. In none of five cases with very large (20 cm or more) leiomyomata uteri was the vascularity rich. The intrinsic vessels were few in two cases and absent in three cases.

CLINICAL FEATURES OF UTERINE LEIOMYOMATA

Asymptomatic Leiomyomata

Most leiomyomata are asymptomatic. Untold numbers of such symptomless leiomyomata are removed surgically by either hysterectomy or myomectomy when they would have been better left undisturbed. The incidence of malignancy in leiomyomata is less than 0.1%, which is lower than the operative mortality rate of hysterectomy in the average hospital; therefore, unless there is some reason to suspect malignant change, the risk of the operation for asymptomatic leiomyomata may exceed the danger of malignancy. A history of rapid growth, however, particularly postmenopausal growth, does indicate removal, even when the tumor produces no symptoms. Signs of rapid enlargement are important in all patients but are even more ominous in older patients. In younger patients, the most common reason for rapid enlargement of a uterus with

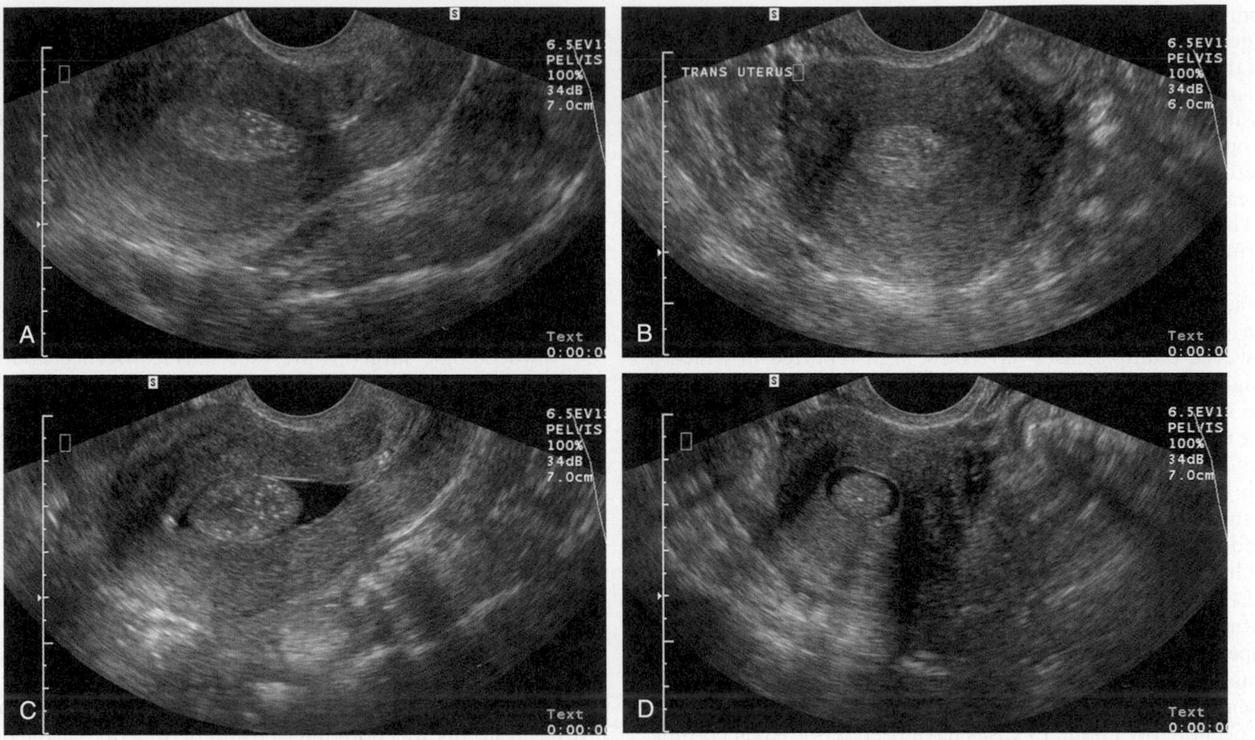

FIGURE 31.9. Sonographic images of a 48-year-old patient with a history of pelvic pain. Both transabdominal and transvaginal images were obtained on cycle day 8. Longitudinal (A) and transversely oriented (B) transvaginal images reveal a suspicious endometrial cavity, suggesting a thickened lining, endometrial polyp, or a submucosal myoma. C and D: Fluid-enhanced sonohysterographic studies clearly demonstrate a mass lesion and not generalized thickening of the endometrial lining. The patient underwent a hysteroscopy and uterine curettage, which revealed a histologically confirmed endometrial polyp. (Images courtesy of Jeff Dicke, M.D.)

leiomyomata is pregnancy. If pregnancy can be ruled out, a leiomyosarcoma may be suspected but is rarely found.

Small leiomyomata that are asymptomatic need only to be observed from time to time, with pelvic examinations perhaps every 6 to 12 months and pelvic ultrasonography when indicated. In the beginning, frequent examination may be indicated to determine the growth rate. Such tumors may remain remarkably constant in size for years. If small leiomyomata are discovered late in menstrual life, it is unusual for symptoms to appear or for surgical treatment to be required. Larger tumors can also be watched safely, but if a policy of watchful waiting is adopted, one should be very sure of the nature of the tumors. If there is uncertainty of the uterine or ovarian origin of a tumor, as may well be the case when the tumor fills the whole pelvis or when a pedunculated tumor is felt in the adnexal region (Fig. 31.10), special diagnostic procedures may be indicated. Pelvic examination by an experienced gynecologist can usually clear up the uncertainty. In difficult cases, an examination under anesthesia may be necessary. Laparoscopy may be of great value in determining the nature of an adnexal mass. Before invasive techniques are used, however, noninvasive diagnostic evaluation should be performed. These include radiographic studies of the abdomen and pelvis, ultrasonography (US), and computed tomography (CT). The characteristic calcification in a leiomyoma may be seen on radiographs. The US and CT features of uterine leiomyomata have been well described. However, mistakes in the interpretation can still be made. Tada and associates reported that 5% of patients given the diagnosis of uterine leiomyomata by CT actually had an ovarian tumor at operation. Therefore, if uncertainty about the diagnosis persists, laparoscopy or laparotomy should still be performed.

When large asymptomatic leiomyomata occur in premenopausal women who have had their families or in whom

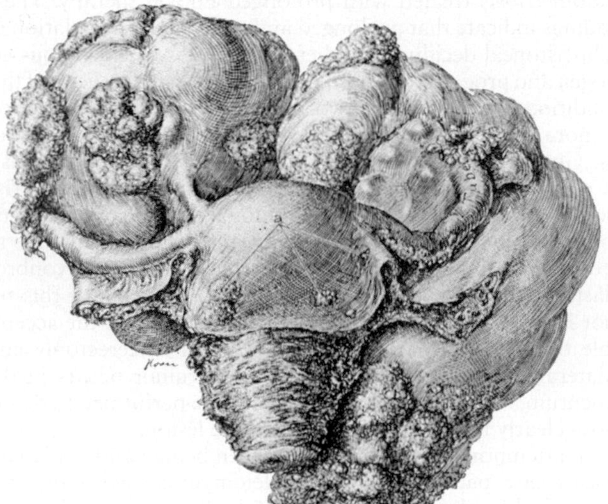

FIGURE 31.10. Although this central pelvic mass may feel like a multiple leiomyomatous uterus on bimanual pelvic examination, it is actually a bilateral ovarian malignancy. Differentiation between these two diagnoses may require special diagnostic procedures.

future childbearing is not important, a recommendation for removal may be made. It is impossible to predict which patients will become symptomatic in the remaining years before menopause. However, such tumors, with additional years to grow, are likely to require surgical removal eventually. Therefore, it is better to remove them when the patient is a good operative risk and when conservation of normal ovaries with a good blood supply can be easily accomplished. Such tumors should usually be 12 to 14 weeks in gestational size or larger. Depending on a variety of factors, either myomectomy or hysterectomy can be recommended to the patient. GnRH agonists may be useful in women approaching menopause to control symptoms or asymptomatic uterine myoma growth until menopause. The regrowth of tumors after the cessation of treatment limits the usefulness of these agents, however. Nakamura and Yoshimura reported their experience with GnRH agonists in the treatment of uterine leiomyomata in perimenopausal women. One third of patients reached menopause after 16 weeks of treatment, thus avoiding the need for surgery.

Reiter and colleagues studied 93 consecutive patients undergoing hysterectomy for leiomyomata. When the uterus was larger than 12 weeks' gestational size, there was no increased incidence of surgical complications compared with women with smaller uteri. On the basis of this small series, the authors concluded that hysterectomy need not be recommended to women with large asymptomatic uterine leiomyomata to avoid a possible increased risk of surgical complications.

There is no uniform size of an asymptomatic leiomyomatous uterus that can be used as an indication for hysterectomy or myomectomy. When size is the only significant indication for surgery in an asymptomatic patient, the location of the tumors is more important than the total uterine mass. When the leiomyomata are located in the cornual area or in the lateral wall of the uterus and obscure the anatomy of the adnexa and broad ligament, the risk of error in the early recognition of an ovarian tumor is greater. In such cases, one must carefully weigh the advantages and disadvantages of the conservative approach to the management of uterine leiomyomata. When adnexal tumors are present, it is critical that the origin of these tumors be confirmed. The diagnostic studies mentioned earlier should be performed to establish clearly that the tumors are of uterine origin before a decision is made to follow up the patient rather than operate. It is unacceptable to wait to see whether an adnexal tumor enlarges before identifying the site of origin of the mass as either uterine or ovarian. Ovarian carcinoma remains the most lethal disease of the female reproductive tract and the most difficult to diagnose early. Every diagnostic and therapeutic effort must be made to avoid errors in the clinical evaluation of pelvic neoplasms (Fig. 31.10). In women who are approaching menopause, relatively large uterine leiomyomata can be kept under observation with the knowledge that after menopause they will not increase in size and may actually regress somewhat. Still, one must be certain that the entire central pelvic mass is a leiomyomatous uterus. Patient management is largely dependent on knowledge of the exact location and size of leiomyomas. Imaging modalities play an important role in determining patient management, especially when differentiating a benign leiomyoma from other pathologic conditions that may require different therapies.

Uterine size as an indication for surgical intervention in women with leiomyomata has been thoughtfully discussed by Friedman and Haas. These authors point out that many gynecologists advocate surgical removal of leiomyomata when the uterus reaches 12 weeks' gestational size or greater, regardless of the presence or absence of significant symptoms. Historical reasons given for surgical intervention include the following:

- The inability to accurately assess the ovaries by examination
- The possible malignancy of the pelvic mass
- The potential for compromise of adjacent organ function if the mass continues to enlarge
- The greater risk of surgical complications if the mass grows to a larger size
- The potential for better fertility if myomectomy is performed when the uterus is smaller
- The possibility of continued growth of uterine leiomyomata if hormone replacement therapy is given after menopause

Friedman and Haas find very little in the literature to support these indications for surgical intervention and believe the availability of modern high-resolution US and magnetic resonance imaging (MRI) allows for expectant management in many patients with large asymptomatic uterine leiomyomata. They prefer to give primary consideration to the presence and severity of myoma-related symptoms in deciding whether surgical intervention is indicated. We believe that such a course of expectant management is appropriate only when there is relative certainty regarding the benign nature of the central pelvic mass and all of its components, and when it is possible to get the patient to return for periodic assessment of gynecologic symptoms and findings on pelvic examination. Repeat MRI may also be required occasionally.

If one elects to observe a patient with a relatively large asymptomatic uterine leiomyoma, it is a good rule to obtain an excretory urogram or renal ultrasound. Everett and Sturgis showed many years ago that ureteral compression at the pelvic brim may occur so that hydroureter and hydronephrosis develop (Fig. 31.11). It is usually the symmetrically enlarged

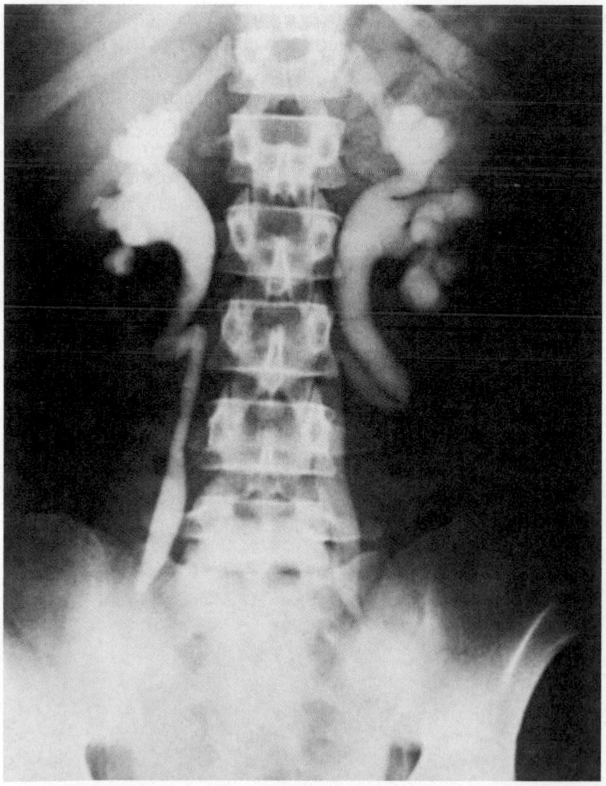

FIGURE 31.11. Bilateral ureteral obstruction and dilatation from pressure of large leiomyomata.

uterus with intramural leiomyomata that extends near or above the umbilicus and rests on the pelvic brim that compresses the ureters, in the same way as a symmetrically enlarged gravid uterus. The process is usually slow and painless even when moderate to severe hydronephrosis has occurred. Pyelographic evidence of kidney damage may be the determining factor in a decision to operate on a patient with an entirely asymptomatic leiomyoma. The irregularly and asymmetrically enlarged uterus with subserous tumors usually does not produce pressure on the ureters.

After menopause, asymptomatic leiomyomata generally should be left undisturbed. Again, the gynecologist must be absolutely certain that an ovarian neoplasm can be ruled out. In the postmenopausal years, shrinkage of myomata and the myometrium occurs. However, the myometrial shrinkage may be disproportionately greater than the myoma shrinkage. Therefore, a myoma in an intramural location before menopause may become a submucous myoma after menopause and then become symptomatic for the first time, usually with postmenopausal bleeding.

In menopausal women, the appearance of even the slightest trace of vaginal bleeding should make one suspect cervical or endometrial malignancy or the possibility of sarcomatous change in the leiomyoma (Figs. 31.12 and 31.13). Careful pelvic examination, Papanicolaou smear, and evaluation of the cervix by colposcopy or biopsy, pelvic US, fractional curettage, and perhaps hysteroscopy should be done. If the bleeding remains unexplained and the presence of atrophic vaginitis or the use of exogenous estrogens has been excluded, the leiomyomatous uterus should be removed because of the risk of sarcomatous change.

Transabdominal and endovaginal US are the standard imaging modalities for the detection of leiomyomas. Pelvic US by transvaginal and transabdominal techniques is most useful because of good patient tolerance, relatively low cost, availability, and accuracy when performed by well-trained and experienced ultrasonographers (Fig. 31.14). Ultrasonography is the most cost-effective screening mechanism for uterine masses suggestive of myomas. Sonographic criteria for diagnosis have been well described. Generally, abdominal US is unable to detect myomas less than 2 cm in diameter. Endovaginal probes have allowed for improved visualization of both the uterus and adnexa. With higher frequencies, sensitivity in the detection of small myomas has substantially increased. In a series evaluated by Fedele and colleagues using endovaginal ultrasound before hysterectomy, submucous leiomyomas were identified with a sensitivity of 100%. Difficulties may arise, however, if myomas are small or pedunculated, patients are obese, or the uterus is retroverted.

Transvaginal fluid-enhanced vaginal probe sonography (sonohysterography) is a useful technique to assess myomata that distort the endometrial cavity. This technique has little to no complications and is generally well tolerated with only mild cramping described by patients. The limitation of detection of leiomyomas with this modality is 0.5 cm diameter. In a study by Hoetzinger, the majority of intrauterine myomata (14 of 16, or 88%) were detected by sonohysterography. Ultrasound transducing catheters have been suggested as a potential tool

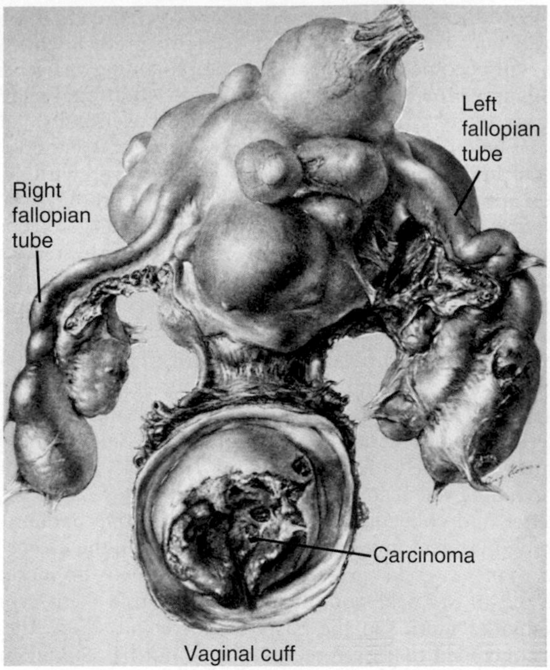

FIGURE 31.13. This specimen shows multiple uterine leiomyomata but also shows chronic pelvic inflammatory disease and cervical carcinoma. Patients with uterine leiomyomata may have abnormal bleeding, but a coexisting cervical carcinoma may also cause bleeding.

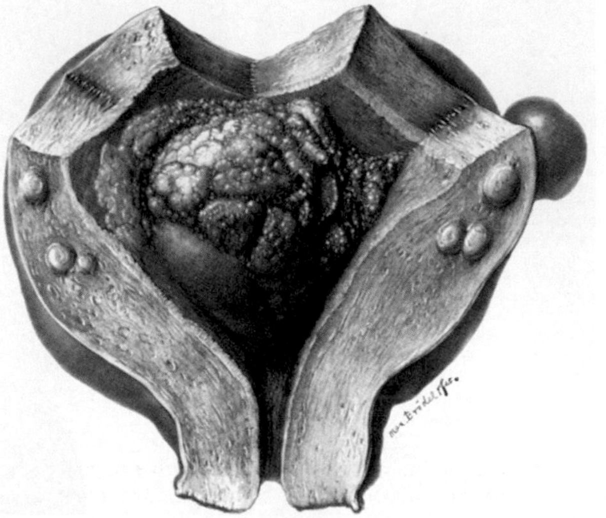

FIGURE 31.12. Adenocarcinoma of the endometrium is present in a symmetrically enlarged leiomyomatous uterus.

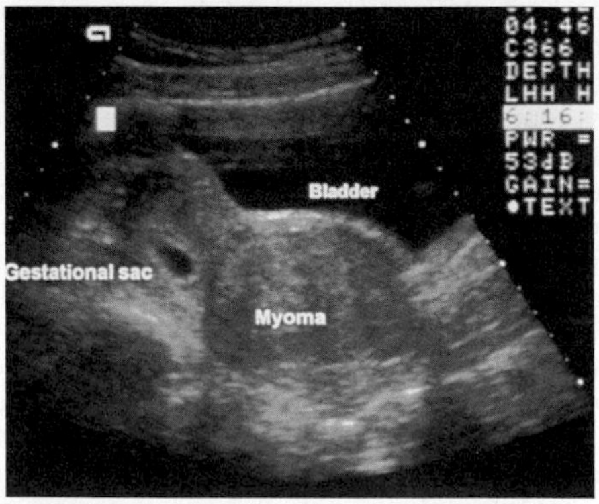

FIGURE 31.14. An ultrasonography study shows a cervical myoma and a very early intrauterine pregnancy.

to supplement abdominal and endovaginal sonography. Three-dimensional data display has recently undergone development and application in sonography; however, the role in evaluation and management of leiomyoma remains unclear (Fig. 31.9).

There is no technique that reliably identifies a leiomyosarcoma. Plain abdominal or pelvic radiographs and hysterosalpingography are older, standard techniques that are still useful in assessing uterine size, calcification in myomata, intrauterine filling defects caused by submucous myomata, and tubal patency. These techniques, combined with US, are the most useful for assessing patients with a central pelvic mass thought to be a leiomyomatous uterus. CA-125 levels may be elevated in women with uterine leiomyomata, but the levels are generally lower than those in patients with ovarian cancer.

Symptomatic Leiomyomata

Less than 50% of patients with uterine leiomyomata have symptoms. Symptoms may be single or multiple and depend on the location, size, and number of tumors present. A clinical and pathologic study of 298 patients with uterine leiomyomata by Persaud and Arjoon revealed no significant relation between the presenting symptoms and the presence of degenerative changes in the tumors. Some form of degeneration was demonstrated in 65% of the specimens, with hyaline degeneration accounting for 63% of all types of degeneration. Hyaline degeneration produces no characteristic symptoms. Symptoms, especially pain and fever, may be present in some patients with red degeneration of a leiomyoma during pregnancy, with torsion and infarction of a subserous pedunculated leiomyoma, or with an infected leiomyoma. A discussion of the signs and symptoms caused by uterine leiomyomata follows.

Abnormal Bleeding

It is surprising but not unusual that even patients with large uterine leiomyomata may have a history of normal menstruation. Such patients should be questioned carefully about recent slight increases in the amount, duration, and frequency of menstruation. Some patients with a history of normal menstruation are found to have iron-deficiency anemia from a gradual increase in menstrual blood loss that even the patient has not recognized. If a case of uterine leiomyomata is to be followed, the patient should be asked to monitor her menstrual blood loss carefully and should be given instructions to keep a menstrual calendar and monthly record of the number of pads or tampons used each day. A more objective measurement of the amount of menstrual blood loss using the method of Hallberg and Nilsson may be helpful in doubtful cases. Iron depletion may not be evident by laboratory determination unless one performs an iron stain of the bone marrow or serum ferritin levels. In the early months of increased menstrual blood loss, the hemoglobin and hematocrit values are normal. Heavy menstruation does not cause anemia until iron stores are first depleted.

Abnormal bleeding occurs in about one third of patients with symptomatic uterine leiomyomata and commonly indicates that treatment is necessary. The menstrual flow is usually heavy (menorrhagia), but it can also be prolonged (metrorrhagia) or both heavy and prolonged (menometrorrhagia). Abnormal bleeding may be associated with submucous, intramural, and subserous tumors, but there is a distinct clinical impression that bleeding is more common and more severe in the presence of submucous tumors. The submucous leiomyoma bleeds freely at menstruation and may also bleed between periods as a result of passive congestion, necrosis, and ulceration of the endometrial surface over the tumor and ulceration of the contralateral uterine surface. If the submucous myoma is pedunculated, there is usually a constant, thin, blood-tinged discharge in addition to the menorrhagia. An intramural tumor that is just beginning to encroach on the uterine cavity can also be responsible for menorrhagia. Intramural leiomyomata near the serosal surface and pedunculated subserous tumors can also be associated with abnormal bleeding. When bleeding occurs with such tumors, however, one should search for some other lesion to account for it. The mere presence of leiomyomata in a woman who has abnormal uterine bleeding is not proof that the leiomyomata are causing the bleeding. This fact is important, particularly when there is intermenstrual bleeding. When a patient with leiomyomata has intermenstrual bleeding, it is a rule in our practice to examine and study the cervix carefully with special diagnostic procedures and to sample and evaluate the uterine cavity before we proceed with treatment of the leiomyomata. If an endometrial or cervical malignancy is detected, the treatment of the leiomyomata may need to be altered.

There are several mechanisms by which leiomyomata can cause abnormal bleeding, although a single specific mechanism may not be apparent in a particular patient. According to Sehgal and Haskins, the surface area of the endometrial cavity in a normal uterus is 15 cm^2. The surface area of the endometrial cavity in the presence of leiomyomata may exceed 200 cm^2. These authors demonstrated a correlation between the severity of the bleeding and the area of endometrial surface. In addition to an increased surface area from which to bleed, the endometrium may demonstrate local hyperestrogenism in areas immediately adjacent to submucous tumors, and endometrial hyperplasia and endometrial polyps are commonly found. Degligdish and Loewenthal noted a broad spectrum of histologic abnormalities in the endometrium associated with leiomyomata, ranging from atrophy to hyperplasia. Thinning and ulceration of the endometrial surface may be present over large submucous tumors; smaller ones may show slight thinning without ulceration. The presence of leiomyomata may interfere with myometrial contractility as well as contractility of the spiral arterioles in the basalis portion of the endometrium. Miller and Ludovici suggested that anovulation and dysfunctional uterine bleeding are more common in the presence of uterine leiomyomata.

Sampson in 1913 was the first to study the blood supply of uterine leiomyomata and its effect on uterine bleeding. More recent studies have been performed by Faulkner and by Farrer-Brown and associates. The most prominent and important change is the presence of endometrial venule ectasia. Tumors that are strategically located in the myometrium may cause obstruction and proximal congestion of veins in the myometrium and endometrium. Thrombosis and sloughing of these large dilated venous channels within the endometrium produce heavy bleeding (Fig. 31.15).

Makarainen and Ylikorkala have presented evidence that further supports the concept that prostanoids play a role in primary menorrhagia. They found that the production of 6-keto-prostaglandin F_1 alpha (6-keto-$PGF_{1\alpha}$), a metabolite of prostacyclin (PGI_2), and thromboxane B_2 (TXB_2), a metabolite of thromboxane A_2 (TXA_2), was normal in menorrhagic endometrium. However, the balance between TXA_2 and PGI_2 shifted to a relative TXA_2 deficiency and was negatively related to blood loss in patients with menorrhagia. Although ibuprofen decreased the blood loss in patients with primary menorrhagia, it failed to reduce myoma-associated menorrhagia. The authors suggest that uterine factors other than prostanoids are more important in causing menorrhagia associated with uterine leiomyomata.

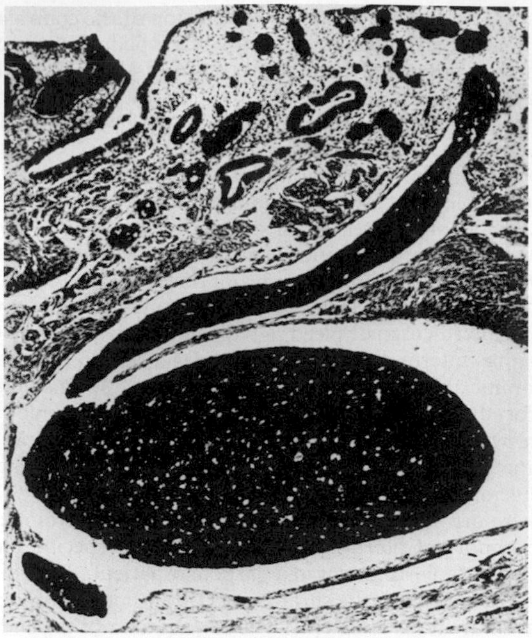

FIGURE 31.15. Dilated endometrial venous space communicating with a grossly enlarged vessel in the inner myometrium of a uterus with submucous leiomyomata. (From Farrer-Brown G, Beilby JO, Tarbit MH. Venous changes in the endometrium of myomatous uteri. *Obstet Gynecol* 1971;83:743.)

In most cases, when bleeding occurs postmenopausally and leiomyomata are discovered on bimanual examination, the bleeding is due to some other factor, such as cervical or endometrial abnormalities, atrophic vaginitis, or exogenous estrogen, and the leiomyomata are purely incidental. Occasionally, however, the postmenopausal leiomyoma can be responsible for the bleeding. As stated earlier, leiomyomata that do not bleed during the menstrual life of the patient have been found to migrate to a submucous position in later years. This occurs because after menopause the myometrium atrophies and the uterine wall becomes thinner. Leiomyomata also shrink somewhat, but not as much as the surrounding myometrium. Thus, a leiomyoma that was intramural before menopause may work itself into a submucous position after menopause, become ulcerated, and bleed. Postmenopausal growth of uterine leiomyomata may indicate malignant change, especially if associated with postmenopausal bleeding. We have rarely observed postmenopausal growth in a leiomyoma without finding malignancy in the tumor; whenever there is enlargement of the leiomyoma after menopause, one should seriously consider the possibility of sarcomatous change and remove the leiomyoma.

Patients with heavy menstruation and uterine leiomyomata should be evaluated for the presence of submucous myomata. Even patients without palpable evidence of uterine leiomyomata or uterine enlargement who have heavy menstruation should be evaluated for the presence of submucous myomata. When endometrial curettage is performed, irregularity of the uterine cavity may suggest the presence of a submucous myoma. However, a submucous myoma may not be detected with the curette. An accurate diagnosis is more likely to be made by hysterosalpingography, conventional transvaginal or transabdominal US, sonohysterography, MRI, or hysteroscopy. Cincinelli and colleagues reported their experience with transabdominal sonohysterography, a technique that involves transabdominal ultrasonographic scanning while 30 mL of sterile isotonic saline is slowly injected into the uterine cavity. According to these investigators, this technique provided the most accurate evaluation of the size of submucous myomata, intracavitary and intramural growth, and location within the uterine cavity, with sensitivity, specificity, and predictive values of 100%.

Pressure

Evidence of pressure on nearby pelvic viscera may be an indication for treatment. The urinary bladder suffers most often from such pressure, giving rise to urgency and frequency of urination and sometimes even urinary incontinence (Fig. 31.16). Although this symptom is common with large leiomyomata, one frequently finds the pelvis filled with leiomyomata when there is no urinary frequency. Occasionally, acute retention of urine or overflow incontinence results from a leiomyoma and necessitates surgical intervention. These effects can occur as a result of rapid interior growth of the leiomyoma with compression of the urethra and bladder neck against the pubic bone. More often, a tumor the size of a 3-month pregnancy may become incarcerated in the cul-de-sac, wedging the cervix forward against the urethra and obstructing the flow of urine through the urethra. A large pedunculated submucous tumor may fill and distend the vagina and press the urethra against the symphysis, causing urinary retention.

As pointed out by Mattingly, one can expect to encounter women who have uterine leiomyomata of significant size and in addition have protrusion of the bladder base and posterior urethra through a widened levator muscle hiatus and a weakened urogenital diaphragm. Both conditions are relatively common. In addition to the usual symptoms produced by the

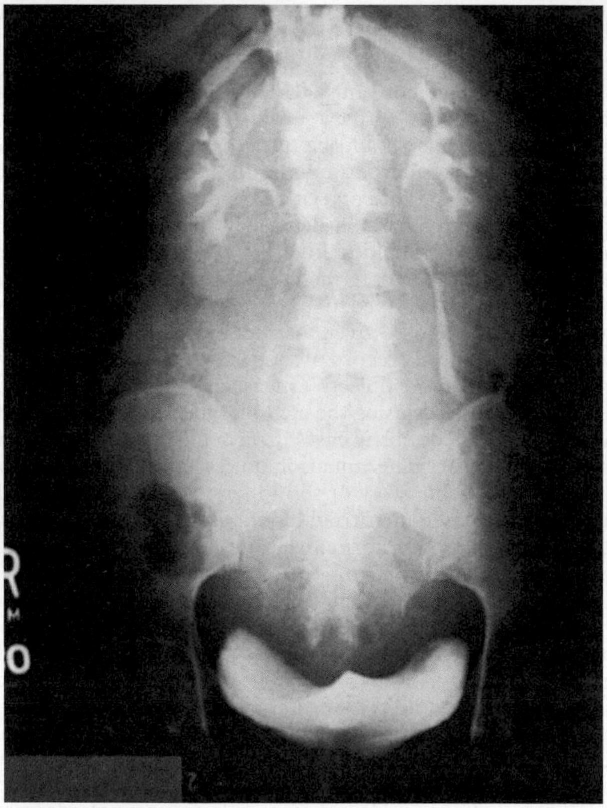

FIGURE 31.16. Cystogram and intravenous pyelogram showing distortion of the bladder by pressure from a leiomyoma.

leiomyomata, socially disabling stress urinary incontinence may be present. When the anterior wall of the uterus is greatly distorted by the presence of these tumors, pressure against the bladder can cause urinary frequency. If anatomic pressure equalization incontinence is also present, it may be aggravated by the increased intravesical pressure caused by the leiomyomata. However, the presence of anatomic stress urinary incontinence has no etiologic relation to the uterine enlargement caused by the leiomyomata.

Silent ureteral obstruction from pressure against the pelvic brim is an uncommon complication of uterine enlargement caused by multiple large leiomyomata. Such an asymptomatic anatomic change occurs more often with a symmetrically enlarged leiomyomatous uterus that becomes large enough to fill the pelvis and compress the ureter against the pelvic sidewalls (Fig. 31.11). Although an infrequent complication, the obstruction can occur in either ureter, depending on the location of the uterine tumors. If there has been no infection or parenchymal damage to the kidney, this anatomic alteration is completely reversible with removal of the uterus and relief of the pressure against the ureter. However, if urinary tract obstruction from leiomyomata has been neglected, uremia may result. Removal of the tumor and relief of obstruction are necessary to restore kidney function. Chronic bladder neck obstruction from uterine leiomyomata can be so severe as to cause a remarkable increase in the thickness of the bladder wall and enlargement of the bladder resembling that seen in men with urethral obstruction from prostatic enlargement. Indeed, in these neglected cases, the bladder may fill the entire lower abdominal wall so that an incision above the umbilicus is required to enter the peritoneal cavity to remove the tumor without injury to the bladder.

The bowel is less apt to show symptoms from pressure than is the bladder, but constipation can be caused and aggravated by pressure of leiomyomata against the rectum. The small intestines can become entwined with subserous pedunculated tumors, causing intermittent intestinal obstruction.

Pain

Abdominal and pelvic pain or discomfort, a feeling of heaviness in the pelvis, and dyspareunia are present in about one third of patients with symptomatic uterine leiomyomata and may be an appropriate reason for intervention. There are several causes of pain with leiomyomata. However, the usual hyaline or cystic degeneration of these tumors does not produce symptoms. In rare instances, pedunculated subserous leiomyomata twist and give rise to a clinical picture of acute abdominal pain, much like that seen with a torsed ovarian tumor. These pedunculated tumors twist more often during pregnancy and after menopause. Acute carneous or red degeneration of a leiomyoma can occur at any period of reproductive life, although pain from this form of degeneration is more common during pregnancy. Dysmenorrhea, acquired in the fourth or fifth decade, may be the outstanding symptom of the growth of leiomyomata. A common symptom complex resulting from leiomyomata at this time of life is menstrual pain coupled with increased menstrual flow. Diffuse adenomyosis can also cause these symptoms, and the differentiation of this condition from a symmetrically enlarged intramural leiomyoma may be extremely difficult and may require MRI. The differentiation may be academic when surgery is planned; however, in cases when uterine artery embolization is considered, this distinction is important because it may be less effective in cases of adenomyosis.

Patients who have uterine leiomyomata and pain may have concomitant pelvic disease such as ovarian pathology, pelvic inflammatory disease, tubal pregnancy, endometriosis, or urinary tract or intestinal pathology, including appendicitis. One must be careful to rule out other pathology that may be obscured by uterine leiomyomata.

Abdominal Distortion

Distortion of the normal abdominal wall contour because of large tumors may justify their removal. Tumors of such size often give rise to other symptoms also, so there is ample reason for surgical interference. However, when no other symptoms are present, one may recommend removal of the tumors if the abdominal distortion is of such a magnitude as to be embarrassing to the patient.

Rapid Growth

Evidence of rapid growth of uterine leiomyomata, as observed by the same examiner over time or as confirmed by US, is an indication for surgical intervention. Such rapid growth in a premenopausal patient is only rarely due to sarcoma. Parker and others reviewed the medical records of 1,332 women admitted for surgical management of uterine leiomyoma. They actually found no correlation between rapid growth and the presence of uterine sarcoma. It may be due to pregnancy or to the use of oral contraceptives containing large amounts of estrogens. In the latter case, these drugs should be discontinued and an alternative method of contraception prescribed. In the postmenopausal patient, however, growth of a uterine leiomyoma is highly suggestive of a malignancy. The malignancy may be a sarcomatous change in the leiomyoma itself, a sarcoma or carcinoma in the endometrium causing uterine enlargement, or an ovarian neoplasm whose estrogen secretion is stimulating enlargement of the leiomyoma or whose growth may be mistaken for rapid enlargement of uterine leiomyomata. Although malignancy is not invariably found, the chances in its favor are so great that one must proceed on the assumption that it exists and should perform dilatation and curettage followed by removal of the enlarged uterus.

Rapid growth of a leiomyomatous uterus is difficult to define in exact terms. Buttram and Reiter have arbitrarily defined it as a gain of 6 weeks or more in gestational size within a year or less. Although this definition could apply in premenopausal women, it might be disastrous to wait for this amount of growth in a postmenopausal woman. It is important to have a definite method of documenting uterine size at periodic intervals. Repeated sounding of the uterine cavity may be of some benefit, although leiomyomatous growth is not always accompanied by concomitant enlargement of the uterine cavity. It is important to document the size of specific leiomyomata or the total uterine size in terms of centimeters or grams of uterine weight rather than in terms of gestational size of the uterus, although the latter method has become quite popular. Changes in a patient's weight can make evaluation of growth more difficult. Ultrasonography is a much more objective way of establishing the size of a uterine leiomyoma in the beginning and, when indicated, of evaluating its rate of growth. There is a need for more information about the natural growth patterns of myomata before and after menopause.

Although leiomyomata can increase dramatically in size during pregnancy, usually there is no appreciable growth. Winer-Muram and coworkers studied 89 pregnant women with uterine leiomyomata documented by US examination. In 83 of the patients, there was no demonstrable increase in the size of the leiomyomata. In six patients, there was an increase in size of up to 4 cm. Those myomata that increase in size during pregnancy will decrease in size a few weeks after the pregnancy is over.

Spontaneous Abortion and Other Pregnancy-Related Problems

Uterine leiomyomata are associated with a significantly increased risk of spontaneous abortion. In a collected series of patients undergoing myomectomy, Buttram and Reiter reported that 41% had spontaneous abortions. This rate was reduced to 19% after myomectomy. Seoud and colleagues did not demonstrate that *in vitro* fertilization live birth rates were improved by myomectomy; however, the authors did note a 50% spontaneous abortion rate in patients with leiomyomata compared with 34% after myomectomy. Various mechanisms have been proposed to explain the occurrence of spontaneous abortion from uteri with leiomyomata. These include disturbances in uterine blood flow, alterations in blood supply to the endometrium, uterine irritability, rapid growth or degeneration of leiomyomata during pregnancy, difficulty in enlargement of the uterine cavity to accommodate for the growth of the fetus and placenta, and interference with proper implantation and placental growth by poorly developed endometrium or by subjacent leiomyomata. Implantation in a thin, poorly vascularized endometrium over a submucous leiomyoma is doomed to failure, because proper growth and development of the embryo and placenta are impossible (Fig. 31.17). Matsunaga and Shiota found a twofold increase in the number of malformed embryos recovered from patients with uterine leiomyomata having artificial termination of pregnancy.

Uterine leiomyomata may also be associated with other obstetrical concerns, including premature delivery, stillbirth, and interstitial pregnancy, as in the case reported by Starks. In a retrospective population-based study by Sheiner and colleagues, obstetrical outcomes appeared to be compromised by uterine leiomyoma. Compared with controls, women with myomas during pregnancy had an increase in intrauterine growth restriction (6.8% vs. 1.9%), placental abruption (2.8% vs. 0.7%), abnormal presentation (16.9% vs. 2.4%), cesarean section rate (57.7% vs. 10.8%), premature rupture of membranes (9.6% vs. 5.5%), and likelihood to receive a blood transfusion (4.2% vs. 1.4%). All of these outcomes were statistically significant ($p < 0.001$). Muram and associates have followed patients with leiomyomata through pregnancy with US. When a leiomyoma was in close proximity to the placental site, an increased incidence of pregnancy-related complications was seen. These were mainly bleeding complications, but pain, premature delivery, and postpartum hemorrhage also occurred. Exacoustos and Rosati reviewed the US scans of 12,708 pregnant patients. Four hundred ninety-two patients had myomata. A statistically significant increased incidence of threatened abortion, threatened preterm delivery, abruptio placentae, and pelvic pain was observed in patients with myomata. Abruptio placentae was particularly evident in women with myoma volumes greater than 200 cm^3, submucosal location, or superimposition of the placenta. The authors suggest that US findings make it possible to identify women at risk for myoma-related complications of pregnancy. Factors responsible for spontaneous abortion in patients without uterine leiomyomata may also be responsible for spontaneous abortion in patients with leiomyomata.

Occasionally, pregnancy causes a remarkable growth of leiomyomata in the same way that the myometrium undergoes hypertrophy in pregnancy. Red or carneous degeneration of leiomyomata during pregnancy is associated with pain, tenderness over the tumor, low-grade fever, and leukocytosis. Management should be expectant with analgesic medications and bed rest. If premature uterine contractions occur, tocolytics may be given. Pain usually subsides within a few days. Operation is not indicated unless it is necessary to rule out other problems that require surgery for relief, because differentiation from appendicitis, placental abruption, torsed adnexa, and other problems may be difficult. After delivery, leiomyomata involute and generally return to their prepregnancy size by the third postpartum month.

Torsion with infarction of subserous pedunculated leiomyomata is more common in pregnancy. A leiomyoma may interfere with labor and delivery by causing an abnormal presentation, by causing dysfunctional labor, or by obstructing the pelvis. A submucous leiomyoma in the lower uterine segment may entrap the placenta, necessitating manual removal. Indeed, furious postpartum hemorrhage can result if a submucous leiomyoma is disturbed at delivery or during exploration of the uterine cavity. Immediate hysterectomy may be necessary to control the bleeding.

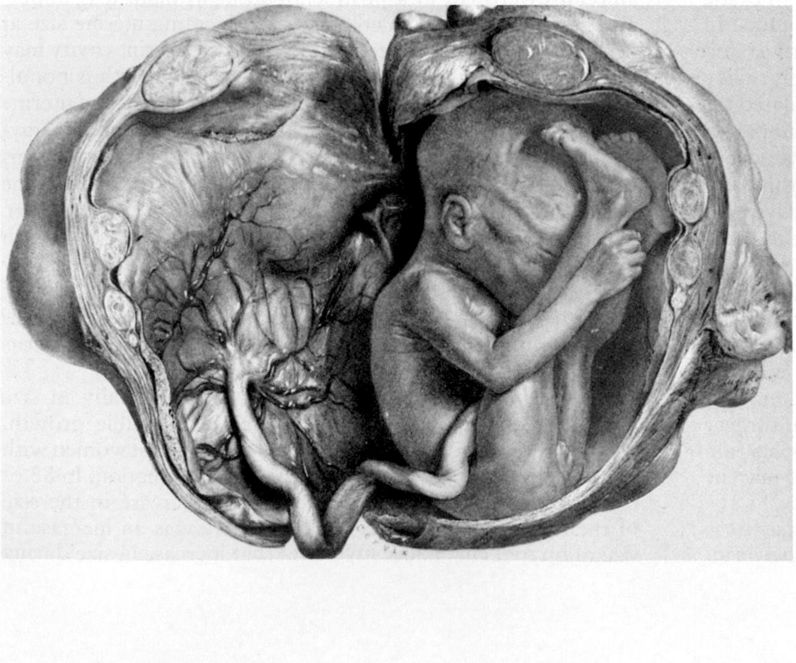

FIGURE 31.17. When the placenta is implanted over a myoma in the uterine wall, the blood supply to the fetus may be tenuous.

Most patients with uterine leiomyomata have no difficulty conceiving and carry their pregnancies to term without complications. The only problem encountered may be a difficulty in estimating gestational age from uterine size because of the presence of leiomyomata.

Infertility

When asymptomatic leiomyomata are discovered in young women, the question of how these tumors relate to sterility and pregnancy usually arises. A number of factors may be responsible for infertility in a patient with uterine leiomyomata. Anovulatory cycles may occur more commonly. There may be interference with sperm transport caused by distortion and an increased surface area within the uterine cavity, impingement of leiomyomata on the endocervical canal or interstitial portion of the fallopian tube, or interference with prostaglandin-induced uterine contractions, which are thought to enhance sperm migration. Endometrial changes (atrophy, ulceration, focal hyperplasia, and polyps), vascular alterations (venous congestion, venule ectasia, impaired blood flow), and enlargement of the uterine cavity may be present. Because uterine leiomyomata occur in later reproductive years, relatively greater difficulty accomplishing conception can be expected in older couples.

The finding of small leiomyomata in sterile women is not an indication for immediate myomectomy. Quite often, an infertile patient with uterine leiomyomata is found to have some other cause of infertility. Tubal inflammatory disease with associated pelvic adhesions is especially common in patients with uterine leiomyomata. Both marital partners should have a complete infertility investigation, and the leiomyomata should be disregarded for a while. The ultimate decision regarding disposal of the tumors depends on their size and location. Usually, small subserous leiomyomata are not considered a factor in infertility. Even if the woman fails to become pregnant, removal of small subserous leiomyomata is not justified. When leiomyomata are intramural or submucous and of significant size, they may well be factors causing the infertility, and a myomectomy may be rewarded with a subsequent pregnancy.

When an unsuspected asymptomatic leiomyomatous uterus of significant size is found in a woman who is planning to become pregnant in the future, great tact is required in describing the problem to the patient. The best surgical and obstetric judgment is needed to make a proper recommendation. Should the patient be discouraged from attempting pregnancy because the risk of complications may be increased? Should a myomectomy be advised before pregnancy is attempted, with the knowledge that postmyomectomy adhesions may cause infertility? Such questions cannot be answered in a stereotypical manner. Each case presents its own problems, and the answers depend on the patient's age, her general physical health, her pelvic findings, and, most important, her own desires. All must be considered before a final recommendation can be made. In general terms, under these circumstances, an attempt to become pregnant will be rewarded with a satisfactory outcome in most cases. If pregnancy does not occur or is not successful, a myomectomy may be advised, but one must keep in mind that all causes of infertility, spontaneous abortion, and other pregnancy-related problems must also be investigated in patients with uterine leiomyomata; uterine leiomyomata represent an infrequent cause of infertility.

Eldar-Geva and colleagues performed a retrospective review of the treatment outcome of 106 assisted reproductive technology cycles in 88 patients with uterine myomata (subserosal, intramuscular without cavity distortion, and submucosal). Patients underwent controlled ovarian hyperstimulation and advanced reproductive technology. Not surprisingly, pregnancy (30.1%) and implantation (15.7%) rates were significantly lower in women with submucosal myomas; however, both pregnancy (16.4%) and implantation (6.4%) rates were also significantly lower in women with intramural myomas. In some advanced assisted reproductive technology patients, this information may influence the decision for surgical intervention regardless of menstrual pattern.

A review of information about infertility and uterine leiomyomata was published by Wallach and Vu, by Vercellini and colleagues, and by Verkauf.

Miscellaneous Signs and Symptoms

A variety of other unusual problems may be associated with uterine leiomyomata and may require treatment. Ascites and uterine inversion have already been mentioned. Sudden intraperitoneal hemorrhage can result from rupture of a dilated vein beneath the serosal surface of a subserous leiomyoma. Although leiomyomata are more often associated with iron-deficiency anemia from chronic uterine blood loss, occasionally patients present with polycythemia. Islands of extramedullary erythropoiesis have been found in leiomyomata. Arteriovenous shunts within the tumors have been found and may be etiologically important in polycythemia. If the tumor obstructs the ureters and causes back pressure on the renal parenchyma, erythropoiesis can be stimulated. Weiss and coworkers and other investigators have found marked erythropoietin activity within uterine leiomyomata. The polycythemia in these cases is cured by hysterectomy.

CHOICE OF TREATMENT FOR UTERINE LEIOMYOMATA

Six hundred fifty thousand hysterectomies are performed annually in the United States. Approximately 33% are performed with uterine leiomyomata as the primary indication. Nearly 35,000 myomectomies were reportedly performed annually in 2001, and it is believed that this number is increasing substantially. There are no statistics to indicate the number of hysteroscopic and laparoscopic myomectomies performed each year. Effective medical therapies are available to use as adjuncts to surgical treatment. Additional radiologic procedures may also be desirous in patients who may not be suitable surgical candidates. However, surgery is the preferred method of therapy in many circumstances.

Hysterectomy (abdominal, vaginal, and laparoscopy assisted) is discussed in Chapters 32A, B, and C. In this chapter, surgical techniques that allow conservation of uterine function are discussed, as are medical therapies that can be used as adjuncts to surgical therapy.

Medical Management of Uterine Leiomyomata

Most (70%–80%) uterine leiomyomata are asymptomatic and are discovered incidentally during a routine pelvic examination. Such patients require an explanation and reassurance and reexamination at periodic intervals. An initial baseline pelvic US examination or MRI study may be indicated for comparison with future examinations and to evaluate the adnexa if the ovaries cannot be felt on pelvic examination. An experienced pelvic examiner can be fairly certain that a central pelvic mass is a leiomyomatous uterus. However, pelvic US examinations and repeat pelvic examinations can add to the certainty of the diagnosis. If the diagnosis remains doubtful, however, visualization of the mass, usually by laparoscopy, may be indicated. Patients with an asymptomatic central pelvic mass should be followed up with periodic pelvic examination only when the mass is benign, usually a leiomyomatous uterus. Otherwise, expectant management is not appropriate.

Effective medical treatment that is likely to result in the permanent cure of uterine leiomyomata is not yet available. Surgical excision by a variety of techniques remains the most effective and widely used method of management for patients with significant symptoms. Medical therapies are available as an adjunct to surgical treatment or as a temporary substitute for definitive surgical treatment. The role of radiologic intervention continues to expand with uterine artery emnolization and recently U.S. Food and Drug Administration (FDA)-approved, MRI-guided, high-frequency focused ultrasonography (HIFUS).

Hormonal therapy for the management of uterine leiomyomata has been the subject of investigation for many years. There is no support for the use of danazol or progestins in view of the disappointing results reported. Antiprogestin therapy with mifepristone (RU-486) for 3 months has been shown by Murphy and colleagues to decrease leiomyoma volume by an average of 49%, with a variation of 0% to 87%. The immunoreactivity of progesterone but not estrogen receptors in the myoma and myometrial tissue was decreased significantly by RU-486 treatment, suggesting that regression of these tumors may be attained through a direct antiprogesterone effect. All patients became amenorrheic. Side effects were mild, and bone density was not diminished. An effective dose to cause a clinically significant (50%) decrease in leiomyoma volume appears to be 25 mg daily. Additional experience is needed to further evaluate these promising results. Reinsch and associates have demonstrated that RU-486 and leuprolide acetate are both effective in decreasing blood flow to the uterus. It is suggested that a decrease in uterine artery blood flow may provide a mechanism for a decrease in uterine size.

Gestrinone, a synthetic derivative of ethinyl-nortestosterone with antiestrogen and antiprogesterone properties, has been shown by Coutinho and associates to induce regression of leiomyomata. The treatment lasted 6 months to 1 year. The best results were obtained when the drug was administered intravaginally. Even the regression of large leiomyomata lasted up to a year after treatment. Side effects, though mildly androgenic, were well tolerated.

Many studies have been performed to investigate the treatment of patients with uterine leiomyomata with GnRH analogs. GnRH analogs bind to GnRH receptors, resulting in a biphasic response: a temporary increase in the levels of gonadotropins and gonadal steroids (agonist phase) is followed by chronic suppression of gonadotropin and gonadal steroid secretion (desensitization phase). In 1 to 3 weeks, a profound hypogonadotropic hypogonadal state begins and exists as long as the treatment lasts, but it is promptly reversed when treatment is discontinued. GnRH agonist treatment results in "medical oophorectomy" and "medical menopause" and is associated with the usual symptoms of a profound hypogonadal state (e.g., hot flashes, insomnia, mood lability, headaches, vaginal dryness, arthralgias, and myalgias). According to Friedman and associates, these adverse effects of treatment are self-limited and disappear within 3 to 6 months of cessation of GnRH agonist treatment. Dawood and colleagues describe a significant reduction in trabecular bone density after 24 weeks of GnRH agonist treatment that may not be completely reversible when treatment is discontinued. A mean reduction in trabecular bone density of 1% per month occurs in women treated for 6 months. Some of this bone loss may be permanent, but some is reversible.

Friedman and colleagues state that the average reduction in uterine and myoma volume is 40% to 50% after 3 to 6 months of GnRH agonist treatment; this is generally confirmed by others. Most of the response occurs in the first 12 weeks, and it is variable and unpredictable.

According to the analysis by these investigators, 4% of patients had an increase in uterine volume ranging from 0.1% to 25%; 24% had decreases in uterine volume ranging from 0.1% to 25%; 51% had decreases in uterine volume ranging from 25.1% to 50%; and 21% had decreases in uterine volume greater than 50%. No factors were found to predict the degree of uterine shrinkage. There were negative correlations with body weight, pretreatment uterine volume, age, height, and serum estradiol concentration.

It is commonly thought that GnRH analogs affect leiomyomata by reducing vascularity and the individual cell size within the tumor. The biochemical changes in leiomyomata obtained from women treated with the GnRH agonist leuprolide acetate depot for 3 months were studied by Rein and coworkers. The concentrations of amino acids contained in collagen were significantly greater in uterine myomata from treated patients than in myomata from placebo-treated controls. These investigators suggest that the reduction in uterine myoma volume associated with GnRH agonist therapy is due primarily to alterations in the extracellular matrix rather than to a reduction in the number or volume of cells in the myoma. Di Lieto and colleagues evaluated the clinical response, immunohistological expression of the angiogenetic growth factors βFGF, VEGF, and PDGF, and vascular changes in uterine leiomyomas from women treated with GnRH agonist. They demonstrated that the GnRH agonist therapy caused a reduction in the synthesis of the three considered growth factors in leiomyomatous cells (βFGF, VEGF, and PDGF). The total number of vessels and angiogenetic vessels was also decreased after treatment with leuprolide acetate for 3 months.

Because uterine leiomyomata are hormone-sensitive neoplasms that can be stimulated to grow by estrogen, some clinicians have been reluctant to prescribe oral contraceptive pills in patients with leiomyomata. However, Friedman and Thomas and others have demonstrated conclusively that oral contraceptives containing 30 to 35 mg of ethinyl estradiol do not cause uterine leiomyomata to increase in size. Therefore, low-dose contraceptives can be used to manage menorrhagia in patients with uterine leiomyomata. Friedman and Thomas demonstrated a significant decrease in the mean duration of menstrual flow and a significant increase in hematocrit values in response to low-dose oral contraceptives in patients with uterine leiomyomata.

When myoma-associated menorrhagia is more severe, GnRH agonist and iron treatment may be more effective than oral contraceptives. In about two thirds of patients, GnRH agonist treatment induces amenorrhea. Most of the remaining patients experience very light, irregular vaginal bleeding or spotting, according to Friedman. A combination of menstrual suppression and iron therapy allows correction of iron deficiency and iron-deficiency anemia during a 6-month treatment period. Ovulatory menses resume 3 to 24 weeks after the last depot GnRH agonist injection. Stovall and associates reported that a GnRH agonist plus iron was more effective than iron alone in treating anemia in patients with leiomyomata and in alleviating menorrhagia. With such effective treatment now available, there is rarely a need to use blood transfusions to correct anemia caused by myoma-associated menorrhagia. Only patients with significant symptoms from severe anemia may require transfusion.

Medical therapy may also be used transiently before surgery. By initiating the medication preoperatively, the maximum decrease in myoma volume may play a role in determining the route of surgery. If a hysterectomy is planned, the pharmacologic effect may facilitate a vaginal hysterectomy when the uterus is of borderline size. Vercellini and colleagues performed a multicenter, prospective, randomized, controlled study to assess if this shrinkage may increase the likelihood of a vaginal procedure. One hundred and twenty-seven premenopausal women with uterine volumes of 12 to 16 weeks were enrolled. After examination and disposition for an abdominal or vaginal hysterectomy, patients were randomized for GnRH therapy. Clinical assessment after the treatment course showed that abdominal hysterectomy was no longer indicated in 25 of 53 (47%) patients. No appreciable difference was found between the groups in postoperative complications. These findings are consistent with previously published studies, as well.

GnRH agonist treatment alone should not be given for periods longer than 6 months. A prolonged hypoestrogenic state is undesirable for a number of reasons, the most important being the loss of trabecular bone. If there are circumstances that require that GnRH treatment be extended beyond 6 months, consideration should be given to adding low-dose steroids after 3 months of GnRH therapy. The usual postmenopausal estrogen-progestin replacement regimen can be prescribed without interfering with the reduction in uterine volume anticipated. Loss of trabecular bone may not be as great. By adding estrogen-progestin replacement to GnRH agonist therapy, the adverse effects of a prolonged hypoestrogenic state may be prevented, and treatment with GnRH agonists may be prolonged. Friedman and colleagues treated 51 premenopausal women with large, symptomatic myomata with leuprolide acetate depot for 104 weeks. After the first 12 weeks, 0.75 mg of estropiptate plus 0.7 mg of norethindrone were added on days 1 through 14 each month. Menorrhagia and other symptoms of uterine leiomyomata were controlled successfully. Hemoglobin and hematocrit levels increased. Symptoms of hypoestrogenism (hot flashes, vaginal dryness) were decreased significantly. Bone density decreased in the first 12 weeks, but only a small additional decrease occurred between weeks 12 and 52.

The use of GnRH analogs in the medical management of uterine leiomyomata is an emerging issue. How valuable it will be remains to be seen. Additional information and experience will define its use more exactly. For example, it may be possible for patients with symptomatic uterine leiomyomata who are approaching menopause to be managed medically through menopause without having a hysterectomy. It may be possible to improve fertility in some patients with uterine leiomyomata by treatment with GnRH analogs without myomectomy. With additional data, these and other questions can be answered.

Vaginal Myomectomy

In 1845, Atlee performed the first successful vaginal myomectomy on a patient with a submucous pedunculated myoma.

When a submucous myoma becomes pedunculated within the uterine cavity, there is a natural tendency for the uterus to try to expel it through the endocervical canal. Eventually, the cervix dilates. Even very large submucous pedunculated myomata can be delivered gradually through a markedly dilated cervix. Because adequate blood circulation through a long pedicle is difficult to maintain, the myoma becomes necrotic and infected (Figs. 31.5 and 31.6).

Patients report cramping lower abdominal pain; pressure and heaviness in the pelvis; a thin, bloody, foul discharge; difficulty with urination; and other symptoms. Episodes of profuse vaginal hemorrhage can occur. Such large submucous myomata may resemble a fetal head.

After satisfactory preoperative preparation, including broad-spectrum antibiotics and correction of anemia, vaginal myomectomy should be performed in the operating room. Morcellation may be required to remove very large tumors in many small pieces. Usually there is very little bleeding. One should avoid too much downward traction on the tumor because the uterine fundus may invert. Eventually, the pedicle is identified. It should be clamped and ligated as high as possible within the uterine cavity. The use of a laparoscopic instrumentation, such as the endoloop, can be advantageous to facilitate safe, secure ligation of the pedicle as high as possible. If ligation of the pedicle is not possible, the clamps can be left in place and safely removed 48 hours later.

Smaller submucous pedunculated myomata can be diagnosed by hysteroscopy, by hysterosalpingography, by US, or at the time of dilation and curettage. They can also be felt on digital exploration through a slightly dilated external cervical os. If the myoma can be grasped with an instrument (ring forceps, Allis clamp, and so forth), it can be removed by twisting it free of its attachment. A tonsil snare can also be used. Bleeding is usually minimal. If brisk bleeding does occur, a 26-French, 30-mL Foley catheter can be inserted through the cervix and inflated for tamponade. If necessary, the cervix can be sutured around the catheter to hold it in place.

To gain access to submucous pedunculated myomata that are higher in the endocervical canal or uterine cavity, special procedures are required. An attempt at hysteroscopic removal may be successful. Alternatively, the cervix can be dilated with instruments or with *Laminaria japonica,* as described by Goldrath. Dührssen incisions can be made in the cervix. Also, the cervix can be incised by having the surgeon perform a vaginal hysterotomy (Fig. 31.18A and B). After the bladder is advanced, the cervix is dilated, and an anterior midline incision is made in the cervix high enough to identify the myoma. The pedicle of the myoma is ligated as high as possible (Figs. 31.18C and D). The incision in the cervix is repaired with 2-0 interrupted delayed-absorbable sutures. The vaginal mucosa is reapproximated with 3-0 delayed-absorbable sutures (Figs. 31.18E and F).

A submucous pedunculated myoma may be solitary, and there may not be other myomata in the uterus. In fact, many patients exhibit no evidence of uterine enlargement. After a successful vaginal myomectomy, most patients are asymptomatic and menstruate normally. A few even become pregnant and deliver vaginally without difficulty. Cervical incompetence has been reported. Hysterectomy or myomectomy is required only for those few patients who have multiple leiomyomata and continue to have significant symptoms.

Excellent results of vaginal removal of submucous pedunculated myomata in 151 patients were reported by Goldrath. Ben-Baruch and coworkers also achieved excellent results in 43 of 46 women in whom vaginal myomectomy was attempted. Vaginal myomectomy is recommended as the most appropriate initial treatment for pedunculated submucous myomata.

Vaginal myomectomy is traditionally used for submucosal myomas; however, it has been described for other myomas. Davies and colleagues reported a prospective study regarding the safety and efficacy of excision of intramural and subserosal leiomyoma by a vaginal route. Preoperative criteria included (i) uterine size less than or equal to 16 weeks' gestation, (ii) good uterine mobility, (iii) adequate vaginal access, (iv) the

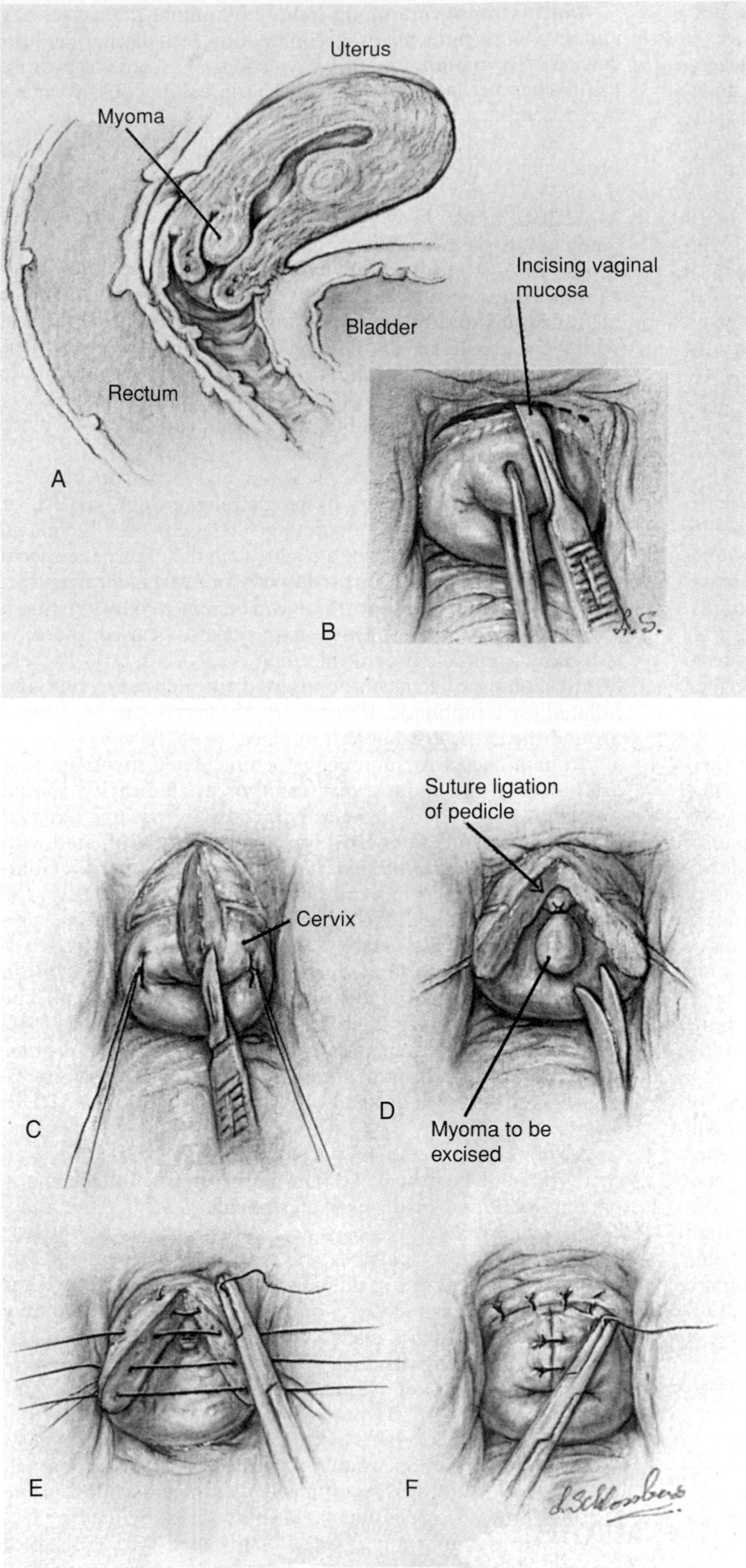

FIGURE 31.18. Transvaginal removal of a pedunculated submucous myoma that presents itself at the external cervical os. **A:** Sagittal view of uterus, demonstrating the location of the myoma originating on the posterior wall of the fundus just above the cervix. **B:** A transverse incision made anteriorly through the vaginal mucosa at the cervicovaginal junction. **C:** After the bladder is advanced bluntly, the cervix is incised anteriorly in the midline. **D:** The myoma and its pedicle are exposed, and the pedicle is suture ligated for hemostasis. **E:** After the myoma is excised, the cervix is reapproximated with interrupted 0-0 absorbable, nonreactive sutures. **F:** The overlying vaginal mucosa is sutured with interrupted 3-0 absorbable sutures.

presence of intramural or subserosal myomas, and (v) the absence of adnexal pathology. Essentially, an open abdominal myomectomy technique was performed through an anterior or posterior colpotomy. The uterus was manipulated to bring the myoma into the colpotomy. The management of 35 women was described. The mean number of myomas removed was 2.5 per patient with mean mass of 113.8 g. Three patients (8.6%) required conversion to a laparotomy. Neither mean blood loss nor length of hospital stay was improved. Additionally, four (11.4%) patients developed pelvic hematomas postoperatively. At this time, this procedure does not seem to provide inherent benefits over an open abdominal myomectomy or a laparoscopic approach. With further review, better outcome data may demonstrate the advantages of this technique.

The tissue removed at vaginal myomectomy must be submitted for pathologic examination to rule out malignancy.

Hysteroscopic Resection of Submucous Myomata

Hysteroscopic resection of submucous myomata was first reported by Neuwirth and Amin in 1976 and was reported again by Neuwirth in 1978. A urologic resectoscope was used. In 1981, Goldrath and associates used "photocoagulation" of the endometrium with the neodymium-doped:yttrium-aluminum-garnet (Nd:YAG) laser to treat patients with menorrhagia. Many subsequent reports by Derman and associates, Donnez and colleagues, Goldenberg and coworkers, Corson, Indman, Hallez, Baggish and associates, Wamsteker and colleagues, and others have confirmed the advantages of hysteroscopic treatment of menorrhagia in women with and without submucous leiomyomata. The menorrhagia associated with submucous myomata can sometimes be managed with oral contraceptives as long as the bleeding is not too severe. A favorable response can also be expected with GnRH analogs, but the menorrhagia usually reappears when the treatment is discontinued. Friedman has reported three cases of severe menorrhagia with resultant anemia requiring transfusions in women with submucous leiomyomata treated with leuprolide acetate. Both oral contraceptives and GnRH analogs are counterproductive in women who are seeking relief from infertility. The uterine cavity can be curetted several times, but the benefit of this procedure is temporary at best.

When hysteroscopic resection of submucous myomata is performed, menorrhagia can be controlled in more than 90% of patients. According to Indman, the mean number of pads used during the heaviest day of menses decreased from 17.8 before treatment to 6.8 after treatment in women undergoing myoma resection only, and from 21.4 to 1.7 pads per day in women whose treatment also included endometrial ablation. Dysmenorrhea was also reduced significantly. Forty-eight of 51 women (94%) with uterine leiomyomata who were seen with menorrhagia were able to avoid major gynecologic surgery for up to 5 years of follow-up. In the report of 156 patients by Derman and associates, 91.3% of patients did not require further surgery after 6 years of follow-up, and 83.9% did not require further surgery after 9 years of follow-up. Further review in recent papers supports Derman's results. Magos and colleagues performed a prospective observational study to identify factors that influence outcomes of hysteroscopic myomectomies by following up patients for almost 8 years. One hundred and twenty-two patients enrolled in the study, and results suggest that hysteroscopic myomectomy is successful in treating menstrual symptoms in four of five cases. In addition, statistical analysis demonstrated that outcome is significantly better when the uterus is only slightly enlarged and if the myoma is mainly submucous in nature.

If endometrial ablation is performed with myoma resection, pregnancy is not likely to occur subsequently. Without simultaneous endometrial ablation, 21 patients became pregnant after myoma resection only, with 18 infants delivered in the series reported by Derman and colleagues. The pregnancy rates among women who wished to conceive varied between 47% and 66% in several reports. These rates are comparable to those reported for abdominal myomectomy.

Donnez and coworkers used a biodegradable GnRH agonist (Zoladex Implant ICI) preoperatively in a series of 60 women with large submucous myomata. Submucous myomectomy by hysteroscopy and Nd:YAG laser was easily performed. In 12 patients, the procedure was accomplished in two stages. Perino and associates used GnRH agonists in 58 women with submucous leiomyomata diagnosed during investigation for infertility or menstrual disorder. There was a significant reduction in operating time, intraoperative bleeding, infusion volume, and failure rate in the treated group compared with the control subjects. Myoma size is reduced and hemoglobin concentration is restored to normal preoperatively. Campo and colleagues collected data on 80 consecutive resectoscopic myomectomies performed on premenopausal women. Forty-two patients did not receive any preoperative medical therapy, whereas 38 patients received 2 months of intramuscular GnRH analog therapy. Perioperative results were recorded followed by a 24-month follow-up period when recurrent symptoms, myoma recurrence, and the need for repeat surgery were collected. Surgical time for the pretreated group was significantly longer than that of the untreated patients. Although GnRH analog pretreatment may be beneficial in improving anemia in some patients, Campo and colleagues did not demonstrate any improvement in short- or long-term outcomes.

When submucous myomata extend deeply into the myometrium, it may not be possible to perform a complete resection for obvious technical reasons. However, it should be possible to remove most irregularities in the uterine cavity and to restore the contour of the cavity to almost normal in most cases. According to Wamsteker and colleagues, hysteroscopic resection of submucous myomata with more than 50% intramural extension should be performed only in selected cases. Repeat procedures may be needed in cases of initial incomplete resection.

To avoid the possibility of inadvertent uterine perforation or to allow its prompt diagnosis if it occurs, hysteroscopic resection is usually performed under laparoscopic guidance. However, as reported by Sullivan and coworkers, laparoscopy may be insufficient to evaluate fully the possible sequelae of uterine perforation. Laparotomy may be necessary to assess the pelvic viscera fully. Letterie and Kramer were able to safely substitute intraoperative transabdominal ultrasonographic guidance for laparoscopy. In their opinion, operative hysteroscopy with intraoperative ultrasonographic guidance provide an accurate and precise method to monitor intrauterine surgery, and it can be used to enhance the performance of hysteroscopic myomectomy and endometrial resection. Intraoperative US guidance provided sufficient details of the relation between the hysteroscope and the myoma and uterine walls to gauge the depth of resection and prevent uterine perforation.

The success and safety of the procedure depend on the experience and skill of the operator. During hysteroscopic resection, vascular spaces are opened in the endometrium and myometrium. Large volumes of fluid are instilled into the uterine cavity. Fluid balance must be monitored carefully by the surgeon and the anesthesiologist to avoid fluid overload.

All tissue must be submitted for pathologic examination. Among 92 patients undergoing hysteroscopic resection in the series reported by Corson and Brooks, two cases of leiomyosarcoma were diagnosed. Leiomyosarcoma is said to be more common in submucous leiomyomata than in intramural or subserous leiomyomata.

As time passes after hysteroscopic resection of submucous myomata, the possibility of recurrent problems increases because of regrowth of myomata. However, this is no more likely to occur than it is with standard abdominal myomectomy. The experience of many investigators has demonstrated that hysteroscopic management of menorrhagia in patients with submucous leiomyomata is a reasonable alternative to classic surgical hysterectomy or myomectomy. The occasional psychological problems and complications of hysterectomy are avoided. An abdominal incision is avoided, there is less discomfort, the procedure can often be performed in an outpatient setting, and the patient can usually resume normal activity after a very brief recovery period.

Hysteroscopic resection of a small submucous myoma is illustrated in Figure 31.19. Details of the indications, technique, complications, and results of hysteroscopic resection are also provided in Chapter 18.

Laparoscopic Myomectomy

When abdominal myomectomy is indicated, the laparoscopic approach can be offered as an alternative to the standard "open" abdominal myomectomy in selected patients. However, this procedure is appropriate in very few patients for several reasons. First, myomectomy is indicated in infertility patients only if there is significant distortion of the uterine wall or endometrial cavity or if there is obstruction or distortion of the fallopian tubes by myomata. Second, myomectomy is indicated in patients who wish to retain their uterus only if the myomata are significantly symptomatic. In both circumstances, the myomata are likely to be multiple and large, and laparoscopic myomectomy should only be considered if the uterine repair is comparable, or superior, to the uterine closure of an abdominal myomectomy.

There are limitations to laparoscopic myomectomy, and these are mostly technical. Myomata in certain locations are difficult to remove. When myomata are large or multiple, or both, operative time and blood loss may be unacceptable. When myomata are embedded deeply in the myometrium, proper repair of the uterine wall may be difficult or impossible, and uterine rupture may occur in a subsequent pregnancy. Retrieval of the resected myomata from the peritoneal cavity can also pose problems. Large myomata must be morcellated into smaller pieces for retrieval. Retrieval through the posterior vaginal fornix or though the abdominal wall requires separate additional incisions, which somewhat defeats the idea of a minimally invasive procedure. Only very skillful laparoscopists should attempt extensive myomectomy through the laparoscope. According to Mais and colleagues, operation time for myomectomy was significantly longer for laparoscopy than for laparotomy when more than four myomata had to be removed and the largest myoma was greater than 6 cm. Dubuisson and coworkers also reinforce the difficulty of the technique by reporting conversion to laparotomy at a rate of 7.5% (93.7% due to operative difficulties) and a complication rate of 3.8%. These authors echo similar intraoperative concerns: (i) the location of the hysterotomy, (ii) the type of hysterotomy, (iii) the uterine suture, and (iv) removal of the myoma. In addition, they report that one third of patients developed adhesions at the uterine scar.

Several technical innovations have been developed to facilitate laparoscopic myomectomy. Electrosurgical and laser techniques are used in ingenious ways. Special traction devices, including corkscrews of various sizes, are required. The operator must be able to provide hemostasis using monopolar

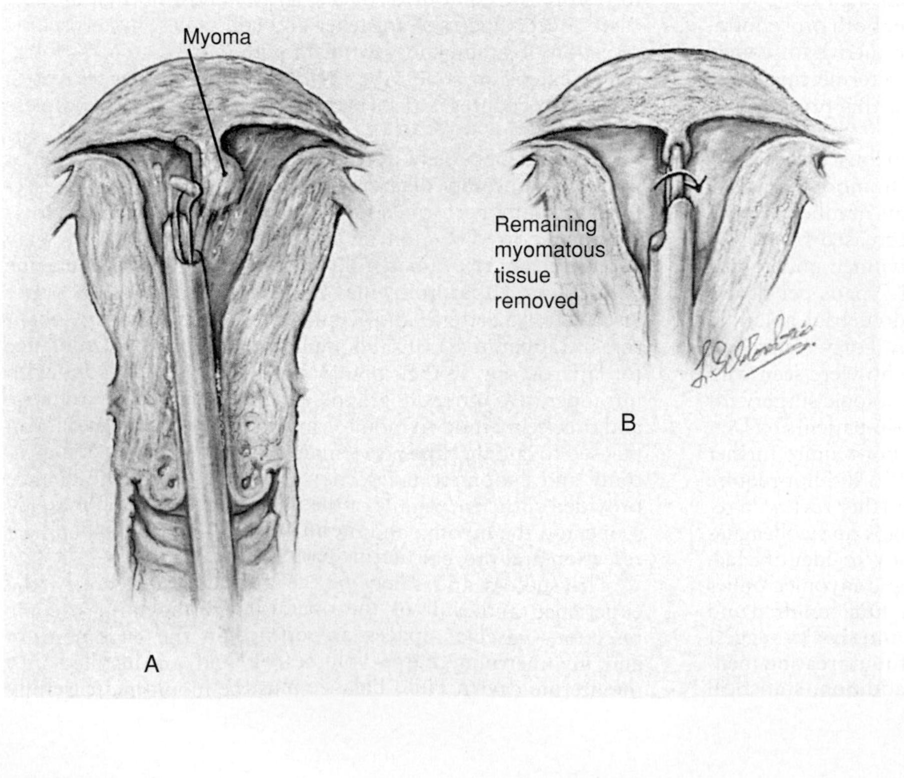

FIGURE 31.19. Hysteroscopic removal of a submucous myoma. **A:** After insertion of the resectoscope, the submucous myoma is removed by progressive shaving. The loop of the resectoscope is placed at the most distant portion of the myoma, and the current is applied as the resectoscope is drawn toward the surgeon. Pressure is exerted by the loop against the myoma with each stroke. **B:** A grasping forceps is used to twist off the remaining tissue once the size has been appreciably reduced.

cutting current and bipolar forceps. The role of the Harmonic Scalpel has also expanded for clean dissection and the potential for less blood loss. Aquadissection can be used to establish planes for dissection between myomata and the surrounding myometrium. Special techniques of approximating myometrium with larger curved needles are used with either intracorpeal or extracorporeal suture tying, depending on the surgeon's expertise. Knowledge of available laparoscopic insteumentaion is essential to maximaize surgical outcome. Autologous blood donation with intraoperative transfusion when necessary reduces the risk of homologous transfusion. Larger myomata can be removed vaginally with morcellation through a posterior colpotomy incision. In cases of myomas of extreme size, Pelosi and colleagues proposed the use of hand-assisted laparoscopy to avoid a laparotomy. This technique allows the insertion of a hand into the abdomen to assist in dissection. This is accomplished through a glove-sized incision at laparoscopy while preserving the pneumoperitoneum. A cylindrical serrated morcellator can also be used to convert smaller myomata to small strips of tissue, which can then be removed abdominally through the trocar sleeve or through a mini-laparotomy incision. Retrieval of all bits and pieces of myoma tissue from the peritoneal cavity can be a tedious challenge. Hirai and colleagues from Japan described a microwave coagulator and electromechanical tissue borer to minimize invasion of the myometrium and abdominal wall. The proposed advantage of this technique is that by morcellating the tissue before removal from the uterus, less myometrial trauma is sustained. Horizontal and perpendicular blades at the tip rotate and hollow out the myoma, allowing large myomas to be removed through a small uterine incision. The authors described the use in five patients with four of the five having myomas weighing less than 170 g. The blood loss and operating time were not substantially different than with conventional abdominal procedures. Long-term data regarding myometrial strength over time and pregnancy outcomes are not yet available. More experience with this procedure is necessary to determine its role in myomectomy.

Another technical innovation called myolysis has been described by Goldfarb and is based on earlier experience in Europe. Either Nd:YAG laser or bipolar needles are used laparoscopically to penetrate the myomata at multiple sites at a 90-degree angle to the uterus. In response to treatment, the myomata ultimately atrophy. The technique is based on the theory that the coagulating effects of lasers or the bipolar needle can necrose myometrial stroma, denature protein, destroy vascularity, and result in substantial shrinkage of myomas when deprived of their blood supply. Goldfarb advises treatment with GnRH agonists before surgery. The ideal candidates for myolysis are perimenopausal women who have symptomatic leiomyomata measuring 3 to 10 cm or uterine size less than 14 weeks' gestation. Goldfarb combines myolysis with endometrial ablation in patients with symptomatic myomas with persistent uterine bleeding. The addition of myolysis to endometrial ablation increased the rate of postsurgical amenorrhea from 36.5% to 57% and second procedures, including hysterectomy, were reduced from 38% to 12.5%. Goldfarb described significant adhesions at follow-up laparoscopy in patients treated with the Nd:YAG laser technique because of excessive serosal injury from multiple punctures. A circumferential technique was later developed to destroy vasculature instead of the myomatous tissue. The devascularized myoma becomes cyanotic, loses viability, and fibroses. Phillips reported on women who underwent elective diagnostic laparoscopy to evaluate adhesions associated with previously performed myolysis. Mean adhesion score was only 1.15 ± 0.6 on a scale of 10.

Zreik and colleagues at Yale University modified the myolysis procedure to include cryotechnology to "freeze" uterine leiomyomas. The technique, *cryomyolysis*, was described in a prospective pilot study of 14 patients. All patients were pretreated with GnRH agonist therapy for 3 months. Thirteen of the 14 endoscopic procedures were performed by laparoscopy and the remaining one by hysteroscopic visualization. Cryoprobe placement was verified, and freezing was performed at an internal probe temperature of −180°C until the ice ball encompassed the entire fibroid or reached maximum size. A thaw cycle was then performed, followed by one more freeze-thaw cycle. A hollow track remained within the frozen myoma after removal of the cryoprobe. MRI studies were used to assess uterine and myoma size. The uterus enlarged by 22% after discontinuation of the GnRH therapy. Myoma volume decreased by 6% over 4 months postoperatively, with some patients having a decrease of more than 50%. Four of six women who underwent second-look office laparoscopy had adhesion formation at freezing sites. The authors attributed risk and severity of adhesion formation to the number of punctures with the cryoprobe. The role of this therapy in conservative treatment of uterine myomata remains to be defined.

Hysteroscopic myomectomy and endometrial resection can be performed simultaneously if submucous myomata are present. In more than 300 myolysis procedures, the author reported minimal morbidity with a 30% to 50% reduction in myoma size beyond the reduction achieved with GnRH agonist treatment. No regrowth occurred after several years of follow-up, even after estrogen replacement therapy. Bipolar coagulation myolysis may be less likely to cause damage to the uterine serosa and less likely to cause adhesion formation postoperatively. According to Goldfarb, "As a same-day procedure, myoma coagulation appears to be an extremely safe alternative to hysterectomy, allowing the patient to avoid major surgery and its subsequent recovery time, while providing an alternative solution for patients with symptomatic leiomyomas."

Nezhat and coworkers used a combination of laparoscopy and minilaparotomy to perform myomectomy in 57 women with uteri at 8 to 26 weeks in gestational size. In this laparoscopically assisted myomectomy procedure, the myomata were removed and the uterus repaired through the minilaparotomy incision. It was technically less difficult than laparoscopic myomectomy and allowed better closure of the uterine defects. This technique may be preferable in the case of large myomas in that it is easier to achieve conventional multilayer suturing and easier to extract myomas.

A significant disadvantage of myomectomy is the risk of postoperative pelvic adhesions. The adhesions may adversely affect fertility, give rise to pain, and increase the risk of ectopic pregnancy or even intestinal obstruction. Several studies have demonstrated that the risk of postoperative adhesions decreases when a laparoscopic approach is used in lieu of an open abdominal approach. Literature review demonstrates that the average rate of postoperative adhesions after laparoscopic myomectomy is 41% versus more than 90% after a myomectomy via laparotomy. Dubuisson and colleagues assessed adhesion formation after laparoscopic myomectomy in a prospective manner. Forty-five patients underwent a second look after laparoscopic myomectomy. Seventy-two sites were evaluated. The overall rate of postoperative adhesions was 35.6% per patient. The rate of adhesions per myomectomy site was 16.7%. The rate of adhesions on the adnexa was 24.4%. Associations with the occurrence of adnexal adhesions included an additional surgical procedure carried out at the same time, the existence of adhesions before the operation, and posterior location of the myoma. Several factors may increase the risk of postoperative adhesion formation after a laparoscopic myomectomy. Recognition of these factors may be helpful in limiting adhesion formation.

The use of uterine suture appears to increase the risk of uterine adhesions. In some studies, the frequency doubled after suturing. The suture induces local tissue ischemia with inflammatory changes, which slow the healing process and induce the formation of adhesions. Contradictory data have been published regarding adhesion formation and the use of bipolar coagulation during a laparoscopic procedure.

The location of the myoma also affects adhesion formation. Adhesions are more likely to form when the myomectomy site is located on the posterior uterine wall. During laparoscopy, a uterine incision must be made over each individual myoma. With laparotomy, a single anterior uterine incision may be used for polymyomectomy, even when posterior myomas are present.

The prior existence of pelvic adhesions significantly increases the risk of postoperative adnexal adhesions, but has not been shown to affect adhesions at the myomectomy site.

Two prospective, randomized controlled studies have evaluated the efficacy of adhesion barriers during laparoscopic myomectomy, and both found intervention to be beneficial. Mais and colleagues evaluated the efficacy of oxidized regenerated cellulose, Interceed, on adhesion formation in a prospective, randomized study of 50 women after laparoscopic myomectomy. Interceed was placed over all incisions and suture material with a 1 cm margin, and the barrier was then moistened with saline. During the second-look laparoscopy, 60% of the Interceed group was free of adhesions compared with only 12% of patients in the control group. Interceed appeared to substantially reduce, but not prevent, adhesions after laparoscopic myomectomy. Pellicano and collaborators showed that hyaluronic acid gel reduced adhesions after laparoscopic myomectomy in a prospective randomized study of 36 infertile women. During second look, 72% of patients were adhesion-free, with hyaluronic acid gel treatment versus an adhesion-free rate of only 22% in the control group.

Multiple published studies (Seracchioli et al., Bulletti et al., Stringer et al., and Campo et al.) suggest that laparoscopic myomectomy may be a viable option for women with leiomyomas and infertility. The best prognosis is for young women with otherwise unexplained infertility and myomas that distort the endometrial cavity. Pregnancy rates and spontaneous abortion rates are comparable to abdominal myomectomy. Data is currently insufficient to determine the appropriate recommendation regarding mode of delivery.

Laparoscopic myomectomy is further discussed in Chapter 17.

Abdominal Myomectomy

The first successful abdominal myomectomy was performed in the United States by the Atlee brothers, Washington and John, in 1844.

The first abdominal multiple myomectomy was performed by W. Alexander of Liverpool in 1898. In the early part of the 20th century, the technique of abdominal myomectomy was refined by many notable gynecologic surgeons, including Kelly, Cullen, Mayo, Rubin, Bonney, and others. The procedure did not gain popularity until the middle of the 20th century. The incidence of complications, including hemorrhage, infection, and postoperative intestinal obstruction from adhesions, was considered to be too high. Advances in surgical techniques to control intraoperative bleeding during myomectomy, along with advances in anesthesia, blood transfusion therapy, and GnRH analogs, have made myomectomy a safe alternative to hysterectomy in women with symptomatic leiomyomata. The number of myomectomies performed in the United States is increasing.

Because myomectomy is rarely an emergency, time is available to prepare the patient for surgery. It is important that she be properly informed of the reasons myomectomy has been recommended. She should understand the nature of the procedure so she can know what to expect and what is expected of her. It is especially important that she be informed of the possibility that intraoperative findings may contraindicate myomectomy and require that hysterectomy be performed instead. For example, myomectomy may not be technically feasible if diffuse leiomyomatosis is found. The technical challenge of removing a large cervical myoma can also preclude myomectomy.

A preoperative hysterosalpingogram may indicate distortion of the fallopian tubes or uterine cavity, findings that are important in planning the technique of myomectomy. An assessment of fallopian tube patency is helpful in predicting fertility. If the tubes are occluded, however, myomectomy is not necessarily contraindicated. According to Seoud and associates, myomectomy does not interfere with *in vitro* fertilization performance in relation to overall and ongoing pregnancy rates. The patient whose tubes are occluded should understand that fertility may not be established by myomectomy, and assisted reproductive technologies may still be required after myomectomy. Tubal reconstruction procedures are uniformly unrewarding when performed at the same time multiple myomectomy is done. Indeed, tubal reconstruction may not always be necessary to establish tubal patency. In a report by Lev-Toaff and associates, nonfilling of the fallopian tubes was present on the preoperative hysterosalpingogram unilaterally in two patients and bilaterally in another two. In all four patients, tubal patency was shown after myomectomy. In the experience of these authors, hysterosalpingography before myomectomy can assist the gynecologic surgeon in planning the surgical approach by showing the presence, size, and location of submucous leiomyomata and concomitant tubal disease.

Imaging modalities such as transabdominal, transvaginal US and MRI play an important role in the management of patients with leiomyomata, especially those patients who are being prepared for myomectomy. As explained by Mayer and Shipilov, US is the preferred method for screening and initial evaluation of the pelvis. In many cases, it is the only imaging study necessary. There are special cases for which US cannot provide all the diagnostic information required. In a study by Schwartz and colleagues, US results were inconclusive in 20% of cases and did not yield a definitive diagnosis in 59% of cases. MRI was more definitive in all cases (Fig. 31.20). The preoperative diagnosis of submucous leiomyomata by MRI may allow hysteroscopic resection and avoid abdominal myomectomy in some cases. Differentiation between uterine leiomyomata and adnexal pathology is more accurate with MRI and thus avoids the need for laparoscopy or laparotomy in some cases (Fig. 31.21). MRI studies can differentiate between uterine leiomyomata, diffuse and localized adenomyosis, and diffuse leiomyomatosis. MRI is the most accurate imaging technique for the detection and localization of leiomyomata (Fig. 31.22). Hricak and coworkers were able to identify accurately by MRI all subserosal (9 of 9), all intramural (37), and 10 of 11 submucosal leiomyomata. Leiomyomata as small as 0.3 cm can be detected. Various degrees of cellularity, degeneration, necrosis, and calcification can be identified by MRI, and sarcomatous change can be suspected. MRI provides imaging planes that are not available on transabdominal or transvaginal US, a feature that permits better visualization of the more lateral and posterior

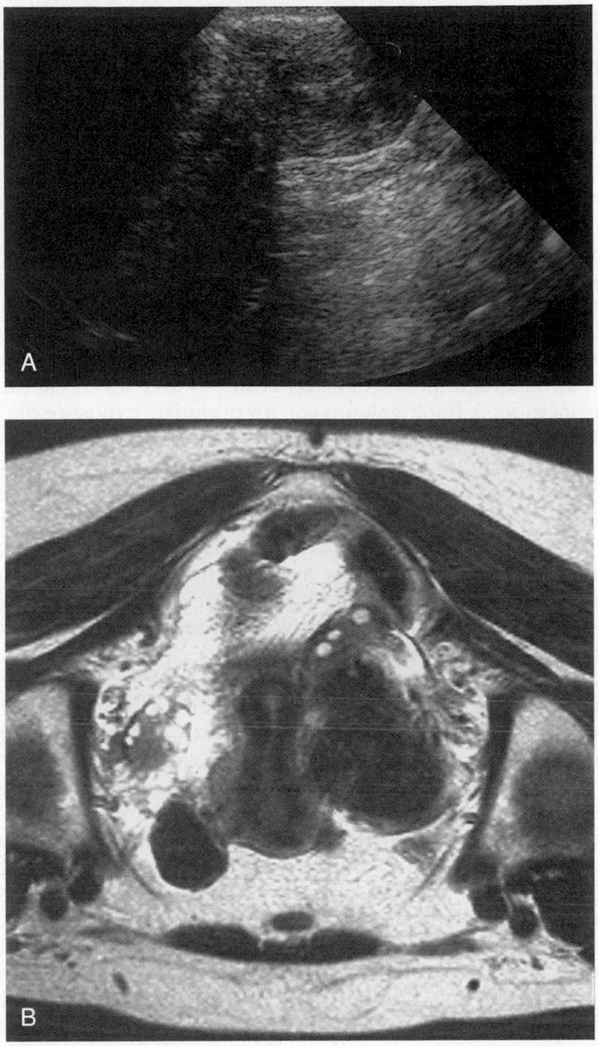

FIGURE 31.20. **A:** The ultrasound evaluation of this patient with a very large leiomyoma was not helpful in delineating the leiomyoma from the adnexa. **B:** The magnetic resonance imaging study demonstrated multiple leiomyomas distinctly separate from the adnexa bilaterally. The ovaries are seen bilaterally with multiple cysts. (Image courtesy of Deborah Baumgarten, M.D.)

areas of the pelvis. MRI is the most accurate method for preoperative localization of leiomyomata and surgical planning for myomectomy. Given the greater costs of MRI, it should be used judiciously. However, as noted by Mayer and Shipilov, the effective cost differential between MRI and US is decreasing.

As discussed by Wiskind and Thompson, one of the most serious risks of surgical bleeding during myomectomy is the risk associated with homologous blood transfusion. The first rule in reducing or eliminating the need for transfusion is to bring the patient to the operating room with the highest possible hemoglobin and hematocrit level. About 30% of myomectomy patients have associated menorrhagia. These small repeated menstrual hemorrhages deplete the body's iron stores over time and eventually result in iron-deficiency anemia of various degrees of severity. Patients scheduled for myomectomy benefit from oral iron supplementation. In a study by Thompson, the liberal use of oral iron therapy preoperatively was shown to decrease the number of blood transfusions on the gynecologic surgical service at the Johns Hopkins Hospital. A blood

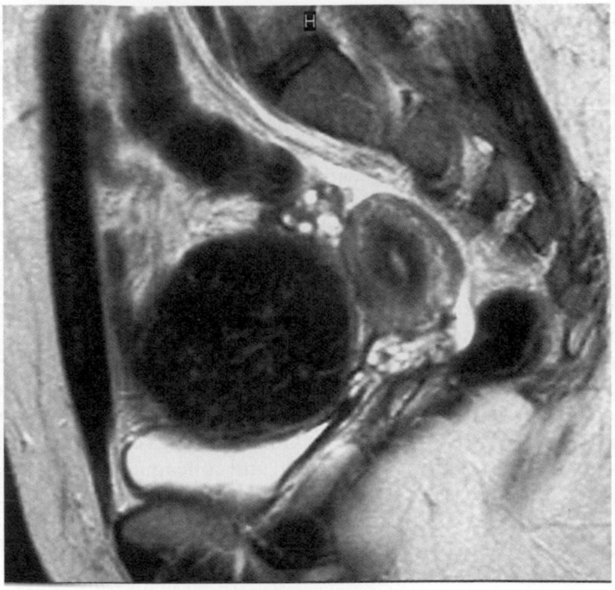

FIGURE 31.21. On magnetic resonance imaging, a large anterior, pedunculated leiomyoma is shown as a separate entity from the ovary in this patient. The ovary is displaced superiorly. (Image courtesy of Deborah Baumgarten, M.D.)

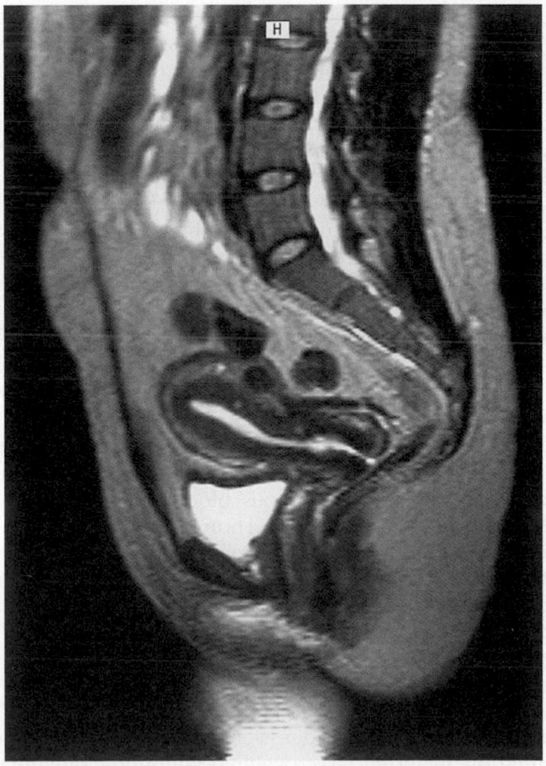

FIGURE 31.22. The location of this small posterior intramural leiomyoma is clearly delineated in this magnetic resonance image. The cervical canal is also easily visible. (Image courtesy of Deborah Baumgarten, M.D.)

transfusion is seldom necessary to correct iron-deficiency anemia in a gynecologic patient. Blood transfusions should generally be reserved for patients with hypovolemic shock or aregenerative forms of anemia. In most other circumstances, elective surgery should be delayed until the anemia has been corrected by oral iron supplementation.

Occasionally, patients with a myomatous uterus have iron-deficiency anemia because of menstrual bleeding that is too heavy or too continuous to allow a response to oral iron therapy. In this situation, it may be beneficial to induce amenorrhea with hormonal therapy to allow the anemia to be corrected more expeditiously. Amenorrhea can be induced with progestational agents such as norethindrone or medroxyprogesterone acetate, with danazol, or with GnRH agonists. Several studies have demonstrated a significant increase in hemoglobin and hematocrit values in patients with leiomyomata treated preoperatively for 8 to 24 weeks with GnRH analogs compared with matched control groups. Friedman and colleagues also found a significant increase in serum iron and total iron-binding capacity in a study group treated with the GnRH agonist leuprolide acetate. In some patients, oral iron was also given. In an evaluation of 265 patients, GnRH agonists plus iron were more effective than iron alone in treating the anemia of patients with uterine leiomyomata, according to Stovall and coworkers. In a double-blind, placebo-controlled, multicenter study, Friedman and associates reported resolution of menorrhagia in 97% of uterine leiomyomata patients treated with GnRH agonists.

Preoperative treatment with GnRH analogs can actually reduce the operative blood loss during myomectomy, according to studies by Friedman and colleagues, Andreyko and coworkers, Moghissi, and others. In a prospective, randomized study of 50 patients undergoing hysterectomy for symptomatic leiomyomata, Stovall and colleagues found a significant decrease in operative blood loss between those patients who received 2 months of leuprolide acetate treatment preoperatively and matched control subjects. An elegant study by Friedman and associates demonstrated a significant decrease in operative blood loss during myomectomy between patients with pretreatment uterine volumes greater than 600 cm^3 who were treated with depot leuprolide acetate for 12 weeks preoperatively and a matched control group. However, there was no significant difference in blood loss between the two groups when patients with smaller uterine volumes (150 to 600 cm^3) were included in the analysis. It has been suggested that the hypoestrogenic environment caused by GnRH analog therapy reduces the vascular supply to uterine leiomyomata. However, even in patients not treated with GnRH agonists, blood flow has been observed to be lower in myomata and adjacent tissue.

Intraoperative autotransfusion and normovolemic hemodilution are also discussed. These techniques of reducing or avoiding the risk of homologous blood transfusion are discussed in detail by Wiskind and Thompson.

Perioperative antimicrobial prophylaxis is indicated with myomectomy. It is preferable to perform the operation in the follicular phase of the menstrual cycle. This avoids the chance of encountering an unknown or unsuspected pregnancy and reduces the problems encountered when a fresh corpus luteum is inadvertently traumatized.

After induction of anesthesia, the patient is placed in Allen universal stirrups, the bladder is emptied, and a careful pelvic examination, including a rectovaginal-abdominal bimanual examination, is performed under anesthesia. Preparation and draping are done to allow access to the vagina and cervix in case it is necessary to place an instrument through the cervix and into the endometrial cavity during the procedure. Cervical dilatation should be done to facilitate postoperative drainage from the endometrial cavity, especially for cases in which the endometrial cavity has been entered during the myomectomy.

Many of the general principles of pelvic surgery are applicable to myomectomy. Perhaps the most important of these is optimum exposure at the operative site. This is accomplished primarily by an adequate incision, but there must also be proper retraction, good lighting, and able assistants. Although a Pfannenstiel incision is considered adequate for myomectomy on a small uterus, we prefer the Maylard incision for larger uteri, even those that exceed a size equivalent to a 12-week pregnancy. A Maylard incision provides excellent exposure throughout the pelvis. Because it is a transverse incision, it is stronger and provides better cosmesis than a vertical midline incision. A Bookwalter retractor optimizes exposure of the operative site. A Pfannenstiel incision can be used for removal of a small solitary myoma.

The importance of adequate exposure cannot be overemphasized. With proper exposure, operative time can be shortened and surgical bleeding can be more easily identified and controlled. Limited exposure may lengthen operative time, increase the risk of inadvertent injury to other pelvic structures, and force abandonment of a myomectomy in favor of a hysterectomy in especially difficult cases.

After the peritoneal cavity is entered, the abdomen is explored as usual. Adhesions in the pelvis must be carefully released or excised so that the intestines can be placed in the upper abdomen and held there with packs. The operation is performed according to microsurgical techniques and principles. For example, the laparotomy packs that are used to hold the intestines in the upper abdomen are placed in plastic bags to reduce the microscopic trauma to peritoneal surfaces caused by regular laparotomy packs. Lintless laparotomy packs are preferred. Several laparotomy packs in plastic bags can be used to fill the cul-de-sac, thus elevating and stabilizing the uterus for easier access. Visualization of the operative site can be improved by the liberal use of suction to remove blood from the field. Suction should be used instead of sponges because it allows for a more accurate determination of blood loss and is less traumatic to tissues.

The operative field is kept moist and free of clots with a solution of lactated Ringer solution containing heparin. Very fine instruments and sutures are used when possible, and tissue is handled gently to avoid unnecessary trauma to serosal surfaces. Traumatic instrumentation (e.g., uterine elevators with teeth, Kocher clamps, or any instrument on the uterine serosa) must be avoided. Sutures on serosal surfaces should be of a fine absorbable nonreactive material. Running suture lines are preferable to avoid extra knot volume, which may contribute to adhesion formation. If pelvic adhesions develop after myomectomy, future fertility may be adversely affected. Performing the operation in a way that minimizes adhesion formation greatly improves the possibility of a successful result.

At this point in the operative procedure, one should pause and evaluate the size, location, and number of myomata present. Special note should be made of their proximity to the endocervical canal, uterine vessels, and fallopian tubes. One must decide if myomectomy is still feasible, how the leiomyomata will be removed (and in what sequence), and how the uterus will be reconstructed.

The conservation of uterine function with myomectomy requires control of bleeding from uterine incisions and myoma beds. Contrary to hysterectomy for leiomyomata, conservation of the uterus requires that the blood supply to the uterus through the uterine and ovarian vessels remain intact.

Removing multiple myomata embedded deeply in a vascular myometrium can result in considerable blood loss. Proper application of special techniques to limit blood loss can allow multiple myomectomies even in uteri up to 20 weeks' pregnancy size if satisfactory reconstruction is possible.

Controlled hypotensive anesthesia has become a useful adjunct to decrease surgical bleeding in selected patients. The main mechanism in the control of operative field bleeding with hypotensive anesthesia is the reduction of venous tone. This can be accomplished by specific vasodilating agents—such as nitroglycerin or sodium nitroprusside, epidural or spinal anesthesia, some inhalation anesthetic agents, and ganglionic blockade—to achieve and maintain a target mean blood pressure of 60 mm Hg. Our experience with this technique has been favorable. Venous bleeding can be further reduced if the patient is placed in a moderate Trendelenburg position. This facilitates venous drainage from the lower extremities and pelvis by gravity and may further reduce the blood pressure at the operative site.

Induced hypotension is contraindicated in patients with cerebrovascular disease, myocardial ischemia, peripheral vascular disease, severe renal or hepatic disease, and hypovolemia. None of these contraindications is seen very often in myomectomy patients. An anesthesiologist experienced with the technique is an essential requirement. The decision to use hypotension should be made jointly by the surgeon and the anesthesiologist. It is essential that the blood pressure be returned to normal before closure of the incision to ensure that adequate surgical hemostasis has been established.

Early proponents of myomectomy focused on methods to temporarily occlude uterine blood flow to control hemorrhage and provide a bloodless operative field. One of the earliest methods was simply to have an assistant grasp the broad ligaments firmly with each hand during myomectomy to impede blood flow through the uterine vessels. In the 1920s, Victor Bonney introduced a specially designed clamp that was placed around the uterine vessels and the round ligaments. The ovarian vessels were occluded with ring forceps. Using this technique, he was able on one occasion to remove more than 200 myomata from a single uterus. Rubin, in 1938, was the first to use an elastic rubber tourniquet through the broad ligament, encircling the cervix and occluding the uterine vessels during myomectomy. Rubber-shod clamps applied to the broad ligaments have also been used to occlude the uterine vessels and control bleeding.

Gynecologic surgeons do not often have the opportunity to use tourniquets to control bleeding; however, a myomectomy is particularly suited to their use. We prefer to use tourniquets fashioned in the manner of a Rumel-type tourniquet, which is used by vascular, thoracic, and trauma surgeons to occlude major vessels. Initially, a small hole is made in an avascular space in the broad ligament on either side of the uterine isthmus just lateral to the uterine vessels. A 5-French pediatric feeding tube is looped around the upper cervix through the holes in the broad ligament, and the two ends of the tube are then threaded through a 4-inch length of 35-French Malecot catheter and held with a clamp. A loop tourniquet can then be placed around each infundibulopelvic ligament through the same holes in the broad ligaments (Fig. 31.23A).

As the tourniquets are being placed, controlled hypotension is induced by the anesthesiology staff. Before the tourniquets are tightened, the location of the uterine arterial blood flow is identified with a sterile Doptone. When everything is in readiness and the plan of operation has been selected by the surgical team, the tourniquets are snugged down and tightened progressively until the uterine arterial flow is no longer audible with the Doptone (Fig. 31.23B). It is very important that the arterial blood flow be occluded. If the venous flow is occluded while the arterial flow remains intact, blood loss could actually be increased with the tourniquets. The mean blood pressure should be reduced to the target hypotensive level (about 60 mm Hg) before the tourniquets are tightened. The higher the blood pressure, the tighter the tourniquets must be to occlude the uterine circulation.

With the combination of properly applied tourniquets and controlled hypotensive anesthesia, the entire circulation to the uterus can be occluded. The myomectomy can then be performed in a bloodless field, greatly facilitating complete removal of all tumors and a neat reconstruction of the uterus (Figs. 31.24 and 31.25). Occasionally, a large cervical or broad ligament myoma prevents placement of the tourniquets. In this situation, the offending tumor should be removed first, the defects repaired when feasible, and the tourniquets applied for the remainder of the multiple myomectomy.

Once the tourniquets are tightened in place, the myomectomy should proceed expeditiously to prevent ischemic damage to the uterus, tubes, and ovaries. The length of time the pelvic structures can be without blood flow before irreversible damage occurs is unknown. We generally do not release the tourniquets until the myomectomy is complete (usually within an hour) and have not experienced any adverse events. Lock also agrees that intermittent release of the tourniquets is unnecessary. However, because the potential for injury does exist, tourniquet time should be monitored and kept to a minimum. The tourniquets should not be tightened until the surgical team is ready to perform the myomectomy. Intermittent release of the tourniquets should be considered if the operating time becomes excessive. We usually release the tourniquets around the ovarian vessels as the uterine serosa is being closed to restore circulation to the tubes and ovaries and to restore some collateral flow to the uterus. After reconstruction of the uterus is complete, the determination of adequate hemostasis in the uterus cannot be made until all the tourniquets are released and the blood pressure has returned to normal. Sometimes additional sutures are required for hemostasis. Before the abdomen is closed, the small holes in the broad ligament are repaired with figure-of-eight sutures.

Tourniquets are not necessary for every myomectomy, especially when the tumors are small or pedunculated. However, they are safe and inexpensive to use and can be of great benefit when large or multiple intramural myomata must be removed. A criticism of uterine tourniquets is that they are traumatic to pelvic structures. Our experience, to the contrary, is that soft plastic tubes used as tourniquets are quite atraumatic. No injuries attributable to these tourniquets have occurred in several hundred cases.

An alternative to the use of tourniquets to control bleeding during myomectomy is the local injection of vasoconstrictive agents. Perhaps the most commonly used agent is vasopressin, a synthetic derivative of the antidiuretic hormone from the posterior lobe of the pituitary gland. In addition to this antidiuretic effect, vasopressin induces smooth muscle contraction of the gastrointestinal tract and the vascular bed. In particular, it has been found to have a potent vasoconstrictor effect on the nonpregnant uterus when injected locally. It has a plasma half-life of 10 to 20 minutes and has been used effectively as a hemostatic agent during myomectomy. Pharmacologic vasoconstriction can be accomplished with vasopressin (antidiuretic hormone), 20 U (Pitressin). Twenty units of vasopressin are diluted in 20 mL of normal saline and injected into the superficial myometrium and serosa overlying the myoma. The effect usually lasts for 30 minutes.

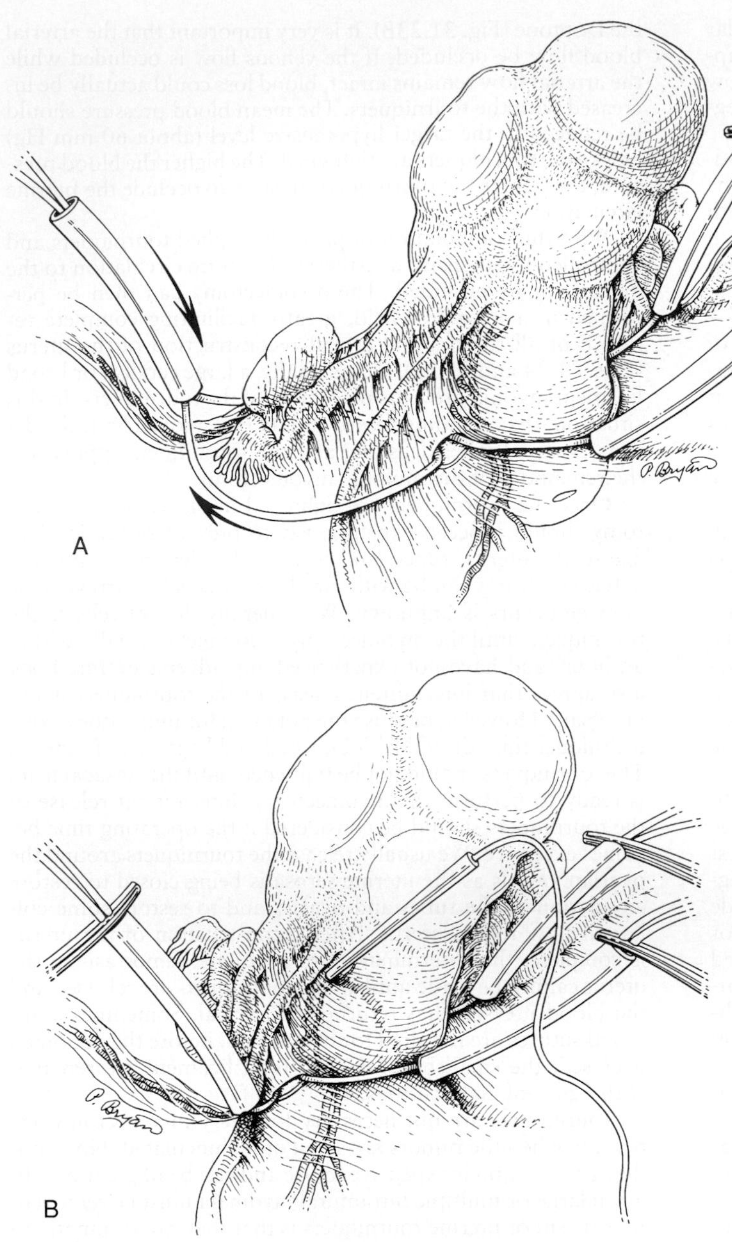

FIGURE 31.23. **A:** Through a small hole in the broad ligament on each side of the uterus, a Rumel tourniquet is placed around the lower uterus and around each infundibulopelvic ligament. **B:** When the tourniquets are tightened sufficiently, the blood flow to the uterus stops. The absence of arterial pulsations can be determined with the sterile Doptone.

Dillon reported that with the use of vasopressin, 72% of patients requiring myomectomy did not need blood replacement compared with control subjects. Frederick and coworkers noted significantly less blood loss compared with an untreated group. Ginsberg and associates compared vasopressin with mechanical vascular occlusion and found that there were no demonstrable differences in blood loss, morbidity, or transfusion requirements between the two techniques. A favorable experience with vasopressin has also been reported by Semm and Mettler.

The weight of evidence in current clinical investigation indicates that vasopressin is as effective as mechanical vascular occlusion in controlling blood loss with myomectomy. Nevertheless, careful dissection around myomata and prompt suturing with exertion of direct pressure to bleeding vessels by the operative assistant are necessary to minimize blood loss. Care should be taken to avoid injecting the solution directly into a vascular channel, and no more than 30 mL per patient is recommended because of potential side effects. Vasopressin should not be used in patients with vascular disease, especially disease of the coronary arteries. Inadvertent intravascular injection can cause anginal pain; larger doses can cause myocardial infarction. Water intoxication can also occur as a result of the antidiuretic effect of vasopressin. This effect is potentiated in patients taking tricyclic antidepressants.

Although late postoperative bleeding does occur with the use of vasopressin, it is not a common complication. Arterial bleeding masked by vasopressin still requires suture ligation. Because of the short half-life of vasopressin, the hemostatic effect is observed only for 20 to 30 minutes and should be over before the incisional closure is started. However, some do claim that vasopressin simply delays bleeding, gives a false sense of security, and is not particularly effective for larger myomata and very extensive myomectomies.

For a variety of reasons, epinephrine as a vasoconstrictive agent is not recommended for use in gynecologic surgery.

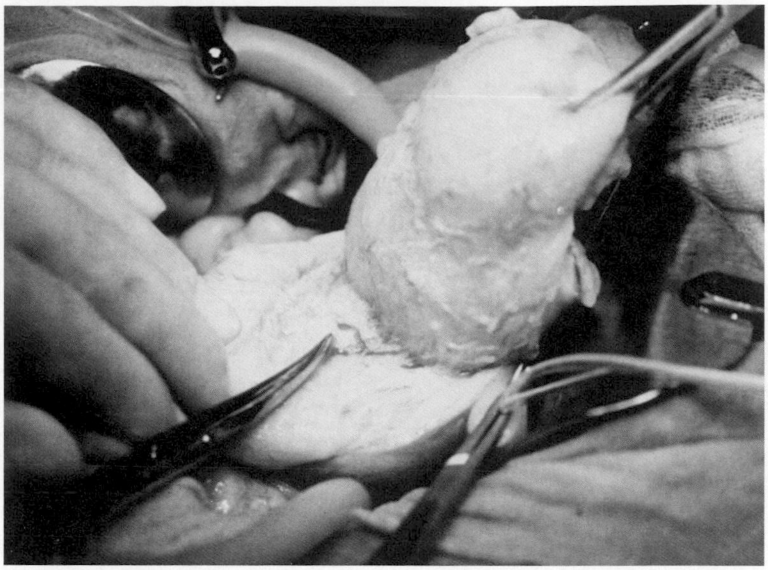

FIGURE 31.24. With tourniquets properly secured, myomectomy can be performed with minimal blood loss. See color version of figure.

Since its introduction into clinical practice in 1972, the CO_2 laser has been touted as a tool that increases surgical precision and decreases bleeding, tissue injury, and adhesion formation. The laser can be used to make a single uterine incision through which multiple myomata are removed. An elliptical incision can also be made around the base of larger myomata to facilitate their removal. Myomata less than 1 cm in diameter can be vaporized directly with the laser, which destroys tissue by vaporizing cellular water. Despite the favorable results reported by Weather, Reyniak and Corenthal, McLaughlin, and Starks, we believe that there is no clear advantage in using the CO_2 laser for abdominal myomectomy, especially considering the added cost to the patient.

Although the methods described earlier to control bleeding during myomectomy are helpful, they cannot substitute for good surgical techniques. Adherence to basic principles is essential for good results. Perhaps the most important of these is careful planning of the uterine incisions. Only a minimal number of incisions should be made. If possible, removal of all leiomyomata should be accomplished through a single incision in the anterior uterine corpus, and in the midline when feasible to avoid the vascular areas of the uterus and broad ligaments laterally. Even intramural leiomyomata in the posterior uterine wall can be removed through anterior incisions. Incisions in the posterior uterine wall may be necessary, however, if posterior subserous tumors are being removed. If posterior uterine incisions are made, adhesions are more likely to develop and will likely involve the tubes and ovaries as well.

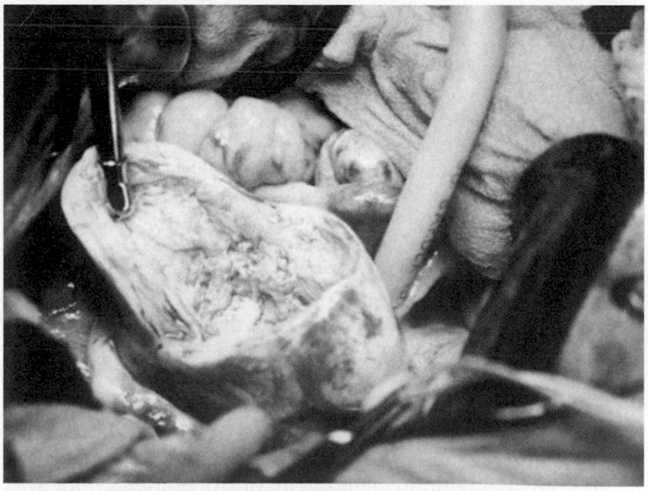

FIGURE 31.25. The use of tourniquets to control bleeding facilitates closure of the myoma bed and uterine incision. See color version of figure.

As many tumors as possible should be removed through a single incision. Methods of removing myomata through a single anterior incision have been described by Bonney. The linear or elliptic incision should usually be over the largest myoma. It should be carried through the superficial myometrium directly into the underlying myoma. The myoma is then grasped with a double-tooth tenaculum or a large Lahey thyroid clamp for traction. The plane of cleavage between the myoma and the surrounding myometrium is easily identified. Sometimes in patients who have been treated with GnRH analogs, the plane of cleavage may seem less distinct. Sharp dissection with the scalpel or Metzenbaum scissors, or blunt dissection with the finger or knife handle, is required to enucleate the myoma from its bed. Sometimes the myoma is larger than expected. It may then be necessary to enlarge the incision or to remove the tumor by morcellation. Other adjacent tumors should be removed through the same incision. Any entry in the endometrial cavity should be noted, and a special attempt should be made to close it with sutures placed in the underlying supporting myometrium. Examples of the step-by-step planning and performance of a multiple myomectomy are illustrated in Figures 31.26 and 31.27.

The muscle fibers and blood vessels surrounding a myoma are compressed by its growth. This compression of surrounding tissue forms a pseudocapsule around the myoma. No large blood vessels enter the myoma, and there is no vascular pedicle. If the dissection can be carried out between the myoma and the pseudocapsule, blood loss can be minimized. If blood vessels are cut or left on the surface of the myoma, it usually means that the dissection has been carried out in an improper plane. Dissection in the proper plane may be more difficult if the patient received GnRH analog therapy preoperatively.

Several ingenious techniques for removing leiomyomata and for repairing defects have been described. For example,

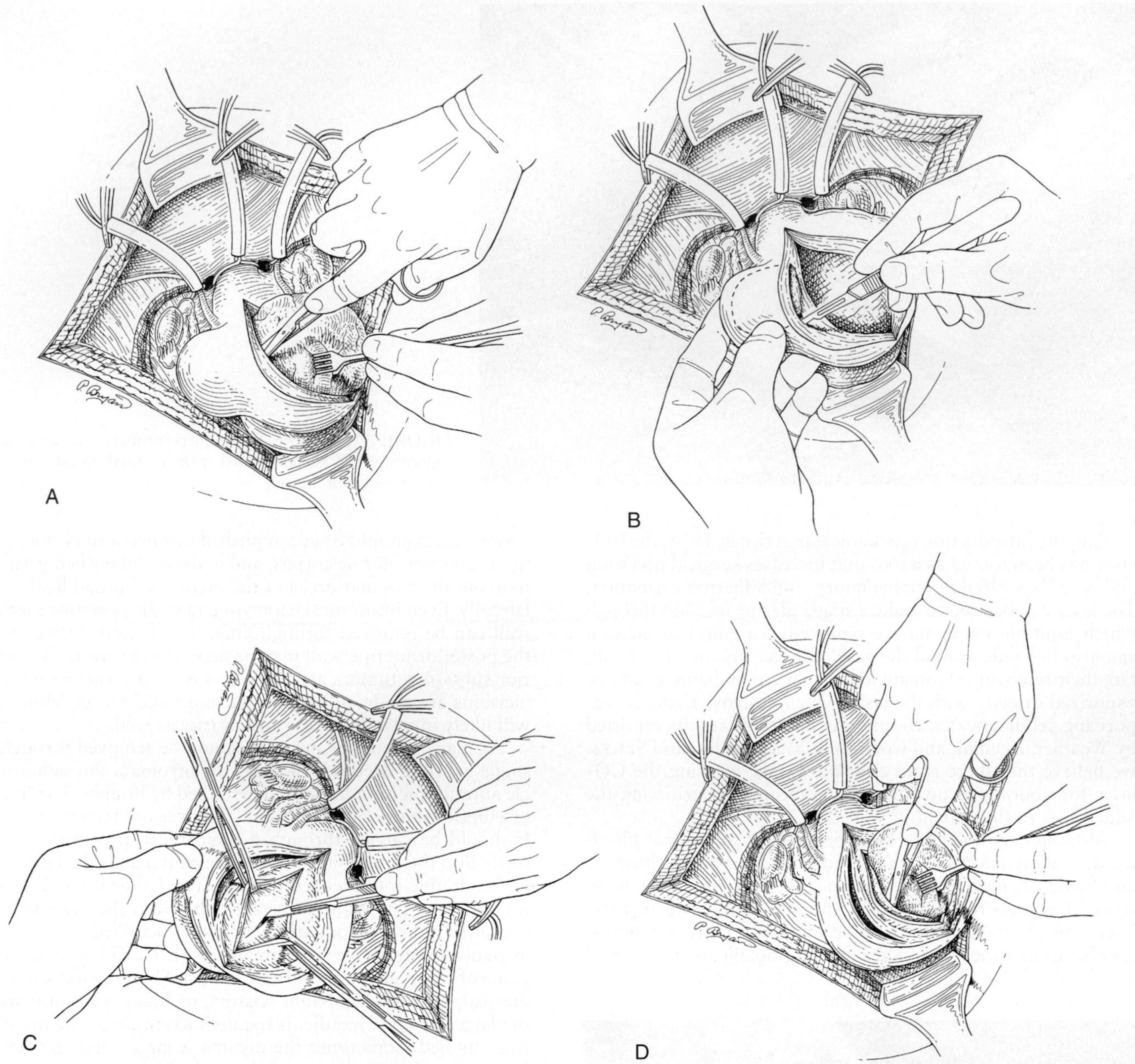

FIGURE 31.26. The sequence of steps in a multiple myomectomy is shown in these illustrations. **A:** Through a transverse Maylard incision, tourniquets are placed to occlude the uterine and ovarian artery flow. Through a single incision in the anterior myometrium, a large anterior myoma is removed first. All other myomas are removed through this incision. **B:** A smaller intramural myoma is removed through the same incision. **C:** To avoid making a separate incision in the posterior uterine wall, a large posterior myoma is removed through the uterine cavity. After an incision has been made through the anterior endometrium, an incision is made in the posterior endometrium directly over the posterior myoma. **D:** The myoma in the posterior uterine wall is dissected from its bed and removed through the uterine cavity. An incision in the posterior uterine serosa is thus avoided. (*Continued*)

Bonney's hood can be used to remove a large leiomyoma in the uterine fundus. The myoma is first exposed through an elliptic incision made transversely across the anterior fundus, taking care to avoid the interstitial portion of the fallopian tube on each side (Fig. 31.28A and B). After the primary tumor is removed (Fig. 31.28C), other leiomyomata can also be removed through the same incision. Excess myometrium can be trimmed away (Fig. 31.28D). Interrupted sutures obliterate the dead space, approximate the myometrium, and accomplish satisfactory hemostasis. The sutures are placed in such a way that the posterior flap of myometrium is folded over the anterior uterine wall and sutured in place, thus fashioning Bonney's hood (Fig. 31.28D).

Meticulous closure of defects from the enucleated myomata is essential to maintain hemostasis postoperatively, but this should be deferred until all the tumors are removed. Hypertrophy of the normal myometrium is always present with uterine leiomyomata. Some of this hypertrophied myometrium is

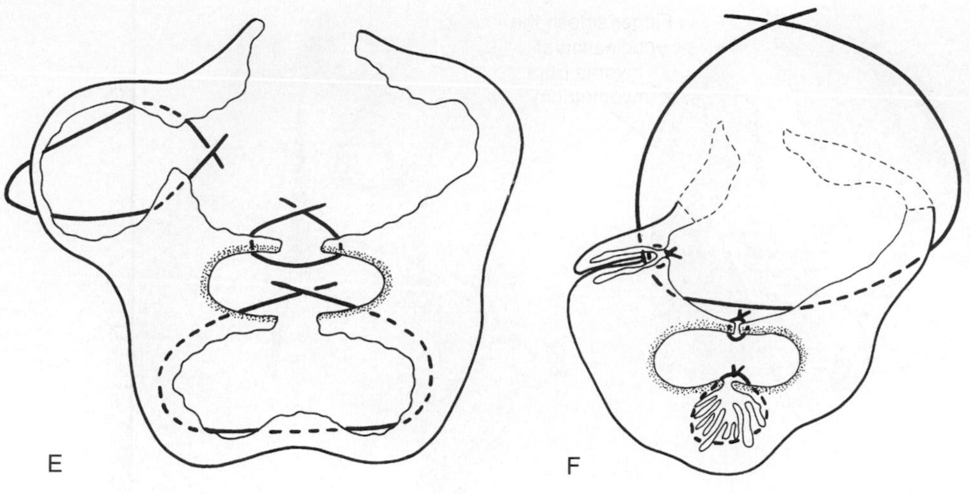

FIGURE 31.26. (*Continued*) **E:** Multiple sutures (2-0 delayed-absorbable) are used to close the defect in the posterior uterine wall first. Incisions in the uterine cavity are closed. Then the defects in the anterior uterine wall are closed. **F:** Trimming excess myometrium from the anterior uterine wall allows a better approximation of the myometrium. The edges of the serosa are closed with a continuous "baseball" stitch with 4-0 delayed-absorbable sutures.

considered excess and can be trimmed to facilitate a more normal reconstruction of the uterus. Involution of the myometrial hypertrophy is expected to occur in the first few months after myomectomy. Therefore, only a small amount of normal myometrial tissue should be removed. In reconstructing the uterus, the surgeon should refer to fixed points such as the attachments of the round ligaments and fallopian tubes on each side of the corpus. Symmetric reconstruction is preferred but is not always possible. The myoma beds are usually closed with interrupted figure-of-eight or mattress 2-0 delayed-absorbable sutures. Large defects can be closed initially with a pursestring suture to obliterate the dead space. Several layers of sutures may be required. One must be careful to avoid occlusion of the uterine vessels, the endocervical canal, or the interstitial portion of the fallopian tubes. Transfundal or transcervical chromotubation to test fallopian tube patency after uterine reconstruction is complete is not usually possible because of leakage of the dye through the myometrial incisions.

In closing a myomectomy incision, the security of the closure comes from sutures placed in the myometrium. If possible, these sutures and knots must not be exposed. In Figure 31.26E and F, several techniques of closing myometrial defects are illustrated. The serosal edge of the uterine incision should be carefully approximated with a continuous 5-0 or 4-0 delayed-absorbable "baseball" stitch.

The tourniquets are removed, the hypotensive anesthesia is reversed, and the uterus is carefully inspected for evidence of bleeding. Additional sutures are sometimes required. If a

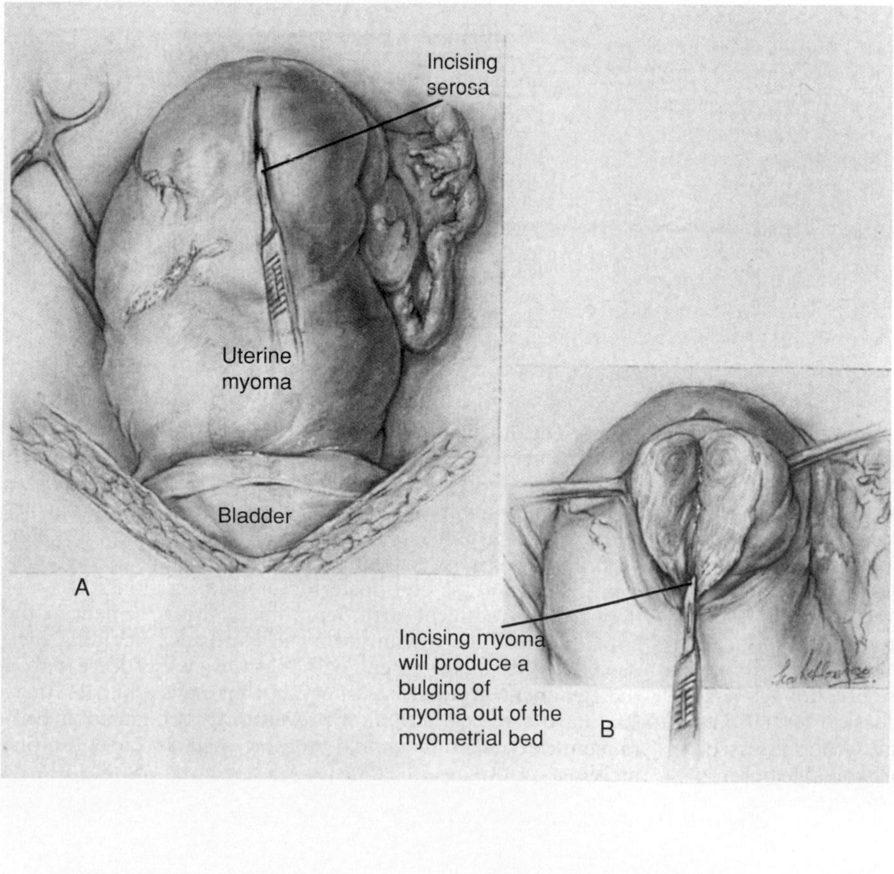

FIGURE 31.27. Techniques of multiple myomectomy. **A:** A vertical incision is made over a myoma on the anterior surface of the fundus as close to the midline as possible. Many myomas can be removed through this single incision. **B:** The incision is extended into the substance of the myoma. (*Continued*)

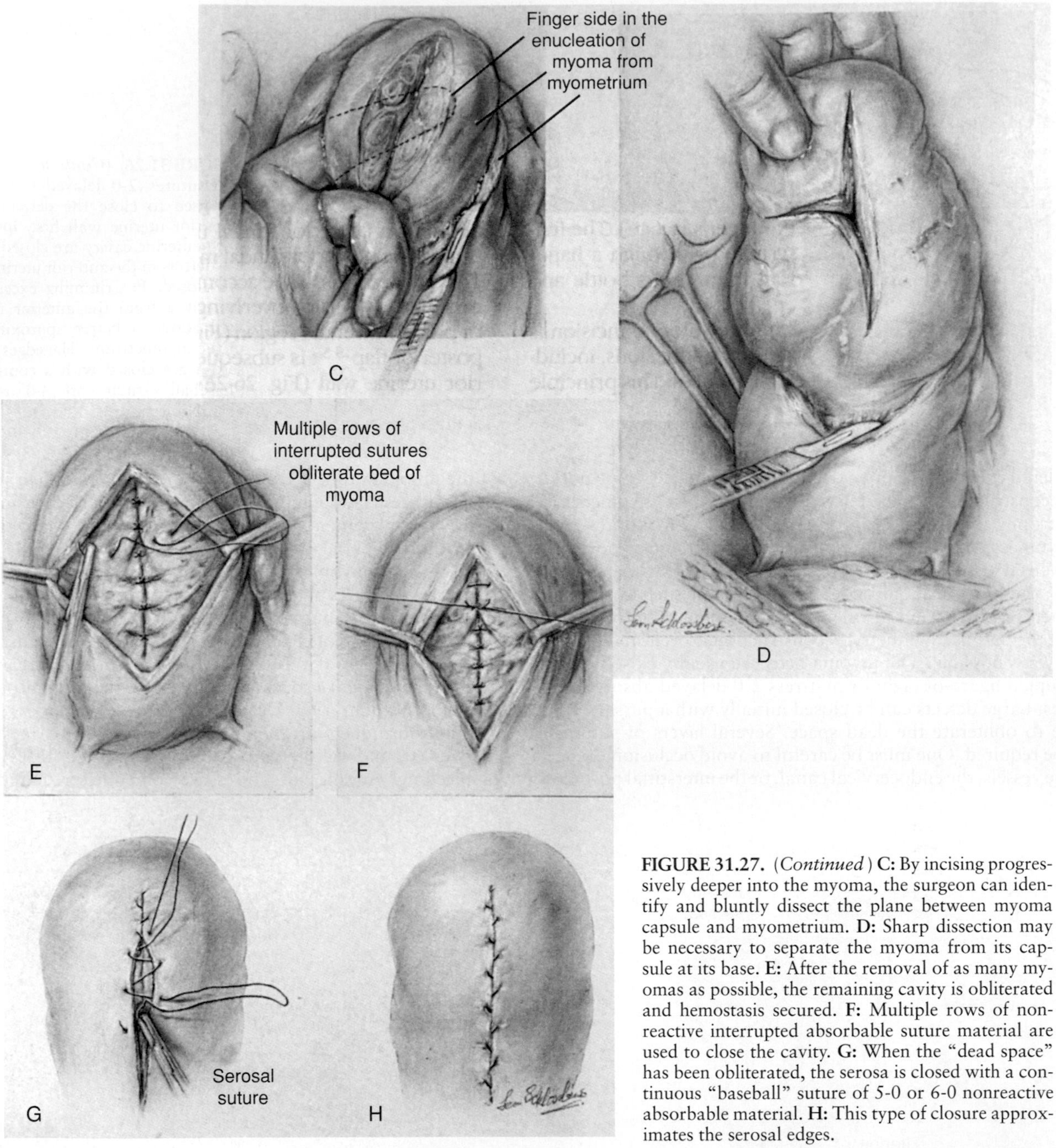

FIGURE 31.27. (*Continued*) **C:** By incising progressively deeper into the myoma, the surgeon can identify and bluntly dissect the plane between myoma capsule and myometrium. **D:** Sharp dissection may be necessary to separate the myoma from its capsule at its base. **E:** After the removal of as many myomas as possible, the remaining cavity is obliterated and hemostasis secured. **F:** Multiple rows of nonreactive interrupted absorbable suture material are used to close the cavity. **G:** When the "dead space" has been obliterated, the serosa is closed with a continuous "baseball" suture of 5-0 or 6-0 nonreactive absorbable material. **H:** This type of closure approximates the serosal edges.

uterine suspension is needed, a modified Coffey or modified Gilliam technique along with uterosacral ligament plication is used.

Adhesion prevention can also be achieved by the use of absorbable or nonabsorbable barriers. The absorbable barrier Interceed (oxidized regenerated cellulose) can be placed over the uterine corpus to protect the tubes and ovaries from denuded peritoneal surfaces and uterine incision. Alternatively, a nonabsorbable barrier, Gore-Tex (polytetrafluoroethylene surgical membrane), can be sutured over the uterine incisions with 7-0 absorbable minimal reactive sutures. The use of Gore-Tex has been associated with a reduction in new adhesion formation. Diamond and the Seprafilm Adhesion Study Group assessed the efficacy of Seprafilm (HAL-F) Bioresorbable Membrane (sodium hyaluronate and carboxymethylcellulose) in reducing the incidence, severity, extent, and area of uterine adhesions after myomectomy. This prospective, randomized, blinded, multicenter study involved an independent gynecologic surgeon's review of each patient's second-look laparoscopy. One hundred and twenty-seven women undergoing uterine myomectomy with at least one posterior uterine incision were randomized to treatment with Seprafilm or no treatment at the completion of the myomectomy. All indices, including incidence, severity, and extent of adhesions, were decreased in the treatment group. This suggests that newer barriers may also have a role in adhesion prevention. Free grafts of peritoneum or omentum should not be used to cover uterine incisions.

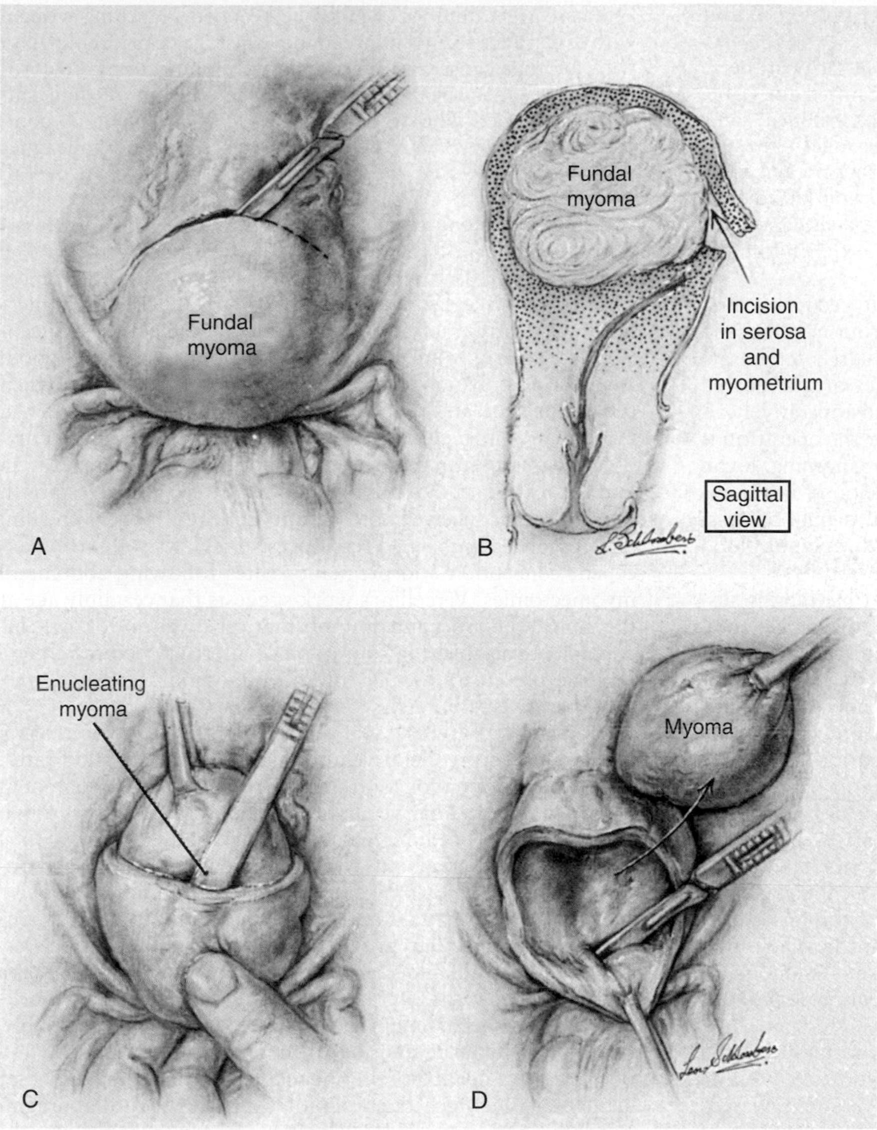

FIGURE 31.28. Technique of myomectomy using an anterior hood incision as described by Bonney. **A:** A transverse incision is made in the anterior fundal wall over the myoma. **B:** Sagittal view of the location of the incision. C and **D:** Using blunt and sharp dissection, the surgeon enucleates the myoma from its bed. Excess hypertrophied myometrium may be trimmed and removed before closure of myometrium and serosa.

In a randomized controlled trial, Imai found fewer adhesions with GnRH analogue pretreatment compared with no treatment after both laparoscopic and abdominal myomectomy. The utility of GnRh analogues in reducing adhesions has also been demonstrated in other clinical and animal studies.

Second-look laparoscopy may be indicated in patients with multiple incisions or in those with posteriorly located incisions adjacent to the adnexa. Early adhesions can be easily lysed, and an additional barrier membrane can be placed. The clinical role of second-look laparoscopy, outside of research, is not well defined, and conflicting studies can be found in the literature regarding the efficacy of this procedure.

A comprehensive review of methods to prevent adhesion formation in gynecologic surgery has been published by Damario and Rock and by diZerega.

Results of Myomectomy

An extensive multiple myomectomy is a major operation with the potential for a higher morbidity than that found with hysterectomy. The major immediate postoperative complications after myomectomy are febrile morbidity and intraperitoneal bleeding.

Postoperative febrile morbidity may be related to extensive tissue trauma or to infection for a variety of reasons. Perioperative antibiotics are routinely given, but antibiotics are not usually continued beyond the day of operation. Any evidence of infection in the recovery period should be treated vigorously and promptly because infection in the operative site may be adhesiogenic and may have devastating effects on future fertility. Unfortunately, subclinical infection in the operative site may not be recognized and therefore may not be treated, but it can also have adverse effects on fertility because of *de novo* adhesion formation. For these reasons, meticulous and sterile surgical technique during myomectomy must be impeccable.

Intraperitoneal bleeding after myomectomy is usually due to failure to achieve hemostasis of the myometrial vessels during closure of the myoma beds and uterine incisions. Although we do use a heparin solution (5,000 U of heparin per 1,000 mL of lactated Ringer solution) for irrigation during myomectomy, there is no evidence to suggest that this contributes to occult intraperitoneal bleeding.

The diagnosis of intraperitoneal bleeding in the postoperative patient may be difficult. The vital signs can remain stable for several hours before rapidly deteriorating. Peritoneal signs are often subtle and may be masked by incisional pain and analgesic medications. In addition, the peritoneal cavity has an enormous capacity for accommodating occult blood loss. Indeed, as much as 3,000 mL of blood can be shed into the peritoneal cavity with only a 1-cm increase in the abdominal radius.

Therefore, patients must be carefully monitored for the first 24 hours after myomectomy. Vital signs are routinely checked every 15 minutes for the first 2 hours after surgery, then every 30 minutes until stable. Subsequently, they are monitored every 2 to 4 hours for the first 24 hours postoperatively. A hematocrit is usually performed 6 hours after the operation is completed and again on the first postoperative morning. It can also be performed whenever there is a suspicion of intraperitoneal bleeding, anemia, or hypovolemia. Any sign of restlessness, tachycardia, or tachypnea may be an indication of blood loss, especially when associated with hypotension.

When occult postoperative intraperitoneal bleeding is suspected, peritoneal lavage can be a valuable diagnostic tool. If the lavage solution yields a red blood cell count of 100,000/mm^3, intraperitoneal bleeding is likely and reexploration is indicated without delay. Lavage is unnecessary when the diagnosis of intraperitoneal bleeding is unequivocal and associated with definite hypovolemia. In this situation, immediate return to the operating room for reexploration is indicated.

Postoperative bleeding after myomectomy can be devastating. Intraoperative control of bleeding during an extensive multiple myomectomy often requires that the uterine blood flow be impeded with tourniquets, clamps, or the local injection of vasoconstrictive agents. However, the demonstration of adequate surgical hemostasis in the uterus cannot be made until the uterine circulation has been fully restored. Assiduous attention to this principle intraoperatively prevents postmyomectomy bleeding in almost all cases.

Reports by Smith and Uhlir, Rosenfield, and LaMorte and associates indicate that the morbidity of myomectomy is no greater than the morbidity of hysterectomy. Verkauf reviewed current published reports and found that the operative risk of myomectomy does not exceed that of hysterectomy. One case of disseminated intravascular coagulation, hemolytic anemia, and acute renal failure associated with extensive multiple myomectomy was reported by Sacks and Hoyne.

Myomectomy has an excellent record in reducing heavy menstruation in patients reporting menorrhagia. In more than 80% of patients, menorrhagia is cured or significantly improved. Pelvic pain and discomfort and dysmenorrhea can also be relieved, but the results are not as dramatic because leiomyomata are often associated with other gynecologic diseases (e.g., endometriosis and pelvic inflammatory disease) that can also cause pelvic pain.

The impact of abdominal myomectomy on infertility is difficult to assess. Other factors besides leiomyomata may be present to a varying degree. The extent to which the uterine cavity or the fallopian tubes are distorted also varies. The percentage of patients in each series who wish to conceive after myomectomy is not the same. There is also considerable variation in the surgical technique and skill of the gynecologic surgeon. Prospective, randomized, controlled studies are lacking. These and other factors make it difficult to assess the impact of abdominal myomectomy on infertility.

There are a number of published reports regarding women who experience recurrent pregnancy wastage or prior infertility with another cause and who undergo myomectomy. According to Verkauf's review, conception occurs in more than half of such women who were not previously pregnant. A comprehensive review of 23 studies by Vercellini and colleagues regarding leiomyomas and reproduction reported an overall conception rate of 57% after myomectomy among prospective studies. Among women with otherwise unexplained infertility, the conception rate was 61% after myomectomy. The conception rate is approximately 53% to 70% after myomectomy for submucous myomas and 58% to 65% after myomectomy with intramural or subserosal leiomyomas. The conception rate among women older than age 35 may not be as good. Also, the postmyomectomy conception rate may be lower when the uterus is greater than 12 weeks' gestational size and when more than four myomata are removed. When abdominal myomectomy includes removal of submucous myomata, Garcia and Tureck report that 53% of patients attempting to establish a pregnancy conceive. Both Li and colleagues and Vercellini and coworkers published retrospective reviews supporting excellent conception and pregnancy rates following abdominal myomectomies. Vercellini's work suggests that certainly age at the time of the procedure is important, as it was one of three independent variables (age, duration of infertility before surgery, and the presence of other infertility factors) associated with postoperative cumulative conception rate.

Buttram and Reiter reviewed 1,914 cases of myomectomy and compared preoperative and postoperative abortion rates. The reduction in abortion rate after myomectomy from 41% to 19% suggests improvement in reproductive salvage through the use of this procedure. According to Verkauf's review, 69.2% of women with previous recurrent pregnancy wastage conceived after myomectomy and had a reduction in fetal loss.

An ultrasonographic study of uterine remodeling after conservative myomectomy was reported by Beyth and associates. There was a gradual decrease in uterine volume in all patients during the 6 months after myomectomy, with the most remarkable decrease occurring in the first 2 to 3 months. Presumably, this represents an involution of myometrial hypertrophy and postoperative healing of uterine incisions. We recommend that all patients use local methods of contraception (diaphragm, condoms, and spermicidal jelly or foam) for at least 3 months to avoid conception until the myomectomy incisions are healed.

Finally, there is the matter of recurrence of myomata after myomectomy. In Verkauf's review, leiomyomata recurred in 7.5% of patients, and 6.8% required reoperation. Most recurrences appeared more than 3 years after myomectomy, thus allowing sufficient time for conception to occur before recurrence. Friedman and associates investigated a concern that GnRH agonist–induced myoma shrinkage would make some small intramural and submucosal tumors "invisible" at myomectomy, causing early "recurrence" of leiomyomata once gonadal suppression ceased and estrogen production returned. In their study, there was no difference in myoma recurrence between women pretreated with GnRH agonists (67%) and those treated with placebo (56%) 27 to 38 months after myomectomy. Their myoma recurrence rate of 61% is much higher than that previously reported in combined myomectomy series. The authors believe that this discrepancy is most likely due to the use of high-resolution US to diagnose small myomata that would otherwise be missed on bimanual examination. Rosetti and colleagues reported long-term follow-up of 81 patients randomized to abdominal or laparoscopic myomectomy plus 84 nonrandomized patients and found similar recurrence rates, 23% and 27% respectively, between the laparoscopic and abdominal myomectomy, with most recurrences seen within 24 months of surgery.

Matta and colleagues reported that after GnRH analog treatment, the US outline of some myomata was lost or obscured. Such myomata are probably more difficult to identify and remove with myomectomy and may be more likely to reappear when GnRH analog treatment is discontinued after myomectomy.

Embolotherapy

With current technology progressing toward less invasive therapies, the minimally invasive procedure of uterine artery embolization (UAE) is gaining popularity. This procedure can potentially obviate the need for surgical procedures in patients who suffer from symptomatic leiomyomas.

In the female genital tract, embolotherapy for control of hemorrhage from malignancy was first reported in the late 1970s. In 1980, Pais and colleagues described successful embolization for postpartum hemorrhage. Many more reports followed in the mid-1980s. In the early 1990s, Ravina and coworkers began using embolotherapy as a preoperative maneuver to decrease intraoperative blood loss during surgery for myomas. The protocol generally included embolization about 24 hours before the surgery; however, some occurred a few days or weeks before surgery. Such an improvement in symptoms occurred that many surgeries were canceled altogether. This serendipitous discovery led to the performance of UAE as a primary procedure. UAE for leiomyomas was first performed in the United States by Goodwin and colleagues in 1995. Since then, several large series have been reported, and experience continues to grow.

UAE is appropriate for patients with symptomatic leiomyomas and a preference for treatment other than surgical treatment. Clinical findings, therapeutic goals, and overall medical conditions factor into the decision making. Several concerns have developed in treating patients who may desire future conception. Hypotheses include reduced fertility as a consequence of injury to the uterus or ovaries, placental insufficiency resulting from inadequate blood flow through the uterus, or uterine rupture during pregnancy from UAE-induced myoma necrosis. A limited number of deliveries have been reported after UAE for uterine myomas. However, embolization therapy appears to increase the risk of preterm delivery and malpresentation compared with laparoscopic myomectomy, and there is a trend toward higher spontaneous abortions and postpartum hemorrhage with UAE. Amenorrhea has been reported in 1% to 2% of patients after UAE; however, some authors have attributed this to the coincidental onset of menopause.

Contraindications to this procedure include pregnancy, active pelvic infection, severe contrast medium allergy, arteriovenous malformations, desire for future pregnancy, a strong suspicion of adenomyosis or pedunculated leiomyoma, and undiagnosed pelvic mass. The technique is generally preceded by preprocedural testing, and patients are pretreated with intravenous antibiotics. Many perform preliminary arteriographic mapping of the pelvis. A review by Hutchins and Worthington-Kirsch provides an excellent description of the procedure.

The technical success rate is consistently reported in the 96% to 98% range with experienced teams. Eighty percent to 90% of embolized patients have reported improvements in menorrhagia, bulk-related symptoms, or both. Reduction in overall uterine volume peaks at more than 60% by 6 to 9 months after the procedure because of the gradual nature of the process. Individual myomas show average volume reductions of 60% to 65%.

The Fibroid Registry for Outcomes Data (FIBROID) was established by the Society of Interventional Radiology and includes 25 core sites and 50 to 60 other participating sites. This clinical registry has enrolled more than 3,300 patients in an effort to obtain rapid and reliable data regarding patient outcomes. Based on 30-day and 1 year data, near 90% of patients responded favorably to UAE. Recurrence of symptoms and repeat procedures occur in about 10% of patients by 3 years. Worthington-Kirsch, a leading member of the steering committee, estimates that by 5 years postprocedure, as many as 20% of patients will have another procedure. Approximately 1,300 to 1,500 patients continue to provide annual data through self-reported questionnaires, permitting continued long-term follow-up of the UAE procedure.

Forty percent of patients develop a syndrome of fever and malaise in the first 10 to 14 days after UAE. This is also associated with leukocytosis. This entity is well described as postembolization syndrome. It is typically self-limited and resolves in 3 to 5 days, and rarely requires treatment except antipyretics. Other complications include those that may be attributed to the angiographic component and target or nontarget organ embolization. Groin infections, groin bleeding or hematoma, contrast-induced renal damage, and vascular damage may be attributed to the angiographic component. Uterine infection or perforation, sexual dysfunction, and myoma sloughing may be attributed to the target organ effects. Reported nontarget organ embolization complications include ovarian sequelae, sciatic nerve effects, and gluteal muscle pain. Current experience confirms a major complication rate of less than 1%.

BEST SURGICAL PRACTICES

- Women with symptomatic or problematic uterine leiomyomas should be considered candidates for surgical or radiologic intervention.
- Management options, including medical, radiologic, and surgical should be discussed with patients, emphasizing risks and benefits of each option.
- Careful preoperative evaluation for women who undergo surgical treatment of leiomyomata should include radiographic evaluation to determine the extent, location, and size of leiomyomata.
- In patients with infertility, myomectomy—performed by either an abdominal or laparoscopic approach—should only be performed after complete evaluation of other potential causes of infertility.
- Adhesion barriers are advantageous in reducing adhesions during both abdominal and laparoscopic myometomy.
- Pregnancy rates and outcomes after laparoscopic myomectomy compare favorably with those after abdominal myomectomy.
- Meticulous repair of the uterine myometrium is essential for patients desiring pregnancy after a myomectomy.
- Hysteroscopic myomectomy is an effective surgical alternative to relieve symptoms associated with submucosal myomas.
- Current information regarding uterine artery embolization (UAE) is promising, but patients should be made aware that limited long-term data are available regarding outcomes, especially relating to fertility and pregnancy.

Bibliography

Adamson G. Myomectomy: GnRH analogs and adhesions. *Prog Clin Biol Res* 1993;381:155.

Aharoni A, Reiter A, Golan D, et al. Patterns of growth of uterine leiomyomata during pregnancy: a prospective longitudinal study. *BJOG* 1988;95:510.

American College of Obstetricians and Gynecologists. ACOG Committee Opinion. Uterine artery embolization. *Obstet Gynecol* 2004;103:403.

Amussat JZ, quoted by Rubin IC. Progress in myomectomy. *Am J Obstet Gynecol* 1942;44:197.

Anderson J, Grine E, Eng CLY, et al. Expression of connexin-43 in human myometrium and leiomyoma. *Am J Obstet Gynecol* 1993;169:1266.

Andreyko J, Blumenfeld Z, Marshall L. Use of an agonistic analog of gonadotropin-releasing hormone (nafarelin) to treat leiomyomas: assessment by magnetic resonance imaging. *Am J Obstet Gynecol* 1988;158:903.

Ariel IM, Trinidad S. Pulmonary metastases from a uterine "leiomyoma." *Am J Obstet Gynecol* 1966;94:110.

Babaknia A, Rock JA, Jones HW Jr. Pregnancy success following abdominal myomectomy for infertility. *Fertil Steril* 1978;30:644.

Baggish MS, Sze EH, Morgan G. Hysteroscopic treatment of symptomatic submucous myomata uteri with the Nd:YAG laser. *J Gynecol Surg* 1989; 5:27.

Bahary CM, Gorodeski IG, Nilly M, et al. Intravascular leiomyomatosis. *Obstet Gynecol* 1982;59:735.

Baines RE. Problems associated with myomectomy in Cape Town. *S Afr Med J* 1971;45:668.

Baird DT, Bramley TA, Hawkins TA, et al. Effect of treatment with LHRH analog Zoladex on binding of oestradiol, progesterone and epidermal growth factor to uterine fibromyomata. *Horm Res* 1989;32:154.

Banner AS, Carrington CB, Emory WB, et al. Efficacy of oophorectomy in lymphangio-leiomyomatosis and benign metastasizing leiomyoma. *N Engl J Med* 1981;305:204.

Beacham WD, Webster HD, Lawson EH, et al. Uterine and/or ovarian tumors weighing 25 pounds or more. *Am J Obstet Gynecol* 1971;109:1153.

Bell SW, Kempson RL, Hendrickson MR. Problematic uterine smooth muscle neoplasm. *Am J Surg Pathol* 1994;18:535.

Ben-Baruch G, Schiff E, Menashe Y, et al. Immediate and late outcome of vaginal myomectomy for prolapsed pedunculated submucous myoma. *Obstet Gynecol* 1988;72:858.

Berkeley AS, DeCherney AH, Polan ML. Abdominal myomectomy and subsequent fertility. *Surg Gynecol Obstet* 1983;156:319.

Beyth Y, Jaffe R, Goldberger S. Uterine remodelling following conservative myomectomy: ultrasonographic evaluation. *Acta Obstet Gynecol Scand* 1992;71:632.

Bonney V. Abdominal myomectomy. In: Berkeley AS, Bonney V, eds. *A textbook of gynaecological surgery*. 5th ed. New York: Paul B. Hoeber; 1948.

Bonney V. The technique and results of myomectomy. *Lancet* 1931;220:171.

Brandon DD, Bethea CL, Strawn EY, et al. Progesterone receptor messenger ribonucleic acid and protein are overexpressed in human leiomyomas. *Am J Obstet Gynecol* 1993;169:78.

Brosens I, Deprest J, Dal Cin P, et al. Clinical significance of cytogenetic abnormalities in uterine myomas. *Fertil Steril* 1998;69:232.

Brown AB, Chamberlain R, TeLinde RW. Myomectomy. *Am J Obstet Gynecol* 1956;71:759.

Brown JM, Malkasian GD, Symmonds RE. Abdominal myomectomy. *Am J Obstet Gynecol* 1967;99:126.

Buchi KA, Keller PJ. Cytoplasmic progestin receptors in myomal and myometrial tissues. *Acta Obstet Gynecol Scand* 1983;62:487.

Buchi KA, Keller PJ. Estrogen receptors in normal and myomatous human uteri. *Gynecol Obstet Invest* 1980;11:59.

Bulletti C, DeZiegler D, Polli V et al. The role of leiomyomas in infertility. *J Am Assoc Gynecol Laparosc* 1999;6:441.

Buttram VC, Reiter RC. Uterine leiomyomata: etiology, symptomatology, and management. *Fertil Steril* 1981;36:433.

Campo S, Campo V, Gambadauro P. Short-term and long-term results of resectoscopic myomectomy with and without pretreatment with GnRH analogs in premenopausal women. *Acta Obstet Gynecol Scand* 2005;84:756.

Campo S, Garcea N. Laparoscopic myomectomy in premenopausal women with and without preoperative treatment with gonadotropin-releasing hormone analogues. *Hum Reprod* 1999;14:44.

Ceccacci L, Jacobs J, Powell A. Leiomyomatosis peritonealis disseminata: report of a case in a non pregnant woman. *Am J Obstet Gynecol* 1982;144:105.

Cincinelli E, Romano F, Anastasio PS, et al. Transabdominal sonohysterography, transvaginal sonography, and hysteroscopy in evaluation of submucous myomas. *Obstet Gynecol* 1995;85:42.

Clark DH, Weed JC. Metastasizing leiomyoma: a case report. *Am J Obstet Gynecol* 1977;127:672.

Cohen LS, Valle RF. Role of vaginal sonography and hysterosonography in the endoscopic treatment of uterine myomas. *Fertil Steril* 2000;73:197.

Cole P, Berlin J. Elective hysterectomy. *Obstet Gynecol* 1977;129:117.

Colgan T, Pendergast S, LeBlanc M. The histopathology of uterine leiomyomas following treatment with gonadotropin-releasing hormone analogs. *Hum Pathol* 1993;24:1073.

Corscaden JA, Singh BP. Leiomyosarcoma of the uterus. *Am J Obstet Gynecol* 1958;75:149.

Corson SL. Hysteroscopic diagnosis and operative therapy of submucous myoma. *Obstet Gynecol Clin North Am* 1995;22:739.

Corson SL, Brooks PG. Resectoscopic myomectomy. *Fertil Steril* 1991;55:1041.

Coutinho E. Treatment of large fibroid with high doses of gestrinone. *Gynecol Obstet Invest* 1990;30:44.

Coutinho E, Boulanger G, Goncalves M. Regression of uterine leiomyomas after treatment with gestrinone, an antiestrogen, antiprogesterone. *Am J Obstet Gynecol* 1986;155:761.

Cramer SF, Meyer JS, Kraner JF, et al. Metastasizing leiomyoma of the uterus: S-phase fraction, estrogen receptor, and ultrastructure. *Cancer* 1980;45:932.

Cramer SF, Patel A. The frequency of uterine leiomyomas. *Am J Clin Pathol* 1990;94:435.

Damario M, Rock J. Methods to prevent postoperative adhesion formation in gynecologic surgery. *J Gynecol Tech* 1995;1:1.

Daniell J, Gurley L. Laparoscopic treatment of clinically significant symptomatic uterine fibroids. *J Gynecol Surg* 1991;7:37.

Darai E, Dechaud H, Benifla JL, et al. Fertility after laparoscopic myomectomy: preliminary results. *Hum Reprod* 1997;12:1931.

Davids A. Myomectomy: surgical techniques and results in a series of 1,150 cases. *Am J Obstet Gynecol* 1952;63:592.

Davies A, Hart R, Magos AL. The excision of uterine fibroids by vaginal myomectomy: a prospective study. *Fertil Steril* 1999;71:961.

Dawood MY, Khan-Dawood FS. Plasma insulin-like growth factor-I, CA-125 estrogen and progesterone in women with leiomyomas. *Fertil Steril* 1994;61:217.

Dawood M, Lewis V, Ramos J. Cortical and trabecular bone mineral content in women with endometriosis: effect of gonadotropin releasing hormone agonist and danazol. *Fertil Steril* 1989;52:21.

DeCherney A, Maheux R, Polan M. A medical treatment for myomata uteri. *Fertil Steril* 1983;39:429.

Degligdish L, Loewenthal M. Endometrial changes associated with myomata of the uterus. *J Clin Pathol* 1970;23:677.

Derman SG, Rehustrom J, Neuwirth RS. The long-term effectiveness of hysteroscopic treatment of menorrhagia and leiomyomas. *Obstet Gynecol* 1991;77:591.

Diamond MP. Reduction of adhesions after uterine myomectomy by Seprafilm membrane (HAL-F): a blinded, prospective, randomized, multicenter clinical study. *Fertil Steril* 1996;66:904.

Di Lieto A, De Falco M, Pollio F, et al. Clinical response, vascular change, and angiogenesis in gonadotropin-releasing hormone analogue-treated women with uterine myomas. *J Soc Gynecol Investig* 2005;12:123.

Dillon T. Control of blood loss during gynecologic surgery. *Obstet Gynecol* 1962;19:428.

diZerega G. Contemporary adhesion prevention. *Fertil Steril* 1994;61:219.

Donnez J, Gillerot S, Bourgoujon D, et al. Neodymium:YAG laser hysteroscopy in large submucous fibroids. *Fertil Steril* 1990;54:999.

Dubuisson JB, Chapron C, Fauconnier A. Laparoscopic myomectomy: operative technique and results. *Ann N Y Acad Sci* 1997;828:326.

Dubuisson JB, Chapron C, Fauconnier A, et al. Laparoscopic myomectomy and myolysis. *Curr Opin Obstet Gynecol* 1997;9:233.

Dubuisson JB, Fauconnier A, Chapron C, et al. Second look after laparoscopic myomectomy. *Hum Reprod* 1998;13:2102.

Dubuisson JB, Lecuru F, Foulot H, et al. Myomectomy by laparoscopy: preliminary report of 43 cases. *Fertil Steril* 1991;56:828.

Edwards DR, Peacock JF. Intravenous leiomyomatosis of the uterus: report of 2 cases. *Obstet Gynecol* 1966;27:176.

Eldar-Geva T, Meagher S, Healy DL, et al. Effect of intramural, subserosal, and submucosal uterine fibroids on the outcome of assisted reproductive technology treatment. *Fertil Steril* 1998;70:687.

Evans AT, Symmonds RE, Gaffey TA. Recurrent pelvic intravenous leiomyomatosis. *Obstet Gynecol* 1981;57:260.

Everett HS, Sturgis WJ. The effect of some common gynecological disorders upon the urinary tract. *Urol Cutan Rev* 1940;44:638.

Exacoustos C, Rosati P. Ultrasound diagnosis of uterine myomas and complications in pregnancy. *Obstet Gynecol* 1993;82:97.

Farber M, Conrad S, Heinrichs WL, et al. Estradiol binding by fibroid tumors and normal myometrium. *Obstet Gynecol* 1972;40:479.

Farquhar C, Vandekerckhove P, Watson A, et al. Barrier agents for preventing adhesions after surgery for subfertility. *Cochrane Database Syst Rev* 2000;4.

Farrer-Brown G, Beilby JO, Tarbit MH. The vascular patterns in myomatous uteri. *J Obstet Gynaecol Br Commonw* 1970;77:967.

Farrer-Brown G, Beilby JO, Tarbit MH. Venous changes in the endometrium of myomatous uteri. *Obstet Gynecol* 1971;38:743.

Faulkner RL. The blood vessels of the myomatous uterus. *Am J Obstet Gynecol* 1944;47:185.

Fedele L, Bianchi S, Dorta M, et al. Transvaginal sonography versus hysteroscopy in the diagnosis of uterine submucous myomas. *Obstet Gynecol* 1991;77:745.

Feeney JG, Basu SB. *Bacteroides* infection in fibroids during the puerperium. *BMJ* 1979;2:1038.

Filiceri M, Hall D, Loughlin J, et al. A conservative approach to the management of uterine leiomyoma: pituitary desensitization by a luteinizing hormone releasing hormone analog. *Am J Obstet Gynecol* 1983;147:726.

Floridon C, Lund N, Thomsen SG. Alternative treatment for symptomatic fibroids. *Curr Opin Obstet Gynecol* 2001;13(5):491.

Frederick J, Fletcher A, Simeon D, et al. Intramyometrial vasopressin as a hemostatic agent. *BJOG* 1994;101:435.

Friedman A. Acute urinary retention after gonadotropin-releasing hormone agonist treatment for leiomyomata uteri. *Fertil Steril* 1993;59:677.

Friedman A. The biochemistry, physiology and pharmacology of gonadotropin releasing hormone (GnRH) and GnRH analogs. In: Barbieri RL, Friedman F, eds. *Gonadotropin releasing hormone analogs: applications in gynecology.* New York: Elsevier; 1991:10.

Friedman A. Use of gonadotropin-releasing hormone agonists before myomectomy. *Clin Obstet Gynecol* 1993;36:650.

Friedman AJ. Vaginal hemorrhage associated with degenerating submucous leiomyomata during leuprolide acetate treatment. *Fertil Steril* 1989;52:152.

Friedman A, Barbieri R, Benacerraf B, et al. Treatment of leiomyomata with intranasal or subcutaneous leuprolide, a gonadotropin-releasing leuprolide, a gonadotropin-releasing hormone agonist. *Fertil Steril* 1987;48:56.

Friedman A, Barbieri R, Doubilet P, et al. A randomized double-blind trial of a gonadotropin-releasing hormone agonist (leuprolide) with or without medroxy progesterone acetate in the treatment of leiomyomata uteri. *Fertil Steril* 1988;49:404.

Friedman A, Daly M, Juneau-Norcross M, et al. Predictors of uterine volume reduction in women with myomas treated with a gonadotropin-releasing hormone agonist. *Fertil Steril* 1992;58:413.

Friedman A, Daly M, Juneau-Norcross M, et al. A prospective randomized trial of gonadotropin-releasing hormone agonist plus estrogen-progestin or progestin "add-back" regimens for women with leiomyomata uteri. *J Clin Endocrinol Metab* 1993;76:1439.

Friedman A, Daly M, Juneau-Norcross M, et al. Recurrence of myomas after myomectomy in women pretreated with leuprolide acetate depot or placebo. *Fertil Steril* 1992;58:205.

Friedman AJ, Haas ST. Should uterine size be an indication for surgical intervention in women with myomas? *Am J Obstet Gynecol* 1993;168:751.

Friedman A, Harrison-Atlas D, Barbieri R, et al. A randomized, placebo-controlled, double-blind study evaluating the efficacy of leuprolide acetate depot in the treatment of uterine leiomyomata. *Fertil Steril* 1989;51:251.

Friedman A, Hoffman D, Canite F, et al, for the Leuprolide Study Group. Treatment of leiomyomata uteri with leuprolide acetate depot: a double-blind, placebo-controlled, multicenter study. *Obstet Gynecol* 1991;77:720.

Friedman A, Juneau-Norcross M, Rein M. Adverse effects of leuprolide acetate depot treatment. *Fertil Steril* 1993;59:448.

Friedman A, Lobel S, Rein M, et al. Efficacy and safety considerations in women with uterine leiomyomas treated with gonadotropin-releasing hormone agonist: the estrogen threshold hypothesis. *Am J Obstet Gynecol* 1990;163:111.

Friedman A, Rein M, Harrison-Atlas D, et al. A randomized, placebo-controlled, double-blind study evaluating leuprolide acetate depot treatment before myomectomy. *Fertil Steril* 1989;52:728.

Friedman A, Thomas P. Does low-dose combination oral contraceptive use affect uterine size or menstrual flow in premenopausal women with leiomyomas? *Obstet Gynecol* 1995;85:631.

Fujita M. Histological and biochemical studies of collagen in human leiomyomas. *Hokkaido Igaku Zasshi* 1985;60:602.

Gabb RG, Stone GM. Uptake and metabolism of tritiated oestradiol and oestrone by human endometrial and myometrial tissue *in vitro*. *J Endocrinol* 1974;62:109.

Gal D, Buchsbaum HJ, Voet R, et al. Massive ascites with uterine leiomyomas and ovarian vein thrombosis. *Am J Obstet Gynecol* 1982;144:729.

Garcia CR, Tureck RW. Submucosal leiomyomas and infertility. *Fertil Steril* 1984;42:16.

Gehlback D, Sousa R, Carpenter S, et al. Abdominal myomectomy in the treatment of infertility. *Int J Obstet Gynecol* 1993;40:45.

Gilbert HA, Kagan AR, Lagasse L. The value of radiation therapy in uterine sarcoma. *Obstet Gynecol* 1975;45:84.

Ginsberg E, Benson C, Garfield J, et al. The effect of operative technique and uterine size on blood loss during myomectomy: a prospective randomized study. *Fertil Steril* 1993;60:956.

Golan A, Bukovsky I, Pansky M, et al. Pre-operative gonadotropin-releasing hormone agonist treatment in surgery for uterine leiomyomata. *Hum Reprod* 1993;8:450.

Goldberg J, Pereira L, Berghella V, et al. Pregnancy outcomes after treatment for fibromyomata: uterine artery embolization versus laparoscopic myomectomy. *Am J Obstet Gynecol* 2004;191:18.

Goldberg MF, Hurt G, Frable WJ. Leiomyomatosis peritonealis disseminata. *Obstet Gynecol* 1977;49:46s.

Goldenberg M, Sivan E, Sharabi Z, et al. Outcome of hysteroscopic resection of submucous myomas for infertility. *Fertil Steril* 1995;64:714.

Goldfarb H. Laparoscopic coagulation of myoma (myolysis). *Obstet Gynecol Clin North Am* 1995;22:807.

Goldfarb HA. Myoma coagulation (myolysis). *Obstet Gynecol Clin North Am* 2000;27:421.

Goldfarb HA. Nd:YAG laser laparoscopic coagulation of symptomatic myomas. *J Reprod Med* 1992;37:636.

Goldfarb HA. Removing uterine fibroids laparoscopically. *Contemp Obstet Gynecol* 1994;39:50.

Goldrath MH. Vaginal removal of the pedunculated submucous myoma: historical observations and development of a new procedure. *J Reprod Med* 1990;35:921.

Goldrath MH, Fuller TA, Segal S. Laser photovaporization of endometrium for the treatment of menorrhagia. *Am J Obstet Gynecol* 1981;140:14.

Goldzieher JW, Maqueo M, Ricaud L, et al. Induction of degenerative changes in uterine myomas by high-dosage progestin therapy. *Am J Obstet Gynecol* 1966;96:1078.

Gomel V. From microsurgery to laparoscopic surgery: a progress. *Fertil Steril* 1995;63:464.

Goodman AL. Progesterone therapy in uterine fibromyoma. *J Clin Endocrinol Metab* 1946;6:402.

Goodwin SC, Vedantham S, McLucas B, et al. Uterine artery embolization for uterine fibroids: results of a pilot study. *J Vasc Interv Radiol* 1997;8:517.

Goustin AS, Leof EB, Shipley GD, et al. Growth factors and cancer. *Cancer Res* 1986;46:1015.

Grow DR, Coddington CC, Hsiu JG, et al. Role of hypoestrogenism or sex steroid antagonism in adhesion formation after myometrial surgery in primates. *Fertil Steril* 1996;66:140.

Gutmann J, Thornton K, Diamond M, et al. Evaluation of leuprolide acetate treatment on histopathology of uterine myomata. *Fertil Steril* 1994;61:622.

Hallberg L, Nilsson L. Determination of menstrual blood loss. *Scand J Clin Lab Invest* 1964;43:352.

Hallez JP. Single-stage hysteroscopic myomectomies: indications, techniques, and results. *Fertil Steril* 1995;63:703.

Hanson H, Rotman C, Rana N, et al. Laparoscopic myomectomy. *Obstet Gynecol* 1992;80:885.

Harris W. Uterine dehiscence following laparoscopic myomectomy. *Obstet Gynecol* 1992;80:545.

Hart R, Molnar BG, Magos A. Long term follow-up of hysteroscopic myomectomy assessed by survival analysis. *BJOG* 1999;106:700.

Healy D, Frazer H, Lawson S. Shrinkage of a uterine fibroid after subcutaneous infusion of a LHRH agonist. *BMJ* 1984;289:1267.

Healy D, Lawson S, Abbott M, et al. Toward removing uterine fibroids without surgery: subcutaneous infusion of a luteinizing hormone-releasing hormone agonist commencing in the luteal phase. *J Clin Endocrinol Metab* 1986;63:619.

Hehenkamp WJ, Volkers NA, Donderwinkel PF, et al. Uterine artery embolization versus hysterectomy for fibroids. *Am J Obstet Gynecol* 2005;193:1618.

Hirai K, Kanaoka Y, Isshiko O, et al. A novel technique for myomectomy: intranodal surgery with an elctromechanical tissue borer. *J Reprod Med* 2000;45:813.

Hoetzinger H. Hysterosonography and hysterography in benign and malignant diseases of the uterus: a comparative *in vitro* study. *J Ultrasound Med* 1991;10:259.

Hoffmann GE, Rao V, Barrows GH, et al. Binding sites for epidermal growth factors in human uterine tissues and leiomyomas. *J Clin Endocrinol Metab* 1984;17:44.

Horstmann JP, Pietra GG, Harman JA, et al. Spontaneous regression of pulmonary leiomyomas during pregnancy. *Cancer* 1977;39:314.

Hricak H, Tscholakoff D, Heinrichs L. Uterine leiomyomas: correlation of MR, histopathological findings, and symptoms. *Radiology* 1986;158:385.

Hunt SH. Fibroid weighing one hundred and forty pounds. *Am J Obstet Gynecol* 1888;21:62.

Hurst BS, Matthews ML, Marshburn PB. Laparoscopic myomectomy for sympotomatic uterine myomas. *Fertil Steril* 2005;83:1.

Hutchins F. Myomectomy after selective preoperative treatment with a gonadotropin-releasing hormone analog. *J Reprod Med* 1992;37:699.

Hutchins FL. Uterine fibroids: diagnosis and indications for treatment. *Obstet Gynecol* 1992;80:545.

Hutchins FL, Worthington-Kirsch R. Embolotherapy for myoma-induced menorrhagia. *Obstet Gynecol Clin North Am* 2000;27:397.

Idelson MG, Davids AM. Metastasis of uterine fibroleiomyomata. *Obstet Gynecol* 1963;21:78.

Imai A, Sugiyama M, Furui T, et al. Gonadotropin-releasing hormone agonist therapy increases peritoneal fibrinolytic activity and prevents adhesion formation after myomectomy. *J Obstet Gynaecol* 2003;23:660.

Indman PD. Hysteroscopic treatment of menorrhagia associated with uterine leiomyomas. *Obstet Gynecol* 1993;81:716.

Ingersoll FM, Malone LJ. Myomectomy: an alternative to hysterectomy. *Arch Surg* 1970;100:557.

Interceed (TC7) Adhesion Barrier Study Group. Prevention of postsurgical adhesions by Interceed (TC7), an absorbable adhesion barrier: a prospective, randomized multicenter clinical study. *Fertil Steril* 1989;51:933.

Irey NS, Norris HJ. Intimal vascular lesions associated with female reproductive steroids. *Arch Pathol* 1973;96:227.

Jones HW Jr, Andrew MC. Congenital anomalies and infertility. In: Ridley JH, ed. *Gynecologic surgery*. 2nd ed. Baltimore: Williams & Wilkins; 1981.

Karlsson S, Persson P. Angiography in uterine and adnexal tumors. *Acta Radiol Diagn* 1980;21:11.

Kastner P, Krust A, Turcotte B, et al. Two distinct estrogen-regulated promotors generate transcripts encoding the two functionally different human progesterone receptor forms A and B. *EMBO J* 1990;9:1603.

Kawaguchi J, Fujii S, Konishi I, et al. Mitotic activity in uterine leiomyomas during the menstrual cycle. *Am J Obstet Gynecol* 1989;160:637.

Kelly HA, Cullen TS. *Myomata of the uterus*. Philadelphia: WB Saunders; 1907.

Kettel L, Murphy A, Morales A, et al. Rapid regression of uterine leiomyomas in response to daily administration of gonadotropin-releasing hormone antagonist. *Fertil Steril* 1993;60:642.

Kiltz R, Rutgers J, Phillips J, et al. Absence of a dose-response effect of leuprolide acetate on leiomyomata uteri size. *Fertil Steril* 1994;61:1021.

Klunder KB, Svanholm H, Frimodt-Moller PC. Uterine bizarre leiomyoma. *Acta Obstet Gynecol Scand* 1982;61:121.

Kornyei J, Csermely T, Szekely JA, et al. Two types of nuclear Ez binding sites in human myometrium and leiomyoma during the menstrual cycle. *Exp Clin Endocrinol* 1986;87:256.

Kumakiri J, Takeuchi H, Kitade M, et al. Pregnancy and delivery after laparoscopic myomectomy. *J Min Inv Gyne* 2005;241.

Kurman RJ, Norris HJ. Mesenchymal tumors of the uterus. VI. Epithelioid smooth muscle tumors including leiomyoblastoma and clear cell leiomyoma. *Cancer* 1976;37:1853.

LaMorte A, Lalwani S, Diamond M. Morbidity associated with myomectomy. *Obstet Gynecol* 1993;82:897.

Lapan B, Solomon L. Diffuse leiomyomatosis of the uterus precluding myomectomy. *Obstet Gynecol* 1979;53:825.

Leibsohn S, D'Ablaing G, Mishell DR, et al. Leiomyosarcoma in a series of hysterectomies performed for presumed uterine leiomyomas. *Am J Obstet Gynecol* 1990;162:968.

Letterie GS, Kramer DJ. Intraoperative ultrasound guidance for intrauterine endoscopic surgery. *Fertil Steril* 1994;62:654.

Lev-Toaff AS, Coleman BG, Arger PH, et al. Leiomyomas in pregnancy: sonographic study. *Radiology* 1987;164:375.

Lev-Toaff A, Karasick S, Toaff M. Hysterosalpingography before and after myomectomy: clinical value and imaging findings. *Am J Radiol* 1993;160:803.

Li TC, Mortimer R, Cooke ID. Myomectomy: a retrospective study to examine reproductive performance before and after surgery. *Hum Reprod* 1999;14:1735.

Ligon AH, Morton CC. Genetics of uterine leiomyomata. *Genes Chromosomes Cancer* 2000;28:235.

Lipschutz A. Experimental fibroids and the antifibromatogenic action of steroid hormones. *JAMA* 1942;120:171.

Lipschutz A, Murillo R, Vargas L. Antitumorigenic action of progesterone. *Lancet* 1939;2:420.

Lock FR. Multiple myomectomy. *Am J Obstet Gynecol* 1969;104:642.

Loeffler FE, Noble AD. Myomectomy at the Chelsea Hospital for Women. *J Obstet Gynaecol Br Commonw* 1970;77:167.

Lumsden MA, West CP, Bromley J, et al. The binding of epidermal growth factor to the human uterus and leiomyomata in women rendered hypo-oestrogenic by continuous administration of an LHRH-agonist. *BJOG* 1988;95:1299.

Magos AL, Bournas N, Sinha R, et al. Vaginal myomectomy. *BJOG* 1994; 101:1092.

Maheux R, Guilloteau C, Lemay A, et al. Luteinizing hormone-releasing hormone agonist and uterine leiomyomata: a pilot study. *Am J Obstet Gynecol* 1985;152:1034.

Maheux R, Guilloteau C, Lemay A, et al. Regression of leiomyomata uteri following hypo-oestrogenism induced by repetitive luteinizing hormone-releasing hormone agonist treatment: preliminary report. *Fertil Steril* 1984;42:644.

Mais V, Ajossa S, Guerriero S, et al. Laparoscopic versus abdominal myomectomy: a prospective, randomized trial to evaluate benefits in early outcome. *Am J Obstet Gynecol* 1996;174:654.

Mais V, Ajossa S, Piras B, et al. Prevention of *de novo* adhesion formation after laparoscopic myomectomy: a randomized trial to evaluate the effectiveness of an oxidized regenerated cellulose absorbable barrier. *Hum Reprod* 1995;10:3133.

Makarainen L, Ylikorkala O. Primary and myoma-associated menorrhagia: role of prostaglandins and effects of ibuprofen. *BJOG* 1986;93:974.

Malone LJ, Ingersoll FM. Myomectomy in infertility. In: Bermen SG, Kistner RW, eds. *Progress in infertility*. Boston: Little, Brown; 1975.

Marschburn PB, Meek JM, Gruber HE, et al. Preoperative leuprolide acetate combined with Interceed optimally reduces uterine adhesions and fibrosis in a rabbit model. *Fertil Steril* 2004;81:194.

Marshall JF, Morris DS. Intravenous leiomyomatosis of the uterus and pelvis: case report. *Ann Surg* 1959;149:126.

Martin JF, Bazin P, Feroldi J, et al. Tumeurs myoides intramurales de l'estomac: considerations microscopiques apropos de 6 cas. *Ann Anat Pathol* 1960;5:484.

Matsunaga E, Shiota K. Ectopic pregnancy and myoma uteri: teratogenic effects and maternal characteristics. *Teratology* 1980;21:61.

Matta W, Shaw R, Hesp R, et al. Reversible trabecular bone density loss following induced hypo-estrogenism with GnRH analog buserelin in premenopausal women. *Clin Endocrinol* 1988;29:45.

Matta W, Stabile I, Shaw RW, et al. Doppler assessment of uterine blood flow changes in patients with fibroids receiving the gonadotropin-releasing hormone agonist buserelin. *Fertil Steril* 1988;49:1083.

Mattingly RF. Large myomata uteri and stress urinary incontinence. In: Nichols DH, ed. *Clinical problems, injuries, and complications of gynecologic surgery*. Baltimore: Williams & Wilkins; 1983.

Mayer D, Shipilov V. Ultrasonography and magnetic resonance imaging of uterine fibroids. *Obstet Gynecol Clin North Am* 1995;22:667.

Mayo WJ. Some observations on the operation of abdominal myomectomy for myomata of the uterus. *Surg Gynecol Obstet* 1911;12:97.

McLaughlin D. Metroplasty and myomectomy with CO_2 laser for maximizing the preservation of normal tissue and minimizing blood loss. *J Reprod Med* 1985;30:1.

McLucas B, Goodwin S, Adler L, et al. Pregnancy following uterine fibroid embolization. *Int J Gynaecol Obstet* 2001;74:1.

Meigs JV. Pelvic tumors other than fibromas of the ovary with ascites and hydrothorax. *Obstet Gynecol* 1954;3:471.

Meloni AM, Surti U, Contento AM, et al. Uterine leiomyomas: cytogenetic and histologic profile. *Obstet Gynecol* 1992;80:209.

Meyer W, Mayer A, Diamond M, et al. Unsuspected leiomyosarcoma: treatment with a gonadotropin-releasing hormone analog. *Obstet Gynecol* 1990;75:529.

Miller NF, Ludovici PP. On the origin and development of uterine fibroids. *Am J Obstet Gynecol* 1955;70:720.

Mixson W, Hammond D. Response of fibromyomas to a progestin. *Am J Obstet Gynecol* 1961;82:754.

Moghissi K. Hormonal therapy before surgical treatment for uterine leiomyomas. *Surg Gynecol Obstet* 1991;172:497.

Montague A, Swartz DP, Woodruff JD. Sarcoma arising in leiomyoma of uterus: factors influencing prognosis. *Am J Obstet Gynecol* 1965;92:421.

Muram D, Gillieson MS, Walters JH. Myomas of the uterus in pregnancy: ultrasonographic follow-up. *Am J Obstet Gynecol* 1980;138:16.

Murphy A, Kettel L, Morales A, et al. Regression of uterine leiomyomata in response to the anti-progesterone RU486. *J Clin Endocrinol Metab* 1993;76:513.

Murphy A, Morales A, Kettel L, et al. Regression of uterine leiomyomata to the antiprogesterone RU486: dose-response effect. *Fertil Steril* 1995;64:187.

Nakamura Y, Yoshimura Y. Treatment of uterine leiomyomas in perimenopausal women with gonadotropin-releasing hormone agonists. *Clin Obstet Gynecol* 1993;36:660.

Nardulli AM, Greene GL, O'Malley BW, et al. Regulation of progesterone receptor messenger ribonucleic acid and protein levels in MCF-cells by estradiol: analysis of estrogen's effect on progesterone receptor synthesis and degradation. *Endocrinology* 1988;122:935.

Nelson WO. Endometrial and myometrial changes including fibromyomatous nodules, induced in the uterus of the guinea pig by the prolonged administration of oestrogenic hormone. *Anat Rec* 1937;68:99.

Neuwirth RS. Hysteroscopic management of symptomatic submucous fibroids. *Obstet Gynecol* 1983;62:509.

Neuwirth RS. A new technique for and additional experience with hysteroscopic resection of submucous fibroids. *Am J Obstet Gynecol* 1978;131:91.

Neuwirth RS, Amin HK. Excision of submucous fibroids with hysteroscopic control. *Am J Obstet Gynecol* 1976;126:95.

Nezhat C, Nezhat F, Bess O, et al. Laparoscopically assisted myomectomy: a report of a new technique in 57 cases. *Int J Fertil* 1994;39:39.

Nisolle M, Smets M, Malvaux V, et al. Laparoscopic myolysis with the Nd:YAG laser. *J Gynecol Surg* 1993;9:95.

Nordic Adhesion Prevention Study Group. The efficacy of Interceed (TC7) for prevention of reformation of postoperative adhesions on ovaries, fallopian tubes, and fimbriae in microsurgical operations for fertility: a multicenter study. *Fertil Steril* 1995;63:709.

Norris HJ, Parmley T. Mesenchymal tumors of the uterus versus intravenous leiomyomatosis: a clinical and pathologic study of 14 cases. *Cancer* 1975;36:2164.

Novak ER. Benign and malignant changes in uterine myomas. *Clin Obstet Gynecol* 1958;1:421.

Otubu JA, Buttram VC, Besch NF, et al. Unconjugated steroids in leiomyomas and tumor bearing myometrium. *Am J Obstet Gynecol* 1982;143:130.

Pais SO, Glickman M, Schwartz PE, et al. Embolization of pelvic arteries for control of postpartum hemorrhage. *Obstet Gynecol* 1980;55:741.

Parazzini F, Negri E, La Vecchia C, et al. Oral contraceptive use and risk of uterine fibroids. *Obstet Gynecol* 1992;79:430.

Parker W. Myomectomy: laparoscopy or laparotomy? *Clin Obstet Gynecol* 1995;38:392.
Parker WH, Fu YS, Berek JS. Uterine sarcomas in patients operated on for presumed leiomyoma and rapidly growing leiomyoma. *Obstet Gynecol* 1994;83:414.
Parmley TH, Woodruff JD, Winn K. Histogenesis of leiomyomatosis peritonealis disseminata (disseminated fibrosing deciduosis). *Obstet Gynecol* 1975;46:511.
Pearce PH. Leiomyomatosis peritonealis disseminata. *Am J Obstet Gynecol* 1982;144:133.
Pelage JP, Jacob D, Fazel A, et al. Midterm results of uterine artery embolization for symptomatic adenomyosis: initial experience. *Radiology* 2005;234: 948.
Pellicano M, Bramante S, Cirillo D, et al. Effectiveness of autocrosslinked hyaluronic acid gel after laparoscopic myomectomy in infertile patients: a prospective, randomized, controlled study. *Fertil Steril* 2003;80:441.
Pelosi MA, Pelosi MA, Eim J. Hand assisted laparoscopy for megamyomectomy. *J Reprod Med* 2000;45:519.
Perino A, Chianchiano N, Petronio M, et al. Role of leuprolide acetate depot in hysteroscopic surgery: a controlled study. *Fertil Steril* 1993;59:507.
Persaud V, Arjoon PD. Uterine leiomyoma: incidence of degenerative change and a correlation of associated symptoms. *Obstet Gynecol* 1970;135:432.
Phillips D. Laparoscopic leiomyoma coagulation (myolysis). *Gynecol Endosc* 1995;4:5.
Pollow K, Geilfub J, Boquoi E, et al. Estrogen and progesterone binding proteins in normal human myometrium. *J Clin Chem Clin Biochem* 1978;16:503.
Prayson RA, Hart W. Pathologic considerations of uterine smooth muscle tumors. *Obstet Gynecol Clin North Am* 1995;22:637.
Ranney B, Frederick I. The occasional need for myomectomy. *Obstet Gynecol* 1979;53:437.
Ravina JH, Aymard A, Ciraru-Vigneron N, et al. Value of preoperative embolization of uterine fibroma: report of a multicenter series of 31 cases. *Contracept Fertil Sex* 1995;23:45.
Ravina JH, Vigneron NC, Aymard A, et al. Pregnancy after embolization of uterine myoma: report of 12 cases. *Fertil Steril* 2000;73:1241.
Razavi MK, Hwang G, Jahed A, et al. Abdominal myomectomy versus uterine fibroid embolization in the treatment of sympotomatic uterine leiomyomas. *AJR Am J Roentgenol* 2003;180:1571.
Reddy VV, Rose LI. Δ^4-3-Ketosteroid 5 α-oxidoreductase in human uterine leiomyoma. *Am J Obstet Gynecol* 1979;135:415.
Reich H. Laparoscopic myomectomy. *Obstet Gynecol Clin North Am* 1995;22: 757.
Rein MS, Barbieri RL, Friedman AJ. Progesterone: a critical role in the pathogenesis of uterine myomas. *Am J Obstet Gynecol* 1995;172:14.
Rein MS, Barbieri RL, Welch W, et al. The concentrations of collagen-associated amino acids are higher in GnRH agonist treated uterine myomas. *Obstet Gynecol* 1993;82:901.
Rein MS, Powell WL, Walters FC, et al. Cytogenetic abnormalities in uterine myomas are associated with myoma size. *Mol Hum Reprod* 1998;4:83.
Reinsch R, Murphy A, Morales A, et al. The effects of RU486 and leuprolide acetate on uterine artery blood flow in the fibroid uterus: a prospective, randomized study. *Am J Obstet Gynecol* 1994;170:1623.
Reiter RC, Wagner PL, Gambone JC. Routine hysterectomy for large asymptomatic uterine leiomyomata: a reappraisal. *Obstet Gynecol* 1992;79: 481.
Reyniak J, Corenthal L. Microsurgical laser techniques for abdominal myomectomy. *Microsurgery* 1987;8:92.
Riley P. Treatment of prolapsed submucous fibroids. *S Afr Med J* 1982;62:22.
Rosenfield DC. Abdominal myomectomy for otherwise unexplained infertility. *Fertil Steril* 1986;46:328.
Ross R, Pike M, Vessey M, et al. Risk factor for uterine fibroids: reduced risk associated with oral contraceptives. *BMJ* 1986;293:359.
Rossetti A, Sizzi O, Soranna L, et al. Long-term results of laparoscopic myomectomy: recurrence rate in comparison with abdominal myomectomy. *Hum Reprod* 2001;16:770.
Rubin I. Progress in myomectomy. Surgical measures and diagnostic aids favoring lower morbidity and mortality. *Am J Obstet Gynecol* 1942;44:196.
Rubin I. Uterine fibromyomas and sterility. *Clin Obstet Gynecol* 1958;1:501.
Sacks P, Hoyne P. Disseminated intravascular coagulation, hemolytic anemia, and acute renal failure associated with multiple myomectomy. *Obstet Gynecol* 1992;79:835.
Sadan O, Vauiddekinge B, Van Gelderen CJ, et al. Oestrogen and progesterone receptor concentrations in leiomyoma and normal myometrium. *Am Clin Biochem* 1987;24:263.
Sampson JA. The influence of myomata on the blood supply of the uterus with special reference to abnormal uterine bleeding. *Surg Gynecol Obstet* 1913;16:144.
Schlaff WD, Zerhoun E, Huth J, et al. A placebo-controlled trial of a depot gonadotropin-releasing hormone analog (leuprolide) in the treatment of uterine leiomyomata. *Obstet Gynecol* 1989;74:856.
Schwartz L, Panageas E, Lange R, et al. Female pelvis: impact of MR imaging on treatment decisions and net cost analysis. *Radiology* 1994;192:55.
Segaloff A, Weed JC, Sternberg WH, et al. The progesterone therapy of human uterine leiomyomas. *J Clin Endocrinol Metab* 1919;9:1273.
Sehgal N, Haskins AL. The mechanism of uterine bleeding in the presence of fibromyomas. *Am J Surg* 1960;26:21.
Semm K, Mettler L. Local infiltration of ornithine 8-vasopressin (POR8) as a vasoconstrictive agent in surgical pelviscopy. *Endoscopy* 1988;20:298.
Seoud M, Patterson R, Muasher S, et al. Effects of myomas or prior myomectomy on *in vitro* fertilization (IVF) performance. *J Assist Reprod Genet* 1992;9:217.
Seracchioli R, Rossi S, Govoni F, et al. Fertility and obstetric outcome after laparoscopic myomectomy of large myomata: a randomized comparison with abdominal myomectomy. *Hum Reprod* 2000;15:2663.
Sheiner E, Bashiri A, Levy A, et al. Obstetric and perinatal outcome of pregnancies with uterine leiomyomas. *J Reprod Med* 2004;49:182.
Singhabhandhu B, Akin JJ Jr, Ridley JH, et al. Giant leiomyoma of the uterus: report of a case and review of the literature. *Am Surg* 1973;39:391.
Smith DC, Uhlir J. Myomectomy as a reproductive procedure. *Am J Obstet Gynecol* 1990;162:1476.
Soules MR, McCarty KS Jr. Leiomyomas: steroid receptor content: variations within normal menstrual cycles. *Am J Obstet Gynecol* 1982;143:6.
Spellacy WN, LeMaire WJ, Buhi WC, et al. Plasma growth hormone and estradiol levels in women with uterine myomas. *Obstet Gynecol* 1972;40:829.
Spies JB, Cooper JM, Worthington-Kirsch R, et al. Outcome of uterine artery embolization and hysterectomy for leiomyomas: results of a multicenter study. *Am J Obstet Gynecol* 2004;191:22.
Spies JB, Myers ER, Worthington-Kirsch R, et al; FIBROID investigators. The FIBROID Registry: symptom and quality-of-life status 1 year after therapy. *Obstet Gynecol* 2005;106:1309.
Starks GC. CO_2 laser myomectomy in an infertile population. *J Reprod Med* 1988;33:184.
Starks GC. Unilateral twin interstitial ectopic pregnancy: a case report. *J Reprod Med* 1980;25:79.
Stovall T. Gonadotropin-releasing hormone agonists: utilization before hysterectomy. *Clin Obstet Gynecol* 1993;36:642.
Stovall T, Ling F, Henry L, et al. A randomized trial evaluating leuprolide acetate before hysterectomy as treatment for leiomyomas. *Am J Obstet Gynecol* 1991;164:1420.
Stovall T, Muneyyirei-Delale O, Summitt R, et al, for the Leuprolide Acetate Study Group. GnRH agonist and iron versus placebo and iron in the anemic patient before surgery for leiomyomas: a randomized controlled trial. *Obstet Gynecol* 1995;86:65.
Stovall TG, Summit RL, Washburn SA, et al. Gonadotropin-releasing hormone agonist before hysterectomy for leiomyomas: results of a multicentre, randomised controlled trial. *BJOG* 1998;105:1148.
Strawn EY, Novy MF, Burry KA, et al. Insulin-like growth factor I promotes leiomyoma cell growth *in vitro*. *Am J Obstet Gynecol* 1995;172:1837.
Stringer NH, Walker JC, Meyer PM. Comparison of 49 laparoscopic myomectomies with 49 open myomectomies. *J Am Assoc Gynecol Laparosc* 1997;4:457.
Sullivan B, Kenney P, Seibel M. Hysteroscopic resection of fibroid with thermal injury to sigmoid. *Obstet Gynecol* 1992;80:546.
Tada S, Tsukioka M, Ishii C, et al. Computed tomographic features of uterine myoma. *J Comput Assist Tomogr* 1981;5:866.
Tamaya T, Fujimoto J, Okada H. Comparison of cellular levels of steroid receptors in uterine leiomyomata and myometrium. *Acta Obstet Gynecol Scand* 1985;64:307.
Thompson J. Anemia due to gynecologic disease. *South Med J* 1957;50:679.
Tierney WN, Ehrlich CE, Bailey JC, et al. Intravenous leiomyomatosis of the uterus with extension into the heart. *Am J Med* 1980;69:471.
Torpin R, Pond E, Peoples WJ. The etiologic and pathologic factors in a series of 1,741 fibromyomas of the uterus. *Am J Obstet Gynecol* 1942;44:569.
Townsend DE, Sparkes RS, Baluda MC, et al. Unicellular histogenesis of uterine leiomyomas as determined by electrophoresis of glucose-6-phosphate dehydrogenase. *Am J Obstet Gynecol* 1970;107:1168.
Tulandi T, Murray C, Guralneck M. Adhesion formation and reproductive outcome after myomectomy and second-look laparoscopy. *Obstet Gynecol* 1993;82:213.
Upadhyaya N, Doddy M, Googe P. Histopathologic changes in leiomyomata treated with leuprolide acetate. *Fertil Steril* 1990;54:811.
Vasserman J, Baracat E, Bondu KC, et al. Vascularization of uterine myomata. *Abstracts of the 12th World Congress of Obstetrics and Gynecology* 1988:108.
Vercellini P, Bocciolone L, Rognoni M, et al. Fibroids and infertility. *Adv Reprod Endocrinol* 1992;4:47.
Vercellini P, Crosignani PG, Mangioni C, et al. Treatment with a gonadotrophin releasing hormone agonist before hysterectomy for leiomyomas: results of a multicentre randomised controlled trial. *BJOG* 1998;105:1148.
Vercellini P, Maddalena S, De Giorgi O, et al. Determinants of reproductive outcome after abdominal myomectomy for infertility. *Fertil Steril* 1999;72: 109.
Vercellini P, Zaina B, Yaylayan L, et al. Hysteroscopic myomectomy: long term effects on menstrual pattern and fertility. *Obstet Gynecol* 1999;94:341.

Verkauf B. Changing trends in treatment of leiomyomata uteri. *Curr Opin Obstet Gynecol* 1993;5:301.

Verkauf B. Myomectomy for fertility enhancement and preservation. *Fertil Steril* 1992;58:1.

Vollenhoven BJ, Lawrence AS, Healy DL. Uterine fibroids: a clinical review. *BJOG* 1990;97:285.

Wallach E, Vu K. Myomata uteri and infertility. *Obstet Gynecol Clin North Am* 1995;22:791.

Wallach EE, Vlahos NF. Uterine myomas: an overview of development, clinical features, and management. *Obstet Gynecol* 2004;104(2):393.

Wamsteker K, Emanuel MH, deKruif JH. Transcervical hysteroscopic resection of submucous fibroids for abnormal uterine bleeding: results regarding the degree of intramural extension. *Obstet Gynecol* 1993;82:736.

Watanabe Y, Nakamura G. Effects of two different doses of leuprolide acetate depot on uterine cavity area in patients with uterine leiomyomata. *Fertil Steril* 1995;63:487.

Weather L. Cardon dioxide laser myomectomy. *J Natl Med Assoc* 1986;78:933.

Weiss DB, Aldor A, Aboulafia Y. Erythrocytosis due to erythropoietin-producing uterine fibromyoma. *Am J Obstet Gynecol* 1975;122:358.

West C, Lumsden M, Lawson S, et al. Shrinkage of uterine fibroids during therapy with goserelin (Zoladex): a luteinizing hormone-releasing hormone agonist administered as a monthly subcutaneous depot. *Fertil Steril* 1987;48:45.

Wilson EA, Yang F, Rees ED. Estradiol and progesterone binding in uterine leiomyomata and in normal uterine tissues. *Obstet Gynecol* 1980;55:20.

Winer-Muram HT, Muram D, Gillieson MS, et al. Uterine myomas in pregnancy. *Can Med Assoc J* 1983;128:949.

Wiskind A, Thompson J. Abdominal myomectomy: reducing the risk of hemorrhage. *Semin Reprod Endocrinol* 1992;10:358.

Wong GC, Muir SJ, Lai AP, et al. Uterine artery embolization: a minimally invasive technique for the treatment of uterine fibroids. *Journal of Women's Health and Gender-Based Medicine* 2000;9:357.

Worthington-Kirsch R, Spies JB, Myers ER, et al; FIBROID investigators. The Fibroid Registry for outcomes data (FIBROID) for uterine embolization: short term outcomes. *Obstet Gynecol* 2005;106:52. Erratum in: *Obstet Gynecol* 2005;106:869.

Wray RC Jr, Dawkins H. Primary smooth muscle tumors of the inferior vena cava. *Ann Surg* 1971;174:1009.

Yamamoto T, Urabe M, Naitoh K, et al. Estrone sulfatase activity in human leiomyoma. *Gynecol Oncol* 1990;37:315.

Ylikorkala O, Kauppila A, Rajala T. Pituitary gonadotrophins and prolactin in patients with endometrial cancer, fibroids or ovarian tumours. *BJOG* 1979;86:901.

Zawin M, McCarthy S, Scoutt LM, et al. High-field MRI and US evaluation of the pelvis in women with leiomyomas. *Magn Reson Imaging* 1990;8:371.

Zreik TG, Rutherford TJ, Palter SF, et al. Cryomyolysis: a new procedure for the conservative treatment of uterine fibroids. *J Am Assoc Gynecol Laparosc* 1998;5:33.

CHAPTER 32A ■ ABDOMINAL HYSTERECTOMY

HOWARD W. JONES III

DEFINITIONS

Incidental oophorectomy—When clinically normal ovaries are removed at the time of a hysterectomy. This is an older term. *Prophylactic oophorectomy* is now preferred.

Prophylactic oophorectomy—The preferred term for removing clinically normal ovaries at the time of hysterectomy. This terminology emphasizes the risk reduction of ovarian and possibly breast cancer as a result of oophorectomy.

Supracervical hysterectomy—Also referred to as a *subtotal hysterectomy*. This operation removes the uterine fundus, transecting the upper portion of the cervix below the level of the uterine vessels. The cervix is left *in situ*.

Trendelenburg position—With the patient on the operating table in the supine position, the head is lowered below the level of the pelvis.

Hysterectomy is the most common operation performed by the gynecologist, and it is the second most common major surgical procedure done in the United States. Only cesarean section is more common. There are many indications for hysterectomy, and the uterus can be removed using any of a variety of techniques and approaches, including abdominal, vaginal, or laparoscopic. In most cases, a total hysterectomy with removal of the uterine corpus and cervix is done; but in recent years, there has been a resurgence in the popularity of supracervical hysterectomy. The ovaries and tubes may or may not be removed along with the uterus, depending on the patient's age and a variety of other factors. The gynecologic surgeon should be not only technically adept at these various procedures, but also should use history, physical examination, and discussion with the patient to match the surgical procedure to the patient to obtain the most satisfactory outcome.

The three sections of this chapter discuss abdominal, vaginal, and laparoscopic hysterectomy.

HISTORY

The history of hysterectomy is long and varied. Although significant advances in the technique of hysterectomy did not occur until the 19th century, earlier attempts are known. Some references to hysterectomy even date to the 5th century B.C., in the time of Hippocrates. The earliest attempts at removal of the uterus were made vaginally for indications of uterine prolapse or uterine inversion. By the 16th century, a number of hysterectomies already had been done in Europe, including Italy, Germany, and Spain. In 1600, Schenck of Grabenberg cataloged 26 cases of vaginal hysterectomy.

Vaginal hysterectomies were done sporadically through the 17th and 18th centuries. In 1810, Wrisberg presented a paper to the Vienna Royal Academy of Medicine recommending vaginal hysterectomy for uterine cancer. Three years later, the German surgeon Langenbeck successfully performed a vaginal hysterectomy for uterine cancer. The first vaginal hysterectomy performed in the United States was in 1829 by John Collins Warren at Harvard University; however, the patient expired on the fourth postoperative day. Three years following Warren's attempt, Herman and Werneberg in Pittsburgh successfully performed a vaginal hysterectomy for uterine cancer. By the late 19th century, techniques for vaginal hysterectomy were systematically studied and developed by Czerny, Billroth, Mikulicz, Schroeder, Kocher, Teuffel, and Spencer Wells.

The earliest abdominal hysterectomy attempts usually involved uterine leiomyomas that had been misdiagnosed as ovarian cysts. In the early 19th century, laparotomy for ovarian cysts still was considered dangerous, despite initial successes by McDowell in the United States and Emiliami in Europe in 1815. Abdominal hysterectomy for any reason was considered impossible to accomplish successfully. Many of the earliest myomectomies involved pedunculated tumors. Washington L. Atlee of Lancaster, Pennsylvania, performed the first successful abdominal myomectomy in 1844; although in a series of 125 surgeries, he did not attempt to remove the uterus.

The first reported abdominal hysterectomy was attempted by Langenbeck in 1825. The 7-minute operation for advanced cervical cancer resulted in the patient's demise several hours later. Abdominal surgery was commonly complicated by postoperative hemorrhage that was often lethal. In the mid-19th century, an English surgeon, A. M. Heath from Manchester, was the first to ligate the uterine arteries, but it would be nearly 50 years before his technique became common practice.

Successful surgery depends on control of bleeding, infection, and pain. Ligatures were known to be used to clamp bleeding vessels as early as 1090, and artery forceps were invented in the mid-16th century by Ambroise Pare. However, information regarding the pathophysiology of hemorrhage, shock, and blood transfusions was not available until the 20th century. The importance of infection control was first recognized by Austrian Ignaz Semmelweiss in his work with childbed fever. His 1840s work was furthered by Joseph Lister in the 1860s, and aided by notable discoveries by Louis Pasteur and Robert Koch. American Crawford W. Long first used ether as anesthesia in 1842, and Scotsman Sir James Y. Simpson initiated use of chloroform in his obstetric practice.

It was not until 1864 that the Frenchman Koeberle introduced his method of securing the large vascular pedicle of the lower uterus with his tool, the serrenoeud. This ligature en masse around the lower uterus with the corpus amputated above was the usual technique of controlling bleeding with hysterectomy in the earliest years. The stump thus formed was such a large mass of tissue that it could not always be safely returned to the peritoneal cavity owing to risk of intraperitoneal bleeding; often the stump was fixed extraperitoneally in the incision so that it could be clamped later if necessary.

W.A. Freund of Germany further refined hysterectomy techniques in 1878 using anesthesia, antiseptic technique, Trendelenburg position, and ligature around ligaments and major vessels. The bladder was dissected from the uterus, and the cardinal and uterosacral ligaments were detached; the pelvic peritoneum then was closed. Late in the 19th century, further refinements were made to abdominal hysterectomy techniques by the surgeons of the Johns Hopkins Hospital, where they reduced their mortality to 5.9%.

In the early decades of the 20th century, hysterectomy became more commonly used as treatment for gynecologic disease and symptoms. Gynecology as a specialty was developing, and little else but surgery was available to gynecologists to help their patients. Major discoveries and concepts of reproductive organ physiology and pathology were just beginning. As surgery became safer, gynecologists concentrated on developing newer surgical procedures. Estrogen and progesterone were not discovered until the late 1920s and early 1930s.

As gynecology matured as a specialty, knowledge of reproductive organ function and disease became more complete. Special and more accurate diagnostic techniques were developed, and effective nonsurgical methods of therapy were discovered. In the modern practice of gynecology, appropriate use of this knowledge and advanced modern diagnostic technologies allow more correct choices of treatment for complicated medical diseases. With proper use of blood transfusions and antibiotics, and with improvements in anesthetic techniques, a hysterectomy can be done safely by the skillful gynecologic surgeon. Mortality from hysterectomy in most medical centers is one to two per 1,000. It is not unusual to report no mortalities in a series of several thousand hysterectomies for benign disease. With the use of prophylactic antibiotics, infectious morbidity has greatly decreased, and overall morbidity rates have been greatly reduced as a result of improved techniques and training.

INCIDENCE

Hysterectomy is a very common surgical procedure. In the United States, more than half a million women undergo hysterectomy each year, and it is estimated that by age 65, one third of women in this country will have had their uterus surgically removed. Annual medical costs related to hysterectomy exceed $5 billion in the United States. However, there are significant variations in hysterectomy rates within the United States and throughout the world. In a study from the Kaiser health care plan in California, Jacobson and colleagues reported an overall hysterectomy rate of 3.41 per 1,000 women older than age 20 in 2003. This is similar but somewhat lower than the rate of 4.7 per 1,000 women reported from Olmsted County, Minnesota, from 1995 to 2002. In a nationwide sample, Farquhar and Steiner reported an overall hysterectomy rate of 5.6 per 1,000 women in the United States in 1997. In Western Australia, Spilsbury and colleagues recently reported an age-standardized rate of 4.8 per 1,000 women. In Italy, Mataria has reported a rate of 3.7, and a very low rate of 1.2 per 1,000 eligible women was reported from Norway.

This variation in rates from one location to another is due to several factors, including patient expectations and availability of medical care. But it is primarily related to the training and practice patterns of the local gynecologic surgeons. In some areas, abnormal uterine bleeding may be managed primarily by hormonal therapy, whereas in other locations, hysterectomy may be quickly recommended. Alternatives to hysterectomy have decreased the rate of hysterectomy in recent years. Systemic hormonal therapies have been effective for managing menorrhagia; recently, a progestational intrauterine system has been shown to be similarly effective. Intrauterine thermal balloons, microwave, and electrical instruments are all effective outpatient techniques for endometrial ablation as an alternative to hysterectomy for symptomatic uterine bleeding. Leiomyomas can now be treated with transcervical hysteroscopic resection and also by transcatheter uterine artery embolization. These new management techniques, together with an overall desire to decrease the use of major surgery, have decreased the use of hysterectomy in recent years.

In addition, today's gynecologic surgeon has several techniques for hysterectomy from which to choose. Although abdominal hysterectomy is still the most commonly used approach, there has been a definite increase in the use of both vaginal and laparoscopic hysterectomy in recent years. Table 32A.1 shows the frequency of the various techniques in recent reports from around the world. For the first time, this edition of the hysterectomy chapter is subdivided into sections on abdominal, vaginal, and laparoscopic hysterectomy. In this section, we will concentrate on the abdominal approach to hysterectomy.

TABLE 32A.1

WORLDWIDE COMPARISON OF HYSTERECTOMY TECHNIQUE

	Abdominal (%)	Vaginal (%)	Laparoscopic (%)
USA, nationwide	63	29	11
USA, California	71	25	4
USA, Minnesota	44	56	<1
England	75	23	1.4
Australia	40	45	15
Denmark	80	14	6
Finland	58	18	24

INDICATIONS FOR HYSTERECTOMY

Table 32A.2 lists commonly accepted indications for hysterectomy. As discussed above, a variety of new surgical and nonsurgical techniques or treatments are now available to manage many of the symptoms or conditions for which hysterectomy has been required in the past. These approaches are often a compromise, and hysterectomy frequently remains the final management option for some patients, such as those who continue to have more bleeding than they are willing to tolerate after transcervical endometrial ablation.

Uterine leiomyoma continues to be the most common indication for hysterectomy. In a study of more than 2 million hysterectomies done in the United States in the 1990s, Farquhar and Steiner reported that leiomyoma was the indication for 40% of all abdominal hysterectomies. Other common indications included endometriosis (12.8%), cancer (12.6%), abnormal bleeding (9.5%), pelvic inflammatory disease (3.7%) and uterine prolapse (3.0%). In contrast, prolapse was the

TABLE 32A.2

INDICATIONS FOR HYSTERECTOMY

Benign disease	Malignant disease
Abnormal bleeding	Cervical intraepithelial neoplasm
Leiomyoma	
Adenomyosis	Invasive cervical cancer
Endometriosis	Atypical endometrial hyperplasia
Pelvic organ prolapse	Endometrial cancer
Pelvic inflammatory disease	Ovarian cancer
	Fallopian tube cancer
Chronic pelvic pain	Gestational trophoblastic tumors
Pregnancy-related conditions	

indication for 44% of all vaginal hysterectomies, and fibroids accounted for only 17%. In their study, abdominal hysterectomy accounted for 63% of all hysterectomies in the United States in 1997, whereas vaginal hysterectomies were done 23% of the time and laparoscopic hysterectomy accounted for 9.9% of the total.

Kovac has shown that vaginal hysterectomy can be safely and effectively performed in most patients for most indications, and many studies have shown that the morbidity and costs are generally lower with vaginal hysterectomy compared with abdominal hysterectomy. However, large leiomyomas, pelvic inflammatory disease, cancer, and most suspicious adnexal masses may still be better approached abdominally. In some cases, hysterectomy may be done in conjunction with other abdominal procedures, such as removal of a benign or malignant ovarian tumor or treatment of chronic pelvic inflammatory disease or endometriosis. There may be no pathologic changes in such a uterus, and some have contended that these are examples of an "unnecessary hysterectomy." This is certainly not true, but it is important that the surgeon clearly explain why the uterus is being removed as a part of the surgical procedure. Because abdominal hysterectomy is the most common major gynecologic operation done in the United States, it is under careful scrutiny by a variety of regulatory agencies and public health care policy groups. The surgeon should carefully evaluate each patient and consider the diagnosis and management options before recommending hysterectomy and, specifically, abdominal hysterectomy. Numerous studies have shown that women who have undergone hysterectomy show a significant improvement in their quality-of-life indices. But care must be taken to make the correct diagnosis, be sure that the patient's condition will benefit from hysterectomy, and recommend the most appropriate type of hysterectomy for that specific patient.

The late Richard W. Te Linde, professor of gynecology at the Johns Hopkins University and the original author of this text, wrote:

> The ease with which the average hysterectomy may be done has proven both a blessing and a curse to womankind. There is no doubt that a hysterectomy done with proper indications may restore a woman to health and even save her life. However, in the practice of gynecology, one has ample opportunity to observe countless women who have been advised to have hysterectomies without proper indications ... I am inclined to believe that the greatest single factor in promoting unnecessary hysterectomies is a lack of understanding of gynecologic pathology. The greatest need today among those who are performing pelvic surgery is a better knowledge of gynecologic pathology.

CHOICE OF APPROACH: ABDOMINAL, VAGINAL, OR LAPAROSCOPIC

Today, there are many different approaches to hysterectomy. The uterus can be removed via the abdominal route, transvaginally, or laparoscopically. Combinations of several techniques can be selected, such as a laparoscopically assisted vaginal hysterectomy. Although abdominal hysterectomy continues to be the most common approach used worldwide, there is good evidence from multiple randomized, prospective trials that vaginal hysterectomy is associated with fewer complications, a shorter hospital stay, a more rapid recovery, and lower overall costs (Table 32A.3). In addition, Kovac and others have shown that most patients who require hysterectomy can have it performed vaginally. Who, then, is a proper candidate for an abdominal hysterectomy? Most patients with gynecologic malignancy are still operated on with an abdominal incision. Although this will undoubtedly continue to be true for women with ovarian cancer who frequently have extensive pelvic and upper abdominal metastases, laparoscopic techniques and more recently robotic surgical techniques are being used more and more frequently in women with endometrial and cervical cancer.

Another indication for abdominal hysterectomy is a large uterus that prevents safe and reasonable vaginal hysterectomy. This is obviously very dependent on the skills and experience of the surgeon, because there are various techniques that allow a very large benign uterus to be removed from below. Nevertheless, most gynecologists would agree that a uterus larger than 12 weeks' gestational size is a reasonable size to qualify for an abdominal approach. The shape and size of the pelvic outlet are also key factors; although the degree of prolapse is not an absolute factor, patients with limited uterine prolapse are

TABLE 32A.3

CHARACTERISTICS OF HYSTERECTOMY BY DIFFERENT APPROACHES

	Abdominal	Vaginal	Laparoscopically assisted vaginal
Number of patients	1,184	530	839
Uterine weight (average)	216 g	113 g	129 g
Operative time (average)	82 min	63 min	102 min
Blood loss[a] (average)	5.35%	5.19%	6.0%
Complications			
Fever 101°F	9.1%	3.2%	2.0%
Transfused	2.5%	0.9%	0.6%
Bowel, bladder or ureteral injury	1.0%	0.9%	0.7%
Death	0	1	0
Hospital stay	60 h	40 h	40 h
Hospital charges	$6,552	$5,879	$6,431

[a]Blood loss is percent change in preoperative versus postoperative hematocrit.

From: Johns DA, Carrera B, Jones J, et al. The medical and economic impact of laparoscopically assisted vaginal hysterectomy in a large, metropolitan, not-for-profit hospital. *Am J Obstet Gynecol* 1995;172:1709, with permission.

more difficult to do transvaginally. Cervical fibroids or cervical enlargement for any reason may compromise vaginal exposure and make it difficult to place clamps laterally.

An unknown adnexal mass, extensive pelvic endometriosis, or adhesions from prior surgery or pelvic infection may also be an indication for an open abdominal approach including a hysterectomy. In some cases, a diagnostic laparoscopy will clarify the situation and may allow the procedure to be converted to a laparoscopically assisted vaginal hysterectomy. A careful preoperative evaluation—starting with a thoughtful history and physical examination and supplemented, where indicated, by imaging studies such as a pelvic ultrasound or computerized tomography scan of the pelvis and abdomen—will usually enable the gynecologist to decide on the most appropriate type of hysterectomy. The diagnosis and reason for the approach selected should be thoroughly explained and discussed with the patient and any appropriate family or friends. In rare cases, the final decision concerning the type of hysterectomy will depend on the findings of the exam under anesthesia or the findings at laparoscopy. In those cases, all the "what ifs . . . " should be carefully reviewed with the patient before the surgery and the family kept informed as decisions are made during surgery.

Subtotal Versus Total Hysterectomy for Benign Conditions

In the United States, and throughout most of the world, hysterectomy—whether done transvaginally or through an abdominal incision—usually includes removal of the cervix. Over the past 50 years, subtotal or supracervical hysterectomy has come to be viewed as a suboptimal procedure reserved for those rare instances when concern over blood loss or anatomic distortion dictates limiting the extent of dissection. Recently, there have been some concerns about a reduced quality of orgasmic function and bladder dysfunction after the cervix has been removed. Much has been written about this in the lay media, and there are undoubtedly some women who develop problems after hysterectomy. However, several recent prospective, randomized studies in the United States and abroad have shown no difference in sexual satisfaction, bowel or bladder function, or vaginal prolapse after simple total hysterectomy compared with supracervical hysterectomy for benign disease. My own clinical experience over 30 years also confirms this impression.

Nonetheless, the routine practice of removing the cervix at the time of hysterectomy for benign disease is now being challenged as many traditional surgical procedures are being modified to accommodate minimally invasive techniques. A new technique of total laparoscopic hysterectomy (as initially described by Semm) involves coring out the endocervical tissue and presumably the squamocolumnar junction area, which should practically eliminate the risk of cervical cancer. More recently, a laparoscopic tissue morcellator has been used to perform a supracervical hysterectomy. However, total laparoscopic hysterectomy has been associated with an increased risk of ureteral and bladder injury so that laparoscopic supracervical hysterectomy has been introduced to avoid these complications. The rapidity of the procedure, the quick postoperative recovery, and the popularity of cervical preservation among the lay public has now resulted in an increased use of abdominal supracervical hysterectomy. There is clearly a market for this procedure, but all of the recent prospective, randomized trials have not found any long-term advantage of supracervical abdominal hysterectomy compared with total abdominal hysterectomy. Further experience will be needed to see if these techniques offer any advantage and if retention of the cervix does not lead to problems with cervical neoplasia or bleeding from the endocervix and lower uterine segment.

Management of Normal Ovaries

Should normal ovaries be removed at the time of hysterectomy for benign disease? The term **prophylactic oophorectomy** is preferred when referring to the removal of clinical normal ovaries at the time of hysterectomy. The use of **incidental oophorectomy** is not recommended because it suggests that an oophorectomy is done without planning or consideration and has no consequences. There is no doubt that bilateral oophorectomy reduces the risk of ovarian cancer and the need for future surgery for benign conditions of the ovaries. However, the ovaries continue to produce low levels of androgens even after the menopause; and although the benefits, if any, of this hormone production are unknown, the psychological effect of oophorectomy on some women is significant.

Prophylactic oophorectomy is done in 50% to 66% of women aged 40 to 65 who undergo hysterectomy in the United States. Averette and Nguyen have estimated that 1,000 of the approximately 24,000 new cases of ovarian cancer in the United States would be prevented if prophylactic bilateral salpingo-oophorectomy was done at the time of hysterectomy on all women older than age 40.

Clearly, there are some significant potential benefits to oophorectomy at the time of any pelvic surgery in women with a known BRCA-1 or BRCA-2 gene mutation, a strong family history of ovarian or breast cancer, or women of Eastern European Jewish heritage.

In a follow-up study of 1,200 women who underwent hysterectomy with at least one ovary retained, Plockinger and Kolbl found that new pathology in the remaining ovary led to reoperation in approximately 4% of the patients. Older data supports this rate of reoperation for problems related to ovaries left behind at operation.

Interestingly, an analysis of the Cancer and Steroid Hormone Study by Irwin and colleagues from the Centers for Disease Control and Prevention (CDC), including women 20 to 54 years old, found a 40% reduction in the risk of ovarian cancer in women who had a hysterectomy *even* with ovarian conservation, unilateral or bilateral. The protection was still present 10 years after surgery (RR = 0.6), but disappeared after two decades. The reason(s) for this risk reduction is unknown, but may be related to the opportunity to examine the ovaries at the time of hysterectomy with removal of those that are abnormal and conservation of those that are grossly normal. Other possible mechanisms include reduction in ovarian blood flow and steroidogenesis after hysterectomy, a higher frequency of previous oral contraceptive use among women who undergo hysterectomy, and protection of ovaries from transtubal migration of potential vaginal carcinogens.

Four case control studies that found a lower risk of ovarian cancer among women who had a history of previous hysterectomy with ovarian conservation have been analyzed by Weiss and Harlow. The authors felt the reduction in ovarian cancer risk was explained by incidental screening for visible ovarian malignancy at the time of hysterectomy in those women in whom the ovaries are not removed. Those women with grossly normal ovaries have a reduced risk of developing symptomatic ovarian cancer over the next few years.

Recent studies also have clearly shown a decrease in the risk of breast cancer in women who have undergone bilateral oophorectomy. This is of particular importance in women from families with a history of ovarian or breast cancer and those with known BRCA gene mutations. In a series of 177 women with BRCA1 or BRCA2 mutations who were enrolled prospectively and followed for up to 6 years, Kauf and associates reported a 4% incidence of breast cancer among the 69 women who underwent prophylactic oophorectomy compared with a 13% incidence among those who elected follow-up surveillance only. In a similar retrospective review of 259 women compared with matched controls, the risk of breast cancer was reduced by 50% in the women who had bilateral oophorectomy. In both series, the risk of peritoneal or ovarian cancer was decreased by 95%.

No studies have examined the operative morbidity of adding oophorectomy at the time of abdominal hysterectomy. There is a slight theoretical risk of ligation or obstruction of the ureter at the time of ligation of the ovarian vessels, but this risk should be very minimal in women with truly normal ovaries who are undergoing abdominal hysterectomy for benign disease. The long-term consequences of the loss of minimal androgen production by the postmenopausal ovary is unknown, but the benefits of hormonal production by the normal premenopausal ovary are significant. Prevention of osteoporosis, urogenital atrophy, skin changes, and possible prevention of arteriosclerotic vascular disease are but some of the known benefits of ovarian estrogens. Clearly, removal of the normal ovaries in a premenopausal woman mandates hormone replacement therapy to prevent these undesirable side effects of the hypoestrogenic state.

However, in a study of 165 premenopausal women who were prescribed estrogen replacement therapy following bilateral oophorectomy, Castelo-Branco and colleagues found that only one third continued their medication for 5 years. Fear of cancer was the most common reason for discontinuation. The anticipated protection from osteoporosis and other consequences of premature menopause that result from oophorectomy may not be effectively prevented by oral hormone replacement therapy because many patients stop or do not take estrogen as prescribed.

Traditionally, many gynecologists have recommended against prophylactic oophorectomy in women younger than the age of 40 and offered oophorectomy to postmenopausal women. There is no consensus for the management of women between 40 and 50. There are no data to support these approaches. It seems reasonable to discuss the possibility of oophorectomy before planned hysterectomy for benign disease in women older than age 45. However, it should be made clear to those women that there are some definite disadvantages to oophorectomy, especially if they will not or cannot use estrogen replacement therapy postoperatively. Each patient brings her own ideas and experiences to this discussion, and the surgeon should try to counsel the patient and her family so she will be happy with her decision about oophorectomy.

PREOPERATIVE COUNSELING

The gynecologist needs to talk with the patient while trying to decide whether a hysterectomy is indicated. Fortunately for the patient and the gynecologist, time for talking is available in almost every instance. A hysterectomy is rarely an emergency. Unfortunately, the time may not be used properly. In a survey of women who underwent hysterectomy, Neefus and Taylor found that there is an urgent need for patient education on the physical, psychological, and sexual aspects of hysterectomy.

Often, the need for hysterectomy is obvious. There is a complete prolapse, or a large and symptomatic leiomyomatous uterus, or a pelvic cancer. Under these and other obvious circumstances, the patient should be told that a hysterectomy is recommended and why. The indication for surgery should be explained clearly and in language that the patient can understand. Treatment alternatives should be mentioned, and the reason to prefer hysterectomy should be explained. Alternative techniques for hysterectomy should be discussed, and the reasons for recommending one approach over another should be explained. The risks, benefits, and side effects, specifically including the possibility of transfusion, must be reviewed, but in such a way that the patient is not unduly alarmed. Then the patient and the physician should spend the time necessary to discuss any questions that the patient may have. Additionally, the patient should be encouraged to discuss details about the operation, how long it will take, the recuperation period in the hospital and at home, whether ovarian function should be conserved, and possible hormone replacement therapy. Patient information pamphlets and videos also are useful for preoperative education. The expectations of the patient and her family are very important in her postoperative view of the success (or failure) of the operation.

Because the uterus is the main organ associated with reproduction, it is an important part of a woman's self-image; in some cultures, a woman's sexuality and reproductive potential are viewed as important parts of her value or status in her family or society as a whole. For these reasons, it is absolutely necessary for the gynecologic surgeon to understand and help patients cope with the emotional turmoil that may accompany hysterectomy. For some women who have had their children and need a hysterectomy for prolonged heavy bleeding and cramping associated with uterine fibroids or those with a diagnosis of endometrial cancer, the indications are clear, the benefits are obvious, and the loss of reproductive capacity often is not of great concern. The emotional stress of hysterectomy on these women is usually minimal, and psychological adjustment often is rapid and complete. However, the young woman needing a hysterectomy for cervical cancer or a ruptured cornual pregnancy may have considerable difficulty adjusting to the loss of her uterus. Even the 32-year-old woman with three children and severe uterovaginal prolapse may not be comfortable with the idea of hysterectomy. The gynecologist must be sensitive to these possible concerns and anxiety. Even when the patient does not express any emotional distress, the gynecologist can provide an opening for the patient to discuss her feelings by statements such as, "Most studies have shown no change in sexuality and sexual function after hysterectomy, but I know many patients have concerns about this. Do you have any questions?" The support of the patient's husband or partner and her family and friends are very useful elements to prevent and manage depression and the emotional stress of hysterectomy. The wise surgeon includes members of this support group in preoperative discussions and encourages them to ask questions or express opinions that actually may be questions or opinions of the patient that she is hesitant to express.

Despite improvements in preoperative counseling in recent years, some women are depressed after hysterectomy. In most instances, this depression is short-lived and self-limiting, but the gynecologist should be alert for severe or prolonged symptoms of continued lack of energy, inability to return to normal activities of daily living, sleep difficulties, or other indicators of depression following surgery. Occasionally, antidepressants and/or psychiatric consultation may be necessary.

The psychological aspects of pelvic surgery are extensively reviewed in Chapter 3.

PREPARATION FOR HYSTERECTOMY

A complete history and physical examination is indicated before any operative procedure. This evaluation is detailed in Chapter 8, but a few points deserve emphasis. Although it is appropriate to ensure that all gynecologic symptoms have been evaluated carefully and a pelvic examination performed, a complete physical evaluation is necessary to be sure the patient can safely tolerate anesthesia and major surgery. Appropriate consultation should be sought where indicated to assure safe anesthesia administration and anticipation of any perioperative medical problems. In addition to a preoperative hematocrit or hemoglobin and other laboratory tests as indicated by the patient's medical condition, it is important to have a recent Pap test to rule out cervical neoplasia. A pregnancy test in reproductive-age women is recommended before surgery.

Preoperative chest x-rays are no longer routinely recommended, but may be indicated in women with a history of cardiorespiratory disease or malignancy. An intravenous pyelogram or computed tomography scan of the abdomen and pelvis may be useful in women with uterine or extrauterine pelvic masses, but these are not indicated routinely.

Although the value of a bowel preparation before simple hysterectomy has been questioned in recent years, we prefer to have the colon evacuated before pelvic surgery to facilitate exposure and reduce trauma to the bowel caused by retraction and packing. We recommend a clear liquid diet on the day before surgery, and 250 cc of oral magnesium citrate is an effective laxative on the afternoon before surgery. A bisacodyl suppository immediately on arising on the morning of surgery will evacuate any residual feces or fluid in the sigmoid and prevent contamination of the field during surgery. A complete mechanical or antibiotic bowel preparation is indicated only when intestinal surgery is a possibility (see Chapter 43).

Surgical site infection risk is decreased by routine use of prophylactic intravenous antibiotics given immediately before induction of anesthesia. First- or second-generation cephalosporins, such as cefazolin or cefoxitin, are commonly used. Recommended antibiotic regimens are shown in Table 32A.4. Prospective, randomized trials have shown a significant reduction in the risk of febrile morbidity and infection in both abdominal and vaginal hysterectomy. Studies have shown no benefit of continuing antibiotics postoperatively, although a second dose of antibiotics generally should be given during hysterectomy procedures that last longer than 3 hours. Some have suggested that bacterial vaginosis increases the risk of postoperative infections after vaginal hysterectomy, but preoperative evaluation and treatment remains controversial. Although povidone-iodine douches and antibiotic scrubs before surgery have been widely used in the past, no added benefit is apparent when perioperative intravenous antibiotics are employed.

If necessary, the pubic and/or vulvar hair should be clipped with an electric clipper or even scissors rather than shaved. The patient should be instructed not to shave the operative site before surgery because it has been shown to increase the risk of wound infection and cellulitis.

TABLE 32A.4

RECOMMENDED PROPHYLACTIC ANTIBIOTIC REGIMENS FOR HYSTERECTOMY

Antibiotic	Dosage	Half-life
Cefoxitin	2 mg IV	0.5–1.1 h
Cefazolin	1–2 g IV	1.2–2.5 h
Cefotetan	1–2 g IV	2.8–4.6 h
For patients with an immediate sensitivity to penicillin		
Metronidazol[a]	1 g IV	6–14 h
OR		
Metronidazole[b] +	1 g IV	
gentamycin or a quinolone	1.5 mg/kg or 500 mg	
OR		
Clindamycin[b]	900 mg IV	2–5 h

IV, intravenously.
[a]American College of Obstetricians and Gynecologists. ACOG Practice Bulletin No. 74. *Antibiotic prophylaxis for gynecologic procedures.* Washington, DC: ACOG;2006.
[b]Surgical Care Improvement Project recommendation, October 2006. Surgical Care Improvement Project. *Prophylactic antibiotic regimen selection for surgery.* Available at: http://www.mediqic.org/scip. Accessed April 16, 2007.

TOTAL ABDOMINAL HYSTERECTOMY: SURGICAL TECHNIQUE

Previous editions of Te Linde's text have described gradually evolving modifications of Edward H. Richardson's technique for abdominal hysterectomy with which thousands of gynecologic surgeons have been trained over the years. The operative technique was first published in 1929, and because Te Linde felt it was a classic, he quoted it word-for-word in the fourth edition of this textbook with two added "modifications." This was the edition on my bedside table when I was a resident. I have had the good fortune to operate with many fine surgeons, including E. Stewart Taylor and Felix Rutledge, and have been challenged by many young residents over the years. These experiences have been further enhanced by discussions of surgical technique with gynecologists from around the world, who have suggested changes or ideas that I have tried and sometimes incorporated into my basic technique for abdominal hysterectomy. Although it is important to learn a basic technique for standard abdominal hysterectomy, every surgeon should be interested in observing new and different techniques or modifications to be tried from time to time when appropriate. As a resident, you should try all of the different techniques used by the different attending physicians, always asking why this clamp is used, that suture or needle is selected, or why the cuff is left open or closed. Having tried many different ideas, each gynecologic surgeon gradually evolves her or his own basic techniques that feel comfortable, work for him or her, and make sense. Because each patient is unique, it also is useful to have experience with different techniques and various modifications of the basic operation so that when the occasion calls for it, an alternative technique that is more suitable for the particular situation can be employed. Our basic technique for abdominal hysterectomy and several modifications are described in the following.

On the day of surgery, the surgeon always attempts to see the patient and her family and supporters before she is brought into the operating room. Although surgery may be routine to the gynecologist, major surgery is often a once-in-a-lifetime, frightening experience for the patient. The calm reassurance of the surgeon and the professional and caring nature of the entire operative team is very helpful to the patient and her family at this point. The focus of attention should be on the patient and her surgery. A certain amount of relaxed chatter about someone's birthday or hospital gossip is reasonable, but the patient should feel that the concentration of the surgical team is focused on the surgery at hand. Remarks about other patients or how the surgeon had to stay up all night with a difficult patient in labor are not appropriate. An equipment problem or technical difficulties that affect the operation certainly should be discussed with the surgeon before starting the procedure; however, it is inappropriate to talk about these in front of the patient. Remarks such as, "The table is broken and won't go down" or "We weren't able to get your favorite retractor today" may not affect the performance of the operation, but such statements just before a patient is ready to be anesthetized may raise serious doubts as to whether the operative team is optimally prepared for this operation and may raise uncomfortable questions later if complications or unexpected results occur.

Positioning

The patient is brought into the operating room and placed in the supine position on the operating table. It is nice to place a warm blanket on the bed immediately before the patient's arrival and to cover the patient with a blanket from the warmer when she is positioned because most operating rooms are somewhat cool and the patient is only lightly clothed.

When the patient has been anesthetized, a careful examination under anesthesia is done. At this point, the surgeon should concentrate on potential problems affecting resectability. Is there nodularity from endometriosis in the cul-de-sac that may make dissection of the rectum off of the posterior cervix difficult? Is the myoma in the broad ligament really wedged into the pelvic sidewall or does it move freely with the uterus? The mobility and descent of the uterus under anesthesia is particularly important when a vaginal hysterectomy is being considered. These potential problems and possible solutions should be considered and possibly discussed with the operative team while the surgeon scrubs.

The vagina and perineum are prepped with antiseptic solutions and a Foley catheter is inserted. I prefer to position the patient supine on the operative table with a soft pillow under her knees to provide gentle flexion. The patient's legs provide a table on which instruments can be placed. Some surgeons prefer the patient to be positioned in the low Allen stirrups with her legs slightly apart. This allows an assistant to stand between the legs and have ready access to the vagina for examination or manipulation, or the urethra for cystoscopy.

The abdomen then is prepped from the anterior thighs to the xiphoid, and sterile drapes are applied. In most instances, abdominal hysterectomy for benign disease can be done through a low transverse incision; most gynecologists prefer a Pfannenstiel incision, which is cosmetically appealing and strong. If more exposure is required, a Cherney or Maylard incision can be used, but a midline incision generally is done if malignant disease is present or exposure to the upper abdomen may be required. The choice of abdominal incision is discussed in Chapter 14.

Once the abdomen is opened, the pelvic pathology is carefully evaluated and the abdomen explored. The operating surgeon should examine the appendix and palpate the upper abdominal organs, including the kidneys, liver, gallbladder, stomach, spleen, diaphragm, and omentum. The retroperitoneal nodes in the pelvic and paraaortic area should be palpated and the area of the pancreas gently examined to identify any abnormalities. The status of these organs should be recorded in the operative note, and an intraoperative consultation may be indicated if abnormalities are identified.

After the abdomen has been explored, a slight Trendelenburg position should be requested, a self-retaining retractor placed, and the bowel packed superiorly to afford good exposure of the pelvis. Any adhesions of the small bowel or rectosigmoid may need to be divided at this time so that the bowel can be mobilized out of the operative field. In relatively thin patients with benign disease, I prefer to use a Kirschner retractor, which is light and simple and provides a choice of several fairly wide, shallow blades that fit on a square frame, allowing adjustable retraction laterally, inferiorly, and superiorly. The cecum and sigmoid are packed first with separate packs, and a third rolled or folded pack is placed in the center behind the superior retractor blade to hold back the small bowel. In larger patients, or patients with a longer midline incision, a Bookwalter or Omni-Tract retractor, with many options of blades and variable positioning, is invaluable. These large retractor systems are screwed onto the operating table and provide excellent retraction in almost any situation. They are particularly useful in obese patients.

Hysterectomy

When the bowel has been packed away and exposure to the pelvis is satisfactory, the round ligaments and uteroovarian ligaments are grasped on each side with a Kocher clamp, elevating the uterus out of the pelvis. In some cases of extensive inflammatory disease, endometriosis, malignancy, or very large fibroids, uterine mobility is limited; but in most benign conditions, uterine mobility is satisfactory. The operator is generally on the patient's left side so that the right-handed surgeon can use her or his dominant hand to extend down into the pelvis. The first assistant is on the opposite side. The uterus is retracted to the patient's left side, and the right round ligament is stretched taunt. A 0 delayed absorbable suture is placed under the round ligament approximately halfway between the uterus and the pelvic sidewall (Fig. 32A.1). The small artery of Sampson runs just under the round ligament and, in many cases, transilluminating this area allows the surgeon to easily visualize the artery and be sure that the suture is passed under it so that the artery will be ligated. A second suture is placed approximately 1 cm medial to the first suture; these two sutures are now tied simultaneously by the surgeon and first assistant. Clamping the round ligament is an extra step that is rarely necessary.

With traction on these sutures, the round ligament is held taunt and divided with Metzenbaum scissors between the two suture ligatures. This opens the retroperitoneal space, which is almost always a free space for blunt dissection, even in the patient with extensive tumor, inflammatory disease, or endometriosis. *If the ovaries are to be removed at the time of hysterectomy*, the peritoneal incision then is extended superiorly, lateral to the ovary and parallel with the infundibulopelvic ligament. The peritoneal incision also can be extended anteriorly down to the bladder reflection, but the peritoneum over

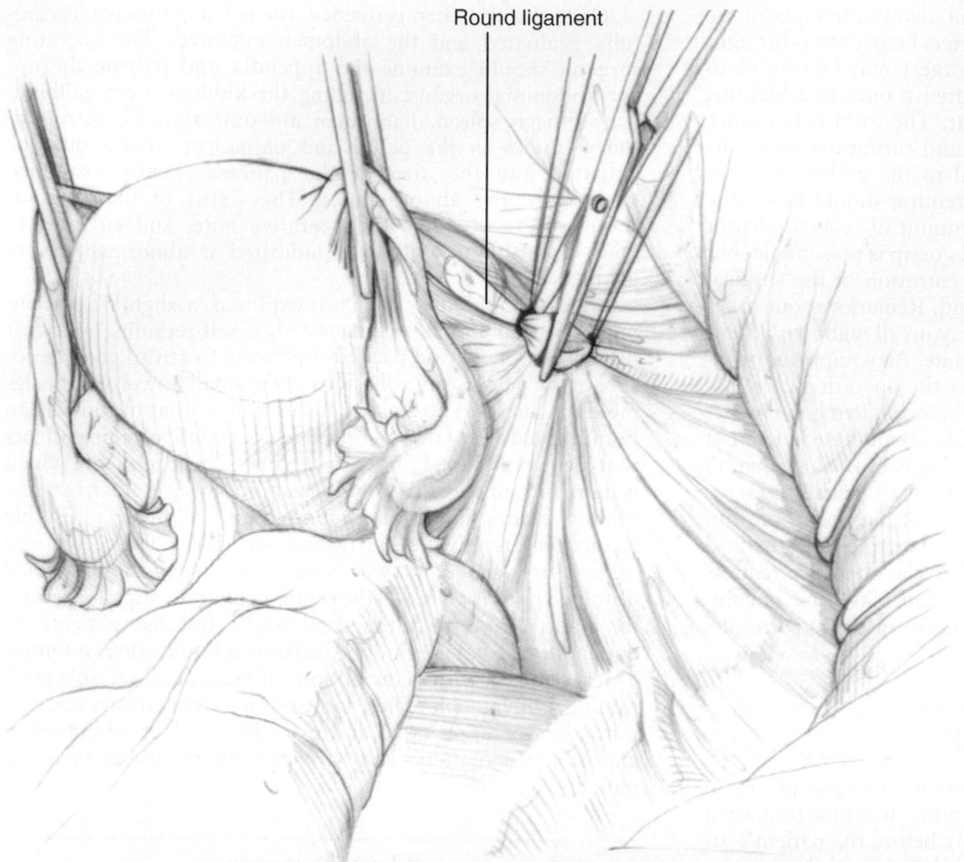

FIGURE 32A.1. The technique of abdominal hysterectomy begins with the round ligament. The ligament is ligated with transfixion sutures, and cut. The broad ligament is opened.

the anterior cervix does not need to be divided at this time because exposure of this area is not yet required and bleeding may be encountered. With the index finger and the tip of the suction or the back of a tissue forceps, the surgeon gently divides the loose areolar tissue of the retroperitoneum, identifying the external iliac artery on the medial surface of the psoas muscle. In most cases, the artery can be identified very easily, and blunt dissection is used to extend the exposure superiorly to the level of the bifurcation of the common iliac artery. The ureter always crosses the pelvic brim at this location and should be identified easily on the inside of the medial leaf of the peritoneum at this point. The internal iliac or hypogastric artery dives into the pelvis at this location parallel to the ureter, and it should be identified also. This retroperitoneal exploration may seem awkward at first, but with practice, the external and internal iliac arteries and ureter can be visualized easily in 10 to 20 seconds.

If the ovary is to be removed, a hole in the peritoneum between the ureter and the ovarian vessels superior to the ovary can be made under direct vision. We use a fairly fine sharp-pointed 9-inch clamp that can be passed gently through the peritoneum from lateral to medial against and between two fingers, supporting the medial side of the peritoneum. Alternatively, the peritoneum may be divided sharply or with the electrosurgical blade. We prefer to use a fairly delicate tonsil clamp on the infundibulopelvic ligament because it reminds us to isolate the vessels and take a fairly small pedicle. If there is significant inflammation or edema, a larger clamp, such as a Heaney clamp, may be used on the infundibulopelvic ligament pedicle (Fig. 32A.2). A second back clamp then is placed distally and the ovarian vessels divided between the two clamps. This pedicle then is ligated with a free-tie, and then a second transfixion suture ligature is placed for safety between the free-tie and the clamp. Zero-gauge delayed absorbable sutures and ties are used throughout. The suture ligature is placed distal to the free-tie so that if the needle happens to puncture one of the ovarian vessels, the vessel has already been ligated by the more proximal free-tie. The back clamp is ligated with a single free-tie, and the posterior peritoneum then is torn or cut above the ureter toward the back of the uterus, mobilizing the ovary, which is then tied to the clamp on the right side of the uterus to keep it from flopping around and obscuring the operative field. The sutures on the round ligaments and infundibulopelvic ligament then are cut. The procedure is repeated on the patient's left side.

If the ovary and tube are to be left in situ *at the time of hysterectomy*, a window in the peritoneum beneath the fallopian tube between the uterus and ovary is made sharply or bluntly, and a heavy clamp—such as a Heaney, Kocher, or similar clamp—is used to clamp the uteroovarian pedicle (Fig. 32A.3, see page 736). The round ligament should not be included in this clamp. The clamp that was initially placed on the round ligament and fallopian tube just lateral to the uterine fundus at the beginning of the procedure serves as the back clamp for this pedicle. The tube and uteroovarian ligament are divided and the pedicle ligated as previously noted with a free-tie followed by a suture ligature. The ovary and tube may be left in the posterior pelvis if exposure is adequate or gently packed in the paracolic gutter, with care being taken to ensure that the blood supply is not compromised.

The next step is the dissection of the bladder from the anterior cervix. At this point, the peritoneum is divided just

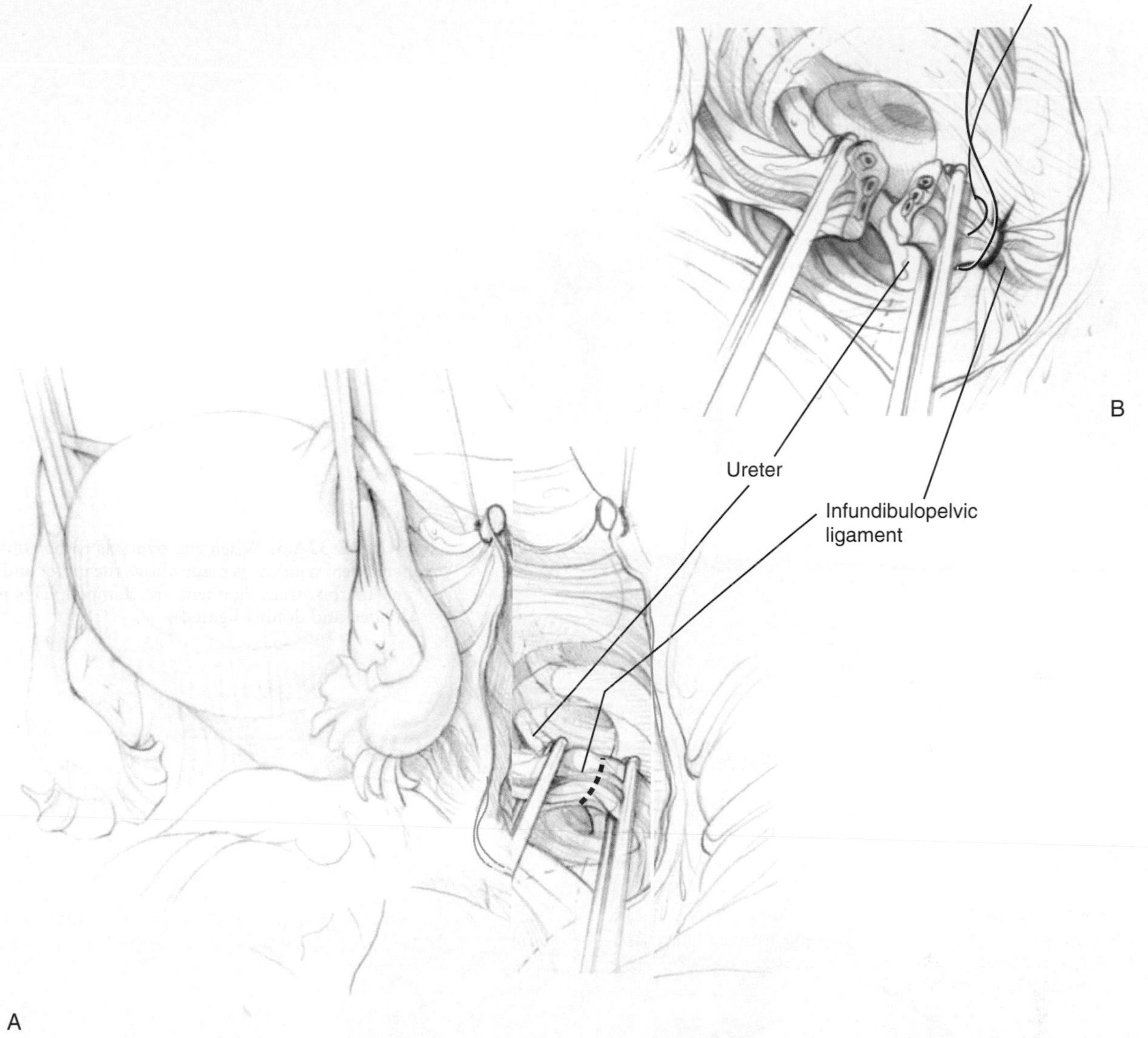

FIGURE 32A.2. A: The infundibulopelvic ligament is doubly clamped, and the ovarian vessels are cut between the clamps. Care is taken to be sure the ureter is clear as the clamps are applied. **B:** The proximal pedicle is ligated with a free tie followed by a transfixion suture ligature.

inferior to its attachment to the lower uterine segment. If the peritoneum is divided 5 to 10 mm below its uterine attachment, it is usually mobile, and an avascular plane of loose areolar tissue can be identified between the posterior bladder wall and the anterior cervix. We begin this dissection sharply using the Metzenbaum scissors. With upward traction on the bladder peritoneum and the uterine fundus stretched tightly out of the pelvis, the tips of the Metzenbaum scissors should rest lightly on the fascia overlying the cervix and small bites used to develop this tissue plane, dissecting the bladder from the anterior cervix (Fig. 32A.4). This dissection should take place over the cervix, because if it is carried too far laterally, bleeding may be encountered, and the uterine vessels or ureters could be injured. Except in patients with a previous cesarean section or an adherent bladder for other reasons, this bladder dissection often can be done bluntly, but it is good practice to do it sharply from time to time so that in those patients in whom the bladder is adherent and sharp dissection is required, the procedure will be familiar. Blunt dissection of the bladder can be accomplished easily by grasping the uterus and lower uterine segment between both hands and gently using the first one or two fingers to advance the bladder, as illustrated in Richardson's classic paper (Fig. 32A.5). It also is possible to grasp the uterus with your dominant hand, placing the thumb in front on the anterior cervix and the fingers behind the uterus. The thumb is gently pushed downward toward the cervix and inferiorly toward the vagina, gently dissecting the bladder off of the cervix and lower uterine segment. With this technique, the pressure is against the cervix rather than against the bladder, which should minimize the risk of bladder injury. Excessive force should not be used. As the bladder is dissected below the cervix, the thumb in front and the fingers behind come into closer opposition because they now have only the vaginal wall between them. The dissection is extended laterally to encompass the full cervix. Usually, it is not necessary to dissect the rectum off of the posterior cul-de-sac; but if adherent rectum prevents good posterior exposure, it should be dissected free after the uterine vessels have been divided.

Once the bladder has been freed from the anterior cervix, the uterine artery and vein are skeletonized (Fig. 32A.6). The

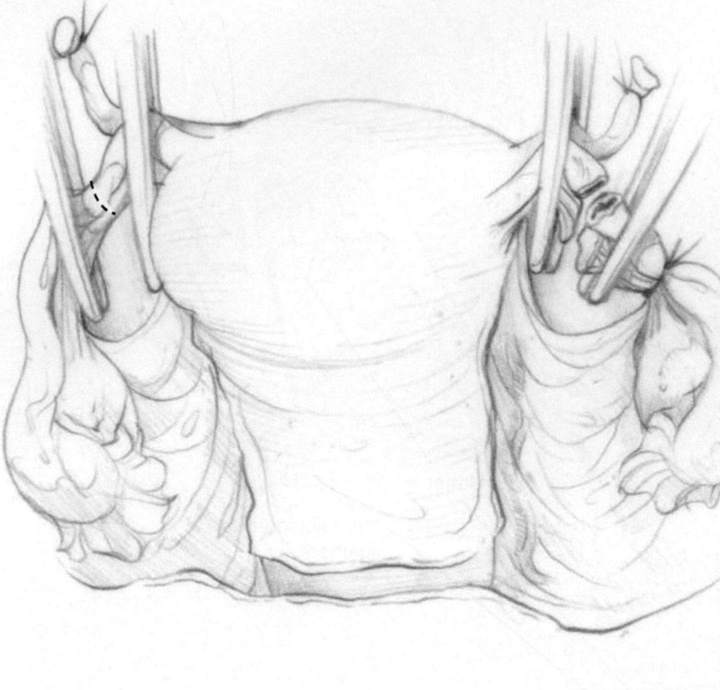

FIGURE 32A.3. When the ovary is to be conserved, a peritoneal window is made above the ureter and the tube and uteroovarian ligament are clamped. This pedicle is divided and doubly ligated.

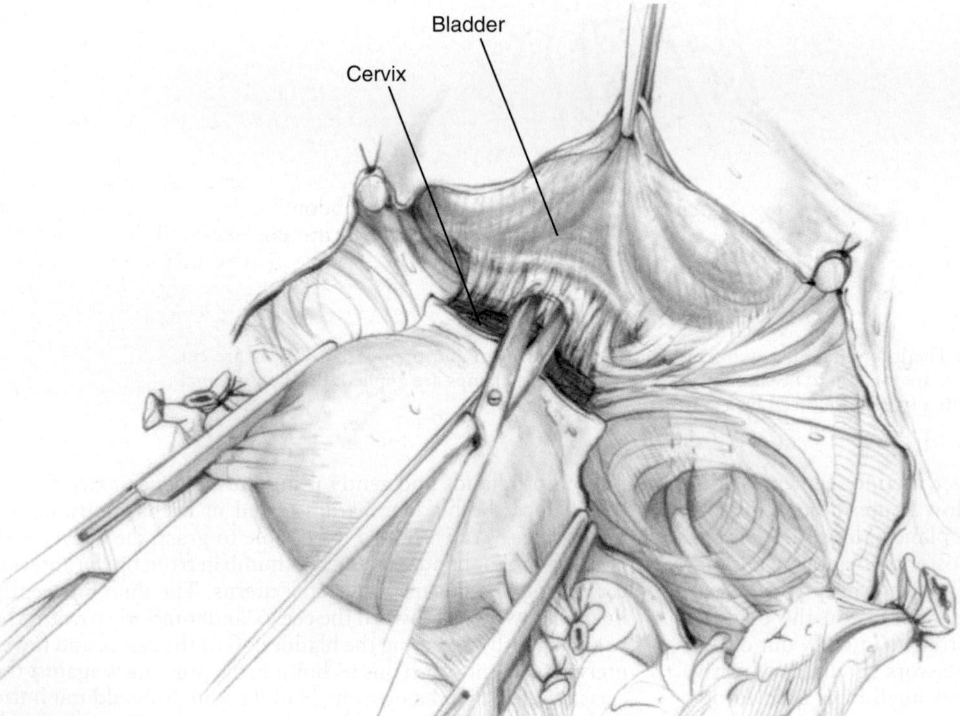

FIGURE 32A.4. The bladder is mobilized inferiorly by sharp dissection away from the cervix. To avoid unnecessary bleeding, this step may be done in stages as necessary.

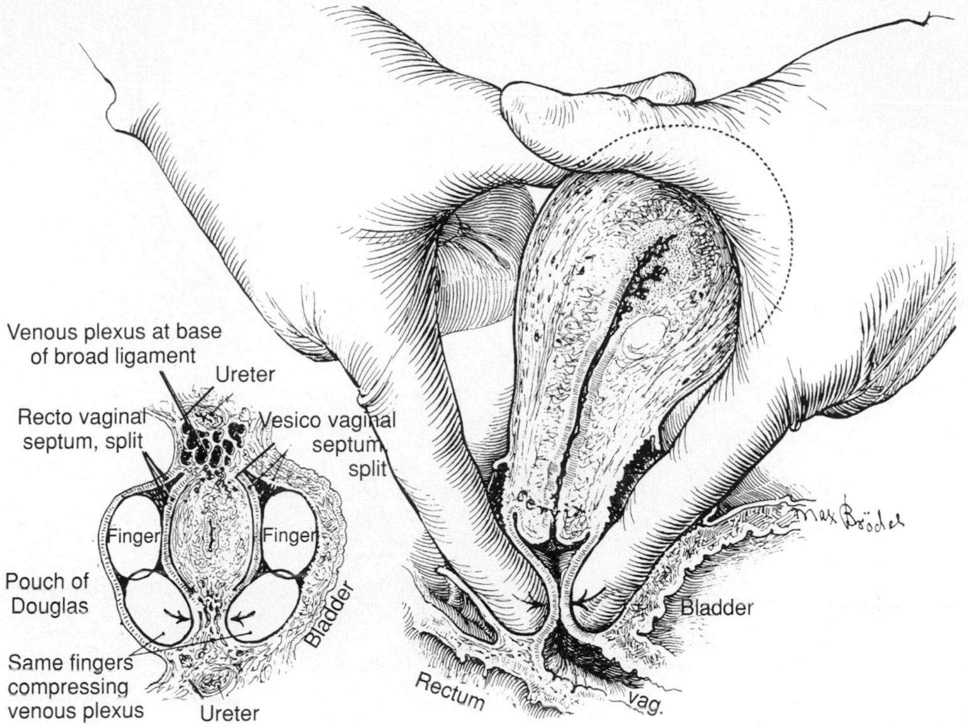

FIGURE 32A.5. The bladder and, if necessary, the rectum can be gently advanced with blunt dissection. The depth of this dissection can be checked by squeezing the anterior and posterior fingers together below the cervix. (From: Richardson EH. A simplified technique for abdominal panhysterectomy. *Surg Gynecol Obstet* 1929;48:248, with permission.)

uterus is pulled sharply to the patient's right side, and the surgeon gently dissects the loose fatty tissue adjacent to the lateral lower uterine segment on the left. The uterine artery is usually found immediately adjacent to the uterus at the level of the internal cervical os. In most patients, the uterine artery is easily exposed by holding the tissue laterally and gently "raking" with the Metzenbaum scissors slightly opened from medial to lateral. "Skeletonizing" the uterine artery and vein allows them to be clamped more accurately; with less adjacent tissue, and a smaller vascular pedicle, which allows more precise and more secure ligation. However, good surgical judgment should be used so that excessive attempts to isolate the vessels do not produce unnecessary bleeding. When the vessels are exposed, a fairly heavy, slightly curved clamp then is used to clamp the vessels just adjacent to the uterus (Fig. 32A.6B). We prefer to use a Heaney, Zeppelin, or Masterson clamp for these pedicles. The tip of the clamp should be around the vessels, and the clamp should come across the pedicle as close to a right angle as possible, rather than at the diagonal, so that the least amount of tissue will be incorporated in the pedicle. The tip of the clamp should not include too much cervical or uterine tissue because this makes application of subsequent clamps more difficult. A second clamp can be placed above the first for added safety, if desired, and a third or back clamp used to prevent annoying back bleeding from the uterus after the vessels have been cut.

If exposure is satisfactory after a single clamp has been placed on the left uterine artery and vein, we skeletonize the uterine vessels on the patient's right side and place a clamp on these vessels as well. If the uterus is small, no back clamp is required because the four major vessels supplying the uterus have now been clamped or ligated. Next, the uterine vessels are cut with scissors or a knife and the pedicle doubly ligated with 0 delayed absorbed sutures. We prefer to use a small tapered point needle (CT-2, Ethicon) for these pedicles because we feel that large needles are more difficult to place in the small confines of the deep pelvis. If a back clamp has been used, it is now ligated and removed so that the field is not obscured by an excessive number of clamps.

Hemostasis should be good at this point. If not, any bleeding should be controlled. The bladder is again checked to ensure it is well below the cervix. If the rectum needs to be dissected from the posterior cervix, this should be done now. This is usually not necessary for a simple abdominal hysterectomy for benign disease. The peritoneum of the posterior cul-de-sac between the uterosacral ligaments can be divided easily, and blunt dissection of the posterior vaginal wall from the anterior rectum usually is easy, although the rectosigmoid occasionally may be densely adherent to the posterior uterine segment or cervix by endometriosis or pelvic inflammatory disease. If the bladder and/or rectum is too densely adherent and there is concern that further attempts at dissection may damage them or cause troublesome bleeding, a supracervical hysterectomy should be considered.

Once the bladder anteriorly and the rectum posteriorly have been freed from the cervix, the uterus is placed on tension, exposing the deeper portions of the broad ligament and pulling the lower uterine segment away from the ureter. A medium-width malleable retractor may be useful to retract the bladder anteriorly; if necessary, a wide malleable retractor in the posterior cul-de-sac will provide deep exposure posteriorly. In most cases, a series of straight Heaney or Zeppelin clamps can now be used to successfully clamp the remaining portion of the broad ligament (Fig. 32A.7). The tips of these clamps should be placed on the lateral portion of the cervix, and the upper portion of the jaw should lie immediately adjacent to the previous pedicle. As the clamp is gently squeezed closed, the tip slides off of the firm cervix, finally closing snugly against the lateral wall of the muscular cervix. By staying close to the cervix in this way, the risk of damaging the ureter, which is not too far away laterally, is minimized. The pedicle then is cut with heavy scissors or a knife. A millimeter or two of tissue may be left

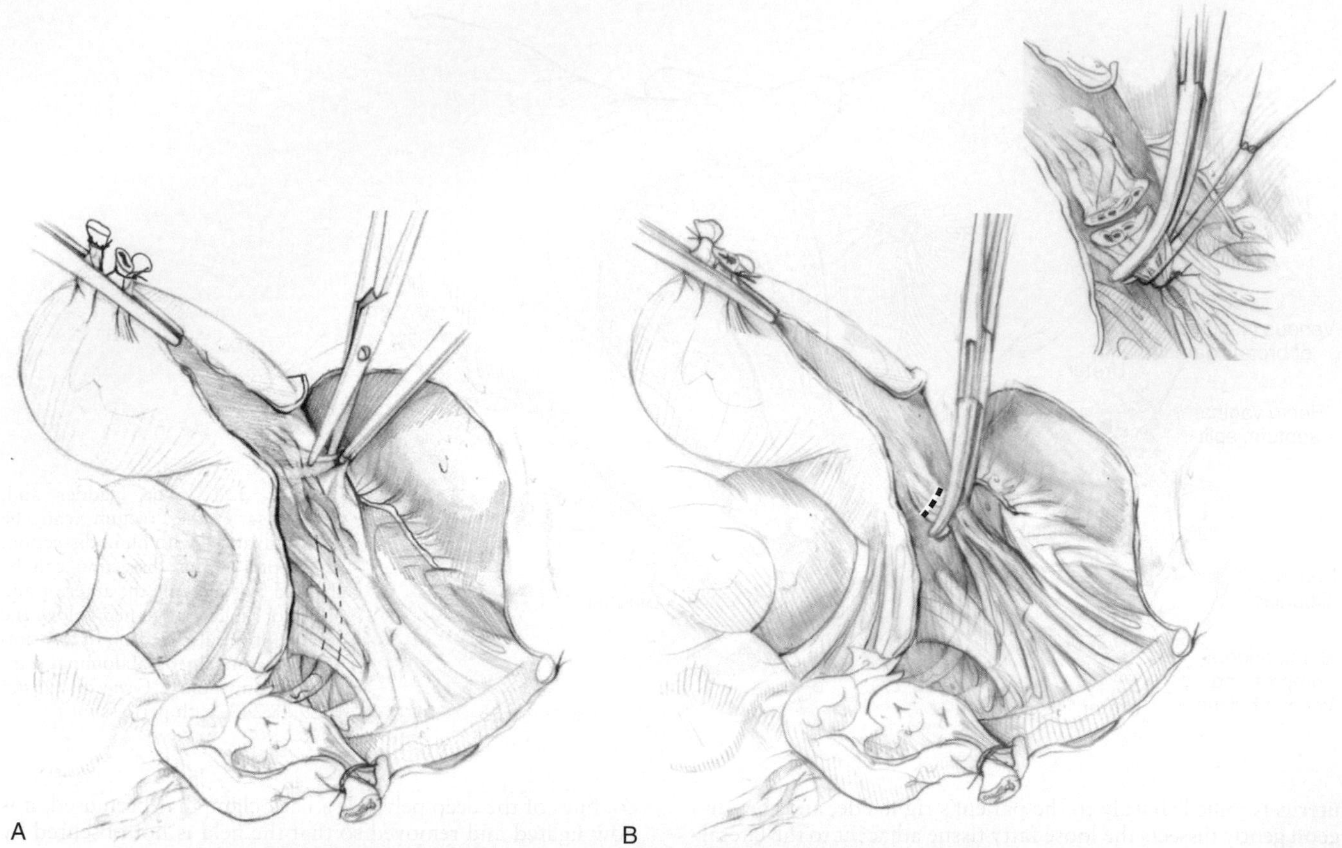

FIGURE 32A.6. A: The uterine vessels are skeletonized. **B:** A curved Haney clamp is used to clamp the uterine vessels immediately adjacent to the uterus. They are ligated by two suture ligatures.

medial to the clamp as insurance, but this is not necessary. The tip of the transfixion suture needle is placed at the lateral tip of the clamp jaw; if the pedicle is longer than 1 cm, we recommend using a Heaney suture ligature so that the upper end of the pedicle is secondarily transfixed to prevent it from slipping out of the ligature. While good exposure is maintained, one or two pedicles are tied on each side, and then the procedure is repeated on the opposite side until the level of the cervical–vaginal junction has been reached. Once again, the bladder and rectum are checked and advanced if necessary to be sure that they are well clear and the anterior and posterior vaginal walls exposed.

Sharply angled large Zeppelin clamps are used to clamp across the vagina below the cervix. These clamps include the base of the cardinal ligaments laterally, the uterosacral ligament posteriorly, and the vaginal wall anteriorly and posteriorly. A clamp is applied from each side; in most cases, the tips of these clamps meet in the middle just below the cervix (Fig. 32A.8). A knife or heavy, sharply angled Jorgenson scissors is used to divide the vagina above these clamps and below the cervix. The uterus is removed and placed in a pan on the back table for later examination. A single figure-of-eight suture is placed between the tips of the two clamps to close the midportion of the vagina. The ends of this suture are held initially and not tied. A Heaney suture ligature is placed on each of the lateral clamps with the second bite going through the uterosacral ligament posteriorly. Inclusion of the uterosacral and cardinal ligament in this pedicle provides excellent support of the vaginal apex. When these lateral sutures have been tied, the figure-of-eight suture in the middle then is tied also. The lateral sutures are cut and the figure-of-eight in the middle of the cuff is held to provide traction on the vaginal apex. With this closed cuff technique, the vagina is never exposed, which reduces contamination of the pelvis. However, there may be instances, such as a large cervical myoma, when there is a very deep vaginal fornix, and a closed technique would remove too much vagina. Entry into the vagina with the electrosurgical blade and then carefully opening the vagina circumferentially under direct vision is an option in such cases. As the vagina is opened, the full-thickness vaginal edges are grasped with Kocher clamps as the dissection proceeds. We generally close the vaginal cuff with a series of figure-of-eight stitches of 0 delayed absorbable suture, taking care to incorporate the uterosacral and cardinal ligaments into the cuff for support. We have not run the vaginal wall with a locking stitch for hemostasis and left the cuff open for drainage (closing the pelvic peritoneum over the open cuff) since the advent of prophylactic antibiotics for hysterectomy many years ago.

In the classic Richardson technique, the peritoneum over the posterior cervix is divided, the peritoneum is dissected off the cul-de-sac, and the rectovaginal septum is entered to reflect the rectum posteriorly. In our experience, this has not been necessary in the vast majority of patients with benign disease. In contrast to the anterior bladder dissection, this posterior peritoneum is much more adherent. There is usually some bleeding associated with this dissection, making it both bloody and time-consuming. With the Richardson technique, the uterosacral ligaments also are clamped separately and subsequently attached to the vaginal cuff for support. In the technique described above, this is accomplished in a single step.

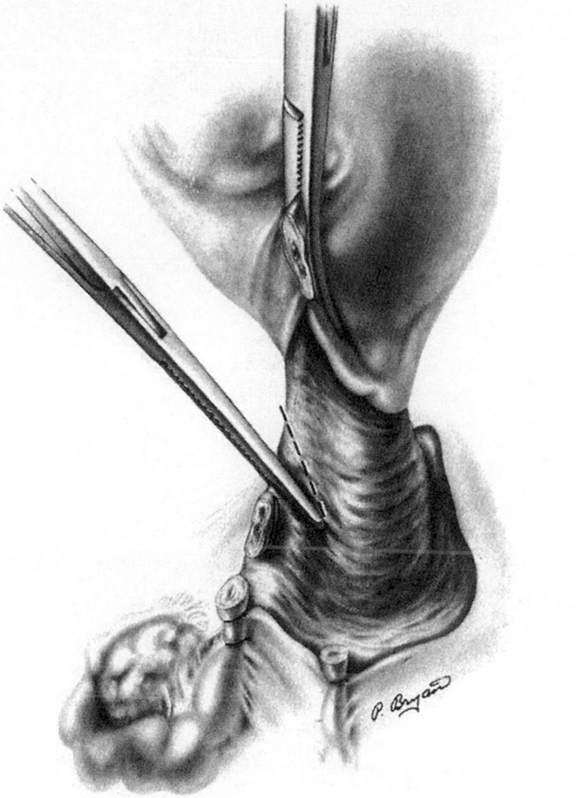

FIGURE 32A.7. After the uterine artery and vein have been ligated, the remaining lower portion of the broad ligament is clamped with a series of straight clamps. The tips are placed on the edge of the cervix and the back of the jaw immediately adjacent to the previous pedicle.

Closure

After the pelvis has been copiously irrigated with warm saline, the pedicles are inspected carefully to be sure that hemostasis is present. Electrocautery or suture ligatures with 3-0 absorbable sutures on fine needles are used to control small bleeders. The location of the ureters, bladder, and major vessels should be known when placing these sutures. Common sites of ureteral injury during abdominal hysterectomy include the infundibulopelvic ligament where the ovarian vessels are ligated; the area of the uterine artery ligation and the bladder base. Distorted anatomy associated with fibroids, endometriosis and malignancy is a signal for special care to avoid ureteral injury. The pelvis is not reperitonealized, but the rectosigmoid colon is gently laid over the vaginal cuff to cover this raw surface and minimize the risk of adhesions. The packs and retractor are removed, the abdomen checked again for hemostasis, and the omentum placed anteriorly to minimize the risk of small bowel adhesions to the abdominal incision. The anterior peritoneum is closed with delayed absorbable suture, although some surgeons today feel that it is unnecessary to close the abdominal peritoneum. The fascial closure should be commensurate with the patient's risk of infection and hernia. Generally, a running monofilament delayed absorbably suture such as PDS (Ethicon) on a larger, curved, tapered needle (CT-1, Ethicon) can be used. If there is a significant risk of dehiscence secondary to infection, obesity, or other medical problems, interrupted sutures or a mass closure technique may be used. Closure techniques are illustrated in Chapter 14. Because patients are often discharged by the third or fourth postoperative day, we generally prefer to close the skin with a subcuticular absorbable suture, which eliminates the necessity for a return to the office for suture or staple removal.

After the patient has been taken to the recovery room, the surgeon should speak with the family, preferably face to face, to assure them that the patient is doing well and to review the operative findings with them. We also strongly recommend that the surgeon ask the circulating nurse to contact the family about once an hour to update them on the progress of the operation during the surgical procedure. This especially is helpful if there were any unknown questions going into the operation (Did the ovaries look normal? Was the endometriosis involving the ureter?). A brief operative note must be immediately recorded in the patient's chart describing the procedure, blood loss, fluid replacement and if any packs or drains were left in the patient. Postoperative orders are written. A careful operative note should be dictated with emphasis on any unusual findings or variations from standard techniques.

SUBTOTAL ABDOMINAL HYSTERECTOMY

The technique of subtotal or supracervical abdominal hysterectomy is similar to the technique for abdominal hysterectomy

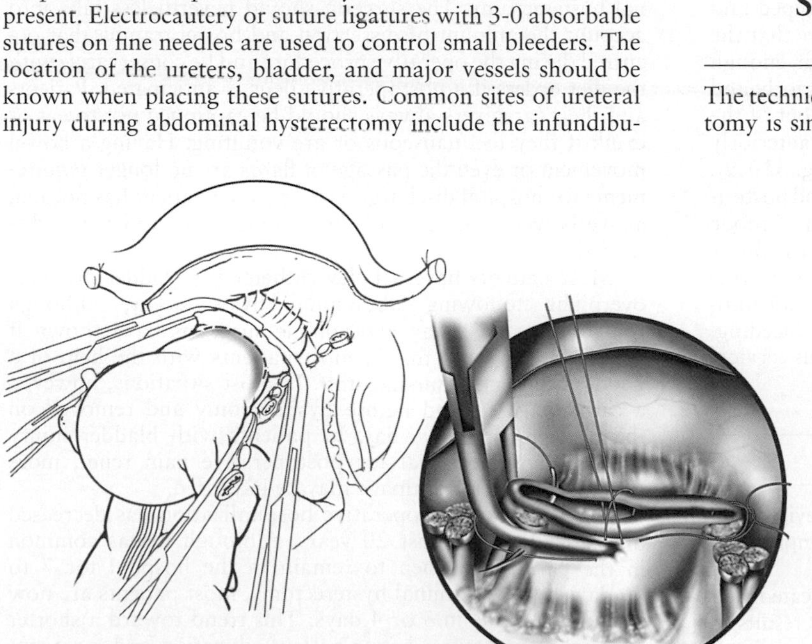

FIGURE 32A.8. **A:** After checking to be sure the bladder and rectum are clear, the vagina is cross clamped with long, sharply curved Zeppelin clamps just below the cervix (*dotted line*). The vagina is divided just above the clamps with a knife or angled scissors. **B:** The vaginal cuff then is closed with a figure-of-eight in the middle and Heaney suture ligatures on the angles, including the uterosacral and cardinal ligaments for support.

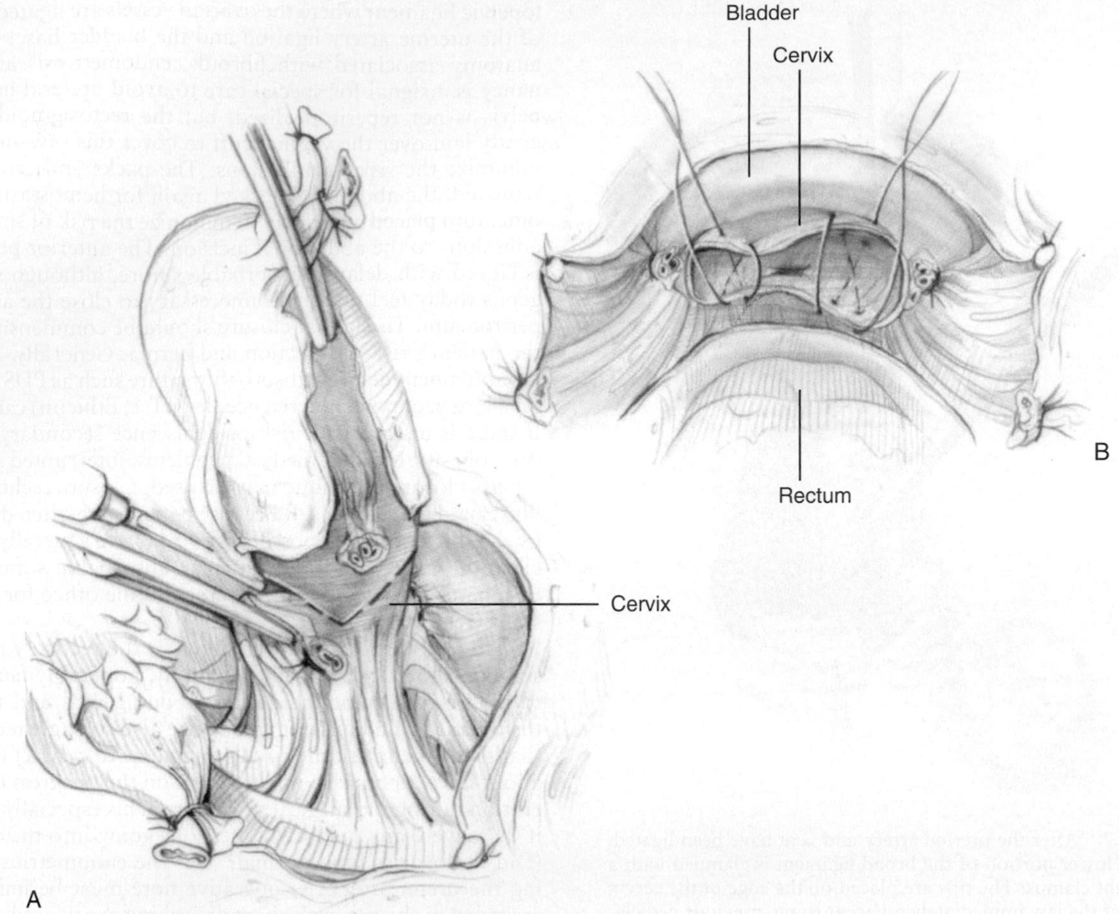

FIGURE 32A.9. Subtotal or supracervical hysterectomy. **A:** After the uterine vessels have been ligated, the fundus is amputated using the electrocautery in a shallow cone-shaped technique. **B:** The cervix or lower uterine segment then is closed with several large figure-of-eight sutures.

as described, until the uterine vessels have been clamped and ligated. At this point, care should be taken to be sure that the bladder and rectum have been advanced at least far enough so that the cervix can be clearly visualized both anteriorly and posteriorly. The uterine fundus is strongly retracted out of the pelvis, and electrocautery is used to cut the cervix anteriorly just above the level of the ligated uterine vessels (Fig. 32A.9). A shallow V-shaped incision is used both anteriorly and posteriorly until the uterine fundus is excised. The "coagulate" mode of the electrosurgical unit is used, and hemostasis usually is excellent. Several generous figure-of-eight sutures on a large needle then are used to close the upper endocervix in a hemostatic fashion. The top of the cervix is checked for bleeding, and the bladder peritoneum may be used to cover this cervical stump to minimize the risk of adhesions.

POSTOPERATIVE CARE

Although routine postoperative care is thoroughly reviewed in Chapter 9, there are several facets that should be emphasized following hysterectomy.

Several studies over the past few years have indicated that early feeding after hysterectomy is safe and actually results in earlier discharge. In many cases, patients are able to tolerate solid food on the first postoperative day following abdominal hysterectomy. The surgeon should nevertheless take into account the amount of dissection and bowel trauma that occurred during the operative procedure and be conservative with the diet orders if a postoperative ileus is anticipated. Patients and their caregivers always should be cautioned not to eat or drink if they feel nauseous or are vomiting. Having a bowel movement or even the passage of flatus are no longer requirements for hospital discharge as long as the patient has normal, active bowel sounds, is tolerating solid food, and is not distended.

Most patients have a Foley catheter for bladder drainage overnight following abdominal hysterectomy, although Richardson and many gynecologic surgeons have shown it is possible to avoid this in most patients with the help of a good, enthusiastic nursing staff. In most situations, however, a catheter is inserted before hysterectomy and removed on the first postoperative day. In patients with bladder injury or continuous epidural for postoperative pain relief, more prolonged catheter drainage may be indicated.

The length of postoperative hospitalization has decreased dramatically in the last 20 years. Although it was common in the past for women to remain in the hospital for 7 to 10 days after abdominal hysterectomy, most patients are now discharged home in 3 or 4 days. This trend toward a shorter hospital stay requires better patient education and a reasonable home environment to which the patient can be safely and

TABLE 32A.5

COMPLICATIONS OF HYSTERECTOMY

Complication	Abdominal	Vaginal	Laparoscopically assisted vaginal
Bleeding			
Hemorrhage	1%–2%	1%–5%	1%
Transfusion	2%–12%	2%–8.3%	1.58%
Infection			
Unexplained fever	10%–20%	5%–8%	2.14%
Operative site	6.6%–24.7%	3.9%–10%	0.54%
Wound	4%–8%	NA	NA
Pelvic	3.2%–10%	3.9%–10%	1.27%
Urinary tract	1.1%–5%	1.7%–5%	0.81%
Pneumonia	0.4%–2.6%	0.29%–2%	0.11%
Injuries			
Bladder	1%–2%	0.5%–1.5%	1%
Bowel	0.1%–1%	0.1%–0.8%	0.1%–1%
Ureter	0.1%–0.5%	0.05%–0.1%	0.19%
Vesicovaginal fistula	0.1%–0.2%	0.1%–0.2%	0.22%
Trocar injuries	—	—	0.5%

From: Harris WJ. Early complications of abdominal and vaginal hysterectomy. *Obstet Gynecol Surv* 1995;50:795, with permission.

comfortably discharged. The surgeon must also carefully evaluate the patient before discharge and resist pressure from insurance companies and hospital administrators when the patient's condition indicates that she is not suitable for an early discharge. The patient and her family must be instructed on proper care. Can she take a bath? Can she go up and down the stairs? Can she pick up her grandchild? How soon can she drive a car? A printed set of instructions for home care as well as answers to frequently asked questions are good ideas. Liberal use of home visiting nurses is also recommended, especially in older or more debilitated patients or in those whose home situation may be less than ideal.

COMPLICATIONS

Complications from hysterectomy can be diagnosed intraoperatively or postoperatively. In a thorough review, Harris found an overall complication rate of up to 50% associated with abdominal hysterectomy, but serious complications requiring reoperation or long-term disability are relatively uncommon. Reoperation rates of 4% to 4.3% have been reported by Gambone and associates and Browne and Frazer. The most common complications include infection, hemorrhage, and injuries to adjacent organs (Table 32A.5). Prevention and management of hemorrhage, infection, and operative injury complications are extensively discussed in several chapters of this text. Good surgical training, proper patient selection, knowledge of the anatomy, and good surgical judgment—which includes knowing your personal skills and limits—are all keys to minimizing complications.

Several factors have been consistently shown to be associated with an increased risk of complications related to hysterectomy. These are increasing age, medical illness, obesity, and malignancy. These conditions are beyond the control of the gynecologic surgeon, but they should be considered in the risk:benefit ratio when considering surgery, and every effort should be made to have the patient in the best possible condition at the time of surgery.

BEST SURGICAL PRACTICES

- Hysterectomy is one of the most common major operations performed in the United States. The most common indications are uterine leiomyoma, endometriosis, abnormal uterine bleeding, and malignancy. There are many techniques to perform a hysterectomy, including abdominal, vaginal, laparoscopic and laparoscopically assisted, total, and subtotal. Before surgery, the surgeon should discuss the indications, other management options, choice of surgical approach, risks and potential complications of surgery, and expected outcomes with the patient and her supporters, and obtain a fully informed operative consent.
- Numerous prospective randomized studies have shown that total abdominal hysterectomy results in the same or better postoperative sexual function, urinary tract and bowel function, and pelvic support as does supracervical hysterectomy.
- Prophylactic antibiotics administered within 1 hour before the initial incision significantly reduces the risk of a surgical site infection. There is no advantage to continuing antibiotics after surgery in an uninfected patient.
- The surgeon and the surgical team should be completely focused on the operation. Thoughtful preoperative preparation, careful surgical technique, well-reasoned judgment intraoperatively, and attentive postoperative care by a well-trained and interactive team will result in the best outcomes. Good communication between all members of the team is of great importance.
- We have found that the surgical techniques described in this chapter has been highly effective, but each surgeon should be familiar with a number of variations of standard hysterectomy technique and use appropriate variations that might suit the anatomy or pathology of a specific patient.

Bibliography

Abdel-Fattah M, Barrington J, Yousef M, et al. Effect of total abdominal hysterectomy on pelvic floor function. *Obstet Gynecol Surv* 2004;59:299.

Alessandri F, Mistrangelo E, Lijoi D, et al. A prospective, randomized trial comparing immediate versus delayed catheter removal following hysterectomy. *Acta Obstet Gynecol Scand* 2006;85:716.

Allen WM, Masters WH. Traumatic laceration of uterine support: the clinical syndrome and the operative treatment. *Am J Obstet Gynecol* 1955;70:500.

American College of Obstetricians and Gynecologists. ACOG Practice Bulletin No. 74. *Antibiotic prophylaxis for gynecologic procedures.* Washington, DC: ACOG;2006.

American College of Obstetricians and Gynecologists. ACOG Technical Bulletin No. 223. *Chronic pelvic pain.* Washington, DC: ACOG;1996.

American College of Obstetricians and Gynecologists. ACOG Practice Bulletin No. 21. *Prevention of deep vein thrombosis and pulmonary embolism.* Washington, DC: ACOG;2000.

American College of Obstetricians and Gynecologists. ACOG Practice Bulletin No. 7. *Prophylactic oophorectomy.* Washington, DC: ACOG;1999.

Aravantinos DJ. Keeping or removing the ovaries at the time of hysterectomy. *Eur J Obstet Gynecol Reprod Biol* 1988;28:146.29A:1231.

Averette HE, Nguyen HN. The role of prophylactic oophorectomy in cancer prevention. *Gynecol Oncol* 1994;55:S38–41.

Babalola EO, Bharucha AE, Schleck CD, et al. Decreasing utilization of hysterectomy: a population-based study in Olmsted County, Minnesota, 1965–2002. *Am J Obstet Gynecol* 2007;196:214.

Berman M, Grosen E. A new method of continuous vaginal cuff closure at abdominal hysterectomy. *Obstet Gynecol* 1994;84:478.

Bernstein S, McGlynn E, Siu A, et al., for the Health Maintenance Organization Quality of Care Consortium. The appropriateness of hysterectomy: a comparison of care in seven health plans. *JAMA* 1993;269:2398.

Black N, Clarke A, Rowe P, et al. A prospective cohort study of the clinical management of total abdominal hysterectomy for benign disease. *J Obstet Gynaecol* 1995;15:394.

Bottle A, Aylin P. Variations in vaginal and abdominal hysterectomy by region and trust in England. *BJOG* 2005;112:326.

Bradham D, Stovall T, Thompson C. Use of GnRH agonist before hysterectomy: a cost simulation. *Obstet Gynecol* 1995;85:401.

Bridgman S, Dobbins J, Casbard A. The VALUE national hysterectomy study: description of the patients and their surgery. *BJOG* 2002;109:302.

Broder MS, Kanouse DE, Mittman BS, et al. The appropriateness of recommendations for hysterectomy. *Obstet Gynecol* 2000;95:199.

Brook R, for the Health Maintenance Organization Quality of Care Consortium. The appropriateness of hysterectomy: a comparison of care in seven health plans. *JAMA* 1993;269:2398.

Brooks P, Clouse J, Morris L. Hysterectomy vs. resectoscopic endometrial ablation for the control of abnormal uterine bleeding: a cost-comparative study. *J Reprod Med* 1994;39:755.

Browne DS, Frazer MI. Hysterectomy revisited. *Aust N Z J Obstet Gynaecol* 1992;31:148.

Bukovsky I, Liftshitz Y, Langer R, et al. Ovarian residual syndrome. *Surg Gynecol Obstet* 1988;167:132.

Cardosi RJ, Hoffman MS. Determining the best route for hysterectomy. *OBG Management* 2002;July:24.

Carenza L. Keeping or removing the ovaries at the time of hysterectomy. *Eur J Obstet Gynecol Reprod Biol* 1988;28:155.

Carlson K, Miller B, Flowler F. The Maine Women's Health Study: I. Outcomes of hysterectomy. *Obstet Gynecol* 1994;83:556.

Carlson K, Miller B, Flowler F. The Maine Women's Health Study: II. Outcomes of non-surgical management of leiomyomas, abnormal bleeding, and chronic pelvic pain. *Obstet Gynecol* 1994;83:566.

Carlson K, Nichols D, Schiff I. Indications for hysterectomy. *N Engl J Med* 1993;328:856.

Castelo-Branco C, Figueras F, Sanjuan A, et al. Long-term compliance with estrogen replacement therapy in surgical postmenopausal women: benefits to bone and analysis of factors associated with discontinuation. *Menopause* 1999;6:307–11.

Clarke A, Black N, Rowe P, et al. Indications for and outcome of total abdominal hysterectomy for benign disease: a prospective cohort study. *BJOG* 1995;102:611.

Dao AH, Cartwright PS. Fallopian tube prolapse following abdominal hysterectomy. *J Tenn Med Assoc* 1987;80:141.

Darai E, Soriano D, Kimata P, et al. Vaginal hysterectomy for enlarged uteri, with or without laparoscopic assistance: randomized study. *Obstet Gynecol* 2001;97:712.

Dexeus S, Munos A, Tusquets JM. Preservation of the ovaries: a controversial subject. *Eur J Obstet Gynecol Reprod Biol* 1988;28:146.

Domengihetti G, Luraschi P, Marazzi A. Hysterectomy and the sex of the gynecologist. *N Engl J Med* 1985;313:1482.

Dorsey J, Steinberg E, Holtz P. Clinical indications for hysterectomy route: patient characteristics or physician preference? *Am J Obstet Gynecol* 1995;173:1452.

Dorsey JH, Holtz PM, Griffiths RI, et al. Costs and charges associated with three alternative techniques of hysterectomy. *N Engl J Med* 1996;335:476.

Drife J. Conserving the cervix at hysterectomy. *BJOG* 1994;101:563.

Ewen S, Sutton C. Initial experience with supracervical laparoscopic hysterectomy and removal of the cervical transformation zone. *BJOG* 1994;101:225.

Farquhar CM, Steiner CA. Hysterectomy rates in the United States 1990–1997. *Obstet Gynecol* 2002;99:229.

Fong YF, Lim FK, Arulkumaran S. Prophylactic oophorectomy: a continuing controversy. *Obstet Gynecol Surv* 1998;53:493.

Franchi M, Ghezzi F, Zanaboni F, et al. Nonclosure of peritoneum at radical abdominal hysterectomy and pelvic node dissection: a randomized study. *Obstet Gynecol* 1997;90:622.

Gambone J, Reiter R, Lench JB, et al. The impact of a quality assurance process on the frequency and confirmation rate of hysterectomy. *Am J Obstet Gynecol* 1990;163:545.

Gambone JC, Reiter RC, Lench JB. Quality assurance indicators and short-term outcome of hysterectomy. *Obstet Gynecol* 1990;76:841.

Garry R. The future of hysterectomy. *BJOG* 2005;112:133.

Garry R. Initial experience with laparoscopic-assisted Doderlein hysterectomy. *BJOG* 1995;102:307.

Gimbel H. Total or subtotal hysterectomy for benign uterine diseases? A meta-analysis. *Acta Obstet Gynecol Scand* 2007;86:133.

Gimbel H, Zobbe V, Andersen BM, et al. Randomised controlled trial of total compared with subtotal hysterectomy with one-year follow up results. *BJOG* 2003;110:1088.

Goldman JA, Feldberg D, Dicker D, et al. Femoral neuropathy subsequent to abdominal hysterectomy: a comparative study. *Eur J Obstet Gynecol Reprod Biol* 1985;20:385.

Griffith-Jones MD, Jarvis GJ, McNamara HM. Adverse urinary symptoms after total abdominal hysterectomy: fact or fiction. *BJU* 1991;67:295.

Hankinson S, Hunter D, Colditz G, et al. Tubal ligation, hysterectomy, and risk of ovarian cancer: a prospective study. *JAMA* 1993;270:2813.

Harris M, Olive D. Changing hysterectomy patterns after introduction of laparoscopically assisted vaginal hysterectomy. *Am J Obstet Gynecol* 1994;171:340.

Harris W. Early complications of abdominal and vaginal hysterectomy. *Obstet Gynecol Surv* 1995;50:795.

Hasson HM. Cervical removal at hysterectomy for benign disease: risks and benefits. *J Reprod Med* 1993;38:781.

Helstrom L, Lundberg PO, Sorbom D, et al. Sexuality after hysterectomy: a factor analysis of women's sexual lives before and after subtotal hysterectomy. *Obstet Gynecol* 1993;81:357.

Hendricks-Mathews M. The importance of assessing a woman's history of sexual abuse before hysterectomy. *J Fam Pract* 1991;32:631.

Hillis S, Marchbanks P, Peterson H. The effectiveness of hysterectomy for chronic pelvic pain. *Obstet Gynecol* 1995;86:941.

Hillis S, Marchbanks P, Peterson H. Uterine size and risks of complications among women undergoing abdominal hysterectomy for leiomyomas. *Obstet Gynecol* 1996;87:539.

Hoffmann M, DeCesare S, Kalter C. Abdominal hysterectomy versus transvaginal morcellation for the removal of enlarged uteri. *Am J Obstet Gynecol* 1994;171:309.

Horbach NS, Lee TTM, Levy BS, et al. Unraveling the myths of laparoscopic supracervical hysterectomy. *Cont OB/GYN* 2006; May:1.

Howard F. The role of laparoscopy in chronic pelvic pain: promise and pitfalls. *Obstet Gynecol Surv* 1993;48:357.

Irwin KL, Weiss NS, Lee NC, et al. Tubal sterilization, hysterectomy, and the subsequent occurrence of epithelial ovarian cancer. *Am J Epidemiol* 1991;134:363–369.

Jacobs I, Oram D. Prevention of ovarian cancer: a survey of the practice of prophylactic oophorectomy by fellows and members of the Royal College of Obstetricians and Gynaecologists. *BJOG* 1989;96:510.

Jacobson GF, Shaber RE, Armstrong MA, et al. Hysterectomy rates for benign indications. *Obstet Gynecol* 2006;107:1278.

Johns D, Carrera B, Jones J, et al. The medical and economic impact of laparoscopically assisted vaginal hysterectomy in a large, metropolitan, not-for-profit hospital. *Am J Obstet Gynecol* 1995;172:1709.

Johnson N, Barlow D, Lethaby A, et al. Surgical approach to hysterectomy for benign gynaecological disease. *Cochrane Database Syst Rev* 2006;19:CD003677.

Kauf ND, Satagopan JM, Robson ME, et al. Risk-reducing salpingo-oophorectomy in women with a BRCA1 or BRCA2 mutation. *N Engl J Med* 2002;356:1609.

Kelly HA. *Operative gynecology.* New York: Appleton; 1896.

Kelly HA, Cullen TS. *Myomata of the uterus.* Philadelphia: WB Saunders;1909.

Kelly HA, Noble CP. *Gynecology and abdominal surgery,* vol. 1. Philadelphia: WB Saunders; 1907.

Kerlikourske K, Brown J, Grady D. Should women with familial ovarian cancer undergo prophylactic oophorectomy? *Obstet Gynecol* 1992;80:700.

Kohli N, Mallipeddi PK, Neff JM, et al. Routine hematocrit after elective gynecologic surgery. *Obstet Gynecol* 2000;95:847.

Kovac SR. Clinical opinion: guidelines for hysterectomy. *Am J Obstet Gynecol* 2004;191:635.

Kovac SR. Hysterectomy outcomes in patients with similar indications. *Obstet Gynecol* 2000;95:787.

Kuppermann M, Varner RE, Summitt RL, et al. Effect of hysterectomy versus medical treatment on health-related quality of life and sexual function. *Obstet Gynecol Surv* 2004;59:706.

Learman LA, Summitt RL Jr, Varner RE, et al. Total or Supracervical Hysterectomy (TOSH) Research Group. A randomized comparison of total or supracervical hysterectomy: surgical complications and clinical outcomes. *Obstet Gynecol* 2003;102:453.

Lofgren M, Poromaa IS, Stjerndahl JH, et al. Postoperative infections and antibiotic prophylaxis for hysterectomy in Sweden: a study by the Swedish National Register for Gynecologic Surgery. *Acta Obstet Gynecol Scand* 2004;83:1202.

Lonnee-Hoffmann RA, Schei B, Eriksson NH. Sexual experience of partners after hysterectomy, comparing subtotal with total abdominal hysterectomy. *Acta Obstet Gynecol Scand* 2006;85:1389.

Luoto R, Kaprio J, Reunanen A, et al. Cardiovascular morbidity in relation to ovarian function after hysterectomy. *Obstet Gynecol* 1995;85:515.

Lynch HT, Lynch PM. Tumor variation in the cancer family syndrome: ovarian cancer. *Am J Surg* 1979;138:439.

Lyons TL. Laparoscopic supracervical hysterectomy. *Obstet Gynecol Clin North Am* 2000;27:441.

Manyonda IT, Welch CR, McWhinney NA, et al. The influence of suture material on vaginal vault granulations following abdominal hysterectomy. *BJOG* 1990;97:608.

Maresh MJ, Metcalfe MA, McPherson K, et al. History of hysterectomy. *West J Surg Obstet Gynecol* 1934;42:2.

Matteson KA, Peipert JF, Hirway P, et al. Factors associated with increased charges for hysterectomy. *Obstet Gynecol* 2006;107:1057.

Miyazawa K. Technique for total abdominal hysterectomy: historical and clinical perspective. *Obstet Gynecol Surv* 1992;47:433–47.

Morgan K, Thomas E. Nerve injury at abdominal hysterectomy. *BJOG* 1995;102:665.

Munro MG. Management of heavy menstrual bleeding: is hysterectomy the radical mastectomy of gynecology? *Clin Obstet Gynecol* 2007;50:324–53.

Muntz HG, Falkenberry S, Fuller AF. Fallopian tube prolapse after hysterectomy: a report of two cases. *J Reprod Med* 1988;33:467.

Myers ER, Steege JF. Risk adjustment for complications of hysterectomy: limitations of routinely collected administrative data. *Am J Obstet Gynecol* 1999;181:567.

Nathorst-Boos J, Fuchs T, von Schoultz B. Consumer's attitude to hysterectomy: the experience of 678 women. *Acta Obstet Gynecol Scand* 1992;71:230.

Neefus MS, Taylor ME. Educational needs of hysterectomy patients. *Patient Coune Health Educ* 1982;4th Quart; 3:105–5.

Neuman M, Beller U, Chetrit A, et al. Prophylactic effect of the open vaginal vault method in reducing febrile morbidity in abdominal hysterectomy. *Surg Gynecol Obstet* 1993;176:591.

Nezhat F, Nezhat C, Gordon S, et al. Laparoscopic versus abdominal hysterectomy. *J Reprod Med* 1992;37:247.

Nichols DH, Randall CL. *Vaginal surgery.* 3rd ed. Baltimore: Williams & Wilkins; 1989.

Nichols DH, Willey PS, Randall CL. Significance of restoration of normal vaginal depth and axis. *Obstet Gynecol* 1970;36:251.

Olsson J, Ellstrom M, Hahlin M. A randomized prospective trial comparing laparoscopic and abdominal hysterectomy. *BJOG* 1996;103:345.

Ostrzenski A. A new, simplified posterior culdoplasty and vaginal vault suspension during abdominal hysterectomy. *Int J Obstet Gynecol* 1995;49:25.

Parazzini F, Negri E, Vecchia C, et al. Hysterectomy, oophorectomy, and subsequent ovarian cancer risk. *Obstet Gynecol* 1993;81:363.

Parys BT, Haylen BT, Hutton JL, et al. The effects of simple hysterectomy on vesicourethral function. *BJU* 1989;64:594.

Peipert JF, Weitzen S, Cruickshank C, et al. Risk factors for febrile morbidity after hysterectomy. *Obstet Gynecol* 2004;103:86.

Pinion S, Parkin D, Abramovich D, et al. Randomized trial of hysterectomy, endometrial ablation, and transcervical endometrial resection for dysfunctional uterine bleeding. *BMJ* 1994;309:979.

Piscitelli J, Bastian L, Wilkes A, et al. Cytologic screening after hysterectomy for benign disease. *Am J Obstet Gynecol* 1995;173:24.

Plockinger B, Kolbl H. Development of ovarian pathology after hysterectomy without oophorectomy. *J Am Coll Surg.* 1994;178:581–5.

Prior A, Stanley K, Smith ARB, et al. Effect of hysterectomy on anorectal and urethrovesical physiology. *Gut* 1992;33:264.

Raju K. A randomized prospective study of laparoscopic vaginal hysterectomy versus abdominal hysterectomy each with bilateral salpingo-oophorectomy. *BJOG* 1994;101:1068.

Ramirez PT, Klemer DP. Vaginal evisceration after hysterectomy: a literature review. *Obstet Gynecol Surv* 2002;57:462.

Rebbeck TR, Lynch HT, Neuhausen SL, et al. Prophylactic oophorectomy in carriers of BRCA1 or BRCA2 mutations. *N Engl J Med* 2002;346:1616.

Redeimeier D, Rozin P, Kahneman D. Understanding patients' decisions: cognitive and emotional perspectives. *JAMA* 1993;270:72.

Reiter R, Gambone J, Lench J. Appropriateness of hysterectomies performed for multiple preoperative indications. *Obstet Gynecol* 1992;80:902.

Reiter R, Wagner P, Gambone J. Routine hysterectomy for large asymptomatic uterine leiomyomata: a reappraisal. *Obstet Gynecol* 1992;79:481.

Ribeiro SC, Ribeiro RM, Santos NC, et al. A randomized study of total abdominal, vaginal and laparoscopic hysterectomy. *Int J Gynecol Obstet* 2003;83:37.

Richardson EH. A simplified technique for abdominal panhysterectomy. *Surg Obstet Gynecol* 1929;48:248.

Richardson R, Bournas N, Magos A. Is laparoscopic hysterectomy a waste of time? *Lancet* 1995;345:36.

Roman L, Morris M, Eifel P, et al. Reasons for inappropriate simple hysterectomy in the presence of invasive cancer of the cervix. *Obstet Gynecol* 1992;79:485.

Rudy D, Bush I. Sexual dysfunction after hysterectomy. *Contemp Obstet Gynecol* 1993;38:39.

Schilling J, Wyss P, Faisst K, et al. Swiss consensus guidelines for hysterectomy. *Int J Gynecol Obstet* 1999;64:297.

Semm K. Endoscopic subtotal hysterectomy without colpotomy: classic intrafascial SEMM hysterectomy. A new method of hysterectomy by pelviscopy, laparotomy, per vaginam or functionally by total uterine mucosal ablation. *Int Surg* 1996;81:362–70.

Sharon A, Auslander R, Brandes-Klein O. Cystoscopy after total or subtotal laparoscopic hysterectomy: the value of a routine procedure. *Obstet Gynecol Surv* 2006;61:511.

Sightler S, Boike G, Estape R, et al. Ovarian cancer in women with prior hysterectomy: a 14-year experience at the University of Miami. *Obstet Gynecol* 1991;78:681.

Speroff T, Dawson NV, Speroff L, et al. A risk-benefit analysis of elective bilateral oophorectomy: effect of changes in compliance with estrogen therapy on outcome. *Am J Obstet Gynecol* 1991;164:165.

Spilsbury K, Semmens JB, Hammond I, et al. Persistent high rates of hysterectomy in Western Australia: a population-based study of 83,000 procedures over 23 years. *BJOG* 2006;113:804.

Stergachis A, Kirkwood KS, Grothaus LC, et al. Tubal sterilization and the long-term risk of hysterectomy. *JAMA* 1990;264:2893.

Storm HH, Clemmenson IH, Manders T, et al. Supravaginal uterine amputation in Denmark 1978–1988 and risk of cancer. *Gynecol Oncol* 1992;45:198.

Stovall T, Muneyyirci-Delale O, Summitt R, et al., for the Leuprolide Acetate Study Group. GnRH agonist and iron versus placebo and iron in the anemic patient before surgery for leiomyomas: a randomized controlled trial. *Obstet Gynecol* 1995;86:65.

Stovall T, Summitt R, Bran D, et al. Outpatient vaginal hysterectomy: a pilot study. *Obstet Gynecol* 1992;80:145.

Stovall T, Summit R, Lipscomb G, et al. Vaginal cuff closure at abdominal hysterectomy: comparing sutures with absorbable staples. *Obstet Gynecol* 1991;78:415.

Surgical Care Improvement Project. *Prophylactic antibiotic regimen selection for surgery.* Available at: http://www.mediqic.org/scip. Accessed April 12, 2007.

Sutton C. Treatment of large uterine fibroids. *BJOG* 1996;103:494.

Symmonds RE, Pettit PDM. Ovarian remnant syndrome. *Obstet Gynecol* 1979;54:174.

Thompson JD, Birch HW. Indications for hysterectomy. *Clin Obstet Gynecol* 1981;24:1245.

Vessy M, Villard-MacKintosh L, McPherson K, et al. The epidemiology of hysterectomy: findings in a large cohort study. *BJOG* 1992;99:402.

Vierhout ME. Influence of nonradical hysterectomy on the function of the lower urinary tract. *Obstet Gynecol Surv* 2001;56:381.

Wall L. A technique for modified McCall culdoplasty at the time of abdominal hysterectomy. *J Am Coll Surg* 1994;178:507.

Watson T. Vaginal cuff closure with abdominal hysterectomy: a new approach. *J Reprod Med* 1994;39:903.

Weiss NS, Harlow BL. Why does hysterectomy without bilateral ooophorectomy influence the subsequent incidence of ovarian cancer? *Am J Epidemiol.* 1986;124:856–8.

Wilcox L, Koonin L, Pokras R, et al. Hysterectomy in the United States, 1988–1990. *Obstet Gynecol* 1994;83:549.

Wingo PA, Huezo CM, Rubin GL, et al. The mortality risk associated with hysterectomy. *Am J Obstet Gynecol* 1985;152:803.

Zakut H, Lotan M, Bracha Y. Vaginal preparation with povidone-iodine before abdominal hysterectomy: a comparison with antibiotic prophylaxis. *Clin Exp Obstet Gynecol* 1987;14:1.

CHAPTER 32B ■ VAGINAL HYSTERECTOMY

S. ROBERT KOVAC

DEFINITIONS

Endopelvic fascia—The layer of visceral endopelvic tissue surrounding the bladder, vagina, and rectum.

Enteroceles—Formed from a separation of the rectovaginal fascia from the pubocervical fascia. Indeed, enteroceles are pelvic hernias that descend through the posterior vaginal fornix. The most common location for an enterocele is the posterior superior vaginal segment.

Intramyometrial coring—A surgical technique for removal of a large uterus during vaginal hysterectomy. After the uterine vessels have been divided, the myometrium can be circumferentially incised with a scalpel placed parallel to the long axis of the uterus and beneath the serosal covering of the uterus. In effect, coring converts a spherical structure into an elongated rod shape, enhancing the surgeon's ability to facilitate uterine removal.

McCall culdoplasty—The most commonly employed technique to close the posterior vaginal cuff.

The technique of operating through the vagina is a prerogative of the gynecologic surgeon. Vaginal surgery is an essential prerequisite in the cultural and surgical training of a qualified gynecologist. However, in the United States, the most common operation gynecologists perform, the hysterectomy, is predominantly done abdominally.

Vaginal hysterectomy is the signature operation of the gynecologic profession. Ample evidence shows that the vaginal approach results in lower morbidity, less pain, more rapid recovery, more rapid return to normal activities, consumption of fewer health care dollars and resources, and a host of other benefits. A gynecologic surgeon should have the ability to perform both abdominal and vaginal hysterectomies. However, vaginal hysterectomy is, and should remain, the hallmark of gynecological extirpative hysterectomy surgery and surgical excellence. Vaginal hysterectomy is the "gold standard" for the surgical removal of the uterus. At minimum, a gynecologic surgeon should perform at least 25% of his/her benign hysterectomies by the vaginal route.

INDICATIONS

With the advent of evidence-based research and outcomes studies, several randomized controlled trials have documented the advantages of the vaginal approach to hysterectomy. A recent Cochrane review concluded that vaginal hysterectomy, rather than abdominal, should be performed whenever technically feasible to reduce complications, shorten hospital stays, and accelerate the patient's return to normal activities. Despite these results, these studies have not stimulated a change in physician practice patterns, which should be expected from this type of objective evidence. Several investigators have addressed the reasons for the continued dominance of the abdominal route for hysterectomy. Johns and colleagues suggested that the route of hysterectomy is usually determined by the skill, experience, and preference of the operating gynecologist. Few other parameters matter. Dorsey and associates stated that the hysterectomy patient is best served by a surgeon who selects the route with which he or she is most comfortable.

Suggesting that the feasibility of performing vaginal hysterectomy may restrict its implementation has always been a concern, especially for surgeons who prefer to use abdominal or laparoscopic techniques. The intent of developing hysterectomy guidelines was to identify when abdominal hysterectomy is truly mandated (Fig. 32B.1). Using these guidelines, expert gynecologic surgeons have achieved vaginal hysterectomy rates in excess of 90%, in contrast to the overall U.S. average of 30%, which includes laparoscopically assisted vaginal hysterectomy.

Vaginal hysterectomy has usually been indicated for women with uterine or pelvic prolapse, and traditional indications for abdominal hysterectomy have included an enlarged uterus, prior pelvic surgery, malignancy, and extrauterine disease, such as endometriosis or pelvic inflammatory disease. We now know that successful vaginal hysterectomy can be done in most of these patients; however, special techniques, such as uterine coring or bivalving, are often helpful, and laparoscopic lymphadenectomy may be required in women with cervical or endometrial cancer. Laparoscopy may also be useful to evaluate an adnexal mass more carefully or the extent of endometriosis before completing the surgery with a vaginal hysterectomy and oophorectomy. Laparoscopy may also be used as an aid to reassure and give confidence to the young vaginal surgeon that extensive adhesions do not exist and the anatomy is relatively normal so that vaginal hysterectomy can be accomplished. With increasing confidence and skill that comes from experience, there are very few patients with indications for hysterectomy in whom the procedure cannot be performed vaginally.

PREOPERATIVE PREPARATION

If the surgeon is concerned about unintentionally injuring the rectum, it is important that he or she have the patient cleanse the rectum with an electrolyte purgative such as GoLYTELY, Nu LYTELY, or CoLyte the evening before surgery. If this concern does not exist, a Fleet's enema is adequate *if* it is given the evening before surgery. Bowel cleansing evacuates solid stool from the rectum, reduces the bacterial load of the intestinal tract, and reduces the incidence of postoperative ileus and constipation.

A single-dose antibiotic as a prophylactic measure, usually a first-generation cephalosporin, should be given within 1 hour before the operation is started. Prophylactic antibiotics have been documented to reduce the risk of postoperative infections. It has been the author's practice during the past 20 years to check the vaginal pH before prepping the patient. If the pH is not normal (3.8–4.2), the normal vaginal ecosystem has been

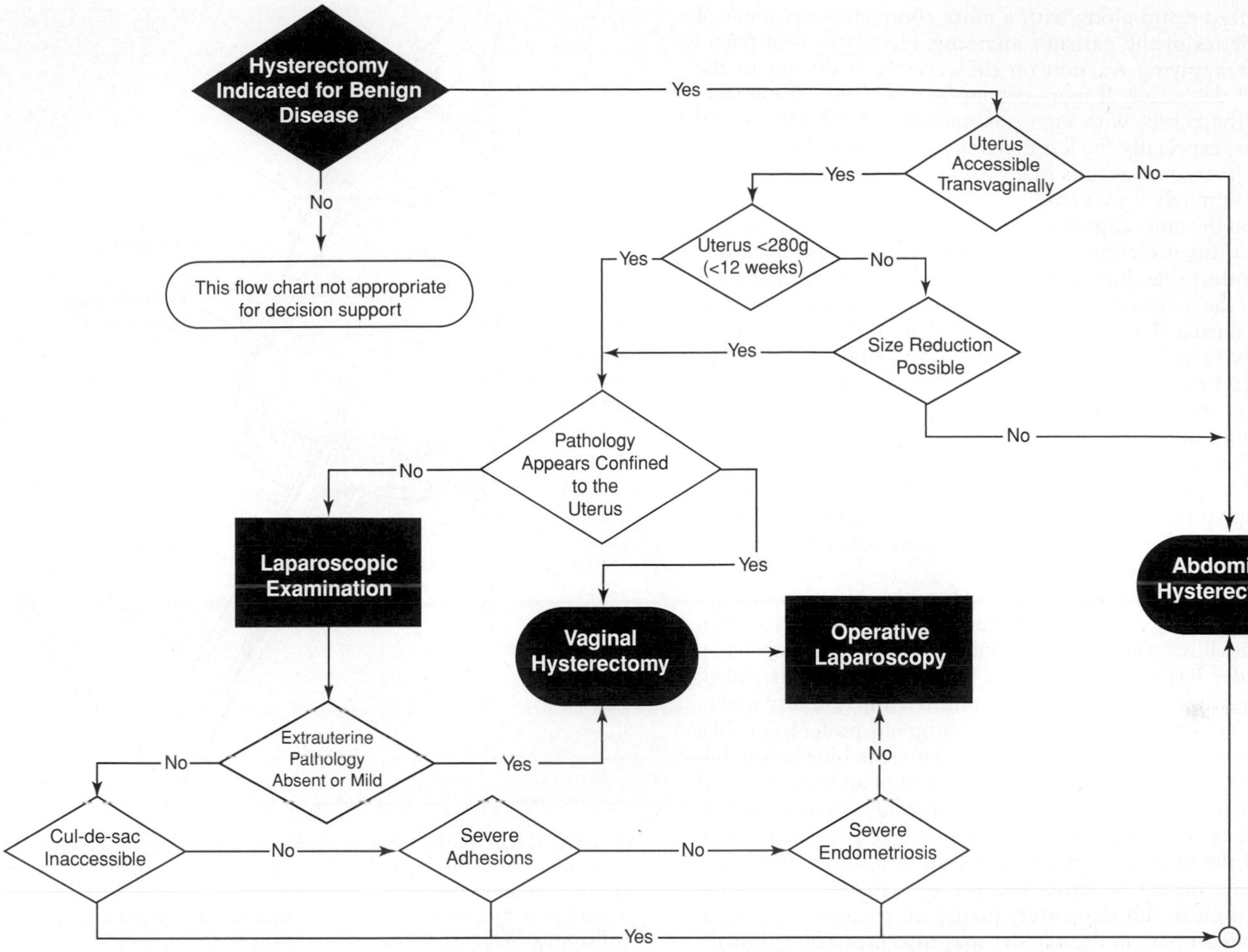

FIGURE 32B.1. Determining the route of hysterectomy. (From Kovac SR, Zimmerman CW, eds. *Advances in reconstructive vaginal surgery.* Philadelphia: Lippincott Williams & Wilkins; 2006;95.)

altered. A vaginal pH in the range of 5.0 or greater suggests the potential for bacterial vaginosis and the likelihood that the facultative bacteria normally present in the vagina at concentrations of 10^3 have reached concentrations of 10^8. This strongly suggests that the vagina is infected before the start of the operation. These patients may not be protected by routine prophylactic antibiotics but may benefit from postoperative therapeutic antibiotics. In such patients, we usually administer 500 mg of metronidazole orally twice daily from the second to the seventh postoperative day. This practice has reduced my postoperative infection rate following vaginal hysterectomy from 9% from 1970 to 1986 to less than 1% from 1987 to present.

Gynecologists have long believed that a Betadine solution used as a preoperative vaginal scrub will remove most potential pathogens in the vagina, but this has recently been questioned. I prefer to prep all patients with 70% ethanol, even in the vagina, and use a self-adherent surgical drape that covers the rectum and conveniently keeps pubic hair and the labia from interfering with the operative field. Shaving of the pubic hair is unnecessary, and shaven patients are more uncomfortable postoperatively. Additionally, the author has always been averse to suturing the labia to the inner thighs.

Copious lavage of the vaginal vault before, during, and after vaginal hysterectomy may also help to prevent postoperative infections by removing bacteria adherent to the vaginal epithelium. Lavage is not used as frequently in the vaginal approach as it should be. Lavage with a lighted irrigation and suction instrument combined can also be used to accomplish this goal.

The type of stirrups used for the lithotomy position is solely at the discretion of the surgeon. No matter what type is used, careful attention is required to protect vulnerable vascular, bony, and neurologic points in the lower extremities. The author prefers the candy cane–type stirrups. The patient should be positioned with the buttocks at the end of the surgical table or just beyond. The table is placed at a zero horizontal position without Trendelenburg. In this manner, the surgeon can look directly into the vagina without having to look over the weighted speculum. Final positioning of the patient should protect the patient, allowing the surgeon to operate comfortably, and provide adequate room for surgical assistants to be effective. Assistants need to stand inside the stirrups to see the operative field to both observe and learn the operation. Pneumatic stockings are also recommended.

OPERATIVE TECHNIQUE

It is valuable to perform an examination under anesthesia before initiating the operation to reconfirm the preoperative exam. Undetected pathology may be appreciated during an anesthetized exam along with a more complete assessment of the subtleties of the patient's anatomy. Placement of a tenaculum for applying traction on the cervix can document the degree of descensus. If more descensus is desired, strong traction on the cervix with vigorous massage of the uterosacral ligaments, especially the left uterosacral ligament, for approximately 30 seconds results in a further descensus of the cervix of approximately 2 to 3 cm.

Although some surgeons prefer to stand during vaginal hysterectomy, my preference is to sit. However, to make the assistants comfortable during the operation, the surgeon's chair is raised so the assistants do not need to bend over but can stand straight during the entire procedure. This surgeon prefers to operate with an instrument tray on his lap, which makes it easier to select the desired instruments during the operation. The number of instruments used during vaginal surgery should be kept at a minimum to prevent instruments from obscuring the surgeon's vision. This author believes that the number of instruments used during any gynecologic operation is inversely proportional to the skill of the surgeon, whereas the quality of instruments is directly proportional. These concepts are especially true in vaginal surgery.

Catheterization of the bladder before the initiation of vaginal hysterectomy is usually at the preference of the surgeon. Sometimes it is easier to identify unintentional cystotomy when the bladder has some urine in it. If the bladder is distended, catheterization of the bladder may improve the visibility within this restricted operative space. Some surgeons prefer to instill a dilute solution of indigo carmine or methylene blue before initiating the operation to ensure recognition of an unanticipated operative injury to the bladder. If a cystotomy occurs, it is best to complete the vaginal hysterectomy before proceeding with repair of the bladder. In many cases, the cystotomy may make the bladder dissection easier because now the location of the bladder is clear and the correct planes more easily visualized. Sometimes a finger in the bladder may also facilitate a difficult dissection. The bladder must be mobilized adequately around the operative injury so that the surgeon can completely evaluate the extent of the cystotomy and be certain that the repair is completed without excess tension on the injured site.

The initial vaginal incision should be made at the border of the vaginal rugae through the full thickness of the vagina (Fig. 32B.2). Unfortunately, it has been taught that the circumscribing incision should be made on the cervix to preserve vaginal length and avoid unintentional entry into the bladder. This is incorrect, because decreased vaginal rugae mark the point where the vagina truly begins. In addition, an incision at the point where the vagina begins appropriately places the mucosal incision closer to the point of entry into the posterior and anterior peritoneum (Fig. 32B.3). An incision in this location allows the surgeon to avoid dissection of the connective tissues between the vagina and the peritoneum, reducing blood loss, because this dissection frequently involves transection of several cervical branches of the uterine artery. Thus, bleeding will be less when the incision is made where the rugae begin or cease to exist.

Julian reported on the benefit of infiltrating the vaginal wall with a mixture of 1:200,000 epinephrine diluted in normal saline to control small blood vessel bleeding from the vagina. Rarely does oozing from the vaginal mucosa result in significant blood loss when the incision is made where the vaginal rugae start. If oozing from the incised edges of the vagina becomes a problem, it is easy to control with electrocautery.

At the beginning of the operation, when the cervix is still within the vagina, it is often difficult to perform a circumscribing incision around the cervix with a scalpel or electrocautery

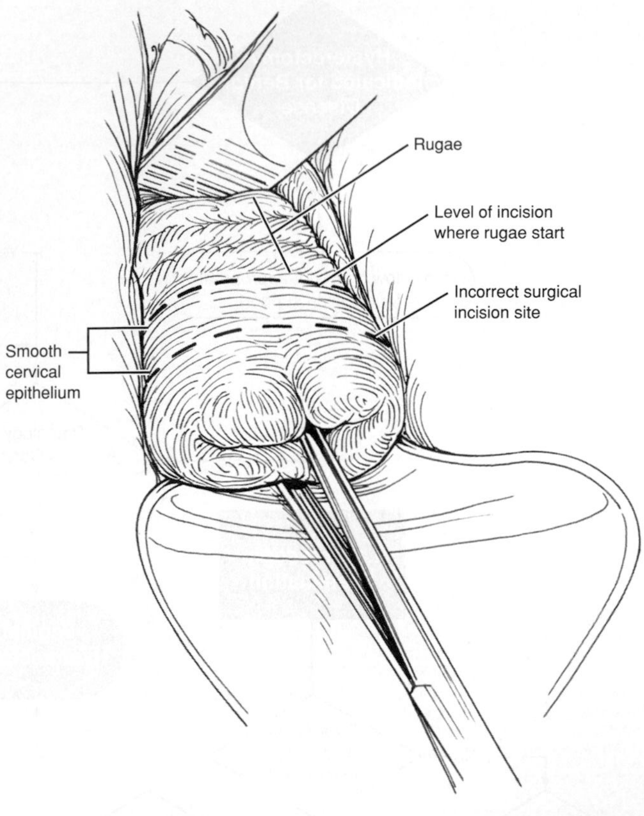

FIGURE 32B.2. Initial incision should be a full-thickness incision at the border where the vaginal rugae begin and the smooth cervical epithelium on the cervix ends. (From Kovac SR, Zimmerman CW, eds. *Advances in reconstructive vaginal surgery.* Philadelphia: Lippincott Williams & Wilkins; 2006.)

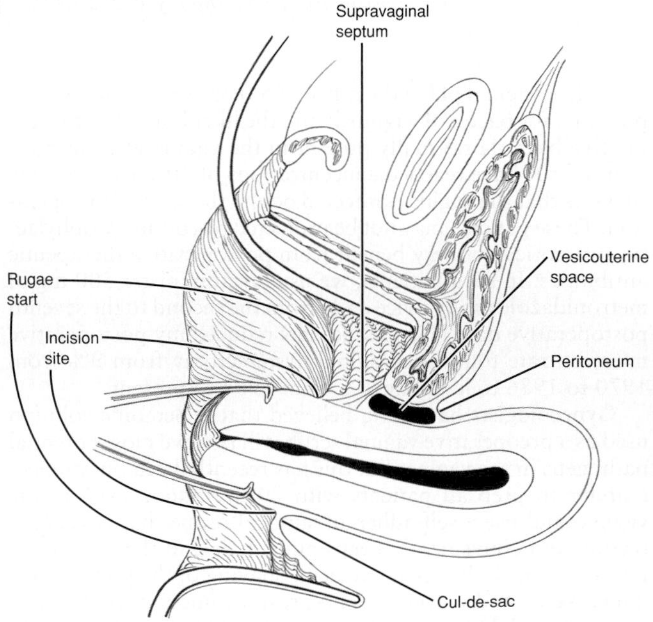

FIGURE 32B.3. Relationship between the vaginal rugae and the anterior and posterior peritoneum. (From Kovac SR, Zimmerman CW, eds. *Advances in reconstructive vaginal surgery.* Philadelphia: Lippincott Williams & Wilkins; 2006).

instrument because it is difficult to maintain either device perpendicular to the circumscribing vaginal incision. This is not a concern when the cervix protrudes from the vagina. However, when the cervix cannot be brought out of the vagina with traction, the initial incision should be made on the anterior vaginal wall from approximately the 10- to 2-o'clock position and on the posterior vaginal wall between the 8- and 4-o'clock positions. These incisions provide adequate space for the subsequent entry into the posterior and anterior peritoneum (Fig. 32B.4A,B).

After completing the vaginal incisions, the cervical tenaculum is replaced on the posterior lip of the cervix with taut traction of the cervix achieved by elevating the tenaculum anteriorly. If the posterior incision in the vagina is placed at the appropriate level where rugae are not present and at the point where the uterosacral ligaments join the cervix, the posterior cul-de-sac and peritoneum can readily be identified with tissue forceps. This is done by putting the subvaginal tissue and accompanying peritoneum on stretch as the peritoneum bulges outward toward the surgeon (Fig. 32B.5). This cannot be overstated. Entry into the posterior peritoneum is best accomplished by an incision directly above the tissue forceps that grasps the outward U-shaped bulge of the peritoneal fold (Fig. 32B.6). If the incision is placed closer to the cervix in an attempt to prevent injury to the rectum, the dissection often proceeds into the posterior cervical stroma. Unfortunately, an incision placed nearer to the cervix frequently results in a retroperitoneal dissection, which continues in this plane and ultimately pushes the peritoneum superiorly and posteriorly, obscuring identification of the peritoneum. Should this occur, the posterior lip of the cervix and vagina can be cut in a vertical direction that exposes the peritoneum at a higher level so it can be recognized and entered directly. This is a cervicocolpotomy (Fig. 32B.7).

The peritoneum is opened with curved scissors, and a long-bladed Steiner Auvard weighted speculum is introduced into the peritoneal cavity. Examination of the cul-de-sac can provide further pathology—such as endometriosis, leiomyomata, or adnexal pathology—that may be encountered later in the operation. Identification of the uterosacral ligaments by palpation can be accomplished during examination of the cul-de-sac through the posterior colpotomy incision. Transection of the uterosacral ligaments is the single most important step in successfully completing a vaginal hysterectomy. It is unnecessary to tag the posterior peritoneum to the vagina, as the edges of the peritoneum do not separate far from its edges. Oozing of blood from this space between the vagina and peritoneum may occur, but placement of a weighted speculum into the posterior peritoneal cavity will compress most bleeding points between the cut edges of the vagina and the peritoneum.

The cervix should then be retracted downward and inferiorly, and the anterior subvaginal tissue, including the supravaginal septum and the bladder, picked up with tissue forceps and elevated in the midline. The supravaginal septum is part of the pericervical ring and is identified and incised using curved scissors with the tips pointing downward. The handles are not

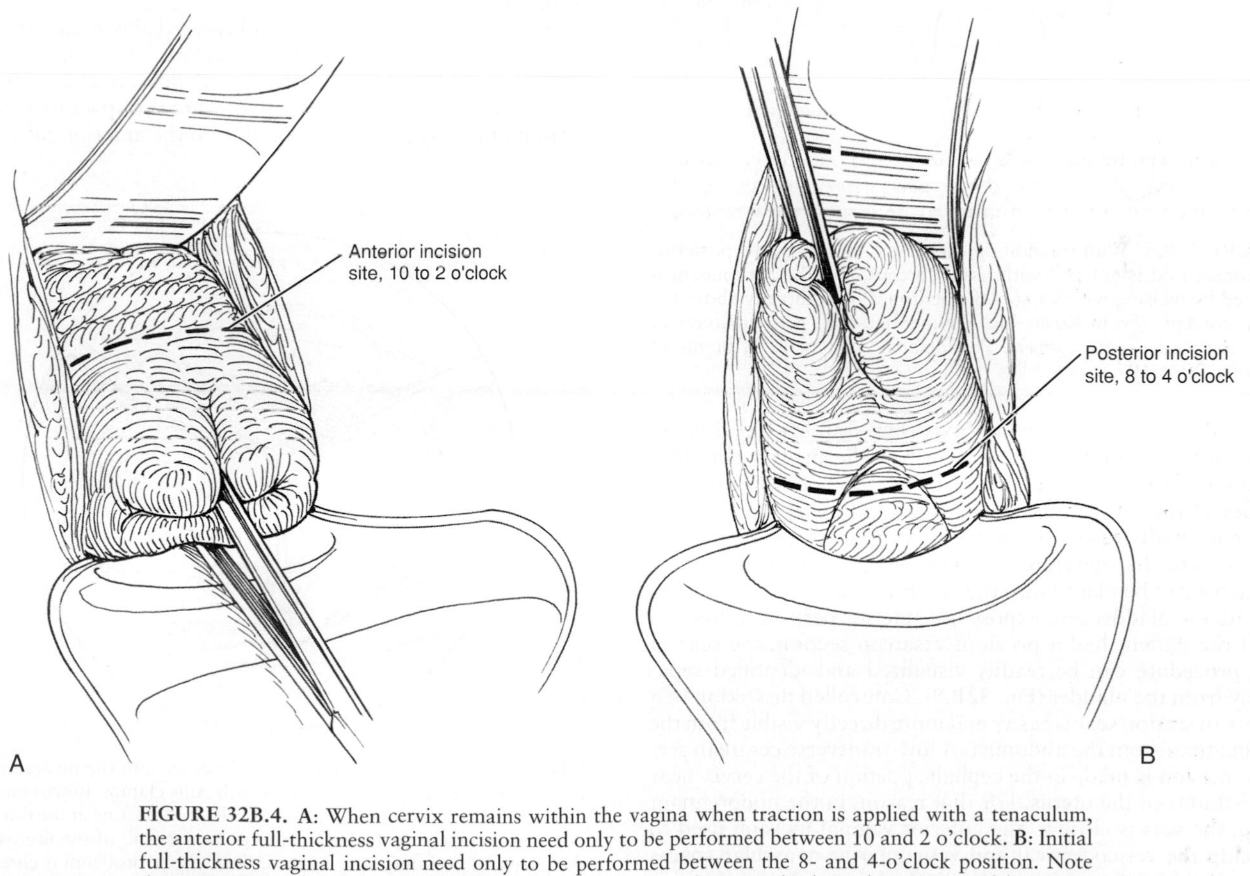

FIGURE 32B.4. **A:** When cervix remains within the vagina when traction is applied with a tenaculum, the anterior full-thickness vaginal incision need only to be performed between 10 and 2 o'clock. **B:** Initial full-thickness vaginal incision need only to be performed between the 8- and 4-o'clock position. Note this incision is placed posteriorly where the vaginal rugae begin and where the uterosacral ligaments attach to the cervix. (From Kovac SR, Zimmerman CW, eds. *Advances in reconstructive vaginal surgery.* Philadelphia: Lippincott Williams & Wilkins; 2006:106.)

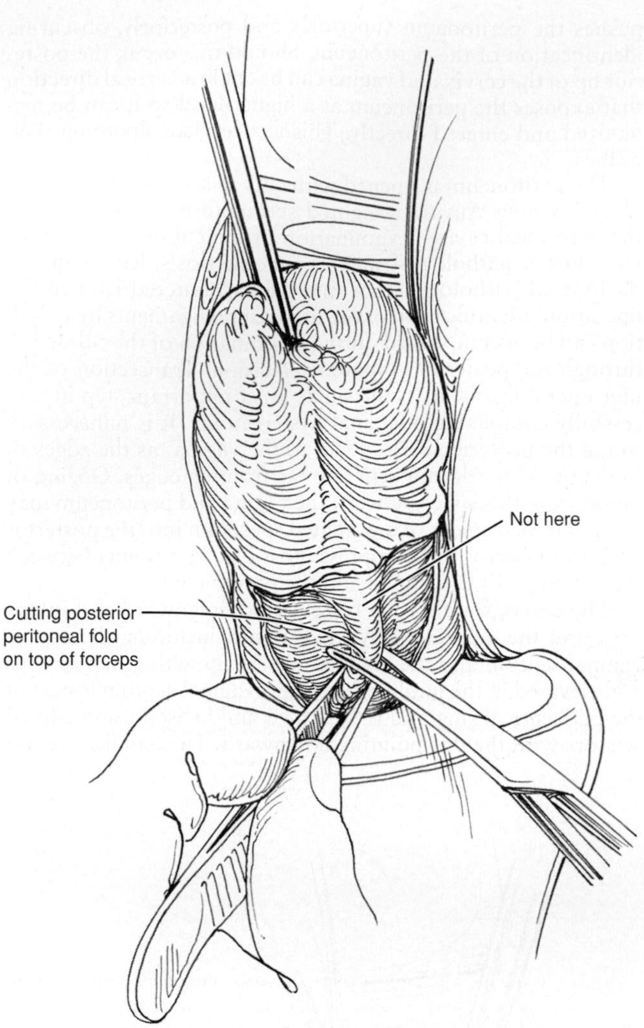

FIGURE 32B.5. With traction on the cervix anteriorly, the posterior peritoneal fold is grasped with tissue forceps, and the peritoneum is entered by incising with scissors the peritoneal fold directly above the tissue forceps. (From Kovac SR, Zimmerman CW, eds. *Advances in reconstructive vaginal surgery.* Philadelphia: Lippincott Williams & Wilkins; 2006:107.)

elevated above the horizontal axis (Fig. 32B.8A,B). This exposes the vesicouterine space, which is the proper avascular cleavage plane to gain access to the anterior peritoneum. The blades of the scissors may then be spread apart, opening the tissue normally fusing the posterior wall of the bladder to the cervix to further develop this space. A lightweight right angle retractor can be placed into the anterior vesicouterine space to elevate the bladder and expose the anterior peritoneal fold.

If the patient had a previous cesarean section, the scar of this procedure can be readily visualized and identified separately from the bladder (Fig. 32B.9). Controlled dissection of a cesarean section scar is easier and more directly visible from the vagina than from the abdomen. A low-transverse cesarean section incision is made in the cephalic portion of the cervix near the isthmus of the uterus. For that reason, in the nonpregnant state, the scar is close to the anterior vaginal incision used to develop the vesicocervical and vesicouterine avascular spaces in vaginal hysterectomy and can be easily seen. A cesarean section scar distorts the anatomy by reducing the vesicouterine space between the scar and the urinary bladder. Further dissec-

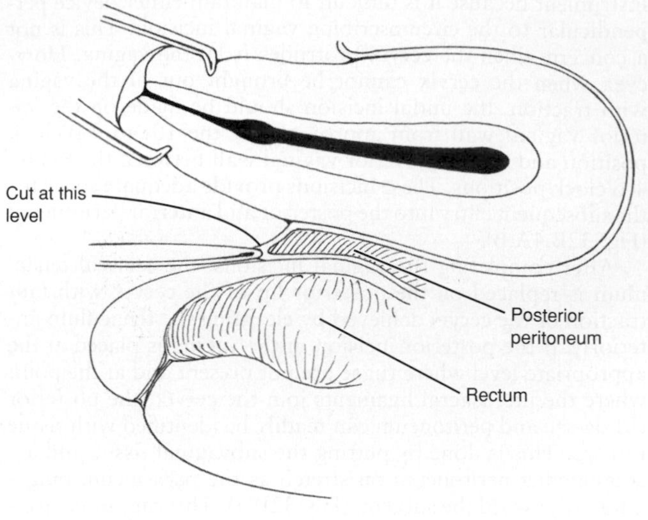

FIGURE 32B.6. Transverse view of entering the peritoneal cavity. (From Kovac SR, Zimmerman CW, eds. *Advances in reconstructive vaginal surgery.* Philadelphia: Lippincott Williams & Wilkins; 2006:107.)

tion above the scar can be performed by identifying the scar, the bladder, and the peritoneum as independent structures. On occasion, it is also possible to dissect under the scar, which keeps the dissection even further from the urinary bladder (Fig. 32B.10).

The peritoneum is grasped and entered above the tissue forceps by a 1-cm opening with the scissors. The shining surface of the peritoneum is recognized, and this opening is further stretched by spreading of the scissors into this space to allow insertion of the right-angle retractor into the anterior cul-de-sac,

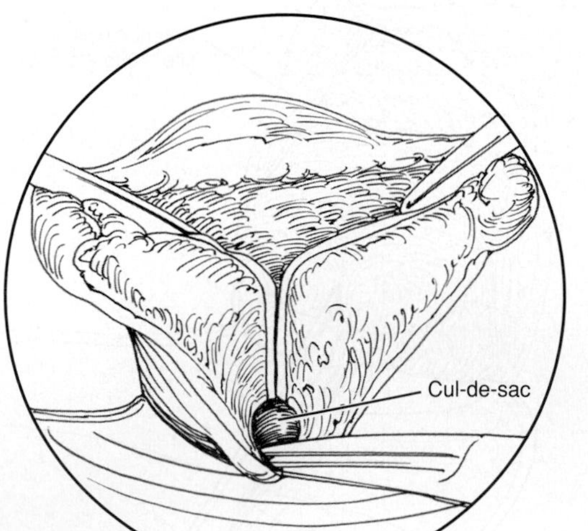

FIGURE 32B.7. Cervical colpotomy for entry into the posterior peritoneum. Posterior cervix is grasped with Allis clamps approximately at 4- and 8-o'clock positions. The cervix is incised starting at the 6-o'clock position and incising the cervix and posterior wall of the uterus until the posterior peritoneum is entered. Once the peritoneum is entered, a weighted speculum is placed into the posterior peritoneal cavity. (From Kovac SR, Zimmerman CW, eds. *Advances in reconstructive vaginal surgery.* Philadelphia: Lippincott Williams & Wilkins; 2006:108.)

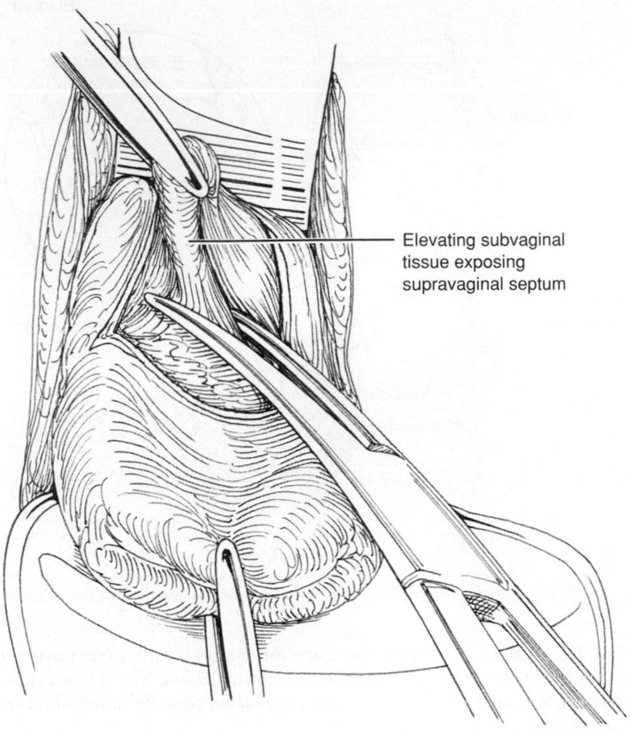

FIGURE 32B.8. Entry into the anterior peritoneum involves incising the supravaginal septum to gain entry into the vesicouterine space. Once the vesicouterine space has been entered, the space is developed by spreading the dissecting scissors for placement of a retractor to elevate the bladder. (From Kovac SR, Zimmerman CW, eds. *Advances in reconstructive vaginal surgery.* Philadelphia: Lippincott Williams & Wilkins; 2006:109.)

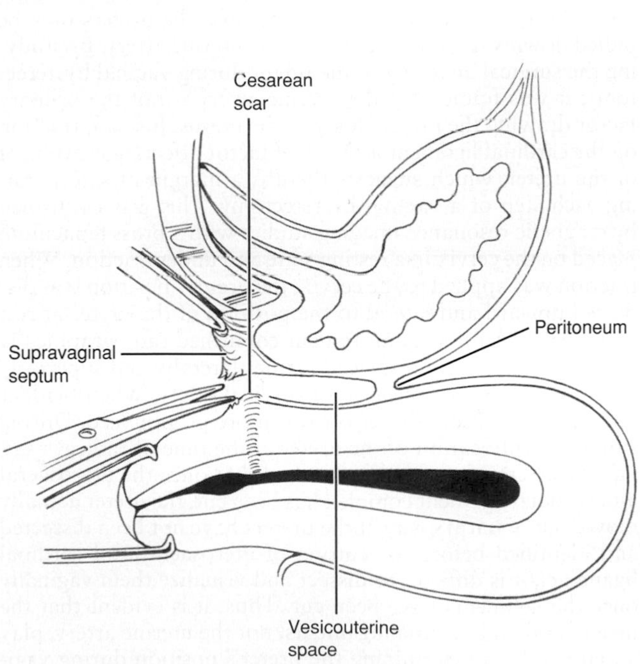

FIGURE 32B.9. Relationship between the supravaginal septum, vesicouterine space, cesarean section scar, and anterior peritoneal fold. (From Kovac SR, Zimmerman CW, eds. *Advances in reconstructive vaginal surgery.* Philadelphia: Lippincott Williams & Wilkins; 2006:109.)

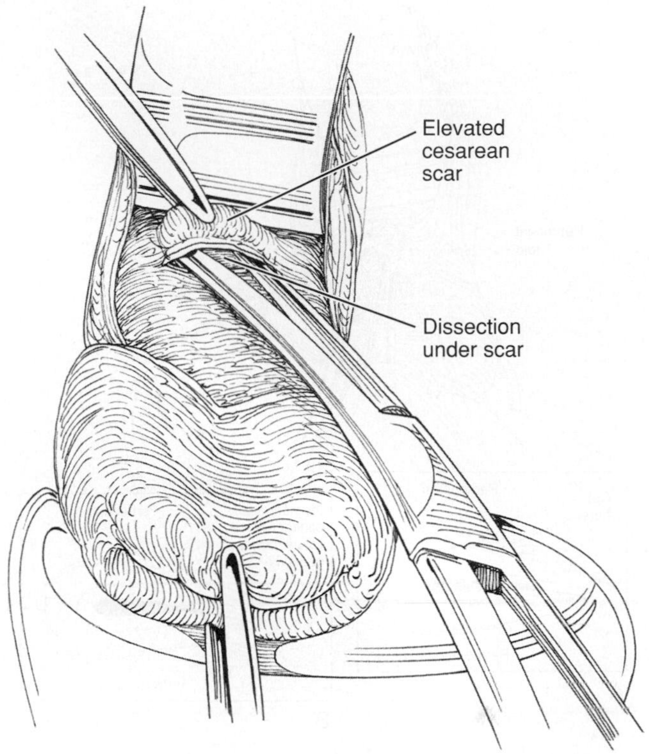

FIGURE 32B.10. Sometimes it is possible to dissect beneath the cesarean section scar to gain entry into the superior part of the vesicouterine space to identify the anterior peritoneal fold. (From Kovac SR, Zimmerman CW, eds. *Advances in reconstructive vaginal surgery.* Philadelphia: Lippincott Williams & Wilkins; 2006:110.)

which remains in this position and elevates the bladder throughout the entire operation. This does not increase the risk of operative injury to the bladder if the surgeon has properly dissected into the vesicouterine space and retracts the bladder superiorly. The anterior peritoneal fold should always be opened under direct vision. Where the tissue forceps actually grasp the fold will determine the best place to enter the peritoneum (Fig. 32B.11A,B).

Because of the surgeon's desire to avoid injury to the bladder, there is the tendency to dissect as far as possible from the bladder. Thus, this may cause him or her to cut into the connective tissue capsule of the cervix, with further retroperitoneal dissection within the connective tissue stroma of the anterior cervix. Similar to the posterior dissection, this is more likely when the initial incision into the vagina is made too close to the cervix. Further dissection beneath the peritoneum covering of the anterior uterine segment results in failure to enter the anatomic plane, the vesicouterine space between the bladder and uterus. Failure to identify this correct tissue plane and/or a lack of caution results in either further retroperitoneal dissection or unintentional bladder penetration. If an injury to the bladder results, it will occur well above the trigone of the bladder and not near the ureteral orifices. This injury is simple to repair after the uterus has been removed. Unintentional operative cystotomy is a risk of any vaginal hysterectomy with any technique. The overall incidence of operative cystotomy while performing and teaching this technique has resulted in an acceptable cystotomy rate of 1.2% with vaginal hysterectomies.

The use of a sponge on the surgeon's finger to push the supravaginal septum and the vesicouterine space superiorly to

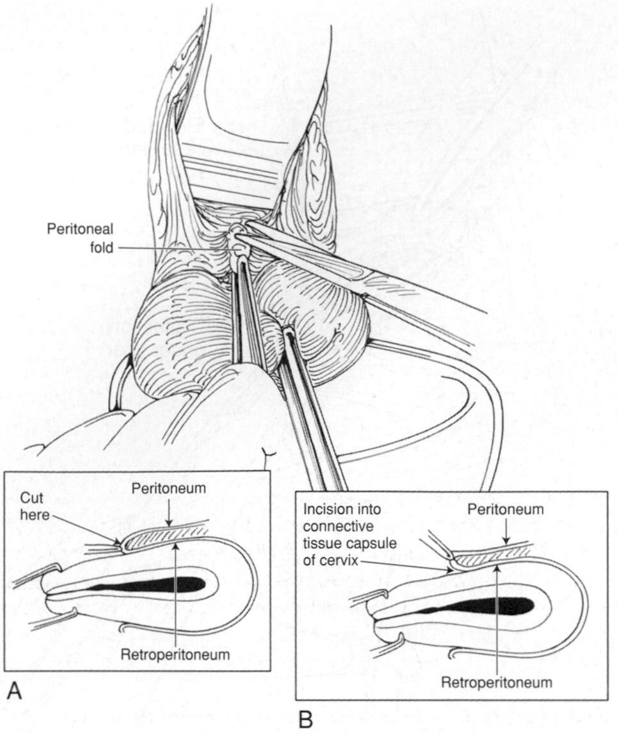

FIGURE 32B.11. Entry into the anterior peritoneum. Peritoneal fold is grasped with tissue forceps and pulled downward. Scissors incise peritoneal fold just above tissue forceps. **Insert A:** Lateral view demonstrating the method for entering the anterior peritoneum. **Insert B:** Retroperitoneal dissection with elevation of the peritoneal fold. (From Kovac SR, Zimmerman CW, eds. *Advances in reconstructive vaginal surgery.* Philadelphia: Lippincott Williams & Wilkins; 2006:110.)

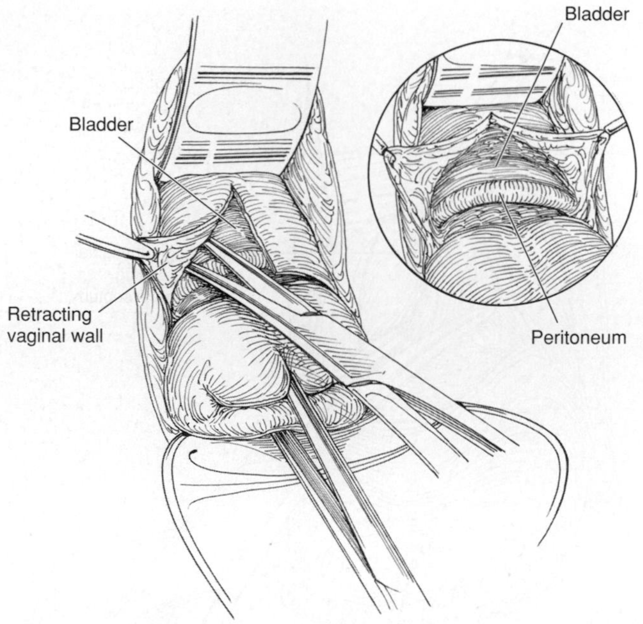

FIGURE 32B.12. Opening the anterior vaginal wall to expose the bladder and anterior peritoneal fold. (From Kovac SR, Zimmerman CW, eds. *Advances in reconstructive vaginal surgery.* Philadelphia: Lippincott Williams & Wilkins:2006.)

expose the anterior peritoneum is frequently taught. This could be considered as more of a technique of *accomplir forcee* (i.e., to accomplish with force) than a surgical dissection, as the cleavage plane becomes indistinguishable from the supravaginal septum up to the anterior peritoneal fold. The risk of tearing the bladder with this technique is potentially increased, especially if the patient had a previous cesarean section. The anterior peritoneum should always be opened under direct vision, never blindly, as unintentional entry into the bladder frequently results from an attempt to enter the peritoneum blindly.

It is not necessary to persist in attempts to open the anterior peritoneum if there is any doubt that the peritoneal fold is not clearly identified. Cutting the uterosacral and cardinal ligaments will bring the uterus closer to both the surgeon and the peritoneal fold, which can be identified and entered at this later point of the operation. The anterior peritoneum can also be safely opened, especially when the uterus is enlarged, with a vertical incision in the vaginal epithelium similar to an anterior colporrhaphy. This allows accurate identification of the bladder from the peritoneal fold (Fig. 32B.12).

After both the posterior and anterior peritoneum are successfully entered, detachment of the uterus from its supportive ligaments can be accomplished. The uterosacral and cardinal ligaments can also be ligated and secured in separate pedicles before attempts to enter the anterior peritoneum. This extraperitoneal approach provides significant additional exposure. Separating the cervix from the paracolpium, along with the resulting descent of the uterus, increases visibility. This exposure is significant and makes the peritoneal identification/entry process less troublesome. Indeed, the uterine artery can also be divided before peritoneal entry, allowing even greater exposure.

The exact location of the ureter during abdominal, laparoscopic, and vaginal hysterectomy is always a concern. Nichols and Randall suggested that the risk of ureteral injury during a vaginal hysterectomy is greater because the ureters may be pulled downward and medially by the uterine artery. By studying the surgical anatomy of the ureter during vaginal hysterectomy, it was found that the uterine artery is not the primary factor drawing the ureter closer to the uterus. Instead, traction on the cardinal ligament is the chief factor affecting movement of the ureter, which suggests there is a margin of safety during each step of a vaginal hysterectomy. This was confirmed by magnetic resonance imaging studies with a brass tenaculum placed on the cervix in a resting state and under traction. When traction was applied to the cervix, the ureter's position was displaced upward and lateral to the position of the ureter at rest (Fig. 32B.13A,B). This movement confirmed radiographically that the ureters were displaced further laterally and superiorly from the cervix to a position of surgical safety. When bladder retraction was used, this effect was more pronounced. During surgical identification of the ureter at the time of radical vaginal hysterectomy, it can be observed that once the uterosacral and cardinal ligament complex has been cut, the ureter actually moves out of harm's way. If the ureters have not been dissected and identified before the cutting of uterosacral and cardinal ligaments, it is difficult to dissect and visualize them vaginally once the ligaments have been cut. Thus, it is evident that the uterosacral and cardinal ligaments, not the uterine artery, play a major role in determining the ureter's position during vaginal hysterectomy. Once these ligaments have been divided, the ureter will retract out of harm's way (Fig. 32B.14A,B).

When possible, I attempt to enter both the posterior and anterior peritoneum before clamping the uterosacral and cardinal ligaments. Placement of a retractor under the bladder also

A

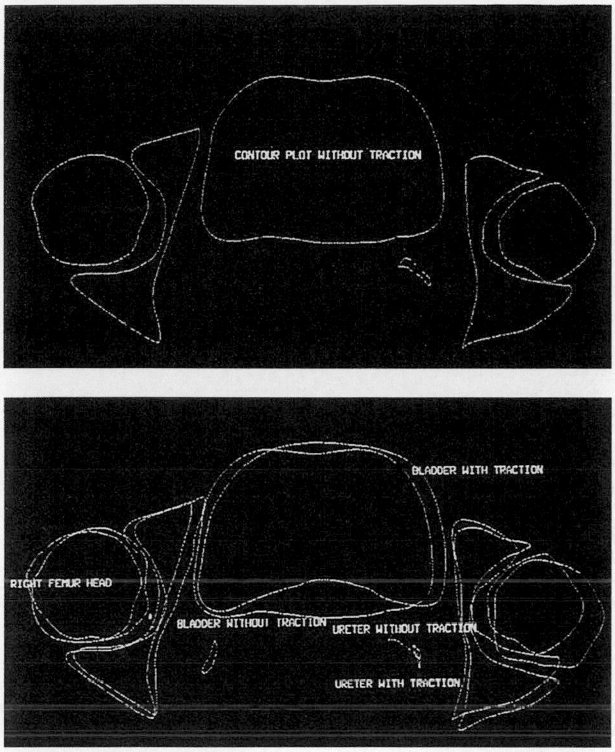

B

FIGURE 32B.13. **A:** Magnetic resonance imaging (MRI) studies of ureteral movement when downward traction is placed on the uterus. Ureter position is seen on the right. **B:** Overlay of MRI films. Traction on the uterus with a brass tenaculum is applied to the cervix. Note indentation to the bladder from the uterus and lateral and upward displacement of the ureter compared with the position of the ureter position without traction to the uterus. (From Kovac SR, Zimmerman CW, eds. *Advances in reconstructive vaginal surgery.* Philadelphia: Lippincott Williams & Wilkins; 2006:112.)

elevates the ureter out of the operative field (Fig. 32B.15A,B). It is recommended that once the retractor is placed under the bladder, it should not be removed during any stage of the vaginal hysterectomy. It was clearly demonstrated in the study of ureteral movement during vaginal hysterectomy that when forceful traction was applied to the uterus during vaginal hysterectomy with no retraction of the bladder, the ureter was pulled medially and potentially placed in harm's way.

If the vaginal mucosa has not been completely circumscribed, once the anterior and posterior peritoneum have been entered, the vaginal incision should be completed by connecting the previous anterior and posterior incisions before the supportive ligaments of the uterus can be clamped. The uterosacral ligaments are clamped with the tip of the clamp, including the lower portion of the cardinal ligaments. The posterior tip of each clamp should be placed within the peritoneal cavity and the anterior tip around the ligament superiorly. The Kovac vaginal hysterectomy clamp (Marina Medical, Hollywood, FL) has less pelvic curve than the Heaney clamp, longer jaws, and two rat-tooth projections within the jaws to prevent slippage of tissue within the clamp (Fig. 32B.16A–C). Rotating the handles of the clamp laterally and superiorly facilitates suturing at the tip of the clamp. This brings the tip of the clamp into full view and exposes a triangular area beneath the clamp for easier retrieval of the needle. I do not believe it is necessary to double clamp each uterine supportive or vascular structures. Each uterosacral ligament is secured by a transfixation suture to the posterolateral surface of the vagina and is tied behind the clamp at about the 4- and 8-o'clock positions. Lateral traction on this suture provides the best exposure to the remaining structures within the broad ligament. This replaces the need for lateral retractors into the vagina, which only expose the lateral vagina and not the broad ligament (Fig. 32B.17). Clamping and tagging the uterosacral ligaments separately allows for their identification, later use in cuff repair, and, if desired, a McCall's culdoplasty at the end of the procedure. The uterosacral ligament pedicle is the only one that needs to be tagged during a vaginal hysterectomy.

After making sure the tips of the clamps are within the posterior peritoneal cavity, the cardinal ligaments are clamped. The anterior peritoneum should not be pulled into this clamp at this point of the operation. Bringing the peritoneal edges together serves to seal off the broad ligament by effectively preventing bleeding from the vascular plexus located within the leaves of the broad ligament. Because the anterior peritoneum usually begins at the level of the uterine vessels, there may not be enough stretchable peritoneum to bring both the anterior and posterior peritoneal surfaces together at the level of the cardinal ligaments. Therefore, to be certain that the surgeon can seal both leaves of the broad ligament together with the uterine artery, it is best to avoid any attempt to bring the peritoneal edges together when the uterosacral or cardinal ligament are clamped (Fig. 32B.18). A simple suture ligature first at the tip and then around the end of the clamp is usually sufficient for hemostasis of the cardinal ligament without the need for transfixation (Fig. 32B.19). This suture ligature is not tagged or held.

At this point, the uterine arteries should become visible on each side of the uterus. They are clamped with one good clamp at a time. This clamp is placed parallel to the uterus as the tip of the clamp secures the uterine artery as it bifurcates into ascending and descending branches (Fig. 32B.19). As traction is placed on the uterus when the artery is cut, there is a definite sensation that the uterus descends; this signifies that the entire uterine artery has been transected, including the ascending and descending branches. If descent of the uterus is not noted, often an additional portion of the uterine artery remains and must be taken with another clamp. A single transfixation is all that is required if only the uterine artery is within the clamp. Limiting the tissue within the clamp to the vascular bundle helps to make the pedicle manageable and the suture ligature more secure. Many surgeons try to include middle portions of the broad ligament with the uterine artery because they feel a need to place clamps on the remaining portions of the broad ligament as they proceed up on each side of the uterus.

Most gynecologic surgeons are comfortable with performing a vaginal hysterectomy to the point of ligating the uterine artery. Beyond this point, many gynecologists wonder if the uterus can be removed vaginally. This is the result of an unfounded belief that continued clamping up each side of the remaining broad ligament is required for successful uterine removal. This is a puzzling idea, because when performing an abdominal hysterectomy, the upper portions of the broad ligament above the uterine vessels are sharply dissected, and no clamps are used. When the vaginal surgeon continues to place clamps above the uterine artery, the space to place each clamp becomes more restrictive, and placing sutures around these clamps becomes more difficult. This problem often spurs comments by surgeons that vaginal hysterectomy is a difficult operation because of restrictive access and visibility. Clamping and suturing of the broad ligament above the uterine artery

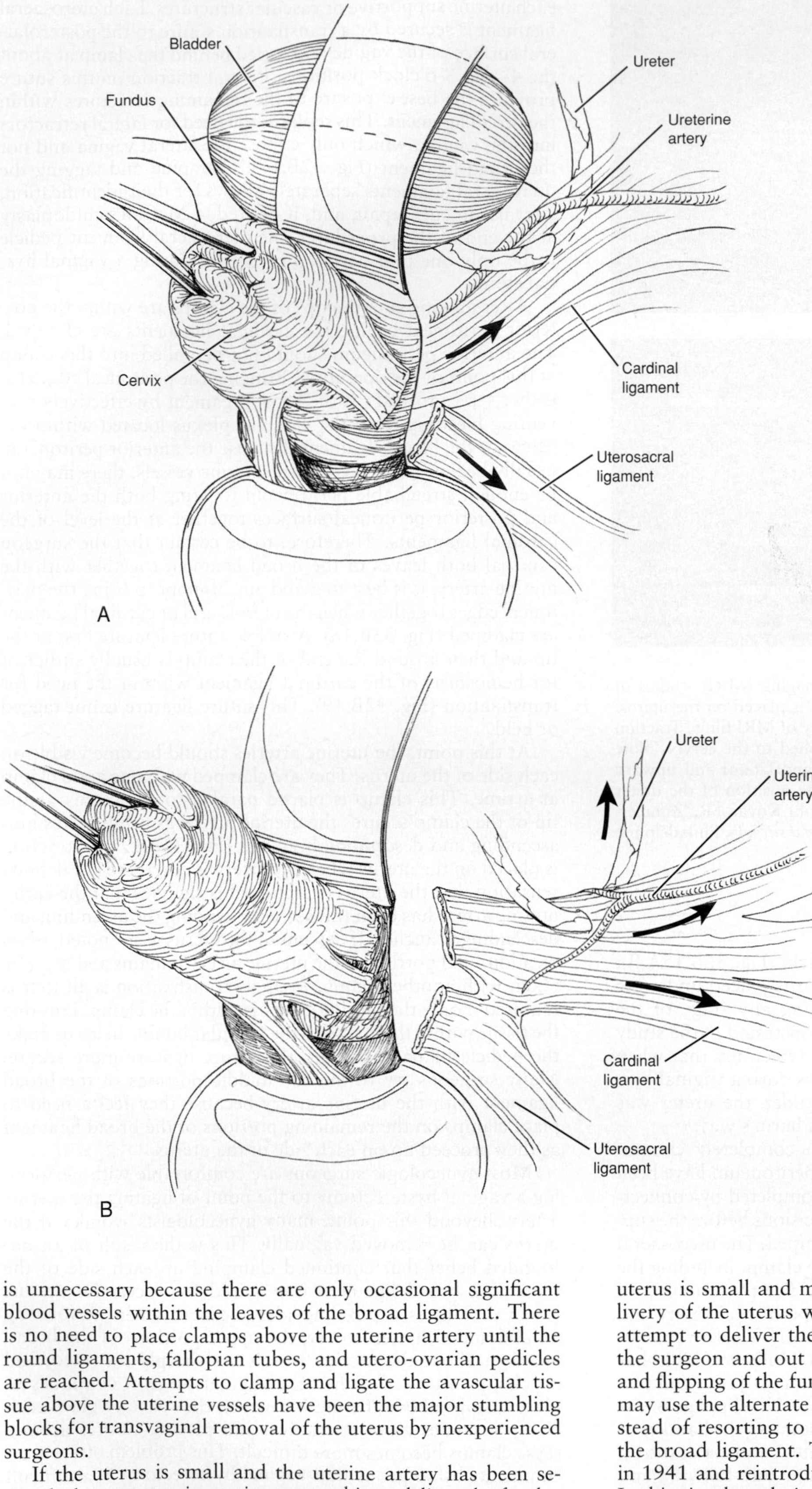

FIGURE 32B.14. A: Transection of the uterosacral ligament returns this structure back to its original position. **B:** After both uterosacral and cardinal ligaments have been transected, ureters are displaced upward and lateral out of harm's way. (From Kovac SR, Zimmerman CW, eds. *Advances in reconstructive vaginal surgery.* Philadelphia: Lippincott Williams & Wilkins; 2006:113.)

is unnecessary because there are only occasional significant blood vessels within the leaves of the broad ligament. There is no need to place clamps above the uterine artery until the round ligaments, fallopian tubes, and utero-ovarian pedicles are reached. Attempts to clamp and ligate the avascular tissue above the uterine vessels have been the major stumbling blocks for transvaginal removal of the uterus by inexperienced surgeons.

If the uterus is small and the uterine artery has been secured, the next step in uterine removal is to deliver the fundus through either the anterior or posterior colpotomy. When the uterus is small and mobile, simple traction may result in delivery of the uterus without the need for "flipping it." In an attempt to deliver the uterus (regardless of the size) closer to the surgeon and out of the vagina when downward traction and flipping of the fundus do not appear possible, the surgeon may use the alternate technique of **intramyometrial coring**, instead of resorting to clamps placed on the upper portions of the broad ligament. This technique was introduced by Lash in 1941 and reintroduced in 1986 for removal of large uteri. In this simple technique, the myometrium can be circumferentially incised with a scalpel placed parallel to the long axis of

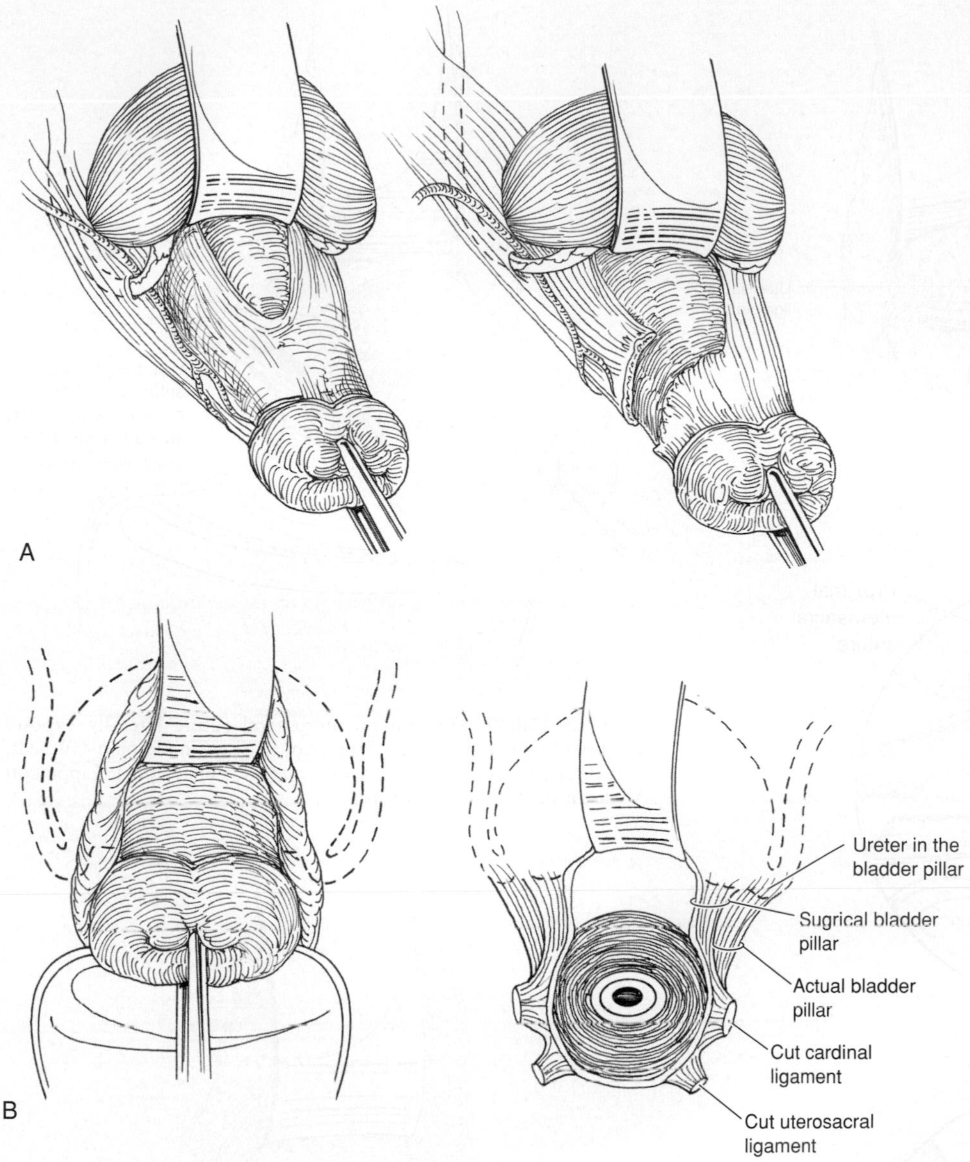

FIGURE 32B.15. A, B: Note elevation of the ureters out of harm's way with upward traction on the bladder during vaginal hysterectomy. (From Kovac SR, Zimmerman CW, eds. *Advances in reconstructive vaginal surgery.* Philadelphia: Lippincott Williams & Wilkins; 2006:114.)

the uterus and beneath the serosal covering of the uterus (Fig. 32B.20A,B). This removes a core inside the uterus without violating the integrity of the endometrial cavity. To facilitate the coring incision, strong traction on the uterus is necessary.

The Lash or coring incision reduces the size of the uterus by decreasing its width, thereby increasing its length, similar to a baby's head as it becomes molded during childbirth. In effect, coring converts a spherical structure into an elongated rod shape, enhancing the surgeon's ability to facilitate transvaginal removal of a wide uterine fundus (Fig. 32B.21A–C). This is a surprisingly bloodless maneuver once the uterine arteries have been secured. Strong traction is placed on the uterus during the coring, which restricts blood flow from the ovarian pedicles.

During the coring procedure, the uterus will begin to descend through the vagina, allowing the surgeon to visualize the cornual portion of the uterus and exposing the utero-ovarian ligament, round ligament, and fallopian tube. Once these structures become visible, the surgeon is assured that the uterus can be removed vaginally. Some surgeons prefer bivalving the uterus, but this can be more cumbersome, as it requires the surgeon to deal with two pieces of the uterus. Once the upper pedicles are visualized, they can either be clamped individually with two clamps or together with one. Depending on the surgeon's preference and experience, a suture placed around the tip of the clamp and tied or transfixed behind is appropriate. This suture is tagged to provide traction on the pedicle and expose the ovary for evaluation or removal, but the ovary should not be removed at this time.

Once the uterus has been removed, it is appropriate to evaluate each pedicle to determine whether bleeding persists. If the ovaries are removed before it is adequately determined that all pedicles are hemostatic, the surgeon may spend considerable operative time finding the source of such bleeding, as it frequently appears to be from a higher point but may actually be from one of the uterine pedicles. Each pedicle can be evaluated by starting at the 12-o'clock position within the peritoneal cavity and proceeding in a clockwise manner. The use of a 4 × 4 sponge folded longitudinally on sponge forceps is most helpful. If brisk bleeding is noted, most often it can be found by

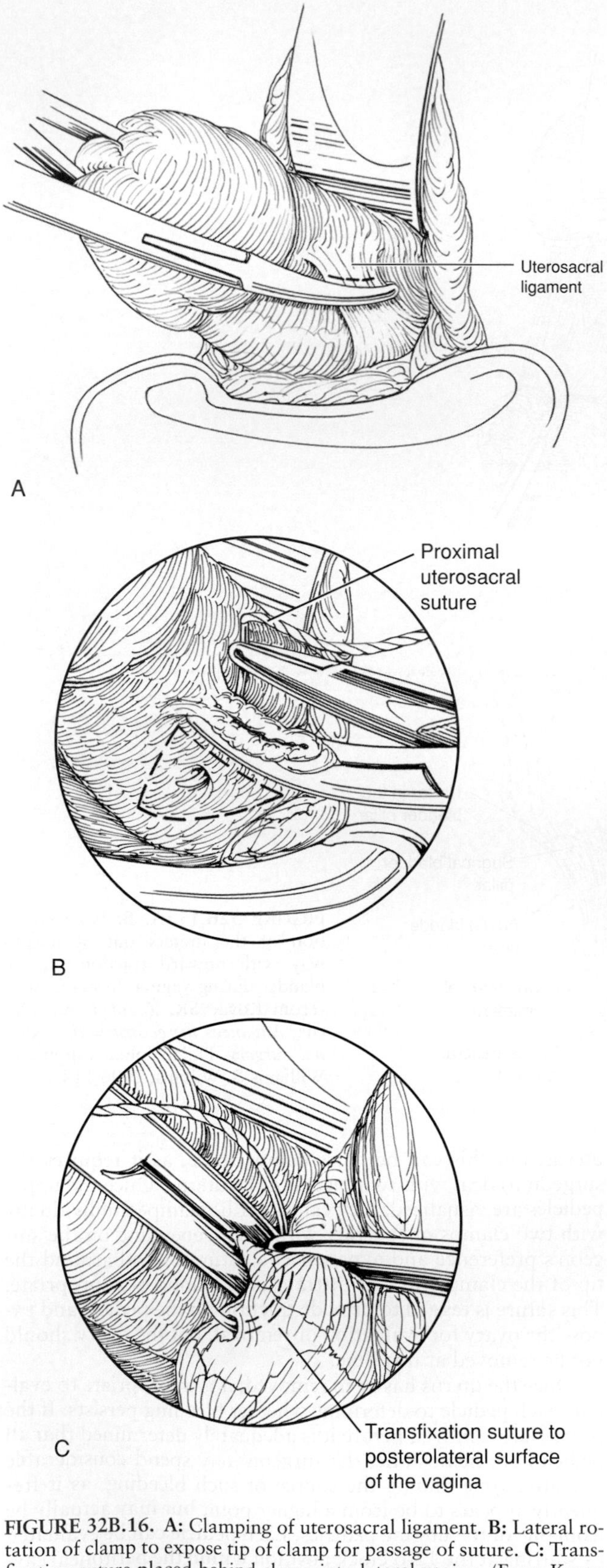

FIGURE 32B.16. A: Clamping of uterosacral ligament. B: Lateral rotation of clamp to expose tip of clamp for passage of suture. C: Transfixation suture placed behind clamp into lateral vagina. (From Kovac SR, Zimmerman CW, eds. *Advances in reconstructive vaginal surgery.* Philadelphia: Lippincott Williams & Wilkins; 2006:115.)

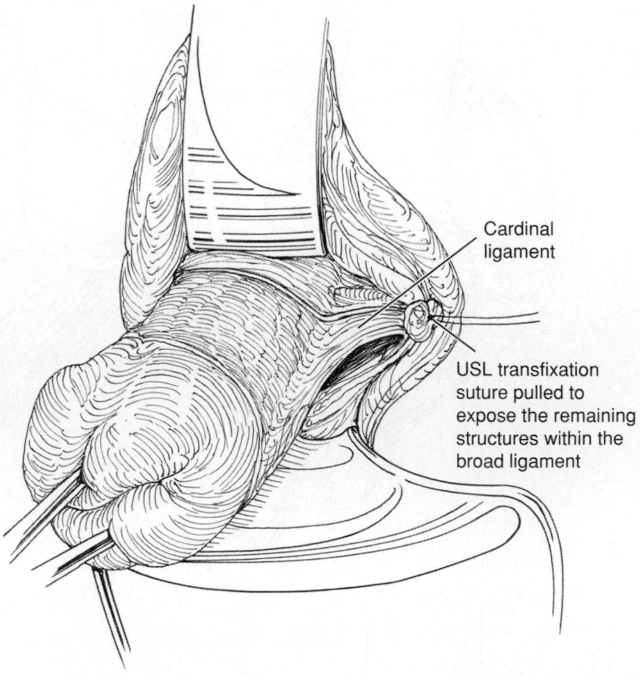

FIGURE 32B.17. Traction on uterosacral suture laterally exposes the broad ligament suture. (From Kovac SR, Zimmerman CW, eds. *Advances in reconstructive vaginal surgery.* Philadelphia: Lippincott Williams & Wilkins; 2006:116.)

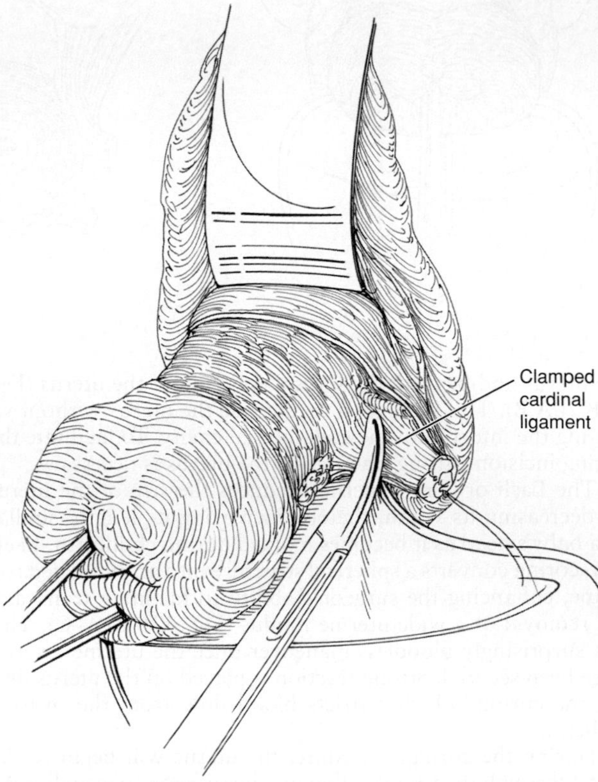

FIGURE 32B.18. Clamping cardinal ligament. Note anterior peritoneum is not included in this clamp. (From Kovac SR, Zimmerman CW, eds. *Advances in reconstructive vaginal surgery.* Philadelphia: Lippincott Williams & Wilkins; 2006:116.)

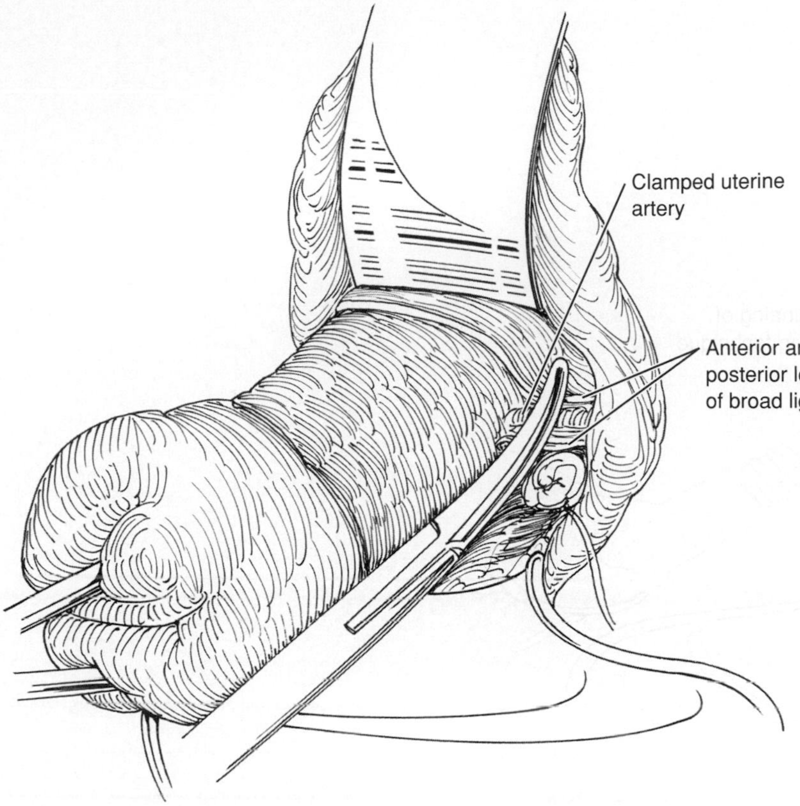

FIGURE 32B.19. Uterine artery clamped with anterior and posterior leaves of the broad ligament included in the clamp. (From Kovac SR, Zimmerman CW, eds. *Advances in reconstructive vaginal surgery.* Philadelphia: Lippincott Williams & Wilkins; 2006:116.)

placing traction on the upper pedicle tags and looking between the uteroovarian and uterine artery pedicles. Bleeding from this area is usually a result of the anastomosis of vessels between the ovarian and uterine artery. Because this is the most frequent site of this type of bleeding, the surgeon should direct his or her search to this area first. Placement of a clamp at the site of bleeding followed by a suture around the clamp or placement of a figure-of-eight suture passed through the vagina into the peritoneum from outward to inward will rapidly control this bleeding (Fig. 32B.22).

If no bleeding points are discovered from any pedicle, the posterior vaginal mucosa will most likely be the source of bleeding. Posterior cuff bleeding may sometimes be rather brisk from the separation of the vagina and the peritoneal edge. It is always more brisk in patients younger than 40 years of age. Before proceeding with any concurrent procedure, it is best to control blood loss from this area with electrosurgery or a running-locked absorbable suture, starting from the left uterosacral ligament tag to the right uterosacral ligament tag. Once this is complete, further examination of the peritoneal cavity should reveal complete hemostasis from all potential bleeding sites.

If only the removal of the uterus has been agreed on by the surgeon and the patient, support of the vaginal apex becomes the next most important decision. If an oophorectomy is planned in conjunction with the hysterectomy, it should be performed at this point.

VAGINAL OOPHORECTOMY

There appears to be some reluctance to combine vaginal hysterectomy with oophorectomy because vaginal oophorectomy is thought to be a risky and difficult procedure. Two factors seem to foster this perception: (i) fear of restricted access to the ovaries and (ii) inadequate visibility of the adnexa during conventional vaginal surgery.

To obtain objective evidence regarding these perceptions, a prospective study was designed by Baden and Walker to determine whether there is adequate visibility and accessibility for transvaginal oophorectomy in most patients undergoing vaginal hysterectomy. After the uterus was removed, accessibility of the ovaries for transvaginal removal was assessed by stretching the infundibulopelvic ligament, placing traction on the suture tag used to ligate the uteroovarian ligament, round ligament, and fallopian tube and grading the position of the ovaries in relation to the long axis of the vagina. The degree of ovarian descent and visibility was graded with a system used to grade pelvic organ prolapse (Fig. 32B.23) (Table 32B.1). The grade corresponded to the minimal degree of descent of either ovary.

To determine what grade would be considered accessible and visible for transvaginal oophorectomy by most gynecologic surgeons, the experience of other surgical specialties was considered. For example, the distance from the hymenal ring to the ischial spine is approximately 8 cm. In dentistry, the distance from the front teeth to the last molar is 6 cm; in otolaryngology, the distance from the front teeth to the tonsil for tonsillectomy is 10 cm. Therefore, it was postulated that any ovary grade I or higher should be visible and accessible for transvaginal removal by most gynecologic surgeons. Of the 875 patients between 29 and 69 years of age who were evaluated for ovarian descent after hysterectomy, 92.9% had ovarian mobility to at least the midportion of the vagina (grade II). In another 4.6%, the ovary could be pulled down outside the hymenal ring (grade II). Only 2.5% of these patients had very little ovarian mobility, which would have made vaginal oophorectomy very difficult (2.4% grade I and 0.1% grade 0). Although this study provided objective evidence that the ovaries may be more visible and accessible for transvaginal removal than previously perceived, there

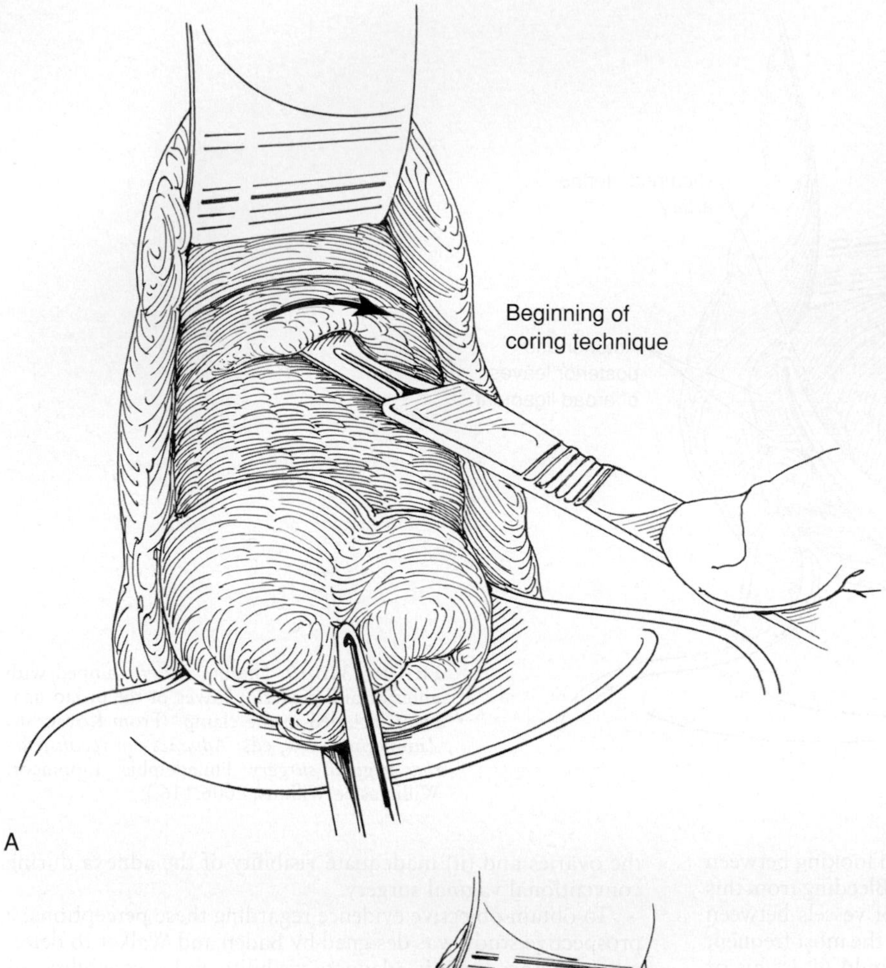

FIGURE 32B.20. A: Coring incision is started just below the serosal covering of the uterus anteriorly. **B:** Coring of a small uterus to facilitate exposure and clamping of the upper pedicle. No sutures were placed above the uterine artery to bring the uterus closer to the surgeon for removal of the uterus. (From Kovac SR, Zimmerman CW, eds. *Advances in reconstructive vaginal surgery.* Philadelphia: Lippincott Williams & Wilkins; 2006:118.)

may be times that the ovary may be inaccessible for transvaginal removal as a result of adhesive disease, endometriosis, suspected significant pathology, or other conditions. However, the ovary should not be considered as completely inaccessible at the start of any vaginal hysterectomy. Smale and colleagues, Davies and associates, and Sheth have reported that planned vaginal salpingo-oophorectomy is successful in 94% to 97% of women undergoing vaginal hysterectomy. The routine use of the laparoscope to perform an oophorectomy before a vaginal hysterectomy has been heralded as safe and comfortable, and has become commonplace. "To be sure we can get the ovaries" is a phrase too often heard worldwide to justify the use of

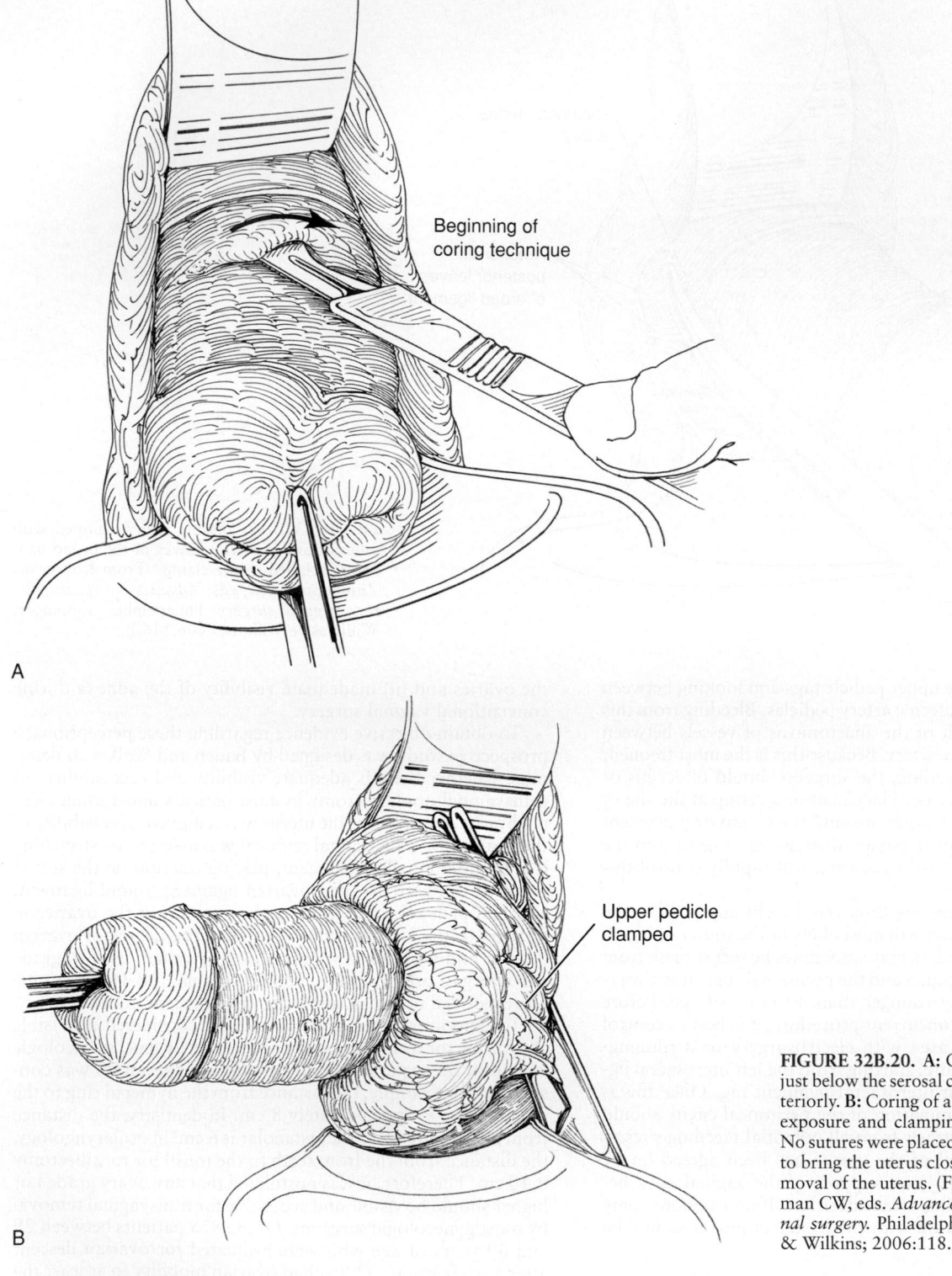

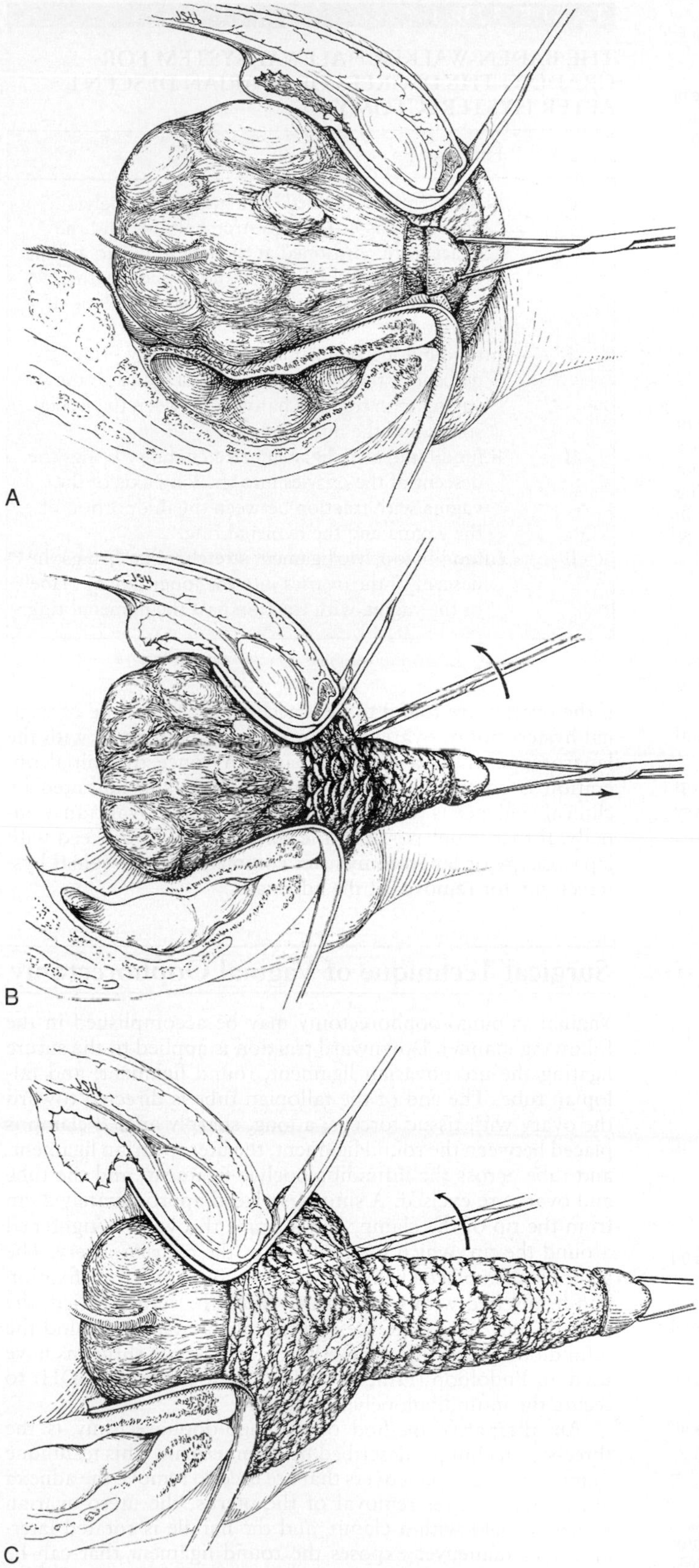

FIGURE 32B.21. **A:** The cervix has been circumscribed through the full thickness of the vagina around the cervix, the posterior and anterior peritoneum entered, and the uterosacral and cardinal ligaments secured. **B:** After ligation of the uterine arteries, an incision is made in a circumferential fashion parallel to the endometrial cavity and into the outer superficial myometrium in the same plane. Constant traction on the tenaculum while coring assists in developing the proper plane. **C:** Continued coring and traction reduces the size of the uterus by exteriorizing the inside of the uterus with an intact endometrial cavity through the introitus. Intramural myomas are sometimes transected during the coring process. (From Kovac SR. Intramyometrial coring as an adjunct to vaginal hysterectomy. *Obstet Gynecol* 1986:76;131.)

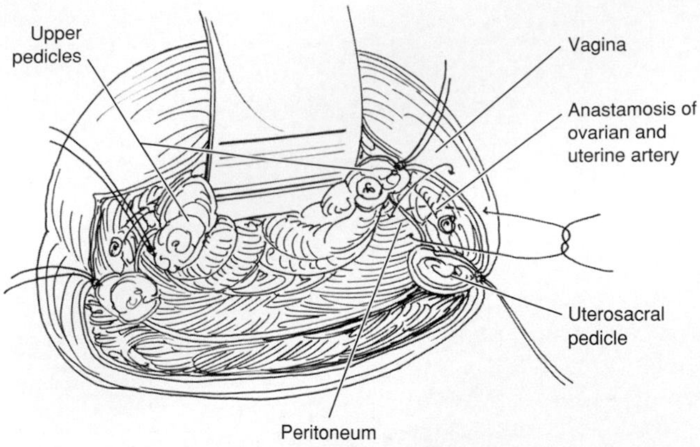

FIGURE 32B.22. Most common source of bleeding after removal of the uterus is the anastomosis between uterine and ovarian arteries. Suture placed through the lateral vagina into the lateral peritoneum in a figure-of-eight fashion and tied resolves most, if not all, bleeding from this area. (From Kovac SR, Zimmerman CW, eds. *Advances in reconstructive vaginal surgery.* Philadelphia: Lippincott Williams & Wilkins; 2006:120.)

TABLE 32B.1

THE BADEN-WALKER HALFWAY SYSTEM FOR GRADING THE DEGREES OF OVARIAN DESCENT AFTER HYSTERECTOMY

Grade	Findings
0	No descent was defined. The infundibulopelvic ligament has little or no stretchability, and the ovaries are positioned at the lateral pelvic wall at or above the ischial spines and cannot, with traction, be brought into the long-axis plane of the vagina.
I	Infundibulopelvic ligament stretchability brings the descent of the ovaries into the long axis of the vagina with traction halfway between the ischial spines and the midvagina.
II	Infundibulopelvic ligament stretchability brings the descent of the ovaries into the long axis of the vagina with traction between the midportion of the vagina and the hymenal ring.
II	Infundibulopelvic ligament stretchability brings the descent of the ovaries into the longitudinal plane of the vagina with traction past the hymenal ring.

abdominal, laparoscopically assisted, or laparoscopic hysterectomy. For too many years, it was believed that the ovaries were inaccessible because they are "too high" for transvaginal removal. This has erroneously guided the selection of abdominal or laparoscopic hysterectomy.

Good surgical practice dictates that objective determination of the visibility and accessibility of the ovaries be the primary criteria for selecting a particular route of oophorectomy. Thus, if the ovaries are found to be inaccessible at the time of vaginal hysterectomy, ovarian removal can be performed with the laparoscope or by a simple laparotomy once the initial operation is complete. The correct paradigm substantiated by clinical evidence is to first attempt ovarian removal transvaginally. If that is not possible, the surgeon should proceed with laparoscopy or laparotomy after completion of a vaginal hysterectomy for removal of the adnexa.

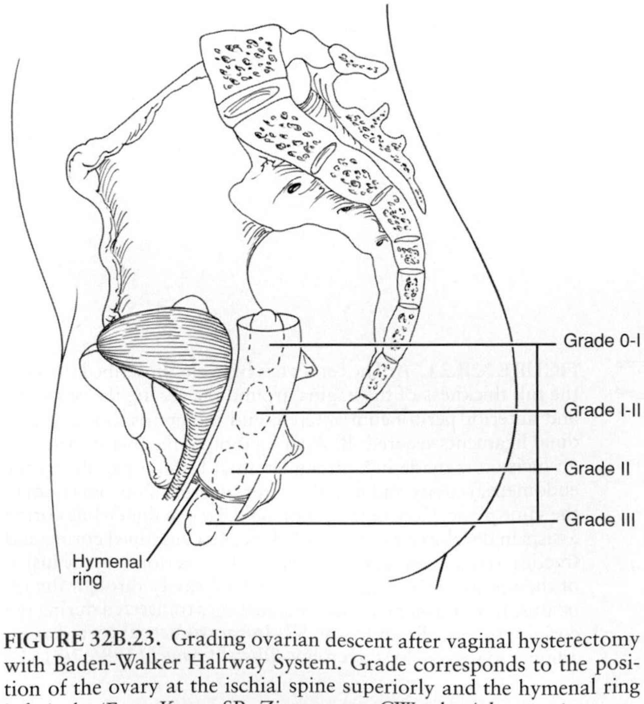

FIGURE 32B.23. Grading ovarian descent after vaginal hysterectomy with Baden-Walker Halfway System. Grade corresponds to the position of the ovary at the ischial spine superiorly and the hymenal ring inferiorly. (From Kovac SR, Zimmerman CW, eds. *Advances in reconstructive vaginal surgery.* Philadelphia: Lippincott Williams & Wilkins; 2006:120.)

Surgical Technique of Vaginal Oophorectomy

Vaginal salpingo-oophorectomy may be accomplished in the following manner. Downward traction is applied to the suture ligating the uteroovarian ligament, round ligament, and fallopian tube. The end of the fallopian tube is directed toward the ovary with tissue forceps; a long, sharply angled clamp is placed between the round ligament, the uteroovarian ligament, and tube across the infundibulopelvic ligament; and the tube and ovary are excised. A suture is placed approximately 2 cm from the tip of the clamp, and a single throw tie is tightened around the tip, which usually secures the ovarian artery. The suture is then placed behind the clamp for suture transfixation and firmly tied with several throws. As the suture is tied, the surgeon can appreciate the security of this suture around the infundibulopelvic ligament. Alternatively, some surgeons have used an Endoloop (Ethicon Endosurgery, Cincinnati, OH) to secure the infundibulopelvic pedicle.

An alternative method of salpingo-oophorectomy is the three-step technique described by Zimmerman. This technique mimics the same maneuvers that are used to remove the adnexa abdominally. After removal of the uterus, the utero-ovarian pedicle is held with a clamp, and the handle is rotated laterally. This maneuver exposes the round ligament that can be clamped, transected, and ligated. Division of the round ligament gives the surgeon access to the retroperitoneal space between the leaves of the broad ligament. Division of this space makes it possible to isolate, clamp, and ligate the mesovarium.

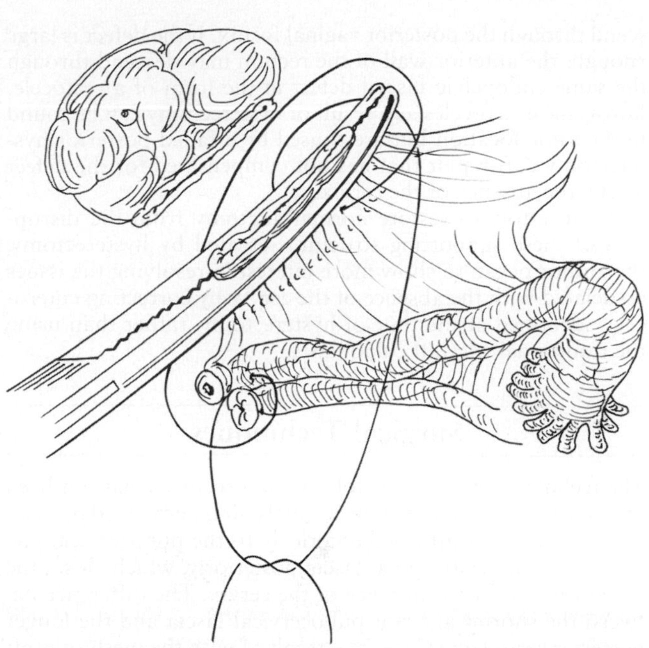

FIGURE 32B.24. The infundibulopelvic ligament has been clamped and the ovary and the tube removed. There is a single penetration of the infundibulopelvic ligament and its midpoint and tied around the end of the clamp. This transfixation suture usually occludes the ovarian artery. The suture is then passed around the end of the clamp and transfixed into the tissues behind the heel of the clamp and tied again. (From Kovac SR, Zimmerman CW, eds. *Advances in reconstructive vaginal surgery.* Philadelphia: Lippincott Williams & Wilkins; 2006:122.)

After division of the mesovarium, the only remaining tissue connected to the adnexa is the infundibulopelvic ligament. This ligament can be clamped and suture ligated or secured with an Endoloop (Fig. 32B.24). Division of the adnexectomy into three manageable steps increases surgical control and decreases the likelihood of a complication during suture application. Transection of the round ligament and mesovarium as separate pedicles significantly increases descent of the adnexa, resulting in increased visibility of the infundibulopelvic ligament.

CLOSURE AND SUPPORT OF THE VAGINAL CUFF

Closure of the peritoneum with vaginal hysterectomy is frequently described as necessary by some surgeons. I have not routinely closed the peritoneum for the past 25 years and have never regretted this sometimes dangerous exercise that results in no benefit to the patient. Leaving the peritoneum open should expose any immediate postoperative bleeding.

The remaining part of the vaginal hysterectomy is to support the vaginal cuff so that an enterocele or vaginal vault prolapse does not occur in later years. Compensation for the connective tissue defect created by the removal of the cervix is best accomplished at the time of hysterectomy. Failure to adequately compensate for the cervical defect may expose the patient to an increased risk for posthysterectomy vaginal vault prolapse in the form of an enterocele or apical anterior vaginal wall prolapse. Enterocele repair and suspension of the prolapsed posthysterectomy vagina are among the most technically demanding of all pelvic surgery procedures. Closure of the cervical defect along with reestablishment of the suspensory axis of the vagina by incorporating the uterosacral ligaments into the cuff are effective prophylaxis reducing the risk of future prolapse.

The incidence of enterocele after hysterectomy can range between 0.1% and 16%. Nichols and Randall described a technique of excising excess peritoneum in the cul-de-sac to prevent future development of an anterior enterocele. Because this technique only removes excess peritoneum and does not address the cause of an enterocele after hysterectomy, subsequent enterocele formation has not been prevented because no musculofascial defect has been corrected or reinforced.

Several other methods to repair the posterior vaginal cuff for prolapse prophylaxis have been described. These procedures emphasize the use of the uterosacral ligaments in any repair. Inclusion of the uterosacral ligaments in cuff repair is very important because of their role as the primary suspensory elements in the vaginal vault. Connecting the uterosacrals to the cuff reestablishes the suspensory axis of the vagina and should be considered during all hysterectomies. The most commonly employed technique to close the posterior vaginal cuff is the McCall culdoplasty. This technique is thought to obliterate the cul-de-sac while it suspends the posterior superior vagina and its fascial attachments to the uterosacral ligaments, bringing these supporting ligaments together in the midline (Fig. 32B.25). This technique was a marked improvement over previous beliefs that the only thing necessary after the uterus was removed was to close the vagina. This resulted in a high incidence of vaginal vault prolapse and associated enterocele formation. I routinely performed the McCall culdoplasty after all

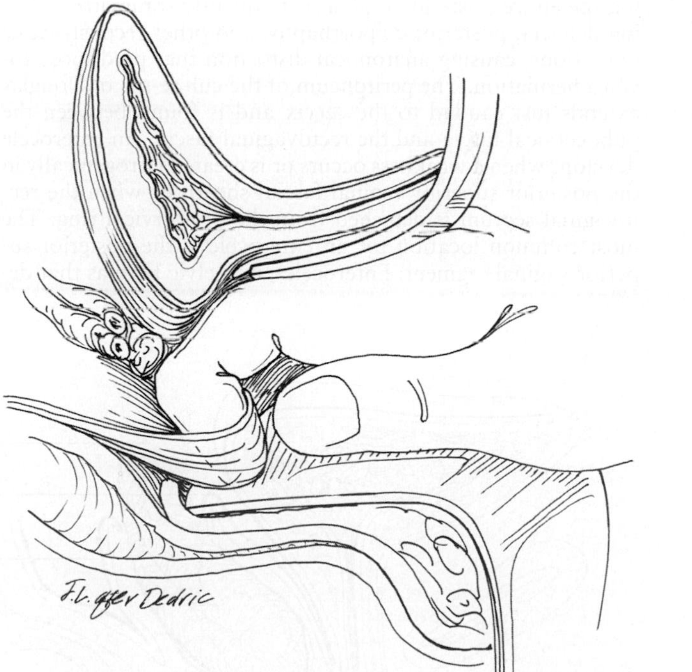

FIGURE 32B.25. Identification of excess peritoneum in cul-de-sac. Excision of excess peritoneum will not prevent future enterocele formation, as the cause of the enterocele is not determined. (From Kovac SR, Zimmerman CW, eds. *Advances in reconstructive vaginal surgery.* Philadelphia: Lippincott Williams & Wilkins; 2006:122.)

vaginal hysterectomies for many years to prevent future vaginal vault prolapse and enterocele formation. Recent advancements in pelvic reconstructive techniques, as well as an understanding of the cause of enteroceles, has brought us to a new method of preventing enteroceles and vault prolapse at the time of hysterectomy, especially with those patients who have a rectocele. Rectoceles result from an apical separation of the rectovaginal fascia from the uterosacral ligaments. This distal apical displacement allows rectoceles and enteroceles to develop contiguously through the same fascial defect. In our experience, enteroceles are routinely associated with rectoceles, which may not have been identified during the vaginal hysterectomy. This suggests that failure to identify and manage the presence of an enterocele at the time of vaginal hysterectomy might be the cause of the increased incidence of enterocele formation discovered in later years.

It is further recognized that enteroceles form as a result of the separation of the rectovaginal fascia from the pubocervical fascia (Fig. 32B.26). As a result of hysterectomy and removal of the cervix, there is an iatrogenic separation of the rectovaginal septum and the fibers that normally connect this structure to the anterior vaginal fascia through the connective tissue that forms the pericervical ring. This separation widens the cul-de-sac and separates the fascial attachments from the posterior vaginal wall and the rectovaginal fascia, thus allowing the peritoneum, with its intraabdominal structures, to protrude through this weakness with any increases in intraabdominal pressure.

Vaginal vault prolapse and enterocele formation differ by anatomy. The upper vagina can be well supported even though an enterocele exists, and vice versa. An enterocele (DeLancey level II of vagina) descends through the weakened floor and fascia of the posterior vaginal segment. Vault prolapse of the superior segment (level I) results from loss of the uterosacral-cardinal ligament support. The rectovaginal fascia, underlying the entire posterior vagina, is frequently traumatized during delivery, posterior colporrhaphy, and other reconstructive operations, causing anatomical distortion that predispose toward herniation. The peritoneum of the cul-de-sac of Douglas extends just caudad to the cervix and is found between the pubocervical fascia and the rectovaginal fascia. An enterocele develops when a weakness occurs or is created iatrogenically in the posterior superior vaginal fascial sheath or when the rectovaginal septum is detached from the pericervical ring. The most common location for an enterocele is the posterior superior vaginal segment. Enteroceles are pelvic hernias that descend through the posterior vaginal fornix. If the defect is large enough, the anterior wall of the rectum may descend through the same endopelvic fascial defect in the form of a rectocele. Iatrogenic enteroceles as a result of hysterectomy can be found in the same location but are caused by a failed posterior hysterectomy cuff repair that has not compensated for the defect left by the absence of the cervix.

In an effort to restore normal anatomy from the disruption of these supporting structures created by hysterectomy, the author began to show more interest in resolving the issues associated with the absence of the cervix by correcting enteroceles identified at the time of hysterectomy, rather than using the traditional McCall culdoplasty.

Surgical Techniques

The techniques used are as follows. If a rectocele has not been identified, management of the vaginal cuff is performed by placing mesh or graft attached anteriorly to the pubocervical fascia and to the rectovaginal fascia posteriorly, which closes the space vacated by the absence of the cervix. The difference between the shorter anterior pubocervical fascia and the longer posterior rectovaginal fascia is resolved with the mesh or graft (Fig. 32B.27). The lateral end of the mesh/graft is attached to the uterosacral ligament at its insertion into the sacral periosteum, a vaginal sacral colpopexy (Fig. 32B.28).

The presence of a rectocele requires the posterior vaginal wall be opened in the midline up to the level of the newly formed cul-de-sac. The defect from separation of the rectovaginal fascia from the uterosacral ligaments is identified. If an enterocele sac is identified, opening of the sac with high ligation of the sac is unnecessary, as the mesothelial lining of the peritoneal sac has little supportive value. The sac is simply pushed upward as a 7 × 10–cm piece of small intestine submucosa (SIS) graft (Cook; Spencer, IN) and is used to reattach the separation of the rectovaginal fascia from the pericervical ring. The central portion of the graft is reattached to the pericervical ring with permanent sutures, as permanent sutures attach the proximal lateral portion of the graft to the uterosacral ligaments or sacrospinous ligaments. The central reattachment of the graft to the pericervical ring corrects the enterocele, as the lateral sutures to the uterosacral or sacrospinous ligaments support the upper vagina to prevent future vault prolapse. The distal end of the graft is

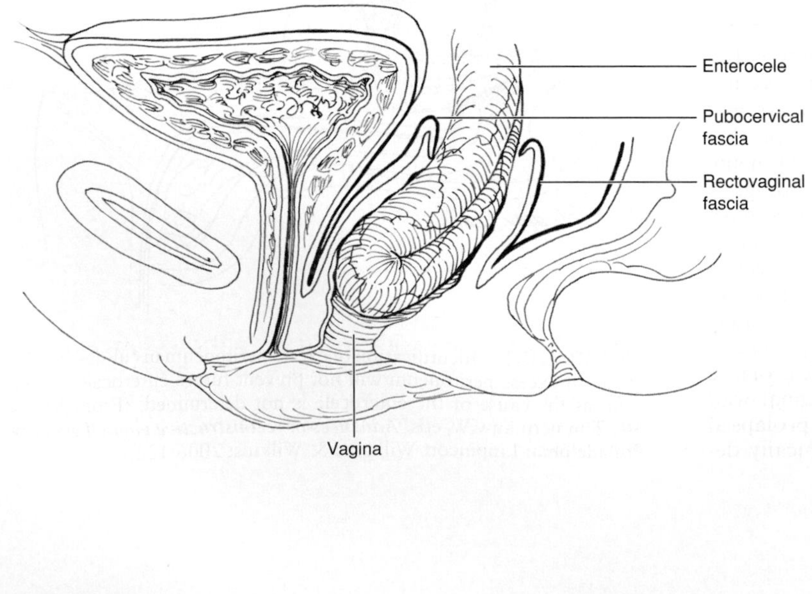

FIGURE 32B.26. Separation of the pubocervical and rectovaginal fascia with enterocele formation. (From Kovac SR, Zimmerman CW, eds. *Advances in reconstructive vaginal surgery.* Philadelphia: Lippincott Williams & Wilkins; 2006:124.)

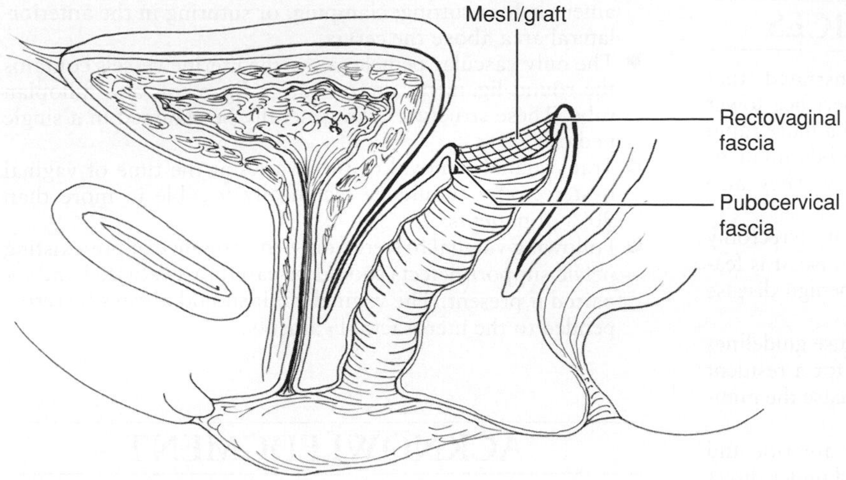

FIGURE 32B.27. Mesh or graft attached to pubocervical fascia anteriorly and rectovaginal fascia posteriorly to compensate for the absence of the cervix. Graft or mesh is attached to the uterosacral of sacrospinous ligaments for prevention of vaginal vault prolapse. (From Kovac SR, Zimmerman CW, eds. *Advances in reconstructive vaginal surgery.* Philadelphia: Lippincott Williams & Wilkins; 2006:125.)

attached to the perineal body. Thus, a new rectovaginal fascia is created, correcting the enterocele and rectocele with its proximal attachment to the pericervical ring and its distal attachment to the perineal body.

The objective in closing the vaginal epithelium is to approximate the cut edges of the vagina together in a smooth line with as little irregularity as possible. This technique will aid in preventing postoperative granulation tissue from forming at the site of vaginal closure. Others have suggested that the vagina should be closed vertically to preserve vaginal length. Cruikshank and Pixley demonstrated that vaginal length depended on the support of the vaginal cuff, not any specific method of epithelial closure. They concluded that as long as there is good vault support, vaginal length is not affected by the orientation of the vaginal mucosal closure. Vertical closure places the scar at the top of the vagina, which may cause hypesthesia during coitus, requiring subsequent scar revision. The author prefers to close the vagina in a transverse direction. If the cuff has been adequately supported, the transverse closure is positioned toward the anterior vagina wall, leaving more depth to the posterior vaginal wall for accommodation with coitus.

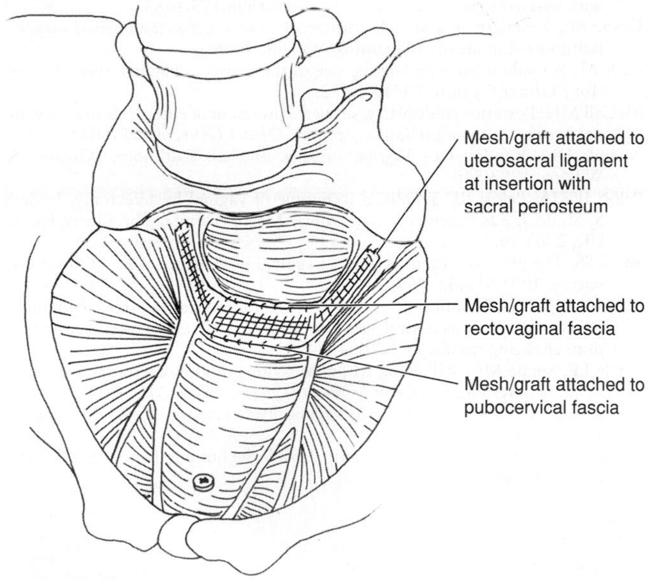

FIGURE 32B.28. Difference between a shorter pubocervical fascia than rectovaginal fascia is resolved with the placement of a graft or mesh to prevent separation of these fascial edges and enterocele formation. (From Kovac SR, Zimmerman CW, eds. *Advances in reconstructive vaginal surgery.* Philadelphia: Lippincott Williams & Wilkins; 2006:125.)

Some investigators have recommended that the vaginal cuff be left open or a drain placed within the vaginal (closure) incision to reduce the morbidity of vaginal cuff cellulitis or abscess formation. With the widespread use of prophylactic antibiotics, there is no longer any need for those techniques. In addition, leaving the cuff open may lead to an increased incidence of enterocele formation and vaginal vault prolapse.

The decision to place packing into the vagina postoperatively is a religious one. A vaginal pack need not be used after vaginal hysterectomy unless concomitant pelvic reconstructive surgery is performed. Complete hemostasis should be achieved after vaginal hysterectomy. Significant postoperative bleeding can rarely occur from a vascular pedicle. If that does occur, it is important to become aware of this problem as soon as possible; vaginal packing will only delay this diagnosis and not prevent the problem. It is important to be aware of postoperative bleeding sooner rather than later while the patient is still hematologically stable, so a pelvic arteriogram may be performed early in the course of such bleeding. The arteriogram may demonstrate the bleeding site and allow arterial occlusion, thus preventing the need for laparotomy.

For some, it is not a routine practice to insert an indwelling transurethral catheter following the removal of a normal-size uterus. Removal of enlarged uterus may cause occasional transient injury to the bladder and transient postoperative voiding problems; therefore, in such patients, bladder drainage is usually suggested, at least overnight.

For 30 years, I have recommended routine cystoscopy following vaginal hysterectomy. Before cystoscopy, 5 cc of indigo carmine is administered intravenously by the anesthesiologist. The strong efflux of blue dye through each ureteral orifice following hysterectomy with or without pelvic reconstruction indicates the integrity of the ureters. Although this may not be necessary with each vaginal hysterectomy, it certainly makes the surgeon more comfortable if the patient reports flank pain the next day.

BEST SURGICAL PRACTICES

- Randomized controlled trials have demonstrated that women treated by vaginal hysterectomy experience lower morbidity, less pain, more rapid recovery, and a more rapid return to normal activities compared with abdominal or laparoscopically assisted vaginal hysterectomy. They also consume fewer health care dollars and resources.
- Using guidelines to determine the route of hysterectomy adopted by the National Guideline Clearinghouse, it is feasible to perform 90% of hysterectomies for benign disease indications via the vaginal route.
- Following the National Guideline Clearinghouse guidelines for selecting the route of hysterectomy, even for a resident training environment, has been shown to decrease the number of abdominal hysterectomies.
- To minimize bladder and rectal injuries, the anterior and posterior peritoneum should always be entered under direct vision.
- The risk of ureteral injury can be minimized by retracting the bladder anteriorly at all times and dividing the cardinal ligament before cutting, clamping, or suturing in the anterior-lateral area above the cervix.
- The only vascular pedicle above the uterine vessels contains the round ligament, utero-ovarian ligament, and fallopian tube. These structures can generally be clamped in a single pedicle.
- Transvaginal removal of the ovaries at the time of vaginal hysterectomy should be technically feasible in more than 90% of patients.
- Following vaginal hysterectomy, the presence of pre-existing pelvic support defects should be carefully evaluated and repaired if present. The vaginal vault should always be resuspended to the uterosacral ligaments.

ACKNOWLEDGMENT

This chapter is based on material from Kovac SR, Zimmerman CW. *Advances in vaginal reconstructive surgery.* Philadelphia: Lippincott; 2007.

Bibliography

Amstey MS, Jones AP. Preparation of the vagina for surgery: a comparison of povidone-iodine and saline solution. *JAMA* 1981;245(8):839.

Baden WF, Walker T. In: Baden WF, Walker T, eds. Fundamentals, symptoms, and classification. *Surgical repair of vaginal defects.* Philadelphia: Lippincott; 1992:51.

Colaco J, Campos AP, Nunes F, et al. Route of hysterectomy: vaginal versus abdominal. *J Pelvic Med Surg* 2003;9(22):69.

Cruikshank SH, Kovac SR. Anatomic changes of the ureter during vaginal hysterectomy. *Contemp Obstet Gynecol* 1993;38:38.

Cruikshank SH, Kovac SR. Role of the uterosacral-cardinal ligament complex in protecting the ureter during vaginal hysterectomy. *Int J Gynaecol Obstet* 1993;40(2):141.

Cruikshank SH, Pixley RL. Methods of vaginal cuff closure and preservation of vaginal depth during transvaginal hysterectomy. *Obstet Gynecol* 1987;70(1):61.

Culligan PJ, Kubik K, Murphy M, et al. A randomized trail that compared povidione iodine and chlorhexidine as antiseptics for vaginal hysterectomy. *Am J Obstet Gynecol* 2005;192(2):422.

Davies A, O'Connor H, Magos AL. A prospective study to evaluate oophorectomy at the time of vaginal hysterectomy. *BJOG* 1996;103(9):915.

Dorsey JH, Steinberg EP, Holtz PM. Clinical indications for hysterectomy route: patient characteristics or physician preference. *Am J Obstet Gynecol* 1995;173(5):1452.

Emergency Care Research Institute (ECRI). Laparoscopy in hysterectomy for benign conditions. *Technology Assessment Custom Report Level 2.* Plymouth Meeting, PA: ECRI; 1995:1.

Garry R, Fountain J, Mason S, et al. The eVALuate study: two parallel randomised trials, one comparing laparoscopic with abdominal hysterectomy, the other comparing laparoscopic with vaginal hysterectomy. *BMJ* 2004;328(7432):129.

Johns DA, Carrera B, Jones J, et al. The medical and economic impact of laparoscopically assisted vaginal hysterectomy in a large, metropolitan, not-for-profit hospital. *Am J Obstet Gynecol* 1995;172(6):1709.

Johnson N, Barlow D, Lethaby A, et al. Surgical approach to hysterectomy for benign gynecological disease. *Cochrane Database Syst Rev* 2005;(1):CD003677.

Julian TM. Vasopressin use during vaginal surgery. *Contemp Obstet Gynecol* 1993;38:82.

Kovac SR. A technique for reducing the risk of intentional cystotomy during vaginal hysterectomy. *J Pelvic Surg* 1999;5:32.

Kovac SR. Intramyometrial coring as an adjunct to vaginal hysterectomy. *Obstet Gynecol* 1986;67(1):131.

Kovac SR, Barhan S, Lister M, et al. Guidelines for the selection of the route of hysterectomy: application in a resident clinic population. *Am J Obstet Gynecol* 2002;187(6):1521.

Kovac SR, Cruikshank SH. Guidelines to determine the route of oophorectomy with hysterectomy. *Am J Obstet Gynecol* 1996;175:1483.

Kovac SR, Zimmerman CW, eds. *Advances in reconstructive vaginal surgery.* Baltimore: Lippincott Williams & Wilkins; 2006.

Lash AF. A method for reducing the size of the uterus in vaginal hysterectomy. *Am J Obstet Gynecol* 1941;42:452.

McCall MH. Posterior culdoplasty, surgical correction of enterocele during vaginal hysterectomy: a preliminary report. *Obstet Gynecol* 1957;10:595.

Nichols DH, Randall CL. *Vaginal surgery.* 2nd ed. Baltimore: Williams & Wilkins; 1983:548.

Pelosi II MA, Pelosi III. Simplified technique of vaginal hysterectomy. In Seth S, Studd J, eds. *Vaginal hysterectomy.* Martin Dunitz, The Livery House UK; 2002:59.

Sheth SS. The place of oophorectomy at vaginal hysterectomy. *Br J Obstet Gynaecol.* 1991:98:662–666.

Sizzi O, Paparella P, Bonito C, et al. Laparoscopic assistance after vaginal hysterectomy and unsuccessful access to the ovaries or failed uterine mobilization: changing trends. *JSLS* 2004;8(4):339.

Smale LE, Smale ML, Wilkening RL, et al. Salpingo-oophorectomy at the time of vaginal hysterectomy. *Am J Obstet Gynecol* 1978;131(2):122.

Zimmerman CW. Oophorectomy at vaginal hysterectomy. *OBG Management* 1990;11:50.

Zimmerman CW. Vaginal hysterectomy: Is skill the limiting factor? *OBG Management* 2006;18:21–31.

CHAPTER 32C ■ LAPAROSCOPIC HYSTERECTOMY

FRED M. HOWARD

DEFINITIONS

Laparoscopically assisted vaginal hysterectomy (LAVH)—Vaginal hysterectomy that is assisted by laparoscopy; the laparoscopic procedures may include adnexectomy and the superior portions of the hysterectomy, but not ligation of the uterine vessels.

Laparoscopic subtotal hysterectomy (LSH)—Hysterectomy that is performed completely by laparoscope; however, the uterine corpus is amputated from the cervix at the level of the isthmus, and the cervical stump will remain *in situ*.

Total laparoscopic hysterectomy (TLH)—Abdominal hysterectomy that is performed completely by laparoscopy with no vaginal component. The vaginal cuff is closed via the laparoscope.

Vaginally assisted laparoscopic hysterectomy (VALH)—Hysterectomy that is performed mostly laparoscopically, including ligation of the uterine vessels. The vaginal portion consists of only the vaginal incision and repair.

There are three major subdivisions of total hysterectomies that involve the use of laparoscopy: laparoscopically assisted vaginal hysterectomy (LAVH), vaginally assisted laparoscopic hysterectomy (VALH), and total laparoscopic hysterectomy (TLH). **LAVH** is a vaginal hysterectomy that is assisted by laparoscopy; the laparoscopic procedures may include adnexectomy and the superior portions of the hysterectomy, but not ligation of the uterine vessels (Fig. 32C.1). Indications for LAVH are known or suspected diseases that preclude a vaginal hysterectomy without assistance laparoscopically; i.e., laparoscopy is used to convert an abdominal hysterectomy into a vaginal hysterectomy. An example might be a patient with extensive peritoneal endometriosis that is not amenable to excision vaginally. In such a case, laparoscopy might be used to excise all of the extrauterine endometriosis, and then a vaginal hysterectomy would be performed. **VALH** is a hysterectomy that is performed mostly laparoscopically, including ligation of the uterine vessels, and the vaginal portion consists of only the vaginal incision and repair (Fig. 32C.2). Generally speaking, the indication for VALH is disease that precludes a vaginal hysterectomy even with laparoscopic assistance and allows a vaginal approach only for colpotomy and repair, either to speed the procedure or because the surgeon lacks the skill to do the colpotomy and vaginal repair laparoscopically. Examples of such cases might be a patient with very restricted gynecologic pelvimetric dimensions and very difficult access to the cervix and upper vagina or a patient with a cervical leiomyoma that precludes access to the uterine artery vaginally. **TLH** is an abdominal hysterectomy performed laparoscopically, in which there is no vaginal component, the colpotomy is made laparoscopically, and the vaginal vault is sutured laparoscopically (Fig. 32C.3). This approach has the same indications as those for abdominal hysterectomy. TLH often is viewed as an alternative to abdominal hysterectomy, but it may be more appropriate to view it as a minimally invasive abdominal hysterectomy. Generally speaking, LAVH, VALH, and TLH are not appropriate when a vaginal hysterectomy is indicated and feasible.

Subtotal, or supracervical, hysterectomy has recently undergone a resurgence of interest. Electromechanical morcellators make it possible to perform subtotal hysterectomy laparoscopically without the need to significantly enlarge the laparoscopic incisions. This is usually termed a *laparoscopic supracervical hysterectomy* (Fig. 32C.4). Whether laparoscopic supracervical hysterectomy is an appropriate substitute for vaginal hysterectomy is debatable.

For research purposes, laparoscopic hysterectomies can be more specifically classified (Table 32C.1), but these classifications have minimal usefulness in clinical practice.

HISTORY

Operative laparoscopy was introduced to gynecological practice by Raoul Palmer, from France. In the late 1950s and early 1960s, Palmer described the use of laparoscopy for adhesiolysis, cyst aspiration, ovarian biopsies, electrocoagulation of endometriosis, and tubal sterilization. Patrick Steptoe, from England, and Hans Frangenheim, from Germany, both of whom studied with Palmer, helped to widely popularize operative laparoscopy in Europe. Melvin Cohen is credited with introducing operative laparoscopy to the United States in 1966, after he returned from visits with Palmer and Steptoe. Initially in the United States, operative laparoscopy consisted primarily of tubal sterilization; its applications grew rapidly to treatment of adnexal disease, ectopic pregnancy, adhesive disease, and endometriosis. Reich and associates published the first case of LAVH in 1989, performing it for the treatment of a patient with endometriosis and leiomyomata. Since that original description, laparoscopy has increased remarkably as a surgical approach to hysterectomy worldwide. From 1990 to 1997, the proportion of hysterectomies performed laparoscopically in the United States increased by 30-fold, from 0.3 to 9.9% (Table 32C.2). Unfortunately, this increase appeared to be the result of laparoscopic assistance of vaginal hysterectomies rather than conversion of abdominal hysterectomies to laparoscopic or vaginal hysterectomies.

INDICATIONS

The indications for hysterectomy already have been discussed in this chapter. The choice of surgical approach—vaginal,

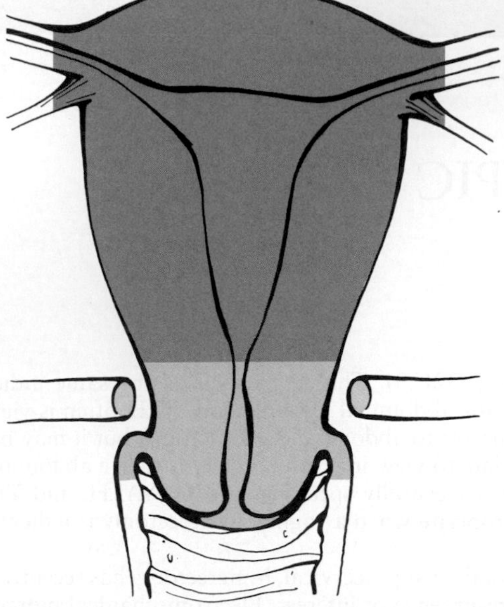

FIGURE 32C.1. Illustration of laparoscopically assisted vaginal hysterectomy (LAVH). With a LAVH, all or none of the superior portion of the hysterectomy, down to but not including ligation of the uterine vessels, may be performed laparoscopically, as illustrated by the darkly shaded portions of the diagram. The colpotomy and ligation of the uterine vessels are performed transvaginally with a LAVH, as illustrated by the lightly shaded portions of the diagram.

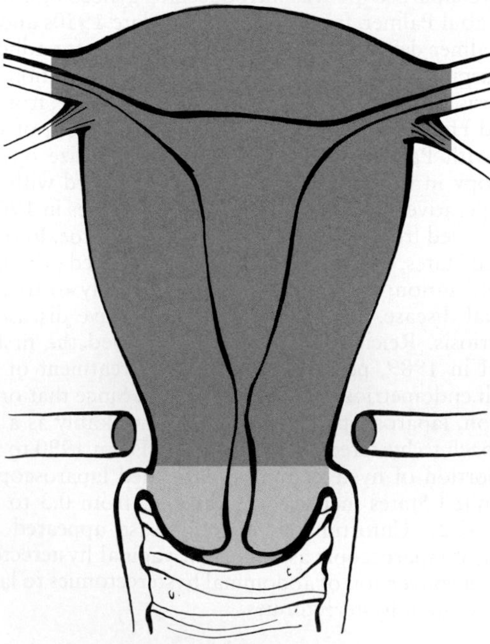

FIGURE 32C.2. Illustration of vaginally assisted laparoscopic hysterectomy (VALH). With a VALH, the superior portion of the hysterectomy down to ligation of the uterine vessels is performed laparoscopically, as illustrated by the darkly shaded portion of the diagram. The colpotomy is performed transvaginally with a VALH, as illustrated by the lightly shaded portion of the diagram.

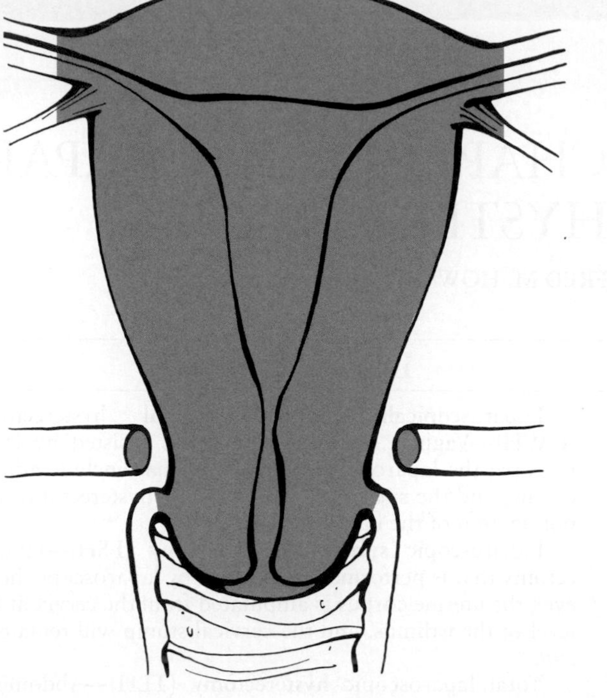

FIGURE 32C.3. Illustration of total laparoscopic hysterectomy (TLH). With a TLH, the hysterectomy is performed completely laparoscopically, as illustrated by the darkly shaded portion of the diagram. None of the surgery is performed transvaginally with a TLH.

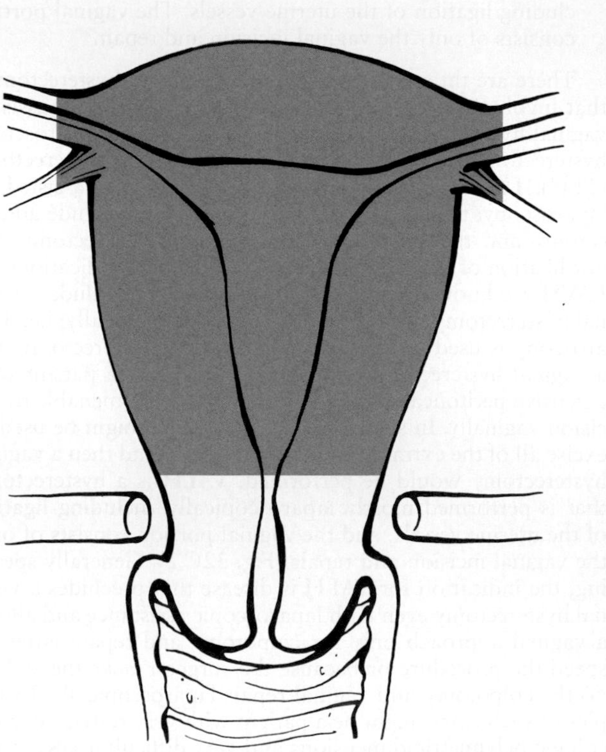

FIGURE 32C.4. Illustration of laparoscopic supracervical hysterectomy (LSH). With an LSH, the hysterectomy is performed completely laparoscopically down to the level of the internal cervical os, as illustrated by the darkly shaded portion of the diagram. The cervix is not removed, and none of the surgery is performed transvaginally with an LSH.

TABLE 32C.1

A PROPOSED STAGING SYSTEM FOR LAPAROSCOPIC HYSTERECTOMIES

Stage	Laparoscopic procedures
0	Diagnostic laparoscopy only; no laparoscopic procedure before vaginal hysterectomy
1	Laparoscopic adhesiolysis or excision of endometriosis
2	One or both adnexa freed laparoscopically
3	Bladder dissected from uterus laparoscopically
4	Uterine arteries transected laparoscopically
5	Anterior or posterior colpotomy or entire uterus freed laparoscopically

From Richardson RE, Bournas N, Magos AL. Is laparoscopic hysterectomy a waste of time? *Lancet* 1995;345:36.

abdominal, or laparoscopic—ideally should be determined by the patient's physical status and pathology, not by the surgeon's needs or skills. The preponderance of abdominal hysterectomies over vaginal and laparoscopic hysterectomies in the United States, however, suggests that the comfort and skill level of the gynecologic surgeon more often dictates the surgical approach than does the patients' underlying indications for hysterectomy (Table 32C.2). There are ample data to suggest that far more hysterectomies could be performed vaginally and that many hysterectomies performed abdominally could be done laparoscopically. Randomized clinical trials support the preferential use of vaginal and laparoscopic approaches over the abdominal approach. It is worthwhile to review details of a few of these trials.

Laparoscopically Assisted Vaginal Hysterectomy versus Total Abdominal Hysterectomy

A well-designed multicenter trial reported by Summitt and colleagues randomized 63 women to LAVH or total abdominal hysterectomy (TAH). LAVH was successfully performed in 31 (91%) of the 34 women randomized to LAVH, confirming the ability to perform LAVH in most women who have contraindications to vaginal hysterectomy. The groups were similar demographically. The outcomes are summarized in Table 32C.3. Operative times averaged 30 minutes longer for LAVH, and estimated blood loss averaged 100 mL greater for TAH, but these differences were not statistically different. Postoperative hematocrits at 2 days were the same for TAH and LAVH. Hospital costs were not different. Overall complications were not statistically different. Two patients who had LAVH incurred incidental cystotomies that were repaired laparoscopically, and one sustained an injury to the abdominal wall inferior epigastric artery that was controlled with suture ligation. Two patients in the TAH group required intraoperative transfusions. Seven patients in the TAH group and one in the LAVH group had some form of postoperative wound complication, and one patient in each group developed pelvic cellulitis postoperatively. More patients in the TAH group (30 of 31) required intramuscular opioids on the day of surgery compared with the LAVH group (26 of 34; $p = .018$). Postoperative recovery was significantly faster with LAVH, with shorter hospital days (2.1 versus 4.1) and fewer convalescent days (28 versus 38).

Another multicenter study from Italy of LAVH compared with TAH enrolled 116 women who were not candidates for total vaginal hysterectomy (TVH). In this trial, there was no difference in operative time between LAVH and TAH, and none of the LAVH cases required conversion to laparotomy (Table 32C.4). There was one intraoperative complication in the LAVH group (a bladder laceration that was repaired laparoscopically) and no intraoperative complications in the TAH group. Postoperative complications in the LAVH group consisted of two cases of febrile morbidity. There were seven cases with postoperative complications in the TAH group. Five patients had postoperative febrile morbidity, and two had postoperative bleeding that required blood transfusions.

A single institution study of LAVH-bilateral salpingo-oophorectomy (BSO) versus TAH-BSO reported by Raju and Auld showed similar results. This was a randomized trial involving 80 women, but obese women and women with uteri greater than 14 weeks' gestational size were excluded from this study. Two (5%) of the LAVH-BSO patients were converted to laparotomy because of bleeding. Although operative time was significantly longer with LAVH-BSO, hospital stay and recovery time were significantly reduced with LAVH-BSO (Table 32C.5).

Vaginally Assisted Laparoscopic Hysterectomy versus Total Abdominal Hysterectomy

A randomized clinical trial of VALH versus TAH showed results similar to those for LAVH versus TAH. This study of 143 women found that 4 (6%) of 71 VALH cases required conversion to laparotomy for completion. In two cases, this was due to large cervical myomas. In one case, each conversion was to repair a laceration to the bladder and because of dense adhesions. Surgical time was significantly longer with VALH (Table 32C.6). Both postoperative hospital stay and the time for convalescence time were significantly shorter with VALH. Pain 2 days postoperatively was significantly less following VALH; 3.6 compared with 4.2 ($p = 0.05$) on a 0 to 7 visual analog scale. It should be noted that this study excluded women with large uteri.

Another trial of VALH, however, specifically selected women with uteri weighing 450 or more grams. This study randomized 60 women to VALH, TAH, or TVH. Two patients required conversion to laparotomy in the planned TVH group (6.6%), and one patient required conversion in the planned

TABLE 32C.2

PROPORTION OF HYSTERECTOMIES PERFORMED LAPAROSCOPICALLY, ABDOMINALLY, VAGINALLY, AND AS SUBTOTALS IN 1990 COMPARED WITH 1997

	1990	1997
Abdominal hysterectomy	73.6	63.0
Vaginal hysterectomy	24.4	23.3
Laparoscopic hysterectomy	0.3	9.9
Subtotal hysterectomy	0.7	2.0

From Farquhar CM, Steiner CA. Hysterectomy rates in the United States 1990–1997. *Obstet Gynecol* 2002;99:229.

TABLE 32C.3

OUTCOMES OF A U.S. MULTICENTER RANDOMIZED CLINICAL TRIAL COMPARING TOTAL ABDOMINAL HYSTERECTOMY (TAH) AND LAPAROSCOPICALLY ASSISTED VAGINAL HYSTERECTOMY (LAVH)

	TAH (N = 31)	LAVH	P value significance
Operative time (min)	146.0 + 69.9 (52–325)	179.8 + 56.4 (80–270)	NS
Estimated blood loss (mL)	660.5 + 610 (100–3,000)	568 + 394 (50–1,600)	NS
Uterine weight (g)	383.9 + 227.8 (70–954)	336.8 + 276.0 (54–1,550)	NS
Postoperative hematocrit	29.3 + 4.3 (21.3–36.8)	29.3 + 4.8 (19.7–37.5)	NS
Hospital days	4.1 + 1.6 (2–9)	2.1 + 1.3 (1–6)	<0.001
Convalescent days	38.0 + 10.8 (15–55)	28.0 + 13.3 (9–70)	0.002
Hospital charges (U.S. dollars)	6,974 + 2,843 (3,183–16,086)	8,161 + 3,600 (3,600–23,591)	NS
Intramuscular opioids day of surgery	30 (97%)	26 (76%)	0.018
Intraoperative complications	2 (6%)	3 (9%)	NS
Postoperative complications	8 (26%)	2 (6%)	0.039
Any complication	10 (32%)	5 (15%)	NS

NS, not significant.
From Summitt RL Jr, Stovall TG, Steege JF, et al. A multicenter randomized comparison of laparoscopically assisted vaginal hysterectomy and abdominal hysterectomy in abdominal hysterectomy candidates. *Obstet Gynecol* 1998;92:321.

TABLE 32C.4

OUTCOMES OF AN ITALIAN MULTICENTER RANDOMIZED CLINICAL TRIAL COMPARING TOTAL ABDOMINAL HYSTERECTOMY (TAH) AND LAPAROSCOPICALLY ASSISTED VAGINAL HYSTERECTOMY (LAVH)

	TAH (N = 58)	LAVH	P value significance
Operative time (min)	91.8 + 26.4	91.1 + 30.2	NS
Uterine weight (g)	352.3 + 165.9	326.4 + 125.8	NS
Estimated blood loss (mL)	353.9 + 254.6	264.7 + 194.4	<0.05
Decrease of hemoglobin g/100 (mL)	1.55 + 1.07	1.09 + 0.97	<0.05
Postoperative hospital days	5.9 + 2.3	4.0 + 1.2	<0.001
Postoperative pain level, day 1	6.3 + 1.6	5.2 + 2.6	<0.05
Postoperative pain level, day 2	4.4 + 1.9	2.3 + 2.3	<0.001
Postoperative pain level, day 3	2.8 + 2.3	1.3 + 1.6	<0.005
Intraoperative complications	0	1	NS
Postoperative complications	7	2	NS

NS, not significant.
From Marana R, Busacca M, Zupi E, et al. Laparoscopically assisted vaginal hysterectomy versus total abdominal hysterectomy: a prospective, randomized, multicenter study. *Am J Obstet Gynecol* 1999;180:270.

TABLE 32C.5

OUTCOMES OF A SINGLE CENTER RANDOMIZED CLINICAL TRIAL COMPARING TOTAL ABDOMINAL HYSTERECTOMY–BILATERAL SALPINGO-OOPHORECTOMY (TAH-BSO) AND LAPAROSCOPICALLY ASSISTED VAGINAL HYSTERECTOMY–BILATERAL SALPINGO-OOPHORECTOMY (LAVH-BSO)

	TAH-BSO (N = 40)	LAVH BSO (N = 40)	P value significance
Operative time (min)	57 (25–151)	100 (61–180)	<0.001
Estimated blood loss (mL)	220 (50–500)	260 (70–700)	NS
Postoperative decrease in hemoglobin (g/L)	1.54 (0.5–3.2)	1.82 (0.1–4.8)	NS
Hospital days	6 (3–13)	3.5 (1–6)	<0.0001
Duration of postoperative analgesia	13.3 (2–38)	6.6 (0–23)	<0.0001
Return to work (days)	21 (7–35)	42 (21–67)	<0.0001
Any complication	1 (2.5%)	0 (15%)	NS

NS, not significant.
From Raju KS, Auld BJ. A randomised prospective study of laparoscopic vaginal hysterectomy versus abdominal hysterectomy each with bilateral salpingo-oophorectomy. *BJOG* 1994;101:1068.

VALH group (3.3%). Uterine sizes greater than 1,100 g were the reasons for conversion in all three cases. The outcome results are summarized in Table 32C.7 and indicate the advantages of vaginal hysterectomy, even with an enlarged uterus.

Another clinical trial of VALH versus TAH was published by Falcone and colleagues and randomized 48 patients (Table 32C.8). One patient (4%) in this study required conversion from VALH to laparotomy because of bleeding. There was one intraoperative complication in the VALH group: a small bowel laceration that did not require a laparotomy for repair. There were no intraoperative complications in the TAH group. Again, results were similar to the previously reviewed trials, with no significant differences in blood loss (based on hematocrits), transfusion rates, or postoperative complications. Hospital stays were shorter and postoperative pain was decreased with VALH. Patients who had VALH returned to work sooner than patients who had TAH.

Total Laparoscopic Hysterectomy versus Total Abdominal Hysterectomy

Perino and associates published a randomized trial of TLH versus TAH in 102 women (Table 32C.9). Uterine size was

TABLE 32C.6

OUTCOMES OF A SINGLE CENTER RANDOMIZED CLINICAL TRIAL COMPARING TOTAL ABDOMINAL HYSTERECTOMY (TAH) AND VAGINALLY ASSISTED LAPAROSCOPIC HYSTERECTOMY (VALH)

	TAH (N = 72)	VALH (N = 71)	P value significance
Surgery time (min)	85 (45–275)	148 (70–240)	<0.001
Postoperative hospital days	4.0 (2–28)	2.0 (1–12)	<0.001
Convalescent days	35 (7–125)	16 (0–74)	<0.001
Decrease in hematocrit	5.6 (0–20)	4.1 (−6.1–12)	
Patients transfused	9 (12.5%)	5 (7.0%)	NS
Units transfused	23	11	<0.001
Complications	24 (33%)	19 (27%)	NS
Hematomas	17	11	
Infections	20	16	
Urinary tract injuries	1	2	

NS, not significant.
From Olsson JH, Ellstrom M, Hahlin M. A randomised prospective trial comparing laparoscopic and abdominal hysterectomy. *BJOG* 1996;103:345.

TABLE 32C.7

OUTCOMES OF A SINGLE CENTER RANDOMIZED CLINICAL TRIAL COMPARING TOTAL ABDOMINAL HYSTERECTOMY (TAH), VAGINALLY ASSISTED LAPAROSCOPIC HYSTERECTOMY (VALH), AND TOTAL VAGINAL HYSTERECTOMY (TVH) IN WOMEN WITH UTERI WEIGHING MORE THAN 450 GRAMS

	TAH (N = 30)	VALH (N = 30)	TVH (N = 30)	P value significance
Operative time (min)	98 ± 16 (85–150)	109 ± 22 (85–175)	93 ± 15 (40–120)	<0.001 <0.001
Estimated blood loss	293 ± 182 (50–750)	343 ± 218 (50–950)	215 ± 134 (50–560)	0.04
Hospital stay	5.0 (4–8)	4.7 (3–7)	4.7 (3–7)	0.003
Return to work	41 ± 10 (26–65)	30 ± 16 (17–42)	29 ± 11 (17–50)	<0.001
Any complication	9 (30%)	6 (20%)	5 (17%)	<.05
Febrile morbidity/infection	8 (27%)	1 (3%)	4 (13%)	
Transfusion	1 (3%)	5 (17%)	1 (3%)	

From Hwang JL, Seow KM, Tsai YL, et al. Comparative study of vaginal, laparoscopically assisted vaginal and abdominal hysterectomies for uterine myoma larger than 6 cm in diameter or uterus weighing at least 450 g: a prospective randomized study. *Acta Obstet Gynecol Scand* 2002;81:1132.

TABLE 32C.8

OUTCOMES OF A SINGLE CENTER RANDOMIZED CLINICAL TRIAL COMPARING TOTAL ABDOMINAL HYSTERECTOMY (TAH) AND VAGINALLY ASSISTED LAPAROSCOPIC HYSTERECTOMY (VALH)

	TAH (N = 21)	VALH (N = 23)	P value significance
Surgery time (min)	130 (97–155)	180 (139–225)	<0.001
Estimated blood loss	250 (150–300)	450 (250–700)	0.003
Postoperative hematocrit	31.2 + 3.2 (23–36)	29.2 + 4.5 (21–36)	NS
Patients transfused	4 (17%)	3 (14%)	NS
Uterine weight (g)	309 (178–636)	370 (195–561)	NS
Any postoperative complication	5	8	NS
Length of hospital stay (days)	2.5 (1.5–2.5)	1.5 (1.0–2.3)	0.038
Length of use of patient controlled analgesia (hours)	36.7 (26.2–45.0)	22.1 (15.9–23.5)	<0.001

NS, not significant.
From Falcone T, Paraiso MF, Mascha E. Prospective randomized clinical trial of laparoscopically assisted vaginal hysterectomy versus total abdominal hysterectomy. *Am J Obstet Gynecol* 1999;180:955.

TABLE 32C.9

OUTCOMES OF A SINGLE CENTER RANDOMIZED CLINICAL TRIAL COMPARING TOTAL ABDOMINAL HYSTERECTOMY (TAH) AND TOTAL LAPAROSCOPIC HYSTERECTOMY (TLH)

	TLH (N = 51)	TAH (N = 51)	P value significance
Operative time (min)	104 + 27	88 + 20	<0.001
Uterine weight (g)	368 + 125	389 + 143	NS
Estimated blood loss (mL)	140 + 42	406 + 104	<0.001
Decrease of hemoglobin (g/100 mL)	0.4 + 0.2	1.6 + 0.4	<0.001
Postoperative stay (days)	2.4 + 0.3	6.2 + 1.9	<0.001
Pain level, day 1	4.1 + 1.2	6.9 + 1.8	<0.001
Pain level, day 2	2.3 + 1.6	5.4 + 1.3	<0.001
Pain level, day 3	1.0 + 0.7	3.1 + 0.9	<0.001
Complications	1	6	NS

NS, not significant.
From Perino A, Cucinella G, Venezia R, et al. Total laparoscopic hysterectomy versus total abdominal hysterectomy: an assessment of the learning curve in a prospective randomized study. *Hum Reprod* 1999;14:2996.

restricted to less than 16 weeks' size in this study. No cases of TLH required conversion to laparotomy. They found that TLH was somewhat slower, requiring on average 16 minutes longer than TAH, but they had significantly lower blood loss, shorter hospital stays, and less postoperative pain with TLH. There were no intraoperative complications in either group. There was one postoperative complication in the TLH group: a ureterovaginal fistula diagnosed 10 days after surgery. There were six postoperative complications in the TAH group: four cases of febrile morbidity and two hematomas, one of which required transfusion.

A clinical trial published by Seracchioli and colleagues selected patients with leiomyomata and uteri estimated to be greater than 14 weeks' gestation in size. A total of 122 women were randomized to either TLH or TAH. One conversion from TLH to laparotomy was necessary because of a bowel injury in a patient with severe adhesions. There were no other complications in the TLH group. One patient in the TAH group had an intraoperative complication: a cystotomy that was repaired immediately. Operative time and blood loss were not different between the two groups in this study (Table 32C.10). Postoperative febrile morbidity, hospital stay, and recovery time were greater in the TAH group. There were six wound infections in the TAH group and none in the TLH group, but this did not reach statistical significance.

In summary, the various types of laparoscopic hysterectomies result in decreased postoperative pain, faster postoperative recovery, less risk of abdominal wall infections, and decreased febrile morbidity and infections when compared with abdominal hysterectomies. Laparoscopic hysterectomies may take longer, but any increase in cost is offset by shorter hospital stays. No increased morbidity that is due to longer operative times has been demonstrated. There are no benefits of TAH over laparoscopic hysterectomy other than a legitimate concern that urinary tract injury may occur more often with laparoscopic hysterectomy. It is unclear if this is experience related rather than being directly related to the surgical approach itself. It is my opinion, based on the quality of the clinical trials available, that whenever possible, a laparoscopic hysterectomy is preferred over an abdominal hysterectomy.

Laparoscopic Subtotal Hysterectomy versus Total Abdominal Hysterectomy or Total Laparoscopic Hysterectomy

The major arguments for subtotal hysterectomy are decreased risk of urinary tract injuries and decreased risk of infection. Randomized trials have been published comparing abdominal subtotal and total hysterectomies, but they provide no evidence of compelling advantages of one procedure over the other. These trials have found no advantage of subtotal hysterectomy on bladder function, vaginal vault prolapse, or sexual satisfaction.

Data from a Danish randomized trial of abdominal subtotal versus total hysterectomies showed a significantly lower proportion of women were incontinent 1 year after total abdominal hysterectomy than after subtotal abdominal hysterectomy (STAH) (9% vs. 18%, respectively; 21% were incontinent preoperatively in each group). At 1 year, there were no statistically significant differences in quality of life, constipation, prolapse of the vaginal or cervical stump, satisfaction with sexual life, or pelvic pain. Vaginal bleeding was present in none of the TAH patients, but was present in 20% of the STAH patients. Operative time was shorter by about 15 minutes with STAH, and median blood loss was 150 mL less. Perioperative and postoperative complications were not different.

A U.S. randomized trial of TAH versus STAH showed no statistically significant differences in procedure time, estimated blood loss, febrile morbidity, urinary tract infections, urinary tract injuries, blood transfusions, return of bladder function, or length of hospital stay. Two-year outcomes for relief of pelvic pain, back pain, pelvic or bladder pressure, prolapse, urinary urgency, incomplete urinary emptying, urinary stress incontinence, or urinary urge incontinence were not different between the two groups. Cyclical bleeding was reported in only 7% of the STAH patients in this study.

A British randomized trial showed that TAH was associated with a statistically significantly longer duration of surgery (12 minutes longer), greater blood loss (100 mL more), more febrile morbidity (19% vs. 6%), and a longer hospital stay

TABLE 32C.10

OUTCOMES OF A RANDOMIZED CLINICAL TRIAL COMPARING TOTAL ABDOMINAL HYSTERECTOMY (TAH) AND TOTAL LAPAROSCOPIC HYSTERECTOMY (TLH) FOR PATIENTS WITH UTERI GREATER THAN 14 WEEKS' GESTATIONAL SIZE

	TAH (N = 62)	LAVHTLH (N = 60)	P value significance
Operative time (min)	89 + 29	95 + 32	NS
Uterine weight (g)	429 + 125	412 + 175	NS
Estimated blood loss (mL)	377 + 225	312 + 182	NS
Decrease of hemoglobin (g/100 mL)	2.3 + 1.8	1.8 + 1.1	NS
Number of transfusions	1	0	NS
Postoperative febrile morbidity	18 (29%)	8 (13%)	<0.05
Hospital stay (hours)	122 + 42	76 + 11	<0.001
Wound infections	6	0	NS
Days of convalescence	36 + 12	22 + 11	<0.001
Complications	1	1	NS

NS, not significant.
From Seracchioli R, Venturoli S, Vianello F, et al. Total laparoscopic hysterectomy compared with abdominal hysterectomy in the presence of a large uterus. *J Am Assoc Gynecol Laparosc* 2002;9:333.

(1 day longer) than was STAH. At 12 months after subtotal hysterectomy, 7% of the women had cyclical vaginal bleeding in this study. There were no differences in bladder function, bowel function, or sexual function between the two groups.

There are no randomized trials, only observational studies, comparing LSH to TLH or LAVH. Results of four such studies are summarized in Table 32C.11. On average, LSH is slightly faster, with slightly less blood loss and shorter hospital stays than LAVH or TLH.

SURGICAL TECHNIQUE

Laparoscopically Assisted Vaginal Hysterectomy

After general anesthesia is induced, the patient is placed in low lithotomy position using Allen-type stirrups. Modern stirrups that allow the legs to be repositioned to full dorsal lithotomy position without the removal of sterile drapes greatly facilitate LAVH. An examination under anesthesia is done with particular attention to evaluation of the pelvic and vaginal dimensions to confirm that the vaginal part of the procedure can be readily performed. Generally the bituberous diameter should be 9 cm or more, the pubic arch 90 degrees or more, and the vaginal apex should be greater than two fingerbreadths (about 4 cm). Although a mobile uterus that descends with traction facilitates the procedure, the vaginal portion of an LAVH can be done as long as the uterine vessels are accessible to clamping and ligation vaginally.

I prefer to position the patient's arms at her side, padding them as necessary and being sure not to hyperextend the elbows or externally rotate the arms. Many anesthesiologists oppose this placement because it makes the intravenous site less easily accessible. If the arms are placed on arm boards, they must be positioned to allow adequate surgical access without hyperextension of the shoulders, to avoid axillary injury. Shoulder braces should generally be avoided; if they are used, adequate padding is important to avoid injury. It is wise for the surgeon to personally supervise positioning of the patient.

After the patient is positioned, the abdomen, perineum, and vagina are prepared and draped. A Foley catheter should be placed. I often prefer a three-way catheter so that sterile infant formula can be instilled into the bladder to aid bladder dissection if it is done laparoscopically. A tenaculum is placed on the cervix, and an intrauterine manipulating device is inserted so that the uterus can be manipulated during the laparoscopy. As an alternative, a laparoscopic tenaculum can be used to manipulate the uterus rather than intrauterine manipulator.

TABLE 32C.11

COMPARISONS OF LAPAROSCOPIC SUBTOTAL HYSTERECTOMIES (LSH) WITH LAPAROSCOPICALLY ASSISTED VAGINAL (LAVH) OR TOTAL LAPAROSCOPIC HYSTERECTOMIES (TLH) FROM FOUR DIFFERENT OBSERVATIONAL STUDIES

	LAVH or TLH	LSH	LAVH or TLH	LSH	LAVH or TLH	LSH	LSH
	OR Time	OR Time	EBL	EBL	Hospital Stay	Hospital Stay	Cyclical Bleeding
El-Mowafi et al.	150	120	149	125	1–2 d	1–2 d	Not reported
Lyons	145	118	250	50	37 h	18 h	—
Richards and Simpkins	117	127	210	179	46 h	34 h	—
Lalonde and Daniell	124	106	245	200	41 h	26 h	10%

OR, operating room; EBL, estimated blood loss.

Usually an umbilical incision is made to allow insertion of a Veress needle or direct insertion of a laparoscopic trocar. If the patient has had a prior laparotomy, however, either a left upper quadrant insertion or an open laparoscopic umbilical insertion is preferred. The abdomen is inflated and distended with carbon dioxide, and the laparoscope is introduced (see Chapter 17). The pelvis should be thoroughly inspected, and the placement of operative trocars should be dictated by the patient's anatomy and pathology. If there is no pathology that requires laparoscopic surgery, no other trocars are needed, and a vaginal hysterectomy can be performed. If laparoscopic surgery is to be done, then two lateral trocars are inserted. Although traditionally these lateral trocars are placed in the lower quadrants, often a more superior placement allows better adnexal and vascular pedicle access. It is crucial that the operative trocars be placed under direct visualization and lateral to the inferior epigastric vessels. The inferior epigastric vessels can almost always be identified and avoided (Fig. 32C.5). If there is extensive pelvic pathology that will require extensive laparoscopic surgery, I prefer to place a fourth trocar ≥6 cm superior to the lower lateral cannula on the primary surgeon's side of the patient (Fig. 32C.6). This allows the primary surgeon to operate with both hands while the assistant can retract with a third instrument (the camera used the fourth port). This greatly facilitates difficult procedures. Although many laparoscopic surgeons add the fourth port suprapubically in the midline, I find this site is not as useful for extensive procedures.

After all extrauterine and extraovarian pathology has been surgically addressed, attention is turned to the hysterectomy. The ligaments and vessels of the pelvis can be coagulated and cut in a number of ways. Although some surgeons use clampless suturing to ligate the ligaments and vessels, most find this slow and cumbersome. The majority of laparoscopic gynecologic surgeons use one of the devices specifically designed for laparoscopic surgery. Bipolar forceps to coagulate and scissors to cut vascular pedicles are inexpensive and readily available. Newer technologies using bipolar electrical energy with feedback control to consistently seal vessels represent an improvement on traditional bipolar forceps. Most of these devices have a built-in cutting blade that speeds the procedure. Trade name examples are Valleylab Ligasure Sealer/Cutter™ and Gyrus PK Cutting Forceps™, both of which are available as 5-mm instruments. Another available technology uses ultrasonic energy to seal and cut tissue and vessels. An example of this type device is the Ethicon Harmonic Scalpel™. Mechanical energy may be used with stapler-cutter devices. Examples are Tyco Endo-GIA™ and Ethicon Endopath ETS™. Clips may also be used. It is important with all of these techniques that tension on vascular pedicles be minimized during coagulation to allow proper vessel sealing.

Usually an LAVH starts the same way as a TAH. The uterus is deviated to one side with the uterine manipulator, and the round ligament on the opposite side is coagulated and cut. The peritoneum of the anterior broad ligament is then dissected and cut in an inferior-medial direction to the midline bladder reflection to start the bladder dissection. If the ovary is to be removed, the peritoneum is also divided cephalad toward the infundibulopelvic ligament. The retroperitoneal space can be opened gently with traction on both sides to allow identification of the ureter either transperitoneally or retroperitoneally. If the ovary is to be removed, then the ureter is identified at the pelvic brim. This is usually easy on the right side, but may be more difficult on the left because of the sigmoid colon. The ovary or fallopian tube is grasped from the contralateral side to expose the infundibulopelvic ligament, and the ovarian artery and vein are ligated and cut. This should be done under full visualization to insure that the ureter and iliac vessels are far from the surgical site. The coagulation and ligation are then carried anteriorly to join the previously ligated area of the round ligament, again insuring that the ureter is in direct view. These procedures then are repeated on the opposite side. The bladder plane can then be sharply dissected if desired, or this can be done transvaginally.

If the ovaries are not to be removed, the proximal fallopian tubes are coagulated and cut several centimeters from the uterus, followed by coagulation and transaction of the uteroovarian ligaments close to the uterus. Often the uteroovarian ligaments are best coagulated and cut from the contralateral cannula site. At this point, the laparoscopic procedure is completed, and the remainder of the operation is done vaginally, exactly as one would perform a standard vaginal hysterectomy. Because the infundibulopelvic ligaments and round ligaments have already been divided via the laparoscope, once the uterine vessels have been ligated from below, there is only minimal fatty, relatively avascular, parametrial tissue to be divided

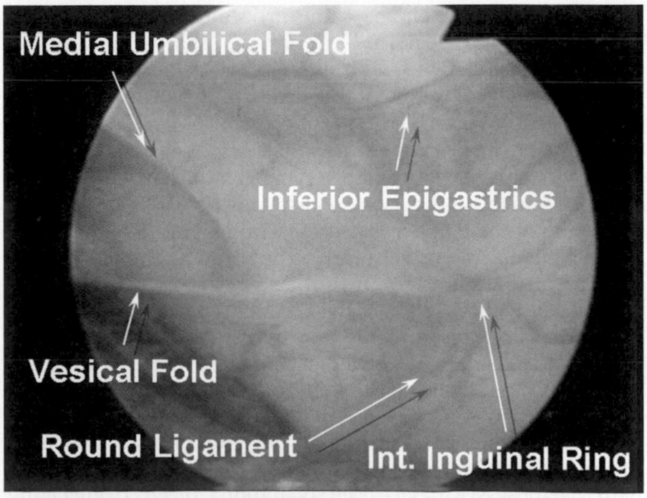

FIGURE 32C.5. Laparoscopic anatomy of the right anterior abdominal wall showing the crucial landmarks for safe placement of lateral operative trocars. The lower abdominal trocars should always be placed under direct visualization and lateral to the inferior epigastric vessels.

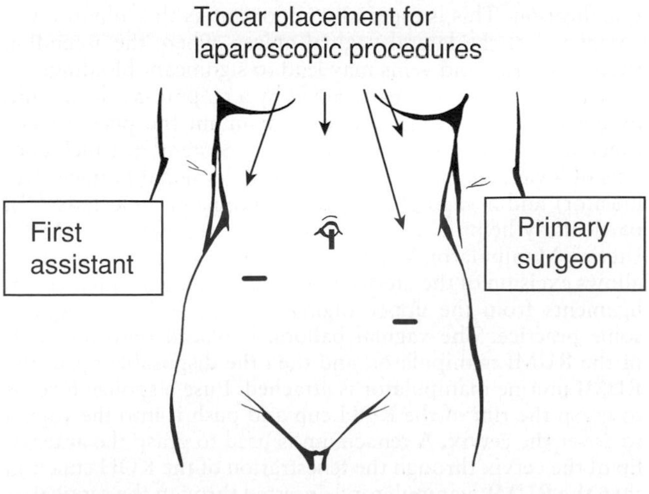

FIGURE 32C.6. An example of placement sites for trocars when there is extensive pelvic pathology. In this example, the primary surgeon is on the patient's left so he or she can operate with both hands while the assistant drives the camera with one hand and assists with the other hand.

before the uterus can be removed. Once the vaginal hysterectomy has been completed and the vagina closed, the laparoscope can be used to check the pelvis for hemostasis before removing the laparoscopic cannulas and closing the laparoscopic incisions.

Vaginally Assisted Laparoscopic Hysterectomy

With VALH, the uterine vessels are coagulated and cut laparoscopically. After completion of the laparoscopic procedures described for LAVH, the bladder is adequately mobilized to allow exposure of the uterine artery and vein. I find that filling the bladder with 100 to 200 mL of infant formula aids the accurate visualization and mobilization of the bladder. Then the uterine vessels are skeletonized by opening the anterior and posterior leafs of the broad ligament. Once this is done, the vessels can be coagulated and cut close to the uterus and well away from the ureters. Moving the uterus laterally and elevating it slightly also aids in protecting the ureters. I find that staplers tend to pull tissue medially at this level, so I prefer not to use them for the uterine vessels.

The legs are then elevated to full dorsal lithotomy, and the colpotomy is performed transvaginally, followed by ligating and cutting the uterosacral ligaments. This allows removal of the uterus, followed by closure of the vagina and the laparoscopic incisions.

Total Laparoscopic Hysterectomy

To perform a TLH, the surgeon continues laparoscopically after ligation of the uterine vessels and adequate mobilization of the bladder by performing anterior and posterior colpotomies. I prefer performing the anterior colpotomy first because subsequent anteversion of the uterus to perform the posterior colpotomy occludes the anterior incision and helps maintain a pneumoperitoneum. The colpotomy incisions can be made with laparoscopic scissors, but most laparoscopic scissors are too delicate to readily cut the thick vaginal tissue. Also, bleeding from the vagina is an issue with this technique. I prefer the use of an ultrasonic device, but electrosurgical incision works well, too. Maintaining hemostasis is important to allow adequate visualization. This is especially important as the colpotomy is completed at the lateral vaginal apices, where the ascending vaginal arteries and veins may lead to significant bleeding.

The colpotomy is greatly aided by a colpotomy device and by a vaginal occluding device to maintain the pneumoperitoneum. I find the KOH Colpotomizer System™, which consists of a vaginal extender (KOH Cup™ Vaginal Fornices Delineator) and a vaginal balloon (Colpopneumo Occluder™), particularly helpful. This system works well with a RUMI™ Uterine Manipulator. When the KOH Cup is fitted properly, it allows excision of the uterus without detaching the uterosacral ligaments from the upper vagina. Using the device requires some practice. The vaginal balloon is placed onto the shaft of the RUMI manipulator, and then the disposable tip to the RUMI uterine manipulator is attached. I use a sponge forceps to grasp the rim of the KOH cup and push it into the vagina to cover the cervix. A tenaculum is used to grasp the anterior lip of the cervix through the fenestration of the KOH cup, and then the RUMI manipulator is inserted through the cervical os and into the KOH cup. When it is time to make the anterior colpotomy, the grip of the RUMI uterine manipulator is rotated counterclockwise and pushed cephalad. This clearly shows the area of the anterior vagina to be incised. The pneumo-occluder balloon is inflated with 60 to 100 cc of saline just before the colpotomy incision is made. It is important that the bladder has been dissected inferiorly to expose 1 to 2 cm of vagina. The RUMI uterine manipulator is then rotated clockwise to antevert the uterus and expose the posterior rim of the KOH cup and direct the site for the posterior colpotomy. Completion of the colpotomy laterally is guided by the KOH cup by moving the uterine manipulator to expose the right and left vaginal fornices. Once the uterus is detached, it may be pulled into the vagina and left there to maintain the pneumoperitoneum while the vagina is closed with interrupted sutures placed laparoscopically.

An example of another technique for aiding in the colpotomy and maintenance of pneumoperitoneum is the McCartney tube (Tyco Healthcare, Inc., Sydney, Australia), which is a disposable silicone tube with a diameter of 45 mm or 35 mm. The vaginal end of the tube is open and is inserted transvaginally to stretch the cervicovaginal junction and aid in identifying the vaginal fornices. The outer end of the tube is covered by a cap containing 5- and 10-mm valves and maintains the pneumoperitoneum when the colpotomy is made. After the uterus is detached, it can be pulled into the tube while the vaginal apex is closed, or the tube can be removed to allow removal of the uterus. Either the uterus can be left in the vagina or the tube replaced to maintain the pneumoperitoneum while the vagina is closed.

It is possible to perform TLH without such devices. Numerous techniques have been described, but an inexpensive technique consists of removing the uterine manipulator when preparing to do the colpotomy (the tenaculum is left on the cervix). A laparoscopic tenaculum is used to move the uterus and expose the vaginal fornices and allow exposure for the colpotomy. Placing a Deaver retractor into the appropriate area of the vaginal fornix may help identify the sites for the anterior and posterior colpotomies. Either a wet towel or wet laparotomy sponge is placed in the vagina to maintain the pneumoperitoneum while the colpotomy is completed. As previously described, once the uterus is detached, it can be placed in the vagina to maintain the pneumoperitoneum while vaginal apex closure is performed.

Laparoscopic Subtotal Hysterectomy

LSH consists of much the same procedure as described for VALH—that is, the uterine arteries are laparoscopically isolated and occluded with a bipolar electricity or ultrasonic vessel sealing device, clips, staples, or sutures. After the uterine vessels are secured, the uterine corpus is amputated from the cervix at the level of the isthmus. Although it may be possible to do this without dissecting the bladder from the lower uterine segment and cervix, realistically, in most cases, some dissection of the bladder is necessary to insure adequate occlusion of the uterine vessels and amputation at the level of the isthmus of the uterus. Many surgeons electrodessicate or excise the epithelium of the cervical canal to decrease the risk of persistent menses postoperatively.

A major challenge with LSH compared with subtotal abdominal hysterectomy is removal of the corpus from the abdominal cavity. Although this can be done by morcellating the uterus through a posterior colpotomy incision, by extension of the umbilical incision, or using a minilaparotomy incision with a hand-assist device, the availability of electromechanical morcellators avoids the need to make additional or larger incisions. Such devices allow relatively rapid removal of the uterine corpus, although large uteri will add significant time to the duration of the procedure.

POSTOPERATIVE CARE

Postoperative care is thoroughly reviewed in Chapter 9. Only aspects specific to laparoscopic hysterectomy will be reviewed in this section.

A diet of the patient's choice may be started immediately after laparoscopic hysterectomy. This has been shown to be safe and allow for same-day or next-day discharge. This recommendation may need to be amended in cases of extensive enterolysis or other tissue dissection or if procedures are performed in addition to the hysterectomy.

A Foley catheter for bladder drainage may be left overnight for patient comfort or convenience, but this is not essential, and the catheter may be removed immediately postoperatively unless there has been bladder injury or extensive dissection.

Limitations on physical activity after laparoscopic hysterectomy are minimal, and most are common sense. Wound infections are uncommon, but keeping the laparoscopic incisions clean and dry for 10 to 14 days seems important. Protection of the vaginal incision is similar to that recommended with total hysterectomy by any technique. In particular, intercourse is best avoided for at least 6 weeks. Otherwise, many women may return to full physical activity within 2 weeks postoperatively after laparoscopic hysterectomy.

COMPLICATIONS

Complications occur with laparoscopic hysterectomy with a frequency similar to that of other surgical approaches to hysterectomy. The common complications—infection, hemorrhage, and injuries to adjacent organs—re the same types as with abdominal or vaginal hysterectomies. Postoperative incisional complications are less common than with abdominal hysterectomy, but laparoscopic hysterectomies may have complications specifically related to insertion of the trocars. These complications and their management are thoroughly discussed in Chapter 17.

BEST SURGICAL PRACTICES

- Preprocedure assessment and counseling are essential elements in a successful laparoscopic hysterectomy. The choice of procedure should be based on the patient's anatomy and pathology. The patient should be thoroughly counseled regarding anticipated outcomes, potential complications, preoperative preparation, and postoperative care.
- Indications for LAVH are known or suspected diseases that preclude a vaginal hysterectomy without assistance laparoscopically; i.e., laparoscopy is used to convert an abdominal hysterectomy into a vaginal hysterectomy.
- Generally speaking, LAVH, VALH, or TLH are not appropriate when a vaginal hysterectomy is indicated and technically feasible.
- Attention to identifying and restoring anatomy is as important in laparoscopic surgery as in any other surgery. The infundibulopelvic ligament and ureter should be clearly identified if the fallopian tube and ovary are to be removed. The uterine arteries should be skeletonized and carefully secured for VALH, TLH, or LSH, with certainty of ureteral location relative to the uterine vessels. The bladder must be identified and sharply dissected from the anterior uterus for LSH and from the cervix and upper vagina for TLH. Filling the bladder with saline, infant formula, or methylene blue may be especially helpful during bladder dissection with VALH and TLH.
- If an energy modality is used to ligate vessels, the surgeon must be knowledgeable about the safe use of the device.
- It is particularly important to prevent bleeding as much as possible during laparoscopic hysterectomy, as the blood absorbs light and hinders full visualization by decreasing light intensity in the surgical field.
- For total laparoscopic hysterectomy, a variety of devices are available to facilitate colpotomy and maintain the pneumoperitoneum.

Bibliography

El Mowafi D, Madkour W, Lall C, et al. Laparoscopic supracervical hysterectomy versus laparoscopic-assisted vaginal hysterectomy. *J Am Assoc Gynecol Laparosc* 2004;11:175.

Falcone T, Paraiso MF, Mascha E. Prospective randomized clinical trial of laparoscopically assisted vaginal hysterectomy versus total abdominal hysterectomy. *Am J Obstet Gynecol* 1999;180:955.

Farquhar CM, Steiner CA. Hysterectomy rates in the United States 1990-1997. *Obstet Gynecol* 2002;99:229.

Gimbel H, Zobbe V, Andersen BM, et al. Randomised controlled trial of total compared with subtotal hysterectomy with one-year follow-up results. *BJOG* 2003;110:1088.

Hwang JL, Seow KM, Tsai YL, et al. Comparative study of vaginal, laparoscopically assisted vaginal and abdominal hysterectomies for uterine myoma larger than 6 cm in diameter or uterus weighing at least 450 g: a prospective randomized study. *Acta Obstet Gynecol Scand* 2002;81:1132.

Kovac SR. Guidelines to determine the role of laparoscopically assisted vaginal hysterectomy. *Am J Obstet Gynecol* 1998;178:1257.

Kovac SR. Transvaginal hysterectomy: rationale and surgical approach. *Obstet Gynecol* 2004;103:1321.

Lalonde CJ, Daniell JF. Early outcomes of laparoscopic-assisted vaginal hysterectomy versus laparoscopic supracervical hysterectomy. *J Am Assoc Gynecol Laparosc* 1996;3:251.

Learman LA, Summitt RL, Jr,Varner RE, et al. A randomized comparison of total or supracervical hysterectomy: surgical complications and clinical outcomes. *Obstet Gynecol* 2003;102:453.

Lyons TL. Laparoscopic supracervical hysterectomy: a comparison of morbidity and mortality results with laparoscopically assisted vaginal hysterectomy. *J Reprod Med* 1993;38:763.

Marana R, Busacca M, Zupi E, et al. Laparoscopically assisted vaginal hysterectomy versus total abdominal hysterectomy: a prospective, randomized, multicenter study. *Am J Obstet Gynecol* 1999;180:270.

McCartney AJ, Obermair A. Total laparoscopic hysterectomy with a transvaginal tube. *J Am Assoc Gynecol Laparosc* 2004;11:79.

Munro MG. Supracervical hysterectomy: . . . a time for reappraisal. *Obstet Gynecol* 1997;89:133.

Olsson JH, Ellstrom M, Hahlin M. A randomised prospective trial comparing laparoscopic and abdominal hysterectomy. *BJOG* 1996;103:345.

Perino A, Cucinella G, Venezia R, et al. Total laparoscopic hysterectomy versus total abdominal hysterectomy: an assessment of the learning curve in a prospective randomized study. *Hum Reprod* 1999;14:2996.

Raju KS, Auld BJ. A randomised prospective study of laparoscopic vaginal hysterectomy versus abdominal hysterectomy each with bilateral salpingo-oophorectomy. *BJOG* 1994;101:1068.

Reich H, DeCaprio J, McGlynn F. Laparoscopic hysterectomy. *J Gynecol Surg* 1989;5:213.

Richards SR, Simpkins S. Laparoscopic supracervical hysterectomy versus laparoscopic-assisted vaginal hysterectomy. *J Am Assoc Gynecol Laparosc* 1995;2:431.

Richardson RE, Bournas N, Magos AL. Is laparoscopic hysterectomy a waste of time? *Lancet* 1995;345:36.

Seracchioli R, Venturoli S, Vianello F, et al. Total laparoscopic hysterectomy compared with abdominal hysterectomy in the presence of a large uterus. *J Am Assoc Gynecol Laparosc* 2002;9:333.

Summitt RL Jr, Stovall TG, Steege JF, et al. A multicenter randomized comparison of laparoscopically assisted vaginal hysterectomy and abdominal hysterectomy in abdominal hysterectomy candidates. *Obstet Gynecol* 1998;92:321.

Thakar R, Ayers S, Clarkson P, et al. Outcomes after total versus subtotal abdominal hysterectomy. *N Engl J Med* 2002;347:1318.

BEST SURGICAL PRACTICES

- Preprocedure assessment and counseling are essential elements in a successful laparoscopic hysterectomy. The choice of procedure should be based on the patient's anatomy and pathology. The patient should be thoroughly counseled regarding anticipated outcomes, potential complications, preoperative preparation, and postoperative care.
- Indications for LAVH are known or suspected diseases that preclude a vaginal hysterectomy without assistance laparoscopically, i.e., laparoscopy is used to convert an abdominal hysterectomy into a vaginal hysterectomy.
- Generally speaking, LAVH, VALH, or TLH are not appropriate when a vaginal hysterectomy is indicated and technically feasible.
- Attention to anatomic and tissue planes is important [illegible]

[illegible]

relative to the uterine vessels. The bladder must be identified and sharply dissected from the anterior uterus for LSH and from the cervix and upper vagina for TLH. Filling the bladder with sterile infant formula or methylene blue may be especially helpful during bladder dissection with VALH and TLH.
- If an energy modality is used to ligate vessels, the surgeon must be knowledgeable about the safe use of the device.
- It is particularly important to prevent bleeding as much as possible during laparoscopic hysterectomy, as the blood absorbs light and hinders full visualization by electrosurgical instruments in the surgical field.
- For total laparoscopic hysterectomy, a variety of devices are available to facilitate colpotomy and manipulation during uterine removal.

POSTOPERATIVE CARE

Postoperative care is thoroughly reviewed in Chapter 9. Only aspects specific to laparoscopic hysterectomy will be reviewed in this section.

A diet at the patient's choice may be started immediately after laparoscopic hysterectomy. This has been shown to be safe and allow for same day or next day discharge. This recommendation may need to be amended in cases of extensive enterolysis or other tissue dissection or if procedures are performed in addition to the hysterectomy.

A Foley catheter for bladder drainage may be left overnight for patient comfort or convenience, but this is not essential, and the catheter may be removed immediately postoperatively unless there has been bladder injury or extensive dissection.

Limitations of physical activity after laparoscopic hysterectomy are minimal, and most are common sense. Wound infec-

[illegible]

return to full physical activity within 2 weeks postoperatively after laparoscopic hysterectomy.

COMPLICATIONS

Complications occur with laparoscopic hysterectomy with a frequency similar to that of other surgical approaches to hysterectomy. The common complications—infection, hemorrhage, and injuries to adjacent organs—are the same types as with abdominal or vaginal hysterectomies. Postoperative incisional complications are less common than with abdominal hysterectomy, but laparoscopic hysterectomies may have complications specifically related to insertion of the trocars. These complications and their management are thoroughly discussed in Chapter 13.

Bibliography

Abel [illegible]
Boike GM, Elfstrand EP, DelPriore G, et al. Laparoscopically assisted vaginal hysterectomy in a university hospital: report of 82 cases and comparison with abdominal and vaginal hysterectomy. [illegible]
[illegible]
[illegible]
[illegible]
[illegible]
Summitt RL, Stovall TG, Steege JF, et al. [illegible]
[illegible]
Clarke [illegible]
[illegible]
[illegible]
Farquhar CM, Steiner CA. Hysterectomy rates in the United States 1990–1997. Obstet Gynecol 2002;99:229. [illegible]
Garry R, Fountain J, Mason S, et al. The eVALuate study: two parallel randomised trials, one comparing laparoscopic with abdominal hysterectomy, the other comparing laparoscopic with vaginal hysterectomy. BMJ 2004;328:129. [illegible]
Hwang JL, Seow KM, Tsai YL, et al. [illegible]
[illegible]
[illegible]

SECTION VI ■ SURGERY FOR OBSTETRICS

CHAPTER 33 ■ MANAGEMENT OF ABORTION

MELISSA J. KOTTKE AND MIMI ZIEMAN*

DEFINITIONS

Abortion—Termination of a pregnancy, whether spontaneous or induced.

Cerclage—A purse-string suture placed around the cervix to treat or prevent premature cervical dilation without labor.

Dilation and curettage—Dilation of the cervix followed by suction or sharp curettage to remove intrauterine contents.

Dilation and evacuation—Termination of pregnancy by wide cervical dilation and evacuation of fetal parts with forceps.

Fetal death—In utero death of fetus after 20 weeks.

Incomplete abortion—Partial expulsion of fetal tissue with open cervical os and products of conception remaining in the uterus.

Induced abortion—Medical or surgical termination of pregnancy.

Manual vacuum aspiration—Uterine evacuation performed with suction generated by a hand-held syringe.

Medical abortion—Use of medications including misoprostol, mifepristone, and methotrexate to terminate a pregnancy.

Spontaneous abortion—Spontaneous expulsion of an embryo or fetus weighing less than 500 g or before 20 weeks' gestation.

Threatened abortion—Vaginal bleeding early in pregnancy with a closed cervix and a potentially viable fetus.

The management of abortion remains a principal focus of gynecology. Several million spontaneous abortions occur annually, and more than 1 million induced abortions are performed each year in the United States. Induced abortion is one of the most frequently performed operations in gynecology and one of the most thoroughly studied. This chapter summarizes the medical and surgical management of abortion. It reviews the incidence, risk factors, and treatment of spontaneous, illegal, and legal abortion. Readers should keep in mind that abortion technology is rapidly evolving, and new protocols may supplant those described here.

SPONTANEOUS ABORTION

Incidence

The World Health Organization (WHO) defines spontaneous abortion as expulsion of an embryo or fetus that weighs 500 g or less. Alternative definitions support a 20-week gestational age limit. The true incidence of spontaneous abortion is uncertain because of the difficulty in recognizing early conceptions and losses. When Edmonds and colleagues monitored urine β-human chorionic gonadotropin (β-hCG) in a cohort of volunteers attempting to conceive, 62% of conceptuses died before 12 weeks' gestation. Most (92%) of these losses occurred before the woman was aware of the pregnancy. A similar study by Wilcox and associates monitored daily urinary β-hCG. They found that 31% of pregnancies resulted in spontaneous abortion after implantation. Approximately 70% of these—therefore, 22% of all losses—were not yet clinically identified. Wang and colleagues published further data in 2003; 8% of all conceptions in their study were recognized pregnancies followed by spontaneous loss. Twenty-six percent of all conceptions in that study were losses before knowledge of the pregnancy.

Overall, reported spontaneous abortion rates in recognized pregnancies are 10% to 20%. The vast majority—approximately 80%—of spontaneous abortions occur before 12 weeks' gestation. The average gestational age for spontaneous abortion of a recognized pregnancy is 9 weeks. However, consideration must be given to the large numbers of losses before detection of pregnancy. From a biological perspective, early pregnancy loss is a common outcome in human reproduction.

Risk Factors

Spontaneous abortion has several important risk factors. Demographic details provide some important nonmodifiable risk factors. The risk increases with advancing maternal age, particularly for women older than 35 years. In a large study published by Nybo Anderson and colleagues, the rates of miscarriage increased with maternal age. Women aged 20 to 30 years, 35 years, 40 years, and 45 years saw a 9% to 17%, 20%, 40%, and 80% miscarriage rate, respectively. Previous studies reported an increase from 12% at ages less than 20 to 26% at age 40. Likewise, the risk increases with advancing paternal age. Race also plays a role. At each stage of pregnancy, women of minority races in the United States have higher rates of spontaneous abortion than do white women.

Independent of the effect of age, the risk of spontaneous abortion changes with previous pregnancy history. Increasing rates of miscarriage are seen with increasing gravidity in some studies. In addition, a history of one or more spontaneous abortions increases the risk of recurrence. This effect is seen at all gestational ages. The risk of spontaneous abortion has been reported to increase with each documented miscarriage in one study, increasing from 20% after one miscarriage to 43% after three or more. Alternatively, the risk for spontaneous abortion

*Updated from a chapter by David A. Grimes.

is lower for a woman who has never had pregnancy or whose last pregnancy was successful. The length of the interval between pregnancies appears to have little impact.

Maternal substance use has been evaluated as a possible risk factor for spontaneous abortion. Smoking may increase the risk of spontaneous abortion. Because smoking is not teratogenic, its effect on spontaneous abortion rates may be via abortion of normal conceptuses. This may be secondary to a vasoconstrictive effect of smoking. In one study, the risk of miscarriage doubled; in other studies, the increase in risk was slight. Recent studies have not confirmed this increased risk. Alcohol consumption is associated with spontaneous abortion as well as teratogenicity. The effects of alcohol on miscarriage rate appear to be greatest for those whose alcohol consumption is greater. Additionally, the risk appears to be greater with increased intake in the earlier gestational ages. Alcohol consumption as a teratogen has a dose-dependent effect and can result in mental retardation, microcephaly, midface hypoplasia, renal, and cardiac defects. Caffeine intake has been evaluated in many studies regarding spontaneous abortion. Several studies have supported an increased risk for spontaneous abortion in women who drank greater than 500 mg—or the equivalence of 5 cups—of coffee per day. However, a recent systematic review by Signorello and McLaughlin indicates that there is insufficient evidence supporting a causal relationship.

Maternal health history and certain diagnoses may lead to increased risk for spontaneous abortion. Women with poorly controlled diabetes have higher levels of pregnancy loss as well as congenital anomalies. There is ongoing research about the effects of thyroid dysfunction on miscarriage. Women with a known hypercoagulable state, including antiphospholipid antibody syndrome, are at increased risk for spontaneous abortion as well as its recurrence.

The presence of uterine anomalies can lead to spontaneous abortion as well. Uterine synechiae, or Asherman syndrome, may permit insufficient surface area to support a pregnancy and lead to miscarriage. Uterine septae and abnormalities of müllerian fusion can also result in spontaneous abortion if the pregnancy implants on the septum and outgrows its blood supply. Although no effect is seen in the first trimester, the incidence of abortion after 13 weeks' gestation may be 20% to 25%. Leiomyomas, specifically submucosal, can interfere with implantation and make sustained pregnancy difficult. Lastly, cervical insufficiency that is due to previous surgery, trauma, or cervical anomaly can lead to pregnancy loss. This will be examined in detail later in this chapter.

Fever in early pregnancy may lead to spontaneous abortion. In one study, rates of spontaneous abortion of euploid conceptuses increased twofold to threefold if fever had preceded the abortion. Alternatively, a second study found no association between febrile episodes and miscarriage. Infection with *Chlamydia trachomatis,* mycoplasmas, or other organisms does not appear to influence spontaneous abortion.

Biologic Role

Spontaneous abortion serves primarily as a quality-control mechanism. The frequency of chromosomal abnormalities in aborted conceptuses is high, ranging from 30% to 61%. In decreasing order of frequency, the most common abnormalities are trisomy, sex chromosome monosomy, and triploidy. The earlier the gestational age at abortion, the higher is the frequency of chromosomal anomaly. Almost all anomalies, including some that would not appear to handicap survival (such as cleft lip), increase the likelihood of spontaneous abortion.

Prevention

It is largely unknown how to reduce the risk of spontaneous abortion. One study by Mills and colleagues indicated that women with diabetes with excellent glycemic control early in pregnancy had the same rate of spontaneous abortion as controls. Optimization of maternal health and avoidance of substances may be advisable for all women to prevent spontaneous abortion as well as encouraging maternal well-being. Studies evaluating use of progesterone support early in pregnancy to reduce the incidence of spontaneous abortion have not shown statistical significance.

Surgery may benefit some women with uterine abnormalities. If uterine synechiae are diagnosed, hysteroscopic lysis of adhesions is recommended. Women with müllerian anomalies who experience spontaneous abortions at 13 weeks' gestation or later may be candidates for reconstructive operations, described elsewhere in this text. Removal of uterine fibroids, if performed only because of infertility, may help little; the effect of myomectomy on spontaneous abortion rates is unknown.

Evaluation and Management

A majority of the time, viability concerns in early pregnancy are preceded by vaginal bleeding. Bleeding in early pregnancy is commonly reported, and ensuring appropriate evaluation and management is essential for women's health. In addition to the history and physical exam, ultrasonography and serial measurement of β-hCG are important diagnostic tools to differentiate a threatened, incomplete, and completed abortion. These are also important in the diagnosis of ectopic pregnancy, as an intrauterine pregnancy identified on ultrasound virtually excludes the diagnosis of ectopic pregnancy.

Increasing use of vaginal ultrasound has improved diagnostic validity, especially at early gestational ages. When an embryo is visible, management is straightforward. Regrettably, most abnormal pregnancies stop developing before an embryo is visible by sonography. Two sonographic criteria have high specificity: a gestation sac at least 13 to 25 mm mean diameter without an embryo and distorted sac shape. On the other hand, the sensitivity of these criteria appears to be low.

Presence of fetal heart activity is more accurate in predicting spontaneous abortion than are morphologic criteria. If an embryo has a crown–rump length of more than 5 mm on transvaginal sonography (or more than 10 mm on transabdominal sonography) but no cardiac activity, the pregnancy is not viable. Several reports concur that once fetal cardiac activity is documented by ultrasonography in the first 12 weeks of pregnancy, the likelihood of spontaneous abortion is low: about 2% to 4.5%. This does not hold true, however, for women older than age 35 or those with a history of recurrent pregnancy loss. Furthermore, the mere presence or absence of fetal cardiac activity may not suffice. Recent studies have evaluated fetal heart rate and its prognosis for early gestations, noting that fetal heart rates less than 100 beats per minute in the embryonic stage is associated with a significantly lower survival rate than those with normal fetal heart rates.

Given the lack of medical need for intervention in early pregnancy failure, physicians need not act on a single abnormal clinical finding, such as a falling β-hCG level or failure to observe fetal cardiac activity. Repeating the ultrasound improves the diagnostic accuracy of this procedure.

The traditional approach to threatened abortion, characterized by uterine bleeding without cervical dilation or expulsion of tissue and demonstration of a potentially viable fetus, has been watchful waiting. Reliably predicting fetal outcomes in such situations is not yet possible, and serial examinations may be necessary to determine viability of a pregnancy that is not actively being passed.

Distinguishing between incomplete (characterized by progressive cervical dilation without complete expulsion of products of conception) and complete abortion is frequently difficult. The woman's description of tissue may not be helpful, and not all women are aware that they should save expelled tissue for the physician's inspection. Likewise, dilation of the cervix, size of the uterus, and presence or absence of bleeding may not indicate whether the abortion is complete or incomplete. Ultrasonography, however, often provides information about the completeness of abortion.

Medical or Surgical Intervention

For women with incomplete abortion and for those with threatened abortion in whom the pregnancy has been judged nonviable, several options are available. Patient preferences should generally determine the management as long as there is hemodynamic stability and absence of infection. One option is to await spontaneous expulsion of the pregnancy. A randomized, controlled trial by Nielsen and Hahlin compared expectant versus surgical management of spontaneous abortion. Most women randomized to expectant management (79%) had completed abortions within 3 days; other outcomes were similar, except for more infections in the group having curettage. An observational study by Luise et al. in 2002 followed nearly 1,100 women with spontaneous abortions expectantly for 4 weeks and found spontaneous resolution in 81%. However, they noted a significantly longer time, approximately 2 weeks, between diagnosis and passage of the pregnancy. They also categorized patients by sonographic criteria, finding that 91% of incomplete abortions resolved spontaneously compared with 66% of anembryonic pregnancies. If choosing expectant management, a woman deserves counseling that several days or weeks may pass before resolution and that medical or surgical intervention may ultimately be necessary. Additionally, women with a diagnosis of anembryonic pregnancy may be counseled that their success rates may be lower with expectant management.

Another option is to expedite the expulsion and still avoid surgery by giving oral or vaginal misoprostol. A randomized controlled trial by Chung et al. found that this medical management was safer than surgical evacuation, although half of those receiving misoprostol subsequently required suction curettage. Several studies have been performed looking at various doses and routes of administration of misoprostol. When misoprostol (600–800 μg) is given vaginally, success rates of 70% to 90% are reported. A recent randomized, controlled multicenter study by Zhang and colleagues comparing medical management with surgical evacuation found an 84% completion rate by day 8 when 800 μg of misoprostol was given vaginally and repeated at 48 hours if passage had not yet occurred. This study reported similar complication rates between the two groups. They also found that 83% of the woman would recommend the medical treatment to others.

However, many women faced with the disappointing diagnosis of a failed pregnancy prefer prompt surgical evacuation. If suction curettage is elected, two other decisions must be made: where the curettage is to occur and by what technique. The choice between outpatient curettage in the physician's office and curettage in an emergency room may depend on the time of day and equipment available. For uncomplicated cases, curettage in an operating room adds to the costs and inconvenience yet offers no medical benefits over outpatient curettage. The choice of evacuation technique depends on the state of the cervix, gestational age, and availability of equipment. Suction curettage is a fast and safe procedure in the first trimester. Practitioners may choose between an electric suction device attached to a rigid or flexible curette or a flexible Karman cannula with syringe as a source of suction. The Karman cannula is portable, inexpensive, and convenient for outpatient use. Both methods are discussed in further detail later in this chapter.

According to a recent metaanalysis, there is insufficient evidence to prescribe one of the above management plans in any given clinical situation. Surgical management is more likely to result in completion than medical management, and medical management is more likely to result in completion than expectant management, but the inverse is true of costs incurred. Patient satisfaction can be seen with any of these management plans. Certainly in the face of severe anemia, hemodynamic instability, or infection, surgical evacuation should be performed. Without these, patient preference should be strongly considered.

Complications and Considerations

Attentive gynecologic care has reduced the risk of complications. Nevertheless, women continue to die from spontaneous abortions. The Centers for Disease Control and Prevention identified 62 maternal deaths from spontaneous abortion in the United States between 1981 and 1991. This represented a case-fatality rate of 0.7 deaths per 100,000 spontaneous abortions. In 2002, there were two maternal deaths that were due to spontaneous abortion. Infection, hemorrhage, and embolism were the leading causes of death. The mortality risk increased with gestational age; women who were older and of minority races also were at increased risk of death.

Spontaneous abortion is a potentially sensitizing event for Rh-negative women. Rates of use of Rh immunoglobulin (RhIG) after spontaneous abortion are significantly lower than after induced abortion. RhIG candidates at 12 weeks' gestation or earlier should receive a 50-μg dose; later abortions mandate a 300-μg dose.

The profound grief that frequently accompanies spontaneous abortion often receives insufficient attention. Women and men experience the stages of grief. Guilt may be a difficult stage to resolve without help, and counseling plays an important role.

FETAL DEATH

Definitions

Physicians often categorize fetal death by gestational age and length of retention of the dead fetus. Death before the 20th week of gestation, or at less than 500 g, is *spontaneous abortion;* thereafter, it is an *antepartum fetal death.* If a dead fetus remains in the uterus for 8 or more weeks, then the term becomes *missed abortion.* However, many use this term to refer to any failed pregnancy that is not promptly expelled. These diagnostic categories all should be viewed as variations of a single obstetric entity: a nonviable or failed pregnancy.

Incidence

Fetal death is uncommon after the first trimester. The 2003 data from the U.S. National Center for Health Statistics shows a fetal death rate of 6.23 per 1,000 live births. The incidence of fetal demise decreases with increasing gestational age. In 2003, greater than 50% of fetal deaths occurred between 20–27 weeks, with over one-third occurring between 20–23 weeks.

Management

Data on the natural history of fetal death are scarce. The uterus expels most dead fetuses within 3 weeks of death. The gestational age, however, influences the probability of expulsion within a given interval: The more remote from term, the longer is the time required.

After confirmation of fetal death, the next, and perhaps most important, step is to counsel the parents. Helping the couple to grieve appropriately can minimize psychological sequelae from this often devastating loss. After these initial steps, subsequent clinical management is largely discretionary. The risk of coagulation defects within 5 weeks of fetal death is minimal, as is the risk of infection, provided the membranes are intact. The emotional burden of carrying a dead fetus, however, often for weeks, can compound the misery experienced by the parents. Thus, although either watchful waiting or uterine evacuation is appropriate, most women opt for intervention.

Two approaches to evacuation exist: surgery or labor induction. The choice between surgery and labor induction should reflect the skill and experience of the physician, the size of the fetus and uterus, the availability of equipment and drugs, and the preference of the woman. Before uterine evacuation by surgery or induction, the physician should confirm that the woman's coagulation system is intact.

Suction curettage is a safe and easy way to evacuate early pregnancies; however, if the pregnancy is more advanced, dilation and evacuation may be necessary. Before dilation and evacuation (D&E), accurate determination of fetal size by ultrasonography is helpful. Both procedures will be detailed later in this chapter. If the patient declines surgical evacuation or if the physician chooses not to perform a D&E procedure, then labor induction can be accomplished in several ways. These include use of misoprostol, vaginal prostaglandin E_2 suppositories, high-dose oxytocin, or intrauterine balloon catheters. Intraamniotic hypertonic abortifacients are inappropriate in the setting of fetal death. Instillation of hypertonic saline may be hazardous because of rapid uptake into the woman's circulation owing to altered membrane permeability.

Complications

Fetal death carries risks of both morbidity and mortality for the woman. The risks of coagulation disorders and infection have received the most attention, yet recent data on their incidence are lacking. The risk of maternal death associated with fetal death is small, although no recent data are available. In the 1970s, the maternal case-fatality rate was estimated to be 4.5 deaths per 100,000 fetal deaths. The risk of maternal death from fetal death increases with maternal age. The risk for women age 35 years and older was 3.6 times that for women aged 15 to 24 years. The most frequent causes of maternal death from fetal death were uterine perforation and coagulopathy. As with all pregnancy terminations, physicians must identify all Rh-negative candidates and give them an appropriate dose of RhIG.

CERVICAL INCOMPETENCE

Incidence

Cervical incompetence is an imprecise term used to explain spontaneous abortions thought to be secondary to cervical factors. Premature cervical dilation without labor is a more descriptive term. Furthermore, it avoids the language "incompetent" which may carry with it some negative inferences for a woman who is having problematic pregnancies.

There is wide disagreement about the case definition and diagnostic criteria, making estimation of incidence difficult. The classic picture: repetitive, painless abortion midpregnancy without associated uterine contractions. Some physicians base their diagnosis on this picture, whereas others rely on tests performed on nonpregnant women. These include passage of an 8-mm Hegar dilator, traction on an intrauterine Foley catheter, or hysterography. These techniques appear to have poor validity.

Significant attention has been paid in recent years to sonographic evaluation of the cervix and its role in prediction of premature cervical dilation. Serial ultrasound examination of the cervix may accurately identify a shortened cervix or funneling of amniotic membranes. It appears that identification of this entity is plagued by low sensitivity and positive predictive values, particularly in low-risk women. However, there may be a role for this evaluation in high-risk women.

The history of unexplained spontaneous abortion without labor in midpregnancy may be the most useful diagnostic criterion, yet its sensitivity and specificity remain unknown. This diagnostic imprecision appears in reported incidence rates. Rates range from 0.05 to 1 per 100 pregnancies. Differences in diagnosis, rather than differences in women, probably account for most of this variation. In 2000, according to the National Center for Health Statistics, 23,000 discharge summaries cited the diagnosis of cervical incompetence.

Risk Factors

The cause of premature cervical dilation without labor is unknown but may be multifactorial. Early theories about this problem focused on cervical trauma, such as conization, laceration, or excessive mechanical dilation. Data are lacking, however, to confirm or refute these. The occurrence of this condition in primigravidas suggests alternative causes. These may include associated uterine anomalies, prenatal exposure to diethylstilbestrol, or abnormal histology of the cervix. In addition, premature cervical dilation without labor may be inheritable.

Management

A variety of approaches have been used to treat premature cervical dilation without labor. The least invasive, bed rest, has been suggested as primary therapy, as well as adjunctive therapy after cerclage. This may be a reasonable approach in terms of hydraulics, although data concerning efficacy are lacking.

A Smith-Hodge pessary can displace the cervix in a posterior direction. Although this approach has received little attention in the United States, it has the appeal of exerting a mechanical effect without requiring an operation.

Surgery is the principal form of therapy for premature cervical dilation without labor in the United States. Several types of cerclage procedures are used; the McDonald and Shirodkar are the most common. Contraindications to cerclage include rupture of membranes, uterine bleeding, uterine contractions, chorioamnionitis, cervical dilation of more than 4 cm, polyhydramnios, or known fetal anomaly.

The Shirodkar operation places a reinforcing band around the cervix beneath the mucosa at the level of the internal os (Figs. 33.1 and 33.2). Spinal or epidural anesthesia is recommended; Trendelenburg positioning and adequate retraction facilitate placement of the suture. The original operation used aneurysm needles to place a band of fascia lata around the cervix; then the knot was tied anteriorly. In recent years, many physicians have used a wide (e.g., 5-mm) Mersilene band swaged onto large atraumatic needles, with the knot tied posteriorly to avoid erosion into the bladder. The cervical canal should remain open 3 to 5 mm. After the band is tied, the band and knot can be secured with several interrupted sutures of silk or other permanent material; the incisions in the mucosa are then closed with absorbable suture, thus burying the band.

The McDonald procedure places a reinforcing purse-string suture around the proximal cervix. Unlike the Shirodkar procedure, however, the McDonald suture is not buried entirely (Fig. 33.3). Instead, several deep penetrations into the cervical stroma are made with a nonabsorbable suture, such as Mersilene. The advantages of this approach compared with the Shirodkar procedure are simplicity, ease of removal, and usefulness when the cervix is effaced or when fetal membranes are bulging. Vaginal discharge may be associated with the exposed suture material. Because the McDonald and Shirodkar procedures have been reported to have similar efficacy, the simplicity and versatility of the McDonald operation make it preferable for most patients in need of cerclage.

Opinions are divided as to whether the cerclage procedure is best performed during or between pregnancies. Studies suggest that the timing of cerclage during pregnancy influences outcome. Cerclage at about 14 weeks' gestation appears preferable. Ideally, fetal viability must be demonstrated and major fetal anomalies ruled out sonographically if possible. If substantial dilation or bulging of fetal membranes has occurred, then the likelihood of a successful cerclage is lessened. An attempt can be made, however, to replace the protruding membranes by means of a sterile Foley catheter. Thereafter, the suture is placed and tied down, and the Foley balloon is deflated and withdrawn.

Postoperative care after cerclage for pregnant women has not been uniform. Although most investigators advise bed rest for several days, and some advocate prophylactic antibiotics, tocolytic drugs, or progesterone, the usefulness of these measures has not been established. The cerclage suture can be removed at 38 weeks' gestation or when fetal pulmonary maturity has been confirmed; it should be removed immediately if membranes rupture or labor starts. Although some physicians leave a well-placed Shirodkar suture in place and deliver infants by cesarean, evidence supporting this course of action is limited.

Intraabdominal cerclage may be appropriate in rare instances. Indications include traumatic cervical laceration, congenital shortening of the cervix, previous failed vaginal

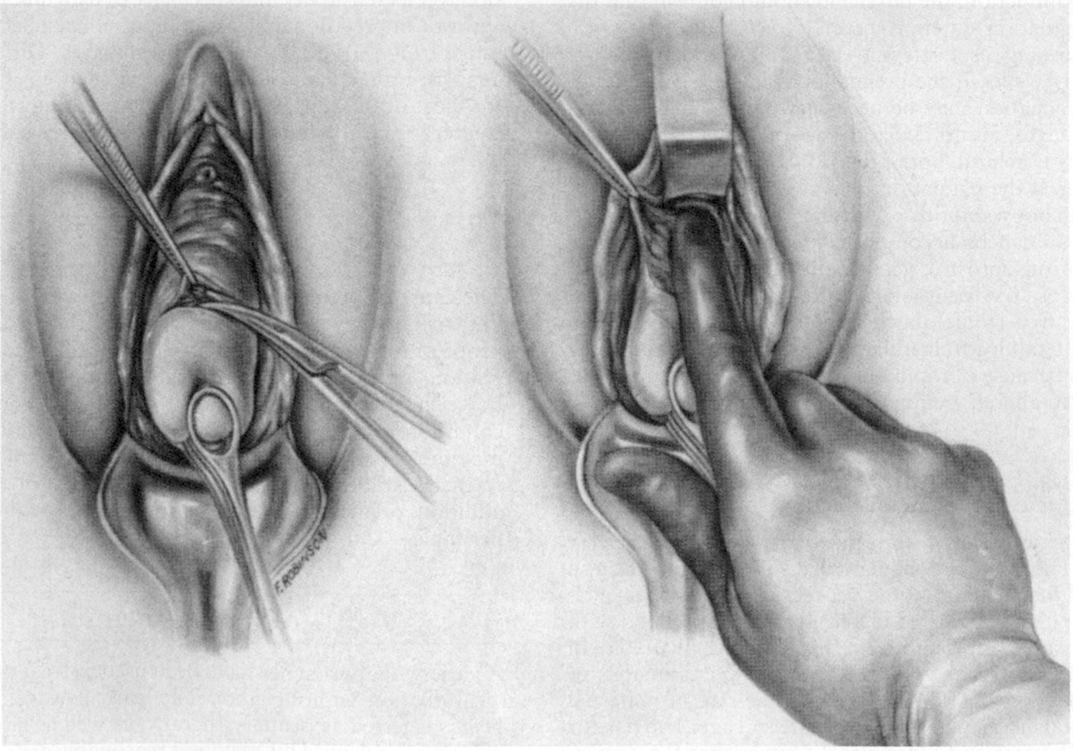

FIGURE 33.1. Shirodkar cerclage operation. **Left:** A transverse incision through the anterior vaginal mucosa at its junction with the cervix. **Right:** The surgeon pushes the bladder cephalad to enable high placement of the suture.

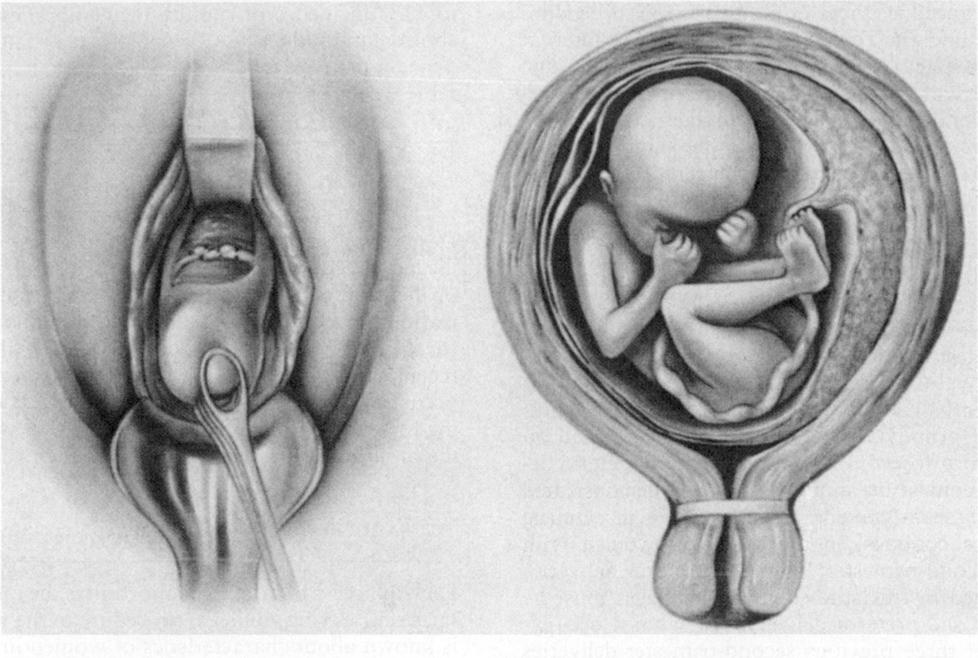

FIGURE 33.2. Shirodkar cerclage operation. **Left:** The encircling suture leaves the cervix with an opening of 3 to 5 mm. The surgeon anchors the suture anteriorly with fine silk. **Right:** Cross section with suture in place.

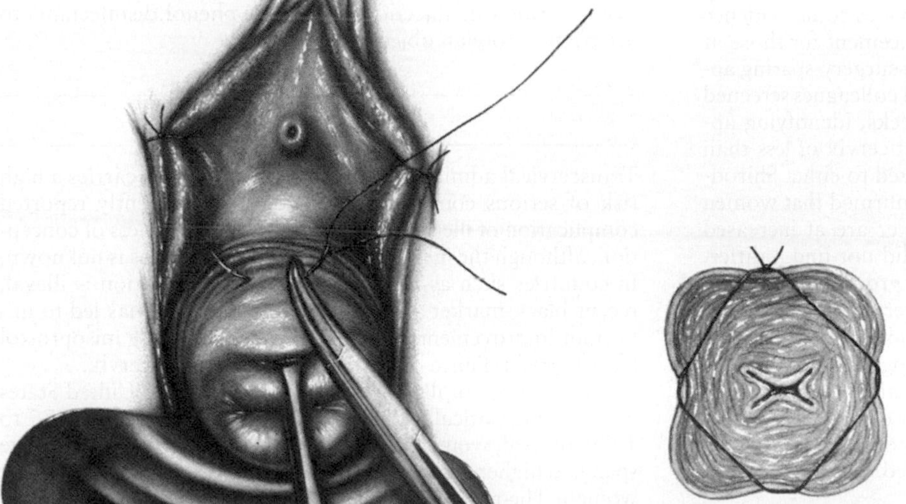

FIGURE 33.3. McDonald cerclage operation. **A:** Four bites taken at the junction of vaginal mucosa and cervix. **B:** A cross section of the cervix with the cerclage in place.

cerclage, and advanced cervical effacement. This procedure places a band around the cervix at the level of the internal os in an avascular space between the branches of the uterine artery. Compared with the vaginal cerclage operations, this procedure has several important disadvantages: two abdominal operations are needed (one to place the suture, one for cesarean delivery), the surgery is performed in a highly vascular area adjacent to the ureters, and the complication rate is higher than with vaginal cerclage. Hence, this approach should be used only when vaginal cerclage has failed or is not feasible.

Consistent with the diagnostic conundrum associated with premature cervical dilation, there remains a challenge in appropriate and effective management recommendations for these patients. The largest randomized trial by the Medical Research Council/Royal College of Obstetricians and Gynaecologists included nearly 1,300 patients. The goal was to evaluate the efficacy of prophylactic cerclage placement based on historical risk factors of second-trimester abortion/preterm delivery or cervical conization/amputation. They demonstrated a significant decrease in preterm delivery (15% in cerclage group vs. 32% in controls) in the subset of women with three previous second-trimester losses or preterm deliveries only. It is estimated in this study that 25 cerclages must be placed to prevent one preterm delivery. For women occupying the stratum of three previous second-trimester deliveries without evidence of labor, a cerclage can be supported by the literature.

The CIPRACT (Cervical Incompetence Prevention Randomized Cerclage Trial) randomly assigned women with a previous preterm delivery to cerclage or bed rest. Secondary randomization occurred as both groups were followed with serial transvaginal ultrasonography. Those in the control group were further randomized if they were noted to develop cervical shortening less than 25 mm at fewer than 27 weeks. This study was small in its subject numbers but identified significantly decreased preterm deliveries and neonatal morbidity in the cerclage group. Additionally, it provides some evidence for serial sonography and late cerclage placement for those at high risk with cervical change, a potentially surgery-sparing approach. In contrast, a large study by To and colleagues screened more than 47,000 women at 22 to 24 weeks, identifying approximately 1% of these with a very short cervix of less than 15 mm. These women were then randomized to either Shirodkar cerclage or observation. This study confirmed that women with shortened cervices in the midtrimester are at increased risk for preterm delivery; however, they did not find a difference between the cerclage or observation group with regards to gestational age at delivery. Several other studies including systematic reviews and metaanalyses do not support cerclage placement based on ultrasonographic findings alone, especially in low-risk women. There is evidence in small studies that support placement of emergency cerclage after clinical cervical dilation can be detected if infection and labor have been ruled out. Larger well-designed studies are needed.

Complications

Complications of cerclage range significantly in their severity. A partial inventory of reported complications includes hemorrhage; rupture of membranes; infection, including chorioamnionitis, abscess, and death; cervical dystocia; uterine rupture; vesicovaginal fistula; and fetal death. Most commonly, rupture of membranes is seen in 0.8% to 18% and chorioamnionitis is seen in 1% to 6.2% of electively placed cerclages. Complications increase when the cerclage is placed emergently, with 0% to 51% incidence of rupture of membranes and 9% to 37% chorioamnionitis.

ILLEGAL ABORTION

Incidence

Despite the availability of legal abortions, small numbers of illegal procedures continue to occur. Estimates of the incidence of illegal abortion in the United States before 1970 or legalization ranged from 200,000 to 1.2 million per year; estimates for the late 1970s ranged from 5,000 to 23,000 per year. More recent estimates are not available. However, illegal abortions occur in large numbers in developing countries, where, according to WHO estimates, 50,000 to 100,000 women continue to die of illegal abortion complications each year.

Risk Factors

Lack of access to safe, legal abortion is the most important risk factor for having an illegal procedure in the world today. Little is known about characteristics of women in the United States who may still obtain illegal abortions.

Techniques

Although a wide variety of illegal abortion methods are used around the world, two methods dominate in the United States: oral abortifacients and intrauterine instrumentation. Orally administered substances include turpentine, laundry bleach, and large doses of quinine: all unsafe. Intrauterine techniques were less common, more effective, and more dangerous; these ranged from intrauterine injection of soap or phenol disinfectants to insertion of foreign objects.

Complications

Transcervical administration of toxic substances carries a high risk of serious complications. The most frequently reported complication of illegal abortion is retained products of conception, although the incidence of such complications is unknown. In countries such as Brazil, where elective abortion is illegal, recent black-market availability of misoprostol has led to important improvements in abortion safety, because misoprostol has reduced reliance on instrumentation of the cervix.

The number of illegal abortion deaths in the United States declined dramatically during the 1970s. During the 1975 to 1979 interval, women in both extremes of the reproductive age span had higher death rates from illegal abortion than did other women. The racial discrepancy in death rate is more striking: The mortality rate for black and Hispanic women is more than 10 times greater than for white women.

As with morbidity, the likelihood of mortality is strongly related to the abortion technique. Of the 17 illegal abortion deaths from 1975 to 1979, only one followed ingestion of an abortifacient (pennyroyal oil). The other deaths were related to intrauterine techniques, ranging from injection of cleaning solutions to insertion of foreign bodies (e.g., catheters, cotton swabs, thermometers, and coat hangers). Sepsis (10 cases) and air embolism (three cases) accounted for most of these deaths.

Management of Septic Abortion

Most women with septic abortion respond rapidly to uterine evacuation plus broad-spectrum antibiotics. Before beginning treatment, intrauterine and blood cultures should be obtained. An upright radiograph of the abdomen may identify a residual foreign body, gas bubbles in the uterus, or free air under the diaphragm; these findings direct management.

Antibiotic administration should begin in the emergency department. Coverage should include Gram-positive, Gram-negative, and anaerobic bacteria. Ideally, in a case of septic abortion, the patient should go directly from the emergency department to the operating room. Peak serum levels of antibiotics will be present within an hour of their administration. Further delay of uterine evacuation is unwarranted and can compromise recovery. Prompt elimination of the necrotic infected tissue is critical. Tissue obtained during curettage should quickly go for microbiologic cultures. The yield of organisms, especially anaerobes, is often higher from a tissue specimen than from a swab inserted into the uterus.

Subsequent management is governed by the response of the woman and by microbiologic findings. All women with septic abortions should be closely observed after surgery, with special attention to vital signs and urine output, to detect incipient shock. Prompt aggressive therapy is essential if septic shock develops. Administration of glucocorticoids is not helpful in this setting.

Postabortal sepsis from *Clostridium perfringens* has become rare. When this infection occurs, however, it can be catastrophic. In the absence of hemolysis, *C. perfringens* bacteremia can be managed by curettage and antibiotics. In the presence of hemolysis, hysterectomy and more aggressive medical therapy are indicated.

LEGAL ABORTION

Incidence

Legal abortion is one of the most frequently performed operations in the United States. In 2000, 1.31 million induced abortions were reported. The national abortion ratio was 245 abortions per 1,000 live births in that year. The abortion rate was 21.3 abortions per 1,000 women age 15 to 44 years. Stated alternatively, about one in four recognized pregnancies ends in induced abortion, and each year, 2% of all women of reproductive age in the United States have an abortion. The numbers of induced abortions have been declining from 1990 to 2002, the most recent year for which data are available.

Demographic Characteristics

The majority of women having induced abortions in the United States tend to be young, white, single, low income, and of low parity. Low-income and black women have higher *rates* of abortion, associated with lack of access to services. Most (59%) abortions took place at 8 weeks' gestation or earlier; 88% occurred at 12 weeks' gestation or earlier. Only 4.3% of procedures were done between 16 and 20 weeks gestation and 1.4% at more than 21 weeks. Before 1990, provision of very early (<6 weeks gestational age) abortions was rare. In 1999, these procedures accounted for 22% of all abortions. Most abortions take place safely in freestanding clinics (93%) and physician's offices (2%). In-hospital procedures (5%) are necessary when women have a higher risk of medical or surgical complications.

Preoperative Considerations

In a recent large study, the reasons most often cited by women for choosing abortion were that having a baby would interfere with her education, work, or ability to care for her other dependents. A majority (73%) could not afford a baby, and almost half were having relationship problems and did not want to be single mothers. Preoperative counseling should include a nonjudgmental discussion of all alternatives available, including continuing the pregnancy and adoption. Abortion procedures are reviewed and compared, including the risks, benefits, and expected experience with each method.

Legal Considerations

It is important for physicians to know the legal restrictions to abortion in their state. State regulations include waiting periods, counseling requirements, parental involvement for minors, and insurance regulations.

Preoperative Medical Evaluation

The preoperative evaluation should include counseling, informed consent, a brief history, and a limited physical examination. The history taking should focus only on relevant data, such as gynecologic problems (e.g., leiomyomas) or medical problems (e.g., cardiac disease, asthma, or drug sensitivities) that might influence the course of the operation. Physical examination should include the heart, lungs, abdomen, and pelvis. Although ultrasonography is not necessary on a routine basis, it is useful if the size, shape, or position of the uterus is unclear. A large survey of abortion providers in the United States reported that 66% of clinics do use ultrasound routinely before first-trimester surgical abortion. In contrast, ultrasound is a routine component of early medical abortions, which requires accurate dating of the gestation. Routine laboratory tests include the hematocrit (or hemoglobin) and Rh type. Many physicians perform a urine pregnancy test on all patients requesting abortion. Screening for chlamydial and gonorrhea need not be routine, but should be targeted. If bacterial vaginosis is detected preoperatively, it should be treated.

Techniques

All methods of abortion fall into two broad categories: surgical and medical. Surgical evacuation includes suction curettage (vacuum aspiration by electric or manual vacuum source), sharp curettage, D&E (defined as transcervical evacuation at 13 menstrual weeks' gestation or later), hysterotomy, and hysterectomy. Medical abortifacients in the United States include uterotonic drugs, such as prostaglandins and oxytocin, the antiprogestin mifepristone, and intrauterine instillation of hypertonic agents, such as saline or urea. Early medical abortion has also begun to play a significant role in provision of abortion, accounting for 6% of procedures in early 2001. In addition, several adjuncts, such as cervical preparation with misoprostol or osmotic dilators, have an important role in abortion practice.

Suction Curettage

Sharp curettage is an obsolete abortion method, supplanted by suction curettage, which usually involves dilation of the cervix, followed by vacuum aspiration at 12 weeks' gestation or earlier. *Menstrual regulation, menstrual extraction,* and *minisuction* are euphemisms for early suction curettage. The more recent term, encompassing this early "regulation" as well as later procedures done by manual vacuum with syringe, is *manual vacuum aspiration* (MVA). This technique uses a plastic cannula as small as 3 mm in diameter, with a self-locking syringe (50–60 cc) as a source of suction (Fig. 33.4). The largest series using MVA in early pregnancy reported a 99% success rate on nearly 2,400 abortions done at less than 6 weeks' gestation. MVA has been shown to be as safe and effective as electric vacuum through 10 weeks' of gestation. For early MVA procedures, dilation is often unnecessary. Consequently, anesthesia may not be necessary, although analgesia can ease the cramping that occurs toward the end of the evacuation. After insertion of the appropriate cannula, the physician attaches the syringe and releases the pinch valve to begin the suctioning. Blood and tissue flow into the syringe. Alternatively, some physicians connect the cannula to the syringe before insertion. The abortion involves rotary and in-and-out cannula movement until the gritty feel of the endometrium occurs. Bubbles appear in the syringe. The physician should not remove the cannula from the uterus while a vacuum exists in the syringe, because the endocervical canal should not be aspirated; likewise, the physician should not advance the plunger of the syringe while the cannula is connected and is within the uterus. Air embolism can result. The syringe and cannula are disposable, although some physicians clean and disinfect the syringe and use it multiple times.

If local anesthesia is to be used alone, no preoperative fasting is necessary, but if conscious sedation is a possibility, the patient should fast for at least 6 hours before the procedure.

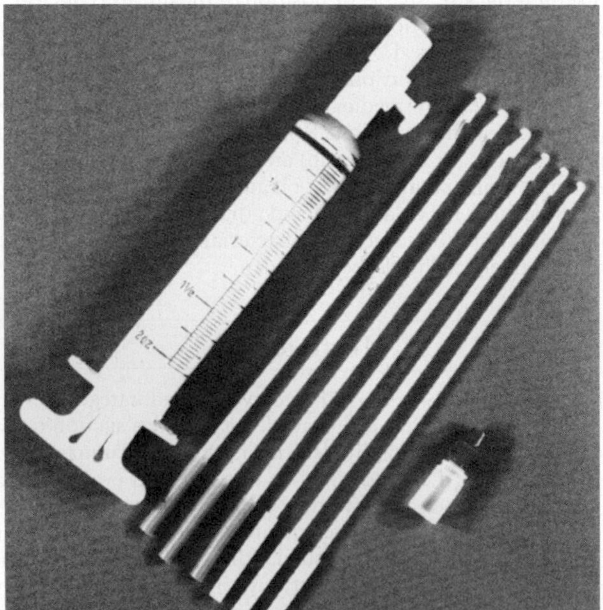

FIGURE 33.4. Karman cannulas, self-locking syringe with pinch valve, and bottle of silicone lubricant. (From: IPAS, Chapel Hill, NC, with permission.)

Similarly, if conscious sedation is used, the patient should be instructed to bring someone with her to escort her home. She should empty her bladder before being placed in the dorsal lithotomy position; catheterization is unnecessary. An antiseptic is applied to the cervix and vagina (e.g., povidone-iodine or chlorhexidine). Routine sterile precautions (e.g., drapes, caps, masks, and gowns) are unnecessary. The physician should use a "no-touch" technique: He or she wears sterile gloves and does not touch those ends and portions of the sterile instruments inserted into the uterus. Use of local anesthesia predominates in the United States. Although local anesthesia does not completely relieve discomfort, it is less expensive and safer than general anesthesia. It is a good general rule, when performing abortions under local anesthesia, to use slow, controlled movements. A support person who can talk to the patient also helps alleviate anxiety and discomfort.

Preoperative Cervical Dilation

Osmotic dilators help to prepare the cervix for curettage abortions (Fig. 33.5). Laminaria are hygroscopic sticks of seaweed that dilate the cervix over several hours. The mode of action is not well understood, but the principal mechanism appears to be desiccation of the cervix. This drying can alter the ratio of collagen to ground substance, thus changing collagen cross-linkages. Alternatively, laminaria can alter the elaboration, release, or degradation of uterine prostaglandins. Laminaria cause the cervix to dilate the areas not in physical contact with the laminaria; whatever the mechanism, it is more complex than mere passive stretching, as used to be thought.

One synthetic osmotic dilator is currently marketed in the United States. Lamicel is a cylinder of polyvinyl alcohol sponge impregnated with magnesium sulfate. It works within several hours and has the advantage of uniform size (either 5- or 3-mm diameter), assured sterility, and easy insertion and removal. Unlike laminaria, the Lamicel device does not assume a rigid hourglass shape that hinders removal.

Osmotic dilators are convenient in an outpatient setting. Placement of laminaria or Lamicel for 3 to 4 hours before abortion frequently dilates the cervix sufficiently for abortion. Women can be sent home with laminaria in place overnight, allowing for maximal dilation. Compared with use of metal dilators, use of laminaria dramatically reduces the risk of cervical

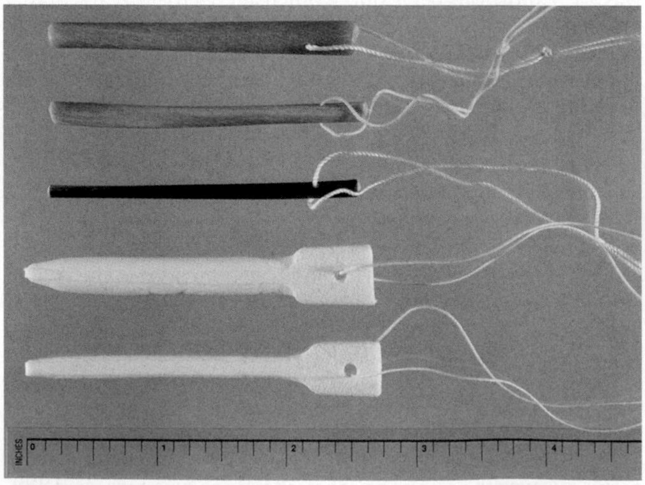

FIGURE 33.5. Osmotic dilators. **Top:** Laminaria of various sizes. **Bottom:** Lamicel in 5- and 3-mm sizes.

injury, requiring suturing and of uterine perforation. This protection against trauma can be especially important for young teenagers with immature cervices who are at increased risk for cervical injury. Disadvantages include the cost, inconvenience, and occasional cramping involved.

Alternatively, preoperative preparation of the cervix with misoprostol can facilitate abortion. Misoprostol, a prostaglandin E derivative, is safe, inexpensive, stable at room temperature, and effective in improving the Bishop score of the cervix. The drug can be given either orally, vaginally, buccally, or sublingually. In general, misoprostol is more effective and better tolerated when given by the vaginal route versus the oral route; this probably relates to different pharmacokinetics when absorbed through the vagina versus through the gut. On the other hand, women often prefer oral to vaginal administration. When placed in the vagina by the physician at the end of the pelvic examination, most patients find this acceptable. A randomized controlled trial by Singh and colleagues suggest that misoprostol 400 μg per vagina 3 to 4 hours before the operation may be the optimal dose. Afterward, the cervix is often dilated sufficiently to operate without further dilation. Ninety-seven percent of women had at least 8 mm cervical dilation. Administration 1 hour before was recently found not to be effective. Disadvantages of cervical preparation with misoprostol include the delay required, spotting and cramping, and occasional abortion in the waiting room. Recent data show an inferior effect of same-day misoprostol for preoperative cervical priming in second-trimester procedures as compared with laminaria administered the day before the procedure.

Paracervical Anesthesia

To perform a paracervical block, the physician should use the smallest volume of the lowest concentration of local anesthetic. Local anesthetics vary in their toxicity; for example, chloroprocaine is substantially less toxic than lidocaine. With lidocaine, a 0.5% concentration is safer than a 1% solution and is equally effective. The total dose of lidocaine should not exceed 2 mg/lb or 300 mg, whichever is less. Maximum is approximately 20 cc of 1% lidocaine or 0.25% bupivacaine for a 50-kg woman, with 10 cc being typically sufficient. Alternatively, use of local anesthesia with vasoconstrictor (e.g., epinephrine 1:200,000) slows systemic absorption of anesthetic and allows a larger total dose, although the epinephrine has additional risks and side effects. Some physicians buffer the lidocaine solution with sodium bicarbonate to decrease burning. Vasovagal episodes occur rarely and can be treated with atropine.

Paracervical anesthesia affords excellent anesthesia regardless of the site of injection. Approaches include infiltration of the cervix at the 12-o'clock position (for application of the tenaculum), then injection at four sites (at the 3-, 5-, 7-, and 9-o'clock positions) or two sites (at the 3- and 9-o'clock positions) at the junction of cervix and vagina. Submucosal injection precludes inadvertent intravascular injection. Slow injection is less painful than rapid injection.

Suction curettage requires few instruments. It is useful to have an ultrasound machine available in case one is not able to enter the uterus or suction adequate tissue. Most physicians prefer to use a bivalve speculum. A speculum with standard-length blades, however, prevents the cervix from being drawn toward the introitus during the procedure and makes the operation more difficult. The commercially available Moore modification of the Graves speculum, which has 1-inch shorter blades of standard width, is excellent. Some physicians prefer an atraumatic tenaculum. Alternatively, having an extra single-toothed tenaculum can sometimes be helpful. If difficulty during dilation occurs, the physician can place the second tenaculum on the posterior cervix to stabilize it. Sounding before the procedure should not be done; there is no need to know where the fundus is at the start of the procedure, and it increases the risk of perforation. If the direction of the cervical canal is in question, then the physician can gently probe with a small dilator. Pratt dilators are preferable to Hegar dilators for abortion because they require less force to dilate the cervix. A useful modification of the Pratt dilators is the Denniston dilator; this is similar to the Pratt dilator but is plastic. Hence, it is light, slightly flexible, and inexpensive, yet it is capable of being autoclaved. Other instruments required for suction curettage include the vacuum machine, hose, swivel handle, and a cannula. Some physicians use a sharp curette to check for completeness at the end of the operation. Use of small (e.g., 8-mm-diameter) Karman-type double-port cannulas provides the same gritty sensation as a metal curette.

Traction on the cervix is important during suction curettage; it both stabilizes the uterus and straightens the angle between cervix and corpus, which should reduce the risk of perforation. The tenaculum should have a firm purchase on the cervix. High vertical placement at the 12-o'clock position, with one tooth in the canal and one on the anterior cervix, almost eliminates the risk of the tenaculum tearing through during dilation. In contrast, a superficial horizontal application of the tenaculum is more likely to allow the tenaculum to pull off. If the uterus is retroverted, some physicians prefer to place the tenaculum on the cervix at the 6-o'clock position (Fig. 33.6). If the puncture site on the cervix bleeds after tenaculum removal, direct pressure stops the bleeding and is preferable to silver nitrate or Monsel solution. While use of the tenaculum straightens the angle of the uterus, the operator must remain cognizant of the anatomy. For an anteverted uterus, instruments used for the

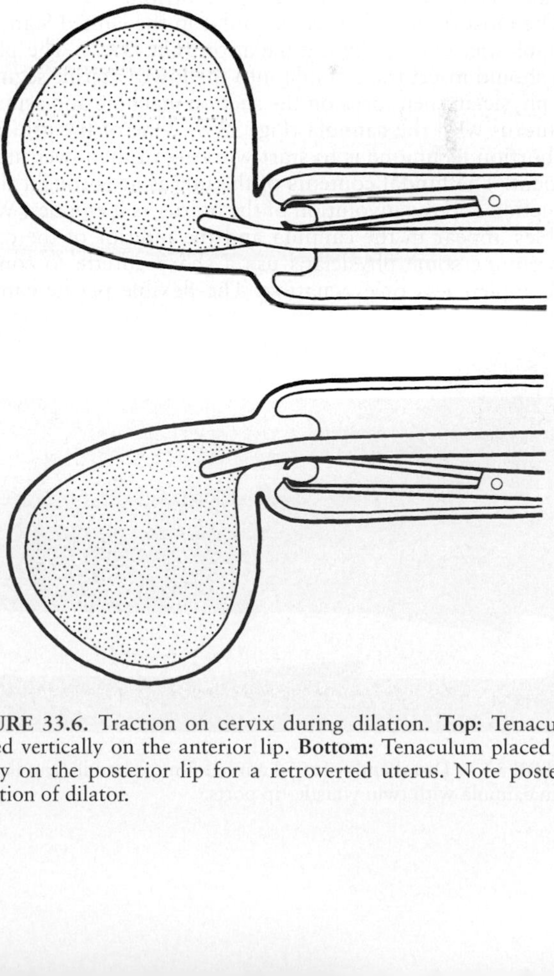

FIGURE 33.6. Traction on cervix during dilation. **Top:** Tenaculum placed vertically on the anterior lip. **Bottom:** Tenaculum placed vertically on the posterior lip for a retroverted uterus. Note posterior direction of dilator.

procedure often need to be at an angle, with the intrauterine tip of the instrument pointing upward. If the instrument was inserted straight back in a patient like this, there would be an increased risk for posterior perforation.

Gentleness is the key to safe cervical dilation. Dilation should allow insertion and rotation of the desired cannula. Pratt dilators are measured in French units, or mm of circumference. Hence, to determine the diameter, the physician needs to divide by pi, or approximately 3. For example, to insert an 8-mm cannula, dilation with Pratt dilators to 25F allows free rotation. The physician should hold the dilator between the thumb and index finger to limit the force applied. In addition, the other fingers can remain extended to prevent plunging forward in case of sudden loss of resistance. Dilation need not start with the smallest dilator on the set; starting with a larger size (e.g., 15F instead of 13F) may reduce the risk of perforating the uterus or creating a false channel.

If more than two fingers of force is necessary during dilation, the physician should stop and reassess the situation, rather than risk injuring the cervix. One option is to use a smaller cannula than originally planned. Alternatively, the physician can pack the cervix with one or more osmotic dilators, interrupt the procedure, then complete the operation several hours later, by which time adequate dilation will have been achieved. Another treatment option is to administer oral or vaginal misoprostol and complete the procedure in several hours. Performance of the procedure in two stages is far preferable to forceful dilation.

After adequate dilation, the physician inserts the cannula. In general, the diameter of the cannula in millimeters should be about one less than the weeks of gestation from last menses. For example, an 8-mm cannula is adequate for evacuating a pregnancy of 9 weeks' gestation. Skilled physicians often prefer to use even smaller cannulas than this guideline suggests; the physician must weigh the advantage of needing less dilation against the potential disadvantages of longer operating time and an increased risk of incomplete abortion.

The most frequently used cannulas in the United States are clear plastic, with a slight angulation (Fig. 33.7). The physician should insert the cannula into the lower uterine segment. The physician then turns on the suction machine and aspirates the uterus with the cannula (Fig. 33.8). One of the principles of abortion technique is to start working in the lower uterine segment. The fundal contents of the uterus are brought down by suction and the involution of the uterus as it empties. When bubbles appear in the cannula and the interior of the cavity feels empty, some physicians use a sharp curette to confirm the completeness of evacuation. The flexible plastic cannula

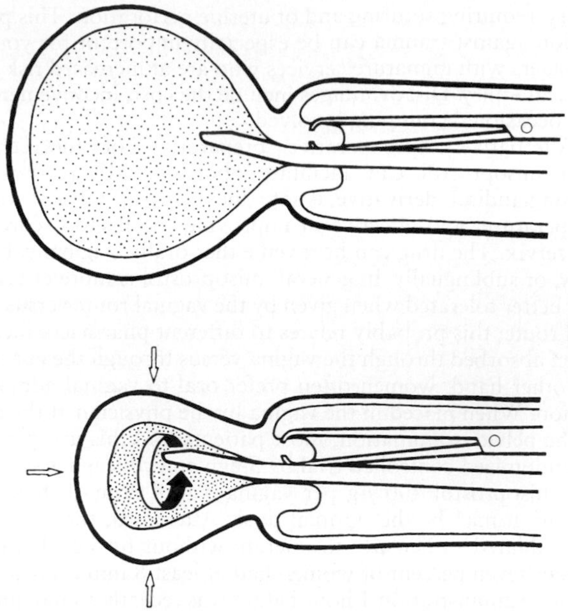

FIGURE 33.8. Uterine aspiration. **Top:** Cannula inserted just beyond internal os. **Bottom:** Aspiration with rotating motion.

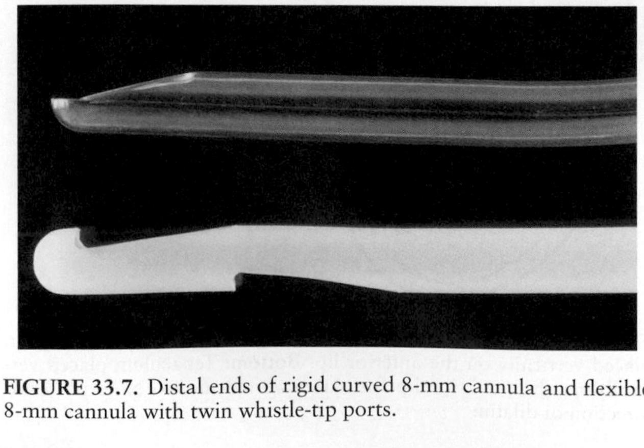

FIGURE 33.7. Distal ends of rigid curved 8-mm cannula and flexible 8-mm cannula with twin whistle-tip ports.

(Fig. 33.7) suctions opposite sides of the cavity simultaneously and provides a distinct gritty sensation when the evacuation is complete. The operation is not finished until the physician or another trained observer has examined the aspirated tissue. This is to confirm the presence of fetal tissue, which usually excludes the possibility of an ectopic pregnancy. Since 1972, more than 20 women in the United States have died from ectopic pregnancies undetected at the time of attempted suction curettage. This tissue inspection will not detect the rare twin ectopic pregnancy, commonly termed "heterotopic."

Pregnancies of 9 weeks' gestation and later will have recognizable fetal parts; earlier pregnancies may not. Identification of chorionic villi and membranes in these earlier pregnancies is essential. The physician rinses the aspirated tissue in a fine-mesh strainer under tap water to remove blood and clots. A glass dish is useful for examining the tissue suspended in water. For early pregnancies, white vinegar (instead of water) may facilitate the recognition of villi. Back lighting from a horizontal x-ray viewing box is especially useful (Fig. 33.9). Villi appear soft, fluffy, and feathery, with discernible finger-like projections; in contrast, decidua appears coarse and shaggy (Fig. 33.10). Amnion and chorion are filmy and transparent; decidua is translucent. With early pregnancies, a magnifying glass, dissecting microscope, colposcope, or standard microscope (3100) can help identify villi (Fig. 33.11). It is essential to learn the difference between the appearance of villi and decidua; this is useful in the management of early pregnancy failure as well as in distinguishing between bleeding from miscarriage from that of an ectopic pregnancy.

When the physician cannot confirm fetal tissue, he or she should reevaluate the patient, with special attention to the adnexa. Repeat aspiration (perhaps with ultrasound guidance) is often appropriate. A sensitive urine pregnancy test or a quantitative β-hCG can be helpful. Ultrasound can sometimes identify a gestational sac. Failure to identify villi in the presence of a positive pregnancy test suggests several possibilities: recent spontaneous abortion, failed attempted abortion, perforation

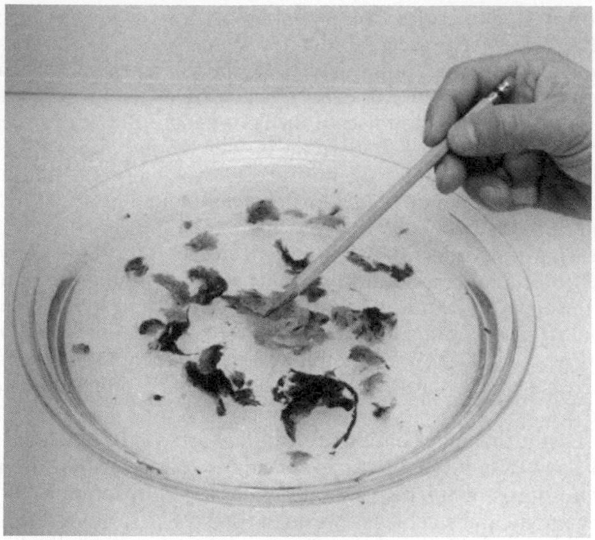

FIGURE 33.9. Examination of aspirated tissue over x-ray viewing box for back lighting.

with aspiration outside the uterus, or ectopic pregnancy. The physician must carefully evaluate these possibilities.

Women with uterine anomalies, such as a bicornuate uterus, have a high risk of failed attempted abortion. Sometimes the unique anatomy makes it difficult to enter the horn with the pregnancy. One useful approach is to perform the aspiration under ultrasound guidance. If the physician can insert a bent sound into the cavity with the pregnancy, he or she can then place the bent sound inside a flexible 8-mm plastic cannula as a stent or guide. With ultrasound guidance, the physician then inserts the cannula into the cavity and removes the sound, connects the cannula adapter, and then aspirates the cavity. Another alternative is to use medical abortion. Rarely, hysterotomy may be needed if curettage and medical abortion fail in the setting of müllerian anomalies.

Postoperative Care

Women should expect some spotting and bleeding after the procedure that improves with time and usually stops by 1 to 2 weeks. They should know to notify the physician with any

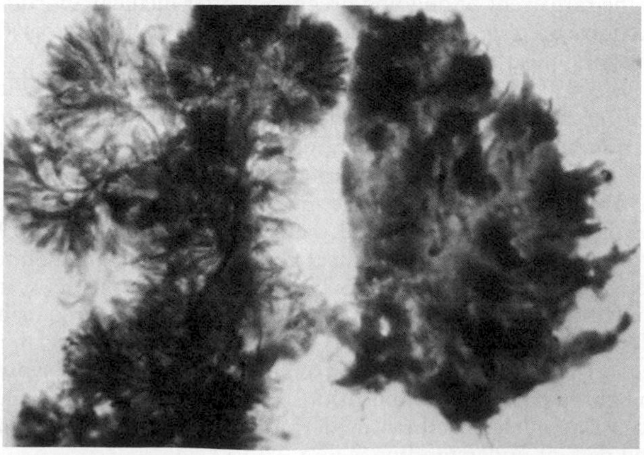

FIGURE 33.10. **Left:** Typical fluffy villi of placenta. **Right:** Shaggy decidua. (From: Munsick RA. Clinical test for placenta in 300 consecutive menstrual aspirations. *Obstet Gynecol* 1982;60:738, with permission.)

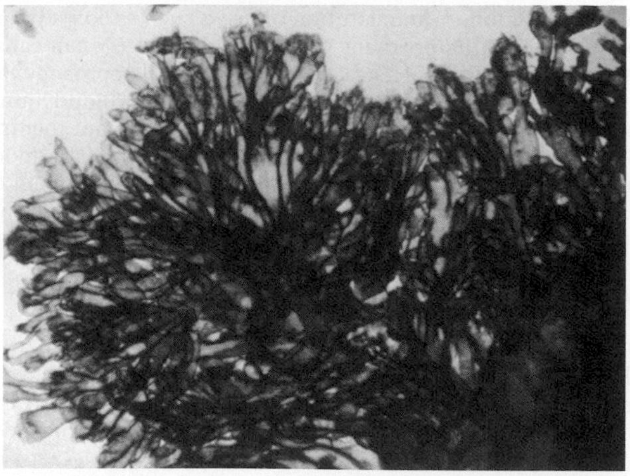

FIGURE 33.11. Wet-mount microscopic appearance of placental villi. (From: Munsick RA. Clinical test for placenta in 300 consecutive menstrual aspirations. *Obstet Gynecol* 1982;60:738, with permission.)

signs of a complication: fever, pain, bleeding more than a period, dizziness or weakness, passage of tissue, and ongoing symptoms of pregnancy. Pregnancy symptoms that do not dissipate within 1 week or normal menses not returning within 6 weeks are reasons to return. They should have 24-hour emergency phone numbers. Any woman whose procedure did not definitely identify tissue should be actively managed to rule out ectopic pregnancy. Women may resume work the day following an abortion or when they feel up to it.

Almost all forms of contraception may be started on the day of an abortion procedure, including the placement of intrauterine devices. Commonly a postoperative visit is scheduled 2 to 3 weeks after the procedure to ensure complete abortion and rule out any complications. It has been suggested that this visit may not be necessary, as women can be trained to return for certain signs and symptoms. Many providers find this visit useful to assess contraceptive use and satisfaction, as well as to provide regular gynecologic care that may not be a routine part of the preoperative abortion care—e.g., cervical cytology. Routine β-hCG testing should not be done at this visit. After an uncomplicated procedure, β-hCG can be detected for a mean of 30 days and up to 60 days. Therefore, it is not useful for ruling out retained tissue and causes confusion when found to be positive.

Use of Oxytocic Agents

The usefulness of administering oxytocic agents during suction curettage is unclear, although administering oxytocin or ergot derivatives reduces blood loss from suction curettage performed under general anesthesia. Although statistically significant, the reduction in blood loss is clinically unimportant. Because blood loss is less with local anesthesia, oxytocic agents probably are not necessary. Although physicians commonly give ergot derivatives by mouth for several days after suction curettage, evidence of the benefit of this practice is lacking, and the drugs cause painful uterine cramping in some women.

Prophylactic Antibiotics

Induced abortion patients should receive prophylactic antibiotics. A metaanalysis of the randomized, controlled trials on this topic by Sawaya and colleagues showed decreased risk for postabortal endometritis for women deemed low and high risk for infection. Administration of drugs such as doxycycline to anxious, fasting pregnant women before surgery can cause nausea and vomiting. Hence, the most practical approach may be to begin a short-course antibiotic with food promptly after the abortion. The choice of antibiotic and duration of therapy is unclear. However, if one administers antibiotics for more than 24 hours, prophylaxis ends and presumptive treatment of *C. trachomatis* begins. In high-risk populations, presumptive treatment of all patients for chlamydia may be a reasonable course of action.

Medical Abortion in Early Pregnancy

The marketing of the antiprogestin mifepristone has opened a new chapter in abortion practice. Mifepristone is a derivative of norethindrone; it binds to the progesterone receptor but does not activate it. When bound, it blocks progesterone activity and acts to alter the decidua, allowing trophoblast separation. This alone can lead to bleeding and *in vivo* prostaglandin release that can cause an abortion in early pregnancy. Mifepristone alone, however, results in completed abortion 64% to 85% of the time. Therefore, the drug is generally followed by a prostaglandin analog to vastly improve the completion rates. The regimen recommended by the distributor and approved by the U.S. Food and Drug Administration (FDA) calls for a single oral dose of mifepristone 600 mg, followed in 48 hours by misoprostol 400 mg orally, both doses given in the clinician's office. This has been approved for use up to 49 days' gestation. Success rates with this regimen range from 92% to 97%.

Several randomized controlled trials have investigated this regimen. Data currently support alternative dosage, route, timing, and gestational age criteria than those established by the FDA and the company guidelines. These changes result in improved efficacy and patient convenience, decreased cost, and sustained safety.

Several studies have shown that 200 mg of mifepristone effect abortion at rates equivalent to 600 mg. El-Rafaey and colleagues first reported this finding in 1995. This was confirmed by a study by WHO, reporting in 2000 that there was found no difference in the completed abortion rate between women given 200 mg of mifepristone compared with those given 600 mg. Additionally, this study included women up to 63 days' gestation. This equivalence in dosing is secondary to nonlinear pharmacokinetics. The binding site for the mifepristone is rapidly saturated. Women given 100 mg, 200 mg, and 800 mg have a peak serum concentration of 2.0 to 2.5 μg/mL approximately 2 hours after ingestion, regardless of dosage given. Therefore, pharmacology and economics support use of 200 mg mifepristone.

Several studies have also investigated misoprostol dosing and route of administration. Vaginal dosing of misoprostol has been shown to increase bioavailability when compared with oral dosing. Furthermore, the gastrointestinal side effects of the medicine are often fewer with this route. Schaff and colleagues compared oral (400 μg and 800 μg) versus vaginal (800 μg) misoprostol following 200 mg mifepristone. They found a statistically significant higher level of completed abortions in those who received vaginal misoprostol compared with either dose of oral misoprostol (84%, 92%, and 96%, respectively). In 2003, WHO published results of a large study comparing vaginal misoprostol with oral/vaginal combinations after mifepristone. There was no difference in completion rates. Recent investigations have focused on administration of misoprostol by the buccal and sublingual routes.

Investigators have also questioned the timing of the misoprostol dosing and where it should be administered. Convention and medication guidelines encourage giving oral misoprostol 48 hours after the mifepristone dose in the clinician's office. However, acceptability of women to self-administer the misoprostol at home has been shown repeatedly. Schaff and colleagues also explored efficacy of different schedules of prostaglandin administration. Following 200 mg of mifepristone, more than 2,000 subjects were randomized to self-administration of 800 μg misoprostol vaginally 24, 48, and 72 hours later. Completed abortions were found in 98%, 98%, and 96%, respectively. Patient satisfaction decreased with increasing time interval. With patient acceptability and convenience of avoiding additional clinic visits, self-administration of misoprostol 24 hours after mifepristone is supported. Recent noninferiority studies suggest that decreasing the time interval further, to 6 to 8 hours after mifepristone, does not significantly decrease efficacy and may decrease some gastrointestinal side effects.

Lastly, the upper limit of gestational age can be extended to 63 days. When mifepristone 200 mg is followed in 48 hours by misoprostol 800 mg vaginally, complete abortion rates 95% or greater can be achieved through 63 days' gestation; this has been supported by several researchers. Some small studies have found success using the combination of mifepristone and misoprostol for gestations up to 91 days; however, most agree that the likelihood of success declines with advancing gestational age.

The National Abortion Federation, Planned Parenthood of America, and many clinicians follow an evidence-based approach to medical abortion. Mifepristone 200 mg is administered orally in the clinician's office to women of 63 days' gestation or less. The patient then self-administers 800 μg misoprostol vaginally 24 hours later. Women undergoing medical abortion who do not bleed within 24 hours of receiving misoprostol should contact their provider, as they may be at higher risk of ectopic pregnancy. If the alternative, evidence-based regimen is chosen, appropriate patient consent and education about variance from the FDA regimen is prudent. With either regimen, women need to be evaluated about 2 weeks after mifepristone administration to confirm by ultrasonography that the pregnancy has ended. An inability to follow up in the time frame specified or in the event of an emergency should preclude provision of a medical abortion. In the few percent of women who fail to abort or who have incomplete abortions, observation, repeated dosing of misoprostol, or completion of the process with a handheld syringe and cannula (Fig. 33.4) are options. If aspiration is chosen, no additional dilation is usually required. Patients should be counseled before starting that in the rare event of ongoing pregnancy after medical abortion, suction curettage is recommended because of the teratogenic effects of misoprostol.

Medical abortion is safe, effective, and well tolerated. With current regimens, cramping and bleeding are common, but infection and bleeding heavy enough to require transfusion are rare. Data collected from postmarketing experience since the FDA approval of mifepristone in the United States in September 2000 have demonstrated the safety. More than 460,000 women have undergone medical abortion in the United States between 2000 and mid-2005. Serious complications have included seventeen ectopic pregnancies, hemorrhage requiring blood transfusion (in $<0.03\%$), and seven serious bacterial infections, including five deaths from *Clostridium sordellii* sepsis. In light of potential complications and the abortion experience occurring outside of the provider's office, thorough counseling and patient understanding is imperative.

Before the marketing of mifepristone in the United States, physicians relied on other medical abortifacient regimens. One regimen included a single intramuscular injection of methotrexate, 50 mg/m^2 body surface area, followed 3 to 7 days later by vaginal administration of misoprostol, 800 μg. The efficacy of the combined regimen was 90%. In a randomized, controlled trial, this regimen proved superior to the same dose of misoprostol given alone. At 49 days' gestation or less, methotrexate and misoprostol can achieve success rates similar to those with mifepristone and misoprostol, but the process is slower with methotrexate. From 20% to 30% of women require 1 to 5 weeks to complete the abortion. On the other hand, methotrexate is much less expensive than is mifepristone. Methotrexate works as an antimetabolite; it continues to be used in the medical management of ectopic pregnancy.

Another alternative is use of misoprostol alone. Varying success rates have been reported with different doses, frequency, and routes of administration. The success rates with misoprostol alone appear lower than when misoprostol is used as an adjunct with mifepristone or methotrexate. Protocols that have achieved a high success rate with misoprostol alone have had high rates of side effects as well, including nausea, vomiting, and diarrhea.

Medical approaches may be especially useful for challenging abortions. These include patients with müllerian anomalies, large cervical leiomyomas, prior failed attempted abortion, or obesity (e.g., 150 kg and more). Should the medical regimen not effect abortion, surgical completion is made substantially easier by this preparation of the cervix.

Dilation and Evacuation

Dilation and evacuation is the generic term for suction curettage abortions at 13 weeks' gestation or later. During the 1970s, D&E emerged as the most frequently used method for second-trimester abortions. The proportion of abortions performed by curettage techniques is inversely related to gestational age (Table 33.1). Even at gestations greater than 20 weeks, D&E remains the dominant method of abortion in the United States. In April 2007, the US Supreme Court upheld a decision to ban an abortion prodedure called D&X, in which there is a partial breech delivery of a fetus and decompression of the calvarium to complete the delivery. The law does not contain an exception to permit the procedure to protect the health and life of the mother. Broader repercussions of this ruling are unknown.

Based on data from the 1970s, D&E is clearly safer than alternative methods through 16 weeks' gestation. At later gestational ages, the distinction blurs between D&E and labor induction methods in terms of morbidity and mortality. Patients often prefer D&E because they avoid experiencing labor. Many physicians have not been surgically trained to provide later D&E procedures. Often the choice of abortion method at this later stage depends on access to abortion services, the presence of skilled personnel, and whether the fetus needs to be intact for autopsy. Some physicians prefer to administer feticidal agents, such as digoxin or potassium chloride, under ultrasound guidance preoperatively. A randomized, controlled trial by Jackson and colleagues found that doing so had no operative benefit. For D&E procedures, accurate determination of gestational age by ultrasound preoperatively is essential. Underestimation of gestational age can lead to inadequate dilation, which complicates the procedure. D&E differs from suction curettage in two principal ways: D&E requires wider cervical dilation, and physicians need forceps to evacuate more advanced pregnancies.

Dilating the cervix to a large diameter over several minutes manually can damage the cervix. Indeed, the first large study of this question revealed a higher incidence of low-birth-weight infants in subsequent desired pregnancies. Hence, D&E procedures beyond about 14 weeks' gestation should use osmotic dilators. Patients must understand that once osmotic dilators have been inserted, the abortion needs completion. Occasionally the patient may abort just from the dilator. Rarely, a patient changes her mind about abortion after placement of an osmotic dilator. Although some women have continued their pregnancies uneventfully after removal of the devices, others have developed infections and/or aborted.

To achieve adequate dilation, many physicians insert osmotic dilators several hours to several days before D&E (Fig. 33.12). For example, five laminaria placed overnight result in 1.5- to 2-cm dilation with minimal or no discomfort for most women. Use of a single Lamicel for about 4 hours produces as much dilation as do several laminaria at 14 to 16 weeks' gestation.

In the 13- to 16-week interval, vacuum alone is adequate; thereafter, forceps extraction predominates. A cannula 14 mm in diameter can evacuate pregnancies through about 16 menstrual weeks' gestation. For later pregnancies, the cannula primarily drains amniotic fluid at the beginning of the evacuation and draws tissue into the lower uterus for forceps extraction. Specially designed forceps for D&E are far superior to standard sponge forceps. As with suction curettage, extraction should occur from the lower uterus to minimize the risks of

TABLE 33.1

PERCENTAGES OF REPORTED LEGAL ABORTIONS AT 13 MENSTRUAL WEEKS' GESTATION AND GREATER, BY METHOD AND GESTATIONAL AGE, SELECTED STATES, UNITED STATES, 2002

	Weeks of gestation		
Type of procedure	13–15	16–20	>21
Curettage (D&E)	99.1	95.7	85.6
Intrauterine instillation	0.2	1.7	1.6
Medical (nonsurgical)	0.2	1.4	3.4
Other	0.5	1.2	9.4
TOTAL	100.0	100.0	100.0

From Strauss LT, Herndon J, Chang J, et al. Abortion surveillance: United States, 2002. In: CDC surveillance summaries, November 25, 2005. *MMWR Morb Mortal Wkly Rep* 2005;54(no. SS-7).

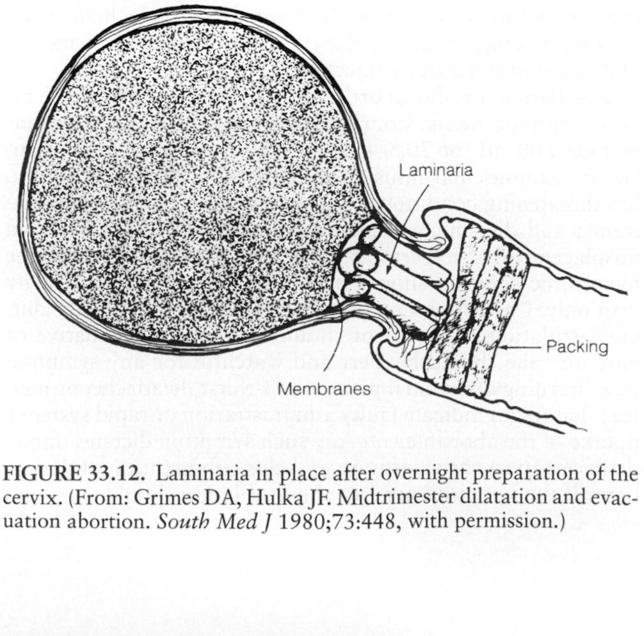

FIGURE 33.12. Laminaria in place after overnight preparation of the cervix. (From: Grimes DA, Hulka JF. Midtrimester dilatation and evacuation abortion. *South Med J* 1980;73:448, with permission.)

perforation. Some physicians use a flexible 8-mm cannula to confirm complete evacuation.

The physician must confirm completion by identifying all major fetal parts (4 extremities, spine, and calvarium). The calvarium is the component most frequently missed during the initial evacuation. Gentle exploration of the fundal and cornual areas with a large curette or forceps usually enables location and removal of the calvarium. Intraoperative ultrasonography can be helpful. If ultrasonography is not available, the physician may be able to remove the speculum and insert one digit into the uterine cavity to locate the missing part.

If the abortion cannot be completed with ease, the physician should interrupt the procedure. A safe and simple remedy is to discontinue the operation and administer intravenous oxytocin to the woman for 2 to 3 hours in the recovery room. After the patient returns to the operating room, the physician usually finds the retained tissue at the internal os, from which it can be easily removed. No D&E abortion needs to finish in a single session; time often helps. Once membranes rupture, the uterus contracts to expel its contents.

In D&E abortions, the skill of the physician is critical. D&E abortion requires specific training that is often not routinely acquired in a U.S. ob/gyn residency. The likelihood that a physician will offer abortion services is highly correlated with whether he or she was trained in residency. The physician should study operative technique. He or she should then observe and assist skilled physicians and then perform D&E procedures only under direct supervision. Use of ultrasound guidance for residents learning D&E was associated with a dramatic lowering of the perforation rate and a reduction in operating time. The gestational age range can advance as skill grows. In summary, D&E is a specialized surgical technique that can be learned with appropriate training.

Labor Induction

Although D&E has supplanted many labor-induction abortions, the need for such abortions continues, particularly at later gestational ages. In contrast to D&E, the proportion of abortions performed by labor induction increases with gestational age (Table 33.1).

Abortifacients include two broad groups: hypertonic solutions (e.g., saline or urea) and uterotonic agents (e.g., oxytocin or misoprostol). The mechanism of action of hypertonic solutions is unclear, but these agents usually result in fetal death from osmotic insult; labor then generally ensues. Uterotonics act directly on the myometrium to stimulate contractions. Prostaglandins available in the United States include misoprostol, prostaglandin E_2 (PGE_2) preparations, and 15-methyl $PGF_{2\alpha}$ for intramuscular injection.

Instillation of the abortifacient hypertonic solutions requires amniocentesis. Common doses of hypertonic solutions include 200 mL of 20% saline or 80 g of urea. Intravascular or intramuscular infusion of hypertonic saline can lead to life-threatening conditions for the mother, including hypernatremia and disseminated intravascular coagulation. To avoid misplacement of hypertonic saline and its consequences, the hypertonic solution should be introduced by a slow gravity drip only. Careful observation of the patient is necessary during instillation. The patient should not receive a sedative or narcotic. She should be alert and watchful for any symptom (e.g., burning abdominal pain, severe thirst, headache, or nausea) that might indicate faulty administration or rapid systemic uptake of the abortifacient. Any such symptom dictates immediate cessation of the infusion and close observation of the patient. If the symptom persists, the instillation should stop, and the physician should choose an alternative method or agent for the abortion.

Use of hypertonic saline or urea is often augmented by placement of osmotic dilators or use of oxytocin secondary to the long induction to abortion time intervals. Because of these increased time intervals, the potential serious side effects of this method, and the development of safe and effective systemic agents, the use of intrauterine instillation techniques have decreased in the past decade. It should be noted that the use of hypertonic solution instillation in the case of fetal demise is not advised secondary to the increased risk for coagulopathy.

The three most common systemic agents for abortion and labor induction include prostaglandin E_2, prostaglandin analog E_1 (misoprostol), and high-dose oxytocin. Administration of prostaglandins or oxytocin has the advantage of simplicity. Amniocentesis is unnecessary, and inadvertent intravascular administration of hypertonic solutions cannot occur. Disadvantages of prostaglandins alone for abortion include a high frequency of nausea, vomiting, and diarrhea. Routine prophylactic use of antiemetics and antidiarrheal drugs can reduce but not eliminate these noxious side effects. Fever occurs in about one third to one half of patients given prostaglandin E_2. Another drawback is that these drugs are not inherently feticidal.

Vaginal PGE_2, a 20-mg suppository is placed in the posterior fornix every 3 to 5 hours; the mean abortion time is 13.4 hours, and 90% of abortions occur within 24 hours. Its efficacy has been evaluated in terminations from 13 to 28 weeks' gestation. Some recommend a smaller dose or avoidance of this drug altogether in later gestations secondary to the increased risk of uterine rupture with advanced gestational age.

Misoprostol as a second-trimester induction agent has received much attention. Its affordability and stability at room temperature make it an appealing option. Currently there is no single misoprostol regimen for recommendation. The first study by Jain and Mishell used 200 μg vaginally every 12 hours, which was found to be as effective as vaginal prostaglandin E_2 suppositories and was associated with fewer side effects. Studies have evaluated dosages from 100 μg to 800 μg with oral, vaginal, and sublingual routes. A review by Ngai and colleagues highlights results of trials comparing various methods. Overall, the use of misoprostol results in very high levels of completed abortion in the second trimester. Time to abortion and side effects must be balanced in decision making about which regimen to use. In general, the higher dose with more frequent dosing schedules results in higher side effects, namely fever. Rigorous trials comparing all methods are lacking.

There appears to be a place for mifepristone in second-trimester inductions, as well as in early terminations. Using misoprostol 36 to 48 hours after administration of mifepristone show improved abortion results. Following 200 mg of mifepristone, Ashok et al. gave 800 μg misoprostol vaginally followed by 400 μg orally every 3 hours, with a maximum of four oral doses. This regimen resulted in 97% successful abortion with a mean induction to abortion time of 6.25 hours (in those that were successful). Of the 1,002 patients in the study, complications were seen in 11. Ten had significant bleeding, and seven required transfusion. One woman had significant hemorrhage and was found to have a myometrial tear upon laparotomy. She had received one dose of prostaglandin. Both mifepristone and misoprostol are not currently labeled for second-trimester termination.

Interest in high-dose oxytocin infusion for abortion has renewed. Oxytocin alone can result in completed abortion 80% to 90% of the time. The frequency of fever, vomiting, and diarrhea was significantly lower with oxytocin compared with prostaglandin E_2 and misoprostol. One regimen includes oxytocin, 50 U in 500 mL of dextrose and normal saline administered intravenously over 3 hours; maintenance fluid (dextrose in normal saline) then follows for 1 hour. In stepwise fashion, the concentration of oxytocin increases by 50 U every 4 hours to a maximum of 300 U/500 mL. The investigators administered oxytocin in isotonic fluid and interrupted the oxytocin infusion every 4 hours for diuresis. With prolonged high-dose oxytocin infusion in hypotonic solutions, water intoxication and death can result.

The decision about labor induction in women with a previous uterine scar remains a difficult one for clinicians. There are reports of uterine rupture with previous cesarean delivery in both misoprostol and prostaglandin E_2. Some have reported uterine rupture rates of approximately 4% in those with previous hysterotomies undergoing medical induction compared with 0.2% in those with unscarred uteri. Conversely, a case series of 100 women at 14 to 28 weeks with previous cesarean delivery undergoing induction with misoprostol reported no uterine ruptures. Further study is necessary. Women with a uterine scar require detailed counseling about the risk of rupture. If induction is chosen, it should be completed in a hospital setting where complications can be managed appropriately.

Direct cervical dilation has been investigated in its role for decreasing the induction interval. Some studies show that osmotic dilators can shorten induction-to-abortion times if placed before the initiation of induction. A study by Borgotta and associates indicates that placement of osmotic dilators at the time of induction may actually prolong the induction process. Further study is needed to answer this question. If induction progress stalls, a metreurynter can be attempted. The physician inserts a sterile Foley catheter with a 30- to 75-mL balloon into the uterus, inflates the balloon with a sterile solution (not air), and ties the catheter to 0.5-kg orthopedic traction at the foot of the bed. A liter bag of intravenous fluids hung over the foot of the bed and tied to the catheter by a string also suffices. This method has the disadvantage of placing a foreign body in the uterus.

Much of the morbidity (and mortality) associated with labor-induction abortion is preventable. Women undergoing labor induction need the same meticulous, attentive obstetric care as do women in labor with childbirth. If the membranes rupture, then labor must conclude within a reasonable period. In many cases, the preferred means of concluding a slow induction abortion is D&E. Twenty-four hours is a reasonable limit for labor-induction abortions. Frequently, the cervix is open several centimeters, and D&E proceeds quickly. Similarly, active management of a retained placenta after abortion prevents morbidity. If spontaneous delivery of the placenta has not occurred after delivery, the placenta should be removed by suction curettage. Notably, misoprostol is associated with a significantly lower rate of retained placenta when compared with prostaglandin E_2 or oxytocin (2% vs. 15%).

Hysterotomy and Hysterectomy

Neither hysterotomy nor hysterectomy should be a primary method of abortion. The morbidity, mortality, expense, and pain associated with these operations are greater than with alternative methods. Hysterotomy for abortion is an archaic operation that should be used only when usual surgical and medical approaches fail. Figure 33.13 depicts a hysterotomy to evacuate a 14-week pregnancy in the left horn of a bicornuate uterus; both labor induction and attempts to enter to pregnant horn through the cervix with ultrasonography and laparoscopy guidance had failed in this primigravida. Hysterectomy is appropriate in rare cases in which preexisting pathology, such as large leiomyomas (Fig. 33.14) or carcinoma *in situ* of the cervix, justify hysterectomy.

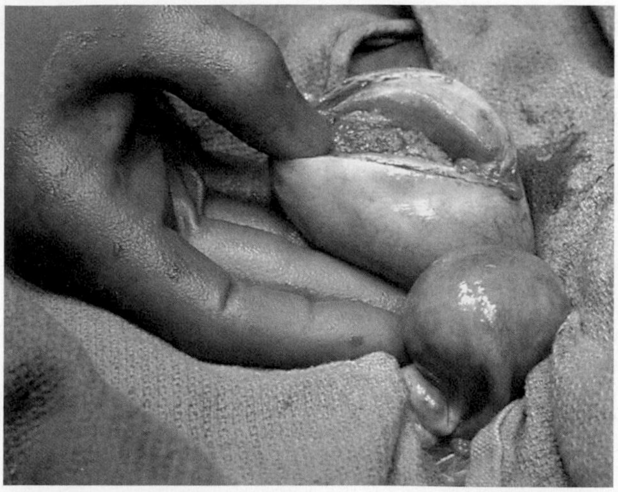

FIGURE 33.13. Hysterotomy incision in left uterine cavity, 14 weeks' gestation, after failed labor-induction abortion and failed attempted dilation and evacuation. Patient had a single cervix and two cavities. Nonpregnant cavity seen at right.

Complications

Morbidity

Legal abortion in the United States is safe. Less than 1 woman in 100 develops a serious complication, and fewer than 1 in 100,000 dies as a result of the operation. This mortality rate is one tenth the rate for women who elect to continue their pregnancy.

Gestational age is one of two important determinants of the likelihood of morbidity. In Table 33.2, which lists serious

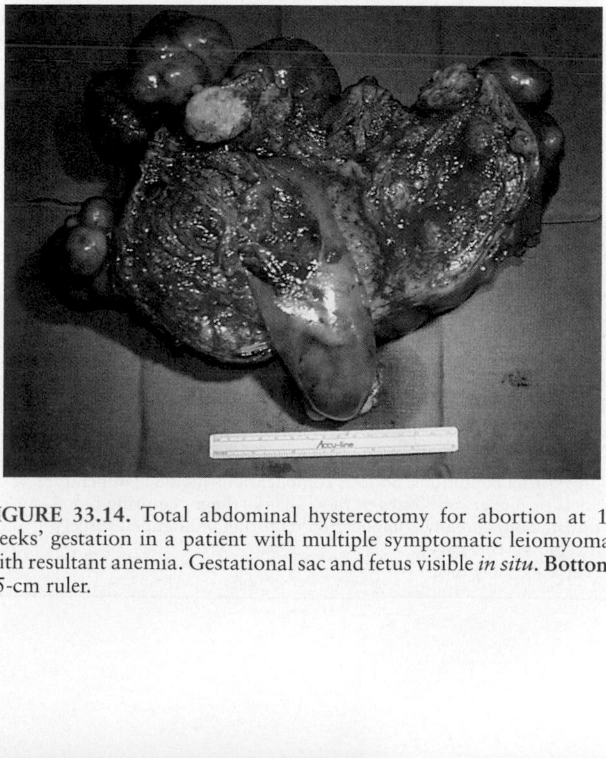

FIGURE 33.14. Total abdominal hysterectomy for abortion at 15 weeks' gestation in a patient with multiple symptomatic leiomyomas with resultant anemia. Gestational sac and fetus visible *in situ*. **Bottom:** 15-cm ruler.

TABLE 33.2

SERIOUS COMPLICATION RATES FOR LEGAL ABORTIONS BY GESTATIONAL AGE: UNITED STATES, 1975–1978[a]

Gestational age (wk)	Rate[b]
6	0.4
7–8	0.2
9–10	0.1
11–12	0.3
13–14	0.6
15–16	1.3
17–20	1.9

[a]For women with follow-up and without concurrent sterilization or preexisting conditions. Serious complications include temperature of 38°C or higher for 3 days or more, hemorrhage requiring blood transfusion, and any complication requiring unintended surgery (excluding curettage).
[b]Per 100 abortions.

complication rates for abortion by gestational age, the term *serious complication rates* is defined as fever of 38°C or higher for 3 or more days, hemorrhage requiring transfusion, or unintended surgery. These data, derived from a 1970s multicenter study including 84,000 abortions, relate to those women without concurrent sterilization or preexisting medical conditions and for whom follow-up information was available. Abortions performed at the 7 to 10 weeks' gestation interval had the lowest incidence of serious complications. Thereafter, complications increased progressively with advancing gestational age. The method of abortion is the second principal determinant of the likelihood of complications. Table 33.3, derived from the same study as Table 33.2, demonstrates that suction curettage is the safest available abortion method. The risk of serious complications with D&E at 13 weeks' gestation or later is higher than that with suction curettage and lower than that with labor-induction abortion.

Abortion complications have three temporal categories: immediate, delayed, and late complications. Immediate complications are those that develop during or within 3 hours of the operation. Delayed complications occur more than 3 hours and

TABLE 33.3

SERIOUS COMPLICATION RATES FOR LEGAL ABORTIONS BY METHOD: UNITED STATES, 1975–1978[a]

Method	Rate[b]
Suction curettage	0.2
Dilation and evacuation	0.7
Saline instillation	2.1
Prostaglandin instillation	2.5
Urea-prostaglandin instillation	1.3

[a]For women with follow-up and without concurrent sterilization or preexisting conditions. Serious complications include temperature of 38°C or higher for 3 days or more, hemorrhage requiring blood transfusion, and any complication requiring unintended surgery (excluding curettage).
[b]Per 100 abortions.

up to 28 days after the procedure. Late complications develop thereafter.

Immediate Complications

Hemorrhage. Reported rates of hemorrhage vary widely, reflecting both diverse definitions (100 to 1,000 mL blood loss) and imprecision in estimating volumes of blood loss. Rates of hemorrhage range from 0.05 to 4.9 per 100 abortions in large case-series reports. The best index of clinically important hemorrhage is probably the rate of blood transfusion. The rate of transfusion associated with suction curettage in a large multicenter study was 0.06 per 100 abortions. For abortions performed later in pregnancy, investigators have reported rates of 0.26 for D&E, 0.32 for urea-prostaglandin, and 1.72 for saline.

Vasopressin administered with paracervical anesthesia decreases blood loss with D&E abortion after 14 weeks' gestation. As little as 4 U (0.2 mL) mixed in with the anesthetic lowers the blood loss significantly; overall, vasopressin lowers fourfold the risk of a hemorrhage of 500 mL or more. It is important to remember to administer vasopressin when opting to administer regional or general anesthesia. In these instances, one would usually forego the paracervical block; however, use of a cervical anesthetic with vasopressin lowers risk of bleeding.

When hemorrhage occurs after suction curettage, it is most often due to uterine atony. Administration of uterotonic agents and manual compression usually resolve the problem. As with labor related atony, methylergonovine maleate may be given (0.2 mg intramuscularly) as well as prostaglandins: carboprost 250 μg intramuscularly or misoprostol 1,000 μg per rectum. Should bleeding persist, assessment of the endometrial cavity by suction curettage should be done to rule out retained tissue. Occasionally, internal compression of the cavity by a large Foley catheter balloon or a vasopressin-soaked pack can be helpful. If these measures fail, uterine artery embolization can be done in a stable patient, with the last resort being hysterectomy.

With the increasing cohort of women who have had cesarean deliveries, the risk of encountering placenta accreta during abortion is increasing as well. In a series of more than 16,000 D&E abortions, the incidence of placenta accreta leading to hysterectomy was 4 per 10,000 cases.

Cervical Injury. Cervical injury encompasses a broad spectrum of trauma. The most common type is a superficial laceration caused by the tenaculum tearing off during dilation. At the other extreme are the cervicovaginal fistula and the longitudinal laceration ascending to the level of the uterine vessels. Rates of cervical injury range from 0.01 to 1.6 per 100 suction curettage abortions. In older studies, the incidence of cervical injury requiring sutures was about 1 per 100 suction curettage abortions.

Several risk factors for cervical injury during suction curettage have emerged. Among factors within the control of the physician, use of laminaria and performance of the abortion by an attending physician (rather than a resident) lower the risk significantly, whereas use of general anesthesia raises the risk significantly. Use of laminaria and performance of the abortion under local anesthesia by an attending physician together yield a 27-fold protective effect. Cervical preparation with misoprostol may confer similar benefits as laminaria, although more extensive experience will be needed to confirm this. Among factors beyond the control of the physician, a history of a prior abortion lowers the risk, and age of 17 years or younger increases the risk.

Acute Hematometra. Also termed the *postabortal syndrome,* acute hematometra is an important complication of suction curettage; its cause is unknown. The incidence of this syndrome ranges from 0.1 to 1.0 per 100 suction curettage abortions, according to the available literature.

Women with this condition develop severe cramping, usually within 2 hours of the abortion. Vaginal bleeding is less than expected. The woman may be weak and sweaty, and her uterus is large and markedly tender. Treatment consists of prompt repeat curettage, usually without anesthesia or dilation. Evacuation of both liquid and clotted blood leads to rapid resolution of the symptoms. The physician can aspirate the blood with a suction cannula, a Karman cannula and syringe, or even a catheter attached to wall suction. Administration of a uterotonic after the repeat evacuation is standard. Whether routine prophylactic use of an oxytocic would reduce the incidence of acute hematometra is unknown.

Anesthesia Complications. Pain experienced during abortion relates not only to the choice of anesthesia but also to the characteristics of the patient. Young women (13 to 17 years old) and those with depression before the abortion report more pain than do other women.

Local anesthesia is safer than general anesthesia for both first- and second-trimester abortions. In an Italian study, use of general anesthesia had a relative risk for all complications combined of 1.8 (95% confidence interval, 1.4 to 2.5). The largest effect occurred with hemorrhage. Similarly, use of general anesthesia for D&E abortion in the United States increases the risk of serious complications. Overall, the attributable risk related to general anesthesia is low, and many women are willing to assume incremental risks in order to have no discomfort during the operation.

Perforation. Perforation is a potentially serious, but infrequent complication of abortion. According to most reports, the incidence of perforation is about 0.2 per 100 suction curettage abortions.

Several risk factors for perforation exist. Performance of a curettage abortion by a resident rather than by an attending physician increases the risk more than fivefold; on the other hand, cervical dilation by laminaria decreases the risk about fivefold. The risk of perforation increases significantly with advancing gestational age. Multiparous women have three times the risk of nulliparous women. The use of routine ultrasound guidance for D&E reduces the risk of perforation.

The two principal dangers of perforation are hemorrhage and damage to the abdominal contents. Lateral perforations in the cervicoisthmic region are particularly hazardous because of the proximity of the uterine vessels. Perforations of the fundus are more likely to be innocuous. Indeed, most perforations are not suspected or detected. In a series of patients undergoing combined abortion and sterilization by laparoscopy, the investigators found a sixfold higher rate of uterine perforation than they had suspected clinically (20 versus 3 per 1,000 abortions).

Not all perforations require treatment. Many suspected or documented perforations require only observation. Perforation with a dilator or sound is unlikely to damage abdominal contents. If the perforation occurs before suction, the procedure can be completed under either ultrasound or laparoscopic guidance with extra observation after the procedure. On the other hand, a recognized perforation with a suction cannula or forceps warrants further surgery to rule out organ injury. It is recommended to administer broad-spectrum prophylactic antibiotics when perforation occurs.

If the physician suspects a perforation, the procedure should stop immediately. If unmanageable hemorrhage, expanding hematoma, or injury to abdominal contents occurs, prompt laparotomy is necessary. In a stable patient, laparoscopy can be useful in documenting perforation and assessing damage; if necessary, the physician can complete the abortion under laparoscopic visualization. Any woman with severe pain within hours after the abortion should be evaluated for possible perforation with bowel injury.

Delayed Complications

Retained Tissue. Although retained tissue after abortion can pass without incident, it can also lead to hemorrhage, infection, or both. This complication occurs infrequently, however. Its incidence after suction curettage abortion is less than 1 per 100 abortions.

This complication usually manifests itself within several days of the abortion. Women present with cramping and bleeding, with or without fever. When women develop pain, bleeding, and low-grade fever after abortion, retained tissue may be present. Prompt administration of antibiotics along with outpatient suction curettage is needed. Close follow-up is necessary.

Infection. Postabortal infection can result simply from the procedure or from retained tissue. The presence of retained products warrants suction curettage. The likelihood of febrile morbidity after abortion depends on the method used. The incidence of fever of 38°C or higher for 1 or more days is usually less than 1 per 100 abortions by suction curettage. Corresponding figures for D&E are 1.5 per 100 abortions; for urea-prostaglandin, 6.3; and for hypertonic saline, 5.0. The organisms responsible for postabortal infection are similar to those responsible for other gynecologic infections.

A number of risk factors for infection exist. Women are at increased risk if they have untreated endocervical gonorrhea or chlamydial infection. Late abortions also increase the risk. Likewise, use of labor-induction abortion instead of D&E and use of local rather than general anesthesia for suction curettage increase the risk. Preoperative prophylactic antibiotics decrease the incidence of infection. Administration of broad-spectrum antibiotics and uterine curettage are the cornerstones of therapy.

Late Complications

Rh Sensitization. Legal abortion is a potentially important cause of Rh sensitization for women at risk. The likelihood of sensitization increases with advancing gestational age (and, hence, larger volumes of fetal erythrocytes). One study has quantified the risk of Rh sensitization from first-trimester suction curettage without RhIG prophylaxis. A total of 3.1% of women whose first pregnancy terminated by suction curettage without RhIG prophylaxis had antibodies in their second pregnancy. Subtracting 0.5% (the percentage of women estimated to have become sensitized primarily during the second pregnancy), the investigators estimated the risk of sensitization from suction curettage to be 2.6%. Thus, on a nationwide basis, the clinical impact of failure to administer RhIG to candidates after abortion may be substantial. Candidates should receive 50 μg of RhIG after abortions performed at 12 weeks' gestation or earlier or 300 μg after abortions performed later in pregnancy.

Adverse Pregnancy Outcomes. Investigators have linked induced abortion with a broad array of adverse reproductive outcomes, ranging from infertility to ectopic pregnancy. Most published reports, however, suffer from serious methodological shortcomings that limit their usefulness. To examine the potential association between first-trimester induced abortion and subsequent reproductive performance, epidemiologists have performed an exhaustive review and analysis of the world literature. This includes more than 150 epidemiologic studies published in 11 languages. The findings of this analysis are largely reassuring. No increase in the risk of secondary infertility and ectopic pregnancy appears, even in studies with substantial power to detect differences in rates. Midtrimester spontaneous abortion is no more common among women who have had one previous abortion than among women pregnant for the first time. Similarly, the risk of premature delivery does not increase for women having undergone induced abortion.

On the other hand, low birth weight is more frequent in first births after abortion by sharp curettage performed under general anesthesia compared with first-pregnancy births. This does not occur after other methods of abortion, such as suction curettage. The question of the effect of repeat induced abortion and second-trimester abortion remains unresolved, but repeat sharp curettage may carry increased risks. First-born infants of women who had one induced abortion have risks of morbidity and mortality similar to those of other first-born children.

Additional studies have corroborated the absence of adverse effects of induced abortion on subsequent reproduction. Outcomes studied included infertility, ectopic pregnancy, spontaneous abortion, and adverse obstetric outcomes. One unresolved issue is placenta previa. Sophisticated studies have found either no or a marginally significant increase in the risk (relative risk, 1.3; 95% confidence interval, 1.0 to 1.6), which was comparable to that with spontaneous abortion.

Induced abortion does not threaten a woman's emotional health. In contrast, the most common emotional reactions to induced abortion are a sense of relief accompanied by sadness and loss. In several studies, abortion appeared to improve the emotional well-being of women by resolving an intense personal crisis. Specifically, claims of a postabortion trauma syndrome lack scientific merit.

The putative association between induced abortion and breast cancer remains controversial. Although a number of case-control studies have found an association, this appears because of recall bias among controls. Women who are well (controls) are less likely to report prior induced abortions than are women with breast cancer (cases). This type of information bias has been documented in studies from Sweden. Two large cohort studies, which are less likely to be biased than are case-control studies, have shown either no effect or a protective effect of induced abortion on later breast cancer. No firm evidence links abortion to other cancers.

Mortality

Since 1972, when the Centers for Disease Control and Prevention first began nationwide surveillance of abortion deaths, the safety of abortion has improved dramatically. As shown in Figure 33.15, the overall death rate fell from 4.1 deaths per 100,000 abortions in 1972 to 0.7 in the data published for the decade between 1988–1997.

The causes of death from legal abortion have changed as well. After abortion became legal in 1973, abortion-related deaths declined because of an increase in the skill and experience of providers. When the abortion surveillance system identified procedures that increased risks, practitioners changed their procedures to increase safety. For example, this led to the decline of instillation procedures identified as riskier in the 1970s and the use of general anesthesia in the 1980s. For the last time period reported, 1988 to 1997, the main causes of death were infection and hemorrhage, which accounted for

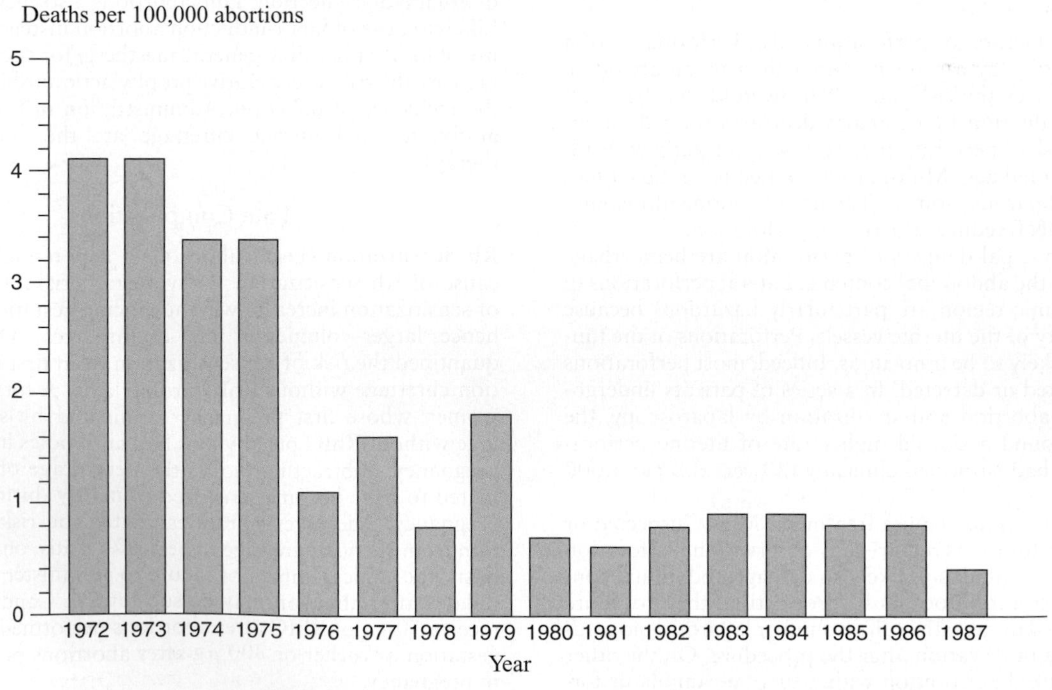

FIGURE 33.15. Case-fatality rates from legal abortion by year, United States, 1972 to 1987. (From: Bartlett LA, Berg CJ, Shulman HB, et al. Risk factors for legal induced abortion-related mortality in the United States. *Obstet Gynecol* 2004;103:729.)

about half of deaths. Embolism, anesthesia, and other causes accounted for the rest.

The risk of death from legal abortion, as reported by Bartlett and colleagues, increases exponentially with increasing gestational age: The earlier the abortion, the safer the abortion (Table 33.4). The risks from 1988 to 1997 (and therefore not including mifepristone abortions) are as follows: The risk with gestational age ≤8 weeks is 1 per million, at 12 weeks is 0.4 per 100,000, at 16 to 20 is 3.4, and at ≥21 weeks is 8.9 per 100,000 procedures (76 times higher than with the earliest procedures). Given the fact that earlier abortions are safer, issues such as access to abortion are medically relevant. These include number of trained providers, cost, and gestational age limit of particular institutions.

The risk of death for women of black and other races was about twice that of white women. For women having second-trimester procedures, mortality rates for D&E were 2.5 times lower than those for instillation and other procedures, although this was not statistically significant. No statistically significant difference in risk related to maternal age or parity was found in this last time period of record.

TABLE 33.4

LEGAL ABORTION CASE-FATALITY RATES AND RELATIVE RISKS BY SELECTED CATEGORIES: UNITED STATES, 1988–1997

Risk category	N[a]	Rate[b]	Relative risk and 95% confidence interval
Age group (y)			
≤19	0.7	20	1.2 (0.6–2.2)
20–24	0.7	29	1.1 (0.6–2.0)
25–29	0.6	18	Referent
30–34	0.9	16	1.5 (0.7–2.9)
≥35	0.8	10	1.3 (0.6–2.9)
Race			
White	38	0.5	Referent
Black and other	56	1.1	2.4 (1.6–3.6)
Parity[c]			
0	16	0.3	Referent
1–2	27	0.5	1.9 (1.0–3.5)
≥3	7	0.5	2.1 (0.9–5.2)
Gestational age (wk)[d]			
≤8	8	0.1	Referent
9–10	5	0.2	1.4 (0.5–4.2)
11–12	6	0.4	3.4 (1.2–9.7)
13–15	15	1.7	14.7 (6.2–34.7)
16–20	19	3.4	29.5 (12.9–67.4)
≥21	15	8.9	76.6 (32.5–180.8)
Time period			
1972–1979	163	2.2	3.1 (2.4–4.0)
1980–1987	80	0.8	1.1 (0.8–1.4)
1988–1997	94	0.7	Referent

[a]Number of legal abortion-related deaths.
[b]Rate of legal abortion deaths as number per 100,000 abortions.
[c]Denominators for calculating rates by parity use previous live-birth data from abortion surveillance. Deaths with unknown parity are excluded.
[d]Deaths with unknown gestational age are excluded.
(From Bartlett LA, Berg CJ, Shulman HB, et al. Risk factors for legal induced abortion-related mortality in the United States. *Obstet Gynecol* 2004;103:729–737.

CONCLUSION

Abortion is the most frequent outcome of human conception; thus, management of abortion and its complications is an important responsibility for physicians. Chromosomal anomalies are the single most important cause of spontaneous abortion. For women with threatened abortion, use of ultrasonography and β-hCG monitoring can help predict the outcome of the pregnancy. Evacuation of the uterus in cases of fetal death is primarily for psychological rather than medical indications; either curettage or labor induction may be appropriate. Premature cervical dilation without labor is a poorly understood cause of spontaneous abortion. There is no uniform case definition and no valid diagnostic test. Randomized clinical trials reveal modest benefit of cervical cerclage on obstetric outcomes.

Small numbers of illegal abortions continue to occur in the United States. Legally induced abortion, however, is one of the most frequently performed—and one of the safest—operations in contemporary practice. Less than 1 per 100 of those having an abortion suffers a major complication, and less than 1 per 100,000 dies from causes associated with the procedure. The marketing of mifepristone in the United States for early abortion has broadened the options available to women, and use of misoprostol for cervical preparation before curettage represents important advances in gynecology.

BEST SURGICAL PRACTICES

- Management of spontaneous abortion includes expectant management, medical management with misoprostol, and suction curettage. Suction can be accomplished with a handheld syringe or an electric vacuum source. Patient preference can direct management plan in most cases.
- Diagnosis of cervical incompetence remains variable in consistency. Cerclage placement can be used in women with a history of repeated premature cervical dilation without labor. The MacDonald and Shirodkar cerclages are most common, with the MacDonald being technically easier to place.
- Septic abortion requires aggressive management. This includes obtaining intrauterine and blood cultures, administration of broad-spectrum antibiotics, and prompt surgical evacuation of the uterus.
- Suction curettage is the most frequent method of legal abortion in the United States. Manual vacuum aspiration is increasing in use. Both may safely be done in outpatient facilities.
- Preoperative medical evaluation for elective abortion should include patient's medical, surgical, and anesthetic history, confirmation of gestational age, and thorough counseling about all available options, including continuing pregnancy, adoption, and medical and surgical abortion. Abortion regulations vary by state and should be followed by providers.
- Cervical dilation necessary for suction curettage can be achieved with osmotic dilators, medical preparation with misoprostol, or manual dilation. If manual dilation is necessary, a variety of dilators are available. Gentle dilation is imperative in prevention of uterine perforation.
- The incidence of retained products of conception after suction curettage can be decreased if aspirated tissue is inspected for presence of fetal tissue or chorionic villi.

- Prophylactic antibiotic use is indicated when instruments are introduced into the uterus, as in suction curettage, manual-vacuum aspiration, and D&E.
- Medical abortion with mifepristone and misoprostol is a safe way to terminate early gestations. Two regimens exist: one approved by the FDA and another that reflects recent evidence in the literature. Either one, with thorough patient counseling, is appropriate. In order to be a candidate for medical abortion, a patient must be able to understand the regimen, have access to emergency care if needed, and be able to follow up to ensure completion of the procedure.
- Second-trimester pregnancy termination can be achieved by surgery with dilation and evacuation (D&E) or with medications to cause labor. D&E is generally safer and faster, but only in the hands of a properly trained physician. Intraoperative ultrasound can decrease operative time as well as complications. Adequate preoperative cervical preparation with laminaria is usually necessary. Special forceps are used to facilitate extraction of later gestations.
- Labor induction can be performed using hypertonic solutions, oxytocin, and prostaglandins ($PGF_{2\alpha}$, PGE_2, and misoprostol). The use of hypertonic solutions has decreased in recent decades because of the safety and ease of alternative medicines. Multiple regimens for prostaglandins exist; currently no one dose or route of administration has proved to be superior. Clinicians must weigh efficacy and speed of abortion against side effects like fever, nausea, vomiting, and diarrhea. Use of prostaglandins in women with scarred uteri remains a controversial topic.
- Complications of abortion include hemorrhage, cervical injury, uterine perforation, retained products, infection, anesthetic complications, and Rh sensitization. Morbidity and mortality from legal abortion is very rare.

Bibliography

Adler NE, David HP, Major BN, et al. Psychological responses after abortion. *Science* 1990;248:41.

Althuisius SM, Dekker GA, Hummel P, et al. Cervical incompetence prevention randomized cerclage trial: emergency cerclage with bed rest versus bed rest alone. *Am J Obstet Gynecol* 2003;189:907.

Althuisius SM, Dekker GA, Hummel P, et al. Final results of the Cervical Incompetence Prevention Randomized Cerclage Trial (CIPRACT): therapeutic cerclage with bed rest versus bed rest alone. *Am J Obstet Gynecol* 2001;185:1106.

Althuisius SM, Dekker GA, Van Geijn HP, et al. Cervical incompetence prevention randomized cerclage trial (CIPRACT): study design and preliminary results. *Am J Obstet Gynecol* 2000;183:823.

American College of Obstetricians and Gynecologists. *Cervical insufficiency.* ACOG Practice Bulletin No. 48. Washington, DC: American College of Obstetricians and Gynecologists; 2003.

American College of Obstetricians and Gynecologists. *Mifepristone for medical pregnancy termination.* ACOG Committee Opinion No. 245. Washington, DC: American College of Obstetricians and Gynecologists; 2000.

Ashok PW, Templeton A, Wagaarachchi PT, et al. Midtrimester medical termination of pregnancy: a review of 1002 consecutive cases. *Contraception* 2004;69:51.

Atrash HK, MacKay HT, Hogue CJR. Ectopic pregnancy concurrent with induced abortion: incidence and mortality. *Am J Obstet Gynecol* 1990;162:726.

Bartlett LA, Berg CJ, Shulman HB, et al. Risk factors for legal induced abortion-related mortality in the United States. *Obstet Gynecol* 2004;103:729.

Blanchard K, Winikoff B, Ellertson C. Misoprostol used alone for the termination of early pregnancy: review of the evidence. *Contraception* 1999;59:209.

Borgiba AF, Rodis JF, Hanlon W, et al. Second-trimester abortion by intramuscular 15-methyl-prostaglandin F_2 or intravaginal prostaglandin E_2 suppositories: a randomized trial. *Obstet Gynecol* 1995;85:697.

Borgotta L, Chen AY, Vragonic O, et al. A randomized controlled trial of addition of laminaria to misoprostol and hypertonic saline for second trimester induction abortion. *Contraception* 2005;72:358.

Bugalho A, Bique C, Almeida L, et al. Pregnancy interruption by vaginal misoprostol. *Gynecol Obstet Invest* 1993;36:226.

Chung TK, Lee DT, Cheung LP, et al. Spontaneous abortion: a randomized, controlled trial comparing surgical evacuation with conservative management using misoprostol. *Fertil Steril* 1999;71:1054.

Cnattinguis S, Signorello LB, Anneren G, et al. Caffeine intake and the risk of first-trimester spontaneous abortion. *N Engl J Med* 2000;343:1839.

Cockwell HA, Smith GN. Cervical incompetence and the role of emergency cerclage. *JOGC* 2005;27:123.

Creinin MD, Edwards J. Early abortion: surgical and medical options. *Curr Probl Obstet Gynecol Fertil* 1997;20:6.

Creinin MD, Fox MC, Teal S, et al. A randomized comparison of misoprostol 6 to 8 hours versus 24 hours after mifepristone for abortion. *Obstet Gynecol* 2004;103:851.

Creinin MD, Vittinghoff E. Methotrexate and misoprostol vs. misoprostol alone for early abortion: a randomized controlled trial. *JAMA* 1994;272:1190.

Creinin MD, Vittinghoff E, Keder L, et al. Methotrexate and misoprostol for early abortion: a multicenter trial. I: Safety and efficacy. *Contraception* 1996;53:321.

Cunningham FG, Leveno KL, Bloom SL, et al. *Williams obstetrics*. McGraw-Hill, New York: 2005.

Daskalakis GJ, Mesogitis SA, Papantoniou NE, et al. Misoprostol for second trimester pregnancy termination in women with prior cesarean section. *BJOG* 2005;115:97.

Doubilet PM, Benson CB, Chow JS. Long-term prognosis of pregnancies complicated by slow embryonic heart rates in early first trimester. *J Ultrasound Med* 1999;18:537.

Doyle NM, Monga, M. Role of ultrasound in screening patients at risk for preterm delivery. *Obstet Gynecol Clin North Am* 2004;31:125.

Edmonds DK, Lindsay KS, Miller JF, et al. Early embryonic mortality in women. *Fertil Steril* 1982;38:447.

Edwards J, Carson SA. New technologies permit safe abortion at less than six weeks' gestation and provide timely detection of ectopic gestation. *Am J Obstet Gynecol* 1997;176:1101.

El-Refaey H, Rajasekar D, Abdalla M, et al. Induction of abortion with mifepristone (RU-486) and oral or vaginal misoprostol. *N Engl J Med* 1995;332:983.

Finer LB, Frohwith LF, Dauphinee LA, et al. Reasons U.S. women have abortions: quantitative and qualitative perspectives. *Perspect Sex Reprod Health* 2005;37(3):110.

Finer LB, Henshaw SK. Abortion incidence and services in the United States in 2000. *Perspect Sex Reprod Health* 2003;35(1):6.

Goldberg AB, Dean G, Kang MS, et al. Manual versus electric vacuum aspiration for early first-trimester abortion: a controlled study of complication rates. *Obstet Gynecol* 2004;103:101.

Goldberg AB, Drey EA, Whitaker AK, et al. Misoprostol compared with laminaria before early second-trimester surgical abortion: a randomized trial. *Obstet Gynecol* 2005;106:234.

Grossman D, Ellertson C, Grimes DA, et al. Routine follow-up visits after first-trimester induced abortion. *Obstet Gynecol* 2004;103:738.

Hamoda H, Ashok PW, Flett GM, et al. Medical abortion at 64 to 91 days of gestation: a review of 483 consecutive cases. *Am J Obstet Gynecol* 2003;188:1315.

Harper CC, Henderson JT, Darney PD. Abortion in the United States. *Annu Rev Public Health* 2005;26:501.

Jackson RA, Teplin VL, Drey EA, et al. Digoxin to facilitate late second-trimester abortion: a randomized, masked, placebo-controlled trial. *Obstet Gynecol* 2001;97:471.

Jain JK, Mishell DR Jr. A comparison of intravaginal misoprostol with prostaglandin E_2 for termination of second-trimester pregnancy. *N Engl J Med* 1994;331:290.

Kochanek KD, Murphy SL, Anderson RN, et al. *Deaths: final data for 2002, National Vital Statistics Report.* Vol. 53, No. 5. Hyattsville, MD: National Center for Health Statistics, 2004.

Koonin LM, Strauss LT, Chrisman CE, et al. Abortion surveillance: United States, 1997. In: CDC Surveillance Summaries, December 8, 2000. *MMWR Morb Mortal Wkly Rep* 2000;49 (no. SS-11):1.

Lawson HW, Frye A, Atrash HK, et al. Abortion mortality, United States, 1972 through 1987. *Am J Obstet Gynecol* 1994;171:1365.

Levi CS, Lyons EA, Zheng XH, et al. Endovaginal US: demonstration of cardiac activity in embryos of less than 5.0 mm in crown-rump length. *Radiology* 1990;176:71.

Lichtenberg ES, Paul M, Jones H. First trimester surgical abortion practices: a survey of National Abortion Federation members. *Contraception* 2001;64(6):345.

Luise C, Jermy K, May C, et al. Outcome of expectant management of spontaneous first trimester miscarriage: observational study. *BMJ* 2002;324:873.

MacDorman MF, Hoyert DL, Martin JA, et al. Fetal and Perinatal Mortality, United States, 2003. National vital statistics reports; Vol 55, no. 6. Hyattsville, MD: National Center for Health Statistics. 2007.

Mills JL, Simpson JL, Driscoll SG, et al. Incidence of spontaneous abortion among normal women and insulin-dependent diabetic women whose pregnancies were identified within 21 days of conception. *N Engl J Med* 1988;319:1618.

MRC/RCOG Working Party on Cervical Cerclage. Final report of the Medical Research Council/Royal College of Obstetricians and Gynaecologists Multicentre Randomized Trial of Cervical Cerclage. *BJOG* 1993;100:516.

National Abortion Federation. *Early medical abortion with mifepristone or methotrexate: overview and protocol recommendations*. Washington, D.C.: National Abortion Federation, 2001.

Ness RB, Grisso JA, Hirshinger, et al. Cocaine and tobacco use and the risk of spontaneous abortion. *N Engl J Med* 1999;340:333.

Newhall EP, Winikoff B. Abortion with mifepristone and misoprostol: regimens, efficacy, acceptability and future directions. *Am J Obstet Gynecol* 2000;183:S44.

Ngai SW, Tang OS, Ho PC. Prostaglandins for induction of second-trimester termination and intrauterine death. *Best Pract Res Clin Obstet Gynaecol* 2003;17:765.

Nielsen S, Hahlin M. Expectant management of first-trimester spontaneous abortion. *Lancet* 1995;345:84.

Nybo Anderson MA, Wohlfahrt J, Christens P, et al. Maternal age and fetal loss: population based register linkage study. *BMJ* 2000;320:1708.

Osborn JF, Arisi E, Spinelli A, et al. General anaesthesia: a risk factor for complication following induced abortion? *Eur J Epidemiol* 1990;6:416.

Owen J, Hauth JC, Winkler CL, et al. Midtrimester pregnancy termination: a randomized trial of prostaglandin E_2 versus concentrated oxytocin. *Am J Obstet Gynecol* 1992;167:1112.

Paul M, Lichtenberg ES, Borgatta L, et al. *A physician's guide to medical and surgical abortion*. New York: Churchill Livingstone, 1999.

Peyron R, Aubeny E, Targosz V, et al. Early termination of pregnancy with mifepristone (RU-486) and the orally active prostaglandin misoprostol. *N Engl J Med* 1993;328:1509.

Rasch V. Cigarette, alcohol, and caffeine consumption: risk factors for spontaneous abortion. *Acta Obstet Gynecol Scand* 2003;82:182.

Rashbaum WK, Gates EJ, Jones J, et al. Placenta accreta encountered during dilation and evacuation in the second trimester. *Obstet Gynecol* 1995;85:701.

Regan L, Braude PR, Trembath PL. Influence of past reproductive performance on risk of spontaneous abortion. *BMJ* 1989;299:541.

Regan L, Rai R. Epidemiology and the medical causes of miscarriage. *Baillieres Best Pract Res Clin Obstet Gynaecol* 2000;14:839.

Remennick LI. Induced abortion as cancer risk factor: a review of epidemiological evidence. *J Epidemiol Community Health* 1990;44:259.

Saraiya M, Green CA, Berg CJ, et al. Spontaneous abortion–related deaths among women in the United States: 1981–1991. *Obstet Gynecol* 1999;94:172.

Sawaya GF, Grady D, Kerlikowske K, et al. Antibiotics at the time of induced abortion: the case for universal prophylaxis based on a meta-analysis. *Obstet Gynecol* 1996;87:884.

Schaff EA, Fielding SL, Westhoff C. Randomized trial of oral versus vaginal misoprostol 2 days after mifepristone 200 mg for abortion up to 63 days of pregnancy. *Contraception* 2002;66:247.

Schaff EA, Fielding SL, Westhoff C, et al. Vaginal misoprostol administered 1, 2, or 3 days after mifepristone for early medical abortion: a randomized trial. *JAMA* 2000;284:1948.

Schaff EA, Wortman M, Eisinger SH, et al. Methotrexate and misoprostol when surgical abortion fails. *Obstet Gynecol* 1996;87:450.

Schreiber C, Creinin MD. Mifepristone in abortion care. *Semin Reprod Med* 2005;23:82.

Sharma S, Refaey H, Stafford M, et al. Oral versus vaginal misoprostol administered one hour before surgical termination of pregnancy: a randomized, controlled study. *BJOG* 2005;112(4):456.

Signorello LB, McLaughlin JK. Maternal caffeine consumption and spontaneous abortion: a review of the epidemiologic evidence. *Epidemiology* 2004;15:229.

Signorello LB, Nordmark A, Granath F, et al. Caffeine metabolism and the risk of spontaneous abortion of normal karyotype fetuses. *Obstet Gynecol* 2001;98:1059.

Singh K, Fong YF, Prasad RN, et al. Randomized trial to determine optimal dose of vaginal misoprostol for preabortion cervical priming. *Obstet Gynecol* 1998;92:795.

Sotiriadis A, Makrydimas G, Papatheodorou S, et al. Expectant, medical, or surgical management of first-trimester miscarriage: a meta-analysis. *Obstet Gynecol* 2005;105:1104.

Stephenson P, Wagner M, Badea M, et al. The public health consequences of restricted induced abortion: lessons from Romania. *Am J Public Health* 1992;82:1328.

Stotland NL. The myth of the abortion trauma syndrome. *JAMA* 1992;268:2078.

Strauss LT, Herndon J, Chang J, et al. Abortion surveillance—United States, 2001. *MMWR Morb Mortal Wkly Rep* 2004;53(9):1.

Strauss LT, Herndon J, Chang J, et al. Abortion surveillance: United States, 2002. In: CDC surveillance summaries, November 25, 2005. *MMWR Morb Mortal Wkly Rep* 2005;54(no. SS-7).

Stubblefield PG, Carr-Ellis S, Borgotta L. Methods for induced abortion. *Obstet Gynecol* 2004;104:174.

Tang OS, Ho PC. Medical abortion in the second trimester. *Best Pract Res Clin Obstet Gynaecol* 2002;16:237.

Taylor VM, Kramer MD, Vaughan TL, et al. Placenta previa in relation to induced and spontaneous abortion: a population-based study. *Obstet Gynecol* 1993;82:88.

To MS, Alfirecvic Z, Heath VC, et al. Cervical cerclage for prevention of preterm delivery in women with short cervix: randomized controlled trial. *Lancet* 2004;363:1849.

Townsend DE, Barbis SD, Mathews RD. Vasopressin and operative hysteroscopy in the management of delayed postabortion and postpartum bleeding. *Am J Obstet Gynecol* 1991;165:616.

Ulmann A, Silvestre L, Chemama L, et al. Medical termination of early pregnancy with mifepristone (RU-486) followed by a prostaglandin analogue: study in 16,369 women. *Acta Obstet Gynecol Scand* 1992;71:278.

Ventura SJ, Abma JC, Mosher WD, et al. Estimated pregnancy rates for the United States, 1990–2000: an update. *Natl Vital Stat Rep* 2004;52(23):1.

Von Hertzen H, Honkanen H, Piaggio G, et al. WHO multinational study of three misoprostol regimens after mifepristone for early medical abortion. I: Efficacy. *BJOG* 2003;110(9):808.

Wilcox AJ, Weinberg CR, O'Connor JF, et al. Incidence of early loss of pregnancy. *N Engl J Med* 1988;319:189.

Wang X, Chen C, Wang L, et al. Conception, early pregnancy loss, and time to clinical pregnancy: a population-based prospective study. *Fertil Steril* 2003,79:577.

Winkler CL, Gray SE, Hauth JC, et al. Mid-second-trimester labor induction: concentrated oxytocin compared with prostaglandin E_2 vaginal suppositories. *Obstet Gynecol* 1991;77:297.

Wisborg K, Kesmodel U, Henriksen TB, et al. A prospective study of maternal smoking and spontaneous abortion. *Acta Obstet Gynecol Scand* 2003;82:936.

World Health Organization. *Medical methods for termination of pregnancy*. WHO technical report series 871. Geneva: World Health Organization, 1997.

Yapar EG, Senoz S, Urkutur M, et al. Second trimester pregnancy termination including fetal death: comparison of five different methods. *Eur J Obstet Gynecol Reprod Biol* 1996;69:97.

Zhang J, Giles JM, Barnhart K, et al. A comparison of medical management with misoprostol and surgical management for early pregnancy failure. *N Engl J Med* 2005;353:761.

Zieman M, Fong SK, Benowitz NL, et al. Absorption kinetics of misoprostol with oral or vaginal administration. *Obstet Gynecol* 1997;90:88.

CHAPTER 34 ■ ECTOPIC PREGNANCY

MARK A. DAMARIO AND JOHN A. ROCK

DEFINITIONS

Abdominal pregnancy—A pregnancy that develops in the peritoneal cavity. Most abdominal pregnancies are secondary, the result of early tubal abortion or rupture with secondary implantation of the pregnancy into the peritoneal cavity. A primary abdominal pregnancy is one that implants directly into the peritoneal cavity.

Arias-Stella reaction—A reaction in endometrial cells associated (but not exclusively) with ectopic pregnancy, showing nuclear enlargement, irregularity, and hyperchromasia with cytoplasmic vacuolization.

β-hCG assay—A quantitative determination of the serum concentration of the human chorionic gonadotropin hormone obtained using a highly sensitive immunoassay that is specific for the β-subunit of human chorionic gonadotropin. Useful in the early diagnosis of ectopic pregnancy.

Cervical pregnancy—A pregnancy developing in the cervical canal below the level of the internal os.

Culdocentesis—Aspiration of fluid from the cul-de-sac (pouch of Douglas) via a needle puncturing the vaginal wall between the uterosacral ligaments.

Dilatation and curettage—A surgical procedure in which the endometrial cavity contents are removed and submitted for histologic study. Useful in the early diagnosis of ectopic pregnancy when β-hCG assays and transvaginal ultrasonography are nondiagnostic and a nonviable pregnancy is suspected.

Ectopic pregnancy—A pregnancy that develops following implantation anywhere other than the endometrial cavity of the uterus.

Heterotopic pregnancy—Combined intrauterine and extrauterine pregnancy.

Interstitial pregnancy—A pregnancy developing in the interstitial portion of the oviduct.

Laparoscopy—A surgical technique that allows for both diagnosis and treatment of an ectopic pregnancy. Remains as the "gold standard" method of diagnosis.

Ovarian pregnancy—A pregnancy developing in the ovary. Criteria for diagnosis includes the following: (i) the ipsilateral tube is intact and clearly separate from the ovary, (ii) the gestational sac definitely occupies the normal position of the ovary, (iii) the sac is connected to the uterus by the uteroovarian ligament, and (iv) ovarian tissue is unquestionably demonstrated in the wall of the sac.

Persistent ectopic pregnancy—Continued presence of viable trophoblastic tissue after conservative surgical treatment of an unruptured ectopic pregnancy. The typical presentation includes persistence of β-hCG concentrations that do not fall appropriately following conservative surgery.

Salpingotomy—Operative opening made in the oviduct that is used to remove an unruptured tubal pregnancy for the purpose of retaining the oviduct.

Salpingectomy—Operative removal of an oviduct.

Serum progesterone assay—A quantitative determination of the serum concentration of progesterone hormone. Useful in the early diagnosis of ectopic pregnancy.

Transvaginal ultrasonography—Ultrasound imaging of the female pelvis using an endoscopic probe placed in the vagina. Useful in the early diagnosis of an ectopic pregnancy.

Tubal pregnancy—The most common type of ectopic pregnancy. May involve the ampullary, fimbrial, or isthmic portion of the oviduct.

Ectopic pregnancy was first recognized in 1693 by Busiere when he was examining the body of a prisoner executed in Paris. Gifford of England made a more complete report in 1731 that described the condition of a fertilized ovum implanted outside the uterine cavity. Ectopic pregnancy has since become recognized as one of the more serious complications of pregnancy. One of the leading causes of maternal morbidity and mortality in the United States, it still accounted for 6% of all maternal deaths from 1991 to 1999, according to the Centers for Disease Control and Prevention (CDC). Despite significant advances in diagnosis and treatment, ectopic pregnancy remains the leading cause of maternal death in the first trimester.

Today, early diagnosis of ectopic pregnancy is possible with highly sensitive and rapid β-human chorionic gonadotropin (β-hCG) assays and the aid of advanced vaginal ultrasonographic equipment. The benefit of early diagnosis is that expectant medical therapy or conservative surgery becomes possible. Conservative management in the case of a small ectopic pregnancy that is present without rupture is usually successful when preservation of the oviduct to maintain or enhance fertility is important. Physicians should maintain a high index of suspicion for ectopic pregnancy and should be cognizant of the importance of early diagnosis and early intervention. This chapter summarizes the contemporary methods for diagnosis and treatment of ectopic pregnancy.

EPIDEMIOLOGY OF ECTOPIC PREGNANCY

Although the total number of pregnancies has declined over the past three decades, the rate of ectopic pregnancy has continued to increase in most western nations. In the United States, the incidence of ectopic pregnancy has increased from 4.5 per 1,000 pregnancies in 1970 to 19.7 per 1,000 pregnancies in 1992 (the last year for which national data are available). In Norway, an increase from 12.5 to 18.0 per 1,000 pregnancies was reported from 1976 to 1993. One contributing factor for the rising ratio of extrauterine to intrauterine pregnancies is felt to be the rising incidence of sexually transmitted diseases as well as the efficacy of modern antibiotic treatments for pelvic inflammatory disease (PID). A second factor may be the increased ability to detect the disease. Although the risk of death from ectopic pregnancy continues to decline among all races and ages in the United States, women of black and other minority races remain at significantly increased risk of death from ectopic pregnancy compared with white women. Although the overall incidence of ectopic pregnancy in the United States during 1970 to 1989 increased approximately fivefold, the risk of death from ectopic pregnancy declined by 90%. This decline in mortality from ectopic pregnancies may be related both to the increased awareness of the condition as well as improved diagnostic and therapeutic methods.

PATHOLOGY

A tubal gestation traditionally has been defined as one that implants and grows within the tubal lumen. Budowick and associates have suggested that tubal implantation actually occurs in the lumen but is soon followed by penetration into the lamina propria and muscularis to become extraluminal. Pauerstein and colleagues demonstrated that trophoblastic infiltration can be predominantly intraluminal or predominantly extraluminal, or, occasionally, mixed. It is impossible to ascertain in the operating room the predominant pattern of growth of a given tubal pregnancy. In any event, fimbrial expression usually is an unacceptable method for removal of ectopic pregnancy. Not only is the method traumatic, but it frequently does not remove all of the trophoblastic tissue. The resultant persistent ectopic pregnancy may therefore require additional therapy.

ETIOLOGY OF ECTOPIC PREGNANCY

Tubal Damage Secondary to Inflammation

Both the increased incidence of sexually transmitted disease resulting in salpingitis and the efficacy of antibiotic therapy in preventing total tubal occlusion after an episode of salpingitis are related to the increasing incidence of ectopic pregnancy. Levin and associates have demonstrated that the risk of ectopic pregnancy is increased in women with a primary history of PID. Westrom compared women with PID confirmed by laparoscopy with healthy women, matched by age and parity, and found a sixfold greater incidence of ectopic pregnancy in women with PID, an alarming rate of 1 ectopic pregnancy out of every 24 gestations. Similar statistics have been reported by other authors. Many of the patients in these studies had received antibiotic treatment for salpingitis.

Before antibiotics became available for the treatment of PID, salpingitis was usually so acute that the inflamed tube became totally occluded, and permanent sterility was the result. Women who attempted to conceive after a pelvic infection were successful less than 40% of the time. Today, the rate of pregnancy exceeds 60% for patients adequately treated with antibiotics. After initial appropriate treatment of an infection with antibiotics, agglutination of the cilia can still occur, and synechial bands can form within the tubal lumen to cause partial tubal obstruction. Westrom has demonstrated by laparoscopy that bilateral tubal occlusion occurs in approximately 12.8% of patients after treatment for the first tubal infection, in 35% after two infections, and in 75% after three or more infections. In addition, Westrom found that approximately 4% of all pregnancies subsequent to salpingitis were ectopic.

Fallopian tubes containing a gestation are frequently normal on macroscopic visualization and gross histologic examination. Vasquez and colleagues, using scanning electron microscopy and light microscopy studies of tubal biopsies from five groups of women, discovered marked differences in their ciliated surfaces. The proportion of ciliated cells was significantly lower in biopsy specimens taken from 25 women with tubal pregnancies as compared with biopsy specimens from seven women with intrauterine pregnancies at the same stage of gestation. Marked deciliation was likewise seen in eight women who had undergone biopsies during tubal reconstructive surgery. In another study, Gerard and colleagues found that seven of ten fallopian tube samples from patients with ectopic pregnancy were PCR positive for *C. trachomatis* DNA. Therefore, the increased occurrence of sexually transmitted diseases contributing to subclinical tubal epithelial damage may be an important contributor to ectopic pregnancy. Comprehensive programs to prevent sexually transmitted diseases undertaken in Sweden and Wisconsin have been found to not only decrease the incidence of *C. trachomatis* infections and other sexually transmitted diseases but also the rate of ectopic pregnancies.

Contraceptive Devices

The use of intrauterine devices (IUDs) has been associated with an increased incidence of ectopic pregnancy. In a summary of published reports on ectopic pregnancy, Tatum and Schmidt observed that 4% of the pregnancies that occurred with an IUD in place were ectopic. In a recent metaanalysis, Mol and associates reported a range of odds ratios from 4.2 to 45 from heterogenous studies of IUD use and ectopic pregnancy. Subtle tubal epithelial damage or actual PID episodes are likely responsible for the observed association between IUDs and ectopic pregnancy.

Oral Contraceptives

The overall risk of an ectopic pregnancy is lowered in women using oral contraceptives. When oral contraceptives fail, however, the risk of an ectopic pregnancy is slightly increased. This increase is presumed secondary to the inhibitory progestin effect on tubal motility. This hypothesis is supported by several studies implicating progestin-only oral contraceptives in the etiology of ectopic pregnancies.

Prior Tubal Surgery

An operative procedure on the oviduct, whether a sterilization procedure or tubal reconstructive surgery, can cause an ectopic pregnancy. The incidence of ectopic pregnancies occurring after neosalpingostomy for distal tubal obstruction ranges from 2% to 18% (Table 34.1). The rate of ectopic pregnancy after a microsurgical reversal of a sterilization procedure is only about 4%, presumably because the tubes have not been damaged by prior infection.

The United States Collaborative Review of Sterilization Working Group followed a total of 10,685 women undergoing tubal sterilization in a multicenter, prospective cohort study. The overall cumulative probability of pregnancy in the study cohort 10 years after sterilization was 18.5 per 1,000 procedures (failure rate of 1.85%). The 10-year cumulative probability of ectopic pregnancy for all methods of tubal sterilization was 7.3 per 1,000 procedures. From these data, one can therefore estimate that in the setting of a positive pregnancy following tubal sterilization, there is an approximately 40%

TABLE 34.1

SUMMARY: ECTOPIC PREGNANCY AFTER TUBAL SURGERY

Procedure	Technique	Total pregnancy (%)	Pregnancy range (%)	Ectopie (%)	Ectopic range (%)
Salpingoscopy	Macrosurgery	42	35–65	3.4	1–20
	Microsurgery	52	31–69	1.8	0–16
Fimbrioplasty	Macrosurgery	42	36–50	14	10–18
	Microsurgery	59	26–68	6	4–11
Neosalpingostomy	Macrosurgery	27	20–38	4.2	2–10
	Microsurgery	26	17–44	7.7	0–18
Tubal anastomosis	Macrosurgery	44	25–83	9.2	0–15
	Microsurgery	62	35–78	2.3	1–6.2
Removal of ectopic pregnancy	Salpingectomy	42	38–49	12	8–17
	Salpingostomy	57	39–73	11	0–20

(Lavy G, Diamond MP, DeCherney AH. Ectopic pregnancy: relationship to tubal reconstructive surgery. *Fertil Steril* 1987;47:543–556.)

risk that the pregnancy will be ectopic. The type of sterilization procedure and age of the patient at the time of sterilization appear to be relevant factors. Women sterilized by bipolar tubal coagulation before the age of 30 years had a probability of ectopic pregnancy that was 27 times as high as that of women of similar age who underwent postpartum partial salpingectomy (31.9 versus 1.2 ectopic pregnancies per 1,000 procedures). In addition, ectopic pregnancy was often seen many years after the sterilization procedure. The annual rates of ectopic pregnancy in the 4th through 10th years after sterilization were no lower than that seen in the first 3 years.

The pathophysiology of ectopic pregnancy after elective tubal sterilization is not clear. It is possible that a tuboperitoneal fistula in a previously coagulated segment of fallopian tube may allow spermatozoa to escape and reach the oocyte. Such fistulas have been demonstrated radiographically by Shah and colleagues in 11% of 150 women after laparoscopic electrocoagulation. Improper surgical technique (such as incomplete coagulation or misplacement of a mechanical device) may also influence the sterilization failure rate and incidence of ectopic pregnancy, although their likelihood is presumably low.

Assisted Reproductive Technologies

Ectopic pregnancies are known to occur with increased frequency after *in vitro* fertilization (IVF) and related techniques. The Society for Assisted Reproductive Technology (SART) reported that 2.1% of pregnancies established after IVF in the United States during 2000 were ectopic. Several theories have been proposed regarding the occurrence of ectopic implantation after transcervical intrauterine embryo transfer. Potential factors include the possibility of direct injection of embryos into the fallopian tube, uterine contractions provoked by the transfer catheter that propel the embryos retrograde, position or depth of the transfer catheter in the uterine cavity, and the volume of transfer medium. Verhulst and colleagues reported that tubal damage was a major risk factor. These researchers found that the ectopic pregnancy rate after IVF was significantly greater in patients with tubal disease (3.65% of pregnancies) than in those without tubal disease (1.19% of pregnancies). Strandell and associates found that a history of a previous ectopic pregnancy and a history of a previous myomectomy also appear to be risk factors for ectopic pregnancies following IVF.

Tummon and coworkers reported a 2% risk of heterotopic pregnancy in women undergoing IVF who had distorted tubal anatomy. This is about 100 to 200 times the reported incidence of combined intrauterine and extrauterine pregnancies occurring spontaneously. These authors also found that the risk of heterotopic pregnancy appeared to increase proportionately with the number of embryos transferred.

Developmental Anomalies

Intramural polyps and tubal diverticula can block or alter tubal transport of fertilized ova. Congenital absence of segments of the fallopian tube with peritoneal fistulas can also predispose to tubal pregnancy. Women exposed to diethylstilbestrol (DES) in utero are at higher risk of ectopic pregnancy. These women may have absent or minimal fimbriae and fallopian tubes that are shorter and thinner than normal.

Other Causal Factors

Several studies have demonstrated that cigarette smoking seems to be an independent, dose-related risk factor for ectopic pregnancy. Other lifestyle factors, such as multiple sex partners and early age at first intercourse, are associated with an increased risk. Vaginal douching has also been associated with a slightly increased risk of ectopic pregnancy, probably by increasing the overall risk of pelvic infections and resultant tubal damage. A summary of risk factors related to ectopic pregnancy is summarized in Table 34.2.

SITES OF ECTOPIC PREGNANCY

About 95% of extrauterine implantations occur in the oviduct. About 55% of these tubal implantations occur in the ampulla, the most common site: Implantation in the isthmic portion accounts for 20% to 25%, implantation in the infundibulum and fimbria accounts for 17%, and implantation in the interstitial segment (cornua) accounts for 2% to 4%. Ectopic implantations occur less often in the ovary, the cervix, and the peritoneal cavity (Fig. 34.1).

Walters and colleagues reported that 16% of tubal pregnancies result from a contralateral ovulation. Transmigration

TABLE 34.2

RISK FACTORS FOR ECTOPIC PREGNANCY

Chronic pelvic inflammatory disease
Prior tubal surgery
Surgical sterilization
Use of an intrauterine device
Previous ectopic pregnancy
Diethylstilbestrol (DES) exposure
Progestin-only contraceptives
Assisted reproductive technologies
Infertility
Developmental tubal anomalies
Multiple sex partners
Early age at first intercourse
Cigarette smoking
Vaginal douching

of the ovum in the peritoneal cavity can occur because the oviducts and ovaries may be situated close together in the cul-de-sac. Alternatively, this phenomenon could also result from transmigration of the embryo through the endometrial cavity into the opposite oviduct.

EFFECTS OF ECTOPIC PREGNANCY ON FUTURE REPRODUCTION

Tubal pregnancy is associated with a poor prognosis for subsequent reproduction. In most cases, an extrauterine pregnancy represents an impairment of the fertilized ovum's ability to migrate through the deep rugae of the oviduct as a result of altered tubal function. The morphologic abnormality is usually bilateral and irreversible, and can produce repeated ectopic pregnancies or permanent sterility. In a 1975 study, Shoen and Nowak concluded that about 70% of patients who have an ectopic first pregnancy are unable to produce a living child. As many as 30% of the patients who have an ectopic first pregnancy will have a repeat ectopic pregnancy, which compares with the total repeat ectopic rate of 10% to 15% for the overall population of reproductive-age women. More than half of the subsequent extrauterine pregnancies will occur within a 2-year period, and 80% will occur within 4 years of the initial ectopic pregnancy. In reviewing the experience of the Kaiser Foundation hospitals, Hallatt reported a 9.2% overall incidence of repeat ectopic pregnancies among 1,330 women who had extrauterine pregnancies. The potential reproductive capacity for a patient who has had an ectopic pregnancy therefore depends on her reproductive history. If an ectopic pregnancy was the result of her first reproductive effort, then the prognosis for future pregnancies is much worse than if the complication occurred after one or more successful pregnancies.

Mueller and associates have estimated that 92% of infertility in women who have had a tubal pregnancy results from tubal damage that is due to the tubal pregnancy itself or other factors that had predisposed to its occurrence. A history of infertility itself is a risk factor for ectopic pregnancy. A twofold increase in the risk of tubal pregnancy exists among infertile women with no evident abnormality during infertility evaluation.

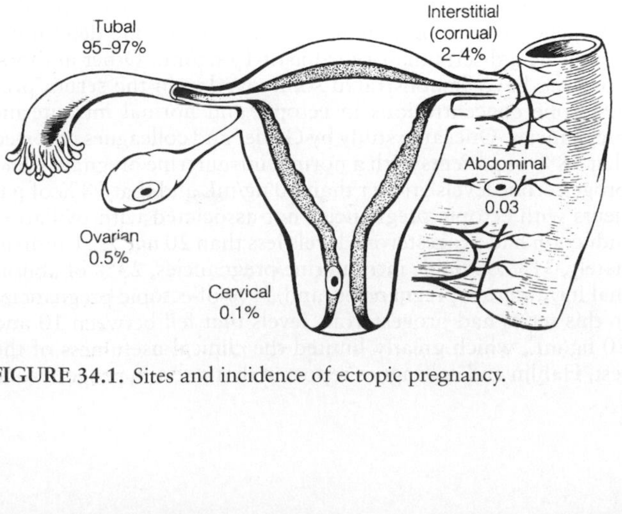

FIGURE 34.1. Sites and incidence of ectopic pregnancy.

TUBAL ECTOPIC PREGNANCY

The morbidity and mortality associated with extrauterine pregnancy are directly related to the length of time required for diagnosis. In a CDC survey, two thirds of all patients who were later proven to have an ectopic pregnancy were previously seen by a physician, and either the diagnosis was deferred or the condition was incorrectly assessed. The mortality rate from an ectopic pregnancy is higher in rural areas, where patients are less likely to receive early medical care.

For a successful outcome, an ectopic pregnancy must be diagnosed early. In some clinics where the condition is treated frequently, more than 50% of cases are diagnosed and treated before tubal rupture occurs. In some cases, however, the symptoms that bring a patient to seek medical care are caused by an already leaking or ruptured ectopic pregnancy. As many as 15% of all tubal pregnancies rupture before the first missed menstrual period, particularly if a patient's usual menstrual pattern is very irregular.

Diagnostic accuracy is often improved in repeat ectopic pregnancies. The vast majority of patients with repeat ectopic pregnancies will be diagnosed and treated before tubal rupture. A difference with a repeat ectopic pregnancy is that the patient herself often raises the question of an extrauterine pregnancy. Being suspicious, the patient may seek medical care earlier and provides a more specific medical history than does a patient experiencing her first ectopic pregnancy. The result is often an earlier diagnosis and an improved chance for a successful outcome.

Some form of vaginal bleeding occurs around the expected time of menses in more than 50% of women with an ectopic pregnancy, so that many patients and their physicians are unaware that a pregnancy has occurred. The vaginal bleeding may be followed by a period of amenorrhea. Clinical symptoms of an ectopic pregnancy usually appear 6 to 10 weeks after the last normal menstrual period.

DIAGNOSIS

Classic Symptoms: Pain, Bleeding, and Adnexal Mass

The classic presentation of pain and uterine bleeding with the finding of an adnexal mass has been the clinical hallmark of an extrauterine pregnancy, but even classic presentations can be misleading. Schwartz and DiPietro observed that of the patients who presented with the classic signs and symptoms, only 14% had an ectopic pregnancy. The severity of the symptoms and signs depends on the stage of the condition, but in the early stages of an ectopic gestation, symptoms are less predictive than in the more advanced stages of the disease. A discrete, unilateral mass separate from the adjacent ovary has been detected in less than one third of all proven ectopic pregnancies. Locating a mass depends on many factors, including the diagnostic skill of the examiner, the degree of pelvic peritonitis present, the presence or absence of tubal rupture, and the degree of stoicism and cooperation of the patient. Even when all factors are optimal, an adnexal mass can be felt in only half of the cases.

Diagnostic Studies

Three major advances have made early diagnosis of extrauterine pregnancy possible: (i) the development of highly sensitive and rapid β-hCG assays; (ii) the ability to use ultrasound to evaluate the uterus and the adnexa (vaginal sonography further increases the accuracy of diagnosis); and (iii) the application of laparoscopy as a diagnostic tool. Culdocentesis or suction curettage, or both, can be useful under certain circumstances (e.g., to help establish the presence of a hemoperitoneum or a nonviable intrauterine pregnancy, respectively). Other newer diagnostic methods, such as serum progesterone assays or color Doppler flow analyses, can also provide useful information.

β-hCG Assays

The principal endocrine marker of pregnancy is human chorionic gonadotropin (hCG), which is synthesized by the trophoblast. Human chorionic gonadotropin is a glycoprotein consisting of two subunits: α and β. The α subunit has significant homology with other glycoprotein hormones, such as follicle-stimulating hormone, luteinizing hormone, and thyroid-stimulating hormone. The β-subunit, on the other hand, is specific to hCG, and antibodies against the β-subunit form the basis for current immunoassays. Current commercial automated β-hCG immunoassays use enzyme fluorimetry, enzyme spectrometry, or chemiluminescence methods, as opposed to the traditional radioimmunoassay methods commonly used in the past. A immunoassay for β-hCG can detect levels of hCG as low as 5 IU/L of serum with less than a 0.2% incidence of false-negative results. β-hCG can be detected in maternal serum as early as 7 to 8 days after ovulation, or approximately the day after blastocyst implantation.

The quantification of serum β-hCG levels is useful in determining the viability of pregnancy. To optimally use β-hCG data in treating a patient with a problematic pregnancy, one should first have a thorough understanding of the particular assay used. The World Health Organization has established reference standards for β-hCG assays. The Third or Fourth International Standards (Third or Fourth IS) are the most commonly used reference standards used by the available commercial kits of today. These standards are roughly equivalent to the First International Reference Preparation (First IRP), but are quite a bit different from the Second International Standard (Second IS). The Second IS contains about 20% intact hCG and was initially developed for use in hCG bioassays. One international unit of β-hCG based on the First IRP is equal to approximately 0.58 IU of β-hCG using the Second IS. Fortunately, the Second IS has been exhausted and is no longer used. The First IRP, Third IS, and Fourth IS are highly purified preparations that were developed to overcome the deficiencies seen in the use of a heterogeneous standard. This notwithstanding, due to the continuing variation of assay methodologies and β-hCG standards, there remains considerable between-method variation in β-hCG assay results.

Serum hCG concentrations increase in an exponential fashion in early pregnancy. During the period of gestation in which the hCG concentration is less than 10,000 IU/L (First IRP), or about 25 to 30 days postovulation, the time required for doubling of hCG levels remains constant, with a mean of 1.9 days. Kadar and colleagues reported that 87% of women with ectopic pregnancies and 15% of women with normal intrauterine pregnancies could expect to have hCG doubling times of more than 2.7 days when the hCG concentration measured less than 6,000 IU/L. The lower limits of the increase in serum hCG for viable intrauterine pregnancies have been established by Barnhart and colleagues in a large cohort study. In this study, the serial β-hCG titres of 287 women who presented with pain and/or bleeding in the first trimester and were ultimately diagnosed with a viable intrauterine pregnancy were evaluated. For viable intrauterine gestations less than 10 weeks from last menstrual period or those with an initial β-hCG titre less than 5,000 mIU/mL, the investigators noted that the curve generated for serial hCG concentrations best fit a log-linear model. Overall, β-hCG concentrations tended to double every 2 days. The median rise of hCG after 1 day was 50% and after 2 days was 124%. The slowest or minimal rise for a normal viable intrauterine pregnancy, however, was 24% at 1 day and 53% at 2 days. Interval β-hCG determinations interpreted within the context of several values can therefore be of prognostic significance in the differentiation between normal intrauterine versus extrauterine pregnancies. A normal rise in hCG production, however, does not always differentiate an ectopic from a viable intrauterine pregnancy. Shepherd and associates reported that, in their experience, a normal rise in hCG production did not reliably differentiate an ectopic from a viable intrauterine pregnancy in the symptomatic patient. Early ectopic pregnancies can initially secrete appropriate amounts of hCG because of a well-vascularized placental bed.

Serum Progesterone Assay

Serum progesterone levels reflect the production of progesterone by the corpus luteum in early pregnancy. During the first 8 to 10 weeks of gestation, serum progesterone concentrations change little; as pregnancy fails, the levels decrease. Matthews and colleagues reported progesterone levels in 29 patients with ectopic pregnancy using a direct radioimmunoassay that offers results within 4 hours. Patients with normal intrauterine pregnancies had serum progesterone levels greater than 20 ng/mL, and all patients with ectopic pregnancies had progesterone levels less than 15 ng/mL. Yeko and associates proposed that all ectopic pregnancies could be potentially diagnosed at the first emergency visit with a single serum progesterone determination using a discriminatory value of 15 ng/mL. Other authors, however, have demonstrated some overlap in the serum progesterone concentrations in ectopic and normal intrauterine pregnancies. One large study by Gelder and colleagues reported that 98% of patients with a normal intrauterine pregnancy had progesterone levels greater than 10 ng/mL and that 98% of patients with ectopic pregnancies not associated with ovulation induction had progesterone levels less than 20 ng/mL. Unfortunately, 31% of viable intrauterine pregnancies, 23% of abnormal intrauterine pregnancies, and 51% of ectopic pregnancies in this series had progesterone levels that fell between 10 and 20 ng/mL, which greatly limited the clinical usefulness of the test. Hahlin and colleagues reported that a serum progesterone value of less than 9.4 ng/mL combined with an abnormal hCG increase had a positive predictive value of 1.0 for pathologic pregnancy. In 1992, Stovall and colleagues reported that in a group of more than 1,000 first-trimester pregnant patients, the lowest serum progesterone level associated with a viable pregnancy was 5.1 ng/mL. Therefore, these investigators established the lower cutoff limit of serum progesterone levels of 5 ng/mL; patients below this threshold had a nonviable pregnancy with 100% certainty and therefore underwent curettage. Patients with serum progesterone levels greater than 25 ng/mL had a 97% likelihood of having a viable intrauterine pregnancy in this study.

Transvaginal Ultrasonography

Pelvic ultrasound has revolutionized the diagnostic process of ectopic pregnancy. Transvaginal ultrasonography, in particular, may identify masses in the adnexa as small as 10 mm in diameter and can provide more detail about the character of the mass than clinical exam (Fig. 34.2). At the same time, transvaginal ultrasonography can evaluate the contents of the endometrial cavity and can document the presence of a viable intrauterine pregnancy with great accuracy. In addition, transvaginal ultrasonography allows for the simultaneous assessment for the presence of free peritoneal fluid.

Transvaginal ultrasonography is usually considered superior to transabdominal ultrasonography in the diagnosis of ectopic pregnancy. Although the latter provides a broader perspective of the abdominal cavity and pelvis, transvaginal ultrasonography generally provides better resolution of the internal female genitalia. A 5-MHz transvaginal transducer allows for a deeper penetration of the pelvis than transducers of higher frequency, whereas a 7.5-MHz transvaginal transducer provides for better near-resolution at the cost of shallower penetration. On rare occasions, an ectopic pregnancy may be located beyond the reach of the transvaginal transducer's scanning field. On these particular occasions, incorporation of transabdominal ultrasonography may be an important adjunctive step.

Jain and colleagues compared endovaginal and transabdominal ultrasound results in 90 patients with a positive serum pregnancy test (Table 34.3). The specific diagnosis of ectopic pregnancy was impossible using only transabdominal ultrasound before 7 gestational weeks. Normal intrauterine pregnancies could be detected earlier with endovaginal ultrasound because the yolk sac, fetal pole, and fetal heart motion could be seen sooner. Fetal heart motion was detected as early as 34 days after the last menstrual period in patients with identifiable fetal poles at the time the crown-to-rump length was 0.3 cm.

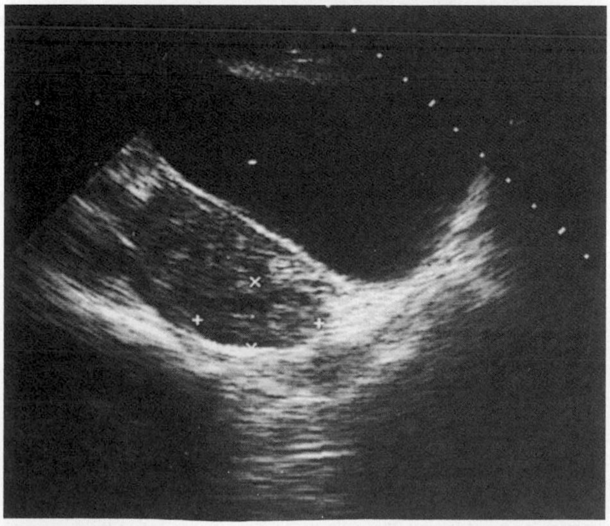

FIGURE 34.2. Tubal ectopic pregnancy documented by endovaginal sonography.

Although diagnosis by transvaginal ultrasound can be quite useful, it may at times be confusing. One problem is that a pseudogestational sac that is due to a decidual cast can be mistaken for an amniotic sac. A useful differentiating feature is the "double-line" image, caused by the faint hypoechoic decidual lining of the uterus and the hyperechogenic rim of the trophoblast surrounding the gestational sac. The double-line image can be seen as early as 5 weeks after the last menstrual period. Even in the presence of the double-line image, however, it is important to further follow the course of pregnancy and subsequently confirm a viable intrauterine pregnancy with the ascertainment of ultrasonographically imaged intrauterine cardiac motion.

Although not always seen, Frates and Laing reported that the presence of a noncystic extraovarian adnexal mass, extrauterine cardiac motion, or a "tubal ring" by transvaginal ultrasonography is highly specific for ectopic pregnancy (98.9%), with a high positive predictive value (96.3%). These authors described that the direct imaging of the ectopic pregnancy using any of these differentiating features is possible in 84% of cases.

Many authors have reported on correlations between threshold levels of hCG above which an intrauterine gestational sac is expected by ultrasonography in a normal pregnancy (discriminatory zone). Early on, Kadar and colleagues described a threshold level of hCG above which an intrauterine gestational sac was expected by abdominal sonography in a normal

TABLE 34.3

PREGNANCY EARLIEST SEEN WITH ULTRASONOGRAPHY

Early intrauterine pregnancy	Endovaginal	Transabdominal
Gestational sac seen		
Gestational sac size	0.5 cm	0.5 cm
Gestational sac age	4.3 wk	4.3 wk
Double decidual outline		
Gestational sac size	0.6–0.7 cm	1.0 cm
Gestational sac age	4.4 wk	5.0 wk
Yolk sac seen		
Gestational sac size	0.7 cm	1.0 cm
Gestational sac age	4.6 wk (34 d)	5.0 wk (35 d)
Fetal pole seen		
Gestational sac size	0.7 cm	1.7 cm
Gestational sac age	4.6 wk	6.0 wk
Fetal heart motion seen		
Crown–rump length	0.3 cm	0.6 cm
Gestational sac age	4.6 wk (34 d)	.5 wk (47 d)

(Jain K, Hamper VM, Sanders RC. Comparison of transvaginal and transabdominal sonography in the detection of early pregnancy and its complications. *Am J Radiol* 1988;151:1139.)

pregnancy (discriminatory zone). This threshold hCG level was initially characterized as a titer of 6,500 IU/L or higher using the First IRP. Presently, transvaginal ultrasonography reliably detects intrauterine gestations as early as 1 week after missed menses (β-hCG >1,500 IU/L; 5–6 weeks' gestation). Barnhart and associates reported that with a β-hCG concentration of 1,500 IU/L or higher, an empty uterus on transvaginal ultrasonography identified an ectopic pregnancy with 100% accuracy. Even using a discriminatory serum β-hCG concentration of 1,000 IU/L, Cacciatore and associates identified an intrauterine gestation in all intrauterine pregnancies and in none of the ectopic pregnancies. Furthermore, these investigators reported that the detection of an adnexal mass in combination with an empty uterus had a sensitivity of 97%, specificity of 99%, positive predictive value of 98%, and negative predictive value of 98%, provided that serum β-hCG concentrations exceeded 1,000 IU/L. The coupling of hCG titers with transvaginal ultrasonographic findings has therefore greatly facilitated the early diagnosis of ectopic gestation. It must be stressed, however, that considering the variations in β-hCG assays, ultrasound equipment, and sonographer experience, each institution must determine their own discriminatory thresholds for the sonographic detection of an intrauterine pregnancy.

The advent of color-flow Doppler technology may even further improve the accuracy of noninvasive diagnostic methods. Kurjak and colleagues reported that ectopic pregnancies are characterized by the identification of peritrophoblastic flow associated with an adnexal mass by color Doppler techniques. Kirchler and coworkers showed that color Doppler qualitative blood flow analyses of the tubal arteries can help localize the side of a tubal ectopic pregnancy. These investigators reported a between-side difference in tubal blood flow of 20% to 45%, with increased blood flow seen on the side of the ectopic pregnancy. Emerson and colleagues demonstrated that color-flow Doppler capability can help differentiate between viable intrauterine pregnancy, completed abortion, incomplete abortion, and ectopic pregnancy by analyzing uterine color Doppler appearance, intrauterine venous flow, the presence or absence of intrauterine peritrophoblastic flow, corpus luteal flow, and the presence or absence of peritrophoblastic flow in the adnexa. Pellerito and associates reported that color-flow imaging increased the sensitivity of detecting an ectopic pregnancy. Of 65 patients with surgically confirmed ectopic pregnancies, 36 (sensitivity 54%) cases were detected by endovaginal sonography alone, whereas 62 (sensitivity 95%) cases were detected by a combination of endovaginal sonography and color-flow imaging.

Dilation and Curettage

At one time, the histologic changes in the endometrium that accompany an ectopic gestation were routinely confirmed by dilatation and curettage (D&C). Today, more accurate diagnostic methods—such as the radioimmunoassay for β-hCG, transvaginal ultrasonography, and laparoscopy—exist. In this setting, a D&C may therefore not always be necessary. If, however, the plateau level of β-hCG is low, a D&C can be helpful to establish the presence of degenerating villi, and if a patient is bleeding excessively, a D&C may also be required. In either case, assessment of the removed material and findings of decidua without chorionic villi suggests the diagnosis of ectopic pregnancy. Such findings do not provide absolute proof, however, because they also occur with spontaneous abortion. To distinguish between an ectopic pregnancy and spontaneous abortion, Stovall and colleagues reported that if β-hCG concentrations did not decline $\geq$15% within 8 to 12 hours following curettage, an ectopic pregnancy was likely.

If available, a frozen section may be obtained immediately after curettage, providing an opportunity to confirm the diagnosis within minutes while the patient is still in the operating room under anesthesia. If no chorionic villi are present, further assessment and treatment by laparoscopy may be undertaken. In a recent report of 87 consecutive frozen section samples taken from uterine curettings, Spandorfer and colleagues found that 93.1% of these specimens were identified correctly after further analyses of the tissue by permanent section.

The atypical epithelial changes of the gestational endometrium in a case of tubal pregnancy were first described by Polak and Wolfe in 1924 and these changes were further expanded on by Arias-Stella in 1954 (Fig. 34.3). These comprise a highly controversial set of histologic criteria that depend, for accuracy, on the precise definition of the particular cell type involved in the morphologic change, together with ill-defined physiologic events that reportedly produce the changes. Arias-Stella and others were convinced that these histologic changes are a progressive phenomenon resulting from the exaggerated proliferative and secretory endometrial responses to the elevated hormonal levels of pregnancy. Lloyd and Fienberg disagreed, maintaining that these endometrial changes are regressive, involutional, and are the result of declining hormonal levels. Whichever hypothesis is ultimately proven, similar endometrial changes may be seen with a normal pregnancy, spontaneous abortion, or ectopic pregnancy. Histologic endometrial criteria, therefore, seems to have limited value in the specific diagnosis of extrauterine pregnancies.

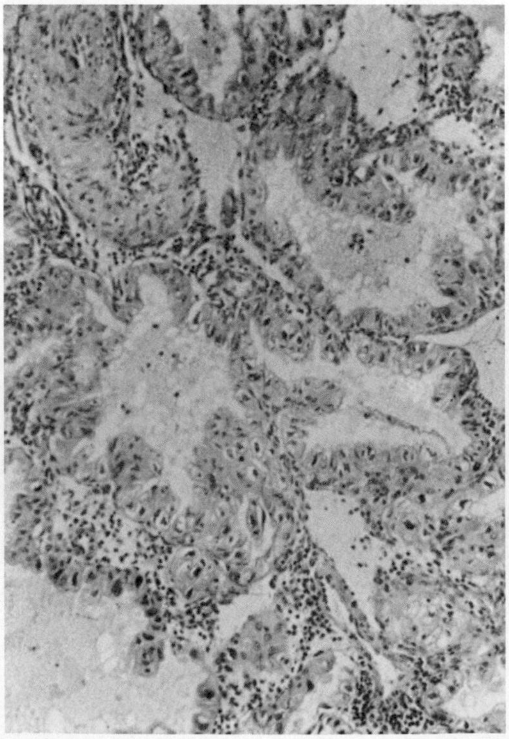

FIGURE 34.3. Arias-Stella reaction in endometrial cells associated with ectopic pregnancy, showing nuclear enlargement, irregularity, and hyperchromasia with cytoplasmic vacuolation.

Culdocentesis

Culdocentesis is a diagnostic tool for identifying the presence of intraperitoneal bleeding. This simple procedure of inserting an 18-gauge spinal needle attached to a 50-mL aspirating syringe into the cul-de-sac between the uterosacral ligaments (Fig. 34.4) provides immediate clinical information when unclotted blood is aspirated from the cul-de-sac. The procedure cannot be used for a definitive diagnosis, of course, because a tubal pregnancy may not have ruptured or leaked into the peritoneal cavity. In addition, a culdocentesis does not provide information concerning whether the blood is from an ectopic pregnancy or from some other cause of intraabdominal bleeding. The rupture of a corpus luteal hemorrhagic cyst, for instance, may cause a similar bleeding pattern.

The availability of sensitive transvaginal ultrasonographic technology presently limits the usefulness of the culdocentesis procedure, such that it is rarely presently performed. Free intraperitoneal blood has a characteristic ultrasonographic appearance and can be seen in nearly all cases in which a significant intraperitoneal hemorrhage has occurred. In the absence of the immediate availability of transvaginal ultrasonography or in an emergency setting, however, a culdocentesis may still be of value.

Laparoscopy

Laparoscopy remains the gold standard in the detection of ectopic pregnancy, although noninvasive diagnostic methods continue to improve. In addition to permitting the diagnosis of an ectopic pregnancy, it enables surgical treatment. Laparoscopy also provides an opportunity to visualize the entire pelvis and other peritoneal organs. In particular, the condition of the unaffected fallopian tube can be assessed, as well as the presence of pelvic adhesions and endometriosis. This information may be particularly valuable for those patients interested in future fertility. The disadvantage of laparoscopy is that it is an invasive procedure that carries some risk of complications. Using standard methods, it requires general anesthesia and an operating room setting, thereby contributing to increased medical costs. Recent investigators, however, have been exploring the potential of "microlaparoscopy," in which improved optics and smaller-diameter laparoscopes and trocars allow for a definitive diagnosis and possible treatment in the nonoperating room setting. Several authors have reported the encouraging use of microlaparoscopy in the office setting, using local rather than general anesthesia. The specific utility of microlaparoscopy, however, for the primary evaluation and treatment of ectopic pregnancy remains to be established.

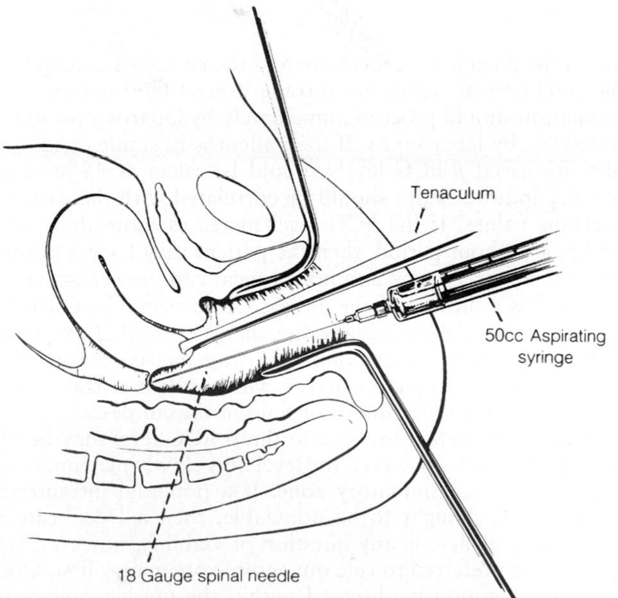

FIGURE 34.4. Culdocentesis. An 18-gauge spinal needle is inserted through the posterior fornix and enters the cul-de-sac between the uterosacral ligaments.

Laparoscopy may be useful when an ectopic pregnancy is suspected but no signs of an ultrasonographically visualized extrauterine gestational sac is evident. This includes situations in which there is an inability to visualize an intrauterine gestational sac and serial β-hCG determinations are rising inappropriately. This also includes situations in which a D&C fails to identify products of conception. One must be careful, however, in settings in which the β-hCG determinations are very low or the gestational age is limited. In these settings, the ectopically implanted gestational mass may be so small that it is still not able to be seen at laparoscopy. The clinician and patient might therefore be falsely reassured by negative laparoscopic findings. All patients without a definitive diagnosis established at laparoscopy should continue to be followed closely.

Other Potential Diagnostic Aids

Gleicher et al. described the use of hysterosalpingography and selective salpingography in differentiating early (biochemical) intrauterine from failing intratubal gestations. A characteristic tubal opacification pattern was seen in the cases of early tubal pregnancy. Confino and coworkers reported that selective salpingography was useful in diagnosing early tubal pregnancies in some patients with equivocal clinical, laboratory, and sonographic findings. In addition, these investigators injected a single dose of methotrexate through the selective salpingography catheter after cannulation of the tubal ostia and identification of a characteristic ampullary radiolucency in seven patients. Each had subsequent complete resolution of the pregnancy without complication. Risquez and colleagues reported the successful visualization of two ectopic pregnancies by transcervical tubal cannulation and falloposcopy. The falloposcope is a microendoscopic instrument 0.5 mm in external diameter that is introduced by a 1-mm coaxial catheter. Although limited by the presence of blood in the tubal lumen, direct visualization of the ectopic pregnancies was accomplished in both cases and confirmed by concurrent laparoscopy. Other investigative teams have explored the potential of other imaging methods, such as magnetic resonance imaging (MRI), in the diagnostic workup for ectopic pregnancy. MRI might be useful if the sonographic image is inconclusive, although it is likely to be rarely needed, particularly if laparoscopy is generally considered in uncertain cases.

Summary of Diagnostic Methods for Detecting Tubal Ectopic Pregnancy

When a patient is seen with a clinical history suggestive of ectopic pregnancy, a careful examination is performed (Fig. 34.5). Quantitative serum β-hCG and rapid serum progesterone levels (if available) are obtained. If the β-hCG titre is positive, a transvaginal ultrasound is performed. If an intrauterine sac is visualized with fetal heart activity, then the diagnosis of

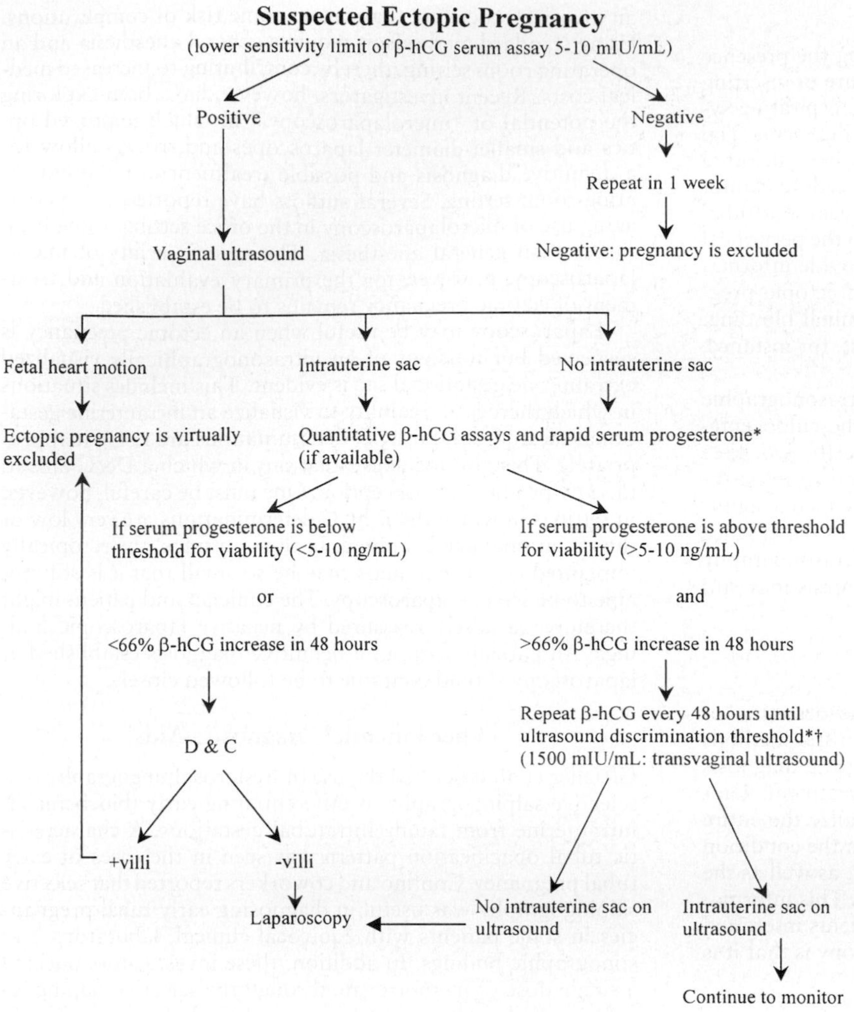

FIGURE 34.5. Evaluation of the stable patient with suspected ectopic pregnancy. Hormonal parameters can vary depending on the assay technique and reference standard used. The discriminatory threshold for sonographic detection of an intrauterine gestational sac must be established by each institution.

intrauterine pregnancy is established. If, however, there are no intrauterine sacs or there is a questionable intrauterine sac without fetal heart activity, then the asymptomatic patient may be expectantly treated awaiting further testing. If the serum progesterone level is, with certainty, below the threshold level for viability, then a uterine curettage can be performed. The subsequent failure to find chorionic villi on curettage is very suggestive, but not diagnostic, of an ectopic pregnancy. If the serum progesterone level is more than 25 ng/mL in the absence of ovulation induction, then there is a strong likelihood that a viable pregnancy is present. If the quantitative serum β-hCG level is above the discriminatory zone for a particular institution and no intrauterine gestational sacs are apparent using transvaginal ultrasonography, then an ectopic pregnancy is likely. The level of hCG at which an intrauterine gestational sac should be visible varies, however, depending on the β-hCG assay and the method of pelvic ultrasonography. Many contemporary investigators report that with transvaginal ultrasonography, an intrauterine gestational sac should be identified at a β-hCG level of 1,500 IU/L (Third or Fourth IS) with high sensitivity and specificity.

Commonly, results from initial testing are equivocal. The ectopic pregnancy can produce a low level of β-hCG from the aborting or degenerating trophoblast. The differential diagnosis should include spontaneous abortion or blighted ovum. When the diagnosis is uncertain and the patient is in an unstable condition or significant intraperitoneal fluid is seen, then evaluation should proceed immediately by laparoscopy and, if necessary, by laparotomy. If the patient is in stable condition, tests for serial β-hCG levels should be taken at 48-hour intervals, and the assays should be correlated with the patient's previous values. If the hCG level increases more than 50% within a 48-hour period, then the patient may have a normal intrauterine pregnancy and nonsurgical care (expectant management) is indicated. If the increase in the serial hCG level is less than 50% of the original value, then a nonviable pregnancy should be suspected. Ultrasound can often then corroborate the diagnosis of an ectopic pregnancy with the demonstration of a gestational sac in the adnexa or fluid in the cul-de-sac.

Initially, a normal increase in the β-hCG level may be observed. Over time, however, the level may slowly plateau, never reaching the discriminatory zone. If a potential intrauterine pregnancy is thought to be nonviable, then a D&C can be performed. If there is any question of viability, however, laparoscopy is preferred to rule out ectopic pregnancy first. Once fetal heart motion is observed within the uterine cavity, the possibility of a tubal ectopic pregnancy is virtually excluded. Certain patients should continue to be observed closely, however, particularly after a superovulation regimen, which is associated with an increased risk of a simultaneous intrauterine and ectopic pregnancy. Nevertheless, the overall risk of the two existing simultaneously even after a superovulation regimen is quite small.

The use of vaginal ultrasonography with improved resolution and the addition of color Doppler flow analysis will invariably further define a lower discriminatory zone in the future. Both modalities appear to complement each other in attaining improved sensitivity and specificity in the diagnosis of ectopic pregnancy. Other investigative diagnostic techniques, such as selective salpingography and falloposcopy, should be considered strictly experimental.

TREATMENT FOR ECTOPIC PREGNANCY

Expectant Therapy

Before the advent of effective therapy for ectopic pregnancy, it was noted that the condition was not uniformly fatal and that some patients had spontaneous resolution of the ectopic gestation, either through spontaneous regression or tubal abortion. The natural history of ectopic pregnancy therefore suggests that a number of tubal pregnancies can resolve without treatment. In 1988, Fernandez and associates reported a spontaneous resolution of ectopic pregnancy in 64% of carefully selected patients. The mean time for resolution was 20 ± 13 days. Spontaneous resolution occurred more frequently when the initial hCG concentration was less than 1,000 IU/L. The authors observed that a β-hCG threshold of 1,000 mIU/mL and a hemoperitoneum of less than 50 mL with a hematosalpinx of less than 2 cm appeared to be most compatible with successful expectant management.

Subsequent larger studies have demonstrated similar results with expectant therapy. Korhonen and colleagues have published the largest series to date. Criteria for patient selection included decreasing β-hCG levels, an absent intrauterine pregnancy by transvaginal ultrasonography, and an adnexal mass of less than 4 cm without an embryonic heartbeat. Seventy-seven (65%) of 118 patients had spontaneous resolution of the ectopic pregnancy. The remaining patients had laparoscopy for either increasing abdominal pain, increasing cul-de-sac fluid volume, or plateauing or increasing β-hCG levels. One patient required a salpingectomy for a ruptured ectopic pregnancy. Similar to other reports, these authors also noted an increased success rate with lower initial β-hCG concentrations.

Medical Treatment

Systemic Medical Therapy

Methotrexate (MTX) is a folic acid antagonist that can be administered to eradicate trophoblastic tissue in an ectopic pregnancy. MTX is the chemotherapeutic agent of choice in the treatment of gestational trophoblastic disease. Long-term follow-up of women who have taken MTX for gestational trophoblastic disease has failed to demonstrate an increase in congenital malformations, spontaneous abortions, or second tumors after chemotherapy.

Tanaka and colleagues reported the first use of systemic MTX for an ectopic pregnancy in 1982. This group successfully treated an interstitial pregnancy with a course of systemic MTX. Shortly thereafter, Farabow and coworkers described the use of systemic MTX in the treatment of a cervical pregnancy. Ory and associates reported the use of high-dose, short-course MTX therapy (plus citrovorum factor) to resolve small unruptured ectopic pregnancies without the need for conservative surgery. Six patients with ampullary pregnancies were treated, and resolution of the ectopic pregnancy was achieved in five patients. Surgical intervention was required in the sixth patient. Two of the five patients who experienced resolution, however, had protracted courses and required blood transfusions. Sauer and associates also reported the use of systemic MTX and citrovorum factor (CF) in 21 patients with ectopic pregnancy. Inclusion criteria included β-hCG levels that were reaching a plateau or slightly rising, laparoscopic confirmation of the ectopic pregnancy, and a tubal diameter of less than 3 cm with the tubal serosa intact and no evidence of bleeding. Treatment consisted of 1.0 mg/kg MTX administered intramuscularly on postoperative days 1, 3, 5, and 7, along with 0.1 mg/kg CF administered intramuscularly on postoperative days 2, 4, 6, and 8. Twenty of 21 pregnancies resolved without the need for laparotomy. Two patients required blood transfusions, including one patient who required laparotomy and salpingectomy for a hemoperitoneum. In both of these cases, fetal heart activity in the adnexa was identified initially on ultrasound examination. This led the authors to suggest that MTX + CF can be safely used in selected cases of unruptured ectopic pregnancies that have not formed fetal elements that can be visualized by ultrasound.

In 1991, Stovall and colleagues reviewed the results of several series of tubal ectopic pregnancies treated with MTX + CF. Of 100 cases, 50 were diagnosed by laparoscopy, and 50 were diagnosed by a nonlaparoscopic algorithm. Complete resolution was achieved in 96 patients over a range of 14 to 92 days. In four patients, laparotomy was necessary because of tubal rupture; in one case, rupture occurred as late as 23 days after MTX administration. In five patients, cardiac activity was observed on ultrasound, and treatment was successful in four of them. Three patients experienced minor side effects. In 49 of 58 (84%) women who underwent subsequent hysterosalpingograms, tubal patency was demonstrated on the ipsilateral side. Of 56 patients desiring to conceive, 37 subsequently became pregnant; 33 of these were intrauterine pregnancies and 4 were repeat ectopic pregnancies.

Stovall and Ling later studied the efficacy and safety of a simplified regimen of single-dose systemic MTX. All patients were diagnosed with a nonlaparoscopic algorithm by the use of serial hCG titers, serum progesterone, transvaginal ultrasonography, and curettage. Patients were treated with a single dose of 50 mg/m^2 MTX intramuscularly if they were hemodynamically stable and the unruptured ectopic pregnancy did not exceed 3.5 cm in diameter. In the initial report, 120 patients were treated, including 14 (11.7%) with visualized cardiac activity. One hundred thirteen (94.2%) patients had complete resolution with treatment, with a mean time to resolution of 35.5 days. Four (3.3%) of the successfully treated patients required a second course of MTX on day 7. Seven (5.8%) patients required surgical management of the ectopic pregnancy, including two of the patients with cardiac activity. No major chemotherapy-related side effects were seen. Posttreatment hysterosalpingograms demonstrated tubal patency on the ipsilateral side in 51 of 62 (82.3%) patients. Of those attempting pregnancy, 79.6% subsequently became pregnant; 87.2% of these were intrauterine and 12.8% were ectopic.

Lipscomb and colleagues further reported on the expanded Memphis cohort of patients treated with single-dose MTX. They used similar inclusion criteria, with the exception of further allowing pregnancies up to 4.0 cm in diameter provided that ectopic cardiac activity was not present. In this series, 287 of 315 (90.1%) patients were successfully treated with MTX. Forty-four patients with positive ectopic cardiac activity were treated with an 87.5% success rate. Of note, however, is that approximately 20% of these patients required more than one cycle of treatment. The authors' protocol reported that following the MTX dosing on day 1, serum chorionic gonadotropin was measured on days 1, 4, and 7. In many patients, they noted that β-hCG levels frequently continued to rise until day 4. If the chorionic gonadotropin levels then declined less than 15% between days 4 and 7, the MTX protocol was repeated. If the levels declined 15% or more between days 4 and 7, serum β-hCG was measured weekly until the level was less than 15 IU/L. If the chorionic gonadotropin level declined less than 15% during any subsequent week of follow-up, the MTX protocol was also then repeated. Other potentially difficult issues with single-dose MTX therapy include the management of "resolution pain" (which may occur in 20% of patients) and the prolonged time to resolution sometimes seen.

A further review of the variables related to the success of single-dose MTX in the treatment of singleton ectopic pregnancy has been compiled. In this review, logistic regression analysis demonstrated that the serum chorionic gonadotropin level before treatment was the only factor that contributed significantly to the failure rate (Table 34.4). Interestingly, the size and volume of the mass, the volume of hematoma, and the presence or absence of free peritoneal blood in the pelvis were not associated with a significant risk of treatment failure.

Use of mifepristone as an adjunct to MTX treatment for ectopic pregnancy has also been assessed in two randomized controlled trials. In the first trial, Gazvani and colleagues reported both treatment approaches were successful, although the time to resolution was significantly faster in the group receiving MTX and mifepristone in comparison to the MTX alone group. In the subsequent, multicenter randomized trial, Rozenberg and colleagues failed to demonstrate an overall benefit from the addition of mifepristone to MTX. These investigators, by contrast, demonstrated a higher efficacy of MTX and mifepristone in the subgroup of patients with higher initial serum progesterone levels ($\geq$10 ng/L). Further studies are needed to define the role of mifepristone in combination with MTX in the treatment of ectopic pregnancy.

MTX has also been used to treat persistent ectopic pregnancy after conservative surgery. In these patients, persistent ectopic pregnancy results from proliferation of residual trophoblastic tissue remaining after a conservative surgical procedure. The trophoblast can be located within the muscular layer of the oviduct or between the muscularis and the serosa such that at the time of salpingotomy, only the portion of the trophoblast within the tubal lumen is removed. In those patients with persistent ectopic pregnancy described in the literature, the majority have been managed by a second operation and salpingectomy. Some patients, however, have been treated with either expectant management or MTX. Hoppe and colleagues have reported the largest MTX experience to date for persistent ectopic pregnancy. These authors noted successful treatment in all 19 patients treated following linear salpingotomy. All patients should therefore have a follow-up β-hCG titer 1 to 2 weeks after conservative surgery. If the titer is elevated, then serial β-hCG titers are indicated. If the titer then continues to fall, the patient can be treated expectantly. If the β-hCG level remains the same or increases, however, consideration should be given to a single dose of MTX or perhaps further surgery to remove the remaining portion of the ectopic pregnancy.

TABLE 34.4

SUCCESS RATES OF METHOTREXATE TREATMENT WITH ECTOPIC PREGNANCIES AS A FUNCTION OF THEIR INITIAL SERUM CHORIONIC GONADOTROPIN CONCENTRATIONS

Serum chorionic gonadotropin concentration (IU/L)	Success rate (95% confidence interval)
>1,000	98 (96–100)
1,000–1,999	93 (85–100)
2,000–4,999	92 (86–97)
5,000–9,999	87 (79–98)
10,000–14,999	82 (65–98)
>15,000	68 (49–88)

(Modified from Lipscomb GH, McCord ML, Stovall TG, et al. Predictors of success of methotrexate treatment in women with tubal ectopic pregnancies. *N Engl J Med* 1999;341:1974.)

Systemic MTX is an alternative that can be used for the treatment of patients with small unruptured ectopic pregnancies or patients with persistent ectopic pregnancies following conservative surgery. Safeguards are necessary to enhance the success and minimize the toxicity of therapy. Patients should be carefully monitored with hematologic indices and liver chemistries. A history of active hepatic, renal, or peptic ulcer disease, elevated baseline liver enzyme concentrations, and thrombocytopenia or neutropenia are contraindications to therapy. Patients should avoid exposure to the sun, because photosensitivity can be a complication. Patients should refrain from sexual intercourse during therapy. Patients should also avoid folate-containing vitamins. Appropriate candidates for systemic medical therapy should also be willing to accept a small risk of tubal rupture and participate in closely monitored follow-up.

Medical Therapy by Local Injection

In 1987, Feichtinger and Kemeter reported the direct injection of MTX under transvaginal ultrasound guidance into an ectopic gestational sac. They instilled 10 mg of MTX and observed resolution of the pregnancy within 2 weeks. Other investigators, including Kojima and colleagues, have reported the successful application of local MTX administered by direct injection at the time of laparoscopy. In 1993, Fernandez and colleagues reported a large series of patients who underwent intratubal MTX at a dose of 1 mg/kg under transvaginal sonographic control. Eighty-three of 100 patients were successfully cured; however, 28 of the 83 successfully cured patients required additional MTX, which was subsequently given intramuscularly.

Direct injection of MTX has theoretic advantages over systemic treatment. The concentration of MTX at the site of implantation is many times higher after local injection than after systemic administration. With less systemic distribution of the drug, a smaller therapeutic dose might be necessary and toxicity would be less. Schiff and associates, however, evaluated the pharmacokinetics of MTX after local tubal injection and found that the peak serum level of MTX after local injection was not significantly lower than that of patients who were treated systemically with a similar dose of the drug. In addition, the success rates in practice appear to be unacceptably low. A review by Carson and Buster revealed that only 83% of the direct tubal injection procedures reported were successful.

Several trials have been conducted evaluating other intratubal agents administered for the treatment of ectopic pregnancy. Studies using prostaglandins (prostaglandin $F_{2\alpha}$, 15-methyl-prostaglandin $F_{2\alpha}$) were discouraging because of poor efficacy and serious adverse effects, including cardiac arrhythmia, malignant hypertension, and gastrointestinal symptoms. Other investigators have studied the use of hyperosmolar glucose, a less toxic agent, injected locally into the gestational sac of the ectopic gestation by either laparoscopy or transvaginal ultrasound-guided needle puncture. Lang and colleagues reported a 92% success rate using hyperosmolar glucose by laparoscopic puncture. Gjelland and associates reported successful treatment in 32 (82%) of 39 patients using local hyperosmolar glucose administered by transvaginal ultrasound guidance. They noted an inverse relationship between initial serum hCG concentrations and successful outcomes. Further larger trials are needed, however, to determine the precise clinical role, if any, of local injection therapies for ectopic pregnancy.

Surgical Treatment

Conservative Surgical Treatment

Conservative management of an unruptured ectopic pregnancy usually consists of one of two possible procedures: linear salpingotomy or segmental resection. A conservative surgical approach is possible when the diagnosis of ectopic pregnancy is made sufficiently early so that rupture of the oviduct has not yet occurred.

Linear Salpingotomy. In women who wish to preserve their fertility, conservative surgery by linear salpingotomy is considered the gold standard for the management of a distal tubal pregnancy. Recent studies have reported that the uninvolved tube may be abnormal, either grossly or subclinically, in at least 50% of cases of ectopic pregnancy. Although there have been no randomized studies comparing the fertility outcome after conservative and radical surgery for ectopic pregnancy, most of the available information suggests that the subsequent intrauterine pregnancy rate is higher after conservative surgery (linear salpingotomy).

In 1898, Kelly was among the first to advocate conservative surgery for tubal gestation. He recommended drainage of the pregnancy per vaginam, particularly for chronic hemorrhage and formation of a pelvic hematoma. More than half a century elapsed before Stromme reported the first successful use of salpingotomy to treat a patient with tubal pregnancy. In 1973, Stromme reported his surgical experience with 36 cases of unruptured tubal pregnancy, 21 of which were treated by conservative salpingotomy. Five were performed when there was only one tube remaining. Only one term pregnancy ensued from the five single-tube procedures, but Stromme's work led to the development of more effective conservative surgical procedures. Stromme reported a rate of 13.5% repeat ectopic pregnancies, which was no higher than the repeat ectopic rate at the time for more radical procedures.

Since the time of Stromme's report, physicians have achieved good success with conservative linear salpingotomy. According to the review by Yao and Tulandi, of the 1,514 patients attempting to conceive following linear salpingotomy, 61.2% had a subsequent intrauterine pregnancy, whereas 15.5% had an ectopic recurrence. On the other hand, only 38.1% of the 3,584 patients attempting to conceive following salpingectomy had a subsequent intrauterine pregnancy, although the ectopic recurrence risk was likewise lower (9.8%). In 1993, Silva and colleagues reported a prospective cohort study in which the intrauterine pregnancy rates were 60.0% and 53.8% and recurrent ectopic rates were 18.3% and 7.7% in the conservative and radical surgery groups, respectively. Many of the available reports on linear salpingotomy unfortunately do not describe the condition of the uninvolved oviduct. Langer and associates did include a description of the uninvolved oviduct in their report of 30 patients undergoing salpingotomy. Of the patients in whom the contralateral tube was normal, 80% subsequently had normal pregnancies. When the contralateral tube was damaged or contained peritubal adhesions, only 11 (55%) patients later achieved a viable pregnancy.

Among recent reports of salpingotomy performed on a single remaining oviduct, an intrauterine pregnancy rate of about 50% has been achieved by several investigators, although the results are quite variable, and some reports have only a limited number of patients treated. The repeat ectopic pregnancy rate in the single-tube salpingotomy patients appears to be about 20%, a slightly higher rate than that in series of patients with both oviducts.

In general, conservative salpingotomy is the preferred treatment for patients who desire further pregnancies. For results to be optimal, the oviduct should be unruptured and without serosal invasion, and the patient should be in a surgically stable condition.

Transabdominal Conservative Procedure. The procedure for linear salpingotomy starts by exposing, elevating, and stabilizing the tube. A linear incision is then made over the distended segment of the tube (Figs. 34.6 and 34.7). The incision is extended through the antimesenteric wall until entry is made into the lumen of the distended oviduct. When gentle pressure is exerted from the opposite side of the tube, the products of gestation are gently expressed from the lumen. Because a certain amount of separation of the trophoblast has usually occurred, the conceptus generally can be easily removed from the lumen. Gentle traction by suction or by forceps teeth can be used if necessary, but care should be taken to avoid trauma to the mucosa. Any remaining fragments of the anchoring trophoblast should be removed by profuse irrigation of the lumen with warm Ringer lactate solution to prevent further damage to the mucosa.

Care must be taken to provide complete hemostasis in the tubal mucosa; failure to do so results in troublesome postoperative bleeding, which can lead to the formation of intraluminal adhesions. The small tubal vessels are easily identified while the tube is being irrigated, and loupe magnifying glasses can be used if necessary for better resolution. An operating microscope is usually not needed.

The mucosal margins are then closed with interrupted sutures, taking care that only the serosa and muscularis are approximated and that there is no undue tension. Care should be taken also to ensure that no suture material is retained on the mucosal surface, because even a small amount can produce a secondary inflammatory reaction with subsequent adhesion formation.

Laparoscopic Conservative Procedure. Currently, most ectopic pregnancies are treated by laparoscopic surgery. In fact, most studies have suggested that laparoscopic surgery is superior to laparotomy in hemodynamically stable patients. Advantages of laparoscopy include lower cost, shorter hospital stay, less surgical blood loss, less analgesia requirement, and a shorter postoperative convalescence. Not all patients, however, may be suitable for laparoscopic treatment. These include patients with an unstable hemodynamic status, those with severe pelvic adhesions, and those with a specific contraindication to laparoscopy.

The presence of a hemoperitoneum should not preclude laparoscopic treatment. Using a large-bore suction irrigator, the blood can be evacuated, and the pelvic organs irrigated with a crystalloid solution. Once the ectopic has been documented, two auxiliary puncture sites are made suprapubically to

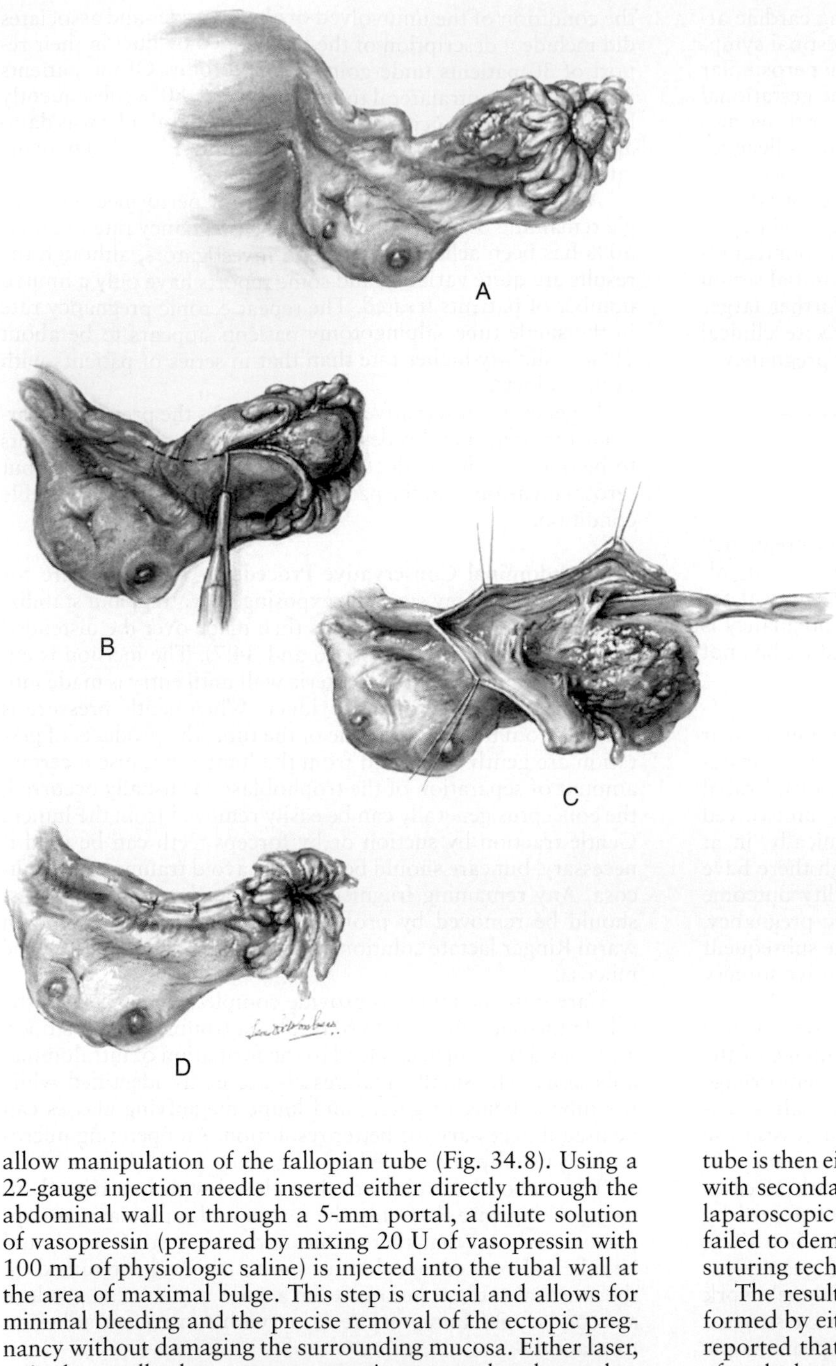

FIGURE 34.6. Removal of ectopic pregnancy of the distal ampulla. **A:** Distal ampulla involved with ectopic pregnancy. **B:** Initial incision on the antimesenteric border. **C:** The gestational contents are carefully removed by use of blunt dissection. **D:** Tubal serosa and muscularis are closed as a single layer with 5-0 nonreactive suture material.

allow manipulation of the fallopian tube (Fig. 34.8). Using a 22-gauge injection needle inserted either directly through the abdominal wall or through a 5-mm portal, a dilute solution of vasopressin (prepared by mixing 20 U of vasopressin with 100 mL of physiologic saline) is injected into the tubal wall at the area of maximal bulge. This step is crucial and allows for minimal bleeding and the precise removal of the ectopic pregnancy without damaging the surrounding mucosa. Either laser, unipolar needle electrocautery, or scissors can than be used to make the salpingotomy incision. It is important to make the incision along the antimesenteric wall of the tube in the area of maximal distension and large enough to allow for complete extrusion of the products of conception without difficulty. It is also important to keep the fallopian tube taut. If the products of conception do not spontaneously extrude following completion of the incision, either hydrodissection or gentle tubal compression with a blunt probe or suction irrigator will usually work. The tissue is then placed in an endoscopic bag and removed from the abdominal cavity. Special care is taken to remove all of the placental tissue as it is known that persistent peritoneal implants of trophoblastic tissue following laparoscopic salpingotomy may occur. After the tissue is removed, the tube is irrigated carefully and checked for hemostasis. The tube is then either left to heal by secondary intention or sutured, with secondary intention being appropriate for most cases. A laparoscopic salpingotomy study by Fujishita and colleagues failed to demonstrate any benefit from suturing over the nonsuturing technique.

The results of salpingotomy are very similar, whether performed by either laparotomy or laparoscopy. Yao and Tulandi reported that among the 811 patients attempting to conceive after the laparotomy approach, the intrauterine pregnancy rate was 61.4%, and the recurrent ectopic pregnancy rate was 15.4%. Similarly, of the 703 patients attempting to conceive following laparoscopy, 61.0% had an intrauterine pregnancy, and 15.5% had a repeat ectopic pregnancy.

Persistent Tubal Ectopic Gestation. Persistent trophoblastic tissue can remain after linear salpingotomy. Although there can be an initial decrease in the β-hCG level after surgery, the level can then slowly rise, ultimately resulting in symptoms. For this reason, it is recommended to obtain weekly β-hCG measurements after linear salpingotomy. Yao and Tulandi reported that persistent ectopic pregnancy was encountered in 8.3% of patients treated by laparoscopic salpingotomy and in 3.9% of patients treated by a similar procedure at laparotomy.

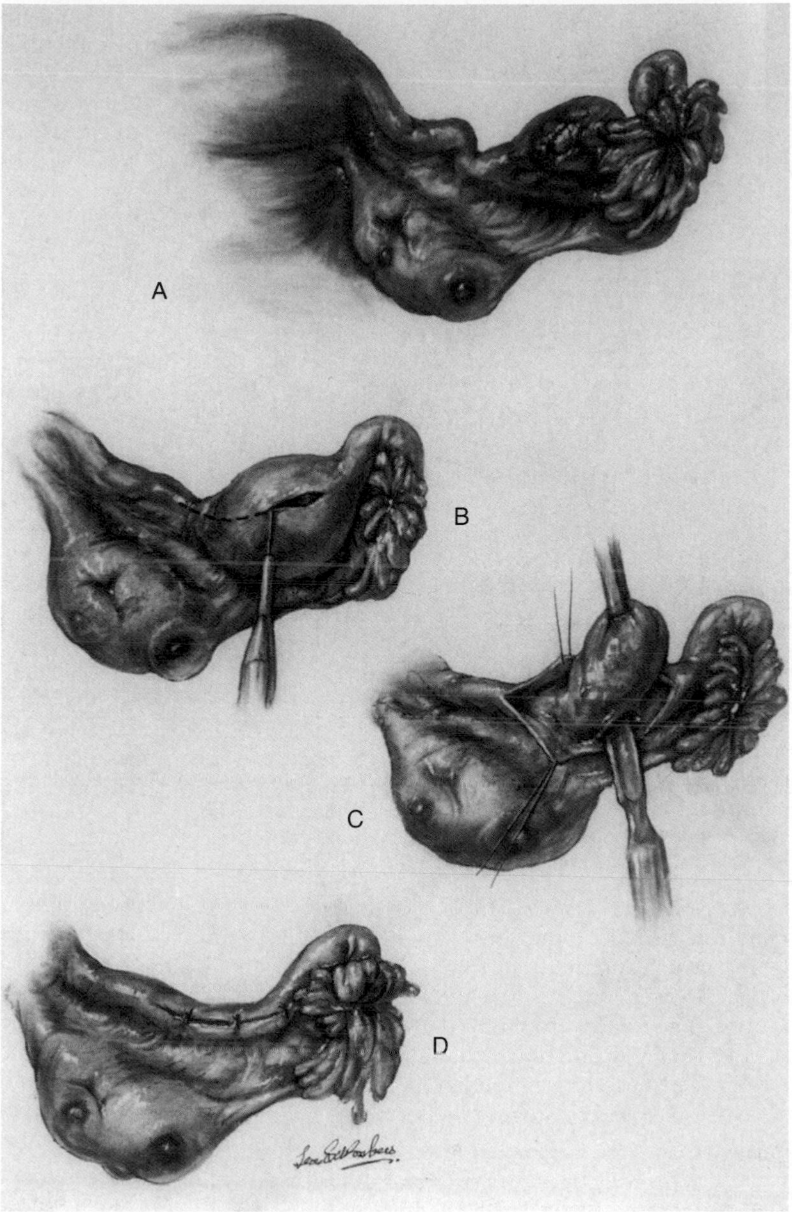

FIGURE 34.7. Removal of a midampullary ectopic pregnancy. **A:** Midampullary ectopic pregnancy. **B:** Antimesenteric incision with fine microdiathermy needle. **C:** The pregnancy is carefully removed by grasping the tissue and lifting while bluntly teasing the trophoblastic tissue away from the endosalpinx. **D:** The serosa and muscularis are closed with interrupted 5-0 nonreactive suture material.

The incidence of persistent ectopic pregnancy following laparoscopy, however, was quite variable, ranging from 3.5% to 20.0%. Pouly and colleagues achieved a relatively low 3.5% incidence of recurrent ectopic pregnancy in the largest series of patients treated to date by laparoscopic salpingotomy. Indeed, in many current practices, the incidence of persistent ectopic pregnancy appears to be low. There is a tendency for persistent trophoblastic tissue to be found in the proximal portion of the tube; therefore, special attention to this area is important. The use of hydrodissection to flush out the gestational products rather than removal of trophoblastic tissue piecemeal with forceps is recommended. One must, however, never assume that the chance for persistent trophoblast is entirely mitigated by the characteristics and ease of the procedure.

Risk factors for persistent ectopic pregnancy include small ectopic pregnancies (<2 cm diameter), early therapy (<42 days from last menstrual period), and high concentrations of β-hCG (>3,000 IU/L by the Third IS) preoperatively. In high-risk cases, a single dose of MTX (1 mg/kg) can be administered postoperatively for prophylaxis. Graczykowski and Mishell demonstrated that the rate of persistent ectopic pregnancy was reduced to a rate of 1.9% using MTX prophylaxis in comparison with a rate of 14.5% among controls. Spandorfer and associates suggested that the postoperative day 1 serum β-hCG concentration can be used as a predictor of persistent ectopic pregnancy. They reported that a day 1 serum β-hCG decrease of <50% from preoperative levels may be predictive of persistent ectopic pregnancy. If day 1 serum β-hCG concentrations decreased >50% of the preoperative value, there was more than an 85% probability that a persistent ectopic pregnancy would not occur.

Options for treatment of persistent ectopic pregnancy include reoperation and medical therapy. The choice of treatment can also include expectant therapy if the patient is asymptomatic and β-hCG levels are not rapidly increasing. MTX appears to be particularly effective in the setting of

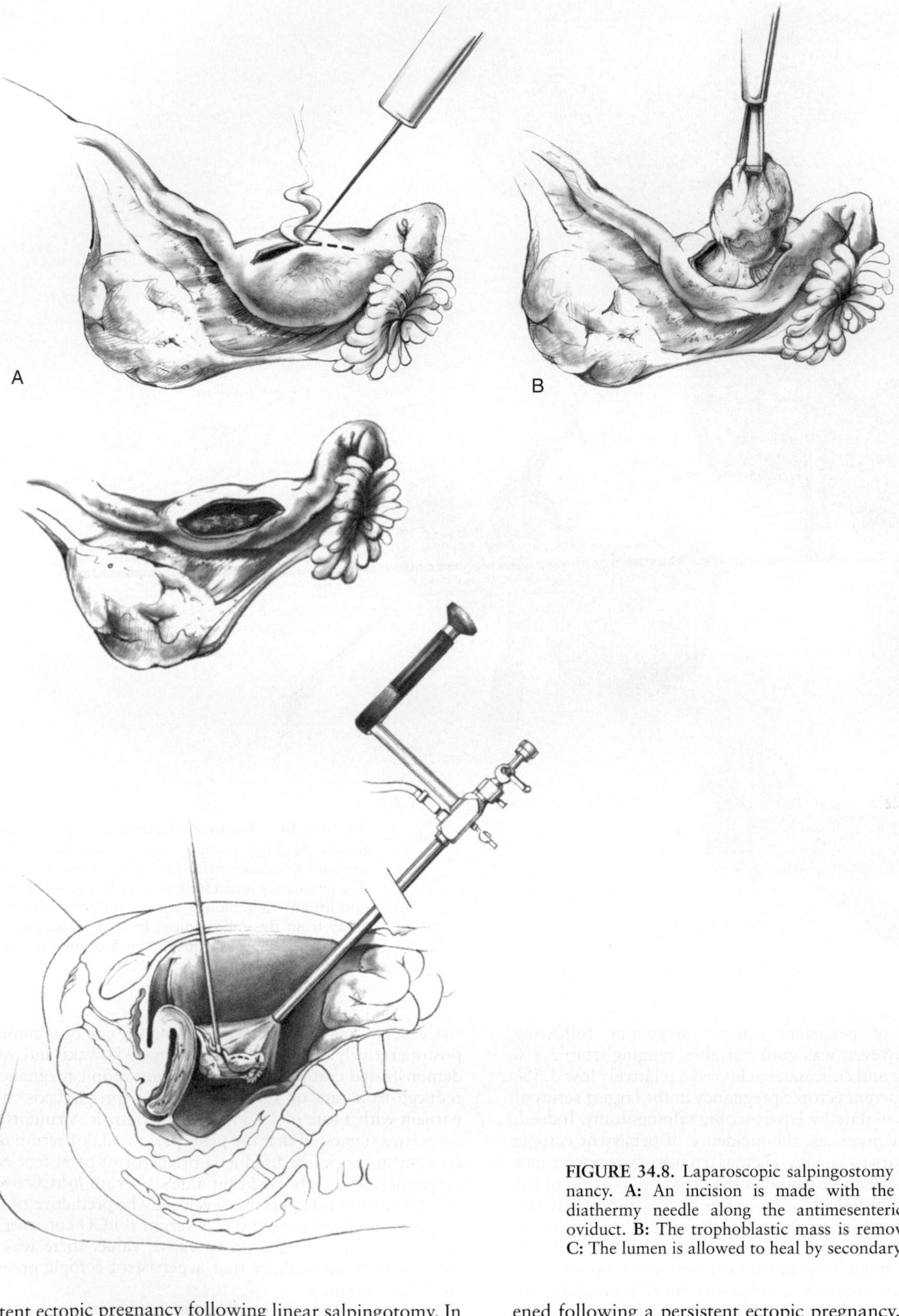

FIGURE 34.8. Laparoscopic salpingostomy for ectopic pregnancy. A: An incision is made with the fine monopolar diathermy needle along the antimesenteric border of the oviduct. B: The trophoblastic mass is removed with forceps. C: The lumen is allowed to heal by secondary intention.

persistent ectopic pregnancy following linear salpingotomy. In the largest series reported to date, all 19 patients with persistent ectopic pregnancies were successfully treated with a single intramuscular dose of systemic MTX (50 mg/m^2). The patient's reproductive prognosis does not appear to be particularly lessened following a persistent ectopic pregnancy. In a review of 50 cases, Seifer and colleagues reported that after 36 months of follow-up, there were 19 (59%) intrauterine pregnancies and no recurrent ectopic pregnancies in 32 such women attempting to conceive.

Because of the chance for persistent ectopic pregnancies to present relatively late following initial appropriate decreases in β-hCG concentrations, it is recommended to obtain weekly β-hCG measurements until they return to the normal range.

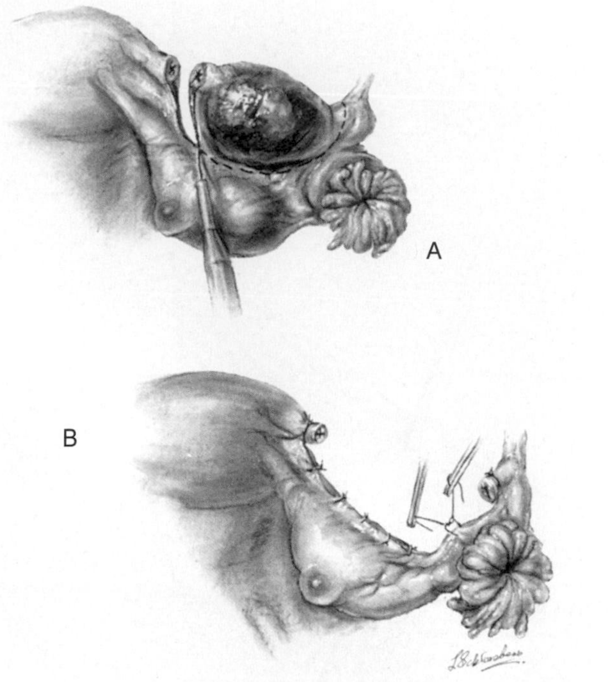

FIGURE 34.9. Segmental resection of midtubal ectopic pregnancy. **A:** A needle cautery is useful to resect the pregnancy. **B:** Care should be taken to approximate the mesosalpinx. Reanastomosis can be performed either immediately or in 3 to 5 months.

Segmental Resection. The optimal surgical approach to the isthmic ectopic pregnancy remains controversial. Three conservative operations have been described: segmental resection of the involved portion of oviduct with primary microsurgical anastomosis, segmental resection with reanastomosis at a later operation, and linear salpingotomy. In Sweden, Swolin initially advocated for segmental resection in 1967. Subsequently, other surgeons, including Stangel and Gomel as well as DeCherney and Boyers, have found segmental resection to be preferable to salpingotomy in most cases of isthmic pregnancy. In the isthmus, the tubal lumen is narrower and the muscularis is thicker than in the ampulla. Thus, the isthmus is more predisposed to severe postoperative damage, and the rate of proximal tubal obstruction seems to be higher following linear salpingotomy.

With segmental resection and end-to-end reanastomosis, the implantation site is removed so that it cannot be involved in a subsequent tubal pregnancy. A more normal architecture for the oviduct is consequently achieved. The anatomic restoration is a time-consuming process requiring special expertise and extensive microsurgical experience; *it should not be undertaken by an inexperienced surgeon.* The success of future pregnancies depends on the skill and precision of technique used in the procedure, and, once begun, the only alternative is total salpingectomy.

Segmental resection is best performed with loupe magnification or the operating microscope; the required microsurgical techniques are identical to those discussed elsewhere in this text. Care must be taken to avoid trauma to the very vascular oviduct; only patients with minimal bleeding should be considered for the operation. The adjacent mesosalpinx must be incised and removed with care to avoid the formation of a hematoma in the broad ligament (Fig. 34.9). The muscularis sutures are placed with use of magnification and no. 6-0 or 7-0 delayed-absorbable material, and the serosa is secondarily supported by additional interrupted sutures. Patency of the oviduct is tested by insufflation of the uterine cavity with indigo carmine dye.

Radical Surgical Treatment

Total salpingectomy is required when a tubal pregnancy has ruptured and a substantial hemoperitoneum has occurred. In these cases, the intraabdominal hemorrhage must be quickly controlled, and a conservative operation should not be attempted. Extensive hemoperitoneum places a patient in serious jeopardy of cardiopulmonary crises.

A salpingectomy may also be indicated for other reasons. These include a recurrent ectopic pregnancy in the same fallopian tube, an ectopic pregnancy in a severely damaged tube, and an ectopic pregnancy in a women who has completed her family.

Some earlier reports advocated for the combined use of a prophylactic oophorectomy with salpingectomy. Theoretically, removal of the ipsilateral ovary would cause the other ovary to ovulate more frequently, perhaps favoring future pregnancy. In reality, the benefits of removal of the contralateral ovary are outweighed by the consideration that any future oophorectomy would then mean castration. The high success rate of IVF is a further incentive to maintain functioning of both ovaries.

As stated earlier, most patients with an ectopic pregnancy currently are candidates for laparoscopic surgery. Radical surgical procedures, such as salpingectomy, are also easily adapted to laparoscopic surgery. Of course, certain patients remain noncandidates for laparoscopic surgery, including those with unstable hemodynamic status or severe pelvic adhesions. The latter patients are still best treated by laparotomy.

At laparotomy, total salpingectomy with partial cornual resection has been criticized for providing a residual sinus tract that allows development of a subsequent interstitial pregnancy. This problem may not lie in the procedure per se, but rather the surgeon's performance of the procedure. Complete peritonealization of the cornual incision and advancement of the round and broad ligaments over the uterine cornua (the modified Coffey technique of uterine suspension) should provide complete protection from recurrent interstitial pregnancy (Fig. 34.10). A too-vigorous resection of the uterine cornua can also cause problems. A residual myometrial defect can cause uterine rupture, interstitial recanalization, or placental encroachment during a subsequent intrauterine pregnancy and should be avoided by making certain that the interstitial resection includes less than one third the thickness of the cornual portion of the myometrium.

Dubuisson and colleagues reported the first large series of patients treated by total salpingectomy at laparoscopy for ampullary ectopic pregnancies. They used a three-puncture laparoscopic technique. They thermocoagulated the tubal isthmus, mesosalpinx, and tubal-ovarian ligament, followed by excision with hook scissors. The tube was subsequently removed with polyp forceps through one of the suprapubic punctures. They reported no immediate complications in 98 patients successfully treated at laparoscopy, although one patient experienced a postoperative deep venous thrombosis. Two patients initially intended for laparoscopy, however, required laparotomy either because of severe pelvic adhesions or significant

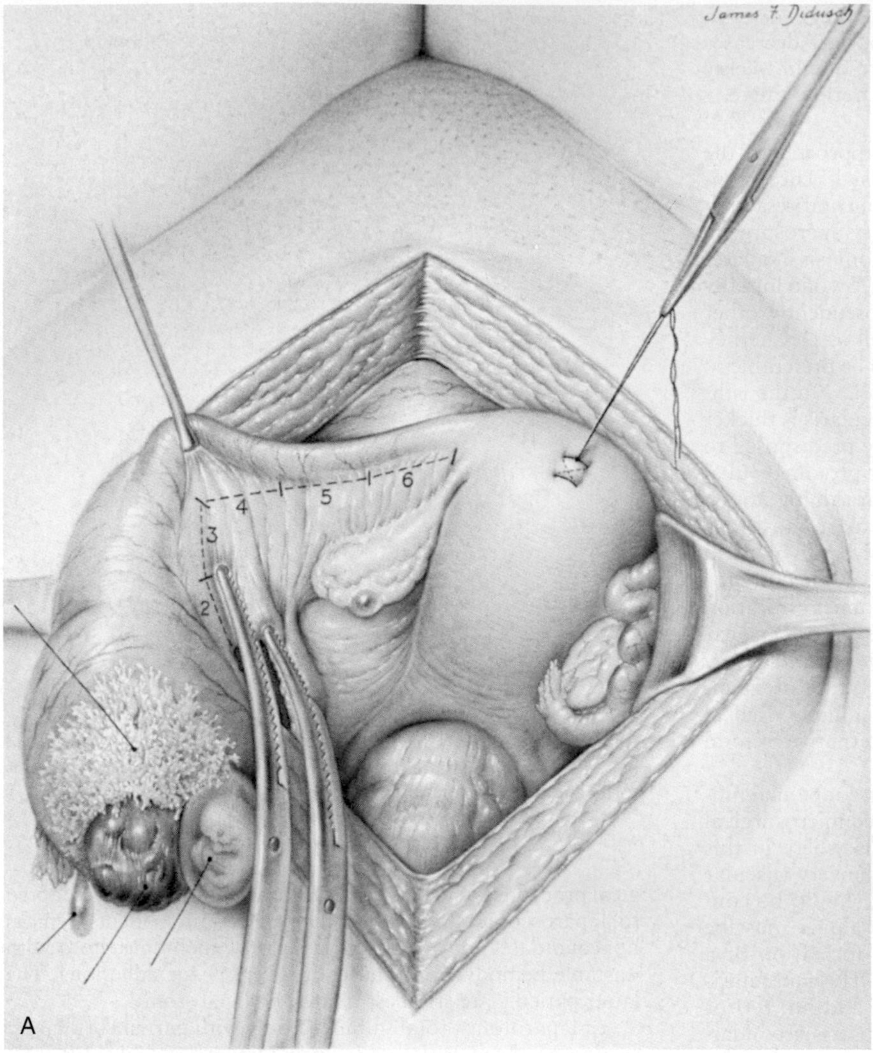

FIGURE 34.10. Salpingectomy for tubal pregnancy. **A:** The tube has been delivered, and the mesosalpinx is being clamped and cut with a succession of Kelly clamps. (*Continued*)

intraperitoneal blood. In a later report, Dubuisson and associates advised opening the tube first to aspirate the trophoblast in cases in which the tube is large to more easily remove the tissue through a 12-mm trocar.

Technique of Salpingectomy at Laparotomy. A suprapubic Pfannenstiel or low midline vertical abdominal incision is used, and the distended tube is elevated. The mesosalpinx is clamped with a succession of Kelly clamps as close to the tube as possible (Fig. 34.10A). The tube is then excised by cutting a small myometrial wedge at the uterine cornu (Fig. 34.10B). Care should be taken to avoid a deep incision into the myometrium. A figure-of-eight mattress suture of no. 0 delayed-absorbable material is used to close the myometrium at the site of the wedge resection. The mesosalpinx is closed with interrupted ligatures of no. 2-0 delayed-absorbable suture. Complete hemostasis is essential to avoid a hematoma of the broad ligament.

The fundus is held forward and the round and broad ligaments are sutured over the uterine cornu (Fig. 34.10C). This procedure, the modified Coffey suspension, accomplishes complete peritonealization. Mattress sutures anchor the broad ligament to the uterus. The no. 0 delayed-absorbable suture first penetrates the broad ligament from its anterior surface, just below the round ligament, at a distance of 2 to 3 cm from the cornu. The next "bite" is taken into the fundus of the uterus, a little posterior and superior to the uterine incision. The suture is then placed through the posterior aspect of the broad ligament, about 1 cm lateral to the previous suture. When this suture is tied, the cornual incision and the mesosalpinx are covered with mesothelium (Fig. 34.10D). If there is excessive tension on this suture, or if peritonealization is incomplete, then supporting sutures can be placed in the myometrium and the round ligament to ensure that the peritonealization suture will remain in place.

Technique of Salpingectomy at Laparoscopy. Several methods have been successfully used for laparoscopic salpingectomy, including endoscopic stapling devices, endocoagulation, bipolar cautery, and pre-tied endoscopic ligatures. Following placement of laparoscopic trocar ports (usually three-puncture technique), irrigation of the pelvis, and the evacuation of all blood clots, the involved tube is then grasped with a toothed grasper. One method then includes cauterizing the tubal-ovarian ligament first with bipolar forceps, followed by transection with scissors (Fig. 34.11) or the blade of a coagulation-cutting

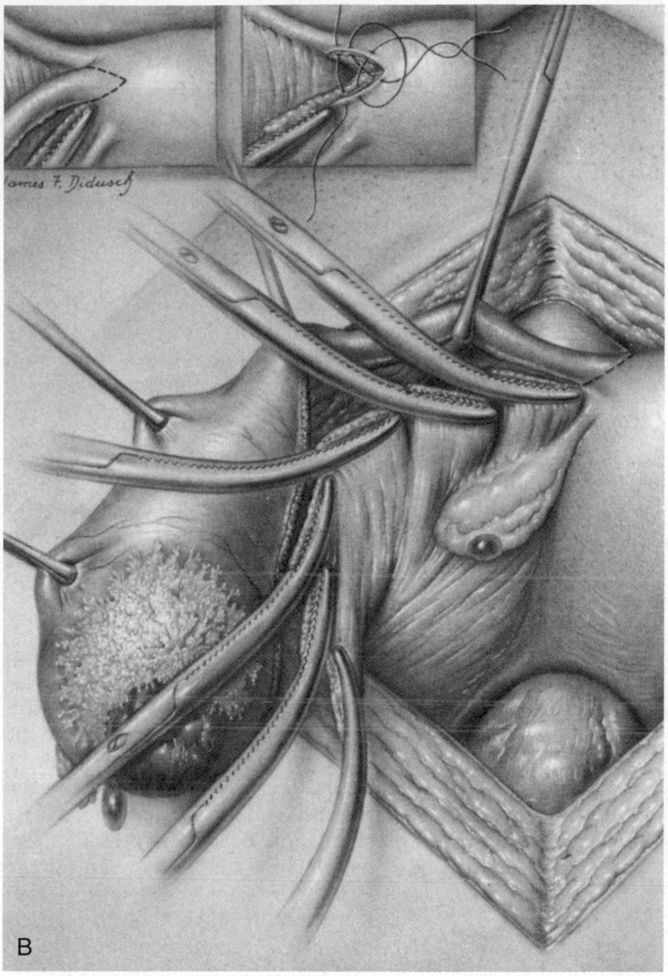

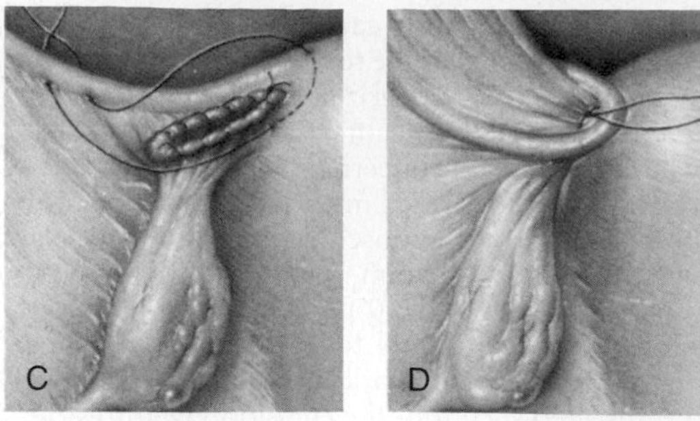

FIGURE 34.10. (*Continued*) **B:** The mesosalpinx has been completely clamped and cut. The dashed line indicates the line of excision of the tube at the cornu. Inset shows the superficial wedge resection of the interstitial portion of the tube and the suture of the cornu. **C:** The method of placing a mattress suture for peritonealization is shown with anchoring of the medial portion of the broad ligament to the uterus, a little posterior and superior to the uterine incision. **D:** Peritonealization is completed by tying the mattress suture, which brings the broad and the round ligaments over the uterine cornu.

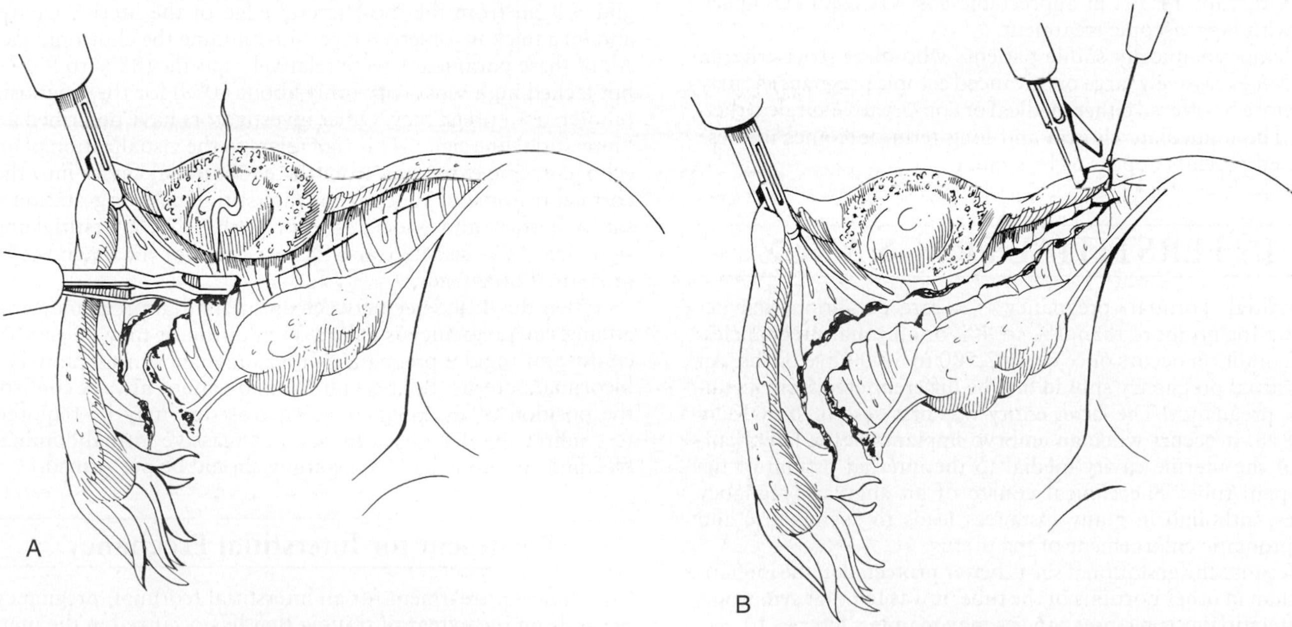

FIGURE 34.11. Techniques of laparoscopic salpingectomy using bipolar cautery and excision.

device. The mesosalpinx is similarly cauterized and transected, taking care to stay as close as possible to the fallopian tube. The proximal tubal isthmus is then cauterized and transected. Care should be taken such that excess cauterization of the uterine cornu does not occur because of concerns about the potential of interstitial sinus tracts or diminished myometrial integrity. The specimen is then placed in an endoscopic specimen retrieval bag and removed through a 12-mm port. Alternatively, the tube can be excised distal to a no. 0 polyglactin 910 (Vicryl) endoloop ligature secured proximal to the ectopic implantation site, although this technique works optimally if the entire mesosalpinx is transected such that the endoloop ligatures can be placed precisely at the tubal insertion at the cornua. Consideration may also be given to covering the proximal tubal pedicle with an absorbable adhesion prevention barrier.

Comparisons of Surgical and Medical Therapy

Several studies have compared conservative laparoscopic treatment with systemic MTX in the management of ectopic pregnancy. Saraj and associates reported a randomized trial comparing single-dose intramuscular MTX (1 mg/kg) with laparoscopic salpingotomy. They reported similar immediate treatment success rates: 94.7% for MTX and 91.4% for laparoscopic salpingotomy. Additional MTX injections were required in 15.8% of women who were randomized to the single-dose MTX group. Initial serum hCG titers were higher for the patients who required additional MTX doses than for those who required only one dose. The mean times for serum progesterone and hCG concentrations to decrease to less than 1.5 ng/mL and 15 IU/L, respectively, were significantly less for laparoscopic salpingotomy. Fernandez and colleagues also reported a randomized trial of conservative laparoscopic treatment and MTX administration (by either transvaginal or intramuscular injection) and found similar immediate treatment success. Additional studies have also suggested that despite the increased number of posttreatment visits that are necessary, MTX therapy results in appreciable cost savings in comparison with laparoscopic treatment.

Hemodynamically stable patients who meet strict criteria, without excessively large or advanced ectopic pregnancies, may therefore be offered either medical or conservative surgical therapy. The immediate clinical and long-term outcomes in these selected patients appear to be similar.

INTERSTITIAL PREGNANCY

Interstitial (cornual) pregnancy is a rare condition that accounts for no more than 2% to 4% of all tubal pregnancies. The condition occurs once every 2,500 to 5,000 live births. An interstitial pregnancy should first be differentiated from an angular pregnancy. The latter entity was first described by Kelly in 1898. It occurs when an embryo implants in the lateral angle of the uterine cavity medial to the internal ostium of the fallopian tube. The clinical course of an angular pregnancy varies, although in many instances leads to asymmetric and symptomatic enlargement of the uterus.

Because the gestational sac is better protected in the interstitial than in other portions of the tube, it was felt that symptoms of interstitial ectopic pregnancies may manifest later (>12 gestational weeks). This general belief has recently been disputed, however, by Tulandi and Al-Jaroudi, who reported the results of an Interstitial Pregnancy Registry sponsored by the Society of Reproductive Surgeons (SRS). In this registry, 14 cases (43.7%) of rupture of interstitial pregnancy was reported, all at the time of initial diagnosis. Pelvic pain and vaginal spotting are common early symptoms. The developing chorionic villi may eventually erode into the blood vessels of the uterine cornu, causing a severe hemorrhage. Because the pregnancy occurs at the most richly vascularized area of the female pelvis—the junction of the uterine and ovarian vessels—rupture usually causes profound and sudden shock.

Before 1893, the only available reports on interstitial pregnancies were from autopsies. Since then, numerous cases have been reported. Most of the same risk factors for interstitial pregnancy are similar to those for ectopic pregnancy in general, including PID, previous pelvic surgery and the use of assisted reproductive technologies. Ipsilateral salpingectomy may be a unique risk factor for interstitial pregnancy, occurring in 37.5% of patients, according to the SRS Interstitial Pregnancy Registry. Earlier diagnosis and more experience in treating this disorder have reduced the present maternal mortality rate to approximately 2% to 2.5% of all interstitial pregnancies.

The diagnosis of interstitial pregnancy is made by critical evaluation of all the criteria used for other types of tubal pregnancy. The presentation often includes acute abdominal pain, intraperitoneal bleeding, a low hematocrit, and a positive serum or urine pregnancy test. Diagnostic tests include the sensitive β-hCG immunoassay and vaginal ultrasonography.

Asymmetry of the uterus, often indicative of an interstitial pregnancy, can be misinterpreted as a pregnancy in a bicornuate uterus or a myoma in a pregnant uterus instead of an interstitial pregnancy. Knowledge of the previous shape of the uterus can help to confirm or exclude the existence of a bicornuate or myomatous uterus. A firm protrusion on the uterus suggests a myoma; a soft, tender asymmetric enlargement suggests an interstitial pregnancy.

Timor-Tritsch and colleagues established transvaginal ultrasonic criteria for interstitial pregnancy. These criteria include: (a) an empty uterine cavity, (b) a chorionic sac seen separately and >1 cm from the most lateral edge of the uterine cavity, and (c) a thick myometrial layer surrounding the chorionic sac. All of these parameters were relatively specific (88% to 93%), but lacked high sensitivity (only about 40%) for the diagnosis of interstitial pregnancy. Other investigators have described an "interstitial line sign." This sign refers to the visualization of an echogenic line extending from the endometrial cavity into the cornual region and abutting the interstitial mass or gestational sac. Ackerman and associates reported that the "interstitial line sign" was 80% sensitive and 98% specific for the diagnosis of interstitial pregnancy.

Often the difference between an interstitial pregnancy and an angular pregnancy is subtle. In addition, it may be easy to confuse an angular pregnancy with a pregnancy in a septated or bicornuate uterus. Because ultrasound cannot always confirm the position of the pregnancy, laparoscopy may be required to confirm the diagnosis. In cases of massive intraabdominal bleeding, an immediate laparotomy should be performed.

Treatment for Interstitial Pregnancy

The choice of treatment for an interstitial (cornual) pregnancy depends on the extent of trauma that has occurred in the uterine wall and on the interest of the patient in preserving her

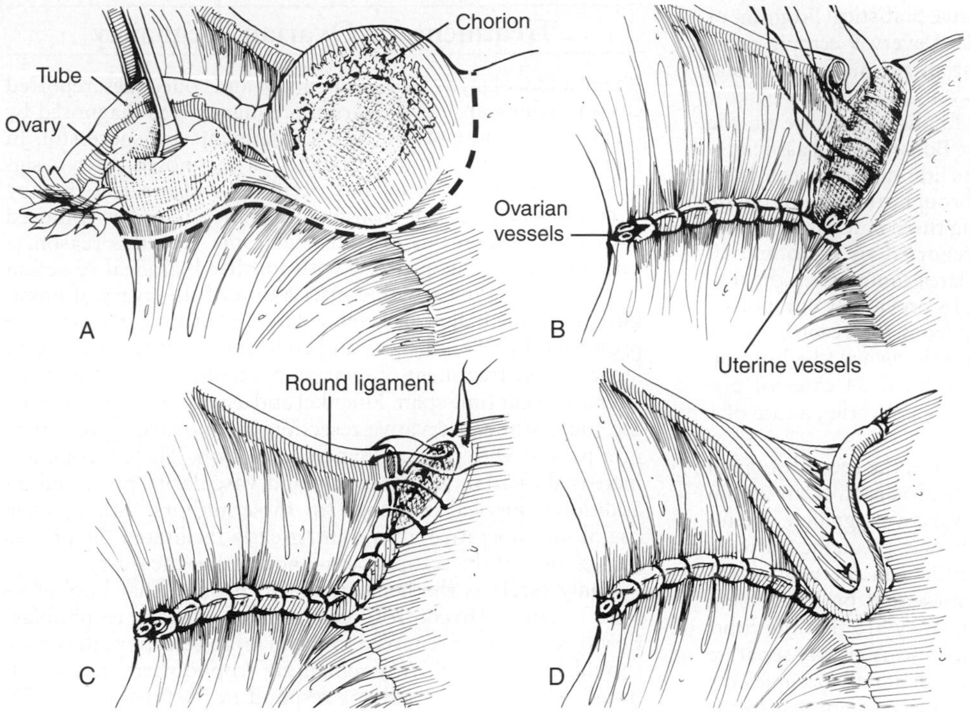

FIGURE 34.12. Salpingo-oophorectomy with resection of interstitial pregnancy. **A:** The dotted line denotes line of excision. **B:** Tube, ovary, and the cornual pregnancy have been excised. Myometrium is being approximated with figure-of-eight sutures of no. 0 delayed-absorbable suture. Note that the uterine vessels have been ligated separately. **C:** The round ligament, which was cut, is being resutured to the cornu. The ovarian vessels have been ligated, and the broad ligament has been closed with a continuous lockstitch. Serosa of the uterine wound is closed with a simple continuous stitch. **D:** The cornual wound is covered with the round and broad ligaments.

childbearing function. Systemic MTX has been used in a limited number of patients with unruptured interstitial pregnancies. Tanaka and coworkers reported the first successful treatment of an interstitial pregnancy with systemic MTX. Since this report, according to Lau and Tulandi, there have been 40 additional published cases of interstitial pregnancies treated with the use of systemic or local MTX, or a combination of both. An overall success rate of 83% was reported.

If an interstitial pregnancy is observed when it is still small, it might be excised using conservative laparoscopic techniques. In their review, Lau and Tulandi noted 22 successful cases of laparoscopic treatment of interstitial pregnancy. Techniques used varied from cornuostomy with careful extraction of the products of conception to a more formal cornual resection. In only one case was bleeding severe enough to require a transfusion. Hemostatic methods have included ligation of the ascending branches of the uterine vessels, intracorporeal and extracorporeal suturing, and surgical stapling. Although the immediate efficacy of laparoscopic conservative procedures for interstitial pregnancy is high, the risk of uterine rupture in a subsequent pregnancy is unknown. Uterine rupture can occur at the site of a previous interstitial pregnancy. Patients treated by conservative laparoscopic techniques should therefore be carefully counseled about this risk. The risk of uterine rupture also emphasizes the importance of proper suturing of the uterine cornu during conservative surgical treatment of an interstitial pregnancy.

For many surgeons, cornual resection and repair of the defect by laparotomy remains the standard conservative surgical procedure for interstitial pregnancy. Provided that uterine rupture has not occurred, this is technically feasible in most cases. Unfortunately, in many cases in which uterine rupture has occurred or a very large interstitial pregnancy is present, a hysterectomy may be required. Hysterectomy remains the treatment of choice for pregnancies advanced to such a stage that repair of the cornu would be technically difficult and medically hazardous.

Excision of Interstitial Pregnancy by Cornual Resection and Salpingectomy

Whenever possible, the ovary should be saved. A cornual resection and salpingectomy is performed by first ligating the ascending uterine vessels where they approach the cornu (Fig. 34.12A). Each is ligated separately with a figure-of-eight suture. One may also consider the use of a dilute solution of vasopressin (prepared with mixing 20 U of vasopressin with 30 mL of physiologic saline) injected in the intended myometrial incisional line to further optimize intraoperative hemostasis. The interstitial pregnancy is excised in a V-shaped manner, and the myometrium is approximated with a figure-of-eight closure using no. 0 delayed-absorbable suture (Fig. 34.12B). The remainder of the fallopian tube is excised. If it becomes necessary, the round ligament can be cut and resutured to the cornu and the uterine serosa by use of interrupted sutures (Fig. 34.12C). The round and broad ligaments are brought over the incision with mattress sutures (the modified Coffey suspension) (Fig. 34.12D), and additional interrupted sutures of no. 2-0 or no. 3-0 delayed-absorbable material can be used to secure the serosa of the round ligament to the serosa of the uterus to maintain the operative site in a permanent retroperitoneal position.

OVARIAN ECTOPIC PREGNANCY

Because IUDs protect the endometrium and, to a lesser extent, the proximal oviducts from implantation, it was expected that when IUDs were introduced, future reports of extrauterine pregnancies might show an increased rate of ovarian involvement. Data from the Cooperative Statistical Program of the Population Council show that 1 of every 9 ectopic pregnancies among IUD users is an ovarian pregnancy. Of total pregnancies among IUD users, 4.3% are extrauterine.

There are several reviews in the English literature on the subject of primary ovarian pregnancy. Boronow and associates summarized 62 cases in a review of the literature between 1950 and 1963. Campbell and associates brought the list up to date through 1973 with 91 cases, including three new cases of their own. Pratt-Thomas and colleagues reported an additional 10 new cases in 1974. Grimes and associates summarized the major reviews through 1980 and added 18 previously unreported cases of primary ovarian pregnancy from the records of six hospitals. Their combined data from this review, the hospital cases, and four other recent reports totaled 34 cases of primary ovarian pregnancy among 236,983 deliveries, a rate of 1 ovarian pregnancy in 7,000 deliveries.

In an intrafollicular ovarian pregnancy, the second stage of meiosis, ovum capacitation, and fertilization each occur within the follicle. Only 15% of cases of ovarian pregnancy are intrafollicular in origin. In an intrafollicular pregnancy, a well-preserved corpus luteum can be identified in the wall of the gestational sac. Four other criteria presented by Spiegelberg for identifying an intrafollicular pregnancy are that the tube, including the fimbria ovarica, is intact and is clearly separate from the ovary; that the gestational sac definitely occupies the normal position of the ovary; that the sac is connected to the uterus by the uteroovarian ligament; and that ovarian tissue is unquestionably demonstrated in the wall of the sac.

Diagnosis of Ovarian Pregnancy

Early diagnosis of an ovarian pregnancy, of all the diagnoses relating to extrauterine gestations, is perhaps the most difficult. As stated previously, the classic symptoms of a tubal gestation are abdominal pain, amenorrhea, and bleeding; however, persistent pelvic pain alone, a symptom not always easily related to its cause, is the most frequent clinical manifestation of an ovarian gestation. Although an adnexal mass is palpable in as many as 60% of ovarian pregnancies, the mass is frequently confused with a leaking corpus luteum hematoma.

All of the test criteria used for diagnosing a tubal pregnancy are helpful in diagnosing a primary ovarian pregnancy. In particular, the highly sensitive β-hCG immunoassay is effective for identifying the presence of low hCG levels. The test can confirm the presence of a gestational process, but knowing the β-hCG level does not help to precisely locate the gestation. Incomplete spontaneous abortion with a leaking corpus luteum hematoma, one of the most common complications of pregnancy, mimics an ovarian pregnancy. In such cases, a D&C will often show the remnants of trophoblastic villi responsible for the low levels of β-hCG.

A tubal pregnancy can easily be ruled out with laparoscopy, but an ovarian pregnancy is sometimes difficult to differentiate from a leaking corpus luteum hematoma by gross appearance. Ultrasonography can be helpful, but only in advanced ovarian pregnancy will the ultrasound image show a discrete gestational sac, therefore confirming an ovarian pregnancy.

Critical evaluation of all of the diagnostic studies, particularly the sensitive β-hCG immunoassay and vaginal ultrasonography, is necessary in making the diagnosis. When the β-hCG is positive, ultrasonography shows no intrauterine gestational sac, and free blood exists in the peritoneal cavity, a laparoscopy should be performed to confirm or refute a diagnosis of suspected ovarian pregnancy.

Treatment for Ovarian Pregnancy

Raziel and Golan, as well as Chelmow and colleagues, reported cases in which an intact ovarian pregnancy was diagnosed by laparoscopy and systemic MTX treatment was successful. In many cases, an ovarian pregnancy is diagnosed after a significant hemoperitoneum has occurred and medical therapy is contraindicated. An ovarian pregnancy is easily confused with a leaking corpus luteum hematoma. For this reason, a safe approach is to proceed with localized surgical resection of the bleeding mass with conservation of the ovary, if possible. Unless the diagnosis is made late, the ovary can usually be preserved. In 1997, Seinera and colleagues reported successful laparoscopic treatment of ovarian pregnancy in eight patients over a 12-year time span. Einenkel and associates even reported the successful conservative resection of an ovarian pregnancy in a patient with ovarian hyperstimulation. The concomitant increased ovarian size, fragility, and vascularity presented an additional surgical challenge for these authors, although the use of intraoperative ultrasound greatly facilitated the precise localization of the ectopic pregnancy within the ovary.

Only rarely is the hemorrhage so profuse that oophorectomy is required to control bleeding. Even if the last trophoblastic villus cannot be removed in the ovarian resection, the ovary should be preserved. Any remaining trophoblastic tissue will usually degenerate rapidly or respond to postoperative MTX therapy and therefore should produce no long-standing clinical problem.

ABDOMINAL ECTOPIC PREGNANCY

An abdominal pregnancy is perhaps both the rarest and the most serious type of extrauterine gestation. Reports of the frequency of abdominal pregnancy vary, ranging from 1 in 3,371 deliveries to greater than 1 in 10,200 deliveries. Stafford and Ragan reported an incidence of 1 abdominal pregnancy in 7,269 deliveries, a figure that is representative of the reports in the literature.

Abdominal pregnancies are classified as primary or secondary. Most are secondary, the result of early tubal abortion or rupture with secondary implantation of the pregnancy into the peritoneal cavity. To be considered a primary abdominal pregnancy, the pregnancy must meet the three criteria defined by Studdiford in 1942:

1. Both tubes and ovaries must be in normal condition with no evidence of recent or remote injury.
2. No evidence of uteroperitoneal fistula should be found.
3. The pregnancy must be related exclusively to the peritoneal surface and be early enough to eliminate the possibility that it is a secondary implantation following a primary implantation in the tube.

Secondary abdominal pregnancy occurs when a tubal gestation attaches itself to other viscera as the enlarging placenta spreads through the wall of the tube or is aborted through the fimbriated end. The placenta probably retains some tubal attachment, which supplies blood for the gestation to continue developing in the new peritoneal site. Rare types of secondary abdominal pregnancies have occurred after spontaneous separation of an old cesarean section scar, after uterine perforation during a therapeutic or elective abortion, and after subtotal or total hysterectomy.

Diagnosis of Abdominal Pregnancy

Early diagnosis of an abdominal pregnancy is difficult but critical, because a catastrophic hemorrhage can result from separation of the placenta later in pregnancy. A history of recurrent abdominal discomfort, fetal movement beneath the abdominal wall, and the presence of fetal movements high in the upper abdomen should alert the clinician to the possibility of an abdominal implantation. Other clinical clues include cessation of fetal movement, vomiting late in pregnancy, fetal malposition, a closed and uneffaced cervix, or the failure of oxytocin to stimulate the gestational mass.

Confirmation of the diagnosis requires demonstration of the fetus outside the uterine cavity. In their review of 199 cases, Costa and colleagues reported that only in 68 cases (40.2%) was a mass adjacent to or distinct from the uterus found. The radiologic finding of fetal small parts in the lateral position overlying the maternal spine was first noted by Weinberg and Sherwin in 1956; this finding is a fairly reliable sign of an abdominal pregnancy. A radiologic examination of the abdomen, including anterior, posterior, and lateral views, is also helpful in defining malposition of the fetus, which is most often discovered to be in the transverse position. Ultrasound, however, is the most effective method for diagnosing an abdominal pregnancy. Ultrasound can usually identify an abdominal gestation as separate from the nonpregnant uterus. Ultrasonography can be expected to have high diagnostic accuracy in most cases. In those cases in which ultrasonography is equivocal, MRI may be useful.

The maternal mortality risk from abdominal pregnancy in the United States is 7.7 times greater than the maternal mortality risk from tubal ectopic pregnancy and 90 times greater than that with intrauterine pregnancy. Reported maternal mortality rates in the literature have varied in the past from 4% to 29%. Maternal morbidity can also be substantial, with high incidences of pelvic abscess, peritonitis, and sepsis caused by retained placental remnants. Rare instances of massive rectal bleeding or rectal passage of fetal bones secondary to the formation of celo-intestinal fistulae have also been reported. Fetal mortality is notoriously high, ranging from 75% to 95% of all cases.

Management of Advanced Abdominal Pregnancy

Recent techniques of fetal monitoring serve as diagnostic adjuncts to the management of the advanced abdominal pregnancy. Fetal assessment—including repeated ultrasonography to measure biparietal diameter, nonstress testing, monitoring of fetal movements, and biophysical profiles—can provide clinical evidence of fetal maturity and fetal welfare. Despite the use of these diagnostic tools, fetal death occurred in all of the 15 cases of abdominal pregnancy reported by Martin and associates. Clark and Jones reported a fetal salvage rate of only 11.4% in a study of 35 advanced abdominal pregnancies.

One of the major factors in fetal survival is the condition of the fetal membranes. If the membranes rupture, the fetus usually dies from respiratory distress in the peritoneal cavity within a short time of the rupture. When the volume of amniotic fluid is significantly decreased or absent, the incidence of fetal malformations increases significantly, pressure deformities occur, and pulmonary hypoplasia precludes the possibility of delivering a viable fetus. In situations in which the pregnancy is advanced and there is sufficient volume of amniotic fluid, there exists a reasonable possibility of a good fetal outcome. In rare instances, there may be justification for postponed surgery to allow for further fetal maturity and a better perinatal prognosis.

Preoperative preparation of a patient with an advanced abdominal pregnancy should include an adequate supply of compatible blood and blood products and appropriate intravenous infusion lines that can deliver large amounts of fluid quickly. The use of a cell-saver or MAST (Military Antishock Trouser) suit has been reported in management of patients experiencing massive hemorrhage and shock. A surgical team should be standing by that is capable of handling the possible bowel, vascular, or genitourinary complications that may arise.

Following incision into the amniotic sac and delivery of the fetus, the management of the placenta still remains a controversial issue. Most clinicians believe the best treatment is to clamp the cord, to leave the placenta *in situ,* and to close the abdomen, but to allow retroperitoneal drainage if possible. The placenta can be removed after complete cessation of function is demonstrated by quantitative β-hCG titers. The placenta should be removed during laparotomy only if it is accessible and if its removal can be accomplished without excessive blood loss. In case of doubt, the placenta should be left in place. Thompson has reported leaving the placenta in the peritoneal cavity for a period of 13 years without physical harm to the patient. MTX has been used occasionally to hasten trophoblastic degeneration, but it leads to the accelerated accumulation of necrotic placental tissue, which may become infected. For this reason, it is currently felt best not to administer MTX in this clinical setting.

CERVICAL ECTOPIC PREGNANCY

The cervix is a rare but hazardous site for placental implantation because the trophoblast can penetrate through the cervical wall and into the uterine blood supply. Cervical gestations have, until recently, received little attention in the literature, but increased awareness of the condition has resulted in a number of recent reports.

The following three criteria for the diagnosis of cervical pregnancy were established by Rubin in 1911:

1. Cervical glands must be opposite the placental attachment.
2. Placental attachment to the cervix must be situated below the entrance of the uterine vessels or below the peritoneal reflection of the anterior and posterior surfaces of the uterus.
3. Fetal elements must be absent from the corpus uteri.

Because strict anatomical and histological criteria necessitate a hysterectomy for a complete study of the entire uterus, Paalman and McElin proposed five more clinically practical criteria for the diagnosis of this condition:

1. Uterine bleeding without cramping pain following a period of amenorrhea
2. A soft, enlarged cervix equal to or larger than the fundus (the "hourglass" uterus)
3. Products of conception entirely confined within and firmly attached to the endocervix
4. A closed internal cervical os
5. A partially opened external cervical os

The incidence of this rare entity varies. The Mayo Clinic reported 1 in 16,000 pregnancies. The highest incidence, 1 in 1,000 pregnancies, was reported from Japan. The high incidence of elective abortion in Japan is probably a factor in the higher rates. Dilatation and curettage (D&C) seems to be

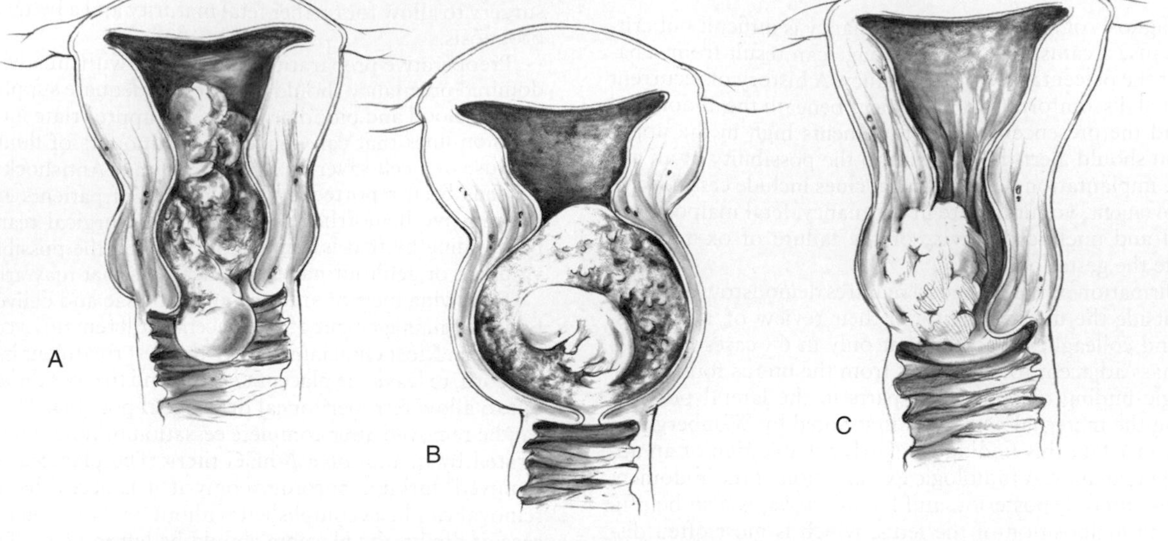

FIGURE 34.13. Differential diagnosis of cervical pregnancy. A: In the cervical phase of uterine abortion, the placenta is mainly within the expanded cervix, and the external and internal ora are dilated. B: In a cervical abortion (abortion into the cervix), because of stenosis of the external os, spontaneous rupture of the cervical wall can cause severe hemorrhage. C: Ragged, friable cervix seen in cervical pregnancy mimics carcinoma of the cervix. (Redrawn from Rothe DJ, Birnbaum SJ. Cervical pregnancy: diagnosis and management. *Obstet Gynecol* 1973;42:675.)

a predisposing factor for cervical pregnancy. Shinagawa and Nagayama noted that in 18 of 19 cases of cervical pregnancy there was a history of legal abortion. In the review by Ushakov and associates, 68.6% of patients with a cervical pregnancy had a previous uterine curettage. It has also been suggested that a previous cesarean section may play a role in the etiology of cervical pregnancy.

Cervical gestation is frequently confused with a neoplastic process because of the marked vascularity and friable appearance of the cervix. Profuse bleeding can occur if the placenta is mistaken for a tumor and a biopsy is taken. A cervical gestation also can be mistaken for a spontaneous abortion in which the products of conception were retained within the cervical canal (Fig. 34.13).

Treatment for Cervical Pregnancy

The treatment for a cervical pregnancy is surgical, and the condition often requires an abdominal hysterectomy. In selected patients, conservative evacuation of an early cervical pregnancy may be accomplished by skillful D&C, although the procedure has the potential to be complicated by profuse hemorrhage. Further preoperative preparations directed to reduce the vascularity of the uterine cervix—such as transvaginal ligation of cervical branches of the uterine arteries, a Shirodkar type cerclage, angiographic uterine artery embolization, or intracervical vasopressin injection—may reduce operative morbidity. In a review by Ushakov and colleagues, of the 16 cases in which one of these methods was employed, 15 had minimal (50–200 mL) blood loss, one patient had a hemorrhage of 1,200 mL requiring transfusion, and no patient required laparotomy or hysterectomy. Among 41 cases in which D&C was performed without cervical preparation, minimal bleeding occurred in just five cases (12.2%), massive bleeding (1,200–5,000 mL) occurred in 70.7%, and hysterectomy was performed in seven cases (17.1%). Laparotomy with bilateral internal iliac artery ligation or bilateral uterine artery ligation was also required in an additional five (12.2%) of these patients. To control postevacuation bleeding, several authors, including Kuppuswami and colleagues and Werberand associates, have described the successful use of a Foley catheter balloon to tamponade the cervical implantation site in patients who continued to have blood loss after cervical pregnancy evacuation. A 26 French Foley catheter with a 30-mL balloon is preferably used and left inflated for 0.5 to 6 days, as clinically indicated.

Medical therapy can also be considered for the primary treatment of cervical pregnancy or as an adjunct to surgical therapy through decreased vascularization of the mass. Kung and Chang reviewed the use of MTX administration for cervical ectopic pregnancy from 1983 to 1997. Among 35 cases of viable cervical ectopic pregnancies <12 weeks' gestation, 63% of patients received either systemic MTX alone or a combination of systemic MTX with a local (intraamniotic or intracervical) injection of either MTX or potassium chloride. Among the 23 cases of nonviable cervical pregnancy <12 weeks' gestation, 96% of women required systemic MTX alone. The ultimate success rate of uterine preservation was similar (94% for the viable pregnancy group; 91% for the nonviable pregnancy group), although the patients in the viable pregnancy group required a significantly higher number of concomitant additional surgical procedures (43% vs. 13%).

HETEROTOPIC PREGNANCY

Heterotopic pregnancy (coexistence of intra- and extrauterine pregnancies) is rare. The incidence has been estimated to be about 1 in 30,000 spontaneous pregnancies. With the use of assisted reproductive technologies, the incidence is higher, as high as 0.75% to 1.5% of pregnancies.

Although the precise cause of a combined pregnancy is frequently obscure, most of the risk factors are the same as those associated with other forms of ectopic pregnancy. The use of ovulation-inducing agents has increased the incidence of multiple gestations and heterotopic pregnancies. Berger and Taymor reported an incidence of combined pregnancy in as many as 1 in 100 stimulated patients. The most common predisposing anatomic finding associated with heterotopic pregnancies is preexisting tubal disease.

Abdominal pain, an adnexal mass, peritoneal irritation, and an enlarged uterus together constitute the major clinical features associated with a heterotopic pregnancy. Additional diagnostic findings include the presence of two corpora lutea found at the time of laparotomy or laparoscopy, hemoperitoneum, acute abdominal pain after the termination of an intrauterine pregnancy, and the persistence of an enlarged uterus with amenorrhea after excision of an ectopic pregnancy.

As opposed to solely extrauterine pregnancies, which are presently diagnosed and treated electively at an early preclinical stage, heterotopic pregnancies are still mostly diagnosed after clinical signs develop. In their review, Rojansky and Schenker report that nearly half of the cases present with rupture, hemorrhage, and emergency intervention. This is due to the fact that serial β-hCG determinations and transvaginal ultrasonography are often not helpful in establishing an early diagnosis of heterotopic pregnancy.

The majority of heterotopic pregnancies consist of a single tubal gestation combined with an intrauterine pregnancy. Rarer varieties include combined cervical-intrauterine, ovarian-intrauterine, abdominal-intrauterine, and interstitial-intrauterine pregnancies.

Treatment for Heterotopic Pregnancy

Laparoscopy has been employed with reasonable success for the treatment of combined tubal and intrauterine pregnancies. Louis-Sylvestre and associates reported treating 13 patients laparoscopically, 10 by salpingectomy and three by salpingostomy. Subsequently, 60% of the patients with a viable intrauterine pregnancy at the time of surgery had a favorable outcome. On the other hand, in cases in which hemodynamic instability or an interstitial-intrauterine pregnancy is present, a laparotomy is indicated. Expectant management does not seem to have a role in the care of a patient with a heterotopic pregnancy. This is due to the fact that the specific course of the extrauterine component can not be monitored by serial β-hCG determinations. Likewise, either local or systemic MTX therapy would be contraindicated in the presence of a viable intrauterine gestation. The use of a local injection of potassium chloride into the extrauterine gestational sac, however, has been used successfully in a few cases. There are very rare cases in which extrauterine abdominal pregnancies progress simultaneously with intrauterine pregnancies to viability. In their review of the world's literature, Reece and associates found only 13 cases in which both pregnancies reached term and both infants were delivered and survived the neonatal period. In the absence of such rare circumstances, the outcome for the intrauterine pregnancy is optimized by immediate therapy of the extrauterine pregnancy.

RH IMMUNOGLOBULIN USE AFTER ECTOPIC PREGNANCY

Grimes has reported that Rh-negative mothers were recognized and administered Rh immunoglobulin in only 36% of cases. Fetomaternal hemorrhage associated with ectopic pregnancy can sensitize Rh-negative women at risk. A dose of 50 μg Rh immunoglobulin is usually sufficient to prevent Rh sensitization.

BEST SURGICAL PRACTICES

- The benefits derived from the early diagnosis of an ectopic pregnancy include the potential use of medical and conservative surgical procedures that optimize future fertility. Early diagnosis may also preclude ectopic pregnancy rupture and therefore result in lower patient morbidity and mortality.
- The astute clinician is aware of the risk factors for ectopic pregnancy, thereby increasing the level of suspicion in the appropriate clinical context. Risk factors for ectopic pregnancy include chronic pelvic inflammatory disease, prior tubal surgery, surgical sterilization, use of an intrauterine device, previous ectopic pregnancy, DES exposure, progestin-only contraceptives, assisted reproductive technologies, infertility, tubal developmental anomalies, multiple sex partners, early age at first intercourse, cigarette smoking, and vaginal douching.
- The classic presentation of pain and uterine bleeding with the finding of an adnexal mass is present in only 14% of patients with ectopic pregnancy. Even when present, these classic signs and symptoms are not entirely specific for ectopic pregnancy.
- Highly sensitive β-hCG assays have greatly aided in the early diagnosis of ectopic pregnancies. Serum hCG concentrations increase in an exponential fashion in early pregnancy. During the period of gestation in which the hCG concentration is less than 10,000 IU/L, the time required for doubling of hCG levels remains consistent, with a mean of 1.9 days. The slowest minimal hCG rise for a normal viable intrauterine pregnancy is 53% in 2 days. Transvaginal ultrasonographic evidence of an intrauterine pregnancy can be expected to be seen with very high sensitivity when β-hCG concentrations exceed 1,500 IU/L.
- Serum progesterone assays are useful in the early diagnosis of an ectopic pregnancy. In one large study, 98% of patients with a normal intrauterine pregnancy had progesterone levels greater than 10 ng/mL, and 98% of patients with an ectopic pregnancy had progesterone levels less than 20 ng/mL. Diagnostic limitations of the serum progesterone assay included the fact that 31% of viable intrauterine pregnancies, 23% of abnormal intrauterine pregnancies, and 51% of ectopic pregnancies had progesterone levels between 10 and 20 ng/mL in this study. In another large trial, the lowest serum progesterone concentration associated with a viable pregnancy was 5.1 ng/mL.
- A dilatation and curettage procedure is helpful when β-hCG assays and transvaginal ultrasonography are nondiagnostic and a nonviable pregnancy is suspected. Appropriate indications include (i) a failure of β-hCG concentration rise of greater than 50% in days, (ii) a serum progesterone level less than 5 ng/mL, and (iii) a failure to visualize an intrauterine gestational sac by transvaginal ultrasonography when the β-hCG concentration exceeds 1,500 IU/L. An ectopic pregnancy is suspected after uterine curettage if chorionic villi are not present on frozen section or if β-hCG concentrations do not fall by at least 15% 8 to 12 hours after the procedure.
- Laparoscopy remains the gold standard for the diagnosis of ectopic pregnancy, although it still has a low rate of false-negative and false-positive outcomes.
- Systemic MTX is an alternative that can be used for the treatment of patients with small, unruptured ectopic pregnancies or patients with persistent ectopic pregnancies

following conservative surgery. A history of active hepatic, renal, or peptic ulcer disease; elevated liver enzyme concentrations; and thrombocytopenia or neutropenia are contraindications to MTX therapy. Appropriate candidates for systemic MTX therapy should be willing to accept a small risk of tubal rupture and participate in closely monitored follow-up.

- In women who wish to preserve their fertility, conservative surgery by linear salpingotomy is the preferred treatment of a distal unruptured tubal pregnancy. Contraindications to conservative tubal surgery include an extensive hemoperitoneum and potentially compromised cardiovascular status, a recurrent ectopic pregnancy in the same fallopian tube, an ectopic pregnancy in a severely damaged tube, and an ectopic pregnancy in a woman who has completed her family.
- Laparoscopic salpingotomy is typically performed through a three-puncture technique. A large-bore suction irrigator is used to evacuate the hemoperitoneum, if present. Once the ectopic pregnancy has been documented, a 22-gauge needle is inserted either through the abdominal wall or through a 5-mm portal to deliver a dilute solution of vasopressin (prepared by mixing 20 U of vasopressin with 100 mL of physiologic saline), which is injected into the antimesenteric tubal wall at the area of maximal bulge. Either laser, unipolar needle electrocautery, or scissors can then be used to make the salpingotomy incision. It is important to make the incision along the antimesenteric wall of the tube in the area of maximal distension and large enough to allow for complete extrusion of the products of conception without difficulty. It is important to keep the fallopian tube taut. If the products of conception do not spontaneously extrude following completion of the incision, either hydrodissection or gentle tubal compression will usually work. The tissue is then placed in an endoscopic bag and removed from the peritoneal cavity. After the tissue is removed, the tube is irrigated carefully and inspected for hemostasis. If hemostasis is present, the tube is then either left to heal by secondary intention or sutured with fine suture. Secondary intention is felt appropriate for most cases.
- Several methods have been successfully used for laparoscopic salpingectomy, including endoscopic stapling devices, endocoagulation, bipolar cautery, as well as the application of pre-tied endoscopic ligatures. Following placement of laparoscopic trocar ports (usually three-puncture technique), irrigation of the pelvis, and the evacuation of all blood clots, the involved tube is grasped with a toothed grasper. One method then includes cauterizing the tubal-ovarian ligament, first with bipolar forceps, followed by transaction with scissors or the blade of a coagulation-cutting device. The mesosalpinx is similarly cauterized and transected, taking care to stay as close as possible to the fallopian tube. The proximal tubal isthmus is then cauterized and transected. Care should be taken such that excess cauterization of the uterine cornu does not occur because of concerns about the potential of interstitial sinus tracts or diminished myometrial integrity. Alternatively, the tube can be excised distal to a no. 0 polyglactin 901 endoloop ligature secured proximal to the ectopic implantation site. This technique works optimally if the entire mesosalpinx is first transected such that the endoloop ligature can be placed precisely at the tubal insertion at the cornu. The specimen is then placed in an endoscopic specimen retrieval bag and removed from the peritoneal cavity. Consideration may be given to covering the proximal tubal pedicle with an absorbable adhesion prevention barrier.
- All Rh-negative patients with an ectopic pregnancy should be offered at least 50 μg of Rh immunoglobulin to prevent Rh sensitization caused by fetomaternal hemorrhage.

Bibliography

Ackerman TE, Levi CS, Dashefsky SM, et al. Interstitial line: sonographic finding in interstitial (cornual) ectopic pregnancy. *Radiology* 1993;189:83.

Ankum WM, Mol BWJ, Van der Veen R, et al. Risk factors for ectopic pregnancy: a meta-analysis. *Fertil Steril* 1996;65:1093.

Arias-Stella J. Atypical endometrial changes associated with the presence of chorionic tissue. *Arch Pathol* 1954;58:112.

Atrash HK, Friede A, Hogue CJR. Abdominal pregnancy in the United States: frequency and maternal mortality. *Obstet Gynecol* 1987;69:333.

Atrash HK, Friede A, Hogue CJ. Ectopic pregnancy mortality in the United States: 1970–1983. *Obstet Gynecol* 1987;70:817.

Auslender R, Arodi J, Pascal B, et al. Interstitial pregnancy: early diagnosis by ultrasonography. *Am J Obstet Gynecol* 1983;146:717.

Barnhart K, Mennuti M, Benjamin J, et al. Prompt diagnosis of ectopic pregnancy in an emergency department setting. *Obstet Gynecol* 1994;84:1010.

Barnhart K, Sammel MD, Rinaudo PF, et al. Symptomatic patients with an early viable intrauterine pregnancy: hCG curves redefined. *Obstet Gynecol* 2004;104:50.

Berger MJ, Taymor ML. Simultaneous intrauterine and tubal pregnancies following ovulation induction. *Am J Obstet Gynecol* 1972;113:812.

Boronow RC, McElin TW, West RH, et al. Ovarian pregnancy: a report of 4 cases and a 13-year survey of the English literature. *Am J Obstet Gynecol* 1965;91:1095.

Budowick M, Johnson TRB Jr, Genadry R, et al. The histopathology of the developing tubal ectopic pregnancy. *Fertil Steril* 1980;34:169.

Cacciatore B, Stenman U, Ylostalo P. Diagnosis of ectopic pregnancy by vaginal ultrasonography in combination with a discriminatory serum hCG level of 1000 IU/L (IRP). *BJOG* 1990;97:904.

Campbell JS, Hacquebard S, Mitton DM, et al. Acute hemoperitoneum, IUD, and occult ovarian pregnancy. *Obstet Gynecol* 1974;43:438.

Carson SA, Buster JE. Ectopic pregnancy. *N Engl J Med* 1993;329:1174.

Centers for Disease Control and Prevention. Current trends ectopic pregnancy—United States, 1990–1992. *MMWR Morb Mortal Wkly Rep* 1995;44:46.

Centers for Disease Control and Prevention. Pregnancy-related mortality surveillance—United States, 1991–1999. *MMWR Morb Mortal Wkly Rep* 2003;52:1.

Chelmow D, Gates E, Penzias AS. Laparoscopic diagnosis and methotrexate treatment of an ovarian pregnancy: a case report. *Fertil Steril* 1994;62:879.

Clark JF, Jones SA. Advanced ectopic pregnancy. *J Reprod Med* 1975;14:30.

Confino E, Binor Z, Molo MW, et al. Selective salpingography for the diagnosis and treatment of early tubal pregnancy. *Fertil Steril* 1994;62:286.

Costa SD, Presley J, Bastert G. Advanced abdominal pregnancy. *Obstet Gynecol Surv* 1991;46:515.

De Voe RW, Pratt JH. Simultaneous intrauterine and extrauterine pregnancy. *Am J Obstet Gynecol* 1948;56:1119.

DeCherney AH, Boyers SP. Isthmic ectopic pregnancy: segmental resection as treatment of choice. *Fertil Steril* 1985;44:307.

Dor J, Seidman DS, Levran D, et al. The incidence of combined intrauterine and extrauterine pregnancy after *in vitro* fertilization and embryo transfer. *Fertil Steril* 1991;55:833.

Dubuisson JB, Aubriot FX, Cardone V. Laparoscopic salpingectomy for tubal pregnancy. *Fertil Steril* 1987;47:225.

Dubuisson JB, Morice P, Chapron C, et al. Salpingectomy: the laparoscopic surgical choice for ectopic pregnancy. *Hum Reprod* 1996;11:1199.

Egger M, Low N, Smith GD, et al. Screening for chlamydia infections and the risk of ectopic pregnancy in a county in Sweden: ecological analysis. *BMJ* 1998;316:1776.

Einenkel J, Baier D, Horn LC, et al. Laparoscopic therapy of an intact primary ovarian pregnancy with ovarian hyperstimulation syndrome: case report. *Hum Reprod* 2000;15:2037.

Emerson DS, Cartier MS, Altieri LA, et al. Diagnostic efficacy of endovaginal color Doppler flow imaging in an ectopic pregnancy screening program. *Radiology* 1992;183:413.

Faber BM, Coddington CC. Microlaparoscopy: a comparative study of diagnostic accuracy. *Fertil Steril* 1997;67:952.

Farabow W, Fulton J, Fletcher V, et al. Cervical pregnancy treated with methotrexate. *N C Med J* 1983;44:91.

Feichtinger W, Kemeter P. Conservative treatment of ectopic pregnancy by transvaginal aspiration under sonographic control and methotrexate injection. *Lancet* 1987;1:381.

Fernandez H, Benifla J-L, Lelaidier C, et al. Methotrexate treatment of ectopic pregnancy: 100 cases treated by primary transvaginal injection under sonographic control. *Fertil Steril* 1993;59:773.

Fernandez H, Capella S, Vincent AY, et al. Randomized trial of conservative laparoscopic treatment and methotrexate administration in ectopic pregnancy and subsequent fertility. *Hum Reprod* 1998;13:3239.

Fernandez H, Rainhorn JD, Papiernik E, et al. Spontaneous resolution of ectopic pregnancy. *Obstet Gynecol* 1988;71:171.

Frates MC, Laing FC. Sonographic evaluation of ectopic pregnancy: an update. *AJR Am J Roentgenol* 1995;165:251.

Fujishita A, Masuzaki H, Khan KN, et al. Laparoscopic salpingotomy for tubal pregnancy: comparison of linear salpingotomy with and without suturing. *Hum Reprod* 2004;19:1195.

Gazvani MR, Baruah DN, Afirevic Z, et al. Mifepristone in combination with methotrexate for the medical treatment of tubal pregnancy: a randomized, controlled trial. *Hum Reprod* 1998;13:1987.

Gelder MS, Boots LR, Younger JB. Use of a single random serum progesterone value as a diagnostic aid for ectopic pregnancy. *Fertil Steril* 1991;55:497.

Gerard HC, Branigan PJ, Balsara GR, et al. Viability of *Chlamydia trachomatis* in fallopian tubes of patients with ectopic pregnancy. *Fertil Steril* 1998;70:945.

Giuliani A, Panzitt T, Schoell W, et al. Severe bleeding from peritoneal implants of trophoblastic tissue after laparoscopic salpingostomy for ectopic pregnancy. *Fertil Steril* 1998;70:369.

Gjelland K, Hordnes K, Tjugum J, et al. Treatment of ectopic pregnancy by local injection of hyperosmolar glucose: a randomized trial comparing administration guided by transvaginal ultrasound or laparoscopy. *Acta Obstet Gynecol Scand* 1995;74:629.

Gleicher N, Parrilli M, Pratt DE. Hysterosalpingography and selective salpingography in the differential diagnosis of chemical intrauterine versus tubal pregnancy. *Fertil Steril* 1992;57:553.

Goldner TE, Lawson HW, Xia Z, et al. Surveillance for ectopic pregnancy-United States, 1970–1989. *MMWR CDC Surveill Summ* 1993;42:73.

Graczykowski JW, Mishell DR. Methotrexate prophylaxis for persistent ectopic pregnancy after conservative treatment by salpingostomy. *Obstet Gynecol* 1997;89:118.

Grimes DA. The morbidity and mortality of pregnancy: still risky business. *Am J Obstet Gynecol* 1995;170:1489.

Grimes DA, Geary FH Jr, Hatcher RA. Rh immunoglobulin utilization after ectopic pregnancy. *Am J Obstet Gynecol* 1981;140:246.

Grimes HG, Nosal RA, Gallagher JC. Ovarian pregnancy: a series of 34 cases. *Obstet Gynecol* 1983;61:174.

Hahlin M, Sjoblom P, Lindblom B. Combined use of progesterone and human chorionic gonadotropin determinations for differential diagnosis of very early pregnancy. *Fertil Steril* 1991;55:492.

Hallatt JG. Tubal conservation in ectopic pregnancy: a study of 200 cases. *Am J Obstet Gynecol* 1986;54:1216–1221.

Hillis SD, Nakashima A, Amsterdam L, et al. The impact of a comprehensive chlamydia prevention program in Wisconsin. *Fam Plann Perspect* 1995;27:108.

Hoppe DE, Bekkar BE, Nager CW. Single-dose systemic methotrexate for the treatment of persistent ectopic pregnancy after conservative surgery. *Obstet Gynecol* 1994;83:51.

Jain K, Hamper VM, Sanders RC. Comparison of transvaginal sonography in the detection of early pregnancy and its complications. *Am J Radiol* 1988;151:1139.

Jauchler GW, Baker RL. Cervical pregnancy: review of the literature and a case report. *Obstet Gynecol* 1970;35:870.

Kadar N, Caldwell BV, Romero R. A method of screening for ectopic pregnancy and its indications. *Obstet Gynecol* 1981;58:162.

Kadar N, DeVore G, Romero R. Discriminatory hCG zone: its use in the sonographic evaluation for ectopic pregnancy. *Obstet Gynecol* 1981;58:156.

Kataoka ML, Togashi K, Kobayashi H, et al. Evaluation of ectopic pregnancy by magnetic resonance imaging. *Hum Reprod* 1999;14:2644.

Kelly H. *Operative gynecology*, vol 2. New York: Appleton; 1898:453.

Kirchler HC, Seebacher S, Alge AA, et al. Early diagnosis of tubal pregnancy: changes in tubal blood flow evaluated by endovaginal color Doppler sonography. *Obstet Gynecol* 1993;82:561.

Kojima E, Abe Y, Morita M, et al. The treatment of unruptured tubal pregnancy with intratubal methotrexate injection under laparoscopic control. *Obstet Gynecol* 1990;75:723.

Korhonen J, Stenman UH, Ylostalo P. Serum human chorionic gonadotropin dynamics during spontaneous resolution of ectopic pregnancy. *Fertil Steril* 1994;61:632.

Kung F-T, Chang S-Y. Efficacy of methotrexate treatment in viable and nonviable cervical pregnancies. *Am J Obstet Gynecol* 1999;181:1438.

Kuppuswami N, Vindekilde J, Sethi CM, et al. Diagnosis and treatment of cervical pregnancy. *Obstet Gynecol* 1983;61:651.

Kurjak A, Zalud I, Schulman H. Ectopic pregnancy: transvaginal color Doppler of trophoblastic flow in questionable adnexa. *J Ultrasound Med* 1991;10: 685.

Lang PF, Tamussino K, Honigi W, et al. Treatment of unruptured tubal pregnancy by laparoscopic instillation of hyperosmolar glucose solution. *Am J Obstet Gynecol* 1992;166:1378.

Langer R, Bukovsky I, Herman A, et al. Conservative surgery for tubal pregnancy. *Fertil Steril* 1982;38:427.

Lau S, Tulandi T. Conservative medical and surgical management of interstitial ectopic pregnancy. *Fertil Steril* 1999;72:207.

Lavy G, Diamond MP, DeCherney AH. Ectopic pregnancy: relationship to tubal reconstructive surgery. *Fertil Steril* 1987;47:543.

Lecuru F, Robin F, Chasset S, et al. Direct cost of single dose methotrexate for unruptured ectopic pregnancy: prospective comparison with laparoscopy. *Eur J Obstet Gynecol Reprod Biol* 2000;88:1.

Levin AA, Schoenbaum SC, Stubblefield PG, et al. Ectopic pregnancy and prior induced abortion. *Am J Public Health* 1982;72:253.

Lipscomb GH, Bran D, McCord ML, et al. Analysis of three hundred fifteen ectopic pregnancies treated with single-dose methotrexate. *Am J Obstet Gynecol* 1998;178:1354.

Lipscomb GH, McCord ML, Stovall TG, et al. Predictors of success of methotrexate treatment in women with tubal ectopic pregnancies. *N Engl J Med* 1999;341:1974.

Louis-Sylvestre C, Morice P, Chapron C, et al. The role of laparoscopy in the diagnosis and management of heterotopic pregnancies. *Hum Reprod* 1997;12:1100.

Lloyd HE, Feinberg R. The Arias-Stella reaction: a non-specific involutional phenomenon in intra- as well as extrauterine pregnancy. *Am J Clin Pathol* 1965;43:428.

Marcus SF, Macnamee M, Brinsden P. Heterotopic pregnancies after in-vitro fertilization and embryo transfer. *Hum Reprod* 1995;10:1232.

Martin JN Jr, Sessums JK, Martin RW, et al. Abdominal pregnancy: current concepts of management. *Obstet Gynecol* 1988;71:549.

Matthews CP, Coulson PB, Weld RA. Serum progesterone levels as an aid in the diagnosis of ectopic pregnancy. *Obstet Gynecol* 1986;68:390.

Mol BMJ, Ankum WM, Bossuyt PMMM, et al. Contraception and the risk of ectopic pregnancy: a meta-analysis. *Contraception* 1995;52:337.

Morlock RJ, Lafata JE, Eisenstein D. Cost-effectiveness of single-dose methotrexate compared with laparoscopic treatment of ectopic pregnancy. *Obstet Gynecol* 2000;95:407.

Mueller BA, Daling JR, Weiss NS, et al. Tubal pregnancy and the risks of subsequent infertility. *Obstet Gynecol* 1987;69:722.

Ory SJ, Villanueva AL, Sand PK, et al. Conservative treatment of ectopic pregnancy with methotrexate. *Am J Obstet Gynecol* 1986;154:1299.

Paalman R, McElin T. Cervical pregnancy. *Am J Obstet Gynecol* 1959;77:1261.

Pauerstein CJ, Hodgson BJ, Kramen MA. The anatomy and physiology of the oviduct. *Obstet Gynecol Annu* 1974;3:137.

Pellerito JS, Taylor KJW, Quedens-Case C, et al. Ectopic pregnancy: evaluation with endovaginal color flow imaging. *Radiology* 1992;183:407.

Peterson HB, Xia Z, Hughes JM, et al. The risk of ectopic pregnancy after tubal sterilization. *N Engl J Med* 1997;336:762.

Peterson HB, Xia Z, Hughes JM, et al. The risk of pregnancy after tubal sterilization: findings from the U.S. Collaborative Review of Sterilization. *Am J Obstet Gynecol* 1996;174:1161.

Polak JO, Wolfe SA. A further study of the origin of uterine bleeding in tubal pregnancy. *Am J Obstet Gynecol* 1924;8:730.

Pouly JL, Mahnes H, Mage G, et al. Conservative laparoscopic treatment of 321 ectopic pregnancies. *Fertil Steril* 1986;46:1093.

Pratt-Thomas HR, White L, Messer HH. Primary ovarian pregnancy: presentation of ten cases including one full-term pregnancy. *South Med J* 1974;67:920.

Raziel A, Golan A. Primary ovarian pregnancy successfully treated with methotrexate [letter; comment]. *Am J Obstet Gynecol* 1993;169:1362.

Reece EA, Petrie RH, Sirmans MF, et al. Combined intrauterine and extrauterine gestations: a review. *Am J Obstet Gynecol* 1983;146:323.

Risquez F, Pennehouat G, Foulot H, et al. Transcervical tubal cannulation and falloposcopy for the management of tubal pregnancy. *Fertil Steril* 1992;7:274.

Risquez F, Pennehoaut G, McCorvey, et al. Diagnostic and operative microlaparoscopy: a preliminary multicentre report. *Hum Reprod* 1997;12:1645.

Rojansky N, Schenker JG. Heterotopic pregnancy and assisted reproduction: an update. *J Assist Reprod Genet* 1996;13:594.

Rothe DJ, Birnbaum SJ. Cervical pregnancy: diagnosis and management. *Obstet Gynecol* 1973;42:675.

Rozenberg P, Chevret S, Camus S, et al. Medical treatment of ectopic pregnancies: a randomized clinical trial comparing methotrexate-mifepristone and methotrexate-placebo. *Hum Reprod* 2003;18:1802.

Rubin IC. Cervical pregnancy. *Surg Gynecol Obstet* 1911;13:625.

Sandberg EC, Pelligra R. The medical antigravity suit for management of surgically uncontrollable bleeding associated with abdominal pregnancy. *Am J Obstet Gynecol* 1983;146:519.

Saraiya M, Berg CJ, Kendrick JS, et al. Cigarette smoking as a risk factor for ectopic pregnancy. *Am J Obstet Gynecol* 1998;178:493.

Saraj AJ, Wilcox JG, Najmabadi S, et al. Resolution of hormonal markers of ectopic gestation: a randomized trial comparing single-dose intramuscular methotrexate with salpingostomy. *Obstet Gynecol* 1998;92:989.
Sauer MV, Gorrill MJ, Rodi LA, et al. Nonsurgical management of unruptured ectopic pregnancy: an extended clinical trial. *Fertil Steril* 1987;48:752.
Schiff E, Shalev E, Bostan M, et al. Pharmacokinetics of methotrexate after local tubal injection for conservative treatment of ectopic pregnancy. *Fertil Steril* 1992;57:688.
Schwartz RO, DiPietro DL. Beta-hCG as a diagnostic aid for suspected ectopic pregnancy. *Obstet Gynecol* 1980;56:197.
Seifer DB, Silva PD, Grainger DA, et al. Reproductive potential after treatment for persistent ectopic pregnancy. *Fertil Steril* 1994;62:194.
Seinera P, DiGregorio A, Arisio R, et al. Ovarian pregnancy and operative laparoscopy: report of eight cases. *Hum Reprod* 1997;12:608.
Shah A, Courey NG, Cunanan RG. Pregnancy following laparoscopic tubal electrocoagulation and excision. *Am J Obstet Gynecol* 1977;129:459.
Shepherd RW, Patton PE, Novy MJ, et al. Serial beta-hCG measurements in the early detection of ectopic pregnancy. *Obstet Gynecol* 1990;75:417.
Shinagawa S, Nagayama M. Cervical pregnancy as a possible sequela of induced abortion: report of 19 cases. *Am J Obstet Gynecol* 1969;105:282.
Shoen JA, Nowak RJ. Repeat ectopic pregnancy: a 16-year clinical survey. *Obstet Gynecol* 1975;45:542.
Silva PD, Schaper AM, Rooney B. Reproductive outcome after 143 laparoscopic procedures for ectopic pregnancy. *Obstet Gynecol* 1993;81:710.
Smith M, Vessey MP, Bounds W, et al. Progestogen-only oral contraception and ectopic gestation. *BMJ* 1974;4:104.
Society for Assisted Reproductive Technology and American Society for Reproductive Medicine. Assisted reproductive technology in the United States: 2000 results generated from the American Society for Reproductive Medicine/Society for Assisted Reproductive Technology Registry. *Fertil Steril* 2004;81:1207.
Spandorfer SD, Menzin A, Barnhart KT, et al. Efficacy of frozen section evaluation of uterine curettings in the diagnosis of ectopic pregnancy. *Am J Obstet Gynecol* 1996;175:603.
Spandorfer SD, Sawin SW, Benjamin I, et al. Postoperative day 1 serum human chorionic gonadotropin level as a predictor of persistent ectopic pregnancy after conservative surgical management. *Fertil Steril* 1997;68:430.
Spiegelberg O. Zur Casuistik den Ovarial-Schwangenschaft. *Arch Gynaek* 1878;13:73.
Stafford JC, Ragan WD. Abdominal pregnancy: review of current management. *Obstet Gynecol* 1977;50:548.
Stangel JJ, Gomel V. Techniques in conservative surgery for tubal gestation. *Clin Obstet Gynecol* 1980;23:1221.
Storeide O, Veholmen M, Eide M, et al. The incidence of ectopic pregnancy in Hordaland county, Norway 1976–1993. *Acta Obstet Gynecol Scand* 1997;76:345.
Stovall TG, Ling FW. Single-dose methotrexate: an expanded clinical trial. *Am J Obstet Gynecol* 1993;168:1759.
Stovall TG, Ling FW, Carson SA, et al. Nonsurgical diagnosis and treatment of tubal pregnancy. *Fertil Steril* 1990;54:537.
Stovall TG, Ling FW, Carson SA, et al. Serum progesterone and uterine curettage in differential diagnosis of ectopic pregnancy. *Fertil Steril* 1992;57:456.
Stovall TG, Ling FW, Gray LA, et al. Methotrexate treatment of unruptured ectopic pregnancy: a report of 100 cases. *Obstet Gynecol* 1991;77:749.
Strandell A, Thorburn J, Hamberger L. Risk factors for ectopic pregnancy in assisted reproduction. *Fertil Steril* 1999;71:282.
Stromme WB. Conservative surgery for ectopic pregnancy: a twenty-year review. *Obstet Gynecol* 1973;41:215.
Stromme WB. Salpingotomy for tubal pregnancy: report of a successful case. *Obstet Gynecol* 1953;1:472.
Studdiford WE. Primary peritoneal pregnancy. *Am J Obstet Gynecol* 1942; 44:487.
Swolin K, Fall M. Ectopic pregnancy; recurrence, postoperative fertility and aspects of treatment based on 182 patients. *Acta Eur Fertil* 1972;3:147.
Tanaka T, Hayashi J, Kutsuzawa T, et al. Treatment of interstitial ectopic pregnancy with methotrexate: report of a successful case. *Fertil Steril* 1982;37:851.
Tatum HJ, Schmidt FH. Contraceptive and sterilization practices and extrauterine pregnancy: a realistic perspective. *Fertil Steril* 1977;28:407.
Thompson LR. Abdominal pregnancy at term with later removal of placenta. *Am J Surg* 1966;111:272.
Timor-Tritsch IE, Monteagudo A, Matera C, et al. Sonographic evolution of cornual pregnancies treated without surgery. *Obstet Gynecol* 1992;79:1044.
Tulandi T, Al-Jaroudi D. Interstitial pregnancy: results from the Society of Reproductive Surgeons Registry. *Obstet Gynecol* 2004;103:47.
Tummon IS, Whitmore NA, Daniel SAJ, et al. Transferring more embryos increases risk of heterotopic pregnancy. *Fertil Steril* 1994;61:1065.
Ushakov FB, Elchalal U, Aceman PJ, et al. Cervical pregnancy: past and future. *Obstet Gynecol Surv* 1996;52:45.
Vasquez G, Winston RML, Brosens IA. Tubal mucosa and ectopic pregnancy. *BJOG* 1983;90:468.
Verhulst G, Camus M, Bollen N, et al. Analysis of the risk factors with regard to the occurrence of ectopic pregnancy after medically assisted procreation. *Hum Reprod* 1993;8:1284.
Walters MD, Eddy C, Pauerstein CJ. The contralateral corpus luteum and tubal pregnancy. *Obstet Gynecol* 1987;70:823.
Weinberg A, Sherwin AS. A new sign in roentgen diagnosis of advanced ectopic pregnancy. *Obstet Gynecol* 1956;7:99.
Weissman A, Fishman A. Uterine rupture following conservative surgery for interstitial pregnancy. *Eur J Obstet Gynecol Reprod Biol* 1992;44:237.
Werber J, Prasadarao PR, Harris VJ. Cervical pregnancy diagnosed by ultrasound. *Radiology* 1983;149:279.
Westrom L. Effect of acute pelvic inflammatory disease on fertility. *Am J Obstet Gynecol* 1975;121:707.
WHO Task Force. A multinational case-control study of ectopic pregnancy. *Clin Reprod Fertil* 1985;3:131.
Yao M, Tulandi T. Current status of surgical and nonsurgical management of ectopic pregnancy. *Fertil Steril* 1997;67:421.
Yeko TR, Gorrill MJ, Hughes LH, et al. Timely diagnosis of early ectopic pregnancy using a single blood progesterone measurement. *Fertil Steril* 1987;48:1048.

CHAPTER 35A ■ OBSTETRIC PROBLEMS

CORNELIA R. GRAVES

DEFINITIONS

B-Lynch stitch—A large mattress suture used to control postpartum hemorrhage following cesarean section delivery. A deep suture is placed vertically on the side of the uterus from 3 cm below the end of the uterine incision to 3 cm above the incision. The suture is then taken over the fundus, and a horizontal bite is taken on the posterior wall of the uterus below the level of the uterine vessels entering the myometrium on the same side as the anterior stitch. The suture is again passed over the fundus on the opposite side, and a deep suture is placed starting 3 cm above the other end of the anterior uterine incision and exiting 3 cm below the incision. This large four-corner mattress suture is then tightly tied down compressing the fundus.

Cervical insufficiency—Premature, painless dilation of the cervix leading to midtrimester delivery if not treated. The etiology of the condition is poorly understood and may be due to prior cervical trauma and/or some inherent cervical defect.

Late postpartum hemorrhage—Hemorrhage occurring more than 24 hours following delivery.

McDonald suture—Surgical treatment for cervical insufficiency. A purse-string suture of heavy caliber is placed around the cervix at the level of the internal os.

Postpartum hemorrhage—Although the clinical significance of postpartum blood loss will vary from one patient to the next, and blood loss during and after delivery is difficulty to estimate accurately, the American College of Obstetricians and Gynecologists has suggested postpartum hemorrhage be defined as blood loss of greater than 500 mL with a vaginal delivery or greater than 1,000 mL with a cesarean section or a 10% drop in the hematocrit.

Shirodkar suture—A thick suture or mesh band is placed submucosally around the cervix to treat cervical insufficiency.

Surgery in the pregnant patient presents several unique challenges. There is, of course, the added complexity of caring for two patients simultaneously. Illness and surgery both affect the fetus as well as the mother, and every decision to recommend surgery and when that surgery should be done requires weighing the risks and advantages to both patients. In many cases, there may be some urgency required to prevent or reduce maternal or fetal morbidity or mortality. In addition, the physiologic and anatomic changes of pregnancy may complicate diagnosis and alter the surgeon's normal operative field so that the size of the uterus and increased vascularity of the pelvis may make it significantly more difficult to perform routine gynecologic procedures.

PHYSIOLOGIC CHANGES

There are a number of physiologic changes that occur during pregnancy. It is important for the surgeon to understand these changes because they may affect laboratory interpretation, blood product replacement, and surgical approach.

Cardiovascular System

Blood volume increases by 45% to 50% at term. Placental hormone production stimulates maternal erythropoiesis, increasing red cell mass by approximately 20%. This results in a functional hemodilution manifested by a physiologic anemia. Therefore, pregnancy should be considered a hypervolemic state. Maternal heart rate increases as early as 7 weeks. In late pregnancy, maternal heart rate is increased by approximately 20% over antepartum values, often resulting in mild tachycardia. The increase in blood volume and heart rate predisposes the parturient to an increased incidence of cardiac ectopy.

Systemic vascular resistance decreases by 20% but gradually increases near term. This results in a decrease in systolic and diastolic blood pressure during pregnancy, with a gradual recovery to nonpregnant values by term. As there is increased pressure in the venous system, there is decreased return from the lower extremities, resulting in dependent edema.

Respiratory System

In pregnancy, minute volume is increased while functional residual volume is decreased. It seems intuitive that lung volume would be decreased during pregnancy, but an increase in minute volume in association with an expansion of the anterior and posterior diameter of the chest results in increased tidal volume, thereby also increasing minute ventilation. These changes result in a compensated respiratory alkalosis. Normal P_{CO_2} in pregnancy ranges from 28 to 35 mm Hg. P_{O_2} is usually greater than or equal to 100 mm Hg. Oxygen consumption and basal metabolic rate are also increased during pregnancy by approximately 20%.

These physiologic changes result in less pulmonary reserve for the acutely ill pregnant patient; therefore, this reduces the time interval from respiratory distress to respiratory failure. Because of this, early intervention for cases of respiratory challenge is mandatory.

Gastrointestinal Tract

During pregnancy, there is a decrease in gastrointestinal motility. This is caused by mechanical changes in the abdomen with the enlarging uterus and smooth muscle relaxation induced by high production of progesterone in pregnancy. Gastric emptying may be delayed for up to 8 hours; therefore, pregnant women should be considered to have a functionally full stomach at all times. In addition, a decrease in large intestine motility may result in constipation severe enough to cause significant abdominal pain.

Coagulation Changes

Pregnancy is a hypercoagulable state. Fibrinogen is increased approximately 30% over baseline values. The hypercoagulable state of pregnancy is associated with increased risk of deep venous thrombosis and pulmonary embolus. This is particularly compounded when bed rest or immobilization occurs during the gestational period.

Renal Changes

Pregnancy increases blood flow to the renal pelvis approximately 50%. This results in an increased glomerulo-filtration rate accompanied by frequent urination. Serum creatinine is approximately 40% less than in a nonpregnant state. Therefore, a creatinine of 1 mg/dL during gestation should be considered abnormal.

Ureteral diameter increases in pregnancy secondary to compression and smooth muscle relaxation. Peristalsis is delayed, and reflux occurs freely from the bladder into the lower ureteral segment. This results in an increased incidence of pyelonephritis during pregnancy, making treatment of significant asymptomatic bacteruria mandatory.

IMAGING TECHNIQUES

The most common imaging technique used during pregnancy is *ultrasound*. Ultrasound is considered safe and primarily is used for fetal assessment. In patients with abdominal pain, an ultrasound should be considered the first-line diagnostic test. During ultrasound, the presence of an intrauterine pregnancy should be documented if possible, and evaluation of the cul-de-sac for fluid, the ureter for dilatation or stones, the gallbladder for the presence of gallstones, and the placenta for abnormalities can be noted.

Magnetic resonance imaging can be also safely used during pregnancy. There are no data to suggest an increased risk from this modality. Magnetic resonance imaging is now used to diagnose fetal abnormalities, especially abnormalities of the central nervous system.

Although there are theoretical risks associated with ionizing radiation, fortunately, most *diagnostic x-ray procedures* are associated with minimal or no risk to the fetus. Existing evidence suggests that there is no increased risk of fetal congenital malformations, growth restriction, or abortion from x-ray procedures that expose the fetus to doses of 5 rads or less. The American College of Obstetricians and Gynecologists has published guidelines regarding diagnostic imaging during pregnancy. Women should be reassured that concern about radiation exposure should not prevent medically indicated diagnostic procedures. It cannot be stressed enough that maternal well-being is of the utmost importance, and appropriate diagnostic procedures should be obtained to facilitate a rapid diagnosis.

POSTPARTUM HEMORRHAGE

Postpartum hemorrhage is poorly defined by estimation of blood loss; therefore, it is difficult, if not impossible, to determine actual or percentage of blood loss at the time of delivery. Additionally, blood volume expansion is variable during pregnancy and can be affected be several factors including hypertension, renal disease, maternal size, and the presence of multifetal gestations. The potential effects of blood loss largely depend on the degree of blood volume expansion. For example, the average blood loss from a cesarean delivery is 1,000 mL. This degree of blood loss is generally well tolerated by the normal pregnant woman. A blood loss of 500 to 750 mL, however, may not be tolerated in a woman with minimal volume expansion, or one who is hemoconcentrated secondary to severe preeclampsia or eclampsia. The American College of Obstetricians and Gynecologists has noted that a number of definitions have been used to define hemorrhage, including a blood loss greater than 500 mL with a vaginal delivery or greater than 1,000 mL during a cesarean section or a drop in hematocrit of 10% regardless of the amount of documented blood loss.

Gilstrap and Ramin have defined clinically significant hemorrhage as that amount of bleeding "that produces signs and symptoms of hemodynamic instability or that is likely to produce such if left unabated."

Incidence and Etiology

Although the exact incidence of hemorrhage associated with pregnancy is unknown, it remains one of the leading causes of maternal mortality in this country. Kaunitz and associates reported that 13% of more than 2,000 maternal deaths were secondary to hemorrhage, and one third of these occurred postpartum. Rochat and colleagues reported a similar incidence of 11% of maternal deaths resulting from hemorrhage.

In a recent randomized trial in the United States, birth weight, labor induction and augmentation, chorioamnionitis, magnesium sulfate use, and previous postpartum hemorrhage were associated with increased risk of postpartum hemorrhage. A large population-based study supported these findings with significant risk factors identified using a multivariable analysis. These risk factors are retained placenta (odds ratio [OR] 3.5; 95% confidence interval [CI], 2.1–5.8), failure to progress during the second stage of labor (OR 3.4; 95% CI, 2.4–4.7), placenta accreta (OR 3.3; 95% CI, 1.7–6.4), lacerations (OR 2.4; 95% CI, 2.0–2.8), instrumental delivery (OR 2.3; 95% CI, 1.6–3.4), large-for-gestational-age newborn (OR 1.9; 95% CI, 1.6–2.4), hypertensive disorders (OR 1.7; 95% CI, 1.2–2.1), induction of labor (OR 1.4; 95% CI, 1.1–1.7), and augmentation of labor with oxytocin (OR 1.4; 95% CI, 1.2–1.7).

Diagnosis and Medical Management

The most important aspects in the management of postpartum hemorrhage are prompt recognition of the condition and ascertainment of its etiology. Recognition is no problem with external bleeding, and such bleeding almost always can be controlled with medical or minor surgical means. Hypotension without obvious external blood loss should serve as a sign of potential internal bleeding, and virtually all such hemorrhage will require a major surgical procedure to arrest the hemorrhage. If the etiology of the hemorrhage is not determined quickly, coagulopathy may complicate the clinical presentation, thereby making diagnosis difficult.

Uterine atony is obvious and easy to diagnose by palpation of the uterus. If atony it not present, the cervix and vagina should be carefully inspected for lacerations. The placenta also should be inspected for missing fragments, and careful manual palpation of the uterine cavity should be performed. If the source of bleeding still is not obvious or if bleeding is seen around venipuncture or catheter sites, then the patient should be evaluated for a coagulopathy. A thrombin-clot (clot retraction test) tube will reveal gross disruption in coagulation within minutes. Useful laboratory tests include prothrombin time, partial thromboplastin time, platelets, fibrinogen, and fibrin degradation product levels. The clinician should note that D-dimer levels may be abnormal during pregnancy even in patients without coagulopathy. Before surgical intervention, an ultrasound examination of the uterine cavity may prove useful for the identification of an accessory placental lobe or fragment.

Except in cases of profuse bleeding, medical management of hemorrhage generally is indicated. The hallmarks of medical management consist of volume replacement and oxytocic agents, including intravenous oxytocin and parenteral methylergonovine and prostaglandins. Volume can be maintained with crystalloid and blood or blood products. Invasive monitoring, such as with a pulmonary artery catheter, generally is not necessary and may be dangerous in the presence of a coagulopathy. Its use should be reserved for those patients who do not respond to usual and expected therapy. As a general rule, monitoring of urine output, vital signs, and oxygen saturation will be sufficient. Volume replacement generally is adequate when the blood pressure is maintained at 90 to 100 mm Hg systolic, pulse rate is less than 100 beats per minute, and urine output is at least 25 to 30 mL per hour. When a patient has required transfusion of significant amounts of packed red blood cells, transfusion of coagulation products should be performed to replace those lost in the hemorrhage. Calcium also should be replaced in these patients because of risk of complications related to hypocalcemia in patients receiving massive transfusions. Coagulation factors should be replaced in patients who receive extensive transfusions with packed red blood cells. Fluid overload generally can be detected with a stethoscope and an oxygen monitor in conjunction with clinical signs and symptoms. Diuretics should only be used to remove excess fluid if the patient becomes hypoxic related to volume overload. A medical management protocol is summarized in Table 35A.1.

Surgical Management

Lower genital tract lacerations usually are best managed by suturing. The rare case of uterine rupture also is managed surgically. Other techniques to control hemorrhage include uterine and uteroovarian artery ligation, hypogastric or internal iliac artery ligation, hysterectomy, or uterine or hypogastric artery embolization.

Uterine packing, which until recently had been abandoned by most clinicians, may allow adequate time for blood and fluid replacement before surgical intervention. Maier described the use of a packing device called a Torpin packer. The device uses a plunger to place several yards of 4-inch-wide gauze into the uterine cavity and has been used successfully to control postpartum hemorrhage. Uterine packing allows time for volume replacement, as well as slowing bleeding enough to allow for surgical techniques short of hysterectomy. In many cases, it may stop the bleeding so that no further treatment is necessary. Other methods of uterine tamponade reported in the literature have included the use of a Foley catheter with a 30- to 50-cc balloon or a Sengstaken-Blakemore tube with the esophageal balloon inflated with 50 cc of normal saline.

The choice of a specific surgical technique to control bleeding depends on several factors, such as the degree of hemorrhage, the condition of the patient, parity, and the desire for future childbearing; although probably the single most important factor is the experience of the surgeon.

TABLE 35A.1

MEDICAL MANAGEMENT PROTOCOL FOR POSTPARTUM HEMORRHAGE

General
Large-bore intravenous line
Foley catheter
Drugs
Oxytocin, dilute solution of 20 U in 1,000 mL of normal saline or Ringer solution, given as IV infusion
Methylergonovine, 0.2 mg IM
15-methyl $PGF_{2\alpha}$, 0.25 mg IM or intramyometrially every 15 to 60 min as indicated
Volume Replacement
Crystalloid, 3 mL/mL of estimated blood loss (maintain urine output $\geq$30 mL/h)
Packed red blood cells
Fresh frozen plasma, platelets, or cryoprecipitate, as indicated

IM, intramuscularly; IV, intravenously.
From: American College of Obstetricians and Gynecologists. *Diagnosis and management of postpartum hemorrhage.* ACOG Technical Bulletin No. 143. Washington, DC: ACOG;1990, with permission.

Arterial Embolization

Angiographically directed arterial embolization has been described for the successful control of obstetric and gynecologic bleeding. Gelfoam, polyvinyl alcohol dehydrated particles, and other substances have been used for such embolizations. Pelage and associates, in two separate reports, describe use of arterial embolization in patients with primary or secondary postpartum hemorrhage, defining primary postpartum hemorrhage as that which occurs within 24 hours after delivery. Twenty-seven women were identified, including two who had already undergone hysterectomy in an unsuccessful attempt to control the hemorrhage. Following transcatheter embolization, immediate decrease or cessation of bleeding occurred in all patients. Two patients required repeat embolization the next day with no further complications. Fourteen women were diagnosed with secondary postpartum hemorrhage after the first 24 hours following delivery. All of these patients had complete resolution of bleeding with embolization with no further complications. Arterial embolization can be performed quickly and safely; therefore, it should be considered in patients with postpartum hemorrhage. There have been reports of successful pregnancies following embolization, which makes it an especially attractive alternative to hysterectomy in the patient who desires preservation of fertility.

Uterine Artery Ligation

Uterine artery ligation is a relatively safe procedure that can be performed by most obstetricians. It also allows for future

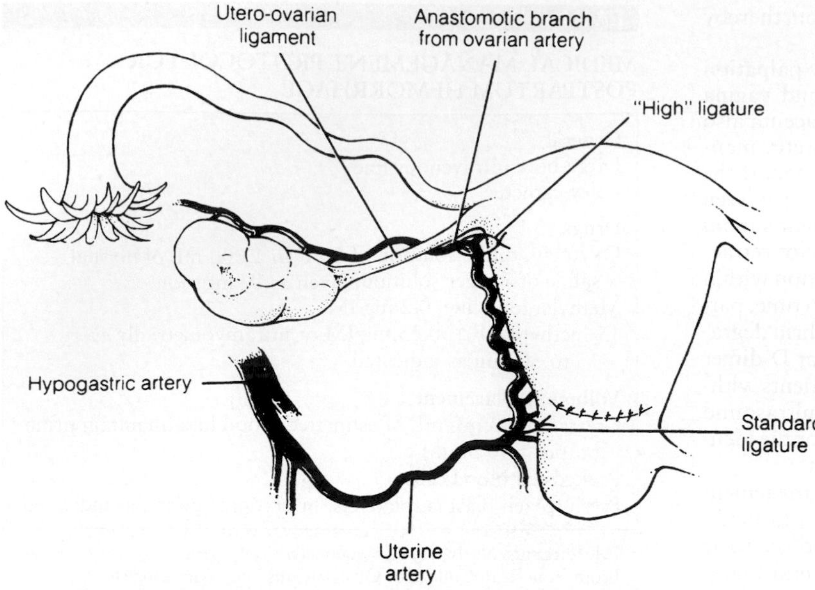

FIGURE 35A.1. Uterine artery ligation. (From: Clark SC, Phelan JP. Surgical control of obstetric hemorrhage. *Contemp Obstet Gynecol* 1984;24:70, with permission.)

childbearing. The technique consists of ligating the uterine artery and vein at the lower uterine segment 2 to 3 cm below the level of the transverse uterine incision. An absorbable ligature is placed 2 to 3 cm medial to the uterine vessels through the myometrium (to obliterate any intramyometrial ascending branches) and then lateral to the vessels through the broad ligament. It is imperative that the bladder be advanced before placement of the suture to prevent bladder injury. Because of collateral flow from the ovarian artery, some recommend that a second ligature be placed at the junction of the uteroovarian ligament and uterus. The technique of uterine artery ligation is shown in Figures 35A.1 and 35A.2.

O'Leary, in a review of 90 women who underwent uterine artery ligation (30 were for uterine atony), reported that only six (7%) procedures resulted in failure. There were no major complications from the procedure itself. In a follow-up review of 265 women who underwent uterine artery ligation, O'Leary reported a greater than 95% success rate.

This technique is most useful (and successful) when hemorrhage is of a moderate degree and originates from the lower uterine segment. Such an example is bleeding from a low placental implantation site. Uterine artery ligation also can prove beneficial for lower segment extensions or lacerations, as well as for a uterine artery laceration itself. Philippe and associates reported a vaginal approach to ligation of the uterine arteries in two patients after vaginal delivery, but a larger case series would have to be performed to determine the feasibility of this approach. B-Lynch and colleagues also described five cases in which hemorrhage was controlled by placing an absorbable suture vertically from 3 cm below the uterine incision to 3 cm above the uterine incision on the right side of the uterus (Fig. 35A.3). The stitch is then taken vertically over the fundus and

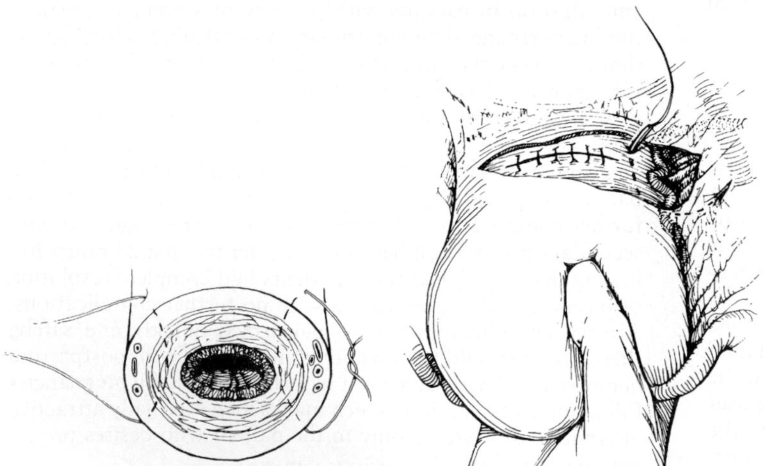

FIGURE 35A.2. Uterine artery ligation. **A:** Lateral view demonstrating ligature placement. **B:** Anatomic relation of ligature to uterine wall and vessels. (From: Floyd RC, Morrison JC. Postpartum hemorrhage. In: Plauche WC, Morrison JC, O'Sullivan MJ, eds. *Surgical obstetrics*. Philadelphia: WB Saunders;1992:272, with permission.)

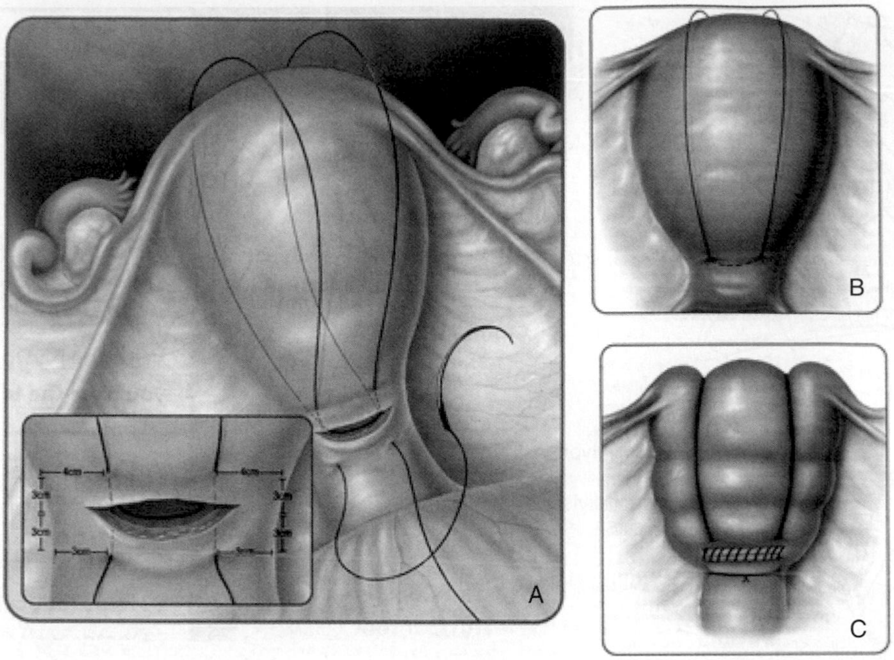

FIGURE 35A.3. Technique of B-Lynch suture placement. **A:** The initial bite is placed anteriorly at one angle of the uterine incision (see inset). **B:** After the anterior B-Lynch suture is placed, the suture is passed over the fundus, a deep transverse bite is taken in the posterior lower uterine segment, and the suture is passed back over the fundus. **C:** The uterine incision is closed, and the B-Lynch suture is tied down. An assistant manually compresses the uterus while the suture is tied.

placed horizontally in the posterior uterus at the same level as the anterior suture. The suture is threaded over the left side of the uterus to place another stitch on the left from 3 cm above the uterine incision to 3 cm below the uterine incision. The long suture is tied, compressing the fundus. A large suture, such as #1 Prolene on a large needle, is used. The uterine incision is closed in the usual fashion (Fig. 35A.3C). There are several case series in the literature supporting the efficacy of the B-Lynch stitch for the treatment of uterine atony. In all series, the suture has been reported to be effective. It has been suggested that the B-Lynch be considered in all cases of severe postpartum hemorrhage before resorting to hysterectomy.

Hypogastric Artery Ligation

The major blood supply to the uterus and pelvis comes from the internal iliac artery, commonly called the hypogastric artery. Bilateral ligation of this artery can effectively control significant bleeding and thus prevent the need for hysterectomy and permanent sterilization. Burchell has aptly described the physiology of internal iliac artery ligation. It appears that ligation of this artery controls bleeding by converting an arterial system into a venous system, which decreases the pulse pressure by as much as 85%. This allows pressure and packing to produce clotting. Hypogastric artery ligation probably interferes little, if at all, with subsequent pregnancies. Mengert and colleagues reported successful pregnancies in five women who had undergone internal iliac artery ligation. This technique also may prove useful for controlling bleeding in patients with large hematomas of the broad ligament or for a lacerated artery that has retracted into the broad ligament. Such vessels or active bleeding sites often are difficult to identify. If the bleeding is from the hypogastric vein, ligation of the hypogastric artery decreases outgoing flow, as well as allowing exposure to the vein.

The technique of hypogastric artery ligation is illustrated in Fig. 35A.4. The peritoneum overlying the common iliac artery is opened by directly cutting on the surface of the artery. The ureter should be identified and retracted medially, if necessary. The sheath covering the internal iliac (hypogastric) artery then can be opened longitudinally. A right-angle clamp is gently passed under the artery in the lateral to medial direction with blunt dissection. Great care must be taken not to perforate the internal iliac vein, and the clamp is passed lateral to medial to avoid injury to the vein by the tip of the clamp. The ligation should be performed about 2 cm distal to the bifurcation to avoid disrupting the posterior division of the hypogastric, which can lead to ischemia and necrosis of the skin and subcutaneous tissue of the gluteus. Two nonabsorbable sutures of 2-0 silk should be used for ligation. It is important that hypogastric artery ligation be performed bilaterally to adequately decrease pressure to the uterus. Clark and associates reported on the successful control of bleeding in 8 (42%) of 19 women who underwent hypogastric artery ligation. In a review of hypogastric artery ligation from three series, Clark reported that this procedure prevented hysterectomy in about half of the cases associated with uterine atony and placenta accreta. Interestingly, in the series by Clark and associates, the success of this procedure did not appear to be related directly to the conditions for which it was performed. It must be noted, however, that the number of patients in each category is small.

Although this procedure is successful in about 50% of the cases and does not interfere with subsequent fertility, it is not technically easy to perform and requires special expertise and skill. Many obstetricians have little, if any, experience with this procedure. Moreover, potential complications of hypogastric artery ligation include laceration of the iliac vein, ligation of the external iliac artery, ureteral injury, and death.

Hysterectomy

Because of the lack of experience and skill with the technique of hypogastric artery ligation, many clinicians prefer to do a hysterectomy to control postpartum hemorrhage. Peripartum hysterectomy is extensively discussed later in this

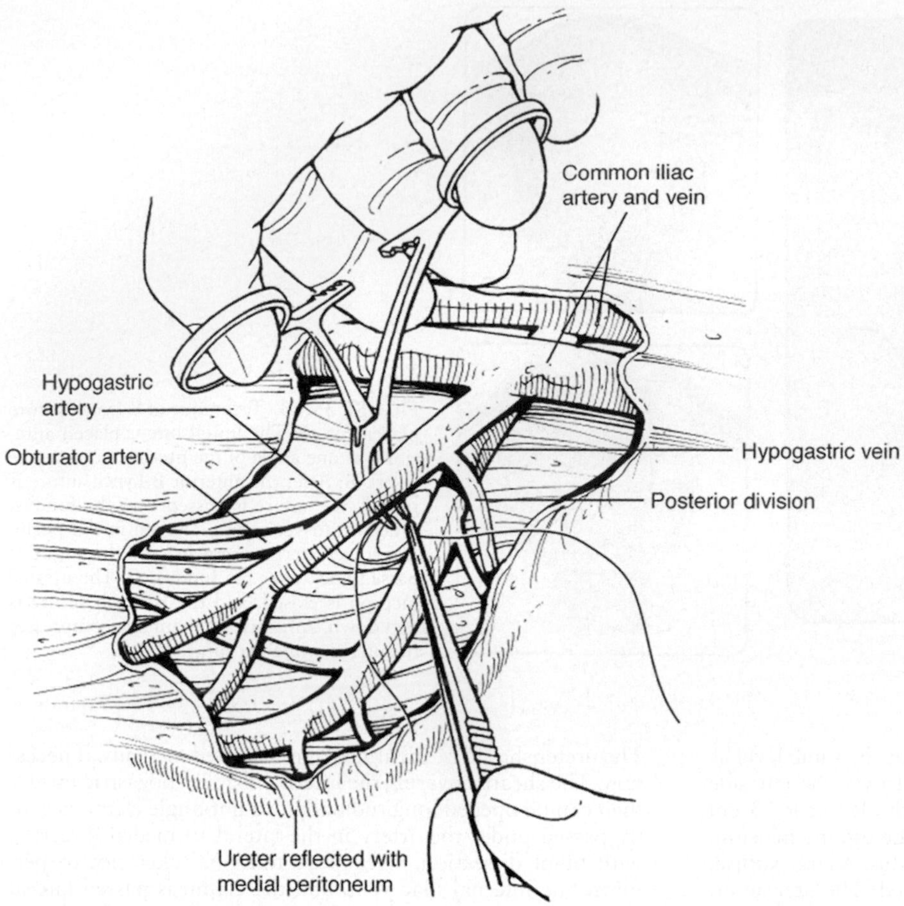

FIGURE 35A.4. Ligation of the right hypogastric artery. The clamp is passed laterally to medial, and the ligature is placed around the anterior division of the hypogastric artery. Note the ureter is attached to the peritoneum, which is reflected medially.

chapter. Hysterectomy usually is the safest procedure and also the quickest that can be performed for refractory bleeding. For example, Clark and associates reported that patients undergoing hypogastric artery ligation who subsequently required hysterectomy had an increased incidence of cardiac arrest secondary to blood loss. The increased morbidity associated with hypogastric artery ligation followed by hysterectomy may be secondary to a delay resulting from attempted conservative management short of hysterectomy. Hypogastric artery ligation was attempted before hysterectomy 64% of the time in nulliparous women, compared with 10% of the time for multiparous patients. Lack of experience with hypogastric artery ligation adds to the overall time required to attempt the procedure and overall blood loss.

In a review of 70 women who underwent emergency hysterectomy for postpartum hemorrhage, Clark and colleagues reported that almost all required blood transfusion, and 50% had postoperative febrile morbidity. The most common indication for hysterectomy in this series was uterine atony, followed by placenta accreta. Of the 70 procedures, 60 were performed after cesarean delivery. Mean operating time was 3.1 hours, and mean blood loss was 3,575 mL.

LATE POSTPARTUM HEMORRHAGE

Late postpartum hemorrhage is that which occurs more than 24 hours after delivery. The etiology of such bleeding includes placental site subinvolution, infection, coagulopathy, and retained products of conception. Initial therapy for this complication is the same as for early hemorrhage. If infection is present, antibiotics should be used. Endometrial curettage may be necessary for retained placental fragments. Angiographic embolization may prove especially useful in the case of late postpartum hemorrhage. Uterine artery ligation, hypogastric artery ligation, and hysterectomy are rarely required for control of late postpartum hemorrhage.

PERIPARTUM HYSTERECTOMY

Horatio Storer performed the first cesarean hysterectomy in 1869. Initially, the procedure was performed only for emergency situations, but in the early 20th century, it became an accepted means of sterilization. In the modern obstetrical age, elective cesarean hysterectomy is rarely performed, except in cases of cervical neoplasia.

Peripartum hysterectomy can be performed in conjunction with a cesarean delivery (e.g., cesarean hysterectomy) or after a vaginal delivery for complications such as postpartum hemorrhage. In a recent review of a nationwide sample of deliveries from 1998 to 2003, Whiteman and colleagues estimated that the rate of peripartum hysterectomy in the Unites States is 0.77 per 1,000 deliveries.

Although there is little controversy regarding peripartum hysterectomy for emergency conditions, there is significant debate in modern obstetrics regarding an elective hysterectomy performed at the time of cesarean delivery. There has been legitimate concern about increased morbidity related to peripartum hysterectomy—including damage to the ureters, bladder, and rectum—and an increased rate of reoperation. However, Plauche has pointed out that morbidity often is associated with the conditions leading to the hysterectomy and not necessarily the procedure itself. Lower morbidities have been reported for elective cesarean hysterectomies when compared with emergency hysterectomies. However, there is inherent bias in these retrospective reviews. Emergent surgery for lifesaving maternal indications would be expected to have higher morbidities, such as blood loss and injury to surrounding structures. Castaneda and colleagues denoted, in a retrospective study, that over the years the indications for peripartum hysterectomy have changed from predominately elective to almost exclusively emergencies. In their data, the average blood loss was 3,009 mL in emergent cases and 1,262 mL in nonemergent cases. They concluded that in current times, peripartum hysterectomy is almost always emergent in nature and associated with a significant blood loss. As might be expected, there are no randomized prospective studies of elective cesarean hysterectomy, and it is unlikely that such a study could ever be done given the ethical dilemma involved.

Emergency Peripartum Hysterectomy

There are several indications for emergency peripartum hysterectomy. The three most common reasons are uterine rupture, abnormal placentation, and uterine atony. Although the exact incidence of emergency peripartum hysterectomy is not known, several authors have reported widely varying rates of 0.004 to 1.5 per 1,000 deliveries.

Obstetric hemorrhage secondary to a variety of etiologies is a common indication reported for peripartum emergency hysterectomy. Clark and associates reviewed 70 cases of emergency hysterectomy for obstetric hemorrhage and found that 60 (86%) of these procedures were performed after cesarean delivery, and 10 (14%) were performed after vaginal delivery. Uterine atony and placenta accreta accounted for almost three fourths of the cases. Other indications were uterine rupture, extension of the uterine incision, and fibroids precluding closure of the uterine incision.

Chestnut and associates reported 44 women undergoing emergency hysterectomy; 20 (45%) procedures were performed for uterine rupture, 7 (16%) were performed for uterine atony, and 4 (9%) were performed for placenta accreta. Other indications included broad ligament hematoma, placenta previa, and chorioamnionitis. Twenty-nine of the cases in this series followed cesarean deliveries, and 15 were postpartum hysterectomies.

In another series of 117 cases of peripartum hysterectomy, Zelop and colleagues reported uterine atony accounted for 25 (21%) of the cases, and most (75, or 64%) were secondary to an abnormally adherent placenta. The rate of emergent hysterectomy increased with increasing parity, placenta previa, and history of previous cesarean section.

It is clear from the literature that abnormal adherent placentation or placenta accreta (with or without hemorrhage) is emerging as the most common condition leading to an emergency hysterectomy. In three studies from 1993 to the present, 156 (56%) of the 279 emergent peripartum hysterectomies were performed for placenta accreta. These studies are outlined in Table 35A.2. The increase in placenta accreta is related to the high rate of cesarean deliveries, which has risen in the United States from 5% in the early 1960s to 30% at the present time. A recent study of more than 60,000 deliveries at the University of Chicago by Wu et al. found that the rate of placenta accreta had increased to 3 per 1,000 deliveries in 2003. They observed that this was directly associated with the increase in cesarean section rate. Placenta previa also is significantly associated with placenta accreta. Zelop et al. reported that the risk of peripartum hysterectomy in women with placenta previa increases from 7 in 1,000 deliveries in nulliparous women to one in four deliveries in women with a history of four or more live births. Clarke and colleagues found that in the presence of a placenta previa, the risk of having placenta accreta increased from 24% in women with one prior cesarean delivery to 67% in women with 3 or more prior cesareans. Zorlu and associates evaluated the indications for emergent hysterectomy in two distinct time periods. Forty-three patients underwent emergent hysterectomy between 1985 and 1989. The incidence of hysterectomy was 1 in 2,495 deliveries, and the indications for hysterectomy included uterine atony (42%), placenta accreta (25.5%), and uterine rupture (21%). Five years later, from 1990 to 1994, the incidence of hysterectomy had decreased by almost 50% to 1 in 4,228 deliveries. In the later time period, the indications for hysterectomy were placenta accreta (41.7%), uterine atony (29.2%), and uterine rupture (20.8%). The authors felt the increase in placenta accreta as an indication for emergent hysterectomy most likely reflected an increase in the cesarean section rate nationwide.

TABLE 35A.2

INDICATIONS FOR EMERGENCY HYSTERECTOMY FOR OBSTETRIC HEMORRHAGE

Indication	Clark et al., 1984	Bakshi et al., 2000	Stanco et al., 1993	Zelop et al., 1993
	($n = 70$)	($n = 39$)	($n = 123$)	($n = 117$)
Uterine atony/hemorrhage	30 (43%)	11 (28%)	44 (35.9%)	25 (21.3%)
Placenta accreta/percreta	21 (30%)	20 (51%)	61 (49%)	75 (64.1%)
Uterine rupture	9 (13%)	5 (15%)	14 (11.5%)	—
Extension of uterine incision	7 (10%)	—	—	—
Leiomyomas	3 (4%)	2 (5%)	3 (2.4%)	—
Uterine infection	—	—	—	17 (14.5%)
Other	—	1 (1%)	1 (1.2%)	—

Elective Cesarean Hysterectomy

Although a number of conditions have been reported as indications for elective cesarean hysterectomy, currently accepted indications are usually limited to microinvasive or invasive cervical cancer. In retrospective reviews that go back to the 1950s and 1960s, sterilization, menstrual abnormalities, and uterine fibroids are listed as indications; however, most practitioners would not consider these appropriate indications for such an invasive surgical procedure in the 21st century.

Morbidity and Mortality of Hysterectomy

The conditions leading to emergency hysterectomy also are responsible for much of the morbidity reported with the procedure. Two other important factors associated with morbidity, both of which are difficult to quantify, are training and experience (or surgical skill) of the surgeon. Chestnut and associates reported statistically significant reductions in operative time, estimated blood loss, intraoperative and total blood replacement, and length of hospital stay if the patient was in the care of an experienced surgeon. It seems reasonable, however, to conclude that morbidity and complications are higher in women undergoing emergency versus elective procedures despite the skill of the surgeon.

Zelop and associates reported 102 (87%) of the patients in their series required transfusion of blood products. Complications of three series, totaling 279 cases of emergency peripartum hysterectomy, are summarized in Table 35A.3. Maternal mortality rates in these studies varied between 0% and 4.5%. As with morbidity, mortality is better correlated with the specific complication than with the hysterectomy per se.

In a review of 80 women undergoing elective cesarean hysterectomy, McNulty reported that only five (6%) experienced febrile morbidity, and 15 (19%) received blood transfusion. Four (5%) women sustained bladder injuries, and four (5%) women developed broad ligament hematomas. Yancey and colleagues compared the outcomes in 43 women undergoing scheduled cesarean hysterectomy with those of 86 women who underwent cesarean delivery and subsequent scheduled hysterectomy. Although women in the cesarean hysterectomy group were more likely to need a blood transfusion than were women in the subsequent hysterectomy group (OR 3.4; 95% CI, 1.4–8.4), they were less likely to have other complications, such as infection (OR 0.34; 95% CI, 0.25–0.45). The overall postoperative complication rate was the same in both groups (51%). Thus, it is likely that elective cesarean hysterectomy is not associated with an increased risk of complications or morbidity compared with a cesarean delivery followed by an elective hysterectomy at a later time. However, in a healthy population, one must weigh the infectious risk of blood transfusion versus the benefit of the combined procedure. As pointed out by Baker and D'Alton, however, there is little doubt that elective cesarean hysterectomy does result in increased morbidity when compared with a cesarean delivery and a tubal ligation.

Emergency Versus Elective Hysterectomy

In two studies comparing emergency with elective peripartum hysterectomy, morbidity was greater with the emergency procedure. Estimated blood loss, number of women transfused, and operating time were all higher in the emergency group. It is important to remember that many of the patients who undergo emergent delivery already had significant blood loss and hemorrhage before the decision being made to proceed with hysterectomy.

Cesarean Hysterectomy Technique

Elective cesarean hysterectomy can be accomplished through either a midline or low transverse (Pfannenstiel) skin incision. Often, it is more prudent to use a midline skin incision in cases of emergency peripartum hysterectomy if one anticipates that a hypogastric artery ligation may be required.

After the cesarean delivery, the placenta is quickly removed unless there is a contraindication to do so. *No attempt is made to remove the placenta in cases of placenta accreta because significant life-threatening hemorrhage can ensue.* In cases of placenta percreta involving the posterior wall of the bladder, a partial cystectomy may be required. In these cases, the bladder trigone and ureteral orifices must be carefully identified, and urologic consultation may be needed. In cases of anterior placenta previa and suspected placenta accreta, it is prudent to arrange for urologic support preoperatively. In cases of suspected accreta, interventional radiology may place bilateral hypogastric artery balloons preoperatively. When inflated, these balloons have significantly decreased operative blood loss in our experience.

The uterine incision can be closed with a running no. 1 suture in a locking fashion. The bladder flap should be dissected

TABLE 35A.3

COMPLICATIONS OF 279 CASES OF EMERGENCY PERIPARTUM HYSTERECTOMY

	Complication Incidence (%)			
	Clark et al. ($n = 70$)	Bakshi et al. ($n = 39$)	Stanco et al. ($n = 123$)	Zelop et al. ($n = 117$)
Infection	50	20.5	9	50
Wound infection	12	—	9	3.4
Blood transfusion	96	80	82	87
Coagulopathy	6	2.5	5.7	27
Urologic injury	4	7.7	13	10.2
Death	1	0	0	0

well down before the start of the hysterectomy. This is best accomplished at the time of the cesarean delivery. The bladder should be dissected off the anterior, lower uterine segment with sharp dissection if firm adhesions are encountered. Firm adhesions often are present in patients who have undergone multiple cesarean deliveries. If bleeding is a problem, further dissection of the bladder from the lower uterine segment can be accomplished after ligation of the uterine artery.

The actual hysterectomy is begun by ligating the round ligament close to the uterus and ligating the distal stump with a 0-Vicryl suture ligature. The vesicouterine serosa, where the bladder was attached before its dissection, then is extended laterally to the severed round ligaments.

The peritoneal incision should be extended superiorly. Because the ureters are dilated in pregnancy, they should be identified quickly to avoid injury. The ureter can be seen crossing the iliac artery at the level of the bifurcation in the medial leaf of the broad ligament and is most easily identified at this location. The uteroovarian ligaments can be secured by first making a "window" through the posterior leaf of the broad ligament and then doubly clamping, cutting, and ligating the uteroovarian ligament bilaterally (Fig. 35A.5). This step is easy and uncomplicated in the nonpregnant patient; but the dilated vasculature of pregnancy requires the surgeon to carefully select a clear window and handle the tissues gently to avoid troublesome bleeding from easily torn veins. The uterine vessels are skeletonized as in the nonpuerperal hysterectomy. These vessels are large and easy to identify. Dissection is made easier with continuous upward traction of the uterus. If possible, the uterine vessels are clamped bilaterally (usually with a Heaney or Zeppelin clamp) before the vessels are cut. If there is room, we prefer to place three large clamps on each side, and divide the pedicle between the first and second clamp (Fig. 35A.6). This provides two clamps on the active vessels for security and one back clamp to prevent back bleeding from the enlarged, blood-engorged uterus. The vascular pedicles are doubly ligated with 0 synthetic absorbable sutures, and we generally prefer to suture ligate the back bleeders also, so that the back camps can be removed from the field. This provides better exposure and reduces the risk of tearing the uterine tissues by excessive traction on these clamps. As with all hysterectomies, care must be exercised in identifying and avoiding the ureter. The next pedicles encountered should be the broad ligament, the base of which is the cardinal ligament. A slightly curved or a straight clamp, whichever fits the anatomy best, can be used for these ligaments. It is better to take several small pedicles instead of one large bite because an excessively large pedicle can slide out of a clamp or suture. This is especially true with the edematous tissues associated with pregnancy. Once the cardinal and uterosacral ligaments have been clamped, cut, and tied at the level of the cervix, the specimen can be removed by clamping across the vagina on each side and incising the vaginal mucosa (Fig. 35A.7). It may be difficult to identify the lower extent of the cervix, especially if the cervix is effaced. The cervix can be grasped with a thumb anteriorly, and the hand wrapping around the cervix with the fingers posteriorly. The cervix is then pinched between the thumb and middle finger as the hand slowly slides down the cervix toward the vagina. Usually, it is possible to feel the lower end of the cervix in this way. If there is any doubt, it may also be helpful to make an incision into

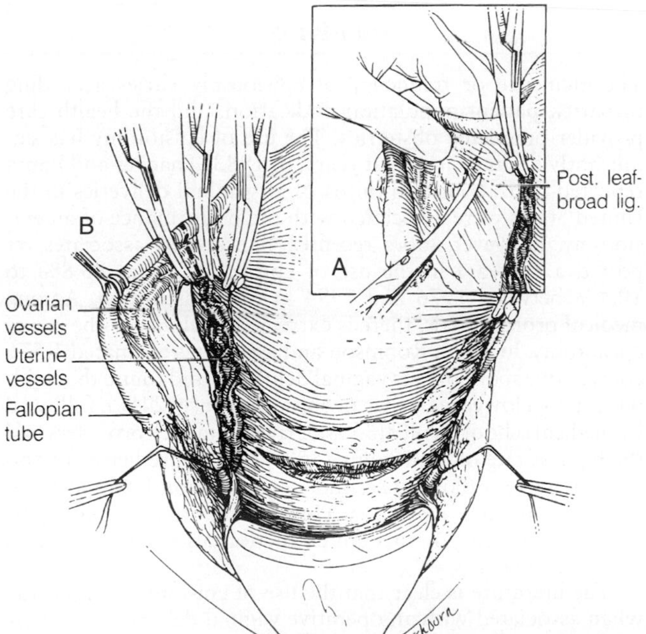

FIGURE 35A.5. **A:** The posterior leaf of the broad ligament adjacent to the uterus is perforated just beneath the fallopian tube, uteroovarian ligaments, and ovarian vessels. **B:** These are then doubly clamped close to the uterus and severed. (From: Cunningham FG, MacDonald PC, Gant NF, et al. Caesarean section and caesarean hysterectomy. In: *Williams Obstetrics*. 19th ed. Norwalk, CT: Appleton & Lange;1993:591, with permission.)

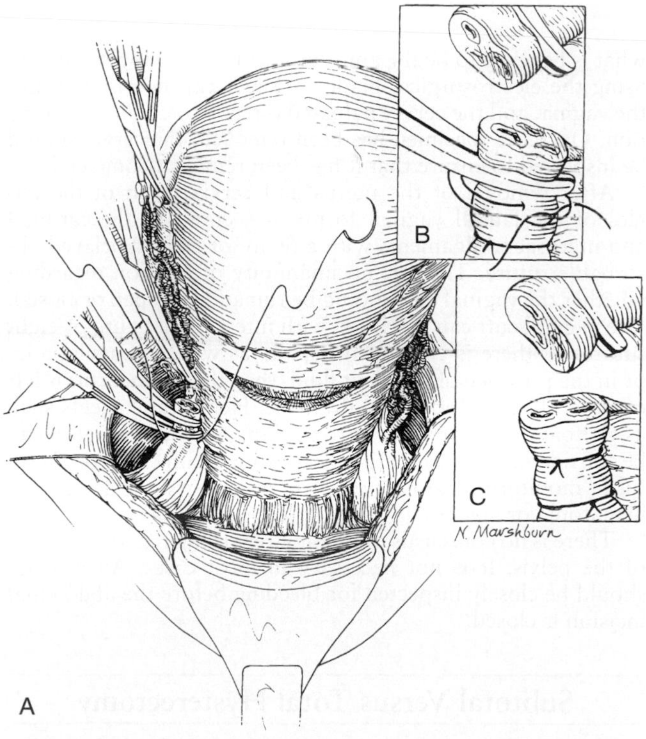

FIGURE 35A.6. **A:** The uterine artery and veins on either side are doubly clamped immediately adjacent to the uterus and divided. **B, C:** The vascular pedicle is doubly suture ligated. (From: Cunningham FG, MacDonald PC, Gant NF, et al. Caesarean section and caesarean hysterectomy. In: *Williams Obstetrics*. 19th ed. Norwalk, CT: Appleton & Lange;1993:591, with permission.)

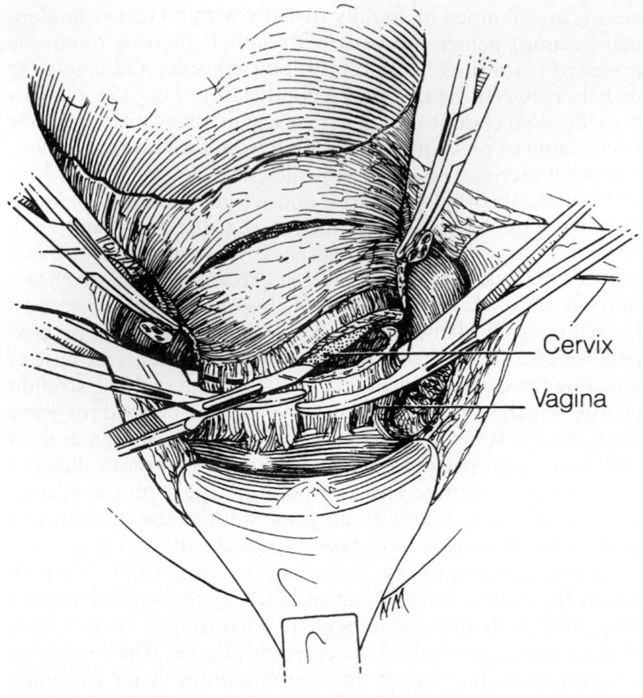

FIGURE 35A.7. A curved clamp is swung in across the lateral vaginal fornix below the level of the cervix, and the tissue is incised medially to the point of the clamp. (From: Cunningham FG, MacDonald PC, Gant NF, et al. Caesarean section and caesarean hysterectomy. In: *Williams Obstetrics*. 19th ed. Norwalk, CT: Appleton & Lange;1993:591, with permission.)

what is believed to be the anterior vagina just below the cervix using the electrosurgical blade. A finger can be inserted into the vagina, and the cervix palpated directly to confirm its location. Once the specimen has been removed, the cervix should be inspected to ensure that it has been removed completely.

After removal of the uterus and cervix, each of the angles of the lateral vaginal fornix is secured to the cardinal and uterosacral ligaments with a figure-of-eight 0 delayed absorbable suture. There is no unanimity of opinion regarding whether the vaginal cuff should be run and left open or closed. The vaginal cuff can be closed with interrupted figure-of-eight sutures. If there is continued oozing, as with a coagulopathy or in the presence of purulent fluid, then the vaginal cuff is left open to allow for adequate drainage. Hemostatic agents such as Gelfoam, with or without topical thrombin, or Surgicel can be considered. An intraperitoneal suction drain can prove helpful in monitoring patients who are at high risk of developing hematoma or abscess.

There is no consensus of opinion regarding reperitonization of the pelvis. It is not necessary in most cases. All pedicles should be closely inspected for bleeding before the abdominal incision is closed.

Subtotal Versus Total Hysterectomy

Some clinicians have a tendency to perform a subtotal or supracervical hysterectomy in most cases of emergency peripartum hysterectomy. There is a general belief that both operating time and blood loss are significantly lower with the subtotal technique. In addition, it is said that the risk of bladder or ureteral injury is less. There is no question that in the select patient who has been or is hemodynamically unstable, it may be prudent to perform a supracervical hysterectomy, especially if all bleeding has been controlled to that point. However, it is necessary to remove the cervix in cases of placenta previa or placenta accreta involving the lower uterine segment.

Despite the reputed advantages of a supracervical hysterectomy, there is evidence that performance of a complete hysterectomy with removal of the cervix adds little to either operating time or blood loss. Clark and associates reported no significant differences in mean values for blood loss and operating time in obstetric patients undergoing emergency total hysterectomy versus supracervical hysterectomy. Mean hospital stay also was not significantly different. However, the women in this study were not randomized to supracervical versus total hysterectomy. In 1998, Zorlu and associates also reported no significant difference between total and supracervical hysterectomy in operative time, blood transfusion, and mean hospital stay. It is important to separate emergency cesarean hysterectomy for hemorrhage, and so on, from elective peripartum hysterectomy for indications such as microinvasive cervical cancer because the blood loss and other morbidity are generally significantly greater for the emergency procedure. A prospective, randomized study would be very helpful.

EPISIOTOMY

An episiotomy is a surgical incision into the perineal body for the purpose of either aiding the actual delivery process or preventing tears and lacerations.

Incidence

The incidence or frequency of episiotomy varies according to parity, patient population, indication, and the health care provider practicing obstetrics. The use of episiotomy has significantly declined in recent years. In 1983, Thacker and Banta reported that about two thirds of all vaginal deliveries in the United States were associated with the performance of an episiotomy. However, more recently, Bansai and associates reported a decrease in the use of episiotomy from 86.8% to 10.4% between 1976 and 1994 at their institution. Among medical professionals, there is extreme variability in the use of episiotomy. In 2000, Robinson and associates evaluated 1,576 consecutive spontaneous vaginal deliveries and found that midwives had a lower incidence of episiotomy use (21%), followed by medical school faculty (33%). Private practice providers had the highest rate of episiotomy (55%). Other predictors of episiotomy were prolonged second stage of labor, fetal macrosomia, and epidural anesthesia. Hueston reported that nulliparity, use of forceps, or vacuum extraction also were predictors of episiotomy.

The literature is clear that the use of episiotomy, especially when associated with an operative vaginal delivery, is directly related to an *increase* in perineal sphincter injury. It has been suggested that given the morbidity associated with these injuries that the combination of these two procedures be avoided, if possible.

Indications

The routine use of episiotomy with vaginal delivery has been strongly challenged. A recent Practice Bulletin from the

American College of Obstetricians and Gynecologists stated that the previously held ideas that episiotomy facilitated vaginal delivery, especially difficult or operative vaginal delivery, or improved neonatal outcome when expeditious delivery was indicated, are *not* supported by current evidence. Studies by Myles and Santolaya and Bodner-Adler and colleagues failed to show any reduction in anal sphincter damage, rectal mucosal tears, or improved neonatal outcomes in women who underwent episiotomy.

In the past, it was thought that episiotomy prevented vaginal and perineal damage that led to subsequent pelvic relaxation. However, there is little evidence to support the premise that "prophylactic" episiotomy prevents cystocele, rectocele, enterocele, uterine prolapse, vaginal prolapse, or stress urinary incontinence. Rockner and associates evaluated pelvic floor muscle strength using vaginal cones and found that women with episiotomies had less strength than those with spontaneous vaginal deliveries. Neural testing of the perineal musculature in other studies showed that the amount of denervation was associated with weight of the baby and the length of the second stage of labor, and was unrelated to episiotomy. Sleep and Grant looked at deliveries in those who restricted use of episiotomy and those who reported liberal use of episiotomy. Over 3 years of follow-up, there was little difference between the two groups in severity of incontinence or the reported incidence of incontinence. These studies indicate that episiotomy does not appear to prevent the physical/anatomic or symptomatic changes of pelvic relaxation.

In addition, there are no good data to support prophylactic episiotomy for the prevention of "trauma" to the fetus, especially the preterm fetus. Although there is no evidence that the risk of shoulder dystocia can be decreased by the use of an episiotomy, many experts feel that a generous episiotomy may help in the management of a shoulder dystocia when it presents.

In summary, current opinion does not support the routine use of episiotomy for vaginal delivery. Previous ideas that suggested episiotomy decreased the risk of perineal injury, reduced trauma of operative delivery, or improved neonatal outcome have not been supported by recent studies. An episiotomy undoubtedly provides more room for a difficult vaginal delivery. Such deliveries are inherently associated with an increased risk of fetal distress and maternal trauma. The obstetrician must individualize each patient and weigh the potential advantages of an episiotomy against the known risks of episiotomy or vaginal delivery without an episiotomy or even cesarean delivery.

Midline Versus Mediolateral Episiotomy

There is little question that the midline perineal incision is easier to perform and repair, and is associated with less postoperative pain than the mediolateral episiotomy. In general, it is also associated with less blood loss and better anatomic results. Midline perineal incisions are used more frequently in the United States, whereas mediolateral episiotomy is used more commonly in Europe. The major disadvantage of midline episiotomy is an increased risk of third- and fourth-degree lacerations. Owen and Hauth report that 20% of primiparous women with a midline episiotomy had a third- or fourth-degree laceration, compared with 9% of women with a mediolateral incision and only 1% when no episiotomy was performed. Of interest, multiparous women with a midline episiotomy had fewer third- and fourth-degree lacerations than those with a mediolateral episiotomy. Although these data appear to favor performing either a mediolateral episiotomy or no episiotomy at all, caution must be exercised when interpreting the data because this was not a randomized, prospective study, and it does not control for possible confounding factors. For example, patients who underwent episiotomy may well have had larger babies, a higher incidence of forceps assistance, or other characteristics resulting in an increased risk of laceration.

Although the mediolateral episiotomy may be associated with fewer third- and fourth-degree lacerations (at least in the primiparous patient) (Table 35A.4), there are several disadvantages to this technique. Blood loss is greater, mediolateral episiotomies are more difficult to repair, and anatomic results may be faulty. Postoperative pain also is more common and can be very troublesome. In the absence of good, prospective, randomized trails, the decision to perform a mediolateral or midline episiotomy must be based on clinical judgment and experience. A mediolateral episiotomy may provide more room for a difficult delivery with a lower risk of third- and fourth-degree laceration, but it also results in more blood loss and a greater risk of long-term dyspareunia.

Episiotomy Repair

An episiotomy can be repaired in numerous ways. One popular method is to close the vaginal mucosa and submucosa with a continuous locking suture of 2-0 synthetic delayed absorbable suture or chromic catgut, followed by closure of the fascia and muscle of the perineal body with three or four interrupted sutures of similar suture material. The skin of the perineum can then be closed with a continuous subcuticular stitch or by interrupted sutures of 3-0 or 4-0 synthetic absorbable or chromic suture through the subcutaneous tissue and skin. In cases of fourth-degree lacerations, it is important to approximate the edges of the rectal mucosa with a running submucosal 3-0 or 4-0 delayed absorbable or chromic suture, followed by a second reinforcement layer of the rectovaginal septal tissue. If the external anal sphincter is severed, it should be carefully reapproximated with several interrupted 2-0 sutures through the muscle and fibrous capsule. The technique for primary episiotomy closure is illustrated later in this chapter and is also discussed in Chapter 40.

TABLE 35A.4

RELATION OF LACERATIONS TO TYPE OF EPISIOTOMY IN 7,675 PRIMIPAROUS WOMEN

	Type of episiotomy		
Laceration type	Midline ($n = 4,822$)	Mediolateral ($n = 79$)	None ($n = 2,774$)
Second-degree	1,425 (30%)	26 (33%)	375 (14%)
Third- or fourth-degree	968 (20%)	7 (9%)	52 (1%)
Other	295 (6%)	7 (9%)	274 (10%)
Totals	2,688 (56%)	40 (51%)	701 (25%)

From: Owen J, Hauth JC. Episiotomy infection and dehiscence. In: Gilstrap LC III, Faro S, eds. *Infections in pregnancy.* New York: Alan R. Liss;1990:61, with permission.

Complications of Episiotomy

Extensions and Fistula Formation

The major complications of episiotomy include infection, hematoma, breakdown, and fistula formation. Probably the single most common complication is extension (i.e., third- or fourth-degree laceration). Extensions in turn can lead to incontinence of flatus and stool, rectovaginal fistula, and infection. The association of extensions with the type of episiotomy has been discussed already. In the report by Harris, 11.6% of the more than 7,000 women with midline episiotomies had a third- or fourth-degree laceration. In the women with these lacerations, 2% subsequently had poor sphincter tone, and 0.1% developed a rectovaginal fistula. Signorello and colleagues performed a retrospective cohort study to evaluate the relationship between midline episiotomy and anal incontinence postpartum. Women with episiotomies had a higher risk of fecal incontinence 3 months and 6 months postpartum. Episiotomy tripled the risk of fecal incontinence at 3 months and 6 months postpartum and doubled the risk of flatus incontinence compared with women with spontaneous lacerations. In a prospective evaluation of 16,583 deliveries, Walsh and colleagues found that 0.56% of deliveries were complicated by third-degree lacerations. Lacerations were not prevented by episiotomy, but were associated with forceps delivery. Of the 81 patients followed, 30 had abnormal anorectal examination; 7% were incontinent of stool, and 12% were incontinent of flatus.

Fistula is fortunately an uncommon complication of episiotomy. Causes include unrecognized lacerations in the rectovaginal septum at the time of episiotomy repair or infected hematoma. Risk factors for fistula formation include obesity, poor hygiene, malnutrition, anemia, history of inflammatory bowel disease, connective tissue disease, or prior exposure to radiation therapy. Half of these fistulae spontaneously heal, but repair should be considered if the patient is very symptomatic.

Dehiscence

The exact incidence of episiotomy dehiscence is unknown, but it appears to occur infrequently. In a review of 390 women with fourth-degree perineal lacerations, 18 (4.6%) experienced a dehiscence, and 11 of these were associated with infection.

Several predisposing factors have been reported to be associated with episiotomy dehiscence, including infection, human papillomavirus, cigarette smoking, hematoma, or trauma. Infection is probably the most common factor. In the study by Ramin and associates, 86% of patients with midline episiotomy dehiscence and 69% of patients with mediolateral episiotomy dehiscence had evidence of infection that was based on the presence of fever or purulent discharge. Infection with human papillomavirus also has been reported by some to be associated with dehiscence. Although inadequate or "faulty" repair has been reported to be associated with dehiscence, this is a rare cause.

Early Repair of Dehiscence. In the past, it has been taught that repair of episiotomy dehiscence should be delayed for several months to allow for revascularization and healing. However, current surgical opinion supported by recent data favors early repair. Delayed repair is an inconvenience for the woman and may be associated with fecal incontinence and loss of sexual function. Delay also can increase the hospital stay, cost, and increase risk of litigation.

There are many advantages to early repair of episiotomy dehiscence. Hauth and colleagues reported on the efficacy and safety of early repair in eight women who had a dehiscence of a fourth-degree midline episiotomy. Early repair was successful in seven of the eight women. One woman developed a pinpoint rectovaginal fistula 4 days after early repair. This was fixed with a 1-cm rectal flap 4 months later.

Monberg and Hammen reported on the successful resuturing of episiotomy breakdown in 20 women with infection, dehiscence, or both. Although four of the women had superficial reseparation, all subsequently healed spontaneously.

Hankins and associates updated the initial report by Hauth and colleagues to include 22 women with dehiscence of an initial fourth-degree repair, four with dehiscence of a third-degree repair and five with breakdown of a mediolateral repair. Initial success of early repair was achieved in 29 (94%) of 31 women. Two women with a pinpoint rectovaginal fistula were subsequently repaired with a rectal flap procedure. Of the 27 women with a follow-up of 1 year or greater, all were continent and had resumption of normal coital activity. The follow-up of the 22 women with early repair of episiotomy dehiscence revealed no complications in 18 patients. Occasional incontinence of flatus and stool, dyspareunia, dyschezia, and numbness occurred in the remaining patients. All of the symptoms resolved by 9 months, except for two patients who had persistent dyspareunia.

Ramin and coworkers reported on the early repair of 34 women with episiotomy dehiscence, most of whom were infected (Table 35A.5). These women received care from a large urban hospital serving primarily an indigent population. The timing of repair for dehiscence ranged from 3 to 13 days. Two women with initial third-degree episiotomy dehiscence had unsuccessful repairs. Thus, successful repairs were accomplished in 32 (94%) of the women. The average time from delivery to subsequent discharge after repair of the dehiscence was 15.5 days. This is similar to the time reported by Hankins and colleagues. This time probably can be shortened significantly with outpatient management of the wound and repair in ambulatory care units.

Secondary Repair Technique. Before attempting a closure, it is important to prepare the wound for repair. The first step is cleaning and debridement of the episiotomy site. This can be

TABLE 35A.5

CHARACTERISTICS OF 34 PATIENTS WITH EPISIOTOMY DEHISCENCE AND SUBSEQUENT EARLY REPAIR

Characteristic	Midline	Mediolateral
Total number of patients	21	13
Type of delivery		
Spontaneous	11	0
Outlet forceps	3	3
Low forceps	7	10
Extension		
None	1	5
Third-degree	9	6
Fourth-degree	11	2
Evidence of infection	18 (86%)	9 (69%)
Early repair failures	1	1

From: Ramin SM, Ramus RM, Little BB, et al. Early repair of episiotomy dehiscence associated with infection. *Am J Obstet Gynecol* 1992;167:1104, with permission.

accomplished either on the ward with intravenous sedation or local anesthesia or in the operating room under regional anesthesia. All necrotic tissue and suture fragments should be removed and the wound irrigated with a diluted povidone-iodine solution or half-strength Dakin's solution. Broad-spectrum antibiotics are indicated for overt infection or significant cellulitis. After initial debridement, the wound should be scrubbed and cleaned at least twice daily. Scrub brushes impregnated with povidone-iodine or gauze dressing pads can be used. A 1% lidocaine jelly is applied to the wound several minutes before cleansing, and analgesics should be used as necessary. The liberal use of sitz baths helps keep the wound clean.

Secondary repair of the episiotomy is not attempted until the wound is free of exudate and covered by granulation tissue. A mechanical bowel preparation with an oral electrolyte solution should be administered the evening before surgery for fourth-degree breakdowns. Prophylactic antibiotics are recommended for all repairs. One to three doses of a first-generation cephalosporin generally proves satisfactory.

The first step in the surgical repair of dehiscence is debridement of granulation tissue and dissection to ensure good tissue mobility. If the anal sphincter muscle has been severed, extensive retraction usually has occurred. It is important to identify the fibrous capsule and mobilize the muscle and capsule for successful reapproximation. If the rectal mucosa has been lacerated, it should be reapproximated as described in this chapter. In a prospective, randomized trial, Fitzpatrick and colleagues compared 55 women who underwent a sphincter overlap procedure with 57 women who underwent staple approximation repair of third-degree lacerations. In this study, there were no significant differences in anal manometry or endoanal ultrasound in the two groups. Therefore, either approach is acceptable. The rest of the closure is the same as for a secondary episiotomy repair. The secondary repair of a fourth-degree episiotomy breakdown is shown in Figures 35A.8 through 35A.11.

Postoperatively, women can be placed on a regular diet if the rectal mucosa is not involved. If the rectal mucosa is involved, a low-residue diet should be used for several days and advanced to a regular diet. Stool softeners may prove useful, but diarrhea should be avoided because of the increased likelihood of infection. Postoperative care should also include sitz baths and a heat lamp.

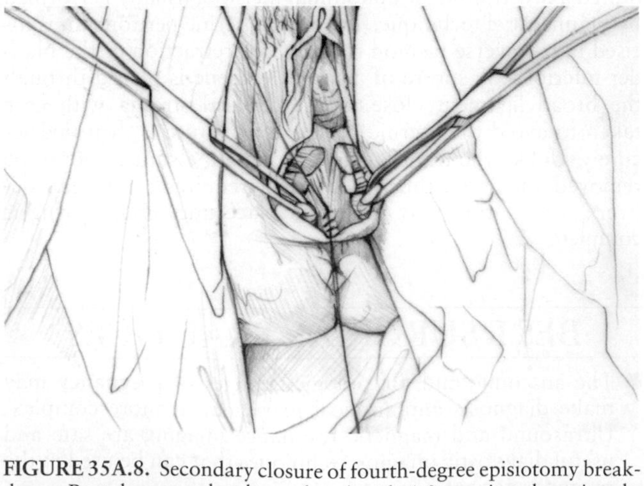

FIGURE 35A.8. Secondary closure of fourth-degree episiotomy breakdown. Rectal mucosa has been closed with 4-0 running chromic submucosal suture and reinforced with a second layer of 3-0 chromic suture through the rectovaginal septum.

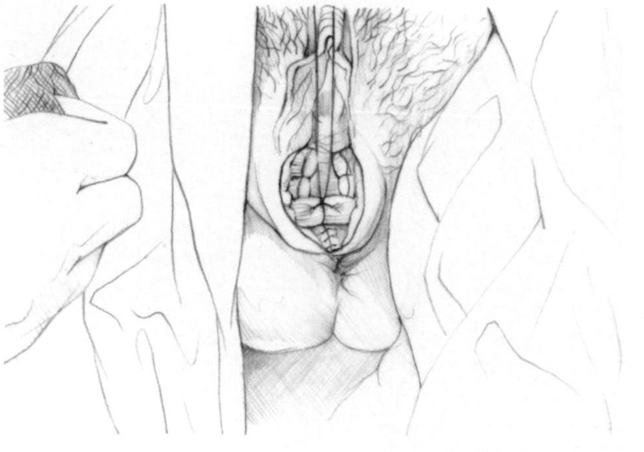

FIGURE 35A.9. The anal sphincter muscle has been reapproximated end to end with several interrupted 2-0 chromic sutures through the muscle and capsule.

The care and repair of a mediolateral episiotomy dehiscence are the same as for a midline repair. More extensive tissue mobilization may be required with the repair of a mediolateral episiotomy dehiscence.

CERVICAL CERCLAGE

Premature dilation of the uterine cervix is a major cause of loss or delivery in midpregnancy. Although the pathophysiology of *cervical insufficiency* is poorly understood and the diagnosis challenging, data are ever involving regarding the management of this complex situation. The concept of cervical insufficiency, its diagnosis, and its management have been well reviewed in a Practice Bulletin issued by the American College of Obstetricians and Gynecologists. Although a variety of diagnostic criteria—including prior midtrimester losses and history of cervical surgery (including loop electrode excision procedure or cone biopsy) and painless dilatation of the cervix—have been used in the past and serve as useful clinical risk factors, today ultrasound monitoring of cervical length and funneling are usually used to make a diagnosis of cervical insufficiency.

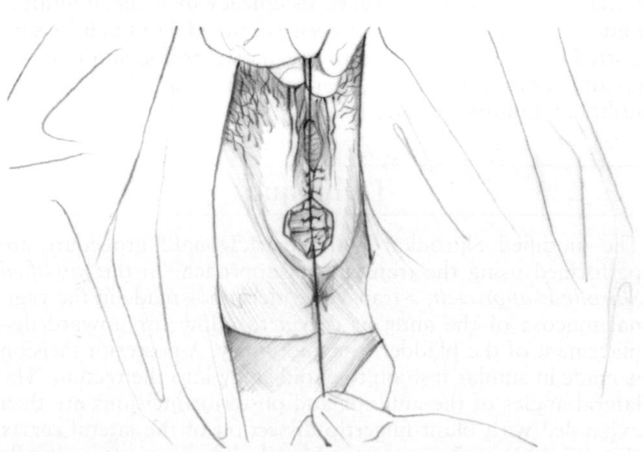

FIGURE 35A.10. The vaginal mucosa and bulbocavernous muscle have been closed with 2-0 chromic suture.

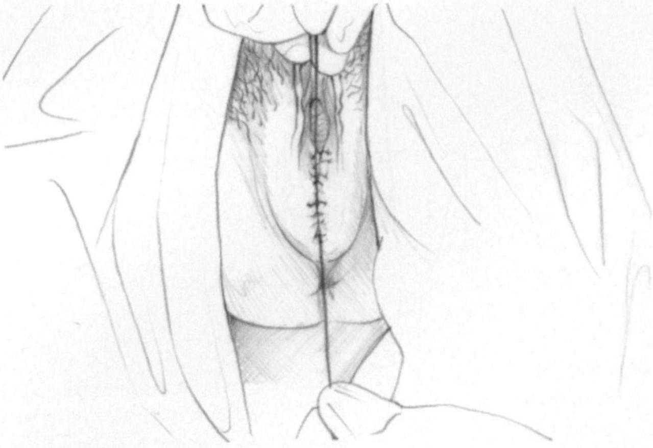

FIGURE 35A.11. Secondary repair of fourth-degree episiotomy dehiscence is completed. (Courtesy of Susan Ramin, University of Texas, Dallas.)

Shirodkar first described cerclage placement in 1955 as a new method to prevent habitual abortion in the second trimester. McDonald, in 1957, reported a simplified technique. The technique for the abdominal approach for cerclage was described by Benson and Durfee in 1965. Data regarding the efficacy of cerclage placement has been conflicting. The Cervical Incompetence Prevention Randomized Cerclage Trial (CIPRACT) concluded that serial ultrasounds for evaluation of cervical insufficiency with secondary intervention is a safe alternative to traditional prophylactic cerclage. Cerclage is rarely performed after 24.5 weeks' gestation because the risks of surgery are outweighed by the benefits of bed rest for a few weeks to achieve improved fetal survival. Zaveri and colleagues noted that transabdominal cerclage may be associated with a lower risk of perinatal death, but has a higher risk of intraoperative complications. Data suggest that an abdominal cerclage may be preferable in patients in whom a transvaginal cerclage has failed. The abdominal approach is also indicated in patients whose cervix has been shortened significantly by cone biopsy or other surgery. Laparoscopic transabdominal suture insertion during and before pregnancy has recently been described. Recent case reports suggest that placement of the abdominal cerclage by a laparoscopic approach is safe and may reduce maternal recovery time; however, its efficacy over the additional abdominal approach has not been examined. Studies have supported the uses of cerclage for pregnancy prolongation in singleton gestations; however, there are conflicting data about its utility in multiple gestations.

Technique

The modified Shirodkar and the McDonald procedure are performed using the transvaginal approach. In the *modified Shirodkar approach*, a transverse incision is made in the vaginal mucosa of the anterior cervix to allow for upward displacement of the bladder to avoid injury. A posterior incision is made in similar fashion to avoid entry into the rectum. The lateral angles of the anterior and posterior incisions are then expanded with blunt fingertip dissection of the lateral cervix (Fig. 35A.12). A 5-mm woven Mersilene tape on a large needle (Ethicon, USA) is then passed through the submucosal tunnel from anterior to posterior on both sides of the cervix. It is preferable to avoid entering the cervical canal because the tape may irritate the fetal membranes; this can be done by placing an index finger in the cervical canal as the needle is passed through the lateral cervix. The lateral cervical mucosa at 3 and 9 o'clock can also be grasped with an Allis clamp or ring forceps as shown in Figure 35A.12 to facilitate placement of the sutures. After the suture is placed on both sides of the cervix, the knot is tied in the posterior defect. The defects are then closed with 3-0 Vicryl in figure-of-eight fashion. We usually leave a whisker of the Mersilene band extending through the closure so that it can be grasped, the suture exposed and cut when the patient goes into labor.

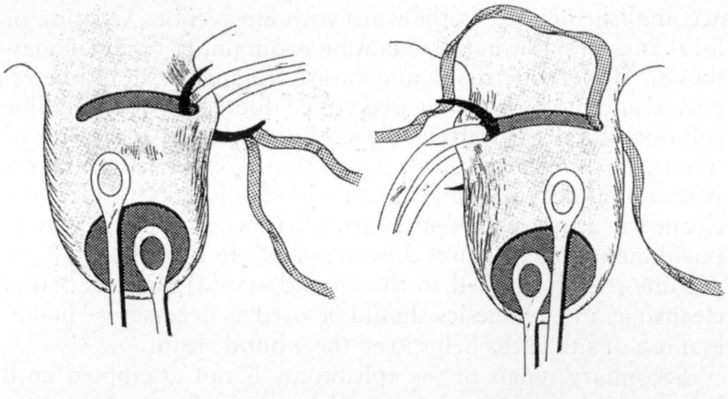

FIGURE 35A.12. Modified Shirodkar cerclage. An incision in the mucosa is made anteriorly and posteriorly to advance the bladder and rectum. A 5-mm Mersilene suture on a large needle is placed in a submucosal tunnel around the cervix and tied posteriorly.

The *McDonald* approach requires no dissection into the cervical tissues. A suture of braided Mersilene or a heavy monofilament suture (Prolene) may be placed around the cervix in purse-string fashion and tied securely (Fig. 35A.13).

Proponents of the modified Shirodkar feel that cervical dissection assists in placing a higher cerclage, but Rozenburg and associates noted that the anterior colpotomy associated with the modified Shirodkar cerclage only increased the distance from the external os by 2.7 mm. Rust and colleagues noted that the length of the cervix below the level of the cerclage does not affect the rate of preterm delivery.

Placement of the *abdominal cerclage* traditionally has required a low transverse abdominal incision, usually performed by Pfannenstiel technique. The vesicouterine peritoneum is incised in transverse fashion to allow for retraction of the bladder inferiorly. A suture of 5-mm Mersilene is placed through the broad ligament close to the cervical stroma with care taken to avoid the uterine vessels. The suture is then tied securely. Unlike the transvaginal cerclage, the suture cannot be removed vaginally; thus, the patient requires a cesarean delivery. This suture may be left in place until childbearing is complete.

BEST SURGICAL PRACTICES

- The anatomic and physiologic changes of pregnancy may make diagnosis and surgical management more complex. Ultrasound and magnetic resonance imaging are safe and useful diagnostic imaging techniques that can be used in the pregnant patient.
- Postpartum hemorrhage may be a life-threatening emergency. It may be due to an obstetric laceration, retained

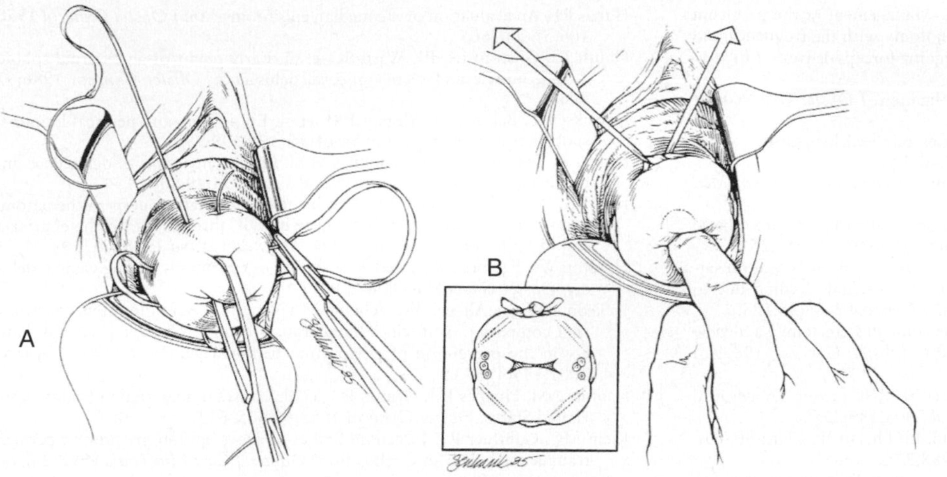

FIGURE 35A.13. Placement of suture for McDonald cervical cerclage. **A:** We use a double-headed Mersilene band with four "bites" in the cervix, avoiding the vessels. **B:** The suture is placed high upon the cervix close to the cervical-vaginal junction, approximately the level of the internal os.

products of conception, uterine atony, or coagulation defects. Aggressive fluid replacement and oxytocic agents are indicated while a diagnostic evaluation is undertaken. Uterine packing has recently been rediscovered as an effective way to treat hemorrhage from uterine atony.

- Transcatheter arterial embolization may be very effective to control postpartum hemorrhage. Bilateral uterine artery or hypogastric artery embolization is recommended. This technique is highly effective, preserves the uterus, and does not preclude future pregnancies.
- Surgical techniques for the management of peripartum hemorrhage include uterine artery ligation, hypogastric artery ligation, B-Lynch compression sutures, and hysterectomy. Emergency hysterectomy for hemorrhage is associated with a significantly increased risk of complications, including urinary tract injury and infection. It is not clear whether elective hysterectomy performed at the time of a scheduled cesarean delivery is associated with increased morbidity, but blood loss and risk of transfusion are increased, and delivery followed by hysterectomy 3 to 6 months later may be considered as an alternative.
- The use of episiotomy has declined significantly in recent years. Recently, studies have not shown any benefit of episiotomy in reducing the risk of third- and fourth-degree lacerations, reducing the risk of long-term pelvic support defects, or improving neonatal outcome. Episiotomy should not be used routinely. Median episiotomy is associated with a higher risk of anal sphincter and rectal injury. Mediolateral episiotomy is associated with increased blood loss and perhaps an increase in postpartum pain and long-term dyspareunia. Repair of episiotomy, especially if there is rectal or sphincter injury, should be done meticulously, using good surgical technique with adequate anesthesia and sterile technique.
- Surgical treatment of cervical insufficiency is complicated by a poor understanding of the pathophysiology of the condition. Painless dilatation and effacement of the cervix in the second trimester, usually documented by ultrasound, is an indication for treatment. Both the McDonald and Shirodkar techniques have been used successfully. An abdominal cerclage may be considered if the cervix has been shortened or damaged by surgery or trauma.

Bibliography

Alamia Jr V, Meyer BA. Peripartum hemorrhage. *Obstet Gynecol Clin North Am* 1999;26:385.

Allahdin S, Aird C, Danielian P. B-Lynch sutures for major primary postpartum haemorrhage at caesarean section. *J Obstet Gynaecol* 2006;26:639.

Allen RE, Hoster GL, Smith ARB, et al. Pelvic floor damage and childbirth: a neurophysiologic study. *BJOG* 1990;97:770.

Althuisius SM, Dekker GA, Hummel P, et al. Cervical in competence prevention randomized cerclage trial. *Am J Obstet Gynecol* 2003;189(4):907–910.

Amant F, Spitz B, Timmerman D, et al. Misoprostol compared with methylergometrine for the prevention of postpartum haemorrhage: a double-blind randomised trial. *BJOG* 1999;106:1066.

American College of Obstetricians and Gynecologists. *Cervical Insufficiency. ACOG Practice Bulletin No. 48.* Washington, DC: ACOG; 2003.

American College of Obstetricians and Gynecologists. *Diagnosis and management of postpartum hemorrhage. ACOG Technical Bulletin No. 76.* Washington, DC: ACOG; 2006.

American College of Obstetricians and Gynecologists. *Episiotomy. ACOG Practice Bulletin No. 71.* Washington, DC: ACOG; 2006.

American College of Obstetricians and Gynecologist. *Guidelines for diagnostic imaging during pregnancy. ACOG Technical Bulletin No. 299.* Washington, DC: ACOG; 2004.

Angioli R, Gomez-Marin O, Cantuaria G, et al. Severe perineal lacerations during vaginal delivery: the University of Miami experience. *Am J Obstet Gynecol* 2000;182:1083.

Arona AJ, Al-Marayati L, Grimes DA, et al. Early secondary repair of third- and fourth-degree perineal lacerations after outpatient wound preparation. *Obstet Gynecol* 1995;86:294.

Argentine Episiotomy Trial Collaborative Group. Routine vs selective episiotomy: a randomised controlled trial. *Lancet* 1993;342:1517.

Baker ER, D'Alton ME. Caesarean section and caesarean hysterectomy. *Clin Obstet Gynecol* 1994;37:806.

Bakshi S, Meyer BA. Indications for and outcomes of emergency peripartum hysterecomy. A five-year review. *J Reprod Med* 2000;45:733–737.

Bamigboye AA, Hofmeyr GJ, Merrell DA. Rectal misoprostol in the prevention of postpartum hemorrhage: a placebo-controlled trial. *Am J Obstet Gynecol* 1998;179:1043.

Bansai RK, Tan WM, Ecker J, et al. Is there a benefit to episiotomy at spontaneous vaginal delivery? A natural experiment. *Am J Obstet Gynecol* 1996;175:897.

Bauman P, Hammond AO, McNeeley SG, et al. Factors associated with anal sphincter laceration in 40,923 primiparous women. *Int Urogynecol J Pelvic Floor Dysfunct* Jan 2007.

Benson RC, Durfee RB. Transabdominal cervico uterine cerclage during pregnancy for the treatment of cervical incompetency. *Obstet Gynecol* 1965;25:145–155.

B-Lynch C, Coker A, Lawai A, et al. The B-Lynch surgical technique for the control of massive postpartum haemorrhage: an alternative to hysterectomy? Five cases reported. *BJOG* 1997;104:372.

Bodner-Adler B, Bodner K, Kimberger O, et al. Management of the perineum during forceps delivery: association of episiotomy with the frequency and severity of perineal trauma in women undergoing forceps delivery. *J Reprod Med* 2003;48:239.

Burchell RC. Physiology of internal iliac artery ligation. *J Obstet Gynaecol Br Commonw* 1968;75:642.

Casele HL, Laifer SA. Successful pregnancy after bilateral hypogastric artery ligation: a case report. *J Reprod Med* 1997;42:306.

Castaneda S, Karrison T, Cibilis LA. Peripartum hysterectomy. *J Perinat Med* 2000;28:472.

Chan C, Razvi K, Tham KF, et al. The use of a Sengstaken-Blakemore tube to control post-partum hemorrhage. *Int J Gynecol Obstet* 1997;58:251.

Chang CY, Wu MT, Shih JC, et al. Preservation of uterine integrity via transarterial embolization under postoperative massive vaginal bleeding due to caesarean section pregnancy. *Taiwan J Obstet Gynecol* 2006;45:183.

Chestnut DH, Eden RD, Gall SA, et al. Peripartum hysterectomy: a review of caesarean and postpartum hysterectomy. *Obstet Gynecol* 1985;65:365.

Christianson LM, Bovbjerg VE, McDavitt EC, et al. Risk factors for perineal injury during delivery. *Am J Obstet Gynecol* 2003;189:255.

Clark SL. Uterine and hypogastric artery ligation. In: Phelan JP, Clark SL, eds. *Caesarean delivery*. New York: Elsevier; 1988:238.

Clark SL, Phelan JP, Yeh SY, et al. Hypogastric artery ligation for obstetric hemorrhage. *Obstet Gynecol* 1985;66:353.

Clark SL, Yeh SY, Phelan JP, et al. Emergency hysterectomy for obstetric hemorrhage. *Obstet Gynecol* 1984;64:376.

Connolly AM, Thorp, Jr JM. Childbirth-related perineal trauma: clinical significance and prevention. *Clin Obstet Gynecol* 1999;42:820.

Craig S, Chau H, Cho H. Treatment of severe postpartum hemorrhage by rectally administered gemeprost pessaries. *J Perinat Med* 1999;27:231.

Cunningham FG, MacDonald PC, Gant NF, et al., eds.Abnormalities of the third stage of labor. In: *Williams obstetrics,* 19th ed. Norwalk, CT: Appleton & Lange, 1993: 615.

Cunningham FG, MacDonald PC, Gant NF, et al., eds. Caesarean section and caesarean hysterectomy. In: *Williams obstetrics,* 19th ed. Norwalk, CT: Appleton & Lange, 1993:591.

Cunningham FG, MacDonald PC, Gant NF, et al., eds. Conduct of normal labor. In: *Williams obstetrics,* 19th ed. Norwalk, CT: Appleton & Lange, 1993: 371.

Cunningham FG, MacDonald PC, Gant NF, et al., eds. Injuries to the birth canal. In: *Williams obstetrics,* 19th ed. Norwalk, CT: Appleton & Lange, 1993: 543.

De Loor JA, van Dam PA. Foley catheters for uncontrollable obstetric or gynecologic hemorrhage. *Obstet Gynecol* 1996;88:737.

Dildy GA, Scott JR, et al. Pelvic pressure pack for catastrophic postpartum hemorrhage. *Obstet Gynecol* 2000;95:7S.

Ding CD, Hsu S, Chu TW, et al. Emergency peripartum hysterectomy in a teaching hospital in Eastern Taiwan. *J Obstet Gynaecol* 2006;26:635.

Eason E, Feldman P. Much ado about a little cut: is episiotomy worthwhile? *Obstet Gynecol* 2000;95:616.

Eason E, Labrecque M, Wells G, et al. Preventing perineal trauma during childbirth: a systematic review. *Obstet Gynecol* 2000;95:464.

Eniola OA, Bewley S, Waterstone M, et al. Obstetric hysterectomy in a population of South East England. *J Obstet Gynaecol* 2006;26:104.

Ferguson II JE, Bourgeois FJ, Underwood PB Jr. B-Lynch suture for postpartum hemorrhage. *Obstet Gynecol* 2000;95:1020.

Fitzpatrick M, Behan M, O'Connell PR, et al. A randomized clinical trial comparing primary overlap with approximation repair of third-degree obstetric tears. *Am J Obstet Gynecol* 2000;183:1220.

Floyd RC, Morrison JC. Postpartum hemorrhage. In: Plauche WC, Morrison JC, O'Sullivan MJ, eds. *Surgical obstetrics*. Philadelphia: WB Saunders; 1992: 272.

Ghomi A, Rodgers B. Laparoscopic abdominal cerclage during pregnancy: a case report and a review of the described operative techniques. *J Minim Invasive Gynecol* 2006;4:337.

Gilstrap LC, Hauth JC, Hankins GDV, et al. Effect of type of anesthesia on blood loss at caesarean section. *Obstet Gynecol* 1987;69:328.

Gilstrap LC, Ramin SM. Postpartum hemorrhage. *Clin Obstet Gynecol* 1994;37:824.

Goldaber KG, Wendel PJ, McIntire D, et al. Postpartum perineal morbidity after fourth-degree perineal repair. *Am J Obstet Gynecol* 1993;168:489.

Gonsoulin W, Kennedy RT, Guidry KH. Elective versus emergency caesarean hysterectomy cases in a residency program setting: a review of 129 cases from 1984 to 1988. *Am J Obstet Gynecol* 1991;165:91.

Handa VL, Harris TA, Ostergard DR. Protecting the pelvic floor: obstetric management to prevent incontinence and pelvic organ prolapse. *Obstet Gynecol* 1996;88:470.

Hankins GDV, Hauth JC, Gilstrap LC III, et al. Early repair of episiotomy dehiscence. *Obstet Gynecol* 1990;75:48.

Hansch E, Chitkara U, McAlpine J, et al. Pelvic arterial embolization for control of obstetric hemorrhage: a five year experience. *Am J Obstet Gynecol* 1999;180:1454.

Harris RE. An evaluation of the median episiotomy. *Am J Obstet Gynecol* 1970; 106(5):660–665.

Hauth JC, Gilstrap LC III, Ward SC, et al. Early repair of an external sphincter ani muscle and rectal mucosal dehiscence. *Obstet Gynecol* 1986;67: 806.

Henriksen T, Bek KM, Hedegaard M, et al. Episiotomy and perineal lesions in spontaneous vaginal deliveries. *BJOG* 1992;99:950.

Homsi R, Daikoku NH, Littlejohn J, et al. Episiotomy: risks of dehiscence and rectovaginal fistula. *Obstet Gynecol Surv* 1994;49:803.

Hsu YR, Wan YL. Successful management of intractable puerperal hematoma and severe postpartum hemorrhage with DIC through transcatheter arterial embolization-two cases. *Acta Obstet Gynecol Scand* 1998;77:129.

Hueston WJ. Factors associated with the use of episiotomy during vaginal delivery. *Obstet Gynecol* 1996;87:1001.

Jackson KW Jr, Allbert JR, Schemmer GK, et al. A randomized controlled trial comparing oxytocin administration before and after placental delivery in the prevention of postpartum hemorrhage. *Am J Obstet Gynecol* 2001;185(4):873.

Kaunitz AM, Hughes JM, Grimes DA, et al. Causes of maternal mortality in the United States. *Obstet Gynecol* 1985;65:605–612.

Klein MC, Gauthier RJ, Jorgensen SH, et al. Does episiotomy prevent perineal trauma and pelvic floor relaxation? Online. *J Curr Clin Trials* 1992; 2 (Document No. 10).

Klein MC, Gauthier RJ, Robbins JM, et al. Relationship of episiotomy to perineal trauma and morbidity, sexual dysfunction, and pelvic floor relaxation. *Am J Obstet Gynecol* 1994;171:591.

Klein MC, Janssen PA, MacWilliam L, et al. Determinants of vaginal-perineal integrity and pelvic floor functioning in childbirth. *Am J Obstet Gynecol* 1997;176:403.

Kovavisarach E. Obstetric hysterectomy: a 14-year experience of Rajavithi Hospital, 1989–2002. *J Med Assoc Thai* 2006;89:1817.

Larsson PG, Platz-Christensen JJ, Bergman B, et al. Advantage or disadvantage of episiotomy compared with spontaneous perineal laceration. *Gynecol Obstet Invest* 1991;31:213.

Lede RL, Belizan JM, Carroli G. Is routine use of episiotomy justified? *Am J Obstet Gynecol* 1996;174:1399.

Liu CM, Hsu JJ, Hsieh TT, et al. Postpartum hemorrhage of the uterine artery rupture. *Acta Obstet Gynecol Scand* 1998;77:695.

Lotgering FK, Gaugler-Senden IP, Lotgering SF. Outcome after transabdominal cervicoisthmic cerclage. *Obstet Gynecol* 2006;107(4):779.

Maier RC. Control of postpartum hemorrhage with uterine packing. *Am J Obstet Gynecol* 1993;169:317.

Marcovici I, Scoccia B. Postpartum hemorrhage and intrauterine balloon tamponade: a report of three cases. *J Reprod Med* 1999;44:122.

McNulty JV. Elective caesarean hysterectomy revisited. *Am J Obstet Gynecol* 1984;149:29.

Mengert WF, Burchell RC, Blumstein RW, et al. Pregnancy of the bilateral ligation after internal iliac and ovarian arteries. *Obstet Gynecol* 1969;34(5):664–666.

Monberg J, Hammen S. Ruptured episiotomies resutured primarily. *Acta Obstet Gynecol Scand* 1987;66:163.

Mousa H, Alfirevic Z. Treatment for primary postpartum haemorrhage. *Cochrane Database Syst Rev* 2007; Jan 24(1):CD003249.

Myers-Helfgott MG, Helfgott AW. Routine use of episiotomy in modern obstetrics: should it be performed. *Obstet Gynecol Clin North Am* 1999;26: 305.

Myles TD, Santolaya J. Maternal and neonatal outcomes in patients with prolonged second stage of labor. *Obstet Gynecol* 2003;102:52–8.

Oei PL, Chua S, Tan L, et al. Arterial embolization for bleeding following hysterectomy for intractable postpartum hemorrhage. *Int J Gynaecol Obstet* 1998;62:83.

O'Leary JA. Stop OB hemorrhage with uterine artery ligation. *Contemp Obstet Gynecol* 1986;28:13.

O'Leary JA. Uterine artery ligation in the control of postcaesarean hemorrhage. *J Reprod Med* 1995;40:189.

Owen J, Andrews WW. Wound complications after caesarean sections. *Clin Obstet Gynecol* 1994;37:842.

Owen J, Hauth JC. Episiotomy infection and dehiscence. In: Gilstrap LC III, Faro S, eds. *Infections in pregnancy*. New York: Alan R. Liss; 1990: 61.

Patino JF, Castro D. Necrotizing lesions of the soft tissue: a review. *World J Surg* 1991;15:235.

Payne TN, Carey JC, Rayburn WF. Prior third- or fourth-degree perineal tears and recurrence risks. *Int J Gynaecol Obstet* 1999;64:55.

Pelage JP, Le Dref O, Mateo J, et al. Life-threatening primary postpartum hemorrhage: treatment with emergency selective arterial embolization. *Radiology* 1999;208:359.

Pelage JP, Soyer P, Repiquet D, et al. Secondary postpartum hemorrhage: treatment with selective arterial embolization. *Radiology* 1999;212:385.

Philippe HJ, d'Oreye D, Lewin D. Vaginal ligature of uterine arteries during postpartum hemorrhage. *Int J Gynaecol Obstet* 1997;56:267.

Plauche WC. Caesarean hysterectomy: indications, technique, and complications. *Clin Obstet Gynecol* 1986;29:318.

Plauche WC. Peripartal hysterectomy. In: Plauche WC, Morrison JC, O'Sullivan MJ, eds. *Surgical obstetrics*. Philadelphia: WB Saunders; 1992:447.

Price N, B-Lynch C. Technical description of the B-Lynch brace suture for treatment of massive postpartum hemorrhage and review of published cases. *Int J Fertil Womens Med* 2005;50:148.

Ramin SM, Gilstrap LC III. Episiotomy and early repair of dehiscence. *Clin Obstet Gynecol* 1994;37:816.

Ramin SM, Ramus RM, Little BB, et al. Early repair of episiotomy dehiscence associated with infection. *Am J Obstet Gynecol* 1992;167:1104.

Reynders FC, Senten L, Tjalma W, et al. Postpartum hemorrhage: practical approach to a life-threatening complication. *Clin Exp Obstet Gynecol* 2006;33:81.

Roberts WE. Emergent obstetric management of postpartum hemorrhage. *Obstet Gynecol Clin North Am* 1995;22:283.

Robinson JN, Norwitz ER, Cohen AP, et al. Episiotomy, operative vaginal delivery, and significant perineal trauma in nulliparous women. *Am J Obstet Gynecol* 1999;181:1180.

Robinson JN, Norwitz ER, Cohen AP, et al. Predictors of episiotomy use at first spontaneous vaginal delivery. *Obstet Gynecol* 2000;96:214.

Rochat RW, Koonin LM, Atrash HK, et al. Maternal mortality in the United States: report from the Maternal Mortality Collaborative. *Obstet Gynecol* 1988;72:91.

Ročkner G, Jonasson A, Blund A. The effect of mediolateral episiotomy at delivery on pelvic floor muscle strength evaluated with vaginal cones. *Acta Obstet Gynecol Scand* 1991;70(1):51–54.

Rozenberg P, Sénat MV, Gillet A, et al. Comparison of two methods of cervical cerclage by ultrasound cervical measurement. *J Matern Fetal Neonatal Med* 2003;13(5):314–317.

Reist OA, Atlas RO, Meyer J, et al. Does cerclage location influence perinatal outcome? *Am J Obstet Gynecol* 2003;189(6):1688–1691.

Selo-Ojeme DO, Okonofua FE. Risk factors for primary postpartum haemorrhage. *Arch Gynecol Obstet* 1997;259:179.

Sheiner E, Sarid L, Levy A, et al. Obstetric risk factors and outcome of pregnancies complicated with early postpartum hemorrhage: a population-based study. *J Matern Fetal Neonatal Med* 2005;18(3):149.

Signorello LB, Harlow BL, Chekos AK, et al. Midline episiotomy and anal incontinence: retrospective cohort study [comment]. *BMJ* 2000;320:86.

Sleep J, Grant A. West Berkshire perineal management trial: three years follow-up. *BMJ* 1987;295:749.

Smith J, Mousa HA. Peripartum hysterectomy for primary postpartum haemorrhage. *J Obstet Gynaecol* 2007;27(1);44.

Snyder RR, Hammond TL, Hankins GDV. Human papillomavirus associated with poor healing of episiotomy repairs. *Obstet Gynecol* 1990;76:664.

Stanco LM, Schrimmer DB, Paul RH, et al. Emergency peripartum hysterectomy and associated risk factors. *Am J Obstet Gynecol* 1993;168:879.

Strickland JL, Griffen WT, Llorens AS, et al. Caesarean hysterectomy: a procedure for modern obstetrics? *South Med J* 1989;82:1245.

Sturdee DW, Rushton DI. Caesarean and post-partum hysterectomy 1968–1983. *BJOG* 1986;93:270.

Thacker SB, Banta HD. Benefits and risks of episiotomy: an interpretive review of the English language literature, 1860–1980. *Obstet Gynecol Surg* 1983;38:322.

Thorp JM Jr, Bowes WA Jr. Episiotomy: can its routine use be defended? *Am J Obstet Gynecol* 1989;160:1027.

Thorp JM Jr, Bowes WA Jr, Brame RG, et al. Selected use of midline episiotomy: effect on perineal trauma. *Obstet Gynecol* 1987;70:260.

Van Selm M, Kanhai HH, Keirse MJ. Preventing the recurrence of atonic postpartum hemorrhage: a double-blind trial. *Acta Obstet Gynecol Scand* 1995;74:270.

Varma A, Gunn J, Gardiner A, et al. Obstetric anal sphincter injury: prospective evaluation of incidence. *Dis Colon Rectum* 1999;42:1537.

Varma A, Gunn J, Lindow SW, et al. Do routinely measured delivery variables predict anal sphincter outcome? *Dis Colon Rectum* 1999;42:1261.

Vedantham S, Goodwin SC, McLucas B, et al. Uterine artery embolization: an underused method of controlling pelvic hemorrhage. *Am J Obstet Gynecol* 1997;176:938.

Viktrup L, Lose G, Rolff M, et al. The symptom of stress incontinence caused by pregnancy or delivery in primiparas. *Obstet Gynecol* 1992;79:945.

Wagaarachchi PT, Fernando L. Fertility following ligation of internal iliac arteries for life-threatening obstetric haemorrhage. *Human Reprod* 2000;15:1311.

Walsh CJ, Mooney EF, Upton GJ, et al. Incidence of third-degree perineal tears in labour and outcome after primary repair. *Br J Surg* 1996;83:218.

Whiteman MK, Kuklina E, Hill SD, et al. Incidence and determinants of peripartum hysterectomy. *Obstet Gynecol* 2006;108:1486.

Woolley RJ. Benefits and risks of episiotomy: a review of the English-language literature since 1980. Part I. *Obstet Gynecol Surv* 1995;50:806.

Woolley RJ. Benefits and risks of episiotomy: a review of the English language literature since 1980. Part II. *Obstet Gynecol Surv* 1995;50:821.

Wu S, Kocherginsky M, Hibbard JU. Abnormal placentation: a 20 year analysis. *Am J Obstet Gynecol* 2005;192(5):1458.

Yancey MK, Harlass FE, Benson W, et al. The perioperative morbidity of scheduled caesarean hysterectomy. *Obstet Gynecol* 1993;81:206.

Zaveri V, Aghajafari F, Amankwah K, et al. Abdominal versus vaginal cerclage after failed transvaginal cerclage: systemic review. *Am J Obstet Gynecol* 2002;187(4):868.

Zelop CM, Harlow BL, Frigoletto FD, et al. Emergency peripartum hysterectomy. *Am J Obstet Gynecol* 1993;168:1443.

Zorlu CG, Turan C, Isik AZ, et al. Emergency hysterectomy in modern obstetric practice: changing clinical perspective in time. *Acta Obstet Gynecol Scand* 1998;77:186.

CHAPTER 35B ■ OVARIAN TUMORS COMPLICATING PREGNANCY

CORNELIA R. GRAVES AND LYNN PARKER

DEFINITIONS

Aminopterin syndrome—Fetal anomalies caused by exposure to antifolate chemotherapy in the first trimester. Multiple fetal anomalies commonly include growth deficiency, craniofacial anomalies, hydrocephalus, mental retardation, and skeletal defects.

Hyperreactio luteinalis—A benign, frequently large (15–20 cm), usually bilateral ovarian enlargement caused by an increased sensitivity to human chorionic gonadotropin (hCG). These masses are composed of numerous luteinized follicular cysts and are more common in conditions in which the hCG is increased (e.g., hydatiform mole, multiple gestation). This condition is benign and will resolve spontaneously after pregnancy.

Luteoma of pregnancy—A solid, usually unilateral ovarian mass found in late pregnancy or at cesarean delivery. It may cause virilization. It is benign and resolves spontaneously after pregnancy.

Pulsatility index (PI)—An arterial waveform index that has shown to be useful in discriminating benign from malignant adnexal masses. A PI >1.0 is almost always associated with a benign mass. A PI <1.0 is suggestive of malignancy but can be seen in a corpus luteum cyst or an inflammatory mass.

The coexistence of an adnexal mass with pregnancy presents problems to both the clinician and the patient, the most serious being that of malignancy. This possibility must be discussed with the patient when obtaining informed consent before surgery. The therapeutic implications of possible hysterectomy with loss of the current pregnancy and loss of future fertility result in an emotionally charged environment because of the young age of the patient and the desire to preserve the pregnancy, as well as her reproductive capacity and ovarian function.

INCIDENCE

Cancer complicates 1:1,000 pregnancies in the United States. The most common malignancies seen in pregnancy include malignant melanoma (2.6:1,000), Hodgkin lymphoma (1:1,000–6,000), breast cancer (1:3,000–10,000), cervical cancer (1.2:10,000), ovarian cancer (1:10,000–100,000), colorectal cancer (1:13,000), and leukemias (1:75,000–100,000).

Benign ovarian tumors complicating pregnancy are more common. The exact incidence, however, depends on whether one considers simple cysts noted on ultrasound examination (1 in 50 live births) or during pelvic examination (1 in 80 live births) or those that ultimately require laparotomy (1 in 1,000–1 in 1,500 live births). Ueda and Ueki reported 106 patients who required ovarian surgery during pregnancy. Of these patients, 29.2% had physiologic ovarian cysts, 66% were benign, and 4.7% were malignant. More recent observations have noted that adnexal masses >5 cm were observed in 0.05% of patients, with 6.8% of masses and 0.0032% of deliveries diagnosed as malignant.

Koonings and colleagues noted the incidence of ovarian tumors complicating cesarean section to be about 1 in 200 cesarean births, and Ballard observed that ovarian tumors complicated termination of pregnancy in 1 of 594 procedures. Hill and colleagues reported that ovarian cysts were diagnosed in 4.1% of second- or third-trimester ultrasounds. Most of these cysts were <3 cm and resolved spontaneously. Eighteen of the 7,996 patients had an exploratory laparotomy, which was equivalent to one surgery in 444 deliveries. All of these lesions were benign on pathologic examination.

DIAGNOSIS

The appropriate diagnosis of ovarian tumors complicating pregnancy depends on the use of certain windows of opportunity. These include the initial pelvic examination in the first trimester, the initial ultrasound, and careful evaluation at the time of operative intervention. A thorough pelvic examination at the time of termination of pregnancy and careful examination of the ovaries at the time of cesarean section or postpartum tubal ligation are other opportunities to evaluate the ovaries.

The increasing (nearly routine) use of ultrasound examination affords an excellent opportunity for the diagnosis of coexistent ovarian pathology; it is for this reason that such an examination should always include the adnexa. The results of ultrasound, although potentially very useful in the relatively rare patient with an ovarian malignancy, may give the clinician a difficult dilemma trying to decide how to proceed when an ovarian cyst is diagnosed in pregnancy.

Perkins and coworkers evaluated 1,001 patients with first-trimester ultrasound and determined that a simple ovarian cyst was seen in 29% of these patients. The incidence of ovarian cysts decreased after 8 weeks, and absence of a cyst was more often associated with blighted ovum.

Resta and coworkers have reported that the upper limits of normal size for the corpus luteum of pregnancy is 2 cm. Most studies evaluating ovarian cysts in pregnancy rely on second-trimester ultrasound characteristics or persistence of a cyst to try to eliminate false-positive results caused by the corpus luteum.

Lavery and colleagues, in a review of 3,918 ultrasound examinations at 20 weeks' gestation, noted cyst formation >2 cm in 2.4% of examinations. Only nine patients (0.23%)

required surgical intervention. Hogston and Lifford, in a review of 26,000 patients who received routine ultrasound, noted an incidence of cyst formation of 0.52%. All complex cysts and those >6 cm were operated on primarily (10%). Eighty-five percent of the remaining patients who were followed conservatively showed a spontaneous resolution, with the exception of five patients who ultimately required laparotomy.

Bromley and Benacerraf evaluated the accuracy of sonographic diagnosis of adnexal masses during pregnancy. They evaluated all patients with an adnexal mass measuring 4 cm or greater noted beyond 12 weeks' gestation. One hundred and thirty-one lesions were noted; of these, 89.3% were accurately diagnosed as benign. Of the 10.7% of lesions with sonographic characteristics of malignancy, 1 of 14 (7%) of these patients had ovarian cancer, for a 0.8% malignancy rate in this study.

Doppler sonography also has been evaluated for use in complex adnexal masses in pregnancy. Wheeler and Fleischer evaluated 34 pregnant patients with complex adnexal masses. Diagnosis made by color Doppler sonography was compared with actual histopathologic diagnosis. Three malignant and five low malignant potential tumors were correctly identified with a sensitivity of 0.89 and a mean pulsatility index (PI) of 0.71. The mean PI for benign lesions was >1, and the negative predictive value for PI >1 was 0.93. The positive predictive value for PI <1 was 0.42, indicating that some benign lesions were incorrectly classified as malignant when a PI <1 is used as a cutoff for possibly malignant tumors. However, color Doppler appears to be highly predictive of a benign lesion when the PI is >1.

From a treatment standpoint, the first trimester is clearly the best time to diagnose an adnexal mass complicating pregnancy. Because tumors are rarely symptomatic during this period, most such tumors are discovered by ultrasound examination (or later, as an incidental finding at cesarean section). With the increasing incidence of ultrasound evaluation and use of cesarean section, recent articles suggest that only about 50% of ovarian tumors complicating pregnancy are symptomatic. When symptomatic, the patient typically presents with abdominal pain, abdominal distention, and vague gastrointestinal symptoms. All these symptoms can be directly attributable to pregnancy itself; therefore, it is not surprising that most pregnant women with these symptoms are not evaluated for an ovarian tumor.

Ovarian tumors complicating pregnancy can be divided into three groups, depending on the severity of presentation.

- Those who are asymptomatic
- Those with symptoms compatible with torsion
- Those with catastrophic presentations consistent with hemorrhage, rupture, and shock

A successful outcome for both mother and fetus depends on a high index of suspicion with early diagnosis. One should consider an ovarian mass in any woman who experiences abdominal pain in pregnancy. Furthermore, torsion, rupture, infection, or hemorrhage of an ovarian tumor should be included in the differential diagnosis of any catastrophic abdominal obstetric event. This is particularly true during times of rapid change in uterine size or position (e.g., 8–16 weeks), during termination of pregnancy, during labor and delivery, or in the immediate postpartum period.

The incidence of torsion complicating an ovarian tumor in the nonpregnant state is about 2%. Torsion complicating an ovarian tumor during pregnancy is much higher, varying from 11% to 50%. Ueda and Ueki report a 21.8% rate of torsion in ovarian tumors in pregnancy. Other recent studies in which there is a high incidence of incidental asymptomatic tumors report much lower incidences of torsion, rupture, and dystocia. Nevertheless, it is clear that the unrecognized symptomatic ovarian tumor complicating pregnancy can become catastrophic, accompanied by hemorrhage, shock, peritonitis, or death. Wang and colleagues retrospectively evaluated 174 patients who underwent surgery for ovarian masses during pregnancy. These patients were divided into two groups: those with emergency surgery (32 patients) and those with elective surgery (142 patients). They found in the emergency surgery group that half of the surgeries occurred in the first trimester; they contributed to 75% of total fetal wastage and 87% of spontaneous fetal loss; and tumor sizes were significantly larger. In their experience, tumors <5 cm in size never caused symptoms requiring surgery. Therefore, size of tumor, ultrasound characteristics, color Doppler flow, as well as symptoms are important in determining the management of pregnant patients with adnexal masses.

PATHOLOGY

Benign neoplasms complicating pregnancy include two tumor-like conditions with which every gynecologist should be familiar. *Hyperreactio luteinalis* (first described by Burger in 1938 as a grossly multicystic, usually bilateral ovarian enlargement, often 15–20 cm in size) is a term used to describe numerous luteinized follicular cysts of the ovary complicating pregnancy (Fig. 35B.1). Microscopically, one notes extensive luteinization of the theca and granulosa cell layers. Bradshaw and associates suggest that the hyperandrogenicity seen in this condition is related to increased ovarian sensitivity to human chorionic gonadotropin (hCG). Therefore, it is seen in conditions in which the hCG is elevated, such as hydatidiform mole, multiple gestations, choriocarcinoma, and erythroblastosis fetalis. Hyperreactio luteinalis also has been associated with normal pregnancy, and, in these patients, it has not been associated with fetal virilization. These tumors spontaneously regress after delivery but may take up to 6 months to resolve. Hyperreactio luteinalis also may occur in subsequent pregnancies.

Luteoma of pregnancy is a specific benign, usually unilateral, solid lutein cell tumor of the ovary found in late pregnancy, often noted at cesarean section (Fig. 35B.2). First described by Sternberg in 1966, this tumor is grossly bosselated, soft, fleshy, yellow, or hemorrhagic. Microscopically, it exhibits an acidophilic granular cytoplasm with sparse lipid formation and a distinctive reticular pattern. It is likely the most common cause of maternal virilization during pregnancy. The etiology is unknown, but theories have included luteinized stromal cells present before pregnancy that respond to hCG or "hyperluteinized" theca cells, granulosa cells, or a combination of the two. Fifty percent of female infants born to virilized mothers with pregnancy luteoma exhibit signs of virilization.

The important clinical implication with both of these lesions is that if they are recognized or suspected, simple biopsy without further surgery is adequate therapy, because both invariably resolve spontaneously.

The most common benign neoplasm of the ovary in pregnancy is the *benign cystic teratoma*, which accounts for about one third of all benign ovarian tumors seen in pregnancy (Fig. 35B.3). The second most common group of ovarian tumors complicating pregnancy is that of cystadenomas. These represent about 15% of tumors (Fig. 35B.4). Endometriomas, simple cysts, corpus luteal cysts, tubal cysts, myomas, and other miscellaneous lesions constitute the remaining types of tumors seen in pregnancy (Table 35B.1).

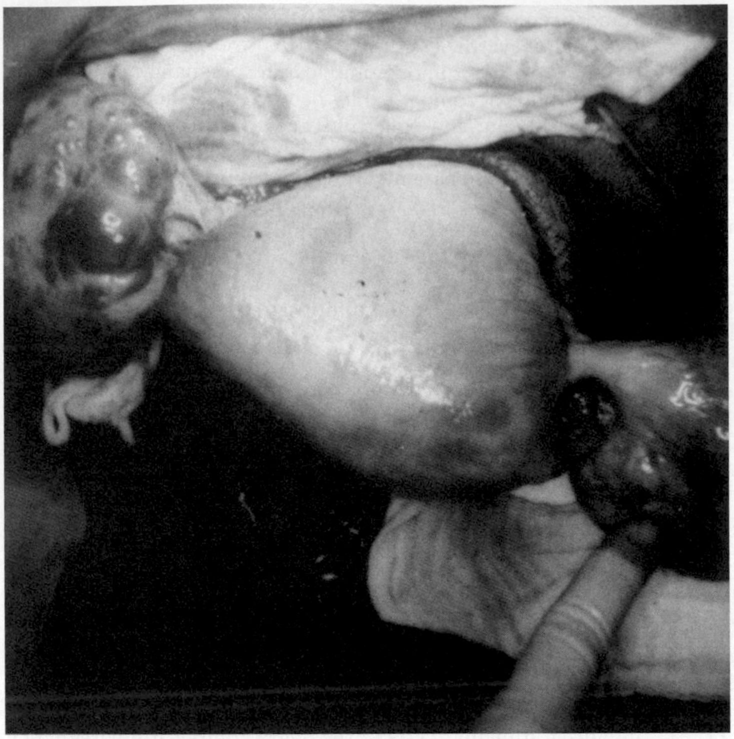

FIGURE 35B.1. Hyperreactio luteinalis (multiple theca luteal cysts) is a tumorlike condition complicating pregnancy. Usually it is bilateral and resolves spontaneously. (Courtesy of David Barclay, Little Rock, AR.)

Malignant ovarian tumors constitute only about 1% to 2% of all adnexal masses that complicate pregnancy and require surgical exploration. The single most common malignant ovarian tumor complicating pregnancy probably is *dysgerminoma*. Malignant tumors of epithelial origin as a group, however, are more common; tumors of low malignant potential occur most frequently (Fig. 35B.5). Sex-cord stromal tumors are the third most common primary malignant ovarian neoplasms, representing about 17% to 20% of such tumors. Krukenberg and other metastatic tumors represent about 12% to 13% of malignant ovarian neoplasms complicating pregnancy.

Whether malignant or benign, most ovarian tumors complicating pregnancy are unilateral. Karlen and associates reported 90% of dysgerminomas in pregnancy to be unilateral, and Young and colleagues reported 35 of 36 sex-cord stromal tumors to be unilateral when complicating pregnancy. Even malignant tumors of epithelial origin noted during pregnancy are unilateral in 90% of cases. The rarer germ cell tumors, such as endodermal sinus tumors, virtually always are unilateral as

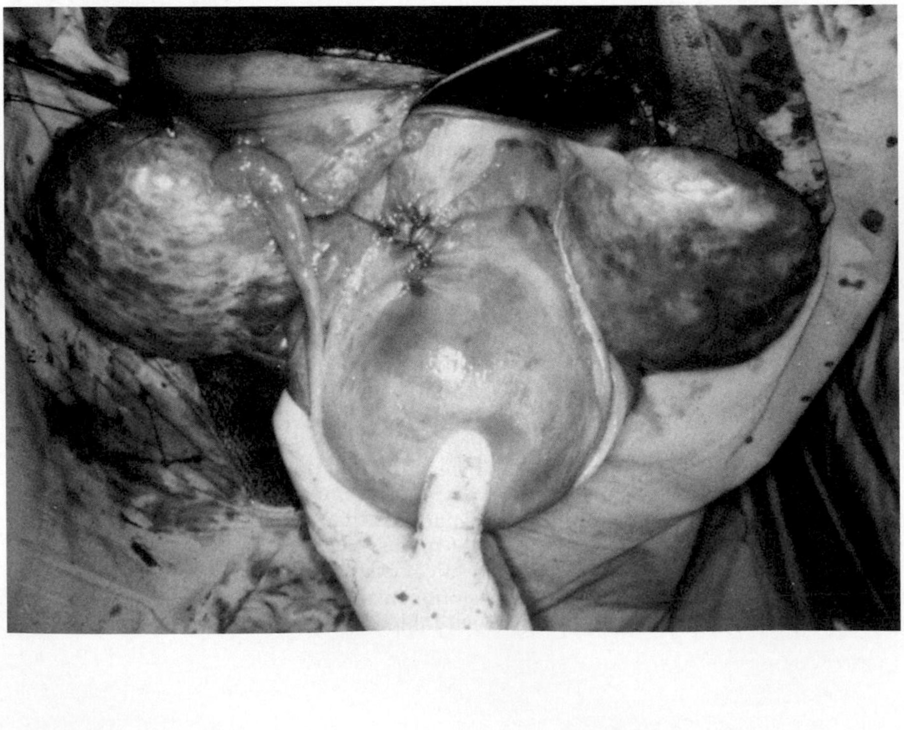

FIGURE 35B.2. Luteoma of pregnancy. Typically occurring late in normal pregnancies and usually unilateral and solid, this lesion resolves spontaneously. (Courtesy of David Barclay, Little Rock, AR.)

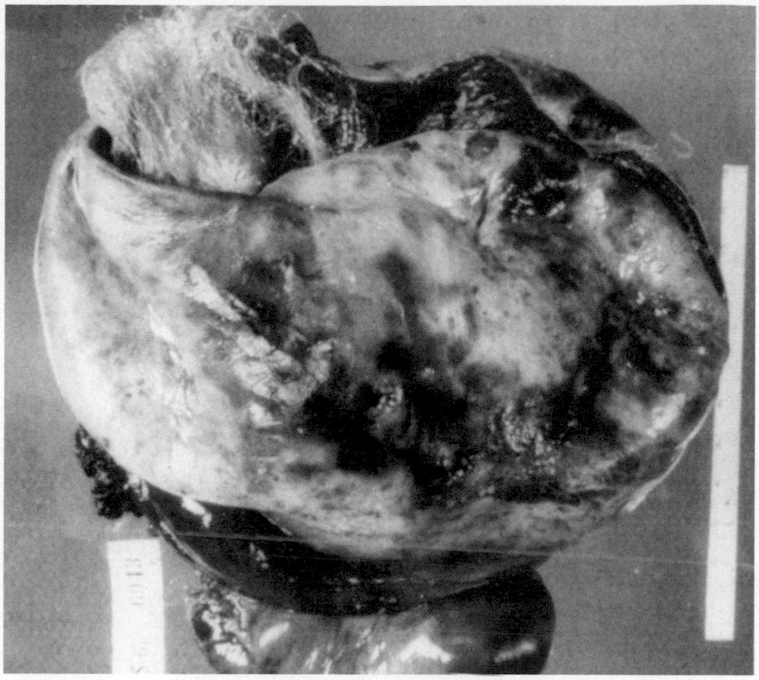

FIGURE 35B.3. The benign cystic teratoma is the most common benign neoplasm of the ovary complicating pregnancy. This tumor has undergone torsion and infarction.

well. It is also interesting that most bilateral tumors occurring in pregnancy are not malignant; these include benign cystic teratoma, endometriosis, and hyperreactio luteinalis. The most common bilateral malignant ovarian tumors are the metastatic Krukenberg types. Somewhat less common are primary malignant tumors of epithelial origin.

Virilization secondary to an ovarian tumor sometimes complicates pregnancy (Fig. 35B.6). The classic painting titled *Magdalena Ventura with Husband and Son,* painted in 1631 by Ribera, documents such a problem (Fig. 35B.7). Magdalena, after having several children, became virilized at age 37, with apparent infertility thereafter. However, when she was 52, a son was born. One would speculate that she probably had an ovarian Sertoli-Leydig cell tumor. Young and colleagues have noted that although about 50% of Sertoli-Leydig cell tumors in the nonpregnant state are functional, only about 15% of those complicating pregnancy result in maternal virilization. They proposed two possible explanations for this apparent decrease in virilization. The first is that the most active of such tumors result in anovulation; therefore, women with virilizing tumors rarely become pregnant. The second is that the placenta may aromatize the tumor-produced androgens into estrogens. In any event, Sertoli-Leydig cell tumors are not the most common tumors in pregnancy associated with virilization. This distinction falls to those tumors associated with a functioning ovarian stroma. The most common virilizing ovarian tumor that complicates

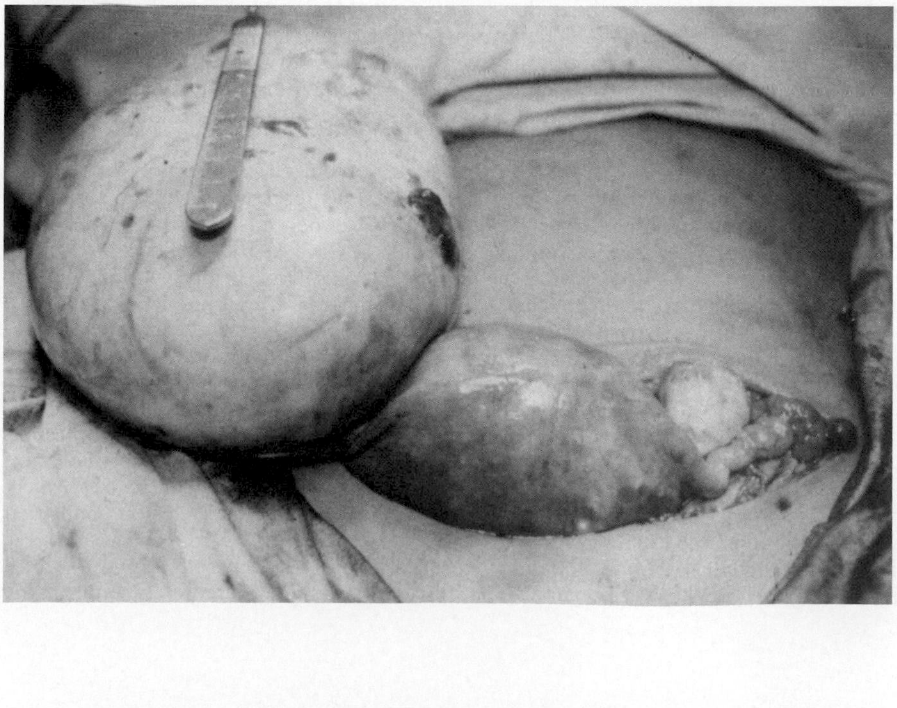

FIGURE 35B.4. A mucinous cystadenoma complicating pregnancy. Tumors of epithelial origin are the second most common benign neoplasm of the ovary complicating pregnancy. Mucinous tumors are relatively more common in pregnancy.

TABLE 35B.1

PATHOLOGY OF PELVIC MASSES COMPLICATING PREGNANCY

	Bromley and Benacerraf $n = 131$	Hill et al. $n = 19$	Wheeler and Fleischer $n = 34$	Ueda and Ueki $n = 106$	Total 290
Dermoid	40	8	8	48	104 (36%)
Endometrioma	15	1	2	10	28 (9.7%)
Functional cysts	14	1	0	6	21 (7.2%)
Cystadenomas	13	4	10	18	45 (15.5%)
Tubal cyst	9	2	0	0	11 (3.8%)
Fibroids	4	0	2	0	6 (2.1%)
Adenocarcinoma of the ovary	1	0	1	2	4 (1.4%)
Corpus luteum	0	2	2	15	19 (6.6%)
Serous cystadenoma/ endometrioma	1	0	0	0	1 (0.3%)
Cystadenofibroma	2	0	0	0	2 (0.6%)
Fibrothecoma	1	0	0	0	1 (0.3%)
Serous	1	0	0	0	1 (0.3%)
cystadenofibroma	1	0	0	0	1 (0.3%)
Dermoid/fibrothecoma	1	0	0	0	1 (0.3%)
Fibroma	0	1	0	4	5 (1.7%)
Tarkov cyst	1	0	0	0	1 (0.3%)
Struma ovarii	2	0	0	0	2 (0.6%)
Luteoma of pregnancy	1	0	1	0	2 (0.6%)
Echinococcal cyst	1	0	0	0	1 (0.3%)
Dysgerminoma	0	0	1	1	2 (0.6%)
Lymphoma	0	0	1	0	1 (0.3%)
Low malignant potential tumors	0	0	6	1	7 (2.4%)
Embryonal carcinoma	0	0	0	1	1 (0.3%)
Normal ovaries	24	0	0	0	

pregnancy is the luteoma, followed by Krukenberg tumors and mucinous epithelial tumors (Table 35B.2).

The clinical implications of virilizing tumors complicating pregnancy are somewhat different from those of such tumors in the nonpregnant state. Virilization usually occurs late in pregnancy, is of short duration, and usually is reversible. The majority of such cases, as mentioned, are secondary to luteoma; therefore, they resolve spontaneously. If sex-cord stromal or epithelial tumors are present, the ultimate outcome remains quite good. However, patients with Krukenberg lesions have a poor outcome.

Malignancies also can be metastatic to the placenta or products of conception. Although this is an uncommon occurrence, tumors that may metastasize to the placenta include malignant melanoma, leukemias and lymphomas, breast carcinoma, lung carcinoma, and some sarcomas.

THERAPY

The first successful oophorectomy for an ovarian tumor complicating pregnancy was performed in 1846 by Bund. Although the woman survived, the fetus aborted at 12 weeks' gestation. At about the same time, J. Marion Sims was the first to successfully remove an ovarian tumor in a pregnant woman and to have both the woman and fetus survive. As late as 1906, McKerran reported a 21% maternal mortality rate and a 50% fetal mortality rate with surgical management of ovarian tumors in pregnancy.

In general, one should avoid elective surgery in the first trimester, because many lesions represent the cystic corpus luteum of pregnancy and resolve spontaneously. Therefore, ultrasound should be repeated in 6 weeks to determine if the mass is persistent before considering surgical intervention. Buttery and colleagues noted an abortion rate of about 30% in those patients operated on in the first trimester, so first-trimester procedures are high risk. Nevertheless, symptomatic, complex, bilateral, and solid tumors should be operated on immediately (Fig. 35B.8). Preoperative evaluation should be limited to careful clinical evaluation and pelvic ultrasound examination. Barium enema, computed tomography, and other such studies are best avoided. Magnetic resonance imaging can be used safely in pregnancy but has not been helpful in evaluation of adnexal masses.

Tumor markers such as CA-125 generally are not helpful in pregnancy, because they can be elevated as a result of the

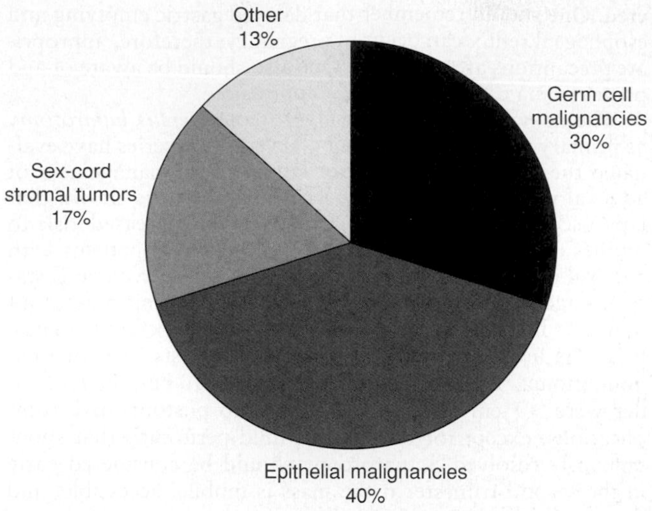

FIGURE 35B.5. The approximate relative frequency of the most common malignant ovarian tumors.

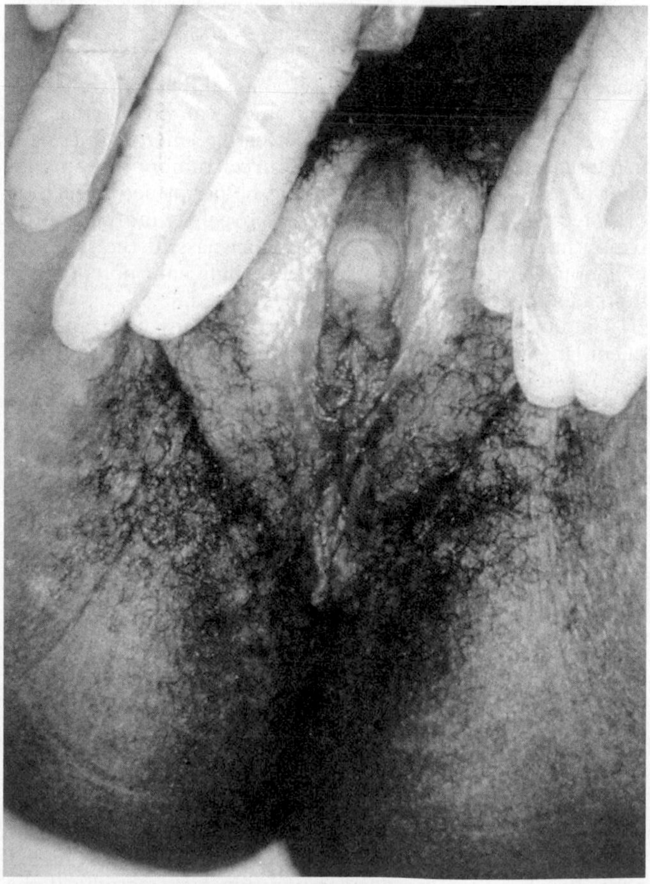

FIGURE 35B.6. Virilization occurring in late pregnancy secondary to a pregnancy luteoma. Note clitoral hypertrophy and hirsutism. (Courtesy of David Barclay, Little Rock, AR.)

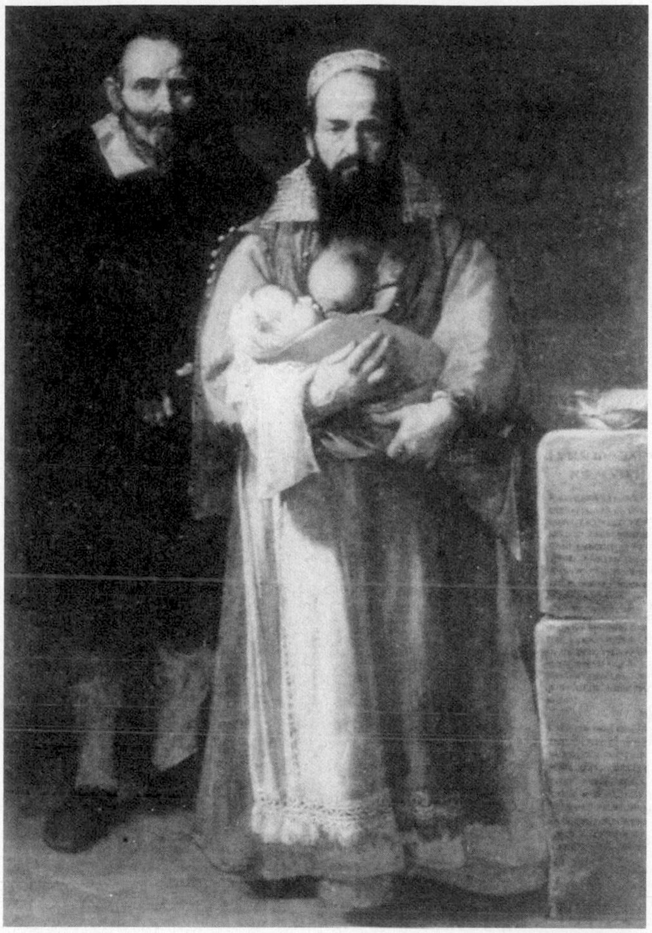

FIGURE 35B.7. The painting by Ribera titled *Magdalena Ventura with Husband and Son.* The most common virilizing tumors of the ovary complicating pregnancy are those with functioning stroma. (Reprinted with permission.)

pregnancy itself. Alpha fetoprotein is heterogenous, and the yolk sac variant can be separated by affinity chromatography to determine if the elevation is due to the yolk sac or liver variant. Lactate dehydrogenase (LDH) can be produced by dysgerminomas. Except in preeclampsia, LDH levels should remain within normal limits in pregnancy.

Wang and colleagues, in their evaluation of surgical management of ovarian masses in pregnancy, found that elective surgery had a much lower rate of fetal wastage and was more likely to occur in the second trimester. Therefore, elective management of adnexal masses in pregnancy appears to be safer than awaiting symptoms or emergency intervention.

The optimum time for surgical intervention is 16 to 18 weeks. In general, the first trimester should be avoided if possible because of the naturally occurring high rate of spontaneous abortion. It is difficult to avoid the conclusion that any pregnancy loss occurring within a short time of surgery is related to the surgery, so that if it is possible to wait until the second trimester, the risk of an unrelated spontaneous abortion is decreased. Patients in whom the asymptomatic mass is noted at or near term may be considered for delivery by cesarean section with careful intraoperative evaluation of the adnexa. Vaginal delivery in this situation has been associated with torsion, rupture, and hemorrhage that can occur during labor or immediately postpartum. The size and ultrasound characteristics of

TABLE 35B.2

DIFFERENTIAL DIAGNOSIS OF VIRILIZING OVARIAN TUMORS ASSOCIATED WITH PREGNANCY[a]

Histologic diagnosis
Luteoma
Hyperreactio luteinalis
Sex-cord disorders
Granulosa theca
Thecomas
Theca-lutein cyst
Sertoli-Leydig
Hilar cell tumor
Hilar cell hyperplasia
Stromal luteomas
Stromal hyperthecosis
Unclassified sex-cord stromal tumors
Other ovarian tumors
Krukenberg tumors
Mucinous cystadenocarcinoma
Dermoid
Brenner tumor

the mass will help to guide the clinician's decision concerning the best route of delivery. Caspi and colleagues described *conservative management* of 63 patients who had dermoid cysts ≤6 cm. None of these patients had an increase in size of the dermoid during pregnancy. In this study, 55 patients had normal vaginal deliveries, and none had complications related to the cyst. They also evaluated the use of *ultrasound guided cyst aspiration* in patients with persistent simple cysts into the second trimester. In this study, 50% of the patients avoided surgical intervention with this procedure. Every case of an adnexal mass should be independently evaluated to determine the best management.

General anesthesia is the anesthesia of choice, although a combination of epidural and general anesthesia can be considered. One should remember that delayed gastric emptying and esophageal reflux can occur in pregnancy; therefore, appropriate precautions are necessary. One also should be aware of and prevent vena caval and aortic compression.

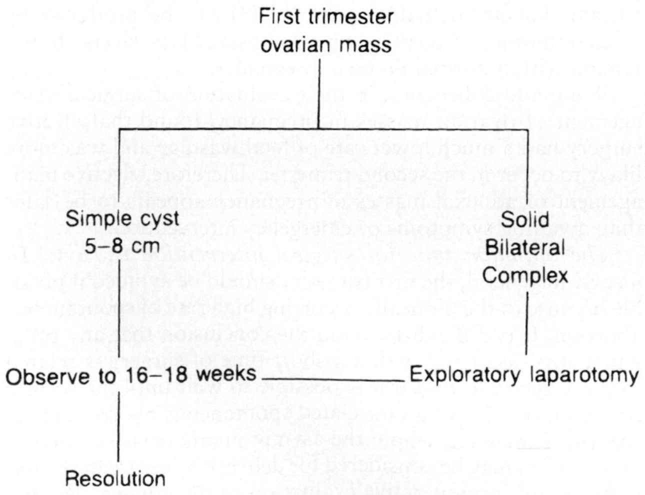

FIGURE 35B.8. Algorithm for the surgical management of ovarian tumors complicating pregnancy in the first trimester. Symptomatic, solid, bilateral, and complex lesions should be operated on when discovered.

The next consideration is *laparoscopy versus laparotomy* as primary surgical management. Several case series have evaluated the safety and efficacy of laparoscopic management of adnexal masses in pregnancy. These studies have shown that laparoscopic surgery can be used without increased risk to mother or fetus. Moore and Smith evaluated 14 patients with adnexal masses treated with laparoscopy. The average gestational age was 16 weeks, with average operating time of 84 minutes. The tumors included three mucinous cystadenomas, three mature teratomas, three functional cysts, and one endometrioma. Three patients had tumors >10 cm; the remainder were >7 cm in size. There were no postoperative complications, except for one case of mild peritonitis that spontaneously resolved. Laparoscopy should be considered early in the second trimester if the mass is mobile, accessible, and does not have characteristics of malignancy such as ascites or carcinomatosis.

If laparotomy is the chosen surgical approach, a vertical incision is preferred, because after 16 weeks' gestation, the ovary is an abdominal rather than pelvic structure. The incision should be placed higher than usual. Thorough gross examination of the lesion, with frozen section—as well as evaluation of the upper abdomen, omentum, and paraaortic nodes—should be performed, along with pelvic washings. The involved ovary should be sent for frozen section to establish a preliminary diagnosis. The contralateral ovary should be carefully inspected. However, biopsy or wedge resection of the contralateral ovary should be avoided if no gross evidence of involvement is present. One possible exception is if the primary tumor is a dysgerminoma, because these tumors can involve the contralateral ovary in a clinically undetectable, microscopic manner. If the patient has a malignant germ cell tumor or low malignant potential tumor, staging should be performed to include omentectomy, peritoneal biopsies, and pelvic and paraaortic lymph node biopsies on the side of the mass. If the tumor is mucinous, either cystadenoma or low malignant potential tumor, an appendectomy should be performed.

The uterus should be handled gently in any case, and frequent irrigation should be used to prevent the tissue from drying. When ovarian cystectomy is required, an internal closure with use of a 5–0 absorbable is recommended. Alternatively, one can decide to perform no closure. The traditional Buxton-type closure should be avoided.

Before the decision is made to perform oophorectomy, one must always consciously exclude hyperreactio luteinalis and luteoma of pregnancy. Furthermore, because most malignant ovarian tumors are unilateral, total abdominal hysterectomy and bilateral salpingectomy are rarely indicated (Fig. 35B.9). Total hysterectomy and removal of ovaries should never be performed on the basis of a frozen section diagnosis of borderline or low-grade malignancy unless the patient has clearly expressed a desire to abort this pregnancy and does not wish to preserve fertility and ovarian function.

When faced with a clearly malignant bilateral or metastatic tumor, one usually treats the patient as if she were nonpregnant, with total hysterectomy, bilateral salpingo-oophorectomy, pelvic and abdominal washings, omentectomy, and pelvic and paraaortic node biopsies. Even with bilateral malignant disease, one can consider omitting hysterectomy if the uterus is not grossly involved, thus allowing preservation of the existing pregnancy, especially because platinum-based chemotherapy can safely be given during pregnancy. Although

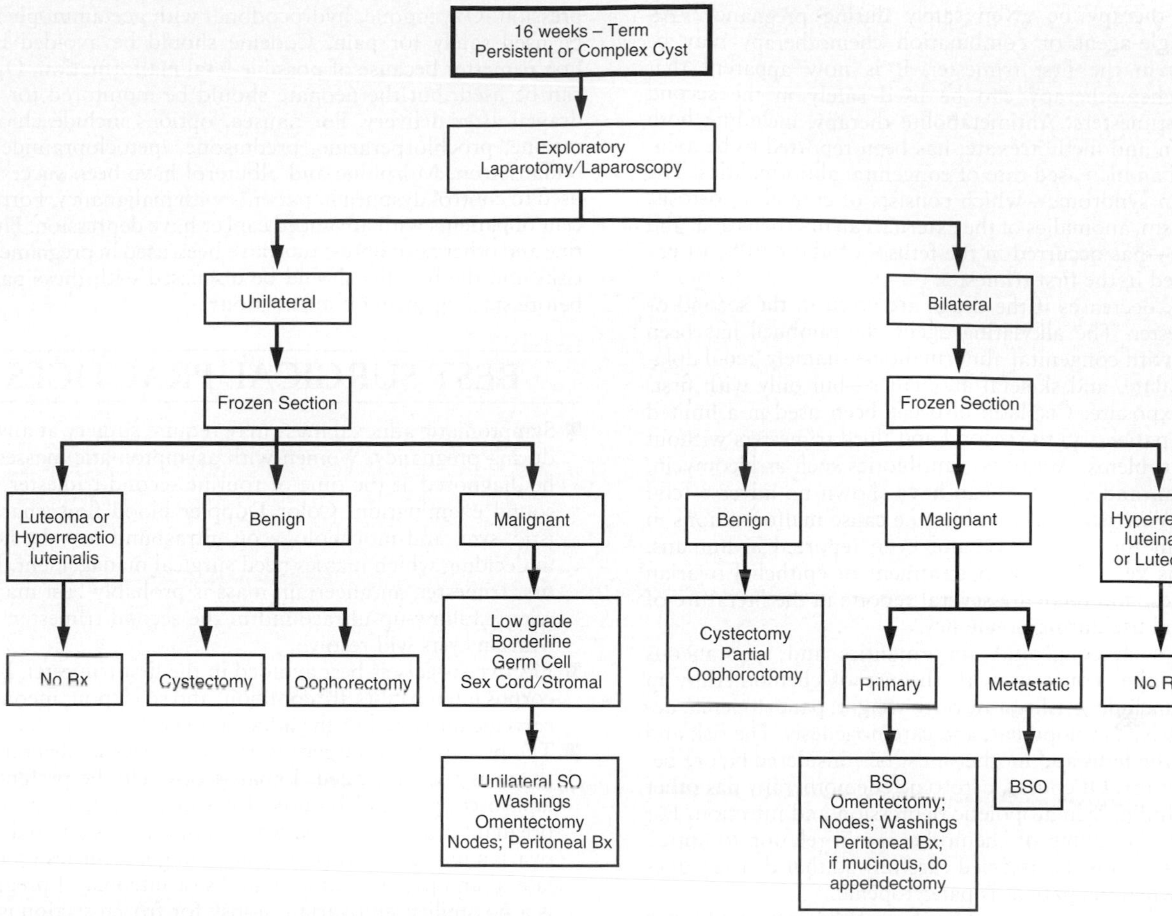

FIGURE 35B.9. Algorithm for the surgical management of ovarian tumors occurring after 16 weeks' gestation. BSO, bilateral salpingo-oophorectomy; SO, salpingo-oophorectomy; TAH, total abdominal hysterectomy; Bx, biopsy; Rx, treatment.

other tumors are known to metastasize rarely to either the placenta or fetus, primary ovarian tumors almost never do so.

All the possible findings at surgery and possible surgical management options should be carefully discussed with the patient, and a good understanding of the planned therapy should be agreed on by all. A careful preoperative note about the discussion should be made in the patient's chart. The family should be informed of the findings and plans during the course of surgery, and consultation should be obtained if necessary.

The role of progesterone to prevent labor in the postoperative period is unclear but should be considered if the surgery occurs in the first trimester. The patient should be monitored for contractions and fetal heart tones checked in the postoperative period. If contractions occur, these can be treated with hydration, sedation, indomethacin (if before 32 weeks), or standard tocolytic therapy.

TREATMENT OUTCOME

Conservative surgical treatment outcome for benign disease should be excellent. With malignant disease, the overall 5-year survival rate depends on stage and cell type. In a classic paper on ovarian cancer in pregnancy, Novak and associates reported a 5-year survival rate of 75% from the Johns Hopkins Hospital. In a review of 27 dysgerminomas, Karlen and associates reported a tendency toward local recurrence with conservative treatment but an overall 5-year survival rate of 90%. Young and coworkers, in a review of 36 sex-cord stromal tumors, noted a 5-year survival rate of 100%, although they cautioned that granulosa cell tumors are prone to late recurrence. However, patients with Krukenberg tumors or metastatic disease have a poor prognosis.

Fetal mortality also should be minimal with early diagnosis and appropriate surgical intervention. Although Karlen and associates reported a fetal mortality rate of 25%, two of the five deaths were secondary to hysterotomy. Young and colleagues reported three fetal deaths in 36 cases, two of which resulted from hysterectomy. Ueda and Ueki reported on 106 surgeries with a spontaneous abortion rate of 10%. Two patients desired termination of pregnancy in the second trimester owing to ovarian diagnosis, and one fetus died despite intensive efforts.

CYTOTOXIC CHEMOTHERAPY DURING PREGNANCY

At no time is the treatment of cancer during pregnancy more complicated than when adjunctive therapy is indicated.

Can such therapy be given safely during pregnancy? Although single-agent or combination chemotherapy may be teratogenic in the first trimester, it is now apparent that cytotoxic chemotherapy can be used safely in the second and third trimesters. Antimetabolite therapy, including both aminopterin and methotrexate, has been reported to be associated with an increased rate of congenital abnormalities. The aminopterin syndrome—which consists of cranial dysostosis, hypertelorism, anomalies of the external ear, micrognathia, and cleft palate—has occurred in the fetuses of about 20% of patients treated in the first trimester.

The risk decreases if the drugs are given in the second or third trimester. The alkylating agent chlorambucil has been associated with congenital abnormalities—namely, renal aplasia, cleft palate, and skeletal anomalies—but only with first-trimester exposure. Cisplatin also has been used in a limited number of patients in the second and third trimesters without apparent problems. Antitumor antibiotics such as bleomycin, doxorubicin, and daunorubicin have shown no adverse fetal outcomes. Vincristine and vinblastine cause malformations in animals, but the effects have not been reported in humans. Paclitaxel is very effective in treatment of epithelial ovarian malignancies, and there are several reports in the literature of its successful use during pregnancy.

Besides such congenital abnormalities and spontaneous abortions, other concerns with the use of chemotherapy in pregnancy include sterility, low birth weight, pancytopenia, delayed cognitive development, and carcinogenesis. The risk and benefits to the fetus and mother must be considered before beginning therapy. Of course, cytotoxic chemotherapy has other effects, including hematopoietic depression and infection. For this reason, the timing of chemotherapy in relation to anticipated delivery must be assessed carefully so that delivery does not occur when the patient is pancytopenic.

Reports in the literature describe safe treatment of germ cell tumors of the ovary with bleomycin, etoposide, and cis-platinum (BEP); vincristine, actinomycin D, and cyclophosphamide (VAC); or vinblastine, bleomycin, and cis-platinum (VPB).

OTHER ISSUES SURROUNDING MALIGNANCY

Symptom control is very important in pregnant patients with malignancy. Symptoms commonly seen in malignancy include pain, nausea, vomiting, anorexia, dyspnea, fatigue, and depression. Oxycodone, hydrocodone, with acetaminophen can be used safely for pain. Codeine should be avoided in the first trimester because of possible fetal malformation. Opiates can be used, but the neonate should be monitored for withdrawal after delivery. For nausea, options include chlorpromazine, prochlorperazine, prednisone, metoclopramide, and ondansetron. Morphine and albuterol have been successfully used to control dyspnea in patients with malignancy. Forty percent of patients with advanced cancer have depression. Fluoxetine and other antidepressants have been used in pregnancy; the risks and the benefits should be discussed with these patients before starting them on medications.

BEST SURGICAL PRACTICES

- Symptomatic adnexal mass may require surgery at any time during pregnancy. Women with asymptomatic masses may be diagnosed at the time of routine second-trimester ultrasound examination. Color Doppler blood flow characteristic, size, and morphology on ultrasound may be helpful in deciding which masses need surgical management. In the first trimester, an uncertain mass is probably best managed with a follow-up ultrasound in the second trimester. Most ovarian cysts will resolve.
- Elective surgery is best avoided in the first trimester. Benign corpus luteum cysts are common, and so is spontaneous miscarriage unrelated to the adnexal mass.
- The best time for surgery is 16 to 18 weeks. General anesthesia is recommended. Laparoscopy may be preferable if laparoscopy would be used for similar findings in a nonpregnant patient. A conservative approach is advised. Most ovarian masses in pregnancy are benign. If the lesion is unilateral and hyperreactio luteinalis or luteoma of pregnancy is a possibility, an ovarian biopsy for frozen section is indicated. Unless obvious metastatic cancer is found, unilateral oophorectomy is indicated. Staging biopsies and washings are done, and final treatment plans are deferred pending a definitive pathology diagnosis.
- Even if unilateral dysgerminoma or a sex-cord stromal tumor is diagnosed, conservative therapy offers a good prognosis. Delivery may be delayed, and further surgery may be unnecessary.
- If metastatic cancer is diagnosed, debulking can be done and the pregnancy continued while the patient is started on chemotherapy. Careful consideration of all options should be discussed with the gynecologic oncologist, the maternal fetal specialist, and the patient and her family.

Bibliography

Agarwal N, Parul K, Bhalta N, et al. Management and outcome of pregnancies complicated with adnexal masses in pregnancy. *Arch Gynecol Obstet* 2003;267:148.

Aiman J. Virilizing ovarian tumors. *Clin J Obstet Gynecol* 1991;34:835.

Borgfeldt C, Iosif C, Masback A. Fertility-sparing surgery and outcome in fertile women with ovarian borderline tumors and epithelial invasive ovarian cancer. *Eur J Obstet Gynecol Reprod Biol* 2006; 134:110–114.

Boulay R, Podczaski E. Ovarian cancer complicating pregnancy. *Obstet Gynecol Clin North Am* 1998;25:385.

Bradshaw KD, Santos-Ramos R, Rawlins SC, et al. Endocrine studies in a pregnancy complicated by ovarian theca lutein cysts and hyperreactio luteinalis. *Obstet Gynecol* 1986;67:66S.

Bromley B, Benacerraf B. Adnexal masses during pregnancy: accuracy of sonographic diagnosis and outcome. *J Ultrasound Med* 1997;16: 447.

Buller RE, Darrow V, Manetta A, et al. Conservative surgical management of dysgerminoma concomitant with pregnancy. *Obstet Gynecol* 1992;79: 887.

Caspi B, Ben-Arie A, Appelman Z, et al. Aspiration of simple pelvic cysts during pregnancy. *Gynecol Obstet Invest* 2000;49:102.

Caspi B, Levi R, Appelman Z, et al. Conservative management of ovarian cystic teratoma during pregnancy and labor. *Am J Obstet Gynecol* 2000;182: 503.

Check JH, Choe JK, Nazari A. Hyperreactio luteinalis despite absence of a corpus luteum and suppressed serum follicle stimulating concentrations in a triplet pregnancy. *Hum Reprod* 2000;15:1043.

De Palma P, Wronski M, Bifernino V, et al. Krukenberg tumor in pregnancy with virilization. *Eur J Gynaecol Oncol* 1995;16:59.

Dgani R, Soham Z, Atar OE, et al. Ovarian carcinoma during pregnancy. *Gynecol Oncol* 1989;33:326.

Dildy GA, Moise KJ, Carpenter RJ, et al. Maternal malignancy metastatic to the products of conception: a review. *Obstet Gynecol Surv* 1989;44:535.

Ebert U, Loffler H, Kirch W. Cytotoxic therapy and pregnancy. *Pharmacol Ther* 1997;74:207.

Elerding SC. Laparoscopic surgery in pregnancy. *Am J Surg* 1993;165:625.

Farahmand SM, Marchetti DL, Asirwatham JE, et al. Ovarian endodermal sinus tumor associated with pregnancy: a review of the literature. *Gynecol Oncol* 1991;41:156.

Ferrandina G, Distefano M, Testa A, et al. Management of an advanced ovarian cancer at 15 weeks of gestation: case report and literature review. *Gynecol Oncol* 2005;97(2):693.

Fleischer AC, Shah DM, Entman SS. Sonographic evaluation of maternal disorders during pregnancy. *Radiol Clin North Am* 1990;28:51.

Frederiksen MC, Casanova L, Schink JC. An elevated maternal serum alphafetoprotein leading to the diagnosis of an immature teratoma. *Int J Gynecol Oncol* 1991;35:343.

Garcia-Bunuel RG, Berek JS, Woodruff JD. Luteomas of pregnancy. *Obstet Gynecol* 1975;45:407.

Ghaemmaghami F, Hasanzadeh M. Good fetal outcome of pregnancies with gynecologic cancer conditions: cases and literature review. *Int J Gynecol Cancer* 2006;16(Suppl 1):225.

Greskovich JF Jr, Macklis RM. Radiation therapy in pregnancy: risk calculation and risk minimization. *Semin Oncol* 2000;27:633.

Giuntoli RL 2nd, Vang RS, Bristow RE. Evaluation and management of adnexal masses during pregnancy. *Clin Obstet Gynecol* 2006;49(3):492.

Henderson CE, Giovanni E, Garfinkel D, et al. Platinum chemotherapy during pregnancy for serous cystadenocarcinoma of the ovary. *Gynecol Oncol* 1993;49:92.

Hermans RH, Fischer DC, van der Putten HW, et al. Adnexal masses in pregnancy. *Onkologie* 2003;26:167.

Hill LM, Connors-Beatty DJ, Nowak A, et al. The role of ultrasonography in the detection and management of adnexal masses during the second and third trimesters of pregnancy. *Am J Obstet Gynecol* 1998;179:703.

Hogston P, Lifford RJ. Ultrasound study of ovarian cysts in pregnancy: prevalence and significance. *BJOG* 1986;93:625.

Hopkins MP, Duchon MA. Adnexal surgery in pregnancy. *J Reprod Med* 1986;31:1035.

Illingworth PJ, Johnstone FD, Steel J, et al. Luteoma of pregnancy: masculinisation of a female fetus prevented by placental aromatisation. *BJOG* 1992;99:1019.

Karlen JR, Akbari A, Cook WA. Dysgerminoma associated with pregnancy. *Obstet Gynecol* 1979;53:330.

Kier R, McCarthy SM, Scoutt LM, et al. Pelvic masses in pregnancy: MR imaging. *Radiology* 1990;176:709.

King LA, Nevin PC, Williams PP, et al. Treatment of advanced epithelial ovarian carcinoma in pregnancy with cisplatin-based chemotherapy. *Gynecol Oncol* 1991;41:78.

Kobayashi H, Yoshida A, Kobayashi M, et al. Changes in size of the functional cyst on ultrasonography during early pregnancy. *Am J Perinatol* 1997;14:1.

Koonings PP, Platt LD, Wallace R. Incidental adnexal neoplasms at caesarean section. *Obstet Gynecol* 1988;72:767.

Leiserowitz GS, Xing G, Cress R, et al. Adnexal masses in pregnancy: how often are they malignant? *Gynecol Oncol* 2006;101:315.

MacDougall M, LeGrand SB, Walsh D. Symptom control in the pregnant cancer patient. *Semin Oncol* 2000;27:704.

Machado F, Vegas C, Leon J, et al. Ovarian cancer during pregnancy: analysis of 15 cases. *Gynecol Oncol* 2007;105:446–450.

Malfetano JH, Goldkrand JW. Cisplatinum combination chemotherapy during pregnancy for advanced epithelial ovarian carcinoma. *Obstet Gynecol* 1990;75:545.

Manganiello PD, Adams LV, Harris RD, et al. *Obstet Gynecol Surv* 1995;50:404.

Mantovani G, Mais V, Parodo G, et al. Use of chemotherapy for ovarian cancer during human pregnancy: case report and literature review. *Eur J Obstet Gynecol Reprod Biol* 2007;131:238.

Marhhom E, Cohen I. Fertility preservation options for women with malignancies. *Obstet Gynecol Surv* 2007;62:58.

Matsuyma T, Tsukamoto N, Matsukuma K, et al. Malignant ovarian tumors associated with pregnancy. *Int J Gynecol Oncol* 1989;28:61.

Mendez LE, Mueller A, Salom E, et al. Paclitaxel and carboplatin chemotherapy administered during pregnancy for advanced epithelial ovarian cancer. *Obstet Gynecol* 2003;102:1200.

Metz SA, Day TG, Pursell SH. Adjuvant chemotherapy in a pregnancy patient with endodermal sinus tumor of the ovary. *Gynecol Oncol* 1989;32:371.

Mooney J, Silva E, Tornos C, et al. Unusual features of serous neoplasms of low malignant potential during pregnancy. *Gynecol Oncol* 1997;65:30.

Moore RD, Smith WG. Laparoscopic management of adnexal masses in pregnant women. *J Reprod Med* 1999;44:97.

Nezhat F, Nezhat C, Silfen SL, et al. Laparoscopic ovarian cystectomy during pregnancy. *J Laparoendosc Surg* 1991;1:161.

Nicklas AH, Baker ME. Imaging strategies in the pregnant cancer patient. *Semin Oncol* 2000;27:623.

Novak ER, Lambrose CD, Woodruff JD. Ovarian tumors in pregnancy. *Obstet Gynecol* 1975;46:401.

Pavlidis NA. Cancer and pregnancy. *Ann Oncol* 2000;11(Suppl 3):247.

Perkins KY, Johnson JL, Kay HH. Simple ovarian cysts: clinical features on a first-trimester ultrasound scan. *J Reprod Med* 1997;42:440.

Piana S, Nogales FF, Corrado S, et al. Pregnancy luteoma with granulosa cell proliferation: an unusual hyperplastic lesion arising in pregnancy and mimicking an ovarian neoplasia. *Pathol Res Pract* 1999;195:859.

Picone O, Lhomme C, Tournaire M, et al. Preservation of pregnancy in a patient with a stage IIIB ovarian epithelial carcinoma diagnosed at 22 weeks of gestation and treated with initial chemotherapy: case report and literature review. *Gynecol Oncol* 2004;94:600.

Rodriguez M, Harrison TA, Nowazki MR, et al. Luteoma of pregnancy presenting with massive ascites and markedly elevated CA-125. *Obstet Gynecol* 1999;94:854.

Sandmeier D, Lobrinus JA, Vial Y, et al. Bilateral Krukenberg tumor of the ovary during pregnancy. *Eur J Gynaecol Oncol* 2000;21:58.

Sasa H, Komatsu Y, Kobayashi M. Ovarian carcinoma in the first trimester. *Int J Gynaecol Obstet* 1998;60:283.

Schapira DV, Chudley AE. Successful pregnancy following continuous treatment with combination chemotherapy before conception and throughout pregnancy. *Cancer* 1984;54:800.

Schmeler KM, Mayo-Smith WW, Peipert JF, et al. Adnexal masses in pregnancy: surgery compared with observation. *Obstet Gynecol* 2005;105:1098.

Schover L. Psychosocial issues associated with cancer in pregnancy. *Semin Oncol* 2000;27:699.

Schwartzberg BS, Conyers JA, Moore JA. First trimester of pregnancy laparoscopic procedures. *Surg Endosc* 1997;11:1216.

Shibahara H, Wakimoto E, Mitsuo M, et al. A case of a patient diagnosed with malignant mixed mullerian tumor of the ovary who conceived after conservative surgery and adjuvant chemotherapy. *Gynecol Oncol* 1997;65:363.

Silva PD, Proto M, Moyer DL, et al. Clinical and ultrastructural findings of an androgenizing Krukenberg tumor in pregnancy. *Obstet Gynecol* 1988;71:432.

Stedman CM, Kline RC. Intraoperative complications and unexpected pathology at the time of c-section. *Obstet Gynecol Clin North Am* 1988;15:745.

Sternberg WH, Barclay DL. Luteoma of pregnancy. *Am J Obstet Gynecol* 1966;95:195.

Tawan K, Baker TH. Ovarian tumors in pregnancy. *J Int Coll Surg* 1964;41:60.

Tewari K, Brewer C, Cappuccini F, et al. Advanced-stage small cell carcinoma of the ovary in pregnancy: long-term survival after surgical debulking and multiagent chemotherapy. *Gynecol Oncol* 1997;66:531.

Tewari K, Cappuccini F, Disaia PJ, et al. Malignant germ cell tumors of the ovary. *Obstet Gynecol* 2000;95:128.

Thornton JF, Wells M. Ovarian cysts in pregnancy: does ultrasound make traditional management inappropriate? *Obstet Gynecol* 1987;69:717.

Ueda M, Ueki M. Ovarian tumors associated with pregnancy. *Int J Gynaecol Obstet* 1996;55:59.

Van der Zee AG, deBruijn HW, Bouma J, et al. Endodermal sinus tumor of the ovary during pregnancy. *Am J Obstet Gynecol* 1991;164:504.

Wang PH, Chao HT, Yuan CC, et al. Ovarian tumors complicating pregnancy: emergency and elective surgery. *J Reprod Med* 1999;44:279.

Weinreb JC, Brown CE, Lowe TW, et al. Pelvic masses in pregnant patients: MR and US imaging. *Radiology* 1986;159:717.

Wheeler TC, Fleischer AC. Complex adnexal mass in pregnancy: predictive value of color Doppler sonography. *J Ultrasound Med* 1997;16:425.

Williams SF, Schilsky RL. Antineoplastic drugs administered during pregnancy. *Semin Oncol* 2000;27:618.

Young RH, Dudley AG, Scully RE. Granulosa cell, Sertoli-Leydig cell, and unclassified sex cord stromal tumors associated with pregnancy: a clinicopathological analysis of thirty-six cases. *Gynecol Oncol* 1984;18:181.

Yuen PM, Chang AMZ. Laparoscopic management of adnexal mass during pregnancy. *Acta Obstet Gynecol Scand* 1997;76:173.

Zanotti KM, Belinson JL, Kennedy AW. Treatment of gynecologic cancers in pregnancy. *Semin Oncol* 2000;27:686.

Zhao XY, Huang HF, Lian LJ, et al. Ovarian cancer in pregnancy: a clinicopathologic analysis of 22 cases and review of the literature. *Int J Gynaecol Cancer* 2006;16:8.

[illegible] RD, Smith [illegible]. [illegible] pregnancy [illegible]. *[illegible] J [illegible]* [illegible].
[illegible] Schwartz [illegible] [illegible] during pregnancy. [illegible] 1994;[illegible].
[illegible] [illegible] the [illegible] [illegible] 2002;[illegible].
[illegible] Landon [illegible], [illegible] [illegible] 1995;[illegible].
[illegible] and pregnancy. [illegible] 20 [illegible] 1998.
[illegible] [illegible] [illegible] 1994;[illegible].
[illegible] pregnancy [illegible] 1996;[illegible].
[illegible] pregnancy [illegible] 2004;[illegible].
[illegible] [illegible] *Obstet Gynecol* [illegible].
[illegible] [illegible] pregnancy [illegible] *Obstet Gynecol* [illegible].
[illegible] [illegible] pregnancy [illegible] *Obstet Gynecol* 1999;[illegible].
[illegible] [illegible] *Obstet Gynecol* 1993;[illegible].
[illegible] pregnancy [illegible] *Am J Obstet Gynecol* 1995;[illegible].
[illegible] [illegible] *Obstet Gynecol* 1996;[illegible].
[illegible] [illegible] 1994;[illegible].
[illegible] [illegible] *Obstet Gynecol* [illegible].
[illegible] [illegible] [illegible] 1995;[illegible].
[illegible] [illegible] *Am J Obstet Gynecol* [illegible].
[illegible] [illegible] pregnancy [illegible] [illegible] 1998;[illegible].
[illegible] [illegible] *Obstet Gynecol* [illegible].
[illegible] [illegible] *Obstet Gynecol* 1988;[illegible].
[illegible] [illegible] pregnancy [illegible] 1985;[illegible].
[illegible] [illegible] 1992;[illegible].
[illegible] [illegible] [illegible].
[illegible] pregnancy [illegible] [illegible].
[illegible] [illegible] *Obstet Gynecol* 1999;[illegible].
[illegible] [illegible] 1998;[illegible].
[illegible] [illegible] *Obstet Gynecol* 2002;[illegible].
[illegible] [illegible] [illegible].

SECTION VII ■ SURGERY FOR CORRECTIONS OF DEFECTS IN PELVIC SUPPORT AND PELVIC FISTULAS

CHAPTER 36A ■ PELVIC ORGAN PROLAPSE: BASIC PRINCIPLES

CARL W. ZIMMERMAN

The judgment as to surgical correction should depend upon a correlation of the history and physical findings. Even marked prolapse in the absence of complaint should rarely be corrected. The patient should ask the gynecologist for relief; the gynecologist should not urge the patient to have corrective surgery if she does not feel sufficiently uncomfortable to request it.

—Richard Te Linde, 1966

DEFINITIONS

Endopelvic fascia—The deep endopelvic connective tissue located between the dependent portion of the pelvic peritoneum and the superior fascia of the pelvic diaphragm. This continuum of tissue serves to support, suspend, and separate the central pelvic organs.

Kegel exercise—Voluntary contraction of the pelvic diaphragm, primarily the puborectalis muscle, and the external anal sphincter.

Interspinous diameter—The distance between the ischial spines and the narrowest diameter in the human pelvis. The components of the deep endopelvic connective tissue suspend the cervix and pericervical ring within this plane in normal anatomy.

Pelvic diaphragm—The skeletal muscles of the pelvic floor and their parietal fasciae. These muscles cover the majority of the pelvic outlet. These muscles originate on the pelvic sidewall and insert on the sacrum, coccyx, or sacrococcygeal raphe.

Rugae—Transverse creases in the vaginal wall that signify the presence of deep endopelvic connective tissue. Conversely, the absence of rugae implies the absence of deep endopelvic connective tissue.

Urogenital hiatus—The large central opening in the pelvic diaphragm. The vagina, urethra, and anus exit the pelvis through this structure.

Uterosacral ligaments—The primary apical suspensory elements of the uterovaginal complex. They extend from the pericervical ring to the presacral periosteum and hold the cervix behind the urogenital hiatus.

Valsalva maneuver—Pressure exerted downward on the pelvic floor by fixing the respiratory diaphragm and the anterior abdominal wall.

BASIC CONCEPTS

Pelvic organ prolapse is the downward displacement of structures that are normally located at the level of or adjacent to the vaginal vault. Because these displacements are each associated with defects in integrated connective tissue structures, they may each be considered a pelvic hernia. These conditions are common and affect a progressively larger percentage of women as age advances. Whereas mortality from this condition is negligible, significant morbidity or deterioration of lifestyle may be associated with prolapse. Women in developed countries who have access to modern health care can benefit from the advances that have been made in treating prolapse. If the problem is viewed from a worldwide perspective, however, the scope of suffering is much greater. In areas of high parity and little or no access to health care, countless women suffer from problems associated with pelvic organ prolapse with no real possibility of resolution. The direct effect that these conditions have on urinary, gastrointestinal, and sexual functions can only be appreciated by those women burdened with these problems on a daily basis.

Treatment of pelvic organ prolapse and the associated symptoms constitutes a major subject in gynecology. Especially in the advanced state, management of these conditions is one of the most challenging problems a pelvic surgeon can face. Indeed, success in treating prolapse is frequently used to judge the overall skill of those surgeons. Providing permanent relief from this classic malady by restoring normal anatomy and maximum physiologic function always tests the ingenuity of gynecologists. As medical sophistication has progressed, so has the ability to understand more completely and better treat pelvic organ prolapse.

A brief review of the history of treatment of prolapse is helpful in understanding modern treatments and current concepts of these conditions. Because it was mentioned in the writings of Hippocrates and Galen, prolapse was clearly known to the ancients. Early treatments may seem quaint by today's standards. Yet some of these interventions continue to be used today. Fortunately, others have not survived. Vaginal packing, tampons, massages, and exercises were used with some success. Other patients were suspended from their feet for a period of 24 hours to treat prolapse. Rodericus A. Castro advised that prolapse should be attacked with a red hot iron as if to burn it, "when fright would cause it to recede into the vagina." Various caustics were used, including silver nitrate, nitric acid, acid nitrate of mercury, hot metal, and sulfuric acid.

Perhaps the first real advance in treatment was the development of pessaries. These devices functioned as trusses. Their fitting and placement became a desirable skill. They continue to bring relief to a large number of women and seldom do any serious harm. They were especially popular in the middle of the 19th century. Some were held in place by waistbands. In some cases, pessaries were deliberately left in place until erosions occurred. The subsequent healing was expected to reduce the caliber of the vagina with scarification adding to support, but serious complications could occur. Reports exist of neglected pessaries being retrieved from the peritoneal cavity and bladder. Fistulae may also occur.

The earliest surgical attempts to relieve prolapse were relatively simple. These procedures included labial suturing and removing portions of the vaginal epithelium to reduce the caliber of the vagina. Although Heming operated on the anterior vaginal wall in 1831, surgery for uterovaginal prolapse was not common until the advent of anesthesia and antisepsis in the middle of the 19th century. The first vaginal hysterectomy for prolapse was performed by Samuel Choppin of New Orleans in 1861. Many years passed before this surgical technique became common. By the beginning of the 20th century, European and American reports of hysterectomy, colporrhaphy, cervical amputation, transposition/interposition operations (Manchester-Fothergill), cervical ligament plications, colpocleisis (LeFort), ventral fixation of the uterus to the abdominal wall, and trachelorrhaphy for procidentia were being published. The timing of this ingenious variety of operations is certainly consistent with the development of anesthesia and various surgical techniques in all fields of medicine.

During the 20th century, advances in understanding and treatment of prolapse have progressed at an ever-increasing rate. In 1909, George R. White of Georgia published an account of cystocele repair using a transvaginal paravaginal approach. His correct perspective on the importance of lateral vaginal support took nearly 50 years to be rediscovered by mainstream gynecologic surgeons. The paravaginal repair was not widely known and accepted at the time because it was overshadowed by the work of Howard A. Kelly of Johns Hopkins. This great and influential surgeon popularized the concept of fascial attenuation. Midline anterior and posterior plications were touted as the correct surgical approach to the problem of prolapse. The Kelly-Kennedy anterior plication and levator ani plication of the posterior vaginal wall remain as commonly performed procedures today, despite the fact that more contemporary surgical techniques described in this chapter more correctly correct the anatomic defects of pelvic prolapse and achieve better clinical results.

In the 1950s, Milton L. McCall of Louisiana developed a culdoplasty technique that emphasized the important suspensory function of the uterosacral ligaments. He believed this operation prevented enteroceles and posthysterectomy vaginal vault prolapse when it was performed at the time of hysterectomy. Currently, the restitution of vaginal vault support at the time of any type of hysterectomy is considered a very important step in prevention of future prolapse.

In the 1960s, Baden and Walker of Texas began to systemize a new defect-specific approach to pelvic organ prolapse repair. Page 1 of their 1992 book, *Surgical Repair of Vaginal Defects,* stated, "In a sense, the defect approach reverses the prior evolution toward 'compensatory' reparative techniques—our goal is to return all vaginal supports to their original anatomic status." Many other surgeons have contributed to this powerful concept of pelvic reconstructive surgery. A. Cullen Richardson and associates of Georgia developed the concept of classifying fascial defects as proximal, distal, central, and lateral. This observation and the teaching of such master surgeons as David H. Nichols of New England encouraged gynecologists to not only identify and repair each vaginal defect but to return support attachments to their original anatomic location. Emphasis was focused on the hernial nature of prolapse and led to the abandonment of absorbable suture in favor of permanent suture in repairs. In the 1990s, pelvic anatomist John O. L. DeLancey of Michigan published a biomechanical analysis of normal vaginal anatomy. His observations have the precision of an engineer's work and identify specific structural goals for each of three vaginal levels of support. Proximal vaginal suspension, midvaginal lateral attachment, and distal vaginal fusion to the perineum and urogenital diaphragm are the basic concepts that modern pelvic surgeons must satisfy to successfully complete a prolapse surgery.

In the 1980s, hernia repair literature began to demonstrate better long-term results with the use of bolsters. For that reason, autografts, allografts, xenografts, and various synthetic meshes are frequently used in today's surgical techniques for prolapse. Debate exists regarding the type, amount, and best location for these materials.

A fusion of anatomic, physiologic, and biomechanical principles has allowed surgeons to offer their patients better treatments for prolapse than have historically been available. This brief and incomplete historical discussion outlines the evolution of our current understanding of a complex topic. Historically ineffective treatments of the presurgical era gave way to surgical approaches for advanced cases. As surgical sophistication has increased, anatomically distorting operations have been replaced by anatomically restoring procedures. Many interesting aspects of the historical development of this subject are described in previous editions of this book and in the bibliographic selections at the end of this section.

A better understanding of a problem always leads to more questions that deserve answers. For example, the process of childbirth is regarded as an important cause of vaginal prolapse. Little or no effort has been made to analyze the forces of childbirth as they relate to specific patterns of damage to the deep endopelvic connective tissue. Delineation of these patterns would assist the surgeon in recognizing defects and undoubtedly improving operative outcome. Precise knowledge of the effects of labor and delivery on the pelvic floor might lead to techniques and decisions designed to reduce the potentially damaging effects of these obstetric events. The concept of prolapse prevention is underused in the practice of gynecology. Teaching patients about physical therapy of the pelvic floor, better lifestyle, and proper evacuation habits should be part of the gynecologist's job. The long-term benefits of an organized program of prolapse prevention have never been evaluated.

Controversy exists as to the best surgical management for specific cases of female pelvic organ prolapse. In fact, now that reparative options are no longer limited to midline plications, more procedures are available than ever before. Vaginal, abdominal, laparoscopic, minimally invasive devices, and combined approaches have their advocates. The necessary randomized trials with matched controls will likely never be done to generate evidence-based outcomes, especially because two of the most powerful variables are surgical skill and experience. The necessary long-term follow-up is rarely available in the pelvic surgery literature. Surgical techniques for prolapse must be carefully evaluated so that anatomic and functional results will continue to improve.

The authors of the various chapters of this section describe interventions and operations that gynecologic surgeons should consider when managing pelvic organ prolapse. Each of these surgeons possesses a combination of operative skill, experience, and special interest in their topics that have led to their selection. The operative techniques presented should be combined with appropriate clinical evaluation and skillful technical performance to obtain maximum benefit for the patients.

ANATOMIC CONSIDERATIONS

The normal position, support, and suspension of the uterus, vagina, bladder, and rectum rely on an interdependent system of bony, muscular, and connective tissue elements. This entire system is three-dimensional, and even subtle alterations in one part may lead to stresses in other parts that eventually lead to failure of normal anatomy. An understanding of normal applied pelvic anatomy is imperative in the repair of pelvic organ prolapse.

The bony pelvis has a central opening that is necessary for reproductive function. During evolutional transition to upright bipedal posture, the potential for prolapse became more likely because of gravitational stress. In the human female, a lordosis of the lumbosacral portion of the spine places the pelvic inlet in an oblique orientation reminiscent of the pelvic posture of a quadruped. The physical result of this shift is that the posterior aspect of the pelvic inlet is approximately 60 degrees above the anterior aspect (Fig. 36A.1). This partially vertical orientation of the pelvic inlet deflects force onto the superior symphysis pubis rather than directly on the pelvic outlet and urogenital hiatus. Consequently, the pelvic outlet is partially shielded from downward stresses in the anatomically normal woman.

The muscles of the pelvic diaphragm primarily provide pelvic support. These muscles form a basin or covering of the pelvic outlet and are often grouped together as the levator ani or levator sling (Fig. 36A.2). Within this diaphragm is the urogenital hiatus, which is large enough to allow childbirth. This large central opening in the muscular pelvic floor explains why prolapse is such a significant problem. The most medial portion of the pelvic diaphragm is formed by the puborectalis, the muscular boundary of the urogenital hiatus. The obstetric axis of the pelvis passes through the urogenital hiatus medial to the puborectalis muscle. In the standing patient, the puborectalis muscle is horizontal and is palpable as a 2- to 2.5-cm band of voluntary muscle on each lateral side of the distal one third of the vagina. When well innervated and contracted, the puborectalis muscle closes the distal vagina and displaces the posterior rectum anteriorly. Forming the bulk of the pelvic diaphragm, the pubococcygeus and iliococcygeus muscles cover the posterior and lateral portions of the pelvic outlet (Fig. 36A.3). The superior insertion of the iliococcygeus muscles is an important landmark in pelvic support anatomy. These insertions are thickenings of the pelvic sidewall parietal fascia that extend from the ischial spines posteriorly to points on the pubic bone known as the pubic tubercles. These lines of insertion are known as the arcus tendineus levator ani or muscular arches (Figs. 36A.4 and 36A.5). Immediately inferior to the muscular arches are thickenings of the parietal fascia of the bellies of the ileococcygeus muscles known as the arcus tendineus fasciae pelvis (fascial arches) or white lines. These structures are

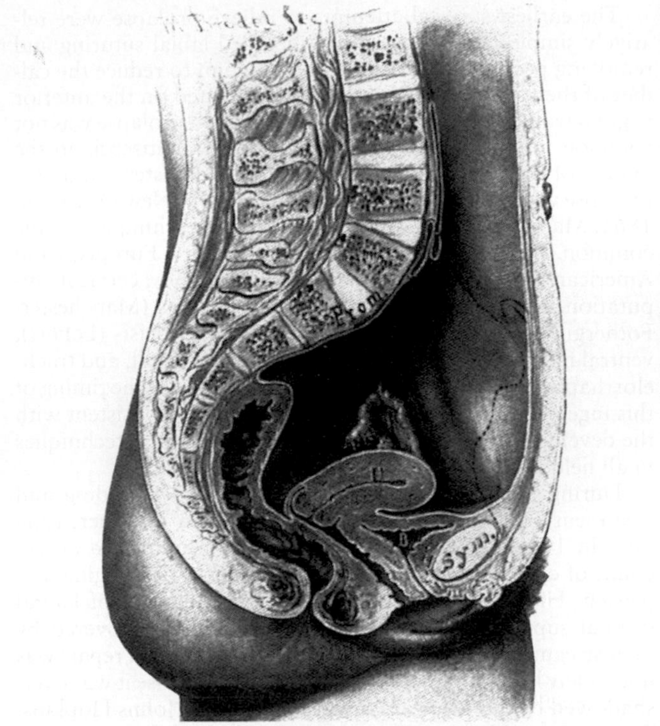

FIGURE 36A.1. The relationship between the pelvic floor and the abdominal cavity. Notice the lordosis of the lumbosacral spine and the almost vertical orientation of the pelvic inlet. (From Kelly HA. *Gynecology.* New York: D. Appleton & Co.; 1928:2. Used with permission of the Department of Art as Applied to Medicine, Johns Hopkins Medical School.)

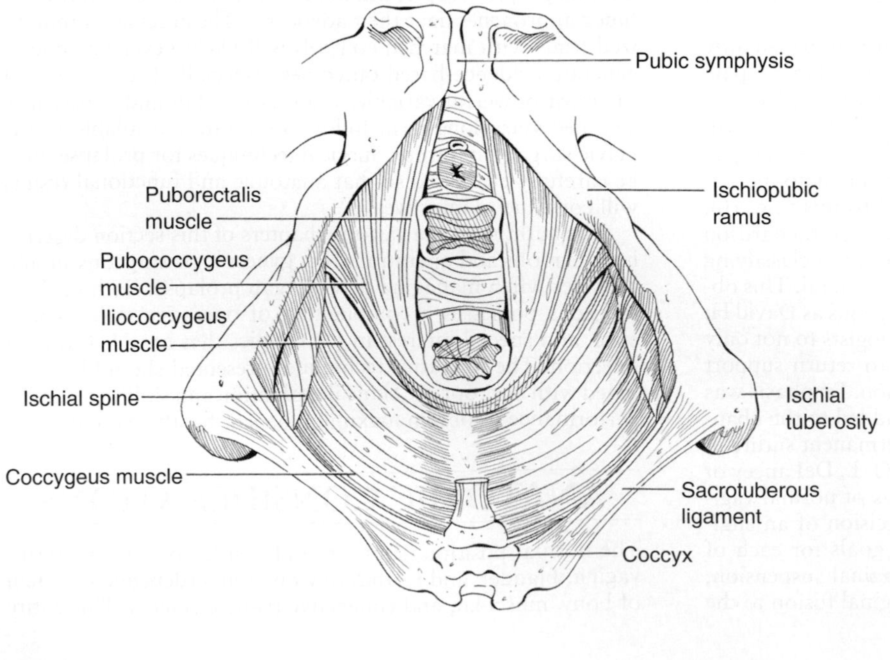

FIGURE 36A.2. The pelvic diaphragm viewed from below.

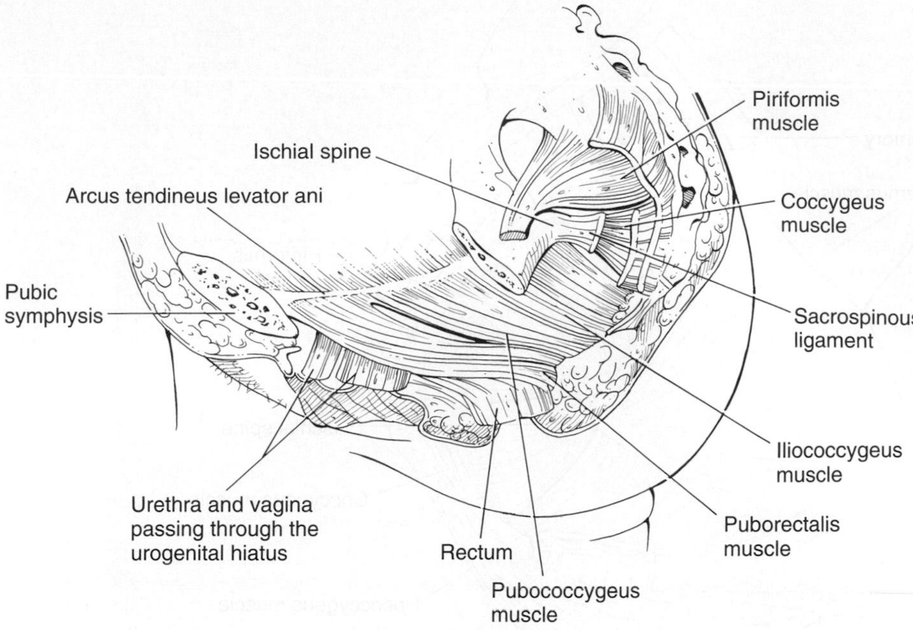

FIGURE 36A.3. Muscles of the pelvic floor, lateral view.

the lateral attachment points for the pubocervical fascia and proximal rectovaginal septum. The white line serves the function of midvaginal lateral support. Paravaginal and proximal pararectal defects are located immediately medial to the white line. In the standing patient, the white line is nearly horizontal; in the lithotomy position, it is nearly vertical.

During paravaginal repair, the white lines are palpable as stringlike structures between the ischial spines and the pubic arch. Another fascial thickening has been described that runs posteriorly from the white line and serves as lateral support for the distal rectovaginal septum of the posterior vagina. This structure has been named the arcus tendineus fasciae rectovaginalis (Fig. 36A.6). The lateral supports of the anterior and posterior vaginal septa merge and are not separate in the proximal half of the vagina. Superior to the muscular arch is the uppermost portion of the obturator internus muscle and the parietal obturator fascia. The obturator internus muscles qualify as pelvic muscles because they form the lateral borders of the upper portion of the pelvic basin inferior to the linea terminalis. Posterior to the iliococcygeus, the pelvic floor is covered by

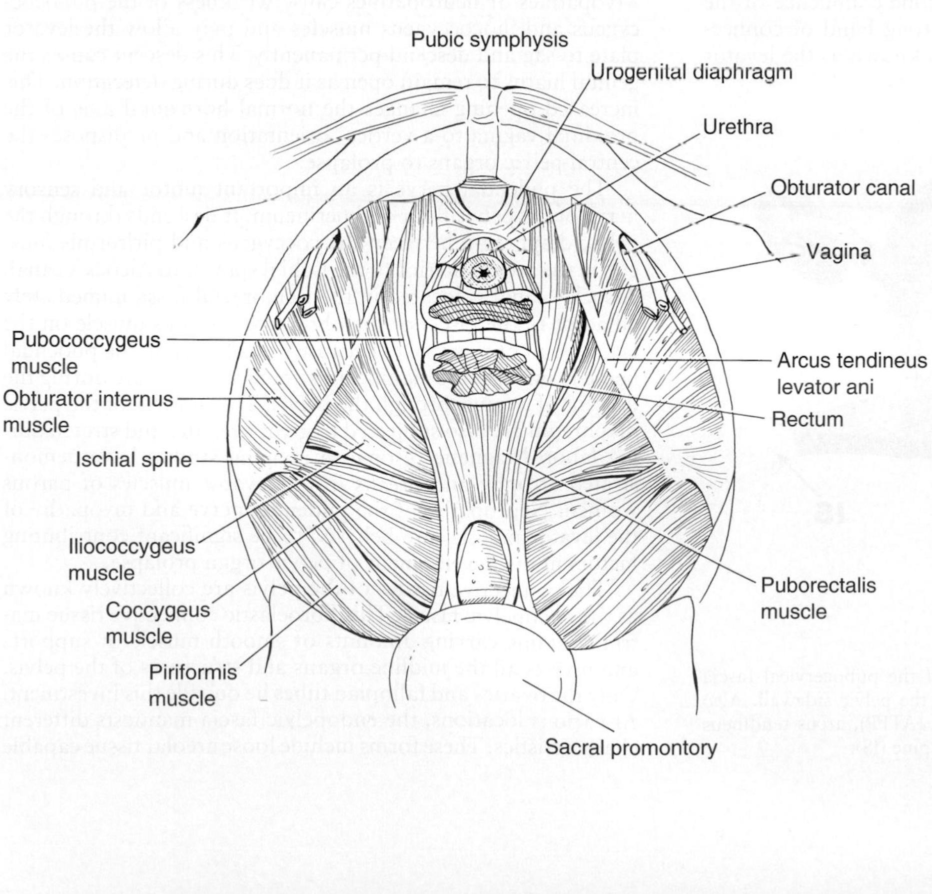

FIGURE 36A.4. The pelvic diaphragm viewed from above.

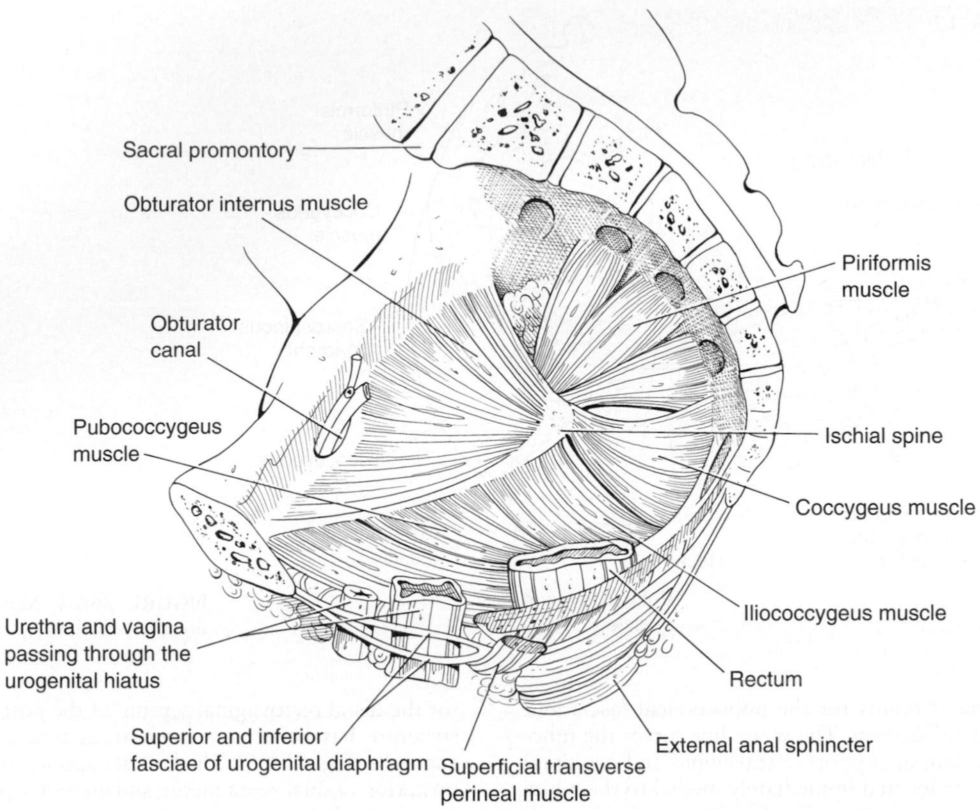

FIGURE 36A.5. Sagittal view of the pelvis.

the coccygeus muscle and the closely associated sacrospinous ligament. These structures pass between the ischial spine and the coccyx. The most posterior portion of the pelvis is covered by the piriformis muscle. The midline confluence of the levator muscles forms a particularly strong band of connective tissue between the coccyx and anus known as the levator plate or sacrococcygeal raphe. This plate is oriented horizontally in the standing patient. The vagina and the rectum are suspended by the endopelvic fascia directly over the levator plate. Myopathies or neuropathies cause weakness of the pubococcygeus and iliococcygeus muscles and may allow the levator plate to sag and descend permanently. This descent causes the genital hiatus to remain open as it does during defecation. This increased opening changes the normal horizontal axis of the proximal vagina to a vertical orientation and predisposes the central pelvic organs to prolapse.

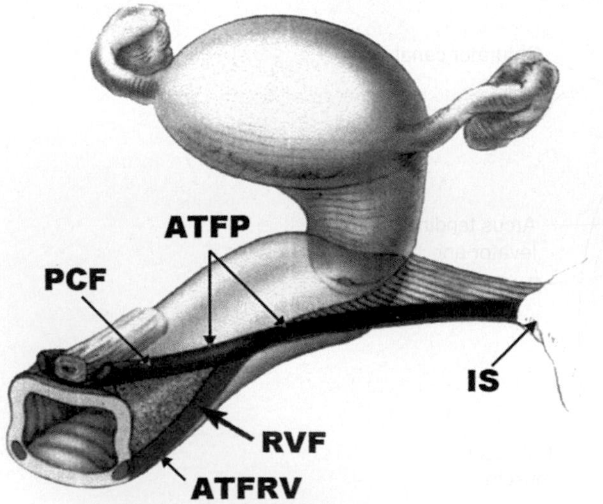

FIGURE 36A.6. The lateral attachments of the pubocervical fascia (PCF) and the rectovaginal fascia (RVF) to the pelvic sidewall. Also shown are the arcus tendineus fascia pelvis (ATFP), arcus tendineus fasciae rectovaginalis (ATFRV), and ischial spine (IS).

The pudendal nerve is an important motor and sensory nerve of the pelvic floor and perineum. It descends through the pelvic diaphragm between the coccygeus and piriformis muscles in the area posterior to the ischial spine into Alcock's canal. Alcock's canal is located in the ischiorectal fossa immediately adjacent to the fascia of the obturator internus muscle on the lateral wall of this space. Because of its location, the pudendal nerve is subjected to significant stretch and pressure during the descent of a fetus through the pelvis. The muscles of the pelvic diaphragm are also subjected to great pressure and stretch during labor. Magnetic resonance imaging studies have demonstrated atrophy and breaks in the levator muscles of parous women. Neuropathy of the pudendal nerve and myopathy of the levator muscles are believed to be significant contributing factors in the development of pelvic organ prolapse.

The connective tissues of the pelvis are collectively known as the endopelvic fascia. This fibroelastic connective tissue matrix contains varying amounts of smooth muscle. It supports and invests all the midline organs and structures of the pelvis. Only the ovaries and fallopian tubes lie outside this investment. At various locations, the endopelvic fascia manifests different characteristics. These forms include loose areolar tissue capable

TABLE 36A.1

PARIETAL PELVIC FASCIAE

Obturator fascia
Particularly well defined in the area superior to the arcus tendineus levator ani and below the linea terminalis. This fascia may represent a vestigial portion of the levator ani whose origin has been lowered through evolution to the level of the muscular arch.

Levator ani fascia (Superior fascia of the pelvic diaphragm)
This fascia is continuous across the pelvic floor, blending laterally with the obturator fascia at the arcus tendineus levator ani and centrally with the levator plate and the visceral fasciae at the urogenital hiatus.

Coccygeus fascia (Sacrospinous ligament)
This important pelvic support structure extends from the ischial spine laterally to the sacrum medially and is an important alternative source of proximal support when the uterosacral ligament is unavailable or insufficient.

Piriformis fascia
This fascia is the thinnest and most posterior of the parietal fasciae of the pelvis.

of distention, neurovascular sheaths, septa and ligaments that support, suspend, and separate the pelvic organs, and dense skeletal muscle investments. In the central pelvis, the visceral peritoneum drapes over the midline structures, dipping into recesses but not descending into direct contact with the muscular pelvic floor. The irregular space between the pelvic diaphragm, the muscular pelvic sidewall, and the visceral peritoneum is the location of the endopelvic fascia (Tables 36A.1–36A.8). The endopelvic fascia may be divided into three parts: parietal fasciae, visceral fasciae, and deep endopelvic connective tissue.

The parietal fasciae of the endopelvic fascia are relatively dense membranes investing the pelvic surface of the skeletal muscles of the pelvic sidewall (Table 36A.1). They are similar in structure, form, and function to other parietal fasciae of the body, such as the rectus abdominis fasciae. At muscular margins, they blend with the various periostea of the bony pelvis.

The visceral pelvic fasciae are loose, highly elastic, and relatively ill-defined encasements of the central pelvic organs, taking the form of sheaths and sleeves (Table 36A.2). These structures allow for the high degree of physiologic distention necessitated by the intestinal, urinary, and reproductive functions of the pelvic organs. The visceral fasciae blend intimately with the organs that they encase.

TABLE 36A.2

VISCERAL PELVIC FASCIAE

Pelvic organs and structures invested by visceral fasciae
Vagina
Uterus
Bladder
Rectum

Pelvic organs and structures not invested by visceral fasciae
Fallopian tubes
Ovaries

The deep endopelvic connective tissue is of central importance in the clinically applied anatomy of the pelvis and is especially significant to the pelvic reconstructive surgeon. This structure is part of a continuum of retroperitoneal connective tissue that extends from the respiratory diaphragm in the upper abdomen to the pelvic diaphragm. Included in this continuum of structures are the mesenteries and ligaments of the upper abdomen. Anatomists debate whether the condensations of this connective tissue should be considered as true ligaments and fasciae. Part of this debate stems from the fact that some of these structures contain a significant muscular component and others serve as neurovascular conduits. Certainly, from a functional standpoint in the pelvis, they meet criteria for being so named. The endopelvic connective tissue is continuous from one part to the other. Separate portions serve different functions, take various forms, and therefore are given different names. The named structures of the deep endopelvic connective tissue include six ligaments, two septa, and one ring. Important anatomic details of these elements are summarized in the following tables.

The six pericervical ligaments form the paracolpium (Tables 36A.3, 36A.4, and 36A.5). The net effect of these structures is the suspension of the cervix in the posterior pelvis and the consequent placement of the vagina directly over the levator plate and away from direct exposure to the urogenital hiatus. In the normal anatomic position, pressure from above tends to close the apical vaginal vault with no tendency toward prolapse.

Two septa or fasciae (Tables 36A.6 and 36A.7) are located within the deep endopelvic connective tissue. These condensations of fibroelastic connective tissue are in close contact with the vaginal epithelium and visceral fasciae of the adjacent

TABLE 36A.3

COMPONENTS OF THE DEEP ENDOPELVIC CONNECTIVE TISSUE: UTEROSACRAL LIGAMENTS

Origin
Periosteum of sacral vertebra 2, 3, and 4

Insertion
The points of insertion are on the posterior and lateral supravaginal cervix at the 5-o'clock and 7-o'clock positions. The ligaments are continuous with and form part of the pericervical ring

Neurologic content
Uterosacral plexus of autonomic nerves

Vascular content
Minimal

Muscular content
Rectouterine muscle

Function
These structures are the primary proximal suspensory elements of the uterovaginal complex. They hold the cervix behind the urogenital hiatus in the posterior pelvis at the level of the ischial spines with the uterus in anteflexion and the vagina suspended over the levator plate.

Synonym
Rectal pillar
At their insertion into the pericervical ring, the uterosacral ligaments blend as continuous structures superiorly and laterally with the cardinal ligaments and distally with the proximal rectovaginal septum

TABLE 36A.4

COMPONENTS OF THE DEEP ENDOPELVIC CONNECTIVE TISSUE: CARDINAL LIGAMENTS

Origin
The hypogastric root with fibrous connections to the lateral abdominal and pelvic walls

Insertion
The points of insertion are on the lateral supravaginal cervix at the 3-o'clock and 9-o'clock positions. This insertion is continuous with and forms part of the pericervical ring.

Neurologic content
Portions of the uterosacral plexus.

Vascular content
Uterine artery and veins

Muscular content
Minimal smooth muscle content with no named component.

Urinary
The distal ureter passes under the uterine artery within the superior portion of the cardinal ligament

Function
These ligaments are the primary vascular conduits of the uterus and vagina, providing lateral stabilization to the cervix at the level of the ischial spines. They are similar in structure, content, and function to the mesenteries of the abdomen.

Synonyms
Mackenrodt's ligament, lateral cervical ligament, and proper cervical ligament

organs. Clinically, they are separate from their adjacent structures. When the septa and their supports are intact, the vaginal and rectal axes have a posterior angle of approximately 130 degrees at the anterior point of their suspension over the levator plate. Distal to the puborectalis muscle, the vagina is nearly vertical as it passes through the urogenital hiatus. The apical or proximal two thirds of the vagina is nearly horizontal and is suspended over the levator plate. The normal vaginal axis is oriented posteriorly toward a point just above the center of the fourth sacral vertebra. This point is the area of the origin of the uterosacral ligaments.

The pericervical ring (Table 36A.8) is the single location where all deep endopelvic connective tissue support structures

TABLE 36A.5

COMPONENTS OF THE DEEP ENDOPELVIC CONNECTIVE TISSUE: PUBOCERVICAL LIGAMENTS

Origin
Inferior surface of the superior pubic ramus medially and the arcus tendineus fascia pelvis laterally

Insertion
The points of insertion are on the anterior and lateral supravaginal cervix at the 11-o'clock and 1-o'clock positions. This insertion is continuous with and forms part of the pericervical ring.

Vascular component
Artery and veins of the bladder pillar

Function
These ligaments are the least well developed of the pericervical ligaments, serving as a vascular conduit and for a minimal degree of cervical stabilization.

Synonym
Bladder pillar

TABLE 36A.6

COMPONENTS OF THE DEEP ENDOPELVIC CONNECTIVE TISSUE: PUBOCERVICAL SEPTUM OR FASCIA

Shape
Trapezoidal with the narrow end located distally

Contents
Fibroelastic connective tissue and smooth muscle

Function
Anterior vaginal support, including support of the bladder

Synonyms
Vesicovaginal septum or fascia, pubovesicocervical septum or fascia

Boundaries
Distal: Pubic tubercles laterally and the pubic arch centrally fusing with the urogenital diaphragm
Lateral: Arcus tendineus fascia pelvis or white line.
Proximal: Pericervical ring centrally and both pubocervical and cardinal ligaments laterally
Superior: Visceral fascia of the bladder
Inferior: Epithelium of the vagina

TABLE 36A.7

COMPONENTS OF THE DEEP ENDOPELVIC CONNECTIVE TISSUE: RECTOVAGINAL SEPTUM OR FASCIA

Shape
Trapezoidal with the narrow end located distally

Contents
Fibroelastic connective tissue and smooth muscle

Function
Posterior vaginal support and suspension, stabilization of the rectum, and perineal suspension. The vaginal suspensory axis consists of the perineum, rectovaginal septum, pericervical ring, uterosacral ligaments, and presacral periosteum. The rectovaginal septum also guides the leading edge of a descending bowel movement into the anus.

Synonym
Denonvilliers' fascia

Boundaries
Distal: Fusion with the proximal perineal body at the central tendon of the perineum.
Lateral: In the distal half of the vagina, the lateral boundary is the arcus tendineus fasciae rectovaginalis; in the proximal half of the vagina, the lateral boundary is the arcus tendineus fascia pelvis.
Proximal: Uterosacral ligaments laterally and the pericervical ring centrally.
Superior: Epithelium of the vagina
Inferior: Visceral fascia of the rectum

TABLE 36A.8

COMPONENTS OF THE DEEP ENDOPELVIC CONNECTIVE TISSUE: PERICERVICAL RING

Shape
Collar of connective tissue encircling the supravaginal cervix

Contents
Fibroelastic connective tissue

Function
Cervical stabilization within the interspinous diameter by connecting with all other named components of the deep endopelvic connective tissue

Synonym
Supravaginal septum

Connections
Anterior: The pericervical ring is located between the base of the bladder and the anterior cervix, where it connects with the pubocervical ligaments at the 11-o'clock and 1-o'clock positions and the proximal pubocervical septum centrally.
Lateral: Cardinal ligaments at the 3-o'clock and 9-o'clock positions
Posterior: The pericervical ring is located between the rectum and the posterior cervix, where it connects with the uterosacral ligaments at the 5-o'clock and 7-o'clock positions and the proximal rectovaginal septum centrally.

converge. *Simply stated, the goal of the defect-specific pelvic reconstructive surgeon is the restitution of the anatomical connections of the pericervical ring.* If the dissection and reconstructive efforts during such a surgery do not extend proximally to the interspinous diameter, the surgery is likely to fail. Because the cervix is located on the anterior vaginal wall, the pubocervical septum is shorter than the rectovaginal septum by a length equal to the diameter of the pericervical ring. If one carries this line of reasoning further, an inherent structural problem is present in the posthysterectomy prolapse patient. If the cervix and its surrounding support tissues are absent, no completely anatomic method to reconstruct the proximal anterior vaginal support exists. Some form of anatomic distortion (e.g., shortening of the vagina or plication) or bolstering is necessary to compensate for this defect. Likely, this dilemma is the

TABLE 36A.9

AVASCULAR SPACES OF THE PELVIS

Prevesical
Paravesical
Vesicovaginal
Vesicocervical
Rectovaginal
Pararectal
Retrorectal

reason that the dominant support defect in the posthysterectomy patient is most frequently in this location.

The three-dimensional structure of the endopelvic fascia has another distinguishing anatomic characteristic that is of interest to the pelvic surgeon. Outside the confines of the named condensations of this tissue are avascular potential spaces (Table 36A.9). When properly used, these spaces give the surgeon access to important support structures deep within the pelvis. Gynecologic oncologists base their surgical training around mastering the surgical manipulation of these spaces, usually from the abdominal approach. These spaces are not only available to the vaginal reconstructive surgeon, but they are also critical in identification of pelvic support landmarks.

DeLancey's biomechanical analysis of normal uterovaginal support by the deep endopelvic connective tissue helps to unify the anatomic principles pertinent to pelvic organ prolapse (Fig. 36A.7). These concepts of support and suspension also help to define a set of goals for the reconstructive surgeon. Each goal must be satisfied for the long-term success of a prolapse surgery. DeLancey divided vaginal support into three levels (Fig. 36A.8). Proximal vaginal level I support is attributed to suspension by the ligaments of the paracolpium. Damage to level I support results in uterovaginal prolapse, posthysterectomy vaginal prolapse, and enterocele. The cause for level I support problems is necessarily at or above the level of the ischial spines. The primary load-bearing elements are the uterosacral ligaments and, to a lesser extent, the cardinal ligaments. This fact is consistent with cadaver observations made many years ago by Mengert showing that prolapse occurred only after 85% of the integrity of the paracolpium was severed. Midvaginal level II support is due to lateral attachment of the fascial septa to

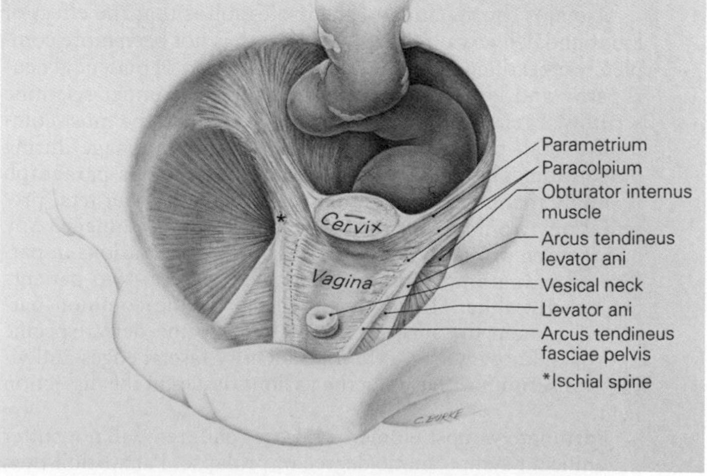

FIGURE 36A.7. Three-dimensional view of the endopelvic fascia. Notice the location of the cervix in the proximal anterior vaginal segment. (From DeLancey JO. Anatomic aspects of vaginal eversion after hysterectomy. *Am J Obstet Gynecol* 1992;166:1717.)

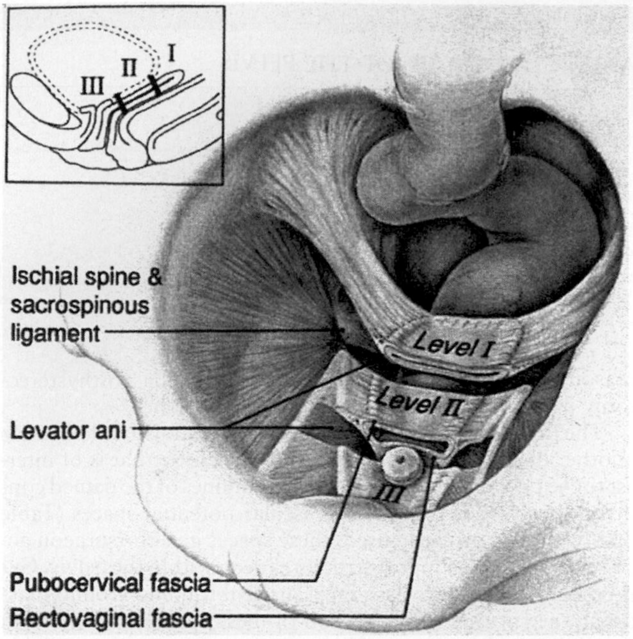

FIGURE 36A.8. The endopelvic fascia of a posthysterectomy patient divided into DeLancey's biomechanical levels: level I—proximal suspension; level II—lateral attachment; level III—distal fusion. (From DeLancey JO. Anatomic aspects of vaginal eversion after hysterectomy. *Am J Obstet Gynecol* 1992;166:1717.)

the pelvic sidewalls. The septa attach to the arcus tendineus fascia pelvis and the arcus tendineus fasciae rectovaginalis. Damage at this level results in paravaginal and pararectal defects. Level III support is attributed to fusion to the urogenital diaphragm anteriorly and to the proximal perineum posteriorly. Damage at these sites results in urinary incontinence anteriorly and in perineal body deficits posteriorly. Cystocele and rectocele are central defects within the fabric of the pubocervical and rectovaginal septa.

ETIOLOGY AND PREVENTION

In the vast majority of women who will develop pelvic organ prolapse, the process begins with their first **vaginal delivery**. Each subsequent vaginal delivery contributes to the likelihood that a clinically symptomatic prolapse will occur. Labor and delivery are certainly desired, necessary, and important physiologic events. Nonetheless, childbirth does have a traumatic aspect by contributing to the development of pelvic organ prolapse. Commonly, many years pass and other factors contribute to the progression of prolapse before such patients present for evaluation.

During labor, the fetal presenting part (about 95% are vertex) must overcome a significant amount of soft tissue resistance presented by the lower uterine segment and cervix, the endopelvic fascia, and the muscular pelvic floor. Because of the lordosis of the lumbosacral spine, the obstetric axis of the pelvis is noticeably angled, differing by 90 degrees between the inlet and outlet. This right angle occurs at the level of the ischial spines and causes the baby's head to extend sharply beginning at the level of the interspinous diameter. Thus, the fetus is driven by strong uterine contractions through a low-velocity, high-pressure, arcing transit through the pelvis. Labor aided by maternal pushing and, at times, by physician traction has a damaging effect on the intricately constructed support structures of the pelvis.

In the initial phase of a nulliparous labor, the fetal head engages, flexes, and descends to a point immediately proximal to the interspinous diameter. Clinical examination at this stage commonly finds the cervix held in a far posterior position as a result of the strength and suspensory function of the uterosacral ligaments. In this situation, great pressure is placed on the anterior vaginal segment. The most common fetal presentation, the left occipitoanterior position, places the rotating arc of the fetal head on the maternal right. As the fetal head overcomes the resistance of the pubocervical septum, significant downward pressure is placed on the maternal right pelvic sidewall. This event likely explains the preponderance of full-length right paravaginal paravesical defects as the most common fascial defect in anterior vaginal relaxation. As further descent occurs, the cervix rotates anteriorly, representing uterosacral ligament damage proximal to the interspinous diameter. The fetus then usually rotates into the occipitoanterior position as it encounters the interspinous diameter. This diameter is the narrowest in the female human pelvis and therefore is the plane of greatest pressure during labor and delivery. The fetal head flexes to allow passage under the pubic symphysis. The anterior sacrococcygeal curvature is concave. As the fetus passes under the pubic arch, this concavity makes it necessary for the fetal head to extend to complete labor. This change in orientation places intense pressure on the posterior pericervical ring. The usual result is further uterosacral stress and a transverse proximal detachment of the rectovaginal septum at its junction with the pericervical ring. As extension of the head progresses, displacement of the rectovaginal septum toward the perineum results in the creation of a nidus for proximal vaginal enterocele and midvaginal rectocele formation. If the rectovaginal septum is displaced far enough distally, pararectal defects form as the septum is sheared away from its lateral attachments. The process of rectovaginal detachment and displacement weakens proximal support for the perineal body and predisposes to perineal descent. Subsequent deliveries progressively contribute damage to the endopelvic fascia. During descent and extension, the fetus passes through the urogenital hiatus. During this process, pressure is transmitted to the levator muscles and the pudendal nerve. If a patient dilates completely, pushes in an attempt to deliver, and then receives a cesarean section, she may have much of the same fascial damage as a woman with a successful vaginal delivery. A nulliparous patient with prolapse would likely suffer from isolated failure of the paracolpium, with the pericervical ring and fascial septa remaining intact.

A major shortcoming of the profession is that the effect of labor and delivery on the female pelvis has not been more completely objectified. Only recently has the study of pudendal neuropathy and levator myopathy been brought under scientific scrutiny. Even less has been done to determine the most common overall patterns of fascial and ligament damage during parturition. The pattern described in the previous paragraph is simply the most common one encountered. Other fetal presentations would result in different patterns of damage. Any experienced prolapse surgeon recognizes the variations in pattern of herniation, leading to the adage that no two patients are exactly alike. However, knowledge of the common pattern does help the surgeon who is new to the defect-specific approach know where to look to identify fascial edges and visually discriminate between the various tissues in the dissection field.

Fortunately, most women who bear children will not suffer a significant symptomatic degree of prolapse. Parturition then is a necessary cause but not a sufficient cause for the vast majority of prolapse cases. Other factors work over time and in combination with the damage caused by childbirth to convert incipient prolapse into a clinically apparent problem.

Prolapse becomes more common with **advancing age**. The likely cause is general weakening of tissues, including the pelvic floor muscles. Passage of time increases the cumulative effect of contributing causes on the pelvic floor. Most cases of prolapse become evident after the age of menopause. Virtually all the tissues of the pelvis possess estrogen receptors, and the **atrophic changes** that occur in the absence of estrogen are a contributing cause for prolapse. With age and a prolonged hypoestrogenic state, osteoporosis may develop. The kyphotic changes in the spine that result from osteoporosis displace the pelvic inlet into a more horizontal plane. This change in the pelvic inlet allows the weight of the abdominal contents to act more directly on the pelvic floor and on the urogenital hiatus.

Lifestyle may contribute to prolapse. Lifting objects heavy enough to require a Valsalva maneuver or fixation of the respiratory diaphragm displaces stress directly down on the pelvic floor. This process may be aided by shoulder, back, and extremity weakness. Defecation or micturition are commonly assisted with straining. This straining occurs when the pelvic diaphragm is intentionally relaxed. This action places substantial force on a passive pelvic floor and open urogenital hiatus several times a day. Straining has essentially the same effect as heavy lifting. Obesity, which is epidemic in the United States, directly increases the load on the pelvic floor and decreases mobility, as well as the ability to do muscle strengthening exercises.

Medical conditions and their complications may contribute to the development of prolapse. A few examples suffice to illustrate how a **chronic medical condition** or the treatments for medical problems may affect the pelvic floor. The natural history of diabetes mellitus includes neuropathy and obesity, both of which contribute to the tendency to prolapse. Chronic cough accompanying asthma, bronchitis, or smoking places repeated stresses on the pelvic floor. The effects of repeated or paroxysmal coughing help to convert incipient prolapse into a clinical problem. Smoking also has antiestrogenic properties, contributes to vascular disease, and creates a chronic hypoxic state. Corticosteroid therapy is used in many chronic medical conditions. The weakening effect of these medications on connective tissue is well known. People with constitutional connective tissue disorders have been shown to be at increased risk for prolapse. Ehlers-Danlos syndrome, for example, is characterized by generalized fascial and connective tissue weaknesses. The pelvic floor is also affected by these deficits. More subtle connective tissue weakness, such as joint hypermobility, has been suspected to increase the long-term risk for prolapse. Development of ascites may cause a rapid increase in the degree of prolapse. This list is by no means complete. Any condition that affects the physical load on the pelvic floor or the integrity of the muscular and connective tissues of the pelvis will increase the likelihood that symptomatic prolapse will develop.

Some medical conditions may reduce the tendency to develop prolapse. This is the case for any condition that causes an inflammatory reaction in the paracervical or parametrial tissues with subsequent tissue fibrosis. Pelvic inflammatory disease, puerperal or postabortal sepsis, endometriosis, and pelvic radiation therapy are conditions that could lead to such a circumstance. Pelvic adhesions, regardless of the cause, might be dense and numerous enough to secondarily suspend a prolapse. Large uterine leiomyomata or other pelvic masses can mechanically prevent the development and descent of prolapse.

The list of contributing causes to pelvic organ prolapse is varied. **Prevention** should begin early in a woman's life and be continued into the later years. Many of the measures discussed as preventions also have a positive effect on a woman's general health. Any discussion of pelvic organ prolapse prevention must include the obstetric management of childbirth. Vaginal delivery undoubtedly has a primary and profound effect on pelvic support anatomy. Debates have occurred for decades about the wisdom of operative vaginal deliveries, optimal length for the second stage of labor, management of macrosomia, usefulness of episiotomy, and multiple other obstetric practices. In truth, little evidence-based information exists regarding these concepts as they relate to the subsequent development of prolapse. The most likely major contributing factor is simply vaginal delivery. The pelvis is contoured so that even in a normal labor and delivery, substantial forces are applied to the endopelvic fascia, muscular floor of the pelvis, and pudendal nerve. The greatest forces generated are at the level of the interspinous diameter. This plane is the location of the singularly important pericervical ring and its junction with every other septa and ligament associated with normal vaginal support and suspension. For example, an episiotomy may shorten the second stage of labor but is unlikely to have any effect on the stresses generated in the interspinous diameter. Does prophylactic cesarean section represent the ultimate in prolapse prevention? This tactic certainly has attained popularity in some parts of the world. One might argue that if vaginal delivery is a necessary cause for prolapse, then this strategy would be preventative. This topic has generated an active and emerging debate in obstetrics and gynecology. Evidence-based resolutions to these questions are unlikely to ever be available. In my opinion, prophylactic cesarean section will never be widely applied. Replacing a desired physiologic process with a major surgery is illogical when the consequence to be prevented is relatively uncommon and not life threatening. However, occasional patients may present convincing arguments in favor of prophylactic cesarean section. The individual practitioner and patient must resolve the course of action in the privacy of the consultation room.

In the adult parous woman, strategies to prevent the development of prolapse center on efforts that decrease physical stress on the urogenital hiatus and strengthen the pelvic floor. Physical therapists have known for years that protection of the lower back is improved by strengthening the shoulder girdle, quadriceps muscles, and abdominal muscles, as well as the muscles of the low back. These same concepts are valid for protection of the pelvic floor. A program of exercise that develops strength in all these muscle groups allows women to accomplish the activities they desire without straining or using the assistance of a Valsalva maneuver. Care must be taken to respect the urogenital hiatus so that during such training, undue stress is not repeatedly placed on the pelvic floor. Likewise, in daily activity, the proper techniques to lift, push, and pull objects should be learned and practiced. The control of obesity must be considered part of the effort to reduce the load placed on the pelvic floor. Osteoporotic spinal changes cause a gradual kyphosis, replacing the normal lumbosacral lordosis. The net effect is to rotate the pelvic brim into a more horizontal position. This shift places more stress on the pelvic floor. Estrogen therapy not only prevents osteoporosis but also has positive effects on the various estrogen-sensitive tissues of the pelvis. Hormone replacement therapy is complicated, controversial, and beyond the scope of this discussion. Other effective treatments for osteoporosis exist.

Pelvic floor strengthening by voluntary contraction of the muscles innervated by the pudendal nerve was popularized by

Arnold Kegel. The associated exercises have been known by his name ever since. Many women know this term because it is used frequently in postpartum instructions. Several different strategies help to remind patients to do their Kegel exercises. One of the most effective techniques is briefly outlined below. The Kegel contraction should be confirmed during a pelvic examination to ensure that the patient understands the correct muscles to contract. Frequently, patients will either perform a Valsalva maneuver or tighten the gluteus maximus muscle instead of the external anal sphincter and levator ani muscles. The proper time to Kegel is after micturition. After the bladder is emptied, the patient is instructed to lean as far forward as her stability allows. While leaning forward, she performs three or more isometric Kegel exercises by tightening the muscles until they voluntarily relax on their own. The dependent portion of a cystocele is below the level of the internal urethral orifice. The forward tilt physically elevates the bladder floor and allows for more complete emptying. The muscular action of the Kegel contractions also aids the process of emptying. Coupling this activity with voiding habituates the patient to perform the exercises several times a day. The result is the combination of more complete emptying and a strengthened pelvic floor, both of which are advantageous for the patient. The patient may then be able to use the Kegel contraction during physical stress to prevent incontinence or to protect against the pelvic floor impact of sudden increases in abdominal pressure. If the patient knows how to use Kegel muscles that are strong and easily controlled, they become an asset in her daily life.

Splinting is particularly effective in alleviating the dysfunctional defecation related to symptomatic rectoceles. If a significant rectocele/enterocele herniation is present, patients frequently experience entrapment of the leading edge of the descending bowel movement. Entrapment leads to straining, which further enhances the entrapment. Often patients in this circumstance will strain until the bowel movement fragments and allows partial defecation and descent of another segment of stool into the rectal pocket. Several trips to the toilet and a large segment of the day may be required to complete this process. This unfortunate problem may be avoided if the patient simply places upward pressure with her finger tips against the perineum or the area lateral to the perineum during the initial urge to defecate. Occasionally, the patient needs to place one or two fingers against the posterior vaginal wall. These maneuvers effectively reduce the rectocele pocket, allowing the stool to evacuate while bypassing the rectocele. This "digital defecation" or splinting technique may avoid surgery and certainly empowers the patient to be in better control of her daily activities. I encourage the use of this technique postoperatively to protect the suspended posterior vaginal segment against undue strain. This protective maneuver is particularly important while acute healing is under way.

Control of chronic diseases and habits are helpful preventative strategies. Effective treatment of persistent cough may decrease incontinence and prevent progression of prolapse. Cessation of smoking certainly may be considered part of the preventative effort. Diabetic complications such as obesity, myopathy, and neuropathy may be prevented by modern management strategies.

The prevention of pelvic organ prolapse involves care of the entire body. A healthy, fit, and well-nourished patient who is aware of ways to actively protect her pelvic floor is less likely to experience this potentially disabling problem. Many of the strategies outlined in this section should be part of the care of patients from their obstetric years onward. Prevention is always preferable to intervention in the operating room.

CLINICAL EVALUATION

The correct management of pelvic organ prolapse depends on a careful evaluation of each patient. Only after a thorough history and physical examination is the practitioner able to develop an effective treatment plan for the individual patient.

The **history** should begin with the patient's perception of the problem. This information helps to determine what specific goals the patient may have. The patient might be afraid that the prolapse could rupture or that it may be caused by a malignant growth. Reassurance may suffice if such ideas are the major concern. Patients may or may not be interested in coital function, further childbearing, or simply knowing that the vagina is present if social circumstances change. Some women have grown accustomed to advanced prolapse and may describe very little inconvenience related to the herniation. These people may simply want to know if the prolapse represents any threat to their longevity. Other women are very conscious of an anatomically minor prolapse or may have pain unrelated to the prolapse. The patient may have unrealistic expectations or may be ready for intervention before the physician's operative criteria are met. In this situation, the pelvic reconstructive surgeon needs to be honest and forthright in discussing what will or will not improve after a surgery. A careful micturition, defecation, and sexual history may be invaluable in developing a treatment plan. Patients must be placed at ease and reassured during the evaluation before a full history concerning the details of pelvic functions can be obtained. Stress, urge, and neurogenic urinary incontinence may be differentiated by history. Obviously, the evaluations and treatments differ for each of these conditions. The complex topic of urinary incontinence is covered in detail elsewhere in this book. The mechanics involved in defecation are important. Determine the number of trips to the toilet and the compensatory measures necessary to complete evacuation. Fecal incontinence is a condition that patients are notoriously reluctant to discuss. This condition may or may not be due to physical damage to the anal continence control mechanism. The patient may be continent or incontinent of gas, liquid, or solids. Each patient may safely be presumed to desire urinary and bowel continence. Marked variation exists in patients' sexual goals. The practitioner should learn about these goals in a respectful and nonjudgmental way. Collecting sexual function information is an art, critical to the development of a management plan.

The past surgical history helps the surgeon assess the status of the patient in general and of the pelvis in particular. Specific interest should be placed on previous attempts to correct pelvic organ prolapse. Before her visit, the patient may be asked to prepare a list of previous surgeries so that none are overlooked. The route of hysterectomy and the indications for the procedure may be helpful. If previous prolapse surgery has been performed, the physician should try to obtain the operative notes. The anatomic details, type of suture used, and other details of the operative technique may help predict problems such as the likely location of anatomic distortion (previous plications) or the location of previously placed foreign bodies (e.g., meshes). Multiple previous attempts at repair necessitate a combination of caution and experience to achieve a successful outcome.

The medical history should be used to determine whether medical conditions exist that would likely interact with surgery or recovery. A complete pelvic reconstructive surgery may last several hours, involve significant blood loss, and require combined vaginal and abdominal approaches. Obviously, the patient needs the physical reserve to withstand this degree of stress. Patients with morbid obesity, limited pulmonary and cardiac function, thromboembolic risks, entrenched tobacco addiction, or limited mobility are not ideal candidates for this type of surgery. A complete list of current medications, including herbals and over-the-counter preparations, and treating physicians is also helpful.

The proper **physical examination** of the prolapse patient requires that the examining physician have a working knowledge of normal pelvic anatomy. Older systems for recording physical findings related to prolapse relied on subjective terms such as *mild, moderate,* and *severe*. These terms have a limited ability to accurately describe prolapse and restrict effective communication between examiners. Two systems are currently in use that encourage a complete prolapse examination and that more objectively record anatomic detail. Each of these systems has strengths and weaknesses. The Baden-Walker Halfway System is user friendly, easy to record, and maximizes the amount of detail that can be recorded in a very brief space. Proponents of this system maintain that the essence of the prolapse examination is recorded after writing six numbers and some editorial notes. Critics note that the abbreviation of detail means that some compromises are made along the way. The second system is the Pelvic Organ Prolapse—Quantification or POP-Q system. This is a more complex system incorporating more specific detail of the physical findings. Even for those clinicians accustomed to its use, the number of measurements needed requires additional time to acquire. The beauty of this system is that, theoretically, physician-to-physician variation is minimized. The POP-Q is currently used in many academic papers on the subject of prolapse. Interested physicians should become familiar with both of these systems. More important than any system is an accurate and anatomically based assessment of the patient at the time of examination.

Baden-Walker Halfway System

The extent of prolapse is recorded using a number (0 to 4) at each of six defined sites in the vagina. There are two sites on the anterior, superior, and posterior walls of the vagina. Table 36A.10 lists the anatomic sites and the associated symptoms. The six numbers are recorded as a measure of descent. For all sites except the perineum, the hymen is used as a fixed anatomic reference point. Zero indicates normal anatomic position for a site, whereas 4 represents maximum prolapse. Between these extremes, the intervening numbers grade descent using a halfway system as illustrated in Figure 36A.9. The examination is performed with the patient straining so that maximum descent is attained. The patient may wish to stand to demonstrate maximum descent.

The perineum is graded using the familiar perineal laceration system used in obstetrics (Fig. 36A.9). The patient is asked to hold or Kegel to evaluate the amount of muscular and fascial compensatory support. Editorial comments may include the site of dominant prolapse, location of scars, palpable plications from previous surgery, and the type of efforts necessary to demonstrate maximum prolapse. Strength of the levator contraction may be recorded as 0 to 4.

TABLE 36A.10

PRIMARY AND SECONDARY SYMPTOMS AT EACH SITE USED IN THE BADEN-WALKER HALFWAY SYSTEM

Anatomic site	Primary symptoms	Secondary symptoms
Urethral	Urinary incontinence	Falling out
Vesical	Voiding difficulties	Falling out
Uterine	Falling out	Heaviness and so forth
Cul-de-sac	Pelvic pressure (standing)	Falling out
Rectal	True bowel pocket	Falling out
Perineal	Anal incontinence	Too loose (gas/feces)

From: Baden WF, Walker T. *Surgical repair of vaginal defects.* Philadelphia: JB Lippincott; 1992:12.

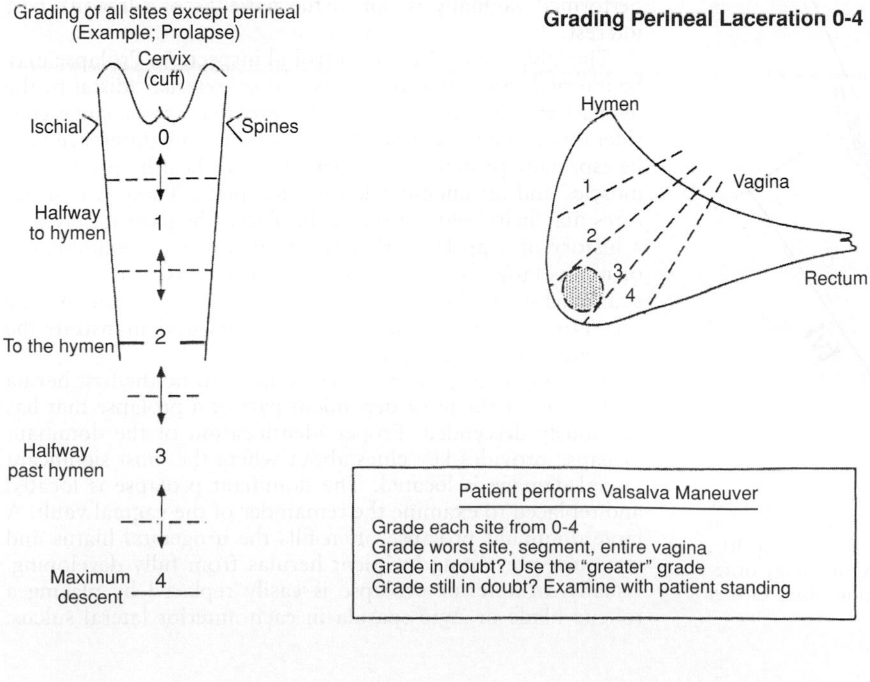

FIGURE 36A.9. Guidelines on how to assign grades in the Baden-Walker Halfway System. (From Baden WF, Walker T. *Surgical repair of vaginal defects.* Philadelphia: JB Lippincott; 1992.)

Example: 12/44/32. A dominant complete apical prolapse is noted with enterocele, significant cystocele and rectocele, and perineal attenuation to the level of the external anal sphincter. 2/4 levator strength is present.

Although this type of notation encodes much information in a small space, no specific location of fascial defects is indicated.

Pelvic Organ Prolapse—Quantification System (POP-Q)

This system was developed as an effort to introduce more objectivity into the quantification of pelvic organ prolapse. For example, measurements in centimeters are used instead of subjective grades. Nine specific measurements are recorded as indicated in Figure 36A.10. Point Aa is defined as being 3 cm proximal to the external urethral meatus on the anterior vaginal wall. Point Ap is defined as being 3 cm proximal to the hymen on the posterior vaginal wall. Points Ba and Bp are defined as points of maximum prolapse excursion on the anterior and posterior vaginal walls, respectively. Measurements are recorded as negative numbers when proximal to the hymen and positive numbers when distal to the hymen. POP-Q sites C and D are identical in location to Baden-Walker sites 3 and 4 in the apical vagina. In addition, measurements of the total vaginal length, genital hiatus, and perineal body are taken. All measurements are recorded on a tic-tac-toe style grid (Fig. 36A.11). When combined with sagittal line drawings, a fairly complete picture of prolapse is attained (Fig. 36A.12). Ordinal stages of pelvic organ prolapse are then assigned from stage 0 (no prolapse) to stage V (complete prolapse) so that the outcome of cases of like magnitude may be compared.

This system is a physical examination tool and does not assign the specific location of fascial defects.

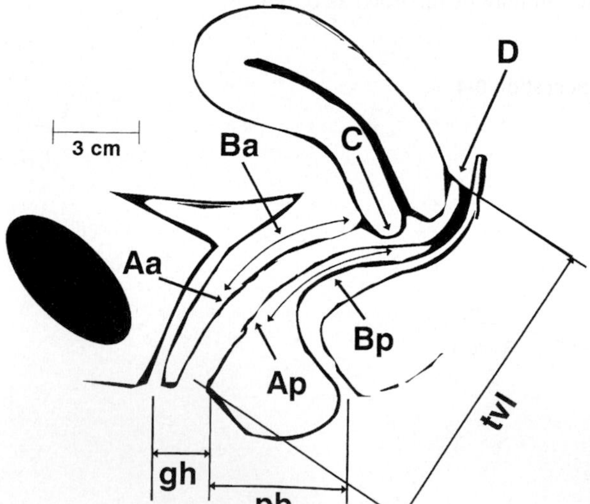

FIGURE 36A.10. The nine specific sites of measurement used in the Pelvic Organ Prolapse—Quantification System (POP-Q). gh, genital hiatus; pb, perineal body; tvl, total vaginal length. (From Bump RC, Mattiasson A, Bø K, et al. The standardization of terminology of female pelvic organ prolapse and pelvic floor dysfunction. *Am J Obstet Gynecol* 1996;175:10.)

anterior wall **Aa**	anterior wall **Ba**	cervix or cuff **C**
genital hiatus **gh**	perineal body **pb**	total vaginal length **tvl**
posterior wall **Ap**	posterior wall **Bp**	posterior fornix **D**

FIGURE 36A.11. The tic-tac-toe grid used to record measurements in the Pelvic Organ Prolapse—Quantification System (POP-Q). (From Bump RC, Mattiasson A, Bø K, et al. The standardization of terminology of female pelvic organ prolapse and pelvic floor dysfunction. *Am J Obstet Gynecol* 1996;175:10.)

Pelvic Examination

After a general physical examination is performed, the prolapse may be evaluated. Any surgical scars on the abdomen should be correlated with the surgical history. Patients frequently forget procedures that may have an impact on the treatment plan. The physician should pay particular attention to the suprapubic region where previous incontinence procedure incisions may be located.

The pelvic examination is initiated with the patient in the lithotomy position. Hip mobility should be evaluated because adequate abduction and flexion of the thighs is required for a vaginal procedure. Thigh and buttock obesity may also be limiting factors. If exposure is limited, an extended procedure performed vaginally is not in the patient's or surgeon's best interest.

The labia are opened for introital inspection. Prolapse may be internal (proximal to the hymen) or external (distal to the hymen) at rest. The extent of the prolapse may change considerably if the patient is asked to strain. This difference may be especially pronounced in patients with healthy pelvic floor muscles and an undescended levator plate. These two structures may help hold a prolapse in place. The patient may give a history of a prolapse that is not apparent on examination or not as large as she describes. In such a case, the patient is examined while she is in the standing position; or she may be asked to perform the maneuvers necessary to demonstrate the full extent of the prolapse.

The dominant prolapse is considered to be the first hernia to descend or the most dependent part of a prolapse that has previously descended. Proper identification of the dominant prolapse provides key clues about where the most significant fascial damage is located. The dominant prolapse is located and replaced to examine the remainder of the vaginal vault. A large dominant prolapse often fills the urogenital hiatus and introitus, preventing incipient hernias from fully developing. Usually an anterior prolapse is easily replaced by placing a tongue blade or Ayre spatula in each anterior lateral sulcus.

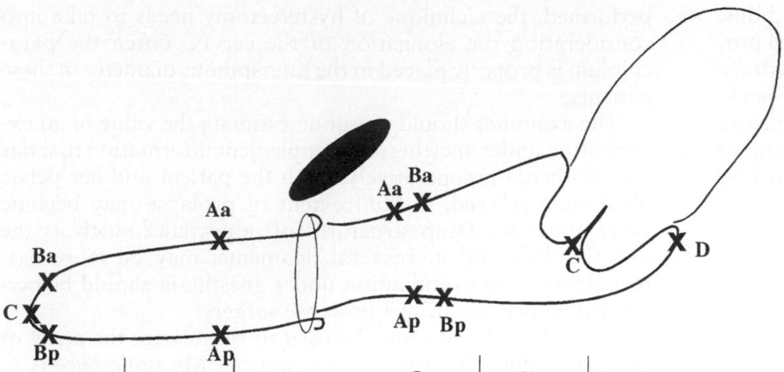

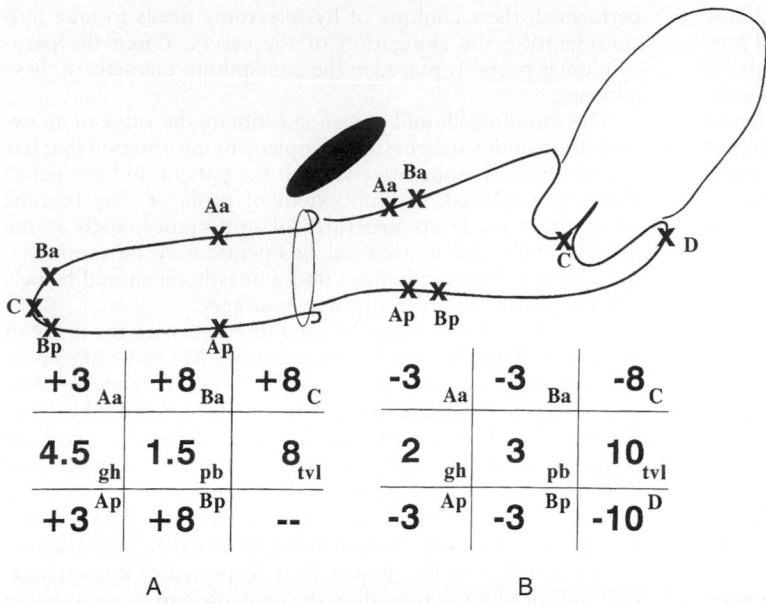

+3 Aa	+8 Ba	+8 C
4.5 gh	1.5 pb	8 tvl
+3 Ap	+8 Bp	--

A

-3 Aa	-3 Ba	-8 C
2 gh	3 pb	10 tvl
-3 Ap	-3 Bp	-10 D

B

FIGURE 36A.12. Two examples of the Pelvic Organ Prolapse—Quantification System (POP-Q). (From Bump RC, Mattiasson A, Bø K, et al. The standardization of terminology of female pelvic organ prolapse and pelvic floor dysfunction. *Am J Obstet Gynecol* 1996;175:10.)

If an apical transverse or lateral paravaginal defect is present, this maneuver replaces the anterior vaginal wall. If this maneuver does not reduce the hernia, a central anterior defect is likely present. A dominant posterior segment prolapse may be replaced with the posterior blade of a disjoined Sims' speculum. A dominant superior segment prolapse may be replaced with a large cotton swab, a sponge stick, or, in advanced cases, by attaching a tenaculum to the cervix. After replacement of the dominant prolapse, the secondary sites of prolapse become more apparent. An isolated single-site prolapse is rare. The location of the cervix or hysterectomy scar helps determine the location of the dominant prolapse. Frequently displaced, either anteriorly or posteriorly, these sites are often not at the most dependent part of the prolapse. The posthysterectomy scar is commonly a transverse fibrous band that may be slightly retracted. To either side of the band are dimples in the epithelium corresponding to the location of the insertion of cardinal and uterosacral ligament remnants. Incomplete evaluation may lead to incomplete repair that results in recurrent prolapse and multiple trips to the operating room. The support structures of all vaginal segments and levels are interdependent. Complete restoration of all defects is necessary for a successful outcome.

Careful inspection of the vaginal epithelium reveals the location of rugae. The presence of these transverse folds implies that endopelvic fascia is adherent to the epithelium in that location. The lateral vaginal sulci are the location of the junction of the pubocervical and rectovaginal septa to their respective lateral arcuate attachments. The pattern of rugae and the condition of the sulci should correlate with the pattern of fascial breaks found at surgery. The vaginal epithelium should also be inspected for atrophy created by the absence of the effects of estrogen. Local or systemic administration of estrogen before surgery assists in dissection and subsequent healing. Occasionally, an external prolapse may develop pressure ulcers as a result of entrapment when the patient is sitting. These lesions must be properly evaluated to rule out malignancy.

Rectovaginal examination assists in the evaluation of the posterior and superior vaginal segments. The uterosacral ligaments may be palpable immediately medial to each ischial spine, especially if the uterus is present. The uterosacral ligaments may be more easily palpated with traction placed on the cervix. Anterior displacement of the rectal examining finger toward the vagina helps to distinguish between rectocele and enterocele. During the rectal examination, the patient is asked to strain. If an enterocele is present, it bulges down in the nonrugated vaginal epithelium proximal to the tip of the examining finger. Palpating the transversely detached proximal edge of the rectovaginal septum is possible during this maneuver. This sharp border may retract distally all the way to the perineum. Perineal descent is also evaluated at the time of rectal examination. The levator plate is immediately posterior to the rectum and should be horizontal and immovable. The perineum is evaluated last. The perineum is triangular in the sagittal plane. The base is on the rectal side, and the apex at the hymen. Perineal attenuation is very common in parous women. Apposition of the thumb of the examining hand while the index finger is in the rectum proximal to the anterior aspect of the external anal sphincter allows for evaluation of the integrity of this muscle. Voluntary contraction of the sphincter may be helpful. The S3 neurologic segment is necessary to contract this muscle and controls the ability to spread and dorsiflex the toes. If the patient cannot perform these tasks, the integrity of that neural segment is in question.

The mechanical strength of the pelvic diaphragm is directly correlated with the ability to voluntarily contract these muscles. This ability is best tested clinically with light pressure placed on the posterior vaginal wall by the examining digits. The patient may need coaching to elicit a response. This time is an excellent opportunity to instruct the patient in the importance of postvoiding Kegel exercises and perineal support (splinting) during defecation.

If muscle activity is elicited, it may be subjectively graded from 0 to 4. If no muscle activity is detected, a more formal neurologic and medical workup should be considered. Pudendal nerve motor latency studies may reveal significant neuropathies. Magnetic resonance imaging of these patients has revealed the presence of advanced muscle atrophy and muscular detachments as well. Neuropathy and myopathy erode the surgeon's ability to correct prolapse. If the patient cannot properly move her toes and cannot contract the levator muscles, a spinal cord or central nervous system lesion must be considered.

The presence of urinary incontinence should be noted during any part of the evaluation of prolapse. In an advanced prolapse, assessment of incontinence should be conducted with the prolapse in a reduced state. A pessary or loose vaginal packing may be helpful in accomplishing this goal. Incontinence may be masked by a hypotonic bladder or reverse kinking of the urethra if a cystocele is large. Repair of a large prolapse may be followed by the appearance of urinary incontinence if the preoperative evaluation is not performed with the prolapse reduced.

When a large prolapse is present, the trigone of the bladder is often located outside the vaginal introitus. In this degree of displacement, one may deduce the location of the trigone as being directly adjacent to the location of a Foley catheter bulb. The course of the ureter in a large prolapse arcs from the superior and lateral aspect of the anterior prolapse to the area of the trigone. The ureter may often be palpated in this location. If the prolapse is chronic and advanced, hydroureter and even hydronephrosis may be present. In this circumstance, the ureters lose their cordlike consistency and are more difficult to palpate or recognize at the time of surgery. A large external prolapse makes the ureter more susceptible to surgical injury. Intraoperative placement of ureteral catheters may be helpful in such a patient. Postoperative documentation of ureteral patency is required.

A patient may present with the cervix near the level of the hymen. If no other signs of prolapse are present, the alert examiner is aware of the possibility of an elongated cervix. Sometimes surgery is not necessary in these patients. If surgery is performed, the technique of hysterectomy needs to take into consideration the elongation of the cervix. Often the paracolpium is properly placed in the interspinous diameter in these patients.

The examiner should not underestimate the value of an examination under anesthesia to supplement information that has been gathered preoperatively. With the patient and her pelvic diaphragm relaxed, the full extent of prolapse may become more apparent. Deep structures of importance, such as the ischial spines and uterosacral ligaments, may be more easily palpated. An examination under anesthesia should be performed before initiating a prolapse surgery.

A number of ways may be used to summarize the array of clinical findings discussed in this section. My preference is to use a pelvic organ prolapse map (Figs. 36A.13 and 36A.14). Key anatomic landmarks are schematically outlined. The three-dimensional structure of the vagina is reduced to two dimensions as if the vagina were divided at the 3-o'clock and 9-o'clock positions. A Baden-Walker profile can be recorded vertically on the map with numbers placed beside the appropriate anatomic location. As seen in Figure 36A.15, fascial defects can be sketched on the map at their suspected or known location. Editorial notes regarding the prolapse can be recorded in the space provided. A POP-Q evaluation may be used as well. The pattern that is noted in Figure 36A.15 is the one most commonly seen in pelvic organ prolapse surgery; however, many variations on this theme are encountered (Fig. 36A.16). Another diagram may be drawn to indicate the exact locations of fascial defects at the time of surgery.

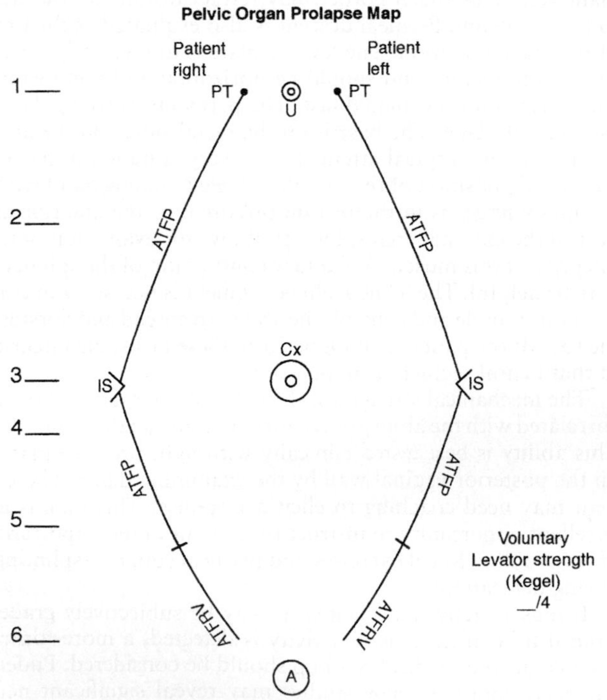

FIGURE 36A.13. Key elements of pelvic support anatomy. Three dimensions are reduced to two by dividing the vagina at the 3-o'clock and 9-o'clock positions. Baden-Walker vaginal support profile sites: 1, urethral; 2, vesical; 3, uterine; 4, cul-de-sac; 5, rectal; 6, perineal. PT, pubic tubercle; ATFP, arcus tendineus fascia pelvis; ATFRV, arcus tendineus fasciae rectovaginalis; IS, ischial spines; U, urethra; Cx, cervix; A, anus.

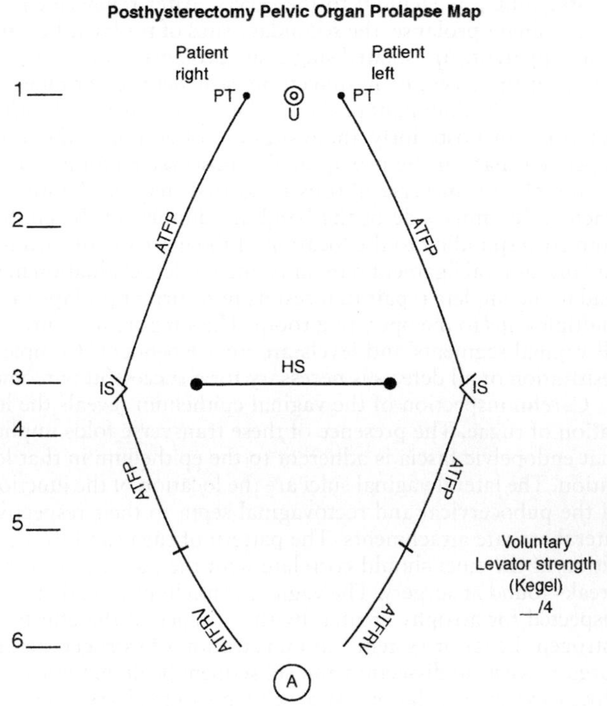

FIGURE 36A.14. Key elements of posthysterectomy pelvic support anatomy. Three dimensions are reduced to two by dividing the vagina at the 3-o'clock and 9-o'clock positions. Baden-Walker vaginal support profile sites: 1, urethral; 2, vesical; 3, uterine; 4, cul-de-sac; 5, rectal; 6, perineal. PT, pubic tubercle; ATFP, arcus tendineus fascia pelvis; ATFRV, arcus tendineus fasciae rectovaginalis; IS, ischial spines; U, urethra; HS, hysterectomy scar; A, anus.

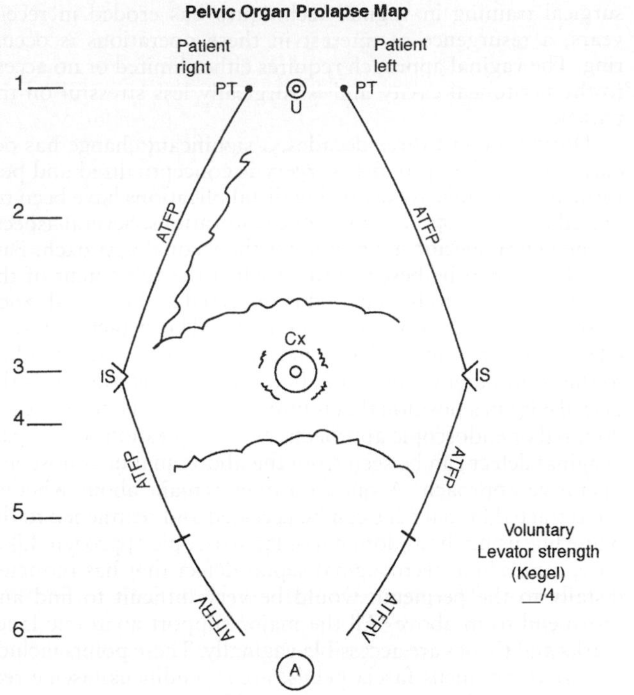

FIGURE 36A.15. The most frequently encountered pattern of fascial damage in pelvic organ prolapse: (1) full-length right paravaginal defect; (2) transverse proximal detachment of the pubocervical septum; (3) transverse proximal detachment of the rectovaginal septum. This pattern of damage is consistent with the mechanics of a left occipitoanterior delivery. Baden-Walker vaginal support profile sites: 1, urethral; 2, vesical; 3, uterine; 4, cul-de-sac; 5, rectal; 6, perineal. PT, pubic tubercle; ATFP, arcus tendineus fascia pelvis; ATFRV, arcus tendineus fasciae rectovaginalis; IS, ischial spines; U, urethra; Cx, cervix; A, anus.

A thorough history and physical examination improves the treatment of the prolapse patient. The physical findings must be recorded in an anatomically accurate and understandable way.

CHOICE OF TREATMENT

> Vaginal reconstructive surgery is concerned with the return of abnormal organ relationships to a usual or normal state. There is no one site or degree of damage that must be repaired or restored; there are many and they occur in various combinations at various times of life, from different etiologic factors, in varying degrees, and with varying degrees of symptoms and disability. (Nichols and Randall, 1989)

Patients with pelvic organ prolapse have highly individualized perceptions of their situation. The single most important concept in the treatment of these conditions is to understand the patient's symptoms, concerns, and limitations related to the prolapse. Her quality of life should be of paramount concern in the decision-making process. The patient's expectations and her ability to tolerate surgery should be expertly evaluated. The physician's job is to educate the patient regarding options of treatment. After informed consent is given, the appropriate course of action is usually obvious to both the doctor and the patient. If the chosen course of action fails or becomes inappropriate over the course of time, the clinical evaluation and decision process can be revisited.

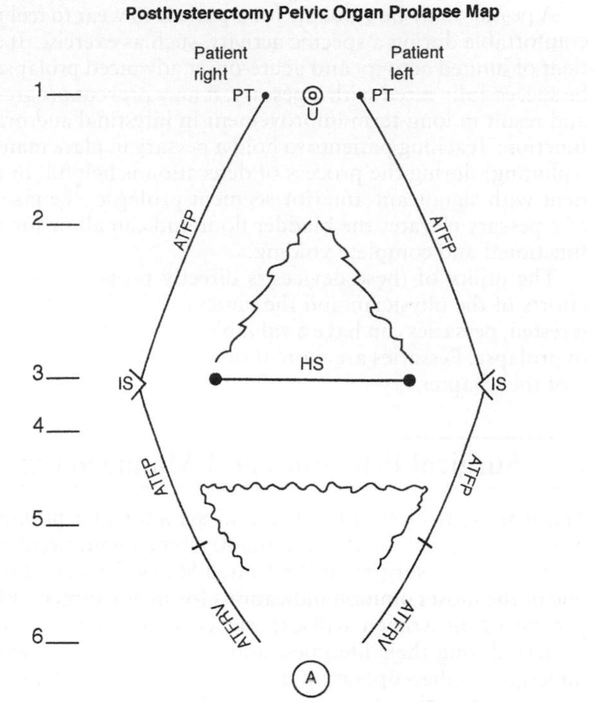

FIGURE 36A.16. An infrequently encountered inverted "V" anterior central fascial defect. Posteriorly, the proximal detachment of the rectovaginal septum has retracted toward the perineum, creating an enterocele and rectocele. Notice the bilateral pararectal defects. Baden-Walker vaginal support profile sites: 1, urethral; 2, vesical; 3, uterine; 4, cul-de-sac; 5, rectal; 6, perineal. PT, pubic tubercle; ATFP, arcus tendineus fascia pelvis; ATFRV, arcus tendineus fasciae rectovaginalis; IS, ischial spines; U, urethra; HS, hysterectomy scar; A, anus.

Nonsurgical Management

Regardless of the degree of prolapse, no surgery should be done unless the patient experiences a sufficient degree of morbidity. Most symptoms relate to quality-of-life issues. Generally, preventative measures should be the most widely applied techniques. Pelvic floor exercises, weight loss, treatment of chronic diseases, physical therapy, cessation of smoking, and estrogen therapy are all considerations in the conservative treatment of pelvic organ prolapse. These interventions have been discussed in the previous section of this chapter and should be used regardless of whether expectant management or surgical intervention is the plan. During expectant management, periodic examinations should be done to determine the status of pelvic organ support and the degree of progression. Symptoms and the ability to participate in daily activities may be reviewed to reinforce the patient's motivation to continue preventative measures.

Pessaries are ingenious devices that have been used for a long time. They were originally the product of an age when surgery was not an option for the prolapse patient. They are available in a variety of shapes and sizes, depending on the needs of the patient. In general, the greater the degree of prolapse and the more strenuous the daily activities of the patient, the less likely it is for a pessary to be a permanent solution. As the prolapse expands, occupies the urogenital hiatus, and dilates the introitus, the pressure of the prolapse tends to expel the pessary.

A pessary may be valuable for a patient to wear to feel more comfortable during a specific activity, such as exercise. If a patient of limited activity and acute-onset advanced prolapse can be successfully fitted with a pessary, it may prevent progression and result in long-term improvement in intestinal and urinary function. Teaching patients to hold a pessary in place manually (splinting) during the process of defecation is helpful. In a patient with significant anterior segment prolapse, the insertion of a pessary elevates the bladder floor and can allow for more functional and complete voiding.

The utility of these devices is directly proportional to the efforts of the physician and the patient. If both parties are interested, pessaries can have a valuable place in the management of prolapse. Pessaries are more thoroughly discussed in Section F of this chapter.

Surgical Principles and Management

The management of advanced and symptomatic prolapse is primarily surgical. In 1997, 226,000 women underwent pelvic organ prolapse surgery in the United States. This condition is one of the most common indications for major surgery. Eleven percent of all women will experience some type of prolapse surgery during their lifetimes, and 30% of these women will undergo another operation for recurrence of prolapse or a complication related to surgery. Prolapse is a high-incidence problem that commands a substantial expenditure of health care dollars. Only those patients who request relief should be considered surgical candidates. Once the decision is made to operate, quality-of-life goals need to be established. If the patient can tolerate a lengthy operation and especially if she desires coital function, a reconstructive operation should be considered. The restoration of normal anatomy (form) maximizes the potential that symptoms and limitations (function) will be corrected or significantly improved. Restoration of normal anatomy automatically addresses the questions of vaginal axis, caliber, and depth. If the patient does not desire coital function, an occlusive procedure, such as colpocleisis, might be the best choice. Colpocleisis with vaginectomy has a very low failure rate, but the end does not justify the means in all patients.

Choosing the correct operation for prolapse is critical for success. The general plan for the procedures that will best correct the problems of the individual patient may be developed from details gathered during the preoperative history and pelvic examination and even the examination under anesthesia. Specific details become evident only during the intraoperative dissection. The goals of the operation are the restoration of normal form and function. Isolated areas of prolapse are uncommon. Childbirth places damaging pressure on all segments of suspension and support during the various phases of labor and delivery. Restricting an operative procedure to the repair of a single dominant or symptomatic site of prolapse simply transfers the physical stress to a different vaginal segment. An incomplete reconstruction may result in a secondary prolapse descending as a new dominant prolapse. Sometimes prolapse can return quickly postoperatively. Perhaps the best known example of this phenomenon was the observation by Burch that many patients developed an enterocele after his anterior urethropexy procedure. An active search for potential and undeveloped defects must be done at the time of prolapse surgery. Site-specific repair of all segments and levels is the best insurance against failure.

The route of operation is a matter of debate. Vaginal surgery is the historical hallmark of the gynecologic surgeon. Although surgical training in vaginal techniques has eroded in recent years, a resurgence of interest in these operations is occurring. The vaginal approach requires either limited or no access to the peritoneal cavity and is surgically less stressful on the patient.

During the last three decades, a significant change has occurred in the way prolapse surgery is conceptualized and performed. Anatomically distorting distal plications have been replaced by defect-specific anatomic restorations. Several aspects of the defect-specific method favor the vaginal approach. Fascial defects can be best identified when the full extent of the vaginal segment to be repaired is dissected and exposed. Such dissections are only possible vaginally. The detached fascial edge of a paravaginal defect may retract across the midline to the contralateral side of the body. This retraction leaves the fascial edge in a position that is impossible to reach from the abdominal or endoscopic approach. No one questions that a paravaginal defect can be seen from the abdominal or endoscopic operative approach. A question does remain about whether the retracted fascial edge can be accessed and reattached to the white line using the abdominal or laparoscopic approach. Likewise, a proximal rectovaginal septal defect that has retracted distally to the perineum would be very difficult to find and resuspend from above. All the major support anatomic landmarks and tissues are accessible vaginally. These points include the arcus tendineus fascia pelvis, arcus tendineus fasciae rectovaginalis, ischial spines, uterosacral ligaments, sacrospinous ligaments, and virtually all components of the deep endopelvic connective tissue. During childbirth, the named components of the endopelvic fascia are displaced away from the interspinous diameter. Reconstructive efforts must be centered in this diameter for a permanently successful outcome. Access to torn fascial edges is best attained by complete dissections of the vesicovaginal and rectovaginal spaces. Midvaginal lateral defects can easily be repaired by this route. Additionally, apical suspension can also be performed to complete the restoration of central pelvic organ suspension. For most primary reconstructions, the vaginal operative route is superior to any other approach. The vaginal route is also preferred for patients with failures from previous operations. This approach is especially useful when a previous operation did not use the defect-specific approach and did not include the use of permanent suture for critical support sites.

The discussion and opinions in the previous paragraph do not preclude the use of abdominal and laparoscopic techniques for certain problems in pelvic reconstructive surgery. Procedures to correct stress urinary incontinence are discussed extensively in Chapter 37. Anterior urethropexy approached through the prevesical space with a suprapubic incision or laparoscopic technique has some advantages when compared with a suburethral sling urethropexy. No iatrogenic paravaginal defect is necessary during anterior urethropexy, for example. Such defects are made with pubovaginal sling procedures of all types. Some intentionally created defects are larger than others. To spend time and effort to reconstruct the pubocervical fascia anatomically from white line to white line and then to destroy part of the paravaginal support intentionally to allow passage of the sling material into the prevesical space does not make good sense. The primary prevesical space approach avoids this destructive necessity. Kelly-Kennedy plications and paravaginal repairs have been shown to be ineffective as incontinence procedures. New minimally invasive sling operations represent an effective totally vaginal operation to cure stress incontinence. Vaginal incontinence operations that avoid iatrogenic paravaginal damage and an abdominal or laparoscopic incision are ideal.

The abdominal approach is useful in some cases of prolapse in which one or more previous pelvic support operations have failed. Abdominal sacral colpopexy is an option in this situation. Colpopexy may be useful in a circumstance in which considerable scar is present from previous surgery. For example, consider a patient with a previous aggressive distal plication and a proximal support failure. Significant fibrolysis would be necessary to gain access to the proximal structures necessary to repair the prolapse. A rescue abdominal sacral colpopexy may more easily and effectively correct the prolapse. Occasional patients whose support has failed following a site-specific operation with permanent suture may also benefit from this operation. Abdominal sacral colpopexy is not a site-specific operation; however, it provides substantial proximal support and protects vaginal length.

During a prolapse surgery, the surgeon may determine that adequate support or repair is not attainable through the primary approach. No harm is done in using a combined approach. If support is not satisfactory after a vaginal procedure, an abdominal sacral colpopexy can be done at that time. Conversely, a vaginal examination should be performed after an abdominal sacral colpopexy to determine if the vaginal axis, caliber, and depth have been restored to an acceptable state. The patient with proper informed consent would likely prefer a combined procedure to subsequent surgery.

Suture selection for pelvic reconstruction has changed with the realization that prolapse surgery is really a series of herniorrhaphies. No surgeon would consider performing a repair of an inguinal or ventral hernia with absorbable suture. In the days of distal plications, the use of absorbable suture was common. Today, fascial defects are repaired with permanent suture. In an attempt to compromise, some surgeons use delayed absorbable sutures. They reason that the suture material is not needed after healing has been completed. No evidence exists in the hernia literature to support the use of anything other than permanent suture for these repairs. Monofilament and polyfilament sutures are acceptable. Monofilament sutures occasionally erode and cause an unpleasant whisker effect in the vagina. If erosion occurs, the suture can be removed. My choice of suture is interwoven braided polyester for fascial repairs. This suture is affordable and easily tied, has no sharp end, and infrequently causes a reaction or erosion.

All prolapse patients should be carefully evaluated for concomitant vaginal, uterine, adnexal, pelvic, or abdominal disease. Coexisting pathology may change the operative approach selected for correction of prolapse. Orthopedic problems and obesity must be factored into the decision-making process because adequate surgical access is important.

Young patients with uterovaginal prolapse may request preservation of their fertility. Unless the problem is severe, these patients should be advised to complete their childbearing so that a definitive operation can be performed. Ring-type pessaries may provide temporary relief. They permit intercourse and may be worn at the discretion of the patient during exercise or strenuous activity and on other occasions. A unilateral sacrospinous ligament fixation with the uterus in place may be beneficial and does not prohibit subsequent vaginal childbirth. Various abdominal or endoscopic uterine suspensions may also be considered. In general, retention of the uterus when a significant degree of prolapse is present compromises the long-term operative result. The cervix limits access to the structures of the paracolpium that are necessary to achieve proper proximal suspension of the vaginal vault. At the same time, removal of the cervix creates an inherent defect in the proximal anterior vaginal wall. The posthysterectomy vault prolapse is in many instances a result of this cervical defect. Care must be taken to compensate for this weakness at the time of hysterectomy. This area is the location of the pericervical ring whose proper attachments are so important to normal vaginal suspension. No totally anatomic method to close this space exists. To achieve a satisfactory result is easier at hysterectomy than at subsequent posthysterectomy repair. Plication of the cardinal ligaments and McCall's culdoplasty are necessary components of hysterectomy cuff repair.

Various grafts, bolsters, and synthetic meshes can be valuable tools in prolapse surgery. For example, in a posthysterectomy prolapse, a small piece of foreign material used to bolster the weak area left by the absence of the cervix may decrease the amount of anatomic distortion needed to support the apical anterior vaginal wall. These materials are useful and necessary in abdominal sacral colpopexy. The overzealous use of grafts and meshes is unnecessary and may predispose to the annoying problems of exposure and erosion. Procedures that require the use of foreign materials to compensate for absent fasciae should be viewed with suspicion. Even in an advanced prolapse, the fascia is present in most cases. Fasciae, unlike muscles, do not atrophy. They may be retracted and scarred but are available for dissection and reattachment if the surgeon is trained in the proper techniques. Bolstering of site-specific repairs is acceptable. At no time should bolsters, grafts, and meshes be used as a substitute for meticulous surgical technique. Foreign materials should be used to strengthen anatomically restorative repairs.

Complications occurred in 15.5% of prolapse surgeries performed in the United States in 1997 (Table 36A.11). The majority of these complications can be addressed in the operating room. Gynecologic surgeons have been well trained to irrigate inside the abdomen. The same principles are applicable when operating vaginally. In the operating room after the surgical prep and draping are completed, a vaginal lavage rinses the vagina of nonadherent bacteria. Intraoperative irrigation at frequent intervals also helps to prevent infection. Irrigation as described and prophylactic antibiotics greatly help reduce the incidence of postoperative infection. A vaginal pack may help initial adherence of the vaginal epithelium to the endopelvic

TABLE 36A.11

FREQUENCY AND PERCENTAGE OF MORBIDITY ASSOCIATED WITH PELVIC ORGAN PROLAPSE SURGERY, 1997

Morbidity	Frequency	Percent of all surgeries[a]
Infections	14,824	5.4
Bleeding complications	13,945	5.4
Surgical injury	9,546	4.2
Pulmonary complications	3,024	1.3
Cardiovascular complications	2,407	1.1
Wound complications	1,368	0.6
Cerebrovascular complications	249	<0.1
Other complications	165	<0.1
Total morbidity	45,528	15.5

[a]N = 225,964 women undergoing prolapse surgery.
From: Brown JS, Waetjen LE, Subak LL, et al. Pelvic organ prolapse in the United States, 1997. *Am J Obstet Gynecol* 2001;186:712. Reprinted with permission.

fascia and may reduce hematoma formation. Packs should be removed the day after surgery.

The pelvis is a busy place anatomically. The deep dissections necessary for the correction of prolapse predispose the patient to injury to adjacent structures. Development of proper surgical planes helps to minimize the potential for such injuries. Vascular injuries are usually immediately apparent and can be corrected during the operation. Intestinal and urinary injuries are often more subtle. The surgeon should not conclude the operative procedure without some reassurance of the integrity of these structures. Cystoscopy is a valuable skill that should be used by the pelvic support surgeon. A high rectal examination may suffice for intestinal reassurance unless damage is suspected higher than the examination extends.

Preoperative and postoperative care is discussed elsewhere in this text. Early ambulation and thrombosis prophylaxis are particularly important in the usual prolapse patient. The patient should be at sexual pelvic rest for approximately 6 weeks. The patient may be quite anxious about sexual activity. Sexual rehabilitation may require time, reassurance, and the helpful advice of the physician. Straining to void and defecate should be minimized. The act of perineal splinting postoperatively helps to protect the perineum from downward displacement during defecation. Lifting should be restricted to those things that can be accomplished with available strength in the shoulders, back, and legs.

The care of patients with pelvic organ prolapse can be equally challenging and rewarding. Attention to the details of anatomy, physical diagnosis, reconstructive surgical techniques, and good medical care will yield the best results.

BEST SURGICAL PRACTICES

- Pelvic organ prolapse affects a patient's quality of life. Any decision regarding treatment of prolapse should ultimately be made with significant input from the patient.
- A careful physical examination documenting the defects in pelvic supportive structures is useful in selecting the appropriate treatment to correct the anatomic defect responsible for the patient's symptoms and physical exam findings.
- Pelvic reconstructive surgeries should be designed to restore maximally the normal biomechanical support and suspension of the central pelvic organs. This concept is called site-specific repair of pelvic support defects. Restoration of normal anatomy maximizes the potential for normal urinary, intestinal, and sexual functions.
- Principles of hernia repair should be followed in prolapse surgery. Use of permanent suture is standard. Judicious use of meshes, bolsters, and grafts may be indicated; however, these products should be used to enhance rather than replace sound surgical technique.
- Complex pelvic surgery and dissection into the deep pelvic spaces require that ureteral patency be documented before leaving the operating room.

Bibliography

Abitbol MM. *Birth and human evolution*. Westport, CT: Bergin & Garvey; 1996.

Baden WF, Walker T. *Surgical repair of vaginal defects*. Philadelphia: JB Lippincott; 1992.

Barber MD, Visco AG, Weidner AC, et al. Bilateral uterosacral ligament vaginal vault suspension with site-specific endopelvic fascia defect repair for treatment of pelvic organ prolapse. *Am J Obstet Gynecol* 2000;183:1402.

Bonney V. An address on genital displacements. *BMJ* 1928;1:432.

Bonney V. The principles that should underlie all operations for prolapse. *J Obstet Gynaecol Br Emp* 1934;41:669.

Bradley CS, Nygaard IE. Vaginal wall descensus and pelvic floor symptoms in older women. *Obstet Gynecol* 2005;106:759.

Brown JS, Waetjen LE, Subak LL, et al. Pelvic organ prolapse in the United States, 1997. *Am J Obstet Gynecol* 2002;186:712.

Brubaker L. Vaginal delivery and the pelvic floor. *Int Urogynecol J* 1998;9:363.

Buller JL, Thompson JR, Cundiff GW. Uterosacral ligament: description of anatomic relationships to optimize surgical safety. *Obstet Gynecol* 2001;97:873.

Bump RC, Mattiasson A, Bø K, et al. The standardization of terminology of female pelvic organ prolapse and pelvic floor dysfunction. *Am J Obstet Gynecol* 1996;175:10.

Bump RC, Norton PA. Epidemiology and natural history of pelvic floor dysfunction. *Obstet Gynecol Clin North Am* 1998;25:723.

Burch JC. Cooper's ligament urethrovesical suspension for stress incontinence. Nine years' experience—results, complications, techniques. *Am J Obstet Gynecol* 2002;187:512, discussion 513.

Clark AL, Gregory T, Smith VJ, et al. Epidemiologic evaluation of reoperation for surgically treated pelvic organ prolapse and urinary incontinence. *Am J Obstet Gynecol* 2003;189:1261.

Clayden CS. The evaluation of pelvic organ prolapse. *J Pelvic Surg* 2004;10:173.

Cunningham F, Gant N, Gilstrap L, et al. *Williams obstetrics*. 21st ed. New York: McGraw-Hill; 2001.

Danforth KN, Townsend MK, Lifford K, et al. Risk factors for urinary incontinence among middle-aged women. *Am J Obstet Gynecol* 2006;194:339.

Davis K, Kumar D, Stanton SL. Pelvic floor dysfunction: the need for a multidisciplinary team approach. *J Pelvic Surg* 2003;9:23.

DeLancey JO. Anatomy and biomechanics of genital prolapse. *Clin Obstet Gynecol* 1993;36:897.

DeLancey JO. Structural anatomy of the posterior pelvic compartment as it relates to rectocele. *Am J Obstet Gynecol* 1999;180:815.

Dietz HP, Lanzarone V. Levator trauma after vaginal delivery. *Obstet Gynecol* 2005;106:707.

Emge LA, Durfee RB. Pelvic organ prolapse: four thousand years of treatment. *Clin Obstet Gynecol* 1966;9:997.

Francis CC. *The human pelvis*. St. Louis: CV Mosby, 1952.

Gershenson DM, ed. Reconstructive pelvic surgery. *Operative Techniques in Gynecologic Surgery* 1996;1:2.

Ghetti C, Gregory WT, Edwards SR, et al. Pelvic organ descent and symptoms of pelvic floor disorders. *Am J Obstet Gynecol* 2005;193:53.

Grody MH. *Benign postreproductive gynecologic surgery*. New York: McGraw-Hill; 1995.

Grody MH, Nyirjesy P, Kelley LM, et al. Paraurethral fascial sling urethropexy and vaginal paravaginal defects cystopexy in the correction of urethrovesical prolapse. *Int Urogynecol J* 1995;6:80.

Handa VL, Garrett E, Hendrix S, et al. Progression and remission of pelvic organ prolapse: a longitudinal study of menopausal women. *Am J Obstet Gynecol* 2004;190:27.

Harris RL, Cundiff GW, Theofrastous JP, et al. The value of intraoperative cystoscopy in urogynecologic and reconstructive pelvic surgery. *Am J Obstet Gynecol* 1997;177:1367.

Hollinshead WH, Rosse C. *Textbook of anatomy*. 4th ed. Philadelphia: Harper & Row; 1985.

Hoyte L, Schierlitz L, Zou K. Two- and 3-dimensional MRI comparison of levator ani structure, volume, and integrity in women with stress incontinence and prolapse. *Am J Obstet Gynecol* 2001;185:11.

Jenkins II VR. Uterosacral ligament fixation for vaginal vault suspension in uterine and vaginal vault prolapse. *Am J Obstet Gynecol* 1997;177:1337.

Kegel AH. Physiologic therapy for urinary stress incontinence. *JAMA* 1952;10:915.

Kovac SR. Guidelines to determine the route of hysterectomy. *Obstet Gynecol* 1995;85:18.

Leffler KS, Thompson JR, Cundiff GW. Attachment of the rectovaginal septum to the pelvic sidewall. *Am J Obstet Gynecol* 2001;185:41.

Lien K-C, Mooney B, DeLancey JO, et al. Levator ani stretch induced by simulated vaginal birth. *Obstet Gynecol* 2004;103:31.

McCall ML. Posterior culdoplasty. *Obstet Gynecol* 1957;10:595.

Mengert WF. Mechanics of uterine support and position. *Am J Obstet Gynecol* 1936;31:775.

Mutone MF, Colin T, Hale DS, et al. Factors which influence the short-term success of pessary management of pelvic organ prolapse. *Am J Obstet Gynecol* 2005;193:89.

Nguyen JK, Lind LR, Choe JY, et al. Lumbosacral spine and pelvic inlet changes associated with pelvic organ prolapse. *Obstet Gynecol* 2000;95:332.

Nichols DH, Clarke-Pearson DL. *Gynecologic, obstetric, and related surgery*. 2nd ed. St. Louis: CV Mosby; 2000.

Nichols DH, Milley PS. Surgical significance of the rectovaginal septum. *Am J Obstet Gynecol* 1970;108:215.

Nichols DH, Milley PS, Randall CL. Significance of restoration of normal vaginal depth and axis. *Obstet Gynecol* 1970;36:251.

Nichols DH, Randal CL. *Vaginal Surgery*. 3rd ed. Baltimore: Lippinecott Williams & Wilkins; 1989.

Nichols DH, Randall CL. *Vaginal surgery*. 4th ed. Baltimore: Williams & Wilkins; 1996.

Peham H, Amreich J. *Operative gynecology*. Philadelphia: JB Lippincott; 1934.

Reiffenstuhl G, Platzer W, Knapstein P-G. *Vaginal operations: surgical anatomy and technique*. 2nd ed. Baltimore: Williams & Wilkins; 1994.

Retzy SS, Rogers RM, Richardson AC. Anatomy of female pelvic support. In: Brubaker LT, Saclarides TJ, eds. *The female pelvic floor: disorders of function and support*. Philadelphia: FA Davis; 1996:3.

Richardson AC, Lyon JB, Williams NL. A new look at pelvic relaxation. *Am J Obstet Gynecol* 1976;126:568.

Shull B. Clinical evaluation and physical examination of the incontinent woman. *J Pelvic Surg* 2000;6:334.

Shull BL, Bachofen C, Coates KW, et al. A transvaginal approach to repair of apical and other associated sites of pelvic organ prolapse with uterosacral ligaments. *Am J Obstet Gynecol* 2000;183:1365.

Singh K, Reid WM, Berger LA. Magnetic resonance imaging of normal levator ani anatomy and function. *Obstet Gynecol* 2002;99:433.

Subak LL, Quesenberry CP, Posner SF, et al. The effect of behavioral therapy on urinary incontinence: a randomized controlled trial. *Obstet Gynecol* 2002;100:72.

Strohbehn K, Ellis JH, Strohbehn JA, et al. Magnetic resonance imaging of the levator ani with anatomic correlation. *Obstet Gynecol* 1996;87:277.

Swift S, Woodman P, O'Boyle A, et al. Pelvic organ support study (POSST): the distribution, clinical definition, and epidemiologic condition of pelvic organ support defects. *Am J Obstet Gynecol* 2005;192:795.

Sze EH, Karram MM. Transvaginal repair of vault prolapse: a review. *Obstet Gynecol* 1997;89:466.

Sze EH, Sherard GB, Dolezal JM. Pregnancy, labor, delivery, and pelvic organ prolapse. *Obstet Gynecol* 2002;100:981.

Te Linde RW. Prolapse of the uterus and allied conditions. *Am J Obstet Gynecol* 1966;94:444.

Toglia MR, DeLancey JO. Anal incontinence and the obstetrician-gynecologist. *Obstet Gynecol* 1994;84:731.

Tunn R, DeLancey JO, Quint EE. Visibility of pelvic organ support system structures in magnetic resonance images without an endovaginal coil. *Am J Obstet Gynecol* 2001;184:1156.

Uhlenhuth E. *Problems in the anatomy of the pelvis*. Philadelphia: JB Lippincott; 1953.

Uhlenhuth E, Nolley GW. Vaginal fascia, a myth? *Obstet Gynecol* 1957;10:349.

Ulfelder H. The mechanism of pelvic support in women: deductions from a study of the comparative anatomy and physiology of the structures involved. *Am J Obstet Gynecol* 1956;72:856.

Wall LL. Birth trauma and the pelvic floor: lessons from the developing world. *J Womens Health* 1999;8:149.

Weber AM, Richter HE. Pelvic organ prolapse. *Obstet Gynecol* 2005;106:615.

Whiteside JL, Weber AM, Meyn LA, et al. Risk factors for prolapse recurrence after vaginal repair. *Am J Obstet Gynecol* 2004;191:1533.

CHAPTER 36B ■ SITE-SPECIFIC REPAIR OF CYSTOURETHROCELE

CARL W. ZIMMERMAN

DEFINITIONS

Arcus tendineus fascia pelvis or white line—A thickening of the parietal fascia of the pelvic sidewall along a line between the ischial spine and pubic tubercle. Along this line, the pubocervical septum attaches to the pelvic sidewall.

Cystocele—A defect within the central pubocervical septum that allows the floor of the bladder to descend. Cystoceles are normally caused by transverse apical defects in the pubocervical septum.

Paravaginal defect—A lateral defect at or near the attachment of the pubocervical septum to the arcus tendineus fascia pelvis. Paravaginal defects create a direct connection between the vesicovaginal space and the paravesical space on the affected side of the patient.

Pericervical ring—The collar of strong connective tissue surrounding the cervix. This is the central support of the vaginal apex to which the cardinal and uterosacral ligaments as well as the anterior pubocervical ligaments and fascia and posterior rectovaginal septum are attached.

Pubocervical septum—A component of the endopelvic fascia composed of fibroelastic connective tissue. This septum separates the vaginal epithelium and the bladder. Defects in the pubocervical septum are associated with anterior vaginal compartment failure.

The anterior compartment of the vagina extends from the pubic symphysis anteriorly to the posterior aspect of the cervix. The lateral boundaries are the white lines or arcus tendineus fasciae pelvis. The anterior vaginal compartment separates the bladder from the lumen of the vagina. Support of the bladder is the function of the pubocervical septum that is part of the deep endopelvic connective tissue. In the anatomically normal woman, the epithelium of the anterior vaginal wall firmly adheres to the pubocervical septum, creating rugae. Rugae are responsible for the finely ridged texture of the vaginal wall. The linear attachment of the pubocervical septum to the white line forms the anterior lateral sulci of the vagina. In the standing woman, the proximal two thirds of the anterior vaginal segment is nearly horizontal. In the lithotomy position, the anterior vaginal wall is oblique, with the apical portion inferior. The cervix and its surrounding ring and ligaments compose the proximal portion of the anterior vaginal segment. As a result, the pubocervical septum is shorter than the rectovaginal septum by the diameter of the cervix. In the absence of the cervix, an inherent defect is present that cannot be repaired in a completely reconstructive fashion. Compensating for the absence of the cervix at the time of hysterectomy is possible by using careful techniques of cuff repair. The failure to correct anatomically for the absent cervix in the posthysterectomy prolapse patient leads to many problems. The correction of the connective tissue defect left by the absence of the cervix is one of the most challenging problems in pelvic reconstructive surgery.

Labor and delivery apply intense pressure to all components of vaginal support and suspension. During descent, flexion, internal rotation, and extension, specific stresses are focused on the pubocervical septum before external rotation and expulsion of the fetus. The damage that results from the passage of a baby through the obstetric axis of the pelvis is the nidus for symptomatic prolapse of the anterior vaginal segment. The named anatomic components of anterior prolapse are cystocele, urethrocele, paravaginal defects, and uterine procidentia. Prolapse may occur without childbirth; however, this clinical circumstance is the exception rather than the rule. Other etiologic factors are normally required for the development of pelvic organ prolapse. These factors include time, age, repeated pelvic stresses, and lack of estrogen.

For most of the 20th century, the assumption was made that during childbirth, gradual attenuation of the endopelvic fascial support structures occurred. Howard Kelly of Baltimore championed this concept. His influence was considerable, and, as a result, surgical repair of a cystocele with anatomically distorting midline anterior plications became the standard of care. The Kelly–Kennedy plication was used to correct the perceived attenuated and stretched support of the bladder and anterior vaginal wall. This method of prolapse correction has been shown to have an unacceptable failure rate and has not proven to be a satisfactory treatment for urinary incontinence. This procedure is seldom used today by pelvic reconstructive surgeons.

In 1909, George White of Georgia noted that the repair of lateral anterior vaginal wall support was sufficient to correct cystocele. His observation remained largely unknown to mainstream gynecologic surgeons until the 1960s. Beginning with observations by Burch and others, the significance and importance of the lateral support of the anterior vagina began to emerge. Burch initially performed his anterior urethropexy using the white line as the ventral attachment point. He quickly abandoned the white line in favor of the more substantial Cooper's ligament. Subsequently, the importance of paravaginal defects in anterior vaginal relaxation has gradually become more and more apparent. Paravaginal defects are created when the pubocervical septum is separated laterally from the arcus tendineus fascia pelvis. A paravaginal defect is a connection between the vesicovaginal space and the paravesical space. A trampoline analogy is useful in illustrating the difference between central and paravaginal defects. A central defect would result from a tear in the fabric of the trampoline. A lateral or paravaginal defect is analogous to unhooking the fabric from the side frame of the trampoline. Either defect results in a failure of the support of the trampoline. The correction of

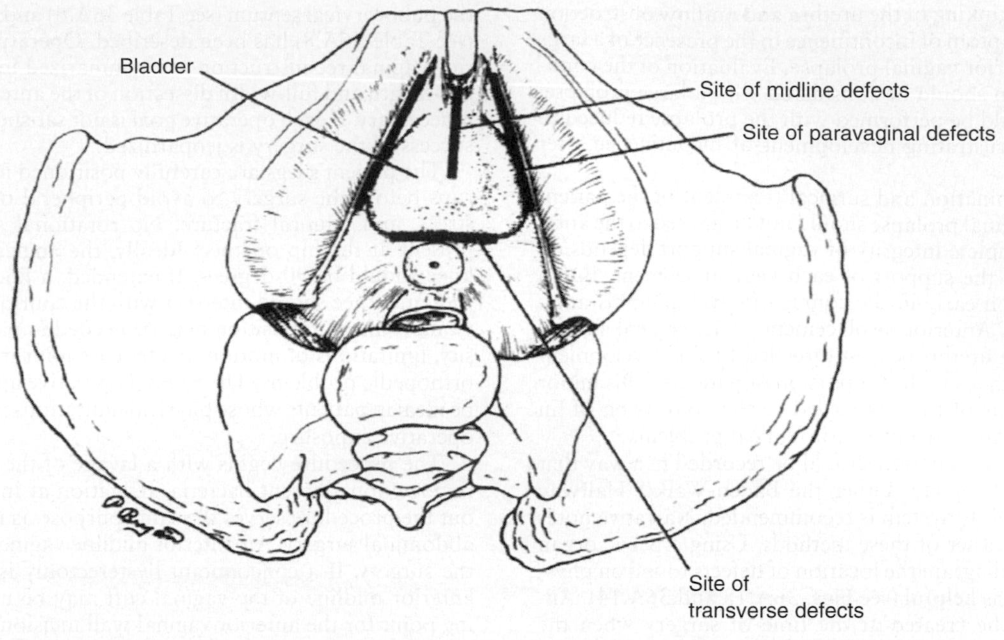

FIGURE 36B.1. The anterior vaginal segment from above. Potential sites of fascial defects are shown in bold lines. (Richardson AC. The rectovaginal septum revisited: its relationship to rectocele and its importance in rectocele repair. *Clin Obstet Gynecol* 1993;36:976.)

lateral defects is now considered to be a necessary component of anterior vaginal reconstruction. In most patients, paravaginal and apical transverse defects are responsible for anterior vaginal prolapse.

A Kelly–Kennedy plication procedure bunches connective tissue in the midline. This operation actually places more stress on paravaginal defects by pulling the detached edge of the pubocervical septum farther away from the pelvic sidewall. Pelvic surgeons have learned how to identify fascial defects. To visually distinguish between the visceral fascia of the bladder wall and the pubocervical septum is possible. The bladder wall is red, distensible, and highly elastic. The pubocervical septum that is part of the deep endopelvic connective tissue is whiter in color, stands out as a separate layer, and, when closely examined, has a coarse fibrous texture. During dissection, if the surgeon irrigates with saline, the color distinction between the visceral fascia of the bladder wall and the pubocervical septum becomes even more apparent.

In the 1970s, A. Cullen Richardson and colleagues of Georgia formally described specific breaks in the deep endopelvic connective tissue (Fig. 36B.1). His observations have been confirmed by others, and these defects are described by their location and direction. For location, the terms *distal, proximal, central,* and *lateral* are used. For direction, the terms *transverse* and *longitudinal* are used. Anatomically specific terms improved the description of fascial defects. In older literature, for example, lateral defects were termed *displacement cystoceles,* and central defects were termed *distention cystoceles.*

The next major conceptual step occurred after the biomechanical observations of DeLancey (see Figs. 36A.7 and 36A.8). He recognized that each portion of the vagina relies on a different biomechanical mechanism to preserve normal anatomy. The proximal one third of the vagina is suspended by the structures of the paracolpium, primarily the uterosacral ligaments (see Fig. 36A.8). The middle one third of the vagina is supported by lateral attachments to the pelvic sidewall at the arcus tendineus fasciae pelvis. The distal one third of the anterior vagina fuses with the relatively immovable urogenital diaphragm. These concepts become very important in site-specific repairs.

Any operation that does not account for the normal attachments at all three DeLancey levels is likely to fail. Specifically, the proximal extent of the operation should extend to the interspinous diameter and include proximal suspension of the pubocervical septum. The lateral extent of the operation should ensure bilateral attachments of the pubocervical septum to the parietal fasciae of the pelvic sidewalls at the white lines. Each lateral attachment should include the entire length of the white line from the ischial spine to the pubic tubercle. Distally, the integrity of the connection between the pubocervical septum and the urogenital diaphragm should be assured. The only way to achieve these goals is a full-length and full-width dissection, followed by a meticulous correction of fascial defects. After the surgeon becomes practiced at detecting these separations, the reattachment becomes a relatively straightforward exercise in reconstruction.

EVALUATION OF THE PATIENT WITH A CYSTOCELE

Cystoceles are common in parous women, and most are asymptomatic. If they are large enough or accompanied by incontinence, the patient will seek surgical relief. Prevention and physical therapy were discussed in the previous section of this chapter. Incontinence is a major presenting symptom in women affected by pelvic support defects. Cystocele and paravaginal repair may improve the symptoms; however, these surgeries do not represent a cure for incontinence. The correction of anterior vaginal defects does play a major role in the treatment of incontinence. Cystocele and paravaginal defects should be corrected at the time of incontinence procedures to improve long-term results. Reverse kinking of the urethra and outflow obstruction may hide the symptom of incontinence in the presence of a large and chronic anterior vaginal prolapse. Evaluation of the continence mechanism should be considered with a large prolapse. This testing should be performed with the prolapse reduced to help avoid the frustrating development of incontinence after prolapse repair.

Physical examination and surgical treatment of the patient with anterior vaginal prolapse should not be limited to the anterior vagina. Complete integrity of vaginal support depends on the normality of the support of each vaginal segment. Burch learned this lesson early in the course of developing his anterior urethropexy. Anterior displacement of the vaginal axis by placement of the urethropexy sutures led to the development of an enterocele in a significant portion of patients. This minor change in the axis of the vagina led to the conversion of an incipient defect into a symptomatic clinical problem.

The physical examination should be recorded in a way that is accurate and complete. Either the Baden-Walker Halfway System or the POP-Q system is recommended. Narrative notes can supplement either of these methods. Using a pelvic organ prolapse map to diagram the location of defects found on physical examination is helpful (see Figs. 36A.13 and 36A.14). Another map may be created at the time of surgery when the defects are actually visualized. The pattern of the presence and absence of rugae is extremely important. Rugae indicate the presence of underlying fascia. In an advanced prolapse, rugae continue to be present even though they may be displaced by the distorted anatomy. Fascia does not atrophy. The most likely place to find rugae in an advanced or chronic prolapse is immediately proximal to the urethra. Both labor and prolapse displace connective tissue structures away from the interspinous diameter in a proximal to distal direction.

Paravaginal defects may be detected by physical examination. A tongue blade or Ayre spatula may be used to replace the anterior lateral sulci. When a paravaginal defect is present, replacement of the sulci causes the anterior vaginal wall to retract into a normal anatomic position. If a central defect is present, a central bulge remains. Removing each of the bolsters in turn may help determine whether paravaginal defects are unilateral or bilateral. In most cases, a right paravaginal defect is present (see Fig. 36A.15). Less commonly, a concomitant or isolated defect is diagnosed on the left. The findings in a defect analysis should correlate with the pattern of rugae.

The location of the cervix or hysterectomy scar is important in determining the location of the dominant prolapse. If the majority of the herniation is anterior to the cervix or hysterectomy scar, the anterior prolapse is dominant. Conversely, if the prolapse is primarily posterior to the cervix or hysterectomy scar, the dominant prolapse is posterior. If the cervix or hysterectomy scar is the most dependent part of the prolapse, the superior segment is dominant. Such observations are important in planning a successful surgery. A large dominant prolapse will fill the urogenital hiatus and prevent any other incipient defect from developing. If only the dominant prolapse is repaired, incipient defects will probably become dominant rapidly. Restitution of all the normal attachments of pelvic organ support is the goal of the pelvic reconstructive surgeon.

SURGICAL TECHNIQUE

The site-specific correction of anterior vaginal defects depends on access to all normal support structures. Complete restoration of the pubocervical septum and of the attachments of the pericervical ring is the surgical goal. The normal anatomy of the pubocervical septum (see Table 36A.6) and pericervical ring (see Table 36A.8) has been described. Operative goals of anterior vaginal reconstruction are summarized in Table 36B.1. A full-length and full-width dissection of the anterior vaginal wall is necessary. If each operative goal is not satisfied, the long-term success of the surgery is jeopardized.

The patient's legs are carefully positioned in adjustable stirrups before the surgery to avoid peripheral neuropathy, joint stress, and femoral fracture. No rotational stress should be present at the hip or knee. Ideally, the angles of the hip and knee should be 90 degrees. If extended, a line connecting the foot and knee should intersect with the contralateral shoulder. Compromises in position may be needed in patients with obesity, limitations of motion, inadequate joint mobility, or other orthopedic problems. The vaginal operative approach may not be ideal in patients whose physical limitations prevent adequate operative exposure.

The procedure begins with a lavage of the vaginal vault to remove nonadherent bacteria. Irrigation at intervals throughout the procedure serves the same purpose as irrigation during abdominal surgery. An anterior midline vaginal incision begins the surgery. If a concomitant hysterectomy is performed, the anterior midline of the vaginal cuff may be used as the starting point for the anterior vaginal wall incision. This maneuver ensures adequate proximal surgical access. In the posthysterectomy patient, the initial incision is made immediately anterior to the hysterectomy scar (Fig. 36B.2). The hysterectomy scar is usually visible as a transverse fibrous band with lateral dimples that signify the location of the remnants of the uterosacral ligaments. The midline incision is extended distally to the plane where the pubocervical septum fuses with the urogenital diaphragm. The goal of the anterior vaginal incision is to allow separation of the epithelium from the underlying deep endopelvic connective tissue (Fig. 36B.3). The plane of separation is continued laterally in each direction to the pelvic sidewall. Separating the deep endopelvic connective tissue from the undersurface of the vaginal epithelium facilitates the dissection. This separation should begin immediately lateral to the line of incision. Once the correct dissection plane is established, the space is avascular and opens to blunt dissection (Fig. 36B.4). According to Uhlenhuth, this plane of dissection is the part of the vesicovaginal space that is below the pubocervical septum. Gynecologic surgeons seldom enter the portion of the vesicovaginal space between the pubocervical septum and the visceral fascia of the bladder. Complete development of the vesicovaginal space allows access to all structures necessary for anterior vaginal reconstruction, except for the prevesical space that is needed for urethropexy.

TABLE 36B.1

OPERATIVE GOALS OF ANTERIOR VAGINAL RECONSTRUCTION

Central: Reconstruct the pubocervical septum or repair of distention cystocele.

Proximal: Reattach the proximal pubocervical septum to the suspensory support of the paracolpium. Rebuild the pericervical ring and compensate for the defect left by the absence of the cervix (DeLancey Level I).

Lateral: Reattach the pubocervical septum to the arcus tendineus fasciae pelvis (white line) or paravaginal repair (DeLancey Level II).

Distal: Urethropexy (DeLancey Level III).

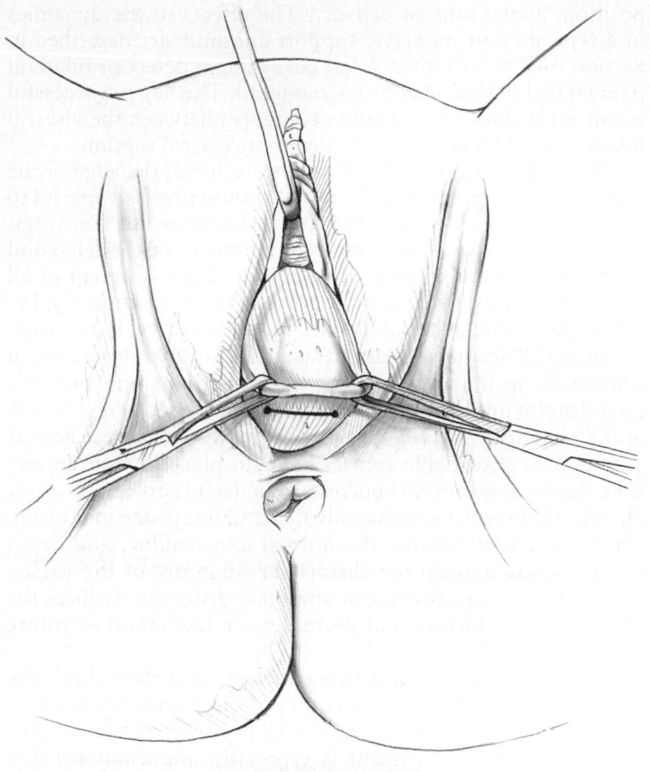

FIGURE 36B.2. A dominant anterior posthysterectomy prolapse is grasped with two Allis clamps. Notice the hysterectomy scar posterior to the clamps. The initial anterior incision will be made in the crease between the clamps.

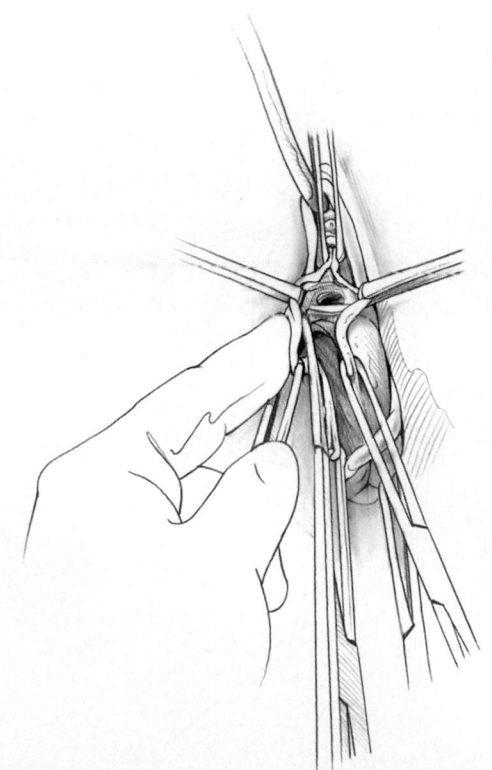

FIGURE 36B.3. The vesicovaginal space is developed by separating the endopelvic connective tissue from the vaginal epithelium.

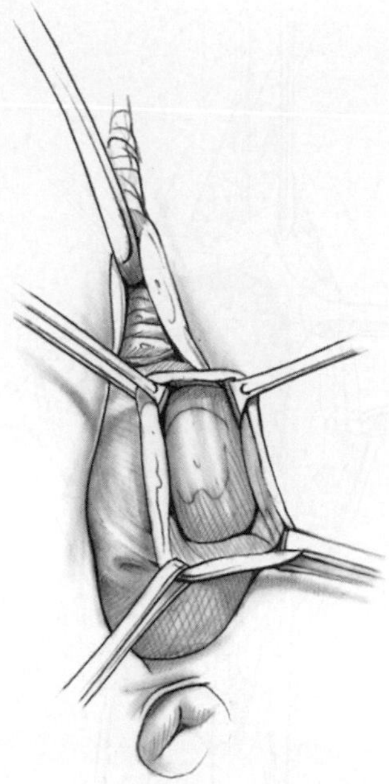

FIGURE 36B.4. Demonstration of the avascular vesicovaginal space.

The arcus tendineus fascia pelvis or white line extends from the ischial spine to the pubic tubercle. In the lithotomy position, the distal end of this structure is approximately 60 degrees above the horizontal plane. The white line may be visible to the surgeon. This structure is the fascial white line, not the arcus tendineus levator ani or muscular white line. The easiest place to palpate the white line is adjacent to its terminus at the ischial spine. Once a suture is placed around the white line and is under slight tension, the entire length of the structure is often palpable. Before initiating a paravaginal repair, the ischial spines must be palpable and accessible at the proximal extent of the dissection.

After the completion of dissection, an inspection may be started for fascial defects (Fig. 36B.5). The visceral fascia of the bladder is red, muscular, and distensible. It has very little tensile strength. The pubocervical septum is whitish, fibrous, strong, and in a different plane than the underlying visceral fascia. Irrigation with saline causes the subtle color difference between the visceral fascia of the bladder and the pubocervical fascia to become more obvious. Careful inspection reveals the presence of fascial edges. These edges are not smooth but are ragged and often beveled or splayed. If the full thickness of the most obvious portion of the fascial edge is grasped with an Allis clamp, the entire length of the defect may become visible (Fig. 36B.6). The fascial edge may retract away from the pelvic sidewall and create a wide paravaginal defect. In an advanced or chronic prolapse, the fascial edge may retract to the contralateral side of the midline.

The ability to recognize fascial defects is acquired during careful dissection and observation. The exact pattern of fascial damage cannot be determined until dissection is completed in the operating room. The most common pattern of anterior fascial damage is a full-length patient right paravaginal defect and a transverse proximal separation of the pubocervical septum from the pericervical ring (see Fig. 36A.15). This pattern of fascial damage is consistent with the physical stress associated with the most common fetal presentation, left occipitoanterior

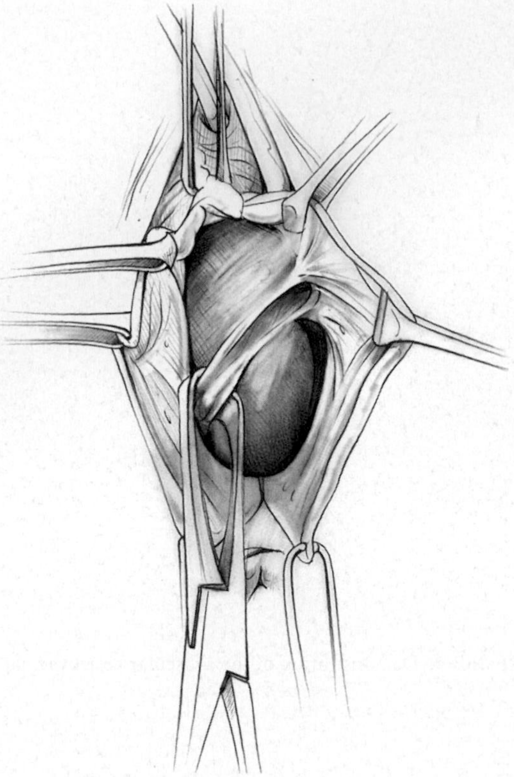

FIGURE 36B.5. Initial identification of the ragged edge of the pubocervical septum. The central Allis clamp is grasping the fascial edge. The right paravaginal defect can be seen in the upper left portion of the incision.

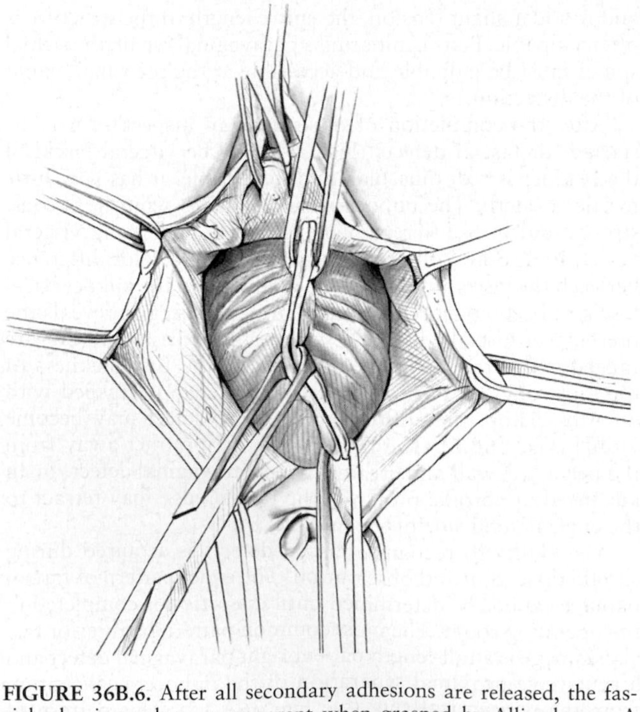

FIGURE 36B.6. After all secondary adhesions are released, the fascial edge is much more apparent when grasped by Allis clamps. A full-length right paravaginal defect is seen with the pubocervical edge retracted to the midline of the body.

position, at the time of delivery. The effects of the dynamics of a typical labor on pelvic support anatomy are described in Section A of this chapter. A left paravaginal defect or bilateral paravaginal defects may be encountered. The key to successful repair is the ability to visually distinguish between the visceral fascia of the bladder wall and the pubocervical septum.

After all the secondary adhesions are freed, the edge of the fully mobilized pubocervical septum should precisely extend to the desired reattachment point: the fascial white line. Paravaginal sutures should connect the arcus tendineus fascia pelvis and lateral edge of the pubocervical septum. The placement of all sutures on a given side should precede tying. Commonly, between three and eight sutures are required for each paravaginal defect. Placement of the paravaginal sutures should begin proximally in the area adjacent to the ischial spine and proceed distally until the defect is completely closed (Figs. 36B.7, 36B.8, and 36B.9). If one accepts the premise that these defects are hernias, absorbable sutures have no place in their correction. Zero-gauge braided polyester is a useful suture; it is a soft and pliable product that is easily tied and not prone to erosion. Anatomic repairs restore the normal axis, caliber, and depth of the vagina and do not distort the anatomy of the vagina (Fig. 36B.10). The absence of anatomic distortion reduces the tension on the sutures and decreases the likelihood of suture erosion.

First, repair the largest lateral defect, and then check the contralateral side to see if the contralateral paravaginal attachment is intact. Checking the proximal portion of the contralateral paravaginal attachment is especially important because closure of the first lateral defect may increase the separation of the pubocervical fascia from the opposite pelvic sidewall, making the defect more apparent. After lateral reattachment has

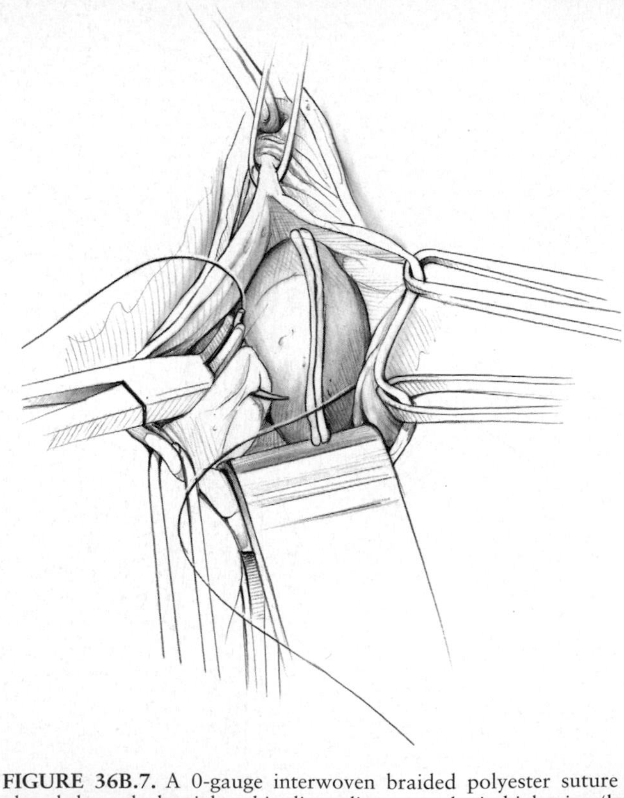

FIGURE 36B.7. A 0-gauge interwoven braided polyester suture is placed through the right white line adjacent to the ischial spine (left-handed surgeon).

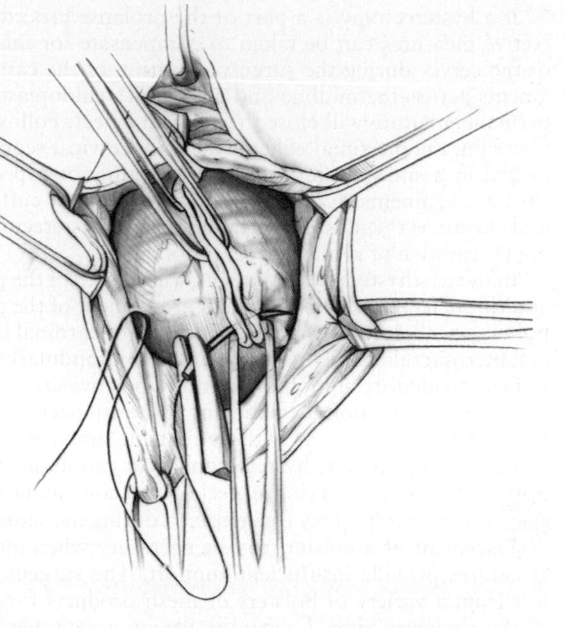

FIGURE 36B.8. The 0-gauge interwoven braided polyester suture from Fig. 36B.7 is passed through the detached edge of the pubocervical fascia to complete the most proximal paravaginal suture. The visceral fascia of the bladder wall is avoided to minimize the potential for urinary injury (left-handed surgeon).

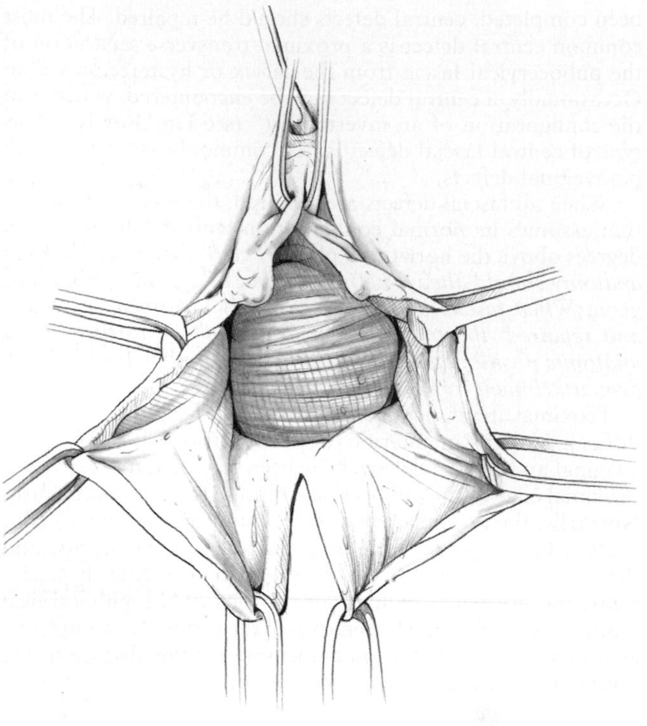

FIGURE 36B.10. After the sutures in Fig. 36B.9 are tied, the pubocervical septum is restored to its normal anatomic location.

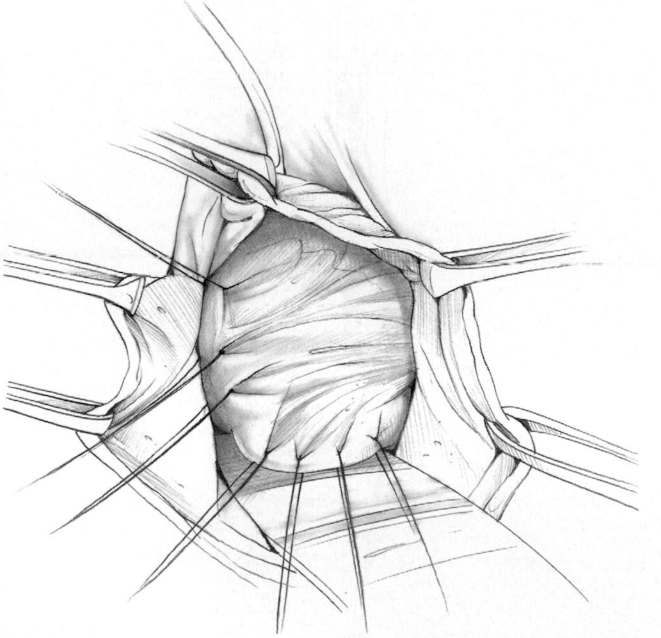

FIGURE 36B.9. Four paravaginal sutures have been placed to completely close the right paravaginal defect. Three sutures have been placed between the proximal edge of the pubocervical septum and the remnants of the hysterectomy scar to close the proximal transverse cystocele.

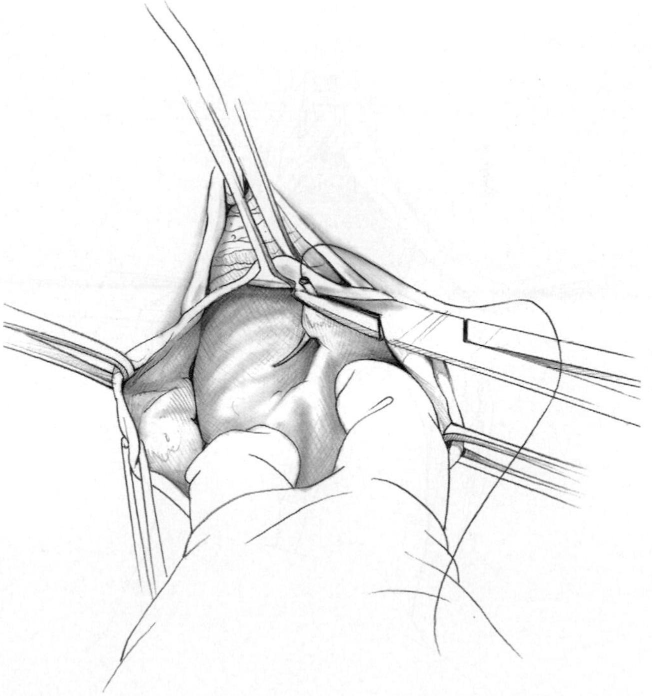

FIGURE 36B.11. A 0-gauge interwoven braided polyester suture is placed in the left white line. This suture will be one of the anchor sutures for the interlocked polyester fiber graft shown in Fig. 36B.12.

been completed, central defects should be repaired. The most common central defect is a proximal transverse separation of the pubocervical fascia from the cervix or hysterectomy scar. Occasionally, a central defect may be encountered, which is in the configuration of an inverted "V" (see Fig. 36A.16). This type of central fascial defect is not commonly associated with paravaginal defects.

When all fascial defects are repaired, the pubocervical septum assumes its normal configuration with the distal end 60 degrees above the horizontal plane. *The restoration of normal anatomy should always be in the mind of the site-specific surgeon. When fascial defects are properly identified, dissected, and repaired, the pubocervical fascia will be in the correct anatomic position as a hammock supporting the bladder with firm attachment to the pelvic sidewalls.*

Proximal attachment of the pubocervical septum is the most difficult problem in anterior vaginal reconstruction. After paravaginal and central defects have been repaired, the transverse proximal edge of the pubocervical septum remains unattached. Normally, the proximal edge of the pubocervical septum connects with the pericervical ring, pubocervical ligaments, and the anterior portion of the cardinal ligaments. After hysterectomy, the normal proximal connections of the pubocervical septum are interrupted by removal of the cervix. No completely anatomic method exists to compensate for the absence of the cervix and to close the defect created by its absence.

If a hysterectomy is a part of the prolapse procedure, corrective measures can be taken to compensate for the absence of the cervix during the surgery. Plication of the cardinal ligaments across the midline and a McCall's culdoplasty with a permanent suture will close the cervical defect. Following this plication, the proximal edge of the pubocervical septum is attached in a site-specific fashion to the anterior aspect of the cardinal ligaments. Careful attention to vaginal cuff support and closure is the most important part of a hysterectomy from the perspective of prolapse prevention.

In the posthysterectomy patient, the closure of the proximal anterior defect and the subsequent attachment of the proximal pubocervical septum are more difficult. The cardinal ligaments and uterosacral ligaments are key anatomic landmarks that are difficult to identify or mobilize during a posthysterectomy anterior vaginal dissection. Attachment of the pubocervical septum to the hysterectomy scar with permanent suture may provide sufficient support. The hysterectomy scar can mimic the function of the pericervical ring, especially if a concomitant vaginal suspension or colpopexy is performed during the same surgery.

Placement of a bolster may be necessary when identifiable structures provide insufficient support. The surgeon may select from a variety of bolsters or mesh products for this part of the reconstruction. I generally use an acceptable biomaterial or a permanent interlocked polyester fiber mesh for this portion of the operation. No definitive evidence exists to show superiority of any specific bolster or graft. The surgeon should choose wisely and never substitute a foreign material for biomechanically sound surgical technique. I do not recommend the use of an extruded polytetrafluoroethylene graft in this area

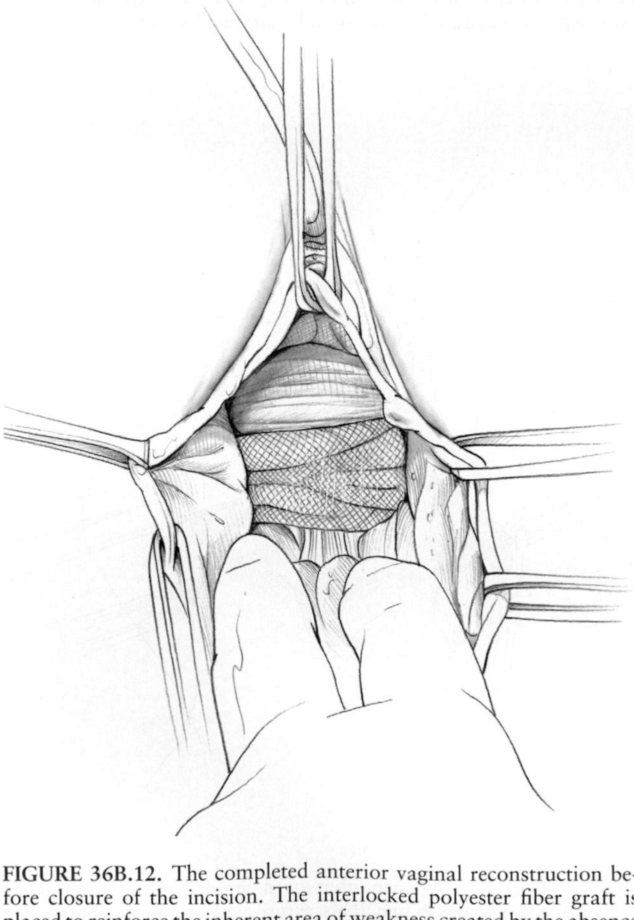

FIGURE 36B.12. The completed anterior vaginal reconstruction before closure of the incision. The interlocked polyester fiber graft is placed to reinforce the inherent area of weakness created by the absence of the cervix. In addition to synthetic material, various autografts, allografts, and xenografts may be chosen to reinforce the apical anterior vaginal segment.

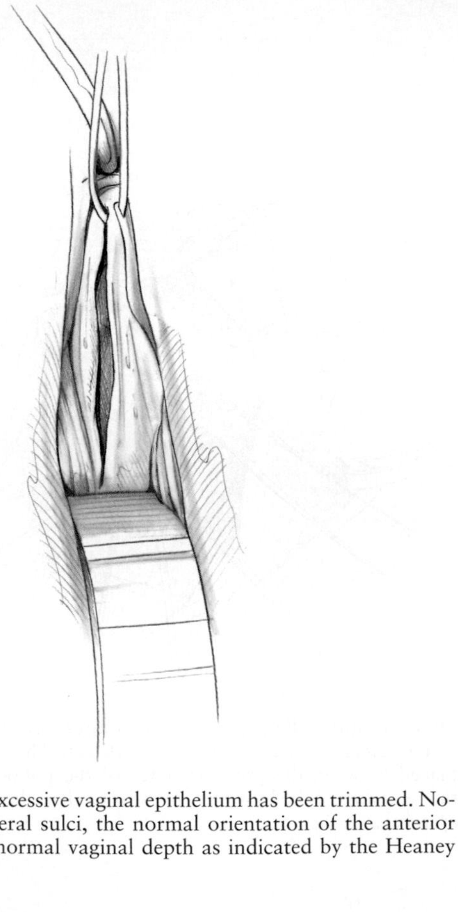

FIGURE 36B.13. Excessive vaginal epithelium has been trimmed. Notice the anterior lateral sulci, the normal orientation of the anterior vaginal plane, and normal vaginal depth as indicated by the Heaney retractor.

because of its tendency to erode when placed in close proximity to the epithelium. A small piece of material, slightly larger than a commemorative postage stamp, adequately covers the defect caused by the absence of the cervix. The bolster should be attached by permanent sutures to both of the white lines in the fashion of a paravaginal repair (Figs. 36B.11 and 36B.12). The middle portion of the bolster may be secured to the underlying tissue to prevent rolling and gathering of the material. Bolsters may also be used to compensate for pubocervical fascia that is significantly scarred or attenuated. Scarring is especially common in a patient who has had more than one previous pelvic support procedure. Scarring and retraction of the pubocervical septum may prevent adequate repair and require the use of a larger bolster.

Excessively distended vaginal epithelium may need to be trimmed. The amount of tissue removed should allow the epithelium to smoothly adhere to the underlying deep endopelvic connective tissue. The vaginal epithelium is not a support structure. Iatrogenic narrowing of the vaginal vault does not increase the likelihood of a successful operation. Absorbable suture is used for epithelial closure. During closure of the incision, attaching the proximal vaginal epithelium to the pubocervical septum near the level of the cuff is helpful. Vaginal packing may help the vaginal epithelium to adhere to the deep endopelvic connective tissue and to prevent venous bleeding or hematoma formation postoperatively.

After reconstruction of the pubocervical septum, both lateral anterior sulci should be visible (Fig. 36B.13). Permanent sutures and bolster material should not be exposed in the vaginal vault. The integrity of the rectum, bladder, and ureters should be confirmed.

The repair of anterior vaginal wall defects has undergone a largely conceptual revision. Anatomically distorting midline plications have been replaced by anatomically restoring operations that resemble herniorrhaphies. Anatomic landmarks define the extent of the components of the surgery. Permanent suture is used for support attachments. Anatomic restoration allows maximum potential for normal urinary, intestinal, and sexual function in the patient. To paraphrase the biological adage: function follows form.

BEST SURGICAL PRACTICES

- Site-specific techniques should be used to restore the anatomy of a prolapsed anterior vaginal segment.
- The pubocervical septum must be dissected completely so that specific fascial defects can be identified and repaired.
- Cystoceles are typically due to apical transverse defects in the pubocervical septum. Central defects in the pubocervical septum are not common or typical.
- The pubocervical septum is shorter than the rectovaginal septum by a length equal to the diameter of the cervix. Complete restoration of the anterior vaginal segment must take into consideration the defect left by the absence of the cervix.
- A cystocele may be due to detachment of the trampolinelike pubovesicle septum from the proximal attachment to the pericervical ring, from the lateral attachments to the white line, or from its distal attachment to the pubic ramus. It can also result from a central tear in the septal fascia itself. Each and every defect must be evaluated and repaired to provide a long-term successful result.

Bibliography

Addison WA, Timmons MC. Abdominal approach to vaginal eversion. *Clin Obstet Gynecol* 1993;36:995.

Aronson MP, ed. Reconstructive pelvic surgery. *Operative Techniques in Gynecologic Surgery* 1996;1:65.

Baden WF, Walker T. *Surgical repair of vaginal defects*. Philadelphia: JB Lippincott; 1992.

Burch JC. Cooper's ligament urethrovesical suspension for stress incontinence. Nine years' experience—results, complications, technique. *Am J Obstet Gynecol* 1968;100:764.

Burch JC. Urethrovaginal fixation to Cooper's ligament for correction of stress incontinence, cystocele, and prolapse. *Am J Obstet Gynecol* 1961;81:281.

DeLancey JO. Fascial and muscular abnormalities in women with urethral hypermobility and anterior vaginal wall prolapse. *Am J Obstet Gynecol* 2002;187:93.

DeLancey JO. Pelvic organ prolapse: clinical management and scientific foundations. *Clin Obstet Gynecol* 1993;36:895.

DeLancey JO. Structural support of the urethra as it relates to stress urinary incontinence: the hammock hypothesis. *Am J Obstet Gynecol* 1994;170:1713.

Grody MH. *Benign postreproductive gynecologic surgery*. New York: McGraw-Hill; 1994.

Kelly HA. Incontinence of urine in women. *Urol Cutan Rev* 1913;17:291.

Pillai-Allen A, Benson JT. Cystocele. In: Brubaker LT, Saclarides TJ, eds. *The female pelvic floor: disorders of function and support*. Philadelphia: FA Davis; 1996:269.

Richardson AC, Lyon JB, Williams NL. A new look at pelvic relaxation. *Am J Obstet Gynecol* 1976;126:568.

Shull BL, Benn SJ, Kuehl TJ. Surgical management of prolapse of the anterior vaginal segment: an analysis of support defects, operative morbidity, and anatomic outcome. *Am J Obstet Gynecol* 1994;171:1429.

Shull BL, Capen CV, Riggs MW, et al. Preoperative and postoperative analysis of site-specific pelvic support defects in 81 women treated with sacrospinous ligament suspension and pelvic reconstruction. *Am J Obstet Gynecol* 1992;166:1764.

Uhlenhuth E. *Problems in the anatomy of the pelvis*. Philadelphia: JB Lippincott; 1953.

Weber AM, Walters MD. Anterior vaginal prolapse: review of anatomy and techniques of surgical repair. *Obstet Gynecol* 1997;89:311.

White GR. An anatomic operation for the cure of cystocele. *Am J Obstet Dis Women Child* 1912;65:286.

White GR. Cystocele: a radical cure by suturing lateral sulci of vagina to white line of pelvic fascia. *JAMA* 1909;53:1707.

Zimmerman CW. New concepts in restoration of the anterior vaginal compartment. *Operative Techniques in Gynecologic Surgery* 2001;6:116.

CHAPTER 36C ■ PARAVAGINAL DEFECT REPAIR

BOBBY SHULL AND PAUL M. YANDELL

DEFINITIONS

Arcus tendineus fascia pelvis—The white line of the pelvic sidewall. This thickening of the pelvic sidewall fascia extends from the ischial spine posteriorly to the pubic tubercle anteriorly. It is the site of lateral attachment of the pubocervical fascia.

Paravaginal defect—When the pubocervical fascia becomes detached from, or torn just medial to, its lateral attachment to the arcus tendineus fascia pelvic (white line).

Pubocervical fascia—A trapezoid-shaped fascia that provides support for the anterior vagina under the bladder. It is attached superiorly to the pericervical ring, distally to the pubic ramus, and laterally to the arcus tendineus fascia pelvis (white line).

HISTORY

In 1909, George R. White quoted Ahlfelt, who said, "the only problem in plastic gynecology left unsolved by the gynecologist of the past century [the 19th century] is that of permanent cure of cystocele." Three years later, in 1912, White reviewed the current theories regarding the etiology of cystocele: overstretching and thinning of the vaginal wall and other supports of the bladder, which allow the bladder to descend in the form of a hernia; stretching of the firm attachment of the bladder to the uterus; and stretching of the ligamentous suspension of the bladder. He rejected each of these theories and also described his autopsy findings regarding the dissection of the anterior vaginal segment. One year before Howard Kelly's report on midline plication of the anterior segment, he discussed vaginal paravaginal repair for the management of certain types of cystocele; however, his theory and recommendation for surgical management did not gain widespread acceptance.

In 1923, Victor Bonney described the "periurethral wedge" that he found attached "to the subpubic angle, the rami of the pubes, and the edges of the levatores ani" and the association between this wedge and the mechanism of continence. Bonney suggested a retropubic repair of the loosened periurethral wedge in the treatment of incontinence. In 1961, Burch reported his experience with colposuspension. He attached the paravaginal fascia to the white line of the pelvis in his first seven patients. Subsequently, he chose Cooper's ligament as the point of fixation. The Burch procedure, as we have come to understand it, no longer uses the white line of the pelvis as a point of fixation. In the next decade, Richardson and colleagues published a "new" and controversial look at pelvic relaxation and its relationship to fascial defects.

ANATOMIC CONCEPTS AND PHYSICAL FINDINGS

Stimulated by the work of Richardson and Baden, we have found it valuable to consider that isolated defects in the anterior compartment not only do occur but must be properly identified and specifically repaired to offer the best opportunity for cure of anatomic and functional symptoms of the anterior vaginal segment. The pubocervical fascia is a trapezoid, part of which was described by Bonney more than 70 years ago. The fascia or fibromuscular tissue of the anterior vagina fuses with the perineal membrane distally, is attached to the arcus tendineus fasciae pelvis from a point just posterior to the pubic ramus to a point just anterior to the ischial spine bilaterally, and is attached to the cervix or to the vaginal cuff and base of the broad ligament and cardinal-uterosacral ligaments (Fig. 36C.1).

There are four clinically identifiable areas in which defects in this support are likely to occur:

- Laterally, where the pubocervical fascia attaches to arcus tendineus fascia pelvis (paravaginal defect)
- Transversely, in front of the cervix where the pubocervical fascia blends into the pericervical ring of fibromuscular tissue, or in the case of a woman who has had a hysterectomy, at the vaginal cuff (transverse defect)
- Centrally, in the area immediately anterior to the vaginal mucosa in between the lateral margins of the pubocervical fascia (midline or central defect)
- Distally, where the urethra perforates the urogenital diaphragm

These isolated defects may occur in combination, requiring the surgeon to identify and repair each defect individually. The clinical evaluation provides clues about the site of the fascial defect. The examination should be performed with the woman in the lithotomy position and the physician using only the posterior blade of the speculum. The patient is asked to strain or bear down maximally while the physician observes the landmarks of the anterior vagina. It is difficult to recognize an abnormal examination without having an understanding of normal. In a woman with normal support and no functional symptoms, there is minimal descent of the urethra and urethrovesical junction on straining. There are lateral sulci in the anterior vagina at the site of attachment of the pubocervical fascia to the arcus tendineus fascia pelvis that extend from the back of the pubic bone to a point just anterior to the ischial spine (Fig. 36C.2). The anterior vaginal wall is normally about a centimeter shorter than the posterior vaginal wall. There are usually rugae in the epithelium overlying the urethra and bladder.

In a woman with paravaginal loss of support, one or both lateral sulci will be lost. Observations by DeLancey have shown

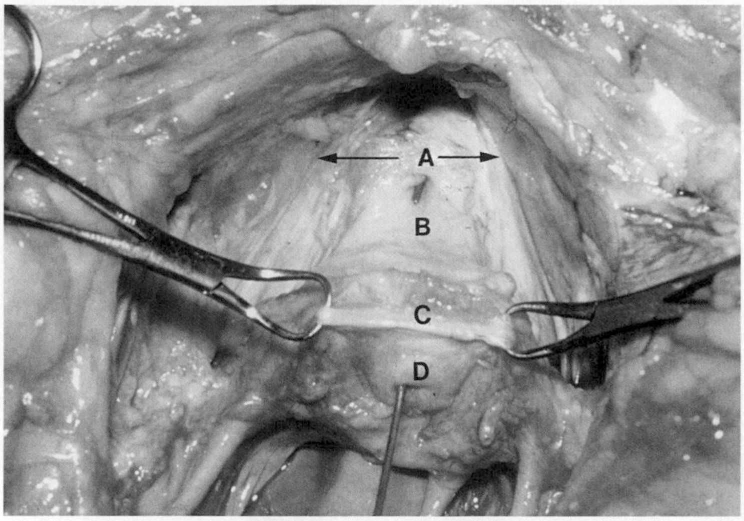

FIGURE 36C.1. An autopsy dissection of the pubocervical fascia. A: Arcus tendineus fasciae pelvis. B: Silver wire through the urethra. C: Towel clamps on the superior portion of the pubocervical fascia. D: Silver wire through the cervix. (From Shull BL. Clinical evaluation of women with pelvic support defects. *Clin Obstet Gynecol* 1993;36:939.)

that defects occur with equal frequency on the left and right sides and are associated with hypermobility of the urethra and urethrovesical junction. When the support defect is predominantly paravesical, the support for the bladder is also poor. Loss of paravaginal support can also be detected during use of the bivalve speculum when the clinician finds that the sides of the vaginal walls collapse through the open sides of the bivalve speculum, obscuring view of the cervix or vaginal apex.

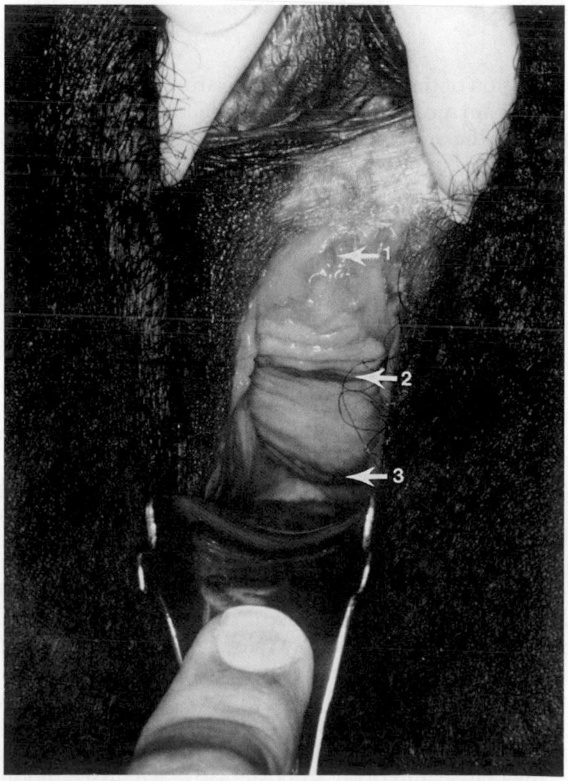

FIGURE 36C.2. Normal support for the urethra (*1*), urethrovesical junction (*2*), and bladder (*3*) in a woman with no functional symptoms. (From Shull BL. Clinical evaluation of women with pelvic support defects. *Clin Obstet Gynecol* 1993;36:939.)

Baden and Walker have recommended the use of a curved ring forceps to elevate the lateral aspects of the anterior vagina to their normal points of attachment along the pelvic sidewall. The curved arms of the ring forceps are directed laterally and posteriorly toward the ischial spines as the patient bears down. When this lateral elevation corrects the support defect, the diagnosis of a paravaginal defect can be made (Fig. 36C.3). If the patient continues to have a bulge of tissue through the open arms of the forceps, she either has a midline loss of support or a combined midline and lateral loss of support. Imaging studies such as magnetic resonance imaging and ultrasound provide details not only about connective tissue support in the pelvis but also about muscle integrity.

Women with complete eversion of the anterior vaginal segment must, by definition, have not only paravaginal loss of support for the urethra, urethrovesical junction, and bladder but also loss of support for the transverse portion of the pubocervical fascia. The eversion may occur in association with procidentia or posthysterectomy vaginal prolapse (Fig. 36C.4). In our own practice, management of the prolapsed anterior vaginal segment is technically the most challenging dilemma because it may require correction of a complex set of problems, including urinary incontinence; incomplete bladder emptying; impaired intravaginal intercourse; symptoms of prolapse, such as pressure, fullness, and a sense of things falling out; or any combination of these. Successful management of prolapse of the anterior vagina should ultimately result in correction of the poor support, maintenance or enhancement of the ability to have intravaginal intercourse, and maintenance or enhancement of urinary continence. A particularly difficult challenge is the patient with complete eversion of the vagina. Vaginal and abdominal operations for the treatment of vaginal vault prolapse are usually successful in suspension of the vaginal cuff. However, a 1992 study found a 15% to 25% incidence of postoperative urinary incontinence and a 15% incidence of persistent or recurrent cystocele.

OPEN RETROPUBIC TECHNIQUE

Paravaginal defects can be surgically repaired through an open retropubic incision, through a vaginal retropubic incision, or laparoscopically. We use the open retropubic repair primarily in the treatment of women who have genuine urinary incontinence associated with paravaginal defects. The operation can

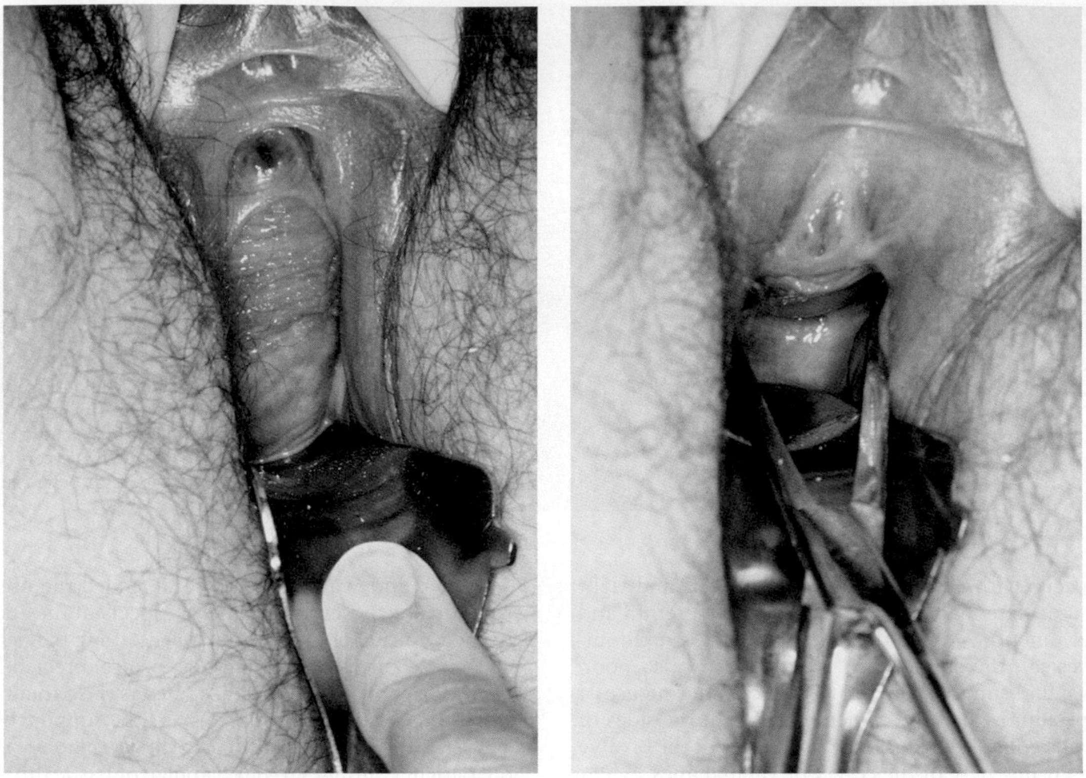

A B

FIGURE 36C.3. **A:** Lateral loss of support with flattening of the urethrovesical junction. **B:** Lateral support with curved forceps restores normal support. (From Shull BL. Clinical evaluation of women with pelvic support defects. *Clin Obstet Gynecol* 1993;36:939.)

be performed with or without hysterectomy. If hysterectomy is performed, we prefer the intrafascial technique and incorporate the cardinal uterosacral ligaments into the angles and the pubocervical and rectovaginal fascia to minimize the occurrence of postoperative enterocele formation. In women with a preoperative enterocele and prior hysterectomy, we repair the enterocele in association with the paravaginal defect repair. The paravaginal repair is performed after completion of the hysterectomy or culdoplasty. The patient's legs are in low leg holders, and she is draped so that there is access to the abdomen as well as to the vaginal canal. A Foley catheter drains the urinary bladder. We prefer a low transverse abdominal incision made about one finger breadth cephalad to the symphysis pubis. The incision is carried to the anterior sheath of the rectus fascia, which is incised sharply. The rectus muscles are reflected laterally. The transversalis fascia is separated from the superior ramus of the pubic bone, and the space of Retzius is entered immediately medial to the superior ramus of pubis on each side. The loose areolar tissue can easily be dissected away from pubic bone by use of either the index finger or a pair of long tissue forceps. The bony landmarks in the pelvis are identified by palpation. The symphysis pubis, the midline landmark, is almost always convex. The pubic bone extends laterally and gently curves posteriorly. The next palpable landmark is the obturator neurovascular canal, which can be felt along the inferior border of the superior ramus of pubis about 7 to 10 cm lateral to the midline. The foramen feels like the buttonhole of a shirt or blouse. About 7 to 8 cm directly dorsal to the obturator canal is the ischial spine. The arcus tendineus fascia pelvis, more commonly known as the white line, extends from the back of the pubic bone to the ischial spine. The arcus is a condensation of the fascia of the obturator internus muscle and the levator ani muscles. The arcus tendineus musculi levator ani demarcates the origin of the pubococcygeal muscle from the inferior ramus of pubis and the condensation of the levator arcus (Fig. 36C.5).

After the bony landmarks have been identified by palpation, we use long tissue forceps to develop the space between the obturator internus fascia and the urethra and bladder. Veins coursing along the inner aspect of the superior ramus of pubis can be a source of troublesome bleeding. It is best not to traumatize them with a retractor or tissue forceps; however, when they bleed, electrocautery promptly controls the bleeding. A set of larger veins that course between the anterior surface of the urethra and the back of the pubic bone can also be the source of considerable bleeding. When they obstruct the dissection or interfere with the operative repair, they should be clipped with silver clips and divided sharply to fall out of the operative field. After the proper cleavage plane has been established, a fluffed-up 4-inch piece of gauze should be placed in the space to rest on the anterior surface of the vagina. Then a small or medium malleable ribbon retractor should be used to hold the bladder and urethra medially while the remaining landmarks are identified by direct visualization. To minimize bleeding, the bladder should never be reflected off of the anterior surface of the vagina. The vessels in the bladder generally course medially to laterally across the operative field. The vessels in the vagina generally course anteriorly to posteriorly. We dissect both the left and the right sides of the space of Retzius before beginning any of the operative repair. We find it helpful to use the long extension for the electrocautery in case it is necessary to cauterize bleeding points.

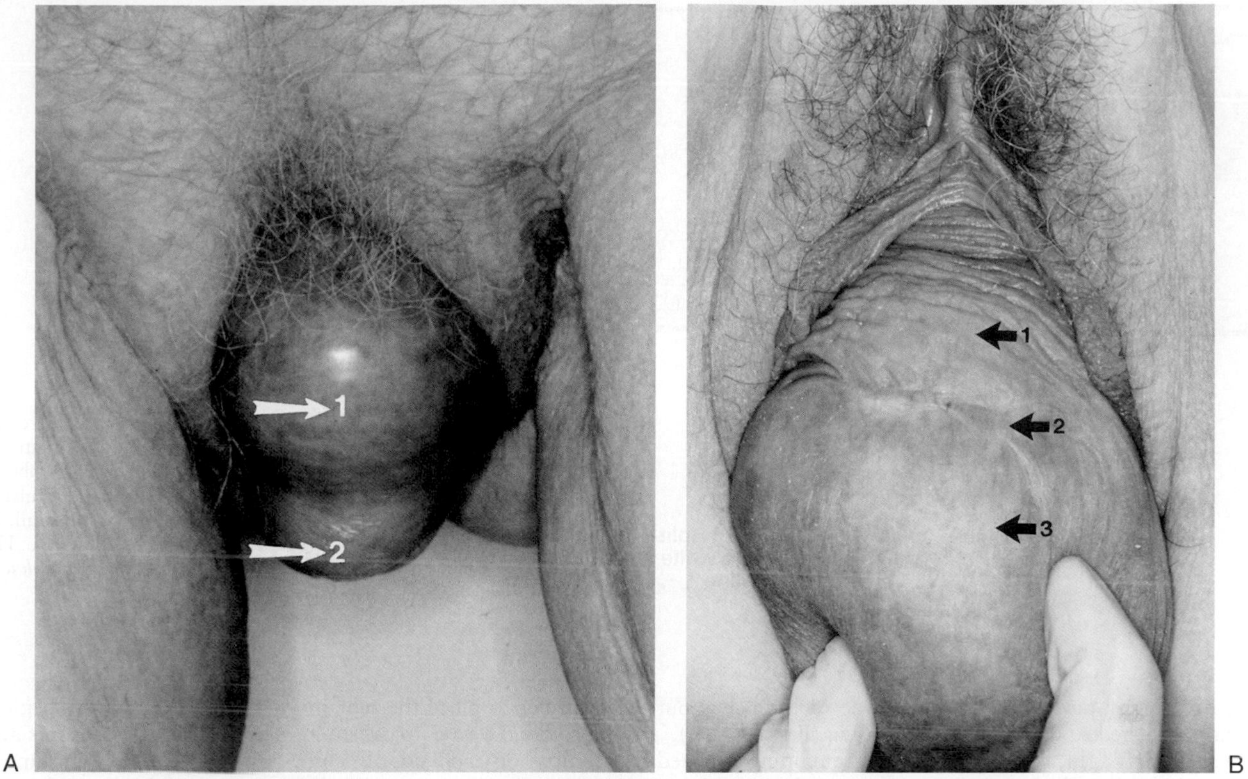

FIGURE 36C.4. **A:** Physical findings in the standing patient who has prolapse of the anterior segment (*1*) as well as uterine prolapse (*2*). **B:** Posthysterectomy prolapse of the anterior vaginal segment (*1*), vaginal cuff (*2*), and enterocele (*3*). (From Shull BL. Clinical evaluation of women with pelvic support defects. *Clin Obstet Gynecol* 1993;36:939.)

The operating surgeon stands on the patient's side opposite to his/her dominant hand. Suturing away from the urethra and bladder to decrease the chance of urologic injury requires backhanding the sutures when sewing at the side of the table on which the surgeon is standing. We prefer to use round tapered needles and 2-0 nonabsorbable suture for the repair. A long needle driver such as is used in chest surgery allows one to reach even the deepest portion of the retropubic space without having a hand directly in the operative field.

Paravaginal defects can occur in one of three different ways (Fig. 36C.6):

1. The entire arcus may remain attached to the pelvic sidewall with the pubocervical fascia breaking away from the arcus (Fig. 36C.6B).

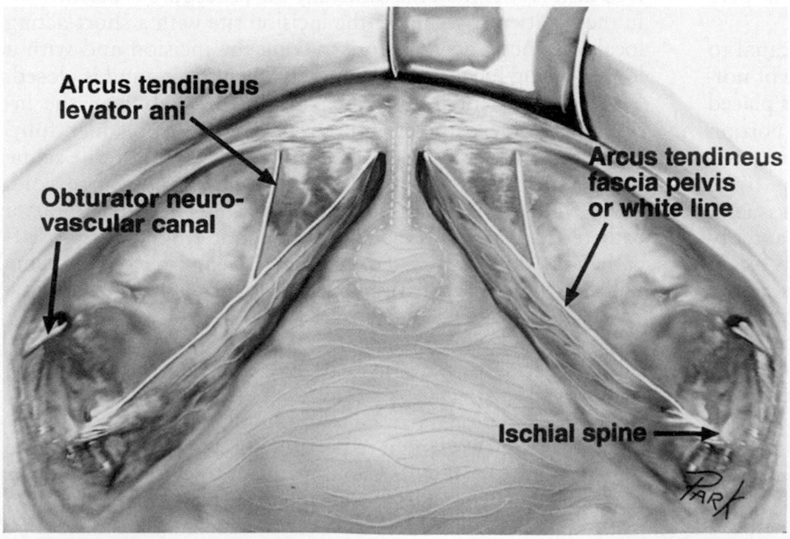

FIGURE 36C.5. The key anatomic landmarks in the space of Retzius in a woman with normal findings. (From Shull BL. How I do abdominal paravaginal repair. *J Pelvic Surg* 1995;1:43.)

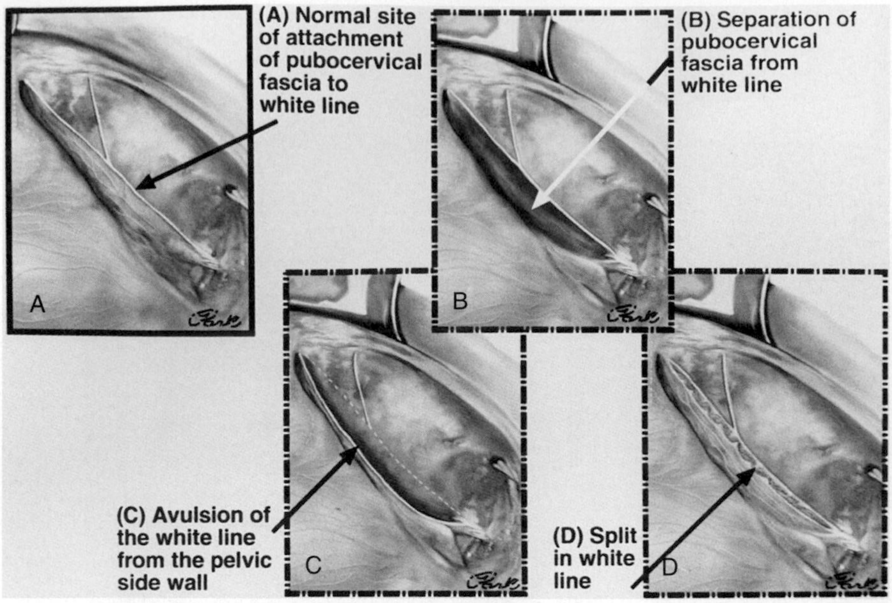

FIGURE 36C.6. Examples of the three types of paravaginal defects. **A:** Normal anatomy on the right side. **B:** Avulsion of the pubocervical fascia from the white line. **C:** Avulsion of the white line from the pelvic sidewall. **D:** A split in the white line. (From Shull BL. How I do abdominal paravaginal repair. *J Pelvic Surg* 1995;1:43.)

2. The arcus may pull away from the side of the pelvis but remain attached to the pubocervical fascia (Fig. 36C.6C).
3. The arcus may split, with a portion of it remaining attached to the sidewall and a portion tearing away but remaining attached to pubocervical fascia (Fig. 36C.6D).

In any circumstance, *the goal of the operative repair is to reattach the pubocervical fascia to the arcus tendineus fasciae pelvis, as well as to the fascia overlying the obturator internus muscle.*

The easiest point of identification of the white line is near its insertion at the back of the pubic bone. Using a pair of tissue forceps to grasp the white line and place it on tension makes it easier to identify the remainder of the white line as it courses toward the ischial spine. The smooth white fibromuscular tissue of the pubocervical fascia is always medial to the white line. The most dependent portion of the operative field is the perivesical space adjacent to the ischial spine. Any bleeding results in the collection of blood in that space; therefore, we prefer to initiate the repair near the vaginal apex while the field is quite dry.

The nondominant hand is placed into the vaginal canal to elevate the periurethral and perivesical tissue to its site of normal attachment along the white line. The first suture is placed near the apex of the vagina through the perivesical portion of the pubocervical fascia. When permanent sutures are used, one should avoid penetration of the vaginal epithelium. If the needle is placed at a right angle to the fibromuscular tissue, it is easier to retrieve and place it through the white line and obturator internus fascia at a point 1 to 2 cm anterior to its origin at the ischial spine. The suture is securely tied with a series of four knots and the excess trimmed. We prefer to place the next suture at the opposite end of the repair through the pubocervical fascia near the distal portion of the urethra. The needle is regrasped and placed through the white line near its origin from the back of the pubic bone. The suture is similarly secured with four knots and the excess cut. At that point, the two extreme ends of the repair have been performed (Fig. 36C.7A). The pubocervical fascia and white line stand out on relief, making it easier to determine the placement of subsequent sutures. I prefer to place the remaining sutures sequentially beginning proximal to the apical stitch. About four to six sutures are required on each side. In some patients, the vascular supply to the vagina is so generous that it is impossible to avoid suturing through or around a vessel. When each suture is tied as placed, significant bleeding is rarely a problem. Bleeding becomes a problem, however, if a needle is placed through a vein and the needle is removed without tying the suture down. Bleeding can also be a problem if one chooses to dissect the bladder or urethra off of the anterior surface of the vagina. When the sutures have all been placed on one side, the suture line adjacent to the urethra and urethrovesical junction is about horizontal to the floor (Fig. 36C.7B). The suture line from the urethrovesical junction to the apex of the vagina angles gently posteriorly. The same sequence of sutures is repeated on the opposite side (Fig. 36.7C). We have used this repair for hundreds of patients over 14 years and have not left a drain in the space of Retzius in a single patient.

In patients who undergo a retropubic repair only, my goal is to dismiss them on the same day the procedure is performed. In these patients, we inject the incision site with a short-acting local anesthetic agent before making the incision and with a longer-acting local anesthetic agent when the wound is closed. When the patient is fully awake and can ambulate, the indwelling Foley catheter is used to empty the bladder fully. Next, the bladder is filled retrograde with 300 mL sterile saline and the catheter is removed. The patient is allowed to void. If she voids more than 150 mL, she is dismissed without a catheter; if not, she is dismissed doing intermittent clean self-catheterization (ICSC). For the last 7 years, all our patients with retropubic repair only have been dismissed on the same day of surgery.

In patients who have more extensive surgery and are admitted overnight, the same catheter management is used the morning following surgery after the patient has breakfast.

In the exceptional patient who cannot perform ICSC, either a family member is taught to perform the catheterization or the patient is dismissed with a Foley catheter to closed drainage. A few days later, the patient returns for retrograde filling and a test of bladder function.

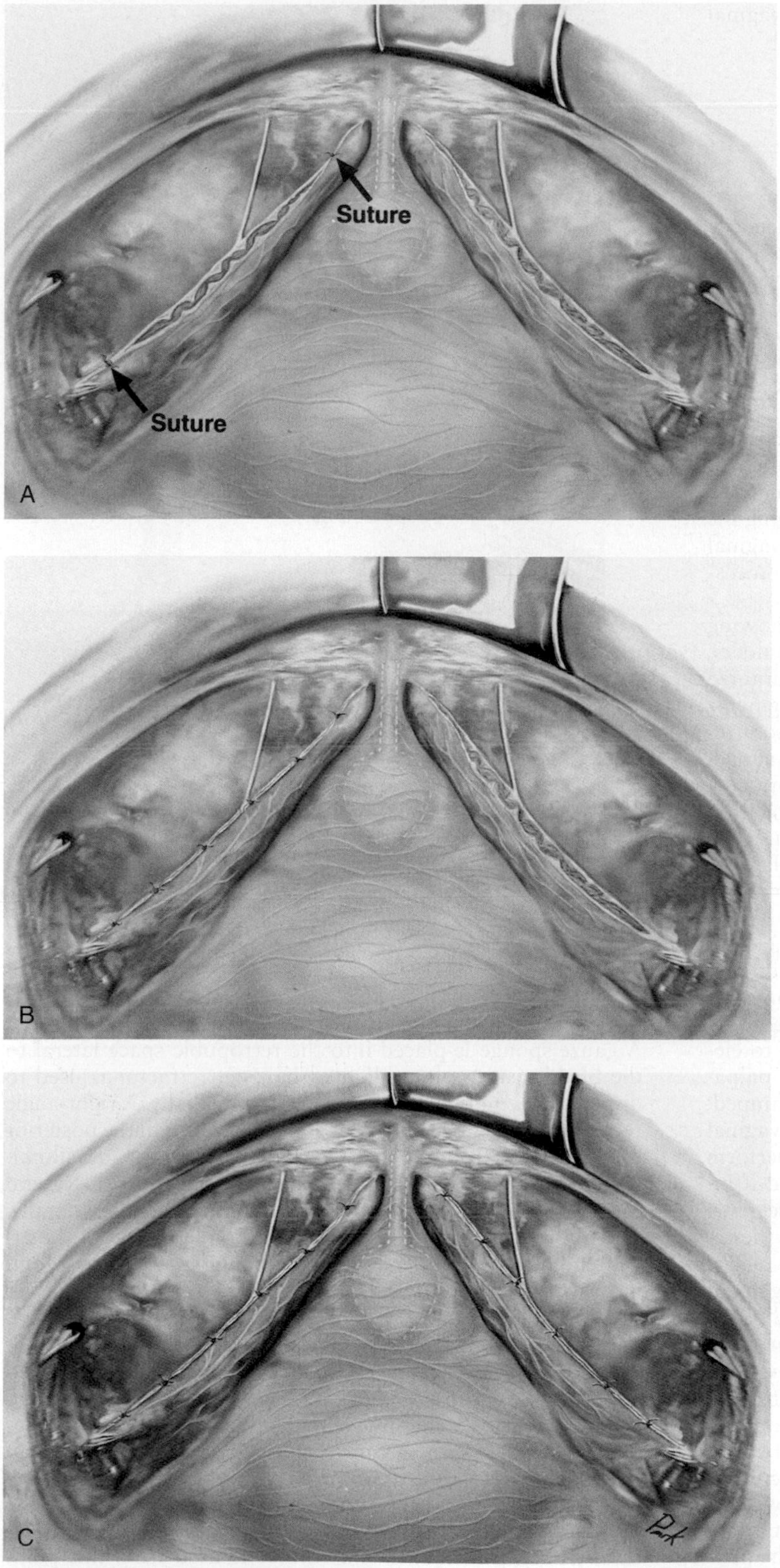

FIGURE 36C.7. **A:** A patient with bilateral paravaginal defects. The repair has been started on the left with sutures at the two extremes of the defect. **B:** The repair is complete on the left side. **C:** Both sides are repaired. (From Shull BL. How I do abdominal paravaginal repair. *J Pelvic Surg* 1995;1:43.)

Some surgeons who treat vaginal eversion by sacral colpopexy have begun to incorporate the paravaginal repair as a part of the total vaginal reconstruction. After completion of the sacral colpopexy, the paravaginal repair is performed as previously described. Others perform a combined Burch procedure and paravaginal repair in association with a sacral colpopexy. After the sacral colpopexy is completed, the sutures adjacent to the urethra and the urethrovesical junction are placed through the Cooper's ligament, as is done in the modified Burch colposuspension. The perivesical loss of support is then repaired with a series of paravaginal sutures.

VAGINAL RETROPUBIC TECHNIQUE

The vaginal approach to the paravaginal repair is particularly helpful in women whose primary symptom is pelvic organ prolapse without significant urinary incontinence. The vaginal approach requires greater technical skills than does the open retropubic repair. It has a limited use for the general gynecologic surgeon. The angle of the subpubic arch is the most important factor affecting access to the retropubic space. In a woman with a subpubic arch that admits three or more finger breadths, several retractors can easily be placed in the retropubic space, making the vaginal approach technically possible. In a woman with prolapse of the anterior segment and a narrow subpubic arch, I prefer a combination approach, managing the defects that can be handled appropriately through a vaginal incision and completing the retropubic repair through a transabdominal incision.

In the vaginal approach to paravaginal repair, the following steps are used. The patient's legs are placed in high leg holders, and she is draped for vaginal surgery. The bladder is drained before the initiation of the surgical procedure. All segments of the vaginal canal area are thoroughly evaluated to confirm the fascial defects. The anterior vaginal segment is examined, specifically to observe loss of lateral sulci, lack of rugation of the epithelium along the base of the bladder, and elongation of the anterior vaginal wall (Fig. 36C.8). Marking sutures are placed through the vaginal epithelium at the level of the urethrovesical junction several millimeters lateral to the normal location of the lateral sulci (Fig. 36C.9). In women who have previously had a hysterectomy, marking sutures are placed at the vaginal apices. In a woman undergoing concomitant hysterectomy, a posterior colpotomy is performed. The anterior epithelium is sharply circumscribed, and an anterior colpotomy is performed by sharp dissection. A retractor is placed to elevate the bladder ventrally. The ureters are identified by palpation. The cardinal-uterosacral ligament pedicles are clamped, divided, and tagged to be used later for support of the vaginal apices. A cross-clamp, cut, and tie technique is used to perform the hysterectomy. Salpingo-oophorectomy is performed if indicated. The cardinal-uterosacral ligament pedicles are sewn into the ipsilateral angles of the vaginal cuff, initiating the reconstructive procedure. At that point, tension can be placed on the cardinal-uterosacral ligament pedicle, and the ligament itself can be palpated as it courses posterior and medial to the ischial spine back to the sacrum. Nonabsorbable sutures are used to initiate the culdoplasty. Regardless of the technique of culdoplasty, the sutures are left untied until the paravaginal dissection and repair have been performed. Tying the culdoplasty sutures at this stage of the operation reduces the field of vision and makes subsequent dissection technically more difficult.

We initiate reconstruction of the anterior segment by placing Allis clamps along the cut edge of the epithelium at about the 3- and 9-o'clock positions. With sharp dissection, the pubocervical fascia is dissected off of the epithelium up to the urethrovesical junction, and the dissection is continued laterally until the index finger can be passed between the vaginal epithelium and the pubocervical fascia into the retropubic space just anterior to the ischial spine. With the index finger in the retropubic space, the dissection is continued anteriorly along the inferior ramus of pubis and medially to the symphysis pubis. Small individual veins may require isolation and ligation. A gauze sponge is placed into the retropubic space lateral to the bladder, and a long, lighted bayonet retractor is used to displace the empty bladder and urethra medially. A right-angle retractor with a fiberoptic light source is placed in the posterior aspect of the retropubic space, providing retraction and illumination. Another right-angle retractor is placed in the lateral aspect of the field, displacing the vaginal epithelium laterally. The obturator internus fascia and the condensation of the arcus tendineus fasciae pelvis are identified first by palpation and next by visualization. With use of a long, straight needle driver and a small, round, tapered needle, the first suture is placed into the tendinous arch and obturator fascia 2 to 3 cm anterior to the ischial spine (Fig. 36C.10). The suture remains armed and is marked with a small clamp. We have found it handy to have a series of six clamps, each identified by one to six pieces of tape, so that sutures can be marked sequentially and can be remembered by the appropriately marked clamp. Traction is placed on the first suture, making it easier to visualize the tendinous arch and to facilitate placement of subsequent sutures. A series of four to six sutures is used from this point anterior to the spine to the attachment of the white line along the posterior aspect of the pubic bone (Fig. 36C.11).

Next, the suture that is placed closest to the posterior surface of the pubic bone is used to penetrate the lateral edge of the periurethral portion of the pubocervical fascia near the midportion of the urethra (Fig. 36C.12). The same suture is then used to penetrate the undersurface of the vaginal

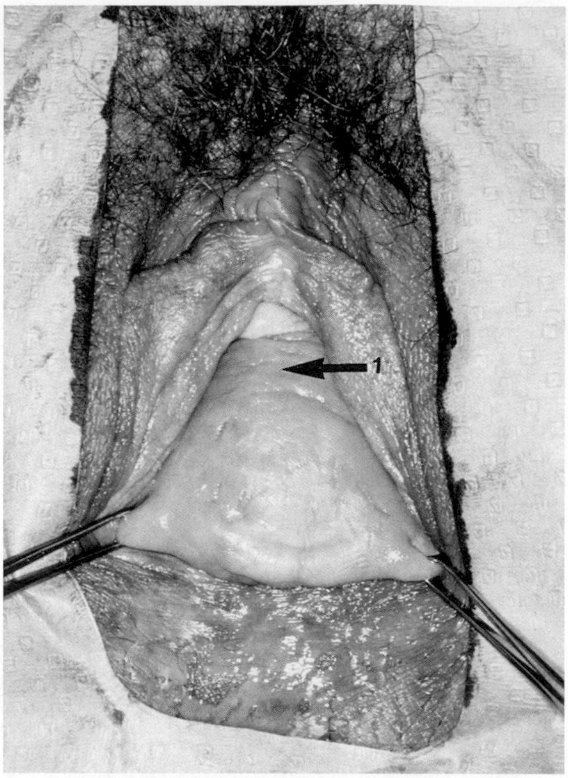

FIGURE 36C.8. A patient with loss of support laterally, centrally, and superiorly. A few rugae can be seen in the upper third of the pubocervical fascia closest to the urethrovesical junction. The remainder of the anterior segment is elongated and has lost its rugae. The apices prolapse less than 1 cm past the hymen. (From Shull BL. Clinical evaluation of women with pelvic support defects. *Clin Obstet Gynecol* 1993;36:939.)

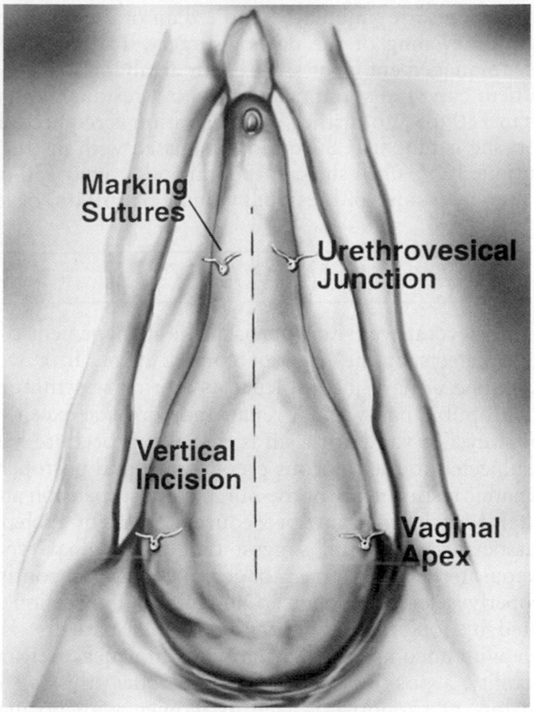

FIGURE 36C.9. A patient with prolapse of the anterior vagina. Marking sutures are at the urethrovesical junction and apices. The dotted line indicates the midline incision to be made. (From Shull BL, Benn SJ, Kuehl TJ. Surgical management of prolapse of the anterior vaginal segment: an analysis of support defects, operative morbidity, and anatomic outcome. *Am J Obstet Gynecol* 1994;171:1429.)

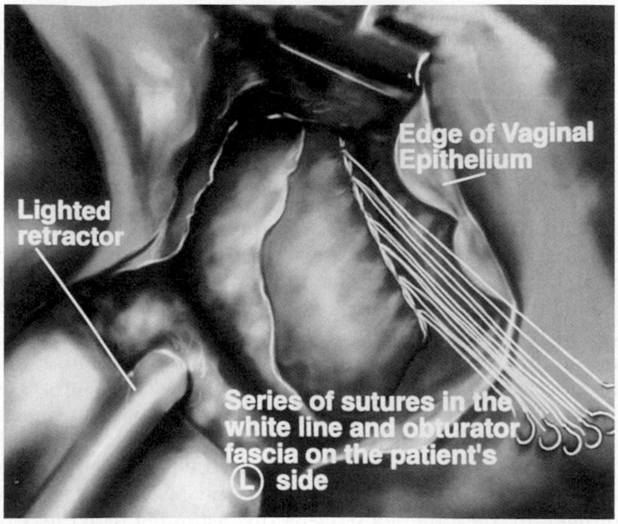

FIGURE 36C.11. A series of sutures has been placed in the arcus tendineus fasciae pelvis from a point ventral to the ischial spine to the back of the pubic bone. (From Shull BL, Benn SJ, Kuehl TJ. Surgical management of prolapse of the anterior vaginal segment: an analysis of support defects, operative morbidity, and anatomic outcome. *Am J Obstet Gynecol* 1994;171:1429.)

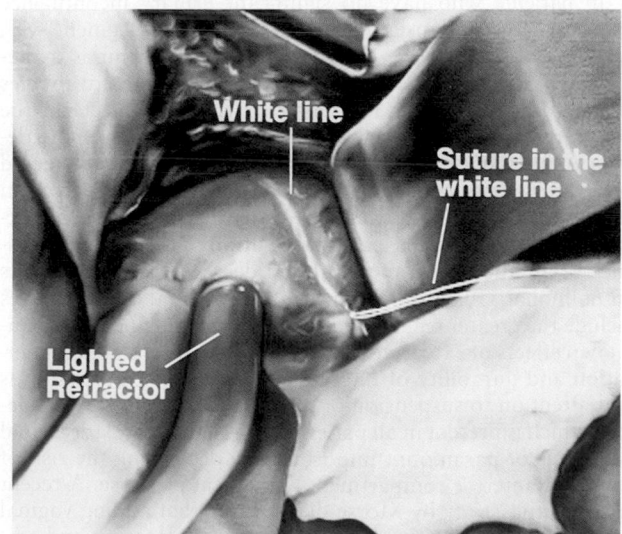

FIGURE 36C.10. A fiber-optic, right-angle retractor is in the retropubic space, retracting the bladder medially and providing illumination to the retropubic space. The suture is through the arcus tendineus fasciae pelvis (white line) about 2 cm ventral to the ischial spine. (From Shull BL, Benn SJ, Kuehl TJ. Surgical management of prolapse of the anterior vaginal segment: an analysis of support defects, operative morbidity, and anatomic outcome. *Am J Obstet Gynecol* 1994;171:1429.)

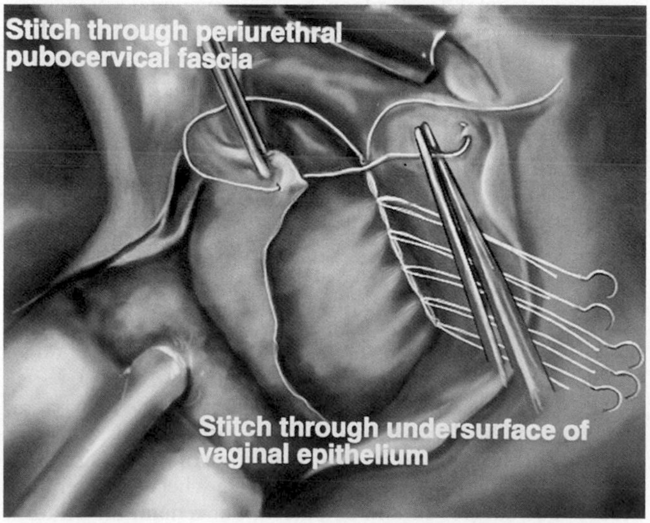

FIGURE 36C.12. The suture in the arcus tendineus fasciae pelvis near the pubic bone is also sewn into the lateral margin on the pubocervical fascia periurethrally and into the undersurface of the vaginal epithelium at the site of the marking suture at the urethrovesical junction. (From Shull BL, Benn SJ, Kuehl TJ. Surgical management of prolapse of the anterior vaginal segment: an analysis of support defects, operative morbidity, and anatomic outcome. *Am J Obstet Gynecol* 1994;171:1429.)

epithelium about halfway between the marking suture of the urethrovesical junction and the urethral meatus. The suture in the vaginal epithelium is placed several centimeters medial to the cut edge. The second suture penetrates the pubocervical fascia near the urethrovesical junction and the undersurface of the vaginal epithelium at the site of the previously placed marking suture. The third suture penetrates the perivesical fascia and the undersurface of the vaginal epithelium. This sequence is repeated until the suture placed closest to the ischial spine is used to secure the most cephalad portion of the pubocervical fascia to the undersurface of the vaginal epithelium near the apex. It is necessary to pick up the lateral edge of the pubocervical fascia to avoid injury to the bladder and urethra as well as to avoid placing undue tension on the anterior segment. It is also necessary to place the sutures in the vaginal epithelium several centimeters away from the cut edges of the midline incision to allow adequate tissue for midline closure. When all sutures are placed with three points of penetration (the white line, pubocervical fascia, and vaginal epithelium), they are tied sequentially beginning with the periurethral suture and ending with the stitch nearest the vaginal apex. A similar procedure is performed on the patient's opposite side. At that point, the bilateral paravaginal defects have been repaired. If a midline defect in pubocervical fascia exists, it is closed with a series of 2-0 interrupted nonabsorbable sutures.

If a hysterectomy has been done, the culdoplasty and peritoneal sutures are tied next, providing depth and support to the posterior portion of the vaginal cuff. Once the culdoplasty sutures have been tied, they are used to attach the transverse or superior portion of the pubocervical fascia to the apex of the vagina. In this manner, the lateral, central, and superior or transverse portions of the pubocervical fascia have been repaired. The cut edges of the anterior epithelium are approximated with interrupted absorbable sutures. Most patients require a posterior colporrhaphy and perineorrhaphy in addition to the anterior vaginal reconstruction. The goals of the reconstructive procedure include establishment of normal support for all segments of the vagina, a posterior axis for the vaginal canal, and vaginal depth adequate for intravaginal intercourse. A gauze pack is placed in the vaginal canal, and a transurethral catheter is used to drain the bladder.

In the patient who has previously had a hysterectomy, the operation is begun by placing marking sutures at the site of the urethrovesical junction near the creation of the new lateral sulci and at the apex of the vagina near the expected approximation of the cuff anterior to the ischial spines. I prefer a vertical incision in the anterior vagina extending from the urethrovesical junction to the apex of the vaginal cuff. Other authors have described bilateral periurethral incisions extending from the urethrovesical junction to a point just anterior to the spine. With use of the single vertical incision, the dissection is continued laterally and superiorly to the vaginal cuff. When an enterocele is present, the sac is opened, and an enterocele repair is performed. I identify the remnants of the uterosacral ligaments at the 4- and 8-o'clock positions and use them to suspend and support the transverse portion of the pubocervical and rectovaginal fascia, closing the space where an enterocele occurs. The sutures should be placed, but remain untied until the anterior dissection and repair have been completed. After the uterosacral sutures have been placed, or in cases in which no enterocele is present, the dissection is continued laterally until the index finger can be placed into the retropubic space just anterior to the ischial spine. The vaginal paravaginal repair, midline and transverse repair, and posterior colporrhaphy and perineorrhaphy are performed as described in the preceding paragraphs.

The patients are ambulated and fed an oral diet on the afternoon or evening of the day of surgery. The transurethral catheter management is the same as for an abdominal repair. If the patient can void spontaneously with a residual volume of less than 150 mL, no further catheterization is required. If she cannot, she is taught ICSC and is dismissed with instructions to continue ICSC until she can spontaneously void 150 mL or more and has a postvoid residual volume of 150 mL or less.

SUMMARY

There are several ways to approach the management of paravaginal defects of the anterior compartment. In a woman with genuine urinary incontinence as a primary symptom, an open retropubic paravaginal repair may provide excellent relief. However, a valid criticism is that this procedure has not been subjected to the rigorous preoperative and postoperative urodynamic testing used for the Burch colposuspension and the Marshall-Marchetti-Krantz procedure. Reports by Richardson and associates and Shull suggest that paravaginal repair is efficacious in the management of genuine urinary incontinence in properly selected patients. Our clinical impression, documented by longitudinal follow-up of our patients, is that women with uncomplicated urinary incontinence, urethral hypermobility, a positive provoked full-bladder stress test, and lateral loss of support—as well as women with no incontinence but paravesical defects and cystocele—are candidates for paravaginal repair. Colombo and associates performed a randomized comparison of the Burch procedure and abdominal paravaginal defect repair for urinary incontinence and reported the Burch procedure was superior for the treatment of urinary incontinence. The patients who underwent a paravaginal repair resumed spontaneous voiding more quickly. Many surgeons now combine the principles of the Burch procedure and the paravaginal defect repair to offer superior results for cure of urinary incontinence as well as correction of anterior support loss.

In patients who have no significant urinary incontinence but who have prolapse of the anterior vaginal segment with paravaginal defects, the vaginal paravaginal repair is a theoretically attractive method of management. The advantages include an opportunity for repair of isolated defects in the pubocervical fascia as well as repair of all other support defects with a single approach. In Shull's series of patients treated with vaginal paravaginal repair, all have had support defects in one or more additional sites. The transvaginal approach is attractive because there is less manipulation of the bowel, avoidance of an abdominal incision, and decreased adverse effects on pulmonary function. However, the potential disadvantages include the greater technical difficulty of the repair and the unknown effects of extensive anterior dissection on bladder innervation and durability of the repair. Our clinical impression is that attention to suspension of the transverse pubocervical defect, which is present in all patients with significant paravaginal defects, is of paramount importance in decreasing the risk of recurrent anterior compartment and apical prolapse. A recent retrospective study by Morse did not find that adding vaginal paravaginal repair to midline pubocervical placation and apical support was superior in terms of anatomic or quality of life outcomes.

BEST SURGICAL PRACTICES

- The goal of the operative repair of a paravaginal defect is to reattach the pubocervical fascia to the arcus tendineus fascia pelvis and to the fascia overlying the obturator internus muscle.

- Using an open retropubic technique, the bony landmarks of the pelvis are identified by palpation; then tissue forceps are used to develop the space between the pelvic sidewall fascia and the bladder and urethra. Care is taken to avoid venous bleeding in this area.
- After the white line and the lateral edge of the pubocervical fascia have been identified, a series of interrupted 2-0 permanent sutures are placed about 1 to 2 cm apart to reapproximate the fascial edge to the white line of the pelvic sidewall fascia.
- When a transvaginal approach is used, the retropublic space is opened and cleared back to the ischial spine and the important landmarks visualized as with an anterior retropublic approach. Starting near the ischial spine, a series of sutures are placed in the white line and held with the needles in place. Then, in reverse order, starting with the most distal suture, a bite is taken in the edge of the pubocervical fascia and the undersurface of the vaginal mucosa. The process is repeated, advancing deeper into the pelvis until the highest suture is placed. The sutures are then tied, starting with the one closest to the vaginal introitus and proceeding to the vaginal apex. The vaginal mucosa is then closed in the midline.
- An indwelling catheter is not used. If patients cannot void spontaneously, they are taught self-intermittent catheterization. They are given a regular diet as desired. If no other surgery has been done, they may be discharged later the same day or the next morning.

Bibliography

Baden WF, Walker T. *Surgical repair of vaginal defects*. Philadelphia: JB Lippincott; 1992.

Bonney V. On diurnal incontinence of urine in women. *J Obstet Gynaecol Br Emp* 1923;30:358.

Burch JC. Cooper's ligament urethrovesical suspension for stress incontinence: nine years' experience—results, complications, technique. *Am J Obstet Gynecol* 1968;100:764.

Burch JC. Urethrovaginal fixation to Cooper's ligament for correction of stress incontinence, cystocele, and prolapse. *Am J Obstet Gynecol* 1961;81:281.

Colombo M, Milani R, Vitobello D, et al. A randomized comparison of Burch colposuspension and abdominal paravaginal defect repair for female stress urinary incontinence. *Am J Obstet Gynecol* 1996;175:78.

DeLancey JO. Pelvic organ prolapse: clinical management and scientific foundations. *Clin Obstet Gynecol* 1993;36:895.

DeLancey JO. Structural support of the urethra as it relates to stress urinary incontinence: the hammock hypothesis. *Am J Obstet Gynecol* 1994;170:1713.

Horbach NS, ed. *Surgery for stress urinary incontinence*. 1997;2:1.

Karram MM. What is the clinical relevance of a paravaginal defect? *Int Urogynecol J* 2004;15:1.

Kovac SR. Follow up of the pubic bone suburethral stabilization sling operation for recurrent urinary incontinence (Kovac procedure). *J Pelvic Surg* 1999;5:156.

Kovac SR, Cruikshank SH. Pubic bone suburethral stabilization sling: an anatomic approach to urinary stress incontinence. *Contemp Obstet Gynecol* 1998;43:52.

Morse AN, O'dell KK, Howard AE, Baker SP, Aronson MP, Young SB. Midline anterior repair alone vs anterior repair plus vaginal paravaginal repair: a comparison of anatomic and quality of life outcomes. *Int Urogynecol J Pelvic Floor Dysfunction*. 2007;18:245–9.

Petrou SP, Franco N. Comparison of techniques for transvaginal and retropubic repair of paravaginal wall defects in the cadaver model. *J Pelvic Surg* 2003;9:15.

Richardson AC, Edmonds PB, Williams NL. Treatment of stress urinary incontinence due to paravaginal fascial defect. *Obstet Gynecol* 1981;57:357.

Richardson AC, Lyon JB, Williams NL. A new look at pelvic relaxation. *Am J Obstet Gynecol* 1976;126:568.

Shull BL. How I do abdominal paravaginal repair. *J Pelvic Surg* 1995;1:43.

Shull BL, Baden WF. A six-year experience with paravaginal defect repair for stress urinary incontinence. *Am J Obstet Gynecol* 1989;160:1432.

Shull BL, Benn SJ, Kuehl TJ. Surgical management of prolapse of the anterior vaginal segment: an analysis of support defects, operative morbidity, and anatomic outcome. *Am J Obstet Gynecol* 1994;171:1429.

Shull BL, Capen CV, Riggs MW, et al. Preoperative and postoperative analysis of site-specific pelvic support defects in 81 women treated with sacrospinous ligament suspension and pelvic reconstruction. *Am J Obstet Gynecol* 1992;166:1764.

White GR. Cystocele. A radical cure by suturing lateral sulci of vagina to white line of pelvic fascia. *JAMA* 1909;53:1707.

Zimmerman CW. Paravaginal repair: restoring the anterior vagina. *OBG Management* 2001;13:18.

CHAPTER 36D ■ POSTERIOR COMPARTMENT DEFECTS

THOMAS M. JULIAN

DEFINITIONS

Anal manometry—A test that uses a pressure-sensitive catheter to measure pressures generated in the anal canal and at the anal sphincter.

Defecography—A fluoroscopy study to assess anatomy by watching the patient evacuate radiopaque dye. It outlines sigmoidocele, enterocele, and rectocele.

Endopelvic fascia—The term used to describe in general all the supporting tissues of the pelvis.

Enterocele, rectocele—The terms historically used to describe protrusion of the vaginal apex with enteric contents or a bulge in the posterior vaginal wall, respectively.

Genital hiatus—The central opening in the pelvic floor through which passes the urethra, vagina, and rectum.

Pelvic floor dysfunction—An all-encompassing term to describe any or all of the patient's symptoms that may be related to pelvic organs. The most common symptoms in the posterior compartment will be those of a mass, the inability to begin emptying or incomplete emptying of the rectum, rectal incontinence, and discomfort or pain. No physical finding on examination is directly related to the degree of patient inconvenience.

Pericervical connective tissue ring—The location where the endopelvic connective tissue support structures become confluent around the cervix and vaginal apex.

Perineal body—A confluence of connective tissue of the bulbocavernosus muscles, transverse perineal muscle, pelvic membrane, anal sphincter, and anchoring sites to the pubic rami, and ischial tuberosities that together make up a central tendineus insertion on the perineum. It is shaped like a pyramid, with the base on the perineum, and extends cephalad 2 to 5 cm to join the rectovaginal septum.

Perineal descent—A bulge in the perineum with straining to below the ischial tuberosities. The total lack of muscular attachment allows the examiner to easily pull the perineum caudally, even against voluntary resistance by the patient.

Posterior colporrhaphy—The operation that divides the epithelium of the posterior vaginal wall and sews together the underlying tissues of the posterior vaginal wall in the midline (plicates), often from the vaginal apex to the perineal body. It is the oldest common operation to repair dysfunction thought to have an anatomic cause related to the posterior vaginal wall.

Posterior vaginal compartment (posterior compartment, posterior segment)—The posterior vaginal compartment encompasses the dorsal wall of the vagina and its supporting structures and therefore extends from the uterosacral and cardinal ligament attachments of the vagina at the pericervical connective tissue ring to the perineal body.

Rectovaginal septum (RVS) or fascia of Denonvilliers—The connective tissue immediately dorsal to the epithelium of the posterior vaginal wall. It is not a histologically distinct structure but rather a confluence of connective tissue that supports and attaches the posterior vaginal wall to the underlying rectum, lateral levator muscle, and perineal body.

Site-specific defect—An anatomic discontinuity in the pelvic connective tissue network that allows the pelvic surgeon to identify and repair a specific break in the connective tissue network of the pelvis.

Uterosacral ligaments—The posterior thickenings of the network of endopelvic connective tissue that extend separately from the midsacrum to the 5- and 7-o'clock positions on the posterior vaginal wall.

With improved understanding of female pelvic floor anatomy and pathophysiology has come change in the gynecologist's treatment of disorders of the posterior vaginal compartment, referred to throughout the remainder of this subchapter as *posterior compartment.* The current concepts used by pelvic reconstructive surgeons are well described by Carl Zimmerman in Chapter 36A. For a better understanding of this subchapter, the reader is advised to read that material before this one.

Students and practitioners interested in pelvic floor dysfunction should no longer consider patient symptoms that seem to be related to the posterior vaginal wall as being caused by a rectocele and curable with posterior colporrhaphy. Leaders in gynecologic surgery are trying to abandon the concept of rectocele and replace it with terms describing specific anatomic defects (site-specific defects).

ANATOMY IN RELATION TO PELVIC REPARATIVE SURGERY

The vagina is a hollow, pliable tube about 9 cm long anteriorly and 11 cm long posteriorly. The caudal 3 cm of the posterior vaginal wall is held in place by connective tissue attachments to the perineal body and ischiopubic rami. The midvagina attaches laterally to the connective tissue covering the medial portion of the ipsilateral levator muscle. The levator covering fuses laterally to the obturator internus fascia and ultimately to the bony pelvic sidewall. The connective tissue immediately dorsal to the epithelium of the posterior vaginal wall is called the rectovaginal septum or the fascia of Denonvilliers. The rectovaginal septum is not a histologically distinct structure but rather a confluence of connective tissue that supports and attaches the posterior vaginal wall to the underlying rectum.

The upper vagina attaches to the uterosacral ligaments on the posterior pericervical connective tissue ring and anterior to pubocervical connective tissue. The uterosacral ligaments are mainly smooth muscle, nerves, blood vessels, and some connective tissue. In the standing position, the uterosacral ligaments are almost vertical in orientation, suspending the vagina as these ligaments fan out in the retroperitoneal space into a broad attachment bilaterally over the second, third, and fourth bony sacral segments.

The cephaladmost posterior compartment is continuous with the apical vaginal compartment. The apical compartment consists of the cervix, located on the anterior vaginal wall, with its attachments to the pubocervical connective tissue anteriorly, the cardinal ligaments laterally, and the uterosacral ligaments posteriorly. The fusion of the cephalad margins of the connective tissue surrounding the cervix and upper vagina make up the pericervical connective tissue ring (Fig. 36D.1).

In posterior segment reparative surgery, the uterosacral ligaments are the major support structure. The contiguity of the connective tissue of the uterosacral ligaments with the connective tissue of the rectovaginal septum and perineal body are the suspensory mechanism holding the vagina in its normal anatomic position.

The Vaginal Axis: The Pelvic Valve Mechanism

The distal one third of the vagina in the standing individual ascends almost vertically, then angles 120 degrees dorsally in its upper two-thirds. This angulation is caused by connective tissue attachments that tether the vagina over the midline levator plate. Held in this position, the vagina will not move caudally through the opening in the pelvic floor called the genital hiatus. If the connective tissue supports do not hold the vagina in this position, the genital hiatus will not be a closed valve but rather a portal for descent of the bladder, uterus, and rectum when intrapelvic/abdominal pressure increases. Current thinking hypothesizes that the pathologic changes in the position of the vagina and contiguous organs, called *urogenital* or *genital prolapse,* results from breaks, attenuation, and/or loss of function in supporting tissues and mechanisms.

Surgery can often correct pathologic anatomic changes and resultant symptoms (pelvic floor dysfunction). When surgery is selected as the treatment, the goal becomes the restoration of the anatomic relationships by either repairing connective tissue supports or by creating a compensatory support mechanism. Although a simple concept, historically, operations did not emphasize repairing an entire connective tissue network, but were incorrectly thought of as organ specific (cystocele, enterocele, rectocele, etc.). Operations were artificially thought of as reinforcing attenuated tissues surrounding organs in contact with the vagina.

In truth, the support for the pelvis is not from ligaments and fascia but a network of connective tissue that intertwines as it surrounds organs. In surgical repair of the female pelvic organ prolapse, the gynecologist uses portions of the entire network of connective tissue, trying to restore the continuity that was lost in those tissues surrounding and supporting the uterus, bladder, vagina, and rectum. The terms *cystocele, rectocele, enterocele, urethrocele,* and *perineocele* do not aid in

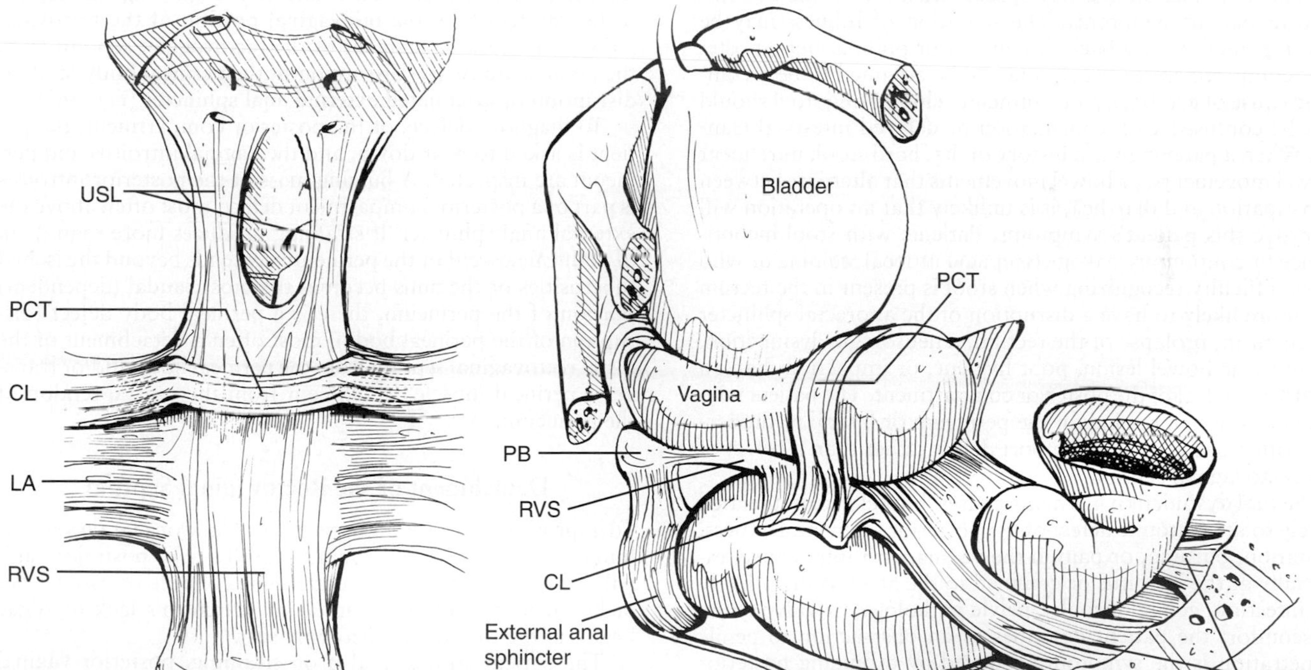

FIGURE 36D.1. The network of pelvic connective tissue. The cephalad posterior compartment is continuous with the apical vaginal compartment at the pericervical connective tissue ring. The pericervical connective tissue (*PCT*) ring is the area around the cervix where there is anteriorly pubocervical connective tissue; laterally the cardinal ligaments (*CL*); and posteriolaterally the uterosacral ligaments (*USL*), which fuse with the rectovaginal septum (RVS), which continues caudally to fuse with the perineal body (*PB*). The connective tissue network is a continuous structure. It is this network (A) that tethers and supports the vagina in its normal axis (B) over the levator ani muscle (*LA*).

understanding the loss of continuity of the connective tissue network. They are not site specific. For many surgeons, the gynecologic conditions traditionally referred to as *enterocele* and *high rectocele* are two separate entities. To the experienced pelvic surgeon, they are the same anatomic defect—detachment (loss of continuity) between the rectovaginal septum and uterosacral ligaments. Later descriptions in this discussion will not describe defects or their repair as isolated phenomena, but will try to integrate what are epiphenomena.

PATIENT SELECTION AND SURGICAL PREPARATION

History

Every surgical procedure should begin, first and always, by determining who would benefit from the operation. In our experience, symptoms of posterior compartment defects include (i) a sensation of fullness or heaviness in the vagina or pelvis made worse by activities that increase intraabdominal pressure, like lifting, exercise, or standing for long periods of time; (ii) bulging mass that increases in prominence with increased activity or as the day progresses; (iii) difficulty initiating stool evacuation from the rectum and anal canal, often accompanied by splinting of stool (placing a finger in the vagina to push stool out the rectum); (iv) feeling of incomplete stool evacuation; and (v) discomfort with intercourse, generally described by the patient as feeling like an obstruction is present.

The examiner should pay special attention to the description of patient symptoms. The sensation of fullness may be accompanied by low back discomfort or pulling, but a posterior compartment defect should not be assumed to be a common cause of low back pain. Difficulty eliminating stool should not be confused with constipation or delayed intestinal transit. When a patient gives a history of dry, hard stool, infrequent bowel movements, or bowel movements that alternate between constipation and diarrhea, it is unlikely that an operation will improve this patient's symptoms. Patients with stool incontinence or continuous leakage (seepage) or fecal staining or who have difficulty recognizing when stool is present in the rectum are more likely to have a disruption of the anorectal sphincter mechanism, prolapse of the rectum, a neurologic dysfunction, an intrinsic bowel lesion, poor hygiene, or impaction than an anatomic defect of the posterior compartment. The patient who splints stool by pressing on the perineum or lateral to the rectum often has a perineal support defect rather than a defect of the rectovaginal septum.

Sexual dysfunction has many causes, but seldom is it related solely to an anatomic defect of the posterior segment. Dryness, irritation, burning, or pain in the vagina with intercourse, especially at the introitus or confined to the apex, is more likely an infection, genital atrophy, pelvic pathology, or vulvodynia. Discomfort the patient describes as an obstruction to penile penetration is the symptom produced by a bulging posterior vaginal wall from retained stool.

Examination

Pelvic examination can be used to diagnose most posterior compartment defects in a manner that allows the examiner to identify a site-specific defect in the continuum of the pelvic connective tissue network. Knowing the underlying anatomic defect allows the surgeon to plan surgery to repair a specific defect. Most defects can be detected during examination with the patient in the dorsolithotomy position. Some examiners recommend that the patient be examined in the standing position with the examiner kneeling on the floor. In the occasional patient in whom I have not been able to find the vaginal compartment defect in the dorsolithotomy position, I have done this—but with limited success.

When a defect cannot be identified, it has been more helpful to us for the examiner to instruct the patient to get up from the examining table, strain on the toilet, perform isometric lifting, or perform whatever maneuver she feels exacerbates her symptoms. The examiner leaves while the patient does this and returns to re-examine after the provocative maneuvers have been completed. If I still cannot find an anatomic defect, the patient leaves the clinic, performs whatever activity brings on the problem and returns for examination later in the day or on another day when symptoms or findings are most prominent.

I find the following examination sequence, a modification of that described by Baden and Walker, essential to diagnose defects and plan treatment. The examination consists of: (i) providing retraction for exposure of the area of the vaginal compartment to be examined; (ii) asking the patient to strain; (iii) determining descending part of the vagina and degree of descent; (iv) simulating normal support using a ring forceps to reduce the defect; and (v) asking the patient to strain again with the ring forceps in place to see if this manual assistance (which simulates surgical repair) corrects the anatomic defect. In general, there are **five defects, which may occur alone or in any combination, that the examiner can identify in the posterior compartment: (i) detachment of the rectovaginal septum from the uterosacral/pericervical connective tissue ring; (ii) central or lateral defects in the midvaginal portion of the rectovaginal septum; (iii) detachment of the rectovaginal septum from the perineal body; (iv) disruption of the perineal body; and (v) disruption or attenuated external anal sphincter** (Fig. 36D.2).

To diagnose defects of the posterior compartment, the patient is asked to bear down, and the vaginal introitus and perineum are inspected. A bulging mass at the posterior introitus is part of a posterior compartment defect, most often above the external anal sphincter. If straining produces more than 2 cm of perineal descent or the perineum descends beyond the ischial tuberosities or the anus becomes the most caudal (dependent) portion of the perineum, there is a perineal body defect (disruption of the perineal body), most often a detachment of the distal rectovaginal septum from the perineal body and/or transverse perineal muscle detachment from the central tendon of the perineum.

Detachment of the Rectovaginal Septum

To improve visualization, the posterior blade of a Graves speculum elevates the anterior vaginal wall. Lack of posterior vaginal wall rugae indicates the underlying connective tissue is detached from the surface epithelium. Often this lack of rugae begins at the top of an episiotomy scar.

The patient strains, and if on straining, posterior vaginal wall descent occurs, there is a posterior compartment defect. If the placement of the posterior speculum blade to the vaginal apex completely reduces the descent, it is likely that the vaginal support defect is apical, involving what has been referred to as an anterior enterocele. This defect is a peritoneal sac containing small bowel, most often adherent to the posterior bladder wall. This defect is most commonly found after a colposuspension procedure.

If the defect is still present, the ring forceps are used to support the posterior vaginal fornix toward the hollow of the

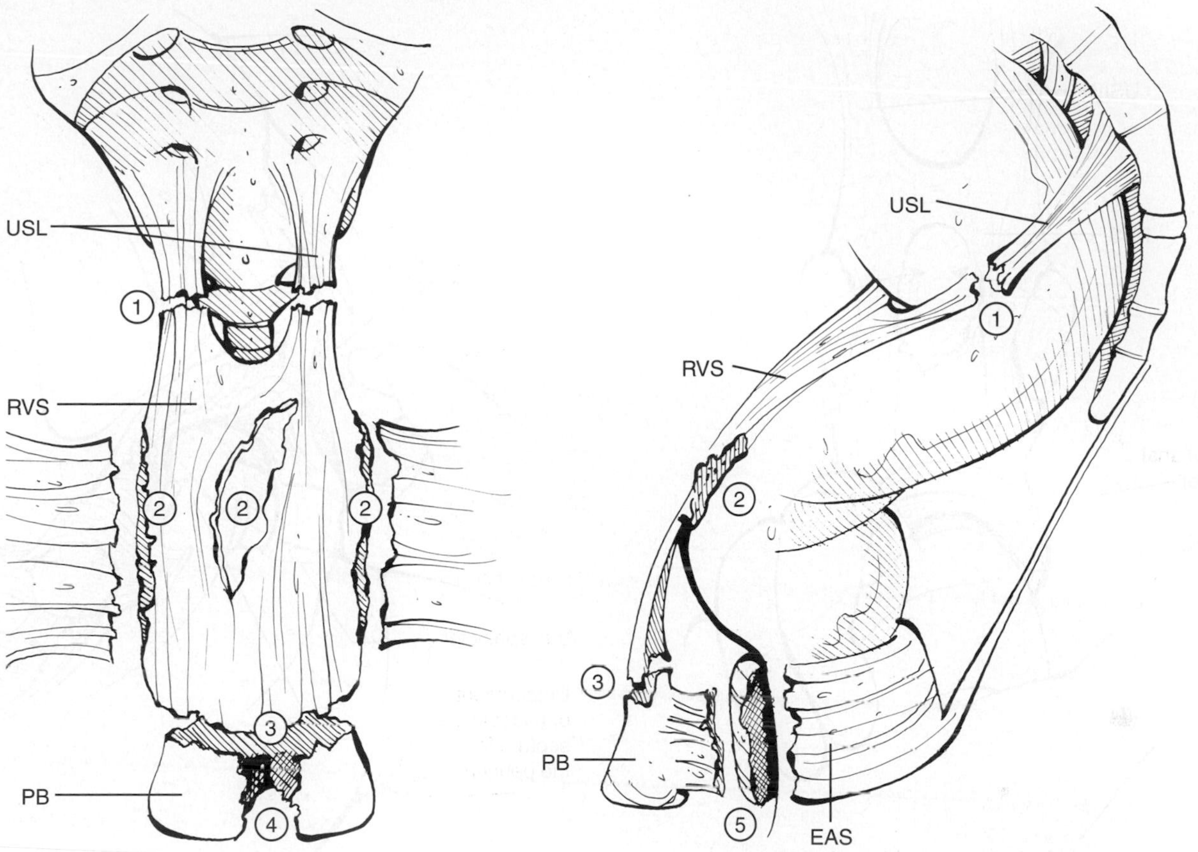

FIGURE 36D.2. There are five general ways to describe defects by site in the posterior compartment. They may occur alone or in any combination. All must be identified for successful reconstruction: (*1*) detachment of the rectovaginal septum from the uterosacral/pericervical connective tissue ring, (*2*) central or lateral defects in the midvaginal portion of the rectovaginal septum, (*3*) detachment of the rectovaginal septum from the perineal body, (*4*) disruption of the perineal body, and (*5*) disruption or attenuation of the external anal sphincter.

sacrum. If on straining, this maneuver reduces the mass in total, the defect is a detachment of the cephalad rectovaginal septum from the uterosacral ligaments. If the mass still bulges, the speculum blade should be placed on the anterior vaginal wall to the apex and the ring forceps on the posterior vaginal wall to the apex, and both are slowly withdrawn. If slow withdrawal immediately produces a bulge that enlarges as the two instruments are withdrawn, there will be a peritoneal sac with small bowel or omentum in addition to detachment of the rectovaginal septum.

As a second maneuver, the presence of this sac can be confirmed on bimanual examination. The examiner inserts one index finger in the patient's rectum and the other index finger in the vagina. The sac can be felt to slide between the examining fingers. As a third maneuver, the rectal examining finger can be inserted as high into the rectal canal as possible, and the examiner determines whether his/her finger enters the bulge. If it does, the mass is rectum alone; if it does not, there is a bowel-containing sac (enterocele) or the very rare entity of sigmoidocele. As mentioned before, there is no anatomic difference between a lack of support of the vaginal apex, traditionally called an enterocele, and the posterior compartment defect referred to as a high rectocele. Both defects result from the rectovaginal septum being detached at the cephalad portion from the pericervical connective tissue ring at the uterosacral ligaments.

Central and Lateral Defects in the Rectovaginal Septum

The midportion of the rectovaginal septum at the posterior cul-de-sac (pouch of Douglas) contains little connective tissue. The rectovaginal septum (thickened connective tissue), therefore, is not palpable centrally between the attachments of the uterosacral ligaments. About 4 cm from the apex, the connective tissue of the rectovaginal septum becomes palpable and extends to the introitus where the last 2 or more centimeters is contiguous with the perineal body.

Detection of tears or detachments of the rectovaginal septum may be done both in the office and at the time of surgery by the examiner placing a finger in the patient's rectum and sweeping widely from lateral to medial along the entire rectovaginal septum (Fig. 36D.3). When the examiner's finger palpates the defect, the digit can be seen to enter the defect, lifting the posterior vaginal wall at the defect site. Lateral defects are detachments of the rectovaginal septum from the levator fascia; central defects are breaks in the rectovaginal septum. Repeating this maneuver in the operating room is essential to find and fix defects in a site specific manner.

Detachment of the Rectovaginal Septum from the Perineal Body

The examiner's index finger is gently moved upward from the external anal sphincter toward the vaginal introitus. If there

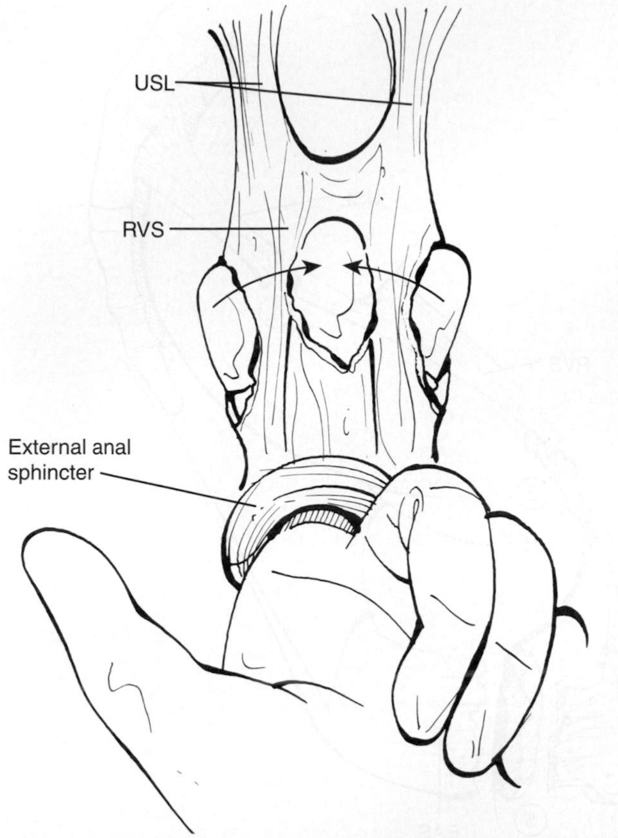

FIGURE 36D.3. Detection of tears or detachments in the rectovaginal septum can be done both in the office and at surgery. The examiner places a finger in the patient's rectum and sweeps widely from lateral to medial along the entire rectovaginal septum. The examining finger palpates the defect and can be seen to enter the defect, lifting the posterior vaginal wall. Lateral defects are detachments of the rectovaginal septum from the medial levator fascia; central defects are openings in the rectovaginal septum.

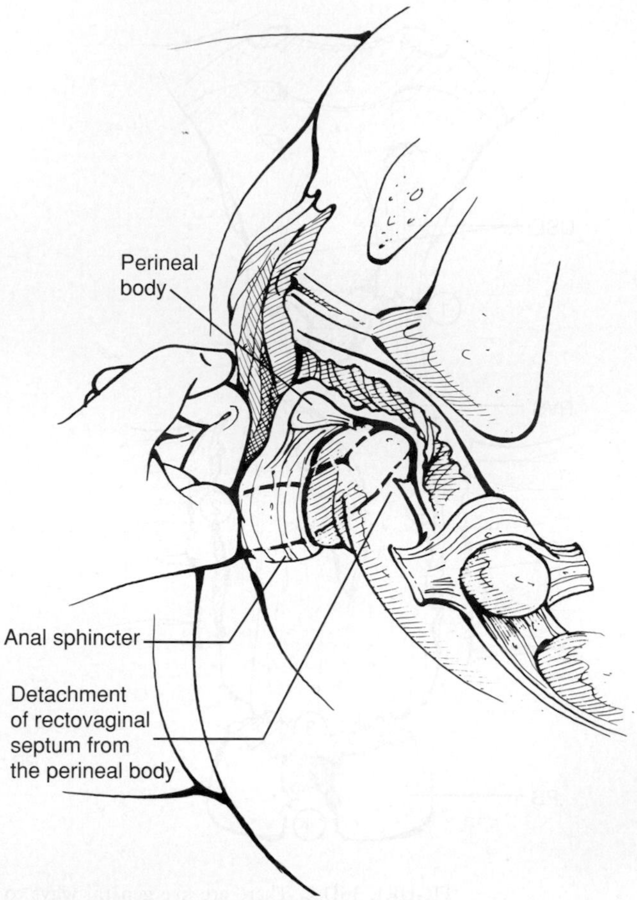

FIGURE 36D.4. Detachment of the perineal body from the rectovaginal septum is shown. The examiner's index finger is gently pushed cephalad from the external anal sphincter with pressure toward the vaginal lumen. If there is a defect at the perineal body attachment to the rectovaginal septum, the examining finger enters the defect.

is a defect at the perineal body attachment of the rectovaginal septum, the examining finger enters the defect (Fig. 36D.4).

Disruption of the Perineal Body

The rectal examining finger applies traction against the rectal side of the perineum with the examiner pulling toward him-/herself. If the perineum is very distensible and can be brought several centimeters caudally while offering little or no resistance when the patient is asked to tighten the perineal muscles, this is perineal descent. Palpating the perineum with the examiner's thumb against the ipsilateral index finger in the patient's rectum often shows that the only palpable structures seem to be the rectal wall and the perineal skin. In the patient with an intact perineal body, the perineal body is largely connective tissue and can be felt as a substantial pyramidal shaped body, 2 to 4 cm wide at its caudal margin and extending cephalad 2 to 5 cm between the vagina and external anal sphincter (Fig. 36D.4).

ADJUNCTIVE TESTING

When symptoms and physical findings are consistent with an anatomic defect, no adjunctive testing is needed before surgery for the patient with a posterior compartment disorder. Adjunctive testing including anal manometry, anal sphincter ultrasound, defecography, electrophysiologic studies, and colonic motility studies have all been reported in these patients in various studies. Anal manometry is used to measure the functional length of the anal canal and the sensation and pressures generated in the anal canal and anal sphincter. Manometry techniques are not standardized, and there is some debate as to what the limits of normal are. Its usefulness may be in identifying patients suspect for bowel storage diseases rather than as a routine diagnostic test.

Defacography is a fluoroscopic study done after ingestion or insertion of radiopaque contrast material. It can be used to outline the anatomy of a rectocele or identify an occult enterocele, sigmoidocele, perineocele, rectal intussusception, rectal prolapse, and paradoxical contracture of the puborectalis muscle during defecation. Studies have shown that interpretation of defacography has a roughly 80% interobserver reliability. Proponents argue that defecography improves the diagnostic ability for the practitioner. There are no studies showing that defacography changes clinical outcomes by changing nonsurgical or surgical management.

Electrophysiological studies of bowel function (electromyography and nerve conduction velocity), especially those measuring individual muscle response, have generally been abandoned by physical therapists and gastroenterologists because of the tests' inability to measure clinically significant parameters. For example, the differences in pudendal nerve latency studies do not directly relate to patient symptomatology or suggest that one type of treatment or procedure is better. The study has some ability to predict the likelihood of surgical success in patients undergoing external anal sphincteroplasty. Imaging with dynamic ultrasound and magnetic resonance imaging seem to show an even greater diagnostic ability to delineate anatomy than defecography.

Ultrasound for the diagnosis of anal sphincter defects offers diagnostic help for the clinician uncertain as to whether patient symptoms relate to a sphincter defect. For a rectocele, it has the same limitation as other radiologic testing.

These techniques and the management of anal incontinence are discussed in Chapter 40.

To summarize diagnosis, a competent, site-specific–directed exam allows the clinician an opportunity to assess the posterior compartment from the retroperitoneum to the perineum. Imaging and electrophysiologic testing is of limited value in a patient with an indicative history and confirmatory physical findings. To routinely add adjunctive diagnostic testing cannot be recommended in everyday practice. Adjunctive testing should rely on the judgment of the clinician. Most of the testing is not cost-efficient, nor has it been shown to improve long-term outcome. For the midposterior compartment (rectocele)—the most common problem the practicing gynecologist will face—defecography parameters, such as size, poor evacuation, barium trapping, and intussusception, have no prognostic value.

It should also be emphasized that an anatomic defect diagnosed either by history and examination or on imaging and physiologic testing often shows no correlation with the degree of patient symptomatology. Large anatomic defects may cause the patient no problem; small ones may be very symptomatic. It remains to the clinician's judgment to decide how much evaluation and treatment is needed. If the clinician cannot do so, consultation should be obtained. The asymptomatic posterior compartment defect needs neither testing nor treatment.

ALTERNATIVE THERAPIES TO SURGERY

When a posterior compartment defect has been diagnosed and the patient seeks relief from the symptoms, the clinician should have a working knowledge of how to manage those symptoms with nonsurgical alternatives. In the case of posterior compartment defects, a pessary may be tried when the symptom is thought to be secondary to a mass lesion. While no pessary is specifically designed for mass lesions in the posterior compartment, those that occupy a larger space within the vagina are most helpful in my own practice—the doughnut, inflatable ball, and cube pessaries.

For symptoms related to difficulty passing stool, a dietary and lifestyle change that includes increasing water, fiber, and exercise may be of benefit. Stool softeners, bulk-forming agents, and, in selected patients, mild laxatives can be added to make stool passage easier. These patients may benefit from counseling to assure them it is not necessary to have a bowel movement daily or even every other day. The patient who spends hours on the toilet straining should be told they may be causing damage to the pudendal nerve and the muscles of the perineum by stretching them with this unrelenting straining. In my experience, convincing the patient of this is difficult, especially in elderly patients.

Discomfort or pain is often difficult to manage nonsurgically. Pain related to intercourse may be managed by treating atrophy, lack of lubrication, or suggesting a change in sexual activity or position. Discomfort exacerbated by activity or prolonged standing can often be alleviated with a pessary. The use of a pessary before considering surgery may be a good diagnostic test to indicate how likely surgery is to help. If the pessary relieves discomfort, surgery is more likely to be beneficial. If it does not, surgery may not be the answer.

Physical therapy and biofeedback have both been shown to improve symptoms from pelvic organ prolapse, especially early stages of pelvic organ prolapse. Its greatest role may be in the treatment of paradoxical contracture of the pelvic floor with attempted defecation and anismus.

SURGERY FOR POSTERIOR COMPARTMENT DEFECTS

Preoperative Counseling

Preoperative counseling entails explaining surgical risks, benefits, and nonsurgical alternatives to the patient. Risks from repair of apical and posterior compartment defects are usually low, but this differs by the route the surgery is performed and the defect repaired. The always-present risks of infection, bleeding, and injury to bladder or bowel vary with the surgical approach taken; whether it is laparoscopy, laparotomy, transvaginal, or transrectal; whether it is simply fixing a detached or torn septum versus a repair that may need to involve bowel resection when rectal intussusception or external prolapse of rectal mucosa is present; or whether graft materials will be necessary.

The most common symptoms reported to the gynecologist are stool retention and discomfort, and the most common defect will be a detachment or a tear of the midrectovaginal septum. A review of the literature shows that there are really very few reports of the long-term success of "rectocele" repair. Studies with a year or more follow-up show success rates of 50% to 80% for treating obstructed defecation, with most tending toward the more favorable of those figures. Failure rates seem to be highest in patients with anismus or other physiologic dysfunction before surgery. The rate of persisting dyspareunia after standard posterior colporrhaphy is quoted as 15%, a figure few share with prospective surgical candidates.

Preoperative Preparation

When performing an operation with even a small risk of entering large or small bowel, many surgeons prefer that the stool be evacuated from the rectum and a single dose of preoperative antibiotic be given. Evacuating the rectal vault with a preoperative Phospho-soda enema or an oral osmotic agent is at the discretion of the surgeon who must consider the risk for causing bacterial contamination and subsequent infection for the surgery being performed. If antibiotics are to be given, they should be chosen as for any operation and given as a single intravenous dose with enough time between administration and the time of incision to ensure adequate serum levels. I check the vaginal pH; if elevated, I do a saline mount to check for bacterial vaginosis and treat with an appropriate regimen.

Positioning, Lighting, and Visualization

For transabdominal repair of the posterior compartment either by laparotomy or laparoscopy, the patient is placed in the low lithotomy position by most gynecologists to allow access to both the abdominal and vaginal fields. For transrectal repair, colorectal surgeons usually place the patient in a jackknife (ventral lithotomy) or kneeling position (using a surgical shelf) to optimize exposure to the perineum and anus. I perform nearly all posterior compartment repairs with the patient in the high dorsolithotomy position with the feet placed in candy-cane stirrups. Many surgeons prefer heavily padded leg rest–type stirrups that do not allow for as much flexion at the hip and provide support at the calf and plantar aspect of the foot, believing that these stirrups have less chance of injury from positioning. Positioning injury has never been a problem for me in thousands of vaginal reparative cases. I feel that candy-cane stirrups allow better visualization and access by assistants. The operator will be seated centrally, and the assistant, either one or two, will stand or sit (their preference) on each side of the operator.

For transvaginal repair of the posterior compartment in my practice, the vaginal and abdominal fields are sterilely prepared. I prefer a plastic drape placed to catch fluid from the cystoscopy that will be part of nearly all our pelvic reparative surgery. The anus is left undraped so that it is accessible for intraoperative rectal examination to aid in defect identification and the placement of our sutures to close fascial defects. I will change the intrarectal examining glove when going from rectum to vagina. Although evidence is insufficient to support or refute this technique, some habits die hard. A drape that comes with a finger cot that allows intrarectal examination during surgery without contamination of the examiner's glove is also available.

Exposure is maintained using mainly self-retaining retractors. A Martin arm is attached to the table to which is affixed a small Deaver retractor that elevates the anterior vaginal wall. A disposable plastic retractor that is a variation of the figure-of-eight–shaped (larger half placed toward the floor) Scott and White retractor is used along with commercially available metal hooks that come attached to stretchable plastic stays that slide into grooves on the two rings of the figure-of-eight retractor. I use self-retaining retractors for several reasons: (i) the exposure is superior to any manual human retraction; (ii) only my hands are directly in front of the wound, making it easier to see and operate; (iii) the countertension from this retractor and the ability to move the eight stays facilitate sharp dissection, which is almost exclusively what I use during the operation; (iv) this system frees the assistant to aid in the operation and mobility to better see the operation (for learning purposes); and (v) self-retaining retractors never complain, fall asleep, or get called to the emergency department or labor and delivery—also big advantages! When used correctly, this setup allows the surgeon to operate with a single scrub assistant without difficulty.

We routinely use a dilute solution of vasopressin, 10 units in 30 mL of normal saline, injected into each compartment to a volume of 8 to 10 mL. I find that this chemical tourniquet controls the minor oozing of blood that often detracts from the operation.

Operative Technique

When only the rectovaginal septum is operated on, an incision is made transversely at the junction of the perineal skin and posterior vaginal wall epithelium. If mesh is to be used, I try to lift up the vaginal epithelium without dividing it, or dividing it cephalad only far enough to provide adequate exposure.

The vaginal epithelium is dissected from the underlying connective tissue in the relatively avascular plane just beneath the epithelium. Dissecting in this plane helps identify the layer that will allow us to see the underlying connective tissue of the rectovaginal septum. Some operators try to dissect the "good stuff" from the underside of the vaginal epithelium. If the tissue that is freed by dividing the epithelium is joined side to side, it covers the true defect(s) rather than allowing the operator to identify them. The space over the rectovaginal septum is opened from the introitus, cephalad to the yellow adipose tissue of the cul-de-sac peritoneum, and laterally out to the area of the junction of the levator and obturator fascia on the pelvic sidewall.

When multiple defects are present in the rectovaginal septum, I usually correct them in the following order: (i) perineal body, (ii) midrectovaginal septum, and (iii) uterosacral ligament attachments to the rectovaginal septum. To identify these intraoperatively, the operator places an index finger in the patient's rectum, and defects are identified with a combination of visualization and palpation similar to that performed during office examination (Fig. 36D.3). It is easier to identify posterior compartment defects intraoperatively with the vaginal epithelium dissected free from the underlying rectovaginal septum. The operator advances the examining finger from the perineal-vaginal junction cephalad to find detachment of the rectovaginal septum at the perineal body, then sweeps laterally to medially on each side of the septum from the levator-obturator junction, and finally palpates and visualizes the vaginal apex connective tissue attachment.

Once identified, these defects are closed by direct approximation of the disrupted connective tissue with interrupted sutures directly along the configuration of the tear. When patient tissues look healthy and seem strong, but just torn, I use 0-polyglycolic acid or polyglactin 910 suture (both delayed absorbable) on a CT-1 or CT-2 needle. These sutures maintain 50% tensile strength at 2 weeks; therefore, successful repair relies on a normal patient healing response. When tissue healing may not be optimal (elderly, immunocompromised, suspected connective tissue compromise, repeat-procedure patients), I close the defects with a permanent suture, such as a coated (polybutilate or silicone), 00-braided, polyester suture on an MO-7 needle. Our needles are swaged on with controlled release, making them easy and quick to use. The CT-2 and MO-7 needles are small, tapered and heavy gauge with a 3/8 curve and fit into small spaces with the ability to penetrate dense tissues. My thinking with the use of permanent suture is that tissue of lesser quality may stay joined together better with a longer period of assisted approximation. Tissue suture purchases are made as deeply into the connective tissue of the rectovaginal septum as possible, avoiding the rectal lumen with assistance from the rectal examining finger.

When the surgeon has a single assistant, the operator grasps each edge of the torn rectovaginal septum after identification with an Allis clamp, starting at the location where the separation is most obvious. Marking with the Allis clamp allows the surgeon to remove the finger from the rectum when closing the defect. Once the most obvious area of the defect is brought together, the defect on either side becomes easier to see, making subsequent tissue purchases similarly easier to place.

I do not use running closures to approximate connective tissue defects. Running closure bunches up tissue and makes for a poorer "fit" that may compromise the vaginal caliber. When closed as described above, the repair is less likely to form the palpable tissue "bridges," often a source of complaint after traditional midline plication repairs. The reason for tissue bridging with traditional posterior colporrhaphy is that some suture purchases when placed will include the disrupted rectovaginal connective tissue and some will not. When "hits" and "misses" occur, bridges are formed (Fig. 36D.5A–D). With site-specific repair (one that repairs the identified connective tissue

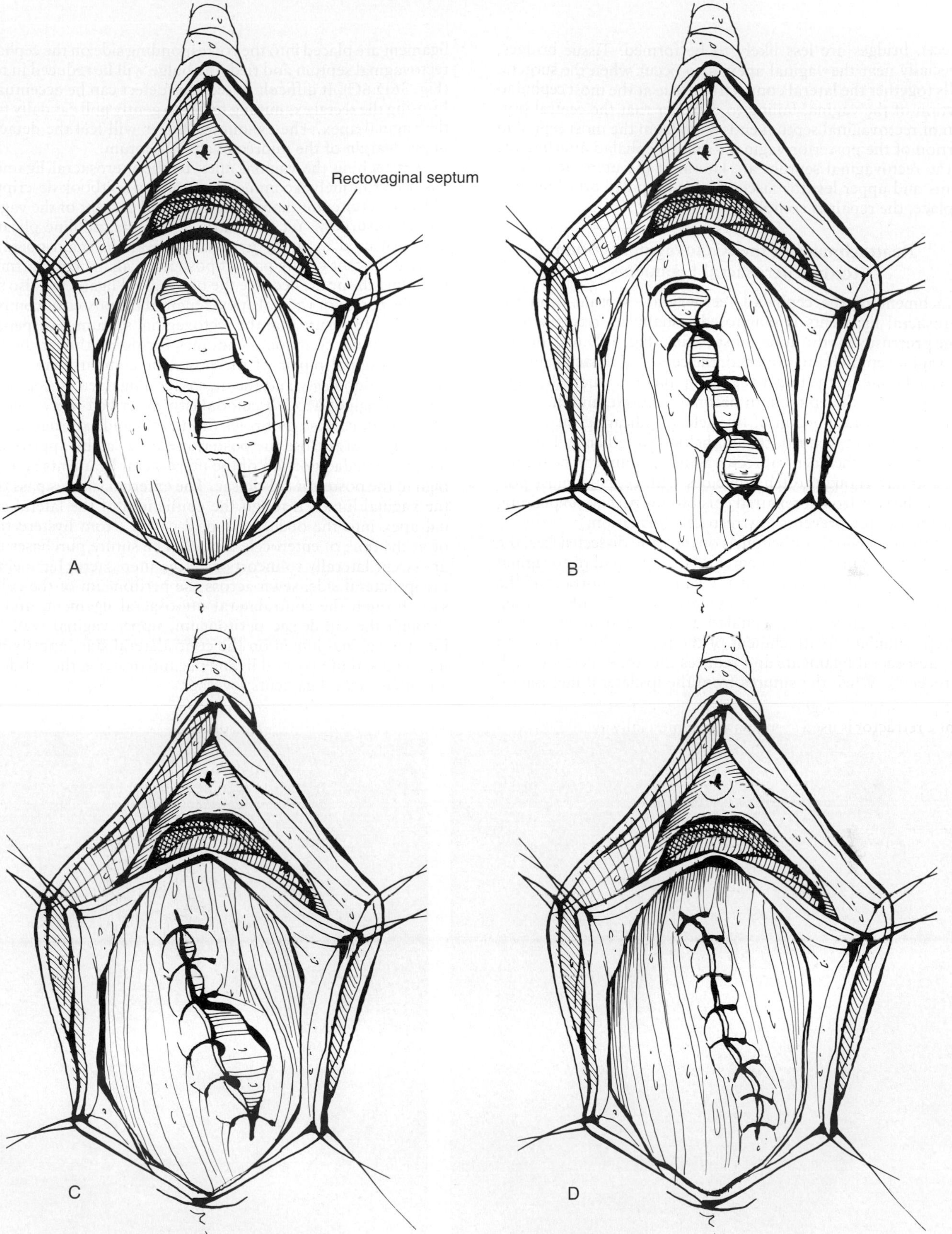

FIGURE 36D.5. The reason for tissue bridging with traditional posterior colporrhaphy is that some suture purchases include each side of the torn rectovaginal connective tissue and some do not. When "hits" and "misses" occur, bridges are produced. **A:** Defect that begins below the cul-de-sac. **B:** The result of a repair that starts too high and uses wide midline suture purchase. **C:** Results from narrow midline purchases. **D:** Site-specific repair.

defect), bridges are less likely to be formed. Tissue bridges, especially near the vaginal apex, also occur when the surgeon pulls together the lateral connective tissue at the most cephalad portion of the vagina, failing to consider that the central portion of rectovaginal septum ends 4 cm from the most cephalad portion of the posterior vaginal fornix. Cephalad attachments of the rectovaginal septum are lateral at the uterosacral ligaments and upper levator fascia. If this cephalad attachment is in place, the repair is complete.

Reattachment of the Rectovaginal Septum to the Uterosacral Ligaments

Detachment of the cephalad rectovaginal septum from the uterosacral ligaments is diagnosed visually by recognizing a large protrusion at the uppermost vagina (Fig. 36D.6A). Before the vaginal epithelium is opened, the cephalad detachment can seen as the site on the intact vaginal epithelium where the vaginal rugae end, the epithelium becomes smooth, and the bulge ends at the distal portion of the defect, indicating there is no connective tissue beneath the epithelium to tether it. This site where the detached central rectovaginal septum can be found, interestingly enough, often coincides with cephaladmost portion of the scar from a repaired episiotomy, perhaps explaining why episiotomy prevents low rectocele formation.

Once the vaginal epithelium is opened and dissected free, the bulge becomes more prominent, and the cephalad rectovaginal septum is readily apparent at the caudalmost portion of the bulge, where its edges can be grasped (Fig. 36D.6B). Pulling the rectovaginal septum cephalad at its lateral margins with forceps simulates reattachment of the rectovaginal septum to the uterosacral ligaments and reduces the upper defect ("high rectocele"). When the sutures from the ipsilateral uterosacral ligament are placed into the corresponding side on the cephalad rectovaginal septum and tied, the bulge will be reduced in total (Fig. 36D.6C). If difficult to see, this defect can be accentuated by using the rectal examining finger to gently pull caudally from the vaginal apex. The examining finger will feel the detached upper margin of the midrectovaginal septum.

Reattaching the vaginal apex to the uterosacral ligaments has been routinely recommended in every textbook description of hysterectomy for many years to avoid descent of the vaginal apex postsurgery. Yet for nearly 100 years, midline plication has been used by many gynecologists as the main operation to treat descent of any part of posterior vaginal compartment, including the apex. Because the uterosacral ligaments also support the posterior vaginal apex, repair of the posterior compartment should ensure that the rectovaginal septum is suspended. The two most common techniques for doing this at the time of transvaginal repair of the posterior compartment are the McCall culdoplasty and the uterosacral ligament suspension.

The original McCall culdoplasty, described in Chapter 37 of this text, consisted of rows of internal and external sutures. Internal sutures close the posterior cul-de-sac by approximating the cephalad portion of the uterosacral ligaments at a level high in the posterior cul-de-sac. The external sutures pass from the vaginal lumen through the epithelium of the lateral vaginal apex into the open peritoneal cavity (from hysterectomy or at the time of enterocele repair). The suture purchases then are swept laterally to incorporate the uterosacral ligament on the ipsilateral side, sewn across the peritoneum of the cul-de-sac, through the contralateral uterosacral ligament, and out through the cul-de-sac peritoneum, upper vaginal wall, and into the vaginal lumen on the contralateral side, approximating the distal uterosacral ligaments and drawing the cul-de-sac and uterosacral ligaments together.

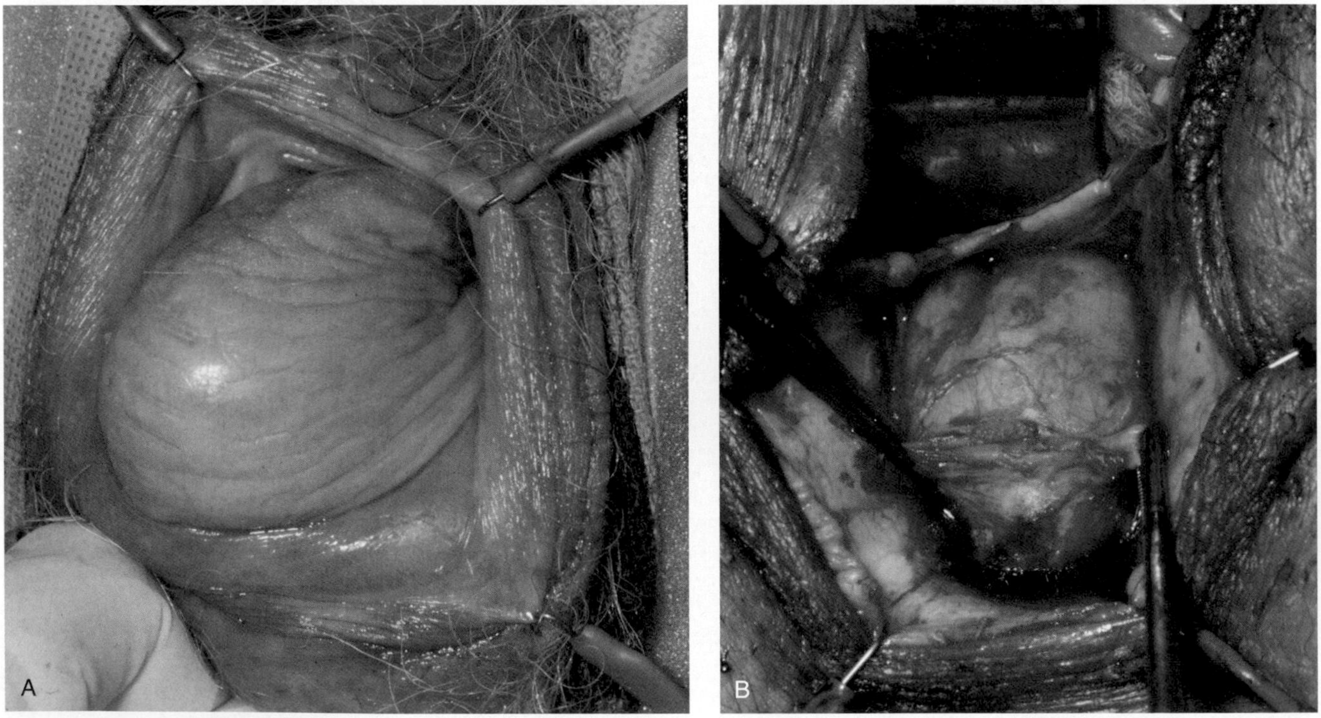

FIGURE 36D.6. Detachment of the cephalad rectovaginal septum from the uterosacral ligaments is diagnosed visually by recognizing a large protrusion at the uppermost vagina (**A**) and grasping the lateral aspects of the detached midportion of the rectovaginal septum that will be present at the caudal portion of the bulge (**B**). Joining the upper rectovaginal septum to the uterosacral ligaments repairs this defect (**C**).

The McCall operation has been successful as an operation for prophylaxis against enterocele formation and descent of the vaginal apex after surgery, a reparative procedure for vault prolapse, and as a rescue operation for recurrent vault prolapse after failed apical suspension surgery. Disadvantages of this operation are entrapment or kinking the ureters, difficulty identifying the uterosacral ligaments, and narrowing of the cephalad vagina.

Recently, many gynecologic surgeons have changed from the McCall culdoplasty to using the uterosacral ligaments for both primary reattachment as a prophylactic measure at the time of hysterectomy and as a reparative technique for posthysterectomy apical compartment prolapse. The most important step in uterosacral ligament suspension, and often the most challenging part of this operation, is identifying the uterosacral ligaments. Identification of the uterosacral ligaments can be done in three ways:

- When the posterior cul-de-sac peritoneum is open with the patient in the dorsolithotomy position, the cul-de-sac peritoneum is grasped and elevated ventrally, placing the uterosacral ligament on tension and allowing visualization and palpation of the ligament through the peritoneal side of the cul-de-sac. This technique is usually combined with palpation of the ureter against the lateral pelvic sidewall to make sure both structures are free.
- The uterosacral ligament is identified anatomically by its position just medial and deep to the ischial spine and by placing a suspension stitch just medial to the ischial spine. This method offers several disadvantages in my opinion. First, the uterosacral ligament is not clearly identified. Second, the placement of the suture at the level of the ischial spine will suspend the vaginal vault no higher than the ischial spine. Some patients' vaginal length is well above this level, and repairing the vault in this manner causes it to droop downward. Third, a deep blind purchase with needle and suture into this tissue may offer support, much like the prespinous fascial suspension described by Meeks and colleagues, but too deep a purchase may penetrate the sacrospinous ligament in its most lateral portion under the coccygeus muscle, going far enough dorsally to injure the pudendal nerve, resulting in postoperative buttock pain. This is one of the reasons sacrospinous ligament fixation sutures are placed two finger breadths medial to the ischial spine.
- The uterosacral ligament is identified by relying on transrectal palpation of the uterosacral ligament as tension is applied on the ipsilateral cu-de-sac. This is the method I use.

Transrectal Identification of the Uterosacral Ligament by Palpation

I use this technique to identify the uterosacral ligament for several reasons.

- With the examiner's finger in the patient's rectum, tension is applied toward the examiner using an Allis clamp on the ipsilateral cul-de-sac (Fig. 36D.7). The surgeon can trace by direct palpation the uterosacral ligament in almost all patients from its disrupted attachment at the vagina to near the sacrum, allowing suspension of the vagina as high as is appropriate based on the length of the vagina to be suspended.
- The uterosacral ligament has characteristic features by palpation; it is very dense, strong, mobile, about the caliber of a pencil, and tracks dorsal and medial to the lateral margin of the midsacrum.

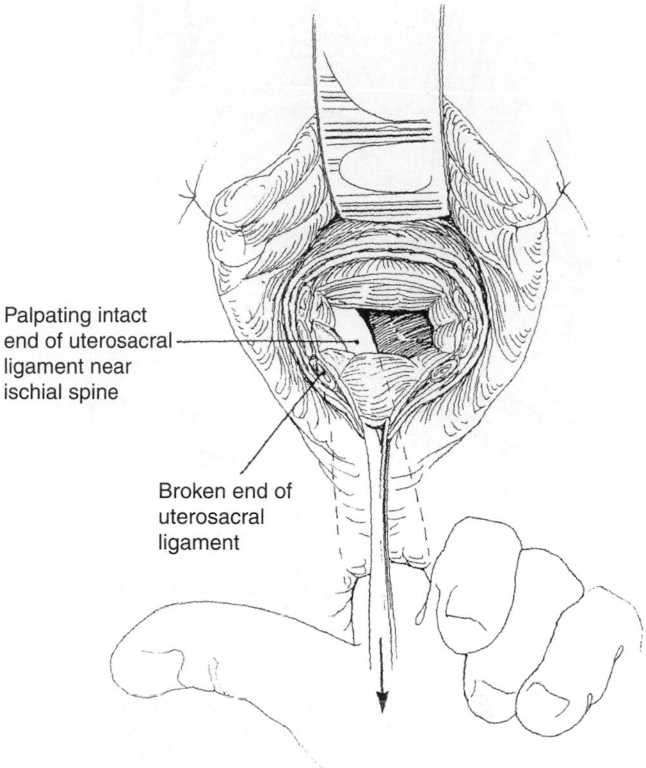

FIGURE 36D.7. With the examiner's finger in the patient's rectum and tension applied on the ipsilateral cul-de-sac, the surgeon directly palpates the uterosacral ligament from its disrupted attachment at the vagina to near the sacrum.

- With the examiner's finger on the ligament, the uterosacral ligament can be grasped with an Allis clamp, and sutures can be placed directly into the body of the ligament at any level. The higher the placement, the farther the ligament is from the ureter. By placing the suture directly into the body of the ligament and always placing the suture from lateral to medial, the surgeon is certain the ureter, which is always lateral to the uterosacral ligament, is not harmed.

I place a cephalad and a caudal suture into the ligament. The higher stitch is used to attach anterior vaginal wall connective tissue to prevent the apical descent of the anterior compartment (high cystocele), the most common compartmental defect found after vaginal reparative surgery. The lower, caudal suture is used to suspend the posterior vaginal wall. I use 00-braided polyester sutures for these stitches to maintain suture integrity for this vital support function. Delayed absorbable suture will have lost most of its tensile strength by the third postoperative week, which is about 2 months short of the time it takes to form maximum tissue strength after an operation.

When not using mesh, the 2-0 braided polyester sutures are tied after the assistant grasps the corresponding site of placement on the vagina and approximates this to the uterosacral ligament it will join. This takes the tension off the suture as it is tied and serves as a check to see how the repair fits the patient. In nearly all cases, this satisfactorily elevates the vaginal cuff and closes the connection of the genital hiatus and pelvis. The anterior and posterior vaginal walls are approximately central with delayed absorbable suture.

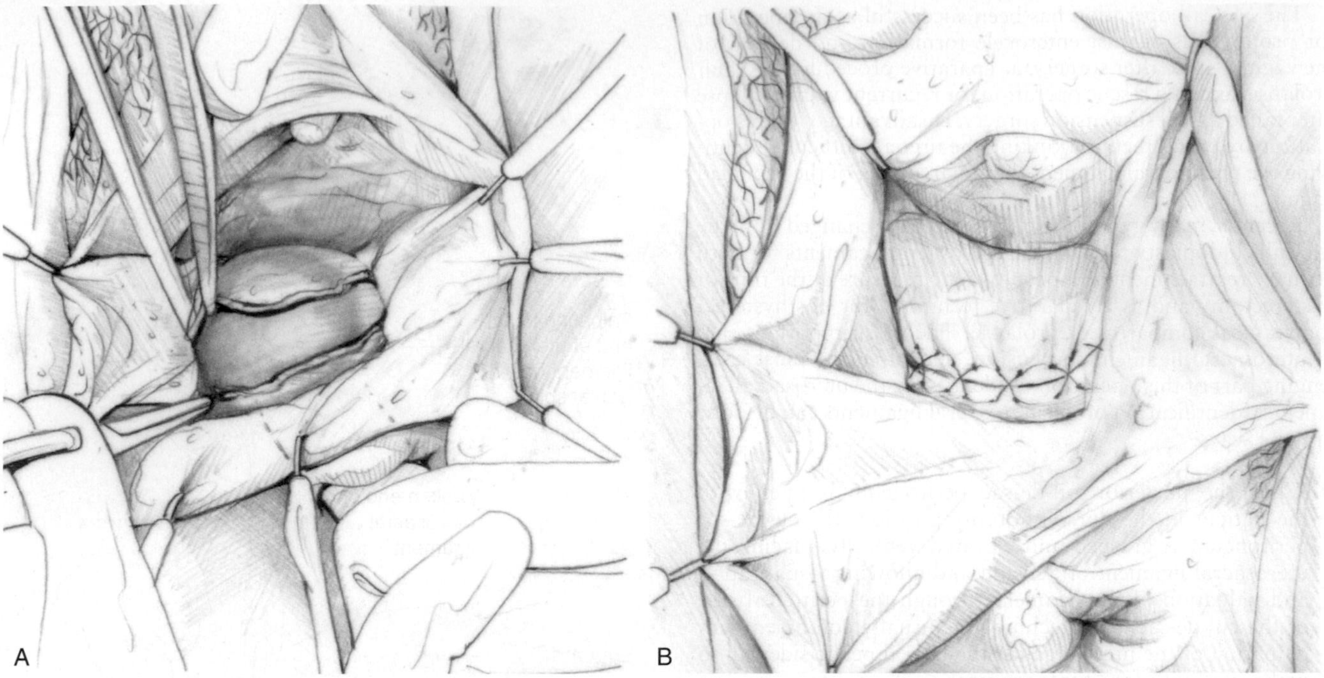

FIGURE 36D.8. The caudalmost portion of the rectovaginal septum must be reattached to the perineal body. This detachment is demonstrated using rectal examination (**A**), and this same view is shown again once the defect has been closed (**B**).

Detachment of the Rectovaginal Septum from the Perineal Body

The caudalmost portion of the rectovaginal septum must be reattached to the perineal body. This defect can easily be felt and seen during rectal examination. The detachment is almost always transverse and right at the level of the perineal body (Fig. 36D.8A). It is closed with interrupted sutures to approximate the two structures (Fig. 36D.8B).

Disruption of the Perineal Body (Perineal Descent Syndrome)

The posterior compartment cannot be repaired completely unless there is a perineal body to which the rectovaginal septum can be attached. I often see disruption of the perineal body presenting as a "failed rectocele repair." The patient still has the symptom of incomplete emptying of stool and often splints the perineum or lateral to the anus to evacuate stool, rather than splinting through the vagina. On examination with the patient bearing down, there may be little or no posterior compartment descent above the vaginal introitus, but the perineum descends, and on palpation, the examiner feels nothing at the perineal body other than rectal mucosa and perineal epithelium.

This posterior compartment defect cannot be repaired by making a small V-shaped incision at the perineum and sewing the skin and superficial connective tissue together or by sewing together the insertions of the bulbocavernosus muscles at the perineum. I have found that the operation performed in this manner often includes a crown stitch, which pulls together the left and right margins of the introitus and results in a ridge. The ridge at the time of intercourse acts like a speed bump and causes dyspareunia. I see this condition several times each year, occurring after perineoplasty and episiotomy repair. I would advise against the crown stitch as a technique to either reduce the caliber of the introitus or lengthen the vaginal canal.

Repair of the perineal body requires reapproximation of the structures that attach at the central tendon of the perineum: the rectovaginal septum, the lateral dorsal bulbocavernosus muscle insertions, the transverse perineal muscle, and the external anal sphincter. The attachments of the perineal body to the inferior pubic rami, ischial tuberosities, and coccyx have always been intact in these patients and require no revision, only a central disruption exists.

To begin the repair, a midline incision from the posterior introitus to the external anal sphincter is made. The skin overlying the perineum is widely dissected until the remnants of the transverse perineal muscle can be seen. Wide deep purchases of these muscles and any overlying connective tissue are taken and tied to approximate these muscles. Most of the time, three to five sutures (2-0 polydioxanone) are required. With the laxity of the perineum, these muscles generally are easily approximated. I will imbricate these muscles with a second layer of interrupted sutures to reinforce the repair. The repair may seem "thick" at this point in the operation, but it will not be as thick at the 6 weeks examination after surgery. I will then make sure the external anal sphincter is attached to the most dorsal portion of the perineal repair with interrupted sutures and that the bulbocavernosus muscles are attached at the ventral and lateral margins of the reapproximated perineal body. When this operation is done correctly, a rectovaginal examination will allow the examiner to feel the pyramid-shaped perineal body, which will now be about 5 cm long and 3 cm thick at its base.

Vaginal/Perineal Closure

It is common for the gynecologic surgeon to "trim excess vaginal epithelium," then close the vaginal epithelium as a midline structure, but I have gotten away from this technique to closing the vaginal epithelium as one would a skin graft. I tack down the undersurface of the lateral margins of the detached vaginal epithelium from apex to perineum, then move medially and put in a second row. This allows the epithelium to be used to cover the repair as it fits, rather than just amputating vaginal epithelium and closing with a running midline suture. It eliminates much dead space and makes a better fit with less trimming and resultant narrowing of the vagina.

Authorities in the past have written that closing this dead space does not allow the vagina to physiologically "slide" one layer over another. There is no evidence to show that this "sliding" phenomenon really takes place. Certainly if one has done enough second and third operations after failed prolapse surgery, one can attest to the fact that the vaginal epithelium may be densely adherent without much movement to facilitate dissection in previously operated areas. Even in the patient who has never been operated on, the caudalmost 4 or 5 cm of the vagina seldom demonstrate a facile cleavage plane and certainly does not slide. The connective tissue from the perineal body is densely intertwined; it is not until several centimeters cephalad during the dissection of the vaginal wall that it separates easily from underlying connective tissue.

Mesh Placement at the Time of Apical Posterior Compartment Repair

In my practice, the most common circumstance for using mesh in posterior compartment repair is suspending the apical compartment and reattaching the rectovaginal septum to the uterosacral ligaments. These two reattachments, traditionally referred to as *repair of a posterior enterocele* and *repair of a high rectocele,* are thought of as separate operations; but in my experience, they are the same.

In repairing these defects, a peritoneal sac containing small intestine, omentum, or sigmoid colon is often found. I isolate this sac by dissecting it free from the surrounding tissues. The sac is opened; the omentum, small bowel, or sigmoid colon is packed out of the sac into the abdominal cavity with a tail sponge or smaller sponge with a suture sewn through it; and the suture is tagged to a surgical clamp. This aids in visualization of the posterior cul-de-sac.

Figure 36D.9A–D shows the repair. The margins of the opened sac are placed on traction using the self-retaining retractor with plastic stays and hooked metal end. This exposes the posterior pelvis. With an examining finger in the patient's rectum, the ipsilateral cul-de-sac is placed on traction and the uterosacral ligament identified, as previously described in this chapter. Two sutures of 2-0 braided polyester are placed through each ligament (Fig. 36D.9A).

After placing the permanent sutures, the cul-de-sac peritoneum is closed at the neck of the sack high in the pelvis, above the cephalad uterosacral stitch of 2-0 braided polyester suture, with a purse-string suture of 0 silk, which is tied after removing the pack (Fig. 36D.9B). The excess peritoneal sac is partially excised. I retain a small area of the sac below the 0-silk purse-string suture to close over the mesh once it is placed. Entering the peritoneum and excising the peritoneal sac, once thought to be crucial to repair of an apical compartment defect containing viscera (enterocele), is probably not necessary because the peritoneal sac and its contents are not the cause of the defect, nor is closure of this sac helpful in restoring anatomic support. I identify the sac and dissect it free to determine if it is an anterior enterocele connected to the posterior bladder wall, which would indicate the need for increased caution in its closure. Reduction of the peritoneal sac also improves surgical visualization. It may well be just as effective to reduce the sac by inverting it and closing over it before the actual surgical repair of the defect.

The repair should reattach the uterosacral ligaments to the rectovaginal septum posteriorly and the pubocervical fascia anteriorly. Doing this suspends the vagina more horizontally over the levator plate, preventing descent of the vagina through the genital hiatus. This is accomplished by sewing the caudal 2-0 braided polyester suture in the uterosacral ligaments into the rectovaginal septum at its lateral margins, not centrally where many surgeons reattach them. I also place the suture into the posterior apical vaginal wall, avoiding penetration into what will be the vaginal lumen. The cephalad permanent suture in the uterosacral ligaments is sewn to the lateral margins of the pubocervical fascia.

In those patients in whom the connective tissue is thought to be inadequate to reattach the uterosacral ligaments to the connective tissue anteriorly and posteriorly, I place the permanent sutures as always, but a 2- to 5-cm elliptical piece of polypropylene mesh is used to fill the space (Fig. 36D.9C). In this repair, it is important to close the peritoneal sac so that bowel does not contact mesh. Mesh and bowel contact induces severe adhesion formation in the abdomen, predisposing to pain, bowel obstruction, and fistula formation. The elliptical piece of polypropylene mesh is sewn to the uterosacral ligaments, one long side of the ellipse to the cephalad 2-0 braided polyester suture and the opposite long side to the caudal uterosacral suture. When tied, they close the space at the top of the apical compartment (Fig. 36D.9D). The remaining edges of the ellipse are sewn into the underlying connective tissue to make sure the mesh lies flat. Within 2 weeks after surgery, native tissue will infiltrate the mesh, and the mesh will be firmly fixed in place.

Laparoscopy and Laparotomy in the Treatment of Posterior Compartment Defects

Transabdominal uterosacral ligament suspension is enjoying a resurgence as the gynecologic surgical community remembers what it seems to have once forgotten: Suspension of the vagina is an important part of vaginal reconstruction, especially after hysterectomy. Reattachment of the uterosacral ligaments to the vaginal vault at hysterectomy has long been described as a preventative measure against vault prolapse and enterocele formation. When the posterior cul-de-sac was considered to be deep, enterocele was prevented by sewing the posterior cul-de-sac closed with either sequential, concentric purse-string sutures placed from the caudal posterior cul-de-sac to the level of the uterosacral ligaments, incorporating peritoneum over the sacrum (Moschowitz procedure), if necessary, or by closing the cul-de-sac by sewing the posterior vaginal wall from its most caudal to most cephalad position to the rectum back to front in parallel rows (Halban culdoplasty). Little data exist measuring the success of these procedures, but they should be fundamentally sound.

Most transabdominal procedures suspend the vaginal apex, but do not deal effectively with the distal one half of the vagina or perineum. With the increasing use of laparoscopic surgery, more surgeons are repairing all compartments of the pelvic floor, including the posterior compartment with laparoscopic techniques. Sacrocolpopexy operations use mainly synthetic mesh grafts to suspend the vaginal apex from near the sacral promontory.

Most surgeons will use a synthetic mesh graft fashioned with a central trunk adjoined to anterior and posterior limbs. The anterior limb is sutured to the anterior vaginal wall dorsal

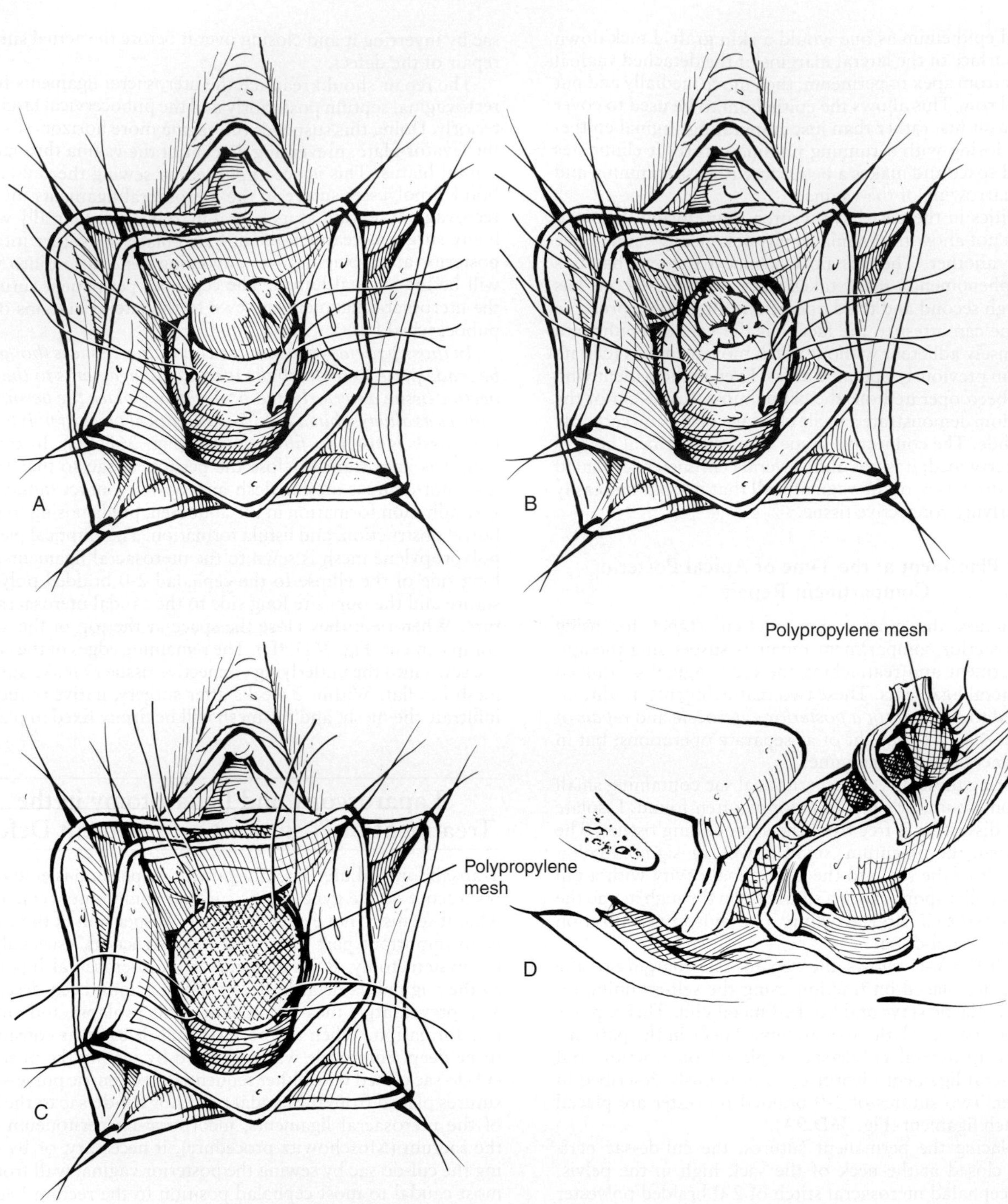

FIGURE 36D.9. When native connective tissue is inadequate to repair the apical defect (enterocele), I place permanent sutures in the uterosacral ligaments after opening and excising the enterocele sack (**A**). I close the enterocele sack neck with a 0-silk purse-string suture (**B**). The four polyester sutures are sewn through a 2- to 5-cm elliptical piece of polypropylene mesh (**C**). When tied, this closes the space at the top of the apical compartment and restores the vaginal axis. The polyester sutures will be sewn to the respective cephalad anterior and posterior vaginal wall connective tissue at the apices, changing the vaginal axis (**D**).

to the freed bladder, and the posterior limb is sutured to the posterior vaginal wall where it has been freed from overlying peritoneum or rectum. The posterior mesh limb can be used to correct posterior compartment defects near the apex and generally caudally to the midvagina. Traditionally, surgeons secure each mesh limb with four to six permanent sutures from the midvagina to the vaginal apex. To correct the most caudal defects, including detachment and/or disruption of the perineal body, surgeons extend the posterior mesh limb to the perineum to perform *sacrocolpoperineopexy*. In addition to being a

21-letter word, this operation is thought to hold the entire posterior compartment from the perineum to the sacrum in place.

Other pelvic reparative surgeons have used a combined transabdominal sacrocolpopexy with transvaginal repair to place the extended posterior mesh limb. Some surgeons will do the sacrocolpoperineopexy to the midvagina and then operate through a transvaginal approach, keeping the surgical fields separate to fix the caudalmost portion of the posterior defects. The number of reports of sacrocolpoperineopexy is limited. Some reports indicate that there is an increased incidence of infection with combined abdominal-perineal procedures using mesh.

COMPLICATIONS

Intraoperative Bleeding

To prevent excess bleeding, I use several techniques. The injection of a dilute solution of vasopressin, 10 units in 30 to 50 mL of normal saline, injected into the area to be dissected immediately before the incision decreases blood loss by about one third, helps clear the operative field of blood for about 75 minutes, and facilitates identification of planes by its hydrodissection effect. Although it was once thought that the use of vasoconstrictors (chemical tourniquets) increases the likelihood of delayed hemorrhage and increases the incidence of postoperative infection, several recent studies have shown the opposite.

The use of sharp dissection, rather than blunt dissection, allows better identification of surgical planes and the small vessels. To control bleeding sites, I use cautery sparingly and rely heavily on fine 3-0 and 4-0 sutures on a small caliber needle (SH-1, RB), theorizing that electrocautery destroys tissue, and the smaller the hole made when suturing to control bleeding, the better hemostasis will be.

To control bleeding from a particular site, I often pack the small area first with thrombin-soaked oxidized cellulose, pack a small sponge over this, and work in another area rather than chase bleeding. Small bleeding areas will stop on their own after this, and I save time (and blood loss) by completing the remainder of the operation while allowing the troublesome ooze to be controlled by packing and thrombin.

Sometimes bleeding from the connective tissue of the rectovaginal septum can be most effectively controlled by using the vaginal epithelial layer as a bolster. We do not sew directly into the rectovaginal septum, but place sutures through the vaginal epithelium into the septum where bleeding occurs and pass the suture back through the vaginal epithelium. This allows the vaginal epithelium to be tied down on top of the bleeding site, using it as an extra tissue bolster to tamponade the bleeding.

Injury to the Rectum

In anticipation of injury to the rectum, many gynecologic surgeons will prepare the bowel or at least the distal bowel with purging regimens, laxatives, or enemas. Although this is commonly done by many gynecologic surgeons for operations in which the incidence of rectal injury is estimated at 1% to 2% of all cases, it is no longer a routine for obstetricians to use enemas before vaginal delivery, in which lacerations of the rectal sphincter and wall are estimated to be 5% of cases.

I do not prep the bowel. I give a single preoperative antibiotic dose, evacuate the distal rectum digitally in the operating room at the time of exam under anesthesia, and repair any rectal injury during surgery by irrigating it, closing it in layers, and having patients use the same stool-softening regimen as I would for any vaginal reparative surgery. It is interesting that the gynecologic surgeon is concerned with entering the rectum and the colorectal surgeon with entering the vagina. Each sees the area that is "not their own" as a contaminated area to be avoided at all cost. Because both specialties have very few rectal complications, it shows us how tradition precludes evidence.

Ureteral Injury

Operations on the posterior compartment may be complicated by ureteral injury. I do cystoscopy after the administration of intravenous indigo carmine dye for nearly all of our vaginal reparative surgery cases, both to teach residents how to do it and because the literature shows some series with very high rates of unrecognized ureteral compromise after gynecologic surgery. In all my years of reparative surgery, I have had only one procedure complicated by ureteral compromise, which was resolved by removing the McCall culdoplasty sutures. However, I do feel cystoscopy is so simple and reassuring that all gynecologists should be able to perform this safety check after every pelvic support operative procedure.

When I cannot demonstrate flow of intravenous indigo carmine dye from a ureter, I give a small dose of furosemide. If unsuccessful, I have retrograde catheters passed. If a catheter can easily be passed 10 cm up from the ureter orifices, injury is unlikely. If the ureteral stent cannot be passed, which is seen in about half the cases of vaginal eversion, retrograde dye studies can be performed in the operating room and patency confirmed radiographically.

The Surgically Small Vagina

During surgery, vaginal caliber and depth should be assessed after each part of the procedure, whether performed on the anterior, apical, or posterior compartment. One of the advantages of site-specific repair is that it seldom results in tissue bridging, vaginal shortening, or reduction of vaginal caliber. When any of these are encountered, there are a number of options available to the surgeon. In the case of bridging, the defect should be rechecked to make sure that the fascial edges are approximated along the defect. If the defect has been closed in a site-specific manner and the vagina still contains palpable bridges, the repair needs to be taken down and either redone or a graft placed where the bridging exists. Graft material may be an autograft, allograft, xenograft, or synthetic graft.

In taking down the repair, the operator needs to determine if the true defect has been closed along lines of tissue breaks. If it has not, it can be closed along these lines, and bridging should be eliminated.

Placing a graft to alleviate bridging requires removing the sutures causing the bridging and identifying the edges of the defect that is not being adequately closed; this results in the pulling together of the tissues involved in the bridge (Fig. 36D. 10A). The defect in the rectovaginal connective tissue is measured and the graft cut to a shape slightly larger than the defect left from bridge removal. For a small defect, I cut a full-thickness skin graft from the thigh or buttock from skin that has been sterilely prepared within the surgical field (Fig. 36D.10B). In harvesting the graft, I follow Langer's lines and choose a site that will not be under pressure during sitting. The graft harvest site is closed with fine absorbable suture and covered with a

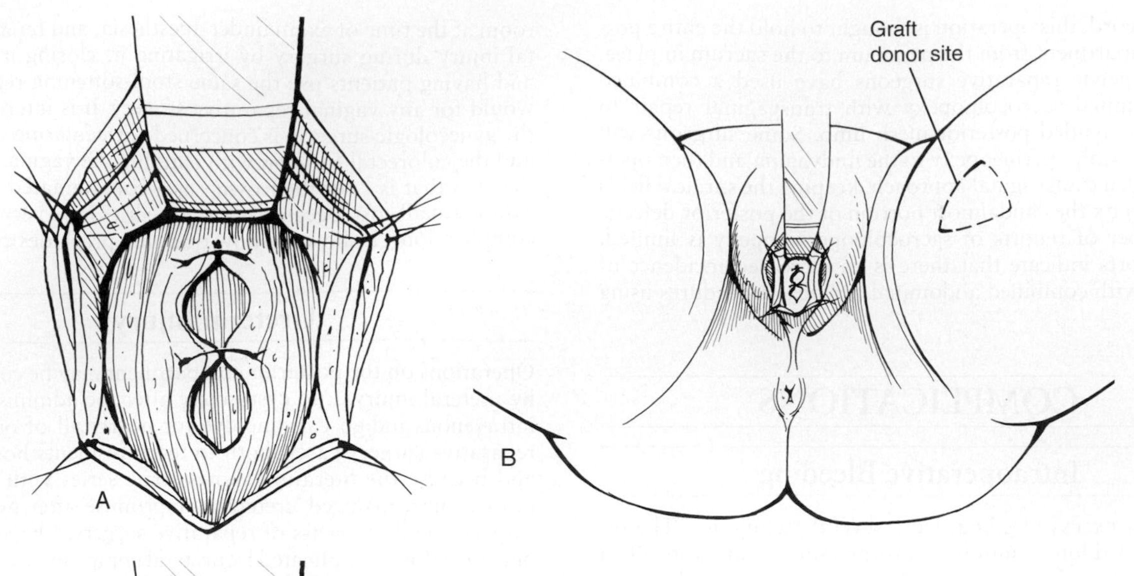

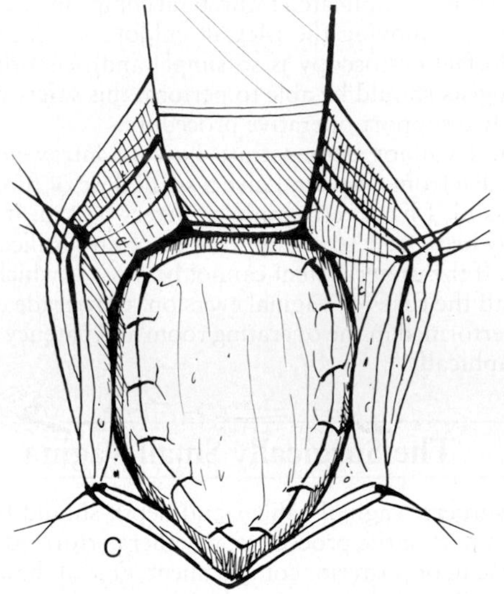

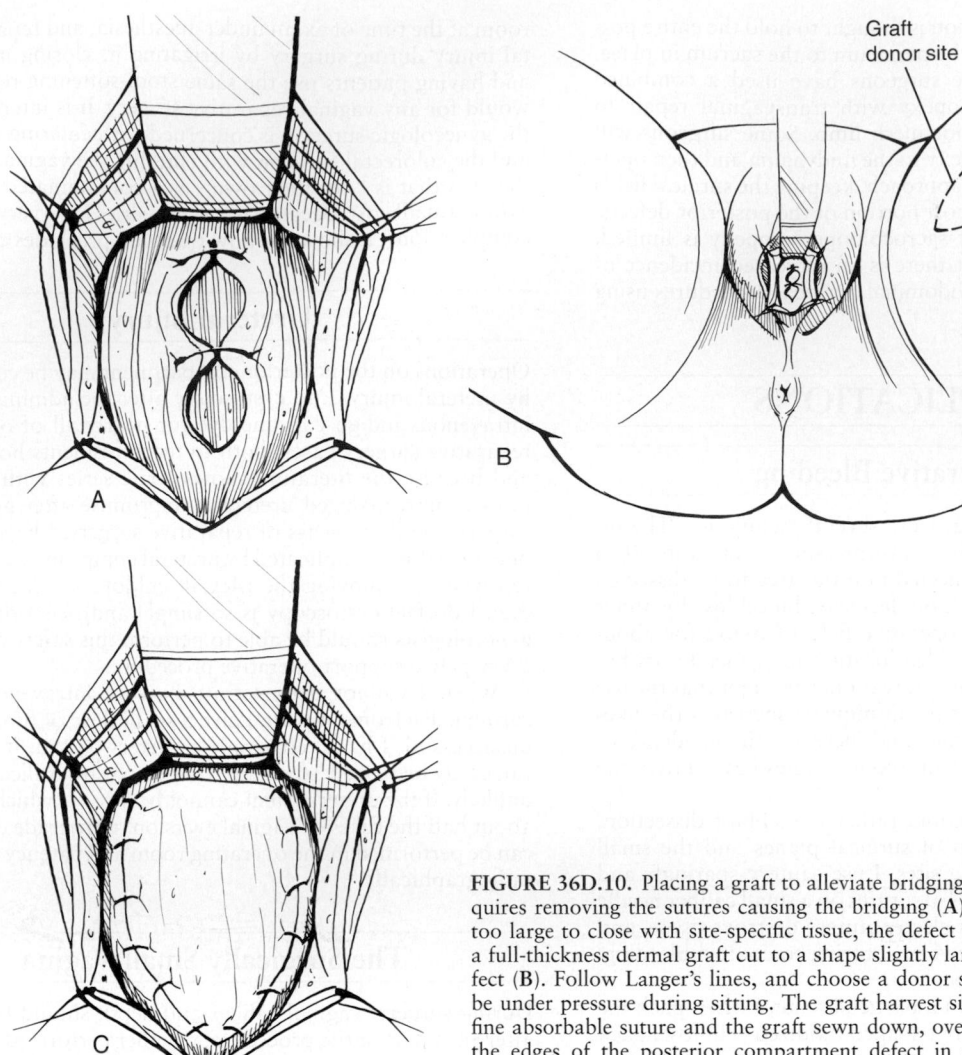

FIGURE 36D.10. Placing a graft to alleviate bridging in the repair requires removing the sutures causing the bridging (**A**). If the defect is too large to close with site-specific tissue, the defect is measured and a full-thickness dermal graft cut to a shape slightly larger than the defect (**B**). Follow Langer's lines, and choose a donor site that will not be under pressure during sitting. The graft harvest site is closed with fine absorbable suture and the graft sewn down, overlapping slightly the edges of the posterior compartment defect in the rectovaginal septum (**C**).

sterile petrolatum-impregnated dressing. The graft material is sewn down along its periphery and overlapping the defect edges (Fig. 36D.10C).

A similar technique is used to place a patch graft when fascial closure narrows the vagina or the vagina is too short. The biggest difference occurs when correcting the short vagina. The graft needed to do this will almost always be larger than can be taken from the buttock or thigh within the operative field, and I will use either a unilateral or bilateral graft from the inguinal areas, much as one would fashion a neovagina.

Using a Graft to Reinforce Posterior Compartment Repair

When native connective tissue or support structures are thought to be of insufficient strength to provide adequate repair, the decision may be to augment or reinforce the entire repair with a graft. In choosing a reparative material, I searched the literature and decided on polypropylene mesh. Since 1988, I have used polypropylene mesh as a reparative material in the posterior compartment in more than 400 cases; including anterior and apical vaginal compartment repairs, in more than 1,500 cases. Polypropylene mesh is preferred because it is readily available in many sizes, soft, easy to shape and handle, relatively inexpensive compared with other graft materials, and consistently strong. It should be realized that in many patients, polypropylene mesh undergoes 10% to 15% shrinkage after placement.

The downside of polypropylene mesh is that it exhibits erosion in 2% to 15% of patients. In my own experience, erosion is twice as likely in the posterior compartment as in the anterior or apical compartment for reasons unknown. Erosion occurs as two types. The first is a simple mesh exposure, usually consisting of small (<1 cm) area. The patient is often asymptomatic but may present with spotting, granulation tissue, pain, or discharge. The second type of erosion presents with a rejectionlike reaction, with an exaggerated inflammatory response associated with a foul-smelling discharge, sometimes pain, and, on exam, a large area of exposure (2 or more cm).

In the case of minimal mesh exposure, the small area can be trimmed in the office with no anesthetic or local anesthesia. I have used scissors and forceps, large Tischler biopsy forceps with colposcopic guidance, or the carbon dioxide laser to trim or remove small areas of erosion. The removal sites in these cases usually heal spontaneously. Mesh erosion characterized by large exposure and/or foul-smelling discharge or pain is treatable only by completely removing the mesh.

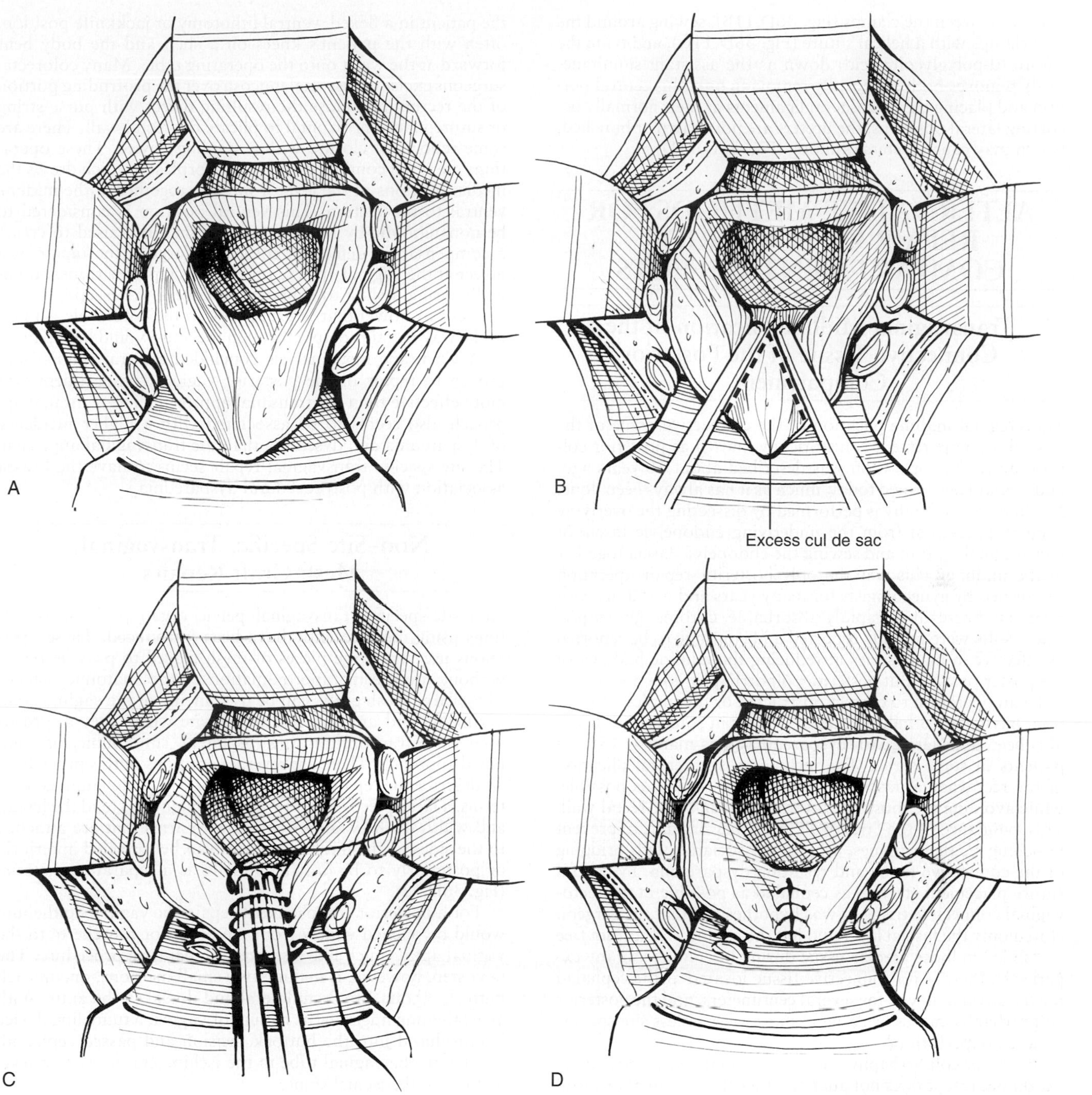

FIGURE 36D.11. If there is redundant posterior cul-de-sac (A) after placement of the uterosacral permanent sutures, I remove it by performing a Torpin culdoplasty rather than obliterate the cul-de-sac by drawing both the uterosacral ligaments and the cul-de-sac peritoneum into a central mass (McCall cul-deplasty). I place two Kocher clamps across the diamond-shaped redundancy (B); excise the cul-sac-between the clamps (B), sewing around the two clamps with a helical suture (C); and tie the suture (0-polyglycolic acid) down as the assistant simultaneously removes both clamps (D).

When true infection is present, which is rare, the mesh can often be removed with little or no dissection.

I have found conservative treatment with cautery, antibiotics, and/or vaginal estrogen cream to be of little value in treating either type of erosion, despite some reports in the literature. I also have patients with small areas of asymptomatic erosion who declined treatment and have had stable mesh exposure for years without problem.

Removing Redundant Cul-de-Sac

When not using mesh, if there is redundant posterior cul-de-sac after placing the 2-0 braided polyester sutures in the uterosacral ligaments and closing the peritoneum, I remove the redundant cul-de-sac. I perform a Torpin culdoplasty, excising only the redundant central portion (Fig. 36D.11A) by placing two Kocher clamps across the diamond-shaped redundancy, excising the cul-sac-between the clamps (Fig. 36D.11B), sewing around the two clamps with a helical suture (Fig. 36D.11C), and tying the suture (0-polyglycolic acid) down as the assistant simultaneously removes both clamps. By removing only this central portion and placing the uterosacral ligaments at their normally occurring lateral positions, the ureters are not drawn or bunched, which may cause ureteral kinking (Fig. 36D.11D).

ALTERNATIVE METHODS FOR REPAIR OF POSTERIOR COMPARTMENT DEFECTS

Transvaginal Midline Plication of the Connective Tissue of the Posterior Compartment

Transvaginal midline plication of the connective tissue of the posterior compartment is historically known as posterior colporrhaphy. The operation was described about 50 years ago, and it is still performed today, much as it has always been done. Midline colporrhaphy is performed by dissecting the overlying vaginal epithelium from the underlying endopelvic fascia of rectovaginal septum and sewing the endopelvic fascia together in the midline. This was the only posterior repair operation performed by gynecologists for many years and was done with relatively fine-caliber, rapidly absorbable, chromic gut suture. The results were initially reported and continue to be reported as effective in many series at reducing the midline budging of the posterior wall. But posterior colporrhaphy does not appear to be an operation to correct obstructed or incomplete defecation, having 40% failure rates at 2 years in some series. It has also been associated with dyspareunia in as many as 15% of patients in some series. The technique is a central plication of the rectovaginal fascia, beginning as cephalad as possible, while avoiding the muscular layer of the vagina or rectal wall. This avoidance of the "true wall" of either organ is to prevent bunching of these tissues, which is associated with bridging of the connective tissue and resulting dyspareunia. By careful suture placement starting as cephalad as possible in the rectovaginal connective tissue, it was hypothesized that the surgeon closed only the fascial layer and left the vagina and rectum free to "slide" in loose areolar tissue during intercourse. In my experience, there is no connective tissue located at the cephalad posterior vaginal wall for several centimeters, and the posterior colporrhaphy causes bridging in most cases unless site-specific repairs are performed.

Posterior colporrhaphy does not eliminate obstructive defecation because it does not anchor either the proximal or distal rectovaginal septum to the uterosacral ligaments or perineal body, leaving what amounts to a reinforced wall of a still-prolapsing organ. When combined with central amputation of the "excess" vaginal wall for midline closure and continuation of a crown stitch joining the dorsalmost portions of the bulbocavernosus muscles and/or the perineal skin, the approximation causes central narrowing of the vagina and a speed bump of perineal skin that partially obstructs the vaginal entrance.

Colorectal Surgeons' Approach to the Posterior Compartment Defect

The surgical repair of a posterior compartment defect by a colorectal surgeon is generally transanal or transperineal with the patient in a flexed, ventral lithotomy or jackknife position, often with the patient's knees on a shelf and the body bent forward at the waist onto the operating table. Many colorectal surgeons excise excess anal mucosa over the protruding portion of the rectum and close the resulting defect with purse-string or suture placed horizontal to plicate the rectal wall. There are some reports of closure with a stapling device. These operations are often combined with a levatorplasty, which draws the medial portions of the levator muscles together in the midline ventral to the rectum. This ventral position is considered to be nonanatomic by many gynecologists but is used to create a compensatory defect. In colorectal surgery, the repair of a defect at the vaginal apex (enterocele) is repaired transabdominally, using a sling to support the viscera or resection of the segment of bowel that is prolapsing in the enterocele, similar to the way rectal prolapse through the anus would be repaired.

A Cochrane metaanalysis concluded the transvaginal approach to repair of the posterior vaginal compartment was more effective than the transanal approach. The transanal approach also seems to be associated with a higher incidence of dyspareunia and dyschezia than the transvaginal approach. The site-specific transvaginal repair seems to have the lowest association with postprocedural dyspareunia.

Non–Site-Specific, Transvaginal, Mesh-Graft Repairs

Non–site-specific transvaginal pelvic organ prolapse operations using mesh recently have been introduced. These operations use very large pieces of mesh placed to provide repair without site-specific approximation of the anatomic defects. These large mesh grafts can be used in any of the vaginal compartments and are tunneled to the site where they are to be used via a transobturator, transgluteal, suprapubic, or combined approach. There are several variations of this procedure. To describe the repairs of the posterior compartment in general terms, a large piece of mesh—large enough to extend the length and width of the vagina—comes with arms that are attached to the sides of the mesh. The arms can be tunneled anteriorly or posteriorly to be drawn caudally as a reparative material (Fig. 36D.12).

For a posterior compartment repair, the vaginal epithelium would be opened widely from the posterior fourchette to the vaginal apex, much like a standard reparative procedure. The next step, however, is making two small incisions, one in each buttock, about 2 to 3 cm lateral and dorsal to the anus. With an examining finger in the rectum or vagina, a tunneling device is introduced into the buttock incision and passed cephalad, parallel to the vaginal tube in the ischiorectal fossa to a level just below the ischial spine.

At this level, the device is turned medially to penetrate the connective tissue of the lateral vaginal wall, entering the deepithelialized vaginal lumen. A piece of polypropylene mesh is attached to the tunneling device within the vaginal lumen. The mesh can be sized to cover just the vaginal apex, the apex to the midvagina on the posterior wall, or from the apex (at the level of the ischial spines) to the perineum. The mesh can be left with or without anchoring, depending on the recommendations of the manufacturer of the device being used. Most mesh grafts are attached at the apex of the vagina but not above the ischial spines.

The lateral arms of the mesh are threaded into the tunneling device and drawn back through the connective tissue lateral to the vaginal wall and below the ischial spine, through ischiorectal fossa, and out the buttock incision. The operator

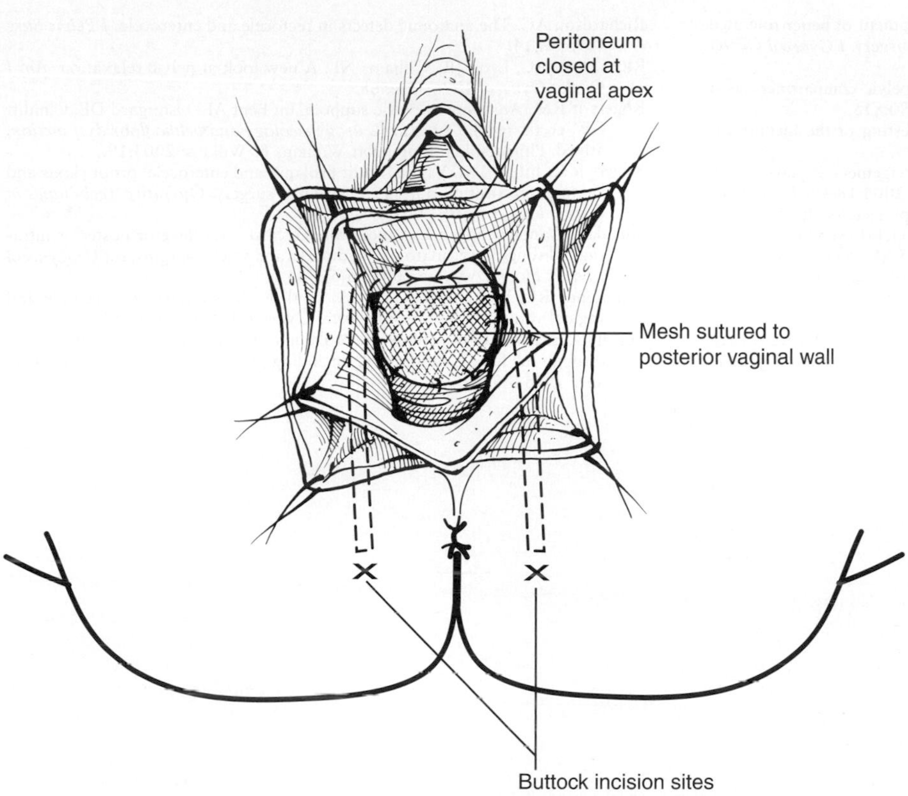

FIGURE 36D.12. A graft, most commonly polypropylene or porcine dermis, is placed over the entire posterior compartment. Introduced through small incisions 2 to 3 cm lateral and dorsal to the anus, a tunneling device is brought up through the buttocks into the ischiorectal space to a level just caudal to the ischial spine. The vaginal wall is penetrated at this point, the tunneling device is threaded with the arm of a precut mesh, and the sling arm is drawn back to the buttock. This is repeated on the opposite side. The central graft is large and can be trimmed so that it attaches to just the apex or to the entire posterior compartment below the opened epithelium. The central graft is sewn into place, and the epithelium closed over it.

then pulls on the mesh arm, and the mesh elevates whatever portion or portions of the posterior compartment to which it is attached. At this point, the mesh can be anchored to the underlying connective tissue of the posterior vaginal wall from apex to perineum and the vaginal wall trimmed and closed or just closed. The mesh arms are trimmed so that they retract back into the subcutaneous tissue of the buttock. Early reports of these large mesh repairs come from outside the United States and appear to be favorable, but long-term results are not yet available at the time of this writing, especially from surgeries done within academic centers.

BEST SURGICAL PRACTICES

- The reparative operation for the posterior compartment should be tailored to fit the needs of the patient.
- Assessing the needs of the patient begins with history and physical examination to determine symptoms and anatomic site-specific defects. Some operations may be better suited to a given patient based on symptoms and findings.
- Understanding of the anatomy and pathophysiology of pelvic organ prolapse has changed and as a result, so has the way we perform surgery to repair it. The gynecologist now in practice will have to learn new surgical techniques to provide the best care possible for patients.
- Site-specific examination of the posterior vaginal compartment from the uterosacral ligaments to the perineum is used to formulate the surgical plan. The surgeon who goes to the operating room with one operation that he/she can perform probably will not be entirely pleased with the long-term results, and neither will the patients.
- Midline plication of the posterior vaginal compartment, or the traditional posterior colporrhaphy, does not anchor either the most cephalad or distal portions of the vagina. Failure to anchor the vaginal apex leads to descent of the apex; failure to anchor the distal vagina may lead to perineal descent syndrome.
- Approximately 20% of posterior vaginal wall repairs are now being performed with augmentation by a graft, with polypropylene mesh being the most common graft material. Although not without complications (exposure, infection, pain, dyspareunia), the use of graft material in gynecologic surgery is likely to become the standard of care for repeat procedures after failed pelvic organ prolapse surgery. Each graft material has its limitations, but gynecologic surgeons will need to become familiar with at least one type of material to use.

Bibliography

Addison WA, Livengood CH 3rd, Sutton GR, et al. Abdominal sacral colpopexy with Mersilene mesh in the retroperitoneal position in the management of post hysterectomy vaginal vault prolapse and enterocele. *Am J Obstet Gynecol* 1985;37(4):140.

Baden WF, Walker T. *Surgical repair of vaginal defects*. Philadelphia: JB Lippincott; 1992:51.

Belot F, Collinet P, Debodinance P, et al. Prosthetic reinforcement by the vaginal approach after surgical repair of pelvic prolapse. *J Gynecol Obstet Biol Reprod* 2005;34(8):763.

Cundiff GW, Wiedner AC, Visco AG, et al. An anatomic and functional assessment of the discrete defect rectocele repair. *Am J Obstet Gynecol* 1998;179:1451.

Debodinance P, Delporte P, Engrand JB, et al. Development of better tolerated prosthetic materials: applications in gynecologic surgery. *J Gynecol Obstet Biol Reprod* 2002;31(6):527.

DeLancey JOL. Structural anatomy of the posterior pelvic compartment as it relates to rectocele. *Am J Obstet Gynecol* 1999;180:815.

Julian TM. Physical examination and pretreatment testing of the incontinent woman. *Clin Obstet Gynecol* 1998;41(3):663.

Maher C, Baessler K, Glazener CM, et al. Surgical management of pelvic organ prolapse in women. *Cochrane Database Syst Rev* 2004;18(4):CD004014.

Marinkovic SP, Stanton SL. Triple compartment prolapse: sacrocolpopexy with anterior and posterior mesh extension. *BJOG* 2003;110(3):323.

McCall ML. Posterior culdoplasty. *Obstet Gynecol* 1957;10:595.

Meeks GR, Washburne JF, McGehee RP, et al. Repair of vaginal vault prolapse by suspension of the vagina to the iliococcygeus (prespinous) fascia. *Am J Obstet Gynecol* 1994;171(6):1444.

Paraiso MF, Falcone T, Walters MD. Laparoscopic surgery for enterocele, vaginal apex prolapse, and rectocele. *Int Urogynecol J Pelvic Floor Dysfunct* 1999;10(4):223.

Richardson AC. The anatomic defects in rectocele and enterocele. *J Pelvic Surg* 1995;1:214.

Richardson AC, Lyon JB, Williams NL. A new look at pelvic relaxation. *Am J Obstet Gynecol* 1976;126:568.

Rogers Jr RM. Anatomy of pelvic support. In: Bent AE, Ostergard DE, Cundiff GW, et al. (eds). *Ostergard's urogynecology and pelvic floor dysfunction.* 5th ed. Philadelphia: Lippincott Williams & Wilkins; 2003:19.

Rogers Jr R, Julian TM. Vaginal vault prolapse and enterocele: prophylaxis and anatomic restitution during transvaginal surgery. *Operative Techniques in Gynecologic Surgery* 2001;6(3):127.

Smajda S, Vanormelingen L, Vandewalle G, et al. Translevator posterior intravaginal slingplasty: anatomic landmarks and safety margins. *Int Urogynecol J Pelvic Floor Dysfunct* 2005;16(5):364.

Symmonds RE, Williams TJ, Lee RA, et al. Posthysterectomy enterocele and vaginal vault prolapse. *Am J Obstet Gynecol* 1981;140(8):852.

Torpin R. Excision of the cul-de-sac of Douglas for the surgical cure of hernias, through the female caudal wall, including prolapse of the uterus. *J Int Coll Surg* 1955;3:322.

CHAPTER 36E ■ VAGINAL VAULT PROLAPSE

STEVEN D. KLEEMAN AND MICKEY M. KARRAM

DEFINITIONS

EEA sizer—One of a series of metal instruments that are used primarily to evaluate the size of the end-to-end anastomosis stapler instrument that is appropriate for a given patient. It is also an excellent instrument for distending and manipulating the vaginal apex from below, allowing the abdominal surgeon to easily feel the vagina and dissect against a firm surface (see Fig. 36E.14).

Levels of support defects (according to DeLancey classification)—Level I: apical defects caused by loss of support of the uterosacral ligaments, paracolpium, and parametrium; Level II: disruption of the normal lateral attachments of the midvagina; and Level III: lower vaginal defects in the perineal body or fusion of the distal urethra to the pubic bone.

Pully stitch—Often used to attach the vaginal apex to the sacrospinous ligament. The suture is passed through the ligament (or other tissue where the final knot is to be located). One end of the suture is then passed through the vaginal apex (or other tissue that is to be approximated or "pulled" next to the first pass). The suture in the vaginal apex is tied with a half hitch. The two free ends of the suture are now tied, and as the knot is tightened down, the vaginal apex is pulled up to the sacrospinous ligament, and the two tissues are then approximated. The pulley stitch reduces the risk of cutting through the tissue as the knot is tightened.

Sacrospinous ligament—A strong ligament that runs within the coccygeus muscle from the ischial spine to the sacrum.

As women live longer and healthier lives, pelvic floor disorders continue to become even more prevalent and are an important health and social issue. It is estimated that by 2030, 63 million women will be 45 years of age or older, and by 2050, 33% of the population will be postmenopausal. The lifetime risk of surgery for pelvic prolapse or incontinence has been estimated at 11%, with a reoperation rate for failure at 29%. The management of pelvic organ prolapse can be difficult because different support defects often coexist. The pelvic surgeon must be adept in the thorough evaluation and management of these issues. An understanding of the anatomy and the relationship of the vagina to surrounding structures is imperative.

Our understanding of pelvic prolapse and the treatment thereof has changed in recent years. It was formerly taught that prolapse resulted from attenuation or stretching of endopelvic fascia. Richardson and colleagues challenged this theory by introducing the concept of discrete breaks in endopelvic fascia. More recently, Richardson and colleagues described apical enterocele as a separation of pubocervical fascia from rectovaginal fascia. This allows peritoneum of an enterocele sac to be in direct contact with vaginal epithelium. This concept has recently been challenged. Microscopic studies of patients with enteroceles have failed to identify peritoneum in contact with vaginal epithelium. Kleeman and colleagues described the microscopic anatomy of the posterior vagina in cadavers without prolapse. Figure 36E.1 shows a microscopic horizontal section of the upper third of the vagina. Identification of all layers fails to reveal a discrete fascial layer. Despite this controversy, the theory proposed by Richardson helps our overall understanding of vaginal support.

DeLancey divided the support of the vagina into three levels. This concept is helpful in understanding normal anatomic relationships and appreciating why certain repairs may work in some patients and not in others. Level I support defects are apical defects caused by loss of support of the uterosacral ligaments, paracolpium, and parametrium. Level II support defects result from disruption of the normal lateral attachment of the midvagina. Level III support defects result from defects in the perineal body or fusion of the distal urethra to the pubic bone (Fig. 36E.2).

The true incidence of vaginal vault prolapse is unknown. However, there is an overall perception that the number of procedures being performed for vaginal vault prolapse is increasing. The main goal of any procedure aimed at suspending the vaginal vault should be to suspend the vaginal vault as near as possible to its normal anatomic position. This should reapproximate the upper vagina in the midline over the levator plate. Distortion of the vaginal vault, whether in an anterior or posterior direction, can lead to a recurrent prolapse opposite the vaginal vault in a significant number of patients.

The ultimate goal of pelvic reconstructive surgery is *to restore anatomy, maintain or restore visceral function, and maintain or restore normal sexual function*. It is extremely important to determine preoperatively whether lower urinary tract dysfunction, sexual dysfunction, and defecatory dysfunction exist. Urinary dysfunction may be masked in patients with advanced pelvic organ prolapse by obstructing or kinking the urethra. Thus, reductive maneuvers aimed at simulating what surgery will accomplish should be used in the hope of identifying those patients who will require an antiincontinence procedure in conjunction with their pelvic reconstructive surgery. It is also important to initiate local estrogen therapy preoperatively in patients who have urogenital atrophy.

Many operations have been described for suspending the prolapsed vaginal vault. There is no general consensus on what is the best procedure. The procedure that the surgeon ultimately chooses is influenced by many factors, including the comfort and skill of the surgeon performing the operation, whether the prolapse is primary or recurrent, the patient's age, state of health, anticipated outcome, sexual activity, and overall state of the tissues. We believe it is important for the surgeon to have a variety of operative approaches available for the individual patient. We prefer to approach most cases transvaginally, reserving abdominal sacral colpopexy for patients who have failed a previous vaginal approach, have a foreshortened

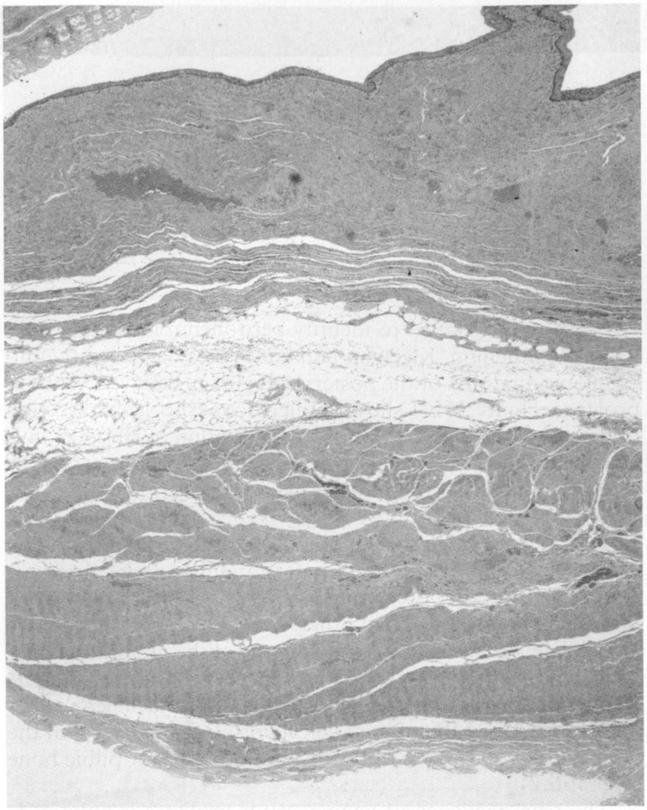

FIGURE 36E.1. Microscopic hematoxylin and eosin stain of the upper third of the vagina. The vaginal epithelium is at the top, and the rectal mucosa at the bottom.

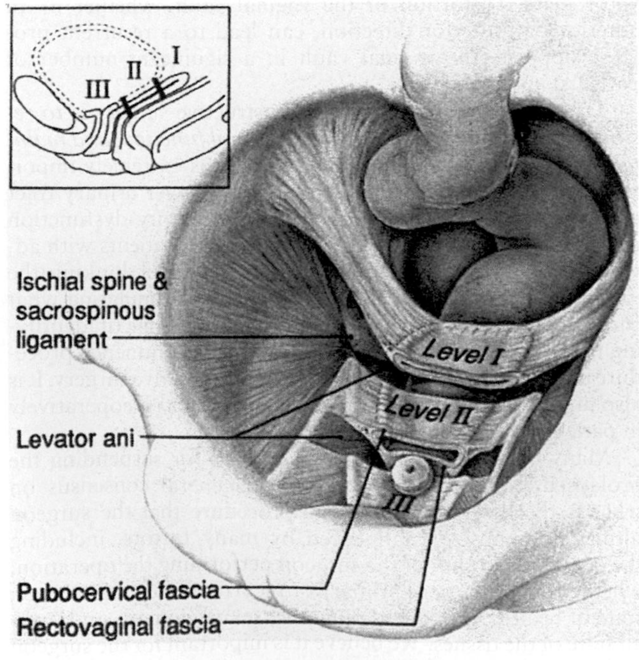

FIGURE 36E.2. Levels of support. DeLancey's biomechanical levels: level I, proximal suspension; level II, lateral attachment; level III, distal fusion. (From DeLancey JOL. Anatomic aspects of vaginal eversion after hysterectomy. *Am J Obstet Gynecol* 1992;166:1717.)

vagina, or in whom a compensatory procedure with the insertion of mesh is necessary to obtain a long-term durable repair. We believe the vaginal approach to pelvic prolapse has the advantage of decreased operative time, decreased incidence of adhesion formation, and quicker recovery time. Obliterative procedures including partial Le Fort colpocleisis and colpectomy; colpocleisis can be used in elderly fragile patients who are no longer sexually active.

VAGINAL PROCEDURES TO SUSPEND THE VAGINAL APEX

McCall Culdoplasty

Several operations have been described and used by surgeons for vaginal vault suspension with correction of concurrent enterocele. McCall (in 1957) described his technique of surgical correction of enterocele at the time of vaginal hysterectomy. He used several nonabsorbable sutures to obliterate the enterocele (internal McCall sutures) by approximating both uterosacral ligaments and several bites of posterior peritoneum together. Delayed absorbable sutures were then inserted through the full thickness of the posterior vagina just lateral to the midline, passed through each uterosacral ligament and back out the posterior vaginal wall. Additional external sutures are placed as required by the amount of prolapse. The internal sutures are then tied, and the external sutures are tied after the vaginal cuff is closed. This simple procedure obliterates the cul-de-sac, supports the vaginal apex, and lengthens the posterior vaginal wall (Fig. 36E.3). McCall originally reported on 45 cases and stated there was no incidence of enterocele recurrence.

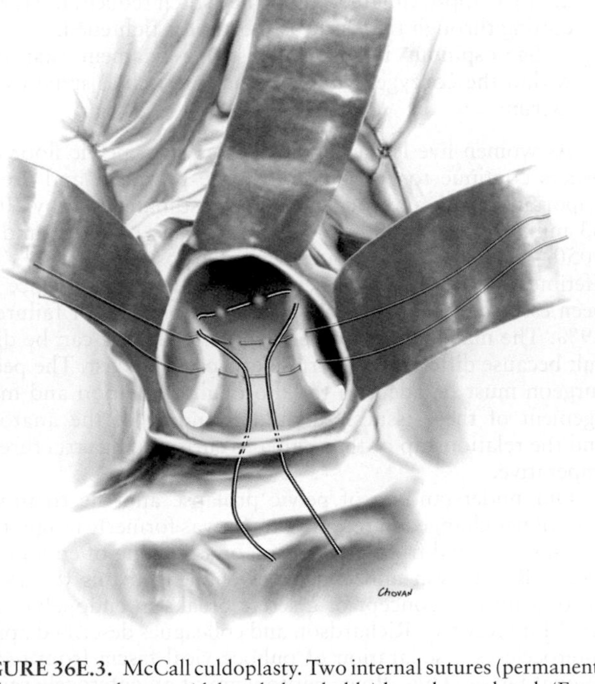

FIGURE 36E.3. McCall culdoplasty. Two internal sutures (permanent) and one external suture (delayed absorbable) have been placed. (From Baggish MS, Karram MM. *Atlas of pelvic anatomy and gynecologic surgery.* New York: Saunders; 2001.)

Several modifications of McCall's technique have been described, most notably the modified endopelvic fascia repair, which was popularized and reported on from the Mayo Clinic. A wedge of vaginal mucosa is removed from the anterior and posterior vaginal wall. This narrows the vault when closed and allows easier access to lateral supports of the vagina (i.e., cardinal and uterosacral ligaments and perirectal fascia). The enterocele sac is then dissected free and excised at the neck. The ureters are identified by palpation bilaterally. One to three internal McCall's sutures are placed as described above. After these sutures are placed and tagged, modified external McCall sutures are placed by passing delayed absorbable sutures through the posterior vaginal wall and peritoneum, through remnants of uterosacral and cardinal ligaments on the patient's left. Several bites of peritoneum overlying the rectosigmoid are taken, and then the right perirectal fascia and uterosacral are incorporated into the suture. Last, the suture is passed back out through the posterior vaginal wall. The number of internal and external sutures placed depends on the size of enterocele and redundancy of the upper vagina (Figs. 36E.4 and 36E.5). A 1998 article by Webb reported on 660 women who underwent primary repair of vaginal vault prolapse. Follow-up was available on 514 of the 660 women. Eighty patients (11.5%) reported a "bulge" or "protrusion" at the time of questioning. Eighty-two percent (385 patients) responded that they were very satisfied or somewhat satisfied with the operation. The most common operative complication was laceration of bowel or rectum in 16 patients (2.3%). Four patients (0.6%) suffered ureteral complication. Three of these were from obstruction, and one developed a ureterovaginal fistula. Nine patients (1.3%) had a vault hematoma, and four (0.6%) had a cuff abscess or infection. Fifteen patients (2.2%) required blood transfusions. Forty-two of the 189 (22%) sexually active women reported dyspareunia.

Sacrospinous Ligament Fixation

To perform sacrospinous ligament fixation, it is imperative that the surgeon be familiar with the anatomy of the sacrospinous ligament complex and of the pararectal space. Obtaining adequate exposure can be difficult, and vascular complications, when encountered, may be life-threatening. The sacrospinous ligament is a cordlike structure that exists within the body of the coccygeus muscle. The sacrospinous ligament attaches medially to the sacrum and coccyx and attaches laterally to the ischial spine. The complex is collectively called the coccygeus-sacrospinous ligament complex (CSSL). The CSSL is best identified by palpating the ischial spine and tracing the fingerlike ligamentous structure medially and posteriorly to the sacrum (Fig. 36E.6). The pudendal nerve and vessels pass directly posterior to the ischial spine. The sciatic nerve lies superior and lateral to the sacrospinous ligament. Superior to the ligament lies the inferior gluteal vessels and the hypogastric venous plexus (Fig. 36E.7). To avoid trauma to these structures, it is important to place the fixation sutures two fingers medial to the ischial spine.

The apex of the vagina is grasped with two Allis clamps so the extent of the prolapse can be assessed. The vagina is then reduced to the sacrospinous ligament. Most surgeons prefer to use the sacrospinous ligament opposite their dominant hand; that is, the right-handed surgeon uses the right sacrospinous ligament, although some surgeons prefer to perform a bilateral fixation. Marking sutures can be used to identify the intended vaginal apex throughout the operation. It may be necessary to choose a different fixation point than the original vaginal cuff scar. This is best illustrated in a patient with a foreshortened anterior segment and a large enterocele. In this case, the

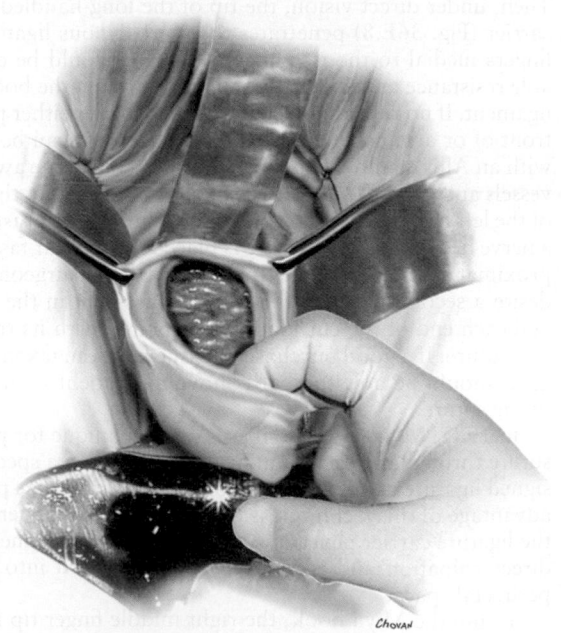

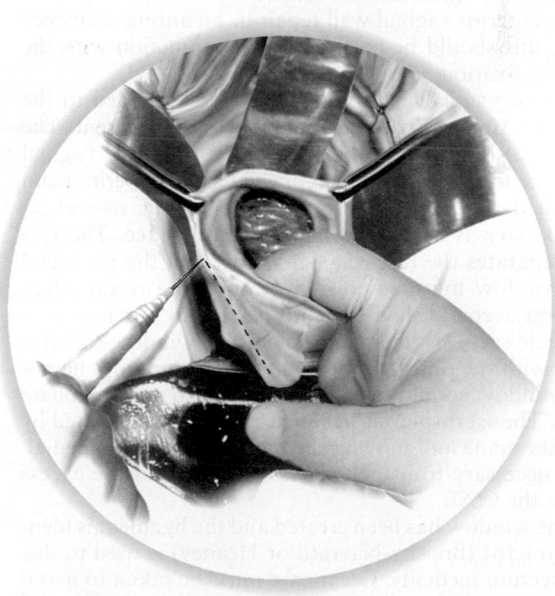

FIGURE 36E.4. Digital palpation of the posterior cul-de-sac and enterocele. Inset: The technique of removal of the redundant wedge of posterior vaginal wall and peritoneum. (From Baggish MS, Karram MM. *Atlas of pelvic anatomy and gynecologic surgery.* New York: Saunders; 2001.)

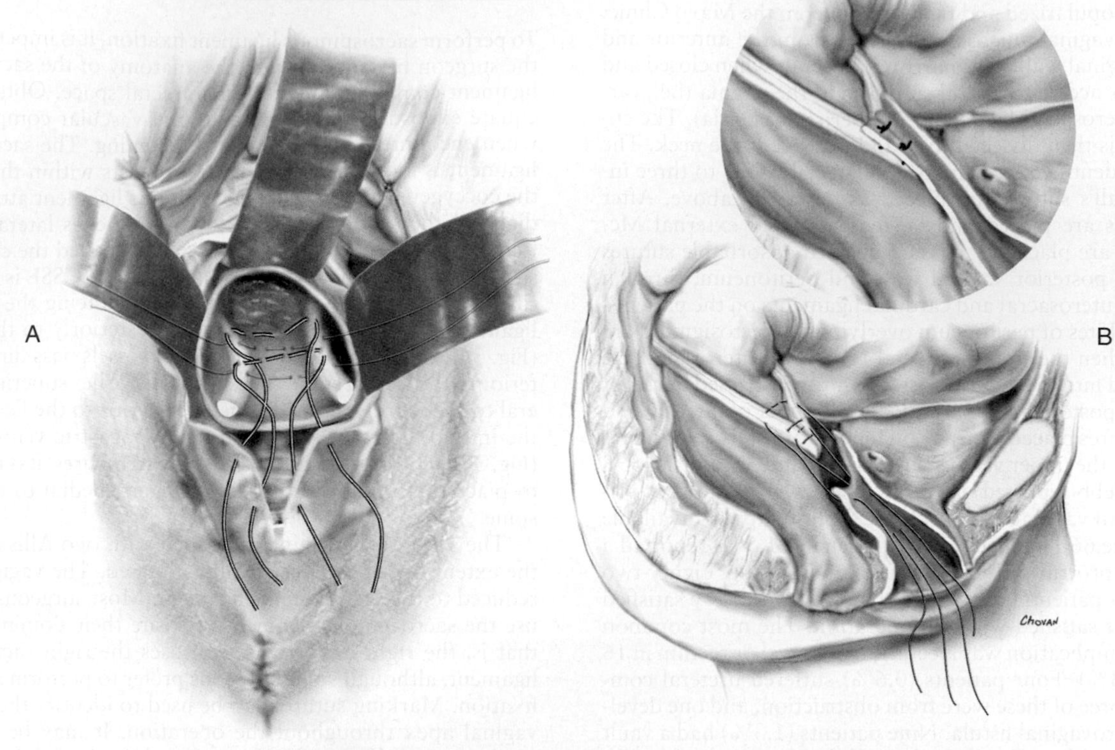

FIGURE 36E.5. A: Placement of internal and external McCall sutures after a wedge of posterior vaginal wall has been removed. **B:** Cross section of the upper vagina and vaginal vault before and after tying of sutures. (From Baggish MS, Karram MM. *Atlas of pelvic anatomy and gynecologic surgery.* New York: Saunders; 2001.)

new fixation point would be moved to an area over the enterocele. It is equally important to access the anterior and posterior segments of the vagina and the genital hiatus. If the patient requires an anterior vaginal wall repair or an antiincontinence procedure, this should be performed in conjunction with the sacrospinous fixation.

A posterior vaginal incision is made and extended to the vaginal apex. Almost always an enterocele sac is present. The enterocele sac should be mobilized off the posterior vaginal wall up to its neck; the sac is then opened and the peritoneum excised. The defect is then closed with purse-string sutures.

The next step is entry into the perirectal space. The rectal pillar separates the rectovaginal space from the perirectal space. A window must be created through the rectal pillar, which is best accomplished by blunt dissection just lateral to the enterocele sac over the ischial spine. The window can also be created with the tips of scissors, a tonsil clamp, or a hemostat. The window should be gently enlarged to accommodate the vagina. The sacrospinous ligament can then be palpated by palpating the spine and moving the fingers dorsal and medial. It may be necessary to use blunt dissection to remove excess tissue from the CSSL.

Once the window has been created and the ligament is identified, a retractor (Breisky-Navratil or Heaney) is used to displace the rectum medially. Great care must be taken to avoid raking the retractor over the anterior surface of the sacrum and causing damage to presacral nerves and vessels. When using the right sacrospinous ligament, the middle and index finger of the left hand are placed on the medial surface of the ischial spine. Then, under direct vision, the tip of the long-handled ligature carrier (Fig. 36E.8) penetrates the sacrospinous ligament two fingers medial to the ischial spine. There should be considerable resistance as the carrier is pushed through the body of the ligament. If no resistance is felt, then the carrier either passed in front of or around the ligament. The ligament can be grasped with an Allis clamp or Babcock to isolate the tissue away from vessels and nerves. After the suture has been passed, the fingers of the left hand are withdrawn. The suture is then grasped with a nerve hook. A second suture is placed in a similar fashion approximately 1 cm medial to the first. If the surgeon doesn't desire a second passage, the suture can be cut in the midline, and each end of the cut loop can be paired with its respective free suture. If a good purchase of tissue has been taken, the surgeon should be able to gently move the patient with traction of the suture.

In 1987, Miyazaki described a new technique for passing a suture through the sacrospinous ligament using a specially designed ligature carrier (Miya hook) (Fig. 36E.9). The proposed advantage of this technique is that it is safer and easier because the ligature carrier penetrates the sacrospinous ligament under direct palpation and is then passed downward into the safe perirectal space.

To use the Miya hook, the right middle finger tip is placed on the sacrospinous ligament, two finger breadths medial to the ischial spine and just below the superior margin. The Miya hook is held closed in the left hand and slid along the palmar surface of the right hand. The point of the hook then comes to rest just beneath the tip of the right middle finger. The handles

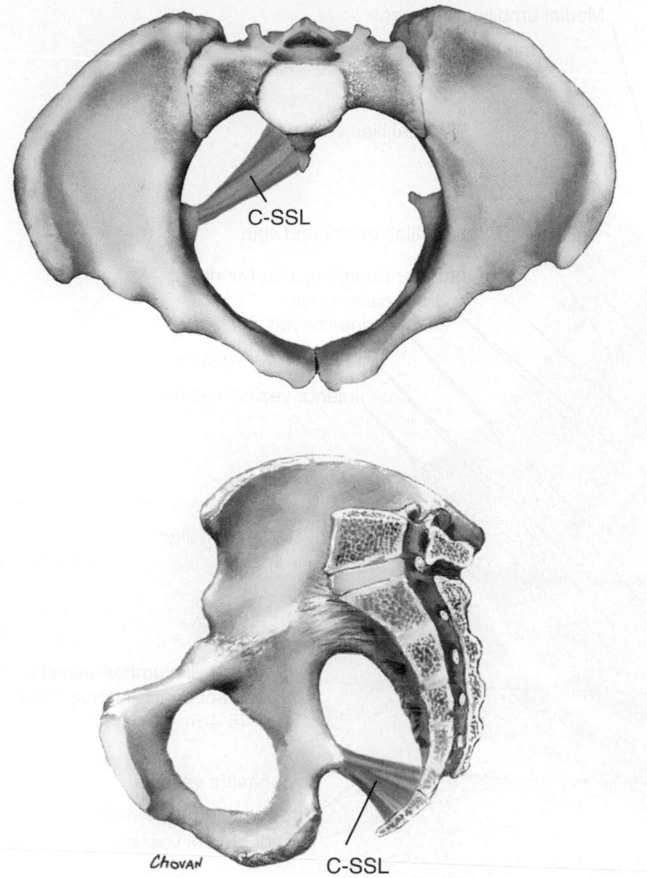

FIGURE 36E.6. The coccygeus-sacrospinous ligament complex (CSSL). Note that the sacrospinous ligament lies within the coccygeus muscle. (From Baggish MS, Karram MM. *Atlas of pelvic anatomy and gynecologic surgery.* New York: Saunders; 2001.)

are opened then lowered to a near horizontal position. The hook point should be at about a 45-degree angle. The tip of the right middle finger then confirms the hook point is placed two finger breadths medial to the ischial spine. The middle and index fingers then apply firm pressure downward just behind the hook hump so the hook penetrates the ligament. One can also place traction with the back of the thumb on the handle to help penetrate the ligament. The surgeon then closes and elevates the handles of the Miya hook and, with the index and middle fingers, clears the tissue from the point so as to make the suture visible. If there is too much tissue in the hook, the surgeon simply backs it out and takes a smaller bite. An assistant can then hold the handle elevated in a closed position. The rectum is held medially by a retractor, and a notched speculum is inserted by palpation underneath the hook point. A nerve hook is then used to retrieve the suture.

Several other instruments have been designed to pass the suture through the ligament. These include the Laurus needle driver and Nichols-Veronikis ligature carrier (Fig. 36E.10). Once the surgeon has the two sutures through the sacrospinous ligament, the vaginal vault can then be suspended. There are two ways for the surgeon to attach the sutures to the vagina. The first is to use a pulley stitch. Here the free end of the suture is threaded through a free needle, sewn into the full thickness of the fibromuscular layer on the undersurface of the vagina (excluding the epithelium), and then tied by a half hitch. Traction on the free end of the suture pulls the vagina directly onto the ligament. A square knot is then used to fix the suture in place. Generally, when using this technique, permanent suture should be used.

The second technique can be used if the vagina is thin or if greater vaginal length is desired. This technique involves passing each end of the sutures through the full thickness of the vagina using 1-0 or 2-0 absorbable suture. The upper portion of the posterior vaginal wall should be closed with interrupted or running 3-0 absorbable sutures before tying the colpopexy sutures (Fig. 36E.11). If the colpopexy sutures are tied before the posterior wall is closed, the visibility of the vault is reduced, and the colporrhaphy sutures are much more difficult to place. The vagina should come into contact with the sacrospinous ligament, especially if absorbable sutures are used. A suture bridge can predispose to recurrent prolapse because a strong scar will not form before suture absorption.

After the colpopexy sutures are tied, a posterior colporrhaphy and perineorrhaphy is done. The vagina is then packed with moist gauze for 24 hours.

The **overall results** from sacrospinous fixation have been good. In 1997, Sze and Karram reviewed the literature on sacrospinous suspension, and of the 1,137 patients available for follow-up, 36 (3%) had recurrent vault prolapse. Ninety-six (8%) had anterior wall prolapse, and 25 (2%) had posterior wall prolapse. Some authors (Sze and Karram in 1997 and Shull and colleagues in 1992) have reported a high incidence of anterior wall prolapse following sacrospinous fixation; others have not. Smilen and colleagues in 1998 compared patients with anterior vaginal wall defects undergoing anterior colporrhaphy with and without sacrospinous fixation with patients with a well-supported anterior vaginal wall who were undergoing pelvic reconstructive procedures with and without sacrospinous fixation. They found no difference between the groups for subsequent anterior wall prolapse during the follow-up period. Three randomized trials evaluating sacrospinous fixation have been reported. Benson and colleagues and Lo and Wang reported higher success rates with abdominal sacral colpopexy than sacrospinous fixation, and Maher and associates reported similar success rates. It has been our experience that this operation does distort the vagina posteriorly and leaves the anterior segment vulnerable to recurrent prolapse. Table 36E.1 reviews published results of sacrospinous ligament suspension.

Complications can occur, and the more common complications are discussed here. It is important to do frequent rectal examinations during this procedure to make sure that no inadvertent proctotomy has occurred. If evidence of suture penetration is evident, the offending suture should be removed and replaced. Lacerations should be closed in a standard two-layer fashion.

Hemorrhage can result from injury to the hypogastric venous plexus, inferior gluteal vessels, and internal pudendal vessels. Injury can occur from overzealous dissection or inappropriate needle passage through the sacrospinous ligament. If bleeding does occur initially, pressure should be applied to the bleeding area. Continued bleeding should be addressed with suture ligation and hemoclips. Because this area is difficult to approach transabdominally, every effort should be made to control bleeding transvaginally. An improperly placed retractor or inattentive assistance can cause damage to the presacral vessels by raking the tip over the bony sacrum.

Stress urinary incontinence may occur postoperatively and is probably the result of straightening of the posterior urethrovesical junction. It is important that all patients have

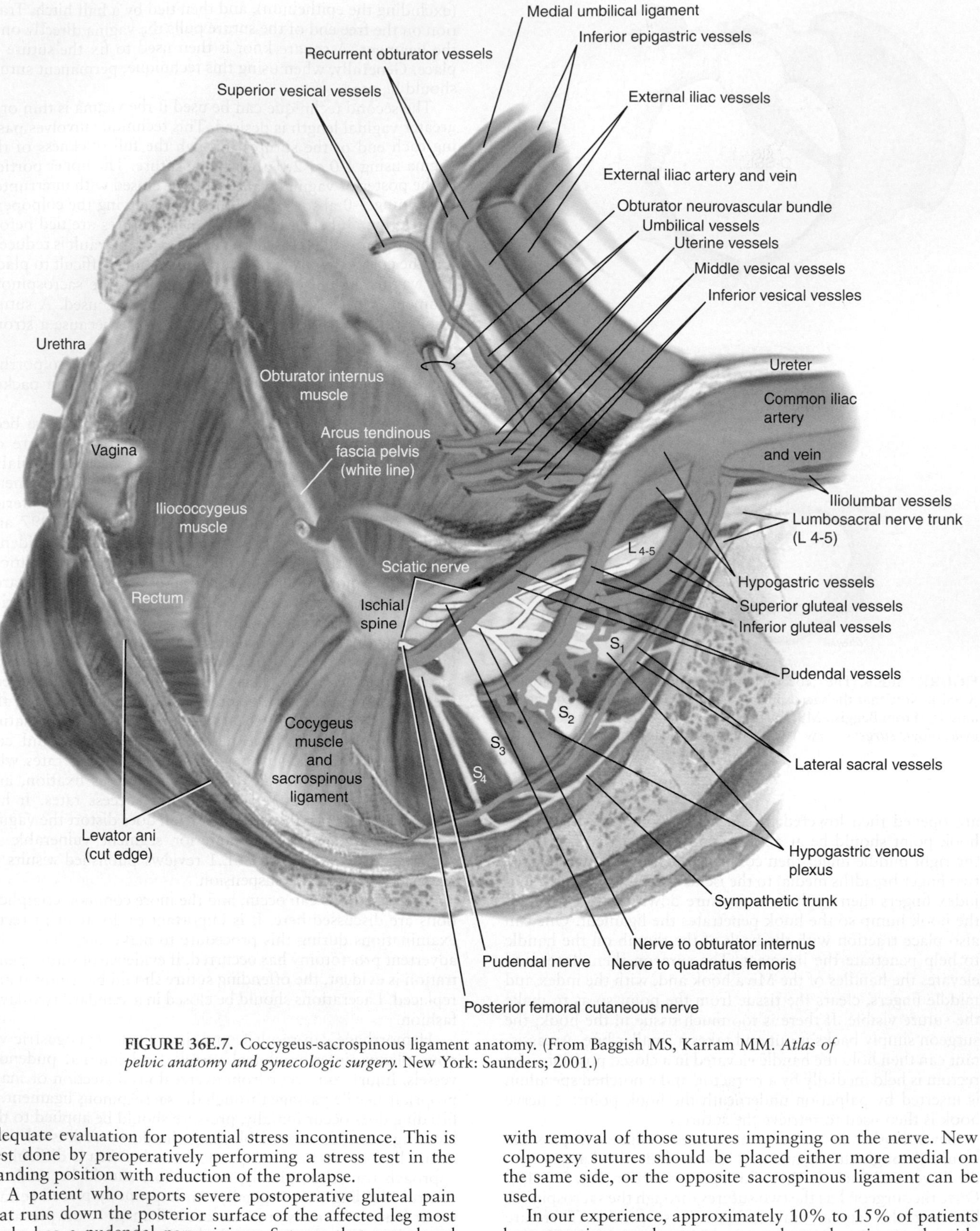

FIGURE 36E.7. Coccygeus-sacrospinous ligament anatomy. (From Baggish MS, Karram MM. *Atlas of pelvic anatomy and gynecologic surgery.* New York: Saunders; 2001.)

adequate evaluation for potential stress incontinence. This is best done by preoperatively performing a stress test in the standing position with reduction of the prolapse.

A patient who reports severe postoperative gluteal pain that runs down the posterior surface of the affected leg most likely has a pudendal nerve injury. Sutures that are placed too close to the ischial spine risk injury to the pudendal nerves and the sciatic nerve. If the patient has evidence of nerve injury, she should immediately undergo reoperation with removal of those sutures impinging on the nerve. New colpopexy sutures should be placed either more medial on the same side, or the opposite sacrospinous ligament can be used.

In our experience, approximately 10% to 15% of patients have transient moderate to severe buttock pain on the side of the sacrospinous suspension. It is usually self-limiting and resolves by 6 weeks postoperatively. Reassurance and antiinflammatory agents are all that are necessary.

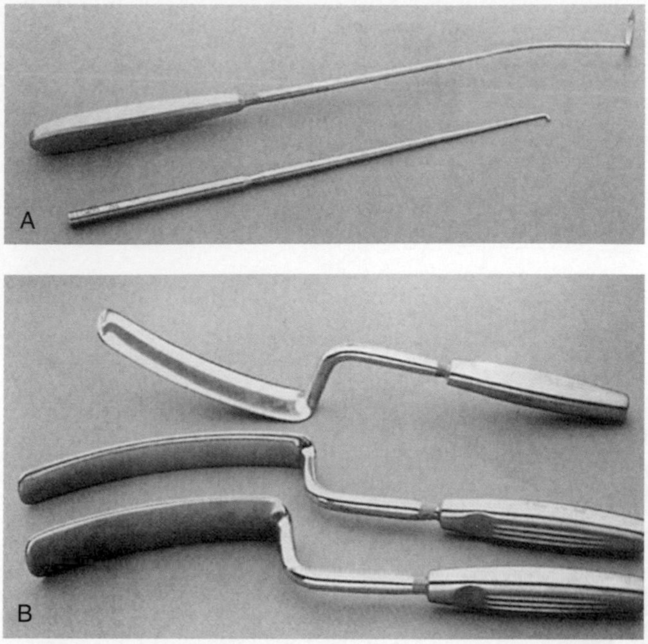

FIGURE 36E.8. **A:** Long-handled Deschamps ligature carrier and nerve hook. Note slight bend near the tip to facilitate suture placement into the coccygeus-sacrospinous ligament complex. **B:** Briesky-Navratil retractors, various sizes. (From Walters MD, Karram MM. *Urogynecology and reconstructive pelvic surgery.* 2nd ed. St. Louis: CV Mosby; 1999.)

Vaginal stenosis can occur if too much vaginal tissue is removed before closing the vaginal incision. An aggressive posterior repair can also cause a constriction ring. If a constriction ring is present while the patient is still under anesthesia, it should be addressed at that time. The colporrhaphy sutures can be removed or lateral-relaxing incisions can be made in the vagina.

High Uterosacral Ligament Suspension with Fibromuscular Vaginal Wall Reconstruction

In 1976, Richardson introduced a new approach to the management of enterocele and vault prolapse. The concept maintains that the endopelvic fascia that surrounds the vagina does not attenuate but breaks at specific points. The reconstruction aims to eliminate the enterocele by using principles of abdominal hernia surgery. This involves identifying the fascial defect, reducing the enterocele sac, and closing the fascial defect. In addition, the vagina is resuspended to its original level I support (the uterosacral ligaments).

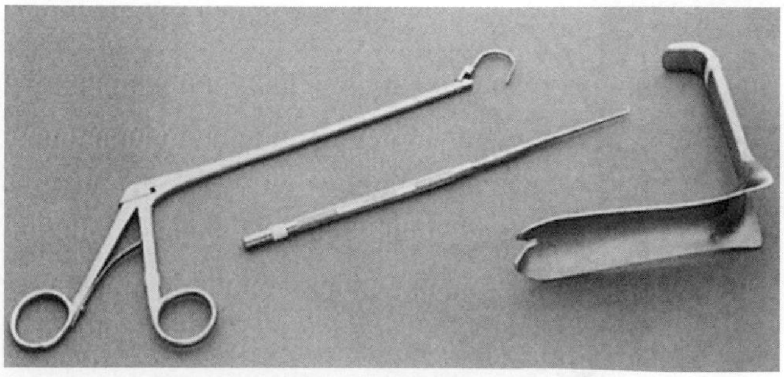

FIGURE 36E.9. Miya hook, notched speculum, and suture hook for use during sacrospinous ligament fixation. (From Walters MD, Karram MM. *Urogynecology and reconstructive pelvic surgery.* 2nd ed. St. Louis: CV Mosby; 1999.)

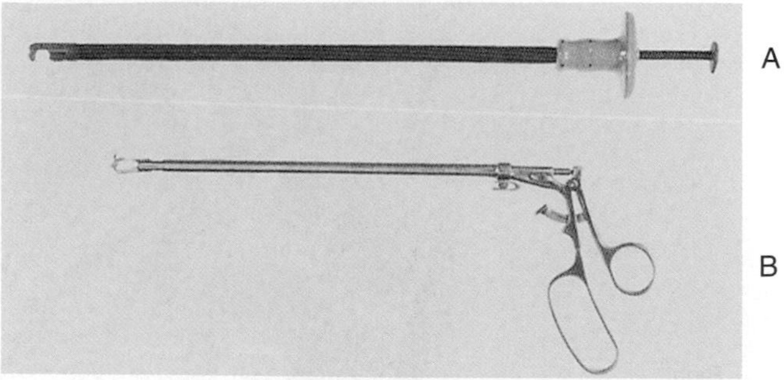

FIGURE 36E.10. Two specially designed instruments to facilitate passage of sutures through the sacrospinous ligament. **A:** Laurus needle driver (Microvasive-Boston Scientific Corporation, Watertown, MA). **B:** Nichols-Voronikis ligature carrier (BEI Medical Systems, Chatsworth, CA). (From Walters MD, Karram MM. *Urogynecology and reconstructive pelvic surgery.* 2nd ed. St. Louis: CV Mosby; 1999.)

Two Allis clamps are used to grasp the vaginal apex. With traction on the Allis clamps, the vaginal epithelium overlying the enterocele is incised. The enterocele sac is then dissected up to the neck of the hernia. The sac is opened, and the cul-de-sac is palpated for adhesions and any unsuspected pathology. If adhesions are present, they should be carefully taken down. The excess peritoneum is excised. A Heaney retractor or Deaver is then placed anteriorly. The abdominal contents are carefully packed away with moist laparotomy sponges. The retractor is withdrawn and then replaced so as to elevate the sponges and abdominal contents out of the pelvis, exposing the cul-de-sac (Fig. 36E.12).

Two Allis clamps are then placed where the remnants of uterosacral ligaments are believed to be, usually the 5-o'clock and 7-o'clock positions. It is sometimes necessary to trim excess vaginal mucosa to facilitate good traction on the uterosacral ligament. With tension on the Allis clamp directed outward, the pelvic sidewalls are palpated. The ischial spine is palpated transperitoneally, and an attempt is made to palpate the ureter. If the uterosacral ligament is difficult to find, the Allis clamp can be repositioned. The ureter is usually found 2 to 5 cm ventral and lateral to the ischial spine. The ureter is best found by applying pressure to the pelvic sidewall with the tip of the index or middle finger and sweeping from an anterior superior to a posterior inferior position.

Initially two or three delayed absorbable sutures are passed through the uterosacral ligament on each side around the level of the ischial spine. The distal remnants of the uterosacral ligaments are plicated across the midline with two to three permanent sutures. Tying of these sutures obliterates any redundant cul-de-sac. The previously placed delayed absorbable sutures are passed through the full thickness of the posterior vaginal wall. The sutures are then tied down, elevating the vault into the hollow of the sacrum. It is imperative to perform cystourethroscopy to evaluate ureteral integrity.

There are three reports to date on the **results** of high uterosacral ligament suspension. In 2000, Shull and colleagues reported on their experience with 298 patients. Thirty-five

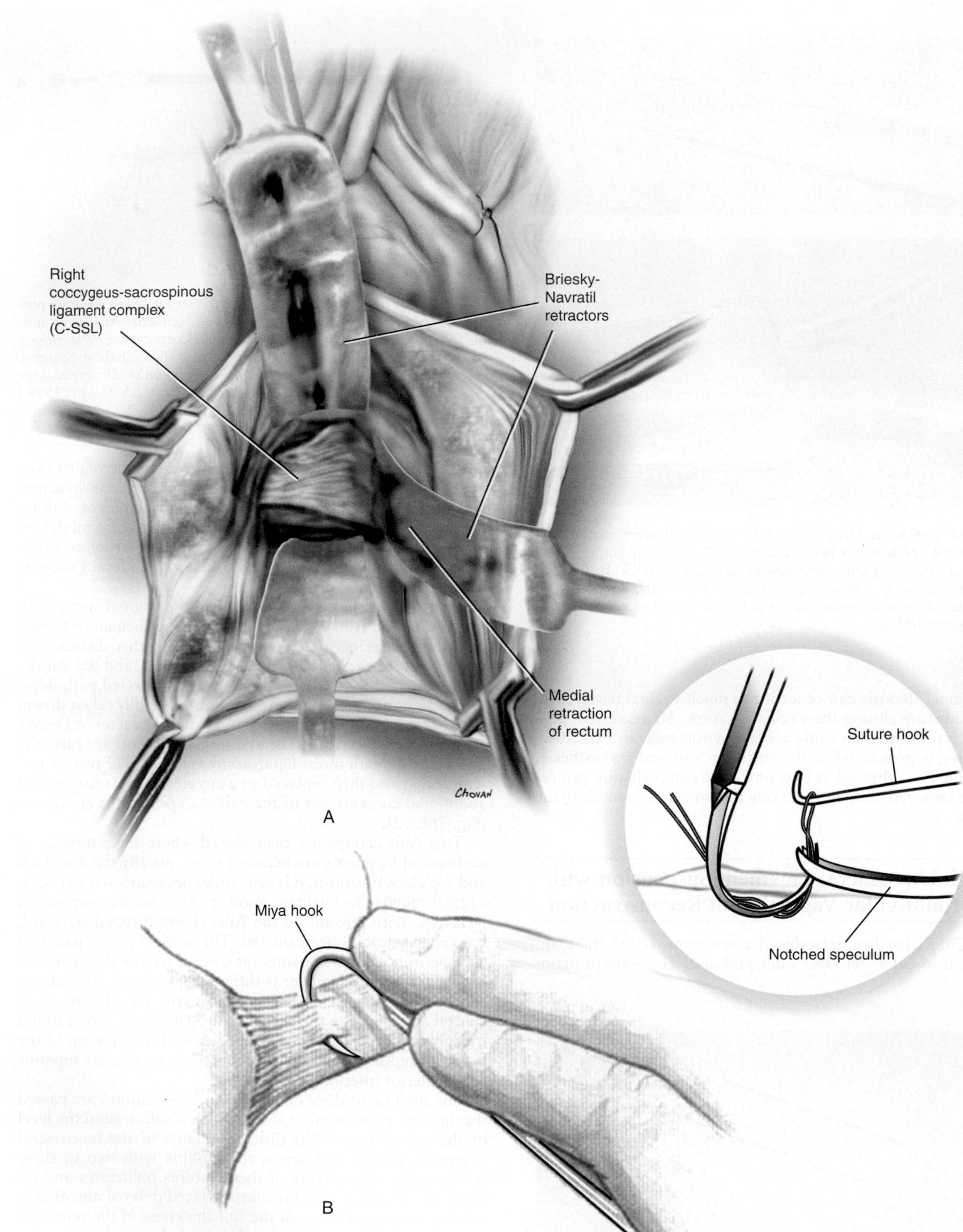

FIGURE 36E.11. A: Briesky-Navratil retractors are used to retract the rectum medially and bladder superiorly and depress the peritoneum. **B:** Technique of passage of a Miya hook through the ligament. **Inset:** Technique of retrieval of the suture. (*Continued*)

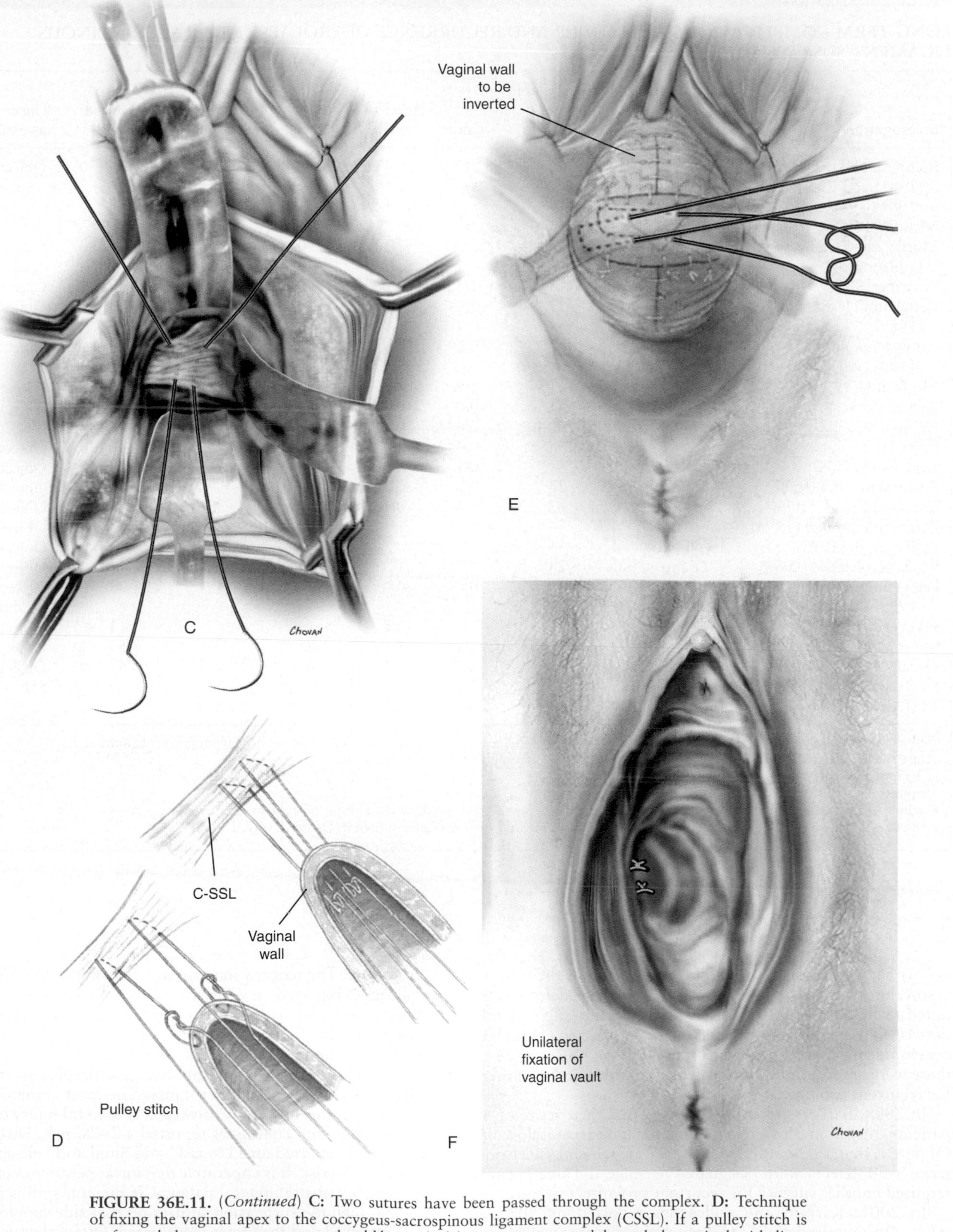

FIGURE 36E.11. (*Continued*) **C:** Two sutures have been passed through the complex. **D:** Technique of fixing the vaginal apex to the coccygeus-sacrospinous ligament complex (CSSL). If a pulley stitch is performed, then permanent sutures should be used. If the sutures are passed through the vaginal epithelium and tied in the vaginal lumen, then delayed absorbable sutures should be used. **E:** The vagina is closed before tying the suspension sutures. **F:** Tied sacrospinous sutures. (From Baggish MS, Karram MM. *Atlas of pelvic anatomy and gynecologic surgery.* New York: Saunders; 2001.)

TABLE 36E.1

LONG-TERM COMPLICATIONS, FOLLOW-UP, AND RECURRENCE OF PROLAPSE AFTER SACROSPINOUS LIGAMENT SUSPENSION

Investigation	Duration of follow-up	No. available for follow-up	Vault	Anterior wall	Posterior wall	Unspecified/ multiple sites	No. cured (%)	Cure assessment[a]
Richter and Albrich (1981) and Richter (1982)	1–10 yr	81	2/2	0/12	0/10		57 (70)	Objective
Nichols (1982)	≥2 yr	163	5/5				158 (97)[b]	
Morley and Delancey (1988)	1 mo–11 yr	92	3/3	2/11	0/0	0/3	75 (82)	Subjective/ Objective
Brown et al. (1989)	8–21 mo	11	1/1	0/0	0/0		10 (91)	Objective
Kettel and Herbertson (1989)	—	31	2/6				25 (81)	Objective
Cruikshank and Cox (1990)	8 mo–3.2 yr	48	0/1	0/5	0/2		40 (83)	Objective
Monk et al. (1991)	1 mo–8.6 yr	61	1/1	0/6	0/2		52 (85)	Objective
Backer (1992)		51	0/0	0/3	0/0		48 (94)	Objective
Heinonen (1992)	6 mo–5.6 yr	22	0/0	0/1	0/2		19 (86)	Objective
Imparato et al. (1992)	—	155	0/4			0/11	140 (90)	Objective
Shull et al. (1992)	2–5 yr	81	0/1	4/20	0/1	0/6	53 (65)	Objective
Kaminski et al. (1993)	—	23	2/2	0/1	0/0		20 (87)	Objective
Carey and Slack (1994)	2 mo–1 yr	63[d]	1/1	0/16	0/0		46 (73)	Objective
Porges and Smilen (1994)	—	76		?/1		0/2	—	Objective
Holley et al. (1995)	15–79 mo	36				0/33[e]	3 (8)	Objective
Sauer and Klutke (1995)	4–26 mo	24	3/5	1/3	0/1		15 (63)	Objective
Peters and Christenson (1995)	Median = 48 mo	30	0/0	0/0	4/6	0/1	23 (77)	Subjective/ Objective
Elkins et al. (1995)	3–6 mo	14		0/2			12 (86)	Objective
Sze et al. (1997)	7–72 mo	75	?/4	?/16	?/1	?/1	53 (71)	Objective
Ozcan et al. (1997)	4–54 mos	54	2/2	3/?	6/?		43 (80)	Objective
Hewson and Hon (1998)	8 mo–5 yr	114	2/2	6/6	?		(80)	Subjective
TOTAL	1 mo–11 yr	1,137	20/36	7/96	4/25	0/57		

[a]Subjective assessment based on telephone interview or questionnaire; objective assessment based on findings from pelvic examination.
[b]Cure rate applies to vaginal vault support only; does not include support defect at other site.
[c]Extrapolated from text.
[d]Includes 11 patients whose uteri were preserved.
[e]Includes 33 patients with anterior vaginal wall defects, three vaginal vault prolapses, and eight posterior vaginal wall relaxations.
From Sze EHM, Karram MM. Vaginal operations to correct vaginal vault prolapse: a review. *Obstet Gynecol* 1997;89:466.

(12%) had evidence of an anterior wall defect in the form of cystocele or urethrocele. However, 25 of these defects were noted to be only grade 1. Eleven (4%) patients subsequently developed posterior wall defects. In all, 38 patients (13%) had development of one or more support defects; however, 24 of these were grade 1 only. Two patients required another surgery for recurrent prolapse.

In 2000, Barber and colleagues reported their series of 46 patients, of whom 39 were available for long-term follow-up. Of note is that 19/26 anterior wall, 5/7 apical, and 13/21 posterior wall defects were designated as stage I. Three patients required another surgery for recurrent prolapse.

In 2001, Karram and colleagues reported on 202 patients. One hundred and sixty-eight patients were available for follow-up either by phone or office visit. Eighty-nine percent of patients indicated that they were happy or satisfied with the procedure. The reoperation rate was 5.5%. In 2006, Silva and colleagues reported on 72 patients who underwent uterosacral vault suspension. Two patients (2.8%) had stage II recurrence of apical prolapse with a mean follow-up of 5.1 years. These results are summarized in Table 36E.2.

Complications included hemorrhage with subsequent transfusion or bowel and bladder injury. The most common complication of this procedure, however, is ureteral injury or kinking. Karram and colleagues reported a 2.4% risk, Barber and colleagues reported an 11% risk, and Shull and colleagues reported a 1% risk. It is imperative that intraoperative cystoscopy be done to ensure ureteral patency. If ureteral spill is not observed, then the suspension sutures on that side should be cut and removed and the ureter reevaluated. Often, the suture can be replaced using a more medial placement into the uterosacral ligament complex.

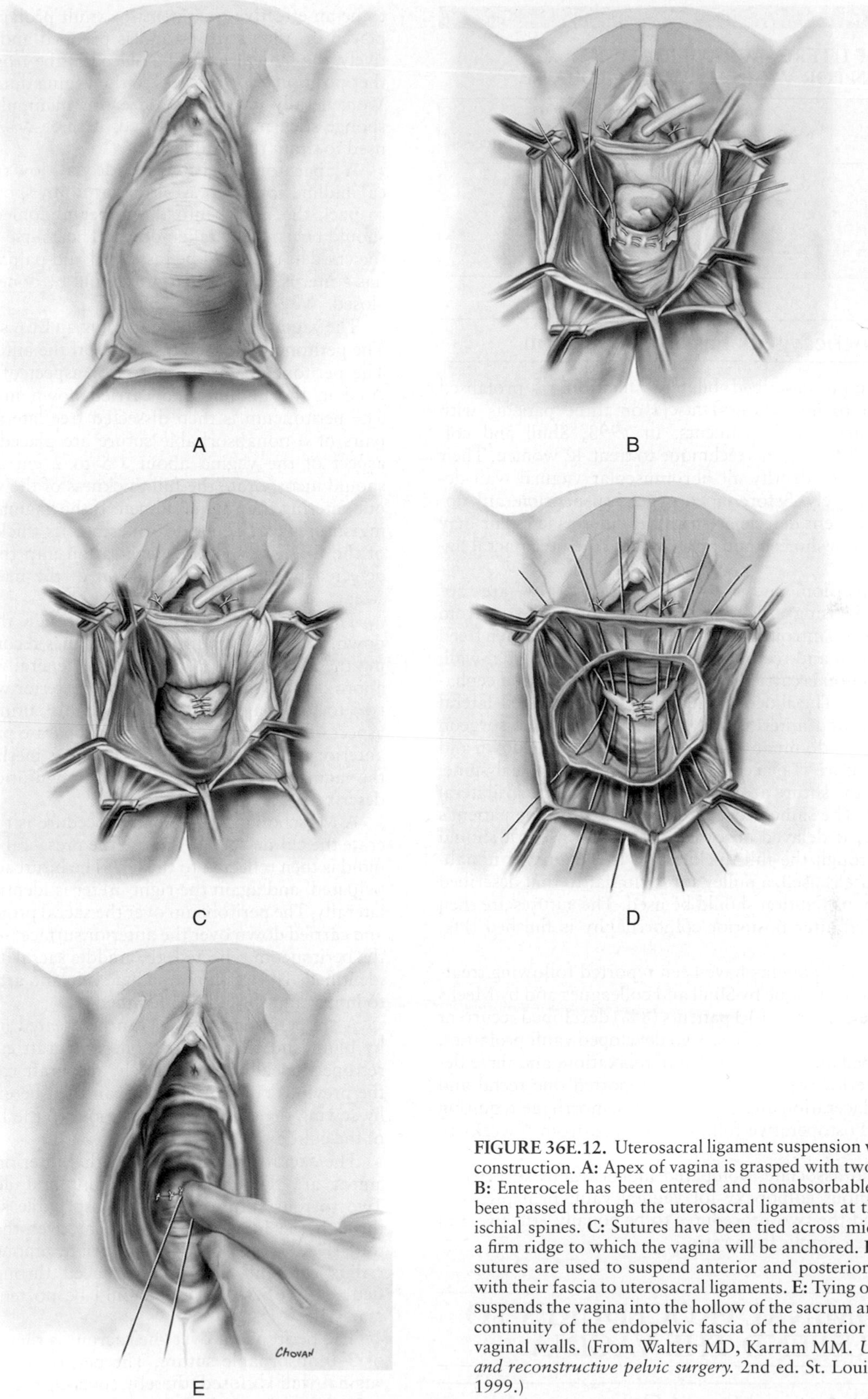

FIGURE 36E.12. Uterosacral ligament suspension with fascial reconstruction. **A:** Apex of vagina is grasped with two Allis clamps. **B:** Enterocele has been entered and nonabsorbable sutures have been passed through the uterosacral ligaments at the level of the ischial spines. **C:** Sutures have been tied across midline, creating a firm ridge to which the vagina will be anchored. **D:** Absorbable sutures are used to suspend anterior and posterior vaginal walls with their fascia to uterosacral ligaments. **E:** Tying of these sutures suspends the vagina into the hollow of the sacrum and restores the continuity of the endopelvic fascia of the anterior and posterior vaginal walls. (From Walters MD, Karram MM. *Urogynecology and reconstructive pelvic surgery.* 2nd ed. St. Louis: CV Mosby; 1999.)

TABLE 36E.2

RESULTS OF UTEROSACRAL LIGAMENT SUSPENSION FOR VAGINAL VAULT PROLAPSE

Author	No. of patients	Follow-up in months (range)	Success
Jenkins 1997	50	6–48	88%
Barber 2001	46	3.5–40	90%
Karram 2001	202	6–36	89.5%
Amundsen et al. 2003	33	6–43	82%

Iliococcygeus Fascia Suspension

In 1963, Inmon described bilateral fixation of prolapsed vaginal vault to iliococcygeal fascia on three patients with inadequate uterosacral ligaments. In 1993, Shull and colleagues reported using this technique to treat 42 women. Their approach was to identify all fibromuscular vaginal wall defects preoperatively. Before iliococcygeus suspension, any anterior compartment defects are fixed. A cul-de-sac repair may be undertaken to shorten and approximate the uterosacral ligaments.

Cuff suspension and posterior colporrhaphy are approached by excising a diamond-shaped section of tissue from the perineum and introitus. The vaginal epithelium is then freed from the rectum and rectovaginal fibromuscular vaginal wall, and the dissection is carried laterally to the levators and cephalad to the cuff. The iliococcygeus muscle is identified lateral to the rectum and anterior to the ischial spine. The surgeon then uses the nondominant hand to press the rectum down and medially. A suture is placed just anterior to the ischial spine. Both ends of the suture are then passed through the ipsilateral vaginal apex. The same procedure is repeated on the patient's opposite side. If delayed absorbable suture is used, it should be passed through the full thickness of the vagina. If nonabsorbable suture is used, a pulley stitch similar to that described for sacrospinous fixation should be used. The sutures are then held to be tied after posterior colporrhaphy is finished (Fig. 36E.13).

A total of 152 patients have been reported following treatment with this technique by Shull and colleagues and by Meeks and colleagues. A total of 13 patients (8%) developed recurrent pelvic prolapse at various sites. Two developed vault prolapses, eight developed anterior vaginal wall relaxation, and three developed posterior wall defects. They reported one rectal and one bladder laceration and two cases of hemorrhage requiring transfusion. Postoperative follow-up ranged from 6 weeks to 5 years.

Maher and associates compared iliococcygeus suspension and sacrospinous colpopexy for vaginal vault prolapse. The authors found the two procedures to be equally effective and have the same complication rates.

ABDOMINAL PROCEDURES TO SUSPEND THE VAGINA

Abdominal Sacral Colpopexy

Suspension of the vagina to the sacral promontory or into the hollow of the sacrum with an intervening mesh has been shown to be an effective treatment for vault prolapse. The patient is placed in Allen stirrups and is prepped and draped. Alternatively, the patient could be placed in the frog-leg position. Either position allows access to the vagina during the operation. We generally use an EEA sizer for manipulation, although a sponge stick may also be used. A three-way Foley catheter is used to drain the bladder.

A laparotomy incision is made via a low transverse or vertical midline approach. Moist laparotomy sponges are then used to pack the bowel into the upper abdomen. Any adhesions should be carefully taken down. The course of the ureters and the cul-de-sac should be inspected and palpated. If the patient has a uterus, a hysterectomy should be done first and the cuff closed.

The vagina is then elevated using an EEA sizer (Fig. 36E.14). The peritoneum is then dissected off the anterior vaginal wall. The peritoneum on the posterior aspect of the vagina is incised in the midline and carried down into the cul-de-sac. The peritoneum is then dissected free laterally. Three to five pairs of 0 nonabsorbable suture are placed on the posterior aspect of the vagina about 1.5 to 2 cm apart. The suture should incorporate the full thickness of the vaginal wall without entering the vaginal lumen. If the vagina is thin, imbricating sutures can be used to increase its thickness. The benefit of the EEA sizer is that penetration into the vagina is easily detected by the tactile sensation of the needle on the metal sizer.

The sutures are then placed through the mesh and tied down. In 1997, Cundiff and colleagues recommended extending the mesh to the perineum. We generally extend the mesh approximately halfway down the posterior wall. We also place two to four pairs of 0 nonabsorbable suture on the anterior aspect of the vagina and attach a separate piece of mesh. This anterior mesh is sewn to the posterior mesh just proximal to the vaginal apex. Other potential configurations have also been described.

A Moschowitz or Halban procedure is then done to obliterate the cul-de-sac. To expose the presacral area, the rectosigmoid is then reflected to the left. The bifurcation of the aorta is palpated, and again the right ureter is identified and retracted laterally. The peritoneum over the sacral promontory is opened and carried down over the anterior surface of the sacrum. With the peritoneum reflected, the middle sacral artery and vein are identified. The left common iliac vein and artery are also prone to injury and should be identified.

A subperitoneal tunnel can be created into the cul-de-sac by blunt and sharp dissection. The graft can then be placed retroperitoneally. Alternatively, the graft can be placed over the previous culdoplasty and can then be extraperitonealized by sewing the serosa of the sigmoid to the lateral peritoneum of the cul-de-sac.

The sacral promontory and the anterior longitudinal ligament are then exposed by blunt and delicate dissection. Two to four sutures of 0 nonabsorbable sutures are placed through the longitudinal ligament over the sacral promontory (Fig. 36E.15). The appropriate amount of graft material is cut, and sutures are placed through the graft and tied (Fig. 36E.16). There should be no tension on the graft material.

The peritoneum over the sacrum is then closed with a 2-0 or 3–0 absorbable suture. The peritoneum over the anterior vaginal wall is closed, thereby covering the mesh. Generally, a paravaginal repair is done and, when indicated, a retropubic urethropexy. Suprapubic telescopy or cystoscopy is performed, and a suprapubic catheter can be placed if desired. The abdomen is then closed.

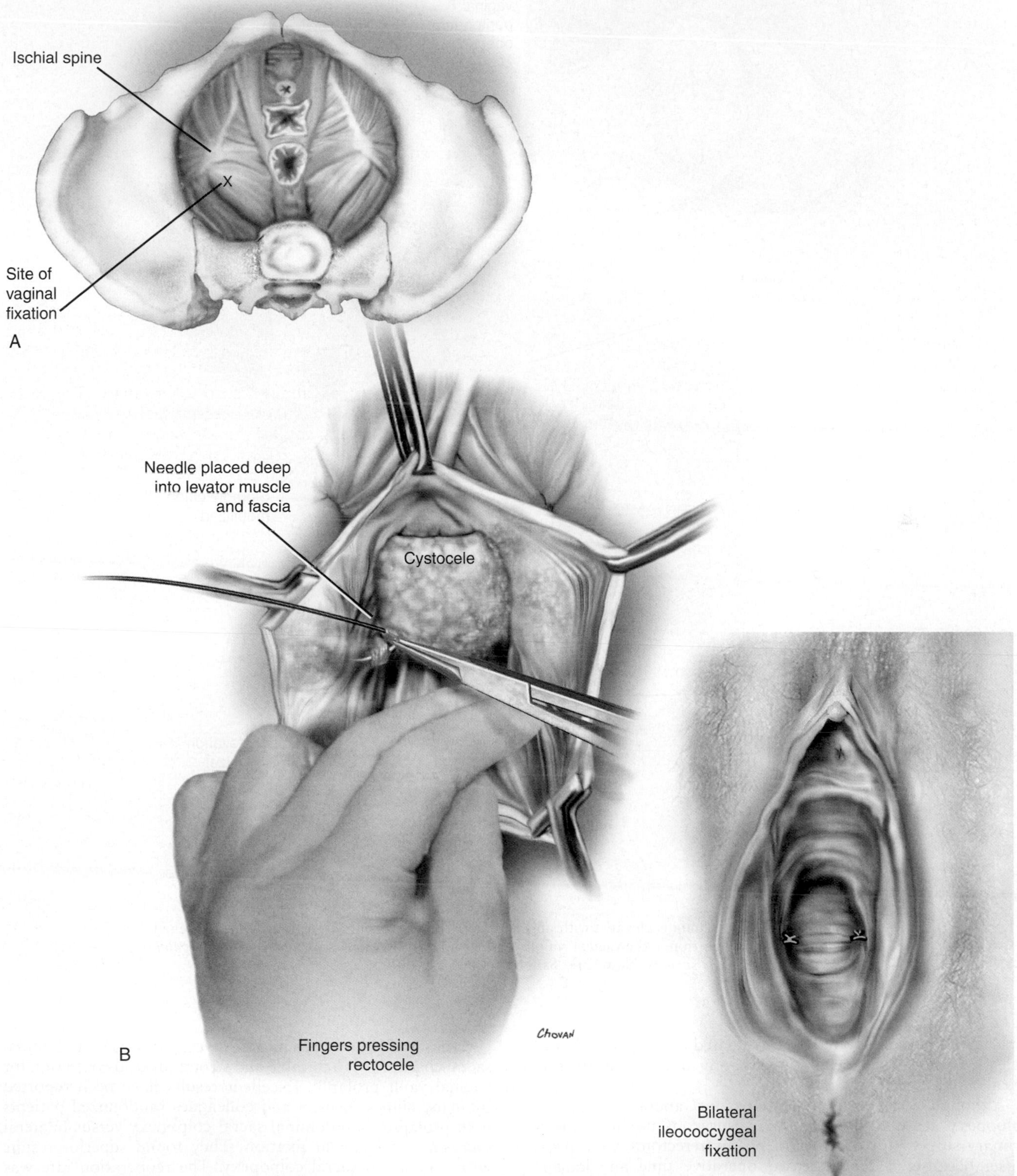

FIGURE 36E.13. Ileococcygeus fascia suspension. **A:** With the surgeon's finger pressing the rectum downward, the right ileococcygeus fascia suture is placed. **Inset:** Approximate location of the ileococcygeus fascia sutures. **B:** Bilateral ileococcygeus fascia suspension. (From Baggish MS, Karram MM. *Atlas of pelvic anatomy and gynecologic surgery.* New York: Saunders; 2001.)

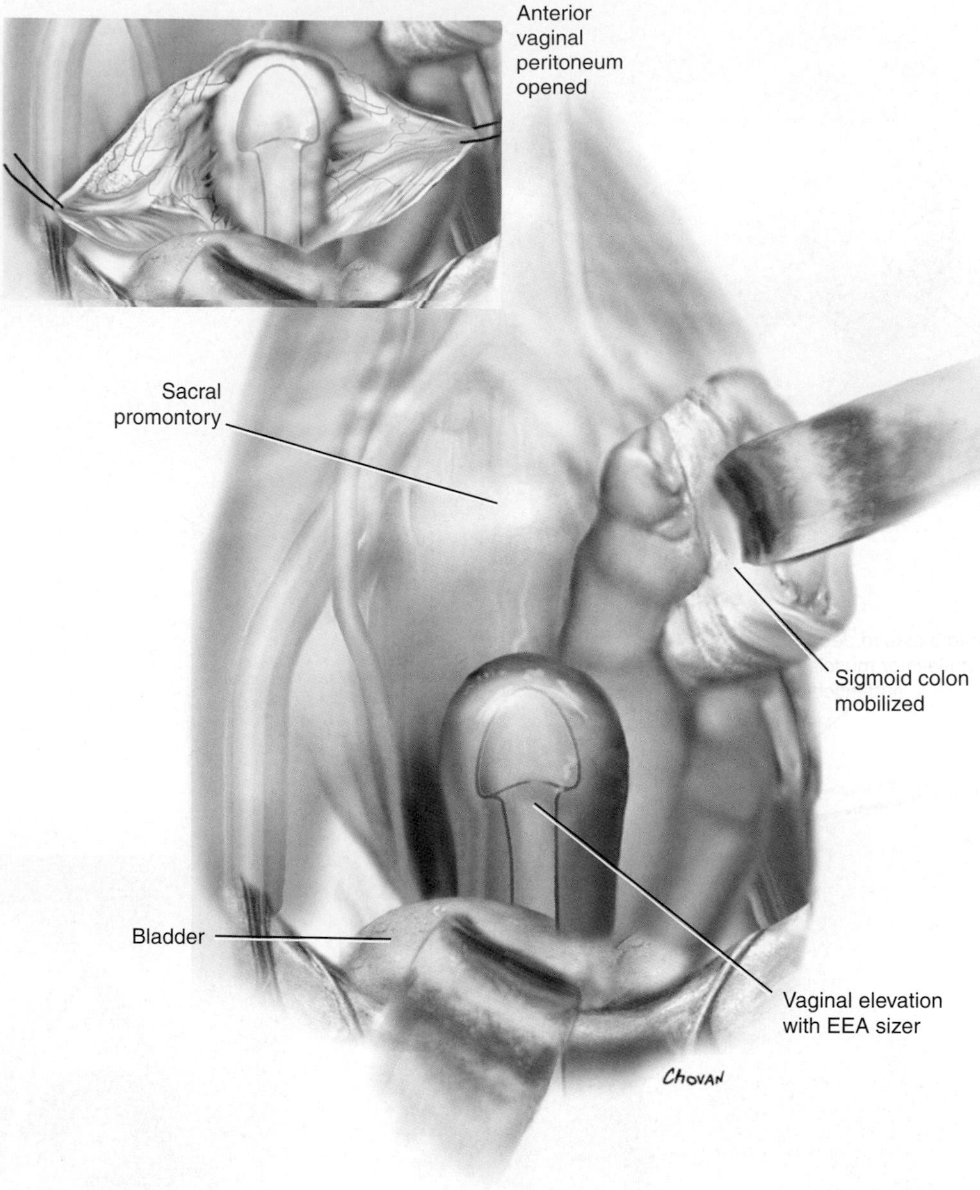

FIGURE 36E.14. The vagina is elevated with an EEA sizer. The peritoneum over the vagina is opened, exposing the muscular portion of the vaginal wall (*inset*). (From Baggish MS, Karram MM. *Atlas of pelvic anatomy and gynecologic surgery.* New York: Saunders; 2001.)

The vagina is inspected and evaluated for any remaining defects. Usually a posterior colporrhaphy and a perineoplasty are also required.

Although the exact **indications** for abdominal sacral colpopexy are controversial, many surgeons use it as their primary surgery for all cases of posthysterectomy vault prolapse. Because of the increased operative time and longer time to recover, we generally use the abdominal approach for young patients with advanced prolapse, patients who have previously failed a vaginal approach, have a foreshortened vagina, or who have other coexisting conditions that predispose to continued marked increases in intraabdominal pressure and therefore possible subsequent failure.

It has been shown by multiple investigators that abdominal sacral colpopexy is a durable and strong surgical correction for vaginal vault prolapse. Excellent **results** have been reported by many clinics. Benson and colleagues randomized patients with prolapse to abdominal sacral colpopexy versus bilateral sacrospinous ligament fixation. They found superior results with abdominal sacral colpopexy. The reoperation rate was 33% in the vaginal group and 16% in the abdominal group. Optimal results were obtained in only 29% of the vaginal group and 58% of the abdominal group. The time of operation was longer for the abdominal group. Lo and Wang also reported higher success rates with abdominal sacral colpopexy than sacrospinous fixation, and Maher and associates reported similar success rates.

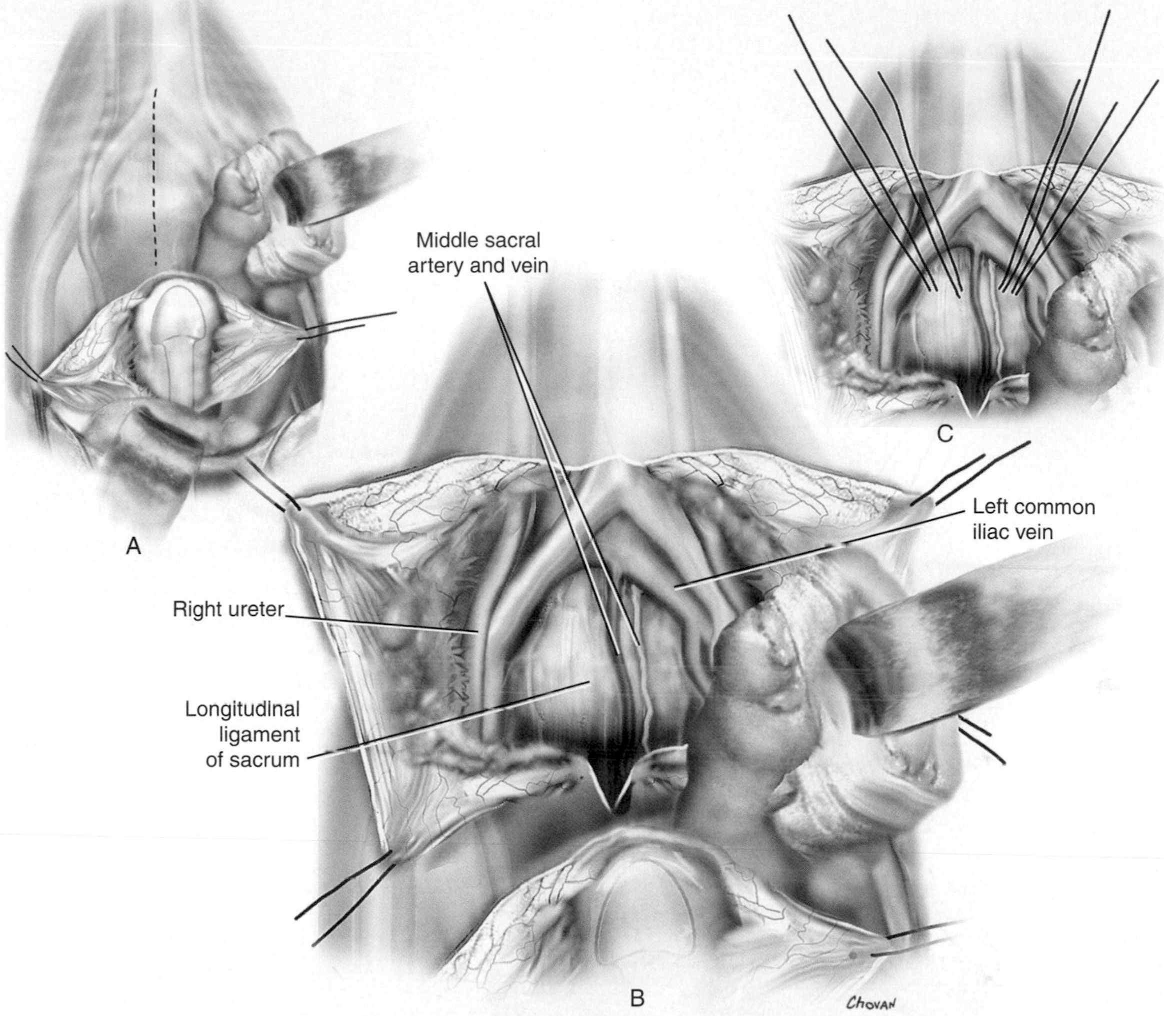

FIGURE 36E.15. Anatomy of the sacral promontory. **A:** Incision into the peritoneum. **B:** Dissection to the longitudinal ligament of the promontory. Note the vascularity of this area. **C:** Placement of permanent sutures through the longitudinal ligament of sacrum. (From Baggish MS, Karram MM. *Atlas of pelvic anatomy and gynecologic surgery.* New York: Saunders; 2001.)

Overall, the long-term results from sacral colpopexy have been very good. Addison and colleagues reported three recurrent prolapses after sacral colpopexy. In two patients, the synthetic mesh had separated from the vaginal wall, and in the third patient, the posterior vaginal wall ruptured distal to the attachment of the mesh. The authors believed that failures can be minimized by performing meticulous culdoplasty and securing the mesh to the culdoplasty with permanent sutures to prevent the dissection of an enterocele. They also recommended attaching the mesh to the vagina at multiple sites. Long-term follow-up is summarized in Table 36E.3.

Intraoperative **complications** are unusual, and injury to bowel, bladder, ureter, and infection, as with all abdominal surgery, have been described. Hemorrhage, especially from presacral vessels, can be life-threatening. Hemostasis can be difficult because damaged presacral vessels tend to retract beneath the bony surface. Sutures, hemoclips, and bone wax should be used initially. If these measures fail, then sterile thumbtacks can be employed. These stainless steel thumbtacks should be placed on the retracted bleeding vessel.

The most common long-term complication has been erosion of synthetic mesh. Kohli and colleagues in 1996 reported an incidence of 7%. Removal of the eroded mesh can be done via an abdominal or vaginal route. We have had good success removing the mesh via the vaginal route. With the patient prepped and draped, as much of the mesh as possible is exposed. The mesh is cut as high as possible and removed. The vaginal edges are then trimmed and closed in layers.

High Uterosacral Ligament Suspension

The vaginal approach of vaginal suspension to the uterosacral ligaments has been described. The same concept can also be used in an abdominal approach. After the abdominal wall has been opened and the bowel has been packed away, the remnants of the uterosacral ligaments are identified and tagged

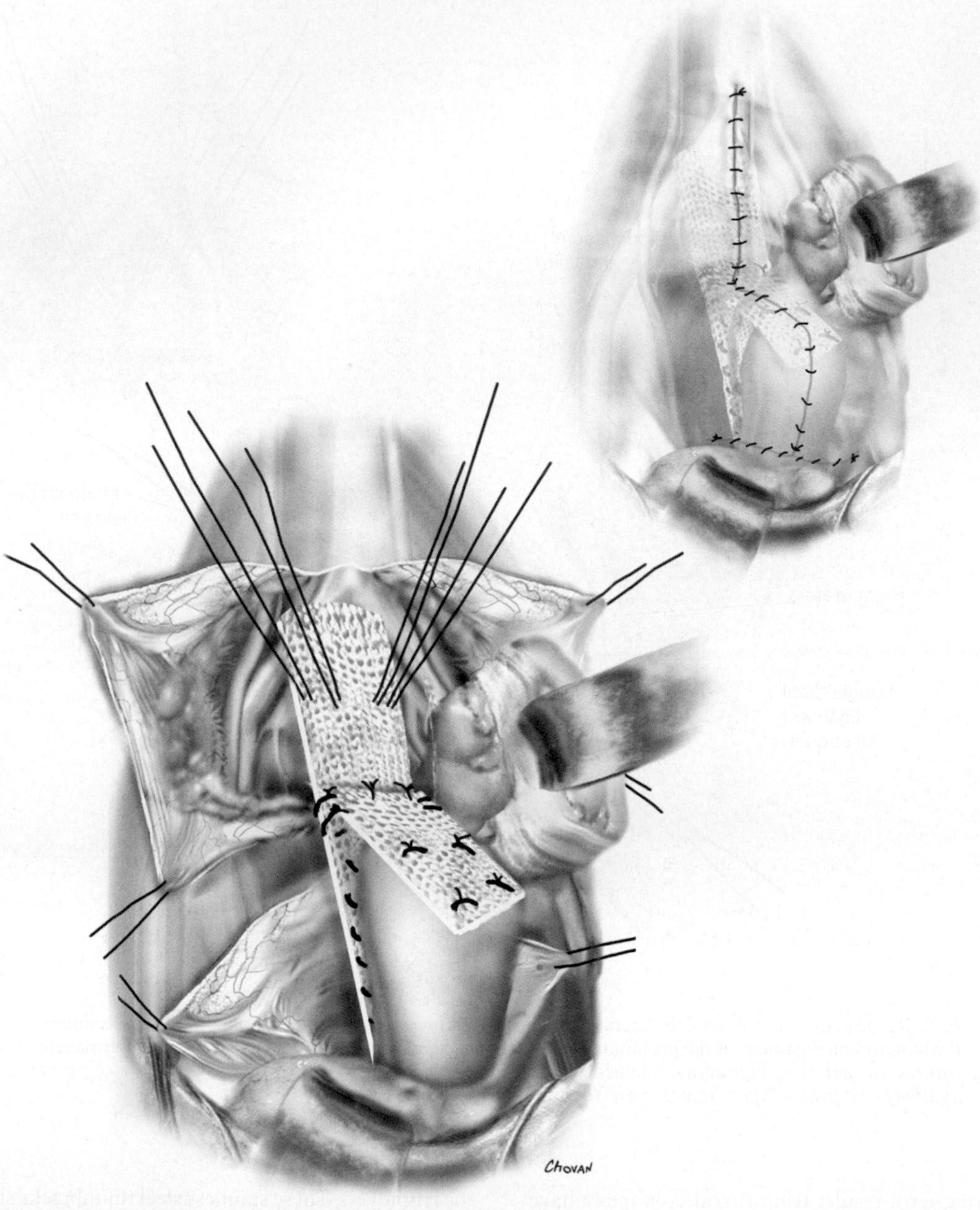

FIGURE 36E.16. Attachment of the mesh to the sacrum. Closure of the peritoneum over the mesh is shown in the inset. (From Baggish MS, Karram MM. *Atlas of pelvic anatomy and gynecologic surgery.* New York: Saunders; 2001.)

with suture near the ischial spine. The ureters are identified bilaterally. The enterocele is then addressed by obliteration of the cul-de-sac. The peritoneum over the vaginal apex is then opened, and the endopelvic fibromuscular vaginal wall is identified and reapproximated to form a continuous covering of endopelvic fibromuscular vaginal wall over the vaginal epithelium. Nonabsorbable sutures are then used to suspend the vagina with the now intact endopelvic fibromuscular vaginal wall to the uterosacral ligaments (Figs. 36E.17 and 36E.18).

Results for the abdominal approach to high uterosacral suspension should be similar to those for the vaginal approach. There are, however, no long-term studies available. Complications are similar to those for the vaginal approach.

LAPAROSCOPIC APPROACH TO VAGINAL SUSPENSION

The techniques and concepts described earlier can also be approached via laparoscopy. The laparoscopic approach to the patient for positioning, port placement, and equipment is described elsewhere. The laparoscopic approach to these

TABLE 36E.3

LONG-TERM FOLLOW-UP AND RECURRENCE OF PROLAPSE AFTER ABDOMINAL SACRAL COLPOPEXY

Investigator	Duration of follow-up (mo)	No. available for follow-up	Vault[a]	Anterior wall[a]	Posterior wall[a]	Unspecified/ multiple sites	No. cured (%)	Cure assessment
Rust et al. (1976)	9–40	12	0/0	0/1	0/0	0/0	12/12 (100)	Objective[b]
Todd (1978)	NA	93	½	0/0	0/1	0/1	91/93 (98)	Objective[b]
Feldman and Birnbaum (1979)	1–48	21	0/1	0/2	0/1	0/1	20/21 (95)	Objective[b]
Cowan and Morgan (1980)	≤60	39	0/1	NA	NA	NA	38/39 (97)	Objective[b]
Addison et al. (1985)	6–126	56	2/2	0/0	0/0	0/0	54/56 (96)	NA
Drutz and Cha (1987)	3–93	15	1/1	0/0	0/2	0/0	14/15 (93)	Objective[b]
Angulo and Kligman (1989)	2–36	18	0/0	NA	NA	NA	18/18 (100)	Objective
Baker et al. (1990)	1–45	59	0/0	0/6	0/4	0/0	51/51 (100)	Subjective/ Objective
Maloney et al. (1990)	12–60	10	0/1	0/0	0/0	0/0	9/10 (90)	NA
Creighton and Stanton (1991)	3–35	23	2/2	0/0	0/0	0/0	21/23 (91)	Objective[b]
Snyder and Krantz (1991)	≥6	116	?/8	NA	NA	?/24	108/116 (93)	Objective
Timmons et al. (1992)	9–216	162	0/1	0/0	3/3	0/0	161/162 (99)	Objective[b]
Imparato et al. (1992)	NA	63	?/4	0/0	0/0	?/10	59/63 (94)	Objective[b]
Traiman et al. (1992)	6–60	11	0/1	NA	NA	NA	10/11 (91)	NA
Iosif (1993)	12–120	40	1/1	0/1	0/2	0/0	39/40 (96)	Objective
Grunberger et al. (1994)	12–240	48	0/3	0/0	0/0	6/6	45/48 (94)	Objective
Virtanen et al. (1994)	12–96	27	0/1	0/1	0/0	0/1	23/27 (85)	Objective
Valaitis and Stanton (1994)	3–91	38	3/3	0/0	0/1	0/0	38/41 (93)	Objective
Van Lindert et al. (1996)	15–63	61	0/0	0/0	0/0	0/2	61/61 (100)	Objective[b]

[a]Denotes the number of patients with recurrent prolapse who underwent surgical repair/number of patients with recurrent prolapse.
[b]Extrapolated from text.
NA, Not available.

procedures requires patience, attention to detail, and the realization that there is a steep learning curve. It is our belief that the operation and subsequent outcomes should not be compromised for the purpose of having achieved the operation by this approach. Therefore, the surgical measures taken to achieve the underlying concepts should not be significantly altered or changed.

ABDOMINAL VERSUS VAGINAL APPROACH TO PELVIC PROLAPSE

Expert opinion differs as to the most appropriate approach to pelvic organ prolapse. There are two randomized controlled trials that evaluate the best approach to prolapse repairs. Benson and associates demonstrated the abdominal sacral colpopexy was more likely to result in an optimal outcome as compared with the vaginal approach using sacrospinous fixation. The vaginal group also underwent needle urethropexy for stress incontinence. Previous authors have shown that retroversion of the vaginal axis predisposes to recurrent anterior vaginal wall prolapse. Maher and colleagues compared abdominal sacral colpopexy to unilateral sacrospinous fixation and found them to be equally effective in the treatment of posthysterectomy vault prolapse. Data from both studies suggest the vaginal route to be safer and require less operative time. It is important to note that in both studies, the authors are in fact comparing a combination of procedures, and this must be taken into account when evaluating this data. It is our opinion that no one surgical approach is appropriate for all patients. Surgeons must be adept at multiple approaches and procedures to effectively care for all patients.

ROLE OF HYSTERECTOMY IN PROLAPSE REPAIRS

Hysterectomy with repair of pelvic support defects is standard practice for most parts of the world. However, more attention has been placed on uterine preservation when undergoing surgery for prolapse repairs. This is probably due to concerns about bowel, bladder, and sexual function following removal of the uterus and the improvement of conservative measures to treat menometrorrhagia. Three studies by Maher and associates, Hefni and colleagues, and van Brummen and associates failed to show a decrease in prolapse recurrence if hysterectomy was performed. There is no evidence that suggests routine hysterectomy improves the outcome of prolapse surgery, and there

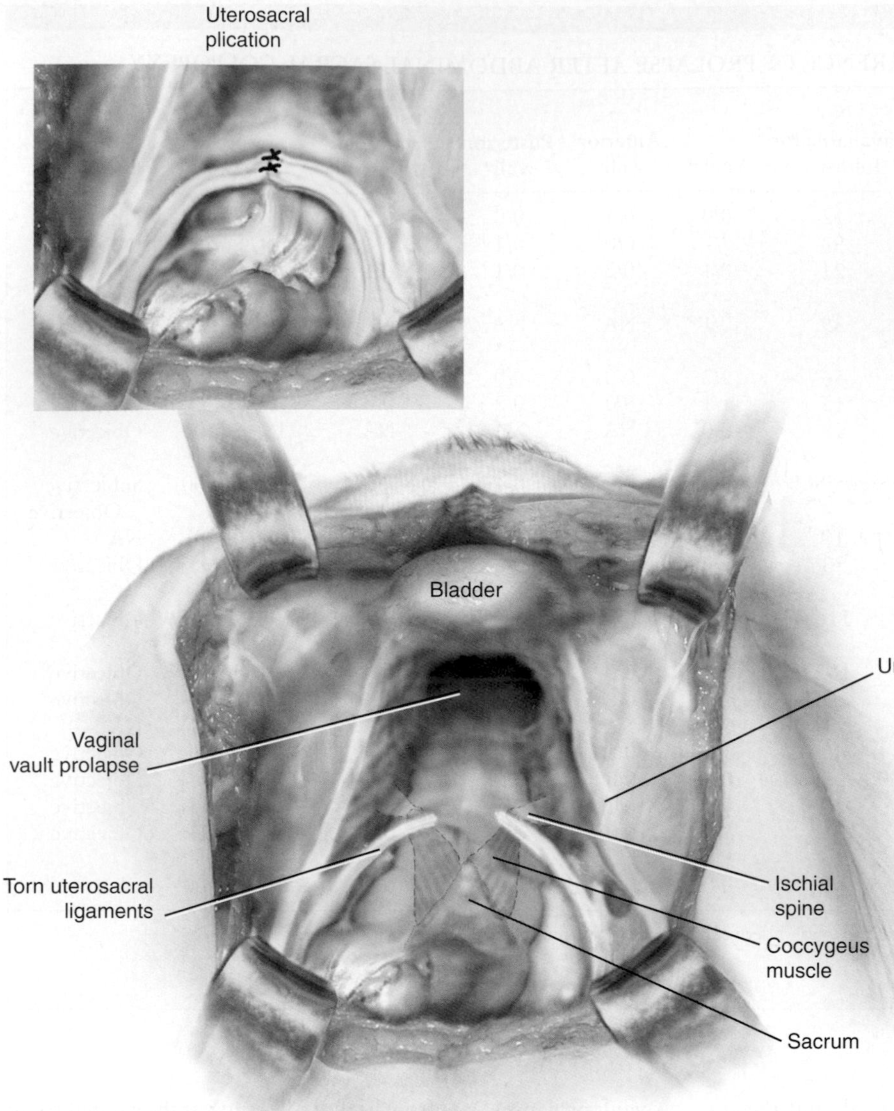

FIGURE 36E.17. Abdominal view of an enterocele and vaginal vault prolapse. Note the broken ends of the uterosacral ligaments at the level of the ischial spine. The inset demonstrates plication of ligaments, creating a firm durable ridge in the hollow of the sacrum to which the vaginal vault will be suspended. (From Baggish MS, Karram MM. *Atlas of pelvic anatomy and gynecologic surgery.* New York: Saunders; 2001.)

are no prospective studies comparing sacralcolpopexy with and without hysterectomy. More research is needed to understand the impact of hysterectomy on anatomic and functional outcomes when performing prolapse surgery.

OBLITERATIVE PROCEDURES

Le Fort Partial Colpocleisis

At times, a patient may be sufficiently bothered by uterovaginal or vault prolapse but they are poor candidates for major reconstructive surgery because of their overall medical condition. An obliterative procedure may then be a good approach for these women. A Le Fort procedure is an option if the patient has her uterus and is no longer sexually active. The rate of postoperative urinary stress incontinence has been reported to be as high as 30% after this procedure, and, because the uterus is retained, it will be difficult to evaluate any future uterine bleeding or cervical pathology. Therefore, endometrial biopsy and Papanicolaou smear must be done before surgery.

The procedure is started by placing the cervix on traction to evert the vagina. The vaginal mucosa is injected with 0.025% Marcaine with 1:200,000 epinephrine just below the epithelium. A Foley catheter with a 30-cc balloon is placed in the bladder for identification of the bladder neck.

A marking pen or scalpel is used to mark out the areas that are to be denuded both anteriorly and posteriorly. The area should extend 2 cm proximal to the tip of the cervix to 4 to 5 cm below the external meatus. A mirror image on the posterior aspect of the cervix should also be marked out.

The previously marked areas are removed by sharp dissection. The surgeon should leave the maximum amount of fibromuscular vaginal wall behind on the bladder and rectum. Hemostasis is an absolute must (Fig. 36E.19).

The cut edges of the anterior and posterior vaginal wall are sewn together with interrupted delayed absorbable sutures. The knot should be turned into the epithelium-lined tunnels that were created bilaterally. The uterus and vaginal apex are

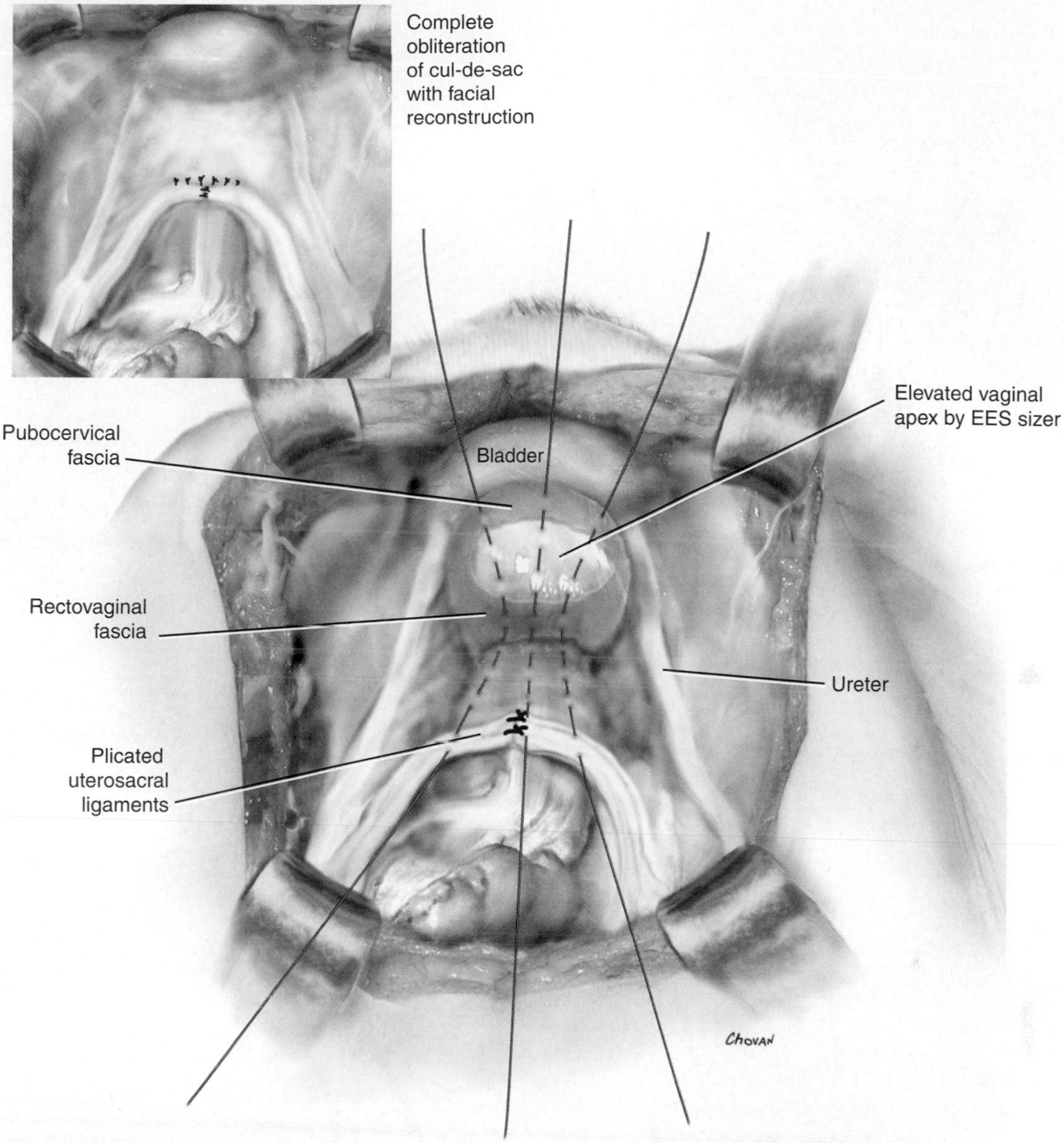

FIGURE 36E.18. Longitudinally placed nonabsorbable sutures are passed through the ridge of uterosacral ligaments, down the cul-de-sac to the edge of the rectovaginal fascia, into the vaginal vault, and finally, through the edge of pubocervical fascia. Tying of the sutures (*inset*) elevates the apex of the vagina to the uterosacral ligaments and reapproximates the pubocervical fascia with the rectovaginal fascia. (From Baggish MS, Karram MM. *Atlas of pelvic anatomy and gynecologic surgery.* New York: Saunders; 2001.)

gradually turned inward. After the vagina has been inverted, the superior and inferior margins of the rectangle can be sutured. A plication of the bladder neck should be routinely performed because of the high incidence of postoperative stress incontinence. Also, because there is no real support to the repair, an aggressive perineorrhaphy should be done to narrow the introitus.

In general, about 90% of patients have relief of symptoms and have good anatomic results. Complete breakdown and recurrence can be expected in 2% to 5% of patients. **Results** are summarized in Table 36E.4.

Early postoperative **complications** include hematoma and infection. These patients typically have other medical problems that may need to be addressed. Goldman and colleagues in 1985 reported on late postoperative complications from a modified Le Fort procedure in 118 patients. Ninety percent of patients had good anatomic results, whereas 85% had relief of symptoms. Two percent to 5% had recurrence of their prolapse, 10.2% developed incontinence or worsening of their incontinence, and 1.8% had late vaginal bleeding.

Colpectomy and Colpocleisis

For patients with posthysterectomy vault prolapse who do not desire coital function and for whom operative time is to be kept

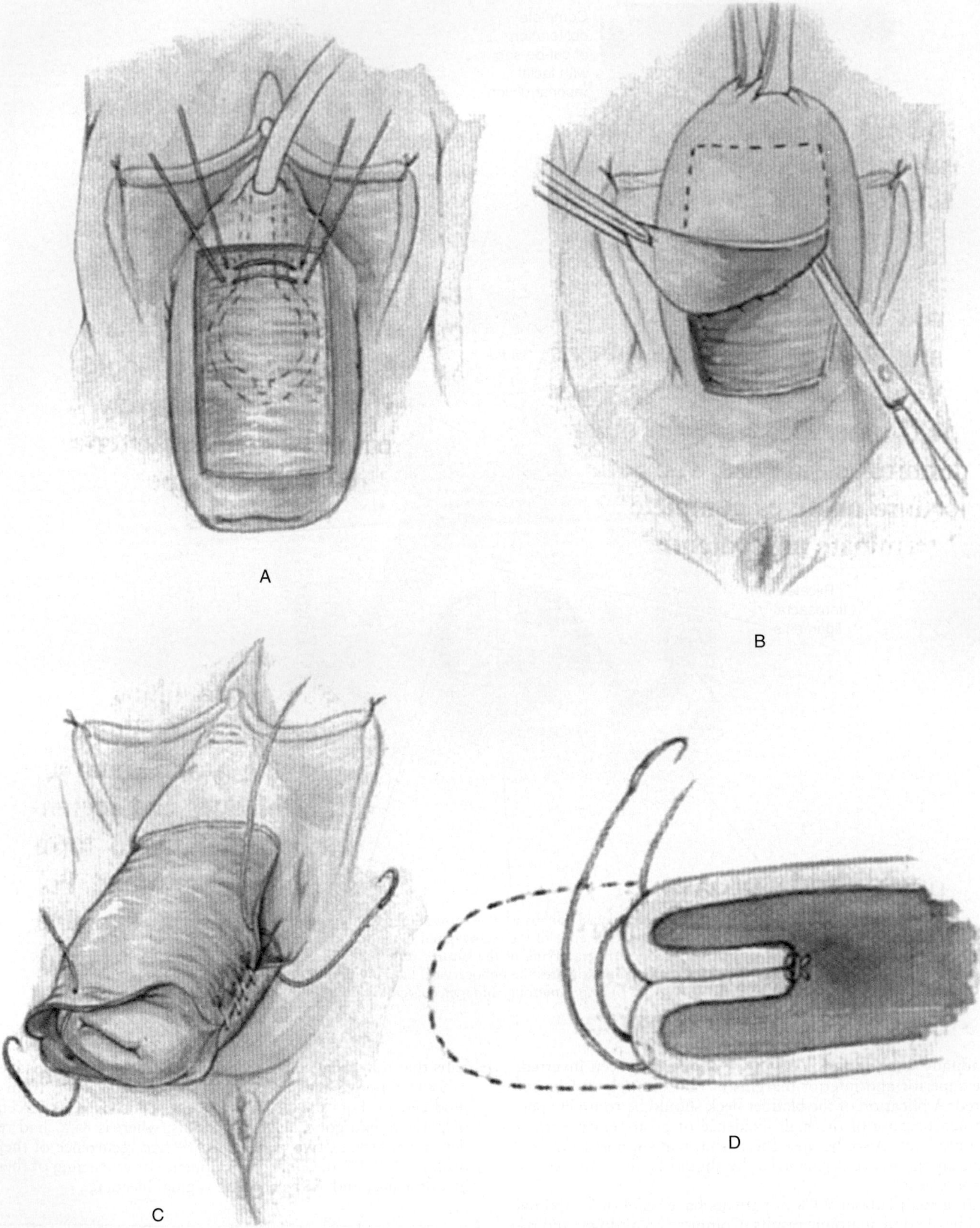

FIGURE 36E.19. Le Fort partial colpocleisis. **A:** The anterior vaginal wall has been removed, and a plication stitch is placed at the bladder neck. **B:** The posterior vaginal wall is removed. **C** and **D:** The cut edge of the anterior vaginal wall is sewn in the cut edge of the posterior vaginal wall in such a way that the uterus and vagina are inverted. (From Baggish MS, Karram MM. *Atlas of pelvic anatomy and gynecologic surgery.* New York: Saunders; 2001.)

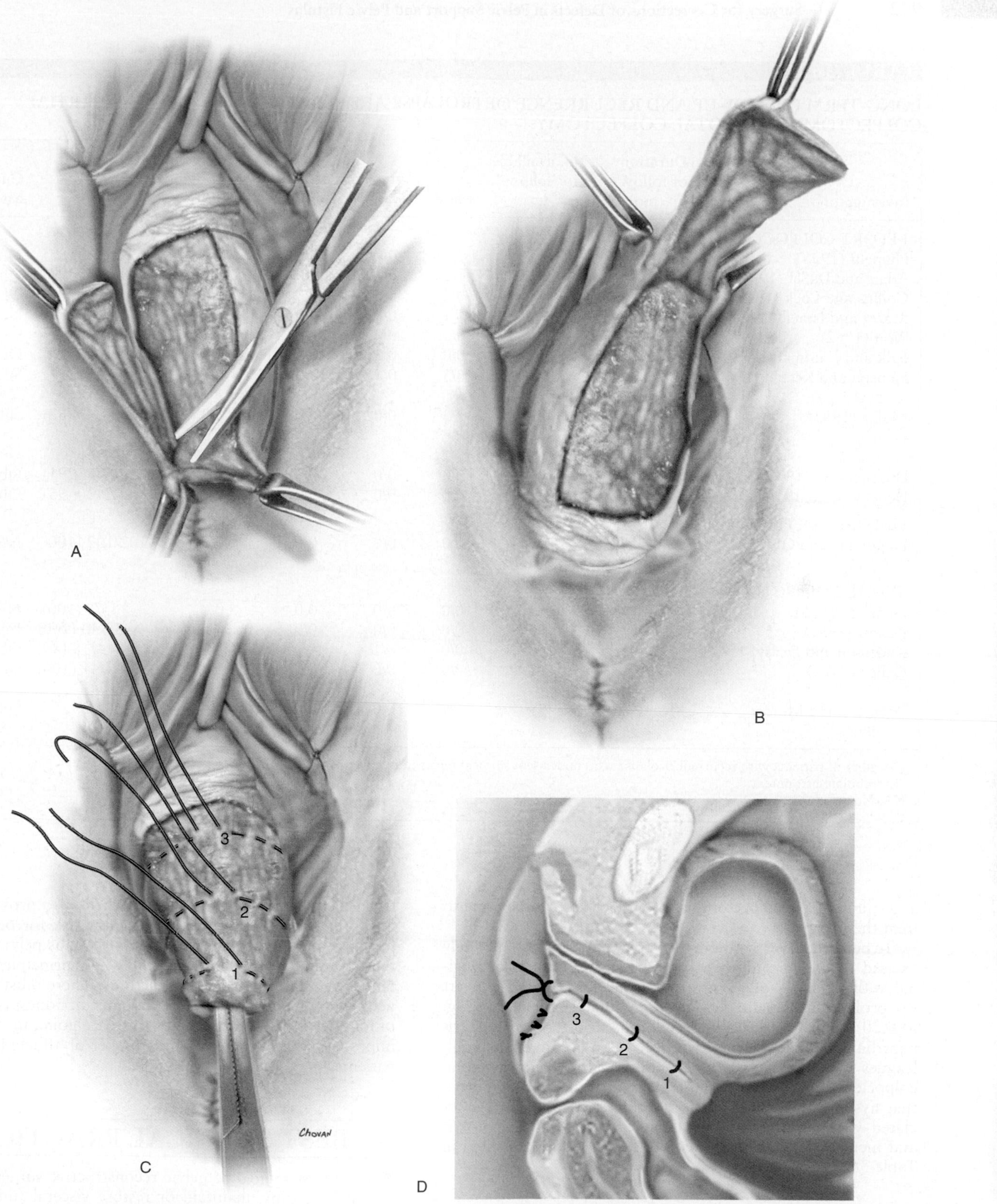

FIGURE 36E.20. Colpectomy and complete colpocleisis. **A** and **B:** After subcutaneous infiltration with lidocaine or bupivacaine hydrochloride in 1/200,000 epinephrine solution, the vagina is circumscribed by an incision at the site of the hymen and marked into quadrants. Each quadrant is removed by sharp dissection. **C:** Purse-string delayed absorbable sutures are placed. The leading edge of the soft tissue is inverted by the tip of a forceps. Purse-string sutures are tied 1 before 2 and 2 before 3, with progressive inversion of the soft tissue before the tying of each suture. **D:** The final relationship is shown in cross section. A perineorrhaphy is also usually performed. (From Baggish MS, Karram MM. *Atlas of pelvic anatomy and gynecologic surgery.* New York: Saunders; 2001.)

TABLE 36E.4

LONG-TERM FOLLOW-UP AND RECURRENCE OF PROLAPSE AFTER LE FORT COLPOCLEISIS, PARTIAL COLPECTOMY, AND TOTAL COLPECTOMY

Investigator	Duration of follow up (mo)	No. available for follow-up	Vault[a]	Anterior wall[a]	Posterior wall[a]	Unspecified/ multiple Sites[a]	No. cured total (%)	Cure assessment
LEFORT COLPOCLEISIS								
Phaneuf (1935)	NA	20	?/2	0/1	0/0	0/0	17/20 (85)	NA
Adair and DaSef (1936)	3–>36	38	0/0	0/2	0/0	1/1	35/38 (92)	Objective[b]
Collins and Lock (1941)	1–48	31	0/2	0/0	0/0	0/0	29/31 (94)	Objective[b]
Mazer and Israel (1948)	24–132	38	1/1	0/0	0/0	0/0	37/38 (97)	NA
Wolf (1952)	NA	13	0/0	0/0	0/0	1/1	12/13 (92)	Objective
Falk and Kaufman (1955)	>24	100	0/0	0/2	0/2	0/0	96/100 (96)	Objective
Hanson and Keettel (1969)	≥60	216	3/3	0/1	?/1	0/8	203/216 (94)	Subjective/ Objective
Ridley (1972)	6–60	17	2/3	0/0	0/0	0/0	14/17 (82)	Subjective/ Objective
Ubachs et al. (1973)	≥36	93	2/3	0/0	0/0	0/5	85/93 (91)	Objective
Denehy et al. (1995)	4–40	20	0/0	0/0	0/0	1/1	19/20 (95)	Objective
PARTIAL COLPECTOMY								
Langmade and Oliver (1986)	12–144	102	0/0	0/0	0/0	0/0	102/102 (100)	NA
TOTAL COLPECTOMY								
Phaneuf (1935)	NA	5	0/0	0/0	0/0	0/0	5/5 (100)	NA
Adams (1951)	12–408	30	0/0	0/0	0/0	0/0	30/30 (100)	NA
Anderson and Deasy (1960)	6–12	18	0/0	0/1	0/1	0/0	16/18 (89)	Objective[b]
Ridley (1972)	6–60	41	0/0	0/0	0/0	0/0	41/41 (100)	Subjective/ Objective
Delancey and Morley (1997)	Mean = 35	33	1/1	0/0	0/0	0/0	32/33 (97)	Subjective/ Objective

[a]Number of patients with recurrent prolapse who underwent surgical repair/number of patients with recurrent prolapse.
[b]Extrapolated from text.
NA, Not available.

at a minimum, a colpectomy and colpocleisis can be done to treat the prolapse.

To perform this operation, the vaginal mucosa is completely excised from the underlying endopelvic fibromuscular vaginal wall. A series of purse-string sutures are used to invert the prolapse and endopelvic fibromuscular vaginal wall (Fig. 36E.20). Once the prolapse is reduced, a posterior colpoperineorrhaphy and levatorplasty is done. Von Pechmann and colleagues reported two cases of rectal prolapse following total colpocleisis in a total of 92 patients. The authors also reported that hysterectomy done at the time of colpectomy was associated with a statistically significant decrease in hematocrit and increase in transfusion requirement. **Results** are listed in Table 36E.4.

CONCLUSION

Our understanding of the anatomy and concepts of pelvic organ prolapse and its treatments are constantly evolving. This evolution will and must continue to facilitate our understanding of the complex and varied etiologies of pelvic organ prolapse. Surgical treatments must restore both anatomic and functional derangements. This evolution will also provide insight into preventive measures for women at risk for pelvic organ prolapse and pelvic floor dysfunction. We, as pelvic surgeons, must continue to evaluate and apply new principles and techniques to established surgical dictums. There must be continued research, education, and a thoughtful, honest comparison of long-term surgical outcomes if we are going to continue to improve our care to a growing number of afflicted but active patients.

BEST SURGICAL PRACTICES

- The ultimate goal of pelvic reconstructive surgery is to restore anatomy, maintain or restore visceral function, and maintain or restore sexual function.
- The McCall culdoplasty and its various modifications are the most commonly used transvaginal techniques to suspend the vaginal apex. Approximately three delayed absorbable sutures are used to plicate the uterosacral ligaments. The Mayo Clinic technique excises a wedge of posterior and anterior vaginal wall, and any enterocele that is present, and includes both the uterosacral and cardinal ligaments for support.

- For significant vaginal prolapse, the sacrospinous ligament fixation is a useful transvaginal technique. Surgeons should be very familiar with the anatomy and experienced with the procedure because injury to the pudendal nerve or vessels can cause serious injury or life-threatening hemorrhage.
- Abdominal sacral colpopexy is a very useful technique if an abdominal approach is indicated for other reasons (adnexal mass) and is preferred by some surgeons for the treatment of recurrent prolapse after a prior surgical failure. We prefer to support the vagina to this longitudinal ligament of the sacrum using synthetic mesh, which is sutured to the anterior and posterior vaginal walls with 0 nonabsorbable sutures.

Bibliography

Adair FL, DaSef L. The LeFort colpocleisis. *Am J Obstet Gynecol* 1936;32: 334.

Adams HD. Total colpocleisis for pelvic eventration. *Surg Gynecol Obstet* 1951;2:321.

Addison WA, Livengood CH, Sutton GP, et al. Abdominal sacral colpopexy with Mersilene mesh in the retroperitoneal position in the management of posthysterectomy vaginal vault prolapse and enterocele. *Am J Obstet Gynecol* 1985;153:140–146.

Addison WA, Timmons MC, Wall LL, et al. Failed abdominal sacral colpopexy: observations and recommendations. *Obstet Gynecol* 1989;74(3 Pt 2):480–483.

Alevizon SJ, Finan MA. Sacrospinous colpopexy: management of postoperative pudendal nerve entrapment. *Obstet Gynecol* 1996;88(4 Pt 2):713–715.

Alsultan H, Suzanne F, Mansoor A, et al. Sacral colpopexy by the abdominal route: possible! *J Gynecol Obstet Biol Reprod (Paris)* 1995;24(4):452–453. French.

Amundsen C, Flynn BJ, Webster G. Anatomical correction of vaginal vault prolapse by uterosacral ligament fixation in women who also require a pubovaginal sling. *J Urol* 2003 May;169(5):1770–4.

Anderson GV, Deasy PP. Hysterocolpectomy. *Obstet Gynecol* 1960;16:344.

Angulo A, Kligman I: Retroperitoneal sacrocolpopexy for correction of prolapse of vaginal vault. *Surg Gynecol Obstet* 1989;169:319.

Backer MH. Success with sacrospinous suspension of the prolapsed vaginal vault. *Surg Gynecol Obstet* 1992;175:419.

Baker KR, Beresford JM, Campbell C: Colposacropexy with Prolene mesh. *Surg Gynecol Obstet* 1990;171:51.

Barber MD, Visco AG, Weidner AC, Amundsen CL, Bump RC. Bilateral uterosacral ligament vaginal vault suspension with site-specific endopelvic fascia defect repair for treatment of pelvic organ prolapse. *Am J Obstet Gynecol Dec* 2000;183(6):1402–10; discussion 1410–1.

Barksdale PA, Elkins TE, Sanders CK, et al. An anatomic approach to pelvic hem orrhage during sacrospinous ligament fixation of the vaginal vault. *Obstet Gynecol* 1998;91(5 Pt 1):715–718.

Barksdale PA, Gasser RF, Gauthier CM, et al. Intraligamentous nerves as a potential source of pain after sacrospinous ligament fixation of the vaginal apex. *Int Urogynecol J Pelvic Floor Dysfunct* 1997;8(3):121–125.

Benson JT, Lucente V, McClellan. Vaginal versus abdominal reconstructive surgery for the treatment of pelvic support defects: a prospective randomized study with long-term outcome evaluation. *AM J Obstet Gynecol* 1996;175:1418.

Bissell D. Fascia lapping as applied to the tissues of the vaginal wall-a misnomer. *Surg Gynecol Obstet* 1929;48:549–550.

Brown WE, Hoffman MS, Bouis PJ, et al: Management of vaginal vault prolapse: retrospective comparison of abdominal versus vaginal approach. *J Fla Med Assoc* 1989;76:249.

Bump RC, Hurt WG, Theofrastous JP, et al. Randomized prospective comparison of needle colposuspension versus endopelvic fascia plication for potential stress incontinence prophylaxis in women undergoing vaginal reconstruction for stage III or IV pelvic organ prolapse. *The Continence Program for Women Research Group. Am J Obstet Gynecol* 1996;175(2):326–333; discussion 333–335.

Cabrera JA, Szekely SJ. Sacrospinous ligament fixation. *Am J Obstet Gynecol* 1990;162(1):295–296.

Gary MP, Slack MC: Transvaginal sacrospinous colpopexy for vault and marked uterovaginal prolapse. *Br J Obstet Gynaecol* 1994;101:536.

Cespedes RD. Anterior approach bilateral sacrospinous ligament fixation for vaginal vault prolapse. *Urology* 2000;56(6 Suppl l):70–75.

Collins CG, Lock FR. The LeFort colpocleisis. *Am J Surg* 1941;53:202.

Colombo M, Milani R. Sacrospinous ligament fixation and modified McCall culdoplasty during vaginal hysterectomy for advanced uterovaginal prolapse. *Am J Obstet Gynecol* 1998;179(1):13–20.

Costantini E, Lombi R, Micheli C, et al. Colposacropexy with Gore-Tex mesh in marked vaginal and uterovaginal prolapse. *Eur Urol* 1998;34(2):111–117.

Cowan W, Morgan HR. Abdominal sacral colpopexy. *Am J Obstet Gynecol* 1980;138(3):348–350.

Creighton SM, Stanton SL: The surgical management of vaginal vault prolapse. *BR J Obstet Gynecol* 1991;98:1150.

Cruikshank SH, Cox DW. Sacrospinous ligament fixation at the time of transvaginal hysterectomy. *Am J Obstet Gynecol* 1990;162(6):1611–1615; discussion 1615–1619.

Cundiff GW, Harris RL, Coates K, et al. Abdominal sacral colpoperineopexy: a new approach for correction of posterior compartment defects and perineal descent associated with vaginal vault prolapse. *Am J Obstet Gynecol* 1997;177(6):1345–1353; discussion 1353–1355.

Delaere K, Moonen W, Debruyne F, et al. Hydronephrosis caused by cystocele. Treatment by colpopexy to sacral promontory. *Urology* 1984;24(4):364–365.

DeLancey JOL. Anatomic aspects of vaginal eversion after hysterectomy. *Am J Obstet Gynecol* 1992;166:1717–1728.

DeLancey JOL, Morley GW. Total colpocleisis for vaginal eversion. *Am J Obstet Gynecol* 1997;176:1228.

DeLancey JOL, Starr RA. Histology of the connection between the vagina and levator ani muscles; implications for urinary tract function. *J Reprod Med* 1990;35:765–771.

Delest A, Cosson M, Doutrelant C, et al. Enterocele Retrospective study of 134 cases: risk factors and comparison between abdominal and perineal routes.. *J Gynecol Obstet Biol Reprod (Paris)* 1996;25(5):464–470. French.

Denehy TR, Choe JY, Gregori CA, et al. Modified LeFort partial colpocleisis with Kelly urethral plication and posterior colpoperineoplasty in the medically compromised elderly: a comparison with vaginal hysterectomy, anterior colporrhaphy, and posterior colpoperineoplasty. *Am J Obstet Gynecol* 1995;173:1697.

Derry DE. On the real nature of the so-called "pelvic fascia."*J Anat* 1907;42: 7–11.

Diana M, Schettini M. Treatment of vaginal vault prolapse with abdominal sacral colpopexy using Prolene mesh. *Minerva Gynecol* 1999;51(9):349–353.

Diana M, Zoppe C, Mastrangeli B. Treatment of vaginal vault prolapse with abdominal sacral colpopexy using Prolene mesh. *Am J Surg* 2000;179(2): 126–128.

Dominguez Vazquez RH, Albarran de Regil CA. Sacro-colpoplexy using Mersilene: report of 12 cases at the General Hospital Zone 7, Monclova, Coahuila. *Ginecol Obstet Mex* 1999;67:13–17. Spanish.

Dorsey JH, Sharp HT. Laparoscopic sacral colpopexy and other procedures for prolapse. *Baillieres Clin Obstet Gynaecol* 1995;9(4):749–756.

Drutz HP, Cha LS: Massive genital and vaginal vault prolapse treated with abdominal-vaginal sacropexy with use of marlex mesh: review of the literature. *Am J Obstet Gynecol* 1987;156:387.

Elkins TE, Hopper JB, Goodfellow K, et al: Initial report of anatomic and clinical comparison of the sacrospinous ligament fixation to the high McCall culdeplasty for vaginal cuff fixation at hysterectomy for uterine prolapse. *J Pelvic Surg* 1995;1:12.

Falk HC, Kaufman SA. Partial colpocleisis: the LeFort procedure. *Obstet Gynecol* 1955;5:617.

Farrell SA, Scotti RJ, Ostergard DR, et al. Massive evisceration: a complication following sacrospinous vaginal vault fixation. *Obstet Gynecol* 1991;78(3 Pt 2):560–562.

Febbraro W, Beucher G, Von Theobald P, et al. Feasibility of bilateral sacrospinous ligament vaginal suspension with a stapler. Prospective studies with the 34 first cases. *J Gynecol Obstet Biol Reprod (Paris)*. 1997; 26(8):815–821. French.

Feldman GB, Birnbaum SJ: Sacral colpopexy for vaginal vault prolapse. *Obstet Gynecol* 1979;53:399.

Fothergill WE. The supports of the pelvic viscera: a review of some recent contributions to pelvic anatomy, with a clinical introduction. *J Obstet Gynaecol Br Emp* 1908;13:18–28.

Fox SD, Stanton SL. Vault prolapse and rectocele: assessment of repair using sacrocolpopexy with mesh interposition. *Br J Obstet Gynaecol* 2000;107 (11):1371–1375.

Funt MI, Thompson JD, Birch H. Normal vaginal axis. *South Med J* 1978;71:1534.

Geomini PM, Brolmann HA, van Binsbergen NJ, et al. Vaginal vault suspension by abdominal sacral colpopexy for prolapse: a follow up study of 40 patients. *Eur J Obstet Gynaecol Reprod Biol* 2001;94(2):234–238.

Given FT, Muhlendorf IK, Browning GM. Vaginal length and sexual function after colpopexy for complete uterovaginal eversion. *Am J Obstet Gynecol* 1993;169(2 Pt l):284–287; discussion 287–288. Review.

Goff BH. An histological study of the perivaginal fascia in a nullipara. *Surg Gynecol Obstet* 1931;52:32–42.

Goff BH. The surgical anatomy of cystocele and urethrocele with special reference to the pubocervical fascia. *Surg Gynecol Obstet* 1948;87:725–734.

Goldman J, Ovadia J, Feldberg D. The Neugebauer-LeFort operation: a review of 118 partial colpocleises. *Eur J Obstet Gynaecol Reprod Biol* 1985;12:31.

Grunberger W, Grunberger V, Wierrani F: Pelvic promontory fixation of the vaginal vault in sixty-two patients with prolapse after hysterectomy. *Surg Gynecol Obstet* 1994;178:69.

Hale DS, Rogers RM. Abdominal sacrospinous ligament colposuspension. *Obstet Gynecol* 1999;94(6):1039–1041.

Hanson GE, Keettel WC. The Neugebauer-LeFort operation: a review of 288 colpocleisis. *Obstet Gynecol* 1979;34:352.

Harer WB. Round ligament synthetic graft colpopexy. *Obstet Gynecol* 1994;83(6):1064–1066.

Heinonen PK. Transvaginal sacrospinous colpopexy for vaginal vault and complete genital prolapse in aged women. *Acta Obstet Gynecol Scand* 1992;71(5):377–381.

Hefni M, El-Toukhy T, Bhaumik J, Katsimanis E. Sacrospinous cervicocolpopexy with uterine conservation for uterovaginal prolapse in elderly women:an evolving concept. *Am J Obstet Gynecol.* 2003 Mar;188(3):645–50.

Hemelt BA, Finan MA. Abdominal sacral colpopexy resulting in a retained sponge. A case report. *J Reprod Med* 1999;44(11):983–985.

Hewson AD. Transvaginal sacrospinous colpopexy for posthysterectomy vault prolapse. *Aust N Z J Obstet Gynaecol* 1998;38(3):318–324.

Holley RL, Varner RE, Gleason BP, et al. Recurrent pelvic support defects after sacrospinous ligament fixation for vaginal vault prolapse. *J Am Coll Surg* 1995;180(4):444–448.

Holley RL, Varner RE, Gleason BP, et al. Sexual function after sacrospinous ligament fixation for vaginal vault prolapse. *J Reprod Med* 1996;41(5):355–358.

Hughes GW, Freeman RM. A modification of the technique of sacrospinous ligament fixation. *Br J Obstet Gynaecol* 1995;102(8):669–670.

Imparato E, Aspesi G, Rovetta E, et al: Surgical management and prevention of vaginal vault prolapse. *Surg Gynecol Obstet* 1992;175:233.

Inmon WB: Pelvic relaxation and repair including prolapse of vagina following hysterectomy. *South Med J* 1963;56:577.

Losif CS. Abdominal sacral colpopexy with use of synthetic mesh. *Acta Obstet Gynecol Scand* 1993;72(3):214–217.

Jenkins. Uterosacral ligament fixation for vaginal vault suspension in uterine and vaginal vault prolapse. *Am J Obstet Gynecol* 1997 Dec;177(6):1337–43.

Kaminski PF, Sorosky JI, Pees RC, et al: Correction of massive vaginal prolapse: an older population. *J Am Geriatr Soc* 1993;41:42.

Karram MM, Goldwasser S, Kleeman S, Steele A, Vassallo B, Walsh P. High uterosacral vaginal vault suspension with fascial reconstruction for vaginal repair of enterocele and vaginal vault prolapse. *Am J Obstet Gynecol* 2001 Dec;185(6):1339–42; discussion 1342–3.

Kettel LM, Hebertson RM. An anatomic evaluation of the sacrospinous ligament colpopexy. *Surg Gynecol Obstet* 1989;168(4):318–322.

Kholi N, Sze E, Karram MM. Incidence of recurrent cystocele after transvaginal needle suspension procedures with and without concomitant anterior colporrhaphy. *Am J Obstet Gynecol* 1996;175(6):1476.

Kleeman SD, Westermann C, Karram MM. Rectoceles and the anatomy of the posteriovaginal wall: revisited. *Am J Obstet Gynecol.* Dec 2005;193(6):2050–5.

Koster H. On the supports of the uterus. *Am J Obstet Gynecol* 1933;25:67–74.

Kulkarni S. Surgery for post-hysterectomy vaginal prolapse. *West Indian Med J* 1993;52(2):65–67.

Lahr SJ, Lahr CJ, Srinivasan A, et al. Operative management of severe constipation. *Am Surg* 1999;65(12):1117–1121; discussion 1122–1123.

Langmade CF, Oliver JA. Partial colpocleisis. *Am J Obstet Gynecol* 1986;154:1200.

Lansman HH. Posthysterectomy vault prolapse: sacral colpopexy with dura mater graft. *Obstet Gynecol* 1984;63(4):577–582.

Lecuru F, Taurelle R, Clouard C, et al. Surgical treatment of genito-urinary prolapses by abdominal approach. Results in a continuous series of 203 operations. *Ann Chir* 1994;48(11):1013–1019. French.

Lee RA, Symmonds RE. Surgical repair of posthysterectomy vault prolapse. *Am J Obstet Gynecol* 1972;112:953.

Lind LR, Choe J, Bhatia NN. An in-line suturing device to simplify sacrospinous vaginal vault suspension. *Obstet Gynecol* 1997;89(1):129–132.

Maher CF, Qatawney AM, Dwyer PL, et al. Abdominal sacral colpopexy or vaginal sacrospinous colpopexy for vaginal vault prolapse: a prospective randomized study. *Am J Obstet Gynecol* 2004;190:20.

Maher CF, Murray CJ, Gary MD, et al. Illiococcygeus or sacrospinous fixation for vaginal vault prolapse. *Obstet Gynecol* 2001;98:40.

Maher CF, Cary MP, Slack MC, Murray CJ, Milligan M, Schluter P. Uterine preservation or hysterectomy at sacrospinous colpopexy for Uterovaginal-prolapse? *Int Urogynecol J Pelvic Floor Dysfunct.* 2001;12(6):381–4.

Maloney JC, Dunton CJ, Smith K: Repair of vaginal vault prolapse with abdominal sacropexy. *J Reprod Med* 1990;35:6.

Mattox TF, Kelly T, Bhatia NN. Modification of the Miya hook in vaginal colpopexy. *J Reprod Med* 1995;40(10):681–683.

Mazor C, Israel SL. The Le Fort colpocleisis: an analysis of 43 operations. *Am J Obstet Gynecol* 1948;56:944.

McCall ML. Posterior culdeplasty. *Obstet Gynecol* 1957;10:595.

Meeks GR, Washburne JF, McGeher RP, et al: Repair of vaginal vault prolapse by suspension of the vagina to iliococcygeus (prespinous) fascia. *Am J Obstet Gynecol* 1994;171:1444.

Meschia M, Bruschi F, Amicarelli F, Pifarotti P, Marchini M, Crosignani PG, Miyazaki FS. Miya hook ligature carrier for sacrospinous ligament suspension. *Obstet Gynecol* 1987;70(2):286–288.

Monk BJ, Ramp JF, Montz FJ, et al: Sacrospinous fixation for vaginal vault prolapse. Complications and results. *J Gynecol Surg* 1991;7:87.

Morley GW. Treatment of uterine and vaginal prolapse. *Clin Obstet Gynecol* 1996;39(4):959–969. Review.

Morley GW, DeLancey JO. Sacrospinous ligament fixation for eversion of the vagina. *Am J Obstet Gynecol* 1988;158(4):872–881.

Nichols DH, Randall CL. *Vaginal surgery,* third ed. Baltimore: Williams & Wilkins, 1989.

Nichols DH. Sacrospinous fixation for massive eversion of the vagina. *Am J Obstet Gynecol* 1982;142:901.

Norton PA. Pelvic floor disorders: the role of fascia and ligaments. *Clin Obstet Gynecol* 1993;36:926–938.

Olsen AL, Smith VJ, Bergstrom JO, et al. Epidemiology of surgically managed pelvic organ prolapse and urinary incontinence. *Obstet Gynecol* 1997;89:501–506.

Ostrzenski A. Laparoscopic colposuspension for total vaginal prolapse. *Int J Gynaecol Obstet* 1996;55(2):147–152.

Ozcan U, Gungor T, Ekin M, et al. Sacrospinous fixation for the prolapsed vaginal vault. *Gynecol Obstet Invest* 1999;47(1):65–68.

Papasakelariou C. Sacrospinous ligament fixation simplified with a new endoscopic suturing device. *J Am Assoc Gynecol Laparosc* 1996;3[Suppl 4]:S38.

Paraiso MF, Ballard LA, Walters MD, et al. Pelvic support defects and visceral and sexual function in woman treated with sacrospinous ligament suspension and pelvic reconstruction. *Am J Obstet Gynecol* 1996;175(6):1523–1530; discussion 1430–1431.

Patsner B. Abdominal sacral colpopexy in patients with gynecologic cancer: report of 25 cases with long-term follow-up and literative review. *Gynecol Oncol* 1999;75(3):504–508.

Patsner B. Mesh erosion into the bladder after abdominal sacral colpopexy. *Obstet Gynecol* 2000;95(6 Pt 2):1029.

Peters WA, Christenson ML. Fixation of the vaginal apex to the coccygeus fascia during repair of vaginal vault eversion with enterocele. *Am J Obstet Gynecol* 1995;172(6):1894–1900; discussion 1900–1902.

Phaneuf LE. The place of colpectomy in the treatment of uterine and vaginal prolapse. *Am J Obstet Gynecol* 1935;30:544.

Pohl JF, Frattarelli JL. Bilateral transvaginal sacrospinous colpopexy: preliminary experience. *Am J Obstet Gynecol* 1997;177(6):1356–1361; discussion 1361–1362.

Porges RF, Smilen SW. Long-term analysis of the surgical management of pelvic support defects. *Am J Obstet Gynecol* 1994;171(6):1518–1526; discussion 1526–1528.

Powell JL, Joseph DB. Abdominal sacral colpopexy for massive genital prolapse. *Prim Care Update Ob Gyns* 1998;5(4):201.

Powell JL, Joseph DB. Abdominal sacral colpopexy in patients with gynecologic cancer and "Burch" not "Birch."*Gynecol Oncol* 2000;77(3):483–484.

Randall C, Nichols D. Surgical treatment of vaginal inversion. *Obstet Gynecol* 1971;38:327.

Raz S, Nitti VW, Bregg KJ. Transvaginal repair of enterocele. *J Urol* 1993;149(4):724–730.

Ricci JV, Lisa JR, Thom CH, et al. The relationship of the vagina to adjacent organs in reconstructive surgery; a histologic study. *Am J Surg* 1947;74:387–410.

Ricci JV, Thom CH. The myth of a surgically useful fascia in vaginal plastic reconstruction. *Q Rev Surg Obstet Gynecol* 1954;2:253–261.

Richardson AC, Edmonds PB, Williams NL. Treatment of stress urinary incontinence due to paravaginal fascial defect. *Obstet Gynecol* 1982;57:357–362.

Richardson AC, Lyon JB, Williams NL. A new look at pelvic relaxation. *Am J Obstet Gynecol* 1976;126:568–573.

Richter K, Albright W: Long-term results following fixation of the vagina on the sacrospinal ligament by the vaginal route. *Am J Obstet Gynecol* 1981;151:811.

Ridley JG. Evaluation of the colpocleisis: a report of fifty-eight cases. *Am J Obstet Gynecol* 1972;113:1114.

Rodau SK, Thomason JL. Vaginal eversion repair. Sacrospinous ligament fixation procedure. *AORN J* 1988;47(2):539, 542–549, 552.

Rose CH, Rowe TF, Cox SM, et al. Uterine prolapse associated with bladder extrophy: surgical management and subsequent pregnancy. *J Matern Fetal Med* 2000;9(2):150–152.

Rust JA, Botte JM, Hewlett RJ. Prolapse of the vaginal vault. Improved

techniques for management of the abdominal approach or vaginal approach. *Am J Obstet Gynecol* 1976;125(6):768–776.
Salvat J, Slamani L, Vincent-Genod A, et al. Sacrospinous ligament fixation by palpation: variation of the Richter procedure. *Eur J Obstet Gynaecol Reprod Biol* 1996;68(1–2):1999–1203.
Sauer HA, Klutke CG. Transvaginal Sacrospinous ligament fixation for treatment of vaginal prolapse. *J Urol* 1995;154(3):1008–1012.
Schettini M, Fortunate P, Gallucci M. Abdominal sacral colpopexy with Prolene mesh. *Int Urogynecol J Pelvic Floor Dysfunct* 1999;10(5):295–299.
Schlesinger RE. Vaginal Sacrospinous ligament fixation with the Autosuture Endostitch device. *Am J Obstet Gynecol* 1997;176(6):1358–1362.
Scotti RJ. Repair of genitourinary prolapse in women. *Curr Opin Obstet Gynecol* 1991;3(3):404–412. Review.
Shafik A, el-Sherif M, Youssef A, et al. Surgical anatomy of the pudendal nerve and its clinical implications. *Clin Anat* 1995;8(2):110–115.
Sharp TR. Sacrospinous suspension made easy. *Obstet Gynecol* 1993;82(5):873–875.
Shull BL, Bachofen C, Coates KW, Kuehl TJ. A transvaginal approach to repair of apical and other associated sites of pelvic organ prolapse with uterosacral ligaments. *Am J Obstet Gynecol* Dec 2000;183(6):1365–73; discussion 1373–4.
Shull BL, Baden WF. A six-year experience with paravaginal defect repair for stress urinary incontinence. *Am J Obstet Gynecol* 1989;160:1432–1435.
Shull BL, Benn SJ, Kuehl TJ. Surgical management of prolapse of the anterior vaginal segment: an analysis of support defects, operative morbidity, and anatomic outcome. *Am J Obstet Gynecol* 1994;171:1429–1439.
Shull BL, Capen CV, Riggs MW, et al. Preoperative and postoperative analysis of site-specific pelvic support defects in 81 women treated with sacrospinous ligament suspension and pelvic reconstruction. *Am J Obstet Gynecol* 1992;166(6 Pt 1):1764–1768; discussion 1768–1771.
Shull BL, Capen CV, Riggs MW, et al: Bilateral attachment of the vaginal cuff to iliococcygeus fascia: an effective method of cuff suspension. *Am J Obstet Gynecol* 1993;168:1669.
Silva WA, Pauls RN, Segal JL, Rooney CM, Kleeman SD, Karram MM. Uterosacral ligament vault suspension: five-year outcomes. *Obstet Gynecol* Aug 2006;108(20:255–63.
Smilen SW, Saini J, Wallach SJ, et al. The risk of cystocele after sacrospinous ligament fixation. *Am J Obstet Gynecol* 1998;179(6 Pt 1):1465–1471; discussion 1471–1472.
Snyder TE, Krantz KE. Abdominal-retroperitoneal sacral colpopexy for the correction of vaginal prolapse. *Obstet Gynecol* 1991;77(6):944–949.
Steiner RA, Healy JC. Patterns of prolapse in women with symptoms of pelvic floor weakness: magnetic resonance imaging and laparoscopic treatment. *Curr Opin Obstet Gynecol* 1998;10(4):295–301. Review.
Symmonds RE, Pratt JH. Vaginal prolapse following hysterectomy. *Am J Obstet Gynecol* 1960;79:899.
Symmonds RE, Williams TJ, Lee RA, et al: Posthysterectomy enterocele and vaginal vault prolapse. *Am J Obstet Gynecol* 1981;140:852, 2981.
Sze E, Karram MM. Vaginal operation to correct vaginal vault prolapse: a review. *Obstet Gynecol* 1997;89:466–475.
Sze E, Miklos J, Partoll L, Karram MM. Sacrospinous ligament fixation with transvaginal needle suspension for advanced pelvic organ prolapse and stress incontinence. *Obstet Gynecol* 1997;89:94–96.
Sze EH, Miklos JR, Partoll L, et al. Sacrospinous ligament fixation with transvaginal needle suspension for advanced pelvic organ prolapse and stress incontinence. *Obstet Gynecol* 1997;89(1):94–96.
Thompson JD, Rock JA, eds. Te Linde's operative gynecology, seventh ed. Philadelphia: JB Lippincott, 1992: 904–914.
Thompson JR, Gibb JS, Genadry R, et al. Anatomy of pelvic arteries adjacent to the sacrospinous ligament: importance of the coccygeal branch of the inferior gluteal artery. *Obstet Gynecol* 1999;94(6):973–977.
Timmons MC, Addison WA, Addison SB, et al. Abdominal sacral colpopexy in 163 women with posthysterectomy vaginal vault prolapse and enterocele. Evolution of operative techniques. *J Reprod Med* 1992;37(4):323–327.
Todd JW: Mesh suspension for vaginal prolapse. *Int Surg* 1978;63:91.
Traiman P, De Luca LA, Silva AA, et al. Abdominal colpopexy for complete prolapse of the vagina. *Int Surg* 1992;77(2):91–95.
Ubachs JMH, Van Sante TJ, Schellekens LA. Partial colpocleisis by a modification of Le Fort's operation. *Obstet Gynecol* 1973;42:415.
Uhlenhuth E, Day EC, Smith RD, et al. The visceral endopelvic fascia and hypogastric sheath. *Surg Gynecol Obstet* 1948;86:9–28.
Unger JB. A persistent sinus tract from the vagina to the sacrum after treatment of mesh erosion by partial removal of a Gore-Tex soft tissue patch. *Am J Obstet Gynecol* 1999;181(3):762–763.
Valaitis SR, Stanton SL: Sacrocolpopexy: a retrospective study of a clinician's experience. *Br J Obstet Gynaecol* 1994;101:518.
van Lindert ACM, Groenendijk AG, Scholten PC, et al: Surgical support and suspension of genital prolapse, including preervation of the uterus, using Gore-tex soft tissue patch. *Eur J Obstet Gynecol Reprod Biol* 1996;50: 133.
Von Pechmann WS, Mutone M, Fyffe J Hale DS. Total colpocleisis with high levator plication for the treatment of advanced pelvic organ prolapse. *Am J Obstet Gynecol* 2003;189:121.
van Brummen HJ, van de Pol G, Aalders CI, Heintz AP, van der Vaart CH. Sacrospinous hysteropexy compared to vaginal hysterectomy as primary surgical treatment for a descensus uteri: effects on urinary symptoms. *Int Urogynecol J Pelvic Floor Dysfunct.* 2003 Nov;14(5):350–5.
Van Lindert AC, Groenendijk AG, Scholten PC, et al. Surgical support and suspension of genital prolapse, including preservation of the uterus, using the Gore-Tex soft tissue patch (a preliminary report). *Eur J Obstet Gynaecol Reprod Biol* 1993;50(2):133–139.
Verdeja AM, Elkins TE, Odoi A, et al. Transvaginal sacrospinous colpopexy: anatomic landmarks to be aware of to minimize complications. *Am J Obstet Gynecol* 1995;173(5):1468–1469.
Veronikis DK, Nichols DH. Ligature carrier specifically designed for transvaginal sacrospinous colpopexy. *Obstet Gynecol* 1997;89(3):478–481.
Virtanen H, Hirvonen T, Makinen J, et al. Outcome of thirty patients who underwent repair of posthysterectomy prolapse of the vaginal vault with abdominal sacral colpopexy. *J Am Coll Surg* 1994;178(3):283–287.
Wall LL. Abdominal-retroperitoneal sacral colpopexy for the correction of vaginal prolapse. *Obstet Gynecol* 1991;78(4):724–726.
Wall LL, Hewitt JK. Voiding function after Burch colposuspension for stress incontinence. *J Reprod Med* 1996;41(3):161–165.
Watson JD. Sacrospinous ligament colpopexy: new instrumentation applied to a standard gynecologic procedure. *Obstet Gynecol* 1996;88(5):883–885.
Webb MJ, Aronson MP, Ferguson LK, Lee RA. Posthysterectomy vaginal vault prolapse: primary repair in 693 patients. *Obstet Gynecol* Aug 1998;92(2):281–5.
Welgoss JA, Vogt VY, McClellan EJ, et al. Relationship between surgically induced neuropathy and outcome of pelvic organ prolapse surgery. *Int Urogynecol J Pelvic Floor Dysfunct* 1999;10(1):11–14.
White GR. Cystocele: A radical cure by suturing lateral sulci of vagina to white line of pelvic fascia. *JAMA* 1909;21:1707–1710.
Winters JC, Cespedes RD, Vanlangendonck R. Abdominal sacral colpopexy and abdominal enterocele repair in the management of vaginal vault prolapse. *Urology* 2000;56[Suppl 6]:55–63.

CHAPTER 36F ■ THE NONSURGICAL MANAGEMENT OF PELVIC ORGAN PROLAPSE: THE USE OF VAGINAL PESSARIES

RONY A. ADAM

DEFINITIONS

Pelvic organ prolapse—Downward displacement of structures that are normally located adjacent to the vaginal vault.

Pelvic Organ Prolapse Quantification (POP-Q) scale—A coring system used to quantify pelvic organ prolapse; see Chapter 36A.

Pessary—A device inserted into the vagina for correction of pelvic organ prolapse.

Splinting—A maneuver that assists with elimination of urine or feces, usually used in cases of pelvic organ prolapse.

Stress urinary incontinence—Leakage of urine with any maneuver that increases intraabdominal pressure (such as a cough or sneeze).

The surgeon who treats patients with pelvic floor defects should also be familiar with the nonsurgical management of these disorders. Although pelvic organ prolapse prevalence has been and continues to rise steadily, pessary use has previously fallen out of favor, with renewed interest having been noted only recently. Vaginal pessaries have been used for the treatment of not only genital prolapse but also urinary incontinence, uterine retroversion, cervical incompetence, and, more recently, local administration of estrogen. Various shapes and sizes allow a variety of pelvic floor defects to be adequately managed without the need for surgery. Although modern pessaries have been used for a long time with an abundance of expert opinion and case reports in the literature, rigorous investigations of these modalities is severely limited, as concluded in a recent Cochrane review. This chapter reviews the available data on pessary use for pelvic organ prolapse, some of the more commonly used pessary types and their proper fitting, subsequent follow-up, and potential complications.

HISTORY

References to female genital prolapse and its treatment can be found as early as 1550 B.C. in ancient Egyptian writings. Hippocrates (400 B.C.) prescribed succussion therapy, in which the patient was hung upside down by her feet and bounced up and down to reduce the prolapsed womb. Hippocrates also advocated inserting half a pomegranate soaked in wine into the vagina. Soranus (98 A.D.) described using pleasant fumigation around the patient's head to entice the prolapse to ascend and foul odors near the vagina to force the organ upward. He also described the use of an astringent solution, manual reduction of the prolapse, and insertion of half a pomegranate dipped in vinegar, if succussion therapy failed. Soranos declared that a surgical procedure be undertaken only if the prolapsed uterus was gangrenous.

By the end of the 16th century, various pessaries of brass and waxed cork were used for uterine prolapse. The late 17th century saw a considerable number of medical therapies and pharmaceutical concoctions promoted for the treatment of genital prolapse, which persisted even into the 18th century. In the mid-19th century, the American Medical Association documented 123 different pessaries. As the safety of surgical procedures has improved and concerns of adverse consequences of pessaries reported, there has been a tendency during the mid-20th century to use pessaries less often in favor of corrective surgery. Modern pessaries are primarily made of silicone, rarely of latex rubber or acrylic. These materials have completely replaced the old Bakelite and hard-rubber types used previously. Silicone is advantageous because it is inert, does not absorb secretions or odors, is flexible yet sturdy, and can be autoclaved for resterilization.

INDICATIONS

The primary indication for fitting a pessary is the nonsurgical relief of symptoms associated with pelvic organ prolapse. This ideally should be achieved without introduction or worsening of urinary incontinence and with minimization of the risk of vaginal mucosal abrasion, erosion, and bleeding. Additionally, pessaries are used for the alleviation of stress incontinence and will be discussed in more detail in Chapter 37.

PESSARY USAGE: PHYSICIAN PERSPECTIVE

Surveys demonstrate that 87% to 98% of gynecologists and/or urogynecologists prescribe pessaries in their practice. Among members of the American Urogynecologic Society (AUGS), 77% of those responding offered pessaries as first-line therapy for pelvic organ prolapse, whereas 12% offered them only to women who are not considered good surgical candidates or those who refused surgery. Among a randomly drawn survey of American College of Obstetricians and Gynecologists (ACOG) members, 20% of gynecologists prescribed pessaries only to patients deemed poor surgical candidates. Some advocate pessaries in patients who have prolapse-related vaginal and/or cervical ulcerations and for mucosal hypertrophy. In the AUGS survey, those who described themselves as gynecologists or urologists (as opposed to urogynecologists or obstetrician-gynecologists) were more likely to offer pessaries only to patients who are poor surgical candidates. Those in practice for more than 20 years were found to be less likely to use pessaries as a first-line management option, preferring to limit their use to nonsurgical patients. In the ACOG members survey, physicians with a self-reported special interest in urogynecology prescribed pessaries more often than those who did not proclaim such an interest, and female physicians were more likely to prescribe pessaries than their male counterparts.

PESSARY USAGE: PATIENT PERSPECTIVE

Only a few recent studies have focused on the efficacy and impact on quality of life that pessaries provide for patients. A cross-sectional study in which all new patients seen in a referral practice were counseled regarding their options found that older patients were 10% more likely to choose a pessary rather than surgery as their initial management option for prolapse. They also found that those patients who had previously undergone surgery for prolapse (all with a different surgeon) were 77% more likely to choose surgery over pessary as their preferred treatment option. Similarly, the greater the degree of prolapse, the more likely patients were to choose surgery over pessary or expectant management.

In a prospective observational study, Clemons and colleagues offered 100 patients a pessary, and 73 of these had a successful initial fitting. Ring pessaries were used in 74% of these 73 patients, and the rest were Gellhorn pessaries. At 2-month follow-up, they found significant resolution of the symptoms of feeling a bulge, pelvic pressure, vaginal discharge, and need for splinting to void or effect a bowel movement. Urinary symptoms of stress incontinence and urge incontinence improved in 45% of patients, and voiding difficulties improved in 53%. On the other hand, *de novo* stress incontinence occurred in 21% of patients with a pessary. Overall, 67 of the 73 women were "very satisfied" or "somewhat satisfied" for a 92% satisfaction rate among those with a successful pessary fitting. Even using an intent-to-treat analysis, 67% of the original 100 women who were fitted for a pessary reported being satisfied. Of the patients who were sexually active before pessary use, 90% were able to continue to have sexual intercourse. Those who could not were the ones fitted with a Gellhorn rather than ring pessary.

A retrospective analysis found that women who wore a pessary for prolapse were more likely to continue than those who wore a pessary for incontinence. They also found that women who reported themselves as sexually active were more likely than those who were not sexually active to continue pessary use regardless of the indication. Age, parity, menopausal status, and previous surgical history were not found to be predictors of pessary continuation.

A small retrospective observational study suggests that 1 year following pessary use, pelvic organ prolapse did not worsen, as evaluated by Pelvic Organ Prolapse Quantification (POP-Q) measurements with Valsalva. The study found that in 4 of 19 (21%) patients, their prolapse improved, and the rest remained unchanged.

SUCCESS AND RISK FACTORS FOR FAILURE

In a prospective study by Wu and colleagues, among 110 women who opted for and were fitted for pessaries as first-line therapy, 81 (74%) were successfully fitted. Characteristics associated with initial failure of pessary fitting included younger age, higher parity, a history of pelvic surgery, and stress incontinence. The degree of pelvic organ prolapse did not predict failure of initial fitting; neither did hormone replacement or the adequacy of the perineal body. In this study, the initial pessary used was a ring or a ring with support in the vast majority of cases (95%), with a cube pessary used for the remaining patients. No differences were noted in efficacy between these different pessary types.

Clemons and colleagues prospectively observed 100 patients who were fitted with ring (with support) or Gellhorn pessaries, with an initial pessary fitting success rate of 94%. However, this declined to 73% when evaluated 2 weeks later. Short vaginal length ($\leq$6 cm) and a wide introitus (4 finger breadths) were associated with failure of pessary fitting. The degree of prolapse, genital hiatus size, and presence of vaginal atrophy were not associated with failure. The same group followed a subset of this cohort—67 women who were satisfied at their 2-month follow-up—for a full year. At the 1-year follow up, 43 patients (64%) continued with pessary use, whereas 16 elected surgery.

Mutone and colleagues, in a retrospective study of 407 patients, reported a lower pessary fitting success rate of 41% when evaluated 3 weeks after the initial fitting. Characteristics associated with failure in this study included prior hysterectomy or surgery for prolapse. There was no association with the type or degree of pelvic organ prolapse. In a retrospective study of 101 patients, Sulak and colleagues reported discontinuation rates using primarily the Gellhorn pessary. The following are the categories reported of the reasons for discontinuation: inconvenience or inadequate relief of symptoms (40%), difficulty in removal (23%), discomfort (13%), patient requesting surgery (13%), pessary fell out (6%), and inability to urinate (5%).

CLINICAL EVALUATION

The patient with pelvic floor dysfunction requires careful evaluation by history and physical examination as outlined in Chapter 36A. Important considerations are assessment of symptoms attributable to prolapse, including pelvic pressure or discomfort, a sensation that something is falling out or protruding, voiding and defecatory symptoms, and urinary incontinence. The clinical evaluation should be aimed at investigating and quantifying the specific pelvic support defects present in terms of anterior, posterior, and apical compartments. The POP-Q scale is a validated and widely accepted measure of the degree of pelvic organ prolapse and includes a measure of vaginal length. Testing for occult stress urinary incontinence by provocative maneuvers with the prolapse reduced using a Sims (or half) speculum helps identify patients who may suffer from urinary leakage associated with pessary use. This may be helpful in the counseling of such a patient and perhaps in choosing a pessary with better support of the bladder neck to prevent such an undesirable outcome.

Evaluation of the vaginal mucosa to assess estrogen status is necessary. The concern for pessary-associated erosion and ulceration in the atrophic vagina leads the vast majority of surveyed AUGS members (94%) to recommend concurrent estrogen replacement therapy in the absence of contraindications. Wu and colleagues reported that the incidence of vaginal abrasions increased as the vaginal epithelium exhibited more atrophy. Furthermore, those that experienced vaginal abrasions were more likely to discontinue pessary use. In my experience, use of vaginal estrogen therapy is the preferred method to treat and prevent vaginal atrophy.

TYPES OF PESSARIES

There have been hundreds of pessaries described throughout the ages. Currently, however, fewer than 20 pessary types are used for prolapse. Some types have been further modified for the nonsurgical management of stress urinary incontinence by increasing support to the bladder neck (Fig. 36F.1).

Of responding AUGS members, 78% tailored their choice of pessary type to the specific pelvic support defect. Of the members who reported using the same pessary for all types of prolapse, the ring was the most commonly used. Most respondents (59%) considered a weak pelvic diaphragm—whereas only 44% considered a prior hysterectomy—as important in the choice of pessary, generally favoring a space-occupying rather than supportive pessary in each of these circumstances. The supportive pessaries were defined as those that were derived by a spring mechanism (ring, Gehrung, lever-type pessaries) and thought to be supported by the symphysis pubis. The space-filling pessaries were defined as supported by the creation of suction between the pessary and the vaginal walls (e.g., cube) or by providing a diameter larger than the genital hiatus (donut, InflatoBall, Shaatz) or by both mechanisms (Gellhorn). Although these categories clearly simplify the analysis of data, such a functional classification has not been studied. It is unclear whether the mechanistic differences inferred by such a classification are indeed valid.

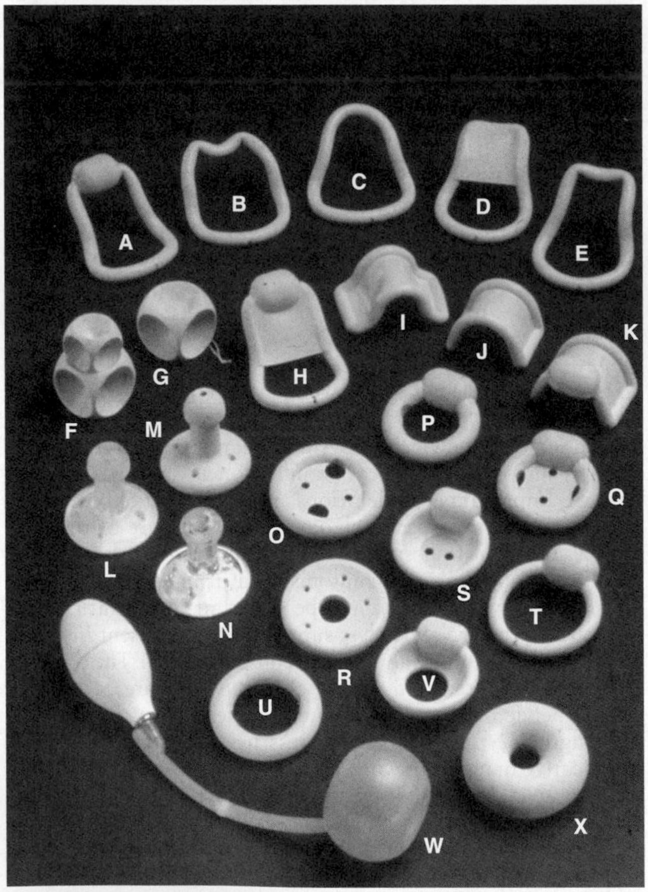

FIGURE 36F.1. Types of pessaries. *A,* Hodge with knob (silicone); *B,* Risser (silicone); *C,* Smith (silicone); *D,* Hodge with support; *E,* Hodge (silicone); *F,* tandem-cube (silicone); *G,* cube (silicone); *H,* Hodge with support plus knob (silicone); *I,* Regula (silicone); *J,* Gehrung (silicone); *K,* Gehrung with knob (silicone); *L,* Gellhorn 95% rigid (silicone); *M,* Gellhorn flexible (silicone); *N,* Gellhorn rigid (silicone); *O,* ring with support (silicone); *P,* ring with knob (silicone); *Q,* ring with support plus knob (silicone); *R,* Shaatz (silicone); *S,* incontinence dish with support (silicone); *T,* ring incontinence (silicone); *U,* ring (silicone); *V,* incontinence dish (silicone); *W,* InflatoBall (latex); *X,* donut (silicone).

Surveys show that the ring pessary is the most commonly used, both among physicians who tailor their pessary choice based on the support defects present and those who use the same pessary for all types of prolapse. It is unclear whether this choice is related to perceived efficacy or issues related to ease of management, patient acceptability, the patient's ability to remove the pessary, or other considerations.

Ring Pessary

The hinged spring circumference of the silicone-coated ring pessary allows for its compression in one direction, which makes for ease of insertion. These pessaries are similar in appearance to the contraceptive diaphragm and thus may be more familiar and acceptable to some patients. It is recommended that once inserted behind the symphysis pubis, the ring be turned 90 degrees because it collapses only along a single axis. The ring with support may provide additional support to a mild anterior vaginal defect and prevents the rare complication of an incarcerated herniated cervix through the open ring. The ring pessary is amenable for self-removal and insertion by the patient. It may be worn during coitus.

Donut Pessary

The silicone donut-shaped pessary may be used for higher degrees of prolapse. It is supported by the levator muscles and fills the upper vagina completely. It is, therefore, considered appropriate for the management of uterovaginal and vaginal vault prolapse. Insertion through the introitus is in the vertical plane, and the pessary is turned to a horizontal plane when inserted beyond the levator muscles. It tends to be difficult for patients to remove this type of pessary by themselves. Coitus is not usually possible with this type of pessary.

The InflatoBall is a variant of the donut pessary. Made out of latex rubber, it can be easily inserted and removed when deflated. When inflated by use of a manual pump, it sits above the levator plate much like the donut pessary, with the valve stem tucked in the vagina (Fig. 36F.2). Because it is made out of latex and therefore absorbs secretions and odors, the InflatoBall should be removed and cleaned every 1 to 2 nights and reinserted in the morning. This pessary's use is contraindicated with a history of latex allergy.

Gellhorn Pessary

The Gellhorn pessary is useful in patients with severe degrees of uterovaginal or vaginal vault prolapse. Support derives from the base that sits above the levator plate and the stem that rests on the distal posterior vagina and perineum (Fig. 36F.3). An adequate perineal body is considered by some important for the effectiveness of this pessary, whereas others believe that suction from the concave base contributes to its support. It is

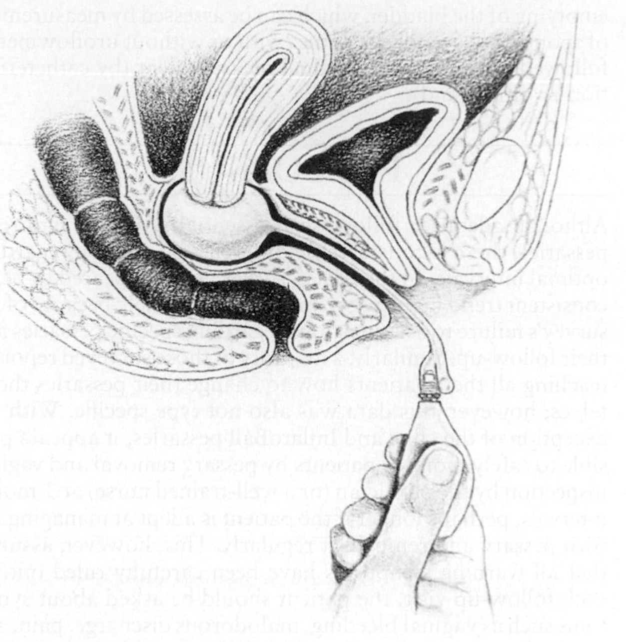

FIGURE 36F.2. InflatoBall pessary being inflated.

highly unlikely that patients will be able to remove and reinsert this pessary. The Gellhorn pessary does not allow comfortable coitus because of its shape.

Shaatz Pessary

The Shaatz has a shape similar to that of the Gellhorn but has no stem. This may facilitate coitus in some patients. Self-management of this pessary is possible.

Cube Pessary

The concave walls of the cube pessary create suction and adhere to the vaginal sidewalls. This characteristic results in effective support for severe uterovaginal or vaginal vault prolapse but can potentially cause ulceration and erosion of the vaginal

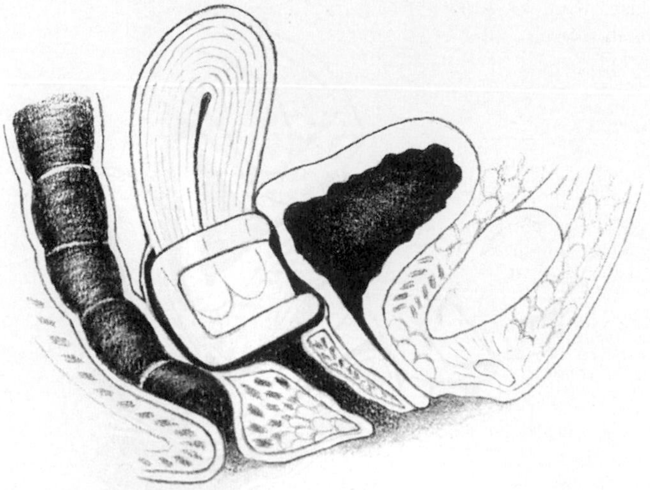

FIGURE 36F.4. Gehrung pessary in place.

mucosa. It is, therefore, recommended to remove this pessary nightly. This is achieved by inserting fingers between the pessary and the vaginal walls to release the suction and grasp the pessary itself (not the string) before pulling it out of the vagina.

Gehrung Pessary

The arch-shaped Gehrung pessary has a pliable metal frame that allows the pessary to be shaped to the patient's dimensions. The heels of the pessary rest on the lateral aspects of the posterior vagina, with the distal arch positioned behind the symphysis pubis (Fig. 36F.4). This underutilized pessary is effective in managing anterior and mild posterior compartment defects. Its shape makes this pessary somewhat difficult to insert but also allows for intercourse.

Lever Pessaries

All lever pessaries in use today are modifications of the original Hodge pessary. The Smith modification is designed to fit a narrow pubic arch, whereas the Risser fits the wider pubic

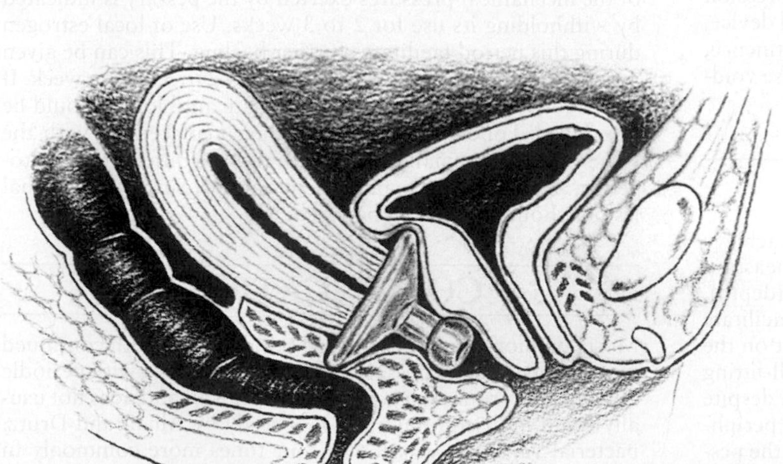

FIGURE 36F.3. Gellhorn placement.

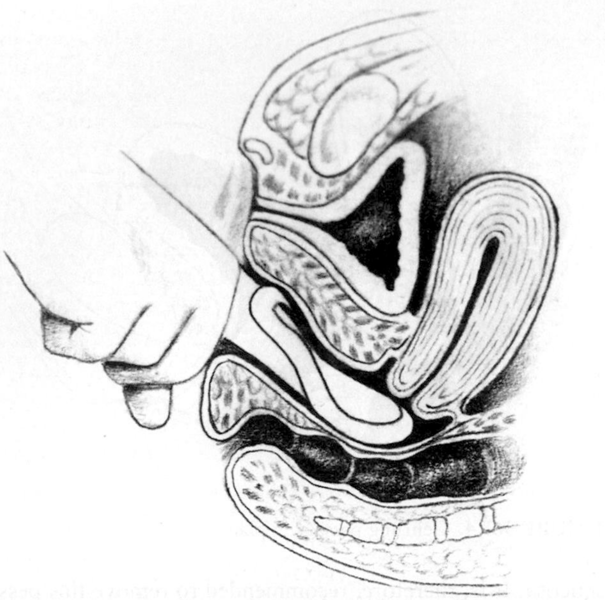

FIGURE 36F.5. Finger guiding the posterior bar of the lever pessary behind the cervix into the posterior fornix. Note the anteverted position of the uterus.

arch. The major function of these pessaries is the management of a retrodisplaced uterus. It has been proposed in the treatment of mild anterior and/or posterior compartment defects, as well as for cervical incompetence during pregnancy. When placing a lever pessary in a patient with uterine retrodisplacement, the uterus must be first manually anteverted (Fig. 36F.5). Lever pessaries can be worn during intercourse and may be self-managed.

Incontinence Pessaries

Many of the previously described pessaries have undergone additional modification to manage concurrent stress urinary incontinence. This usually involves the addition of a knob that is positioned under the urethra at the level of the bladder neck to help prevent its descent and facilitate temporary compression of the urethra with effort. These pessaries and the Introl device, which is solely designed for treatment of stress incontinence, may be somewhat uncomfortable and occasionally cause voiding dysfunction.

INITIAL FITTING

Pessary fittings are by trial and error. It is possible to achieve a good approximation regarding proper fit by digital measurement of the genital hiatus (width) and vaginal length (depth). Several sizes and pessary types should be available to facilitate a proper fit. A small amount of water-soluble lubricant on the leading edge of the pessary facilitates insertion. A well-fitting pessary should be comfortable to wear and be retained despite ambulation and straining. Digital palpation around the periphery ensures that a finger can be easily inserted between the pessary and the vaginal wall. The distal portion of the pessary should rest behind the symphysis or on the perineal body, depending on the pessary type. It should also allow for adequate emptying of the bladder, which can be assessed by measurement of spontaneous voided volume (with or without uroflowmetry) followed by a postvoid residual measurement (by catheterization or ultrasound).

FOLLOW-UP

Although adequate follow-up is essential given the nature of pessaries, there is considerable difference of opinion regarding optimal intervals. In the AUGS survey, there appeared to be no consistent trend in the regimens used, most likely because of the survey's failure to ask questions regarding specific pessaries and their follow-up. Similarly, a majority of those surveyed reported teaching all their patients how to change their pessaries themselves; however, this data was also not type specific. With the exception of the cube and InflatoBall pessaries, it appears possible to safely monitor patients by pessary removal and vaginal inspection by the physician (or a well-trained nurse) at 3-month intervals, perhaps longer if the patient is adept at managing her own pessary and removes it regularly. This, however, assumes that all warning symptoms have been carefully ruled out. At each follow-up visit, the patient should be asked about symptoms such as vaginal bleeding, malodorous discharge, pain, and discomfort. Symptoms of voiding difficulty with the pessary in place should be elicited, as well as any symptoms or signs of urinary tract infection.

At the set intervals determined by the patient and her care provider, the pessary is palpated to verify proper positioning and lack of undue tension on the vaginal walls. It is then gently removed with the aid of a water-soluble lubricant, and the vaginal and cervical surfaces are carefully inspected for any signs of erosion or abrasion. Suspicious lesions should be carefully inspected and biopsy considered. If the patient is satisfied with her pessary, it is reinserted if the inspection is negative. Voiding function should be assessed with the pessary in place if there is a concern regarding voiding function or if urinary tract infection has occurred since the last follow-up.

Presence of a new vaginal erosion may present a clinical dilemma because prolapse-associated erosion is considered by some an indication for pessary use rather than a contraindication. If, however, such an erosion or serious abrasion is diagnosed after pessary insertion but was not present before, the erosion is probably related to pressure from the pessary. Relief of the mechanical pressures exerted by the pessary is indicated by withholding its use for 2 to 3 weeks. Use of local estrogen during this period facilitates further healing. This can be given as 0.5- to 1-g applicatorful intravaginally 2 to 3 times a week. If infectious vaginitis is noted, appropriate antibiotics should be prescribed. Following mucosal healing, replacement with the same or a slightly smaller pessary, or trying a different type altogether, are reasonable management options. Suspicious vaginal lesions should always be biopsied.

COMPLICATIONS

Most commonly, a discharge and odor develop with continued wearing of a vaginal pessary. This is often treated with periodic douching or Trimo-San gel (Cooper Surgical) and does not usually result in discontinuation. In a study by Alnaif and Drutz, bacterial vaginosis was found four times more commonly in pessary users.

Mucosal erosion and abrasions of the vagina and/or cervix are more common with cube and Gellhorn pessaries. They are also more likely in patients who do not remove and reinsert their own pessary, as well as women with untreated vaginal atrophy. Recurrent erosions despite multiple attempts at pessary fitting with an adequately estrogenized vagina should prompt discontinuation of this mode of therapy. Pessary incarceration within the vagina with formation of vaginal adhesions has been described. Removal is facilitated by application of estrogen cream for several days.

Although rare, serious complications have been reported, mainly with the pessary that has been neglected, sometimes for many years. These complications include infections, fistulas, and even complete erosion with transmigration of the pessary into the bladder or the rectum. Herniation and incarceration of the cervix and even small bowel through neglected ring pessaries have been described. Unilateral and bilateral hydronephrosis with urosepsis and uremia have also been reported.

Chronic irritation associated with prolonged, uninterrupted pessary use has been associated with vaginal cancer. The literature comprises case reports that preclude the assumption of a causal relationship between pessary use and vaginal cancer. It appears to be more likely in the patient with a pessary neglected for many years and perhaps with older pessaries made of rubber. Pessaries used in practice today are primarily made of inert medical grade silicone, which may further reduce the risk of vaginal cancer.

SUMMARY

Although vaginal pessaries have been used throughout the millennia, their use has not been intensely studied. They remain a useful alternative either as initial management or reserved for those patients who are otherwise not candidates or do not desire surgery. This requires frank discussion with the patient regarding potential risks and benefits of all the proposed management options before she makes a decision. Pessary types may, at the discretion of the physician, be chosen for specific pelvic support defects. Although follow-up regimens may be individualized, adequate follow-up and treatment of vaginal atrophy are important to prevent the minor and major complications that can be associated with pessary use. The available evidence suggests that most patients who wish to proceed with pessary use as initial management can be successfully fitted.

BEST SURGICAL PRACTICES

- Nonsurgical management of pelvic organ prolapse should be considered in all patients with symptomatic prolapse.
- Indications for insertion of a vaginal pessary include symptomatic prolapse, urinary incontinence, uterine retroversion, or cervical incompetence.
- When using a pessary, care should be taken to avoid worsening stress urinary incontinence after placement.
- Intent to continue vaginal intercourse does not preclude use of a pessary.
- Evaluation of the vaginal mucosa should be performed before pessary placement. Atrophic vaginitis can increase the risk of pessary complications.
- Choice of pessary is highly individualized and will be guided by the type and severity of prolapse, desire to have intercourse, and the practitioner's preference.
- Patients should be followed closely after pessary placement and should be examined at regular intervals. Patients should be asked about vaginal bleeding, malodorous discharge, pain, voiding difficulty, or symptoms of a urinary tract infection.
- At each follow-up visit, the pessary should be removed and the vagina and cervix inspected for signs of erosion or abrasion. Suspicious vaginal lesions should be biopsied.
- Common complications of long-term pessary use include discharge and mucosal erosion/abrasion. Erosions or abrasions can often be addressed by local estrogen treatment or a change in pessary type.
- Serious complications of pessary use are usually only seen in patients with neglected pessaries and can include infection, fistulas, complete erosions, or incarceration.

Bibliography

Adams E, Thomson A, Maher C, et al. Mechanical devices for pelvic organ prolapse in women. *Cochrane Database Syst Rev* 2004;2:CD004010.

Alnaif B, Drutz HP. Bacterial vaginosis increases in pessary users. *Int Urogynecol J* 2000;11:219.

Bash KL. Review of vaginal pessaries. *Obstet Gynecol Surv* 2000;55:455.

Benson RC. Pessaries: past and present. Paper presented at: the Postgraduate Course in Obstetrics and Gynecology; 1959; Iowa City, IA.

Bhatia NN, Bergman A, Gunning JE. Urodynamic effects of a vaginal pessary in women with stress urinary incontinence. *Am J Obstet Gynecol* 1983;147:876.

Brincat C, Kenton K, Fitzgerald MP, et al. Sexual activity predicts continued pessary use. *Am J Obstet Gynecol* 2004;191:198.

Chow SH, LaSalle MD, Rosenberg GS. Urinary incontinence secondary to vaginal pessary. *Urology* 1997;49:458.

Clemons JL, Aguilar VC, Sokol ER, et al. Patient characteristics that are associated with continued pessary use versus surgery after 1 year. *Am J Obstet Gynecol* 2004;191:159.

Clemons JL, Aguilar VC, Tillinghast TA, et al. Patient satisfaction and changes in prolapse and urinary symptoms in women who were fitted successfully with a pessary for pelvic organ prolapse. *Am J Obstet Gynecol* 2004;190:1025.

Clemons JL, Aguilar VC, Tillinghast TA, et al. Risk factors associated with an unsuccessful pessary fitting trial in women with pelvic organ prolapse. *Am J Obstet Gynecol* 2004;190:345.

Cundiff GW, Weidner AC, Visco AG, et al. A survey of pessary use by members of the American Urogynecologic Society. *Obstet Gynecol* 2000;95:931.

Emge LA, Durfee RB. Pelvic organ prolapse: four thousand years of treatment. *Clin Obstet Gynecol* 1966;9:997.

Handa VL, Jones M. Do pessaries prevent the progression of pelvic organ prolapse? *Int Urogynecol J* 2002;13:349.

Heit M, Rosenquist C, Culligan P, et al. Predicting treatment choice for patients with pelvic organ prolapse. *Obstet Gynecol* 2003;101:1279.

Jay GD, Kinkead T, Hopkins T et al. Obstructive uropathy from uterine prolapse: a preventable problem in the elderly. *J Am Geriatr Soc* 1992;40:1156.

Morley GW. Treatment of uterine and vaginal prolapse. *Clin Obstet Gynecol* 1996;39:959.

Mutone MF, Terry C, Hale DS, et al. Factors which influence the short-term success of pessary management of pelvic organ prolapse. *Am J Obstet Gynecol* 2005:193:89.

Poma PA. Nonsurgical management of genital prolapse: a review and recommendations for clinical practice. *J Reprod Med* 2000;45:789.

Pott-Grinstein E, Newcomer JR. Gynecologists' patterns of prescribing pessaries. *J Reprod Med* 2001;46:205.

Russell JK. The dangerous vaginal pessary. *BMJ* 1961;2:1595.

Sulak PJ, Kuehl TJ, Shull BL. Vaginal pessaries and their use in pelvic relaxation. *J Reprod Med* 1993;38:919.

Wu V, Farrell SA, Baskett TF, et al. A simplified protocol for pessary management. *Obstet Gynecol* 1997;90:990.

Zeitlin MP, Lebherz TB. Pessaries in the geriatric patient. *J Am Geriatr Soc* 1992;40:635.

CHAPTER 37 ■ STRESS URINARY INCONTINENCE

ALFRED E. BENT

DEFINITIONS

Cystometrics—Tests of bladder function, including bladder sensation, capacity, and compliance. These tests may be simple clinical evaluations of bladder filling and emptying or may involve electronic measurement of bladder, urethral, and intraabdominal pressures.

Hypermobile stress incontinence—Stress incontinence caused by loss of anatomic support of the urethra and bladder base.

Intrinsic sphincter deficiency—Urinary incontinence that is due to dysfunction of the urethral sphincter mechanism.

Stress urinary incontinence—Involuntary leakage of urine from the urethra caused by increased intraabdominal pressure (coughing, straining, etc.).

Urodynamic stress incontinence—Involuntary leakage of urine during increased abdominal pressure in the absence of a detrusor contraction.

Urinary incontinence is a condition that affects 30% to 40% of older American women, with the majority afflicted with stress urinary incontinence (SUI). Conservative therapy helps a large number of these patients but cures relatively few. Surgical approaches for SUI have become more and more common, and have moved to delivery through minimally invasive surgical techniques. The purpose of this chapter is to detail the required evaluation before surgical intervention, then describe the surgical procedures used most effectively, along with the indications, results, and complications.

Stress urinary incontinence is defined by the International Continence Society as a condition defined by urodynamic observations associated with characteristic signs or symptoms. *Urodynamic stress incontinence* is defined as the involuntary leakage of urine during increased abdominal pressure in the absence of a detrusor contraction. Under the category of lower urinary tract symptoms, SUI is a storage disorder for which the characteristic symptom is the involuntary leakage of urine on effort or exertion, or on sneezing or coughing. The sign of SUI is the observation of involuntary leakage from the urethra synchronous with exertion or effort, such as sneezing or coughing. Current terminology refers to the condition described by both symptoms and urodynamic findings.

Stress incontinence has been divided into **hypermobile stress incontinence**, caused by anatomic defects, and **intrinsic sphincter deficiency**, with incontinence resulting from a poorly functioning urethra. This separation has become less distinct with time. SUI may include a wide spectrum of varying degrees of disruption of normal anatomy causing hypermobility or, somewhat paradoxically, scarring and fixation of these same tissues. Urethral sphincter function may be minimally altered so as not to be discernable on testing, or it may be severe. Most experts in the field are of the opinion that there is a contribution of each kind of dysfunction in most patients. The development of SUI has been attributed to a number of causes, with childbearing thought to be a dominant role in altering structural function (Table 37.1).

INITIAL EVALUATION

In 1996, the Agency for Health Care Policy and Research published its consensus guidelines for the evaluation and management of urinary incontinence. These recommendations from a panel of experts include the following: a thorough history (including voiding diary), physical examination, postvoid residual, and urinalysis.

More recently, the 3rd International Consultation on Incontinence held in Monaco (June 26–29, 2004) has published a series of management algorithms, including one for women with incontinence. The basic evaluation includes history; urinary symptom assessment, including a frequency-volume chart and questionnaire; assessment of quality of life and desire for treatment; cough stress test; urinalysis; assessment of voluntary pelvic floor contraction; and assessment of postvoid residual urine.

INITIAL MANAGEMENT

The recommendations for initial management do not require detailed testing, but treatment is based on a presumptive diagnosis of SUI. The first-line therapies commence with lifestyle interventions, which include weight reduction, smoking cessation, and dietary and fluid modification. Estrogen deficiency requires treatment followed by reassessment. Supervised pelvic floor muscle training and bladder training are recommended. The key word here is *supervised*. Patients will not and can not manage the proper therapy on their own. An appropriate duration of therapy is 8 to 12 weeks before reassessment for further treatment. Vaginal support devices can be included in the treatment options, depending on availability of the product, ability of the patient to manage the product, patient acceptance, and cost. In Europe, there is drug therapy available in the form of a dual serotonin and noradrenalin reuptake inhibitor, which has well-documented efficacy in large placebo-controlled drug studies.

EVALUATION BEFORE SURGERY

The American College of Obstetricians and Gynecologists Practice Bulletin issued in 2005 describes the evaluation of patients with symptoms of SUI. In addition to a focused history and

TABLE 37.1

FACTORS CONTRIBUTING TO STRESS URINARY INCONTINENCE

Factor	Possible mechanisms
Childbirth	Disruption of normal anatomy Pelvic nerve injury
Aging	Estrogen deficiency Tissue degradation Peripheral neuropathy
Iatrogenic: postsurgery	Disruption of normal anatomy Pelvic nerve injury Loss of tissue elasticity Loss of vascular cushion
Chronic obstructive pulmonary disease, chronic heavy lifting Chronic constipation	Straining causing stresses on normal anatomy and pelvic nerve injury
Iatrogenic: medication side effect	Loss of urethral tone
Pelvic radiation	Peripheral neuropathy Loss of tissue elasticity Loss of vascular cushion
Obesity	Increased intraabdominal pressure causing stresses on normal anatomy and pelvic nerve injury
Neurogenic disease	Loss of normal reflexes, pelvic floor tone, and urethral tone
Congenitally poor tissues: • Connective tissue disorder • Genetic predisposition	Poor anatomic integrity

TABLE 37.2

ACOG GUIDELINES FOR PRIMARY SURGERY FOR STRESS URINARY INCONTINENCE

Confirmation of indication	Actions before the procedure
Documentation of stress incontinence Identify and manage transient causes of stress incontinence Demonstrate stress loss and confirm low residual urine	Document normal voiding habits Document normal neurological examination Document absence of prior incontinence or radical surgery Document absence of pregnancy Counsel patient regarding alternative therapy

ACOG, American College of Obstetricians and Gynecologists.

physical examination, a urine culture, urine analysis, and renal function blood tests are indicated. Office evaluation of bladder filling and voiding should be done, and specialized tests of bladder function, including cystometry and cystourethroscopy, may be helpful in some patients. Guidelines for operating on patients with urethral hypermobility–type stress incontinence are shown in Table 37.2. This criteria set does not include urodynamic evaluation. The guidelines from the International Consultation on Incontinence recommended urodynamics to diagnose the type of incontinence. Urethral function testing by urethral pressure profile or leak-point pressure was optional. Basically, the recommendation is that in addition to the basic evaluation already completed, a cystometrogram is recommended to diagnose detrusor overactivity or stress incontinence.

The patient having a primary repair for SUI should have detailed history, physical examination with assessment for prolapse, frequency-volume chart (voiding diary), symptom questionnaire, urinalysis, assessment of bladder-neck mobility (Q-tip test or imaging), and residual urine determination. Bladder-neck mobility can be assessed by inserting a lubricated Q-tip into the urethra to the bladder neck and assessing for movement greater than 30 degrees from horizontal with straining. In the patient who has symptoms that are mixed (stress and urge) or whose voiding diary does not fit a pattern of pure stress incontinence, further evaluation is indicated.

The patient who has failed prior surgery or who has symptoms other than straightforward stress incontinence merits urodynamic evaluation and cystoscopy before surgery. Other options include imaging or videourodynamics.

SURGICAL TECHNIQUES FOR THE TREATMENT OF STRESS INCONTINENCE

More than 200 procedures have been described in the literature for the treatment of stress incontinence (Table 37.3). This reflects a combination of the alteration of techniques and approaches of established and effective procedures and the introduction of newer technologies and materials. In today's surgical practice, it is well established that performing an anterior repair or Kelly plication for the treatment of SUI is substandard compared with more effective procedures. This procedure was described in the 19th century; although it remains a recognized therapy for central defect cystocele, the most current international recommendation for use in patients with stress incontinence is in women who prefer to sacrifice some chance of becoming continent for a reduced chance of complication. Because of significant recurrence rates at even 1 and 2 years of follow-up, long-needle procedures—such as the Peyera, Stamey, or Raz procedures—are not recommended. Currently, the two primary forms of surgery for SUI are retropubic urethropexy and sling procedures. Injection of urethral bulking agents also is used as a less invasive intervention for SUI in certain patients. A comprehensive listing is provided in Table 37.3, but the procedures presented in detail will be those in current widespread use.

Retropubic Urethropexy

The gold-standard surgical treatment of SUI in patients with a mobile bladder neck and normally functioning urethra has been accomplished through a retropubic approach using either

TABLE 37.3

TIME LINE OF SIGNIFICANT SURGICAL PROCEDURES FOR STRESS INCONTINENCE

Anterior repair
- Schultz 1870—anterior repair
- Kelly plication 1913—wedge of tissue to support ureterovesical junction
- Ingelman Sundberg 1951–1952—bulbocavernosus

Sling
- von Giordano, 1907—gracilis muscle
- Goebell 1910—pyramidalis muscle
- Frangenheim 1914—abdominal wall fascia with pyramidalis
- Stoeckel 1917—same as Frangenheim
- Price 1933—fascia lata
- Aldridge 1942—rectus fascia
- Ridley 1974—description of sling in textbook
- Zoedler 1961—gauze hammock synthetic sling

Paravaginal repair
- White 1909—original description
- Richardson 1981—renewal of White technique

Retropubic
- Marshall-Marchetti-Krantz 1949
- Burch 1968
- Tanagho 1976—Burch modification
- Vancaillie 1991—laparoscopic Burch

Needle suspension
- Pereyra 1959
- Stamey 1973
- Raz 1981
- Gittes 1987

Periurethral bulking
- McGuire 1994—Contigen® injection

Tension-free synthetic tape
- Ulmsten and colleagues 1996—TVT (tension-free tape)
- DeLorme 2001—Transobturator tension-free tape

a Burch retropubic urethropexy or Marshall-Marchetti-Krantz (MMK) procedure. Although retropubic urethropexy has been widely used and is very effective, the newer midurethral, tension-free sling procedures are very popular, effective, and easier to perform.

The traditional approach to the retropubic space has been through a low transverse incision, which has gradually diminished in size to a minilaparotomy-type approach (Fig. 37.1). A Foley catheter keeps the bladder empty and helps identify the bladder neck. Entry into the peritoneal cavity is avoided unless there is a surgical indication. After opening the rectus fascia, the rectus muscles are separated, and then gentle downward pressure just behind and lateral to the symphysis allows approach to the pelvic sidewall and endopelvic fascia. If there has been prior surgery in this area, sharp dissection is required to separate the rectus muscle from the underlying preperitoneal tissue and bladder. Depending on the incision size, a self-retaining retractor may be used. The bladder is retracted superiorly with the aid of a moist pack, and the inferior part of the incision is retracted to expose the bladder. Following exposure of the retropubic space, the bladder neck is identified by palpation of a Foley catheter bulb, and it may be marked with hemoclips if desired. The anatomic landmarks and points of attachment of endopelvic fascia can then be identified (Fig. 37.2).

When performing a Burch retropubic urethropexy, the paraurethral tissue is exposed either with a "daisy sponge" (three 4 × 4 sponges on a sponge stick) or by using a moist sponge and narrow retractor. The best instrument for this is a Miyazaki all-purpose lighted retractor. The paraurethral areas may be cleared of fat that overlies the pubocervical fascia (fibromuscular layer of the vagina). The pubocervical tissue is elevated with a vaginal finger, and the overlying tissue and bladder are mobilized medially and superiorly away from the site of suture placement using a small dissecting sponge or "peanut" (Fig. 37.3). The large veins in this area are avoided, if possible, but may require control with suture, hemoclips, or cautery. The most important aspects of the development of the retropubic space dissection are exposure and retraction, and identification of the white endopelvic fascia (also called pubocervical fascia or fibromuscular layer of the vagina). Permanent sutures are placed on either side and 2 cm lateral to the urethra into the endopelvic fascia (avoiding full thickness), one set at the bladder neck and the second set at midurethra (Figs. 37.4 and 37.5). One or both arms of each suture are sutured through the ipsilateral Cooper's ligament and then tied from inferior to superior with an assistant elevating the vagina (Fig. 37.6).

An MMK procedure is performed by identifying the urethra with the aid of the Foley catheter (Fig. 37.7). Sutures are placed on either side of the urethra in a paraurethral location quite close to the urethra (Fig. 37.8). Bilateral permanent sutures are placed at the bladder neck and usually at least one set is placed just distal to this. These sutures are attached to the fibrocartilage of the symphysis pubis. Some surgeons open the bladder dome to locate the bladder neck by direct vision for exact suture placement at the bladder neck.

The aim of both procedures is to reestablish the intraabdominal location of the proximal urethra and urethrovesical junction, and to minimize descent of the bladder neck or urethrovesical junction, thus allowing normal pressure transmission to this crucial area during times of increased intraabdominal pressure. Cure rates for these procedures range from 85% to 90% at 1 to 5 years and greater than 70% at 10 years.

These procedures can be performed in concert with an abdominal hysterectomy or alone through a retropubic approach without opening the peritoneal cavity. Minilaparotomy techniques allow incisions as small as 5 cm to accomplish the suspension.

Laparoscopic Burch urethropexy became very popular in the mid-1990s. The approach could be either intraabdominal or extraperitoneal, and numerous modifications to the original Burch procedure were described, including using only two sutures; substituting mesh; or using tacks, anchors, and other tools to elevate the bladder neck. These variations significantly lowered cure rates as compared with traditional open urethropexy. Placement of four permanent sutures identical to an open procedure, though, has yielded similar 1- and 2-year cure rates as an open Burch (93% and 89%, respectively). In a prospective randomized trial of 62 laparoscopic and 28 open Burch procedures followed by urodynamics at 1 year, the cure rates were 93% for the laparoscopic and 88% for the open group. However, the more recent introduction of tension-free tape procedures made the use of laparoscopic Burch markedly less frequent, and it is now generally performed only with other intraabdominal reconstructive surgery.

Another procedure in the category of a retropubic approach is the paravaginal defect repair, first described by White and revitalized with Richardson and Shull. However, this procedure is for correction of lateral defect cystocele and not for treatment of SUI.

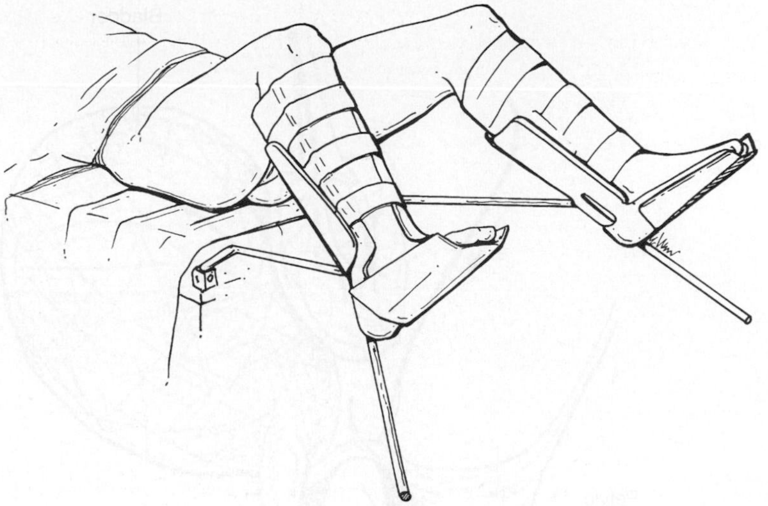

FIGURE 37.1. Positioning the patient for retropubic urethropexy in Allen universal stirrups to allow vaginal and abdominal access.

Tension-free Midurethral Slings

Tension-free slings are surgical procedures using a polypropylene mesh to support the midurethra without tension, a technique first described by Ulmsten and colleagues. Long-term follow-up has been reported with cure rates of approximately 85%. The original technique uses a retropubic approach, but the transobturator approach is fast becoming the most common tension-free sling technique performed worldwide for primary SUI. The appeal of a tension-free midurethral sling is that it is an effective, minimally invasive technique using local anesthetic and intravenous sedation in a day-surgery setting.

Many products are now marketed for this type of sling (Table 37.4). Some surgeons fashion their own sling from polypropylene soft mesh and place it without the aid of specially devised needles and kits. The manufactured products have a protective plastic sheath, allowing easy movement and adjustment of the sling under the urethra (Fig. 37.9).

The anesthetic for the procedure is injected as a solution of lidocaine hydrochloride diluted to 0.25% (1/4%) strength. Because the approximate maximum safe dose is 30 mL of a 1% solution, the 0.25% (1/4%) solution will provide 120 mL. Epinephrine may be used in the mixture, and with an original concentration of 1/100,000, the dilution ends up as 1/400,000. Alternatively, bupivacaine HCl may be used for local infiltration. The maximum dose of bupivacaine is 225 mg

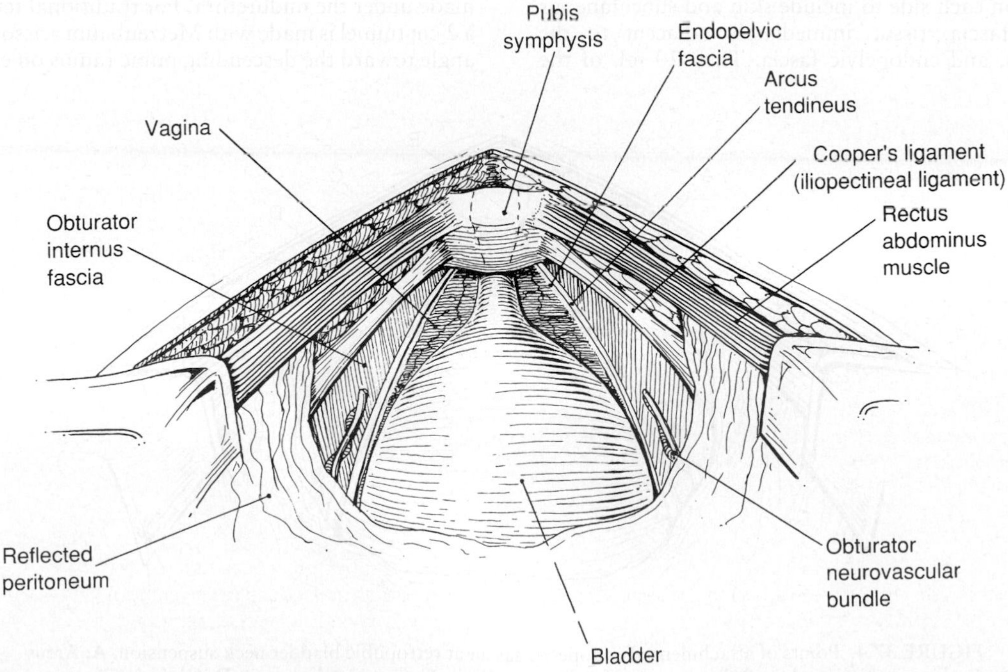

FIGURE 37.2. Anatomic landmarks in the space of Retzius.

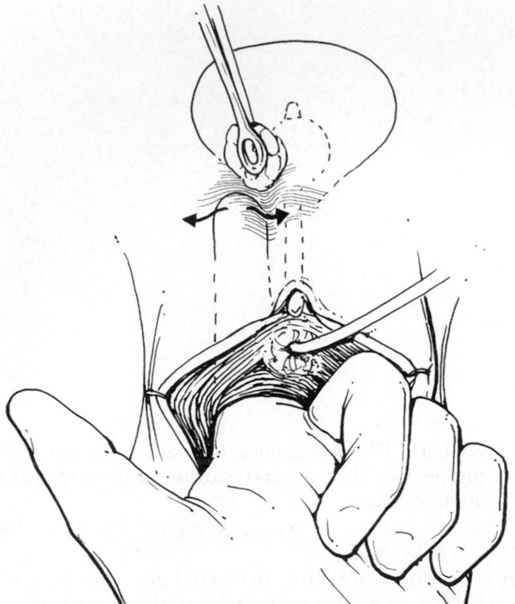

FIGURE 37.3. Dissection of bladder medially to expose endopelvic fascia. The finger of the vaginal hand elevates the vagina while the instrument pushes medially against the finger.

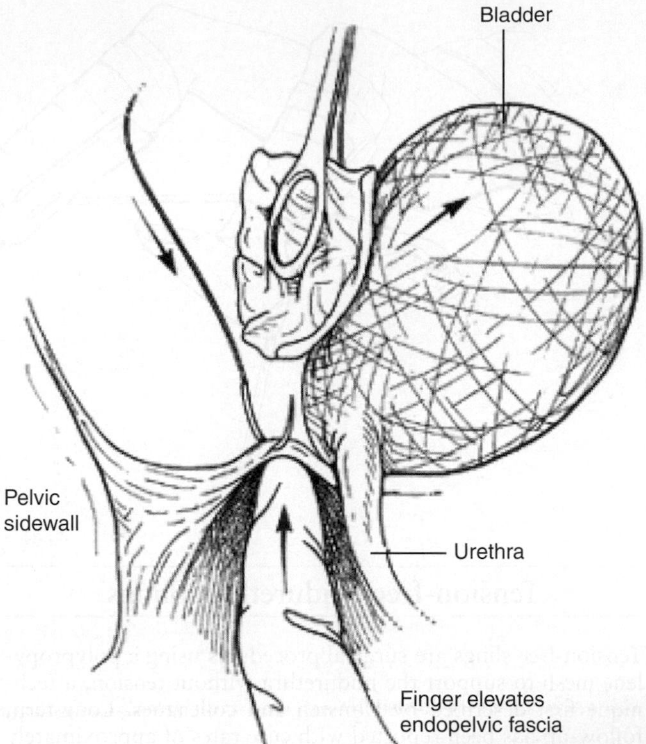

FIGURE 37.5. Medial displacement of the bladder for Burch suture placement. (From Robinson D, Norton PA. Diagnosis and management of urinary incontinence. In: William WM, Stovall TB, eds. *Gynecologic surgery.* New York: Churchill Livingstone; 1996:713.)

with epinephrine and 175 mg without epinephrine. In the traditional tension-free tape, 30 mL of solution is injected suprapubically on each side to include skin and subcutaneous tissues, rectus fascia, tissue immediately adjacent to the symphysis pubis, and endopelvic fascia. Then 20 mL of the solution is placed bilaterally by a vaginal approach, extending laterally from the midline into the endopelvic fascia and under the descending pubic rami. Five to 10 mL is placed under the midurethra. The bladder is emptied. A 1- to 2-cm incision is made under the midurethra. For traditional tension-free tapes, a 2 cm tunnel is made with Metzenbaum scissors at a 45-degree angle toward the descending pubic ramus on each side. A rigid

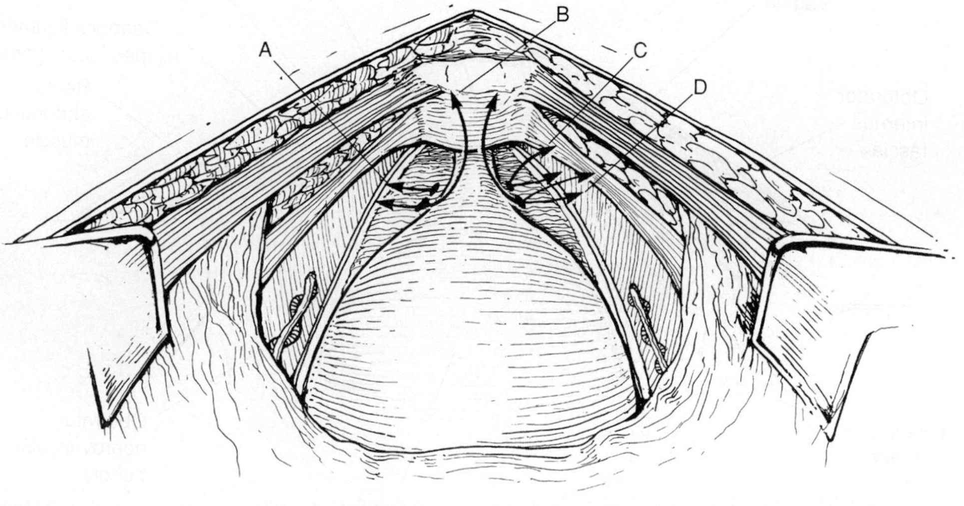

FIGURE 37.4. Points of attachment of endopelvic fascia at retropubic bladder neck suspension. A: Arcus tendineous fascia pelvis. B: Periosteum of pubic symphysis. C: Cooper's ligament. D: Obturator internus fascia.

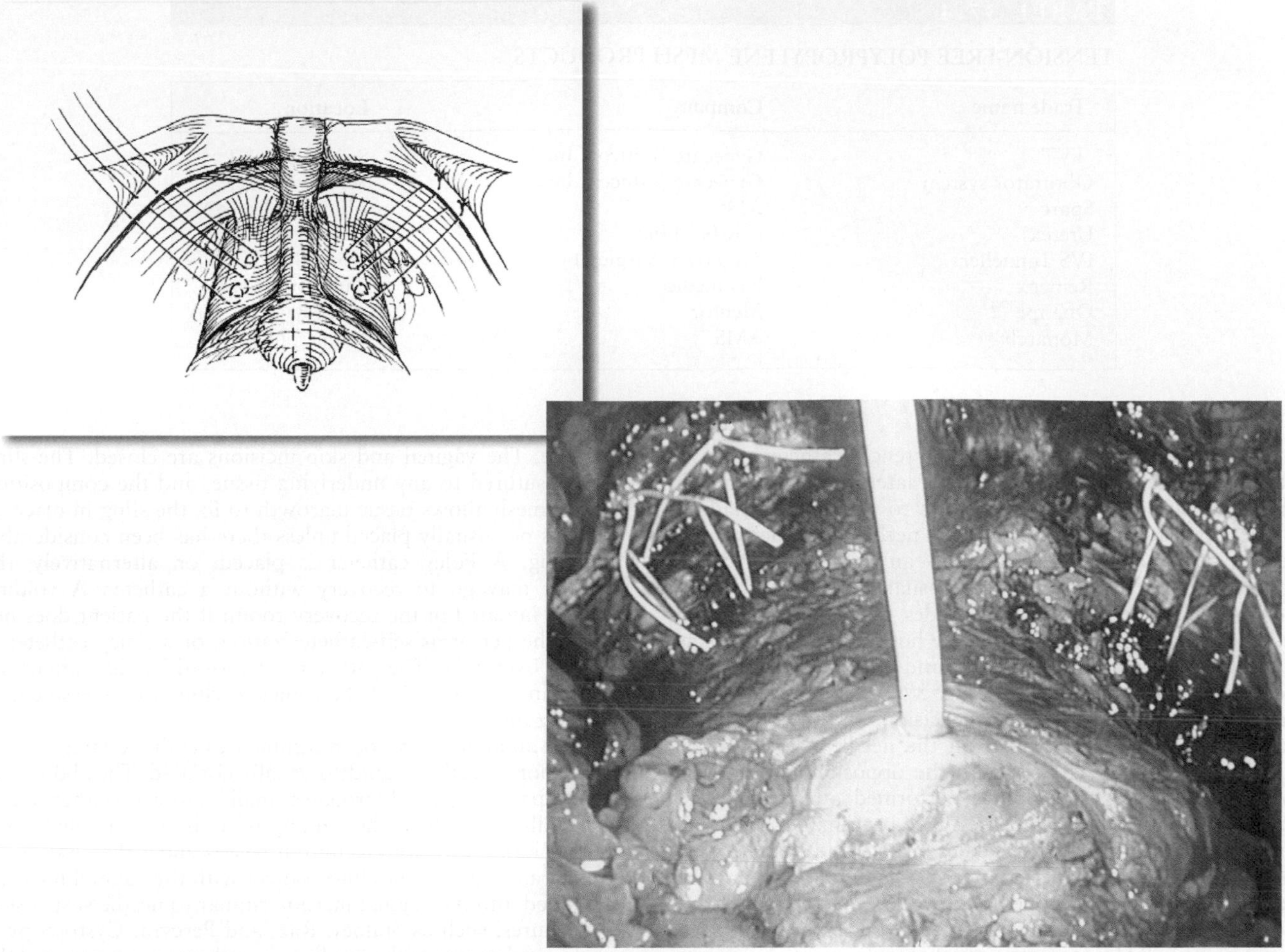

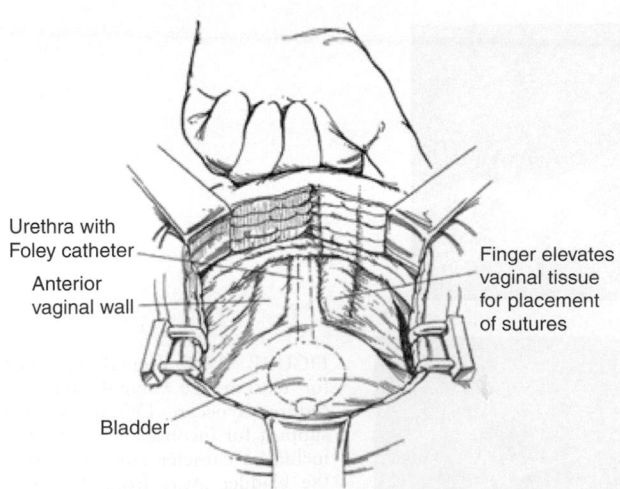

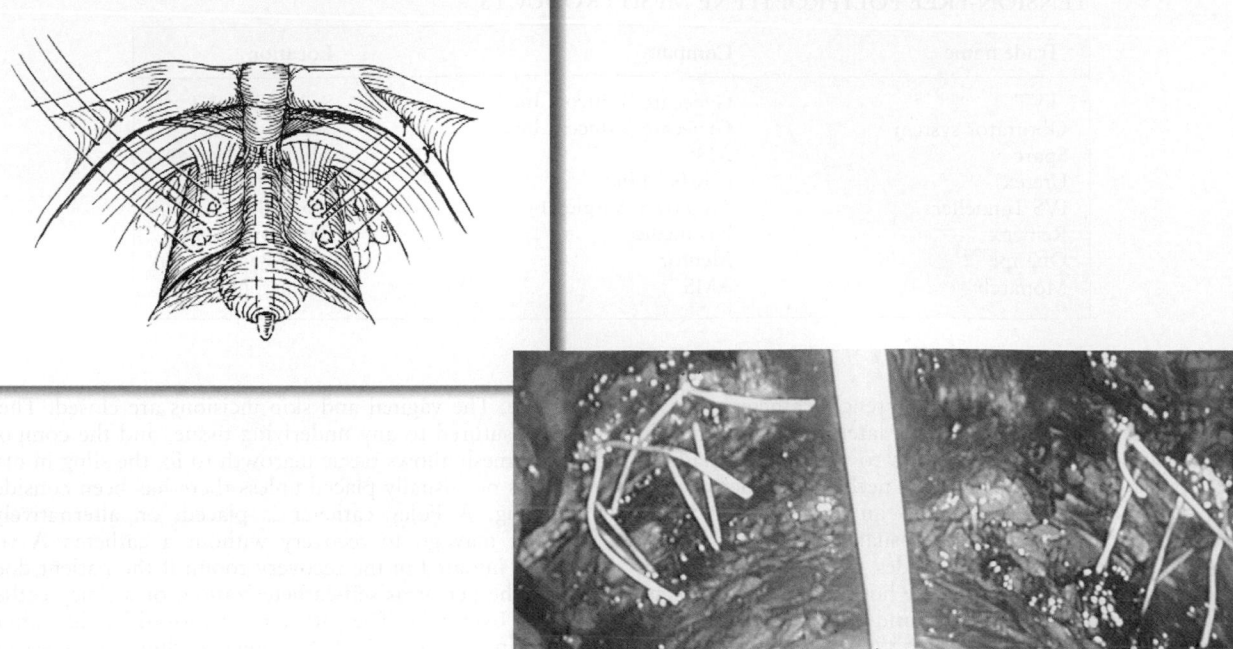

FIGURE 37.6. Placement of Burch colposuspension sutures. Sutures are placed in the endopelvic fascia, then passed through Cooper's ligament and tied.

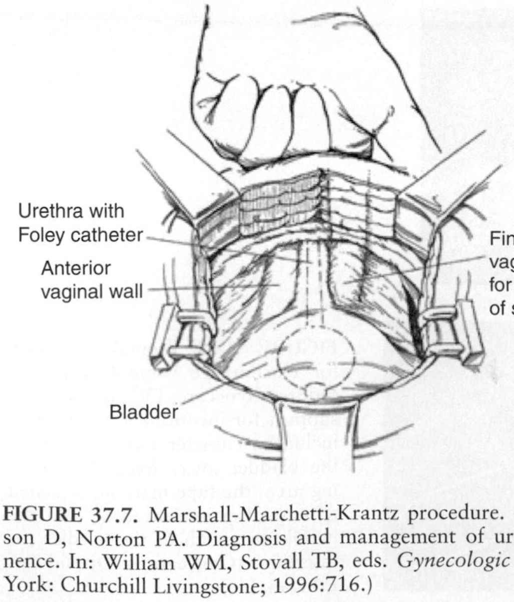

FIGURE 37.7. Marshall-Marchetti-Krantz procedure. (From Robinson D, Norton PA. Diagnosis and management of urinary incontinence. In: William WM, Stovall TB, eds. *Gynecologic surgery.* New York: Churchill Livingstone; 1996:716.)

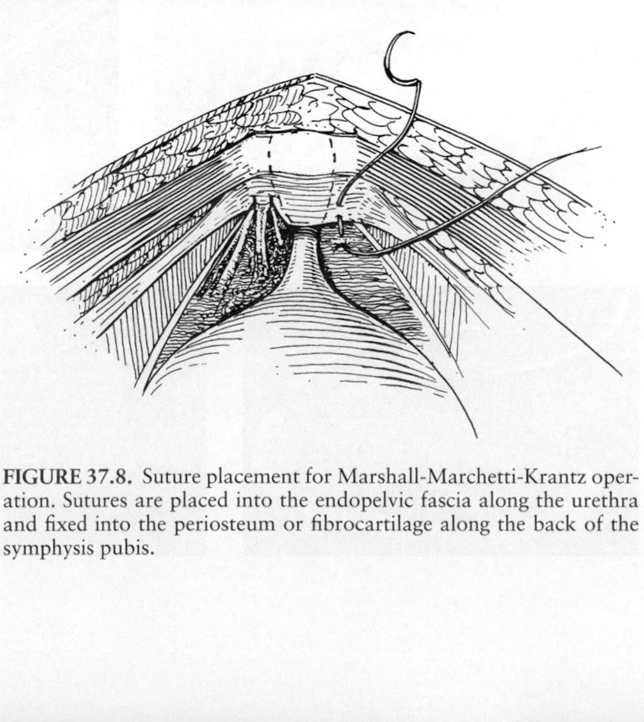

FIGURE 37.8. Suture placement for Marshall-Marchetti-Krantz operation. Sutures are placed into the endopelvic fascia along the urethra and fixed into the periosteum or fibrocartilage along the back of the symphysis pubis.

TABLE 37.4

TENSION-FREE POLYPROPYLENE MESH PRODUCTS

Trade name	Company	Location
TVT	Gynecare (Ethicon, Inc.)	Somerville, NJ
Obturator system	Gynecare (Ethicon, Inc.)	Somerville, NJ
Sparc	AMS	Minneapolis, MN
Uretex	C R Bard Inc.	Covington, GA
IVS Tunneller	Tyco (U.S. Surgical)	Norwalk, CT
Remeex	Neomedic	Barcelona, Spain
ObTape^{TM}	Mentor	Santa Barbara, CA
Monarch	AMS	Minnetonka, MN

catheter guide is placed in a 18 French catheter; this is placed into the urethra and directed laterally to the side on which the surgeon is working so as to deviate the bladder to the opposite side. The delivery needle with detachable handle is placed into the tunnel by an initial lateral direction, then directed toward the ipsilateral shoulder while the opposite-hand index finger guides the needle under the descending pubic ramus. The needle hugs the pubic ramus as the endopelvic fascia is penetrated, and then is advanced until the tip appears suprapubically (Fig. 37.10). The needle tip is passed just through a 5-mm skin incision, and the detachable handle is removed and placed on the needle passer for the other side. The tape is passed on the opposite side, and the handle removed. Cystoscopy is performed after each pass, or, alternatively, after both passes have been made. If there is no bladder perforation, the needles are advanced and pulled completely through the suprapubic area while viewing the bladder with the cystoscope. The needles are removed from the sling device. The sling with protective sheath is tightened over a number 8 Hegar dilator or other instrument. A clamp is positioned to grasp only the plastic sheath, and, while tension is maintained on the Hegar dilator to prevent the sling from becoming too tight, the plastic sheaths are gently pulled free from the mesh. The excess sling arms are cut flush to the skin surface. The vaginal and skin incisions are closed. The sling is not sutured to any underlying tissue, and the composition of the mesh allows tissue ingrowth to fix the sling in place. A pack is not usually placed unless there has been considerable bleeding. A Foley catheter is placed; or, alternatively, the patient may go to recovery without a catheter. A voiding trial is initiated in the recovery room; if the patient does not pass, she performs self-catheterization, or a Foley catheter is placed overnight. The catheter is removed by the patient the following morning, and she comes to clinic for assessment of voiding function.

The abdominal approach commences with the same vaginal dissection. A catheter guide is usually not used. The abdominal needle passer is passed through a small incision on either side of the midline just above the symphysis pubis and is guided along the back of the symphysis until it passes under the descending pubic ramus and comes into contact with the vaginal finger. It is guided into the vaginal incision similar to needle suspension procedures, such as Stamey, Raz, and Pereyra. Cystoscopy is performed to ensure the needle passers have not penetrated the bladder. The mesh is attached to the needle passers and pulled from the vaginal incision through the retropubic space to the abdominal site. The remainder of the procedure is the same as the vaginal route. Complications are similar to tension-free

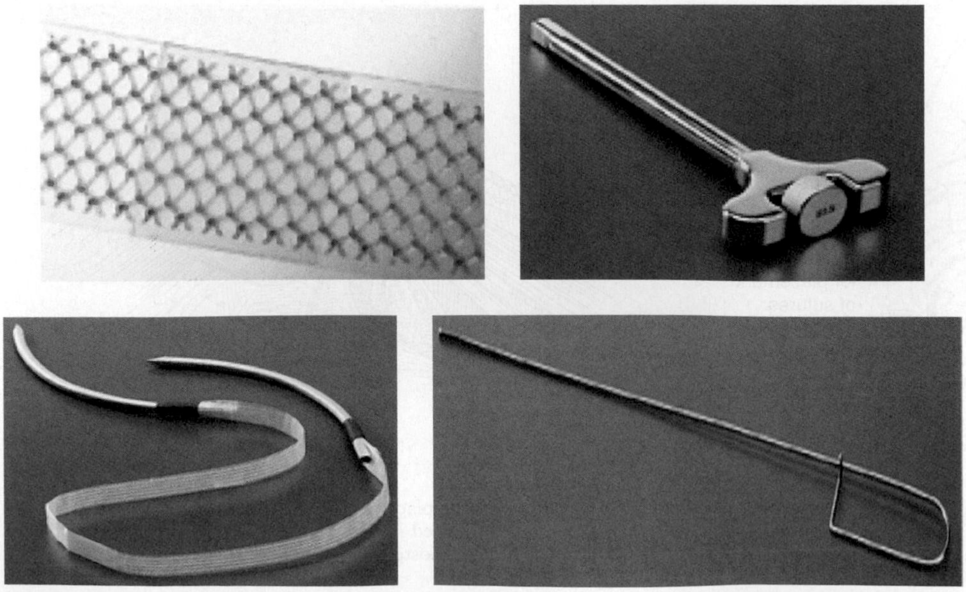

FIGURE 37.9. Vaginal approach for tension-free vaginal tape procedure. Gynecare TVT tension-free support for incontinence. Materials include a catheter guide to retract the bladder away from the working area, the tape material attached to two insertions needles, and the handle to attach to the needles for insertion. (Gynecare, a Division of Ethicon, Inc).

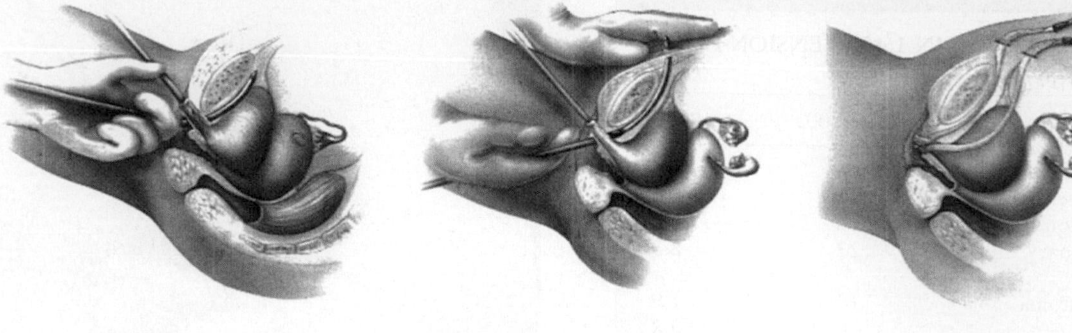

FIGURE 37.10. Insertion of vaginal tension-free tape. **A:** Vaginal guidance of needle under descending pubic ramus along back of symphysis. **B:** Pressure over skin of abdomen to allow needle to penetrate abdominal skin. **C:** Both needles passed through retropubic space and resting on abdomen. (With permission: Klutke J, Klutke C. The promise of tension-free vaginal tape for SUI. *Contemporary Urology® Archive*. 2000; October: Figures 4, 6, and 7.)

vaginal tape (TVT) except for fewer described severe problems with vascular or bowel injury. Bladder perforation occurs with equal frequency.

The most serious complications after the first 500,000 cases of TVT procedures are shown in Table 37.5. There were seven deaths from that group, which included five after undiagnosed bowel perforation, one from uncontrolled bleeding in the retropubic space in a woman with a bleeding disorder, and one after a bowel perforation in which no additional information could be obtained. Major vascular injury may be prevented by using universal Allen stirrups. The insertion needle must not stray laterally. Smaller venous channels are frequently penetrated and are managed by pressure for 5 minutes or placement of a vaginal pack. Moderate bleeding may be controlled by a Foley catheter with 50 mL in the balloon to tamponade the bleeder against a pack in the vagina. Occasionally, a retropubic space hematoma will develop; but it is self-limited, and the usual treatment is observation. Bladder perforation occurs 2% to 4% of the time and is usually managed by withdrawal and reinsertion of the needle. When this occurs, a Foley catheter is recommended for 1 to 2 days, and antibiotic coverage provided. Bladder perforation may be prevented by infiltration of the dilute local anesthetic in large volume amounts, keeping the bladder empty, and directing the bladder away from the operative site with the rigid catheter guide. Bowel perforation may be prevented by imaging prospective patients who have had prior retropubic surgery and who may have bowel adherent in the cul-de-sac in close proximity to the retropubic area.

Frequent delayed complications include voiding dysfunction, urgency, and urinary tract infection (Table 37.6). About half of patients will void by the time of discharge from day surgery, and most are voiding well by the following day. There is a 2% to 5% persistent urinary retention rate, and these patients require sling revision. This is best performed in the first 4 to 6 weeks after surgery before advanced scarring around the mesh. The tape has usually migrated somewhat proximally along the urethra and needs to be exposed by sharp dissection, then loosened or cut to allow retraction of the mesh away from the underside of the urethra. Continence is maintained in most patients, and the release of the sling allows normal voiding in most cases. Urinary tract infection may be prevented by preoperative antibiotics, but there is still a 7% to 8% incidence of urinary tract infection in the first 2 months postoperatively. Urgency with some urge incontinence occurs in 10% to 12%; although time resolves a lot of this, a number of patients require medical intervention. Release or loosening of the sling may help resolve severe urgency symptoms. Mesh erosion is a delayed complication, occurring in 1% of patients, and usually is managed by excision of the exposed mesh and resuture of the vagina.

The **transobturator approach** (TOT) theoretically has safety factors that may make it preferable to the original TVT

TABLE 37.5

REPORTED MAJOR TENSION-FREE VAGINAL TAPE COMPLICATIONS[a] BASED ON 500,000 CASES

Complication	United States	Outside United States	Total	Percent
Vascular injury	7	37	44	0.009
Vaginal mesh exposure	43	17	60	0.012
Urethral erosion	20	0	20	0.004
Bowel perforation[b]	16	12	28	0.006
Nerve injury	3	1	4	0.0008
Urinary retention	48	45	93	0.019
Hematoma formation	4	16	20	0.004

[a]Gynecare report to Food and Drug Administration as of September 26, 2003.
[b]Seven deaths have been reported, six associated with bowel perforation.

TABLE 37.6

MINOR COMPLICATIONS IN 1,455 TENSION-FREE VAGINAL TAPE CASES[a]

Incidence	N/1,000	Percent
Minor voiding difficulty	76	7.6
Urinary tract infection	41	4.1
Bladder perforation	38	3.8
Postoperative urinary retention	23	2.3
Retropubic hematoma	19	1.9
Wound infection	8	0.8

From Kuuva N, Nilsson CG. *Acta Obstet Gynecol Scand* 2002;81:72.
[a]A nationwide analysis of complications associated with the tension-free vaginal tape.

approach. It is placed more horizontally and should interfere with voiding even less than a TVT. Local infiltration of dilute lidocaine or Marcaine is carried out along the tracks of needle passes. There are two basic types of transobturator surgeries for stress incontinence. One is an outside-in technique, which emphasizes speed, safety, and ease of placement. The vaginal incision needs to be large enough to insert a finger to reach to the ischiopubic ramus, and the thumb of the same hand grasps the outline of the ramus in the genitofemoral fold between labium majus and the thigh. A point in the groin fold level with the clitoris is selected and a 5-mm incision made on each side. The needle passer is inserted perpendicularly and guided by the finger until it penetrates the obturator membrane (Fig. 37.11). The needle is then rotated under the pubic ramus, and the vaginal index finger guides it into the vaginal incision. The tightening of the sling is the same as the TVT.

The **inside-out TOT** starts with local infiltration of dilute anesthetic. The incision may be slightly smaller than the outside-in TOT. Scissor dissection proceeds on one side until the obturator membrane is penetrated with the scissor tips. A metal winged guide is placed into the defect in the obturator membrane. The needle passer is placed along the direction of the winged guide and then rotated while the handle is moved inferiorly to a vertical position. The needle passer exits 1 cm lateral to the groin fold about 2 cm superior to the urethral meatus and parallel to the clitoris. The tape is retrieved, and tightening follows the same pattern as with the technique described above. The same-day patient attempts to void in recovery; if unsuccessful, she uses self-catheterization or has a Foley placed overnight.

The transobturator tape does not have a retropubic passage and therefore avoids the major complications of retroperitoneal vascular injury, bowel injury, and bladder perforation. Because of the horizontal placement for TOT, the incidence of postoperative voiding dysfunction is considered to be less, though no large randomized trial has definitively shown this (Fig. 37.12). There remains the possibility of damage to the obturator vessels and nerve during passage of the needle, but this can be avoided by following the procedure as described. There have been isolated reports of bladder perforation, and it may still be appropriate to carry out cystoscopy with urethral inspection at the end of the procedure, especially in women with significant prolapse. There are still the same complications of bleeding, hematoma, dysuria, urgency, and bladder infections as with TVT. Abscess formation in the ischiorectal fossa has been reported, but it is very uncommon. Occasionally, there is persisting groin pain or irritation with movement.

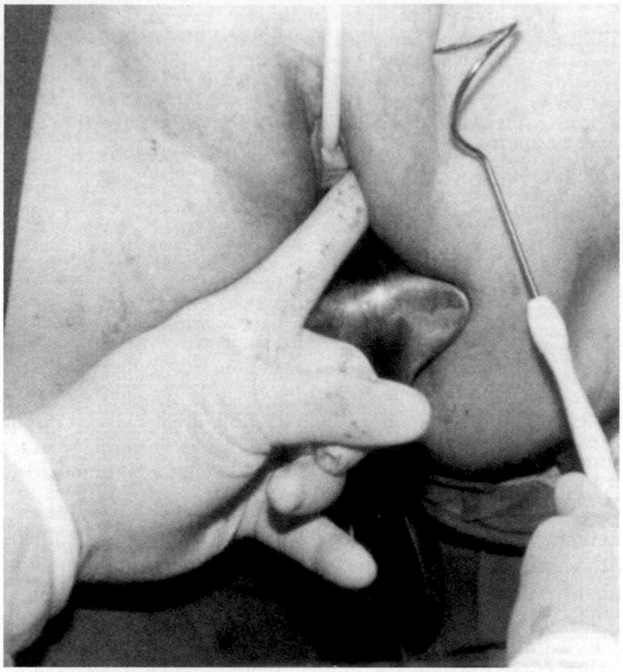

FIGURE 37.11. Transobturator tension-free tape (TOT) approach. The finger is placed in the vaginal dissection into the space of Retzius while the thumb hooks the tissue at the genital-crural fold. The specialized needle is passed from either outside to inside, or vice versa, and the tape is attached and pulled through the space. (With permission: Pelosi MA II, Pelosi MA III. New transobturator sling reduces risk of injury. *ObGyn Management* 2003;15:17.)

The tension-free sling is thought to work by forming a solid buttress under the midurethra, allowing the mobile bladder neck to descend and rotate with increased intraabdominal pressure, and compress the urethra against the sling. Most efficacy reports are in the 85% range for both TVT and TOT procedures, and this can safely be quoted to patients in preoperative discussion.

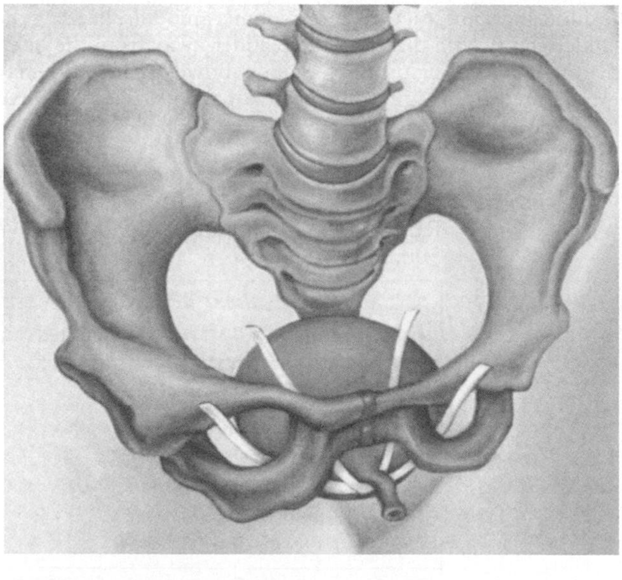

FIGURE 37.12. Comparison of retropubic and transobturator placement of TVT and TOT. The TOT is more horizontal and may therefore have less voiding dysfunction.

When the tension-free tape procedures are done in conjunction with other pelvic floor surgery, it does not seem to matter as to the order in which things are done. The tape can be laid in position initially and then the rest of the procedures completed and the tape tightened at the end of the case. If there is a lot of bleeding from dissection for the tape, this can cause some delay and interference with the rest of the case. The other way is to do all the other procedures, and then place the tape at the end. Any anterior vaginal wall dissection should not extend closer than 2 cm to the urethral meatus, thus leaving room for the tape dissection. If a colpocleisis is performed, the tape has to be placed before obliterating the anterior wall.

Suburethral Slings

The concept of placing a material under the urethra and suspending it to the abdominal tissues was introduced as early as 1907 when Giordano used gracilis muscle transposed beneath the bladder neck. Goebell (1910) used pyramidalis muscles transposed through the space of Retzius, and first Frangenheim (1914) and then Stoeckel (1917) described using a strip of anterior abdominal fascia with the pyramidalis muscles. Price (1933) harvested fascia lata, which he passed beneath the urethra and then retropubically, and attached it to the anterior rectus fascia on either side of the midline. This technique and its modifications became known as the Goebell-Stoeckel-Frangenheim procedure, or fascia lata sling, but the named surgeons never used fascia lata. Aldridge (1942) used strips of rectus fascia from a transverse abdominal incision, passed them retropubically, and secured them beneath the urethra. McGuire and Lytton (1978) described a sling procedure using rectus fascia supported by sutures extending through the space of Retzius and attached to the rectus fascia. This procedure and its modifications are referred to as a rectus sling.

The sling acts like a hammock under the bladder neck to both elevate the urethrovesical junction into an intraabdominal location and to provide partial compression of the urethra. These techniques differ from the modern tension-free procedures because the ends of the sling or suspending sutures are fixed to the rectus fascia. During periods of increased abdominal pressure, the abdominal wall moves outward and the sling is drawn upward. This compresses the urethra and increases intraurethral resistance. Variations of the sling procedure in which the ends of the sling are attached to an immovable tissue (Cooper's ligament or bone anchors in the pubic symphysis) do not allow upward displacement of the sling and urethra during straining. In these operations, the sling is thought to create a secure platform of urethral support. Increases in intraabdominal pressure press the urethra downward against the sling, thereby compressing the urethra from both above and below. It is this compression of the urethra that is believed to lead to increases in urethral resistance and a resolution of stress incontinence. However, the potential for excess compression of the urethra also contributes to the most common complications of the sling procedure: voiding dysfunction.

The intervening 100 years have provided time for development of many materials and techniques for sling surgery. The autologous tissues have included rectus fascia, fascia lata, vagina, gracilis muscle, round ligaments, pyramidalis muscle, and rectus muscle. Because of additional operative time and morbidity to harvest autologous materials, many substitute materials were used and evaluated. Synthetic materials are now almost completely confined to polypropylene mesh. Biomaterials have included human-derived dermal and fascial tissues, with fascia lata composing most of the active use. Allograft fascia materials have been in use for more than 25 years but have to be harvested, processed, preserved, and distributed by tissue banks regulated by the American Association of Tissue Banks. Xenograft materials are mostly porcine dermis and bovine pericardium.

Surgeons who prefer an autologous sling use either rectus fascia or fascia lata. Rectus fascia is harvested at the time of a suprapubic incision by excising a strip of rectus fascia and closing the residual defect. A 4- to 5-cm incision easily allows harvest of a fascial strip 2 cm wide and 8 to 10 cm long (Fig. 37.13). A fascial closure suture is placed beyond the harvest site on both sides and a strip of rectus fascia developed medially from each side. The graft is wrapped in saline-soaked gauze or placed in an antibiotic solution. The fascia is mobilized sharply off the underlying muscle to avoid tension in the closure. The rectus fascia is cleared of fat just above the symphysis pubis on either side to allow for fixation of the sling.

Alternatively, fascia lata may be harvested from the lateral aspect of the thigh (Fig. 37.14) using a Masson stripper or a Crawford fascial stripper. Alternatively, the fascia may be excised directly. The Masson stripper comes in 1-cm and 2-cm sizes and can remove a strip up to 3 cm in width and 20 cm long. The Crawford stripper can remove a strip 1 cm wide and 20 cm long.

Harvest is accomplished with the patient supported leaning to one side and the leg positioned on a pillow (Fig. 37.15). The iliotibial fan of fascia is palpated over the lateral thigh near the knee. A vertical or transverse incision is made 2 to 3 cm above the knee over the fascia and the fascia lata cleaned with a gauze-tipped finger. Two incisions are made in the fascia, 1.5 to 2 cm apart, and the fascia lata transected 3 to 4 cm superior to its attachment into the lateral condyle of the femur. The distal 4 to 5 cm of fascia is mobilized with sharp dissection and the free end threaded into the Masson or Crawford fascial stripper and held firmly with straight Kocher clamps. The fascia is freed superiorly from attachments by passing a long forceps (handle end) over the superior and inferior surfaces of the fascia. The stripper is then advanced parallel to the fascia lata fibers, toward the greater trochanter of the hip (Fig. 37.16). The Masson stripper has an inner and outer component, and the outer

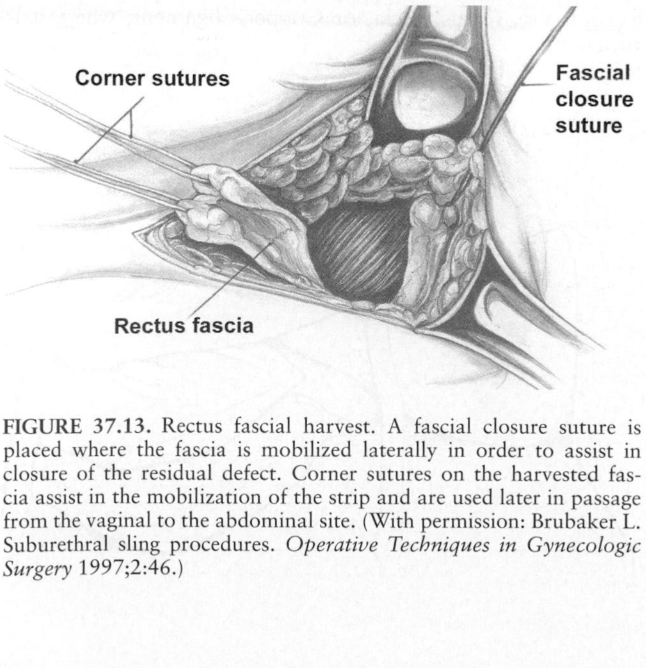

FIGURE 37.13. Rectus fascial harvest. A fascial closure suture is placed where the fascia is mobilized laterally in order to assist in closure of the residual defect. Corner sutures on the harvested fascia assist in the mobilization of the strip and are used later in passage from the vaginal to the abdominal site. (With permission: Brubaker L. Suburethral sling procedures. *Operative Techniques in Gynecologic Surgery* 1997;2:46.)

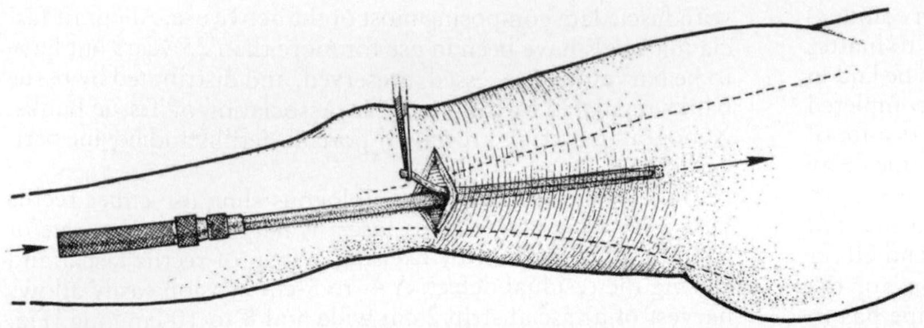

FIGURE 37.14. Masson fascial stripper. (With permission: Ridley JH. Surgery for stress urinary incontinence. In: Ridley JH, ed. *Gynecologic surgery: errors, safeguards, salvage*. Baltimore: Williams & Wilkins; 1974:135.)

sheath is disengaged and advanced briskly or turned over the inner portion, which severs the fascia at the uppermost area of the leg. The Crawford stripper requires a pulley action to advance a cutter at the end of the instrument to cut the fascial strip. The 1-cm-wide strip obtained with the Crawford stripper requires a second pass to get a second strip if a full-length sling is desired, and the two are sutured together, overlapping in the center 2 or 3 cm, to make that area thicker as well as wider. The open technique requires two vertical incisions separated by an intact skin area at least the size of each incision. The fascia lata is dissected free from the muscle underneath, and elevation of the skin bridge allows dissection to the higher incision. The fascia is cut 2 to 3 cm wide, and the uppermost end is severed to procure the strip. The fascial defect is not closed, but a pressure dressing is usually applied, and the skin may be closed with a subcuticular suture.

Sling length has varied in the many procedures described. A patch sling is several cm in length, but the tails of the sling do not perforate the endopelvic fascia into the retropubic space. The patch is suspended by permanent sutures and allows harvest of small amounts of tissue, but there is little *in situ* scarring and fixation of the fascial material. A full-length sling passes underneath the urethra, through the endopelvic fascia and retropubic space, all the way to the point of fixation, where it is secured with sutures. Usually the fixation point is rectus fascia. A half sling (7 cm length or more) extends into the retropubic space through the endopelvic fascia and is attached by sutures secured to the tails to suspend the material to the appropriate fixation site, usually the rectus fascia. This has become the most common sling length when using autologous materials. A full-length sling extends all the way to the fixation site, rectus fascia, or Cooper's ligament, where it is attached.

The abdominal dissection is performed through a 4- to 5-cm incision (unless the patient is obese) usually placed 2 cm above the symphysis pubis, but not in the crease of the panniculus. The fascia is cleared of fat and subcutaneous tissues at sites 2 cm above the symphysis and 2 cm lateral to the midline, where the sling arms or sutures will be passed through the fascia. If an instrument is used to grasp the sling or suture tails (as opposed to a needle passer technique using Pereyra or Stamey needles), then a small 0.5- to 1-cm incision is made in the full-thickness rectus fascia. If rectus fascia has been harvested, the remaining lower margin of fascia is cleared of fat and subcutaneous tissue.

The retropubic space may be opened, especially in cases in which there has been previous retropubic surgery. If necessary, the bladder can be opened at the dome to facilitate sharp dissection of the bladder away from the sidewall of the pelvis. In this technique, a finger can be placed through the abdominal incision reaching to the level of the endopelvic fascia. The vaginal dissection extends to the same level, and the sling material can easily be passed from vaginal to abdominal surgeon without concern regarding placement of the sling in the bladder or through a segment of bowel. This can still be accomplished through a small (5-cm) skin incision.

The vaginal dissection commences with an inverted U or 2-cm midline incision along the anterior vaginal wall. The epithelium is dissected off the fibromuscular layer laterally until access through the endopelvic fascia is readily available beneath the descending pubic ramus. The epithelial flap may be left thick to protect against poor healing of the vaginal epithelium over the sling material. The fibromuscular layer does not need to be plicated unless extra thickness is desired under a synthetic sling or there is a central anterior vaginal wall defect. Sharp dissection to the level of the pubic ramus allows easy access to perforate the endopelvic fascia sharply or bluntly,

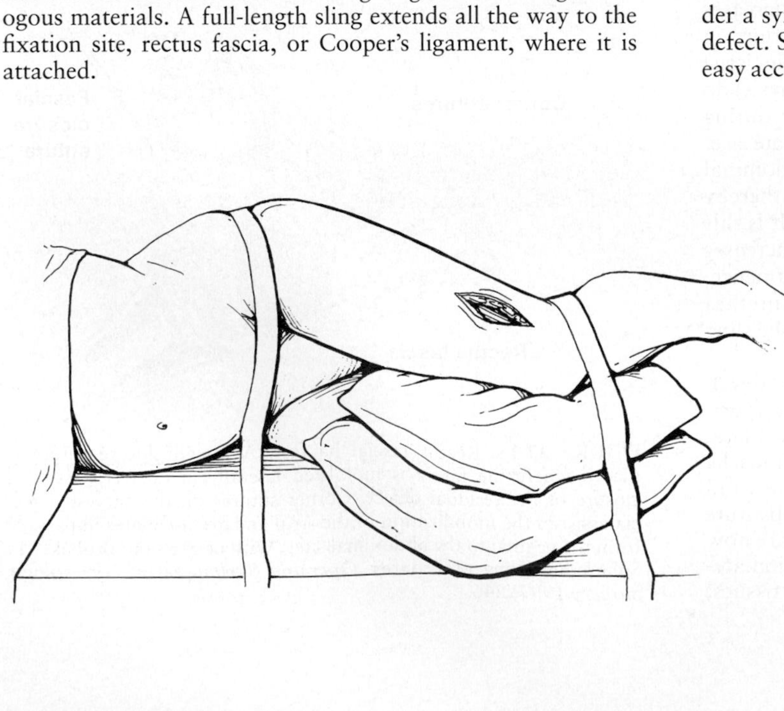

FIGURE 37.15. Patient positioning for fascia lata harvest. An incision is made over the fascia lata approximately 3 to 4 cm above the knee.

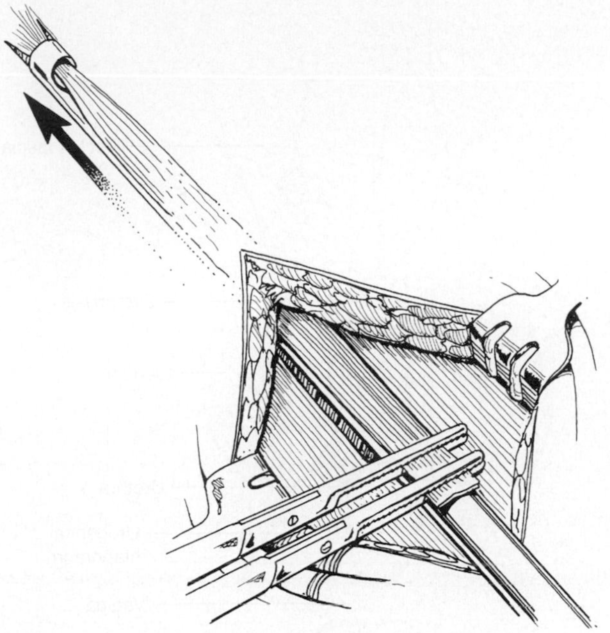

FIGURE 37.16. Harvesting fascia lata. With the fascial end secured by Kocher clamps, the stripper is slowly advanced parallel to the fascia lata fibers, shearing off a long strip of fascia.

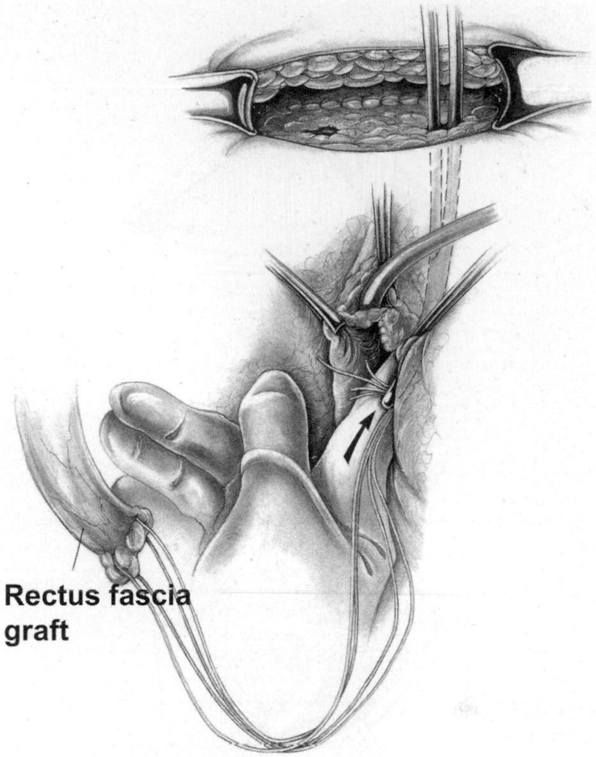

FIGURE 37.18. Passage of sling material through the space of Retzius from vaginal to abdominal site. Rectus fascia partial sling with attached sutures. (With permission: Brubaker L. Suburethral sling procedures. *Operative Techniques in Gynecologic Surgery* 1997;2:48.)

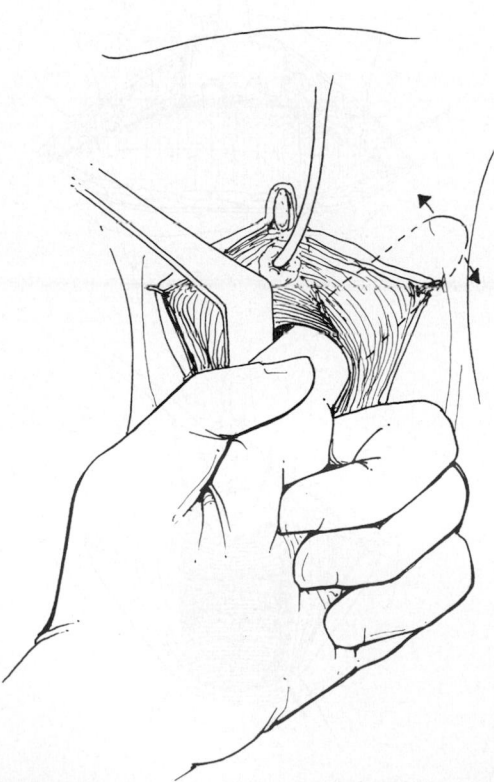

FIGURE 37.17. Perforation of the endopelvic fascia to open the space of Retzius and mobilize the periurethral tissues.

directing the instrument or finger toward the ipsilateral shoulder (Fig. 37.17). Some surgeons do not enter the retropubic space when placing a sling. Others use a finger to guide an instrument or needle pass from the abdominal to the vaginal incision, and this is the recommended technique. The instrument is directed through the abdominal incision and directed toward the back of the symphysis pubis. A finger placed in the vaginal dissection reaches to the retropubic space to meet the advancing clamp or needle to minimize the distance of blind passage (Figs. 37.18 and 37.19). Cystoscopy ensures bladder integrity and ureteral function. The sling is sutured to the pubocervical fascia under the mid- to proximal urethra to prevent movement from the placement site. A Foley catheter bulb marks the bladder neck. Historically, the position of the sling was bladder neck and proximal urethra (Fig. 37.20). With the introduction of the tension-free tape procedures at the midurethra, a number of surgeons have also moved traditional suburethral sling placement more distally to override the midurethra. A broad-based sling is considered preferable to a narrow band of material.

The most common fixation site is rectus fascia (Fig. 37.21). The arms of the sling or suspending sutures may be secured together loosely over the rectus fascia without actually being sutured to the fascia. Cooper's ligament can also be used to support the sling arms. Bone anchors allow alternative fixation to a solid structure, although there is no evidence that weak rectus fascia attachment is a cause of procedure failure. The sutures or sling tails are placed through the fascia and tied with 1 to 3 finger breadths between the tissue and the sutures or sling. The object is to leave the sling loose.

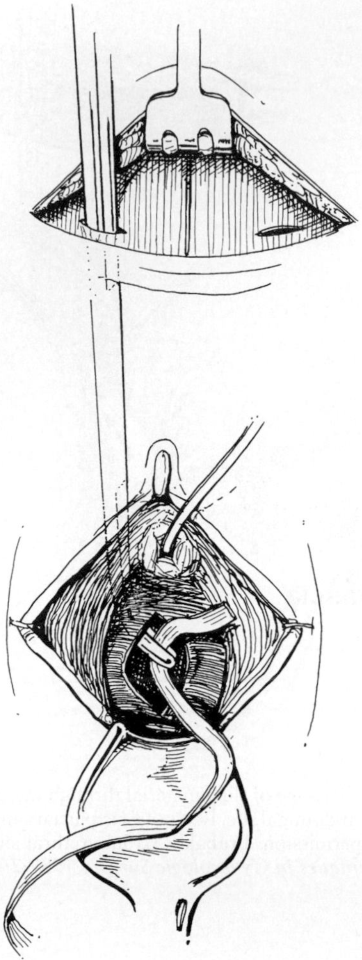

FIGURE 37.19. Passage of fascia lata strip through space of Retzius. Under guidance from the surgeon's hand in the vaginal incision through the endopelvic fascia into the space of Retzius, a clamp is passed from the abdominal incision to the vaginal incision. The end of the fascia is grasped and retrieved to the abdominal site.

Bladder drainage techniques include suprapubic catheter, Foley catheter, or intermittent self-catheterization. Most often, a Foley catheter is left overnight and then removed the following day, allowing the patient the opportunity to void. Postvoid residual urine determinations are measured by bladder scan or catheterization; if voiding is not adequate, the Foley catheter may be reinserted or self-catheterization used. There is no uniform residual urine determination considered normal, but it should be less than 200 mL, with a reasonable voided amount equal to or two times greater than the residual amount.

Hospital length of stay is variable but often is only 1 day. Patients should avoid strenuous exercise and heavy lifting for 3 months. Intercourse and vaginal inserts should be avoided until there is good vaginal healing. There is no need to restrict showers or shallow tub baths.

Complications (Table 37.7) are addressed before surgery by use of preoperative antibiotics to prevent infection and use of compression stockings or heparin to prevent deep venous thrombosis (DVT). Early mobilization and use of an incentive spirometer help avoid DVT and respiratory problems. The

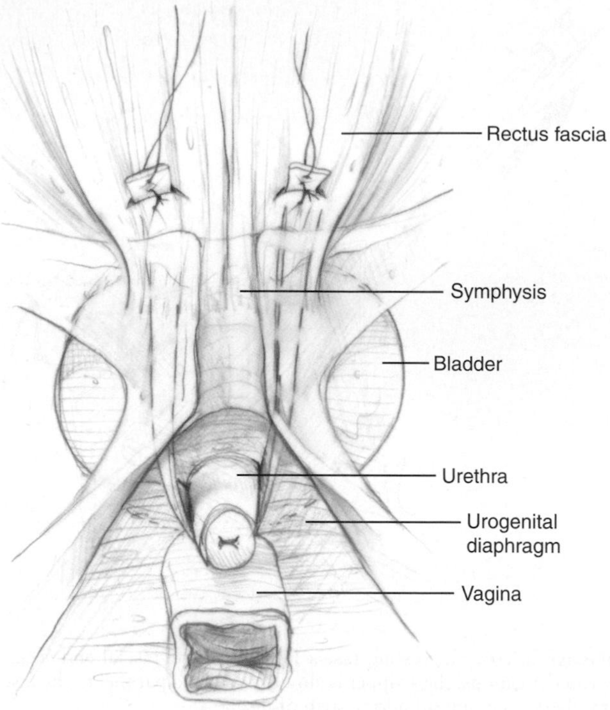

FIGURE 37.20. Sling positioned at proximal urethra, extending through the space of Retzius, and fixed to the rectus fascia.

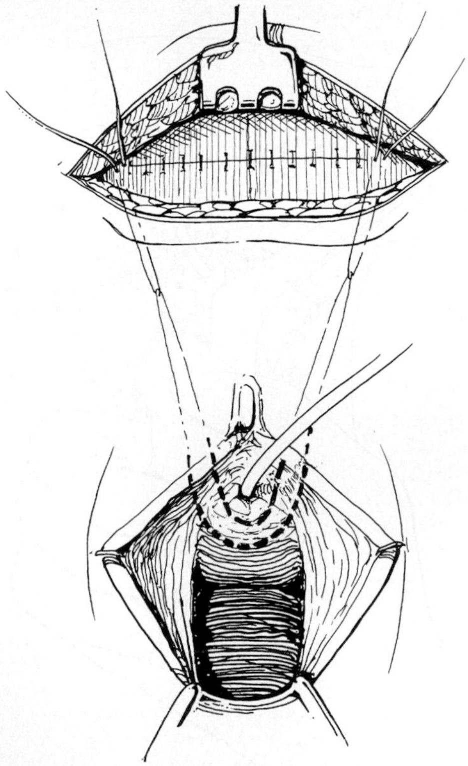

FIGURE 37.21. Rectus sling. Sutures sewn into each end of the fascial strip are passed through the space of Retzius on each side and secured to the rectus fascia.

TABLE 37.7

COMPLICATIONS OF CONVENTIONAL SUBURETHRAL SLINGS

Complication	Frequency (%)	Resolution
Bleeding with vaginal dissection	20	Pressure, cautery, suture, packing
Retropubic space bleeding	5–10	Spontaneous absorption
Bladder perforation	1–2	Replace sling, leave catheter 2 to 3 days
Infection—wound	<5	Eventual healing
Wound seroma—leg or abdomen	3–5	Closed drainage
Infection—urine	20	No long-term sequelae
Retropubic space hematoma	2	Slow resorption
Retropubic space abscess	Infrequent	Drainage: open vs. imaging technique
Blood clot (deep venous thrombosis)	2–30	Aggressive treatment, prevention
Respiratory problem	2–5	Incentive spirometer, physiotherapy
Vaginal breakdown over sling	1–2	Soaks, local irrigation, antibiotics
Mesh erosion	5–25	Local excision, revision, and resuture
Voiding dysfunction	2.5–24	Patience, self-catheterization, medication
Obstructed voiding	1–2	Sling release
De novo urge incontinence	3–23	Bladder retraining, medication
Persistent urge incontinence	26–60	Bladder retraining, medication
Urethral erosion	Rare	Sling removal; surgical repair

usual intraoperative complication of surgery is bleeding. Large veins under the descending pubic ramus may be avulsed during the vaginal portion of the procedure, and there are often vessels on the medial side of the vaginal dissection into the retropubic space. The latter ones can be isolated and cauterized or sutured, but the ones under the pubic ramus are best controlled by pressure, completion of the procedure, and placement of a vaginal pack. Large vessels of the pelvis are seldom penetrated by instruments or sling. The sling may be passed through the bladder and may have to be removed and repassed. On rare occasions, the sling or a suprapubic catheter may be placed through a portion of bowel, and recognition of this complication can be delayed. Temperature elevation is rare but may be caused by atelectasis, pneumonia, and hematoma in the early postoperative period. Cystitis, pyelonephritis, bowel injury, and wound infection are not usually obvious for a few days. Voiding function and possible bladder overdistension must be monitored carefully.

Short-term complications include continued voiding difficulty, bladder infection, and overactive bladder symptoms. A wound seroma or infection may occur at either the abdominal incision site or at the fascial harvest site. If a significant hematoma has occurred in either the abdominal incision or retropubic space, abscess formation may follow. Vaginal healing may be compromised by delayed healing of the anterior vaginal wall, oozing or bleeding from the suture sites, and failure of the incision to close properly over the sling.

Long-term complications include voiding dysfunction, overactive bladder symptoms, and procedure failure. If the patient is unable to void at all, the sling may need to be incised. The occurrence of a vaginal erosion is usually a delayed event with synthetic materials, and this area of incomplete healing can be difficult to resolve.

The cure rate for sling procedures is more than 80% for all procedures, primary and repeat. Traditional suburethral sling procedures have long-term durability, effectiveness in cases with impaired urethral sphincter function or restricted mobility of the bladder neck, and applicability to primary cases with minimal risk of complications.

Periurethral Bulking Procedures

The major impetus for use of periurethral bulking in the United States came in 1993 when the U.S. Food and Drug Administration approved the use of Contigen®. This was followed in July 1994 by Medicare's approved payment for the service based on a number of criteria. These criteria were altered in 1996 and included the presence immobility of the bladder neck, as well as a leak point pressure less than 100 cm of water. The ideal patient is one who meets the above criteria with a fixed bladder neck (Q-tip straining angle 40 degrees or less), who is medically compromised and/or elderly, and in whom an operative intervention may offer too much risk. Also, some patients prefer to use a less invasive technique. There are still little data on effectiveness of minimally invasive midurethral slings in patients who have a scarred bladder neck; although a traditional suburethral sling has a very good cure rate, it is invasive and is associated with greater risk and complications.

The ideal material is biocompatible, nonimmunologic, and hypoallergenic. It should be inexpensive and easy to inject, and it should not migrate. Materials approved for use or in studies are shown in Table 37.8. Methods of injection include periurethral, transurethral through the cystoscope, or transurethral using an injector device that fits in the urethra. The ideal setting for injection is the office or clinic. No preoperative sedation is

TABLE 37.8

PERIURETHRAL BULKING AGENTS IN NORTH AMERICA

Trade name	Company	Approval
Contigen®	C R Bard Inc., Atlanta, GA	1993
Durasphere®	Boston Scientific, Boston, MA Carbon Medical Technologies Inc., St. Paul, MN	1999
Tegress	C R Bard Inc., Atlanta, GA	2004
Macroplastique®	Uroplasty, Minneapolis, MN	FDA trials ongoing[a] Approval in Canada
Zuidex™	Q-med, Uppsala, Sweden	FDA trial ongoing[b]
Coaptite®	Genesis Medical Ltd, London, UK	FDA trials ongoing[c]
Permacol™	TSL, Aldershot, Hampshire, UK	FDA trials starting

FDA, U.S. Food and Drug Administration.
[a]Ghoniem G. Transurethral Macroplastique® injection for treatment of female stress urinary incontinence: office-based technique. Paper presented at: International Urogynecological Association 28th Annual Meeting; October 2003; Buenos Aires, Argentina (abstract 36).
[b]Larsson G, Fienu Jonesson A, Farrelly E, et al. Efficacy and safety of dextranomer/hyaluronic acid via a novel applicator (Zuidex®) in the treatment of stress urinary incontinence. Paper presented at: International Continence Society 33rd Annual Meeting; October 2003; Florence, Italy (abstract 400).
[c]Dmochowski, Appell R, Klimberg I, et al. Initial clinical results from Coaptite® injection for stress urinary incontinence comparative clinical study. Paper presented at: International Continence Society 32nd Annual Meeting; September 2002; Heidelberg, Germany (abstract 282).

required. The injection is performed in a sterilized field by using no-touch technique.

Periurethral Injection

The patient empties her bladder and is placed in lithotomy position. Local anesthesia using 0.5 to 1.0 mL of lidocaine hydrochloride is injected 0.5 cm on either side of the urethral meatus (Fig. 37.22). Under endoscopic guidance, lidocaine 1% solution is injected parallel to the urethra in small amounts until the proximal urethra is reached and the needle or injection can be seen distending an area 1 cm distal to the bladder neck. The syringe with lidocaine is replaced with a syringe of bulking agent, and the material is injected until the entire syringe has been injected or there has been adequate effect noted with urethral bulking. The process is repeated on the opposite site, but the second side is more difficult to inject because of the distortion caused by the initial injection (Fig. 37.23).

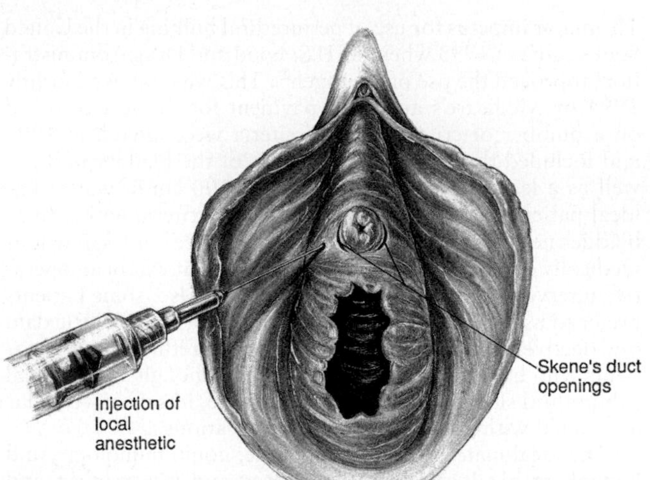

FIGURE 37.22. Periurethral bulking technique. Injection of local anesthetic lateral to Skene duct openings. (With permission: Bent AE. Periurethral collagen injections. *Operative Techniques in Gynecologic Surgery* 1997;2:52.)

Transurethral Injection

The transurethral method is best accomplished using a cystoscope with a 12-degree or 25-degree lens. The sheath has no fenestration, and the operating channel allows the passage of a disposable injection needle with a guide or a reusable needle. Alternatively, a spring-loaded mechanism is favored by some operators. The needle is prefilled with lidocaine 1% solution, the syringe with bulking material is attached, and the cystoscope with injection needle retracted is placed into the bladder. The bladder neck is identified, and the scope is withdrawn to visualize the proximal urethra. The usual injection sites are 3 and 9 o'clock, but this can be varied depending on user preference and number of injection sites selected (up to four). The injection needle is advanced into the urethra submucosa approximately 2 cm distal to the bladder neck (Fig. 37.24), and the injection of material is preceded by the small amount of local anesthetic solution. The needle is advanced 1 cm, and the bulking material is injected. The injection needle is flushed with lidocaine at the first site, and then the second site is selected.

A pressure system is required for transurethral injection of Macroplastique. Injection needles vary in diameter according to the ease of injection of the selected material.

An insertion device is available for Macroplastique and for Zuidex. Transurethral injection is facilitated without

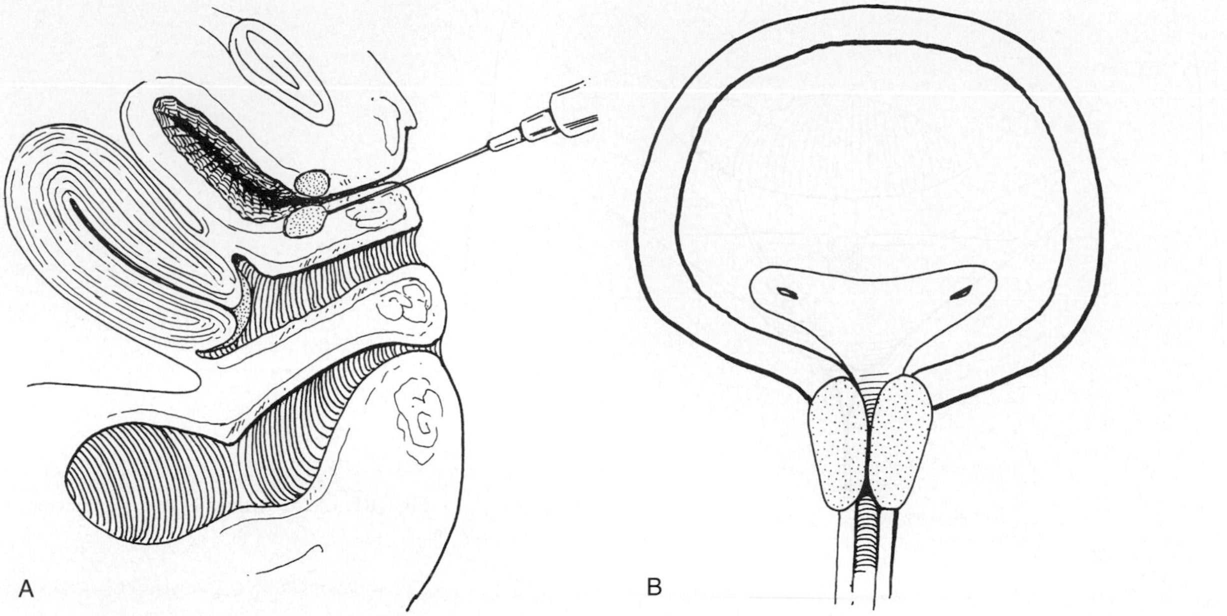

FIGURE 37.23. **A:** Periurethral injection at the bladder neck. **B:** Bulking of bladder neck and proximal urethra.

visualization of the injection site. The device has four angled ports for four needles; after measurement of the urethral length, the device is inserted into the urethra to allow placement of the material at the desired submucosal depth in the mid- to proximal urethra. The efficacy reports are still in early stages, and

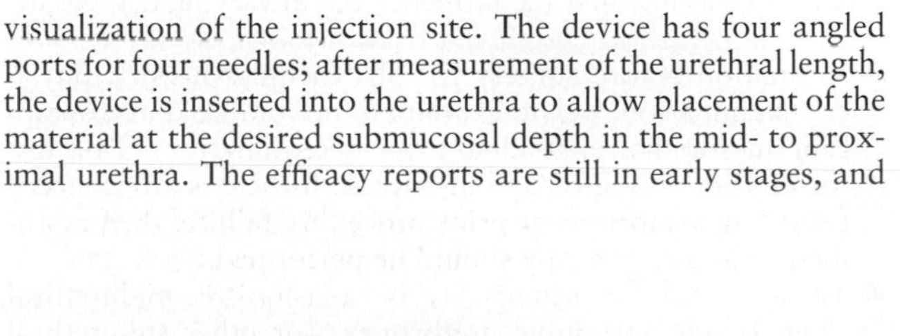

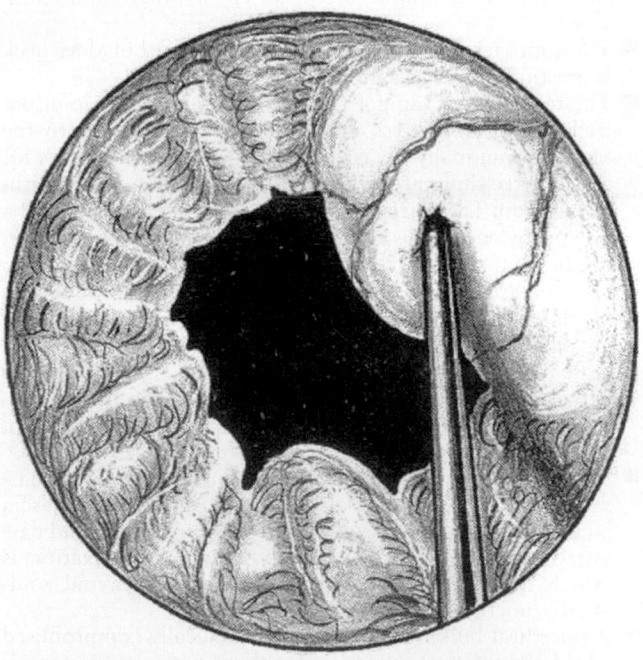

FIGURE 37.24. Transurethral needle placement in urethral submucosa. (With permission: Bent AE. Periurethral collagen injections. *Operative Techniques in Gynecologic Surgery* 1997;2:54.)

the more traditional injection techniques are the current recommendation.

After injection, the patient may have urethral burning that lasts for only part of a day and can be controlled with phenazopyridine (Pyridium). Antibiotics are prescribed for 1 to 2 days after injection because the rate of urinary tract infection is high. The patient attempts voiding after the injection, and she should be prepared to stay in the clinic area for 1 to 2 hours to allow the initial swelling from the injection to diminish. If the patient is unable to void or she has a high residual urine, she either needs to be instructed in self-catheterization or have a small catheter (8 to 10 French Foley) placed, using no more than 5 mL in the balloon. Patients should be called or seen the day following the injection to be sure there is no continuing problem. At follow-up, assessment is made for voiding function, urinary tract infection, and swelling at the injection site. Effectiveness is assessed, and overactive bladder symptoms are managed as appropriate.

One or two injections may be required to obtain a satisfactory result; if there is no improvement at that point, additional injections are not indicated. The success rate is generally quoted to be about 70%. Most injections last 6 months to 2 years and then have to be repeated. There is no limit to the number of injections provided that improvement occurs after each injection and lasts a reasonable period of time. There is no advantage of any particular bulking agent, and selection is usually based on operator experience, ease of injection, cost, and availability of the product.

ARTIFICIAL URINARY SPHINCTER

The ultimate treatment of urinary incontinence secondary to intrinsic sphincter deficiency is implantation of an artificial urinary sphincter. The device consists of a small inflatable cuff, a pump (which usually is implanted within one of the labia

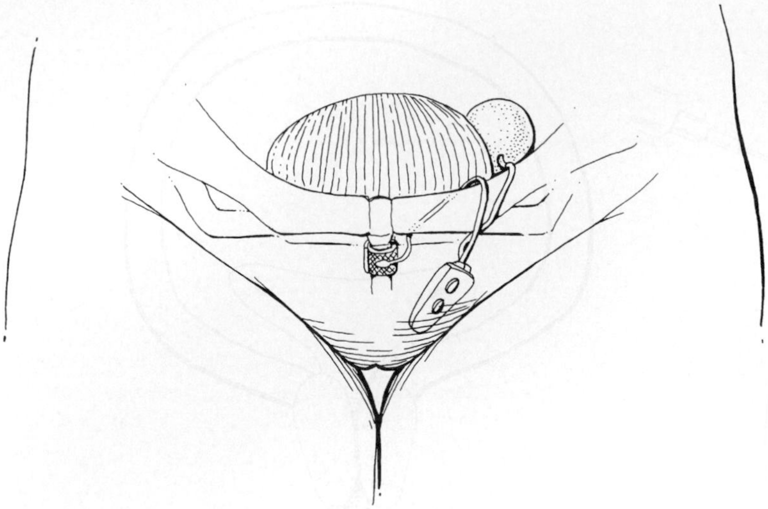

FIGURE 37.25. Artificial urinary sphincter.

majora), and a reservoir, which is placed in the abdomen beneath the fascia (Fig. 37.25). The cuff is placed around the bladder neck and proximal urethra usually through a combined vaginal and abdominal approach. After allowing 6 weeks for healing to take place, the cuff is inflated to compress the urethra. Once inflated, the cuff maintains urethral closure until the patient needs to void. The patient deflates the cuff by squeezing the labial pump, moving fluid from the cuff into the reservoir. After voiding, the cuff automatically reinflates from the reservoir over 1 or 2 minutes and remains closed until the pump is reactivated.

There are a number of complications related to artificial urinary sphincter, including cuff erosion, infection, and device failure. The device is not indicated as a primary treatment for SUI and should only be inserted by an experienced surgical team working in an isolated and controlled operative environment.

SUMMARY

The surgical management of SUI has developed over almost 100 years. Only recently have randomized controlled trials been conducted, and new procedures are often introduced with little long-term efficacy or complication risk data. One of the problems has been the numerous modifications surgeons like to make on other procedures, thus producing yet another new approach.

More recently, instrument manufacturers have introduced a multitude of new instruments and new tape materials for the tension-free midurethral tape procedures with very little clinical data to support their safety or efficacy, much less any comparison with older, established procedures or equipment. The basic evaluation of incontinence includes history, physical examination, measurement of postvoid residual urine, and urinalysis. Preoperative assessment may include a measure of urethral mobility, 24-hour voiding diary, cough stress test, symptom questionnaire, and cystometry. Long-term data indicate the Burch colposuspension and tension-free tapes have similar cure rates. Anterior repair, needle procedures, and paravaginal repairs are not indicated for SUI.

BEST SURGICAL PRACTICES

- There are two types of SUI: hypermobility (or anatomic) and intrinsic sphincter deficiency. Most patients have elements of both causes for their incontinence but in varying degrees for each.
- Evaluation before surgery for SUI includes history, physical examination, pelvic examination, voiding diary, symptom questionnaire, residual urine determination, Q-tip test for urethral mobility, and urinalysis. If there is any concern regarding symptoms or prior procedure failure, then cystometrics and cystoscopy should be performed.
- The approach for primary SUI is a tension-free midurethral sling, Burch retropubic urethropexy, or other suburethral sling.
- The approach for recurrent SUI and a scarred bladder neck is most often a suburethral sling.
- The tension-free vaginal tape procedures have revolutionized surgery for stress incontinence, bringing it into the realm of minimally invasive day surgery. The principles for tension-free slings are to place them at the midurethra without tension. There are numerous brands, but the essence is a polypropylene mesh sling, 1 cm in width, placed by insertion needles and small incisions. Cystoscopy is recommended to assure there is no bladder injury. There are suprapubic as well as transobturator techniques without obvious proven advantages of one kind over another. The cure rates are all close to 85%. The procedures may be combined with other pelvic floor reconstructive surgery. Complications are minimal and include voiding dysfunction, overactive bladder, and mesh erosion.
- Standard suburethral slings are best performed with harvested autologous materials, either rectus fascia or fascia lata. The vaginal dissection should allow minimal blind passage from the vaginal to the abdominal site. Fixation is loosely accomplished to rectus fascia so as to avoid voiding dysfunction.
- Periurethral bulking has a place in medically compromised or elderly patients, especially for those with severe incontinence and minimal mobility of the bladder neck, i.e., Q-tip test <40 degrees straining.

Bibliography

Abrams P, Andersson KE, Brubaker L, et al. Recommendations of the International Scientific Committee. In Abrams P, Cardozo L, Khoury S, et al., eds. *Incontinence*. Paris: Health Publications Ltd; 2005:1606.

Abrams P, Cardozo L, Fall M, et al. The standardization of terminology of lower urinary tract function: report from the standardization sub-committee of the International Continence Society. *Am J Obstet Gynecol* 2002;187(1): 116.

Alcalay M, Monga A, Stanton S. Burch colposuspension: a 10–20 year follow up. *BJOG* 1995;102:740.

Aldridge AH. Transplantation of fascia for relief urinary stress incontinence. *Am J Obstet Gynecol* 1942;44:398.

American College of Obstetricians and Gynecologists. ACOG Practice Bulletin Number 63. Urinary incontinence in women: clinical management guidelines for obstetricians–gynecologists. Washington, DC: ACOG; June 2005.

American College of Obstetricians and Gynecologists, Committee on Quality Assessment. ACOG Criteria Set: Surgery for genuine stress incontinence due to urethral hypermobility (no. 4). Washington, DC: ACOG;1995.

Appell RA, McGuire EJ, DeRidder PA, et al. Summary of effectiveness and safety in the prospective, open, multicenter investigation of collagen implant for incontinence due to intrinsic sphincteric deficiency in females. *J Urol* 1994;151:418 (abst).

Beck RP, Grove D, Arnusch D, et al. Recurrent urinary stress incontinence treated by the fascia lata sling procedure. *Am J Obstet Gynecol* 1974;120:613.

Bent AE. Periurethral collagen injections. *Operative Techniques in Gynecologic Surgery* 1997;2:51.

Blaivas JG, Jacobs BZ. Pubovaginal sling in the treatment of complicated stress incontinence. *J Urol* 1991;145:1214.

Brubaker L. Suburethral sling procedures. *Operative Techniques in Gynecologic Surgery* 1997;2:44.

Bump RC, Norton PA. Epidemiology and natural history of pelvic floor dysfunction. *Obstet Gynecol Clin* 1998;25(4):723.

Burch JC. Cooper's ligament urethrovesical suspension for stress incontinence: nine years' experience—results, complications, technique. *Am J Obstet Gynecol* 1968;100:764.

Burch JC. Urethrovaginal fixation to Cooper's ligament for correction of stress incontinence, cystocele, and prolapse. *Am J Obstet Gynecol* 1961;81:281.

DeLancey JOL. Structural support of the urethra as it relates to stress incontinence: the hammock hypothesis. *Am J Obstet Gynecol* 1994;170:1713.

DeLorme E. Transobturator urethral suspension: mini-invasive procedure in the treatment of stress urinary incontinence in women. *Prog Urol* 2001;11:1306.

de Tayrac R, Deffieux X, Droopy S, et al. A prospective randomized trial comparing tension-free vaginal tape and transobturator suburethral tape for surgical treatment of stress urinary incontinence. *Am J Obstet Gynecol* 2004;190:602.

Fantl JA, Newman DK, Colling J, et al. *Urinary incontinence in adults: acute and chronic management*. Clinical Practice Guideline, No. 2, 1996 Update. Rockville, MD: U.S. Department of Health and Human Services. Public Health Service, Agency for Health Care Policy and Research. AHCPR Publication No. 96-0682, March 1996.

Frangenheim P. Zu operative behandlung der inkontinenz der mannlichen harnohre. *Ver Dtsch Ges Chir* 1914;43:149.

Gittes RF, Loughlin KR. No-incision pubovaginal suspension for stress incontinence. *J Urol* 1987;138:568.

Glazner CM. Anterior vaginal repair for urinary incontinence in women. *Cochrane Database Syst Rev* 2000;2:CD001755.

Goebell R. Zur operativen beseitigung der angeborenen. *Incontinentia Vesicae Z Gynakol Urol* 1910;2:187.

Gross M, Appell RA. Periurethral injections. In: Bent AE, Ostergard DR, Cundiff GW, et al., eds. *Ostergard's urogynecology and pelvic floor dysfunction*. 5th ed. Philadelphia: Lippincott Williams & Wilkins; 2003:495.

Ingleman-Sundberg A. Urinary incontinence in women excluding fistulas. *Acta Obstet Gynecol Scand*. 1952:31:266.

Jarvis GJ. Surgery for genuine stress incontinence. *BJOG* 1994;101:371.

Karram MM, Segal JL, Vassallo BJ, et al. Complications and untoward effects of the tension-free vaginal tape procedure. *Obstet Gynecol* 2003;101:929.

Kelly HA. Incontinence of urine in women. *Urol Cutan Rev* 1913; 17:291.

Kubic K, Horbach NS. Suburethral sling procedures and treatment of complicated stress incontinence. In: Bent AE, Ostergard DR, Cundiff GW, et al., eds. *Ostergard's urogynecology and pelvic floor dysfunction*. 5th ed. Philadelphia: Lippincott Williams & Wilkins; 2003:469.

Kuuva N, Nilsson CO. A nationwide analysis of complications associated with the tension free vaginal tape (TVT) procedure. *Acta Obstet Gynecol Scand* 2002; 81:72

Leach GE, Dmochowski RR, Appell RA, et al. Female Stress Urinary Incontinence Clinical Guidelines Panel summary report on surgical management of female stress urinary incontinence. *J Urol* 1997;158:875.

Mainprize TC, Drutz HP. The Marshall-Marchetti-Krantz procedure: a critical review. *Obstet Gynecol Surv* 1988;43:724.

Marshall VF, Marchetti AA, Krantz KE. The correction of stress incontinence by simple vesicourethral suspension. *Surg Gynecol Obstet* 1949;88:509.

McGuire EJ, Lytton B. Pubovaginal sling procedure for stress incontinence. *J Urol* 1978;119:82.

McGuire EJ, Appell RA. Transurethral collagen injection for urinary incontinence. *Urology* 1994;43:413.

Medicare Coverage Issues Manual. Incontinence Control Devices. Department of Health and Human Services, Health Care Financing Administration, June 1994, Transmittal No. 70. Section 65–69.

Medicare Coverage Issues Manual. Incontinence Control Devices. Department of Health and Human Services, Health Care Financing Administration, September 1996, Transmittal No. 89. Section 65–69.

Nilsson CG, Kuuva N, Falconer C, et al. Long-term results of the tension-free vaginal tape (TVT) procedure for surgical treatment of female stress urinary incontinence. *Int Urogynecol J* 2001;12(Suppl 2):S5.

Nilsson CG, Rezapour M, Falconer C. 7 year follow-up of the tension free vaginal tape procedure. *Int Urogynecol J* 2003;14(Suppl 1):35.

Paraiso MFR, Walters MD, Karram MM, et al. Laparoscopic Burch colposuspension versus the tension-free vaginal tape procedure: a randomized clinical trial. *Obstet Gynecol* 2004.

Pereyra AJ. A simplified surgical procedure for the correction of stress incontinence in women. *West J Surg* 1959;67:223.

Price PB. Plastic operations for incontinence of urine and fesces. *Arch Surg* 1933;26:1043.

Raz S. Modified bladder neck suspension for female stress incontinence. *Urology* 1981;17:82.

Richardson AC, Lyon J, Williams N. A new look at pelvic relaxation. *Am J Obstet Gynecol* 1976;126:568.

Richardson AC, Edmonds PB, Williams NL. Treatment of stress urinary incontinence due to paravaginal fascial defect. *Obstet Gynecol* 1981;57:357.

Ridley JH. Surgery for stress incontinence. In: Ridley JH. *Gynecologic surgery: errors, safeguards, salvage*. Baltimore: Williams & Wilkins; 1974:114.

Ridley JH. Surgical treatment of stress urinary incontinence in women. *J Med Assoc Ga* 1955;44:135.

Ross JW. Multichannel urodynamic evaluation of laparoscopic Burch colposuspension for genuine stress incontinence. *Obstet Gynecol* 1998;91:55.

Schultze BS. The pathology and treatment of displacements of the uterus. Translated from German by J J Macan. D Appleton. New York, 1888

Shull BL, Baden WF. A six-year experience with paravaginal defect repair for stress urinary incontinence. *Am J Obstet Gynecol* 1989;160:1432.

Smith ARB, Daneshgari F, Dmochowski et al. Surgery for urinary incontinence in women. In: Abrams P, Cardozo L, Khoury S, et al., eds. *3rd International Consultation on Incontinence*. Paris: Health Publications Ltd; 2005; 1297.

Smith ARB, Hosker GL, Warrell DW. The role of partial denervation of the pelvic floor in the aetiology of genitourinary prolapse and stress incontinence of urine: a neurophysiological study. *BJOG* 1989;96;24.

Stamey TA. Endoscopic suspension of the vesical neck for urinary incontinence. *Surg Gynecol Obstet* 1973;136:547.

Stoeckel W. Uber die verwendung der musculi pyridimale beider operative behandlung der incontinentia urinae. *Gynakol* 1917;41:11.

Summit RL, Lucente V, Karram MM, et al. Randomized comparison of laparoscopic and transabdominal Burch urethropexy for the treatment of genuine stress incontinence. *Obstet Gynecol* 2000;95(Suppl):2S.

Tanagho EA. Colpocystourethropexy: the way we do it. *J Urol* 1976;116:751.

U.S. Food and Drug Administration. The FDA interagency guidelines for human tissue intended for transplantation. *Fed Reg* 1993;58:65514.

Ulmsten U, Henricksson L, Johnson P, et al. An ambulatory surgical procedure under local anesthesia for treatment of female urinary incontinence. *Int Urogynecol J* 1996;7:81.

Vancaillie TG, Schuessler W. Laparoscopic bladder neck suspension. *J Laparoendosc Surg* 1991;1:169.

Von Giordano D. 20 ieme Congres *Franc de Chirug*. 1907;p 506.

Wheeless CR Jr. *Atlas of pelvic surgery*. 3rd ed. Baltimore: Williams & Wilkins; 1997:125.

White GR. Cystocele: a radical cure by suturing lateral sulci of vagina to white line of pelvic fascia. *JAMA* 1909;21:1707.

Zoedler D. Zur operative behandlung der weiblichen stress inkontinenz. *Z Urol* 1961;54:355.

CHAPTER 38 ■ OPERATIVE INJURIES TO THE URETER

PAUL UNDERWOOD, JR.

DEFINITIONS

Cystotomy—Incision into the urinary bladder.

Spatulate—To incise the cut end of a tubular structure longitudinally and splay it open to allow creation of an elliptical anastomosis of greater circumference than would be possible with conventional transverse or oblique end-to-end anastomoses.

Ureteroileoneocystomy—Restoration of the continuity of the urinary tract by anastomosis of the upper segment of a partially destroyed ureter to a segment of ileum, the lower end of which is then implanted into the bladder.

Ureteroureterostomy—Establishment of an anastomosis between the two ureters or between two segments of the same ureter.

Ureteroneocystotomy—An operation whereby a ureter is implanted into the bladder.

Ureteral injuries have been recognized as a potential complication of gynecologic surgical procedures since the inception of our discipline. Over the years, numerous unique surgical modifications of procedures have been offered with the specific intent of decreasing the probability of ureteral injury. Despite these efforts, ureteral injury remains a very real complication of abdominal-pelvic surgery in the female patient, affecting as many as 1.79% of women taken to the operating theater for pelvic surgery, although the accepted incidence is about 0.35% to 0.4%. The risk depends on the procedure performed and the skill and experience of the surgeon. Therefore, it is important for the gynecologic surgeon to be cognizant of ways to minimize the occurrence of these potentially disastrous complications, as well as facile in the diagnosis and management of such an injury should it occur.

The goals of this chapter are to (a) outline the functional anatomy of the ureter and illustrate how this leads to the ureter being in harm's way during gynecologic surgery, (b) review the unique issues surrounding ureteral injury during the performance of specific groups of gynecologic surgical procedures, and (c) summarize the basic principles of injury avoidance and, should injury occur, recognition and management.

FUNCTIONAL ANATOMY OF THE URETER

When viewed in cross section, the ureter can be divided into distinct layers: the lumen with transitional epithelium; the mucosa—the muscular layer—which is made up of longitudinal, circular, and spiral smooth muscle fibers; and the adventitia, which contains an intercommunicating network of blood vessels. The peritoneum lies over the ureter, making it a completely retroperitoneal structure (Fig. 38.1).

In normal adults, the ureter is between 25 and 30 cm in length from the renal pelvis to the trigone of the bladder. By convention, the ureter is divided into the abdominal and pelvic segments by the pelvic brim; each of these components if approximately 12 to 15 cm in length.

The abdominal ureter runs along the ventral surface of the psoas muscle and posterior to the ovarian vessels to the level of the pelvic brim. The right ureter lies slightly lateral to the inferior vena cava and descends into the pelvis over the common iliac artery at approximately the site of the latter's bifurcation. On rare incidences, the right ureter can be over the vena cava; therefore, if one is performing a paraaortic node sampling, the ureter must be identified before removing any nodes. The left ureter runs lateral to the aorta and posterior to the inferior mesenteric artery, ovarian vessels, and colon. The left ureter mirrors the right at the pelvic brim, entering the pelvis over the bifurcation of the left common iliac artery. The left ureter often is obscured by the sigmoid colon at the pelvic brim (Fig. 38.2).

There is little variance between the positions taken by the pelvic ureters. They descend into the posterior lateral pelvis lateral to the sacrum and immediately ventral to internal iliac (hypogastric) artery. The ureters then deviate medially and course medial to the internal iliac artery and its anterior branches. The ureters subsequently pass beneath the uterine artery (often referred to as *water under the bridge*). At this point, it is approximately 1.5 cm lateral to the cervix, and this is the site of entrance into the paracervical tissues. The ureter passes through this paracervical tissue often referred to as "the tunnel" of the cardinal ligament/anterior bladder pillar (also referred to as the web or the tunnel of Wertheim). Once through this tunnel, the ureter travels medially and anteriorly over the vaginal fornix to enter the trigone of the bladder.

When inflammatory or adhesive changes are not present, the ureters can usually be visualized through the peritoneum from the pelvic brim to this parametrial tissue. Once the ureters have entered this tunnel, they cannot be easily seen or palpated; if identification is required, they must be mobilized out of this tissue. Although the peristaltic activity that occurs in the normal ureter may be helpful in its identification, it is not uncommon that the ureter, following any degree of trauma, will have transient paralysis. Therefore, the skill of definitely identifying the ureter is based on its anatomy, not its motion. The ureter is unique in that it has a "snap" feeling when passed between ones fingers. This may be helpful in massively obese women with poor exposure. This "snap" will also permit one to follow the ureter to the tunnel without actually exposing it. Having defined the general anatomy of the ureter, one must appreciate

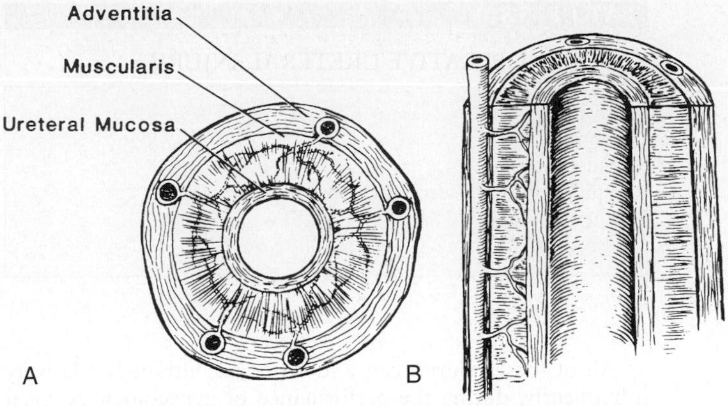

FIGURE 38.1. Cross-sectional (A) and sagittal (B) views of the longitudinal arteries and veins in the adventitia. These arteries and veins provide the important collateral circulation along the course of the ureter.

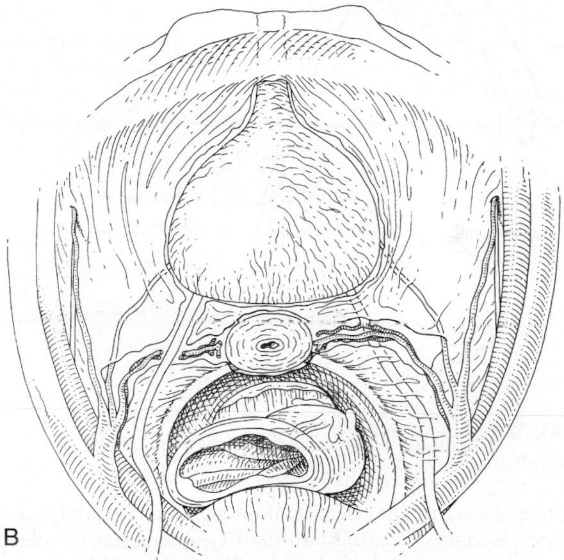

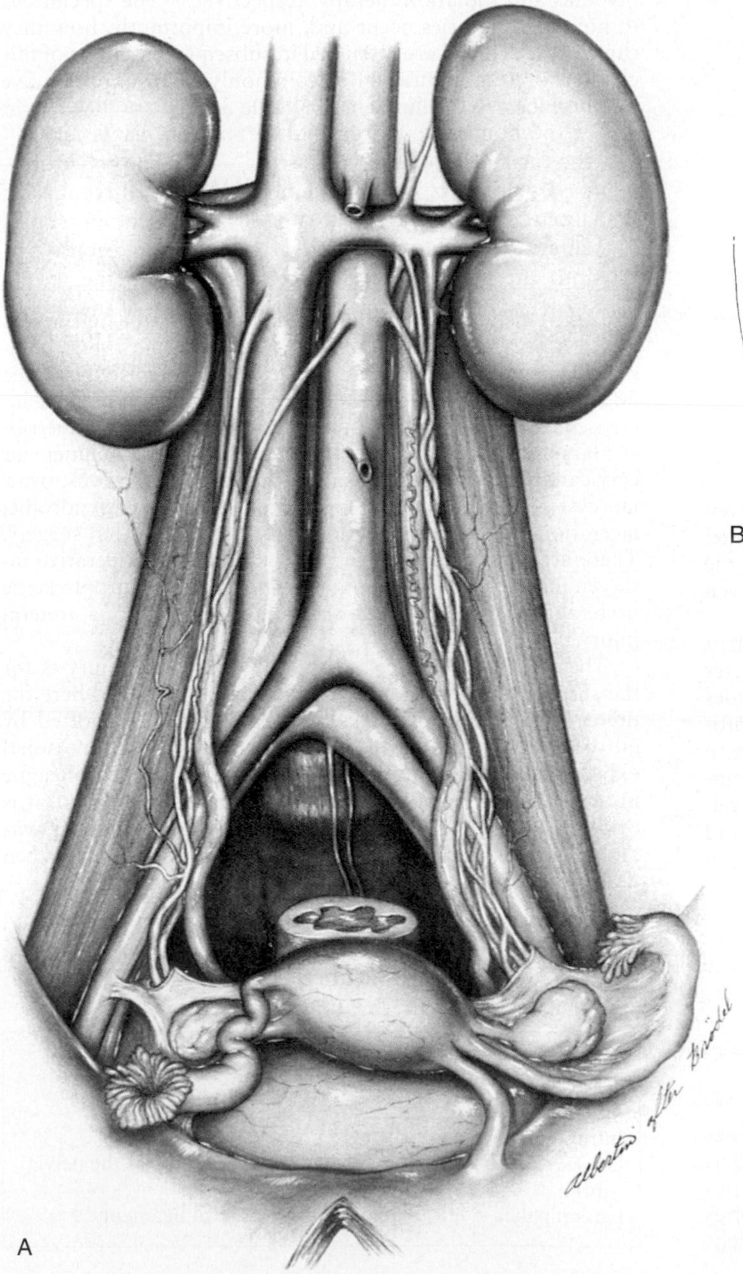

FIGURE 38.2. A: Abdominal and pelvic portions of the ureter showing relation to aorta, psoas muscle, vena cava, and common iliac artery and vein. B: Pelvic portion of the ureter showing its course along the sidewall of the pelvis and its relation to the common iliac vessels, hypogastric vessels, uterosacral ligaments, uterine vessels, and cervix.

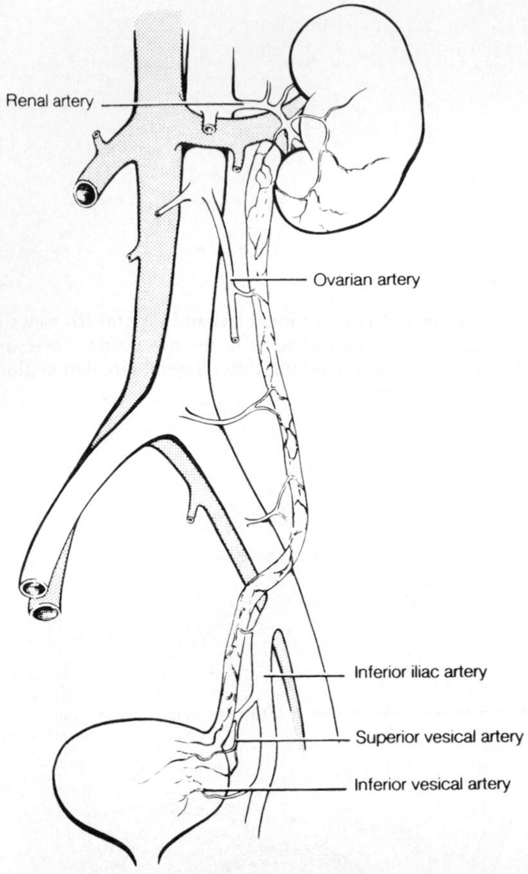

FIGURE 38.3. Blood supply of the ureter.

that there is a significant degree of interpatient variability, even in the pelvis that is free of inflammatory, infectious, neoplastic, congenital, or postsurgical changes. Direct visualization of the ureter is the only sure way to know its location in any given patient.

The ureter obtains blood supply from every vessel that it transverses (Fig. 38.3). The small vessels that nourish the ureter are interconnected by a lush network of anastomosing arcades within the adventitial sheath. It is this vigorous and multi-origin blood supply that helps to make the ureter resistant to devascularization, even when it has been stripped of the surrounding ureteral sheath. Yet, although the ureter may be relatively difficult to devascularize, such injuries can occur and are more likely to happen if one fails to remember the origin of the blood supply, as illustrated in Figure 38.3. Cephalad to the pelvic brim, the blood supply enters from the medial side; therefore, dissection and mobilization should be carried out from the lateral aspect of the ureter. The inverse is true below the pelvic brim.

URETERAL INJURY

Thompson, in preceding editions of this test, listed six types of operative ureteral injuries, which are shown in Table 38.1. Other authors have proposed that avulsion and stretch injuries also be listed as separate types, although these two categories are included under "transaction" and "ischemia," respectively.

TABLE 38.1

TYPES OF OPERATIVE URETERAL INJURIES

Crushing
Ligation
Transection
Angulation (with secondary obstruction)
Ischemia
Resection

All of these injuries can and do occur, although relatively infrequently, during the performance of gynecologic surgical procedures. Additionally, angulation and ischemia can be the sequelae of nonsurgical processes (e.g., broad ligament cervical myomas and radiation therapy, respectively). The specifics as to how these injuries occur and, more importantly, how they can be best avoided are discussed in subsequent sections of this chapter. Ureteral injuries most commonly occur at one of five different locales, as illustrated in Table 38.2.

GENERAL PRINCIPLES OF PREVENTION AND MANAGEMENT

It is extremely important to be cognizant of the settings in which a ureteral injury is more likely to occur. Several common elements associated with ureteral injury are listed in Table 38.3. Among the clinical diagnoses that put the ureter at increased risk during gynecologic surgery are severe endometriosis; large fibroids, especially lower uterine broad ligament or cervical fibroids; large adnexal masses; dense adhesions; ovarian cyst adherent to peritoneum; residual ovarian syndrome; lacerations at cesarean section; and radical cancer surgery. There are no data supporting the belief that preoperative intravenous pyelogram, computed tomography, or prophylactic ureteral stint placement decreases the probability of a ureteral injury.

The most important way to prevent ureteral injury is for the surgeon to constantly and unequivocally know where the ureter is located at all times. Not only is this supported by all of the references in this chapter, but also by my personal experience. Often when we are called to assist a colleague in an operation in which a ureteral injury has occurred. it is evident that the surgeon did not know where the ureter was and, therefore, clamped, ligated, incised, or transected it. When

TABLE 38.2

COMMON SITES OF URETERAL INJURIES

Cardinal ligament where the ureter crosses under the uterine artery
Tunnel of Wertheim
Intramural portion of the ureter
Dorsal to the infundibulopelvic ligament near or at the pelvic brim
Lateral pelvic sidewall above the uterosacral ligament

TABLE 38.3

URETERAL INJURY ASSOCIATED WITH GYNECOLOGIC SURGERY: "MOST COMMONS"

Most common site: Pelvic brim near the infundibulopelvic ligament
Most common procedure: Simple abdominal hysterectomy
Most common type of injury: Obstruction
Most common "activity" leading to injury: Attempts to obtain hemostasis
Most common time of diagnosis: None: 50-50 split between intraoperative and postoperative
Most common long-term sequelae: None

dissecting a ureter from its location, try to stay outside the adventitial sheath. This will decrease the probability of devascularization and subsequent ischemia. This cannot always be accomplished, particularly in those settings in which there is a malignancy, significant scarring and fibrosis that accompany endometriosis, or prior pelvic radiation. However, because of its rich longitudinal blood supply, the ureter usually survives. Finally, when using instruments that transmit energy to the tissues (e.g., electrocoagulation, whether monopolar or bipolar, argon beam coagulator or laser), the surgeon should know the zone of thermal injury for that instrument at that power setting. Although the mean distance of thermal damage with most of these instruments is approximately 2 mm, it may be as much as 5 mm; therefore, the use of such energy sources near the ureter has the potential for unrecognized injury and delayed necrosis.

Every obstetrician and gynecologist performing pelvic surgery must know how to enter the retroperitoneal space and identify the ureter. Starting at the round ligament, cut the peritoneum lateral to the ovarian vessels to the colon at the pelvic brim (Fig. 38.4). There is nothing one can injure or cause to bleed in this zone. Bluntly dissect the ovary and its vessels medially to enter this posterior retroperitoneal space. The large vessels and pelvic sidewall will be lateral and easily identified by palpation and visualization. The ureter will be seen adhered loosely to the medial peritoneum. It always crosses over the iliac artery at this pelvic brim just where the internal iliac artery arises. Gently caress the ureter with the sucker or pickups, and it will further identify itself with a peristaltic movement. In massively obese women with poor exposure, place your index finger in this retroperitoneal space and your thumb outside the peritoneum. The ureter can be identified by a distinct "snap" or "click" between one's fingers. Once identified, the ureter can easily be followed by using blunt dissection with a right angle clamp all the way to the uterine artery. Between the uterine artery and bladder, it can usually be followed by the palpation and "snap" technique previously described.

SPECIFIC HIGH-RISK PROCEDURES FOR URETERAL INJURIES

Laparoscopy-Associated Ureteral Injuries

Ureteral injuries at the time of laparoscopy are very uncommon, occurring in approximately 0.3% to 0.4% of all cases. Laparoscopic ureteral injuries are unique when compared with

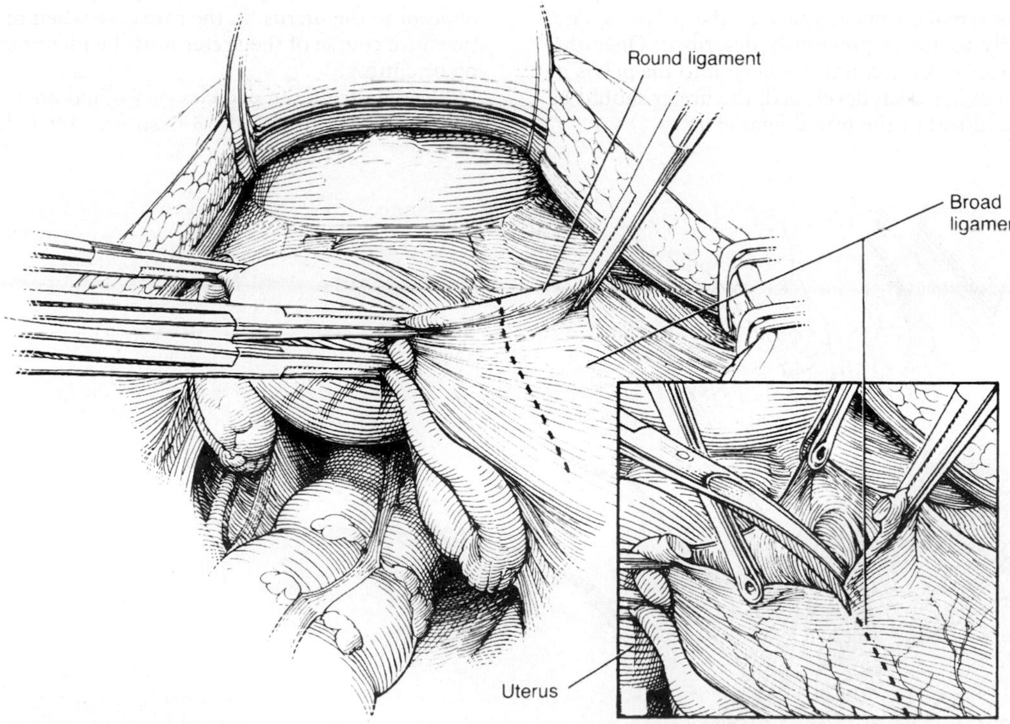

FIGURE 38.4. The initial step for ureteral identification is clamping and cutting of the round ligament. The loose areolar tissue is dissected and the ureter identified on the medial leaf of the broad ligament peritoneum.

open injuries from two potentially complicating realities. First, these injuries are more likely to be the result of a thermal injury than incision, transaction, or encroachment/ligation. Second, ureteral injuries in association with laparoscopy are more likely to be diagnosed 2 to 5 days after the surgery. This delay in diagnosis decreases the probability of a successful immediate primary repair and increases the risk of a long-term complication. The ureter is most commonly injured during laparoscopic hysterectomy when the uterine vessels are stapled or electrocoagulated. Another common site of injury is when the infundibulopelvic ligament is transected. When performing laparoscopic surgery near the pelvic wall or cul-de-sac, it is imperative to know the location of the ureter. Extreme caution should be used with cautery or laser near or over the ureter. It can usually be seen and followed through the peritoneum; but when not visible, it should be identified retroperitoneally and followed down to the site of operative interest. When primary injury is recognized, laparoscopic repair can be successfully performed by an experienced laparoscopist.

Complex Adnexectomy

Ureteral injury at the time of complex adnexectomy is worthy of specific comment because (a) it is in this setting that the ureter is commonly injured, and (b) these injuries can be avoided by using the retroperitoneal approach as previously described.

Every obstetrical or gynecological surgeon must be able to quickly and safely enter the retroperitoneum. This surgical skill is necessary to (a) access the pelvic vessels for the purpose of establishing hemostasis and (b) use the retroperitoneum as an adhesion- and pathology-free "space" in which to operate. Access is obtained most commonly for the latter purpose. Entrance into this retroperitoneal space in the pelvis is safe, easy, and extremely useful as previously described. Once this retroperitoneal space (which continues deep into the pelvis as the pararectal space) has been developed, the ureter should be visible on the medial leaf of the broad ligament.

If an adnexal mass is adherent to the medial leaf of the broad ligament or pelvic peritoneum overlying the ureter, the ureter can safely be dissected laterally from the peritoneum. Once the ureter has been mobilized and is out of harm's way, resection of inflamed, scarred, or fibrotic peritoneum with the overlying adherent mass can safely be performed (Fig. 38.5). There are rare instances when it is impossible to mobilize the ureter from the pathology. In this setting, the surgeon must decide whether to leave a little tumor or endometriosis on the ureter, risking subsequent obstruction, or resect a segment of ureter and repair accordingly.

Abdominal Hysterectomy

Ureteral injury during resection of an adnexal mass usually results from surgical trauma to the ureter between the level of the pelvic brim to the tunnel of Wertheim. When discussing ureteral injuries associated with the performance of an abdominal hysterectomy, the focus of our attention is on where the ureter enters the tunnel under the uterine artery, lateral to the uterosacral ligaments, until the ureter terminates in the bladder. When performing an abdominal hysterectomy for benign disease, there are two situations that are particularly high risk for a ureteral injury: (i) a lower uterine segment or cervical fibroid protruding into the broad ligament or (ii) bleeding from pedicles, especially at the vaginal corners.

With a broad ligament fibroid, the ureter can be anterior, lateral, or posterior to the fibroid. The clamp, cut, suture technique around the fibroid is too dangerous for injury. I prefer a myomectomy by an incision adjacent to the uterus or cervix. One can do this with no risk of ureteral injury by staying within the myometrial capsule of the fibroid. Bleeding may occur, but once the fibroid is out, bleeding is easily controlled by clamping adjacent to the uterus. In the rare case when this is impossible, the entire course of the ureter must be identified before clamping or cutting.

Bleeding from the pedicles or vaginal angle should be controlled by a "superficial" 3-0 suture. One should place the

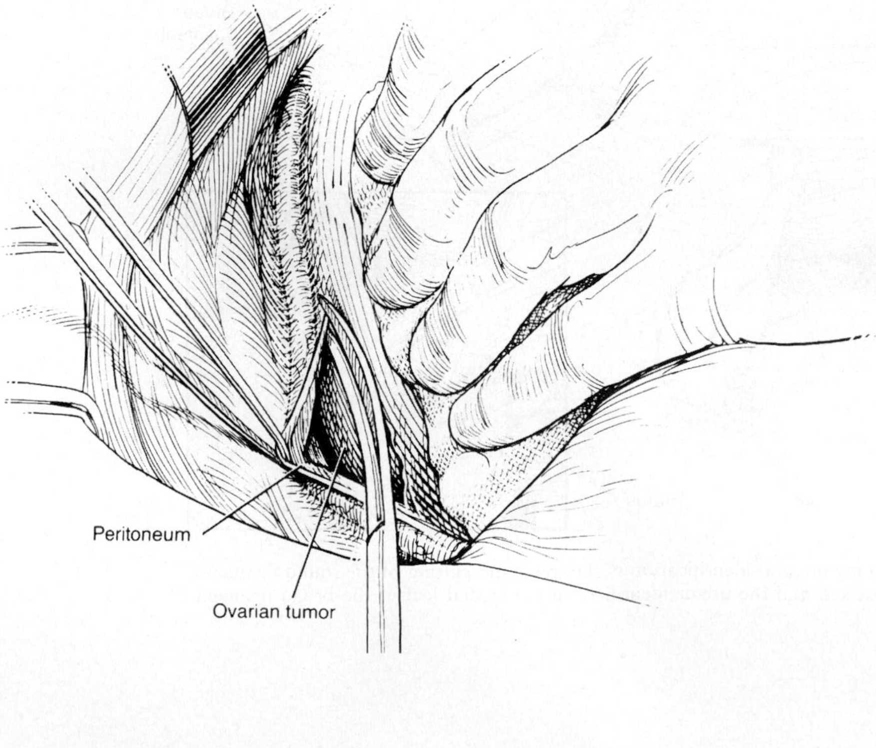

FIGURE 38.5. The ureter is dissected away from the peritoneum to permit resecting of ovarian mass/remnant.

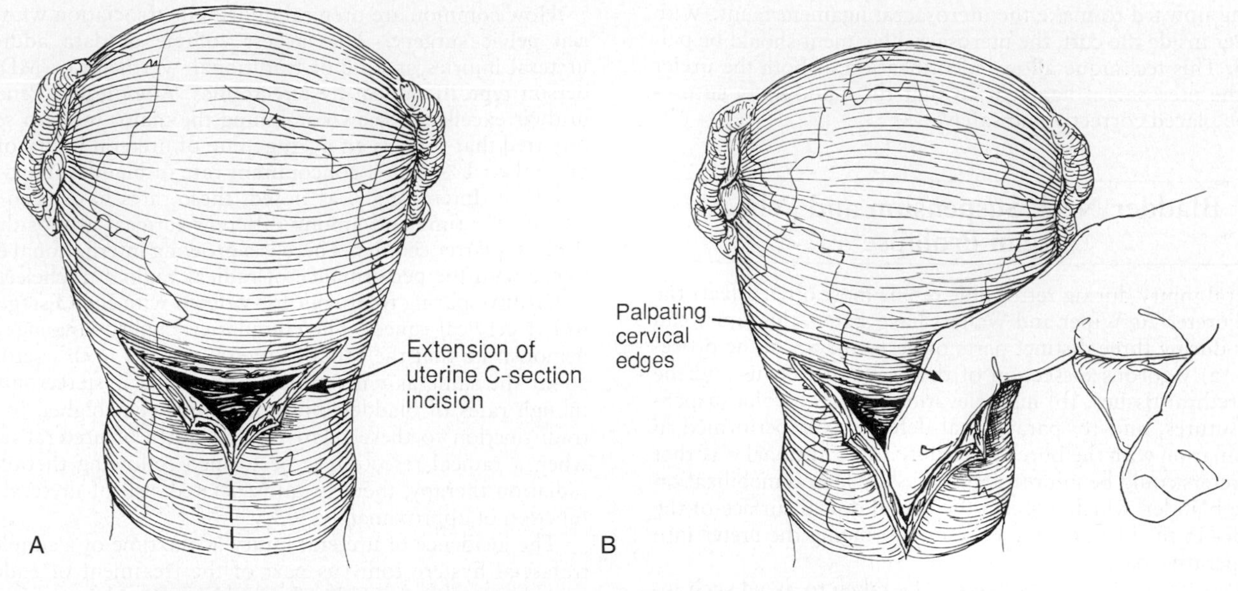

FIGURE 38.6. Avoiding ureteral injury with removal of the cervix at cesarean hysterectomy. **A:** Extension of uterine cesarean section incision downward in the midline of the anterior cervix. **B:** Palpating cervical edges internally.

suture very superficially so that it cannot be around the ureter, which is "very close" once the tissues have retracted. It is that deep suture that gets the ureter here.

To avoid ureteral injury, an "intrafascial hysterectomy" technique was used in the past. In this technique, a plane within the myometrium of the lower uterine segment and cervix is developed once the uterine vessels have been ligated. This technique is illustrated in Chapter 32A. It is rarely used today because it results in increased blood loss; however, it theoretically reduces the risk of injury to the distal ureter.

If one is fearful that the ureter is ligated or injured on one side, it is easy to answer the question. Find the ureter at the common iliac artery, place it on stretch, and insert a 21-gauge "butterfly" needle into its lumen—just like an IV. Inject 5 to 10 cc methylene blue stained saline directly into the lumen of the ureter. If the ureter is intact, blue stain is seen in the Foley catheter verifying an open ureter. If the ureter has a leak, blue stain will be seen in the pelvis. If the ureter enlarges and no blue stain is seen in the Foley, the ureter is ligated and needs appropriate repair. I have done this many, many times and never seen a complication secondary to it.

Cesarean Hysterectomy

I feel this special situation is worthy of comment, even though it is relatively uncommon. The location of the ureter is a frequent cause of intraoperative consultations to advanced pelvic surgeons during the course of cesarean hysterectomy, which is often bloody and where distorted anatomy is almost always present. An easy way to avoid ureteral injuries is to simply perform a supracervical hysterectomy; however, some surgeons find this a suboptimal choice. Therefore, in addition to the techniques outlined to this point, a hysterotomy incision can be extended caudally toward the cervix (Fig. 38.6). This permits the relatively easy placement of the forefinger into the endocervical canal and upper vagina, allowing tactile as well as visual guidance for the cervical-vaginal junction. With your finger in place, it is simple to identify where to place a clamp adjacent to the cervix.

Vaginal Hysterectomy

Ureteral injury during a vaginal hysterectomy is remarkably uncommon because of traction on the cervix, which pulls the uterus farther from the ureter. However, a culdoplasty frequently is part of the reconstructive phase of the procedure, and this places the ureter at risk. There are maneuvers that can be taken to minimize the probability of injuring a ureter. Palpatory ureteral identification via the vaginal approach is one useful step (Fig. 38.7). Another technique is placing an Allis clamp on the vaginal cuff in the area of the uterosacral ligament and

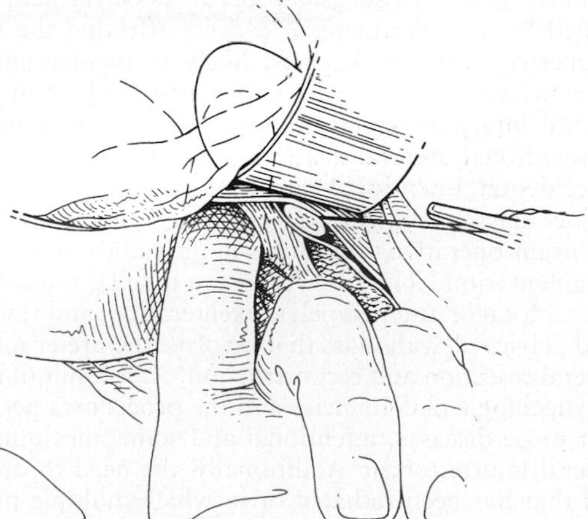

FIGURE 38.7. During vaginal hysterectomy, the ureter can be felt against a metal retractor placed in the paravesical space.

pulling upward to make the uterosacral ligament taunt. With a finger inside the cuff, the uterosacral ligament should be palpated. This technique allows identification of both the ureter and the uterosacral ligament so that the culdoplasty sutures can be placed correctly and safely.

Bladder Neck Suspension and Pelvic Organ Prolapse

Ureteral injury during retropubic repair most often affects the distal ureter. As Wiper and Walters have stated, this injury can occur during three distinct parts of performance of the procedure: (a) vigorous dissection of the space of Retzius and the periurethral tissues, (b) high elevation of Burch colposuspension sutures, and (c) paravaginal defect repair performed in combination with the Burch procedure. An additional way that the ureters could be injured is by excessive lateral mobilization of the bladder, which exposes the actual dorsal surface of the bladder in the vicinity of the trigone, bringing the ureter into the operative field.

There are specific steps that can be taken to avoid such injuries. Dissection into and through the space of Retzius should be done under direct visualization, remaining as close to the symphysis pubis as possible. The amount of dissection that occurs over the lateral paravaginal tissues should be kept to the minimal amount needed to guarantee accurate and appropriate placement of the sutures. Marked lateral mobilization of the bladder off of the underlying vagina potentially exposes the ureters. The urethrovesical junction must not be elevated as high as possible. Unquestionably, this can cause kinking not only of the urethra but also the ureters in certain patients.

Ureteral injury at time of surgical correction of pelvic organ prolapse is relatively common. The method of ureteral injury may result from direct ligation or, more likely, from kinking as the redundant tissues are plicated. Many surgeons who specialize in this type of surgery recommend that cystoscopy with intravenous indigo carmine be routinely performed during these procedures to check for ureteral integrity.

Radical Pelvic Surgery

Of all the groups of surgical procedures performed, those performed for the treatment of cancers affecting the female reproductive tract are the most likely to involve either intentional ureteral surgery or have the highest risk of an associated ureteral injury. It is very important to differentiate between an intentional ureteral disruption and one that is unintended or accidental. Intentional cutting of the ureter or entry into the bladder may be an integral part of performing many of the most important operative procedures in the radical pelvic surgeon's armamentarium. The MD Anderson type IV radical hysterectomy, a total or anterior pelvic exenteration, and resection of a fixed pelvic sidewall mass that involves the ureter may include ureteral resection and reconstruction. As a result of the nature of gynecologic malignancies and the procedures performed to treat those diseases, intentional and sometimes unintentional ureteral injuries occur. Additionally, the need to operate in a field that has been radiated or in which multiple prior surgical procedures have been performed compounds the cofactors that put the ureter at risk. It is evident that the radical pelvic surgeon must not only be a scholar of pelvic anatomy, but also have judgment skills as to how and when to attack a problem to minimize the probability of inducing a ureteral injury.

How common are ureteral injuries in association with radical pelvic surgery? The largest volume of data addresses ureteral injuries at time of traditional Wertheim or MD Anderson type III radical hysterectomies. Angioli and Penalver, in their excellent review combining the major modern series, reported that there is an average rate of ureteral injury of just more than 1% with a concomitant rate of bladder injury that is similar. Interestingly, as noted, these rates have been consistent over time and among different surgical groups during the last quarter century. There is a growing international experience with the performance of radical vaginal trachelectomy as fertility-sparing treatment for women with FIGO stage IA1 to IB1 cervical cancer. The cumulative English-language data demonstrate that the rate of ureteral injuries in this setting is about the same as with radical abdominal hysterectomy, although rates of bladder injury are somewhat higher. In contradistinction to these relatively low rates of ureteral injury, when a radical resection is performed following therapeutic radiation therapy, there is an associated risk of ureteral dysfunction of approximately 30%.

The incidence of ureteral injury at the time of a simple extrafascial hysterectomy as part of the treatment of endometrial cancer is low and similar to that when hysterectomy is performed for nonmalignant disease. Ureteral injuries in association with lymph node dissections, sampling, or when performing "radical" oophorectomies are remarkably uncommon when those injuries that occur near the entrance to and through the tunnel of Wertheim are excluded from the data. The reader is referred to the appropriate chapters within this text for more details concerning ureteral injury and its prevention during surgery for gynecologic malignancies.

DIAGNOSING URETERAL INJURY

In most instances, the symptoms and findings associated with an intraoperative ureteral injury that are not appreciated at the time of surgery are subtle and may be overlooked. Signs and symptoms such as unilateral cramping, flank pain, unexplained temperature elevation, ascites, retroperitoneal fluid collection, and unusual delay in return of bowel function (ileus) should lead one to consider an investigation into the integrity and function of the ureter, depending on the degree of suspicion of the surgeon. From a laboratory perspective, relatively inconsequential rises in serum creatinine (as little as 0.8 mg/dL) may be related to unilateral ureteral ligation. In contrast, it is unlikely that specific urinary tract symptomatology—such as the frank draining of urine from a drain, vagina, or abdominal incision—would be ignored. In all instances, when a patient reports a watery vaginal discharge following a hysterectomy, urinary tract injury must be investigated. A ureteral fistula may be suspected if there is urine leakage from the vagina; however, a bladder or urethral fistula is more common, depending on the type of surgery. *Several simple tests can differentiate between a ureteral and bladder fistula.* The bladder is filled with 200 cc saline stained with 1 to 3 cc methylene blue. If blue fluid comes out of the vagina, there is a bladder injury. If the watery discharge does not stain, inject 5 cc indigo carmine intravenously. If within 5 to 10 minutes the fluid turns blue, a ureteral fistula is present. If neither procedure results in bluish drainage fluid, check the creatinine level of the fluid. If it is the same as serum levels, the drainage is peritoneal fluid or lymph. If it is urine, the creatinine level will be 10 or greater. These simple, rapid tests will usually answer the problem.

If there is any significant degree of suspicion that a ureteral injury has occurred, further evaluation must be undertaken expeditiously. If there is concern of ureteral ligation, a noninvasive renal ultrasound showing hydronephrosis or hydroureter is fast, inexpensive, and accurate. In the past, these investigations began with the performance of an intravenous pyelogram. However, in the modern era, urinary tract imaging is usually done by computed tomography (CT) scan. The CT scan with contrast can give the same information regarding the integrity and function of the renal collecting system while offering the advantage of identifying urinomas, ascites, or changes in the postoperative anatomy of the surrounding structures. When the serum creatinine is elevated, intravenous contrast can cause significant renal damage, so a contrasted CT scan in contraindicated in these circumstances. A renal/proximal ureter ultrasound would be preferable in this situation.

MANAGEMENT OF URETERAL INJURY

It is an oversimplification to state that every specific type of ureteral injury can be managed by a specific and universally applicable way. Unique variables among patients play an important role in deciding which approach is best for a given setting. Nevertheless, general guidelines and techniques may be helpful. General recommendations for the management of ureteral injuries identified at the time of surgery are outlined in Table 38.4.

One of the most controversial issues regarding the management of ureteral injuries diagnosed in the postoperative period is how long one should wait before attempting repair. Some form of immediate intervention must be undertaken no matter what type of injury has occurred. If there is an obstruction without intraperitoneal or retroperitoneal leakage of urine, an immediate (same-day) attempt at ureteral stint placement should be undertaken. It is important to appreciate that the higher the grade of obstruction, the less likely that a retrograde stint can be placed successfully. In those instances in which a retrograde stint cannot be placed, a percutaneous nephrostomy must be immediately carried out. A percutaneous nephrostomy usually can be done under fluoroscopic guidance by the interventional radiologist without too much difficulty. Any delay in relieving the obstruction can translate into loss of renal parenchyma.

If there is no obstruction of the ureter but there is leakage of urine, whether the leakage is draining extracorporeally or not, I similarly recommend that a percutaneous nephrostomy be performed. Once drainage of urine has been (re)established by the nephrostomy stint, the next decision is when surgical intervention should be undertaken. Some believe that for those women with high-grade obstructions, an attempt at surgical deligation or performance of the appropriate repair as described later in this chapter (which is unlikely to be successful) should be undertaken as soon as can be scheduled electively. If the nephrostomy is functioning well, this is not an emergency; therefore, most believe that a workup to localize the site of obstruction or leakage should be completed, the patient stabilized, and any appropriate consultation obtained. If diagnosed immediately postoperatively, the best chance of healing with primary repair is reoperation within 24 to 48 hours. However, most injuries are diagnosed later, and edema, necrosis, and tissue reaction reduces the possibility of immediate successful primary repair and dictates delayed repair. By waiting several weeks, the postoperative inflammatory changes will resolve making repair easier.

In those instances in which there is no major degree of obstruction and the obstruction is not the result of a “permanent” agent (metal clip or suture), or when only a ureteral leak occurs, a period of watchful waiting may be tried in the hope of avoiding surgical intervention entirely. If there is a ureteral leak, delay is advised only if a ureteral stint can be placed that stops the leakage.

If a ureteral leak has been identified postoperatively and the leak has developed in the setting of prior pelvic radiation, then an aggressive attempt at percutaneous nephrostomy diversion should be undertaken. A period of many months should be allowed to pass before reevaluating the patient radiographically to determine whether the leak has spontaneously healed. Although it is less likely that spontaneous closure will take place, the complex and risky nature of surgical correction in the radiated pelvis demands, in the patient’s best interest, that the maximal attempt for spontaneous healing be allowed before any attempt at surgical repair. The site of ureteral repair should incorporate a functional blood supply. Therefore, the success of an ureteroneocystostomy is very low. This may be the one time an ureteroureterostomy above the irradiated pelvis is indicated. Omental wrap at the anastomotic site will improve blood supply.

TABLE 38.4

GENERAL GUIDELINES FOR MANAGEMENT OF URETERAL INJURIES IDENTIFIED AT TIME OF SURGERY

Ureteral ligation: Deligation, assessment of viability, stint placement
Partial transaction: Primary repair over ureteral stint
Total transaction
Uncomplicated upper and middle thirds: Ureteroureterostomy over ureteral stint
Complicated upper and middle thirds: Ureteroileal interposition
Lower third: Ureteroneocystostomy with psoas hitch over ureteral stint
Thermal injury: Resection with management as per a transection

Ureteral Ligation

Complete ureteral ligation can occur, but it is much more common that the ureter will be angulated or kinked by the placement of a suture that is either within the paraureteral tissue or partially placed through the ureter. If kinked, which is probably much more common than has been recognized, the first management approach would be to attempt to pass a ureteral catheter. This may be done via the classic approach from below, but in recent years, a percutaneous nephrostomy can be done by the interventional radiologist. The dilated renal pelvis, which results from the distal ureteral obstruction, often simplifies the percutaneous nephrostomy. Once the nephrostomy tube is in place, contrast can be injected to see if even a small trickle of dye gets past the obstruction into the bladder. If there is any opening, an attempt is made to pass a thin guidewire through the nephrostomy tube, down the ureter, and past the obstruction into the bladder. If successful, larger catheters can be passed over the guidewire. Finally, a double-J stent with one end in the bladder and the other in the real pelvis can be left in place for 6 to 8 weeks until the sutures responsible for the ureteral obstruction have dissolved. If the obstruction is too tight to be stented, a nephrostomy has been done to protect renal function until definitive surgery can be done to relieve the obstruction.

In those instances in which the ureter has been either partially or totally ligated and the obstruction cannot be bypassed and dilated, surgical ureterolysis is indicated. At reoperation, this ureter should be dissected free down to the point of obstruction, generally starting at the pelvic brim. The surgeon must be completely confident that the ureter is viable. There is no perfect way to guarantee this. Blanching and blood flow through the vessels in the adventitial sheath, ureteral peristalsis, and lack of discoloration are all valuable, although imperfect, measures. Usually, to be safe, the segment of the ureter about which there is concern should be stented, and, if believed dead, resected. Placement of a ureteral stent will also help to identify the site of obstruction. A ureteral stent can be inserted one of three ways: via ureterostomy, cystoscopy, or cystostomy. We strongly favor cystotomy. Performing a ureterostomy when one is not required produces an unnecessary site for stenosis or a leak. Cystoscopy requires additional time, instrumentation, repositioning, and prepping of the patient if she has not been placed in the dorsal low-lithotomy position from the beginning of the case. Opening the dome of the bladder in an extraperitoneal (preperitoneal via the space of Retzius) fashion is easy, safe, and efficient. We prefer the use of a no. 7 French double J ureteral stent over a guidewire. The use of a right-angle clamp to manipulate the wire makes placement quite easy. The cystotomy is closed in two layers of absorbable suture: (a) the urothelium and (b) the detrusor muscle in a running Lembert technique.

Partial Ureteral Transection

Repair of a partial transection (buttonhole) is probably the easiest and fastest of all the ureteral injuries to manage. Because the ureterotomy already has occurred, if it is believed a stent is needed, it can be placed up and down through the ureterotomy. If it is a small hole, a stent is not necessary. The ureter is repaired using small absorbable interrupted sutures. *Excessive suture placement should be avoided.* It is uncommon that more than two or three individual sutures are needed. Unless there is distal obstruction or the ureter has been devascularized, healing is usually rapid and complete. Additional suture placement does not increase the probability of adequate watertight closure and simply increases the probability of infection, ischemia, and scar formation. A closed suction drain should be placed at the base of the repair.

Total Transection

Uncomplicated Upper and Middle Thirds

A transaction of the ureter in its upper or middle thirds occurs in association with the performance of a paraaortic lymph node dissection or colonic resection. When this type of injury occurs, an end-to-end ureteroureterostomy over a ureteral stent is the recommended method of repair. The rules regarding performance of the ureteroureterostomy are the same as for the repair of the primary subtotal transaction: a limited number of sutures using small-gauge absorbable suture are placed over a ureteral stent, and the site of the repair is drained using a closed suction drain (Fig 38.8). There are two major modifications that we recommend. First, the surgeon should be assured that the ureteroureterostomy is completely tension free. Extra length of the ureter can be obtained by either mobilizing the kidney or mobilizing the distal ureter. The latter is usually preferable. Second, we recommend that both ends (proximal and distal) of the ureteroureterostomy site be spatulated. When the spatulating incision is made, care must be taken to assure that the blood vessels running in the ureteral sheath are not transected. If this occurs, the advantages of increasing the lumen size at the site of the ureteroureterostomy are probably offset by the possibility of a devascularization injury and subsequent sloughing of the site of repair. The vessels in the ureteral adventitial sheath usually can be visualized. Of course, the spatulation should be done on opposing sides of the proximal and distal ureter so as to facilitate a watertight seal.

Complicated Upper and Middle Thirds

By convention, complicated upper- and middle-third ureteral injuries are those in which one has resected a sizable segment of the ureter, and it can not be brought together in a tension-free fashion using either proximal or distal mobilization techniques as described. Although there are really two ways to effect repair (transureteroureterostomy and ureteroenteroneocystomy), most argue against the performance of the first technique. By definition, this places both urinary drainage systems with injuries and, therefore, at risk. For this reason, transureteroureterostomy has generally been abandoned and remains of historical interest only. Therefore, it is ureteroenteroneocystomy, in the form of an ureteroileal interposition, that most call standard for management of such an injury.

Ureteroileal interposition is a relatively easy procedure to perform. A healthy and mobile segment of the distal ileum is identified and the vascular arcades assured to be adequate for viability. We prefer to perform this resection using linear stapling devices. The ileum is repaired with a side-to-side stapled anastomosis before the performance of the ureteral repair. Once the bowel has been reanastomosed and packed off, the proximal end of the isolated loop of ileum is opened and all metal staples excised. A ureteral-ileal end-to-side anastomosis is performed over a ureteral stent or infant feeding tube. The ureter is spatulated, and the full thickness of the ureter is pulled through a hole made in the antimesenteric wall of the ileal segment. The full-thickness ureter is splayed open inside of the ileal segment using a small-gauge suture. In addition, the seromuscular portion of the ureter is attached to the serosa of the ileal segment so that the intra-ileal anastomosis is completely tension free. Unless a "pigtail" stent is used, the stent must be fixed with a catgut suture to the bowel lumen to prevent expulsion by normal ureteral peristalsis. After the proximal ureteroileal anastomosis is completed, the patent lumen of the proximal end of the ileal segment is closed. Either PGA staples (our preference) or a two-layer hand-sewn technique can be used. Closing the ileum with metal staples is not an acceptable option because of the potential for stone formation on the permanent foreign body that is exposed to urine. The distal end of the ileal segment is then opened and the staple line removed. The distal end of the ileal segment and ureteral stent are then inserted directly into the bladder. The interposed ileal segment should be trimmed to an appropriate length that is neither too long and redundant or too short so that there is tension on the anastomoses. The edges of the distal ileal segment are pulled through an incision in the dome of the bladder and sutured to the bladder mucosa with 3-0 delayed absorbable sutures placed via another incision in the bladder done. A series of 2-0 delayed absorbable sutures are then used to secure the serosa of the bowel to the outside serosa and muscularis of the bladder

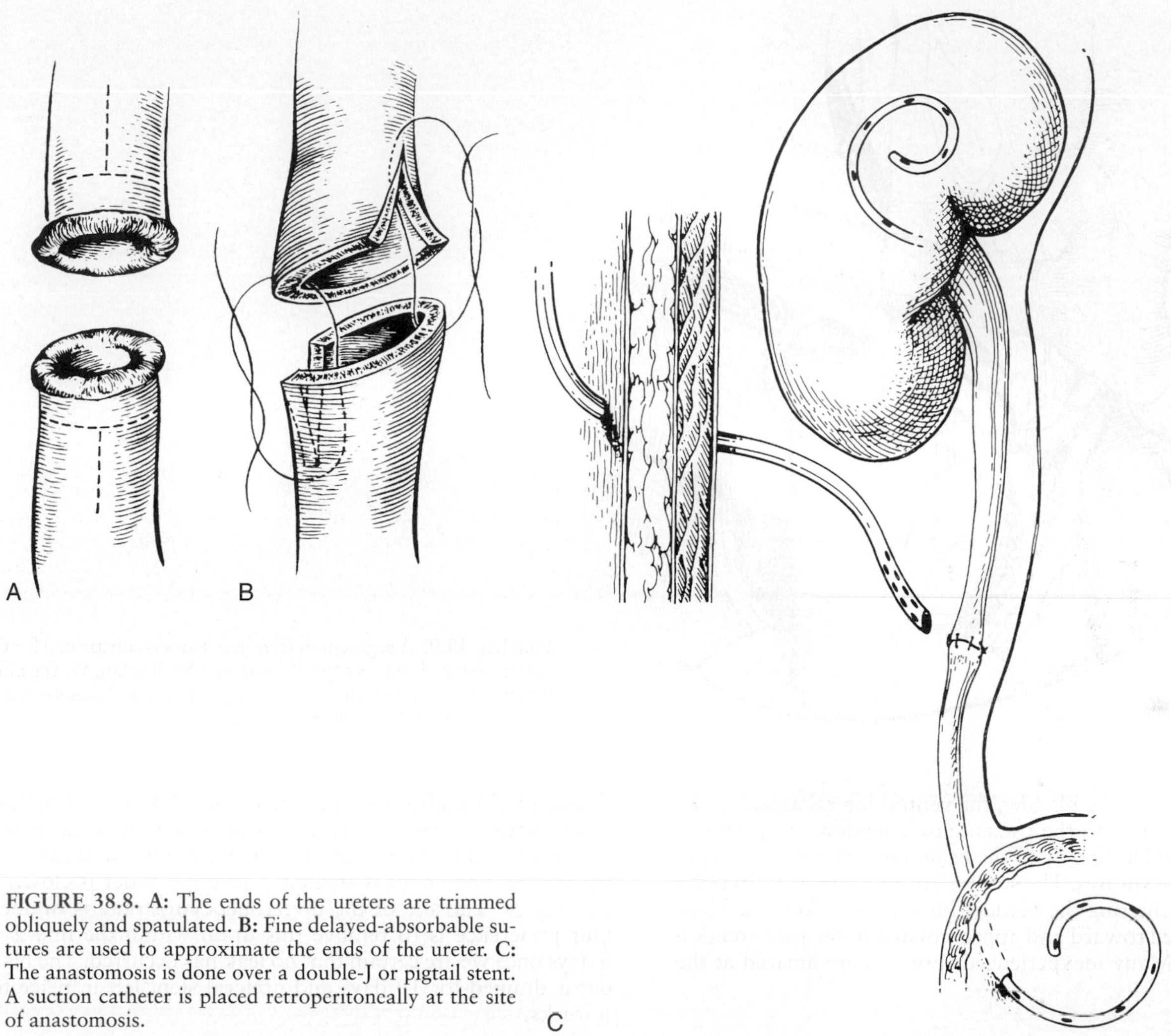

FIGURE 38.8. **A:** The ends of the ureters are trimmed obliquely and spatulated. **B:** Fine delayed-absorbable sutures are used to approximate the ends of the ureter. **C:** The anastomosis is done over a double-J or pigtail stent. A suction catheter is placed retroperitoneally at the site of anastomosis.

(Fig. 38.9). This "ileal conduit" may be secured to the psoas muscle fascia to minimize tension on that bowel segment mesentery and potential tension on the proximal ureteroileal anastomosis that may result from the effect of gravity when the patient is in an upright position. The ureteral stent should remain *in vivo* for at least 6 weeks. A cystoureterogram to identify any persistent occult leaks is recommended before removing the stent.

Lower Third of Ureter

Following a ureteral transaction within 6 cm of the ureterovesical junction or at the time of any resection of the lower third of the ureter, there must be a serious concern that vascularity of the distal remaining ureteral segment has been seriously compromised. Usually, it is possible to mobilize the bladder and do a direct ureteroneocystostomy so that there is no reason to take a risk with a possibly compromised distal ureter. The standard for repair in these situations has become the ureteroneocystostomy over a ureteral stent. A psoas hitch may be necessary for the ureter to reach the bladder. As with the performance of the ileal interposition, this is not a technically difficult procedure. There is a very high probability of a successful outcome if a meticulous focus on surgical technique is maintained. The first step in performing the ureteroneocystostomy is to tie off the distal segment of the ureter that is still attached to the bladder. Because the lumen of the remaining distal ureter is not in contact with the sutures, a permanent material can be used for the ligation. If a psoas hitch is required, the entire ventral surface of the bladder is freed from its areolar attachment in the retropubic space. This facilitates mobilization of the bladder toward the proximal ureter and can be done with no functional risk for the bladder as long as the dorsal lateral blood supply is left intact. Once the bladder has been fully mobilized, a cystotomy in the bladder dome is performed. The cystotomy incision should be at 90 degrees to the direction desired to elongate the bladder. After the ureterostomy has been done, the incision is then closed at right angles to the way it was opened (the two ends of the incision are closed together as the middle of the closure and the middle of the incision becomes the end of the closure). This will elongate the bladder toward the shortened ureter helping to avoid tension on the ureteral anatomosis. The ureteroneocystostomy is performed using the same technique for anastomosis as described in the discussion of the ileal interposition procedure. The site where the ureter should be drawn into the bladder usually is self-evident. We attempt to place this attachment on the posterior aspect of the bladder dome, some distance from the trigone so as to minimize any potential stenosis or injury to the contralateral ureteral orifice. Using direct tactile and visual guidance, with the primary

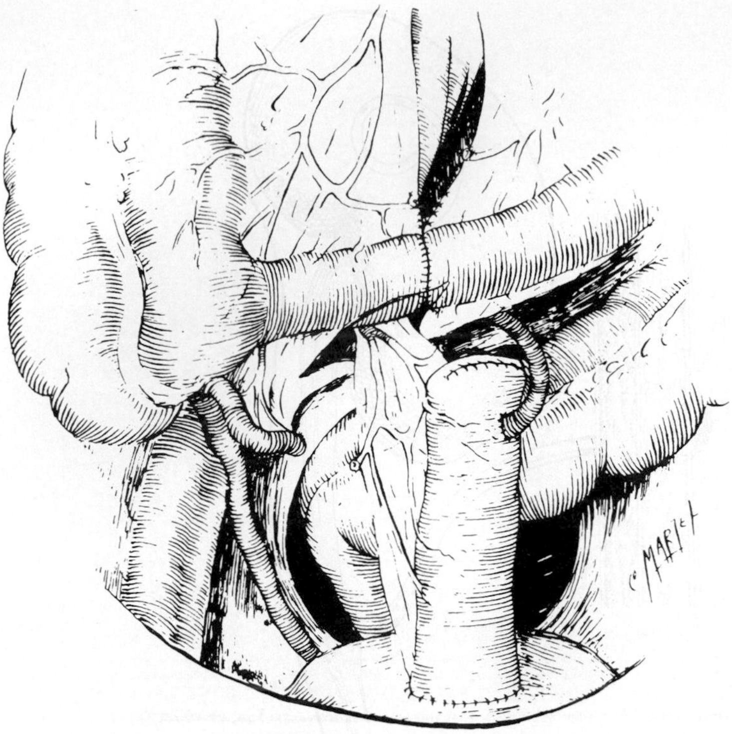

FIGURE 38.9. A segment of terminal ileum is substituted for the lower ureter. (From: Krupp P, Hoffman M, Roeling W. Terminal ileum as ureteral muscle: relationship to intubated ureterostomy. *J Urol* 1955;73:47, with permission.)

surgeon's finger in the bladder, the ventral-lateral aspect of the bladder is attached to the psoas muscle tendon. We prefer to attach the bladder directly to the psoas tendon using two separate permanent sutures. The sutures are attached to the bladder wall without entering the bladder lumen. Therefore, the bladder is elongated toward and approximated to the psoas tendon (Fig. 38.10). Many inexperienced surgeons are amazed at the degree of elongation that can be obtained and the length of the ureterovesicular gap that can be bridged if there has been a thorough bladder mobilization in the retropubic and paravesical spaces. The ureter is stented, and the bladder is closed in two layers. The site of the ureteroneocystostomy is drained. Our preference is to remove this drain within the first 2 to 3 days once we are certain that no leak has occurred. The bladder is drained for 10 days and ureteral stent left in place for 6 weeks.

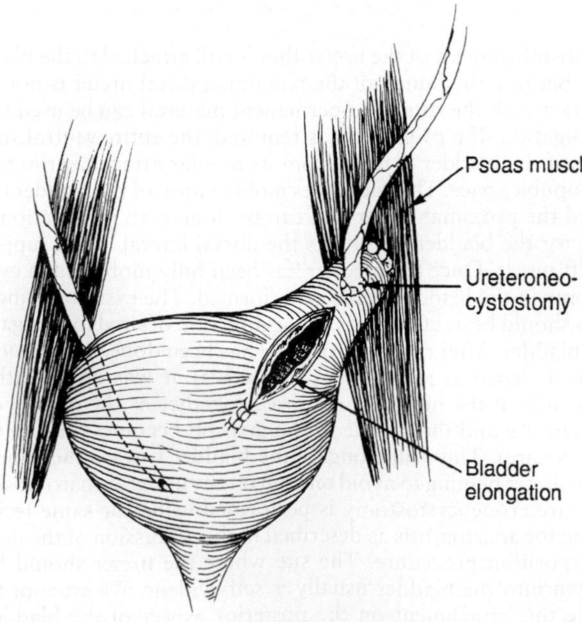

FIGURE 38.10. Bladder elongation performed to allow a tension-free ureteroneocystostomy. The bladder is anchored to the psoas muscle to avoid tension.

SUMMARY

Ureteral injuries can be expected, and, although unpleasant, they are a reality in the life of the active gynecologic surgeon. The vast majority of these misadventures can be avoided by constant reflection on the location of the ureter and meticulous attention to optimal surgical technique. Should ureteral injury occur, an optimal outcome is the result of accurately diagnosing the type of injury and its location; protecting the kidney by nephrostomy, retrograde stenting, or prompt reoperation; and, finally, by correcting the ureteral injury by appropriate surgical or nonsurgical techniques.

BEST SURGICAL PRACTICES

- The pelvic surgeon must always be aware of the location of the ureters in relation to the operative field.
- The most common sites of ureteral injuries are within the cardinal ligament where the ureter crosses under the uterine artery, in the tunnel of Wertheim, in the intramural portion of the ureter dorsal to the infundibulopelvic ligament near or at the pelvic brim, and lateral on the pelvic sidewall above the uterosacral ligament.

- Abdominal hysterectomy is the most common gynecologic surgery resulting in operative injury to the ureter. The two high-risk areas for ureteral injuries during abdominal hysterectomies for benign disease are lower-uterine-segment or cervical fibroids protruding into the broad ligament or bleeding from pedicles, especially at the vaginal corners.
- Postoperatively signs and symptoms of ureteral injury include unilateral cramping, flank pain, unexplained temperature elevation, ascites, retroperitoneal fluid collection, and unusual delay in return of bowel function.
- A test to differentiate between bladder and ureteral fistulae is instillation of 200 cc saline stained with 1 to 3 cc methylene blue in the bladder. If blue fluid is visualized from the vagina, it is a bladder injury. If the discharge does not stain, inject IV 5 cc indigo carmine. If within 5 to 10 minutes the fluid turns blue, it is a ureteral fistula. If neither stains, the drainage may be peritoneal fluid or lymph.
- Complete or partial ureteral ligation at the same time of surgery should be treated with confirmation of ureteral viability and diversion with ureteral stent placement via cystostomy. Postoperatively, a stent may be placed via nephrostomy or cystoscopy.
- The standard repair following ureteral transection within 6 cm of the ureterovesical junction is ureteroneocystostomy.
- Should ureteral injury occur, an optimal outcome is the result of accurately diagnosing the type of injury and its location; protecting the kidney by nephrostomy, retrograde stenting, or prompt reoperation; and, finally, by correcting the ureteral injury by appropriate surgical or nonsurgical techniques.

Bibliography

Angioli R, Penalver M. Ureteral injury at time of radical pelvic surgery. *Oper Tech Gynecol Surg* 1998;43:132.

Barber MD, Visco AG, Weider AC, et al. Bilateral uterosacral ligament vaginal vault suspension with site-specific endopelvic fascia defect repair for treatment of pelvic organ prolapse. *Am J Obstet Gynecol* 2000;183:1402.

Bristow RE, Smith-Sehdev AE, Kaufman HS, et al. Ablation of metastatic ovarian carcinoma with the argon beam coagulator: pathologic analysis of tumor destruction. *Gynecol Oncol* 2001;83:49.

Cornella JL, Lee RA. Management of ureteral injury at complex adnexectomy. *Oper Tech Gynecol Surg* 1998;3:97.

Cornella JL, Walter A. Prevention and early recognition of ureteral injuries at vaginal hysterectomy. *Oper Technol Gynecol Surg* 1998;3:115.

Covens A, Shaw P, Murphy J, et al. Is radical trachelectomy a safe alternative to radical hysterectomy for patients with stage I A-B carcinoma of the cervix? *Cancer* 1999;86:2273.

Daly JW, Higgens KA. Injury to the ureter during gynecologic surgical procedures. *Surg Gynecol Obstet* 1988;167:19.

Dargent D, Martin X, Sacchetoni A, et al. Laparoscopic vaginal radical trachelectomy. *Cancer* 2000;88:1877.

Drake MJ, Noble JG. Ureteric trauma in gynecologic surgery. *Int Urogynecol J Pelvic Floor Dysfunct* 1998;9:108.

Ehrlich RM, Skinner DG. Complications of transureteroureterostomy. *J Urol* 1975;113:467.

Elkins TE. Ureteral injury at time of abdominal hysterectomy for benign disease. *Oper Tech Gynecol Surg* 1998;3:108.

Eriksen BC, Hagen B, Kik-Nes SH, et al. Long term effectiveness of the Burch colposuspension in female urinary stress incontinence. *Acta Obstet Gynecol Scand* 1990;69:45.

Goldstein SL, Harold KL, Lentzner A, et al. Comparison of thermal spread after ureteral ligation with the laparo-sonic ultrasonic sheers and the ligature system. *J Laparoendosc Adv Surg Tech A* 2002;12:61.

Gomel V, James C. Intraoperative management of ureteral injury during operative laparoscopy. *Fertil Steril* 1997;55:416.

Goodno JA Jr, Powers TW, Harris VD. Ureteral injury in gynecologic surgery: a ten-year review in a community hospital. *Am J Obstet Gynecol* 1995;172:1817.

Haney NS. Technique of vaginal hysterectomy. *Surg Clin North Am* 1942;22:73.

Harkk-Siren P, Kurki T. A nationwide analysis of laparoscopic complications. *Obstet Gynecol* 1997;89:108.

Harris RL, Cundiff GW, Theofratous JP, et al. The value of intraoperative cystoscopy in urogynecologic and reconstructive surgery. *Am J Obstet Gynecol* 1997;177:1367.

Karram M, Goldwasser S, Kleeman S, et al. High ureteral sacral vaginal vault suspension with fascial reconstruction for vaginal repair of enterocele and vaginal vault prolapse. *Am J Obstet Gynecol* 2001;185:1339.

Klutke JJ, Klutke CG, Hsieh G. Bladder injury during the Burch retropubic urethropexy: is routine cystoscopy necessary? *Tech Urol* 1998;4:145.

Koelliker SL, Cronann JJ. Acute urinary tract obstruction: imaging update. *Urol Clin North Am* 1997;24:571.

Kuno K, Menzin A, Kauder HH, et al. Prophylactic ureteral catheterization in gynecologic surgery. *Urology* 1998;52:1004.

Liapis A, Bakas P, Giannopoulos V, et al. Ureteral injuries during gynecologic surgery. *Int Urogynecol J Pelvic Floor Dysfunct* 2001;12:391.

Mainprize TC, Drutz HP. The Marshall-Marchetti-Krantz procedure: critical review. *Obstet Gynecol Surv* 1988;43:724.

Mann WJ, Arato M, Patsner B, et al. Ureteral injuries in an obstetrics and gynecology training program: etiology and management. *Obstet Gynecol* 1988;72:82.

Mariotti G, Natale F, Trucchi A, et al. Ureteral injuries during gynecologic procedures. *Minerva Urol Nefrol* 1997;49:95.

Mattingly RF, Borkow HL. Acute operative injury to the lower urinary tract. *Clin Obstet Gynecol* 1978;5:123.

Meirow D, Moriel EZ, Zilberman M, et al. Evaluation and treatment of iatrogenic ureteral injuries during obstetrics and gynecologic operations for non-malignant conditions. *J Am Coll Surg* 1994;178:144.

Miklos JR, Kohli N. Laparoscopic paravaginal repair plus Burch colposuspension: review and descriptive technique. *Urology* 2000;56:64.

Modi P, Goel R, Dodiya S. Laparoscopic ureteroneocystostomy for distal ureteral injury. *J Urol* 2005;66(4):751.

Monk BJ, Solkh S, Johnson MT, et al. Radical hysterectomy after pelvic irradiation in patients with high risk cervical cancer or uterine sarcoma: morbidity and outcome. *Eur J Gynaecol Oncol* 1993;14:506.

Munro M. Ureteral injury associated with gynecologic laparoscopy. *Oper Tech Gynecol Surg* 1998;3:84.

Neuman M, Eidelman A, Langer R, et al. Iatrogenic injuries to the ureter during gynecologic and obstetric operations. *Surg Gynecol Obstet* 1991;173:268.

Nezhat C, Nezhat F. Laparoscopic repair of ureter resected during operative laparoscopy. *Obstet Gynecol* 1992;80:543.

Nezhat C, Nezhat FR, Nezhat F. Laparoscopic ureteroneocystostomy vesicopsoas hitch for infiltrative ureteral endometriosis. *Fertil Steril* 1999;71:376.

Oh BR, Kwon DD, Park KS, et al. Late presentation of ureteral injury after laparoscopic surgery. *Obstet Gynecol* 2000;95:337.

Piver M, Rutledge F, Smith J. Five classes of extended hysterectomy for women with cervical cancer. *Obstet Gynecol* 1974;44:265.

Plante M, Roy M. Radical trachelectomy. *Oper Tech Gynecol Surg* 1997;2:187.

Rosen DM, Korda AR, Waugh RC. Ureteric injury at Burch colposuspension: four case reports and literature review. *Aust N Z J Obstet Gynecol* 1996;36:354.

Saidi MH, Sadler RK, Vanvaillie TG, et al. Diagnosis and management of serious urinary complications after major operative laparoscopy. *Obstet Gynecol* 1996;87:272.

Sandoz IL, Paul DP, MacFarlane CA. Complications of transureteroureterostomy. *J Urol* 1977;117:39.

Selzman AA, Spirnak JP. Iatrogenic ureteral injuries: a 20-year experience in treating 165 injuries. *J Urol* 1996;155:878.

Speights SE, Moore RD, Miklos JR. Frequency of lower urinary tract injury at laparoscopic Burch and paravaginal repair. *J Am Assoc Gynecol Laparosc* 2000;7:515.

Te Linde RW. Cancer of the cervix uteri. In: Te Linde RW, ed. *Operative gynecology*. Philadelphia: JB Lippincott, 1946:386.

Thompson JD. Operative injuries to the ureter: prevention, recognition, and management. In: Rock JA, Thompson JD, eds. *Te Linde's operative gynecology*.. 8th ed Philadelphia: JB Lippincott, 1997: 1135.

Vabili B, Chesson RR, Kyle BL, et al. The incidence of urinary tract injury during hysterectomy and a prospective analysis based on universal cystoscopy. *Am J Obstet Gynecol* 2005;192(5):1599.

Webb JA. Ultrasonography and Doppler studies in the diagnosis of renal obstruction. *BJU Int* 2000;86(Suppl 1):25.

Wiper DW, Walters MD. Ureteral injury at time of bladder neck suspension. *Oper Tech Gynecol Surg* 1998;3:126.

Woodland MB. Ureter injury during laparoscopy-assisted vaginal hysterectomy with the endoscopic linear stapler. *Am J Obstet Gynecol* 1992;167:756.

Yossepowitch O, Lifshitz DA, Dekel Y, et al. Predicting the success of retrograde stenting for managing ureteral obstruction. *J Urol* 2001;166:1746.

CHAPTER 39 ■ VESICOVAGINAL FISTULA AND URETHROVAGINAL FISTULA

G. RODNEY MEEKS AND TED M. ROTH

DEFINITIONS

Interposition graft—Placement of tissue to enhance tissue bulk or vascularity in an effort to enhance success of repair.

Latzko repair—A vaginal technique for repair of a vesicovaginal fistula at the apex of the vagina that includes partial colpocleisis.

O'Conor repair—An abdominal technique for repair of vesicovaginal fistula that uses cystotomy, separation of the vagina and bladder, excision of the fistula tract, and layer closure of the bladder and vagina.

Urethrovaginal fistula—An abnormal communication between urethra and vagina.

Vesicovaginal fistula—An abnormal communication between bladder and vagina.

Although it is difficult to accurately gauge the incidence of genitourinary fistulae in the United States, the majority result from gynecologic surgery, specifically total abdominal hysterectomy, urogynecologic procedures, radiation therapy, or complications of parturition. Prolonged obstructed labor remains the most common cause of destruction of the urethra and base of the bladder in developing countries, where good medical care is limited. When a fistula becomes symptomatic depends on its cause, location, and size. Differences of opinion have developed regarding timing and route of repair; however, success of fistula repair ultimately depends on a surgeon's experience, judgment, and appropriateness of technique.

HISTORICAL SURVEY

Vesicovaginal fistulae (VVF) have occurred since the beginning of recorded time. Professor Derry, of the medical faculty at Fouad I University in Egypt, discovered a large VVF in the mummy of Henhenit, a lady in the court of Mentuhotep of the Eleventh Dynasty who reigned about 2050 B.C. He found the pelvis was considerably contracted in the transverse diameter, and there was a through-and-through tear of the perineum. The Kahun papyrus, which refers back to 2000 B.C. and generally is thought to contain the earliest gynecologic references, and the Eber's papyrus, from about 1500 B.C., make no mention of VVF. The Talmud, likewise, fails to give any evidence that ancient Hebrew physicians were cognizant of this malady. The first record of a VVF is found in the writings of ancient Hindu medicine, the Vedas and Upavedas. Avicenna, a Persian physician, was the first known writer to mention the occurrence of a VVF. He also recognized the association between such a lesion and labor. The delayed recognition of VVF as a clinical entity may be related to the prolonged influence of Arab physicians from 600 to 1600 A.D., who regarded postmortem examinations sinful, and, as men, were forbidden by religious tenets from practicing obstetrics and gynecology.

In 1663, Hendrik Von Roonhuysen published his *Medico-Chirurgical Observations about the Infirmities of Women.* His innovations for the management of VVF included proper exposure with a speculum, marginal denudation of the fistula, and approximation of the denuded edges with "stitching needles made of stiff swan's quills." No figures or postoperative results were presented. Posthumously published in 1752, Johann Fatio described the first reported cures using Von Roonhuysen's technique.

A new era in the surgical treatment of VVF occurred in the 19th century. In 1834, de Lamballe was the first to emphasize tension-free closures. He also noted that newly acquired fistulae without evidence of induration at the edges might be cured by prolonged catheterization alone. De Lamballe also made attempts to cure VVF with pedicle flaps from labia, buttocks, and thigh. Simon of Darmstadt, a colleague of de Lamballe, suggested transverse colpocleisis in those cases that defied previous attempts at closure. Although this procedure was fraught with complications, partial colpocleisis was later espoused by Latzko to cure posthysterectomy fistulae.

In 1852, Marion Sims published his classic work, which formally established the technique of VVF repair. His contribution to this endeavor is recognized by the recent republication of his original paper. Although many of his innovations were not new, he attained greater success than anyone else, and his personality helped in bringing public attention to the treatment of women's diseases. Although Sims's only innovation was the use of silver wire suture, he standardized and defined the surgical principles of vesicovaginal repair that are used to this day. The ethics surrounding Sims's seminal work have recently been reviewed. The fact that his original subjects were slaves leads to a question of ethical treatment of women who had minimal, if any, personal autonomy. It is generally believed that Sims was trying to enhance the lives of these women and was in concert with accepted mores.

As laparotomy became safer, many surgeons developed abdominal techniques for VVF repair. Trendelenburg, in 1881 to 1890, described opening the bladder suprapubically, freeing the bladder wall, and closing the defect. Maisonneuve and Mackenrodt independently described separating the bladder from the vaginal mucosa and suturing each as an individual layer. These principles remain foundations for modern closure techniques.

In 1896, Kelly described a vaginal method of closing a large bladder defect. The bladder is freed away from the cervix to the level of the visceral peritoneum and closed. He also advocated the use of preoperative ureteral catheterization to minimize risk of ureteral injury, a technique first championed by Pawlik in 1882. By 1906, when Kelly described a suprapubic route for repair of VVF, at least 12 different surgical approaches had been detailed.

In 1942, Latzko described, in detail, the principles of his transvaginal operation, based on the work by Simon, which is considered by some to be the gold standard for the surgical management of posthysterectomy VVF. Latzko reported that 29 of 31 cases of VVF treated by his method of partial colpocleisis were cured. The outcomes are impressive considering that the majority of these patients had antecedent radical abdominal hysterectomy for cervial cancer.

ETIOLOGY/EPIDEMIOLOGY

The etiology of urogenital fistulae may be categorized as congenital or acquired, the latter being associated with childbirth, gynecologic surgery, malignancy, and radiation therapy. When VVF occurs in childhood, antecedent events include penetrating trauma, retained or neglected foreign bodies, and genitourinary surgery. Congenital VVFs are extremely rare, and most coexist with other congenital urinary tract abnormalities. In one small series, seven of nine were associated with other genitourinary malformations. This chapter focuses on acquired VVF.

Much of the literature consists of retrospective case series and reflects the experience of a particular surgeon or fistula center. During a 15-year period of review, 303 women with genitourinary fistulae were seen at the Mayo Clinic (of whom 280 underwent surgical repair). Of the 190 patients with *vesicovaginal fistulae,* gynecologic surgery was responsible for 145 (82%) of the fistulae, 19 (11%) were from obstetric procedures, 13 (7%) followed treatment for malignant disease, and 5 (3%) were from trauma. Similarly, Goodwin and Scardino found 74% of their cases to be of gynecologic origin, 14% of urologic origin, and 12% from radiation injury.

Culture and geography are reflected in the frequencies and etiologies of VVFs. In England, Kelly found that 95% of the VVF occurred with nonobstetric causes. In contradistinction, obstructed labor caused 98% of the VVF in Nigeria. In developing countries, obstetric trauma remains the leading cause of VVF. Most often the inciting event is prolonged and obstructed labor, which results in pressure necrosis. Introital stenosis secondary to female circumcision, cephalopelvic disproportion (from inadequate pelvic dimensions associated childbearing at a very early age), an android pelvis, malnutrition, orthopedic disorders including rickets, and hydrocephalus contribute to dystocia. Fistulae may be caused by the misuse of forceps, destructive instruments used to deliver stillborn infants, or surgical abortion. Symphysiotomy and the postpartum use of intravaginal caustic agents also have a role. A large series of VVF details 1,443 cases in northern Nigeria between 1969 and 1980. Eighty-three percent resulted from prolonged, obstructed labor, and 13% resulted from *gishiri* cuts, a traditional tribal practice of cutting the anterior vagina with a razor blade to treat a variety of conditions, including obstructed labor, infertility, dyspareunia, backache, and goiter. Only 1% of fistulae in this study were associated with antecedent surgery.

The need to continue to implement health education programs in underdeveloped countries has been emphasized. So serious is the problem that a National Task Force on VVF was formed in Nigeria in 1990. The purpose of the task force is to prevent VVF through public awareness campaigns, education, and advocacy for women's medical and surgical services. In this population, there can be grave social consequences of VVF, including divorce, poverty, depression, and societal isolation.

Premature childbearing as a result of early adolescent marriage continues to be epidemic in Africa. In sub-Saharan Africa, nearly 50% of the women are married by age 18, many by age 15 or younger. A recent case-control study from Ojanuga and Ekwempu in Katsina, Nigeria, found that primiparous girls who married during early adolescence were more likely to experience VVF than those who married at an older age. Uneducated women and those married to men who were unskilled laborers were 14 times more likely to sustain a VVF than their cohorts. In contrast, Hilton and Ward, in a review of 2,979 fistula repairs in 2,484 patients from southern Nigeria, found that fistula patients were older and of higher parity. These women appeared to have a higher literacy rate and were more likely to remain in a married relationship despite being symptomatic with a VVF. Ibrahim and colleagues described 31 women treated over a 12-month period in a university teaching hospital in Sokoto, Nigeria. In contrast to previous reports, all cases were directly caused by obstructed labor, and none of the patients had undergone traditional surgical practices of *gishiri* or ritual circumcision. Because of variations in the populations studied, patient selection, and techniques employed, the rates of successful repair of VVF are difficult to compare.

In countries with more modern obstetric care, the most common cause of VVF remains injury at the time of gynecologic or urological surgery. Predisposing risk factors for VVF include a history of pelvic irradiation, cesarean section, endometriosis, prior pelvic surgery, pelvic inflammatory disease, diabetes mellitus, concurrent infection, vasculopathies, and tobacco abuse. Patients undergoing total abdominal hysterectomy are a particular risk. Although the incidence of VVF after hysterectomy is approximately one in 1,300 surgeries, there are only a few "large" series on which to base reliable estimates of risk. In a series of 17 cases of posthysterectomy fistulae reported over a 15-year period from Dublin, the risk of VVF was 1 in 605 for total abdominal hysterectomy, 1 in 571 for vaginal hysterectomy, and 1 in 81 for radical hysterectomy.

Using data from the National Patient Insurance Association in Finland, Harkki-Siren and associates reviewed the incidence of urinary tract injury on a national scale. During the study period, 62,379 hysterectomies were performed and 142 urinary tract injuries recorded. The incidence of bladder injury was 1.3 per 1,000 hysterectomies. The incidence of VVF was one in 1,200 procedures; 1 in 455 after laparoscopic hysterectomy, 1 in 958 after total abdominal hysterectomy, and 1 in 5,636 after vaginal hysterectomy. Risk of ureteral injury was seven times greater with laparoscopic procedures than with open procedures. A recent series of 100 total laparoscopic hysterectomies included two VVF among the reported complications.

The underlying mechanism of posthysterectomy fistula formation is probably multifactorial, but actual etiologies remain enigmatic. Cystotomy at the time of hysterectomy has been thought to be associated with an increased risk of VVF. Armenakas and colleagues reviewed 65 patients in whom intraoperative bladder cystotomy was identified and in whom immediate repair was accomplished. With prompt intraoperative recognition, the success rate for immediate repair was 98.4%. Therefore, simple cystotomy is an uncommon culprit if repaired immediately. However, an unrecognized cystotomy or partial tear of the bladder muscularis may lead to a fistula. In some cases, a fistula may arise from avascular necrosis secondary to crush injury. Meeks and associates, in a rabbit model, demonstrated that suture material intentionally placed through the vaginal cuff and the bladder was not associated with the development of fistulae. Similar findings have been described in a canine model.

Bladder injury and urogenital fistulae are known complications of incontinence surgery. Synthetic sling materials are prone to infection and erosion. Kobashi and colleagues reviewed cases in which sling removal was required after the use of a woven polyester sling treated with pressure-injected bovine collagen. Over a 2-year period, 34 women required sling removal, and 6 had a urethrovaginal fistulae. Although periurethral injectable materials are thought of as being relatively innocuous, at least two reports have linked the placement of periurethral collagen to the development of bladder neck fistulae in women with normal anatomy and following ileal bladder substitution.

Radiation-induced fistulae occasionally are associated with treatment for carcinoma of the cervix or other pelvic malignancies. However, fistulae are much less common with today's planning techniques. Radiation-induced VVF formation does not always correlate with the absolute dose and distribution of radiation, or with the patient's weight or age; this suggests that some women are more sensitive to radiation therapy than others. Healthy tissues of the anterior vaginal wall tolerate radiation doses as high as 8,000 rads. Fistulae may appear during the course of radiotherapy (usually from necrosis of the tumor itself) or remote from completion of therapy. Endarteritis obliterans progresses during the first 2 years and may lead to ischemic changes that result in the delayed occurrence of a fistula. In planning repair, recurrent malignancy must be excluded with biopsies of the fistula margins. Because of decreased vascularity of the adjacent tissue, healing is impaired, and techniques incorporating revascularization must be considered when planning repair of a radiation-induced fistula.

There are "fascinoma" case reports of VVF caused by vaginal foreign bodies, forgotten pessaries, direct trauma from masturbation or automobile accidents, tuberculosis, schistosomiasis, bladder calculi, endometriosis, syphilis, and lymphogranuloma venereum, as well as from idiopathic congenital causes. Approach to management cannot be generalized in these situations. Care must be individualized in these situations. Isolated reports in the literature may help guide management of these unique problems.

Urethrovaginal fistulae are uncommon and usually occur after surgery for urethral diverticulum, anterior vaginal wall prolapse, or urinary incontinence, and after radiation therapy. In these cases, the most common causes include tissue ischemia, problems related to healing, or radiation necrosis. Operative vaginal delivery also is a risk factor for the development of a urethrovaginal fistula. Pressure necrosis, resulting in a urethrovaginal fistula, can occur with a prolonged indwelling transurethral catheter. Urethrovaginal fistulae also may be congenital, although these are extremely rare.

Vesicouterine and *vesicocervical fistulae* are rare. They are usually complications of cesarean section. The clinical presentation may be similar to VVF, with urine egressing through the vagina. The examination fails to reveal a vaginal fistula, however, and rarely urine trickles down through the os. Cyclic hematuria (menouria) is common. An abdominal approach with interposition graft is favored for repair, using the techniques for VVF.

PREVENTION

Many of the techniques advocated to reduce the incidence of fistulae are directed toward protecting the bladder during hysterectomy. The base of the bladder rests on the anterior lower uterine isthmus and the cervix, whereas the trigone is caudad to the internal os. The bladder is subjected to trauma during dissection from the cervix and upper vagina. A fistula following injury in this area will be found in the posterior wall of the bladder superior to the interureteric ridge in almost all cases. Because the trigone overlies the upper one third of the anterior vagina, it is unlikely to be injured because dissection at this level is rarely needed during hysterectomy for benign conditions. Bladder injury associated with supracervical hysterectomy is rare because bladder dissection is minimal. Harkki-Siren and colleagues reported no VVFs in their review of 1,000 consecutive supracervical hysterectomies.

Tancer, in a retrospective study of 151 urogenital fistulae, found that 91% of the fistulae occurred after gynecologic procedures. Total hysterectomy was the most common antecedent procedure ($n = 110$), resulting in a vault fistula. Seventy percent occurred in the absence of factors that typically place the patient at risk. Based on these observations, Tancer made suggestions on avoiding injury to the bladder during total abdominal hysterectomy. These include the use of a two-way indwelling catheter, sharp dissection to isolate the bladder, an extraperitoneal cystotomy when the dissection is difficult, retrograde filling of the bladder when injury is suspected, and repair of an overt bladder injury only after mobilization of the injured area. Retrograde filling of the bladder also may help define the border of a bladder otherwise distorted or displaced by prior surgery or a lower uterine segment fibroid.

An intrafascial technique for removing the cervix at hysterectomy also may protect the bladder. The vesicocervical space must be completely developed, and the bladder must be thoroughly mobilized inferiorly and laterally. Before the cardinal ligament pedicles are developed and before the anterior vagina is incised, an inverted "T" or "V" incision is made in the pubocervical fascia. The fascia is separated from the cervix and upper anterior vagina. The exposed vaginal epithelium can be entered directly. In theory, the bladder has been mobilized from the site of entry into the vagina and is less likely to be compromised because it rests on the dissected fascia. Constant traction of the uterus cephalad and gentle caudad traction on the bladder allows placement of clamps and sutures without injuring the bladder. In a recent review of 867 women who underwent intrafascial abdominal hysterectomy, there was a bladder injury incidence of 0.4%. This compares with a 1% rate of bladder injury during total abdominal hysterectomy. Because there are no prospective clinical trials comparing these techniques, conclusions are impossible.

CYSTOTOMY AND REPAIR

The principles and technique of repairing a cystotomy are the same regardless of the inciting event. The margins of the wound should be delineated carefully to assess the extent of injury and prevent injury to the ureters. The closure is started slightly beyond the poles of the defect. Closure may be accomplished with interrupted or continuous sutures. The authors prefer to leave the sutures long at the poles to help with orientation and subsequent suture placement. Choice of suture for repair of the urinary tract has been studied based on calculus formation. When a permanent suture penetrates the urothelium, it creates a nidus for encrustation and stone formation. Although numerous studies show that permanent sutures should be avoided, a clear choice among available absorbable suture has not evolved. Indeed, the risk of stone formation seems to be equivalent for chromic catgut, polyglactin, polydioxanone, and polyglyconate. Poliglecaprone also has been touted by its manufacturer as an option for urinary tract repair, but data to support this use is limited. Therefore, suture preference for VVF repair and other urinary tract surgery is physician dependent. Suture of 2-0 or 3-0 caliber is most commonly recommended. A point of contention is whether the bladder mucosa

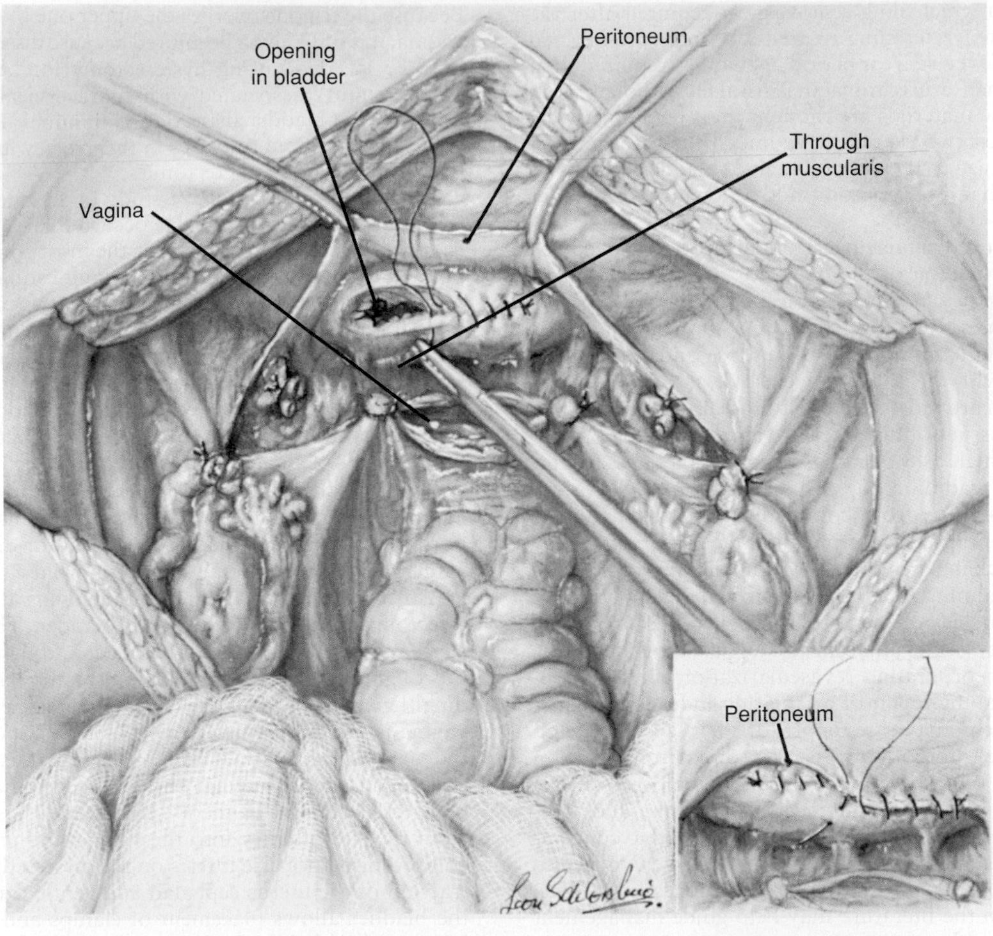

FIGURE 39.1. Closure of cystotomy associated with total abdominal hysterectomy. The bladder mucosa is closed with a continuous delayed-absorbable suture. The suture may invert the mucosa or may be through and through the mucosa. A second row of suture is placed in the musculofascial layer of the bladder to support the initial layer. The bladder peritoneum may be sutured over the operative site to protect it from postoperative pelvic cellulitis to further prevent leakage into the vagina. The edge of the bladder peritoneum also may be sutured to the anterior vaginal cuff.

should be penetrated with the suture or if the sutures should be placed so as to entropion the edges of the wound. Benefits of the former include ease of suture placement and possibly improved hemostasis of the wound edges. The possibility of stone formation secondary to foreign body reaction is a drawback to "through-and-through" suture placement. Subsequent rows of continuous or interrupted sutures are placed in the musculofascial tissues to imbricate initial layers. If cystotomy occurs at the time of laparotomy in addition to the repair, a flap of peritoneum or omentum may be mobilized for further buttressing (Fig. 39.1). A watertight closure is assured by instilling 200 cc of sterile baby's formula or dilute methylene blue via a transurethral catheter. Ureteral patency, integrity of the bladder repair, and hemostasis may be assessed with cystoscopy. Decisions regarding postoperative drainage of cystotomies depend on the extent of the injury, factors that may delay healing, and the security of the closure. Following cystotomy at the time of vaginal hysterectomy or intraperitoneal injuries, the bladder is drained for 7 to 10 days. If the injury occurs extraperitoneally, the bladder may be drained for as little as 2 days. Before removing the catheter, some advocate obtaining a cystogram to evaluate the integrity of the bladder.

Although in theory, intraoperative recognition and repair may avert the formation of a VVF, Tancer noted more than 21% of patients formed a VVF despite immediate repair of intraoperative cystotomy at the time of hysterectomy.

CLINICAL PRESENTATION OF A FISTULA

The most common presenting feature of a VVF is continuous leakage of urine from the vagina. When VVF follows gynecologic surgery, urinary leakage is most commonly recognized in the first 10 days after operation and less commonly, between the 10th and 20th postoperative days. Rarely does incontinence develop later. In the case of posthysterectomy VVF, onset of symptoms and early diagnosis may be delayed by postoperative vaginal cuff edema. In rare cases, it may be difficult to distinguish urine loss secondary to a VVF and other forms of urinary incontinence.

The size and location of the fistula determines the degree of leakage. Patients with small fistulae may void normal amounts of urine and notice only slight position-dependent drainage.

Alternatively, they may experience leakage only at maximal bladder capacity. The patient may present with recurrent cystitis or pyelonephritis; unexplained fever; hematuria; flank, vaginal, or suprapubic pain; and abnormal urinary stream. Women with larger fistulae may not be able to collect enough urine intravesically to void normally. Irritation of the vagina, vulvar mucosa, and perineum follows, and women report a foul ammoniacal odor. As urea is split by vaginal flora, the vaginal pH becomes alkaline, which precipitates greenish-gray phosphate crystals in the vagina and on the vulva. These crystals serve to further irritate what already may be compromised tissue. Large vaginal encrustations are seen with fistulae secondary to neglected vaginal foreign bodies. This constant leakage of urine may make the patient a social recluse; disrupt sexual relations; and lead to depression, low self-esteem, and insomnia. Steady incontinence of urine leads the majority of patients to use a variety of protective methods, including rubber sheets to protect bedding, diapers or rubber pants to protect clothing, and continence pad products.

Kursh and associates examined the records of 12 patients who had VVF develop after total abdominal hysterectomy. Most of the patients had excessive postoperative abdominal pain, distention or paralytic ileus, or both. Hematuria and symptoms of bladder irritability were also noted in women who suffered a fistula. A prolonged, postoperative fever and increased white blood cell count occurred more often in the fistula group. The clinical features described are seen with an unrecognized bladder injury resulting in intraperitoneal extravasation of urine.

EVALUATION OF A VESICOVAGINAL FISTULA

Even though a diagnosis is obvious in many patients, a thorough urologic investigation is mandatory, especially to rule out coexistent fistulae. In a series of 43 patients with VVF, Goodwin and Scardino found 12% to have an associated ureterovaginal fistula. Lee and associates found 10 of 53 patients (19%) with urethrovaginal fistulae also had a separate VVF.

An evaluation begins with a history and physical examination facilitated by use of a speculum, good lighting, and positioning. A history of large-volume vaginal leakage with no voided urine suggests a sizable defect, whereas lesser vaginal fluid drainage associated with regular voiding raises the possibility of a small VVF or one that only leaks intermittently. Small volumes of drainage may be associated with a vesicouterine or vesicocervical fistula. Only rarely is urine seen actually coming from the cervical os. Vaginal fluid may be collected for measurement of urea concentration to confirm that it is urine as opposed to peritoneal fluid or ascites. Urinalysis and urine culture may identify the presence of a concomitant infection. Intravenous urography may aid in localizing the fistula, assessing ureteral anatomy, and determining the adequacy of renal function. Leakage from the vagina both during and after voiding suggests a urethrovaginal fistula. These fistulae usually are easily distinguished on examination. Otherwise, a double balloon Tratner catheter may be used to perform positive pressure urethrography with contrast medium.

Dye flowing into the vagina demonstrates the fistula. Dye tests traditionally have been performed to evaluate patients for a urinary tract fistula. With the patient in lithotomy position for a pelvic examination, a transurethral catheter is placed and a speculum is inserted into the vagina to facilitate inspection. In the case of a larger VVF, urine is encountered immediately; in most cases, the fistula itself is visualized and the diagnosis confirmed. In the event that the fistula is not easily visualized, the vaginal apex is sponged dry, and 100 cc of a dilute solution of methylene blue or indigo carmine is instilled in the bladder via a Foley catheter. This is done with the speculum in place and the vaginal cuff or cervix and upper vagina in full view. Appearance of blue dye indicates a vesical fistula. The vaginal apex should be carefully scrutinized to identify the site of the fistula. If no dye is seen, it is possible that the open speculum is occluding the fistula. In this situation, the speculum should be slowly rotated, partially closed, and slowly withdrawn to see if dye begins to leak into the vagina as the speculum blades are repositioned. If dye is still not seen in the vagina, a tampon is inserted, and the patient is asked to sit up and ambulate for 15 or 20 minutes. With the patient on the examining table once again, the tampon is carefully removed. If blue dye stains the end adjacent to the vaginal apex, a small VVF probably is present. If the distal end of the tampon near the vaginal introitus is blue, urethral integrity may be compromised. If the tampon is wet with urine, but not blue, a ureterovaginal fistula is likely. The patient's symptoms of vaginal fluid leakage may result from leakage of urine from the ureter with pooling in the vagina and subsequent loss of this urine from the vagina when the patient changes position or moves about.

When the tampon does not stain blue with retrograde bladder filling, further dye studies may be done to demonstrate a ureterovaginal fistula. The bladder is emptied and flushed with saline, and 2 cc of sterile methylene blue or indigo carmine is injected intravenously. An alternate method is administration of phenazopyridine hydrochloride orally. One advantage of phenazopyridine is ease of administration. A second is that it stains urine an orange color, which eliminates any confusion with blue in the bladder. With either option, a fresh tampon is inserted and left in place for 15 minutes. If the upper end of the new tampon is stained, a ureterovaginal fistula is probably present. The vaginal apex is inspected carefully. Leakage of dye from one side of the postoperative vaginal apex strongly suggests the ipsilateral ureter is most likely the site of the fistula, but this is not definitive. An intravenous urogram or retrograde pyelogram is indicated not only to confirm the side of involvement but also the level of the fistula.

Before any attempt at surgical repair, all patients should undergo cystourethroscopy, with careful attention paid to the bladder neck, ureteral orifices, and urethra. The exact location of the fistula in relation to the ureteral orifices, its size, and its possible underlying cause should be determined. Additional fistulous communications need to be excluded to reduce the risk of surgical failure. Larger fistulae may prohibit or cause difficulty in performing liquid-based cystoscopy. In that case, the vagina may be packed with gauze to limit egress of fluid. Alternatively, the bladder may be allowed to fill with air and dry cystoscopy performed with the patient in a jackknife or knee-chest position. Carbon dioxide also may be used as a distention medium.

The ureteral orifices should be identified and evaluated. Urine fails to spurt through the orifice of a damaged or obstructed ureter. On rare occasions, a compromised ureter continues to spurt urine from the ureteral orifice. With a previously ligated ureter or damaged kidney, the ureters may look atrophic, and no urine flow is seen. Attempts to pass a ureteral catheter usually fail when the tip reaches the point of obstruction. A retrograde pyelogram sometimes is needed to fully evaluate the ureter. A ureterovaginal fistula is associated commonly with hydronephrosis and hydroureter because stenosis of the ureter occurs at the site of the injury. Scarring at the edges of a VVF in the region of the ureteral orifice also may lead to ureteral stenosis and proximal dilatation. Further discussion of the differential diagnosis of ureteral fistula is found in Chapter 39.

Although novel radiologic techniques are proving useful in other fields of medicine, their efficacy in the diagnosis of urogenital fistula does not surpass traditional methods. The use of computed tomography (CT) with intravaginal contrast has been reported with limited success. CT may be more helpful in evaluating for coexistent disease involving the upper tracts before surgical correction. Recently, color Doppler ultrasound with contrast media has been described as a diagnostic tool. Sonography was positive in 11 of 12 (92%) patients with VVF. (A jet phenomenon was demonstrated through the bladder wall, in the direction of the vagina, which was distinguishable from ureteral flow.) All patients were known to have fistulae before enrollment into these studies, and specificity of color Doppler for detection of VVF cannot be calculated. In fact, 100% were shown to have a fistula with dye tests. The benefits of color Doppler are that is it easy to learn, noninvasive, results in no radiation exposure, and can evaluate the distance from the fistula to the ureteral orifices. Abulafia and colleagues described the diagnostic use of transperineal ultrasound in a woman who was unable to undergo cystoscopy secondary to urethral obstruction. Currently available ultrasonography and CT are unlikely to replace the traditional diagnostic methods of intravenous urography, retrograde pyelograms, and cystoscopy.

Preoperative urodynamic testing is defended by some authors. Hilton argues for its use before surgical repair of urogenital fistulae to establish the presence of abnormal lower urinary tract function. In his series of the 38 patients, 47% had genuine stress incontinence, 40% showed detrusor instability, and 17% had impaired bladder compliance. The overall incidence of functional abnormality was highest in the patients with urethral or bladder neck fistulae. Most patients became continent after surgical treatment of the fistulae. Those who had urethral or bladder neck fistulae had more residual detrusor instability. Thomas and Williams argue that documenting abnormal urodynamic findings may protect the surgeon medicolegally and prepare patients for a less than perfect outcome. However, for the typical vaginal repair of a posthysterectomy VVF, *de novo* detrusor instability is rare.

Anatomic Considerations

Posthysterectomy fistulae are usually supratrigonal and medial to both ureteral orifices. Vaginally, this corresponds to the cuff. Fistulae from obstetric causes are typically larger, more distal, and may be associated with urethral injury. Obstetric fistulae have been classified according to their anatomic location in relation to the cervix. They may have a single channel or multiple channels. There may be a single orifice on one side that tracks to multiple orifices on the other side, although this presentation is very unusual (Fig. 39.2). Cystourethroscopy and possible hysteroscopy are absolutely indicated before surgical repair to delineate the anatomy of the fistula or fistulae.

Preoperative Care

Cystitis, vaginitis, and perineal dermatitis should be treated with the appropriate antibiotic. Acute cystitis is uncommon in conjunction with a VVF; therefore, suppressive antibiotic therapy is unnecessary unless upper tract infection is suspected. Perineal care is important and makes the patient more comfortable and tolerant of delayed closure. Frequent pad changes are required to minimize inflammation, edema, and vulvar irritation. Incontinence products are much preferred over menstrual hygiene products because incontinence products are designed for the larger volume associated with drainage of urine and the low viscosity of urine. Zinc oxide ointment or a cream containing lanolin may be especially helpful in the treatment of perineal and vulvar dermatitis. Inventive collection and drainage

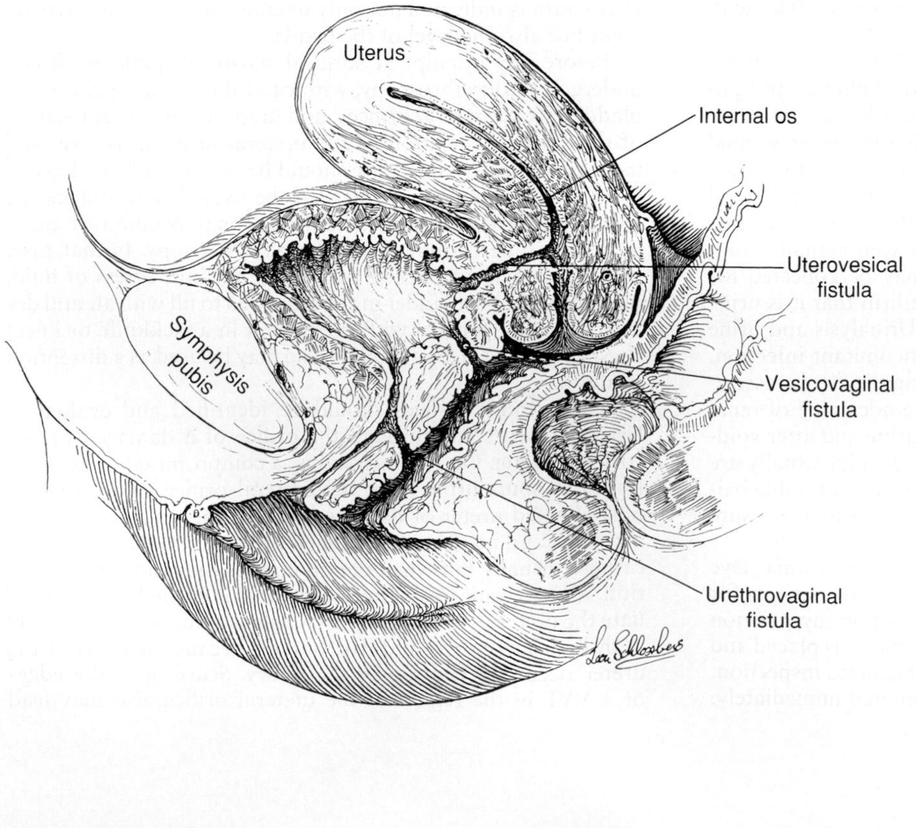

FIGURE 39.2. Sagittal section showing vesicocervical, vesicovaginal, and urethrovaginal fistulae.

systems have been described for this purpose as well. Green and Philips described using dental prosthetic techniques to create a vaginal appliance to control urinary incontinence resulting from a VVF. Another system has been fashioned by gluing a Pezzer catheter to a fitted contraceptive diaphragm with rubber cement (Fig. 39.3). This device traps urine in the vagina and diverts it to a collecting leg bag. It may be worn for the weeks or months before repair is carried out.

Every attempt should be made to divert the urinary stream to protect the perineum and allow the fistula margins to mature. In fact, fistulae <5 mm in greatest dimension may close with catheter drainage alone. In a series of urogenital fistulae referred to a tertiary unit, 7% closed without the need for surgery (Hilton, unpublished data).

Medical therapy as an adjunct to surgery also is important. In the case of the malnourished patient, healing is improved if nutrition needs are optimized and anemia corrected before surgery. Some have described the preoperative use of steroids to reduce tissue inflammation. Despite earlier reports of efficacy, no convincing evidence exists that steroid therapy improves tissue quality before closure or that repair is more likely to be successful. In theory, steroid therapy could even interfere with healing when an early repair is attempted. The authors do not use steroids as an adjunct for these reasons. Estrogen therapy may be used to improve tissue thickness and vascularity provided there are no contraindications. Hyperbaric oxygen has been described as an adjuvant to surgery for radiation-induced fistulae.

Timing of Repair

The timing of repair remains controversial. The traditional belief is to wait a minimum of 3 to 6 months after the inciting event or the last attempt at repair. The delay allows the inflammatory or necrotic fistula margins that are thought to be responsible for surgical failure to resolve and the outcome of cancer therapy to be reevaluated. This interim period of waiting is often very distressing for the patient. O'Conor has said, "A surgeon must stand firm in his conviction that an impatient patient is easier to manage than a surgical failure." Wein and colleagues have attributed surgical failures to an inadequate delay until repair. Lee and associates recommended delaying surgery to increase the success rate of the first attempt at repair. Symmonds recommends generally waiting 3 to 4 months for the tissues to "clean up," lose their edema, and obtain good vascularity and pliability. In a series from Duke University Medical Center, Iselin and colleagues had a 100% cure rate with an average time to repair of 16 weeks.

Transvaginal repair of VVF within a few weeks of diagnosis was first reported in 1960 by Collins and associates. Patients received 100 mg of cortisone three times daily for 10 to 12 days preoperatively. Of 15 patients without a history of pelvic malignancy or radiation therapy, 13 (87%) had successful repairs. In this series, 3 of 5 (60%) patients with cervical cancer and radiation-induced fistulae had recurrences within a brief postoperative period. Eleven years later, these same authors reported a 28% failure rate in a series of 38 patients, all of whom had a transvaginal repair and preoperative steroids within 60 days after diagnosis. The experience with steroids and early closure was again updated in 1984 as O'Quin in an abstract for the Society of Pelvic Surgeons with a series of 54 patients, 11% of whom required a second procedure for successful repair.

Because reported series of early repair with steroid therapy do not show superior results, the use of steroids as an adjunct is no longer accepted. Persky and associates, also advocates for early repair, reported a series of seven patients who all underwent successful transvesical repair using interposition grafts of peritoneum or omentum within 10 weeks of the antecedent surgery. Cruikshank also had success in 10 of 11

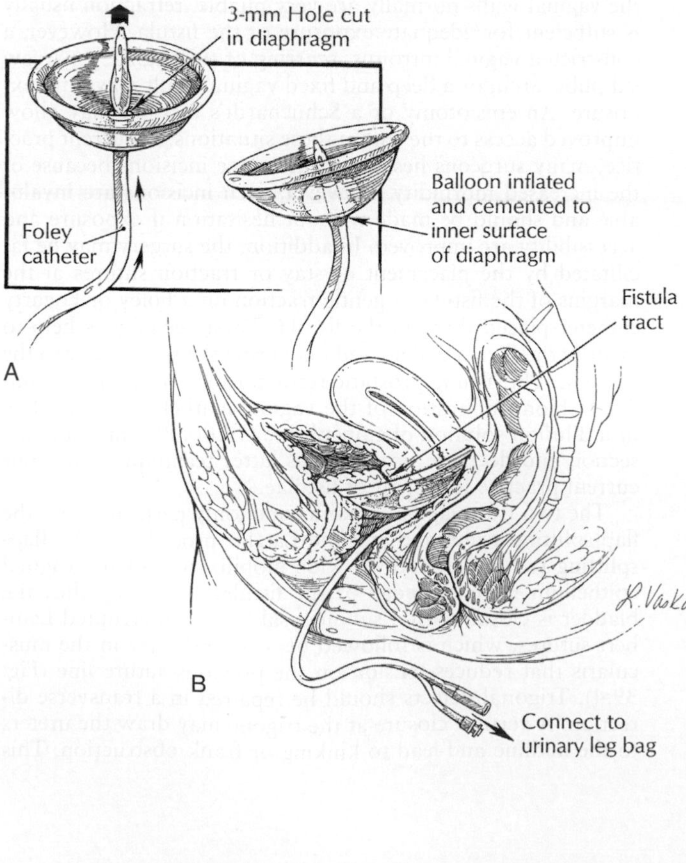

FIGURE 39.3. Vaginal appliance for collecting urine from urinary tract fistula. **A:** The tip of a urinary catheter has been placed through a small opening in the center of a contraceptive diaphragm. The catheter balloon is inflated and cemented to the inner surface of the diaphragm. **B:** The appliance is inserted so the diaphragm covers the fistula. The catheter exits the vagina and is connected to a collection bag. The figure shows the uterus in place, but the appliance is effective in a patient who has had hysterectomy. (Reproduced with permission: Nichols DH, Randall CL. *Vaginal surgery.* 4th ed. Baltimore, MD: 1996:437.)

fistulae in his series repaired between 10 and 35 days after a hysterectomy. None of these latter series used preoperative steroid therapy.

Treatment should be tailored to the individual patient. If the fistula is recognized within the first 48 hours postoperatively, the tissue should be more mobile, have less inflammation, and be amenable to early repair. Fistulae arising later usually are complicated by significant edema, inflammation, and induration. An interval of 3 months from injury to repair in obstetric and surgical fistulae allows inflammation and edema to resolve. As long as 1 year may be required for improvement in the tissues in radiation-induced fistulae before repair; that is, it is difficult to determine accurately when radiation necrosis has run its course. The outcome of prolonged catheterization alone for small fistulae is unpredictable. Large fistulae may be easier to repair once the tract is allowed to scar and edema resolves. On the other hand, the delay of closure may have a significant negative impact on a patient's quality of life.

The principles outlined for VVF repair also are applicable to urethrovaginal fistulae. Because the urethra has a minimum of redundant tissue with which to work, the tissues must be as near to normal as possible before a repair is undertaken. A delay of several months usually is recommended to allow tissues to completely heal and for inflammation to resolve.

SURGICAL TECHNIQUE: VESICOVAGINAL FISTULA

Surgery is the mainstay of therapy for urogenital fistulae. Following the tenets of Sims, Symmonds proposed several surgical principles to improve the success rate of fistula repair: (a) wide mobilization of the vaginal epithelium to expose the bladder; (b) excision of all scar tissue, even at the risk of increasing the size of the fistula in an attempt to create a "fresh bladder injury" (this recommendation is not universally endorsed); (c) a tension-free layered closure of the bladder and the vagina; (d) nontraumatizing technique; (e) good hemostasis; and (f) bladder drainage postoperatively. These principles are the same for fistulae involving the urethra. Although most authors agree that the best chance at closure of the fistula is the primary attempt, staged procedures have been described. Unfortunately, no controlled trials of route or timing of repair are available to guide management, and the general view is for individualized management.

In most cases, the gynecologic surgeon will favor the vaginal approach, which avoids the potential morbidity associated with abdominal surgery and is believed to provide a quicker recovery and a more cosmetic result. Because it does not require a laparotomy, it is considered to be easier, safer, and more comfortable for the patient. Success rates of 98% and 100% have been reported in two of the larger series. Although an abdominal approach has traditionally been favored for larger fistulae, fistulae located high on the posterior wall, fistulae adjacent to the ureters, and concurrent intraabdominal pathology, the usual postsurgical fistula is low in the bladder and easily accessible in the anterior vaginal wall. However, an attempted vaginal repair of a fistula high in an immobile vaginal vault may be limited by visibility and lead to a less than satisfactory result. The abdominal route of repair offers benefit in this circumstance.

Involvement of the ureter also may require an abdominal approach to facilitate ureteral reimplantation. Laparotomy is necessary in fistulae requiring bowel for augmentation cystoplasty. In certain circumstances, a combined vaginal and abdominal approach may be helpful. The authors have described a combined approach to the repair of a large fistula secondary to a vaginal foreign body that involved the trigone.

There is no consensus concerning the need to excise the fistulous tract. Some authors advocate its total removal, whereas others prefer to merely debride the margins, thereby avoiding an increase in the size of the defect. Iselin and associates advocate the excision of the fistula tract and vaginal cuff scar. This step enables the surgeon to suture viable tissues in every layer to promote wound healing, obviating the need for interpositional flaps or grafts. They reported a 100% cure rate on first attempt. In their series of 65 transvaginal repairs, Raz and associates did not excise the fistula tract in any patient and had no apparent adverse effects. Cruikshank did not excise the tract in a series of 11 patients and had a 100% cure rate. Zacharin warns that excision of the fistula scar markedly increases the risk of operative failure. Elkins and colleagues and Lawson also advised against excising the tract in large obstetric fistulae.

APPROACH FOR VESICOVAGINAL FISTULA REPAIR

Patient positioning for greater visualization of the fistula edges is a matter of physician preference and some debate. Most prefer lithotomy position for a typical fistula at the vaginal cuff. However, Elkins and others feel that adequate visualization, especially of the proximal urethra and bladder neck, can best be achieved by the knee-chest or Lawson position. Dropping the head of the table and elevating the buttocks may further facilitate exposure.

Technical difficulties encountered at surgery are likely to be avoided by optimal exposure and accessibility of the fistula rather than a change in specific instrumentation. Because the vaginal walls normally are very pliable, retraction usually is sufficient for adequate exposure of the fistula. However, a constricted vaginal introitus, scarring of the vagina, a narrow subpubic arch, or a deep and fixed vaginal vault may limit exposure. An episiotomy or a Schuchardt's incision may allow improved access to the cuff in these situations. In current practice, many surgeons hesitate to use these incisions because of the increased morbidity. However, such incisions are invaluable and should be made without hesitation if exposure and accessibility are improved. In addition, the surgery may be facilitated by the placement of stay or traction sutures at the margins of the fistula or gentle traction on a Foley or Fogarty catheter placed through the fistula. These techniques help to identify the fistula's edges and may bring the tract closer to the surgeon. The Young prostatic retractor may be used in a similar fashion. Infiltration of the vaginal epithelium with saline or a dilution solution of epinephrine (1:200,000) may aid dissection and decrease oozing. This latter technique is not our current practice for repair of fistulae.

The two transvaginal repairs commonly performed are the flap-splitting technique and the Latzko procedure. The **flap-splitting technique** involves wide mobilization of the vaginal epithelium from the edge of the fistula. Following this, the bladder is closed with a submucosal line of interrupted Lembert sutures, which is followed by a second layer in the muscularis that reduces tension on the previous suture line (Fig. 39.4). Trigonal defects should be repaired in a transverse direction. A vertical closure at the trigone may draw the ureters to the midline and lead to kinking or frank obstruction. This

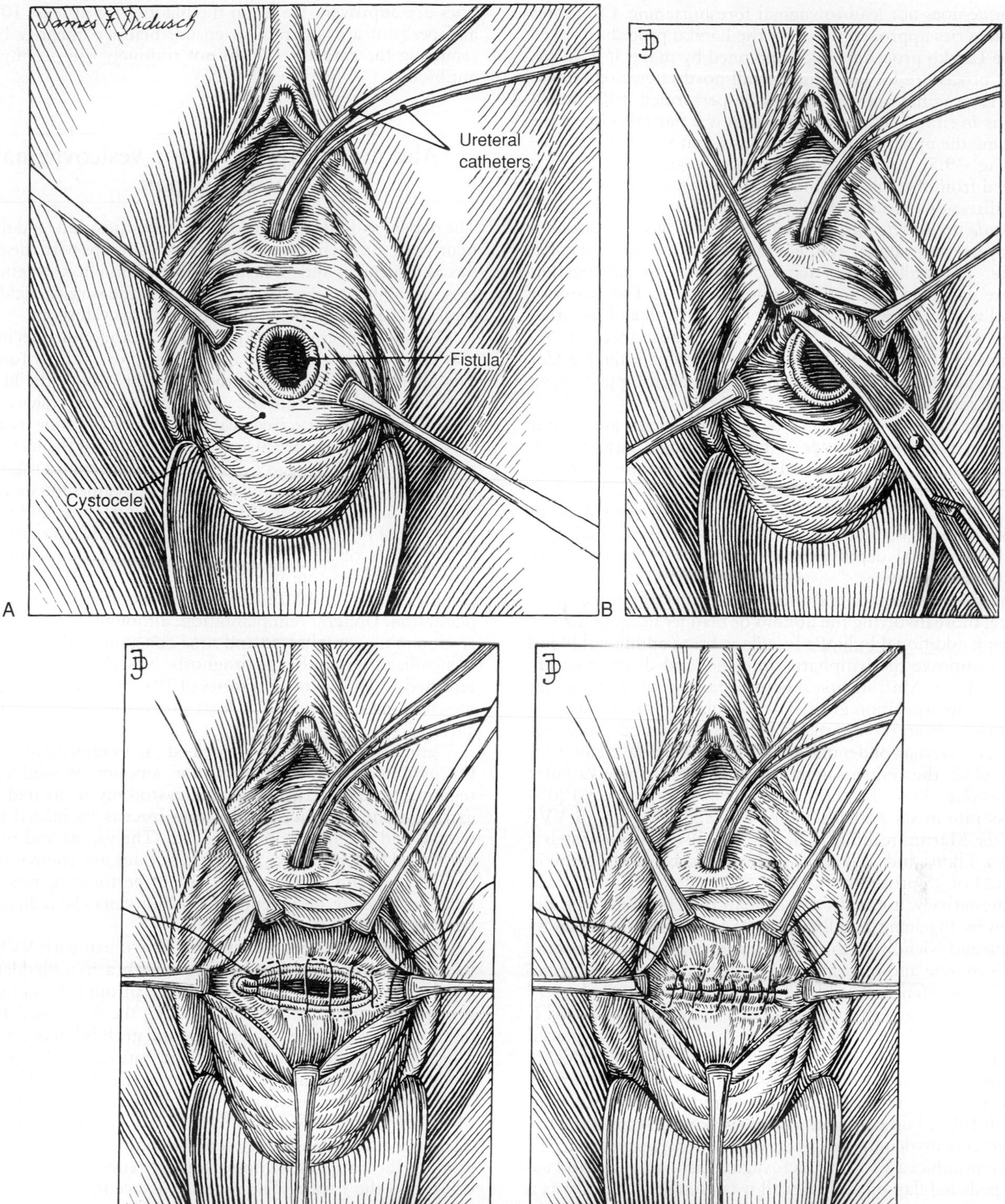

FIGURE 39.4. Flap-splitting closure of a simple vesicovaginal fistula. **A:** Ureters have been catheterized. An incision through the vaginal epithelium is made circumferentially around the fistula. **B:** The vaginal epithelium is widely mobilized from the bladder. The scarred fistula tract should be excised. **C:** A continuous (or interrupted) delayed-absorbable suture inverts the mucosa into the bladder. **D:** A second suture line is placed in the musculofascial layer to reinforce the first. Vaginal epithelium is trimmed and approximated.

technique does not lead to vaginal foreshortening. Cure rates in some series approach those for the Latzko procedure.

The **Latzko procedure** is championed by many. It is an excellent procedure for correcting small posthysterectomy fistulae at the vaginal apex. It cannot be performed if the cervix remains *in situ*. The Latzko operation is a partial colpocleisis involving the upper 2 to 3 cm of vagina that surrounds the fistula (Fig. 39.5). An elliptical portion of vaginal epithelium is stripped from the anterior and posterior fascia at least 2.5 cm in all directions around the fistula tract. *The vesical edges of the fistula are not denuded.* The pubovesical fascia is closed in two layers, and vaginal epithelium is closed using interrupted sutures. The walls have a natural tendency to fall together and are easily approximated without tension. The posterior vaginal wall becomes the posterior bladder wall and reepithelializes with urothelium. Theoretically, because there are no sutures in the bladder wall with a Latzko repair, the bladder wall can fill without tension, obviating the need for prolonged catheterization.

Success rates for the Latzko partial colpocleisis are greater than 89% at the first attempt. Other advantages include short operating time, minimal blood loss, and low postoperative morbidity. Because posthysterectomy fistulae are almost always small and high in the vagina, the loss of vaginal depth and interference with sexual function should be minimal. Furthermore, vaginal depth expands once the patient resumes intercourse.

Interposition flaps or **grafts** may be used in large or recurrent fistulae, those involving the urethra or bladder neck, or fistulae requiring additional bulk. Pedicle flaps bring additional blood supply, improve the lymphatic drainage, and distance suture lines. In 1928, Martius first described the use of the labial fat pad as an interposition graft. The vascular supply to the graft inferiorly is from the internal pudendal artery and superiorly from the external pudendal artery. In mobilizing a labial fat pad pedicle, the surgeon must preserve one of these vascular bundles (Fig. 39.6). Birkhoff and colleagues reported a 100% success rate in six patients with transvaginal repairs of VVF using the Martius technique. In a series mostly of postobstetric injuries, Elkins and colleagues reported a successful closure in 96% (24 of 25 procedures).

Alternatively, a gracilis muscle flap may be used. First described by Ingelman-Sundberg in 1954, and later modified by Hamlin and Nicholson, the technique involves dissection of the gracilis muscle and separation of its attachment to the medial condyle of the femur. The blood supply from the femoral artery is preserved. The graft may be rotated or advanced directly. It is then tunneled under the labia at the introitus and placed over the fistula. The gracilis muscle provides a bulky closure to urogenital fistulae with new tissue and a new blood supply, which may be particularly useful in postradiation or large, traumatic fistulae. Fujiwara and associates have described the use of a gracilis myocutaneous graft in a patient with concurrent radiation-induced VVF and rectovaginal fistulae. A method using a pedicled flap of vaginal wall was presented recently as a case report by Hurley and Previte. Although the results were good in this case, a subvaginal cyst may develop in the buried vaginal tissue.

Regardless of the route of repair for VVF, the closure should be watertight. The integrity of the repair may be tested during surgery by filling the bladder with 200 cc of fluid colored with methylene blue or indigo carmine. We prefer to leave a pack in the vagina 24 hours postoperatively and drain the bladder with a suprapubic catheter. The bladder can be drained for as little as 2 days or as long as 3 weeks. The need for a cystogram before discontinuing drainage and the benefit of prophylactic antibiotics are unproven. We drain the bladder for at least 10 days and perform a cystogram to ensure bladder integrity before removing the catheter. We do not routinely use prophylactic antibiotics.

Abdominal Approach for Vesicovaginal Fistula Repair

The patient should be in the low lithotomy position, and the patient's legs should be placed in universal stirrups with the thighs flexed 15 degrees and abducted slightly. This allows vaginal access, the ability to elevate the fistula into the surgical field with a vaginal hand, and the ability to perform cystoscopy.

O'Conor and coworkers pioneered an abdominal technique that can be performed extraperitoneally or intraperitoneally. The bladder is bisected, and the posterior wall of the bladder is widely mobilized from the vagina through the vesicovaginal space. The fistula is excised, leaving margins of viable tissue for closure. Stay sutures are placed on either side of the incision to facilitate exposure (Fig. 39.7). Both the bladder and vagina are closed in layers. Mondet and coworkers documented successful outcome in 85% (24 of 28) of patients after transperitoneal-transvesical repair of VVF (after O'Conor). It is notable that in this series of 28 VVF, 33% required ureteral reimplantation. The success rate was 87.5% for simple VVFs, 71% for complex VVFs, and 80% for fistulae requiring ureteral reimplantation. Ureteral reimplantation, although it makes the operation more complicated and time-consuming, does not seem to significantly worsen the prognosis. Nesrallah and associates reported 100% success in a series of 29 women with VVF, 34% of whom had undergone at least one prior attempt at fistula closure.

Cetin and colleagues described a modification of the O'Conor technique that limits the amount of bladder dissection. A small vertical anterior cystotomy is created in an extraperitoneal fashion. The fistula tract is mobilized to the wound and circumferentially excised. The vagina and bladder are closed in separate layers. Success rates are comparable to the O'Conor and Latzko techniques. By performing the surgery extraperitoneally, perioperative morbidity may be reduced and recovery time shortened.

Vyas and associates reported on 22 women with VVF who were treated by patching the fistula with a free bladder mucosal graft. After exposing the defect through a suprapubic cystotomy, the urothelium surrounding the fistula is debrided but not excised. A free bladder mucosal graft is harvested from a healthy portion of the bladder and sutured to the denuded bladder with interrupted sutures over the fistula. The bladder is drained for 3 weeks to allow the donor site to reepithelialize and the cystotomy to heal. Advantages include a reduced need for extensive dissection and the ability to tailor the graft to the patient's anatomy and proximity to the ureteral orifices to the fistula. The repair was accomplished without the need of ureteroneocystomy, and 90% of the women were cured.

The use of vascularized tissue grafts is helpful in assuring a successful abdominal repair. Omental flaps are excellent in this regard. In fact, one third of omental aprons may reach the deep pelvis without creating a flap. The omentum has a dual blood supply and may be mobilized based on either the right or left gastroepiploic arteries. A laparoscopic approach has even been described. Rectus muscles also have been used as grafts for abdominal repairs. A recent review by Evans and colleagues evaluated the use of interposition grafts for VVFs of benign and

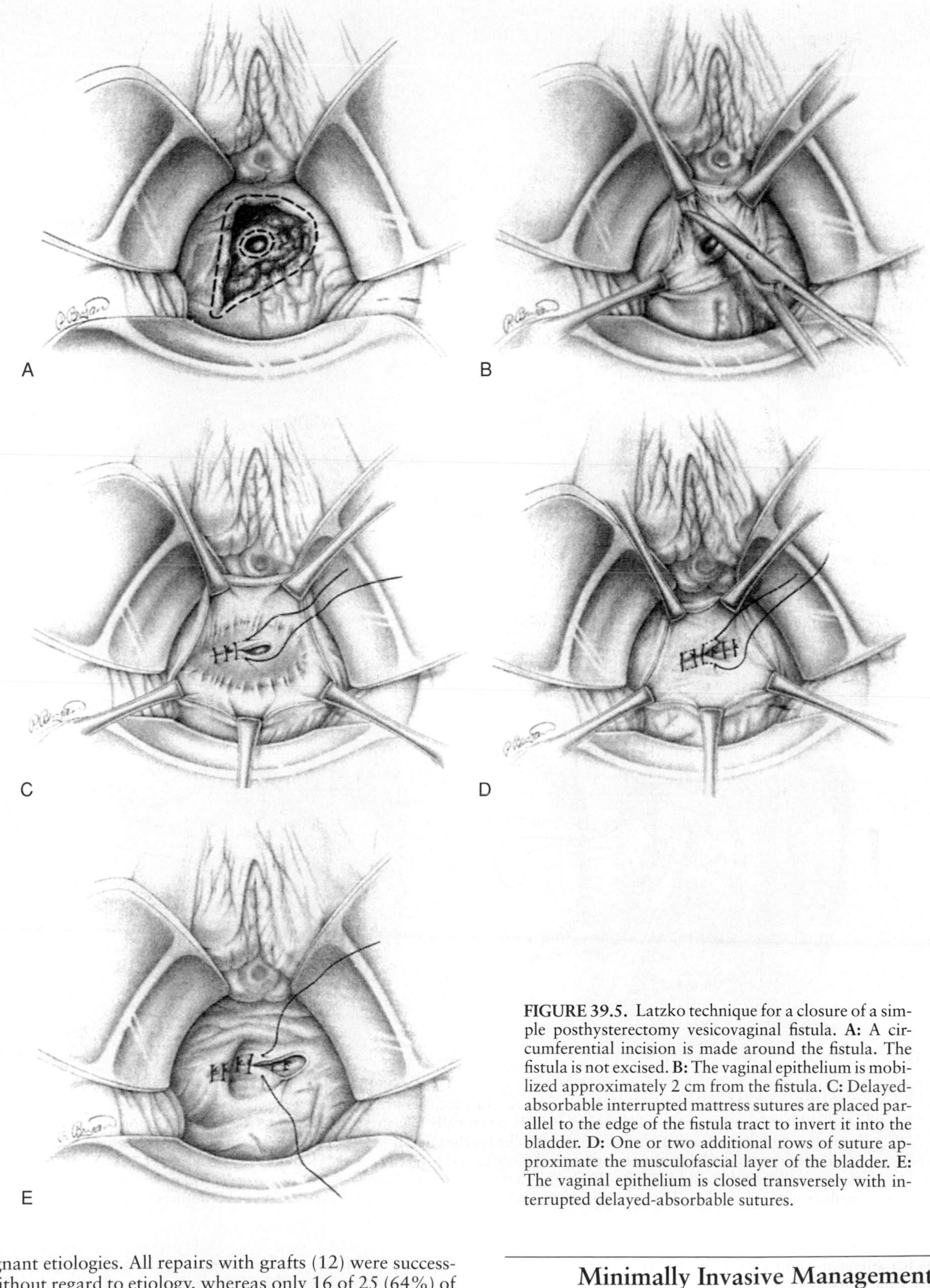

FIGURE 39.5. Latzko technique for a closure of a simple posthysterectomy vesicovaginal fistula. **A:** A circumferential incision is made around the fistula. The fistula is not excised. **B:** The vaginal epithelium is mobilized approximately 2 cm from the fistula. **C:** Delayed-absorbable interrupted mattress sutures are placed parallel to the edge of the fistula tract to invert it into the bladder. **D:** One or two additional rows of suture approximate the musculofascial layer of the bladder. **E:** The vaginal epithelium is closed transversely with interrupted delayed-absorbable sutures.

malignant etiologies. All repairs with grafts (12) were successful without regard to etiology, whereas only 16 of 25 (64%) of repairs without grafts were successful. The authors concluded that transabdominal VVF repairs should be performed with an interposition flap regardless of the appearance of healthy surrounding tissues and etiology.

Minimally Invasive Management

Minimally invasive approaches center on the use of endoscopy and natural orifice access. Sotelo and associates described laparoscopic repair of VVF in 15 patients who had clear

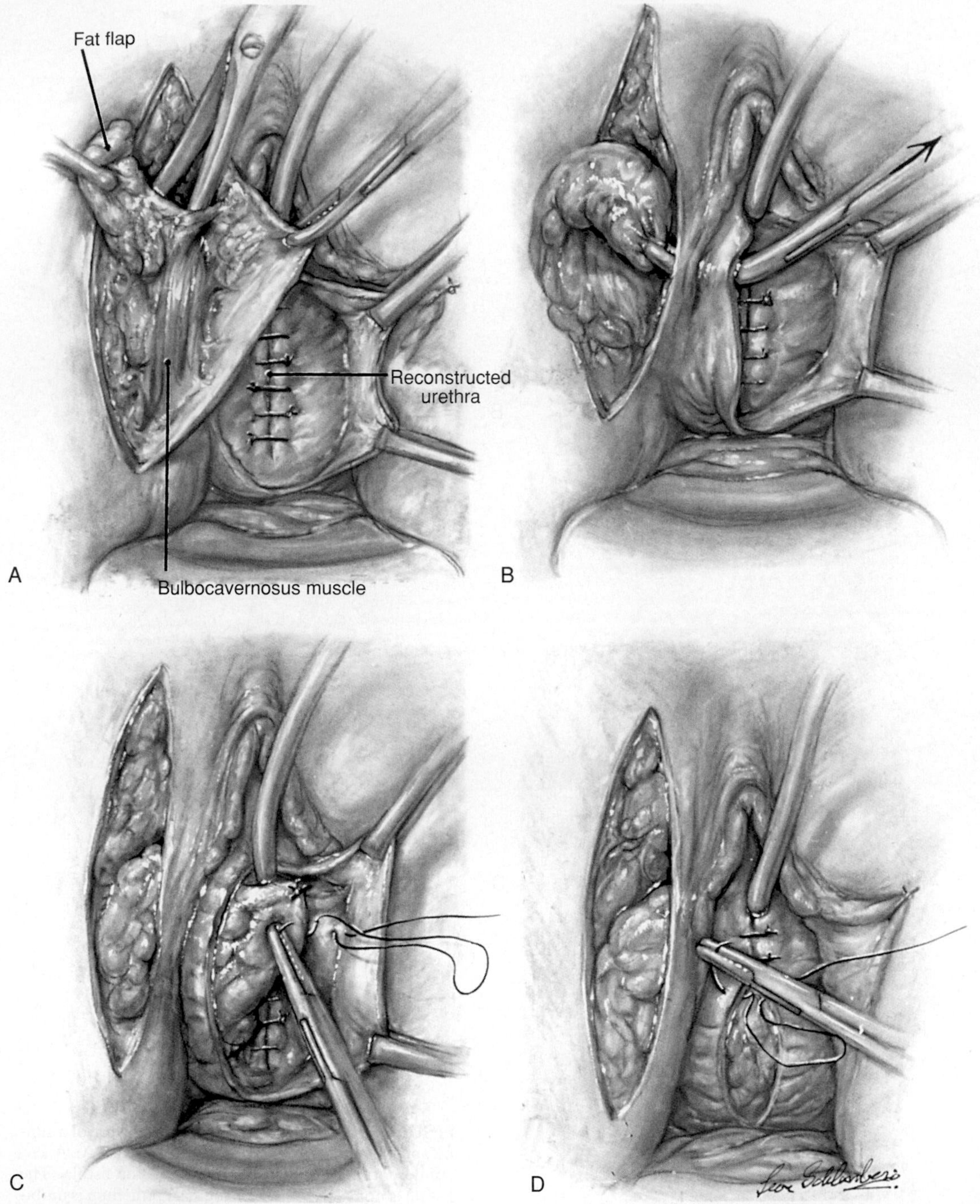

FIGURE 39.6. Martius bulbocavernosus fat pad graft for urethrovaginal or vesicovaginal fistula repair. **A:** The lateral margin of the labia majora is incised vertically. The fat pad adjacent to the bulbocavernosus muscle is mobilized, leaving a broad pedicle attached at the inferior pole. **B, C:** The fat pad is drawn through a tunnel beneath the labia minor and vaginal mucosa and sutured with delayed-absorbable sutures to the fascia of the urethra and bladder. **D:** The vaginal mucosa is mobilized widely to permit closure over the pedicle without tension. The vulvar incision is closed with interrupted delayed-absorbable sutures.

indications for surgical treatment. Hysterectomy was the prior surgery in 14 patients (93%).

The technique involved cystoscopy, catheterization of the VVF, laparoscopic cystotomy, dissection of the vesicovaginal space, opening and excising the fistulous tract, cystotomy and colpotomy closure, and use of an interposition graft. None of the cases required conversion to laparotomy. Operative time, hospital stay, and duration of bladder drainage were comparable to open techniques. Only 1 of 14 patients (7%) had a recurrent postoperative fistula. Chibber and colleagues also reported excellent results when the O'Conor technique is performed via the laparoscopic

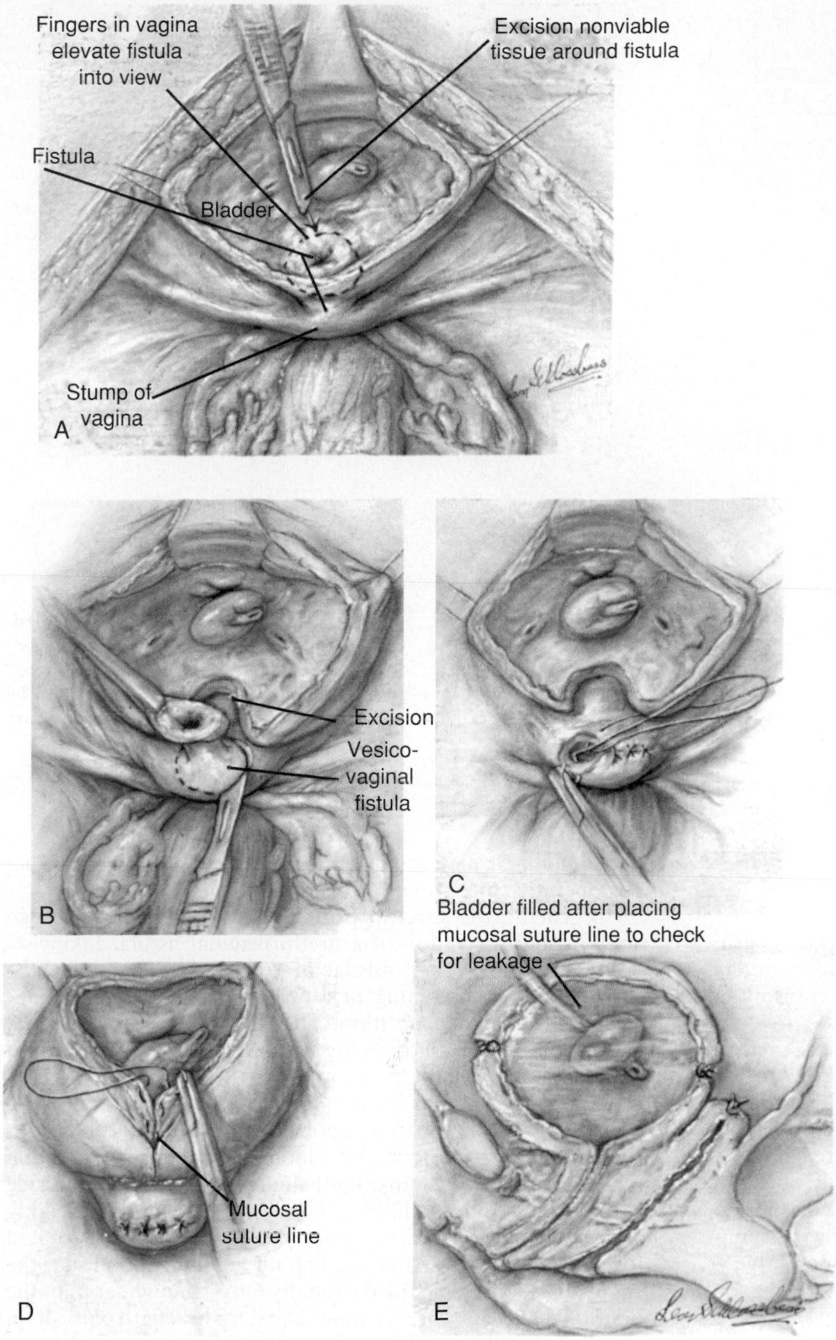

FIGURE 39.7. Transabdominal, transvesical closure of vesicovaginal fistula. **A:** A longitudinal incision is placed in the bladder dome. **B:** The incision is extended around the fistula. The fistulous tract and its vaginal orifice are completely excised. **C:** Interrupted delayed-absorbable sutures are used to close the vagina in one or two layers. **D:** Continuous delayed-absorbable suture closes the bladder mucosa longitudinally. **E:** A suprapubic catheter is placed into the bladder in an extraperitoneal location. (*Continued*)

approach. McKay has described successful repair of VVF using transurethral suture cystorrhaphy. A 5-mm laparoscopic sleeve, for passage of the suture, is inserted alongside a 17F cystourethroscope with a 30-degree lens. Extracorporeal knot tying similar to other endoscopic suturing techniques is used.

Techniques that do not require suture have been used because of the difficulty of extracorporeal knot tying. Successful occlusion of a VVF with fibrin glue was first reported by Pettersson and colleagues in 1979. Because the patient also had continuous bladder drainage for 8 weeks, some questioned the etiology of the success. Recently, Sharma and colleagues reported successful treatment of urinary tract fistulas in eight patients who underwent a single endoscopic injection of fibrin glue. Retrograde endoscopic injection of fibrin glue would appear to offer an efficacious alternative to traditional options for small defects and may avoid the morbidity of open surgery. Electrosurgical fulguration of small VVF followed by continuous drainage has been reported to be successful by Stovsky and associates and Falk and Orkin. Recently, Dogra and Nabi described the use of an endoscopic Nd-YAG laser to fulgurate a small 2- to 3-mm posthysterectomy VVF. They refer to the procedure as a "laser welding." Whether the denuded tract closed spontaneously after the 3-week period of continuous drainage or was truly welded remains a matter of conjecture.

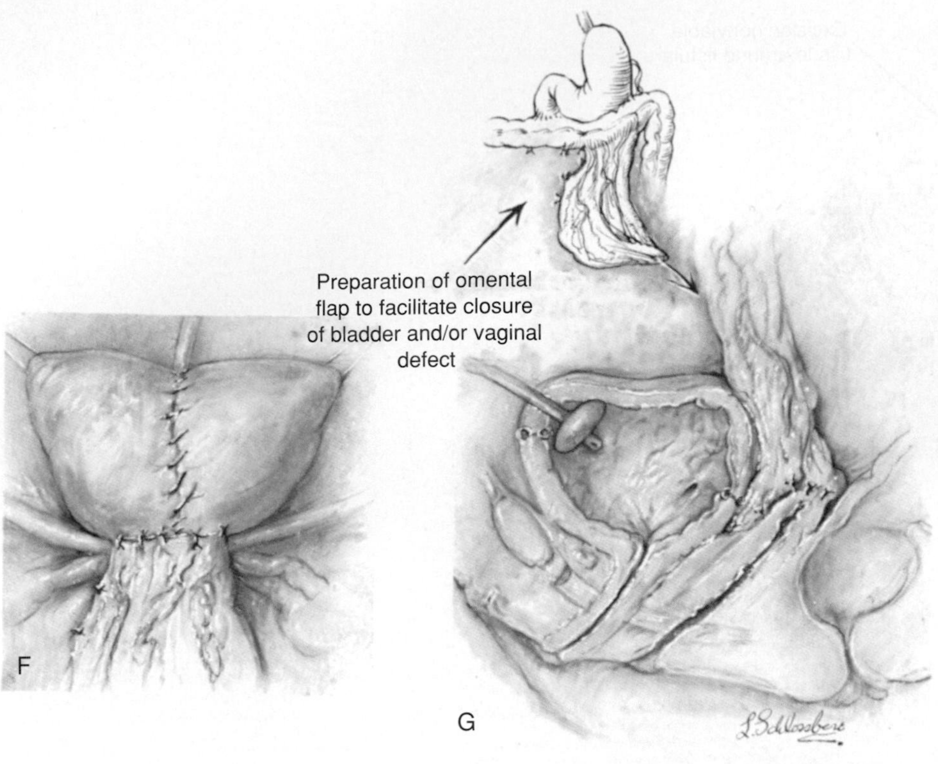

FIGURE 39.7. (*Continued*) **F:** The bladder muscularis is closed with delayed-absorbable continuous or interrupted sutures. **G:** An omental "J" flap can be interposed between the bladder closure and the vaginal closure.

Urethrovaginal Fistula

Damage to the urethra that leads to loss of structural integrity is fortunately uncommon. Parturition, gynecologic surgery, pelvic radiotherapy, pelvic trauma, and sexually transmitted infections that are associated with tissue destruction are common antecedent events. Complications of surgery for urethral diverticulum, cystocele, or urethral hypermobility head the list and account for more than 90% of urethrovaginal fistulae. Indeed, some 15% to 20% of women who have surgery to remove a suburethral diverticulum develop a fistula. The remainder is preceded by intrapartum obstetric events, especially operative vaginal delivery, pelvic radiotherapy, and traumatic disruption.

A urethrovaginal fistula may present with a variety of symptoms, but new onset urinary incontinence is almost always the trigger for diagnostic evaluation. Fistulae involving the proximal urethra and bladder neck present similarly to VVF. Midurethra fistulae may present with stress incontinence, recurrent cystitis, or no symptoms. Patients with distal fistulae may be asymptomatic or report a spraying urinary stream. The algorithm for evaluation of fistula is similar without regard to its etiology.

Most fistulae are easily seen on physical examination. However, when inspection does not reveal the fistula, additional studies are needed. A double balloon urethrogram may reveal an otherwise undemonstrated fistula by increasing pressure in the urethra and forcing fluid through the opening. Because urethrovaginal fistula may be complex and associated with injuries to bladder and ureters, the integrity of the entire urinary tract must be assessed with radiographic imaging, such as cystogram, voiding cystourethrogram, and intravenous pyelogram. The location of the fistula and its relationship to the urethrovesical junction is assessed with cystourethroscopy. Knowing the relationship of the fistula to the bladder neck and to the point of maximum urethral pressure will help predict postoperative incontinence.

In general, the surgical principles for repair of VVF also apply to the correction of a urethrovaginal fistula. Likewise, because urethrovaginal fistulae are relatively uncommon, the surgical approach, timing of repair, and postoperative management lack standardization. The repair of a urethrovaginal fistula is more difficult than for simple VVF. Extensive urethral loss and lack of viable tissue may make conventional layered closures impractical, if not impossible. The success rate of urethrovaginal fistula repair is reported to be 73% to 100%.

Urethral reconstruction of a large defect begins by making a U-shaped flap of vaginal epithelium exposing the underside of the trigone and sphincter. The length of the flap roughly approximates the length of a normal urethra. The flap is rotated forward (Fig. 39.8). After the flap of vagina is mobilized, the vaginal incision is extended caudally 6 to 7 mm wider than the urethral defect and for a distance equal to the length of the flap. The vagina is then mobilized laterally.

The original flap is rotated so that the raw edges of the flap may be sutured to the denuded area of the urethral remnant. When this step is completed on both sides, an epithelial-lined conduit is formed that serves as a neourethra. Because the pedicles are relatively long, they are very susceptible to ischemia and subsequent necrosis. Thus, a layer of paraurethral fascia is plicated beneath the new urethra for support and additional blood supply. Two or three deep sutures are placed in the region of the sphincter and, when tied, will tighten the internal orifice. Approximation of the lateral edges of vaginal epithelium buries the newly constructed urethra and completely closes the wound.

Symmonds described another technique for urethral reconstruction in which an incision is made in the anterior vaginal wall and is extended around the margins of the urethral defect. No more than 2 mm of vaginal epithelium remains attached to

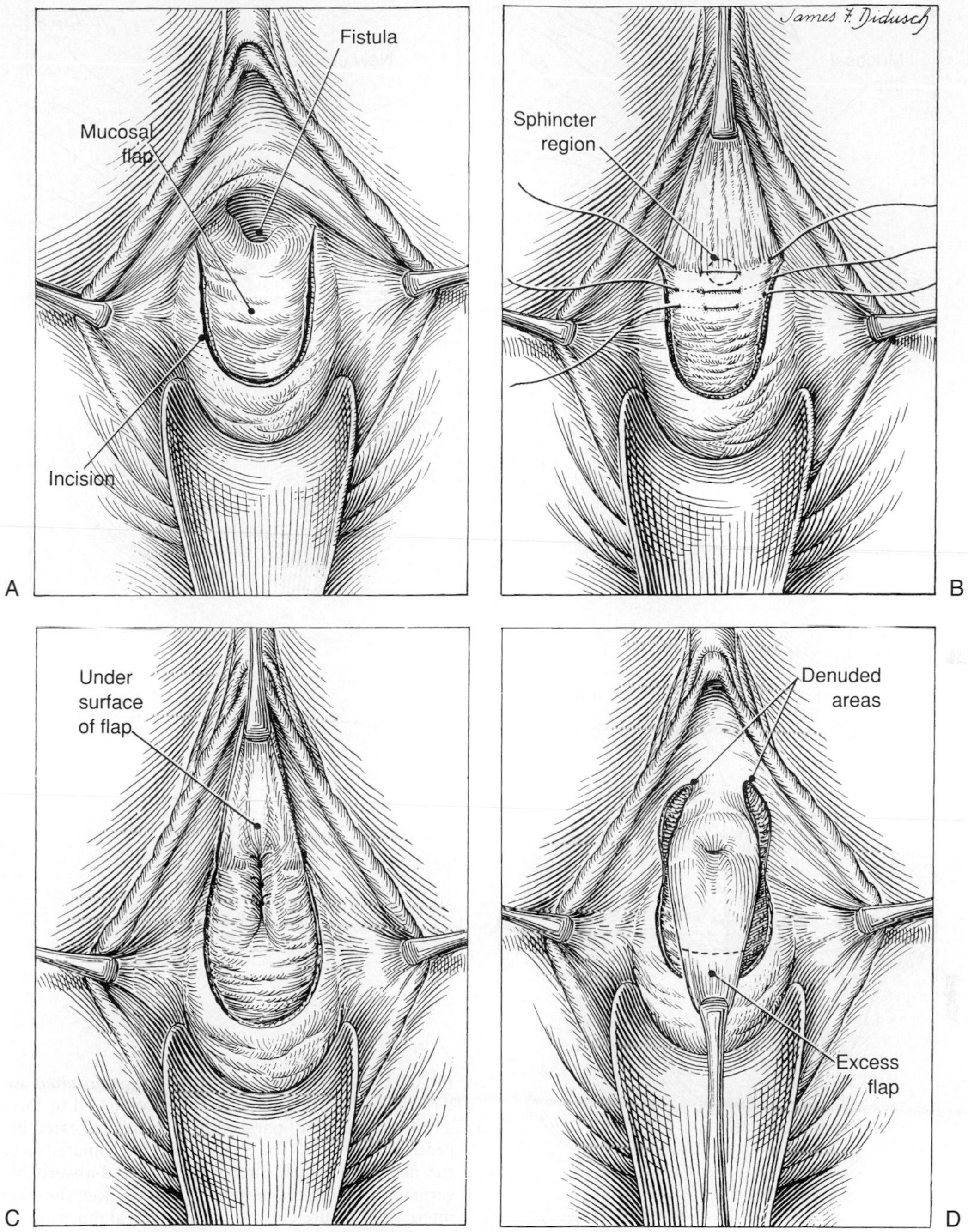

FIGURE 39.8. Reconstruction of urethra and repair of sphincter. **A:** A U-shaped incision is made through the vaginal epithelium. **B:** The flap is mobilized and rotated over the fistula. **C:** Three interrupted sutures of delayed-absorbable suture are placed in the sphincter region, and the tissue inverted. **D:** The mucosal flap is pulled downward, and the incision is extended on both sides. (*Continued*)

the urethral walls. Sharp dissection frees the edges of the retracted urethra while protecting its paraurethral blood supply. Enough urethral tissue must be mobilized to permit tension-free approximation of the edges over a 12F catheter (Fig. 39.9). The fascia adjacent to the newly created urethral tube is freed with sharp dissection, avoiding deep lateral dissection that disrupts the blood supply. Sutures are placed through the fascia on each side of the urethra. Each suture is held until placement of its counterpoint. The lower strand of the pair is tied across the urethral floor, as are the upper strands. Alternatively, vertical mattress sutures may be used to approximate the fascia to support the urethral wall. The vaginal mucosa is closed without tension. The small caliber urethra created by this technique may aid in establishing continence.

Numerous pedicle grafts have been described as sources of tissue to reconstruct a destroyed urethra. These include pedicles mobilized from vaginal epithelium, skin from the vulvar skin, skin of the buttock, and labia minora. Pedicles from the

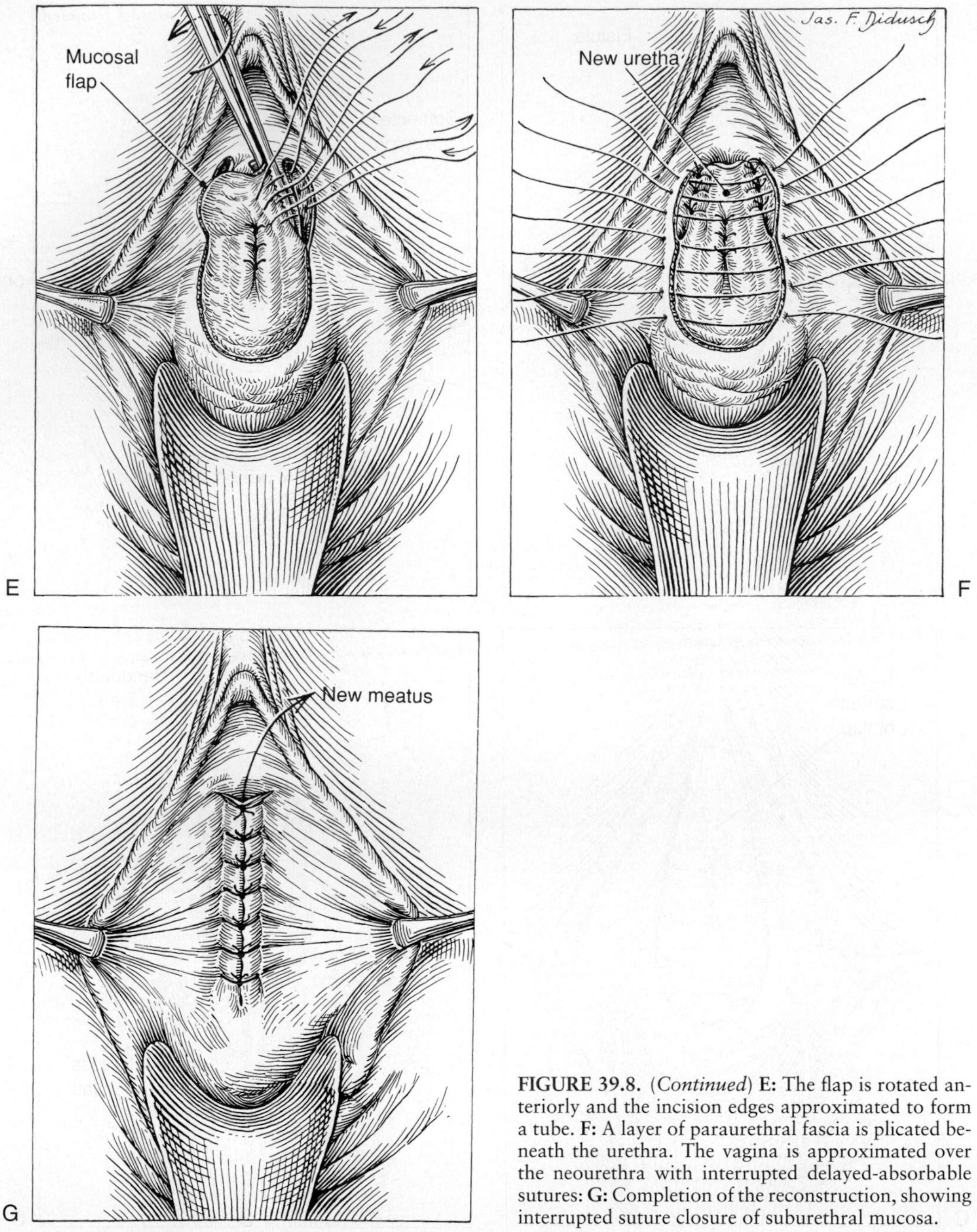

FIGURE 39.8. (*Continued*) **E:** The flap is rotated anteriorly and the incision edges approximated to form a tube. **F:** A layer of paraurethral fascia is plicated beneath the urethra. The vagina is approximated over the neourethra with interrupted delayed-absorbable sutures: **G:** Completion of the reconstruction, showing interrupted suture closure of suburethral mucosa.

buttock have been advocated for especially large defects. The anterior bladder wall can be mobilized via a retropubic approach through the vagina and used to fashion a neourethra. An alternative method is to harvest patch grafts from the detrusor and to use the patch to form a tubular structure. Not enough data is available to prove that one of these techniques has a clear advantage over another. Therefore, use of these grafts is individualized to meet individual patient needs.

When using an abdominal approach, the urethra may be reconstructed using the bladder. Fernandes has reported tubularizing an anterior advancement flap of bladder to reconstruct an entire urethra. Omo-Dare has used patch grafts of bladder mucosa for urethral reconstruction after gonococcal stricture with some success. The use of a tubularized rectus abdominis muscle flap has also been described in a series of refractory urethrovaginal fistula patients, all of whom had undergone at least one unsuccessful repair incorporating a Martius graft.

A pedicle graft may be appropriate to eliminate tissue tension, fill a defect in the vagina, reestablish vascularity, and enhance cosmesis. For the most part, Martius grafts are used for this purpose. The principles are similar to when they are used for VVF.

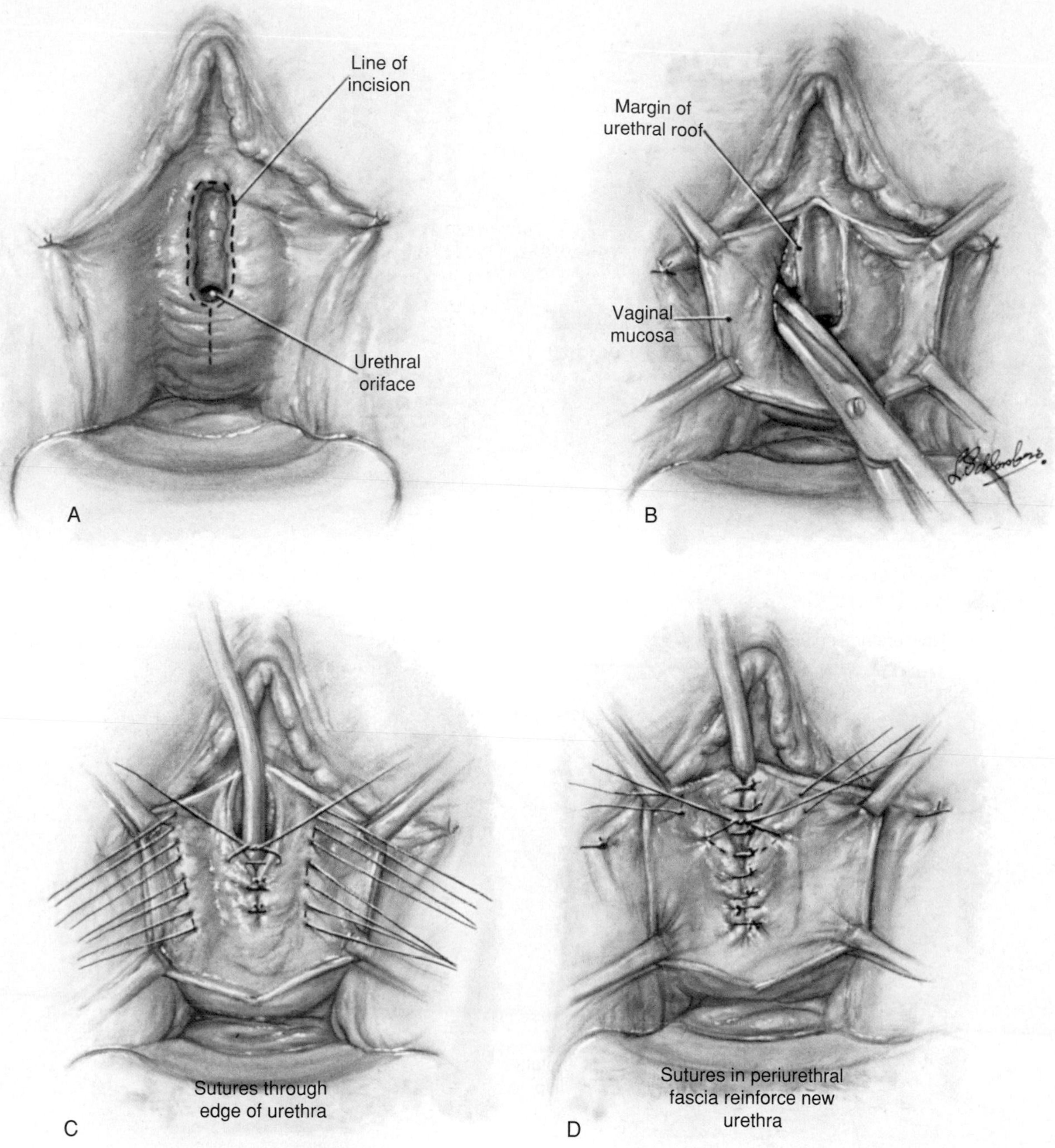

FIGURE 39.9. Reconstruction of total or partial loss of the urethral floor. **A:** A line of incision is made along the margins of the roof of the urethra and extended to the bladder base. **B:** The urethral margins and fascia are mobilized from the vagina to permit tension-free approximation of the urethral mucosa. **C:** Urethral edges are approximated over a 12F catheter with interrupted delayed-absorbable sutures. Mobilized urethral fascia is sutured on each side of the total length of the urethra. **D:** The lower strand of each suture is tied beneath the urethral floor, and the upper strands of the two sutures are used to pull the fascia beneath the urethra, where they are tied. (*Continued*)

Urinary Diversion and Reconstructive Techniques

In irreparable or recurrent urinary tract fistulas and cloacal defects following high-dose irradiation therapy for gynecologic malignancies, urinary diversion is the last resort to achieve a socially acceptable solution. An early technique of urinary diversion was implantation of the ureters into the sigmoid colon. Kidney failure, metabolic and electrolyte disturbance, and increased risk of colon cancer at the site of ureteral anastomosis led to its disfavor. Ureterosigmoid implantations are rarely performed in the United States but continue to be used in developing countries. Ureteral implantation into an isolated ileal loop

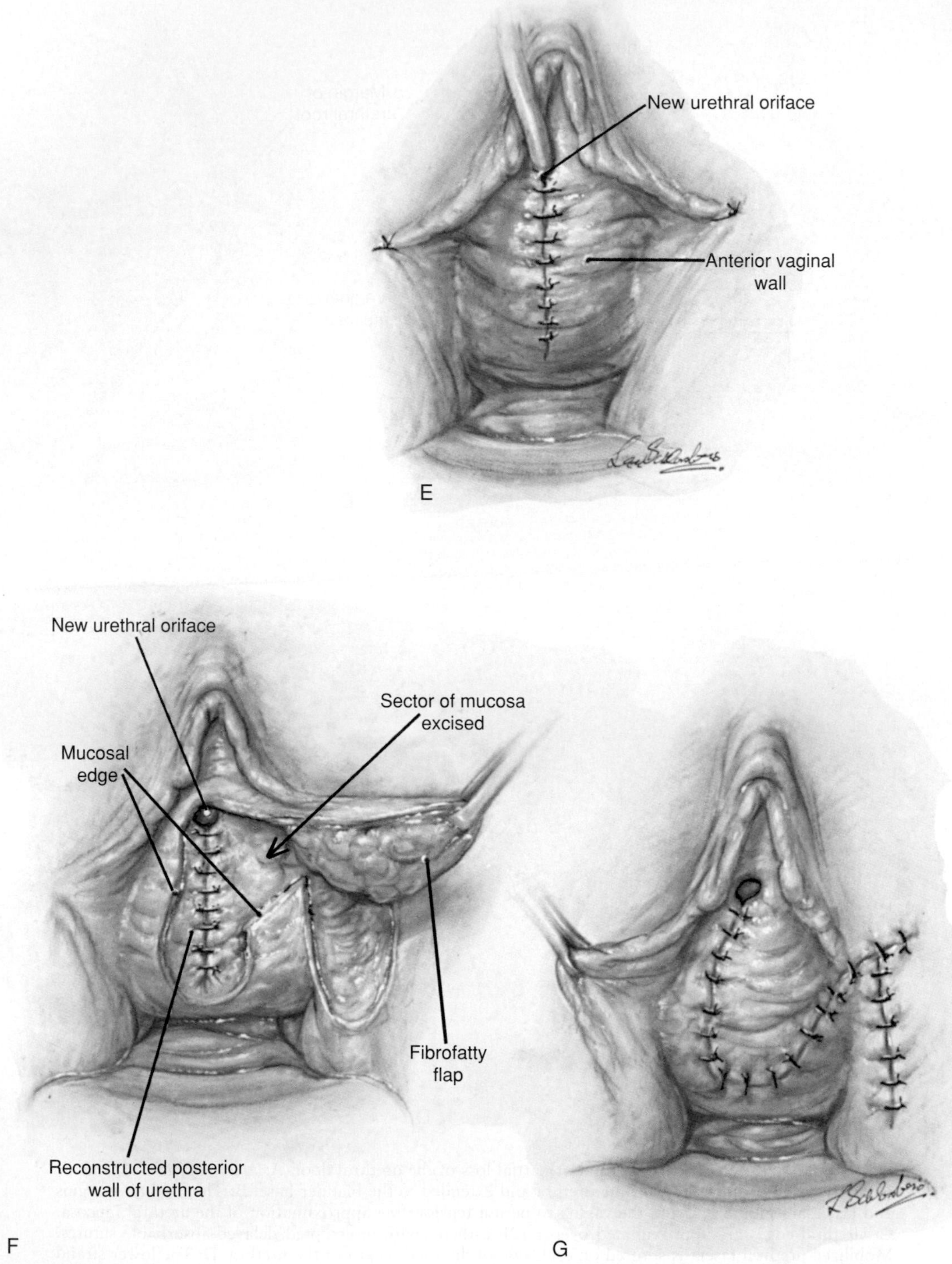

FIGURE 39.9. (*Continued*) **E:** The vaginal mucosa is closed without tension. **F:** For additional reinforcement, a U-shaped labial fat pad can be developed along the labia, leaving a broad pedicle superiorly. The vaginal mucosa between the urethral operative site and the labial graft is resected. **G:** The skin margins of the labial graft are sutured to the vaginal margins. The labial defect is closed.

or into a continent colon or ileal pouch is now the preferred method for fistulae that are irreparable. Leissner and coworkers have reported the use of the Mainz III colon pouch for continent diversion. This group has also described the construction of a neovagina from redundant bladder or colon following urinary diversion.

POSTOPERATIVE CARE

Postoperative care issues center on urinary drainage and resumption of coitus. Duration of urinary drainage and choice of transurethral or suprapubic routes are influenced by geography, culture, complexity of the fistula, and the technique used. The surgeon should tailor the length of time for drainage and route of drainage to the individual patient. Transurethral drainage for 10 to 14 days with an overall success rate of 70% was reported by Elkins and colleagues in a series of 36 obstetrical fistulae. Tancer, in his series of Latzko closures, described removing the transurethral catheter on the first or second postoperative day. His rationale was that the suture line is not part of the bladder. Therefore, distention of the bladder should not place tension on the suture line. All patients remained dry.

Symmonds has recommended suprapubic catheters for distal fistulae involving the urethra or bladder neck. He argues that a transurethral catheter should not be used because of the proximity to the suture line and the risk of disrupting the wound. We prefer suprapubic catheters to facilitate voiding trials.

Excellent hydration will ensure irrigation of the bladder and help to prevent clots that could obstruct the catheter, leading to unwanted excessive bladder distention and potential disruption of suture lines. As long as bladder drainage is adequate, prolonged bed rest and patient positioning in bed probably make little difference. Some surgeons advocate obtaining a cystogram to evaluate the integrity of the bladder before discontinuing bladder drainage. Although we have recently endorsed this approach, no data is available to show its benefit.

Resumption of sexual activity is a question following every gynecologic surgical procedure. For all of its relevance, this question has been addressed only minimally. Following an abdominal hysterectomy, a 4- to 6-week period is often recommended before a patient resumes normal activities, including sexual intercourse, without restrictions. This time frame may have more to do with the abdominal incision than the vaginal cuff incision. It would seem that healing of the vaginal cuff incision and an incision in the vagina associated with an uncomplicated vaginal fistula should be comparable. Lacking formal studies for guidance, the authors recommend waiting 6 weeks before subjecting the vagina to the rigors of coitus. In larger and more complicated repairs, the delay before resuming sexual activity must be individualized.

Incontinence after Fistula Repair

The occurrence of stress incontinence in patients after the successful repair of obstetric VVF has been long recognized and is estimated to occur in as many as 12% of such patients. Indeed, successful anatomic restoration of the urethra is not synonymous with restoration of physiologic function. Preoperative urodynamics have not predicted which patients go on to suffer stress incontinence after fistula repair. Sphincter involvement and the degree of tissue loss seem to be a better indicator of postoperative urinary incontinence. Waaldijk documented the subjective occurrence of stress incontinence after repair of fistulae of varying types. He described incontinence in 1% of cases without sphincter involvement in the fistula, 13% with sphincter involvement but with no additional tissue loss, and 16% with both sphincter involvement and tissue loss. In contrast, Hilton found that the incidence of urodynamically proven genuine stress incontinence associated with fistulae before repair was generally higher. He reported incontinence in 75% (9 of 12) with sphincter involvement and 36% (5 of 14) without such involvement. In Hilton's series, all patients who reported urgency after repair of their fistulae had abnormal cystometry preoperatively. Thus, there was no evidence of *de novo* detrusor instability after surgery.

The extent of scarring in the area of the bladder neck and urethra may present a challenge to conventional techniques for surgical correction of stress incontinence. Furthermore, many authors have advocated that concomitant retropubic suspensions be avoided for fear of devascularizing or disrupting the suburethral repair. Birkhoff and colleagues and Hilton believe that the reestablishment of continence is facilitated by the use of the Martius interposition flap. In addition, Gray found that 50% of patients in his review were incontinent postoperatively without this added intervention.

Periurethral injections traditionally have been appropriate in intrinsic sphincter deficiency with a relatively fixed or immobile bladder neck. This technique recently has been reported with initial short-term success in the stress incontinent, post-fistula patient. Falandry has had some success with a modified needle suspension procedure in a group of 49 patients. Sixty-three percent were continent at a mean follow-up of 2 years.

CONCLUSION

The literature on urogenital fistulae is extensive but largely based on small case series and individual surgeon's or fistula center's experience with a particular technique. The principles of fistula surgery are well established: visualization of the tract, a tension-free watertight closure, assurance of adequate vascular supply to the repair, and appropriate bladder drainage. The diagnosis of the condition traditionally has been based on clinical methods and confirmation with dye tests. Modern imaging techniques are increasingly being used in novel ways in other fields, but their utility in the detection of urogenital fistulae does not surpass conventional methods for urinary fistula. Radiographing imaging—including pyelogram, cystogram, and voiding cystourethrogram—is used to assess the complexity of the fistula and potential involvement of the ureters. Preoperative cystourethroscopy should be used to evaluate the anatomic relationship of the fistula.

Optimal management regarding timing of repair and surgical approach remains undecided. Laparoscopic repair of VVF is a feasible and efficacious minimally invasive alternative for its management. Minimally invasive approaches seem most appropriate for small, uncomplicated fistulae. Obstetric fistulae remain common in developing countries where access to adequate health care is limited, and fistulae in industrialized nations typically occur after gynecologic surgery.

The role of bladder injury antecedent to fistula formation seems obvious; thus, much of the effort in preventing VVF relies on protecting the bladder at the time of surgery or delivery. The risk of bladder injury is substantially higher at laparoscopic surgery and antiincontinence surgery. Despite preventive measures and good surgical technique, these injuries still occur. Even when cystotomy is recognized and repaired, a fistula may arise. Because fistula formation is multifactorial, defining the benefit of individual preventive strategies is virtually impossible.

BEST SURGICAL PRACTICES

- Transvaginal repair is the preferred method of repair whenever possible for both vesicovaginal and urethrovaginal fistula. We favor the Latzko technique for repair of uncomplicated posthysterectomy VVF. This technique is associated with an extremely high success rate, low morbidity, and rapid return to routine daily activities. The location of the urethrovaginal fistula and the degree of tissue loss will dictate the approach to repair.
- Interposition grafts can be used for tissue bulk and as a source of neovascularity. They may also be used to expand the vagina when caliber or depth is compromised. They may also enhance postoperative continence.
- The abdominal approach should be reserved for situations in which access to the fistula is limited. When the abdominal approach is chosen, the O'Conor technique as modified by Cetin and associates is a technique favored by many surgeons. An interposition graft of peritoneum or omentum seems to enhance overall success.

ACKNOWLEDGMENT

The authors wish to thank Dr. John Thompson for his enormous contribution to the previous editions of this text.

Bibliography

Abulafia O, Cohen HL, Zinn DL, et al. Transperineal ultrasonographic diagnosis of vesicovaginal fistula. *J Ultrasound Med* 1998;17:333.

Armenakas NA, Pareek G, Fracchia JA. Iatrogenic bladder perforations: long term follow-up of 65 patients. *J Urol* 2005;174(4 Pt 1):1299.

Asanuma H, Nakai H, Shishido S, et al. Congenital vesicovaginal fistula. *Int J Urol* 2000;7:195.

Billmeyer BR, Nygaard IE, Kreder KJ. Ureterouterine and vesicourethrovaginal fistulae as a complication of cesarean section. *J Urol* 2001;165:1212.

Birkhoff JD, Wechsler M, Romas NA. Urinary fistulae: vaginal repair using a labial fat pad. *J Urol* 1977;117:595.

Bruce R, El-Galley R, Galloway N. Use of rectus abdominis muscle flap for the treatment of complex and refractory urethrovaginal fistulae. *J Urol* 2000;163:1212.

Carlin B, Klutke C. Development of urethrovaginal fistula following periurethral collagen injection. *J Urol* 2000;164:124.

Cetin S, Yazicioglu A, Ozgur S, et al. Vesicovaginal fistula repair: a simple suprapubic transvesical approach. *Int Urol Nephrol* 1988;20:265.

Chibber PJ, Shah HN, Jain P. Laparoscopic O'Conor's repair for vesico-vaginal and vesico-uterine fistulae. *BJU Int* 2005;96(1):183.

Collins CG, Collins JH, Harrison BR, et al. Early repair of vesicovaginal fistula. *Am J Obstet Gynecol* 1971;111:524.

Collins CG, Pent D, Jones FB. Results of early repair of vesicovaginal fistula with preliminary cortisone treatment. *Am J Obstet Gynecol* 1960;80:1005–12.

Collins CG, Collins JH, Harrison BR, Nicholls RA, Hoffman ES, Krupp PJ. Early repair of vesicovaginal fistula. *Am J Obstet Gynecol* 1971 Oct 15;111(4):524–8.

Conde-Agudelo A. Intrafascial abdominal hysterectomy: outcomes and complications of 867 operations. *Int J Gynaecol Obstet* 2000;68:233.

Cruikshank SH. Early closure of posthysterectomy vesicovaginal fistulae. *South Med J* 1988;81:1525.

De Lamballe J. *Traite des fistules vescio-uterines*. Paris: Bailliere; 1852.

Dogra PN, Nabi G. Laser welding of vesicovaginal fistula. *Int Urogynecol J Pelvic Floor Dys* 2001;12:69.

Dolan LM, Easwaran SP, Hilton P. Congenital vesicovaginal fistula in association with hypoplastic kidney and uterus didelphys. *Urology* 2004;63(1):175.

Dotters DJ, Droegemueller W. Diaphragm catheters for vesicovaginal fistula management. *Contemp Obstet Gynecol* 1992;36:45.

Elkins TE, DeLancey JOL, McGuire EJ. The use of modified martius graft as an adjunctive technique in vesicovaginal and rectovaginal fistula repair. *Obstet Gynecol* 1990;75:727.

Elkins TE, Drescher C, Martey JO, et al. Vesicovaginal fistula revisited. *Obstet Gynecol* 1988;72:307.

Evans DH, Madjar S, Politano VA, et al. Interposition flaps in transabdominal vesicovaginal fistula repairs: are they really necessary? *Urology* 2001;57:670.

Falandry L. Vaginal route treatment for residual incontinence after closing an obstetrical fistula: a series of 49 cases (French). *J Gynecol Obstet Biol Reprod* 2000;29:393.

Falk H, Orkin L. Nonsurgical closure of vesicovaginal fistulae. *Obstet Gynecol* 1957;9:538.

Falk HC, Tancer ML. After office hours: vesicovaginal fistula. *Obstet Gynecol* 1954;3:337.

Fatio J. *Helvetisch-vernunstige Wehenmutter.* (op. posthum.) Basel: 1752.

Fernandes M, Lavengood RW Jr, Ward JN, Draper JW. Reconstruction of lower ureter and urethra, and closure of vesicovaginal fistula and other bladder defects. Various uses of bladder flap. *Urology* 1973 May;1(5):444–52.

Fujiwara K, Koshima I, Tanaka K. Radiation-induced vesico-vaginal fistula successfully repaired using a gracilis myocutaneous flap. *Int J Clin Oncol* 2000;5:338.

Goodwin WE, Scardino PT. Vesicovaginal and ureterovaginal fistulae: a summary of 25 years experience. *J Urol* 1980;123:370.

Gray LA. Urethrovaginal fistulae. *Am J Obstet Gynecol* 1968;101:28.

Green DE, Philips GL. Case report: vaginal prosthesis for control of vesicovaginal fistula. *Gynecol Oncol* 1986;23:119.

Grody MH, Nyirjesy P, Chatwani A. Intravesical foreign body and vesicovaginal fistula: a rare complication of a neglected pessary. *Int Urogynecol J Pelvic Floor Dysfunc* 1999;10:407.

Hamlin RH, Nicholson EC. Reconstruction of urethra totally destroyed in labour. *Br Med J.* 1969 Apr 19;2 (5650):147–50.

Hanai T, Miyatake R, Kato Y, et al. Vesicovaginal fistula due to a vaginal foreign body: a case report. *Acta Urol Jpn* 2000;46:141.

Harkki-Siren P, Sjoberg J, Titinen A. Urinary tract injuries after hysterectomy. *Obstet Gynecol* 1998;92:113.

Hendren WH. Construction of female urethra from vaginal wall and a perineal flap. *J Urol* 1980;123:657.

Hilton P. Urodynamic findings in patients with urogenital fistulae. *BJU Int* 1998;81:539.

Hilton P. Vesico-vaginal fistula: new perspectives. *Curr Opin Obstet Gynecol* 2001;13:513.

Hilton P, Ward A. Epidemiological and surgical aspects of urogenital fistulae: a review of 25 years experience in south-east Nigeria. *Int Urogynecol J Pelvic Floor Dysfunct* 1998;9:189.

Hilton P, Ward A, Molloy M, et al. Periurethral injection of autologous fat for the treatment of post-fistula repair stress incontinence: a preliminary report. *Int Urogynecol J Pelvic Floor Dysfunct* 1998;9:118.

Huang S, Yao B, Chou C. Transvaginal ultrasonographic findings in vesicovaginal fistula. *J Clin Ultrasound* 1996;24:209.

Hurley LJ, Previte SR. Vaginal pedicled flap for closure of vesicovaginal fistula. *Urology* 2000;56:856.

Ibrahim T, Sadiq A, Daniel S. Characteristics of VVF patients as seen at the specialist hospital Sokoto, Nigeria. *West Afr Med J* 2000;19:59.

Iselin CE, Aslan P, Webster GD. Transvaginal repair of vesicovaginal fistulae after hysterectomy by vaginal cuff excision. *J Urol* 1998;160:728.

Kelly J. Vesicovaginal and rectovaginal fistulae. *J R Soc Med* 1992;85:257.

Kelly HA. The suprapubic route for vesicovaginal fistulae. *Trans Am Gynecol Soc* 1906;31:25.

Kelly HA. The treatment of large vesicovaginal fistulae. *Bull Johns Hopkins Hosp* 1896;7:29.

Kobashi KC, Dmochowski R, Mee SL. Erosion of woven polyester pubovaginal sling. *J Urol* 1999;162:2070.

Kuhlman JE, Fishman EK. CT evaluation of enterovaginal and vesicovaginal fistulae. *J Comput Assist Tomogr* 1990;14:390.

Kursh ED, Morse RM, Resnick MI, et al. Prevention of the development of a vesicovaginal fistula. *Surg Gynecol Obstet* 1988;166(5):409.

Latzko W. Behandlung hochsitzender Blasen und Mastdarmscheiden Fisteln nach Uterus Extirpation mit hohom Scheidenverschluss. *Zentralbl Gynakol* 1914;38:906.

Latzko W. Postoperative vesicovaginal fistulae: genesis and therapy. *Am J Surg* 1942;58:211.

Lawson J. Vaginal fistulae. *J R Soc Med.* 1992 May; 85(5): 254–6. No abstract available.

Leach GE. Urethrovaginal fistula repair with Martius labial fat pad graft. *Urol Clin North Am* 1991;18:409.

Lee RA, Symmonds RE, Williams TJ. Current status of genitourinary fistula. *Obstet Gynecol* 1988;72:313.

Leissner J, Black P, Filipas D, et al. Vaginal reconstruction using the bladder and/or rectal walls in patients with radiation-induced fistulae. *Gynecol Oncol* 2000;78:356.

Leissner J, Black P, Fisch M, et al. Colon pouch (Mainz pouch III) for continent urinary diversion after pelvic irradiation. *Urology* 2000;56:798.

Leng WW, Amundsen CL, McGuire EJ. Management of female genitourinary fistulae: transvesical or transvaginal approach? *J Urol* 1998;160:728.

Mackenrodt A. Die operative Heilung grosser Blasencheiden-fisteln. *Zentralbl Gynak* 1894;18:180.

Madjar S, Gousse A. Postirradiation vesicovaginal fistula completely resolved with conservative treatment. *Int Urogynecol J Pelvic Floor Dysfunct* 2001;12:405.

Maisonneuve JG. *Clinique chirurgicale.* Paris: F Savy, 1863.

Martius H. Die operative Wiederherstellung der vollkommen fehlenden Harnrohre und des Schiessmuskels derselben. *Zentralbl Gynakol* 1928;52:480.

Martius H. *Gynecologic operations and their topographic-anatomic fundamentals.* Chicago: SB Debour, 1939.

McKay HA. Vesicovaginal and vesicocutaneous fistulae: transurethral suture cystorrhaphy as a minimally invasive alternative. *J Endourol* 2004;18(5):487.

Meeks GR, Sams JO, Field K, et al. Formation of vesicovaginal fistula: the role of suture placement into the bladder during closure of the vaginal cuff after transabdominal hysterectomy. *Am J Obstet Gynecol* 1997;177:1298.

Miklos JR, Sobolewski C, Lucente V. Laparoscopic management of recurrent vesicovaginal fistula. *Int Urogynecol J Pelvic Floor Dysfunct* 1999;10:116.

Moir JC. Vesicovaginal fistula as seen in Britain. *J Obstet Gynaecol Br Commonw* 1973;80:598.

Mondet F, Chartier-Kastler EJ, Conort P, et al. Anatomic and functional results of transperitoneal-transvesical vesicovaginal fistula repair. *Urology* 2001;58:882.

Morita T, Tokue A. Successful endoscopic closure of radiation induced vesicovaginal fistula with fibrin glue and bovine collagen. *J Urol* 1999;162:1689.

Mulvey S, Foley M, Kelly DG, et al. Urinary tract fistulae following gynecological surgery. *J Obstet Gynecol* 1998;18:369.

Nesrallah LJ, Srougi M, Gittes RF, et al. The O'Conor technique: the gold standard for supratrigonal vesicovaginal fistula repair. *J Urol* 1999;161:566.

O'Conor VJ Jr. Review of experience with vesicovaginal fistula repair. *J Urol* 1980;123:367.

O'Conor VJ Jr, Sokol JK, Bulkley GJ, et al. Suprapubic closure of vesicovaginal fistula. *J Urol* 1973;109:51.

Ojanuga D, Ekwempu CC. An investigation of sociomedical risk factors associated with vaginal fistula in northern Nigeria. *Women Health* 1999;28:103.

O'Leary JP. J. Marion Sims: a defense of the father of gynecology. *South Med J* 2004;97(5):427.

Omo-Dare P. Reconstruction of the urethra for stricture: description and evaluation of a technique. *J Urol* 1970;103:69.

O'Quin A. Early closure of vesicovaginal fistulae. *Abstract Soc Pelvic Surgeons* 1984.

Osterhage HR, Grun BR, Judmann G, et al. Experimental comparison of Maxon and chromic catgut in suturing of the urinary bladder. (German). *Urologe A* 1988;27(1):61.

Ottesen M, Moller C, Kehlet H, et al. Substantial variability in postoperative treatment, and convalescence recommendations following vaginal repair: a nationwide questionnaire study. *Acta Obstet Gynecol Scand* 2001;80(11): 1062.

Pawlik C. Ueberdie Operation der Blasenscheidenfisteln. *Ztschr F Gerburtsh U Gynakol* 1882;8:22.

Persky L, Forsythe WE, Herman G. Vesicovaginal fistulae in childhood. *Urology* 1980;15:36.

Pettersson S, Hedelin H, Jansson I, et al. Fibrin occlusion of a vesicovaginal fistula. *Lancet* 1979;28:933.

Portilla E, Ramos A, Ramos L, et al. A model of suture-induced urolithiasis with urographic control in the bladder of the rat. *J Invest Surg* 1999;12(4): 205.

Pruthi R, Petrus C, Bundrick WJ. New onset vesicovaginal fistula after transurethral collagen injection in women who underwent cystectomy and orthotopic neobladder creation: presentation and definitive treatment. *J Urol* 2000;164:1638.

Ralph G, Tamussino K, Litchtenegger W, et al. Urological complications after radical hysterectomy with or without radiotherapy for cervical cancer. *Arch Gynecol Obstet* 1990;248:61.

Ramaiah KS, Kumar S. Vesicovaginal fistula following masturbation managed conservatively. *Aust N Z J Obstet Gynecol* 1998;38(4):475.

Raz S, Bregg KJ, Nitti VW, et al. Transvaginal repair of vesicovaginal fistula using a peritoneal flap. *J Urol* 1993;156:56.

Roth TM, Meeks GR, Blythe J, et al. Massive vesicovaginal fistula associated with a vaginal foreign body: a combined abdominal vaginal repair with gracilis muscle interposition flap. *J Pelvic Med Surg* 2003;9(1):19.

Sartin JS. J. Marion Sims, the father of gynecology: hero or villain? *South Med J* 2004;97(5):500.

Schmidt JD, Buchsbaum HJ. Transverse colon conduit diversion. *Urol Clin North Am* 1986;13:233.

Schoenrock GJ, Cianci P. Treatment of radiation cystitis with hyperbaric oxygen. *Urology* 1986;27:271.

Sharma SK, Madhusudnan P, Kumar A, et al. Vesicovaginal fistulae of uncommon etiology. *J Urol* 1987;137:280.

Sharma SK, Perry KT, Turk TM: Endoscopic injection of fibrin glue for the treatment of urinary-tract pathology. *J Endourol* 2005;19(3):419.

Sims JM. On the treatment of vesico-vaginal fistula (classic articles in *Urogynecology*). *Int Urogynecol J Pelvic Floor Dysfunct* 1998;9:236.

Sims JM. On the treatment of vesicovaginal fistulae. *Am J Med Sci* 1852; 23:59.

Sotelo R, Mariano MB, Garcia-Segui A, et al. Laparoscopic repair of vesicovaginal fistula. *J Urol* 2005;173(5):1615.

Stewart DW, Buffington PJ, Wacksman J. Suture material in bladder surgery. *J Urol* 1990;143(6):1261.

Stovsky MD, Ignatoff JM, Blum MD, et al. Use of electrocoagulation in the treatment of vesicovaginal fistulae. *J Urol* 1994;152:1443.

Symmonds RE, Hill LM. Loss of urethra: a report on 50 patients. *Am J Obstet Gynecol* 1978;130:130.

Tancer ML. Observations on prevention and management of vesicovaginal fistula after total hysterectomy. *Surg Gynecol Obstet* 1992;175:501.

Thomas K, Williams G. Medicolegal aspects of vesicovaginal fistulae. *BJU Int* 2000;86:354.

Trendelenberg F. *Uber blasenscheidenfisteloperationen.* Leipzig: Samml Klin Vortrage, 1890.

Volkmer BG, Kuefer R, Nesslauer T, et al. Colour Doppler ultrasound in vesicovaginal fistulae. *Ultrasound Med Biol* 2000;26:771.

Von Roonhuysen H. *Medico-chirurgical observations.* London: Moses Pitt at the Angel, 1676.

Vyas N, Nandi PR, Mahmood M, et al. Bladder mucosal autografts for repair of vesicovaginal fistula. *BJOG* 2005;112(1):112.

Waaldijk K. *The surgical management of bladder fistula in 775 women in Northern Nigeria.* Nymegen: Benda BV; 1989.

Wein AJ, Malloy TR, Carpiniello VL, et al. Repair of vesicovaginal and ureterovaginal fistulae by a suprapubic transvesical approach. *Surg Gynecol Obstet* 1980;150:57.

Yeoum SG, Park CS. Adjustment after a hysterectomy (Korean). *Taehan Kanho Hakhoe Chi* 2005;35(6):1174.

Zacharin RF. A history of obstetric vesicovaginal fistula. *Aust N Z J Surg* 2000 Dec; 70(12):851–4.

CHAPTER 40 ■ ANAL INCONTINENCE AND RECTOVAGINAL FISTULAS

MICHAEL P. ARONSON AND RAYMOND A. LEE

DEFINITIONS

Anal incontinence—Involuntary loss through the anus of flatus, liquid, or solid stool that is perceived as a social or hygienic problem.

External anal sphincter—Striated muscle sphincter, under voluntary control, that is responsible for much of the squeeze pressure in the anal canal.

Extra-anal incontinence—Involuntary loss through a fistula of flatus, liquid, or solid stool.

Fecal incontinence—Involuntary loss through the anus of liquid or solid stool only; excludes flatal incontinence.

Internal anal sphincter—Thickened continuation of the circular smooth muscle layer of the bowel, under autonomic control, that is responsible for much of the resting pressure in the anal canal.

Puborectalis muscle—Striated muscle medial portion of the levator ani that is responsible for maintaining and increasing the anorectal angle and contributes to the squeeze pressure in the anal canal.

Rectovaginal fistula—Epithelial lined connection between the rectosigmoid or anal canal and the vagina or perineum.

No symptom of pelvic floor dysfunction is more debilitating or has greater psychosocial impact on a woman than that of anal incontinence. The inability to control solid stool, liquid, or gas can have a devastating effect on a woman's feelings of self-worth, sexuality, and ability to be an active social participant in her community. The evaluation and treatment of the anally incontinent patient is a challenging but rewarding task because relief of these symptoms can greatly improve the quality of a patient's life. Because the problem of anal incontinence is multifactorial, the approach to the problem is often multidisciplinary, involving health care providers from gynecology, colorectal surgery, and gastroenterology, as well as nutrition and physical therapy. Anal incontinence is part of a spectrum of disorders of defecatory function that includes constipation, incomplete evacuation of the bowels, urgency, frequency, and painful defecation. Outcomes of treatments should be understood in terms of their impact on a patient's symptoms and quality of life, not purely on anatomic results.

Although anal incontinence has a major impact on a patient's quality of life, most individuals are reticent to discuss this symptom with their health care providers. Johanson and Laferty report that more than 50% of women with anal incontinence will never present to a health care provider with their problem. The prevalence of both anal and fecal incontinence is difficult to establish as there has been a lack of uniform definitions used in past studies. The 3rd International Consultation on Incontinence in Monaco in 2004 defined anal incontinence as involuntary loss of flatus, liquid, or solid stool that is perceived as a social or hygienic problem. Fecal incontinence excludes flatal incontinence and represents the loss of liquid or solid stool only. Boreham and colleagues, in a multicenter study of 457 consecutive women presenting for routine general gynecologic care, found anal incontinence in 28.4% with irritable bowel syndrome, constipation, age, and body mass index identified as significant risk factors. In a questionnaire study designed to reflect the age and sex distribution of the adult population of Germany, Giebel and associates found anal incontinence in 19.6% and fecal incontinence in 4.8% (specifically incontinence of solid stool). In a review, Macmillan and colleagues found the prevalence of fecal incontinence to be between 2% and 13% of community-dwelling adults.

There are no data regarding the incidence of anal incontinence in the community-dwelling population, but Chassagne and associates reported on an elderly, long-term-care facility population. They enrolled 1,186 individuals 60 years of age or older who did not have anal incontinence. After 10 months, 20% had developed anal incontinence. They identified five significant risk factors: history of urinary incontinence, neurologic disease, poor mobility, severe cognitive decline, and age older than 70 years.

It is well established that the presence of anal incontinence is associated with the presence of urinary incontinence as well as pelvic organ prolapse. The connective tissue and muscular and neurologic elements of the pelvic floor function in concert with the organs they support as an interdependent unit to provide multiple functions simultaneously. In a cross-sectional community-based study involving 762 randomly selected women age 50 or older, Roberts and colleagues found 15% had anal incontinence, 48% had urinary incontinence, and 9% had both. Viewed another way, 60% of those with anal incontinence had concurrent urinary incontinence. Among patients presenting to a urogynecology clinic for evaluation of urinary incontinence, a high proportion have dual incontinence, defined as concurrent urinary and anal incontinence. Leroi and associates (1999) found 28% of 409 patients in France, and Gordon and colleagues found 29% of 283 consecutive patients in Israel, had dual incontinence. Nichols and coworkers looked at 100 patients with stage II or greater pelvic organ prolapse and/or urinary incontinence. Fifty-four percent had concomitant anal incontinence, and 52% had anal sphincter defects by ultrasound. Clearly because the pelvic floor uses some common elements in maintaining support and continence of feces and urine, it follows that injury to one mechanism could simultaneously affect the other.

An important development has been the beginning of an understanding of the relationship of vaginal birth to the problem of anal incontinence. In a review, Sultan and associates noted a reported 6.6% to 14% prevalence of anal incontinence in vaginally parous women. In a more recent prospective study of 949 consecutive women delivering vaginally, Eason and colleagues found at 3 months postpartum that 26% percent had anal incontinence and 3% had fecal incontinence. As tools for treatment of this problem have limited success, it becomes apparent that future research should focus on the prevention of childbirth injuries that can contribute to anal incontinence.

In this chapter, we examine the anal continence mechanism in an effort to understand how damage may be sustained. Particular emphasis is placed on the effect of childbirth on the anatomic and neurologic aspects of that mechanism. We then review the evaluation of the anally incontinent patient as well as medical and surgical treatment options. Finally, we consider the etiology, evaluation, and techniques for surgical repair of extraanal incontinence of feces through a rectovaginal fistula.

ANAL CONTINENCE MECHANISM

Normal anal continence requires the coordinated control of the multiple synergistic elements summarized in Table 40.1. An anatomically and neurologically intact anal sphincter complex is necessary to keep the anal canal closed effectively. Intact reflex arcs and anorectal sensation are necessary for the individual to perceive rectal filling and discriminate the nature of the rectal contents. Intact motor enervation is essential so that the sphincter mechanism can respond appropriately to the increased need for anal closure such as during straining or coughing. The puborectalis muscle sling must be anatomically and neurologically intact to create an anorectal angle. The puborectalis muscle must be capable of reflexive contraction at the moment of need to increase that angle and move rectal contents off the sphincter complex into a capacious and distensible rectal reservoir. Last, gastrointestinal considerations such as colonic motility and stool consistency need to be reasonable for maintenance of continence. The complete interrelated mechanisms of defecation and anal control are more easily visualized once the principal elements of the anatomy related to continence are delineated.

Anatomy of the Anal Canal and Related Structures

The anal and rectal regions of the lower colon share a common embryologic origin: the posterior portion of the endoderm of the cloaca. During the development of these regions, the terminal end of the alimentary canal is surrounded by muscular sphincters of somatic origin. Thus, the anorectal region is composed of both visceral and somatic components. The visceral components include the rectum, internal anal sphincter, and lining of the upper part of the anal canal. The voluntary or somatic components are the epithelium of the lower part of the anal canal as well as the striated muscles of the pelvic floor and the external anal sphincter. The rectal mucosa consists of mucus-secreting columnar goblet cells, which invaginate to form tubular glands. The mucosa is surrounded by a muscularis mucosa and an inner circular layer of smooth muscle. This circular smooth muscle layer thickens distally to become the internal anal sphincter. An outer longitudinal layer of smooth muscle transitions distally into fibrous fascicles that travel between the internal and external anal sphincter and insert into the perianal skin, thus anchoring the sphincter complex and creating the puckering effect seen on clinical examination.

TABLE 40.1

MECHANISMS OF ANAL CONTINENCE

Anatomic
Anal sphincter mechanisms
Puborectalis sling/anorectal angle
Neurologic
Intact pudendal enervation
Anorectal reflex and sensory mechanisms
Functional
Stool volume and consistency
Colonic transit time
Rectal capacity, distensibility and tone

The anal canal in the female is approximately 2.5 to 4 cm in length and normally remains completely collapsed because of the tonic contractions of the sphincters. Posterior to the anal canal is the coccyx, from which it is separated by intervening fibrofatty tissue. The levator ani muscles are posterior to the canal until it opens onto the perineal skin. The levator muscles also separate the lateral boundary of the anal canal from the ischiorectal fossa, through which pass the important nerves, lymphatics, and blood supply of the terminal rectum, anal canal, and perineum. The canal is fused anteriorly with the lower portion of the rectovaginal septum and perineal body (Fig. 40.1).

The lining of the anal canal is nonuniform. The proximal 1 cm is lined by rectal-type columnar mucosa, followed by modified or stratified columnar epithelium for about 1.5 cm. The distal half of the anal canal is lined by squamous epithelium, which is richly supplied by branches of the inferior hemorrhoidal nerves and is exquisitely sensitive. The anal mucosa, like the rectum, is also surrounded by the inner circular layer of smooth muscle, which is in turn surrounded by the outer longitudinal layer. The main blood supply to the rectum and anal canal is from branches of the superior and inferior hemorrhoidal arteries.

The anatomic sphincter mechanism of the anal canal has been a matter of controversy since first described by Galen almost 2,000 years ago. It is most often thought of as consisting of three separate anatomic structures: the internal anal sphincter, the external anal sphincter, and the action of the most medial portion of the levator ani, the puborectalis muscle (Fig. 40.2). The circular smooth muscle layer of the rectal wall, which is under autonomic control, thickens at the proximal anal canal to form the internal anal sphincter. It can be identified on dissection or at the time of third- or fourth-degree obstetric laceration repair as a thick, fibrous, white layer between the anal mucosa and the external anal sphincter. The internal sphincter accounts for about 70% of the resting tone of the anal canal and is innervated by the autonomic nervous system, providing continuous involuntary muscle tone. The remainder of the resting tone of the anal canal is thought to be provided by the slow twitch fibers of the external sphincter and the hemorrhoidal complexes.

The portions of the anal continence mechanism that are under voluntary control are the striated muscles of the external anal sphincter complex and the medial puborectalis portion of the pubococcygeus muscle, which courses behind the anorectum in a slinglike fashion. Unlike most other striated muscles, the external anal sphincter and the puborectalis muscle

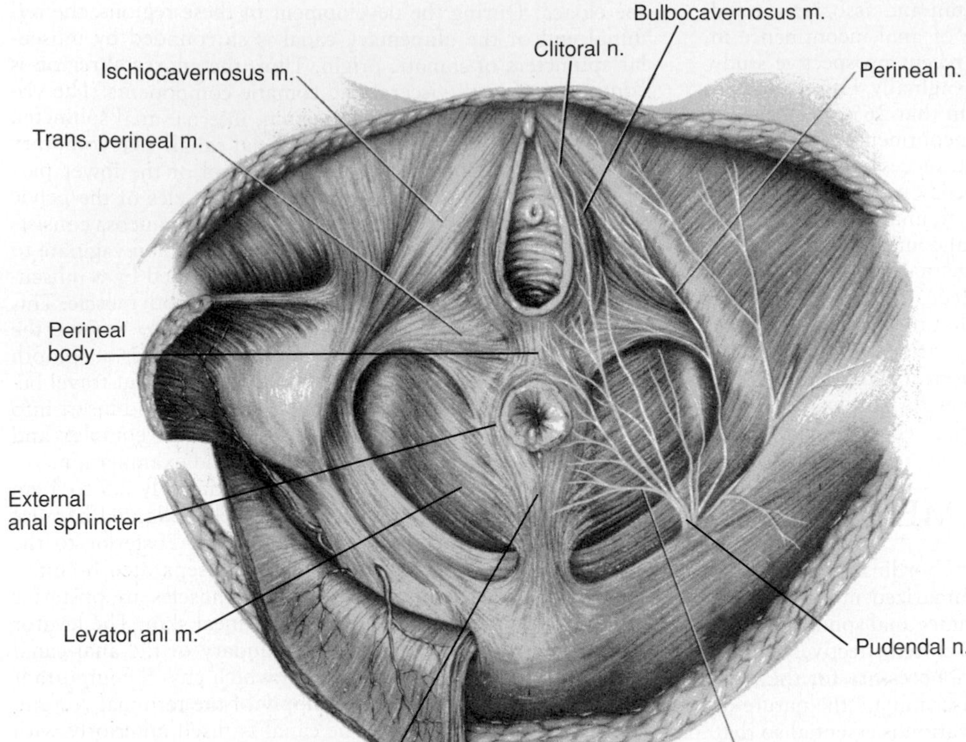

FIGURE 40.1. Location of the anal sphincter in relation to other structures of the female pelvic floor.

maintain a constant muscular tone that is directly proportional to the volume of rectal contents. The tone of the puborectalis muscle wrapping around posterior to the junction of the rectum and the anal canal produces what is called the anorectal angle. The fibers of pubococcygeus that do not wrap around go on to form the fibrinous anococcygeal raphe, often referred to as the levator plate, which inserts onto the last two segments of the coccyx. Willful contraction of structurally and neurologically intact puborectalis and pubococcygeus muscles, along with the rest of the levator sling, can increase the anorectal angle and support the levator plate and the rectal reservoir above it in a horizontal axis to aid in maintenance of continence.

The external anal sphincter complex is thought by different anatomists to be composed of one, two, or three parts. Most anatomists agree, however, that the entire external anal sphincter complex is enervated by perineal branches of the pudendal nerves emanating from S2–4. Although some authors refer to a three-part sphincter as having superficial, medial, and deep portions (Fig. 40.2), clinically the entire external sphincter responds to the same enervation and functions as a single

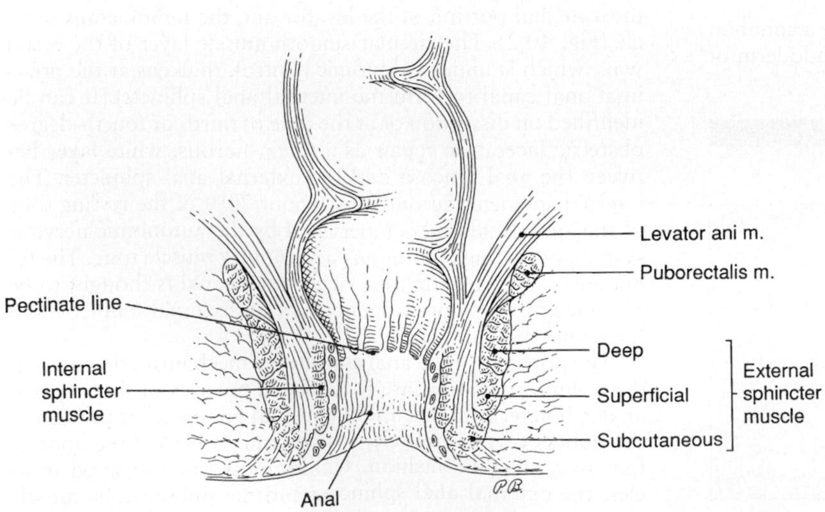

FIGURE 40.2. Diagrammatic illustration of the anal canal and sphincters.

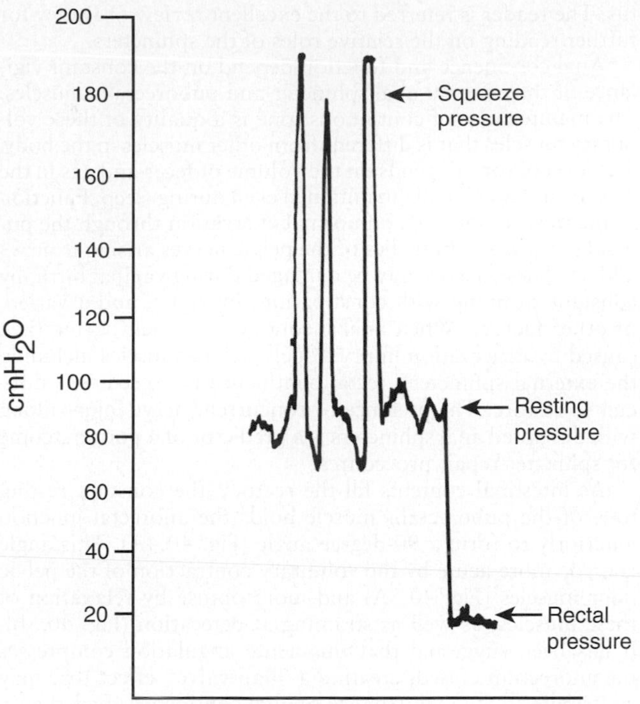

FIGURE 40.3. Anal manometry demonstrating pressures in the anal canal. Rectal pressure reflects intraabdominal baseline pressure recorded in the rectal reservoir. Resting pressure essentially reflects the effect of the involuntary, smooth-muscle internal anal sphincter. Squeeze pressure largely reflects the transient contractile effort of the voluntary, striated external anal sphincter.

unit. The subcutaneous part of the external sphincter is small and inserts in the perianal skin. The superficial part is more substantial and is attached posteriorly through the anococcygeal raphe to the coccyx. The deep portion is intimately related to the puborectalis muscle posteriorly, where its fibers loop around the anorectal junction. The external anal sphincter and puborectalis muscle are responsible for most of the voluntary squeeze pressure that is exerted in the anal canal (Fig. 40.3).

To review, the puborectalis muscle originates from the pubic bone on either side of the midline, passes behind the vagina and rectum, and fuses posteriorly behind the anorectal junction to form a U-shaped sling around the rectum. Some fibers interdigitate with the walls of the anal canal (Fig. 40.4). The constant resting tone of the puborectalis muscle pulls the anorectal junction anteriorly to create an approximately 90-degree angle between the rectum and anal canal, thereby maintaining anorectal continence of solid stool by closing the rectal inlet. Both the puborectalis muscle and the external anal sphincter contain a majority of type I (slow-twitch) muscle fibers that are ideally suited to maintaining constant tone over time. Each muscle also contains a smaller portion of type II (fast-twitch) fibers, which allow them to respond quickly during sudden increases in intraabdominal pressure. The external anal sphincter is enervated by branches of the pudendal nerve (S2–4). The puborectalis muscle is enervated directly by the S3–4 pelvic nerves, as well as possibly by collateral branches of the pudendal nerve.

Classically, the female anal sphincter complex has been thought of as forming a broad band of tissue posteriorly but narrowing to a small tubular bundle of tissue anteriorly within the perineal body. In the past, the internal sphincter has most often been portrayed as a minor structure. These concepts came from many centuries of anatomic study of cadavers augmented by observations in the delivery room, at the time of third- and fourth-degree laceration repairs, of the transected ends of the anterior portion retracted into round holes in the perineal body. In the recent past, it has become possible to view this anatomy undisturbed in living, continent, nulliparous subjects with magnetic resonance imaging (MRI). In an early MRI study, Aronson and colleagues found the shape of the combined internal and external anal sphincter complex to be nearly cylindrical as it encircles the anal canal. Measured in the midline, the anterior portion of the anal sphincter complex appeared as a broad band of tissue, not a narrow tube. In this study, 54% of the anterior thickness was smooth muscle of the internal anal sphincter. Subsequent studies, including the cadaver studies of DeLancey et al. (1997), found a similar shape with a substantial contribution from the internal anal sphincter. This substantial anterior anal sphincter length and thickness, as well as the contribution from the internal sphincter, is important to keep in mind during primary repair of obstetric lacerations as well as in surgical

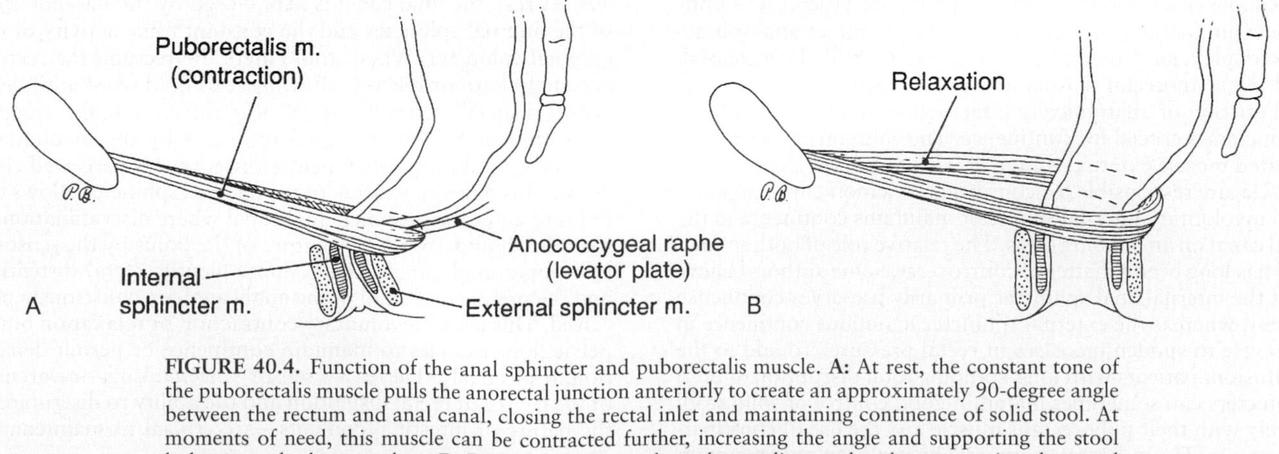

FIGURE 40.4. Function of the anal sphincter and puborectalis muscle. A: At rest, the constant tone of the puborectalis muscle pulls the anorectal junction anteriorly to create an approximately 90-degree angle between the rectum and anal canal, closing the rectal inlet and maintaining continence of solid stool. At moments of need, this muscle can be contracted further, increasing the angle and supporting the stool bolus over the levator plate. B: During defecation, the puborectalis muscle relaxes, opening the rectal inlet, while intestinal peristalsis and the voluntary increase in intraabdominal pressure move stool into the anal canal. The anorectal angle is decreased and the stool bolus is lined up over the anal canal.

correction of anal incontinence secondary to a chronic perineal laceration.

The tone of the levator ani muscle is stabilized by the skeletal muscles of the anterior compartment of the urogenital diaphragm, and by the bulbocavernosus and transversus perinei muscles, which have a common insertion into the central perineal body between the anus and vaginal introitus. The perineal body is an important anatomic structure that is closely associated with the external anal sphincter and anal canal, and includes the insertion of two components of the transverse perineal muscles: a superficial and a deep muscle layer, both composed of striated muscle. The central raphe of the perineal body serves as a pivotal point tying in the transverse perineal musculature, the terminal end of the bulbocavernosus muscles, the external anal sphincter, and, to an extent, the medial aspect of the levator ani or the puborectalis muscles (Fig. 40.1). Trauma or separation of the perineal raphe causes relaxation of the perineal body, which is attached to the external anal sphincter. The resulting alteration of attachment may contribute to loss of control of both liquid stool and gas.

Physiology of Anal Continence

Anal continence is dependent on the complex interaction of many physiologic and anatomic factors. Often the focus is on the anatomic and neurologic aspects of continence that obstetricians see damaged in the labor room and attempt to repair. However, many factors essential to continence are actually quite distant from the pelvic floor. They can include problems with stool volume and consistency, colonic transit time, rectal capacity, and rectal distensibility. For example, a severe malabsorption syndrome delivering massive quantities of stool of a liquid consistency that is difficult to manage can overwhelm even a normally adequate continence mechanism. The rectum also needs to be capacious and distensible to serve as a storage vessel so that the timing of defecation may be consciously deferred. A patient with a radiation-damaged and fibrotic rectum may lose that capacity. An individual must also possess adequate mental faculties to recognize the need for evacuation, as well as sufficient mobility to transfer to an appropriate location for willful defecation to remain continent. Although the relative importance of these factors has not been defined, it seems clear that for the normal patient with a normal consistency and quantity of stool and a capacious, compliant, and evacuable rectal reservoir, three factors are crucial for continence: an anatomically and neurologically intact anal sphincter complex, an anorectal angle that can willfully be increased, and intact anorectal sensory and reflex mechanisms.

Function of anatomically intact external and internal anal sphincters is crucial for continence. The voluntarily controlled, striated muscle external sphincter, along with the puborectalis muscle, are responsible for continence at a moment of urgency. The involuntary internal sphincter maintains continence in the anal canal on an ongoing basis. The relative role of both sphincters has long been a matter of controversy. Some authors believe that the internal anal sphincter primarily preserves continence at rest, whereas the external sphincter maintains continence in response to sudden increases in rectal pressure. To add to the confusion, patients with long-standing total disruption of both sphincters can sometimes maintain good control of solid stool purely with their puborectalis muscle and the use of constipating agents. The puborectalis muscle by itself can only maintain continence of solid feces; the internal and external sphincters in the anal canal maintain continence of liquid stool and flatus. The reader is referred to the excellent review of Dalley for further reading on the relative roles of the sphincters.

Anal continence and function depend on the constant vigilance of the external anal sphincter and puborectalis muscles. The maintenance of continuous tone is a quality of these voluntary muscles that is different from other muscles in the body. The level of tone depends on the volume of feces and gas in the rectum and is normally maintained even during sleep. Function of the muscles depends on normal enervation through the pudendal nerve and branches of the pelvic nerves arising from S3 and S4. These nerves may be damaged during vaginal birth, by constant straining with constipation, by aging, and a variety of other factors. When anal incontinence is neurogenic (i.e., caused by denervation injury of pelvic floor muscles including the external sphincter), rectal continence is exceedingly difficult to restore. The presence of concurrent nerve injury along with disrupted anal sphincters is a predictor of a poor outcome for sphincter repair procedures.

As intestinal contents fill the rectum, the constant resting tone of the puborectalis muscle holds the anorectal junction anteriorly to form a 90-degree angle (Fig. 40.4A). This angle is made more acute by the voluntary contraction of the pelvic floor muscles (Fig. 40.5A) and more obtuse by relaxation of these muscles, as well as straining at defecation (Fig. 40.5B). It has been suggested that this acute angulation compresses the anorectum closed, creating a "flap-valve" effect that may contribute to the maintenance of anal continence. This theory has been questioned. Defecography studies have not confirmed the relationship of the anorectal angle to anal continence, just as the surgical restoration of the normal anorectal junction angle with a Parks postanal repair, or retrorectal levatorplasty, has not been consistently associated with the return of continence.

For defecation to occur, the puborectalis muscle must voluntarily relax while intestinal peristalsis and a voluntary increase in intraabdominal pressure allow the stool to move downward into the anal canal (Figs. 40.4B and 40.5B). Of note is when denervation of the pelvic floor musculature occurs, the muscles relax, lining up the rectum over the fatigable sphincter complex just as during an act of normal defecation. This relationship is unfavorable to continence and may contribute to incontinence, especially in patients with compromised sphincter function.

The internal and external sphincters maintain continence below the level of the puborectalis muscle. As discussed, they are particularly important in the control of liquid stool and gas. At rest, the anal canal is kept closed by the baseline tone of the internal sphincter and the constant tonic activity of the external sphincter. When stool enters the rectum, the rectum accommodates or relaxes, allowing it to hold stool until defecation is socially convenient. Stool in the rectum also triggers relaxation of the internal anal sphincter by the involuntary rectoanal inhibitory reflex before distention is perceived (Fig. 40.6). This reflex relaxation of the internal sphincter allows the bolus to enter the proximal anal canal where discrimination of the solid, liquid, or gaseous nature of the bolus by the sensory-rich upper anal canal occurs. Subsequently, rectal distention and the presence of stool in the anal canal are consciously perceived. This leads to voluntary contraction or relaxation of the pelvic floor muscles to maintain continence or permit defecation, respectively. These two sensory mechanisms—awareness of the degree of rectal distention and the ability to discriminate the nature of intestinal contents—are crucial to maintenance of continence.

As rectal filling continues, the internal sphincter contracts once again to facilitate anal closure. If defecation or passage

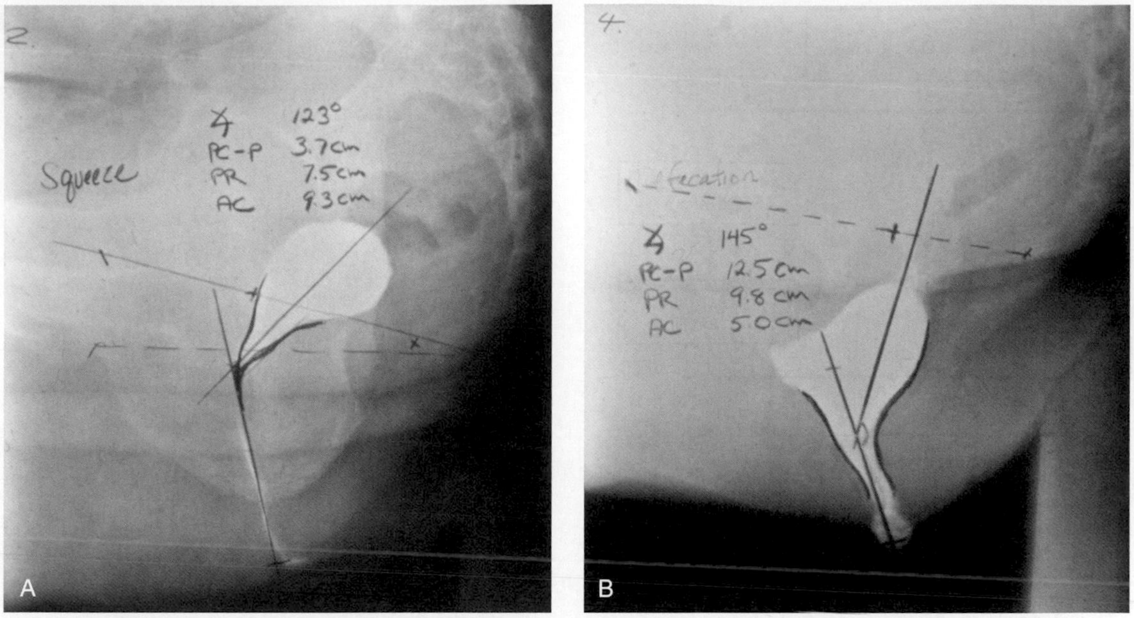

FIGURE 40.5. **A:** Lateral defecography of normal continent patient deferring defecation by contracting puborectalis sling, increasing anorectal angle, and exerting squeeze pressure in anal canal. Note how barium bolus is supported over levator plate and away from the fatigable anal sphincter complex. **B:** Lateral defecography of normal continent patient willfully defecating by relaxing puborectalis sling, decreasing anorectal angle, and decreasing pressure in the anal canal. Note how barium bolus becomes lined up over anal canal.

of gas is inconvenient, the external sphincter and puborectalis muscle can be firmly contracted. This helps force rectal contents back into a capacious and distensible rectal reservoir supported over the levator plate. Striated muscle, such as the external sphincter and puborectalis, can only be contracted maximally for approximately 1 minute; by the end of 3 minutes, most of the force of contraction is diminished (Fig. 40.7). Injury to the internal sphincter that results in loss of tonicity of the anal canal may permit the involuntary passage of liquid stool and gas. Such an injury is particularly noticeable when the urge to defecate is persistent from a bolus of fecal material in the terminal rectum and when the voluntary contraction of the external sphincter and puborectalis muscle wanes.

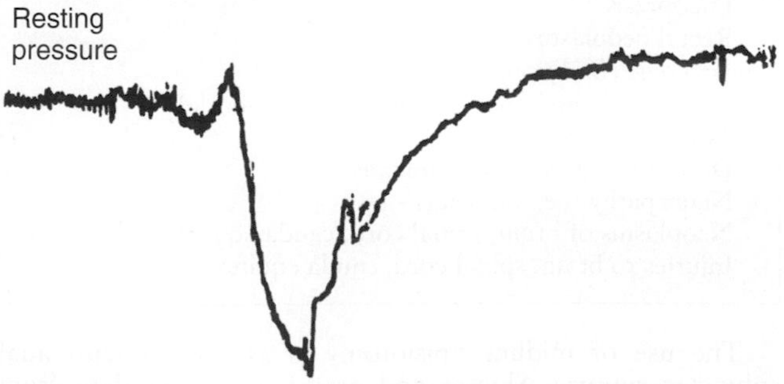

FIGURE 40.6. Rectoanal inhibitory reflex. Arrival of stool in the rectum triggers reflex relaxation of the internal anal sphincter, allowing the bolus to enter the proximal anal canal, where discrimination of the solid, liquid, or gaseous nature of the bolus by the sensory-rich upper anal canal occurs.

CAUSES OF ANAL INCONTINENCE

The Effects of Vaginal Birth

Although numerous causes of anal incontinence are summarized in, a major factor is obstetric injury to the pelvic floor in healthy adult women. Vaginal birth may compromise the continence mechanism by direct anatomic injury to the anal sphincters, puborectalis sling, perineal muscles, and perineal fascia. DeLancey and associates (2003) and Dietz and Lanzarone demonstrate—in MRI and ultrasound studies, respectively—significant damage to the puborectalis sling associated with vaginal birth. Kearney and colleagues show an association of these defects with use of forceps (odds ratio [OR] 14.7), anal sphincter rupture (OR 8.1), and use of episiotomy (OR 3.1). Nerve injury may occur in some women as well and play a significant role. These injuries, either separately or in combination, can lead to some degree of anal incontinence. Other risk factors have been also defined. In a study of identical twin sisters, Abramov and associates identify age, menopause, obesity, parity, and stress urinary incontinence as major associated risk factors for anal incontinence.

Third- or fourth-degree obstetrical laceration of the anal sphincter complex is highly associated with subsequent development of anal incontinence. In a population-based, retrospective look at more than 2 million vaginal deliveries, Handa and coworkers found an anal sphincter laceration rate of 5.85% when preterm births, breech deliveries, stillbirths, and multiple gestations were excluded. Numerous case control studies report 6% to 44% of patients, after obstetric injury to the anal sphincter, have some degree of anal incontinence despite immediate surgical repair. Sultan and colleagues (1993) prospectively studied 202 consecutive pregnant women with multiple

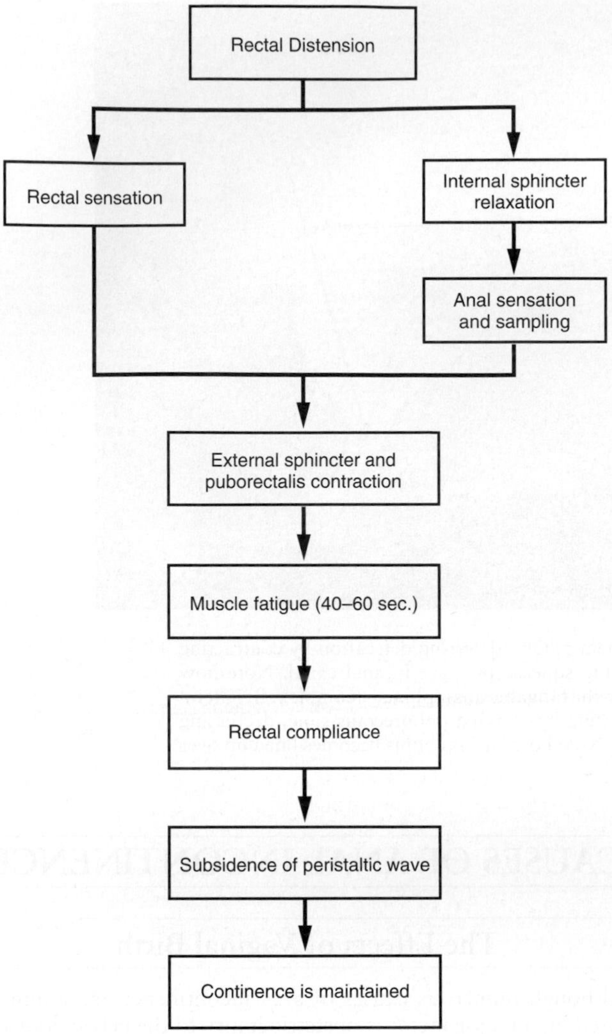

FIGURE 40.7. Algorithm for anal continence mechanism.

modalities and found that although none of the nulliparas entering the study had a sphincter defect before delivery, 35% of primiparous women and 44% of multiparous women who delivered vaginally had an internal and/or external anal sphincter defect present postpartum. They found that anal incontinence in their study population was significantly associated with the presence of a sphincter defect. In a study of 808 vaginally delivered women in Sweden, Zetterstrom and associates found sphincter tears detected at delivery to be associated with nulliparity (OR 9.8), midline episiotomy (OR 5.5), fundal pressure (OR 4.6), postmaturity (OR 2.5), and increased fetal weight (OR 1.3). Of their subjects with primarily repaired sphincters, 54% reported at least "mild" anal incontinence at 5 months, and 41% still had symptoms at 9 months postpartum. In a 10-year follow-up of anal sphincter injuries, Fornell and associates found that subjective and objective anal function after injury deteriorates further over time and with subsequent deliveries. However, Nygaard and colleagues found, in a 30-year retrospective cohort study, that differences in anal incontinence between women with sphincter rupture, those with episiotomy and no rupture, and those who had cesarean delivery decrease with time from delivery to the point of equivalence.

TABLE 40.2

CAUSES OF ANAL INCONTINENCE

ABNORMAL PELVIC FLOOR
Congenital anorectal malformations
Obstetric injury
Third- of fourth-degree perineal lacerations
Episiotomy breakdown
Forceps delivery
Operative procedures
Colpoperineorrhaphy
Vulvectomy
Difficult hysterectomy
Colpotomy drainage of pelvic abscess
Excision of Bartholin gland
Hemorrhoidectomy
Trauma
Impalement
Pelvic fracture
Foreign body
Anal intercourse
Inflammatory bowel disease
Crohn disease
Tuberculosis
Granulomatous venereal disease
Ulcerative colitis
Diverticulitis
Perirectal abscess
Malignancy
Carcinoma of the cervix
Carcinoma of the vagina
Carcinoma of the vulva
Carcinoma of the rectum
Pelvic floor denervation (idiopathic neurogenic incontinence)
Vaginal delivery
Chronic straining at stool
Rectal
Aging
NORMAL PELVIC FLOOR
Diarrheal states
Infectious diarrhea
Inflammatory bowel disease
Short-gut syndrome
Laxative abuse
Radiation enteritis
Overflow
Impaction
Encopresis
Rectal neoplasms
Neurologic conditions
Congenital anomalies (i.e., myelomeningocele)
Multiple sclerosis
Dementia, stroke, tabes dorsalis
Neuropathy (i.e., diabetes)
Neoplasms of brain, spinal cord, cauda equina
Injuries to brain, spinal cord, cauda equina

The use of midline episiotomy is associated with anal sphincter rupture. Shiono and associates, using data from the Collaborative Perinatal Project, reported that midline episiotomy was associated with statistically significant 4.2-fold and 12.8-fold increases in the risk of third- and fourth-degree lacerations among primiparous and multiparous women, respectively. Studies by Green and Soohoo, Wilcox and colleagues, Thorp and associates, as well as others, suggest that midline episiotomy is associated with third- or fourth-degree laceration even when other factors are controlled for. The Collaborative Perinatal Project data indicate that 10% of women who had a midline episiotomy had a severe laceration. Shiono and associates believe that the risks and benefits of midline episiotomy as practiced in the United States should be reevaluated, especially in view of the observation that midline episiotomy may cause, rather than prevent, lacerations. Mediolateral episiotomy results in less risk of sphincter trauma but is not widely practiced in the United States. Sartore and colleagues have observed that mediolateral episiotomy is associated with lower subsequent pelvic floor muscle strength compared with spontaneous perineal lacerations. Data from Sultan and colleagues (1993) and others suggest an association between sphincter rupture and the use of forceps, to a greater degree than with the use of vacuum, for assisted delivery.

The obstetric repair of a third- or fourth-degree laceration represents a primary surgical procedure that has significant implications for the patient's quality of life. Because many patients are left with some degree of incontinence, attention has begun to focus on the repair procedure itself. These lacerations often are repaired at odd hours by individuals of varying experience in the delivery room, where conditions such as lighting, exposure, anesthesia, and asepsis are less than optimal. The standard repair is taught most often as an end-to-end repair of a narrow tube of external anal sphincter with little attention being paid to possible internal sphincter damage. Evaluations of patients treated with current repair techniques have demonstrated unsatisfactory outcomes. Poen and colleagues reported on long-term clinical and functional results of standard primary repair of third-degree lacerations. They found significantly diminished squeeze pressures and increased first sensation of filling and anal mucosal electrosensitivity compared with controls. Forty percent of their study population had anal incontinence 5 years after repair. Eighty-eight percent of these subjects had a sphincter defect on anal endosonography. In a prospective cohort study of women after primary repair of anal sphincter laceration, Kammerer-Doak and colleagues found significantly decreased resting and squeeze pressures in study subjects versus controls. Forty percent of study subjects were found to have sphincter defects present on ultrasound despite primary repair, and a trend toward continued anorectal dysfunction was found in the laceration group.

The idea of a different repair using an overlapping technique for the external anal sphincter with a separate repair of the internal anal sphincter is the subject of some research interest at present. Sultan et al. (1999) published an initial experience with such a repair in 32 patients performed by two experienced surgeons with the patient moved to a well-lit operating room and given adequate anesthesia and antibiotics. At follow-up, all had apparent healing, 8% encountered incontinence of flatus, 15% had persistent external sphincter defects on ultrasound, and 44% had persistent internal sphincter defects. Fitzpatrick and associates prospectively randomized 112 primiparas who suffered a third-degree laceration to overlapping versus approximation repair. At 3 months, they found no statistically significant difference in incontinence scores, anal manometry, or endoanal ultrasound. Interestingly, 66% of all subjects had a residual full-thickness defect present in their external anal sphincter regardless of type of primary repair. Most recently, Fernando and colleagues, in a randomized controlled trial, found that primary overlapping repair of the external anal sphincter with separate repair of the internal sphincter when needed was associated with a significantly lower rate of fecal incontinence (0% vs. 24%), fecal urgency (3.7% vs. 32%), and perineal pain (0% vs. 20%) compared with an end-to-end approach. In general, most of these studies imply that results of obstetric sphincteric rupture repair may be improved by optimizing standard surgical considerations, including lighting, exposure, adequate anesthesia, use of antibiotics, and proper aseptic surgical technique.

On occasion, the rectal mucosal portion of a repair will break down, which can result in rectovaginal fistula. In Hibbard's series of 24 rectovaginal fistulae and 27 chronic perineal lacerations, 47 (92%) were caused by obstetric trauma. Even meticulously repaired lacerations will occasionally completely break down. This leaves the patient with an open cloacal deformity. Anal incontinence usually is a problem for these patients until the tissues are healed sufficiently to allow secondary repair. Repairs that appear on the surface to have healed satisfactorily may have some internal persistent structural defects, such as partial separation of the sphincter muscle fibers, revealed by ultrasound. The clinical significance of these small defects is not clear.

Another potential cause of persistent incontinence, even after successful anatomic repair of the anal sphincter, is denervation injury to the sphincter muscles. Snooks and colleagues (1984) demonstrated that there is physiologic evidence of denervation of the sphincter in 60% of patients with anal incontinence and an obstetric tear. In women who did not sustain any injury to the external sphincter during delivery, 42% had evidence of denervation. These denervation injuries were strongly associated with a prolonged second stage of labor, forceps delivery, and a large fetus, suggesting that the mode of injury of the pelvic nerves may be from stretching of the nerves during descent of the pelvic floor, from ischemic injury, or from direct compression of the nerves. Most of these individuals reenervate their pelvic floor over the first 6 months postpartum with improvement in their anal function, but many do not regain full neurologic function. At present, there is no way to predict who will sustain damage or who will regain function. Much of what used to be termed "idiopathic" anal incontinence is now understood to be neurogenic anal incontinence.

Other Causes

A promoter of anal incontinence over time is the fact that the normal process of aging results in decreased efficiency of the anal sphincter complex. Haadem and associates showed a natural decline with aging in resting and squeeze pressures in the anal canal of continent subjects. With increasing age, the internal sphincter generates a lower resting pressure, and the proportion of fibrous tissue increases. The squeeze pressure able to be exerted by the external sphincter suffers a natural decline as well. Increasing age also is associated with prolonged pudendal nerve terminal motor latencies (PNTMLs) and elevated rectal and anal sensory thresholds. Because of this, many patients with damaged continence mechanisms may be able to compensate for a period of time, but they go on to decompensate secondary to these age-related changes and become incontinent.

Functional problems of the bowel, such as constipation or diarrhea, can result in incontinence. Chronic constipation with its repeated straining at stool can cause stretch-induced injury to pudendal enervation. Overall, the most common cause of anal incontinence in the elderly, particularly those who are institutionalized, is fecal impaction with overflow incontinence. A diarrheal state can result in anal incontinence even in a patient with normal anorectal function, owing to the presence of large quantities of liquid stool that may overwhelm a normally functional mechanism. Neurologic disorders affecting sphincter control also may result in anal incontinence. Usually, the neurologic defect is widespread, and anal incontinence is but one manifestation.

Traumatic injury, more often a side-straddle injury in young girls, may result in simple or extensive laceration of the perineum. The extent of the injury may be difficult to determine because of pain, fear, edema, hemorrhage, and hematoma formation. Examination under anesthesia is advisable so that appropriate repair can be made, looking carefully for lacerations of the anal sphincter and rectum as well as other structures. Hematoma dissection above the levator muscles must be ruled out with pelvic ultrasound and with careful rectovaginal examination under anesthesia. Above the levator muscles, there is nothing to impede the progression of a hematoma until the diaphragm is reached.

Rectal trauma from operative procedures can affect rectal capacity and compromise anal continence or perhaps lead to extraanal incontinence through a rectovaginal fistula. Entry into the rectum may occur during posterior colpoperineorrhaphy, especially when the anterior rectal wall and posterior vaginal skin are closely adherent with little, if any, intervening connective tissue. Such an enterotomy should be repaired transversely if longitudinal closure would compromise rectal capacity. A difficult hysterectomy, either abdominal or vaginal, may result in injury to the rectum, especially when dissection behind the cervix is difficult because of dense adhesions, indurated tissue from infection, or involvement of the cul-de-sac and anterior rectal wall with endometriosis. If the rectal defect does not heal properly or is not closed properly, a high rectovaginal fistula may develop through the newly closed vaginal apex. Partial excision of anal sphincter and other muscles involved in maintaining anal continence may be required in extensive vulvectomy for cancer resulting in anal incontinence, as reported by Berek and others. Injury to the anterior rectal wall may occur during hemorrhoidectomy, excision of a Bartholin's gland, or colpotomy for pelvic abscess drainage.

Forty to sixty percent of patients with rectal or rectal mucosal prolapse also have some degree of anal incontinence. Although this was originally thought to be secondary to a dilatation effect on the internal anal sphincter, there is often evidence of associated neurogenic damage to the external sphincter muscles as well. This has been confirmed by studies demonstrating prolonged PNTMLs in these patients. These individuals may present with a patulous anal sphincter, passive stretching of the puborectalis muscles, and a long history of straining with constipation. The tissue prolapse may be related to prolapsing internal hemorrhoidal tissue, rectal mucosa, or complete (full-thickness) rectal prolapse. Questions such as the frequency of occurrence of the prolapse, association with activity or defecation, estimated distance of the prolapsed tissue from the anus, spontaneous or manual reducibility, and history of incarceration may be helpful in better defining the type of problem. Patients may have relatively occult prolapse of tissue, which can manifest as mucous or brownish staining in the undergarments with occasional blood.

On physical examination, it is important to note the following: a patulous anus, which may indicate that chronic tissue prolapse has been occurring. The presence of enlarged external hemorrhoidal tissue may suggest the presence of enlarged internal hemorrhoidal complexes; however, they may be found in relative isolation and may be mistaken as prolapsed tissue. Patients should be asked to bear down as if defecating to manifest any prolapsed tissue. Concentric circular folds and a large protruding mass suggest the presence of complete prolapse, which often extends well beyond the anus. Noncircumferential folds may be either mucosal prolapse or hemorrhoidal tissue. If the patient's history suggests the presence of prolapse and it is not visualized with the patient in the left lateral or lithotomy position, it is often helpful to have the patient sit on a commode with subsequent examination in this position. Correction of prolapsing tissue such as hemorrhoids may lead to improvement in anal continence, if this is the primary cause of the problem. In patients with complete rectal prolapse undergoing surgical repair, the rate of some degree of residual incontinence ranges from 40% to 90%, depending on the type of repair used.

Crohn disease is the most important of the variety of inflammatory bowel diseases that may cause extraanal incontinence through a rectovaginal fistulae. Among 138 patients with rectovaginal fistulae seen at Duke University Medical Center, Bandy and associates reported that 15 (11%) were caused by Crohn disease. The diagnosis, perioperative management, and surgical technique chosen for these patients constitute a special challenge for the gynecologic surgeon. Crohn disease must be considered as a possible cause of rectovaginal fistula in any patient in whom other causes are not clear, particularly if the fistula orifice is tender to palpation. Crohn disease also should be considered in the patient who has failed multiple attempts at fistula repair because the fistula tends to recur at the operative site in these individuals.

The role of diverticulitis as a cause of sigmoidovaginal fistulae has been highlighted by Tancer and Veridiano, who report on 130 such cases. These fistulae usually present with a malodorous vaginal discharge in women older than 50 years of age, some years after a hysterectomy. Such fistulae commonly develop between the inflamed bowel segment and the apical vaginal scar from the previous hysterectomy, although they may infrequently occur through a retained cervix. Often, the diverticular disease is silent and is only discovered with further investigations of the fistula tract. A diverticular abscess may have formed and found drainage though the path of least resistance, which in this case is the thinned out scar of the vaginal cuff.

Malignant tumors may erode through the tissues between the vagina and the rectum. When a patient with tumor involvement of the rectovaginal wall receives radiation, sloughing of the tumor may result in a rectovaginal fistula. Radiation also may cause a rectovaginal fistula without tumor erosion.

Rarely, anal incontinence may be congenital, as seen in one of 5,000 newborn girls who have an imperforate anus with associated fecal incontinence through a congenital rectovaginal or rectoperineal fistula. Total rectal agenesis is rare. Paul and Lloyd reported hindgut duplication with a congenital rectovaginal fistula; however, most anal incontinence is acquired. Finally, although anal incontinence may be termed idiopathic in about 10% of women, the mechanism of incontinence in these women is usually secondary to pelvic floor denervation.

In summary, although an intact and functional anal sphincter complex and puborectalis sling are important in the maintenance of anal continence, it must be remembered that a variety of other factors are involved, including intact anorectal sensation and reflexes, rectal capacity and distensibility, reasonable colonic transit time, appropriate stool volume and consistency, and adequate patient mental function and mobility.

EVALUATION OF ANAL INCONTINENCE

A careful history and physical examination are vital to eliciting the presence of, delineating the cause of, and guiding the management of anal incontinence. Judiciously used, diagnostic tests such as anal endosonography, anal manometry, pelvic floor electromyography (EMG), PNTMLs, and defecography can be useful as well. In addition, anal endosonography and defecography may uncover anatomic defects and gastrointestinal abnormalities not previously appreciated by physical examination alone. All of these objective studies are valuable as research tools and have done much to increase our understanding of anorectal anatomy and function; however, their precise clinical role still remains somewhat unclear. Many of the above studies are most useful in patients with idiopathic anal incontinence or persistent incontinence after a failed surgical repair.

History and Physical Examination

Patients are reticent to discuss problems of anal incontinence. A survey of 666 patients in a general gynecologic outpatient clinic in Switzerland by Faltin and colleagues found that 5.6% had anal incontinence. Of those individuals, only 20% had ever reported this symptom to a health care provider. For this reason, patients should always be asked during a history about specific symptoms of anal incontinence in a nonthreatening way that helps them overcome feelings of embarrassment and invites discussion.

Once a history of defecatory dysfunction is elicited, the examiner should attempt to differentiate true incontinence from other conditions. A symptom diary can be useful both for diagnosis as well as monitoring progress during treatment. Perianal leakage of material other than stool can occur because of prolapsing hemorrhoids, anorectal neoplasms, or sexually transmitted diseases. Poor hygienic practice can lead to patients noting fecal staining after bowel movements that does not truly represent anal incontinence. Anorectal frequency and urgency without the loss of bowel contents may occur in patients with inflammatory bowel disease, irritable bowel syndrome, and prior pelvic irradiation. In patients for whom the diagnosis is in doubt, the ability to retain an enema argues strongly against severe anal sphincter weakness.

The severity and impact of anal incontinence on a patient's quality of life can be assessed and quantified with validated questionnaires such as the Fecal Incontinence Severity Index, Modified Manchester Health Questionnaire, and the Fecal Incontinence Quality of Life Scale. Dietary habits should be discussed. Screening for associated medical conditions such as diabetes mellitus, neurologic problems, and medication use should be included in the initial evaluation. Past surgical and obstetric history should be carefully reviewed for any prior gastrointestinal or anorectal surgery, number of vaginal deliveries, a history of prolonged labor, use of forceps, and significant perineal lacerations.

Physical examination should include a general screening neurologic examination to identify occult neurologic disease. (Anal incontinence is rarely the presenting symptom in patients with spinal cord lesions.) Pelvic examination should include a careful inspection of the posterior vaginal wall, perineum, anal sphincter, anal canal, and rectum, including assessment of the patient's function as well as anatomy. A patulous anus indicates a major loss of sphincter function and can be associated with rectal prolapse. Most obstetric injuries are associated with an anterior segmental defect in the external anal sphincter and may appear as the loss of the perineal body, loss of the corrugated appearance surrounding the anus, or attenuation of the rectovaginal septum in some instances. In more subtle cases in which the perineal body appears intact but the external sphincter is actually separated, there may be only the dimples of the laterally retracted ends of the anal sphincter muscles apparent. This produces a "dovetail" appearance, as described by Toglia and DeLancey, in which the normal radial distribution of the anal creases is absent anteriorly but is present laterally and inferiorly. If there is a question as to the presence of a segmental defect, endoanal or transperineal ultrasound can be useful in delineating the anatomy. Next, a screening evaluation of the perineal reflexes to assess the integrity of the S2–4 dermatomes should be performed. Perception of pinpoint and light touch over the perineal skin and buttocks can be tested easily with the broken end of a wooden cotton swab or a safety pin. Light stroking of the inferolateral margin of the labia majora should cause a reflex contraction of the bulbocavernosus muscle within the labia. The anal wink reflex can be elicited by lightly stroking the perianal skin or touching it with a pin to cause a reflex contraction of the external anal sphincter. Asking the patient to cough also should elicit the reflex contraction of the external anal sphincter. With both of these maneuvers, the anal canal should constrict concentrically owing to contraction of the external sphincter, and the anus should be pulled inward secondary to the contraction of the puborectalis muscle. In women with separation of the external anal sphincter, voluntary contraction of the pelvic floor muscles can cause an accentuation in the lateral perineal dimpling of the retracted ends. In patients with a denervated sphincter, there is no retraction of the anal skin during voluntary contraction. Patients who demonstrate abnormalities of these pelvic floor reflexes may require more in-depth neurologic evaluation.

Extraanal incontinence may result from a fistulous tract. A rectovaginal fistula is usually easily diagnosed by careful inspection of the posterior vaginal wall. By spreading the labia, a low fistula can be revealed, usually involving the area of a previous episiotomy or obstetric laceration. A high fistula can be seen using a bivalve speculum and often appears at the vaginal cuff scar. A straight-handled speculum can be useful as it can be rotated to allow full visualization of both the anterior and posterior vaginal walls. The vaginal opening of a fistula may be localized by the presence of feces in the vagina or by the dark red rectal mucosa seen protruding at the fistulous opening contrasting with the lighter vaginal mucosa. Colposcopic examination of the vagina sometimes assists in the identification of a small fistula orifice. When the fistula is small, it may be difficult to locate both the vaginal and rectal ends of the fistula, but both orifices must be located for complete care to be given. A small probe can be pushed gently from the vaginal side of the fistula and the tip felt on a rectally placed finger. Instillation of methylene blue through the vaginal orifice of the fistula may aid in the proctoscopic visualization of the rectal orifice. Carey describes the following examination technique to identify a suspected rectovaginal fistula. A Foley catheter with a 10-mL balloon is inserted into the anus while the posterior vaginal wall is painted with a concentrated solution of soap and water, or, alternatively, the vagina can be filled with water. As the rectum is distended with air by a syringe attached to the Foley catheter, the vaginal orifice of the fistula may be localized by the presence of bubbles forming at the fistula site. A small probe may then be passed along the fistula tract.

Alternatively, when a rectovaginal fistula is suspected but cannot be identified, radiologic studies such as a vaginogram or fistulogram may identify a fistulous tract. These studies are superior to barium enema for identifying a fistula because they use a thin, water-soluble radioopaque medium rather than a thick barium solution. As such, although fistulae occasionally may be identified by barium enema, the intraluminal pressure of the bowel often is inadequate to force the barium solution through a small fistula opening. In addition, the presence of barium in the lower bowel may obscure a fistula tract.

When a rectovaginal fistula is diagnosed, it is important to complete a thorough assessment of the anal sphincter and pelvic floor as well because these patients may have multiple defects. If not properly evaluated preoperatively, the patient may undergo successful repair of her fistula only to become anally incontinent postoperatively. Her compromised sphincter function may have been adequate preoperatively when excess pressure was bypassing the sphincter through the fistula. After her fistula is repaired and the full force of rectal contents is delivered to the sphincter complex, there may not be adequate function to maintain continence. A full treatment of rectovaginal fistula management appears later in this chapter.

A thorough digital rectal examination should be performed. Any rectal mass must be noted and the stool consistency assessed. A gross assessment of the patient's resting and squeeze pressures within the anal canal and her ability to contract her levator ani muscles should be included. Anal sphincter tone should be evaluated with the patient at rest and during sphincter contraction. An anterior sphincter defect may be easily detectable as the loss of the palpable muscular ring within the perineal body. Even in the absence of external anal sphincter muscle anteriorly, a scarified band of tissue can remain that completes the contractile ring and helps the patient maintain continence. Next, the anorectal axis can be assessed. On rectal examination, the puborectalis muscle is palpable posteriorly at the junction between the rectum and the anal canal. By directing the examining finger posteriorly, the angle between the anus and rectum can be estimated and should approximate 90 degrees in a normal woman. More important, when the patient is asked to squeeze the sphincter, the puborectalis muscle should pull the examiner's finger anteriorly toward the pubic bone.

The cause of anal incontinence can be identified in most cases by using these guidelines for careful evaluation of the perineum, posterior vaginal wall, pelvic floor muscles, external anal sphincter, and rectum. In the young parous patient, obstetric injury to the anterior anal sphincter complex is most often apparent on physical examination. One exception is the integrity of the internal anal sphincter. It cannot be assessed adequately by physical examination alone, but can be determined by radiologic and physiologic tests. A defect of the internal sphincter can be assumed, however, if there is significant thinning of the rectovaginal septum. In many of these cases, both the internal and external anal sphincters are injured. Certainly, the patient with a cloacal deformity by definition has a segmental defect in both sphincters. From a practical and technical viewpoint, the internal anal sphincter cannot be repaired unless the external sphincter also is repaired. Surgery is rarely effective for an isolated defect of the internal sphincter. When surgical repair of the external anal sphincter is indicated, however, one should consider repairing defects in the internal sphincter as well.

Testing

Clearly, many patients will have a diagnosis and be ready to proceed to treatment after their history and physical examination. For others, the picture will be less clear. There may be questions about a particular patient that thoughtful use of testing can answer. Is a segmental defect present in the internal or external anal sphincter? What is the functional status within the anal canal? Is rectal sensation normal? Is the enervation to the striated musculature of the continent mechanism intact? How does the patient actually defecate: Are rectoceles, enteroceles, or sigmoidoceles interfering? Is intussusception involved? Judicious use of testing based on the information needed to arrive at an accurate diagnosis and to plan successful treatment can be important.

Anal Imaging

Endoanal, transvaginal, and transperineal ultrasound techniques have made it simple and relatively inexpensive to identify defects in both the internal and external anal sphincters. These defects can go clinically unrecognized, but may be amenable to surgical repair. Anal endosonography is one radiologic technique for assessing posttraumatic defects of the internal and external anal sphincters. High-resolution images of the separate sphincter muscles are obtained using a rotating endoprobe, and anatomic defects can be identified as a loss of continuity of the muscle rings (Fig. 40.8). Several studies have found that anal endosonography correlates well with needle EMG mapping of sphincter defects, manometric mapping of sphincter defects, and intraoperative findings. Ultrasound is less time-consuming than EMG or manometry and much more comfortable for the patient. Other studies have established that transvaginal ultrasound is equally efficacious to endoanal ultrasound in identifying sphincter defects. Peschers and colleagues described normal sphincter and puborectalis anatomy as well as defects in both the internal and external sphincters using exoanal ultrasonography: a conventional 5-MHz convex transducer placed on the perineum. Ultrasound currently is the study of choice for establishing the presence or absence of a segmental anal sphincter defect. The approach chosen—endoanal,

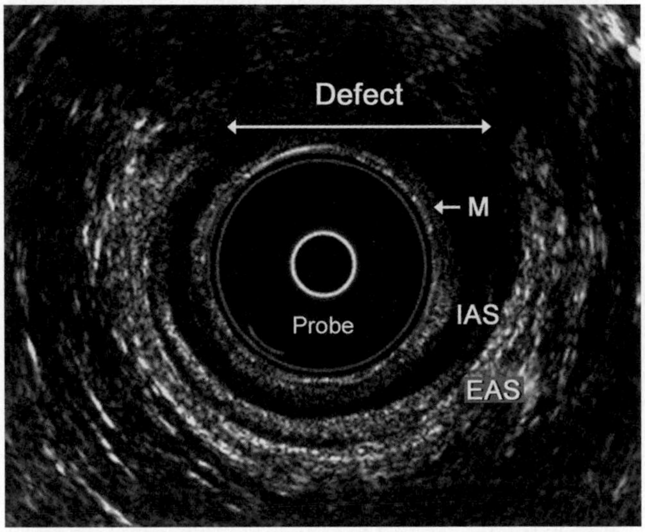

FIGURE 40.8. Endoanal ultrasound image of an anally incontinent patient with a segmental external anal sphincter defect. *Probe*, endoanal ultrasound probe; *M*, anal mucosa; *IAS*, internal anal sphincter; *EAS*, external anal sphincter; *defect*, segmental defect of external anal sphincter. (Photograph courtesy of Justin A. Maykel, MD.)

transvaginal, or transperineal—may depend on the equipment available and operator expertise.

Endoanal ultrasound identifies anatomic defects or thinning of the internal anal sphincter, but Heyer and associates showed that interpretation of external sphincter images is much more subjective and confounded by normal anatomic variations in the external anal sphincter. Indeed, the external anal sphincter and perirectal fat are both echogenic and frequently indistinguishable; the external sphincter may be asymmetrical in the upper anal canal, particularly in women. A new imaging modality with better soft-tissue definition may be desirable. MRI may prove to be superior to endoanal ultrasound because of high tissue contrast between the external anal sphincter and the perirectal fat. DeSouza and associates reported 100% concordance between MRI performed with an endoanal coil and surgical findings for presence, size, and location of anal sphincter tears in seven patients with obstetric trauma. Additionally, Lienemann and colleagues and Healy and associates have demonstrated that MRI also can define dynamic pelvic floor motion during defecation and squeeze. Rapid image acquisition is crucial for optimal visualization of dynamic motion, particularly because patients cannot maintain rectal expulsion or puborectalis contraction for more than 15 to 30 seconds. Prospective comparisons of endoanal MRI to endoanal ultrasound and barium defecography in anally incontinent subjects are in progress.

Although MRI is very effective at delineating the soft-tissue anatomy related to anal continence—whether it is performed with a body coil, phased array coil, endovaginal coil, or endoanal coil—the high cost of scanning, limited access to scanners, and the complexity of the examination itself keep MRI largely a research modality at present. This is especially true because ultrasound is now relatively inexpensive, widely available, and easy for the patient. MRI's exquisite soft-tissue differentiation and capability for multiplanar imaging makes it an excellent research modality for studying these structures undisturbed in living patients. Its clinical role in relation to anal incontinence is emerging.

Anal Manometry

Anal manometry provides information regarding function, sensation, compliance, and the presence of intact reflexes within the anal canal and distal rectum. The first part of this test is essentially a pressure profile of the anal canal, providing information on the functional status of the internal and external anal sphincters. Some computer-based, multichannel manometry equipment can provide graphic cross-sectional analysis of the anal canal to help detect the presence of segmental sphincter defects.

The test usually is performed with the patient in the left lateral decubitus position without any special bowel preparation. There are many different protocols for performing anal manometry. Most commonly, a fluid-filled pressure catheter with radial side ports located 90 degrees apart circumferentially is connected to pressure transducers, and a recording device is used to measure the anal canal pressures during rest and during voluntary contraction of the anal sphincter (Fig. 40.9). These pressures may be recorded either as the pressure catheter is slowly pulled through the anal canal—a station pull-through technique—or at static points along the anal canal as the pressure catheter is pulled out in certain increments, usually every 0.5 cm. The average pressure measured at rest in the anal canal

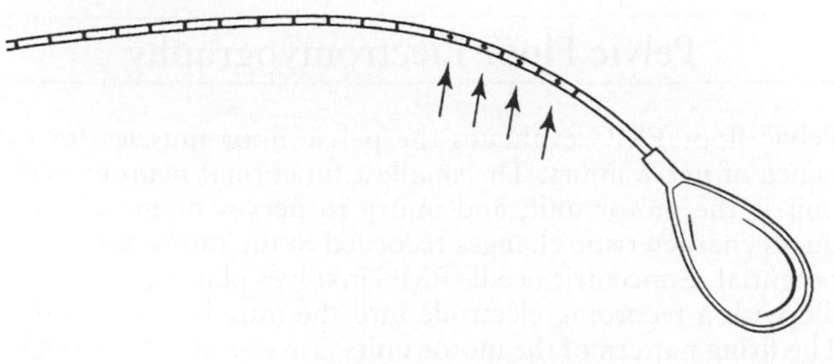

FIGURE 40.9. Anal manometry perfusion catheter. An open-tipped perfusion catheter with radial side ports located every 0.5 cm (*arrows*) records anorectal pressures. Distention of the balloon at the end of the catheter is used to determine rectal sensory thresholds and to elicit the rectoanal inhibitory reflex.

is the resting pressure, and the highest pressure recorded along the anal canal with the patient at rest is the maximum resting pressure. The increase in pressure over the basal canal pressure initiated by voluntary contraction of the anal sphincter is the squeeze pressure, and the highest such increment is the maximum squeeze pressure. The resting anal canal length is measured from the point at which the anal sphincter pressure continuously exceeds the average intrarectal pressure by 4 mm Hg. The resting pressure is largely a reflection of the internal anal sphincter function, whereas the squeeze pressure reflects the strength of the external anal sphincter voluntary contraction (Fig. 40.3).

A second part of anal manometry testing is the evaluation of rectal sensation. A balloon is placed in the rectum and incrementally distended. The minimum perceived volume, the volume causing the urge to defecate, and the maximum tolerable volume are recorded. Measurements of pressures within the balloon allow the calculation of rectal compliance. The presence of a reflex rectal contraction after a bolus of air is introduced into the balloon, followed by the return to normal baseline pressures as the rectum accommodates, also is noted. Most healthy patients have a minimal perceived volume of about 30 cc and a maximum tolerable volume of about 300 to 350 cc, although this can be highly variable. When the rectal capacity is 200 cc, however, proctitis is often found.

"Normal" range for maximum resting pressure is 40 to 80 cmH_2O and for maximum squeeze pressure is 100 to 200 cmH_2O; however, there is tremendous overlap in values between patients who are continent and those who are incontinent. As a group, incontinent patients have lower values on anal manometry testing than continent patients, although there is no discriminatory level that can be used to predict incontinence. It has been suggested that patients with a maximum resting pressure of <20 cmH_2O and a maximum squeeze pressure of >40 cmH_2O are unlikely to be continent. Sentovich and colleagues found decreased resting and squeeze pressures in 90% of patients with a history of anal sphincter injury. Poen and associates found significantly decreased maximum squeeze pressures and also found first sensation of filling to be significantly increased in 40 subjects who had third-degree lacerations primarily repaired compared with controls. They also found that 35 (88% percent) of these subjects still had sphincter defects present on endoanal ultrasound despite apparently successful healing of their repair. Gearhart and colleagues were unable to demonstrate any single preoperative manometric parameter that was predictive of outcome following sphincteroplasty.

Pelvic Floor Electromyography

Pelvic floor EMG evaluates the pelvic floor muscles for evidence of nerve injury. The smallest functional neuromuscular unit is the motor unit, and injury to nerves or muscles produces characteristic changes recorded in the motor unit action potential. Concentric needle EMG involves placing a small needle with a recording electrode into the muscle being studied. The firing pattern of the motor units is assessed as the needle is being inserted, during spontaneous muscle activity, and during maximum voluntary contraction of the muscle. The characteristics of the recordings can then be evaluated. Single-fiber EMG allows the recording of action potentials from individual muscle fibers of a motor unit. When nerve injury occurs, there is often reenervation but with a change in fiber density. The reenervation is more diffuse and results in less effective muscle contraction than the original active enervation. When these studies indicate nerve reenervation, therefore, it reflects prior nerve damage that has healed. Needle EMG studies also can be used to map specific anatomic defects of the external anal sphincter but, as stated previously, this function currently is more often fulfilled by ultrasound studies.

Nerve conduction velocities, which are the actual speed of conduction of the action potential along the nerve, are another measure of nerve function. The nerve conduction velocity can be calculated by measuring the nerve latency, which is the delay between the stimulation of the nerve at a specific point and the response in the target muscle supplied by the nerve. Standardized latencies for most peripheral nerves have been established. Evaluation of PNTML, as developed by Snooks and colleagues, is of interest in patients with anal incontinence. The pudendal nerve is stimulated as it courses behind the ischial spine into Alcock's canal, and the time is measured until a response is detected in the external anal sphincter. Prolonged PNTMLs indicate nerve damage; however, this test only reflects the conduction time of the healthiest axon remaining in a nerve. Therefore, normal PNTMLs do not confirm a lack of damage to the whole nerve, only that at least one axon remains intact that can conduct a response normally. Cheong and colleagues found pudendal neuropathy in 36% (21% bilateral, 15% unilateral) of 225 patients (174 women) presenting with anal incontinence. Osterberg and associates found a correlation between fiber density and clinical and manometric variables in 72 incontinent patients (63 women), but failed to find a correlation with PNTML. Vaccaro and coworkers found pudendal neuropathy to be an age-related phenomenon in patients with anal incontinence and constipation. A finding of prolonged PNTML may be of clinical significance; however, normal PNTMLs do not exclude the possibility of neurologic damage. Although PNTML testing is in use by many centers, it may lack sensitivity and specificity for detection of external anal sphincter weakness caused by pudendal nerve damage. The American Gastroenterological Association's (AGA) medical position statement on anorectal testing techniques states that "although interesting from a research point of view, the clinical usefulness of this test is controversial.... The PNTML cannot be recommended for evaluation of patients with fecal incontinence."

Although suggestion of neurologic injury may be identified by careful physical examination, neither ultrasound nor anal manometry is helpful in identifying neuropathic patients. Identification of such patients is important. In the presence of neurologic damage, patients are less likely to have a good functional response to operations designed to restore anal incontinence, even when the anatomic result appears completely successful. Knowledge of a patient's pelvic floor neurologic status can be particularly useful for counseling her on what to expect after surgical repair. Although the presence of pudendal neuropathy implies a poorer prognosis for the potential sphincteroplasty patient, it does not mean that many such patients could not derive significant improvement in their continence. Chen and colleagues found in a small group of patients undergoing sphincteroplasty that, based on continence scores, the one patient with no neuropathy had an excellent result; of seven patients with unilateral pudendal neuropathy, 70% had a good to excellent result and 30% had a fair to poor result; whereas in four patients with bilateral neuropathy, half had a good to excellent result and the other half scored fair to poor.

Defecography

Defecography is a radiologic evaluation of the lower gastrointestinal tract. It was used initially in the evaluation of patients with defecation disorders; but more recently, it has been used as part of the evaluation of anal incontinence. The rectum of the patient is filled with a barium-oatmeal or potato starch paste mixed to a consistency to approximate semisolid stool. The patient then is seated on a special commode chair and asked to defecate during fluoroscopy. Lateral radiographs usually are taken before, during, and after evacuation of the rectum (Fig. 40.5). Alternatively, cinedefecography can be performed, which is a videotaped dynamic fluoroscopic study.

The anorectal angle can be observed, as can the effect of willful contraction of the puborectalis muscle on this angle. It also provides information about rectal emptying and the mobility of the rectal wall. Anatomic abnormalities of the gastrointestinal tract not previously identified, such as intussusception, rectal prolapse, and rectal ulcers, can be detected by defecography. Now it is possible to perform a triple contrast study wherein the rectosigmoid, small bowel, and bladder are all opacified with contrast. These studies often reveal disturbances of dynamic pelvic floor motion and interaction of support defects in more than one compartment, for example, rectoceles, sigmoidoceles, enteroceles, and cystoceles.

In relation to anal incontinence, however, the clinical relevance of many of these findings is questionable because there are no findings that are specific for anal incontinence. Many anatomic abnormalities are also found in asymptomatic controls. Although the anorectal angle may be more obtuse in incontinent patients both at rest and during squeezing than in continent patients, recent studies have questioned the significance of the anorectal angle because of the wide overlap in measurements between the two groups. In addition, there is a significant intraobserver variation in the measurement of the anorectal angle from the same set of radiographic films among different radiologists. Last, surgical restoration of the angle with a postanal repair, or retrorectal levatorplasty, is poorly correlated with a return of continence. Therefore, the role of defecography in the evaluation of patients with anal incontinence is unclear.

In summary, because anal continence depends on multiple mechanisms, no one test is ideal for clinical evaluation of the incontinent patient. There is not a standard testing protocol for the anally incontinent patient. Testing should be individualized. Studies should be obtained only to gather specific information needed in the evaluation of an individual patient. Procedures thought by the AGA to be of value in selected patients follow: (a) symptom diary for diagnosis and monitoring of progress; (b) digital examination for basic qualitative assessment of resting and squeeze pressures; (c) anal ultrasound to assess anatomic integrity of the sphincters; (d) anorectal manometry to define sphincter weakness and predict response to biofeedback training; (e) rectal and anal sensory testing; and (f) testing of rectal compliance. Procedures of possible value for an individual patient might include (a) surface EMG for evaluation of sphincter function and evacuation proctography or (b) cinedefecography, when rectal prolapse is suspected. Testing procedures that are controversial for the clinical evaluation of anally incontinent individuals at present include (a) PNTML testing for assessment of pudendal nerve function and (b) MRI, because of its expense.

NONSURGICAL THERAPY OF ANAL INCONTINENCE

The goal of nonsurgical therapies is to minimize the threat to continence from intestinal contents by managing stool consistency and maximizing the patient's remaining levator ani and sphincter function. Because surgical therapy has less than perfect outcomes, strong consideration should be given to trying to optimize a patient's function before the decision for surgery is made. Dietary manipulations and pharmacologic agents may reduce flatus and liquid stools, and pelvic floor exercises, biofeedback therapy, and electrical stimulation facilitate optimization of anal sphincter and levator ani function. To reduce the challenge to the sphincter mechanism, all conditions producing diarrheal states, such as inflammatory bowel disease and malabsorption syndromes, should be treated directly. For constipated patients, a high-fiber diet and the addition of an osmotic laxative (e.g., sorbitol) may produce soft, formed stools that are more easily managed by a compromised sphincter mechanism. Conversely, for patients with diarrhea, a low-residue diet to reduce stool bulk and constipating agents such as loperamide or diphenoxylate with atropine often are helpful. Patients should avoid foods that cause intestinal hypermotility as well as carbonated beverages and foods that tend to produce flatus. Many patients learn on their own that constipation helps them with continence and maintain themselves in a constipated state for many years before presenting to a health care practitioner. Santoro and associates studied amitriptyline for both its ability to slow colonic transit time resulting in a firmer stool that is passed less frequently, as well as improve pressure dynamics in the rectal reservoir. They found significant improvement in symptoms as well as manometric parameters in the study group. In some patients, a system of planned defecation with the use of glycerol suppositories or a daily tap water enema may leave the rectum clean between evacuations and decrease incontinence episodes.

Pelvic floor rehabilitation through physiotherapy with biofeedback, pelvic floor exercises, and electrical stimulation may help improve anal sphincter and pelvic floor function. These techniques are particularly helpful in patients with mild pelvic floor denervation to maximize the strength and function of the sphincter mechanism and levator sling. Rehabilitation techniques may be useful as an initial conservative measure in patients with recent obstetric trauma and evidence of pelvic floor nerve injury. Some reenervation tends to occur over the first 6 months postpartum in these patients. Those who are not able to willfully contract their pelvic floor muscles immediately postpartum because of transient nerve injury may best benefit from electrical stimulation techniques. Pelvic floor rehabilitation may be useful preoperatively to try to maximize the outcome of a subsequent surgical repair. Patients who are improved but not totally continent after surgical repair also may benefit from these techniques to restore their margin of continence.

Pelvic floor exercises, similar to the Kegel exercises performed to improve urinary incontinence and pelvic support, may improve the functioning tone of the external anal sphincter. Biofeedback therapy using an anal balloon or plug electrode can facilitate the proper muscle contraction by measuring the strength of the sphincter contraction and by providing the patient with a visual demonstration of muscle function. Biofeedback therapy also has the advantage of being able to train patients to perceive decreasing volumes of air in the rectum and to coordinate this with the contraction of the external anal sphincter. Biofeedback therapy has been reported to improve anal incontinence in 50% to 90% of patients treated, with most studies showing improvement in about 80% of patients. Some effects of biofeedback training may be long lasting in relation to anal incontinence. Enck and associates studied anally incontinent patients treated with biofeedback versus controls almost 10 years after treatment ended. They did not find a lasting difference in prevalence of anal incontinence, but did find a significant difference in severity of incontinence measured in number and frequency of incontinent episodes. The success of biofeedback therapy seems primarily dependent on the improvement in rectal sensation; manometric studies have not consistently shown an increase in sphincter pressures after therapy. Suitable candidates for biofeedback therapy must have some degree of rectal sensation and be able to contract the anal sphincter voluntarily.

Transanal electrical stimulation can be used as an adjunct to pelvic floor exercises in patients who are unable to contract their pelvic floor muscles or who are unsuccessful with biofeedback therapy alone. An anal probe connected to a neuromuscular stimulation unit delivers a preset voltage to the external anal sphincter to induce contraction of the striated sphincter muscles. This technique causes minimal patient discomfort and has been associated with a significant increase in the maximum squeeze pressure following therapy, with subsequent improvement in partial anal incontinence. It has not been successful in patients with major incontinence of solid stool. Transanal electrical stimulation also is unlikely to be successful in patients with a severely denervated anal sphincter because of the degree of irreparable end-organ damage.

SURGICAL THERAPY FOR ANAL INCONTINENCE

Surgical procedures for anal incontinence are measured by their impact on an individual's symptoms and quality of life. Cure (i.e., total continence of solid, liquid, and gas) is rarely achieved. Papers that discuss surgical results for anal incontinence procedures most often use significant improvement on an incontinence scoring system scale as their criterion for success.

Most patients with anal incontinence who see an obstetrician-gynecologist present with a specific anatomic defect resulting from obstetric or postoperative trauma. These patients suffer from a long-standing disruption of the perineal body and anterior anal sphincter complex often called a chronic perineal laceration (Fig. 40.10). Approaches to the surgical repair of this problem are discussed at length in this chapter. Treatment of patients with idiopathic, neurogenic, or recurrent incontinence without an anatomic defect requires more specialized care and more advanced procedures. These patients are most often referred to a colorectal surgeon or proctologist with a special interest in this area. Although a full discussion of

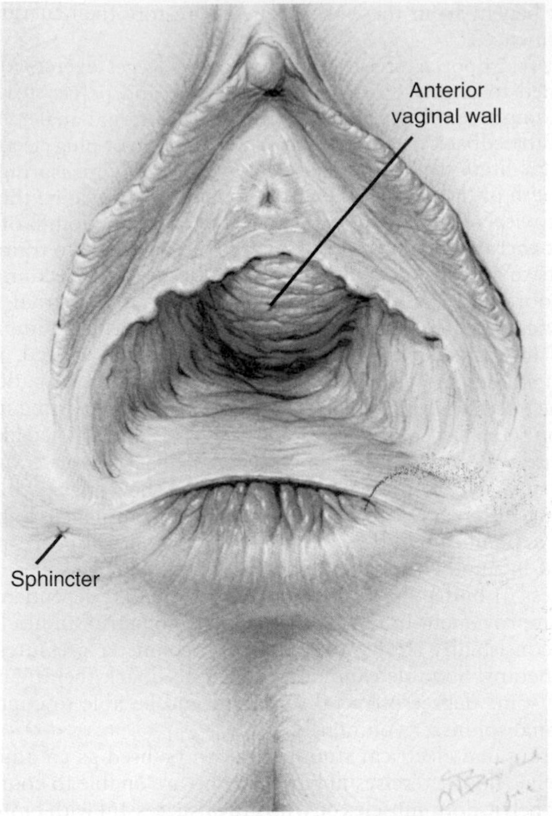

FIGURE 40.10. Chronic perineal laceration. Long-standing disruption of the perineal body and anterior anal sphincter complex usually secondary to obstetric trauma in the past. When the posterior vaginal wall heals directly to the anterior rectal wall above the hymenal ring, this is termed a *cloacal deformity.* Note the dimples on either side of the anal opening owing to the retraction of the ends of the torn external sphincter.

these more difficult patients is beyond the scope of this chapter, some background is given for perspective at the end of this section.

Regardless of which surgical approach is chosen, *a preoperative mechanical bowel preparation* is important. An oral bowel preparation should be given the evening before surgery is scheduled. If such a preparation is given the day of surgery, the patient may still be releasing stool during the operation. Although the patient may be given three doses of oral erythromycin, 500 mg, and neomycin, 1 g, the day before surgery, this may not be necessary in all patients.

The optimal postoperative diet for these patients is a matter of much controversy and little data. Decades ago, these patients were given diverting colostomies to keep the fecal stream away from the repair until healing was complete. Patients would then have another procedure to close their colostomy. Most postoperative feeding regimens are based on the concept of keeping fecal material from the repair site for at least 4 to 5 days until the mucosal suture line has healed adequately and the reparative process is well established. A regimen of clear liquids for 3 to 5 days, with progression to a soft, low-residue diet for the next several weeks, can be given. Constipating agents are sometimes used immediately postoperatively, but should not be used for a prolonged period of time because one wants the first bowel movement to be soft so as not to distend the repair. The use of an elemental liquid diet for 1 week postoperatively can be useful, but is poorly tolerated by many patients and can lead to diarrhea in some. Alternatively, fiber supplementation and adequate hydration can be used to give patients more bulky but deformable stool so as to not traumatize the repair. Stool softeners and a high-fiber diet are advisable for 6 weeks postoperatively.

Over the decades, many surgical approaches to anal incontinence have been tried and found to have less than encouraging results. In the mid-1970s, Sir Allan Parks proposed the postanal repair operation to treat idiopathic anal incontinence. The concept was to plicate the levator ani together behind the anorectal junction to increase the anorectal angle and augment what was proposed as a "flap valve" mechanism for continence involving the levator plate. Since that time, the idea of a flap valve mechanism has been discredited. Keighley studied 105 patients who underwent this operation. With a follow-up of at least 6 months, he found that two-thirds had regained continence. Long-term results of the postanal repair have been disappointing. Matsuoka and colleagues found postanal repair successful in 7 of 20 (35%) patients based on a significant decrease in incontinence scores after a mean follow-up of 3 years. Setti Carraro and associates studied 34 postanal repair patients with a mean follow-up of 6.2 years. They found that only 9 (26%) had continence of solid and liquids and 5 of the 9 still leaked flatus. Recognizing that improvement may be a significant goal, it is important to note that 28 of the 34 subjects assessed their outcome as improved, with the remainder relating no change.

A total pelvic floor repair operation has been proposed that involves a postanal repair, a plication of the levator muscles anterior to the rectum, and a sphincteroplasty. This operation was studied by Deen and colleagues (1993) in a prospective, randomized trial. A total pelvic repair was compared with anterior levator plication plus sphincteroplasty alone as well as with postanal repair alone. They found at 6 and 24 months a significantly better outcome for the total pelvic repair than for either of the other two procedures.

Chronic Perineal Laceration

In most cases of chronic perineal laceration with long-standing disruption of the anterior anal sphincter complex, classic symptoms include the progressive loss of control of gas and feces from the anus. The severity of symptoms generally varies with the degree of perineal laceration and sphincter loss. If the puborectalis muscle is left intact and is well innervated and functional, it can provide sufficient muscular contraction to permit control of feces when the patient is constipated or when the stool is of normal consistency. Such patients quickly learn this and maintain a constipated state to decrease their symptoms. If the entire perineal body is disrupted, including the internal and external anal sphincters, and the posterior vaginal wall heals directly to the anterior rectal wall above the level of the hymenal ring, then the patient is said to have a cloacal deformity (Fig. 40.10).

If repair at the time of delivery breaks down, it has traditionally been taught that a second attempt should be deferred for a minimum of 8 weeks to provide sufficient time for resolution of the inflammatory response, return of an adequate blood supply to the margins of the defect, and return of optimum viability of the perineal tissues. This delay also may allow time for some reenervation to occur if the injury also was associated with pelvic floor denervation injury. A careful physical examination and, perhaps, a proctoscopic examination, should precede the second attempt so that the presence of an occult rectovaginal fistula can be excluded.

To avoid 2 months of uncomfortable symptoms, some surgeons have advocated an earlier repair. The results of early repair of an external anal sphincter and rectal mucosal dehiscence were first reported in 1986 by Hauth and associates. Each patient was seen within 10 days of delivery with dehiscence of a repaired fourth-degree laceration. Patients underwent preoperative mechanical bowel preparation on admission, preoperative wound cleansing and debridement appropriate to the extent of superficial inflammation and necrosis, and preoperative intravenous antibiotic therapy. A range of 1 to 6 days elapsed to allow preparation of the wound area before a layered closure was performed. The bowel was rested for 10 days after the repair. Seven of eight cases were successfully repaired, with complete healing, normal external sphincter function, and no dyspareunia. Similar good results with early repair of dehiscence of fourth-degree episiotomy in 22 patients were reported by Hankins and colleagues. The average hospital stay for debridement, intravenous antibiotic therapy, and repair was 15 days. Two patients developed pinpoint rectovaginal fistulae after early repair. Secondary repair in both cases was successful. Good results of early repair of dehiscence after mediolateral episiotomies, as opposed to midline episiotomies, have been reported by Monberg and Hammen.

A number of techniques have been described over the past 100 years for reconstruction of a complete chronic perineal laceration, including the layered method of repair, the Warren flap procedure, and the Noble-Mengert-Fish operation. Today, some form of layered method of repair is performed most often. If the anorectal mucosa is intact and the injury is largely limited to the anal sphincter complex and perineal body, repair consists of anal sphincteroplasty with extensive perineorrhaphy. If the injury extends into the anal canal and involves the anorectal mucosa, this approach would essentially recreate a fresh fourth-degree perineal laceration, which would then be repaired in a standard layered fashion. Therefore, the initial layer of such a repair would include a suture line in the anorectal mucosa. This was a major disadvantage to the layered approach in these patients in the preantibiotic era. Today this does not represent a significant problem, although infectious complications do occur.

The Warren flap method, first described in 1882, avoids a mucosal incision in the anus, provides a pedicle graft of vaginal mucosa for enlargement of the perineal skin, and provides a more cosmetic result to the perineal body. However, the Warren technique offers no particular improvement in the correction of the muscular defect that produced the anal incontinence. The major advantage of the procedure is that a suture line is not created in the anal mucosa. With the Warren technique, the vaginal mucosa is turned backward and used as the new portion of the anterior wall at the end of the anal canal. The anal sphincter is then reapproximated over the inner portion of the vaginal flap, which remains attached to the anal mucosa. The Warren flap procedure is still used, although less frequently than when first described.

The Noble operation, or anal pull-through procedure, as it is more commonly called, also avoids creating a suture line in the anal mucosa. The procedure was described originally in 1902 by Noble, but received little attention until described again independently by Mengert and Fish in 1955. Noble's original claims for the operation in the surgical era before the availability of antibiotics, blood banks, and modern advances in general anesthesia included (a) elimination of the danger of infection or fecal matter from the rectum in the surgical wound, (b) avoidance of the tediousness of dissecting a vaginal flap, (c) minimal blood loss, and (d) uniformly good results. The most important advantage was the absence of a suture line in the anterior rectal wall. Although performed much less frequently than a layered approach today, interest in this operation remains, particularly for the treatment of rectovaginal fistula. Veronikas and associates reported a 94% anatomic success rate and 77% excellent functional success rate in 34 patients treated with this operation for primary and persistent rectovaginal fistulae.

Regardless of which approach is taken to repair a chronic perineal laceration in the patient with anal incontinence, it is the sphincteroplasty itself that is the keystone to the repair. Below we discuss techniques of anal sphincteroplasty as well as approaches to overall repair of a chronic perineal laceration. The surgeon should keep in mind that the anal sphincteroplasty may be the most important part of the overall repair, especially when transanal incontinence is part of the indication for the operation.

Anal Sphincteroplasty

The anal sphincter complex is a surgical challenge to repair because both the internal and external sphincters have a constant tone that begins pulling against the healing area almost immediately. Functional results from this surgery are far from perfect. The overlapping repair was proposed for the external anal sphincter in the hopes that the scarified ends of the torn sphincter would bolster support for the reparative sutures and not allow them to pull through, resulting in a better anatomic result and, it is hoped, better functional results. The advantage in terms of outcome seems to favor the overlapping approach over the end-to-end approximation method; however, more data clearly are needed in this area. Past studies of these operations are difficult to evaluate because the criteria for what constitutes success or cure often are poorly defined. Total continence of solid stool, liquid, and gas is not often achieved. Again, improvement in continence and quality of life may represent the best outcome measure.

Blaisdell, in an older report, and Arnaud and associates more recently, reported success rates of approximately 60% using the end-to-end approach. Using the overlapping technique, Sitzler and Thomson reported a 74% success rate in 27 women, most of whom had obstetric sphincter injuries. The continence rates after anal sphincteroplasty appear to diminish with time. Rothbarth and colleagues reported on 39 patients who had obstetric injuries and underwent overlapping sphincteroplasty. Their success rates were 77%, 67%, and 62% at 3, 9, and 12 months, respectively.

Three long-term follow-up studies of the degree and quality of continence after overlapping sphincteroplasties reflect the difficulty of the task at hand. Malouf and associates studied patients with a minimum of 5 years follow-up (median 77 months) and found that 23 of 46 patients (50%) had a successful outcome defined as no further surgery and episodes of urge fecal incontinence occurring once a month or less. Of the 23 patients judged to have a successful outcome, 15 had passive soiling, 17 had fecal urgency, 19 were incontinent of solid and liquid stool, and none were fully continent of stool and flatus. Halverson and Hull found in patients with a median follow-up of more than 5 years that 54% were incontinent of solid or liquid stool, and 14% remained totally continent. Gutierrez and colleagues reported on 130 patients with a median follow-up of 10 years. Sixty-one percent continued to have incontinence or required further surgery. Eight patients were totally continent.

The success rates for anal sphincter repair in patients with concurrent pudendal neuropathy are much lower than for those with intact enervation. Gilliland and colleagues looked at a large group of patients who had undergone an overlapping sphincteroplasty with a median follow-up of 2.4 years. They found that 62% of 59 patients with normal pudendal function had a successful outcome, compared with only 17% of the 12 patients with unilateral or bilateral prolonged PNTMLs. Karoui and associates found success rates to deteriorate with time and reported that poor results also were associated with the presence of an internal sphincter defect.

The importance of the internal anal sphincter to continence is a subject of recent interest. It has long been known that this structure contributes most of the resting tone in the anal canal and helps to maintain our day-to-day continence. Purposeful lateral disruption of the internal sphincter to aid with anal fissure healing has been shown to be associated with the development of at least transient incontinence. Vaizey and associates have identified primary degeneration of the internal sphincter as an independent cause of passive anal incontinence in some women with normal neurologic function and no obstetric trauma. It follows that repair of a disrupted internal sphincter should contribute to continence.

Little attention has been paid in the past to repair of the internal sphincter either at the time of initial obstetric injury or at the time of reconstruction of a long-standing injury. Repair of this smooth muscle structure that is tonically contracting against the suture line is more of a challenge in the healing phase than it is to actually accomplish in the operating room. Preliminary reports regarding this repair are mixed. Abou-Zeid reported on eight patients (two women) who had their ultrasonically established internal sphincter defects repaired end to end with 2-0 polyglactic acid sutures. At a median follow-up of 15 months, all were improved, and two achieved full continence. On the other hand, Leroi and associates (1997) reported on five patients with persistent incontinence after surgery that affected the internal sphincter. Three patients felt improved, but none were fully continent. All had persistent defects on ultrasound postoperatively. Three had improvement of their resting pressure, but only one was in the normal range. In a randomized trial addressing internal sphincter repair during total pelvic floor repair for anal incontinence, Deen and colleagues (1995) showed no differences in resting and squeeze pressures or in symptom relief.

Layered Method of Repair of Chronic Perineal Laceration

A transverse or crescent perineal incision is used at the junction of the posterior vaginal wall and anal mucosa. The lateral margins of the incision are extended to the region of the perineal dimple created by the retracted external sphincter, and a midline incision is made along the lower half of the posterior vaginal wall (Fig. 40.11A).

The edges of the vaginal and rectal mucosa are grasped separately with Allis clamps, and the anterior rectal wall is separated in the midline from the posterior vaginal wall with careful scissors dissection. The dissection is carried laterally by sharp dissection to the region of the external anal sphincter. The internal anal sphincter, which is the thickened distal condensation of the circular smooth muscle layer of the rectum, can be seen between the external anal sphincter and the anorectal mucosa as an area of white fibrous tissue (Fig. 40.11B). Meticulous hemostasis and wide mobilization to allow closure without tension are crucial to success with this operation.

A fibrous scar that is retracted lateral to the wall of the anal canal (Fig. 40.11B) often identifies the external sphincter. The exact anatomic margins of the external sphincter frequently are difficult to ascertain. A nerve stimulator can be used to identify contractile skeletal muscle. Alternatively, the Allis clamps containing the ends of the external sphincter can be brought together in the midline and a circumferential sphincter tested for by inserting a double-gloved index finger into the rectum. If necessary, the clamps should be readjusted to incorporate more of the retracted muscle bundles until the constricted effect of the reapproximated sphincter can be demonstrated.

All scar tissue is excised from the margins of the anorectal mucosa, and the defect in the anal mucosa is closed using a continuous or interrupted suture of 3-0 delayed-absorbable material. A running suture may have the advantage of distributing tension along the entire suture line and helping prevent a gap in the closure that could occur from ischemia if an interrupted suture is tied too tight. A submucosally placed suture is ideal. Sometimes this tissue is quite friable, and a full-thickness suturing of the mucosa is the safest method.

After the mucosal margins are approximated, a second supporting layer inverts the initial mucosal suture line. This layer often has been thought of in the past as "perirectal fascia," but in fact it is the thickened downward continuation of the circular smooth muscle layer of the rectum that is the internal anal sphincter. This appears as a white smooth layer of tissue between the anorectal mucosal closure and the external anal sphincter (Fig. 40.11C). Care should be taken in reapproximating this layer over a length of 3 to 5 cm as this muscle is responsible for most of the resting pressure in what is normally a 4-cm high-pressure zone in the anal canal. This layer also serves to imbricate and isolate the mucosal layer and take tension off of it to help it heal and seal against infection.

In an approximation-type external anal sphincteroplasty, the external anal sphincter ends are completely trimmed of scar tissue and united in the midline with interrupted 0 or 2-0 delayed-absorbable sutures. Although some surgeons prefer a permanent suture, such as a braided silicone-treated polyester, a delayed-absorbable monofilament suture such as polydioxanone has the advantage of maintaining excellent tensile strength for an extended period while avoiding the presence of a permanent foreign body. This becomes particularly important in the event of wound infection. Four or five sutures are used to approximate the sphincter muscle. These can be placed 1 cm apart, full thickness, with the nondominant index finger in the anal canal to aid in acquiring excellent purchase on both ends while assuring no penetration of the anal canal itself.

In an overlapping approach to the external anal sphincter, the scarified ends of the sphincter are important to the repair itself and are left in place. The concept of the overlapping sphincteroplasty is to use the scarred ends of the torn sphincter to help hold the sutures that reconstitute the circumferential sphincter. The ends are widely mobilized with the scar tissue left on. Care should be taken to not dissect beyond the 3- and 9-o'clock position because the pudendal enervation to the sphincter enters laterally. The external sphincter then is brought together over

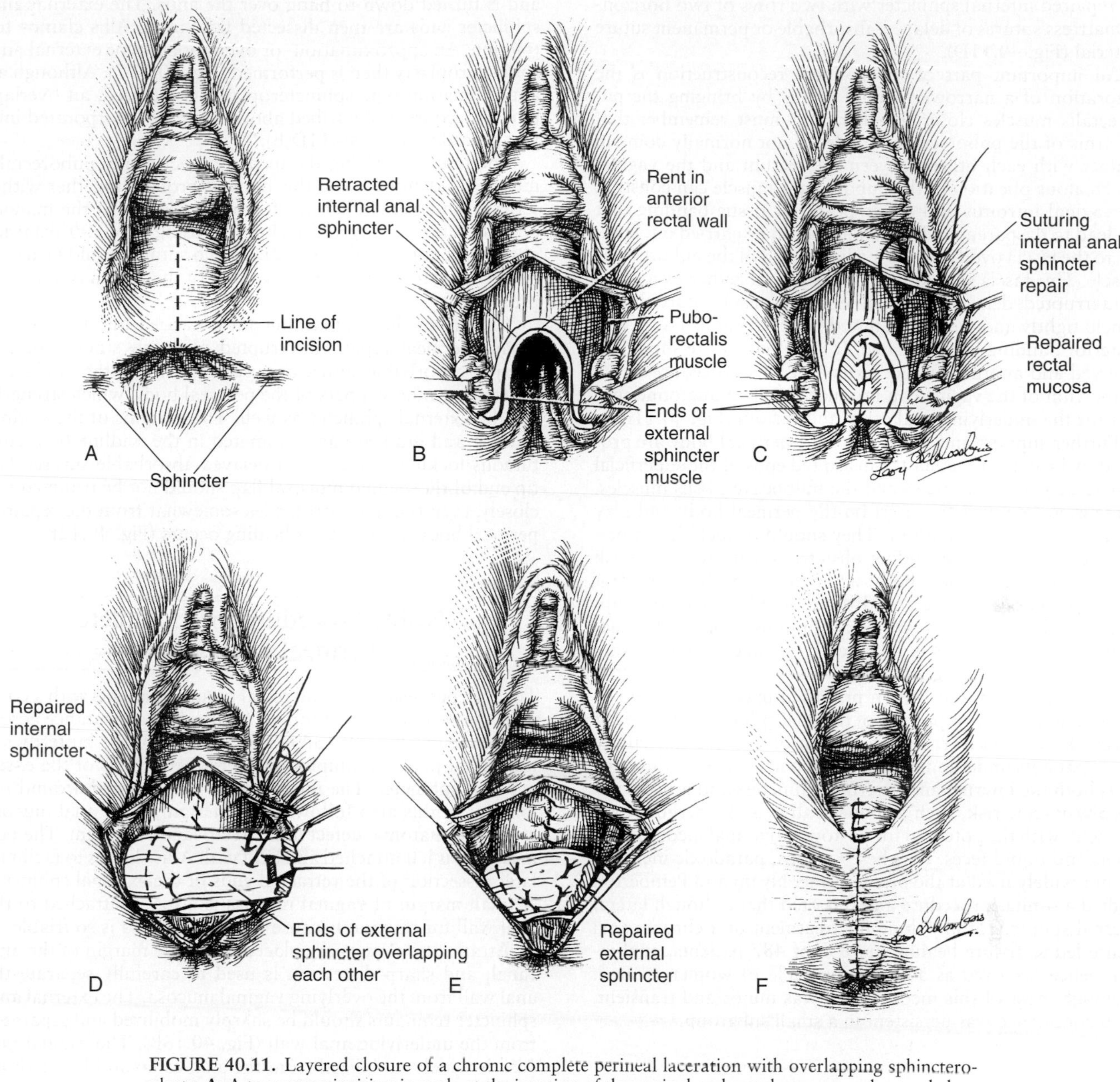

FIGURE 40.11. Layered closure of a chronic complete perineal laceration with overlapping sphinctero-plasty. **A:** A transverse incision is made at the junction of the vaginal and rectal mucosa and extended up the midline of the posterior vaginal wall. **B:** The rectal wall has been separated from the posterior vaginal wall with careful sharp dissection. The ends of the external sphincter have been identified and grasped with Allis clamps. The internal anal sphincter can be seen between the external anal sphincter and the anorectal mucosa as an area of white fibrous tissue. **C:** The defect in the anal mucosa has been closed with a continuous 3-0 delayed-absorbable suture. The internal anal sphincter then is reapproximated over a length of 3 to 5 cm. This layer also serves to imbricate and isolate the mucosal layer and take tension off of it to help it heal and seal against infection. **D:** The ends of the external anal sphincter are widely mobilized with the scar tissue left on. Care should be taken not to dissect beyond the 3- and 9-o'clock position as that is where the pudendal enervation to the sphincter enters laterally. The external sphincter then is brought together over the repaired internal sphincter with two rows of two horizontal mattress sutures of delayed-absorbable or permanent suture material. **E:** After the external sphincter has been repaired, the genital hiatus is narrowed by bringing the puborectalis muscles closer together with interrupted delayed-absorbable sutures placed in the fascia overlying them. **F:** The bulbocavernosus and superficial transverse perinei muscles have been reattached to the perineal body, and the vaginal mucosa was closed with a continuous locking stitch of 3-0 delayed-absorbable suture that was continued subcuticularly to approximate the perineal skin.

the repaired internal sphincter with two rows of two horizontal mattress sutures of delayed-absorbable or permanent suture material (Fig. 40.11D).

An important part of the perineal reconstruction is the restoration of a narrower genital hiatus by bringing the puborectalis muscles closer together. One must remember that the arms of the puborectalis muscle do not normally come in contact with each other between the rectum and the vagina. Overzealous plication of the puborectalis muscle can constrict the vaginal introitus and create posterior tissue banding that can lead to dyspareunia. Dissection should be carried out laterally to the fascia overlying the medial border of the puborectalis muscle. This fascia should then be brought together by a series of interrupted, delayed-absorbable sutures. Each suture should be held tightly and the vagina tested before tying to assure that posterior banding is not created. If it is, that suture should be removed and another placed. Extending this procedure to the midportion of the vagina can produce excellent anatomic support for the underlying anal canal and rectum (Fig. 40.11E).

Further support and elevation of the perineal body are provided by bringing together the disrupted ends of the superficial transverse perineal muscles and the bulbocavernosus muscles. These muscles normally insert on the perineal body and play a part in pelvic floor support. They should be included in perineal reconstruction, including obstetric repair, to reestablish and support the perineal body. After this step, the redundant vaginal mucosa is excised, and the remaining mucosa is approximated in the midline with a continuous 2- or 3-0 delayed-absorbable suture. This is followed by a subcuticular closure of the perineal skin (Fig. 40.11F).

In 1937, Miller and Brown proposed making a paradoxic incision in the inferior portion of the anal sphincter at the 5- or 7-o'clock position to relax the tension on the anterior suture line in patients undergoing sphincter repair. The procedure disrupts both the internal and external sphincters and is not without physiologic risk, such as poor healing and scarring of the sphincter with the potential for postoperative anal incontinence of gas and liquid feces. For these reasons, paradoxic incisions are not widely used at the present time. Nyam and Pemberton studied a similar procedure and reported that although lateral internal sphincterotomy done for treatment of a chronic anal fissure led to fissure healing in 96% of 487 patients, anal incontinence occurred as a sequela in 53% of women treated. Although most of this incontinence was minor and transient, the incontinence was persistent in a small subgroup.

Warren Flap Operation for Complete Third-Degree Tear

An inverted V-shaped incision is made in the posterior vaginal mucosa, outlining the flap that is to be turned down. The lower ends of the incision should be just lateral to the dimples caused by retracted sphincter ends (Fig. 40.12A). The length of the flap should measure a minimum of 3 cm to provide sufficient vaginal mucosa to be incorporated into the anal canal and cover the reconstructed perineal body.

Taking care to avoid injuring the bowel wall, the surgeon dissects the flap of mucosa free from the top downward (Fig. 40.12B), stopping short of the margin between the vaginal and anal mucosa. If this margin is perforated, then the blood supply to the mucosal flap is compromised, thereby nullifying the advantage of the flap technique. The properly demarcated flap allows the areas overlying the sphincter ends to be denuded. The flap is grasped with two mucosal Allis clamps and is turned down to hang over the anus. The external anal sphincter ends are then dissected free, using Allis clamps for traction. An approximation- or overlapping-type external anal sphincteroplasty then is performed (Fig. 40.12C). Although an approximation-type sphincteroplasty is pictured, an overlapping procedure as described above could be incorporated into this procedure (Fig. 40.11D,E).

The fascia overlying the medial aspect of the puborectalis muscles is identified, and this tissue is brought together with a series of interrupted sutures for reinforcement in the manner described for the layered technique, using 0 or 2-0 delayed-absorbable sutures (Fig. 40.12D). Each suture should be tested before tying to assure that the caliber of the vagina is not compromised.

Closure of the vaginal mucosa is carried out as in an ordinary perineal repair. Interrupted plication stitches of 2-0 delayed-absorbable suture are used to advance the fascia and shorten the muscle fibers of the perineal body, which strengthens the external sphincter as well. The margins of the vaginal mucosa and graft are approximated in the midline by a continuous locking stitch of 3-0 delayed-absorbable suture. The tip end of the vaginal mucosal flap should not be trimmed too closely, even though it protrudes somewhat from the repaired perineal body. It retracts as healing occurs (Fig. 40.12E).

Noble Procedure for Complete Perineal Laceration

The torn perineal, anal, and rectal tissue in patients with a complete perineal laceration form a "butterfly" appearance across the perineum (Fig. 40.13A). The "wings" of the butterfly are the lateral perineal dimples of the retracted ends of the external anal sphincter. The initial incision is outlined around the margins of this area following the margin of the anal mucosa along the anatomic defect in the rectovaginal septum. The perineal skin is left attached and held with Allis clamps to facilitate later dissection of the retracted ends of the external sphincter. A small margin of vaginal mucosa is also left attached to the anal wall for traction because the anal mucosa is so friable.

Atraumatic clamps are placed along the margin of the anal canal, and sharp dissection is used to carefully separate the anal wall from the overlying vaginal mucosa. The external anal sphincter remnants should be sharply mobilized and separated from the underlying anal wall (Fig. 40.13B). The vaginal mucosa is widely mobilized from the anal canal and lower rectal wall laterally to the underlying levator muscles and proximally into the middle or upper one third. Adequate mobilization of the anterior anorectal wall allows it to be pulled outside the margin of the anal orifice without difficulty, thus avoiding sutures in the anorectal canal.

Once the ends of the external anal sphincter are mobilized to meet in the midline with traction on the Allis clamps, the overlying skin previously left attached is excised, and the sphincter ends are approximated end to end in the midline (Fig. 40.13C). Alternatively, one could perform an overlapping sphincteroplasty as previously described (Fig. 40.11D,E). Several of these sphincteroplasty sutures also should include the muscular layers of the anterior rectal wall to prevent it from retracting inward and to avoid tension on the suture line between the advanced anterior anorectal wall and the perineal skin. The genital hiatus should be narrowed by bringing the puborectalis muscles closer together as previously described (Fig. 40.13D). The transverse perineal muscles and the inferior margins of the bulbocavernosus muscles then are

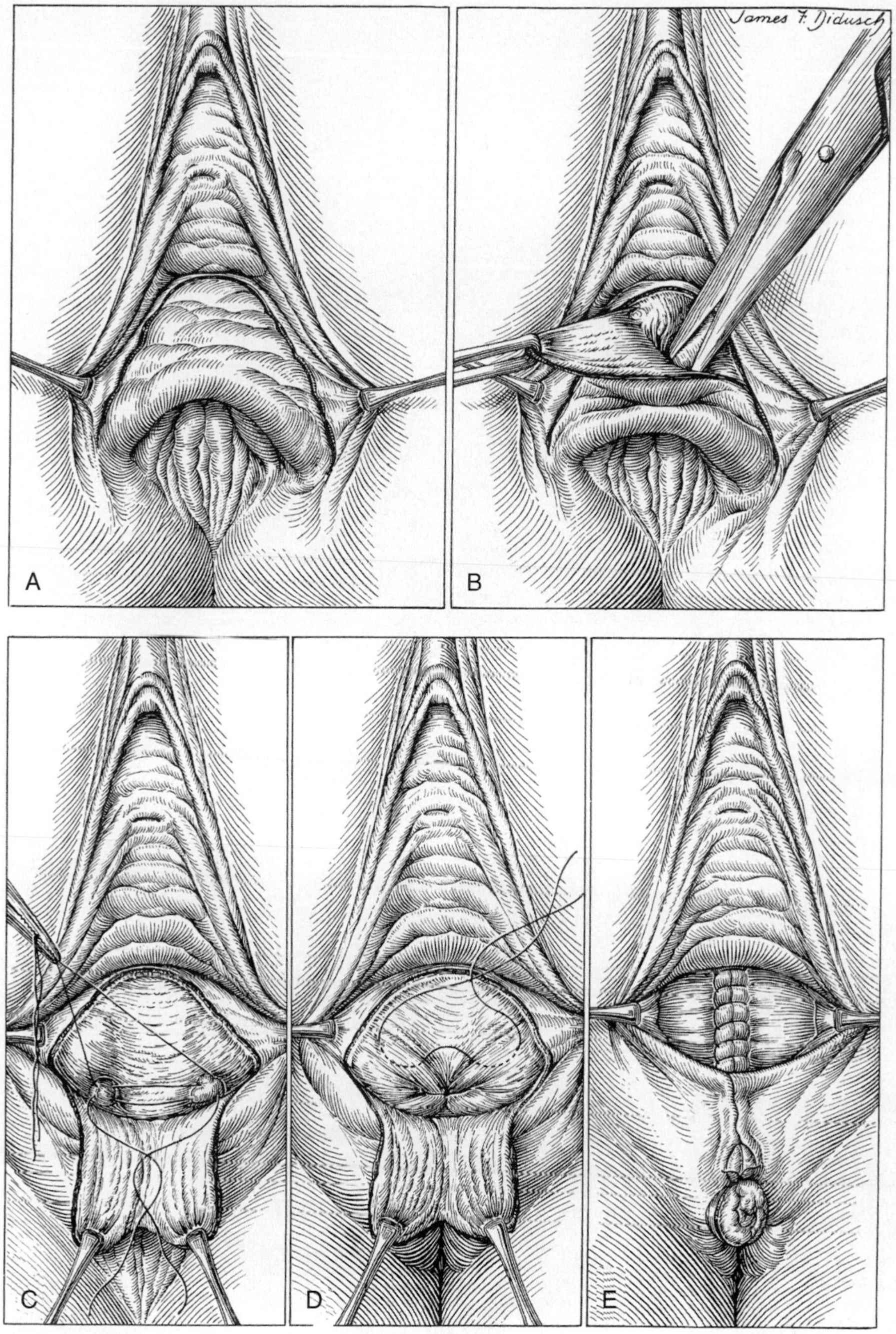

FIGURE 40.12. Warren flap operation for complete perineal laceration. **A:** The line of incision outlines the flap of vaginal mucosa. **B:** The flap is dissected free and turned back. **C:** The flap is retracted downward. The ends of the sphincter are delivered and are either sutured end to end as pictured or with an overlapping technique as described. **D:** The external sphincter has been repaired, and the puborectalis muscles are then brought closer together taking care to not create a posterior band of tissue. **E:** The vaginal incision is closed with a continuous locking stitch that is continued subcuticularly over the perineum. The margins of the flap are included in the continuous suture, which may temporarily create a peaked appearance in the perineal skin. If the margins of the vaginal mucosal flap are redundant, it may be trimmed.

reapproximated, further reconstituting and supporting the perineal body.

The vaginal mucosa is trimmed, if necessary, and the margins of the posterior vaginal wall are approximated with a continuous locking stitch of 3-0 delayed-absorbable suture. The continuous suture closing the posterior vaginal mucosa is carried over the perineal body as a subcuticular stitch, and the perianal skin then is approximated at the midline. The mobilized anterior wall of the anal canal is drawn outside the reconstructed anal orifice and sutured without tension to the perianal skin (Fig. 40.13E). The excess anal mucosa is trimmed. Care should be taken to remove as little of the distal anal canal as possible because this tissue contains the internal anal sphincter. Vertical mattress sutures of 3-0 delayed-absorbable suture are used to approximate the broad surface of the anal submucosa to the perianal skin. Any residual separation of the margins of the anal mucosa and perianal skin can be approximated with interrupted sutures.

Muscle Transposition, Artificial Sphincters, Diversion, and Other Procedures

The following advanced procedures are largely reserved for patients with difficult anal incontinence problems or multiple operative failures. Muscle transposition procedures exist

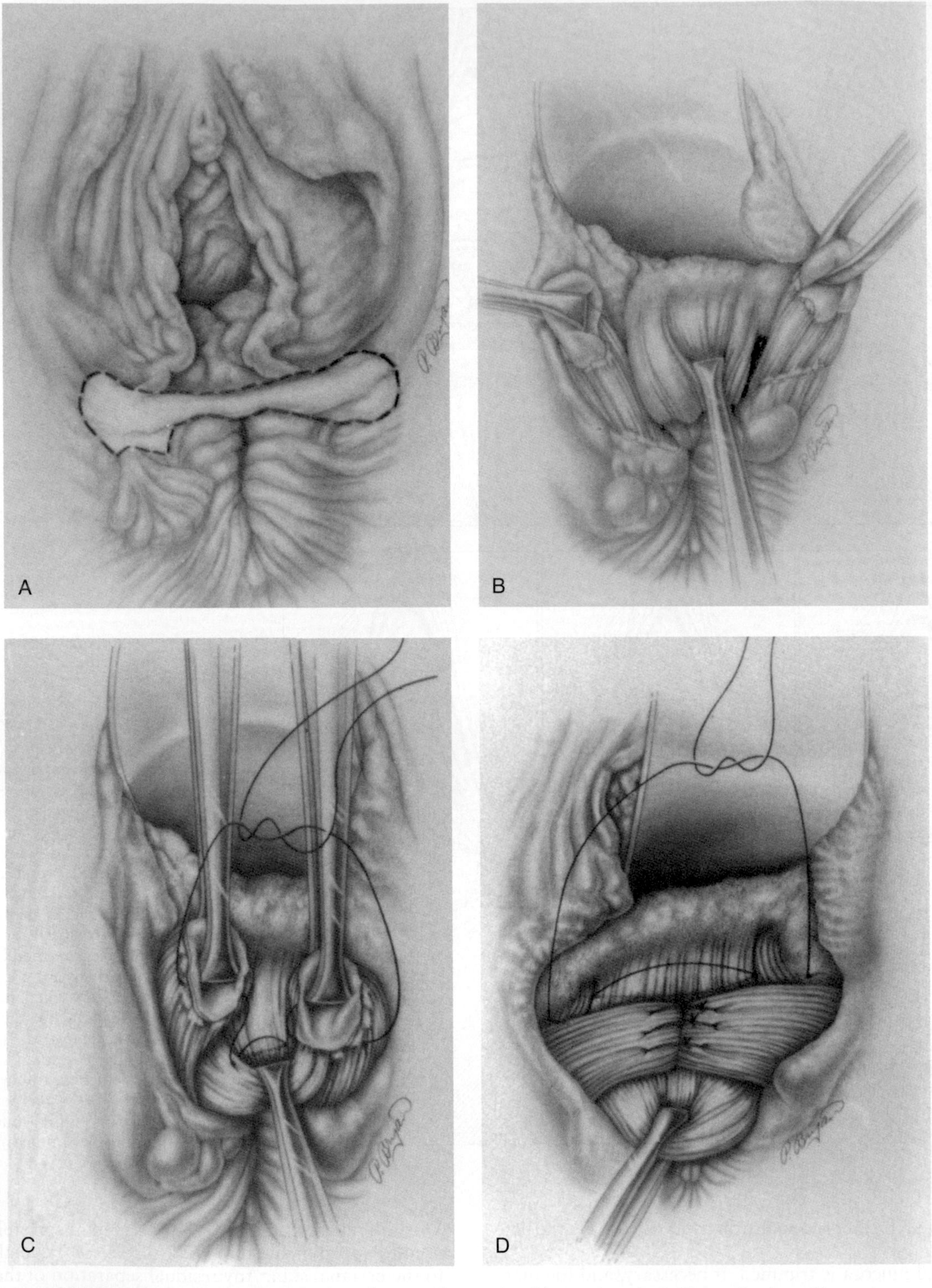

FIGURE 40.13. The Noble operation for complete perineal laceration. **A:** A "butterfly-shaped" scar is noted across the perineum, where there are torn perineal, anal, and rectal tissues. The ends of the external anal sphincter can be recognized by lateral perineal dimpling. **B:** The anterior rectal wall is mobilized extensively from the posterior vaginal wall to allow it to be pulled down without tension. The wings of the butterfly are left attached to facilitate dissection of the retracted ends of the sphincter. **C:** Ends of the anal sphincter are trimmed and sutured together and to the pararectal fascia of the advanced anterior rectal wall. Several delayed-absorbable sutures are used. **D:** The levator muscles and pararectal fascia are brought closer together in the midline. (*Continued*)

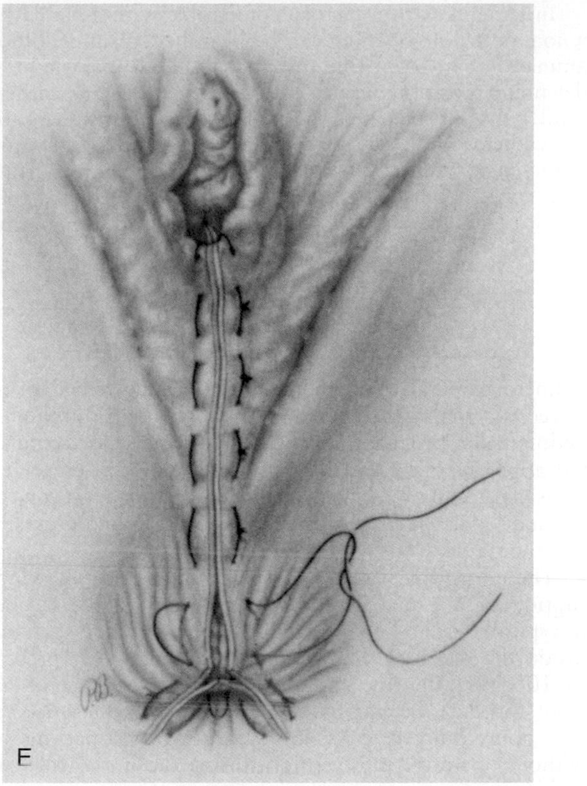

FIGURE 40.13. (*Continued*) E: The transverse perineal muscles and the inferior margins of the bulbocavernosus muscles are brought together to reconstitute the perineal body and the vaginal mucosa and perineal skin are closed. The mobilized anterior wall of the anal canal is sutured without tension to the perineal skin.

in which the gracilis muscle, sartorius muscle, or gluteus muscle are swung as flaps to encircle the anal canal. Dynamic muscle plasty procedures involve stimulation of this muscle with an intramuscular neurostimulator to induce it to convert to the characteristics of normal external anal sphincter muscle. The muscle is continuously stimulated at a low frequency for 8 to 10 weeks until the transformation from a fast-twitch to a slow-twitch muscle has been achieved. At this point, the frequency of stimulation is increased so that the muscle contracts around the anal canal and occludes it continuously. When the patient wishes to defecate, the pulse generator can be turned off by a magnet. Once defecation is complete, the stimulator can be turned on again by the magnet. In a series of 20 patients reported by Hallan and associates, 12 have a functioning neoanal sphincter. Madoff and colleagues (1999) found a 70% reduction in solid stool incontinence in two thirds of patients undergoing a dynamic graciloplasty. However, one third of these patients experienced a major wound complication with their surgery. Penninckx studied 60 consecutive patients undergoing dynamic graciloplasty. The operation failed in 27, 7 of whom went on to have stoma construction. There were 75 complications that required 61 reoperations in 44 patients.

Some investigators have used an artificial urinary sphincter around the anal canal in patients with severe anal incontinence. Although the initial results were good in a small series of patients, cuff erosion into the anal canal and infection have been significant problems that have caused a number of the sphincters to be removed. In a small randomized controlled trial of artificial sphincter versus supportive care, O'Brien and associates found a significant improvement in continence scores in the operative group. However, they concluded that because of morbidity, between 15% and 30% may require subsequent removal of the device. For the patient with uncontrollable anal incontinence that cannot be addressed by any other procedure, a diverting colostomy may be a more manageable and preferable alternative to constant perineal soiling with the hygienic and social problems it brings. Stoma problems, however, occur in as many as one quarter of patients.

Sacral nerve root stimulation, originally performed for treating urinary retention and urge urinary incontinence resistant to medical therapy, may show some promise for anal incontinence for patients with anatomically intact but functionally deficient sphincters. In 34 patients who underwent implantation during a multicenter trial, Matzel and colleagues found that frequency of incontinent episodes per week fell from 16.4 to 3.1 at 12 months and 2.0 at 24 months. Mean number of days per week with incontinent episodes decreased from 4.5 to 1.4 to 1.2 at the same intervals. Scant data exist at the time of this writing regarding other investigational approaches, such as delivery of radiofrequency energy to the anorectal junction and injecting bulking agents into the intersphincteric space to treat internal anal sphincter defects.

RECTOVAGINAL FISTULAE

A rectovaginal fistula resulting in extraanal fecal incontinence is a distressing condition for the patient and a challenge to her physician. Most fistulae actually arise in the anal canal beginning distal to the pectinate line (Fig. 40.2) and should more accurately be considered anovaginal fistulae. The result of this condition often is the uncontrolled passage of flatus or stool from the anorectal canal through the fistulous tract into the vagina. It can be a socially disabling condition. Further, the difficulties of treatment leading to failure (contaminated operative site, high-pressure anal canal, usually without diversion) challenge both the patience of the affected individuals and the surgeon's skill.

There are several classifications systems for rectovaginal fistulae. We have favored that of low (vaginal opening near the posterior fourchette), mid (from the level of the cervix to just superior to the posterior fourchette), and high (the fistula is in the area of the posterior fornix).

Etiology

Although there are many different causes of rectovaginal fistulae (Table 40.3), numerous series report that obstetric trauma is the cause for the majority of them. Rectovaginal fistulae usually arise as a complication of a repaired fourth-degree perineal tear. Venkatesh and colleagues reported that even though this sequence of events may be the most common, only 0.1% of vaginal deliveries result in fistula formation. Risk factors for development of a rectovaginal fistula in association with vaginal deliveries include prolonged labor, difficult forceps delivery, shoulder dystocia, and a midline episiotomy.

A rectovaginal fistula may develop as a result of direct surgical injury to the rectum or vagina, ischemia, or postoperative infection. Other less common causes include blunt instrumentation or penetrating trauma caused by an accident.

TABLE 40.3

CAUSES OF RECTOVAGINAL FISTULA

Congenital
Acquired
Trauma
Obstetric
Operative
Violent
Infectious
Inflammatory bowel disease
Radiation
Carcinoma

Occasionally, rectovaginal fistulae follow an infectious process such as a perianal abscess or an infected Bartholin duct cyst abscess. The most common cause of high rectovaginal fistulae is repeated bouts of diverticulitis with abscess formation followed by development of a sigmoidovaginal fistula or a combined sigmoidovesicovaginal fistula. Inflammatory bowel disease such as ulcerative colitis or Crohn disease may result in complex rectovaginal fistulae. Crohn disease is a transmural condition that often results in a rectovaginal fistula.

Radiation is a relatively infrequent cause of fistula formation, usually beginning as a proctitis with ulceration and fistula formation followed by a stricture. Fistulae may occur several years after completion of radiation therapy. Primary or metastatic disease in surrounding organs (rectum, cervix, uterus, or vagina) may result in rectovaginal fistulae. Because congenital rectovaginal fistula is usually managed at a young age and is associated with other anomalies, it is usually not managed by the gynecologic surgeon.

Clinical Evaluation

The most common symptoms are the passage of flatus and stool into the vagina. The severity of those symptoms may be affected by the size of the fistula and its number. There is usually a foul-smelling vaginal discharge with periodic, uncontrolled escape of gas. Occasionally, the fistula may develop immediately. More commonly, it appears 7 to 10 days after delivery. The breakdown of a primary repair, inadequate repair, or infection at the primary site may explain this delayed presentation. Because of the unpredictable condition and the desire to have more children, the patient may not seek medical attention for some time. Diarrhea, rectal bleeding, mucus discharge, and abdominal pain are caused by the underlying status of the bowel and do not result from the fistula per se.

The history frequently suggests the underlying cause of the fistula and may greatly influence the timing and route of repair. On physical examination, the location, size, and number of openings can be identified. The route of the fistula may be outlined by the passage of a thin probe from the vagina through the fistulous tract into the anal or rectal canal. Placing an examining finger in the rectum aids this process. Contraction of the puborectalis and external anal sphincter should be evaluated for competency. The perineal body is examined, and the tissues about the fistula are delineated to gain more insight into the cause of the underlying fistula. A proctosigmoidoscopic examination usually is done to ensure that the mucosa of the intestinal tract is normal.

In patients with a history compatible with a fistula but in whom no fistula opening can be identified, a simple office examination can be helpful. With the patient in a slight Trendelenburg position with a size 20 Foley urinary catheter, a 5-mL balloon is placed in the anal canal. Air is instilled through the catheter while the water-filled or soap-covered vagina is observed for any escape of air bubbles originating from the anal canal. Contrast studies are necessary to define the sigmoidovaginal fistula or fistulae associated with primary bowel disease.

Surgical Management

Numerous operative procedures have been described for repair of rectovaginal fistula, including transvaginal, transanal, and abdominal approaches. Gynecologists usually use a transvaginal approach, whereas colon and rectal surgeons prefer the transanal technique. The determining factors to be considered include the cause of the fistula, its location and accessibility, and the status of the anal sphincter.

The most typical rectovaginal fistula is one following disruption of a primary repair of a fourth-degree laceration. It typically occurs low along the rectovaginal septum just inside the external anal sphincter. Generally, it presents 6 to 10 days after the initial repair with passage of air or stool through the vagina. Venkatesh and colleagues report that approximately 50% of these small fistulae may heal without operative intervention during the first 6 to 8 weeks postpartum.

Early Repair

As previously mentioned, Hankins and colleagues described early repair of carefully selected rectovaginal fistulae and episiotomy breakdowns using a technique of early return to the operating room for debridement followed by daily cleansing of the wound area. After a 6- to 7-day interval, their patients were returned to the operating room for surgical repair of the fistula. With this approach, successful healing occurred in 90% of their patients. We prefer to wait 8 to 12 weeks to allow the surrounding inflammation to resolve before surgical intervention. Preoperative mechanical bowel preparation should be given. On the morning of operation, tap water enemas can be given until clear.

Appropriate treatment of a rectovaginal fistula requires consideration of the cause and location of the fistula and the condition of the involved tissues. For fistulae located in the lower portion of the anal canal, we prefer to use the lithotomy position to carry out the operative repair. For fistulae at the very apex of the vagina, an abdominal approach generally is required.

Low Rectovaginal Fistula: Technique of Repair

A transvaginal technique for small rectovaginal fistula repair involves a circular incision about the fistulous opening (Fig. 40.14). With traction on the vaginal wall and countertraction applied to the edge of the fistulous tract, the vagina is separated from the underlying rectal wall with sharp dissection, and this proceeds circumferentially (Fig. 40.15). This wide mobilization permits later approximation of the fresh injury free of tension.

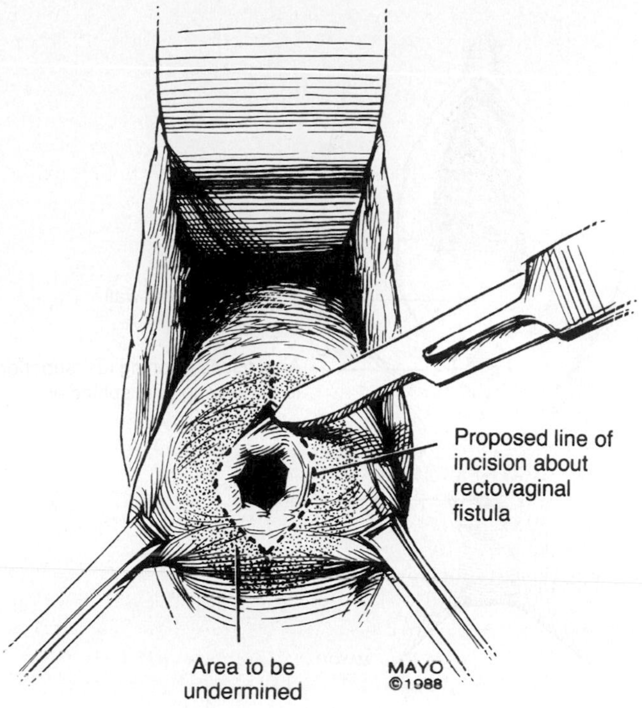

FIGURE 40.14. Small rectovaginal fistula with proposed line of initial incision.

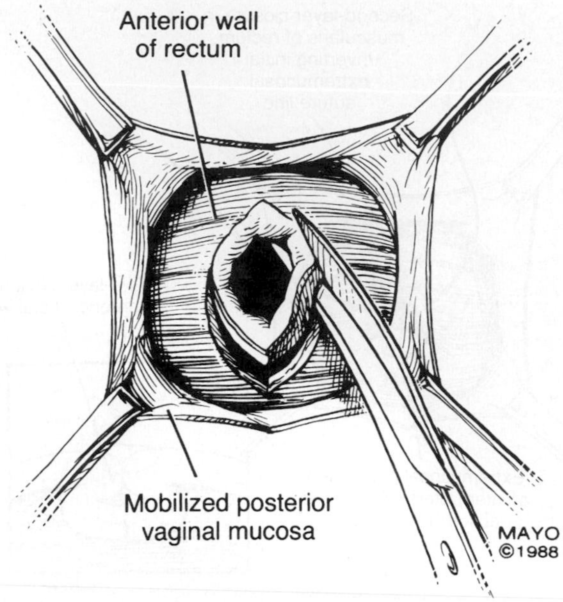

FIGURE 40.16. Excision of fistulous tract.

Once the vaginal walls are mobilized from the underlying rectum, the entire fistulous tract is excised to include a small rim of the rectal mucosa (Fig. 40.16), converting the fistula to a fresh injury. With the surgeon's nondominant index finger lifting and supporting the anterior rectal wall, the initial sutures are placed extramucosally, including a portion of the muscularis and submucosa, with 3-0 delayed-absorbable sutures (Fig. 40.17). We frequently place all sutures throughout the length of the fistula, after which they are individually tied in the order in which they were placed. The initial suture line begins and is extended a full 5 to 8 mm above and below the site of the fistulous tract to assure complete closure. A second layer

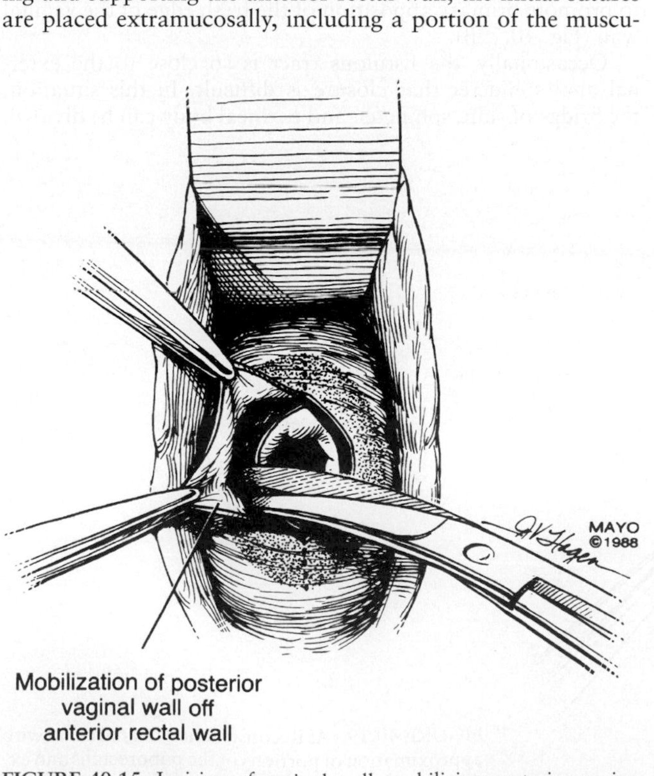

FIGURE 40.15. Incision of vaginal wall, mobilizing posterior vagina from underlying anterior anal canal.

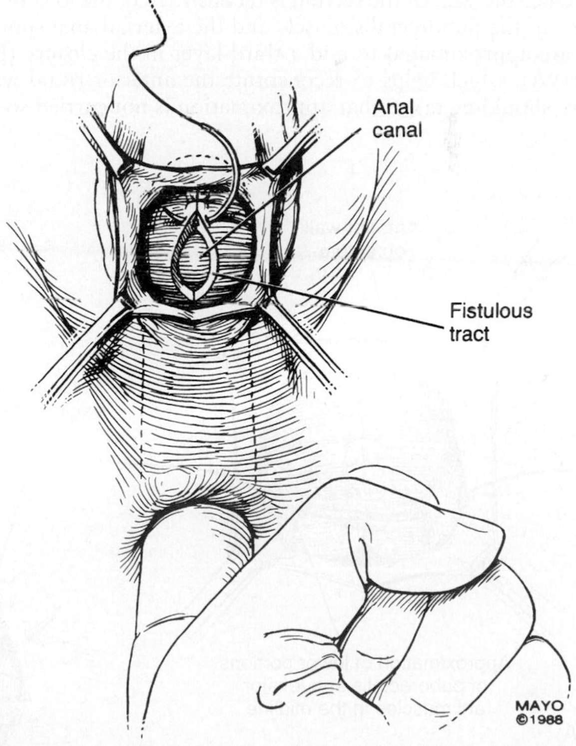

FIGURE 40.17. Extramucosal placement of sutures in wall of anterior anal canal.

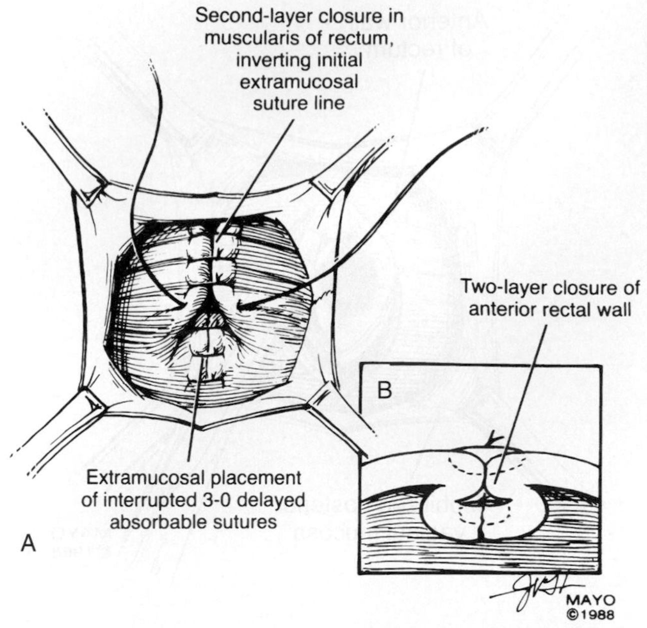

FIGURE 40.18. **A:** Inversion of initial suture line with approximation of muscularis of the anal canal. This thickened smooth muscle layer is the internal anal sphincter. **B:** Side view representing closure of the first and second layers in the anal canal.

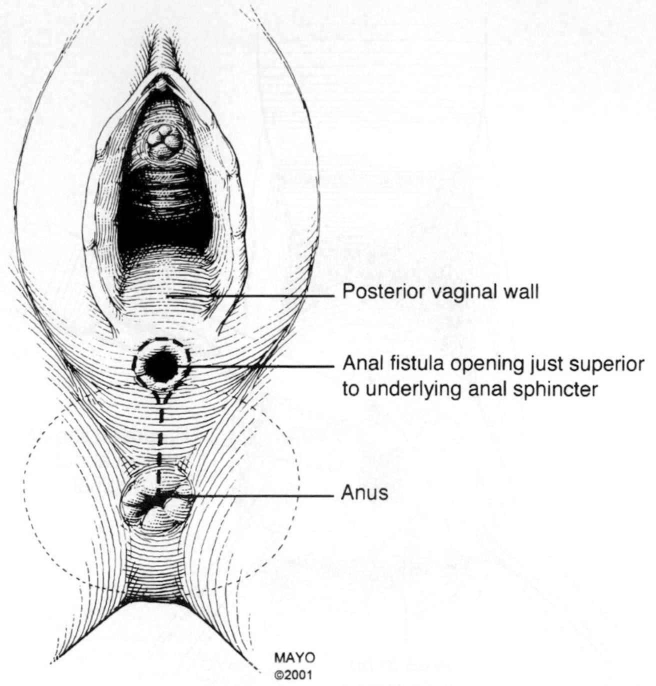

FIGURE 40.20. Proposed incision of perineal body and posterior vaginal wall with excision of fistulous tract.

(Fig. 40.18) begins 5 mm above the previously closed suture line and extends 5 mm distal to the fistulous closure, inverting the initial suture line into the rectum, and no sutures are located within the rectal lumen.

Once the wall of the rectum is reconstructed, the lower portions of the puborectalis muscle and the external anal sphincter are approximated to add a third layer in the closure (Fig. 40.19A), which helps to reconstitute the anterior rectal wall. Care should be taken that approximation is not carried so far superiorly that it results in a transverse bar across the posterior vaginal wall, which may lead to dyspareunia. Once the muscular walls are approximated, the vaginal wall is approximated with 3-0 delayed-absorbable sutures, accurately placed so as to promote primary apposition of the fresh edge of the vaginal wall (Fig. 40.19B).

Occasionally, the fistulous tract is so close to the external anal sphincter that closure is difficult. In this situation, the bridge of skin, sphincter, and perineal body can be divided,

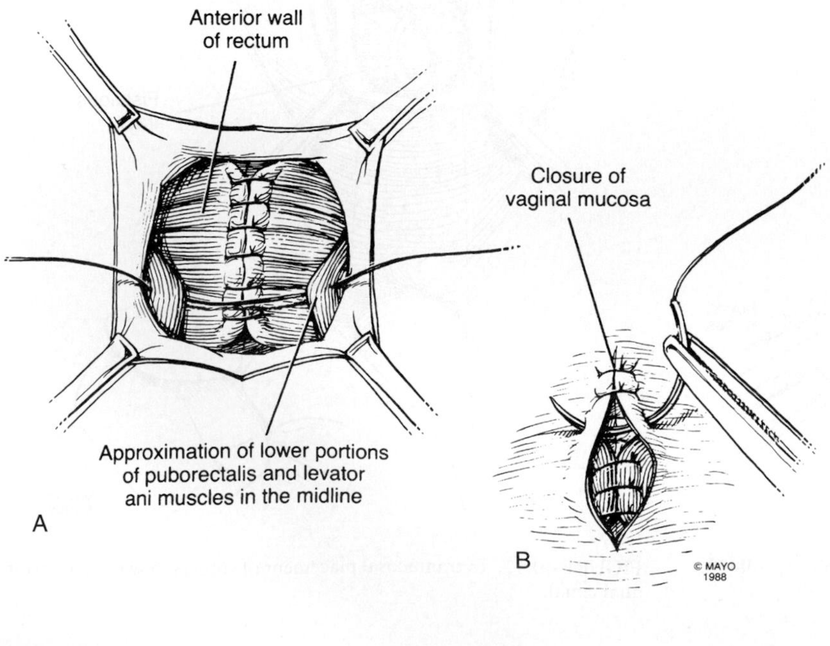

FIGURE 40.19. **A:** Reconstruction of anal canal with approximation of portions of the puborectalis and external anal sphincter. **B:** Interrupted sutures approximating posterior vaginal wall.

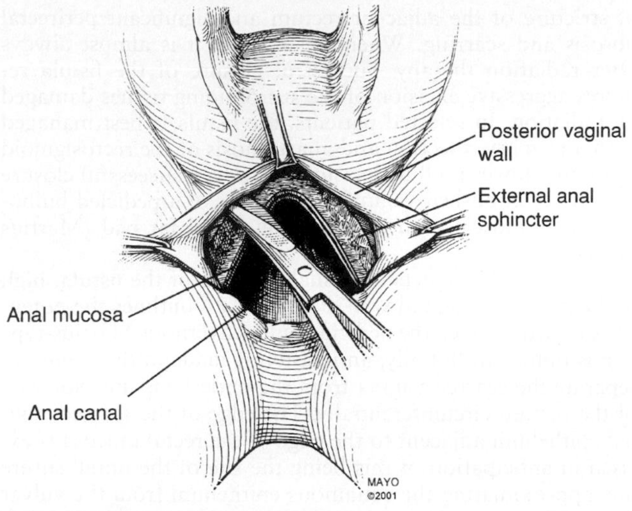

FIGURE 40.21. Mobilization of posterior vagina off anterior anal canal with conversion of rectovaginal fistula to fourth-degree injury.

and the fistula is thus essentially converted to a fourth degree tear (Fig. 40.20). The fistulous tract is excised, and the posterior vaginal wall is mobilized from the anterior anal wall (Fig. 40.21). The anal canal is then reconstructed with interrupted or running fine delayed-absorbable sutures approximating the mucosa of the anal canal. This initial suture line then is inverted with a second layer of interrupted fine delayed-absorbable sutures approximating the retracted tissues of the internal anal sphincter, resulting in reconstruction of the anal canal (Fig. 40.22). The retracted ends of the external anal sphincter are approximated in the midline in an end-to-end fashion with fine delayed-absorbable sutures (Fig. 40.23). This results in a snug closure that is resistant to the passage of the surgeon's little finger. Alternatively, at this point one could perform an overlapping sphincteroplasty as described earlier (Fig. 40.11D,E). The perineal body is reconstructed in such a

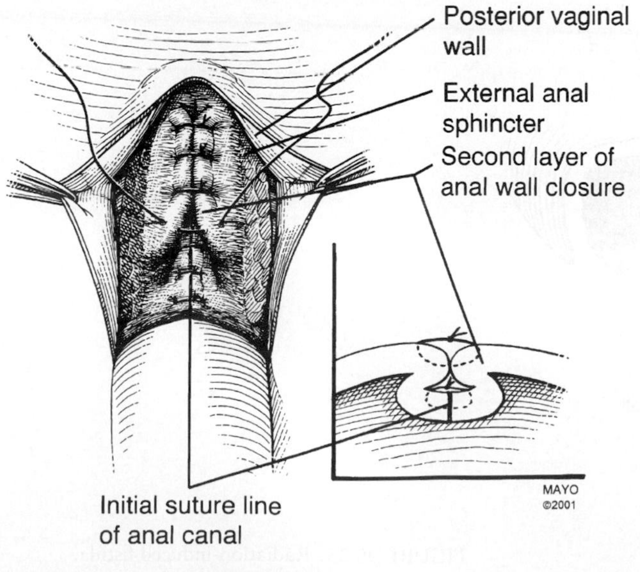

FIGURE 40.22. Two-layer reconstruction of anal canal.

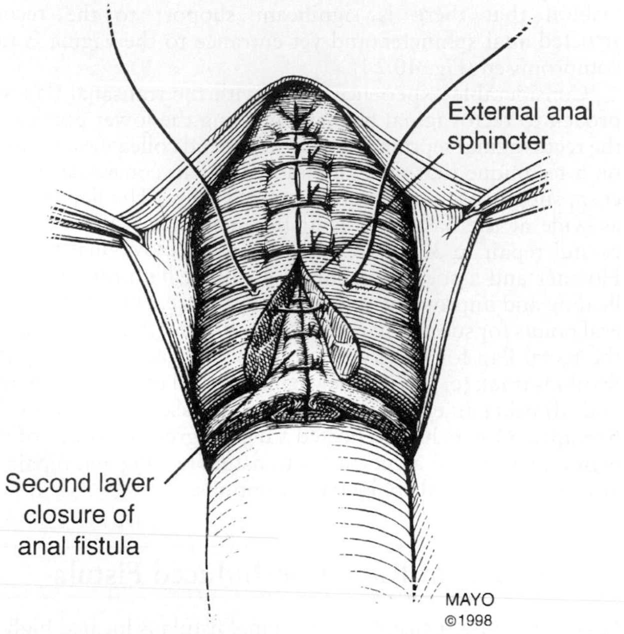

FIGURE 40.23. Reanastomosis of retracted external anal sphincter with surgeon's left index finger in the anal canal.

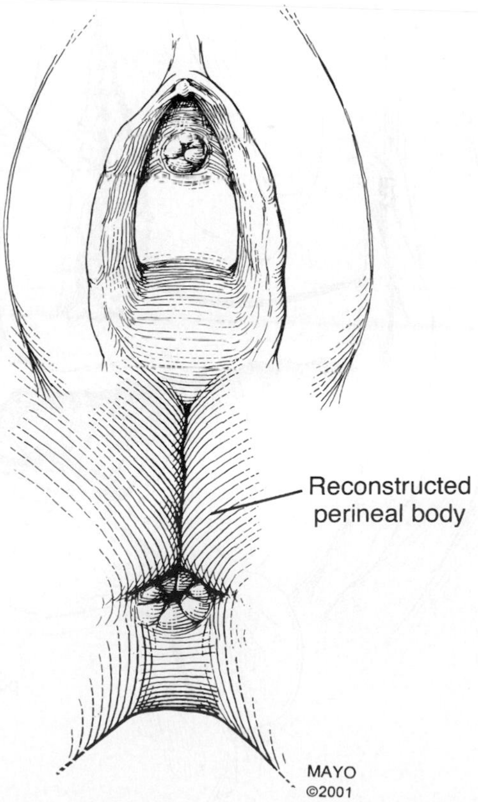

FIGURE 40.24. Reconstructed perineal body with subcuticular approximation of skin of perineum.

fashion that there is significant support to the reconstructed anal sphincter, and yet entrance to the vagina is not compromised (Fig. 40.24).

Considerable experience exists with the transanal flap approach to rectovaginal fistulae involving the lower portion of the rectovaginal septum. Rothenberger and colleagues reported on a technique that uses an endorectal flap consisting of mucosa, submucosa, and circular muscle fibers. The flap is twice as wide at the base as it is at the apex. They achieved successful repair in 32 of 35 patients with rectovaginal fistulae. Hoexter and associates reported a similar high rate of fistula healing and improvement in anal continence, emphasizing several points for successful repair via endorectal flap: (a) elevating the rectal flap for at least 4 cm to the fistula, (b) excising the fistulous tract, (c) leaving the vaginal wound open for drainage, and (d) using an elliptic flap to avoid devascularization of the flap apex. Others have reported a high degree of efficacy of the endorectal flap for achieving both fistula healing and repair of any associated anal sphincter disruptions.

Repair of Radiation-Induced Fistula

Less commonly, a sizable rectovaginal fistula is located high in the posterior vaginal wall, frequently associated with a degree of stricture of the adjacent rectum and significant perirectal fibrosis and scarring. When this occurs, it is almost always after radiation therapy. Successful closure of the fistula requires aggressive excision of the surrounding tissues damaged by radiation. In selected patients, the fistula is best managed with a primary resection and anastomosis of the rectosigmoid through a lower midline incision. However, successful closure can be accomplished vaginally by means of a pedicled bulbocavernous muscle with an overlying labial fat pad (Martius procedure).

Figure 40.25 depicts the usual location of the fistula, high in the posterior vaginal wall. Figure 40.26 outlines the potential sites from which the pedicled bulbocavernous Martius-type flap is obtained. Initially, an incision is made in the vagina to separate the scarred vagina from the underlying anterior wall of the rectum circumferentially. The edge of the scarred vaginal epithelium adjacent to the edge of the rectal mucosa is excised in anticipation of this being the site of the initial suture line approximating the squamous epithelium from the vulvar flap to the rectum in order to fill the defect in the rectum. With a Mayo scissors, a subcutaneous tunnel is made from the labium majus to the fistula under the labium and vaginal mucosa (Fig. 40.27). The free end of the muscle is guided through the subcutaneous tunnel with a single absorbable suture placed along its edge to assist in passage through the tunnel. The

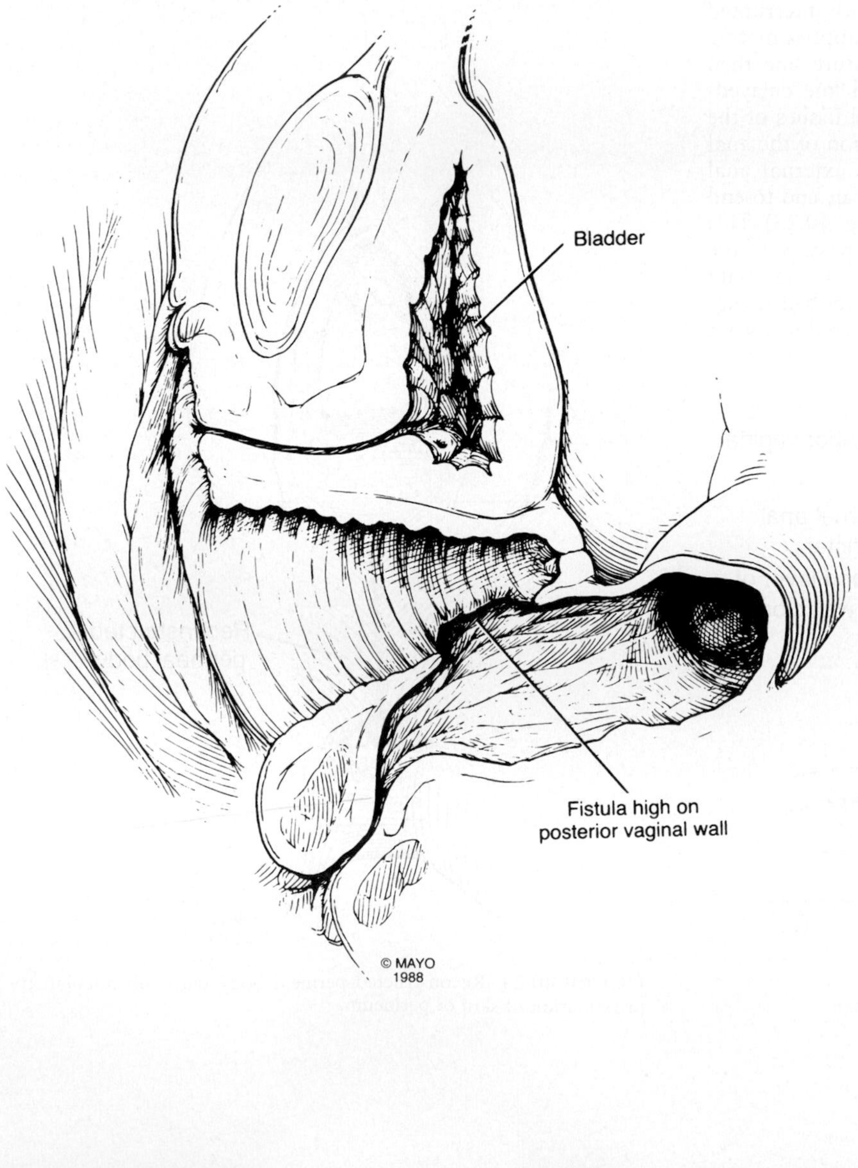

FIGURE 40.25. Radiation-induced fistula.

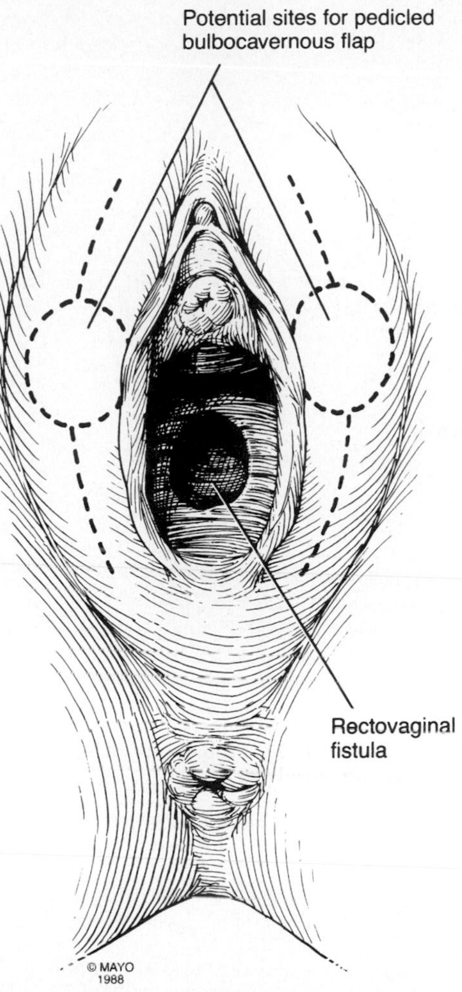

FIGURE 40.26. Proposed sites to harvest skin and subcutaneous tissue in preparation to fill hole of rectovaginal fistula.

rectal defect is such that it cannot be closed primarily. Thus, the edge of the squamous epithelium from the vulvar graft is sutured to the edge of the rectal mucosa with 4-0 delayed-absorbable sutures. Occasionally, a Schuchardt incision is required in the vagina to obtain adequate exposure for the dissection.

The pedicled graft is used to close the fistulous defect, beginning at the 3-o'clock position, in a synchronous fashion such that the entire edge of the fistulous tract is in immediate proximity to the edge of the skin from the vulva (Fig. 40.28). Once in place, the muscle and subcutaneous tissue of the graft are sutured to the surrounding connective tissue.

To provide coverage for the exposed Martius flap, which has been inserted as a plug into the rectum, a similar pedicled graft is developed from the patient's right side; this is placed so that the skin of the vulva is approximated to the skin of the vagina (Fig. 40.29). The edges are placed such that there is no exposed source for granulation tissue (Fig. 40.30).

A small suction catheter is placed between the two pedicled grafts and brought out through a stab wound lateral to the perineal incision. The vulvar incision is closed in layers, the skin approximated with fine interrupted delayed-absorbable suture. In patients requiring a pedicled graft, the repair may result in a narrowing of the vagina and a degree of stenosis. This results not only from the encroachment on the vaginal lumen by the pedicled grafts but also from the associated contracture caused by the underlying cause of the fistula: pelvic radiation. There is a tendency for further contracture and stenosis of the vagina, which may result in significant dyspareunia or apareunia.

Boronow has used bulbocavernosus-labial tissue graft to successfully treat radiation-induced rectovaginal fistulae. He reported on 25 radiation-induced vaginal fistulae in 22 patients. There were 16 rectovaginal fistulae, 3 vesicovaginal fistulae, and 3 combined vesicovaginal and rectovaginal fistulae. Successful closure was accomplished in 84% of the patients with rectovaginal fistulae.

Sigmoidovaginal Fistula: Sigmoid Resection with Sigmoidorectostomy

Fistulae between the sigmoid colon and vagina occur infrequently, but the overwhelming majority result from diverticulitis of the sigmoid colon (Fig. 40.31) in a patient who has previously had a hysterectomy. Generally, the sequence of events consists of the patient experiencing repeated bouts of acute diverticulitis that finally result in perforation of a diverticulum and abscess formation with a fistulous tract communicating to the vagina. Passage of fecal material or gas through the vagina in the absence of a rectal communication should lead one to suspect a fistula arising from the sigmoid colon or small intestine. A proctoscopic examination should be done, although often it is impossible to visualize the fistulous orifice because of narrowing or fixation resulting from the inflammatory condition. Surgical intervention is indicated for a sigmoidovaginal fistula that is large enough to permit the passage of fecal material. In a few selected patients, a colostomy may be the only treatment, or the fistula may be divided and the sigmoidal defect closed with or without a temporary colostomy. In the overwhelming majority of patients, we prefer a sigmoid resection with primary anastomosis and closure of the opening into the vagina. The need for a temporary protective colostomy is determined on an individual basis.

Hartmann Procedure

Under some circumstances, the infected, inflammatory process is such that the sigmoid mass may be excised, but a primary anastomosis is ill advised. It may be more appropriate to excise the diseased colon, close the fistula in the vagina, leaving the defunctionalized rectal stump in the pelvis for later reanastamosis (Fig. 40.32). Omentum and a suction drain are usually placed over the stump. The distal end of the descending colon is brought out as a colostomy, which is matured at that time. Later, usually after 2 to 3 months, reoperation can be done through the previous incision. Placement of a gauze pack in the vagina and an EEA sizer in the anal stump will help to identify these structures. Once identified, the descending colon is freed from the splenic flexure in a sufficient fashion to permit the primary descending colorectostomy in a noninfected field as a closing step in this two-stage procedure.

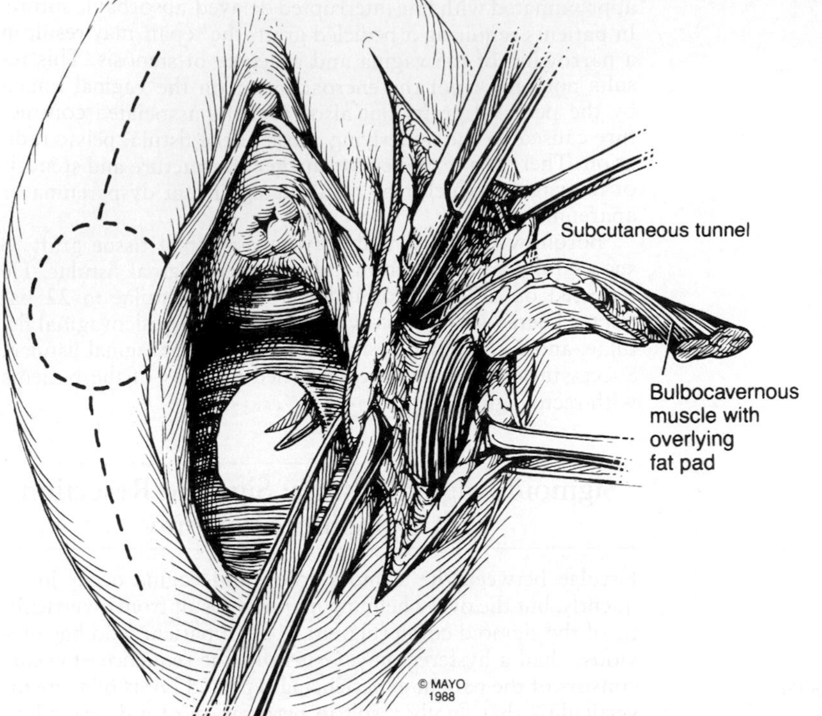

FIGURE 40.27. Mobilization of bulbocavernosus muscle with overlying fat pad.

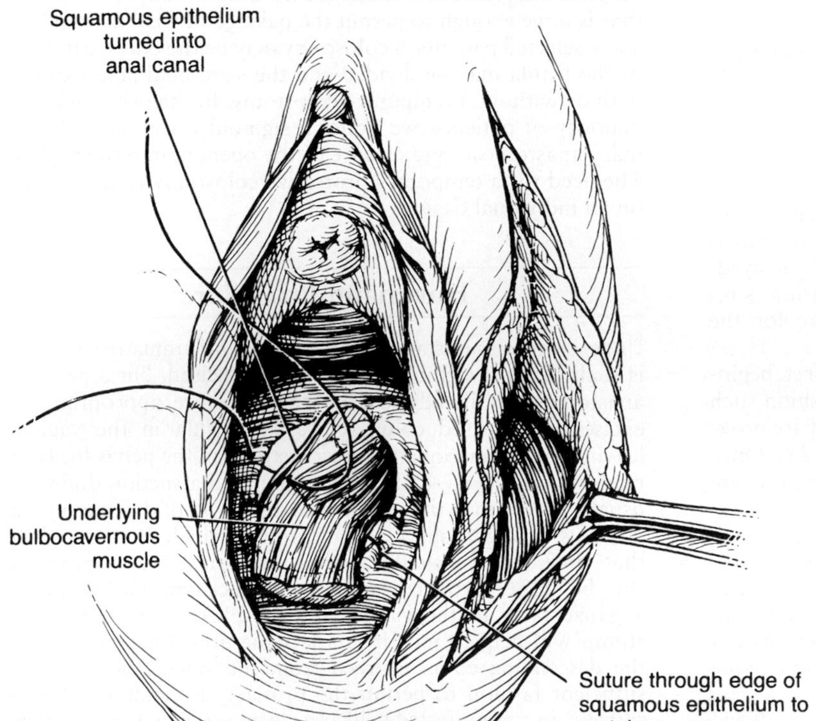

FIGURE 40.28. Suture fixation of pedicled skin to rectal mucosa.

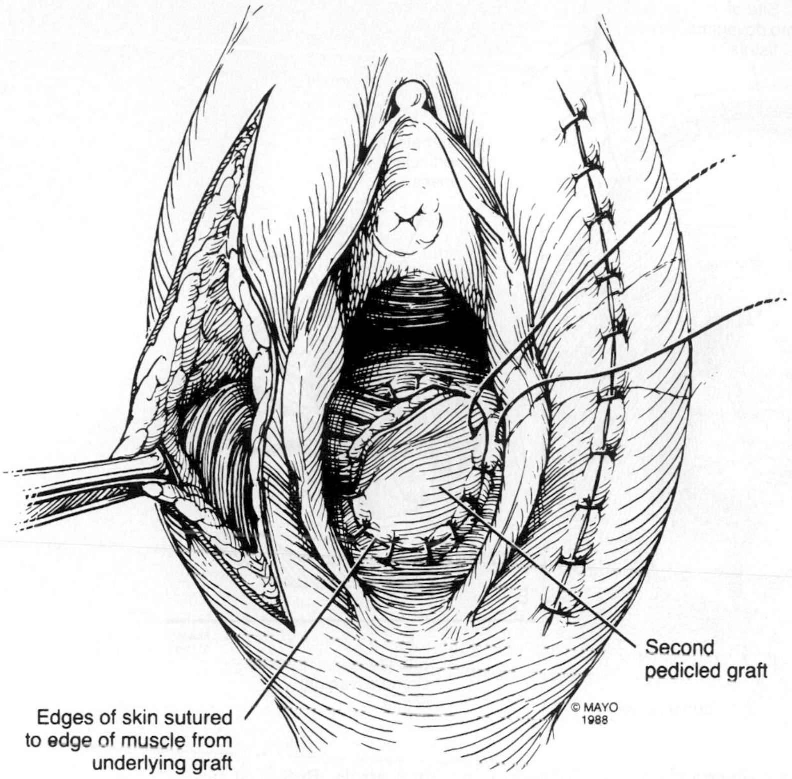

FIGURE 40.29. Approximation of the skin of the vulvar flap to the skin of the vaginal wall.

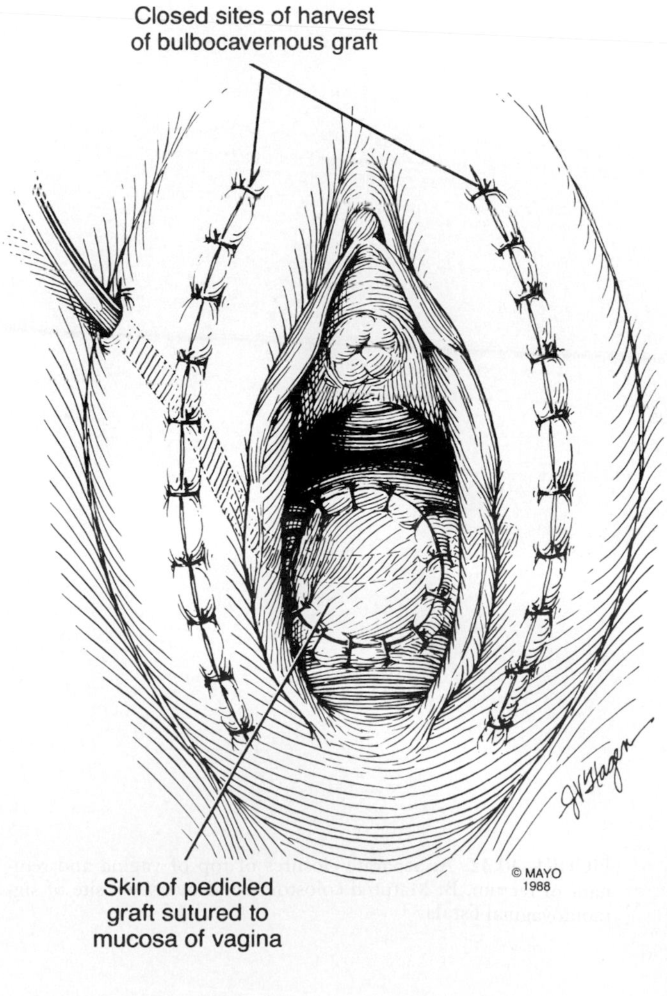

FIGURE 40.30. Reconstructed perineum in completed repair of fistula.

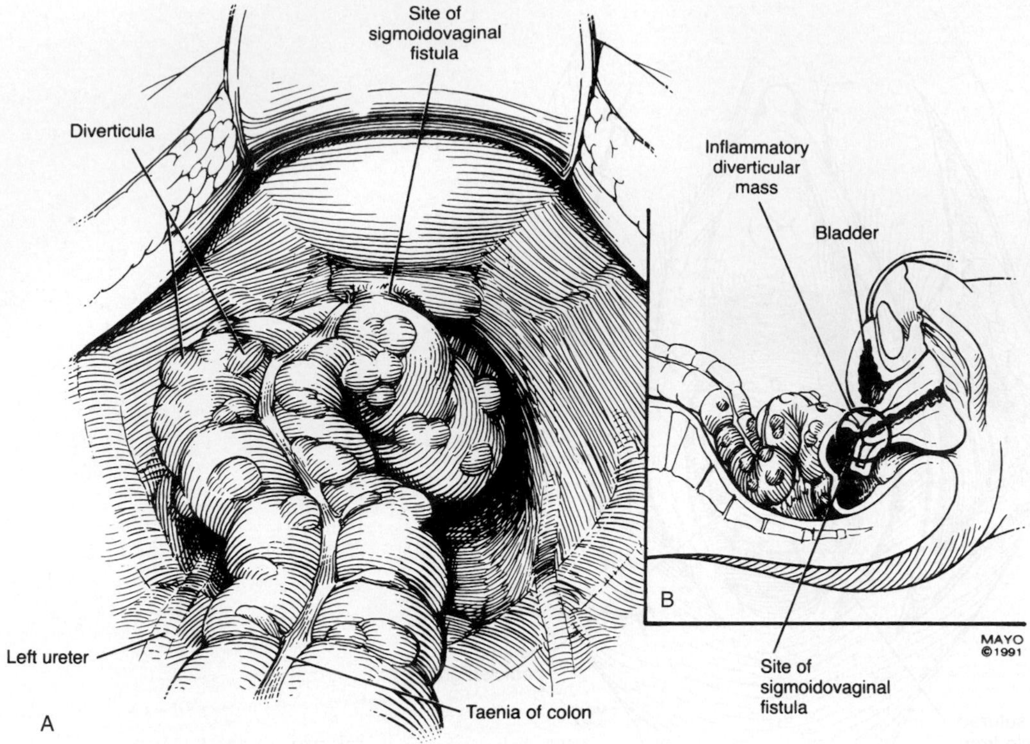

FIGURE 40.31. **A:** Sigmoid with multiple diverticula and site of sigmoidovaginal fistula. **B:** Site of sigmoidovaginal fistula at apex of vagina.

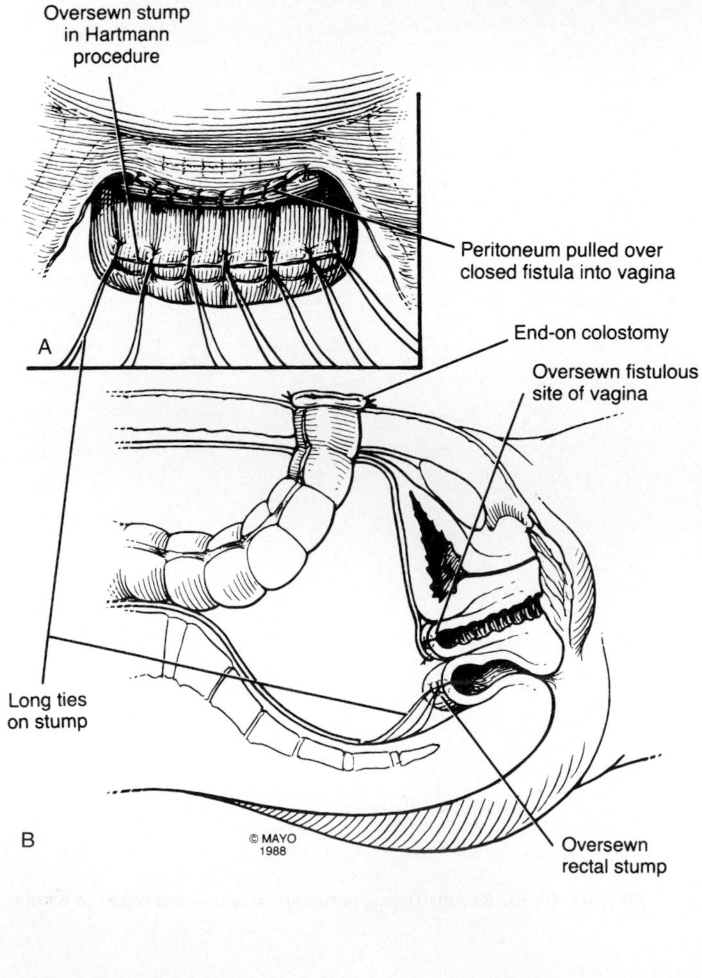

FIGURE 40.32. **A:** Separate closures of top of vagina and remnant of rectum. **B:** Matured colostomy and oversewn site of sigmoidovaginal fistula.

SUMMARY

The management of the anally incontinent patient is a complex undertaking whether that incontinence is transanal or extraanal through a rectovaginal fistula. Care must be taken in the assessment and diagnosis of these patients with testing judiciously used where it will provide clinically useful information. Because surgical results in anally incontinent patients are less than perfect, consideration should be given to initially trying nonsurgical management. In those who fail conservative therapy, and in those who go directly to surgical therapy, a thoughtful preoperative workup with extensive preoperative counseling regarding expectations and possible outcomes is crucial for the ultimate satisfaction of the patient. Surgery for anal incontinence and rectovaginal fistula repair requires thorough surgical planning, careful attention to detail, and a meticulous operative technique to provide the patient with optimal results.

BEST SURGICAL PRACTICES

- Preoperative evaluation of the anally incontinent patient should include a careful assessment of her symptoms and their impact on her quality of life.
- Success of surgical procedures for anal incontinence should be thought of, and explained preoperatively to patients, in terms of improvement rather than "cure."
- Consideration should be given to extensive use of nonsurgical therapy before a decision for surgery is made.
- Judicious use of preoperative testing can aid in identifying patients most likely to achieve benefit from surgery.
- Mechanical bowel preparation, perioperative antibiotic prophylaxis, and attention to postoperative diet and stool consistency management are important.
- The anal sphincteroplasty is the most important part of any perineal reconstruction for the patient with anal incontinence.
- Current data suggest that an overlapping sphincter repair may yield greater functional improvement than an end-to-end sphincter reapproximation.
- Rectovaginal fistula repair requires careful attention to sharp dissection, gentle tissue handling, wide mobilization, meticulous hemostasis, and a tension-free closure.

ACKNOWLEDGMENT

The authors would like to thank Craig A. Paterson, MD, Justin A. Maykel, MD, and Allison E. Howard, BS, for their invaluable contributions to this chapter.

Bibliography

Aartsen EJ, Sindram IS. Repair of the radiation induced rectovaginal fistula without or with interposition of the bulbocavernosus muscle (Martius procedure). *Eur J Surg Oncol* 1988;14:171.

Abou-Zeid AA. Preliminary experience in management of fecal incontinence caused by internal anal sphincter injury. *Dis Colon Rectum* 2000;43(2):198.

Abramov Y, Sand PK, Botros SM, et al. Risk factors for female anal incontinence: new insight through Evanston-Northwestern twin sisters study. *Obstet Gynecol* 2005;106:726.

Abrams P, Cardozo L, Khoury S, et al., eds. *Incontinence*. 3rd International Consultation on Incontinence, Monaco 2004. Pub Health Publications Ltd.; 2005:286.

Allen RE, Hosker GL, Smith ARB, et al. Pelvic floor damage and childbirth: a neurophysiological study. *BJOG* 1990;97:770.

American Gastroenterological Association Medical Position Statement on Anorectal Testing Techniques. *Gastroenterology* 1999;116:732.

Arnaud A, Sarles JC, Sielezneff I, et al. Sphincter repair without overlapping for fecal incontinence. *Dis Colon Rectum* 1991;34:744.

Aronson MP, Lee RA, Berquist TH. Anatomy of anal sphincters and related structures in continent women studied with magnetic resonance imaging. *Obstet Gynecol* 1990;76:846.

Ayoub SF. Anatomy of the external anal sphincter in man. *Acta Anat* 1979;105:25.

Bandy LC, Addison A, Parker RT. Surgical management of rectovaginal fistulas in Crohn's disease. *Am J Obstet Gynecol* 1983;147:359.

Bartolo DCC, Roe AM, Locke-Edmunds JC, et al. Flap-valve theory of anorectal incontinence. *Br J Surg* 1986;73:1012.

Barton JR. A rectovaginal fistula cured. *Am J Med Sci* 1840;26:305.

Berek JS, Lagasse LD, Hacker NF, et al. Levator ani transposition for anal incompetence secondary to sphincter damage. *Obstet Gynecol* 1982;59:108.

Bielefeldt K, Enck P, Erckenbrecht JF. Sensory and motor function in the maintenance of anal continence. *Dis Colon Rectum* 1990;33:674.

Bielefeldt K, Enck P, Zamboglou N, et al. Anorectal manometry and defecography in the diagnosis of fecal incontinence. *J Clin Gastroenterol* 1991;13:661.

Birnhaum W. A method of repair for a common type of traumatic incontinence of the anal sphincter. *Surg Gynecol Obstet* 1948;87:716.

Blaisdell PC. Repair of the incontinent sphincter ani. *Surg Gynecol Obstet* 1940;70:692.

Boreham MK, Richter HE, Kenton KE, et al. Anal incontinence in women presenting for gynecologic care: prevalence, risk factors, and impact on quality of life. *Am J Obstet Gynecol* 2004;192:1637.

Boronow RC. Repair of the radiation-induced vaginal fistula using the Martius technique. *World J Surg* 1986;10:237.

Carey JC. A new method of diagnosing rectovaginal fistula: a case report. *J Reprod Med* 1988;33:789.

Chassagne P, Landrin I, Neveu C, et al. Fecal incontinence in the institutionalized elderly: incidence, risk factors, and prognosis. *J Urol* 1999;161(6):1813.

Chen AS, Luchtefeld MA, Senagore AJ, et al. Pudendal nerve latency. Does it predict outcome of anal sphincter repair? *J Clin Gastroenterol* 1998;27(2):108.

Cheong DM, Vaccaro CA, Salanga VD, et al. Electrodiagnostic evaluation of fecal incontinence [Published erratum appears in *Muscle Nerve* 1995;18(11):1368]. *JAMA* 1995;274(7):559.

Christiansen J, Sparso B. Treatment of anal incontinence by an implantable prosthetic anal sphincter. *Ann Surg* 1992;215:383.

Cundiff GW, Nygaard I, Bland DR, et al. Proceedings of the American Urogynecologic Society Multidisciplinary Symposium on Defecatory Disorders. *Eur J Obstet Gynecol Reprod Biol* 2000;89(2):159.

Dalley AF II. The riddle of the sphincters: the morphophysiology of the anorectal mechanism reviewed. *Am J Surg* 1987;53:298. [Published erratum appears in *Am J Surg* 1987;53:398.]

Deen KI, Kumar D, Williams JG, et al. Randomized trial of internal anal sphincter plication with pelvic floor repair for neuropathic fecal incontinence. *Dis Colon Rectum* 1995;38:14.

Deen KI, Oya M, Ortiz J, et al. Randomized trial comparing three forms of pelvic floor repair for neuropathic faecal incontinence. *Br J Surg* 1993;80:794.

DeLancey JOL, Hurd WW. Size of the urogenital hiatus in the levator ani muscles in normal women and women with pelvic organ prolapse. *Obstet Gynecol* 1998;91:364.

DeLancey JO, Kearney R, Chou Q, et al. The appearance of levator ani muscle abnormalities in magnetic resonance images after vaginal delivery. *Obstet Gynecol* 2003;101(1):46.

DeLancey JOL, Toglia MR, Perucchini D. Internal and external anal sphincter anatomy as it relates to midline obstetric lacerations. *Obstet Gynecol* 1997;90:924.

DeSouza NM, Puni R, Zbar A, et al. MR imaging of the anal sphincter in multiparous women using an endoanal coil: correlation with in vitro anatomy and appearances in fecal incontinence. *Am J Roentgenol* 1996;167:1465.

Dietz HP, Lanzarone V. Levator trauma after vaginal delivery. *Obstet Gynecol* 2005;106:707.

Eason E, Labrecque M, Marcoux S, et al. Anal incontinence after childbirth. *CMAJ* 2002;166(3):326.

Elkins TE, DeLancey JOL, McGuire EJ. The use of modified Martius graft as an adjunctive technique in vesicovaginal and rectovaginal fistula repair. *Obstet Gynecol* 1990;75:727.

Enck P, Daublin G, Lubke HJ, et al. Long-term efficacy of biofeedback training for fecal incontinence. *Dis Colon Rectum* 1995;38(4):370.

Faltin DL, Sangalli MR, Curtin F, et al. Prevalence of anal incontinence and other anorectal symptoms in women. *Int Urogynecol J* 2001;12:117.

Felt-Bersma RJF, Luth WJ, Janssen JJWM. Defecography in patients with anorectal disorders: which findings are clinically relevant? *Dis Colon Rectum* 1990;33:277.

Fernando RJ, Sultan AH, Kettle C, et al. Repair techniques for obstetric anal sphincter injuries: a randomized controlled trial. *Obstet Gynecol* 2006;107:1261.

Fitzpatrick M, Behan M, O'Connell PR, et al. A randomized clinical trial comparing primary overlap with approximation repair of third degree obstetric tears. *Am J Obstet Gynecol* 2000;183(5):1220.

Fornell EU, Matthiesen L, Sjödahl R, et al. Obstetric anal sphincter injury ten years after: subjective and objective long term effects. *BJOG* 2005;112:312.

Gaston EA. Physiology of faecal continence. *Surg Gynaecol Obstet* 1948;87:280.

Gearhart S, Hull T, Floruta C, et al. Anal manometric parameters: predictors of outcome following anal sphincter repair? *J Gastrointest Surg* 2005;9(1):115.

Giebel GD, Lefering R, Troidl H, et al. Prevalence of fecal incontinence: what can be expected?. *Dis Colon Rectum* 1998;41(6):705.

Gilliland R, Altomare DF, Moreira H, et al. Pudendal neuropathy is predictive of failure following anterior overlapping sphincteroplasty. *Dis Colon Rectum* 1998;41(12):1516.

Goligher JC, Leacock AG, Brossy JJ. Surgical anatomy of anal canal. *Br J Surg* 1955;43:51.

Gordon D, Groutz A, Goldman G, et al. Anal incontinence: prevalence among female patients attending a urogynecologic clinic. *AJR Am J Roentgenol* 1999;173(1):179.

Green JR, Soohoo SL. Factors associated with rectal injury in spontaneous deliveries. *Obstet Gynecol* 1989;73:732.

Gutierrez AB, Madoff RD, Lowry AC, et al. Long term results of anal sphincteroplasty. *Dis Colon Rectum* 2004;47:727.

Haadem K, Dahlström JA, Ling L. Anal sphincter competence in healthy women: clinical implications of age and other factors. *Obstet Gynecol* 1991;78:823.

Hallan RI, George B, Williams NS. Anal sphincter function: fecal incontinence and its treatment. *Surg Annual* 1993;25:85.

Halversen AL, Hull TL. Long-term outcomes of overlapping anal sphincter repair. *Dis Colon Rectum* 2002;45:345.

Handa VL, Danielsen BH, Gilbert WM. Obstetric anal sphincter lacerations. *Obstet Gynecol* 2001;98(2):225.

Hankins GDV, Hauth JC, Gilstrap LC, et al. Early repair of episiotomy dehiscence. *Obstet Gynecol* 1990;75:48.

Hauth JC, Gilstrap LC, Ward SC, et al. Early repair of an external sphincter ani muscle and rectal mucosal dehiscence. *Obstet Gynecol* 1986;67:806.

Healy JC, Halligan S, Reznek RH, et al. Dynamic MR imaging compared with evacuation proctography when evaluating anorectal configuration and pelvic floor movement. *AJR Am J Roentgenol* 1997;169:775.

Heyer T, Enck P, Grantke B, et al. Anal endosonography: are morphometric measurements of the anal sphincter reproducible?. *Gastroenterology* 1995;108:A613.

Hibbard LT. Surgical management of rectovaginal fistulas and complete perineal tears. *Am J Obstet Gynecol* 1978;130:139.

Hoexter B, Labow SB, Moseson MD. Transanal rectovaginal fistula repair. *Dis Colon Rectum* 1985;28:572.

Ingleman-Sundberg A. Transplantation of the levator muscles in the repair of complete tear and rectovaginal fistula. *Acta Chir Scand* 1947;96:313.

Jackson SL, Weber AM, Hull TL, et al. Fecal incontinence in women with urinary incontinence and pelvic organ prolapse. *Obstet Gynecol* 1997;89:423.

Jacobs PPM, Scheuer M, Kuijpers JHC. Obstetric fecal incontinence: role of pelvic floor denervation and results of delayed sphincter repair. *Dis Colon Rectum* 1990;33:494.

Johanson JF, Laferty J. Epidemiology of fecal incontinence: the silent affliction. *Am J Gastroenterol* 1996;91:33.

Jorge JM, Wexner SD. Etiology and management of fecal incontinence. *Dis Colon Rectum* 1993;36:77.

Kamm MA. Obstetric damage and faecal incontinence. *Lancet* 1994;344:730.

Kammerer-Doak DN, Wesol AB, Rogers RG, et al. A prospective cohort study of women after primary repair of obstetric anal sphincter laceration. *Am J Obstet Gynecol* 1999;181(6):1317.

Karoui S, Leroi AM, Koning E, et al. Results of sphincteroplasty in 86 patients with anal incontinence. *Ann Surg* 2000;232(1):143.

Kearney R, Miller JM, Ashton-Miller JA, et al. Obstetric factors associated with levator ani muscle injury after vaginal birth. *Obstet Gynecol* 2006;107:144.

Keighley MR. Postanal repair for faecal incontinence. *J R Soc Med* 1984;77(4):285.

Kodner IJ, Mazor A, Shemesh EI, et al. Endorectal advancement flap repair of rectovaginal and other complicated anorectal fistulas. *Surgery* 1993;114:682.

Kuijpers HC, Scheuer M. Disorders of impaired fecal control: a clinical and manometric study. *Dis Colon Rectum* 1990;33:207.

Kwon S, Visco AG, Fitzgerald MP et al. Validity and reliability of the Modified Manchester Health Questionnaire in assessing patients with fecal incontinence. *Dis Colon Rectum* 2005;48(2):323.

Laurberg S, Swash M, Henry MM. Delayed external sphincter repair for obstetric tear. *Br J Surg* 1988;75:786.

Law PJ, Kamm MA, Bartram CI. A comparison between electromyography and anal endosonography in mapping external anal sphincter defects. *Dis Colon Rectum* 1990;33:370.

Law PJ, Kamm MA, Bartram CI. Anal endosonography in the investigation of faecal incontinence. *Br J Surg* 1991;78:312.

Lee RA, ed. *Atlas of gynecologic surgery*. Philadelphia: WB Saunders, 1992.

Leroi AM, Kamm MA, Weber J, et al. Internal anal sphincter repair. *Int J Colorectal Dis* 1997;12(4):243.

Leroi AM, Weber J, Menard JF, et al. Prevalence of anal incontinence in 409 patients investigated for stress urinary incontinence. *Obstet Gynecol* 1999;94(5Pt1):689.

Levy E. Anorectal musculature. *Am J Surg* 1936;34:141.

Lienemann A, Anthuber C, Baron A, et al. Dynamic MR colpocystorectography assessing pelvic-floor descent. *Eur J Radiol* 1997;7:1309.

Lowry AC, Thorson AG, Rothenberger DA, et al. Repair of simple rectovaginal fistulas: influence of previous repairs. *Dis Colon Rectum* 1988;31:676.

Macmillan AK, Arend MB, Merrie AE, et al. The prevalence of fecal incontinence in community-dwelling adults: a systematic review of the literature. *Dis Colon Rectum* 2004;47:1341.

Madoff RD, Rosen HR, Baeten CG, et al. Safety and efficacy of dynamic muscleplasty for anal incontinence: lessons from a prospective, multicenter trial. *Eur J Radiol* 1999;9(3):436.

Madoff RD, Williams JG, Caushaj PF. Fecal incontinence. *N Engl J Med* 1992;326:1002.

Malouf AJ, Norton CS, Engel AF, et al. Long-term results of overlapping anterior anal-sphincter repair for obstetric trauma. *Lancet* 2000;355(9200):260.

Malouf AJ, Vaizey CJ, Nicholls RJ, et al. Permanent sacral nerve stimulation for fecal incontinence. *Dis Colon Rectum* 2000;43(8):1100.

Martius H. Die operative Wiederherstel-lung der vollkommen fehlenden. Harnrohare und des Schliessmuskels derselben. *Zentralb Gynakol* 1928;52:480.

Matsuoka H, Mavrantonis C, Wexner SD, et al. Postanal repair for fecal incontinence—is it worthwhile? *Dis Colon Rectum* 2000;43(11):1561.

Matzel KE, Kamm MA, Stosser M, et al. Sacral spinal nerve stimulation for faecal incontinence: multicentre study. *Lancet* 2004;363(9417):1270.

Mazier WP, Senagore AJ, Schiesel EC. Operative repair of anovaginal and rectovaginal fistulas. *Dis Colon Rectum* 1995;38:4.

McIntosh LJ, Frahm JD, Mallett VT. Pelvic floor rehabilitation in the treatment of incontinence. *J Reprod Med* 1993;38:662.

Mengert WF, Fish SA. Anterior rectal wall advancement. *Obstet Gynecol* 1955;5:262.

Miller NF, Brown W. The surgical treatment of complete perineal tears in the female. *Am J Obstet Gynecol* 1937;34:196.

Milligan ETC, Morgan CN. Surgical anatomy of the anal canal, with special reference to anorectal fistulae. *Lancet* 1934;2:1150.

Miner PB, Donnelly TC, Read NW. Investigation of mode of action of biofeedback in treatment of fecal incontinence. *Dig Dis Sci* 1990;35:1291.

Monberg J, Hammen S. Ruptured episiotomies resutured primarily. *Acta Obstet Gynecol Scand* 1987;66:163.

Nichols CM, Gill EJ, Nguyen T, et al. Anal sphincter injury in women with pelvic floor disorders. *Obstet Gynecol* 2004;104:690.

Nielsen MB, Buron B, Christiansen J, et al. Defecographic findings in patients with anal incontinence and constipation and their relation to rectal emptying. *Dis Colon Rectum* 1993;36:806.

Nielsen MB, Hauge C, Pedersen JF, et al. Endosonographic evaluation of patients with anal incontinence: findings and influence on surgical management. *Am J Radiol* 1993;160:771.

Nivatvongs S, Stern HS, Fryd DS. The length of the anal canal. *Dis Colon Rectum* 1981;24:600.

Noble GH. A new technique for complete laceration of the perineum designed for the purpose of eliminating infection from the rectum. *Trans Am Gynecol Soc* 1902;27:357.

Nyam DC, Pemberton JH. Long-term results of lateral internal sphincterotomy for chronic anal fissure with particular reference to incidence of fecal incontinence. *Neurourol Urodyn* 1999;18(6):579.

Nygaard IE, Roa SS, Dawson JD. Anal incontinence after anal sphincter disruption: a 30-year retrospective cohort study. *Obstet Gynecol* 1997;89(6):896.

O'Brien PE, Dixon JB, Skinner S, et al. A prospective, randomized, controlled clinical trial of placement of the artificial bowel sphincter for the control of fecal incontinence. *Dis Colon Rectum* 2004;47(11):1852.

Osterberg A, Graf W, Edebol Eeg-Olofsson K, et al. Results of neurophysiologic evaluation in fecal incontinence. *Dis Colon Rectum* 2000;43(9):1256.

Parks AG. Anorectal incontinence. *Proc R Soc Med* 1975;68:21.

Parks TG. The usefulness of tests in anorectal disease. *World J Surg* 1992;16:804.

Paul DJ, Lloyd TV. Hindgut duplication with rectovaginal fistula. *Obstet Gynecol* 1979;54:390.

Pemberton JH, Kelly KA. Achieving enteric continence: principles and applications. *Mayo Clin Proc* 1986;61:586.

Penninckx F. Belgian experience with dynamic graciloplasty for faecal incontinence. *Br J Surg* 2004;91(7):872.

Pescatori M, Pavesio R, Anastasio G, et al. Transanal electrostimulation for fecal incontinence: clinical, psychologic, and manometric prospective study. *Dis Colon Rectum* 1991;34:540.

Peschers UM, DeLancey JO, Schaer GN, et al. Exoanal ultrasound of the anal sphincter: normal anatomy and sphincter defects. *Dis Colon Rectum* 1997;40(12):1430.
Poen AC, Felt-Bersma RJ, Strijers RL, et al. Third-degree obstetric perineal tear: long-term clinical and functional results after primary repair. *Br J Surg* 1998;85(10):1433.
Roberts RO, Jacobsen SJ, Reilly WT, et al. Prevalence of combined fecal and urinary incontinence: a community-based study. *Dis Colon Rectum* 1999;42(7):857.
Rock JA, Woodruff JD. Surgical correction of a rectovaginal fistula. *Int J Gynecol Obstet* 1982;20:413.
Rockwood TH, Church JM, Fleshman JW, et al. Fecal Incontinence Quality of Life Scale: quality of life instrument for patients with fecal incontinence. *Dis Colon Rectum* 2000;43(6):813.
Rosenshein NB, Genadry RR, Woodruff JD. An anatomic classification of recto-vaginal septal defects. *Am J Obstet Gynecol* 1980;137:439.
Rothbarth J, Bemelman WA, Mierjerink WJ, et al. Long-term results of anterior anal sphincteroplasty repair for fecal incontinence due to obstetric injury/with invited commentaries. *Dig Surg* 2000;17(4):390.
Rothenberger DA, Goldberg SM. The management of rectovaginal fistulae. *Surg Clin North Am* 1983;63:61.
Rothenberger DA, Christenson CE, Balcos EG, et al. Endorectal advancement flap for treatment of simple rectovaginal fistula. *Dis Colon Rectum* 1982;25:297.
Sandridge DA, Thorp JM. Vaginal endosonography in the assessment of the anorectum. *Obstet Gynecol* 1995;86:1007.
Sangwan YP, Coller JA, Barrett RC, et al. Unilateral pudendal neuropathy: impact on outcome of anal sphincter repair. *Dis Colon Rectum* 1996;39:686.
Santoro GA, Eitan BZ, Pryde A, et al. Open study of low-dose amitriptyline in the treatment of patients with idiopathic fecal incontinence. *Dis Colon Rectum* 2000;43(12):1676.
Sartore A, DeSeta F, Maso G, et al. The effects of mediolateral episiotomy on pelvic floor function after vaginal delivery. *Obstet Gynecol* 2004;103:669.
Sentovich SM, Blatchford GJ, Rivela LJ, et al. Diagnosing anal sphincter injury with transanal ultrasound and manometry. *Elder Care* 1997–1998;9(6 Suppl):3.
Setti Carraro P, Kamm MA, Nicholls RJ. Long-term results of postanal repair for neurogenic faecal incontinence. *Br J Surg* 1994;81:140.
Shafik A, Doss S. Surgical anatomy of the somatic terminal enervation to the anal and urethral sphincters: role in anal and urethral surgery. *J Urol* 1999;161(1):85.
Shiono P, Klehanoff MA, Carey JC. Midline episiotomies: more harm than good? *Obstet Gynecol* 1990;75:765.
Sitzler PJ, Thomson JP. Overlap repair of damaged anal sphincter: a single surgeon's series. *Dis Colon Rectum* 1996;39:1356.
Snooks SJ, Henry MM. Faecal incontinence due to external anal sphincter division in childbirth is associated with damage to the enervation of the pelvic floor musculature: a double pathology. *BJOG* 1985;92:824.
Snooks SJ, Henry MM, Swash M. Anorectal incontinence and rectal prolapse: differential assessment of the enervation to puborectalis and external anal sphincter muscles. *Gut* 1985;26:470.
Snooks SJ, Swash M, Setchell M, et al. Injury to enervation of pelvic floor sphincter musculature in childbirth. *Lancet* 1984;2:546.
Soffer EE, Hull T. Fecal incontinence: a practical approach to evaluation and treatment. *Am J Gastroenterol* 2000;95(8):1873.
Sorensen M, Tetzschner T, Rasmussen OO, et al. Sphincter rupture in childbirth. *Br J Surg* 1993;80:392.
Stewart LK, Wilson SR. Transvaginal sonography of the anal sphincter: reliable, or not? *J Am Geriatr Soc* 1999;47(7):837.
Strohbehn K, Ellis JH, Strohbehn JA, et al. MRI of the levator ani with anatomic correlation. *Obstet Gynecol* 1996;87:277.
Sultan AH. Anal incontinence after childbirth. *Curr Opinion Obstet Gynecol* 1997;9:320.
Sultan AH, Kamm MA, Hudson CN, et al. Anal-sphincter disruption during vaginal delivery. *N Engl J Med* 1993;329:1905.
Sultan AH, Monga AK, Kumar D, et al. Primary repair of obstetric anal sphincter rupture using the overlap technique. *BJOG* 1999;106(4):318.
Swash M, Snooks SJ, Henry MM. A unifying concept of pelvic floor disorders and incontinence. *J R Soc Med* 1985;78:906.
Tancer ML, Veridiano NP. Genital fistulas secondary to diverticular disease of the sigmoid colon. *Obstet Gynecol Surv* 1996;51:67.
Thacker SB, Banta HD. Benefits and risks of episiotomy: an interpretive review of the English language literature, 1860–1980. *Obstet Gynecol Surv* 1983;38:322.
Thorp JM, Bowes WA, Brame RG, et al. Selected use of midline episiotomy: effect on perineal trauma. *Obstet Gynecol* 1987;70:260.
Tjandra JJ, Lim JF, Hiscock R, et al. Injectable silicone biomaterial for fecal incontinence caused by internal anal sphincter dysfunction is effective. *Dis Colon Rectum* 2004;47:2138.
Tjandra JJ, Milsom JW, Schroeder T, et al. Endoluminal ultrasound is preferable to electromyography in mapping anal sphincter defects. *Dis Colon Rectum* 1993;36:689.
Toglia MR, DeLancey JOL. Anal incontinence and the obstetrician-gynecologist. *Obstet Gynecol* 1994;84:731.
Uhlenhuth E, Wolfe WM, Smith EM, et al. The rectogenital septum. *Surg Gynecol Obstet* 1948;76:148.
Vaccaro CA, Cheong DM, Wexner SD, et al. Pudendal neuropathy in evacuatory disorders. *Dis Colon Rectum* 1995;38(2):166.
Vaizey CJ, Kamm MA, Bartram CI. Primary degeneration of the internal anal sphincter as a cause of passive faecal incontinence. *Lancet* 1997;349(9052):612.
Varma A, Gunn J, Gardiner A, et al. Obstetric anal sphincter injury: prospective evaluation of incidence. *Am J Obstet Gynecol* 2000;182(1 Pt 1):S1.
Venkatesh KS, Ramanujam PS, Larson DM, et al. Anorectal complications of vaginal delivery. *Dis Colon Rectum* 1989;32:1039.
Vernava AM III, Longo WE, Daniel GL. Pudendal neuropathy and the importance of EMG evaluation of fecal incontinence. *Dis Colon Rectum* 1993;36:23.
Veronikas DK, Nichols DH, Spino C. The Noble-Mengert-Fish operation revisited: a composite approach for persistent rectovaginal fistulas and complex perineal defects. *Am J Obstet Gynecol* 1998;179:1411.
Wall LL. The muscles of the pelvic floor. *Clin Obstet Gynecol* 1993;36:910.
Warren JC. A new method of operation for the relief of rupture of the perineum through the sphincter and rectum. *Trans Am Gynecol Soc* 1882;7:322.
Watts JD, Rothenberger DA, Buls JG, et al. The management of procidentia: 30 years' experience. *Dis Colon Rectum* 1985;28(2):96–102.
Wilcox LS, Strobino DM, Baruffi G, et al. Episiotomy and its role in the incidence of perineal lacerations in a maternity center and a tertiary hospital obstetric service. *Am J Obstet Gynecol* 1989;160:1047.
Williams JG, Wong WD, Jensen L, et al. Incontinence and rectal prolapse: a prospective manometric study. *Dis Colon Rectum* 1991;34:209.
Wise WE, Aguilar PS, Padmanabhan A, et al. Surgical treatment of low rectovaginal fistulas. *Dis Colon Rectum* 1991;34:271.
Wiskind AK, Thompson MD. Transverse transperineal repair of rectovaginal fistulas in the lower vagina. *Am J Obstet Gynecol* 1992;167:694.
Zetterstrom J, Lopez A, Anzen B, et al. Anal sphincter tears at vaginal delivery: risk factors and clinical outcome of primary repair. *Obstet Gynecol* 1999;94(1):21.

[illegible]

[illegible]

[illegible]

SECTION VIII ■ RELATED SURGERY

CHAPTER 41 ■ BREAST DISEASES: BENIGN AND MALIGNANT

VICTORIA L. GREEN

DEFINITIONS

Axillary lymph node dissection—Removal of all or part of the lymph nodes in the axilla to examine microscopically for carcinomatous implants.

Axillary tail of Spence—A lateral projection of glandular breast tissue extending from the upper, outer portion of the breast toward the axilla.

BRCA—Currently one of two tumor suppressor genes (BRCA1 and BRCA 2) that tend to be associated with an increased risk of certain cancers, especially breast and ovarian cancers when the gene is in a mutated (abnormal) form. Accounts for 40% to 50% of inherited susceptibility to breast cancer; however, there are other less common mutated genes that also affect cancer risk.

Cooper's ligaments—Fibrous septa connecting the skin to the underlying pectoralis fascia. Involvement in a carcinomatous process may lead to contraction of the ligament and result in dimpling of the overlying skin.

Core biopsy—Procedure that involves obtaining a cylindrical specimen of tissue for microscopic analysis through a hollow needle, usually 8- to 14-gauge. A histologic sample is obtained rather than a cytologic sample as with fine-needle aspiration.

Cystosarcoma phyllodes—Rare, usually slow-growing circumscribed or infiltrating fibroepithelial breast tumor that resembles a fibroadenoma but may be partly cystic. The stroma is cellular and resembles a fibrosarcoma. The tumor is usually benign, but occasionally may be malignant and metastasize.

Cytologic evaluation—Evaluation of a cellular sample for microscopic evaluation to determine the presence or absence of a cancerous condition.

Diagnostic mammogram—Imaging in a women with symptoms, which may include a mammogram, sonogram, and/or examination by a radiologist.

Digital mammography—An imaging technique that stores an x-ray image as a computer image rather than on the usual x-ray film.

Ductal carcinoma in situ (DCIS)—Histologically variable collection of carcinomas of the lactiferous ducts that have not spread beyond the basement membrane but have the potential of becoming invasive and spreading to other tissues.

Ductogram (galactogram)—A test used in the evaluation of nipple discharge in which a radioopaque dye is instilled through a fine plastic tube placed into the ductal opening of the nipple, the outline of which is displayed on x-ray.

Fibrocystic lesions—Refers to a broad spectrum of heterogeneous benign histopathologic changes in the breast associated with stromal fibrosis and with variable degrees of intraductal epithelial hyperplasia and sclerosing adenosis.

Fine-needle aspiration—Process of obtaining a specimen of cells and tissue for microscopic examination by applying suction through a fine needle (usually 21- to 23-gauge) attached to a syringe. May be therapeutic in drainage of a fluid-filled cyst. Ultrasound guidance may be helpful but is not necessary. A cytologic sample is obtained rather than a histologic sample as through a core biopsy or excisional biopsy. Sometimes called *fine-needle aspiration biopsy.*

Genetic counseling—Guidance provided by a medical professional typically to individuals with an increased risk of harboring genes that may increase their risk for developing cancer or producing an offspring having a genetic disorder. Includes providing information and advice concerning the probability of disease, diagnostic testing, and available options/treatments.

Hormone receptor assay—Evaluation of a breast tumor to determine if it is likely to be affected by/responsive to hormones (generally estrogen, progesterone, and human epidermal growth factor 2 [HER2]).

Immunohistochemistry (immunocytochemistry)—Use of antibodies to detect specific chemical antigens in cells or tissue samples evaluated under the microscope.

Intraductal papilloma—Generally benign breast mass that is usually microscopic but may grow to 2 to 3 mm in diameter. The lesion may present with spontaneous unilateral bloody nipple discharge.

Lobular carcinoma *in situ*—Early type of breast cancer developing within the lobules that does not penetrate through the basement membrane.

Lumpectomy—Surgical excision of a margin of normal breast tissue (preferably 1–2 cm) surrounding a breast carcinoma usually less than 4 cm in diameter. Often a component of breast-conserving therapy, which may also include removal of axillary lymph nodes and radiation therapy.

Macrocalcifications—Large, coarse calcium deposits that are often caused by noncancerous processes/conditions, such as aging of the breast arteries, old injuries, or inflammation. Common in women older than the age of 50.

Mammography—Special imaging examination of the breasts using x-ray.

Magnetic resonance imaging (MRI)—A noninvasive imaging technique that generates computerized images of internal body tissues and is based on nuclear magnetic resonance of atoms within the body induced by the application of radio waves. A large magnet polarizes hydrogen atoms in the tissues and then monitors the summation of the spinning energies within living cells.

Mastectomy—Surgical removal of all or part of the breast tissue; may be associated with removal of lymph nodes and muscles.

Microcalcifications—Tiny specks of calcium in the breast that may appear alone or in clusters. To judge the likelihood of malignant change, a radiologist uses the shape and appearance of the clusters on mammography. Specks of deodorant may be mistaken for calcifications and thus should not be used before a mammogram.

Modified radical mastectomy—Removal of the breast tissue and only the fascia over the pectoralis major muscle.

Montgomery glands/tubercles—Accessory glands located at the periphery of the areola. They are intermediate glands in between sebaceous glands and true mammary glands, and thus may secrete milk.

Paget disease—Rare breast carcinoma often mistaken for eczema, dermatitis, or mastitis of the nipple. May or may not be associated with an underlying mass lesion.

Partial or segmental mastectomy—A type of surgery that removes only the part of the breast in which the cancer is located and a margin of normal breast tissue surrounding the tumor.

Polymastia—More than two breasts.

Polythelia—More than two nipples.

Positron emission tomography—Highly specialized imaging technique using short-lived radioactive substances with formation of tomographic images by computer analysis of photons detected from annihilation of positrons emitted by radionuclides incorporated into biochemical substances. The scanner uses integrated x-ray and computing equipment.

Prophylactic mastectomy—Procedure performed before any evidence of cancer is found for the purpose of preventing cancer.

Quadrantectomy—Partial mastectomy in which the quarter of the breast that contains a tumor is removed.

Radical mastectomy—En bloc removal of the breast tissue; associated skin, nipple, areola, axillary lymph nodes; and the underlying pectoralis major and minor muscles.

Screening mammography—Breast imaging based on guidelines to detect cancer early in symptomatic women.

Sentinel lymph node biopsy—Currently considered conventional treatment in certain categories of breast cancer patients for initial evaluation of the axilla. The surgeon uses either blue dye and/or a radioisotope tracer injected into the tumor site at the time of surgery. The first (sentinel) node that picks up the dye is removed and biopsied. If the node is cancer-free, further lymph node evaluation is terminated.

Simple mastectomy—Removal of the breast tissue and associated skin, nipple, and areola, but without removing the underlying muscle or fascial tissue. May be used as a prophylactic procedure. Also called *total mastectomy.*

Stereotactic needle biopsy—Use of mammogram images taken at two angles to map the exact location of a (usually nonpalpable) mass by computers. The patient lies face down on a table with the breast hanging through an aperture in the table.

Subcutaneous mastectomy—Excision of breast tissue by undermining the skin, thus preserving the cosmetic appearance and form of the nipple, areola, and skin. Appears to have been abandoned as a procedure for prophylactic mastectomy.

Thermography—Imaging technique in which cutaneous temperatures of the breast or infrared radiation from the breast are measured through electronic detectors to diagnose breast disorders.

TNM staging—A system of clinicopathologic evaluation of tumors based on the extent of tumor involvement in the primary site (T), lymph nodes (N), and metastasis (M).

TRAM flap—Muscle flap procedure using the transverse rectus abdominis muscle as a method of breast reconstruction.

Triple test—Not an actual test, but a correlation of the results of the breast physical examination, mammogram, and tissue sampling technique to determine the malignant potential of a lesion. If all agree that the lesion is benign, there is a high likelihood of correlation with a benign result.

Ultrasound (sonography)—Imaging technique that uses high-frequency sound-wave transmission through tissues to outline organs. No radiation is used.

The specialty of obstetrics and gynecology is devoted to the health care of women throughout their lifetime. Concerns about breast health are common to women from puberty to menopause, therefore obstetrician/gynecologists are becoming increasingly involved in not only the detection of breast masses but also the diagnosis, evaluation, and treatment of such lesions. Although the etiology of most breast symptoms is a benign disorder, the fear of cancer is often the motivating factor for women seeking attention. Breast cancer remains the most common cancer in women, with the American Cancer Society (ACS) estimating more than 211,000 cases in the United States in 2005. Although mortality from breast cancer is decreasing, cancer of the breast remains second only to lung cancer in cancer deaths in women, making it an especially dreadful adversary. Advances in treatment modalities, genetic predisposition, and chemoprevention have thrust breast health issues into the forefront of the media and medical technology. The zeal to achieve the ideal cure or prevention strategy persists unabated in the medical profession and remains an ongoing challenge. A thorough understanding of the diagnosis and management of breast disease, as well as an appreciation of contemporary treatment options, are essential for the practicing gynecologist.

The purpose of this chapter is to review breast embryology, anatomy, and pathology and to examine strategies for the diagnosis, management, and treatment of breast conditions. The role of the women's health clinician in breast cancer detection, therapy, assessment of risk factors, genetic testing, and chemoprevention is also discussed. The woman in whom breast cancer develops requires a multidisciplinary team. The gynecologist must be a knowledgeable participant in her treatment plan.

EMBRYOLOGY

The breasts, or mammary glands, begin embryologic differentiation in the fifth or sixth week of fetal development. Two ventral bands of thickened ectoderm (known as mammary ridges or "milk lines") develop and extend from the area of the future axilla at the base of the forelimb to the future inguinal region of the hind limb (Fig. 41.1). With normal regression of the ridges (which occurs shortly after the sixth week of fetal development), only one gland persists on each side, at the level of the thorax. This process is similar in both sexes. Accessory mammary glands (polymastia) or accessory nipples (polythelia) may result along the original mammary ridge with failure of normal regression. This minor congenital anomaly may occur in both sexes with an estimated frequency of about 1%.

Ingrowth of the remaining ectoderm into the underlying mesenchyme initiates the development of the primary and secondary bud of the mammary gland. Canalization of these

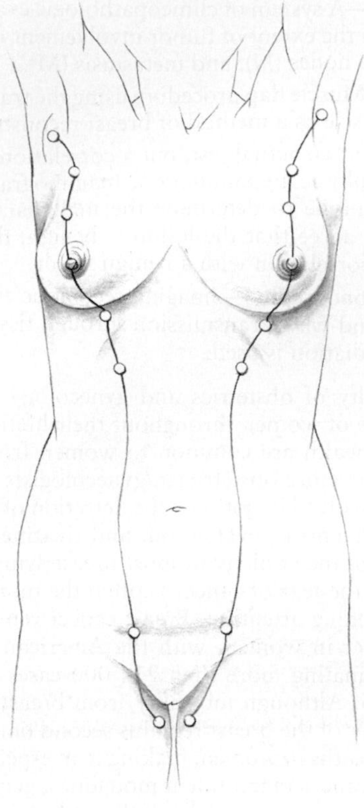

FIGURE 41.1. Mammary milk line.

epithelial cords (under the influence of placental sex steroids) during the third trimester marks the development of the lactiferous ductal system. Proliferation of basal mesenchymal cells and smooth muscle development initiates transformation into the fully formed nipple. Failure of elevation of the nipple above the skin level occurs in 2% to 4% of the population, resulting in inverted nipples.

Anatomy

The breast, or mammary gland, is a highly modified sudoriferous gland situated between two layers of superficial fascia on the pectoralis major, serratus anterior, and external oblique muscles. It is bordered by the second rib superiorly, the sternum medially, the sixth intercostal space inferiorly, and the midaxillary line laterally. It is composed of several lobes, with the greatest volume of glandular tissue located in the upper outer quadrant. Fibrous septa, called *suspensory* or *Cooper's ligaments,* interdigitate between the parenchymal tissues to connect the two fascial planes. The ligaments permit mobility of the breast on the anterior thoracic wall while also providing structural support (Fig. 41.2).

The breast lobes are arranged in a radial pattern and contain many lobules. Each lobule consists of 10 to 100 alveoli or tubulosaccular secretory units (Fig. 41.3). Breast cancer is thought to originate in these units, also called *terminal duct lobular units.* Each lobe terminates in a lactiferous duct, which opens onto the nipple. Beneath the areola, each lactiferous duct features a dilated portion called the *lactiferous sinus.* Inspissation of material in the lactiferous sinus may account for galactoceles.

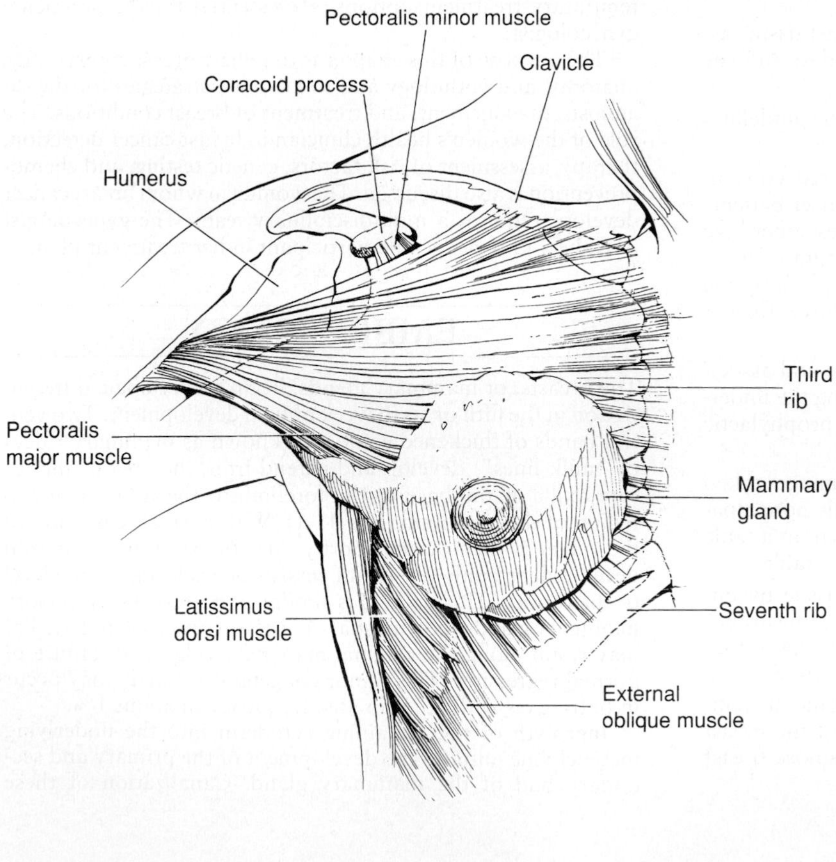

FIGURE 41.2. Topography of the breast. The breast lies approximately over the midportion of the hemithorax with the tail extending toward the axilla. Ramifications also penetrate the interstices of the underlying muscle. These extensions and the close adherence of the skin to subcutaneous breast tissue make complete subcutaneous mastectomy nearly impossible.

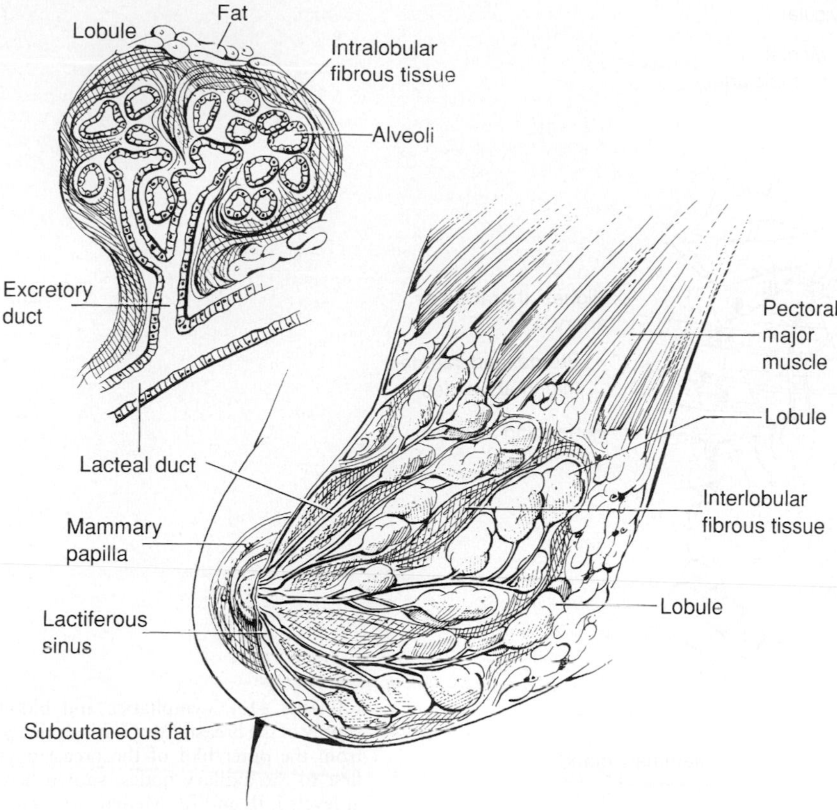

FIGURE 41.3. Internal structure of the breast. The breast is a large apocrine gland. The secreting parenchyma is composed of lobules containing acini, fat, and fibrous tissue. The ducts drain centrally toward large lacunae located directly beneath the nipple. These act as reservoirs until they receive the impetus for ejection.

The epidermis of the nipple and areola is highly pigmented. Additional increased pigmentation and size of the nipple–areolar complex is noted in pregnancy. The nipple contains the only muscle "within" the breast tissue. The areola consists of many sweat, sebaceous, and accessory glands. During pregnancy, accessory glands called *Montgomery tubercles* become prominent.

The breast tissue is well supplied by an extensive arterial and venous system. The anterior perforating branches of the internal thoracic (internal mammary) artery supplies the medial and central aspect of the breast. The upper outer quadrant is supplied by the lateral thoracic artery, a branch of the axillary artery. The two vessels combined provide the major blood supply to the nipple. Other vessels supplying the breast include the anterior and lateral branches of the intercostals, other branches of the axillary artery (including the pectoral branch of the thoracoacromial artery), and the subscapular and thoracodorsal arteries.

Venous and lymphatic drainage of the breast follows the course of the superficial and deeper arteries. Principal venous drainage goes to the internal thoracic vein medially, to the axillary vein superolaterally, and by way of the intercostal veins to the vertebral and azygous veins posteriorly. This drainage pathway accounts for the frequent sites of metastases, as breast cancer enters the venous system and metastasizes to the lungs by way of the axillary or intercostal veins or to thoracic, abdominal, and pelvic organs by way of the vertebral vein. Similarly, the primary lymph node drainage is initially into the axillary region, but additional drainage can precede to the infraclavicular and mediastinal (parasternal) areas, thus suggesting the need to extend the routine breast examination to the bony borders to ensure adequate coverage of these potential cancer-bearing areas. The lymphatic plexus has deep and superficial drainage pathways. Lymphatic drainage from the deep lesions is directed toward the axilla and the axillary nodes, although all breast quadrants contribute lymph to the medial parasternal lymph nodes. This lymphatic plexus is divided into levels based on their relation to the pectoralis minor muscle. Level I nodes are located lateral to the muscle, and level III nodes are located medially. Level II nodes are located deep or posterior to the pectoralis minor muscle (Fig. 41.4).

LIFE CYCLE CHANGES

The development and physiologic functioning of the breast is orchestrated by the anterior lobe of the pituitary gland and the ovaries. This development is a lifelong process that begins in utero. Transient enlargement of the breast bud and associated milklike nipple secretion ("witches milk") may occur in both newborn girls and boys as a result of transplacental transfer of maternal hormones (primarily estrogen). The fluid secretion may appear for a week postpartum, but subsequent involution of the tissue results by the third or fourth week postpartum.

Breast development occurs during thelarche, which signifies the beginning of puberty. This stage typically begins between 9 and 10 years of age, but may begin as early as 8 years in some girls, with ethnic and environmental factors accounting for the variation. Before the transformation that occurs at puberty, the function and histology of the human breast is identical in boys and girls. However, at puberty in girls, the rudimentary gland buds proliferate and increase in size, and the nipple and areola become pigmented. The ductal system develops as a consequence of estrogen stimulation, and the lobular-alveolar system develops in response to progesterone secretion. The first

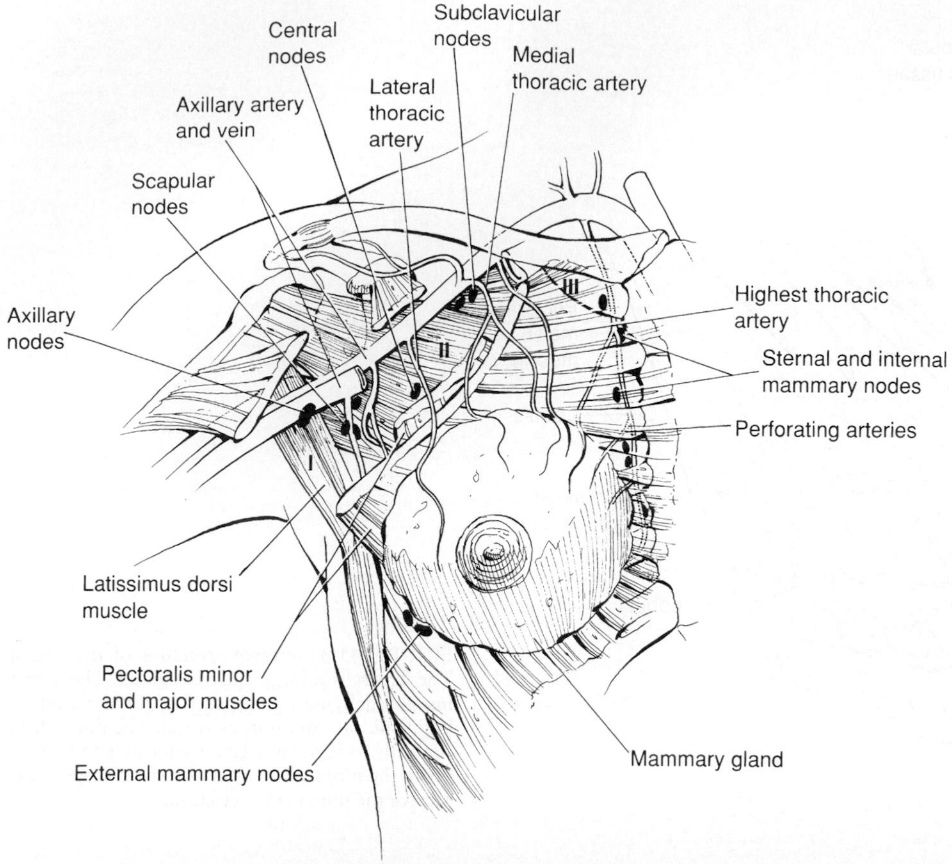

FIGURE 41.4. Lymphatics and blood supply of the breast. Lymphatic drainage from the outer half of the breast goes first to the axillary nodes, shown here at levels I, II, and III. Medial lesions are more likely to metastasize first to the internal mammary chain.

visible manifestation of this hormonal response is a symmetric palpable enlargement beneath the nipple.

Menstruation, pregnancy, and menopause are additional sentinel events in the cycle of breast development. Before the onset of menstruation, breast transformation begins with ductal branching and proliferation of interductal stroma. With each menstrual cycle, ductal proliferation occurs under the influence of estrogen. Proliferation of the terminal duct structure and increased mitotic activity in the basal epithelial cells occur in the secretory phase under the influence of progesterone. Stromal proliferation and edema, in response to the hormonal milieu, accounts for the sense of fullness or tenderness experienced premenstrually. The decrease in hormones that occurs with menstruation signals disappearance of stromal edema, desquamation of epithelial cells, atrophy of intralobular connective tissue, and overall shrinkage in the size of the ducts.

Further maturation of the breast occurs with pregnancy. Significant development of glandular tissues and decrease in the surrounding stroma portends reversal of the stromal glandular relation seen before this stage. After pregnancy, these changes regress but do not return completely to their prepregnancy state. Menopause heralds a further reduction and shrinkage of the ducts, gland buds, and surrounding stroma.

Lactation

Hormonal and structural changes, which prime the breast for future milk production, occur during pregnancy. As previously occurred during puberty, increased estrogen and progesterone secretion in early pregnancy results in ductal development and maturation as well as enlargement of lobular size. During the latter half of pregnancy, glandular epithelium is transformed into secretory epithelium in response to insulin, thyroxine, growth hormone, and corticosteroids. Human placental lactogen and prolactin also play critical roles in breast development during pregnancy. Paradoxically, despite considerable increases in prolactin, its functioning is inhibited at the alveolar level by progesterone. Thus, lactation (the process of mature milk secretion) does not occur until the rapid decline of estrogen and progesterone that occurs with delivery, although colostrum leakage may be seen in the second half of pregnancy.

Stimulation of the afferent neural arc suppresses prolactin inhibitory factor (PIF), allowing release of prolactin-releasing factor (PRF) and further elevation of the prolactin concentration. Breast suckling stimulates the neural arc, as do auditory (infant crying) and visual stimuli. PIF is thought to be dopamine, and PRF is thought to be thyroid-releasing hormone or thyrotropin-releasing hormone. Additionally, stimulation of the neural arc triggers release of oxytocin by involving the paraventricular and supraoptic nuclei of the hypothalamus. Oxytocin release from the posterior pituitary induces contraction of the myoepithelial cells surrounding the nipple ducts, resulting in milk ejection or letdown. Continued suckling induces additional prolactin secretion and replenishment of the milk supply; however, this can be modified by psychological stress, pain, or fatigue, resulting in a decreased milk output. Discontinuation of suckling results in increased levels of PIF, which inhibit prolactin production. Ultimately, lactation ceases, with resultant decrease in size of the alveoli.

PATHOLOGY

Table 41.1 lists the basic anatomic structures and the most commonly associated pathologic abnormalities. A brief review of pathology of the breast follows.

Congenital Anomalies

Congenital abnormalities affecting the breast anlage include amastia, hypertrophy, asymmetry, and congenital inversion of the nipples. Additionally, supernumerary nipples or breasts may be seen—the result of persistence of epidermal thickenings along the milk line.

Inflammation

Acute mastitis or breast abscesses may develop during nursing or with other dermatologic conditions of the nipples. The breast is vulnerable to bacterial infection from tears or fissures in the nipples. The offending bacterium in puerperal mastitis is most commonly *Staphylococcus aureus* and *Streptococcus*. Treatment includes continued emptying of breast milk, either through nursing or pumping, and use of warm or cold compresses. The most effective broad-spectrum antibiotics are dicloxacillin or a first-generation cephalosporin for 10 days. For those with penicillin allergies, erythromycin may be substituted.

Nonpuerperal mastitis is often associated with a sticky, multicolored discharge and is noted in individuals who are immunocompromised (e.g., diabetic patients), people who have undergone radiation treatment, and those who have an autoimmune disorder. Purulent discharges generally respond to antibiotics, but an abscess requires incision and drainage for complete resolution.

Duct ectasia is characterized by dilation of the ducts, inspissation of breast secretions, and marked periductal and interstitial chronic granulomatous inflammatory reaction. It is often association with a multicolored, sticky, spontaneous, bilateral nipple discharge coming from multiple ducts. It is most commonly seen in women in the fifth or sixth decade of life; however, the etiology is unknown. Periductal inflammation may result in nipple inversion, areolar thickening, and a breast mass that can mimic a cancer or nonpuerperal abscess. This condition is discussed further under the section on nipple discharge.

Galactocele occurs as a result of overdistention of lactiferous ducts with resultant inspissation of milk. It usually presents as a firm nontender mass in the outer quadrants of the breast, away from the areolar margin.

TABLE 41.1

ANATOMICAL LOCATION OF COMMON BREAST LESIONS

Anatomic structures	Lesions
Nipple and areola	Nipple adenoma
Lactiferous ducts	Duct ectasia
	Intraductal papilloma
	Subareolar abscess
Terminal ductal lobular unit	Cysts
	Sclerosing adenosis
	Small ductal papilloma
	Hyperplasia
	Atypical hyperplasia
	Carcinoma
Lobular stroma	Fibroadenoma
	Phyllodes tumor
Interlobular stroma	Fat necrosis
	Lipoma
	Fibrous tumor
	PASH
	Sarcoma
	Fibromatosis

Adapted from Kumar V, Abbas A, Fausto N, eds. *Robbins & Cotran: Pathologic basis of disease*, 7th ed. Philadelphia: Elsevier Saunders, 2005.

Fibrocystic Changes

Fibrocystic change (FCC) of the breast is the most frequently encountered benign breast disorder. It occurs most often in reproductive women between the ages of 30 and 50 years. It also occurs in approximately 10% of women younger than 21 years of age; therefore, breast symptoms in adolescence must not be ignored. Fibrocystic condition does not increase the risk of developing breast cancer, but it does often make the physical examination of the patient more difficult (Fig. 41.5).

In 85% to 90% of cases of significant FCC, breast discom fort is the leading symptom. Women often present with a history of bilateral, menstrually related, painful, tender, and nodular breasts, most often localized to the upper outer quadrants. Typically, the pain is most severe just before menses as a result of the normal physiologic stromal edema and ductal dilation.

The breast is normally an inhomogeneous appendage with uneven distribution of adipose and fibrous tissue. It is estimated that at least 50% of women have palpably irregular breasts. This "normal" anatomic asymmetry leads to physiologic inhomogeneity, irregularity, or lumpiness in some women. Nodularity, particularly as it waxes and wanes during the menstrual

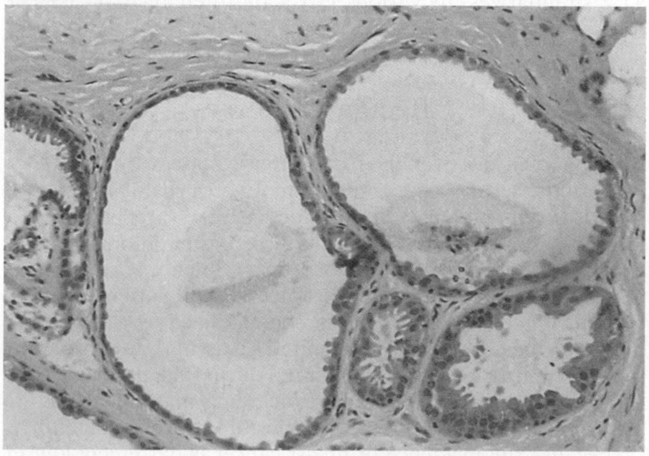

FIGURE 41.5. Histologic section of fibrocystic changes with cyst formation and at right lower corner apocrine metaplasia (H&E ×120). (Courtesy of Taalat Tadros, MD, Emory University, School of Medicine, Atlanta, GA.)

cycle, is a physiologic process. This nodularity and irregularity is often mistaken for a dominant breast mass. Evaluation of FCC, thus, creates a difficult dilemma for physicians. Providers must carefully decide whether their findings represent a dominant mass or an exaggeration of normal breast tissue associated with the "nodularity" of FCC.

Dominant masses may represent a variety of benign and malignant processes, including fibroadenomas, macrocysts, prominent areas of FCC, fat necrosis, abscesses, or carcinoma. Dominant masses are distinguished by their persistence throughout the menstrual cycle and palpable difference on examination from the surrounding breast parenchyma. Often, evaluation of the contralateral breast assists in determination of whether an anatomic variation is a mass or normal breast tissue. However, any concern should be referred for evaluation, or a repeat examination may be performed after a menstrual cycle to detect persistence. A delay of 1 to 2 months in a reproductive age woman is acceptable; however, a shorter-term follow-up is preferable in a menopausal woman because of the higher frequency of breast cancer in this age group. Breast masses are often easier to appreciate in postmenopausal women because of atrophy of the surrounding nodular glandular elements. A *positive* mammogram is helpful. Conversely, a negative mammogram does not obviate the need to evaluate a mass by fine-needle aspiration (FNA) or a histologic method of biopsy as there is a 10% to 15% false-negative rate for mammography.

Fibrocystic change is a term proposed by the ACS. The terminology encompasses several histopathologic categories, including macrocyst formation, hyperplasia of ductal epithelium, apocrine metaplasia, papillomatosis, duct ectasia, sclerosing adenosis, and stromal fibrosis, thus leading to significant confusion. Reporting criteria for pathologists may include all or only some of these groups. It is important to know whether *severe* ductal hyperplasia is included in the pathologist's category of FCC because this variant increases a patient's risk of subsequent development of breast carcinoma by three- to fivefold.

Conversely, mild hyperplasia (which may also be included in the FCC categorization) does not increase a patient's risk of breast cancer development. Practitioners should attempt to describe exactly what they are feeling rather than use the undefined FCC term in the clinical arena. This term is not *clinically* meaningful in that it designates a heterogeneous group of processes, some pathologic and some physiologic. Treatment options for FCC-induced mastalgia are discussed later. Table 41.2 summarizes the various FCCs and their relative risks of breast cancer.

TABLE 41.2

BREAST LESIONS AND RELATIVE RISK OF DEVELOPING INVASIVE BREAST CARCINOMA

Pathologic lesions	Relative risk
Nonproliferative breast changes	
Cysts	No increased risk
Fibrocystic changes	
Apocrine metaplasia	
Duct ectasia	
Fibroadenoma without complex features	
Adenosis	
Hyperplasia—mild	
Proliferative disease without atypia	1.5–2.0
Sclerosing adenosis	
Papilloma	
Radial scar (complex sclerosing lesion)	
Fibroadenoma with complex features	
Hyperplasia (moderate to florid)	
Proliferative disease with atypia	4.0–5.0
Atypical ductal hyperplasia	
Atypical lobular hyperplasia	
Carcinoma *in situ*	8–10
Lobular carcinoma *in situ*	
Ductal carcinoma *in situ* (low grade)	

Adapted from Kumar V, Abbas A, Fausto N, eds. *Robbins & Cotran: Pathologic basis of disease,* 7th ed. Philadelphia: Elsevier Saunders, 2005.

Benign Tumors

Most women discover their own breast masses by chance or by periodic self-breast examination. Two thirds of the masses found during a woman's reproductive years are benign and include cystic changes, fibroadenomas, and papillomas. However, 50% of the palpable masses in perimenopausal women and the majority of lesions in postmenopausal patients are malignant. Once a lesion has been characterized as a mass or a lump, further evaluation is required. This may involve additional examinations at optimal times during the patient's menstrual cycle; radiologic imaging, including mammography or ultrasound; FNA/core biopsy; or referral for excisional biopsy.

Because the incidence of breast cancer is extremely low in patients younger than 20 years, patients in this age group who have solid masses less than 2 cm who have low clinical suspicion by physical examination and ultrasonography can be monitored without biopsy at the discretion of the physician, although surgical consultation is often recommended. However, the ability of the patient to follow up and other risk factors for breast cancer should be considered.

Gross cysts or macrocysts may be silent or painful, single or multiple, and may be associated with a green-brown nipple discharge (although a thorough evaluation of the nipple discharge should occur despite the presumption of its origin). Of course, any dominant mass must be differentiated from a cancerous process.

Fibroadenomas are the most common benign tumors of the female breast and represent the most common breast tumor in women younger than 25 years of age. These tumors are often clinically painless, well circumscribed, and freely movable with a rounded configuration. They are usually rubbery or firm, but when calcified, they may present as a stony hard mass. Multiple fibroadenomas may develop simultaneously or successively in one or both breasts in 10% to 15% of cases. Growth of the fibrous stromal and glandular tissue is thought to be the result of an unopposed estrogenic influence on susceptible tissue, aberrations of normal breast development, or the product of hyperplastic processes, rather than a true neoplasm. These tumors often contain estrogen receptors; hence, they may fluctuate in size with the menstrual cycle or increase in size during pregnancy. They routinely involute with menopause. They are uncommonly associated with carcinoma, but, rarely, *in situ* lobular or ductal carcinomas arise in or involve fibroadenomas (Fig. 41.6).

Fibroadenomas infrequently grow to be very large (10–15 cm in diameter). These are called *giant fibroadenomas*, although most are excised at 2 to 4 cm. When morphologic changes such as leaflike clefts and "slits" are present, these fibroadenomas are called *phyllodes tumors* (formerly known

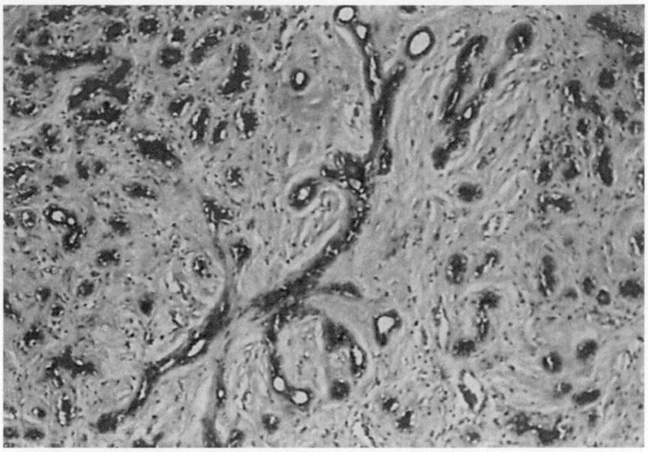

FIGURE 41.6. Histologic section of fibroadenoma with cellular stroma (in a pericanalicular pattern), ducts maintain patency (H&E ×240) (Courtesy of Taalat Tadros, MD, Emory University, School of Medicine, Atlanta, GA.)

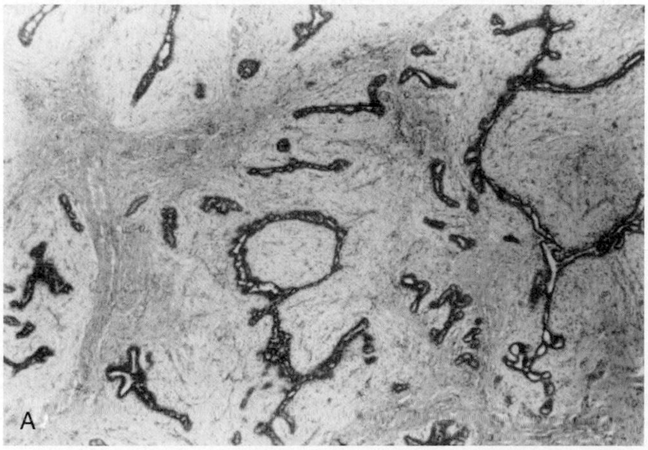

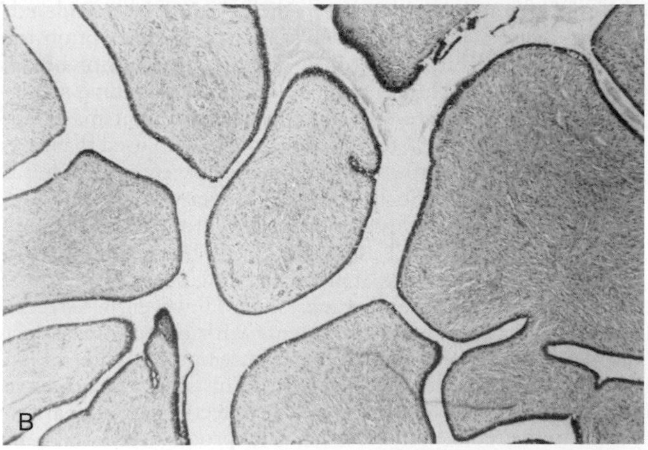

FIGURE 41.7. Benign tumors. **A:** A circumscribed breast tumor from a young patient illustrates fibroadenoma. A mixture of benign epithelial and stromal components is seen. **B:** Phyllodes tumor of the breast showing a pattern superficially similar to that of (**A**). It is distinguished by its leaflike pattern of stromal growth in cystic spaces. The stroma is also markedly cellular. This tumor, although structurally benign, is capable of recurrence. (Courtesy of Bhagirath Majmudar, MD, Emory University School of Medicine, Atlanta, GA.)

as *cystosarcoma phyllodes*). These can be benign or malignant lesions. Histologic examination reveals that these lesions have a more cellular stroma, rarely display a prominent pericanalicular growth pattern, and tend to occur in an older age group (Fig. 41.7).

Management of fibroadenomas is varied. The key to management in all clinical situations is individualization. In women younger than 25 years who have fibroadenomas diagnosed by concurring physical examination, sonography, and FNA ("modified" triple test), the risk of missing breast cancer is 1 in 229 to 1 in 700. This risk remains very low in women younger than 35 years who also have the battery of tests. Fibroadenomas do not regress spontaneously and tend to enlarge with time. Because of the low probability of cancer, conservatism is particularly acceptable in women younger than age 25 years if the fibroadenoma is small, not increasing in size, or is not psychologically disturbing. Mammography is an integral part of the evaluation in women older than 30 years (or younger depending on risk factors and clinical suspicion). Lesions greater than 2 to 3 cm should probably be evaluated for excision.

Some authors promote excision of all fibroadenomas, regardless of histology. Clearly, if the FNA cytology reveals atypia or hyperplasia, excisional biopsy should be performed. Small, asymptomatic, mammographically detected fibroadenomas proven by FNA or core biopsy may be watched depending on clinical duration and patient risk factors. Although fibroadenomas may be suspected on the basis of their clinical presentation, a final diagnosis cannot be made without histologic or cytologic confirmation.

Intraductal papilloma and breast cancer are discussed later in this chapter.

COMMON BREAST SYMPTOMS

Mastalgia

Pain is a common and enigmatic condition experienced by 70% of women younger than 55 years and accounting for nearly 50% of breast related visits to the physician's office. Research into the treatment of breast pain is difficult to interpret as a result of the heterogeneous nature of the pain, the fact that symptoms generally resolve spontaneously within a short time, and because typically, one fifth of patients respond to placebo. Because of the subjective nature of the problem and difficulty in quantification, it was often ignored as a psychoneurotic disorder, although nearly 10% of breast cancer patients have pain as the initial presenting symptom (yet breast pain alone is rarely a presenting symptom of cancer). The histopathologic correlation and optimal treatment of mastalgia are still inadequately defined.

Breast pain may be divided into cyclic, noncyclic, and extramammary categories. A careful history should include the use of pain charts (particularly in patients with persistent or recalcitrant symptoms), documenting exactly when pain occurs during the month and the exact nature of the discomfort. The Cardiff Breast Pain Chart, visual analog scales, and the McGill Pain Questionnaire are frequently used to quantify pain. In addition, a thorough physical examination and radiologic procedures (when appropriate) can assist in distinguishing these three groups. Delineation is important as presenting symptoms, spontaneous remission rates, and likelihood of response to treatment differs for these categories.

Cyclic breast pain usually starts during the luteal phase of the menstrual cycle and may crescendo until the onset of menses, when it dissipates. Conversely, some pain may be present at low levels during the entire cycle with premenstrual intensification of symptoms. Cyclic mastalgia typically involves bilateral upper outer quadrants of the breast diffusely, but may be more severe in one breast than the other and is often attributed to FCC. The mechanism of pain is not understood, although there is some evidence that this could be related to a decreased progesterone:estrogen ratio during the luteal phase of the menstrual cycle, increased levels of saturated fats, reduced proportions of essential fatty acids, or an unusually high reactive state in the body's regulation of normal cyclic prolactin release. Because so many women experience asymmetric discomfort, it is unlikely that the sole basis of the monthly pain is hormonal or dietary.

Although mastalgia may be the presenting symptom, most patients are concerned with the possibility of cancer. Therefore, for the majority of patients without a dominant mass, reassurance is often sufficient without the need for medical intervention. Appropriate assessment should be performed, which may include examination, sonography, mammography (depending on age and risk factors), pregnancy testing, and/or frequent follow-up.

Those with severe and protracted symptoms that blanket everyday life, interfering with normal enjoyment and disrupting daily routine, merit treatment. One study showed that mastalgia hampers sexual activity in 48% of women, physical recreation in 37%, social endeavors in 12%, sleep in 10%, and work/school activity in 6%. Thus, breast pain affects not only the individual sufferer but the patient's family and society at large.

Numerous nonpharmacologic methods have been promoted to ameliorate cyclic breast pain. These have included relaxation training, acupuncture, increasing soy or iodine intake, decreasing methylxanthine intake (coffee, tea, chocolate, cola beverages), promoting weight loss (low-fat diet), and taking diuretics (on the hypothesis that fluid retention is the basis of the pain), but scientific support for these methods is lacking or inconsistent. However, given the well-documented health benefits of caffeine avoidance and weight loss, as well as its low cost and few side effects, health care practitioners may want to suggest these measures, especially in those with symptomatic disease and moderate to heavy intake of caffeine. Anecdotal evidence exists for the use of ginseng tea, vitamin A, vitamin B complex, and a supportive brassiere, but the extent to which these methods are effective is unclear, and placebo controlled trials have not confirmed these results. Depending on severity, acetaminophen or nonsteroidal antiinflammatory drugs (NSAIDs) may be helpful. Additionally, topical NSAIDs have shown some effectiveness.

Several hormonal methods for treatment of cyclic breast pain have been advocated. No regimen is 100% effective, and some have a significant placebo response rate. Currently, danazol, an antigonadotropin, is considered the most efficacious (response rates near 75%–92%) and is the only medication approved by the Food and Drug Administration (FDA) for this problem. However, nearly 30% of patients experience the androgenic side effects of hirsutism, deepening voice, and amenorrhea, thereby limiting its widespread acceptance. Thus, it is not routinely recommended as a first-line therapy and should be reserved for patients whose pain is strongly affecting their lifestyle. Treatment should begin at 100 to 200 mg/day, with eventual tapering to lower dose or alternate-day administration. Many patients may not experience relief until 400 mg/day is given. Recommendations on the length of treatment vary from 2 to 6 months. Upon discontinuation, the dose should be tapered to prevent rapid withdrawal. As with all hormonal medication, discontinuation may cause resumption of symptoms.

Because doses less than 400 mg/day do not ensure inhibition of ovulation, an effective method of mechanical/barrier contraception (as it may interfere with oral contraception) should be given to avert possible teratogenic effects of the drug. Luteal phase-only danazol (200 mg/day) is an alternative treatment regimen that appears to be highly effective for the relief of premenstrual mastalgia. This regimen is associated with few side effects, but further study is necessary to ascertain whether such a regimen avoids potentially detrimental effects on lipid status.

Bromocriptine (Parlodel, Sandoz) is an ergot alkaloid that acts as a dopaminergic agonist on the hypothalamic-pituitary axis and has been effective for mastalgia in 40% to 88% of patients. The dosage of bromocriptine is similar to that discussed later in the section on nipple discharge. However, one third of patients experience side effects, and 30% relapse once treatment is discontinued. Side effects may be minimized with use of an incremental dosing regimen, with stepwise increases during a period of 2 weeks. Medication is usually discontinued after 2 months to review symptoms.

Evening primrose oil (EPO) (gamma-linolenic acid) is advocated by many as initial therapy for breast pain. At 3 to 4 g/day, EPO has been noted to have an overall useful response rate of 44% to 97% in some groups of women. Side effects were found in 2% to 12%, but all were insignificant. Yet a randomized double-blind trial comparing EPO and fish oil showed no difference in response rate; thus, data are conflicting. Gamma-linolenic acid is a precursor of the unsaturated fatty acids and is essential for the production of beneficial prostaglandins in the body. Several hypotheses have been espoused to explain the effects, including modification of membrane fluidity and lipid-associated receptors, changes in the inositol cycle, or diminishing response of the breasts to cyclic hormone activity. Yet, the delayed effectiveness (4 months) and the potential gastrointestinal and abortifacient side effects suggest caution in its use, especially in women desiring pregnancy. Moreover, physicians must be cognizant that herbal agents and nutritional supplements are not standardized or monitored for adulteration; thus, potential interaction with other medicinals must be considered.

Oral contraceptive pills (OCPs) may be a good option for patients seeking birth control in addition to relief of breast symptoms. Earlier studies (which used pills containing significantly higher progesterone contents) indicate that mastalgia was suppressed in 70% to 90% of patients who used the medication for 3 to 6 months. Maximum effects were noted after 2 years of use, but significant decreases in symptoms were noted after 1 year of use. Symptoms recur in up to 40% of patients when the high-dose OCP is discontinued. There is limited research on the effectiveness of the current low-dose formulations of OCPs in the treatment of mastalgia. However, in a recent study by Leonardi, 60% of patients with chronic mastalgia showed a reduction or improvement in symptoms while taking a low-dose formulation for 3 months. This study did not have a placebo group for comparison. The effectiveness appears to be due to the reduced ovarian estradiol production and the alteration of breast estrogen receptors caused by the progestin component of the pill. Although the older formulations appear to have some benefit, the new low-dose estrogen, patches, and the phased estrogen and progesterone dosage medications should be evaluated in a prospective trial to determine their effectiveness in the treatment of severe mastalgia. Topical, oral, and parenteral progestogens have also been studied for treatment of breast pain with variable results.

Tamoxifen (20 mg/day) has also been successful in the treatment of mastalgia. It has been heralded as the most effective and least toxic agent for the treatment of severe chronic breast pain. In one study comparing tamoxifen, danazol, and placebo, tamoxifen had the greatest pain relief score, with nearly 75% of those receiving tamoxifen having significant pain relief compared with 65% with danazol and 38% with placebo. Twelve months after treatment was discontinued, 53% of women who received tamoxifen were still free of symptoms, compared with 37% of the danazol-treated patients and none of the placebo-treated patients. Lower dosages (10 mg/day) appear to have significantly fewer side effects and to be as effective in pain control as the higher dosages (20 mg/day). The metabolic effects on bone, mineral metabolism, and lipid profile were insignificant after 3 months of treatment. The effectiveness appears to be due to a reduction in nuclear volume and mitotic activity of the epithelium even when administered only in the luteal phase. However, lack of evidence of the long-term consequences of treatment (particularly deep venous thrombosis and endometrial adenocarcinoma) portends caution in implementation of its use in benign breast disease. Toremifene citrate, a new member of the family of selective estrogen receptor modulators (SERMs), has been shown to have a better safety profile than tamoxifen, as well as efficacy in treatment of mastalgia in a double-blind, randomized, placebo controlled study. Adverse events were similar to that in the placebo group, except vaginal discharge was increased in this short-term study.

Vitamin E at dosages of 600 to 1,200 international units (IU)/day has been associated with a 41% response rate. However, lower dosages have usually been recommended. The mechanism of action is unknown but is proposed to include its potential to alter steroidal hormone production (dehydroepiandrosterone or progesterone), to correct abnormal serum cholesterol-lipoprotein distribution, and to function as an antioxidant (which appears to neutralize free radicals, thereby preventing cell damage and subsequent malignant transformation). Data are inconsistent regarding vitamin E and cardiovascular risk. Recent epidemiologic data indicate an inverse association between cardiovascular risk and vitamin E intake, but other studies indicate benefit for vitamin E in prevention of heart disease, cancer, and dementia. Two randomized controlled trials in women older than 45 years (using 600 IU/every other day) and in elderly patients with cardiovascular disease or diabetes (using 400 IU/day) have shown no benefit in prevention of major cardiovascular events or cancer. Germane to this discussion was the discovery that vitamin E slightly increased the risk of heart failure (5.8% compared with 4.2% hospitalizations for heart failure) at a dosage of 400 IU/day in elderly patients with chronic disease. Thus, researchers are now recommending that vitamin E doses be limited to less than 400 IU/day. Although myocardial infarction prevention is likely not a role for vitamin E, there is strong evidence from other studies that moderately high doses may have other important health roles, including delaying the onset of macular degeneration (a major cause of early blindness) and boosting the immune system in the elderly. Moreover, it is currently being studied by the National Institutes of Health (NIH) in 35,000 men in the Selenium and Vitamin E Cancer Prevention Trial (SELECT) for the delay/prevention of prostate cancer at dosages of 400 IU. Thus, determinative data is needed regarding the proper use and dosage of this method.

Dietary flaxseed has also resulted in significant reduction in symptoms of severe cyclic mastalgia in a 3-month, double-blind, randomized clinical trial. Women consuming a single daily muffin containing 25 g of ground flaxseed had improvement in symptoms. Flaxseed is a rich source of lignan precursors with antiestrogenic and antiproliferative effects.

Several investigations of depot gonadotropin-releasing hormone (GnRH) treatment used for 3 to 6 months reported improvements in clinical mastalgia that was recurrent or refractory to other hormonal drugs. Studies have shown a 53% complete response rate in premenopausal patients with clinical, histologic, and ultrasonographic evidence of fibrocystic mastopathy and mastalgia after treatment with GnRH analogs. A statistically significant partial response was observed in 45% of patients. A recent randomized placebo controlled multicenter study of goserelin revealed a 67% improvement in the mean breast pain score compared with 35% improvement in the placebo group. When administered long term, GnRH analogs result in marked reductions in blood levels of estradiol, progesterone, androgens, and prolactin. However, side effects of vaginal dryness, hot flushes, decreased libido, oily skin or hair, and decreased breast size are seen. Thus, this regimen should be reserved for patients with symptoms refractory to other forms of treatment. Potentially, goserelin could be used to induce a rapid relief of symptoms, with subsequent maintenance using alternative (lower side-effect profile) therapies. Further studies are required to determine the optimal length of treatment and the adverse effects on bone density and lipid metabolism generated by estrogen deficiency in premenopausal women. Decline in trabecular bone mineral density is as high as 6% within 6 months, although usually reversible. Estrogen or progestin "add-back" therapies and bisphosphonates have been used in the treatment of endometriosis with GnRH analogs to minimize vasomotor symptoms and loss of bone mineral density.

Noncyclic mastalgia is seen less often than the cyclic variety. This form of mastalgia is usually anatomic in nature rather than hormonal. Although rare, it can be a sign of cancer and thus always demands an extensive breast examination and possible follow-up or consultation. Common causes include trauma, pregnancy, mastitis, thrombophlebitis, benign tumors, macrocysts, sports injury, and postsurgical biopsy. However, frequently the cause is unknown. Many of the previously discussed regimens have shown efficacy in treatment of noncyclic mastalgia but at a lower rate.

Exercise may result in excessive breast motion, leading to breast pain. Because the female breast contains minimal intrinsic structural support, breast motion is often difficult to reduce. It is suggested that the primary anatomic support for the breast is the Cooper's ligaments, but their true functional properties are unknown. Studies indicate a sports bra provides superior support for the breast in relation to the amplitude of movement, deceleration forces on the breast, and perceived pain when compared with fashion bras, crop tops, and bare-breasted motion.

Nipple pain or itching may be caused by a physiologic result of anatomic growth (in pubescent girls), local skin dryness, eczema, or allergic reaction to clothing or clothes detergent. Symptomatic relief measures can include the use of antipruritic creams or ointments, such as calamine lotion, or other oils that enhance skin moisture, such as vitamin E oil. On the other hand, unilateral nipple itching must be viewed with suspicion so as not to miss the diagnosis of Paget disease. Paget disease often presents as a scaly pruritic nipple rash that is often mistakenly diagnosed as eczema. Nipple symptoms that do not resolve after 1 to 2 weeks of treatment require biopsy to rule out Paget disease. The skin presentation is often not associated with an underlying mass, so a heightened suspicion must always be present (Fig. 41.8).

Nonbreast sources that mimic breast pain include costochondritis, pleuritis, muscle pain including fibromyalgia,

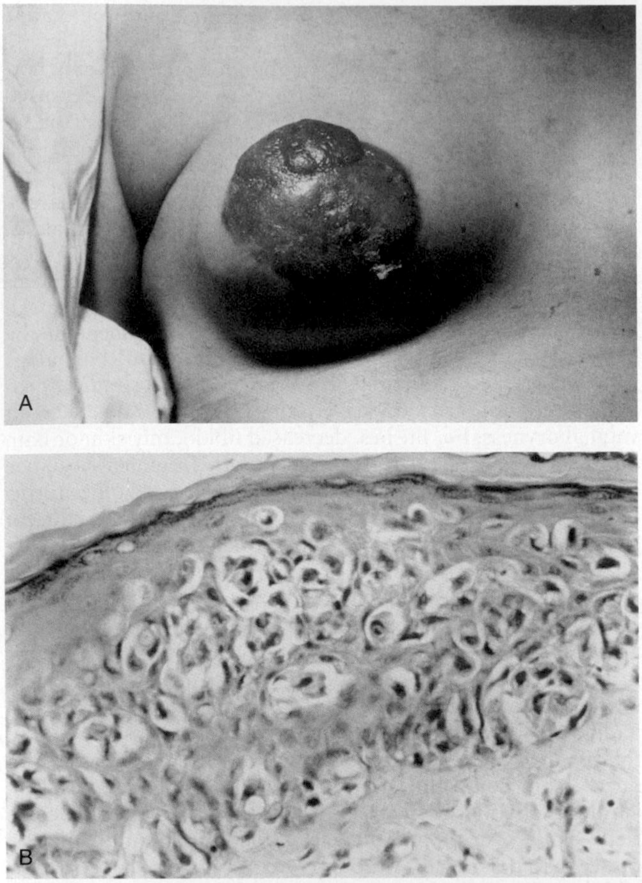

FIGURE 41.8. Paget disease. A: Right breast showing an extensive area of erythema with a nodular surface suggesting Paget disease. B: Skin biopsy specimen from a patient with Paget disease shows intraepidermal collections of anaplastic cells (Paget cells) arranged singly and in microclusters. (Courtesy of Bhagirath Majmudar, MD, Emory University School of Medicine, Atlanta, GA.)

Tietze syndrome, fractured rib, cervical radiculopathy, angina, cholecystitis or cholelithiasis, hiatal hernia, and peptic ulcer disease.

Nipple Discharge

Any breast symptom has the potential for creating an enormous amount of anxiety for patients. Nipple discharge is the third most common reason for women to consult their physicians regarding a breast problem and is responsible for 7% of breast operations. Reports of nipple discharge not only account for 3% to 6% of office visits for women with breast symptoms, but also occur in 10% to 50% of women with benign breast disease and in 10% to 15% of women with breast cancer.

Almost one half of women in their reproductive years can manually *express* one or more drops of nonpathologic liquid from the breast; conversely, *spontaneous* discharge from the nipples is uncommon. The practice of squeezing the nipple either during breast self-examination (BSE), clinical breast examination (CBE), or sexual and physical activity can elicit fluid from women of all ages and is thus divisive. This outcome is the basis for suggesting that one should not attempt to elicit nipple discharge during an examination of an asymptomatic patient because pathologic discharge is likely to occur spontaneously without nipple manipulation. However, if nipple discharge is a symptom, the breast examination must include "milking" of the breast toward the nipple to delineate the exact ductal source of the problem.

Galactorrhea

Secretions from the breast may be divided into milky (galactorrhea) and nonmilky discharge with physiologic and pathologic etiologies in each category. Other investigators classify secretion from the nipples according to color, cellularity, and biology. Galactorrhea, which is the nonpuerperal secretion of breast milk, must be separated from other types of nipple discharge. This may be done by viewing a sample, under low-power magnification, for multiple fat droplets of various sizes. If the secretion does not contain fat droplets, it is not (by definition) galactorrhea and must be evaluated by other criteria. Galactorrhea usually results in bilateral nipple discharge from multiple ducts and is unassociated with a mass. On the contrary, pathologic sources of nipple discharge may be characterized by unilateral discharge from a single duct with an associated mass in some cases. Also, nipple discharge in women older than 50 years is of concern. Pathologic sources of galactorrhea include medications, hypothalamic lesions or dysfunction, thyroid disorders, Forbes-Albright syndrome, chest lesion (chest trauma, burns, herpes zoster, lung cancer), renal disease, pituitary prolactin-secreting tumors, and nonpituitary prolactin-producing tumors (lung, kidney, craniopharyngioma).

Although many hormones are involved in normal lactation and galactorrhea, prolactin is the most significant. Prolactin was isolated in 1971 and is secreted by the anterior pituitary, the chorion of pregnancy, and by decidual and endometrial tissue. Prolactin (like luteinizing hormone) is secreted in a pulsatile fashion throughout the day with a circadian rhythm. Normal values generally range between 0 and 20 ng/mL.

The most common cause of physiologic nipple discharge is pregnancy, when prolactin values increase to 100 to 200 ng/mL as early as the 10th week of gestation. Lactation does not occur until after delivery because the peripheral action of prolactin is inhibited by estrogen and progesterone. During the process of suckling, prolactin increases to 300 to 600 ng/mL. After 6 months postpartum, there is no longer an increase from baseline associated with suckling. Therefore, amenorrhea, galactorrhea, or hyperprolactinemia more than 6 months after delivery is not physiologic. Any duration of galactorrhea demands evaluation in a nulliparous woman and, if at least 12 months have elapsed since the last pregnancy or weaning, in a parous woman.

The differential diagnosis of galactorrhea (excluding physiologic lactation) is a complex clinical challenge resulting from multiple factors involved in the control of prolactin release. A thorough and detailed history and physical examination are necessary to discern the cause. Prolactin itself, PIF, and PRFs are the major substances involved in prolactin homeostasis. Thus, the pathologic cause of nipple discharge can be easily comprehended with an awareness of the release–inhibition pathway.

To be significant, a discharge should be spontaneous, persistent, and nonlactational. The most common source of galactorrhea is consumed medication; thus, a thorough review of the patient's medication list is an essential element of the initial evaluation. Tranquilizers and antidepressant medications block the dopamine receptor, whereas antihypertensive agents, such as reserpine and methyldopa (Aldomet), inhibit the synthesis of dopamine. Opiates (including heroin), amphetamines, marijuana, phenothiazines, and anesthesia suppress dopamine release. OCPs may lead to milk secretion via hypothalamic suppression from excessive estrogen. This may result in reduction of PIF and release of pituitary prolactin by direct stimulation of pituitary lactotrophs. In one study, about 40% of women taking low-dose OCPs had modest elevations of prolactin (20 to 40 ng/mL), although other research has yielded conflicting results.

Once medications and manual breast stimulation have been ruled out, the other sources of galactorrhea are less common. Stimulation of neurogenic reflexes results in hypothalamic reduction of PIF and hyperprolactinemia. This is the mechanism found to be operational with prolonged stimulation of the breast, thoracotomy scars, cervical spinal lesions, and herpes zoster. Hypothyroidism is the cause of hyperprolactinemia in 5% to 10% of cases. Hypothyroidism results in diminished circulating levels of thyroid hormone and consequently excess hypothalamic thyrotropin-releasing hormone (TRH). TRH acts as a PRF with resultant hyperprolactinemia. Because prolactin is predominantly excreted or cleared by the kidney, chronic renal failure results in hyperprolactinemia in 25% of affected patients. Lastly, Chiari-Frommel and Forbes-Albright syndromes result in amenorrhea after pregnancy and galactorrhea secondary to a pituitary tumor.

Hyperprolactinemia with normal thyroid and renal function studies, as well as a normal chest and breast examination, may indicate a pituitary or hypothalamic problem. Prolactin-producing tumors, such as microadenomas and macroadenomas, account for a small percentage of cases. Evaluation of visual fields and a neurologic examination may be necessary. Imaging studies of the sella turcica, pituitary gland, and hypothalamic area are helpful to delineate problems. Previous routine use of the coned-down view of the sella turcica has been surpassed by magnetic resonance imaging (MRI) and computed axial tomographic (CT) at some institutions. MRI provides better resolution, detects smaller lesions, and does not use radiation; however, it is much more costly than the sella turcica study. If the prolactin level is greater than 60 ng/mL, an imaging study should always be performed. However, with only mild elevation of the prolactin level (20 to 60 ng/mL), some investigators advise that imaging is unwarranted if there is more than a threefold (i.e., 200%) increase in prolactin after a TRH stimulation test. The reliability of this test is not supported in all circles; thus, many recommend a CT scan or MRI study for all patients who have persistently elevated prolactin levels.

Treatment of microadenomas (smaller than 1 cm) and macroadenomas (larger than 1 cm in diameter) is controversial. Depending on several factors, investigators promote surveillance, bromocriptine, or transsphenoidal resection. Prolactin-producing microadenomas rarely progress to macroadenoma size. Most are exceedingly slow growing or stable, which accounts for the recommendation for surveillance in most cases. Bromocriptine shrinks tumors and can prevent growth, although complete elimination of the tumor does not usually occur. Discontinuation of the drug usually leads to rapid regrowth. Transsphenoidal microsurgery is a safe procedure, but there is a high rate of recurrence.

Positive cytology is helpful in diagnosis, but negative cytology should not delay further evaluation. Discharge cultures may be useful as duct ectasia commonly is associated with *Enterococcus,* anaerobic *Streptococcus, Staphylococcus aureus,* and *Bacteroides* species; however, whether infection is the primary cause or a secondary supercontamination is unknown. If results of all tests are negative except for an elevated prolactin level, a provisional diagnosis of a dysfunction of the hypothalamus can be made. Small pituitary tumors may be missed; accordingly, a prolactin level should be obtained every 6 months. Repeat imaging, visual field, and neurologic examinations should be performed if an increase in the prolactin level is noted. However, a tumor may increase without a concomitant rise in the prolactin level.

If galactorrhea persists despite a normal prolactin level, normal examination, and negative imaging studies, the condition is called *idiopathic galactorrhea.* This may be caused by excessive sensitivity of the breasts to normal levels of circulating prolactin, intermittent elevations of prolactin, excess sleep-induced prolactin secretion, or elevated biologically active prolactin, which is not immunoreactive or detectable by current methods. Although androgens, danazol, and combined OCPs have been used for this purpose, the effectiveness of these drugs has been limited. The most common treatment for galactorrhea has been bromocriptine (Parlodel), a dopamine agonist. This drug has received negative publicity because there is an increased risk of hypertensive crises and strokes in postpartal women who use the medication. However, its use in women who are not recently pregnant or lactating continues to be recommended. Treatment begins with 1.25 mg orally twice daily and is increased to 2.5 mg orally twice daily once the patient is able to tolerate the side effects. Primary side effects include nausea and hypotension, which can be alleviated by administering the medication vaginally. Typical use of bromocriptine is for 2 years, followed by a period of cessation to determine whether symptoms return. It is prudent for the practitioner who prescribes bromocriptine to be aware of any government, manufacturer, or health advocate updates on the use of this drug.

Nonmilky Nipple Discharge

Nonmilky nipple discharge is often divided into bloody and nonbloody categories (with physiologic and pathologic sources in each). Tests such as hemoccult or urine dipstick may be helpful to discover occult blood in the secreted fluid, but results should be scrutinized in the face of severe inflammation, which may lead to false-positive results. Additionally, although breast cancer presents as nipple discharge in 5% to 15% of cases, only 2% to 3% of *bloody* nipple discharges are associated with a malignancy. Breast cancer may also be associated with a watery or serous discharge; hence, no single piece of information can lead to a definitive diagnosis.

Physiologic causes of nonmilky, nonbloody nipple discharge include manual stimulation and poorly fitting brassiere as described earlier. Common causes of pathologic bloody nipple discharge include duct ectasia, mastitis, and intraductal papilloma (IDP).

Duct ectasia may present with a bloody nipple discharge, although more commonly a multicolored discharge is seen. Duct ectasia, without an associated mass, generally does not require more than symptomatic treatment, emphasizing gentle washing and application of moist packs. However, surgery may be appropriate in the presence of a mass, serosanguineous discharge, or excessive discomfort.

Mastitis, eczema, periareolar abscesses, and insect bites may present with purulent nipple discharge. Mastitis is discussed earlier under "Inflammation."

IDP is the most common cause of bloody nipple discharge and may also be associated with nipple retraction. It usually presents as a small, solitary, nonmalignant papillary growth of the dilated portion of the lactiferous duct, and clinically is rarely more than 1 cm in diameter. Although it is usually not cancerous, hyperplastic changes may be associated; thus, an IDP should be treated by excision through a circumareolar incision to rule out a malignancy. The surgical significance of nipple discharge rests on its frequency of association with cancer or precancerous mastopathy.

Bloody nipple discharge may be seen during the third trimester of pregnancy and while breast feeding is becoming established. It typically subsides within 2 months. Evaluation with cytology is often unproductive. However, discharge lasting more than 2 months, associated with a mass, deriving from a single duct, or in older women requires more definitive evaluation. Moreover, unilateral or bilateral bloody nipple discharge may be elicited immediately after pregnancy in the absence of significant breast pathology. The phenomenon is likely due to the development of delicate, easily traumatized capillary networks within the ducts. If a breast mass is not found by physical examination or sonography, regular follow-up should be continued because the condition usually disappears shortly after delivery. If a mass is present, FNA or CNB should be performed.

Physical examination, mammography, or galactography and sonography may be used to delineate the exact nature, location, and extent of the lesion preoperatively. Galactography involves cannulation of the discharge-producing duct with a small catheter or needle and injection of a water-soluble contrast agent in the duct. Ductal-orientated sonography uses modern high-resolution techniques to visualize the mammary ducts in detail. These procedures may be complementary in that cases of ductal abnormalities have been missed by sonography yet visualized by galactography. However, researchers caution that modern galactography has a high false-negative rate, so it does not reliably exclude intraductal pathology and is, therefore, not a substitute for surgery in patients with pathologic discharge. Ultrasound may be used in pregnancy to delineate a mass. However, if there is a high suspicion for cancer, a shielded mammogram should be ordered.

Fiberoptic ductoscopy is an emerging technique allowing direct visualization of the ductal system of the breast through nipple orifice exploration. When this procedure was applied to women with nipple discharge, an 83% positive predictive value was noted. The positive predictive value was increased to 86% with the addition of ductal washings to obtain exfoliated cells for evaluation at the time of the ductoscopy. MRI has also been shown to be of diagnostic value, but it is not as informative as regular galactography. Both modalities may offer safe alternatives to galactography in guiding subsequent breast surgery in the treatment of nipple discharge.

If imaging studies were unable to preoperatively identify the specific ductal source of nipple discharge, surgical exploration may be required. Skin hooks are used to lift the skin flaps for easier visualization and exploration. The affected duct is identified and excised. Hemostasis and closure techniques are similar to those used with excisional breast biopsies.

Papanicolaou and associates advocated cytologic analysis of breast secretions. Floria and associates concur, finding cytologic analysis in addition to galactography useful in identifying minimal breast cancer and in detecting premalignant lesions such as papillomatosis in patients with a nipple discharge but without a breast lump. Immunologic tests may also be performed on secreted fluid to detect high levels of carcinoembryonic antigen, indicating a latent malignancy. Conversely, Leis reported a false-negative rate for cytologic evaluation to be 16.4%. Because of the high false-negative rate, evaluation of a suspicious nipple discharge must continue despite negative cytology results.

Breast carcinoma and precancerous changes are thought to begin in the lining of the milk duct or terminal duct lobular unit, yet, until recently, we have not had direct access to this area for pathologic correlation other than by blindly removing tissue by core biopsy or FNA. Ductal lavage is a minimally invasive method of collecting ductal epithelial cells for cytologic evaluation currently under investigation at several institutions. In a clinical trial of 507 high-risk women, cells collected through ductal lavage were shown to detect the presence of precancerous and cancerous changes in 20% of the women. The presence of these changes correlated with a fivefold to 18-fold increase in the risk of developing breast cancer, depending on family history and the patient's risk of breast cancer development as determined by the Gail model. However, sensitivity in detection of invasive and *in situ* breast carcinoma is low and thus the initial fervor over this procedure is waning except when used for proteomic analysis. Ductal lavage may not only be a helpful adjunct to determine which high-risk women require closer, more active management, but it may also be used to track cell status in particular ducts over time. Additionally, proteomic analysis of ductal lavage fluid may provide answers regarding tumor markers or patient response to treatments. Because breast cancer is known to develop over time and to be present nearly 6 years before earliest detection on mammography, availability of this technique is surmised to provide practitioners with a tool to detect precancerous and cancerous breast cells *before* they become palpable cancers that can be imaged, thus allowing closer surveillance, surgical intervention, or chemoprevention. Investigational protocol eligibility often includes (i) women with a prior history of breast cancer; (ii) women at high risk for development of breast cancer as defined by Gail Index score, family history, BRCA mutation, or atypical hyperplasia; and (iii) those with persistent or bloody nipple discharge. Incorporation of ductal lavage into an examination of nipple discharge should not replace other standard evaluations. In studies combining CBE, mammography, MRI, and ductal lavage, ductal lavage was noted to detect atypia in an individual with a normal MRI and mammogram. However, additional research is needed to determine the role, sensitivity, and specificity of this method. Additionally, the significance of detection of high-risk lesions in decreasing breast cancer morbidity must be ascertained.

Ductal lavage involves placing a special suction cup over the nipple and applying negative pressure to collect the nipple aspirate fluid (NAF) (Fig. 41.9). A microcatheter is then inserted through the nipple orifice, into the identified fluid-yielding ducts. After saline infusion, the ductal fluid is withdrawn and sent for cytologic analysis. In preliminary trials, 79% of subjects yielded NAF, although this rate may be influenced by race and age, in that women older than 50 years, African American, Mexican American, and Asian women typically yielded less NAF. The phase of the menstrual cycle, a history of pregnancy, or use of OCPs did not significantly affect the availability of NAF. Hormone replacement therapy (HRT) in postmenopausal women tended to increase the amount of NAF obtained.

DIAGNOSIS

Breast cancer accounts for 30% of all cancers in women and 15% of deaths from cancer. Although mortality rates from breast cancer are continuing to decline, incidence rates among certain subgroups (Asian Pacific Islander women) are increasing. Gynecologists are in a crucial position for coordination of ongoing medical care for patients with breast problems. Breast symptoms are appropriately evaluated by a breast-oriented history, physical examination, cytology studies, and imaging techniques. If the diagnosis is in doubt, open surgical biopsy provides the definitive histologic diagnosis.

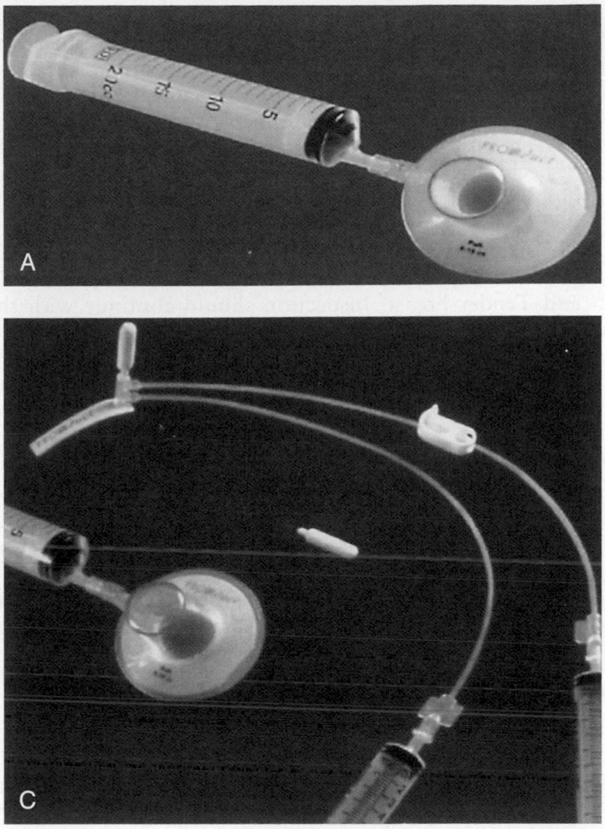

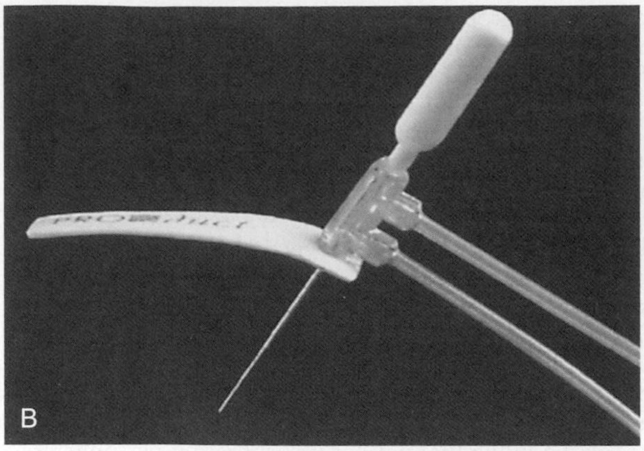

FIGURE 41.9. A: Pro-Duct breast aspirator. B: Breast micro-catheter. C: Devices used in ductal lavage.

History

A thorough history is a vital aspect of the initial evaluation. However, breast cancer cannot be excluded by any single fact within the patient's history; rather, the history focuses attention on additional information. The practitioner should obtain detailed information about the patient's symptom and other pertinent related positive and negative symptoms. The information necessary to assess breast health includes age, menstrual, gynecologic, sexual, reproductive, and lactation history, and any family history of breast or ovarian disorders (including age at onset/diagnosis). Because of recent advances in genetic etiologies, be sure to include cancer assessment of the maternal *and* paternal family history. In addition, a total body review of systems (e.g., headache, blurred vision for macroadenomas) should be focused on the patient's symptom. Of vital importance are the following:

- Menopause status
- Timing and specific nature of symptoms
- Cyclic changes
- Onset, duration, and growth pattern of any masses
- Presence of pain
- Attempted and successful relief measures
- Alleviating and aggravating factors
- Use of HRT or OCPs
- Presence or absence of risk factors for breast cancer

All previous breast diagnostic and surgical procedures should be documented. Past medical and surgical history, as well as current medications and social history (including smoking, alcohol, and educational level), should also be reviewed. Because most breast symptoms in reproductive-aged women are due to a benign cause, reassurance may be an important aspect in reducing anxiety. However, the practitioner should notify the patient of any concerns regarding the history and examination to ensure that the patient understands the significance of follow-up and does not misconstrue the practitioner's reassurance to mean the diagnostic workup is completed.

Self-Breast Examination

Mammography remains the gold standard for early detection of breast carcinoma, but this technique it is not 100% effective. CBE and BSE are important facets of a breast screening program. Controversy exists regarding the utility of routine BSE for increasing the rate of breast cancer detection. Studies yield conflicting results. The research has been hampered by differing BSE education strategies, schedules of performance, and control groups. Although the results are often incongruous, some authors have found a 34% reduction in nodal involvement and increased survival in women performing BSE compared with women who do not. In addition, 70% to 90% of masses are first detected by the women themselves. In a randomized trial in Russia, more cancers were found in the instruction group than in the control group (RR 1.24, 95% CI 1.09–1.41), whereas this was not the case in Shanghai. Conversely, a study from Shanghai of more than 250,000 women, who were randomized to no instruction or to intensive BSE instruction, failed to demonstrate any difference in the number of cancers detected or in the stage or size at which they were found (RR 0.97, 95% CI 0.88–1.06). No reduction in mortality was seen, but more than twice as many benign lesions were found in the self-examination group. Yet, these trials review BSE *instruction*, not the *practice* of BSE, as this information could not be reliably obtained from self-report. Accordingly, promotion of BSE as a single screening method is often not recommended. These findings require assessment, but to negate BSE as an important component of overall personal health care seems inappropriate if there is any possibility that it will affect the survival rate in women. In breast disease, wherein early detection is so clearly related to improved survival, the value of these relatively simple, economical, and minimally inconvenient techniques cannot be overemphasized. With this in mind, the American College of Obstetricians and Gynecologists (ACOG) and the ACS continue to recommend BSE be performed monthly beginning at age 20.

Clearly, discussion of BSE must include the benefits and limitations for the individual patient incorporating personal risk factors. Effective instruction of patients in the technique of BSE incorporates description of the procedure while the patient views the health care provider's performance of the examination. Additionally, having the patient reiterate her understanding of what has been taught and then demonstrating her mastery of the technique using manufactured breast models further solidifies compliance. The patient should understand the significance of breast inspection in various positions as well as the utility of breast palpation in the standing as well as supine positions. The circular method of breast palpation is routinely the easiest to master, although for patients with pendulous breasts, positional changes to ensure positioning of the breast tissue on the chest wall must be emphasized. The best time to perform the examination is usually the week after the menses, although menopausal women should pick a convenient time of the month, such as their birth date or the first of each month. After hysterectomy, patients with continued estrogenic support of the ovaries should observe for breast fullness or tenderness. Breast examination should then be performed 7 to 10 days after maximal breast symptoms.

Clinical Breast Examination

As with BSE, the utility of routine CBE in asymptomatic women has been questioned. Query into its reliability and efficacy has been propagated; however, there is greater scientific support for CBE. The Canadian Health Insurance Plan noted a 70% reduction in mortality from breast cancer as a result of physical examination. Although inferior to mammography, CBE has a sensitivity of 57% to 70% in detecting breast cancer. In addition, the ACS recommends annual CBE of women age 40 years and older and CBE every 3 years for women ages 20 to 39. Strategies to improve a practitioner's ability to detect a mass include increasing the time devoted to the examination, using a technique with variable degrees of pressure, and developing a systematic, consistent search mode. The size of the lesion, of course, is also correlated with the practitioner's ability to detect the mass.

To capture any benefit from early detection, CBE should be a routine part of the examination of gynecologic and obstetrics patients. Obstetrician/gynecologists should not abdicate their responsibilities by relying on previous examinations performed by other specialists. The practitioner must also be concerned with protecting himself or herself from future lawsuits that are due to errors of omission.

At least 3 to 5 minutes should be devoted to the CBE to improve mass detection. As with the BSE, CBE should be performed approximately 1 week after the end of the menstrual cycle to diminish the impact of luteal phase breast vascular or lymph congestion, which can obscure mass detection. Each portion of the breast examination should be performed with the patient in both the sitting and supine positions because positional changes often expose a lesion that was otherwise masked by the patient's normal anatomic variations.

The initial part of the examination should focus on breast inspection, viewing for symmetry, skin retraction, rashes, and nipple retraction or deviation (Fig. 41.10). Use of the acronym BREAST may assist providers in remembering critical physical signs associated with advanced breast cancer, including **B**reast mass, **R**etraction, **E**dema, **A**xillary mass, **S**caly nipple, and **T**ender breast. Inspection should continue with the patient's arms raised overhead. Not only does this allow visualization of the lateral aspects of the breast (which are often obscured by excess arm girth), but also provides a complete view of the skin on the undersurface of the breast (inframammary ridge). Again, asymmetry and skin changes are sought. Inspection continues with placing the patient's hands behind her head with elbows retracted or placing her hands on her hips while contracting the pectoralis muscles. In patients with rheumatoid arthritis or other conditions preventing pressure on the hip joint, other more comfortable options may be used. One may have the patient either grasp her fingertips at a level near the waistline while pulling laterally or press her palms together while extended above the head. Because the breast lies on the pectoralis muscle and Cooper's ligaments are attached to the muscle and the skin, tension on the muscle accentuates carcinoma invading these structures. The clinician should always survey the breast for nipple retraction or inversion, which can result from carcinomatous invasion of the tissue beneath the nipple (Fig. 41.11). Nipple inversion is significant only when developed secondarily and unilaterally. If gentle manual eversion may be accomplished, the inversion is generally a normal variation.

Another position for breast inspection that is especially helpful in women with pendulous breasts is to have the woman lean forward while placing her hands on the practitioner's shoulders. Palpation of the breast in this position (while the breast tissue is away from the chest wall) is helpful to differentiate *chest wall* pain from true *breast* pain.

Next, the axilla is evaluated for masses. To allow proper assessment of the axilla for all positions, the patient's shoulder girdle must be relaxed.

Inspection of the breast is followed by palpation. The patient should be properly gowned, with only the area being examined exposed. The patient must be positioned (by tilting her hips and torso) to allow the portion of the breast tissue being examined to lie directly upon the chest wall. For patients with pendulous breasts, this may require three to four positional changes for each breast. The pads of the fingers (and not the finger tips) are the most sensitive and should be used in examination. Three circular motions are made with three levels of pressure (superficial, medium, and firm) on each 1-cm square area of the breast. Not only does this improve mass detection but it also prevents masking a mass through excessive pressure.

To adequately evaluate the axilla in the supine position, the arm should be extended at a 90-degree angle from the chest wall. This maneuver relaxes the area to be examined for a more thorough evaluation. Next, the patient should be placed in a comfortable supine position with her arm—on the same side as the breast being examined—raised above her head to evenly distribute the breast over the chest wall, thereby making its deeper regions accessible. The circular pattern is the most frequently used; however, the "vertical-strip" pattern is espoused as the most sensitive technique and thus endorsed by the Centers for Disease Control and Prevention and the ACS. Oregon

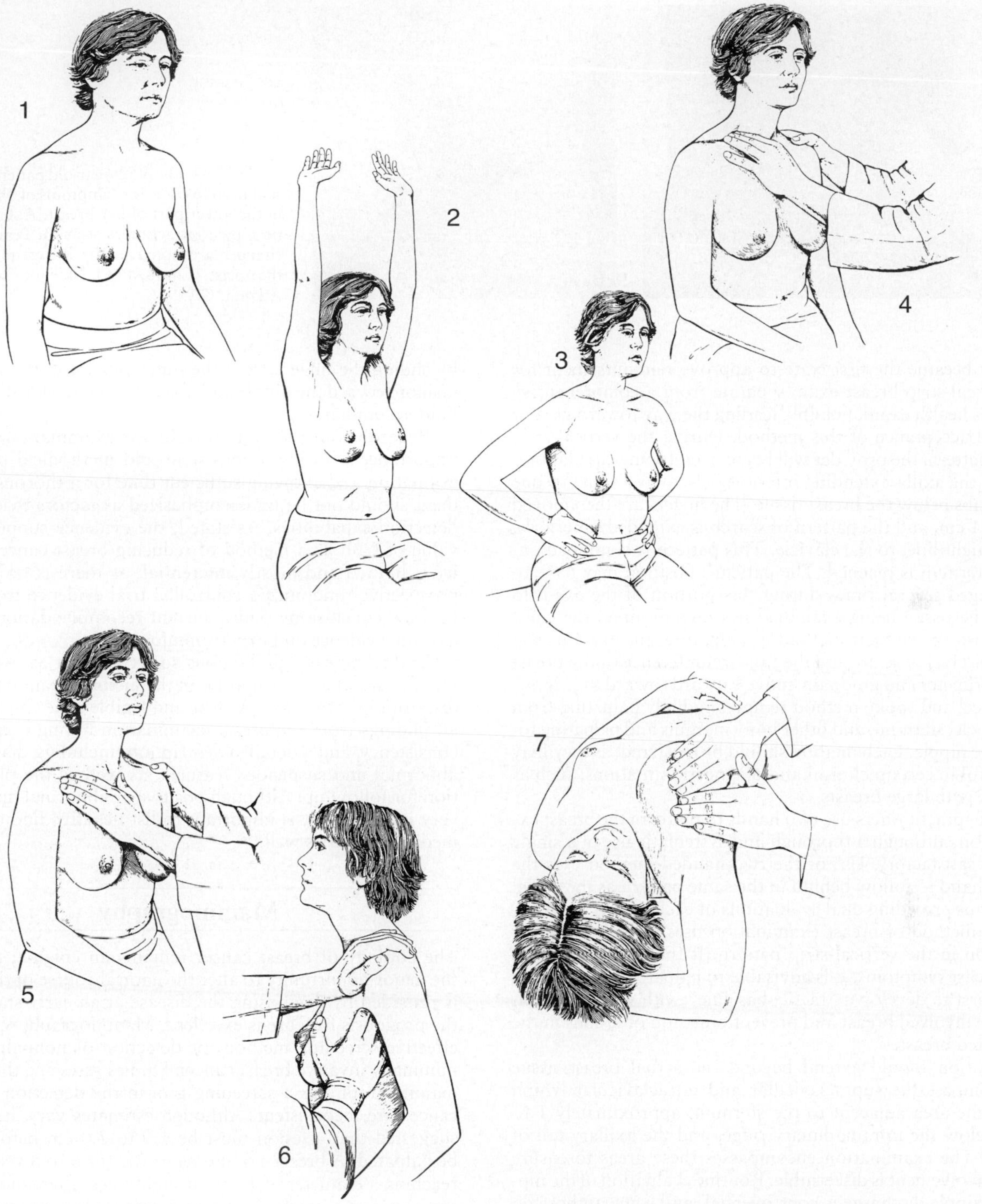

FIGURE 41.10. *(1)* Examination of the breasts begins with inspection. The patient is disrobed to the waist and comfortably seated facing the examiner. Asymmetry, prominent veins, and skin changes may be signs of disease. (*2*) The patient raises her arms above her head, thereby altering the position of the breasts. Immobility or abnormal cutaneous attachments may become evident. (*3*) Inward pressure on the hips tenses the pectoralis major muscle. Abnormal attachments to its overlying fascia and skin can produce retraction or dimpling of the skin. (*4*) Supraclavicular lymph nodes are examined by palpation. (*5*) The deltopectoral triangle is palpated for evidence of infraclavicular nodal enlargement. (*6*) Each axilla is examined for nodal enlargement. Proper placement of the examiner's hands and of the patient's arm is important. (*7*) Thorough palpatory examination of the entire breast for masses is performed with the patient in the supine position. A fine rotational movement of the hands is useful to appreciate the consistency of the underlying tissues. The examiner should check for nipple discharge by compressing the ducts in a clockwise manner toward the nipple. (From Scott JR, DiSaia PJ, Hammond CB, et al. *Danforth's obstetrics and gynecology,* 7th ed. Philadelphia: JB Lippincott, 1994:700.)

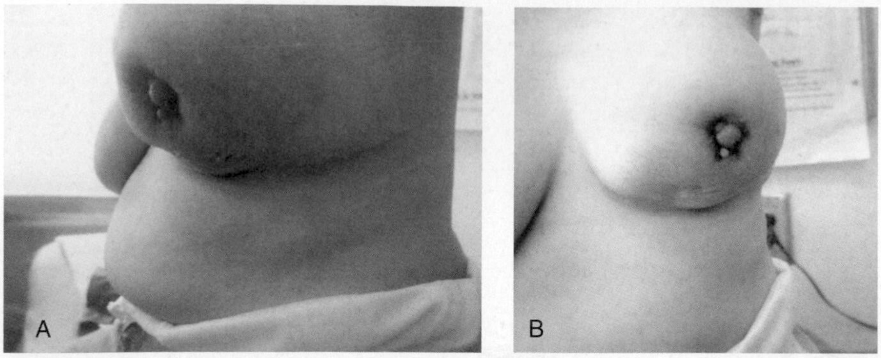

FIGURE 41.11. A 52-year-old patient with presentation to clinic for symptoms of "hardening" in the lower part of her breast. **A:** Characteristic nipple retraction is seen. **B:** Peau d'orange changes are noted in the lower quadrants of the breast. (Courtesy of Jacqueline Foster, PA-C, Atlanta, GA.)

recently became the first state to approve reimbursement for the vertical-strip breast exam separate from a comprehensive women's health exam, possibly leading the way toward greater national acceptance of this method. During the vertical-strip search pattern, the provider will begin overlapping circular motions in the axilla extending inferiorly (1 cm at a time) to one to two ribs below the breast tissue. The fingers are then moved inward 1 cm, and the pattern of search is extended superiorly, in a straight line, to the clavicle. This pattern is continued until the sternum is reached. The patient's position may have to be changed several times during this portion of the exam to assure the tissue being examined lies directly upon the chest wall. With the circular method of palpation, the examination proceeds clockwise around the full circumference of the breast at its perimeter and gradually moves inward toward the nipple. The wheel and spoke method requires radially palpating from the clavicle, sternum, and other bony margins and palpating toward the nipple. Each method should be mastered, as they may be helpful in certain clinical and diagnostic situations, such as patients with large breasts.

Many practitioners use two hands to perform the breast examination, although a thorough and systematic use of a single hand is satisfactory. Use of the two-handed method uses the second hand to follow behind in the same pattern as the initial hand, thus providing dual evaluations of each area. The Mammocare method of breast examination uses a single hand for palpation in the vertical-strip pattern. If the patient presents with breast symptoms, it is advisable to palpate the unaffected breast first to develop a "tactile baseline" with which to compare the involved breast and prevent omission of lesions in the unaffected breast.

Palpation should extend beyond the actual breast tissue to encompass the supraclavicular and infraclavicular lymph nodes, the area adjacent to the sternum, approximately 1 to 2 cm below the inframammary ridge, and the axillary tail of Spence. The examination encompasses these areas to ensure nodal involvement is discernible. Routine evaluation of the nipple for nipple discharge is controversial, and some authors do not recommend this as a routine portion of the breast examination in women without symptoms. It is well known that excessive breast manipulation can lead to a nipple discharge. If one does exclude this as a routine part of the examination, a *detailed* history should be obtained to rule out any nipple symptoms. Patients often have such symptoms but forget to relate this information to the practitioner, particularly if they have experienced the symptoms for an extended period of time. Squeezing the nipple may actually obstruct the ductal orifice and impede any discharge from coming to the surface. Using a milking technique improves the examiner's ability to elicit a nipple discharge. Each quadrant of the breast is "milked" by sliding the fingers from the outer quadrant in a clockwise fashion toward the nipple and documenting the location of any fluid accumulation.

Regardless of the pattern of breast examination used, the importance of using a consistent and methodical pattern of evaluation and allowing sufficient time for a thorough assessment should not be underemphasized as factors that increase detection capabilities. As stated, the evidence supporting the value of CBE as a method of reducing breast cancer mortality is limited and mostly inferential, as there is no definitive prospective randomized controlled trial evidence from which to draw conclusions. Thus, current recommendations rely on existing evidence and expert opinion.

In this increasingly litigious society, breast assessment demands careful documentation of the history, examination, and disposition of the case. A clear and legible note should record all findings from the breast examination noting texture, size, consistency, and a detailed description (including diagrams) of abnormal and suspicious features, as well as the plan of action for follow-up. Although positive or abnormal findings are very important, it is important to list negative findings in the medical record as well.

Mammography

The etiology of breast cancer remains an enigma; therefore, the major opportunity to alter the natural course of the disease is provided by diagnosing the disease at an early stage, when the prognosis for cure is excellent. Mammography is the most effective screening method for detection of nonpalpable and minimally invasive breast cancer. Studies assessing the value of mammography as a screening tool in the detection of breast cancer are inconsistent. Although estimates vary, it has been suggested that a lesion must be 1.0 to 2.0 cm before it may be palpated. A breast carcinoma grows for 6 to 8 years before reaching a diameter of 1 cm. In slightly less than another year, the carcinoma reaches 2 cm in diameter. It is estimated that, on the average, a mammogram detects a breast cancer 2 years before it is palpable.

Routinely, a false-negative rate of 10% to 15% is quoted; therefore, a normal mammographic examination does not rule out the presence of breast cancer (Table 41.3). Thus, a palpable mass requires further evaluation despite a "negative" mammographic examination. Dense parenchymal tissue is the principal cause of false-negative mammograms. Other sources of error include misjudging a well-circumscribed carcinoma for a benign mass, misconstruing malignant calcifications for benign aberrations, not recognizing the indirect signs of malignancy such as asymmetry, and faulty radiographic technique.

TABLE 41.3

REASONS FOR FALSE-NEGATIVE MAMMOGRAMS

Failure to image the region of interest
Poor image quality
Errors of perception
Breast cancer indistinguishable from normal breast tissue

Guidelines promulgated by the American College of Radiology Mammography Accreditation Program have significantly reduced this latter problem. In some studies, HRT reduced the sensitivity of mammographic screening and may undermine the capacity of population-based mammographic screening programs to achieve their potential mortality benefit. For instance, in one research paper, among women who were diagnosed with cancer in the 2-year mammography screening interval, HRT users were more likely to have a false-negative result than nonusers (OR, 1.60; 95% CI, 1.04–2.21). However, among women who did not have cancer diagnosed in the interval, HRT users were more likely to have a false-positive result (adjusted OR, 1.12; CI, 1.05–1.19).

It is important to forewarn patients that adequate breast compression is essential to improved radiographic technique and to deliver a high-quality mammogram. Compression holds the breast motionless, decreasing artifact; separates tissues to disclose small lesions; improves image quality by decreasing radiation scatter; and reduces the radiation dose by decreasing breast thickness.

Widespread use of this imaging test, in conjunction with improved treatment, may be responsible for the recent decline in number of deaths from breast cancer. Not only does mammographic imaging enable the detection of nonpalpable breast cancer, but early detection also permits breast conservation surgery (BCS). Moreover, it has been suggested that substantially greater reductions in mortality would have resulted if more rigorous screening guidelines were in place. These results have been achieved while maintaining acceptably low rates of recall for additional imaging after basic screening examination (10% for the initial prevalence screening and 5% for subsequent incidence screenings) as well as maintaining false-positive biopsy rates for nonpalpable lesions that are lower than those for lesions found at clinical examination. Positive predictive values for lesions for which biopsy is recommended on the basis of mammographic findings range from 25% for women in the fifth decade of life to 50% for women in the eighth decade of life, which are all within an acceptable range (Fig. 41.12).

Mammography serves multiple purposes in the evaluation of women's breast health. It is useful not only for screening but also in evaluating lesions identified by clinical symptoms (e.g., nipple discharge) or physical examination (e.g., a palpable mass or "suspicious" examination), called a *diagnostic mammogram.* Screening mammography is provided to an asymptomatic patient, is used as a baseline against which future mammograms can be compared, and may often be performed without the presence of a radiologist. On the other hand, a diagnostic mammogram is administered to a patient with symptoms or a breast mass. The diagnostic examination includes not only the craniocaudal and mediolateral view of the routine screening mammogram, but also may include additional views, as well as ultrasound and physical examination by the radiologist. Additionally, when a lesion is found in one breast, mammography is used to detect further lesions in the ipsilateral or contralateral breast, which ultimately may modify the treatment plan.

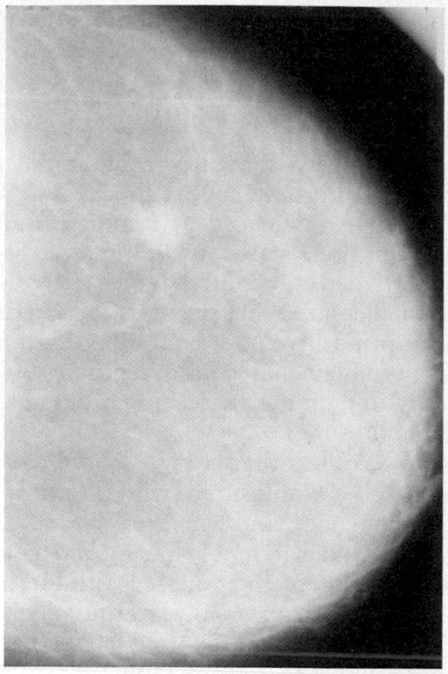

FIGURE 41.12. Mammogram of a 44-year-old woman with breast carcinoma in the upper quadrant. Characteristic features of spiculations interdigitating into the surrounding tissue and irregular margins are seen.

In detection of breast cancer, there are several mammographic characteristics of malignancy, which include the presence of a mass, architectural distortion, asymmetrical density, and microcalcifications. Malignant lesions generally display more of these pathognomonic mammographic appearances than do benign lesions, but benign lesions may have similar features. Calcification in the breast can be benign or malignant. Round, smooth calcium deposits of uniform size generally tend to be associated with benign processes, whereas branching and polymorphic calcifications suggest the possibility of malignancy. The presence of clusters of microcalcifications in a small geographic area is also a suspicious finding. Microcalcifications play an important role in the early detection of breast cancer. However, calcifications occur in fewer than half of nonpalpable cases, and fewer than half of these calcified lesions demonstrate the classic appearances suggestive of malignancy. The calcifications of FCCs often mimic those of malignancy, leading to unavoidable false-positive mammograms. Calcificlike deposits in the skin secondary to tattoos, deodorants, ointments, or sebaceous gland secretions can also be mistaken for malignancy. Therefore, clustered microcalcifications are a sensitive but not a specific sign of malignancy.

The radiation risks associated with x-ray mammography are considered negligible. Contemporary roentgenogram units, specifically designed for breast imaging, use the most advanced technology to obtain images of the highest quality with a considerable decrease in radiation dose to probably less than 0.2 to 0.3 rads (2–3 cGy). Information from the Breast Cancer Detection Demonstration Project, sponsored by the ACS and the National Cancer Institute (NCI), indicates an even lower average midbreast dose of 0.08 rads. To put radiation risk in perspective, data presented by the National Council on Radiation Protection illustrate that mammographic examination of

100,000 women at age 45 years would *theoretically* result in the eventual loss of one life.

Screening Guidelines

Mammography has been shown in randomized trials to reduce breast cancer mortality by as much as 25%. Survival from breast cancer is influenced by tumor size, degree of invasion, and lymph node status at the time of diagnosis. The advantage of early detection and diagnosis is reduced mortality because of smaller-sized cancers, more localized lesions with a lower percent of positive nodes, and increased feasibility of BCS. Clearly this fundamental tenet accentuates the importance of compliance with radiologic screening programs and knowledge of guidelines.

Women who have less than a high school education, who are a minority, who are uninsured, who do not speak English as their primary language, and who are socioeconomically disadvantaged are less likely to report having had a mammogram. According to data from the National Health Interview Survey, fewer than 60% of women age 50 years and older and 45% of women age 70 years and older reported having had a mammogram in the preceding 1 to 2 years. Only 38% of women aged 50 years and older with low income and 42% of those with less than a high school education had a recent mammogram. Clearly, efforts to increase screening should specifically target older women and socioeconomically disadvantaged women, who are at the highest risk for underutilization of mammograms.

Randomized controlled trials (RCTs) have demonstrated a decreased mortality rate in women who received mammography at age 50 to 69. However, a metaanalysis by Olsen and Gotzsche demonstrated no reduction of breast cancer mortality when incorporating only two of the existing RCTs of screening mammography—indicting that the then additional five trials had serious methodological flaws and excluded their results. Yet, a review specifically of the Health Insurance Plan of Greater New York (HIP) screening trials and both Canadian National Breast Screening Studies (CNBSS1 and CNBSS2) documented improved mortality in screen-detected cancers compared with those detected symptomatically. In the HIP trail, 76% of screen-detected cancers were stage I, compared with 51% of interval/incident cancers (cancers detected within less than 1 year or more than 1 year after the last negative screen) and 49% of cancers in the control (no screening mammography). Those unscreened and women who failed to attend their screenings had the highest percentage of stage III/IV cancers (14% and 22%, respectively). Likewise, in the CNBSS 1, 55% of screen-detected cancers, 40% of interval/incidence cancers, and 47% of cancers in the control group were stage I. In CNBSS 2, 62% of screen-detected cancers, 44% of interval/incident cancers, and 47% of cancers in the control group were state I. Although adjusted for lead-time bias, tumor sizes were smaller in the screening groups, and there were significantly higher proportions of negative lymph nodes among women with screen-detected cancers. The survival advantage seems to arise from the mammogram's tendency to detect less aggressive, more slow-growing, and thus less biologically lethal tumors than those discovered symptomatically. However, despite this benefit, fewer than 40%, even among this age group of women, had had a mammogram in the past year.

The controversy regarding screening in women younger than 50 years of age is multifold. Reduction of mortality rates as a result of screening is a subject of debate, the cost-effectiveness when compared with that in older women is unknown, and, finally, the frequency of screening intervals has become a point of disagreement among the committees that issue imaging guidelines. Authors have argued that mammograms performed in women younger than 50 years are not useful because younger women have more radiographically dense breast tissue that obscures abnormalities (Fig. 41.13). Some investigators have advocated yearly mammograms for all women 40 to 49 years old because breast cancer is often more aggressive and faster growing in younger women. The benefit of mammography in women age 40 to 49 years is less clear than for those age 50 and older. However, with mounting years of follow-up, evidence of a benefit for women in their 40s has increased, and studies show that regular mammograms reduce the death rate from breast cancer in this age group by about 17% to 23%. However, some trials with significant numbers still fail to show benefit in this age group. Nevertheless, NCI and the U.S. Preventive Services Task Force recommend screening with mammography beginning at age 40 in women of average risk for breast cancer. ACOG and the ACS continue to recommend offering screening mammography for women 40 to 49 years of age and annually for women older than 50 years. (Tables 41.4 and 41.5). Women who are at higher-than-average risk of breast cancer should seek expert medical advice about earlier screening and the frequency of screening (Table 41.6). Although there are insufficient data regarding women age

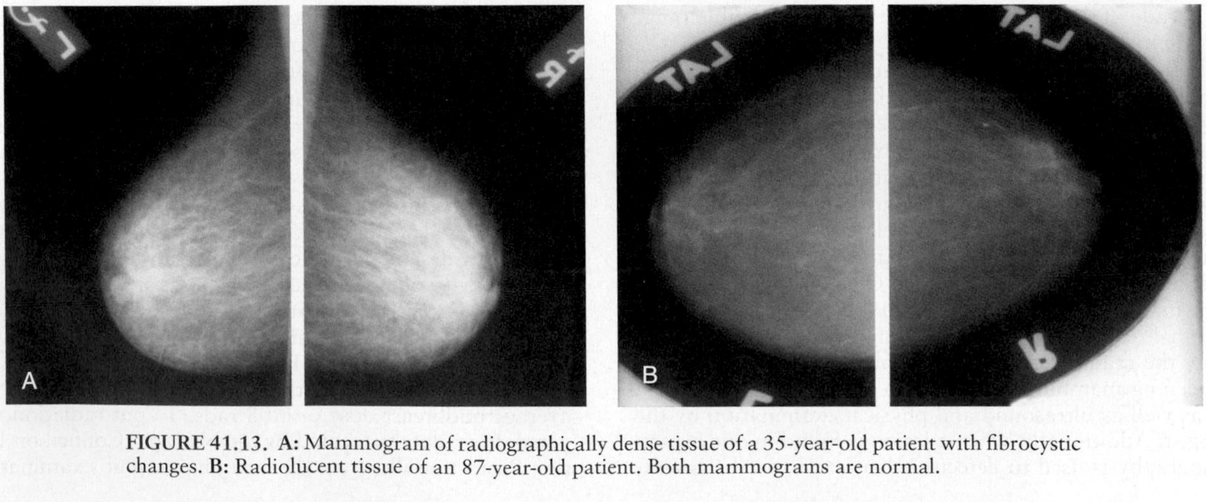

FIGURE 41.13. A: Mammogram of radiographically dense tissue of a 35-year-old patient with fibrocystic changes. **B:** Radiolucent tissue of an 87-year-old patient. Both mammograms are normal.

TABLE 41.4

AMERICAN COLLEGE OF OBSTETRICS AND GYNECOLOGY: BREAST CANCER SCREENING GUIDELINES, 2000

Average Risk (asymptomatic)
Age 20–39
BSE—monthly
CBE—yearly
Age 40–49
BSE—monthly
CBE—yearly
Mammography every 1–2 years[a]
Age 50 and over
BSE—monthly
CBE—yearly
Mammography—yearly

[a]Unless mammographic or physical findings suggest more frequent evaluation.
BSE, breast self-examination; CBE, clinical breast examination.
Modified from the American College of Obstetricians and Gynecologists. *Primary and preventive care: periodic assessments.* ACOG Committee Opinion 246. Washington, DC: ACOG; 2000.

TABLE 41.5

AMERICAN CANCER SOCIETY GUIDELINES FOR EARLY BREAST CANCER DETECTION, 2003

Average Risk (asymptomatic)
Age 20–40
BSE—monthly (optional)
CBE every 1–3 years
Age older than 40
BSE—monthly (optional)
CBE annual or biannual
Mammography annually

BSE, breast self-examination; CBE, clinical breast examination.
Modified from Smith RA, Saslow D, Sawyer KA, et al. American Cancer Society guidelines for breast cancer screening: update 2003. *CA Cancer J Clin* 2003;53(3):141.

TABLE 41.6

BREAST CANCER SURVEILLANCE FOR WOMEN WITH BRCA1 AND BRCA2

Age 18–20
BSE—monthly
Beginning between 20 and 35 years
CBE semiannually
Beginning between 25 and 35 years
Mammography annually

BSE, breast self-examination; CBE, clinical breast examination.
Modified from The NCCN 2003 genetic/familial high-risk assessment clinical practice guidelines in oncology, version 1, 2003. Available at: http://www.nccn.org. Accessed October 2004.

70 years and older, the incidence of breast cancer does increase with age. Therefore, ACOG continues to recommend annual screening in this age group.

In general, clinicians should have a detailed conversation regarding the present knowledge and the risks and benefits of screening for each individual woman.

Digital Mammography

Many exciting developments are occurring in breast imaging. Although mammography still remains the gold standard for breast cancer screening and diagnosis, it often cannot differentiate benign from malignant disease and is less accurate in patients with dense glandular breasts, with diffuse involvement of the breast with tumor, and in those taking HRT. Ten percent to 20% of breast cancers detectable by physical examination are not visible radiographically. Furthermore, of the women who are referred for biopsy based on mammographic findings, only 20% to 40% of lesions actually prove to be malignant. Clearly, there is room for improvement in both breast cancer detection and lesion characterization.

Digital mammography (DM) is a rapidly evolving technology offering improved efficiency of absorption of x-ray photons, as well as greater contrast resolution, especially in dense breast tissue. Systems are based on the absorption of x-rays by a phosphor material with subsequent conversion of the absorbed energy to electronic charge. The charge signal is then digitized and stored as a matrix in computer memory to represent the image.

The recently reported DMIST trial (Digital Mammographic Imaging Screening Trial) evaluated 49,528 asymptomatic women in the United States and Canada with both digital and film mammography. The overall diagnostic accuracy of digital and film mammography was similar for screen detection of breast cancer, but DM was more accurate in women younger than age 50 years, women with radiographically dense breasts, and pre- or perimenopausal women. Additional data indicate digital systems may be superior to conventional film-screen mammography in detection of microcalcifications, which are the earliest evidence of minimal breast cancer. Other studies have shown inferior sensitivity of DM compared with conventional film screen mammography but significantly lowered recall rates.

DM offers further technologic advancements. Computer-aided diagnosis (CAD) is the detection of a potential abnormality by means of computer analysis of the mammogram; that is, a second reading by a computer. Information of this kind can be supplied to radiologists to help improve their diagnostic performance. Several investigators have demonstrated improved radiologist performance in lesion detection and characterization when a CAD system is used. The CAD enhancement of DM appears highly promising; however, further clinical studies are needed to evaluate the relative efficacy of different CAD methods. Moreover, the medicolegal status of CAD is uncertain at present and needs to be clarified.

Because digital images can be readily transmitted electronically for remote interpretation and consultation, DM holds the promise of telemammography. DM also allows for stereoradiography or *stereomammography,* in which two images of the breast are taken at slightly different angles and later "fused" to provide greater perception of the relative depths of structures within the image. Additionally, DM can be used to combine several single images into a three-dimensional image called *tomosynthesis.* Both techniques have been proposed as solutions to the problem of false-negative conventional screen-film mammography due to masking from overlying structures, particularly in very dense breast tissue. During tomosynthesis, multiple images are acquired as the x-ray tube rotates in an arc above the breast and detector. By manipulating the digital image, any plane in the breast can be easily displayed. Preliminary data have shown breast tomosynthesis to be equivalent or superior to conventional diagnostic mammography in small numbers of women. Ultimately such systems may substantially improve diagnostic accuracy. A multicenter validation study is planned.

Dual-energy mammography is another technology that becomes practical once the image is digitized. This technique provides another approach to the problem of overlying breast tissue masking lesion detection. With this method, two exposures of the breast are made at substantially different x-ray spectra. Weighted subtraction of one image from the other provides additional information about breast tissue composition. Specifically, it may render calcifications more obvious in dense breast tissue.

DM offers other benefits, including diagnostic signs that are identical for interpretation of screen-film mammography and DM, which could facilitate the transition from one system to the other. Another variation, *mammoscintigraphy,* may be helpful in identifying drug-resistant tumors before therapy. Although DM may reduce some costs by eliminating film and film processing chemicals, decreasing film storage space, and reducing film library staff, immediate cost savings are unlikely. Substantial capital equipment costs are necessary in that the DM systems cost four to five times that of conventional mammography units.

Major technical challenges remain, and further clinical studies are necessary to determine the actual clinical value of this modality as a probable adjunct to conventional mammography, primarily in the area of dense breast tissue. Moreover, measuring cost-effectiveness of this evolving technology and the effect on quality-of-life issues (because of the expected reduction of false-positives) will be critical in clinical assessment.

Ultrasound

Ultrasound imaging of the breast has been an extremely valuable addition to the breast-imaging armamentarium. Ultrasound is currently used to assist in differentiation of benign and malignant lesions, to distinguish cystic from solid masses (95% accuracy, 96.9% sensitivity, and 98.4% specificity), and to guide aspirations and biopsies in mammographically detected nonpalpable lesions, thus likely preventing unnecessary open biopsy (Fig. 41.14). Moreover, this technique is useful in intraoperative surgical margin evaluation and staging of breast cancer. The rate of inadequate samples in ultrasound-guided FNA was 0% for malignant lesions and 28.4% for benign (primarily because of the decreased cellularity of benign fibrous lesions) in a recent research study.

In younger women, sonography has evolved into a highly specialized imaging technique useful as primary imaging modality in this population, as well as in pregnant and lactating women. An ultrasonically detected cyst in a young woman may allow deference of mammography and prevent unnecessary x-ray exposure. However, a normal sonogram at any age should not prevent further evaluation of an abnormal physical finding. Conversely, if a nonpalpable solid mass is detected by sonography but is not clearly seen on a mammogram, biopsy or needle localization must be performed during real-time sonographic imaging (Fig. 41.15). The benefits of this diagnostic technique include the absence of radiation, noninvasive technique, lack of morbidity, and ease of repeated examinations.

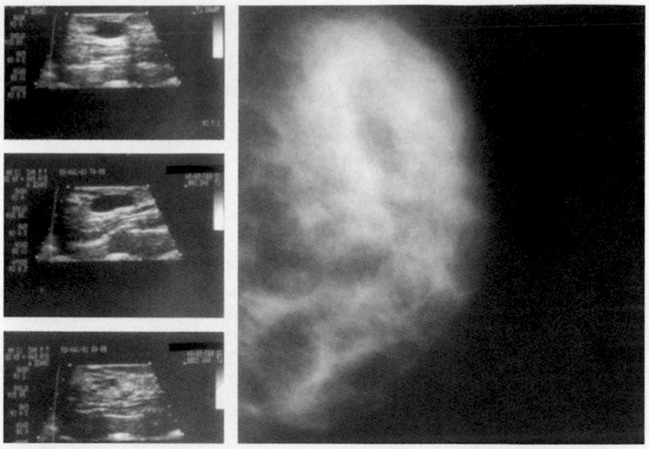

FIGURE 41.14. Ultrasound of a benign cyst in a patient with a "normal" mammogram. The mammogram did not detect the cyst because of the density of the tissue. The cyst shows the typical characteristics of transmission, homogenous internal features without "debris," and smooth margins. The compressibility of the cyst can be seen in the second ultrasound screen.

Unfortunately, breast ultrasound in its current state is extremely inefficient in detecting malignancy and is thus not suitable as a method of breast cancer screening (Fig. 41.16). In one study, only 44% of the mammographically detected nonpalpable lesions and 37% of the cancers could be visualized by high-frequency ultrasound. Ultrasound also has a low capacity for detecting small lesions or small aggregate groups of calcifications, which may be evidence of early breast carcinoma. However, newer sonographic techniques of spatial compound imaging, tissue harmonics imaging, and three-dimensional imaging in breast disorders do not appear to offer improved accuracy or diagnostic value over current methods. Because breast cancer control can be achieved only by early diagnosis of minimal breast cancer, diagnostic ultrasound in its present state

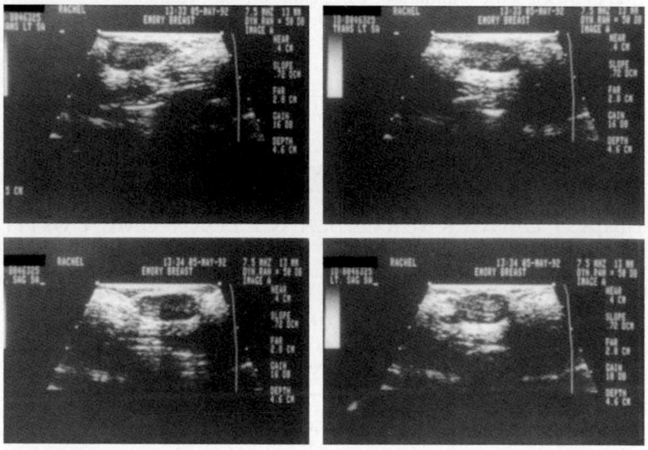

FIGURE 41.15. Ultrasound of a 27-year-old patient presenting with breast mass. Mammogram shows inhomogeneous internal structure, without through transmission, and indistinct margins on the lower border. Thus, if the typical features of a cyst are not met, ultrasound should not be used to delineate the mass further. Fine-needle aspiration showed fibroadenoma.

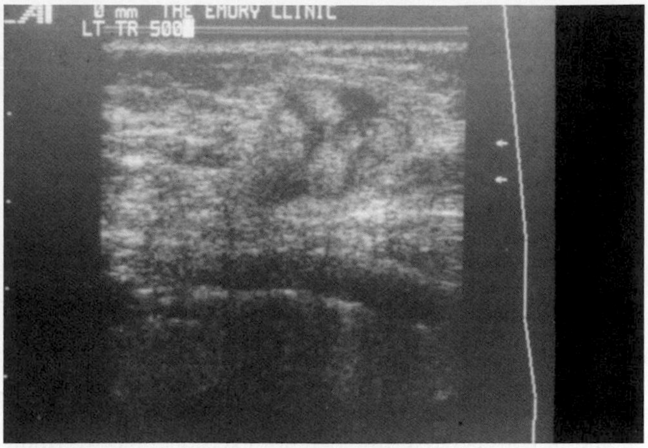

FIGURE 41.16. Ultrasound of a palpable mass in a 39-year-old patient that was not seen on mammography. Typical features of a cyst are not seen. Fine-needle aspiration showed invasive ductal carcinoma.

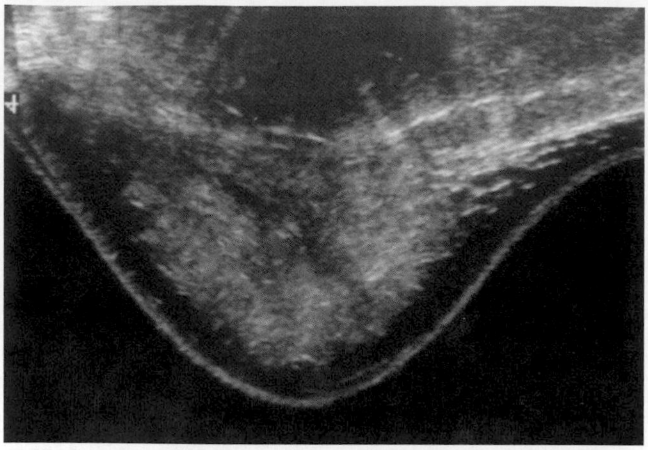

FIGURE 41.17. Magnetic resonance imaging (MRI) study of a 32-year-old patient with a normal examination. MRI results were normal. The patient was reporting breast pain.

of development is incapable of accomplishing this task. However, there is renewed interest in evaluating ultrasound as a potential adjunctive screening tool in women with radiographically dense breasts when the detection benefit of supplemental sonography increased with increasing grades of breast density. Moreover, some authors consider ultrasound significantly better than mammography for detecting invasive breast cancer, especially in certain subpopulations. False-positives appear to be increased; thus, minimizing unnecessary patient anxiety and costs are critical goals of any new screening procedure. Authors caution use of screening sonography only for practitioners experienced in breast sonography, with comprehensive discussion with the patient to consider the risk of a false-positive examination and understanding that early detection may or may not be of benefit to her if a cancer is found. As an RCT with mortality as an end point may be unethical, weighing *potential* risks and benefits with each patient is vital.

Blood flow in malignant breast lesions is considerably increased because of vascular proliferation. Doppler flow ultrasonography can detect increased blood flow and has the potential to distinguish benign from malignant lesions. As a rule, malignant lesions produce Doppler signals of higher frequency and amplitude during continuous flow through diastole. Presently, Doppler flow analysis is not sensitive enough to be used as a tool for distinguishing malignant from benign tissue, but it offers potential for advancement in the field.

Magnetic Resonance Imaging

MRI is emerging as perhaps the most promising imaging modality as an adjunct for breast cancer detection to date (Fig. 41.17). Interventional MRI machines have produced unique opportunities for image-guided surgery. MRI has excellent sensitivity in demonstrating invasive breast cancer that is both mammographically and clinically occult, especially in dense breast tissue, but it has a low specificity (ranging from only 37% to 97%). Moreover, its sensitivity in noninvasive lesions, such as ductal carcinoma *in situ,* has been reported as low as 40%, possibly secondary to more variable angiogenesis in these lesions. Nevertheless, contrast-enhanced MRI may be used in monitoring chemotherapeutic responses in breast cancer, in the preoperative evaluation of patients being considered for BCS, and intraoperatively to define the margins of the lesion and ensure complete excision. Published results, although from studies with relatively small numbers of patients and small numbers of cancers, have shown robust data for screening women at high risk for breast cancer based on genetic mutation or strong family history of breast cancer. The Magnetic Resonance Imaging for Breast Screening (MARIBS) researchers reported MRI to be nearly twice as sensitive as mammography for detecting breast cancers in this subgroup of patients. In total, MRI detected 77% of cancers, and mammography detected 40%. Combined, the two methods produced a sensitivity of 94%, yet 25% of cancers in younger women and 10% in older women were missed. Studies combining MRI with mammography, ultrasound, and CBE have also shown improved detection of cancers with MRI (77% vs. 36%, 33%, and 9.1%, respectively). Combined the modalities had a sensitivity of 95% versus 45% for mammography and CBE combined.

This imaging modality has considerable benefits, including absence of ionizing radiation and lack of known radiobiologic hazards, but it is time-consuming and expensive, and it lacks sufficient resolution for the identification of small lesions. It is also especially deficient in detecting the aggregates of small calcifications that may be evidence of early carcinoma, and it possesses significant overlap in contrast enhancement kinetics and morphologic features of benign and malignant lesions, which severely limits its usefulness as a screening method. MRI, though, seems to be the most accurate method for detection of breast implant integrity. Although MRI screening appears to be feasible in the high-risk populations, further clinical investigation is needed to address the issue of cost-effectiveness and to define the technical requirements for optimal imaging, interpretation criteria, and clinical indications for which MRI should be used as an adjunct to conventional imaging methods.

Positron Emission Tomography

Oncologic breast imaging using positron emission tomography (PET) scanning is a noninvasive nuclear medicine imaging modality rapidly gaining acceptance. Fluorodeoxyglucose is the most commonly used agent, which is a short-lived positron-emitting radiopharmaceutical with increased activity in neoplastic and other rapidly dividing cells. PET scans may be able to assist in distinguishing scar or benign tissue from active malignancy; detect metastatic disease in normal-size lymph nodes; detect locoregional recurrence or distant metastases; identify patients with dense breast or fibrosis from radiotherapy; verify inconclusive results from other imaging modalities; and assess early tumor treatment response. Studies have demonstrated improved tumor detection with PET scans but reduced sensitivity for identification of masses less than 1 cm.

Other modalities, such as CT mammography and Sestamibi scintimammography, are being used in limited situations as an adjunct to mammography with increased diagnostic precision.

Fine-Needle Aspiration

FNA or fine-needle aspiration biopsy was first reported by Martin and Ellis at Sloan-Kettering Cancer Center in 1930 and is now an established diagnostic method in evaluation of palpable breast lesions. In response to the increasing frequency with which women are consulting their obstetrician-gynecologists about concerns related to their breasts, the American Board of Obstetrics and Gynecology (ABOG) has promulgated specific educational requirements for resident training in the various aspects of diagnosing and treating breast disease. Technical proficiency in this procedure is essential for the proper evaluation, treatment, and further definition of a palpable lesion.

FNA is recognized as highly accurate and cost-effective when used in conjunction with clinical examination and imaging as part of the triple test. The "triple test" consists of tissue sampling, mammography, and CBE. If all components of the triple test are benign/negative, the chance of breast cancer is low (0.7%). Yet, if each aspect is suggestive of cancer, the risk of breast cancer is very high (99%). Alone, FNA is relatively accurate but has a false-negative rate as high as 20%. The false-negative rate is highest in detection of lobular cancers and carcinoma *in situ*. However, FNA has a sensitivity of 96% and specificity of 98% (similar to core biopsies), as well as a 99% positive predictive value and 94% negative predictive value and an overall efficacy of 97%.

FNA provides a cytologic rather than histologic sample for review. Thus, limitations include inability to distinguish invasive from *in situ* carcinoma. Use of FNA or core needle biopsy as the initial diagnostic testing remains controversial and is left to the clinician. However, FNA has multiple advantages (Table 41.7) over excisional biopsy and is helpful in confirming the clinical impression of both benign and malignant breast disease. Nevertheless, a negative cytologic report, as with a negative mammographic report, must not be relied on to rule out malignancy in a clinically suspicious lesion and thus should not preclude further evaluation. Any clinically suspicious mass in a patient with negative FNA findings requires additional evaluation, including core biopsy or excisional biopsy, or other methods of detection should be performed. If breast cancer or a *specific* benign condition (e.g., apocrine metaplasia or fibroadenoma) is not detected by FNA (or is inconsistent with the triple test), core biopsy or excisional biopsy is warranted. A positive finding of malignant cells expedites evaluation and allows early selection of appropriate therapy before further surgical intervention. When cyst aspiration is performed, the fluid may be discarded if it is clear (transparent and not bloody) and the mass disappears. If the cyst aspirate is bloody or the mass does not disappear, the patient should be considered a candidate for excisional biopsy. Additionally, if the cyst recurs after aspiration, excisional biopsy is warranted.

The recommendations of the National Cancer Institute Consensus Conference include use of FNA for sufficiently defined palpable breast masses of clinical or patient concern, persistent or suspicious masses in patients with increased family risk factors, evaluation of nonpalpable mammographically suspicious breast lesions, or low risk for malignancy lesions when recommended follow-up with imaging is not feasible or accepted by the patient. FNA should not be used for investigation of microcalcifications but may be used under ultrasound or stereotactic guidance to investigate densities presumed to be nonmalignant. Doubtful densities are best assessed by core biopsy.

FNA is an easily mastered technique, but the adequacy of specimens is improved with experience and training (Fig. 41.18). Procedure risks include infection, bleeding, and bruising at the site. Because the chest wall is immediately beneath the site, pneumothorax has been listed as a potential complication. The small size of the needle and assuring the mass is stabilized over a rib during the procedure significantly decreases this complication.

After the procedure is explained to the patient and consent has been obtained, the skin is cleansed. The lesion is identified and stabilized, preferably over a rib, between the fingers of the nondominant hand (Fig. 41.19). The instrument table should be prepared for easy access because the nondominant hand should not be removed (once it has been placed alongside the mass) until the procedure is completed (Table 41.8). Stabilization of the hand throughout the procedure prevents frequent "loss" of the mass and repeated attempts to locate the targeted structure.

If anesthesia is desired, a small wheal is placed in the skin over the mass, assuring excess local anesthesia does not obscure the mass. A 21- to 23-gauge needle with a clear hub attached to a 10- to 20-mL syringe is then inserted into the central portion of the mass. Increasing the needle gauge does not necessarily increase the sample size. In fact, the larger the needle, the more blood aspirated, and the greater the likelihood of hematoma formation. A pistol-grip holder may also be used, as the mechanics of hand motion are often easier with the holder. Mastery of both techniques (with the holder and without) is recommended because not all institutions have this equipment. If a holder is not used, two fingers are placed under the piston of the syringe, and the thumb is used against the body of the syringe to pull the piston toward the examiner, applying negative pressure. With use of the holder, the grips of the holder are pulled together to apply negative pressure.

TABLE 41.7

ADVANTAGES OF FINE-NEEDLE ASPIRATION

Outpatient procedure
Minimal discomfort
Anesthesia not required (though often used)
Negligible complication rate
Rapid diagnosis
Both diagnostic and therapeutic for breast cysts
Low false-negative rate

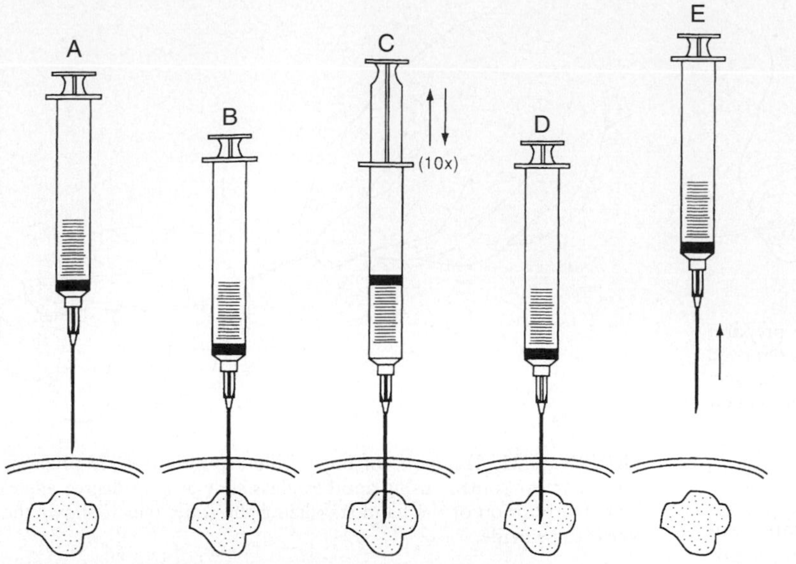

FIGURE 41.18. Overview of fine-needle aspiration. **A:** The mass is located. **B:** The needle is inserted into the mass without negative pressure. **C:** Negative pressure is applied while the needle is moved in an up-and-down fashion within the mass. **D:** Negative pressure is released. **E:** The needle is removed from the mass.

The lesion is sampled by moving the needle up and down within the mass several times. Several passes should be made into every portion of the mass to prevent false-negative samples. If the lesion is cystic, liquid material is seen in the hub of the needle and possibly the body of the syringe. With a solid mass, one may not see evidence of cellular material in the hub.

After complete sampling along each axis of the mass, suction is released and the needle is removed from the lesion. Releasing the suction *before* removing the needle is a critical aspect of this procedure. Continued negative pressure upon removing the needle (without release of suction) results in aspiration of the specimen into the body of the syringe, from which it is difficult to retrieve. Once the needle is removed, pressure is applied to the puncture site (by an assistant or the patient). Significant bleeding from the site of the needle puncture is often characteristic of carcinoma or an inflammatory lesion, although benign conditions and bleeding diathesis may also result in this complication. The patient usually does not require any dressing or bandage on completion of the procedure.

The material should be expelled onto a glass slide (frosted ends facing up toward the practitioner) with the needle bevel facing down to prevent scatter of the specimen (Figs. 41.20–41.23). To release additional sample, the needle is detached, air is drawn into the syringe, the needle is reattached, and further expulsive efforts are accomplished. The "detach, draw air, and reattach" portion is repeated until all the cellular material has been expelled.

Complete aspiration of a cystic mass should always be attempted because at follow-up it will be difficult to determine whether the fluid has reaccumulated or is a remnant from the prior procedure. This becomes important, because reaccumulated fluid in a cyst should be referred for excisional biopsy (Table 41.9).

FIGURE 41.19. Technique of fine-needle aspiration. The mass is stabilized with the nondominant hand (preferably over a rib). After the needle is inserted into the mass, negative pressure is applied.

TABLE 41.8

EQUIPMENT FOR FINE-NEEDLE ASPIRATION

Fine-needle aspiration gun or 10- to 20-cc syringe
21- to 23-gauge needle with *clear* hub
Syringe holder (if desired)
Clear frosted-end glass slides
Alcohol/Betadine pads
Fixative (if desired)
Gauze pads
Adhesive bandage
Toluidine blue if immediate microscopic examination desired
Local anesthesia if desired

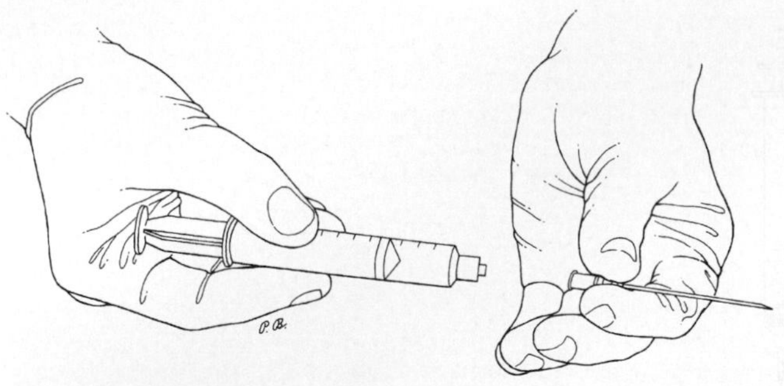

FIGURE 41.20. Technique of fine-needle aspiration—slide preparation. After the needle is removed from the mass, the needle is removed from the syringe and air is aspirated into the syringe. This avoids suctioning cellular material from the needle into the syringe; the cellular material should stay within the needle.

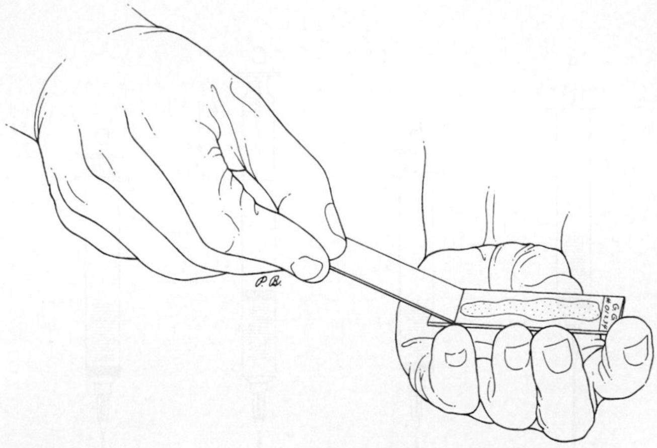

FIGURE 41.22. Technique of fine-needle aspiration—slide preparation. A smear is made using another glass slide at a 45-degree angle. Note the position of the hand stabilizing the slide, which allows the smear to be made.

Cells air dry quickly, so it is crucial that immediate fixation with 95% ethanol or a spray fixative occur after smearing. The examiner must provide the cytopathologist with an accurate clinical history, including age, clinical examination, and whether the patient is pregnant or lactating, because this information is crucial in interpretation of the sample. Figures 41.24 through 41.26 demonstrate examples of FNA cytology. With adequate sampling, HER2/neu, estrogen, and progesterone receptor status may be determined. FNA can produce bleeding into the breast tissue and a hematoma formation beneath the surface, which can complicate mammographic interpretation. For this reason, mammograms (and probably ultrasounds) should be performed either before the FNA procedure or at least 2 weeks afterward.

Random periareolar fine-needle aspiration (RFNA), a modification of FNA, has been espoused as a risk assessment technique to determine an individual's risk for development of breast cancer and as a tool to measure response to preventive measures. It has also been shown to be effective in evaluating breast lesions for high-risk tumor markers. Trials are under way comparing RFNA and ductal lavage; however, there are currently insufficient data to recommend either method as an independent screening modality or in combination with screening mammography.

Core Needle Breast Biopsy

It is estimated that approximately 1 million breast biopsies are performed yearly to diagnose approximately 200,000 breast cancers. Percutaneous core needle biopsy (CNB) may spare many of these women the need for more deforming, invasive, and expensive surgical procedures. With this procedure, a histopathologic diagnosis may be obtained compared with cytologic evaluation with FNA. Studies indicate a high degree of accuracy (98% positive predictive value and 80% negative predictive value), sensitivity of 89%, and specificity of 100% in confirming malignant invasion. False-negative results may occur, but false-positive results are rare except with radial scars. Increasing the number of core specimens by taking samples

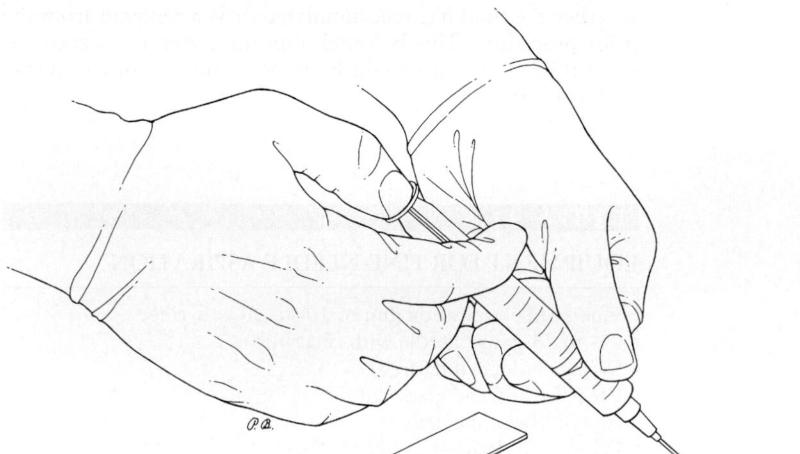

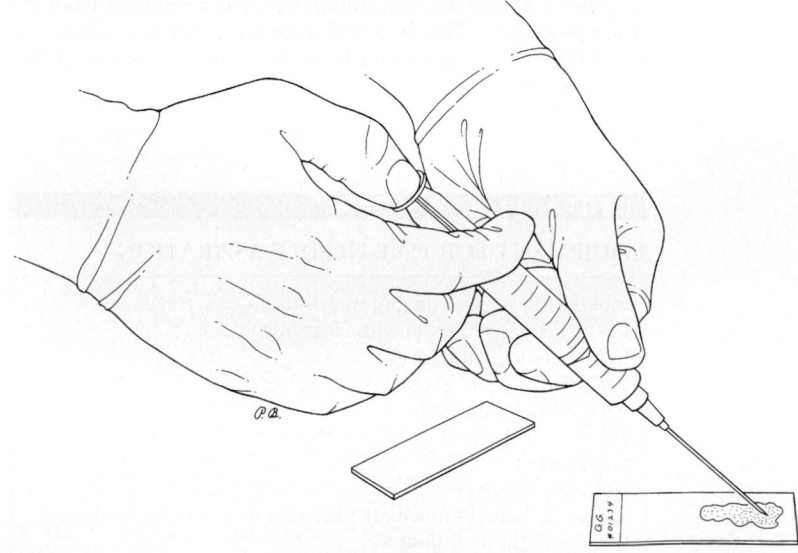

FIGURE 41.21. Technique of fine-needle aspiration—slide preparation. Cellular material is ejected onto a labeled slide.

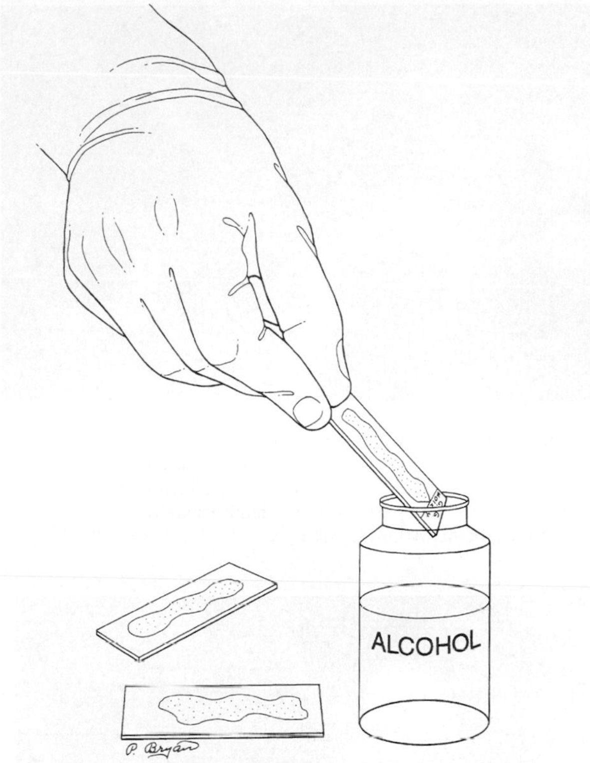

FIGURE 41.23. Technique of fine-needle aspiration—slide preparation. The slide is fixed as rapidly as possible to avoid air drying. Usually, two to three slides can be made from one fine-needle aspiration attempt. The technique chosen for slide preparation depends on the desire of the pathologist

from several locations in the lesion may increase the representativeness of the specimens.

CNB may be performed under tactile, stereotactic, or ultrasound guidance. Less tissue is removed during CNB compared with excisional biopsy, resulting in no deformity in the breast and minimal to no scarring on subsequent mammograms. Another advantage is the ability to distinguish between invasive and intraductal carcinoma (unlike FNA). Because special training is not required to interpret the histologic material obtained from CNB, this obviates the need for the special skills of a cytopathologist needed for FNA. One disadvantage of CNB is that local anesthesia is needed because of the large size of the needle (generally 8- to 18-gauge).

This biopsy procedure is often used in the assessment of BI-RADS category 4 lesions (Table 41.10). If core biopsy of a category 4 lesion yields a benign diagnosis concordant with the imaging characteristics, the woman is usually spared the diagnostic surgical biopsy. Although most often performed for nonpalpable lesions, percutaneous imaging–guided core biopsy can also be helpful in the evaluation of palpable breast masses, particularly for those that are deep, mobile, or vaguely palpable.

Stereotactic CNB requires dedicated equipment but may be helpful in evaluating suspicious mammographic findings, particularly in nonpalpable lesions. Ultrasound-guided CNB has several advantages, including real-time visualization of the needle, lack of ionizing radiation, accessibility to all parts of the breast and axilla, multipurpose use of equipment, and lower cost. However, it is limited in detection of lesions less than 1 cm and has decreased sensitivity in detection of microcalcifications. Vacuum-assisted and Mammotome devices may improve tissue sampling by obtaining larger and more intact samples. The choice depends on several factors, including equipment availability, lesion visibility and accessibility, and preferences of the radiologist and the patient.

After administration of local anesthesia, the area is cleaned. As the core needle is introduced into the mass, the tissue inside the core of the needle is cut from the surrounding tissue as the outer sheath is advanced. After removal of the sheath and core needle, a pressure dressing is applied. This procedure may obviate the need for needle localization surgical biopsy, and studies indicate similar sensitivity and lower cost. The histologic core specimen may be used to determine hormone receptor status and to study other tumor markers using immunohistochemistry.

TABLE 41.9

REQUIRES OPEN BIOPSY

Bloody or serosanguineous fluid on aspiration
Failure of mass to disappear on fluid aspiration
Recurrence of cyst after aspiration
Bloody nipple discharge
Nipple excoriation
Skin edema and erythema suspicious of inflammatory breast carcinoma

Open Surgical Biopsy

Open surgical biopsy includes excisional and incisional techniques. Incisional biopsy is a diagnostic procedure reserved for masses that are too large to be completely excised. There are currently few indications for the use of incisional biopsy because FNA and CNB usually provide sufficient tissue to make a diagnosis with less morbidity and lower cost. Conversely, excisional biopsy refers to the removal of all gross evidence of disease, usually with a small rim of normal breast tissue, and is the definitive procedure for some benign breast masses. Excisional biopsy is usually an outpatient procedure performed under local anesthesia with intravenous sedation as needed.

Some authors recommend beginning the procedure by marking the incisional site with the patient in the sitting position. Conversely, others recommend locating the lesion with the patient in the same position in which the surgery is to be performed. This marking should be performed before injection of any anesthesia because the anesthetic may obliterate the outlines of the mass. Circumareolar incisions are the most ideal cosmetically and heal well. They are attempted for most benign masses despite having to tunnel a short distance to reach the lesion. This should not be done with suspected malignant lesions to prevent the spread of tumor cells along the tunnel, thus prohibiting breast-conserving therapy in the future. On the other hand, Langer or curvilinear lines (following the anatomic skin lines) may be used depending on the location of the lesion. Langer's lines may be defined by gently pinching the skin over the mass and noting the outline. Radial incisions are made over the axilla and inframammary portions of the breast but are ill-advised in the upper portions of the breast because of possible contracture and asymmetric cosmetic result. It is important

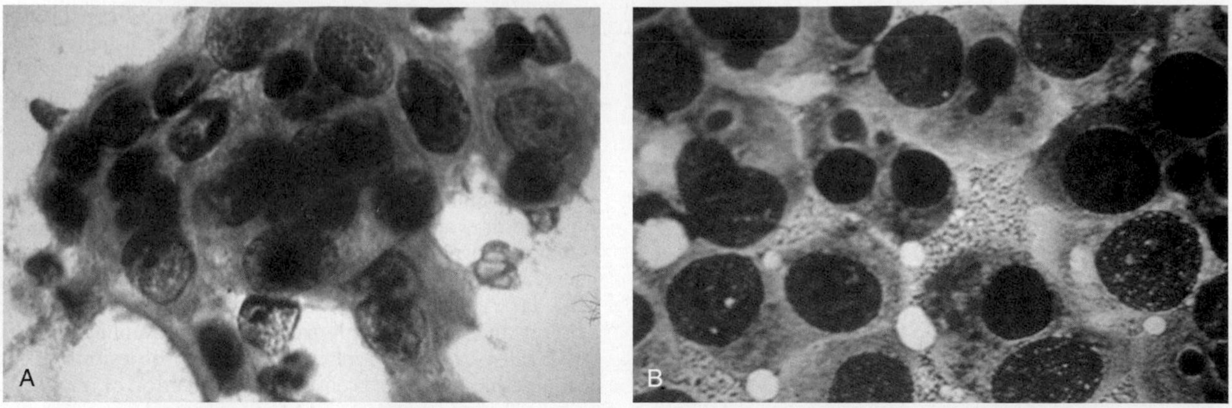

FIGURE 41.24. Fine-needle aspiration of ductal carcinoma. **A:** Smears are cellular with loosely cohesive cells arranged in a malignant cluster. Cells demonstrate clumping of chromatin and irregular nucleoli (Papanicolaou stain ×240). **B:** Single malignant cells with absence of myoepithelial cells are viewed using Diff-Quik stain (×400). Diff-Quik stains are air dried, thus the chromatin pattern is less demonstrative. (Courtesy of Taalat Tadros, MD, Emory University, School of Medicine, Atlanta, GA.)

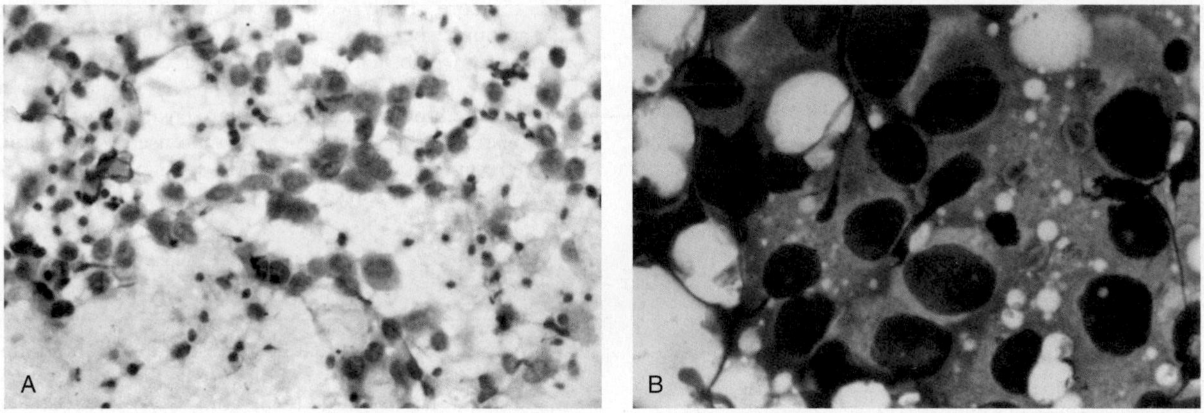

FIGURE 41.25. Fine-needle aspiration of medullary carcinoma. The smears are cellular. **A:** Loosely syncytial malignant aggregates (Papanicolaou stain ×240). **B:** Single malignant cells with benign lymphoid cells noted in the background (Diff-Quik ×400). (Courtesy of Taalat Tadros, MD, Emory University, School of Medicine, Atlanta, GA.)

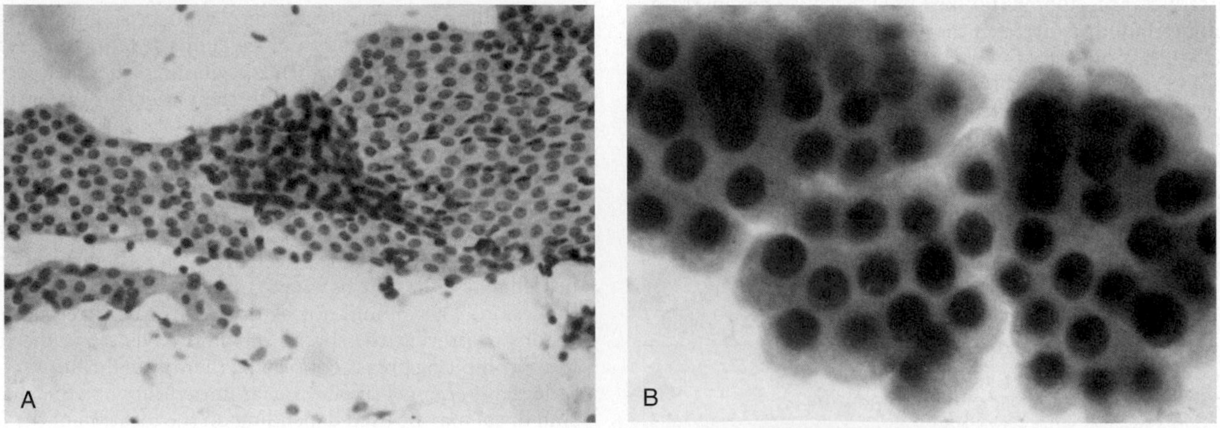

FIGURE 41.26. Fine-needle aspiration of fibrocystic change. **A:** View of uniform ductal cells in right upper quadrant with honeycomb pattern. Characteristic adherent bipolar naked nuclei of myoepithelial cells are noted. Stripped nuclei are seen in the background (Papanicolaou stain ×240). **B:** A flat sheet of apocrine cells are seen in this view. Cells have abundant granular cytoplasm, and the nuclei have prominent nucleoli (Papanicolaou stain ×240). (Courtesy of Taalat Tadros, MD, Emory University, School of Medicine, Atlanta, GA.)

TABLE 41.10

BREAST IMAGING REPORTING AND DATA SYSTEM (BI-RADS)

Category assessment	Category	Follow-up
1	Negative	Routine (annual)
2	Benign	
3	Probable benign	Short interval follow-up at 6 months for ipsilateral breast, followed by both breasts at 1, 2, 3 years after initial mammogram.
4	Suspicious for malignancy	Biopsy
5	Highly suggestive of malignancy	

to keep biopsy incisions within the boundaries of the future mastectomy or wide local excision site, which may be required for definitive treatment.

After marking the site of the lesion, the patient is placed supine with her arm extended comfortably on an arm board. In draping the patient, the nipple should be kept in view for orientation during surgery. Local anesthesia without epinephrine is infiltrated at the incision site and deeply around the mass. Very small masses may be obscured, however, by the use of large amounts of local anesthesia. The absence of epinephrine permits immediate visualization of blood loss, which helps in obtaining adequate hemostasis (rather than oozing later when the anesthetic has worn off, resulting in unsightly hematomas). The incision is made with a no. 15 knife blade and carried through the skin and subcutaneous tissue to the lesion (Fig. 41.27). Sharp dissection is used to develop the skin flaps to achieve better exposure. Blunt dissection increases adhesions and inflammation. The edges of the incision are retracted with skin hooks. Instruments that will crush the tissue are never used so as to prevent cutting the tumor into smaller pieces, thus making excision more difficult, or to prevent tumor seeding. The mass may be gently grasped with suture for traction while excision is performed with sharp dissection. Cautery should be used *only* for hemostasis, not for excision of the mass, because heat may distort estrogen and progesterone receptor evaluation and margin delineation. If malignancy is suspected, the biopsy specimen should include a margin of normal tissue around the mass. Furthermore, estrogen and progesterone receptor status and human epidermal growth factor receptor 2 protein (HER2/neu) evaluation is critical. Ideally, the pathology department should receive the specimen on ice, because room temperature (heat) can damage the estrogen and progesterone receptors.

Closure of the defect left by the excised mass (dead space) is discouraged because of the increased risk of infection from suture placement and the potential for skin distortion. If a large defect is obtained, a minimum number of sutures should be used, and drainage of the site bears additional significance. A subcuticular closure with 4-0 or 5-0 absorbable material using Steri-Strips is generally performed. Alternatively, nonabsorbable suture can be used and removed 1 or 2 weeks postoperatively. To prevent hematoma formation, a snugly placed elastic dressing is applied for 24 to 48 hours. A bra should then be worn continuously for 3 to 7 days to minimize the risk of bleeding and discomfort. The patient should avoid heavy lifting with the affected arm and strenuous activity for 3 to 7 days.

Needle localization excisional biopsy is performed for suspicious nonpalpable abnormalities seen on mammography. In the radiology suite, under local anesthesia, the lesion is identified by fluoroscopy, and a needle is placed near it. A hooked wire is inserted through the needle and located just beneath the lesion. After the needle is removed, the wire is stabilized on the skin, and the patient is transported to the operating suite for surgical excision. Incisions similar to those used for excisional biopsy are made, and the suspected abnormality and the wire are excised. Radiographic studies are performed on the specimen to ensure that the lesion originally noted on mammography has been excised in its entirety. This procedure can be done under local anesthesia in an outpatient setting. The complications are similar to those of excisional biopsies, including bleeding, hematoma formation, and infection (cellulitis, abscess). Improvements in CNB (either stereotactic or ultrasound-guided) has made this procedure less necessary.

BREAST CANCER

The risk of breast cancer has reached epidemic proportions, affecting one in eight women who live to the age of 85 years. Its incidence is more that two times that of all female pelvic cancers combined, and it is probably the most feared disease by women today. The increasing lifetime risk for development of breast cancer may be attributed to early detection of prevalent cases, primarily because of the increased use of mammographic screening, and lower mortality that is due to causes other than breast cancer. A millennium of scientific inquiry, theoretical investigation, and systematic experimentation has only now begun to provide the medical profession with prevention strategies for women at high risk.

Thus, breast cancer remains a leading cause of cancer-related mortality, with estimates that more than 40,000 women will die of this disease. Men are not immune; 1,500 new cases of male breast cancer were expected to be diagnosed in 2005. There is good news, though, in that the incidence rates appear to have leveled off in the 1990s after increasing about 4% per year in the 1980s. Additionally, mortality rates have declined since 1992, with the largest decreases noted in younger women (both black and white).

Epidemiology of Breast Cancer

The etiology of breast cancer is multifactorial and, although numerous risk factors have been identified, they only account for 21% of the risk of breast cancer in women age 30 to

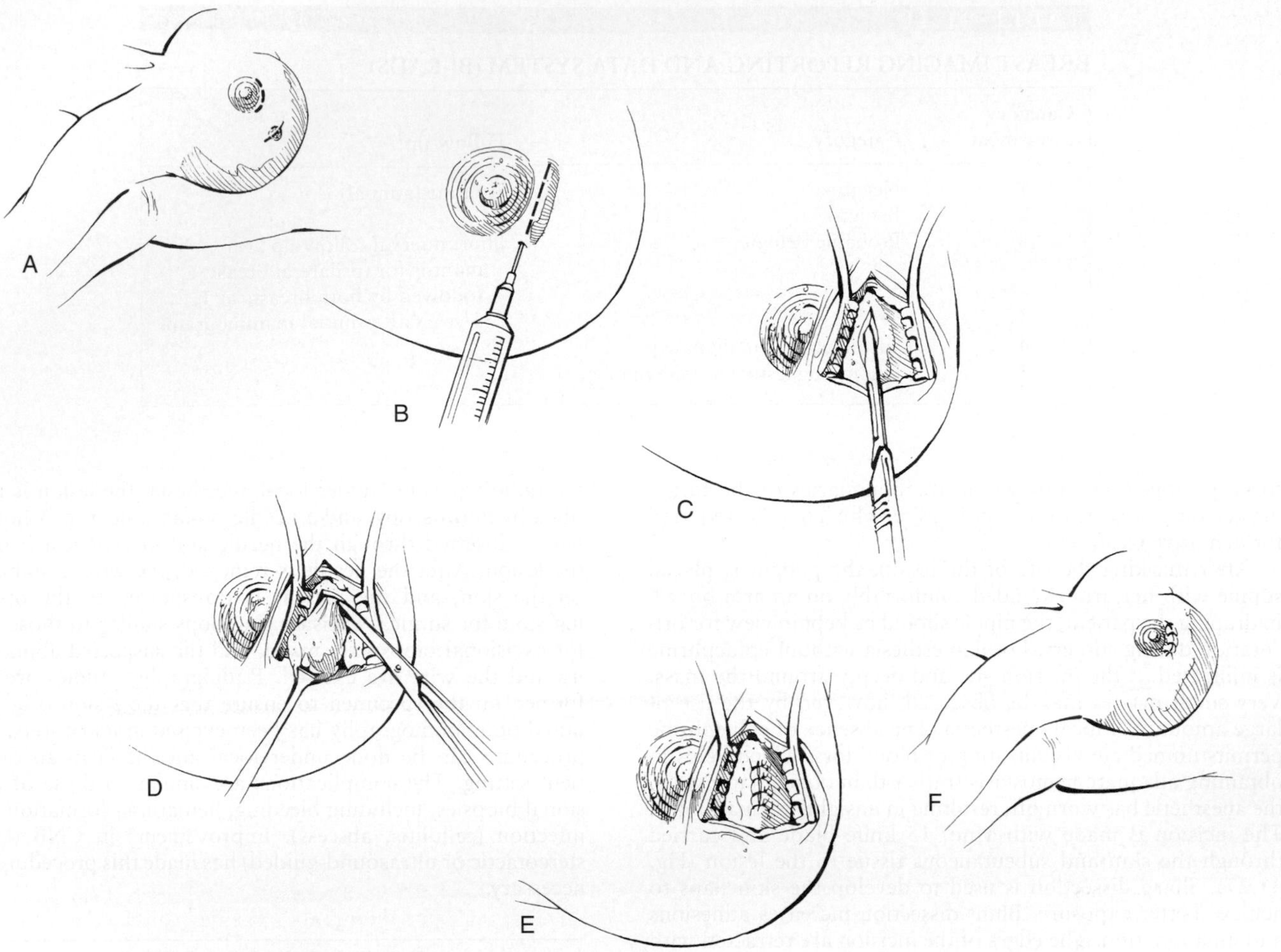

FIGURE 41.27. Technique of excisional biopsy. **A:** For cosmetic reasons, circumareolar incisions are preferable when the lesion is thought to be within 2 or 3 cm of the areola. Not more than one half of the areolar margin should be incised. A curved incision parallel to the areola is made over lesions further out from the center. When malignant disease is strongly suspected, the surgeon should attempt to avoid the probable path of the subsequent mastectomy incision. **B:** An intradermal wheal is raised along the path of the proposed incision using 1% lidocaine and a hypodermic (no. 25) needle. From the wheal, deeper injections of anesthetic are made around the circumference of the lesion and beneath it. **C:** The incision is carried down through the dense subcutaneous tissue and into the lobule containing the lesion. Self-retaining retractors are helpful when an assistant is not available. **D:** If the lesion is small or easily mobilized, it should be sharply dissected and excised with a thin margin of adjacent tissue. **E:** The lobular defect is sutured with fine absorbable suture material if the closure places no tension on the overlying skin. Bleeding is controlled with absorbable ligatures or electrocoagulation. Absolute hemostasis is essential. **F:** The skin is closed with interrupted 4-0 or 5-0 silk or nylon sutures. Drainage is seldom necessary. A pressure dressing for 24 to 48 hours is desirable if a significant amount of dead space has been left behind.

54 years and only 29% in women age 55 to 84 years. Furthermore, nearly three fourths of women with breast cancer have no identifiable risk factors other than sex and age; thus, all women should be considered at risk.

Previously identified risk factors for breast cancer include increasing age, nulliparity, delayed childbearing (childbirth before age 18 years portends one third the risk of breast cancer than in a woman delivering at age 35 years), personal or family history of breast cancer, benign proliferative breast disease, obesity in postmenopausal women, a long menstrual history (menarche before age 12 and late menopause), and higher education and socioeconomic status. Lactation has been shown in observational studies to decrease the risk of breast cancer. Other factors—such as fat intake, previous abortions, smoking, prior placental weight, and alcohol intake—have all been suggested to contribute to breast cancer risks, but the associations either show no effect or remain inconclusive, inconsistent, and controversial.

Family History

Family history is the most widely recognized breast cancer risk factor. First-degree female relatives of women with breast carcinoma have two to three times the general population risk of developing the disease. The risk increases even more if the affected relative was premenopausal with bilateral breast disease on diagnosis (eightfold increased risk) compared with a postmenopausal affected relative with only unilateral disease (onefold to twofold increased risk). Centers for Disease

Control and Prevention data indicate a 2.3 relative risk for patients with an affected mother or sister or daughter (first degree) and a 1.5 relative risk for patients with an affected aunt, niece, or grandmother (second degree). The risk for patients with both an affected mother and sister has been listed between a twofold and 14-fold increase. A family history of male breast cancer significantly increases the likelihood of detecting a BRCA gene in the proband. Moreover, a family history of ovarian cancer (especially in a relative who also had breast cancer) greatly increases the likelihood of an inherited genetic etiology.

Ethnicity

Breast cancer incidence and mortality rates vary among racial and ethnic groups. For all ages combined, white women are more likely to develop breast cancer, yet African-American women are more likely to die of breast cancer. Native Americans have the lowest incidence of breast cancer, nearly one third the risk of white women. In addition, Native American and Asian women have approximately one third the mortality of African-American women. Although Hispanic women appear to have a lower incidence of breast cancer (compared with Caucasian women), some studies have shown a greater proportion of this ethnic group to be less than 50 years of age at diagnosis, to present with larger tumors, and to have a greater likelihood of being estrogen receptor (ER) negative (when compared with Caucasian women). Individuals of Ashkenazi Jewish ancestry have a higher likelihood of harboring one of the founder mutations of BRCA1 and -2 when combined with other risk factors.

Genetic Predisposition and Hereditary Breast Cancer

The past decade has witnessed an explosion of knowledge in the field of cancer genetics and inherited susceptibility to cancer syndromes. It has been estimated that approximately 5% to 10% of breast cancers are inherited in an autosomal dominant pattern. Breast cancer susceptibility genes, BRCA1 and BRCA2, were discovered in the early 1990s and mapped to chromosome 17q and 13q, respectively. In 1996, commercially available DNA-based carrier detection became available, opening up a quandary for women at risk for inherited forms of breast cancer. Because these tests are expensive, often difficult to interpret, and documented to have a significant psychologic impact for both positive and negative test results—as well as placing healthy individuals at risk for insurance and employment discrimination—the decision to undergo testing must be made after a thorough and informed discussion between the physician and the patient. Thus, testing is reserved for research settings and is not yet suited for wide-scale screening.

The only currently known BRCA genes are BRCA1 and BRCA2, thus the discussion herein is based only on these mutations. There are more than 1,000 different mutations in BRCA1 and -2. BRCA1 mutation is believed to account for nearly half of all inherited breast cancer cases and nearly 90% of the hereditary ovarian cancer cases. Similarly, BRCA2 mutations are responsible for approximately 40% of familial breast cancer and 5% to 10% of familial ovarian cancer. Li-Fraumeni syndrome, p53 mutations, Hras, ataxia-telangiectasia, and as yet undetected genes appear to account for the other cases of inherited breast cancer.

Initial studies suggest that the lifetime risk of developing breast cancer in families with BRCA1 was approximately 80% to 90%, whereas the risk of ovarian cancer was approximately 30% to 60%. It is estimated, based on data from families linked to BRCA1, that 50% of female mutation carriers will develop breast cancer by age 50 years (compared with 1.7% in the general population) and 85% by age 70 years (compared with 11% in the general population at age 70 years). Pedigree analysis in BRCA2 carriers has identified a similar risk of development of female breast cancer to that seen with BRCA1 mutations. However, the risk of ovarian cancer for carriers of BRCA2 mutations is only 10%. Based on this information, the overall lifetime risk of developing breast *or* ovarian cancer is nearly 100%. Population-based studies (versus studies based on specific families), however, suggest that the *actual* overall lifetime cancer risk of mutation carriers is closer to 56% for breast cancer and 16% for ovarian cancer. It is unclear whether these inconsistent results are related to the populations tested, to the size of the studies, or, perhaps, to differences in penetrance between different mutations. Further longitudinal studies may resolve this question.

BRCA mutation carriers not only have an increased overall risk of developing cancer, but commonly have a younger age at onset and a greater probability of second tumors. Accordingly, although the inherited mutations account for only 5% to 10% of all breast cancers, they account for nearly 25% of breast cancer cases diagnosed before the age of 30.

Not only are the BRCA genes associated with increased risk of female malignancies, they have also been shown to be a marker for hereditary cancer syndromes in men. Male breast cancer is much more common in BRCA2 families than in the general population. Five to fifteen percent of male breast cancer is associated with BRCA2 mutations, with recent data indicating an association with BRCA1 mutations as well. Male carriers of BRCA2 mutations have a 6% lifetime risk for the development of breast cancer compared with 0.1% in the general population.

In addition, other malignancies are increased in BRCA2 carriers, such as laryngeal, prostate, gallbladder, stomach, melanoma, primary peritoneal, and pancreatic cancer. Hence, the BRCA mutation may be transferred to a woman through a male relative. However, a male carrier of a BRCA1 mutation is much more likely to be cancer-free than is a woman who carries the same mutation. And, although a family history of breast cancer places a mutation carrier at increased risk not only for breast cancer but also for ovarian cancer, her brother will be at similarly increased risk for prostate cancer. It is therefore important to elicit a history of *all* related malignancies, not just a family history of breast and ovarian cancer. Patients are often unaware that the risk of transmission of a BRCA mutation is equally high from the paternal side and do not volunteer information about cancers from that side. Episodes of malignancies from both sides of the families must be elicited, including age at onset, bilaterality, and history of multiple primary cancers in an individual in the family.

BRCA1 and BRCA2 are believed to be tumor suppressor genes. Inactivation of tumor suppressor genes is almost a universal step in the development of a wide range of cancers in humans and experimental animals. In individuals who are not genetically at increased risk for cancer, environmental mutagenesis with time can result in inactivation of both gene copies. In individuals who have inherited a mutation in one of these tumor suppressor genes, the probability of acquiring additional mutations to produce cancer is significantly increased.

Histologic differences in the hereditary breast cancers compared with the sporadic cancers may account for the earlier presentation of cancer in mutation carriers. It has been reported that BRCA1-associated breast cancers are characterized by higher-grade medullary features, overexpression of p53, aneuploidy, and high proliferation index relative to sporadic breast cancers. Essinger and colleagues noted that 19% of BRCA1 cancers were of the medullary variety, as compared with none in the sporadic cases, suggesting that medullary cancer alone may be an indication for susceptibility testing. Additionally, BRCA1-associated cancers are ER negative 65% to 80% of the time, compared with a rate of 25% to 35% in sporadic cancers. In contrast, the excess of ER-negative tumors is not demonstrated in the BRCA2-associated cancers. Moreover, the clinicopathologic characteristics of BRCA2-associated cancers are similar to sporadic breast cancers with the suggestion of higher grades. However, a number of studies have found no differences between prognosis in BRCA-associated cancers and sporadic cancers. Thus, the issue remains unresolved and suggests the need for longitudinal studies to ferret out this needed information.

The frequency of a BRCA1 mutation in the general population is estimated to be 1 in 500 to 1 in 1,000 (with BRCA2 mutations occurring somewhat less), although it appears to be higher in certain ethnic groups, such as Ashkenazi Jews, in whom it is estimated to be 1%. In the Ashkenazi Jewish population (of eastern or central European origin), three different founder mutations have been identified: 185delAG and 5382insC in BRCA1 and 6174delT in BRCA2. Estimates indicate that 1 in 40 Ashkenazi individuals carry one of these founder mutations, and they are responsible for 25% of the early-onset breast cancer in this population. Current investigations indicate the estimated gene frequency in the general population may be artificially high because of ascertainment bias in the initial studies of high-risk families.

Testing for BRCA1 and BRCA2

Our knowledge regarding BRCA mutations is far from complete, and many incongruencies form the basis of our present information. The decision to proceed with genetic testing for BRCA1 or BRCA2 mutations is complex. Considerable caution must be used in counseling patients because definitive data are limited. Therefore, genetic counseling is an essential element of breast cancer susceptibility testing. The ability to reassure those with negative tests is limited by the possible existence of other—as yet undiscovered—genes. Nonpenetrance of the gene may make pedigree interpretation difficult in that absence of cancer in a parent cannot necessarily be interpreted to mean that the children are not at risk.

A history of multiple affected first-degree relatives, bilateral disease, early or premenopausal age at onset, male breast cancer, and a family history of both ovarian and breast cancer increases the probability of having an inherited predisposition to breast cancer.

It is preferable to test an *affected* family member to document the particular familial BRCA1 or BRCA2 mutation. A negative result in the proband is most meaningful in a situation in which the family member has previously tested positive. In the absence of the detectable mutation in the proband, the patient may be reassured that she does not have the high risk of cancer seen in her family. She should be counseled, however, that she still has the baseline risk of cancer seen in the general population (one in eight for women who live to age 85 years) and that she should continue usual care, such as mammography and breast examination. On the other hand, if the family member with cancer has not or cannot be tested, the interpretation of a negative result is more problematic. Either (i) a BRCA mutation is present but was not detected by the test (possibly because of the testing modality or polymorphisms); (ii) a BRCA mutation is present in the family but was not inherited by the proband; (iii) there is no BRCA mutation, but another gene mutation exists (as yet unidentified or related to a regulatory gene); or (iv) the proband does not have inherited breast cancer predisposition, nor do other family members. In the last case, again, the woman still has a risk equal to the general population for sporadic forms of breast cancer. One study showed that one third of mutations detected involved deletions that are not currently detected by conventional techniques. In summary, present techniques do not identify all disease-causing mutations, and patients need to be informed of the limitations of the present technology.

Hormonal Replacement Therapy

No issue related to breast cancer risk has been fraught with as much controversy as has the use of exogenous hormones. The extensive research conducted to answer this question has expanded the debate rather than resolved it.

Currently, nearly 42 million American women are postmenopausal, and this number is predicted to increase to 62 million by 2020. Before the Women's Health Initiative study, nearly 40% of postmenopausal women in the United States used HRT; thus, the association of breast cancer with the use of HRT received considerable attention in the medical and lay press.

Initial case control studies did not find an increased risk of breast cancer associated with the use of HRT, but these studies were limited by statistical power and methodological problems. A review of the epidemiologic studies on postmenopausal hormone therapy and the risk of breast cancer also failed to provide definitive evidence regarding this issue because results are inconsistent. The Nurses Health Study (69,586 participants) and the Collaborative Group on Hormonal Factors in Breast Cancer refute previous data and indicate that current users of HRT have a relative risk of 1.33 of developing breast cancer but note no increased risk with past use. The shear number of participants warrants giving great credibility to these findings. In addition, four subsequent metaanalyses note a slight increased risk in long-term users of HRT (>15 years), although here also there are conflicting results, affected by dosage and duration of HRT use. In contrast, the Four State Case Control Study and the Iowa Women's Health Study showed no change in the risk of breast cancer diagnosis with long-term current use. Note that metaanalyses have the same flaws in methodology and bias as the initial epidemiologic studies on which they are based. Pooling several groups of data does not remove this problem; thus, this information should be viewed with caution. Nevertheless, the trend propels one to consider these findings when making recommendations to patients.

The Women's Health Initiative was a randomized primary prevention trial and persists as pivotal study of this decade. There were 16,608 postmenopausal women aged 50 to 79 with intact uteri at baseline recruited. After slightly more than 5 years of follow-up, the risk of coronary heart disease (CHD) (nonfatal myocardial infarction and CHD death) increased by 29%, breast cancer by 26%, and stroke by 41%, and the risk of pulmonary embolism doubled. Conversely, the risks of hip fractures and colorectal cancer were decreased by more than 30%. Absolute excess risks per 10,000 person years attributable to estrogen plus progestin were seven more CHD events, eight more strokes, eight more pulmonary embolisms, and eight more invasive breast cancers, whereas absolute risk reductions per 10,000 person years were six fewer colorectal cancers and five fewer hip fractures. Based on this information, the combined arm of the study was halted; however, the estrogen-only arm continued, showing no increased risk of breast cancer. Rectifying these data is difficult. Many have criticized this study, as the age of initiation of HRT use was greater than generally used, body mass index (BMI) stratification showed greater risk in obese women, and more than half of the women had other risk factors for cardiac disease, including smoking, diabetes, hypertension, hypercholesterolemia, or prior coronary event. Many have speculated that because the study closed after an average 5 years of follow-up, possibly the detected breast cancers were present *before* patient accrual into the study. Detailed discussions with patients regarding this information is necessary.

On the other hand, additional data are being compiled showing benefits to HRT when breast cancer is diagnosed. Survival data indicate that the risk of mortality from breast cancer was decreased among women who were using HRT at the time of diagnosis compared with age-matched nonusers. HRT user-associated cancers were more likely to be less advanced clinically and more likely to be ER positive. Possibly this information supports the idea that the increased risk of breast cancer diagnosis among users of HRT may result from detection bias, wherein participants were more likely to see a physician regularly and have regular breast examination and mammography.

In summary, medical studies over the preceding 25 years contain conflicting information regarding HRT use in postmenopausal women. Sufficient evidence exists to indicate an increased risk of breast cancer associated with postmenopausal estrogen use. Patients must consider this possibility in their informed decision making. In addition, the role these agents may play in the development of cancers in genetically predisposed women has to be evaluated. Although HRT use can improve the quality of life for postmenopausal women, it should not be initiated solely for the purpose of prevention of CHD events and should be used for the shortest duration possible for amelioration of menopausal symptoms.

Oral Contraceptive Medications

OCPs are used by nearly 11 million women worldwide and are the second most popular contraceptive method available (surpassed only by female sterilization). Since its approval by the FDA in 1960, OCPs have become one of the most extensively studied medications ever prescribed. Recent studies relating OCPs to breast cancer have yielded conflicting results, thus the issue continues to be controversial. Interestingly, OCPs have been shown to decrease the risk of ovarian cancer. This creates a quandary for their use in BRCA mutation carriers, who are at increased risk for both breast and ovarian cancer.

Case control studies, including the Cancer and Steroid Hormone Study, initially showed no overall association between OCP use and the development of breast cancer. However, the enrollees were not representative of the current OCP user who is younger, uses OCPs for longer duration, and delays initial versus subsequent pregnancies. Reanalysis of the data shows a correlation between certain subgroups and an increased risk of development of breast cancer, specifically among women using OCPs before their first full-term pregnancy, women age 25 to 34, and long-term users. By age 50 years, the cumulative risk is the same in users and nonusers, and there is no evidence of increased overall breast cancer risk, even with prolonged duration of use. Although incongruous, it may be that estrogen in OCPs stimulates breast cancer, promotes its growth, and makes it detectable, so that it is more likely to be diagnosed while the OCP user is younger, yet without conferring an increase in overall lifetime risk. Another possibility is that the increased risk seen in these analyses represents detection bias—that is, women taking OCPs are more likely to have breast examinations and thus are more likely to have the diagnosis made while they are younger. Furthermore, the Nurses Health Study, a prospective cohort study of more than 100,000 female nurses in the United States, showed no increased risk of breast cancer or breast cancer mortality in past users of OCPs. In a metaanalysis of 54 studies, a relative risk of 1.24 was associated with current use of OCPs ($p = 0.001$). The risk was elevated for 10 years after use of oral contraceptives was discontinued but was not influenced by a family history of breast cancer, which contrasts with the 2000 study mentioned below. In many of these studies, the increased risk was noted only in women taking OCPs before 1975 when formulations were likely to contain higher dosages of estrogen and progesterone than that in OCPs today.

Studies specifically of women at high risk for breast cancer have also generated contradictory results. In women with a family history of breast cancer and OCP use, a 1989 study by Murray (with more than 4,500 women) showed no association with subsequent development of breast cancer. Conversely, a study published in 2000 involving 426 families (3,300 women with a positive family history for breast or ovarian cancer) revealed a threefold increased risk of development of breast cancer in those with a family history compared with those without such history who also used OCPs. However, other authors belie the strength of the study and indicate they would continue to support use of low-dose formulations in women with a family history of breast cancer unless the cancer history was compelling.

Additionally, Narod and colleagues showed that OCP use may provide a reduction in the risk of ovarian cancer specifically in women harboring BRCA1 and -2 germline mutations. Marchbanks and associates showed that neither use of OCPs nor the initiation of OCP use at a young age was associated with an increased risk of breast cancer in women with a family history of breast cancer.

The purported associations must be placed in perspective, though. It is evident that case control studies have inferior methodological strength compared with the gold standard of RCTs. The conclusions may be imprecise because of the low numbers of participants in some studies. Also, studies have not included current low-dose formulations in wide scale, but have been based on previous high-dose OCPs, which clearly may confer higher risk. Finally, studies often include women with a family history of *both* ovarian and breast cancer, whereas there is evidence that OCPs actually decrease the risk of ovarian and endometrial cancer in the general population.

Overall, it appears that long-term use of OCPs is associated with a modest increase in the risk of early-onset breast cancer in the general population and a decrease in the risk of ovarian cancer (at least 50% reduction in an unselected population of women). As patients carrying the BRCA gene have a 50% to 80% lifetime risk of developing breast cancer and a 25% to 45% lifetime risk of ovarian cancer, OCP use may create a quandary. Narod and associates found an increased risk of early-onset breast cancer among BRCA1 mutation carriers who first used OCPs before 1975, who used them before age 30, or who used them for 5 or more years. OCP use did not appear to be associated with the risk of breast cancer in BRCA2 carriers, although data for this group were limited. However, the same author found OCP use may reduce the risk of ovarian cancer in both BRCA1 and BRCA2 mutation carriers. The author suggests that OCP use after age 30 is not likely to increase the risk of breast cancer among BRCA1 mutation carriers and can be used safely to reduce the risk of ovarian cancer.

Mammographic Breast Density

Assessing the impact of breast density on breast cancer risk is hampered by data comparisons derived by applying differing mammographic screening intervals and by improvements in radiographic technology that may hinder our ability to accurately analyze and generalize the information. Nonetheless, women with greater mammographic breast density have been reported to have a four- to sixfold increased risk of breast cancer. This relationship has also been shown in differing ethnic groups. Increased density impairs the detection of breast masses, increases interval cancers, and produces false-positive recalls with the associated patient psychological stress and elevated costs of care. The likelihood of dense breasts increases with nulliparity, older age at first birth, and current use of postmenopausal hormone therapy (about 25% of women taking combined HRT have increased density in their breast tissue) and decreases with advancing age and increasing body weight. The correlation with nulliparity supports the assertion that early pregnancy produces structural change in the breast tissue that persists throughout life and is associated with resistance to proliferation.

Moreover, hormonal agents associated with increased breast cancer risk (estrogen and estrogen with progestin) likewise increase breast density, whereas hormonal agents that decrease risk (tamoxifen and raloxifene) likewise decrease breast density. The breast is rapidly responsive either to initiation or discontinuation of hormones, with increases in mammographic density noted largely within the first year and decrease in density occurring in as little as 2 weeks after withdrawal. In postmenopausal women on HRT (especially continuous combined as opposed to sequential regimens), many studies have indicated a 5% to 20% decreased mammographic sensitivity in hormone users with dense breasts. Yet current evidence does not explain whether the increased density associated with hormone therapy specifically changes an individual's risk of breast cancer development. In an effort to influence a women's risk of developing breast cancer, antiestrogens such as tamoxifen have been shown to decrease breast density. In one study, this was associated with a decreased rate for breast cancer development, although the confidence intervals were broad. This seems appealing, but if women with dense breast tissue are at increased risk as a result of genetic predisposition, then reducing breast density may not reduce breast cancer risk. Further study is necessary to elucidate a resolution to this issue.

Breast Cancer Risk Assessment

Several algorithms have been developed to estimate a woman's risk of developing breast cancer, with the best known of these being the Gail and Claus models. The Gail Model Risk Assessment Tool (Fig. 41.28) incorporates the patient's race, current age, age at menarche and first live birth, number of first-degree relatives with breast cancer, number of previous breast biopsies, and histology (as modified) results in generating an estimate of breast cancer risk. Limitations of this model include inclusion of only first-degree relatives, lack of information on the age at diagnosis or Ashkenazi Jewish background and lack of inclusion of a history of ovarian cancer. Conversely, the Claus model, using fewer categories, incorporates maternal and paternal breast cancer family history, first- and second-degree relatives, and the relative's age at cancer diagnosis. Although helpful in diagnosis, models are often inapplicable to the proband. In particular, the Gail model cannot be used for women younger than 35 years of age and is less accurate in women who do not obtain annual mammograms. Moreover, studies have shown that the Gail model underestimates risk in women with a personal history of breast cancer and those who are BRCA positive. Concordance of the two models is only fair, but only the Gail model has been clinically validated.

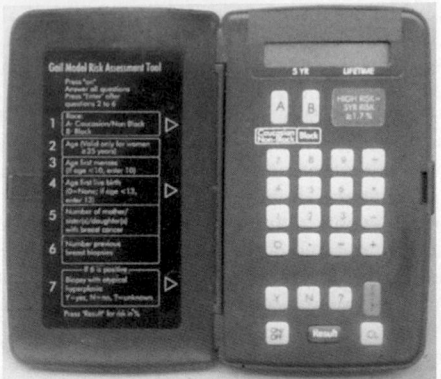

FIGURE 41.28. Gail model risk-assessment tool.

The BRCAPRO model developed by Parmigiani and colleagues, provides estimates of the likelihood of harboring the BRCA mutation. This model incorporates information regarding relatives diagnosed with early-onset breast cancer, male breast cancer, and ovarian cancer. As these women are at risk for breast and ovarian cancer, incorporating their information into the ROCA (risk of ovarian cancer algorithm) model may be helpful, with initial studies showing specificity of 99% and positive predictive value of 19%. Counseling must stress that these figures are estimates and not absolute risks, and thus balance the magnitude of risk for the individual patient.

Breast Cancer Risk Reduction

Risk reduction options in women at increased risk for breast cancer include increased cancer surveillance, chemoprevention, lifestyle modifications, and prophylactic (or risk-reducing) surgeries (mastectomy and/or oophorectomy).

Increased Surveillance

In a consensus statement by the Cancer Genetics Study Consortium (CGSC), it is recommended that carriers of BRCA mutations have vigilant surveillance through monthly self-examination beginning in early adulthood (18–21 years), annual or semiannual CBE, and annual mammography starting at age 25 to 30 years.

The benefit of close follow-up alone for women at increased risk of breast cancer seems questionable from National Surgical Adjuvant Breast Project (NSABP) P-1 data, wherein, despite the close follow-up mandated by the trial, fully 25% of the cancers found were greater than 2 cm in diameter and 29% node positive. Thus, it is not clear whether close clinical and yearly mammographic follow-up of women at high risk secondary to a family history or those harboring a BRCA1 and BRCA2 mutation will reduce mortality from breast cancer.

Although the 1994 NIH Consensus Development Conference concluded that "there is no evidence available as yet that the current screening modalities of CA125 and transvaginal ultrasonography can be effectively used for widespread disease screening," these currently available screening tests may be applicable to patients at risk for hereditary ovarian cancer syndromes with appropriate counseling.

Chemoprevention

Chemoprevention became an option for risk reduction based on information from the Breast Cancer Prevention Trial (BCPT), which was launched in 1992. This clinical trial (NSABP P-1) randomized 13,207 healthy women at increased risk for breast cancer (based on Gail model score >1.66, age older than 60 years, or history of lobular carcinoma *in situ*) in a double-blind fashion to receive either placebo or tamoxifen 20 mg/day. The short-term risk of invasive breast cancer was reduced by 43% and that of noninvasive cancer reduced by 37%, particularly in women with a history of atypical hyperplasia ($p < 0.00001$). Tamoxifen significantly reduced the rate of ER-positive tumors but had no effect on ER-negative tumors. However, as anticipated from the experience of women taking tamoxifen for breast cancer treatment, the drug was associated with an increased risk of thromboembolic disease, endometrial cancer, and cataracts. However, a decreased rate of fractures was noted. The earlier results of this trial prompted approval of tamoxifen by the FDA for use in the reduction of breast cancer incidence in 1998, despite two other negative trials from Europe. Several factors may account for the discrepancy, including dissimilar inclusion criteria, the length of treatment, and the length of follow-up.

The International Breast Intervention Study (IBIS 1) closely replicated the findings of the BCPT. In this trial, nearly 7,200 women aged 35 to 70 were randomized to receive tamoxifen or placebo. Women enrolled had a fourfold increased risk of breast cancer compared with the general population, in most cases based on family history. A 32% reduction was noted in the group receiving tamoxifen.

It is unclear how effective tamoxifen is in reducing breast cancer risk in women with hereditary breast cancer. Because the majority of cancers in BRCA1 mutation carriers are ER negative, one would not expect tamoxifen to be effective. However, BRCA2 carriers often have ER-positive tumors and thus are more likely to be responsive to tamoxifen chemoprophylaxis. Conversely, bilateral oophorectomy (which also affects the estrogen load) has been shown to reduce the risk of both ovarian and breast cancer (by 50%) in BRCA1 carriers.

Despite benefit seen in use of tamoxifen for chemoprevention, many eligible women are not accessing its use, usually because concerns about side effects. One such side effect includes hot flashes, which recent information indicates are not controlled by the addition of hormone therapy.

Raloxifene hydrochloride is a SERM that has antiestrogenic effects on breast and endometrial tissue and estrogenic effects on bone, lipid metabolism, and blood clotting. Raloxifene binds to estrogen receptors to competitively block estrogen-induced DNA transcription in the breast and endometrium. Because raloxifene does not increase the risk of endometrial cancer as seen with tamoxifen, it is particularly attractive as a preventive strategy in reducing the incidence of breast cancer. Raloxifene is being studied in the second NSABP prevention trial, the STAR (Study of Tamoxifen and Raloxifene) trial. This trial enrolled 6,139 postmenopausal women at increased risk for breast cancer in the first year. The study is designed to determine whether raloxifene (60 mg/day) is as effective as tamoxifen in reducing breast cancer risk. The results of this trial should be available in 2006. Results from the multicenter, randomized, double-blind Multiple Outcomes of Raloxifene Evaluation (MORE) trial revealed a 76% decreased risk of breast cancer among postmenopausal women with osteoporosis during 3 years of treatment with raloxifene; however, no objective tumor response was noted in patients with metastatic breast cancer in a phase II clinical trial. The trial was not accrued with breast cancer as a primary end point; thus, additional information is necessary to determine the possible benefits of this SERM over tamoxifen.

Many clinical trials are ongoing to determine additional effective options in the arena of chemoprevention. Based on benefits over tamoxifen noted in early breast cancer patients, aromatase inhibitors are being reviewed. Moreover, interest in using suppressants of prostaglandin synthesis has been stimulated by epidemiological observations that the use of aspirin and other NSAIDs is associated with a reduced incidence of breast cancer by nearly 30%. In preclinical models, COX-2 inhibitors reduced the incidence and growth of ER-positive tumors. Moreover, an additive effect with aromatase inhibitors in preventing tumor growth was also seen. NSAIDs function through inhibition of the cyclooxygenase enzyme (COX). The COX-2 enzyme is induced in both *in situ* and invasive breast cancers resulting in overexpression. COX-2 catalyzes the conversion of arachidonic acid to prostaglandin E_2. This prostaglandin in turn up-regulates a number of intracellular growth pathways, resulting in increased angiogenesis, induction of aromatase activity, cell growth, and division. It is postulated that inhibition of COX-2 may have a general anticancer effect via decreased blood vessel formation, decreased cell growth, and enhanced apoptosis, as has been seen in mammary carcinogenesis in rats. It remains to be seen if these findings can be extrapolated to humans, possibly resulting in modulation of a critical step in the initiation and promotion as well as progression of breast cancer. Overshadowing the magnitude of breast cancer reduction, however, are recent concerns regarding cardiovascular risks associated with this class of medications. Two randomized trials have yielded conflicting results. Born out of the premise that much of the gastrointestinal toxicity appeared to be related to COX-1 (which predominates in the gastric mucosa and yields protective prostaglandins), pharmaceutical efforts were rekindled toward development of a COX-2 inhibitor as an antiinflammatory agent without gastric toxicity. The Vioxx Gastrointestinal Outcomes Research Study (VIGOR: 8,076 patients) showed the relative risk of developing a cardiovascular event was nearly twofold greater in the COX-2 inhibitor rofecoxib compared with naproxen. The Celecoxib Long-term Arthritis Safety Study (CLASS; 8,059 patients) revealed no significant difference in cardiovascular event rates between celecoxib and NSAIDs. Of note, the annualized myocardial infarction rates for COX-2 inhibitors in both trials were significantly higher than that in the placebo group of a recent metaanalysis of prevention trials. Additional data reported at the European Congress on Rheumatology about a cohort of 651,000 adult patients featuring nearly 2.4 million patient years of follow-up support the notion that non–COX-2 inhibitor NSAIDS may have equivalent effectiveness in causing myocardial infarction as compared with COX-2 inhibitors (except rofecoxib, which has a higher rate than other noncoxibs). Thus, the available data raise a cautionary flag about the risk of cardiovascular events with COX-2 inhibitors and have prompted a black box warning by the FDA. Many ongoing prevention trials involving COX-2 inhibitors have consequently been placed on hold, and those continuing may now have difficulty accruing additional patients. Accordingly, additional trials using COX-2 inhibitors may be difficult to attain, although further analysis of prospective data is needed to characterize the magnitude of cardiovascular risk and breast cancer risk reduction. Trials such as PRECISION (Prospective Randomized Evaluation of Celecoxib Integrated Safety vs. Ibuprofen or Naproxen) was recently opened to evaluate this issue with the anticipated accrual of 20,000 patients. Results are expected in 2009.

Lipophilic statins (atrovastatin, simvastatin, lovastatin), which more readily permeate cell and nuclear membranes (which in theory should enhance full expression of the statins' pleiotropic benefits), have been shown to reduce the likelihood of developing ER-negative breast cancer. Mouse studies, which laid the groundwork for these studies, also showed that lipophilic statins conferred protection against ER-negative murine breast carcinoma. Based on these encouraging results and the statins' remarkably good safety profile, studies are developing to review these statins' role in breast cancer prevention.

Lifestyle Modification

Although heredity may be the strongest risk for development of breast and ovarian cancer syndromes, reproductive risk factors may be modifiable. Early age of first live birth and increased parity appear to lower the risk of breast cancer development. Use of fertility drugs and ovulation induction may need to be reevaluated. OCP use appears to increase the risk of breast cancer but decreases the risk of ovarian cancer. Modification of diet, alcohol consumption, exercise, or lactation is unlikely to have profound alterations, especially on genetically determined breast cancer risk. There are few prospective, randomized controlled studies that directly address breast cancer risk modification in women with hereditary breast cancer syndromes.

Prophylactic Surgeries

Prophylactic oophorectomy and mastectomy are attempts to remove at-risk healthy tissue before the onset of cancer. However, neither approach removes all the risk. Furthermore, there are undoubtedly modifying genes and environmental factors that play a role in the onset of carcinogenesis, but for BRCA1 and BRCA2 mutation carriers, these remain unknown.

Even though these women's greatest concern may be breast cancer, gynecologists should advise that they are also at risk for ovarian cancer and can substantially reduce risk by undergoing risk-reduction surgery. Analysis of case control data from women with a BRCA mutation demonstrated not only a 90% reduction in ovarian cancer risk but also a 60% reduction in breast cancer risk with bilateral prophylactic oophorectomy (BPO), especially when performed at an early age. Delaying BPO until age 40 years had minimal effect on the magnitude of risk reduction, suggesting that delaying surgery until after the completion of childbearing is a reasonable approach. Metcalfe and colleagues examined women with BRCA1 and -2 and a history of stage I or II breast cancer, and found that 10% developed an ovarian, fallopian tube, or peritoneal carcinoma. The median time was 8.1 years from the development of breast cancer to the development of ovarian cancer. Additionally, studies have shown that use of short-term hormone replacement (2–3 years) to abrogate immediate symptoms of surgically induced menopause in those BRCA mutation carriers undergoing BPO does not negate the protective effect of BPO on subsequent breast cancer risk.

Many prefer the terminology *risk reducing salpingo-oophorectomy* (RRSO) rather than BPO. General obstetricians/gynecologists are increasingly called on to perform this procedure. A number of studies have discovered that mutation carriers who undergo RRSO are at increased risk for occult malignancies already existing in the ovaries and fallopian tubes that are removed prophylactically. These studies recommend use of a specific surgical approach and pathologic examination of specimens. Powell and colleagues found an increased number of occult malignancies with this strategy: (i) complete removal of ovaries *and* fallopian tubes, (ii) serial histologic sectioning of both ovaries and fallopian tubes, (iii) peritoneal and omental biopsies, and (iv) peritoneal washings for cytology. Of 67 procedures, 7 (10.4%) occult malignancies were discovered: 4 in the fallopian tubes and 3 in the ovaries. Six of the occult malignancies were microscopic. Most importantly, physicians need to speak with the pathologist. For most benign cases in which the ovaries and fallopian tubes look grossly normal, pathologists take a single representative section of each ovary and fallopian tube for histologic diagnosis. However, in these high-risk cases, complete serial sectioning of ovaries and fallopian tubes is absolutely necessary to rule out microscopic cancer. Removal of the uterus should be based on other indications.

Prophylactic mastectomy has long been considered a potential approach to reducing the risk of breast cancer. A retrospective study by the Mayo Clinic reviewed women who underwent bilateral prophylactic subcutaneous mastectomy because of a strong family history of breast cancer. The authors demonstrated a 90% reduction in the risk of breast cancer and decreased mortality during 14 years of follow-up. Of interest, unsuspected cancers were found in the prophylactic mastectomy specimens. The costs (both emotional and financial) and benefits of these options must be carefully explained to the individual.

Initially, subcutaneous mastectomy was performed wherein breast tissue is removed with preservation of the nipple–areolar complex; however, subsequent cases of breast cancer development were noted. This procedure has been largely abandoned because only 90% to 95% of the breast parenchyma is removed, residual ductal tissue remains adherent to the undersurface of the nipple–areolar complex, and nipple sensation is not preserved. Conversely, simple or total mastectomy (skin-sparing removal of the breast tissue) has supplanted the subcutaneous procedure, because the cosmetic result after this procedure is excellent. Total mastectomy reduces the amount of breast tissue remaining postoperatively; however, cases of breast cancer after this procedure have been reported.

Although there is limited data regarding the efficacy of prophylactic surgery, statistical models suggest that certain woman at high risk for development of breast or ovarian cancer may gain 2.9 to 5.3 years of life expectancy by undergoing prophylactic mastectomies as well as 0.3 to 1.7 years in life expectancy with prophylactic oophorectomy. To place this gain in perspective, studies of mammography in normal risk women have life expectancy gains of less than 0.7 years. Whereas prophylactic surgery is not a panacea for women with a genetic predisposition for cancer, identification of the women at high risk and counseling of her options is an important aspect of her care. Prophylactic surgery may be a reasonable approach for women at substantially high risk for breast cancer who are willing to accept its irreversible consequence.

Staging

Partly as a result of widespread adherence to mammographic screening, breast cancer is being detected at earlier stages.

TABLE 41.11

STAGING FOR BREAST CARCINOMA

6th edition

The Staging of Cancer

Staging for Breast Carcinoma

DEFINITIONS:

PRIMARY TUMOR (T)

Definitions for classifying the primary tumor (T) are the same for clinical and for pathologic classification. If the measurement is made by physical examination, the examiner will use the major headings (T1, T2, or T3). If other measurements, such as mammographic or pathologic measurements are used, the subsets of T1 can be used. Tumors should be measured to the nearest 0.1 cm increment.

TX	Primary tumor cannot be assessed
T0	No evidence of primary tumor
Tis	Carcinoma in situ
(DCIS)	Ductal carcinoma in situ
(LCIS)	Lobular carcinoma in situ
(Paget)	Paget disease of the nipple with no tumor

Paget disease associated with a tumor is classified according to the size of the tumor.

T1	Tumor 2 cm or less in greatest dimension
T1mic	Microinvasion 0.1 cm or less in greatest dimension
T1a	Tumor more than 0.1 cm but not more than 0.5 cm in greatest dimension
T1b	More than 0.5 cm but not more than 1 cm in greatest dimension
T1c	More than 1 cm but not more than 2 cm in greatest dimension
T2	Tumor more than 2 cm but not more than 5 cm in greatest dimension
T3	Tumor more than 5 cm in greatest dimension
T4	Tumor of any size with direct extension to (a) chest wall or (b) skin, only as described below
T4a	Extension to chest wall, not including pectoralis muscle
T4b	Edema (including peau d'orange) or ulceration of the skin of breast, or satellite skin nodules confined to the same breast
T4c	Both T4a and T4b
T4d	Inflammatory carcinoma

Nearly 64% of white women and 53% of African-American women are presenting with localized disease. A critical aspect of breast cancer treatment is full knowledge of the extent of disease and microscopic features that contribute to the determination of the stage of disease, assist in the estimation of the risk of recurrence, and yield information predictive of tumor response. Breast cancer is staged clinically according to tumor size, regional lymph node involvement, and distant metastasis (TNM classification) (Table 41.11). The American Joint Committee on Cancer staging was modified in 2003 to incorporate a reclassification of nodal status by the number of involved lymph nodes and use of sentinel lymph node biopsy, distinguishing between micrometastases and isolated tumor cells on the basis of size and histologic evidence of malignant activity and change in staging if clavicular or internal mammary nodes are involved. These changes dramatically affect stage-specific survival.

Complete staging includes a thorough history, physical examination, bilateral mammography (ultrasound as necessary), pretreatment chest radiograph, and routine blood studies,

TABLE 41.11

STAGING FOR BREAST CARCINOMA (*Continued*)

REGIONAL LYMPH NODES (N)

Clinical

NX	Regional lymph nodes cannot be assessed (e.g., previously removed)
N0	No regional lymph node metastasis
N1	Metastasis to movable ipsilateral axillary lymph node(s)
N2	Metastases in ipsilateral axillary lymph nodes fixed or matted, or in clinically apparrent* ipsilateral internal mammary nodes in the *absence* of clinically evident axillary lymph node metastasis
N2a	Metastasis in ipsilateral axillary lymph nodes fixed to one another (matted) or to other structures
N2b	Metastasis only in clinically apparent* ipsilateral internal mammary nodes and in the *absence* of clinically evident axillary lymph node metastasis
N3	Metastasis in ipsilateral infraclavicular lymph node(s) with or without axillary lymph node involvement, or in clinically apparent* ipsilateral internal mammary lymph node(s) and in the *presence* of clinically evident axillary lymph node metastasis; or metastasis in ipsilateral supraclavicular lymph node(s) with or without axillary or internal mammary lymph node involvement
N3a	Metastasis in ipsilateral infraclavicular lymph node(s)
N3b	Metastasis in ipsilateral internal mammary lymph node(s) and axillary lymph node(s)
N3c	Metastasis in ipsilateral supraclavicular lymph node(s)

*Clinically apparent *is defined as detected by imaging studies (excluding lymphoscintigraphy) or by clinical examination or grossly visible pathologically.*

Pathologic (pN)[a]

pNX	Regional lymph nodes cannot be assessed (e.g., previously removed, or not removed for pathologic study)
pN0	No regional lymph node metastasis histologically, no additional examination for isolated tumor cells (ITC)

Isolated tumor cells (ITC) are defined as single tumor cells or small cell clusters not greater than 0.2 mm, usually detected only by immunobisiochemical (IHC) or molecular methods but which may be verified on H&E stains. ITCs do not usually show evidence of malignant activity, e.g., proliferation or stromal reaction.

pN0(i–)	No regional lymph node metastasis histologically, negative IHC
pN0(i+)	No regional lymph node metastasis histologically, positive IHC, no IHC cluster greater than 0.2 mm
pN0(mol–)	No regional lymph node metastasis histologically, negative molecular findings (RT•PCR)[b]

including hematology and liver panels. Pathology slides should be reviewed, and of course ER, PR, and HER2 status should be determined. Breast MRI may be considered for BCS for preoperative evaluation of the extent of disease and detection of mammographically occult disease in the breast; however, decision making should include tissue sampling of suspicious areas. Routine bone scan is not cost-effective in that only 0.6% of asymptomatic patients have a positive bone scan. However, bone scans may be helpful if patients experience localized symptoms, elevated alkaline phosphatase, or otherwise are at increased risk for metastasis. In addition, abdominal imaging is optional in early-stage disease but maybe helpful if elevated alkaline phosphatase, abnormal liver function tests, or advanced disease (stage III or above) is present.

Mammography is essential to adequate staging, even in the most obvious cases. Synchronous cancer is present in 4% to 5% of patients, and multicentric disease may be discovered in the involved breast. Furthermore, the clinical nodal status is often incorrect, with a false-positive and false-negative rate of approximately 25%. The pathologic stage of the primary lesion

TABLE 41.11

STAGING FOR BREAST CARCINOMA (*Continued*)

pN0(mol+)	No regional lymph node metastasis histologically, positive molecular findings (RT-PCR)[b]

[a]Classification is based on axillary lymph node dissection with or without sentinel lymph node dissection. Classification based solely on sentinel lymph node dissection without subsequent axillary lymph node dissection is designated (sn) for "sentinel node," e.g., pN0(i+) (sn).

bRT-PCR: reverse transcriptase/polymerase chain reaction.

pN1	Metastasis in 1 to 3 axillary lymph nodes, and/or in internal mammary nodes with microscopic disease detected by sentinel lymph node dissection but not clinically apparent**
pN1ml	Micrometastasis (greater than 0.2 mm, none greater than 2.0 mm)
pN1a	Metastasis in 1 to 3 axillary lymph nodes
pN1b	Metastasis in internal mammary nodes with microscopic disease detected by sentinel lymph node dissection but not clinically apparent**
pN1c	Metastasis in 1 to 3 axillary lymph nodes and in internal mammary lymph nodes with microscopic disease detected by sentinel lymph node dissection but not clinically apparent.** (If associated with greater than 3 positive axillary lymph nodes, the internal mammary nodes are classified as pN3b to reflect increased tumor burden)
pN2	Metastasis in 4 to 9 axillary lymph nodes, or in clinically apparent* internal mammary lymph nodes in the *absence* of axillary lymph node metastasis
pN2a	Metastasis in 4 to 9 axillary lymph nodes (at least one tumor deposit greater than 0.2 mm)
pN2b	Metastasis in clinically apparent* internal mammary lymph nodes in the *absence* of axillary lymph node metastasis
pN3	Metastasis in 10 or more axillary lymph nodes, or in infraclavicular lymph nodes, or in clinically apparent* ipsilateral internal mammary lymph nodes in the *presence* of 1 or more positive axillary lymph nodes; or in more than 3 axillary lymph nodes with clinically negative microscopic metastasis in internal mammary lymph nodes; or in ipsilateral supraclavicular lymph nodes
pN3a	Metastasis in 10 or more axillary lymph nodes (at least one tumor deposit greater than 2.0 mm), or metastasis to the infraclavicular lymph nodes
pN3b	Metastasis in clinically apparent* ipsilateral internal mammary lymph nodes in the *presence* of 1 or more positive axillary lymph nodes; or in more than 3 axillary lymph nodes and in internal mammary lymph nodes with microscopic disease detected by sentinel lymph node dissection but not clinically apparent**
pN3c	Metastasis in ipsilateral supraclavicular lymph nodes

*Clinically apparent *is defined as detected by imaging studies (excluding lymphoscintigraphy) or by clinical examination.*

*Not clinically apparent *is defined as not detected by imaging studies (excluding lymphoscintigraphy) or by clinical examination.*

based on histologic examination at the time of surgery is the main determinant of actuarial survival of the patient.

Staging is reflective of 5-year survival rates. The 5-year survival rate for localized breast cancer has increased from 72% in the 1940s to nearly 98%. If the cancer has spread regionally, however, the survival rate is 81%. There is a significant decrease in survival to 26% for women with distant spread. African-American women have a lower overall 5-year survival rate compared with Caucasian women (76.7% vs. 90.3%). This is surmised to be reflective of fewer presenting with early-stage disease or premature termination of chemotherapy. A better understanding of the determinants of suboptimal

TABLE 41.11

STAGING FOR BREAST CARCINOMA (*Continued*)

DISTANT METASTASIS (M)

MX	Distant metastasis cannot be assessed
M0	No distant metastasis
M1	Distant metastasis

STAGE GROUPING

Stage 0	Tis	N0	M0
Stage I	T1*	N0	M0
Stage IIA	T0	N1	M0
	T1*	N1	M0
	T2	N0	M0
Stage IIB	T2	N1	M0
	T3	N0	M0
Stage IIIA	T0	N2	M0
	T1*	N2	M0
	T2	N2	M0
	T3	N1	M0
	T3	N2	M0
Stage IIIB	T4	N0	M0
	T4	N1	M0
	T4	N2	M0
Stage IIIC	Any T	N3	M0
Stage IV	Any T	Any N	M1

**T1 includes T1mic.*

Stage designation may be changed if post-surgical imaging studies reveal the presence of distant metastasis, provided that the studies are carried out within 4 months of diagnosis in the absence of disease progression and provided that the patient has not received neoadjuvant therapy.

AMERICAN SOCIETY OF CLINICAL ONCOLOGY

No. 3485.22-Rev. 1/03

From Greene FL, Page DL, Fleming ID, et al. *AJCC cancer staging manual*, 6th ed. New York; Springer; 2002, with permission.

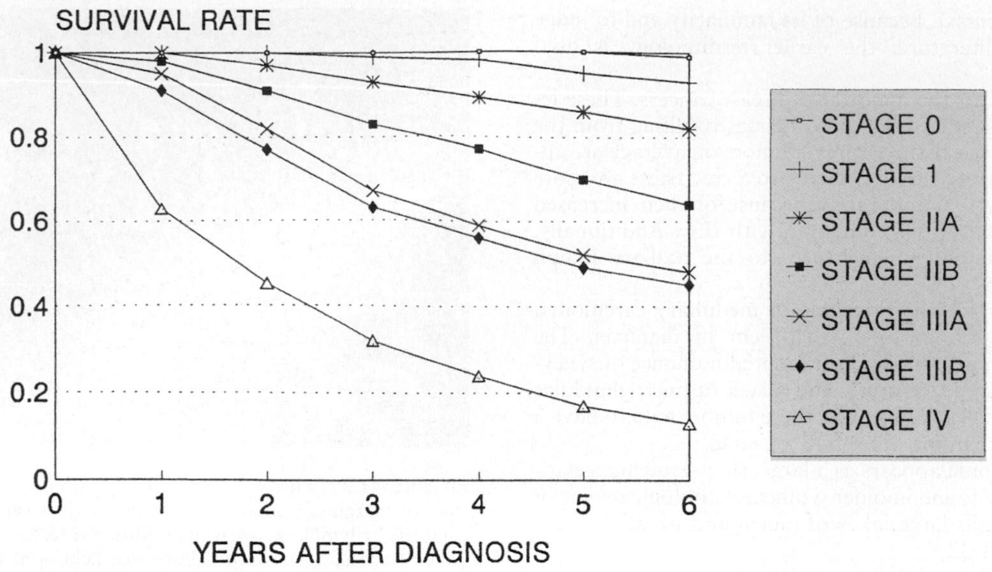

FIGURE 41.29. Relative survival rates according to stage of disease.

treatment may lead to interventions that can reduce racial disparities and improve breast cancer outcomes for all women (Fig. 41.29).

Pathology

Cancers of the mammary gland comprise a histologically heterogeneous group of tumors. More than 90% of breast cancers arise with the ducts. Infiltrating or invasive ductal carcinoma (IDC) is by far the most common histologic pattern of breast cancer seen, constituting 68% of cases (Fig. 41.30). Infiltrating lobular carcinoma (ILC) is the second most frequent cancer of the breast at 6.3% incidence. Other histologic subtypes include medullary carcinoma (2.8%), mucinous adenocarcinoma (2.2%), comedocarcinoma (1.4%), and Paget disease (1.1%). Papillary carcinoma, tubular adenocarcinoma, and inflammatory carcinoma each have an incidence of less than 1%. Inflammatory carcinoma is by far the most aggressive of the histologic types and has the poorest 5-year rate of 18%.

Terminology, however, has been confusing in that nearly three fourths of infiltrating carcinomas of the breast have been included in the imprecise category of *infiltrating ductal* or *adenocarcinoma, not otherwise specified.* Much of the terminology of breast cancer is divided into lobular and ductal, based principally on historical perspectives. Initially, early classifications used the term *lobular* to refer to lobular carcinoma *in situ,* and those without a lobular pattern were referred to as *ductal*; hence, the term *ductal* has no specific meaning. In fact, the majority of breast cancers originate in the terminal duct lobular unit, but these terms have impelling familiarity and are thus the basis of much of the scientific literature. Some authors promote the histologic classification that recognized special types of mammary carcinoma defined in terms of specific histologic criteria (lobular, tubular, medullary, and

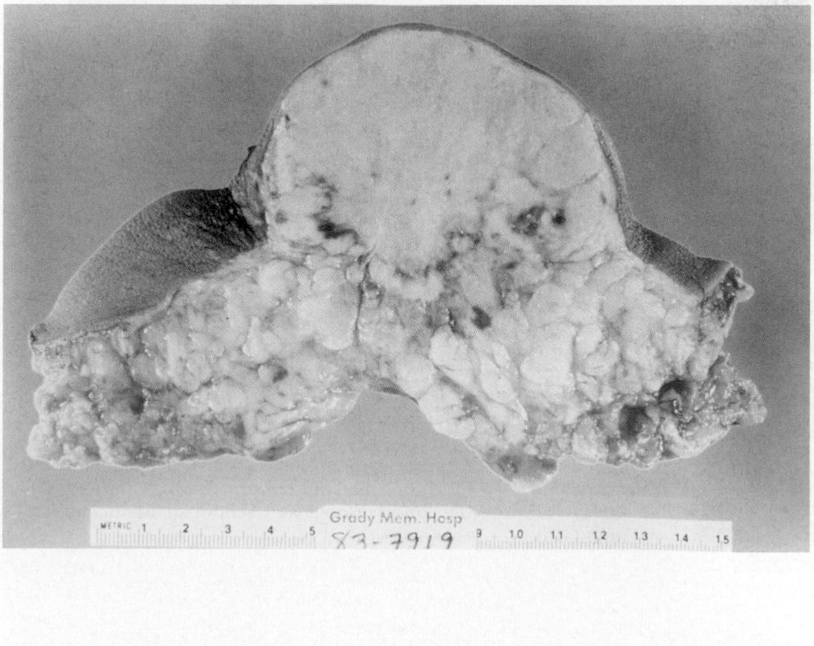

FIGURE 41.30. Invasive breast cancer. This mastectomy specimen shows a large tumor growing under the epidermis above and invading the soft tissue below. Foci of hemorrhage (*black areas*) are seen in the tumor.

mucinous carcinomas). Because of its familiarity and to judge against current literature, the earlier terminology is used herein.

IDC accounts for the majority of breast cancers. These lesions usually present as stony hard masses resulting from the density of the fibrous tissue stroma. Tumors on average are approximately 2 cm and rarely exceed 4 to 5 cm. These are more often detected by mammography because of their increased frequency of calcifications compared with ILC. Additionally, this variant commonly metastasizes to the axillary lymph nodes.

Fleshy tumors are characteristic of medullary carcinoma, which can measure up to 5 to 10 cm in diameter. The histopathologic appearance exhibits a predominance of syncytial cells, lymphocytic infiltrate, and a lack of microglandular structure (Fig. 41.31). As a group, these tumors tend to have a better prognosis than the other IDC variants.

Colloid carcinoma appears as a large, slow-growing, gelatinous mass usually found in older women. Pathologic review of the specimen reveals large lakes of mucin and isolated tumor groupings (Fig. 41.32).

Paget disease is another form of IDC that originates in the excretory ducts of the breast. Involvement of the nipple–areolar complex may result in a firm consistency of the nipple, inflammation, ulceration, edema, and "weeping" of the skin. Characteristic Paget cells appear in the epidermis as large anaplastic cells surrounded by a clear halo. Paget may present solely with skin changes and the absence of an underlying mass. Thus, any nipple rash or skin changes that do not resolve with symptomatic treatment in a few weeks should be evaluated with dermatologic punch biopsy.

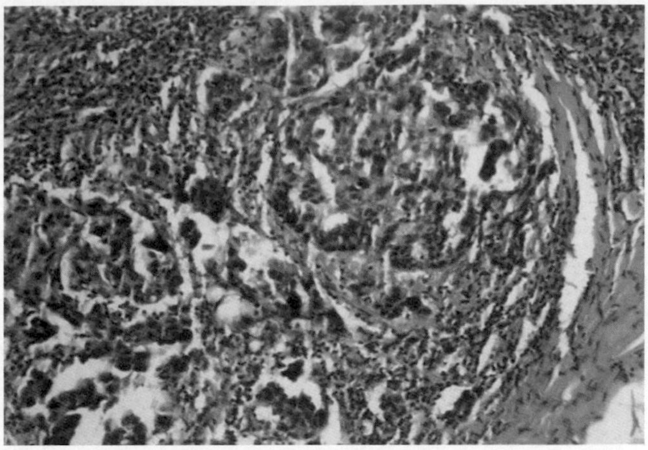

FIGURE 41.31. Histologic section of medullary carcinoma showing smooth margins, primitive malignant cells in syncytial growth surrounded by lymphoplasmacytic infiltrate (H&E ×240). (Courtesy of Taalat Tadros, MD, Emory University, School of Medicine, Atlanta, GA.)

Finally, ILC arises from the terminal ductules of the breast and tends to be multifocal within the same breast as well as frequently bilateral. Involvement of the contralateral breast occurs in 20% of cases. Histologically, loosely, dispersed single-cell columns form strands of infiltrating tumor cells (Fig. 41.33).

In situ or noninvasive histologic variants of breast cancer also exist. Coincident with the widespread use of screening

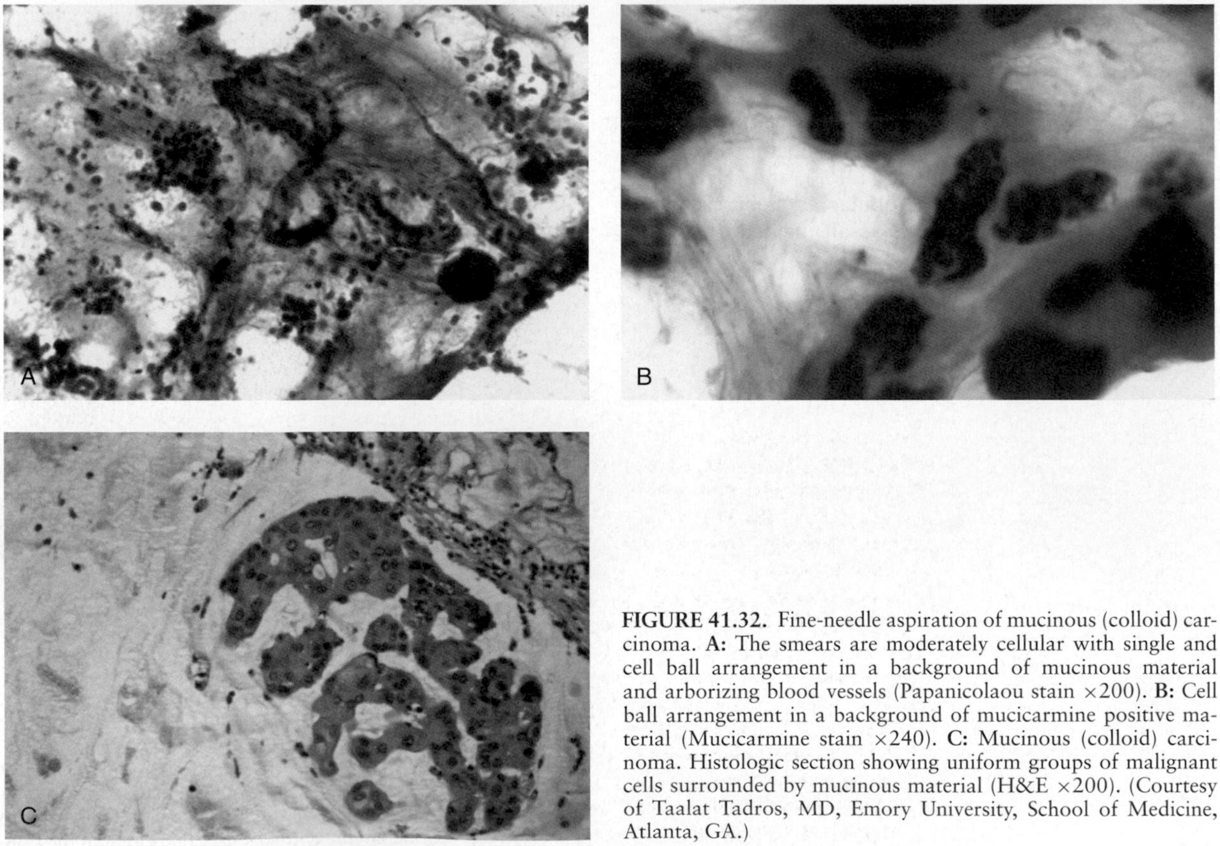

FIGURE 41.32. Fine-needle aspiration of mucinous (colloid) carcinoma. **A:** The smears are moderately cellular with single and cell ball arrangement in a background of mucinous material and arborizing blood vessels (Papanicolaou stain ×200). **B:** Cell ball arrangement in a background of mucicarmine positive material (Mucicarmine stain ×240). **C:** Mucinous (colloid) carcinoma. Histologic section showing uniform groups of malignant cells surrounded by mucinous material (H&E ×200). (Courtesy of Taalat Tadros, MD, Emory University, School of Medicine, Atlanta, GA.)

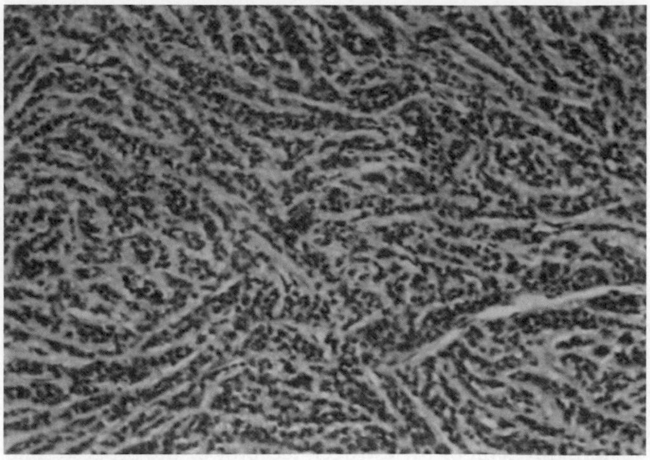

FIGURE 41.33. Histology of infiltrating lobular carcinoma, showing characteristic single small malignant cells in an Indian file pattern. Cells are diffusely infiltrating the stroma (H&E ×240). (Courtesy of Taalat Tadros, MD, Emory University, School of Medicine, Atlanta, GA.)

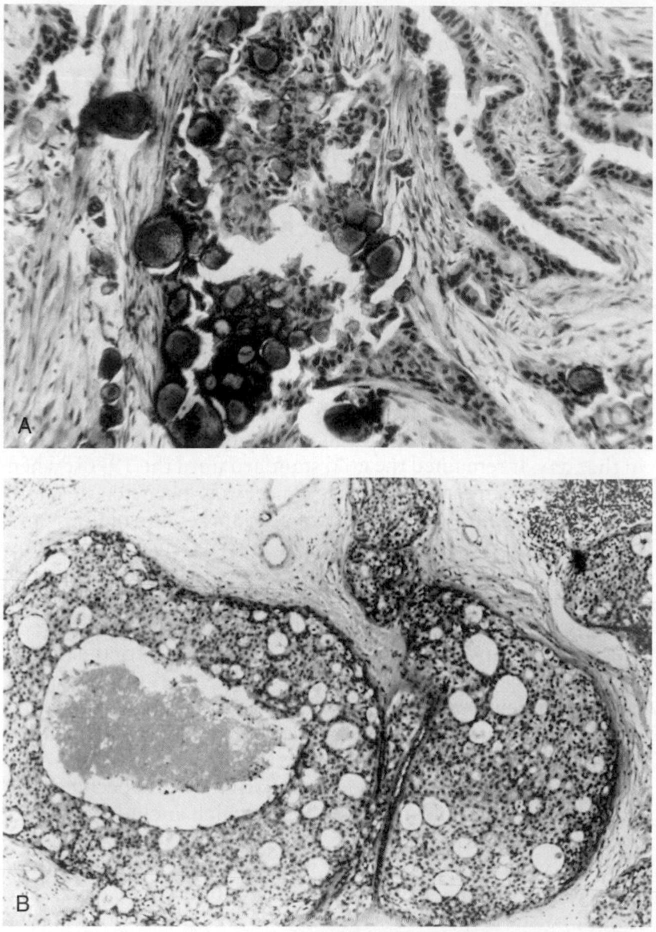

FIGURE 41.34. Ductal carcinoma *in situ*. **A:** A dilated duct is filled with proliferating atypical ductal cells interspersed with multiple microcalcifications. The microcalcifications were identified by mammogram. **B:** Ductal carcinoma *in situ* with central necrosis suggesting a comedo pattern.

mammography, there has been a shift in the stage at presentation of breast cancer toward earlier-stage disease, particularly for ductal carcinoma *in situ* (DCIS) (Fig. 41.34). Data from Surveillance, Epidemiology, and End Results (SEER) shows nearly 300% change in incidence of DCIS in women age 50 years and older and greater than 100% increase in the incidence of stage I disease in the same group. The percentage of change was more pronounced in African-American women than in white women. DCIS is a nonobligatory precursor to IDC with variable rates of progression, depending on histology, size, and margin status. DCIS refers to lesions with proliferation of malignant cells within the ductal system of the breast but without invasion of the stromal tissue (basement membrane). This category represents 20% of all newly diagnosed breast cancers with a 20-year survival rate of 97%. In at least 90% of patients, the diagnosis is made with mammography. Only about 10% of patients have a palpable mass. Because of the controversy as to the potential for progression of DCIS to IDC, optimal management is one of the biggest challenges in breast disease faced by clinicians. Although DCIS is a preinvasive form of breast cancer and is not life threatening, treatment options may include lumpectomy, mastectomy, radiotherapy, and/or tamoxifen. Current treatment modalities may be overly aggressive because many cases of DCIS may not recur or progress to invasive cancer. Conservative contemporary treatments include lumpectomy with breast irradiation, generally excluding axillary lymph node dissection. Evidence is accumulating that DCIS <2 cm may not require irradiation. However, sentinel lymph node biopsy may be useful in evaluating large or high-grade lesions because of the increased risk of undetected microinvasion. Historically, multicentricity was used to justify mastectomy for DCIS. In the literature, estimates of multicentricity in DCIS range widely, from 2% to 78% depending on the definition and mode of detection. Until we are better able to identify those patients at low risk for progression, it is unlikely that current treatment will change. Genomics holds great promise in this regard, yet prospective studies with long-term follow-up will be needed before treatment can be personalized for individual subsets.

Lobular carcinoma *in situ* (LCIS) refers to proliferation of cells within the breast lobules. LCIS is considered a predictive marker of future cancer rather than a cancer precursor. It is usually found *incidentally* by microscopy at the time of breast biopsy performed for another indication and does not present characteristic clinical or mammographic findings. It is typically multicentric and has a sevenfold to 10-fold increased risk of subsequent invasive breast cancer, which is typically ductal carcinoma. Studies of women with LCIS managed with biopsy alone demonstrate a risk of cancer development of approximately 1% per year.

Breast cancer may present with a firm consistency, fixed position (lack of mobility), dimpling or retraction of the overlying skin, nipple retraction, and irregular shape. Peau d'orange skin changes are associated with obstruction of the lymphatics and associated edema. This characteristic feature is not always associated with breast cancer and may be seen with mastitis. IDC frequently metastasizes to bone, lung, liver, or brain, whereas ILC more often metastasizes to meningeal serosal surfaces. On the other hand, inflammatory cancer causes extensive swelling, redness, and tenderness, which is often mistaken for a hematoma or abscess.

In general, breast cancer is slightly more common in the left breast than in the right. In most women, the left breast is slightly larger than the right. The upper outer quadrant is more frequently involved in malignant changes (this is the site of the highest distribution of breast tissue), with the central and subareolar regions being second.

TREATMENT

Surgical Techniques

The first recorded operative treatment for breast cancer was in the Greco-Roman period 220 B.C. by a Greek physician named Leonides. A century ago, William Halsted published his first paper on the radical mastectomy for the control of breast cancer. This procedure was very extensive, including removal of the breast tissue en bloc, pectoralis muscles, and axillary lymph nodes to achieve superior local and regional control of disease in that day. It remained the gold standard until the 1970s, when the trend in surgery for breast cancer has been to use more limited procedures. Taking into account comorbidities and the patient's preferences, treatment may involve lumpectomy (local removal of the tumor); mastectomy (surgical removal of all the breast tissue); sentinel lymph node biopsy and/or axillary lymphadenectomy; radiation therapy; chemotherapy; or hormone therapy based on the stage and histology of the tumor, completeness of removal (i.e., status of the margins of the surgical specimen), and prognostic factors, including lymph node involvement, tumor size and grade, hormone receptor status, HER2-neu status, and S-phase fraction.

Currently, long-term updates of original prospective clinical trials have confirmed that BCS, which includes lumpectomy, postoperative radiation therapy, and surgical axillary staging (when appropriate), is the appropriate primary therapy for most women with stage I and II breast cancer. The largest of the BCS trials, NSABP B-06, reviewed women over 15 years and proved the equivalence of the treatments. Other studies have shown congruent results demonstrating no statistically significant differences between rates of local and regional recurrences, distant metastasis, and overall survival between mastectomy and BCS with early-stage disease. Tumor recurrence is 40% with BCS but is decreased to 10% with the addition of radiation therapy, which is similar to treatment with modified radical mastectomy. The appropriate candidate for mastectomy is primarily the patient in whom it is evident that BCS will not control the primary tumor. Cosmetic factors are important, but the primary concern is adequate removal of the primary tumor with pathologically negative margins. One other concern with respect to BCS is the necessity for radiation therapy and continued intense surveillance. For this reason, patients with certain medical conditions, such as active or preexisting collagen vascular disease, may not be candidates for BCS, because these patients have been shown to have poor tolerance to radiation in the breast and chest wall areas (Tables 41.12 and 41.13). Complete axillary dissection continues to assume a position of diminishing importance in the treatment of breast carcinoma but remains controversial. As the role for systemic therapy even in patients with negative nodes expands, some investigators have stated that not all patients require an axillary dissection, but 30% of patients with no palpable lymph nodes (clinically negative axilla) have been found to have histologically positive lymph nodes. Because axillary nodal status is the best established indicator of their risk for systemic relapse, the potential of the more limited sentinel lymph node evaluation is evident (discussed below).

For patients with negative axillary involvement, the tumor size and histologic grade are the most useful prognostic factors.

TABLE 41.12

ABSOLUTE CONTRAINDICATIONS TO BREAST CONSERVATION SURGERY

Prior moderate- or high-dose radiation therapy to the breast/chest wall
Pregnancy (as required radiation therapy is contraindicated)
Diffuse suspicious or malignant-appearing microcalcifications on mammography
Multicentric/widespread disease
Positive pathologic margin (reexcision may be an option)

Among patients with invasive tumors of less than 1 cm in greatest diameter, the 5-year disease-free survival rate is more than 90%. Expression of the estrogen receptor or the progesterone receptor is associated with a better prognosis, primarily attributable to the responsiveness of these tumors to antiestrogen therapies, for example, tamoxifen and aromatase inhibitors.

HER2 amplification has been associated with a poor prognosis; however, the role of HER2/neu as a prognostic factor remains controversial. The role of HER2 as a predictor of response to chemotherapy is discussed in the section on tumor-specific therapies.

There is no clear evidence to suggest that women with breast cancer associated with a BRCA1 or BRCA2 mutation should be managed differently from those with sporadic cancers. BCS remains the standard of care for women with early-stage sporadic breast cancer and is routinely offered to mutation carriers who have been diagnosed with breast cancer. BRCA mutation carriers are at increased risk for contralateral breast cancers; this risk may be as high as 60%. Thus, questions exist regarding optimal surgical management. Researchers question whether these patients may benefit from an ipsilateral mastectomy on the affected breast and contralateral prophylactic mastectomy on the unaffected breast. Thus, advance knowledge of one's BRCA status may be important in determining surgical options.

Image-Guided Ablation Techniques

Ablative procedures can be performed in the office or ambulatory surgical setting and may offer patients an alternative to surgical excision. Ablative techniques were initially used on metastatic hepatic tumors with success; thus, similar technology is now being applied to the treatment of breast disease. Ablative therapy uses radiofrequency, cryoablation, laser, microwave, and focused ultrasound in clinical protocols as a minimally invasive treatment modality for small malignant and benign breast tumors. Data are available that demonstrate

TABLE 41.13

RELATIVE CONTRAINDICATIONS TO BREAST CONSERVATION SURGERY

Large tumor/breast ratio (cosmetic result)
Large breast size (difficult to radiate)
Focally positive pathologic margins
Active connective tissues disease involving the skin (especially scleroderma and lupus)

variable success in tissue destruction using different modalities. Long-term follow up data regarding local effects on the breast tissue or recurrence rates of cancer are not available, and local breast changes may pose a diagnostic dilemma in future trials to distinguish recurrent cancer from scar or fat necrosis.

Sentinel Lymph Node Biopsy

The status of axillary nodes is one of the most well-established prognostic indicators for systemic relapse used to select patient subgroups for adjuvant chemotherapy. Patients with involvement of the lymph nodes have a 60% to 70% risk for relapse within 5 years, whereas 70% to 80% of patients with negative nodes are cured by local therapy. Yet currently, there is no evidence that axillary lymph node dissection (ALND) improves survival, thus diminishing its importance. ALND, however, is an effective staging procedure and may be essential for local control of disease in the axilla. In general, the standard treatment of the axilla involves level I and level II axillary lymph nodes. This is extended to level III only if gross disease is apparent for treatment of stages I, IIA, and IIb cancer.

The prior standard of care for surgical management of invasive disease was complete excision of the tumor by either mastectomy or lumpectomy followed by ALND. Based on information gathered from treatment of melanomas, it was established that the first lymph node (the sentinel node) to receive drainage from the primary tumor can be used to predict the presence or absence of tumor in the remainder of the lymph nodes. Published and unpublished results in breast carcinoma surgery support the same concept for axillary node breast metastases. Intraoperative lymphatic mapping and sentinel lymph node biopsy (SLNB) has emerged as an alternative to routine ALND in clinically node-negative early breast cancer and represents a major new opportunity obviating the need for more invasive surgical management of many tumors. Lymphatic mapping with selective lymphadenectomy is an attractive approach in breast cancer patients because it may lead to a substantial reduction in the need for axillary node dissection without compromising survival and regional control and without loss of prognostic staging information, thus translating into a significant reduction in patient morbidity and medical expenses. SLNB is highly accurate and sensitive in patients with small tumors, and no false-negative SLNB has been reported for a breast cancer smaller than 1.0 to 1.5 cm, resulting in a negative predictive value of 100%. In the future, axillary dissection might be avoided in patients who have no metastatic involvement of the sentinel lymph node; however, if the sentinel lymph node cannot be identified or is positive for metastasis, a formal ALND should be performed (or in some cases, axillary radiation therapy administered).

The surgeon can use two techniques to find the node. The technique of intraoperative sentinel lymph node mapping was pioneered by Giuliano and is performed using a blue dye injected peritumorally, which stains the lymphatic duct (Fig. 41.35). After 5 minutes, blue dye can be visualized traversing afferent lymphatics and collecting in an sentinel lymph node through an axillary incision at the tumor site. There is a 93.5% success rate in identifying an axillary node as the sentinel node. The false-negative rate has been 0%. Alternatively,

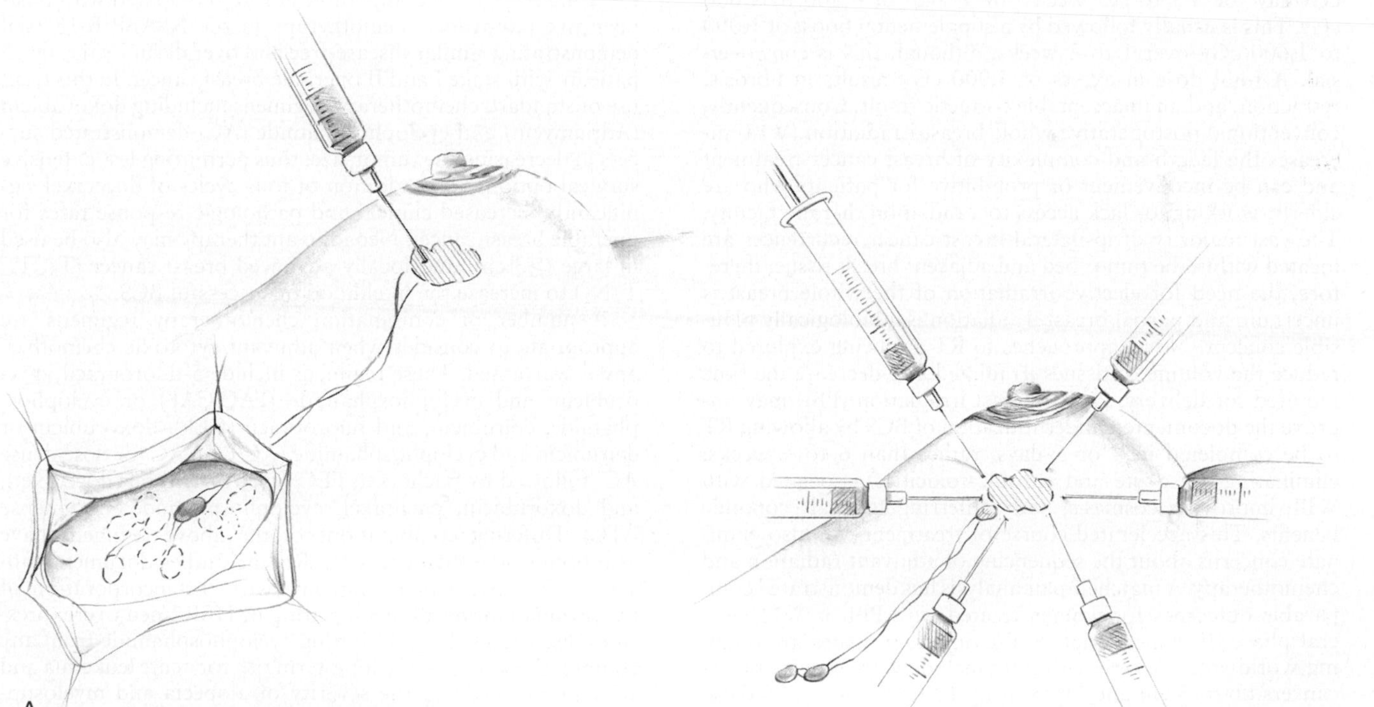

FIGURE 41.35. Sentinel lymph node mapping. **A:** Schematic diagram depicting the transit of blue dye, injected into the primary breast cancer, to the sentinel lymph node. **B:** Injection technique for lymphatic mapping and sentinel lymphadenectomy showing peritumoral injection. For a palpable lesion, dye is injected into the breast parenchyma around the tumor. If the tumor has previously been removed, dye is injected into the wall of the biopsy cavity.

a lymph node–seeking radioactive tracer (^{99m}Tc) migrates from the tumor site (when injected into the breast parenchyma) to the sentinel node and enables its retrieval with the use of a gamma detection probe. Blue dye and lymphoscintigraphy are complementary techniques, and optimal localization is achieved when the two methods are used together. Several authors have achieved greater than 95% success rate and quote a sensitivity of 98% when the procedures are used complementarily. Other variations of the procedure have been espoused, including the addition of ultrasound to the protocol and endoscopic axillary clearance after liposuction.

Radiation

The role of radiation therapy (RT) in breast cancer treatment has been more clearly defined in the last 2 decades. RT may be applied to invasive and noninvasive disease. It is a standard component of BCS and has been shown to be of benefit postmastectomy in patients with large tumor burdens or more than four positive lymph nodes.

Recent results from an Intergroup study found lower rates of recurrence in the radiation arm but no differences in survival or disease-free survival in a group of women with early-stage breast cancer older than age 70 when randomized to receive whole breast irradiation plus tamoxifen or tamoxifen alone. Thus, women older than 70 with early-stage ER-positive disease and negative lymph nodes may be treated without breast irradiation in conjunction with BCS. RT should begin as soon as the wounds of surgery are healed and may be given concurrently with certain chemotherapy regimens. It is generally agreed that the breast should be treated with 180 to 200 cGy/day for 4.5 to 5.5 weeks for a total of 4,500 to 5,000 cGy. This is usually followed by a supplemental boost of 1,000 to 1,600 cGy over 1 to 2 weeks, although this is controversial. A total dose in excess of 5,000 cGy results in fibrosis, retraction, and an unacceptable cosmetic result. Consequently, conventional postoperative whole breast irradiation (WBI) increases the length and complexity of breast cancer treatment and can be inconvenient or prohibitive for patients who are elderly, working, or lack access to a radiation therapy facility. The vast majority of ipsilateral breast cancer recurrences are located within the tumor bed and adjacent breast tissue; therefore, the need for elective irradiation of the whole breast is uncertain, and partial breast irradiation is a biologically plausible concept. Novel approaches to RT are being explored to reduce the volume of tissues irradiated and decrease the time required for delivery. Partial breast irradiation (PBI) may improve the documented underutilization of BCS by allowing RT to be completed in 4 or 5 days, rather than 6 to 7 weeks; eliminating the acute and chronic toxicities associated with WBI; improving cosmesis; and conferring societal economic benefits. This accelerated course of treatment can also eliminate concerns about the sequencing of adjuvant radiation and chemotherapy. A matched-pair analysis has demonstrated comparable outcomes for women treated with PBI or WBI. Several phase III clinical trials evaluating these issues are ongoing worldwide. Criteria currently include women with breast cancers up to 3 cm and DCIS using 10 fractions over 5 days. Before PBI can be routinely incorporated into clinical practice, appropriate patient selection, optimal fractionation schedules, and PBI techniques must be determined, as well as establishment of long-term efficacy, rates of locoregional recurrence, survival rates, cosmesis, and patient satisfaction. Options for PBI currently include interstitial catheter brachytherapy and balloon-based intracavitary brachytherapy (MammoSite, Alpharetta, GA). Additional trials are focusing on intraoperative radiation therapy, three-dimensional conformal RT, and other novel techniques.

Radiation is also useful in the palliative treatment of bone pain in advanced metastatic disease. Complications of radiation therapy include fatigue and development of dry skin, erythema or tanning, edema, and muscle stiffness within the tissues encompassed by the radiation beam. After completion of the irradiation treatment, most patients recover their normal skin color and texture within a few weeks, but edema can take much longer to resolve. Late complications from RT are unusual, including a very low incidence of rib fracture, radiation pneumonitis, brachyplexopathy, and pericarditis in cases of left-sided lesions. In the overwhelming majority of cases, a return to normal is the rule.

Systemic Therapy

Therapeutic options for patients with noninvasive or invasive breast cancer are complex and varied. Use of additional systemic therapy is based on the patient's likelihood of recurrence and predicted response to hormonal or chemotherapy. This can be estimated with use of an online model, ADJUVANTONLINE!. In addition, newer molecular techniques, including proteomic and genomic analysis, are being developed that may add greater specificity to treatment decisions.

Cytotoxic Chemotherapy

Neoadjuvant (preoperative) chemotherapy is increasingly used, presumably associated with eradication of micrometastatic disease, and has shown comparable efficacy compared with postoperative (adjuvant) chemotherapy in the NSABP B-18 trial demonstrating similar disease-free and overall survival rates in patients with stage I and II operable breast cancer. In this trial, use of standard chemotherapy regimens including doxorubicin (Adriamycin) and cyclophosphamide (AC) demonstrated success in decreasing the tumor size, thus permitting less extensive surgical options. The addition of four cycles of docetaxel significantly increased clinical and pathologic response rates for operable breast cancer. Neoadjuvant therapy may also be used in large ($\geq$3 cm) and locally advanced breast cancer (T_3, T_4, T_xN_2) to increase the likelihood of successful BCS.

A number of combination chemotherapy regimens are appropriate to consider when adjuvant cytotoxic chemotherapy is warranted. These regimens include 5-fluorouracil, doxorubicin, and cyclophosphamide (FAC/CAF) or cyclophosphamide, epirubicin, and fluorouracil (CEF); doxorubicin or epirubicin and cyclophosphamide (AC/EC); AC (or dose dense AC) followed by paclitaxel; FEC (with or without docetaxel); and doxorubicin, paclitaxel, cyclophosphamide (dose-dense ATC). Differing combinations of the above regimens have also been studied with success. Recent studies document substantial improvement in outcome with the incorporation of trastuzumab in the adjuvant setting of HER2/neu overexpression (discussed below). Omitting cyclophosphamide from any combination obviates the long-term risk for acute leukemia and substantially reduces the severity of alopecia and myelosuppression; thus, it is a better tolerated regimen. Fifty percent to 80% of women have an objective response to FAC, and 40% to 60% have an objective response to CMF (cyclophosphamide, methotrexate and fluorouracil). Studies of CMF chemotherapy versus no chemotherapy have shown disease-free and overall survival advantages with CMF chemotherapy. Regimens containing anthracyclines (doxorubicin or epirubicin) were superior to CMF in the Early Breast Cancer Trialists' Collaborative Group overview. These chemotherapy regimens may cause short-term complications, including nausea, vomiting, myelosuppression, alopecia, and weight gain. Use of anthracycline-based chemotherapy has the long-term risks of chemotherapy-induced ovarian ablation (70%), cardiac dysfunction, premature menopause, and secondary malignancies. Node-positive patients may benefit from the addition of paclitaxel to the AC regimen; therefore, until other studies are analyzed, treating node-positive patients with four cycles of AC (or CAF) followed by four cycles of paclitaxel is reasonable.

Common toxicities include nausea, vomiting, alopecia, fatigue, mucositis, weight gain, premature menopause, neuropathy (taxanes), and myalgias (taxanes). Less common toxicities include febrile neutropenia (common with TAC) thrombosis, hemorrhagic complications, cardiomyopathy (anthracyclines), and secondary leukemia.

Adjuvant therapy has also been proven to have added benefit for node-negative patients with breast cancer. Zambetti and colleagues found adjuvant chemotherapy increases disease-free survival in 85% of patients compared with 42% of untreated control subjects. Similar values have been verified in other studies. The goal is to determine which node-negative patients are at high risk for recurrence to avoid further unnecessary treatment in patients already cured of their disease.

Several prognostic factors are currently used to predict risk of relapse or death from breast cancer. The strongest are patient age, comorbidity, the number of involved lymph nodes, tumor diameter/grade, and receptor status. Other less well-established prognosticators include S-phase fraction (an indicator of proliferative capacity), HER2/neu overexpression, histology, nuclear grade, and DNA aneuploidy. The innovative technique of DNA microarray is poised to revolutionize the treatment of breast cancer patients. Classification systems of breast cancer subtypes have been developed by gene expression profile. In retrospective analysis, these subtypes have shown differing relapse-free and overall survival, thus permitting both prognostic and predictive functions. Additionally, a multigene assay using reverse transcription polymerase chain reaction on RNA isolated from paraffin-embedded tissue was able to identify prognostic subsets and to predict responsiveness to both tamoxifen and CMF or methotrexate/5-fluorouracil/leucovorin chemotherapy.

Thus, node-negative women with moderately or poorly differentiated invasive tumors of larger than 1 cm and negative hormone receptors should be offered chemotherapy. Because the risk for node-negative patients with well-differentiated tumors of less than 1 cm in size is 10% or less, adjuvant chemotherapy is not recommended. In addition to chemotherapy, patients who are premenopausal (or younger than 50 years of age) with negative nodes and ER-positive tumors should be considered for a 5-year course of tamoxifen because even in node-negative patients, 30% of patients have a relapse in 5 years. The treatment of postmenopausal patients with negative nodes and hormone receptor–positive tumors is evolving. Randomized clinical trials showed that chemotherapy plus tamoxifen yields better survival rates than tamoxifen alone, but the absolute benefit is small and the use of chemotherapy in this setting should be individualized. Recent data on trends in breast cancer treatment indicates an increasing proportion of women receiving both chemotherapy and tamoxifen with ER-positive tumors and positive lymph node status as recommended by evidence-based guidelines from the NIH. However, use of concurrent therapy remained relatively low among women aged 65 and older, who were more likely to receive tamoxifen only. The international consensus panel recommends hormonal therapy as the treatment of choice for ER-positive women with limited disease regardless of menopausal status, tumor size, or axillary involvement, especially for patients who are asymptomatic or are of advanced age. Hormone receptor status determines the likelihood that a patient will respond to hormonal therapy, with 75% to 80% of patients with estrogen receptor/progesterone receptor–positive tumors showing an objective response. Even patients with ER/progesterone receptor–negative tumors had a 10% objective response rate.

Hormonal Therapy

Breast cancers are often exquisitely sensitive to endocrine manipulation, thus laying the foundation for the success of antiestrogens in the fight against cancer. Endocrine therapies have been a critical factor in the dramatic decline in mortality from this disease in both the United Kingdom and the United States. Since the introduction of tamoxifen in the 1970s, endocrine therapy for breast cancer has enjoyed a remarkable renaissance with the generation of data touting the benefits of aromatase inhibitors in hormone responsive breast cancer treatment as well.

Selective Estrogen Receptor Modulators

Tamoxifen citrate has been shown to be of immense significance in the battle against breast cancer. Tamoxifen has demonstrated benefit when used alone or in combination with chemotherapy in the treatment of advanced breast cancer and has proven efficacy in reducing tumor recurrence, prolonging disease-free survival, and lowering the incidence of contralateral second primary breast cancer by nearly 40% when administered as postoperative adjuvant therapy in stages I and II disease. The improved effectiveness of tamoxifen in this setting prompted its use in the preventive setting in the NSABP P-1 and BCPT trials (discussed earlier under "Chemoprevention"). Although relatively well tolerated compared with cytotoxic chemotherapy, tamoxifen is beset with side effects, particularly hot flashes (30%), vaginal discharge, vaginal bleeding, endometrial cancer, and thromboembolic events. However, it has been suggested that for every endometrial cancer death, 80 breast cancer deaths have been averted with the use of tamoxifen.

SERMs were first evaluated in the 1960s as nonsteroidal antiestrogens. This group of drugs showed potent antifertility activity in rats, but paradoxically proved to be an inducer of ovulation in subfertile women. Clomiphene is a SERM that remains a vital part of the regimen for ovulation induction. Further study was commenced based on the compound's multifaceted actions on different types of receptors. Ancillary studies in this group of drugs focused on treatments for advanced breast cancer; however, only tamoxifen was investigated further because of its high potency, efficacy, and modest side effects.

The strategic application of these medications was first noted in long-term adjuvant treatment of node-positive and node-negative, ER-positive breast cancers. Tamoxifen decreases the serum levels of total cholesterol by 13% and those of low-density lipoprotein cholesterol by 19%. Therefore, tamoxifen has the added benefit of maintaining bone density and reducing the risk of myocardial infarction in postmenopausal women. Thus, despite known benefits of aromatase inhibitors, tamoxifen may remain the standard in patients with osteopenia or osteoporosis.

Several new SERMs are under investigation. Raloxifene has shown benefit for breast cancer prevention in postmenopausal women with osteoporosis; clinical trials are ongoing. Toremifene (Fareston® has shown efficacy similar to tamoxifen and may be a reasonable first-line alternative. Because of substantial cross-resistance between toremifene and tamoxifen, there is no role in patients who have tumors resistant to tamoxifen. Droloxifene and idoxifene have had minimal evaluation but show binding affinity to ER-positive breast cancers and response rates of 0% to 70%.

Aromatase Inhibitors

Aromatase inhibitors (AIs)—generally anastrozole, letrozole, and exemestane—have made an exciting contribution to the management of hormone-responsive breast cancer. A plethora of studies has shown the superiority of AIs over tamoxifen in postmenopausal patients with ER-positive tumors. Current therapy in these patients may include tamoxifen for 5 years, AI for 5 years, combination of tamoxifen and AI for 5 years, and addition of AI for 5 years at the end of the tamoxifen treatment.

AIs function through inhibition of aromatization, thus blocking the enzyme that catalyzes the final and rate-limiting step in the synthesis of estrogens. Currently, studies are noting benefit primarily in postmenopausal women in whom production of aromatase in nonovarian tissues in the periphery (such as adipose tissue, adrenal gland, and muscle) are the dominant sources of estrogen. Now in their third generation, AIs (specifically anastrozole) have proven superior to tamoxifen in a RCT (ATAC—Arimidex, tamoxifen, alone or in combination trial) of treatment of 9,366 postmenopausal women with localized breast cancer with respect to disease-free survival, time to recurrence, incidence of contralateral breast primary tumors as first events, and a number of important tolerability parameters. Additionally, fewer patient withdrawals from the study occurred with anastrozole than with tamoxifen as anastrozole was associated with fewer side effects than tamoxifen, particularly vascular and gynecologic events, including thromboembolism, hot flashes, vaginal bleeding, endometrial cancer, and vaginal discharge. Yet arthralgias and fractures were increased. Anastrozole now offers a choice for postmenopausal patients with hormone-responsive tumors, although longer follow-up will enable a more definitive benefit/risk assessment. Furthermore, AIs are being studied in premenopausal patients and in the chemoprevention setting.

An additional RCT comparing letrozole to placebo in 5,187 postmenopausal women with hormone-sensitive early-stage breast cancer *after* 5 years with tamoxifen showed improved disease-free survival and decreased recurrences in the letrozole group compared with placebo. Before this finding, there was no additional standard treatment *after* the tamoxifen therapy to prevent recurrences. A recent update of the trial indicates substantial clinical benefit even following a 1- to 5-year hiatus after 5 years of adjuvant tamoxifen in disease-free survival, distant disease-free survival, and overall survival. Furthermore, switching to anastrazole or exemestane in the middle of the standard 5-year tamoxifen treatment has also shown improved disease-free survival over continuation of tamoxifen. Thus, women's health practitioners must become knowledgeable regarding current patterns of breast cancer treatment and have a thorough discussion with their medical oncologists, thereby referring women appropriately (who may have missed or been reluctant to continue oncologic care but still follow for gynecologic care) for additional care. Researchers are following these women to ascertain long-term effects on bones and lipids. Current evidence is inconclusive regarding the use of bisphosphonates to prevent bone loss in patients taking AIs, although studies are under way to evaluate this possibility.

Letrozole has also shown effectiveness in ovulation induction and is one of the only safe options for breast cancer patients wishing to undergo *in vitro* fertilization and ovarian stimulation to freeze embryos before their cancer therapy. Although the product's label has always stated a contraindication in premenopausal women because of "the potential for maternal and fetal toxicity," many intrauterine insemination programs have replaced the standard clomiphene citrate with letrozole because of its superior pregnancy success rates and ability to decrease gonadotropin requirements. However, a small, unpublished Canadian study presented at the conjoint annual meeting of the American Society for Reproductive Medicine and the Canadian Fertility and Andrology Society warned that the drug may be associated with congenital anomalies, which prompted the pharmaceutical company to send letters to health care professionals regarding this information. However, many fertility experts suggest caution in interpreting the results, as a higher-than-normal dose of letrozole was used (5 mg rather than 2.5 mg) and may portend the dubious consequences.

Additional Treatments

Ovarian ablation has been shown to reduce the risk of tumor recurrence and death in women younger than 50 years, at least in the absence of adjuvant chemotherapy. The combination of oophorectomy and chemotherapy was as effective as either treatment alone in premenopausal women, but the invasive nature of surgical feminine castration has limited its use in the United States. In addition, tamoxifen is effective in premenopausal women, and no randomized trial has shown the superiority of oophorectomy over tamoxifen.

Luteinizing hormone-releasing hormone analogs are an alternative to oophorectomy. These agents induce a "chemical castration" and are effective for premenopausal patients with metastatic breast cancer. Interest in the integration of the luteinizing hormone-releasing hormone agonist goserelin and leuprolide in the adjuvant setting is increasing and occurring in many practices. Large randomized trials are under way.

Tumor-Specific Therapies

New, innovative treatment strategies are clearly needed to capitalize on and continually improve breast cancer outcomes. Overexpression of HER2/neu in primary breast carcinomas induces cell transformation and has been shown to correlate with unfavorable tumor biology and a significantly worse clinical prognosis for patients with breast cancer. Amplification or overexpression of this protein is noted in 10% to 30% of human breast tumors and in 9% to 32% of ovarian cancer cases. These tumors tend to grow faster and are generally more likely to recur than tumors that do not overproduce HER2. Trastuzumab (Herceptin) is an FDA-approved monoclonal immunoglobulin G1 antibody that inhibits human epidermal growth factor receptor 2 (HER2) with high affinity for the HER2/neu receptor and has been shown to be a potent weapon against the recurrence of cancer cells that amplify HER2. Trastuzumab significantly inhibits the growth of breast tumors with high levels of the HER2 protein when administered alone or in combination with paclitaxel or carboplatin and has been shown to improve the overall response in women with metastatic breast cancer. A recent clinical trial evaluated women with early-stage disease receiving doxorubicin, cyclophosphamide followed by paclitaxel versus doxorubicin, cyclophosphamide followed by paclitaxel and trastuzumab. Those patients receiving trastuzumab in combination with standard combination chemotherapy had a 52% statistically significant reduction in disease recurrence and 33% reduction in mortality compared with patients treated with chemotherapy alone. Overexpression of this gene product also predicts *resistance* to tamoxifen therapy. Currently, trastuzumab prolongs survival in metastatic breast cancer patients whose tumors overexpress the HER2/neu protein. Its effect on ovarian cancer is investigational at present.

Trastuzumab has few additional side effects, apart from cardiac toxicity in patients concurrently receiving anthracyclines. Thus, careful cardiac monitoring is required in these patients to detect reduction in left ventricular ejection fraction as congestive heart failure rates ranged from 0.5% to 4.1% in several trials. It is thus reasonable for trastuzumab to become a treatment option in early or metastatic breast cancer. Several institutions routinely incorporate HER2/neu status testing into the assessment of all patients with invasive breast disease. Additional approaches are being investigated as possible therapeutic strategies targeting HER2, including growth inhibitory antibodies, which can be used alone or in combination with standard chemotherapeutics; receptor inhibitors, developed to block receptor activity because phosphorylation is the key event leading to activation and initiation of the signaling pathway; and active immunotherapy, because the HER2 oncoprotein is immunogenic in some breast carcinoma patients. Unanswered questions include the appropriate duration and dose of therapy, and whether cardiotoxicity is reversible, especially if doxorubicin is not used.

CARE FOR BREAST CANCER SURVIVORS

Follow-Up

The risk of recurrent disease in the contralateral breast is estimated at 30% for patients with *in situ* carcinoma and 5% to 10% with invasive cancer. In addition, patients receiving definitive treatment for breast cancer have a 16% risk at 3 years of developing a second *primary* site of cancer, including the contralateral breast, ovaries, endometrium, and large intestine. Thus, recommended breast cancer surveillance guidelines include a thorough history and physical examination every 3 to 6 months for 3 years, every 6 to 12 months for 2 years, then annually. A review of systems should elicit symptoms in the breast and at those sites where recurrences frequently occur, such as nodal disease, lung, bone, liver, adrenal gland, and ovary. A focused history should include information on weight loss, local or distant skin changes (radiation effects or breast skin changes—ipsilateral and contralateral), mental status changes, headache or sensory deficits, pleuritic chest pain, shortness of breath, bone pain, changes in bowel function and melena or blood in the stools, and abnormal rectal or vaginal secretions. Physical examination should incorporate an evaluation of the remaining breast tissue and lymph node–bearing areas, range of motion of the upper extremity, and increasing arm girth, which may indicate onset of lymphedema or axillary recurrence. Examinations of the chest and abdomen are performed to search for evidence of pleural effusions or hepatomegaly. A mammogram, pelvic examination, and Pap test should be performed annually. Routine radiological studies (bone scan, CT, chest x-ray) or laboratory testing (liver function tests, complete blood count, tumor markers) is not recommended except based on symptomatology in that no survival advantage is conferred by detecting asymptomatic disease; however, institutional policies may differ. Many surgeons continue to recommend yearly complete blood counts and chemistry panels as well as chest radiograph despite evidence of specificity in detection of metastatic disease. One series indicated less than 18% specificity for routine testing.

Those with initial advanced disease should have regularly scheduled visits at 3-month intervals for their lifetime. Others recommend visits every 3 months for 3 to 5 years, then every 6 months thereafter for patients with advanced disease.

Women with DCIS require physical examination every 6 months for 5 years and then annually, as well as yearly diagnostic mammography.

Hormone Replacement Therapy

As more breast cancers are detected at an earlier stage, resulting in increased survival, there is a wealth of attention directed toward use of HRT in breast cancer survivors. Many authors sanction use of HRT for menopausal breast cancer survivors who are disease-free and have symptomatic estrogen deficiency, especially after the first 2 years when the risk of recurrence is decreased. Furthermore, patients with localized node-negative breast cancers who are at low risk for recurrent disease may be excellent candidates for long-term replacement. ACOG recommends HRT use with a treatment plan that includes dietary control, exercise, smoking cessation, reduction of alcohol consumption, and weight reduction when appropriate. Women with unexplained vaginal bleeding, acute vascular thrombosis, or significant liver function impairment would remain ineligible for use. All women should be carefully and completely counseled regarding the potential, albeit unproven, risks of disease recurrence.

Gabapentin has also been shown in a randomized double-blind placebo controlled trial of 420 women to control hot flashes in breast cancer patients at 900 mg/day, demonstrating greater reduction in the posttreatment hot flash severity score compared with placebo and lower doses of gabapentin (Neurontin). Gabapentin is approved for the treatment of epileptic seizures but often used for treatment of migraine headaches, restless legs syndrome, and bipolar disorder. Additionally, venlafaxine appears to be an effective treatment for hot flashes.

Pregnancy after Treatment for Breast Cancer

Although oncologists generally caution patients to avoid pregnancy until 2 years after completing treatment for breast cancer, several investigators have not shown any adverse effects or decreased survival for women who become pregnant after cancer therapy. Moreover, although lactation is decreased in the treated breast, radiation therapy appears to have no effect on the contralateral breast. Increased rates of stillbirth, preterm birth, and low birth weight portend a suboptimal intrauterine environment, but the infants are otherwise unaffected.

BREAST CANCER AND PREGNANCY

Breast cancer is estimated to occur in 1 in 3,000 to 1 in 10,000 and have an incidence of 0.2% to 3.8% of pregnancies. Pregnancy-associated breast cancer is defined as that occurring during pregnancy or within 1 year after delivery. Breast cancer diagnosed in pregnancy has an overall inferior prognosis as it tends to be diagnosed at a more advanced stage;

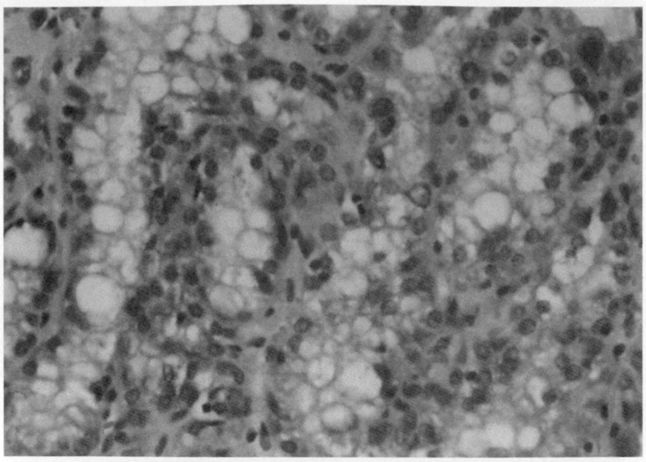

FIGURE 41.36. Lactating adenoma. Uniform cells have large nuclei and abundant vacuolated cytoplasm. Secretory material (milk) is present in the lumens (not seen in this figure).

however, when patients are categorized according to age, stage at presentation, and lymph node status, prognosis and survival is similar in pregnant and nonpregnant patients. The intense hormonal milieu normally associated with pregnancy triggers progressive increases in breast volume and firmness as pregnancy advances, thus making physical examination of the breast increasingly difficult. Nevertheless, a complete CBE would be performed on the initial visit of a pregnant or lactating patient. The associated physiologic edema and intensification of growth in the ductal and lobular system makes both physical and radiologic examination of the multinodular consistency of the breast challenging and may obscure early abnormalities, both benign and malignant. Consequently, women considering pregnancy near the age of 40 or older should consider having their screening mammogram before attempting to conceive (Fig. 41.36).

The evaluation, diagnosis, and treatment of a breast mass in a pregnant patient is unchanged from their nonpregnant counterparts. The conventional diagnostic modalities may be performed—including FNA, ultrasonography, CNB under local anesthesia, or excisional biopsy under local or general anesthesia—without adverse sequelae. However, additional false-positive FNA results may occur as a function of the increased cellularity and frequent mitosis that can occur normally during gestation. Core biopsies are more accurate, but milk fistulas—a complication seen in surgical biopsy—have been reported. The finding of a thickness or a possible mass usually requires a short interval follow-up and examination because the mass may feel similar to normal hypertrophic thickness as pregnancy advances. A mass that appears to "disappear" as pregnancy advances could actually be obscured by the normal changes in pregnancy and represent an ongoing developing breast carcinoma. For this reason, ultrasound may be used to evaluate an area that is "negative" on examination but was previously thought to harbor a mass lesion. Breast ultrasonography during pregnancy is safe and helpful in differentiating between cystic and solid masses. However, ultrasound is less specific in distinguishing benign solid masses from malignant masses. Conversely, MRI has been used in pregnancy and seems safe for fetuses because it does not expose them to ionizing radiation, although the safety committee indicates that the safety during pregnancy has not been proven. Recent reports on its use for fetal imaging in prenatal diagnosis contain limited follow-up of the infants, but no untoward effects have been reported. MRI may be particularly useful for the diagnosis or confirmation of bone, liver, or even brain metastases in the staging of patients, although head CT scans with abdominal shielding yield only small amounts of fetal exposure.

If an area is suspicious for malignancy, a shielded mammogram should be obtained during pregnancy; however, shielding cannot completely prevent internal radiation scatter dose to the fetus. Large doses may result in intrauterine growth retardation, mental retardation, and prematurity. If mammography is necessary in lactating women, it should be performed immediately after emptying the breast by nursing or pumping.

Any dominant mass should be evaluated as it would be in the nonpregnant patient to prevent diagnostic delay. Screening mammography may be deferred to limit fetal exposure but should be obtained without hesitation if the lesion requires additional evaluation. Radiation exposure to the fetus during mammography is estimated at less than 10 mrad, depending on the gestational age, with increasing dose as the gravid fundus grows closer to the targeted breast tissue.

The risk for teratogenicity in subsequent fetal development may discourage the institution of therapy for cancer in pregnant women; however, established surgical and adjunctive therapies should be undertaken. Therapeutic termination does not appear to affect the survival in early-stage breast carcinoma and is therefore not advocated. Indeed, the possibility of a detrimental effect on survival has been suggested. Modified radical mastectomy is the optimal treatment for local management of stage I and II. BCS is contraindicated in the first and second trimester because of the effect of the required adjunctive radiation on the fetus. The survival risk to the mother prompted by delaying radiation therapy until after delivery is not known. In the first trimester, particularly during fetal organogenesis, both irradiation and chemotherapy—especially with folate antagonists—are contraindicated. There are scattered case reports of normal, well babies both in all of these treatment circumstances, but the risks to the fetus are significant. Concerns continue to be raised about the future neurologic development and potential subsequent increased risk for childhood cancers among these newborns exposed to radiation; reliable long-term data are unavailable. Thus individualized counseling should be provided in a compassionate, caring forum considering the patients psychosocial situation, anxieties, and future expectations.

If the diagnosis is made during the third trimester, the patient may elect to be observed until delivery, when prompt treatment is initiated. Adjuvant therapy may also be delayed until delivery as long as the risks are exhaustively discussed with the patient. As in the nonpregnant patient, most recurrences occur within 2 years of treatment; therefore, patients with breast cancer are advised to delay pregnancy for 2 to 3 years, and effective nonhormonal birth control should be administered. However, studies have not shown an adverse effect of subsequent pregnancy even in patients with positive axillary nodes or patients whose pregnancy occurred earlier than 2 years after completion of treatment. If nodal involvement is found, studies have indicated no adverse effects of the frequent forms of chemotherapy in the second or third trimesters, although long-term effects on the fetus are unknown. Methotrexate, taxanes, and tamoxifen should be avoided during pregnancy until further studies are available. Detailed studies of transplacental passage of chemotherapeutic agents to fetuses are also not available. The potential adverse effects of antineoplastic agents on fetuses and neonates include immediate effects (such as spontaneous abortion, teratogenesis, and organ damage) and delayed effects (such as growth retardation and gonadal dysfunction). Chemotherapy administration during the first trimester is associated with an increased incidence of stillbirths and congenital malformations. The risk of fetal malformation when chemotherapy is instituted in the first trimester is 12% compared with no increased risk with chemotherapeutic administration in the second and third trimester.

Staging procedures for breast cancer are often considered inappropriate in the gravid patient, but there are no contraindications for chest radiography performed with abdominal and pelvic shielding. In late pregnancy, the fetal shield may obscure the lower lung parenchyma; however, exposing third-trimester fetuses to chest radiography presents no great concern. Alkaline phosphatase is elevated in normal pregnancy, making its use in evaluation of bone metastasis ineffectual. Conventional radiography, excluding the pelvis and abdomen (e.g., skull and long bones), can be performed. No adequate substitute for bone scanning exists, although articles have promoted certain modifications of the bone-scanning technique for pregnant patients. Because the incidence of bone metastasis is very low in stage I and II disease, bone scanning can usually be avoided. On the other hand, in clinical stage III disease, in which the possibility of bone metastasis is increased, treatment methods differ and may weigh in favor of provision of the test.

Whereas other human malignancies—including melanoma, hematopoietic malignancies, hepatoma, and choriocarcinoma—have been reported to cause fetal metastases, breast cancer has not. On the contrary, placental metastases from breast cancer and other solid tumors have been reported. Because half of these patients did not have visible lesions, microscopic examination of the placenta is warranted.

Rarely, breast fibroadenomas may infarct during pregnancy. These cases warrant close microscopic review because they may mimic carcinomas.

RISK MANAGEMENT AND PROFESSIONAL LIABILITY

Associated with the increased involvement in evaluation of diseases of the breast comes attached potential liability. Although medicolegal concerns should never alter one's method of practice, gynecologists must be cognizant of the legal environment. The special challenge of these cases derives from the emotionally charged nature of the cancer diagnosis, combined with high public expectations as to the current capability of breast cancer screening and treatment outcome. In this litigious society, nearly 80% of board-certified obstetricians/gynecologists in the United States have been sued for alleged malpractice. The most recent ACOG Professional Liability survey listed failure to diagnose breast cancer as the second leading primary allegation in claims against gynecologists (second only to surgical injury). Specifically, failure to diagnose breast cancer accounted for 33% of these claims, with failure to diagnose cervical (7.4%) and ovarian cancers (7.3%) running a far second and third. According to the Physician's Insurers Association of America, failure to diagnose cancer is the second most expensive condition to indemnify with an average payment of $212,894.

Health care providers encounter a wide variety of legal issues with regard to patients with breast disorders, including liability for alleged misdiagnosis, delayed diagnosis of breast cancer, failure to obtain informed consent, and improper treatment of breast disease. Contextual legal issues other than medical malpractice often affect the care of breast disorders. For example, many state legislatures have mandated informed consent requirements for those treating patients with breast cancer. Finally, legislation and litigation regarding insurance coverage for mammography screening, managed care policies, and new breast cancer treatments are becoming increasingly common. The idea that physicians would not be brought into suits against Health Maintenance Organizations (HMO) and pharmaceutical companies has drastically changed, with more private doctors becoming involved in lawsuits against corporate entities.

Analysis of the paid malpractice claims revealed women who were relatively young for the diagnosis of breast cancer (60% were younger than 50 years of age) and a high occurrence of false-negative mammogram results (nearly 80% of the claims had negative or equivocal mammogram results) were overrepresented. The average length of diagnostic delay was 14 months, with the average malpractice award or settlement increasing with longer periods of delay. The average indemnity payment increased by 36%. Interestingly, radiologists have surpassed gynecologists as the most frequently sued practitioner for delayed diagnosis, accounting for 24% of claims (gynecologists accounted for 23%). Specifically, this is a significant change from the previous study, wherein gynecologists accounted for 39% of the claims and radiologists for 11%. In 1995, family practitioners accounted for 17%, surgical specialties for 14%, internal medicine for 4%, and pathologists for 2%.

Historically, U.S. jurisdictions used a "but for" test to establish legal, or proximate, causation. Causation in legal terminology signifies that the practitioner's action (e.g., delayed diagnosis) must have an association with the resultant injury (development of breast cancer) that is sufficiently close to hold the practitioner liable for damages. Under the "but for" test, malpractice damages are not awarded unless a better outcome was probable, better than even, or more likely than not, absent the actions of the practitioner. Under this test, only actions that possibly or with a likelihood of 50% *or greater* result in the alleged injury are deemed sufficient to make the practitioner liable for damages.

Historically, the "but for" standard was the most frequently used test of causation; however, this standard has been replaced in most states by causation theories that allow recovery in circumstances in which the probability that the negligent action led to patient injury is *less than* 50%. For instance, the "substantial factor" test permits recovery when the negligent behavior is a substantial factor in producing injury, even if the plaintiff's chance at a better outcome absent the actions of the practitioner was less than 50-50. A distinct, but related, alternative causation standard is the "loss of a chance" theory. Many states have adopted this theory as a standard. In those jurisdictions, a physician may be held liable for actions that deny the patient *some* chance or prospect of a better outcome. For instance, a delayed diagnosis that reduced a patient's chance of survival from 39% to 24% would preclude a verdict in favor of the physician in a "loss of a chance" state. Recovery would not be possible in a jurisdiction that followed the traditional "but for" causation analysis, in which, as in this scenario, there was less than a probable impact on outcome. Hence, the particular causation standard that a jurisdiction follows can have an enormous impact on the outcome of a medical malpractice liability case.

Medical malpractice cases based on delayed diagnosis are usually barred after the statute of limitations has run except under the Continuous Treatment Doctrine. Here the statute of limitations is tolled until the end of a course of treatment, when the course of treatment, which includes the wrongful acts or omissions, has run continuously and is related to the same original condition or symptom. The purpose of the doctrine to "maintain the physician-patient relationship in the belief that the most efficacious medical care will be obtained when the attending physician remains on a case from onset to cure." It is essential to establish a course of treatment with respect to the condition that gives rise to the lawsuit for this doctrine to apply. Accordingly, "Where the physician and patient reasonably intend the patient's uninterrupted reliance upon the physicians' observation, directions, concern and responsibility for overseeing the patient's progress," the requirements of the continuous treatment doctrine are satisfied.

Hereditary cancer litigation may evolve into the new frontier of medical litigation. Allegations include failure to diagnose, failure to consider patient's genealogy, failure to inform other family members (one must be cognizant of Health Insurance Portability and Accountability Act [HIPAA] considerations), and failure to offer testing. This has already occurred in obstetrics with Tay-Sachs testing. Physicians should familiarize themselves with risk assessment models or refer patients when susceptibility testing is deemed appropriate. Counseling must stress these figures are estimates and not absolute risks, and thus balance the magnitude of risk for the individual patient. Clinicians must also become familiar with the eligibility criteria for breast cancer susceptibility gene testing, the principles of genetic counseling, options available to those at high risk, and follow-up of patients at high risk.

As proffered by one expert, "The price of skill in the diagnosis of breast carcinoma is a kind of eternal vigilance based upon an awareness that any indication of disease in the breast may be due to carcinoma."

The most common reason underlying delay in diagnosis was physical examination findings that did not impress the physician (35%). Other reasons included failure to follow up in a timely fashion (31%), negative/misread mammogram (26%/23%), failure to perform a biopsy (23%), delayed/failure to consult (16%), failure to order/react to mammogram (11%/12%), communication failure (11%), and poor clinical examination (10%). Because mammography has a 15% to 20% false-negative rate, the practitioner should not rely on a "negative" mammogram in the face of a dominant lesion or suspicious examination. However, because mammography may not detect neoplastic changes in the breast until the cancer has been developing for 6 years, some lesions will not be seen on mammography in retrospect, some should be considered as subthreshold, and some are appropriately classified as missed.

The significance of medicolegal issues in the arena of breast cancer compels practitioners to develop risk-management techniques that incorporate policies for reducing malpractice liability risk. The old adage "Good medicine is good law" is apropos as the guiding principles for care of women with breast disorders, which must be grounded in medical science and sound clinical judgment.

Patient education and effective communication are key components of good clinical care and effective risk management. Inadequate or lack of informed consent is a pervasive issue in allegations against obstetricians and gynecologists. Physicians have been sued despite "successful" breast cancer surgery for breaching the physician's duty in failing to obtain informed consent. Additionally, one should not underemphasize significant diagnostic or therapeutic uncertainty in critical clinical decisions while maintaining an optimistic tenor in the doctor–patient relationship. This prevents the patient from misconstruing the importance or true implications of returning for follow-up examinations, repeat diagnostic tests, or other procedures. The clinician should allow the patient to participate in the decision-making process.

The best defense is an adequate record. For women with breast symptoms, the medical record should include a description and diagram of findings from the history and physical examination that will allow effective comparison during follow-up examinations. The chart notation "breasts okay" or "breasts normal" is not adequate chart documentation for a woman who presents with breast symptoms. The use of a printed encounter form designed specifically for breast symptoms may facilitate suitable chart documentation. Documentation of a dominant mass, which may be measured or diagrammed, requires evaluation and resolution. Practitioners should make a record of each visit and any changes that occurred in the interval from the previous checkup. The results of any diagnostic tests should be documented, including patient notification and discussion. Clinicians should also record the rationale and factors of importance in their decision making in the medical record. If, ultimately, the patient's clinical course is unfavorable, prior documentation of the clinical reasoning may prove that the action taken was appropriate in light of the information available at the time.

The desired follow-up visits in women with breast symptoms should be explicit and clear. Scheduled appointment dates are preferable to patient-initiated ("PRN") follow-up. Continuity of care for breast symptoms must be carefully ensured, even when other medical problems or referred specialists become interposed. An extra effort to dispatch reminder telephone calls and letters are appropriate for patients with particularly suspicious clinical presentations who do not follow up for appointments. If a referral is made, follow-up is necessary to ensure the patient has seen the appropriate consultant, and a copy of their recommendations should be made a part of the chart.

CONCLUSION

The epidemic of breast cancer represents a significant public health problem affecting a large number of women. As obstetricians/gynecologists continue to care for women and expand their primary care function, we must remain knowledgeable of the changes in the field of breast disease. Advanced technology has improved the ability to define risk status and identify women with genetic predisposition to breast cancer development. Increased access to and use of screening mammography have been instrumental in decreasing the mortality rate associated with breast cancer by identifying earlier stage disease. Although changes in mammographic screening have occurred, a consensus on the evaluation of women younger than 50 years is controversial. Further radiologic technology in the arena of DM may provide an alternative or adjunct to current conventional screen film, especially in subpopulations of women such as those with dense breasts and/or perimenopausal status. Although the impact of OCPs and HRT on the risk of breast cancer continues to be debated, the information must be used to provide informed consent for patients while continuing to keep an eye on the horizon for supplementary information. Medicolegal concerns will continue to hover, but an accurate assessment and attention to testing and follow-up will decrease the delayed diagnosis in the future. Ultimately, reaching all segments of the population with comprehensive prevention, early detection, and treatment services could reduce cancer incidence and mortality even further, thus decreasing disparities. Continued monitoring and preparation in ensuring uniformly high standards of care is an important aspect of future national policy goals.

BEST SURGICAL PRACTICES

- Lumpectomy plus irradiation has been shown in RCT to be equally efficacious as modified radical mastectomy for treatment of stage I and II disease.
- Iatrogenic pneumothorax is a potentially dangerous, although rare, complication of FNA, which may be reduced by stabilizing the lesion over a rib before needle introduction.
- Positioning of the patient at the margin of the exam table for an FNA is helpful to improve access to breast structures.
- Care must be taking in performing CNB to avoid advancing the cutting needle beyond the suspect mass, lest the contiguous normal breast or chest wall be injured or implanted with malignant cells.
- Vacuum-assisted CNB technique using a no. 11-gauge needle is becoming the method of choice for stereotactic and ultrasound biopsies with placement of a radiopaque clip.
- Risk-reducing breast procedures include total mastectomy (removal of the skin overlying the breast, the breast tissue, and the nipple/areola complex), skin-sparing mastectomy (resection of the nipple/areola complex and the biopsy scar, and removal of the breast parenchyma), and subcutaneous mastectomy (removal of most of the breast tissue with preservation of the nipple/areola complex). Breast cancers have been noted after subcutaneous mastectomy, but additional studies are needed.
- Masses within 2 cm of the areolar margin may be best dissected through a circumareolar incision at the areolar margin.
- The most cosmetically acceptable scars result from incisions that follow the contour of Langer's lines.
- The most unfavorable incisions for mastectomy are the transverse or vertical incisions. Moreover, asymmetric incisions always accentuate the deformity.
- Closure of mastectomy incisions with decreased tension is improved by undermining the attached skin flaps 3 to 4 cm.
- It is best to keep biopsy incisions within the boundaries of "potential" incisions for future mastectomy or wide local excision should those therapies be required for definitive treatment.
- Use of tissue expanders has become the predominant means of breast reconstruction in patients who have not had extensive skin removal.
- Risk-reducing salpingo-oophorectomy should include complete removal of the ovaries *and* fallopian tubes with serial sectioning by the pathologist.

Bibliography

Abati A, Simsir A. Breast fine needle aspiration biopsy: prevailing recommendations and contemporary practices. *Clin Lab Med* 2005;25:631.

Agency for Healthcare Research and Quality. *Screening for breast cancer: recommendations and rational*. Rockville, MD: Agency for Healthcare Research and Quality; 2002.

American Academy of Pediatrics and American College of Obstetricians and Gynecologists. Anatomy and physiology of lactation. In: *Breastfeeding handbook for physicians*. Washington DC: AAP and ACOG; 2006.

ATAC Trialists' Group. Results of the ATAC (Arimidex, tamoxifen, alone or in combination) trial after completion of 5 years of adjuvant treatment for breast cancer. *Lancet* 2005;365:60.

Barrios R, Dalai D, Reamers RA, et al. Meta-analysis; high dosage vitamin E supplementation may increase all-cause mortality. *Ann Intern Med* 2005;142(1):37.

Bassa P, Kim EE, Inoue T, et al. Evaluation of preoperative chemotherapy using PET with fluorine-18-flurodeoxy-D-glucose to predict the pathologic response of breast cancer to primary chemotherapy. *J Clin Oncol* 2000;18:1676.

Benson SRC, Blue J, Judd K, et al. Ultrasound is now better than mammography for the detection of invasive breast cancer. *Am J Surg* 2004;188: 381.

Berry DA, Iversen ES Jr, Guddbjartsson DF, et al. BRCAPRO validation, sensitivity of genetic testing of BRCA1/BRCA2, and prevalence of other breast cancer susceptibility genes. *J Clin Oncol* 2002;20:2701.

Blommers J, de Lange-De Klerk ES, Kuik DJ, et al. Evening primrose oil and fish oil for severe chronic mastalgia: a randomized, double blind, controlled trial. *Am J Obstet Gynecol* 2002;187:1389.

Boccardo F, Rubagotti A, Puntoni M, et al. Switching to anastrozole versus continued tamoxifen treatment of early breast cancer: preliminary results of the Italian tamoxifen anastrozole trial. *J Clin Oncol* 2005;23: 5138.

Bombardier C, Laine L, Reicin A, et al. Comparison of upper gastrointestinal toxicity of rofecoxib and naproxen in patients with rheumatoid arthritis. *N Engl J Med* 2000;343:1520.

The Breast International Group (BIG) 1-98 Collaborative Group. A comparison of letrozole and tamoxifen in postmenopausal women with early breast cancer. *N Engl J Med* 2005;353:2747.

Cassidy A, Bingham S, Setchell KD. Biological effects of a diet of soy protein rich in isoflavones on the menstrual cycle of premenopausal women. *Am J Clin Nutr* 1994;60:333.

Collaborative Group on Hormonal Factors in Breast Cancer. Breast cancer and hormonal contraceptives: collaborative reanalysis of individual data on 53,297 women with breast cancer and 100,239 women without breast cancer from 54 epidemiological studies. *Lancet* 1996;347:1713.

Coombes RC, Hall E, Gibson LJ, et al. A randomized trial of exemestane after two to three years of tamoxifen therapy in postmenopausal women with primary breast cancer. *N Engl J Med* 2004;350:1081.

Cuzick J, Forbes J, Edwards R, et al. First results from the IBIS 1: a randomized prevention trial. *Lancet* 2002;360:817.

Davies G, Martin LA, Sacks N, et al. Cyclooxytenase-2 (COX-2), aromatase and breast cancer: a possible role for COX-2 inhibitors in breast cancer chemoprevention. *Ann Oncol* 2002;13:669.

Domchek SM, Eisen A, Calzone K, et al. Application of breast cancer risk prediction models in clinical practice. *J Clin Oncol* 2005;21(4):593.

Early Breast Cancer Trialists Collaborative Group. Effects of chemotherapy and hormonal therapy for early breast cancer on recurrence and 15 year survival: an overview of the randomized trials. *Lancet* 2005;365:1687.

Edwards BK, Brown ML, Wingo PA, et al. Annual report to the nation on the status of cancer, 1975–2002, featuring population-based trends in cancer treatment. *J Natl Cancer Inst* 2005;97(19):140.

Fabian CJ, Kamel S, Kimler DR, et al. Potential use of biomarkers in breast cancer risk assessment and chemoprevention trials. *Breast J* 1995;1:236.

Fentiman IS, Caleffi M, Hamed H, et al. Dosage and duration of tamoxifen treatment for mastalgia: a controlled trial. *Br J Surg* 1988;75(9):845.

Fisher B, Costantino JP, Wickerham DL, et al. Tamoxifen for prevention of breast cancer: current status of the national surgical adjuvant breast and bowel project P1 study. *J Natl Cancer Inst* 2005;97(22):1652.

Freer TW, Ulissey MR. Screening mammography with computer-aided detection: prospective study of 12,860 patients in a community breast center. *Radiology* 2001;220(3):781.

GEMB Group. Tamoxifen therapy for cyclical mastalgia: a dose randomized trial. *Breast* 1997;5:212.

Gong C, Song E, Jia W, et al. A double blind randomized controlled trial of toremifen therapy for mastalgia. *Arch Surg* 2006;141:43.

Goss PE, Ingle JN, Martino S, et al. A randomized trial of letrozole in postmenopausal women after five years of tamoxifen therapy for early stage breast cancer. *N Engl J Med* 2003;349(19):1793.

Goss PE, Ingle JN, Martino S, et al. Randomized trials of letrozole following tamoxifen as extended adjuvant therapy in receptor-positive breast cancer: updated findings from NCIC CTG MA 17. *J Natl Cancer Inst* 2005;97(7): 1262.

Gotzsche PC, Olsen O. Is screening for breast cancer with mammography justifiable?. *Lancet* 2000;355(9198):129.

Green VL. Breast cancer screening. In: Bieber EJ, Horowitz I, Sanfilippo J, eds. *Clinical gynecology*. Philadelphia: Elsevier Inc.; 2006.

Hartman AR, Daniel BL, Kurian AW, et al. Breast magnetic resonance image screening and ductal lavage in women at high genetic risk for breast carcinoma. *Cancer* 2004;100(3):479.

Hindle WH, Gonzalez S. Diagnosis and treatment of invasive breast cancer during pregnancy and lactation. *Clin Obstet Gynecol* 2002;45(3):770.

Hippisley-Cox J, Coupland C. Risk of myocardial infarction in patients taking cycloxygenase-2 inhibitors or conventional non-steroidal anti-inflammatory drugs: population based nested case-control analysis. *BMJ* 2005;330(7504):1366.

Holmes MD, Chen WY, Feskanich D, et al. Physical activity and survival after breast cancer diagnosis. *JAMA* 2005;293(20):2479.

Hutcheon AW, Heys SD, Sarkar TK, and the Aberdeen Breast Group. Neoadjuvant docetaxel in locally advanced breast cancer. *Breast Cancer Res Treat* 2003;79(suppl 1):S19.

Ingram DM, Hickling C, West L, et al. A double blind randomized controlled trial of isoflavones in the treatment of cyclical mastalgia. *Breast* 2002;11(2):170.

Jakesz R, Jonat W, Gnant M, et al. Switching of postmenopausal women with endocrine-responsive early breast cancer to anastrazole after 2 years' adjuvant tamoxifen: combined results of ABCSG trial 8 and ARNO 95 trial. *Lancet* 2005;366:455.

Kauff ND, Satagopan JM, Robson ME, et al. Risk reducing salpingo-oophorectomy in women with a BRCA1 or BRCA2 mutation. *N Engl J Med* 2002;346:1609.

Kessler JH. The effect of supraphysiologic levels of iodine on patients with cyclic mastalgia. *Breast J* 2004;10(4):328.

King MC, Wieand S, Hale K, et al. National Surgical Adjuvant Breast and Bowel Project. Tamoxifen and breast cancer incidence among women with inherited mutations in BRCA1 and BRCA2: National Surgical Adjuvant Breast and Bowel Project (NSABP-P1) Breast Cancer Prevention Trial. *JAMA* 2001;286(18):2251.

Klein EA. Selenium and vitamin E cancer prevention trial. *Ann N Y Acad Sci* 2004;1031:234.

Klimberg VS, Harms SE, Henry-Tillman RS. Not all MRI techniques are created equal. *Ann Surg Oncol* 2000;7:404.

Kosters JP, Gotzsche PC. Regular self-examination or clinical examination for early detection of breast cancer. *Cochrane Database Syst Rev* 2003;(2):CD003373 .

Krag D, Weaver D, Ashikaga T, et al. The sentinel mode in breast cancer: a multicenter validation study. *N Engl J Med* 1998;339:941.

Larfeniere R. Bloody nipple discharge during pregnancy: a rationale for conservative treatment. *J Surg Oncol* 1990;43:228.

Larsson L, Anderson I, Bjurstam N, et al. Update overview of the Swedish randomized trails in breast cancer screening with mammography: age group 40–49 at randomization. *J Natl Cancer Inst Monogr* 1997;22:57.

Leach MO, Boggis CRM, Dixon AK, et al. MARIBS Study Group. Screening with magnetic resonance imaging and mammography of a UK population at high familial risk of breast cancer: a prospective multicenter cohort study (MARIBS). *Lancet* 2005;365:1769.

Lee IM, Cook NR, Gaziano JM, et al. Vitamin E in the primary prevention of cardiovascular disease and cancer: the women's health study: a randomized controlled trial. *JAMA* 2005;294(1):56.

Leonardi M. [Hormonal contraception and benign breast disease. Evaluation of a treatment protocol for chronic mastopathy with mastalgia. *Minerva Ginecol* 1997;49(6):271.

Lewin JM, D'Orsi CJ, Hendrick RE, et al. Clinical comparison of full-field digital mammography and screen-film mammography for detection of breast cancer. *AJR Am J Roentgenol* 2002;179:671.

Lonn E, Bosch J, Yusuf S, et al. and The HOPE and HOPE-TOO Trial Investigators. Effect of long-term vitamin E supplementation on cardiovascular events and cancer: a randomized controlled trial. *JAMA* 2005;293:1338.

Loprinzi CL, Kugler JW, Sloan JA, et al. Venlafaxine in management of hot flashes in survivors of breast cancer: a randomized controlled trial. *Lancet* 2000;356:2059.

Mansel RE, Goyal A, Preece P, et al. European randomized, multicenter study of goserelin (Zoladex) in the management of mastalgia. *Am J Obstet Gynecol* 2004;191:1942.

McDonald S, Saslow D, Alciati MH. Performance and reporting of clinical breast examination: a review of the literature. *CA Cancer J Clin* 2004;54:345.

Menon U, Skates SJ, Lewis S, et al. Prospective study using the risk of ovarian cancer algorithm to screen for ovarian cancer. *J Clin Oncol* 2005;23(31):7919.

Metcalfe KA, Lynch HT, Ghadirian P, et al. The risk of ovarian cancer after breast cancer in BRCA1 and BRCA2 carriers. *Gynecol Oncol* 2005;96:222.

Miller AB, Baines CJ, To T, et al. Canadian National Breast Screening Study. Breast cancer detection and death rates among women aged 40–49 years. *CMAJ* 1992;147:1459.

Millet AV, Dribas FM. Clinical management of breast pain: a review. *Obstet Gynecol Surv* 2002;57(7):451,

Mitwally MF, Biljan MM, Casper RF. Pregnancy outcome after the use of an aromatase inhibitor for ovarian stimulation. *Am J Obstet Gynecol* 2005;192:381.

Mukherjee D, Nissen SE, Topol EJ. Risk of cardiovascular events associated with selective COX-2 inhibitors. *JAMA* 2001;286(8):954.

Narod SA, Dube M, Klijn J, et al. Oral contraceptives and the risk of breast cancer in BRCA1 and BRCA2 mutation carriers. *J Natl Cancer Inst* 2002;94(23):1773.

Narod SA, Risch H, Moslehi R, et al. Oral contraceptives and the risk of hereditary ovarian cancer. *N Engl J Med* 1998;339(7):424.

National Cancer Institute Office of Communications/Mass Media Branch. *NCI statement on mammography screening*. Bethesda, MD: National Institutes of Health; 2002.

National Comprehensive Cancer Network. Clinical Practice Guidelines in Oncology – NCCN 2004. at http://www.nccn.org.

NIH Consensus development conference on adjuvant therapy for breast cancer. Bethesda, MD: National Institutes of Health, 2000.

Oktay K, Buyuk E, Libertella N, et al. Fertility preservation in breast cancer patients: a prospective controlled comparison of ovarian stimulation with tamoxifen and letrozole for embryo cryopreservation. *J Clin Oncol* 2005;23:4347.

Olsen O, Gotzsche PC. Cochrane review on screening for breast cancer with mammography. *Lancet* 2001;358:1340.

O'Meara ES, Rossing MA, Daling JR, et al. Hormone replacement therapy after diagnosis of breast cancer in relation to recurrence and mortality. *J Natl Cancer Inst* 2001;93:754.

Paik S, Shak S, Tang G, et al. A multigene assay to predict recurrence of tamoxifen-treated, node negative breast cancer. *N Engl J Med* 2004; 351(27):2817.

Pandya KJ, Morrow GR, Roscoe JA, et al. Gabapentin for hot flashes in 420 women with breast cancer: a randomized double blind placebo controlled trial. *Lancet* 2005;366:818.

Parmigiani G, Berry D, Aguilar O. Determining carrier probabilities for breast cancer-susceptibility genes BRCA1 and BRCA2. *Am J Hum Genet* 1998;62:145,

Peto R, Boreham J, Clark M, et al. UK and USA breast cancer deaths down 25% in year 2000 at ages 20–69 years. *Lancet* 2000;355:1822.

Pisano ED, Gatsonis C, Hendrick E, et al. Diagnostic performance of digital versus film mammography for breast cancer screening. *N Engl J Med* 2005;353(17):1773.

Powell CB, Kenley E, Chen LM, et al. Risk-reducing salpingo-oophorectomy in BRCA mutation carriers: role of serial sectioning in the detection of occult malignancy. *J Clin Oncol* 2005;23:127.

Prentice RL, Caan B, Chlebowski RT, et al. Low-fat dietary pattern and risk of invasive breast cancer; the women's health initiative randomized controlled dietary modification trial. *JAMA* 2006;295(6):629.

Ravdin PM, Siminoff LA, Davis GJ, et al. Computer program to assist in making decisions about adjuvant therapy for women with early breast cancer. *J Clin Oncol* 2001;19(4):980.

Rebbeck TR, Friebel T, Lynch HT, et al. Bilateral prophylactic mastectomy reduces breast cancer risk in BRCA1 and BRCA2 mutation carriers: the PROSE study group. *J Clin Oncol* 2004;22(6):1055.

Rebbeck TR, Friebel T, Watner T, et al. Effect of short-term hormone replacement therapy on breast cancer risk reduction after bilateral prophylactic oophorectomy in BRCA1 or BRCA2 mutation carriers: the PROSE study group. *J Clin Oncol* 2005;23:7804.

Rebbeck TR, Lynch HT, Neuhausen SL, et al. Prophylactic oophorectomy in carriers of BRCA1 or BRCA2 mutations. *N Engl J Med* 2002;346:1616.

Ries LAG, Eisner MP, Kosary CL, et al. SEER Cancer Statistics review, 1975–2002, National Cancer Institute, Bethesda, MD, http://seer.cancer.gov/csr/1975_202/, based on November 2004 SEER data submission, posted to the SEER website 2005.

Romond EH, Perez EA, Bryant J, et al. Trastuzumab plus chemotherapy for operable HER2 positive breast cancer. *N Engl J Med* 2005;353(16):1673.

Rutter CM, Mandelson MT, Laya MB, et al. Changes in breast density associated with initiation, discontinuation and continuing use of hormone replacement therapy. *JAMA* 2001;285(2):171.

Saslow D, Hannan J, Osuch J, et al. Clinical breast examination: practical recommendations for optimizing performance and reporting. *CA Cancer J Clin* 2004;54:327.

Shen Y, Yang Y, Inoue LY, et al. Role of detection method in predicting breast cancer survival: analysis of randomized screening trials. *J Natl Cancer Inst* 2005;97(16):1195.

Silverstein FE, Faich G, Goldstein JL, et al. for the Celecoxib Long-term Arthritis Safety Study. Gastrointestinal toxicity with celecoxib vs. nonsteroidal anti-inflammatory drugs for osteoarthritis and rheumatoid arthritis: the CLASS study: a randomized controlled trial. *JAMA* 2000;284:1247.

Singletary SE, Allred C, Ashlet P, et al. Revision of the American Joint Committee on Cancer staging system for breast cancer. *J Clin Oncol* 2002;20(17):3628.

Smith RL, Purthi S, Fitzpatrick LA. Evaluation and management of breast pain. *Mayo Clin Proc* 2004;79:353.

Smith S. Full field breast tomosynthesis. *Radiology Management* 2005;27(5):25.

Speroff L. Clinical implications of hormone-induced breast density. *Menopausal Medicine* 2005;13(2):1.

Surrey ES. Add-Back Consensus Working Group. Add-back therapy and gonadotropin-releasing hormone agonists in the treatment of patients with endometriosis: can a consensus be reached?. *Fertil Steril* 1999;71:420.

Tabbara SO, Frost AR, Stoler MH, et al. Changing trends in breast fine needle aspiration: results of the Papanicolaou Society of Cytopathology Survey. *Diagn Cytopathol* 2000;22:126.

Ueda T, Yokoyama Y, Irahara M, et al. Influence of psychological stress on suckling induced pulsatile oxytocin release. *Obstet Gynecol* 1994;84:259.

Vacek PM, Geller BM. A prospective study of breast cancer risk using routine mammographic breast density measurements. *Cancer Epidemiol Biomarkers Prev* 2004;13:715.

Van't Veer LJ, Dai H, Van de Vijver MJ, et al. Gene expression profiling predict clinical outcome in breast cancer. *Nature* 2002;415(6871):530.

Veronesi U, Paganelli G, Viale G, et al. A randomized comparison of sentinel-node biopsy with routine axillary dissection in breast cancer. *N Engl J Med* 2003;349(6):546.

Vetto JR, Pomiier RF, Schmidt WA, et al. Diagnosis of palpable breast lesions in younger women by the modified triple test is accurate and cost effective. *Arch Surg* 1996;131(9):967.

Vicini FA, Kestin L, Chen P, et al. Limited-field radiation therapy in the management of early state breast cancer. *J Natl Cancer Inst* 2003;95(16):1205.

Warner E, Plewes DB, Hill KA, et al. Surveillance of BRCA1 and BECA2 mutation carriers with magnetic resonance imaging, ultrasound, mammography and clinical breast examination. *JAMA* 2004;292(11):1317.

Warner E, Plewes DB, Shumak RS, et al. Comparison of breast magnetic resonance imaging, mammography and ultrasound for surveillance of women at high risk for hereditary breast cancer. *J Clin Oncol* 2001;19:3524.

Weir HK, Thun MJ, Hankey BF, et al. Annual report to the nation on the status of cancer, 1975–2000, featuring the uses of surveillance data for cancer prevention and control. *J Natl Cancer Inst* 2003;95(17):1276.

Whittemore AS, Harris R, Itnyre J. Collaborative Ovarian Cancer Group. Characteristics relating to ovarian cancer risk; collaborative analysis of 12 US case-control studies. II. Invasive epithelial ovarian cancers in white women. *Am J Epidemiol* 1992;136:1184.

Woodward WA, Strom EA, Tucker SL, et al. Changes in the 2003 American Joint Committee on Cancer staging for breast cancer dramatically affect stage-specific survival. *J Clin Oncol* 2003;21(17):3244.

Writing Group for the Women's Health Initiative. Risks and benefits of combined estrogen and progestin in healthy postmenopausal women: principal results for the Women's Health Initiative randomized controlled trial. *JAMA* 2002;288:321.

CHAPTER 42 ■ THE VERMIFORM APPENDIX IN RELATION TO GYNECOLOGY

BARRY K. JARNAGIN

DEFINITIONS

Appendicitis—Inflammation of the appendix, usually initiated by obstruction of the appendiceal lumen and subsequent production of frank pus; obstruction may be caused by hyperplasia of lymphoid follicles in response to systemic infectious disease, by bacterial enterocolitis, by a fecalith, by a tumor or other invasive process, or by a foreign body.

Incidental appendectomy—Prophylactic removal of the normal-appearing appendix during surgery for another condition.

McBurney's point—Located at the junction of the middle and lateral thirds of a line drawn from the umbilicus to right anterolateral spine.

Obturator sign—Increased pain in the right lower abdomen when passively flexing the hip.

Psoas sign—Increased pain as the right leg is extended at the hip when the patient is in the left lateral decubitus position.

Rovsing sign—Pain in the right lower quadrant when pressure is applied to the left lower quadrant.

Appendectomy is the most common surgical procedure performed on an emergency basis and the most common cause of abdominal pain requiring surgery. The differential diagnosis of lower abdominal pain not only includes acute appendicitis, but many gynecologic problems, such as pelvic inflammatory disease, ectopic pregnancy, ovarian torsion, and ruptured ovarian cyst. Therefore, the differential diagnosis of lower abdominal pain is one of the most common and difficult diagnoses that the gynecologist is called on to make. It is a serious undertaking and one in which a mistake could be fatal.

Individuals have a 7% lifetime risk of developing appendicitis. In the United States, reports show that approximately 300,000 operations are done per year, with the greatest incidence in the second and third decade of life. Although the overall mortality rate with appropriate and timely treatment is much less than 1%, it remains approximately 5% to 15% in the elderly. The higher mortality and morbidity rate in the elderly is caused by the increased difficulty in diagnosing appendicitis in older people, which leads to a higher rate of perforation. The incidence of perforation in patients ranges from 17% to 40%, with a median of 20%. The perforation rate in the elderly patient is significantly higher, with rates as high as 60% to 70% reported. Several factors contribute to this, including significant delay in seeking care, nonspecificity of the presenting symptoms and signs, diminished febrile response, and fewer abnormalities in laboratory parameters, such as the white blood cell count. Although the mortality rate for acute appendicitis is less than 0.1%, the mortality rate for gangrenous appendicitis is about 0.6%, and the mortality rate for perforated appendicitis is 5%. Death usually is the result of uncontrollable sepsis with generalized peritonitis, intraabdominal abscesses, intestinal obstruction, pyelonephritis, and Gram-negative septicemia. The overall morbidity rate is about 15% to 20% in most reports of appendicitis, with wound infection from a gangrenous or perforated appendix being the most common complication. Preoperative antibiotic therapy has greatly improved the morbidity rate, but perforation of the appendix is not prevented by antibiotics. Nor has the incidence of perforation decreased in recent years. Acute inflammation of the appendix commonly extends to the right adnexa (Fig. 42.1) and can involve the left as well when a large periappendiceal abscess develops in the pelvis. When the appendix ruptures, bilateral tubal adhesions commonly occur that may result in sterility or tubal pregnancy as a sequela. Incidental appendectomy at the time of other pelvic surgery remains controversial, but proponents argue that appendectomy simplifies the differential diagnosis of lower abdominal pain and prevents the possibility of a ruptured appendix in the future. This controversy is discussed later in the chapter.

HISTORY

The first known surgical removal of the appendix occurred in December 1735 when Claudius Amyand operated on an 11-year-old boy with a longstanding scrotal hernia and fecal fistula. He found a perforated appendix in the hernia sac and removed it. The fistula closed, and the boy recovered. The first known successful appendectomy for acute appendicitis was performed in 1880 by Lawson Tait, the renowned British abdominal and gynecologic surgeon who was also the first to operate successfully on a patient with a ruptured tubal pregnancy.

The recognition of appendicitis as a significant problem necessitating surgical removal was described by Fitz in 1886 and McBurney in 1889. Fitz described the sequence of appendiceal inflammation, perforation, abscess formation, and peritonitis.

In 1905, Kelly and Hurdon coauthored a beautifully illustrated book titled *The Vermiform Appendix and Its Diseases.* The book is unexcelled in its definition of the pathology, clinical manifestations, and natural history of appendicitis and its complications. There have been numerous reviews through the years since that time.

ANATOMY AND FUNCTION OF THE APPENDIX

The base of the appendix arises from the inferior wall of the cecum about 2.5 cm from the ileocecal valve. The taeniae coli of the cecum form the outer longitudinal muscle of the

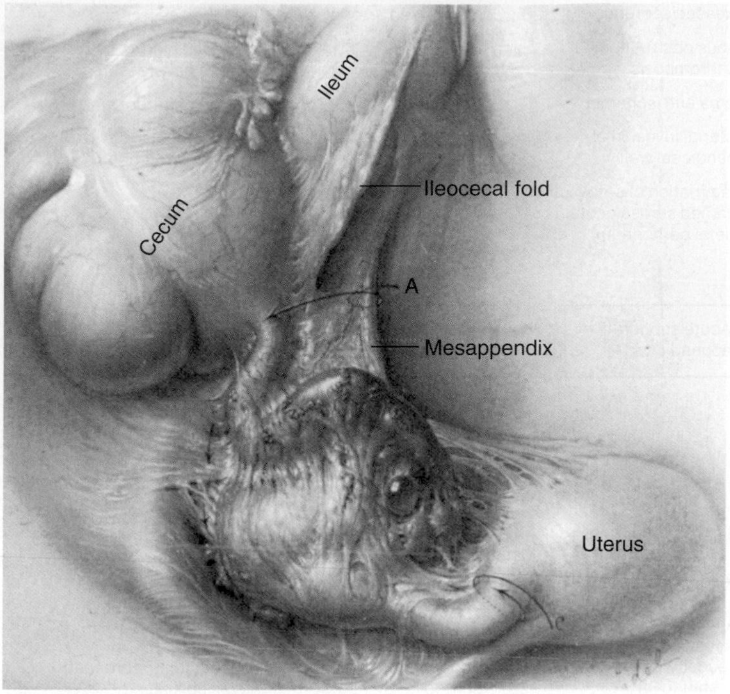

FIGURE 42.1. As illustrated in this original Max Broedel drawing, inflammatory disease of the appendix can involve the fallopian tube or vice versa. Extensive adhesions can form. The tube and the appendix can be removed as a single mass.

appendix and, therefore, can be followed inferiorly to help locate an appendix that is hidden. The appendiceal tip is found most commonly in a retrocecal position (65% of cases). Signs and symptoms of appendicitis may vary depending on the location of the appendix. The main blood supply to the appendix, the appendicular artery, is a branch of the ileocolic artery and is located in the mesoappendix. The base of the appendix is supplied by a branch of the posterior cecal artery.

The appendiceal wall is composed of smooth muscle; the narrow lumen is lined by colonic mucosa. A large number of submucosal lymphoid follicles are found in the appendix in teenagers and young adults. This number declines rapidly after 30 years of age. These lymphoid follicles function in the gut-associated lymphoid tissue secretory globulin immune system, but their function is not indispensable in the secretory immune system of the gut.

Anatomists have questioned the purpose of the appendix since its initial description. Leonardo da Vinci considered the appendix to serve and protect the cecum from rupture by too great an accumulation of "superfluous wind" because it had the ability to dilate and contract. Current belief is that the appendix is a vestigial organ with no function in humans. The appendix is absent in carnivores such as the dog, wolf, tiger, and lion. In herbivores, a long and well-developed cecum is noted. In omnivores, which include apes and humans, a portion of the cecum is smaller in diameter with a prominent lymphoid aggregation susceptible to inflammation or atrophy. The preserve of lymphoid aggregation has led to the hypothesis that the appendix has a role in immune surveillance of the gut. Others postulate an exocrine function to assist in the digestion of plants. In a 24-hour period, the adult human appendix produces a maximum of 2 mL of fluid containing mucin, amylase, and proteolytic enzymes. It is unlikely that this volume aids substantially in digestion. A pressure gradient normally exists along the long axis and prohibits the entrance of food or other intestinal contents into the lumen of the appendix.

ACUTE APPENDICITIS

Acute appendicitis is initiated by an obstruction of the appendiceal lumen. The obstruction can be caused by hyperplasia of lymphoid follicles of the appendix as part of a generalized response of lymphoid tissue to a systemic infectious disease, by bacterial enterocolitis, or by a fecalith, a foreign body, or intestinal parasites in the appendiceal lumen. An increase in intraluminal pressure distal to the obstruction from increased mucus secretion is followed by an increase in bacteria and, finally, the production of frank pus. The appendix becomes swollen, and the appendiceal wall becomes edematous from obstruction of lymphatic and venous drainage. Ulceration of the mucosa allows invasion of the wall by bacteria. Further progression causes venous thrombosis and obstruction of blood flow through the appendiceal artery. Because this is an end artery, no collateral circulation is available to prevent ischemic necrosis and gangrene with eventual rupture of the wall. Escape of bacteria through the perforation causes peritonitis. Unless necrosis of the base of the appendix occurs, continued fecal contamination of the peritoneal cavity is prevented by the initial blockage of the appendiceal lumen. The infection in the right lower quadrant can be walled off efficiently in young, healthy patients. In women, this abscess usually involves the right adnexal organs to some extent. Generalized peritonitis may ensue in advanced age or in the presence of reduced host resistance from other illnesses or immunosuppression. A correlation between the clinical course and pathologic progress of appendicitis is illustrated in Figure 42.2.

Diagnosis of Acute Appendicitis

The diagnosis of acute appendicitis is based primarily on history and physical examination, although today computed

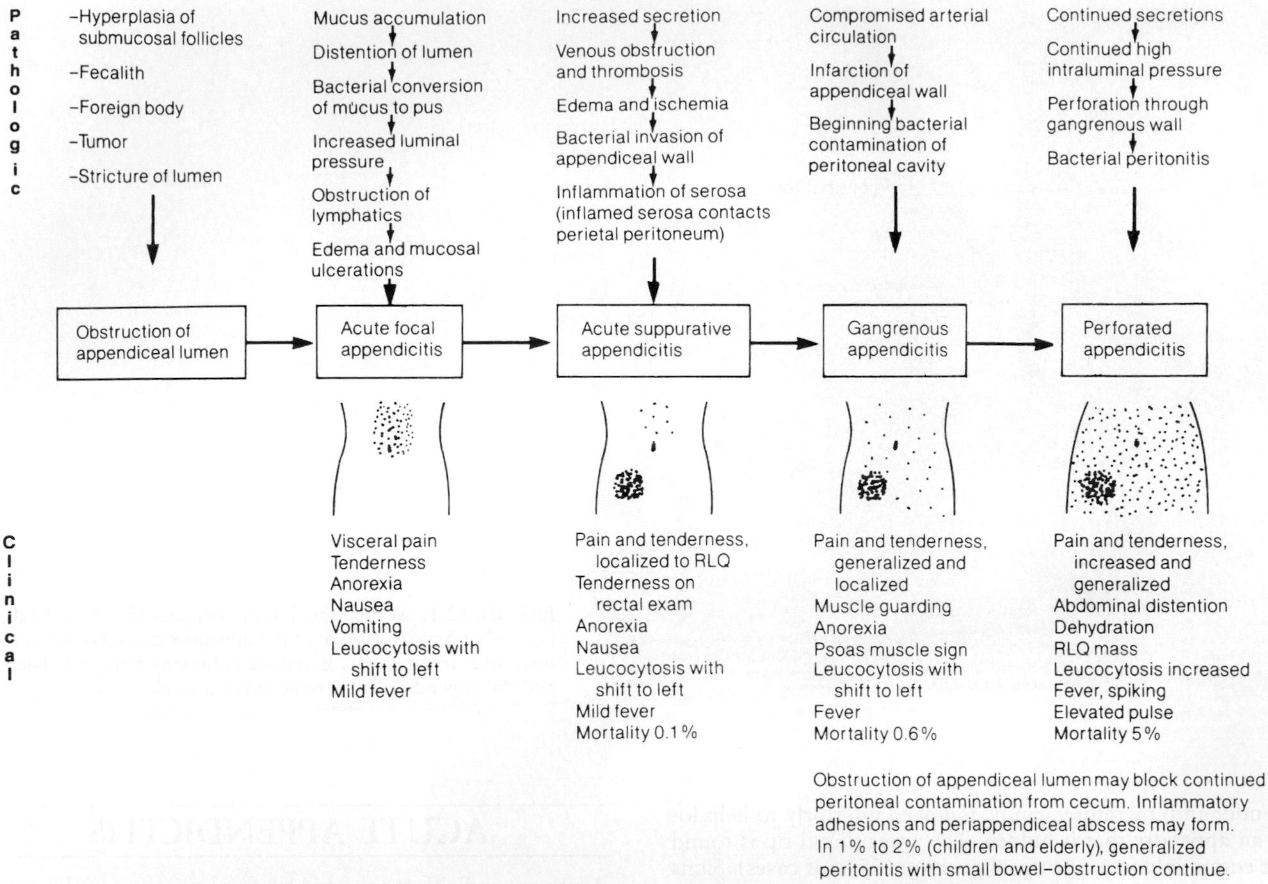

FIGURE 42.2. The clinical-pathologic correlations of appendicitis. RLQ, right lower quadrant. (From: Sabiston DC Jr, ed. *Textbook of surgery.* Philadelphia: WB Saunders, 1991, with permission.)

tomography (CT) scan of the abdomen is a very helpful imaging modality. All symptoms and signs should be listed, and careful evaluation must be done with assignment of different weights to each as appropriate to the clinical setting. Pain is present in 95% of patients and is the most consistent symptom. The typical pain of acute appendicitis is diffuse and mild and initially located in the epigastrium and periumbilical region. Once local peritonitis occurs, the maximum tenderness usually is located in the region of the appendix. Anorexia, nausea, and occasional vomiting usually are present. (The diagnosis of appendicitis is in doubt if vomiting occurs first.) This classic sequence can be found in 50% of patients. However, it should be emphasized that the typical presentation is absent in the remaining 50%. Atypically, pain can be localized in the right lower quadrant in the beginning, or it can remain diffuse throughout the abdomen. Although the location of the cecum is constant, the inflamed appendiceal tip may be located in the right upper quadrant, in the cul-de-sac, or anywhere in between. The location and magnitude of the pain may vary with the position of the appendix and age of the patient. Elderly patients may have less severe pain and delayed localization in the right lower quadrant. Indeed, appendicitis in the elderly presents a real challenge to early diagnosis, because very few clinical findings may be present. This is the reason for the higher incidence of appendiceal perforation and, consequently, the higher morbidity and mortality in older patients, as confirmed in the 1986 report by Lau and associates.

In infants and children, the diagnosis is also more difficult, and the incidence of appendiceal perforation higher. Improvement in the results for these two age groups depends on a higher index of suspicion and a lower threshold for intervention, which inevitably results in the removal of a larger number of normal appendixes. Improved diagnosis with ultrasound and CT scanning may decrease the incidence of appendiceal rupture and also the frequency of exploratory laparotomy for what turns out to be a normal appendix. However, removal of a normal appendix in a symptomatic patient who is thought to have appendicitis, a potentially lethal disease, should not be considered an unnecessary operation. The number of elderly patients and children who die of appendicitis because of failure to operate early enough when the diagnosis is in doubt is much higher than the number of patients who die from a complication following removal of a normal appendix. The morbidity of negative laparoscopy or laparotomy is minimal and is much more acceptable than the significantly higher morbidity of a perforated appendix. Unfortunately, after 60 years of age, about 50% of patients are found to have a ruptured appendix when the operation is finally done. The mortality rate in these patients is 5%; however, this represents more than 50% of all deaths from appendicitis.

Twelve to forty-eight hours usually elapse from the onset of symptoms until the patient consults her physician. On physical examination, patients with appendicitis classically have tenderness to direct palpation, rebound tenderness, and muscle guarding in the right lower quadrant over the point where the inflamed appendiceal serosa is in contact with the parietal peritoneum, often at McBurney's point, which is located at the junction of the middle and lateral thirds of a line drawn from the umbilicus to the right anterosuperior spine. The Rovsing sign (pain in the right lower quadrant when pressure is applied in the left lower quadrant) as well as psoas and obturator muscle signs may be positive. A positive psoas sign is increased pain as the right leg is extended at the hip when the patient is in the left lateral decubitus position, indicating irritation of the psoas muscle by the inflamed appendix. A positive obturator sign is increased pain in the right lower abdomen when passively flexing the right hip and knee and internally rotating the leg at the hip, indicating irritation of the obturator muscle. Rectal and pelvic examinations always should be done and often reveal tenderness high on the right side of the pelvis. Pelvic inflammatory disease is almost always associated with bilateral adnexal tenderness. A pelvic mass from an inflamed appendix sometimes can be felt on pelvic examination. A tender, unilateral adnexal mass also may be found in a patient with ovarian torsion, but ultrasound should help make the diagnosis. As the disease progresses to gangrene and appendiceal rupture, a mass consisting of inflammatory adhesions, omentum, indurated bowel, mesentery, and pockets of purulent exudate usually can be felt in the right lower quadrant or right adnexa. Tenderness and muscle rigidity are more pronounced. If the infection fails to localize, generalized peritonitis ensues with diffuse tenderness, guarding, distention, ileus, dehydration, tachycardia, and spiking fever. All these signs may be less apparent in the elderly. Several studies over the past few decades have evaluated the clinical presentation of patients with acute appendicitis. A summary of the common history and physical findings is shown in Table 42.1.

Laboratory and Radiology Diagnosis

Minimal investigation is required when the history and physical examination are definitive. About two thirds of patients with appendicitis have an elevated white blood cell (WBC) count of greater than 10,000 WBC/mL. However, an elevated WBC is also found in acute pelvic inflammatory disease, diverticulitis, pyelonephritis, and in many patients with ovarian torsion. In elderly patients, however, the white cell count may be elevated only slightly or not at all, even though the differential count is abnormal. The erythrocyte sedimentation rate is elevated when the appendix is severely inflamed, but this is a very nonspecific test. Some white cells and red cells may be present in the urine of patients with appendicitis, although significant bacteriuria suggests a urinary tract infection is a more likely diagnosis.

CT is usually the initial imaging technique used in emergency departments in the United States today. CT imaging has a 90% sensitivity for detecting intraabdominal inflammation. A specific diagnosis can be made in 80% of these patients. A normal appendix may be difficult to locate on CT examination and may require extra scans at finer intervals. Appendicoliths are seen in one fourth of all people as a ringlike or homogenous calcified density on CT. Specific CT findings of appendicitis become more prominent with advanced diseases, including a distended, thick-walled, edematous appendix seen as a target structure (Fig. 42.3). Other findings include inflammatory streaking of surrounding fat and the presence of an appendicolith. CT findings suggestive of appendicitis include a pericecal phlegmon or abscess and small amounts of right lower quadrant intraabdominal free air that signals perforation.

Ultrasound may also be a valuable adjunct to physical examination in young women with pelvic or lower quadrant pain. Graded abdominal compression is used to displace the cecum and ascending colon, exposing the retrocecal area and pelvis. A typical "target appearance" identifies the appendix by characteristic changes within its wall (Fig. 42.4). Findings associated with appendicitis include wall thickening beyond the normal 8 to 10 mm, luminal distention, lack of compressibility, and localized pain and tenderness at the site of the visualized appendix. Advanced cases are noted by asymmetric wall thickening, abscess formation, associated free intraperitoneal fluid, surrounding tissue edema, and decreased local tenderness to compression. The sensitivity of ultrasound in the diagnosis of appendicitis from several centers has been reported to be as high as 80%, with a specificity as high as 90%.

Standard abdominal radiography may show a calcified fecalith in the right lower quadrant along with a paucity of gas in the right lower quadrant of the abdomen. A loss of the right

TABLE 42.1

SUMMARY OF CLINICAL EXAMINATION OPERATING CHARACTERISTICS FOR APPENDICITIS

Procedure	Sensitivity	Specificity	LR+ (95% CI)	LR- (95% CI)
Right lower quadrant pain	0.81	0.53	7.31–8.46	0–0.28
Rigidity	0.27	0.83	3.76 (2.96–4.78)	0.82 (0.79–0.85)
Migration	0.64	0.82	3.18 (2.41–4.21)	0.50 (0.42–0.59)
Pain before vomiting	1.00	0.64	2.76 (1.94–3.94)	—
Psoas sign	0.16	0.95	2.38 (1.21–4.67)	0.90 (0.83–0.98)
Fever	0.67	0.79	1.94 (1.63–2.32)	0.58 (0.51–0.67)
Rebound tenderness test	0.63	0.69	1.10–6.30	0–0.86
Guarding	0.74	0.57	1.65–1.78	0–0.54
No similar pain previously	0.81	0.41	1.50 (1.36–1.66)	0.323 (0.246–0.424)
Rectal tenderness	0.41	0.77	0.83–5.34	0.36–1.15
Anorexia	0.68	0.36	1.27 (1.16–1.38)	0.64 (0.54–0.75)
Nausea	0.58	0.37	0.69–1.20	0.70–0.84
Vomiting	0.51	0.45	0.92 (0.82–1.04)	1.12 (0.95–1.33)

LR, likelihood ratio; CI, confidence interval.
Source: Wagner JM, McKinney WP, Carpenter JL. Does this patient have appendicitis? *JAMA* 1996;276:1589, with permission.

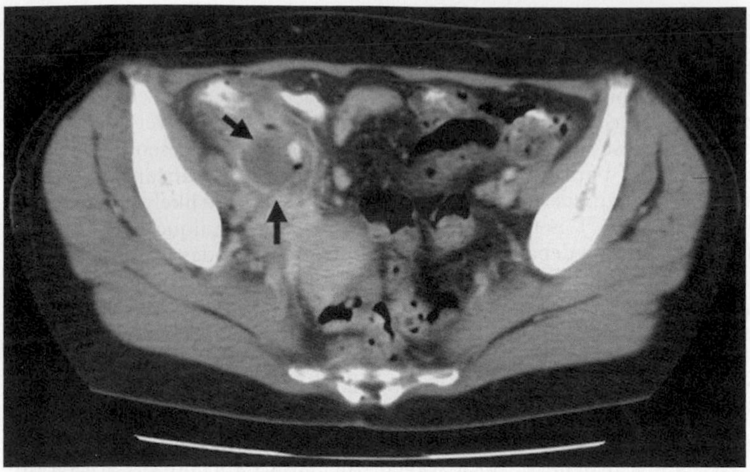

FIGURE 42.3. Computed tomography of appendiceal abscess. Note complex fluid mass with an enhancing rim in the right lower quadrant. (Courtesy of Ronald Arildsen, MD, Vanderbilt University.)

psoas shadow may be noted and represents late appendicitis with retroperitoneal inflammation. A perforated or gangrenous appendix may exhibit extraabdominal gas on radiographs, but this occurs in only 1% of cases. A sentinel loop ileus or a soft-tissue mass with or without gas bubbles also be may seen in advanced cases.

Barium contrast studies remain a simple, safe, and readily available test that may be helpful. However, ultrasound and CT examinations now are preferred. A barium study assures luminal patency of the appendix, colonic wall for mass effects or secondary effects of appendicitis, and right colonic or terminal ileal mucosal disease that may simulate appendicitis. When the barium contrast fills the appendix, a diagnosis of acute appendicitis is very unlikely but not impossible. Up to 10% to 20% of normal appendices do not fill during a barium study.

Laparoscopy can be both diagnostic and therapeutic for acute appendicitis. Some have advocated diagnostic laparoscopy in all women presenting with symptoms associated with acute appendicitis to reduce unnecessary appendectomy while also examining for gynecologic pathologies. The diagnostic error of presumed appendicitis in young, adult women in the reproductive years is 35% to 50%. According to Leape and Romanofsky, and Deutech and associates, about one third of patients who underwent laparoscopy for suspected appendicitis did not have appendicitis.

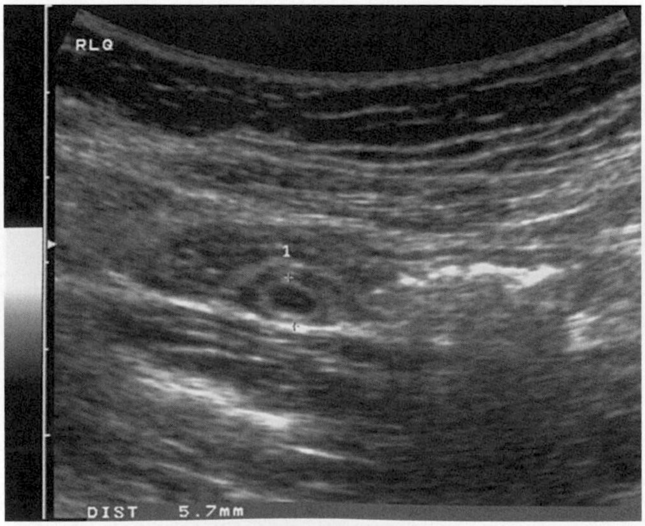

FIGURE 42.4. Transabdominal ultrasound of acute appendicitis. Note the "targetlike" appearance produced by the thickened, inflamed wall of the appendix. (Courtesy of Arthur Fleischer, MD, Vanderbilt University.)

Because there is no single diagnostic test for acute appendicitis that is accurate and applicable to the general population, most physicians agree with Levine and associates that a decrease in the number of negative explorations is most likely to be achieved by sound clinical judgment supplemented by basic laboratory and radiologic studies. Using this standard classical approach assiduously, these authors reported negative laparotomy in only 7.4% of 282 patients with a preoperative diagnosis of suspected appendicitis. Most patients with the classic pattern of migratory abdominal pain, direct and rebound tenderness in the right lower abdominal quadrant, and increased metamyelocytes in the peripheral blood smear require prompt operation. However, when there is an atypical presentation in a young adult women, close in-hospital observation may be indicated to allow progression of the clinical picture and complete the radiologic workup. Simultaneous evaluation by the general surgeon and gynecologist is also of benefit in improving diagnostic accuracy.

Laparoscopy may be indicated in problem patients. In almost all circumstances, a laparoscopy with negative findings is preferred to expectantly watching the appendix rupture or pelvic inflammatory disease progress untreated. An unnecessary delay increases the likelihood of perforation, increasing morbidity and mortality. In the younger patient, it also increases the risk of pelvic adhesions, infertility, and chronic pain. When surgery is performed within 24 hours of the onset of symptoms, less than 20% of appendixes are perforated, compared with more than 70% when operation is delayed more than 48 hours after symptoms began. A delay in diagnosis in pregnant patients has especially devastating effects on the outcome. A proper evaluation of clinical presentation allows the index of suspicion to be set at the proper level so that a threshold for intervention can be reached before the appendix ruptures. According to Condon and Telford,

> The removal of a normal appendix in appropriate clinical circumstances never constitutes an unnecessary appendectomy. A policy of active surgical intervention on the basis of minimal clinical suspicion has been demonstrated to reduce both the morbidity and mortality of appendicitis. Watching and waiting, however careful it may be, runs the risk of increasing both morbidity and mortality.

Treatment of Acute Appendicitis

There is general agreement that the treatment of acute appendicitis is appendectomy. Clinical experience and numerous reports on mortality clearly show the advantage of early operation. The current operative mortality without perforation is essentially nil, and only 3% of patients have postoperative complications. After perforation, the overall mortality rate is less than 5%, but more than 30% of patients have postoperative complications. These statistics have improved with the use of antibiotics and earlier intervention.

The patient with appendicitis should not be rushed to the operating room without adequate hydration and antibiotic treatment. Most surgeons use short-course (<24 hours) antimicrobial prophylaxis. One common combination is cefazolin and metronidazole to cover Gram-negative, -positive, and anaerobic bacteria. Recent studies have recommended monotherapy with a second-generation, broad-spectrum cephalosporin such as cefotetan for patients undergoing surgery. Antibiotics have been shown to be effective in reducing the incidence of postoperative wound infections if started preoperatively. Antibiotics can be discontinued immediately following surgery if the appendix is not gangrenous or perforated. However, if the appendix has ruptured, many surgeons switch to triple antibiotic therapy including ampicillin, metronidazole, and gentamicin to encompass a wide spectrum of enteric bacteria. Intravenous antibiotic therapy should be continued until the patient is well on the way to recovery, which is usually 3 to 5 days.

Postoperatively, if the appendix is not ruptured, the patient usually is discharged within 24 hours. However, if the appendix was ruptured or gangrenous, supportive treatment is continued in the ill patient. Food and fluid by mouth are restricted. Nasogastric suction is rarely used today. Wound infection is the most common complication after appendectomy. Other more serious complications include pelvic, subphrenic, and intraabdominal abscess; fecal fistula; peritonitis; pyelonephritis; venous thrombosis; and intestinal obstruction. Septicemia, pneumonia, septic shock, renal failure, and pulmonary embolus can lead to death in the most advanced or neglected cases.

It is relatively safe to remove the appendix in virtually any patient. However, if there are significant medical contraindications to surgery in a nontoxic patient with a clear diagnosis of an appendiceal abscess, a nonoperative approach can be considered. If a distinct mass in the right iliac fossa is palpated and the patient has no systemic manifestations, the patient is kept nil per os (NPO) while intravenous fluids and broad-spectrum antibiotics are given to cover enteric organisms. The patient should be kept under close observation with the pulse closely followed because tachycardia is one of the first signs of sepsis. Other clinical parameters to follow include change in pain quality, white blood cell counts, differential counts, and serial radiologic evaluations, including ultrasound and/or CT. Failure to respond to therapy after 24 to 48 hours indicates that operative intervention should be reconsidered. Patients with well-formed periappendiceal abscesses can undergo CT-guided placement of pigtail drainage catheters to help resolve the abscess more rapidly, rather than depending on the abscess to drain internally into the cecum. If the abscess is palpable, it is usually large and should be drained. Limitations of percutaneous drainage include the inadequacy of draining multiloculated abscesses, inaccessible location, and possible need for anesthesia. Periappendiceal abscesses usually resolve in 10 to 14 days without appendectomy or drainage. Most surgeons wait 6 to 12 weeks after nonoperative therapy to perform an interval appendectomy. Technical difficulties during interval appendectomy may be minimal but can be extreme, depending on the nature of the initial abscess.

Laparoscopic Technique

Since it was first described by Semm in 1983, laparoscopic appendectomy has gained acceptance as both a diagnostic and treatment method for acute appendicitis. Many studies have demonstrated that a videolaparoscopic approach to acute appendicitis is safe and effective for the experienced endoscopist. The laparoscopic approach offers many potential advantages, including less surgical tissue trauma, a better postoperative course, the ability to explore the entire abdominal cavity, assessment for the existence of associated pathologies, better cosmetic results, and a rapid return to normal activity. The ability to completely evaluate the pelvis and the entire peritoneal cavity when a healthy appendix is found is extremely important for the gynecologist in light of the other conditions that mimic appendicitis in women, such as adnexitis, endometriosis, ovarian cysts, ectopic pregnancies, and even cholecystitis.

Removing a normal appendix during laparoscopic evaluation for suspected acute appendicitis can be performed with no added morbidity or increased length of hospitalization as compared with diagnostic laparoscopy. Initially, there were some concerns about an increased risk of intraabdominal abscess formation following laparoscopic surgery for acute appendicitis, possibly secondary to peritoneal insufflation spreading local infection throughout the abdominal cavity and the carbon dioxide pneumoperitoneum creating a favorable environment for the survival of virulent anaerobic bacteria. However, many studies comparing open versus laparoscopic appendectomies have shown a lower morbidity rate with laparoscopy. The laparoscopic approach offers the advantage of shorter hospitalization and less morbidity, with a lower rate of abdominal wall infection. There is no significant difference in the rate of abscess formation in patients with perforated appendicitis. The interval until the patient may return to work is shortened and postoperative pain is decreased with the laparoscopic approach, and the quality of life appears to improve faster than when the traditional open approach is used. Obese patients may benefit substantially from the laparoscopic approach as it obviates the problems of a large incision, strong retraction, prolonged surgery, and wound infection that are associated with open surgery in the obese.

The disadvantages of the laparoscopic approach have been longer duration of surgery and higher costs. However, the length of surgery has been significantly reduced with improved surgical skills and experience. Also, the immediate cost difference appears to be diminished with the use of reusable laparoscopic equipment, and when the more rapid return to work and other activities is included, the laparoscopic approach turns out to be extremely cost-effective. It is increasingly recommended as the procedure of choice for the diagnosis and treatment of suspected acute appendicitis.

The operation is conducted under general anesthesia with endotracheal intubation and muscle relaxation to allow controlled ventilation after the patient has been positioned in the modified dorsal lithotomy position with low stirrups. The position of the patient may be adjusted with Trendelenburg tilt or tilting the table to the left to optimize visualization of the appendix and better exposure to the structures on the right side of the pelvis and the right iliac fossa. The stomach and bladder are decompressed to minimize risk of injury during trocar insertion

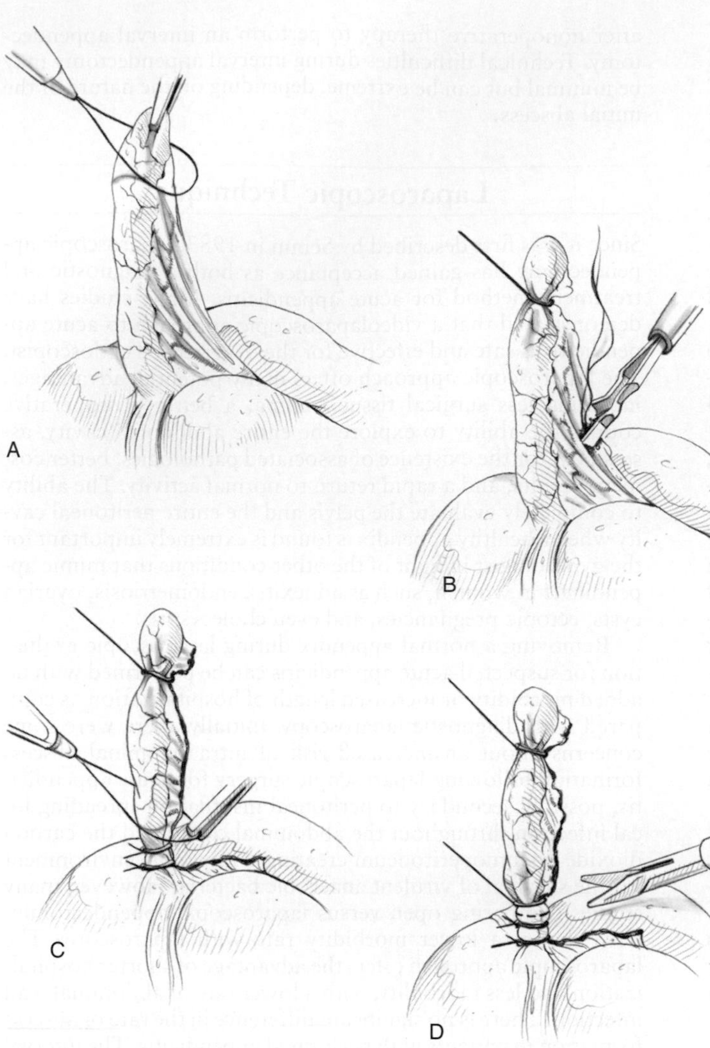

FIGURE 42.5. Laparoscopic appendectomy technique. **A:** The appendix is elevated with atraumatic forceps, and a pretied suture loop is placed around the distal end to provide traction. **B:** The mesoappendix is divided using cautery. Clips or the harmonic scalpel also can be used. **C:** The skeletonized base of the appendix is then crushed with forceps to empty its contents, and three ligatures are placed around the base. **D:** The appendix is divided, leaving two absorbable ligatures on the stump.

and allow optimal visualization of the operative field. Initially, an open or closed laparoscopic trocar insertion technique is used to place a 5- or 10-mm laparoscope. After viewing the location of the appendix, the accessory trocars can be placed in several different ways, again depending on the preference of the surgeon and anatomy of the appendix. We prefer placing the accessory trocars in the right and left lower quadrants and then one in the midline two finger breadths above the symphysis pubis. This places the trocars in positions familiar to the gynecologist and results in cosmetically appealing incisions. Atraumatic forceps are used through the lower right trocar to secure the tip of the appendix. If the appendix is markedly swollen, a pretied surgical loop can be placed at the tip and used for traction (Fig. 42.5). The appendix is elevated and retracted toward the pelvis, keeping the mesoappendix stretched. Adhesions can be separated from the appendix with sharp or blunt dissection. Dense and vascular adhesions require bipolar cautery, the harmonic scalpel, or clips. The appendix is skeletonized and isolated from the mesoappendix with bipolar cautery. (Metal clips, unipolar cautery, and the harmonic shears also may be used.) Special attention should be given to the appendicular artery that is located near the base of the appendix. The base of the appendix is secured by various methods: (a) three metal clips or three Endoloops with transection between them so that two ligatures remain at the base of the appendix, (b) the use of bipolar coagulation and resection, (c) the use of mechanical cutting and stapling devices, and (d) the use of endoloops with which self-locking extracorporeal slip-knots or normal surgical knots are made. Mechanical suturing devices can be used offering a secure and technically easy method, but this is an expensive option. We prefer the Endoloop technique using no. 1 chromic sutures. After isolating the appendix, two chromic Endoloop ties are placed securely at the base of the appendix. The area distal to the ties is then milked, and the third Endoloop is placed 2 to 4 mm from the other ties. The appendix can be excised with scissors or harmonic scalpel and removed through the larger trocar under direct visualization. The appendix can be placed in an endobag or surgical glove when there is the possibility of rupture. Some advocate cauterizing the stump; however, this can cause necrosis of the cecum at the site of the ligature on the appendicular stump and result in a subsequent cecal fistula. Care should be taken to remove the entire appendix because appendicitis of the appendicular stump has been reported. A total appendectomy can be achieved by ensuring that the mesoappendix is cleared off the base of the appendix until the three taenia on the cecum can be identified clearly. Stump invagination is not necessary and not performed routinely by this author because of the reasons previously discussed. If the surgeon desires to bury the stump, it is performed in a fashion similar to the open technique using no. 0 chromic catgut suture and one extracorporal knot. Careful irrigation and suction is performed after removal of the appendix.

The procedure is terminated in the usual laparoscopic fashion, with the trocars removed and the scope skin incision closed with 4-0 delayed absorbable sutures or Steri-strips. The fascia at the 10-mm incision must be closed with 0 or 2-0 delayed absorbable sutures. The postoperative course and hospital stay varies with the pathology and need for antibiotic coverage. Hospitalization generally is not required after uncomplicated laparoscopic appendectomy for an unruptured appendix. If the appendix is perforated at the base, the cecal strip would require suturing. If the appendix cannot be identified within an abscess cavity, the surgeon may either place a closed suction drain and plan an interval appendectomy, or convert to an open procedure.

Open Technique

The standard management of appendicitis has been open appendectomy by way of a limited right lower quadrant incision. The surgeon should note the point of maximal tenderness before anesthesia and attempt to palpate masses after anesthesia. McBurney's point, at the junction of the middle and lateral thirds of a line drawn from the umbilicus to the right anterosuperior iliac spine, does not universally mark the tip of the appendix. In general, an inferior incision below the area of maximal tenderness helps in rotating the cecum into the wound. The McBurney incision is the classical oblique appendectomy incision through McBurney's point to the lateral edge of the rectus sheath; it can be extended into the lateral rectus sheath, if necessary. It is quite cosmetically acceptable when healed (Fig. 42.6). Alternatively, a skin line or transverse incision placed 1 to 2 cm medial to the anterosuperior iliac spine can be used. Both incisions generally are performed with a muscle-splitting technique through all layers lateral to the rectus abdominis muscle as entrance into the abdomen is gained. A low, horizontal skin incision also can be used and is possibly more cosmetic. The incision is continued through the superficial fascia until the external oblique muscle aponeurosis is exposed. The fibers of the aponeurosis are opened sharply, and the muscle fibers are bluntly separated, as are the fibers of the internal oblique and transverse abdominis muscles. The peritoneum is incised, and cultures can be obtained. The cecum is mobilized into the wound, and the appendix is mobilized as adhesions are bluntly and/or sharply dissected. The base of the appendix always lies at the confluence of the taeniae. When the appendix is mobile, the mesoappendix can be grasped near the tip of the appendix with a Kelly clamp and the appendix can be supported with a Babcock clamp near its base (Fig. 42.7). The mesoappendix can be ligated en masse with no. 3-0 absorbable suture if the pedicle is not too large or edematous. If this is not feasible, it is clamped and ligated with a succession of small bites with hemostats or Kelly clamps. Ligation of the mesoappendix usually is performed from the distal tip to the base of the appendix, but sometimes reversing the sequence can facilitate appendectomy. It may be appropriate to pass one suture into the musculature of the cecal wall and mesoappendix at the base of the appendix to ligate the accessory branch of the posterior cecal artery securely. Packs should be placed around the appendix to isolate it from the operative field. The appendix is double clamped with straight hemostats across the base, leaving sufficient space between clamps to permit passage of the

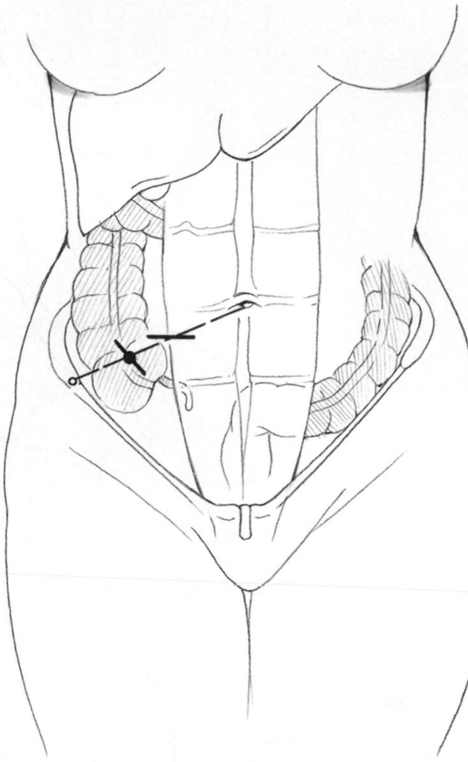

FIGURE 42.6. Common incisions for appendectomy. The classic McBurney incision over the cecum is not as easily extended to perform gynecologic procedures if needed.

cautery or scalpel. The space between clamps can be crushed or milked before clamping to minimize contamination into the peritoneal cavity. The appendix is amputated with the scalpel or with cautery, and the appendix and the attached clamp are dropped into a small basin to avoid contamination. The appendiceal stump is then doubly ligated with 2-0 absorbable or delayed absorbable suture. The appendiceal stump may be cauterized to prevent mucocele formation or inverted with a purse-string suture or Z-stitch in the cecum. If this is done, a purse-string suture of medium silk is placed around the base of the appendix. The circumference of the purse-string suture should be large enough to permit easy inversion of the stump. A half-knot is placed in the silk; after the appendix is amputated, the stump is inverted, and the purse string is drawn tight. The site of the inversion should be covered with mesoappendix or any convenient flap of fat. However, inversion of the stump is no longer considered necessary by many authors. It is not recommended when the appendix is inflamed. An abscess can form in the cecal wall, or a space-occupying mass may be seen in the cecum on barium enema leading to diagnostic confusion. Copious irrigation with saline or antibiotic solution should be performed in cases of perforated appendicitis to reduce the risk of a pelvic or subhepatic abscess. The peritoneum and muscular fasciae are usually closed with a running absorbable suture. The skin can be closed in nonperforated cases of appendicitis, but delayed primary closure is routine in cases of ruptured appendicitis. Skin mattress sutures can be placed and left untied until the third to fifth postoperative day. If the wound is clean, the skin sutures are tied and adhesive strips placed. If the wound is not healthy, it should not be closed but packed with wet to dry dressings and allowed to granulate from the

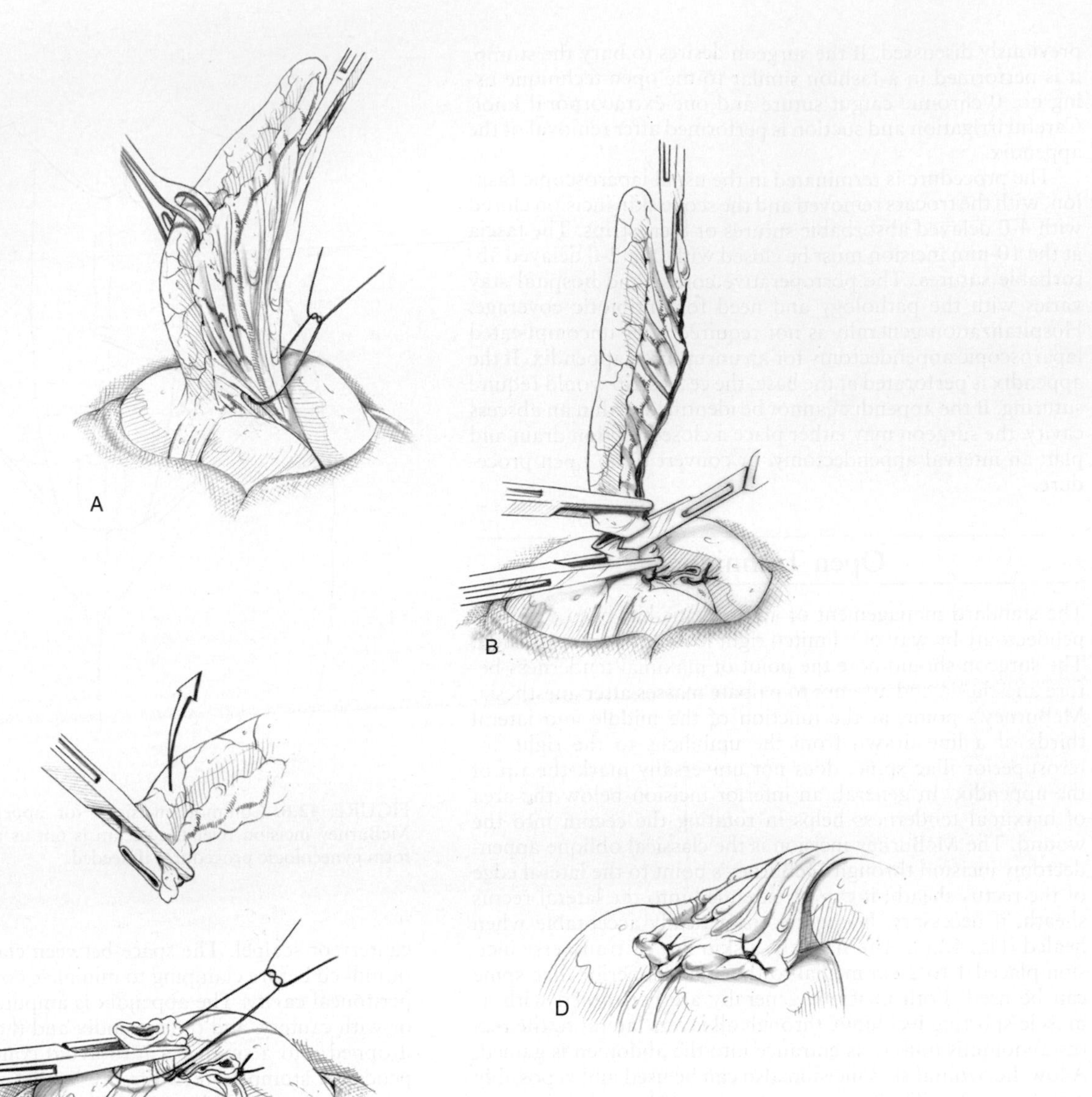

FIGURE 42.7. Technique of open appendectomy. A: The appendix is elevated by a Babcock clamp, and the mesoappendix is ligated. Alternatively, small clamps may be used to clamp, cut, and tie the mesoappendix. B: The operative field is isolated with gauze packs, and the appendix is cross-clamped and divided between the two closely placed clamps. C: The stump of the appendix is ligated with a 2.0 absorbable ligature. D: The stump is usually cauterized and covered with the adjacent mesoappendix.

bottom until healing is complete, which may take approximately 1 month.

APPENDICITIS IN PREGNANCY

In 1898, Hancock reported the first case of appendicitis complicating pregnancy. Appendectomy is the most common nonobstetrical operative intervention in the pregnant patient. The reported incidence of appendicitis in pregnancy varies from 1 in 355 to 1 in 11,479 deliveries. If ectopic pregnancy is excluded, appendicitis is responsible for about 75% of all cases of an acute abdomen during pregnancy. The incidence of acute appendicitis does not seem to be increased during pregnancy above that of the nonpregnant state, but the diagnosis often is delayed. Acute appendicitis occurs more often during the second trimester (50%) than during the first (10%) or third trimester (35%). Five percent of cases occur during labor or in puerperium. Although pregnancy does not appear to increase the incidence of appendicitis, it does increase the difficulty of diagnosis. This is because many abdominal symptoms are considered "normal" during pregnancy. Added to this are the anatomic changes in the location of the appendix. Baer and associates showed by repeat roentgenographic studies throughout pregnancy and the puerperium that the appendix rotated in a counterclockwise direction, with the tip displaced near the right kidney at term. The base of the appendix underwent upward and outward displacement after the third month, caused by the enlarging uterus, and reached the level of the iliac crest at the end of the sixth month. After the seventh month of pregnancy, in 88% of their cases, the appendix was found above the iliac crest. However, in interpreting these findings in relation to abdominal pain and tenderness, one must remember that in dealing with an abnormal appendix in which previous attacks of appendicitis may have occurred, adhesions can fix it in a low position and do not permit its upward displacement.

Ultrasound may be particularly useful in the diagnosis in pregnancy; but as noted, it may not be located in its normal, nonpregnant, right lower quadrant location. The most important step for the clinician is to consider the diagnosis of appendicitis in pregnancy.

The incidence of gangrenous and perforated appendix has been reported to be twice as high in pregnant patients as in women who are not pregnant and is highest in advanced pregnancy. In a pregnant patient, the omentum may not be able to reach the site of infection and perform its walling off function efficiently. If rupture is followed by abscess formation, the uterus is always a part of the abscess wall because of its proximity. Generalized peritonitis without abscess is more common in advanced pregnancy and is a serious threat to the expectant mother and her unborn child. The speed of onset and spread of peritonitis in pregnant patients can be insidious and strikingly rapid. The patient can become seriously ill and appear moribund within 24 hours. Peritonitis increases uterine irritability and the risk of preterm labor. Premature labor and delivery are the most serious fetal risks with up to 30% fetal mortality reported if perforation occurs. Maternal complications include wound infections, pelvic abscess, peritonitis, and pulmonary complications.

Treatment of Appendicitis in Pregnancy

Immediate operation is the treatment for acute appendicitis in pregnancy, regardless of the duration of pregnancy. Preoperative measures to improve the patient's condition should be brief and intensive. Although antibiotics may not be needed in simple acute appendicitis, antibiotic therapy should be initiated 30 minutes before surgery so that an adequate level can be present in the tissues when the incision is made. When a gangrenous or perforated appendix is found, antibiotics with broad-spectrum bacterial coverage should be continued or initiated immediately in both the pregnant and nonpregnant patient. One may choose to give cefoxitin and metronidazole. In the more serious cases, triple antibiotic therapy with ampicillin, gentamicin, and clindamycin should be used.

In this inflammatory environment, some suggest the use of nonsteroidal antiinflammatory drugs, such as indomethacin or ibuprofen, for tocolysis. Intravenous magnesium sulfate also can be used. Although the use of tocolytic agents to combat premature labor might seem reasonable, they should be used only in patients who are hemodynamically stable because they can increase pulmonary edema. As pointed out by deVeciana and associates, injudicious fluid management and tocolytic use can greatly increase the risk of pulmonary complications with antepartum appendicitis, especially in a third-trimester patient with a perforated appendix. Spontaneous premature labor is more likely when the appendix has ruptured. Tocolytic agents are the most dangerous in the patients who need them the most.

Delay in operating also can stem from concern about what harm the operation will do to the pregnancy, with the consequent desire to operate only when acute appendicitis is definitely present. Such a delay only increases the risk of perforation with its attendant problems for both mother and fetus. Proper removal of a normal appendix found at operation for suspected appendicitis rarely is associated with preterm labor, so the benefits clearly outweigh the minimal risks.

The anesthetic should be planned and administered to avoid hypotension and hypoxia. If the pregnancy is 3 months or less in duration, the appendix can be removed through the usual gridiron McBurney or Rockey-Davis incision. The more advanced the pregnancy, the higher should be the incision. If a midline incision is not used, it is important to center the incision over the point of maximum tenderness, which usually means using a high transverse muscle-cutting or a right paramedian incision. Tilting the patient to her left side minimizes displacement and handling of the uterus and relives the compression of the vena cava by the gravid uterus. The appendectomy should be done as quickly and atraumatically as possible, and the patient should be given intensive antibiotic therapy. In the case of appendiceal rupture with or without frank abscess formation, the patient should be treated immediately, in the same way as in the nonpregnant state, with the understanding that premature labor usually occurs as a result of the infection. Cesarean section should not be performed at that time of appendectomy with or without rupture to avoid infection in the newborn and postoperative endometritis and parametritis. Cesarean section in the third-trimester patient with appendicitis is indicated only for strict obstetric reasons. Some authors have advised that a cesarean section hysterectomy be performed to control the spread of infection into the uterus and broad ligaments.

Laparoscopic management of appendicitis now has been described with good results. The open laparoscopic technique is used, and all reports have shown success during all trimesters without complications. Some argue that the laparoscopic approach exposes the fetus to excessive risks from trocar placement and CO_2 insufflation. Others, however, note that laparoscopy expands the ability to explore the abdomen with less uterine manipulation and offers an increased ability for irrigation. Further, it increases the ability to locate the appendix and results in relatively small incisions compared with the open technique.

INCIDENTAL APPENDECTOMY IN GYNECOLOGIC AND OBSTETRIC SURGERY

Incidental appendectomy refers to the prophylactic removal of the normal-appearing appendix during surgery for another condition. In 1905, Howard Kelly of Johns Hopkins argued against incidental appendectomy because he felt it increased operative risk for the unproved benefit of reduction in the morbidity of acute appendicitis. He reported a survey of prominent surgeons of the day in which 37% said that they routinely performed incidental appendectomy. However, delayed diagnosis and a significant morbidity and even mortality associated with appendicitis in those days led Fischer in 1909 and Goldspohn in 1911 to endorse incidental appendectomy during other abdominal operations. However, the risk of morbidity and mortality have been substantially reduced in the past 50 years, and presently the use of incidental appendectomy at the time of gynecologic surgery is controversial. The decision to resect the appendix during routine gynecologic procedures depends on the risk:benefit ratio. It is estimated that at 60 years of age, about 125 incidental appendectomies need to be performed to prevent one case of appendicitis, 250 to prevent one ruptured appendix, and 5,000 to prevent one death. These benefits are greater in younger women in whom acute appendicitis is more common.

There are potential risks of the surgery. These include bleeding and hematoma formation, adhesion formation with subsequent intestinal obstruction, blowout of the appendiceal stump with abscess or fecal fistula or both, and others. However, in a careful review of the literature, Snyder and Selanders concluded that there was no statistically significant increase in morbidity or mortality when incidental appendectomy is performed at the time of routine abdominal hysterectomy, salpingectomy, tubal ligation, or cesarean section. Good judgment must be exercised and good technique used in performance of the procedure, and circumstances should be favorable, including satisfactory condition of the patient during the operation, satisfactory tolerance of the anesthesia, and easy exposure of the appendix. If the patient has lost a great deal of blood or the operation has been unusually prolonged, appendectomy should be performed only when significant pathology of the appendix is found. Incidental appendectomy should not be performed in the presence of bowel obstruction or when severe postoperative ileus is likely.

One of the main advantages of incidental appendectomy is to eliminate the appendix from consideration when a patient presents subsequently with perplexing pelvic or abdominal pain. In addition to preventing appendicitis in future years, incidental appendectomy offers the advantage of removing unsuspected pathology. In a retrospective study of 260 women with pelvic or right iliac fossa pain, Lynch and coworkers reported that 90% of the women who had appendectomy in addition to hysterectomy, oophorectomy, or other gynecologic surgery reported relief of symptoms, compared with only 49% in the group who did not have an appendectomy. Quite probably all these appendices did not look grossly normal, and this was not a prospective, randomized study; however, a significant incidence of "chronic obstructive appendicitis," endometriosis, and granuloma were found on microscopic examination of the removed appendices. Among the pathologic findings in clinically normal-appearing appendixes are acute, subacute, and chronic appendicitis, carcinoid tumors, and endometriosis. Others have reported that about 10% of incidental appendectomy specimens show significant pathology. The incidence obviously depends on the definition of "incidental" and how carefully the appendix is examined by the pathologist.

Ectopic pregnancy and endometriosis have been reported in association with appendicitis. Panganiban and Cornog reported that 4 of 31 patients with endometriosis of the appendix had symptoms of appendicitis. The appendix is a common site of involvement in patients with pelvic endometriosis, although endometriosis is rarely confined only to the appendix. Pittaway found endometriosis in 13% of appendixes removed from patients with pelvic endometriosis at the Johns Hopkins Hospital. In 38%, the appendix was grossly normal when histologic evidence of endometriosis was found. The author concluded from the study that (a) appendectomy is warranted in patients who are not interested in having children and are undergoing definitive surgery for endometriosis, and (b) appendectomy should be done when the appendix is abnormal, even in patients with endometriosis who are undergoing surgery to restore fertility.

The appendix is the most common site for carcinoid tumors, with an incidence of 0.03% of all appendixes removed. Almost all appendiceal carcinoids are benign. It is rare for the carcinoid syndrome to be present. In Waters' series of 830 patients in whom elective appendectomy was performed, six appendiceal carcinoid tumors were suspected or diagnosed on gross surgical appearance.

In summary, there are three main reasons to perform incidental appendectomy:

1. To reduce the risk of future mortality and morbidity from appendicitis, including possible infertility after a perforated appendix
2. To eliminate undiagnosed incidental pathology in the appendix
3. To eliminate the appendix from diagnostic consideration when the patient has abdominal or pelvic symptoms in the immediate postoperative period and in future years

The incidence of appendicitis decreases with increasing age. The risk is greatest in girls 15 to 19 years old, and 70% of acute appendicitis occurs in patients younger than age 30. However, the rate of perforation increases with advancing age; in women older than age 65, perforation occurs about 50% of the time. Using life table analysis, Snyder and Selanders estimated that for girls 15 to 19 years old, 1,000 incidental appendectomies would prevent 52 cases of appendicitis, 5 of which would be ruptured. For women 35 to 39 years old, 24 cases of appendicitis would be prevented by 1,000 incidental appendectomies; for patients 60 to 64 years old, only 8 cases of acute appendicitis would be prevented, but 4 of these would rupture before diagnosis.

Studies show that incidental appendectomy is far more commonly done in women, probably because they more often have abdominal or pelvic surgical procedures, such as hysterectomy, oophorectomy, or cholecystectomy. It is also more commonly done in women 35 to 55 years old, probably for the same reason.

In a careful analysis of the potential cost savings of incidental appendectomy, Wang and Sax evaluated the impact of laparoscopy and managed care on this question. They reasoned that many of the primary procedures performed at the time of incidental appendectomy were now done via the laparoscope (laparoscopically assisted vaginal hysterectomy and laparoscopic cholecystectomy). Taking into account long-term risk of appendicitis and complication, as well as various fee schedules and other surgical costs, they calculated that laparoscopic incidental appendectomy was not cost-effective at any age. Because there is very minimal cost associated with slightly increased operating time and a few sutures, with open appendectomy there are more cost savings for women younger than 30 years when incidental appendectomy is done as part of an open abdominal procedure. With the frequent changes in managed care plans and strong pressure to minimize costs, they felt there was no incentive to spend money today (for incidental appendectomy) with the hope of saving money in the future (decreased risk of appendicitis at a later time).

Analyzing the various factors, it is easy to see why incidental appendectomy remains controversial. Many experts have suggested that it is most appropriate for women younger than 30 or 35 years, especially if they have a history of pelvic pain, pelvic inflammatory disease, or endometriosis. Because of the low risk of appendicitis, many experts do not recommend incidental appendectomy for women older than 50 years. In women between ages 35 and 50 who are undergoing gynecologic surgery, the status of the abdomen and pelvis, diagnosis, overall condition of the patient, and appearance of the appendix and surrounding structures all should be taken into account when deciding on the advisability of incidental appendectomy. The possibility of appendectomy should be discussed with the patient during the preoperative period and the benefits and risks explained. Informed consent should be documented in the chart. At the time of surgery, the appendix should be carefully examined; if abnormal or involved with the pelvic disease process, it should be removed. Women with mucinous ovarian tumor should have an appendectomy if possible to rule out an appendiceal primary.

BEST SURGICAL PRACTICE

- Appendicitis is the most common cause of acute abdominal pain requiring surgery, with a 7% lifetime risk. The mortality rate of appendicitis is 0.1%, which increases to 5% with perforation. There is an elevated mortality rate of 5% to 15% in the elderly population, mainly because of the difficultly in diagnosing the condition in this group. The morbidity rate of appendicitis, which is mainly due to infection, is 15% to 20% but has been greatly improved with the use of perioperative antibiotics.
- Acute appendicitis is diagnosed primarily on physical examination, and 50% of patients present with the classic sequence of anorexia, nausea, and vomiting. Other potential findings include tenderness at McBurney's point, a positive Rovsing sign, a positive psoas sign, or a positive obturator sign. A pelvic exam should always be performed to rule out gynecologic causes. Ultrasound and computed tomography have assisted in more accurate diagnosis and thus have contributed to decreased rates of rupture and exploratory laparotomy.
- The standard treatment for acute appendicitis is appendectomy, and the operative mortality without perforation is close to zero. Preoperative use of broad-spectrum antibiotics is important in reducing associated morbidity, and continuation of the regimen postoperatively should be considered in cases of appendiceal rupture. Common complications of appendectomy include wound infection, abscess or fistula formation, peritonitis, pyelonephritis, venous thrombosis, and intestinal obstruction.
- Standard management of appendicitis has been with open laparotomy per variations of a right lower quadrant incision. Alternatively, laparoscopy is an option. When performed by an experienced surgeon, the latter offers many potential advantages, including decreased surgical morbidity. Laparoscopic assessment of the peritoneal cavity may prove especially useful for the gynecologist, as many other abdominopelvic conditions can mimic appendicitis.
- Appendectomy is the most common nonobstetrical operative intervention in the pregnant patient and occurs most frequently in the second trimester. Diagnosis, which may be improved through ultrasonography, can be more challenging as a result of displacement of the appendix by the gravid uterus. The incidence of perforation and its repercussions, including an increased risk of preterm labor, is twice as high in pregnancy. Immediate operation is the treatment, regardless of duration of the pregnancy.
- Incidental appendectomy refers to the prophylactic removal of the normal-appearing appendix during surgery for another condition. The appropriateness of this procedure is widely debated and should be judged on a case-by-case basis.

Bibliography

Affleck D, Handraham D, et al. The laparoscopic management of appendicitis and chololithiasis during pregnancy. *Am J Surg* 1999;178:523.

Aluarez C, Voitk A. The road to ambulatory laparoscopic management of perforated appendicitis. *Am J Surg* 2000;179:63.

American College of Obstetrians and Gynecologists. *Incidental appendectomy. ACOG Committee Opinion No. 164*. Washington, DC: 1995.

Anderson B, Niclen T. Appendicitis in pregnancy: diagnosis, management and complications. *Acta Obstet Gynecol Scand* 1999;78:758.

Andersson REB, Lambe M. Incidence of appendicitis during pregnancy. *Int J Epidemiol* 2001;30:1281.

Attwood SA, Hifi AK, Murphy PG. A prospective randomized trial of laparoscopic versus open appendectomy. *Surgery* 1992;112:497.

Azaro E, Amaral P, Ettinger J, et al. Laparoscopic versus open appendectomy: a comparative study. *J Soc Laparoendosc Surg* 1999;3:279.

Bickell NA, Aufses AH Jr, Rohas M, et al. How time affects the risk of rupture in appendicitis. *J Am Coll Surg* 2006;202:401.

Birchard KR, Brown MA, Hyslop WB, et al. MRI of acute abdominal and pelvic pain in pregnant patients. *AJR Am J Roentgenol* 2005;184:452.

Byrne DS, Bell G, Morrice JJ, et al. Technique for laparoscopic appendicectomy. *Br J Surg* 1992;79:574.

Chung R, Rowland D, Li P, et al. A meta-analysis of randomized controlled trials of laparoscopic versus conventional appendectomy. *Am J Surg* 1999;177:250.

Condon RE, Telford GL. Appendicitis. In: Sabiston DC Jr, ed. *Textbook of surgery*. Philadelphia: WB Saunders; 1991.

Deutsch AA, Zelikovsky A, Reiss R. Laparoscopy in the prevention of unnecessary appendectomies: a prospective study. *Br J Surg* 1982;69:336–337.

deVeciana M, Towers CV, Major CA, et al. Pulmonary injury associated with appendicitis in pregnancy: who is at risk?. *Am J Obstet Gynecol* 1994;171:1008.

El Ghoneimi A, Valla JS, Limmone B, et al. Laparoscopic appendectomy in children: report of 1,379 cases. *J Pediatr Surg* 1994;29:86.

Engstrom L, Fenyo G. Appendectomy: assessment of stump invagination versus simple ligation: a prospective randomized trial. *Br J Surg* 1985;72:971.

Farquharson RG. Acute appendicitis in pregnancy. *Scott Med J* 1980;25:36.

Fingerhut A, Millat B, Borne F. Laparoscopic versus open appendectomy: time to decide. *World J Surg* 1999;23:835.

Fitz RH. Perforating inflammation of the vermiform appendix, with special reference to its early diagnosis and treatment. *Trans Assoc Am Phys* 1886;1:107.

Flancbaum L, Nosher JL, Brolin RE. Percutaneous catheter drainage of abdominal abscesses associated with perforated viscus. *Ann Surg* 1990;56:52.

Flum DR, McClure TD, Morris A, et al. Misdiagnosis of appendicitis and the use of diagnostic imaging. *J Am Coll Surg* 2005;201:933.

Fontanelli R, Paladini D, Raspagliesi F, et al. The role of appendectomy in surgical procedures of ovarian cancer. *Gynecol Oncol* 1992;46:42.

Forsell P, Pieper R. Infertility in young women due to perforated appendicitis?. *Acta Chir Scand* 1986;5:30(suppl):53.

Frazee RC, Roberts JW, Symmonds RE, et al. A prospective randomized trial comparing open versus laparoscopic appendectomy. *Ann Surg* 1994;219:725.

Fritts LL, Orlando R III. Laparoscopy appendectomy: a safety and cost analysis. *Arch Surg* 1993;128:521.

Geerdsen JP. Sterility: a delayed complication after appendicitis acuta perforata in girls. *Nord Med* 1988;103:62.

Grubham J, Sutton C, Nicholson M. A case for the removal of the "normal" appendix at laparoscopy for suspected acute appendicitis. *Ann R Coll Surg Engl* 1999;81:279.

Halvorsen AC, Brandt B, Andreasen JJ. Acute appendicitis in pregnancy: complications and subsequent management. *Eur J Surg* 1992;158:603.

Halvorsen AC, Brandt B, Andreasen JJ, et al. Pregnancy complicated by acute appendicitis: commentary. *Acta Obstet Gynecol Scand* 1991;70:183.

Hellberg A, Rudberg C, Kullman E, et al. Prospective randomized multicentre study of laparoscopic versus open appendicectomy. *Br J Surg* 1999;86:48.

Herczeg J, Kovacs L, Kerseru T. Premature labour and coincident acute appendicitis not resolved by beta mimetic but surgical treatment. *Acta Obstet Gynecol Scand* 1983;62:373.

Horowitz MD, Gomez GA, Santiesteban R, et al. Acute appendicitis during pregnancy. *Arch Surg* 1985;120:1362.

Isaacs JH, Knaus JV. The detection of non-genital pelvic tumors mimicking gynecologic disease. *Surg Gynecol Obstet* 1981;153:74.

Jadallah FA, Abdul-Ghani AA, Tibblin S. Diagnostic laparoscopy reduces unnecessary appendectomy in fertile women. *Eur J Surg* 1994;160:41.

Katkhouda N, Mason RJ, Towfigh S, et al. Laparoscopic versus open appendectomy: a prospective randomized double-blind study. *Ann Surg* 2005;242:439.

Kelly HA, Hurdon E. *The vermiform appendix and its diseases*. Philadelphia: WB Saunders; 1905.

Khalili T, Hiatt J, Savar A, et al. Perforated appendicitis is not contraindicated to laparoscopy. *Am Surg* 1999;65:965.

Kraemer M, Ohmann C, Leppert R, et al. Macroscopic assessment of the appendix at diagnostic laparoscopy is reliable. *Surg Endosc* 2000;14:625.

Krukowski ZH, Irwin ST, Denholm S, et al. Preventing wound infection after appendicectomy: a review. *Br J Surg* 1988;75:1023.

Kum CK, Ngoi SS, Goh PY, et al. Randomized controlled trial comparing laparoscopic and open appendectomy. *Br J Surg* 1993;80:1599.

Kum CK, Sim EK, Goh PY, et al. Diagnostic laparoscopy: reducing the number of normal appendectomies. *Dis Colon Rectum* 1993;36:763.

Langman J, Rowland R, Vernon-Roberts B. Endometriosis of the appendix. *Br J Surg* 1981;68:121.

Lau WY, Fan ST, Yiu TF, et al. Acute appendicitis in the elderly. In: Schwarts SI, ed. *The year book of surgery*. Chicago: Year Book; 1986.

Leape LL, Ramenofsky ML. Laparoscopy for guestionable appendicitis: can it reduce the negative appendectomy rate? *Ann Surg* 1980; 191:410–413.

Lechmann-Wfflenbrock E, Miecke H, Riedel HH. Sequelae of appendectomy, with special reference to intraabdominal adhesions, chronic abdominal pain, and infertility. *Gynecol Obstet Invest* 1990;29:241.

Lemieur T, Rodriguez J, Jacobs D, et al. Wound management in perforated appendicitis. *Am Surg* 1999;65:439.

Levine JS, Gomez GA, Dove DB, et al. Negative appendix with suspected appendicitis: an update. *South Med J* 1986;79:177.

Lim HK, Bae SH, Seo GS. Diagnosis of acute appendicitis in pregnant women: value of sonography. *AJR Am J Roentgenol* 1992;159:539.

Lynch CB, Sinha P, Jalloh S. Incidental appendectomy during gynecological surgery. *Int J Gynecol Obstet* 1997;59:261.

Mahmoodian S. Appendicitis complicating pregnancy. *South Med J* 1992;85:19.

Mangi A, Berger D. Stump appendicitis. *Am Surg* 2000;66:739.

Mazze RI, Kallen B. Appendectomy during pregnancy: a Swedish registry study of 778 cases. *Obstet Gynecol* 1991;77:835.

McAnena OJ, Austin O, O'Connell PR, et al. Laparoscopic versus open appendicectomy: a prospective evaluation. *Br J Surg* 1992;79:818.

McBurney C. Experience with early operative interference in cases of disease of the vermiform appendix. *N Y Med J* 1889;50:676.

McGee TM. Acute appendicitis in pregnancy. *Aust N Z J Obstet Gynecol* 1989;29:378.

Meynaud-Kraemer L, Cohn C, Vergnon P, et al. Wound infection in open versus laparoscopic appendectomy: a meta-analysis. *Int J Technol Assess Health Care* 1999;15:380.

Morrow CP. Is incidental appendectomy a safe practice? (editor's comments) In: Mishell DR, ed. *The year book of obstetrics and gynecology*. Chicago: Year Book; 1990.

Mourad J, Eliott JP, Erickson L, et al. Appendicitis in pregnancy: new information that contradicts long-held clinical beliefs. *Am J Obstet Gynecol* 2000;182:1027.

Mueller BA, Daling JR, Moore DE, et al. Appendectomy and the risk of tubal infertility. *N Engl J Med* 1986;315:1506.

Nakhgevany KB, Clarke LE. Acute appendicitis in women of child-bearing age. *Arch Surg* 1986;121:1053.

Nauta RJ, Magnant C. Observation versus operation for abdominal pain in the right lower quadrant. *Am J Surg* 1986;151:746.

Nezhat C, Nezhat F. Incidental appendectomy during videolaseroscopy. *Am J Obstet Gynecol* 1991;165:559.

Nguyen D, Silen W, Hodin R. Appendectomy in the pre- and post-laparoscopic eras. *J Gastroenterol Surg* 1999;3:67.

Olsen JB, Myre CJ, Haahr PE. Randomized study of the value of laparoscopy before appendectomy. *Br J Surg* 1993;80:922.

Ozmen M, Zulfikaroglu B, Tanik A, et al. Laparoscopic versus open appendectomy: prospective randomized trials. *Surg Laparosc Endosc Percutan Technol* 1999;9:187.

Oto A, Ernst RD, Shah R, et al. Right-lower-quadrant pain and suspected appendicitis in pregnancy women: evaluation with MR imaging—Initial experience. *Radiology* 2005;234:445.

Parsons AK, Sauer MV, Parsons MT, et al. Appendectomy at cesarean section: a prospective study. *Obstet Gynecol* 1986;68:479.

Paterson-Brown S, Thompson JN, Eckersley JRT, et al. Which patient with suspected appendicitis should undergo laparoscopy?. *Br Med J* 1988;296: 1363.

Pier A, Gotz F, Bacher C. Laparoscopic appendectomy in 625 cases: from innovation to routine. *Surg Laparosc Endosc* 1991;1:8.

Pittaway ED. Appendectomy in the surgical treatment of endometriosis. *Obstet Gynecol* 1983;61:421.

Pun P, McGuinness EPJ, Guiney EJ. Fertility following perforated appendicitis in girls. *J Pediatr Surg* 1989;24:547.

Rose PG, Reale FR, Fisher A, et al. Appendectomy in primary and secondary staging operations for ovarian malignancy. *Obstet Gynecol* 1991;77: 116.

Sauerland S, Lefering R, Neugebauer EA. Laparoscopic versus open surgery for suspected appendicitis (Cochrane Review). *Chochrane Database Syst Rev* 2002;CD001546.

Schirmer BD, Schmieg RE Jr, Dix J, et al. Laparoscopic versus traditional appendectomy for suspected appendicitis. *Am J Surg* 1993;165:670.

Schreiber JH. Early experience with laparoscopic appendectomy in women. *Surg Endoscop* 1987;1:211.

Schreiber JH. Results of outpatient laparoscopic appendectomy in women. *Endoscopy* 1994;26:292.

Semm K. Endoscopic appendectomy. *Endoscopy* 1983;15:59.

Spirtos NM, Eisenkop SM, Spirtos TW, et al. Laparoscopy: a diagnostic aid in cases of suspected appendicitis. Its use in women of reproductive age. *Am J Obstet Gynecol* 1987;154:90.

Snyder TE, Selanders JR. Incidental appendectomy—yes or no?. A retrospective case study and review of the literature. *Infect Dis Obstet Gynecol* 1998;6:30.

Sugimoto T, Edwards D. Incidence and costs of incidental appendectomy as a preventive measure. *Am J Public Health* 1987;77:471.

Tamir IL, Bongard FS, Klein SR. Acute appendicitis in the pregnant patient. *Am J Surg* 1990;160:57.

Temple L, Litwin D, McLeod R. A meta-analysis of laparoscopic versus open appendectomy in patients suspected of having acute appendicitis. *Can J Surg* 1999;42:377.

Terasawa T, Blackmore CC, Bent S, et al. Systematic review: computed tomography and ultrasonography to detect acute appendicitis in adults and adolescents. *Ann Intern Med* 2004;141:537.

Wagner J, McKinney W, Carpenter J. Does this patient have appendicitis?. *JAMA* 1996;276:1589.

Wang HT, Sax HC. Incidental appendectomy in the era of managed care and laparoscopy. *J Am Coll Surg* 2001;192:182.

Wittich A, DeSantis R, Lockrow E. Appendectomy during pregnancy: a survey of two army medical activities. *Mil Med* 1999;164:671.

Wu JM, Chen KH, Lin HF, et al. Laparoscopic appendectomy in pregnancy. *J Laparoendosc Adv Surg Tech A* 2005;15:447.

Udwadia T, Udwadia R. How we do it: laparoscopic appendicectomy. *Natl Med J India* 1999;12:281.

Yao C, Lin C, Yang C. Laparoscopic appendectomy for ruptured appendicitis. *Surg Laparosc Endosc Percutan Technol* 1999;9:271.

CHAPTER 43 ■ INTESTINAL TRACT IN GYNECOLOGIC SURGERY

KELLY L. MOLPUS

DEFINITIONS

Abdominal hernia—Defect in the fascia through which peritoneum-encased viscera may protrude.

Adhesion—Intraperitoneal scar tissue that connects opposing peritoneal and/or serosal surfaces.

Anastomosis—Surgical communication created between two segments of the gastrointestinal tract.

Anastomotic bursting pressure—Experimental measure of the magnitude of intraluminal pressure required to disrupt the bowel wall at the site of anastomosis.

Antimesenteric edge—Anatomical edge along the intestine opposite to where the mesentery is attached.

Bacterial translocation—In the setting of intestinal obstruction, the process whereby enteric bacteria traverse the damaged bowel wall to seed the peritoneal cavity.

Bezoar—Concretion formed within the alimentary canal due to ingestion of nondigestible substances.

Blind loop syndrome—Progressive symptomatic dilation of a nonfunctioning bowel segment, such as may occur when a large segment of cecum persists distal to an ileo-ascending anastomosis.

Bowel prep—Preoperative cleansing of the intestinal tract with cathartics to reduce enteric volume and antibiotics to decrease colonic flora.

Bridge—Apparatus secured between the abdominal wall and exteriorized bowel loop to provide support until tissue healing secures the stoma in place.

Cheatle slit—A longitudinal full-thickness incision made in the antimesenteric bowel wall to increase the diameter of the anastomosis.

Closed loop obstruction—Isolated segment of bowel with diminished influx and efflux of enteric content at risk for distention and perforation.

Closed techniques—Generalized term to include methods of gastrointestinal anastomosis in which the lumens of the involved segments are not exposed.

Colocolostomy—Communication and/or surgical anastomosis between two segments of the large intestine.

Colostomy—Segment of large bowel exteriorized through the abdominal wall to divert fecal output.

Crohn's disease—An inflammatory process of uncertain etiology that adversely affects the colon and intermittent segments of small intestine (regional enteritis) and manifests clinically as recurrent diarrhea, intestinal cramping, and weight loss.

Dehiscence—Postoperative wound separation that most commonly involves the skin and subcutaneous tissue (superficial or incomplete) or, less commonly, the fascia (deep or complete).

EndoGIA—General term for endoscopic stapling instrument used during laparoscopic gastrointestinal procedures.

End-to-end (EEA) stapler—Surgical stapling instrument designed to join the ends of two bowel segments of similar diameter.

Enteral nutrition—Use of the gut to provide nutrition.

Enteroenterostomy—Communication and/or surgical anastomosis between two segments of small intestine.

Enterostomal therapist—Nurse with specialized training in ostomy-related issues, who is an invaluable resource in providing perioperative counseling, education, and clinical care.

Enterotomy—Full-thickness opening in the small bowel wall.

Evisceration—An acute full-thickness wound disruption through which abdominal contents extrude.

Fistula—Abnormal communication between two organ systems that have no inherent anatomical connection (i.e., enterocutaneous, rectovaginal, vesicovaginal, or enterovesical fistula).

Gastrocolic ligament—Intraabdominal fibroadipose tissue that arises from the greater curvature of the stomach and fuses with the greater omentum along the transverse colon.

Gastrointestinal anastomosis (GIA) stapler—General term for surgical stapling instrument used during open gastrointestinal procedures.

Gastrostomy—Artificial opening in the stomach for the purpose of decompression, nutrition, or anastomosis.

Greater omentum—Intraabdominal fibroadipose tissue that arises from the inferior surface of the transverse colon.

Haustra—Widely spaced, transverse, partially encircling folds within the wall of the colon.

Ileocecal valve—Functional communication between the terminal ileum and cecum that facilitates forward motility of digestive contents.

Ileocolonic anastomosis—Surgical communication established between the ileum and colon.

Ileostomy—Segment of ileum exteriorized through the abdominal wall to divert enteric output.

Ileus—Mechanical dysfunction in which the normal anterograde gastrointestinal peristalsis is temporarily disrupted.

Incarceration—Extrusion of a hernia sac that becomes edematous, entrapped, and at risk for vascular compromise (strangulation).

Inferior mesenteric artery—Major artery arising from the abdominal aorta that supplies the left colon via left colic and sigmoid arteries.

Inflammatory bowel disease—A general descriptive term referring to any inflammatory condition of the intestines, including Crohn's disease and ulcerative colitis.

Intestinal adaptation—Subsequent to small bowel resection, compensatory mechanisms whereby the absorptive capacity and surface area of the remaining small intestine increase over time.

Jejunostomy—Artificial opening in the jejunum for the purpose of decompression, nutrition, or anastomosis.

Loop ileostomy, loop colostomy—Intact segment of ileum, or nonretroperitonealized large bowel, which is exteriorized and opened to divert the digestive output.

Marginal artery of Drummond—Mesenteric artery that establishes vascular communication from the cecum to the rectum and gives off numerous terminal vasa recta.

Maturation of stoma—Process of opening the exteriorized intestine and suturing the everted bowel edge to the skin of the abdominal wall.

Meckel's diverticulum—Residual portion of the vitelline (yolk) duct located along the antimesenteric border of the distal ileum that may cause acute symptoms that are due to inflammation, hemorrhage, or obstruction.

Mesenteric border—Anatomical edge along the intestine where blood supply is derived via the attached mesentery.

Mesentery—Dual layer of peritoneum and fibroadipose tissue, attached to the posterior abdominal wall, which carries the arteriovenous and lymphatic structures to and from the intestines.

Nasogastric decompression—Use of a tube passed through the nose into the stomach for the purpose of removing air and gastric content via suction.

Neovascularization—Process whereby blood and oxygen delivery to tissue is increased via the proliferation of new blood vessels.

Ogilvie's syndrome—Acute colonic pseudoobstruction resulting from dysfunction of colonic peristalsis that may be clinically indistinguishable from a large bowel obstruction.

Omental flap—Surgical rotation of the infracolic omentum to a specific area to increase blood supply to that area.

Open techniques—Generalized term to include methods of gastrointestinal anastomosis in which the lumens of the involved segments are exposed.

Ostomy—Any artificial opening in the gastrointestinal tract.

Parenteral nutrition—Use of an alternative route to the gut for provision of nutrition (i.e., intravenous infusion).

Perforation—Spontaneous full-thickness defect in the gastrointestinal tract with resultant intraperitoneal efflux of bacteria and digestive content.

Peristalsis—Normal anterograde movement of digestive content via rhythmic circular contractions and relaxations of the intestinal wall musculature.

Plicae circulares (valvulae conniventes)—Numerous closely spaced, transverse, encircling folds within the wall of the small intestine.

Short bowel syndrome—Insufficient nutrient absorption to meet the body's metabolic requirements as a result of extensive intestinal resection and/or inadequate function of intact bowel.

Small bowel obstruction—Partial or complete impedance to the anterograde movement of enteric content through the small bowel that is due to extrinsic or intrinsic compromise of the lumen.

Stoma—Terminal segment of intestine that is exteriorized and secured to the abdominal wall, through which digestive output is diverted.

Stoma appliance—Fitted wafer adherent to the skin surrounding the stoma that serves as an attachment site for the collection bag.

Stricture—Circumferential narrowing of the intestinal lumen.

Stricturoplasty—Procedure in which the bowel wall is opened longitudinally and closed transversely for the purpose of creating a wider lumen.

Submucosa—Tissue layer within the bowel wall that provides the greatest strength during reparative healing.

Superior mesenteric artery—Major artery arising from the abdominal aorta that supplies blood to the entire small intestine, as well as the right and middle colon.

Teniae coli—Three distinct muscle fiber bands that run longitudinally within the wall of the large intestine.

Ulcerative colitis—A chronic condition of uncertain etiology that adversely affects the colon and rectum via ulceration, and manifests clinically as pain, bleeding, diarrhea, and weight loss.

Vasa recta—Small arcading vessels that terminate directly into the wall of the small or large intestine.

Volvulus—An acute malrotation of the bowel that causes intestinal obstruction.

White line of Toldt—Peritoneal reflection that runs lateral and parallel to the ascending and descending colon that is used to guide dissection for colon mobilization.

INTRODUCTION

An indistinguishable overlap exists such that women may present with clinical signs and symptoms that are common to both primary gynecologic and digestive disorders. Intestinal disorders may be found intraoperatively at the time of gynecologic procedures. Additionally, gynecologic conditions may adversely affect the gastrointestinal tract. The gynecologic surgeon should have a basic understanding of the anatomy and physiology of the intestinal tract and should possess the fundamental skills necessary to recognize and correct common conditions affecting the digestive system. Meticulous dissection and cautious handling of tissues reduce the occurrence of intestinal injury and the risk of postoperative complications.

GASTROINTESTINAL DISORDERS THAT MIMIC GYNECOLOGIC PROBLEMS

Diverticulitis

Colonic diverticulitis may be confused with pelvic inflammatory disease (PID). These two processes generally do not occur in the same age group; however, rarely diverticulitis may occur in women younger than age 40 years. Patients with acute diverticulitis present with pain, altered bowel function, fever, and leukocytosis. Tenderness and guarding are usually localized to the left lower quadrant. One in five patients with acute diverticulitis also has signs and symptoms of colonic obstruction. Treatment for unruptured diverticulitis and PID are similar, and include intravenous fluid resuscitation, bowel rest, and broad-spectrum antibiotic coverage for anaerobes, Gram-negative rods, and enterococci.

Diagnostic computed tomography (CT) scan clarifies whether a pericolonic abscess is present, and CT-directed drainage of an abscess expedites recovery and avoids surgical exploration in most cases. Nasogastric decompression is necessary in the setting of obstruction. If obstructive symptoms persist, or if bowel perforation has occurred, surgical exploration is warranted. If bowel perforation results in generalized peritonitis, consideration is given to diverting colostomy, with extensive irrigation and drainage of the peritoneal cavity.

Appendicitis

Perhaps one of the most frequently encountered diagnostic dilemmas is that of acute appendicitis versus PID. Appendicitis is most frequently seen during the second and third decades of life, which coincides with that of reproductive-aged women at risk for PID. Whereas cervical motion tenderness is helpful in the diagnosis of PID and right-sided pain on rectal examination is helpful in the diagnosis of appendicitis, neither is pathognomonic. Peritoneal irritation from any source can be elicited by manipulation of the pelvic organs, so that manual manipulation of the cervix elicits an intensely painful response (cervical motion tenderness) in women with either PID or appendicitis. Similarly, rectal examination may illicit pain in a woman who has PID. Acute appendicitis may be overlooked by clinicians who assume the ailment is PID after finding cervical motion tenderness.

Progressive anorexia and lateralization of pain (vague periumbilical discomfort that intensifies over time while gravitating toward McBurney's point) raise suspicion for appendicitis. A history of prior PID, multiple sex partners, recent acquisition of a new sex partner, recent menses, and physical findings of a purulent cervical discharge suggest PID. Radiographic studies may be needed to clarify the diagnosis because acute appendicitis is a surgical emergency; PID, however, is usually treated with broad-spectrum antibiotics and supportive care. Spiral CT scan has gained acceptance as an accurate determinant of the appendiceal anatomy. Contrasted CT imaging is also invaluable in the diagnosis of pelvic abscess. Bilateral pelvic abscesses are more characteristics of PID than an appendiceal process.

Meckel's Diverticulum

Meckel's diverticulum represents a residual portion of the vitelline (yolk) duct and is present in 1% of women. Diverticula average 5 cm in length and are located along the antimesenteric border of the ileum within 2 feet of the ileocecal valve. They are lined by ileal-type mucosa, but at least one in five cases has ectopic pancreatic or gastric tissue. Acute symptoms result from inflammation, hemorrhage, or obstruction in approximately 5% to 16% of cases, with hemorrhage being most common. Inflammation and hemorrhage result from gastric acid secretion, and obstruction follows intussusception or torsion. Presenting signs and symptoms may mimic acute appendicitis or PID, but may not localize in the right lower quadrant.

Most complications from Meckel's diverticula are during early childhood, and the likelihood of problems significantly decreases with advancing age. Accordingly, most surgeons believe routine resection of an asymptomatic Meckel's diverticulum in adulthood is unnecessary. Some recommend prophylactic removal if encountered during surgery, because morbidity associated with resection is low. It is generally agreed, however, that resection should be undertaken if the individual has previously been symptomatic, if the diverticulum is unusually long or has a narrow neck, or if thickening at the tip suggests ectopic gastric mucosa. Resection is accomplished by excising the base of the diverticulum with transverse closure of the enterotomy. Care is taken to avoid unnecessary resection of bowel wall to prevent luminal narrowing. Alternatively, transection may be completed via an automated stapler secured across the diverticular base.

Volvulus

Sigmoid volvulus is an acute malrotation that presents with sudden onset of intense pain, similar to that of ovarian torsion. Volvulus is generally accompanied by obstipation, abdominal pain, and distention. Nausea and vomiting may occur. Volvulus is most commonly seen after the age of 60 years; however, cases in young individuals have been reported. Flat-plate abdominal radiographic features are that of a markedly dilated, gas-filled sigmoid colon. Barium enema shows a tapered obstruction at the rectosigmoid junction with a typical bird's beak deformity. Sigmoid volvulus can usually be corrected nonoperatively with sigmoidoscopy or cautious barium enema. If volvulus is discovered at the time of surgery, initial management consists of untwisting the loop of bowel and observing for viability. Resection is infrequently necessary and should be reserved for devitalized bowel. Cecal volvulus is rare and tends to occur in the elderly population. This too is best managed by derotation, and resection is reserved for nonviability.

Pelvic Malignancies

Colorectal carcinomas may be difficult to distinguish from other pelvic malignancies. Advanced colorectal carcinoma may invade the vagina and/or bladder, producing symptoms suggestive of a gynecologic or urologic problem. Advanced ovarian, cervical, and endometrial cancers may also invade the bowel leading to rectal bleeding. Resultant inflammation, tissue necrosis, and abscess formation contribute to the diagnostic dilemma. Historical information, thorough physical examination, colonoscopy or barium enema, cystoscopy, CT scan, and tissue biopsy can clarify the origin of pelvic malignancies in most cases.

Inflammatory Bowel Disease

Inflammatory bowel disease includes Crohn's disease (regional enteritis) and ulcerative colitis. Crohn's disease is an inflammatory process of uncertain etiology that usually involves the small bowel. It most frequently occurs in young adults with symptomatic onset during the late teens, but may occur at any age. Those affected have intermittent diarrhea, intestinal cramping, and weight loss. The extent of intestinal symptoms generally enables the clinician to distinguish inflammatory bowel disease from PID. Clinical findings, such as a functional ovarian cyst, may lead to overdiagnosis of a gynecologic disorder and result in unnecessary surgery. Gynecologic surgery is best avoided if possible in Crohn's patients because of the high risk of intestinal complications, even if the bowel is uninjured.

Medical management is the mainstay of treatment because there is a high recurrence rate that follows surgical resection. Therapy consists of bowel rest, total parenteral nutrition, and antiinflammatory medication such as sulfasalazine and corticosteroids. Surgery is reserved for patients whose disease is complicated by obstruction, perforation, fistula, or hemorrhage. Affected areas of the small intestine may be interspersed by normal segments of bowel. The appearance of Crohn's intestine is thickened walls with dull, purple-red discoloration, inflammatory exudate, and adherent mesenteric fat. If surgical resection is necessary, only the involved segments of bowel are removed. Management of women with inflammatory bowel disease should be left to specialists in the field.

Because of the high rate of anastomotic dehiscence following resections for Crohn's disease, some surgeons advocate stricturoplasty as an alternative to resection. Stricturoplasty is accomplished by opening the bowel longitudinally and closing transversely, creating a wider lumen. The appendix is eventually affected by Crohn's disease and ulcerative colitis in 25% and 50% of cases, respectively. Prophylactic appendectomy may be considered if the terminal ileum and cecum are not involved by active disease at the time of exploration. Fistulae (i.e., enterocutaneous, enterovaginal, enterovesical) are frequently associated with inflammatory bowel disease and its surgical management. Surgical correction is reserved for problematic fistulae that fail to respond to extended medical management. The intestinal defect, as the source of fistulous drainage, must be corrected for any chance of successful resolution.

Ulcerative colitis is a chronic illness of uncertain etiology characterized by ulcerative lesions of the colon and rectum. Clinical symptoms are pain, bleeding, and diarrhea. Additional manifestations are weight loss, anemia, mucosal crypt abscesses, inflammatory pseudopolyps, and low serum protein. Ulcerative colitis is infrequently complicated by toxic megacolon, peritonitis, and colon cancer.

Hemorrhoids

It has been said of hemorrhoids that few human afflictions cause greater distress without posing threat to life. Hemorrhoids are dilated perianal and rectal veins. Chronic pressure causes distention and loss of resistance in the venous wall, resulting in varices. The collection of blood further draws fluids into the dilated perianal skin. Internal hemorrhoids protrude into the rectal lumen and cause painless bleeding, which may be severe. Larger internal hemorrhoids can protrude through the anus, resulting in pain, itching, and burning. Spasm of the external sphincter may constrict the hemorrhoid, resulting in strangulation, necrosis, and extreme discomfort. This process is recognized clinically as thrombosed hemorrhoids, which are not actually thrombosed vessels but rather perianal hematomas. An understanding of the Bartholin's gland anatomy helps delineate a Bartholin's abscess from hemorrhoidal inflammation or a perirectal abscess.

If thrombosed hemorrhoids are recognized during the first 3 days of onset, incision and drainage or excision with primary closure are acceptable treatments. Excision is favored in most cases because excision reduces the chance of recurrence, has less postoperative bleeding, and avoids development of skin tags. Protruding symptomatic hemorrhoids can be excised by the radial hemorrhoidectomy technique. Removal of excessive anoderm predisposes to anal stricture and should be avoided. Regular postoperative bowel function and follow-up digital examinations are helpful in reducing stricture formation. Techniques of elastic ligation have also been developed and modified for selected use in the management of hemorrhoids. Symptomatic hemorrhoids persisting more than 72 hours may best be treated nonoperatively. Nonoperative intervention includes fiber laxatives, sitz baths, antiinflammatory medication, and topical steroids. Care is taken in the use of topical anesthetic ointments because these may worsen symptoms in some patients. Perianal lidocaine injection can alleviate sphincter spasm in markedly symptomatic individuals.

GYNECOLOGIC CONDITIONS THAT AFFECT THE GASTROINTESTINAL TRACT

Extensive endometriosis may involve the small or large intestine. Inflammation from small bowel endometriosis may result in adhesions with painful peristalsis and intermittent or complete obstruction. Rectal implants and invasive endometriosis can manifest clinically as cyclic pain, intermittent diarrhea, bleeding, and pain associated with bowel movements. Rectovaginal endometriosis can cause perineal discomfort and a tender palpable mass on rectovaginal examination, which could mimic a perirectal abscess.

Pregnancy, either ectopic or intrauterine, must be considered in any symptomatic woman of reproductive age. Serum beta human chorionic gonadotropin (β-hCG) can be obtained rapidly in most hospital settings to rule out pregnancy. Tuboovarian abscess and adnexal torsion are often difficult to distinguish from inflammatory gastrointestinal conditions such as appendicitis or diverticulitis. All of these conditions may cause fever, nausea, anorexia, diarrhea, pain, and leukocytosis. Gynecologic infections may also adversely affect the intestinal tract, causing inflammation, adhesions, and obstruction. The fundamental history and physical examination help clarify the situation and separate gynecologic from gastrointestinal disorders in most cases.

PREOPERATIVE CONSIDERATIONS

Preoperative Bowel Prep

The objectives of preoperative bowel prep are to reduce enteric volume and bacterial load. Potential benefits include better operative handling and exposure, reduced infectious complications, and enhanced anastomotic healing. Efficient mechanical bowel prep does eliminate stool and gas from the colon, thus improving exposure and making it easier to pack the bowel out of the operative field. Mechanical cleansing also allows for better visibility during intraoperative colonoscopy, if needed. Various bowel preps have been proposed and used, including mechanical cleansing alone versus mechanical prep plus oral antibiotics, with or without parenteral antibiotics. In the past, such agents as castor oil, senna, bisacodyl, and magnesium citrate were used, but frequently resulted in inadequate bowel cleansing. Large volumes of isotonic solution and osmotic agents such as mannitol were more effective in bowel preparation; however, the prohibitive side effects included electrolyte and fluid abnormalities, nausea, vomiting, and abdominal distention.

Newer mechanical preparations usually consist of either polyethylene glycol or sodium phosphate. Polyethylene glycol is an effective, osmotically balanced solution that causes fewer electrolyte and fluid abnormalities. The major disadvantage is that 4 L must be consumed. Many patients are unable to complete this prep because of the large volume and the resultant gastrointestinal symptoms. Sodium phosphate has the advantage of being an effective cathartic while only requiring

90 cc of oral liquid. In randomized clinical trials comparing polyethylene glycol with sodium phosphate, patients who took sodium phosphate had significantly less trouble drinking the solution and reported less abdominal discomfort. Sodium phosphate provided a significantly better prep for colonoscopy. This trend was also observed in surgical patients, although not statistically significant. Polyethylene glycol and sodium phosphate should be used cautiously in debilitated patients and those with cirrhosis, renal impairment, electrolyte abnormalities, or ascites. They should not be used in patients with renal failure, congenital megacolon, bowel obstruction, or congestive heart failure.

Nonabsorbable or minimally absorbed oral antibiotics have traditionally been used in bowel preparation to reduce the intraluminal colonic flora. It is presumed that reduction in the bacterial load causes less peritoneal contamination and complications if the bowel is opened during surgery. Following colorectal surgery, cultures from wound infections and intraperitoneal abscesses most commonly reveal aerobic bacteria and other coliforms, such *as Escherichia coli, Streptococcus faecalis, Pseudomonas, Klebsiella,* and *Proteus,* and anaerobes such as *Bacteroides* and *Clostridia*. In some randomized trials of oral preoperative neomycin and erythromycin compared with no oral antibiotics, the infection rate was significantly decreased. The patients studied had also been given a mechanical prep plus intravenous antibiotics. Other clinical studies have not shown an additional benefit to oral antibiotics when intravenous antibiotics are used. Similarly, oral antibiotics alone have not been proven to be superior to intravenous antibiotics alone for infection prophylaxis. Oral ciprofloxacin compared with no oral antibiotic has been noted to reduce postoperative infections. Metronidazole with either erythromycin or neomycin has also been effectively used. There are no data to support that one regimen is superior to another.

The literature is inconclusive as to whether bowel prep consistently reduces operative morbidity. There are few randomized trials comparing mechanical bowel preparation with no preparation. The utility of bowel prep is called into question with collective retrospective data from trauma surgeries involving colonic injury and from emergent colorectal surgery for bowel obstruction. A review of 2,964 unprepped patients who underwent primary repair of colon injury reported an anastomotic leak rate of only 2.3%. Some studies have suggested that bowel prep may actually increase the risk of intraoperative spillage and anastomotic leak. A metaanalysis of seven randomized clinical trials, including 1,297 patients, showed a leak rate of 5.6% in patients given a bowel prep compared with 2.8% in those with no prep ($p = 0.03$).

Despite lack of consistent evidence supporting reduced morbidity, there is a general consensus regarding the potential benefit, such that the majority of gynecologic oncologists, surgical oncologists, and colorectal surgeons continue to recommend preoperative bowel prep. In selected patients, the bowel prep regimen that we prefer is summarized in Table 43.1.

Positioning the Patient

Examination under anesthesia facilitates evaluation of anatomy and may clarify the likelihood of intestinal involvement by disease. Low dorsal lithotomy position is used if there is an expectation of possible rectosigmoid resection and anastomosis. Proper positioning reduces the risk of injury. The anesthetized patient is placed with her hips at the end of the table and buttocks extending several centimeters beyond the table end. Padding is secured below the coccyx to avoid pressure point injury. Careful positioning ensures the thighs are slightly flexed and the weight of the legs is distributed evenly, with

TABLE 43.1

BOWEL PREPARATION FOR SURGERY

Your surgery is planned for:
Day__________ Date__________ Time__________

Follow these instructions on the day before surgery
Day__________ Date__________

6:00 A.M. Only clear liquid foods today. Clear liquid foods would include beef or chicken broth, plain Jell-O, hot tea, Popsicles, 7-Up, or clear fruit juices. Do not eat or drink any milk products. Do not eat or drink anything you cannot see through. Do not drink any alcoholic beverages.
10:00 A.M. Take one Reglan 10-mg pill. This will help keep your stomach from being upset by the other medicines. You may repeat this every 4 hours if needed for nausea.
11:00 A.M. (1) Drink 1/2 of the 3-ounce bottle of Fleet Phospho-Soda. This is a strong laxative and will cause you to have diarrhea. (2) Take one of each of the antibiotic pills, Neomycin and Flagyl.
2:00 P.M. Take one Reglan 10-mg pill.
3:00 P.M. (1) Drink the second 1/2 of the bottle of Fleet Phospho-Soda. (2) Take the second dose of each of the antibiotic pills, Neomycin and Flagyl.
6:00 P.M. Take one Reglan 10-mg pill.
7:00 P.M. Take the third dose of each of the antibiotic pills, Neomycin and Flagyl.
12:00 midnight. No eating, drinking, or smoking between now and surgery.

We understand this bowel prep may be difficult for you. However, we strongly encourage you to follow all of these steps as outlined. Proper bowel prep may help maximize your effective healing and minimize your chance of problems after surgery.
If you have any questions about these instructions, please call our office.

no pressure points from the stirrups. Lithotomy position also allows access for intraoperative pelvic examination and provides easy exposure to assess bladder or rectal integrity after pelvic dissection. Additionally, a surgeon can be positioned between the stirrups to elevate the vaginal apex or assist with a rectal anastomosis, or to enable dissection in the paraaortic and upper abdominal areas.

INTRAOPERATIVE CONSIDERATIONS

Lysis of Adhesions

Intraperitoneal adhesions are fibrous bands of scar tissue that connect opposing peritoneal and/or serosal surfaces. Adhesions may be associated with prior surgical procedures, trauma, irradiation, infection, bleeding, or chemical irritants. Prior abdominal or pelvic surgery is the most frequently noted predisposing factor. After surgery, desiccated tissue surfaces in direct opposition are those at greatest risk for adhesion formation. History alone is not predictive in that certain individuals have adhesions without identifiable predisposing factors. Others have a predilection for an exaggerated healing response and excessive adhesion formation.

Adhesiolysis may be necessary to mobilize the bowel, expose the surgical field, and circumvent obstruction. Constricting adhesive bands require transection. It is best to start with translucent adhesions that can be sharply lysed without difficulty. As adhesions become more dense, efforts are made to isolate a window such that an index finger and thumb can be placed behind and in front of the adhesions, respectively. Gentle blunt tissue dissection by rubbing the index finger and thumb back and forth helps to identify translucent adhesive bands that can be sharply lysed. There is often a recognizable white line between adhesions and their peritoneal attachment, which identifies a safe tissue plane for dissection (Fig. 43.1). Another plane ideal for sharp dissection is one followed in close parallel proximity to a recognizable structure, such as along a loop of small bowel.

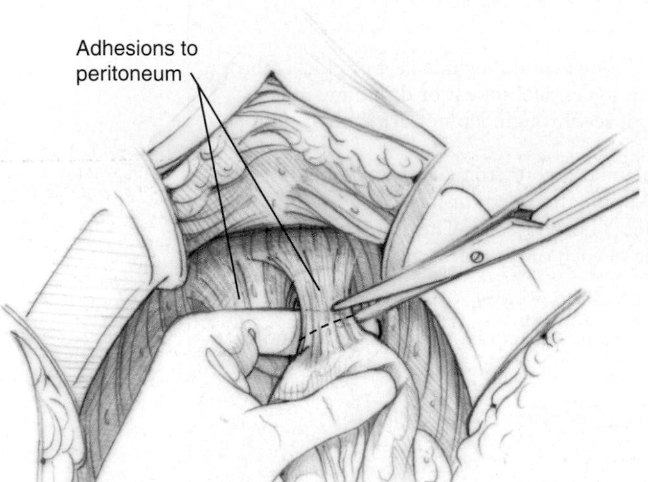

FIGURE 43.1. Traction-countertraction gives good exposure of an abdominal adhesion, which is lysed with scissors.

Inadvertent tissue injury is less likely with adhesiolysis close to the bowel wall than with cutting through the center of dense adhesions. Controlled traction and countertraction facilitates isolation and dissection, but excessive force is avoided. With dense adhesive bands, excessive force may literally tear a hole in the bowel wall, which may go unrecognized during surgery.

Intestinal Injury in Open Gynecologic Surgery

Enterotomy refers to a full-thickness opening in the bowel wall such that the lumen is entered. Enterotomy may be an incidental occurrence during dissection or an intentional orchestrated maneuver during gastrointestinal surgery. Inadvertent enterotomies are best avoided by cautious entry into the peritoneal cavity and meticulous dissection of adhesions.

Adequate visualization and access are necessary for safe adhesiolysis. Ongoing visual and manual bowel inspection is advisable to ensure there is no compromise to wall integrity. If an inadvertent enterotomy occurs, the affected bowel must be mobilized from surrounding tissues to allow adequate exposure and a tension-free repair. Although it is generally best to repair an enterotomy immediately, if the dissection is particularly difficult, it is advisable to finish the dissection so the extent of injuries can be assessed and the best plan for repair of any and all injuries can be accomplished. The initial impression of a single enterotomy can be incorrect. Mobilization of tissues from the surrounding area may demonstrate multiple enterotomies within a single bowel segment or involvement of more than one loop of bowel (Fig. 43.2).

If an enterotomy is not immediately repaired, it should be marked with a suture of 3-0 silk tied loosely with the tails left long for easy identification. Eventual suture repair should be accomplished in a transverse direction to avoid excess narrowing of the lumen. This is most important in the small bowel. Staple repair is also acceptable if luminal diameter is not compromised. If multiple enterotomies occur within a localized segment of small bowel, the best plan may be to resect the damaged segment rather than individually repair three or four injuries. Resection of an affected bowel segment may also be necessary if greater than 50% of the circumference is injured, if irregular edges preclude repair, if the blood supply is compromised, or if repair would result in excessive luminal narrowing.

In general, small bowel injury with intraperitoneal contamination by enteric content is associated with less morbidity than a similar occurrence in the large bowel. Historically, large bowel injury (colotomy) with gross intraperitoneal contamination has been managed by diverting colostomy, with delayed surgical repair and colostomy closure after several months. Collective clinical experience from scheduled procedures and trauma surgeries has demonstrated that immediate repair without colostomy is associated with acceptably low morbidity. Suture and staple closure techniques, as well as segmental resection with anastomosis, have been successfully used. Furthermore, some studies suggest that immediate recognition and repair of intestinal injury is associated with less morbidity than the diversion techniques previously thought to be mandatory.

Aggressive peritoneal irrigation and administration of intravenous broad-spectrum antibiotics reduce bacterial count. Peritoneal drains should not be placed in the immediate vicinity of an anastomosis, because this can actually impede healing. However, there may be therapeutic benefit from suction drains in dependent regions, such as the pelvis and paracolic gutters, which prevent accumulation of fluid. A diverting colostomy is indicated when a full-thickness colonic injury occurs in those who have undergone irradiation, who are profoundly

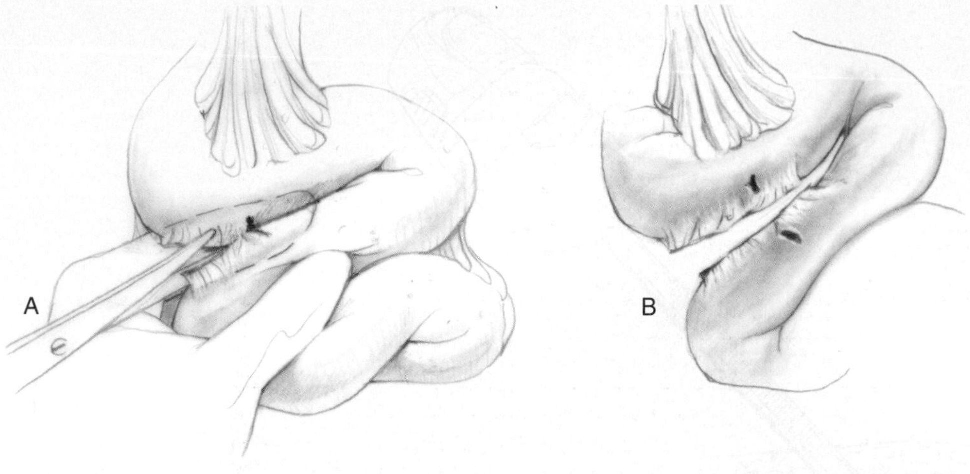

FIGURE 43.2. Sharp dissection of a loop of bowel containing an enterotomy is made to ascertain whether there is one enterotomy or two enterotomies. Note that it appears that there is only one enterotomy (**A**); however, after dissection of adhesions (**B**), two enterotomies are apparent.

malnourished, or whose condition is unstable from shock or sepsis.

Intestinal Injury during Endoscopic Procedures

Historically, most intestinal injuries in gynecologic surgery have occurred during open abdominal procedures. Exponential growth in the number of laparoscopic cases, however, has shifted the spectrum of risk. Gastrointestinal injury during laparoscopy most commonly occurs during initial peritoneal entry. Injury can occur from use of a scalpel, insufflating needle, trocar, or blunt dissection. Use of the open (Hasson) technique does not prevent bowel injuries. Good clinical judgment is necessary to determine which patients are appropriate candidates for laparoscopy. Previous surgeries, inflammatory conditions, and prior irradiation increase risk of injury from enteric adhesions, which fix intestine to the abdominal wall. Oxygenating the patient via bag-mask in preparation for intubation can distend the stomach below the level of the umbilicus, placing it at risk for injury. Nasogastric decompression before introduction of a Veress needle or trocar reduces this risk. In the presence of enteric adhesions, the laparoscopic trocar can be inadvertently placed into the stomach, transverse colon, or small intestine. Perforation is suspected by nonvisualization of intraperitoneal structures, identification of intraluminal tissue, and reflux of enteric content. If perforation occurs, it is prudent to leave the trocar in position, as it is much easier to recognize injuries using the trocar as a guide to the affected anatomy (Fig. 43.3). If the extent of injury cannot be determined, or the necessary repair cannot be accomplished via laparoscopy, then a laparotomy should be performed.

Cautery or sharp dissection can result in enterotomy, which commonly occurs during adhesiolysis. The skill and comfort level of the laparoscopic surgeon determines whether the defect can be successfully repaired via endoscopy or whether laparotomy is required. The most serious laparoscopic intestinal injuries are those that go unrecognized at the time of surgery. Thermal injury from electrocautery or laser can have a potentially disastrous outcome. With electrosurgical injury, a progressive zone of tissue destruction extends well beyond the area of thermal contact, resulting in tissue necrosis and perforation 72 to 96 hours after surgery. Perforation may be signaled by high fever, leukocytosis, nausea, vomiting, and a generalized ill appearance. Signs of peritonitis are present on examination. Flat-plate x-ray studies may be of limited benefit in the early postoperative period, because intraperitoneal air can persist for 7 days following surgery. CT scan using water-soluble contrast is better suited for this evaluation and should demonstrate extravasation of contrast material into the peritoneal cavity with possible abscess formation.

If perforation is suspected or confirmed, urgent exploration is warranted. Hypovolemia, electrolyte abnormalities, and anemia should be aggressively corrected. Broad-spectrum antibiotics are administered, and nasogastric decompression is performed as the patient is prepared for surgery. At surgery, aggressive irrigation is necessary to enhance visibility. Copious enteric exudate causes a profound inflammatory response and generalized matting together of intraperitoneal content. Inspection of the small bowel is initiated at the ileocecal junction and is continued proximally in a hand-over-hand fashion. Careful examination of the bowel and mesentery is continued to the ligament of Treitz, followed by thorough inspection of the large intestine. The stomach and proximal small bowel are also inspected. In contrast to sharp enterotomy, which can be repaired primarily, significant thermal injury is best corrected by resection of affected bowel. At the very least, a wide margin of bowel wall is removed beyond any visible thermal injury. Because of enteric contamination, other necrotic tissues, such as fulgurated endometriotic implants, are at high risk for abscess formation and should be excised.

Intestinal Injury during Uterine Curettage and Other Gynecologic Procedures

It is estimated that most uterine perforations go unrecognized; therefore, injury to pelvic viscera may also go unrecognized. If fundal perforation occurs during sharp or suction curettage, intestine and mesentery can be drawn into the uterine cavity by the curette. Evisceration as a consequence most commonly occurs during dilatation and curettage of the gravid uterus. Tactile feedback may suggest products of conception, when in fact prolapsed abdominal viscera are being curetted (Fig. 43.4). Recognition of this injury warrants immediate surgical exploration. With the abdomen open, the bowel is retrieved by gentle traction from above. The surgical objectives are to control hemorrhage from the uterine injury thoroughly inspect the bowel, repair injuries, and complete the uterine

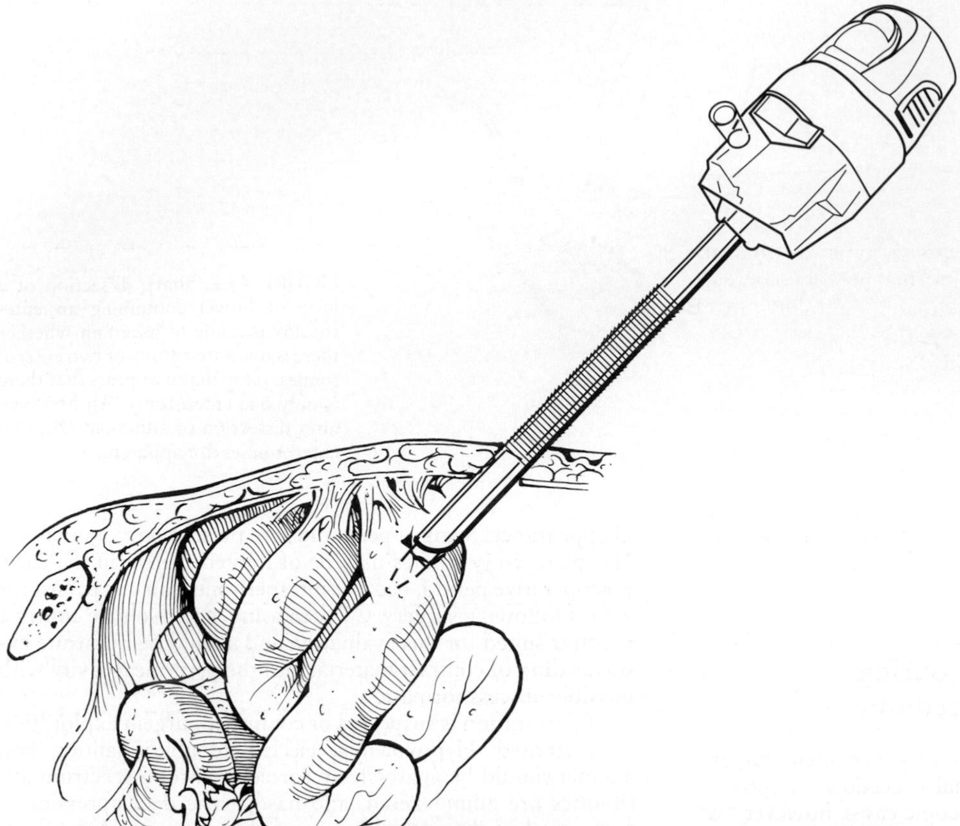

FIGURE 43.3. Perforation of trocar into small bowel.

evacuation. In women of reproductive age, hysterectomy is avoided unless uterine preservation poses a significant threat to her health.

Intestinal injury has been associated with a vast array of other gynecologic procedures, including those generally considered to be minor outpatient surgeries. For example, rectal lacerations and thermal injuries have occurred during cervical conization and loop electrosurgical excision procedure, respectively. Intestinal perforations and obstructions have resulted from placement of tension-free vaginal tape. A variety of pelvic reconstructive grafts have reportedly eroded into the small or large bowel, and intestinal perforations have resulted from extrauterine migration of an intrauterine contraceptive device. Accordingly, the gynecologic surgeon should be cognizant of possible intestinal ramifications of his/her operative endeavors.

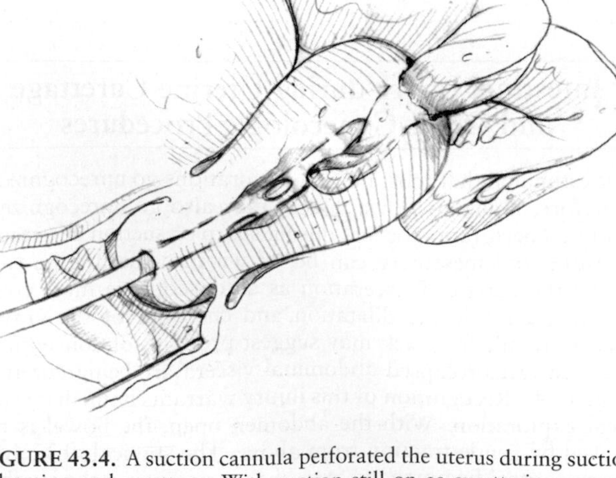

FIGURE 43.4. A suction cannula perforated the uterus during suction dilatation and curettage. With suction still on as curette is removed, the bowel is drawn through the uterus and vagina.

Radiation Injury

Radiation therapy for gynecologic cancers can cause intestinal injuries that require surgical correction. Also, damage from prior irradiation contributes to complications during other surgical procedures. The intestinal tract is adversely affected by radiation during treatment and soon thereafter (acute injury) and/or remote from treatment (late injury). The acute phase is associated with small bowel irritability, cramping, and diarrhea, with onset generally 2 to 3 weeks after initiation of therapy. Injury to the large bowel manifests acutely as proctosigmoiditis, with resultant pain, tenesmus, frequent bowel movements, and bleeding. Low-residue diet, antispasmodics, and antiinflammatories are helpful in uncomplicated cases. In more severe cases, debilitating symptoms can adversely affect lifestyle. Intestinal adhesions, fibrosis, obstruction, perforation, abscess, and fistulae are potential late complications.

Surgery in previously irradiated patients warrants special attention and is best performed by those experienced in this regard. Whenever possible, the surgical incision is made in a location beyond the radiation field. Extensive lysis of adhesions is best avoided, and dissection should be confined to the minimum area necessary to complete the surgical objectives. If obstruction occurs, consideration is given to intestinal bypass as opposed to extensive mobilization. Resection is avoided unless the anastomosis can be completed with nonirradiated bowel segments. This objective is often theoretical, because damaged bowel may appear normal and yet have significant microscopic endarteritis and vasculature obliteration. The characteristic pale, thickened bowel wall, telangiectatic vessels, and strictured lumen need not be present to indicate significant radiation injury. If resection is unavoidable, the suture line can be reinforced by wrapping the anastomosis with omentum, which elicits support of exogenous blood supply.

A vesicovaginal or rectovaginal fistula may develop if there is extensive damage to the intervening tissue. The time course of fistula occurrence is usually between 6 and 24 months after therapy, but it may present years after irradiation. The mechanism of late radiation injuries is believed to be obliterative vascular injury with compromised blood flow and tissue necrosis. Postirradiation rectovaginal fistulae are complex problems that rarely heal with simple excision, mobilization, and closure, such that they are probably best corrected using a three-staged approach. First, a diverting ileostomy or colostomy is performed to redirect the colonic content, reduce bacterial infiltration, and allow resolution of inflammation. Several months later, the objectives of the second surgery are complete resection of the fistulous tract and surrounding damaged tissue plus neovascularization via an omental flap or myocutaneous graft. The goal of the eventual third surgery is reversal of the diverting ostomy to reestablish normal intestinal continuity.

POSTOPERATIVE CONSIDERATIONS

Nasogastric Decompression

Some surgeons use routine postoperative nasogastric decompression to reduce nausea, vomiting, and abdominal distention and to enable healing of bowel anastomoses. These prophylactic objectives differ from the therapeutic goals of nasogastric decompression used to alleviate symptoms and expedite recovery from an existing ileus or small bowel obstruction. The literature, however, does not support routine postoperative use. Nasogastric tubes increase patient discomfort and increase the occurrence of sinus infections and epistaxis. A meta-analysis of selective versus routine nasogastric decompression after elective laparotomy included 26 trials and 3,964 patients. Routine postoperative decompression was associated with an increased incidence of pneumonia, atelectasis, and fever. Abdominal distention and vomiting were increased in selectively treated patients who did not have nasogastric tubes, and eventual tube insertion was required in 5% to 7% of patients in this group. Nasogastric tube reinsertion was required in 2% of routinely decompressed patients. There was no significant difference in the occurrence of wound infections, wound dehiscence, or anastomotic leaks. The authors of this analysis concluded that through the selective use of nasogastric decompression, only 1 in 20 patients require a nasogastric tube.

Early Postoperative Feeding

There is a wide spectrum of practice patterns among surgeons regarding postoperative diet. For many decades, the conventional approach has been to wait for auscultation of bowel sounds before providing clear liquids and to wait for the occurrence of flatus before giving solid food. Inpatient managed care pressures and successful outpatient recovery following laparoscopic procedures have challenged clinicians to reevaluate traditional postoperative feeding regimens. Current trends are toward much more aggressive early postoperative feeding, even in the setting of bowel resection and anastomosis. Some randomized clinical trials have shown early feeding to be associated with increased frequency of nausea and vomiting, whereas others have shown no difference. The overall rates of ileus, anastomotic complications, and times required for return of bowel function are generally comparable. Early postoperative feeding, however, has not consistently resulted in shorter average length of hospital stay.

Supplemental Nutrition

Perioperative nutritional support is indicated in patients who have been without nutrition for more than 7 days, in patients who are malnourished (weight loss exceeds 15% of usual weight), and when expected duration of recovery is longer than 10 days. Total parenteral nutrition (TPN) has extended the lives of numerous surgical patients and enabled the resumption of normal lifestyle in many. Long-term parenteral nutrition, however, has morbidity that is not insignificant. The need for indwelling central venous access puts patients at risk for catheter sepsis and other catheter-related complications. Metabolic derangements and pancreatic or hepatic dysfunction are common. Intestinal mucosal atrophy results from nonuse in patients who are reliant solely on parenteral nutrition.

Use of the gut for nutrition is advisable whenever possible. The advantages of enteral tube feeding over TPN include no requirement for venous access, enhanced intestinal lymphatic function, reversal of mucosal atrophy, decreased risk of bacterial translocation, and stimulation of intestinal adaptation. Adaptation is the process whereby the villous height and crypt depth increase, with gradual bowel dilation and lengthening, resulting in increased absorptive surface area. Enteral feeding is not indicated in patients with a nonfunctional intestinal tract or intestinal obstruction, or in those at high risk for aspiration.

Acute Gastric Distention

Acute gastric distention results from inhibition of gastric peristalsis. Postoperative gastric distention more commonly occurs after surgical manipulation in the vicinity of the stomach. Patients at increased risk are those who are diabetic, elderly, or medically debilitated. Short-term postoperative nasogastric decompression can prevent and manage this problem in those who are at high risk. Stimulatory agents such as metoclopramide may expedite gastric emptying in the nonobstructed patient.

Ileus

Postoperative ileus is a mechanical dysfunction in which the normal anterograde gastrointestinal peristalsis is disrupted.

Ileus may involve any segment of the digestive tract, including the stomach, small bowel, or colon. In fact, ileus is most frequently a large bowel dysfunction in that the colon is generally the last segment in the gastrointestinal tract to regain function after pelvic surgery. Postoperatively, the stomach and small intestine usually resume activity within 8 hours. At times, active small bowel peristalsis is noted at the conclusion of even complex abdominal procedures. In contrast, the colon may take 48 to 72 hours to regain function. Colonic dysfunction generally resolves from proximal to distal, such that rectosigmoid activity is the last to return.

Factors that predispose to ileus or worsen the severity of ileus include dehydration, electrolyte abnormalities, diabetes, chronic laxative use, bowel manipulation during surgery, extensive retroperitoneal dissection, general anesthetic agents, narcotic analgesics, immobility, urinary or gastrointestinal leak, peritonitis, abscess, and hematoma. Some degree of adynamic ileus results from all intraabdominal procedures. With return of bowel function, peristaltic pains are often severe, such that many patients describe them as being worse than surgical pain. Normal recovery of bowel function is evident by gradual increase in appetite, tolerance of oral nutrition, and flatus.

Delay in bowel function, worsening gas pains, nausea, and vomiting are suggestive of a clinically significant ileus. Physical examination confirms abdominal distention with diffuse discomfort, hypoactive bowel sounds, and tympanic percussion. Correction of contributing factors and supportive care are the cornerstones of management. Therapeutic interventions include bowel rest, intravenous hydration, correction of electrolytes (i.e., potassium, sodium, and magnesium), physical activity, and judicious use of narcotic analgesia. If good bowel sounds for 24 hours or more suggest that colonic dysfunction is a predominant underlying factor, colonic stimulation (e.g., docusate sodium suppository or enema) may be helpful. Patients with vomiting, those not responding to supportive measures, and those with evidence of gastric or small bowel dilatations on x-ray study benefit from nasogastric decompression. Decompression is generally continued until flatus ensues and abdominal distention resolves.

Adynamic ileus must be distinguished from a mechanical small bowel obstruction. If the patient has not passed flatus within 4 to 5 days or does not respond to conservative measures, then the possibility of a mechanical small bowel obstruction should be considered. Early in the disease process, radiographs may provide little assistance in clarifying the diagnosis because the changes of postoperative ileus and early obstruction are similar. However, after 3 to 5 days, plain abdominal radiographs with supine, upright, and/or lateral recumbent views will help distinguish ileus from mechanical small bowel obstruction. The typical radiographic pattern of an ileus is that of intermittent air found throughout the gastrointestinal tract, including the colon and rectum. Upright views may show air-fluid levels within the small bowel and stomach, and, on occasion, the transverse colon (Fig. 43.5). In contrast, radiographic characteristics of mechanical small bowel obstruction include proximal distended loops with a paucity or absence of gas in the colon. The dilated small bowel loops with air-fluid levels may follow a stair-step pattern from the right lower quadrant to the left upper quadrant in parallel with the anatomic base of the small bowel mesentery.

With intermittent or partial small bowel obstruction, some gas is seen in the colon. Conversely, if the obstruction is in the proximal small bowel, there may be no distended loops at all. Radiographic studies can at times clarify the type of obstruction (mechanical vs. nonmechanical), the extent of obstruction (partial vs. complete), and the location of obstruction (stomach vs. small bowel vs. colon). If the diagnosis remains unclear, a water-soluble contrasted CT scan or gastrointestinal study with small bowel follow-through can clarify the situation and localize the point of obstruction if present. Contrast material may also stimulate peristalsis and has been reportedly therapeutic in some cases of paralytic ileus.

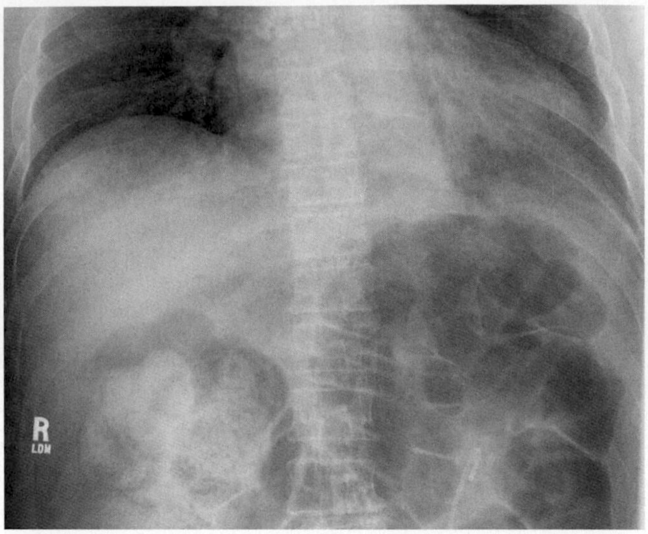

FIGURE 43.5. Plain x-ray view of dilated colon in postoperative ileus.

Small Bowel Obstruction

Intraperitoneal adhesions are the most common etiology of intestinal obstruction. Malignancies and hernias are also frequent extrinsic causes. An estimated 85% of all small bowel obstructions are secondary to one of these three conditions. Intraluminal causes include tumors, polyps, gallstones, and bezoars. Obstructive intramural strictures can complicate irradiation or inflammatory bowel disease.

Early postoperative obstruction deserves a trial of nonsurgical management. Nasogastric decompression, supportive care, and correction of underlying contributing factors are as described for adynamic ileus. Supine position with legs flexed helps relax rectus abdominis muscles to facilitate examination. Early in the course of obstruction, there may be minimal to absent distention. Proximal obstruction may also manifest with minimal abdominal distention. High-pitched bowel sounds with metallic tones and rushes are suggestive of an obstructive process. Hypoactive or absent bowel sounds are more suggestive of paralytic ileus. Hypoactive bowel sounds may also occur with intestinal fatigue from long-standing obstruction, closed loop obstruction, or pseudoobstruction. Fewer than half of obstructed patients manifest the classic triad of rebound tenderness, guarding, and rigidity. Also, the physical findings of focal tenderness and guarding are neither sensitive nor specific in confirming underlying obstruction or ischemia.

The duration of asymptomatic intervals between peristaltic pains may suggest the level of obstruction. Peristaltic waves tend to be 3 to 5 minutes apart in high obstruction, whereas in distal obstruction, 10 to 15 minutes may lapse between episodes. On flat-plate abdominal x-ray, small bowel distended by gas outlines the valvulae conniventes (plicae circulares), which traverse the entire diameter of the dilated bowel lumen.

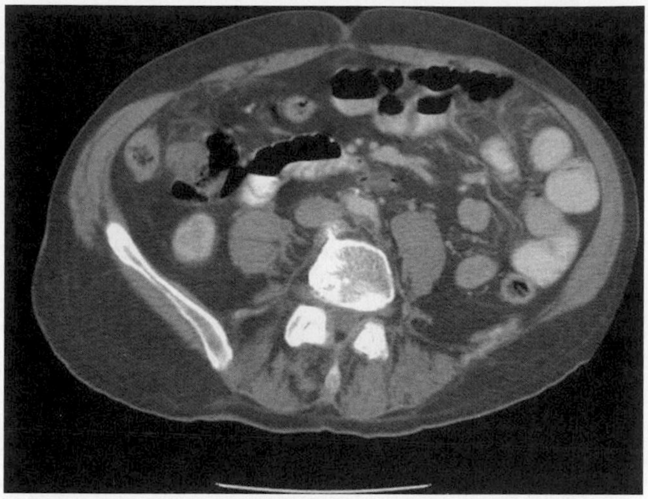

FIGURE 43.6. Computed tomography scan of small bowel obstruction; air-fluid levels in dilated small bowel.

Valvulae conniventes are closely spaced and may appear to interdigitate. In contrast, distended colon highlights the haustra, which partially traverse the bowel lumen and are spaced more widely apart. The central abdomen is occupied by distended small bowel loops, whereas the abdominal periphery houses the colon. In the decompressed patient, character of gastric aspirate suggests the potential anatomic site of obstruction. Gastric outlet obstruction produces clear gastric secretions. Bilious output is suggestive of obstruction in the proximal to mid small bowel, or a colonic obstruction with a competent ileocecal valve. Feculent drainage is characteristic of a distal small bowel obstruction or colonic obstruction with an incompetent ileocecal valve.

Intestinal obstruction leads to an accumulation of intraluminal fluid and gas with distention proximal to the occlusion (Fig 43.6). It is estimated that more than 70% of air in the gastrointestinal tract is from swallowing. Accordingly, distention is significantly worsened by swallowed air. With progressing distention comes tension and venous compression. Arterial inflow continues, resulting in blood accumulation within the bowel wall and lumen. Protein-rich fluid exudes from the capillaries, adding to tissue edema. Malabsorption combined with intestinal secretion further exacerbates intraluminal fluid collection. In the setting of complete obstruction, up to 7 to 8 L of fluid can accumulate, including 50% of plasma volume and 30% of circulating blood volume. Mucosal integrity is disrupted, and enteric bacteria traverse the defective bowel wall, seeding the peritoneum. If the process goes uncorrected, intestinal viability is irreversibly damaged as tissue necrosis ensues.

If a decision is made for operative intervention, preparation concentrates on correction of hypovolemia, anemia, and electrolyte imbalances. Broad-spectrum antibiotics may suppress bacterial translocation and delay intestinal ischemia. Upon exploration, the point of obstruction is identified and corrected. All necrotic bowel must be resected. It is not always possible, however, to discern the viability of bowel in the setting of obstruction. Visible characteristics—such as tissue color, extent of edema, and peristalsis—are not consistently reliable. Active bleeding from the cut bowel edge is a more accurate indicator. Intraoperative Doppler testing of the antimesenteric border should provide characteristic arterial pulsations. Absent Doppler sounds do not necessarily indicate inadequate arterial blood flow. In this setting, viability can be confirmed by intravenous 10% fluorescein (15 mg/kg), followed in 10 minutes by Wood's lamp illumination. Observation of bowel wall fluorescence suggests adequate blood flow to support anastomotic healing. Bowel segments that are less than 2 cm in length with no fluorescence can be preserved, but should not be included in the anastomosis. Larger areas of nonfluorescence suggest ischemia and likely require resection.

Large Bowel Obstruction

The vast majority of large bowel obstructions are due to malignancy or inflammatory conditions. This is in contrast to small bowel obstructions, for which adhesions are the principal etiology. The gynecologic surgeon may encounter large bowel obstruction from a primary colon or a gynecologic malignancy, ulcerative colitis, diverticular disease, pelvis abscess, or radiation injury. The onset of most colonic obstructions is insidious because of gradual luminal narrowing, which manifests clinically as decreased caliber stools, constipation, and bleeding. Progressive obstruction leads to obstipation, abdominal distention, colicky pain, nausea, and vomiting. Radiographic studies reveal a dilated colon proximal to the point of obstruction (Fig. 43.7). If the ileocecal valve is incompetent, the distention extends proximally into the small bowel, as evidenced by dilated bowel loops with air-fluid levels. A more serious closed loop obstruction occurs when the ileocecal valve is competent. The cecum is commonly involved; as cecal dilation exceeds 10 to 12 cm, the risk of perforation increases significantly. Preoperative endoscopy or water-soluble contrast study can clarify the etiology and location of obstruction. Barium enema should not be performed in the setting of acute obstruction or suspected perforation to avoid barium peritonitis. If necessary, any viable segment of large bowel proximal to the point of obstruction can be exteriorized as a colostomy.

Ogilvie Syndrome

Ogilvie syndrome (acute colonic pseudoobstruction) is a dysfunction of colonic peristalsis. Clinical presentation may be

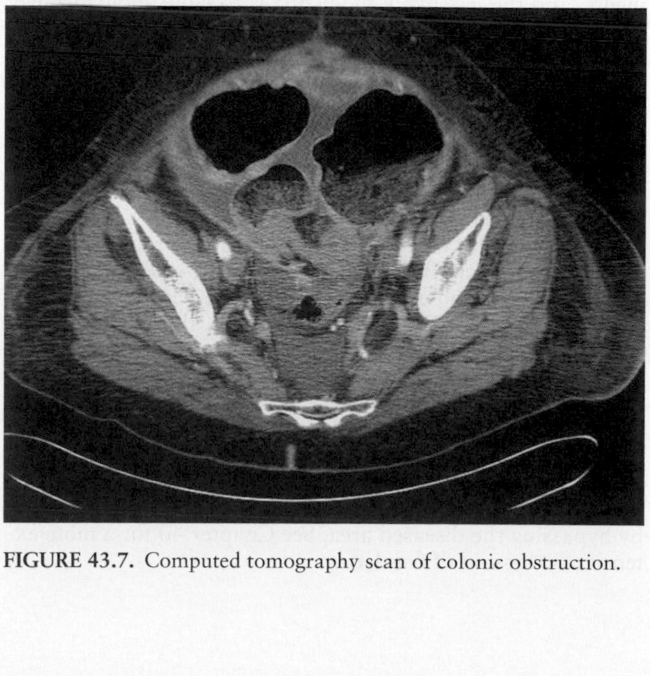

FIGURE 43.7. Computed tomography scan of colonic obstruction.

indistinguishable from a large bowel obstruction. The mechanism of colonic pseudoobstruction is theorized to be an imbalance between the proximal and distal colonic innervation. Parasympathetic innervation from the vagus nerve supplies the colon proximal to the splenic flexure. In contrast, the left colon receives parasympathetic innervation from the sacral plexus (S2–S4). Most commonly, only the right colon is dilated. Ogilvie syndrome is seen more commonly in elderly and debilitated patients and in those who are on narcotics and phenothiazine or tricyclic antidepressants. Supportive care includes hydration, correction of electrolyte abnormalities, and gastrointestinal decompression (nasogastric tube, rectal tube). Sequential radiographs are used to monitor cecal dilation to assess the risk of perforation. Endoscopic decompression or tube cecostomy are preferred alternatives to exploration, because surgical morbidity is significant. If necessary, intraoperative colonic decompression can be accomplished using an 18-gauge needle passed obliquely through the taenia coli and attached to suction. Decompression facilitates exteriorization of the bowel for diverting colostomy, if necessary.

Fistulae

Postoperative intestinal fistulae are an especially challenging problem for patients and clinicians. An enterocutaneous or enterovaginal fistula may be difficult to confirm, even when clinical findings are strongly suggestive of a fistulous communication. The high-pressure bowel defect may be small with only intermittent drainage, thus obscuring localization. Oral administration of charcoal or of brilliant blue or carmine red dye confirms the diagnosis if characteristic color change is observed in the effluent. Clarification of the fistulous tract can be aided by a fistulogram. Contrast material is injected transcutaneously, and the pattern of flow is evaluated radiographically. Excessive force during injection is avoided to prevent dislodgment of the bowel from its adherence to the abdominal or vaginal wall.

Initial nonoperative management of fistulae in selected cases has gained wide acceptance. The fundamentals of conservative management include correction of underlying inflammatory processes and electrolyte abnormalities, nutritional support, and maintenance of adequate hydration. The more proximal the fistula, the greater the potential for physiologic derangements, and the less likely the fistula is to close spontaneously with conservative management. Gastric, duodenal, and proximal jejunal fistulae can cause potentially fatal physiologic disturbances and thus require prompt intervention. Distal ileal or colonic fistulae are generally well tolerated and tend to close spontaneously if predisposing factors are circumvented. There must be no abscess, peritonitis, distal bowel obstruction, or foreign body within the fistulous tract. Prior irradiation is likely to preclude spontaneous healing.

Approximately two thirds of distal fistulae are expected to heal within 6 weeks if no complicating factors persist. A fistula that persists beyond 6 weeks is unlikely to heal without operative intervention. Depending on the clinical situation, it may be reasonable to wait an additional 1 to 2 months to optimize nutritional status and allow for resolution of inflammation. The appropriate time for surgical intervention must be individualized. The surgical objectives are to completely excise the fistulous tract and resect the affected bowel segment whenever possible. In certain circumstances, such as irradiated bowel or extensive adhesions, the fistula could be more aptly addressed by bypassing the diseased area. See Chapter 40 for a more extensive discussion of fistulae.

Dehiscence and Evisceration

Dehiscence implies postoperative wound separation and most commonly involves only the skin and subcutaneous tissue (superficial or incomplete dehiscence). Complete (deep) wound dehiscence refers to separation of the fascia and usually manifests with skin and subcutaneous disruption as well. Fascial disruption generally occurs between the fifth and tenth postoperative day, and is estimated to occur in approximately 1 in 200 high-risk patients. Complete dehiscence is most frequently associated with suture tearing through the tissue and is suspected in the setting of copious serous or serosanguineous drainage from the abdominal wound. The incision is explored with a sterile swab or gloved finger to assess for fascial defects. A small defect (1 to 2 cm) in an otherwise intact fascia with no associated bowel extrusion may be reapproximated with an interrupted fascial suture. Larger fascial defects and all defects with bowel herniation (evisceration) require immediate surgical attention.

Evisceration is an acute full-thickness wound disruption through which abdominal contents extrude and most commonly includes loops of distal small bowel and omentum. Evisceration is rare following laparoscopic procedures but should be suspected with a palpable or visible hernia defect and serosanguineous fluid drainage. Concomitant problems may include abnormal bowel function, nausea, vomiting, or evidence of bowel incarceration. CT and ultrasound imaging are useful if the diagnosis is uncertain. In preparing the eviscerated patient for surgery, she is kept in supine position, and the exposed bowel is covered with towels moistened by sterile saline or povidone-iodine solution. If accomplished without difficulty, eviscerated organs should be cautiously replaced back into the abdomen. The protective towels can be secured using a sterile plastic drape and reinforced with an abdominal binder. Broad-spectrum antibiotics are administered, and steps are taken to correct fluid and electrolyte abnormalities. Sedatives and analgesics can reduce intraperitoneal pressure. Intraoperatively, all layers of the wound are inspected for infection, and devitalized abdominal wall tissue is sharply debrided. The bowel and mesentery are inspected for injury, viability, hemostasis, and obstruction. The peritoneal contents are copiously irrigated. Bowel resection is generally not necessary, but it may be required if obstruction or ischemia is present.

Vaginal Evisceration

Protrusion of viscera through the vagina (Fig. 43.8) has been reported in association with surgery, enterocele, trauma, Valsalva maneuver, coitus, radiation, and foreign bodies. Small bowel and mesentery are most commonly involved, but evisceration may also include large bowel and omentum. Approximately two thirds of reported cases have occurred in patients with a history of prior surgery for pelvic relaxation or in the setting of symptomatic enterocele. Prior hysterectomy is a factor in only half of reported cases. This distressing situation tends to occur outside of the hospital setting, and bacterial contamination is inevitable. Severe abdominal pain may indicate mesenteric compromise. Surgical preparation is similar to that for an abdominal evisceration, but in contrast, it is best to resist preoperative attempts at replacing the bowel through the vagina. Surgical management should be via exploratory laparotomy. During exploration, the eviscerated contents are replaced into the peritoneal cavity with a combination of gentle traction from above and guidance from below. Copious intraperitoneal irrigation and broad-spectrum antibiotics are

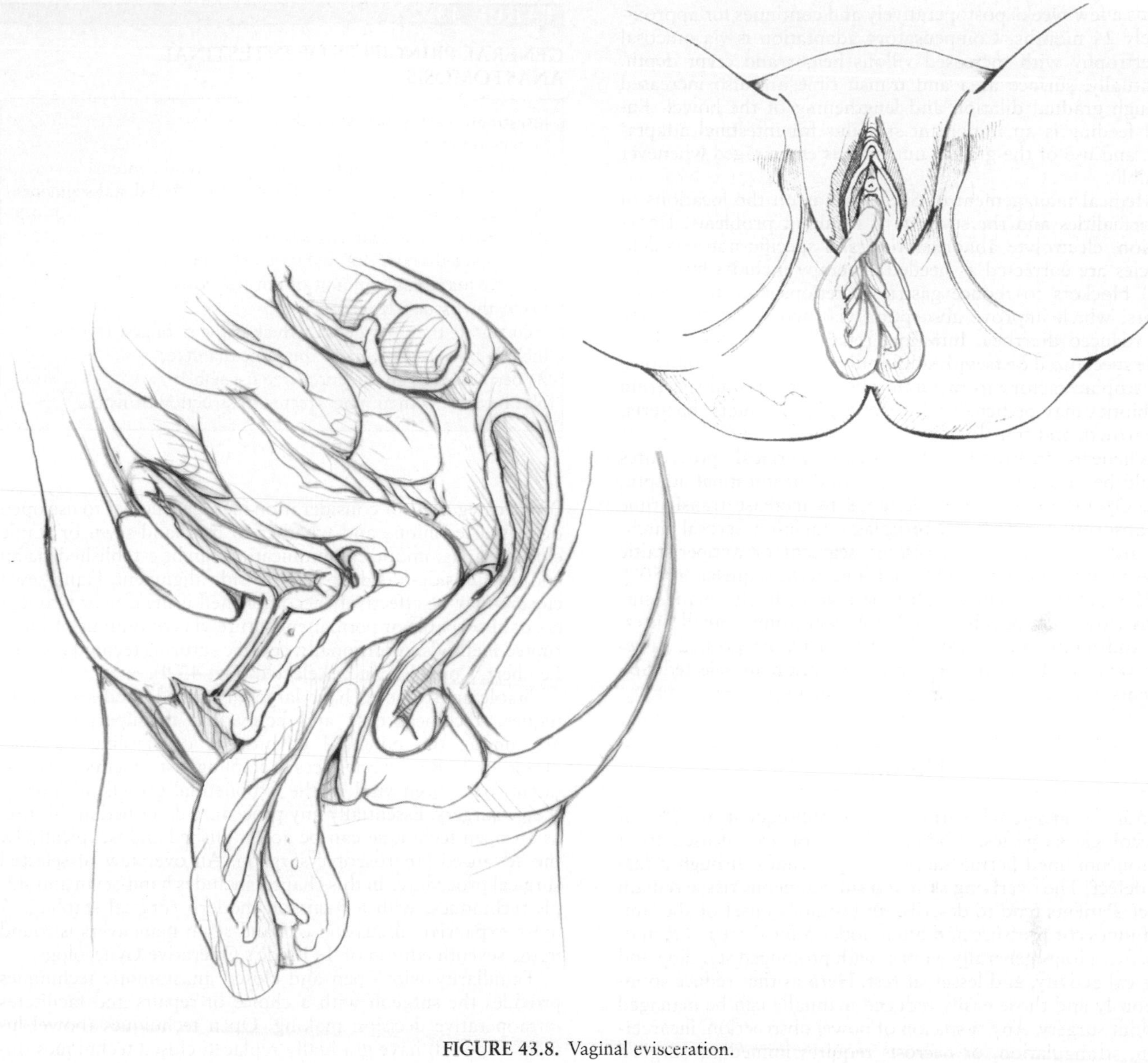

FIGURE 43.8. Vaginal evisceration.

used. Careful inspection of the bowel and mesentery are necessary to identify and repair injuries and to ensure viability. Severely damaged or obstructed bowel requires resection.

Short Bowel Syndrome

Short bowel syndrome (SBS) results from loss of significant bowel length or inadequate function of normal-length bowel. The net result is insufficient nutrient absorption necessary to meet the body's metabolic requirements. Causes include extensive surgical resection, regional enteritis (Crohn's disease), and radiation injury. An increasingly frequent etiology of SBS is reexploration subsequent to prior abdominal procedures. Extensive bowel resection is most often necessary as a result of postoperative adhesions or volvulus. In a 20-year review from the University of Nebraska Medical Center, 25% of adult SBS cases were attributed to secondary surgeries. Initial operations included colectomy, hysterectomy, appendectomy, gastric bypass, and others, with hysterectomy being the second-most-common predisposing procedure.

In women, the average length of small bowel is approximately 600 cm (range 350–700 cm). Some authors define SBS as having less than 200 cm of functional small intestine. In general, 50% of the small bowel can be resected without long-term impairment of nutritional status, as long as there is normal function in the remainder of the bowel. Severe nutritional deficiencies will likely result with loss of two thirds to three fourths of the small intestine. Malabsorption manifests as diarrhea, dehydration, weight loss, metabolic derangements, nutrient deficits, low serum protein, and anemia (iron, folate, and B_{12}).

Therapy for SBS begins with preemptive planning. A concerted effort is made to preserve as much small bowel and colon as possible at the time of any surgical resection. Preemptive strategies include steps taken to prevent adhesions, to avoid technical errors, and to act expeditiously on potentially ischemic bowel. After undergoing an intestinal resection, the remaining small bowel has adaptation capacity that begins a few weeks postoperatively and continues for approximately 24 months. Compensatory adaptation is via mucosal hypertrophy with increased villous height and crypt depth. Eventually, surface area and transit time are also increased through gradual dilation and lengthening of the bowel. Enteral feeding is an important stimulus for intestinal adaptation, and use of the gut for nutrition is encouraged whenever possible.

Medical management of SBS depends on the locations of abnormalities and the severity of resultant problems. Dehydration, electrolyte abnormalities, and specific nutrient deficiencies are corrected as needed. Therapy includes histamine (H2) blockers to reduce gastric secretions and antimotility agents, which improve absorption via increased transit time and reduced diarrhea. Intestinal rehabilitation programs include specialized diets with soluble fiber, rehydration solutions, and trophic factors to facilitate absorption. Broad-spectrum antibiotics may be beneficial in patients with enteric bacterial overgrowth and translocation.

Whenever reasonable, therapeutic surgical procedures should be delayed until after the period of intestinal adaptation. Operative maneuvers designed to increase transit time and absorption include stricturoplasty, tapering, serosal patching, and interposing of a colonic segment or antiperistaltic small bowel segment. Additional long-term sequelae in 50% of SBS patients include gallstones; accordingly, many surgeons advocate prophylactic cholecystectomy. Small intestine and multivisceral transplantation have progressed in recent years to be a viable treatment option in selected SBS patients.

Hernias

Ventral or incisional hernias occur subsequent to 1% of gynecologic surgeries. Abdominal viscera are encased by a peritoneum-lined hernia sac, which protrudes through a fascial defect. The overlying skin and subcutaneous tissue remain intact. Patients tend to describe an insidious onset of abdominal fullness or pressure and often notice a focal area of distention. Symptoms generally worsen with prolonged standing and physical activity, and lessen at rest. Hernias that reduce spontaneously and those easily reduced manually can be managed without surgery. Any suspicion of bowel obstruction, incarceration, strangulation, or necrosis requires immediate surgical evaluation. The surgical objectives are to isolate and resect the hernia sac, reduce the sac contents, lyse pertinent adhesions, and inspect the viscera to ensure gastrointestinal integrity. Resection may be necessary to alleviate intestinal obstruction or remove severely damaged bowel. Before closure, steps are taken to acquire hemostasis, control infection, excise preexisting scar tissue, and mobilize the abdominal wall to enable a tension-free fascial approximation.

OPERATIVE TECHNIQUES

General Principles

Numerous variations exist on bowel resection and anastomotic techniques. Discussed in this text are some of the more commonly used methods, instruments, and materials. This review is by no means exhaustive, given the vast array of reported options on this theme. Strict adherence to the fundamental principles of anastomosis is more important to successful healing than are the specific techniques or materials used (Table 43.2).

TABLE 43.2

GENERAL PRINCIPLES OF INTESTINAL ANASTOMOSIS

Intestinal anastomosis should:
Be tension free
Avoid intraperitoneal spill of gastrointestinal content
Incorporate healthy tissue in the proximal and distal segments
Preserve adequate lumen
Be hemostatic and watertight/airtight
Be completed under optimal surgical exposure
Preserve maximum amount of normal bowel
Invert the tissue edges
Incorporate the submucosa, which is the strongest layer
Include bowel segments of the same diameter
Be performed in an infection-free tissue bed
Not be done with an uncorrected obstruction or fistula

Broad categories for consideration include whether to use open or closed technique and whether to use hand-sewn or staple closure. Anastomotic communication can be established via an end-to-end, side-to-side, or end-to-side alignment. Hand-sewn closure may be effectively accomplished using one or two layers of absorbable or permanent suture via continuous or interrupted methods. Additionally, specific suturing techniques (i.e., Lembert, Connell) can be selected (Fig. 43.9).

Staple anastomoses have largely replaced hand-sewn techniques. Technical ease and equivalent to superior results are among the potential advantages of stapling methods (Table 43.3). Recent advances in stapling instruments and techniques have been vital to the exponential growth in laparoscopic surgery. Essentially any procedure described in this text as an open technique can be accomplished endoscopically by the advanced laparoscopic surgeon. An overview of selected surgical procedures in this chapter includes hand-sewn and staple techniques, with a focus on modern surgical stapling. A more expansive discussion of hand-sewn maneuvers is found in the seventh edition of Te Linde's Operative Gynecology.

Familiarity with open and closed anastomotic techniques provides the surgeon with a choice of repairs and facilitates intraoperative decision making. Open techniques (bowel lumens exposed) have gradually replaced closed techniques (lumens occluded) in most circumstances. Morbidity associated with open techniques is acceptably low. The extent of intraperitoneal spill can generally be controlled with aggressive preoperative bowel prep and atraumatic bowel clamps. Closed techniques are potentially advantageous in reducing complications from unprepped bowel and with anastomosis involving the colon.

Angiogenesis at the anastomotic margins begins within the first 72 hours of surgery if not impeded by infection or inflammation. The most important strength layer of the bowel wall is the submucosa, which must be incorporated into any anastomosis. Collagen is believed to be the single most important contributor to submucosal strength. The maximum anastomotic bursting pressure reflects the pressure required to disrupt an anastomosis and has been used experimentally to assess the strength of healing. The bursting pressure of an anastomosis increases rapidly during the early postoperative period. Sixty percent of the surrounding bowel wall strength is reached by postoperative day 3 to 4, and pressure tolerated by the anastomotic site approximates 100% of that tolerated by intact bowel wall by postoperative day 7. The ideal suture material should provide maximum strength during the

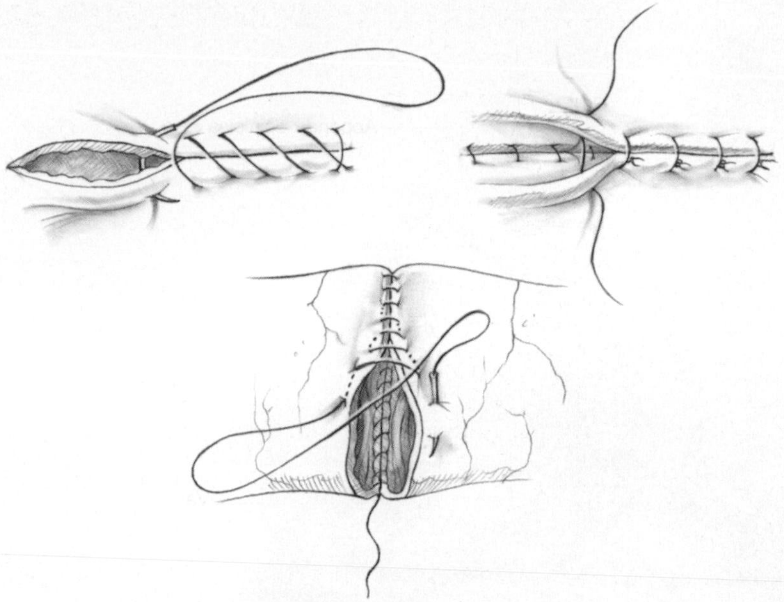

FIGURE 43.9. Commonly used suture techniques for intestinal anastomosis: continuous over-and-over suture (**A**), interrupted Lembert suture (**B**), and Connell continuous suture (**C**). Adapted from Cohen Z, Sullivan B. Intestinal anastomosis. In: Wilmore DW, Cheung LY, Harken AM, et al., eds. *ACS surgery: principles and practice*. New York: WEBMD; 2002; 803.

lag phase of wound healing with minimal tissue reaction and inflammation. Although the perfect suture material is yet to be identified, modern monofilament and coated braided sutures represent progress toward this goal.

Double-layer intestinal closures have long been touted as more secure than single-layer closures. The traditional anastomosis includes a running inner layer of 3-0 chromic cat gut (absorbable) and an interrupted outer layer of 3-0 silk (nonabsorbable). Extensive clinical evidence, however, suggests single-layer closure to be equivalent and may offer some advantages over double-layer anastomosis. Comparative animal studies have demonstrated more rapid vascularization and mucosal healing, and greater early anastomotic strength associated with single-layer repair. Double-layer closures, along with traditional sutures such as cat gut and silk, are associated with greater inflammation, reduced microneoangiogenesis, and less blood flow across the anastomosis. A single-layer reapproximation generally causes less narrowing of the intestinal lumen and can be accomplished in less time. When done properly, all hand-sewn techniques result in an inverted suture line.

TABLE 43.3

STAPLE TECHNIQUES

Advantages	Disadvantages
Better blood flow and oxygen delivery across the anastomotic line	Greater expense with stapling instruments
Less operative time required	Everted tissue edges using some techniques
Uniform staple placement an inherent design of surgical staplers	Dependence on equipment that could malfunction
Less luminal narrowing	Staple lines may be less resistant to tension injury
Technically easier to learn and perform in most cases	Technically difficult to align the surgical staplers in some anatomic locations

Either continuous or interrupted closures can be used for intestinal anastomosis. Continuous technique is rapid and has the potential advantage of a more even tension distribution along the suture line. In comparing running versus interrupted closure, animal studies have also shown reduced tissue oxygen tension, impaired collagen synthesis, and increased anastomotic complications using running closure. To date, however, randomized clinical trials are lacking, and retrospective studies show no consistent benefit of one technique over the other. Clinical and subclinical anastomotic leak rates, associated morbidity, and length of hospitalization are generally equivalent, even for high-risk patients (e.g., patients with prior radiation therapy, malnutrition, or carcinomatosis).

SURGERY ON THE SMALL INTESTINE

Blood Supply to the Small Intestine

The small bowel receives its arterial blood supply from the superior mesenteric artery (SMA), which arises from the ventral surface of the abdominal aorta (Fig. 43.10). In addition to the small bowel, the SMA also gives rise to the middle and right colic arteries, which supply those regions of the colon. The most proximal small bowel is supported by the common inferior pancreaticoduodenal artery from the SMA. Arising from the left side of the SMA is a series of jejunal and ileal arteries that branch to form anastomotic arcades. Primary arcades terminate directly into the small bowel via vasa recta or extend to form secondary, tertiary, and quaternary arcades that eventually give rise to terminal vasa recta. Avascular spaces between the vasa recta are known as windows of Deaver. In general, up to 8 cm of small intestine can remain viable distal to the closest vasa recta because of intramural vascular communications.

The ileocolic artery arises from the right side of the SMA and traverses the base of the mesentery to form a loop anastomosis with the SMA in the region of the terminal ileum. This loop encircles an area devoid of vessels known as the avascular space of Treves. The arterial blood supply to the distal ileum is considered tenuous because of a decreased number of

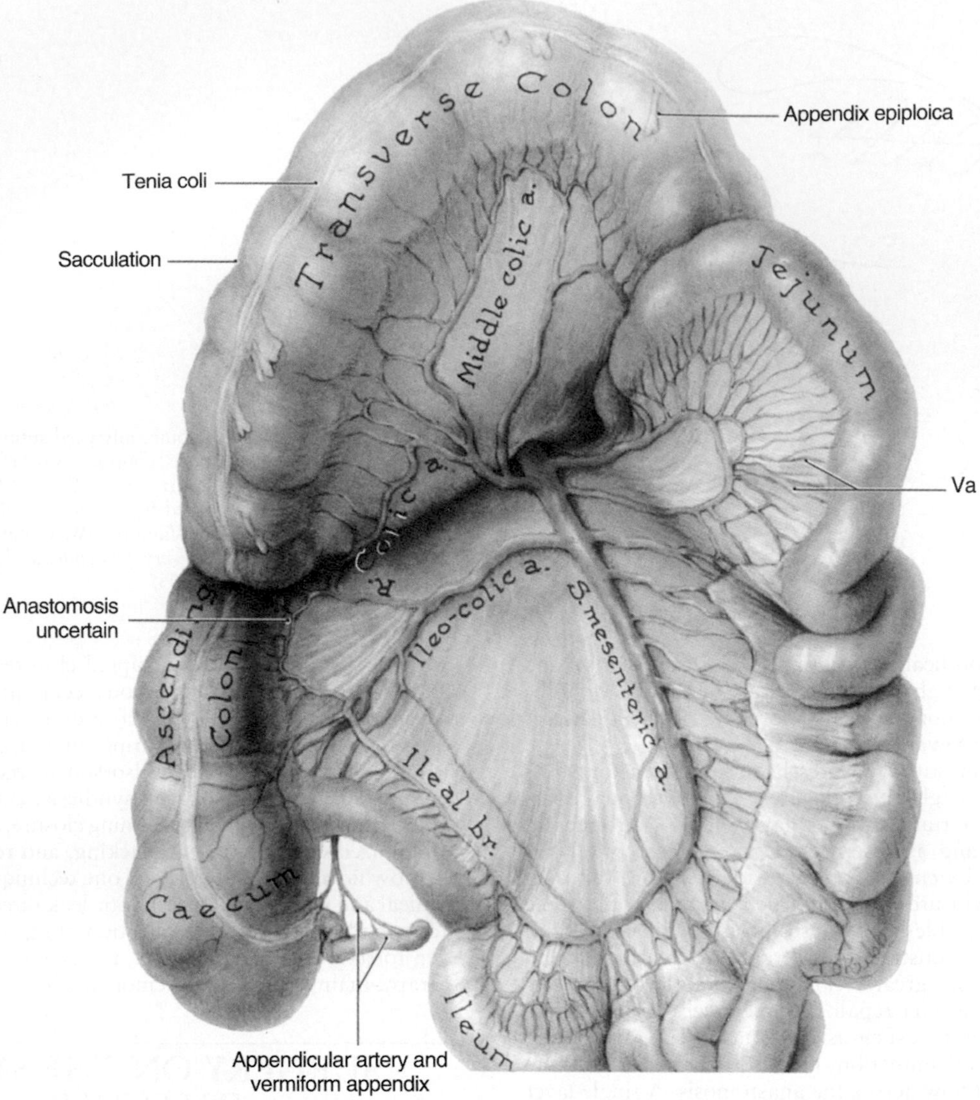

FIGURE 43.10. Intestinal blood supply: superior mesenteric artery. The peritoneum is in part stripped off. Observe the following: (*1*) The superior mesenteric artery, which ends by anastomosing with the ileal branch of the ileocolic artery. (*2*) Its branches: from its left side, (*a*) 12 or more jejunal and ileal branches. These anastomose to form arcades from which vasa recta pass to the small gut. From its right side, (*b*) the middle colic, the ileocolic, and commonly, but not here, an independent right colic artery. These anastomose to form a marginal artery (labeled in Fig. 43.14) from which vasa recta pass to the large gut. (*c*) The two inferior pancreaticoduodenal arteries (not in view) arise from the main artery either directly or in conjunction with the first jejunal branch. (*3*) Taeniae coli, sacculations, and appendices epiploicae distinguish the large gut from the smooth-walled small gut.

vasa recta from only primary vascular arcades. Because of the uncertain vascular status in this area, it is recommended that 10 cm of terminal ileum also be removed during cecal resection to improve the anastomotic blood supply.

Small Bowel Resection

It is important to resect only the length of bowel necessary to adequately address the disease process, thereby sparing as much normal intestine as possible. For benign disease, bowel transection sites are located just proximal and distal to the abnormal segment. Moist laparotomy pads are positioned to isolate the surgical field from the remaining peritoneal contents. At the proposed transection sites, blunt dissection is used to make a small opening through the avascular mesenteric window adjacent to the bowel wall. The staple cartridge half of the gastrointestinal anastomotic (GIA) stapler is passed through the proximal mesenteric defect, perpendicular to the axis of the bowel. The anvil half is placed across the bowel and aligned with the cartridge. This effectively occludes the bowel as the GIA stapler is closed. Proper positioning is confirmed, and the stapler is fired by steady forward motion on the pusher-bar knife assembly. Upon release of the assembly and opening of the GIA handles, two double-staggered staple lines are noted with the intervening bowel transected. The

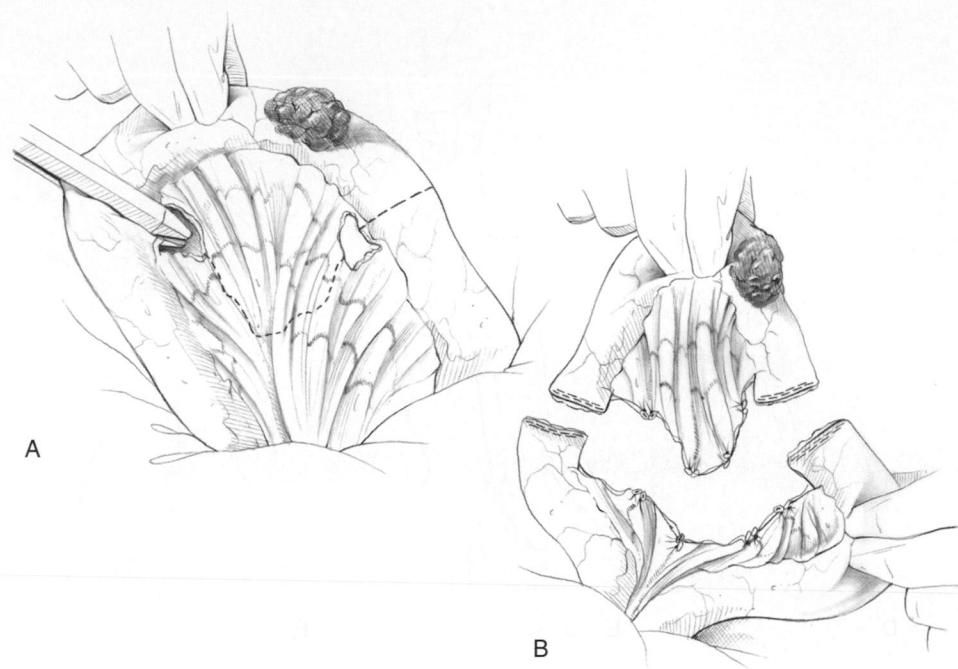

FIGURE 43.11. Small bowel resection with side-to-side (functional end-to-end) staple anastomosis. **A:** The two halves of the gastrointestinal anastomotic (GIA) stapler are passed through the mesenteric window and secured across the bowel. **B:** The GIA stapler has been fired proximal and distal to the abnormal bowel. Staggered double staple lines are noted to occlude each segment. Extent of mesenteric resection is tailored to the case-specific disease process. (*Continued*)

same steps are carried out at the distal site for transection (Fig. 43.11).

For benign disease, the mesenteric resection can be carried out in close proximity to the bowel, with no need to remove an intervening wedge. The objective is to preserve as much intact mesenteric blood supply as possible. The peritoneum overlying the mesentery is opened with cautery. Visual inspection and transillumination help to identify mesenteric vessels, which are clamped, cut, and suture-ligated using 2-0 silk ligatures. Division of the mesentery completes the resection. In preparation for anastomosis, tissue attachments are cleared 5 mm from both stapled bowel edges to avoid incorporation of mesenteric fat.

Staple Anastomosis

Staple end-to-end anastomosis in the small bowel is rarely used because of excess narrowing of the lumen. More favorable are the staple side-to-side anastomotic techniques that are functionally likened to an end-to-end anastomosis. Staple end-to-end techniques are more aptly used to create an anastomosis between two segments of large bowel following transverse colectomy or rectosigmoid resection.

Side-to-Side (Functional End-to-End) Staple Anastomosis

The side-to-side functional end-to-end staple techniques have gained wide acceptance because of the technical ease, availability of reliable instruments, and capacity to join bowel lumens of different diameters. Following resection, the occluded bowel ends are juxtaposed with the antimesenteric edges aligned in parallel along a distance of approximately 8 cm. This alignment is secured by a seromuscular 3-0 silk suture placed at the proximal end. Mayo scissors are used to excise a full-thickness oblique segment from the antimesenteric corner of each staple-occluded bowel segment. The anvil half of the GIA stapler and the cartridge half are inserted into each enterotomy (Fig. 43.11). The stapler is secured into position by closing the lock lever such that the antimesenteric borders are aligned. Proper positioning is confirmed, and the instrument is fired by sliding the pusher-bar knife assembly forward, and then returning it to the neutral position. This maneuver delivers two double-staggered staple rows and cuts the intervening bowel walls. The GIA instrument is disengaged and removed. The resultant enteroenterostomy is inspected to ensure patency, viability, and hemostasis.

The open bowel edges are grasped with Allis clamps, and a linear thoracoabdominal (TA) stapler is placed across the common lumen, ensuring that full-thickness bowel wall is circumferentially elevated above the staple line. After releasing the safety, the TA stapler is fired via steady closing grip on the handles. Excess tissue above the edge of the stapler is excised, and the instrument is released. Luminal capacity is evaluated by transmural palpation between the thumb and index finger, moving in a circular motion to outline the two layers of bowel wall (in contrast to the four palpable layers proximal to the common lumen). Oversewing the staple line is unnecessary unless there is concern regarding the anastomotic integrity.

An open variation of this technique is such that after resection, the ends of the *in situ* bowel are not occluded. Atraumatic bowel clamps, protective moist laparotomy pads, irrigation, and povidone-iodine–soaked gauze reduce enteric contamination. The antimesenteric borders are aligned and secured as described above. The anvil half of the GIA stapler is introduced through one open bowel lumen, and the cartridge half is introduced through the other. The GIA stapler is locked and fired along the antimesenteric borders, and the TA stapler is used to close the resultant common enterotomy. These staple techniques are also ideal for joining bowel segments of discordant diameters (i.e., ileocolonic anastomosis). The ileum and colon are aligned and secured in parallel along their antimesenteric borders. An enterotomy and colotomy are made

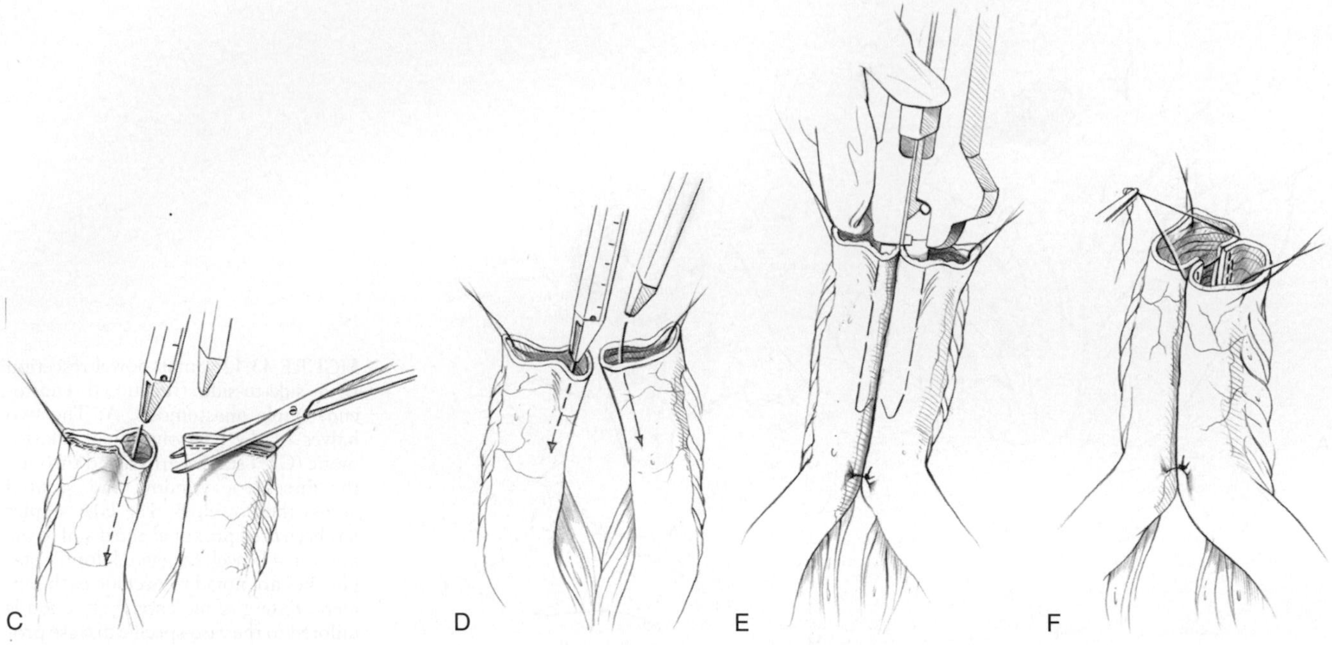

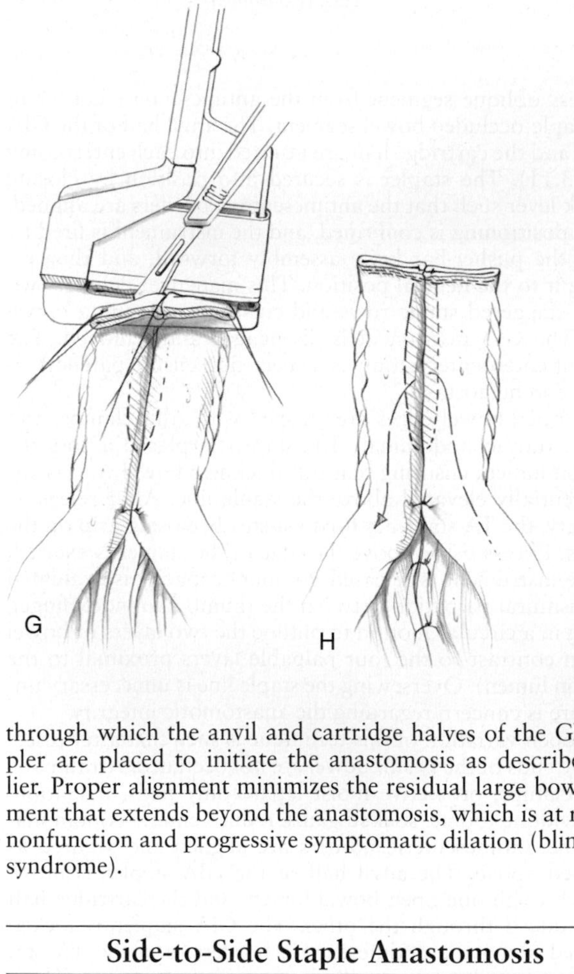

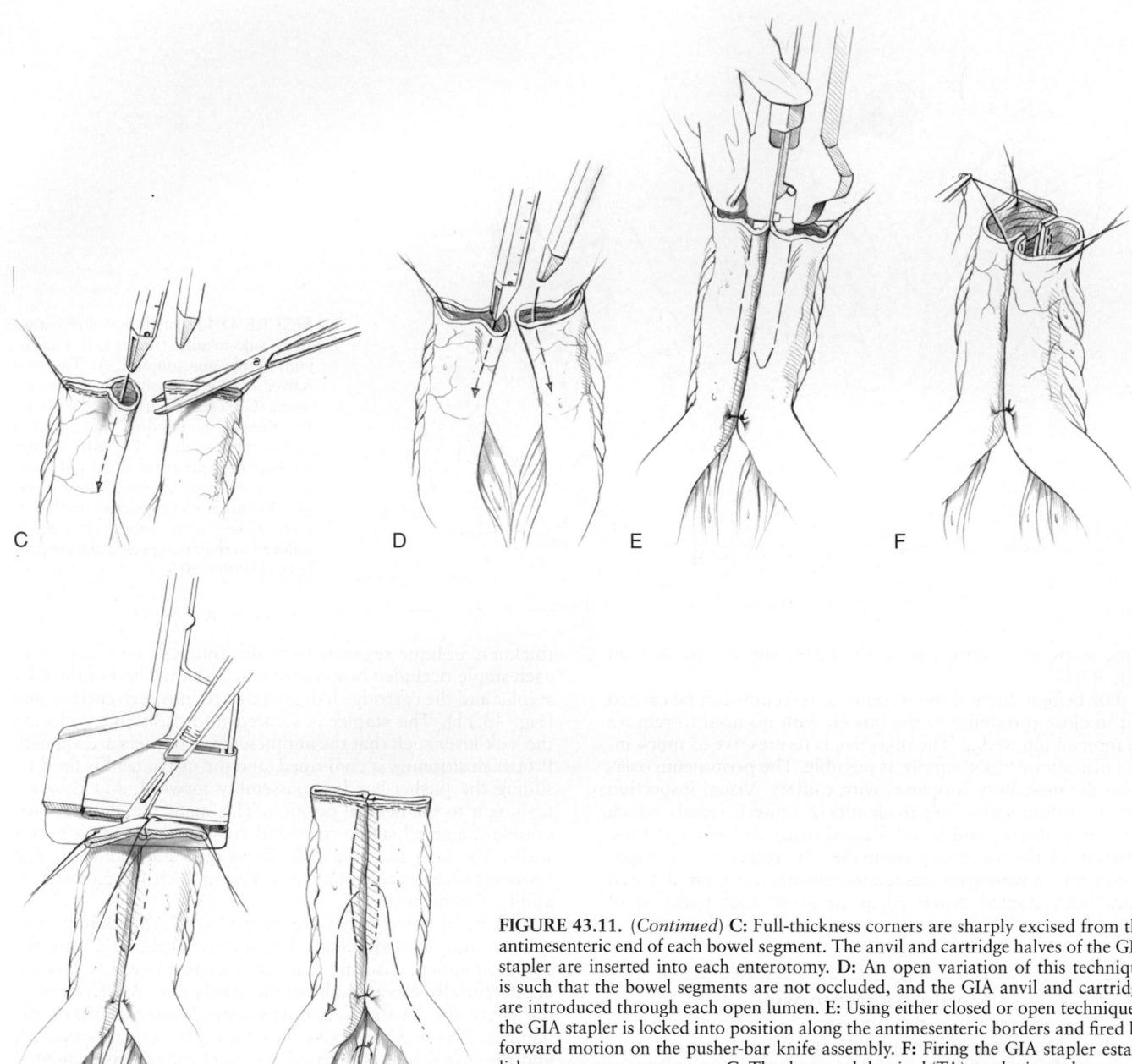

FIGURE 43.11. (*Continued*) **C:** Full-thickness corners are sharply excised from the antimesenteric end of each bowel segment. The anvil and cartridge halves of the GIA stapler are inserted into each enterotomy. **D:** An open variation of this technique is such that the bowel segments are not occluded, and the GIA anvil and cartridge are introduced through each open lumen. **E:** Using either closed or open techniques, the GIA stapler is locked into position along the antimesenteric borders and fired by forward motion on the pusher-bar knife assembly. **F:** Firing the GIA stapler establishes a common enterotomy. **G:** The thoracoabdominal (TA) stapler is used to secure the open ends. Full-thickness bowel wall is circumferentially elevated above the staple line before firing. **H:** Shown is the resultant side-to-side functional end-to-end anastomosis. The mesenteric defect is closed with interrupted 3-0 silk sutures.

through which the anvil and cartridge halves of the GIA stapler are placed to initiate the anastomosis as described earlier. Proper alignment minimizes the residual large bowel segment that extends beyond the anastomosis, which is at risk for nonfunction and progressive symptomatic dilation (blind loop syndrome).

Side-to-Side Staple Anastomosis

Side-to-side techniques are less commonly used than they once were and have largely been replaced by end-to-end or functional end-to-end anastomoses. Nevertheless, side-to-side techniques are an effective means of reanastomosis, and they can be used to bypass an obstructed intestinal segment. Either hand-sewn or staple closure may be used. The antimesenteric borders are aligned, and the bowel segments are overlapped along 8 cm and secured into position such that the stapled bowel edges are at opposite ends of this alignment. Subsequent steps taken for the staple method are as previously described.

End-to-End Hand-Sewn Double-Layer Anastomosis

In performing an end-to-end anastomosis, it is desirable to have adequate and equivalent lumens in both the proximal and distal segments. The diameter of any lumen can be increased

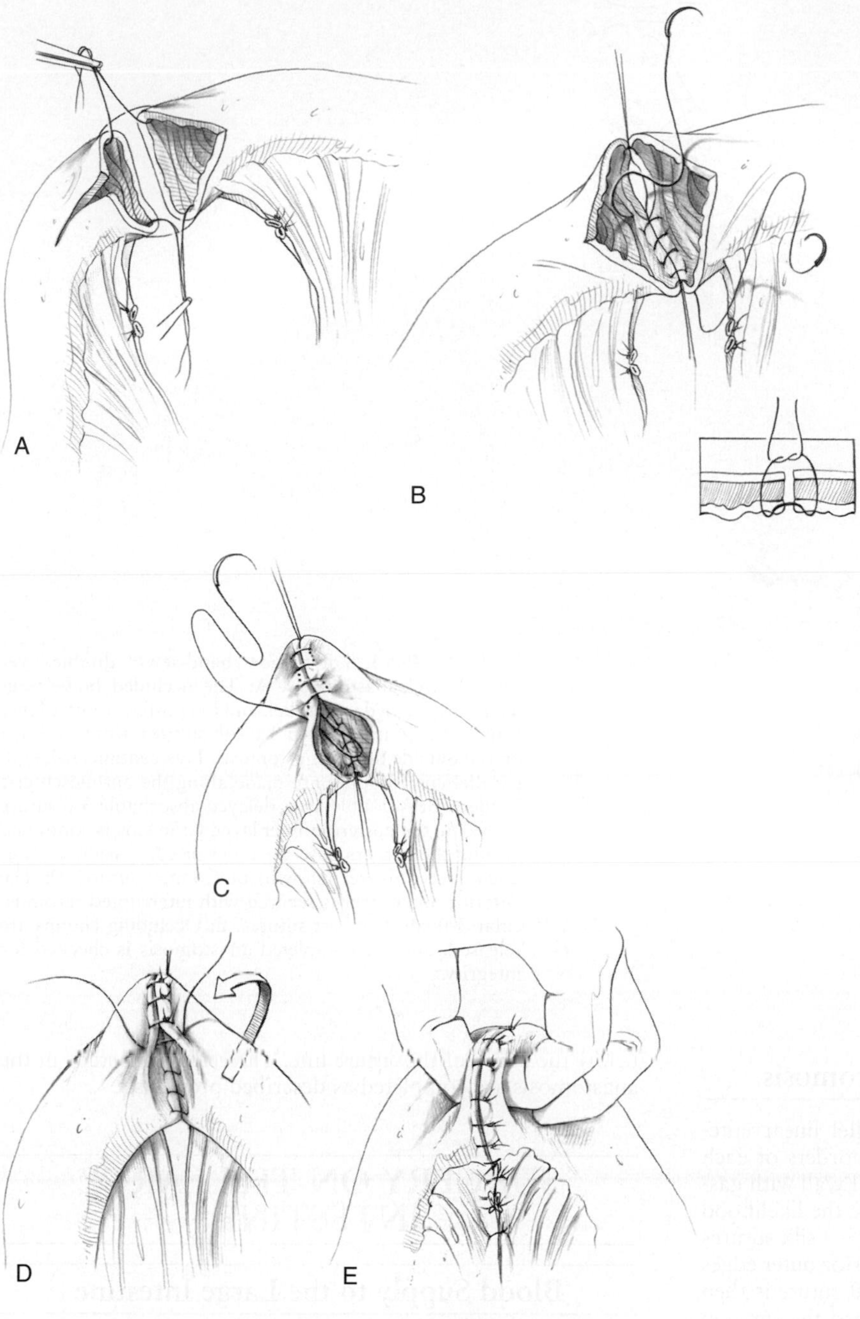

FIGURE 43.12. End-to-end hand-seven double-layer small bowel anastomosis. **A:** The bowel segments are aligned end to end and secured by stay sutures placed midway between the mesenteric and antimesenteric borders. Each luminal diameter is increased via a linear incision along the antimesenteric border (Cheatle slit). **B:** The inner running layer is started on the mesenteric (posterior) bowel edges. A double-arm needle facilitates bidirectional sewing as the closure continues around the corners onto the antimesenteric (anterior) edges. **C:** The anterior inner layer is completed in a continuous over-and-over or Connell suture (shown). **D:** The bowel is rotated 180 degrees to expose the posterior wall. Interrupted seromuscular 3-0 silk sutures are placed to finish the posterior outer layer. **E:** The bowel is rotated back into its normal alignment, and the anterior outer layer is closed with interrupted silk sutures. The mesenteric defect is reapproximated, and the adequacy of the lumen is assessed. **Inset:** Conventional inner layer inverting technique.

by transecting the bowel obliquely or via linear incision along the antimesenteric border (Cheatle slit). Atraumatic linen-shod or rubber-shod intestinal clamps are placed across the proximal and distal bowel to decrease intestinal spill. The bowel segments and mesenteries are aligned and secured by 3-0 silk seromuscular sutures placed midway between the mesenteric and antimesenteric borders. The traditional two-layer anastomosis includes a running inner layer of 3-0 chromic catgut and an outer layer of interrupted 3-0 silk sutures (Fig. 43.12).

The inner layer is closed first, starting on the mesenteric (posterior) bowel edges and continuing the closure around to incorporate the antimesenteric (anterior) edges. This is best accomplished with a double-arm needle, sewing in both directions. Suturing begins on the mucosal side, passing from in to out, and then out to in, bringing the inverted bowel edges together. Full-thickness tissue bites are initiated approximately 3 mm from the edge and advanced approximately 3 mm between throws. After circumferential closure, the knot is tied toward the lumen, and the bowel is rotated 180 degrees to expose the posterior wall. Rotation is facilitated by passing one stay suture through the mesenteric defect, with sustained counterclockwise rotational traction on both stay sutures. Interrupted seromuscular 3-0 silk sutures are placed to complete the mesenteric (posterior) outer layer. The bowel is rotated back 180 degrees into its normal anatomic position, and the anterior outer layer is lastly closed with interrupted silk Lembert sutures. If the bowel cannot be rotated, the mesenteric (posterior) outer segment must be sewn first.

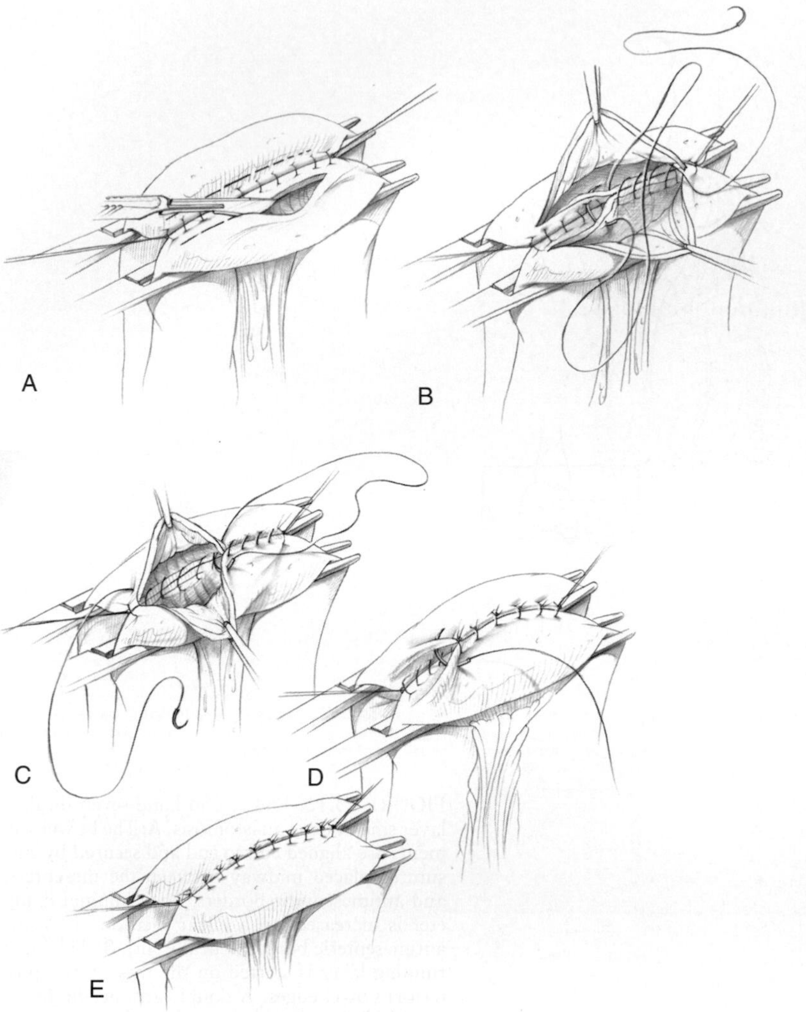

FIGURE 43.13. Side-to-side hand-sewn double-layer small bowel anastomosis. **A:** The occluded bowel segments are aligned in parallel, and the posterior outer layer is placed with interrupted 3-0 silk sutures. Knots are tied on the outside of the anastomosis. Five-centimeter-length parallel enterotomies are made along the antimesenteric borders. **B:** A double-arm, delayed absorbable 3-0 suture is used on the posterior inner layer. **C:** Sewing is continued around the corners onto the anterior edges using continuous over-and-over (shown) or Connell suture. **D:** The anterior outer layer is secured with interrupted seromuscular 3-0 silk Lembert sutures. **E:** Occluding clamps are released, and the completed anastomosis is checked for integrity.

Side-to-Side Hand-Sewn Anastomosis

For hand-sewn technique, 5 cm–length parallel linear enterotomies are made along the antimesenteric borders of each bowel segment. Elevation of the anterior bowel wall with gastrointestinal forceps during incision will reduce the likelihood of posterior wall injury. A row of interrupted 3-0 silk sutures are placed in Lembert fashion to join the posterior outer edges of the enterotomies. A running absorbable 3-0 suture is then used on the posterior inner layer sewing toward the surgeon and continuing around to the anterior edges of the enterotomies. A second posterior inner layer suture or a double-arm suture is continued away from the surgeon around the far end of the enterotomies. Suturing is continued along the anterior inner layer using the continuous over-and-over or Connell suture. The two suture ends are tied together across the anastomosis. The final anterior outer layer is placed using interrupted seromuscular sutures of 3-0 silk in Lembert fashion. Stay sutures are secured or removed, and the anastomosis is checked for integrity.

As a modification to the aforementioned procedure, the initial posterior layer of interrupted 3-0 silk Lembert sutures are placed before performing the enterotomies (Fig. 43.13). Silk sutures are placed such that the knots are secured on the outside. Parallel enterotomies are made approximately 4 mm above and below the edges of the suture line. The remaining steps in the anastomosis are completed as described previously.

SURGERY ON THE LARGE INTESTINE

Blood Supply to the Large Intestine

The SMA arises from the abdominal aorta and gives rise to the ileocolic, right colic, and middle colic arteries, which supply the right and transverse portions of the colon (Fig. 43.10). The inferior mesenteric artery (IMA) also arises from the abdominal aorta and gives off the left colic and sigmoid branches, which supply the descending and sigmoid colon. Each of these major vessels divides into numerous smaller branches, forming an anastomotic arcade that communicates from the cecum to the rectum via the marginal artery of Drummond. The marginal artery gives off numerous terminal vasa recta that directly supply the colon (Fig. 43.14). Arterial perfusion is thus preserved to any segment of the colon as long as the marginal artery is not disrupted. The marginal artery, however, is absent at the hepatic or splenic flexure in 1% to 2% of the population. This anatomic inconsistency most often affects the left side, such

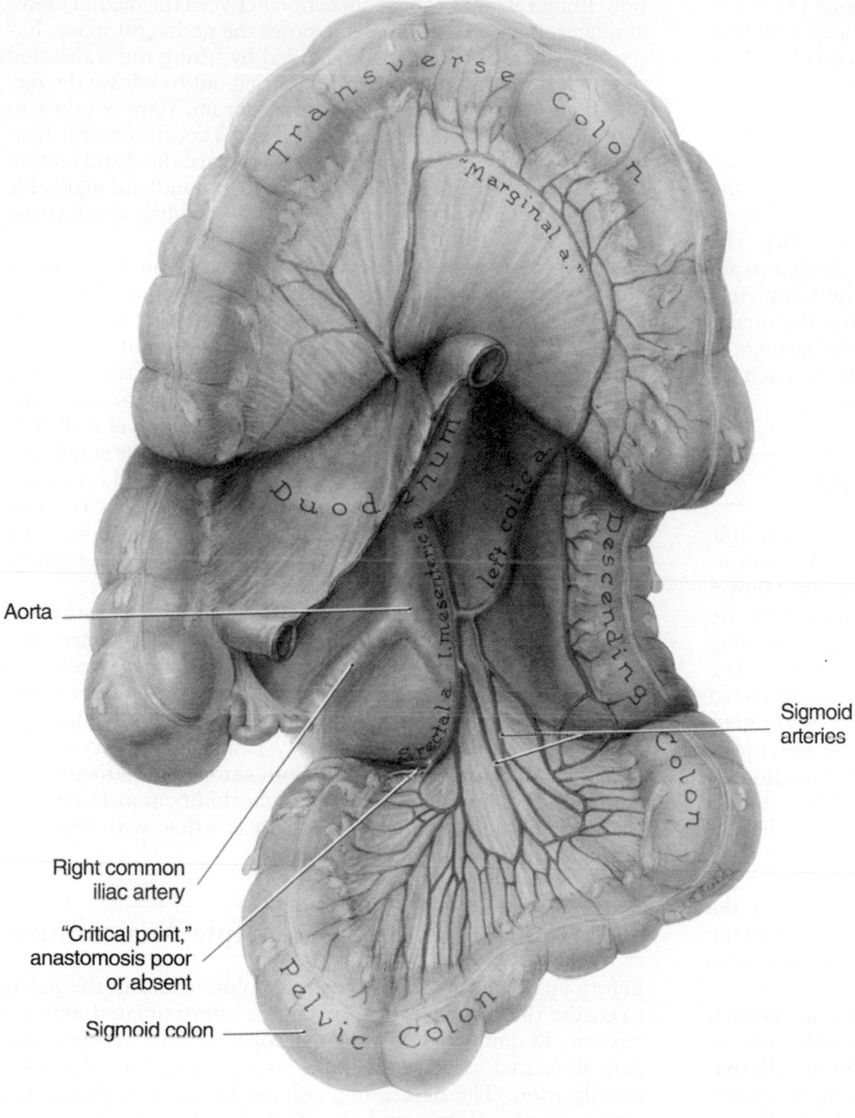

FIGURE 43.14. Intestinal blood supply: inferior mesenteric artery. The mesentery has been cut at its root and discarded with the jejunum and ileum. Observe the following: (*1*) The inferior mesenteric artery arising 1 to 1½ inches above the bifurcation of the aorta. On crossing the left common iliac artery, it becomes the superior rectal (hemorrhoidal) artery. (*2*) Its branches: (*a*) a single (superior) left colic artery and (*b*) several sigmoid arteries (inferior left colic arteries) springing from its left side. In this specimen, the two lowest sigmoid arteries spring from the superior rectal artery. The point at which the last sigmoid artery leaves the superior rectal artery is known as the critical point of Sudeck.

that colon resection in this area should include removal of the splenic flexure. Again noted is the tenuous ileocolic blood supply, such that if the cecum is resected, 10 cm of terminal ileum should also be removed. The rectum derives its oxygenation from the IMA via the superior rectal artery and from the hypogastric artery via the middle and inferior rectal arteries. An elaborate anastomotic lattice with other pelvic vessels encircles the rectum and anus.

Large Bowel Resection

The principles important in large bowel resection and anastomosis are essentially the same as those described previously for the small bowel. Segmental colon resection in gynecologic surgery is most commonly necessary because of malignancy or radiation injury. The gynecologic surgeon may also encounter benign conditions that require resection, such as severe endometriosis, diverticular disease, extensive adhesions, or nonreparable colonic injury. Large bowel resection for benign gynecologic conditions does not require segmental wedge resection of the mesentery. The integrity of the marginal artery is protected when the mesentery is transected close to the bowel wall through the vasa recta.

Mobilization of the Colon

The majority of large bowel resections require some degree of mobilization to ensure a tension-free anastomosis. The general objectives of colon mobilization are to gain retroperitoneal access and transect avascular attachments from the splenic and/or hepatic flexures. If needed, additional mobility is acquired via transecting the gastrocolic ligament. This also provides entry into the lesser omental sac, which facilitates resection of the gastrocolic ligament and infracolic omentum if necessary. Also, the inferior mesenteric artery can usually be sacrificed without significant compromise because of the rich vascular network surrounding the rectum. Mobilization can be carried out before or after the segmental colon resection, depending on the clinical situation.

To free the right colon, retroperitoneal dissection is initiated at the base of the cecum and continued lateral and parallel to the ascending colon along the white line of Toldt. This is aided by medial traction on the ascending colon. The hepatocystocolic ligament is transected as dissection is carried into Morison's pouch and along the proximal transverse colon. Mobilization of the left colon is initiated at the most distal site of retroperitonealized sigmoid colon, which is usually located at the pelvic brim. With medial retraction on the bowel, a peritoneal incision is made lateral and parallel to the descending colon. Dissection is continued around the splenic flexure as the lienocolic and phrenicocolic ligaments are transected. Excessive traction is avoided to prevent splenic capsule injury. The left lateral portion of the gastrocolic ligament is divided to access the lesser omental sac. This ligament can be completely transected along the transverse colon by dividing the omental vessels. If necessary, division of the gastrocolic ligament is accomplished along the greater curvature of the stomach by dividing the gastroepiploic and short gastric vessels.

End-to-End Staple Anastomosis

Transverse colon resection is used as an illustrative example of this technique. After completing the resection and mobilization of the left and right colon, the proximal and distal bowel edges are brought into close opposition. Their mesenteries are aligned, and seromuscular 3-0 silk sutures are placed, dividing the bowel circumference into equal one-third segments. The mesenteric (posterior) segment of the anastomosis is completed first. Bowel rotation of 180 degrees is facilitated by counterclockwise passage of one stay suture through the mesenteric defect, with continued counterclockwise rotational traction on the adjacent stay suture. Allis clamps are used to lift both full-thickness bowel walls into the noncutting TA stapler. The stapler is positioned such that the staple line extends just beyond the lateral edge of both stay sutures. Steady closing grip secures the device into position. After confirming proper placement, the safety latch is released, and firm closure of the handles fires the staple line. Excess tissue is sharply excised, and the stapler is released (Fig. 43.15).

The bowel is rotated back 180 degrees to its normal anatomic alignment. The two remaining equilateral segments are stapled from the serosal side in similar fashion. Alternatively, if the bowel is not easily rotated, the mesenteric (posterior) segment can be stapled first from the mucosal side. The remaining segments are closed from the serosal side as described earlier. Slight overlap of adjoining staple lines ensures complete closure without hindering anastomotic healing. Adequacy of the lumen, integrity of repair, and hemostasis are confirmed before closing the mesenteric defect.

Sigmoid Resection

The appropriate site for sigmoid transection is identified proximal to the area of diseased bowel. A small mesenteric opening is made adjacent to the colon, through which the GIA cartridge is introduced. The GIA anvil is placed across the bowel, and the stapler is secured and fired, resulting in a transected sigmoid with occluded proximal and distal segments. Moist laparotomy towels are used to pack the proximal segment above the surgical field. The mesenteric peritoneum is opened adjacent to the bowel, and the incision is continued parallel to the sigmoid as the mesentery transitions from a medial to a posterior insertion (Fig. 43.16). Mesenteric vessels are clamped, cut, and secured with 2-0 silk ligatures. The rectovaginal space is opened between the uterosacral ligaments with cautery and sharp dissection. Blunt retroperitoneal dissection between the medial ureter and lateral hypogastric vessel exposes the perirectal space. Entry into the retrorectal space is aided by lifting the transected sigmoid. Retrorectal dissection is carried out to release the rectum from its attachments along the sacrum. Care is taken to avoid laceration of the presacral veins. The uterosacral ligaments are transected to gain exposure toward the distal rectum as the ureters are retracted laterally with a handheld malleable retractor. The rectal stalks are secured by dividing and ligating the posterior portion of the cardinal ligaments.

The extent of required dissection depends on the location and severity of disease. For nonmalignant pathology, dissection below the pelvic peritoneal reflection and levator ani is rarely necessary and may actually disrupt the blood supply. When normal rectum has been isolated below the diseased segment, the rectosigmoid resection can be completed. Pericolonic tissue attachments are cleared to expose smooth bowel wall. The TA stapler is guided across the rectum, ensuring the staple line incorporates only the rectum. The stapler is locked into position, checked for proper alignment, and fired by firm closure of the handles. Occluding clamps are placed across the bowel just above the staple line, and sharp dissection is used to transect the rectum and complete the resection.

The number of total laparoscopic sigmoid resections and hand-assisted laparoscopic sigmoid resections has increased significantly in recent years. Reports of clinical experience to date suggest comparable morbidity in comparison to open procedures, and endoscopic resection may offer the advantage of more rapid postoperative recovery. Timing of surgery is also an important factor to consider. For example, in patients with a history of diverticular disease, the morbidity associated with elective sigmoid resection is reportedly less than with resection during an acute bout of diverticulitis.

Rectosigmoid End-to-End Staple Anastomosis

Before anastomosis, the descending colon is laid in the pelvis to ensure the colon and rectum can be approximated without tension. Redundant laxity of the colon should be observed. Any resistance or tension indicates the need for additional mobilization. The descending colonic lumen is occluded via an atraumatic clamp, and the staple line is sharply excised. The appropriate diameter end-to-end anastomosis (EEA) stapler is selected based on the largest EEA obturator that can be placed into the lumen without undue stretch on the bowel wall. One milligram (one ampule) of intravenous glucagon causes relaxation of the muscularis and allows more accurate sizing.

Various designs of the EEA stapler exist, but generally the proximal portion consists of an anvil with a spike. An auto purse string or hand-sewn purse string is placed circumferentially around the open end of the descending colon. The anvil is positioned within the lumen, and the purse string is secured around the base of the spike, the tip of which is directed toward the rectal stump. The anus is digitally dilated, and the lubricated shaft of the EEA stapler is introduced into the anal canal. The shaft is visually and manually guided to the apex of the rectal stump. Clockwise rotation of the central wing nut advances the sharp trocar to pierce the apex of the rectal stump. The trocar is removed, leaving the hollow center shaft of the EEA in place through the rectum. The anvil spike from the descending colon is guided into the hollow center shaft of the rectal stump until it locks into place (Fig. 43.17). The central wing nut is further rotated clockwise until the indicator line

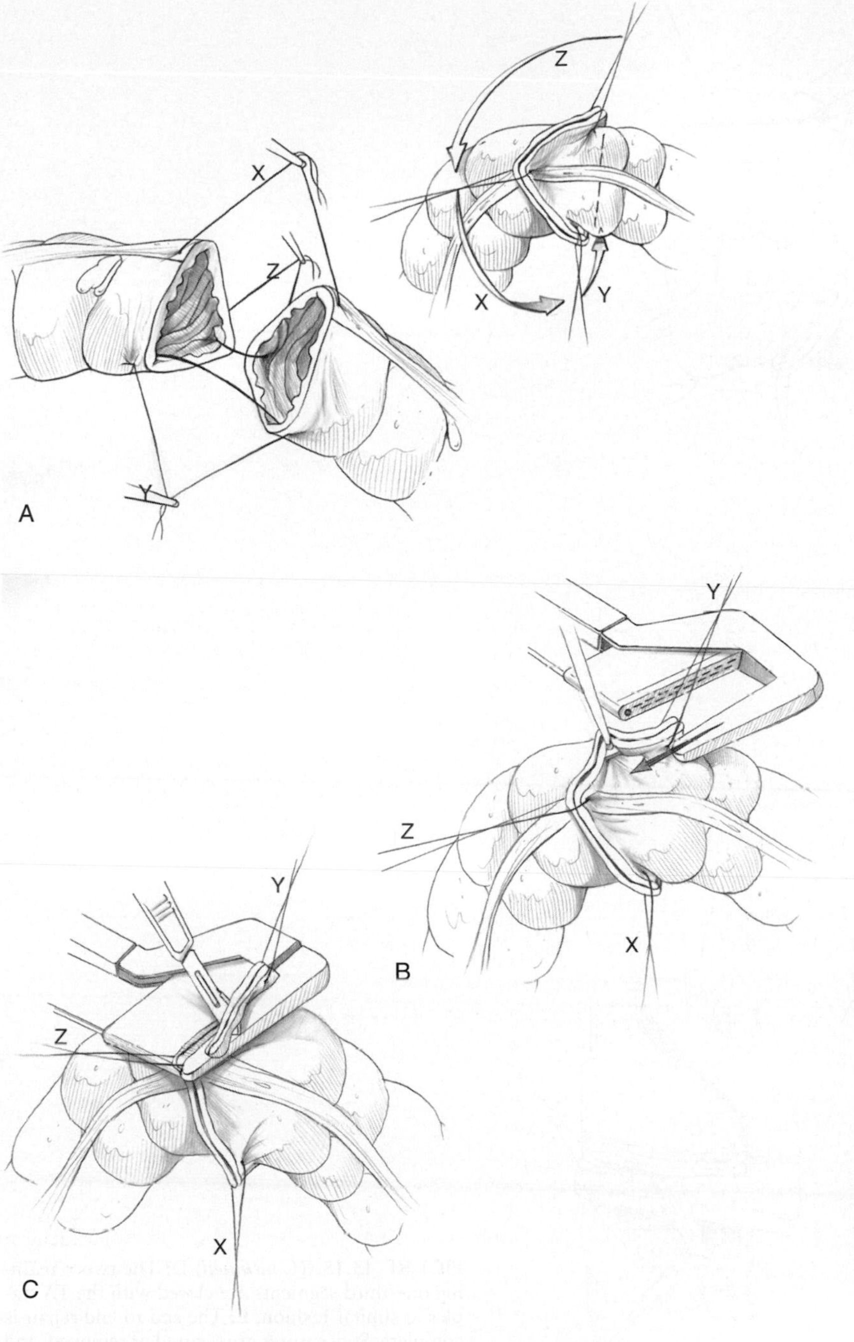

FIGURE 43.15. End-to-end colon staple anastomosis. **A:** The colon segments are aligned end-to-end, and 3-0 silk sutures are placed to divide the bowel circumference into equal one-third segments. **Inset:** The mesenteric (posterior) bowel edges are joined first. The bowel is rotated 180 degrees counterclockwise. This is done by passing stay suture (*y*) through the mesenteric defect, with continued counterclockwise rotational traction on sutures (*z*) and (*y*). **B:** The thoracoabdominal (TA) stapler is used to close the posterior segments. Full-thickness bowel walls are lifted above the staple line with Allis clamps. **C:** After firing the stapler, excess tissue is sharply excised. The bowel is then rotated 180 degrees clockwise into its normal alignment. (*Continued*)

is readily visible in the indicator window. This rotation draws the rectum and sigmoid colon into direct opposition. Normal anatomic alignment of the mesentery is confirmed. The safety is released, and steady, firm closure of the handles fires the instrument. The handles are released, and the central wing nut is rotated counterclockwise two complete turns. A gentle rocking motion back and forth frees the instrument tip from the anastomosis, as the EEA shaft is slowly withdrawn from the rectum.

The anastomotic integrity is confirmed through a series of checks. First, the staple line is visually and manually inspected. Second, the EEA instrument is inspected for two complete 360-degree tissue rings. This confirms circumferential stapling and resection of both the colonic and rectal segments. Third, the pelvis is filled with sterile crystalloid, and a rigid sigmoidoscope is used to insufflate the bowel. Manual occlusion of the proximal sigmoid ensures adequate testing pressure across the anastomosis. The anastomosis is observed while underwater, looking for air bubbles that would indicate an anastomotic leak (Fig. 43.18). Rigid sigmoidoscopy also allows direct internal inspection of the staple line. If any of these methods suggest an incomplete anastomosis, the area in question is reinforced with interrupted 3-0 silk sutures, and the integrity is retested. Care is taken to avoid vascular compromise as the mesenteric defect is closed with interrupted sutures.

Postanastomotic morbidity and symptoms are largely related to the amount of residual rectum at the time of repair. Patients with a high colorectal anastomosis (11 cm or more

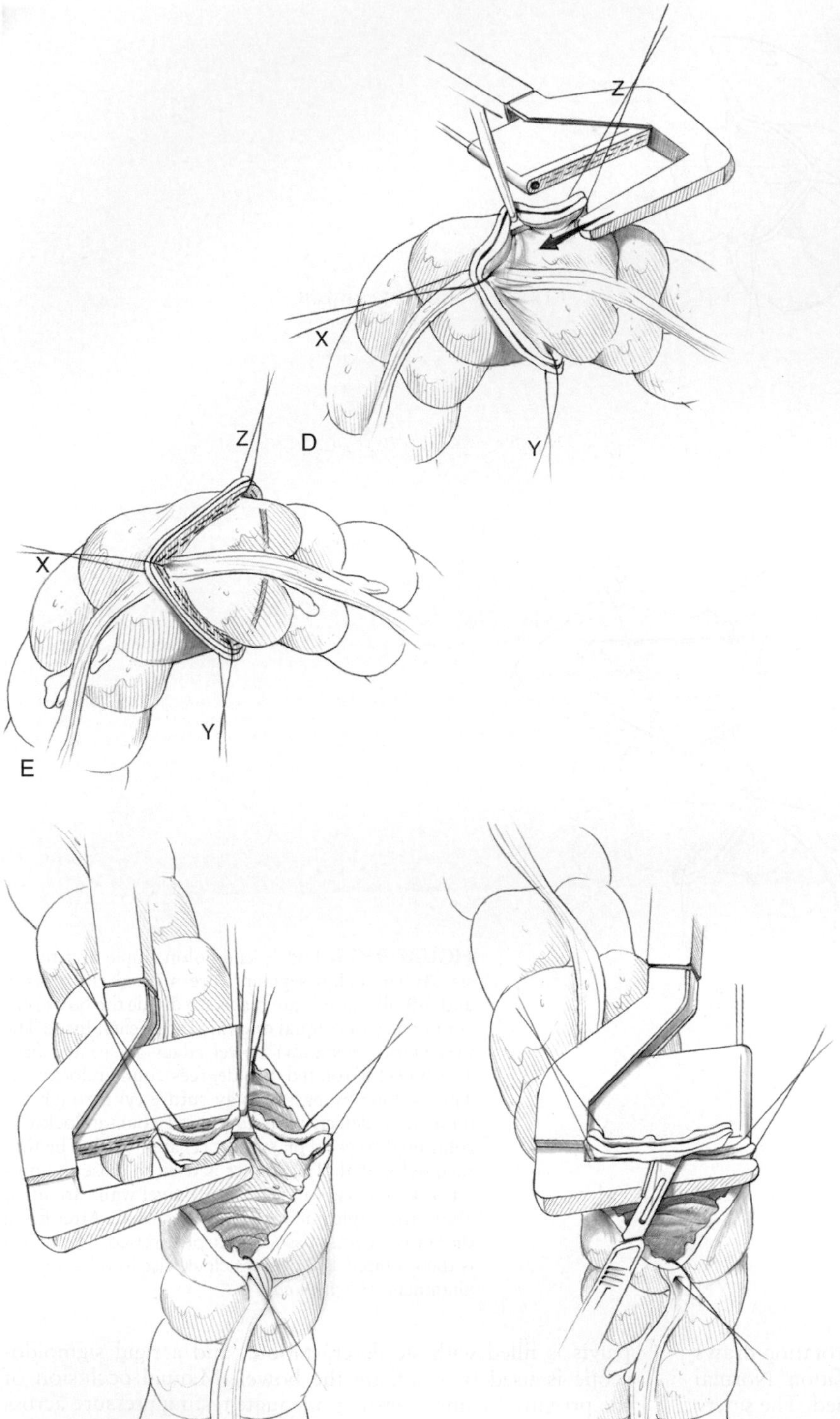

FIGURE 43.15. (*Continued*) **D:** The two remaining one-third segments are closed with the TA stapler in similar fashion. **E:** The end-to-end repair is complete. Stay sutures are secured or removed, and the anastomosis is evaluated for integrity. Alternative method: **F:** If the bowel cannot be effectively rotated, the mesenteric (posterior) one-third segment is closed first, using the TA stapler applied to the mucosal surfaces. **G:** Excessive tissue is sharply excised. The two remaining one-third segments are closed from the serosal surfaces as described.

above the anal verge) have relatively low morbidity and excellent functional results. Those who have undergone a low anastomosis (between 7 and 11 cm) have intermediate levels of morbidity, but generally have satisfactory functional results after several months of physiologic adaptation. In contrast, patients with a very low colorectal anastomosis (less than 7 cm from the anal verge) are at highest risk for complications, including anastomotic leak. These patients are also more likely to have chronic symptoms of gastrointestinal frequency, urgency, and incontinence. The sigmoid J-pouch for rectosigmoid anastomosis provides a reservoir that may decrease the frequency of stools and reduce the incidence of incontinence (Fig. 43.19). Accordingly, the J-pouch is considered if resection leaves less than 7 cm of rectum and if the colon is redundant enough to

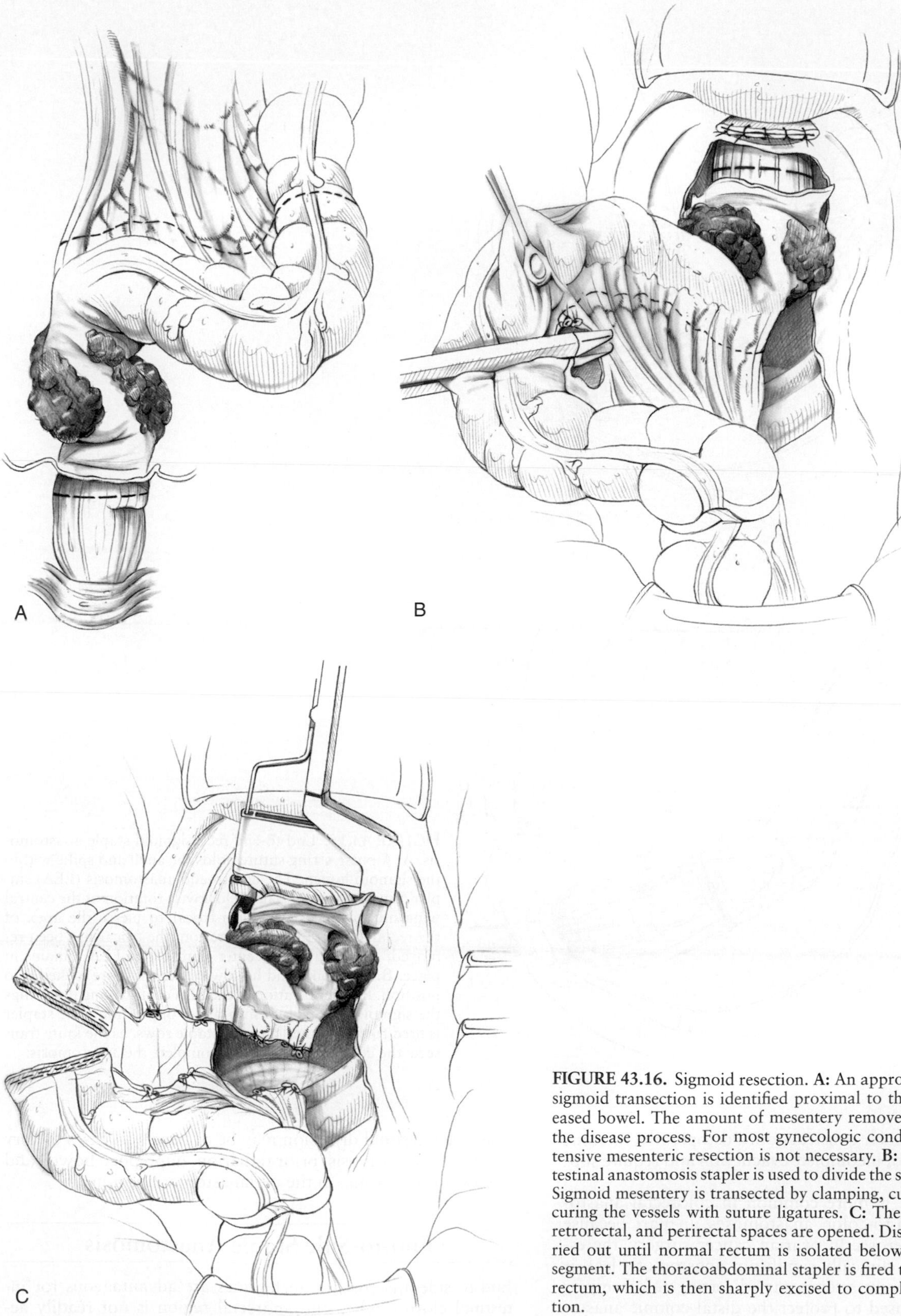

FIGURE 43.16. Sigmoid resection. **A:** An appropriate site for sigmoid transection is identified proximal to the area of diseased bowel. The amount of mesentery removed depends on the disease process. For most gynecologic conditions, an extensive mesenteric resection is not necessary. **B:** The gastrointestinal anastomosis stapler is used to divide the sigmoid colon. Sigmoid mesentery is transected by clamping, cutting, and securing the vessels with suture ligatures. **C:** The rectovaginal, retrorectal, and perirectal spaces are opened. Dissection is carried out until normal rectum is isolated below the diseased segment. The thoracoabdominal stapler is fired to occlude the rectum, which is then sharply excised to complete the resection.

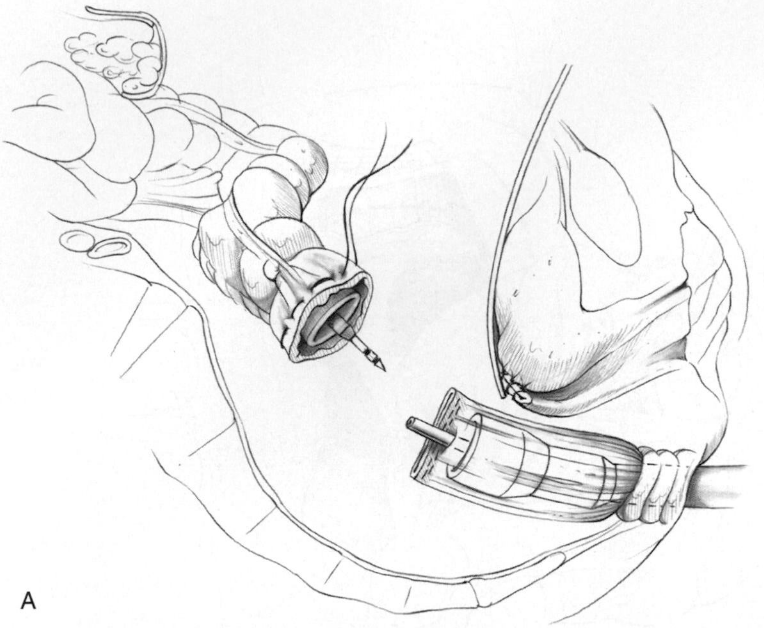

A

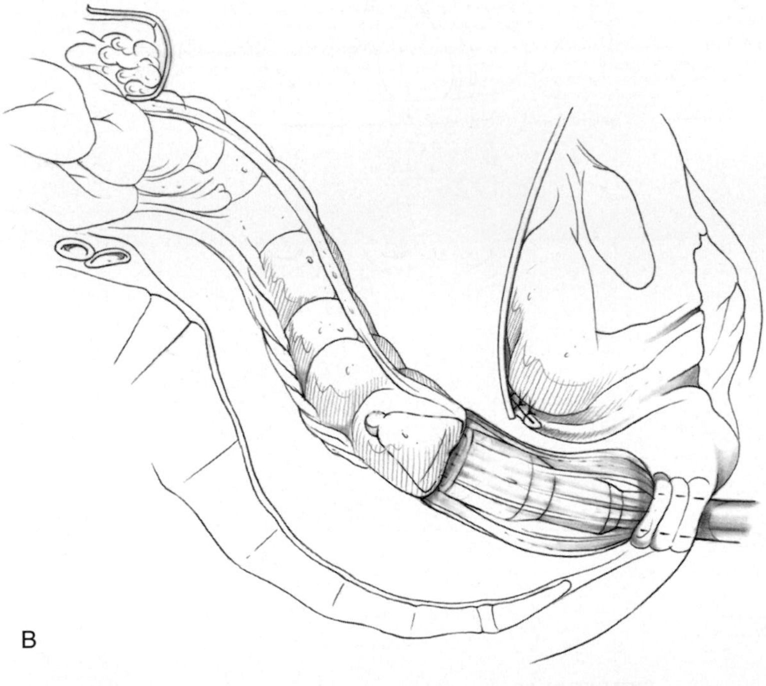

B

FIGURE 43.17. End-to-end rectosigmoid staple anastomosis. **A:** A purse-string suture holds the anvil and spike within the sigmoid lumen. The end-to-end anastomosis (EEA) stapler is inserted transanally. Clockwise rotation of the central wing nut advances the sharp trocar to pierce the apex of the rectal stump. In this illustration, the trocar has been removed, and the hollow center shaft of the EEA remains in place. **B:** The spike and hollow center shaft are locked into position. Further rotation of the EEA central wing nut brings the sigmoid and rectum into direct opposition. The stapler is fired to deliver dual circular staple rows, as the knife transects the central tissue core to complete the anastomosis.

allow tension-free pouch construction. Postoperatively, some patients have a sense of incomplete evacuation and require suppositories or enemas.

Anastomotic leak is more common in colorectal anastomoses than in colon-to-colon anastomoses, in part because the rectum has no serosa. In ovarian cancer surgery, the estimated incidence of clinically significant anastomotic leak is 3% to 5%. Traditionally, a temporary diverting colostomy or ileostomy has been used to protect the distal colonic anastomosis. Clinical studies do not support the notion that routine protective intestinal diversion reduces the risk of anastomotic breakdown. Diversion of fecal contents, however, may reduce the severity of infectious complications if a leak occurs. Selective intestinal diversion may be of benefit in cases of very low rectal anastomosis, prior radiation, unprepped bowel, and abscess or hematoma in the perianastomotic region.

End-to-Side Staple Anastomosis

End-to-side anastomotic techniques are advantageous for intestinal closure when the anorectal region is not readily accessible (e.g., supine position) or when access is not necessary to complete the closure (e.g., ileocolonic or high rectosigmoid anastomosis). A high rectosigmoid repair is used for illustrative purposes. Following sigmoid resection, a small colotomy

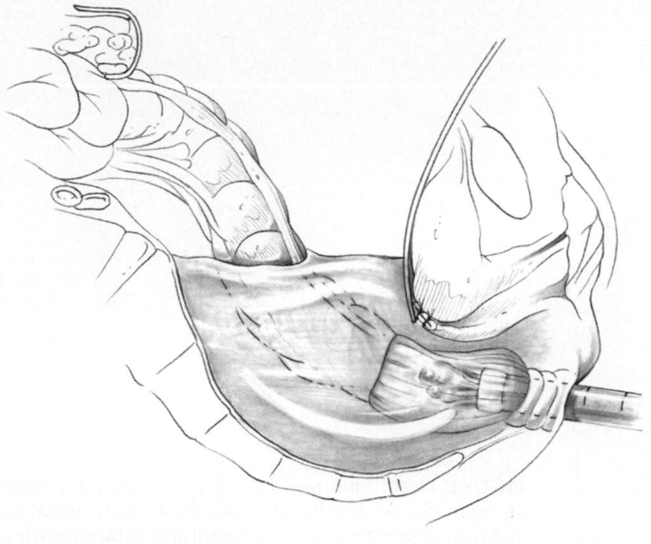

FIGURE 43.18. Testing the anastomotic integrity. The pelvis is filled with sterile crystalloid. The descending colon is manually occluded as air is insufflated via a rigid sigmoidoscope to create pressure across the anastomosis. Holding the anastomosis under water, it is examined for air bubbles that would suggest an anastomotic leak.

is made 3 to 4 cm from the end of the descending colon. The EEA instrument is introduced through the open lumen, and the hollow center shaft is advanced through the colotomy. The instrument is positioned such that the tip of the EEA rests perpendicular to bowel wall. A purse-string suture is used to secure the anvil spike within the rectal lumen. The end of the rectum is brought into close proximity with the side of the descending colon as the anvil spike is secured into the EEA hollow center shaft. Clockwise rotation of the central wing nut brings the bowel edges into direct opposition. Rotation is continued until adequate closure is confirmed via the indicator window. The stapler is fired by closing the instrument grips. Counterclockwise rotation of the wing nut, followed by a subtle back-and-forth rocking motion, frees the instrument from the staple line. The open end of the descending colon is repaired using the TA stapler as previously described, and the integrity of the anastomosis is assessed.

End-to-End Hand-Sewn Single-Layer Colon Anastomosis

Before the common availability of surgical staplers, intestinal anastomoses were accomplished using hand-sewn techniques. Suture is still preferred over staple repair by some surgeons. Anastomosis can be accomplished using a single layer of delayed absorbable monofilament suture (small or large intestine) or nonabsorbable suture for large bowel (i.e., 4-0 polypropylene). The continuous closure has been proven efficacious in colon-to-colon repair and is used for this illustration. The bowel segments and mesenteric edges are aligned and secured with stay sutures. Suturing begins on the mesenteric (posterior) mucosal edges and is facilitated by a double-arm needle. The running stitch is carried out such that the needle enters near the transected mucosal edge and passes obliquely through the bowel wall to exit the serosa approximately 5 mm from the edge. The needle is passed through the adjoining segment in

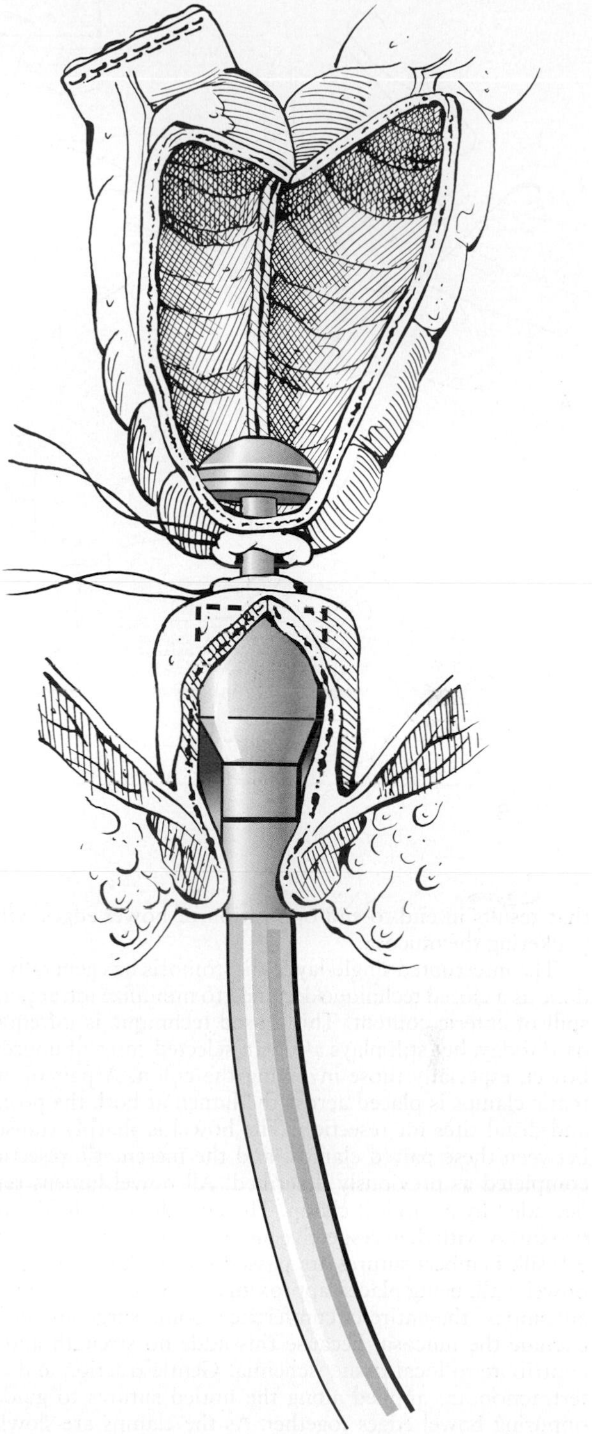

FIGURE 43.19. Rectal J-pouch coloproctostomy.

the same oblique fashion. Sequential tissue bites are placed 2 to 3 mm apart. This effectively inverts the bowel wall as the running suture is secured (Fig. 43.20). Bidirectional suturing is continued around the corners onto the antimesenteric (anterior) surfaces, which are closed from the serosal side. The Gambee single-layer technique is an equally effective method

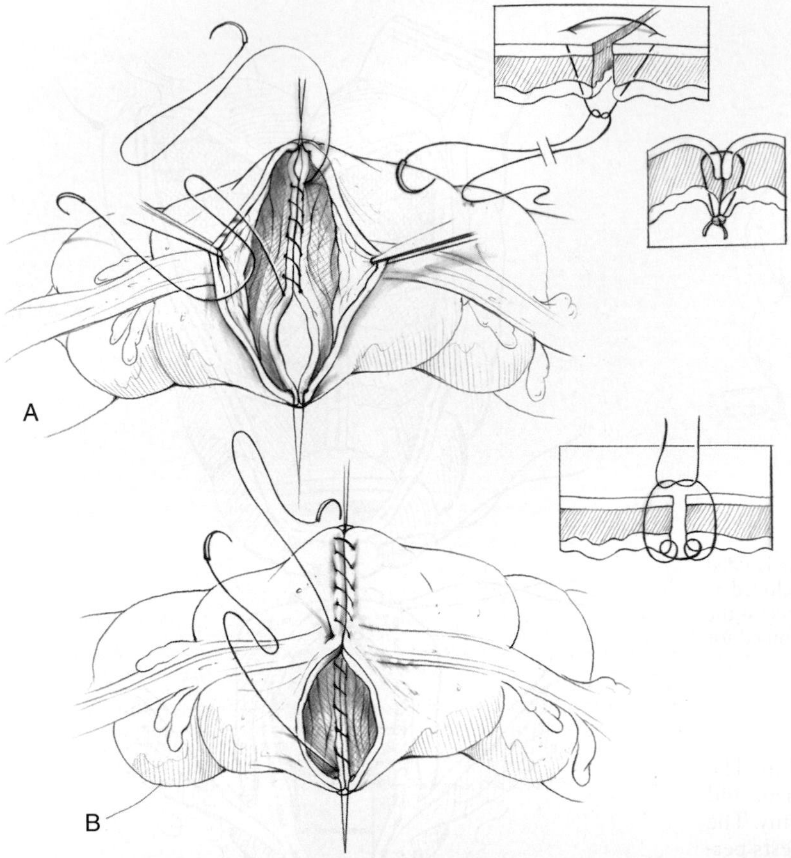

FIGURE 43.20. End-to-end hand-sewn single-layer colon anastomosis. **A:** The bowel edges are brought together, and their alignment is stabilized with stay sutures. Sewing is started on the mucosal surfaces of the posterior bowel edges. A double-arm suture enables bidirectional sewing in a continuous fashion. **Insets:** The needle enters near the transected mucosal edge and passes obliquely through the bowel wall to exit 5 mm from the serosal edge. The needle is passed through the adjoining segment in the same oblique fashion, which inverts the tissue edges as the running suture is secured. **B:** Suturing is continued around the corners onto the anterior edges, which are closed from the serosal side. **Inset:** Alternative method of single-layer closure is the Gambee technique, which results in end-to-end opposition of the tissue edges without puckering the mucosa.

that results in end-to-end opposition of bowel edges without puckering the mucosa.

The interrupted single-layer anastomosis has generally been done as a closed technique designed to minimize intraoperative spill of enteric content. This closed technique is infrequently used today, but still plays a role in selected cases of unprepped bowel, especially those involving the colon. A pair of atraumatic clamps is placed across the lumen at both the proximal and distal sites for resection. The bowel is sharply transected between these paired clamps, and the mesenteric resection is completed as previously described. All bowel lumens remain occluded by a surgical clamp. The cut edges are held in close proximity with their respective mesenteries aligned. Interrupted 3-0 silk Lembert sutures are passed full thickness through the bowel wall, being placed approximately 3 mm apart until they encompass the entire circumference. Some surgeons prefer to exclude the mucosa, because this adds no strength and may contribute to local tissue ischemia. Gentle traction and countertraction are applied along the untied sutures to guide the opposing bowel edges together. As the clamps are slowly removed, the sutures are tied. Patency of the lumen is assessed, and any insecure anastomotic areas are reinforced with additional sutures.

Colostomy

A colostomy should include tension-free bowel with uncompromised blood supply. The colon remains viable only about 2 cm beyond the closest intact vasa recta. The abdominal wall aperture must be generous enough to allow easy passage of the bowel with its intact mesentery, because even mild constriction may result in venous congestion, tissue edema, and necrosis. In gynecologic surgery, temporary colonic diversion may be necessary because of severe radiation injury (proctosigmoiditis), distal obstruction, perforation, or fistula. Permanent colostomy may be required if the rectum has been completely resected or is unacceptable for anastomosis. A diverting colostomy can also provide emergent decompression in the setting of complete large bowel obstruction at risk for perforation.

Perioperative Considerations

Preoperative consultation with an enterostomal therapist is very important in the perioperative planning and care. Counseling sessions, reading materials, support groups, and contact with other ostomy patients provide educational and emotional benefit. In nonemergent cases, the stoma appliance can be worn preoperatively to determine appropriate positioning and clarify postoperative expectations. The stoma should be located in an area that is easily seen and reached by the patient (Fig. 43.21). The tentative stoma site is marked preoperatively with indelible ink. As a general guide, a line is drawn connecting the anterior-superior iliac spine to the umbilicus, and the colostomy is exteriorized through the rectus muscles at some point along this line. Placement is avoided within skin folds, surgical scars, and the umbilicus because the appliance will not seal securely with these skin irregularities.

Postoperatively, the enterostomal therapist can assist in teaching the patient independent ostomy care. Daily inspection is important to ensure tissue viability, adequate function,

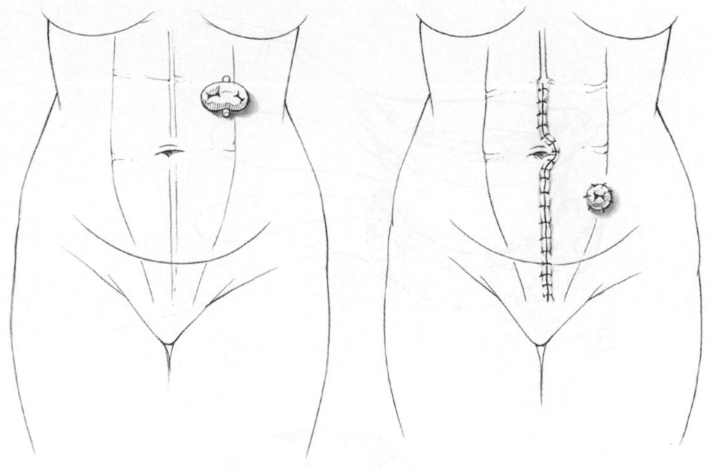

FIGURE 43.21. Positioning the stoma. A: Shown is a transverse loop colostomy positioned in the left upper abdomen. B: An end colostomy located in the left lower abdomen. As a guide, a line can be drawn to connect the umbilicus with the anterior-superior iliac spine, along which the end colostomy is positioned. The stoma is exteriorized through the rectus abdominis muscle and secured to skin that is devoid of folds or surgical scars.

and nonretraction of the stoma. If tissue viability is in question, closer investigation under bright light is warranted. Insertion of a glass test tube or syringe with penlight transillumination allows for an easy bedside inspection of the internal bowel wall. If tissue viability remains uncertain, an anoscope or sigmoidoscope can be used. Focal ischemia is suggested if the mucosa is gray or dusky in appearance. Tissue necrosis distal to the skin edge may be safely observed and reevaluated after tissue sloughing has occurred. Surgical correction is generally unnecessary in this setting. Deeper and more extensive necrosis indicates compromised blood flow and the need for colostomy revision. Excessive retraction, stricture, or peristomal herniation may also require surgical correction.

Some patients with an end sigmoid or descending colostomy prefer irrigation management over a collection appliance. Motivation, capacity for self-care, and relatively normal preoperative bowel function are requisite. Irrigation is started early in the postoperative period and is continued on a daily basis thereafter. The eventual goal is fecal continence between irrigations. Irrigation can also help reduce stoma odor and flatus, which can be further suppressed with a charcoal-based stoma cap. Some patients will develop predictable evacuation patterns such that irrigation is eventually not required. Others will be satisfied with the security of a continuous appliance.

End Colostomy Technique

Efforts are made to create the stoma at the site marked on the abdominal wall preoperatively. The bowel selected for use should be adequately mobilized so the distal end can be brought beyond the abdominal wall by several centimeters. To fashion the abdominal wall aperture, a 3-cm diameter circle is drawn on the skin at the marked site. Symmetry is aided by a circular guide such as the flat, round end of a 60-cc syringe plunger. Dissection is carried through the skin and subcutaneous tissue to the level of the rectus fascia. A core of subcutaneous adipose tissue is not necessarily removed. Cruciate incisions are made in the anterior rectus sheath, with each incision being approximately 4 cm in length. The rectus muscle fibers are bluntly separated until the posterior rectus sheath and peritoneum are reached, through which similar cruciate incisions are made. When separating the rectus abdominis muscle, care is taken to avoid injury of the inferior epigastric vessels. All layers of the abdominal aperture are manually dilated and should easily admit three fingers without stricture.

A Babcock clamp is inserted through the aperture to grasp the colon for exteriorization. The bowel is brought through the abdominal wall, such that the occluded end rests easily above the skin surface without tension. Large epiploic appendices can be removed with electrocautery if needed to ease exteriorization. Tissue viability is assessed to ensure uncompromised blood flow. Interrupted 3-0 silk seromuscular sutures are fixed to the posterior and anterior rectus sheaths to secure the alignment and reduce the chance of retraction or herniation. The lateral paracolic gutter is obliterated to prevent small bowel herniation. Maturation of the stoma is deferred until after the abdomen is closed.

Any remaining surgical objectives are completed, and the peritoneal cavity is irrigated and checked for hemostasis. The intraabdominal and extraabdominal bowel is again inspected before closing the surgical wound. After closure, the incision is protected with collodion or sterile towels. The exteriorized colon is opened, and the cut edges are observed for bleeding to ensure viability. Excessive bowel is trimmed such that approximately 2 to 3 cm remain above the skin surface. If viability is questionable, the edges are trimmed further until adequate blood flow is confirmed.

The stoma is matured using interrupted delayed absorbable sutures (3-0 polyglycolic acid). Stitches are initiated at the skin surface and carried in and out through the seromuscular bowel wall approximately 2 cm from the distal end and then full thickness through the cut bowel edge (Fig. 43.22). Sutures are placed circumferentially at about 5-mm intervals. As the sutures are tied, the everted bowel wall is folded back on itself. The result is a slightly protruding stoma that enables a better appliance fit and is less prone to retraction. In patients with a thick abdominal wall, it may not be possible to evert the stoma. In this scenario, a stoma flush with the skin surface is matured by securing the skin to full-thickness bowel edge using interrupted sutures. The appliance is fashioned and secured intraoperatively.

Diverting Loop Colostomy

A loop colostomy is technically less difficult to create and/or reverse than an end colostomy. This is a good technique when a temporary diverting colostomy is needed, and it can often be accomplished through a single incision. Readily mobile transverse or sigmoid colon is preferred. As a general rule, the loop colostomy is fashioned from the most distal site along the bowel

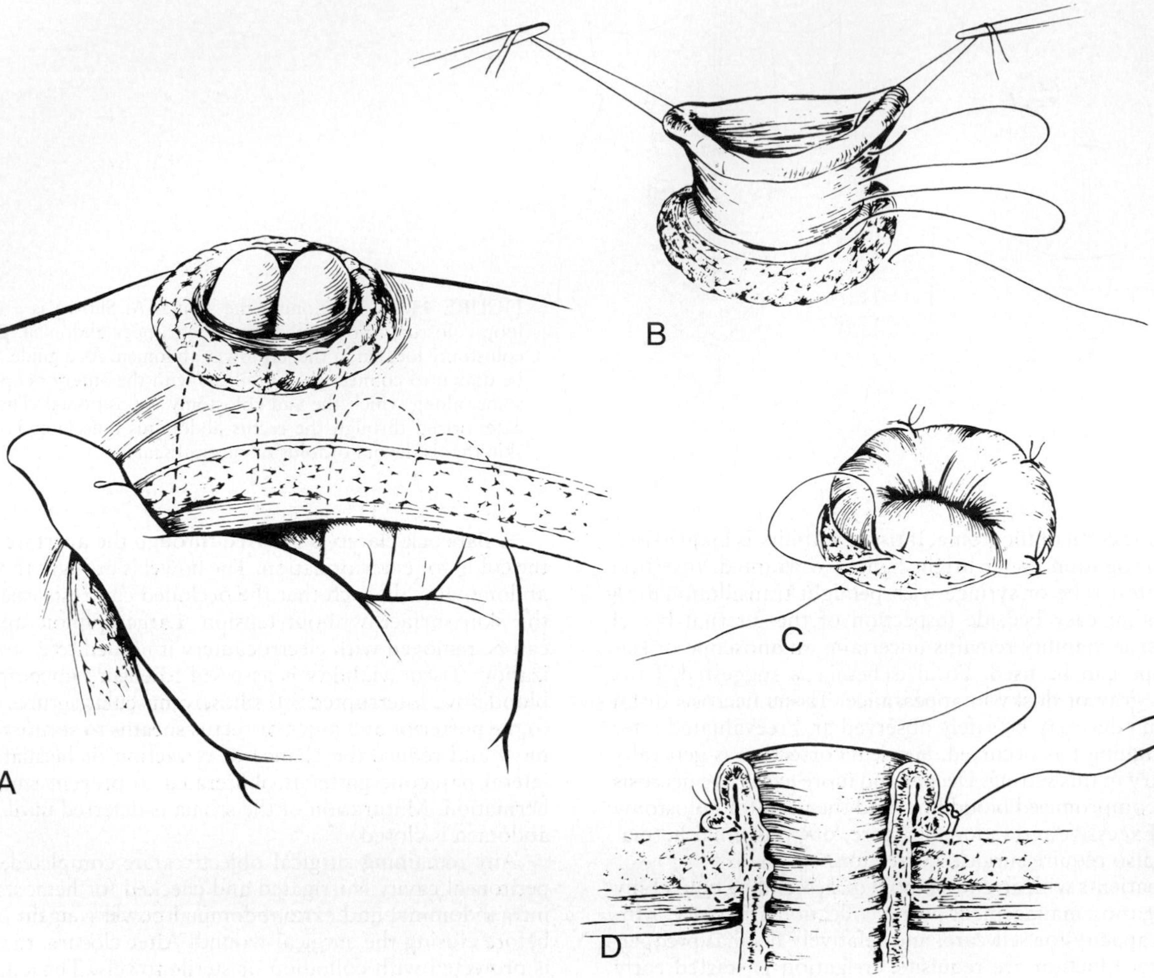

FIGURE 43.22. End colostomy. Technique for creating a bowel stoma that is elevated from the skin surface. This everted stoma is developed by excising a 3-cm circumferential segment of abdominal wall (A), anchoring the skin margin with the adjacent wall of the exteriorized bowel (B), and approximating the mucosal edge of the bowel to the skin (C). The cross-sectional view demonstrates how the bowel wall is anchored to the skin margin to prevent retraction (D).

that can be effectively used. Factors to consider are that the transverse colon is generally outside of the previous surgical or radiation field and the transverse colon has a lower bacterial count than the more distal colon. Alternatively, use of the sigmoid preserves a greater length of intact bowel. The traditional loop colostomy is described for illustrative purposes and uses the transverse colon with the stoma created in the left upper quadrant.

In comparison to an end colostomy, a larger aperture is required to bring two full segments of colon and intervening mesentery through the abdominal wall. A stoma site is selected overlying the rectus muscle, which avoids skin folds, surgical scars, and the umbilicus. A transverse incision is carried down through the anterior rectus fascia. Two evenly spaced, perpendicular fascial incisions can be used to increase the diameter of this aperture. The rectus muscle fibers are bluntly separated, and the posterior rectus sheath and peritoneum are incised in a manner similar to that of the anterior fascia. The opening is manually dilated and should easily admit four fingers without stricture.

The transverse colon is identified by the presence of teniae and the omental attachment. Once isolated, the bowel is followed in a hand-over-hand fashion until the most distal yet readily mobile segment is brought through the abdominal wall. Lifting the loop is simplified by using a half-inch diameter Penrose drain passed under the intestine. A bridge device is also passed through the adjacent mesenteric window and positioned onto the skin, thereby supporting the bowel loop above the skin surface. Fascial supporting sutures are generally not necessary as the normal healing process scars the stoma into position. Any extra length of the abdominal incision is closed. The stoma is matured by a sharp longitudinal incision through the teniae that is extended to within 1.0 cm of the skin edge at both ends. The stoma edges are everted and secured with interrupted skin to full-thickness bowel sutures using 3-0 delayed absorbable material (Fig. 43.23).

The traditional Hollister bridge frequently precludes a secure appliance fit. A number of various supporting devices have been used effectively. We prefer a supporting bridge fashioned from a 20-French thoracostomy tube. A segment of about 20 cm length is cut and passed through the mesenteric window underneath the bowel. The ends are brought together over the bowel and sutured together to form a loop. This method requires no skin sutures, does not interfere with application of

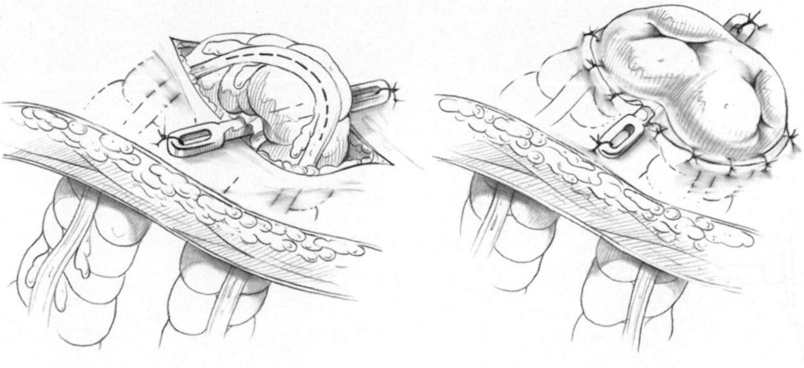

FIGURE 43.23. Transverse loop colostomy. A: An isolated loop of transverse colon is held above the skin surface by a supporting bridge. The bowel is opened via sharp incision through the tenia. B: The stoma is matured using interrupted 3-0 delayed absorbable sutures, which are placed from skin to full-thickness bowel edge.

the collecting bag, and permits secure adherence between the stoma wafer and skin. After adequate healing (10 to 14 days), the bridge is easily removed by cutting the suture to open the loop and withdraw the tube.

Variations of the loop colostomy include the double-barrel colostomy, in which the bowel is transected and both stomas are matured. An end colostomy with mucous fistula is used in the setting of distal obstruction, because the decompression provided by the mucous fistula avoids a closed loop obstruction. When the mucous fistula is placed immediately adjacent to the end colostomy, it is known as an end loop or terminal loop colostomy.

GASTRIC PROCEDURE

Open Gastrostomy

A gastrostomy tube avoids prolonged nasogastric intubation when long-term gastric decompression is needed. This access route can also be used for enteral hydration, nutrition, and medication administration in patients who have an intact intestinal tract. Gastrostomy is avoided in obtunded patients and those with massive ascites, esophageal varices, coagulopathy, or extensive tumor that precludes tension-free placement. Commercially available gastrostomy tubes generally have an inflatable balloon tip that secures the tube within the stomach. Other catheters such as a Foley, Robinson, or Malecot may also suffice.

The technique of open gastrostomy begins with ensuring that there is adequate mobilization to bring the stomach wall into direct opposition with the abdominal wall. An insertion site is chosen in the midanterior gastric wall, away from the short gastric vessels. Cautery or sharp dissection is used to make a small puncture. Injury to the posterior gastric wall is avoided by making the gastrotomy directly over a nasogastric tube, which is secured into position with handheld traction. A stab incision is made through the skin of the left upper abdomen. A narrow clamp is passed from peritoneum through skin, and the tip of the gastrostomy tube is grasped and brought through the abdominal wall. The tube is guided into the stomach through the gastrotomy and secured in place with two purse-string sutures of 2-0 delayed absorbable or nonabsorbable material. The inner purse-string suture is first secured. The gastric wall is then elevated and held in position using Babcock clamps as the outer purse-string suture is tied securely around the tube in Stamm fashion. If a balloon apparatus is used, it is inflated with approximately 10 cc of fluid. Traction on the gastrostomy tube elevates the stomach wall into direct contact with the abdominal wall. The stomach is secured in place using interrupted 2-0 delayed absorbable sutures. The tube can be further secured at the skin surface using nonabsorbable suture. Similar techniques are also used to decompress the intestinal tract at other anatomic locations, such as via a tube jejunostomy.

This open technique can also be used for gastroduodenal tube insertion. Commercially available catheters (Moss gastrostomy tube, Moss Tubes, West Sand Lake, NY) have proximal ports for gastric decompression and distal ports to deliver enteral nutrition (Fig. 43.24). Intraoperatively, the tube is manually guided through the pylorus into the duodenum. Advantages of small bowel enteral nutrition include less gastroesophageal reflux and aspiration in comparison with gastric feedings. This also allows simultaneous enteral nutrition while decompressing the stomach. Such feedings are, however, more likely to cause cramping, abdominal distention, and rapid transit with diarrhea.

If a permanent gastrostomy is intended at the time of surgery, consideration is given to a gastric flap procedure. With this approach, a portion of the stomach wall is incorporated into the stoma. An inverted U-shaped flap is raised from the anterior stomach wall, with the base located near the greater curvature. An adequate flap reduces gastric reflux onto the skin and should be 6 cm in width by 10 cm in length. The flap is closed around the gastrostomy catheter in continuum with the gastric closure, using two layers of delayed absorbable suture. The distal end of the flap is exteriorized and matured as a stoma.

Postoperatively, the gastrostomy tube is attached to low wall suction (≤80 mm Hg) and irrigated frequently. The catheter is generally not removed before the fourth postoperative week to ensure adequate healing between the gastric wall and peritoneum. When the tube is discontinued, gastric leaking tends to persist for several days until the defect closes. Occasionally, a gastrocutaneous fistula persists, which could require surgical closure. A long-term indwelling gastrostomy tube is replaced every 2 to 3 months to maintain adequate function. This is accomplished by decompressing the balloon and removing the old tube, with immediate replacement of a new tube through the mature tract.

Excessive tension can cause tissue ischemia and necrosis. Conversely, an inadequate seal between the stomach and abdominal wall can lead to intraperitoneal leakage of gastric content with resultant abscess and/or peritonitis. Surgical exploration is necessary if the leak cannot be corrected by increasing balloon tension against the undersurface of the abdominal wall. Other potential gastrostomy complications include bleeding, tube malfunction, skin irritation, infection, and migration through the pylorus or gastroesophageal junction.

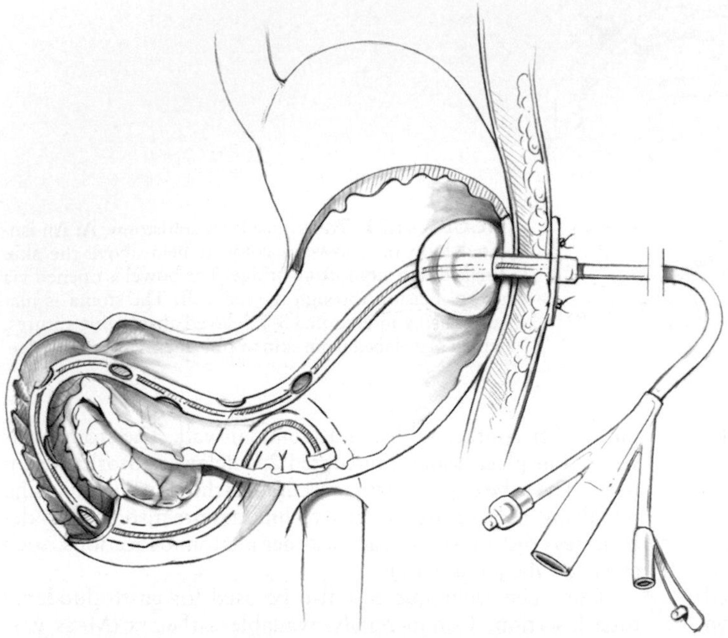

FIGURE 43.24. Gastrostomy tube. The gastric wall and abdominal wall are juxtaposed and held into position via balloon apparatus and suture fixation. Shown is a gastrostomy tube with proximal ports for gastric decompression and distal ports for enteral nutrition (i.e., Moss gastrostomy tube, Moss Tubes, West Sand Lake, NY).

Endoscopic Gastric Procedures

Percutaneous procedures are currently available for patients in need of gastrostomy who are not undergoing laparotomy. Percutaneous endoscopic gastrostomy (PEG) and percutaneous endoscopic jejunostomy (PEJ) are performed under local anesthesia with intravenous sedation. The PEG tube is placed via endoscopic gastric insufflation and transillumination to guide percutaneous needle and guide wire placement through the abdominal wall. An introducer is passed transcutaneously into the stomach over the guide wire. The introducer is withdrawn, leaving a sheath through which the gastrostomy tube is inserted. As the sheath is peeled away, traction on the tube draws the flange and stomach wall into direct contact with the abdominal wall. Another external flange or fixation suture is used to secure the apparatus into position. Using similar endoscopic techniques, a jejunostomy tube can be guided through the pylorus and duodenum, into the jejunum.

BEST SURGICAL PRACTICES

- The gynecologic surgeon should have a basic understanding of the anatomy and physiology of the intestinal tract and should possess the fundamental skills necessary to recognize and correct common conditions affecting the digestive system.
- Peritoneal irritation from any source can be elicited by manipulation of the pelvic organs, such that manual manipulation of the cervix can create an intensely painful response (cervical motion tenderness) in women with either PID or appendicitis.
- Medical management is the cornerstone of treatment for inflammatory bowel disease (Crohn's disease and ulcerative colitis), as intestinal surgery is reserved for obstruction, perforation, fistula, or hemorrhage. Elective gynecologic surgery is best avoided in patients with Crohn's disease or ulcerative colitis because of the high risk of intestinal complications.
- In previously irradiated patients, elective surgical procedures within the radiation field should not be attempted.
- The objectives of preoperative bowel prep are to reduce enteric volume and bacterial load. The literature, however, is inconclusive regarding the effectiveness of preoperative bowel prep in reducing infectious complications and facilitating anastomotic healing.
- Prior gynecologic surgery is the most frequently noted predisposing factor to intraperitoneal adhesions, with other risk factors being trauma, irradiation, infection, bleeding, and chemical irritants. An estimated 85% of all small bowel obstructions are secondary to intraperitoneal adhesions, malignancies, or hernias, with the most common etiology being adhesions.
- The vast majority of large bowel obstructions are caused by malignancies or inflammatory conditions. In the setting of a large bowel obstruction, the risk of perforation increases significantly as the cecum is dilated beyond 10 to 12 cm. Barium enema should not be performed in the setting of acute colonic obstruction or suspected perforation to avoid barium peritonitis.
- If intestinal perforation occurs during introduction of a laparoscopic needle or trocar, it is prudent to leave the instrument in position to guide identification of the affected anatomy. Thermal injury from electrocautery or laser results in a progressive zone of tissue destruction that extends well beyond the area of thermal contact, resulting in tissue necrosis and perforation 72 to 96 hours after surgery. In contrast to sharp enterotomy, which can be repaired primarily, significant thermal injury is best corrected by resection of the affected bowel segment.
- Enterotomies are best avoided by cautious entry into the peritoneal cavity and meticulous dissection of adhesions. If an inadvertent enterotomy occurs, the affected bowel is mobilized from surrounding tissues to allow adequate exposure and a tension-free repair. Resection of an affected bowel segment may be necessary if the blood supply is compromised, if greater than 50% of the circumference is injured, if irregular edges preclude reapproximation, or if repair would result in excessive luminal narrowing. Immediate repair of a large

bowel injury is associated with acceptably low morbidity and does not usually require a diverting colostomy. A diverting colostomy is indicated when a full-thickness colonic injury occurs in someone who has previously been irradiated, or who is profoundly malnourished, or who is unstable from shock or sepsis.

- Peritoneal drains should not be placed in the immediate vicinity of an anastomosis as this can impede healing.
- Current trends are toward much more aggressive early postoperative feeding, even in the setting of bowel resection and anastomosis. Use of the gut for nutrition is advisable whenever possible. Perioperative nutritional support is indicated in patients who have been without nutrition for more than 7 days before surgery, in those who are malnourished (weight loss exceeds 15% of usual weight), and in those whose expected duration of recovery is longer than 10 days.
- Therapeutic nasogastric decompression is indicated in symptomatic patients with an ileus who are perpetually nauseated, markedly distended, actively vomiting, and/or who are not responding to supportive measures. Decompression is generally continued until consistent flatus ensues and abdominal distention resolves. The typical radiographic pattern of an ileus is that of air-fluid levels in the stomach and small bowel with intermittent air throughout the entire gastrointestinal tract. In contrast to an ileus, radiographic characteristics of mechanical small bowel obstruction include proximal distended bowel loops with a paucity or absence of gas in the colon.
- Fewer than half of obstructed patients manifest the classic triad of rebound tenderness, guarding, and rigidity.
- If no complicating factors persist, approximately two thirds of distal intestinal fistulae are expected to heal within 6 weeks from nonoperative management. The more proximal the fistula, the greater the potential for physiologic derangements, and the less likely the chance of spontaneous closure. The fundamentals of conservative fistulae management include correction of electrolyte abnormalities, resolution of underlying inflammatory processes, maintenance of adequate hydration, and nutritional support.
- Short bowel syndrome occurs when there is insufficient nutrient absorption to meet the body's metabolic requirements because of extensive bowel resection or inadequate function of normal-length bowel. In general, 50% of the small bowel (300 cm on average) can be resected without long-term impairment of nutritional status as long as there is normal function in the remainder of the intestine. For approximately 24 months after an intestinal resection, the remaining small bowel undergoes adaptation to increase the functional surface area via increasing villous height and crypt depth, and through gradual dilation and lengthening of the bowel.
- Strict adherence to the fundamental principles of anastomosis is more important to successful healing than are the specific techniques or materials used. Open anastomotic techniques (bowel lumens exposed) have gradually replaced closed techniques (lumens occluded) in most circumstances because of technical ease and acceptably low morbidity. The most important strength layer of the bowel wall is the submucosa, which must be incorporated into any anastomosis. Sixty percent of the bowel wall strength is reached by postoperative day 3 to 4, and pressure tolerated by the anastomotic site approximates 100% of that tolerated by intact bowel wall as of postoperative day 7. Clinical evidence suggests that single-layer anastomosis is equivalent to double-layer closure and may provide some advantages.
- In general, as much as 8 cm of small intestine can remain viable distal to the closest vasa recta because of intramural vascular communications. It is recommended that ~10 cm of terminal ileum be removed during right colon resection because of the tenuous blood supply of the distal ileum. It is important to resect only the length of bowel necessary to adequately address the disease process. The diameter of any lumen can be increased by transecting the bowel obliquely or via linear incision along the antimesenteric border (Cheatle slit).
- Arterial perfusion can generally be preserved to any segment of the colon as long as the marginal artery of Drummond is not disrupted. The integrity of the marginal artery is protected when the mesentery is transected close to the bowel wall through the vasa recta. The marginal artery is absent at the hepatic flexure, or more commonly the splenic flexure, in 1% to 2% of the population. Colon resection near the splenic flexure should include removal of the flexure due to the arterial inconsistency in that region. The inferior mesenteric artery (IMA) can be sacrificed during rectosigmoid resection, without significant compromise, because of collateral circulation from the middle and inferior rectal arteries. The colon remains viable only 2 cm beyond the closest intact vasa recta. Subsequent to a rectosigmoid resection, morbidity is inversely related to the length of intact rectum at the time of repair.
- Preoperative consultation with an enterostomal therapist enhances surgical planning, patient education, and postoperative care. As a general guide, a line is drawn connecting the anterior-superior iliac spine to the umbilicus, and the colostomy is exteriorized through the rectus muscles at some point along this line. The stoma is secured in an area that is easily seen and reached by the patient, and placement is avoided within skin folds, surgical scars, or the umbilicus.
- A loop colostomy is technically less difficult to create and/or to reverse than an end colostomy and can often be accomplished through a single incision. An end colostomy is more satisfactory from a long-term-care standpoint because it is generally smaller, easier to fit with an appliance, and usually more distal, resulting in formed stools. Maturation of the stoma is deferred until after the abdomen is closed.

Bibliography

Bahadursingh AM, Virgo KS, Kaminski DL, et al. Spectrum of disease and outcome of complicated diverticular disease. *Am J Surg* 2003;186(6):696.

Brage M, Gianotti L, Gentilini O, et al. Feeding the gut early after digestive surgery: results of a nine year experience. *Clin Nutr* 2002;21(1):59.

Beart RW, Kelly KA. Randomized prospective evaluation of the EEA stapler for colorectal anastomoses. *Am J Surg* 1981;141:143.

Brennan SS, Pickford IR, Evans M, et al. Staples or sutures for colonic anastomosis—a controlled clinical trial. *Br J Surg* 1982;69:722.

Bucher P, Mermillod B, Gervaz P, et al. Mechanical bowel preparation for elective colorectal surgery: a meta-analysis. *Arch Surg* 2004;139(12):1359.

Byrne TA, Wilmore DW, Iyer K, et al. Growth hormone, glutamine, and an optimal diet reduces parenteral nutrition in patients with short bowel syndrome:

a prospective, randomized, placebo-controlled, double-blind clinical trial. *Ann Surg* 2005;242(5):655.
Carey LC, Fabri PJ. The intestinal tract in relation to gynecology. In: Thompson JD, Rock JA, eds. *Te Linde's operative gynecology*. 7th ed. Philadelphia: JB Lippincott; 1992; 1017.
Cheatham ML, Chapman WC, Key SP, et al. A meta-analysis of selective versus routine nasogastric decompression after elective laparotomy. *Ann Surg* 1995;221(5):469; discussion 476.
Chung RS. Blood flow in colonic anastomoses: effect of stapling and suturing. *Ann Surg* 1987;206:335.
Cohen Z, Sullivan B. Intestinal anastomosis. In: Wilmore DW, Cheung LY, Harken AM, et al., eds. *ACS surgery: principles and practice*. New York: WEBMD; 2002; 803.
Curran TJ, Borzotta AP. Complications of primary repair of colon injury: literature review of 2,964 cases. *Am J Surg* 1999;177:42.
Eskelinen M, Ikonen J, Lipponen P. Contributions of history-taking, physical examination and computer assistance to diagnose acute small bowel obstruction: a prospective study of 1333 patients with acute abdominal pain. *Scand J Gastroenterol* 1994;29:715.
Falcone RE, Wanamaker SR, Santanello SA, et al. Colorectal trauma: primary repair or anastomosis with intracolonic bypass vs. ostomy. *Dis Colon Rectum* 1992;35(10):957.
Fanning J, Andrews S. Early postoperative feeding after major gynecologic surgery: evidence-based scientific medicine. *Am J Obstet Gynecol* 2001;185(1):1.
Feo CV, Romanini B, Sortini D, et al. Early oral feeding after colorectal resection: a randomized controlled study. *ANZ J Surg* 2004;74(5):298.
Gambee LP, Garnojobst W, Harwick CE. Ten years experience with a single layer anastomosis in colon surgery. *Am J Surg* 1956;92:222.
Gillette-Cloven N, Burger RA, Monk BJ, et al. Bowel resection at the time of primary cytoreduction for epithelial ovarian cancer. *J Am Coll Surg* 2001;193:626.
Gonzalez R, Smith CD, Mattar SG, et al. Laparoscopic vs open resection for the treatment of diverticular disease. *Surg Endosc* 2004;18(2):276.
Helton WS. Intestinal obstruction. In: Wilmore DW, Cheung LY, Harken Am, et al., eds. *ACS surgery: principles and practice*. New York: WEBMD; 2002; 263.
Hesp F, Hendriks T, Lubbers EJ, et al. Wound healing in the intestinal wall: a comparison between experimental ileal and colonic anastomosis. *Dis Colon Rectum* 1984;24:99.
Jaeger W, Ackermann S, Kessler H, et al. The effect of bowel resection on survival in advanced epithelial ovarian cancer. *Gynecol Oncol* 2001;83:286.
Levine JH, Longo WE, Pruitt C, et al. Management of selected rectal injuries by primary repair. *Am J Surg* 1996;172(5):575; discussion 578.
Lynch AC, Delaney CP, Senagore AJ, et al. Clinical outcome and factors predictive of recurrence after enterocutaneous fistula surgery. *Ann Surg* 2004;240(5):825.
MacMillan SL, Kammerer-Doak D, Rogers RG, et al. Early feeding and the incidence of gastrointestinal symptoms after major gynecologic surgery. *Obstet Gynecol* 2000;96(4):604.
Matarese LE, O'Keefe SJ, Kandil HM, et al. Short bowel syndrome: clinical guidelines for nutrition management. *Nutr Clin Pract* 2005;20(5):493.
Miettinen RP, Laitinen ST, Makela JT, et al. Bowel preparation with oral polyethylene glycol electrolyte solution vs. no preparation in elective open colorectal surgery: prospective, randomized study. *Dis Colon Rectum* 2000;43:669.
Mirhashemi R, Averette HE, Estape R, et al. Low colorectal anastomosis after radical pelvic surgery: a risk factor analysis. *Am J Obstet Gynecol* 2000;183:1375.
Mitchell GW Jr. Evisceration and repair of ventral hernias. In: Nichols DM, ed. *Gynecologic and obstetrical surgery*. St. Louis: Mosby–Year Book; 1993; 197.
Molpus KL. The intestinal tract in gynecologic surgery. In: Rock JA, Jones HW III, eds. *Te Linde's operative gynecology*. 9th ed. Philadelphia: Lippincott Williams & Williams; 2003;1239.
Monk BJ, Berman ML, Montz FJ. Adhesions after extensive gynecologic surgery: clinical significance, etiology, and prevention. *Am J Obstet Gynecol* 1994;170:1396.
Morrow CP, Curtin JP. Surgical anatomy. In: *Gynecologic cancer surgery*. Philadelphia: Churchill Livingstone; 1996; 67.
Morrow CP, Curtin JP. Surgery on the intestinal tract. In: *Gynecologic cancer surgery*. Philadelphia: Churchill Livingstone; 1996; 181.
Mourton SM, Temple LK, Abu-Rustum NR, et al. Morbidity of rectosigmoid resection and primary anastomosis in patients undergoing primary cytoreductive surgery for advanced epithelial ovarian cancer. *Gynecol Oncol* 2005;99(3):608.
Obermair A, Hagenauer S, Tamandl D, et al. Safety and efficacy of low anterior en bloc resection as part of cytoreductive surgery for patients with ovarian cancer. *Gynecol Oncol* 2001;83(1):115.
Oliveira L, Wexner SD, Daniel N, et al. Mechanical bowel preparation for elective colorectal surgery: a prospective, randomized, surgeon-blinded trial comparing sodium phosphate and polyethylene glycol-based oral lavage solutions. *Dis Colon Rectum* 1997;40:585.
Park JJ, Wolff BG, Tollefson MK, et al. Meckel diverticulum: the Mayo Clinic experience with 1476 patients (1950–2002). *Ann Surg* 2005;241(3):529.
Pessaux P, Muscari F, Ouellet JF, et al. Risk factors for mortality and morbidity after elective sigmoid resection for diverticulitis: prospective multicenter multivariate analysis of 582 patients. *World J Surg* 2004;28(1):92.
Pearl ML, Frandina M, Mahler L, et al. A randomized controlled trial of a regular diet as the first meal in gynecologic oncology patients undergoing intraabdominal surgery. *Obstet Gynecol* 2002;100:230.
Rex D. Should we colonoscope women with gynecologic cancer? *Am J Gastroenterol* 2000;95(3):812.
Santos JC Jr, Batista J, Sirimarco MT, et al. Prospective randomized trial of mechanical bowel preparation in patients undergoing elective colorectal surgery. *Br J Surg* 1994;81:1673.
Schrock TR. Colorectal procedures. In: Wilmore DW, Cheung LY, Harken AM, et al., eds. *ACS surgery: principles and practice*. New York: WEBMD; 2002.
Schwartz SI. Small intestinal surgery incidental to gynecologic procedures. In: Nichols DH, ed. *Gynecologic and obstetric surgery*. St. Louis: Mosby–Year Book; 1993; 925.
Schwartz SI. Surgery of the colon, incidental to gynecologic surgery. In: Nichols DH, ed. *Gynecologic and obstetric surgery*. St. Louis: Mosby–Year Book; 1993; 935.
Stewart BT, Woods RJ, Collopy BT, et al. Early feeding after elective open colorectal resections: a prospective randomized trial. *Aust N Z J Surg* 1998;68(2):125.
Tamussino KF, Lim PC, Webb MJ, et al. Gastrointestinal surgery in patients with ovarian cancer. *Gynecol Oncol* 2001;80(1):79.
Thompson JS, DiBaise JK, Iyer KR, et al. Postoperative short bowel syndrome. *J Am Coll Surg* 2005;201(1):85.
Van Der Krabben AA, Dijkstra FR, Nieuwenhuijzen M, et al. Morbidity and mortality of inadvertent enterotomy during adhesiotomy. *Br J Surg* 2000;87(4):467.
Wheeless Jr CR. The intestinal tract in gynecologic surgery. In: Rock JA, Thompson JD, eds. *Te Linde's operative gynecology*. 8th ed. Philadelphia: Lippincott-Raven; 1996.
Zmora O, Mahajna A, Bar-Zakai B, et al. Colon and rectal surgery without mechanical bowel preparation: a randomized prospective trial. *Ann Surg* 2003;237(3):363.

CHAPTER 44 ■ NONGYNECOLOGIC CONDITIONS ENCOUNTERED BY THE GYNECOLOGIC SURGEON

JAMES R. DOLAN AND MICHAEL D. MOEN

DEFINITIONS

Air contrast barium enema—Sometimes called a "double-contrast" barium enema. The colon is filled with barium, and x-ray films are taken. The barium is then allowed to empty, leaving a thin film on the internal bowel wall. The colon is filled with air, making the colonic mucosa more easily seen. This is especially useful for diagnosis of polyps and inflammatory bowel disease.

Carcinoembryonic antigen (CEA)—A glycoprotein tumor marker that is elevated in the serum of many patients with colorectal cancer. It may also be elevated in patients with lung cancer. It is often elevated in patients who smoke cigarettes.

Hartmann procedure—The colon is divided or resected and an end colostomy is brought up. The distal colonic stump is stapled or sewn closed and left *in situ* in the pelvis.

Methyl methacrylate—Cement used to anchor orthopedic screws or implants to bony structures. Excess cement may form a hard mass adjacent to the site of application, and this new mass may create a diagnostic dilemma.

Protrusio acetabuli—Inward protrusion of the femor head through the inner wall of the acetabulum. This may be palpated as a hard pelvic wall mass. This condition can occur with rheumatoid arthritis, osteomalacia, Marfan syndrome, and other conditions.

Women of all ages look to their gynecologist to diagnose and treat problems that arise within the pelvis. Because the pelvis contains multiple organ systems, it is possible the gynecologic surgeon will unexpectedly encounter a nongynecologic condition. It is extremely important, therefore, that the gynecologic surgeon be aware of the various conditions that may be present in the pelvis and search for them preoperatively. This chapter discusses the various diagnostic tools available that may help to identify these conditions preoperatively and reviews intraoperative strategies when these conditions are encountered.

PREOPERATIVE DIAGNOSTIC EVALUATION

A careful history and physical examination combined with routine laboratory data remain the cornerstone of the preliminary evaluation. Although nongynecologic pelvic disorders can occur at any age, they most often are found in the obese or elderly patient with an ill-defined pelvic mass. The symptoms often are vague and may be minimized, particularly in elderly patients, who can have a high threshold for pain.

Gastrointestinal Disease

Symptoms such as pelvic pain, low-grade fever, change in bowel habits, or bloody stools should arouse suspicion of intestinal pathology. In such instances, a gastrointestinal evaluation is essential before laparotomy.

A pelvic examination may reveal a right or left adnexal mass that may seem to be an inflammatory or neoplastic disorder of the tube or ovary or both, but this may not be the true situation. Line drawings and representative computed tomography scanning (CT scans) depict various intestinal disorders that may easily be mistaken for ovarian or tubal pathology (Figs. 44.1–44.5). The digital rectal exam and testing stool for the presence of occult blood should be a routine component of every physical exam. Although the guaiac test (hemoccult slide) may be of some aid as a screening test for asymptomatic patients, it is not reliable in symptomatic patients. Approximately 50% of patients with documented colorectal cancer have a negative fecal hemoccult test. This is consistent with the intermittent bleeding patterns of these tumors and, if negative, may give the physician a false sense of security.

Preoperative evaluation should include lower gastrointestinal radiologic studies and possibly a colonoscopic examination, especially in patients with gastrointestinal symptoms. The gynecologic surgeon should be aware that radiologic studies of the colon can be in error from 10% of the time in cooperative and well-prepared patients to as often as 50% in uncooperative or improperly prepared patients. A large number of colon lesions are missed on radiologic examination because they are mistaken for fecal material or are hidden by fecal material. This is particularly true when a single-contrast barium enema is used. For this reason, it is vital that the gynecologic surgeon make certain that the patient is properly prepared for the radiologic studies and that they are of the air-contrast type. Without air contrast, the colonic mucosa cannot be adequately outlined. Even if the air-contrast barium enema is performed, a conscientious gynecologist should carefully and critically review the films with the radiologist before surgery is undertaken.

To ensure that the colon is properly prepared, the patient should be given instructions on how to clean the colon before the radiologic studies. On the day before the test, a regular breakfast is advised, but only clear liquids for lunch and dinner. Although cathartics and cleansing enemas are acceptable, the colon is best prepared by using an isotonic lavage solution (such as GoLYTELY or Colyte), which washes the colon clean. The

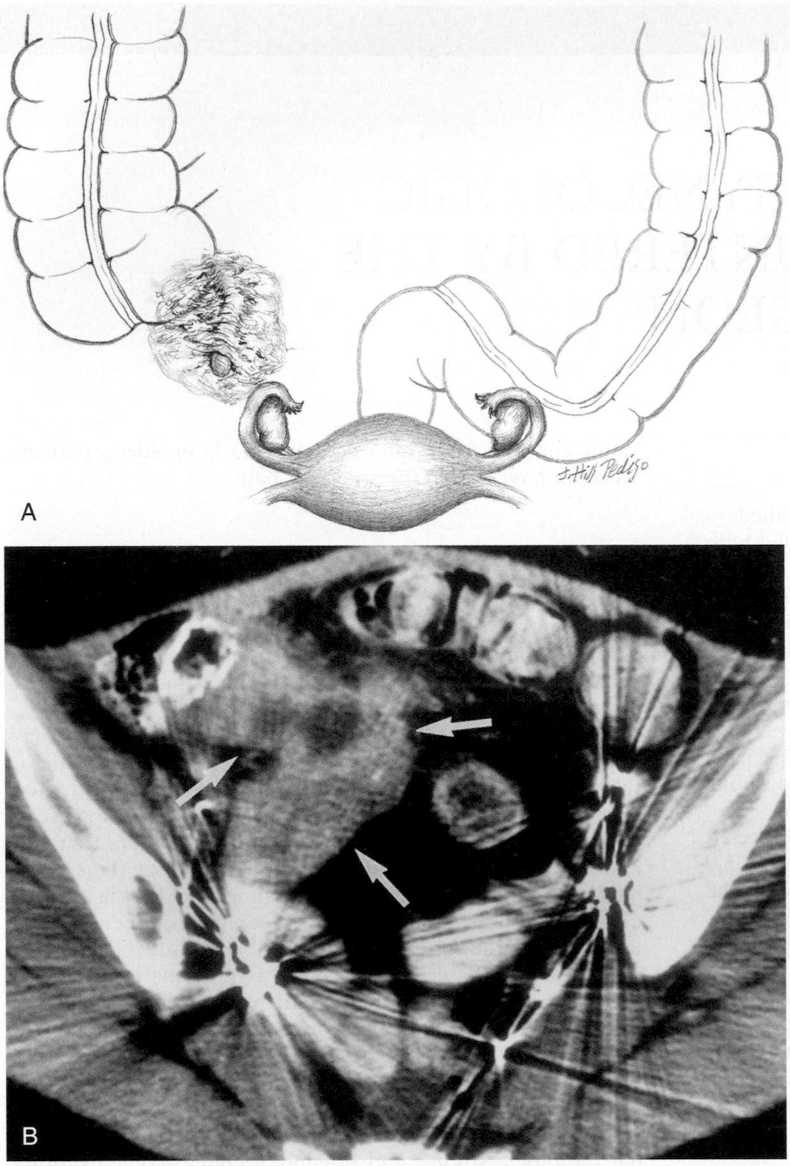

FIGURE 44.1. Appendiceal abscess. **A:** On bimanual examination, this abscess is felt to be slightly higher in the pelvis but can be mistaken for an adnexal condition. **B:** Computed tomography (CT) image shows inhomogeneous abscess (*arrows*) in the right side of the pelvis. Hemoclip artifact is also present. (Courtesy of T. Demos, Maywood, IL.)

solution is begun at noon on the day before the test, with the patient drinking 8 to 16 ounces every 10 to 15 minutes until the rectal discharge is clear. This usually requires 2 to 4 quarts of solution. After midnight, the patient should not have anything to eat or drink. Early on the morning of the test, a 10-mg bisacodyl suppository (Dulcolax) should be inserted into the rectum.

In addition to being an invaluable aid in the detection of colon cancer and diverticulitis, the barium enema may detect appendicitis or an appendiceal abscess. Additionally, CT studies may be of tremendous benefit in delineating small bowel, colon, cecal, or appendiceal pathology. Figures 44.6 through 44.9 are examples of colonic pathology diagnosed by barium enema and CT studies.

Laparoscopy can be used to distinguish gynecologic disease and ileitis from appendicitis. If the diagnosis of appendicitis is made, laparoscopic appendectomy using ligatures or stapling devices can be performed.

Although the value of digital rectal examination and sigmoidoscopy in detecting lesions of the rectum and sigmoid cannot be overemphasized, the changing distribution of colon cancer makes colonoscopy more important in the diagnostic workup. Cohn and Nance have noted that the incidence of left-sided colon and rectal cancer in their 1950–1954 series was 78.6%, and right-sided colon and rectal cancer was 21.4%. In their 1975–1979 series, the incidence of left colon and rectal cancer had dropped to 68.4%, and the incidence of right-sided colon cancers had increased to 31.6%. McCallion and colleagues reported an increase in proximal colon cancers from 23.5% in 1970 to 36.7% between 1990 and 1997. If symptoms suggest colon pathology, even if the barium enema is reported normal, colonoscopy is indicated.

Unusual small bowel lesions may present as a pelvic mass; thus, small-bowel barium-contrast radiologic studies and CT scans often are helpful. CT scans are particularly useful in delineating mesenteric cysts (Fig. 44.10), volvulus of the small bowel, small bowel intussusception (Fig. 44.11), and Crohn's disease of the ileum (Fig. 44.12), any one of which may prolapse into the pelvis and be mistaken for gynecologic pathology. Gastrointestinal stromal tumors (previously termed *leiomyomas* or

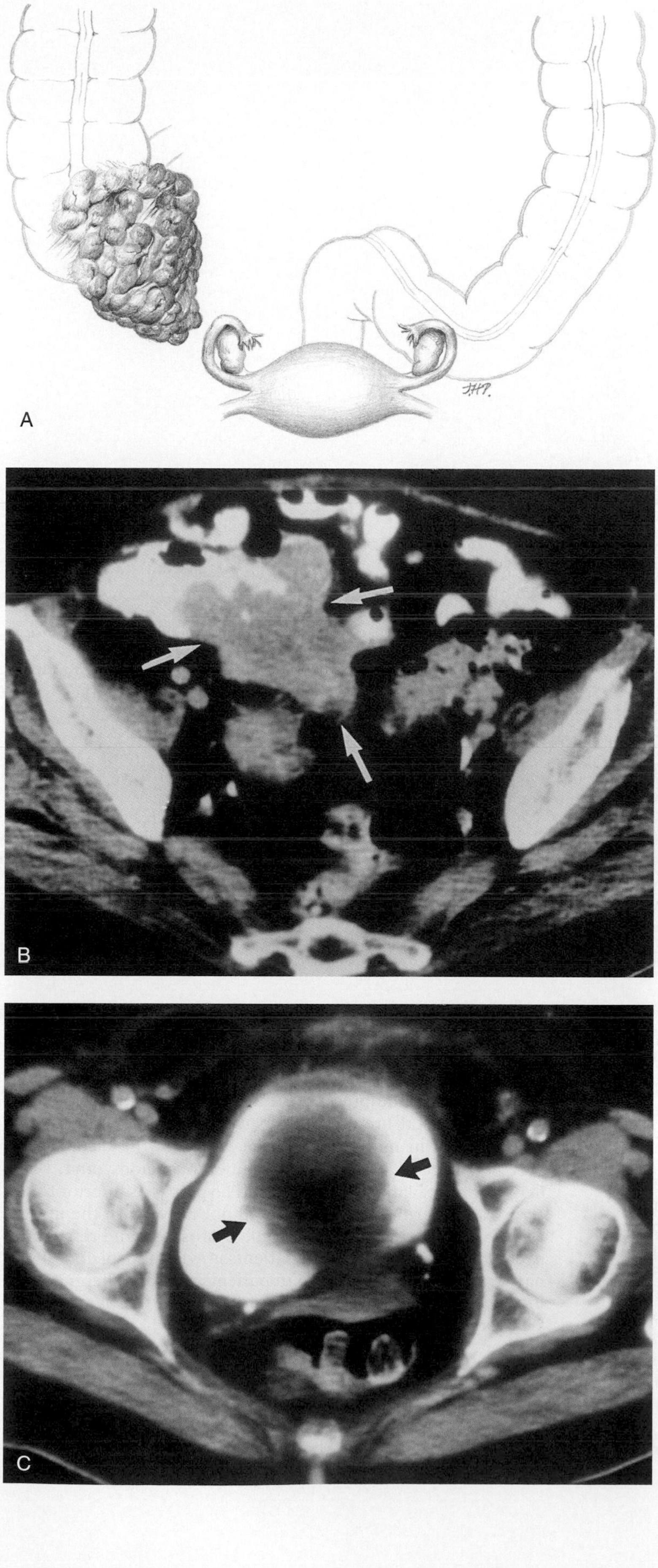

FIGURE 44.2. Cecal carcinoma. **A:** A cecal carcinoma encroaching on the right adnexa can be mistaken for an adnexal condition. **B:** CT image shows a large neoplasm (*arrows*) extending from the cecum. **C:** CT image through the opacified urinary bladder shows invasions by the cecal neoplasm (*arrows*). (Courtesy of T. Demos, Maywood, IL.)

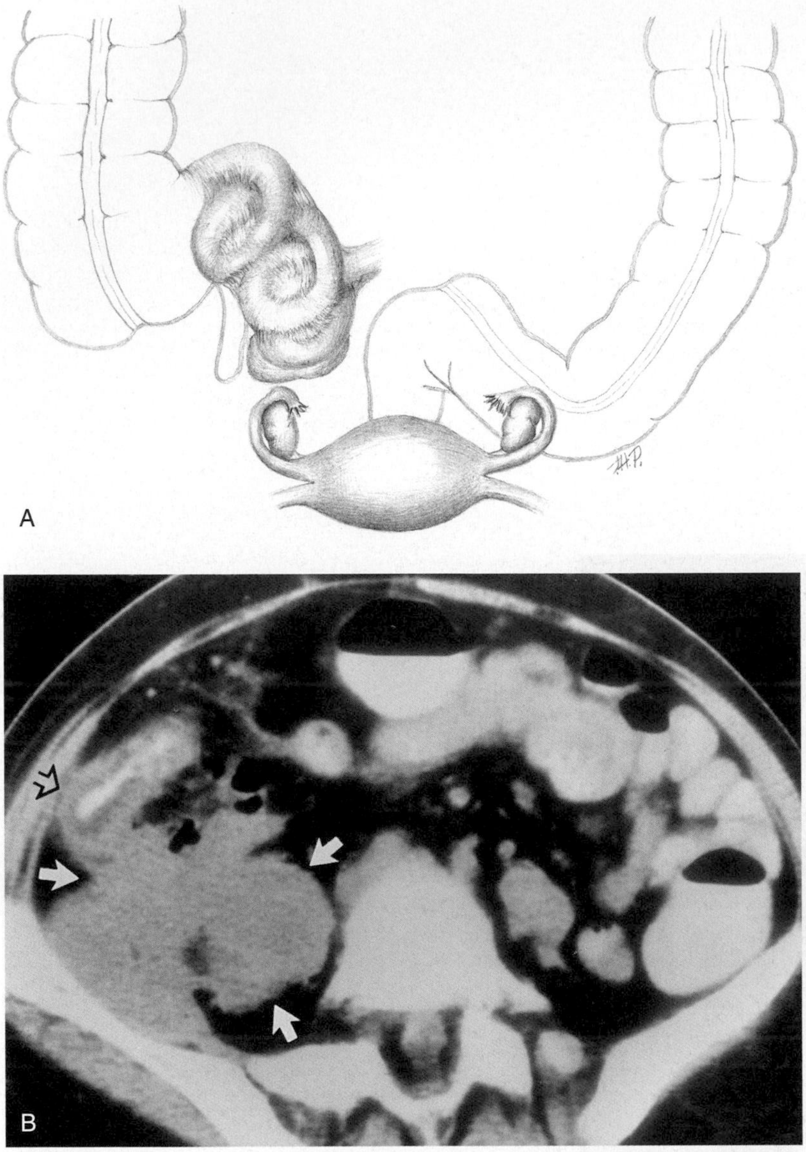

FIGURE 44.3. Crohn's disease with pelvic abscess. **A:** A conglutinant mass of small bowel adjacent to the right tube and ovary is Crohn disease and can suggest inflammatory adnexal disease. **B:** CT image shows a pelvic abscess (*closed arrows*) involving the iliacus and psoas muscles. The wall of the distal ileum (*open arrows*) is thickened because of Crohn disease. (Courtesy of T. Demos, Maywood, IL.)

leiomyosarcomas) may occur in the small bowel and present as a solid pelvic mass, which easily could be mistaken for a pedunculated uterine leiomyoma. These tumors appear as solid masses adjacent to normal bowel on CT scan.

Urologic Tumors

Urinary conditions that occur concomitant with or mimicking gynecologic disease include pelvic kidney, carcinoma of the distal ureter, tumors of the bladder wall, hemangiopericytoma posterior to the bladder, and bladder cancers (Fig. 44.13). Figure 44.14 is a CT scan of a large urachal cyst. A routine urinalysis that reveals hematuria should alert the gynecologist to the possibility of urinary tract disease. A urine culture should be obtained; if an infection is present, the hematuria should clear after a course of antibiotic therapy. For those patients without infection or with persistent hematuria following antibiotic therapy, a cystoscopy and radiologic imaging of the upper urinary tract (intravenous pyelogram, CT scan, or renal ultrasound) are warranted.

A CT scan of the urinary tract before laparotomy in a patient with a pelvic mass may be helpful in diagnosing nongynecologic conditions. It establishes the function of the kidneys and determines the presence of a pelvic kidney or a partially obstructed distal ureter. When performing a bimanual examination, bear in mind that a large tumor of the distal ureter may be confused with an intraligamentous leiomyoma. Bladder tumors or bladder stones should be palpable anterior to the cervix and uterine fundus, and will not move with the uterus, as does an anterior uterine fibroid. Cystoscopy and retrograde pyelography are indicated in patients in whom suspicion of urinary tract disease is high and in patients who are allergic to the intravenous contrast media used for excretory urography and CT studies.

Retroperitoneal Tumors

Although gastrointestinal tract disease is the most frequent pathology mistaken for gynecologic disease, retroperitoneal

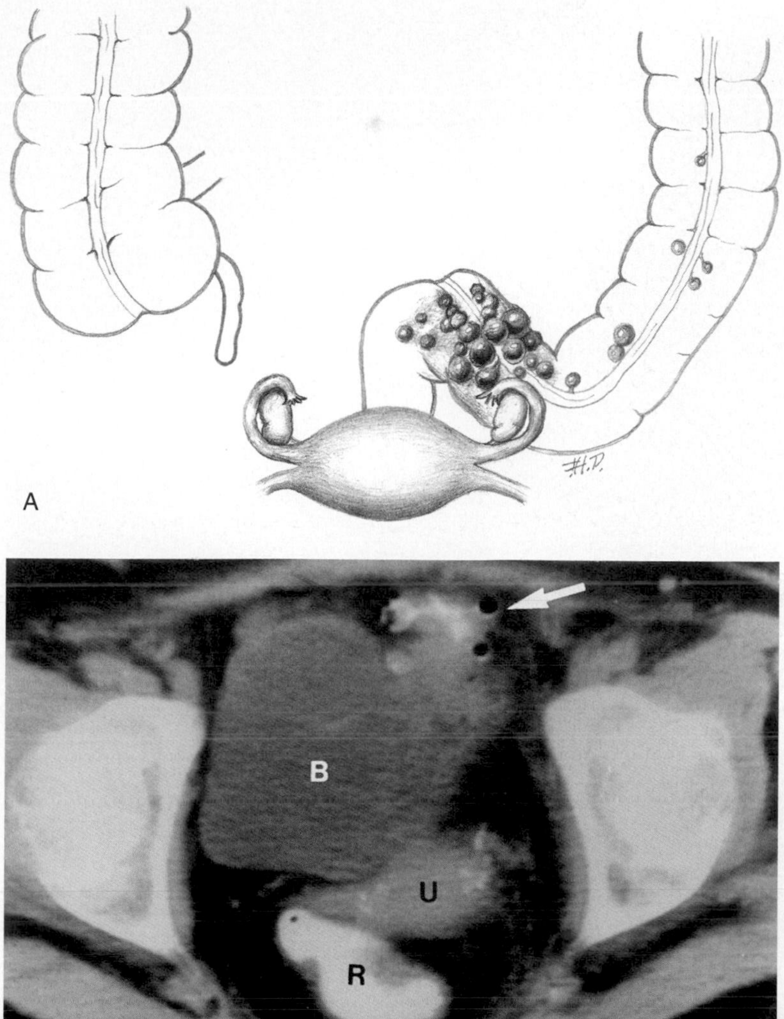

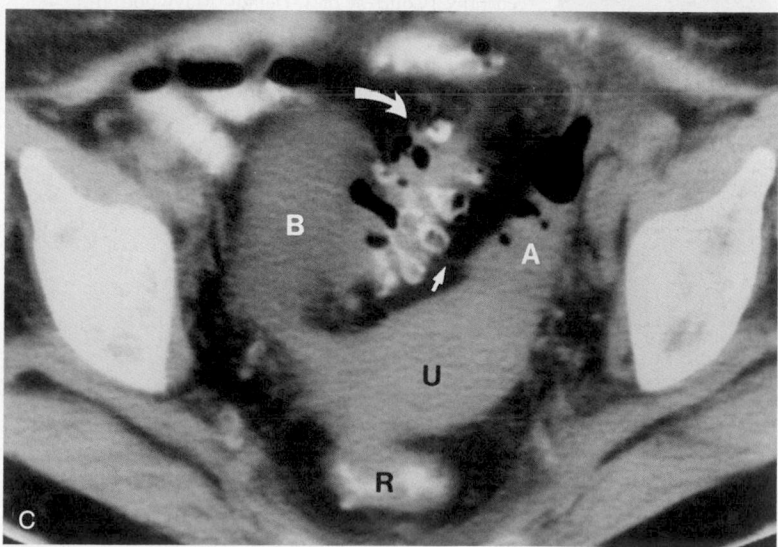

FIGURE 44.4. Sigmoid diverticulitis with abscess. **A:** This is easily confused with a left adnexal pathologic condition. **B:** CT image low in pelvis shows sigmoid diverticula (*arrow*) with infiltration of adjacent fat. **C:** CT image at a higher level shows sigmoid diverticula (*arrow*) and a small sinus tract (*straight arrow*) leading to an abscess (*A*), which contains fluid and gas. The abscess is inseparable from the uterus (*U*). B, bladder; R, rectum. (Courtesy of T. Demos, Maywood, IL.)

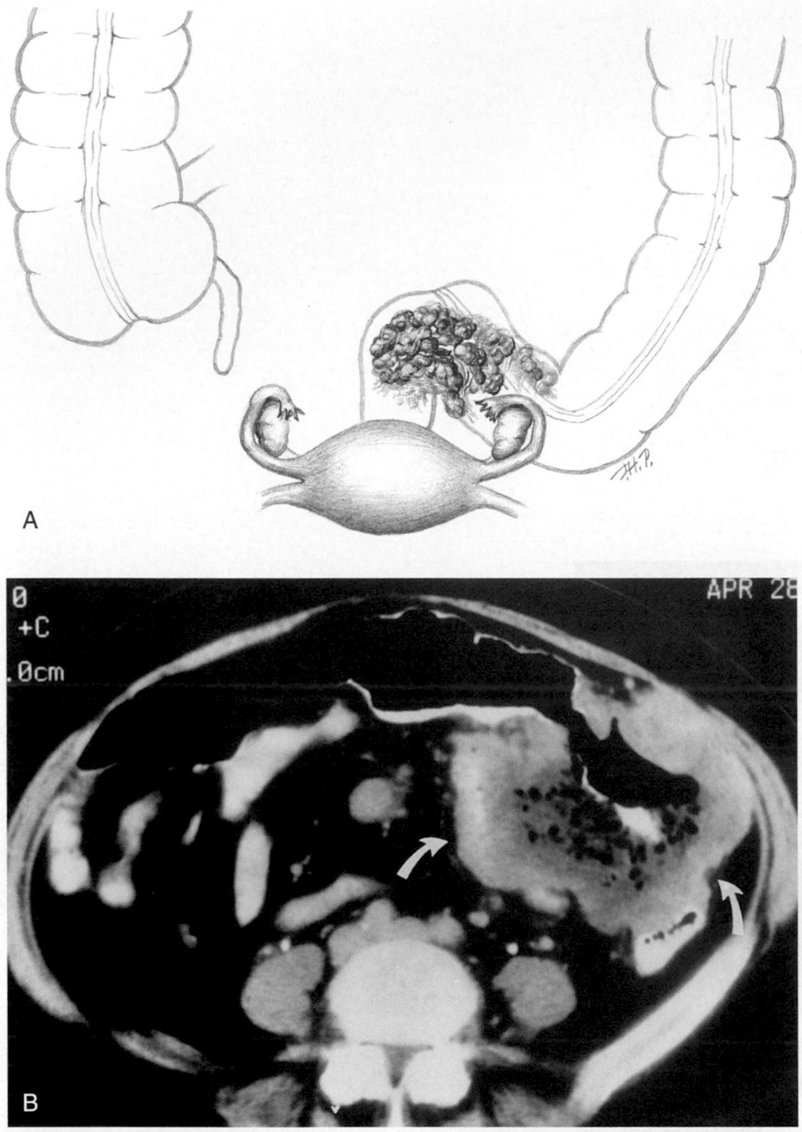

FIGURE 44.5. Rectosigmoid carcinoma. **A:** This tumor may encroach on the left adnexa and be mistaken for gynecologic disease. **B:** CT image shows a large sigmoid carcinoma (*arrows*) containing a necrotic tumor and gas centrally. (Courtesy of T. Demos, Maywood, IL.)

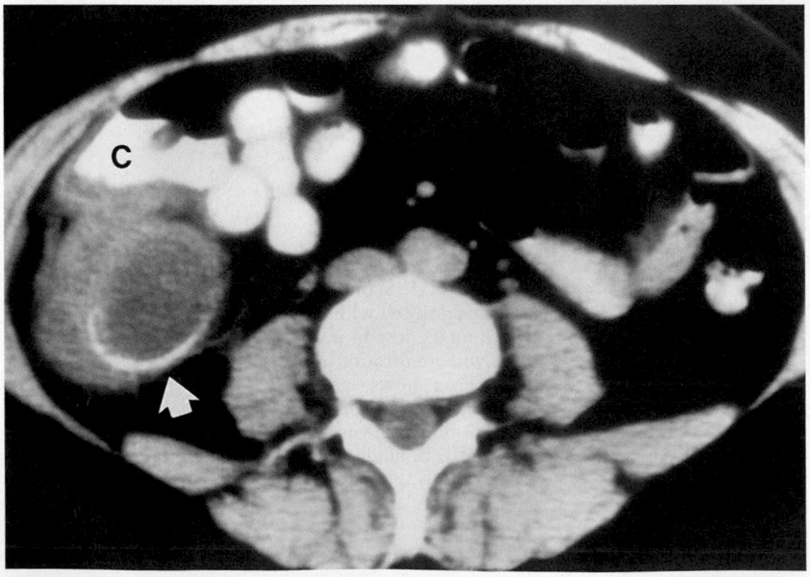

FIGURE 44.6. Infected mucocele of the appendix. CT image shows a mucocele (*arrow*), which has a thin rim of calcification and indents the cecum (*C*). (Courtesy of T. Demos, Maywood, IL.)

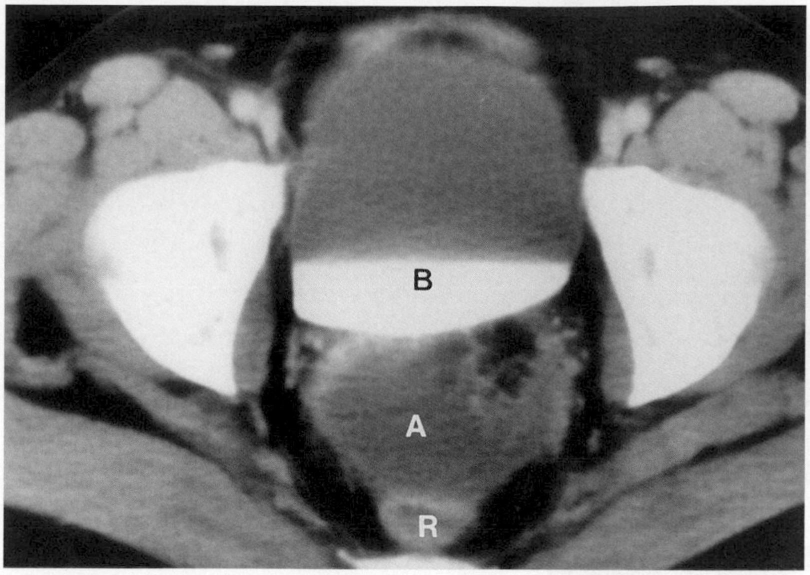

FIGURE 44.7. Appendicitis with pouch of Douglas abscess. CT image shows a large abscess (*A*) between the rectum (*R*) and the bladder (*B*). (Courtesy of T. Demos, Maywood, IL.)

tumors occur often enough within the pelvis that the gynecologic surgeon must keep such tumors in mind, especially when dealing with vague or unusual pelvic symptoms and physical findings. Beck reported on seven collected series of retroperitoneal tumors and noted that the major symptoms include abdominal pain, abdominal mass or swelling, and weight loss or anorexia, or both. The symptoms depend on the location of the tumor in the retroperitoneal space. Retroperitoneal tumors in the pelvis may become manifest earlier than those in the abdomen because the bony confines of the pelvis cause pressure on adjacent organs earlier than in the upper abdomen. Sarcomas of the pelvic or buttocks muscles or bone will usually present with hip pain and leg edema.

Abnormal findings noted on an excretory urogram and on upper and lower gastrointestinal x-ray studies may be secondary to extrinsic involvement rather than intrinsic pathology. The most reliable tools for diagnosing retroperitoneal tumors are CT scanning and magnetic resonance imaging (MRI).

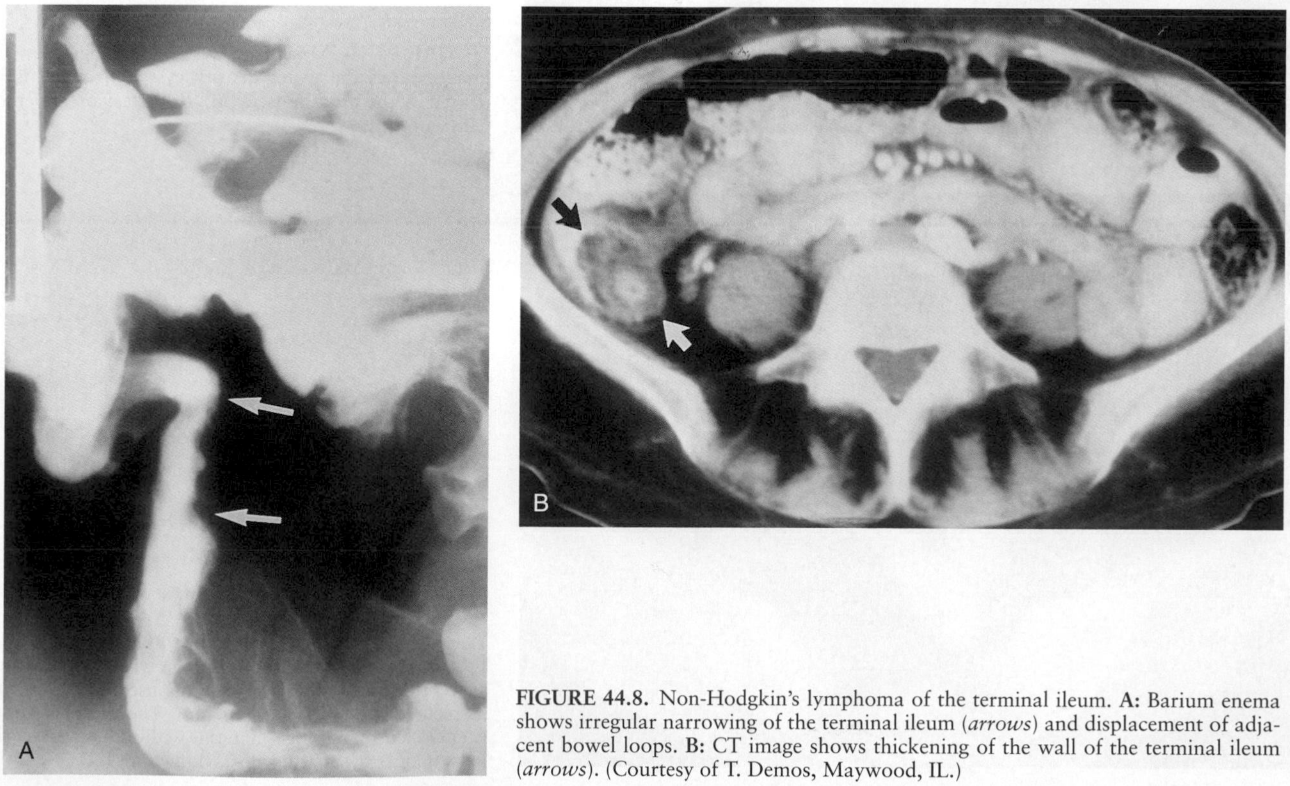

FIGURE 44.8. Non-Hodgkin's lymphoma of the terminal ileum. **A:** Barium enema shows irregular narrowing of the terminal ileum (*arrows*) and displacement of adjacent bowel loops. **B:** CT image shows thickening of the wall of the terminal ileum (*arrows*). (Courtesy of T. Demos, Maywood, IL.)

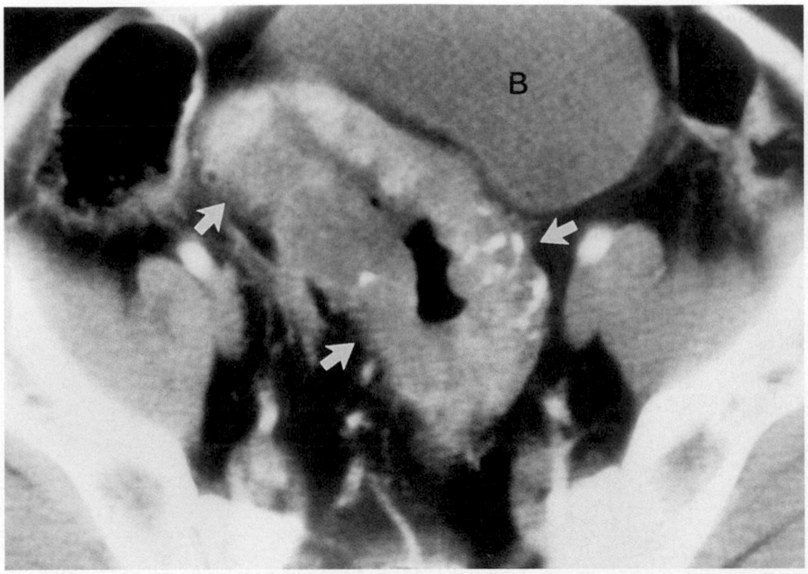

FIGURE 44.9. Ulcerative colitis with sigmoid carcinoma. CT image shows circumferential sigmoid tumor (*arrows*), which indents the bladder (*B*). (Courtesy of T. Demos, Maywood, IL.)

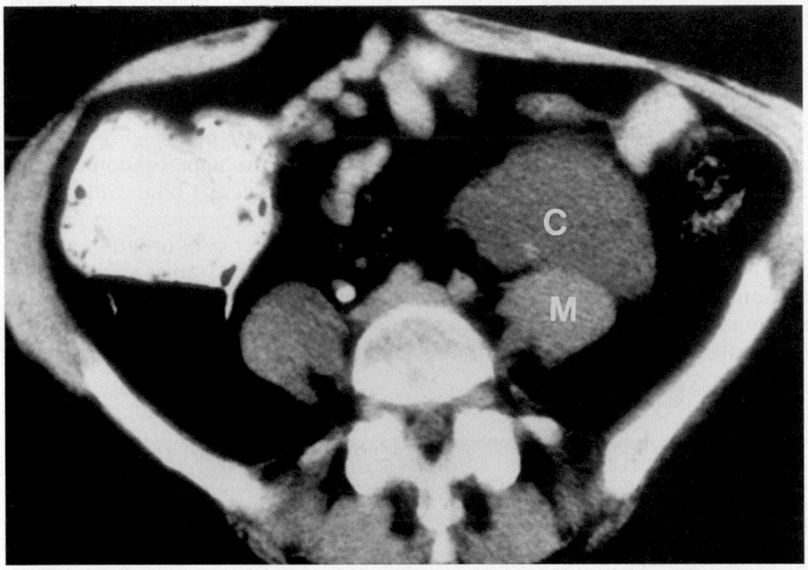

FIGURE 44.10. Mesenteric cyst (lymphangioma). CT image shows the water density cyst (*C*), which is indented by the psoas muscle (*M*). (Courtesy of T. Demos, Maywood, IL.)

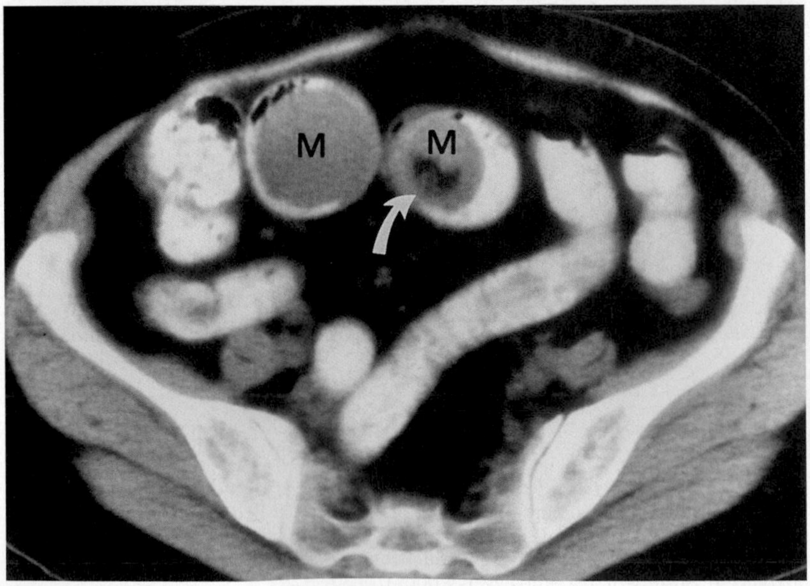

FIGURE 44.11. Small bowel polyp with ileoileal intussusception. CT image shows intussusceptum (*M*) with associated mesenteric fat (*arrow*). The intussusceptum is encircled by contrast material within the intussuscipiens. (Courtesy of T. Demos, Maywood, IL.)

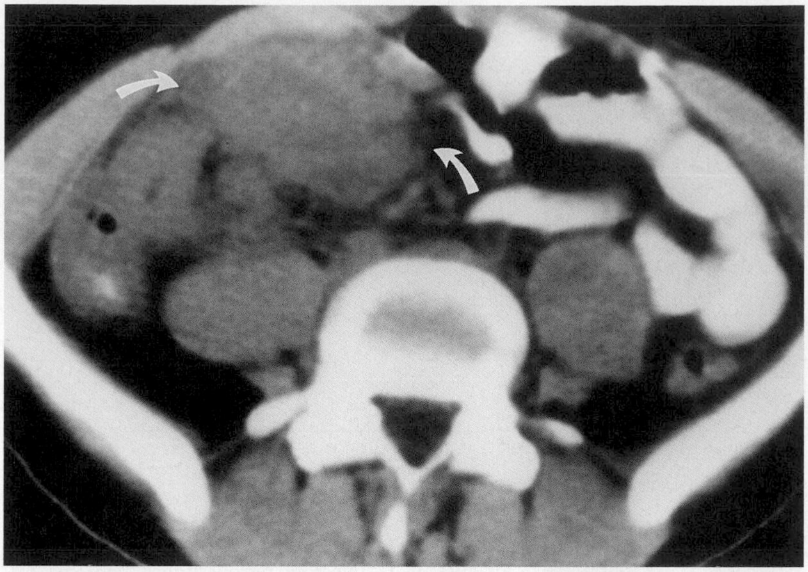

FIGURE 44.12. Crohn's disease with pelvic abscess. CT image shows an inhomogeneous lesion (*arrows*) displacing the opacified intestine. This abscess cannot be differentiated from a phlegmon. (Courtesy of T. Demos, Maywood, IL.)

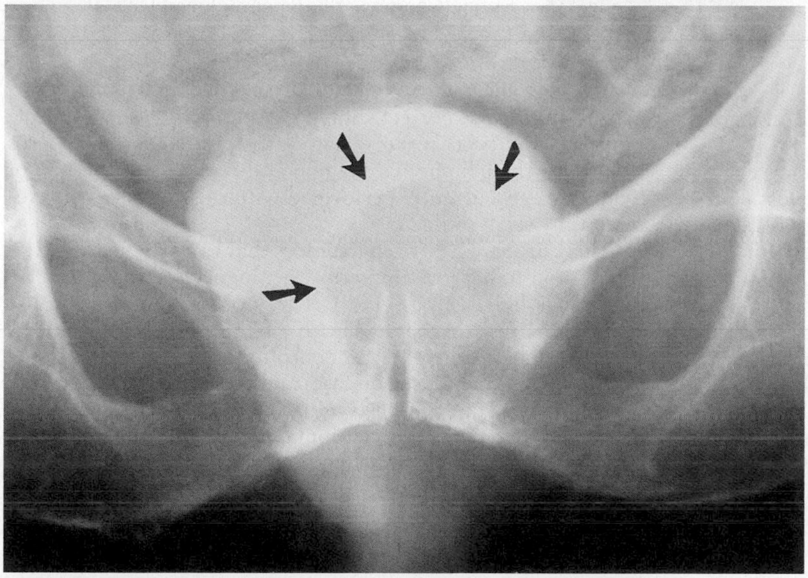

FIGURE 44.13. Urinary bladder carcinoma. Intravenous urogram shows inferior displacement of the bladder because of a cystocele. The bladder tumor produces a lobulated filling defect (*arrows*). (Courtesy of T. Demos, Maywood, IL.)

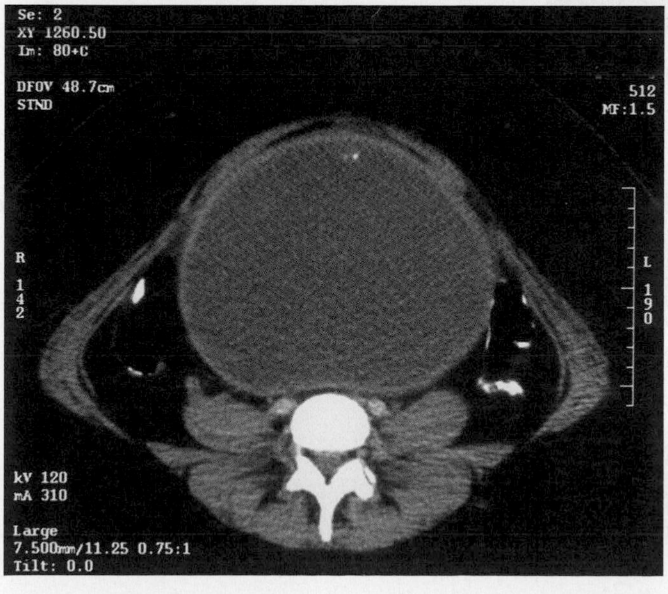

FIGURE 44.14. CT image of a large midline mass in a 25-year-old patient that on final pathology was a necrotic benign urachal cyst. (Courtesy of J. Dolan, Park Ridge, IL.)

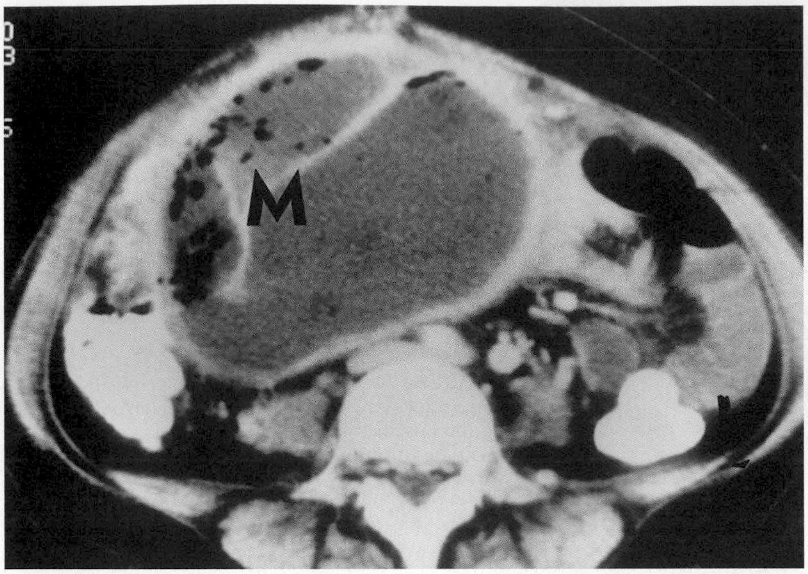

FIGURE 44.15. Necrotic retroperitoneal teratoma. CT image shows a large septate mass (*M*), which contains fluid and gas. Opacified intestine is draped around the lesion. (Courtesy of R. Benjoya, Libertyville, IL.)

Figures 44.15 through 44.17 demonstrate CT and MRI images of retroperitoneal pathology.

If the tumor is a lymphoma, a careful history may elicit reports of fever, night sweats, pruritus, and weight loss. On physical examination, patients with a lymphoma may have skin nodules, enlarged lymph nodes, liver and spleen enlargement, and areas of joint or bone tenderness. On pelvic examination, large external iliac lymph nodes may be mistaken for an adnexal mass, but careful examination will often reveal that these firm, smooth masses bulge outward from the pelvic sidewall, where they are firmly fixed and the uterus remains viable. There is no nodular tumor or inflammatory induration in the cul-de-sac. Figure 44.18 illustrates a CT image of a patient with an ilealcecal lymphoma and mesenteric adenopathy. A biopsy of a peripheral lymph node or skin nodule may establish the diagnosis of lymphoma and allow enough tissue for proper characterization of the correct subtype. Additionally, a core needle biopsy of the bone marrow can be helpful as a staging procedure for the lymphoma. Staging and response to therapy of lymphomas is currently performed with positron emission tomography scans and CT.

There are rare neurogenic tumors that can arise in the pelvis in addition to very rare anterior meningoceles and arachnoid cysts (Figs. 44.19 and 44.20). The most common are those that arise from the nerve sheath of the obturator or sacral nerve complex, which are the neurofibromas (often associated with von Recklinghausen disease) and the neurilemmomas. Tumors may develop from the sympathetic nervous system of the pelvis and include ganglioneuroma, sympathicoblastoma, and neuroblastoma. As with the lymphomas noted above, a firmly fixed mass bulging outward from the pelvic sidewall is often palpable on pelvic examination.

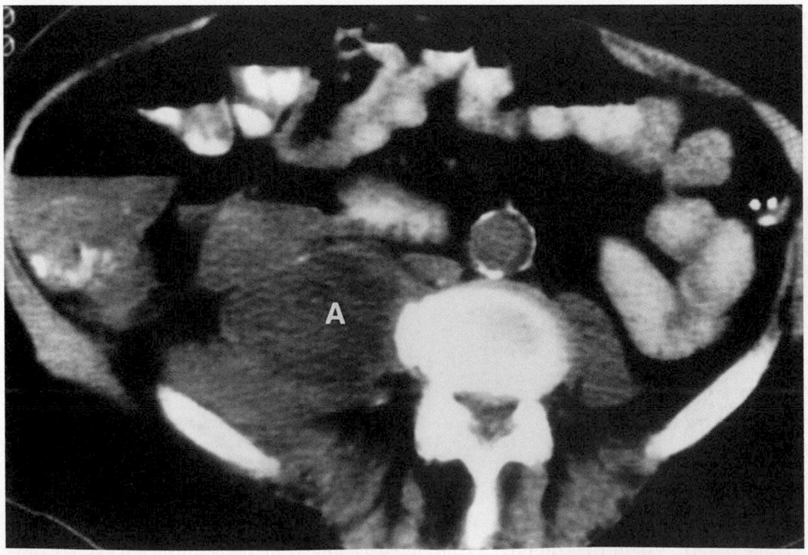

FIGURE 44.16. Large psoas abscess. CT image shows a large low-density psoas abscess (*A*). (Courtesy of T. Demos, Maywood, IL.)

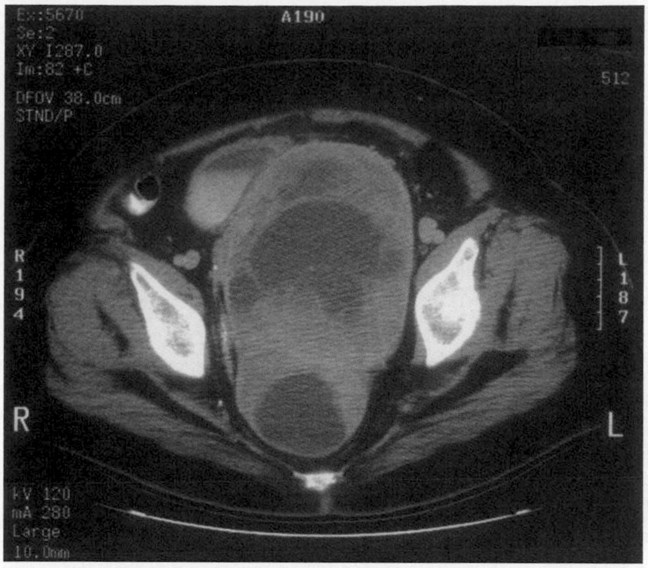

FIGURE 44.17. CT image of a large retroperitoneal pelvic schwannoma. Note displacement of the bladder anteriorly. (Courtesy of J. Dolan, Park Ridge, IL.)

Soft-tissue sarcomas may occur anywhere in the retroperitoneal space. According to Adam and associates, these tumors are diagnosed most easily by CT scan, but ultrasonography, arteriography, and venography may be useful. Figure 44.21 demonstrates an intravenous urogram of a large pelvic neurofibroma with sarcomatous degeneration. Figure 44.22 demonstrates a CT scan of a large neurofibrosarcoma in the right sciatic notch in a 25-year-old patient with von Recklinghausen disease.

Lewis and colleagues reported on 500 patients with retroperitoneal sarcomas and found the most common were liposarcomas and leiomyosarcomas. Survival was inversely related to tumor size, and complete surgical resection with a tumor-free margin offered the best survival.

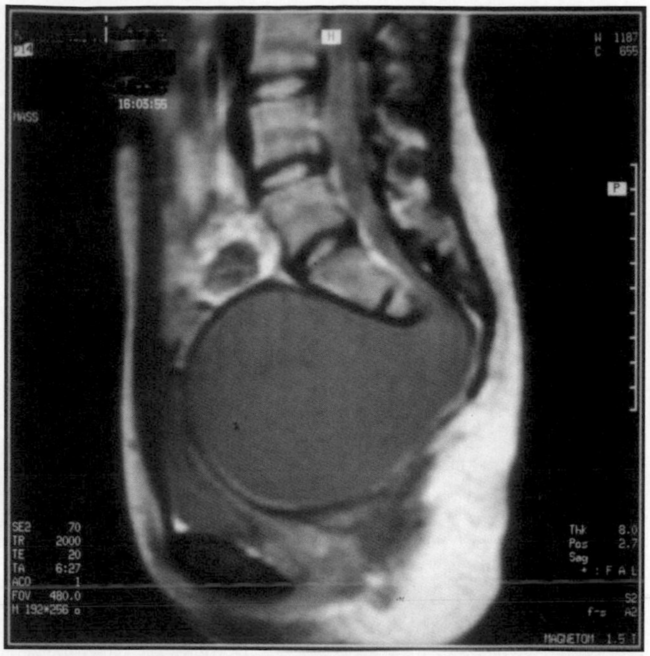

FIGURE 44.19. MRI image of a large anterior meningocele in an 18-year-old patient with chronic headache following Valsalva and squatting. The patient also noted constipation, urinary difficulties, and low-back pain. (Courtesy of J. Dolan, Park Ridge, IL.)

Orthopedic Disorders

Disorders that may arise from the bony pelvis include those that are congenital, iatrogenic, metabolic, or septic, as well as fractures and tumors. The congenital or developmental abnormalities include anterior sacral meningocele (discussed above), spondylolisthesis, and sacrococcygeal teratomas. Spondylolisthesis is a slow, forward displacement of the lumbar spine over

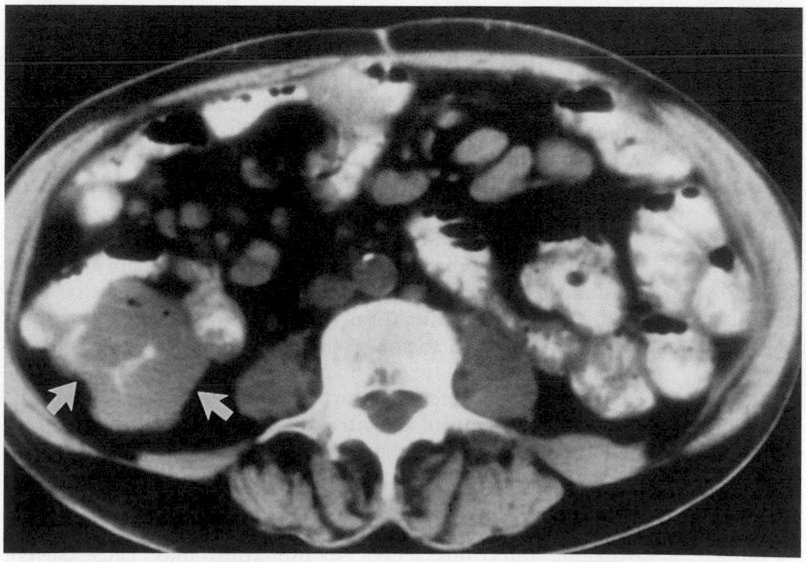

FIGURE 44.18. Ileocecal non-Hodgkin's lymphoma with mesenteric adenopathy. CT image shows an ileocecal mass (*arrows*). There are numerous oval, enlarged mesenteric lymph nodes between opacified loops of intestine. (Courtesy of T. Demos, Maywood, IL.)

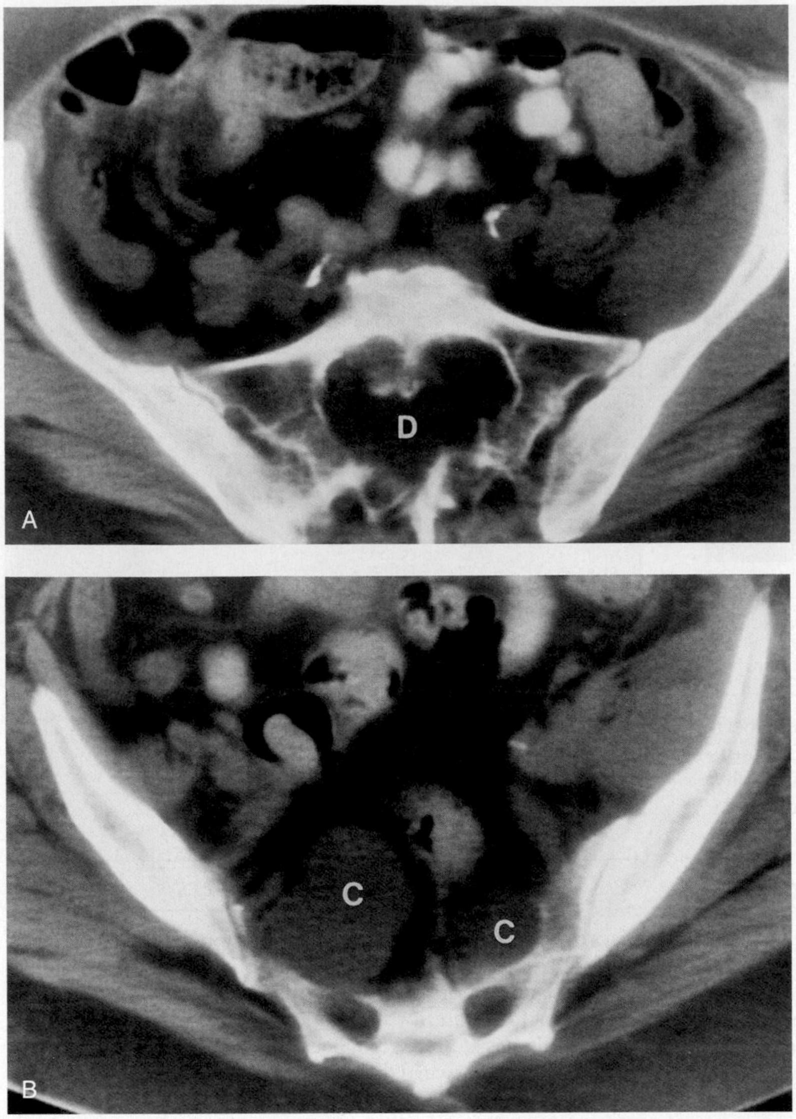

FIGURE 44.20. Arachnoid cysts. **A:** CT image shows a central defect (*D*) of the sacrum. **B:** A more inferior CT image shows water density arachnoid cysts (*C*) bulging into the pelvis. (Courtesy of T. Demos, Maywood, IL.)

the sacrum. The degree of slip usually is not severe enough to cause significant impairment. If the entire fifth lumbar vertebra is displaced forward of the sacrum (spondyloptosis), severe narrowing of the anteroposterior diameter of the pelvis and displacement of the pelvic viscera are noted. Pelvic examination is significantly abnormal. A pelvic radiograph or CT defines the problem.

Sacrococcygeal teratomas usually are diagnosed by age 2 or 3, but occasionally the dermoid forms are not discovered until early adulthood. These anomalies are four times more common in women, and malignant forms are more common in adults. Such lesions usually can be defined by ultrasonography and CT (Fig. 44.23).

Total hip arthroplasty has become commonplace since it was introduced in the 1960s. In some earlier cases, the inner wall of the acetabulum was penetrated, allowing the cement (methyl methacrylate) to flow into the pelvis to improve fixation. The cement produces a bony, hard mass fixed to the pelvic wall that varies in size, shape, and convolution. If such a mass is encountered on pelvic examination, it may well represent a challenging diagnostic problem. Patients with prior total hip arthroplasty may develop an intrapelvic protrusion of the acetabular cup caused by trauma or weakness of the inner wall. This protrusion may be seen as a mass fixed to the pelvic sidewall, causing confusion and difficulty with diagnosis. Only a high degree of suspicion can alert the examining gynecologist that the hard, nodular fixed pelvic mass is, indeed, a cementing substance that should not be disturbed.

Certain metabolic disorders of the skeletal system can cause gradual development of pelvic deformities that may be confusing on pelvic examination. With bone deficiency, sometimes there is inward protrusion of the femoral head through the inner acetabular wall (protrusio acetabuli). Other causes of protrusion acetabuli include Marfan syndrome, Paget disease of the bone, rheumatoid arthritis, and osteomalacia.

Fungal, parasitic, and pyogenic afflictions of the bony pelvis can cause the development of soft tissue masses that may be difficult to diagnose. Most of these cases present as acute, painful infectious processes, but some develop as subacute or chronic pyogenic infections. Pelvic examination may cause severe

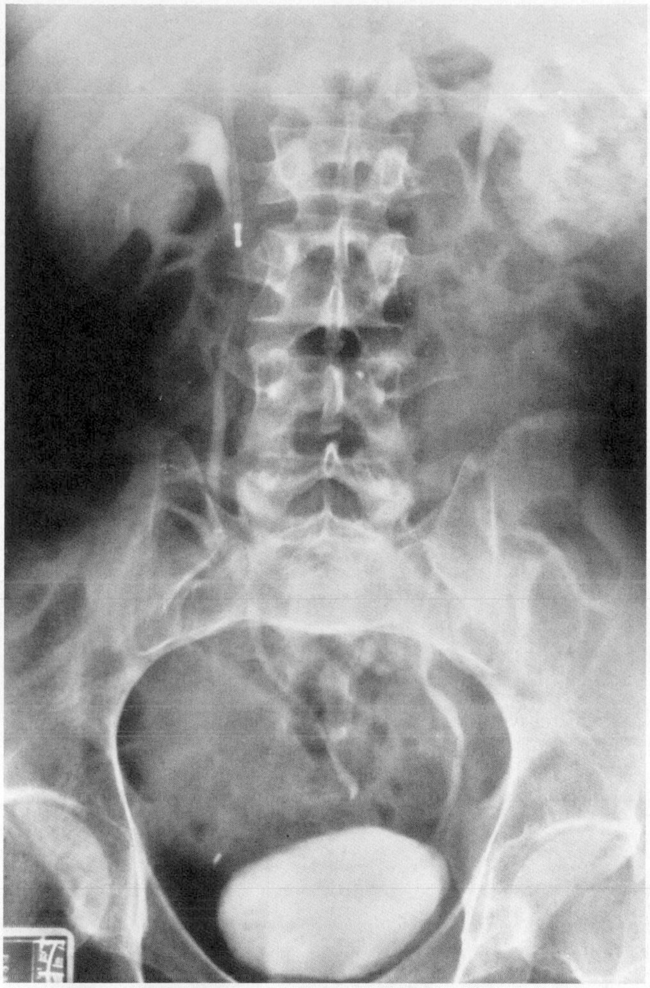

FIGURE 44.21. Neurofibromatosis with pelvic sarcoma. Intravenous urogram shows the distal right ureter displaced by a soft-tissue mass within the pelvis. (There is a ventriculoperitoneal shunt extending to the right upper quadrant.) (Courtesy of T. Demos, Maywood, IL.)

discomfort and produce findings suggestive of a deep fullness or masses on either pelvic sidewall. Sometimes such infections present as a presacral abscess. There usually is an associated tenderness over the sacroiliac joints and both buttocks.

A rather common cause of intrapelvic distortion is a residual bony deformity resulting from a pelvic fracture. These are often the result of an automobile accident or other major trauma. Radiologic examination of the pelvis reveals the cause of the unusual findings.

Primary bone tumors that involve the pelvis are quite rare except for those on the anterior sacrum. The sacrum is the primary site of more than 50% of chordomas (malignant) and 6% of giant cell tumors (benign). These tumors usually may be discovered on pelvic or rectal examination. Urinary frequency and constipation are common presenting symptoms. Radiographic studies of the pelvis usually are sufficient for diagnosis, and a technetium 99 bone scan may demonstrate bone destruction not apparent on the radiographic films. MRI gives far better detail to delineate bone and nerve involvement.

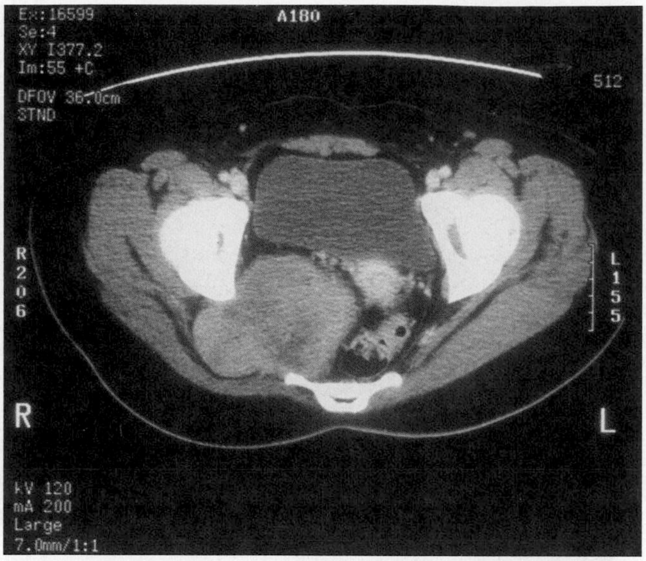

FIGURE 44.22. Retroperitoneal sarcoma. Demonstrates a CT scan of a large neurofibrosarcoma originating from the right sciatic nerve. Note intrapelvic and extrapelvic extension through the sciatic notch with displacement of the rectum laterally. (Courtesy of J. Dolan, Park Ridge, IL.)

Vascular Considerations

Two significant vascular lesions of the pelvis are iliac aneurysms and arteriovenous fistulas. Isolated iliac aneurysms are rare, but many patients with abdominal aortic aneurysms have associated iliac aneurysms. They are more common on the common iliac and hypogastric arteries and very rare on the external iliac artery. Most iliac aneurysms remain asymptomatic until rupture unless they impinge on adjacent structures. Diagnosis of iliac artery aneurysms is difficult, but ultrasonography and CT scanning occasionally detect these vascular conditions. Figure 44.24A shows a barium enema with extrinsic pressure on the colon by the iliac aneurysm. Figure 44.24B demonstrates an iliac arterial aneurysm on CT scan. Contrast angiography is necessary to formulate the therapeutic plan.

Pelvic arteriography is a valuable part of preoperative evaluation of unusual pelvic tumors or findings. Although pelvic arteriography is not often necessary, it helps to delineate a highly vascular tumor. Hasty exploration without knowledge of the source of the blood supply of the tumor could lead to uncontrollable hemorrhage.

Aneurysms that are symptomatic because of local factors or because of distal emboli should be carefully evaluated. Growing aneurysms should almost always be resected. Internal iliac aneurysms are usually not resected but are treated by simple ligation.

Metastatic Lesions to the Pelvis

The ovary is a frequent recipient of metastases from numerous primary sites. In comparison with the ovary, solitary extragenital metastases to the fallopian tubes or uterus are rare. Although statistics vary, probably 5% to 10% of all ovarian tumors are metastatic in origin. The most common metastases to the ovary are from the colon, stomach, breast, and the uterus.

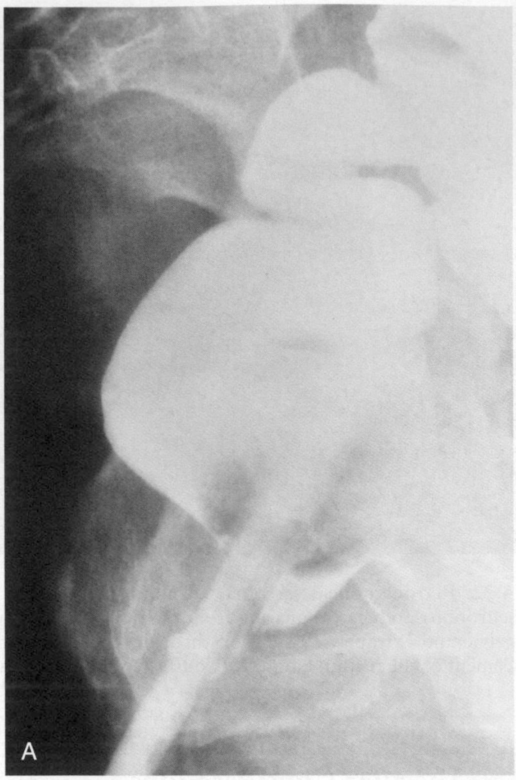

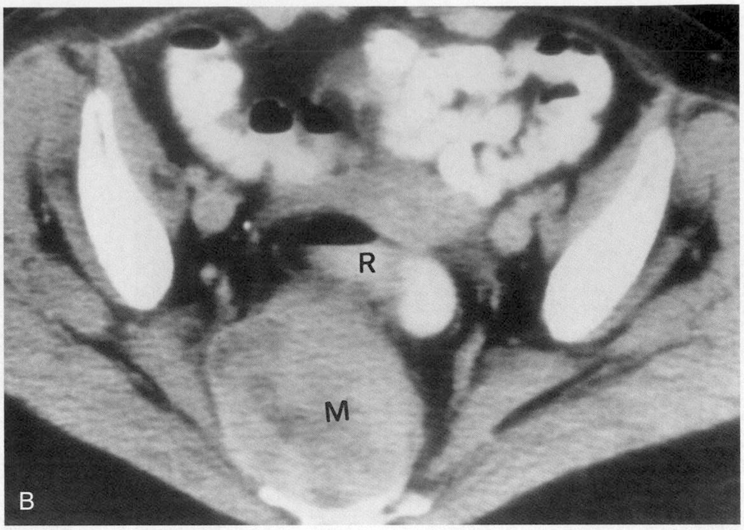

FIGURE 44.23. Presacral teratoma. CT image shows a soft tissue mass (*M*), which deforms the sacrum and displaces the rectum (*R*) anteriorly. (Courtesy of K. Baliga, Rockford, IL.)

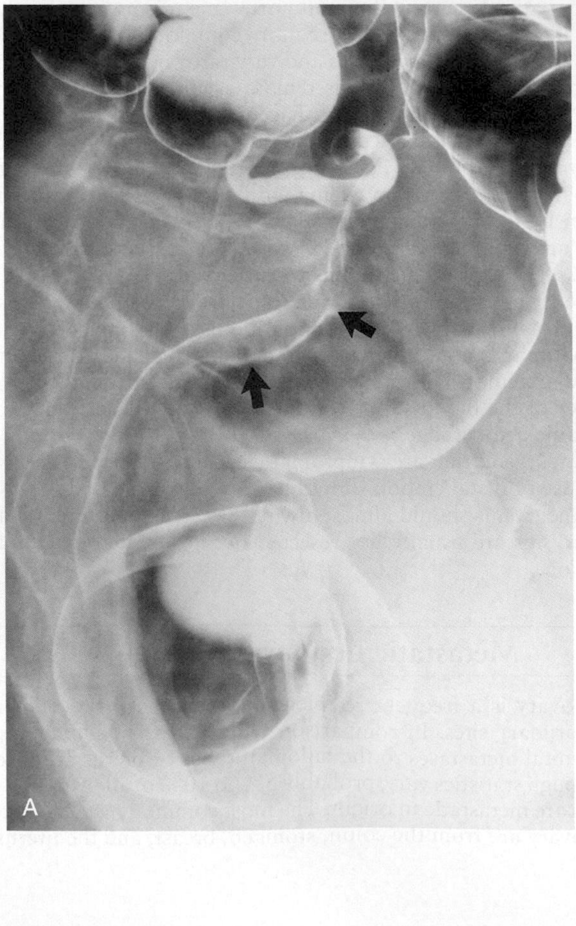

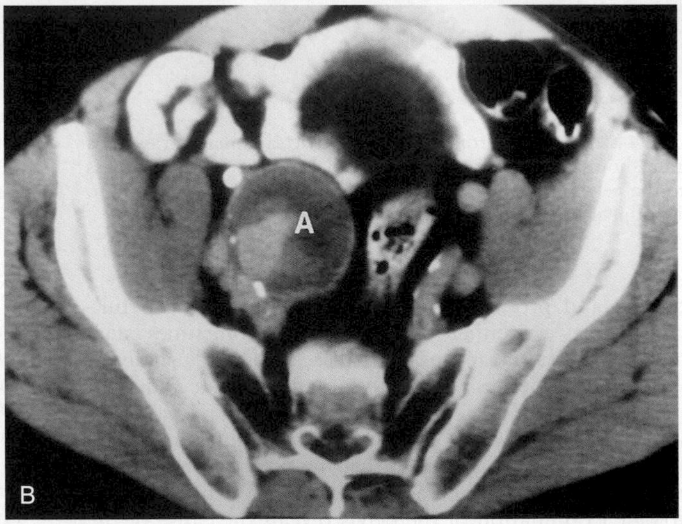

FIGURE 44.24. Iliac artery aneurysm. **A:** Barium enema shows extrinsic filling defect (*arrows*) of the rectosigmoid. **B:** CT image shows an iliac artery aneurysm (*A*), which contains a clot. Adjacent bowel is displaced. (Courtesy of T. Demos, Maywood, IL.)

The functional ovary seems particularly prone to extragenital metastatic disease. The possibility of an extragenital primary cancer with metastases to one or both ovaries should always be considered and can usually be ruled out by a careful preoperative history, physical examination, and appropriate imaging. When the ovarian metastases are from the gastrointestinal tract, they are almost always bilateral. When the ovarian metastases are from gastrointestinal cancer, both ovaries usually become symmetrically enlarged while retaining their shape and capsular integrity.

Nonsurgical Acute Abdomen

There are a number of nonsurgical causes of acute abdominal pain that may be mistaken for a gynecologic problem. *Sickle cell anemia* is one of these conditions. Such patients may have attacks of bone and joint pain, but also may suffer abdominal pain. The major disabilities suffered by patients with sickle cell anemia are related to painful vasoocclusive crises and occlusion of the microvasculature by the sickling phenomenon. Precipitating factors are infection, hypoxia, dehydration, and acidosis. A careful history and laboratory testing for sickle cells and hemoglobin S usually establish the diagnosis.

Recurrent attacks of abdominal pain occur with *acute porphyria*. This disease is an autosomal dominant condition and is most common in women in the third and fourth decades of life. Abdominal tenderness is much less than would be expected, considering the severity of pain. Activation of the disease is related to factors such as medications, infections, low-calorie diets, and steroid hormones. Fever and leukocytosis may be present, and abdominal radiologic studies show distended loops of bowel. Diagnosis is made by a history of similar attacks and by the quantitative detection of excessive porphobilinogen and aminolevulinate in a 24-hour urine collection.

Other nonsurgical causes of abdominal pain include familial Mediterranean fever, lower-lobe pneumonia, rectus sheath hematoma (frequently preceded by a paroxysm of coughing), pyelonephritis, and acute viral gastroenteritis.

PREOPERATIVE PREPARATION

Preparation of the patient for pelvic surgery begins with the establishment of as accurate a diagnosis as possible. Because an absolute diagnosis is not always possible, the extent of the surgery is difficult and sometimes impossible to determine. Thus, when major pelvic surgery is anticipated, it is imperative that the patient (and often the family) be as well informed as possible. If the patient understands that bowel or bladder resection may be needed, requiring a colostomy, ileostomy, or urinary conduit, she will be much better prepared to cope with these problems postoperatively. It cannot be overemphasized that despite extensive diagnostic strides, it is not always possible to know what the findings might be until the abdomen is opened. It is prudent to advise the patient and the family that intraoperative consultation with other surgical subspecialists may be necessary. If consultation is likely, it is very appropriate for the patient to meet these specialists before the contemplated surgery.

Preoperative Bowel Preparation

If there is a possibility that a portion of the colon will be opened or resected, bowel preparation should be carried out. We prefer a combined mechanical and antibiotic bowel preparation. The most commonly used bowel prep is an isotonic lavage solution such as GoLYTELY or Colyte.

The patient may have a light lunch of a high-protein, low-residue diet and clear liquid dinner the day before surgery. To achieve sufficient cleansing of the colon, approximately 4 L of solution must be ingested over a 4-hour period. We usually have patients begin the Colyte at around noon the day before surgery and ask that they drink 8 to 16 ounces every 10 to 15 minutes. Most surgeons also use a combination of oral antibiotics, erythromycin base (1 g) and neomycin (1 g) at 1 P.M., 2 P.M., and 11 P.M. the day before the operation. Additionally, broad-spectrum intravenous antibiotics are given preoperatively and may be continued after surgery if there is gross contamination or if an infectious process is encountered.

Additional Preoperative Preparation

If the patient is nutritionally depleted because of extrinsic or intrinsic bowel obstruction or dysfunction, preoperative nutritional support is indicated, usually by instituting total parenteral nutrition. Dehydrated patients undergoing bowel preparation should be given intravenous fluids and appropriate electrolytes for 16 to 24 hours before major pelvic surgery. This is particularly important in the older patient.

Prior bleeding problems must be investigated. Patients on broad-spectrum antibiotics and those with multiple or prolonged bowel prep for imaging studies, colonoscopy, or surgery may have a prolonged prothrombin time secondary to depressed vitamin K absorption. Such patients usually respond well to vitamin K in doses of 10 mg/day for 2 days preoperatively. Some medications, such as aspirin and coumarin, may be forgotten by the patient, and the physician should ask specifically about recent use of these medications.

Patients receiving chronic corticosteroids will need additional corticosteroids during surgery. Postoperatively, the corticosteroids are tapered down over 4 to 5 days to their usual maintenance dose.

Patients with cardiopulmonary problems should have maximum pulmonary preparation. Smoking should be stopped several days before surgery. If possible, pulmonary toilet with chest physiotherapy and incentive spirometry can begin when preoperative workup takes place. Preoperative consultation with anesthesiologists, pulmonologists, and cardiologists may be appropriate for the elderly patient and patients with multiple concomitant severe medical problems.

INTRAOPERATIVE MANAGEMENT OF NONGYNECOLOGIC PELVIC DISORDERS

After a thorough history and physical examination and a meticulous diagnostic laboratory workup, most nongynecologic conditions should have been diagnosed, or at least highly suspected, before laparotomy. However, situations may still arise that are outside the purview of the gynecologic surgeon, and intraoperative consultation is indicated.

Once the abdomen has been opened, a thorough evaluation of the upper abdomen and the pelvis is necessary. If the upper abdomen is normal, the upper abdominal contents should be packed away with laparotomy pads and the patient placed in

Trendelenburg position. Next, the pelvic findings are assessed and the problem analyzed, with the tissues being put in as near an anatomically normal position as possible. If dense adhesions are present, these should be lysed by sharp dissection. If the disease involves the uterus or fallopian tubes and ovaries with extension into the surrounding organs, the appropriate surgery to remove the diseased organs should be undertaken. Depending on the pathology, this may be within the gynecologist's expertise; if not, another surgical specialist should be consulted.

If the findings are not gynecologic in nature, then a determination of the problem is essential. The most common nongynecologic condition encountered is disease of the gastrointestinal tract, including colon cancer and a diverticular abscess. If the colon and small bowel are normal, the gynecologic surgeon must consider retroperitoneal tumors or pathology of the distal ureter or urinary bladder. If the patient has had an adequate bowel preparation and has been apprised of the various possibilities (i.e., colostomy, bowel resection, urinary diversion, excessive blood loss, and possibly prolonged hospital stay), then definitive surgery should be carried out. If these precautions have not been taken preoperatively, the abdomen should be closed; the surgeon must explain to the patient and family the diagnosis and plans for further management, including consultation and referral.

Gastrointestinal Disease

Appendicitis

Appendicitis frequently involves gynecologic conditions in the differential diagnosis. It is discussed in Chapter 42.

Diverticulitis

The usual therapy for diverticulitis is medical. Most patients with acute diverticulitis should be hospitalized for bowel rest, intravenous fluids, and broad-spectrum antibiotics. Repeated attacks of diverticulitis in the same area generally require surgical resection. Severe attacks with acute peritoneal signs, fistula formation, suspected abscess, or perforation require intravenous antibiotics directed against Gram-negative anaerobic bacteria, followed by surgical drainage or resection.

In operating on a patient for what was presumed to be recurring attacks of pelvic inflammatory disease or an ovarian mass, the gynecologist may find a portion of the rectosigmoid colon involved with diverticulitis. If the colon has been preoperatively prepared and cleansed, the patient may undergo elective resection of the involved segment of colon and a primary anastomosis with a very low operative risk. On the other hand, if there is acute inflammation with evidence of perforation, fistula, obstruction, or bleeding, the diseased colon must be mobilized and resected. The proximal colon is brought out as an end colostomy, and the distal rectal segment is closed (Hartmann procedure). The colon may be reanastomosed 2 to 3 months after recovery.

Cancer of the Colon and Rectum

Cancer of the colon is predominantly a disease of older people, but it can occur at any age. It is important to remember that the incidence of right-sided colon cancer is steadily increasing. Radical surgical removal of the primary lesion is the only acceptable curative therapy. If a colon cancer is found unexpectedly and the bowel has had both mechanical and antibiotic preparation, an appropriate resection should be carried out by a surgeon experienced in colorectal surgery. A carcinoembryonic (CEA) blood sample should be obtained. This is helpful when follow-up CEA levels are obtained. If the patient has not had suitable bowel preparation, or if a surgeon experienced in colorectal surgery is not available, the abdomen should be closed and definitive surgery performed at a later date. The resection includes the entire segment of the involved portion of the colon and its associated lymphovascular pedicle up to the level of its takeoff from the aorta for left colon lesions or to the mesenteric vessels for right colon lesions. Primary resection and anastomosis of right colon lesions may be carried out even in the absence of prior bowel preparation with a very low incidence of postoperative infection.

Crohn's Disease

Crohn's disease (regional enteritis) is a chronic inflammatory disorder of the gastrointestinal tract of unknown cause. Because it usually involves the terminal ileum and proximal colon, it may easily be mistaken by history and pelvic examination as an inflammatory process of the appendix, fallopian tube, or ovary. The most common symptom is right lower quadrant pain that usually is associated with fever, diarrhea without blood, weight loss, fatigability, and a tender, palpable abdominal mass. The disease most commonly has its onset in the young, but there appears to be an increased incidence in people after age 60. The complications of the disease are often local, resulting from intestinal inflammation and involvement of adjacent viscera. Intestinal obstruction, fistula formation, right ureteral obstruction and hydronephrosis, malabsorption, anorexia, and intestinal perforation with abscess formation are all possible manifestations and complications of this disease. Endoscopic exam of the colon and radiologic studies of the bowel are most important in establishing the diagnosis of inflammatory bowel disease. At laparotomy, the finding of thickened mesentery with growth of mesenteric fat ("fat wrapping") around the circumference of leathery fibrotic bowel is almost always pathognomonic of Crohn's disease. Intraoperative management of incidentally discovered Crohn's disease depends on the indication for operation and the experience of the surgeon. Patients explored for pelvic inflammatory disease who are found to have perforated Crohn's disease need resection, possibly including an ileostomy. Like complicated diverticular disease, these resections can be quite challenging and hazardous for the occasional surgeon. Patients explored for a mass and found to have diseased terminal ileum without perforation may be resected in some cases (if there is evidence of proximal obstruction), or the patient may be closed and further examinations carried out. Most patients with small-bowel disease can have endoscopic biopsy to confirm the diagnosis and then are managed medically. Surgery is held in reserve until complications (stricture, obstruction, abscess) develop. Current surgical management of Crohn's disease involves very conservative resections, preserving bowel length to avoid short-bowel syndrome, caused by repeated resections of progressively involved bowel. Crohn's disease is not cured surgically and recurs in more than 75% of patients with ileocecal Crohn's disease, the most common site of the disease. Bypass procedures for obstructing Crohn's disease are of historical interest only; current surgical treatment involves resection or stricturoplasty.

Metastatic Carcinoma of the Ovaries

Metastatic carcinoma to the endometrium or fallopian tube from distant sites may occur, but this is relatively rare and does not present a surgical dilemma to the gynecologist. The uterus, tubes, and ovaries are removed, and the presence of metastatic lesions most often is discovered in the pathology laboratory.

The ovaries, on the other hand, are a frequent site of metastases from cancer originating in many different organs, including the breast, stomach, pancreas, and colon. It has been reported by Israel and colleagues and by Webb and coworkers that young women are more prone to metastatic carcinoma than to primary ovarian cancer and that one half of all women with ovarian metastases are premenopausal.

In most situations, ovarian metastases can be regarded as a local manifestation of generalized carcinomatosis, and extensive resection is not indicated. Ovarian metastases from the colon may have a better prognosis if aggressive resection is undertaken, providing all gross tumor can be extirpated. Morrow and Enker have noted that the most important discriminant of survival in patients with metastatic ovarian disease from colorectal cancer was whether the patient could be surgically rendered free of gross disease. In their series, the mean survival rate for patients rendered free of gross disease was 48 months, compared with 8 months for all other patients. Thus, significant palliation is achieved by removing large tumor masses in and around the ovaries. Aggressive resection seems justified if such a lesion is encountered by the gynecologic surgeon, particularly if the metastases represents a late recurrence of colon cancer.

Urologic Disease

The most common retroperitoneal urologic mass to be encountered is a pelvic or horseshoe kidney. It is important to realize that pelvic and horseshoe kidneys have an arterial supply that courses much more anteriorly than the normal kidney, and their collecting system lies anteriorly as well, exposing both to risk of injury. An attempt should be made to identify a renal pelvis or ureter if the retroperitoneal mass appears to be a kidney. Aspiration with a 22-gauge needle may reveal the presence of urine within the mass. Excretory urography can be performed during surgery by intravenously injecting 50 to 100 mL of contrast material and taking a 10- to 20-minute supine film. An alternative is to inject 5 to 10 mL of indigo carmine intravenously and obtain an aspirate from the suspected renal pelvis 5 to 10 minutes later. The presence of blue or green urine confirms that the mass is a functioning kidney. One cannot rely on palpation of the ipsilateral or contralateral side to ascertain that a kidney is present. According to Schuster, "palpating the kidney" was done in almost all the reported cases of removal of a solitary pelvic kidney, and the surgeon thought a normal kidney was present in its usual proper position. If the surgeon unwittingly attempts to remove a pelvic kidney, bleeding will become profuse as the "tumor mass" is entered. If the tumor mass is recognized as a kidney, the injured kidney usually can be repaired. Packing the wound will stop some of the small bleeders and control massive bleeding until the situation can be evaluated. If the vascular pedicle can be located, vascular clamps can be placed across the vessels and left for 30 minutes without harm to the kidney. The intrarenal blood vessels need to be individually ligated. Electrocautery will not stop parenchymal bleeding and may increase it. If defects in the collecting system are noted, these defects should be repaired with fine absorbable suture.

Tumors of the lower third of the ureter are five times more frequent than ureteral tumors of the upper third of the ureter. Although ureteral tumors normally are quite small, they may be large and infiltrate the surrounding tissue. When they infiltrate the surrounding tissues and are firm, theoretically they may be palpated on bimanual examination and mistaken for an adnexal or pelvic mass. The treatment of ureteral tumors traditionally has been nephroureterectomy with removal of the entire renal unit and ureter. Some authors believe that a more conservative approach—involving local resection of the tumor and cuff of the bladder with reimplantation of the ureter and preservation of the renal unit—is acceptable.

If an adequate preoperative workup has been carried out, it is unlikely that an unsuspected cancer of the bladder will be encountered. The surgeon may encounter a paraganglioma of the bladder wall invading adjacent loops of small bowel that had been mistaken for a leiomyoma or an adnexal mass. These tumors usually are benign and can be managed by resection of the involved portion of the bladder wall and small bowel. Hemangiopericytomas posterior to the bladder require total resection of the tumor mass.

Retroperitoneal Tumors

Although retroperitoneal tumors are relatively rare, the pelvic surgeon should be prepared to deal with them. Primary retroperitoneal tumors arise from retroperitoneal tissue that does not represent growth from another body organ in the retroperitoneum. Ackerman has compiled and classified a lengthy list of all the possible retroperitoneal tumors. *There is virtually no retroperitoneal tumor that should be resected if found unexpectedly at the time of operation for other pelvic disease.* Retroperitoneal sarcomas, teratomas, sacral chordomas, and anterior meningoceles all need careful preresection imaging and very specialized surgical techniques. Anterior meningoceles are best treated by neurosurgeons via a posterior transsacral laminectomy. Anterior abdominal management should be avoided because it carries a much higher risk of complications and meningitis. Even biopsy can cause severe bleeding, and retroperitoneal masses should not be biopsied without intraoperative consultation with the appropriate consultant scrubbed in. If the appropriate consultant is not available, it is more judicious to close the abdomen than to venture into a difficult retroperitoneal tumor.

SUMMARY

A thorough history, a physical examination, and appropriate laboratory and imaging procedures usually detect unsuspected pathology before laparotomy. Even if a thorough workup suggests gynecologic pathology, bowel preparation and a thorough discussion with the patient of problems that may be encountered will prevent many otherwise difficult, if not impossible, situations. Because gastrointestinal disease most often is the unexpected pathology, the gynecologist should be aware of the correct management of these disorders. Urinary tract pathology and retroperitoneal tumors should also be familiar to the gynecologic surgeon. Surgical management of retroperitoneal tumors requires a thorough knowledge of the retroperitoneal space and typically requires consultation with appropriate specialists if successful surgery is to be achieved.

BEST SURGICAL PRACTICES

- The pelvic surgeon must give careful consideration to the broad differential diagnosis of possible nongynecologic causes of a pelvic mass. Particular attention to the gastrointestinal tract is extremely important since the gastrointestinal tract is the most common nongynecologic source of a pelvic mass.

- When the diagnosis of a pelvic mass is uncertain, thorough evaluation of the gastrointestinal tract and urologic system before surgery using modern imaging techniques and endoscopy to further delineate normal from abnormal structures is often necessary.
- Thorough bowel preparation and consideration of cystoscopy with ureteral stent placement is helpful if there is a high degree of suspicion of potential secondary or possibly primary involvement of these organ systems.
- Intraoperative evaluation should entail complete and thorough assessment of the entire abdominal cavity, including the upper abdomen as well as the pelvis. The choice of the operative incision should also be predicated on the likelihood for need of exposure or access to the upper abdomen.
- Judicious use of nongynecologic surgical consultations is advised whenever the preoperative assessment or the intraoperative evaluation determine that the pelvic mass is nongynecologic in origin.
- Unknown retroperitoneal masses should be biopsied only with extreme caution. Resection of an unknown peritoneal mass is not recommended. Neurologic tumors or masses that present in the retroperitoneum are best approached by an intradisciplinary team frequently consisting of neurosurgeons, vascular surgeons, general surgeons, orthopedic surgeons, and the gynecologic surgeon.

ACKNOWLEDGMENT

Special thanks and acknowledgment to our mentor, John H. Isaacs, M.D.

Bibliography

Ackerman LV. Tumors of the retroperitoneum mesentery and peritoneum. In: Armed Forces Institute of Pathology. *Atlas of tumor pathology.* Section VI, Fascicles 23 & 24. Washington, DC: Armed Forces Institute of Pathology; 1954.

Adam YG, Halevy A, Reif R. Primary retroperitoneal soft tissue sarcomas. *J Surg Oncol* 1984;25:8.

Aufses AH. The surgery of granulomatous inflammatory bowel disease. In: *Current problems in surgery*. Chicago: Year Book Publishers; 1983; 755.

Bader I, Akhter N, Haq A, et al. Anterior sacral meningomyelocele with sacrococcygeal teratoma. *J Coll Phys Surg Pakistan* 2004;14(5):302.

Bartlett JG, Condon RE, Gorbach SL, et al. Veterans Administration cooperative study on bowel preparation for elective colorectal operations: impact of oral antibiotic regimen on colonic flora, wound irrigation cultures, and bacteriology of septic complications. *Ann Surg* 1978;188:249.

Beck HH. Retroperitoneal tumors: diagnosis and treatment. In: Isaacs JH, Byrne MP, eds. *Pelvic surgery: a multidisciplinary approach*. Mt. Kisco, NY: Futura Publishing Co.; 1987:91.

Chappins CW, Cohn I Jr. Acute colonic diverticulitis. *Surg Clin North Am* 1988;68:301.

Clarke JS, Condon RE, Bartlett JG, et al. Preoperative oral antibiotics reduce septic complications of colon operations. *Ann Surg* 1977;186:251.

Cohn I, Nance JC. The colon and rectum. In: Sabiston DC Jr, ed. *Textbook of surgery*. Philadelphia: WB Saunders; 1986:1004.

Condon RE. Appendicitis. In: Sabiston DC Jr, ed. *Textbook of surgery*. Philadelphia: WB Saunders; 1986:967.

Desnick RJ, Anderson K. Disorders of heme-biosynthesis: The porphyrias in hematology: Basic principles and practices. R Hoffman, EJ Benz, and SJ Shattil, et al., eds. New York: Churchill Livingstone; 1991:350.

Drennan DB. Orthopedic lesions. In: Isaacs JH, Byrne MP, eds. *Pelvic surgery: a multidisciplinary approach*. Mt. Kisco, NY: Futura Publishing Co.; 1987:173.

Drucker WR. Crohn's disease (regional enteritis). In: Sabiston DC Jr, ed. *Textbook of surgery*. Philadelphia: WB Saunders; 1986:914.

Forget BG. Sickle cell anemia and associated hemoglobinopathies. In: Wyngaarden JB, Smith LH Jr, Bennett JC, eds. *Cecil textbook of medicine*. 19th ed. Philadelphia: WB Saunders; 1992:888.

Francis RB Jr, Johnson CS. Vascular occlusion in sickle cell disease: current concepts and unanswered questions. *Blood* 1991;77:1405.

Glickman RM. Inflammatory bowel disease. In: Isselbacher KJ, Braunwald E, Wilson JD, et al., eds. *Harrison's principles of internal medicine*. 13th ed. New York: McGraw-Hill; 1994:1403.

Hricak H. MRI of the female pelvis: a review. *AJR Am J Roentgenol* 1986;146:1115.

Hunter VP, Burke TW, Crooks LA. Retroperitoneal nerve sheath tumors: an unusual cause of pelvic mass. *Obstet Gynecol* 1988;71:1050.

Israel SL, Helsel EV, Hansman DH. The challenge of metastatic ovarian carcinoma. *Am J Obstet Gynecol* 1965;93:1094.

Knaus JV, Barber HRK. Metastatic lesions presenting as pelvic mass. In: Isaacs JH, Byrne MP, eds. *Pelvic surgery: a multidisciplinary approach*. Mt. Kisco, NY: Futura Publishing Co.; 1987:69.

Kodner IJ, Fry RD, Fleshman JW, et al. Colon, rectum, and anus. In: Schwartz SI, Shires GT, Spencer FC, et al., eds. *Principles of surgery*. 6th ed. New York: McGraw-Hill; 1994:1191.

LaMont JT, Isselbacher KJ. Diseases of the small and large intestine. In: Isselbacher KJ, Braunwald E, Wilson JD, et al., eds. *Harrison's principles of internal medicine*. 13th ed. New York: McGraw-Hill; 1994: 1417.

Lewis JJ, Leung D, Woodruff JM, et al. Retroperitoneal soft-tissue sarcoma: analysis of 500 patients treated and followed at a single institution. *Ann Surg* 1998;228:355.

Mayer RJ. Tumors of the large and small intestine. In: Isselbacher KJ, Braunwald E, Wilson JD, et al., eds. *Harrison's principles of internal medicine*. 13th ed. New York: McGraw-Hill; 1994:1424.

McCallion K, Mitchell RMS, Wilson RH, et al. Flexible sigmoidoscopy and the changing distribution of colorectal cancer: implications for screening. *Gut* 2001;48:522.

Miller RE. The clean colon. *Gastroenterology* 1976;70:289.

Miller RE. Detection of colon carcinoma and the barium enema. *JAMA* 1974;230:1195.

Morrow W, Enker WE. Late ovarian metastases in carcinoma of the colon and rectum. *Arch Surg* 1984;119:1385.

Paulson DF. The urinary system. In: Sabiston DC Jr, ed. *Textbook of surgery*. Philadelphia: WB Saunders; 1986:1658.

Pickelman J. Gastrointestinal pathology. In: Isaacs JH, Byrne MP, eds. *Pelvic surgery: a multidisciplinary approach*. Mt. Kisco, NY: Futura Publishing Co.; 1987:57.

Podolsky DK. Inflammatory bowel disease. *N Engl J Med* 1991;325:928.

Rajagopalon AE, Mason JH, Kennedy M, et al. The value of the barium enema in the diagnosis of acute appendicitis. *Arch Surg* 1977;112: 531.

Raval B, Allan N, St. Ville E. Use of computed tomography in appendicitis: technique, findings, and pitfalls. *J Comput Tomogr* 1987;11:17.

Schuster G. Urologic disease. In: Isaacs JH, Byrne MP, eds. *Pelvic surgery: a multidisciplinary approach*. Mt. Kisco, NY: Futura Publishing Co.; 1987: 150.

Schwartz SI. Appendix. In: Schwartz SI, Shires GT, Spencer FC, et al., eds. *Principles of surgery*. 6th ed. New York: McGraw-Hill; 1994:1307.

Sleisenger MH. Miscellaneous inflammatory diseases of the intestine. In: Wyngaarden JB, Smith LH Jr, Bennett LC, eds. *Cecil textbook of medicine*. 19th ed. Philadelphia: WB Saunders; 1992:746.

Swamy S, Edwin P, Philip B, et al. Anterior sacral meningocele—as part of the currarino triad. *Ind J Radiol Imag* 2003;13(2):207.

Symmonds RE. Preface. In: Isaacs JH, Byrne MP, eds. *Pelvic surgery: a multidisciplinary approach*. Mt. Kisco, NY: Futura Publishing Co.; 1987: vi.

Webb MJ, Decker DG, Mussey E. Cancer metastatic to the ovary, factors influencing survival. *Obstet Gynecol* 1975;45:391.

Wright DG. Familial Mediterranean fever. In: Wyngaarden JB, Smith LH Jr, Bennett LC, eds. *Cecil textbook of medicine*. 19th ed. Philadelphia: WB Saunders; 1992:1140.

SECTION IX ■ GYNECOLOGIC ONCOLOGY

CHAPTER 45 ■ MALIGNANCIES OF THE VULVA

MITCHEL S. HOFFMAN

DEFINITIONS

Lymphoscintigraphy—A nuclear medicine study examining the distribution of uptake of radiocolloid (injected peritumorally) into the lymphatic system.

Modified radical vulvectomy—Radical removal of the portion of the vulva containing the tumor with approximately a 2-cm margin.

Radical vulvectomy—Removal of the vulvar soft tissue. The lateral borders are the labiocrural folds. The anterior border is located in the mons pubis. The posterior border is across the perineal body. The medial borders are within the vestibule.

Sentinel lymph node—The concept of a sentinel lymph node in the context of malignancy relies on the presumption that this lymph node(s) is the initial site of metastatic disease and that the histology of the sentinel lymph node reflects the histology of the rest of the lymph nodes in the basin.

Superficial inguinal lymphadenectomy—Removal of the inguinal lymph nodes superficial to the cribriform fascia, mainly associated with the great saphenous and superficial epigastric veins.

Carcinoma of the vulva is an uncommon malignancy accounting for 0.5% of all female cancers in the United States and 2% of all female genital malignancies. It is predominantly a disease of older women. In this country as a whole, the steady increase in life expectancy has brought carcinoma of the vulva into a place of more importance among gynecologic malignancies. The predominant histologic type is squamous cell carcinoma, which accounts for about 90% of the tumors in most series. This malignancy metastasizes primarily through the lymphatic system in an orderly manner through the superficial inguinal, deep inguinal, and pelvic lymph nodes. During the first half of the 20th century, the absolute 5-year survival rate for carcinoma of the vulva was 15%. During the late 19th and early 20th centuries, principles of surgical oncology were developed and put into clinical practice. The application of these surgical principles to the treatment of vulvar cancer resulted in a significant improvement in survival. The survival of patients with invasive squamous cell carcinoma of the vulva is dependent on a number of histopathologic factors, but it most closely relates to the pathologic status of the inguinal lymph nodes. Until the early 1980s, patients with invasive carcinoma of the vulva were routinely treated with radical vulvectomy and bilateral inguinofemoral and pelvic lymphadenectomy. Accumulation of data on vulvar cancer during the mid- to late-20th century led to earlier diagnosis and a better understanding of the nature and modes of spread of this disease. Especially over the past 2 decades, treatment of this malignancy has undergone a number of significant modifications that are applicable to most patients.

This chapter first reviews the epidemiology, clinical characteristics, staging, and prognostic factors for invasive carcinoma of the vulva. The broad spectrum of treatment of this disease is then reviewed with an emphasis on the surgical treatment. Finally, histologic variants of vulvar malignancy and their treatment are discussed individually.

EPIDEMIOLOGY

Invasive squamous cell carcinoma of the vulva is typically a disease of postmenopausal women, with a median age at diagnosis of about 65 years. However, the age range is wide, and some data suggest an increasing incidence in younger women. This has been attributed to some extent to the human papillomavirus. Human papillomavirus does not appear to play a significant role in the epidemiology of invasive squamous cell carcinoma of the vulva in older women, who frequently have coexistent lichen sclerosis (Fig. 45.1).

The other sexually transmitted factors that have been epidemiologically associated with vulvar cancer are the granulomatous venereal diseases, especially in countries where these are prevalent.

Vulvar carcinoma *in situ* (Fig. 45.2A–B), like cervical carcinoma *in situ,* is considered a precursor to invasive disease, although the risk of progression appears to be lower. There are no substantial long-term natural history studies of untreated patients. Although Jones and Rowan found in seven of eight women with untreated vulvar intraepithelial neoplasia (VIN) that invasive cancer developed within 8 years, three other studies found progression rates of 5% to 16%. In a recent systematic review of 3,322 published patients, 8 of 88 untreated women with VIN 3 progressed to invasive cancer in 12 to 96 months. Occult invasion has been discovered in 16% to 22% of patients undergoing excision of VIN 3 (although it was only 3.2% in the systematic review). The risk for invasive cancer may be greater with perianal location, increased age, immunosuppression, and previous radiotherapy. Vulvar carcinoma *in situ* tends to be multifocal with a lower risk of invasive cancer in younger women, but it tends to be unifocal with a higher risk of invasive disease in older women. Most patients with VIN 3 should be treated, and long-term follow-up is mandatory. Although progression of VIN from grade 1 to grade 2 and grade 3 has been demonstrated, in the absence of atypical changes, other vulvar epithelial abnormalities do not appear to have significant precancerous potential. Patients who have cervical neoplasia are at increased risk for developing vulvar neoplasia, and vice versa. This so-called field phenomenon should heighten the physician's surveillance for the development of other lesions once a lower genital tract neoplasm occurs.

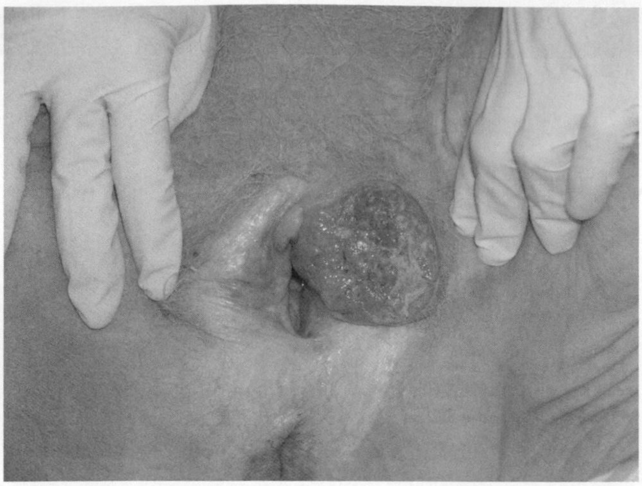

FIGURE 45.1. Vulvar cancer arising in a background of lichen sclerosis.

Hypertension and diabetes mellitus are common in patients with invasive vulvar cancer, but this may simply be related to the elderly population affected. The associations of vulvar cancer with obesity and cigarette smoking are also unclear. There does not appear to be any significant association with parity or race. One group that does appear to be at increased risk for the development of invasive vulvar cancer is chronically immunosuppressed women.

CLINICAL PRESENTATION

The most common initial symptom of vulvar cancer is pruritus vulvae, which may be of long duration. Vulvar pain, discharge, and bleeding are less commonly reported. The patient often becomes aware of a lesion on her vulva; but despite the superficial nature of the lesion, delay in seeking medical help is common. Physician delay has also been commonly reported, often related to prolonged medical treatment before a biopsy is done. These findings underscore the need for patient and physician education with regard to the early diagnosis of carcinoma of the vulva and the importance of having a biopsy diagnosis before treating vulvar lesions. Biopsy of the vulva is a simple procedure that can be performed in the physician's office (see Chapter 23).

Invasive squamous cell carcinoma of the vulva involves the labia majora in about two thirds of patients. The remaining tumors involve the clitoris, labia minora or posterior fourchette, and perineum. These cancers can be exophytic, ulcerating, or flat (Figs. 45.3–45.5).

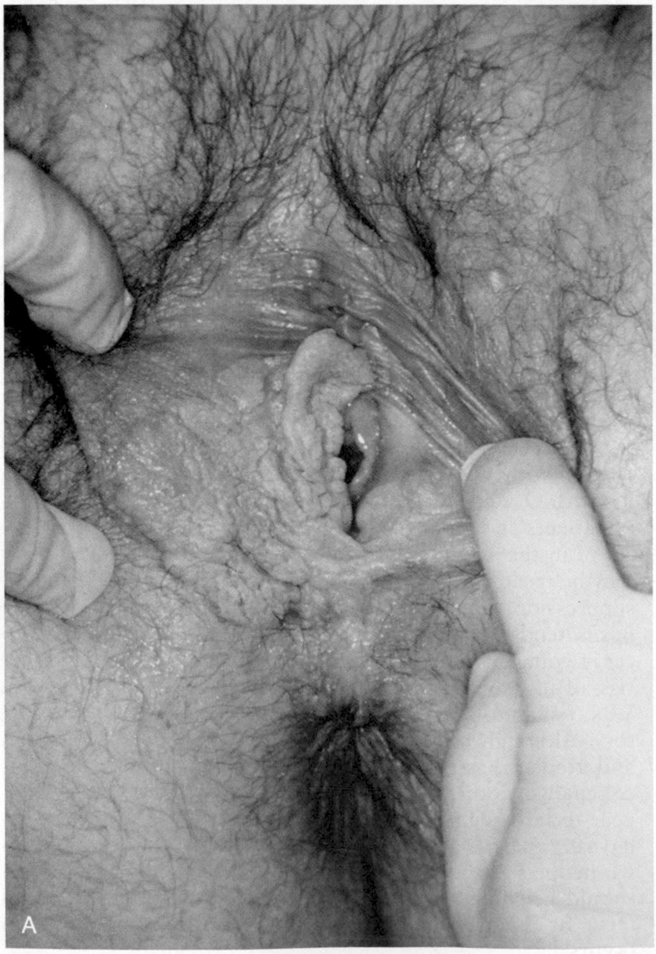

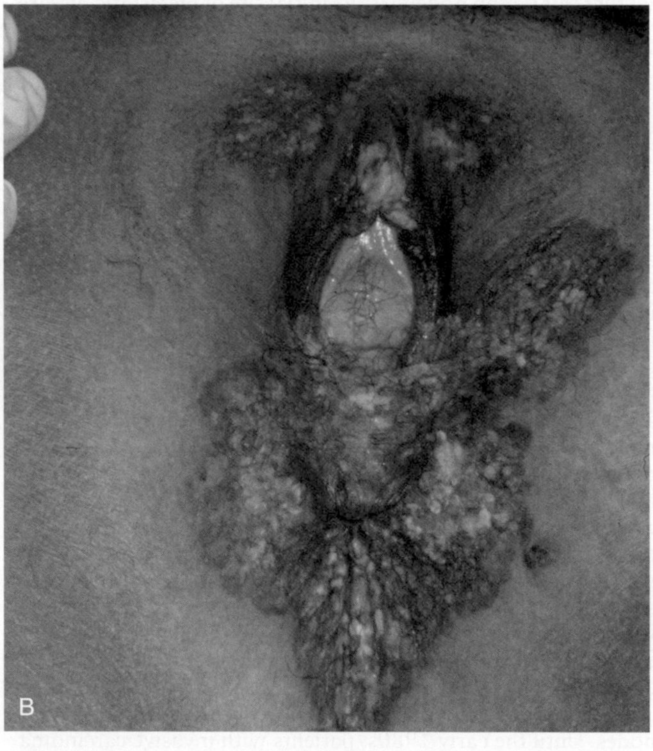

FIGURE 45.2. A and B: Carcinoma *in situ* of the vulva.

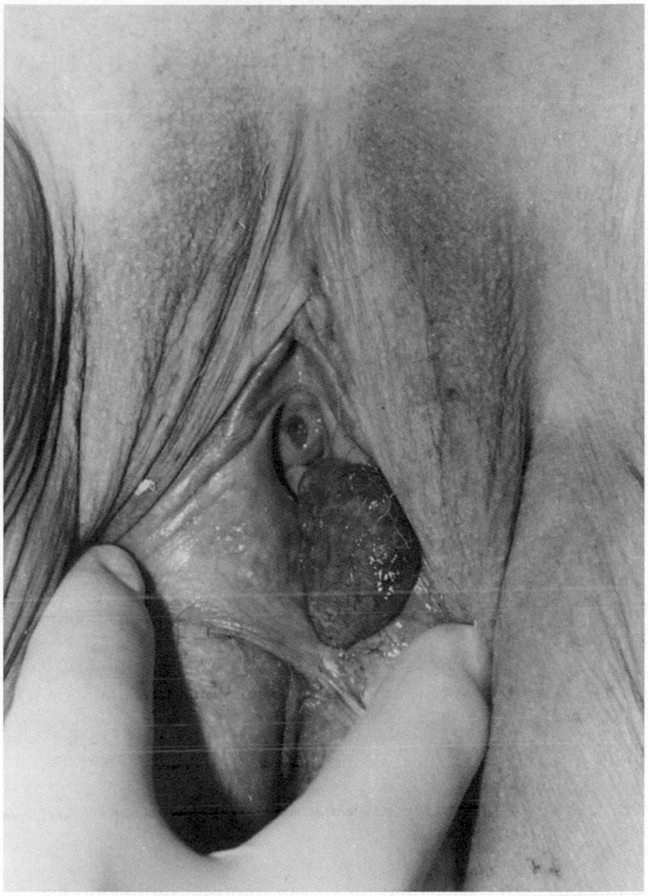

FIGURE 45.3. Exophytic vulvar cancer.

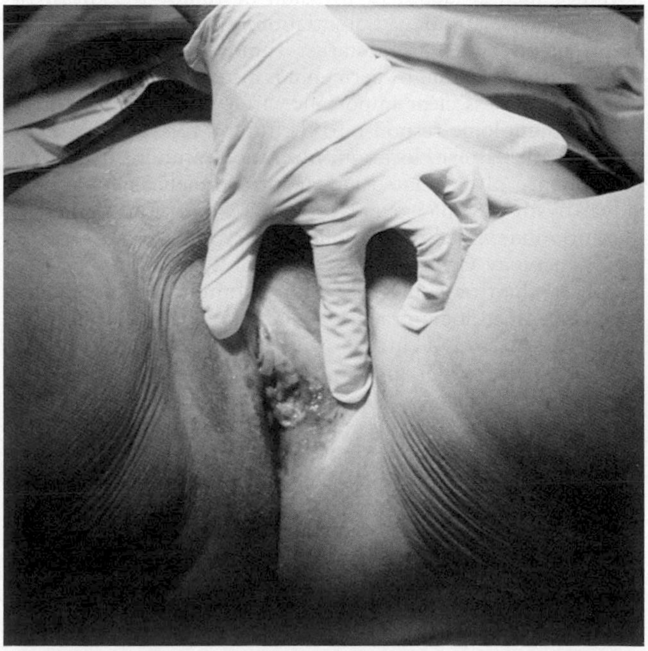

FIGURE 45.4. Ulcerating vulvar cancer.

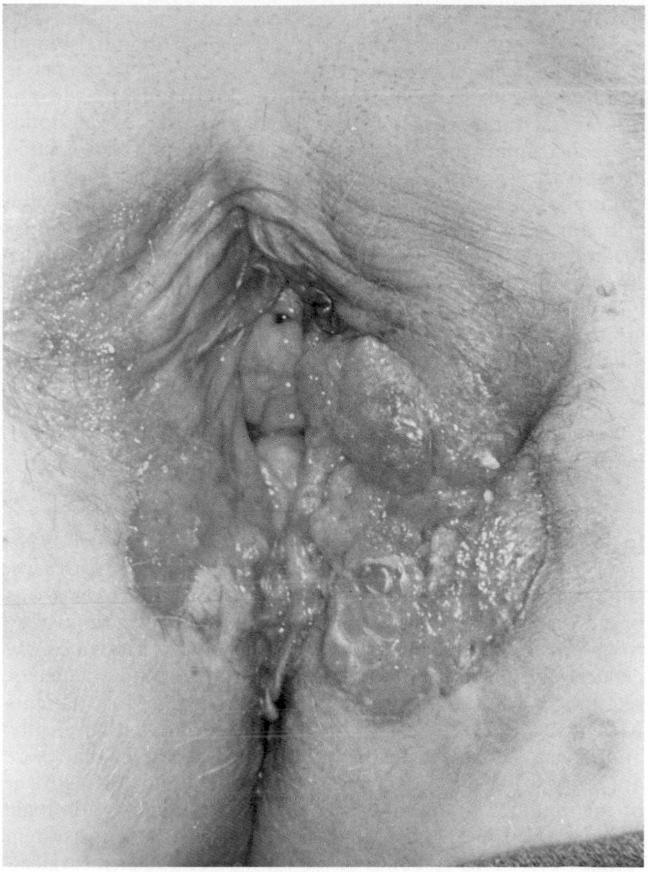

FIGURE 45.5. Flat vulvar cancer.

HISTOLOGY

Squamous cell carcinoma accounts for about 90% of the invasive vulvar malignancies in most large series. Melanoma is the second most common histologic type, accounting for 5% to 10% of vulvar cancers. Some of the less common vulvar malignancies include Bartholin carcinoma (with most of these being adenocarcinoma or squamous carcinoma), basal cell carcinoma, verrucous carcinoma, adenocarcinoma, invasive Paget disease, and sarcomas. This chapter mainly deals with invasive squamous cell carcinoma, followed by a discussion of the less common vulvar malignancies.

ROUTES OF SPREAD

Squamous cell carcinoma of the vulva can spread by local extension to involve the vagina, urethra, anus, or pubic bone. Metastasis from the primary site can occur by the lymphatic or the vascular system, but, by far, the most common is the lymphatic route. The lymphatics of the labia communicate to the inguinal lymph nodes. The lymphatics of the perianal area drain in a similar manner, but lesions that extensively involve the anus or rectovaginal septum can drain directly into the pelvic lymph nodes. Although there are channels that interconnect the clitoris to the deep pelvic nodes, it appears that they are of minimal clinical significance. The lymphatics of the vulva are numerous and tend to cross the midline. The regional lymph nodes include the superficial inguinal lymph nodes, the deep inguinal femoral lymph nodes, and the pelvic lymph nodes (external iliac, obturator, internal iliac, and common iliac lymph nodes). The superficial inguinal lymph nodes are the primary nodal group of the vulva and are located around the saphenous, superficial epigastric, and superficial circumflex iliac veins. These lymph nodes drain through the cribriform fascia to the femoral lymph nodes, which are mainly located medial to the femoral vein. Drainage from here is under the inguinal ligament into the pelvic lymph nodes. The pelvic lymph nodes are virtually never positive in the absence of inguinofemoral lymph node metastases. Overall, 20% to 40% of all patients with invasive squamous cell carcinoma of the vulva have lymph node metastases.

STAGING

In 1979, the International Federation of Gynecology and Obstetrics (FIGO) approved a clinical classification for invasive squamous cell carcinoma of the vulva (Table 45.1). This was based on an analysis of tumor (T) by size and location; node (N) status by palpation; distant metastases (M) as assessed by general and pelvic examination; evaluation of the bladder or rectum, or both; and radiologic investigation. Most patients with invasive carcinoma of the vulva are treated surgically, and it was recognized through a number of studies that there are substantial discrepancies between the clinical assessment of the inguinal lymph node status and the surgical pathologic findings. In 1988, FIGO approved a surgical staging system (Table 45.2). This system is based on well-established surgical-pathologic prognostic criteria. In 1995, stage I was divided into A and B based on a depth of invasion less or greater than 1 mm.

PROGNOSTIC FACTORS

Invasive squamous cell carcinoma of the vulva has a relatively low propensity for distant metastases. Recurrences tend to be local or regional, and even unremitting disease tends to remain locoregional for long periods of time. The dominant prognostic factor in this disease is the status of the inguinofemoral lymph nodes. Further definition of prognosis includes evaluation of a number of factors relating to the regional lymph nodes. In addition, several prognostic factors related to the primary tumor have been delineated. These primary tumor characteristics have been correlated with the likelihood of regional nodal involvement and/or risk of local recurrence.

Primary tumor factors that appear to have prognostic importance include depth of invasion or tumor thickness, tumor diameter, tumor differentiation, lymph-vascular space involvement, and margin status. Tumor involvement of the distal urethra, vagina, or perineum is also an adverse prognostic factor. Of less clear importance are cytologic grading, the local immunologic response to the tumor, tumor volume, tumor growth pattern, location, ulceration, amount of keratin, the presence of associated vulvar intraepithelial neoplasia or vulvar dystrophy, p53 overexpression, DNA ploidy, and proliferation index. Sedlis and colleagues reported on a Gynecologic Oncology Group (GOG) study of 272 patients with lesions less than or equal to 5 mm in tumor thickness. They found that histologic grade, capillarylike space involvement, tumor thickness, and clitoral or perineal location were all significant predictors of groin node metastases. A subsequent GOG study reported by Homesley and associates on 588 evaluable patients with invasive carcinoma found lymph-vascular space involvement, GOG tumor differentiation, age, and tumor thickness to be significant independent risk factors for groin node metastases. A few of the primary tumor characteristics, such as tumor diameter and lymph-vascular space involvement, may be significant independent predictors of survival. Other factors may be predictive of an increased risk of local recurrence, including margin status, large tumor size, and deep invasion.

A few histologic variants have been described that have been associated with a favorable prognosis, including verrucous

TABLE 45.1

CLINICAL STAGING OF INVASIVE CANCER OF THE VULVA

Stage I	All lesions confined to vulva, with maximal diameter of 2 cm or less and no suspicious groin nodes.
Stage II	All lesions confined to vulva, with diameter greater than 2 cm and no suspicious groin nodes.
Stage III	Lesions extending beyond vulva but without grossly positive groin nodes. Lesions of any size confined to vulva, with suspicious groin nodes.
Stage IV	Lesions involving mucosa of rectum, bladder, or urethra, or involving bone. All cases with distant or palpable deep pelvic metastases.

TABLE 45.2

FIGO STAGING OF INVASIVE CANCER OF THE VULVA

Stage 0	Carcinoma *in situ,* intraepithelial carcinoma
Stage I	Tumor confined to the vulva or perineum, or both; 2 cm or less in greatest dimension (no nodal metastasis)
Stage IA	Stromal invasion no greater than 1.0 mm[a]
Stage IB	Stromal invasion greater than 1.0 mm
Stage II	Tumor confined to the vulva or perineum, or both; more than 2 cm in greatest dimension (no nodal metastasis)
Stage III	Tumor of any size with one or both of the following: Adjacent spread to the lower urethra, vagina, or anus; Unilateral regional lymph node metastasis
Stage IVA	Tumor invades any of the following: upper urethra, bladder mucosa, rectal mucosa, or pelvic bone; or bilateral regional node metastasis
Stage IVB, any T, any N, MI	Any distant metastasis including pelvic lymph nodes

FIGO, International Federation of Gynecology and Obstetrics; T, tumor; N, groin lymph nodes; MI, distant metastasis.
[a]The depth of invasion is defined as the measurement of the tumor from the epithelial-stromal junction of the adjacent most superficial dermal papilla to the deepest point of invasion.

carcinoma (discussed later), warty carcinoma, carcinoma *in situ* with early stromal invasion, and keratoacanthoma.

The status of the groin nodes is clearly the most important prognostic factor for patients with invasive squamous cell carcinoma of the vulva. The overall 5-year survival rate for all treated patients is about 60%, with a corrected 5-year survival rate of about 70%. In the GOG study previously mentioned, 65.5% of the patients had negative groin nodes and 34.5% had positive nodes; this is consistent with my own experience and with other reports in the literature. In the GOG report, the survival rate was 90.9% for patients with negative lymph nodes and 57.7% for patients with positive lymph nodes, again consistent with the other reports in the literature. When the pelvic lymph nodes are known to be positive, the survival rate decreases to about 20%.

Further definition of prognosis is achieved by examining a number of variables related to the lymph node metastases; the most significant of these is the number of nodes involved. Other factors that have been reported to be prognostically significant include bilateral involvement, extracapsular extension, clinical nodal status, size of the metastatic deposit inside the lymph node, percentage of nodal replacement, nodal immune response, and location of the metastasis within the lymph node. Several studies have shown that when only one lymph node is involved, survival is still quite good; it decreases drastically with metastases to three or more nodes or with bilateral nodal involvement. In the 1991 GOG report, the relative survival rate was 75.2% when one or two nodes were involved and decreased to 36.1% when three or more nodes were involved. The survival rate was 70.7% with unilateral involvement versus 25.4% with bilateral involvement. On the basis of limited data from a few studies, it appears that large nodal diameter, extensive nodal replacement, and especially extracapsular extension of a lymph node metastasis are adverse prognostic factors. In a report by Origoni and colleagues in 1992 that was based on 53 vulvar cancer patients with groin node metastases, the survival rate varied from 90.9% when the diameter of the metastasis was less than 5 mm to 20% when it was larger than 15 mm, and from 85.7% to 25% when the metastases were intracapsular and extracapsular, respectively. Especially important are the data from the 19 patients in that study with a single positive node. For these patients, the 5-year cancer-related survival rate was 90% when the metastasis diameter was less than 5 mm versus 37.5% when it was 15 mm, and 85.7% when the metastasis was intracapsular versus 20% when it was extracapsular. Results from a study by Paladini and associates were similar; they reported that patients with intracapsular metastases tended to have recurrence at distant sites, whereas patients with extracapsular nodal disease were more likely to have local or groin recurrence. Both of the previously mentioned studies also revealed that a lack of active immune response within the lymph node metastases was an adverse prognostic factor. A 1995 study from the Netherlands (van der Velden and colleagues) found a predominantly distant failure pattern in a subgroup of patients with extranodal spread, multiple positive lymph nodes, and lymph nodes replaced greater than 50% by tumor. Hoffman and coworkers studied 48 patients with groin node metastases and reported prognostic significance for the size and number of the nodal metastases, but they found that the immune response and the location of the metastasis within the lymph node were much less important. Groin nodes that are both clinically and surgically positive may also portend a worse prognosis, which is probably a reflection of the factors mentioned earlier.

PRETREATMENT INVESTIGATION

Patients with carcinoma of the vulva are generally elderly and often have coexisting medical problems. A thorough preoperative evaluation by internal medicine and anesthesiology consultants is essential in the care of these patients. As previously discussed, these women have an increased incidence of cervical and vaginal neoplasia, which may be coexistent. Therefore, careful examination of these areas preoperatively is important. Beyond physical examination and a chest radiograph, routine studies to rule out metastases are not indicated except in the presence of locally advanced disease. Cystoscopy, intravenous pyelography, or proctoscopy (or all three) is indicated if it appears that locally advanced cancer may be involving the bladder, bladder base, or rectum. Imaging the tumor with magnetic resonance imaging (MRI) or computed tomography (CT) may help to determine resectability and treatment planning. When a locally advanced tumor or obvious inguinal lymph node metastases is noted, CT of the groins, pelvis, and abdomen is suggested. This aids in determining the resectability of the tumor and metastases, extension to the pelvic lymph nodes, and distant metastases (Fig. 45.6).

TREATMENT OF INVASIVE SQUAMOUS CELL CARCINOMA OF THE VULVA

Invasive squamous cell carcinoma of the vulva is a heterogeneous group of tumors requiring considerable flexibility in the approaches to treatment. Dating back to the favorable reports of Taussig in 1940 and Way in 1948, radical vulvectomy with bilateral inguinal lymphadenectomy performed by en bloc excision became the standard therapy applied to most patients with carcinoma of the vulva. This operation involves radical removal of the entire vulva, the mons pubis, the inguinofemoral lymph nodes, and often the pelvic lymph nodes. A large surgical defect is created that is generally closed under tension with a high subsequent breakdown rate and marked disfigurement

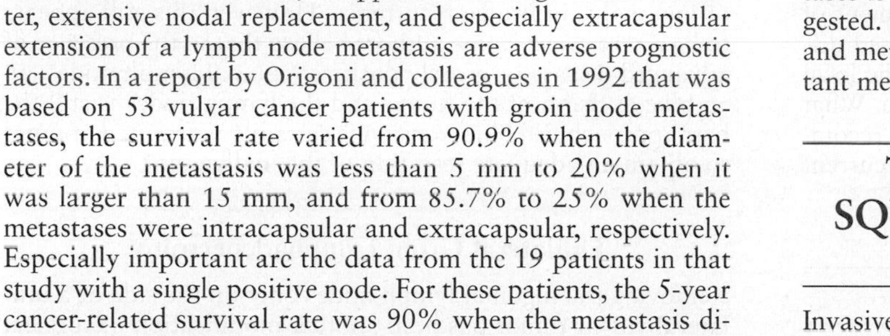

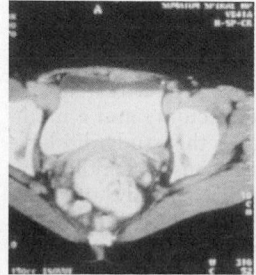

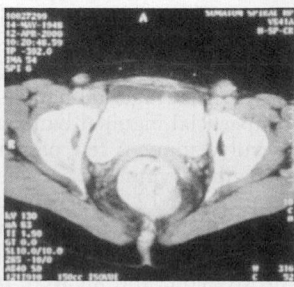

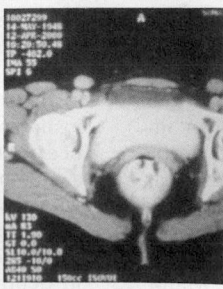

FIGURE 45.6. Patient had bilateral clinically positive inguinal lymph nodes. CT scan demonstrates their relationship to the femoral vessels and additional lymph node metastases above these.

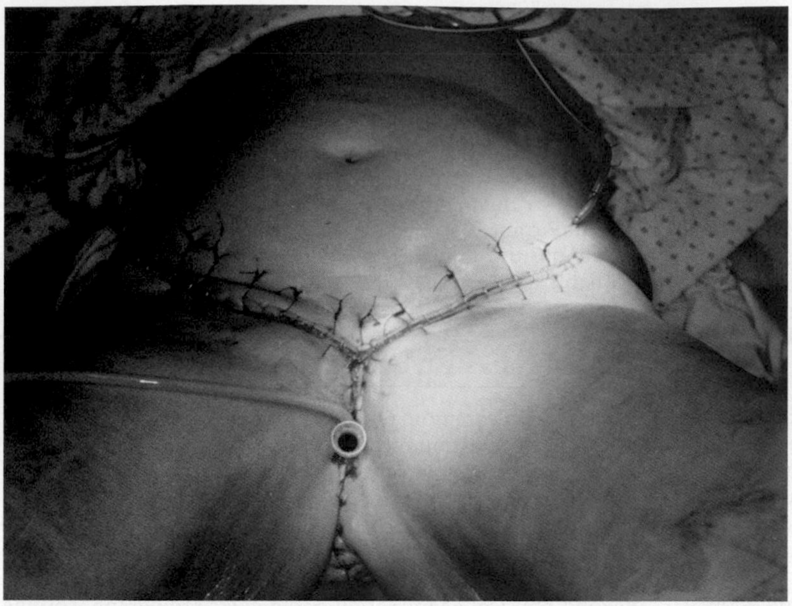

FIGURE 45.7. Closure of en bloc radical vulvectomy with bilateral inguinofemoral lymphadenectomy. Foley catheter and vaginal stent are in place.

of the genital area (Fig. 45.7). Important concerns with this approach for the treatment of vulvar cancer have led to a number of modifications, especially over the past 25 years (Fig. 45.8). Some of these concerns include the high rate and the severity of wound complications and the psychosexual effects of radical removal of the vulvar tissues. Other potential problems related to the en-bloc radical resection include urinary or fecal incontinence and vaginal relaxation, the overtreatment of early cancer, the inadequate treatment of more advanced disease, and the lack of attention directed specifically at the local vulvar lesion to ensure an adequate margin of resection. What I wish to emphasize in this section are some treatment recommendations based on my own experience as well as current literature on the subject.

Regional Nodal Management

It should be kept in mind that certain vulvar cancers, by virtue of their anatomic extent, may have access to lymphatics that bypass the groins. These include tumors that extensively involve the anus (particularly the anal canal or its surrounding tissue), the rectovaginal septum, the vagina above the lower third, and the proximal urethra.

Separate Incisions

Although reported earlier by Kehrer, Taussig, Byron and associates, and Ballon and Lamb, it was only after later reports by Hacker and colleagues, DiSaia and associates, and others that separate incisions for the vulvar and inguinal phases of the operation came into increasing use (Fig. 45.8B). This was the most important modification of the classic en bloc excision. The separation of incisions results in a significant reduction in wound morbidity. Importantly, the separation allows for increased flexibility in the modification of the two aspects of the operation (regional and local). The report by Hacker and colleagues in 1981 consisted of 100 patients in whom three separate incisions were used to perform the bilateral inguinofemoral lymphadenectomy and radical vulvectomy, leaving a bridge of tissue between the incisions and sparing the mons pubis. Major groin wound breakdown occurred in 14 patients, which was a considerable reduction from the 50% or higher groin wound breakdown rate generally seen with the en bloc excision. In this report, there were no isolated recurrences in either the groin or the inguinal skin bridge. There were two recurrences in the inguinal skin bridge associated with other recurrence sites; both patients originally had positive inguinal lymph nodes. In addition to these two patients, there have been other isolated reports of inguinal skin bridge recurrence. However, this still appears to be a rare event. Some authors believe that in the presence of advanced disease or grossly positive inguinal lymph nodes, an en bloc excision of the tumor and the lymph nodes is still the best approach. En bloc excision is certainly warranted at times to obtain an adequate resection of the malignancy.

Unilateral Groin Lymphadenectomy

Removing the inguinal lymph nodes only on the side of a unilateral vulvar tumor has been another modification of surgical treatment that has been used for selected patients (Fig. 45.8C). In 1981, Iversen reported on 53 women with unilateral tumors and lymph node metastases. Eighty-three percent of these patients had only one positive ipsilateral node, 15% had bilateral positive nodes, and one patient had contralateral positive lymph nodes only. Other retrospective studies have confirmed these results. It has been the opinion of a number of authors that capillary or lymphatic space involvement by tumor may increase the risk of contralateral nodal metastases. Patients with tumors approaching the midline or involving more medial structures (perineum, clitoral hood or clitoris, vagina, and labia minora) are at increased risk for contralateral lymph node metastases. The issue of unilateral groin lymphadenectomy was studied to some extent in 1992 by Stehman and associates in a GOG study. Briefly, patients with early disease and negative ipsilateral superficial inguinal lymph nodes were treated with ipsilateral superficial inguinal lymphadenectomy and a modified radical vulvectomy. A few patients in this study did have a bilateral inguinal lymphadenectomy because of midline involvement. A total of 121 patients were in the study, and 3 experienced contralateral inguinal lymph node recurrences. The vulvar lesions of these 3 patients ranged from 0.6 to 2.5 mm in depth of invasion, and all were poorly differentiated. Although lesion location was not given for these three cases,

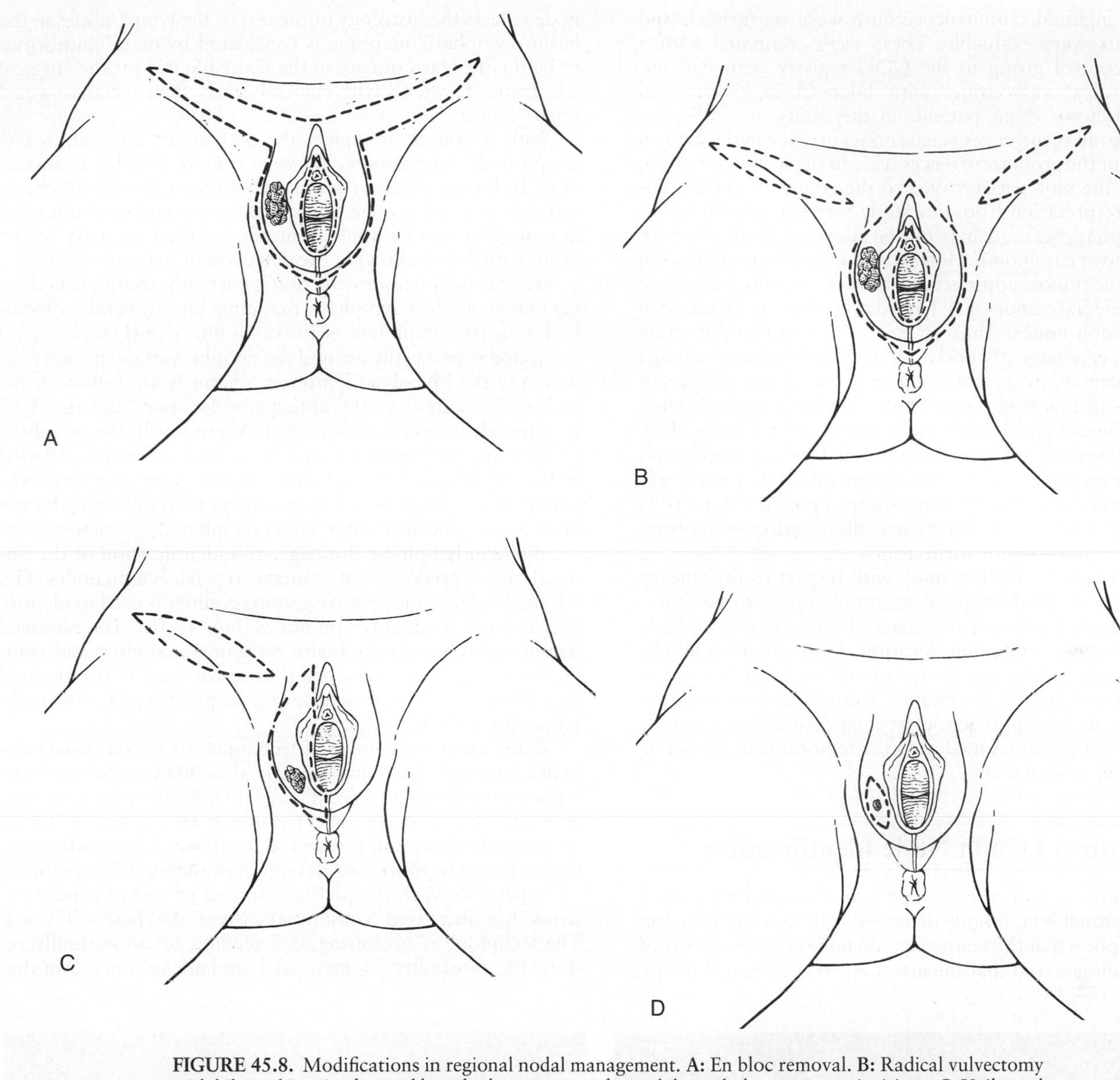

FIGURE 45.8. Modifications in regional nodal management. **A:** En bloc removal. **B:** Radical vulvectomy with bilateral inguinofemoral lymphadenectomy performed through three separate incisions. **C:** Unilateral lymphadenectomy for a well-lateralized lesion. **D:** Early lesion with lymphadenectomy omitted.

a large percentage of patients included in this study had lesions approaching the midline, as defined by involvement of the labia minora. Tumors with capillary or lymphatic space involvement were excluded from this study. The role of unilateral inguinal lymphadenectomy in the management of invasive squamous cell carcinoma of the vulva requires further evaluation; at present, it appears to be a reasonable approach in a patient with a well-lateralized early tumor that is well differentiated, with no capillary or lymphatic space involvement, and with negative ipsilateral inguinal lymph nodes.

Superficial Inguinal Lymphadenectomy

A more limited resection of the inguinal lymph nodes in the management of superficially invasive vulvar cancer was reported by DiSaia and coworkers in 1979. The dissection they described is aimed at removal of the superficial lymph nodes above the cribriform fascia, mainly associated with the great saphenous and superficial epigastric veins. These lymph nodes are sent for frozen section analysis. If results are positive, a complete bilateral inguinofemoral lymphadenectomy is performed. In the 1979 study, DiSaia and colleagues also reported 79 cases of invasive squamous cell carcinoma of the vulva treated with radical vulvectomy and bilateral inguinal lymphadenectomy. In these cases, it was noted that the deep femoral lymph nodes were never positive in the absence of positive superficial inguinal lymph nodes. The purpose of this modification is to reduce the morbidity of the inguinal lymphadenectomy. The dissection is less radical and resulted in only one groin breakdown in the 18 patients in the series of DiSaia and associates. The series was updated in 1989 and reported no groin recurrences in 50 patients, 42 of whom had been followed for a median of 36 months. The previously mentioned GOG study specifically studied the issue of superficial inguinal lymphadenectomy in patients with early carcinoma of the vulva. The study group included clinical stage I patients with tumor invasion of 5 mm or less and no capillary or lymphatic space involvement. A modified radical vulvectomy and ipsilateral superficial inguinal lymphadenectomy were performed, and 121 patients were evaluable. These were compared with a historical control group in the GOG registry who had undergone radical vulvectomy with bilateral inguinofemoral lymphadenectomy. Nine patients in this study, or 7.3%, experienced groin recurrences versus no recurrence in the control group. Six of the groin recurrences were in the ipsilateral groin, and five of the nine patients died of the recurrent vulvar cancer. The interpretation from this study was that superficial inguinal lymphadenectomy may not be adequate treatment even for early vulvar carcinoma. However, in a number of patients in this study, the tumors approached the midline; there is evidence that more medial tumors may have direct drainage to the deep inguinal lymph nodes. Another area of concern in this study is the high percentage of poorly differentiated tumors—almost twice as many as in the control group. Six of the nine groin recurrences in this study were from the poorly differentiated tumors. Whether poorly differentiated tumors are more likely to metastasize to deep inguinal or contralateral inguinal lymph nodes deserves further study. Subsequent additional retrospective data from large cancer centers also report a 5% to 10% incidence of groin relapse in patients with negative nodes from superficial inguinal lymphadenectomy.

Factors requiring further study with respect to the efficacy of superficial inguinal lymphadenectomy appear to be tumor grade, depth of invasion, the presence of capillary or lymphatic space involvement, and tumor location. The patients should be those generally at low risk for lymph node metastases with a tumor confined to the labia majora. Until further information is available on this approach, extending dissection to include removal of lymph nodes medial to the femoral vein should be considered in most patients.

Sentinel Lymph Node Identification

A large number of reports have been published over the past 15 years on sentinel lymph node detection. The concept relies on the presumption that the sentinel lymph node is the initial site of metastatic disease and that the histology of the sentinel lymph node reflects the histology of the rest of the lymph nodes in the basin. Lymphatic mapping is considered by many authorities to be the standard of care in the United States for the surgical treatment of patients with clinically early-stage melanoma and breast cancer.

With lymphatic mapping, the pathologist has only a few lymph nodes to examine, allowing a more detailed examination. Techniques such as serial sectioning, immunohistochemical staining, and reverse transcriptase–polymerase chain reaction analysis can be applied, increasing the sensitivity of the examination and allowing the detection of micrometastases.

Sentinel lymph node detection is currently accomplished using two methods of lymphatic mapping: blue dye and radiocolloid. One to 2 milliliters of isosulfan blue dye (Lymphazurin) is injected superficially around the periphery of the primary tumor, and the blue-dyed lymphatic channels are followed. An incision is made over the anticipated location, and the dyed lymph node or nodes are removed. Alternatively, the periphery of the tumor is injected with 400 mCi of technetium-labeled sulfur colloid 2 to 4 hours before surgery. A preoperative technetium scan is done, which may be helpful in confirming lymph node uptake, localization of target lymph nodes, unilateral versus bilateral lymphatic drainage, and identification of the unusual case of predominant drainage to pelvic lymph nodes (Fig. 45.9A–B). An intraoperative gamma counter is used to identify one or more sentinel lymph nodes (Fig. 45.10). The removed lymph nodes are checked with the gamma counter, and complete removal is assured when the radioactivity in the inguinal area returns to background levels. In practice, the two techniques are complementary.

When using the combined technique for vulvar cancer patients, lymphatic mapping is nearly always successful in identifying sentinel lymph nodes (Fig. 45.11). Further, the false negative rate (based on standard pathology) is very low. A formal lymph node dissection is reserved for those cases in which the sentinel node is positive or has not been successfully identified.

Experience with lymphatic mapping of vulvar cancer patients has increased substantially over the past 10 years. The technique is promising as a method to substantially reduce the morbidity of inguinal lymphadenectomy. Another

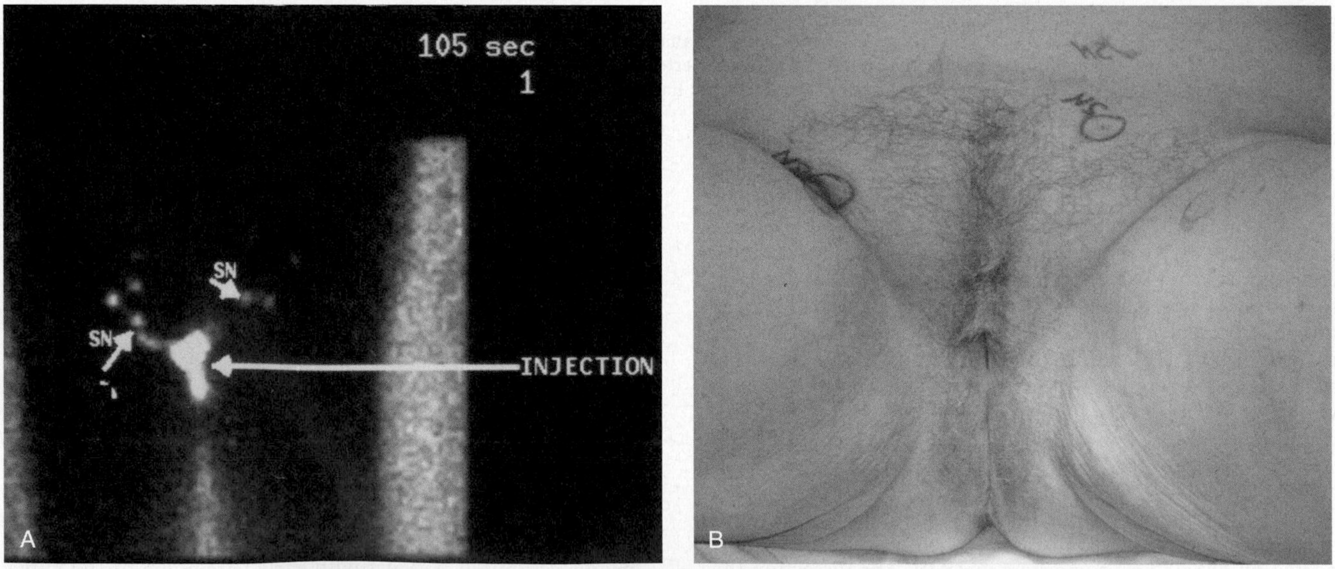

FIGURE 45.9. A: Preoperative technetium scan to evaluate lymphatic drainage and sentinel lymph nodes. B: Skin marked overlying the region of lymphoscintigraphy-identified sentinel lymph nodes.

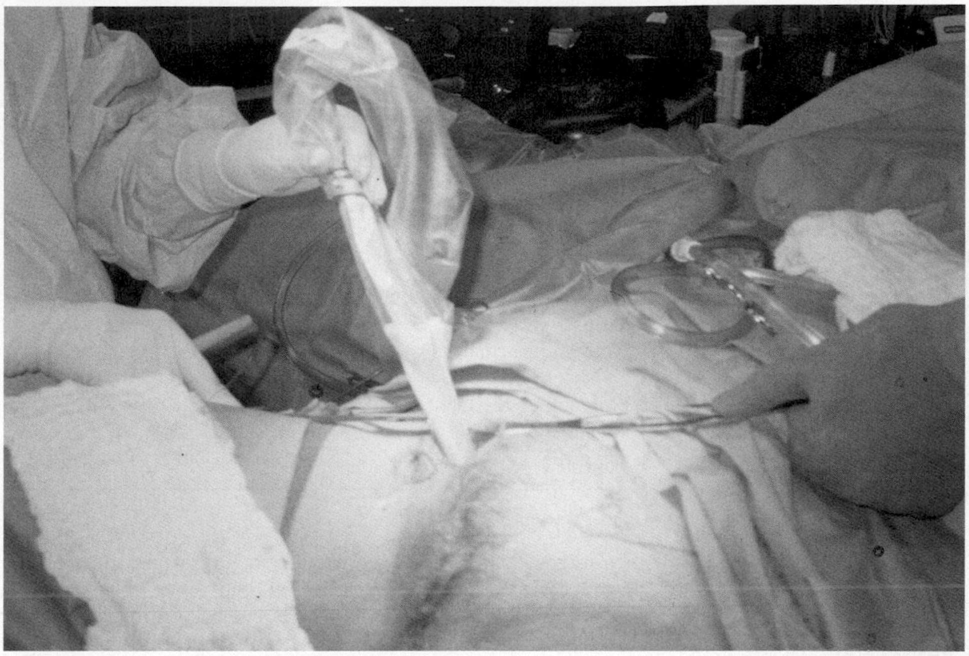

FIGURE 45.10. Intraoperative use of the gamma probe to identify sentinel inguinal lymph nodes.

important benefit may be more reliable clearance of at-risk lymph nodes. Injection of radiocolloid is best done 2 to 4 hours before surgery, but this is painful. Many unanswered questions remain, including who the best candidates are for the technique, the role of frozen section, the role of immunohistochemistry, the role of lymphoscintigraphy, the reliability of an isolated lymphoscintigraphy-directed unilateral negative sentinel node with a midline lesion, the role of ultrasound, management of a patient with a microscopically positive sentinel lymph node, the incidence of "skip" metastases, the reliability of lymphatic mapping after prior excisional biopsy, and the optimal lymphatic mapping methodology for vulvar cancer patients.

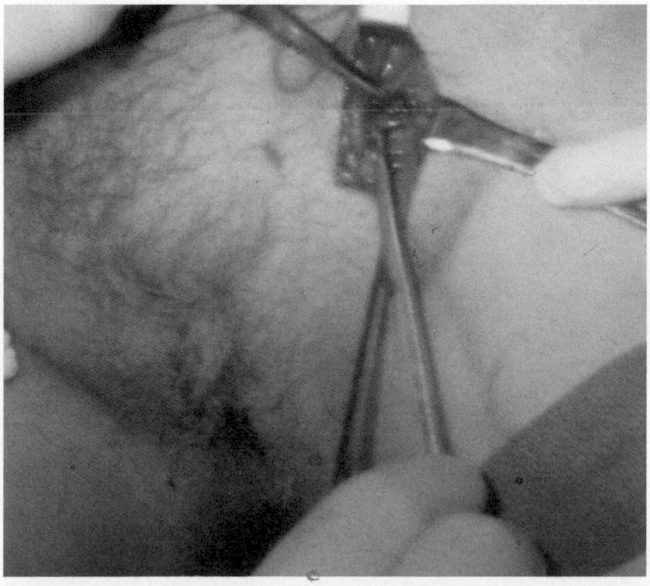

FIGURE 45.11. "Blue" lymph node found with the help of the gamma probe.

Pelvic Lymph Nodes

During the late 1970s and early 1980s, several studies were published showing that carcinoma of the vulva metastasizes to the inguinofemoral lymph nodes before spreading to the pelvic lymph nodes. Extension of the groin lymphadenectomy to include removal of the pelvic lymph nodes continued to be performed in selected patients with positive inguinofemoral lymph nodes. A number of studies also showed that the 5-year survival rate of vulvar cancer patients with positive pelvic lymph nodes is less than 20%. A 1986 study by the GOG directed by Homesley compared pelvic lymph node dissection with groin and pelvic radiotherapy in patients with positive inguinofemoral lymph nodes. The study included 114 patients and showed no difference in morbidity between the two treatment arms and a better 2-year survival rate in the radiotherapy group (68% versus 54%). The improved survival was seen in those patients with suspicious or grossly positive lymph nodes or those with more than one positive groin lymph node. There was no evidence that groin radiation therapy was beneficial to those patients with occult metastases and only one positive groin node. Review of the pattern of recurrence in that study suggested that adjuvant radiation was more effective largely because groin recurrences were reduced. A recent report described laparoscopic pelvic lymphadenectomy as a method to potentially avoid pelvic radiotherapy in patients with positive groin lymph nodes. The value of removing positive pelvic lymph nodes before radiotherapy is unknown. In a patient with obvious inguinal lymph node metastases who is otherwise suitable for surgical resection, consideration may be given to extending the dissection and removing enlarged pelvic lymph nodes. Preoperative CT may help with such a decision (Fig. 45.6).

Primary Inguinal Radiotherapy

The use of elective radiotherapy to the groins in the place of bilateral inguinofemoral lymphadenectomy offers the potential for avoiding operative morbidity. The method is believed to be appropriate only in the absence of clinically suspicious lymph nodes. Frischbier and Thomsen reported on this method for the treatment of 118 patients and reported a 70% survival rate for the N0, N1 group. Henderson and colleagues used the method for 91 N0, N1 patients with minimum morbidity. In that series, there were no groin recurrences in the radiotherapy field and two outside the field. In addition, there are extensive supporting data on elective nodal radiation for other sites, including the cervix, endometrium, vulva (pelvic), and head and neck. This issue was later addressed in another GOG study by Stehman and coworkers in 1992 in which there was a randomization of patients with nonsuspicious groin lymph nodes to radical vulvectomy plus bilateral inguinofemoral lymphadenectomy, or radical vulvectomy plus radiation therapy to the groins bilaterally. This study was closed early because of a high incidence of recurrence in the radiated groins and reduced survival (in the first 49 evaluable patients, there were five groin recurrences in the irradiated patients and no groin failures in the operated group). Upon review, however, it was believed that the radiation program used in the study may not have provided an adequate dose to the depth where the lymph nodes were located. The role of elective primary groin radiotherapy in the management of invasive squamous cell carcinoma of the vulva, therefore, remains unclear.

Omitting Groin Dissection for Superficial Disease

Extensive data support the contention that a subset of early vulvar carcinomas (carefully studied pathologically) can be identified that have an extremely low risk of nodal involvement. In another GOG study reported by Sedlis and associates, a subgroup (63 of 272) of patients with early disease was identified as having a zero incidence of lymph node metastases. This subset included nonmidline tumors with no capillary or lymphatic space involvement that were well differentiated or were grade 2 and limited to 2 mm in thickness. Other factors that have been studied for the purpose of identifying a low-risk group include tumor volume (which does not appear to have received further attention since Wilkinson's report in 1985), tumors that are largely carcinoma *in situ* with very early stromal invasion and with a pushing rather than an infiltrative pattern, tumor diameter, squamous cell type, the presence of an inflammatory response, and tumor ploidy.

There seems to be general agreement that the patients for whom it would be most reasonable to omit the lymphadenectomy are those with tumor invasion less than or equal to 1 mm. The risk of lymph node metastases in this group of patients is about 1% (Table 45.3). Based on this, FIGO stage I was divided into stages IA and IB. As reported in the literature, three of five patients with nodal disease or nodal recurrence in association with tumor invasion less than or equal to 1 mm had poorly differentiated cancers (Table 45.4). Thus, certain high-risk patients with superficially invasive tumors should still undergo a groin node dissection. These include women with suspicious lymph nodes, poorly differentiated tumors, tumors with capillary or lymphatic space involvement, and perhaps those with multiple foci or broad areas of invasion, or aneuploidy. Meanwhile, it is important to remember that in the report by Sedlis and colleagues on 272 patients with invasion of 5 mm or less, the groin nodes were positive in approximately 20%.

TABLE 45.3

INVASION OF LESS THAN 1 MILLIMETER: NODAL DISEASE

Investigator	Patients	Positive nodes
Wilkinson, 1985	115	0
Hacker et al., 1984	34	0
Parker et al., 1975	19	0
Magrina et al., 1979	19	0
Struyk et al., 1989	11	0
Sedlis et al., 1987	32	1
Ross and Ehrmann, 1987	17	0
Kelley et al., 1992	24	1
Stehman et al., 1992	13	1
Magrina et al., 2000	40	0
TOTALS	324	3 (1%)

Modifications in Management of the Vulvar Phase of Treatment

The main type of morbidity relating to a radical vulvectomy is subsequent sexual dysfunction and a sense of disfigurement. In some cases, there may also be compromised function of the anus or urethra. Additional types of morbidity are encountered in the treatment of locally advanced tumors because of the extensive therapy required. In a 1979 study, DiSaia and colleagues reported complete preservation of sexual function in 17 of 18 patients who underwent wide local excision for

TABLE 45.4

INVASION OF LESS THAN 1 MILLIMETER: NODAL DISEASE

Investigator	Patient age (y)	Tumor size (cm)	Grade	Tumor depth (mm)	Capillary or lymphatic space involvement	Months[a]	Status (mo of follow-up)
Sedlis et al., 1987	61	2.5	4[b]	1	(2)	0	NA
Atamdede and Hoogerland, 1989	75	1.0	1	0.72	(2)	13	AWD
van der Velden et al., 1992	84	1.0	3	0.3	(2)	20	DOD
Kelley et al., 1992	52	NA	NA	<1	NA	31	A (27)
Stehman et al., 1992	57	2.0	3	0.6	(2)	26	A (35)

NA, not available; AWD, alive with disease; DOD, dead of disease; A, alive.
[a]Months to diagnosis of nodal disease.
[b]Gynecologic Oncology Group grading system.

early invasive tumors. They also reported that preservation of the mons pubis as well as the major portion of the superior aspect of the vulva resulted in an appreciably more satisfactory cosmetic result. There is little additional information in the literature on sexual function as it relates to modifications of radical vulvectomy. It seems reasonable to assume, however, that the sparing of as much normal vulvar tissue as possible is less likely to produce sexual dysfunction and a sense of disfigurement than is radical vulvectomy. Modified radical vulvectomy is an ambiguously defined operation that generally refers to radical removal of the portion of the vulva containing the tumor (Fig. 45.12). Recommendations have included 1- to 3-cm skin margins for the treatment of well-localized, unifocal lesions.

The chief concerns with a modified radical vulvectomy are the possibility of an increased risk of local recurrence and later an increased risk of a second primary vulvar cancer. Multicentricity has been reported to occur in 20% to 28% of invasive squamous cell carcinomas of the vulva (Fig. 45.13). Ross and Ehrmann reported 15 of 64 stage I patients as having microscopic multifocal disease and 3 of 64 patients with grossly multifocal disease. There may be an ongoing occult process within the vulva of patients with vulvar carcinoma, and biochemical abnormalities have been demonstrated in normal-appearing epithelium adjacent to malignancy. In the report by Ross and Ehrmann, occult microscopic multifocal disease appeared in the immediate vicinity of the grossly evident tumor as surface noncontiguity of the primary lesion. Occult microscopic disease away from the primary tumor has not been reported, and the concern that microscopic multicentric foci might be left behind as a result of a modified operation does not appear to be valid. The potential for local microscopic noncontiguity of the tumor, however, would indicate the importance of an adequate tumor margin. In fact, two studies reported a higher local recurrence rate when the resected tumor-free margin was less than 1 cm. For most well-demarcated vulvar cancers, the gross and microscopic borders of the tumor correlate. One study found that ulcerative tumors with an infiltrative pattern of invasion involving mucosal epithelium may be more likely to extend beyond what is grossly apparent. Simonsen and colleagues noted that in many radical vulvectomies, margins are close. Iversen suggested that the goal in treating the primary tumor in vulvar squamous cell carcinoma of all stages should be adequate margins rather than removal of the entire vulva. Hacker and colleagues compared radical vulvectomy with wide local excision in the treatment of superficially invasive squamous cell carcinoma of the vulva. Fifty-six patients underwent radical vulvectomy and 28 patients underwent wide local excision. The local recurrence rate of 4% was identical in both groups. A later review by Hacker and van der Velden of literature regarding patients with vulvar cancer 2 cm or less in diameter showed a local invasive recurrence rate of 7.2% for 165 patients treated with radical local excision versus 6.3% for 365 patients treated with radical vulvectomy. In a comparative study at my institution of 45 patients who underwent radical vulvectomy and 45 patients who underwent

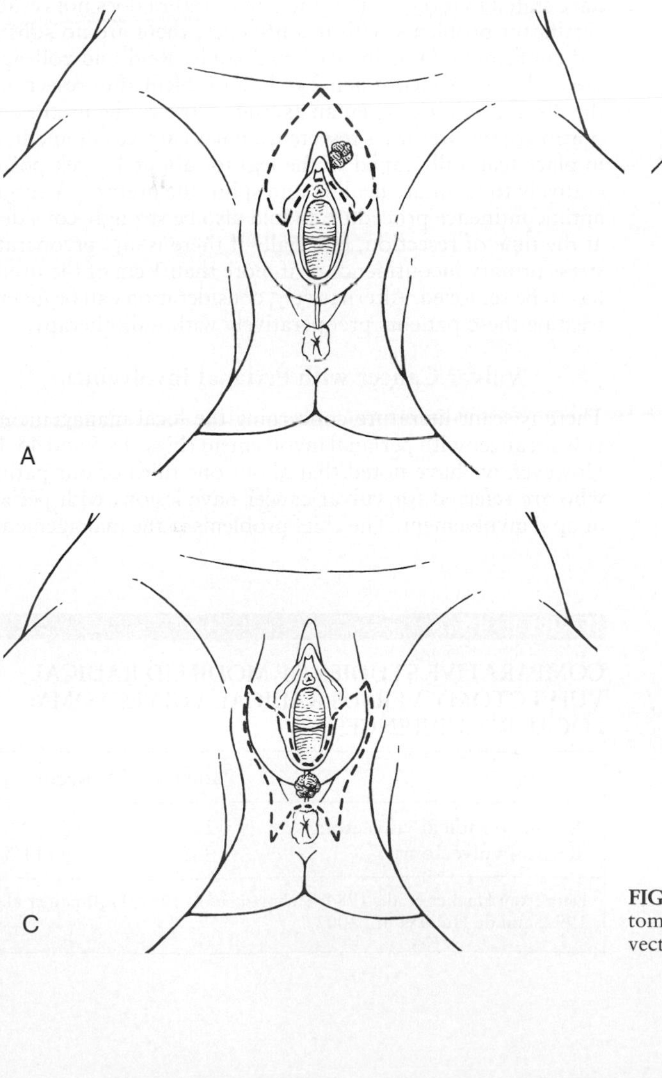

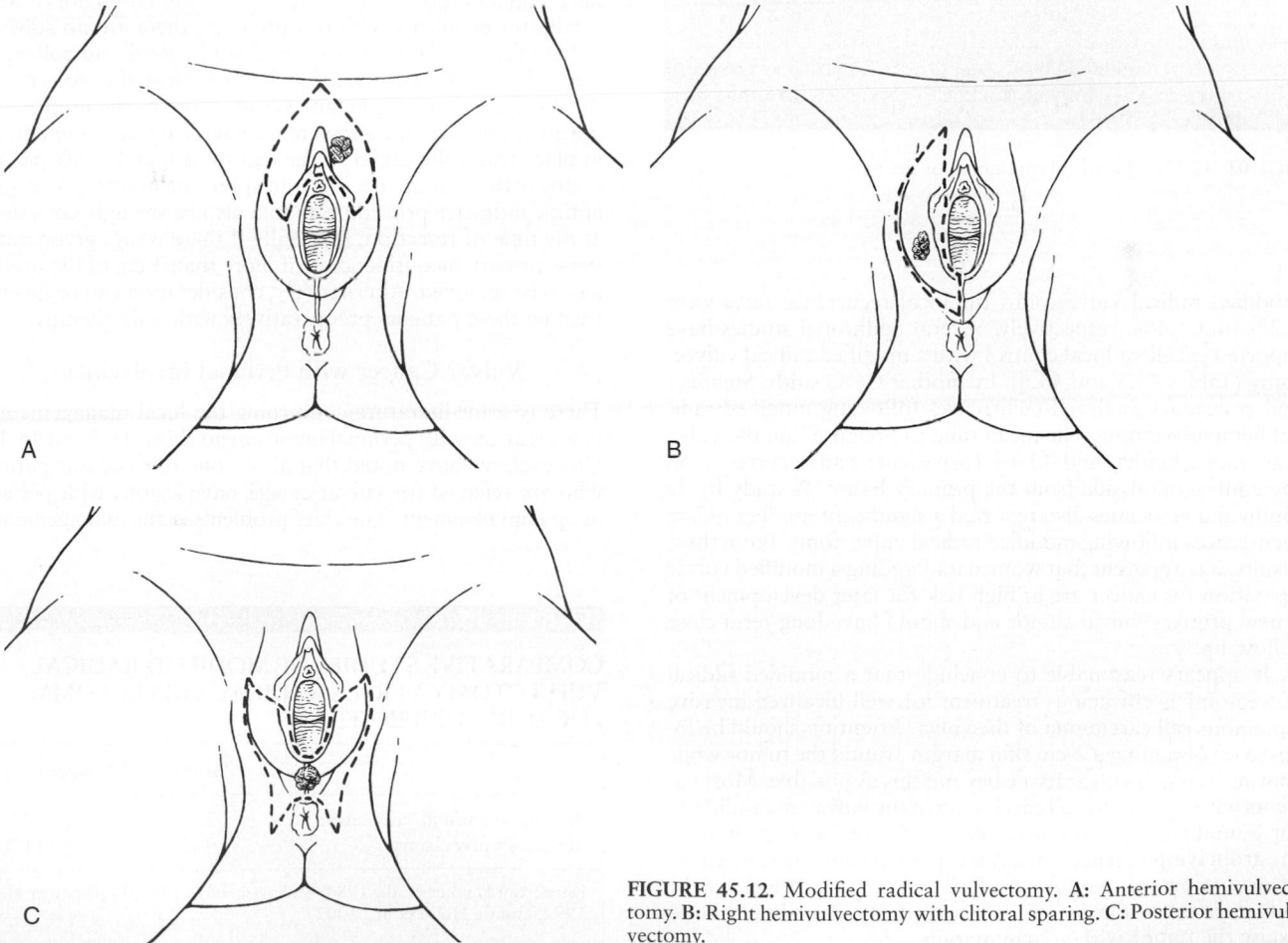

FIGURE 45.12. Modified radical vulvectomy. **A:** Anterior hemivulvectomy. **B:** Right hemivulvectomy with clitoral sparing. **C:** Posterior hemivulvectomy.

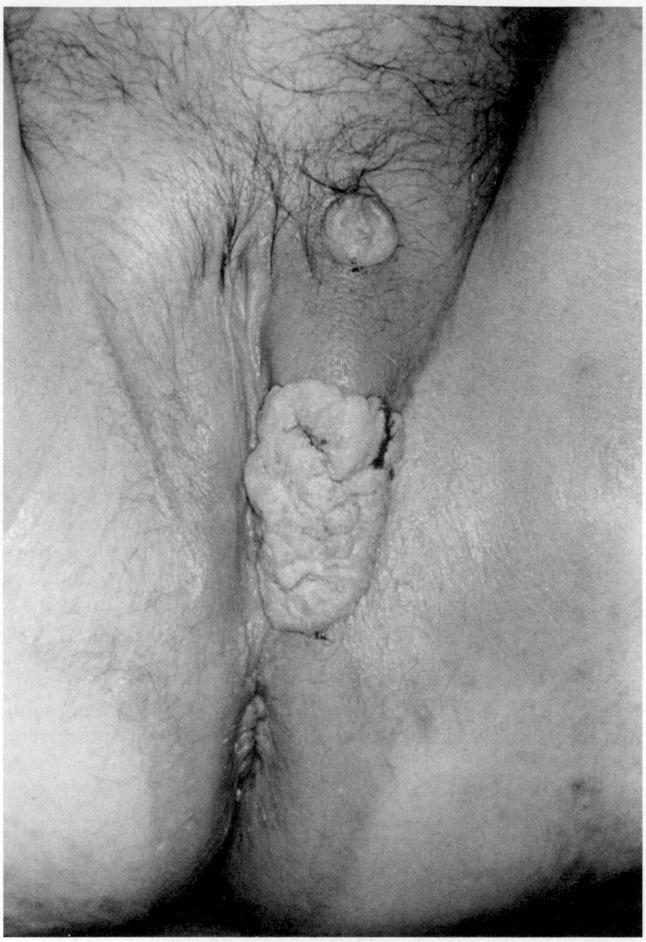

FIGURE 45.13. Multifocal carcinoma of the vulva.

modified radical vulvectomy, the local recurrence rates were 2.2% and 4.4%, respectively. Several additional studies have reported excellent local control with a modified radical vulvectomy (Tables 45.5 and 45.6). In another GOG study, Stehman and colleagues analyzed recurrences following modified radical hemivulvectomy. The mean time to "relapse" on the vulva was 43.4 months, and 11 of 18 patients had recurrence on the contralateral side from the primary lesion. A study by de Hullu and associates also reported a significant number of late recurrences following modified radical vulvectomy. From these results, it is apparent that women undergoing a modified vulvar operation for cancer are at high risk for later development of a new primary vulvar tumor and should have long-term close follow-up.

It appears reasonable to conclude that a modified radical vulvectomy is efficacious treatment for well-localized invasive squamous cell carcinoma of the vulva. Attention should be focused on obtaining a 2-cm skin margin around the tumor while sparing as much vulvar tissue beyond this as possible. Most patients with squamous cell carcinoma of the vulva are candidates for a modified radical vulvectomy performed separately from the groin lymphadenectomy. A few patients, however, by virtue of disease extent, require a radical vulvectomy. Whatever the vulvar phase of the operation is called, the aim should be to excise the tumor with a 2-cm margin.

TABLE 45.5

MODIFIED RADICAL VULVECTOMY LITERATURE: LOCAL RECURRENCE

	Patients	Local recurrence	Minimum follow-up (mo)
DiSaia et al., 1979	18	0	7
Hacker et al., 1984	28	1 (4%)	24
Burrell et al., 1988	28	0	16
Berman et al., 1989	50	4 (8%)	12
Sutton et al., 1991	56	7 (12%)	1
Stehman et al., 1992	121	10 (8%)	36
Hoffman et al., 1992	45	1 (2%)	12
Lin et al., 1992	12	2 (13%)	24
Andrews et al., 1994	28	2 (7%)	12
Burke et al., 1995	76	9 (12%)	NA
de Hullu et al., 2002	85	7 (8%)	NA
TOTALS	547	43 (8%)	

NA, not available.

Partial Urethral Resection

Because of tumor proximity, it is occasionally necessary to remove a portion of the urethra to obtain an adequate resection of a vulvar carcinoma (Fig. 45.14A–C). Although several authors have stated that removal of the outer urethra does not result in significant problems with incontinence, there are no substantial confirming data. In one small study, Reid and colleagues did find urinary incontinence to be a problem after resection of the distal urethra or even an excision close to the urethra. If a portion of the urethra is resected, a Foley catheter should be left in place (carefully taped to the leg) for about 1 week postoperatively to facilitate healing and splint the urethra. A surgical antiincontinence procedure should also be strongly considered at the time of resection, especially if there is any preoperative stress urinary incontinence or if more than 1 cm of the urethra has to be removed. Alternatively, consideration can be given to treating these patients preoperatively with radiotherapy.

Vulvar Cancer with Perianal Involvement

There is scant literature concerning the local management of vulvar cancer with perianal involvement (Figs. 45.5 and 45.15). However, we have noted that about one third of our patients who are referred for vulvar cancer have lesions with perianal or anal involvement. The chief problems in the management of

TABLE 45.6

COMPARATIVE STUDIES OF MODIFIED RADICAL VULVECTOMY VERSUS RADICAL VULVECTOMY: LOCAL RECURRENCE

	Patients	Recurrence
Modified radical vulvectomy	263	35 (13%)
Radical vulvectomy	343	39 (11%)

Data from Hacker et al., 1984; Stehman et al., 1992; Hoffman et al., 1992; and de Hullu et al., 2002.

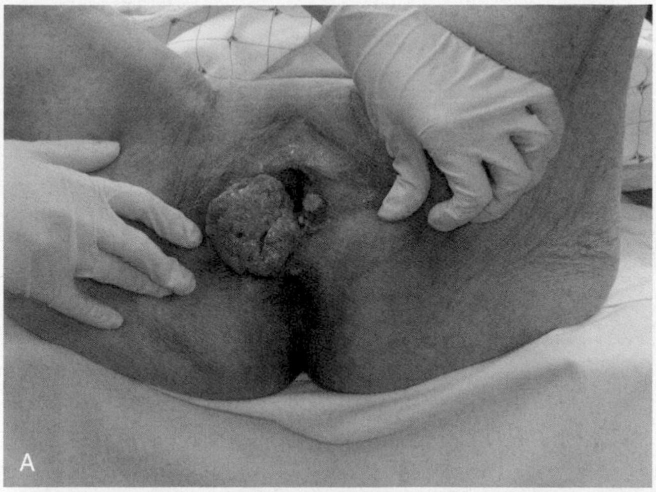

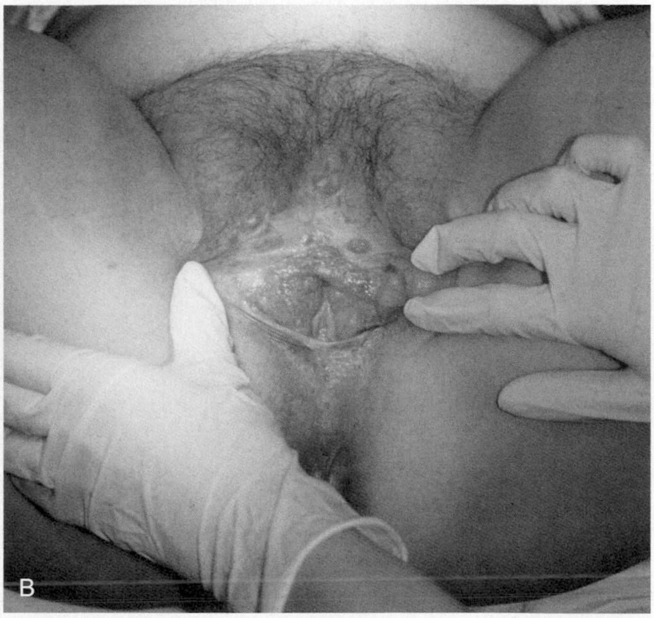

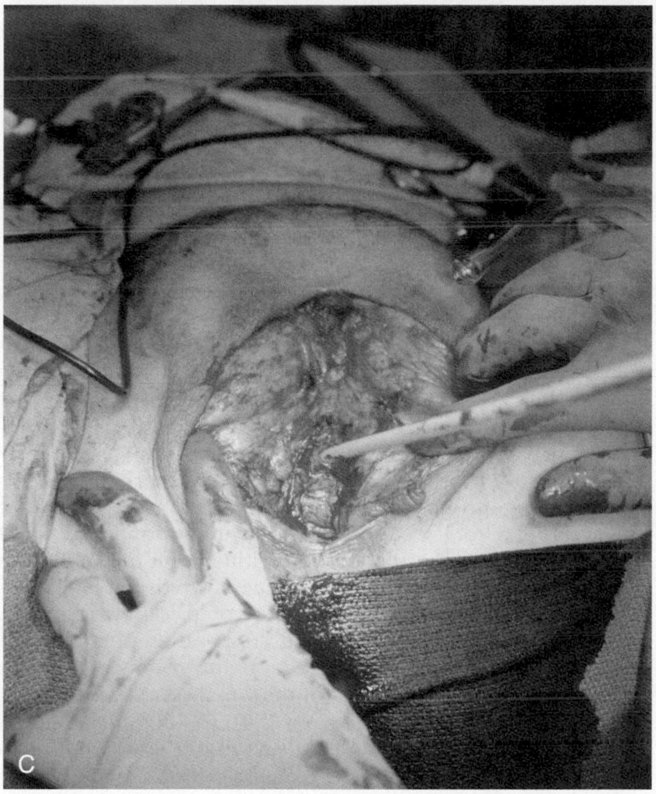

FIGURE 45.14. A–B: Vulvar cancer in close proximity to the urethra. **C:** Modified radical vulvectomy with resection of the distal urethra.

patients with these tumors are the difficulty in obtaining adequate surgical margins on the resection while attempting to preserve anal sphincter function, and deciding on which patients would be better treated either with a more radical excision and colostomy or with preoperative radiotherapy (Fig. 45.16). In our experience with vulvar carcinoma, partial resection of the external anal sphincter in combination with radical local resection of perianal tissue is associated with a significant rate of subsequent fecal incontinence. Careful sphincter reapproximation and levator muscle plication are done in an effort to minimize incontinence. Other important measures include good bowel preparation preoperatively, prophylactic antibiotics, and careful postoperative bowel management. In addition, we have had good results with the use of cutaneous rhomboid flaps in the reconstruction of the perineum and perianal area. These flaps allow for reconstruction of a perineal body, they bring tissue with a good blood supply into the area that promotes healing, and they allow closure of the wound without tension on the anus. As with urethral involvement, an option for these patients is preoperative radiotherapy.

LOCALLY ADVANCED DISEASE

About 30% to 40% of vulvar cancers have FIGO (clinical) stage III or IV disease. Although surgical staging was introduced by FIGO in 1988 and hard data on this system are still in relatively short supply, a review of our own patients suggests that this percentage probably still holds. We have considered carcinoma of the vulva to be locally advanced when the

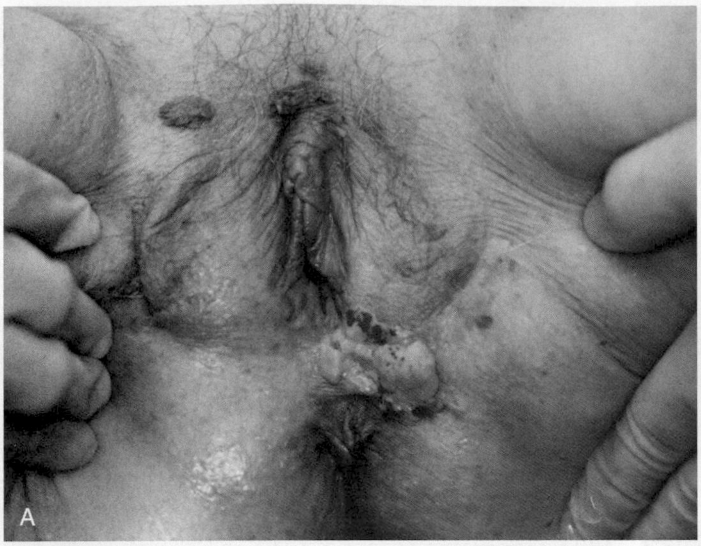

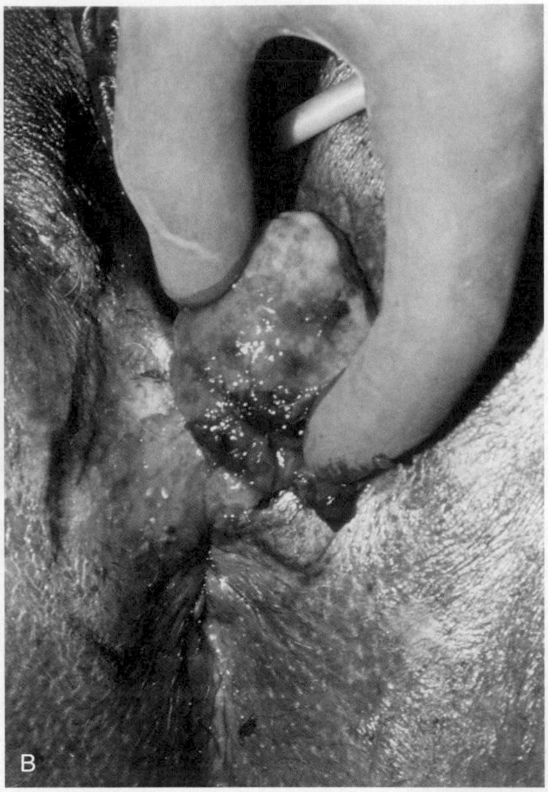

FIGURE 45.15. Perianal carcinoma. **A:** Slightly raised, superficially invasive perianal carcinoma. **B:** Exophytic, polypoid perianal carcinoma.

primary or recurring tumor cannot be locally managed by a radical vulvar resection (Fig. 45.17A–C). Current approaches to the treatment of locally advanced vulvar cancer include ultraradical surgery, radiotherapy, or a combination of treatment modalities. This section reviews the current approaches to the treatment of locally advanced vulvar cancer.

Ultraradical Surgery

Ultraradical surgery has been used for patients with clinically resectable vulvar lesions and has generally consisted of a radical vulvar operation extended to include the anorectum and/or the lower urinary tract. This has included resection of bone in a few reports (Fig. 45.18). Inguinofemoral and pelvic lymphadenectomies are usually performed as well (Fig. 45.19).

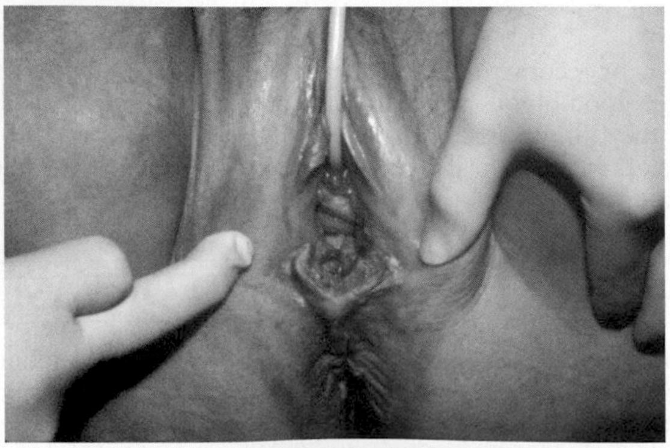

FIGURE 45.16. Perineal carcinoma encroaching upon the anus. See color version of figure.

In some cases, resection can be limited to partial removal of the urethra, anus, or anterior rectal wall. Subsequent incontinence may occur, but this can be prevented to some degree by reconstructive efforts. Reid and associates reported problems with urinary incontinence in 4 of 4 patients who underwent resection of 1 to 1.5 cm of the distal urethra and in 2 of 14 patients who underwent resection within 1 cm of the urethra for carcinoma of the vulva. The value of urethral reconstruction in this setting is uncertain, but it would seem worthwhile. Three recent studies have reported preservation of anal continence after partial sphincter resection and reconstruction for posteriorly located carcinoma of the vulva.

The cumulative literature from 1970 to 2006 includes 163 vulvar cancer "exenteration" patients (Table 45.7). The postoperative mortality rate ranges from 0% to 20%, with a mean of about 4%. The cumulative disease-free survival rate for these patients is 46%. In those series that have included an analysis, the survival has correlated well with the status of the regional lymph nodes. Most studies have not differentiated inguinal and pelvic lymph nodes. There have been very few survivors with positive nodes, either in our series or elsewhere. Although not well addressed in the literature, there is also significant physical and psychological morbidity resulting from these operations as a result of the extensive nature of the surgery and the need for a permanent colostomy and/or urostomy. It appears that the use of a combination of treatment modalities avoids the need for such extensive surgery in many of these patients (see later text). Likely in large part related to this, utilization of the "ultraradical" surgical approach for primary management of locally advanced vulvar cancer appears to have markedly decreased over the past decade. It may be reasonable to confine the use of ultraradical surgery to highly selected patients with

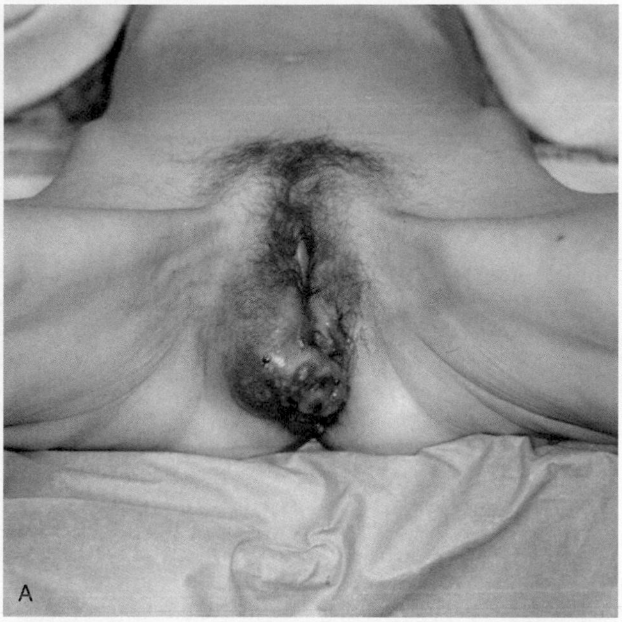

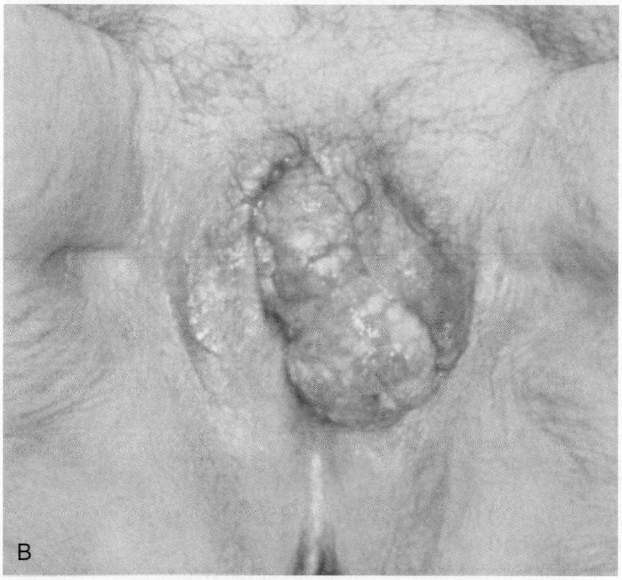

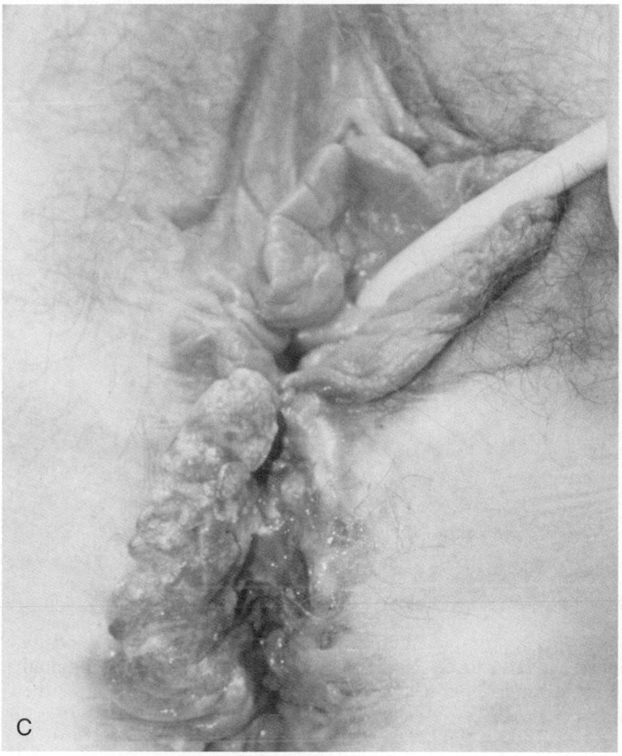

FIGURE 45.17. **A:** Locally advanced vulvar carcinoma. The lesion extensively involved the anus and lower rectovaginal septum but was mobile. There was no suspicious adenopathy. **B:** Large and locally extensive vulvar cancer. **C:** Vulvar cancer extensively involving perineum and anus.

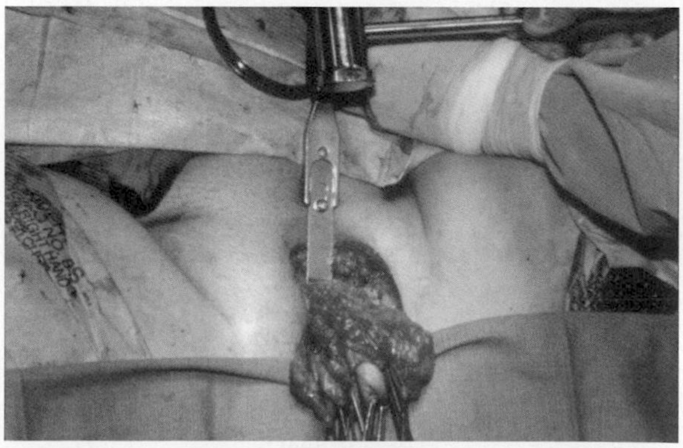

FIGURE 45.18. Locally advanced vulvar tumor fixed to the periosteum of the pubic bone. This portion of the bone is being removed with the tumor using a Richardson osteotome.

clearly respectable lesions who have negative—or perhaps one or two microscopically positive—regional lymph nodes. It may be the only option for a patient who has previously received radiotherapy to the region (Fig. 45.20).

Radiotherapy

The role of primary radiotherapy as the sole method of treatment for carcinoma of the vulva remains unclear, but may be the only option available when the patient presents with unresectable disease. The literature concerning the use of radiotherapy for this disease consists of retrospective studies with small numbers of patients (many of whom were medically infirm or had locally advanced disease) who were treated with a variety of radiotherapy techniques (Table 45.8). Overall, this information is difficult to interpret. The older literature is discouraging in terms of both low cure rates and vulvar skin intolerance.

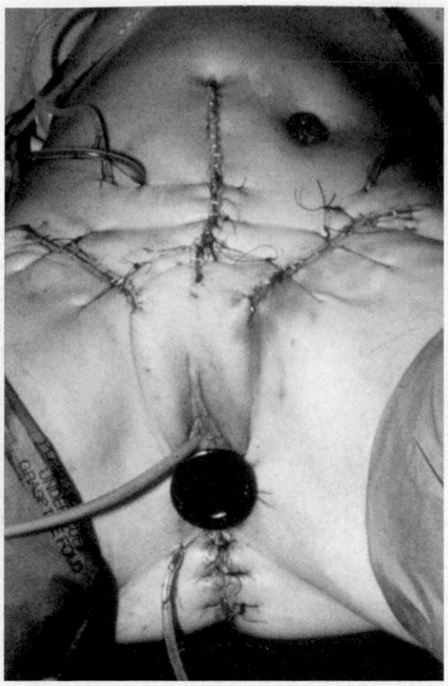

FIGURE 45.19. Completed posterior pelvic exenteration for a locally advanced vulvar cancer. Note the end-sigmoid colostomy, inguinal incisions, extended perineal incision, and a Young's dilator in the vagina.

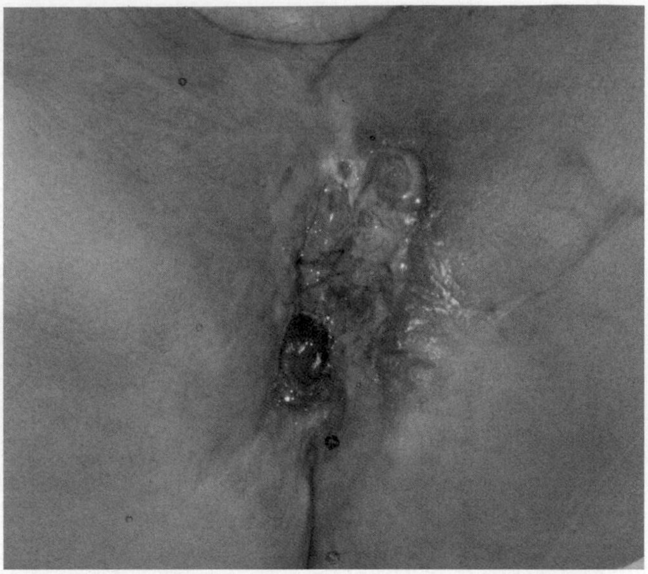

FIGURE 45.20. Carcinoma of the vulva recurring after previous radiotherapy and radical vulvectomy.

Contemporary literature with use of high-energy radiotherapy with its relative skin-sparing effects as well as the use of modern radiotherapy techniques has been more encouraging. Whether normal bladder and bowel function is preserved with this type of treatment is difficult to determine.

The optimal techniques for radiotherapeutic treatment of carcinoma of the vulva have not been well defined. In the more recent literature, teletherapy has been administered to the whole pelvis, including the vulva and the groins, at a dose of 45 to 55 Gy. It is not uncommon for patients to require treatment interruption because of vulvitis. The treatment regimen has been modified in some studies, with only brachytherapy or palliative treatment used. A few studies have described the use of a direct perineal portal. We reported a series of 10 patients with locally advanced vulvovaginal malignancy treated mainly with teletherapy followed by interstitial needles (Fig. 45.21) to the local tumor bed for a tumor dose of 70 to 90 Gy. The therapy was highly morbid, with six patients developing severe radionecrosis (Fig. 45.22). Treatment fields, the role of interstitial radiotherapy, the overall dose, and the integration of combination treatment with chemotherapy or surgery, or both, are among the issues to be studied. Preliminary results suggest that radiotherapy (possibly combined with chemotherapy) followed

TABLE 45.7

POSTOPERATIVE MORTALITY AND SURVIVAL OF PATIENTS WITH ADVANCED VULVAR CANCER TREATED BY ULTRARADICAL SURGERY

Investigator	Patients	Postoperative mortality	Disease-free survivors
Rutledge et al., 1970	13	0	10 (3 yr)
Thornton and Flanagan, 1973	12	1	4 (7 mo–9.5 yr)
Kaplan and Kaufman, 1975	9	1	4 (5+ yr)
Krupp et al., 1975	13	2	3 (1.5–15 yr)
Adams and Daly, 1979	5	1	3 (10–41 mo)
Benedet et al., 1979	5	0	1 (>5+ yr)
Phillips et al., 1981	12	1	5 (52–153 mos)
Cavanagh and Shepherd, 1982	13	1	5 (>5+ yr)
King et al., 1989	7	0	3 (9 mo–18 yr)
Hopkins and Morley, 1992	19	0	10 (5 yr)
Grimshaw et al., 1991	23	0	15 (4–136 mo)
Miller and Morris, 1992	21	0	9 (5 yr)
Hoffman et al., 1993	11	0	6 (30–84 mo)
Miller et al., 1995	21	0	7 (70% primary, 38% recurrent)
TOTALS	163	7 (4.3%)	76 (46%)

TABLE 45.8

RADIATION ALONE FOR VULVAR CANCER, 1970 TO PRESENT

Investigator	Technique	Stage	Dose (Gy)	L/R control (%)	Follow-up (yr)	Serious complication rate (%)
Frischbier and Thomsen, 1971	MeV E	III-II III-IV	45–54	23/33 (70) 33/85 (39)	5	8
Backstrom et al., 1972	^{60}Co	IV	52–69	7/19 (36)	5	NA
Helgason et al., 1972	ORTH, ^{60}Co + RI	I-IV Recurrence	15–58 30	16/29 (55) 4/24 (17)	2–5 3	—
Kuipers, 1975	MeV	EI-II III-IV	60–80	3/11 (27) 12/37 (32)	5	— 12
Jafari and Magalotti, 1981	^{60}Co, t-Ces	II-IV	30–60	7/8 (88)	1–11	2
Pirtoli and Rottoli, 1982	ORTH	I-IV	45–85	17/36 (47)	5	18
Miyazawa et al., 1983	Betratron + implant	III-IV Recurrence	40–50 50–80	2/12 (17) 2/10 (20)	2–11	—
Prempree and Amornmarn, 1984	^{60}Co, MeV E + RI	Limited Extensive	40–60 + 15–55	8/8 (100) 0/13 (0)	>5	37
Carlino et al., 1984	Betratron + Ir I	I-IV	NG	2/8 (25)	<1	0
Fairey et al., 1985	^{60}Co	I-II Local recurrence	50–55	3/6 (50)	>3	22
	Palliative			2/9 (22)		
			30	19/40 (48)		25
Pao et al., 1988	Meg	III-IV	7.5–78	2/5 (40)	4	—
Slevin and Pointon, 1989	I ± Meg	I-IV Recurrence	45–55	23/58 (40)	NA	5
	Palliative					
Hoffman et al., 1990	Meg + Ir I	III-IV, Recurrence	44–90	8/10 (80)	1–4	60
Perez et al., 1993	Meg ± Ir I	I-IV, Recurrence	50–70	NA/33	NA	25
Tewari et al., 1999	Meg + Ir I	III-IV, Recurrence	24–55[a]	11/11 (100)	0.75–6.5	18

L/R, local/regional; MeV, million electron volts; E, electrons; ^{60}C, cobalt-60; ORTH, orthovoltage; RI, radium implant; t-Ces, teletherapy cesium; IrI, iridium implant; Meg, megavoltage; NG, not given; NA, not availble.
[a]Interstitial dose only.

by a more limited resection is more efficacious than radiotherapy alone. These treatment methods are discussed in the next two sections.

Preoperative Radiotherapy

From the work of Boronow and others, data confirm that megavoltage radiotherapy can cause marked regression of even locally advanced vulvar carcinoma to the point to which a more limited resection can be undertaken (often with an improved resection margin) with sparing of organ function and improved quality of life. In an update of his study in 1987, Boronow reported that, of 48 bladders and 48 rectums at risk, one bladder and two rectums were lost because of local failure, and one bladder and one rectum were lost because of radiation injury. The report did not mention other types of bladder or bowel morbidity. Of 40 patients who underwent vulvectomy, 17 contained no identifiable residual cancer. There were no reported problems with wound healing. Similar results have been reported in other studies (Table 45.9). In these studies, survival with locally advanced disease so far has been comparable to that with ultraradical surgery. Again, the optimal radiotherapeutic techniques for such treatment are not well defined. Boronow's group generally used a combination of external beam radiation and intracavitary brachytherapy, delivering a mean vaginal surface maximum dose of 86.26 Gy. His group and others have also used preoperative external beam therapy only, generally delivering a dose of about 50 Gy to the whole pelvis, including the vulva and groins. Surgery has generally been performed 2 to 6 weeks after completion of radiotherapy. Boronow and associates reported 42.5% of

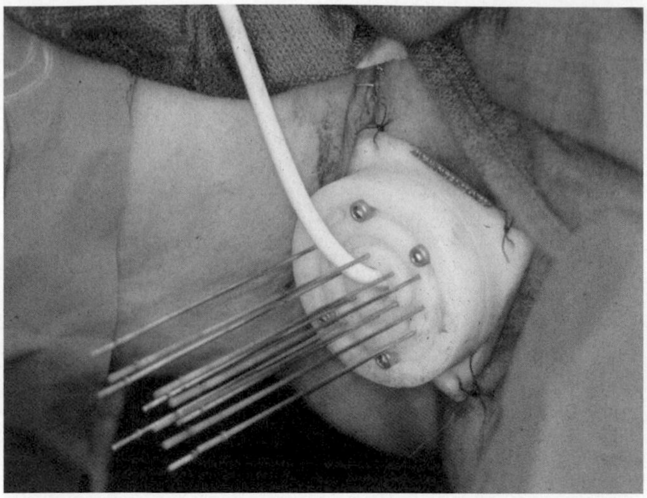

FIGURE 45.21. Interstitial needle implant into the vulvar tumor bed.

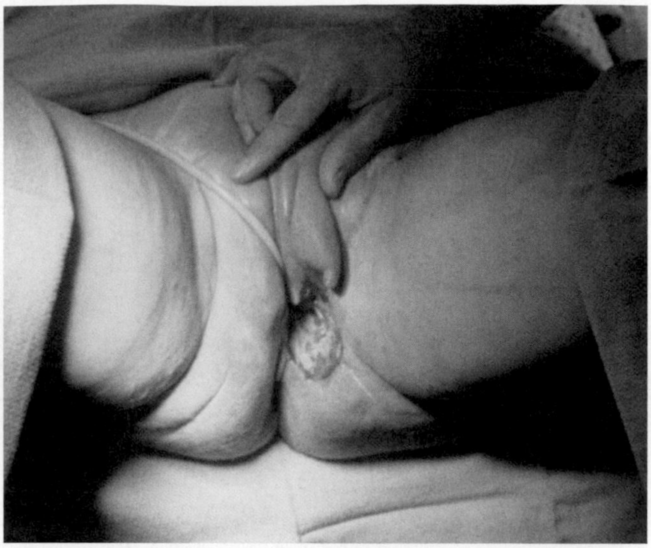

FIGURE 45.22. Radionecrosis with large ulcer.

vulvectomy specimens and Hacker and colleagues reported 4 of 7 (57%) vulvectomy specimens to be negative for residual tumor.

Chemoradiotherapy

As with preoperative radiotherapy, combined chemoradiotherapy with or without resection has been used increasingly over the past 25 years with promising results in squamous cell carcinomas of several different primary sites. This approach has been particularly successful in the treatment of squamous cell carcinoma of the anus. This type of carcinoma may be somewhat analogous to carcinoma of the vulva in terms of location and, in some instances, preservation of the anus. Although the cumulative data on this type of treatment for carcinoma of the vulva is quite limited, the results are promising.

The most commonly used chemotherapeutic agents are 5-fluorouracil, mitomycin-C, and cisplatin. Chemotherapy has been combined with external radiotherapy administered in a manner similar to that described in the previous sections. Most data have been accumulated over the past 20 years with the use of regimens similar to those used at other sites. Results suggest a high rate of local control for locally advanced or recurrent disease (Table 45.10). However, an increase in the degree of local morbidity is seen with this type of therapy. Most of these patients develop a moderate amount of mucositis in the vulvovaginal area (Fig. 45.23). This leads to dysuria and generalized pelvic and perineal discomfort. An indwelling catheter (suprapubic in some cases) and the use of various perianal and rectal preparations help ease the discomfort, although treatment interruption is necessary at times. The GOG investigated the use of chemoradiotherapy for the treatment of advanced squamous cell carcinoma of the vulva. Results from this study are included in Table 45.10 and confirm those reported by the other investigators.

Neoadjuvant Chemotherapy

A large number of pilot studies in the recent literature have reported on the use of neoadjuvant chemotherapy (NACT)

TABLE 45.9

PREOPERATIVE RADIOTHERAPY FOR CARCINOMA OF THE VULVA

Investigator	Patients	Stage	Survival rate (%)	Survival	Severe complications (%)
Boronow et al., 1987	48	III, IV, Recurrent	72	4–168 mo	23
Acosta et al., 1978	14	II-III	71	2 mo–8 yr	14
Jafari and Magalotti, 1981	4	II-III	100	4–5 yr	0
Hacker et al., 1984	8	IV	62.5	15 mo–10 yr	12
Carlino et al., 1984	6	II-III	66.6	15 mo	NA
Fairey et al., 1985	7	I-IV	86	13 mo–3 yr	14
Pao et al., 1988	2	I, III	100	1–2 yr	0
Rotmensch et al., 1990	16	III, IV	45	12–72 mo	4
TOTALS	105		69		19

NA, not available.

TABLE 45.10

RESULTS OF CHEMORADIOTHERAPY WITH AND WITHOUT RESECTION

Investigator	Radiotherapy (Gy)	Stage	Chemotherapy	Surgery	Proportion of patients with local control	Severe complications (%)
Kalra et al., 1981	^{60}Co (30)	III	Mit-C, 5FU	RV, GND (-)	1/1	0
Iversen, 1982	Meg (30–40)	Inoperable/ Recurrent	Bleo	2 RV, GND	4/15 (26%) 1–4	40
Nori et al., 1983	Meg (34–58)	III-IV, Recurrent	Flagyl	1 vulv	5/6 (83%) 1–3	0
Levin et al., 1986	Meg (18–45)	T3N1-T4N0	Mit-C, 5FU	4 RV	5/5 1–25 mo	17
Lovett et al., 1987	Meg (40 ± I)	III, IV	DDP, 5FU	NA	1/2 10 mo	NA
Evans et al., 1988	Meg (20–64 ± I)	NA	Mit-C, 5FU	NA	4/4 > 18 mo	NA
Thomas et al., 1989	Meg (40–64)	1.3–9 cm	5FU ± Mit-C	5 LE	7/9 (77%) 5–43 mo	9
	Recurrent 1.5–12 cm				8/12 (66%) 5–45 mo	
Whitaker et al., 1990	Meg (25–45)	III, IV, Recurrent	Mit-C, 5FU	2 RV	3/12 6–9 mo	25
Carson et al., 1990	Meg (45–50)	III, IV, Recurrent	5FU, Mit-C DDP	4 RV, 3 LE	6/8 (75%)	12.5
Podczaski et al., 1990	Meg (51 + H)	IV	5FU, DDP	RV	1/1 8 mo	0
Berek et al., 1991	Meg (44–54)	III, IV	DDP, 5FU	3 RV, 1 PE	10/12 7–60 mo	0
Russel et al., 1992	Meg (46–78)	III, IV[a]	5FU ± DDP	1 RV	20/25 (80%) 2–52 mo	8
Scheistroen et al., 1993	Meg (9–45)	III, IV[a]	Bleo	4 RV	6/20 (30%) 7–60 mo	30
Koh et al., 1993	Meg (34–70)	III, IV,[a] Recurrent	5FU	9 LE, 2 RV, 1 PE	11/20 (55%) 14–75 mo	5
Sebag-Montefiore et al., 1994	Meg (45–50)	III, IV, Recurrent	Mit-C, 5FU	8 RV	17/32 3–40 mo	11
Whalen et al., 1995	Meg (45–50 ± I)	II, III[b]	Mit-C, 5FU	6 LE	14/19 11–72 mo	0
Eifel et al., 1995	Meg (40–50)	Recurrent-T4N3	DDP, 5FU	6 LE, 1 RV, 1 PE, 3 GND	4/12 (33%) 17–37 mo	17
Lupi et al., 1996	Meg (NG)	Recurrent-T4N2	Mit-C, 5FU	18 RV, 11 LE, 29 GND	25/31 (80%) 22–90 mo	20
Landoni et al., 1996	Meg (54)	II, III, IV,[a] Recurrent	Mit-C, 5FU	39 RV, 30 GND	47/58 (82%) 4–48 mo	20
Cunningham et al., 1997	Meg (50–65)	III, IV[a]	DDP, 5FU	NG	9/14 (64%) 7–81 mo	23
Moore et al., 1998	Meg (41–50)	III, IV[a]	DDP, 5FU	24 LE, 24 RV, 2 PE	60/71 (84%) 22–72 mo	21
Montana et al., 2000	Meg (47)	N2/N3 nodes	DDP, 5FU	34 LE, 37 GND	28/38 (74%) 56–89 mo	47
Mulayim et al., 2004	Meg (45–62)	T3, T3N1	Mit-C, 5FU		Surgery: none; 5/6 13–74 mo	17

^{60}C, cobalt-60; Mit-C, mitomycin-C; 5FU, 5-fluorouracil; Bleo, bleomycin; DDP, cisplatin; RV, radical vulvectomy; GND, inguinal lymphadenectomy; Meg, megavoltage; vulv, vulvectomy; LE, local excision; PE, posterior exenteration; H, hyperthermia; I, implant; NG, not given; NA, not available.
[a]1988 staging.
[b]1992 staging.

in cervical cancer. The planned course of chemotherapy has been followed by surgery, radiotherapy, or both. Reported response rates have been high, and preliminary results with NACT followed by radical surgery are somewhat encouraging.

In 1993, Benedetti-Panici and colleagues reported the results of a pilot study using NACT followed by surgery in patients with locally advanced carcinoma of the vulva. Twenty-one patients with FIGO stage IVA (clinical) were treated. Chemotherapy consisted of cisplatin, 100 mg/m^2 intravenously on day 1; bleomycin, 15 mg intravenously on days 1 and 8; and methotrexate, 300 mg/m^2 intravenously plus citrovorum factor rescue dose on day 8, repeated every 21 days for two to three cycles. A partial response was observed in the primary tumor in two patients, and progression of disease was seen in two other patients. Eleven complete and three partial responses

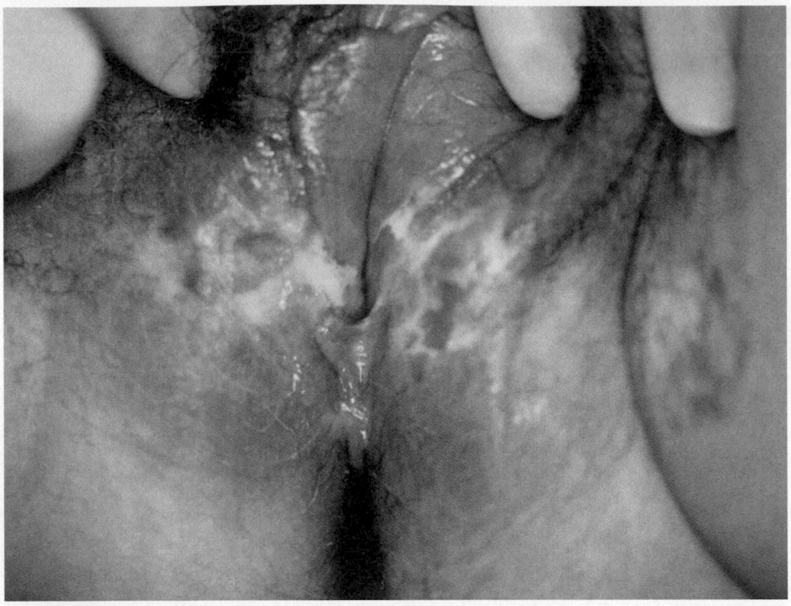

FIGURE 45.23. Desquamative vulvitis and mucositis during chemoradiotherapy.

were noted in the patients with nodal disease. On pathologic examination of the 19 patients undergoing resection, 15 had inguinal lymph node metastases and 9 of these had pelvic lymph node metastases. Local control was achieved in 12 of 21 (57%) of the patients (3 to 37 months), and the 3-year corrected survival rate was 24%.

The study just discussed does not suggest any benefit of NACT over the previously described treatment approaches, and the authors of that report subsequently have used the chemoradiotherapeutic approach. Two European cooperative studies used bleomycin, methotrexate, and CCNU and reported similar results.

Treatment of Locally Advanced Disease: Summary

Ultraradical surgery appears to be a reasonable treatment option for selected patients with locally advanced but resectable carcinoma of the vulva, especially in the absence of nodal metastases. The role of radiotherapy in the treatment of this malignancy is still being defined. In our experience, teletherapy combined with interstitial needles for locally advanced carcinoma of the vulva appears to be effective but associated with extensive morbidity. With the use of more modern treatment techniques and better definition of the optimal delivery of radiotherapy to the vulva, the role of this modality has been expanded. A modified course of radiotherapy used in combination with other treatment modalities appears to be more efficacious than radiotherapy alone in the treatment of this disease. Combined treatment modalities for this disease present an important form of management. Especially in patients with locally unresectable disease, initial treatment with external radiation therapy possibly combined with chemotherapy appears to be the most reasonable approach. With the use of radiologic techniques and perhaps random biopsies, an additional treatment course could be planned. Careful planning of how much surgery may be necessary or how much volume needs additional radiation therapy may contribute to an overall decrease in morbidity in these patients.

Management of the regional lymph nodes in the context of combined treatment modalities has been variable and, by necessity, highly individualized.

The management of locally advanced vulvar cancer continues to evolve as reports of small series of these patients accumulate. Considering the relative paucity of data and the rarity and heterogeneity of these tumors, no clear-cut management guidelines can be constructed. It seems reasonable to individualize the management of these patients, carefully considering all of the various treatment modalities available.

RECURRENT SQUAMOUS CELL CARCINOMA OF THE VULVA

About 15% to 40% of patients with squamous cell carcinoma of the vulva develop recurrence after treatment. As discussed previously, the incidence of recurrence is influenced by a number of factors, including the original stage of the disease, the depth of invasion, and the regional lymph node status. About 70% of recurrences have a local component, and 55% to 90% of these are isolated local recurrences (Fig. 45.24A–B). This is more likely to occur in the patient with negative lymph nodes at initial treatment. For patients with recurrent squamous cell carcinoma of the vulva, recurrence site is the strongest predictor of outcome. Only with an isolated local recurrence is there a reasonable expectation of successful salvage therapy (Table 45.11).

The presence of inguinal nodal metastases, especially when multiple, bilateral, or extranodal, predisposes the patient to recurrence within the groin or pelvis and systemically. The prognosis for a patient with regional or systemic recurrence is poor. Regional recurrences do not lend themselves well to salvage resection, radiotherapy is not very effective against grossly recurrent disease, and there is no effective systemic therapy. A small percentage of patients with groin recurrence can be salvaged with resection followed by radiotherapy.

Certain factors predispose the patient to develop local recurrence, including a close resection margin (less than 1 cm), deep invasion, and a large tumor size. When a patient develops

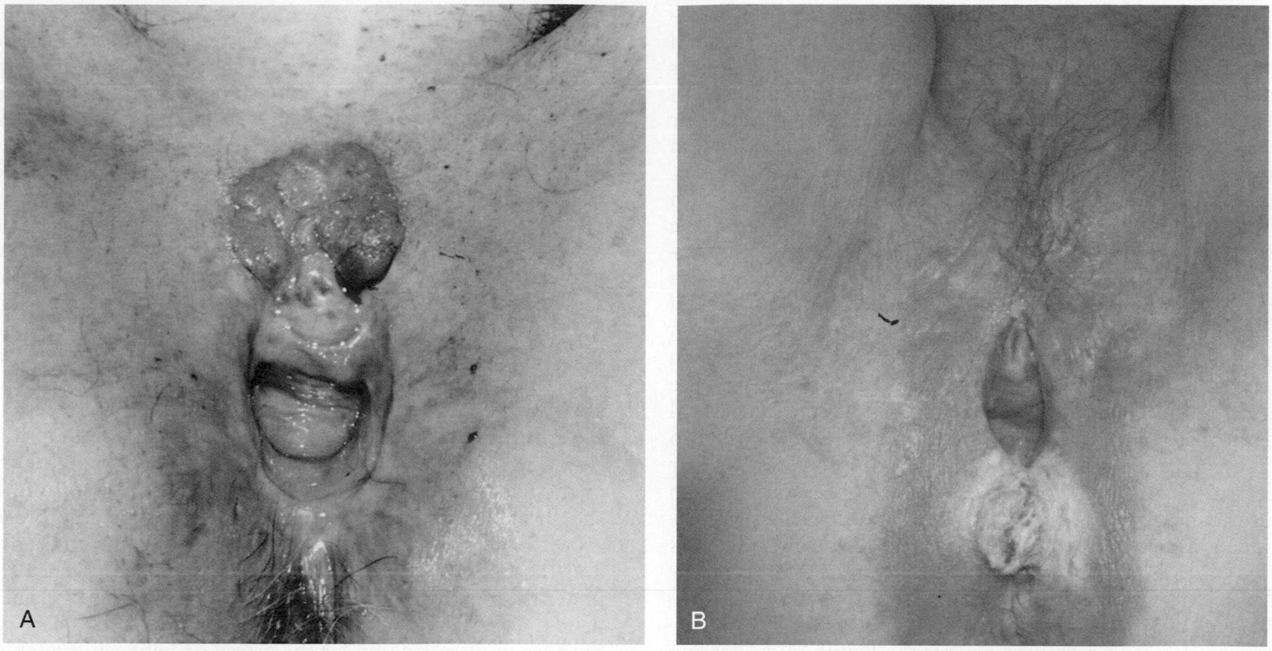

FIGURE 45.24. A: Local recurrence around urethral meatus. B: Local recurrence in the perianal region.

an isolated local recurrence, the reported salvage rate ranges from 40% to 80%. Treatment depends on the individual situation. When feasible, radical resection is performed. Otherwise, the best approach is probably preoperative radiotherapy with or without chemotherapy followed by resection.

TABLE 45.11

VULVAR RECURRENCE SITE AND SALVAGE RATE

Investigator	Patients	Local recurrence only (%)	Groin (± local)	Pelvis (± local)
Buchler et al., 1979	27	13/18 (72)	0/7	1/2
Podratz et al., 1982	59	15/30 (50)	NA	NA
Simonsen, 1984	41	11/29 (38)	1/12	—
Prempree and Amornmarn, 1984[a]	21	6/12 (50)	2/5	0/4
Hopkins et al., 1990	34	19/24 (79)	0/10	—
Tilmans et al., 1992	40	9/17 (53)	2/12	1/11
Piura et al., 1993	73	24/39 (61)	NA	NA
Stehman et al., 1996	37	13/21 (62)	0/12	—
Maggino et al., 2000	187	56/94 (60)	8/33	0/10
TOTALS	519	166/284 (58)	13/91	2/27

NA, not available.
[a]All patients treated with radiotherapy only.

Operative Techniques

Radical Vulvectomy with Bilateral Inguinofemoral Lymphadenectomy

The patient is placed in the "ski position" in adjustable stirrups so that the legs can be elevated to high lithotomy during the perineal phase of the operation.

The radical vulvectomy with bilateral inguinofemoral lymphadenectomy is ideally performed with the use of two teams, and dissection of each groin is performed simultaneously. A crescent-shaped incision is made starting about 2 to 4 cm medial and about 2 cm caudal to the anterior superior iliac spine (Fig. 45.25). The incision gradually curves downward

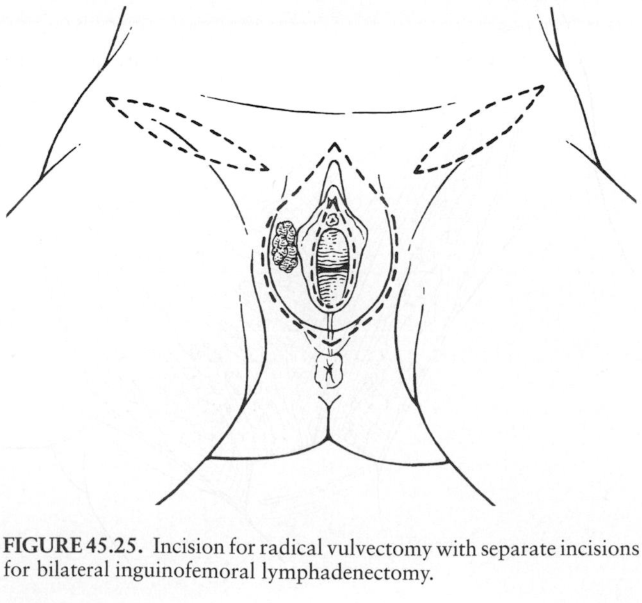

FIGURE 45.25. Incision for radical vulvectomy with separate incisions for bilateral inguinofemoral lymphadenectomy.

just above the superior border of the inguinal ligament medially to the inguinal ring or about 2 cm below and 2 cm medial to the pubic tubercle. Unless there is a large clitoral lesion or palpably suspicious nodes, the mons pubis is spared, and separate incisions with a skin bridge are made as illustrated. For anterior lesions, such as those involving the clitoris, a portion of the mons pubis is included in the resection and the lymphadenectomy on one or both sides may be done en bloc with the radical vulvectomy as illustrated in Figure 45.8A. From the lateral points, caudal incisions are carried medially so as to excise a strip of skin (optional) 2 to 4 cm in width. Excising an ellipse of skin may reduce the likelihood of skin necrosis and facilitate more complete dissection of the groin. This incision is designed to extend from just below the fossa ovalis (this can generally be identified clinically as the area just medial to the femoral pulsation in the groin) to the top of the labiocrural fold above a point just medial to the external inguinal ring. In the presence of grossly positive inguinal lymph nodes, a wider resection of both the groin skin and fat is necessary to help ensure adequate tumor clearance. The separate groin skin incision may also be done vertically (with the leg), centered across the fossa ovalis and about halfway between the femoral artery and pubic tubercle.

Leaving a layer of subcutaneous tissue with the skin, the superior incision is undermined so that the lymph node–bearing adipose tissue above the inguinal ligament and around the superficial circumflex iliac, as well as the superficial epigastric vessels, are included with the resection. These vessels are ligated as they are encountered. The superior dissection over the groin area is carried down to the superior border of the inguinal ligament. The midline aspect of the superior flap can be mobilized off the pubic bone and rectus fascia at this point to facilitate later closure of the wound without tension. Dissection of the block of inguinal tissue is carried inferiorly off of the inguinal ligament. The lateral corner is dissected medially off of the sartorius fascia (Fig. 45.26). The inferior flap of the lower incision is also mobilized, especially medially, and the saphenous vein is identified as it enters the region of the femoral triangle (Figs. 45.27–45.29). Accessory saphenous veins can also be seen entering this area. The long saphenous vein is isolated and ligated with a free-tie and a transfixion ligature of 2-0 polyglactin (Vicryl). The vein with its surrounding block of lymph node–bearing tissue is dissected superiorly off of the sartorius and adductor fascia. Dissection of the block of inguinal tissue is continued from the three sides toward the fossa ovalis. As this area is approached, the overlying cribriform fascia is recognized, and the femoral artery pulsation can be palpated in the lateral aspect. En bloc dissection continues and includes the contents of the fossa ovalis (Fig. 45.30). The area under the fascia lateral to the femoral artery should be left undisturbed. There are no lymph nodes of consequence here, and avoidance of this area prevents injury to the femoral nerve and possibly reduces subsequent lymphedema. Rather, resection of the cribriform fascia begins over the area of femoral pulsation, exposing the underlying femoral vessels. A few small branches of the femoral nerve are sacrificed during this dissection. The sheath of the femoral artery is incised along its anteromedial aspect from somewhere between the base of the fossa ovalis and the apex of the femoral triangle to its emergence from under the inguinal ligament. Branches, such as the external pudendal artery, are ligated as they are encountered. There is no purpose in dissecting under the artery or between the femoral artery and vein. Rather, the dissection that has been performed over the top of the artery is continued over the top of the vein, mobilizing the specimen to the medial aspect of the femoral vein. During this process, the saphenofemoral venous junction is identified, ligated with a 2-0 silk free-tie followed by a suture ligature for security, and transected, thus removing several centimeters of the saphenous vein with the specimen (Figs. 45.31 and 45.32).

An alternative method, as long as there are no adherent suspicious lymph nodes, is to dissect the saphenous vein free of the specimen so that it can be preserved, potentially reducing the risk of subsequent leg edema. Complete

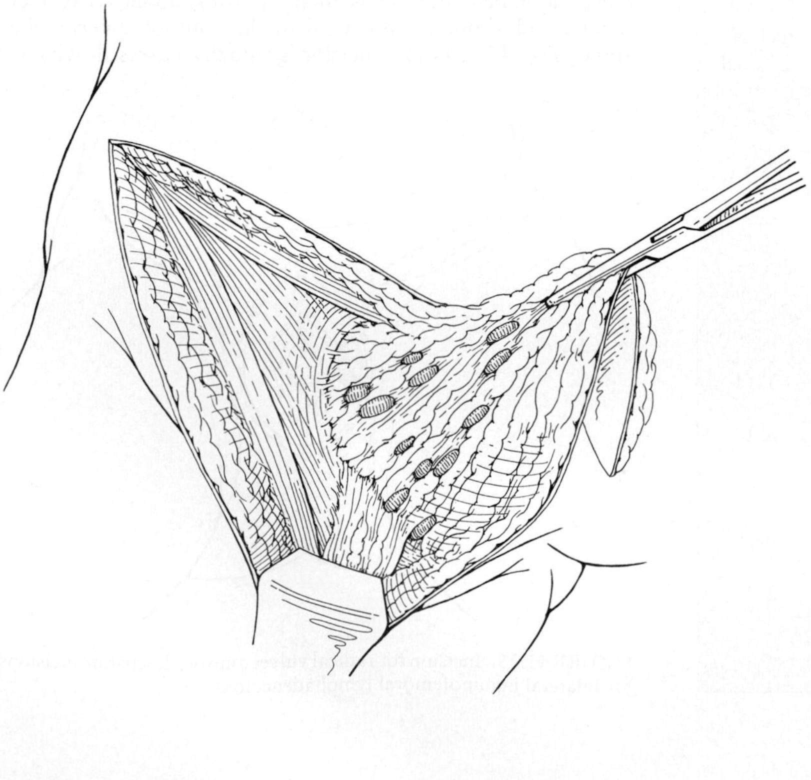

FIGURE 45.26. Corner of groin specimen dissected up medially off sartorius muscle. Lateral portion of fossa ovalis and cribriform fascia are exposed.

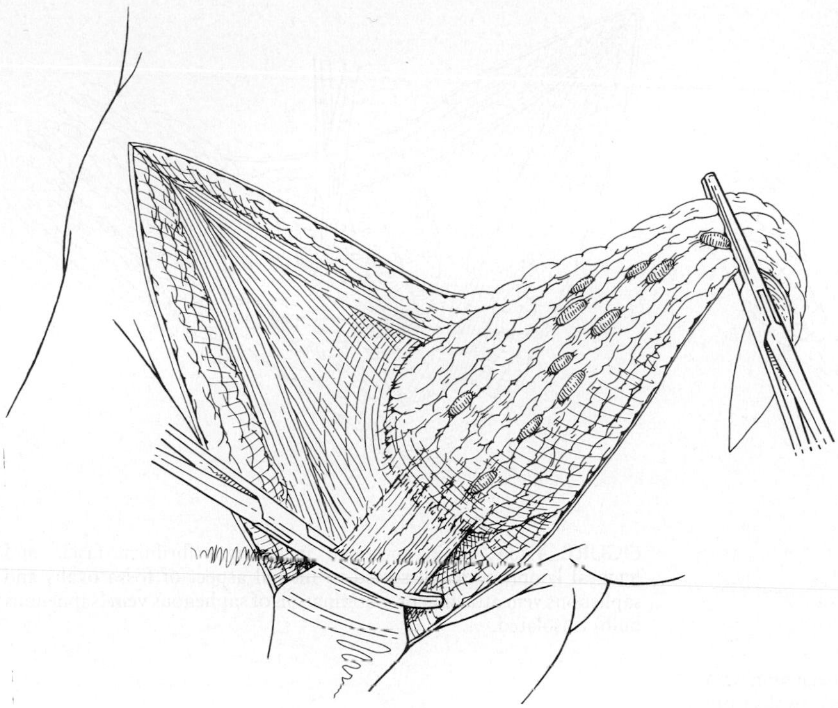

FIGURE 45.27. Block of lymph node–bearing tissue overlying saphenous vein has been mobilized and clamped inferiorly.

dissection of the space medial to the vein is important because this is where most of the femoral groin nodes are located. The specimen is freed from the femoral vein medially, from the inguinal ligament superiorly, and from the underlying pectineal fascia. Dissection is continued toward and off of the adductor longus fascia until the labiocrural fold is reached.

To protect the femoral vessels in the event of subsequent wound breakdown, the sartorius muscle can be transposed over them at this point. Alternatively, the vessels can be covered by a variety of other materials or simple approximation of musculofascial tissues. To accomplish sartorius transposition, the muscle is divided with cautery at its tendinous attachment to the anterior superior iliac spine. The proximal end of the muscle is then mobilized and transposed so that it covers the femoral vessels. It is sutured at this location to the inguinal ligament and pectineal fascia with 0 polyglactin (Fig. 45.33). We have largely discontinued the practice of transposing the sartorius

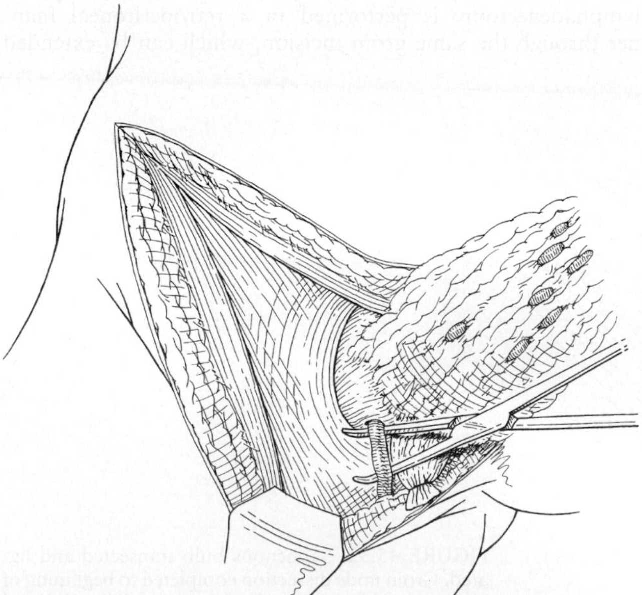

FIGURE 45.28. Segment of saphenous vein in groin is isolated.

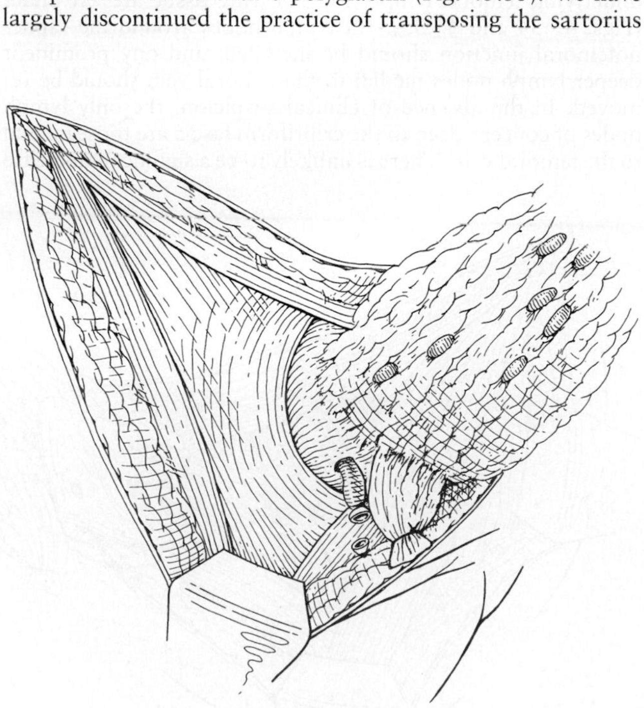

FIGURE 45.29. Saphenous vein has been transected and ligated near its entrance into the femoral triangle.

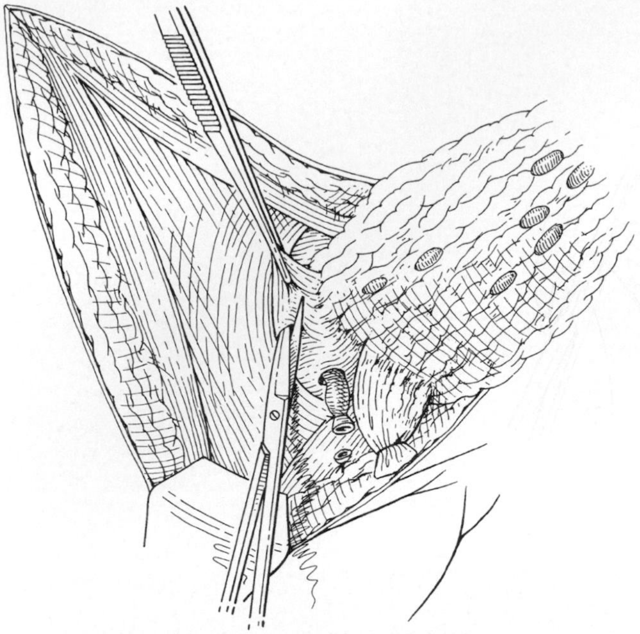

FIGURE 45.30. Dissection of the femoral lymph nodes beginning with separation of the cribriform fascia and contents of the fossa ovalis from the anterior aspect of the femoral artery.

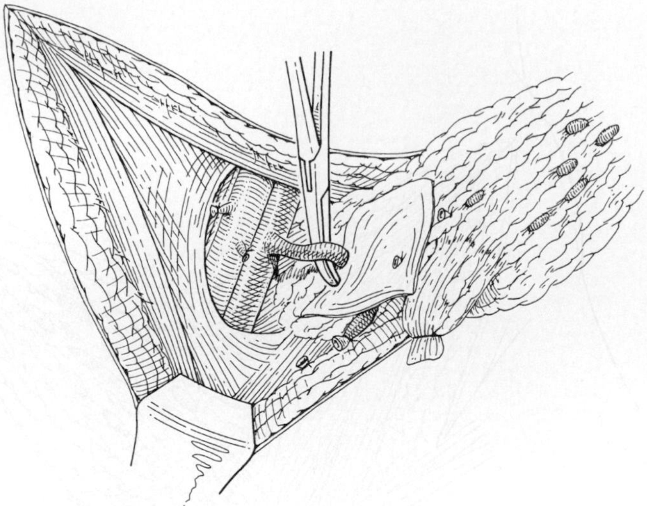

FIGURE 45.31. Groin specimen including cribriform fascia and femoral lymph nodes dissected to medial aspect of fossa ovalis and saphenous vein attachment. Termination of saphenous vein (saphenous bulb) is isolated.

muscles because of the improved healing of these wounds and less radical dissection.

If a superficial inguinal lymphadenectomy has been chosen (also generally done through separate incisions), the same general dissection is done except that the cribriform fascia and underlying femoral lymph node–bearing tissue are left intact (Figs. 45.34 and 45.35). All lymph nodes around the saphenofemoral junction should be included, and any prominent deeper lymph nodes medial to the femoral vein should be removed. In the absence of clinical suspicion, the only lymph nodes of concern deep to the cribriform fascia are those medial to the femoral vein. There is unlikely to be a significant increase in morbidity by extending the dissection to include removal of these femoral lymph nodes. There is not an apparent major distinction between this dissection and a contemporary formal inguinofemoral lymphadenectomy.

If a prominent femoral lymph node can be identified at the most superior aspect of the dissection in the space just medial to the femoral vein (Cloquet node or node of Rosenmüller), this can be used as a sentinel lymph node when deciding on the risk of pelvic lymph node metastases. When such a lymph node is positive, a search should be made for further nodes above this by carrying the dissection up the femoral ring under the inguinal ligament.

A pelvic lymphadenectomy, when chosen, is done immediately after completion of the groin dissection. The pelvic lymphadenectomy is performed in a retroperitoneal manner through the same groin incision, which can be extended

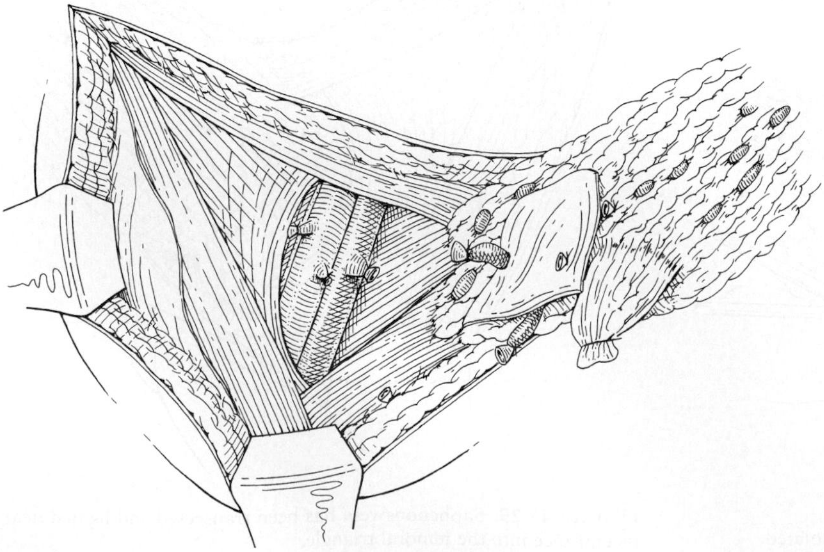

FIGURE 45.32. Saphenous bulb transected and ligated. Groin node dissection completed to beginning of planned vulvectomy incision. Fossa medial to femoral vein and overlying the pectineus muscle has been cleared of lymph node–bearing tissue.

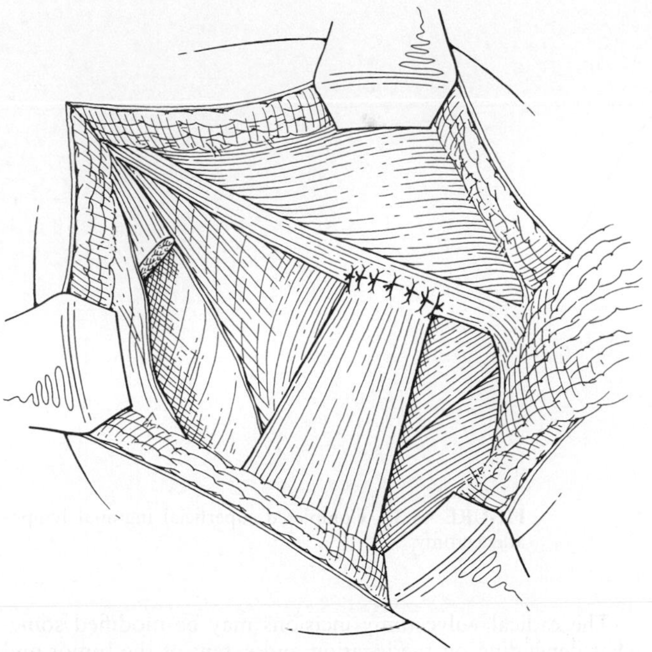

FIGURE 45.33. Transposed sartorius muscle.

laterally and superiorly (in a "J" or vertical manner), if necessary. About 2 cm above and parallel to the inguinal ligament, an incision is made through the external oblique, internal oblique, and transversalis musculofascial layers (Fig. 45.36). The retroperitoneal space is then opened bluntly, mobilizing the peritoneum and ureter medially. It is necessary to ligate and transect the inferior epigastric vessels and round ligament to fully develop this space. A self-retaining retractor or handheld retractors can be used for adequate exposure of the retroperitoneal space. The pararectal and paravesical spaces are opened bluntly, fully exposing the iliac vessels and obturator fossa. All (or suspicious) lymph node–bearing tissue from the external iliac and internal iliac vessels and the superficial obturator fossa is removed. Separate pelvic Jackson-Pratt drains can be placed at the discretion of the surgeon. The incised musculofascial tissues are closed in a single layer with no. 1 synthetic, absorbable, monofilament sutures. Special attention is paid to closure of the internal inguinal ring with 2-0 silk sutures. The wounds are irrigated, and hemostasis is secured. When performed through separate incisions, the groin wounds are closed at this point.

Soft, active suction drains are placed in each groin and are brought out through separate stab wounds superolaterally. The groin wound may be approximated with a large mass closure using no. 2 polypropylene vertical mattress retention sutures (Fig. 45.37A). Three to five sutures are placed on each side. Each suture starts several centimeters from the edge of the superior flap, with a bite then taken of the underlying inguinal ligament. This is designed to close the dead space under the superior flap. Under the inferior flap, a bite of sartorius, adductor, or pectineal fascia is taken (with care taken to avoid injury to the femoral vessels and nerve), followed by placement of the suture from inside to out through the inferior flap several centimeters from the edge. Again, this is designed to close the dead space of the inferior flap and, once pulled together, to close the dead space of the midline wound. Going back from inferior to superior, a small bite of each skin edge is then taken, which is designed to approximate these edges. The sutures are not tied until all have been placed. The sutures are tied somewhat loosely, with only enough tension to bring the wound together (Fig. 45.37B). The skin is further closed with stainless steel staples (Fig. 45.37C). When there has been less extensive dissection, the groin wound may be closed with 2-0 polyglycolic acid suture, approximating first the dead space with interrupted sutures and then the skin with vertical mattress or subcuticular sutures. En bloc groin incisions are closed in an identical manner, but this is delayed until completion of the entire resection. With separate incisions, the medial aspects of the groin wounds are under much less tension and are easily closed because of preservation of the inguinal skin bridge. Separation of the groin and vulvar wounds and especially closure without tension are the factors thought to be largely responsible for the reduced wound complications seen with the three-incision technique.

After completion of the inguinofemoral lymphadenectomy, attention is turned to the radical vulvectomy. The surgeon may elect to change the position of the legs to high lithotomy;

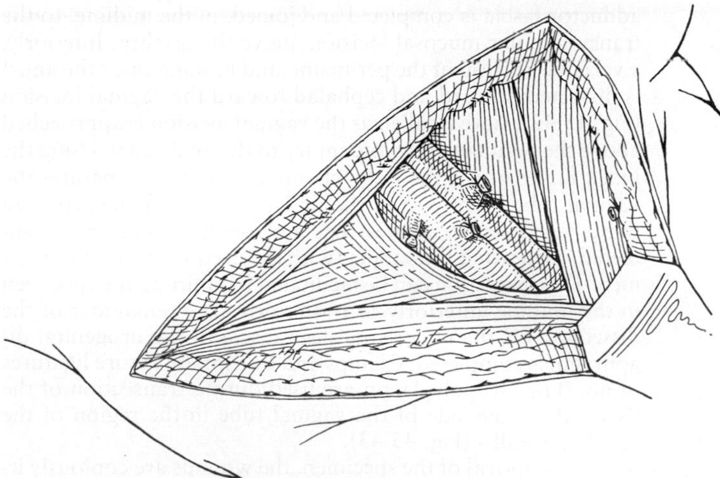

FIGURE 45.34. Inguinofemoral lymphadenectomy completed through a separate incision.

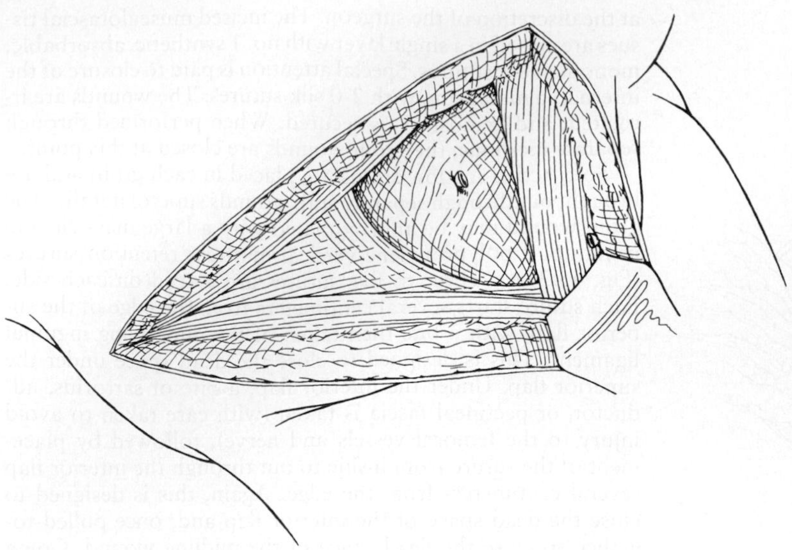

FIGURE 45.35. Completed superficial inguinal lymphadenectomy.

"high-low" Allen-Brown stirrups are useful for this purpose (for a difficult perineal dissection, high lithotomy with sling stirrups is preferred). With en bloc resection, the inguinal specimens are mobilized toward the vulva as just described (Fig. 45.38). From the point of completion of the inferior inguinal dissections, incisions are continued down along the labiocrural folds on each side and across the perineum, where they meet. A medial mucosal incision is made along the introitus extending through the anterior vestibule and around the urethral meatus.

When radical vulvectomy is performed through a separate vulvar incision, the same labiocrural, posterior, and mucosal incisions are used and the same vulvar tissue is excised (Fig. 45.39). The superior incision extends from the top of the labiocrural folds as an inverted V, with the point above the base of the clitoris. As previously discussed, a variable amount of superior tissue (i.e., mons pubis) is removed, depending on the location and size of the lesion.

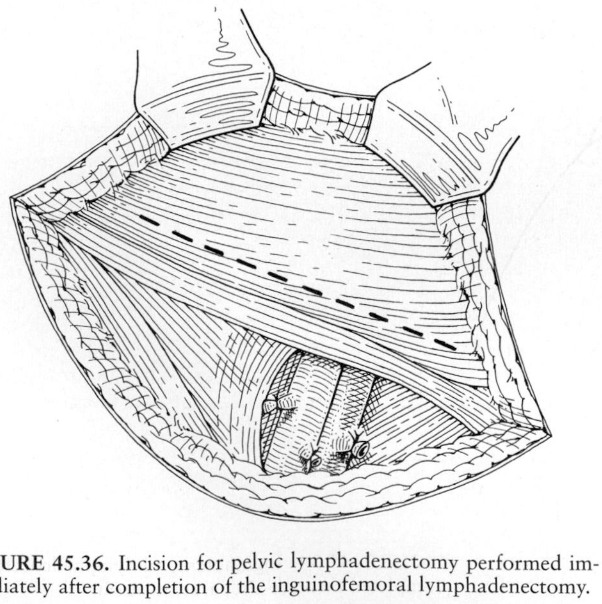

FIGURE 45.36. Incision for pelvic lymphadenectomy performed immediately after completion of the inguinofemoral lymphadenectomy.

The radical vulvectomy incisions may be modified somewhat depending on the location and extent of the tumor and the condition of the remaining vulvar skin. The surgeon should attempt to attain at least a 2-cm margin of normal-appearing skin or mucosa around the tumor. To accomplish this, it may be necessary to excise a portion of vagina, anus, or distal urethra. For an anterior lesion, it is reasonable to spare the perineal body; but for a posterior lesion, it is important to incorporate radical resection of this area. For a lesion (especially superficial) in proximity to the urethral meatus or anus, it is reasonable to limit the margin of resection to 1 cm (but not less) to preserve these structures and their function.

The labiocrural incisions are extended to the lateral margins of the deep fascia of the urogenital diaphragm (Fig. 45.40). The internal pudendal vessels are ligated as they are encountered entering the vulva at about the 4 o'clock and 8 o'clock positions. Superiorly, the specimen is dissected off the pubic periosteum and adductor fascia. The vascular base of the clitoris is clamped and transected, and a transfixion suture ligature is placed (Fig. 45.41). If deemed necessary, the attachment of the ischiocavernosus muscles can also be transected at this level. Dissection of the superior portion of the vulva off of the pubic bone and adductor fascia is completed and joined, in the midline, to the transvestibular mucosal incision above the urethra. Inferiorly, a variable portion of the perineum (and in some cases the anus) is dissected upward and cephalad toward the vaginal incision (Fig. 45.42). Care is taken as the vaginal incision is approached above the perineum to avoid injury to the anal canal. Using the index finger or a large Kelly clamp, the surgeon separates the vaginal tube bluntly from the underlying soft tissue cephalad to the vestibular structures. The mucosal incision is then completed, separating the vagina (with the urethra) from the specimen. This dissection can be facilitated by splitting the specimen in the midline anteriorly or posteriorly. The remainder of the dissection off the underlying deep fascia of the urogenital diaphragm is completed. Clamps and transfixion suture ligatures of no. 0 or 2-0 polyglactin are used during transection of the tissue along the side of the vaginal tube in the region of the vestibular bulbs (Fig. 45.43).

After removal of the specimen, the wounds are copiously irrigated with antibiotic solution, and hemostasis is secured (Fig. 45.44). After en bloc resection, the superior abdominal wall flap and the groin and vulvar thigh flaps are further mobilized

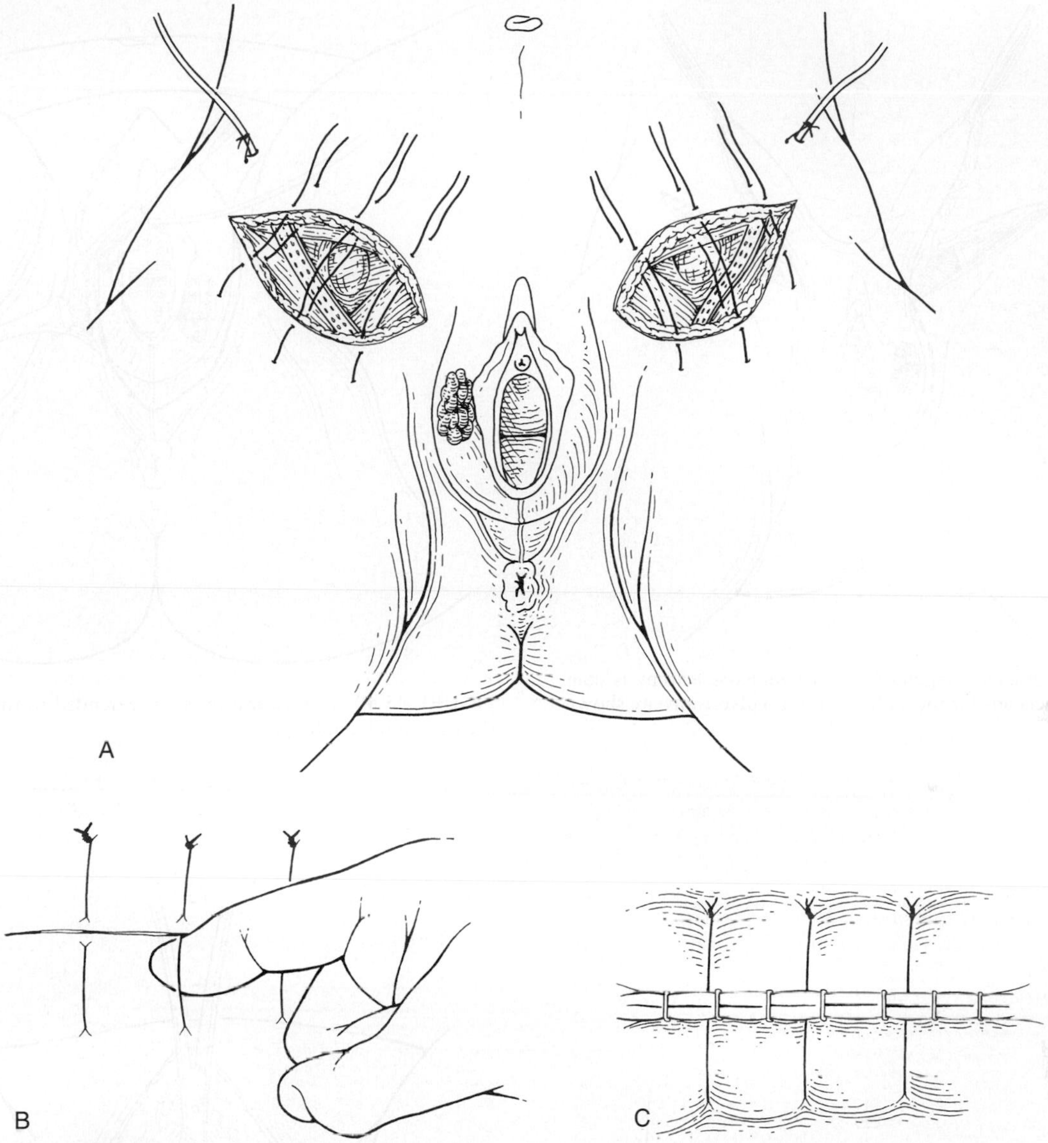

FIGURE 45.37. A: Large block closure of groin wounds (separate in this case) with vertical mattress retention sutures. Note drains in place. **B:** The groin closure sutures are tied somewhat loosely. **C:** Groin closure completed with stainless steel skin staples.

as necessary to achieve closure of the wounds without tension. Any ischemic-appearing skin is excised. It is very useful, especially if there is an element of vaginal relaxation, to mobilize the lower vagina to facilitate wound closure. Any pelvic relaxation defects (i.e., cystocele, rectocele, loss of the posterior urethrovesical angle) are repaired at this time. To the extent that it is necessary or possible, the perineal body is also reinforced or reconstructed at this time.

The vulvar wound and the perineal area are closed with vertical mattress 2-0 delayed-absorbable sutures (Fig. 45.45). Depending on the amount of tissue that has been removed, the superior portion of an en bloc wound may be difficult to close. When done through a separate incision, closure of the vulvar wound is under much less tension, again because of preservation of the inguinal skin bridges. Careful attention must be paid to closure of the periurethral area. The urethra should be secured on a straight course without tension. A hood of skin above the urethra is also avoided because this can obstruct the path of the urinary stream and cause spraying.

As previously discussed, it is reasonable in most patients to manage the vulvar lesion locally with a modified radical vulvectomy. This operation consists of radical removal of the portion of the vulva containing the tumor. It is performed with the techniques described earlier except that the excision is basically limited to removal of that particular part of the vulva. The lateral and deep tumor margins are not compromised by this operation. After the surgeon carefully demarcates a 2-cm radius of normal skin or mucosa around the tumor, an encompassing incision is designed that will readily close and be as cosmetically acceptable as possible (Figs. 45.12, 45.46, and 45.47).

Postoperative Care. After closure, silver sulfadiazine (Silvadene, Hoechst Marion Roussel) cream is applied to the

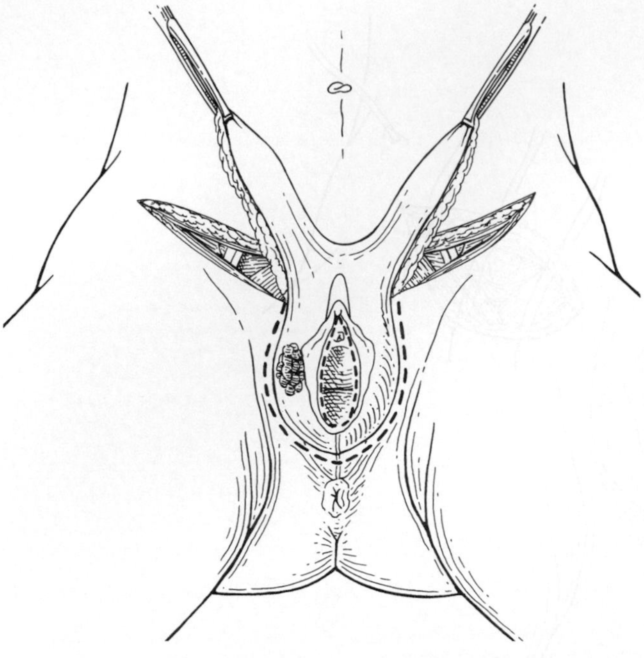

FIGURE 45.38. Bilateral inguinofemoral lymphadenectomy is complete. Planned incisions for the en bloc radical vulvectomy are shown.

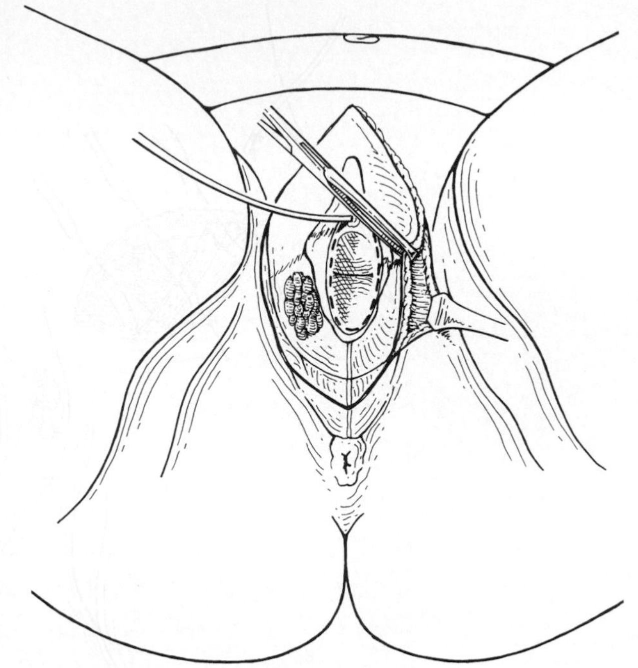

FIGURE 45.40. Labiocrural incisions extended to the deep fascia of the urogenital diaphragm.

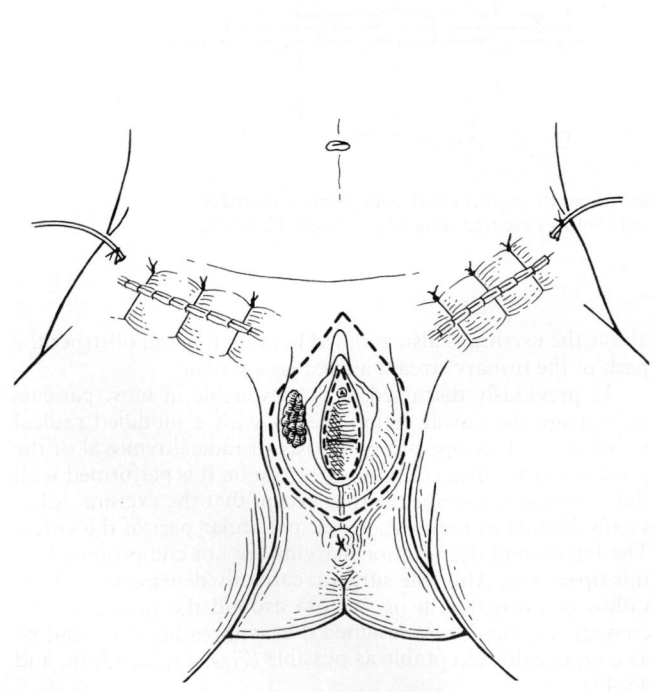

FIGURE 45.39. Bilateral inguinofemoral lymphadenectomy through separate incisions is completed, and wounds are closed. Separate incisions for radical vulvectomy are marked.

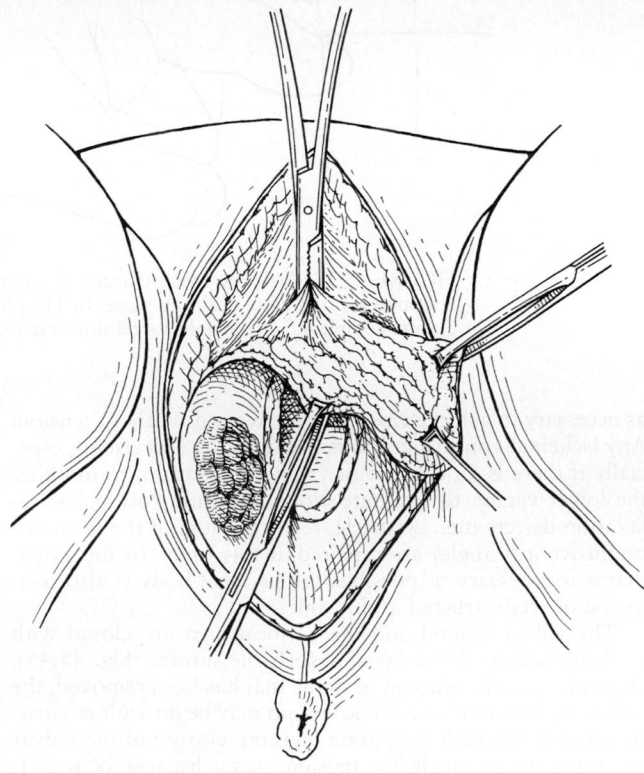

FIGURE 45.41. Dissection proceeds dorsally off of the pubic bone. The vascular base of the clitoris clamped, followed by transection and ligation.

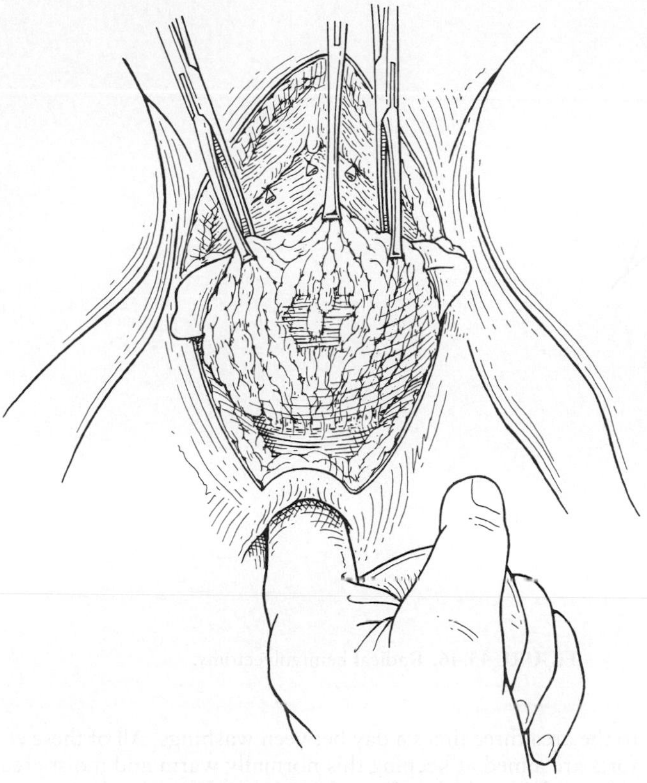

FIGURE 45.42. Perineal body and posterior vulvar tissues are dissected away from the anus.

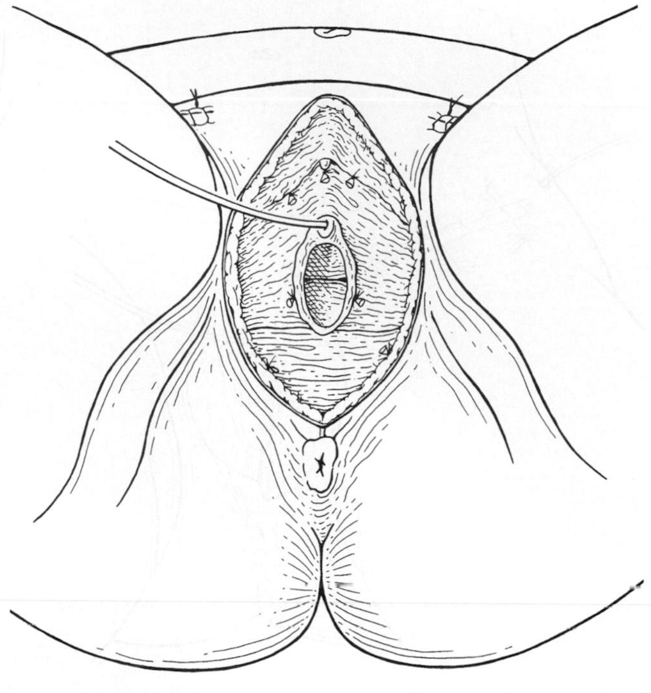

FIGURE 45.44. Radical vulvectomy resection is completed.

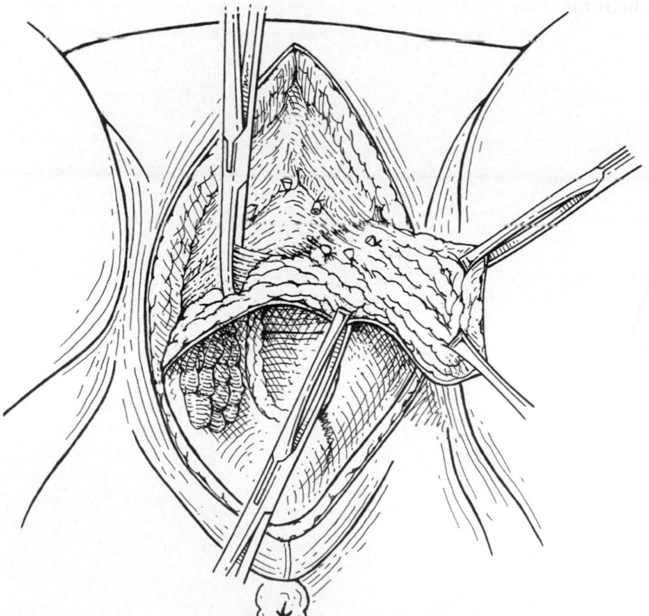

FIGURE 45.43. The vascular vestibular tissue along the sides of the vaginal tube is clamped. Transection and suture ligation follow.

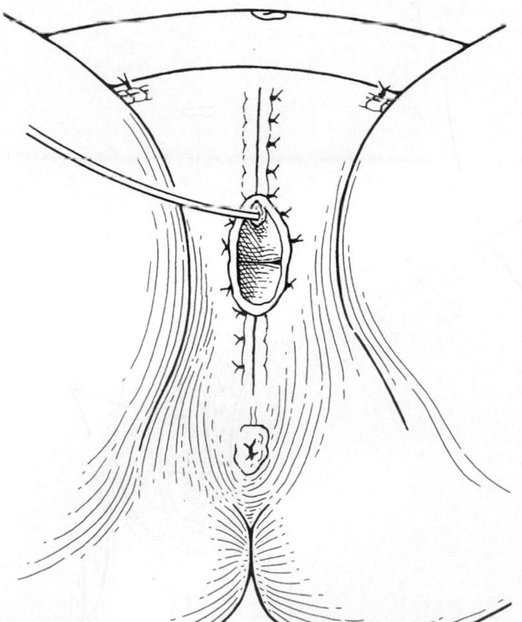

FIGURE 45.45. Closure of the vulvar wound is completed.

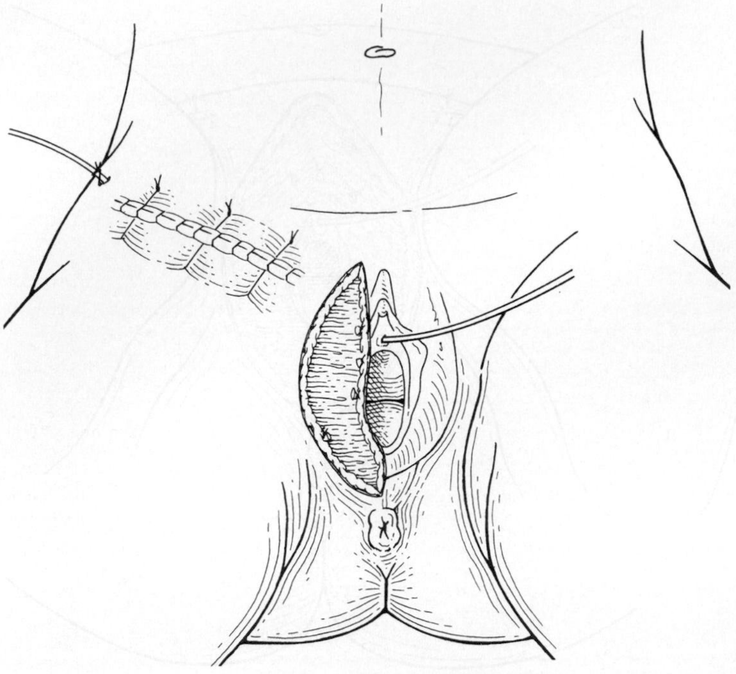

FIGURE 45.46. Radical hemivulvectomy.

perineal wound, and a light dressing is placed. In the recovery room, ice is applied to the vulvar wound, and this is continued off and on for 48 to 72 hours. On postoperative day 3 or 4, the patient is started on a regimen of cleansing the vulvar wound with a showerhead, followed immediately by complete drying of the area with a blow dryer using cool air. This is done three times a day and as needed (i.e., after a liquid bowel movement) and is continued until the wounds are healed. If moisture in the wound is a problem despite this regimen, other useful measures include placing a roll of gauze between the legs and against the wound between washings, increasing the frequency of washings, not wearing an undergarment, and applying a heat lamp to the area three times a day between washings. All of these efforts are aimed at keeping this normally warm and moist area clean and dry, which reduces the risk of infection and promotes healing. Intermittently leaving the legs slightly apart to air (the immodest position) is also beneficial. The patient should also avoid sitting on the healing wound.

If the vulvar wound is left open, postoperative management is the same except that silver sulfadiazine cream is applied after each showerhead, blow drying until there is good granulation tissue formation. In addition, these women are seen more frequently in the office to ensure good wound care and healing.

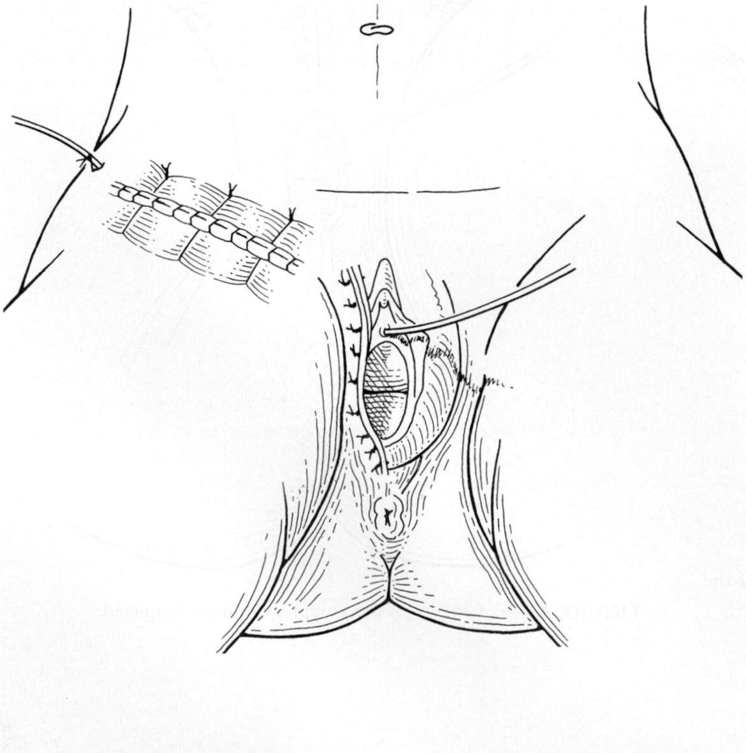

FIGURE 45.47. Closure of hemivulvectomy wound.

Drains are removed on the second or third day. A compression dressing (rolled gauze and an abdominal binder) is maintained on the groins for an additional 24 to 48 hours to prevent lymphocyst formation. Compression boots are continued during this time, and care is taken to avoid marked femoral vein compression.

A prophylactic antibiotic is continued for 24 hours, and Jobst compression boots plus prophylactic dose fractionated heparin are used until the patient is ambulating. If the wounds are closed under tension, ambulation is restricted for 3 to 5 days, and the patient is instructed to avoid leg abduction when getting into and out of bed. A no. 18 Foley catheter is left in place for 3 to 5 days to act as a stent and divert urine while the urethra is healing. Depending on the degree of perineal or perianal resection, several days of bowel rest may be indicated, with or without a constipating agent, followed by a stool softener.

Especially when lymph node dissection has been extensive or radiotherapy is planned, long-term use of fitted graduated compression stockings may be beneficial.

Reconstructive Techniques for the Vulva and Groin

After radical resection for carcinoma of the vulva, the wounds can generally be closed primarily. This is greatly facilitated when the incisions are modified somewhat (as with sparing of the mons pubis), and especially when separate incisions are used. When an extensive resection is necessary, it may not be possible to close the wound primarily, or at least not without considerable tension. This is often the case after resection of a recurrent tumor, where previous radical surgery has already left a paucity of tissue. If the area was treated previously with radiotherapy, then closure may be difficult because of the lack of elasticity of the fibrotic tissue and because of radiation-induced healing impairment. Under these various circumstances, closure of the incisions and healing can be facilitated by a variety of reconstructive procedures. Other potential benefits of such reconstruction include maintenance of anal, urethral, and sexual function and a more cosmetically acceptable result. However, leaving the wound open is sometimes the best option, and healing by secondary intention is usually quite satisfactory.

Closure of groin and vulvar wounds using reconstructive techniques involves moving a block of expendable tissue (with its blood supply intact) from some nearby site into the deficient area. The mobilized block of tissue is commonly referred to as a flap. Flaps are classified according to what layers of tissue they include and according to their blood supply. The types of flaps that have been useful in reconstruction of the vulva and groin are full-thickness skin (random and arterial based), fasciocutaneous, and myocutaneous flaps. Some flaps remain completely attached at their base and are rotated into the defect, whereas others are partially separated from the base and are transposed as an island of tissue.

A full-thickness skin flap involves rotating an adjacent block of skin with its underlying subcutaneous tissue into the defect. The flap is mobilized from the donor site but remains attached at its base; through this base travels the arterial and venous circulation. The blood supply of the flap may be random, or it may depend on a specifically planned arterial source. A random flap relies on the many small musculocutaneous perforating vessels that are retained through the base. For this reason, the subcutaneous layer must be kept thick, and the length of the flap should not be much greater than the width of the base (1.0 to 1.5 times greater). This is the type of flap most commonly used for reconstruction of a radical vulvectomy wound. The healing of such flaps is less reliable in patients with impaired wound healing ability, such as those with diabetes, heavy tobacco users, those with vascular disease, and patients who have previously received radiation therapy to the region.

A few specific arterial-based full-thickness skin flaps, sometimes called axial flaps, have been used for reconstruction in vulvar cancer patients. Arterial sources of these flaps have included the internal pudendal, circumflex iliac, superficial circumflex iliac, superficial inferior epigastric, superficial branch of the deep external pudendal, and superficial external pudendal arteries. With some of these arterial flaps, the deep fascia must be carefully mobilized with the subcutaneous tissue to maintain an adequate blood supply. The main advantage of an arterial flap, because of the good arterial blood supply, is that it can be considerably longer than a random flap. However, these flaps are technically more difficult to construct and have a low margin for error in terms of compromising blood supply.

As previously mentioned, some full-thickness skin flaps are designed to include the deep fascia taken off the underlying muscle. These are known as fasciocutaneous flaps, and they are more reliable than random cutaneous flaps because the preserved fascial layer provides additional musculocutaneous perforators along its length. A fasciocutaneous flap can also be relatively long and is transposable as an island of tissue. Some fasciocutaneous flaps have a designated arterial blood supply. Locally useful fasciocutaneous flaps include the pudendal thigh, superior medial thigh, inferior gluteal, and island groin flaps.

A myocutaneous flap makes use of an expendable muscle with its intact overlying fascia and cutaneous tissue. The use of these flaps for vulvovaginal reconstruction began after the 1976 report by McCraw and colleagues. A substantial blood supply is preserved through a narrow pedicle connected to the muscle, which allows the flap to be transposed as an island with a wide arc of rotation. Another advantage of a myocutaneous flap is the capacity to bring tissue into the defect that has a blood supply separate and independent from that of the operative site. This makes these flaps particularly valuable in the reconstruction of heavily radiated tissues. These flaps are also somewhat bulky and have the ability to fill a large tissue defect. The main disadvantage of myocutaneous flaps is that they are technically demanding, and the survival ability of some of these flaps is somewhat tenuous.

The difficulties resulting from a large wound created by an extensive radical vulvectomy with bilateral inguinofemoral lymphadenectomy were previously discussed. Reconstruction of these wounds with bilateral tensor fascia lata (TFL) myocutaneous flaps has been reported. The TFL originates from the anterior superior iliac spine. It inserts into the fascia lata and is supplied by the lateral femoral circumflex artery. The base is just lateral to the groin wound, into which the flap is directly rotated. The flaps are easily made long enough to reach and close the often large area created by resection of the mons pubis and anterior vulva. A TFL myocutaneous flap is also useful for reconstruction of the groin after extensive resection for recurrent disease (Fig. 45.48).

The rectus abdominis myocutaneous flap, based on the inferior epigastric artery, is also useful for reconstruction of a large groin defect. The block of tissue based on this muscle is taken from the abdominal wall, and the muscle is divided at the superior border of the flap. The island of cutaneous tissue is completely mobilized with its carefully preserved attachment to the muscle, and this is further mobilized inferiorly. This allows the island flap to rotate down easily into the groin (or vulva) through a generous subcutaneous tunnel. The rectus abdominis myocutaneous flap is also suitable for the reconstruction of large vulvar wounds (Fig. 45.49).

I commonly use flaps for vulvar wound reconstruction after radical resection of cancer involving the perineal or perianal

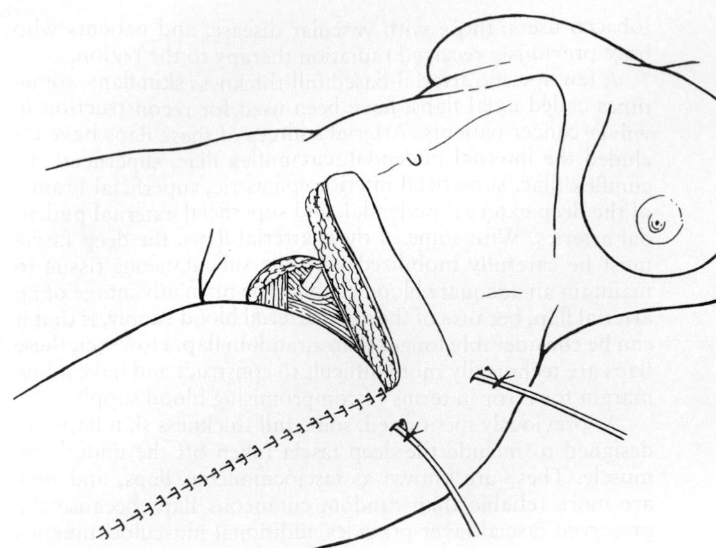

FIGURE 45.48. Tensor fascia lata flap being rotated to close a large groin wound.

tissues. Such a resection removes the entire perineal body as well as portions of the superficial muscles and leaves a large defect that is difficult to close (Fig. 45.50). Poor healing of this area may significantly compromise both anal and coital function. The use of flaps for such a defect allows closure without tension and brings tissue with a good blood supply into the area, which promotes healing and helps recreate a perineal body. Preventing tension on the anal apparatus helps promote healing of its associated reconstructed musculature and helps preserve its function. Reconstruction of a perineal body separates the vagina from fecal contamination and helps create a smooth and less scarred platform for intercourse. For reconstruction of such defects, we prefer to use local, full-thickness rhomboid skin flaps (Figs. 45.51–45.54). Closure of a larger defect involving the perineal or perianal and vulvar areas may be better accomplished with gluteal thigh fasciocutaneous, gluteus maximus myocutaneous, or gracilis myocutaneous flaps.

Closure of a heavily radiated wound should be accomplished with a block of relatively unradiated tissue, the blood supply to which is unlikely to have been significantly compromised by the prior treatment. In general, myocutaneous flaps are better for this purpose.

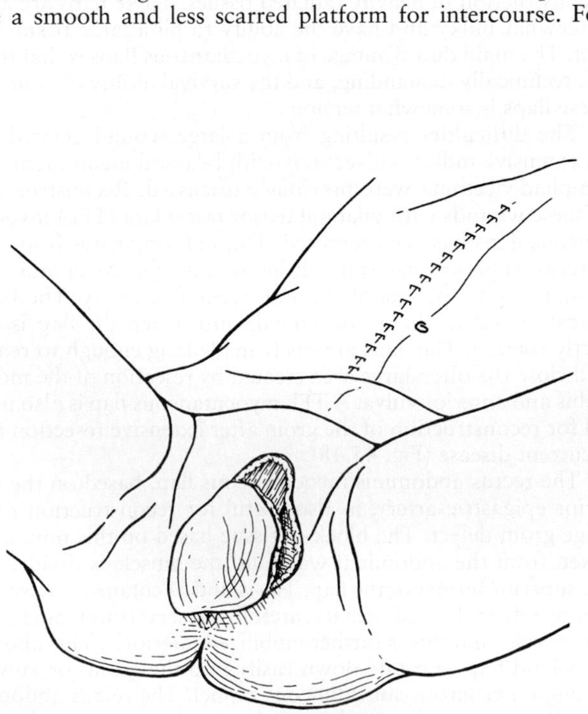

FIGURE 45.49. Rectus abdominis myocutaneous flap is brought through a subcutaneous tunnel to close a large perineal wound.

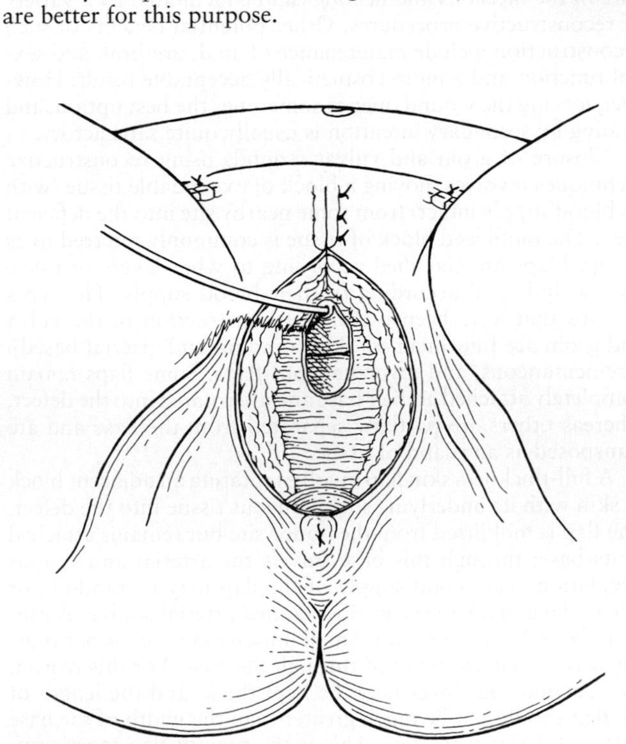

FIGURE 45.50. Extensive posterior vulvar resection leaves a large defect between the anus and the introitus.

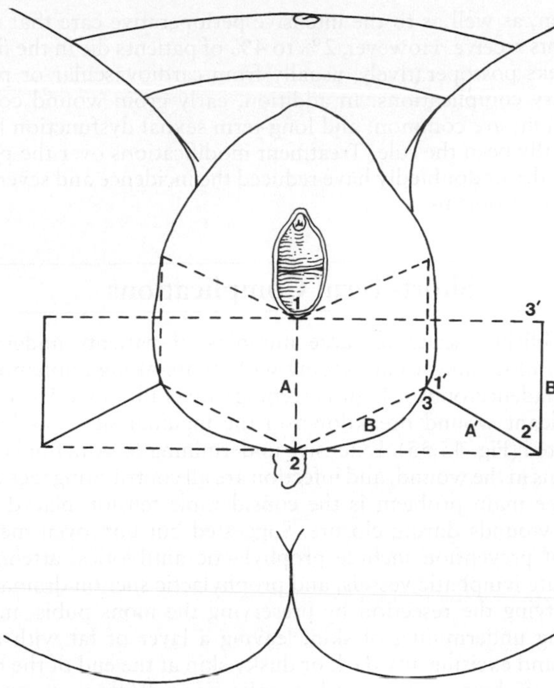

FIGURE 45.51. Planning rhomboid flap. Defect is divided into two rhomboids. Configuration and measurement of the flap are based on this rhomboid defect, as shown. Numbers and letters indicate proposed location of flap in reconstructed site.

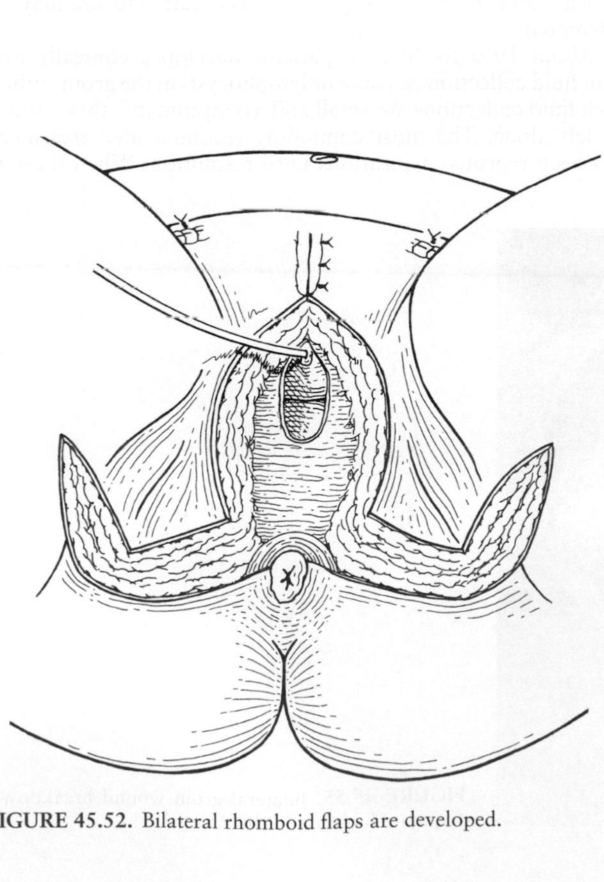

FIGURE 45.52. Bilateral rhomboid flaps are developed.

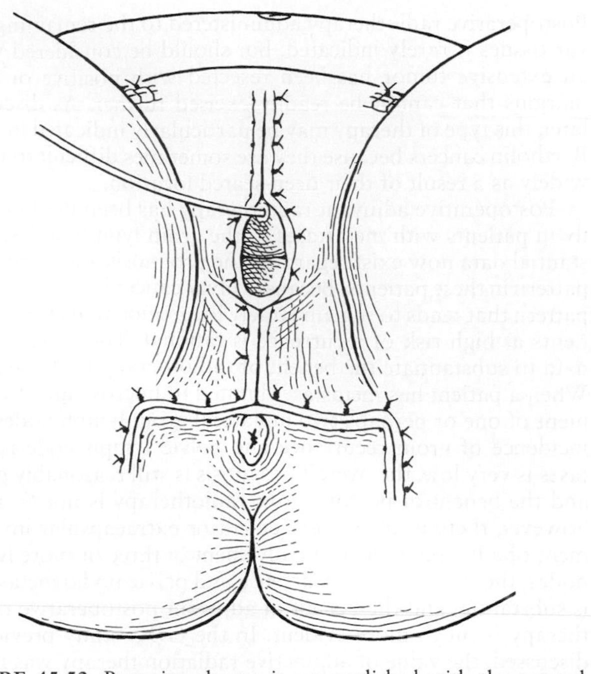

FIGURE 45.53. Posterior closure is accomplished with the rotated flaps.

Many other flaps have been reported to be useful for groin and vulvar reconstruction and may be used depending on the individual situation and preference of the surgeon.

POSTOPERATIVE ADJUVANT THERAPY

This section deals with adjuvant therapy following radical or modified radical vulvectomy with inguinofemoral lymphadenectomy. The role of adjuvant therapy in the management of locally advanced vulvar cancer is discussed elsewhere in this chapter. Other than with locally advanced disease, preoperative adjuvant therapy has generally not been used or recommended.

Postoperatively, the only adjuvant therapy that appears to be of value is radiotherapy (+/– chemotherapy). This can consist of radiotherapy to the local area of primary tumor resection, to the groins, to the pelvic nodal areas, or to all three.

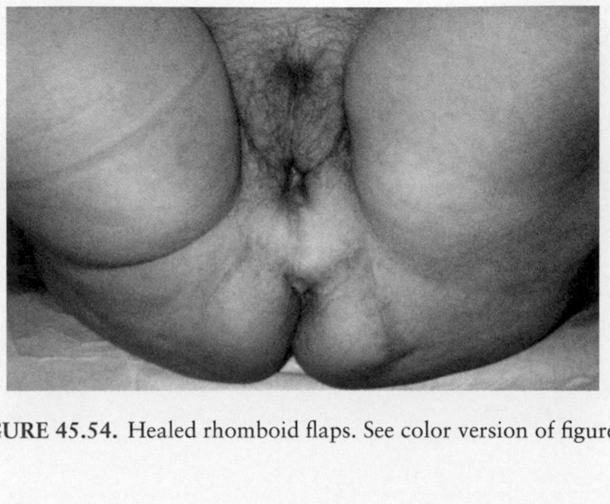

FIGURE 45.54. Healed rhomboid flaps. See color version of figure.

Postoperative radiotherapy administered to the remaining vulvar tissues is rarely indicated, but should be considered when an extensive tumor has been resected with positive or close margins that cannot be readily excised further. As discussed later, this type of therapy may be particularly indicated in some Bartholin cancers because they are sometimes difficult to resect widely as a result of their deep-seated location.

Postoperative adjuvant radiotherapy has been used primarily in patients with metastases to the groin lymph nodes. Substantial data now exist regarding the prognosis and recurrence pattern in these patients. Because vulvar cancer has a recurrence pattern that tends to remain largely locoregional, its use for patients at high risk of recurrence is rational. There are further data to substantiate the benefit of radiotherapy in this setting. When a patient has metastases limited to microscopic involvement of one or perhaps two unilateral groin lymph nodes, the incidence of groin recurrence and pelvic lymph node metastases is very low, the overall prognosis is still reasonably good, and the benefit of postoperative radiotherapy is not great. If, however, there is gross replacement or extracapsular involvement of a lymph node, or involvement of three or more lymph nodes, the risk of groin recurrence and pelvic nodal metastases is substantial and the benefit of adjuvant postoperative radiotherapy is much more evident. In the GOG study previously discussed, the value of adjunctive radiation therapy was in the reduction of groin recurrences. When such treatment is anticipated, placement of metal clips to localize metastatic sites may aid the radiation oncologist in treatment planning. Postoperative adjuvant chemotherapy, either alone or in combination with radiotherapy, has not been extensively studied, but it is unlikely to be of substantial benefit with use of the currently available agents.

MORTALITY AND MORBIDITY OF RADICAL VULVAR SURGERY

Even though most patients affected by invasive carcinoma of the vulva are elderly, radical vulvar surgery is generally well tolerated. This is attributed to the external nature of the operation, as well as to the intensive perioperative care that the patients receive. However, 2% to 4% of patients die in the first 4 weeks postoperatively, usually from cardiovascular or pulmonary complications. In addition, early groin wound complications are common, and long-term sexual dysfunction has generally been the rule. Treatment modifications over the past 3 decades undoubtedly have reduced the incidence and severity of these problems

Short-Term Complications

In published series of large numbers of patients undergoing en bloc radical vulvectomy with bilateral inguinofemoral lymphadenectomy, a high percentage (overall about 50%) of significant wound breakdown in the inguinal sites has been reported (Fig. 45.55). Extensive undermining of skin, fluid collections in the wound, and infection are all contributing factors, but the main problem is the considerable tension placed on these wounds during closure. Suggested but unproven methods of prevention include prophylactic antibiotics, attempts to ligate lymphatic vessels, and prophylactic suction drainage. Modifying the resection by preserving the mons pubis, minimizing undermining of skin, leaving a layer of fat with the skin, and excising any dark or dusky skin at the end of the operation reduce groin wound complications. With more extensive resection, plastic reconstruction (such as with TFL flaps) is also likely to be helpful. However, the single most effective method of reducing groin wound breakdown (to around 20%) has been the use of separate incisions, as previously discussed. Management of groin wound breakdown is similar to that of other wounds, with debridement and wet-to-dry dressings. During debridement, the surgeon must be cognizant of the femoral vessels. If infection has completely cleared, the wound is clean, and the tissues are pliable, secondary closure may be attempted.

About 10% to 20% of patients develop a clinically evident fluid collection (seroma or lymphocyst) in the groin. When such fluid collections are small and asymptomatic, they should be left alone. The most commonly recommended treatment has been repeated aspirations until resolution. When there is

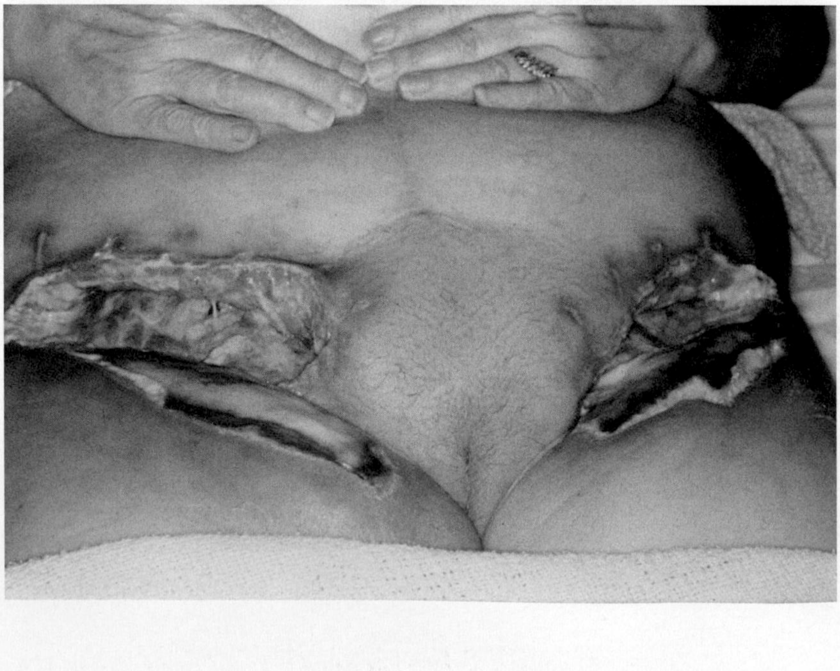

FIGURE 45.55. Bilateral groin wound breakdown (separate incisions in this case).

infection, prompt hospitalization with drainage and intravenous antibiotics is necessary. For persistent collections, we prefer reinstitution of suction drainage combined with pressure. Sclerotherapy is another option. If the problem is recalcitrant, the best course of action is to open and pack the cavity.

Femoral nerve injury is a rare but potentially debilitating complication of inguinofemoral lymphadenectomy. Not uncommonly, a few sensory branches are sacrificed, resulting in numbness or paresthesia of the anterior thigh. However, surgical injury of a major portion of the nerve lateral to the artery results in significant and potentially permanent difficulty with ambulation. As previously discussed, this complication is prevented by avoiding dissection on the lateral side of the femoral artery.

Urinary tract infection is common in these patients and generally resolves with antibiotics or catheter removal. However, elderly women sometimes tolerate urosepsis poorly and become profoundly ill. A diligent search for urinary tract infection, treatment of the infection, and removal of the Foley catheter as soon as is practical are important measures in these patients.

In the past, large series of patients undergoing en bloc radical vulvectomy with bilateral inguinofemoral lymphadenectomy reported a 1% to 2% incidence of severe postoperative hemorrhage from femoral vessel rupture. This was related to the extensive wound breakdown that occurred in a high percentage of these patients, with associated infection and necrosis involving the exposed and denuded femoral vessel walls. Coverage of the vessels by transposition of the sartorius muscle largely prevented this complication. With the use of separate incisions as well as other techniques that have reduced groin wound breakdown, and with avoidance of vessel skeletonization, postoperative femoral vessel rupture is now exceedingly rare.

Patients who have undergone radical vulvectomy with bilateral inguinofemoral lymphadenectomy are at high risk for thromboembolic complications because most are elderly and have coexisting medical problems, malignancy, and femoral vein trauma, and have undergone prolonged surgery and prolonged bed rest. If prophylaxis fails, then treatment is promptly begun with heparin.

Rarely, a rectovaginal fistula develops days to weeks after radical vulvectomy. Prevention of this complication is based on preoperative evacuation of the colon, careful surgical dissection of this area, and prompt recognition of rectal entry. Surgical repair of the fistula is carried out once the area has healed and regained its elasticity.

Osteitis pubis and osteomyelitis are rare complications that may not become symptomatic until several weeks after radical vulvectomy. The patient reports pain over the pubic bone and difficulty with ambulation, which may become chronic and debilitating. This complication is more likely to develop if the periosteum is traumatized, although this is not always avoidable. Extensive use of the cautery on the periosteum should be avoided. The mainstay of treatment is bed rest and nonsteroidal antiinflammatory drugs. Even more rarely, frank osteomyelitis of the pubic bone develops. This is a serious condition that requires debridement and drainage of the bone, along with prolonged antibiotic therapy.

Late Complications

After groin node dissection, it is not uncommon for a patient to develop some degree of lower extremity edema. It is most often transient or mild, but persists chronically as a significant problem in about 10% of patients. Factors that have been implicated as contributing to this complication include the performance of a pelvic lymphadenectomy, groin radiotherapy, major groin wound breakdown, postoperative lower extremity lymphangitis, sartorius muscle transposition, and preoperative lymphangiography. Suggested methods for reducing this problem include limiting the groin dissection to the sentinel lymph nodes when feasible, confining femoral lymphadenectomy to the medial side of the femoral vein, preserving the fascia lata, avoiding pelvic lymphadenectomy, using adjuvant radiotherapy in a more tailored and selective manner, sparing the saphenous vein, wearing fitted support stockings prophylactically for the first 6 months to 1 year after surgery, using a low-dose prophylactic antibiotic to prevent lower extremity lymphangitis, and treating lymphangitis promptly with antibiotics when it occurs (Fig. 45.56). Management of lymphedema begins with patient education, avoidance of trauma to the affected leg, and meticulous skin and nail care. Constricting clothing or jewelry should be avoided. A treatment program with a physical therapist specifically trained in lymphedema management is particularly helpful. Components of management include intermittent leg elevation, manual lymphatic drainage (massage) combined with bandaging, a carefully tailored moderate exercise program, carefully fitted compression stockings, and a carefully fitted pneumatic compression device. There is no effective pharmacologic therapy, and lymphangioplasty remains investigational. Some lymphedema patients occasionally

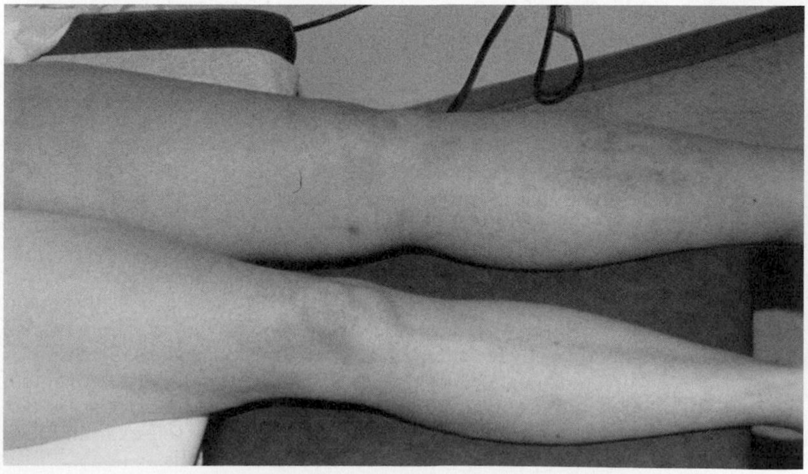

FIGURE 45.56. Lymphedema with lymphangitis of the left leg.

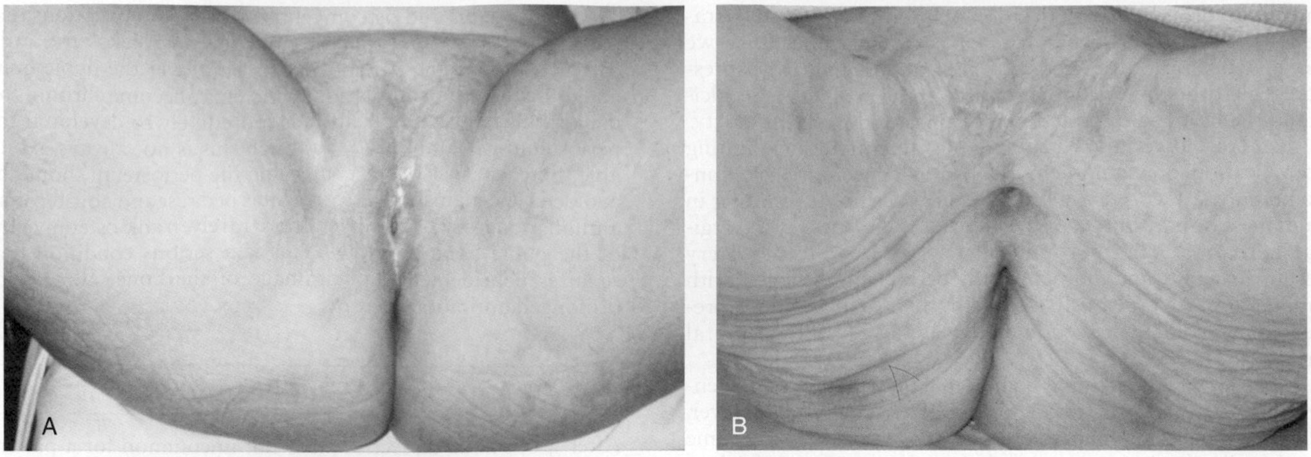

FIGURE 45.57. A–B: Marked introital stenosis following radical vulvectomy.

develop lymphangitis, which presents with fever, pain, and redness of the involved extremity. This condition is treated promptly with an intravenous antibiotic that covers streptococci.

A few good studies on sexual dysfunction after radical vulvectomy have been published. Generally, the capacity for intercourse remains. However, patients experience a marked sense of disfigurement and a reduction in genital sensitivity. Dyspareunia can occur as a result of stenosis or scar tissue (Fig. 45.57A–B), and these problems may be surgically treatable. Some patients remain orgasmic. There is evidence to suggest that a modified radical vulvectomy, especially with preservation of the anterior vulvar structures, helps maintain sexual function. It does seem reasonable to assume that sparing of as much normal vulvar tissue as possible is less likely to produce sexual dysfunction and a sense of disfigurement than is radical resection.

During follow-up of radical vulvectomy patients, it is not uncommon to discover pelvic relaxation (cystocele or rectocele) (Fig. 45.58). This may be related to resection of the perineal body with the attendant loss of its support functions, or it may simply be a result of aging. If the patient's medical condition and extent of cancer surgery permit, any stress urinary incontinence or defects in vaginal support should be repaired at the time of radical vulvectomy because they are likely to worsen subsequently.

Spraying or misdirection of the urinary stream is related to poor alignment of the urethra, a hood of periclitoral tissue obstructing the path of the urinary stream (Fig. 45.57), or asymmetry created by a hemivulvectomy. Digital manipulation or the use of an applied collection or directing device is useful, but in some cases minor surgical revision is necessary.

Rarely, after inguinofemoral lymphadenectomy, a femoral or inguinal hernia develops. When a hernia or any apparent weakness of the femoral or inguinal canal is noted at the time of surgery, it should be repaired at that time. Avoiding incision of the inguinal ligament is also important in the prevention of this complication.

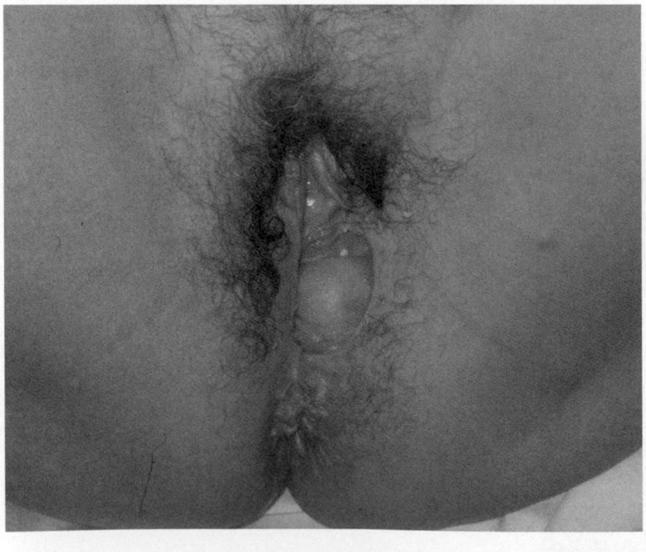

FIGURE 45.58. Large rectocele that developed after a modified radical vulvectomy.

Follow-Up

Following completion of treatment for vulvar cancer, long-term follow-up is warranted. It is reasonable to examine these women at least every 6 months for the first 5 years and annually thereafter. Some women are at higher risk for recurrence or have ongoing problems, and more frequent office visits may be warranted.

Follow-up is directed at early detection of recurrence (or later, a new primary vulvar tumor), identification and management of treatment-related complications, and surveillance for associated malignancies.

As previously discussed, it is only with local recurrence of vulvar cancer that there is a reasonable expectation for effective salvage treatment.

Approximately 10% to 15% of women treated for vulvar cancer will develop an isolated local recurrence or a subsequent new primary vulvar tumor, well more than half of whom receive effective salvage therapy. During follow-up visits, attention is directed at careful inspection and palpation of the vulvovaginal area and groins. Annual cervical or vaginal cuff cytology is also recommended. Patients are encouraged to do self-examinations and promptly report new symptoms or lesions.

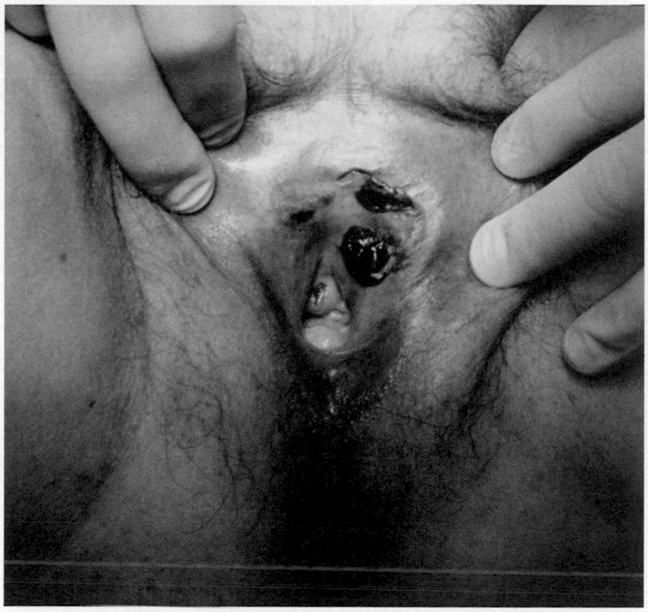

FIGURE 45.59. Melanoma of the vulva. Multifocal, darkly pigmented lesions are in the anterior vestibule.

VULVAR MELANOMA

Melanoma is the second most common histologic type of malignancy of the vulva, but still accounts for only 5% to 10% of vulvar cancers (Fig. 45.59). This lesion occurs predominantly in white women in the seventh decade, and although the vulva covers only 1% to 2% of the body surface, vulvar melanoma accounts for 3% to 5% of malignant melanomas in women. The most common presenting symptoms are bleeding, a lump or changing mole, and pruritus or irritation. In a small percentage of patients, there is a family history of melanoma. Melanoma of the vulva is uncommon, so most of the literature on the subject consists of retrospective studies of small numbers of patients. For this reason, the behavior of this tumor is difficult to define, and a rationale for treatment continues to evolve. However, it seems clear that the pattern of regional metastases is the same as that for squamous cell carcinoma; the behavior of the tumor is predicted best by a microstaging system. Importantly, the behavior of vulvar melanoma appears to be very similar to that of cutaneous melanomas in general.

Based on information that has accumulated over the past 3 decades, the treatment of vulvar melanoma is individualized based on clinical-pathologic factors, including microstaging, and modeled using experience derived from cutaneous melanomas in general.

What Do We Know about Cutaneous Melanoma?

Important areas of information that can be extrapolated from the general melanoma literature include individualization of management based primarily on microstaging, determination of what constitutes an adequate margin of resection, and definition of which groups of patients might benefit from an elective regional lymph node dissection.

Clark's classification had been used extensively for the microstaging of melanomas, with division into five levels of invasion (Fig. 45.60). Subsequently, Breslow's classification—based on millimeters of invasion from the upper granular layer of the epidermis to the deepest point of invasion—has become widely used. According to this method, tumor confined to a depth of 0.76 mm or less is generally within the epidermis and behaves as carcinoma *in situ*. Invasion of 0.76 to 1.49 mm is considered superficial; 1.5 to 4 mm, intermediate; and greater than 4 mm, deep. Some tumors can be quite superficial in measurement and yet be deep melanomas according to Clark's classification.

Over the past 3 decades, the independent prognostic factors in cutaneous melanoma have been well defined. For the

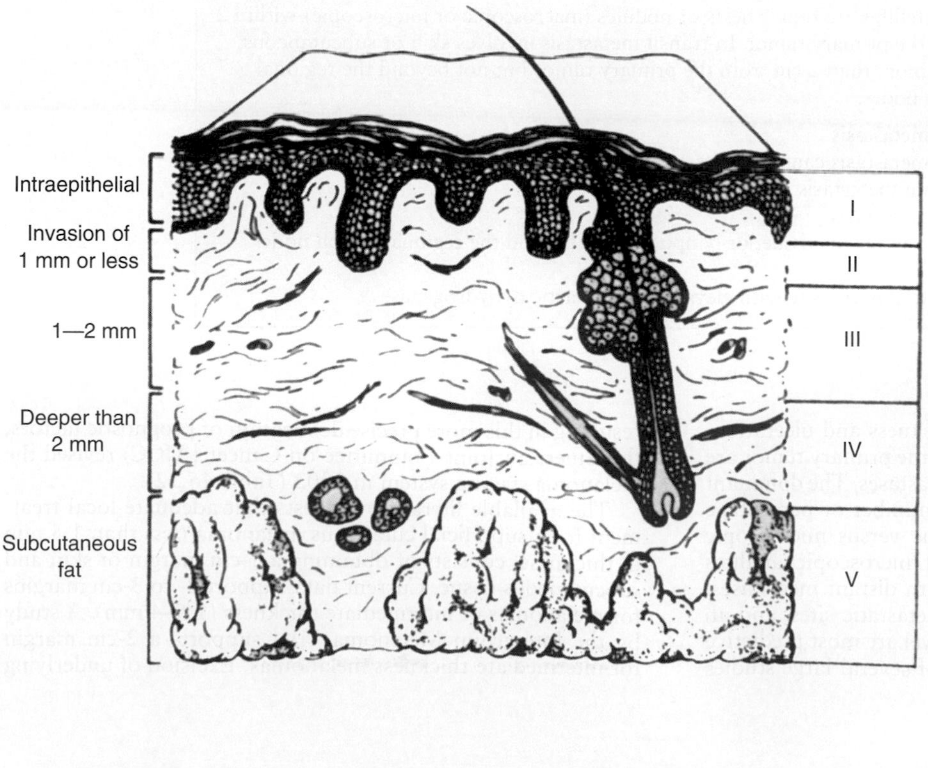

FIGURE 45.60. Levels of involvement of vulvar melanoma (Left, Chung; right, Clark). Level I (melanoma confined to the surface epithelium and pilar sheath) and level V (tumor extension into the underlying adipose tissue) are the same as Clark's levels I and V. Levels II, III, and IV are determined by measurements from the granular layer of the vulvar skin or the outermost epithelial layer of the squamous mucosa. (Chung AF, Woodruff JM, Lewis JL Jr. Malignant melanoma of the vulva: a report of 44 cases. *Obstet Gynecol* 1975;45:638.)

TABLE 45.12

TNM STAGING SYSTEM OF THE AMERICAN JOINT COMMITTEE ON CANCER

pT	**Primary tumor**
pTX	Primary tumor cannot be assessed
pT0	No evidence of primary tumor
pTis	Melanoma *in situ* (Clark level I) (atypical melanocytic hyperplasia, severe melanocytic dysplasia, not an invasive malignant lesion)
pT1	**Tumor 1 mm or less in thickness**
pT1a	Clark level II or III, without ulceration
pT1b	Clark level IV or V, or with ulceration
pT2	Tumor more than 1 mm but not more than 2 mm in thickness
pT2a	Without ulceration
pT2b	With ulceration
pT3	Tumor more than 2 mm but not more than 4 mm in thickness
pT3a	Without ulceration
pT3b	With ulceration
pT4	Tumor more than 4 mm in thickness
pT4a	Without ulceration
pT4b	With ulceration
pN	**Regional lymph nodes**
pN0	No regional lymph node metastatis
NX	Regional lymph nodes cannot be assessed
	Histologic examination of a regional lymphadenectomy specimen ordinarily includes six or more lymph nodes. If the lymph nodes are negative, but the number ordinarily examined is not met, classify as pN0. Classification based solely on sentinel node biopsy without subsequent axillary lymph node dissection is designated (sn) for sentinel node, e.g., pN1 (sn).
pN1	Metastasis in one regional lyph node
pN1a	Only microscopic metastasis (clinically occult)
pN1b	Macroscopic metastasis (clinically apparent)
pN2	Metastasis in two or three regional lymph nodes or intralymphatic regional metastasis
pN2a	Only microscopic nodal metastasis
pN2b	Macroscopic nodal metastasis
pN2c	Satellite or in-transit metastasis without regional nodal metastasis
pN3	Metastasis in four or more regional lymph nodes, or matted metastastic regional lymph nodes, or satellite or in-transit metastasis with metastasis in regional lymph node(s)
	Note: Satellites are tumor nests or nodules (macroscopic or microscopic) within 2 cm of the primary tumor. In-transit metastasis involves skin or subcutaneous tissue more than 2 cm from the primary tumor but not beyond the regional lymph nodes.
M	**Distant metastasis**
MX	Distant metastasis cannot be assessed
M0	No distant metastasis
M1	Distant metastasis
M1a	Skin, subcutaneous tissue, or lymph node(s) beyond the regional lymph nodes
M1b	Lung
M1c	Other sites, or any site with elevated serum lactic dyhydrogenase

primary tumor, these include tumor thickness and ulceration. Clinical or microscopic satellites around the primary tumor are considered to be in-transit lymphatic metastases. The dominant regional prognostic factors include the number or percentage of metastatic lymph nodes, macroscopic versus microscopic metastases, and the presence of clinical or microscopic satellites around a primary tumor. In patients with distant metastases, the site of metastases, the number of metastatic sites, and an elevated serum lactate dehydrogenase level are most predictive of poor survival. Based on the results of several large studies resulting in this more precise delineation of prognostic factors, the American Joint Committee on Cancer (AJCC) revised the melanoma staging system in 2002 (Table 45.12).

The available literature suggests that adequate local treatment for a superficial cutaneous melanoma (less than 1.5 mm in thickness) consists of obtaining a 1-cm margin of skin and subcutaneous tissue. Current data support 2- to 3-cm margins for melanomas of intermediate thickness (1.5–4 mm). A study by the Intergroup Melanoma Trial supports a 2-cm margin for intermediate-thickness melanomas. Excision of underlying fascia continues to be controversial. The local management of deep (greater than 4 mm) melanomas is less clear. The risk of metastatic disease in these patients is high, which lessens the impact of local therapy.

It is generally agreed that melanomas less than 0.76 mm in thickness are associated with a very low risk of lymph node metastases, and elective regional lymph node dissection is not indicated in this group. However, recent evidence suggests that subsets of these patients with adverse prognostic factors should be offered sentinel lymph node biopsy. Patients with melanomas greater than 4 mm in thickness have a high risk of both regional and systemic metastases, and they are less likely to benefit from elective lymph node dissection. There is significant controversy, however, about the benefit of prophylactic lymphadenectomy in patients with intermediate-thickness melanomas. The results of some retrospective studies have shown a beneficial effect of elective lymph node dissection on the survival of these patients. Two prospective studies, one from the Mayo Clinic and one multiinstitutional study directed by the World Health Organization, did not show any significant effect of elective lymph node dissection on survival. However, problems cited with these two studies have included the small numbers of intermediate-thickness melanomas and an imbalance of prognostic factors. In an Intergroup Melanoma Trial, patients with melanomas 1 to 4 mm thick on the trunk or proximal extremities were randomized to wide local excision with elective lymph node dissection versus wide local excision only. Overall survival was not significantly different. However, two subsets of patients had a significantly better overall 5-year survival rate with elective lymph node dissection. These subsets included patients age 60 years or younger and patients with a tumor thickness of 1.1 to 2.0 mm.

Intraoperative lymphatic mapping and sentinel lymph node biopsy were discussed earlier. Detection of occult melanoma cells by a more detailed examination of the sentinel nodes does correlate with recurrence and overall survival, and the information is potentially useful in the decision regarding adjuvant therapy. Since these techniques have come into more widespread use, recommendations regarding elective lymph node dissection are being reconsidered.

What Do We Know about Vulvar Melanoma?

As pointed out by Chung and colleagues, Clark's microstaging system for melanoma may be less suitable for vulvar tumors because of the lack of a well-defined papillary dermis in much of the vulvar skin and its virtual absence in the mucosal areas. Chung and associates proposed an alternative microstaging system (Fig. 45.60), which combines aspects of the Clark and Breslow systems. Because of the large percentage of vulvar melanomas that arise from or include mucosal membranes, caution is warranted in extrapolating data from squamous cell carcinoma of the vulva and from cutaneous melanoma in general. However, many of the tumors only superficially extend onto mucosal surfaces; until further data are available, it does appear reasonable to consider the available data on cutaneous melanoma and the data on squamous cell carcinoma of the vulva when managing a vulvar melanoma. Factors besides depth of invasion that seem to have an impact on the incidence of nodal metastases and survival include the AJCC stage, the presence of satellite lesions, tumor ulceration, central tumor location, tumor size, and capillary or lymphatic space involvement. The presence of any metastases indicates high-risk disease, although some studies report a few patients with positive groin nodes to be long-term survivors. In a retrospective report on 75 patients from the Norwegian Radium Institute, Scheistroen and associates identified nodal metastasis, angioinvasion, tumor thickness greater than 5 mm, clitoral or multifocal involvement, and aneuploidy as high-risk factors.

Diagnosis

When a vulvar melanoma is suspected, the diagnosis is best confirmed by an excisional biopsy. This allows pathologic evaluation of the entire lesion and therefore the most complete information on which to base definitive treatment. If the lesion is large, a generous incisional biopsy specimen is obtained from what appears to be the most significant portion of the lesion. Workup of the patient with a clinically localized vulvar melanoma need only consist of a careful history and physical examination, a chest radiograph, and a serum lactate dehydrogenase level. Depending on the results of these evaluations, further studies may be indicated.

Treatment

As with squamous cell carcinoma, the main modification in the local management of vulvar melanomas has been to tailor the resection to the individual lesion. Accordingly, some patients still require radical vulvectomy or even more extensive surgery. For many patients, however, the local treatment consists of a wide or radical local excision. For apparently localized lesions amenable to local removal, margin size should probably be that which is appropriate for a cutaneous melanoma, based on the depth of invasion of the melanoma as determined from the excisional biopsy. As with vulvar tumors in general, the excision is also tailored to the local vulvar anatomy. The frequent encroachment on midline vulvar structures by the melanoma creates difficulty in obtaining adequate margins while avoiding compromise of urinary or bowel function. The appropriate margin size of mucosally involved areas is much more difficult to define but should probably be at least the same as that for the cutaneous margin. The surgeon must frequently remove the clitoris, a portion of the distal vagina, or part of the distal urethra—or all three. Because of the propensity for early hematogenous spread in patients with deeply invasive tumors, ultraradical resection is rarely, if ever, indicated. Trials are being carried out to determine the benefit of adjuvant systemic therapy (see later text).

Modifications of the regional nodal management of vulvar melanoma have also paralleled those for squamous cell carcinoma of the vulva and cutaneous melanoma. The same arguments regarding elective lymph node dissection for cutaneous melanoma apply to vulvar melanoma. Inguinal-femoral lymphadenectomy is not generally recommended for very superficial or deeply invasive vulvar melanoma. Nodal metastases are rarely found in lesions with less than 0.76-mm invasion, and systemic disease is usually present in women with a depth of invasion greater than 4 mm. In melanomas with depth of invasion between 0.75 and 4 mm, the data are unclear, and many experts continue to recommend regional lymphadenectomy in these patients. As with issues surrounding local tumor management, there is a small amount of literature supporting some of these concepts with site-specific vulvar melanoma data, including the possible benefit from elective lymph node dissection and removal of clinically positive lymph nodes. The overall incidence of lymph node metastases in vulvar melanoma patients is reported to be around 30%. As with squamous cell carcinoma, pelvic lymphadenectomy does not appear to be warranted for a melanoma confined to the vulva with negative inguinal lymph nodes. The role of pelvic lymphadenectomy in patients with positive inguinal lymph nodes is unclear; considering the poor prognosis, the value would be very limited. The value of elective radiotherapy to the regional lymph nodes in melanoma patients is not known, so it should be used cautiously. If, during follow-up, isolated metastases appear in an undissected groin, they should be excised.

For patients in whom high-risk features have been identified after primary surgical therapy (e.g., positive lymph nodes, deep invasion), effective adjuvant treatment has not yet been identified. Radiotherapy may improve locoregional control of disease. One randomized study (mostly stage III resected cutaneous melanoma) demonstrated improved disease-free and overall survival with adjuvant interferon α-2b. Recurrent or metastatic disease carries a very poor prognosis in vulvar melanoma patients. Systemic therapy is of limited palliative benefit and most commonly consists of immunotherapy, chemotherapy (dacarbazine [DTIC]), hormonal therapy (tamoxifen), or all three.

Results

Overall, about one third of vulvar melanoma patients survive 5 years. This rate is lower than that reported for patients with squamous cell carcinoma of the vulva and with cutaneous melanoma in general. The worse prognosis has been attributed to an older age and a large percentage of deeply invasive and generally more advanced tumors at the time of diagnosis. According to several reports, survival of vulvar melanoma patients does correlate closely with depth of invasion. Other factors include the worse prognosis associated with mucosal melanomas in general and the difficulty in obtaining an adequate resection for the more centrally located tumors. Local recurrence is a common problem after removal of vulvar melanoma and tends to occur on the medial margin of resection. Local recurrence is reported to occur in about one third of patients, and the prognosis for these women is poor. Local tumor control and survival are reduced with more central and deeply invasive tumors. The presence of lymph node metastases also carries a poor prognosis, which has been correlated with the extent and number of lymph nodes involved. When the inguinal lymph nodes are positive, the reported survival rate is in the range of 10% to 31%. Vulvar melanoma has a propensity for late recurrence, and 5-year survival may not be an accurate predictor of cure in these patients.

BARTHOLIN GLAND CARCINOMA

A malignancy can arise from the Bartholin gland or duct, with most of the cancers being adenocarcinoma or squamous cell carcinoma. Other much rarer histologic types include transitional cell carcinoma, mixed carcinoma, and sarcoma. Bartholin carcinoma accounts for only 1% to 2% of vulvar malignancies, and, in some cases, a Bartholin origin is not clear-cut. Several criteria have been described to define a primary Bartholin malignancy, including anatomic position consistent with a Bartholin tumor, intact overlying skin, areas of apparent transition from normal to neoplastic elements, involvement of areas of the Bartholin gland with an origin histologically compatible with the gland, and no evidence of any other primary cancer. Although some of these criteria may not be met in an individual case, the tumor should at least be in a location consistent with a Bartholin tumor. As with the other rare types of vulvar malignancy, the available information on Bartholin malignancy is derived from retrospective studies of small series of patients.

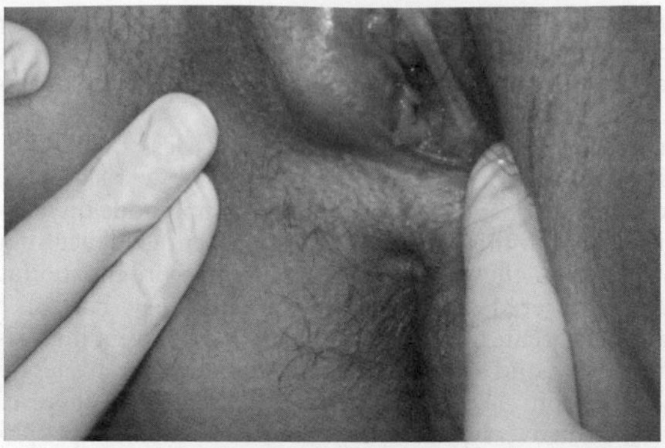

FIGURE 45.61. Right Bartholin gland carcinoma. See color version of figure.

Diagnosis

Bartholin carcinoma should be suspected when a tumor is noted in the region of the Bartholin gland, particularly in a woman older than 40 years of age (Fig. 45.61). The average age at diagnosis is about 50 years, but there is a wide age range. Many studies report a significant delay in diagnosis, attributed both to the deep-seated location of the tumor and to frequent misdiagnosis and treatment as a Bartholin abscess. When a woman presents with a Bartholin mass, biopsy or excision should be considered if she is older than 40 years of age, if the mass is suspicious, or when an apparently benign process does not resolve promptly with conservative therapy. Fine-needle aspiration for cytologic examination may be useful in some cases.

Treatment

Because of their deep location in the vulva, Bartholin malignancies tend to invade the ischiorectal fossa, close to the anorectum, or close to the pubic ramus (or all three) before they are diagnosed. These cancers also can erode through the overlying skin. Radical excision with an adequate margin tends to be more difficult with Bartholin malignancies. As with other vulvar cancers, surgical resection should be aimed at adequate resection of the tumor. Depending on the tumor extent, local resection must consist of at least a radical hemivulvectomy, but it may need to include removal of portions of vagina, levator ani, ischiorectal fat, perineal body, anal sphincter, anorectum, pubic bone, or all of these. In locally advanced but respectable cases, exenterative surgery or multimodality therapy may be necessary.

In relation to the difficulty in obtaining an adequate local resection, Copeland and associates reported improved local control with the administration of adjuvant postoperative radiotherapy. This is especially appropriate in the presence of close or positive margins. However, external radiotherapy alone should not be expected to control gross residual disease.

At the time of diagnosis, inguinal lymph node metastases are present in about half of patients with a Bartholin carcinoma. This propensity for lymphatic spread has been attributed to the frequent delay in diagnosis and the more advanced local extent of these tumors. The pattern of lymphatic spread is the same as that for other vulvar malignancies, primarily to the ipsilateral inguinofemoral lymph nodes. There are not enough data on which to base a reasonable estimate of the risk of metastases to the contralateral groin nodes. As with other vulvar cancers, if positive nodes are found, dissection of the opposite groin or radiotherapy to the inguinal and pelvic nodal basins, or both, may be warranted. Inguinal lymphadenectomy in these patients appears to be both prognostic and therapeutic.

Local, regional, and distant recurrences are common with Bartholin malignancies, and overall survival rate is lower than that for carcinoma of the vulva in general. Copeland and associates reported on a series of 36 patients with this cancer. The local recurrence rate was 2 of 12 (17%) for patients treated with hemivulvectomy (with or without radiotherapy) and 5 of 24 (21%) for patients treated with radical vulvectomy.

Adenoid Cystic Carcinoma

Adenoid cystic carcinoma accounts for about 15% of Bartholin gland carcinomas. As seen with electron microscopy, the tumor contains glandlike lumens filled with eosinophilic material derived from basement membrane, so it is of squamous cell origin. The behavior of this rare malignancy appears to be different from that of other Bartholin and vulvar cancers and to be similar to that of adenoid cystic carcinomas arising from other sites, such as the salivary gland. These vulvar tumors have a high local recurrence rate and a propensity for hematogenous metastases usually developing subsequent to local recurrence. Both local recurrences and metastases can be slowly progressive over a period of years but are not very responsive to radiotherapy or chemotherapy. In view of the difficulty in obtaining adequate surgical margins with Bartholin malignancies in general, and the high local recurrence rate and uncertain sensitivity to radiotherapy with adenoid cystic carcinoma in particular, a concerted effort to obtain at least 2-cm margins should be made when resecting this tumor. Postoperative adjuvant radiotherapy for close or positive margins did appear to be of possible benefit in another 1986 report by Copeland and colleagues and in the report by Rosenberg and associates. From the scant information available, inguinal lymph node metastases occur less frequently with this tumor and have all been ipsilateral. The prognostic and therapeutic value of lymphadenectomy in these patients remains to be defined. The role of adjuvant postoperative chemotherapy for this malignancy also deserves further study.

BASAL CELL CARCINOMA

Although basal cell carcinoma is the most common malignancy of the skin, basal cell carcinoma of the vulva is a rarely reported tumor. Approximately 250 cases have been reported in the literature, and basal cell carcinoma constitutes 2% to 3% of vulvar cancers. The cause is unknown, but there is frequently a history of chronic vulvar irritation. This lesion shares many features with vulvar squamous cell carcinoma. The average age of patients at diagnosis is 65 years, and there is a predilection for white women. Common symptoms include chronic pruritus vulvae and the presence of a mass. Authors have repeatedly reported a delay in diagnosis. Most basal cell carcinomas occur on the labia majora and, less commonly, on the labia minora, urethral meatus, and prepuce of the clitoris. The gross appearance is variable. Tumor size has ranged from 0.2 to 13 cm in greatest diameter, averaging 1.5 to 2 cm. There are also reports of multifocal lesions.

As many as 20% of patients with vulvar basal cell carcinoma have a history of other primary cancers. These other cancers have infrequently included coexistent melanoma or squamous cell carcinoma. Keratinization and mature squamous differentiation are commonly found in basal cell carcinomas and do not alter the prognosis. These lesions must be carefully distinguished from the rarer basosquamous carcinoma, which contains a malignant squamous component. This has been estimated to occur in 3% to 5% of basal cell carcinomas. Careful histologic evaluation of the biopsy material is necessary to rule out a malignant squamous component. With the exception of very large lesions, this is best accomplished by excisional biopsy.

One of the subtypes of basal cell carcinoma, adenoid basal cell carcinoma, must be differentiated from the more aggressive adenoid cystic carcinoma arising in a Bartholin gland or in the skin of the vulva. Merino and colleagues have suggested clinical and histologic criteria for this distinction.

In 1977, Safai and Good reviewed the literature and found 109 cases of basal cell carcinoma of the skin with metastases. These are rare cases, with an incidence of less than 0.1%. Basosquamous carcinoma of the skin, including the vulva, is a more aggressive neoplasm, with the squamous component metastasizing. Basal cell carcinoma of the vulva is also an indolent, locally invasive lesion that rarely metastasizes. There are only ten well-documented cases of metastatic basal cell carcinoma of the vulva in the literature. Nine of these 10 have been lymphatic metastases. When a patient with basal cell carcinoma has suspicious inguinal lymph nodes, these lymph nodes should probably be removed, especially if the vulvar tumor is large or locally advanced. If the inguinal lymph nodes are not suspicious, they can be removed if they become suspicious during follow-up.

Treatment

Most authorities agree that the treatment of choice for vulvar basal cell carcinoma is wide local excision including a generous amount of underlying subcutaneous tissue. For a multifocal lesion, complete vulvectomy may be appropriate. If a malignant squamous component is present, however, then treatment is the same as that for invasive squamous cell carcinoma of the vulva as outlined above. There is little information available on the use of radiotherapy or chemotherapy in the treatment of primary or metastatic basal cell carcinoma of the vulva, but there is one report of a locally advanced lesion that had a complete response to radiotherapy. Close follow-up is essential, because the local recurrence rate has been reported to be 10% to 21.5%.

Prognosis

The overall prognosis for patients with vulvar basal cell carcinoma is difficult to ascertain. In a review by Breen and colleagues, there was a 5-year survival rate of about 64%. However, they were unable to find documentation for a single death directly related to recurrent or residual basal cell carcinoma. Rather, they attributed the deaths to old age, attrition, and overzealous therapy.

The prognosis for the rare metastatic basal cell carcinoma of the vulva is even more difficult to predict. Sworn and coworkers concluded that the prognosis is similar to that for basal cell carcinoma at other skin sites. With basal cell carcinoma elsewhere on the skin, the mean survival after discovery of metastatic disease has been reported to be 10 to 14 months. However, Conway and Hugo reported prolonged survival if only regional lymph nodes are involved.

SARCOMA OF THE VULVA

Primary sarcoma constitutes 1% to 3% of all vulvar malignancies. The literature consists of case reports and small series of patients, often with very limited follow-up. In addition, this is a heterogeneous group because of the variety of histologic types and their associated differences in behavior. Hence, the natural history and appropriate treatment of these tumors have not been well defined.

Leiomyosarcoma

The most common histologic type of primary vulvar sarcoma is leiomyosarcoma. Most of these patients are in the age range of 40 to 50 years, but a few are younger (one patient was 17). At least three cases of pregnant women with leiomyosarcoma have been reported. According to the descriptions, most patients present with an enlarging mass in the labia majora or Bartholin region (Fig. 45.62A–B). Like tumors at other sites, smooth-muscle tumors of the vulva appear to have a range of appearances and behavior, from benign to malignant. Tavassoli and Norris reported 32 smooth-muscle tumors of the vulva and attempted to delineate the histologic features that might relate to prognosis. They believed that their analysis was impeded by small numbers of patients in subgroups and by varied adequacy of excision. According to their results, prognosis was best predicted by three main determinants (size, tumor contour, and mitotic activity). Neoplasms greater than 5 cm that have infiltrating margins and five or more mitotic figures per 10 high-power fields are likely to recur unless controlled by total excision. It was also determined that lesions larger than 5 cm with infiltrative margins and prominent mitotic activity have a more aggressive behavior as the number of mitotic figures increases. The significance of mitotic activity could not be fully evaluated because of the small number of cases with intermediate grades of mitotic activity and because of other factors. The degree of cellular atypism did not correlate well with the mitotic activity or with recurrence. In 1996, Nielsen and colleagues proposed similar prognostic criteria but included cytologic atypia. In keeping with a range of behaviors, according to the available reports, vulvar leiomyosarcomas may do

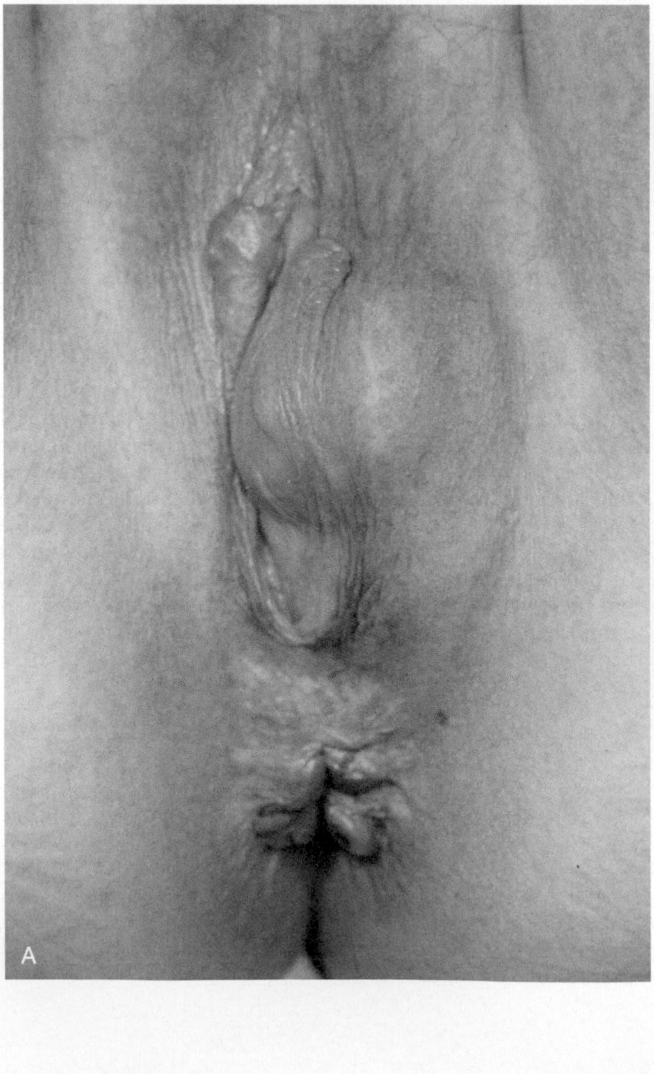

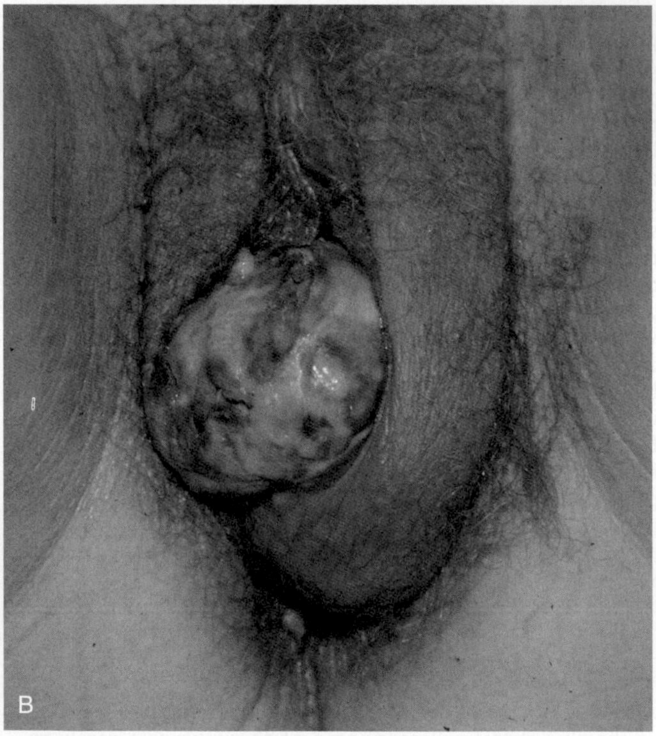

FIGURE 45.62. **A:** A tumor in the left labia majora determined to be a low-grade leiomyosarcoma. **B:** Leiomyosarcoma of the vulva breaking through the overlying skin.

well with adequate excision, may follow a slowly progressive course, or may rapidly progress to fatality. Local recurrences are common, and several authors have recommended early radical excision of these tumors to improve treatment results. As with the other genital tract sarcomas, there is a propensity for hematogenous metastases that may develop early. From the few studies reporting long-term follow-up, it appears that only about half of these patients are 5-year survivors. Information regarding the propensity of these tumors to metastasize to the regional lymph nodes and the prognostic and therapeutic value of inguinal lymphadenectomy is scant. On the basis of general knowledge of the behavior of these types of sarcomas, the regional lymph nodes are probably at minimal risk with a low-grade tumor. In patients with high-grade tumors, removal of regional lymph nodes is probably of prognostic value only, although control of disease in the groin is a consideration. In a fit patient with a high-risk but apparently localized tumor, inguinal lymphadenectomy seems reasonable. Radiotherapy has been used in only a few cases with mixed results. Postoperative adjuvant radiotherapy to the pelvis (including the perineum) may be worthwhile in selected cases to improve local control. As with other genital tract leiomyosarcomas, chemotherapy has been of limited palliative benefit.

Six cases of myxoid leiomyosarcoma of the vulva have been reported. All were managed by local resection. Three experienced local recurrence that responded well to repeat excision. From available follow-up, five of the six remained alive without evidence of active cancer at 25 to 83 months.

Other Sarcomas

According to our review, 14 cases of *dermatofibrosarcoma protuberans* (DFSP) of the vulva have been reported. These patients ranged in age from 37 to 87 years and presented with a tumor characteristic of DFSP at other sites. The tumors range in maximum diameter from 1 to 8 cm and are multinodular, firm, seemingly well-circumscribed masses. The mass is reportedly mobile but fixed to the overlying skin from which it originated. The clinical impression of a mobile, well-circumscribed mass is apparently misleading, because fine microscopic projections of the tumor have been shown to extend well beyond the apparent mass. This explains the marked tendency of this tumor to recur locally and the need for wide (3 cm has been recommended) surgical margins. Intraoperative frozen section analysis of margins has also been recommended. Despite this tendency for local recurrence, DFSP behaves like a low-grade sarcoma that rarely metastasizes. In the absence of suspicious lymph nodes, a lymphadenectomy is not warranted. Hematogenous metastases may be seen after multiple local recurrences. Local radiotherapy has not been useful for these tumors, but may be of benefit as adjuvant postoperative treatment for a close resection margin. With adequate resection, the overall prognosis for DFSP of the vulva should be good. Two cases of a fibrosarcoma arising in a vulvar DFSP have been reported, but the clinical behavior and prognosis for such tumors appear to be the same as those for DFSP alone.

Six cases of *malignant fibrous histiocytoma* of the vulva have been reported. The age range of these patients is 38 to 79 years. Five of the six tumors were on the labia majora, and the sixth was vulvovaginal. Based on these few reports and the more abundant literature on malignant fibrous histiocytoma at other sites, recommended treatment includes radical excision of the tumor with an inguinal lymphadenectomy. Adjuvant radiotherapy and chemotherapy may have a role, and the one vulvovaginal tumor reported was without evidence of recurrence 6 years after sequential chemotherapy and radiotherapy.

We found five reports of *pure fibrosarcoma* of the vulva. Two of these patients died with disseminated disease at 3 weeks and 16 months after diagnosis, and one patient had inguinal lymph node metastases but was without evidence of recurrence at 48 months. According to the general literature on fibrosarcomas, the malignant potential varies depending on the tissue of origin and the histologic pattern (cellularity, mitotic activity). Three of the four reported patients who were treated developed local recurrences (two of them repetitive), which is in agreement with the general behavior reported for these tumors. Again, the importance of wide excision at the time of primary treatment is emphasized. Fibrosarcoma is reported to only rarely metastasize to lymph nodes; however, as previously pointed out, one of the five described cases did have an isolated lymphatic metastasis.

Nineteen *primary epithelioid sarcomas* of the vulva have been reported. Nine of the women were 31 years of age or younger, and five of the lesions arose on the labium majus. Seven of the patients developed repetitive local recurrences (generally in the form of multiple subcutaneous nodules) and coincident or subsequent hematogenous or lymphatic metastases, or both, and died over the course of months to years. This tumor apparently penetrates along soft tissue planes, and there is reported difficulty in delineating tumor extent. Radical excision with wide, clear margins seems to be the most reasonable initial treatment. Regional lymphadenectomy should be considered on an individual basis.

A few malignant *rhabdoid tumors* of the vulva have also been reported. There is apparent difficulty distinguishing this malignancy histologically from epithelioid sarcoma. Both tumors present similarly as a benign-appearing labial mass in young women. Malignant rhabdoid tumors may follow an even more aggressive course.

Although sarcomas constitute only a small percentage of vulvar malignancies in general, they account for most vulvar cancers in children and young women. Overall, pediatric vulvovaginal *rhabdomyosarcoma* has a good prognosis and greatly reduced treatment morbidity because of the efficacy of combined treatment modalities (especially chemotherapy and brachytherapy). Rhabdomyosarcoma arising in older women and other histologic variants of rhabdomyosarcoma may not be so amenable to therapy.

At least 100 cases of *aggressive angiomyxoma* involving the female pelvis or perineum, or both, have been described, and at least 14 of these primarily involved the vulva. It is an unusual tumor derived from fibroblasts or myofibroblasts with nuclei that have no atypical features or mitotic activity. The tumor appears to be locally invasive and spreads by direct extension only. Local recurrences are common, although there have been no reported deaths attributable to this tumor. The mainstay of treatment is wide excision both primarily and for recurrences. Response to gonadotropin-releasing hormone has been reported.

Isolated reports of a variety of other types of sarcomas arising in the vulva have been published. Treatment of these various sarcomas must be individualized according to the scant literature available, the potential aggressiveness of the malignancy as suggested by the pathologist, and the individual situation.

PAGET DISEASE OF THE VULVA

Paget disease is classified, according to location, as mammary or extramammary disease. The original lesion described by

Paget is a skin (nipple and areola) lesion related to an underlying invasive ductal adenocarcinoma. Extramammary Paget disease most commonly involves the anogenital region, appearing as a patchy, reddish and whitish, velvety, and eczematous lesion (Fig. 45.63). Patients with Paget disease of the vulva are usually white, postmenopausal women who report localized itching and burning.

Paget disease of the vulva is of apocrine origin and is confined to the epithelium in most cases. However, invasive disease is present in about 15% to 25% of cases, either as a result of direct invasion through the basement membrane or, less commonly, because of the presence of an underlying apocrine gland adenocarcinoma. Histologically, intraepithelial Paget disease appears as large, pale cells, often in nests at the tips of the rete ridges (Figs. 45.64 and 45.65). The cells are often seen infiltrating upward in the epithelium, which is hyperkeratotic. The Paget cells can be located within any of the skin adnexa.

Vulvar Paget disease occurs with other malignancies in about 25% of patients; the most common of these is breast carcinoma. Other commonly associated malignancies are basal cell, rectal, and genitourinary carcinomas. When Paget disease involves the anus, there is a very high incidence of coexisting rectal cancer. Part of the preoperative workup should be directed at screening for these malignancies. Wilkinson and Brown proposed a classification of vulvar Paget disease as primary or secondary (involvement of the vulvar skin by a noncutaneous internal neoplasm). They subclassified primary disease according to the presence of invasive cancer and subclassified secondary disease according to tumor origin. They report that secondary vulvar Paget disease is always intraepithelial.

When a patient is diagnosed with Paget disease of the vulva, the area of involvement should be carefully inspected and palpated to detect areas suspicious for invasive cancer. If the disease clinically appears to be intraepithelial, a wide local excision is performed, including a small amount of subcutaneous tissue. A well-known characteristic of intraepithelial Paget disease is histologic extension far beyond that which is clinically apparent. Intraoperative assessment of margins with frozen sections may be helpful (Fig. 45.63B–D). Other methods that have been reported to be useful in ensuring clear margins include preoperative biopsies, Mohs micrographic surgery, and fluorescein dye with ultraviolet light. Colposcopy and toluidine blue staining are not helpful, according to Friedrich and colleagues. An experimental technique reported to be potentially useful in evaluating histologically negative margins is the application of a panel of monoclonal antibodies that may detect occult Paget cells.

When intraepithelial Paget disease extends far beyond that which is clinically apparent, very extensive excision is necessary to obtain clear margins. Primary closure of vulvar wounds is desirable, but may not be possible. Reported means of dealing with such cases include skin grafting and laser vaporization of the occult disease (guided by peripheral biopsies). There are a few reports of Paget disease recurring within a skin graft. Topical 5-fluorouracil or bleomycin, administered either preoperatively or postoperatively, has also been used to treat the clinically negative disease. If it appears that excision of persistently positive margins may prevent primary closure, it is not unreasonable to close the wound and follow the patient closely.

After excision of intraepithelial Paget disease of the vulva, local recurrence develops in about one third of patients (Fig. 45.66). This tends to take the form of multiple recurrences over a prolonged period of time. In some studies, recurrence risk has been correlated with excisional margin status, but it also has been pointed out that the initial disease in some cases is multifocal. Of particular concern are a few reports of patients whose recurrent lesions eventually became invasive. Whether such instances are preventable by diligently eradicating the full histologic extent of the disease is not known.

When vulvar Paget disease is found to contain an invasive component, the treatment is radical surgery, as for squamous cell carcinoma. Overall, these patients have a high incidence of inguinal lymph node metastases with an associated poor prognosis. The role of adjuvant therapy in these patients is unclear.

Management of recurrent intraepithelial Paget disease of the vulva is similar to that of the primary lesion, with excision of at least the clinically evident disease.

VERRUCOUS CARCINOMA OF THE VULVA

Verrucous carcinoma of the vulva is a rare variant of squamous cell carcinoma, with about 50 cases reported in the literature. This tumor was first described in the oral cavity by Ackerman in 1948 and most commonly occurs in the oral cavity, larynx, and anogenital region. The mean age of the women diagnosed with this malignancy of the vulva is about 50 years. The reported tumors have ranged from 1 to 10 cm in maximum diameter and appear as a slow-growing, cauliflowerlike tumor (Fig. 45.67). Characteristically, verrucous cancers have well-demarcated borders that are pushing rather than infiltrating. Verrucous carcinoma can be confused with condyloma; when an apparent condyloma (especially when large and in an older woman) does not respond to the usual conservative measures, it should be excised. About one third of patients with vulvar verrucous carcinoma have a history of genital warts, and human papillomavirus (HPV) has been detected in some lesions, the most common type being HPV-6.

The diagnosis of verrucous carcinoma requires a large (preferably excisional) biopsy that must include the base of the lesion. Verrucous carcinoma can also be confused with so-called warty carcinoma, another variant of well-differentiated squamous cell carcinoma that tends to remain *in situ* or superficially infiltrating. Differentiation of these two entities is not of great importance because both have a very low incidence of metastases, and treatment is essentially the same.

Verrucous carcinoma is rarely associated with metastatic disease, and many of the reports of such spread have shown histologic evidence of nests of squamous cell carcinoma invading the stroma beneath the tumor. Some authors have suggested that if areas of distinct invasion are found beneath a verrucous lesion, the behavior may be more aggressive, and treatment should be more radical. Inflammatory enlargement of the inguinal lymph nodes has been a frequently reported finding with verrucous carcinoma of the vulva.

It is generally agreed that the main treatment of verrucous carcinoma of the vulva is excision with free margins. How radical this resection should be is unclear, but local recurrences have not been uncommon (Fig. 45.68). Local lesions have had a good initial response to radiation therapy but a high rate of subsequent recurrence and about a 30% incidence of anaplastic transformation with associated aggressive behavior. The few reported cases of metastatic verrucous carcinoma of the genital tract have followed radiotherapy. However, many

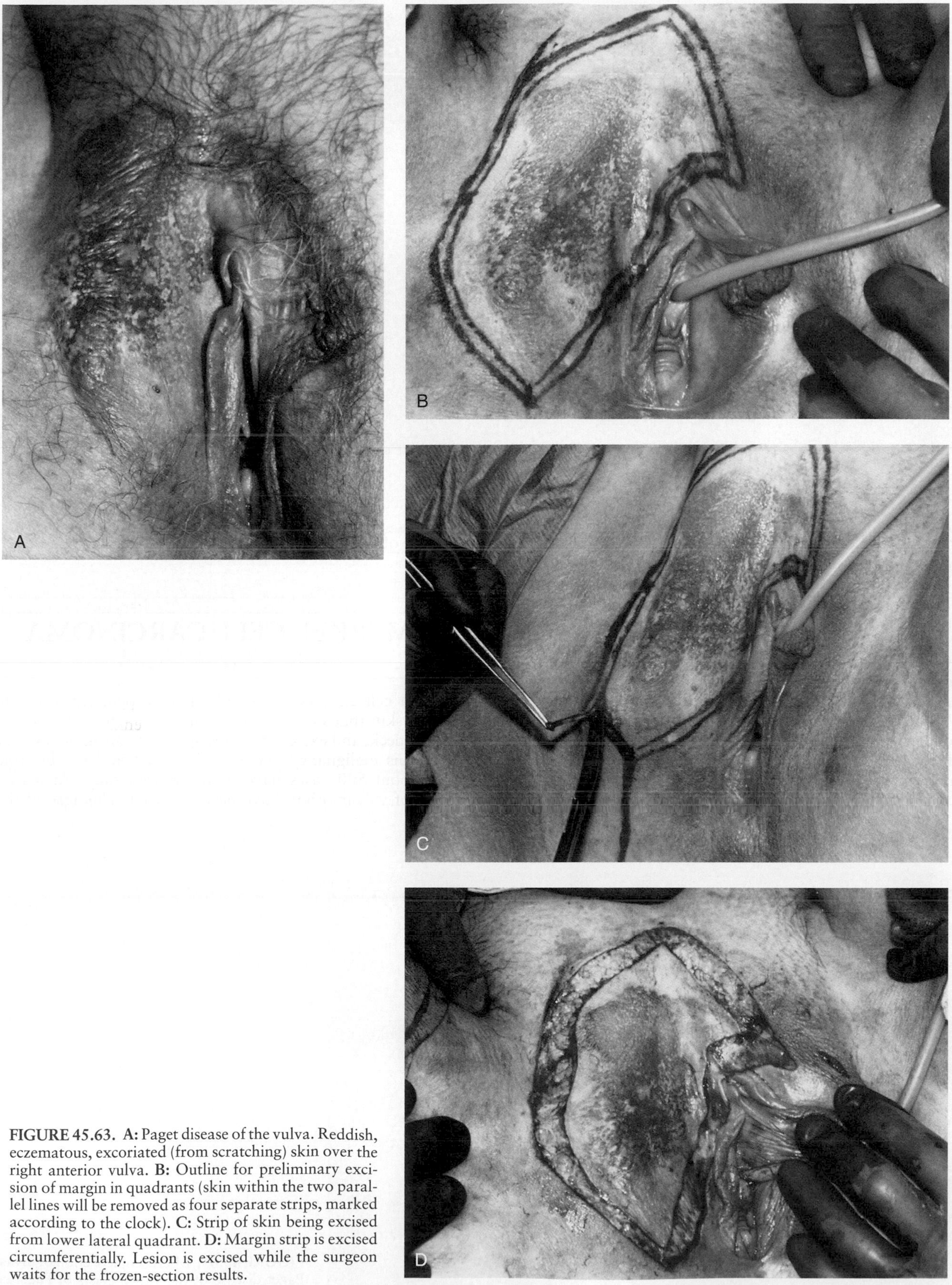

FIGURE 45.63. **A:** Paget disease of the vulva. Reddish, eczematous, excoriated (from scratching) skin over the right anterior vulva. **B:** Outline for preliminary excision of margin in quadrants (skin within the two parallel lines will be removed as four separate strips, marked according to the clock). **C:** Strip of skin being excised from lower lateral quadrant. **D:** Margin strip is excised circumferentially. Lesion is excised while the surgeon waits for the frozen-section results.

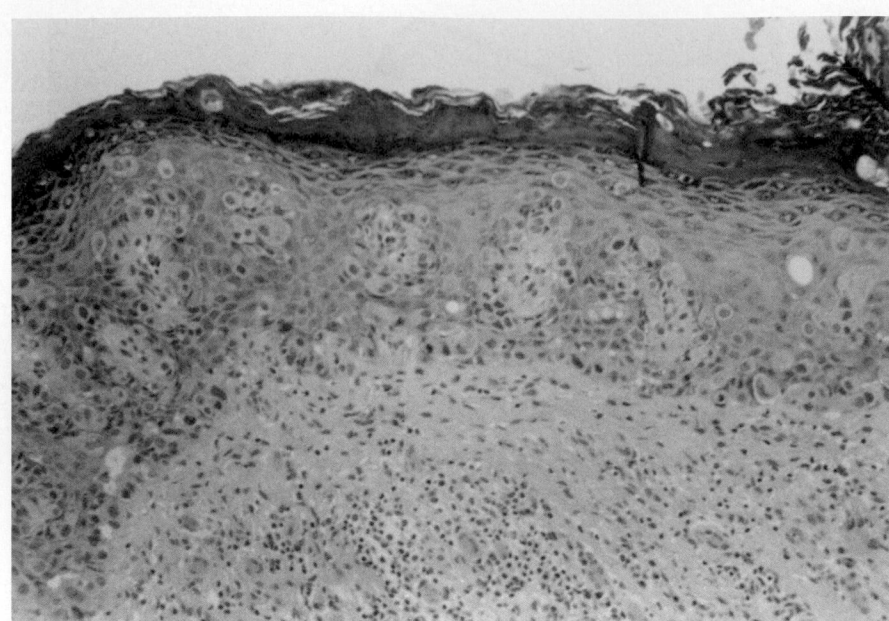

FIGURE 45.64. Microscopic section of intraepithelial Paget disease of the vulva. Nests of large, pale cells infiltrate upward in the epithelium, which is hyperkeratotic.

tumors have been successfully treated with a combination of surgery and radiotherapy; when a tumor is locally advanced, this seems to be a reasonable treatment. Inguinal lymphadenectomy may be indicated in patients with large tumors, in patients with persistence or recurrence of disease, especially after radiotherapy, and in patients with infiltrating cancer beyond very early invasion below the verrucous tumor. Biopsy specimens may be obtained of enlarged lymph nodes thought to be inflammatory.

Verrucous carcinoma of the vulva has been associated with second malignant tumors, most commonly of the cervix, breast, and anogenital skin. Although verrucous carcinoma of the genital tract is a slow-growing tumor that rarely metastasizes, a 1988 review by Andersen and Sorensen reported that 26.1% of the patients with this type of carcinoma had died of disease.

MERKEL CELL CARCINOMA OF THE VULVA

Merkel cell cancers are small-cell (neuroendocrine) tumors of the skin that occur most commonly in sun-exposed areas (head, neck, and extremities) and behave in an aggressive manner. This malignancy was first described in 1972 by Toker, and about 500 cases have been reported since. At least 11 cases of vulvar origin have been reported. The ages of these

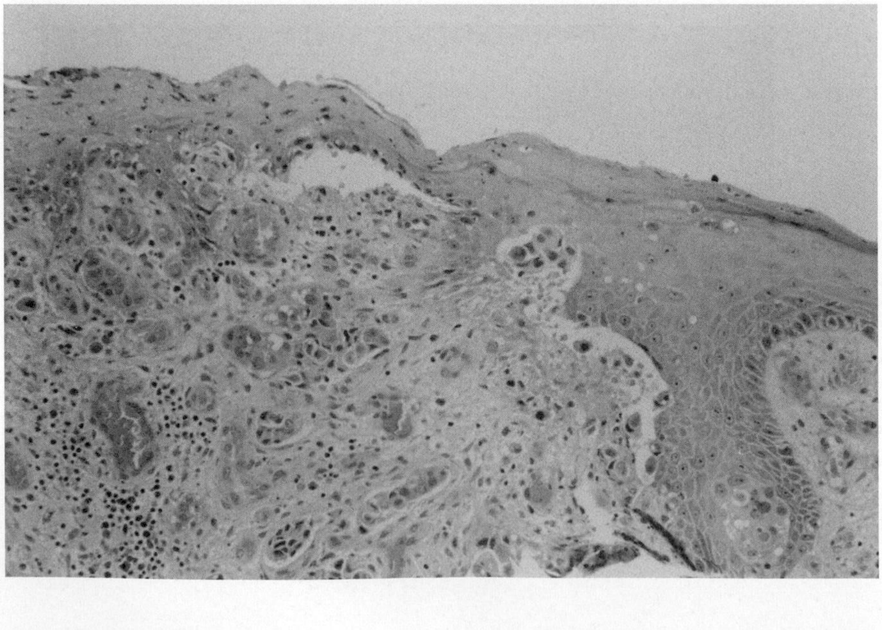

FIGURE 45.65. Microscopic section of invasive Paget disease of the vulva. Nests of Paget cells infiltrate the stroma.

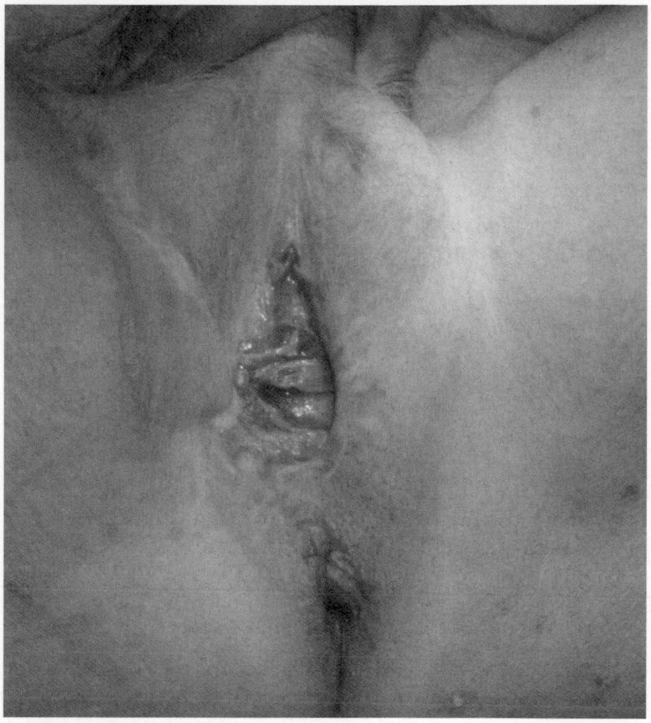

FIGURE 45.66. Recurrent Paget disease of the vulva.

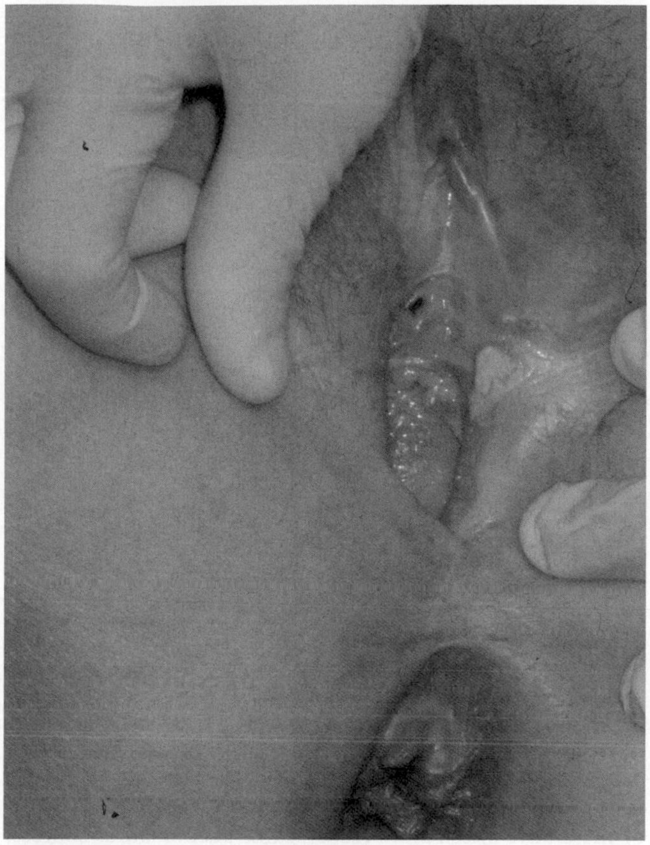

FIGURE 45.68. Recurrent verrucous carcinoma of the vulva.

10 patients ranged from 28 to 74 years, and the tumors occurred in all regions of the vulva (three in the Bartholin gland). When originating from the vulva, Merkel cell carcinoma has behaved in a highly aggressive manner (even more so than Merkel cell tumors in general), with nine patients having regional lymph node metastases. At least seven had distant metastases and died within 2.5 years of diagnosis. Surgery and radiotherapy appear to be of value for local control only, and as yet no effective systemic treatment exists. As in the treatment of small-cell carcinoma of the lung, etoposide and cisplatin have been used for a few cases of Merkel cell carcinoma, with good responses. Three of the vulvar cases were treated with this regimen. Two progressed, and one had a partial response of very short duration.

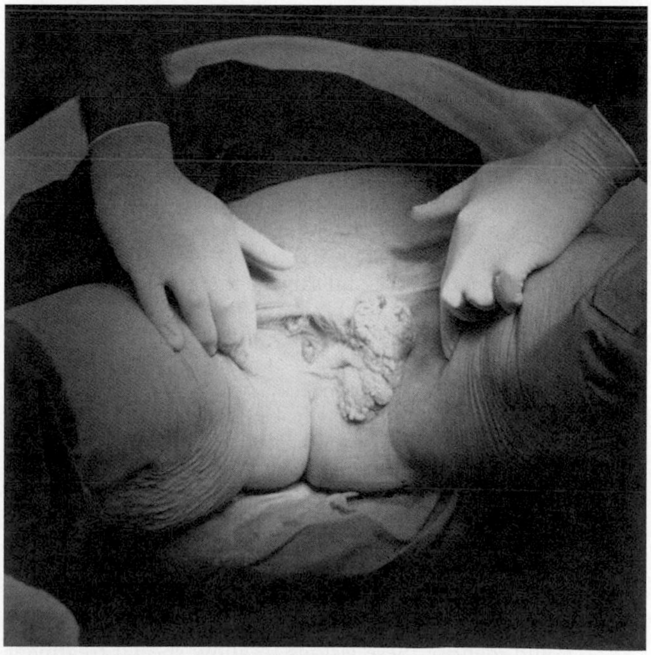

FIGURE 45.67. Verrucous carcinoma of the vulva. A large cauliflowerlike tumor arising from the left labia majora.

SUPERNUMERARY MAMMARY ADENOCARCINOMA

Ectopic breast tissue in the vulva is very rare, but at least nine cases of mammary-type adenocarcinoma arising in the vulva have been reported. These patients ranged in age from 49 to 71 years, and five of the nine presented with an asymptomatic vulvar nodule. Only one of the patients had evidence of primary breast cancer, but rather than representing metastatic disease, the vulvar lesion appeared to be primary from ectopic tissue. The diagnosis of vulvar mammary adenocarcinoma is based primarily on the histologic pattern of the vulvar tumor. Other criteria can include the finding of adjacent normal mammary glandular elements (one case of adjacent *in situ* malignancy), the presence of estrogen or progesterone receptor positivity, positivity for common breast markers, and ruling out an origin from skin appendages.

One of the nine patients died of disease without treatment 1 month after diagnosis. The patient with coexistent primary breast carcinoma died of widespread metastatic (including cerebral) disease 22 months after the diagnosis. One patient had 2 of 10 positive ipsilateral inguinal lymph nodes and was placed on tamoxifen postoperatively; this patient remained without evidence of recurrence at 1 year. A fourth patient had extensive nodal metastases at the time of diagnosis, subsequently developed distant metastases, and died of disease 27 months after diagnosis despite chemotherapy. A fifth patient had 4 of 11 positive ipsilateral inguinal lymph nodes and was placed on tamoxifen postoperatively. After 2 years of disease-free survival, the patient stopped taking the tamoxifen and presented 4 months later with bony metastases. After radiotherapy and reinstitution of tamoxifen, she was disease-free at 1 year of follow-up. A sixth patient had microscopic involvement in 1 of 14 ipsilateral lymph nodes. She received adjuvant chemotherapy with a plan for subsequent radiotherapy and tamoxifen. Follow-up was not available for the other three patients, but two of the three had undergone an inguinal lymphadenectomy, and in both cases there were positive lymph nodes.

Beyond surgical treatment, such a rare patient might be considered for adjuvant therapy (especially with metastatic disease) such as radiotherapy, tamoxifen (if estrogen receptor-positive), or chemotherapy.

OTHER REPORTED VULVAR MALIGNANCIES

There are scattered reports of a variety of adenocarcinomas arising in the vulva other than those previously discussed. Most of these have arisen from recognizable adenomatous sources, such as adnexal structures and endometriosis. There are five reports of malignancy arising in the vulva from isolated foci of extraovarian endometriosis; four were clear-cell adenocarcinoma, and the fifth was an endometrial stromal sarcoma. There are also rare reports of vulvar sebaceous carcinoma, apocrine gland carcinoma, mucinous carcinoma, lymphoma, and a peripheral primitive neuroectodermal tumor.

At least four endodermal sinus tumors of the vulva have been reported. The ages of these patients were 22 months, 2 years, 15 years, and 26 years, and all four presented with a painless vulvar mass. Three of the four patients died of metastatic disease 6, 11, and 23 months after diagnosis. The 2-year-old patient remains without evidence of recurrence 5.5 years after local excision.

A variety of metastatic lesions to the vulva have been documented, most commonly from the gynecologic tract. Nongynecologic metastatic disease to the vulva is rare, with isolated reports of primary sites such as the urinary tract, colorectum, skin (melanoma), non-Hodgkin's lymphoma, lung and breast.

BEST SURGICAL PRACTICES

- Prognostic Factors
  - The dominant prognostic factor for invasive squamous cell carcinoma of the vulva is the status of the inguinofemoral lymph nodes.
  - Primary tumor factors that appear to have prognostic importance include depth of invasion or tumor thickness, tumor diameter, tumor differentiation, lymph-vascular space involvement, and margin status.
- Pretreatment Investigation
  - A biopsy confirming the presence of invasive cancer is necessary before any therapy. Because of the frequent advanced age and coexisting medical problems typical of women with vulvar cancer, a thorough preoperative evaluation by internal medicine and anesthesiology consultants should be considered. Sophisticated radiologic evaluation is only of potential benefit in the presence of locoregionally advanced disease.
- Treatment of Invasive Squamous Cell Carcinoma of the Vulva
  - *Unilateral groin lymphadenectomy.* Limiting inguinofemoral lymphadenectomy to the ipsilateral side appears to be a reasonable approach in a patient with a well-lateralized early tumor that is well differentiated, with no lymph-vascular space involvement, and with negative ipsilateral inguinal lymph nodes.
  - *Superficial inguinal lymphadenectomy.* In patients with early invasive squamous cell carcinoma of the vulva, removal of the lymph nodes superficial to the cribriform fascia may result in a lower incidence of wound complications and subsequent lymphedema. The approach has been widely used in recent years, but there is some concern that the risk of groin recurrences is higher than standard inguinal/femoral lymphadenectomy.
  - *Sentinel lymph node identification.* Preliminary results suggest that lymphatic mapping with a combination of isosulfan blue dye and technetium-labeled sulfur colloid followed by sentinel lymph node dissection is applicable to a large percentage of women with early invasive squamous cell carcinoma of the vulva. However, many questions require further investigation to better define the usefulness of the sentinel lymph node approach in women with vulvar cancer.
  - *Pelvic lymph nodes.* Pelvic lymphadenectomy is not indicated in most patients with vulvar cancer. Pelvic radiation therapy is usually administered in patients with positive groin nodes, but surgical resection of enlarged pelvic nodes may be considered.
- Locally Advanced Vulvar Cancer
  - About 30% to 40% of vulvar cancers are locally advanced. Current approaches to the treatment of locally advanced vulvar cancer include ultraradical surgery, radiotherapy, or a combination of treatment modalities.
- Recurrent Squamous Cell Carcinoma of the Vulva
  - About 15% to 40% of patients with squamous cell carcinoma of the vulva develop recurrence after treatment. Only with an isolated local recurrence is there reasonable expectation of successful salvage therapy (preferably resection).
- Reconstructive Techniques for the Vulva and Groin
  - When an extensive resection of a vulvar malignancy or a groin node metastasis is necessary, it may not be possible to close the wound primarily. Under these circumstances, closure of the incision and healing can be facilitated by a variety of reconstructive procedures. Leaving the wound open is another reasonable option.
- Uncommon Histologic Types
  - Melanoma, basal cell carcinoma, cancers of the Bartholin gland, invasive Paget disease, and other uncommon or rare vulvar tumors are often managed differently from squamous cell carcinoma. A biopsy of the lesion should identify these lesions to allow special treatment planning.

Bibliography

Abrao FS, Baracat EC, Marques AF, et al. Carcinoma of the vulva: clinicopathologic factors involved in inguinal and pelvic lymph node metastasis. *J Reprod Med* 1990;35:1113.

Achauer BM, Braly P, Berman ML, et al. Immediate vaginal reconstruction following resection for malignancy using the gluteal thigh flap. *Gynecol Oncol* 1984;19:79.

Ackerman LV. Verrucous carcinoma of the oral cavity. *Surgery* 1948;23:670.

Acosta AA, Given FT, Frazier AB, et al. Preoperative radiation therapy in the management of squamous cell carcinoma of the vulva: preliminary report. *Am J Obstet Gynecol* 1978;132:198.

Adams J, Daly JW. Proctectomy combined with vulvectomy for carcinoma of the vulva. *Obstet Gynecol* 1979;54:643.

Adelson MD, Miranda FR, Strumpf KB. Necrotizing fasciitis: a complication of squamous cell carcinoma of the vulva. *Gynecol Oncol* 1991;42:98.

Agarossi A, Vago L, Lazzarin A, et al. Vulvar Kaposi's sarcoma. A case report [Letter]. *Ann Oncol* 1991;2:609.

Agress R, Figge DC, Tamimi H, et al. Dermatofibrosarcoma protuberans of the vulva. *Gynecol Oncol* 1983;16:288.

Al-Ghamdi A, Freedman D, Miller D, et al. Vulvar squamous cell carcinoma in young women: a clinicopathologic study of 21 cases. *Gynecol Oncol* 2002;84:94.

Andersen ES, Sorensen IM. Verrucous carcinoma of the female genital tract: report of a case and review of the literature. *Gynecol Oncol* 1988;30:427.

Andersen WA, Franquemont DW, Williams J, et al. Vulvar squamous cell carcinoma and papillomaviruses: two separate entities? *Am J Obstet Gynecol* 1991;165:329.

Anderson BL. Sexual functioning complications in women with gynecologic cancer: outcomes and direction for prevention. *Cancer* 1987;60:2123.

Andreasson B, Moth J, Jensen SB, et al. Sexual function and somatopsychic reactions in vulvectomy operated women and their partners. *Acta Obstet Gynecol Scand* 1986;65:7.

Andreasson B, Nyboe J. Predictive factors with reference to low risk of metastases in squamous carcinoma of the vulva region. *Gynecol Oncol* 1985;21:196.

Andreasson B, Nyboe J. Value of prognostic parameters in squamous cell carcinoma of the vulva. *Gynecol Oncol* 1985;22:341.

Andreasson B, Visfeldt J, Bock JE, et al. Value of four models for selecting patients for local excision of invasive squamous cell carcinoma of the vulva. *J Reprod Med* 1990;35:1041.

Andrews SJ, Williams BT, DePriest PD, et al. Therapeutic implications of lymph nodal spread in lateral T1 and T2 squamous cell carcinoma of the vulva. *Gynecol Oncol* 1994;55:41.

Ansink AC, Sie-Go DMDS, van der Velden J, et al. Identification of sentinel lymph nodes in vulvar carcinoma patients with the aid of a patent blue V injection. *Cancer* 1999;86:652.

Ansink A, van der Velden J. Surgical interventions for early squamous cell carcinoma of the vulva (Cochrane Review). In: *The Cochrane Library*, Issue 4, 2002. Oxford: Update Software.

Anthony JP, Mathes SJ, Hoffman WY. Immediate flap coverage in the treatment of large surgical defects after tumor resection. *Surg Gynecol Obstet* 1993;176:355.

Atamdede F, Hoogerland D. Regional lymph node recurrence following local excision for microinvasive vulvar carcinoma. *Gynecol Oncol* 1989;34:125.

Atlante G, Lombardi A, Mariani L, et al. Carcinoma of the vulva (1981–85): analysis of a radio-surgical approach. *Eur J Gynaecol Oncol* 1989;10:341.

Auger M, Colgan TJ. Detection of metastatic vulvar and cervical squamous carcinoma in regional lymph nodes by use of a polyclonal keratin antibody. *Int J Gynecol Pathol* 1990;9:337.

Ayhan A, Tuncer R, Tuncer ZS, et al. Risk factors for groin node metastasis in squamous carcinoma of the vulva: a multivariate analysis of 39 cases. *Eur J Obstet Gynecol Reprod Biol* 1993;48:33.

Baachi CE, Goldfogel GA, Greer BE, et al. Paget's disease and melanoma of the vulva. *Gynecol Oncol* 1992;46:216.

Bachrendtz H, Einhorn N, Pettersson F, et al. Paget's disease of the vulva: the Radiumhemmet series 1975–1990. *Int J Gynecol Cancer* 1994;4:1.

Backstrom A, Edsmyr F, Wicklund H. Radiotherapy of carcinoma of the vulva. *Acta Obstet Gynecol Scand* 1972;51:109.

Bailey CL, Sankey HZ, Donovan JT, et al. Primary breast cancer of the vulva. *Gynecol Oncol* 1993;50:379.

Baird WL, Hester TR, Nahai F, et al. Management of perineal wounds following abdominoperineal resection with inferior gluteal flaps. *Arch Surg* 1990;125:1486.

Bakri YN, Akhtar M, El-Senoussi M, et al. Vulvar sarcoma: a report of four cases. *Gynecol Oncol* 1992;46:384.

Balat O, Edwards C, Delclos L. Complications following combined surgery (radical vulvectomy versus wide local excision) and radiotherapy for the treatment of carcinoma of the vulva: report of 73 patients. *Eur J Gynaecol Oncol* 2000;21(5):501.

Balch CM, Buzaid AC, Atkins MB. A new American Joint Committee on Cancer staging system for cutaneous melanoma. *Cancer* 2000;88:1484.

Balch CM, Buzaid AC, Soong SJ, et al. Final version of the American Joint Committee on cancer staging system for cutaneous melanoma. *J Clin Oncol* 2001;19:3635.

Balch CM, Soong SJ, Bartolucci AA, et al. Efficacy of an elective regional lymph node dissection of 1 to 4 mm thick melanomas for patients 60 years of age or younger. *Ann Surg* 1996;224:255.

Balch CM, Soong S-J, Milton GW, et al. A comparison of prognostic factors and surgical results in 1,786 patients with localized (stage 1) melanoma treated in Alabama, USA, and New South Wales, Australia. *Ann Surg* 1982;196:677.

Balch CM, Urist MM, Karakousis CP, et al. Efficacy of 2-cm surgical margins for intermediate-thickness melanomas (1 to 4 mm): results of a multi-institutional randomized surgical trial. *Ann Surg* 1993;218:262.

Ballon SC, Lamb EJ. Separate inguinal incisions in the treatment of carcinoma of the vulva. *Surg Gynecol Obstet* 1975;140:81.

Baltzer J, Kurzl RY, Lohe KJ, et al. Melanoma of the vulva. *J Reprod Med* 1986;31:825.

Barbero M, Micheletti L, Preti M, et al. Biologic behavior of vulvar intraepithelial neoplasia: histologic and clinical parameters. *J Reprod Med* 1993;38:108.

Barclay DL, Collins CG, Macey HB Jr. Cancer of the Bartholin gland: a review and report of 8 cases. *Obstet Gynecol* 1964;24:329.

Barnhill DR, Boling R, Nobles W, et al. Vulvar dermatofibrosarcoma protuberans. *Gynecol Oncol* 1988;30:149.

Barnhill DR, Hoskins WJ, Metz P. Use of the rhomboid flap after partial vulvectomy. *Obstet Gynecol* 1983;62:444.

Barton DPJ, Berman C, Cavanagh D, et al. Lymphoscintigraphy in vulvar cancer: a pilot study. *Gynecol Oncol* 1992;46:341.

Barton DP, Hoffman MS, Roberts WS, et al. Use of local flaps in the preservation of fecal continence following resection of perianal neoplasias. *Int J Gynecol Cancer* 1992;3:318.

Benedet JL, Miller DM, Ehlen TG, et al. Basal cell carcinoma of the vulva: clinical features and treatment results in 28 patients. *Obstet Gynecol* 1997;90:765.

Benedet JL, Turlo M, Fairey RN, et al. Squamous carcinoma of the vulva: results of treatment, 1938 to 1976. *Am J Obstet Gynecol* 1979;134:201.

Benedetti-Panici P, Greggi S, Scambia G, et al. Cisplatin (P), bleomycin (B) and methotrexate (M) preoperative chemotherapy in locally advanced vulvar carcinoma. *Gynecol Oncol* 1993;50:49.

Ben-Izhak O, Levy R, Weill S, et al. Anorectal malignant melanoma: a clinicopathologic study, including immunohistochemistry and DNA flow cytometry. *Cancer* 1997;79:18.

Berek JS, Heaps JM, Fu YS, et al. Concurrent cisplatin and 5-FU chemotherapy and external radiation for primary treatment of advanced stage squamous carcinoma of the vulva. *Gynecol Oncol* 1991;40:171(abst).

Bergen S, DiSaia PJ, Liao SY, et al. Conservative management of extramammary Paget's disease of the vulva. *Gynecol Oncol* 1989;33:151.

Berman ML, Soper JT, Creasman WT, et al. Conservative surgical management of superficially invasive stage 1 vulvar carcinoma. *Gynecol Oncol* 1989;35:352.

Bertani A, Riccio M, Belligolli A. Vulval reconstruction after cancer excision: the island groin flap technique. *Br J Plast Surg* 1990;43:159.

Binder SW, Huang I, Fu YS, et al. Risk factors for the development of lymph node metastasis in vulvar squamous carcinoma. *Gynecol Oncol* 1990;37:9.

Bjerregaard B, Andreasson B, Visfeldt J, et al. The significance of histology and morphometry in predicting lymph node metastases in patients with squamous cell carcinoma of the vulva. *Gynecol Oncol* 1993;50:323.

Bleicher RJ, Essner R, Foshag LJ, et al. Role of sentinel lymphadenectomy in thin invasive cutaneous melanomas. *J Clin Oncol* 2003;21:1326.

Bock J, Andreasson B, Thorn A, et al. Dermatofibrosarcoma protuberans of the vulva. *Gynecol Oncol* 1985;20:129.

Borgno G, Micheletti L, Barbero M, et al. Topographic distribution of groin lymph nodes. *J Reprod Med* 1990;35:1127.

Boronow RC, Hickman BT, Reagan MT, et al. Combined therapy as an alternative to exenteration for locally advanced vulvovaginal cancer. II. Results, complications, and dosimetric and surgical considerations. *Am J Clin Oncol* 1987;10:171.

Bosquet JG, Magrina JF, Gaffey TA, et al. Long-term survival and disease recurrence in patients with primary squamous cell carcinoma of the vulva. *Gynecol Oncol* 2005;97:828.

Bottles K, Lacey CG, Goldberg J, et al. Merkel cell carcinoma of the vulva. *Obstet Gynecol* 1984;63:61S.

Bouma J, Dankert J. Recurrent acute leg cellulitis in patients after radical vulvectomy. *Gynecol Oncol* 1988;29:50.

Boutselis JG. Radical vulvectomy for invasive squamous cell carcinoma of the vulva. *Obstet Gynecol* 1972;39:827.

Boyce J, Fruchter RG, Kasambilides E, et al. Prognostic factors in carcinoma of the vulva. *Gynecol Oncol* 1985;20:364.
Bradgate MG, Rollason TP, McConkey CC, et al. Malignant melanoma of the vulva: a clinico-pathological study of 50 women. *BJOG* 1990;97:124.
Brand A, Covert A. Malignant rhabdoid tumor of the vulva: case report and review of the literature with emphasis on clinical management and outcome. *Gynecol Oncol* 2001;80:99.
Breen JL, Neubecker RD, Greenwald E, et al. Basal cell carcinoma of the vulva. *Obstet Gynecol* 1975;46:122.
Brennan MJ, Miller LT. Overview of treatment options and review of the current role and use of compression garments, intermittent pumps, and exercise in the management of lymphedema. *Cancer* 1998;83:2821.
Breslow A. Thickness, cross-sectional areas, and depth of invasion in the prognosis of cutaneous melanoma. *Ann Surg* 1970;172:902.
Breslow A, Macht SD. Optimal size of margins for thin cutaneous melanoma. *Surg Gynecol Obstet* 1977;145:691.
Brisigotti M, Moreno A, Murcia C, et al. Verrucous carcinoma of the vulva: a clinicopathologic and immunohistochemical study of five cases. *Int J Gynecol Pathol* 1989;8:1.
Brooks JJ, LiVolsi VA. Liposarcoma presenting on the vulva. *Am J Obstet Gynecol* 1987;156:73.
Brunschwig A, Brockunier A Jr. Surgical treatment of squamous cell carcinoma of the vulva. *Obstet Gynecol* 1967;29:362.
Bryson SC, Dembo AJ, Colgan TJ, et al. Invasive squamous cell carcinoma of the vulva. Defining low and high risk groups for recurrence. *Int J Gynecol Cancer* 1991;1:25.
Buchler DA, Kline JC, Tunca JC, et al. Treatment of recurrent carcinoma of the vulva. *Gynecol Oncol* 1979;8:180.
Buhl A, Landow S, Lee YC, et al. Microcystic adnexal carcinoma of the vulva. *Gynecol Oncol* 2001;82:571.
Burger MPM, Hollema H, Emanuels AG, et al. The importance of the groin node status for the survival of T1 and T2 vulvar carcinoma patients. *Gynecol Oncol* 1995;57:327.
Burke TW, Levenback C, Coleman RL, et al. Surgical therapy of T1 and T2 vulvar carcinoma: further experience with radical wide excision and selective inguinal lymphadenectomy. *Gynecol Oncol* 1995;57:215.
Burke TW, Morris M, Levenback C, et al. Closure of complex vulvar defects using local rhomboid flaps. *Obstet Gynecol* 1994;84:1043.
Burke TW, Morris M, Roh RS, et al. Perineal reconstruction using single gracilis myocutaneous flaps. *Gynecol Oncol* 1995;57:221.
Burke TW, Stringer A, Gershenson DM, et al. Radical wide excision and selective inguinal node dissection for squamous cell carcinoma of the vulva. *Gynecol Oncol* 1990;38:328.
Burrell MO, Franklin EW III, Campion MJ, et al. The modified radical vulvectomy with groin dissection: an eight-year experience. *Am J Obstet Gynecol* 1988;159:715.
Buscema J, Naghashfar S, Sawada E, et al. The predominance of human papillomavirus type 16 in vulvar neoplasia. *Obstet Gynecol* 1988;71:601.
Buscema J, Stern J, Woodruff JD. The significance of histologic alterations adjacent to invasive vulvar carcinoma. *Am J Obstet Gynecol* 1980;137:902.
Buscema J, Woodruff JD. Progressive histobiologic alteration in the development of vulvar cancer. *Am J Obstet Gynecol* 1980;138:146.
Buzaid AC, Tinoco LA, Jendiroba D, et al. Prognostic value of size of lymph node metastases in patients with cutaneous melanoma. *J Clin Oncol* 1995;13:2361.
Byron RL, Lamb EJ, Yonemoto RH, et al. Radical inguinal node dissection in the treatment of cancer. *Surg Gynecol Obstet* 1962;114:401.
Cady B. Sentinel lymph node procedure in squamous cell carcinoma of the vulva. *J Clin Oncol* 2000;18(15):2795.
Calabro A, Singletary E, Balch CM. Patterns of relapse in 1001 consecutive patients with melanoma nodal metastases. *Arch Surg* 1989;124:1051.
Calame RJ. Pelvic relaxation as a complication of radical vulvectomy. *Obstet Gynecol* 1980;55:716.
Camacho-Martinez F, Moreno JC, Sanchez-Conejo MJ, et al. International dermatosurgery: advancement local flaps in the reconstructive treatment of vulvar carcinoma. *J Dermatol Surg Oncol* 1983;9:748.
Cardosi RJ, Speights A, Fiorica JV, et al. Bartholin's gland carcinoma: a 15-year experience. *Gynecol Oncol* 2001;82:247.
Carlino G, Parisi S, Montemaggi P, et al. Interstitial radiotherapy with Ir in vulvar cancer. *Eur J Gynaecol Oncol* 1984;3:183.
Carlson JW, McGlennen RC, Gomez R, et al. Sebaceous carcinoma of the vulva: a case report and review of the literature. *Gynecol Oncol* 1996;60:489.
Carson LF, Twiggs LB, Adcock LL, et al. Multimodality therapy for advanced and recurrent vulvar squamous cell carcinoma: a pilot project. *J Reprod Med* 1990;35:1029.
Carter J, Carlson J, Fowler J, et al. Invasive tumors in young women—a disease of the immunosuppressed? *Gynecol Oncol* 1993;51:307.
Castaldo TW, Petrilli ES, Ballon SC, et al. Endodermal sinus tumor of the clitoris. *Gynecol Oncol* 1980;9:376.
Cavanagh D, Beasley J, Ostapowicz F. Radical operation for carcinoma of the vulva: a new approach to wound healing. *J Obstet Gynaecol Br Commonw* 1970;77:1037.
Cavanagh D, Desai S. Invasive carcinoma of the vulva. *Aust N Z J Obstet Gynaecol* 1968;8:171.
Cavanagh D, Fiorica J, Hoffman MS, et al. Invasive carcinoma of the vulva: changing trends in surgical management. *Am J Obstet Gynecol* 1990;163:1007.
Cavanagh D, Hovadhanakul P, Taylor HB. Invasive carcinomas of the vulva: current view on diagnosis and treatment. *Mo Med* 1976;73:129.
Cavanagh D, Roberts WS, Bryson SCP, et al. Changing trends in the surgical treatment of invasive carcinoma of the vulva. *Surg Gynecol Obstet* 1986;162:164.
Cavanagh D, Shepherd JH. The place of pelvic exenteration in the primary management of advanced carcinoma of the vulva. *Gynecol Oncol* 1982;13:318.
Chafe W, Fowler WC, Walton LA, et al. Radical vulvectomy with use of tensor fascia lata myocutaneous flap. *Am J Obstet Gynecol* 1983;145:207.
Chafe W, Richards A, Morgan L, et al. Unrecognized invasive carcinoma in vulvar intraepithelial neoplasia (VIN). *Gynecol Oncol* 1988;31:154.
Chamlian DL, Taylor HB. Primary carcinoma of the Bartholin's gland: a report of 24 patients. *Obstet Gynecol* 1972;39:489.
Chan JK, Sugiyama V, Tajalli TR, et al. Conservative clitoral preservation surgery in the treatment of vulvar squamous cell carcinoma. *Gynecol Oncol* 2004;95:152.
Chandeying V, Sutthijumroon S, Tungphaisal S. Merkel cell carcinoma of the vulva: a case report. *Asia-Oceania J Obstet Gynaecol* 1989;15:261.
Chapman GW Jr, Benda J, Lifshitz S. Adenoid cystic carcinoma of the vulva with lung metastases: a case report. *J Reprod Med* 1985;30:217.
Chen KTK. Merkel's cell (neuroendocrine) carcinoma of the vulva. *Cancer* 1994;73:2186.
Chen L, Schink JC, Panares BN, et al. Resection of a giant aggressive angiomyxoma in the Philippines. *Gynecol Oncol* 1998;70:435.
Cheung TH, Chan MK, Chang A. Aggressive angiomyxoma of the female perineum: case reports. *Aust N Z J Obstet Gynaecol* 1991;31:285.
Cho D, Buscema J, Rosenshein N, et al. Primary breast cancer of the vulva. *Obstet Gynecol* 1985;66[Suppl]:79.
Christophersen W, Buchsbaum HJ, Voet R, et al. Radical vulvectomy and bilateral groin lymphadenectomy utilizing separate groin incisions: report of a case with recurrence in the intervening skin bridge. *Gynecol Oncol* 1985;21:247.
Chu J, Tamimi HK, Figge DC. Femoral node metastases with negative superficial inguinal nodes in early vulvar cancer. *Am J Obstet Gynecol* 1981;140:337.
Chung AF, Woodruff JM, Lewis JL. Malignant melanoma of the vulva: a report of 44 cases. *Obstet Gynecol* 1975;45:638.
Clark WH, From L, Bernardino EA, et al. The histogenesis and biologic behavior of primary human melanomas of the skin. *Cancer Res* 1969;29:705.
Coates AS, Ingvar CL, Petersen-Schaefer K, et al. Elective lymph node dissection in patients with primary melanoma of the trunk and limbs treated at the Sydney Melanoma Unit from 1960 to 1991. *J Am Coll Surg* 1995;180:402.
Cohen R, Margolius KA, Guidozzi F. Non-gynaecological metastases to the vulva and vagina. *S Afr Med J* 1988;73:159.
Coldiron BM, Goldsmith BA, Robinson JK. Surgical treatment of extramammary Paget's disease: a report of six cases and a reexamination of Mohs micrographic surgery compared with conventional surgical excision. *Cancer* 1991;67:933.
Collins CG, Lee FYL, Roman-Lopez JJ. Invasive carcinoma of the vulva with lymph node metastases. *Am J Obstet Gynecol* 1971;109:446.
Conway H, Hugo NE. Metastatic basal cell carcinoma. *Am J Surg* 1965;110:620.
Copas P, Dyer M, Comas FV, et al. Spindle cell carcinoma of the vulva. *Diagn Gynecol Obstet* 1982;4:235.
Copeland LJ, Cleary K, Sneige N, et al. Neuroendocrine (Merkel cell) carcinoma of the vulva: a case report and review of the literature. *Gynecol Oncol* 1985;22:367.
Copeland LJ, Sneige N, Gershenson DM, et al. Adenoid cystic carcinoma of Bartholin's gland. *Obstet Gynecol* 1986;67:115.
Copeland LJ, Sneige N, Gershenson DM, et al. Bartholin gland carcinoma. *Obstet Gynecol* 1986;67:794.
Corney RH, Everett H, Howells A, et al. Psychosocial adjustment following major gynaecological surgery for carcinoma of the cervix and vulva. *J Psychosom Res* 1992;36:561.
Creasman WT. New gynecologic cancer staging. *Obstet Gynecol* 1990;75:287.
Creasman WT. New gynecologic cancer staging. *Gynecol Oncol* 1995;58:157.
Creasman WT, Gallager HS, Rutledge F. Paget's disease of the vulva. *Gynecol Oncol* 1975;3:133.
Creasman WT, Phillips JL, Menck HR. A survey of hospital management practices for vulvar melanoma. *J Am Coll Surg* 1999;188:670.
Creasman WT, Phillips JL, Menck HR. The national cancer database report on early stage invasive vulvar carcinoma. *Cancer* 1997;80:505.
Crowley NJ, Seigler HF. The role of elective lymph node dissection in the management of patients with thick cutaneous melanoma. *Cancer* 1990;66:2522.
Crowther ME, Shepherd JH, Fisher C. Verrucous carcinoma of the vulva containing human papillomavirus-11: case report. *BJOG* 1988;95:414.
Crum CP. Carcinoma of the vulva: epidemiology and pathogenesis. *Obstet Gynecol* 1992;79:448.
Crum CP, Liskow A, Petras P, et al. Vulva intraepithelial neoplasia (severe atypia

and carcinoma in situ): a clinicopathologic analysis of 41 cases. *Cancer* 1984;54:1429.
Cruz-Jimenez PR, Abell MR. Cutaneous basal cell carcinoma of the vulva. *Cancer* 1975;36:1860.
Cunningham MJ, Goyer RP, Gibbons SK, et al. Primary radiation, cisplatin, and 5-fluororacil for advanced squamous carcinoma of the vulva. *Gynecol Oncol* 1997;66:258.
Curry SL, Wharton JT, Rutledge F. Positive lymph nodes in vulvar squamous carcinoma. *Gynecol Oncol* 1980;9:63.
Curtin JP, Rubin SC, Jones WB, et al. Paget's disease of the vulva. *Gynecol Oncol* 1990;39:374.
Curtin JP, Saigo P, Slucher B, et al. Soft-tissue sarcoma of the vagina and vulva: a clinicopathologic study. *Obstet Gynecol* 1995;86:269.
Daly JW, Million RR. Radical vulvectomy combined with elective node irradiation for TXNO squamous carcinoma of the vulva. *Cancer* 1974;34:161.
Davos I, Abell MR. Soft tissue sarcomas of the vulva. *Gynecol Oncol* 1976;4:70.
de Hullu JA, Hollema H, Hoekstra HJ, et al. Vulvar melanoma. Is there a role for sentinel lymph node biopsy? *Cancer* 2002;94:486.
de Hullu JA, Hollema H, Lolkema S, et al. Vulvar carcinoma: the price of less radical surgery. *Cancer* 2002;95:2331.
de Hullu JA, Hollema H, Piers DA, et al. Sentinel lymph node procedure is highly accurate in squamous cell carcinoma of the vulva. *J Clin Oncol* 2000;18:2811.
de Hullu JA, Oonk MHM, Ansink AC, et al. Pitfalls in the sentinel lymph nodes procedure in vulvar cancer. *Gynecol Oncol* 2004;94:10.
DeCesare SL, Fiorica JV, Roberts WS, et al. A pilot study utilizing intraoperative lymphoscintigraphy for identification of the sentinel lymph nodes in vulvar cancer. *Gynecol Oncol* 1997;66:425.
Dehner LP. Metastatic and secondary tumors of the vulva. *Obstet Gynecol* 1973;42:47.
Demian SDE, Bushkin FL, Echevarria RA. Perineural invasion and anaplastic transformation of verrucous carcinoma. *Cancer* 1973;32:395.
Deppe G, Cohen C, Bruckner H. Chemotherapy of squamous cell carcinoma of the vulva: a review. *Gynecol Oncol* 1979;7:345.
Deppe G, Malviya VK, Smith PE, et al. Limb salvage in recurrent vulvar carcinoma after rupture of femoral artery. *Gynecol Oncol* 1984;19:120.
Di Bonito L, Patriarca S, Falconieri G. Aggressive "breast-like" adenocarcinoma of vulva. *Pathol Res Pract* 1992;188:211.
DiSaia PJ. The case against the surgical concept of en bloc dissection for certain malignancies of the reproductive tract. *Cancer* 1987;60:2025.
DiSaia PJ. Management of superficially invasive vulvar carcinoma. *Clin Obstet Gynecol* 1985;28:196.
DiSaia PJ, Creasman WT, Rich WM. An alternative approach to early cancer of the vulva. *Am J Obstet Gynecol* 1979;133:825.
DiSaia PJ, Dorion GE, Cappuccini F, et al. A report of two cases of recurrent Paget's disease of the vulva in a split-thickness graft and its possible pathogenesis—labeled "retrodissemination." *Gynecol Oncol* 1995;57:109.
DiSaia PJ, Rutledge F, Smith JP. Sarcoma of the vulva: report of 12 patients. *Obstet Gynecol* 1971;38:180.
Dolan JR, McCall AR, Gooneratne S, et al. DNA ploidy, proliferation index, grade and stage as prognostic factors for vulvar squamous cell carcinomas. *Gynecol Oncol* 1993;48:232.
Donaldson ES, Powell DE, Hanson MB, et al. Prognostic parameters in invasive vulvar cancer. *Gynecol Oncol* 1981;11:184.
Downs LS Jr, Ghosh K, Dusenbery KE, et al. Stage IV carcinoma of the Bartholin gland managed with primary chemoradiation. *Gynecol Oncol* 2002;87:210.
Dubreuilh W. Paget's disease of the vulva. *Br J Dermatol* 1901;13:1407.
Dudley AG, Young RH, Lawrence WD, et al. Endodermal sinus tumor of the vulva in an infant. *Obstet Gynecol* 1983;61:76S.
Dudzinski MR, Askin FB, Fowler WC. Giant basal cell carcinoma of the vulva. *Obstet Gynecol* 1984;63:57S.
Echt ML, Finan MA, Hoffman MS, et al. Detection of sentinel lymph nodes with Lymphazurin in cervical, uterine, and vulvar malignancies. *South Med J* 1999;92:204.
Egwuatu VE, Ejeckam GC, Okaro JM. Burkett's lymphoma of the vulva. Case report. *BJOG* 1980;87:827.
Eifel PJ, Morris M, Burke TW, et al. Prolonged continuous infusion cisplatin and 5-fluorouracil with radiation for locally advanced carcinoma of the vulva. *Gynecol Oncol* 1995;59:51.
Elchalal U, Dgani R, Zosmer A, et al. Malignant fibrous histiocytoma of the vagina and vulva successfully treated by combined chemotherapy and radiotherapy. *Gynecol Oncol* 1991;42:91.
Elit L, Hancock G, Carey M, et al. Comparing the morbidity of single versus separate incision surgical approaches to vulvar cancer. *J Gynecol Tech* 1999;5:147.
Elsandabesee D, Sharma B, Preston J, et al. Sclerotherapy with bleomycin for recurrent massive inguinal lymphoceles following partial vulvectomy and bilateral lymphadenectomy—case report and literature review. *Gynecol Oncol* 2004;92:716.
Enker WE, Heilwell M, Janov AJ, et al. Improved survival in epidermoid carcinoma of the anus in association with preoperative multidisciplinary therapy. *Arch Surg* 1986;121:1386.
Eriksson JE, Eldh J, Peterson LE. Surgical treatment of carcinoma of the clitoris. *Gynecol Oncol* 1984;17:291.
Evans LS, Kersh CR, Constable WC, et al. Concomitant 5-fluorouracil, mitomycin-C and radiotherapy for advanced gynecologic malignancies. *Int J Radiat Oncol Biol Phys* 1988;15:901.
Ewing TL. Paget's disease of the vulva treated by combined surgery and laser. *Gynecol Oncol* 1991;43:137.
Fairey RN, Mackay PA, Benedet JL, et al. Radiation treatment of carcinoma of the vulva: 1950–1980. *Am J Obstet Gynecol* 1985;151:591.
Fanning J, Lambert L, Hale T, et al. Paget's disease of the vulva: prevalence of associated vulvar adenocarcinoma, invasive Paget's disease, and recurrence after surgical excision. *Am J Obstet Gynecol* 1999;180:24.
Farias-Eisner R, Cirisano FD, Grouse D, et al. Conservative and individualized surgery for early squamous carcinoma of the vulva: the treatment of choice for stage I and II (T1–2, N0–1,M0) disease. *Gynecol Oncol* 1994;53:55.
Feuer GA, Shevchuk M, Calanog A. Vulvar Paget's disease: the need to exclude an invasive lesion. *Gynecol Oncol* 1990;38:81.
Figge DC, Tamimi HK, Greer BE. Lymphatic spread in carcinoma of the vulva. *Am J Obstet Gynecol* 1985;152:387.
Finon MA, Fiorica JV, Roberts WS, et al. Artificial dura film for femoral vessel coverage after inguinofemoral lymphadenectomy. *Gynecol Oncol* 1994;55:333.
Fioretti P, Gadducci A, Prato B, et al. The influence of some prognostic factors on the clinical outcome of patients with squamous cell carcinoma of the vulva. *Eur J Gynaecol Oncol* 1992;13:97.
Fiorica JV, Cavanagh D, Roberts WS, et al. Carcinoma-in-situ of the vulva: twenty-four years' experience. *South Med J* 1988;81:589.
Fiorica JV, Roberts WS, LaPolla JP, et al. Femoral vessel coverage with dura mater after inguinofemoral lymphadenectomy. *Gynecol Oncol* 1991;42:217.
Fishman DA, Chambers SK, Schwartz PE, et al. Extramammary Paget's disease of the vulva. *Gynecol Oncol* 1995;56:266.
Flamant F, Gerbaulte A, Nihoul-Fekete C, et al. Long-term sequelae of conservative treatment by surgery, brachytherapy, and chemotherapy for vulval and vaginal rhabdomyosarcoma in children. *J Clin Oncol* 1990;8:1847.
Flannelly GM, Foley ME, Lenehan PM, et al. En bloc radical vulvectomy and lymphadenectomy with modifications of separate groin incisions. *Obstet Gynecol* 1992;79:307.
Fletcher CD, Tsang WY, Fisher C, et al. Angiomyofibroblastoma of the vulva: a benign neoplasm distinct from aggressive angiomyxoma. *Am J Surg Pathol* 1992;16:373.
Fons G, ter Rahe B, Sloof G, et al. Failure in the detection of the sentinel lymph node with a combined technique of radioactive tracer and blue dye in a patient with cancer of the vulva and a single positive lymph node. *Gynecol Oncol* 2004;92:981.
Franklin EW, Bostwick J III, Burrell MO, et al. Reconstructive techniques in radical pelvic surgery. *Am J Obstet Gynecol* 1977;129:285.
Frankman O. Stage III squamous cell carcinoma of the vulva: results of a Swedish study. *J Reprod Med* 1991;36:108.
Frankman O, Kabulski Z, Nilsson B, et al. Prognostic factors in invasive squamous cell carcinoma of the vulva. *Int J Gynecol Obstet* 1991;36:219.
Friedrich E, Wilkinson E, Steingraeber P, et al. Paget's disease of the vulva and carcinoma of the breast. *Obstet Gynecol* 1975;46:130.
Friedrich EG, Wilkinson EJ, Fu YS. Carcinoma in situ of the vulva: a continuing challenge. *Am J Obstet Gynecol* 1980;136:830.
Frischbier HJ, Thomsen K. Treatment of cancer of the vulva with high-energy electrons. *Am J Obstet Gynecol* 1971;111:431.
Frumovitz M, Ramirez PT, Tortolero-Luna G, et al. Characteristics of recurrence in patients who underwent lymphatic mapping for vulvar cancer. *Gynecol Oncol* 2004;92:205.
Gadducci A, De Punzio C, Facchini V, et al. The therapy of verrucous carcinoma of the vulva: observations on three cases. *Eur J Gynaecol Oncol* 1989;10:284.
Gallousis S. Verrucous carcinoma: report of three vulvar cases and review of the literature. *Obstet Gynecol* 1972;40:502.
Ganjei P, Giraldo KA, Lampe B, et al. Vulvar Paget's disease: is immunocytochemistry helpful in assessing the surgical margins? *J Reprod Med* 1990;35:1002.
Garbe C, Buttner P, Bertz J, et al. Primary cutaneous melanoma: identification of prognostic groups and estimation of individual prognosis for 5093 patients. *Cancer* 1995;75:2484.
Garcia C, Boronow RC. Carcinoma of the vulva—anatomic and histologic prognostic facts. *South Med J* 1972;65:237.
Genton CY, Maroni ES. Vulval liposarcoma. *Arch Gynecol* 1987;240:63.
George M, Durrant KR, Mangioni C, et al. Bleomycin (BLM), methotrexate (MTX) and CCNU as neoadjuvant treatment of carcinoma of the vulva. Second International Congress on Neo-Adjuvant Chemotherapy, February 19–21, Paris, 1988:67(abst).
Gershenwald JE, Thompson W, Mansfield PF, et al. Multi-institutional melanoma lymphatic mapping experience: the prognostic value of sentinel lymph node status in 612 stage I or II melanoma patients. *J Clin Oncol* 1999;17:976.
Ghamande SA, Kasznica J, Griffiths CT, et al. Mucinous adenocarcinomas of the vulva. *Gynecol Oncol* 1995;57:117.

Gil-Moreno A, Garcia-Jimenez A, Gonzalez-Bosquet J, et al. Merkel cell carcinoma of the vulva. *Gynecol Oncol* 1997;64:526.
Gleeson NC, Hoffman MS, Cavanagh D. Isolated skin bridge metastasis following modified radical vulvectomy and bilateral inguinofemoral lymphadenectomy. *Int J Gynecol Cancer* 1994;4:356.
Gleeson NC, Ruffolo EH, Hoffman MS, et al. Basal cell carcinoma of the vulva with groin node metastasis. *Gynecol Oncol* 1994;53:366.
Goldberg MI, Rothfleisch S. The tensor fascia lata myocutaneous flap in gynecologic oncology. *Gynecol Oncol* 1981;12:41.
Gordinier ME, Malpica A, Burke TW, et al. Groin recurrence in patients with vulvar cancer with negative nodes on superficial inguinal lymphadenectomy. *Gynecol Oncol* 2003;90:625.
Gordinier ME, Steinhoff MM, Hogan JW, et al. S-Phase fraction, p53, and HER-2/neu status as predictors of nodal metastasis in early vulvar cancer. *Gynecol Oncol* 1997;67:200.
Gould N, Kamelle S, Tillmanns T, et al. Predictors of complications after inguinal lymphadenectomy. *Gynecol Oncol* 2001;82:329.
Graziottin A, Maggino T, Francia G, et al. Non mutilant radical vulvectomy vs radical vulvectomy. *Eur J Gynaecol Oncol* 1983;4:128.
Green H. Adenocarcinoma of supernumerary breast of the labia majora in a case of epidermoid carcinoma of the vulva. *Am J Obstet Gynecol* 1936;32:660.
Green TH Jr, Ulfelder H, Meigs JV. Epidermoid carcinoma of the vulva: an analysis of 238 cases. Parts I and II. *Am J Obstet Gynecol* 1958;75:834.
Greenall MJ, Quan SHQ, Stearns MW, et al. Epidermoid cancer of the anal margin: pathologic features, treatment and clinical results. *Am J Surg* 1985;149:95.
Grimshaw RN, Aswad SG, Monaghan JM. The role of anovulvectomy in locally advanced carcinoma of the vulva. *Int Gynecol Cancer* 1991;1:15.
Grimshaw RN, Murdoch JB, Monaghan JM. Radical vulvectomy and bilateral inguino-femoral lymphadenectomy through separate incisions: experience with 100 cases. *Int J Gynecol Cancer* 1993;3:18.
Guerry R, Pratt-Thomas HR. Carcinoma of supernumerary breast of vulva with bilateral mammary cancer. *Cancer* 1976;38:2570.
Guidozzi F, Sadan O, Koller AB, et al. Combined chemotherapy and irradiation therapy after radical surgery for leiomyosarcoma of the vulva. *S Afr Med J* 1987;71:327.
Hacker NF, Berek JS, Juillard GJF, et al. Preoperative radiation therapy for locally advanced vulvar cancer. *Cancer* 1984;54:2056.
Hacker NF, Berek JS, Lagasse LD, et al. Individualization of treatment for stage 1 squamous cell vulvar carcinoma. *Obstet Gynecol* 1984;63:155.
Hacker NF, Berek JS, Lagasse LD, et al. Management of regional lymph nodes and their prognostic influence in vulvar cancer. *Obstet Gynecol* 1983;61:408.
Hacker NF, Leuchter RS, Berek JS, et al. Radical vulvectomy and bilateral inguinal lymphadenectomy through separate groin incisions. *Obstet Gynecol* 1981;58:574.
Hacker NF, Nieberg RK, Berek JS, et al. Superficially invasive vulvar cancer with nodal metastases. *Gynecol Oncol* 1983;15:65.
Hacker NF, van der Velden J. Conservative management of early vulvar cancer. *Cancer* 1993;71:1673.
Hall DJ, Grimes MM, Coplerud DR. Epithelioid sarcoma of the vulva: case report. *Gynecol Oncol* 1980;9:237.
Hall JSE, Amin UF. Fibrosarcoma of the vulva: case report and discussion. *Int Surg* 1981;66:185.
Har-Shai Y, Hirshowitz B, Marcovich A, et al. Blood supply and innervation of the supermedial thigh flap employed in one-stage reconstruction of the scrotum and vulva: an anatomical study. *Ann Plast Surg* 1984;13:504.
Hart WR, Millman RB. Progression of intraepithelial Paget's disease of the vulva to invasive carcinoma. *Cancer* 1977;40:2333.
Heaps JM, Fu YS, Montz FJ, et al. Surgical-pathologic variables predictive of local recurrence in squamous cell carcinoma of the vulva. *Gynecol Oncol* 1990;38:309.
Helgason NM, Haas AC, Latourette HB. Radiation therapy in carcinoma of the vulva: a review of 53 patients. *Cancer* 1972;30:997.
Helm CW, Hatch K, Austin JM, et al. A matched comparison of single and triple incision techniques for surgical treatment of carcinoma of the vulva. *Gynecol Oncol* 1992;46:150.
Helm CW, Hatch KD, Partridge EE, et al. The rhomboid transposition flap for repair of the perineal defect after radical vulvar surgery. *Gynecol Oncol* 1993;50:164.
Henderson RH, Parsons JT, Morgan L, et al. Elective ilioinguinal lymph node irradiation. *Int J Radiat Oncol Biol Phys* 1984;10:811.
Hendrix RC, Behrman SJ. Adenocarcinoma arising in a supernumerary mammary gland in the vulva. *Obstet Gynecol* 1956;8:238.
Hensley GT, Friedrich EG. Malignant fibroxanthoma: a sarcoma of the vulva. *Am J Obstet Gynecol* 1973;116:289.
Herod JJ, Shafi MI, Rollason TP, et al. Vulvar intraepithelial neoplasia: long term follow-up of treated and untreated women. *BJOG* 1996;103:446.
Herod JJO, Shafi MI, Rollason TP, et al. Vulvar intraepithelial neoplasia with superficially invasive carcinoma of the vulva. *BJOG* 1996;103:453.
Hilgers RD, Pai R, Bartow SA, et al. Aggressive angiomyxoma of the vulva. *Obstet Gynecol* 1986;68S:60.
Hitchcock CL, Bland KI, Laney RG III, et al. Neuroendocrine (Merkel cell) carcinoma of the skin: its natural history, diagnosis and treatment. *Ann Surg* 1988;207:201.
Hoffman JS, Kumar NB, Morley GW. Microinvasive squamous carcinoma of the vulva: search for a definition. *Obstet Gynecol* 1983;61:615.
Hoffman JS, Kumar NB, Morley GW. Prognostic significance of groin lymph node metastases in squamous carcinoma of the vulva. *Obstet Gynecol* 1985;66:402.
Hoffman MS, Cavanagh D, Roberts WS, et al. Ultraradical surgery for advanced carcinoma of the vulva: an update. *Int J Gynecol Cancer* 1993;3:369.
Hoffman MS, Greenberg S, Greenberg H, et al. The use of interstitial needles for the treatment of advanced or recurrent vulvar and distal vaginal malignancy. *Am J Obstet Gynecol* 1990;162:1278.
Hoffman MS, Greenberg H, Roberts WS, et al. Management of locally advanced squamous cell carcinoma of the vulva. *J Gynecol Surg* 1991;7:175.
Hoffman MS, Gunasekaran S, Arango H, et al. Lateral microscopic extension of squamous cell carcinoma of the vulva. *Gynecol Oncol* 1999;73:72.
Hoffman MS, LaPolla JP, Roberts WS, et al. Use of local flaps for primary anal reconstruction following perianal resection for neoplasia. *Gynecol Oncol* 1990;36:348.
Hoffman MS, Mark JE, Cavanagh D. A management scheme for postoperative groin lymphocysts. *Gynecol Oncol* 1995;56:262.
Hoffman MS, Roberts WS, Finan MA, et al. A comparative study of radical vulvectomy and modified radical vulvectomy for the treatment of invasive squamous cell carcinoma of the vulva. *Gynecol Oncol* 1992;45:192.
Hoffman MS, Roberts WR, LaPolla JP, et al. Carcinoma of the vulva involving the perianal or anal skin. *Gynecol Oncol* 1989;35:215.
Hoffman MS, Roberts WS, LaPolla JP, et al. Recent modifications in the treatment of invasive squamous cell carcinoma of the vulva. *Obstet Gynecol Surv* 1989;44:227.
Hoffman MS, Roberts WS, Ruffolo EH. Basal cell carcinoma of the vulva with inguinal lymph node metastases. *Gynecol Oncol* 1988;29:113.
Homesley HD, Bundy BN, Sedlis A, et al. Assessment of current International Federation of Gynecology and Obstetrics staging of vulvar carcinoma relative to prognostic factors for survival (a Gynecologic Oncology Group study). *Am J Obstet Gynecol* 1991;164:997.
Homesley HD, Bundy BN, Sedlis A, et al. Prognostic factors for groin node metastasis in squamous cell carcinoma of the vulva (a Gynecologic Oncology Group study). *Gynecol Oncol* 1993;49:279.
Homesley HD, Bundy BN, Sedlis A, et al. Radiation therapy versus pelvic node resection for carcinoma of the vulva with positive groin nodes. *Obstet Gynecol* 1986;68:733.
Hopkins MP, Morley GW. Pelvic exenteration for the treatment of vulvar cancer. *Cancer* 1992;70:2835.
Hopkins MP, Reid GC, Johnston CM, et al. A comparison of staging systems for squamous cell carcinoma of the vulva. *Gynecol Oncol* 1992;47:34.
Hopkins MP, Reid GC, Morley GW. Radical vulvectomy; the decision for the incision. *Cancer* 1993;72:799.
Hopkins MP, Reid GC, Morley GW. The surgical management of recurrent squamous cell carcinoma of the vulva. *Obstet Gynecol* 1990;75:1001.
Hopkins MP, Reid GC, Vettrano I, et al. Squamous cell carcinoma of the vulva: prognostic factors influencing survival. *Gynecol Oncol* 1991;43:113.
Hording U, Junge J, Poulsen H, et al. Vulvar intraepithelial neoplasia III: a viral disease of undetermined potential. *Gynecol Oncol* 1995;56:276.
Hoyme UB, Tamimi HK, Eschenbach DA, et al. Osteomyelitis pubis after radical gynecologic operations. *Obstet Gynecol* 1984;63:47.
Husseinzadeh N, Recinto C. Frequency of invasive cancer in surgically excised vulvar lesions with intraepithelial neoplasia (VIN 3). *Gynecol Oncol* 1999;73:119.
Husseinzadeh N, Wesseler T, Newman N, et al. Neuroendocrine (Merkel cell) carcinoma of the vulva. *Gynecol Oncol* 1988;29:105.
Husseinzadeh N, Wesseler T, Schneider D, et al. Prognostic factors and the significance of cytologic grading in invasive squamous cell carcinoma of the vulva: a clinicopathologic study. *Gynecol Oncol* 1990;36:192.
Hyde SE, Ansink AC, Burger MPM, et al. The impact of performance status on survival in patients of 80 years and older with vulvar cancer. *Gynecol Oncol* 2002;84:388.
Imachi M, Tsukamoto N, Kamura T, et al. Alveolar rhabdomyosarcoma of the vulva: report of two cases. *Acta Cytol* 1991;35:345.
Imachi M, Tsukamoto N, Shigematsu T, et al. Cytologic diagnosis of primary adenocarcinoma of Bartholin's gland: a case report. *Acta Cytol* 1992;36:167.
International Federation of Obstetricians and Gynecologists Committee on Gynecologic Oncology. Changes in staging of cancer of the vulva and of the endometrium. *Int J Gynaecol Obstet* 1989;28:189.
International Society of Lymphology Executive Committee. Diagnosis and treatment of peripheral lymphedema. Consensus document of the International Society of Lymphology Executive Committee. *Lymphology* 1995;28:113.
Irvin WP, Cathro HP, Grosh WW, et al. Primary breast carcinoma of the vulva: a case report and literature review. *Gynecol Oncol* 1999;73:155.
Irvin Jr WP, Legallo RL, Stoler MH, et al. Vulvar melanoma: a retrospective analysis and literature review. *Gynecol Oncol* 2001;83:457.
Irvin W, Pelkey T, Rice L, et al. Endometrial stromal sarcoma of the vulva arising

in extraovarian endometriosis: a case report and literature review. *Gynecol Oncol* 1998;71:313.
Isaacs JH. Verrucous carcinoma of the female genital tract. *Gynecol Oncol* 1976;4:259.
Itala J, de Paola GR, Gomez-Rueda N, et al. Melanoma of the vulva: the experience of the University of Buenos Aires. *J Reprod Med* 1986;31:836.
Iversen T. Irradiation and bleomycin in the treatment of inoperable vulvar carcinoma. *Acta Obstet Gynecol Scand* 1982;61:195.
Iversen T. New approaches to the treatment of squamous cell carcinoma of the vulva. In: Pitkin RM, Scott JR, Kaufman RH, et al., eds. *Clinical obstetrics and gynecology*, vol. 28. Philadelphia: Harper & Row; 1985:204.
Iversen T. Squamous cell carcinoma of the vulva: localization of the primary tumor and lymph node metastases. *Acta Obstet Gynecol Scand* 1981;60:211.
Iversen T. The value of groin palpation in epidermoid carcinoma of the vulva. *Gynecol Oncol* 1981;12:291.
Iversen T, Aalders JG, Christensen A, et al. Squamous cell carcinoma of the vulva: a review of 424 patients, 1956–1974. *Gynecol Oncol* 1983;9:271.
Iversen T, Aas M. Lymph drainage from the vulva. *Gynecol Oncol* 1983;16:179.
Iversen T, Abeler V, Aalders J. Individualized treatment of stage 1 carcinoma of the vulva. *Obstet Gynecol* 1981;57:85.
Jackson KS, Das N, Naik NDR, et al. Contralateral groin node metastasis following ipsilateral groin node dissection in vulval cancer: a case report. *Gynecol Oncol* 2003;89:529.
Jafari K, Magalotti M. Radiation therapy in carcinoma of the vulva. *Cancer* 1981;47:686.
Japaze H, Dinh TV, Woodruff JD. Verrucous carcinoma of the vulva: study of 24 cases. *Obstet Gynecol* 1982;60:462.
Jaramillo BA, Ganjei P, Averette HE, et al. Malignant melanoma of the vulva. *Obstet Gynecol* 1985;66:398.
Johnson TL, Kumar NB, White CD, et al. Prognostic features of vulvar melanoma: a clinicopathologic analysis. *Int J Gynecol Pathol* 1986;5:110.
Jones MA, Mann EW, Caldwell CL, et al. Small cell neuroendocrine carcinoma of Bartholin's gland. *Am J Clin Pathol* 1990;94:439.
Jones RW, Baranyai J, Stables S. Trends in squamous cell carcinoma of the vulva: the influence of vulvar intraepithelial neoplasia. *Obstet Gynecol* 1997;90:448.
Jones RW, Rowan DM. Vulvar intraepithelial neoplasia III: a clinical study of the outcome in 113 cases with relation to the later development of invasive vulvar carcinoma. *Obstet Gynecol* 1994;84:741.
Judson PL, Jonson AL, Paley PJ, et al. A prospective, randomized study analyzing sartorius transposition following inguinal-femoral lymphadenectomy. *Gynecol Oncol* 2004;95:226.
Julian CG, Callison J, Woodruff JD. Plastic management of extensive vulvar defects. *Obstet Gynecol* 1971;38:193.
Kadar N, Nelson JH. Sling operation for total incontinence following radical vulvectomy. *Obstet Gynecol* 1984;64[Suppl]:85.
Kalra JK, Grossman AM, Krumholz BA, et al. Preoperative chemoradiotherapy for carcinoma of the vulva. *Gynecol Oncol* 1981;12:256.
Kaplan AL, Kaufman RH. Management of advanced carcinoma of the vulva. *Gynecol Oncol* 1975;3:220.
Karakousis CP, Emrich LJ. Tumor thickness and prognosis in clinical stage I malignant melanoma. *Cancer* 1989;64:1432.
Kehrer E. Soll das vulvakarzinom operiert oder bestrahlt werden? *Geburtsch & Franuenk* 1918;48:346.
Kelley JL III, Burke TW, Tornos C, et al. Minimally invasive vulvar carcinoma: an indication for conservative surgical therapy. *Gynecol Oncol* 1992;44:240.
Kennedy JC, Majmuder B. Primary adenocarcinoma of the vulva, possibly cloacogenic: a report of two cases. *J Reprod Med* 1993;38:113.
Keys H. Gynecologic Oncology Group randomized trials of combined technique therapy for vulvar cancer. *Cancer* 1993;71:1691.
Khansur T, Sanders J, Das SK. Evaluation of staging workup in malignant melanoma. *Arch Surg* 1989;24:847.
Khoury-Collado F, Elliott KS, et al. Merkel cell carcinoma of the Bartholin's gland. *Gynecol Oncol* 2005;97:928.
Kim SH, Garcia C, Rodriguez J, et al. Prognosis of thick cutaneous melanoma. *J Am Coll Surg* 1999;188:241.
King LA, Downey GO, Savage JE, et al. Resection of the pubic bone as an adjunct to management of primary, recurrent and metastatic pelvic malignancies. *Obstet Gynecol* 1989;73:1022.
Kirby TO, Rocconi RP, Numnum TM, et al. Outcomes of stage I/II vulvar cancer patients after negative superficial inguinal lymphadenectomy. *Gynecol Oncol* 2005;98:309.
Kirkwood JM, Strawderman MH, Ernstoff MS, et al. Interferon alfa-2b adjuvant therapy of high risk resected cutaneous melanoma: the Eastern Cooperative Oncology Group Trial EST 1684. *J Clin Oncol* 1996;14:7.
Kirschner CV, Yordan EL, Geest KD, et al. Smoking, obesity, and survival in squamous cell carcinoma of the vulva. *Gynecol Oncol* 1995;56:79.
Klemm P, Marnitz S, Köhler C, et al. Clinical implication of laparoscopic pelvic lymphadenectomy in patients with vulvar cancer and positive groin nodes. *Gynecol Oncol* 2005;99:101.
Knapstein PG. Reconstructive procedures following extended vulvectomy. In: Knapstein PG, diRe F, DiSaia P, et al., eds. *Malignancies of the vulva*. New York: Theime Medical Publishers; 1991.
Kneale BL. Microinvasive cancer of the vulva: report of the International Society for the Study of Vulvar Disease Task Force, VIIth Congress. *J Reprod Med* 1984;29:454.
Kodama S, Kaneko T, Saito M, et al. A clinicopathologic study of 30 patients with Paget's disease of the vulva. *Gynecol Oncol* 1995;56:63.
Koh W-J, Wallace III J, Greer BE, et al. Combined radiotherapy and chemotherapy in the management of local-regional advanced vulvar cancer. *Int J Rad Oncol Biol Phys* 1993;26:809.
Konefka T, Senkus E, Emerich J, et al. Epithelial sarcoma of the Bartholin's gland primarily diagnosed as vulvar sarcoma. *Gynecol Oncol* 1994;54:393.
Krag Miller LB, Nygaard Nielsen M, Trolle C. Leiomyosarcoma vulvae. *Acta Obstet Gynecol Scand* 1990;69:187.
Krupp PJ, Bohm JW. Lymph gland metastases in invasive squamous cell cancer of the vulva. *Am J Obstet Gynecol* 1978;130:943.
Krupp PJ, Lee FY, Bohm JW, et al. Prognostic parameters and clinical staging criteria in epidermoid carcinoma of the vulva. *Obstet Gynecol* 1975;46:84.
Kuipers T. Carcinoma of the vulva. *Radiol Clin* 1975;44:475.
Kuller JA, Zucker PK, Peng TC. Vulvar leiomyosarcoma in pregnancy. *Am J Obstet Gynecol* 1990;162:164.
Kuppers V, Stiller M, Somville T, et al. Risk factors for recurrent VIN: role of multifocality and grade of disease. *J Reprod Med* 1997;42:138.
Kurzl R, Messerer D. Prognostic factors in squamous cell carcinoma of the vulva: a multivariate analysis. *Gynecol Oncol* 1989;32:143.
Lambrou NC, Mirhashemi R, Wolfson A, et al. Malignant peripheral nerve sheath tumor of the vulva: a multimodal treatment approach. *Gynecol Oncol* 2002;85:365.
Landoni F, Maneo A, Zanetta G, et al. Concurrent preoperative chemotherapy with 5-fluororacil and mitomycin-C and radiotherapy (FUMIR) followed by limited surgery in locally advanced and recurrent vulvar carcinoma. *Gynecol Oncol* 1996;61:321.
Landoni F, Proserpio M, Maneo A, et al. Skin flap reconstruction of the perineal defect after radical vulvar surgery. *J Gynecol Surg* 1995;11:165.
Landthaler M, Braun-Falco O, Leitl A, et al. Excisional biopsy as the first therapeutic procedure versus primary wide excision of malignant melanoma. *Cancer* 1989;64:1612.
Lataifeh I, Nascimento MC, Nicklin JL, et al. Patterns of recurrence and disease-free survival in advanced squamous cell carcinoma of the vulva. *Gynecol Oncol* 2004;95:701.
Lavie O, Comerci G, Daras V, et al. Thrombocytosis in women with vulvar carcinoma. *Gynecol Oncol* 1999;72:82.
Lawton FG, Hacker NF. Surgery for invasive gynecologic cancer in the elderly female population. *Obstet Gynecol* 1990;76:287.
Lawton G, Rasque H, Ariyan S. Preservation of muscle fascia to decrease lymphedema after complete axillary and ilioinguinofemoral lymphadenectomy for melanoma. *J Am Coll Surg* 2002;195:339.
Leake JF, Buscema J, Cho KR, et al. Dermatofibrosarcoma protuberans of the vulva. *Gynecol Oncol* 1991;41:245.
Leiserowitz GS, Russell AH, Kinney WK, et al. Prophylactic chemoradiation of inguinofemoral lymph nodes in patients with locally extensive vulvar cancer. *Gynecol Oncol* 1997;66:509.
Leiter U, Buettner PG, Eigentler TK, et al. Prognostic factors of thin cutaneous melanoma: an analysis of the central malignant melanoma registry of the German dermatological society. *J Clin Oncol* 2004;22:3660.
Lenaz MP, Nguyen TC, Hewett WJ. Leiomyosarcoma of the vulva. *Conn Med* 1987;51:705.
Lens MB, Dawes M, Goodacre T, et al. Elective lymph node dissection in patients with melanoma: systemic review and meta-analysis of randomized controlled trials. *Arch Surg* 2002;137:458.
Lens MB, Dawes M, Goodacre T, et al. Excision margins in the treatment of primary cutaneous melanoma: a systematic review of randomized controlled trials comparing narrow vs. wide excision. *Arch Surg* 2002;137:1101.
Leuchter RS, Hacker NF, Voet RL, et al. Primary carcinoma of the Bartholin gland: a report of 14 cases and review of the literature. *Obstet Gynecol* 1982;60:361.
Levenback C, Burke TW, Gershenson DM, et al. Intraoperative lymphatic mapping for vulvar cancer. *Obstet Gynecol* 1994;84:163.
Levenback C, Coleman RL, Burke TW, et al. Intraoperative lymphatic mapping and sentinel node identification with blue dye in patients with vulvar cancer. *Gynecol Oncol* 2001;83:276.
Levenback C, Morris M, Burke TW, et al. Groin dissection practices among gynecologic oncologists treating early vulvar cancer. *Gynecol Oncol* 1996;62:73.
Levin M, Pakarakas RM, Chang HA, et al. Primary breast carcinoma of the vulva: a case report and review of the literature. *Gynecol Oncol* 1995;56:448.
Levin W, Rad FF, Goldberg G, et al. The use of concomitant chemotherapy and radiotherapy prior to surgery in advanced stage carcinoma of the vulva. *Gynecol Oncol* 1986;25:20.
Lewandowski G, O'Toole RV, Delgado G, et al. Carcinoma of the vulva: significance of surgical margin involvement in assessing prognosis. *J Reprod Med* 1989;34:884.

Lin JY, DuBeshter B, Angel C, et al. Morbidity and recurrence with modifications of radical vulvectomy and groin dissection. *Gynecol Oncol* 1992;47:80.

Loree TR, Hempling RE, Eltabbakh GH, et al. The inferior gluteal flap in the difficult vulvar and perineal reconstruction. *Gynecol Oncol* 1997;66:429.

Loret de Mola Jr, Hudock PA, Steinetz C, et al. Merkel cell carcinoma of the vulva. *Gynecol Oncol* 1993;51:272.

Lotem M, Anteby S, Peretz T, et al. Mucosal melanoma of the female genital tract is a multifocal disorder. *Gynecol Oncol* 2003;88:45.

Lovett RD, Kuske RR, Perez CA, et al. Preliminary evaluation of toxicity and tumor response to radiotherapy with cisplatin and 5-fluorouracil for advanced or recurrent gynecologic malignancies. *Int J Radiat Oncol Biol Phys* 1987;13:129.

Lupi G, Raspagliesi F, Zucali R, et al. Combined preoperative chemoradiotherapy followed by radical surgery in locally advanced vulvar carcinoma. *Cancer* 1996;77:1472.

Mader MH, Friedrich EG Jr. Vulvar metastasis of breast carcinoma: a case report. *J Reprod Med* 1982;27:169.

Maggino T, Landoni F, Sartori E, et al. Patterns of recurrence in patients with squamous cell carcinoma of the vulva: a multicenter CTF study. *Cancer* 2000;89:116.

Magrina JF, Gonzalez-Bosquet J, Weaver AL, et al. Squamous cell carcinoma of the vulva stage 1A: long-term results. *Gynecol Oncol* 2000;76:24.

Magrina JF, Webb MJ, Gaffey TA, et al. Stage 1 squamous cell cancer of the vulva. *Am J Obstet Gynecol* 1979;134:453.

Malfetano J, Piver MS, Tsukada Y. Stage III and IV squamous cell carcinomas of the vulva. *Gynecol Oncol* 1986;23:192.

Malfetano JH, Piver MS, Tsukada Y, et al. Univariate and multivariate analyses of 5-year survival, recurrence, and inguinal node metastases in stage I and II vulvar carcinoma. *J Surg Oncol* 1985;30:124.

Mariani L, Conti L, Atlante G, et al. Vulvar squamous carcinoma: prognostic role of DNA context. *Gynecol Oncol* 1998;71:159.

Marsden DE, Hacker NF. Urinary problems following simple and radical vulvectomy. *J Gynecol Oncol* 2002;7:61.

Massad LS, DeGeest K. Multimodality therapy for carcinoma of the Bartholin gland. *Gynecol Oncol* 1999;75:305.

Matias C, Nunes JF, Vicente LF, et al. Primary malignant rhabdoid tumour of the vulva. *Histopathology* 1990;17:576.

Mayer AR, Rodriguez RL. Vulvar reconstruction using a pedicle flap based on the superficial external pudendal artery. *Obstet Gynecol* 1991;78[Suppl]:964.

Mazouni C, Morice P, Duvillard P, et al. Contralateral groin recurrence in patients with stage 1 Bartholin's gland squamous cell carcinoma and negative ipsilateral nodes: report on two cases and implications for lymphadenectomy. *Gynecol Oncol* 2004;94:843.

McCall AR, Olson MC, Potkui RK. The variation of inguinal lymph node depth in adult women and its importance in planning elective irradiation for vulvar cancer. *Cancer* 1995;75:2286.

McClay EF, Mastrangello MJ, Sprandio JD, et al. The importance of tamoxifen to a cisplatin-containing regimen in the treatment of metastatic melanoma. *Cancer* 1989;63:1292.

McClintock J, Hoffman MS, Fiorica JV, et al. Vulvar melanoma: a retrospective review of prognostic factors and outcome. *J Gynecol Surg* 1998;14:25.

McCraw JB, Massey FM, Shaklin KD, et al. Vaginal reconstruction with gracilis myocutaneous flaps. *Plast Reconstr Surg* 1976;58:176.

McKee PH, Hertogs KT. Endocervical adenocarcinoma and vulvar Paget's disease: a significant association. *Br J Dermatol* 1980;103:443.

McKinnon JG, Yu XQ, McCarthy WH, et al. Prognosis for patients with thin cutaneous melanoma: long term survival data from the New South Wales Central Cancer Registry and the Sydney Melanoma Unit. *Cancer* 2003;98:1223.

Mendenhall WM, Zlotecki RA, Scarborough MT. Dermatofibrosarcoma protuberans. *Cancer* 2004;101:2503.

Menzin AW, DeRisi D, Smilari TF, et al. Lobular breast carcinoma metastatic to the vulva: a case report and literature review. *Gynecol Oncol* 1998;69:84.

Merino MJ, LiVolsi VA, Schwartz PE, et al. Adenoid basal cell carcinoma of the vulva. *Int J Gynecol Pathol* 1982;1:299.

Mesko JD, Gates H, McDonald TW, et al. Clear cell ("mesonephroid") adenocarcinoma of the vulva arising in endometriosis: a case report. *Gynecol Oncol* 1988;29:385.

Messing MJ, Gallup DG. Carcinoma of the vulva in young women. *Obstet Gynecol* 1995;86:51.

Messing MJ, Richardson MS, Smith MT, et al. Metastatic clear-cell hidradenocarcinoma of the vulva. *Gynecol Oncol* 1994;48:264.

Micheletti L, Preti M, Zola P, et al. A proposed glossary of terminology related to the surgical treatment of vulvar carcinoma. *Cancer* 1998;83:1369.

Microinvasive cancer of the vulva: report of the ISSVD Task Force. *J Reprod Med* 1984;29:454.

Miller B, Morris M, Levenback C, et al. Pelvic exenteration for primary and recurrent vulvar cancer. *Gynecol Oncol* 1995;58:202.

Misas JE, Cold CJ, Hall FW. Vulvar Paget's disease: fluorescein-aided visualization of margins. *Obstet Gynecol* 1991;97:156.

Misas JE, Larson JE, Podczaski E, et al. Recurrent Paget's disease of the vulva in a split-thickness graft. *Obstet Gynecol* 1990;76:543.

Mitchell MF, Prasad CJ, Silva EG, et al. Second genital primary squamous neoplasms in vulvar carcinoma: viral and histopathologic correlates. *Obstet Gynecol* 1993;81:13.

Miyazawa K, Nori D, Hilaris BS, et al. Role of radiation therapy in the treatment of advanced vulvar carcinoma. *J Reprod Med* 1983;28:539.

Modesitt SC, Waters AB, Walton L, et al. Vulvar intraepithelial neoplasia III: occult cancer and the impact of margin status on recurrence. *Obstet Gynecol* 1998;92:962.

Moller LBK, Nielsen MN, Trolle C. Leiomyosarcoma vulvae. *Acta Obstet Gynecol Scand* 1990;69:187.

Monaghan JM, Hammond IG. Pelvic node dissection in the treatment of vulval carcinoma: is it necessary? *BJOG* 1984;91:270.

Monk BJ, Burger RA, Fritz L, et al. Prognostic significance of human papillomavirus DNA in vulvar carcinoma. *Obstet Gynecol* 1995;85:709.

Montana GS, Thomas GM, Moore DH, et al. Preoperative chemo-radiation for carcinoma of the vulva with N2/N3 nodes: a gynecologic oncology group study. *Int J Radiat Oncol Biol Phys* 2000;48:1007.

Moore HD, Thomas GM, Montana GS, et al. Preoperative chemoradiation for advanced vulvar cancer: A phase II study of the Gynecol. Oncol. group. *Int J Radiat Oncol Biol Phys* 1998;42:79–85.

Moore RG, DePasquale SE, Steinhoff MM, et al. Sentinel node identification and the ability to detect metastatic tumor to inguinal lymph nodes in squamous cell cancer of the vulva. *Gynecol Oncol* 2003;89:475.

Moore RG, Granai CO, Gajewski W, et al. Pathologic evaluation of inguinal sentinel lymph nodes in vulvar cancer patients: a comparison of immunohistochemical staining versus ultrastaging with hematoxylin and eosin staining. *Gynecol Oncol* 2003;91:378.

Moore RG, Steinhoff MM, Granai CO, et al. Vulvar epithelioid sarcoma in pregnancy. *Gynecol Oncol* 2002;85:218.

Poirer M, Traser R, Meterission S. Case 1. Aggressive angiomyxoma of the pelvis: response to leutinizing hormone-releasing hormone agonist. *J Clin Oncol* 2003;21(18):3535–3536.

Morley GW. Cancer of the vulva: a review. *Cancer* 1981;48[Suppl 2]:597.

Morley GW. Infiltrative carcinoma of the vulva: results of surgical treatment. *Am J Obstet Gynecol* 1976;124:874.

Morrow CP, DiSaia PJ. Malignant melanoma of the female genitalia: a clinical analysis. *Obstet Gynecol Surv* 1976;31:233.

Mulayim N, Silver DF, Ocal IT, et al. Vulvar basal cell carcinoma: two unusual presentations and review of the literature. *Gynecol Oncol* 2002;85:532.

Mulayim N, Silver DF, Schwartz PE, et al. Chemoradiation with 5-fluorouracil and mitomycin C in the treatment of vulvar squamous cell carcinoma. *Gynecol Oncol* 2004;93:659.

Nahai F. The tensor fascia lata flap. *Clin Plast Surg* 1980;7:51.

National Comprehensive Cancer Network (NCCN) melanoma practice guidelines. *Oncology* 1998;*NCCN Proc* 3:153.

National Institutes of Health Consensus Development Panel on Early Melanoma. Diagnosis and treatment of early melanoma. *JAMA* 1992;268:1314.

Ndubisi B, Kaminski PF, Olt G, et al. Staging and recurrence of disease in squamous cell carcinoma of the vulva. *Gynecol Oncol* 1995;59:34.

Newman PL, Fletcher CDM. Smooth muscle tumors of the external genitalia: clinicopathological analysis of a series. *Histopathology* 1991;18:523.

Nicklin JL, Hacker NF, Heintze SW, et al. An anatomical study of inguinal lymph node topography and clinical implications for the surgical management of vulvar cancer. *Int J Gynecol Cancer* 1995;5:128.

Nielsen GP, Rosenberg AE, Koerner FC, et al. Smooth-muscle tumors of the vulva: a clinicopathological study of 25 cases and review of the literature. *Am J Surg Pathol* 1996;20:779.

Nobler MP. Efficacy of a perineal teletherapy portal in the management of vulvar and vaginal cancer. *Ther Radiol* 1972;103:393.

Nori D, Cain JM, Hilaris BS, et al. Metronidazole as a radiosensitizer and high-dose radiation in advanced vulvovaginal malignancies: a pilot study. *Gynecol Oncol* 1983;16:117.

Odongo FN, Ojwang SB. Verrucous carcinoma of the vulva: report of two cases managed at Kenyetta National Hospital, and literature review. *East Afr Med J* 1990;67:830.

Ogino M, Sakamoto T, Inoue J, et al. Reconstruction of surgical defects using the gluteus maximus myocutaneous flap following radical vulvectomy. *Asia-Oceania J Obstet Gynaecol* 1992;18:23.

Oonk MHM, de Hullu JA, Hollema H, et al. The value of routine follow-up in patients treated for carcinoma of the vulva. *Cancer* 2003;98:2624.

Origoni M, Sideri M, Garsia S, et al. Prognostic value of pathological patterns of lymph node positivity in squamous cell carcinoma of the vulva stage III and IVA FIGO. *Gynecol Oncol* 1992;45:313.

Paget J. On disease of the mammary areola preceding cancer of the mammary gland. *St Barth Hosp Reports* 1874;10:87.

Paladini D, Cross O, Lopes A, et al. Prognostic significance of lymph node variables in squamous cell carcinoma of the vulva. *Cancer* 1994;74:2491.

Paley PJ, Johnson PR, Adcock LL, et al. The effect of sartorius transposition on wound morbidity following inguinal-femoral lymphadenectomy. *Gynecol Oncol* 1997;64:237.

Pao WM, Perez CA, Kuske RR, et al. Radiation therapy and conservation surgery for primary and recurrent carcinoma of the vulva: report of 40 patients

and a review of the literature. *Int J Radiat Oncol Biol Phys* 1988;14: 1123.
Parazzini F, Vecchia CL, Garsia S, et al. Determinants of invasive vulvar cancer risk: an Italian case-control study. *Gynecol Oncol* 1993;48:50.
Parker RT, Duncan I, Rampone J, et al. Operative management of early invasive epidermoid carcinoma of the vulva. *Am J Obstet Gynecol* 1975;123:349.
Parmley T, Woodruff J, Julian C. Invasive vulvar Paget's disease. *Obstet Gynecol* 1975;46:341.
Parry-Jones E. Lymphatics of the vulva. *J Obstet Gynaecol Br Commonw* 1963;70:751.
Partridge EE, Murad R, Shingleton HM, et al. Verrucous lesions of the female genitalia. II. Verrucous carcinoma. *Am J Obstet Gynecol* 1980;137:419.
Patsner B, Hetzler P. Post-radical vulvectomy reconstruction using the inferiorly based transverse rectus abdominis (TRAM) flap: a preliminary experience. *Gynecol Oncol* 1994;55:78.
Patsner B, Mann WJ Jr. Radical vulvectomy and "sneak" superficial inguinal lymphadenectomy with a single elliptic incision. *Am J Obstet Gynecol* 1988;158:464.
Patsner B, Mann WJ. Serum squamous cell carcinoma antigen levels in patients with invasive squamous vulvar and vaginal cancer: a preliminary report. *Gynecol Oncol* 1989;33:323.
Pelosi G, Martignoni G, Bonetti F. Intraductal carcinoma of mammary-type apocrine epithelium arising within a papillary hydradenoma of the vulva: report of a case and review of the literature. *Arch Pathol Lab Med* 1991;115: 1249.
Perez CA, Grigsby PW, Galakatos A, et al. Radiation therapy in management of carcinoma of the vulva with emphasis on conservation therapy. *Cancer* 1993;71:3707.
Perez CA, Kraus FT, Evans JC, et al. Anaplastic transformation in verrucous carcinoma of the oral cavity after radiation therapy. *Radiology* 1966;86:108.
Perrone T, Swanson PE, Twiggs L, et al. Malignant rhabdoid tumor of the vulva: is distinction from epithelioid sarcoma possible? *Am J Surg Pathol* 1989;13:848.
Perrone T, Twiggs LB, Adcock LL, et al. Vulvar basal cell carcinoma: an infrequently metastasizing neoplasm. *Int J Gynecol Pathol* 1987;6:152.
Petry KU, Kochel H, Bode U, et al. Human papillomavirus is associated with the frequent detection of warty and basaloid high-grade neoplasia of the vulva and cervical neoplasia among immunocompromised women. *Gynecol Oncol* 1996;60:30.
Phillips B, Buchsbaum HJ, Lifshitz S. Pelvic exenteration for vulvovaginal carcinoma. *Am J Obstet Gynecol* 1981;141:1038.
Phillips GL, Bundy BN, Okagaki T, et al. Malignant melanoma of the vulva treated by radical hemivulvectomy. *Cancer* 1994;73:2626.
Phillips GL, Twiggs LB, Okagaki T. Vulvar melanoma: a microstaging study. *Gynecol Oncol* 1982;14:80.
Pickel H. Early stromal invasion of the vulva. *Eur J Gynaecol Oncol* 1989;10:97.
Pinto AP, Signorello LB, Crum CP, et al. Squamous cell carcinoma of the vulva in Brazil: prognostic importance of host and viral variables. *Gynecol Oncol* 1999;74:61.
Pirtoli L, Rottoli ML. Results of radiation therapy for vulvar carcinoma. *Acta Radiol Oncol* 1982;21:45.
Piura B, Masotina A, Murdoch J, et al. Recurrent squamous cell carcinoma of the vulva: a study of 73 cases. *Gynecol Oncol* 1993;48:189.
Piver MS, Barlow JJ, Wang JJ, et al. Combined radical surgery, radiation therapy and chemotherapy in infants with vulvo-vaginal and embryonal rhabdomyosarcoma. *Obstet Gynecol* 1973;42:522.
Piver MS, Xynos FP. Pelvic lymphadenectomy in women with carcinoma of the clitoris. *Obstet Gynecol* 1977;49:592.
Plentl AA, Friedman EA. Clinical significance of vulvar lymphatics. Lymphatic system of the female genitalia: the morphologic basis of oncologic diagnosis and therapy. In: Plentl AA, Friedman EA. *Major problems in obstetrics and gynecology*, vol. 2. Philadelphia, WB Saunders; 1971:27.
Plouffe K Jr, Tulandi T, Rosenberg A, et al. Non-Hodgkin's lymphoma in Bartholin's gland: case report and review of literature. *Am J Obstet Gynecol* 1984;148:608.
Podczaski E, Stryker J, Banducci D, et al. Multimodality approach to a massive carcinoma of the vulva. *Eur J Gynecol Oncol* 1990;11:415.
Podratz KC, Gaffey TA, Symmonds RE, et al. Melanoma of the vulva: an update. *Gynecol Oncol* 1983;16:153.
Podratz KC, Symmonds RE, Taylor WF. Carcinoma of the vulva: analysis of treatment failures. *Am J Obstet Gynecol* 1982;143:340.
Podratz KC, Symmonds RE, Taylor WF, et al. Carcinoma of the vulva: analysis of treatment and survival. *Obstet Gynecol* 1983;61:63.
Potkul RK, Barnes WA, Barter JF, et al. Vulvar reconstruction using a mons pubis pedicle flap. *Gynecol Oncol* 1994;55:21.
Powell JL, Donovan JT, Reed WP. Hip disarticulation for recurrent vulvar cancer in the groin. *Gynecol Oncol* 1992;47:110.
Prempree T, Amornmarn R. Radiation treatment of recurrent carcinoma of the vulva. *Cancer* 1984;54:1943.
Preti M, Ronco G, Ghiringhello B, et al. Recurrent squamous cell carcinoma of the vulva: clinicopathologic determinants identifying low risk patients. *Cancer* 2000;88:1869.
Proffitt SD, Spooner TR, Kosek JC. Origin of undifferentiated neoplasm from verrucous carcinoma of the oral cavity following irradiation. *Cancer* 1970;26:389.
Puig-Tintoré LM, Ordi J, Vidal-Sicart S, et al. Further data on the usefulness of sentinel lymph node identification and ultrastaging in vulvar squamous cell carcinoma. *Gynecol Oncol* 2003;88:29.
Raber G, Mempel V, Jackisch C, et al. Malignant melanoma of the vulva: report of 89 patients. *Cancer* 1996;78:2353.
Ragnarsson-Olding B, Johansson H, Rutqvist L-E, et al. Malignant melanoma of the vulva and vagina: trends in incidence, age distribution, and long-term survival among 245 consecutive cases in Sweden 1960–1984. *Cancer* 1993;71:1983.
Ragnarsson-Olding BK, Kanter-Lewensohn LR, Lagerlof B, et al. Malignant melanoma of the vulva in a nationwide, 25-year study of 219 Swedish females: clinical observations and histopathologic features. *Cancer* 1999;86:1273.
Ragnarsson-Olding BK, Nilsson BR, Kanter-Lewensohn LR, et al. Malignant melanoma of the vulva in a nationwide, 25-year study of 219 Swedish females: predictors of survival. *Cancer* 1999;86:1285.
Reid GC, Delancey JOL, Hopkins MP, et al. Urinary incontinence following radical vulvectomy. *Obstet Gynecol* 1990;75:852.
Reid R. Local and distant skin flaps in the reconstruction of vulvar deformities. *Am J Obstet Gynecol* 1997;177:1372.
Reintgen DS, Cox EB, McCarty KS, et al. Efficacy of elective lymph node dissection in patients with intermediate thickness primary melanoma. *Ann Surg* 1983;198:379.
Remmenga S, Barnhill D, Nash J, et al. Radical vulvectomy with partial rectal resection and temporary colostomy as primary therapy for selected patients with vulvar carcinoma. *Obstet Gynecol* 1991;77:577.
Ribaldone R, Piantanida P, Surico D, et al. Aggressive angiomyxoma of the vulva. *Gynecol Oncol* 2004;95:724.
Roberts WS, Hoffman MS, LaPolla JP, et al. Management of radionecrosis of the vulva and distal vagina. *Am J Obstet Gynecol* 1991;164:1235.
Roberts WS, Kavanagh JJ, Greenberg H, et al. Concomitant radiation therapy and chemotherapy in the treatment of advanced squamous carcinoma of the lower female genital tract. *Gynecol Oncol* 1989;34:183.
Rockson SG, Miller LT, Senie R, et al. Workgroup III: diagnosis and management of lymphedema. *Cancer* 1998;83:2882.
Rodriguez A, Isaac MA, Hidalgo E, et al. Villoglandular adenocarcinoma of the vulva. *Gynecol Oncol* 2001;83:409.
Rogo KO, Andersson R, Adbom G, et al. Conservative surgery for vulvovaginal melanoma. *Eur J Gynaecol Oncol* 1991;12:113.
Rose PG, Piver S, Tsukada Y, et al. Conservative therapy for melanoma of the vulva. *Am J Obstet Gynecol* 1988;159:52.
Rose PG, Roman LD, Reale FR, et al. Primary adenocarcinoma of the breast arising in the vulva. *Obstet Gynecol* 1990;76:537.
Rose PG, Tak WK, Reale FR, et al. Adenoid cystic carcinoma of the vulva: a radiosensitive tumor. *Gynecol Oncol* 1991;43:81.
Rosen C, Malmstrom H. Invasive cancer of the vulva. *Gynecol Oncol* 1997;65:213.
Rosenberg P, Simonsen E, Risberg B. Adenoid cystic carcinoma of Bartholin's gland: a report of five new cases treated with surgery and radiotherapy. *Gynecol Oncol* 1988;34:145.
Ross MJ, Ehrmann RL. Histologic prognosticators in stage I squamous cell carcinoma of the vulva. *Obstet Gynecol* 1987;70:774.
Rotmensch J, Rubin SJ, Sutton HG, et al. Preoperative radiotherapy followed by radical vulvectomy with inguinal lymphadenectomy for advanced vulvar carcinomas. *Gynecol Oncol* 1990;36:181.
Rouzier R, Haddad B, Dubernard G, et al. Inguinofemoral dissection for carcinoma of the vulva: effect of modifications of extent and technique on morbidity and survival. *J Am Coll Surg* 2003;196:442.
Rowley KC, Gallion HH, Donaldson ES, et al. Prognostic factors in early vulvar cancer. *Gynecol Oncol* 1988;31:43.
Russel AH, Mesic JB, Scudder SA, et al. Synchronous radiation and cytotoxic chemotherapy for locally advanced or recurrent squamous cancer of the vulva. *Gynecol Oncol* 1992;47:14.
Rutledge F, Smith JP, Franklin EW. Carcinoma of the vulva. *Am J Obstet Gynecol* 1970;106:1117.
Rutledge FN, Mitchell MF, Munsell MF, et al. Prognostic indicators for invasive carcinoma of the vulva. *Gynecol Oncol* 1991;42:239.
Safai B, Good RA. Basal cell carcinoma with metastasis. *Arch Pathol Lab Med* 1977;101:327.
Salti GI, Kansagra A, Warso MA, et al. Clinical node-negative thick melanoma. *Arch Surg* 2002;137:291.
Santala M, Suonio S, Syrjanen K, et al. Malignant fibrous histiocytoma of the vulva. *Gynecol Oncol* 1987;27:121.
Scheistroen M, Tropé C. Combined bleomycin and irradiation in preoperative treatment of advanced squamous cell carcinoma of the vulva. *Acta Oncol* 1993;32:657.
Scheistroen M, Tropé C, Kaern J, et al. Malignant melanoma of the vulva: evaluation of prognostic factors with emphasis on DNA ploidy in 75 patients. *Cancer* 1995;75:72.

Scheistroen M, Tropé C, Kaern J, et al. Malignant melanoma of the vulva FIGO stage 1: evaluation of prognostic factors in 43 patients with emphasis on DNA ploidy and surgical treatment. *Gynecol Oncol* 1996;61:253.
Scherr GR, d'Ablaing G, Ouzounian JG. Peripheral primitive neuroectodermal tumor of the vulva. *Gynecol Oncol* 1994;54:254.
Schulz MJ, Penalver M. Recurrent vulvar carcinoma in the intervening tissue bridge in early invasive stage I disease treated by radical vulvectomy and bilateral groin dissection through separate incisions. *Gynecol Oncol* 1989;35:383.
Scurry J, Brand A, Planner R, et al. Vulvar Merkel cell tumor with glandular and squamous differentiation. *Gynecol Oncol* 1996;62:292.
Sebag-Montefiore DJ, McLean C, Arnott SJ, et al. Treatment of advanced carcinoma of the vulva with chemoradiotherapy: can extensive surgery be avoided? *Int J Gynecol Cancer* 1994;4:150.
Sedlis A, Homesley H, Bundy BN, et al. Positive groin lymph nodes in superficial squamous cell vulvar cancer. *Am J Obstet Gynecol* 1987;156:1159.
Selman TJ, Luesley DM, Acheson N, et al. A systematic review of the accuracy of diagnostic tests for inguinal lymph node status in vulvar cancer. *Gynecol Oncol* 2005;99:206.
Shanbour KA, Mannel RS, Morris PC, et al. Comparison of clinical versus surgical staging systems in vulvar cancer. *Obstet Gynecol* 1992;80:927.
Shen JT, D'ablaing G, Morrow CP. Alveolar soft part sarcoma of the vulva: report of first case and review of literature. *Gynecol Oncol* 1982;13:120.
Shepherd JH, Van Dam PA, Jobling TW, et al. The use of rectus abdominis myocutaneous flaps following excision of vulvar cancer. *BJOG* 1990;97:1020.
Shivers SC, Wang X, Li W, et al. Molecular staging of malignant melanoma: correlation with clinical outcome. *JAMA* 1998;280:1410.
Shutze WP, Gleysteen JJ. Perianal Paget's disease. Classification and review of management: report of two cases. *Dis Colon Rectum* 1990;33:502.
Siller BS, Alvarez RD, Conner WD, et al. T2/3 vulva cancer: a case-control study of triple incision versus en bloc radical vulvectomy and inguinal lymphadenectomy. *Gynecol Oncol* 1995;57:335.
Sim FH, Taylor WF, Ivins JC, et al. A prospective randomized study of the efficacy of routine elective lymphadenectomy in the management of malignant melanoma. *Cancer* 1978;41:948.
Simon KE, Dutcher JP, Runowicz CD, et al. Adenocarcinoma arising in vulvar breast tissue. *Cancer* 1988;62:2234.
Simonsen E. Invasive squamous cell carcinoma of the vulva. *Ann Chir Gynaecol* 1984;73:331.
Simonsen E. Treatment of recurrent squamous cell carcinoma of the vulva. *Acta Radiol Oncol* 1984;23:345.
Simonsen E, Johnsson JE, Tropé C, et al. Stage I squamous cell carcinoma of the vulva. *Acta Radiol Oncol* 1984;23:443.
Singhal RM, Narayana A. Malignant melanoma of the vulva: response to radiation. *Br J Radiol* 1991;64:846.
Singletary SE, Shallenberger R, Guinee VF. Surgical management of groin nodal metastases from primary melanoma of the lower extremity. *Surg Gynecol Obstet* 1992;174:195.
Slevin NJ, Pointon RCS. Radical radiotherapy for carcinoma of the vulva. *Br J Radiol* 1989;62:145.
Sliutz G, Reinthaller A, Lantzsch T, et al. Lymphatic mapping of sentinel nodes in early vulvar cancer. *Gynecol Oncol* 2002;84:449.
Smith HO, Worrell RV, Smith AY, et al. Aggressive angiomyxoma of the female pelvis and perineum: review of the literature. *Gynecol Oncol* 1991;42:79.
Snijders-Keilholz T, Trimbos JB, Hermans J, et al. Management of vulvar carcinoma radiation toxicity, results and failure analysis in 44 patients (1980–1989). *Acta Obstet Gynecol Scand* 1993;72:668.
Soergel TM, Doering DL, O'Connor D. Metastatic dermatofibrosarcoma protuberans of the vulva. *Gynecol Oncol* 1998;71:320.
Soltan M. Dermatofibrosarcoma protuberans of the vulva. *BJOG* 1981;88:203.
Soper JT, Elbendary AA, Hurteau JA, et al. Bulbocavernosus myocutaneous flap for perineal reconstruction. *J Gynecol Tech* 1996;2:141.
Stacy D, Burrell MO, Franklin EW III. Extramammary Paget's disease of the vulva and anus: use of intraoperative frozen-section margins. *Am J Obstet Gynecol* 1986;155:519.
Steeper TA, Rosai J. Aggressive angiomyxoma of the female pelvis and perineum: report of nine cases of a distinctive type of gynecologic soft-tissue neoplasm. *Am J Surg Pathol* 1983;7:463.
Stehman FB, Bundy BN, Ball H, et al. Sites of failure and times to failure in carcinoma of the vulva treated conservatively: a Gynecologic Oncology Group study. *Am J Obstet Gynecol* 1996;174:1128.
Stehman FB, Bundy BN, Dvoretsky PM, et al. Early stage I carcinoma of the vulva treated with ipsilateral superficial inguinal lymphadenectomy and modified radical hemivulvectomy: a prospective study of the Gynecologic Oncology Group. *Obstet Gynecol* 1992;79:490.
Stehman FB, Bundy BN, Thomas G, et al. Groin dissection versus groin radiation in carcinoma of the vulva: a Gynecologic Oncology Group study. *Int J Radiat Oncol Biol Phys* 1992;24:389.
Struyk APHB, Bouma JJ, van Lindert ACM, et al. Early stage cancer of the vulva: a pilot investigation on cancer of the Vulvain Gynecologic Oncology Centres in the Netherlands. Proceedings of the second meeting of the International Gynecologic Cancer Society, Toronto, 1989:303.
Sturgeon SR, Brinton LA, Devesa SS, et al. In situ and invasive vulvar cancer incidence trends (1973 to 1987). *Am J Obstet Gynecol* 1992;166:1482.
Sturgeon SR, Curtis RE, Johnson K, et al. Second primary cancers after vulvar and vaginal cancers. *Am J Obstet Gynecol* 1996;174:929.
Sutton GP, Miser MR, Stehman FB, et al. Trends in the operative management of invasive squamous carcinoma of the vulva at Indiana University, 1974 to 1988. *Am J Obstet Gynecol* 1991;164:1472.
Sworn MJ, Hammond GT, Buchanan R. Metastatic basal cell carcinoma of the vulva: a case report. *BJOG* 1979;86:332.
Sykiotis C, Vitoratos N, Kalabokis D, et al. Dermatofibrosarcoma protuberans of the vulva. *J Gynecol Surg* 1999;15:149.
Tamussino KF, Bader AA, Lax SF, et al. Groin recurrence after micrometastasis in a sentinel lymph node in a patient with vulvar cancer. *Gynecol Oncol* 2002;86:99.
Tan GW, Lim-Tan SK, Salmon YM. Epithelioid sarcoma of the vulva. *Singapore Med J* 1989;30:308.
Tateo A, Tateo S, Bernasconi C, et al. Use of V-Y flap for vulvar reconstruction. *Gynecol Oncol* 1996;62:203.
Taussig FJ. Cancer of the vulva: an analysis of 155 cases. *Am J Obstet Gynecol* 1940;40:764.
Tavassoli FA, Norris HJ. Smooth muscle tumors of the vulva. *Obstet Gynecol* 1979;53:213.
Tawfik O, Huntrakoon M, Collins J, et al. Leiomyosarcoma of the vulva: report of a case. *Gynecol Oncol* 1994;54:242.
Taylor RN, Bottles K, Miller TR, et al. Malignant fibrous histiocytoma of the vulva. *Obstet Gynecol* 1985;66:145.
Tebes S, Cardosi R, Hoffman M. Paget's disease of the vulva. *Am J Obstet Gynecol* 2002;187:281.
Terada KY, Coel M, Ko P, et al. Combined use of intraoperative lymphatic mapping and lymphoscintigraphy in the management of squamous cell cancer of the vulva. *Gynecol Oncol* 1998;70:65.
Terada KY, Shimizu DM, Wong JH. Sentinel node dissection and ultrastaging in squamous cell cancer of the vulva. *Gynecol Oncol* 2000;76:40.
Tewari K, Cappuccini F, Syed N, et al. Interstitial brachytherapy in the treatment of advanced and recurrent vulvar cancer. *Am J Obstet Gynecol* 1999;181:91.
Thomas G, Dembo A, DePetrillo A, et al. Concurrent radiation and chemotherapy in vulvar carcinoma. *Gynecol Oncol* 1989;34:263.
Thornton WN, Flanagan WC. Pelvic exenteration in the treatment of advanced malignancy of the vulva. *Am J Obstet Gynecol* 1973;117:774.
Tilmans AS, Sutton GP, Look KY, et al. Recurrent squamous carcinoma of the vulva. *Am J Obstet Gynecol* 1992;167:1383.
Tjalma WAA, Colpaert CGA. Myoxoid leiomyosarcoma of the vulva. *Gynecol Oncol* 2005;96:548.
Tjalma WAA, Hauben EI, Deprez SME, et al. Epithelioid sarcoma of the vulva. *Gynecol Oncol* 1999;73:160.
Toker C. Trabecular carcinoma of the skin. *Arch Dermatol* 1972;105:107.
Trelford JD, Deer DA, Ordorica E, et al. Ten-year prospective study in a management change of vulvar carcinoma. *Am J Obstet Gynecol* 1984;150:288.
Trimble CL, Hildesheim A, Brinton LA, et al. Heterogeneous etiology of squamous carcinoma of the vulva. *Obstet Gynecol* 1996;87:59.
Trimble EL, Lewis JL Jr, Williams LL, et al. Management of vulvar melanoma. *Gynecol Oncol* 1992;45:254.
Ulbright TM, Brokaw SA, Stehman FB, et al. Epithelioid sarcoma of the vulva: evidence suggesting a more aggressive behavior than extra-genital epithelioid sarcoma. *Cancer* 1983;52:1462.
Ungerleider RS, Donaldson SS, Warnke RA, et al. Endodermal sinus tumor: the Stanford experience and the first reported case arising in the vulva. *Cancer* 1978;41:1627.
Valentine BH, Arena B, Green E. Laser ablation of recurrent Paget's disease of vulva and perineum. *J Gynecol Surg* 1992;8:21.
van der Griend MD, Burda P, Ferrier AJ. Angiomyofibroblastoma of the vulva. *Gynecol Oncol* 1994;54:389.
van der Velden J, Kooyman CD, Van Lindert ACM, et al. A stage IA vulvar carcinoma with an inguinal lymph node recurrence after local excision: a case report and literature review. *Int J Gynecol Cancer* 1992;2:157.
van der Velden J, van Lindert ACM, Lammes FB, et al. Extracapsular growth of lymph node metastases in squamous cell carcinoma of the vulva: the impact on recurrence and survival. *Cancer* 1995;75:2885.
van Seters M, van Beurden M, de Craen AJM. Is the assumed natural history of vulvar intraepithelial neoplasia III based on enough evidence? A systematic review of 3322 published patients. *Gynecol Oncol* 2005;97:645.
Veronesi U, Adamus J, Bandiera DC, et al. Inefficacy of immediate node dissection in stage I melanoma of the limbs. *N Engl J Med* 1977;297:627.
Veronesi U, Cascinelli N. Narrow excision (1-cm margin): a safe procedure for thin cutaneous melanoma. *Arch Surg* 1991;126:438.
Veronesi U, Cascinelli N, Adamus J, et al. Thin stage I primary cutaneous malignant melanoma: comparison of excision with margins of 1 and 3 cm. *N Engl J Med* 1988;318:1159.
Visco AG, Del Priore G. Postmenopausal Bartholin gland enlargement: a hospital-based cancer risk assessment. *Obstet Gynecol* 1996;87:286.

Wagenaar HC, Colombo N, Vergote I, et al. Bleomycin, methotrexate, and CCNU in locally advanced or recurrent, inoperable, squamous-cell carcinoma of the vulva: an EORTC gynaecological cancer cooperative group study. *Gynecol Oncol* 2001;81:348.

Waibel M, Richter K, Von Lengerken W, et al. Merkel cell carcinoma (neuro-endocrine carcinoma) in uncommon skin location, immunohistochemical and lectinhistochemical findings. *Zentralbl Pathol* 1991;137:140.

Watring WG, Roberts JA, Lagasse LD, et al. Treatment of recurrent Paget's disease of the vulva with topical bleomycin. *Cancer* 1978;41:10.

Way S. The anatomy of the lymphatic drainage of the vulva and its influence on the radical operation for carcinoma. *Ann R Coll Surg Engl* 1948;3:187.

Way S, Benedet JL. Involvement of inguinal lymph nodes in carcinoma of the vulva. *Gynecol Oncol* 1973;1:119.

Weikel W, Hoffmann M, Steiner E, et al. Reconstructive surgery following resection of primary vulvar cancers. *Gynecol Oncol* 2005;99:92.

Weissmann D, Amenta PS, Kantor GR. Vulvar epithelioid sarcoma metastatic to the scalp: a case report and review of the literature. *Am J Dermatopathol* 1990;12:462.

Whalen SA, Slater JD, Wagner RJ, et al. Concurrent radiation therapy and chemotherapy in the treatment of primary squamous cell carcinoma of the vulva. *Cancer* 1995;75:2289.

Wharton JT, Gallager S, Rutledge FN. Microinvasive carcinoma of the vulva. *Am J Obstet Gynecol* 1974;118:159.

Wheeless CR Jr, McGibbon B, Dorsey JH, et al. Gracilis myocutaneous flap in reconstruction of the vulva and female perineum. *Obstet Gynecol* 1979;54:97.

Wheelock JB, Goplerud DR, Dunn L, et al. Primary carcinoma of the Bartholin gland: a report of ten cases. *Obstet Gynecol* 1984;63:820.

Whitaker SJ, Kirkbride P, Arnott SJ, et al. A pilot study of chemoradiotherapy in advanced carcinoma of the vulva. *BJOG* 1990;97:436.

Wick MR, Goellner JR, Wolfe JT, et al. Vulvar sweat gland carcinomas. *Arch Pathol Lab Med* 1985;109:43.

Wilkinson EJ. Superficially invasive carcinoma of the vulva. *Clin Obstet Gynecol* 1985;28:188.

Wilkinson EJ, Brown HM. Vulvar Paget disease of urothelial origin: a report of three cases and a proposed classification of vulvar Paget disease. *Human Pathol* 2002;33:549.

Wilkinson EJ, Kneale B, Lynch PJ. Report of the ISSVD Terminology Committee. *J Reprod Med* 1986;31:973.

Winkelmann SE, Llorens AS. Case report: metastatic basal cell carcinoma of the vulva. *Gynecol Oncol* 1990;38:138.

Woolcott RJ, Henry RJ, Houghton CR. Malignant melanoma of the vulva: Australian experience. *J Reprod Med* 1988;33:699.

Zaidi SNH, Conner MG. Primary vulvar adenocarcinoma of cloacogenic origin. *South Med J* 2001;94:744.

Zaino RJ, Husseinzadeh N, Nahhas W, et al. Epithelial alterations in proximity to invasive squamous carcinoma of the vulva. *Int J Gynecol Pathol* 1982;1:173.

Zapas JL, Coley HC, Beam SL, et al. The risk of regional lymph node metastases in patients with melanoma less than 1.0 mm thick: recommendations for sentinel lymph node biopsy. *J Am Coll Surg* 2003;197:403.

Zerner J, Fenn ME. Basal cell carcinoma of the vulva. *Int J Gynaecol Obstet* 1979;17:203.

Zettersten E, Sagebiel RW, Miller III Jr, et al. Prognostic factors in patients with thick cutaneous melanoma (.4 mm). *Cancer* 2002;94:1049.

Zhang SH, Sood AK, Sorosky JI, et al. Preservation of the saphenous vein during inguinal lymphadenectomy decreases morbidity in patients with carcinoma of the vulva. *Cancer* 2000;89(7):1520.

CHAPTER 46 ■ CERVICAL CANCER PRECURSORS AND THEIR MANAGEMENT

HOWARD W. JONES III

DEFINITIONS

The Bethesda System (TBS)—Another classification system that was introduced in 1991 for grading cytologic abnormalities. It has also been used for histologic diagnoses. *Low-grade squamous intraepithelial lesion (LSIL)* = mild dysplasia/human papillomavirus changes. *High-grade squamous intraepithelial lesion (HSIL)* = moderate/severe dysplasia or carcinoma *in situ*.

Carcinoma *in situ*—A histopathologic diagnosis involving severe epithelial atypia. In the cervix, the full thickness of the cervical epithelium is atypical, but the basement membrane remains intact. Despite the confusing name, the lesion is not a cancer. It does not metastasize.

Cervical cytology—A diagnostic technique that involves microscopic examination of individual cells or cell clusters scraped, brushed, or washed from the surface of the cervix and stained with Papanicolaou's stain. The nuclear characteristic and the nuclear/cytoplasmic ratio are used to diagnose the degree of cervical abnormality present. It is a common screening test for cervical cancer.

Cervical dysplasia—Dysplasia is a pathologic term to indicate noninvasive epithelial atypia that involves various degrees of the cervical epithelium. By convention, in *mild dysplasia*, the nuclear atypia, mitoses, and cellular irregularity involved the lower one third of the squamous epithelium. When the atypia involves the middle third, the diagnosis is *moderate dysplasia*; in *severe dysplasia*, the upper one third of the epithelial layer is involved. A full-thickness change is called *carcinoma in situ*.

Cervical intraepithelial neoplasia (CIN)—A cytologic and histologic classification of preinvasive cervical atypias or neoplastic changes. In general, CIN 1 = mild dysplasia, CIN 2 = moderate dysplasia, and CIN 3 = severe dysplasia/carcinoma *in situ*.

Colposcopy—A diagnostic technique in which the examiner visualizes the cervix and other areas of the lower genital tract with a low-power (3–15×) binocular scope. The surface contour, vascular pattern, and staining pattern with dilute acetic acid and Lugol's iodine allow the experienced colposcopist to diagnose the severity and extent of cervical abnormality and to select a location for biopsy confirmation.

LEEP—Loop electrosurgical excision procedure; also called a LLETZ (large loop excision of the transformation zone). A thin wire electrosurgical loop electrode of 1 to 2.5 cm in diameter is used to excise the transformation zone under local anesthesia.

Squamocolumnar junction—The junction between the squamous and columnar epithelium on the cervix. Although it is found in the area of the external cervical os in most women during the reproductive years, it is a dynamic, ever-changing location.

Transformation zone—A colposcopic term for the area of cellular change that is observed adjacent to the squamocolumnar junction.

Although cellular atypia adjacent to invasive squamous cell cancers of the cervix has long been recognized, it was not until the 1950s that *carcinoma in situ* of the cervix was characterized and its preinvasive potential became accepted. In their 1952 publication, Galvin, Jones, and Te Linde described their observations of the natural history of carcinoma *in situ*. Their report confirmed and advanced previous studies by Thomas Cullen and Pemberton and Smith. The concept of a clearly identifiable preinvasive neoplastic change in the cervical epithelium represented a major breakthrough in an understanding of the development and natural history of cervical cancer. However, it was the parallel development of *cervical cytology* that provided a technique that made this concept clinically useful. Because these preinvasive epithelial changes are asymptomatic and essentially unrecognizable on gross inspection or palpation, the concept of a preinvasive lesion was not particularly useful to the clinician until it was shown such lesions could be diagnosed by cervical cytology. The introduction of practical cytology by Papanicolaou and Traut in 1943 and its later widespread adaptation into clinical practice represented the second major development in cervical cancer preventions. These developments have been further assisted by the use of *colposcopy*, which allows the clinician to visually identify these preinvasive lesions on the cervix, determine their extent, and select a site for biopsy confirmation. Once the extent and severity of the lesion have been evaluated and invasive cancer has been ruled out, these preinvasive epithelial changes can usually be treated with simple, inexpensive conservative techniques with preservation of fertility. These developments have led to a dramatic 70% reduction in cervical cancer deaths in the United States over the past 50 years. In addition, the intense study of these preinvasive cervical epithelial changes have enabled us to understand the mechanisms of the development of cervical cancer and the role of human papillomavirus.

This chapter discusses the cytologic, histologic, and molecular changes that occur in the cervix as cervical cancer develops and how these preinvasive lesions can be diagnosed and treated.

TERMINOLOGY

Although *carcinoma in situ* became well recognized as a full-thickness epithelial change without stromal invasion, the terminology and clinical significance of adjacent, less-than-full-thickness atypia was uncertain. In 1956, Reagan and Hamonic introduced the term *dysplasia* to designate these cervical epithelial abnormalities that were characterized by cytologic atypia, increased mitotic activity, and loss of polarity. If these basoid changes involved only the basal one third of the epithelium, they were referred to as *mild dysplasia.* Changes extending into the middle third of the cervical epithelium were classified as *moderate dysplasia,* and when more than two thirds of the epithelium was involved, the lesion was designated *severe dysplasia.* At its first international meeting in 1961, the International Congress on Exfoliative Cytology accepted the following definition: "Only those cases should be classified as *carcinoma in situ* which, in the absence of invasion, show as surface lining epithelium in which, throughout its whole thickness, no differentiation takes place. The process may involve the lining of the cervical glands without thereby creating a new group. It is recognized that the cells of the uppermost layers may show some slight flattening." At this same meeting, dysplasia was defined as "all other disturbances of differentiation of the squamous epithelium of surface and glands. They may be characterized as of high or low degrees, terms that are preferable to 'suspicious' and 'nonsuspicious' as the proposed terms describe the histological appearance and do not express an opinion." It generally was assumed that these lesions represented a spectrum of disease and that the more severe abnormalities were more likely to progress to invasive cancer and to do so in a shorter period of time. However, it was not until the studies of Barron and Richart and later of Nasiell and colleagues that the natural history of these preinvasive lesions became well understood.

The original cytologic classification introduced by Papanicolaou used a four- or five-step "class" designation, in which "class 1" was normal or benign and "class 5" was suspicious of invasive cancer. This terminology was replaced gradually by the histologic terms of *mild, moderate,* or *severe dysplasia* and *carcinoma in situ,* although various modifications were formally or informally introduced and adopted in the United States and throughout the world. One of the most important values of an accurately defined and widely accepted terminology is that it allows investigators and clinicians to accurately observe and classify the natural history of a disease or lesion and the effect of various treatments on the outcome and to communicate these findings to others. Over time, it became clear that histopathologists and cytopathologists could not accurately and reproducibly differentiate between severe dysplasia and carcinoma *in situ.* In addition, clinicians managed these two lesions in a similar fashion. Therefore, in 1976, Richart proposed the terminology of *cervical intraepithelial neoplasia* (*CIN*), which combined the categories of severe dysplasia and carcinoma *in situ* into the term *CIN 3.* Cervical intraepithelial neoplasia, grade 1 (CIN 1) was essentially the same as mild dysplasia, and CIN 2 was similar to moderate dysplasia. But CIN 3 combined severe dysplasia and carcinoma *in situ,* thus simplifying the classification from four categories to three (Table 46.1). This practical terminology was favored by clinicians and widely adopted throughout the world. It has been used for both cytologic and histologic diagnoses.

However, as the role of human papillomavirus (HPV) in cervical neoplasia became more evident and the difficulties of intraobserver variation with a lack of reproducibility of cytologic diagnoses became better accepted, another change in terminology was undertaken. At a series of conferences held at the National Cancer Institute in Bethesda, Maryland, *The Bethesda System* was introduced and first published in 1991 and subsequently updated and revised in 2001 (Table 46.2). These conferences clarified a number of ill defined or previously undefined problems with cytologic diagnoses, such as what constituted an adequate specimen for accurate interpretation. It tried to eliminate the term *atypia,* which had become increasingly used to designate a wide range of nonspecific changes that were clinically confusing. The Bethesda System combined HPV cytopathologic effects, often referred to as *koilocytosis,* with mild dysplasia or CIN 1 into a category called *low-grade squamous intraepithelial lesion* (LSIL). More significant lesions—including moderate and severe dysplasia and carcinoma *in situ,* or CIN 2 and 3—were combined into *high-grade squamous intraepithelial lesion* (HSIL). Pap tests with "cellular abnormalities that are more marked than those attributable to reactive changes but that quantitatively or qualitatively fall short of a definitive diagnosis of squamous intraepithelial lesion" are placed in a category called *atypical squamous cells* (ASC). These specimens may be further categorized as *of undetermined significance* (ASC-US) or *cannot exclude high grade* (ASC-H). This latter category, together with more specific diagnostic terminology for glandular abnormalities, were new additions in the 2001 revision of the Bethesda System. Although the Bethesda System terminology for reporting the results of cervical cytology has been almost universally accepted in the United States and is used in many other countries, other terminology and definitions are used in Great Britain, Germany, Australia, and other countries, which creates some difficulty in publishing and understanding scientific studies from different countries.

In the United States, a typical laboratory that processes cervical cytology from an average, generally low-risk population reports epithelial cell abnormalities in about 5% to 6% of patients. Usually one half to two thirds of these abnormalities are ASC (2%–4%), whereas 1% to 2% are LSIL and 0.5% to 1.0% are HSIL diagnoses, with occasional glandular cell abnormalities. The ratio of ASC to SIL diagnoses should be between 2:1 and 3:1 for most cytology laboratories.

The Bethesda System was designed and published to be used for cytologic diagnoses; however, it has been applied increasingly to histologic or tissue diagnoses. This is advantageous in that it provides uniform terminology for both cytology and cervical biopsies. However, by combining moderate dysplasia, severe dysplasia, and carcinoma *in situ,* it lacks the imagined specificity that is occasionally helpful in clinical management decisions. The word *imagined* is used intentionally because many studies have shown that there is a significant lack of reproducibility in the diagnoses of various grades of dysplasia and even carcinoma *in situ.* There is no clear dividing line between the different cytologic or histologic grades of cervical epithelial atypias, lesions, or neoplasias, and the diagnosis

TABLE 46.1

THE CHANGING TERMINOLOGY OF CERVICAL CYTOLOGY

Dysplasia	CIN	Bethesda[a]
Mild	Grade 1	Low-grade SIL
Moderate	Grade 2	High-grade SIL
Severe	Grade 3	High-grade SIL
Carcinoma *in situ*	Grade 3	High-grade SIL

[a]The Bethesda System classification of low-grade SIL includes both CIN 1 and HPV changes.
SIL, squamous intraepithelial lesion; CIN, cervical intraepithelial neoplasia; HPV, human papillomavirus.

TABLE 46.2

THE BETHESDA SYSTEM OF CYTOLOGIC CLASSIFICATION

The 2001 Bethesda System (Abridged)

SPECIMEN ADEQUACY

Satisfactory for evaluation (*note presence/absence of endocervical/transformation zone component*)

Unsatisfactory for evaluation . . . (*specify reason*)

- Specimen rejected/not processed (*specify reason*)
- Specimen processed and examined, but unsatisfactory for evaluation of epithelial abnormality because of (*specify reason*)

GENERAL CATEGORIZATION (OPTIONAL)

Negative for intraepithelial lesion or malignancy

Epithelial cell abnormality

Other

INTERPRETATION/RESULT

Negative for Intraepithelial Lesion or Malignancy

Organisms

- *Trichomonas vaginalis*
- Fungal organisms morphologically consistent with *Candida* species
- Shift in flora suggestive of bacterial vaginosis
- Bacteria morphologically consistent with *Actinomyces* species
- Cellular changes consistent with herpes simplex virus

Other nonneoplastic findings (*Optional to report; list not comprehensive*)

- Reactive cellular changes associated with inflammation (includes typical repair), radiation, intrauterine contraceptive device
- Glandular cells status posthysterectomy
- Atrophy

Epithelial Cell Abnormalities

- Squamous cell
  - Atypical squamous cells (ASC)
    - Of undetermined significance (ASC-US)
    - Cannot exclude high-grade squamous intraepithelial lesion (HSIL) (ASC-H)
  - Low-grade squamous intraepithelial lesion (LSIL)
    - Encompassing human papillomavirus/mild dysplasia/cervical intraepithelial neoplasia (CIN) 1
  - High-grade squamous intraepithelial lesion (HSIL)
    - Encompassing moderate and severe dysplasia, carcinoma *in situ,* CIN 2 and CIN 3
  - Squamous cell carcinoma
- Glandular cell
  - Atypical glandular cells (AGC) (*specify endocervical, endometrial, or not otherwise specified*)
  - Atypical glandular cells, favor neoplastic (*specify endocervical or not otherwise specified*)
  - Endocervical adenocarcinoma *in situ* (AIS)
  - Adenocarcinoma

Other (*List not comprehensive*)

- Endometrial cells in a woman ≥40 years of age

AUTOMATED REVIEW AND ANCILLARY TESTING (INCLUDE AS APPROPRIATE)

EDUCATIONAL NOTES AND SUGGESTIONS (OPTIONAL)

on the Papanicolaou or biopsy report is a general impression, not a precise predictor of the benign or malignant behavior of the cervical epithelium sampled. Nevertheless, many clinicians would favor conservative follow-up only in an 18-year-old with CIN 2 or moderate dysplasia, but a diagnosis of CIN 3 or severe dysplasia would make the same clinicians favor treatment. Both diagnoses fit into the HSIL category, and this creates a problem of possible overtreatment or overevaluation for some patients with a cytologic or histologic diagnosis of HSIL. The clinician's desire for a precise cytologic or histologic diagnosis that accurately predicts the likelihood of a given lesion to progress to invasive cancer cannot be satisfied by even the most experienced and expert pathologist. However, molecular markers, including HPV and P-16 testing, provide hope for more specific clinical predictors in the future.

EPIDEMIOLOGY

In 1842, Rigoni-Stern noted that cervical cancer was found in married women, but was virtually absent in celibate groups such as Catholic nuns. This observation was one of the earliest epidemiologic studies of any cancer. Others noted that cervical cancer was almost never found in virginal women and that a woman's risk of developing cervical cancer was directly related to the number of male sex partners she had had. Subsequent epidemiologic studies reported that early age at first sexual intercourse, low socioeconomic status, cigarette smoking, and early age at first pregnancy increased a woman's risk of cervical neoplasia. More recently, it became obvious that immunosuppression from any cause, including infection with human immunodeficiency virus (HIV), substantially increased a woman's risk of cervical neoplasia. Oral contraceptive use has been reported to increase a woman's risk of cervical cancer as well, but the odds ratios are relatively low, and it is difficult to control for confounding factors.

Many of these epidemiologic studies have shown a pattern of cervical cancer that is typical for a sexually transmitted infection. For this reason, investigators focused on etiologic agents that might be passed by intimate sexual contact. Virtually every sexually transmitted agent has been studied for its relation to cervical neoplasia, including *Chlamydia,* gonorrhea, *Gardnerella, Mycoplasma, Trichomonas,* and herpes simplex virus (HSV).

As the epidemiologists studied the lifestyle characteristics of women with cervical cancer and cytopathologists described the microscopic morphologic transition of the cervical epithelium, clinicians were observing certain abnormalities on the cervix in patients with the preinvasive changes of cervical dysplasia. First popularized by Hinselmann in Germany, the *colposcope* is a magnifying instrument used to examine the cervix. With the colposcope, vascular changes and other epithelial patterns were recognized and correlated with the cytologic and histologic changes that were being described. These early neoplastic changes were most prominent adjacent to the squamocolumnar junction (SCJ), and this area was called the *transformation zone.* With time, colposcopic patterns associated with the developing stages of dysplasia and early invasive cancer were identified and described by Mestwerdt, Wespi, Kolstad, Stafl, Barghardt, Coupez, Coppelson, and others. In 1974, Stafl and Mattingly brilliantly synthesized these observations and the work of the epidemiologists and proposed a theory of the development of cervical cancer (Fig. 46.1). They did not know the identity of the environmental carcinogen that they presumed was sexually transmitted, but they proposed a framework that has been enormously useful for the clinician.

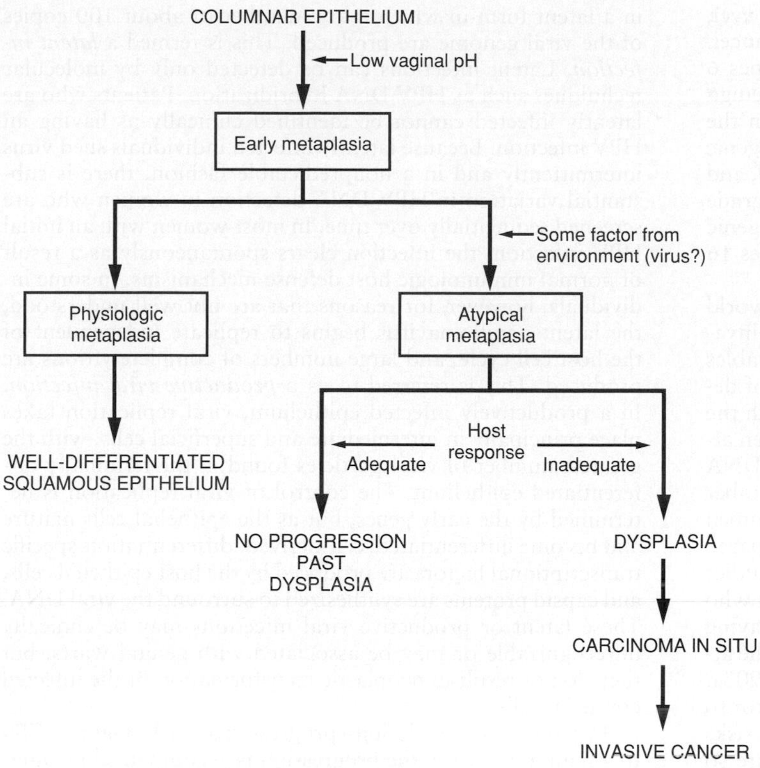

FIGURE 46.1. Diagrammatic illustration of the theory of development of cervical neoplasia proposed by Stafl and Mattingly. (From Stafl A, Mattingly. Vaginal adenosis: a precancerous lesion? *Am J Obstet Gynecol* 1974:120:666.)

In 1976, Meisels and Fortin—and in 1977, Purola and Savia—reported finding HPV in the nuclei of dysplastic squamous epithelial cells, particularly those that had koilocytotic features. These observations were confirmed by a number of other investigators, and it was suggested by zur Hausen that this virus might be important etiologically in cervical carcinogenesis. Using electron microscopy and antibodies to the HPV capsid protein, several investigators identified viral particles or HPV-related antigens in CIN. They were particularly prevalent in low-grade lesions and became less frequently observed in cells associated with higher-grade lesions. These observations strongly implicated HPV as a possible etiologic agent in cervical neoplasia and led to an explosion of molecular and clinical studies of HPV and its related lesions.

HUMAN PAPILLOMAVIRUSES

Human papillomaviruses are members of a large family of viruses known as the *Papovaviridae*. This includes another oncogenic DNA virus, the simian virus 40 (SV40), as well as the polyomavirus. All the viruses in this group are DNA tumor viruses. Although they have dissimilar DNA base-pair sequences and dissimilar capsular antigens, they appear to produce neoplasms through similar mechanisms. The papillomaviruses have a tightly coiled, circular, double-stranded DNA molecule about 8,000 base pairs in length. The complete virion consists of a DNA core and a surrounding protein capsid that measures about 45 to 55 nm in diameter. The capsid has an icosahedral shape. Papillomaviruses are found throughout the animal kingdom and infect not only humans but cattle, rabbits, dogs, deer, monkeys, and birds. The viruses are highly species specific. Cross-infections between species have not been reported. Unlike many viruses that infect humans and that are classified by their surface antigens, the papillomaviruses are classified according to their DNA base-pair sequence. The degree of relatedness is determined by the degree of hybridization homology.

Although in animals papillomaviruses can infect both epithelial cells and fibroblasts, the human papillomavirus is an exclusively epitheliotropic virus that produces alterations in the supporting structures solely as a secondary effect related to infection of the epithelium. HPV infects virtually all surface epithelia, including the skin and mucous membranes. The infected epithelium is characterized by epithelial proliferation at the infected site, by various degrees of epithelial thickening, and by papillomatosis.

At least 100 HPV types have been identified; about 25 of these affect the male and female anogenital tract. The most prevalent anogenital HPVs can be divided into three groups that are predictive of their ability to produce neoplasia (Table 46.3). Low-risk HPV types are commonly associated with

TABLE 46.3

ANOGENITAL HPV TYPES[a]

Low-risk types	6, 11, 40, 42, 43, 44, 53, 54, 61, 72, 73, 81
High-risk types	16, 18, 31, 33, 35, 39, 45, 51, 52, 56, 58, 59, 68, 82
Possible high-risk types	26, 66, 73

[a]Adapted from Munoz N, Bosch FX, de Sanjose S, et al. Epidemiologic classification of human papillomavirus types associated with cervical cancer. *N Engl J Med* 2003;348:518.
From Clinical Uses of Human Papillomavirus (HPV) DNA Testing. ASCCP, 2004

cellular changes described as CIN 1, but they rarely, if ever, are associated with high-grade dysplasia or invasive cancer. They may also be associated with condyloma. HPV types 6 and 11 are responsible for approximately 90% of all benign genital warts (condyloma) seen in the United States. On the other hand, the anogenital HPV types with a high oncogenic risk are types 16, 18, 31, 33, 35, 39, 45, 51, 52, 56, 58, 59, and 68. HPVs in this risk group are overrepresented in high-grade lesions. The group with a low oncogenic risk or no oncogenic risk includes HPV types 6, 11, 42, 43, and 44. HPV types 16 and 18 are very-high-risk cervical cancer viruses.

Recent epidemiologic studies from all parts of the world have shown that almost all high-grade CIN lesions and invasive cancers contain HPV DNA. In addition, the covariables that have traditionally been associated with a high risk of developing cervical neoplasia are also highly correlated with the presence of HPV DNA. In a relatively large study of women attending a university health clinic, it was found that HPV DNA positivity was strongly correlated with an increasing number of sexual partners; the prevalence of HPV infection in women with 10 or more lifetime sexual partners was 69%, compared with 21% in women with only a single sexual partner. In studies by Schiffman and colleagues, it was reported that women who are HPV DNA positive have a relative risk of 40% of having an abnormal Papanicolaou smear. He also reported that the attributable risk of HPV in such populations is greater than 90%. The only other covariable that was a significant contributor to risk was cigarette smoking. He also noted that "relative risks and attributable risks of this strength and consistency are so rare that the statistical association of HPV and cervical neoplasia is beyond question" and that "the epidemiological data support a central, causal role for genital HPV infection in the etiology of cervical neoplasia."

In a compilation of worldwide data, Clifford and colleagues reported that HPV-16 was found in about 50% of all invasive cervical cancers studied, and HPV-18 was found in approximately 12%. Women with an HPV-16 genital infection are 435 times more likely to develop invasive cervical cancer than women with no HPV infection. The enormous magnitude of this risk can be appreciated when one considers that the risk of endometrial cancer associated with unopposed estrogen is about eightfold, and cigarette smokers have an approximately 20-fold risk of lung cancer. The overwhelming risk of cervical cancer in women with high-risk HPV types is one of several lines of evidence that link HPV to cervical cancer. Thus, *the clinical, histologic, molecular, and epidemiologic data all support HPV as the causative agent for most, if not all, epithelial cancer of the cervix.*

Human Papillomavirus Genome and the Mechanism of Carcinogenesis

The HPV genome has been very well studied and is relevant to this chapter because the molecular mechanisms involved have allowed scientists and clinicians to understand the process of malignant transformation and thus develop diagnostic tests and prophylactic vaccines to screen for and, it is hoped, prevent cervical cancer.

The papillomavirus infects only epithelium. In the cervix, viral access also occurs via microtrauma to the thin, immature portions of the transformation zone adjacent to the SCJ, where the metaplastic squamous epithelium consists principally of immature basal- and parabasal-type cells. When a mitotically active epithelial cell is infected, the virus may remain in the cell in a latent form in which a low number of about 100 copies of the viral genome are produced. This is termed a *latent infection.* Latent infections can be detected only by molecular techniques such as HPV DNA hybridization. Patients who are latently infected cannot be identified clinically as having an HPV infection. Because latently infected individuals shed virus intermittently and in a nonpredictable fashion, there is substantial variation in HPV DNA detection in women who are screened sequentially over time. In most women with an initial HPV infection, the infection clears spontaneously as a result of normal immunologic host defense mechanisms. In some individuals, however, for reasons that are not well understood, the latent papillomavirus begins to replicate independent of the host cell cycle, and large numbers of complete virions are produced. This is referred to as a *productive viral infection.* In a productively infected epithelium, viral replication takes place principally in intermediate and superficial cells, with the greatest number of viral particles found in the terminally differentiated epithelium. The control of viral replication is determined by the early genes, but as the epithelial cells mature and become differentiated, cell-derived, differentiation-specific transcriptional factors are produced by the host epithelial cells, and capsid proteins are synthesized to surround the viral DNA. These latent or productive viral infections may be clinically unrecognizable or may be associated with genital warts, but they do not result in neoplastic transformation of the infected epithelial cells.

In patients whose lesions progress from a low-grade CIN to a high-grade CIN, the progression is accompanied by alterations in the virus-host interaction. These interactions appear to be critical to the transformation of normal epithelial cells to neoplastic cells. The key alteration seems to be the integration of the viral DNA into host chromosomes. Because the episomal (nonchromosomal) virus that is found in latently or productively infected cells is in a circular form and because the DNA in the host chromosomes is linear, a change in the physical state of the virus must take place before the viral DNA can be integrated into the host chromosome. What initiates this change and the mechanism by which it occurs is not yet understood, but the circular strand of viral DNA is opened and the linear DNA can be spliced into the host DNA. It can then use the protein production apparatus of the transformed host cell.

The viral genome of HPV can be divided into three regions: the upstream regulatory region (URR), the early region, and the late region (Fig. 46.2). The URR is a noncoding region that has as its major functions the regulation of viral replication and the transcription of downstream sequences in the early region. The early and the late region both contain a series of open reading frames (ORFs), linear sequences that lack stop codons and hence are potentially transcribable into proteins. The early region transcribes proteins that are important in the early life cycle of the virus and interact with the cellular genome to program the host cell to produce new viral DNA. The late region, as the name implies, encodes for capsid proteins that surround the DNA core to produce the infectious unit: the complete virion.

Six different ORFs have been identified in the early region of HPV. They are designated E_1, E_2, E_4, E_5, E_6, and E_7. These viral genes are extremely important because they control the process of viral replication, they encode for the maintenance of a high intracellular viral copy number, and they encode for the genes whose transcription produces the oncogenic proteins that transform the normal cervical cells into neoplastic cells. The E_6 and E_7 ORFs encode for two highly oncogenic proteins by which the oncogenic HPV types transform normal cervical cells into neoplastic cells. In laboratory experiments, the E_7

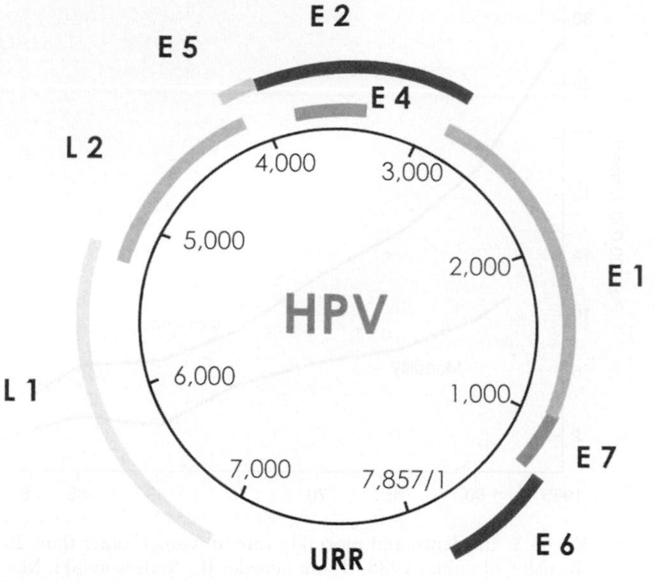

FIGURE 46.2. Schematic representation of the circular HPV genome. Transcription by the "early" (E_{1-7} or nonstructural) genes and the "late" (capsid protein) genes is controlled by the upstream regulatory region (URR). (From Munoz N, Catellsague X, de Gonzalez AB, et al. *Vaccine* 2006;24S3:2.)

protein binds to the pRB protein, which in turn triggers E_2F transcription factor, which leads to the production of proteins required for cellular DNA synthesis. By this mechanism, the virus takes over control of the infected epithelial cell and uses its synthetic mechanism to produce new viral DNA and viral proteins. This out-of-sequence initiation of new (viral) DNA synthesis by the HPV E_7 protein would ordinarily lead to activation of epithelial cell p53 protein, an important protector of the normal cell cycle. In such circumstances, p53 would initiate the process of apoptosis leading to death of the epithelial cell, thus halting the hijacked DNA synthetic mechanism. However, the HPV E_6 protein targets p53 for proteolytic degradation, allowing oncogenic HPV types to bypass this key cellular control mechanism.

The late-region ORFs, designated L_1 and L_2, are transcribed late in the replication cycle and encode for major and minor capsid proteins. The L_1-encoded protein predominates in the capsid, is highly conserved among papillomaviruses, and is similar in all HPV types. On the other hand, the L_2-encoded protein is highly variable between different HPV types and largely accounts for the differences in antigenicity from one HPV type to another. *The current prophylactic HPV vaccines are targeted against these HPV capsid proteins and thus are HPV-type specific.* All the proteins that are transcribed in the late region appear to be regulated by cell-derived transcriptional proteins that are produced only by squamous epithelial cells undergoing terminal maturation. The quantity of L_1- and L_2-encoded capsid proteins is highly correlated with terminal maturation of the epithelium. Well-differentiated HPV-induced lesions, such as condylomata, are generally rich in L_1- and L_2-encoded proteins, whereas high-grade CIN lesions, which tend to be highly undifferentiated, contain only small quantities of capsid proteins.

Since the importance of HPV in the etiology of cervical neoplasia has become more certain, various investigators have suggested that a vaccine against papillomavirus might prevent infection and perhaps even eliminate the virus in already infected individuals. This idea of immunization against HPV type 16 was tested in a clinical trial by Koutsky and colleagues, who prospectively randomized almost 2,400 young women who tested negative for HPV type 16 infection, immunized half with three doses of viruslike particle vaccine, and treated the other half with placebo. The patients were then followed up for a median of 17 months, and the risk of developing a persistent HPV type 16 infection was 3.8 per 100 women-years in the placebo group compared with 0 in the vaccinated patients (p >0.001). CIN developed in nine women in the placebo group, whereas there was no instance of CIN among the vaccinated women.

Natural History of Human Papillomavirus Infections

For centuries, clinicians have speculated that cervical cancer was caused by some infectious agent transmitted by intimate sexual contact. We have seen how many investigators have shown that this agent is HPV. But although it is true that all women with cervical cancer have been infected with HPV, most women with an HPV infection *do not* develop cervical cancer. Infections with HPV are very common in young sexually active women throughout the world. In a study of 60 college women, Brown and associates found that 28% were infected with HPV at the time they entered college. These women were closely followed and tested at frequent intervals. Four years later, when they left college, 40% tested positive for HPV. However, the interval examinations showed that most women cleared their infection and later become positive again following exposure to a new boyfriend. Overall, 82% of these women tested positive for HPV, and 77% tested positive for high-risk oncogenic HPV during the 5 years of the study. In other studies of young women, similar results have been found, and it appears that most women clear their infections within 12 months or so. On average, about 50% of women who test positive for HPV will test negative at 6 months, about 70% will be negative at 12 months, and by 24 months, only 8% to 20% remain positive. It seems as if the highly oncogenic types 16 and 18 are more slowly cleared than the less oncogenic HPV types.

It has been observed that women with transient HPV infection have a much lower risk of developing high-grade CIN. Although women with transient infections may develop cervical abnormalities that result in abnormal Pap tests and even colposcopic abnormalities, these are usually low-grade lesions and often clear spontaneously. Approximately 50% of women with a diagnosis of CIN 1 will resolve their lesions over 2 years without any active therapy. Women with highly oncogenic HPV types are more likely to have persistent infections, and they are at increased risk to develop high-grade CIN. In an analysis of HPV screening data of more than 20,000 women in the Portland, Oregon, area, Khan and colleagues found that women who had a negative Pap test and tested negative for any HPV had a less than 1% risk of developing CIN 3 within 10 years of follow-up. This contrasted sharply with women who had a negative Pap but who tested positive for HPV-16 on study entry; they had a 17.3% risk of developing CIN 3 or greater during the next 10 years. The risk of CIN 3 was 11.8%; for those who tested positive for other HPV types, the risk was only 3%. At least half of these women develop high-grade CIN within 24 months, so the rate of progression may be relatively rapid in some patients.

The patient's immune system clearly plays an important and yet poorly understood role in the clearance or progression of

HPV. Women with impaired immunocompetence, such as those infected with HIV, and women who are immunosuppressed by various medications or chronic disease have a higher rate and, perhaps, more rapid progression of CIN that may make it more difficult to achieve a long-term cure.

Human Papillomavirus Vaccine

The immunogenicity of the virus and the development of antibodies with clearance of detectable virus in many women suggested the possibility of developing a vaccine against HPV. Prophylactic vaccines against HPV-16 and -18 and -6 and -11 have been clinically tested and are highly effective in HPV-naïve women. These have been introduced and are available in many countries, including the United States. Very few serious adverse side effects have been noted. However, it must be remembered that the current vaccines are effective only for preventing cancer and high-grade CIN related to HPV-16 or -18. Although these two viral types cause approximately 70% of all cervical cancer, several other viral types (31, 33, 45, and others) are responsible for almost a third of cervical cancer. In addition, women who have already been exposed to HPV-16 or -18 will not be protected by the vaccine. Continued cervical cancer screening will certainly be required for the foreseeable future.

SCREENING FOR CERVICAL NEOPLASIA

Cervical Cytology

After the introduction of cervical cytology for cervical cancer screening more than 50 years ago, multiple screening programs from all parts of the world have reported decreased rates of invasive cervical cancer and decreased death rates from a malignancy that had previously been the number-one worldwide cause of cancer deaths in women. Yet, even today, cervical cancer remains one of the leading causes of death for women in developing nations where Papanicolaou smear screening programs are nonexistent. The cervical screening program in the Province of British Columbia, Canada, is one of many examples of how effective cervical cytology screening can be. Since the implementation of a population-based Papanicolaou smear screening program in 1949, the incidence rate of invasive cervical cancer has decreased from more than 30 per 100,000 women to less than 5, and the mortality rate has decreased from 12 to about 3 per 100,000 (Fig. 46.3). These excellent results have been obtained through a combination of a population-based program with a central registry that notifies women every 3 years that their screening visit is due and follows up to be sure they do not default (a "call and recall" system); an excellent central cytology laboratory with well-trained clinicians to obtain the smears; and a network of colposcopy follow-up clinics where women with abnormal results are evaluated and treated. The program is well organized, with quality control built in at every level, and funding for this preventive health service and any follow-up or treatment required is universally provided to all residents of the province. All of these elements are required to achieve excellent results from a screening program.

Despite the effectiveness of this and other cervical cytology screening programs, there are several limitations of Papanicolaou smear screening. A single Pap smear has a sensitivity of only about 50% to 60%. This means that a single test will

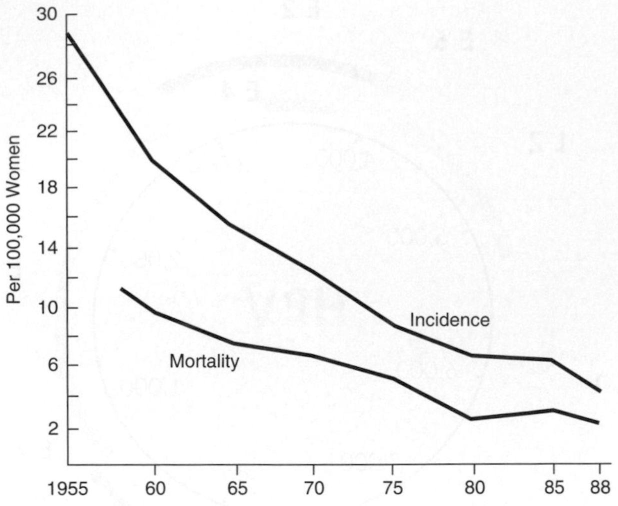

FIGURE 46.3. Incidence and mortality rate in women older than 20 years. British Columbia, 1988. (From Benedet JL, Anderson GH, Matisic JP. A comprehensive program for cervical cancer detection and management. *Am J Obstet Gynecol* 1992;166:1254.)

not detect a cervical lesion in many women. However, the slow progression of CIN before the development of an invasive cancer provides the opportunity for multiple screening cytologies over a period of years. So even with limited sensitivity, if three consecutive tests are negative, there is less than a 1% chance that the patient will have a high-grade cervical abnormality.

A false-negative Papanicolaou smear may result from either screening or interpretation problems. Screening problems include lesions that do not shed cells or that are not sampled by the clinician. Or, sometimes, the diagnostic cells are not transferred from the spatula or collection device to the glass slide. Rarely, the slide preparation or staining is unsatisfactory. In other patients, problems with interpretation include failure to identify abnormal cells or misinterpretation of cells that are diagnosed as reactive or metaplastic when a dysplastic lesion exists. Various studies have shown that women who are diagnosed with invasive cervical cancer after a reportedly "negative" Papanicolaou smear most often have abnormal cells on review of their slides. The diagnostic cells may be few in number or obscured by blood or inflammatory changes. It is unfortunate that litigation over the "missed diagnosis" of cervical neoplasia is such a common problem for cytology laboratories in the United States. The threat of a lawsuit may cause cytologists and cytopathologists to "overcall" a diagnosis and the gynecologist to recommend colposcopy and possibly cervical biopsy in a patient with any hint of abnormality. This not only increases the anxiety and morbidity associated with cervical cancer screening, but it also increases the costs.

Liquid-Based, Thin-Layer Cytology

To decrease the false-negative rate of cervical cytology, attempts have been made to improve both specimen collection and quality and to reduce errors of interpretation. Over the past several years, several liquid-based techniques have been approved by the Food and Drug Administration in the United States. These techniques differ from the conventional method of Papanicolaou smear collection in several ways. Once the clinician obtains a scraping of the SCJ and transformation zone area of the exocervix, the spatula and brush are dipped and agitated in a small bottle of fixative solution to elute the cells rather than being smeared on a glass slide. This bottle is then labeled and sent to the cytology laboratory rather than sending a slide. Once in the lab, a machine prepares a slide containing about 40,000 representative epithelial cells in a thin layer. The slide is then stained with the conventional Papanicolaou stain and reviewed by the cytologists and cytopathologist. Several studies have shown that more diagnostic cervical cells are collected by this liquid-based technique and that the slides prepared from this sample provide a "cleaner" appearance with less clumping, blood, and inflammatory changes, thus providing a better specimen and, it is hoped, a better interpretation. In a review, Dunton found that thin-layer, liquid-based cytology resulted in significantly fewer unsatisfactory or "satisfactory, but limited by" specimens and that more patients were diagnosed with both low- and high-grade lesions. The Agency for Healthcare Research and Quality evaluated the literature available and concluded, "The relative true-positive rate for ThinPrep compared to conventional cytology is 1.13, suggesting a modestly higher sensitivity with ThinPrep, the relative false-positive rate is 1.12, suggesting a modestly lower specificity." This new technology costs more money than the conventional Papanicolaou smear, but theoretical analysis suggests that these costs are balanced by the possibility of less frequent screening intervals made possible by a more sensitive test. Liquid-based cytology reduces the rate of false-negative results from both screening and interpretation errors.

Computer-Assisted Diagnosis

It has long been believed that optical scanning by computer could be used for Papanicolaou smear interpretation, but differences in staining and the overlap of cells has made practical application very difficult. However, in the past several years, two different computer-based systems for cervical cytology use have been approved by the Food and Drug Administration. The widespread use of liquid-based cervical cytology specimens has greatly enhanced the applicability of these optical image recognition systems. Although the initial cost of these computer-based systems is large, considerable savings should be realized by the around-the-clock work and a reduced need for cytotechnologists, who could concentrate on the diagnostic evaluation of high-risk slides identified by the computer on primary screening. More clinical experience with these techniques is needed, but early results are promising.

Visual Inspection

Although colposcopy has been used for cervical cancer screening in some areas of Europe and South America, it is time-consuming, it requires well-trained clinicians, and it is expensive in most countries. However, simple visual inspection of the cervix after application of acetic acid has been effectively used in resource-poor settings for cervical cancer screening. Areas of cervical dysplasia turn white after application of acetic acid, and inspection of the cervix using handheld 3× magnifying lenses can identify many CIN lesions. This technique, commonly referred to as VIA (visual inspection with acetic acid), has been effectively used in areas of Africa, India, and China. Nurses or even health care technicians can be trained to use the technique and do biopsies or refer women with suspicious lesions for more extensive evaluation. Although VIA is not as specific as cytology, it is almost as sensitive and does not require several visits or the considerable infrastructure needed by cytologic screening.

Human Papillomavirus Testing

With the knowledge that significant cervical neoplasia is always associated with HPV, it has been suggested that HPV testing could be used to screen women for cervical neoplasia. HPV testing in the past has been inaccurate, and the complex laboratory techniques were not conducive to large-volume clinical work. However, with the newer second-generation hybrid capture techniques, these problems seem to have been solved. Current technology uses DNA hybridization and quantification by a chemiluminescence reaction to identify the presence of any of 13 different, high-risk HPV subtypes. Indeed, HPV testing was demonstrated to be more sensitive than traditional Pap smear or liquid-based cytology in a study by Schiffman and colleagues. In a trial of 1,119 high-risk women in Costa Rica, HPV testing demonstrated an 88% sensitivity to detect high-grade lesions compared with a Papanicolaou test sensitivity of 77.7%. Twelve percent of the women screened were HPV positive and were referred for colposcopy as compared with a 6.9% referral rate with Papanicolaou smear screening. In a similar trial from South Africa, Wright and colleagues instructed patients on self-collection of vaginal samples and were able to detect high-risk HPV DNA in 66% of the patients with high-grade lesions. This was almost identical to the 68% pickup rate of abnormal cytology collected at the time of a pelvic examination by a clinician. High-risk HPV was detected in 84% of the specimens obtained by the clinician during a pelvic examination. However, in high-risk, sexually active populations, many women with a subclinical HPV infection clear the virus without ever developing cervical neoplasia. In the South African trial, 15% of the women who tested positive for HPV had no identifiable cervical lesion. Nevertheless, HPV testing is easy to perform and is a relatively inexpensive test that can be automated in the laboratory and requires no interpretation (a problem with the Papanicolaou test). These advantages must be weighted against its lack of specificity for high-grade lesions; however, it may be of particular benefit in resource-poor settings where cytology laboratories are not available. Many studies from various parts of the world have confirmed the excellent sensitivity of HPV screening for cervical cancer, but its lack of specificity compared with cytology remains a problem.

Several approaches have been suggested to improve the specificity of HPV testing. Because the prevalence of HPV infection in most populations decreases dramatically after age 30 or 35, it has been suggested that HPV screening would be more specific for cervical neoplasia in the population. Indeed, when Cuzick and associates screened a series of 10,358 women older than age 30, they found a sensitivity of 97.1% and a specificity of 93.3% for detecting CIN 2 or worse. Only 7.5% required referral for colposcopy.

Even better specificity and improved sensitivity can be achieved by combining HPV testing with cervical cytology. Several large studies from Europe, America, Africa, and China were reviewed by Wright and associates in 2004. They found that the combination of HPV testing plus cytology produced a sensitivity of more than 95% for detecting CIN 2 or greater in most studies. Even more important, when cytology was added to HPV testing, the specificity was better than 90% in most studies. Both sensitivity and specificity were better with the combination of the two tests than with either one alone. The problem with this, of course, is the cost. Theoretical analysis indicates that in the United States, if HPV testing and cervical cytology were done in women older than age 30, and if both tests were done only every 3 years if they were both negative, screening for CIN 2 or greater would be more sensitive and less expensive than conventional Pap smears every year or liquid-based cytology every other year. The American College of Obstetricians and Gynecologists recognized this in their 2003 Cervical Cytology Screening Practice Bulletin. Management of women with a normal Pap but who test positive for high-risk HPV is still somewhat controversial, but it is probably reasonable to rescreen them again in 6 to 12 months.

EVALUATION OF ABNORMAL CYTOLOGY

Following the announcement of the 2001 Bethesda System terminology for reporting the results of cervical cytology, the American Society of Colposcopy and Cervical Pathology sponsored a 3-day consensus conference to develop management guidelines. These guidelines were revised at another Consensus Conference held in 2006. The guidelines, which are evidence based and carefully crafted to include almost all situations, were published by Wright and colleagues in 2007. It is important for the clinician to distinguish between cytologic or Papanicolaou smear diagnosis and biopsy or histologic diagnosis. In this subsection, the evaluation of cytologic abnormalities are discussed; in the following subsection, the management of patients with biopsy-proven abnormalities is presented. In both sections, high-grade abnormalities are discussed first because they are the least controversial and most important. Treatment rarely is initiated based on the results of cervical cytology alone. The Papanicolaou smear result, colposcopic impression, and biopsy diagnosis should all be in general agreement, although it is common that they vary slightly on the grade of abnormality.

High-Grade Squamous Intraepithelial Lesions

Approximately 0.5% of all Papanicolaou smears are diagnosed as HSIL (Fig. 46.4). When these patients are evaluated, more than 70% will have biopsy-proven moderate dysplasia (CIN 2) or worse, and 1% to 2% will have an invasive cancer. Because high-grade abnormalities may progress to invasive cancer or, indeed, be associated with an already existing invasive cancer, women with an HSIL cytologic diagnosis should be referred for colposcopic evaluation.

In many cases, biopsy confirmation of the lesion will be done by loop electrode excision procedure (LEEP) of the whole transformation zone, which serves as both a diagnostic and a treatment procedure. This is particularly important in large, high-grade lesions because the colposcopic diagnosis of microinvasive cancer is difficult. Unless excision and histologic study of the whole transformation zone is done, microinvasive cancer may be missed.

If a woman with an HSIL Papanicolaou smear does not have a high-grade lesion identified on colposcopy of the cervix and upper vagina, an endocervical curettage (ECC) should be done. If the origin of the HSIL Papanicolaou finding is still not identified, the clinician should request a review of the cytology, ECC, and any cervical biopsies. If the cytopathologist still believes that a high-grade lesion exists that has not been identified by biopsy, then the cervix and vagina should be reexamined and a LEEP or cone biopsy done, especially if the SCJ cannot be visualized. Consultation with an expert colposcopist should be considered.

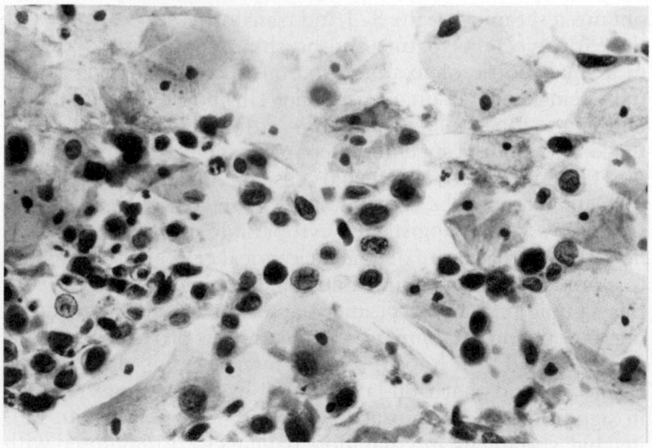

FIGURE 46.4. Papanicolaou smear showing high-grade cervical intraepithelial neoplasia. Normal superficial cells contain small, pyknotic, regular nuclei. Abnormal cells exfoliated from high-grade lesions are of the neoplastic basal and parabasal types, have an altered nuclear:cytoplasmic ratio, and contain very hyperchromatic, irregularly shaped, pleomorphic nuclei with a dense, abnormal chromatin pattern.

Low-Grade Squamous Intraepithelial Lesion

Of all Papanicolaou smear diagnoses, about 1.5% to 2.0% are LSIL. Between 15% and 30% of these women have moderate dysplasia or worse, and 1 to 2 per 1,000 have invasive cancer (Fig. 46.5). Although the risk of a significant lesion is lower in these women, referral for colposcopic evaluation is still recommended.

There are many treatment options for women with mild dysplasia (CIN 1) on colposcopically directed biopsy. But

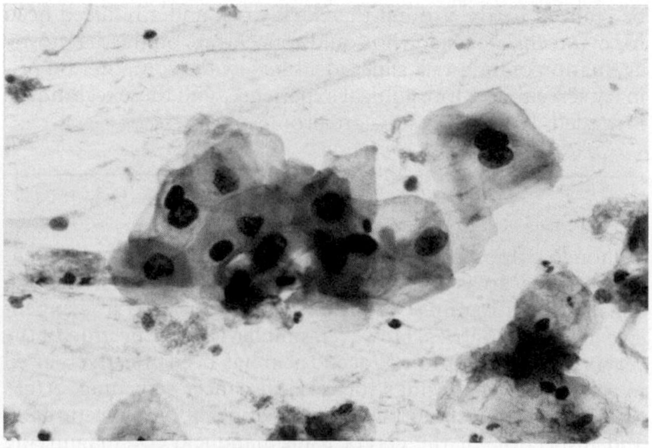

FIGURE 46.5. Papanicolaou smear showing low-grade cervical intraepithelial neoplasia. A cluster of superficial squamous cells containing hyperchromatic, atypical nuclei is seen. Several cells are binucleated. The cells with perinuclear clearing and nuclear atypia are referred to as koilocytes. These changes are characteristic of a productive human papillomavirus infection of the genital tract mucosa.

because of the wide possibility of diagnosis in women with an LSIL Papanicolaou finding, colposcopic evaluation and biopsy confirmation of the diagnosis is indicated. In a patient with no visible lesion on the exocervix and vagina to explain the abnormal Pap test, an ECC may be useful.

When no lesion to explain the LSIL Papanicolaou finding can be found, the evaluation can be repeated in 4 to 6 months, a LEEP can be done, or consultation with a more experienced colposcopist can be requested. In postmenopausal women, atrophy can cause minor cellular atypia, which can produce an LSIL Papanicolaou finding, so treatment with topical estrogen for 2 months may be helpful before repeating the cytologic study. HPV testing in these patients may be helpful.

Atypical Squamous Cells

A diagnosis of ASC is the most common abnormal Papanicolaou diagnosis, occurring in 2.5% to 5.0% of all Papanicolaou smears. Careful evaluation of women with an ASC-US diagnosis will identify 5% to 10% with a biopsy diagnosis of high-grade CIN. Although the incidence of CIN 3 may be low in women who are initially diagnosed with an ASC-US Pap, because of the large number of women who have ASC-US diagnoses, the total number with a final diagnosis of CIN 3 is large. In a review of 46,000 Paps, Kinney and associates reported 39% of the women with a final diagnosis of CIN 3 initially presented with an ASC-US Pap; more than the 31% who presented with an HSIL Pap. Although the risk of a high-grade cervical lesion is low in patients with an ASC-US Pap, because the number of patients in this category is so large, there are a significant number who will need further evaluation and treatment. Even so, immediate referral to colposcopy for all these patients *is not cost-effective* because there are so many women with no significant cervical abnormalities. A second option is to bring these patients back for *repeat Pap testing in 4 to 6 months*. This can lead to a delay in diagnosis, and it is not unusual for 20% or more of these patients to be lost to follow-up, producing an even greater delay.

The third management option for women with an ASC-US Pap finding is *triage by HPV testing*. Several large prospective studies have demonstrated the effectiveness of this approach. In a National Cancer Institute–sponsored randomized trial, Schiffman and colleagues randomized a group of 4,500 women with ASC-US Papanicolaou findings to immediate colposcopy, follow-up every 6 months until two consecutive ASC-US Paps, or HPV triage. All women were eventually colposcoped and treated by LEEP at 24 months if they had not already been diagnosed and treated for CIN earlier. In this study, HPV testing identified 95% of the patients with CIN 3 or greater and required colposcopy in only 55% of the patients. The follow-up arm was able to identify only 85% of the patients with a high-grade lesion and referred 60% for colposcopy. Even though the immediate colposcopy group should diagnose almost 100% of the CIN 3 lesions, it is very expensive in the United States, where colposcopy charges are three to four times greater than an HPV test. In locations where the cost of colposcopy is relatively less than HPV testing, immediate referral for colposcopy may be a more cost-effective management option.

Patients with a Papanicolaou diagnosis of ASC-H should be referred for colposcopy because they have a 15% to 35% risk of having moderate dysplasia or worse. Even if colposcopic evaluation, including an ECC, is negative, these patients need to be followed up carefully. HPV testing for triage in these patients is not cost-effective and not recommended; 65% to 85% of such patients test positive for high-risk HPV.

Glandular Abnormalities

In the 2001 Bethesda System, there are four categories under the classification of glandular cell abnormalities. These include atypical glandular cells (AGC), atypical glandular cells–favor neoplastic, endocervical adenocarcinoma *in situ* (AIS), and adenocarcinoma. The cytologist should state if possible whether the glandular cells are endocervical, endometrial, or not otherwise specified. Although it may be helpful for the clinician in the future, the experience with the different categories is still limited, and it remains to be proven whether cytology can reliably differentiate between glandular dysplasia and AIS—and, indeed, between AIS and invasive adenocarcinoma.

Therefore, all patients with abnormal glandular cells on Pap test should be referred for further evaluation. Follow-up studies show that 35% to 50% of these patients have a lesion and that most actually have squamous *not* glandular CIN (Fig. 46.6). A few have endocervical glandular dysplasia or AIS, and a few have endometrial hyperplasia or adenocarcinoma. Endocervical glandular neoplasia is also HPV related so that it is often accompanied by a squamous dysplasia. For this reason, the diagnosis of moderate squamous dysplasia on the exocervix in a woman with an AGC Papanicolaou smear does not rule out an accompanying glandular lesion. The workup should be continued to rule out the possibility of a glandular abnormality. The association of HPV, especially type 18, suggests that HPV testing might also serve as a useful triage step in the evaluation of women with AGC findings, but this concept has not yet been proven clinically.

Evaluation of the patient with an AGC Papanicolaou finding usually involves a colposcopic examination and an ECC, whether or not the SCJ can be visualized. An endometrial biopsy is indicated in women older than age 35 or in women with abnormal bleeding. If the ECC is positive for a glandular abnormality, a cone biopsy is indicated. Even though some experts are able to adequately excise endocervical glandular lesions with a LEEP specimen, we find that a LEEP often

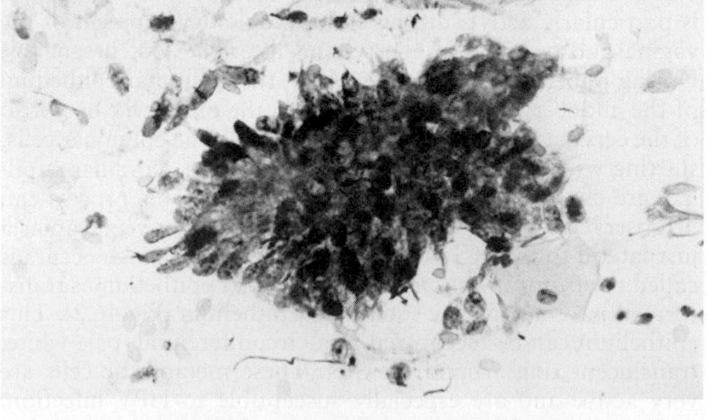

FIGURE 46.6. Papanicolaou smear showing adenocarcinoma *in situ*. A cluster of atypical endocervical cells with a feathered border and cytologically atypical nuclei characteristic of adenocarcinoma *in situ* is seen. Cells exfoliated from adenocarcinoma *in situ* tend to occur in clumps, which should raise the suspicion that a glandular neoplasm may be present.

provides a specimen that is not deep enough and the deep endocervical margin is positive. We recommend a traditional, deep, wide, cold-knife cone biopsy under anesthesia in the operating room for the definitive evaluation of endocervical glandular abnormalities. If the ECC is negative and the colposcopic examination is normal, the Papanicolaou diagnosis should be reviewed. Management options include a repeat Papanicolaou test with or without colposcopy, ECC in 4 to 6 months, or cone biopsy if suspicion of a cervical lesion is high. A pelvic ultrasound should help identify glandular lesions of the uterine corpus, fallopian tube, or ovary.

Abnormal Papanicolaou Diagnosis in Pregnancy

The pregnant woman with an abnormal Papanicolaou finding generally is evaluated by colposcopic examination and directed biopsy if a high-grade lesion is suspected. The goal of evaluation of the pregnant patient with CIN is to rule out invasive cancer. CIN is not treated in pregnancy but is followed up until the postpartum period, when the patient is reevaluated and managed as indicated by the biopsy results and her social situation. During pregnancy, most clinicians do a cervical biopsy to confirm the diagnosis only if a high-grade lesion is suspected, although some recommend a confirming biopsy in all patients with a colposcopically visible lesion. The pregnant cervix is very vascular, especially in the last trimester, so a biopsy may bleed profusely, and cervical trauma can initiate uterine contractions. An ECC is contraindicated in pregnancy. Rarely, a cone biopsy is required in pregnancy to rule out invasive cancer when colposcopy with directed biopsy does not eliminate that possibility. This can be a difficult and potentially bloody procedure and should be undertaken by an experienced gynecologist only after all other avenues to rule out invasion have been exhausted.

Colposcopy

Clinicians have observed that the earliest and most severe epithelial changes on the cervix occur adjacent to the SCJ on the cervix. Anatomic studies have shown that the location of the SCJ is not fixed and changes during a woman's life. Under the influence of the vaginal pH, columnar cells on the exocervix are transformed into squamous cells by a process called *metaplasia*. There are three times in a woman's life that metaplasia is particularly active: during embryologic development of the vagina and cervix, at puberty, and after the first pregnancy. During puberty and after pregnancy, the columnar epithelium of the endocervix is everted out onto the exocervix or portio of the cervix, and metaplasia is stimulated. The columnar cells, starting with the epithelium on the tips of the glandular papillae, are changed into squamous epithelium. This process can be observed with the colposcope. The area of active metaplasia just lateral to the SCJ where this metaplastic change occurs is called the *transformation zone*—columnar epithelium is transformed into metaplastic squamous epithelium (Fig.46.2). This epithelium can be recognized as a circumferential, pale white, translucent ring around the SCJ. These metaplastic cells are very active and are especially susceptible to HPV infection. As described earlier, certain oncogenic HPV types may infect and transform these epithelial cells, and the resulting increased mitotic activity and DNA density can be identified as white epithelium following application of 3% to 5% acetic acid to the cervix. As CIN develops, vascular changes occur, and these may be recognized as punctation or mosaic. If the lesion progresses, bizarre vascular changes can be seen. These atypical vessels have grossly abnormal architecture and are colposcopic hallmarks of invasive cancer.

A standard colposcopic examination involves careful inspection of the cervix with both low- and high-power magnification after application of normal saline and then 3% to 5% acetic acid. After examination with the standard white light, a green filter may be used on the light source to increase the contrast of the red blood vessels and help clarify any vascular changes present. Lugol's iodine solution may also be used to stain the cervix to clarify areas of dysplasia, metaplasia, or columnar epithelium.

To evaluate the cervix for abnormal squamous epithelium, all of the squamous epithelium needs to be examined. Therefore, for the examination to be *adequate* or satisfactory, the entire SCJ must be visualized. Once the adequacy of the examination has been evaluated, a careful systematic evaluation of the cervix and upper vagina is performed, concentrating on the *transformation zone* adjacent to the SCJ. Areas of white epithelium, punctation, and mosaic are noted. The severity of any lesions seen are graded based on the whiteness of the epithelium, the intercapillary distance in vascular lesions, the sharpness of the lesion border, and the surface contour (flat, ulcerated, or raised). The staining characteristics of the lesion with Lugol's iodine has also been used to grade CIN.

Once a lesion has been identified, the most severely abnormal area or areas are selected, and a colposcopically directed biopsy is done. Although experienced colposcopists can often accurately grade the cervical dysplasia based on examination alone, a histologic diagnosis based on one or more cervical biopsies is the gold standard for determining the final diagnosis of the cervical lesion.

These general guidelines should be helpful in most cases, but there are many special situations—including the evaluation of adolescents and postmenopausal patients—in which alternative management plans may be more suitable. More extensive management guidelines are available on the American Society for Colposcopy and Cervical Pathology Web site, *www.asccp.org*, where the most recent guidelines are available.

MANAGEMENT OF CERVICAL INTRAEPITHELIAL NEOPLASIA

The management of CIN or cervical dysplasia is almost always based on a colposcopically directed biopsy of the lesion rather than just the Papanicolaou or cytologic diagnosis or even the colposcopic impression. If there is a significant discrepancy between these diagnoses, the clinician should review the whole diagnostic evaluation to be sure that cervical cancer is not being undertreated or that benign cervical inflammation, viral effect, metaplasia, or atrophy is not being overtreated. In addition to the biopsy diagnosis of the cervical lesion, the social situation of the patient often plays an important part in management decisions. For example, a 32-year-old mother of three with a two-quadrant CIN 2 lesion should probably be treated with LEEP or cryotherapy, whereas the same lesion in a 21-year-old unmarried student might well be watched for 12 months or so in hope that it will regress and no cervical tissue will have to be removed or destroyed.

Treatment Indications

It is difficult, if not impossible, to write out a complete set of guidelines that encompasses every clinical situation. An updated set of management guidelines arrived at by a Consensus Conference sponsored by the American Society for Colposcopy and Cervical Pathology is available online at *www.asccp.org*. The preceding sections on the natural history of the transformation zone and CIN need to be applied to the specific patient and the various management options reviewed to select the best plan for that patient. In many cases, the patient's personal preference may tip the balance in the decision to treat or follow a lesion. Insurance coverage, school vacations, and equipment availability may also influence the choice or timing of treatment.

CIN 1—Mild Dysplasia

Reviews by Oster and, more recently, Nuovo and colleagues have shown that during 12 to 24 months of follow-up, regression occurs with no treatment in about 50% of women with a cervical biopsy showing CIN 1 (Table 46.4). Current management guidelines for the management of biopsy-confirmed CIN 1 strongly recommend conservative follow-up with no therapeutic intervention. Although good data do not exist, larger lesions and lesions that have persisted for a longer time are probably less likely to regress spontaneously. Because the treatment options are the same and chance of complete cure approaches 100% for CIN 1, 2, or 3, the consequences of progression within the grades of CIN are minimal. It is therefore reasonable to manage a patient with CIN 1 by observation alone. Prolonged follow-up of CIN 1 (Fig. 46.7) without biopsy confirmation is not recommended because cytology and colposcopy are not sufficiently accurate to confidently rule out a more severe lesion. The only two risks to this approach are that invasive cancer already exists and has been missed on the diagnostic evaluation of this patient or that the patient becomes lost to follow-up and does not reappear until her condition has progressed to invasive cancer. These risks are minimal, but should be considered for each patient at each visit. In almost all series in which women with low-grade cervical abnormalities have been followed up with no treatment, invasive cancer has eventually been diagnosed in a few patients even under the careful follow-up protocol of a clinical study.

For this reason and because treatment is relatively easy with limited patient inconvenience, side effects, complications, and costs, CIN 1 lesions in women who have completed their families, who have three- or four-quadrant lesions, or who have had a lesion for 12 months or longer may be considered for treatment. These low-grade abnormalities have cure rates of 90% or better with LEEP, cryotherapy, or CO_2 laser vaporization. Cryotherapy may result in less cervical destruction and be associated with a slightly lower risk of pregnancy complications than excisional techniques. Traditional cold-knife cone biopsy is probably associated with more morbidity and cost than is warranted by a diagnosis of CIN 1.

TABLE 46.4

NATURAL HISTORY OF CIN: LITERATURE REVIEW

	Patients	Regress	Persist	Progress to CIN 3	Progress to invasive cancer
CIN 1	4,504	57%	32%	11%	1%
CIN 2	2,247	43%	35%	22%	5%
CIN 3	767	32%	>56%	—	0.12%

CIN, cervical intraepithelial neoplasia.

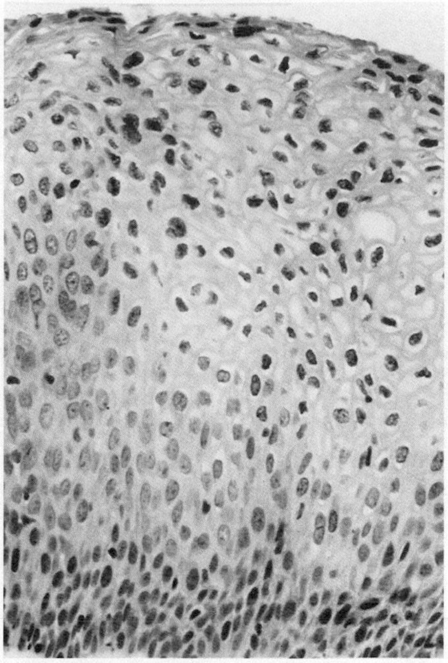

FIGURE 46.7. Histologic section of low-grade cervical intraepithelial neoplasia. A productive human papillomavirus infection in the cervical epithelium is characterized by cytologic atypia and hyperchromasia (heteroploidy), binucleated cells (lack of cytokinesis), and koilocytosis (binding of filaggrin). No other agent produces these changes, which are diagnostic.

Although patients with "atypical metaplasia" or chronic cervicitis have been treated with cautery or cryotherapy in the past, these are not generally indications for treatment under modern guidelines.

CIN 2 or 3—Moderate or Severe Dysplasia, Carcinoma *In Situ*

Patients with a biopsy diagnosis of CIN 2 or 3 (Fig. 46.8) have a less than 50% chance of regression and a significant chance of progression to carcinoma *in situ,* so treatment is usually recommended. Adolescents, pregnant women, and women who previously have been treated for CIN should probably be followed up conservatively without treatment. There is an increasing tendency for conservative follow-up alone in young women with CIN 2 lesions.

Although treatment of these lesions can be successful using either ablative or excisional techniques, high-grade lesions bordering on invasive cancer are best managed by excision, which provides a tissue specimen for examination by the pathologist. In several large series of LEEP specimens, a few invasive cancers that had been unsuspected were diagnosed on histopathologic examination of the excised transformation zone. Cryotherapy or laser vaporization of undiagnosed invasive cancer could result in progression, resulting in a deeply invasive cancer that remains untreated for several months or even several years. In the past and in some limited resource settings, ablative therapy has been or still continues to be used successfully in women with high-grade lesions, but the risk of undiagnosed invasive lesions makes this approach less than ideal.

A cold-knife cone biopsy in the operating room under anesthesia is indicated when cytology, colposcopy, or directed punch biopsy suggests superficially invasive cancer. Negative margins and a large specimen in one piece that can be well oriented are essential for an accurate and complete diagnosis of

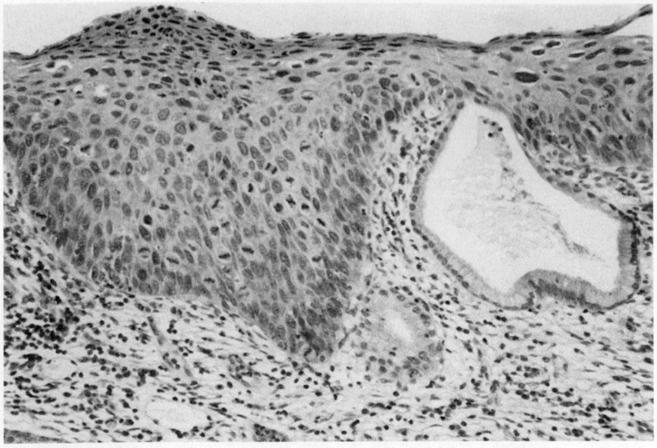

FIGURE 46.8. Histologic section of high-grade cervical intraepithelial neoplasia. This lesion has some features of low-grade cervical intraepithelial neoplasia but also contains abnormal mitotic figures—a diagnostic feature of an aneuploid, high-grade, human papillomavirus–related lesion.

microinvasive cervical cancer (Fig. 46.9). A final diagnosis of microinvasive cervical cancer cannot be made on punch biopsy or ECC. It is necessary to examine tissue on all sides of the microinvasive focus to be sure more deeply invasive disease does not exist adjacent to the focal area sampled by punch biopsy or ECC. If a grossly visible lesion on the cervix is seen, a simple punch biopsy may confirm the diagnosis of invasive cancer. A cone biopsy is not needed in these patients.

Adenocarcinoma *In Situ* or Glandular Dysplasia

These diagnoses also require a cone or large biopsy of the endocervical epithelium and stroma with negative margins for diagnosis. An ECC or punch biopsy is inadequate to rule out a

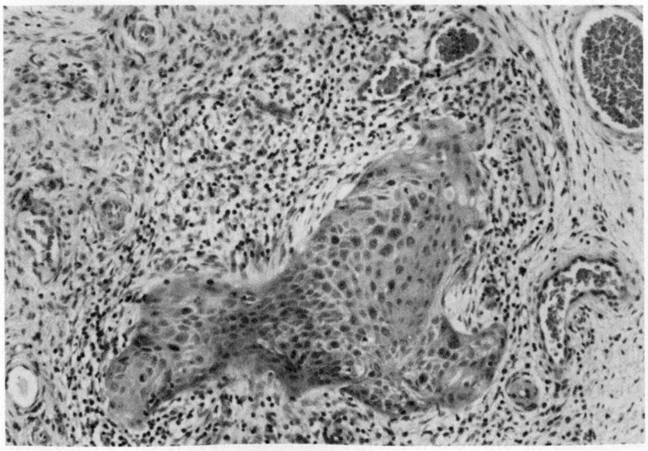

FIGURE 46.9. Histologic section of microinvasive squamous cell carcinoma. In microinvasive cancer, tongues of neoplastic epithelium extend through the plane of the basal lamina to split collagen bundles as they penetrate the cervical stroma, creating an irregular outline. Early invasion is commonly accompanied by a local inflammatory response.

more extensive, possibly invasive, lesion. These lesions may be multifocal. As previously noted, most experts favor cold-knife cone biopsy for the evaluation of glandular lesions.

The standard of care for AIS of the cervix in the United States is still simple hysterectomy, although there is increasing acceptance of cone biopsy alone for these patients. If cone biopsy is used as definitive management of AIS, the margins should be negative, and enough sections of the specimen need to have been studied to be confident that an early invasive adenocarcinoma does not coexist. Glandular dysplasia can also be managed by cone biopsy if the margins are clear, but there are few data on this subject.

Treatment Techniques

In general, treatment techniques can be divided into ablative and excisional. Destructive methods such as cryotherapy, CO_2 laser ablation, and electrocautery rely on an accurate colposcopically directed biopsy diagnosis because no tissue specimen is provided by the treatment procedure. On the other hand, punch biopsy, LEEP, and cone biopsy all provide a specimen, so these techniques are both diagnostic and therapeutic.

Punch Biopsy as Therapy

In most developed countries, women are highly screened and invasive cancers are uncommon, particularly in younger age groups. High-grade CIN is relatively uncommon, and most lesions that are detected are low-grade CINs found as incident cases. Because most of the cases of CIN are low-grade lesions that have developed between screening visits, the lesions tend to be small, to be located at the SCJ, and to occur in younger, often nulliparous women. For patients with a single, focal lesion, simple removal of the lesion with one or two punch biopsies may result in a cure. In the patient with a focal lesion, this approach may be worth a try. Theoretically, the entire transformation zone should be destroyed or removed, but in some patients, these small biopsies clear the abnormalities. The inflammatory healing response to the cervical biopsy may stimulate a response in the tissue surrounding the biopsy, resulting in improvement of adjacent areas. Whether these women would have cleared the lesion even without a biopsy can be debated.

Cryotherapy

Cryosurgery is a destructive technique that was introduced to gynecologists in the late 1960s to treat CIN. The cryosurgical instruments use nitrous oxide or carbon dioxide as a refrigerant to lower the temperature of the tissue below –22°C and to produce cell death by intracellular and extracellular water crystallization. The refrigerant is applied to the cervix with a cryoprobe, which is placed in contact with the cervical epithelium. As the gas is circulated through the cryoprobe, it withdraws heat from the cervix until freezing temperatures occur. The cervix and cryoprobe generally reach a steady state after about 3 minutes of freezing, at which time the amount of heat brought to the cervix by the vascular supply balances the amount of heat withdrawn from the cervix by the evaporating cryogenic gas.

Tens of thousands of patients have been treated with cryotherapy, which has proved to be a predictable, reliable treatment technique with limited side effects and morbidity. Cryotherapy is used principally in patients whose lesions are confined to the exocervix because the depth of cryodestruction seldom exceeds 5 mm. The cure rates are dependent on the size of the lesion. They generally average about 90% for lesions involving one quadrant, but only 75% for lesions involving three or more quadrants. Cryocurability is not related to the histologic grade of the lesion, except as histologic grade influences lesional size and distribution. Opinions differ as to whether a single freeze-thaw cycle or a double freeze-thaw cycle is the optimal approach, but there appears to be no difference in cure rates between the two approaches.

The most important end point in cryotherapy is that the ice ball should extend well past the edge of the lesion. A minimum margin of 5 mm is recommended. The incidental, small CIN lesions can be treated adequately by cryotherapy with a single cryoprobe application. When multiple probe placements are required to cover the lesion, cryotherapy may not be the best treatment. It is generally useful to apply acetic acid and Lugol's to the cervix before cryotherapy to reestablish the size and distribution of the lesion. Application of a thin film of lubricant jelly to the probe will eliminate "air gaps" and improve the thermal contact with the surface of the cervix, resulting in a more uniform and effective cryotherapy treatment.

Patients treated with cryotherapy may experience minor cramping during the procedure but otherwise the treatment is not painful. Thus, it is generally not necessary to anesthetize the cervix or give the patient premedication. During the 2 weeks after cryosurgery, about 20% of patients experience a profuse watery discharge that may require wearing a pad. Some patients experience light spotting, particularly 12 to 15 days after cryotherapy, when the eschar begins to separate from the treated area. Infections following cervical cryotherapy are rare but can occur, especially in women who already have a subclinical endometritis or salpingitis.

Long-term complications of cryotherapy are minimal and consist principally of cervical stenosis in 1% to 4% of patients. Several studies have reported that there is no change in fertility and that pregnancy complications seldom occur, except in patients who have excessive cervical fibrosis and in whom cervical dystocia may be a problem. Postcryotherapeutic healing is rapid (it is generally completed within 12 weeks) and usually restores the SCJ to be coincident with the external os. It is important, however, that the flat or shallow cone cryoprobe be used for treatment, because cryoprobes that have deep endocervical extensions may lead to a high rate of cervical stenosis. In many patients, the SCJ will not be visible after the cervix has healed following cryotherapy. Cryosurgery is a safe, useful, inexpensive procedure that should be considered for any patient (particularly young and nulliparous patients) with CIN 1 or 2 confined to one or two quadrants of the exocervix.

Carbon Dioxide Laser

The CO_2 laser is another useful treatment modality for the management of CIN lesions. The CO_2 laser is used to ablate CIN in patients whose lesion is confined to the portio and in whom invasive cancer has been ruled out by colposcopically directed biopsies and ECC. This laser is an instrument that produces a high-intensity columnar beam of light that can be concentrated to a small spot where it produces a small footprint and a high-power density. This concentration of energy vaporizes the tissue by rapidly boiling the intracellular water, causing the cells to explode. The CO_2 laser can be used to ablate tissue or to cut, depending on the spot size and the power density. When the energy is concentrated on an extremely small spot, the light beam penetrates the tissue deeply and rapidly. It can be used as a knife to excise a lesion, although this requires considerable skill and experience as well as an expensive laser. Surgical excision using the CO_2 laser is not often used for CIN these days. When the laser beam is defocused to spread the energy over a larger area but while it still retains sufficient power density to produce cellular destruction, it can be used to evaporate tissues fairly rapidly.

The CO_2 laser has the following advantages: it can be used for either cutting or ablation; the healing after laser surgery is rapid; and there are minimal side effects, including limited vaginal discharge. Patients treated with the CO_2 laser generally have less cervical narrowing and a lower stenosis rate than those treated with cryotherapy. There is no diminution of fertility, and there are no obstetric complications after laser treatment. The major disadvantages of the laser are (i) its acquisition expense; (ii) the time required to acquire and maintain laser skills, particularly for excisional laser conization; and (iii) the relatively high maintenance cost of the instrument. Use of the CO_2 laser for the management of CIN has decreased dramatically since the introduction of LEEP.

Loop Electrosurgical Excision

LEEP was introduced in the United Kingdom by Prendeville as large loop excision of the transformation zone (LLETZ). The technique uses a modification of a small electrosurgical wire loop biopsy instrument originally developed by Cartier in France. LEEP was introduced in North America in the early 1990s and, as in Europe, rapidly became the procedure of choice for the management of CIN. It is usually done under local anesthesia as an outpatient or clinic procedure.

Although low-grade lesions can readily be treated with cryotherapy, many gynecologists choose LEEP excision instead because of its ease of use, its limited morbidity, and the fact that it provides a specimen. Caution is advised in choosing LEEP for small lesions in women who have only small areas of CIN in a small, nulliparous cervix because it is possible to produce irreversible cervical damage. With few exceptions, all high-grade lesions should be removed with use of an excisional, rather than an ablative, procedure.

LEEP takes advantage of the properties of modern, solid-state, electrosurgical generators coupled with loop electrodes made with a thin stainless steel or tungsten wire to excise areas of CIN (Fig. 46.10). It is also possible to electrocoagulate tissue with a 5-mm ball electrode. LEEP is used under colposcopic control and has the advantage of being a diagnostic and therapeutic procedure at the same time. The fact that a tissue specimen is provided makes the procedure particularly useful in ruling out early invasive cancer and in identifying unsuspected AIS. Many authors have reported that 0.4% to 0.6% of cases diagnosed as CIN by colposcopy, punch biopsies, and ECC in fact have invasive cancer or AIS in the LEEP specimen.

Because LEEP is easy to learn, easy to teach, and easy to apply, it can be used to treat patients with high-grade CIN without the disadvantages and great cost of cold-knife conization. The major advantage of LEEP over conventional cold-knife conization is that the procedure can be performed under colposcopic control and the margins can be examined colposcopically after the initial excisions are completed. This gives the operator the opportunity to reexcise additional tissue if it is found colposcopically that residual CIN remains. For LEEP to be used effectively, the extent of excision and the choice of electrodes must be tailored to the size and distribution of the lesion (Fig. 46.11). If the lesion is present on both the portio and the canal, a "cowboy hat" or "top hat" combined endocervical-portio excision is appropriate. The first pass removes the exocervical lesion with a wide, shallow loop, and a second pass with a smaller electrode excises the endocervical canal. The use of extremely large electrodes may lead to inadvertent cervical amputations and significant reproductive and obstetric morbidity.

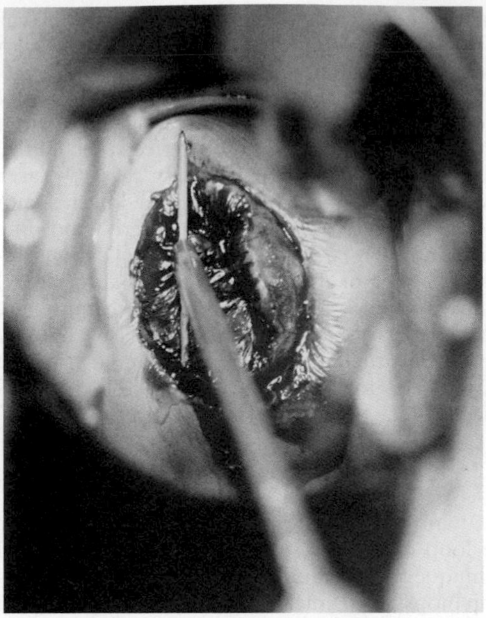

FIGURE 46.10. Loop electrosurgical excision procedure. Endosurgical loop is passed through a Lugol-stained cervix from right to left. Note cut surface of cervical stroma from the 12-o'clock to the 6-o'clock position. Also note lack of charring so commonly seen with laser ablation.

The complications of LEEP are similar to those of cone biopsy or laser ablation of cervical dysplasia. Significant bleeding at the time of cervical LEEP is uncommon but can occur, and the surgical team and the clinic need to be prepared and equipped for such a situation. Hemorrhage requiring special techniques to control is more common if a larger loop is used, if epinephrine or some vasoconstrictive agent is not injected in the cervix locally, or if the vagina is accidentally lacerated with the electrode. The first step in controlling hemorrhage is the same as for any surgical bleeding: Apply direct pressure to stop the bleeding. This can be done with a large cotton-tipped swab or a gauze or cotton balls grasped in the tip of a ring forceps. After the blood is cleared away and the cervix visualized, the swab is carefully rolled off the bleeding site and the ball electrocautery used to vigorously coagulate the bleeder. More pressure is applied for 2 minutes or so, and the cautery reapplied, if necessary. Sometimes an additional injection of epinephrine will be helpful. Bleeding from the cervix can also be temporally controlled by clamping the cervical lip with a ring forceps. If these simple techniques do not work, the situation should be completely reevaluated. Is the patient stable and comfortable? Does she need a paracervical block? Should we start an intravenous line? Do we need suction to evacuate the blood? Do I have adequate assistance, adequate exposure, adequate lighting? Can this be controlled in an outpatient setting, or should the cervix be packed and the patient transported to a hospital?

With a paracervical block, more local anesthesia in the cervix, and/or systemic sedation, a large figure-of-eight hemostatic suture in the cervix will usually control the bleeding. For those situations, the clinic should be equipped with a long 12-inch needle holder and long 12-inch tissue forceps with teeth. We use a 0-gauge delayed absorbable suture on a 1-inch curved, taper-point needle. An emergency tray with this equipment should always be available in an outpatient area where cervical biopsies and LEEP are done. Suction equipment and equipment to start an intravenous line should also be available.

Infection in the cervix or an ascending endometritis, parametritis, or salpingitis can occasionally be seen following LEEP, but they are rare and usually represent a flare-up of an already existing subclinical infection. Long-term complications include cervical incompetence and cervical stenosis, which are relatively uncommon but can have serious implications.

Although cervical incompetence leading to premature cervical dilation and delivery in subsequent pregnancies has been a well-known complication of traditional cold-knife cone biopsy for many years, it was not until the large metaanalysis of

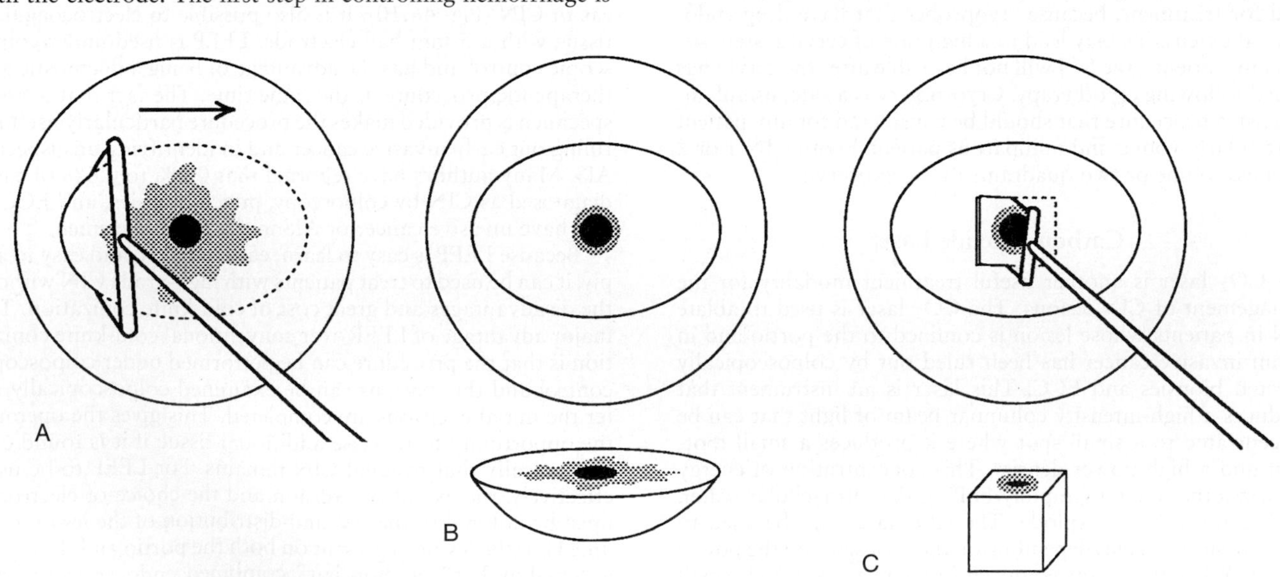

FIGURE 46.11. Diagram of approach to loop excision of small portio lesion, which can be removed by a single pass (**A**) of the 2-cm × 7-mm exoloop. **B:** Note the shallow dish configuration of the removed tissue. After the exocervical excision is completed, the canal is recolposcoped after additional acetic acid is applied. If residual disease is found in the canal, it can be removed by a second pass with a smaller loop (**C**). (From Wright TC, Richart RM, Ferenczy A. *Electrosurgery for HPV-related diseases of the anogenital tract.* New York: ArthurVision; 1992.)

Kyrgion and colleagues that the risk of LEEP was well accepted. In this analysis of 27 studies that examined pregnancy outcomes after excisional cone biopsy by cold knife, LEEP, or laser, the authors concluded that all excisional techniques resulted in a roughly doubled rate of premature delivery. Patients treated with a LEEP greater than 1 cm deep had a higher incidence of prematurity. There was no increase in neonatal morbidity or mortality. In a large prospective follow-up study from Denmark, Nohr and colleagues found a 3.5% incidence of preterm birth (<37 weeks) among untreated women compared with 6.6% for women after a LEEP. The problem is somewhat confused by another large epidemiologic study of 5,548 births in Australia by Bruinsma and associates. These authors found that women with cervical dysplasia had a higher incidence of prematurity than the general population. But even within the cohort of women with dysplasia, those who had an excisional treatment procedure had a 1.23-fold increased risk of a premature birth. However, when adjustments were made for other associated risks—such as prior spontaneous abortions, illicit drug use during pregnancy, and another major medical condition—cervical excisional procedures were no longer associated with an increased risk of prematurity. These studies suggest that for a variety of reasons, women who undergo LEEP or cone are at an increased risk to delivery prematurely with subsequent pregnancies, but that serious neonatal complications are not increased.

The overall "cure" rate of LEEP is about 95%, but the incidence of persistent disease is related to the anatomy of the lesion. Lesions that involve the exocervix, no matter how severe, are easily visualized and can usually be excised successfully under direct vision. However, lesions that extend into the endocervical canal are more difficult because the upper extent of the lesion may not be easily seen, and it is more difficult to visually guide the depth of excision. However, even with a histologically involved margin, immediate reexcision is not necessary (unless possible invasive cancer might be present). Healing of the cone bed and the electrosurgical injury of the margin often results in destruction of a minimal rim of residual dysplasia. Repeat excision is necessary only when residual disease is documented at the 4- to 6-month follow-up.

See and Treat. Because LEEP is a simple procedure that can be used for both diagnosis and treatment during a single office visit, its use has been recommended in the so-called see-and-treat mode. With this application, patients who are detected as having an abnormal Papanicolaou smear are seen for colposcopy, and when a clear-cut colposcopically visible lesion is present, the lesion is removed in its entirety with use of the loop electrode. The patient does not first have to undergo cervical biopsies and an ECC.

The advantages to this approach are that the procedure is done in one office visit, thus reducing patient anxiety by eliminating the need to wait for a diagnosis to be rendered and to then return for additional treatment. If used appropriately, it may save time and money. The disadvantage to this approach is that the colposcopic appearance of squamous metaplasia, repair, or other minor changes may mimic CIN, leading to inappropriate excision of benign epithelium. For see and treat to be used effectively and appropriately, the colposcopist must be certain that the colposcopic changes that are seen are sufficiently characteristic that a diagnosis of an HPV-related high-grade CIN lesion can be assured. Under these circumstances, see and treat may be the procedure of choice. Spitzer and colleagues have shown that in an inner-city clinic, the LEEP see-and-treat approach is highly beneficial and provides the opportunity to treat patients with significant lesions who might otherwise not return for their scheduled therapeutic follow-up visits.

Cervical Conization

Traditional cold-knife conization has been used successfully for generations to excise lesions that extend into the endocervical canal or to rule out invasive cancer. Hot cautery was used in the past to remove a cone-shaped piece of tissue from an inflamed, hypertrophic, chronically infected cervix. A standard surgical scalpel is more appropriate for the excision of CIN, and, thus, the term *cold knife* was introduced to differentiate these two procedures. A more or less cone-shaped biopsy can be excised from the cervix using a sharply focused laser beam or an electrosurgical wire as well as a scalpel. The laser is very expensive and requires considerable operator experience to be used effectively. The electrosurgical wire is quite effective and hemostatic. Both techniques often result in some thermal artifact, which may make interpretation of the surgical margins difficult.

A cervical cone biopsy is generally planned to be both diagnostic and therapeutic, and the technique is widely understood and practiced. We recommend cone biopsy for endocervical glandular lesions and for suspected microinvasion because accurate diagnosis of these lesions requires a large, deep tissue specimen with negative margins. A large cold-knife cone biopsy is also recommended for treatment of persistent or recurrent CIN after failure of LEEP or ablation. The cone usually is performed in an operating room under anesthesia; thus, it is expensive.

The size and shape of the cone specimen to be excised will vary depending on the location of the cervical lesion and the size of the patient's cervix. Although most glandular lesions are located within a few millimeters of the SCJ, a cone biopsy for a glandular abnormality needs to go deeply into the cervix to include most of the length of the cervical canal. On the other hand, a clearly visible lesion on the exocervix in a 28-year-old woman with a Pap test, biopsy, or colposcopic exam showing possible microinvasion needs a wide—but not so deep—cone. Colposcopic examination and Lugol's stain will help the surgeon determine the size and location of the lesion to be excised. After a careful examination under anesthesia, a gentle vaginal prep is done. The cervix should not be scrubbed too vigorously or the surface epithelium containing the intraepithelial lesion will be wiped away.

To decrease blood loss, the cervix is injected with a vasoconstrictive agent. We usually use a commercially available mixture of local anesthetic (lidocaine) with 1:100,000 epinephrine. Acute hypertension can be caused by this drug, and its use should be considered and discussed with the anesthesiologist. Approximately 1.5 cc is injected directly into the cervix, where the incision will be made at 12, 2, 3, 6, 8, and 10 o'clock. This is a total of 9 to 10 cc, and it should cause some "ballooning" up and blanching of the cervix. Although deep lateral sutures in the side of the cervix at 3 and 9 o'clock have been said to decrease blood loss by ligating the descending branch of the uterine artery, there is no evidence that this reduces bleeding with a cone biopsy.

The cervix is then restained with Lugol's solution to outline the lesion, and a scalpel is used to cut the cone. The cervix can be stabilized with a tenaculum placed high on the anterior lip away from the anticipated line of excision. Sometimes two tenacula are better, or the lateral stay sutures described above may be used if the cervix is very large or the vagina is small. We prefer a pointed no. 11 scalpel blade, but a large no. 10 blade or a smaller no. 15 is the choice of other surgeons. Some experts will use a bare electrosurgical wire or thin pointed electrosurgical blade. Still others have used a sharply focused laser beam to cut the cone biopsy. Each technique can be used with good success. As the cone is cut, it is retracted to the opposite side to provide visibility at the base of the incision. If possible, the cone should be symmetrical around the endocervical canal with the apex in the canal. It is desirable to remove the specimen intact as one piece and mark it with a suture at 10 or 6 o'clock so that the pathologist can orient any positive margins or foci of invasive cancer.

There are several ways to manage the cone bed once the specimen has been removed. If bleeding is minimal, bleeders may be cauterized and the cone bed left open to granulate. This may result in a visible SCJ more frequently than if the bed is sutured. If there is more bleeding, the bleeders may be cauterized as before; but the cone bed can be closed with a running locked suture placed from just lateral to the cone edge to deep in the cervical stroma by the canal. This is run circumferentially around the cervix—often called a "baseball stick," because it is similar to the strong stitches used to sew the leather cover on a baseball. This is the most hemostatic way to close the cone bed. Finally, there is the classic Sturmdoff suture illustrated in Figure 46.12. The anterior and posterior cervical mucosa are pulled in to cover the cone defect. This is the most aesthetically pleasing closure, but in many cases, the SCJ cannot be seen after the cervix is healed.

The complications of cold-knife cone biopsy are similar but perhaps somewhat more common than those with LEEP because the specimen is larger. Significant bleeding may occur in the first 24 hours or 10 to 21 days after surgery when the sutures dissolve. Five to 10% of patients will require reevaluation, packing, or suturing after cold-knife cone biopsy, and occasional patients will require a transfusion. Cervical stenosis occurs in about 3% of patients. This is more common if the patient is not having monthly menstrual periods. This risk of premature labor and delivery caused by an excisional cone biopsy has already been discussed in the section on LEEP. The size of the cone is related to the risk of premature labor. The larger the cone, the greater the risk.

As with LEEP, the success of cone biopsy in the treatment of CIN is directly related to the incidence of positive margins. Persistence or recurrence of CIN after cold-knife cone biopsy is usually quoted at 5% to 10%; but as smaller lesions that do not extend into the canal are done by the simpler, less expensive LEEP, lesions with a higher risk of failure are left to be treated by cold-knife cone biopsy.

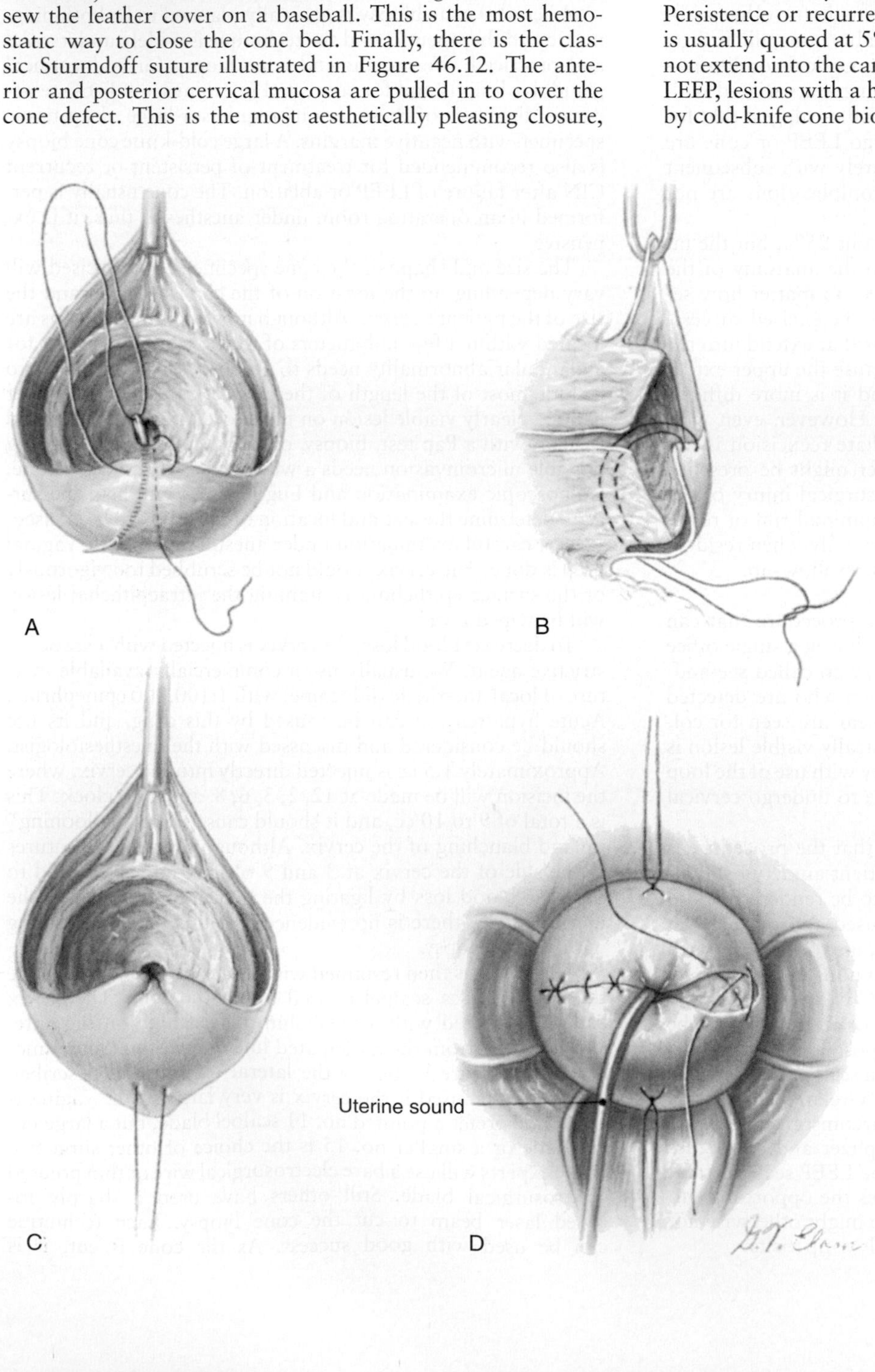

FIGURE 46.12. **A:** Mattress suture is placed as in Sturmdorf tracheloplasty. **B:** Method of action of suture in drawing the flap into the canal. **C:** The lower flap has been pulled into position. **D:** Anterior and posterior flaps have been drawn into the canal. Lateral mucosa wounds are being sutured.

BEST SURGICAL PRACTICES

- The identification of a preinvasive lesion that precedes the development of invasive cancer of the cervix and development of screening tests and diagnostic procedures that allow the clinician to screen for, diagnose, and treat these precursor lesions has greatly reduced the incidence of cervical cancer worldwide.
- It is now well established that cells adjacent to the squamocolumnar junction of the cervix become infected by HPV, which may produce a malignant transformation. These transformed cells may eventually progress through various degrees of dysplasia or cervical intraepithelial neoplasia to invasive cervical cancer. The viral subtype, the immunologic competence of the patient, and various associated events or activities such as cigarette smoking all influence the risk of progression to invasive cancer.
- Effective screening for cervical cancer and its precursor lesions has been done in many areas of the world using cervical cytology. With an organized system of testing every 3 to 5 years and with good diagnostic follow-up and treatment, cervical cancer death rates have been reduced by more than 70%. Visual inspection using acetic acid (VIA) and HPV testing have been introduced in recent years and are also effective screening techniques in certain circumstances.
- Following identification of a significant abnormality (LSIL or ASC-US/HPV positive in the U.S.) by screening techniques, the patient is evaluated by colposcopy and directed biopsy to determine the actual diagnosis and extent of disease.
- At least 50% of women with a diagnosis of mild dysplasia will resolve spontaneously within 2 years. Therefore, conservative follow-up is the recommended initial management for most patients with biopsy-confirmed low-grade lesions. In young women and women in whom future fertility is important, conservative management may be considered in higher-grade lesions. As a general rule, a biopsy diagnosis of CIN 3 or severe dysplasia indicates a cervical lesion that should be treated. Excisional techniques such as loop electrosurgical excision procedure (LEEP) is recommended in high-grade lesions because excision provides histologic confirmation that invasive cancer is not present.
- Traditional cold-knife cone biopsy of the cervix should be used for patients who might have microinvasive cancer or those with a glandular lesion. Cone biopsy under general anesthesia provides a large, deep specimen that can be well oriented and has a better chance of a clear margin.
- Many different treatment techniques are available for cervical dysplasia. In general, ablative or destructive techniques such as cryotherapy or laser ablation are less injurious to the cervix and have a lower risk of cervical incompetence in future pregnancies. Excisional techniques such as LEEP provide a specimen for histologic confirmation of the diagnosis. The severity and size of the lesion—together with the desire for future pregnancy and the training of the surgeon and availability of the equipment—all help to guide the choice of treatment technique.

Bibliography

Agency for Health Care Policy and Research. *Evaluation of cervical cytology. AHCPR Publication No. 99-E010.* Rockville, MD: AHCPR; 1999.

American College of Obstetricians and Gynecologists. *Cervical cytology screening. ACOG Practice Bulletin No. 45.* Washington, DC: ACOG; 2003.

Anderson GH, Benedet JL, Le Riche JC, et al. Invasive cancer of the cervix in British Columbia: a review of the demography and screening histories of 427 cases seen from 1985–88. *Obstet Gynecol* 1992;80:1.

Barron BA, Richart RM. A statistical model of the natural history of cervical carcinoma based on a prospective study of 557 cases. *J Natl Cancer Inst* 1968;41:1343.

Belinson J, Qiao YL, Pretorius R, et al. Shanxi Province Cervical Cancer Screening Study: a cross-sectional comparative trial of multiple techniques to detect cervical neoplasia. *Gynecol Oncol* 2001;83:3429.

Benedet JL, Anderson GH, Boyes DA. Colposcopic accuracy in the diagnosis of microinvasive and occult invasive carcinoma of the cervix. *Obstet Gynecol* 1985;65:557.

Benedet JL, Anderson GH, Matisic JP. A comprehensive program for cervical cancer detection and management. *Am J Obstet Gynecol* 1992;166:1254.

Berstein SJ, Sanchez-Ramos L, Ndubisi B. Liquid-based cervical cytologic smear study and conventional Papanicolaou smears: a metaanalysis of prospective studies comparing cytologic diagnosis and sample adequacy. *Am J Obstet Gynecol* 2001;185:308.

Brown DR, Shew ML, Qadadri B, et al. A longitudinal study of genital human papillomavirus infection in a cohort of closely followed adolescent women. *J Infect Dis* 2005;191.2:182.

Bruinsma F, Lumley J, Tan J, et al. Precancerous changes in the cervix and risk of subsequent preterm birth. *BJOG* 2007;114:70–80.

Burghardt E, Pickel H, Girardi F (eds). Colposcopy-Cervical Pathology, 3rd ed. Stuttgart, New York: Thieme, 1998.

Cartier R, Cartier I. Practical Colposcopy, 3rd ed. Paris: Laboratorie Cartier, 1993.

Chanen W. Electrocoagulation diathermy. *Ballieres Clin Obstet Gynaecol* 1995;9:157.

Clavel C, Masure M, Bory JP, et al. Human papillomavirus testing in primary screening for the detection of high-grade cervical lesions: as study of 7932 women. *Br J Cancer* 2001;89:1616.

Clifford G, Franceschi S, Diaz M, et al. Chapter 3: HPV type-distribution in women with and without cervical neoplastic diseases. *Vaccine* 2006; 24S3:S326–S344.

Coppleson M, Pixley E, Reid BL. Colposcopy. A Scientific and Practical Approach to the Cervix in Health and Disease. Springfield: Thomas, 1971.

Creasman WT, Weed JC Jr, Curry SL, et al. Efficacy of cryosurgical treatment of severe cervical intraepithelial neoplasia. *Obstet Gynecol* 1973;41:501.

Cuzick J, Mayrand MH, Ronco G, et al. New dimensions in cervical cancer screening. *Vaccine* 2006;24S3:90.

Cuzick J, Szarewski A, Cubie H, et al. Management of women who test positive for high-risk types of human papillomavirus: the HART study. *Lancet* 2003;362:1871.

Denny L, Kuhn L, Pollack A, et al. Evaluation of alternative methods of cervical cancer screening for resource-poor settings. *Cancer* 2000;89:826.

Denny L, Quinn M, Sankaranarayanan R. Screening for cervical cancer in developing countries. *Vaccine* 2006;24S3:71.

Duncan IA. Cold coagulation. *Ballieres Clin Obstet Gynaecol* 1995;9:145.

Galvin GA, Jones HW Jr, Te Linde RW. Clinical relationship of carcinoma in situ and invasive carcinoma of the cervix. *JAMA* 1952;149:744.

Goldie JS, Kuhn L, Denny L, et al. Policy analysis of cervical cancer screening strategies in low-source settings: clinical benefits and cost-effectiveness. *JAMA* 2001;285:3107.

Gram IT, Austin H, Stalsberg H. Cigarette smoking and the incidence of cervical intraepithelial neoplasia grade 3 and cancer of the cervix. *Am J Epidemiol* 1992;135:341.

Gram IT, Macaluso M, Stalsberg H. Incidence of cervical intraepithelial neoplasia grade III, and cancer of the cervix uteri following a negative Pap-smear in an opportunistic screening. *Acta Obstet Gynecol Scand* 1998;77:228.

Grohs HK, Husain OAN, eds. *Automated cervical cancer screening.* New York: Igaku-Shoin, 1994.

Guijon FB, Paraskevas M, Brunham R. The association of sexually transmitted diseases with cervical intraepithelial neoplasia: a case control study. *Am J Obstet Gynecol* 1985;151:185.

Hallam NF, West J, Harper C, et al. Large loop excision of the transformation zone (LLETZ) as an alternative to both local ablative and cone biopsy treatment: a series of 1,000 patients. *J Gynecol Surg* 1993;9:77.

Hinselmann H. Colposcopy (with a section on colpophotography by A. Schmitt). Wuppertal-Elberfeld, Girardet, 1955.

Ho GYF, Bierman R, Beardsley L. Natural history of cervicovaginal papillomavirus infection in young women. *N Engl J Med* 1998;338:423.

Jones HW III. Cervical intraepithelial neoplasia. *Bailliere's Clin Obstet Gynaecol* 1995;9(1):.

Khan MJ, Castle PE, Lorincz AT, et al. The elevated 10-year risk of cervical

precancer and cancer in women with human papillomavirus (HPV) type 16 or 18 and the possible utility of type-specific HPV testing in clinical practice. *J Natl Cancer Inst* 2005;97:1072.
Kinney WK, Manos MM, Hurley LB, et al. Where's the high-grade cervical neoplasia?. The importance of minimally abnormal Papanicolaou diagnoses. *Obstet Gynecol* 1998;91:973.
Kitchener HC, Castle PE, Cox JT. Achievements and limitations of cervical cytology screening. *Vaccine* 2006;24S3:53.
Kiviat NB, Koutsky LA, Paavonen JA, et al. Prevalence of genital papillomavirus infection among women attending a college student health clinic or an STD clinic. *J Infect Dis* 1989;159:293, 302.
Kolstad P, Klem V. Long-term follow-up of 1121 cases of carcinoma in situ. *Obstet Gynecol* 1979;48:125.
Kolstad P, Stafl A (eds). Atlas of Colposcopy. Oslo, Bergen, Tromso:Scandinavian University Books, 1972.
Koss LG. *Diagnostic cytology and its histopathologic basis*. Philadelphia: JB Lippincott; 1992.
Koss LG, Stewart FW, Foote FW, et al. Some histological aspects of behavior of epidermoid carcinoma in situ and related lesions of the uterine cervix. *Cancer* 1963;16:1160.
Koutsky LA, Ault KA, Wheeler CM, et al. A controlled trial of a human papillomavirus type 16 vaccine. *N Engl J Med* 2002;347:1645.
Koutsky LA, Harper DM. Current findings from prophylactic HPV vaccine trials. *Vaccine* 2006;24S3:114.
Kottmeier HL. Evolution et traitment des epitheliomas. *Rev Fr Gynecol Obstet* 1961;56:821.
Kyaer SK, van den Brule AJ, Paull G, et al. Type specific persistence of high-risk human papillomavirus (HPV) as indicator of high grade cervical squamous intraepithelial lesions in young women: population based prospective follow up study. *BMJ* 2002;325:572.
Kyrgiou M, Koliopoulos P, Martin-Hirsch P, et al. Obstetric outcomes after conservative treatment for intraepithelial or early invasive cervical lesions: systematic review and meta-analysis. *Lancet* 2006; 367.9509:489.
Luesley DM, Cullimore J, Redman CW, et al. Loop diathermy excision of the cervical transformation zone in patients with abnormal cervical smears. *BMJ* 1990;300:1690.
Mandelblatt JS, Lawrence WF, Womack SM, et al. Benefits and cost of using HPV testing to screen for cervical cancer. *JAMA* 2002;287:23721.
McIndoe WA, McLean MR, Jones RW, et al. The invasive potential of carcinoma in situ of the cervix. *Obstet Gynecol* 1984;64:451.
Meisels A, Fortin R. Condylomatous lesions of the cervix and vagina. I: Cytologic pattern. *Acta Cytol* 1976;20:505.
Meisels A, Fortin R, Roy M. Condylomatous lesions of the cervix. II: Cytologic, colposcopic, and histopathologic study. *Acta Cytol* 1977;21:379.
Mestwerdt G, Wespi HJ. Atlas der Kolposkopie, 3rd ed. Stuttgart: Fisher, 1961.
Montz FJ, Frederick KM, Farber L, et al. Impact of increasing Papanicolaou test sensitivity and compliance: a modeled cost and outcomes analysis. *Obstet Gynecol* 2001;97:781.
Moscicki A-B, Palefsky J, Gonzales J, et al. Colposcopic and histologic findings and human papillomavirus (HPV) DNA test variability in young women positive for HPV DNA. *J Infect Dis* 1992;166:951.
Moscicki A-B, Shiboski S, Broering J, et al. The natural history of human papillomavirus infection as measured by repeated DNA testing in adolescent and young women. *J Pediatr* 1998;132:277.
Munoz N, Bosch FX, de Sanjose S, et al. Epidemiologic classification of human papillomavirus types associated with cervical cancer. *N Engl J Med* 2003;348:518.
Munoz N, Catellsague X, de Gonzalez AB, et al. HPV in the etiology of human cancer. *Vaccine* 2006;24S3:1.
Nanda K, McCrory D, Myers ER, et al. Accuracy of the Papanicolaou test in screening for and follow-up of cervical cytologic abnormalities: a systematic review. *Ann Intern Med* 2000;132:810.
Nasiell K, Nasiell M, Vaclavinkova V. Behavior of moderate cervical dysplasia during long-term follow-up. *Obstet Gynecol* 1983;61:609.
Nasiell K, Roger V, Nasiell M. Behavior of mild cervical dysplasia during long-term follow-up. *Obstet Gynecol* 1986;67:665.
Nohr B, Tabor A, Frederiksen K, et al. Loop electrosurgical excision of the cervix and the subsequent risk of preterm delivery. *Acta Obstet Gynecol* 2007; 86:596–603.
Nuovo J, Melnikow J, Willan AR, et al. Treatment outcomes for squamous intraepithelial lesions. *Int J Gynecol Obstet* 2000;68:25.
Oster AC. Natural history of cervical intraepithelial neoplasia: a critical review. *Int J Gynecol Pathol* 1993;12:186.
Papanicolaou GN, Traut HF. *Diagnosis of uterine cancer by the vaginal smear*. New York: Commonwealth Fund; 1943.
Patnick J, Monsonego J, de Wolf C, et al. ESGO consensus document on cervical cancer screening. *Eur J Gynaecol Oncol* 2001;22:99.
Pemberton FA, Smith GV. The early diagnosis and prevention of carcinoma of the cervix: a clinical pathologic study of borderline cases treated at the Free Hospital for Women. *Am J Obstet Gynecol* 1929;17:165.
Prendiville W, Cullimore J, Norman S. Large loop excision of the transformation zone (LLETZ). A new method of management for women with cervical intraepithelial neoplasia. *BJOG* 1989; 57:145.
Purola E, Savia E. Cytology of gynecologic condyloma acuminatum. *Acta Cytol* 1977;21:26–31.
Reagan JW, Hamonic MJ. The cellular pathology in carcinoma in situ: a cyto-histopathological correlation. *Cancer* 1956;9:385.
Reid R, Greenberg M, Jenson AB, et al. Sexually-transmitted papillomaviral infections. I: The anatomic distribution and pathologic grade of neoplastic lesions associated with different viral types. *Am J Obstet Gynecol* 1987;156: 212.
Richart RM. A modified terminology for cervical intraepithelial neoplasia. *Obstet Gynecol* 1990;75:131.
Richart, RM. Cervical intraepithelial neoplasia. In: Sommers SC (ed): Pathology Annual 1973; New York: Appleton-Century Crofts, 1973, p. 301.
Richart RM, Wright TC. The pathology of cervical neoplasia. In: Luesley D, Jordan J, Richart RM, eds. *Intraepithelial neoplasia of the lower genital tract*. New York: Churchill Livingstone; 1995:19.
Rigoni-Stern D. Fatti statistici relativi alle malattie cancerose. *Gior Serv Progr Pathol Terap* 1842;2:507.
Russell J, Crothers BA, Kaplan KJ, et al. Current cervical screening technology considerations: liquid-based cytology and automated screening. *Clin Obstet Gynecol* 2005;48:108–19.
Saslow D, Runowicz CD, Solomon D, et al. American Cancer Society guideline for the early detection of cervical neoplasia and cancer. *CA Cancer J Clin* 2002;52:342.
Schiffman M, Herrero R, Hildesheim A, et al. HPV DNA testing in cervical cancer screening: results from women in a high-risk province of Costa Rica. *JAMA* 2000;283:87.
Schiffman M, Kjaer SK. Natural history of anogenital human papillomavirus infection and neoplasia. *J Natl Cancer Inst Monogr* 2003;31:14.
Solomon D, Davey D, Kurman R, et al. The 2001 Bethesda System: terminology for reporting results of cervical cytology. *JAMA* 2002;287:2114.
Solomon D, Nayar R, eds. *The Bethesda System for reporting cervical cytology*. 2nd ed. New York: Springer-Verlag; 2004.
Solomon D, Schiffman M, Tarone R. Comparison of three management strategies for patients with atypical squamous cells of undetermined significance: Baseline results from a randomized trial. *J Natl Cancer Inst* 2001;93: 293–9.
Spitzer M, Chernys AE, Seltzer VI. The use of large loop excision of the transformation zone in an inner city population. *Obstet Gynecol* 1993;82:731.
Stafl A, Mattingly. Vaginal adenosis: a precancerous lesion?. *Am J Obstet Gynecol* 1974:120:666.
Teale G, Moffitt DD, Mann CH, et al. Management guidelines for women with normal colposcopy after low grade cervical abnormalities: population study. *BMJ* 2000;320:1693.
Weid GL. *Proceedings of the First International Congress on Exfoliative Cytology*. Philadelphia: JB Lippincott; 1961.
Werness BA, Levine AJ, Howley PM. Association of human papillomavirus types 16 and 18 proteins with p53. *Science* 1990;248:76.
Wilbur DC, Norton MK. The primary screening clinical trials of the TriPath AutoPap system. *Epidemiology* 2002;13:S30.
Wilbur DC, Prey MU, Miller WM, et al. Detection of high grade squamous intraepithelial lesions and tumors using the AutoPap system: results of a primary screening clinical trial. *Cancer* 1999;87:354.
Willet GD, Kurman RJ, Reid R. Correlation of the histological appearance of intraepithelial neoplasia of the cervix with human papillomavirus types. *Int J Gynecol Pathol* 1989;8:18.
Wright TC Jr, Cox JT. Clinical uses of human papillomavirus (HPV) DNA testing. American Society for Colposcopy and Cervical Pathology, 2004.
Wright TC Jr, Cox JT, Massad LW, et al. 2001 consensus guidelines for the management of women with cervical cytological abnormalities. *JAMA* 2002;287:2120.
Wright TC Jr, Denny L, Kuhn L, et al. HPV DNA testing of self-collected vaginal samples compared with cytologic screening to detect cervical cancer. *JAMA* 2000;283:81.
Wright TC, Ellerbrock TV, Chiasson MA, et al. Cervical intraepithelial neoplasia in women infected with human immunodeficiency virus: prevalence, risk factors, and validity of Papanicolaou smears. *Obstet Gynecol* 1994;84:591.
Wright TC Jr, Massad LS, Dunton CJ, Spitzer M, Wilkinson EJ, Solomon D; 2006 American Society for Colposcopy and Cervical Pathology-sponsored Consensus Conference. 2006 consensus guidelines for the management of women with abnormal cervical cancer screening tests. *Am J Obstet Gynecol* 2007;197:346–55.
Wright TC, Schiffman M. Adding a test for human papillomavirus DNA to cervical-cancer screening. *New Engl J Med* 2003;348:489.
Wright TC, Schiffman M, Solomon D, et al. Interim guidance for the use of human papillomavirus DNA testing as an adjunct to cervical cytology for screening. *Obstet Gynecol* 2004;103:304.
zur Hausen H. Human papillomaviruses and their possible role in squamous cell carcinomas. *Curr Top Microbiol Immunol* 1977;78:1.
zur Hausen H. Human papillomaviruses in the pathogenesis of anogenital cancer. *Virology* 1991;184:9.
zur Hausen H. Papillomaviruses and cancer: from basic studies to clinical application. *Nat Rev Cancer* 2002;2:342.
zur Hausen H. Papillomaviruses in human cancer. *Cancer* 1987;59:1692.

CHAPTER 47 ■ CANCER OF THE CERVIX

DENNIS S. CHI, NADEEM R. ABU-RUSTUM, MARIE PLANTE, AND MICHEL ROY

DEFINITIONS

FIGO staging—The International Federation of Gynecology and Obstetrics (FIGO) has defined staging of gynecologic cancers for more than 50 years. The cancer stage defines the extent of disease at diagnosis before treatment. FIGO staging is used worldwide to compare clinical experience and results of treatment.

Lymph-vascular space invasion (LVSI)—Small endothelial-lined vessels within the cervical stroma may be either lymphatic vessels or small capillaries. On histologic examination of a surgical specimen, tumor cells or clusters of tumor cells are sometimes seen in these vessels. Tumor invasion or involvement of these lymph-vascular spaces is generally believed to increase the risk of nodal metastases and worsen prognosis.

Parametrium—Connective tissue lateral to the cervix and uterus within the broad ligament.

Pararectal space—The avascular space in the posterior-lateral pelvis. It is bounded medially by the rectum, laterally by the pelvic wall, posteriorly by the presacral fascia, and anteriorly by the broad ligament and cardinal ligament.

Paravisical space—The avascular space in the anterior-lateral pelvis bounded by bladder mediall, the pelvic sidewall laterally and anteriorly, and the broad ligament and cardinal ligament posteriorly.

SEER Database—The Surveillance, Epidemiology and End Results Database is managed by the United States National Cancer Institute. It collects data from population-based tumor registries around the country that represent a cross section of 23% of the population.

Sentinel lymph node—The sentinel node is the first node involved in lymphatic metastases from the primary cancer. The sentinal node concept holds that lymph node metastasis occur in an orderly, stepwise progression so that if the first or *sentinal node* is negative, then no other nodes are involved with metastatic cancer. Because cervical cancer is a midline tumor that may spread to either side and perhaps by more than one lymphatic pathway, it has not yet been proven whether the concept of the sentinel lymph node is applicable in this cancer.

In the first half of the 20th century, more women died from cervical cancer in the United States than from any other cancer. With the introduction of the Papanicolaou (Pap) smear in the 1940s, the early detection and treatment of preinvasive disease became possible. Consequently, both the incidence and mortality rates that are due to invasive cervical cancer in the United States declined approximately 75% by the end of the 20th century. The American Cancer Society estimates that in 2007, approximately 11,000 women will be diagnosed with cervical cancer. This represents a 15% decrease compared with the 13,000 estimated cases diagnosed in 2002. It is also estimated that 3,700 women will succumb to the disease in 2006 as compared with 4,100 in 2002. Based on these figures, cervical cancer currently ranks as the third most common female genital tract malignancy in the United States (behind uterine corpus and ovarian cancer) and the third most common cause of gynecologic cancer death.

Worldwide, however, more than 370,000 cases are diagnosed annually, leading to approximately 190,000 deaths. This makes cervical cancer not only the most common gynecologic malignancy, but also the third most frequently diagnosed cancer in women (behind breast and colorectal cancer). In general terms, the disease is much more common in developing countries. Overall, 78% of cases occur in these areas. In developing countries, cervical cancer accounts for 15% of female malignancies, carrying a lifetime risk of about 3%. In contrast, in developed countries, cervical cancer accounts for only 4.4% of female malignancies, with a lifetime risk of 1.1%. The highest incidence rates are observed in Latin America, the Caribbean, sub-Saharan Africa, and Southern and Southeast Asia. In developed countries, the incidence rates generally are low, with age-standardized rates less than 14 per 100,000. This geographical disparity is felt to be related to the presence or absence of effective screening programs, because epidemiologic and biologic studies have not shown significant differences in tumor biology in countries with high rates of cervical cancer.

STAGING OF CERVICAL CANCER

In 1937, the Health Organization of the League of Nations adopted a clinical classification system for cervical cancer. Cervical cancer was the first cancer to be so classified. In 1950, this classification was modified to include preinvasive (*in situ*) cervical cancer, which was designated stage 0. New recommendations for the clinical classification of carcinoma of the cervix were adopted by the General Assembly of the International Federation of Gynecology and Obstetrics (FIGO) in 1961, and several other modifications have been made since then. The general use of this classification abroad and in the United States has been extremely helpful in reporting and comparing results of various modalities of therapy. Descriptions of the clinical stages in carcinoma of the cervix uteri as updated by FIGO in 1995 appear in Table 47.1. Although the TNM (tumor, regional nodes, and metastasis) staging system is included for completeness, most clinicians use the FIGO staging.

Stages II, III, and IV have remained essentially unchanged through the various modifications (Fig. 47.1). The major redefinition and refinements have occurred in stage I disease. Microinvasive (stage IA) carcinoma has been subdivided into stage IA1 and IA2 based on the depth of cervical stromal invasion by carcinoma. Stage IB has been subdivided into stage IB1 and IB2 based on the size of the clinical lesion.

TABLE 47.1

STAGING OF CARCINOMA OF THE CERVIX UTERI (FIGO, 1995)

TNM classification		
Primary tumor (T)	FIGO classification	Definition
TX	C	Primary tumor cannot be assessed
T0	C	No evidence of primary tumor
Tis	0	Carcinoma *in situ,* intraepithelial carcinoma
T1	I	Cervical carcinoma confined to cervix (extension to the corpus should be disregarded)
T1a	IA	Invasive carcinoma, diagnosed microscopically only. All gross lesions, even with superficial invasion, are stage IB cancers. Invasion is limited to measured stromal invasion with maximum depth of 5 mm and maximum width of 7 mm.[a]
T1a1	IA1	Minimal microscopically evident stromal invasion. Measured stromal invasion with maximum depth of 3 mm and maximum width of 7 mm
T1a2	IA2	Measured stromal invasion with depth from 3B5 mm and maximum width of 7 mm
T1b	IB	Clinical lesions confined to the cervix or preclinical lesions >stage IA
	IB1	Clinical lesions no >4 cm in size
	IB2	Clinical lesions >4 cm in size
T2	II	Cervical carcinoma invades beyond the uterus but not to the pelvic wall or to the lower third of the vagina
T2a	IIA	No obvious parametrial invasion
T2b	IIB	Obvious parametrial invasion
T3	III	Extends to the pelvic wall or involves lower third of the vagina or causes hydronephrosis or nonfunctioning kidney
T3a	IIIA	Tumor involves the lower third of the vagina. No extension to the pelvic wall
T3b	IIIB	Tumor extends to the pelvic wall or causes hydronephrosis or nonfunctioning kidney
T4	IV	Carcinoma extends beyond the true pelvis or has clinically involved the mucosa of the bladder or rectum. A bullous edema as such does not permit a case to be alotted to stage IV
T4a	IVA	Spread of the growth to adjacent organs
T4b	IVB	Spread to distant organs

[a]The depth of invasion should not be more than 5 mm taken from the base of the epithelium, either surface or glandular, from which it originates. Vascular space involvement, either venous or lymphatic, should not alter the staging.
FIGO, International Federation of Gynecology and Obstetrics; TNM, tumor, regional nodes, and metastasis.

HISTOPATHOLOGY

The principal histologic type of invasive cervical cancer, occurring in about 80% to 90% of cases, is the *squamous* (*epidermoid*) lesion. In 1923, Martzloff classified these squamous tumors into three main histologic subtypes and grades. Grade 1 tumors contain well-differentiated spinal cells, keratin, and squamous pearls (Fig. 47.2A). Grade 2 tumors, the most common, are predominantly composed of transitional cells of the large-cell nonkeratinizing type (Fig. 47.2B). Grade 3 tumors, the least common, are poorly differentiated small-basal-cell–type tumors (Fig. 47.2C). The classification of Martzloff did not prove to be clinically useful, mainly because biopsies taken from different areas of the same tumor often show different degrees of differentiation and different predominant cell types. Martzloff's work did stimulate Broders, Wentz and Reagan, and others to continue to categorize the histologic types and degree of differentiation of squamous cell cervical tumors and to study their clinical behavior and response to treatment. The histologic classification of squamous cell tumor types introduced in 1959 by Wentz and Reagan sometimes is used in pathology reports. However, Willen and coworkers were unable to confirm a predictive value for survival from the Wentz-Reagan classification. Similarly, most recent studies, including those by the Gynecologic Oncology Group (GOG), have shown the use of grading of squamous carcinomas to be of little predictive value.

A rare form of squamous cell cancer of the cervix is a *verrucous carcinoma.* It is a very well-differentiated squamous cell carcinoma with extensive keratinization that usually presents as a large bulky tumor of the cervix and often is confused with giant condylomas, such as those seen on the vulva. There is a sharp line between the tumor and underlying cervical stroma. Verrucous carcinoma has been shown to be associated with human papillomavirus (HPV) infection. Although metastatic disease is rare, this tumor has been said to become more virulent if treated with irradiation. Goldberger and coworkers reported an unusually aggressive verrucous carcinoma of the cervix. According to deJesus and coworkers, at least 49 cases of this tumor have been reported in the female genital tract, sometimes as verrucous carcinoma and sometimes as squamous papillary tumor.

Adenocarcinomas of the cervix are becoming more common, especially in younger women. In a review of the Surveillance, Epidemiology, and End Results (SEER) Cancer Incidence Public-Use database from 1973 to 1996, Smith and colleagues reported that although the age-adjusted incidence rates per 100,000 for all invasive cervical cancers and squamous cell cancers decreased by 37% and 42%, respectively, the rates for

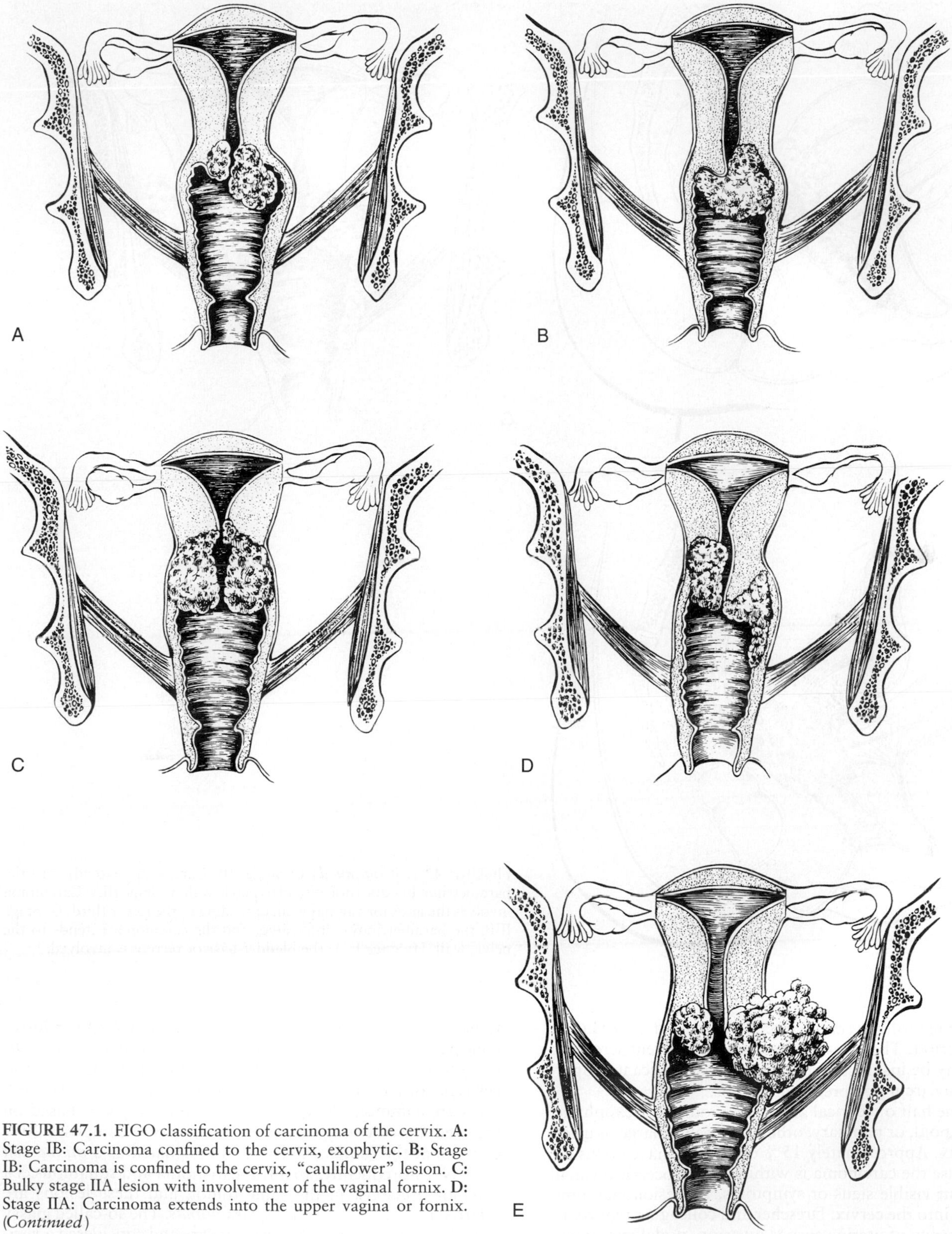

FIGURE 47.1. FIGO classification of carcinoma of the cervix. **A:** Stage IB: Carcinoma confined to the cervix, exophytic. **B:** Stage IB: Carcinoma is confined to the cervix, "cauliflower" lesion. **C:** Bulky stage IIA lesion with involvement of the vaginal fornix. **D:** Stage IIA: Carcinoma extends into the upper vagina or fornix. (*Continued*)

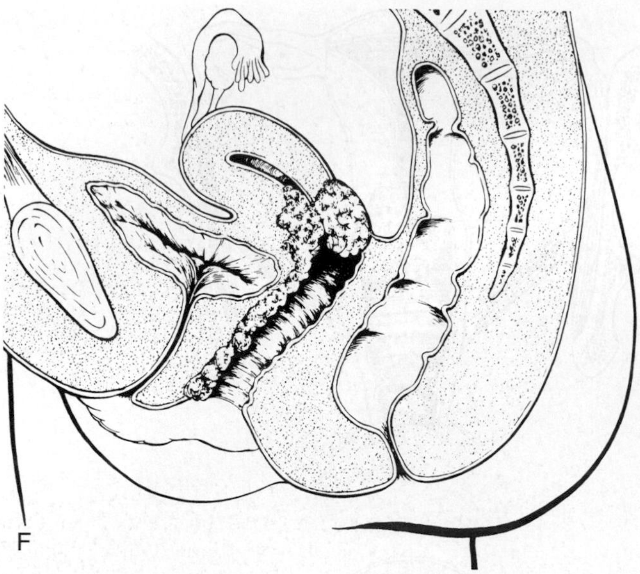

F

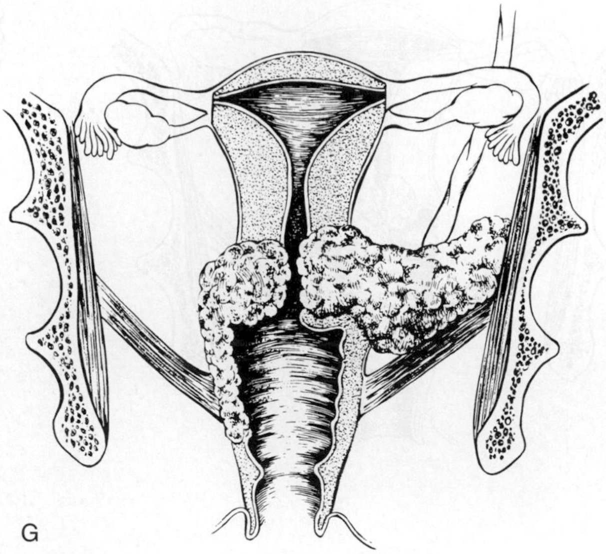

G

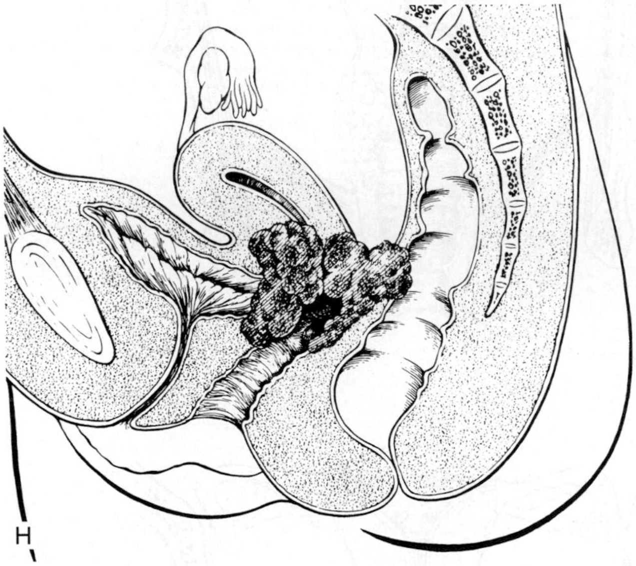

H

FIGURE 47.1. (*Continued*) **E:** Stage IIB: Carcinoma extends into the parametrium but does not extend to pelvic wall. **F:** Stage IIIA: Carcinoma involves the anterior vaginal wall, extending to the lower third. **G:** Stage IIIB: the parametrium is infiltrated, and the carcinoma extends to the pelvic wall. **H:** Stage IVA: the bladder base or rectum is involved.

adenocarcinoma of the cervix actually increased 29% during the study period. These results suggest that current screening practices may be insufficient in detecting a significant proportion of adenocarcinoma precursor lesions.

About one half of cervical adenocarcinomas are exophytic, usually polypoid, or papillary; others diffusely enlarge or ulcerate the cervix. Approximately 15% of patients have no visible lesion because the carcinoma is within the endocervical canal. Even without visible signs or symptoms, the lesion may infiltrate deeply into the cervix. Drescher and colleagues reported a higher frequency of uterine corpus invasion, nodal metastasis, and ascites in 26 patients with cervical adenocarcinoma compared with 139 cases of squamous cell carcinoma. More recent studies have reached contradictory conclusions regarding the prognostic significance of this histology.

In addition to pure (endocervical) adenocarcinoma (Fig. 47.3), cervical adenocarcinomas can exhibit a variety of patterns and can be composed of diverse cell types. Other histologic patterns include *adenoma malignum*, *endometrioid*, *clear-cell*, *serous*, and *mesonephric*. Different histologic patterns and cell types often appear in the same cervical tumor. Because mixtures are common, the designation of tumor type is based on the predominant component. If a second type composes 20% or more of the tumor, the lesion is designated as a *mixed-cell type*. Not infrequently, an adenocarcinoma and squamous cell carcinoma coexist in the same tumor, and these lesions are referred to as *adenosquamous carcinomas*. The so-called glassy cell adenocarcinoma of the cervix is rare and considered a variant of poorly differentiated adenosquamous carcinoma. It is known to be especially aggressive, with frequent early distant metastasis. *Clear-cell adenocarcinoma* of the cervix can occur in the presence or absence of intrauterine exposure to diethylstilbestrol. Saigo and coworkers found that the endometrioid pattern was associated with a more favorable prognosis than

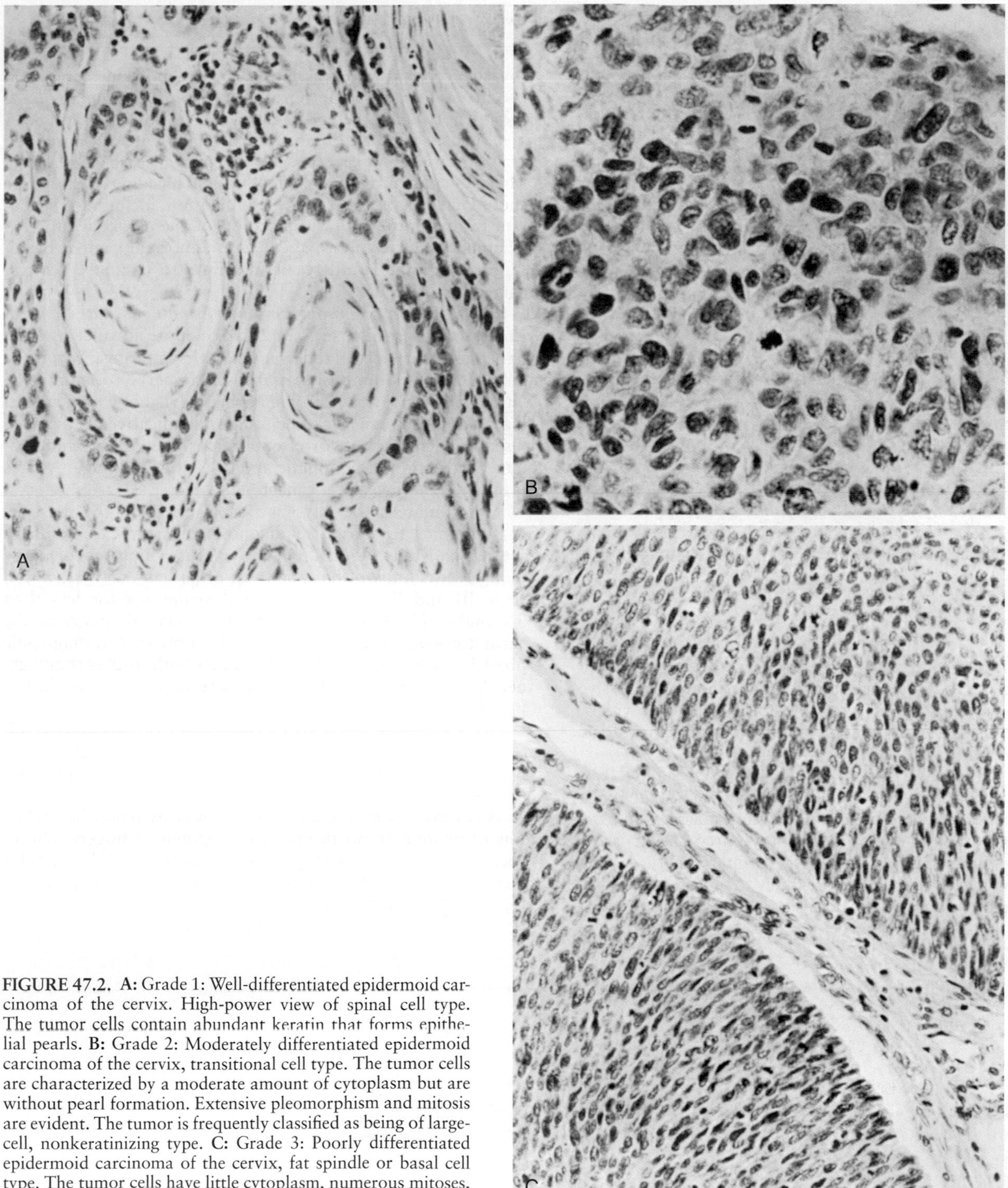

FIGURE 47.2. **A:** Grade 1: Well-differentiated epidermoid carcinoma of the cervix. High-power view of spinal cell type. The tumor cells contain abundant keratin that forms epithelial pearls. **B:** Grade 2: Moderately differentiated epidermoid carcinoma of the cervix, transitional cell type. The tumor cells are characterized by a moderate amount of cytoplasm but are without pearl formation. Extensive pleomorphism and mitosis are evident. The tumor is frequently classified as being of large-cell, nonkeratinizing type. **C:** Grade 3: Poorly differentiated epidermoid carcinoma of the cervix, fat spindle or basal cell type. The tumor cells have little cytoplasm, numerous mitoses, and no keratin or epithelial pearls.

any other histologic type of cervical adenocarcinoma; however, other authors believe that the subpatterns have no prognostic significance.

The early classifications of squamous cell carcinoma of the cervix proposed by Martzloff and others divided these tumors into three categories: keratinizing squamous cell carcinoma, large-cell nonkeratinizing squamous cell carcinoma, and small-cell carcinoma. Over the years, however, it became apparent that the group designated as *small-cell carcinoma* was composed of a heterogeneous group of tumors, many of which displayed neuroendocrine differentiation. Recent changes in the nomenclature have led to the subdivision of these *neuroendocrine tumors* into typical carcinoid, atypical carcinoid, large-cell neuroendocrine carcinoma, and small-cell carcinoma. Typical carcinoid and atypical carcinoid tumors are rare in the cervix; therefore, their clinical and

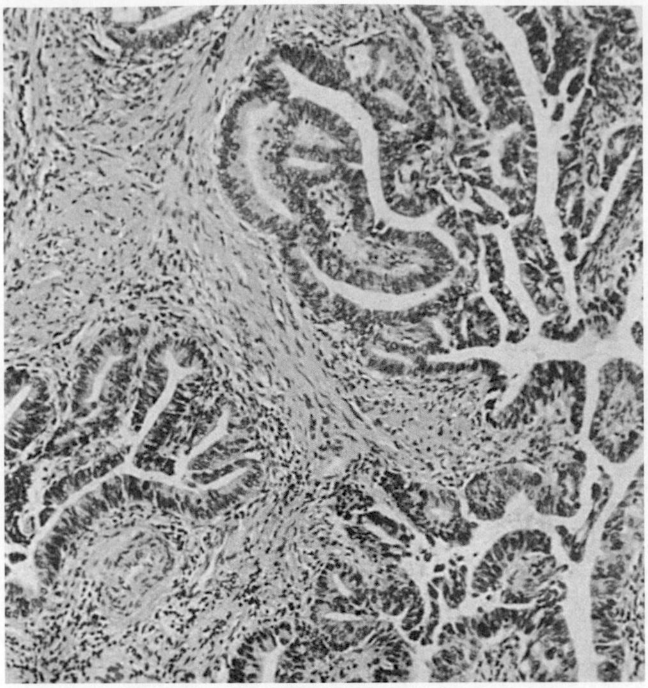

FIGURE 47.3. Adenocarcinoma of the cervix.

pathologic features have not been well characterized. Large-cell neuroendocrine and small-cell carcinomas are highly aggressive neoplasms, with a propensity to metastasize early and widely. Usual methods of therapy are not effective for these histologic types.

Various *cervical sarcomas* have been described by Rotmensch and coworkers. These tumors constitute less than 0.5% of all cervical cancers and include adenosarcomas, leiomyosarcomas, carcinosarcomas, and rhabdomyosarcomas. It is extremely rare for a lymphoma to develop primarily in the cervix, but lymphoma in the cervix is more likely to represent evidence of generalized lymphomatous disease.

CLINICAL PRESENTATION

Invasive cervical cancer is more likely than its intraepithelial precursors to cause symptoms such as *abnormal vaginal bleeding* (menorrhagia, metrorrhagia, postcoital bleeding, or postmenopausal bleeding). Many patients have a profuse and often malodorous discharge, especially when the disease is advanced. Thus, any patient with abnormal vaginal bleeding or discharge should have a complete pelvic examination, including a speculum examination with visualization of the cervix. Failure to examine the cervix in a patient with abnormal vaginal bleeding or discharge could result in failure to diagnose cervical cancer.

Pain is not a common symptom in patients with cervical cancer unless the disease is advanced. In more advanced stages, patients may report bladder and rectal symptoms. When the disease involves lumbosacral and sciatic nerve roots and the lateral pelvic sidewall, chronic boring pelvic bone pain radiating down the leg can be excruciating and indicative of advanced disease. Edema of the lower extremities likewise indicates tumor obstruction of lymphatic and/or venous drainage. Ascites is uncommon in cervical cancer.

Unfortunately, the physician cannot rely on the presence of symptoms to lead to a diagnosis of early carcinoma of the cervix. Many women remain without symptoms for many months. It is known that one third of patients with advanced stage III and IV disease have had symptoms for less than 3 months. The only way to diagnose cervical cancer in the earliest possible stages is to routinely apply special diagnostic procedures to large groups of women with and without gynecologic symptoms. This means screening the adult female population with Pap smears.

Invasive cervical lesions can be exophytic, infiltrative, ulcerative, or occult. The size of the visible lesion on the cervix may not correlate well with the extent or depth of invasion (Fig. 47.4).

An everted exophytic carcinomatous growth may be friable. Bits of tissue may break off on the examining fingers. On inspection, the friable exophytic cancer shows a rough, granular bleeding surface that can be sloughing and infected, with a foul-smelling discharge.

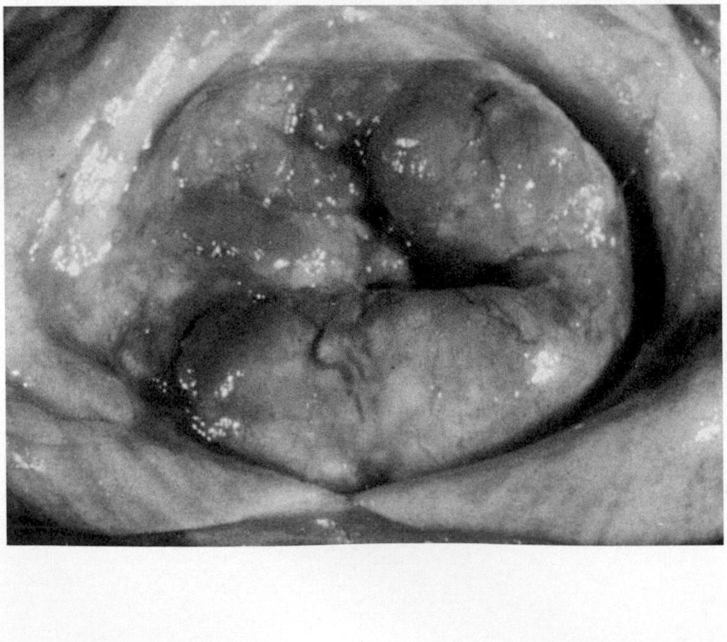

FIGURE 47.4. Squamous cell carcinoma, cervix uteri, FIGO stage IIA.

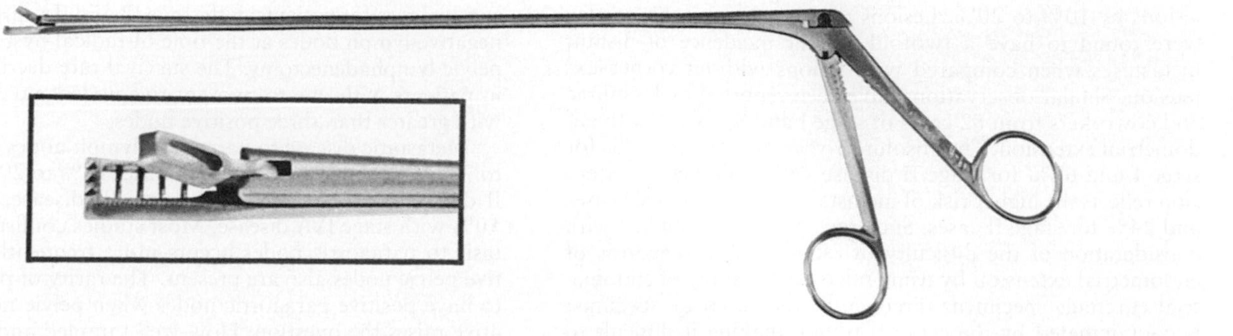

FIGURE 47.5. Kevorkian square-jawed cervical biopsy forceps.

A tumor that develops beneath the mucosa of the exocervix and infiltrates the cervical stroma usually causes cervical enlargement. The surface of the cervix may feel smooth, but the cervical consistency to palpation is firm or nodular. It is characteristic of cervical cancers that develop in the endocervical canal to cause cervical enlargement and a firm cervical consistency before breaking through the mucosa of the exocervix to cause a lesion. This also is characteristic of many cervical cancers that develop in postmenopausal women. In fact, it is possible, although uncommon, for a cervical cancer that is developing high in the endocervical canal to invade the parametrial tissue and even obstruct the ureters before causing a visible cervical lesion. An ulcerative lesion can look like a fairly clean punched-out ulcer, but more commonly it is an irregular crater with a necrotic bleeding base and a foul-smelling discharge.

Any grossly visible lesion of the cervix should be considered suspicious for cancer, and biopsy should be performed. Good visualization with a speculum and adequate illumination are essential. A Pap smear should be taken even though it can be less accurate in the presence of a grossly visible cervical lesion.

Colposcopic examination is neither needed nor particularly effective for a gross cervical lesion, but can be helpful when there is a small surface lesion to identify the most abnormal area for directed biopsies. The primary benefit of colposcopy is in visualizing noninvasive, precursor, or minimally invasive lesions that cannot be visualized without magnification.

Cervical biopsy techniques are discussed in Chapter 46. Biopsies can be undertaken with any of a number of special instruments: the Kevorkian (Fig. 47.5), Younge, or Gaylor biopsy forceps are particularly functional for taking an adequate biopsy specimen. It is important to obtain a specimen where frank stromal invasion can be demonstrated, not from the exophytic portion where no benign stroma is present. Surgical conization under anesthesia is unnecessary when a grossly visible lesion is present; indeed, it is contraindicated in the presence of a gross lesion because it has the potential of delaying the initiation of definitive treatment. Iodine (Schiller) staining can be used to demarcate the vaginal margins of a neoplastic area from adjacent normal epithelium. All of these procedures, as well as the popular loop diathermy conizations, can be done in the outpatient setting. It is rarely necessary to take the patient to the operating room to diagnose cervical cancer. If an anesthetic is deemed necessary for some other reason, a careful pelvic examination under anesthesia, biopsy of any vaginal lesions, cervical and uterine sounding, cystoscopy and proctoscopy (if warranted), and even uterine curettage can be done. Useful information to plan treatment thus can be obtained.

PROGNOSTIC FACTORS

Several factors have been reported to affect prognosis in cervical cancer. However, the most important determinant of prognosis remains FIGO clinical stage. Based on studies by Piver and colleagues, van Nagell and associates, Delgado and coworkers, and numerous others that demonstrated the prognostic significance of depth of cervical stromal invasion and tumor size in early-stage disease, FIGO incorporated these factors into its current clinical staging system by subdividing stage I. The 5-year survival rates by stage as reported by FIGO in the most recent report are shown in Table 47.2.

In addition to FIGO stage, other reported prognostic factors include endometrial cavity extension, regional (pelvic) and distant (paraaortic) lymph node metastases, histologic tumor grade, and lymphovascular space invasion (LVSI).

Uterine corpus and endometrial cavity extension from primary cervical cancer was originally thought to be a poor-prognosis factor. The original League of Nations classification of 1937 included such lesions in the stage II category. Over the years, classification of the disease based on extension to the uterine corpus or endometrial cavity has gradually been discounted. These lesions, classified as stage IC in 1950, were included in the broad category of stage IB in 1961. Despite the change in classification, there is still some concern about patients whose tumor extends into the corpus of the uterus. Evidence from Washington University reported by Perez and coworkers showed that tumor extension into the endometrial cavity lowers the 5-year survival rate of stage IB and IIA

TABLE 47.2

FIVE-YEAR SURVIVAL BY FIGO STAGE

Stage	Number of patients	Five-year survival rate (%)
Ia1	860	98.7
Ia2	227	95.9
IB1	2,530	88.0
IB2	950	78.8
IIA	881	68.8
IIB	2,375	64.7
IIIA	160	40.4
IIIB	1,949	43.3
IVA	245	19.5
IVB	189	15.0

International Federation of Gynecology and Obstetrics.

lesions by 10% to 20%. Lesions that involve the corpus also were found to have a twofold greater incidence of distant metastases when compared with lesions without corpus extension. Similar observations have been reported by Prempree and coworkers from 82 cases of stage I and II disease with endometrial extension. The absolute 5-year cure rates of 68% for stage I and 62% for stage II disease with endometrial extension reflects the higher risk of metastases: 20% for stage I cases and 24% for stage II cases. Such reports must be studied with consideration of the difficulty of establishing a diagnosis of endometrial extension by using microscopic study of endometrial curettage specimens. Frequently, the curettage specimen is contaminated by the cervical tumor, making it difficult to be certain about endometrial extension. Treatment planning is not altered by such observations, nor is a fractional curettage recommended as part of pretreatment evaluation.

Lymph node metastases, either regional (pelvic) or to higher-level (common iliac and paraaortic) lymph nodes, have proved to be one of the most reliable prognostic factors for patients with cervical cancer (Fig. 47.6). The frequency of metastases to pelvic lymph nodes is about 0% to 0.5% for patients with stage IA1; 7% to 9% for stage IA2; 12% to 20% for stage IB; 20% to 38% for stage IIA; 16% to 36% for stage IIB; 35% for stage III; and 50% for stage IV. Preoperative detection of positive pelvic and paraaortic lymph nodes is unreliable, even with newer radiologic imaging techniques. Detection of positive lymph nodes is more accurately determined when lymphadenectomy is used in preoperative staging or treatment. Although Kolstad showed that when intraoperative lymphography is used, 15% to 25% more patients with stage IB disease are found to have positive regional lymph nodes, this technique is rarely used outside the research setting.

When patients with stage IB cervical cancer are primarily treated with radical hysterectomy and pelvic lymphadenectomy, the 5-year cure rate is about 90% if there are no lymph node metastases. However, if metastatic disease to lymph nodes is detected, the 5-year cure rate falls to about 65% to 80%. The number of positive nodes also influences prognosis. In a review of the literature before the current standard of postoperative concurrent chemoradiation therapy, Hoskins reported an 83% survival rate for patients with stage IB and IIA disease who had negative lymph nodes at the time of radical hysterectomy and pelvic lymphadenectomy. The survival rate decreased to 57% in patients with one to two positive nodes and 31% in those with greater than three positive nodes.

Metastatic disease to paraaortic lymph nodes occurs in 4% to 7% of patients with stage I disease, 15% to 20% with stage II disease, 25% to 30% with stage III disease, and 30% to 50% with stage IVA disease. Most studies confirm that metastasis to paraaortic nodes occurs more frequently when positive pelvic nodes also are present. The rarity of patients found to have positive paraaortic nodes when pelvic nodes are negative raises the question: How well sampled and/or sectioned were the pelvic nodes? Even with extended-field radiation therapy, the 5-year survival rate for patients with metastases to the paraaortic nodes is only about 25% to 35%.

Histologic tumor grade has been reported to affect prognosis. Early studies by Chung and coworkers and van Nagell and colleagues demonstrated a poorer prognosis among patients with poorly differentiated tumors. However, more recent studies by Zaino and GOG have shown the grading of squamous tumors to be of little predictive value in cervical carcinoma. Shingleton and Orr reviewed nine publications that reported on 3,761 patients with predominantly squamous cell carcinoma. Twenty-eight different factors were evaluated for prognostic significance. *On multivariate analysis, tumor volume, lymph node metastasis, parametrial invasion, and LVSI were found to be significant independent prognostic factors, but patient age and tumor grade were not.*

On the other hand, tumor differentiation may have a significant prognostic role in adenocarcinoma of the cervix. Shingleton and Orr also reviewed eight studies containing 577 patients with adenocarcinoma of the cervix. As with squamous cell carcinoma, the strongest independent prognostic variables were tumor size and nodal metastasis. However, unlike with squamous cell carcinoma, tumor grade appeared to have prognostic significance.

Several investigators, including Swan and Roddick, Wheeless and Graham, and Julian and coworkers, have drawn attention to the fact that when there is a mixture of

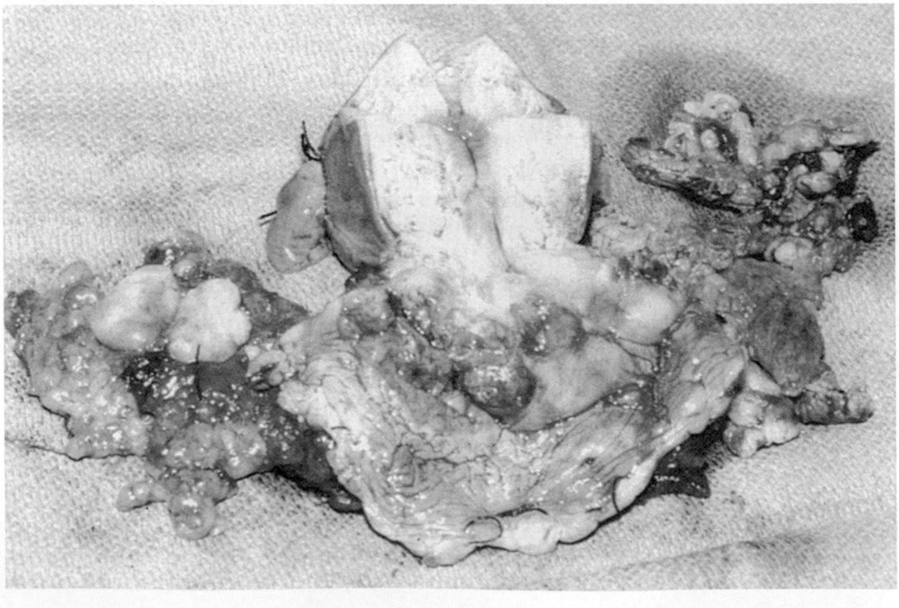

FIGURE 47.6. Squamous cell carcinoma, cervix uteri, FIGO stage IIA, with gross metastatic tumor in a right parametrial lymph node.

adenocarcinomatous and squamous elements—so-called adenosquamous tumors—the prognosis is poor and the incidence of pelvic lymph node metastases is high. Histologic combinations should be considered when comparing the prognoses of adenocarcinoma and squamous cancers of the cervix. The literature is mixed on the overall issue of whether adenocarcinoma in general and adenosquamous cancers in specific are more virulent and less curable than their squamous counterparts. Stehman and colleagues performed a multivariate analysis of prognostic variables for 626 patients with locally advanced cervical carcinoma treated with radiation therapy on three GOG protocols. Histologic cell type was not found to be a significant prognostic factor. A national pattern of care and evaluation study of the American College of Surgeons also failed to report statistically different 5-year survival rates for squamous and adenocarcinoma, regardless of type of therapy chosen.

In a GOG prospective study of 645 patients with stage IB squamous cell carcinoma of the cervix treated with radical hysterectomy and pelvic lymphadenectomy, Delgado and colleagues identified three independent risk factors in relation to disease-free survival: the depth of invasion, the size of the tumor, and LVSI. The disease-free interval was 89% for those patients without LVSI compared with 77% for those found to have LVSI. Although not all studies have found LVSI to be an independent prognostic factor, as stated, in a review of nine studies (including the study by Delgado et al.) containing 3,761 patients, Shingleton and Orr found LVSI to be a significant independent prognostic factor on multivariate analysis. The incidence of LVSI in early-stage lesions varies widely, depending on multiple factors, including the number of sections of the cervix prepared, the depth of stromal invasion, and the interest of the examining pathologist.

Observations from Austria and Germany indicate that there is considerable variation in the frequency with which LVSI is recognized by the pathologist. In a combined study of more than 1,000 patients at three different reference centers (Graz, Munich, and Erlangen), Burghardt and associates reported the frequency with which LVSI was identified ranged from 9% in Munich, where only blood vessel involvement was so classified, to 43% in Graz, where it was classified as capillarylike space involvement. At the third center, Erlangen, the corresponding value was intermediate at 23%. Such variations in histopathologic criteria may well contribute to some of the controversy that exists regarding the prognostic significance of LVSI.

To this point, this discussion of prognostic factors has included only anatomic and morphologic factors. Peipert and associates emphasize that cancer, including cervical cancer, has both form and function. Accordingly, other clinical variables, such as patient's symptoms, symptom severity, and comorbidity, affect the survival rate of patients with invasive cervical cancer. Unless these variables are suitably included, prognostic estimates based on morphology alone are imprecise, and therapeutic evaluations can be misleading. According to Rutledge and associates, there is no consistent effect of age on survival rate in patients treated for cervical cancer. Younger patients with early-stage disease seemed to survive longer than older patients, but the tendency reversed when disease was advanced.

PRETREATMENT EVALUATION

When a diagnosis of invasive cervical cancer has been established histologically, the clinician should perform an evaluation of all pelvic organs to determine whether the tumor is confined to the cervix or has extended to the adjacent vagina, parametrium, endometrial cavity, bladder, ureters, or rectum. According to the FIGO guidelines for clinical staging, diagnostic studies may include intravenous urography (IVU), cystoscopic examination of the bladder and urethra, a proctosigmoidoscopic study, a barium enema (BE), and in the case of early-stage disease, a colposcopic study of the vagina and the vaginal fornices. Colposcopic findings may be used for assigning a stage to the tumor (for instance, FIGO stage IIA), but the results must be confirmed by biopsy. Chest radiographs and electrocardiographic studies are used to determine cardiopulmonary disease, particularly in the older patient. Pulmonary function studies can be important, especially for evaluating patients who are candidates for extensive surgery.

When studies detect ureteral obstruction, a tumor is classified as a stage IIIB lesion, regardless of the size of the primary lesion. Ureteral obstruction, either hydronephrosis or nonfunction of the kidney, is well established as an indicator of poor prognosis, as recognized in the FIGO classification. Retrograde pyelography can be performed after the ureteral obstruction is located for further evaluation; however, it is not routinely recommended. Kidney function studies such as serum creatinine and creatinine clearance provide important baseline information before treatment; complete urinalysis is useful for detecting the presence of albumin or white and red blood cells and renal tubular casts.

In women with bulky or advanced-stage tumors, the bladder mucosa also should be inspected cystoscopically for possible bullous edema, which indicates lymphatic obstruction within the bladder wall. Evidence of tumor in the bladder must be confirmed by biopsy before the lesion can be classified as stage IVA. Rectal mucosal lesions also require a biopsy via proctosigmoidoscopy, because they can be related to an inflammatory process rather than to the cervical tumor.

A pelvic examination must be performed as part of the staging process, and it may be necessary to have the patient completely relaxed by general anesthesia. In as many as 20% of patients, the initial clinical classification of the disease based on office evaluation has been proven to be incorrect based on findings at the time of pelvic examination under anesthesia. Such an examination can reveal a more advanced stage of the disease than was originally found; additional biopsies (if indicated) or fractional curettage can be done as well as colposcopy, cystoscopy, and proctosigmoidoscopy. In today's health care climate however, the cost of a separate examination under anesthesia may need to be reserved for only the most problematic cases.

Pretreatment pedal lymphangiography has been used in the past to detect pelvic and paraaortic lymph node metastases, but the procedure is tedious and associated with many false-negative and -positive findings. When compared with lymphadenectomy, positive lymphangiograms have an accuracy rate of less than 75% and a false-negative rate as high as 50%. Furthermore, a lymphangiogram only detects metastatic lesions when the parenchyma of the lymph node has become distorted, by which time the lesions are macroscopic. The procedure thus is not recommended for routine use in the pretreatment evaluation of cervical cancer patients.

Surgical experience from pelvic lymphadenectomy has confirmed an error rate of 15% to 25% in the clinical staging of patients with stage IB or II lesions. In 10% to 30% of cases with stage II or III tumors, in addition to positive findings of occult pelvic lymph nodes, other metastases may be found in the paraaortic nodes. Unfortunately, pelvic examinations and clinical staging as defined by FIGO cannot detect such metastases. Consequently, there is a growing body of literature showing the superiority of cross-sectional imaging (computed tomography [CT] and magnetic resonance imaging [MRI]) over clinical staging in delineating the extent of disease in patients with cervical cancer. As stated earlier, official FIGO guidelines do not incorporate the use of either CT or MRI findings into the staging of cervical cancer. This is due to FIGO guidelines that staging methods should be universally available so that staging can be a standardized means of communication between different institutions worldwide. However, as knowledge of prognostic factors and the value of cross-sectional imaging have accumulated, its use in treatment planning has increased despite the lack of change in the official FIGO clinical staging guidelines.

In a Patterns of Care Study conducted between 1978 and 1988, Montana et al. reported a decrease in the use of IVU (86% to 42%) and BE (58% to 32%) in the staging of cervical cancer patients. During the same time period, the use of CT scan increased from 6% to 70%. In another Patterns of Care Study in the United States recently reported by Amendola and colleagues, the use of lymphangiography, IVU, and BE had fallen to 1% in the pretreatment evaluation of patients with clinical FIGO stage IB1 or greater cervical cancer who were scheduled for surgery.

The greatest value of CT scan in the pretreatment evaluation of patients with cervical cancer is in the assessment of advanced disease (stage IIB and greater) and in the detection and biopsy of suspected lymph node metastasis. The treatment plan for patients with locally advanced disease must be modified if retroperitoneal lymph node involvement and/or distant metastasis are discovered. A metaanalysis by Schneidler et al. reported a positive predictive value of 61% for CT scan in the pretreatment evaluation of nodal disease in cervical cancer. Moreover, in experienced hands, fine-needle aspiration of retroperitoneal nodes with CT scan guidance has an accuracy rate of 80% to 95%. When the aspiration study unequivocally shows malignant cells, a surgical biopsy need not be performed. This information is most valuable in patients who have metastasis to the paraaortic nodes, because these patients would need the pelvic radiation fields extended to incorporate the involved region if there is no other evidence of distant metastasis.

TABLE 47.3

GENERAL TREATMENT SCHEMA FOR INVASIVE CERVICAL CARCINOMA[a]

Disease stage	Treatment
Stage IA1	Simple hysterectomy, abdominal or vaginal, or cervical conization
Stages IA2,[b] IIA, IB1, and nonbulky IIA	Radical (class III)[c] hysterectomy or trachelectomy[d], bilateral pelvic lymphadenectomy with postoperative irradiation, plus or minus concurrent chemotherapy in selected high-risk patients
Stages IB2 and bulky IIA[e]	Full external and intracavitary pelvic irradiation with concurrent chemotherapy (± extrafascial hysterectomy) or radical abdominal hysterectomy and pelvic (± periaortic lymphadenectomy)
Stages IIB to IVA[f]	Full external and intracavitary pelvic irradiation with concurrent chemotherapy
Stage IVB	Palliative chemotherapy

[a]For individual patients, recommendations for treatment can vary, depending on the clinical circumstances.
[b]Some authorities recommend modified (class II) radical hysterectomy, bilateral pelvic lymphadenectomy for stage IA2 disease.
[c]Refer to Figure 47.7.
[d]In highly selected cases.
[e]Some authorities recommend simple hysterectomy in addition to radiation/chemotherapy for stage IB2 and bulky stage IIA disease.
[f]A patient with a stage IVA lesion that extends only in the anterior or posterior direction may be a candidate for pelvic exenteration.

SURGICAL TREATMENT OF EARLY-STAGE CERVICAL CANCER

Based on the pretreatment evaluation of the patient, including the prognostic factors of tumor size, clinical stage of the disease, and risk of pelvic node metastases, a treatment schema can be developed for invasive cervical cancer as shown in Table 47.3. Almost all patients are treated with either primary surgery or primary radiation therapy with concurrent chemotherapy. Some patients are appropriately treated with combinations of all three. The standard management of patients with early cervical carcinoma is surgical removal of the cervix. The extent of resection of the surrounding tissue depends on the size of the lesion and the depth of cervical stromal invasion.

Stage IA1 Disease

The exact definition of early-stage cervical cancer has been debated for several decades. This is illustrated by the fact that FIGO changed the definition of early-stage cervical cancer at least five times from 1960 to 1995. In 1985, FIGO defined stage IA cervical cancer as that which invaded the cervical stroma to a maximal depth of 5 mm with no greater than 7 mm of horizontal spread. In 1995, FIGO made its most recent revision in the cervical cancer staging system. After an extensive evaluation of the data in the literature, as well as seeking advice from specialty societies and individuals worldwide, FIGO changed the definition of stage IA1 disease to lesions that invaded the cervical stroma ≤3 mm in depth and ≤7 mm in width. Stage IA2 includes patients with >3 mm but <5 mm invasion and ≤7 mm lateral extent.

In an exhaustive review of the literature, Ostor identified 31 studies spanning the years 1976 to 1993 that reported on 3,598 patients with squamous cell carcinoma of the cervix and ≤3 mm stromal invasion. Although not all patients had lymph nodes removed as part of their treatment, the calculated incidence of lymph node metastasis in this group of patients was <1%.

Diagnosis

Microinvasive carcinoma cannot be diagnosed from a punch biopsy because adjacent areas may contain more advanced tumor; conization is required for definitive diagnosis in this situation. The accuracy of the diagnosis depends on the adequacy of the cone and the adequacy of the pathologic examination of the cone. The entire cone should be blocked so that an adequate number of histologic sections can be taken from each block. If the diagnosis is still not certain, more sections should be made. Although some experts can obtain a large tissue specimen with negative margins using loop electrosurgical excision techniques for a satisfactory diagnosis of microinvasive cancer, a traditional cold-knife cone biopsy in the operating room under anesthesia is often preferable. This is thoroughly discussed in Chapter 46.

Treatment

In 1996, the National Institutes of Health (NIH) invited an international panel of experts to develop a consensus conference statement on cervical cancer. After an extensive literature review and presentation of the scientific evidence, they concluded that patients who have squamous cell carcinoma of the cervix with ≤3 mm stromal invasion and negative conization margins have virtually a 100% cure rate when treated with simple hysterectomy or conization alone. However, for patients treated by conization alone, both the internal conization margin and the postconization endocervical curettage must be negative for cancer and dysplasia, because the risk of residual invasive cancer is significantly increased if either the margin or the curettage is positive. The choice of therapy should be influenced by the patient's desire to maintain fertility. Although LVSI generally is considered to be an adverse prognostic factor in cervical cancer, its prognostic significance in stage IA1 disease is uncertain. Because of this uncertainty, some clinicians suggested that the presence of LVSI in stage IA1 disease might be more appropriately treated with radical hysterectomy or radiation therapy.

Recurrence in the vaginal vault usually is the result of failing to accurately define the extent of the lesion and the presence of involvement of adjacent vaginal mucosa. This usually can be prevented with a careful colposcopic examination before hysterectomy. If vaginal fornices are involved, partial vaginectomy is easier to perform with hysterectomy if the operation is done vaginally (Fig. 47.7). Alternatively, if the woman is not a good surgical candidate, radiation therapy (usually in the form of brachytherapy alone) can be selected.

Increased infection morbidity has been reported with intracavitary irradiation of a recently coned cervix. The cervix must be allowed to heal completely before intracervical irradiation. The survival rates for microinvasive disease (all treatments) should reach 98% to 99% if patients are adequately studied and properly treated.

Contrary to its squamous cell counterpart, the currently favored treatment for early invasive adenocarcinomas of the cervix is radical surgery or radiation therapy. Only a few studies of microinvasive adenocarcinoma of the cervix have been done. Webb and colleagues recently reviewed the SEER Public-Use Database to identify 131 cases of cervical adenocarcinoma with 3 mm or less stromal invasion. Fifty patients had a radical hysterectomy and pelvic lymph node dissection, and none were found to have lymph node metastasis. Furthermore, there were no deaths among the 54 patients treated with simple hysterectomy alone. Others have reported a 0% rate of lymph node metastasis with depths of stromal invasion of up to 5 and 12 mm. However, bilateral pelvic lymph node metastases have been reported with as little as 2.5 mm of stromal invasion. Furthermore, Elliot and associates reported a case of lymph node metastasis with cervical adenocarcinoma with <1 mm invasion and a second case of recurrence and death after radical hysterectomy and pelvic lymphadenectomy in a patient with 1.8 mm of stromal invasion. More information is needed before sound recommendations regarding conservative treatment options for microinvasive adenocarcinoma can be made.

Hysterectomy after Conization

To evaluate the extent of an early lesion, cervical conization occasionally is required. If simple extrafascial hysterectomy is subsequently chosen as the definitive surgical treatment, the operation should be done within 48 hours of the conization or delayed until the cervix has healed, usually about 4 to 6 weeks later. If the hysterectomy is done after 48 hours and before the cervix has healed, the risk of serious postoperative infectious morbidity is increased. However, a radical abdominal hysterectomy and bilateral pelvic lymphadenectomy can be done at almost any time after cervical conization, even before the cervix is completely healed, without increasing the risk of serious postoperative infectious morbidity. The reason for this difference is not clear, but may be related to the fact that indurated and possibly infected paracervical and parametrial tissue is actually removed when a radical hysterectomy is done.

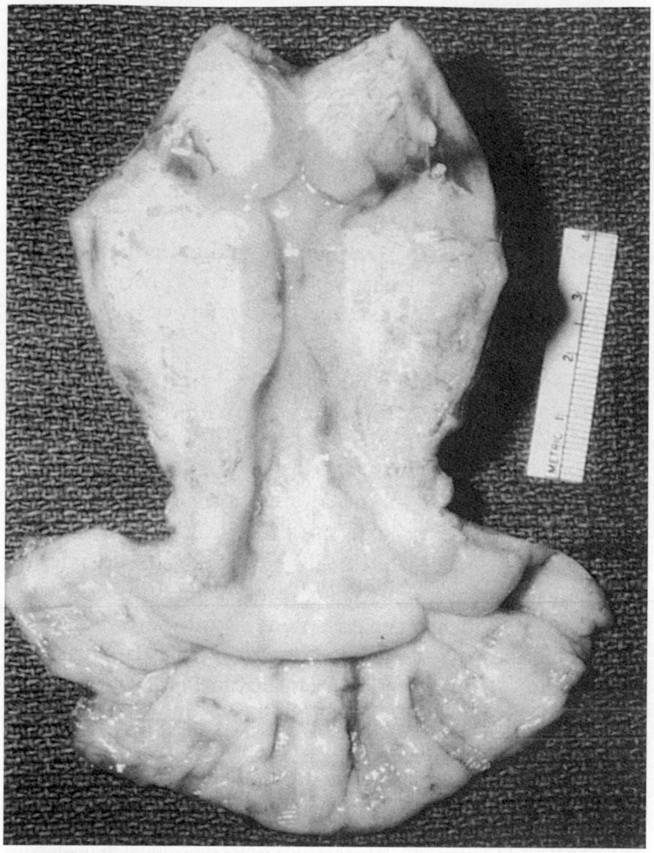

FIGURE 47.7. Vaginal hysterectomy and partial vaginectomy specimen from patient with squamous cell carcinoma, cervix uteri, FIGO stage IA1, with extension to adjacent vaginal fornix. Note uniform width of vaginal cuff.

Stages IA2, IB1, and Nonbulky (≤4 cm) IIA Disease

The recommended treatment by the NIH Consensus Conference for patients with stage IA2 disease is primary radical or modified radical hysterectomy with bilateral pelvic lymphadenectomy or primary radiation therapy because the risk of nodal metastases is 4% to 10% in these patients. Again, the diagnosis of both stage IA1 and IA2 disease should be based on microscopic examination of removed tissue, preferably a conization or large-loop excision specimen, which must include the entire lesion. For stage IA2 disease, the depth of invasion should not be more than 5 mm taken from the base of the epithelium, either surface or glandular, from which it originates. The second dimension, the horizontal spread, must not exceed

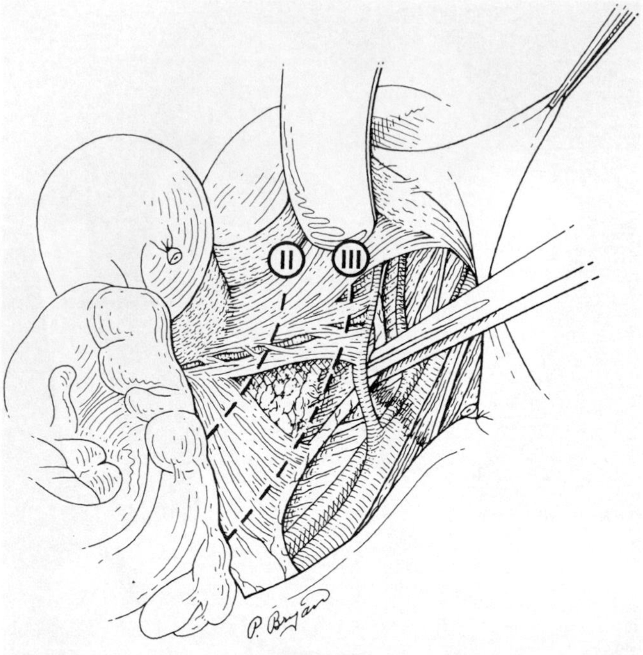

FIGURE 47.8. The cardinal ligament is excised medially in women with microscopic lesions (class II operation) or laterally in those with larger-volume lesions (class III operation). (Modified from: Piver MS, Rutledge F, Smith JP. Five classes of extended hysterectomy for women with cervical cancer. *Obstet Gynecol* 1974;44:265, with permission.)

7 mm. Vascular space involvement, either venous or lymphatic, should not alter the staging but should be specifically recorded. The remaining stage I cases should be allotted to stage IB. All grossly visible lesions are defined as stage IB.

For stage IA2 disease, standard treatment is class III radical hysterectomy with bilateral pelvic lymphadenectomy; however, some authors recommend a class II modified radical hysterectomy (Fig. 47.8). The class II hysterectomy removes the medial half of the cardinal and uterosacral ligaments, ligating the uterine artery at the ureter. This more conservative operation has been used by some authors in the past 3 decades to excise small primary tumors while reducing the partial bladder denervation associated with the complete excision of the cardinal and uterosacral ligaments required for a class III hysterectomy. Five-year survival rates of 97% to 98% have been reported for patients with small cervical lesions treated with class II hysterectomy. The role of the class II modified radical hysterectomy was recently evaluated in a randomized, prospective study reported by Landoni and colleagues. Two hundred forty-three patients with FIGO stages IB and IIA were randomized to either class II or III hysterectomy. The recurrence-free and overall survivals were similar between the two groups. Patients treated with type II radical hysterectomy had a statistically significant reduction in operative time and postoperative morbidity, particularly bladder dysfunction. However, given the relatively high cure rate for early cervical cancer treated by radical hysterectomy, larger trials are necessary to prove equivalence in survival between the two types of hysterectomy. As stated by Rose, larger trials are required before we can accept these results as the new standard of care. The estimated extent of tissue resection in surgical procedures for early cervical cancer is summarized in Table 47.4.

RADICAL HYSTERECTOMY

Historical Points in the Development of Radical Surgery for Cervical Cancer

Although the first truly radical hysterectomy for cervical cancer was performed by John Clark while still a resident trainee at the Johns Hopkins Hospital in 1895, the procedure is linked in perpetuity to Wertheim of Vienna, who reported his series of 500 cases of radical extended abdominal hysterectomy and partial lymphadenectomy performed from 1898 until 1911. Despite the skill and enthusiasm of Wertheim, Schauta (who

TABLE 47.4

COMPARISON OF EXTENT OF RESECTION FOR SURGICAL PROCEDURES TO TREAT EARLY-STAGE CERVICAL CANCER

Tissue	Cervical conization	Total abdominal/vaginal hysterectomy	Modified radical hysterectomy	Radical abdominal hysterectomy	Radical vaginal trachelectomy	Radical vaginal hysterectomy
Cervix uteri	Partially removed	Completely removed	Completely removed	Completely removed	Majority removed	Completely removed
Corpus uteri	Preserved	Completely removed	Completely removed	Completely removed	Preserved removed	Completely removed
Ovaries and tubes	Preserved	Preserved	Preserved	Preserved	Preserved	Preserved
Parametria and paracolpos	Preserved	Preserved	Removed at level of ureter	Removed lateral to ureter	Partially removed	Removed at level of ureter
Uterine vessels	Preserved	Ligated at level of cervical internal os	Ligated at level of ureter	Ligated at origin from hypogastric vessels	Descending cervicovaginal branch ligated	Ligated at level of ureter
Uterosacral ligaments	Preserved	Ligated at uterus	Divided midway to rectum	Divided near rectum	Partially removed	Partially removed
Vaginal cuff	Preserved	None removed	1–2 cm removed	≥2 cm removed	1–2 cm removed	≥2 cm removed

developed the vaginal radical hysterectomy), Okabayashi, and others, radical surgery was fraught with significant operative morbidity and mortality. The introduction of radium brought irradiation to the forefront of primary treatment for carcinoma of the cervix for the next several decades.

In the United States, Joe V. Meigs reintroduced radical hysterectomy as the treatment of choice, publishing a series of 344 cases in 1945. Until formalization of training fellowships in gynecologic oncology in the early 1970s, many outstanding gynecologic surgeons in the United States (Parsons, Ulfelder, Green, and many others) made important contributions and modifications in the radical surgical approach that have markedly decreased complications while preserving the cure rate. Today, proficient performance of the radical hysterectomy is the benchmark of the gynecologic oncology surgeon.

Patient Selection for Radical Hysterectomy

Simple hysterectomy is not adequate treatment for stage IB cervical cancer. In 1943, Jones and Jones reported a 5-year survival rate of only 41.6% in patients who had been treated for stage I cervical cancer with simple hysterectomy only. Such poor results also have been reported by Schmidt and others. When more than FIGO stage IA1 invasive cervical cancer is a surprise finding in a simple hysterectomy specimen, additional therapy—usually radiation therapy with or without chemotherapy—should be given postoperatively. Suggested indications for radical abdominal hysterectomy are summarized in Table 47.5.

Although radical hysterectomy and pelvic lymphadenectomy occasionally are used to treat patients with adenocarcinoma of the endometrium with involvement of the cervical stroma (stage IIB) and, rarely, patients who have a small cervical cancer that persists or recurs in the cervix after primary radiation therapy, in this chapter emphasis is given to the use of the operation as primary treatment for invasive cervical cancer.

In most institutions, the majority of patients with stages IA2, IB1, and nonbulky IIA cervical cancer are offered radical abdominal hysterectomy and bilateral pelvic lymphadenectomy as primary treatment.

TABLE 47.5

INDICATION FOR RADICAL ABDOMINAL HYSTERECTOMY

Indication	Extent of disease
Invasive cervical cancer	Stage IA1 with lymphvascular invasion Stage IA2 Stage IB1 Stage IB2 (selected) Stage IIA (selected)
Invasive vaginal cancer	Stage I–II (limited to upper one third of vagina, usually involving posterior vaginal fornix)
Endometrial carcinoma	Clinical stage IIB (gross cervical invasion)
Persistent or recurrent cervical cancer after radiotherapy	Clinically limited to cervix or proximal vaginal fornix

Patients with bulky stage IB disease (currently FIGO stage IB2) have traditionally been treated with radical hysterectomy and bilateral pelvic lymphadenectomy or primary radiation therapy with equivalent survivals. However, patients with these larger lesions treated surgically have a very high risk of having lymph node metastasis or close resection margins, which are often reasons for postoperative pelvic radiation treatment. Landoni and colleagues performed a randomized trial of radical hysterectomy and pelvic lymphadenectomy versus pelvic radiation therapy for stage IB to IIA cervical cancer. Patients randomized to the surgery arm who had pathologic risk factors, such as lymph node metastasis, received adjuvant radiation therapy. Of the 55 patients with tumors >4 cm, 46 (84%) required postoperative irradiation. The disease-free and overall survival for these patients treated with surgery and radiation therapy was the same as that for patients with bulky tumors treated with radiation therapy alone; however, the combination therapy significantly increased morbidity. Subsequently, a randomized trial performed by the GOG has demonstrated the benefit of the addition of cisplatin chemotherapy to pelvic radiation followed by extrafascial hysterectomy in this group of patients. Therefore, many experts feel that patients with FIGO stage IB2 and bulky IIA cervical cancer are best treated with concomitant cisplatin chemotherapy and radiation therapy followed by extrafascial hysterectomy.

In this country, patients with stage IIB invasive cervical cancer usually are excluded from primary treatment with surgery. They are usually treated with concomitant radiation therapy and chemotherapy.

The clinical significance of parametrial involvement dates from the early studies of Kundrat and Sampson. Kundrat, working in Wertheim's clinic, studied more than 21,000 serial microscopic sections of the parametrium, finding that the parametrium of one or both sides was involved in 44 of 80 patients. In a similar study at the Johns Hopkins Hospital, Sampson pointed out that the parametrium could feel indurated and yet shows no evidence of cancer. Also, the parametrium can feel normal and yet contain cancer. Sampson emphasized that only by the microscope can the surgeon exclude cancer involvement of the parametrium. More recently, Inoue and Okumura found parametrial extension in 7% of stage IB patients and in only 34% of stage IIB patients. Burghardt and Pickel found true parametrial involvement in only 19% of stage IIB patients. Matsuyama and coworkers found no parametrial cancer in 58% of stage IIB patients. These studies were based on careful examination of microscopic sections and reemphasize the difficulty of being certain about parametrial extension from pelvic examination alone, emphasizing the shortcomings of a clinical staging system. Inoue and Okumura studied 628 operative specimens from patients treated with radical hysterectomy and lymphadenectomy and found that parametrial extension is an important factor in the number of positive lymph nodes found and in patient survival. If there is suspicion of spread into the parametrial tissues by examination, CT scan, or MRI scan, it is reasonable to offer radiation therapy with concomitant chemotherapy as primary treatment (despite the fact that the official FIGO stage should remain unchanged).

The major point to be emphasized is that the gynecologic surgeon should not attempt to treat a patient with a large cervical tumor with primary radical surgery unless there is reasonable assurance that the operation will result in the complete removal of the central tumor with an adequate margin of tumor-free tissue around it. The surgeon should not operate on patients with the idea that radiation therapy with or without chemotherapy can be used postoperatively to eliminate residual fragments of tumor tissue left behind after incomplete resection. Such patients usually are better treated with concurrent pelvic radiation and chemotherapy from the beginning.

Primary radical surgical treatment is not contraindicated in any histologic type of cervical cancer. Shingleton and coworkers have suggested that the survival of patients with stage I adenocarcinoma of the cervix is better with surgery than with irradiation. Patients with stage I adenosquamous cancer, clear-cell cancer, and undifferentiated adenocarcinoma have a poorer prognosis, regardless of the method of treatment chosen, and therefore are often considered for adjuvant radiation therapy and/or chemotherapy after primary surgery.

Patients considered for radical hysterectomy must be acceptable candidates for an operation and free of serious medical problems that contraindicate extensive surgery. In former years, some institutions limited radical surgery as primary treatment to premenopausal women so that ovarian function might be conserved. As experience has accumulated, it has become apparent that the operation is also well tolerated by older women. In a study of 45 women aged 65 years and older with cervical cancer, Fuchtner and associates concluded that age alone should not be a contraindication to extensive hysterectomy in the elderly patient with American Society of Anesthesiologists physical status I to III. Kinney and coworkers reported their experience with the Wertheim operation in a geriatric population. Thirty-eight selected women between 65 and 89 years of age (median age, 69 years) were compared with 320 patients younger than age 65. The survival rates were almost identical in the two groups. Perioperative morbidity was minimally increased in the geriatric group. Geisler and Geisler recently compared the outcomes after radical hysterectomy and pelvic lymphadenectomy of 62 patients older than age 65 to 124 matched controls age 50 or younger. Even using this relatively younger cohort for comparison, there were no significant differences in operative mortality or morbidity. However, to achieve such excellent results in older women, Kinney and coworkers pointed out that "meticulous surgical technique, high-quality ancillary services, and support from internal medicine and anesthesia services" are required. Such extended supportive care is not available in every hospital.

Extreme obesity (especially morbid obesity) presents especially difficult technical problems when radical surgery is chosen for primary treatment. Not only is the performance of the operation less satisfactory, but also there may be an increased risk of wound dehiscence and evisceration, postoperative infection, intraoperative hemorrhage, pulmonary embolus, pulmonary atelectasis, and anesthesia-related and other problems. Unfortunately, primary treatment with radiation therapy with or without chemotherapy also is frequently less than satisfactory in extremely obese patients.

Studies by Soisson and Levrant compared outcomes after radical hysterectomy for cervical cancer in obese versus nonobese women. They found that survival was not compromised and the incidence of serious complications was not increased in obese patients. However, in obese women, the authors reported that the operative technique is more difficult, the procedure lasts longer, and the surgery is associated with greater blood loss. Cohn and colleagues recently reported their results with radical hysterectomy for cervical cancer in 46 obese women. The median body mass index was 36 kg/m^2 and the median weight was 95 kg. Nine patients (20%) experienced postoperative morbidity, mostly related to wound complications. No patient developed a fistula. Massi and associates have reported that the Schauta-Amreich vaginal hysterectomy can be used as an alternative to the radical abdominal hysterectomy in the presence of obesity or elevated surgical risks.

According to Shingleton, primary treatment with radical surgery paradoxically also can be riskier in very thin patients because of a higher incidence of fistula. It is speculated that easy exposure and lack of excess fatty tissue in these patients may result in removing essential vasculature around the ureters and bladder, resulting in ischemic necrosis. A thin patient has less fat around the pelvic vessels and in the lymph fields; thus, the surgeon should be satisfied to remove less tissue in an operation that will still be adequate in a thin patient.

The management of the *pregnant patient* diagnosed with invasive cervical carcinoma is perplexing. First, a decision must be made to either save the pregnancy or treat the cancer. Pregnancy is not a contraindication to primary treatment of stage IB or IIA carcinoma of the cervix with radical surgery (Fig. 47.9). In 1974, Sall and coworkers reported on 29 patients with stage IB carcinoma of the cervix in pregnancy treated with radical hysterectomy and pelvic lymphadenectomy. At the time of publication, 28 patients were alive and well, and 23 patients had been followed for more than 5 years. There were no

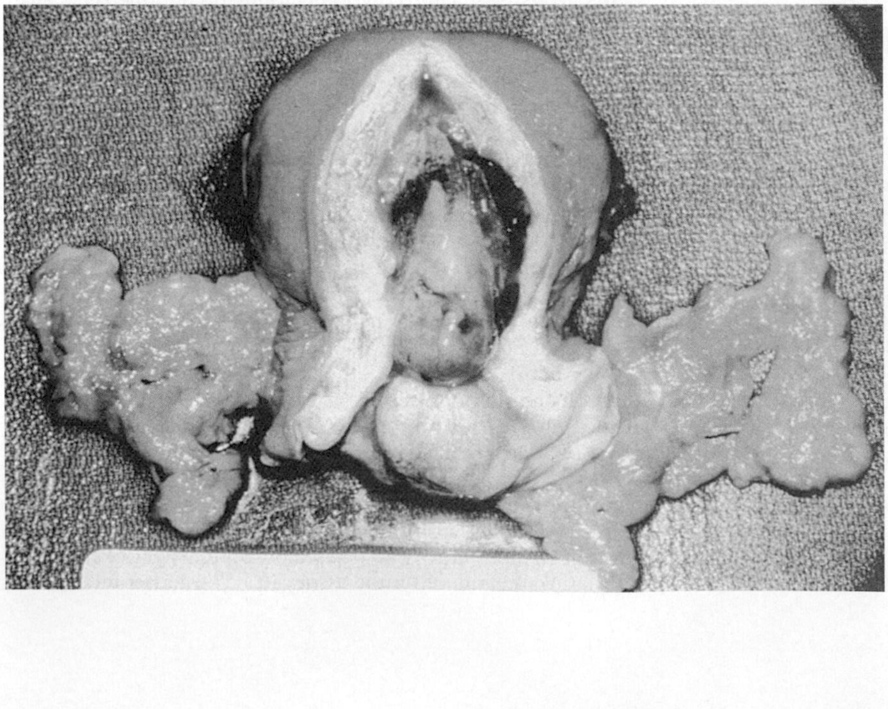

FIGURE 47.9. Squamous cell carcinoma, cervix uteri, FIGO stage IB with intrauterine pregnancy, 16 weeks (lymphadenectomy specimen not included).

fistulas or major complications. Others have confirmed 5-year survival rates of 85% to 95% for patients treated with radical surgery for stage IB cervical cancer in pregnancy. Funnell and associates, operating on 17 pregnant patients, suggested that the associated pregnancy changes facilitated the surgical dissection. Sood and colleagues performed a case-control study comparing the outcomes after radical hysterectomy and pelvic lymphadenectomy for 26 pregnant versus 26 nonpregnant patients. Operative times and postoperative complication rates were similar between the two groups. There was a statistically significant increase in blood loss at the time of surgery for pregnant patients; however, there was no difference in the frequency of blood transfusion. Eleven patients underwent surgical treatment in the third trimester of pregnancy with a mean planned delay in therapy of 16 weeks. None of the patients with the planned delay in therapy developed recurrent disease. The authors concluded that surgical management of early cervical cancer is safe during pregnancy. In select obstetric patients who desire to maintain their pregnancies, Sood and colleagues agree with the conclusions of Greer and coworkers that planned delay in therapy to increase the likelihood of fetal maturity is safe for early stage I squamous cell cancers diagnosed in the late second and early third trimester. All other patients should be treated promptly in an attempt to cure the cancer.

Finally, based on data from Orr, Chapman, and others, extensive parametrectomy and pelvic lymphadenectomy appear to be appropriate management for selected patients found to have *unexpected invasive cancer of the cervix on pathologic examination of a uterus removed for benign conditions.* Low morbidity rates and acceptable rates of long-term disease-free survival have been reported. However, pelvic irradiation is usually recommended for these patients.

Advantages of Radical Surgery as Primary Treatment for Invasive Cervical Cancer

The most important considerations in choosing a method of therapy for any cancer are, first, effectiveness of the treatment in curing the disease and, second, mortality and morbidity rates associated with the treatment plan. For the indications listed previously, the cure rates of primary radiation therapy and primary extensive surgery are about equal. The modern mortality rates also are about equal. Both modalities of therapy have a list of complications unique to each that seem about equal. There are, however, important major and minor advantages of primary radical surgery over irradiation for early-stage disease, some of which are discussed in the following sections.

Accurate Evaluation of Extent of Disease

The findings at operation and from careful pathologic examination of the surgical specimen can be immensely helpful in selecting high-risk patients for adjuvant postoperative radiation therapy, chemotherapy, or both. Most patients with FIGO stages IA2, IB1, and nonbulky IIA disease are not found to have high-risk factors and thus are spared the potential morbidity associated with whole pelvic radiation therapy. Furthermore, the findings at operation and careful pathologic examination of the surgical specimen can be helpful in determining prognosis and in identifying patients at greatest risk for persistence or recurrence of disease. Such high-risk patients may require additional therapy.

In addition to an accurate assessment of the extent of the cervical cancer, primary surgical treatment allows for discovery of other intraabdominal incidental conditions and diseases entirely unrelated to the cancer. Ovarian malignancies, pelvic tuberculosis, sigmoid diverticulitis, cholelithiasis, and other diseases and conditions may be encountered at the time of operation.

Preservation of Ovarian Function

When primary radiation therapy with or without chemotherapy is used to treat invasive cervical cancer in premenopausal women, premature loss of ovarian function is an unfortunate and inevitable result. When primary surgery is used instead, the function of normal ovaries can be conserved. Sutton and associates analyzed the incidence of ovarian metastasis for 991 patients with stage IB carcinoma of the cervix treated with radical hysterectomy and pelvic lymphadenectomy on a prospective GOG protocol. Ovarian spread was found in 4 of 770 patients (0.5%) with squamous cell carcinoma and in 2 of 121 patients (1.7%) with adenocarcinoma. The difference was not statistically significant. All six patients with ovarian metastases had other evidence of extracervical disease. This study confirmed that ovarian metastasis is rare in patients with stage IB cervical cancer and extremely rare in the absence of other evidence of extracervical disease.

Although the incidence of ovarian metastasis is slightly higher in women with adenocarcinoma of the cervix as compared with squamous cell carcinoma, ovarian conservation should still be considered, especially in young women. Brand and Berek reported no ovarian metastases in more than 60 patients with adenocarcinoma of the cervix treated with radical surgery. Angel and associates found no ovarian metastases in 41 patients with adenocarcinoma of the cervix who underwent oophorectomy. Greer and coworkers treated 55 patients with stage IB adenocarcinoma of the cervix with radical hysterectomy and pelvic lymphadenectomy. Ninety-one percent had ovarian preservation, and there was no evidence that this contributed to tumor recurrence. Hopkins and coworkers found that the best cumulative 5-year survival rate (93%) with cervical adenocarcinoma was in patients treated by radical hysterectomy without bilateral salpingo-oophorectomy and concluded that "ovarian conservation seems to be an acceptable alternative to bilateral salpingo-oophorectomy" in young patients.

Some authors have advocated transposing the ovaries into the paracolic gutters at the time of radical hysterectomy in premenopausal women to protect the ovaries from radiation damage should postoperative pelvic radiation therapy be needed. The technique used for ovarian transposition was described by Husseinzadeh and coworkers. However, in the series reported by Chambers and coworkers, there was a threefold increase in symptomatic benign ovarian cyst formation with lateral ovarian transposition compared with those who did not have their ovaries transposed. Furthermore, Anderson and coworkers reported that only four of 24 patients (17%) who had ovarian transposition retained ovarian function after postoperative radiation therapy. Moreover, after transposition, 17.6% of patients required surgical treatment for ovarian-associated pain or cysts. These data raise the question of whether paracolic gutter transposition actually achieves its goal of protecting the ovaries.

Sexual Function

Studies of the effect of surgical and radiation treatment for cervical carcinoma on sexual function have been published by Seibel and coworkers from Emory University and by others. Among patients treated with radiation, there are decreases in sexual enjoyment, ability to attain orgasm, frequency of intercourse, and desire for intercourse. Marked alterations can be seen and felt in the upper vagina and paravaginal tissues. The vagina usually is shorter from stenosis. The upper vagina is less pliable. Tissues are fixed and firm. The vaginal mucosa is thin, smooth, and dry with a tendency to split and bleed with slight trauma. Some of these changes are made more pronounced in young women because of hypoestrogenism from radiation-induced premature menopause. They are not completely reversed by intravaginal or oral administration of estrogen. Such functional and anatomic changes are not seen nearly as frequently in patients treated with primary extensive surgery. Even if the vagina has been surgically shortened by several centimeters with primary surgery, it remains soft, pliable, moist, and functional. Unfortunately, in those women who undergo postoperative adjuvant pelvic irradiation, some of this advantage is lost.

Fewer Late Recurrences and Complications

Late recurrences after treatment for cervical cancer are almost never seen after primary radical surgery. They occur more often when patients are treated with primary radiation therapy. The same can be said for complications of treatment. Because of the gradual and progressive obliterative endarteritis produced by irradiating tissue, complications resulting from ischemic changes (e.g., cystitis, proctitis, enteritis, colpocleisis, pyelonephritis) can be seen many years after radiation treatment. Late onset of complications after primary radical hysterectomy and pelvic lymphadenectomy are unusual. These points are especially important when selecting a method of primary treatment for young women.

Psychological Benefits

There are probably important psychological benefits of primary treatment with radical surgery compared with radiation therapy. Most patients prefer to have the tumor removed and are especially encouraged when the surgeon can report that "the cancer is out" and that no evidence of metastatic disease was found at operation. Radiation therapy carries an unfortunate connotation in some patients who feel that it is the treatment of last resort, that the treatments are actually "cooking" the tissues in the pelvis, that the tumor is still there (albeit treated), or that irradiation can cause other cancers. All gynecologic surgeons have heard the disappointment patients express when they are told that they cannot be treated with an operation. Some patients continue to request an operation even after they have completed radiation therapy.

Justification for Pelvic Lymphadenectomy

Historically, there was competition between gynecologic surgeons who advocated radical vaginal hysterectomy without lymphadenectomy and those who advocated radical abdominal hysterectomy with lymphadenectomy. The advocates of extensive vaginal hysterectomy without lymphadenectomy (the Schauta-Amreich-Navratil operation) argued that their patients had fewer postoperative complications (especially urinary fistulas), a lower operative mortality rate, and a cure rate that was almost equal to that achieved by an abdominal operation that included lymphadenectomy. Furthermore, they pointed out that pelvic lymphadenectomy is an incomplete operation at best in that removal of all pelvic lymph nodes that can possibly be involved with metastatic tumor is technically impossible. This is especially true of those inferior gluteal nodes that are located in the region of the ischial spine, as pointed out by Reiffenstuhl. However, even Navratil stated in 1965 that "indications for the Schauta operation must take the lymph node problem into account." Later he performed extraperitoneal pelvic lymphadenectomy with the Schauta operation in all cases of stage I and II that were locally advanced, as did Mitra.

In recent years, the operative mortality and complication rates in patients who have undergone radical abdominal hysterectomy and bilateral pelvic lymphadenectomy have significantly decreased. Operative mortality and fistulas occur in <1% and about 2% of patients, respectively. Therefore, one purported disadvantage of radical hysterectomy (high morbidity) has essentially been removed, and the surgeon can concentrate on the question of whether lymphadenectomy adds anything to the possibility of cure. If a pelvic lymphadenectomy is not done in patients who have a radical hysterectomy for cervical cancer, at least 15% to 20% of patients (those with positive nodes) will be inadequately treated for their disease (unless perhaps all patients receive postoperative pelvic irradiation). In our judgment, it is better to do a pelvic lymphadenectomy in all patients and then give postoperative radiation therapy selectively than to avoid a lymphadenectomy and give postoperative radiation therapy to all patients.

It is the opinion of some that pelvic lymphadenectomy is of no value in those 80% to 90% of patients who have negative lymph nodes. We disagree with this view. We believe that lymphadenectomy is helpful in achieving an adequate central dissection around the cervical tumor, the most important part of the operation. This is especially true of that part of the lymphadenectomy that involves removal of tissue from around the hypogastric vessels, from the obturator fossa, and from the lower presacral region. Admittedly, dissection of lymph nodes from the common iliac vessels and from the paraaortic region does not add to the completeness of the central dissection. Removal of these and other nodes, however, is helpful in prognosis and in identifying patients at greater risk for persistent disease who might receive adjuvant postoperative radiation therapy to the pelvis and perhaps to extended fields along the aorta. Although we seldom dissect and remove the highest paraaortic lymph nodes, we do remove the lower paraaortic nodes around and just above the aortic bifurcation. If pelvic lymph nodes involved with tumor are found during the operation, a concerted effort is made to do a more complete paraaortic dissection. Although it is possible for paraaortic nodes to be directly involved without involvement of pelvic nodes, this is extremely rare. For the group of patients who usually would be chosen for treatment with primary radical surgery, routine extensive paraaortic lymph node dissection would not result in a therapeutic benefit very often. Podczaski and coworkers found positive paraaortic lymph nodes in 7 of 52 patients (13.4%) with stage IB and IIA disease. Twenty-eight of the 52 patients, however, had bulky tumors >5 cm in greatest diameter. Currently, such patients are considered by many gynecologic oncologists not to be appropriate candidates for treatment with primary radical surgery. Patsner and coworkers performed paraaortic lymph node sampling in patients with small (tumor ≤3 cm) stage IB cervical cancer. Only 2 of the 125 patients who underwent radical hysterectomy, bilateral pelvic lymphadenectomy, and paraaortic node sampling had metastases to the paraaortic nodes. No patient had gross paraaortic nodal involvement, and both patients with microscopic paraaortic nodal metastases had grossly positive pelvic nodal involvement. These investigators recommended that paraaortic sampling in patients with small stage IB cervical tumors be restricted to patients with suspicious or positive pelvic or paraaortic nodes. The

TABLE 47.6

SQUAMOUS CELL CARCINOMA OF THE CERVIX: DOSE–TUMOR–VOLUME RELATION[a]

Tumor volume (cm)	Dose (Gy)
<2	50
2	60
2–4	70
4–6	75–89
6	80–100

[a] Average radiation dose required to obtain 90% control in area treated.
From: Shingleton HM, Orr JW. *Cancer of the cervix: diagnosis and treatment.* New York: Churchill Livingstone, 1987:174, with permission.

paraaortic region should be carefully palpated and any enlarged or firm nodes removed, but the gynecologic surgeon should be aware of the added morbidity associated with comprehensive paraaortic lymphadenectomy.

A study reported by Downey and colleagues provides indirect evidence that postoperative pelvic irradiation is more effective in controlling disease after pelvic lymphadenectomy has removed clinically positive lymph nodes that contain metastatic tumor. The amount of irradiation required to eliminate tumor in lymph nodes is directly related to the volume of tumor present (Table 47.6). Thus, removing the larger nodes involved with tumor increases the probability of control of tumor with irradiation. Patients in this study who underwent resection of large positive pelvic nodes followed by postoperative extended-field irradiation had a surprisingly high 5-year recurrence-free survival rate of 51%. The advantages of surgical debulking of positive lymph nodes also was discussed by Potish and coworkers in a later study from the same center. No patient with unresectable pelvic nodes survived 5 years. In 84% (49/58) of cases with grossly positive pelvic nodes, the nodes were able to be debulked. The 5-year actuarial relapse-free survival rates were the same for patients with only microscopically involved pelvic node metastases (56%) and for patients with grossly involved but surgically resected pelvic node metastases (57%). All patients with positive pelvic nodes received postoperative irradiation to the pelvis and paraaortic nodes. These authors believe that surgical debulking of grossly involved pelvic lymph nodes to microscopic residual disease can improve the chance of control with postoperative irradiation.

PERTINENT PELVIC ANATOMY

Arterial and Venous Anatomy

Although the lower portions of the aorta and vena cava are frequently incorporated into the operative field of the pelvic lymphadenectomy, the major operative dissection includes the common iliac, external iliac, and hypogastric (also known as the internal iliac) arteries and veins and their various branches and tributaries. The abdominal aorta emerges through the aortic hiatus of the diaphragm at the lower border of the last thoracic vertebra and descends along the ventral surface of the vertebral column, where it bifurcates into the left and right common iliac arteries at the fourth lumbar vertebra (Fig. 47.10). This is an important anatomic landmark because the bifurcation at L4 lies directly beneath the umbilicus in most cases. Therefore, an abdominal midline incision that provides surgical exposure to the lower aorta needs to be extended somewhat above the umbilicus. The right common iliac artery crosses the upper portion of the left common iliac vein at the aortic bifurcation. This segment of the venous drainage of the left side of the pelvis joins with the right common iliac vein to form the vena cava, which lies directly along the right side of the aorta and on the right lateral side of the bodies of the lumbar vertebrae in its retroperitoneal course through the abdomen.

Both common iliac arteries continue along the medial border of the psoas muscle to the pelvic brim, where they divide into external iliac and hypogastric vessels. As shown in Fig. 47.10, this important vascular division marks the site where the ureters enter the pelvis from the abdomen, usually overlying the terminal end of the common iliac artery on the left and commonly crossing the actual bifurcation of the artery on the right. Both external iliac arteries pass beneath the inguinal ligament to proceed into the leg as the femoral artery. The external iliac artery makes no direct vascular contribution to the pelvis, although there is a fairly consistent arterial branch to the ureter from the midportion of the common iliac artery.

The external iliac vein emerges from beneath the inguinal ligament, where it courses along the lateral pelvic brim on the medial side of the artery until it reaches the proximal segment. Here, the vein passes directly beneath the artery at the bifurcation of the common iliac artery and then passes along the lateral side of the upper half of the artery. It then joins the left common iliac vein to become the inferior vena cava at the fifth lumbar vertebra. In dissecting the lymph nodes along the external iliac vessels, these anatomic landmarks are important to avoid trauma to the wall of the vein as it deviates from the medial to the lateral side of the arterial tree.

The hypogastric artery provides the major blood supply to the pelvic viscera. For descriptive purposes, it is conveniently divided into an anterior and a posterior division. The important branches of the hypogastric artery are shown in Figs. 47.11 and 47.12.

A fairly consistent arterial branch to the ureter arises from the hypogastric artery near the common iliac bifurcation. This vessel passes medially to the ureter and should be preserved, if possible, during the dissection of the hypogastric vessels. The posterior division of the hypogastric artery continues beneath the coccygeus muscle through the ischiorectal fossa, where it becomes the internal pudendal artery to supply the perineum and vulva.

The major blood supply to the pelvic viscera is derived from the anterior division of the hypogastric artery. Figure 47.11 shows the anterior division, which gives off the uterine artery before continuing along the posterolateral pelvic wall to supply the superior and inferior vesical branches to the bladder. The anterior division then continues as the obliterated umbilical artery as it passes cephalad along the inferior surface of the rectus muscle to the umbilicus. In dissecting along the hypogastric artery in a caudad direction, the uterine artery is the first vessel encountered; it emanates from the medial side of the vessel. Passing more inferiorly and medially is the middle hemorrhoidal artery, which supplies a major segment of the rectum and communicates with the superior hemorrhoidal (from the inferior mesenteric) and the inferior hemorrhoidal (from the internal pudendal) arteries.

The hypogastric vein and its tributaries course along the pelvic floor and medial side of the artery to drain the pelvis in close relation to the arterial blood supply. Its extensive anatomic variations and its location along the pelvic sidewall

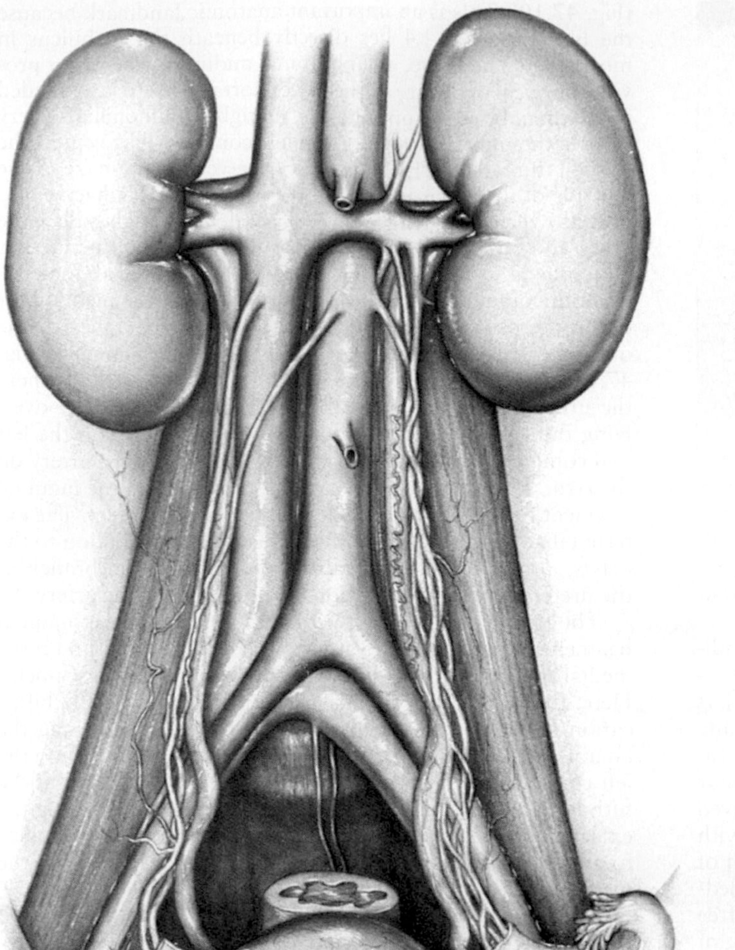

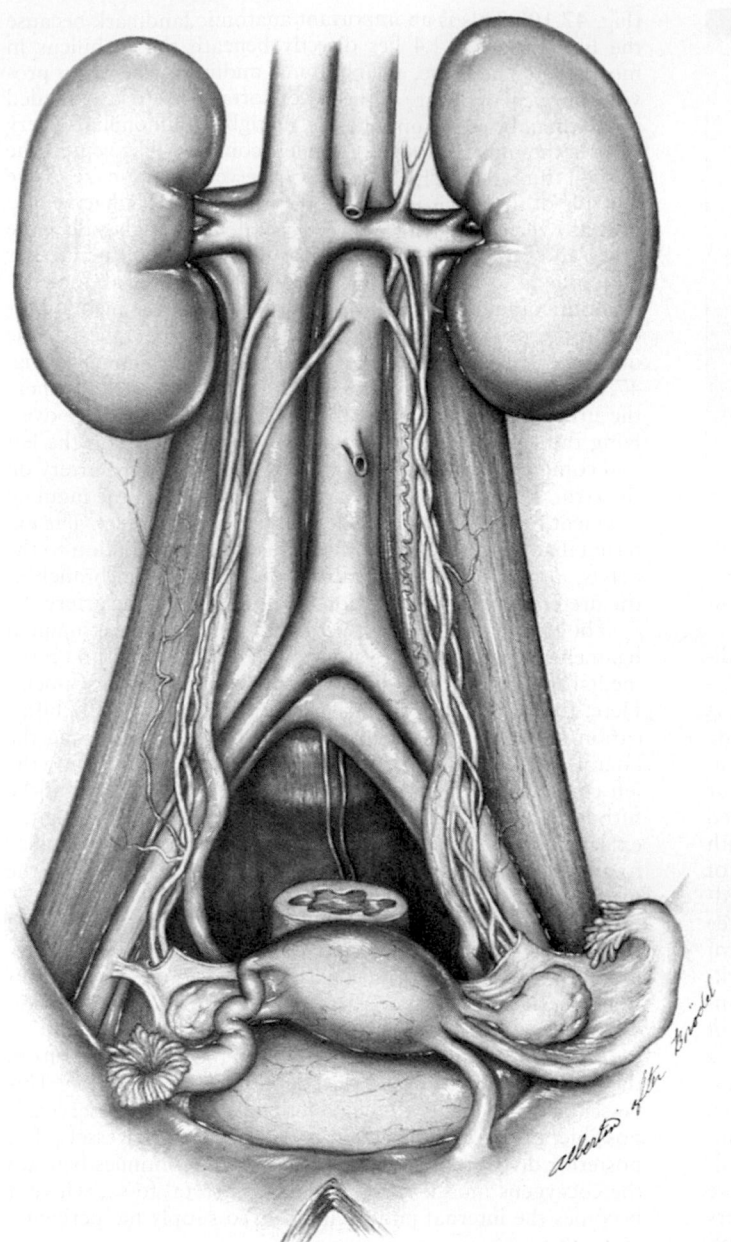

FIGURE 47.10. Abdominal and pelvic anatomy, showing the anatomic relations of the aorta, vena cava, iliac vessels, and ureters. Note the arteriovenous crossing of the right common iliac artery and the left iliac vein.

and floor place these tortuous, thin-walled veins in a precarious and vulnerable position for trauma during deep dissection of the pelvis. As shown in Fig. 47.12, the delicate tributaries of the trunk of the hypogastric vein extend into sacral foramina and pass beneath nerve fibers and muscles within the pelvis, so that their identity during the dissection of the pelvis frequently is obscured. The continuation of the hypogastric vein, in association with the artery, beneath the coccygeus muscle is a frequent site of bleeding when dissection is undertaken along the pelvic floor. When this occurs, it is difficult to identify the vessel because it retracts beneath the margins of the muscle.

The profuse collateral blood supply to the ureter is an important anatomic safeguard that protects its pelvic segment from ischemic necrosis as a result of radical hysterectomy (Fig. 47.13). The ureter has the advantage of a multiple-source blood supply. This favorable collateral circulation permits interruption of small arteries and veins deep in the pelvis during extensive dissection of the base of the broad ligament without producing a significant incidence of ischemic necrosis and fistula formation. The freely anastomosing arterial and venous network that courses along the longitudinal surface of the ureter in its adventitial layer is supplied in its superior segment by branches from the renal and ovarian arteries. The middle segment of the ureter derives its blood supply directly from aortic branches and from a vessel from the common iliac artery. As the ureter enters the pelvis and courses along the lateral pelvic wall, it receives arterial branches from the uterine, vaginal, middle hemorrhoidal, and vesical arteries. As it approaches the trigone of the bladder, it has a rich arteriovenous collateral circulation from the arterial branches to the vagina and base of the bladder. Protection of this important vascular network is important for the integrity of the terminal ureter during extensive dissection of the cardinal ligament. Preservation of the lateral aspect of the posterior segment of the

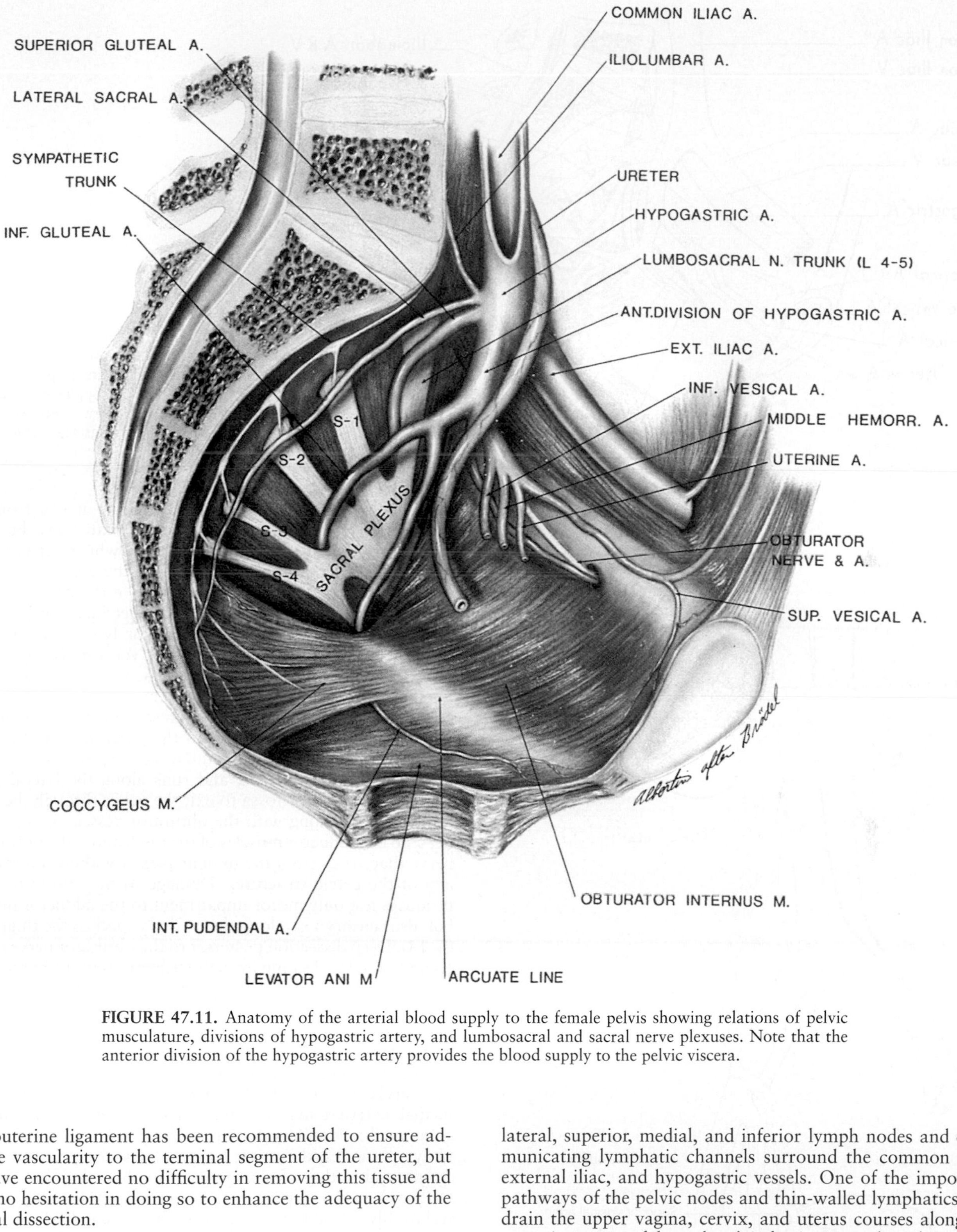

FIGURE 47.11. Anatomy of the arterial blood supply to the female pelvis showing relations of pelvic musculature, divisions of hypogastric artery, and lumbosacral and sacral nerve plexuses. Note that the anterior division of the hypogastric artery provides the blood supply to the pelvic viscera.

vesicouterine ligament has been recommended to ensure adequate vascularity to the terminal segment of the ureter, but we have encountered no difficulty in removing this tissue and have no hesitation in doing so to enhance the adequacy of the central dissection.

Lymphatic Anatomy

The lymphatic drainage of the pelvis follows the course of the arterial and venous blood supply. Although there are multiple variations in the lymphatic anatomy of the pelvis, in general, lateral, superior, medial, and inferior lymph nodes and communicating lymphatic channels surround the common iliac, external iliac, and hypogastric vessels. One of the important pathways of the pelvic nodes and thin-walled lymphatics that drain the upper vagina, cervix, and uterus courses along the posterior aspect of the endopelvic fascia. Here, the pelvic nodes pass through the uterosacral ligament area and terminate in lymph nodes along the lateral aspect of the sacrum. These nodes communicate freely with lymphatic channels from the bifurcation of the common iliac artery near the lateral sacral and ischiosacral fossae. These can be difficult nodes to resect because they are closely attached to the thin-walled tributaries

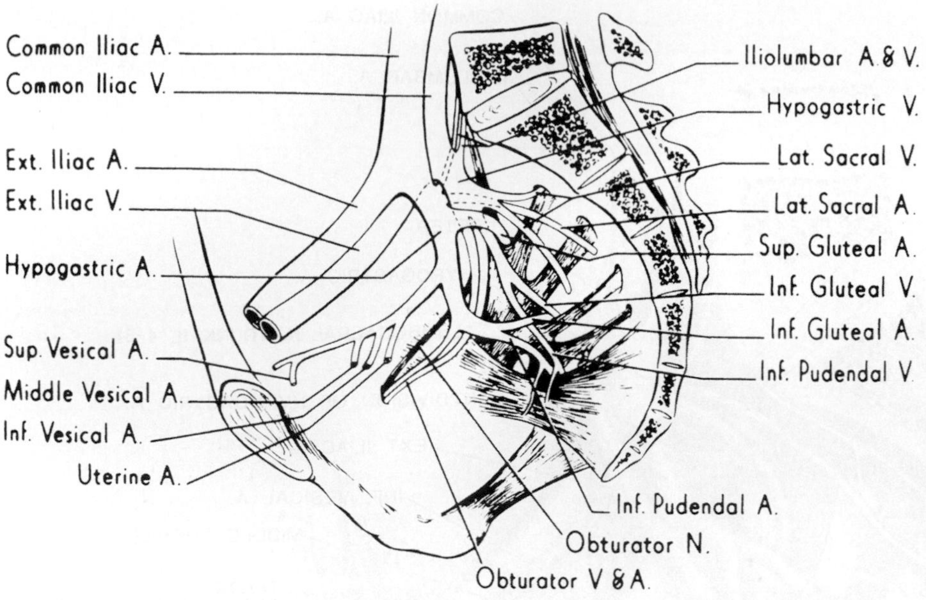

FIGURE 47.12. Anatomy of hypogastric vein. (From: Thompson JD. Extensive hysterectomy and bilateral pelvic lymphadenectomy. In: Coppleson M, ed. *Gynecologic Oncology.* 2nd ed. New York: Churchill Livingstone, 1992, with permission.)

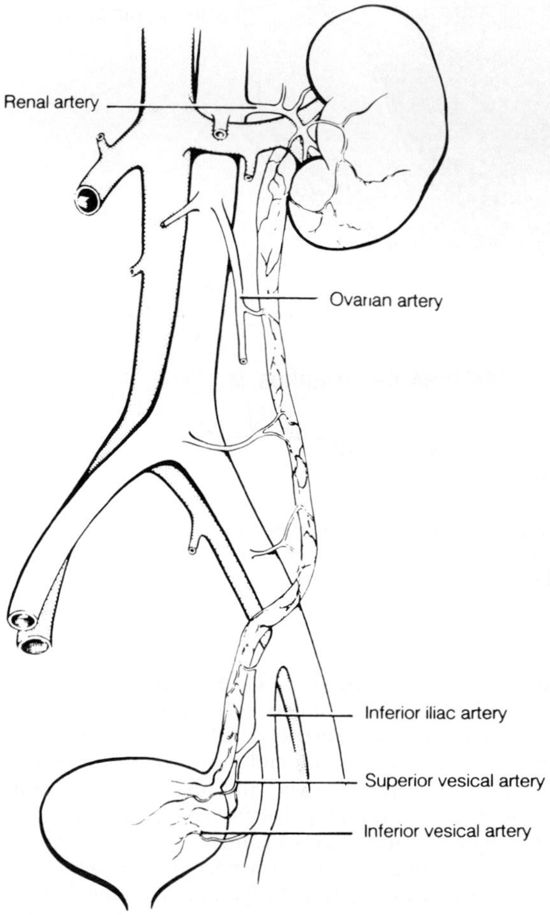

FIGURE 47.13. Blood supply of the ureter showing multiple sources of collateral arterial circulation.

of the hypogastric vein. In dissecting the nodes from the bifurcation of the common iliac vessels, care must be taken to avoid injury to the hypogastric vein, which extends from beneath the artery on the medial side in this area.

The most direct lymphatic drainage of the cervix and upper vagina is through the lateral parametrium (cardinal ligament) to the hypogastric and obturator lymphatics. Because of the presence of obscure obturator veins and multiple venous tributaries from the hypogastric vein along the pelvic floor, the obturator dissection can be associated with troublesome venous bleeding. Injury also can occur to the obturator nerve, which arises from the anterior division of the second, third, and fourth lumbar nerves; enters the pelvis through the psoas muscle; and runs along the lateral pelvic wall in the obturator fossa to exit the pelvis through the obturator foramen along with the obturator vessels. It is a motor nerve to the adductor muscles of the thigh and is the only motor nerve that arises from the lumbar plexus without innervating any of the pelvic structures. Damage to the obturator nerve produces not only motor impairment to the adductor muscles but also sensory loss along the medial aspect of the thigh (Fig. 47.14). Deep dissection posterior to the obturator nerve can be complicated by bleeding from the tributaries of the hypogastric and obturator veins so that dissection in this area, if necessary, must be done with great care, using clips on the small vessels and compression for troublesome venous bleeding.

Reiffenstuhl, in his classic study of the lymphatics of the female genital organs, describes efferent lymph channels from the cervix to the interiliac lymph nodes, the lateral and medial external iliac lymph nodes, the lateral and medial common iliac lymph nodes, the sacral lymph nodes, the subaortic lymph nodes, the aortic lymph nodes, the superior gluteal lymph nodes, the inferior gluteal lymph nodes, and the rectal lymph nodes. Of these, the inferior gluteal nodes are not technically possible to remove with the standard approach. This is because the nodes lie around the ischial spine in proximity to the inferior gluteal artery and pudendal artery and nerve. An imposing network of veins also surrounds the inferior gluteal nodes. They are thin walled, easy to damage, difficult to expose, and difficult to control when damaged. Reiffenstuhl's concepts of the lymphatic drainage of the cervix are partially shown in Fig. 47.15.

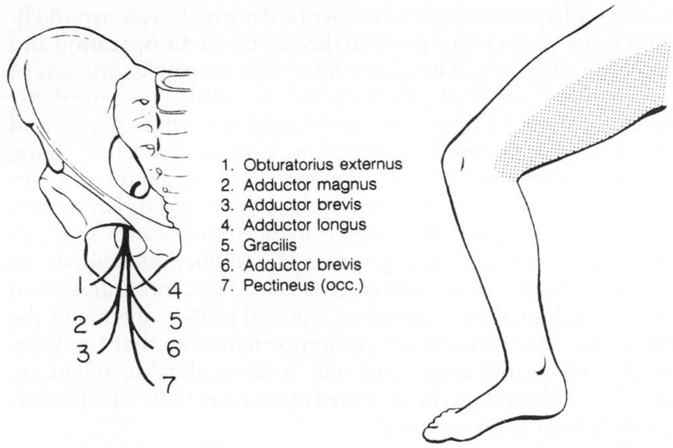

FIGURE 47.14. Obturator nerve (L2 through L4): motor and sensory innervation.

Sentinel lymph node studies in women with cervical cancer are also adding to our knowledge of the lymphatic drainage *in vivo,* and identification of sentinel lymph nodes with blue dye and technicium injections is feasible with very low morbidity. These sentinel lymph nodes can be submitted for ultrastaging with immunohistochemistry staining and may help in the postoperative management of cases. Further evaluation is needed to see if sentinel lymph node identification can potentially replace complete pelvic lymphadenectomy. This might reduce the total operative time as well as some perioperative complications and long-term complications, such as the risk of postoperative leg lymphedema, which is occasionally seen in patients undergoing pelvic lymphadenectomy.

CONCEPT OF RADICAL ABDOMINAL HYSTERECTOMY AND BILATERAL PELVIC LYMPHADENECTOMY

There are several variations of hysterectomy used in the management of cervical carcinoma. The description of the five

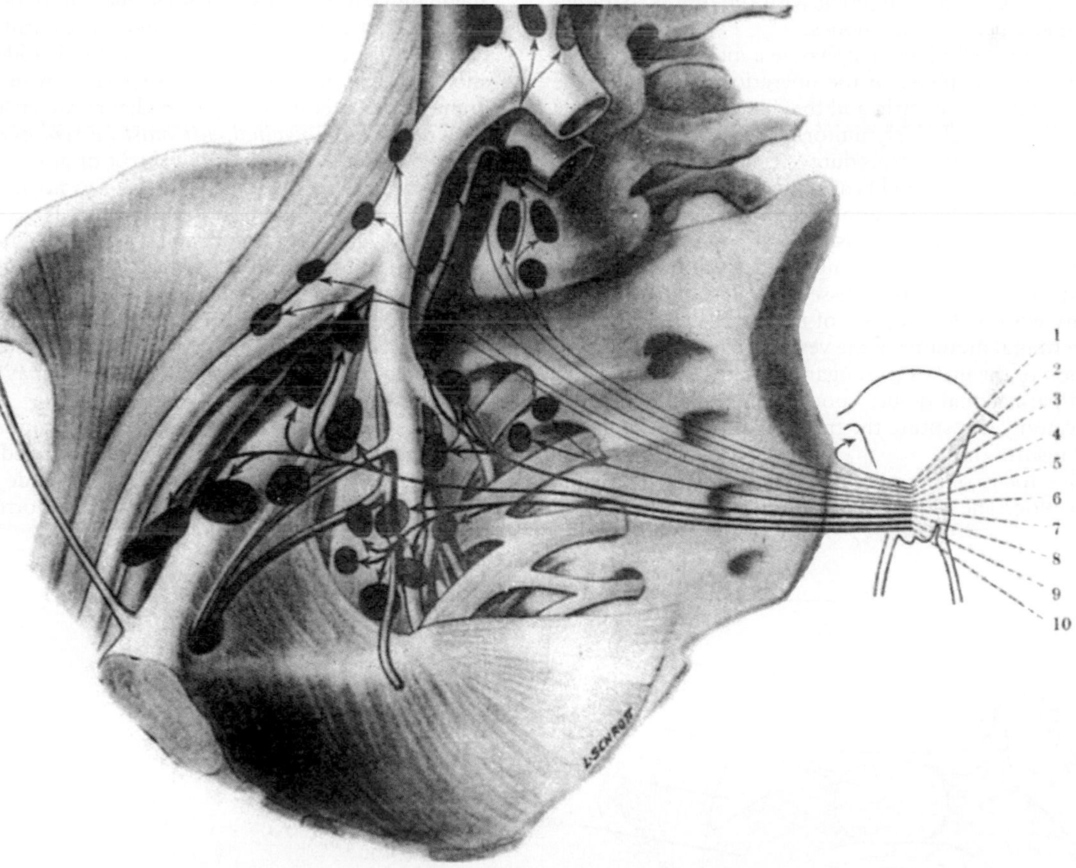

FIGURE 47.15. The regional lymph node stations of the uterine cervix. Channels 8, 9, and 10 (indicated by especially heavy lines) lead to those regional lymph node stations most frequently reached by the efferent lymph vessels of the cervix. Nonetheless, it is necessary to remember that carcinoma cells also can reach the pelvic lymph nodes by way of channels 1 through 7, without previous interruption, to (*1*) rectal, (*2*) subaortic (promontorial), (*3*) aortic, (*4*) medial common iliac, (*5*) lateral common iliac, (*6*) lateral external iliac, (*7*) sacral, (*8*) superior gluteal, (*9*) interiliac, and (*10*) inferior gluteal lymph nodes. (From: Reiffenstuhl G. *The lymphatics of the female genital organs.* Philadelphia: JB Lippincott, 1964, with permission.)

classes of hysterectomy by Piver and colleagues has found general acceptance. The first three classes are used in the primary treatment of cervical carcinoma, whereas the last two classes are generally reserved for patients with recurrent disease. The class I hysterectomy is a simple extrafascial total hysterectomy. It is used as primary treatment for stage IA1 disease and after concurrent chemotherapy and radiation therapy for stage IB2 and bulky stage IIA cervical carcinoma. The class II hysterectomy (Fig. 47.8), also known as a modified radical hysterectomy, removes a more generous vaginal cuff, ligates the uterine artery on the medial side of the ureter (but does not dissect the ureter from the vesicouterine ligament), and removes the inner one third to one half of the cardinal ligament. As previously stated, some authors recommend the performance of the class II hysterectomy for stage IA2 cervical carcinoma. The class III operation is the classic Meigs procedure, with removal of all of the parametrium and paravaginal tissue in addition to the pelvic lymph nodes (Fig. 47.8). A more extensive procedure is performed in the class IV radical hysterectomy, in which the ureter is completely dissected from the cardinal and vesicouterine ligaments, the superior vesical artery is sacrificed, and three fourths of the vagina is removed as well as the uterus and parametria, along with a complete lymphadenectomy. A far more extensive procedure is done with the class V radical hysterectomy, in which the terminal ureter or a segment of the bladder or rectum is removed along with the uterus, parametria, adnexa, and pelvic lymph nodes.

Although many techniques emphasize a more or less extensive dissection in one phase of the operation or another, the management of the parametria and the dissection of the pelvic lymph nodes appear relatively uniform. Because the most serious complication of this procedure is related to ureteral fistulas and stenosis, many modifications have been undertaken to ensure an adequate blood supply to the terminal ureter. We agree that the terminal ureter must have a good blood supply and believe that this can be accomplished without jeopardizing the adequacy of the central dissection. The classic radical hysterectomy with wide resection of the parametrium, dissection of the terminal ureter from the vesicouterine ligament, and wide resection of the uterosacral ligaments, upper 2 to 3 cm of vagina, and paravaginal tissues, along with a thorough pelvic lymphadenectomy, constitute the traditional procedure that is used in our institution.

The major focus of the operation is the adequacy of the central dissection. The central cervical tumor must be removed with an adequate margin of uninvolved normal tissue around it. This is the most crucial point in the success of the operation and has been emphasized by many of the famous pelvic surgeons of former years, especially Parsons and Navratil. The central dissection can be facilitated by developing the pelvic spaces and using proper planes for dissection. Correct dissection along natural rather than artificial connective tissue planes and correct development of the pelvic spaces (paravesical, pararectal, vesicocervical, and rectovaginal) avoid unnecessary injury to pelvic vessels, keep blood loss to a minimum, and facilitate an adequate central dissection (Fig. 47.16). The central dissection also is facilitated by a complete removal of the contents of the obturator fossa (except the obturator nerve) so that branches of the hypogastric artery and vein in the cardinal ligament are clearly visible and can be dissected away from their attachments to the lateral pelvic sidewall.

The importance of an adequate central dissection also was emphasized by Girardi and coworkers. By studying surgical specimens processed according to the giant-section technique of Burghardt and Pickel, parametrial lymph nodes were found in 280 (78%) of the 359 surgical specimens from radical hysterectomies. Metastases to parametrial nodes were found in 63 (22.5%) of these 280 specimens. The lymphatic drainage from the cervix to the pelvic lymph nodes runs through the parametrium, and deposits of tumor often are found there. An adequate central dissection must include removal of a wide margin of parametrial tissue around the central tumor and total removal of the parametria from the bladder, the rectum, and the lateral pelvic wall because positive lymph nodes can be found in the lateral as well as medial parametrium.

When a large vaginal cuff must be removed because of a bulky cervical tumor or involvement of adjacent vaginal mucosa, starting the operation from below may facilitate the central dissection. Sometimes, a bulky lesion is excised and fulgurated transvaginally. The formation of the vaginal cuff is done in a manner similar to that in the Schauta-Amreich procedure. The vaginal incision is made around the entire circumference of the vagina, mobilizing the vaginal cuff from paravaginal tissue. Further dissection into the paravesical space, vesicocervical space, and rectovaginal space from below may be easier than from above.

Superior to the midcommon iliac arteries and in the paraaortic region, lymph nodes are sampled in selected patients (usually stage IB1 and IIA). A special effort is made to remove any nodes that look or feel suspicious. The paraaortic lymph nodes

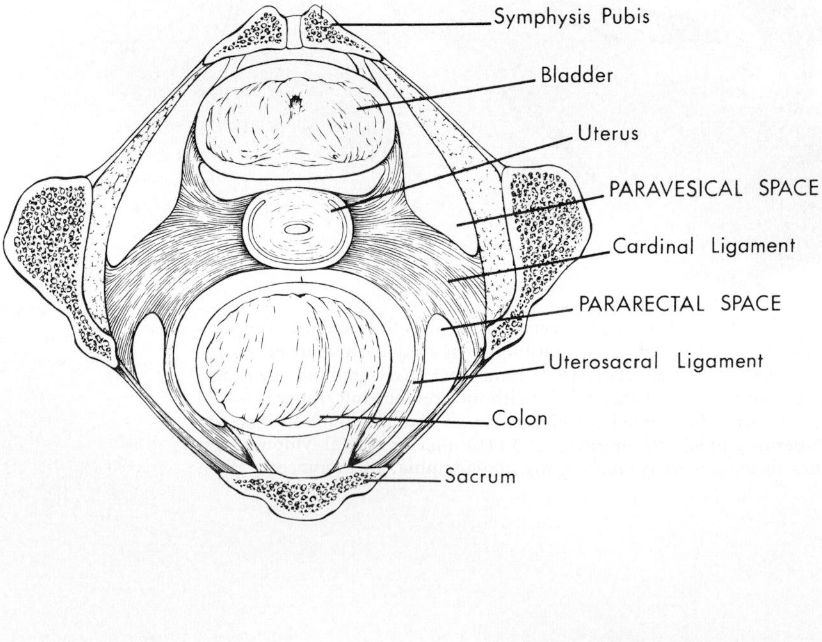

FIGURE 47.16. Cross section of pelvis showing paravesical and pararectal space. The base of the broad ligament (cardinal ligament) extends to the lateral pelvic wall and contains the major lymphatics draining the cervix.

then are sent for frozen section analysis. Approximately 5% to 10% of stage IB patients have paraaortic lymph node metastasis. Metastasis to the paraaortic lymph nodes is considered by many gynecologic oncologists as a contraindication to radical hysterectomy. These patients are currently being treated with extended-field radiation therapy with concurrent chemotherapy.

RADICAL ABDOMINAL HYSTERECTOMY SURGICAL TECHNIQUE

Preoperative Evaluation and Preparation

After the initial history and physical examination have indicated the possibility of primary treatment with radical hysterectomy and pelvic lymphadenectomy, the usual preoperative evaluation common before any extensive operation is indicated. We also recommend a chest x-ray to screen for cardiac or pulmonary disease as well as the very low risk of pulmonary metastases.

Contrary to the frequent practice of doing all possible tests on every patient, it is our practice to be selective and to do only those tests and procedures that are expected to yield useful information. It is not necessary (and indeed may be inappropriate) to subject every patient to a long list of preoperative procedures that are expensive and exhausting and have little, if any, expectation of providing useful information. Indeed, it is most unfortunate when a test or procedure yields questionable or suspicious findings that require one or more additional studies that, after delay, discomfort, and expense turn out to be negative or even perhaps nondiagnostic. Good judgment from an experienced clinician is usually the most helpful.

A young, healthy patient with a small cervical lesion requires an admission history and physical examination, chest radiograph and routine laboratory studies, and anesthesia consultation. If the patient is older, has medical complications, or has a larger or undifferentiated cervical lesion, the preoperative workup and preparation may be more involved and thorough. Although an intravenous pyelogram provides good visualization of the course and number of ureters, if radiologic evaluation of the abdomen and pelvis is being considered, most surgeons obtain a CT scan of the abdomen and pelvis, which also shows the course and number of ureters and also may provide additional information about nodal or other metastases. However, because of the uncertainty of enlarged nodes on CT scan, patients with clinical stage IB1 disease and enlarged pelvic nodes on CT scan would not make us cancel the surgical approach in favor of radiation therapy.

Larger lesions or those more likely to have metastases may be investigated by pelvic and abdominal CT scan or magnetic resonance scans, but we have rarely found those to be helpful in women with small cervical cancers. They may be most helpful when the clinician is undecided regarding whether primary surgery or radiation is the best management option—a clean, normal study may be reassuring that primary surgery is the way to go, whereas suspicious, enlarged nodes in a woman with a 4-cm cervical lesion helps make the decision to recommend radiation. Likewise, cystoscopy or proctoscopy are rarely indicated or helpful in the preoperative evaluation of early-stage cervical cancer. As much as possible should be done on an outpatient basis before admission to the hospital.

Bowel Preparation

In our institution, patients are asked to start a liquid diet 24 hours before surgery. They also are given a mechanical bowel preparation and sometimes oral antibiotics if significant peritoneal adhesions are anticipated or there is a history of previous pelvic surgery or radiation. An intestinal tube for suction is not necessary.

Positioning and Incision

Multiple approaches to performing a radical abdominal hysterectomy and bilateral pelvic lymphadenectomy have been described. The traditional transperitoneal approach has been used in our institution for many years with satisfactory results. The transverse Maylard or Cherney incisions are used by some, whereas others prefer midline incisions. Orr and Scribner have reported shorter hospital stays when a Pfannenstiel incision is used. Currie has presented and published a film using a transverse cosmetic incision with vertical fascial entry for selected patients.

After anesthesia is induced, some surgeons prefer that the patient be placed comfortably in stirrups with the buttocks brought to the edge of the "broken" table. Pneumatic compression devices are placed on both lower extremities and the knees are separated about 90 degrees. The thighs are elevated only 15 to 20 degrees relative to the abdomen. Care is taken to avoid pressure on the peroneal nerves in the legs. Proponents of this position claim several advantages. There is less strain on the patient's lumbosacral spine when the thighs are slightly flexed. This is especially important for patients with lumbosacral back problems. It is possible to have a second assistant stand at the foot of the table between the patient's legs. His or her participation in the operation is greatly facilitated by being closer to the operative field. Finally, in this position, the urethral orifice, vaginal introitus, and anal orifice are all available for instrumentation in case this is necessary to clarify anatomy.

After the patient is positioned on the operating table, a careful rectovaginal-abdominal pelvic examination is done. This can be followed by cystoscopy or proctosigmoidoscopy if desired. It may be necessary to shave a small amount of the escutcheon, but vulvar hair is not shaved completely. The skin is prepared from the rib margin to the midthigh, with special attention given to the umbilicus, perineum, and vagina. The patient is draped, a transurethral Foley catheter is inserted into the bladder, and the operation is begun.

When operating abdominally, the exposure achieved depends on the choice of incision, the method of retracting, the placement and intensity of overhead lights, and the participation of willing and skillful assistants. Suction should be available to keep the field as dry as possible and is preferred over sponges for two reasons. First, sponges are more traumatic to delicate serosal surfaces and other tissues. Second, a determination of the amount of blood lost can be more accurate if the largest percentage has been suctioned from the operative field into a calibrated bottle and measured.

It usually is possible (and always desirable) to keep the number of clamps in the operative field to an absolute minimum. If the field is cluttered with clamps, the operator cannot see well to operate. There is an unfortunate tendency for gynecologic surgeons to use instruments that are too short. Pedicle clamps, tissue forceps, dissecting scissors, needle holders, and all other instruments must be longer when operating deep in the pelvis and when operating on obese patients. The handles of the instruments must come all the way out and above the level of the incision so that they do not interfere with the operator's vision.

Evaluation at Laparotomy

As stated, the operation is initiated through a low transverse (Maylard, Cherney, Pfannenstiel) or a low midline incision. In most patients, the umbilicus identifies the location of the bifurcation of the aorta; therefore, extension of the incision about 2 to 3 cm above the umbilicus is recommended for adequate exposure of this area if a lower midline incision is used. The midline incision is protected by a moist pack beneath each arm of the self-retaining retractor to avoid excessive compression of the epigastric vessels that course beneath the rectus muscles. In case of a lengthy operative procedure, the mechanical retractors are released at periodic intervals to improve circulation through the abdominal musculature. The bladder is decompressed by an indwelling catheter throughout the procedure to facilitate exposure and maintain an accurate record of urine output.

Before initiating the pelvic procedure, the abdominal viscera and parietal peritoneum of the abdominal cavity are evaluated meticulously for possible evidence of metastatic tumor. The superior and inferior surfaces of the liver are carefully palpated, as is the region of the celiac plexus. The undersurface of the diaphragm is particularly vulnerable to metastases, especially the right hemidiaphragm, where the paraaortic lymphatics pass from the abdominal cavity into the mediastinum. The mesentery of the large and small bowel and the serosal surface of the bowel along with the omentum should be examined carefully for evidence of metastatic tumor. The kidneys are examined and the retroperitoneal space along the aorta and vena cava is palpated assiduously because these are the major sites of extrapelvic spread of cervical cancer. It is well known that 15% or more of paraaortic node metastases are occult; therefore, even the most unsuspecting node should be removed and evaluated histologically by frozen-section study for possible metastatic tumor. Therefore, it is our practice to sample any paracaval or paraaortic node that is identifiable before initiating the procedure and send it for frozen section analysis. If there is histopathologic evidence of unsuspected, metastatic tumor in a paraaortic lymph node, we generally do not proceed with a radical hysterectomy, and the operation is abandoned. These patients are currently being treated with concurrent chemotherapy and extended-field radiation therapy.

Peritoneal washings for cytologic examination usually are not obtained because the yield is low and the prognostic significance is undetermined.

At this point in the procedure, any adhesions in the pelvis are lysed, and the intestines are placed in the upper abdomen and held there with moist packs. A suitable self-retaining retractor can be used. If Bookwalter, Turner-Warwick, or Balfour retractors are used in a lower midline incision, care must be taken to avoid compression of the femoral nerves by the lateral blades.

Evaluation of the extent of the pelvic tumor is carried out at this time by examining the course of the lymphatic drainage of the pelvis, which is carefully palpated along the pelvic vessels. When enlarged or clinically suspicious nodes are found, they are removed and immediately sent for frozen-section study while further evaluation of the pelvis is undertaken. The paravesical and pararectal spaces are important anatomic landmarks. When developed, they provide an opportunity for thorough exploration of the intervening base of the broad ligament (Fig. 47.16). Tumor can extend into the base of the broad ligament without detection of anatomic evidence of disease before operation. This step, therefore, is a safeguard in determining the possible extension of tumor beyond the cervix and into the immediate paracervical tissues. When there is evidence of extracervical disease, we may abandon the surgical procedure unless there is clear evidence that the disease can be removed cleanly. In either case, full pelvic irradiation is indicated. Certainly, the lateral pelvic wall must be free of tumor. When the central tumor is clearly resectable, we do not hesitate to complete the operation, even if there is evidence of metastatic disease in the pelvic lymph nodes.

A decision must be made about conservation or removal of the tubes and ovaries before the pelvic planes and spaces are developed. If normal ovaries are conserved in premenopausal patients, the tubes usually also are left in. After the round ligaments are clamped, cut, and ligated, the uteroovarian ligaments and medial fallopian tubes are clamped and doubly ligated. The infundibulopelvic ligaments are carefully mobilized, and the adnexal organs are packed out of the operative field with the intestines.

Development of Paravesical Space

The anterior leaf of the broad ligament forms the roof of the *paravesical space* and blends with the bladder peritoneum medially and the parietal peritoneum laterally. This deep fossa beneath the peritoneal covering is composed of loose connective tissue and fat. It occupies the area between the bladder and the retropubic space medially, with the pelvic sidewall and obturator muscle forming the lateral boundaries. The superior boundary is formed by the cardinal ligament, whereas the floor is composed of the levator ani muscle. After clamping and ligating the round ligament about midway along its course, the anterior leaf of the broad ligament is opened in an inferior direction, passing well into the pelvis before diverting the incision medially to reflect the bladder peritoneum from the lower uterine segment (Fig. 47.17A). The paravesical space can be entered without difficulty with gentle digital pressure, making certain that the dissection is initiated between the external iliac vein laterally and the obliterated hypogastric artery (lateral umbilical ligament) medially. The dissection is carried all the way down to the levator ani muscle (Fig. 47.17B). There are no major blood vessels in this potential space, although occasionally an aberrant obturator vessel emerges from the inferior epigastric artery and courses along the posterior aspect of the pubic bone to the obturator space. With gentle digital dissection, the pelvic floor can be palpated and the posterior aspect of the space can be identified, including the anterior margin of the cardinal ligament.

Development of Pararectal Space

The *pararectal space* lies beneath the pelvic peritoneum and extends between the cardinal ligament laterally and the uterosacral ligament medially. It can be entered by extending the incision in the anterior leaf of the broad ligament in a cephalic direction along the lateral margin of the infundibulopelvic ligament (Fig. 47.18A). By retracting the infundibulopelvic ligament and displacing the uterus medially, the uterosacral ligament is placed on a stretch, and the pararectal space is widened. Dissection of this space is much more precarious than that of the paravesical space. Unskilled dissection in this area frequently is associated with troublesome bleeding. The medial border of the fossa is bounded by the uterosacral ligament and rectum, and the lateral border is formed superiorly by the piriformis muscle and inferiorly by the levator

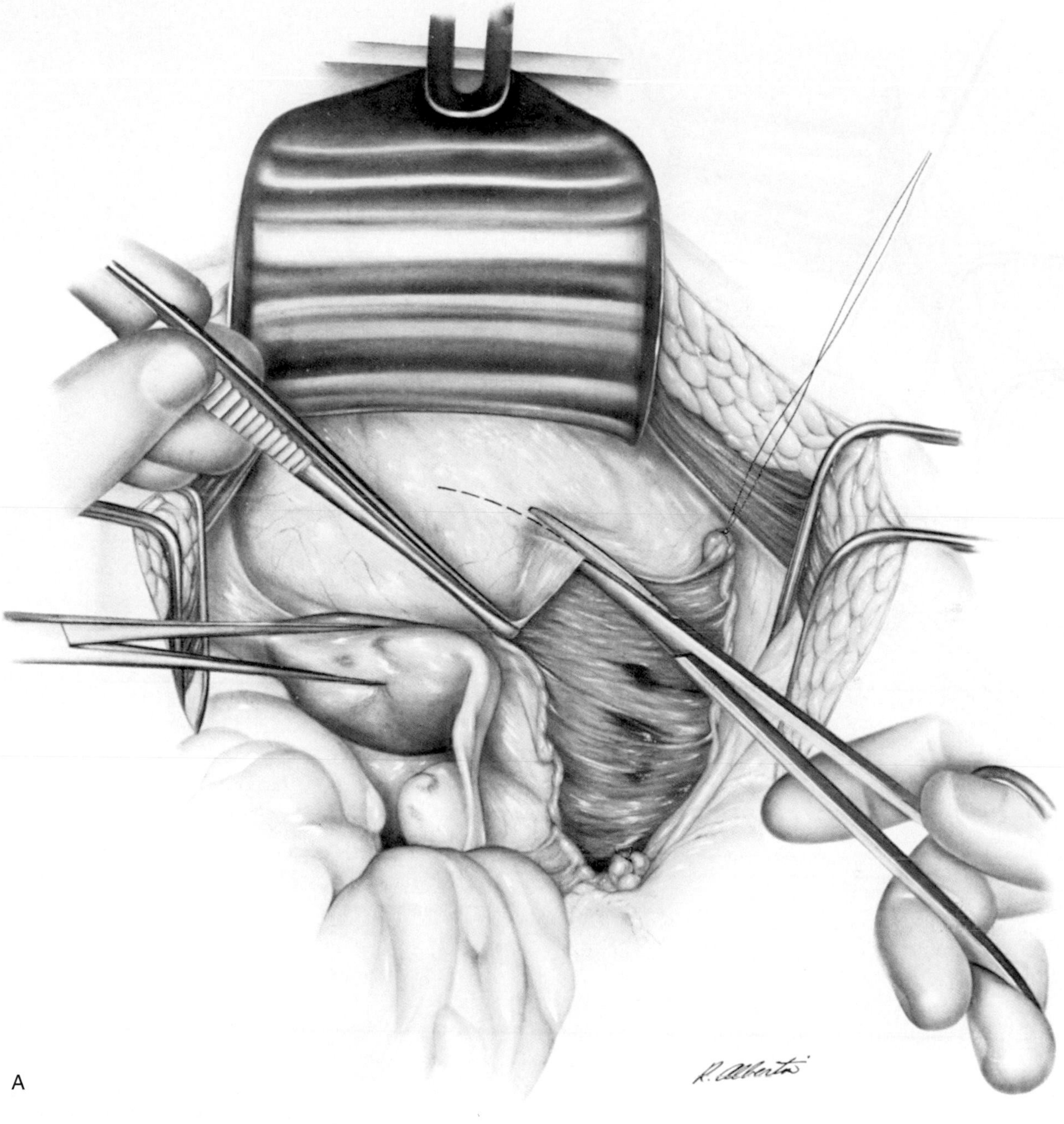

FIGURE 47.17. **A:** Opening the anterior leaf of the broad ligament after ligation of the right round ligament and infundibulopelvic ligament. *(Continued)*

muscle. The sacrum forms the posterior margin of the space, and the ureter is attached to the peritoneum along the roof of the space before entering the medial aspect of the cardinal ligament. The hypogastric artery and vein are located in the deeper aspect of the pararectal space along the levator ani muscle. The cardinal ligament forms the caudal and lateral borders of this important area. Entry into the pararectal space must be made cautiously (Fig. 47.18A) with medial displacement of the ureter and its attached peritoneum. A point between the ureter, which is attached to the medial leaf of peritoneum, and the hypogastric artery is selected. Blunt dissection should be used in this area, and careful handling of tissue is imperative to avoid unnecessary damage to small veins deep in this fossa. When the examining finger reaches the pelvic floor and levator ani muscle, the fossa narrows, and care must be taken to avoid damage to the lateral sacral and hemorrhoidal vessels. The dissection is carried vertically downward for a short distance. The further development of the space then changes to an inferior and caudad direction lateral to the rectum. If the development of the space is difficult, it should be delayed until a later time in the operation. When the paravesical and pararectal spaces have been dissected (Fig. 47.18B), the pelvic floor and cardinal ligament easily can be identified and palpated. In the absence of demonstrable tumor extension, the case is

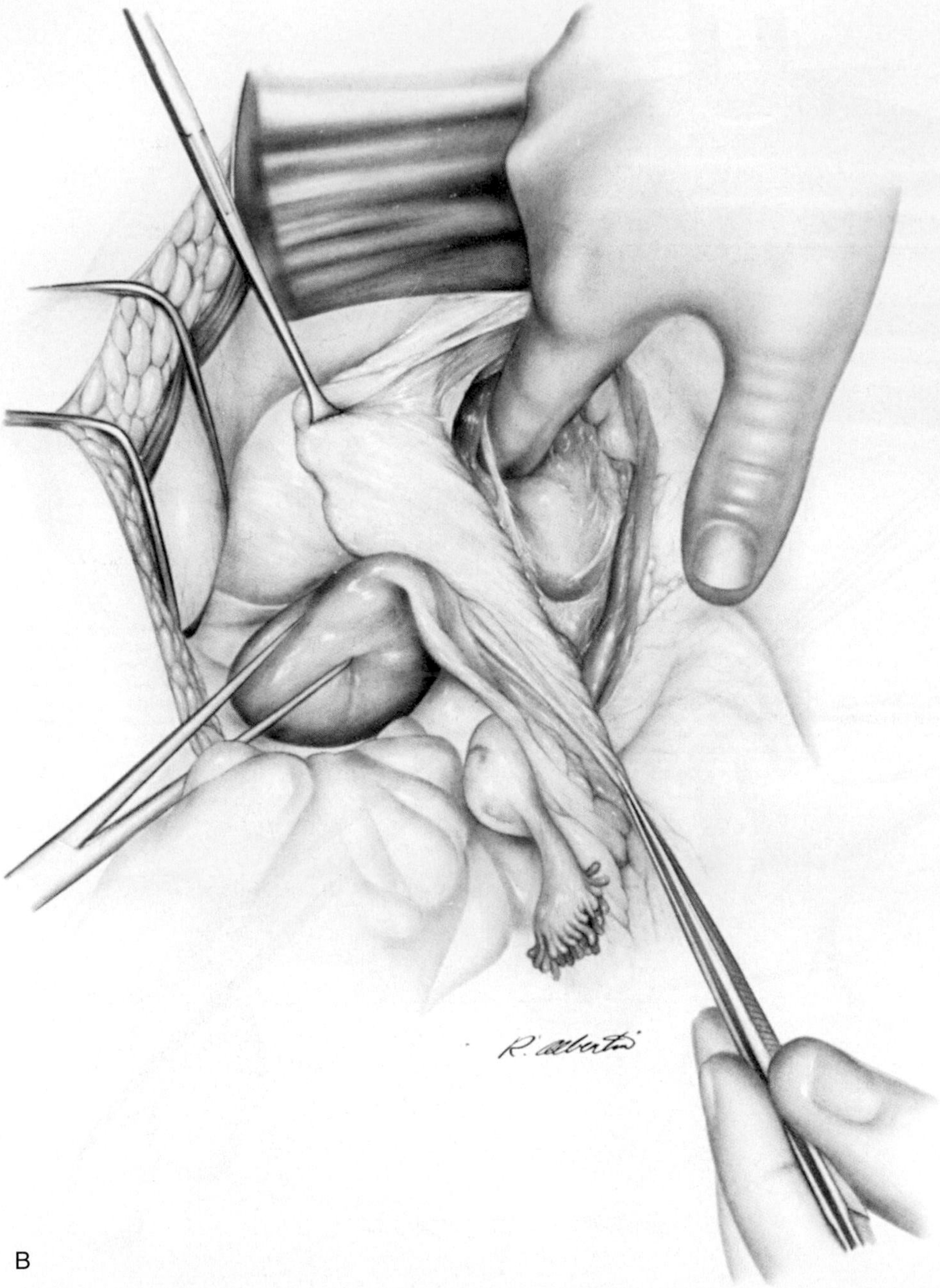

B

FIGURE 47.17. (*Continued*) **B:** Development of paravesical space.

considered operable, and the lymph node dissection is initiated at this time.

Pelvic Lymphadenectomy

Dissection of the lymphatic tissue along the iliac vessels can begin in the region of the bifurcation of the common iliac artery and extend superiorly to the bifurcation of the aorta and inferiorly to the inguinal ligament and deep circumflex iliac vein, or it can begin at another point along the course of the iliac vessels. The opening of the posterior peritoneal leaf of the broad ligament must be extended to the area of the pelvic brim, where the ureter is easily identified as it enters the pelvis at the bifurcation of the common iliac artery. This dissection is made easier if the infundibulopelvic ligament has been ligated and divided; however, the ligament and ovarian vessels can be retracted medially if the adnexa are preserved. The ovary and tube also can be detached from the uterine corpus and gently tucked beneath the retractor above. In dissecting the presacral area in the angle of the bifurcation of the aorta, care must be taken to avoid bleeding from the middle sacral vessels as well as from the proximal part of the left external iliac vein, which courses through this retroperitoneal space. It is best to occlude the middle sacral vessels with smaller vascular clips as they are identified, and if traumatized, the venous bleeding can be controlled with positive pressure against the sacrum and with vascular clips. The lymphatic tissue along the common iliac vessels

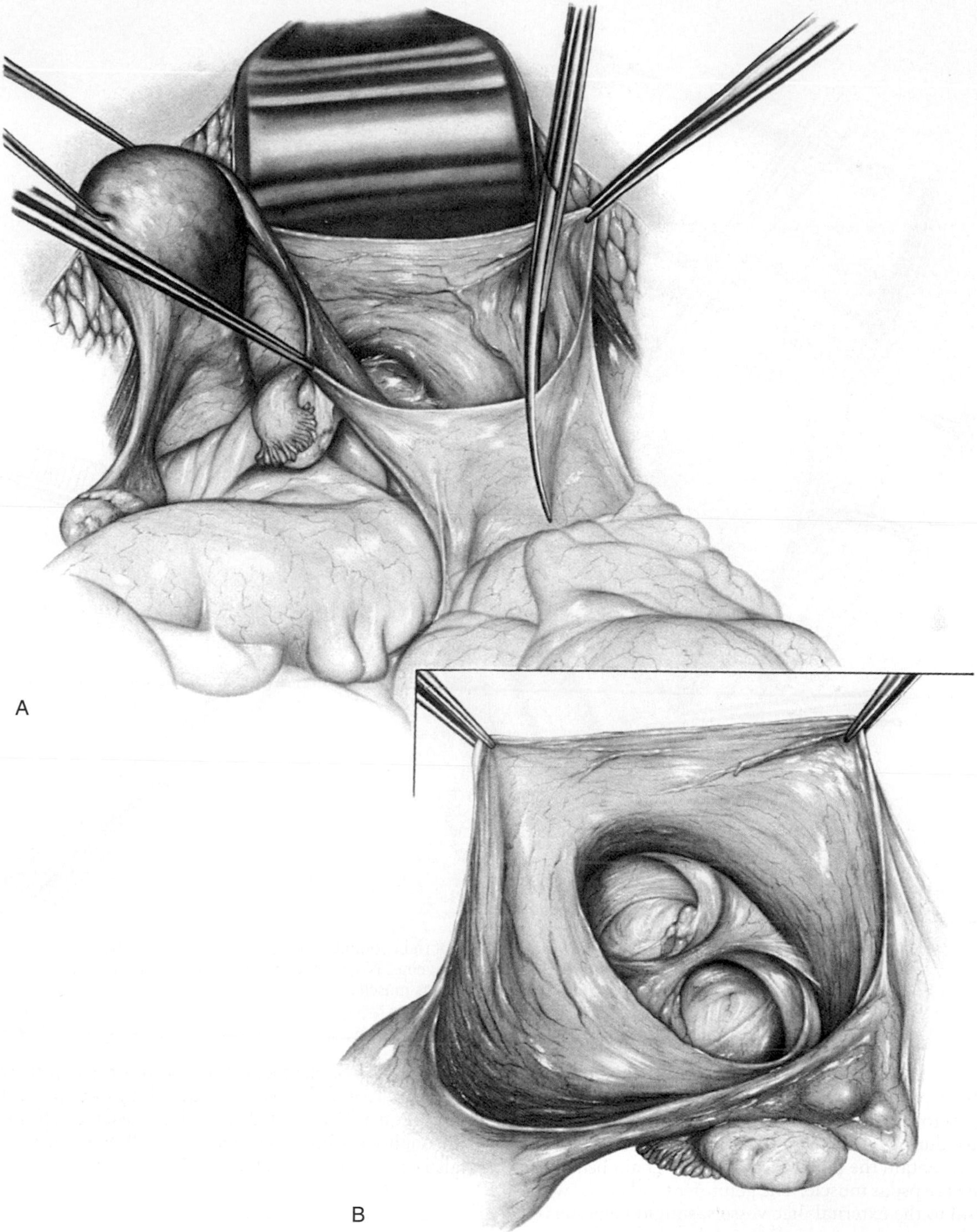

FIGURE 47.18. **A:** Extending the incision in the anterior leaf of the broad ligament in a cephalic direction along the lateral margin of the right infundibulopelvic ligament. **B:** Paravesical and pararectal fossae, with intervening base of broad ligament attached to pelvic floor and lateral pelvic wall.

is removed by sharp dissection with the points of the Metzenbaum scissors directed upward, while special care is taken to avoid trauma to the ureter (Fig. 47.19). The ureter is reflected medially during the dissection of the common iliac vessels and left attached to the parietal peritoneum to maintain its blood supply.

It is important to remove the loose areolar tissue and fascial sheath from the iliac vessels; however, to avoid trauma to the intima or wall of the vessels (particularly the veins), the surgeon should not attempt to skeletonize the pelvic vessels to the point of producing a pearl-white vascular tree. If there is tumor in the adventitia of the vessel wall, the patient probably will

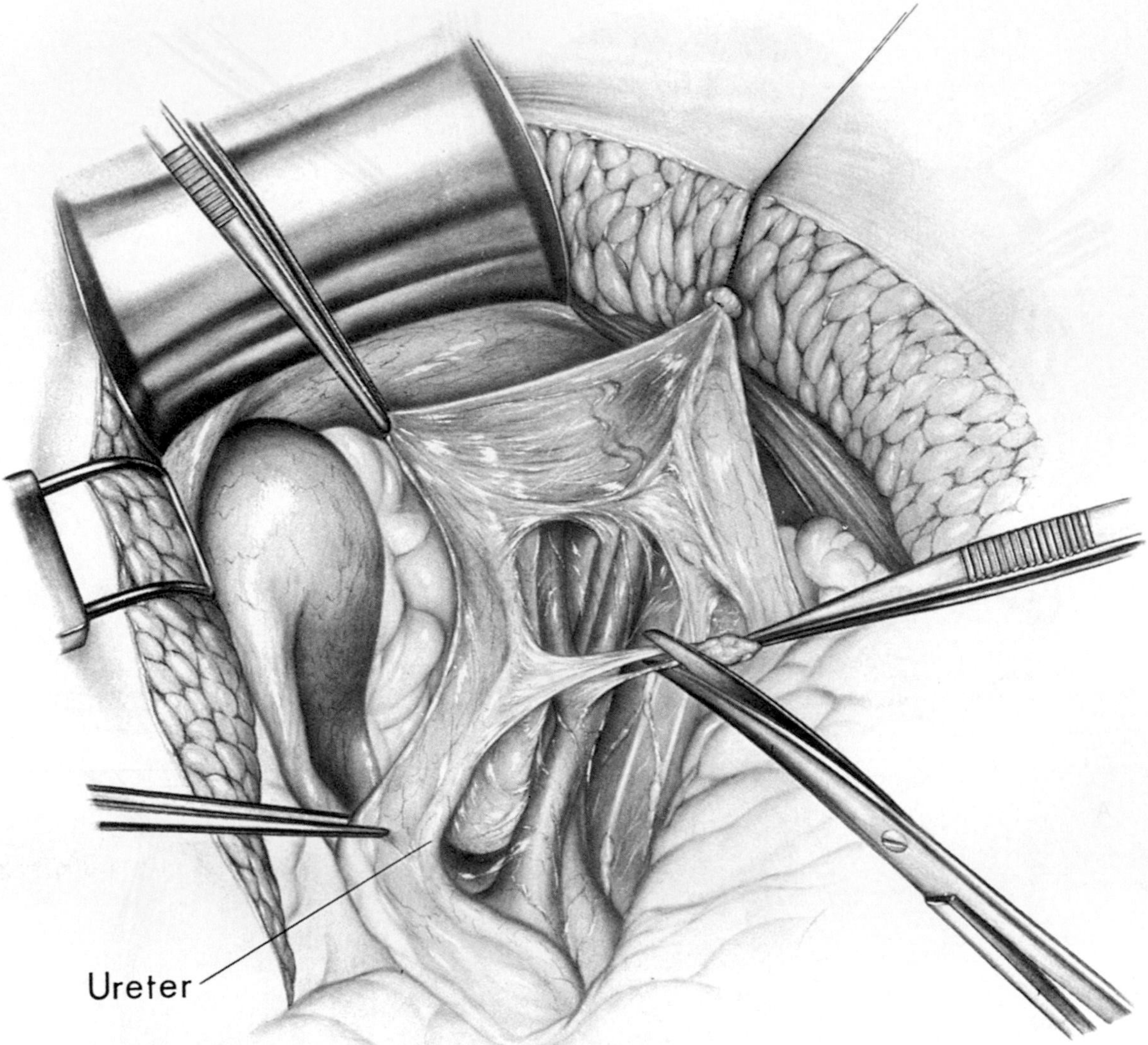

FIGURE 47.19. Pelvic lymphadenectomy with dissection of right common iliac vessels and their branches, including the external iliac and hypogastric arteries and veins. Note attachment of ureter to parietal peritoneum. The genitofemoral nerve courses along the psoas muscle.

not be cured by this procedure; consequently, such compulsive surgical efforts produce far more complications than benefits. It is important to rotate the vessels medially and laterally with a vein retractor during the dissection of the common and external iliac trunks to obtain the posterior lymphatic chain behind the vessels along the psoas muscle. The genitofemoral nerve, which is seen lateral to the external iliac vessels, should be preserved, if possible, because damage to this peripheral nerve occasionally produces postoperative discomfort in the groin and medial aspect of the thigh.

The external iliac vessels are carefully dissected down to the point where the deep circumflex iliac vein crosses over the external iliac artery. At this point, care must be taken to avoid injury to the inferior epigastric artery and vein, which arise from the anterior and medial side of the iliac vessels and course along the anterior peritoneum onto the lower abdominal wall. The surgeon also must be cognizant of the anomalous obturator artery and vein, which can arise from the lower portion of the external iliac or inferior epigastric vessels and course over the pelvic sidewall into the obturator space. If accidentally traumatized, they should be ligated at their point of origin from the artery or vein. To avoid bleeding in the obturator space, these vessels are frequently occluded with small vascular clips as they pass through the obturator space, regardless of their origin. Clips also can be used to occlude the lymphatic channels coming into the pelvis from the leg.

The obturator space is entered by reflecting the external iliac vessels medially away from the psoas muscle and freeing the areolar tissue that lies directly between these vessels and the lateral pelvic wall (Fig. 47.20A), usually with blunt dissection. Once the space has been entered and the adjacent tissue cleaned from the external iliac vessels, the artery and vein are released and gently retracted laterally with a vein retractor, and the obturator space is clearly exposed. The lymphatic and areolar tissue are dissected from the obturator space to the region of the pelvic floor, with particular care taken to avoid trauma to the obturator nerve and vessels (Fig. 47.20B). The dissection is continued by removing all of the nodes below the bifurcation of the iliac vessels, including the hypogastric nodes and the nodes in the obturator fossa. A lymph node may be encountered in

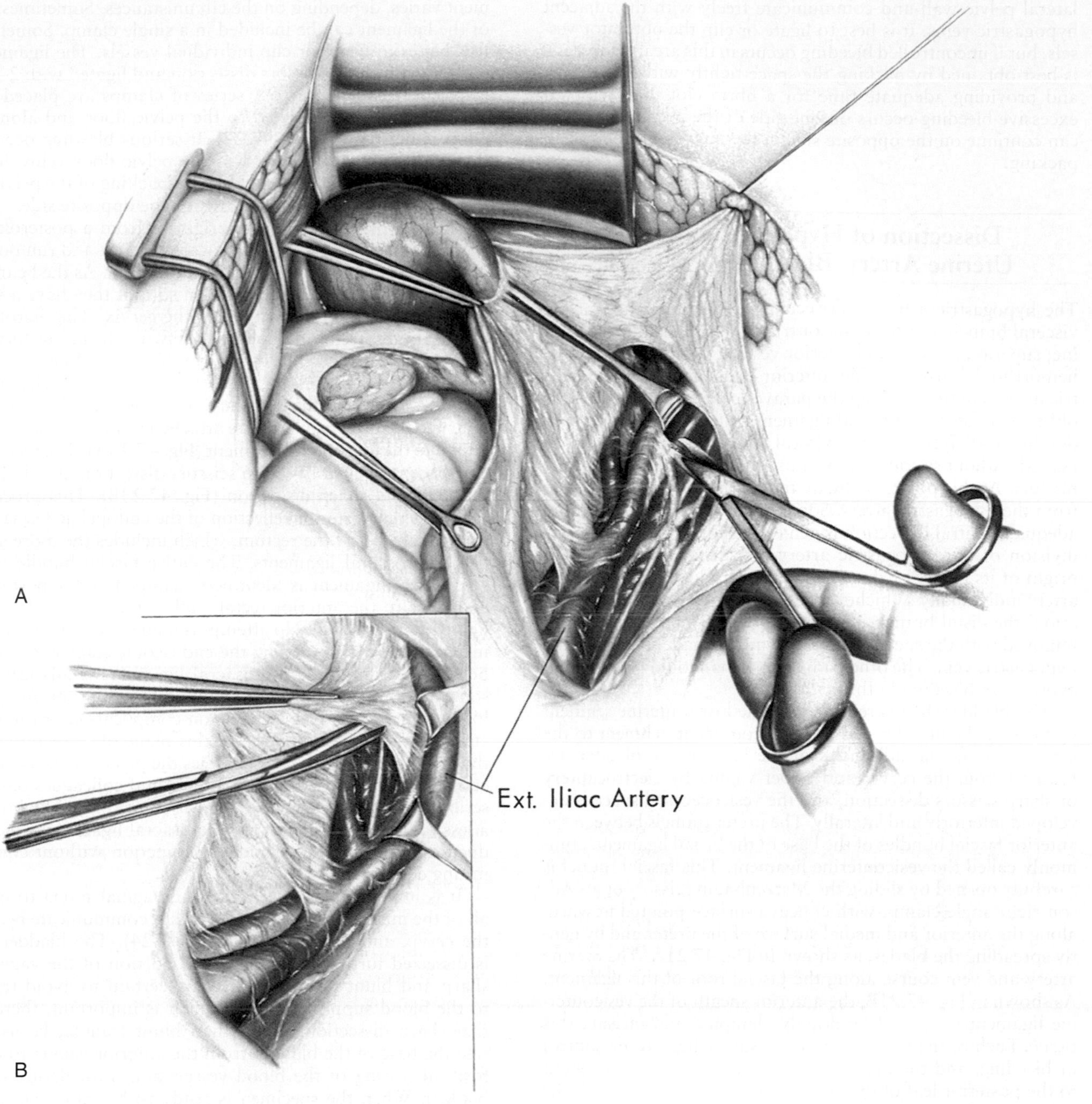

FIGURE 47.20. **A:** Entry into obturator space by medial reflection of external iliac vessels. **B:** Dissection of obturator fossa, demonstrating obturator nerve with areolar tissue attached superiorly to external iliac vessels.

the angle formed by the external iliac and hypogastric arteries and must be carefully dissected out, avoiding trauma to the adjacent hypogastric vein.

Retraction of the common iliac artery and vein medially exposes a group of lymph nodes that should be removed carefully. These lymph nodes are the lateral common iliac nodes. There is danger of venous bleeding in this area. When this area has been cleared, the surgeon can see the obturator nerve entering the obturator fossa through the body of the psoas muscle. The nerve roots of the lumbosacral plexus also are exposed. Particular care must be exercised in the dissection of the lateral sacral and sacroiliac plexus, just medial to the hypogastric artery and vein, near their origin. The rich arcade of small arteries and veins increases the risk of bleeding in this area. When the vessels retract into the sacral foramen, control of bleeding becomes difficult.

The obturator artery can be identified as it courses along the lateral pelvic wall adjacent to the obturator nerve. The nerve, artery, and vein advance toward the obturator foramen, through which they leave the pelvis. Care must be taken to avoid trauma to all of the structures, particularly the obturator veins, which have a rich anastomotic network against the lateral pelvic wall and communicate freely with the adjacent hypogastric veins. It is best to ligate or clip the obturator vessels, but if uncontrolled bleeding occurs in this area, hemostasis is best obtained by packing the space tightly with a hot pack and providing adequate time for a fibrin clot to develop. If excessive bleeding occurs on one side of the pelvis, dissection can continue on the opposite side in the interim after pressure packing.

Dissection of Hypogastric Artery, Uterine Artery, Bladder, and Ureter

The hypogastric artery is dissected with identification of the visceral branches of the anterior trunk, which include the uterine; superior, middle, and inferior vesical; vaginal; and middle hemorrhoidal arteries. The anterior division of the hypogastric artery continues along the paravesical fossa to become the obliterated lateral umbilical ligament beneath the anterior abdominal wall. If the superior vesical artery is damaged, it can be ligated without serious compromise to the blood supply of the bladder. At this point, we ligate the uterine artery at its origin from the hypogastric artery. Some authors believe that a more adequate central dissection is achieved by ligating the anterior division of the hypogastric artery just distal to the point of origin of its posterior division rather than ligating the uterine artery individually. Whichever vessel is chosen, after double ligation, the distal branches traversing the cardinal ligament are removed with the specimen. No attempt is made to remove the hypogastric vein. The other, adjacent veins should be ligated to avoid brisk bleeding in this area.

The bladder then is reflected off the lower uterine segment by incising the bladder peritoneum from its attachment to the uterus. The fascial adhesions of the base of the bladder are released from the cervix and upper vagina by electrocautery or sharp scissors dissection, and the vesicocervical space is developed inferiorly and laterally. The ureter tunnels between the anterior fascial bundles of the base of the broad ligament, commonly called the vesicouterine ligament. This fascial tunnel is carefully opened by sliding the Metzenbaum scissors or an Adson right-angle clamp, with concave surface pointed upward, along the anterior and medial surface of the ureter and by gently spreading the blades, as shown in Fig. 47.21A. The uterine artery and vein course along the fascial roof of this ligament. As shown in Fig. 47.21B, the anterior sheath of the vesicouterine ligament is opened by doubly clamping and incising this tissue. Each of the fascial bundles is suture ligated for control of bleeding, and the ureter is dissected free of its attachment to the posterior leaf of the vesicouterine ligament. As with the pelvic vessels, care must be taken to prevent damage to the adventitia and muscular wall of the ureter, which contain nutrient vessels from the collateral circulation. In the event that the blood supply to the ureter is compromised by thrombosis or trauma to the veins, fistula formation is a serious and frequent complication. The ureter is gently retracted with an umbilical tape or vein retractor. If forceps are used to handle the ureter, they should gently grasp only the adventitia.

Dissection of Cardinal Ligament

The base of the broad ligament (the cardinal ligament) then can be excised from its attachment at the lateral pelvic wall. The technique of clamping and ligating the vascular cardinal ligament varies, depending on the circumstances. Sometimes, part of the ligament can be included in a single clamp. Sometimes, it is better to ligate or clip individual vessels. The ligament is excised with sharp scissors dissection and ligated with 2–0 delayed absorbable suture. A series of clamps are placed until the dissection is completed to the pelvic floor and along the paravaginal tissues (Fig. 47.22). If serious bleeding occurs in this region owing to trauma to the pelvic floor veins, hemostatic control is best obtained by firm packing of the pelvis and shifting the dissection temporarily to the opposite side.

The uterosacral ligaments originate from a posterolateral position on the cervix where they are thickest and run posteriorly to the anterolateral aspect of the rectum. As the ligaments approach the rectum, they broaden so that they have a wider attachment to the rectum than to the cervix. The uterosacral ligaments are stretched by sharply drawing the uterus forward. The peritoneal reflection of the cul-de-sac of Douglas then is incised, leaving a small segment of peritoneum attached to the anterior surface of the rectum. Care must be taken to avoid injury to the ureters, which are attached to the peritoneum just lateral to the uterosacral ligament (Fig. 47.23A). The rectovaginal space is opened by sharp scissors dissection and deepened by blunt and sharp dissection (Fig. 47.23B). This procedure separates the posterior reflection of the endopelvic fascia from the lateral wall of the rectum, which includes the more superficial uterosacral ligaments. The entire fascial bundle of the uterosacral ligament is identified, clamped as far posteriorly and close to the anterior rectal wall as possible, and cut and ligated (Fig. 47.23C). No attempt is made to divide the attachments to the sacrum. Using the endoscopic stapler to transect both the cardinal and uterosacral ligaments is advocated by some authors to significantly reduce operating time and blood loss without any adverse effects on complication or tumor recurrence rates. Continuation of this plane of dissection along the posterior endopelvic fascia frees the posterior aspect of the cervix from the pelvic floor. Trimbos and colleagues have described a "nerve sparing" radical hysterectomy that involves a less radical dissection of the uterosacral ligament, which reduces the incidence of bladder dysfunction without compromising cure rates.

It is important to dissect the paravaginal fascia to obtain all of the microlymphatic channels that communicate between the cervix and upper vagina (Fig. 47.24). The bladder then is dissected further from the upper portion of the vagina by sharp and blunt dissection, making certain to avoid trauma to the blood supply of this organ. It is important, therefore, that sharp dissection, rather than blunt trauma, be used to free the base of the bladder from the anterior vagina to avoid forceful tearing of the blood vessels and musculature of the bladder. When the specimen is ready to be removed, a long right-angled Wertheim clamp is placed across the vagina below the cervix (not shown) to avoid gross spillage of tumor cells into the pelvis. The specimen then is removed by dividing the vagina above clamps placed on the lateral vaginal angles (Fig. 47.25).

Closure

The vaginal angles are suture ligated separately to secure hemostasis, and then the remaining cuff is closed in an anterior-to-posterior direction using a continuous locking 2–0 delayed absorbable suture. No additional attempt is made to support the vaginal vault because all of the fascial support of the uterus and vagina has been removed. The remaining vagina, which

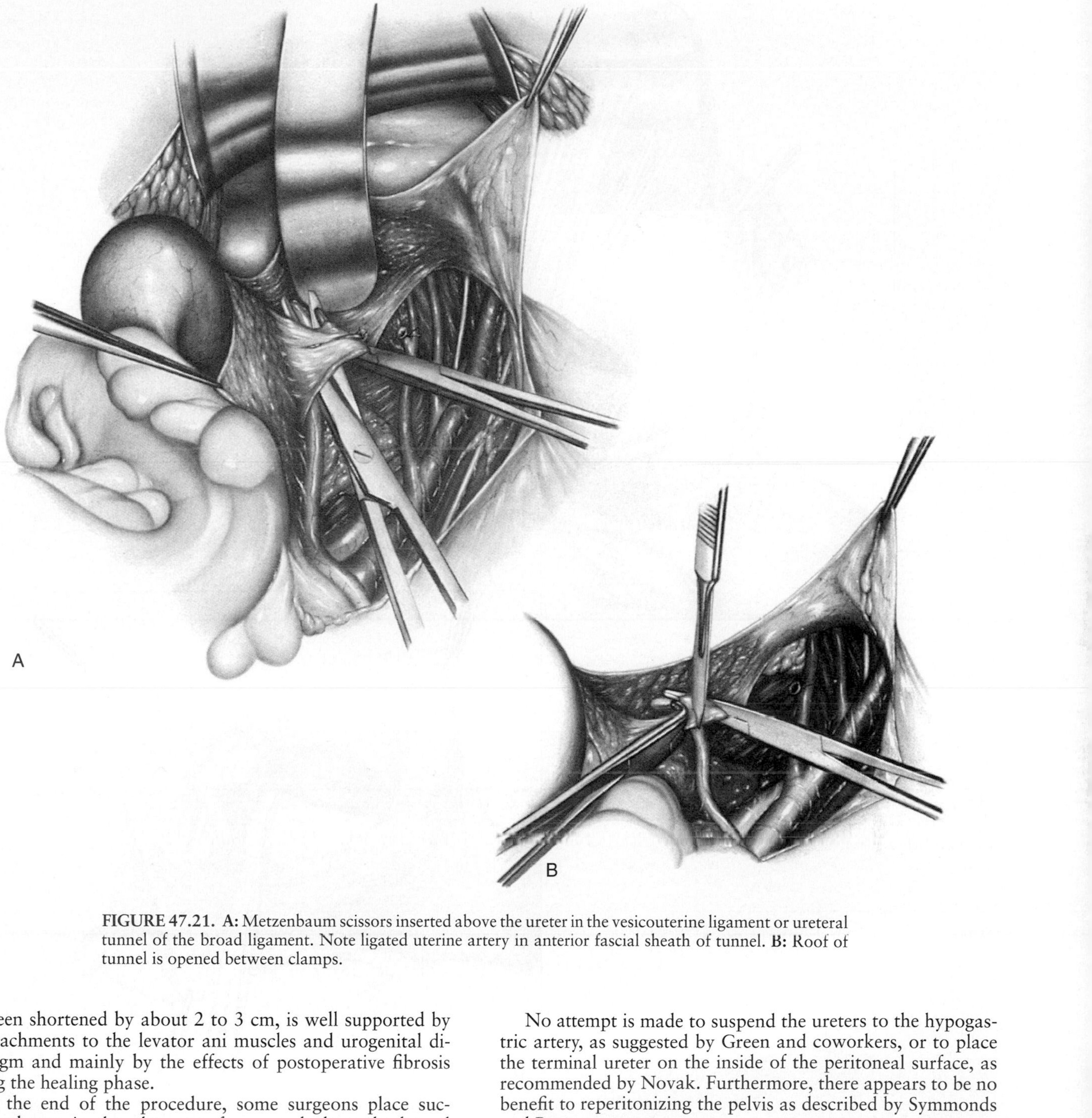

FIGURE 47.21. A: Metzenbaum scissors inserted above the ureter in the vesicouterine ligament or ureteral tunnel of the broad ligament. Note ligated uterine artery in anterior fascial sheath of tunnel. **B:** Roof of tunnel is opened between clamps.

has been shortened by about 2 to 3 cm, is well supported by its attachments to the levator ani muscles and urogenital diaphragm and mainly by the effects of postoperative fibrosis during the healing phase.

At the end of the procedure, some surgeons place suction catheters in the obturator fossae and along the lateral pelvic walls and bring them out through stab wounds in the lower abdomen. After the abdomen is closed, these catheters are connected to intermittent, low-suction drainage units. Traditionally, these drains were thought to be effective in preventing pelvic infection and fistula and lymphocyst formation. However, recent retrospective and prospective studies have demonstrated that the incidence of these complications is minimal and the same whether or not drains are used. Therefore, many gynecologic oncologists no longer use pelvic drains.

No attempt is made to suspend the ureters to the hypogastric artery, as suggested by Green and coworkers, or to place the terminal ureter on the inside of the peritoneal surface, as recommended by Novak. Furthermore, there appears to be no benefit to reperitonizing the pelvis as described by Symmonds and Pratt.

If the tubes and ovaries are to be transposed out of the pelvis, a tunnel is dissected beneath the peritoneum laterally and superiorly toward each lateral gutter. An incision in the peritoneum is made as high as possible at the top of the tunnel. The adnexal structures are guided through the tunnel and through the incision at the top of the tunnel, making absolutely certain that the ovarian vessels in the infundibulopelvic ligament are not twisted. Permanent suture material is used to suture the tuboovarian pedicle as high as possible to the peritoneum and underlying muscle. Two large metal clips also are placed across

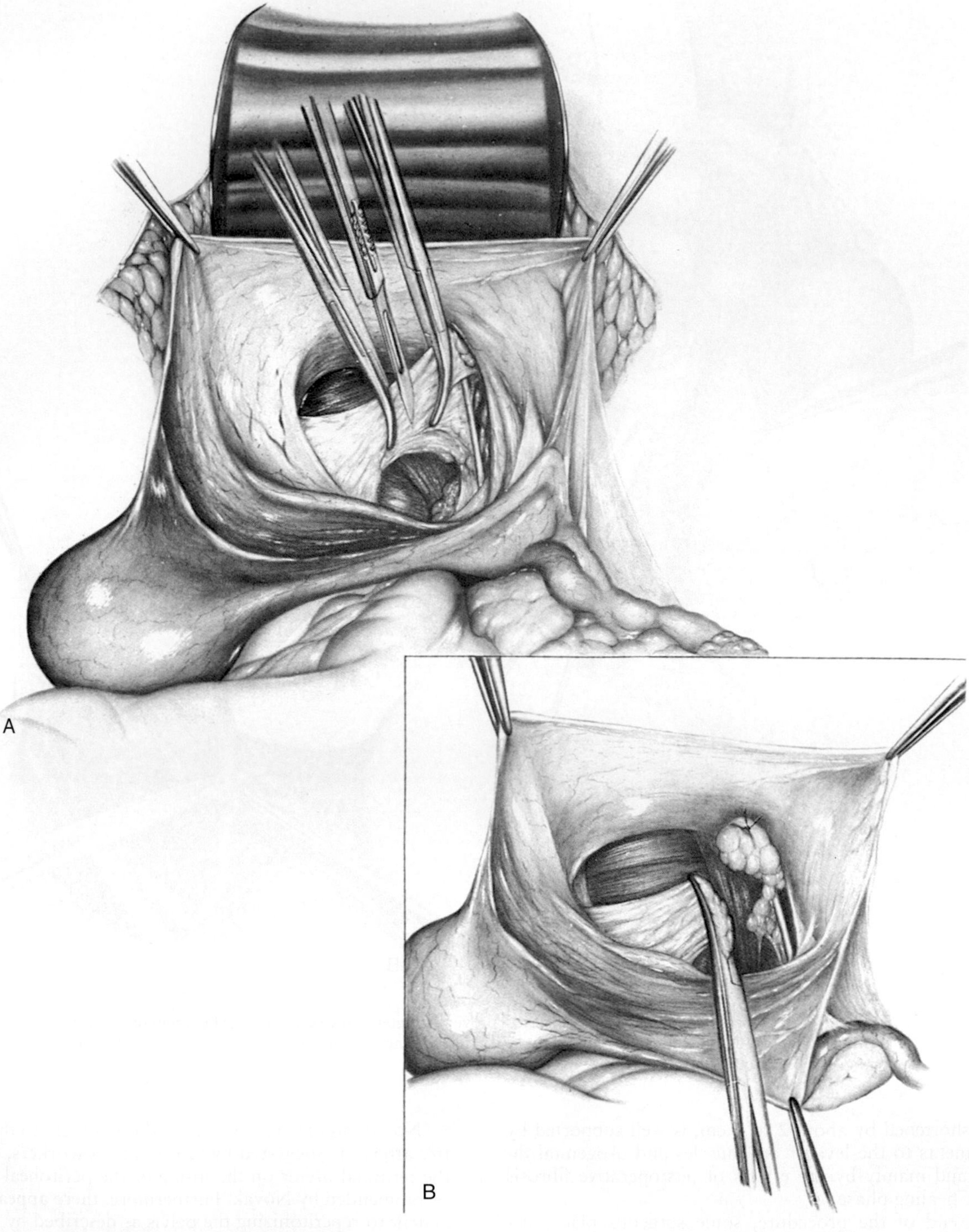

FIGURE 47.22. A: Clamping and incision of lateral portion of cardinal ligament adjacent to the lateral pelvic wall. B: Excised ligament showing pelvic floor and levator muscles. Dissected obturator nerve is seen in obturator space.

the pedicle to identify later the location of the ovaries with an abdominal radiograph. This ovarian suspension is done when there is a reasonable chance that a patient will need postoperative pelvic irradiation (Figs. 47.26 and 47.27). In most operations, however, the tubes and ovaries can be left in their natural positions in the pelvis.

FERTILITY-SPARING RADICAL ABDOMINAL TRACHELECTOMY

Historically, the recommended surgical treatment for a stage IA2–IB1 cervical cancer is a total radical hysterectomy and

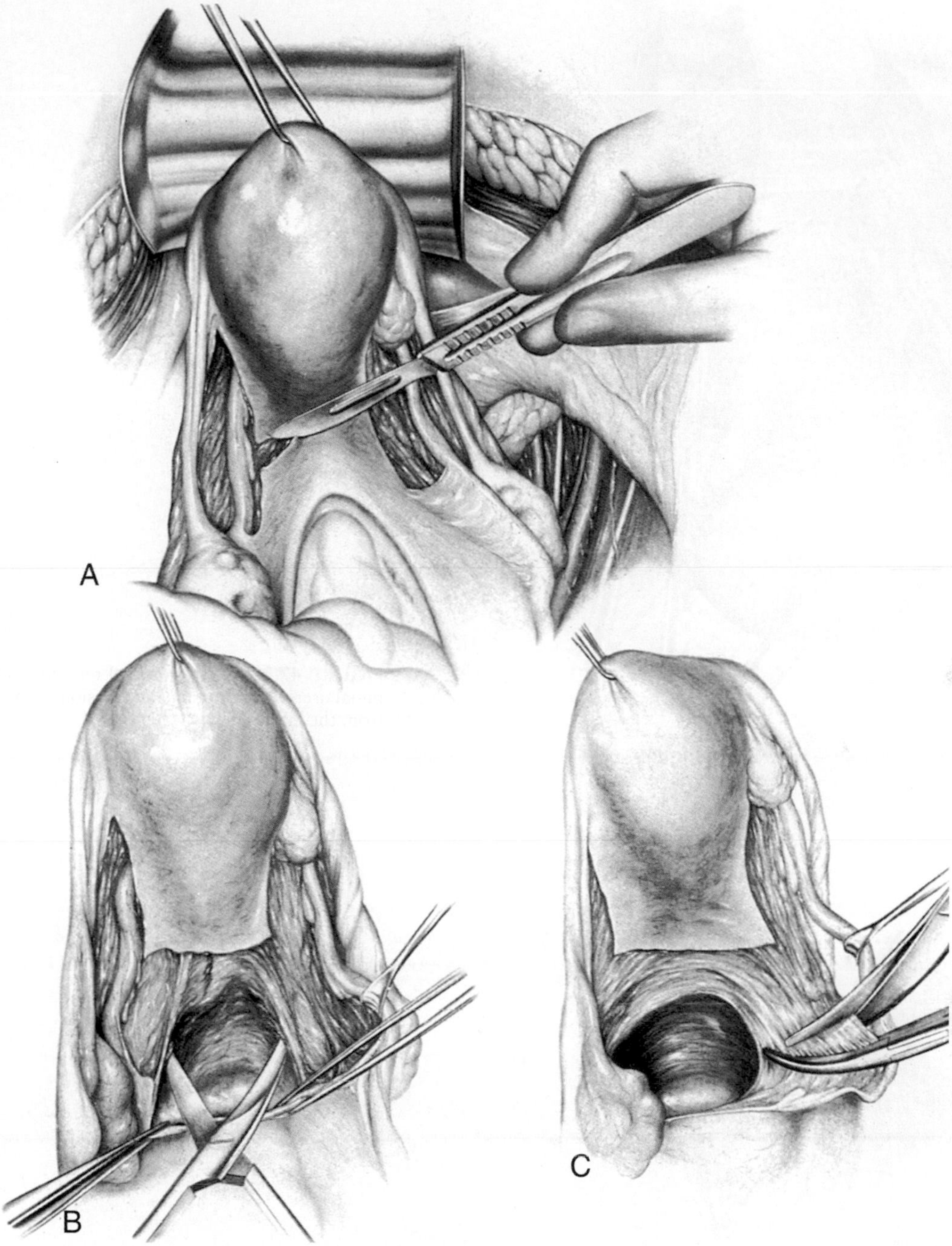

FIGURE 47.23. **A:** Cutting the cul-de-sac peritoneum as it reflects onto the rectum. Ureters course laterally, devoid of peritoneum. **B:** Dissection of the rectovaginal septum with development of rectal stalks (uterosacral ligaments). **C:** Clamping the uterosacral ligament. Ureter is gently retracted to avoid trauma.

pelvic lymphadenectomy. This operation is very effective at treating early-stage cervical cancer; however, infertility is one of the serious and inevitable consequences of treatment. Partial radical organ resection has been accepted in many solid tumors, such as partial gastrectomy, nephrectomy, pneumonectomy, and colectomy to treat malignancies affecting these organs. In gynecologic oncology, partial organ resection with radical abdominal or vaginal trachelectomy and pelvic lymph node dissection are relatively new techniques used in women with early cervical cancer who wish to retain fertility (Table 47.7). This operation and technique are to be distinguished from the radical abdominal trachelectomy, which is commonly used for resection of cervical stump malignancy following a previous supracervical hysterectomy in the setting in which fertility preservation is not an issue.

Technique

A laparotomy and a bilateral complete pelvic lymphadenectomy are performed in a similar manner to patients undergoing a radical abdominal hysterectomy. The limits of nodal

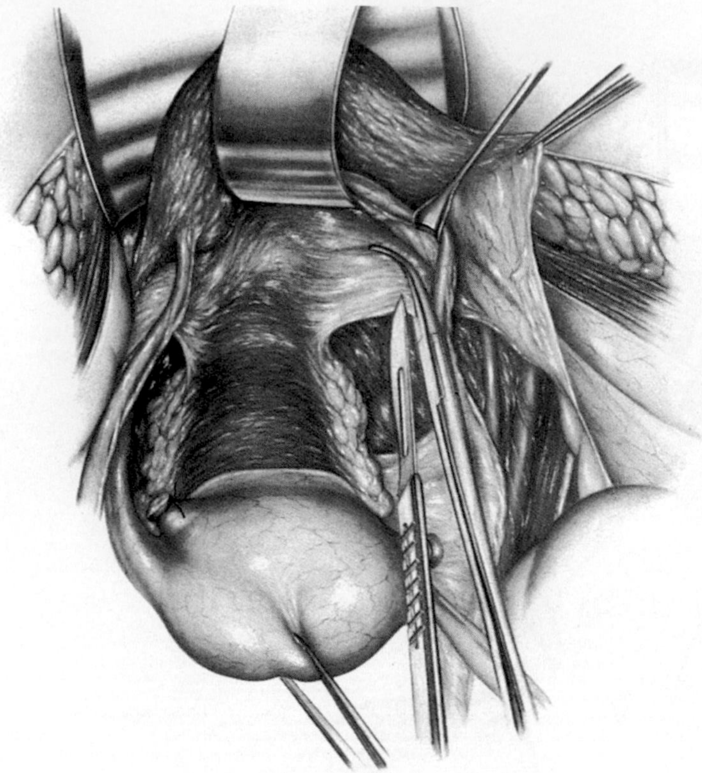

FIGURE 47.24. Dissection and retraction of bladder and terminal ureter from vagina and excision of the paravaginal fascia from the lateral pelvic wall.

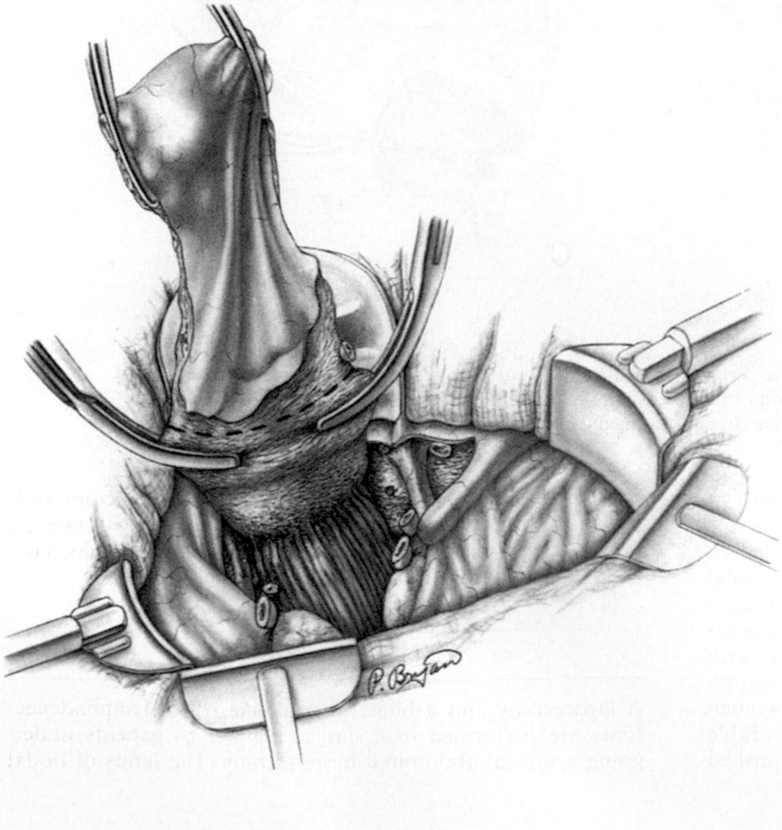

FIGURE 47.25. After clamping and ligating paravaginal tissue laterally, an incision is made in the vagina several centimeters below the cervix.

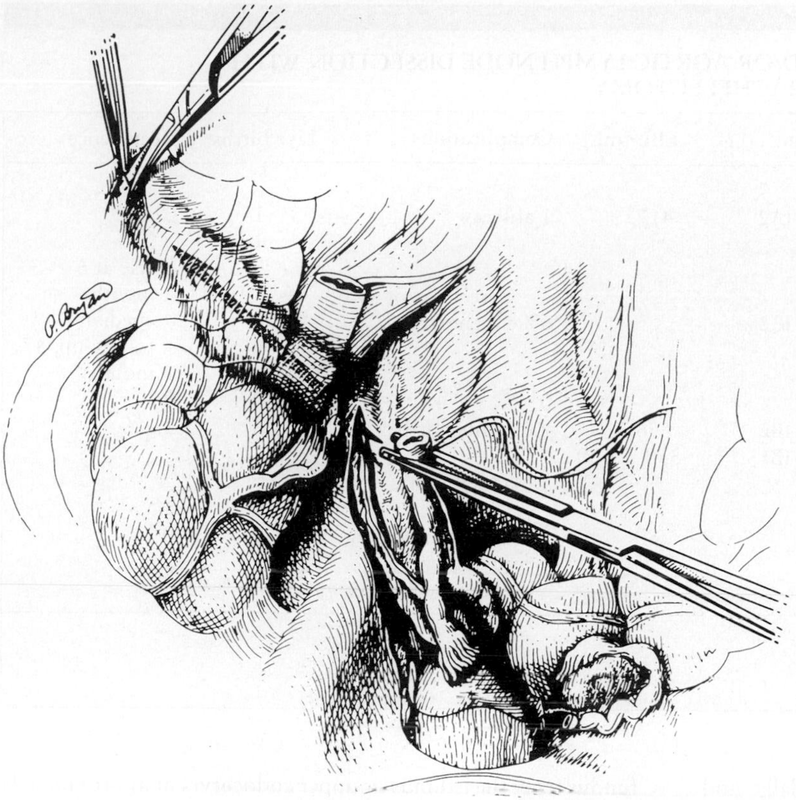

FIGURE 47.26. If the ovaries are to be suspended, a tunnel can be made under the peritoneum and the cecum on the right. The tube and ovary are guided through the tunnel to the new position in the right colic gutter above the pelvis.

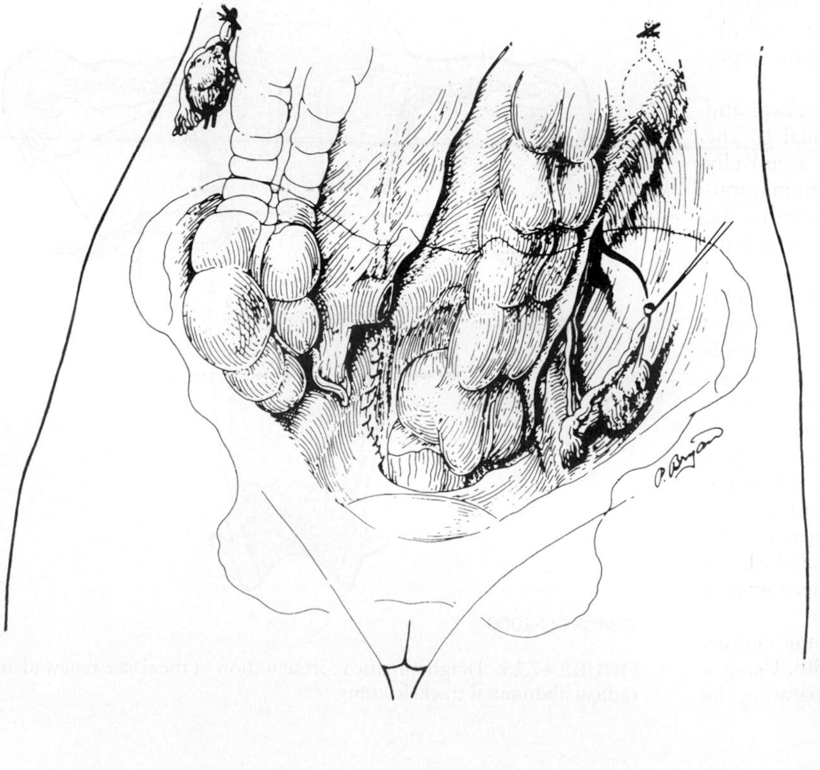

FIGURE 47.27. A similar procedure can be performed on the left. The ovarian vessels should not be twisted. Metal clips are placed on the pedicles to allow later identification with abdominal radiograph.

TABLE 47.7

SUMMARY OF SERIES DESCRIBING PELVIC AND/OR AORTIC LYMPH NODE DISSECTION WITH FERTILITY-SPARING RADICAL ABDOMINAL TRACHELECTOMY

Author	N[a]	Age (years)[b]	Stage	EBL (mL)	Complications	Live births[a]	Recurrence
Smith et al. 1997	1		IB				
Rodriguez et al. 2001	3	26.3	IA1–IA2	417	1 abscess	1	0
Palfalvi 2003	1		IB1			1	
Del Priore et al. 2004	1	28	IB1				Pelvic at 6 months
Ungar et al. 2005	33	30.5	IA2–IB2		6% amenorrhea	2	0, median follow-up, 47 months
Abu-Rustum et al. 2005	2	7	IB1		0	0	0
Ungar et al. 2006	91	30.7	IA2–IB2	656	4.8% amenorrhea	6	2.4%
Cibula et al. 2005	3		IA2–IB1	350–3,500	1 ileus 1 bladder atony		
Bader et al. 2005	1	34	IB1			0	1
Abu-Rustum et al. 2006	5	36	IB1	280	1 needed completion hysterectomy for positive margin	0	0

EBL, estimated blood loss.
[a]Some patients may be reported more than once.
[b]Mean when calculated.

dissection are the deep circumflex iliac vein caudally and the proximal common iliac artery cephalad. Any suspicious lymph nodes were sent for frozen-section analysis. It was our intent to abandon a fertility-sparing approach if positive lymph nodes were identified. Sentinel lymph node biopsy followed by a complete pelvic lymphadenectomy is also a reasonable option and may allow for pathologic ultrastaging of these sentinel nodes. The removal of paraaortic nodes is also considered for lesions stage IB1 or greater.

The intent of the radical abdominal trachelectomy was to resect the cervix, upper 1 to 2 cm of the vagina, parametrium, and paracolpos in a similar manner to a type III radical abdominal hysterectomy but sparing the uterine fundus or corpus (Figs. 47.28 and 47.29).

The procedure is begun by developing the paravesical and pararectal spaces and dissecting the bladder caudal to the midvagina. The round ligaments are divided, and large Kelly clamps are placed on the medial round ligaments to manipulate the uterus. Care is taken not to destroy the cornu or the uteroovarian pedicles. The infundibulopelvic ligaments with ovarian blood supply are kept intact. Care is also taken not to injure the fallopian tubes or disrupt the uteroovarian ligament.

The uterine vessels are then ligated and divided at their origin from the hypogastric vessels. The parametria and paracolpos with uterine vessels are mobilized medially with the specimen, and a complete ureterolysis is performed similar to a type III radical abdominal hysterectomy. The posterior cul de sac peritoneum is incised and the uterosacral ligament divided; similarly, the parametria and paracolpos are divided. Using a vaginal cylinder (Apple Medical Corporation; Marlborough, MA), the desired length of vaginectomy is performed, and the specimen is completely separated from the vagina and placed in the midpelvis, keeping its attachment to the uteroovarian ligaments.

The lower uterine segment is then estimated, and clamps are placed at the level of the internal os (Fig. 47.30). Using a knife, the radical trachelectomy is completed by separating the fundus from the isthmus or upper endocervix at approximately 5 mm below the level of the internal os, if possible (Figs. 47.31 and 47.32).

The uterine fundus with preserved attachments to the uteroovarian ligaments, placed in the superior part of the pelvis, and the specimen, consisting of radical trachelectomy and parametria with suture marking the vaginal cuff at

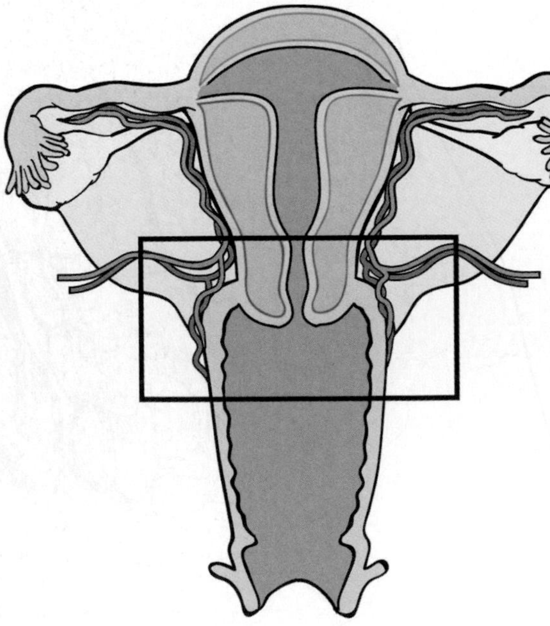

FIGURE 47.28. Diagrammatic representation of the tissue renewed at radical abdominal trachelectomy.

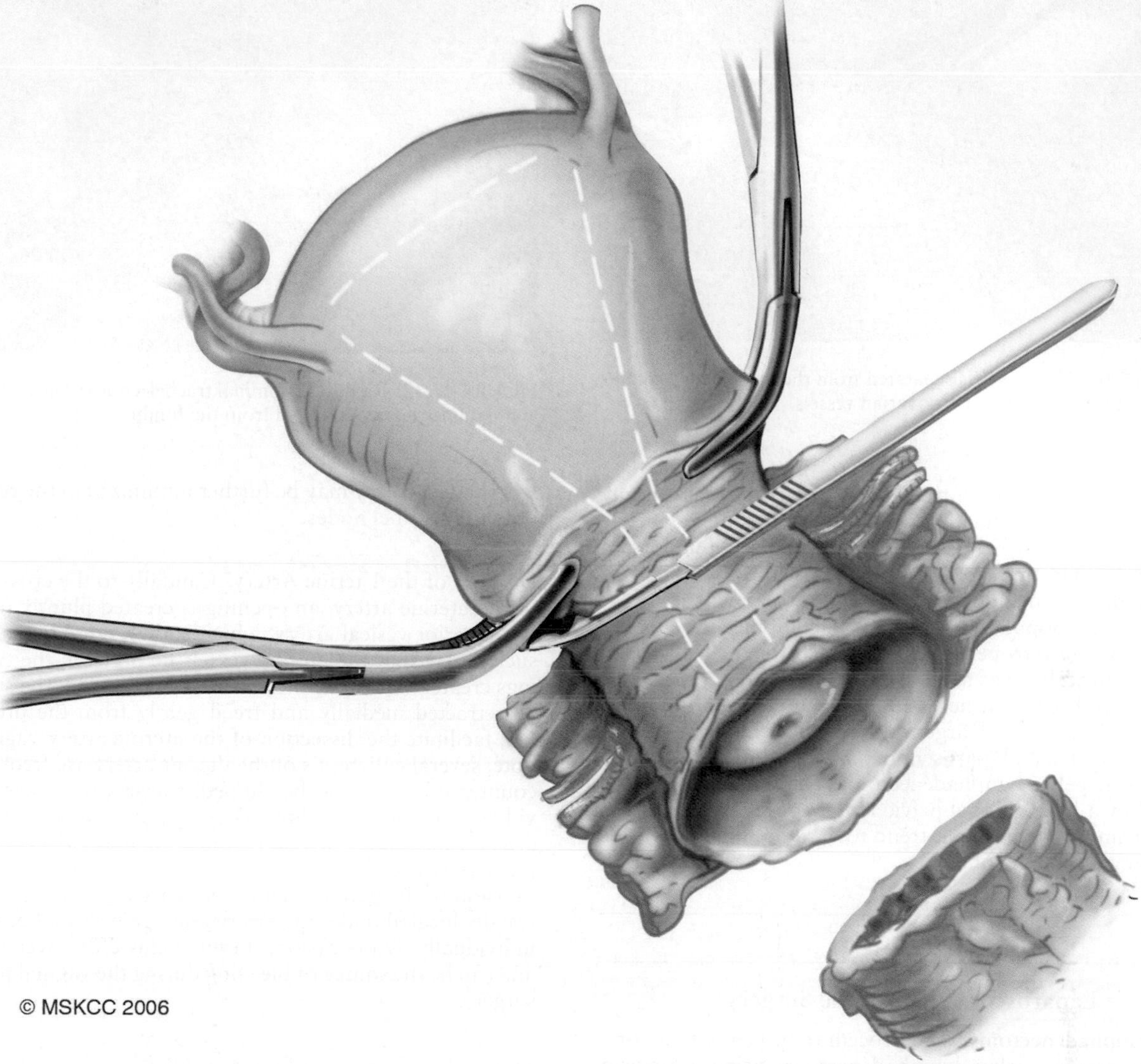

FIGURE 47.29. The intent of the radical abdominal trachelectomy is to resect the cervix, upper 1 to 2 cm of the vagina, parametrium, and paracolpos in a similar manner to a type III radical abdominal hysterectomy but sparing the uterine corpus.

12 o'clock, is sent for frozen-section evaluation of its endocervical margin. The uterine fundus is inspected and curettage of the endometrial cavity is performed as well as a shave disc margin on the remaining cervical tissue, which is sent for frozen-section analysis (Fig. 47.33). This is performed to ensure that the reconstructed uterus to vagina is disease free. A frozen-section analysis is also obtained on the distal vaginal margin, if clinically indicated.

If all frozen sections tested are benign and at least a 5-mm clear margin is obtained on the endocervical edge, a permanent cerclage with no. 0 Ethibond (knot tied posteriorly) may be placed before the reconstruction (Fig. 47.34). A cerclage was placed in three cases in this series. The uterus is then reattached to the upper vagina with six to eight no. 2–0 absorbable sutures (Figs. 47.35–47.37). No drains are placed. Standard antibiotic prophylaxis and routine postoperative care is prescribed.

An alternative approach would be to separate the fundus from the cervix before the colpotomy, pack the fundus with the intact uteroovarian blood supply in the upper pelvis, place retraction clamps on the cervix, and perform the radical trachelectomy. The role of cystourethroscopy with bilateral temporary ureteral catheterization is optional.

LAPAROSCOPICALLY ASSISTED RADICAL VAGINAL HYSTERECTOMY (SCHAUTA)

History

The "extended" hysterectomy performed vaginally for the treatment of cervical cancer was invented by Schauta in Austria in 1901. A few years earlier, in 1898, also in Austria, Wertheim had reported on the abdominal extended hysterectomy. The

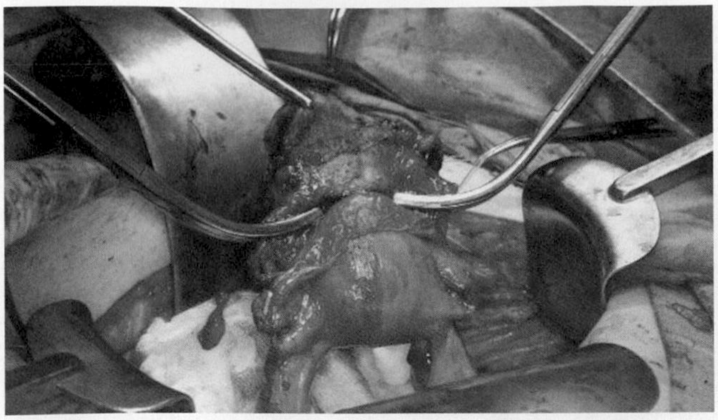

FIGURE 47.30. The uterus is separated from the vagina and remains attached to the adnexa and uteroovarian vessels.

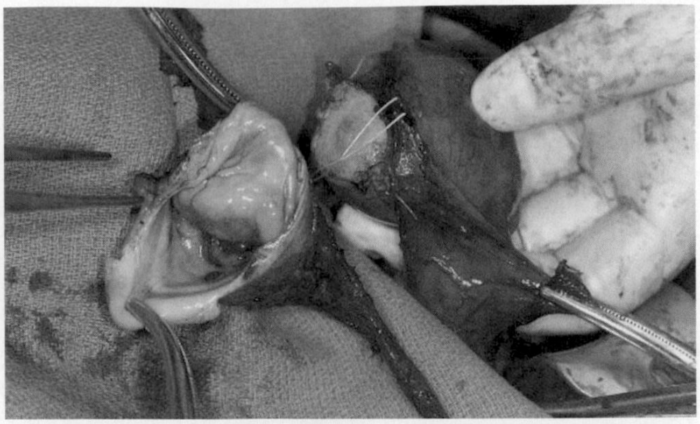

FIGURE 47.32. Radical abdominal trachelectomy: The cervical tissue and parametria are separated from the fundus.

mortality and morbidity of the Wertheim method was initially much higher, but it had the advantage of including a pelvic lymphadenectomy, which is now appreciated as an important and necessary part of the procedure. Because the initial Schauta operation did not include the lymph node assessment, it gradually became less popular. In 1959, Mitra combined the Schauta operation with a retroperitoneal approach for the pelvic lymphadenectomy. This was a clever idea, but it did not gain a lot of acceptance because it necessitated bilateral flank incisions. More recently, in 1987, Dargent revived the Schauta operation by combining it with laparoscopic surgery, allowing thorough and complete pelvic lymphadenectomy. The Schauta operation preceded by a laparoscopic pelvic lymphadenectomy is thus a perfect example of the recent trend toward minimally invasive surgery in gynecologic oncology.

Technique

Laparoscopic Part of the Surgery

Pelvic Lymphadenectomy. The procedure begins with a complete laparoscopic pelvic lymphadenectomy using a 4-trocar technique as detailed in the laparoscopic surgical staging section below. In the future, if sentinel lymph node mapping proves acceptable to gynecologic oncologists, the extent of the lymphadenectomy may be further minimized to the removal of only the sentinel nodes.

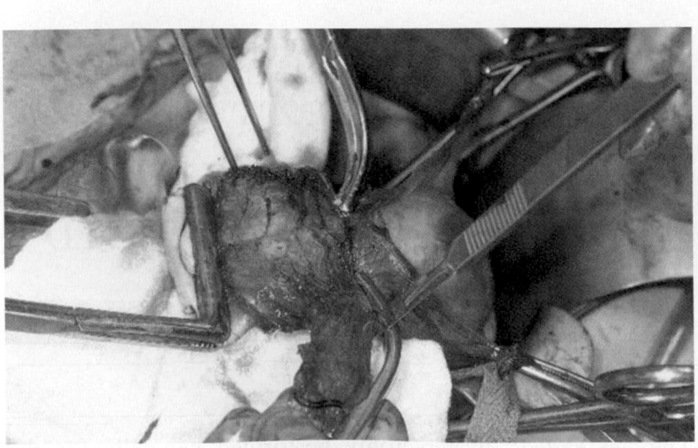

FIGURE 47.31. The radical abdominal trachelectomy incision is done at or just below the internal os, ideally preserving 5 mm or so of upper endocervix.

Division of the Uterine Artery. Caudally to the crossing point of the uterine artery, an opening is created bluntly just under the superior vesical artery, which is then retracted laterally in such a way that the uterine vessels lie between the two openings created. Once the uterine artery is divided, the stump can be retracted medially and freed gently from the ureter. This will facilitate the dissection of the uterine artery vaginally. Of note, several collaterals of the uterine artery are frequently encountered and should be clipped, excised, or cauterized individually to avoid bleeding. The vaginal branch of the uterine artery is also frequently seen appearing under the excised uterine artery. It can be divided now or later during the vaginal excision of the parametrial tissue. Lastly, the uterine veins are usually located under the artery and again should be managed individually. On occasion, uterine veins cross over the ureter and can be the source of bleeding during the vaginal part of the surgery.

Vaginal Part of the Surgery

The vaginal part of the surgery can be divided into five steps: (i) vaginal cuff preparation, (ii) anterior phase (opening of the vesicouterine space and paravesical space, and mobilization and dissection of the ureter), (iii) posterior phase (opening of the cul-de-sac and pararectal space and excision of the paracolpos), (iv) lateral phase (excision of the parametrium), and (v) excision of the specimen and closure.

Vaginal Cuff Preparation. Because the radical vaginal hysterectomy is primarily offered to women with cervical lesions less than 3 cm, it is rarely necessary to remove more than 1 cm of vaginal mucosa. A rim of vaginal mucosa is delineated circumferentially clockwise around the cervix with six to eight straight Kocher clamps placed at regular intervals, about 1 cm below the cervix (Fig. 47.38).

To reduce bleeding from the edges of the vaginal mucosa, a 10- to 20-cc solution of xylocaine 1% mixed with epinephrine 1:100,000 is injected between each Kocher clamp, then a circumferential incision is made with the scalpel just above the Kocher clamp (Fig. 47.39). The anterior and posterior edges of the vaginal mucosa are grasped with four to six Chrobak clamps to completely cover the cervix.

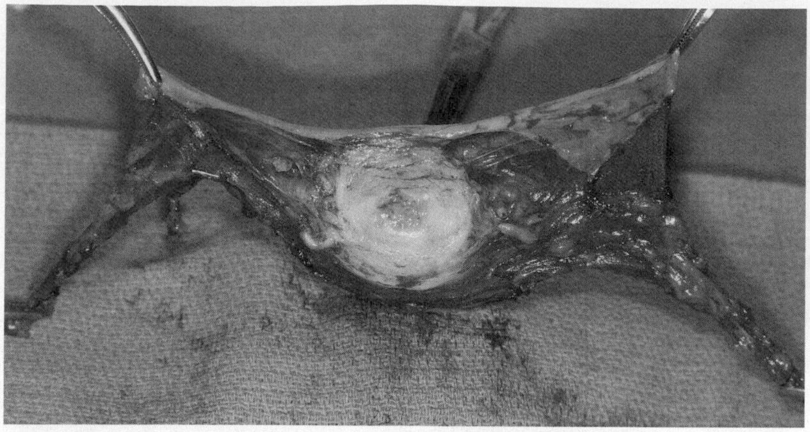

FIGURE 47.33. Radical abdominal trachelectomy specimen showing endocervical margin and uterine vessels with parametria. Endometrial and upper endocervical curettage as well as a shave margin on the remaining uterine tissue is sent for frozen-section analysis before reconstruction.

Anterior Phase (Described for the Patient's Right Side)

Opening of the vesicouterine space. While pulling the specimen slightly downward with the Chrobak clamps, a single-tooth forceps is used to hold and retract the anterior vaginal mucosa, which usually creates a triangular fold indicating where to cut (Fig. 47.40). The vesicouterine space is opened with Metzenbaum scissors held perpendicular to the cervix in the midline to avoid bleeding from the bladder pillars laterally. The space is further defined and stretched by gentle dissection with the index finger. Care is taken not to enter the anterior peritoneum as in a simple vaginal hysterectomy as it makes identification of the bladder base and ureters more difficult. If entered correctly, the space should be avascular, and the anterior surface of the endocervix and isthmus should be easily identified without resistance. If a resistance is felt, it usually means that the plane of dissection is either too posterior and that the surgeon is digging into the endocervix, or too anterior, which carries a risk of damage to the bladder. For that reason, the bladder base should be carefully delineated. In patients who have had a recent conization, there may be substantial fibrosis and scarring between the cervix and the bladder base. The opening of the vesicouterine space may be particularly difficult in those cases. In such situations, a metal bladder catheter introduced in the urethra may be used to locate the bladder base and facilitate its mobilization. Once clearly identified, the vesicouterine space is stretched upward with a narrow Deaver retractor, showing the intact peritoneum (Fig. 47.41).

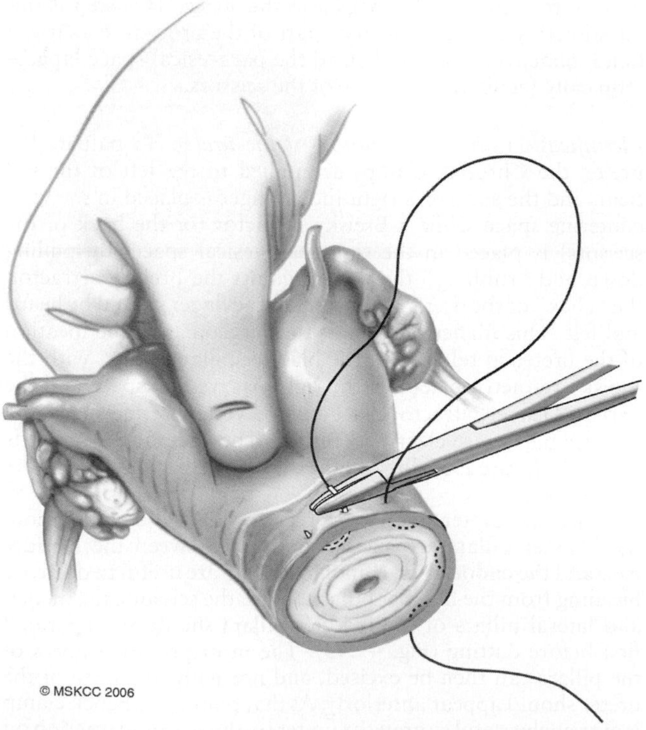

FIGURE 47.34. A permanent cerclage with no. 0 Ethibond is placed and the knot tied posteriorly.

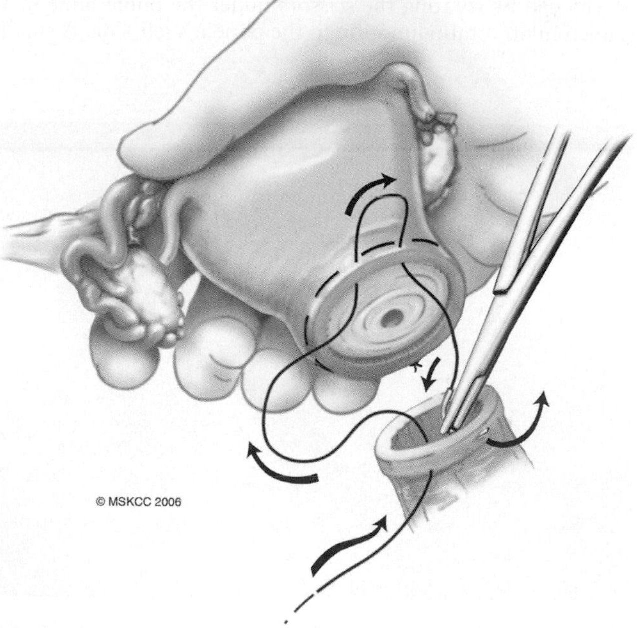

FIGURE 47.35. Reconstruction of the uterine corpus to upper vagina after the cerclage is placed.

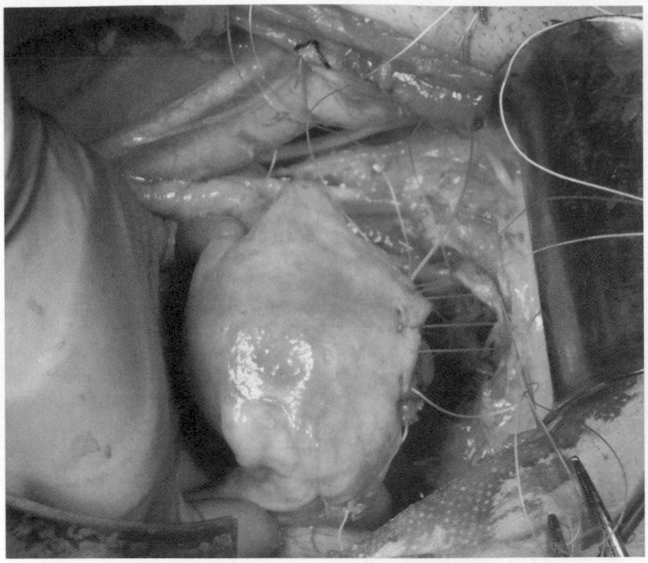

FIGURE 47.36. The uterine fundus is reattached to the vaginal apex with six to eight interrupted no. 2–0 absorbable sutures.

Opening of the paravesical space. To open the right paravesical space, the Chrobak clamps are slightly pulled toward the patient's right side. Straight Kocher clamps are placed onto the vaginal mucosa at 11 and 9 o'clock and stretched out (this is where the 12 o'clock mark made earlier is useful). This maneuver defines a triangle formed by the bladder pillars, the vaginal mucosa, and the Chrobak clamps. An areolar opening is seen just medial and slightly anterior to the 9 o'clock clamp, indicating where to enter to define the paravesical space. The space is blindly entered by opening and closing Metzenbaum scissors, with the tips pointing upward and outward in an oblique axis. If entered correctly, the space should be avascular and the scissors should slide inside easily. Once entered, the space is widened by rotating the scissors under the pubic bone in a semicircular, rotating motion to the patient's left side. A small Breisky retractor is then placed in the space. This step is unquestionably the most "scary" part of the procedure as it is a blind maneuver. Having defined the paravesical space laparoscopically facilitates the entry of the scissors.

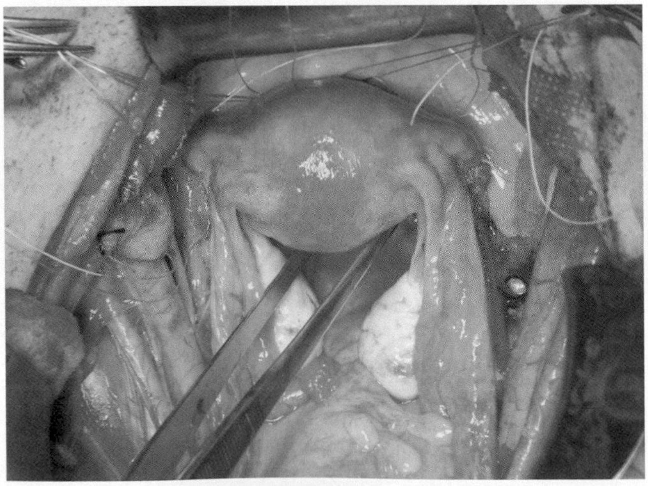

FIGURE 47.37. The reconstructed fundus with remaining blood supply from the intact uteroovarian ligaments: uterine serosa without evidence of fundal ischemia.

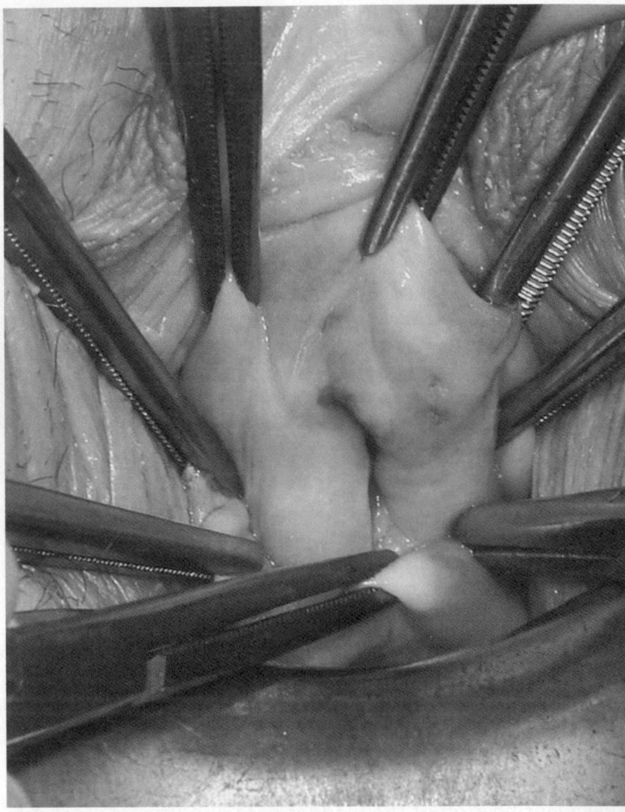

FIGURE 47.38. A vaginal cuff is prepared to remove about 1 to 2 cm of vaginal mucosa.

Identification and mobilization of the ureter. To palpate the ureter, the Chrobak clamps are pulled to the left of the patient, and the surgeon's right index finger is placed in the vesicouterine space while a Breisky retractor (or the back of the scissors) is placed in the right paravesical space. By pulling down and "rubbing" the finger against the Breisky retractor, the "click" of the ureter rolling under the finger should be heard and felt. This maneuver orients the surgeon as to the location of the ureter in relation to the bladder pillars. Next, with the Breisky retractor placed in the right paravesical space and the narrow Deaver retractor placed in the vesicouterine space, the bladder pillars are clearly identified. The knee of the ureter is normally located on the lateral aspect of the bladder pillars (Fig. 47.42).

Once the ureter has been precisely located by palpation, the bladder pillars are excised midway between the bladder base and the endocervix. (Bipolar scissors are useful to decrease bleeding from the bladder pillars.) With the scissors, the medial and lateral pillars of the bladder pillars should be separated first before cutting (Fig. 47.43). The most proximal fibers of the pillars can then be excised, and normally, the knee of the ureter should appear anteriorly. At that point, a Babcock clamp is extremely useful to grab the ureter to allow a good traction on it and to constantly keep it under direct visualization. Once the ureter is clearly identified, the medial and lateral bladder pillars

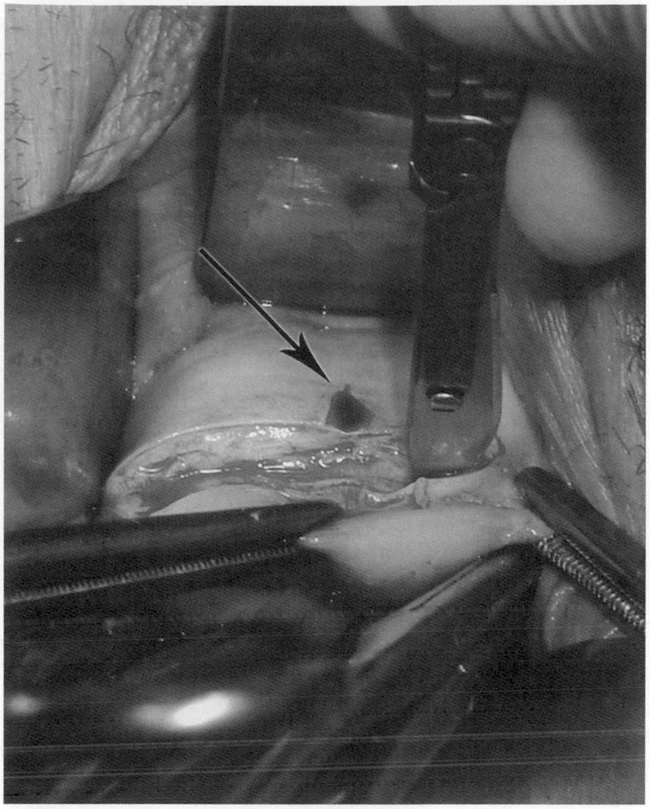

FIGURE 47.39. Section of the anterior vaginal mucosa, with the 12 o'clock mark (*arrow*).

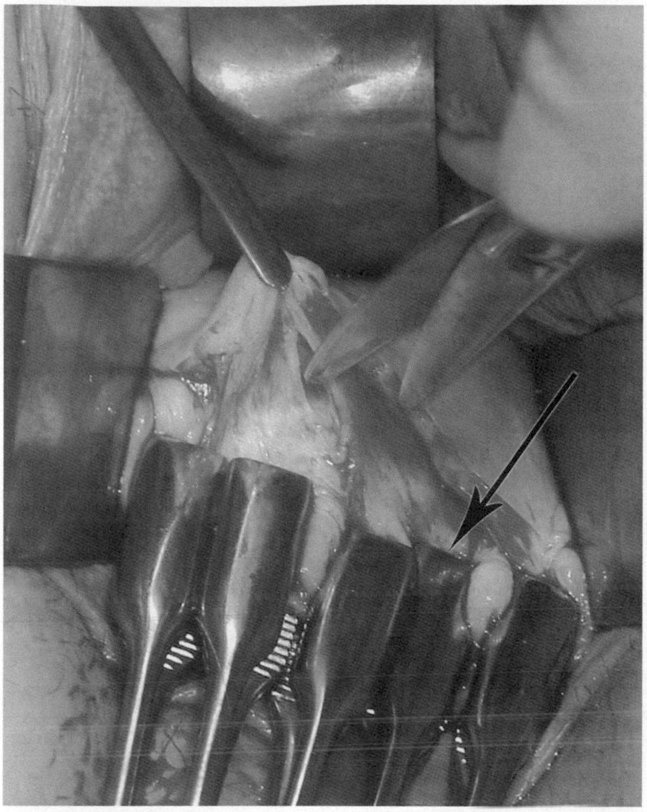

FIGURE 47.40. Opening of the vesicouterine space, with the Chrobak clamps pulling the vaginal cuff.

are safely excised. If the ureter is not seen unequivocally, it should be palpated again to relocate its position before cutting the pillars.

Dissection of the ureter. Once the ureter is clearly identified and placed under traction with a Babcock clamp, it is possible to dissect the ureter. (It is easier if part of the unroofing has been done laparoscopically.) The uterine vessels are usually seen just under the knee of the ureter (Fig. 47.44). With a Kelly clamp, the vessels are pulled down from under the ureter, while at the same time, Metzenbaum scissors are used to free the filmy attachments and allow mobilization of the ureter upward. The uterine artery can be drawn completely into the operative field along with the clips (if they have been used laparoscopically to divide the uterine artery).

Posterior Phase (Described for the Patient's Right Side)

Opening of the cul-de-sac. Chrobak clamps are sharply angulated anteriorly and the posterior cul-de-sac is opened using Metzenbaum scissors as for a simple vaginal hysterectomy. Once entered, the space is stretched laterally to allow placement of a retractor.

Opening of the pararectal space and excision of the uterosacral ligaments. Using Metzenbaum scissors, the pararectal space is defined by opening a space just lateral to the peritoneal folds of the uterosacral ligaments. The medial or rectouterine fibers of the uterosacral ligaments are separated and excised.

Excision of the paracolpos. To complete the posterior phase preparation, the paracolpos is excised. The paracolpos is in fact the inferior border of the parametrium. With the Chrobak clamps rotated to the left, the paracolpos is clamped just medial to the vaginal mucosa, excised, and ligated.

Lateral Phase (Excision of the Parametrium). Before clamping the parametrium, the paravesical space and the ureter should be relocated. The space is verified by palpation with the finger, and a Breisky retractor is replaced in the paravesical space. The ureter should be readily visible and placed under traction with a Babcock clamp. While the Chrobak clamps are pulled and rotated to the patient's left side, a curved Heaney clamp is placed proximally on the parametrium, then a second clamp is placed higher and more lateral to obtain wider parametrium. The second Heaney clamp should be placed at the contact of the knee of the ureter, which can be further dissected if needed (Fig. 47.45). The parametrial tissue is excised and ligated.

Once completed on the other side, the uterus can now be tilted backward and should only be held by the ovarian ligaments (if the adnexae are preserved) or by residual peritoneal attachments. These can be clamped, excised, and ligated. The specimen is removed (Fig. 47.46).

Closure. In general, an attempt is made to include the anterior and posterior pelvic peritoneum along with the vaginal mucosa. Interrupted figures-of-eight of Vicyl 2–0 sutures are used for the closure, starting with the lateral angles. No drains are left in place except for the Foley catheter.

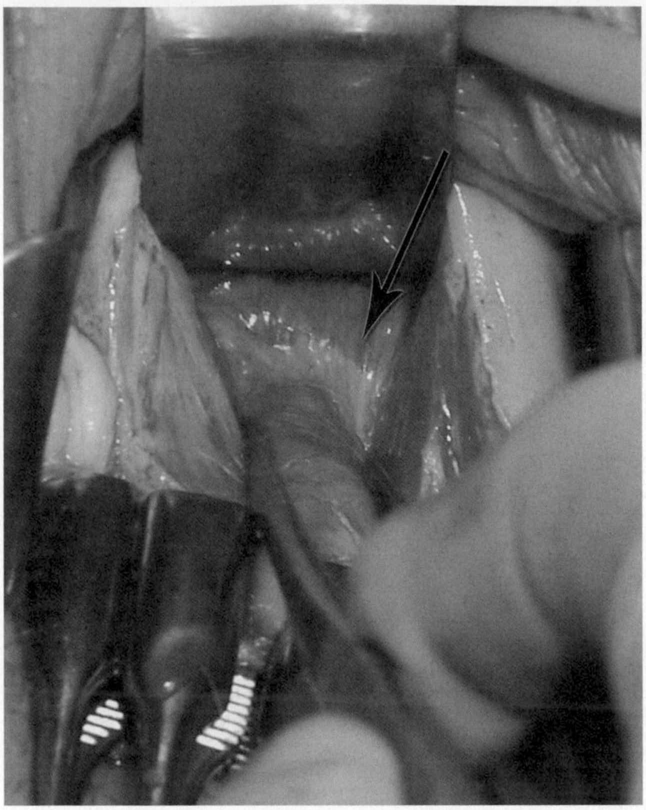

FIGURE 47.41. The vesicovaginal space is open. showing the intact peritoneum (*arrow*).

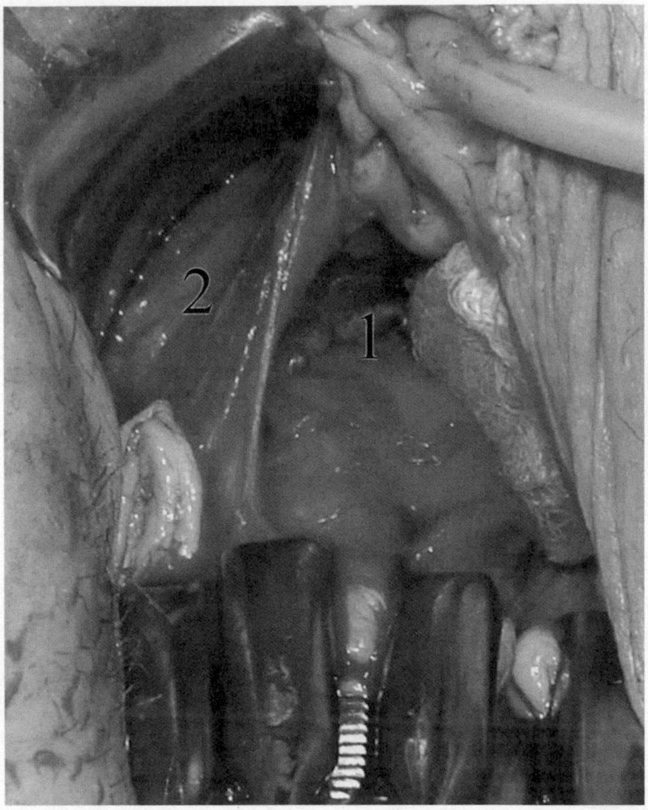

FIGURE 47.42. The right bladder pillars separate the vesicouterine (*1*) and the right paravesical (*2*) spaces.

Results

Over the last 2 decades, data have been accumulating in the literature to indicate that the laparoscopically assisted radical vaginal hysterectomy is a safe procedure, with an overall low morbidity rate. Several studies—including those of Jackson and associates, Malur and colleagues, Nam and coworkers, Renaud and associates, Roy and colleagues, and Steed and coworkers—compared laparotomy (LAP) versus laparoscopically assisted vaginal (LAV) route. In general, the data suggest that the operative time is longer for the LAV group, but blood loss, transfusion rate, and hospital stay are significantly lower. The lymph node yield is similar between the two groups. Malur even reported a higher lymph node count in the LAV group. Intraoperative complication rate appears to be higher in the LAV group, probably related in part to the initial learning curve. In the study by Steed and coworkers, most of the complications were related to bladder and ureteral injuries. However, postoperative complications, such as wound infection and bleeding, tend to be higher in the LAP group. Jackson and associates reported the incidence of bladder and bowel dysfunction to be less in the LAV group, whereas Steed and coworkers found the opposite. Renaud and associates reported that the conversion rate to laparotomy is low. Importantly, there does not appear to be a statistically significant difference in recurrence rate and overall survival, suggesting that the radicality of the vaginal approach is adequate. However, Nam and coworkers noted a higher recurrence rate in the LAV group in patients with larger tumor volume and concluded that the vaginal approach should be restricted to patients with small tumor (<2 cm).

For larger-sized lesions, Possover and colleagues and Querleu have described a technique to provide extended radicality comparable to that of a type III radical hysterectomy with the idea that it may reduce long-term lateropelvic recurrences. However, the more radical the hysterectomy, the more side effects there are on the bladder and bowel function. In recent years, attention has been paid to this matter, and laparoscopic nerve-sparing surgical techniques have been developed by Querleu and associates to reduce these side effects. However, this extensive paracervical and parametrial dissection is of limited value in patients with small lesions (measuring <2 cm), as the risk of lateropelvic recurrence is low.

LAPAROSCOPICALLY-ASSISTED RADICAL VAGINAL TRACHELECTOMY (DARGENT PROCEDURE)

History

In 1987, Dargent proposed a modification of the Schauta-Amreich radical vaginal hysterectomy to preserve the body of the uterus and thus the reproductive function. The procedure, the radical vaginal trachelectomy, today known as the *Dargent procedure,* implies the removal of the cervix along with the proximal portion of the parametrium and is preceded by a complete laparoscopic pelvic lymph node dissection. After

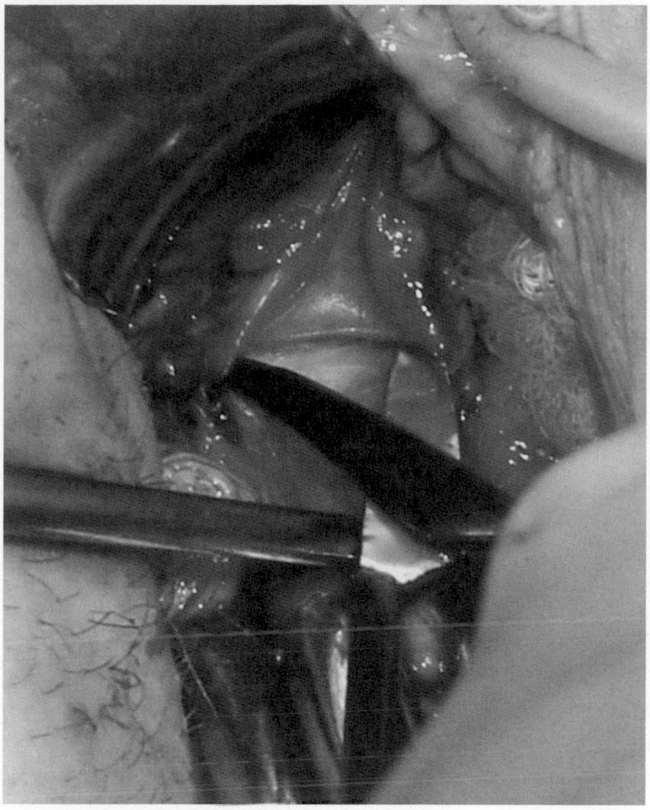

FIGURE 47.43. The ureter is localized by opening the bladdar pillars.

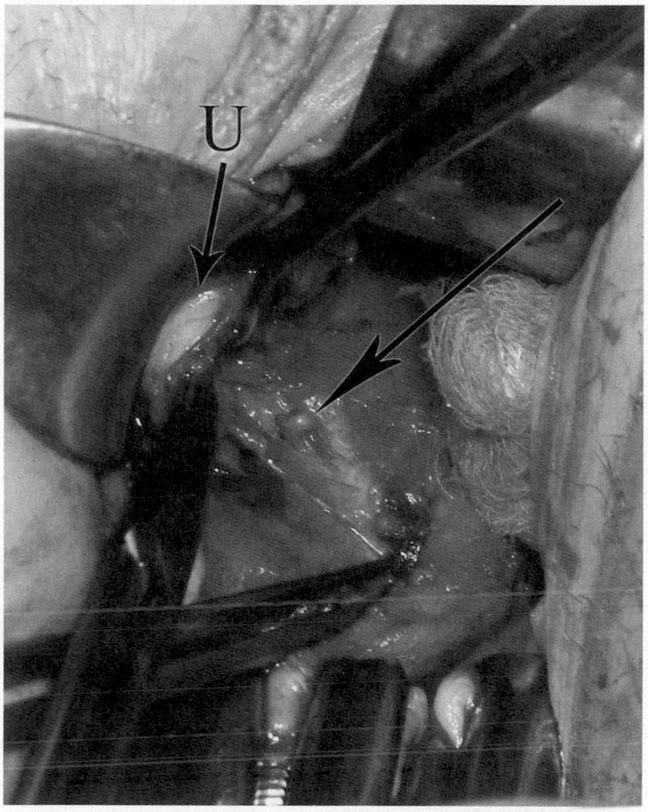

FIGURE 47.44. After dissection of the ureter (*U*), the uterine vessels are seen underneath (*arrow*).

nearly 2 decades, the accumulating experience worldwide summarized by Plante and coworkers suggests that the oncologic outcomes with this conservative procedure are comparable to those obtained following a radical hysterectomy for similarly sized lesions. Obstetrical outcomes are also very encouraging.

Indications

Eligibility criteria for this conservative procedure were initially proposed by Roy and Plante in 1998 and, for the most part, have remained unchanged thus far.

1. Desire to preserve fertility
2. No clinical evidence of impaired fertility (relative contraindication)
3. Lesion size lesser or equal to 2.5 cm
4. FIGO stage IA1 with presence of vascular space invasion, IA2 and IB1
5. Squamous cell or adenocarcinoma
6. No involvement of the upper endocervical canal as determined by colposcopy or MRI
7. No metastasis to regional lymph nodes

The procedure can be offered to women older than age 40, understanding that the fertility potential is obviously reduced, or to women who already have children, as they may wish to have other children in the future. Sonoda and colleagues reviewed the Memorial Sloan-Kettering Cancer Center experience over the course of 10 years and noted that 43% of their patients who underwent a radical hysterectomy for early-stage cervical cancer were younger than 40 years old; of those, 48% would have met the eligibility criteria for a radical trachelectomy. Therefore, a substantial proportion of young women with cervical cancer are potential candidates for this fertility-preservation alternative.

Technique

The laparoscopic part of the procedure is identical to that of the Schauta except that the uterine arteries are obviously not excised. The first three steps of the vaginal part of the surgery are also identical to the Schauta operation (vaginal cuff preparation, anterior phase, and posterior phase). The initial part of the lateral phase—i.e., excision of the parametrium—is also identical; however, only the descending branch of the uterine artery is excised. The excision of the trachelectomy specimen and closure also differ from the Schauta operation and will be detailed here.

Lateral Phase (Described for the Patient's Left Side)

Ligation of the Cervicovaginal Artery. As opposed to the Schauta operation, in which the uterine artery is clamped at its origin, pulled down, and unroofed from under the ureter, the cross of the uterine artery is actually preserved in the case of a trachelectomy to maintain optimal vascularization of the uterus in the event of a future pregnancy. Therefore, only the cervicovaginal or descending branch of the uterine artery is excised. So, after precise localization of the isthmus and the cross of the uterine artery, the cervicovaginal artery is clamped with

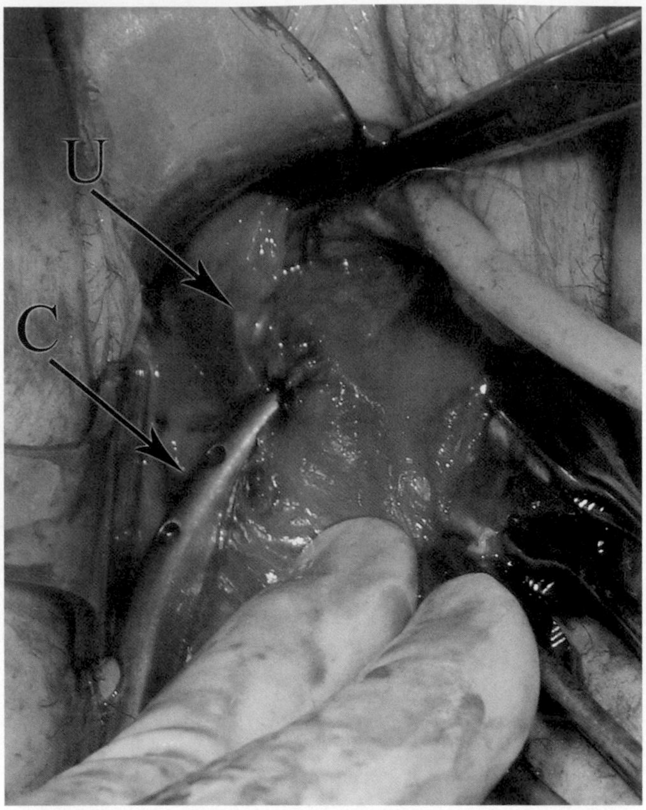

FIGURE 47.45. A clamp (C) has been applied to the right parametrium, very close to the ureter (*U*).

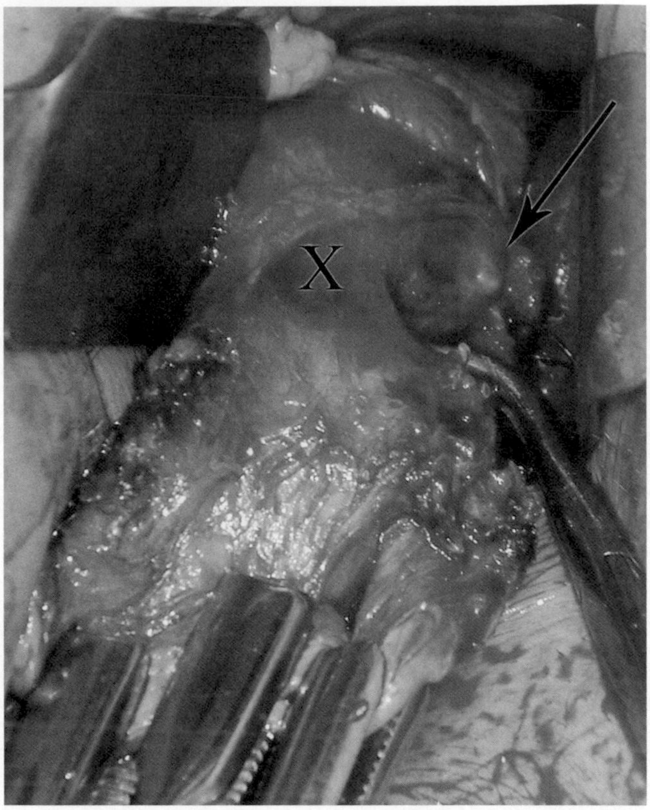

FIGURE 47.47. A clamp is applied just under the arch of the left uterine artery (*arrow*). The uterine isthnic area is visible (*X*).

a right-angle clamp placed at 90 degrees and directly applied to the isthmus (Fig. 47.47); then it is sectioned and ligated.

Excision of the Specimen and Closure. The uterine isthmus and endocervix are precisely located by palpating the uterus anteriorly and posteriorly. The cervix is amputated with a scalpel held perpendicular to the specimen about 1 cm distal to the isthmus (Fig. 47.48). As the specimen is excised, the cervical os appears gradually, and the anterior lip can be grasped with a straight Kocher clamp. Care is taken not to angulate the scalpel to avoid removing too much cervix posteriorly. The specimen is completely excised in one piece to facilitate the pathological evaluation of the margins.

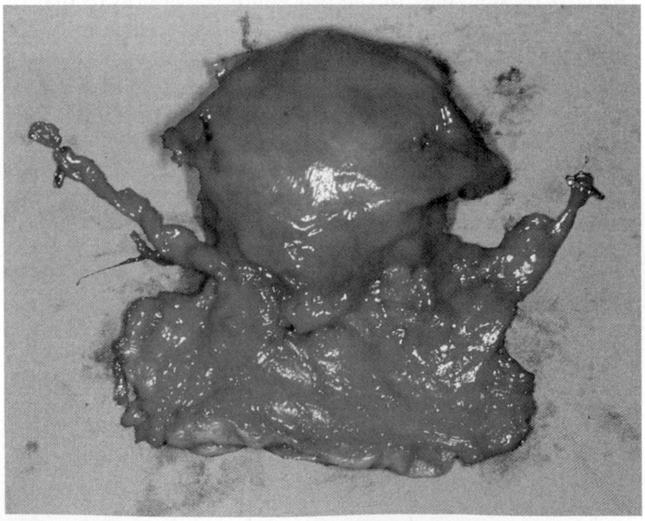

FIGURE 47.46. Specimen with parametrium and uterine arteries.

Ideally, the specimen should be at least 1 to 2 cm wide, with 1 cm of vaginal mucosa and 1 to 2 cm of parametrium (Fig. 47.49A-B). When there is no clinical evidence of residual tumor, a frozen-section analysis is not performed. The specimen is kept intact for final analysis and will be processed as a cone specimen. However, in patients with a visible lesion, the trachelectomy specimen is sent for immediate frozen-section analysis to assess the level of the tumor in relation to the endocervical resection margin. At least 8 to 10 mm of tumor-free tissue should be obtained between the level of the tumor and the endocervical resection margin; otherwise, additional endocervix should be removed or the trachelectomy should be completed by a radical vaginal hysterectomy (Schauta). It is thus extremely important to ask the pathologist to do a frozen-section analysis of the cervix with a section made longitudinally from the ectocervix to the endocervix to evaluate the distance between the most cephalad edge of the tumor and the endocervical resection margin. A permanent cerclage is placed at the level of the isthmus using a nonresorbable Prolene or Ethibond 0 suture starting posteriorly at 6 o'clock to have the knot lying posteriorly. The sutures should not be placed too deeply into the cervical stroma, as the cerclage can eventually erode into the endocervical canal and be expelled. When tying the

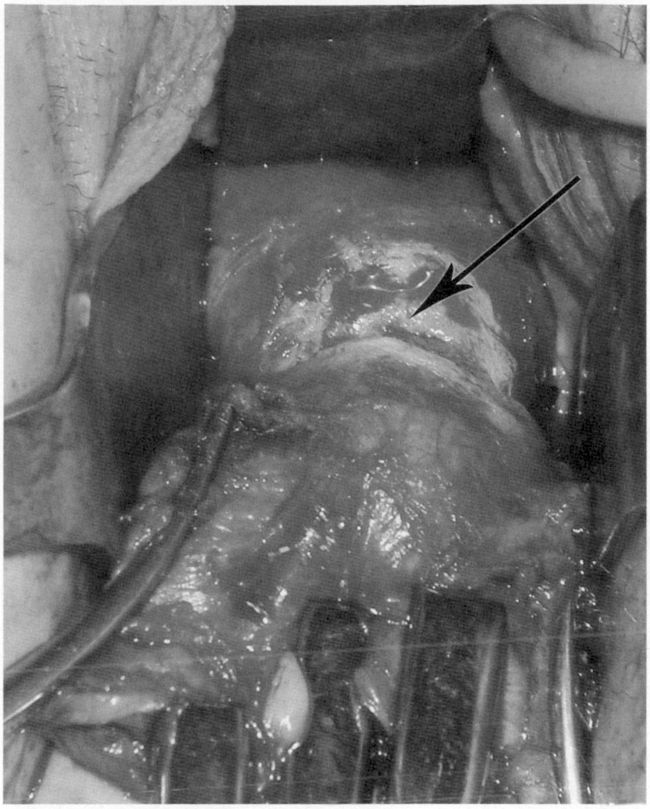

FIGURE 47.48. Section of the cervix 1 cm below the isthmis. The endocervical canal is visible (*arrow*).

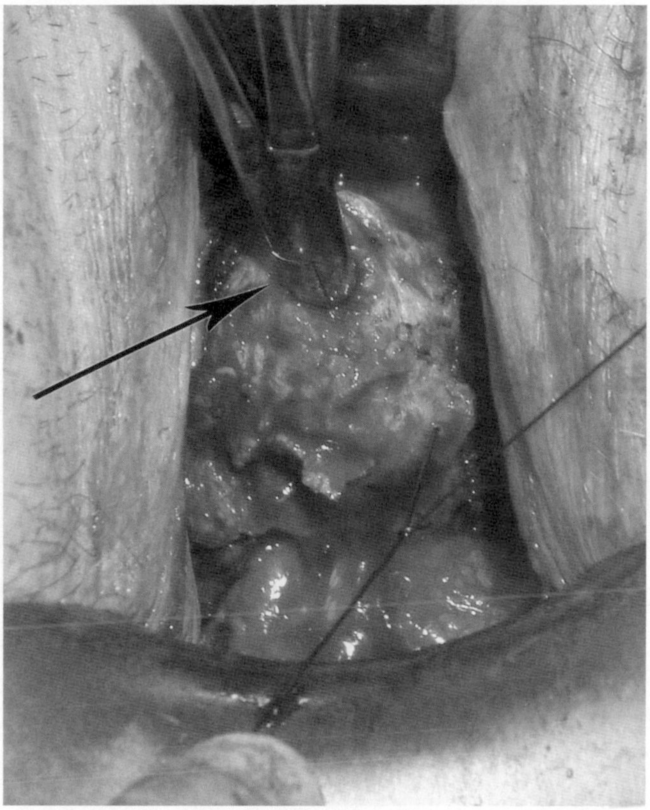

FIGURE 47.50. A cerclage is put in place and ligated posteriorly with a dilator (*arrow*) in the cervical canal.

cerclage knot, a uterine probe can be placed in the cervical os to avoid tightening the knot too much, as this may cause cervical stenosis (Fig. 47.50).

The Dargent procedure is completed by reapproximating the edges of the vaginal mucosa to the new exocervix. This is accomplished with interrupted figures-of-eight sutures of 2–0 Vicryl. It is easier to begin with the sutures at 12 and 6 o'clock first. The lateral sutures are then placed separately to include the anterior and posterior vaginal mucosa only. Although easy to do, the closure of the vaginal mucosa is an extremely important step of the procedure, and care should be taken not to bury the cervical opening into folds of redundant vaginal

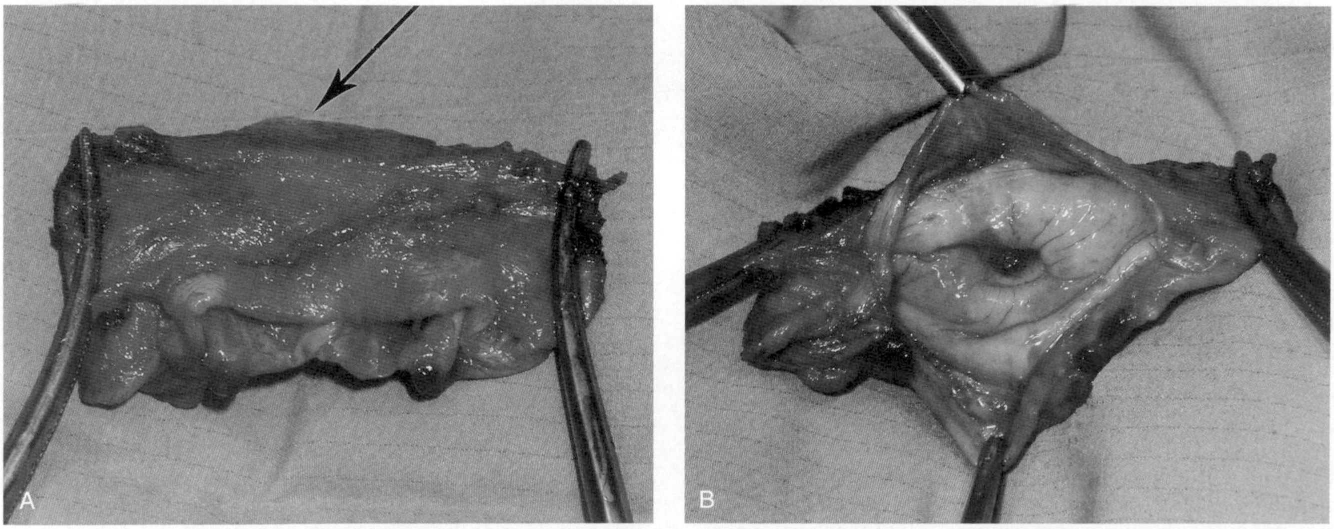

FIGURE 47.49. A and B: The specimen with its parametrium. The superior endocervical canal is shown (*arrow*).

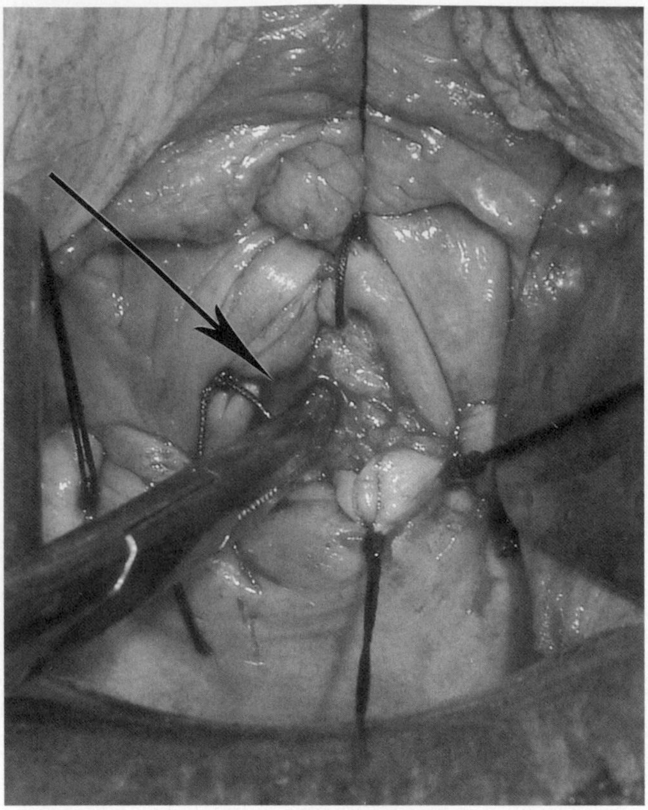

FIGURE 47.51. Suturing the vaginal mucosa to the cervical stroma. A clamp (*arrow*) is indicating the endocervical canal.

mucosa (Fig. 47.51). The new exocervix should remain accessible for monitoring with colposcopic examination and cytology.

At the end of the trachelectomy procedure, laparoscopy is performed to verify hemostasis in the pelvis and the integrity of the pelvic structures. No drains or packings are left.

Oncologic Outcome

Data are accumulating worldwide indicating that the oncologic outcome following the radical trachelectomy is comparable to the outcome following a radical hysterectomy for similar-size lesions. Indeed, several large series totaling more than 600 cases consistently report a recurrence rate of less than 4% and a death rate of less than 2% (Table 47.8). Plante and colleagues have noted that the size of the lesion (≥2 cm) and the presence of LVSI seem to be the most important risk factors for recurrences. The recent work of Hertel and coworkers also suggests that adenocarcinomas may carry a higher risk of recurrence.

Morice and associates have noted unusual sites of recurrences, such as in the vesicovaginal septum and in the bladder, which suggests that very meticulous surgical technique should be observed to avoid entering the wrong planes of dissection and potentially disseminating tumor cells at the time of the procedure. Piketty recently reported a recurrence in the ovary in a patient with an adenocarcinoma. Only two recurrences have been reported so far on the residual cervix itself. The first one was reported by Bali and occurred nearly 7 years following the initial surgery. It is unclear whether it truly represents a recurrence or a new primary. The other one was reported by Bader and coworkers; it occurred 6 months postabdominal trachelectomy and was picked up on routine Pap smear. A radical hysterectomy was performed and disclosed a 3-mm recurrence (or persistence) in the cervix.

TABLE 47.8

ONCOLOGIC OUTCOME POST RADICAL TRACHELECTOMY

Authors	Number	Recurrences	Deaths
Plante and Roy	100	2 (2.0%)[a]	1 (1.0%)
Covens and Steed	121	7 (5.8%)	4 (3.3%)
Shepherd et al.	112	3 (2.7%)	2 (1.8%)
Hertel et al.	100	4 (4.0%)	2 (2.0%)
Dargent and Mathevet	95	4 (4.2%)[a]	3 (3.1%)
Ungar et al.[b]	91	2 (2.2%)	0
Total	619	22 (3.5%)	12 (1.9%)

[a] Excluding one case of neuroendocrine tumor.
[b] Abdominal radical trachelectomy.

Ungar and associates and del Priore and colleagues have reported two recurrences following the abdominal radical trachelectomy procedure, and both were in patients with bulky lesions: One had a 3.8-cm lesion, and she recurred within 4 months of the surgery with a 6-cm lesion; the other had a 5-cm glassy-cell adenocarcinoma and recurred 14 months after surgery. Strict selection criteria are extremely important to lower the risks of recurrences. Further experience will determine if the abdominal radical trachelectomy is safe in bulky lesions. Another alternative for patients with larger lesions is the use of neoadjuvant chemotherapy to reduce the size of the tumor followed by a fertility-preserving radical trachelectomy. Plante and coworkers have recently published their preliminary experience with three cases. All have had a complete pathological response to the chemotherapy with no residual cancer in the surgical specimen. Obviously, this approach is currently experimental but has potential merits and deserves further investigation.

Shepherd recommends regular follow-up posttrachelectomies, including a colposcopic examination, cytology, and rectovaginal examination every 3 to 4 months for the first 2 to 3 years, every 6 months for the next 2 years, and yearly thereafter. Unfortunately, colposcopy and cytologies are frequently unsatisfactory after trachelectomy because the squamous columnar junction is often not visualized and the cytology frequently contains only squamous cells. Conversely, atypical glandular cells from the lower uterine segment are commonly picked up on the smear and misinterpreted as suspicious for recurrence. Singh and coworkers have reported their experience with nearly 200 smears posttrachelectomy and concluded that a high proportion of the smears were unsatisfactory; 2% of the smears were reported as suspicious and in fact represented atypical endometrial cells, but two patients recurred and retrospectively had abnormal smears long before the recurrence was diagnosed. Reports of cytology posttrachelectomy should thus be interpreted with caution. Shepherd and coworkers recommend the use of an endocervical cytobrush for the cytology and an MRI at 6, 12, and 24 months postsurgery. The superb work by Sahdev and associates emphasizes the fact that radiologists interpreting those MRIs should be very well aware of the anatomical changes posttrachelectomy, as some of the changes may be misinterpreted as cancer recurrences.

Obstetric Outcome

The collected data on obstetric outcome are also very promising. As can be seen in Table 47.9, there have been more than 220 pregnancies reported from the same group of investigators. In general, the rate of first-trimester miscarriage does not seem to be higher than in the general population at approximately 16%. It is interesting to note that even though women undergoing the radical trachelectomy procedure do so to preserve their fertility, there is a surprising 4% rate of elective pregnancy termination. The rate of second-trimester losses is higher than in the general population (8%). Overall, 66% to 75% of all pregnancies reach the third trimester. Of those, approximately 15% will end with significant prematurity at less than 32 weeks of gestation. Luckily, less than 10% will deliver before 28 weeks, when most of the severe neonatal morbidities and mortalities occur. Of note, multiple pregnancies appear to be at a particularly high risk of severe prematurity posttrachelectomy, and this should be taken into consideration when discussing *in vitro* fertilization in patients with infertility. Overall, 85% of the pregnancies reaching the third trimester will evolve normally beyond 32 weeks, and the majority will actually deliver at term (>37 weeks of gestation). The work of Klemm and colleagues suggests that there is no evidence that birth weight of newborns delivered from women who had a trachelectomy is lower. They showed that the vascular flow to the uterine artery before and after vaginal trachelectomy is well preserved.

The etiology of the second-trimester losses and the preterm deliveries is thought to be either mechanical and/or infectious. Indeed, the short cervix probably does not offer as much support to the lower uterine segment. As the uterus enlarges and gets heavier, the cervix is more likely to dilate prematurely. However, the main etiology is felt to be infectious. Indeed, the shortened cervix after the trachelectomy procedure seems to prevent the formation of an efficacious mucus plug. The mucus plug is thought to play an important role as a physiological barrier between the vaginal flora and the membranes to prevent ascending infections. Hence, the subclinical chorioamnionitis is thought to be responsible for the premature rupture of membranes and premature labor. Plante and associates have proposed some guidelines for the follow-up of these high-risk pregnancies. A consultation with a specialist in fetal-maternal medicine is recommended. The value of prophylactic antibiotic coverage—as well as steroid injections to accelerate fetal lung maturity near term—is unclear, although Shepherd and colleagues strongly recommend it. The work of Berghella and coworkers has shown that serial transvaginal ultrasound is the best modality for the follow-up of cervical length in the general obstetric population and has been used in the follow-up of pregnant women posttrachelectomy. If the pregnancy evolves normally, delivery is planned at 38 to 39 weeks of gestation. Because of the permanent cerclage, women should be delivered by elective cesarean section.

Outcomes of pregnancy following an abdominal trachelectomy also appear promising. Although the numbers are smaller, Ungar and coworkers have reported 10 pregnancies so far, with results comparable to pregnancies after the vaginal approach. There was a concern that ligating the uterine arteries at the time of the procedure might have an impact on the vascularization of the uterus and potentially lead to intrauterine growth retardation. So far, the data seem reassuring in that regard.

Conclusion

Based on the collected data available thus far, the radical trachelectomy procedure truly offers a valuable alternative to young women with small, early-stage cervical cancer who wish to preserve their fertility potential. Oncologic outcomes are comparable to standard radical hysterectomy for similar-size lesions, and the complication rate is low. Pregnancies are definitely possible after this procedure, and overall obstetrical outcome is good despite the rate of second-trimester loss and premature delivery. In the last 2 to 3 decades, there has been a tremendous shift toward minimally invasive surgical techniques in gynecologic oncology. Laparoscopic and radical vaginal surgeries have revolutionized the surgical management of cervical cancer. The radical trachelectomy procedure (Dargent operation)

TABLE 47.9

OBSTETRICAL OUTCOME POST–RADICAL TRACHELECTOMY

Author	Pregancy	T-1[a] miscarriage	TAB[b]	T-2 miscarriage	T-3 delivery	Delivery <32 wks	Delivery >32 wks
Plante and Roy	59	10 (16%)	3 (4%)	2 (5%)	44 (75%)	3 (7%)	41 (93%)
Dargent and Mathevet	56	11 (18%)[c]	3 (5%)	8 (14%)	34 (61%)	5 (15%)	29 (85%)
Shepherd et al.	52	15 (29%)	2 (4%)	7 (13%)	28 (54%)	7 (25%)	21 (75%)
Covens and Bernardini	45	8 (16%)	0	3 (7%)	34 (77%)	6 (18%)[d]	28 (82%)
Hertel et al.[e]	14	1 (7%)	2 (14%)	0	11 (78%)	3 (27%)	8 (73%)
Ungar et al.[f]	10	4 (40%)	0	0	6 (60%)	1 (17%)	5 (83%)
Total	236	49 (20%)	10 (4%)	20 (8%)	157 (66%)	25 (15%)	132 (85%)

[a]T-1, first trimester; T-2, second trimester ; T-3, third trimester.
[b]TAB, therapeutic abortions.
[c]Includes two ectopic.
[d]Includes six sets of twins.
[e]Personal communication, April 2006.
[f]Abdominal radical trachelectomy.

is unquestionably the most important surgical development in the treatment of early-stage cervical cancer in the last century.

LAPAROSCOPIC RADICAL HYSTERECTOMY WITH PELVIC AND AORTIC LYMPHADENECTOMY

Laparoscopic radical hysterectomy with pelvic and aortic lymph node dissection was first reported by Nezhat in 1992. This technically challenging procedure initially was received with caution by gynecologic oncologists who have used the abdominal radical hysterectomy as the traditional approach for decades. So far, no randomized trials are available for comparing these two surgical approaches; however, more than 150 patients have been reported with encouraging results. So far, the largest series reported has been by Spirtos and associates, who described 78 consecutive patients, all with early cervical cancer and a Quetelet body mass index <35, who underwent the procedure. In all, 94% of the procedures were completed laparoscopically with an average operative time of 205 minutes and an average blood loss of 225 mL, with only one patient (1.3%) requiring transfusion. There was one ureterovaginal fistula documented. The average lymph node count was 34, with 11.5% of patients having positive lymph nodes. Three patients (3.8%) had close or positive surgical margins, and 5.1% recurred with a minimum of 3-year follow-up. Table 47.10 summarizes reports on laparoscopic radical hysterectomy with pelvic and aortic lymphadenectomy.

Laparoscopic Radical Hysterectomy Technique

One technique of laparoscopic radical hysterectomy is well described by Spirtos and associates and Chen and colleagues. The laparoscopic approach uses different surgical instruments and techniques than the classic approach to accomplish the same procedure performed via laparotomy. The technique of laparoscopic radical hysterectomy described in this section relies on the use of the 10-mm argon beam coagulator (ABC) and the 12-mm endoscopic stapler. Four trocars are needed with the camera in the umbilical site and the ABC in the suprapubic site. The retroperitoneum is opened and the round ligaments coagulated. The paravesical and pararectal spaces are developed with the ABC, and the ureter is clearly identified. Resection of the adnexa are managed on an individual basis as per the open approach. The uterine artery is identified after developing the pararectal and paravesical spaces, and the umbilical ligament is isolated. The uterine artery and vein are stapled with the endoscopic stapler in one or two separate applications. The bladder flap then is developed. The posterior cul-de-sac peritoneum is incised and the rectouterine ligaments exposed. The ureter is then unroofed from the parametria by placing medial traction on the stapled uterine artery stump, and the bladder is dissected further inferiorly. The uterosacral/rectouterine ligaments are stapled or coagulated and the ureter is retracted laterally to

TABLE 47.10

SUMMARY OF REPORTS ON LAPAROSCOPIC RADICAL HYSTERECTOMY AND PELVIC LYMPHADENECTOMY WITH OR WITHOUT PARAAORTIC AORTIC LYMPHADENECTOMY

Author	N[a]	PLN	ORT (min)	EBL (mL)	LOS (days)	Complications	Recurrences
Nezhat et al. 1992, 1993	7	22	315	30–250	2.1	None	None
Sedlacek et al. 1994, 1995	14	16	420	334	5.5	1 VVF, 1 ureteral injury	—
Ting 1994	4	8	330–480	150–500	—	None	—
Osterzenski 1996	6	—	280	—	2–6	1 hydronephrosis	—
Spirtos et al. 1996	10	18.3	253	300	3.2	None	—
Kim and Moon 1998	18	22	363	619	—	None	—
Hsieh et al. 1998	8	—	—		6.5	None	1 distant
Spirtos 2002	78	23.8	205	250	2.9	1.3% transfusion, 3 cystotomies, 1 UVF, 1 DVT 5 conversions	8 (10.3%)
Lee 2002	12	19.2	235	428	6.8	2 transfusion	None at 1 year
Lin 2003	10	—	—	250	4.1	None	—
Obemair 2003	55	—	210	200	5	3 vascular, 1 nerve, 1 fistula	None
Pomel 2003	50	13.2	258	—	7.5	1 bladder fistula, 1 ureter stenosis	5-year survival 96%
Abu-Rustum 2003	19	25.5	371	301	4.5	1 transfusion, 2 conversion, 1 fever	None
Gil-Moreno 2005	27	19.1	—	400	5	—	None

N, number of patients; PLN, mean pelvic lymph nodes; ORT, mean operating room time; EBL, mean estimated blood loss; LOS, mean hospital stay; VVF, vesicovaginal fistula; UVF, ureterovaginal fistula; DVT, deep venous thrombosis.
[a]Some patients may be reported more than once.

resect the desired length of parametria with the stapler. Anterior colpotomy is performed at the desired vaginal length. A vaginal probe facilitates stretching the vagina for easier incision. The remaining parametria and paracolpos are resected with the ABC and staplers. The specimen is removed vaginally with a single tooth tenaculum, and the vaginal cuff is closed laparoscopically with endoscopic sutures or the endostich. The placement of ureteral catheters or stents to facilitate ureteric manipulation is optional. The pelvic and aortic lymphadenectomy is performed as described in the preceding. Pelvic drains usually are not necessary, and a suprapubic catheter is optional.

LAPAROSCOPIC SURGICAL STAGING

Currently available clinical staging methods and imaging studies are not completely accurate in the detection of pelvic and aortic lymph node metastasis from cervical cancer, and pathologic evaluation of retroperitoneal lymph nodes remains the gold standard for establishing metastasis. In addition, identifying retroperitoneal nodal metastasis may alter the overall therapeutic approach and affect the patient's prognosis.

Laparoscopic surgical staging with pelvic and aortic lymph node dissection for cervical cancer was initially reported by Querleu in France. Since this initial report, many investigators have adopted the laparoscopic pretreatment surgical approach and continue to modify the technical details of the procedure. It is well established at this point that transperitoneal or extraperitoneal laparoscopic pelvic and aortic lymph node dissection for cervical cancer, in experienced hands, is feasible, yields similar results as the open approach, and is associated with low morbidity. Furthermore, this approach may provide valuable information that is not available using clinical staging techniques. Computed tomography was able to detect retroperitoneal nodal metastasis in only 17% to 57% of cervical cancer patients staged laparoscopically. Table 47.11 summarizes selected reports on laparoscopic pelvic and aortic lymph node dissection in the management of stage I to IV cervical cancer.

Laparoscopic Surgical Staging Technique

The technique of laparoscopic surgical staging continues to evolve as experience with this minimally invasive approach increases. There are two main approaches: the transperitoneal approach and the extraperitoneal approach (popularized by Querleu and Dargent from France). For the transperitoneal approach, four laparoscopic trocars usually are needed (Fig. 47.52): 10-mm trocars in the umbilical and suprapubic regions and 5-mm trocars just medial to the iliac crest on each side. For the aortic nodal dissection, the laparoscope is placed in the suprapubic region, and the monitors are moved cephalad. For the pelvic lymphadenectomy, the laparoscope is placed in the umbilical region, and the monitors are placed caudal. A variety of endoscopic tools may be used with similar results. The selection usually is based on the surgeon's preference and experience. Both monopolar and bipolar currents are available, and a wide variety of endoscopic dissecting instruments, clip appliers, and specimen retrieval devices are available. The 10-mm argon beam coagulator (ABC, Conmed, Utica, NY) is ideal in this setting. It works both as a dissector and a coagulator. A retroperitoneal nodal dissection may be satisfactorily completed in the majority of cases with the aid of a tissue grasper and an endoscopic clip applier. The right aortic nodal tissue is approached via a retroperitoneal incision over the right common iliac artery. The right ureter and ovarian vessels are identified, and the nodal tissue over the inferior vena cava is removed. The left aortic nodal tissue may be approached via the same incision. The inferior mesenteric artery, left ureter, and

TABLE 47.11

SUMMARY OF PRETREATMENT LAPAROSCOPIC PELVIC AND AORTIC LYMPH NODE DISSECTION IN THE MANAGEMENT OF STAGE I TO IV CERVICAL CANCER

Author	*n*	Stage	PLN (% +)	PAN (% +)	ORT	HD	Complications
Querleu, 1991	39	IB–IIB	8.7 (12.8%)	—	90	1	3 Minor
Childers, 1993	18	IB–IVA	31.4 (both) (33.3%)	(6.2%)	75–175	1.5	Not significant
Fowler, 1993	12	IB	23.5 (16.7%)	6.5 (0%)	373 With laparotomy	7.4 With laparotomy	2 Minor
Su, 1995	38	—	15	—	77	—	1 Vascular 1 Ureteral
Recio, 1996	12	IB2	18 (25%)	7 (0%)	176	1	Not significant
Chu, 1997	67	IA2–IIIB	26.7 (12.8%)	8 (35.7%)	93	2	1 Vascular
Possover, 1998	26	IIB–IIIB	15.3 (11.5%)	6.8 (7.7%)	162	3.2	1 Vascular
Vidaurreta, 1999	84	IB2–IV	18.5 (45.2%)	—	108	1–2	1 Vascular
Schlaerth, 1999	40	IA–IIA	32.1	12.1	—	—	—
Querleu, 2000	53	≥IB2	With common iliac	20.7 (32%)	126	1–2	1 Ureteral
Altgassen, 2000	108	IA1–IVB	21–24.3	5.1–10.6	Aortic: 35–73 Pelvic: 61–70	—	3 Vascular
11 Reports	497	I–IV	9–32 (24%–25%)	6–21 (19%–20%)	120	1–2	1%–2% Vascular 0.4% Ureteral

HD, mean hospital stay in days; *n*, number of patients; ORT, mean operating room time in minutes; PAN, mean aortic lymph nodes; PLN, mean pelvic lymph nodes.

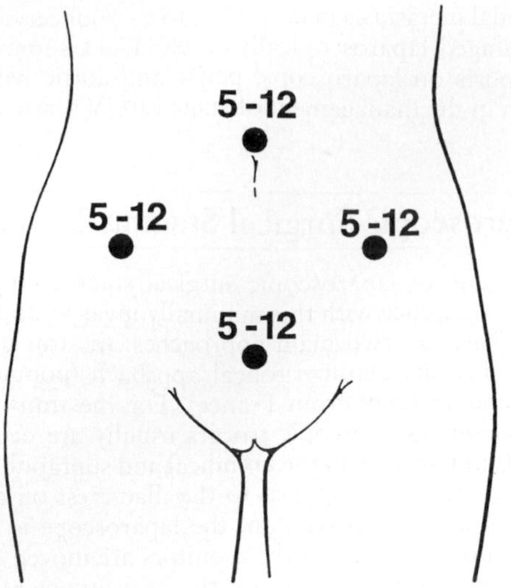

FIGURE 47.52. The transperitoneal minimally invasive approach for laparoscopic surgical staging. Four laparoscopic trocars usually are needed. Figure © MSKCC, 2002.

left ovarian vessels are identified, and the nodal tissue over the left aortic region is removed.

Dissection above the inferior mesenteric artery to include the infrarenal nodal regions may be accomplished through a similar approach, and a left-sided laparoscopic suprarenal retrocrural paraaortic lymphadenectomy in advanced cervical cancer has been described.

PATHOLOGIC EXAMINATION OF THE OPERATIVE SPECIMEN

Considerable useful information about the extent of the disease can be obtained by a careful pathologic examination of the operative specimen. This is helpful in determining prognosis but is also absolutely essential to the identification of patients at greater risk for persistent disease so that additional therapy and close surveillance can be provided. Even though the operator may be fatigued at the end of the operation, he or she should consider accompanying the specimen to the pathology laboratory, where it can be examined with the pathologist before it is placed in fixative and sectioned. Another alternative is to call the pathologist to the operation room for a joint examination of the specimen while the surgical incisions are being closed. The gynecologic surgeon then can point to worrisome parts of the specimen; such information assists the pathologist in taking sections. Critical margins of dissection can be pointed out and stained with India ink so that they can be seen on microscopic slides. The primary cervical tumor should be measured as accurately as possible so that at least an estimate of its size and volume can be recorded. Numerous microscopic sections of the cervix with adjacent vaginal cuff; lower uterine segment; and paravaginal, paracervical, and parametrial tissue should be examined to show the cell type, degree of differentiation, depth of stromal invasion, and presence or absence of invasion of lymphatic and vascular spaces. It is important to know not only the depth of invasion but also the thickness of the uninvolved fibromuscular stroma of the cervix, as pointed out by Kishi and coworkers. These authors found that the nodal metastasis and 5-year cancer death rates were 7% and 8%, respectively, in patients with uninvolved fibromuscular stroma thickness >3 mm, and 37% and 26%, respectively, in patients with the thickness <3 mm. Furthermore, GOG has demonstrated that the percentage of invasion of tumor into the cervical stroma is an independent prognostic factor and is used to help determine the need for postoperative adjuvant treatment.

Unfortunately, the exquisite giant-section technique of pathologic examination used by Burghardt and coworkers is not available in any U.S. pathology laboratory. These authors measured ratio of tumor size to the size of the cervix. The incidence of lymph node involvement increased with tumor size, reaching a maximum of 68.3% in the group with a ratio from 70% to 80% of cervical anatomic involvement. Surprisingly, direct spread into the parametrium seldom was found, even when large tumors were found to occupy the entire cervix. This finding is contrary to that of Bleker and coworkers, who found 16.8% unrecognized parametrial tumor involvement in patients with stage IB and IIA lesions. The 5-year survival rate fell with parametrial involvement.

Thorough examination of the lymphadenectomy specimens must be done. Tumor metastasis to lymph nodes affects patient survival adversely and is an indication for postoperative adjuvant therapy. In patients with positive nodes, the pathologic examination should report whether the metastatic disease is microscopic or macroscopic, single or multiple, unilateral or bilateral. The location of lymph nodes positive for tumor also should be reported because the prognosis is especially poor in patients with positive common iliac or paraaortic nodes. The usual standard technique of pathologic examination of lymphadenectomy specimens involves removal of visible and palpable nodes from fatty tissue, with bisection of each node for microscopic examination. This standard technique may not be adequate for an accurate assessment of lymph node metastases. A significant increase in positive findings can be obtained if special pathologic examination techniques are used, as demonstrated by To and coworkers, Ahrens and Tschoke, and Wilkinson and Hause. With their technique of dissection of lymph nodes at multiple levels before paraffin embedding, To and coworkers showed that 9% of patients originally reported to have negative nodes actually had positive nodes.

An accurate assessment of the extent of disease by a careful pathology examination of the operative specimen is imperative in deciding whether additional treatment is needed. Indeed, it is such an important component in the surgical management of patients with cervical cancer that these patients should be operated on only in hospitals where such expert specimen evaluation is available.

POSTOPERATIVE COMPLICATIONS

Bladder

Neurogenic Dysfunction

A radical hysterectomy substantially denervates the bladder and upper urethra; the more extensive the dissection, the greater the degree of interference with their function. Parasympathetic and sympathetic nerve fibers to and from the bladder and urethra are removed, along with paracervical, paravaginal, cardinal ligament tissues, and pelvic lymph nodes. All patients have some degree of bladder dysfunction; the incidence of significant bladder dysfunction can be as high as 50%.

Studies have demonstrated that the bladder initially can be hypertonic, with decreased bladder capacity, increased resting pressure, and increased residual urine volume. Many patients have difficulty initiating micturition and experience a loss of sensation of bladder fullness. Using sensitive urodynamic instrumentation, Scotti and coworkers found a variety of abnormalities, including obstructive voiding patterns, immediate and delayed loss of compliance, sensory losses, and genuine stress incontinence. Some patients had complete absence of bladder contractions during voiding. Although these findings are quite compelling, Lin and associates recently reported normal preoperative urodynamic findings in only 17% of 210 patients with cervical cancer scheduled to undergo radical hysterectomy.

Mundy and Sasaki and coworkers have suggested that the posterior part of the cardinal ligament (pars nervosa) contains the major part of the parasympathetic and sympathetic nerve supply to the bladder and urethra and that its removal is responsible for postoperative bladder dysfunction. Sasaki and coworkers demonstrated that removal of the anterior cardinal ligament (pars vasculosa) with preservation of the pars nervosa reduces the incidence of postoperative bladder dysfunction. The work of Kadar and coworkers and that of Asmussen and Ulmsten suggests that the nerve supply to the bladder and urethra can be spared without compromising the necessary extensive dissection and tissue removal around the central disease, thus sparing many patients the loss of urethrovesical function. Kuwabara and colleagues recently reported a decrease in bladder dysfunction by using a technique of intraoperative electrical stimulation to identify and preserve the vesical nerve branches. These nerve-sparing modifications have not been widely adopted by gynecologic oncologists in the United States because of a concern that this same cardinal ligament tissue also carries lymphatic channels draining the cervix and should be removed in a complete central dissection. However, Trimbos and colleagues, from the Netherlands, have reported no increase in recurrence or decreased survival in a series of patients treated with nerve-sparing radical hysterectomy.

Techniques of managing the postoperative bladder have varied widely. Duration of catheter drainage, suprapubic versus transurethral drainage, the value of self-catheterization, and the value of cystometric studies have all been debated as described by Bandy and coworkers. These authors also found that patients receiving postoperative adjunctive pelvic radiation had significantly more contracted and unstable bladders than patients treated with surgery alone. Proper management of the bladder in the first several weeks after operation is essential to avoid overdistention. The duration of postoperative bladder catheterization has decreased in recent years. Chamberlin and investigators reported a contemporary median indwelling catheter duration of 6 days compared with 30 days in historical controls with no increase in complication rates.

Although some clinicians leave an indwelling catheter or suprapubic tube in place 2 to 3 weeks, we prefer continuous transurethral catheter drainage until the patient is ready for discharge, which is usually about 4 to 7 days after surgery. Early postoperative intravenous pyelography (IVP) in the absence of intraoperative urinary tract injury or clinical symptoms suggestive of injury is not indicated; moreover, an abnormal early IVP is not predictive of subsequent urinary tract dysfunction. When the patient is ready for discharge, the catheter is removed, and postvoid residuals are checked with a bladder ultrasound scan (transurethral catheterization also can be used). If the postvoid residual volume is below 50 to 75 mL and the volume of urine spontaneously voided is greater than the postvoid residual, then the patient is allowed to leave the hospital without an indwelling catheter. She must be thoroughly schooled in the importance of not allowing her bladder to become overdistended. Allowing the bladder to overdistend, especially in the early postoperative recovery period, can result in a flaccid bladder from stretching and decompensation of the detrusor muscle, prolongation of bladder dysfunction with high residual urine volumes, and the likelihood of urinary infections. Patients who have unacceptable postvoid residuals are best managed with prolonged indwelling catheter drainage for several weeks before attempting removal. If a serious episode of overdistention of the bladder ever occurs, continuous indwelling catheter drainage should be reinstituted, sometimes for several weeks, with the hope that permanent impairment of bladder function can be avoided. Urinary tract infections can occur in conjunction with bladder dysfunction and should be looked for with periodic urinalysis and culture and treated with appropriate antibiotics. Patients should be encouraged to maintain a urine output above 2,000 mL per day to avoid urinary tract infection.

In most patients, a satisfactory voiding pattern can be established within several months. Urodynamic studies, however, can show some evidence of slight and persistent chronic bladder dysfunction for several years. Fraser stated that 20% of his patients continued to report changes in bladder sensation as long as 5 to 15 years after operation. In many patients who have had properly performed radical hysterectomy and pelvic lymphadenectomy, it is inevitable that bladder function will never be completely normal again. With proper postoperative bladder care and rehabilitation, however, function should be satisfactory in most patients at the end of the first year. According to Fishman and coworkers, 35% of patients continued to express unhappiness at the extent and effect of their postoperative urinary dysfunction.

Vesicovaginal Fistula

In the absence of prior pelvic irradiation, bladder ischemia and vesicovaginal fistula are infrequent complications of this procedure. Vesicovaginal fistulas occur in less than 1% of patients (Table 47.12). Nearly one third of urinary tract fistulas following surgery heal spontaneously, as compared with none if adjuvant radiation therapy is given. The management of vesicovaginal fistulas is discussed in Chapter 39.

Ureter

Clark, working at the Johns Hopkins Hospital, published one of the first descriptions of radical hysterectomy for cervical cancer in 1895. Sampson, working in the same institution during the same time, recognized that injury to the ureter was the most serious problem associated with primary radical surgery for this disease. His publications on ureteral anatomy and blood supply and the relation between the ureter and gynecologic disease are classic and pertinent today. Devascularization and ischemic necrosis of the wall of the terminal ureter has proved to be one of the more serious complications of this operation. Wertheim found this complication to be one of the more serious sequelae. In Meigs's clinic, there was a 12.5% significant ureteral complication rate, including an 8.5% incidence of ureterovaginal fistulas and a 4% incidence of ureteral stricture.

For many years, gynecologic surgeons have attempted to lower the rate of ureteral complications with special techniques. Novak, from Yugoslavia, reduced the incidence of ureteral fistulas to 2% after primary radical surgery by placing

TABLE 47.12

URINARY FISTULAS IN NONIRRADIATED PATIENTS TREATED BY RADICAL ABDOMINAL HYSTERECTOMY

Investigators	Number of patients	Ureteral fistula (%)	Vesical fistula (%)
Kaser et al., 1973	717	3.3	0.6
Park et al., 1973	156	0	0
Hoskins et al., 1976	224	1.3	0.45
Morley and Seski, 1976	208	4.8	0.5
Sail et al., 1979	349	2.0	0.8
Webb and Symmonds, 1979	423	1.4	0.7
Benedet et al., 1980	241	1.2	0.4
Langley et al., 1980	284	5.6	1.4
Lerner et al., 1980	108	0.9	0
Bostofte et al., 1981	479	3.8	1.4
Powell et al., 1981	135	1.5	0
Zander et al., 1981	1,092	1.4	0.3
Gitsch et al., 1984	187	0.5	NS
Shingleton, 1985	444	1.4	0.23
Artman et al., 1987	153	1.3	1.3
Larson et al., 1987	233	0.8	NS
Ralph et al., 1988	320	1.9	2.5
Lee et al., 1989	954	1.2	1.2
Kenter et al., 1989	213	3.3	3.3
Burghardt et al., 1989	325	2.5	2.8
Massi et al., 1993	228	0.9	0.4
TOTAL	7,473	2.0	0.9

NS, no sample.
From: Shingleton HM, Orr JW Jr, eds. *Cancer of the cervix*. Philadelphia: JB Lippincott, 1995, with permission.

the dissected pelvic ureter on the inside (peritoneal surface) of the pelvic peritoneum and by preserving the lateral mesentery to the terminal ureter. Green and coworkers suggested that the terminal ureter should be lifted out of the accumulated fluid in the retroperitoneal space by suturing it to the obliterated hypogastric artery. Ohkawa developed a procedure that attempted to elevate and isolate the ureter from the infected retroperitoneal fluid and also to develop a new blood supply to the terminal ureter by placing it in a peritoneal envelope from the pelvic brim to the bladder. Blythe and coworkers compared this technique with simple retroperitoneal suction drainage first advised by Symmonds and Pratt. They found that ureteral obstruction and ureterovaginal fistulas occurred twice as often and that the operative time was extended 45 minutes to 1 hour with the Ohkawa technique. More recently, Patsner and others have recommended the routine use of the omental J-flap (omentopexy) at the conclusion of radical hysterectomy and pelvic lymphadenectomy as an effective means of minimizing urinary tract fistulas.

Given a normal unirradiated ureter, we believe that the incidence of ureteral fistulas and permanent stenosis can be kept below 1% with meticulous intraoperative management of the ureter by a technically skillful operator who can prevent vascular trauma to the periureteral sheath and injury to the muscularis of the ureter.

Some temporary postoperative changes in ureteral function are an almost inevitable result of radical hysterectomy, as pointed out by Gal and Buchsbaum. Using special static and cinefluoroscopic IVP techniques, these authors found ureteral dilation in 87% of patients in the first week after surgery. In most cases, by 6 weeks after surgery, the dilation had regressed and the pyelograms had returned to normal. Peristalsis was altered in the distal ureter, which appeared as a rigid conduit during the first postoperative week. Peristalsis had returned 1 month later. These changes may explain the increased frequency of urinary tract infections after radical hysterectomy and the possibility of permanent ureteral stenosis if radiation, serious infection, or lymphocyst formation is superimposed.

Table 47.12 shows the frequency of urinary fistulas in a collected series of 7,473 nonirradiated patients treated by radical hysterectomy as compiled by Shingleton and Orr. The management of ureterovaginal fistulas is discussed in Chapter 39.

Retroperitoneal Spaces

Traditionally, a closed system of constant suction was placed in the retroperitoneal spaces on each side at the end of the procedure. These drains were thought to be effective for reducing the risk of pelvic infection, fistula, and lymphocyst formation. However, recent retrospective and prospective studies have demonstrated that the incidence of these complications is not decreased in patients who have retroperitoneal drains placed compared with those who do not. Furthermore, the drains may actually increase infectious complications.

Therefore, we do not routinely place drains in the retroperitoneal spaces.

Whether drains are placed or not, a small percentage of patients develop lymphocysts. A lymphocyst becomes obvious by symptoms and examination in the weeks after radical hysterectomy and pelvic lymphadenectomy. It may be small and asymptomatic. Most patients with large lymphocysts report lower abdominal discomfort on the same side with radiation to the back, hip, or thigh. Some edema of the lower extremity on the same side may be present. Evidence of ureteral obstruction may be found on IVP.

Small lymphocysts that do not cause ureteral obstruction can be observed without treatment. Large symptomatic lymphocysts and those that cause ureteral obstruction should be aspirated. CT-directed needle aspiration can be done with local anesthesia and repeated as needed. The fluid should be submitted for cytologic examination and culture. It is seldom necessary to perform open drainage of a lymphocyst. Mann and coworkers reported successful sclerosis of a recurrent lymphocyst by injection of a solution of tetracycline. Others have used povidone-iodine sclerosis.

Infection

Historically, patients were treated with antibiotics only if postoperative infection occurred. However, antibiotic prophylaxis has been associated with decreased febrile morbidity and decreased rates of serious infections in women undergoing radical abdominal hysterectomy. Furthermore, Orr and colleagues have demonstrated that a single dose of prophylactic antibiotic is as effective as a multiple-dose regimen and lessens patient exposure and cost. Thus, the prophylactic use of broad-spectrum antibiotics with both aerobic and anaerobic coverage has proved to be a useful addition to the surgical armamentarium.

We initiate single-agent broad-spectrum antibiotic coverage immediately before surgery. The administration of the drug is timed to allow adequate distribution before incision. During an extended operation, if the antibiotic given has a short half-life, a second dose is administered.

When secondary infection occurs despite the use of prophylactic antibiotics, the appropriate cultures are obtained, and bacteria-specific antibiotic therapy is chosen.

Venous Thrombosis and Pulmonary Embolus

Patients who undergo radical pelvic surgery fulfill the components of Virchow's triad and are at high risk for the development of venous thrombosis of the lower extremities and thromboembolic phenomena. Factors such as postoperative alteration of blood coagulation, trauma to the vein wall, and venous stasis are recognizable features of this type of surgery. In particular, pelvic lymphadenectomy invariably produces some trauma to the vein wall during the mobilization of the vessel and resection of the adherent lymphatic tissue. One of the biologic effects of radical surgery is the occurrence of local tissue necrosis during healing. This results in the release of tissue thromboplastin into the circulation, which contributes to venous thrombosis by acceleration of the clotting mechanism. The release of thromboplastin from the intima of the vein wall also provides an excellent nidus for the formation of fibrin, particularly in an area of the venous system where there is alteration in venous flow with stagnation of blood. This is frequently seen behind the valves of the veins of the lower extremity, where silent thrombosis is common. Prolonged immobilization of the lower extremities during a lengthy operative procedure is responsible for intraoperative venous stasis and clot formation. There is evidence to document that postoperative thrombosis of the lower extremity is a result of the surgical procedure in more than 50% of cases. The prevention, diagnosis, and treatment of venous thromboembolic events is extensively discussed in Chapter 9.

Efforts to decrease the frequency of this complication initially used prophylactic low-dose heparin, 5,000 U subcutaneously, three times daily, beginning 2 hours before surgery, and given every 8 hours thereafter for the subsequent 5 postoperative days. By using perioperative heparin alone, the incidence of deep vein thrombosis in a study by Kakkar and associates was decreased from 24.6% in the untreated control group to 7.7% in the heparin-treated group of surgical cases. More impressive was the observation in a subsequent study by the same investigators that 16 patients in the control group, as compared with only 2 patients in the heparin-treated group, were found on autopsy study to have died of acute, massive pulmonary embolism.

We use intermittent pneumatic calf compression beginning in the operating room and continuing whenever the patient is in bed until she is discharged. These compression boots are used not only in our patients undergoing radical hysterectomy but in all our patients undergoing major gynecologic surgical procedures. In very high-risk patients, we add prophylactic low-molecular-weight heparin.

Approximately 3% to 5% of patients with occult venous thrombosis of the lower extremities develop pulmonary emboli. Unfortunately, more than half of the cases of fatal pulmonary embolism occur in patients with silent venous thrombosis and without any clinical evidence of this complication before the acute pulmonary catastrophe. When evidence of venous thrombosis of the lower extremity is verified, full anticoagulation therapy is required for prevention of pulmonary embolism. However, the decision about how soon after radical surgery it is safe to fully anticoagulate a patient may be very difficult. In the rare case that a pulmonary embolus occurs after full anticoagulation has been achieved, it is necessary to prevent further migration of clot to the lung by either inferior vena cava ligation or the use of an intracaval Silastic umbrella. These complications are rare, but the sinister effects of thromboembolism must be carefully evaluated on a daily basis, and a high index of suspicion needs to be maintained in this high-risk group of patients.

Hemorrhage

Intraoperative and postoperative pelvic hemorrhages also are discussed in Chapter 19.

Intraoperative Bleeding

Despite the surgeon's adequate technical skills and careful dissection, serious hemorrhage can suddenly appear, especially during retroperitoneal dissections on the lateral pelvic sidewalls and around the sacrum. When it happens, it is hoped that the operative field will not be cluttered with clamps; exposure, lighting, and suction will be adequate; the patient's condition will be stable; and anesthesia will be sufficient to maintain good relaxation. If the bleeding vessel cannot be clamped quickly, the simplest and most effective method of controlling the bleeding is provided by pressure applied by the index finger of the gloved hand. With cessation of bleeding, the operative site can be cleared of accumulated blood by suctioning, exposure of the area can be improved, and the surgeon can gain a few moments to evaluate the situation and choose the best possible course of action. Arterial bleeding is easy to identify and control with clips, clamps, or ligatures. The difficult problem with hemorrhage in the pelvis comes from lacerations of deep pelvic veins that are fragile, tortuous, distended, sometimes hidden or retracted from view, and sometimes held open by attachment of the vein wall to surrounding tissue. Blood returning through the lacerated vein can come from multiple sources unavailable for ligation. Placing clamps or sutures blindly is dangerous and can even make the problem worse. Sometimes, digital pressure for at least 7 minutes is the most effective procedure to control venous bleeding. Sometimes, additional careful dissection in the area is required to free the vessel above and below the bleeding point to allow more precise clipping or suture ligation. A cardinal rule in dissecting in the pelvis is to avoid creating a deep hole, the bottom of which cannot be exposed in case a deep vein is lacerated. This is the reason that dissection of the pararectal space, for instance, should not be forced if it does not develop easily.

Whenever an extensive pelvic dissection is anticipated, preparations should be made in advance in case severe intraoperative bleeding is suddenly encountered. Adequate quantities of blood should be available to replace lost volume. More blood should be requested in advance of its need, if possible. A responsible member of the operating team or anesthesia team should be assigned the task of monitoring blood loss, blood replacement, and urine output. When bleeding is profuse, in the excitement of the moment, it is possible to lose count of the number of units of whole blood, blood components, crystalloids, and other fluids that have been given and how much blood has been lost. A dependable route for administering blood must be maintained. Without it, rapid blood replacement is not possible. If massive hemorrhage occurs or if even a possibility of its occurrence exists, a Swan-Ganz or similar catheter should be placed for better monitoring of physiologic functions and blood replacement. In extreme cases in which no other vessels are available for rapid intraoperative blood volume replacement, transfusions can be given under pressure directly into the common iliac artery, with the needle pointed in the direction of the heart.

The most frequent site of troublesome intraoperative bleeding during radical hysterectomy occurs from the pelvic floor veins in the dissection of the cardinal ligament and the hypogastric vessels. The collateral venous circulation of the hypogastric veins is an ever-present source of potential hemorrhage owing to difficulty in identification of these vessels as they course among muscle bundles and fascial planes on the pelvic floor. The pararectal fossa, cardinal ligament, and presacral and paraaortic areas are frequent sites of venous bleeding. Therefore, meticulous dissection is important to avoid these complications. When venous bleeding does occur, it can be difficult to identify the site of the lacerated vein. In these circumstances, it is important to use compression of the pelvic floor veins by either a sponge stick or finger held in place for several minutes, or to use an abdominal pack placed firmly against the site of bleeding for a similar length of time. In these cases, it is advisable to keep pressure on the vein until full control of the bleeding has been established, in the meantime dissecting in other places in the pelvis. Only when the wall of a major pelvic vein has been severely traumatized and has retracted out of the operative field is there a serious problem in reestablishing hemostasis. In contrast to arterial bleeding, hemorrhage from deep pelvic veins is seldom improved by hypogastric artery ligation, owing to the extensive collateral venous circulation to the pelvis from the lower extremity and vena cava. It occasionally is beneficial to ligate the anterior division of both hypogastric arteries to determine whether interruption of the major arterial blood supply to the pelvis can reduce the venous bleeding. When more extensive trauma to the wall of the external or common iliac vein has occurred, it is necessary to place vascular clamps above and below the area of injury and to repair the defect with fine vascular sutures.

Postoperative Hemorrhage

This condition is a rare complication of radical pelvic surgery. Because all of the blood supply to the pelvis has been skeletonized as part of the operative procedure, it is exceedingly rare for secondary hemorrhage to occur unless there has been uncontrolled bleeding at the completion of the operation. In these cases, the pelvis usually is packed with multiple gauze packs, with one end exteriorized through the open vagina. Tamponade of the pelvis by means of an umbrella or parachute gauze pack and external ring (see Chapter 19) has been advocated by some when there is persistent venous oozing in the pelvis at the completion of the operation. Pelvic packs should be advanced within 24 to 48 hours and removed shortly thereafter to avoid ascending infection from the vagina.

In certain cases of postoperative hemorrhage, selective embolization by invasive radiographic techniques can prevent reoperation.

Neuropathies

Nerve injury with radical hysterectomy was reviewed by Hoffman and coworkers, who reported its infrequent occurrence. The most important injuries are to the femoral, obturator, peroneal, sciatic, genitofemoral, ilioinguinal, iliohypogastric, lateral femoral cutaneous, and pudendal nerves. Awareness of the anatomic location of these nerves in the operative field, careful surgical technique in dissection and securing hemostasis, careful placement of self-retaining retractors, and careful positioning of patients in stirrups prevent most nerve injuries. Fortunately, most nerve injuries are not associated with serious or permanent disability.

However, injury to the obturator nerve can lead to difficulty with adduction of the lower extremity. Obturator nerve injuries are the most common neurologic injuries, and they occur most frequently during the removal of the obturator lymph nodes from the obturator fossa. If the nerve is transected, it should be repaired as described by Vasilev.

Rectum

Although much less frequent than bladder dysfunction, both acute and chronic rectal dysfunction may occur following radical hysterectomy. The rectal dysfunction is characterized by difficulty with defecation and loss of defecation urge. Barnes and associates reported that postoperative anorectal manometry studies were abnormal in all patients studied, suggesting disruption of the spinal reflex arcs controlling rectal emptying, possibly secondary to partial denervation of the rectum. Dietary fiber modifications and rectal stimulation with suppositories over several weeks or months are effective in addressing these problems.

ADJUVANT THERAPY IN CONJUNCTION WITH RADICAL SURGERY

Postoperative Pelvic Irradiation

External-beam radiation therapy is used in the postoperative period as an adjunct to radical abdominal hysterectomy and bilateral pelvic lymphadenectomy in selected cases. It is given selectively to patients considered to be at high risk for persistent disease based on operative findings and careful study of the surgical specimens. Previously, if only one or two lymph nodes show micrometastases, postoperative irradiation may not be given. However, when several nodes are involved, the risk of persistent disease is greater, and postoperative irradiation is usually given; it can be extended as high as T12 if proximal common iliac or paraaortic nodes are involved with metastatic disease. However, nodal metastasis is not the only risk factor for recurrence, and other local tumor-related factors may be indicators of high-risk tumors that may warrant adjuvant radiation therapy.

Sedlis and associates—in a GOG randomized trial of pelvic radiation therapy versus no further therapy in selected patients with stage IB carcinoma of the cervix with negative lymph nodes after radical hysterectomy and pelvic lymphadenectomy—evaluated the benefits and risk of adjuvant pelvic radiation therapy aimed at reducing recurrence in this group of patients. In this study, 277 eligible patients were entered with at least two of the following tumor-related risk factors: greater than one third stromal invasion, capillary lymphatic space involvement, or large clinical tumor diameter. Table 47.13 summarizes the eligibility criteria: Of the 277 patients, 137 were randomized to pelvic radiation therapy and 140 to no further treatment. Twenty-one (15%) in the radiation-therapy group and 39 (28%) in the no-further-treatment group had a cancer recurrence, 18 of whom were vaginal/pelvic in the radiation-therapy, with 27 in the no-further-treatment group. Life table analysis indicated a statistically significant (47%) reduction in risk of recurrence (relative risk $= 0.53$, $p = 0.008$, one-tail) among the radiation-therapy group, with recurrence-free rates at 2 years of 88% versus 79% for the radiation-therapy and no-further-treatment groups, respectively. Toxicity was generally acceptable, with severe or life-threatening urologic adverse effects occurring in four (3.1%) in the radiation-therapy group and two (1.4%) in the control group. The authors concluded that adjuvant pelvic radiation therapy following radical surgery in selected women with stage IB cervical cancer reduces the number of recurrences at the cost of 6% grade 3 and 4 adverse events versus 2.1% in the control group.

Many physicians use these data to identify node-negative patients with local risk factors following radical hysterectomy and pelvic lymphadenectomy to prescribe adjuvant radiation therapy.

If invasive cervical cancer is unexpectedly found after a simple hysterectomy has been done, postoperative pelvic radiation therapy is recommended. Survival rates in these patients have improved with the advent of megavoltage irradiation, as reported by Andras and coworkers, Davy and coworkers, and Papavasilou and coworkers. Heller and coworkers reported 35 patients with invasive cervical carcinoma discovered *in uteri* removed for benign conditions. All patients received postoperative radiation therapy; patients with presumed stage IB disease had a corrected 5-year survival rate of 78%, and those with presumed stage IIB disease had a corrected 5-year survival rate of 67%.

TABLE 47.13

ELIGIBILITY CRITERIA FOR RADIATION THERAPY AFTER RADICAL HYSTERECTOMY IN NODE-NEGATIVE PATIENTS

CLVI	Stromal invasion	Tumor size (cm)
+	Deep one third	Any
+	Middle one third	≥2
+	Superficial one third	≥5
−	Middle or deep one third	≥4

From: Sedlis A, Bundy BN, Rotman MZ, et al. A randomized trial of pelvic radiation therapy versus no further therapy in selected patients with stage IB carcinoma of the cervix after radical hysterectomy and pelvic lymph adenectomy: a Gynecologic Oncology Group Study. *Gynecol Oncol* 1999;73:177–183, with permission.

Postoperative Adjuvant Chemoradiation

After radical surgery in high-risk, early-stage cancer of the cervix, Peters and colleagues reported a phase III trial of adjunctive concurrent chemotherapy and pelvic radiation therapy compared with pelvic radiation therapy alone. In all, 243 assessable patients with clinical stage IA (2), IB, and IIA carcinoma of the cervix, initially treated with radical hysterectomy and pelvic lymphadenectomy, and who had positive pelvic lymph nodes and/or positive margins and/or microscopic involvement of the parametrium were evaluated. Patients were randomized to receive platinum-based chemoradiation or radiation only. Patients in each group received 49.3 Gy radiation therapy in 29 fractions to a standard pelvic field. Chemotherapy consisted of cisplatin 70 mg/m^2 and a 96-hour infusion of fluorouracil 1,000 mg/m^2 day every 3 weeks for four cycles, with the first and second cycles given concurrent to radiation therapy.

Progression-free and overall survival are significantly better in women receiving chemoradiation. The projected progression-free survival at 4 years was 63% with radiation therapy alone and 80% with chemoradiation. The projected overall survival rate at 4 years is 71% with adjuvant radiation therapy and 81% with adjuvant chemoradiation. However, grade 3 and 4 hematologic and gastrointestinal toxicity were more frequent in the chemoradiation group.

The authors concluded that the addition of concurrent cisplatin-based chemotherapy to radiation significantly improves progression-free and overall survival for high-risk, early-stage patients who undergo radical hysterectomy and pelvic lymphadenectomy for carcinoma of the cervix and are found to have positive pelvic lymph nodes and/or positive margins and/or microscopic involvement of the parametrium. Although the data from this study are compelling, use of this regimen should be undertaken only with understanding of the toxicities encountered.

The data from this randomized trial and the Sedlis trial currently provide practical guidelines for eligibility of patients for adjuvant chemoradiation following primary radical hysterectomy and pelvic lymphadenectomy.

Postoperative Extended-Field Irradiation or Chemoradiation

In selected cases, with multiple positive pelvic nodes, metastasis to common iliac nodes, or aortic nodal metastasis, patients are treated with pelvic and extended-field radiation to include the paraaortic lymph chain. To numerous previous studies can be added two studies from Japan that describe the results of paraaortic nodal irradiation in the treatment of cervical cancer. Inoue and Morita (1988) administered extended-field radiation after extensive surgery to 76 patients with aortic nodal metastases. Two patients developed severe intestinal complications that required reoperation. Postoperative extended-field irradiation improved the survival rate of patients with four or more positive nodes from 39% to 69%, as well as the survival rate of patients with unresectable nodes from 0% to 44%. The authors concluded that postoperative extended-field irradiation can control the distant spread by way of lymphatic routes and can increase the survival time of patients. In addition, 86 patients with cervical cancer were treated with paraaortic nodal irradiation by Horii and coworkers (1988). None of the patients developed severe complications from the treatment. Based on their selection criteria for paraaortic nodal irradiation, the authors found a statistically significant improvement in the prognosis for the treated group.

In 1987, Jones reported on a collected series of 332 patients with paraaortic lymph node metastases who received extended-field radiation. Twenty-six percent were long-term survivors. Although it is true that most patients with positive paraaortic lymph nodes die of their disease (probably because systemic disease is already present), it also is clear that some patients are curable with extended-field radiation or chemoradiation, especially if the nodes are involved with only microscopic disease. The surgeon must anticipate a 10% incidence of enteric complications even with doses limited to 5,000 cGy. Again, micrometastatic disease is more likely to be eradicated by a dose of paraaortic radiation that can be tolerated by the patient. Patients with paraaortic nodes that contain a large volume of tumor are not likely to be cured, even with a dose of paraaortic radiation that exceeds 5,000 cGy, unless the bulky nodes are excised before the irradiation.

Extended-field chemoradiation also may be used. The GOG reported on a multicenter trial of chemoradiation therapy to evaluate the feasibility of extended-field radiation therapy with 5-fluorouracil (5-FU) and cisplatin, and to determine the progression-free interval, overall survival, and recurrence sites in patients with biopsy-confirmed paraaortic node metastases from cervical carcinoma. In all, 86 evaluable stage I to IV patients with aortic metastases were reported. Radiation therapy doses were 4,500 cGy to paraaortic nodes, and concomitant chemotherapy consisted of 5-FU 1,000 mg/m^2 per day for 96 hours and cisplatin 50 mg/m^2 in weeks 1 and 5.

Initial sites of recurrence were pelvis alone, 20.9%; distant metastases only, 31.4%; and pelvic plus distant metastases, 10.5%. The 3-year overall and progression-free survival rates were 39% and 34%, respectively, for the entire group. Overall survival was stage I, 50%; stage II, 39%; and stage III/IVA, 38%.

GOG grade 3 and 4 acute toxicity was gastrointestinal (18.6%) and hematologic (15.1%). Late morbidity actuarial risk of 14% at 4 years primarily involved the rectum. The authors concluded that extended-field radiation therapy with 5-FU and cisplatin chemotherapy was feasible in a multicenter clinical trial, that a progression-free survival of 33% at 3 years suggests that a proportion of patients achieve control of advanced pelvic disease, and that not all patients with paraaortic metastases have systemic disease. This points to the importance of assessment and treatment of paraaortic metastases.

Adjuvant Postoperative Chemotherapy

Few studies of adjuvant chemotherapy following radical hysterectomy have been done. Wertheim et al. from Memorial Sloan-Kettering Cancer Center (MSKCC) in 1985 reported on a pilot study of adjuvant chemotherapy with cisplatin and bleomycin and pelvic radiation therapy in patients with cervical cancer at high risk of recurrence after radical hysterectomy and pelvic lymphadenectomy.

The continuous disease-free survival rate for the 32 evaluable patients was 84% at a median follow-up time of 28 months. In addition, the complications of this treatment program were not significantly greater than those observed in prior studies using the combination of surgery and adjuvant radiation therapy without chemotherapy. When compared with the results from historical controls in a large series of similar patients at the same institution, the results in this pilot study were encouraging and appeared to justify a randomized prospective clinical trial.

Two randomized trials have attempted to clarify the role of adjuvant postoperative chemotherapy. In 1992, Tattersall and colleagues reported a randomized trial comparing standard pelvic radiation therapy versus three cycles of combination chemotherapy with cisplatin, vinblastine, and bleomycin followed by pelvic radiation therapy. No difference in disease-free or overall survival emerged between the two treatment groups. Relapse was more common in patients with nonsquamous tumors (44%) and in those with metastases in several pelvic lymph nodes.

In 1996, Curtin et al. from MSKCC reported on a prospective multicenter randomized phase III trial of adjuvant chemotherapy versus chemotherapy plus pelvic irradiation for high-risk stage IB to IIA cervical cancer patients after radical hysterectomy and pelvic lymphadenectomy. The objective was to compare the clinical efficacy of adjuvant chemotherapy alone versus chemotherapy plus whole pelvic radiation therapy on recurrence rates, patterns of recurrence, and survival of patients after radical hysterectomy and pelvic lymphadenectomy for cervical cancer at high risk for recurrence.

Risk factors included deep cervical invasion, tumor >4 cm, parametrial involvement, nonsquamous histology, and/or pelvic lymph node metastasis. Chemotherapy consisted of cisplatin and bleomycin alone or in combination with whole-pelvic radiation therapy. Eighty-nine patients were entered, 19 had recurrences, and 16 died. Nine of 44 (20%) patients receiving chemotherapy alone recurred compared with 10 of 45 (22%) patients receiving chemotherapy and radiation ($p =$ NS). Patterns of recurrence were statistically similar between the two treatment arms, even among the subgroup of patients with more than three risk factors. In addition, both regimens were well tolerated. The authors concluded that recurrence rates and patterns of recurrences (local, regional, or distant) were not influenced by the addition of radiation therapy.

However, in view of the more recent randomized trial of adjuvant chemoradiation, most high-risk patients with nodal metastasis will probably be offered adjuvant platinum-based chemoradiation. Whether weekly cisplatin or other platinum-based regimes are the optimal choice remains to be determined.

FOLLOW-UP AFTER RADICAL SURGERY FOR CERVICAL CANCER

Despite carefully planned and executed radical surgery for early-stage cervical cancer, 5% to 20% of patients in various series show evidence of recurrent or persistent tumor. About half occur in the first year after treatment. Almost all occur within the first 3 years. Few occur later. Recurrences many years later are extremely rare after primary surgical treatment and are more likely to be seen in patients treated with primary radiation therapy.

Persistent or recurrent disease after primary radical surgery may represent incomplete resection of the central tumor undetected at operation or by the pathologist's examination of the surgical specimen. Microscopic metastatic involvement of lymph nodes may be undetected by incomplete pathologic examination or these nodes may be left behind by incomplete lymphadenectomy. Viable tumor cells in small numbers may escape by way of lymphatics or vascular channels to distant sites and overcome host resistance. Probably in as many as 10% of patients with persistent disease, recurrence may result from continued growth of unrecognized intraperitoneal spread of tumor.

After the immediate postoperative recovery is completed, patients are scheduled for regular follow-up examinations, which vary depending on circumstances. Patients who are at greater risk for recurrence should be followed especially closely at frequent intervals. These usually are the same patients who have been given postoperative therapy, including patients with metastatic disease in lymph nodes and/or parametria, close surgical margins, large-volume cervical tumors, deep cervical stromal invasion, and lymphatic and/or vascular channel involvement. The frequency of examination varies somewhat from patient to patient. Most patients are seen every 3 months during the first 3 years after primary treatment, every 6 months during the fourth and fifth years, and every 6 months to 1 year thereafter. Patients are instructed to report unusual signs or symptoms (e.g., vaginal bleeding or discharge, leg swelling, discomfort in the pelvis, discomfort or swelling in the legs, difficulty with urination or defecation, enlarged neck or groin nodes) at any time they appear. Krebs and coworkers, however, reported that 25% of their patients did not have symptoms when persistent disease was diagnosed. In the study reported by Larson and coworkers, 37% did not have symptoms.

A follow-up examination should include palpation of the neck for enlarged lymph nodes, abdominal and leg examination, and a speculum and bimanual rectovaginal pelvic examination. A vaginal cytology smear is performed with each visit. Computed tomography scan of the abdomen and pelvis, proctosigmoidoscopy, cystoscopy, IVP, and biopsy (needle, punch, or both) of any suspicious lesions may be required, depending on the patient's symptoms and examination findings. These special diagnostic procedures are not done routinely as part of postoperative follow-up surveillance in patients without symptoms. Positive findings are rare unless the patient has symptoms. For example, IVP seldom shows ureteral obstruction in a patient who does not also have symptoms of persistent pelvic sidewall disease and is, therefore, not routinely done at specific intervals. It is in the patient's best interest to have follow-up examinations done in the same center in which her treatment was administered. Findings at each visit must be compared with previous information all the way back to her original presentation.

Soisson and coworkers reported a comparison of symptoms, physical examination, and vaginal cytology in the detection of recurrent cervical carcinoma after radical hysterectomy. The study group consisted of 203 women with stage IB and IIA cervical cancer followed at the Duke University Medical Center. Thirty-one (15%) patients developed recurrence. For the detection of recurrent tumor, vaginal cytology had a sensitivity and specificity of 13% and 100%, pelvic or general physical examination 58% and 96%, and the presence of suspicious symptoms 71% and 95%, respectively. Ninety-four percent of all patients with recurrent tumor had at least one abnormal surveillance index. Another Duke study by Weber and associates found that MRI correctly demonstrated the extent of recurrence in 18 of 21 cases.

Regular pelvic examinations and vaginal cytology smears may detect a central pelvic recurrence early. This can be a great advantage. Just as it is important to detect the original cancer in the earliest stage possible so that the patient can have the best possible chance of cure, it also is important to detect persistent disease at the earliest possible moment, for the same reason. For example, Jobsen and coworkers reported on the use of radiation therapy to treat locoregional recurrence of carcinoma of the cervix after primary surgery. The overall 5-year survival rate was 44%. Response to radiation therapy was strongly correlated with tumor volume, providing additional supportive evidence to the idea that persistent disease should be diagnosed as early as possible and, it is hoped, when the volume of persistent tumor is still small and responsive.

Patients with recurrent or persistent cancer of the uterine cervix after initial radiation therapy can have radical surgery provided the disease is limited and judged to be surgically resectable. Usually some type of pelvic exenteration is required to resect the recurrent tumor with negative margins. In carefully selected patients with centrally recurrent disease, 5-year survivals of 40% to 60% have been reported. Pelvic exenteration is discussed in Chapter 50.

Tumor ulceration in the upper vagina can produce vaginal discharge and spotting, a palpable tumor mass, and induration and nodularity of tissue extending to the pelvic sidewalls. Pain may not be present unless the tumor involves nerve roots. Symptoms related to urination and defecation can result from pressure, infection, or tumor involvement of the bladder and rectum. Either unilateral or bilateral edema of the lower extremities or unilateral or bilateral hydroureter and hydronephrosis can be an ominous sign of persistent disease, but these also can be the result of a combination of the effects of radical surgery and postoperative irradiation. When initially diagnosed, recurrences are central in about one fourth of patients, involve the pelvic sidewall in one fourth, and involve distant sites in one fourth; the remaining one fourth of patients have multiple sites of involvement.

About 20% to 25% of patients with recurrence after primary radical surgery still can be cured. The best chance of cure is in patients who had no postoperative radiation treatment and no metastatic disease to pelvic lymph nodes and in whom persistent disease is limited to the central pelvis. A combination of total pelvic irradiation plus vaginal brachytherapy can be effective in controlling the disease. The addition of concurrent platinum-based chemotherapy also should be considered.

Chemotherapy can be given for palliation when there is evidence of unresectable persistent disease in the pelvis in patients who have already received postoperative pelvic radiation, or when there is metastatic disease in distant sites.

Because recurrence or persistence of cervical cancer after treatment is difficult but important to detect as early as possible, attempts have been made to use a serum marker that would monitor the course of the disease. Kato and Torigoe isolated a squamous cell carcinoma antigen from cervical carcinoma tissue. A squamous cell carcinoma antigen radioimmunoassay kit, developed by Abbott Laboratories (Abbott Park, Illinois), has been tested, but the role of this antigen in the follow-up of patients with cervical carcinoma is yet to be determined.

Although the early detection of persistence is the primary purpose of and justification for follow-up visits, assessment of urinary tract function also is important. Particular attention should be paid to bladder function and maintaining a satisfactory voiding pattern. Urinary tract infection should be diagnosed and treated promptly. If ureteral stenosis impairs renal function, early intervention can be successful in avoiding nephrectomy. This is more likely to be seen in patients who receive a combination of radical surgery and irradiation as primary treatment.

Rehabilitation of sexual function after surgical therapy for cervical cancer usually is easily done by the patient and her partner but is more difficult if the vagina and paravaginal tissues have received heavy doses of radiation or if the patient has lost ovarian function as a result of treatment. The gynecologic surgeon should inquire about sexual problems and should give advice and permission when needed. Counseling, including instruction in the technique of alternative means of sexual gratification, may be needed. If ovarian function has been lost as a result of treatment, estrogen replacement therapy should be provided, even though symptoms of hypoestrogenism are not present. If normal ovaries were conserved, their function should be monitored with periodic follicle-stimulating hormone and estrogen levels so that estrogen replacement can be discussed when ovaries cease functioning in future years. There may be other contraindications to estrogen replacement therapy in patients treated for cervical cancer, but a history of treatment for cervical cancer is not one of them.

And finally, patients who have been treated for cervical cancer are at greater risk for developing other primary cancers at different sites, especially if the treatment included irradiation. Detection of other primary cancers should be part of posttreatment follow-up. This subject has been studied by Hoffman and coworkers, Buchler, and others. Axelrod and coworkers reported that 3.9% of patients with invasive cervical cancer had second primaries. In 1987, Arneson and Kao reported that 61 new primary cancers were detected among 718 patients with invasive cervical cancer who had been studied from 1955 to 1979.

RADIATION THERAPY

Although radical hysterectomy is generally recommended for women with early-stage cervical cancer who can tolerate the surgery, women with Stage IIB or more advanced disease are usually treated with radiation therapy. Radiation is also appropriate for women who are poor surgical candidates because of medical conditions or age.

Inonizing radiation can destroy tumor and cure cancer effectively. Radiation therapy for cervical cancer is usually delivered by two techniques. *Intracavitary therapy* or *brachytherapy* is administered by placing a radioactive element—such as radium, cesium, or iridium—in close contact with the tumor. This produces a very effective, high-dose local treatment, but the dose rate delivered falls off very sharply as the distance away from the radioactive source increases. This is called "the inverse square law." The radiation dose delivered to a given point is equal to 1 divided by the square of the distance away from the radiation source (dose = 1/distance^2). Because of the rapid decrease in the dose, it is necessary to treat potential pelvic lymph node metastases and large primary cervical cancer with *external beam radiation*. This type of radiation was originally produced by modified diagnostic x-ray machines, but now special high-energy linear accelerators or betatrons are used. These machines are capable of delivering a uniform dose of radiation across the whole pelvis or even an extended field to include the paraaortic lymph nodes.

The use of radiation for the treatment of cervical cancer followed very shortly after the discovery of radium by Marie and Pierre Curie. Beginning in 1903, several methods of intracavitary therapy were developed, including the Stockholm technique from the Radiumhemmet; the Paris technique, designed at the Curie Foundation; and the Manchester technique from England. The Stockholm radium technique consisted of high-intensity central irradiation, repeated two or three times within 3 weeks, whereas the Paris technique used low-intensity central irradiation, continuously delivered over 1 week. The Manchester technique, derived from the Paris method, used low-dosage rates that required at least two separate intracervical insertions of radiation sources. Other radioactive elements, including cesium and iridium, have replaced radium in central brachytherapy for cervical cancer.

The traditional brachytherapy systems for cervical cancer have been low-dose-rate systems delivering 0.4 to 2 Gy per hour, and typical implants have been of 24- to 72-hour durations. More recently, high-dose-rate systems have been employed capable of delivering dose rates of more than 0.2 Gy per minute, thereby allowing treatments of only a few minutes' duration and adaptable to the outpatient—rather than the inpatient—setting. A comparison of 5-year survival rates of the two systems by clinical stage documents the usefulness of the newer system (Table 47.14).

With the establishment of the roentgen as a defined unit of radiation exposure (Stockholm, 1921), it became possible to measure the quantity of irradiation delivered to the tumor. Although many clinicians are most familiar with the dosing measure of rads, modern therapy is calculated in grays (Gy) [1 Gy = 100 rads; 1 centigray (1 cGy) = 1 rad]. High-energy, external-beam radiation sources, ranging to 25 mV for the betatron and linear accelerator, have significantly reduced the complication rates after radiation therapy and have improved the cure rates. An intracavitary pelvic dosage derived from the gamma rays of radium or cesium is complementary to the megavoltage external-beam irradiation to ensure tumoricidal dosages to the cervix, broad ligaments, and lateral pelvic walls. Extended fields of external radiation can deliver therapy to common iliac and aortic nodal tissues.

The balance between enough radiation to destroy the tumor and too much radiation (which results in damage to adjacent normal tissues such as the bladder, vagina, or rectum) is sometimes difficult to achieve. It requires using the correct combination of brachytherapy with external radiation therapy. Treatment planning has been enormously improved in recent years because of the integration of imaging techniques (such as CT scanners) with computer programs that can calculate the dose to the tumor volume and adjacent normal tissues, which helps the radiation oncologist maximize the tumor dose while minimizing the damage to nearby organs.

Survival rates of irradiation and primary surgery can be compared by analyzing the reports from patients treated for stage I cervical cancer. Patients treated by irradiation have an average 5-year survival rate essentially identical to the survival rate for those who undergo radical surgery (Table 47.15).

In the United States, radical hysterectomy generally is recommended for women with stage IA2 and IB1 cervical cancer who are good operative risks, especially if they are

TABLE 47.14

5-YEAR SURVIVAL RATES OF PATIENTS WITH STAGE I CANCER OF THE CERVIX BY TREATMENT MODALITY

Investigators	Number of patients	5-Year survival rate (%)
SURGERY		
Morley and Seski, 1976	149	91.3
Zander et al., 1981	747	84.5
Noguchi, 1987	191	85.3
Barber, 1988	273	78.8
Carenza, 1988	105	85.7
Fuller et al., 1989	285	86.0
Kentler, 1989	178	87.0
Lee, 1989	237	86.1
Monaghan, 1990	494	83.0
Hopkins, 1991	213	89.0
Alvarez, 1991	401	85.0
Burghardt, 1992	443	83.4
Massi, 1993	211	75.8
TOTAL	3,526	84.2
RADIOTHERAPY		
Madowski et al., 1962	442	81.3
Kottmeier, 1964	611	89.5
Crawford et al., 1965	63	46.0
Masubuchi et al., 1969	152	88.2
Marcial, 1970	41	87.0
Neinminen and Pollanen, 1970	77	70.0
Fletcher, 1971	549	91.5
Newton, 1975	61	74.0
Einhorn, 1975	60	88.0
Petersson, 1987	160	76.9
TOTAL	2,196	85.1

premenopausal. Women with larger tumors and those who are at risk for surgical complications generally are referred for radiation therapy.

SUMMARY

Many improvements have been made in the operative technique of the radical hysterectomy and lymphadenectomy since its original description. The incidence of complications after this procedure has decreased during the past 75 years, and the survival rates have increased. The operation has achieved its peak of clinical usefulness during this period and is now considered to be the principal method of treatment of early invasive carcinoma of the cervix. Among the better surgical institutions, the meticulous execution of this operative procedure has reduced the incidence of complications to an acceptable and infrequent occurrence. In medical centers in which the operation is performed well, the 5-year cure rate for stage IB1 carcinoma of the cervix is more than 90%. Newer laparoscopic approaches are promising, with comparable cure rates and the potential to retain fertility in carefully selected patients. Radical vaginal trachelectomy has proven safe and effective for selected patients with small tumors who wish to preserve their fertility.

Comparative studies with primary radiation therapy have demonstrated an equal cure rate with primary radical surgery

TABLE 47.15

HIGH DOSE RATE (HDR) VERSUS LOW-DOSE-RATE (LDR) INTRACAVITARY BRACHYTHERAPY FOR CARCINOMA OF THE CERVIX, 1979 TO 1981

Stage	Number of patients (HDR/LDR)	5-year survival rate (%) HDR	LDR
I	160/422	76.9	71.6
II	358/796	58.1	54.4
III	386/588	38.1	38.4
IV	66/50	15.2	10. 0

From: Annual report on the results of treatment in gynecological cancer. In: Pettersson F, ed. *Twentieth volume statements of results obtained in patients treated in 1979–81, including 5-year survival up to 1986*. Stockholm: International Federation of Gynecology and Obstetrics, 1987:52, with permission.

in the treatment of early-stage disease. However, the complications of irradiation are far more difficult to manage than are those of primary surgery. In young women, when preservation of ovarian function is important, primary surgery is a preferable choice of treatment.

The major limiting factor in the long-term surgical cure of cervical cancer is related to the spread of the disease at the time of initiation of treatment. Historically, in cases in which pelvic lymph nodes were positive for metastatic tumor, the 5-year cure rate was reduced to about 60%. However, numerous recently reported prospective, randomized trials have demonstrated the benefit of concurrent chemotherapy and radiation therapy in various settings. In the management of high-risk patients after radical hysterectomy and pelvic lymphadenectomy, including those with positive nodes, the reported 4-year disease-free survival is 80%.

It is important to understand that it is the individual surgical expertise that offers the highest cure rate and lowest incidence of complications to the patient with invasive carcinoma of the cervix. One of the greatest errors in clinical judgment is made by the gynecologist who attempts a radical hysterectomy and pelvic lymph node dissection without adequate surgical training and experience. Unless the pelvic surgeon is performing this type of surgery regularly in a well-staffed medical center with trained assistants, he or she would be well advised to refer the patient to an established cancer center. From the patient's point of view, the initial treatment, whether primary surgery or irradiation, provides the best chance for long-term cure of this disease. It would be to her advantage to have the treatment conducted in the most expert hands because secondary treatment for recurrent disease offers only limited potential long-term cure.

The gynecologic surgeon who becomes thoroughly familiar with the pathology and natural history of cervical cancer, who appreciates the history of the development of radical hysterectomy and pelvic lymphadenectomy as primary treatment of the disease, and who then thoroughly masters the technical details of performing the operation can feel enormous pride in his or her achievement because there is no greater challenge in gynecologic surgery and no greater personal satisfaction than that which comes to those who are able to perform the operation correctly and save a woman from the intense suffering and undignified death that cervical cancer can cause.

BEST SURGICAL PRACTICES

- Invasive cancer of the cervix is predominantly of squamous histology. Adenocarcinoma is increasingly common and now accounts for up to 20% of the lesions in some series. Adenosquamous, clear-cell, and small-cell neuroendocrine histology are seen infrequently. Tumor grade is not prognostically significant.
- Although most women with early-stage cancer are asymptomatic, patients with larger tumors may have vaginal discharge, vaginal bleeding (especially postcoital bleeding), and eventually pelvic or low-back or hip pain. Leg edema and ureteral obstruction are signs of advanced disease.
- A careful and thorough staging workup should be done after a diagnosis is made. This evaluation of the extent of disease is very important for treatment planning and prognosis. FIGO staging should be used, but the metastatic workup should not be limited by FIGO's restrictive guidelines.
- Patients with microinvasion (stage IA1) are generally treated with cone biopsy or simple hysterectomy. Patients with stage IA2 disease should be treated by radical hysterectomy with pelvic lymphadenectomy. Most of these patients can be adequately treated by a modified radical hysterectomy (class II), but women with larger tumors and lymph-vascular space involvement may benefit from a traditional (class III) radical hysterectomy.
- In the United States, most women with stage IB1 and stage IIA cervical cancer are treated with radical surgery. Women with larger, higher-stage tumors are usually treated with radiation therapy plus adjuvant chemotherapy. Women who are poor surgical risks are also usually treated with radiation ± chemotherapy. The main advantage of surgery compared with radiation is the preservation of ovarian function, which is most advantageous in younger patients. There is also less risk of upper vaginal stenosis and dysparunia following surgery. Bladder and rectal dysfunction and, rarely, fistulas occur with both surgery and radiation. Surgical complications tend to occur in the perioperative period, whereas complications and side effects from radiation are often delayed and long lasting.
- Radical surgery for cervical cancer requires training, experience, and good ancillary support. This means well-trained operating room personnel, surgical assistants, and anesthesia staff—as well as adequate radiology, intensive care, and consulting physicians—need to be a regular part of the patient care team.
- In a radical hysterectomy for stage IB cervical cancer, we do not routinely do a paraaortic lymphadenectomy, but any palpable nodes are removed and sent for frozen section. The surgical procedure is abandoned if aortic lymph node metastases are identified.
- Radical hysterectomy for cervical cancer can be done using the classic abdominal approach, a vaginal approach (Schauta), or a total laparoscopic approach. There are advantages and disadvantages to each of these techniques, but overall survival appears to be similar. The basic technique is the same.
- In recent years, a fertility-sparing radical trachelectomy with laparoscopic lymphadenectomy has been described by Dargent. Women with stage IA and early IB1 tumors who wish to preserve fertility have been treated successfully, and the cure rates appear to be comparable to more radical surgery. More that 200 successful pregnancies following Dargent's operation have been reported.

Bibliography

Abu-Rustum NR, Hoskins WJ. Radical abdominal hysterectomy. *Surg Clin North Am* 2001;81(4):815.

Abu-Rustum NR, Lee S, Correa A, et al. Compliance with and acute hematologic toxic effects of chemoradiation in indigent women with cervical cancer. *Gynecol Oncol* 2001;81(1):88.

Abu-Rustum NR, Lee S, Massad LS. Screening for HIV infection in indigent women with newly diagnosed cervical cancer. *J Acquir Immune Defic Syndr* 2001;27(1):95.

Abu-Rustum NR, Lee S, Massad LS. Topotecan for recurrent cervical cancer after platinum-based therapy. *Int J Gynecol Cancer* 2000;10(4):285.

Abu-Rustum NR, Rajbhandari D, Glusman S, et al. Acute lower extremity paralysis following radiation therapy for cervical cancer. *Gynecol Oncol* 1999;75(1):152.

Abu-Rustum NR, Sonoda Y, Black D, et al. Fertility-sparing radical abdominal trachelectomy for cervical carcinoma: technique and review of the literature. *Gynecol Oncol* 2006;103:1083.

Abu-Rustum NR, Su W, Levine DA, et al. Pediatric radical abdominal trachelectomy for cervical clear cell carcinoma: a novel surgical approach. *Gynecol Oncol* 2005;97:296.

Ahrens CA, Tschoke S. Lvmphknotenbefunde nach Wertheim Meigscher operation. *Geburtshilfe Frauenheilkd* 1961;21:219.

Albores-Saavedra J, Gersell D, Gilks CB, et al. Terminology of endocrine tumors of the uterine cervix: results of a workshop sponsored by the College of American Pathologists and the National Cancer Institute. *Arch Pathol Lab Med* 1997;121:34.

Alexander-Sefre F, Chee N, Spencer C, et al. Surgical morbidity associated with radical trachelectomy and radical hysterectomy. *Gynecol Oncol* 2006;101:450.

Altgassen C, Possover M, Krause N, et al. Establishing a new technique of laparoscopic pelvic and paraaortic lymphadenectomy. *Obstet Gynecol* 2000;95(3):348.

Alvarez RD, Potter ME, Soong S-J, et al. Rationale for using pathologic tumor dimensions and nodal status to sub-classify treated stage IB cervical cancer patients. *Gynecol Oncol* 1991;43:108.

Amendola MA, Hricak H, Mitchell DG, et al. Utilization of diagnostic studies in the pretreatment evaluation of invasive cervical cancer in the United States: results of intergroup protocol ACRIN 6651/GOG 183. *J Clin Oncol* 2005;23(30):7454.

Anderson B, LaPolla J, Turner D, et al. Ovarian transposition in cervical cancer. *Gynecol Oncol* 1993;40:206.

Andras EJ, Hetcher EH, Rutledge F: Radiotherapy of carcinoma of the cervix following simple hysterectomy. *Am J Obstet Gynecol* 1973;115(5): 647–655.

Angel C, DuBeshter B, Lin JY. Clinical presentation and management of stage 1 cervical adenocarcinoma: a 25-year experience. *Gynecol Oncol* 1992;44: 71.

Bader AA, Tamussino KF, Moinfar F, et al. Isolated recurrence at the residual uterine cervix after abdominal radical trachelectomy for early cervical cancer. *Gynecol Oncol* 2005;99:785.

Balega J, Michael H, Hurteau JA, et al. The risk of nodal metastasis in early adenocarcinoma of the uterine cervix. *Gynecol Oncol* 2000;76:235(abstr).

Bandy LC, Clarke-Pearson DL, Soper JT, et al. Long-term effects on bladder function of radical hysterectomy with and without postoperative radiation. *Gynecol Oncol* 1987;26:160.

Barber HRK. Cervical cancer: pelvic and paraaortic lymph nodes sampling and its consequences. *Baillieres Clin Obstet Gynaecol* 1988;2:768.

Barnes W, Waggoner S, Delgado G, et al. Manometric characterization of rectal dysfunction following radical hysterectomy. *Gynecol Oncol* 1991;42:116.

Behbakht K, Abu-Rustum NR, Lee S, et al. Characteristics and survival of cervical cancer patients managed at adjacent urban public and university medical centers. *Gynecol Oncol* 2001;81(1):40.

Bellomi M, Bonomo G, Landoni F, et al. Accuracy of computed tomography and magnetic resonance imaging in the detection of lymph node involvement in cervix carcinoma. *Eur Radiol* 2005;15:2469.

Benedet JL, Anderson GH. Stage IA carcinoma of the cervix revisited. *Obstet Gynecol* 1996;87:1052.

Benedet JL, Odicino F, Maisonneuve P, et al. Carcinoma of the cervix uteri. *Int J Gynaecol Obstet* 2003;83:41.

Berman ML, Keys H, Creasman W, et al. Survival and patterns of recurrence in cervical cancer metastatic to periaortic lymph nodes: a Gynecologic Oncology Group study. *Gynecol Oncol* 1984;19:8.

Bernardini M, Barrett J, Seaward G, et al. Pregnancy outcome in patients post radical trachelectomy. *Am J Obstet Gynecol* 2003;189:1378.

Bleker OP, Ketting BW, van Wayjen-Eecen B, et al. The significance of microscopic involvement of the parametrium and or pelvic lymph nodes in cervical cancer stages IB and IIA. *Gynecol Oncol* 1983;6:56.

Blythe JG, Hodel KA, Wahl TP. A comparison between peritoneal sheathing of the ureters (Ohkawa technique) and retroperitoneal pelvic suction drainage in the prevention of ureteral damage during radical abdominal hysterectomy. *Gynecol Oncol* 1988;30:222.

Bonney V. The results of 500 cases of Wertheim's operation for carcinoma of the cervix. *J Obstet Gynaecol Br Emp* 1941;48:421.

Brewer CA, Chan J, Kurosaki T, et al. Radical hysterectomy with the endoscopic stapler. *Gynecol Oncol* 1998;71:50.

Broders AC. The grading of carcinoma. *Minn Med* 1925;8:726.

Buchsbaum HJ. Extrapelvic lymph node metastases in cervical carcinoma. *Am J Obstet Gynecol* 1979;133:814.

Buller RE, Tamir IL, DiSaia PJ, et al. Early evaluation of the urinary tract following radical hysterectomy: structure and function relationships. *Obstet Gynecol* 1991;78:840.

Burghardt E, Baltzer J, Tulusan AH, et al. Results of surgical treatment of 1028 cervical cancers studied with volumetry. *Cancer* 1992;70:648.

Burghardt E, Pickel H, Haas J, et al. Prognostic factors and operative treatment of stages IB to IIB cervical cancer. *Am J Obstet Gynecol* 1987;156:988.

Carter J, Rowland K, Chi D, et al. Gynecologic cancer treatment and the impact of cancer-related infertility. *Gynecol Oncol* 2005;97:90.

Chamberlin DH, Hopkins MP, Roberts JA, et al. The effects of early removal of indwelling urinary catheter after radical hysterectomy. *Gynecol Oncol* 1991;43:98.

Chambers SK, Chambers JT, Holm C, et al. Sequelae of lateral ovarian transposition in unirradiated cervical cancer patients. *Gynecol Oncol* 1990;39:155.

Chapman JA, Mannel RS, DiSaia PJ, et al. Surgical treatment of unexpected invasive cervical cancer found at total hysterectomy. *Obstet Gynecol* 1992;80:931.

Chen MD, Spirtos NM, Lim PC. Laparoscopic radical hysterectomy. *CME J Gynecol Oncol* 2001;1:110.

Chi DS. Laparoscopy in gynecologic malignancies. *Oncology (Huntington)* 1999;13(6):773.

Childers JM, Hatch K, Surwit EA. The role of laparoscopic lymphadenectomy in the management of cervical carcinoma. *Gynecol Oncol* 1992;47(1):38.

Chu KK, Chang SD, Chen FP, et al. Laparoscopic surgical staging in cervical cancer-preliminary experience among Chinese. *Gynecol Oncol* 1997;64(1):49.

Cibula D, Ungar L, Svarovsky J, et al. Abdominal radical trachelectomy-technique and experience. *Ceska Gynekol* 2005;70:117.

Clark JG. A more radical method of performing hysterectomy for cancer of the uterus. *Bull Johns Hopkins Hosp* 1895;6:120.

Clarke-Pearson DL, Jelovsek FR, Creasman WT. Thromboembolism complicating surgery for cervical and uterine malignancy: incidence, risk factors, and prophylaxis. *Obstet Gynecol* 1983;61:87.

Clarke-Pearson DL, Synan IS, Dodge R, et al. A randomized trial of low-dose heparin and intermittent pneumatic calf compression for the prevention of deep venous thrombosis after gynecologic oncology surgery. *Am J Obstet Gynecol* 1993;168:1146.

Cohn DE, Swisher EM, Herzog TJ, et al. Radical hysterectomy for cervical cancer in obese women. *Obstet Gynecol* 2000;96:727.

Corney RH, Crowther ME, Everett H, et al. Psychosexual dysfunction in women with gynaecological cancer following radical pelvic surgery. *BJOG* 1993;100:73.

Covens A. Preserving fertility in early cervical cancer with radical trachelectomy. *Contemp Obstet Gynecol* 2003;48:46.

Covens A, Shaw P, Murphy J, et al. Is radical trachelectomy a safe alternative to radical hysterectomy for patients with stage IA-B carcinoma of the cervix? *Cancer* 1999;86(11):2273.

Creasman WT. New gynecologic cancer staging [editorial]. *Gynecol Oncol* 1995;58:157.

Creasman WT, Zaino RJ, Major FJ, et al. Early invasive carcinoma of the cervix (3 to 5 mm invasion): risk factors and prognosis. A Gynecologic Oncology Group study. *Am J Obstet Gynecol* 1998;178:62.

Currie JL. *A cosmetically-pleasing transverse incision for pelvic surgery.* ACOG Film Library, 1996.

Curtin JP, Hoskins WJ, Venkatraman ES, et al. Adjuvant chemotherapy versus chemotherapy plus pelvic irradiation for high-risk cervical cancer patients after radical hysterectomy and pelvic lymphadenectomy (RH-PLND): a randomized phase III trial. *Gynecol Oncol* 1996;61(1):3.

Dargent D. A new future for Schauta's operation through pre-surgical retroperitoneal pelviscopy. *Eur J Gynecol Oncol* 1987;8:292.

Dargent D. Using radical trachelectomy to preserve fertility in early invasive cervical cancer. *Contemp Ob/Gyn* 2000;45:23.

Dargent D, Ansquer Y, Mathevet P. Technical development and results of left extraperitoneal laparoscopic paraaortic lymphadenectomy for cervical cancer. *Gynecol Oncol* 2000;77(1):87.

Dargent D, Brun JL, Roy M. La trachctomie rgie (T.E.). Une alternative hysterectomy radicale dans le traitement des cancers infiltrants doppler la face externe du col utn. *J Obstet Gynecol* 1994;2:292.

Dargent D, Brun JL, Roy M, et al. Pregnancies following radical trachelectomy for invasive cervical cancer. *Gynecol Oncol* 1994;52:105(abstr).

Dargent D, Franzosi F, Ansquer Y, et al. Extended trachelectomy relapse: plea for patient involvement in the medical decision. *Bull Cancer* 2002;89:1027.

Dargent D, Martin X, Sacchetoni A, et al. Laparoscopic vaginal radical trachelectomy: a treatment to preserve the fertility of cervical carcinoma patients. *Cancer* 2000;88(8):1877.

Dargent D, Mathevet P. Schauta's vaginal hysterectomy combined with laparoscopic lymphadenectomy. *Baillieres Clin Obstet Gynaecol* 1995;9(4):691.

Dary M, Bentzen H, Jahren R. Simple hysterectomy in the presence of invasive cervical cancer. *Acta Obstet Gynecol Scand* 1977;56(2):105–108.

Delgado G, Bundy BN, Zaino R, et al. Prospective surgical-pathological study of disease-free interval in patients with stage IB squamous cell carcinoma of the cervix: a Gynecologic Oncology Group study. *Gynecol Oncol* 1990;38:352.

Del Priore G, Ungar L, Richard Smith J, Heller PB. Regarding "First case of a centropelvic recurrence after radical trachelectomy: literature review and implications for the preoperative selection of patients" [Letter]. *Gynecol Oncol* 2004;95:414.

Downey GO, Potish RA, Adcock LL, et al. Pretreatment surgical staging in cervical carcinoma: therapeutic efficacy of pelvic lymph node resection. *Am J Obstet Gynecol* 1989;160:1055.

Drescher CW, Hopkins MP, Roberts JA. Comparison of the pattern of metastatic spread of squamous cell cancer and adenocarcinoma of the uterine cervix. *Gynecol Oncol* 1989;33:340.

Eifel PJ, Burke TW, Morris M, et al. Adenocarcinoma as an independent risk factor for disease recurrence in patients with stage IB cervical carcinoma. *Gynecol Oncol* 1995;59:38.

Elliott P, Coppleson M, Russell P, et al. Early invasive (FIGO stage IA) carcinoma of the uterine cervix: a clinico-pathologic study of 475 cases. *Int J Gynecol Cancer* 2000;10:42.

Ellsworth LR, Allen HH, Nisker JA. Ovarian function after radical hysterectomy for stage IB carcinoma of the cervix. *Am J Obstet Gynecol* 1983;145:185.

Estape R, Angioli R, Wagman F, et al. Significance of intraperitoneal cytology in patients undergoing radical hysterectomy. *Gynecol Oncol* 1998;68:169.

Fanning J, Kraus K. Surgical stapling technique for radical hysterectomy: survival, recurrence, and late complications. *Gynecol Oncol* 2000;79:281.

Fernando JN, Moskovic E, Fryatt I, et al. Is there a role for lymphography in the management of early-stage carcinoma of the cervix? *Br J Radiol* 1994;67:1052.

Fowler JM, Carter JR, Carlson JW, et al. Lymph node yield from laparoscopic lymphadenectomy in cervical cancer: a comparative study. *Gynecol Oncol* 1993;51(2):187.

Franchi M, Ghezzi F, Zanaboni F, et al. Nonclosure of peritoneum at radical abdominal hysterectomy and pelvic node dissection: a randomized study. *Obstet Gynecol* 1997;90:622.

Freund WA. Method of complete removal of the uterus. *Am J Obstet Gynecol* 1879;7:200.

Fuchtner C, Manetta A, Walker JL, et al. Radical hysterectomy in the elderly patient: analysis of morbidity. *Am J Obstet Gynecol* 1992;166:593.

Fuller AF Jr, Elliott N, Kosloff C, et al. Determinants of increased risk for recurrence in patients undergoing radical hysterectomy for stage IB and IIA carcinoma of the cervix. *Gynecol Oncol* 1989;33:34.

Gallion HH, van Nagell JR Jr, Donaldson ES, et al. Combined radiation therapy and extrafascial hysterectomy in the treatment of stage IB barrel-shaped cervical cancer. *Cancer* 1985;56:262.

Gallup DG, Jordan GH, Talledo OE. Extraperitoneal lymph node dissections with use of a midline incision on patients with female genital cancer. *Am J Obstet Gynecol* 1986;155:559.

Geisler JP, Geisler HE. Radical hysterectomy in the elderly female: a comparison to patients age 50 or younger. *Gynecol Oncol* 2001;80:258.

Gilks CB, Young RH, Gersell D, et al. Large cell neuroendocrine carcinoma of the uterine cervix: a clinicopathologic study of 12 cases. *Am J Surg Pathol* 1997;21:905.

Gilliland JD, Spies JB, Brown SB, et al. Lymphoceles: percutaneous treatment with povidone-iodine sclerosis. *Radiology* 1989;171:227.

Girardi F, Lichtenegger W, Tamussino K, et al. The importance of parametrial lymph nodes in the treatment of cervical cancer. *Gynecol Oncol* 1989;34:206.

Green TH Jr, Meigs JV, Ulfelder H, et al. Urologic complications of radical Wertheim hysterectomy: incidence, etiology, management and prevention. *Obstet Gynecol* 1962;20:293.

Greer BE, Easterling TR, McLennan DA, et al. Fetal and maternal considerations in the management of stage I-B cervical cancer during pregnancy. *Gynecol Oncol* 1989;34:61.

Greer BE, Figge DC, Tamimi HK, et al. Stage IB adenocarcinoma of the cervix treated by radical hysterectomy and pelvic lymph node dissection. *Am J Obstet Gynecol* 1989;160:1509.

Griffenberg L, Morris M, Atkinson N, et al. The effect of dietary fiber on bowel function following radical hysterectomy. *Gynecol Oncol* 1997;66:417.

Hatch KD, Hallum AV 3rd, Nour M. New surgical approaches to treatment of cervical cancer. *J Natl Cancer Inst Monogr* 1996;21:71.

Heller PB, Barnhill DR, Mayer AR, et al. Cervical carcinoma found incidentally in a uterus removed for benign indications. *Obstet Gynecol* 1986;67(2): 187–190.

Hertel H, Kohler C, Hillemanns P, et al. Radical vaginal trachelectomy (RVT) combined with laparoscopic pelvic lymphadenectomy: prospective multicenter study of 100 patients with early cervical cancer. *Gynecol Oncol* 2006;103:506–511.

Hoffman MS, Parsons M, Gunasekaran S, et al. Distal external iliac lymph nodes in early cervical cancer. *Obstet Gynecol* 1999;94:391.

Hoffman MS, Roberts WS, Cavanagh D. Neuropathies associated with radical pelvic surgery for gynecologic cancer. *Gynecol Oncol* 1988;31:462.

Hoffman MS, Roberts WS, Cavanagh D. Second pelvic malignancies following radiation therapy for cervical cancer. *Obstet Gynecol Surv* 1985;40:611.

Hopkins MP, Morley GW. The prognosis and management of cervical cancer associated with pregnancy. *Obstet Gynecol* 1992;80:9.

Hopkins MP, Schmidt RW, Roberts JA, et al. The prognosis and treatment of stage adenocarcinoma of the cervix. *Obstet Gynecol* 1988;72:915.

Horii T, Mitsumoto T, Noda K. Significance of paraaortic node irradiation in the treatment of cervical cancer. *Gynecol Oncol* 1988;31:371.

Hoskins WJ. Prognostic factors for risk of recurrence in stages IB and IIA cervical cancer. *Baillieres Clin Obstet Gynecol* 1988;2:817.

Hsieh YY, Lin WC, Chang CC, et al. Laparoscopic radical hysterectomy with low paraaortic, subaortic and pelvic lymphadenectomy: results of short-term follow-up. *J Reprod Med* 1998;43(6):528.

Jackson KS, Das N, Naik R, et al. Laparoscopically assisted radical vaginal hysterectomy vs. radical abdominal hysterectomy for cervical cancer: a match controlled study. *Gynecol Oncol* 2004;95:655.

Jensen JK, Lucci JA, DiSaia PH, et al. To drain or not to drain: a retrospective study of closed-suction drainage following radical hysterectomy with pelvic lymphadenectomy. *Gynecol Oncol* 1993;512:46.

Jones HW, Jones GES. Panhysterectomy versus irradiation in early cancer of the cervix. *JAMA* 1943;122:930.

Jones WB. Surgical approaches for advanced or recurrent cancer of the cervix. *Cancer* 1987;60:2094.

Kadar N. Laparoscopic vaginal radical hysterectomy: an operative technique and its evolution. *Gynaecol Endosc* 1994;3:109.

Keys HM, Bundy BN, Stehman FB, et al. Cisplatin, radiation, and adjuvant hysterectomy compared with radiation and adjuvant hysterectomy for bulky stage IB cervical carcinoma. *N Engl J Med* 1999;340:1154.

Kilgore LC, Soong S-J, Gore H, et al. Analysis of prognostic features in adenocarcinoma of the cervix. *Gynecol Oncol* 1988;31:137.

Kim DH, Moon JS. Laparoscopic radical hysterectomy with pelvic lymphadenectomy for early, invasive cervical carcinoma. *J Am Assoc Gynecol Laparosc* 1998;5(4):411.

Kim SH, Choi BI, Han JK, et al. Preoperative staging of uterine cervical carcinoma: comparison of CT and MR imaging in 99 patients. *J Comput Assist Tomogr* 1993;17:633.

Kinney WK, Egorshin EV, Podratz KC. Wertheim hysterectomy in the geriatric population. *Gynecol Oncol* 1988;31:227.

Klemm P, Tozzi R, Kohler C, et al. Does radical trachelectomy influence uterine blood supply? *Gynecol Oncol* 2005;96:283.

Kolstad P. Follow-up study of 232 patients with stage Ia1 and 411 patients with stage Ia2 squamous cell carcinoma of the cervix (microinvasive carcinoma). *Gynecol Oncol* 1989;33:265.

Kurman RJ, Norris HJ, Wilkinson F. *Atlas of tumor pathology, tumors of the cervix, vagina, and vulva,* third series, fascicle 4. Washington, DC: Armed Forces Institute of Pathology, 1992.

Kuwabara Y, Suzuki M, Hashimoto M, et al. New method to prevent bladder dysfunction after radical hysterectomy for uterine cervical cancer. *J Obstet Gynaecol Res* 2000;26:1.

Lagasse LD, Creasman WT, Shingleton HM, et al. Results and complications of operative staging in cervical cancer: experience of the Gynecologic Oncology Group. *Gynecol Oncol* 1980;9:90.

Landoni F, Maneo A, Cormio G, et al. Class II versus class III radical hysterectomy in stage IB-IIA cervical cancer: a prospective randomized study. *Gynecol Oncol* 2001;80:3.

Larson DM, Copeland LJ, Malone JM Jr, et al. Diagnosis of recurrent cervical carcinoma after radical hysterectomy. *Obstet Gynecol* 1988;71:6.

Larson DM, Malone JM Jr, Copeland LJ, et al. Ureteral assessment after radical hysterectomy. *Obstet Gynecol* 1987;69:612.

Latzko W, Schiffmann J. Klinisches and anatomisches zur radikaloperation des gebarmutterkrebses. *Zentralbl Gynakol* 1919;43:715.

Levrant SG, Fruchter RG, Maiman M. Radical hysterectomy for cervical cancer: morbidity and survival in relation to weight and age. *Gynecol Oncol* 1992;45:317.

Lin HH, Yu HJ, Sheu BC, et al. Importance of urodynamic study before radical hysterectomy for cervical cancer. *Gynecol Oncol* 2001;81:270.

Look KY, Brunetto VL, Clarke-Pearson DL, et al. An analysis of cell type in patients with surgically staged IB carcinoma of the cervix: a Gynecologic Oncology Group study. *Gynecol Oncol* 1996;63:304.

Lopes AD, Hall JR, Monaghan JM. Drainage following radical hysterectomy and pelvic lymphadenectomy: dogma or need? *Obstet Gynecol* 1995;86:960.

Lovecchio JL, Averette HE, Donato D, et al. Five-year survival of patients with periaortic nodal metastasis in clinical stage IB and IIA cervical cancer. *Gynecol Oncol* 1989;34:43.

Malur S, Possover M, Schneider A. Laparoscopically assisted radical vaginal versus radical abdominal hysterectomy type II in patients with cervical cancer. *Surg Endosc* 2001;15:289.

Mann WJ, Vogel F, Patsner B, et al. Management of lymphocysts after radical gynecologic surgery. *Gynecol Oncol* 1989;33:248.

Martzloff KH. Carcinoma of the cervix uteri: a pathological and clinical study with particular reference to the relative malignancy of the neoplastic process as indicated by the predominant type of cancer cell. *Bull Johns Hopkins Hosp* 1923;34:141.

Massi G, Savino L, Susini T. Schauta-Amreich vaginal hysterectomy and Wertheim-Meigs abdominal hysterectomy in the treatment of cervical cancer: a retrospective analysis. *Am J Obstet Gynecol* 1993;168:928.

Mathevet P, Laszlo de Kaszon E, Dargent D. Fertility preservation in early cervical cancer. *Gynecol Obstet Fertil* 2003;31:706.

Maxwell GL, Synan I, Dodge R, et al. A prospective randomized comparison of pneumatic compression and low-molecular-weight heparin in the post-operative prophylaxis of gynecologic oncology patients. *Gynecol Oncol* 2001;80:284(abstr).

McCall ML, Keaty EC, Thompson JD. Conservation of ovarian tissue in the treatment of carcinoma of the cervix with radical surgery. *Am J Obstet Gynecol* 1958;75:590.

McIntyre JF, Eifel PJ, Levenback C, et al. Ureteral stricture as a late complication of radiotherapy for stage IB carcinoma of the uterine cervix. *Cancer* 1995;75:836.

Meigs JV. The Wertheim operation for carcinoma of the cervix. *Am J Obstet Gynecol* 1945;49:542.

Mitra S. Radikale vaginale hysterektomie and extraperitoneale lymphadenektomie bei rvixkrebs. *Zentralbl Gynakol* 1951;73:574.

Montana GS, Hanlon AL, Brickner TJ, et al. Carcinoma of the cervix: patterns of care studies; review of 1978, 1983 and 1988–1989 surveys. *Int J Radiat Oncol Biol Phys* 1995;32:1481.

Moore DH, Fowler WC, Walton LA, et al. Morbidity of lymph node sampling in cancers of the uterine corpus and cervix. *Obstet Gynecol* 1989;74: 180.

Morice P, Dargent D, Haie-Meder C, et al. First case of a centropelvic recurrence after radical trachelectomy: literature review and implications for the preoperative selection of patients. *Gynecol Oncol* 2004;92:1002.

Morris M, Eifel PJ, Lu J, et al. Pelvic radiation with concurrent chemotherapy versus pelvic and paraaortic radiation for high-risk cervical cancer: a randomized radiation therapy oncology group clinical trial. *N Engl J Med* 1999;340:1137.

Morris PC, Haugen J, Anderson B, et al. The significance of peritoneal cytology in stage IB cervical cancer. *Obstet Gynecol* 1992;80:196.

Morrow CP. Panel report: is pelvic radiation beneficial in the postoperative management of stage IB squamous-cell carcinoma of the cervix with pelvic node metastases treated by radical hysterectomy and pelvic lymphadenectomy? *Gynecol Oncol* 1980;10:105.

Nagarsheth NP, Maxwell GL, Bentley RC, et al. Bilateral pelvic lymph node metastases in a case of FIGO stage IA1 adenocarcinoma of the cervix. *Gynecol Oncol* 2000;77:467.

Nahhas WA, Abt AB, Mortel R. Stage IB glassy cell carcinoma of the cervix with ovarian metastases. *Gynecol Oncol* 1977;5:87.

Nam JH, Kim JH, Kim DY, et al. Comparative study of laparoscopico-vaginal radical hysterectomy and abdominal radical hysterectomy in patients with early cervical cancer. *Gynecol Oncol* 2004;92:277.

Navratil E. Indications and results of the vaginal and abdominal radical operation in the treatment of carcinoma of the cervix. *J Int Coll Surg* 1965;43:82.

Nezhat CR, Nezhat FR, Burrell MO, et al. Laparoscopic radical hysterectomy and laparoscopically assisted vaginal radical hysterectomy with pelvic and paraaortic node dissection. *J Gynecol Surg* 1993;9(2):105.

Nori D, Valentine E, Hilaris BS. The role of paraaortic node irradiation in the treatment of cancer of the cervix. *Int J Radiat Oncol Biol Phys* 1985;11:1469.

Okabayashi H. Radical abdominal hysterectomy for cancer of the cervix uteri. *Surg Gynecol Obstet* 1921;33:335.

Orr JW Jr, Orr PJ, Bolen DD, et al. Radical hysterectomy: does the type of incision matter? *Am J Obstet Gynecol* 1995;173:399.

Ostor AG. Pandora's box or Ariadne's thread? Definition and prognostic significance of microinvasion in the uterine cervix. Squamous lesions. *Pathol Ann* 1995;30:103.

Ostor AG, Rome R, Zuinn M. Microinvasive adenocarcinoma of the cervix: a clinicopathologic study of 77 women. *Obstet Gynecol* 1997;89:88.

Owens S, Roberts WS, Fiorica JV, et al. Ovarian management at the time of radical hysterectomy for cancer of the cervix. *Gynecol Oncol* 1989;35: 349.

Papavasiliou C, Yiogarakis D, Pappas J, et al. Treatment of cervical carcinoma by total hysterectomy and postoperative external irradiation. *Int J Radiat Oncol Biol Phys* 1980;6(7):871–874.

Patsner B. Closed-suction drainage verus no drainage following radical abdominal hysterectomy with pelvic lymphadenectomy for stage IB cervical cancer. *Gynecol Oncol* 1995;57:232.

Patsner B. Radical abdominal hysterectomy using the ENDO-GIA stapler: a report of 150 cases and literature review. *Eur J Gynaecol Oncol* 1998;19:215.

Patsner B, Hackett TE. Use of the omental J-flap for prevention of postoperative complications following radical abdominal hysterectomy: report of 140 cases and review of the literature. *Gynecol Oncol* 1997;65:405.

Patsner B, Sedlacek TV, Lovecchio JL. Paraaortic node sampling in small (3-cm or less) stage IB invasive cervical cancer. *Gynecol Oncol* 1992; 44:53.

Peipert JF, Wells CK, Schwartz PE, et al. Prognostic value of clinical variables in invasive cervical cancer. *Obstet Gynecol* 1994;84:746.

Peters WA 3rd, Liu PY, Barrett RJ 2nd, et al. Concurrent chemotherapy and pelvic radiation therapy compared with pelvic radiation therapy alone as adjuvant therapy after radical surgery in high-risk early-stage cancer of the cervix. *J Clin Oncol* 2000;18(8):1606.

Piver MS, Rutledge F, Smith JP. Five classes of extended hysterectomy for women with cervical cancer. *Obstet Gynecol* 1974;44:265.

Plante M, Lau S, Brydon L, et al. Neoadjuvant chemotherapy followed by vaginal radical trachelectomy in bulky stage IB1 cervical cancer: case report. *Gynecol Oncol* 2006;101:367.

Plante M, Renaud MC, Harel F, et al. Vaginal radical trachelectomy: an oncologically safe fertility-preserving surgery. An updated series of 72 cases and review of the literature. *Gynecol Oncol* 2004;94:614.

Plante M, Renaud MC, Hoskins IA, et al. Vaginal radical trachelectomy: a valuable fertility-preserving option in the management of early-stage cervical cancer. A series of 50 pregnancies and review of the literature. *Gynecol Oncol* 2005;98:3.

Plante M, Renaud MC, Roy M. Sentinel node evaluation in gynecologic cancer. *Oncology* 2004;18:75.

Plante M, Roy M. Radical trachelectomy. *Oper Tech Gynecol Surg* 1997;3(3):187.

Possover M, Krause N, Drahonovsky J, et al. Left-sided suprarenal retrocrural paraaortic lymphadenectomy in advanced cervical cancer by laparoscopy. *Gynecol Oncol* 1998;71(2):219.

Possover M, Krause N, Kuhne-Heid R, et al. Laparoscopic assistance for extended radicality of radical vaginal hysterectomy: description of a technique. *Gynecol Oncol* 1998;70:94.

Possover M, Krause N, Plaul K, et al. Laparoscopic paraaortic and pelvic lymphadenectomy: experience with 150 patients and review of the literature. *Gynecol Oncol* 1998;71(1):19.

Potish RA, Downey GO, Adcock LL, et al. The role of surgical debulking in cancer of the uterine cervix. *Int J Radiat Oncol Biol Phys* 1989;17: 979.

Querleu D. Laparoscopically assisted radical vaginal hysterectomy. *Gynecol Oncol* 1993;51(2):248.

Querleu D, Dargent D, Ansquer Y, et al. Extraperitoneal endosurgical aortic and common iliac dissection in the staging of bulky or advanced cervical carcinomas. *Cancer* 2000;88(8):1883.

Querleu D, Leblanc E, Cartron G, et al. Audit of preoperative and early complications of laparoscopic lymph node dissection in 1000 gynecologic cancer patients. *Am J Obstet Gynecol* 2006;195:1287.

Querleu D, Leblanc E, Castelain B. Laparoscopic pelvic lymphadenectomy in the staging of early carcinoma of the cervix. *Am J Obstet Gynecol* 1991;164(2):579.

Querleu D, Narducci F, Poulard V, et al. Modified radical vaginal hysterectomy with or without laparoscopic nerve-sparing dissection: a comparative study. *Gynecol Oncol* 2002;85:154.

Ralph G, Tamussino K, Lichtenegger W. Urological complications after radical hysterectomy with or without radiotherapy for cervical cancer. *Arch Gynecol Obstet* 1990;248:61.

Recio FO, Piver MS, Hempling RE. Pretreatment transperitoneal laparoscopic staging pelvic and paraaortic lymphadenectomy in large (> or = 5 cm) stage IB2 cervical carcinoma: report of a pilot study. *Gynecol Oncol* 1996;63(3):333.

Reiffenstuhl G. *The lymphatics of the female genital organs.* Philadelphia: JB Lippincott; 1964.

Renaud MC, Plante M, Roy M. Combined laparoscopic and vaginal radical surgery in cervical cancer. *Gynecol Oncol* 2000;79(1):59.

Rodriguez M, Guimares O, Rose PG. Radical abdominal trachelectomy and pelvic lymphadenectomy with uterine conservation and subsequent pregnancy in the treatment of early invasive cervical cancer. *Am J Obstet Gynecol* 2001;185:370.

Rose PG. Type II radical hysterectomy: evaluating its role in cervical cancer [Editorial]. *Gynecol Oncol* 2001;80:1.

Rose PG, Bundy BN, Watkins EB, et al. Concurrent cisplatin-based radiotherapy and chemotherapy for locally advanced cervical cancer. *N Engl J Med* 1999;340:1144.

Rose PG, Lappas T. Analysis of cost effectiveness of concurrent cisplatin-based chemoradiation in cervical cancer: implications from five randomized trials. *Gynecol Oncol* 2000;78:3.

Roy M, Plante M. Pregnancies after radical vaginal trachelectomy for early-stage cervical cancer. *Am J Obstet Gynecol* 1998;179(6):1491.

Roy M, Plante M, Renaud MC, et al. Vaginal radical hysterectomy versus abdominal radical hysterectomy in the treatment of early-stage cervical cancer. *Gynecol Oncol* 1996;62(3):336.

Russell AH, Anderson M, Walter J, et al. The integration of computed tomography and magnetic resonance imaging in treatment planning for gynecologic cancer. *Clin Obstet Gynecol* 1992;35:55.

Rutledge FN, Fletcher GH, MacDonald RJ. Pelvic lymphadenectomy as an adjunct to radiation therapy in treatment for cancer of the cervix. *Am J Roentgenol Radium Ther Nucl Med* 1965;93:607.

Rutledge FN, Mitchell MF, Munsell M, et al. Youth as a prognostic factor in carcinoma of the cervix: a matched analysis. *Gynecol Oncol* 1992;44:123.

Sahdev A, Jones J, Shepherd JH, et al. MR imaging appearances of the female pelvis after trachelectomy. *Radiographics* 2005;25:41.

Sampson JA. A careful study of the parametrium in twenty-seven cases of carcinoma cervices uteri and its clinical significance. *Am J Obstet* 1906;54:433.

Sardi J, Vidaurreta J, Bermudez A, et al. Laparoscopically assisted Schauta operation: learning experience at the Gynecologic Oncology Unit, Buenos Aires University Hospital. *Gynecol Oncol* 1999;75(3):361.

Schellhas HF. Extraperitoneal paraaortic node sampling in small stage IB invasive cervical cancer. *Gynecol Oncol* 1992;44:53.

Schneider A, Possover M, Kamprath S, et al. Laparoscopy-assisted radical vaginal hysterectomy modified according to Schauta-Stoeckel. *Obstet Gynecol* 1996;88(6):1057.

Schneidler J, Hricak H, Yu KK, et al. Radiologic evaluation of lymph nodes in patients with cervical cancer: meta analysis. *JAMA* 1997;278:1096.

Scotti RJ, Bergman A, Bhatia NN, et al. Urodynamic changes in urethrovesical function after radical hysterectomy. *Obstet Gynecol* 1986;68:111.

Sedlacek TV, Campion MJ, Reich H, et al. Laparoscopic radical hysterectomy: a feasibility study. *Gynecol Oncol* 1995;56:126(abstr).

Sedlis A, Bundy BN, Rotman MZ, et al. A randomized trial of pelvic radiation therapy versus no further therapy in selected patients with stage IB carcinoma of the cervix after radical hysterectomy and pelvic lymphadenectomy: a Gynecologic Oncology Group Study. *Gynecol Oncol* 1999;73(2):177.

Seibel MM, Freeman MG, Graves WL. The effect of surgical and radiation treatment for cervical carcinoma on sexual function. *South Med J* 1982;75:1195.

Sheets EE, Berman ML, Hrountas CK, et al. Surgically treated, early stage neuroendocrine small-cell cervical carcinoma. *Obstet Gynecol* 1988;71:10.

Shepherd JH, Crawford RA, Oram DH. Radical trachelectomy: a way to preserve fertility in the treatment of early cervical cancer. *BJOG* 1998;105(8):912.

Shepherd JH, Mould T, Oram DH. Radical trachelectomy in early stage carcinoma of the cervix: outcome as judged by recurrence and fertility rates. *BJOG* 2001;108(8):882.

Shepherd JH, Spencer C, Herod J, et al. Radical vaginal trachelectomy as a fertility-sparing procedure in women with early-stage cervical cancer-cumulative pregnancy rate in a series of 123 women. *BJOG* 2006;113:719.

Shingleton HM, Bell MC, Fremgen A, et al. Is there really a difference in survival of women with early stage squamous cell carcinoma, adenocarcinoma and adenosquamous cell carcinoma of the cervix? *Cancer* 1995;76:1948.

Shingleton HM, Orr JW, eds. *Cancer of the cervix.* Philadelphia: JB Lippincott; 1995.

Shingleton HM, Soong SJ, Gelder MS, et al. Clinical and histopathologic factors predicting recurrence and survival after pelvic exenteration for cancer of the cervix. *Obstet Gynecol* 1989;73:1027.

Singh N, Titmuss E, Aleong JC, et al. A review of post-trachelectomy isthmic and vaginal smear cytology. *Cytopathology* 2004;15:97.

Smith HO, Tiffany MF, Qualls CR, et al. The rising incidence of adenocarcinoma relative to squamous cell carcinoma of the uterine cervix in the United States—a 24-year population-based study. *Gynecol Oncol* 2000;78:97.

Smith JR, Boyle DC, Corless DJ, et al. Abdominal radical trachelectomy: a new surgical technique for the conservative management of cervical carcinoma. *BJOG* 1997;104:1196.

Soisson AP, Geszler G, Soper JT, et al. A comparison of symptomatology, physical examination, and vaginal cytology in the detection of recurrent cervical carcinoma after radical hysterectomy. *Obstet Gynecol* 1990;76:106.

Soisson AP, Soper JT, Berchuck A, et al. Radical hysterectomy in obese women. *Obstet Gynecol* 1992;80:940.

Sonoda Y, Abu-Rustum NR, Gemignani ML, et al. A fertility-sparing alternative to radical hysterectomy: how many patients may be eligible? *Gynecol Oncol* 2004;95:534.

Sood AK, Sorosky JI, Krogman S, et al. Surgical management of cervical cancer complicating pregnancy: a case-control study. *Gynecol Oncol* 1996;63:294.

Spirtos NM, Eisenkop SM, Schlaerth JB, et al. Laparoscopic radical hysterectomy (type III) with aortic and pelvic lymphadenectomy: surgical morbidity and intermediate-term follow-up. *Gynecol Oncol* 2000;76:232(abstr).

Spirtos NM, Schlaerth JB, Kimball RE, et al. Laparoscopic radical hysterectomy (type III) with aortic and pelvic lymphadenectomy. *Am J Obstet Gynecol* 1996;174(6):1763.

Spirtos NM, Schlaerth JB, Spirtos TW, et al. Laparoscopic bilateral pelvic and paraaortic lymph node sampling: an evolving technique. *Am J Obstet Gynecol* 1995;173(1):105.

Stallworthy J. Radical surgery following radiation treatment for cervical carcinoma. *Ann R Coll Surg Engl* 1964;34:161.

Steed H, Covens A. Radical vaginal trachelectomy and laparoscopic pelvic lymphadenectomy for preservation of fertility. *Postgrad Obstet Gynecol* 2003;23:1.

Steed H, Rosen B, Murphy J et al. A comparison of laparascopic-assisted radical vaginal hysterectomy and radical abdominal hysterectomy in the treatment of cervical cancer. *Gynecol Oncol* 2004;93:588.

Stehman FB, Bundy BN, DiSaia PJ, et al. Carcinoma of the cervix treated with radiation therapy I: a multi-variate analysis of prognostic variables in the gynecologic oncology group. *Cancer* 1991;67:2776.

Stryker JA, Mortel R. Survival following extended field irradiation in carcinoma of cervix metastatic to paraaortic lymph nodes. *Gynecol Oncol* 2000;79:399.

Su TH, Wang KG, Yang YC, et al. Laparoscopic paraaortic lymph node sampling in the staging of invasive cervical carcinoma: including a comparative study of 21 laparotomy cases. *Int J Gynaecol Obstet* 1995;49(3):311.

Sutton G, Bundy B, Delgado G, et al. Ovarian metastases in stage IB carcinoma of the cervix. *Am J Obstet Gynecol* 1992;166:50.

Symmonds RE, Pratt JH. Prevention of fistulas and lymphocysts in radical hysterectomy: preliminary report of a new technique. *Obstet Gynecol* 1961;17:57.

Tattersall MH, Ramirez C, Coppleson M. A randomized trial of adjuvant chemotherapy after radical hysterectomy in stage Ib-IIa cervical cancer patients with pelvic lymph node metastases. *Gynecol Oncol* 1992;46(2): 176.

Trimbos JB, Franchi M, Zanaboni F, et al. "State of the art" of radical hysterectomy: current practice in European oncology centers. *Eur J Cancer* 2004;40:375.

Trimbos JB, Maas CP, Deruiter MC, et al. A nerve-sparing radical hysterectomy: guidelines and feasibility in Western patients. *Int J Gynecol Cancer* 2001;11:180.

Underwood PB Jr, Lutz MH, Smoak DL. Ureteral injury following irradiation therapy for carcinoma of the cervix. *Obstet Gynecol* 1977;49:663.

Ungar L, Palfalvi L, Hogg R, et al. Abdominal radical trachelectomy: a fertility-preserving option for women with early cervical cancer. *BJOG* 2005;112:366.

Ungar L, Palfalvi L, Smith JR, et al. Update on and long term follow-up of 91 abdominal radical trachelectomies. *Gynecol Oncol* 2006;101:S20(abst).

van Nagell JR Jr, Donaldson ES, Parker JC, et al. The prognostic significance of pelvic lymph node morphology in carcinoma of the uterine cervix. *Cancer* 1977;39:2624.

Varia MA, Bundy BN, Deppe G, et al. Cervical carcinoma metastatic to paraaortic nodes: extended field radiation therapy with concomitant 5-fluorouracil and cisplatin chemotherapy: a Gynecologic Oncology Group study. *Int J Radiat Oncol Biol Phys* 1998;42(5):1015.

Vasilev SA. Obturator nerve injury: a review of management options. *Gynecol Oncol* 1994;53:152.

Vidaurreta J, Bermudez A, di Paola G, et al. Laparoscopic staging in locally advanced cervical carcinoma: a new possible philosophy? *Gynecol Oncol* 1999;75(3):366.

Wagenaar HC, Trimbos JB, Postema S et al. Tumor diameter and volume assessed by magnetic resonance imaging in the prediction of outcome for invasive cervical cancer. *Gynecol Oncol* 2001;82:474.

Weber TM, Sostman HD, Spirtzer CE, et al. Cervical carcinoma: determination of current tumor extent versus radiation changes with MR imaging. *Radiology* 1995;194:135.

Weiser EB, Bundy BN, Hoskins WJ, et al. Extraperitoneal versus transperitoneal selective paraaortic lymphadenectomy in the pretreatment surgical staging of advanced cervical carcinoma (Gynecologic Oncology Group Study). *Gynecol Oncol* 1989;33:283.

Wentz WB, Reagan JW. Survival in cervical cancer with respect to cell type. *Cancer* 1959;12:384.

Wertheim E. *Die erweiterte abdominale operation bei carcinoma colli uteri (auf grund von 500 fallen)*. Berlin: Urban; 1911.

Wertheim E. Discussion on the diagnosis and treatment of carcinoma of the uterus. *BMJ* 1905;2:689.

Wertheim E. The extended abdominal operation for carcinoma of the cervix. *Am J Obstet Gynecol* 1912;66:169.

Wertheim E. Zur frag der radikaloperation beim uteruskrebs. *Arch Gynakol* 1900;61:627.

Wertheim MS, Hakes TB, Daghestani AN, et al. A pilot study of adjuvant therapy in patients with cervical cancer and pelvic lymphadenectomy. *J Clin Oncol* 1985;3(7):912.

Whitney CW, Sause W, Bundy BN, et al. Randomized comparison of fluorouracil plus cisplatin versus hydroxyurea as an adjunct to radiation therapy in stage IIB-IVA carcinoma of the cervix with negative paraaortic lymph nodes: a Gynecologic Oncology Group and Southwest Oncology Group study. *J Clin Oncol* 1999;17:1339.

Wilkinson EJ, Hause L. Probability in lymph node sectioning. *Cancer* 1974;33:1269.

Zaino RJ, Ward S, Delgado G, et al. Histopathologic predictors of the behavior of surgically treated stage IB squamous cell carcinoma of the cervix: a GOG study. *Cancer* 1990;69:1750.

CHAPTER 48 ■ ENDOMETRIAL CANCER

MARTA ANN CRISPENS

DEFINITIONS

Endometrial cancer staging—Consists of pelvic peritoneal washings, hysterectomy, bilateral salpingo-oophorectomy, pelvic and paraaortic lymph node dissection, performed either by laparotomy or by laparoscopy.

Hereditary nonpolyposis colon cancer syndrome (HNPCC)—A hereditary cancer syndrome caused by inactivation of one of several DNA-mismatch repair genes. Patients are at increased risk of colon, endometrial, ovarian, ureteral, or small bowel cancers. The lifetime risk of endometrial cancer in women with HNPCC is 40% to 60%. In approximately half of women with HNPCC, the endometrial cancer will occur before the colon cancer.

Type I endometrial cancer—Endometrial cancers that are typically of endometrioid pathology, low grade, and diagnosed at early stage and that have an excellent prognosis. These tumors are typically associated with exposure to unopposed estrogen. They account for approximately 90% of endometrial cancers.

Type II endometrial cancer—Endometrial cancers that are typically high grade and often of papillary serous or clear-cell pathology. They tend to be diagnosed at a later stage, but have a poor prognosis even if diagnosed at an early stage.

The management of endometrial cancer has changed significantly over the last 40 to 50 years. During the 1970s, endometrial cancer was clinically staged. Patients with early-stage disease were treated with preoperative packing of the endometrial cavity with radiation sources, Heyman's capsules, and followed by hysterectomy. In 1988, the International Federation of Gynecology and Obstetrics (FIGO) approved a surgical staging system for endometrial cancer. This acknowledged the shift to surgery as primary therapy, with pelvic radiotherapy being used postoperatively as adjuvant therapy for women at increased risk for recurrence. The last decade has seen a gradual move away from the use of adjuvant pelvic radiotherapy in patients who have been fully surgically staged. Laparoscopic surgery is becoming more important in the treatment of this disease.

In 1983, Bokhman described two pathogenetic types of endometrial cancer. Type I tumors account for approximately 90% of endometrial cancers and are associated with exposure to unopposed estrogen. They are typically of endometrioid pathology, low grade, diagnosed at early stage, and have an excellent prognosis. Type II tumors are high grade and often have papillary serous or clear-cell pathology. They tend to be diagnosed at a later stage, but have a poor prognosis even if diagnosed at an early stage. There is a clear difference in the molecular biology of these tumors. Type I tumors may be associated with a number of genetic changes, including microsatellite instability (17%), inactivation of the PTEN tumor suppressor gene (55%), mutational activation of the K-ras oncogene (13%–26%), and gain of function mutation of the β-catenin gene (25%–38%). Type II tumors are characterized by aneuploidy and inactivating mutations of p53.

EPIDEMIOLOGY

According to American Cancer Society (ACS) estimates, endometrial cancer remains the most common of the gynecologic malignancies in the United States, with 41,200 new cases anticipated in 2006. This makes it the fourth most common cancer occurring in women, behind only breast, lung, and colorectal cancer. It is estimated that there will be 7,350 deaths resulting from endometrial cancer in 2006. That most women with newly diagnosed endometrial cancer can expect a good prognosis is due to the fact that endometrial cancer is usually diagnosed at an early stage, when it is readily treatable with surgery alone. However, there remain a few patients with endometrial cancer who present with high-risk histologic subtypes or advanced-stage disease, in whom the prognosis is more guarded. The current FIGO staging system for endometrial cancer is shown in Table 48.1.

For the years 1993 to 1995, FIGO evaluated the outcomes of 6,260 patients worldwide, of whom 5,694 patients had surgical staging data available. Of these, 3,996 (70%) were stage I, 709 (12%) were stage II, 758 (13%) were stage III, and 231 (4%) were stage IV. The overall 5-year survival for all patients with endometrial cancer was 76.6%. Among surgically staged patients, 5-year survival was 87.4% for patients with stage I disease, 76.3% for patients with stage II disease, 56.6% for patients with stage III disease, and 17.8% for patients with stage IV disease.

The Surveillance, Epidemiology, and End Results (SEER) Program of the National Cancer Institute tracks cancer incidence and mortality in the United States. SEER uses a three-tier staging system encompassing localized disease, which is limited to the organ in which the tumor arose; regional disease, which has spread beyond the primary site to nearby organs, tissues, or lymph nodes; and distant disease, which has spread from the primary site to distant organs or tissues. According to SEER data for the years 1995 to 2002 in the United States, 71% of patients had localized disease, 16% of patients had regional disease, 8% of patients had distant disease, and 4% of patients were unstaged. Overall 5-year survival for patients with localized disease was 96%, for patients with regional disease was 66%, for patients with distant disease was 26%, and for patients with unstaged disease was 57%.

In the United States, there is a significant disparity in the survival of African American women as compared with white women with endometrial cancer. According to SEER data, for the years 1994 to 2003, the age-adjusted total U.S. mortality rate from cancers of the uterus was approximately 7 per 100,000 for African American women, but only about 4 per 100,000 for white women. A number of explanations have been proposed for this racial disparity. Some have proposed

TABLE 48.1

FIGO STAGING OF CARCINOMA OF THE CORPUS UTERI, 1988

Stage IA	Tumor limited to the endometrium
Stage IB	Invasion to less than half of the myometrium
Stage IC	Invasion equal to or more than half of the myometrium
Stage IIA	Endocervical glandular involvement only
Stage IIB	Cervical stromal invasion
Stage IIIA	Tumor invades the serosa of the corpus uteri and/or adnexa and/or positive cytological findings
Stage IIIB	Vaginal metastases
Stage IVA	Tumor invasion of bladder and/or bowel mucosa
Stage IVB	Distant metastases, including intraabdominal metastasis and/or inguinal lymph nodes
Histopathology: degree of differentiation	
Grade 1	5% or less of a solid growth pattern
Grade 2	6%–50% of a solid growth pattern
Grade 3	More than 50% of a solid growth pattern

Notable nuclear atypia, inappropriate for the architectural grade, raises the grade of a grade 1 or grade 2 tumor by 1.

Uterine papillary serous carcinomas and clear-cell carcinomas of the endometrium are always high grade tumors, by definition.

FIGO, International Federation of Obstetrics and Gynecology.

that it is due to limited access to care for African American women. Others have suggested that there is an increased incidence of high-risk histologic subtypes and potential adverse molecular features among African American women as compared with white women.

In a review of data from the National Cancer Data Base from 1988 to 1994 by Hicks and colleagues, endometrial cancer was diagnosed in 52,307 non-Hispanic white and 3,226 African American women. Despite a lower incidence of endometrial cancer among African American women as compared with white women, African American women had a higher mortality rate. For the years 1988 to 1989, the 5-year overall relative survival rate for African American women in this study was 55%, as compared with 86% for white women. Among African American women, the tumors were generally diagnosed at later stage, were higher grade, and were more likely to be of an aggressive histologic subtype. The authors found that African American women were treated less often at every stage and were less frequently treated surgically than white women. This study strongly suggested that the poorer outcomes of African American women with endometrial cancer were due to racial disparities in treatment.

A subsequent review by Randall and Armstrong also demonstrated that African American women had a higher risk of death from endometrial cancer and were less likely to be treated surgically than white women. Even when controlling for tumor and sociodemographic factors, African American women had a hazard ratio for death from endometrial cancer of 1.8.

Other authors have suggested that the difference in survival between African American and white women is, in part, due to differences in tumor biology. Clifford and associates evaluated the incidence of overexpression of p53, a genetic alteration associated with the more aggressive type II endometrial cancers, in women with stage I endometrial adenocarcinoma. They found that p53 overexpression was three times more common among African American women than in white women.

Schimp and coworkers have recently confirmed an increased incidence of p53 overexpression among African American women as compared with white women. Although they found that this correlated with an increased rate of type II endometrial cancers among African American women, they saw no difference in survival between African American and white women when adjusting for tumor type. Finally, in a study performed at the Memorial Sloan Kettering Cancer Institute, the gene expression profiles of endometrial cancers from African American and white women were compared. The two groups were matched for stage, grade, and histologic subtype. These investigators found no statistically significant difference in the gene expression profiles between these two groups.

The Gynecologic Oncology Group (GOG) has performed a retrospective analysis comparing the outcomes of 169 African American women to 982 white women with stage III, IV, or recurrent endometrial cancer being treated on one of four clinical trials. These trials evaluated the use of various chemotherapy regimens in the treatment of advanced stage or recurrent endometrial cancer. African American women were more likely than white women to have papillary serous histology, stage IV disease, and higher tumor grade. Even though the two groups of patients received similar treatment, survival among African American women was worse, suggesting some contribution of socioeconomic, biologic, or cultural factors in the poorer outcomes of these women. These data taken together suggest that there are both biologic and sociologic issues involved in the survival disparity noted between African American and white women with endometrial cancer.

RISK FACTORS

There are no clear risk factors for type II endometrial cancers. Type I endometrial cancers are usually related to exposure to unopposed estrogen, whether exogenous or endogenous. Risk factors for type I tumors are summarized in Table 48.2.

TABLE 48.2

RISK FACTORS FOR THE DEVELOPMENT OF ENDOMETRIAL CANCER

INCREASED RISK
Increasing age
Residence in North America or Northern Europe
Higher socioeconomic status
Higher level of education
White race
Nulliparity
Infertility
Menstrual irregularities
Early menarche
Late menopause
Treatment with unopposed estrogen
Tamoxifen use
Anovulatory disorders, such as polycystic ovarian syndrome
Estrogen-producing tumors, such as granulosa-theca cell tumors
Obesity
Hypertension
Diabetes
High-fat diet
Hereditary nonpolyposis colon cancer syndrome (HNPCC)
DECREASED RISK
Oral contraceptive use
Nonmedicated plastic or copper intrauterine device (IUD) use
Consumption of some phytoestrogens, such as isoflavones and lignans
Diet rich in fruits, vegetables, and fiber
Physical activity
Cigarette smoking

Endometrial cancer incidence increases with age, until about 70 years, when rates begin to decline. Living in North America or Northern Europe and higher levels of income and education are associated with an increased risk of endometrial cancer. Endometrial cancer incidence is higher among whites than among African Americans, as already discussed.

Reproductive factors can be associated with an increased risk of endometrial cancer. Endometrial cancer risk is increased in women who are nulliparous, infertile, or have menstrual irregularities. Early onset of menarche or late age at menopause is also associated with an increased risk of endometrial cancer.

Estrogen replacement therapy is clearly associated with an increased risk of endometrial cancer. A metaanalysis that combined data from both case-control and cohort studies found a 2.3-fold increased risk of endometrial cancer among women who had ever used estrogen replacement therapy as compared with never users. The risk increases with increasing estrogen dose and increasing duration of estrogen use. The risk can be reduced by the concurrent use of cyclic or continuous progestin.

The use of tamoxifen by postmenopausal women for the prevention or treatment of breast cancer is associated with an increased risk of endometrial cancer and uterine sarcomas. However, this small increased risk of uterine cancer is outweighed by the survival benefit of tamoxifen use among women with breast cancer. As compared with other endometrial cancers, tamoxifen-related endometrial cancers are not associated with an increased incidence of adverse prognostic features. There is no known increased risk of endometrial cancers among premenopausal women using tamoxifen. The role of aromatase inhibitors for the adjuvant treatment of breast cancer, either alone or in combination with tamoxifen, is currently being investigated in multiple clinical trials. There is no increased risk of endometrial cancer associated with the use of aromatase inhibitors.

The ovaries may be a source of unopposed estrogen in women with anovulatory disorders, such as polycystic ovarian syndrome (PCOS). In a retrospective study of 128 women with endometrial cancer, Pillay and colleagues found that among women younger than 50 years old, PCOS was significantly more prevalent among women with endometrial cancer than among normal controls. They observed no relationship between PCOS and endometrial cancer in postmenopausal women. Premenopausal women with PCOS should be counseled on the risk of endometrial cancer and the importance of hormonal therapy to maintain regular menstrual cycles. The optimal regimen of progestin treatment is unknown. Estrogen-producing tumors, such as granulosa cell tumors of the ovary, may be another source of endogenous, unopposed estrogen.

Obesity is associated with an increased risk of endometrial cancer. Obesity increases circulating estrogens that are due to peripheral conversion of adrenal androgens to estrogens by the aromatase enzyme in adipocytes. Obesity also causes a decrease in serum sex hormone–binding globulin (SHBG) levels, leading to an increase in the amount of estrogen available to bind to its receptor. Diabetes has been found to be a risk factor for endometrial cancer independent of obesity. The exact mechanism is unknown but may be due to increased estrogen levels in diabetic women, hyperinsulinemia, or elevated levels of insulinlike growth factor-I (IGF-I).

Conversely, factors that decrease exposure to unopposed estrogens decrease the risk of endometrial cancer. The Cancer and Steroid Hormone Study demonstrated that 12 months of oral contraceptive use decreased the risk of endometrial cancer by 40% and that the effect persisted for at least 15 years after the cessation of use. Smoking also decreases the risk of endometrial cancer. The exact mechanism is unknown. It may be due to alterations in estrogen metabolism, a reduction in body weight among smokers, or an earlier age at menopause among smokers. However, smoking cannot be recommended as a chemopreventive measure for endometrial cancer.

A number of studies have suggested a protective effect of intrauterine device (IUD) use on the risk of endometrial cancer. A large case-control study of 2,416 women in Shanghai, China, demonstrated an approximately 50% reduction in the risk of endometrial cancer among women who had ever used an IUD. Several other studies have shown either a statistically significant decrease or a nonstatistically significant trend toward a decrease in endometrial cancer risk among users of nonmedicated plastic or copper IUDs. The effect of progestin-containing IUDs is unknown.

Some phytoestrogens, weakly estrogenic compounds found in plants, may also decrease the risk of endometrial cancer. These compounds include the isoflavones, which are found in soybeans, and the lignans, which are found in whole grains, seeds, and dried fruit. There are likely multiple mechanisms by which this effect may occur. First, these compounds stimulate the production of SHBG. Estrogen in the circulation that is bound to SHBG is not available to bind to cellular estrogen receptors, resulting in a decrease in the amount of bioavailable estrogen in the circulation. Phytoestrogens also directly bind to the estrogen receptor, which blocks the binding of other estrogens. Phytoestrogens have such a weak estrogenic effect that this binding effectively decreases the growth and proliferation of estrogen-dependent cells. Finally, phytoestrogens may inhibit the aromatase enzyme in adipose tissue. A study by

Goodman and colleagues found that greater consumption of tofu with or without other soy products was associated with a 50% reduction in endometrial cancer risk. Another retrospective, case-control trial found that consumption of isoflavones and lignans was inversely associated with the risk of endometrial cancer.

More generally, a high-fat diet is associated with an increased risk of endometrial cancer. Conversely, diets rich in fruits and vegetables are associated with a decreased risk of endometrial cancer. Some studies have suggested that exercise may reduce the risk of endometrial cancer, even after controlling for the effects of body mass index and caloric intake.

Endometrial cancer is one of the components of the hereditary nonpolyposis colon cancer syndrome (HNPCC). The lifetime risk of endometrial cancer in women with HNPCC is 40% to 60%. This syndrome is caused by inactivation of one of several genes involved in DNA-mismatch repair. A family history of colon, endometrial, ovarian, ureteral, or small bowel malignancy should prompt the clinician to consider referral of the patient for genetic counseling and possible genetic testing. Patients with HNPCC may consider chemoprevention with oral contraceptives, increased surveillance with serial endometrial biopsies or transvaginal pelvic ultrasounds, or risk-reducing surgery with hysterectomy and bilateral salpingo-oophorectomy.

PROGNOSTIC FEATURES

The prognostic features for endometrial cancer have been well defined (Table 48.3). These include race, FIGO stage, depth of myometrial invasion, cervical or adnexal involvement, positive pelvic washings, metastasis to pelvic or paraaortic lymph nodes, histologic subtype, tumor grade, presence of lymph-vascular space invasion, and DNA aneuploidy. Of these factors, FIGO stage is the most important. For women with stage I endometrial cancers, prognosis depends primarily on tumor grade, histologic subtype, and depth of myometrial invasion.

Although positive pelvic peritoneal washings result in upstaging of patients to stage IIIA, the presence of positive pelvic peritoneal washings in the absence of other sites of metastasis probably does not have any adverse prognostic significance. Kasamatsu and colleagues found that in 280 women with surgically staged endometrial cancer, the presence of positive peritoneal cytology alone did not affect patient outcome. Instead, positive peritoneal cytology probably acts only to worsen the adverse prognosis of patients with other sites of metastatic disease. Thus, many patients with positive peritoneal cytology as their only site of metastatic disease do not receive additional treatment postoperatively.

TABLE 48.3

PROGNOSTIC FEATURES FOR ENDOMETRIAL CANCER

Race
FIGO stage
Depth of myometrial invasion[a]
Tumor grade[a]
Histologic subtype[a]
Cervical involvement
Adnexal involvement
Positive pelvic washings
Metastases to the pelvic or paraaortic lymph nodes
Lymph-vascular space invasion
DNA aneuploidy

FIGO, International Federation of Obstetrics and Gynecology.
[a]Denotes prognostic features that are most important in patients with endometrial cancers confined to the uterus.

SCREENING FOR ENDOMETRIAL CANCER

The 2006 ACS guidelines for the early detection of cancer recommend that for average-risk, asymptomatic individuals, endometrial cancer screening should consist of education of women at the time of menopause regarding the risks and symptoms of endometrial cancer. Women should be strongly encouraged to report any unexpected bleeding or spotting to their physicians. Likewise, routine screening of asymptomatic women for endometrial cancer or its precursors is not recommended by the American College of Obstetricians and Gynecologists (ACOG).

Even women at mildly increased risk for endometrial cancer because of a history of unopposed estrogen therapy, tamoxifen use, late menopause, nulliparity, infertility, anovulation, obesity, diabetes, or hypertension do not benefit from routine screening for endometrial cancer, beyond the reporting of symptoms. The ACS recommends that women at high risk for endometrial cancer, such as women known or at substantial risk to be a carrier of an HNPCC mutation, should begin annual testing for endometrial cancer, usually with an endometrial biopsy, at the age of 35. However, this recommendation is based on expert opinion. There is no scientific evidence that this approach will result in earlier diagnosis or improved outcomes for these women.

Rijcken and associates reported on a screening program using annual transvaginal pelvic ultrasonography in 41 women who had known mismatch repair gene mutations or who were members of high-risk families. Seventeen of 179 transvaginal ultrasounds were abnormal, leading to the performance of an endometrial biopsy. Three patients were found to have complex endometrial hyperplasia with atypia. One patient with stage IB, grade 2 endometrioid endometrial adenocarcinoma was diagnosed when the patient presented with interval reports of vaginal bleeding 8 months after having a normal ultrasound. In another trial, transvaginal pelvic ultrasound was offered to women with or at risk of having HNPCC. Results were available from 269 women with a total of 825.7 years of risk. Two cases of endometrial cancer were diagnosed, but neither was detected by surveillance scanning. Both patients developed abnormal bleeding and were found to have early-stage endometrial cancers. The findings of these two studies emphasize the importance of patient report and prompt physician evaluation of abnormal uterine bleeding for the early diagnosis of endometrial cancer, particularly in high-risk patients.

EVALUATION OF THE SYMPTOMATIC PATIENT

Abnormal uterine bleeding is the most common presenting symptom of endometrial cancer. In a review of the pathologic findings among women with postmenopausal bleeding, Gredmark and colleagues found that the risk of adenomatous endometrial hyperplasia or cancer in a woman with postmenopausal bleeding is approximately 18%. The risk of malignancy increased with increasing age, with the peak incidence of endometrial cancer occurring in women between 65 and 69 years of age. The most common cause of postmenopausal bleeding was endometrial atrophy, which was identified in 50% of the patients. All patients with postmenopausal bleeding should undergo evaluation for possible endometrial cancer.

Endometrial cancer can also occur in premenopausal women and may present with heavy or irregular vaginal bleeding. Any women age 35 or older with abnormal bleeding should have endometrial sampling performed. Young women with risk factors for endometrial cancer, such as obesity or anovulation, should also undergo endometrial sampling. A 25-year-old woman who experienced menarche at age 12, is obese, and has polycystic ovarian syndrome will already have experienced more than 10 years of exposure to unopposed estrogen.

There are multiple options for the evaluation of a woman with postmenopausal bleeding. One approach is to perform an office endometrial biopsy. This is typically accomplished with a Pipelle instrument, which is a disposable plastic catheter that can be placed through the cervix into the endometrial cavity for the aspiration of endometrial cells. Its use may occasionally require the placement of a single-toothed tenaculum on the cervix for countertraction or gentle cervical dilatation.

In a metaanalysis comparing endometrial sampling techniques, the Pipelle was found to be the most accurate. Among postmenopausal women, the sensitivity for detection of atypical endometrial hyperplasia was 81% and for the detection of endometrial cancer was 99.6%. The sensitivity of the device for the detection of endometrial cancer among premenopausal women was 91%. The specificity of the Pipelle device for the diagnosis of endometrial hyperplasia or malignancy was 98%. From 0 to 54% of patients will have failure of endometrial sampling. Farrell and coworkers have reported a 20% incidence of uterine pathology after an "insufficient" endometrial biopsy, with 3% of these patients having malignancy.

Another option for the evaluation of postmenopausal bleeding is transvaginal pelvic ultrasound to evaluate the endometrial stripe thickness. Gupta and associates in a metaanalysis found that among postmenopausal women with an endometrial stripe thickness of 5 mm or less, the risk of endometrial pathology was approximately 2.5%. These patients can be observed. If the patient has an endometrial stripe thickness of greater than 5 mm, she should undergo endometrial sampling.

Dilatation and curettage (D&C) in the operating room has been considered the gold standard for endometrial sampling. However, even D&C fails to sample the entire endometrial cavity. Stock and Kanbour performed prehysterectomy D&Cs and found that in approximately 60% of patients, less than half of the endometrium had been sampled. There are limited data regarding the sensitivity and specificity of D&C for the diagnosis of endometrial hyperplasia and malignancy. However, studies have suggested that D&C may have a false-negative rate of as much as 10%. Thus, women with persistent postmenopausal bleeding despite a negative prior workup should undergo reevaluation.

Authors differ as to whether the addition of hysteroscopy improves the accuracy of D&C in the detection of endometrial neoplasia. Hysteroscopy may aid in the identification of other uterine pathology, such as polyps or submucous myomas, and in the identification of small, focal lesions. Patients with endometrial cancer who undergo hysteroscopy may be more likely to have positive pelvic peritoneal washings than those

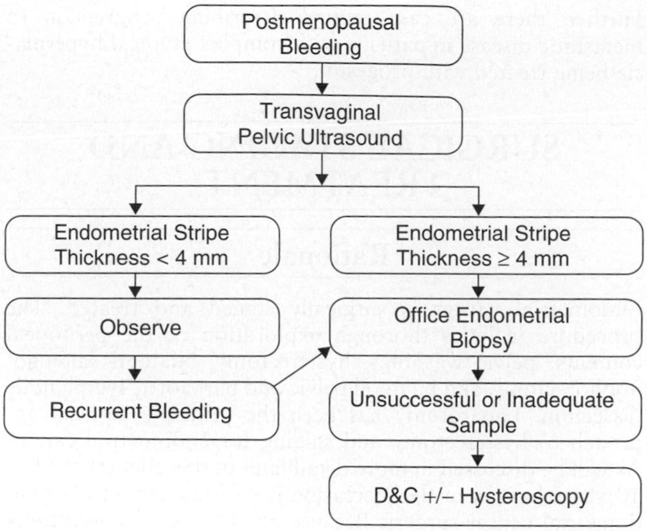

FIGURE 48.1. Algorithm for the evaluation of postmenopausal bleeding (Adapted from Moodley M, Roberts C. Clinical pathway for the evaluation of postmenopausal bleeding with an emphasis on endometrial cancer detection. *J Obstet Gynaecol* 2004;24:736.)

who do not undergo hysteroscopy. There is currently no evidence that this results in decreased survival.

The most clinically and cost-effective sequence or combination of tests for the evaluation of postmenopausal bleeding has not been defined. Clark and colleagues performed a decision analysis comparing twelve different strategies for the evaluation of postmenopausal bleeding. They found that initial evaluation with either an office endometrial biopsy or a transvaginal pelvic ultrasound, with a normal endometrial stripe thickness being defined as 4 mm or less, was the most cost-effective strategy.

Based on a review of the literature, Moodley and Roberts recommended that transvaginal pelvic ultrasonography should be the first step in the evaluation of postmenopausal bleeding, with an endometrial stripe thickness of less than 4 mm being defined as normal. They recommended office endometrial biopsy for those patients with an endometrial stripe thickness of less than 4 mm who were at high risk for endometrial cancer or who had persistent bleeding and for all patients with an endometrial stripe thickness greater than or equal to 4 mm. D&C was reserved for patients in whom office endometrial biopsy could not be successfully performed or resulted in an inadequate sample (Fig. 48.1).

ENDOMETRIAL HYPERPLASIA

Complex atypical hyperplasia of the endometrium is a premalignant condition. Kurman and coworkers found that 29% of patients with complex atypical hyperplasia who went untreated progressed to cancer. Treatment usually consists of hysterectomy with or without bilateral salpingo-oophorectomy. For young women who wish to retain their fertility or patients with comorbid conditions precluding surgery, treatment with systemic progestin or a progestin-containing IUD can be considered. This approach requires close follow-up and appropriate counseling of the patient regarding the risks. A more thorough sampling of the endometrium by D&C will identify endometrial cancer in approximately 42% of patients with a biopsy diagnosis of complex atypical endometrial hyperplasia.

Further, there are case reports describing progression to metastatic disease in patients with complex atypical hyperplasia being treated with progestin.

SURGICAL STAGING AND TREATMENT

Rationale

Endometrial cancer is surgically staged and treated. The procedure includes thorough exploration of the peritoneal contents, pelvic washings, hysterectomy, bilateral salpingo-oophorectomy, and bilateral pelvic and paraaortic lymph node dissection. Laparotomy has been the principle surgical approach to hysterectomy and staging for endometrial cancer. As will be discussed in more detail later in this chapter, the last 10 years have seen the increasing use of laparoscopy for endometrial cancer surgery. Because laparoscopic hysterectomy and lymph node dissection techniques are discussed in detail elsewhere in this textbook, the discussion below will focus on open techniques.

Type I endometrial cancers have three main patterns of spread: by direct extension, to regional lymph nodes, and hematogenously. The most common mechanism of spread for type I endometrial cancer is by direct extension, invading into the myometrium or by extension to the adjacent cervix. Hematogenous metastasis tends to occur late in the course of the disease. Type II endometrial cancers, particularly uterine papillary serous carcinomas, may also metastasize within the peritoneal cavity, similar to ovarian carcinomas.

Endometrial carcinoma spreads through three separate lymphatic pathways: Paracervical and parametrial lymphatics drain to the pelvic lymph nodes, ovarian lymphatics drain to the paraaortic lymph nodes, and round ligament lymphatics drain to the inguinal lymph nodes (Fig. 48.2). The lymphatic drainage of the uterine fundus and cervix directs most of the metastases to the pelvic lymph nodes. Although the paraaortic lymph nodes may be primary metastatic sites via spread through the infundibulopelvic ligament lymphatics, it is rare for an endometrial cancer patient to have isolated paraaortic lymph node metastases without concomitant pelvic lymph node metastases. Boronow and colleagues found that the incidence of isolated paraaortic lymph node metastases was only 1.5%.

GOG performed a large, prospective evaluation of the prognostic features associated with lymph node metastases in patients with apparent early-stage endometrial cancers. The presence of these features define a population of patients with endometrial cancers of intermediate risk, who have an approximately 15% to 20% chance of recurrence. This group included patients with grade 3 tumors with invasion of the inner one third of the myometrium, grade 2 or 3 tumors with invasion of the middle one third of the myometrium, cancer of any grade with invasion of the outer one third of the myometrium, presence of lymph-vascular space invasion, and/or extension to the cervix. Until recently, these patients were often treated with postoperative adjuvant pelvic radiotherapy. Although radiotherapy reduces the risk of pelvic recurrence, it has not been shown to improve survival in these patients.

In the past, the need for surgical staging with pelvic and paraaortic lymphadenectomy was determined based on pre- and intraoperative assessment of tumor grade and depth of invasion, as these are the factors most predictive of the risk of lymph node metastasis. Recently, there has been a shift toward

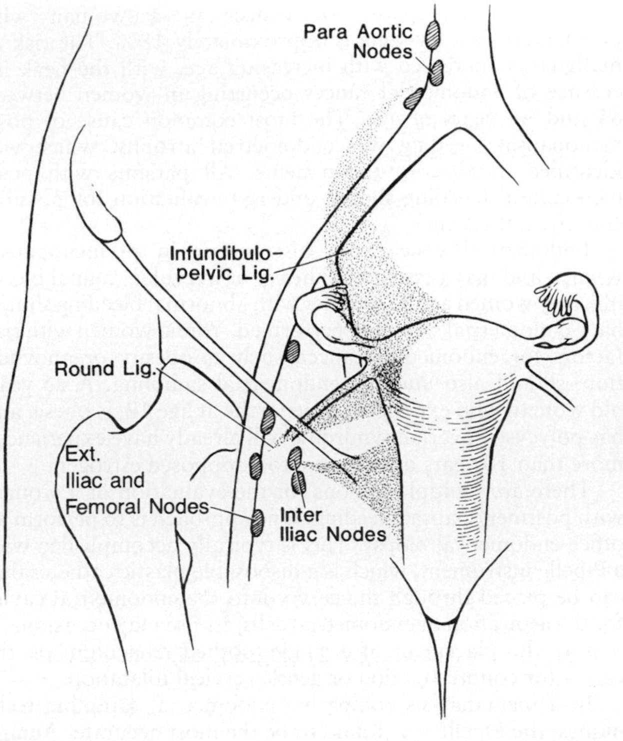

FIGURE 48.2. Lymphatic pathways of tumor spread of endometrial carcinoma to pelvic and extrapelvic nodes.

the routine staging of the majority of patients with endometrial cancer. This has occurred for two reasons. First, pre- and intraoperative assessment of tumor stage and grade has been demonstrated to be inaccurate. Second, routine performance of lymphadenectomy in patients with early-stage endometrial cancer has been shown to improve survival. Patients with negative pelvic and paraaortic lymph nodes may be able to avoid pelvic radiotherapy and its attendant morbidity.

Many authors have demonstrated the inaccuracy of pre- and intraoperative evaluation of the stage and grade of endometrial cancers. Eltabakkh and colleagues performed a retrospective analysis of 182 women with endometrial cancer who had a preoperative endometrial biopsy showing grade 1 disease. Among these patients, 30% had grade 2 or 3 tumors on final pathology, and 12.6% had stage III or IV disease diagnosed at surgery.

In a retrospective series of 153 patients, Frumovitz and associates have reported on the poor sensitivity and specificity of preoperative histology and intraoperative assessment of gross depth of tumor invasion in predicting the final histologic diagnosis of patients with endometrial cancer. They found that 25% to 30% of patients were upstaged based on final pathology. The exact rate of upstaging depended on whether stage IB, grade 2 tumors were considered clinically significant disease that would result in performance of pelvic and paraaortic lymphadenectomy, if that diagnosis were known intraoperatively.

Kilgore and coworkers were the first to suggest that lymphadenectomy might have a therapeutic effect for patients with endometrial cancer. They evaluated the outcomes of 649 patients surgically managed for endometrial cancer. In this study, 212 patients had pelvic lymph nodes sampled from at least four separate sites (multiple-site lymph node sampling), 205 patients had pelvic lymph nodes sampled from fewer than four sites (limited-site lymph node sampling), and 208 patients had no pelvic lymph nodes sampled. Patients undergoing multiple-site lymph node sampling had a survival of approximately 85%, whereas patients in whom pelvic lymph nodes were not sampled had a survival of approximately 65%, a statistically significant difference ($p = 0.0027$). This survival advantage for patients with multiple-site lymph node sampling persisted even in a subgroup analysis of patients treated with postoperative whole-pelvic radiotherapy.

The impact of routine surgical staging on the treatment of 181 women with a preoperative diagnosis of grade 1 endometrioid adenocarcinoma of the endometrium was evaluated by Ben-Shachar and coworkers. Surgical staging was performed in 82% of cases and was omitted only when the disease was apparently confined to the endometrium and the surgical risk was high. High-risk uterine features—including greater than one half myometrial invasion, grade 3 tumors, high-risk histologic variants, and/or cervical extension—were identified in 26% of patients. Lymph node metastases were identified in 3.9% of patients. Overall, the findings of the surgical staging procedure significantly affected postoperative treatment decisions in 29% of patients. This includes 12% of patients who were determined to need adjuvant therapy and 17% of patients who were able to forego external-beam whole-pelvic radiotherapy or chemotherapy. The incidence of severe surgical complications in the surgically staged group was 3.2%.

Pelvic and paraaortic lymph node sampling in patients with endometrial cancer is not associated with a significant increase in surgical morbidity. Homesley and colleagues compared the outcomes of 196 patients undergoing hysterectomy with pelvic and paraaortic lymph node sampling for endometrial cancer with those of 104 patients who underwent hysterectomy alone. They found an increased operative time and higher blood loss among women undergoing lymph node dissection, but no difference in the rate of transfusion. Other complications were found to be primarily related to other factors, such as patient age and weight. Chuang and associates reported a series of 295 patients with endometrial cancer, 193 (65%) of whom had lymph node sampling performed. They noted two intraoperative injuries (one ureteral transection and one major venous laceration) that apparently were repaired without sequelae. They believed that the information gained from the dissection greatly outweighed the operative risk.

What constitutes an adequate lymphadenectomy? In Kilgore and colleague's study from the University of Alabama at Birmingham, the median number of lymph nodes removed was 11. In the study by Chuang and associates, the lymph node–bearing areas at risk were divided into 10 lymphatic zones: right and left paraaortic, common iliac, external iliac, hypogastric, and obturator. Patients who had lymph nodes removed from at least three zones, including one paraaortic and at least one pelvic site on each side, had a mean of 6.2 sites biopsied, with an average yield of nine lymph nodes per patient. In this group, there were no recurrences at retroperitoneal lymph node sites.

Chan and colleagues performed a retrospective review of the SEER database. They found that for patients with intermediate and high-risk endometrial cancers—defined as stage IB, grade 3 and stage IC to IV of all grades—a more extensive lymph node dissection was associated with improved 5-year disease-specific survival, ranging from 75% for patients with only one lymph node removed to 86.8% in patients with greater than 20 lymph nodes removed ($p < 0.01$). Likewise, Lutman and associates reported that a lymph node count greater than or equal to 12 was an important prognostic variable in patients with FIGO stage I and II endometrial cancer with high-risk histology, which was defined as patients with grade 3 tumors or those with papillary serous or clear-cell tumors.

Certain medical problems may alter the safety of the pelvic and paraaortic lymphadenectomy. In patients with medical comorbidities, the small added time and blood loss required to perform bilateral pelvic and paraaortic lymph node sampling may be prohibitive. Additionally, in very obese patients, exposure may be compromised. No attempt at lymph node removal should be undertaken if adequate exposure is not possible.

Preoperative Assessment and Preparation

As noted above, many patients with endometrial cancer may be older and have multiple medical comorbidities. Thus, preoperative preparation is important. All patients should have a thorough history and physical examination. The history should assess the length and severity of the patient's bleeding or other presenting symptoms. It should also assess for symptoms of metastatic disease, such as abdominal or pelvic pain, changes in bowel or bladder function, lower extremity pain or swelling, abdominal bloating, early satiety, shortness or breath, or cough. Previous medical history and symptoms suggestive of occult cardiopulmonary disease or other medical illnesses should be ascertained. Careful attention should be paid to the family history, as endometrial cancer may develop before colon cancer in 50% of women with HNPCC.

The physical examination should focus on assessment for supraclavicular and inguinal lymphadenopathy, abdominal distension or fluid wave suggestive of ascites, abdominal masses, and lower extremity edema. On pelvic examination, close attention should be paid to possible vaginal or cervical extension of disease. Uterine size and mobility, the presence of adnexal masses, parametrial extension, and cul-de-sac nodularity should be assessed.

Basic laboratory evaluation should include a hematocrit and type and screen. CA-125 testing is not indicated, except in patients with uterine papillary serous carcinoma. A chest x-ray should be performed both to rule out lung metastases and evaluate for concurrent pulmonary disease. An electrocardiogram will be needed in most patients for preoperative assessment for potential cardiac disease. Extensive preoperative radiographic assessment for metastatic disease with computed tomography (CT), magnetic resonance imaging (MRI), or positron emission tomography (PET) is not indicated, unless the history or physical examination are suggestive of distant disease. This would be most likely to occur in patients with uterine papillary serous or clear-cell carcinomas. Other preoperative testing should be performed as dictated by the patient's history and physical findings, and may include complete blood count, electrolytes, and assessment of hepatic and renal function. For patients with multiple medical comorbidities, preoperative cardiac, pulmonary, or other medical consultation may be necessary. In such patients, preoperative consultation with the anesthesiologist may also be of benefit.

Once a patient has completed her preoperative evaluation and has been cleared for surgery, she should be recounseled regarding her options for therapy, including surgical therapy; primary pelvic radiotherapy, which is usually reserved for patients who are not good candidates for surgery; and no therapy. Patients should be thoroughly counseled on the indications, risks, and benefits of surgery; that there is no guarantee as to outcome; and that further therapy in the form of additional surgery, chemotherapy, or radiotherapy may be necessary. The patient and her family should be given the opportunity to have all of their questions answered. Written informed consent should be signed.

Preoperative preparation of the patient who is to undergo lymphadenectomy should include a mechanical bowel preparation to decompress the small bowel. Standard preoperative antibiotic prophylaxis for hysterectomy should be used, typically with cefazolin 1 to 2 g intravenously given 30 minutes before incision. Metronidazole can be used in patients with a history of immediate hypersensitivity reaction to penicillin.

High-risk features for thromboembolism in patients undergoing gynecologic surgery include patients older than 40 years with any of the following: history of prior deep venous thrombosis or pulmonary embolism, varicose veins, infection, malignancy, estrogen therapy, obesity, or prolonged surgery. Without prophylaxis, these patients have a risk of deep venous thrombosis of 40% to 70% and of pulmonary embolism of 1% to 5%. Thus, all patients undergoing surgery for endometrial cancer should receive thromboembolism prophylaxis with low-dose heparin 5,000 units every 8 hours, low-molecular-weight heparin with enoxaparin 40 mg daily or daltaperin 5,000 units daily, or pneumatic compression devices. For patients at highest risk, double prophylaxis with pneumatic compression devices and either low-dose heparin or low-molecular-weight heparin can be considered, but there are no prospective data to indicate that combination therapy is more effective than single modality therapy.

Surgical Technique: Laparotomy

Before taking the patient to the operating room, the patient should confirm the surgical site (abdomen), and this should be marked according to hospital protocol. Once in the operating room, a time-out is performed as per hospital protocol to ensure the correct patient and procedure. After the induction of anesthesia, the patient should be positioned for surgery. Some surgeons prefer the supine position for hysterectomy. It does avoid the risk of neurologic injury that can rarely occur with lithotomy position in Allen stirrups. Many gynecologic oncologists will place the patient in the lithotomy position because of the ready access to the paraaortic lymph nodes that can be achieved with the surgeon between the patient's legs.

The abdomen is usually opened through a vertical midline lower abdominal incision. This is preferable to a low transverse incision, such as a Pfannenstiel incision, because it allows for better access to the paraaortic lymph nodes. In morbidly obese patients, a paramedian or high transverse incision is sometimes used to keep the incision out of the pannus and reduce the risk of infection. Occasionally, panniculectomy in conjunction with hysterectomy may be performed.

On entering the abdominal cavity, *peritoneal washings are obtained*. The operator washes the pelvic organs with 50 to 100 mL of saline. The fluid is gently agitated, then aspirated from the posterior cul-de-sac, mixed with heparin, and submitted for cytologic evaluation. The presence of malignant cells in the washings is an adverse prognostic feature.

Next, the *peritoneal cavity is carefully explored*. The approach to abdominal exploration should be systematic. Explore the pelvis last, so as not to be distracted by findings there. Exploration of the upper abdomen is facilitated by having the assistant elevate the anterior abdominal wall at the apex of the incision using a large Richardson retractor. The omentum is brought into the field and carefully examined for metastatic implants. The upper abdominal contents—including the anterior surface of the stomach, the surface of the liver, and the gallbladder—can be visualized. Starting on the right, the operator's hand is used to palpate the peritoneum of the anterior abdominal wall and the paracolic gutter. As the hand moves superiorly, the kidney can be palpated. Then, palpate the gallbladder, right lobe of the liver, and right hemidiaphragm. The operator then explores the left upper abdomen, including the left diaphragm, left lobe of the liver, spleen, and stomach, including the pylorus. Finally, follow the left anterior abdominal wall and paracolic gutter inferiorly back to the pelvis, palpating the left kidney in the process. At this point, the cecum is identified, and the appendix can be examined. The small bowel is run from the ileocecal valve to the ligament of Treitz. With the bowel on the surface of the abdomen, palpation of the retroperitoneum is facilitated. Start superiorly with the pancreas, and continue inferiorly to palpate the paraaortic lymph nodes. Continue the nodal palpation to the pelvic lymph nodes bilaterally. The small bowel is returned to the abdomen. The large bowel is run *in situ*. Finally, while retracting the small bowel into the upper abdomen, the pelvis is carefully explored. Assess the pelvic peritoneum, with careful attention to the cul-de-sac peritoneum, for implants. Note the size and mobility of the uterus. Assess the ovaries and fallopian tubes for any masses or implants.

Once the peritoneal exploration is completed, a self-retaining retractor can be placed, and the bowel can be packed into the upper abdomen with the assistance of moist laparotomy sponges. This is assisted with the use of gentle Trendelenburg positioning. Care must be taken with the use of a self-retaining retractor to keep the blades off the psoas muscles to avoid injury to the femoral nerves.

The uterine cornua are grasped bilaterally with long Kelly or similar clamps, occluding the fallopian tubes. This allows for manipulation of the uterus during the *hysterectomy* while preventing efflux of malignant cells via the tubes during the course of the procedure. To avoid contamination of the field by malignant cells from the interior of the uterus, a tenaculum, Leahy, or other perforating clamp should not be placed on the uterine fundus.

On either side, the round ligament is ligated and transected. The pelvic sidewall peritoneum is then incised approximately 1 cm lateral and parallel to the infundibulopelvic ligament. The retroperitoneal space can be bluntly dissected to reveal the course of the ureter through the pelvis. The ureter lies on the medial peritoneal leaf. It is at its most superficial—therefore, easiest to identify—as it crosses the bifurcation of the common iliac artery at the pelvic brim. A common mistake is to look for the ureter deep in the pelvis, where it can be confused with the superior vesical artery. A helpful anatomic point is that the superior vesical artery will be seen to rise out of the retroperitoneum as it is followed distally, whereas the ureter will tend to course more deeply in the retroperitoneum as it is followed distally. The ureter can be positively identified by visualizing its distinct peristalsis. When palpated between the operator's fingers, it gives a "popping" sensation, like a rubber band.

Once the ureter has been clearly identified, the infundibulopelvic ligament can be identified coursing anterior and parallel. It should be isolated by making a window in the posterior leaf of the broad ligament between the infundibulopelvic ligament and the ureter. Ideally, this should be performed under direct visualization so as to avoid injury to the vessels within or to the ureter. The infundibulopelvic ligament is doubly clamped using Haney clamps, transected and doubly ligated. The uteroovarian ligament is skeletonized back to the uterus. The adnexa should not be amputated unless there is an adnexal mass preventing access to the pelvis. Again, this is to prevent spillage of tumor cells into the peritoneal cavity. The adnexa can be suspended off of the Kelly clamp on either uterine cornua to keep them out of the way during the hysterectomy.

The vesicouterine peritoneum is incised, and the bladder can be dissected sharply off the lower uterine segment and cervix. Blunt dissection should be avoided because of the risk of injury to the bladder. The operator should attempt to keep the dissection in the fine areolar tissue between the bladder and the cervix. If there is difficulty with the bladder dissection, the bladder can be dissected down just far enough to allow the uterine artery pedicles to be taken. After the initial pedicles are taken, the bladder dissection often becomes easier. The bladder flap is advanced through the course of the hysterectomy, as necessary.

The uterine arteries are now skeletonized to isolate the vessels. The pedicles on both sides are clamped simultaneously, obviating the need to place a back clamp. The uterine artery pedicle is clamped with a Heaney clamp, placing the tip perpendicular to the cervix. The pedicle is transected on the clamp with curved scissors, then ligated. Straight Ballentine clamps are then used to clamp serially down the cardinal ligaments bilaterally. Each pedicle should be approximately 1 to 1.5 cm in length. Smaller pedicles allow for the ureter to effectively fall away with each bite and allow for better hemostasis. In taking the uterine artery and cardinal ligament pedicles, the clamp should be placed just against the cervix, not "rolled off" the cervix. The practice of rolling the clamp off the cervix may cause the lateral cervix to be caught in the clamp, with risk of leaving residual cervix. Be sure that each clamp is placed medial to the last pedicle so as to not clamp the ureter. The uterosacral ligaments can be clamped, cut, and ligated separately. Often, this is best done with a curved Haney clamp.

When the cervicovaginal junction is reached, either a right-angled Zeppelin clamp or a curved Heaney clamp, depending on the size of the cervix and vagina, is used to clamp across the upper vagina from either side, approximately 1 cm below the cervix. The specimen—consisting of uterus, cervix, bilateral fallopian tubes, and bilateral ovaries—is now amputated with curved scissors. A figure-of-eight suture is placed through the vaginal apex between the two clamps and held, to decrease contamination of the peritoneal cavity with the contents of the vagina and to decrease bleeding. The lateral pedicles are sutured with Heaney sutures, and the suture in the middle of the vagina is tied. Any remaining open vagina is closed with figure-of-eight sutures. The pelvis is copiously irrigated, and hemostasis is assured. The pelvis should be carefully examined to be sure that there has been no injury to the surrounding pelvic organs, particularly the bladder, rectum, and ureters.

Attention can now be turned to the *pelvic and paraaortic lymphadenectomy*. The bowel will need to be packed to the opposite side of the dissection. The peritoneum should be incised superiorly along the white line of Toldt. The colon can then be mobilized bluntly anteriorly and medially. The paravesical space can be opened by bluntly dissecting the bladder off the pubic ramus, staying lateral to the superior vesical artery. The pararectal space is opened by bluntly dissecting between the ureter and hypogastric artery.

The colon and ureter can be retracted with a large Deaver retractor, which should be oriented toward the contralateral shoulder. Sharp dissection with Metzenbaum scissors with hemoclips for hemostasis can be used to excise the fatty, lymph node–bearing tissues in the pelvis. This should include the tissues anterior and medial to the common iliac artery, anterior and medial to the external iliac artery, medial to the external iliac vein, and anterior to the hypogastric artery, extending distally along the superior vesical artery. The inferior margin of the dissection is the point at which the circumflex iliac vein crosses over the external iliac artery. The external iliac vein is retracted anteriorly with a vein retractor. Blunt dissection is performed within the obturator space to reveal the course of the obturator nerve. The lymph nodes anterior to the obturator nerve are removed.

The left paraaortic lymph node dissection is extended from the level of the bifurcation of the common iliac artery superiorly along the lateral aspect of the aorta. Care must be taken not to extend the dissection too far posteriorly, where the lumbar arteries arise from the aorta. On the right, the paraaortic lymph node dissection is performed superiorly, along the anterior surface of the inferior vena cava. Small, perforating vessels are numerous on both sides, so careful hemostasis as the dissection proceeds is important. Because paraaortic lymph node metastases from the uterus usually represent direct extension from pelvic lymph node metastasis, it is usually necessary to extend the dissection only to the level of the inferior mesenteric artery.

Special Situations

Uterine papillary serous carcinomas behave in a manner similar to ovarian cancers, demonstrating spread within the peritoneal cavity even when the primary tumor is confined to the endometrium. Goff and associates evaluated the patterns of spread in patients with noninvasive uterine papillary serous carcinomas and found that with complete surgical staging, 36% of patients were found to have lymph node metastases and 43% of patients were found to have intraperitoneal metastases. Chan and coworkers found that 25% of patients with noninvasive uterine papillary serous carcinomas had occult omental disease. Thus, *staging of patients with uterine papillary serous carcinoma* should include hysterectomy with bilateral salpingo-oophorectomy, peritoneal washings and biopsies, bilateral pelvic and paraaortic lymph node dissection, and omentectomy, as is typically performed for ovarian cancer.

For patients with *stage IIB endometrial cancers with a bulky cervix*, there is a risk of parametrial extension, as for primary cervical carcinomas. Further, it can sometimes be difficult to distinguish between a primary endometrial adenocarcinoma with extension to the cervix versus a primary cervical adenocarcinoma that may extend into the lower uterine segment or above. These patients may be treated similarly to cervical cancer patients with a radical hysterectomy and pelvic and paraaortic lymphadenectomy. Five-year survival rates of 90% to 94% have been reported for this treatment strategy.

The alternative is to treat these patients with preoperative external beam whole-pelvic radiotherapy and intracavitary brachytherapy followed by completion hysterectomy with bilateral salpingo-oophorectomy. Completion hysterectomy is necessary, as radiotherapy is not as effective in treating disease in the uterine corpus as in the uterine cervix. Reisinger and colleagues reported a 5-year actuarial survival of 82% in patients with endometrioid histology treated with this strategy. Patients with high-risk histologic subtypes had only a 38% 5-year actuarial survival, with a high incidence of recurrence in the upper abdomen.

In *patients with stage III or IV endometrial cancers*, tumor debulking may be of benefit. Goff and associates reported on 47 patients with stage IV endometrial cancer. Overall median survival for these patients was 12 months. Among those patients who underwent successful cytoreduction, overall median survival was 18 months as compared with 8 months among patients who did not undergo surgery ($p = 0.0001$). Similarly, Chi and colleagues showed that among 55 patients with stage IV endometrial cancer, overall median survival was 31 months for those whose disease could be optimally cytoreduced to less than or equal to 2 cm residual disease, 12 months for those whose disease was suboptimally cytoreduced, and 3 months for those whose disease was unresectable (p <0.01).

Lambrou and colleagues also evaluated the efficacy and safety of cytoreductive surgery in patients with stage III and IV endometrial cancer. They excluded patients with uterine papillary serous carcinomas and clear-cell carcinomas. They found that optimal cytoreduction to less than or equal to 2 cm maximal residual disease was possible in 72% of their patients. Overall median survival was 17.8 months for patients undergoing optimal cytoreduction and only 6.7 months for patients who could not be optimally cytoreduced ($p = 0.001$). Further, they observed that the proportion of patients having major postoperative complications was actually higher among those who were suboptimally cytoreduced as compared with those who were not, 37.5% versus 7.25%, respectively ($p = 0.005$).

Bristow and coworkers evaluated the survival benefit of lymph node debulking among patients with stage IIIC endometrial cancer. All patients had macroscopic spread to pelvic lymph nodes, and approximately 50% had macroscopic involvement of the paraaortic lymph nodes. Disease-specific survival was 37.5 months among patients whose involved lymph nodes could be completely resected as compared with 8.8 months among patients whose involved lymph nodes could not be completely resected ($p = 0.006$).

Role of Laparoscopy

Multiple surgeons have published data demonstrating the feasibility of laparoscopic staging and treatment of endometrial cancer. These studies consistently demonstrate that the laparoscopic approach is associated with significantly decreased blood loss and shorter hospital stays when compared with open laparotomy. Postoperative complication rates of patients undergoing laparoscopy are typically reported as comparable to or lower than those of patients undergoing laparotomy. The overall cost of laparoscopy has been shown to be equal to or lower than that for laparotomy. Although laparoscopy is associated with increased equipment costs, this is balanced by the increased hospital costs of patients undergoing laparotomy. Short-term quality of life has been shown to be improved in patients undergoing laparoscopy, with decreased need for pain medications postoperatively and faster return to work.

Despite the apparent benefits of laparoscopy, gynecologic oncologists in the United States have been slow to embrace this surgical approach. In fact, most of the United States data regarding the use of laparoscopy for the treatment of endometrial cancer comes from a very limited number of surgeons and centers, who have developed special expertise in this technique. For these individuals, operative times are only slightly longer than for laparotomy, and rates of conversion to laparotomy are low—generally 5% or less. Unfortunately, the experience of these few individuals and centers has not been generalizable within the United States.

The GOG Lap 2 study was a multicenter, randomized trial comparing treatment of endometrial cancer performed by laparoscopy versus laparotomy. Although the results of this study have not yet been published in a peer review journal, the results presented in abstract form are revealing. This study enrolled 2,616 patients, 990 of whom were randomized to laparotomy and 1,696 of whom were randomized to laparoscopy. Although this study confirmed previous reports of generally good outcomes for patients undergoing laparoscopy, there was a 23% conversion rate to laparotomy. The reasons for this are unclear. It is probably largely due to the experience and expertise of the surgeons. Both Eltabbakh and Holub and colleagues have described the significant learning curve for this technique. Patient selection may also be a factor, although laparoscopic management of early-stage endometrial cancer has been shown to be feasible even in the elderly and the obese.

The most important factor in assessing the appropriateness of the use of laparoscopy in the staging and treatment of endometrial cancer is survival. Eltabbakh performed a retrospective review of women presenting with FIGO stage I endometrial cancer. He identified 100 women who underwent laparoscopy and 86 who underwent laparotomy. There was no difference in outcomes. The 5-year disease-free survival was 90% for those women treated by laparoscopy and 92% for those women who underwent laparotomy. In univariate and multivariate analysis, surgical stage, tumor grade, and tumor histology—but not surgical approach—were predictors of survival. In retrospective analyses, Holub and associates, Magrina, and Obermair and colleagues have all confirmed the finding of no difference in the recurrence and survival rates of women treated for early-stage endometrial cancer by laparoscopic surgery as compared with women treated with a conventional open surgical approach. A prospective, randomized trial evaluating disease-free survival among women with early endometrial cancer treated with laparoscopy versus laparotomy is currently ongoing in Australia.

Although some authors have suggested that laparoscopy, rather than laparotomy, should be considered the standard surgical approach for endometrial cancer, it is important to keep in mind that laparotomy and laparoscopy are only methods of abdominal entry. The surgical management of early-stage endometrial cancer should include hysterectomy, bilateral salpingo-oophorectomy, pelvic and paraaortic lymph node dissection, and pelvic washings. The surgeon must choose the approach that allows him or her to best care for the patient with the least risk of complications. Although for certain surgeons this may be laparoscopy, there are many surgeons for whom laparotomy remains the best and safest approach. On the other hand, it is incumbent on all surgeons to continue to advance our skills throughout our surgical careers so that we may provide the most effective and safest surgical management for our patients. The best approach to the surgical management of endometrial cancer is likely only to continue to evolve with the introduction of robotics and other new surgical technologies.

RADIATION THERAPY

At the present time, radiation therapy is rarely used as the primary or sole treatment modality for women with endometrial cancer. The goal of postoperative radiotherapy in patients with endometrial cancer is to treat the pelvic lymph node beds with external-beam whole-pelvic radiotherapy and upper vagina with vaginal vault brachytherapy. This has been demonstrated to decrease the risk of local recurrence, but not to improve survival. With the increasing use of surgical staging with pelvic and paraaortic lymph node dissection, the use of adjuvant pelvic radiotherapy has decreased.

Patients with low-risk endometrial cancers, stage IA or IB, grade 1 or 2, require no additional treatment postoperatively. The PORTEC trial was a randomized trial of postoperative radiotherapy versus observation in 714 patients with stage IB, grade 2 or 3 and IC, grade 1 or 2 endometrial cancer who had undergone hysterectomy with bilateral salpingo-oophorectomy. These patients had not undergone lymph node dissection. At 10 years, the pelvic failure rate was 5% in the patients who received pelvic radiotherapy and 14% among

controls ($p < 0.0001$). However, there was no statistically significant difference in survival, with an overall survival of 66% among patients who received pelvic radiotherapy and 73% among controls ($p = 0.09$).

Straughn and colleagues performed a retrospective review of 613 patients with stage I endometrial cancer who had undergone comprehensive surgical staging. Among 325 patients with stage IB disease, 321 did not receive pelvic radiotherapy. Fifteen (5%) of these patients recurred. All nine local recurrences were salvaged. There were 77 patients with stage IC disease, of whom 53 (69%) did not receive pelvic radiotherapy. Four (8%) patients recurred, and three of them were salvaged. For all stage I patients, the 5-year disease-free survival was 93% and overall survival was 98%. These authors concluded that pelvic radiotherapy is not needed in patients who have undergone comprehensive surgical staging because of the low risk of recurrence and high salvage rate with subsequent therapy.

In a follow-up to this study, Straughn and colleagues subsequently evaluated an expanded cohort of 220 patients with stage IC endometrial cancer. Ninety-nine (45%) patients were treated with radiotherapy—either external beam whole pelvic, vaginal cuff brachytherapy, or both—and 121 (55%) patients were observed. There was no statistically significant difference in the recurrence rate between the two groups. The overall 5-year survival was 92% for the patients who received radiotherapy and 90% for those who were observed. There was noted to be an improved 5-year disease-free survival of 93% among the radiated patients as compared with 75% among those who were observed. The overall salvage rate for patients who recurred was 64%.

In a separate report from the PORTEC trial, there were 99 evaluable patients with stage IC, grade 3 endometrial cancers. All of these patients were treated with pelvic radiotherapy. The 5-year overall survival for this group was 58%, which is significantly lower than that found by Straughn and colleagues among patients with stage IC disease. It is important to remember that patients in the PORTEC trial did not undergo pelvic and paraaortic lymph node dissection. The difference in survival noted is likely largely due to upstaging of patients with microscopic lymph node metastases in the Straughn series. However, it is important to note that the use of pelvic radiotherapy in the PORTEC trial did not salvage these unstaged patients, again suggesting a therapeutic role for pelvic and paraaortic lymphadenectomy. Because of the higher risk of recurrence among patients with stage IC disease, particularly those with grade 3 disease, these patients are often considered for adjuvant postoperative radiotherapy, even after complete surgical staging.

Pelvic radiotherapy does carry a significant risk of complications. Among the randomized patients in the PORTEC trial, 5-year complication rates were 17% in the radiated patients and 4% in the controls, with all severe complications (3%) occurring in the radiated group.

Patients with pelvic and/or paraaortic lymph node metastases are usually treated with postoperative radiotherapy directed to the involved nodal basins. Nelson and associates reported a 5-year disease-free survival rate of 72% for patients with pelvic lymph node metastases treated with pelvic or whole-abdominal radiotherapy. Rose and coworkers demonstrated improved survival for patients with paraaortic lymph node metastases who were treated with paraaortic radiotherapy as compared with those who were not treated with paraaortic radiation.

The optimum postoperative treatment for patients with *uterine papillary serous carcinoma* remains controversial. Both whole-abdominal radiotherapy and platinum-based chemotherapy have been used. The prognosis for this disease is poor, and adjuvant therapy is often recommended, even for patients with early-stage disease.

Patients stage I or II endometrial cancers who are not surgical candidates because of medical comorbidities are sometimes treated with primary pelvic radiotherapy. In a review of the experience at Yale from 1975 to 1992, 3.5% of all patients with stage I or II endometrial cancer were deemed medically inoperable and treated with pelvic radiotherapy alone. The 5-year disease-specific survival rate for inoperable patients with stage I disease was 80%, which was significantly less than that for operable patients at 98%. Notably, the overall 5-year survival of medically inoperable patients was only 30%, as compared with 88% for operable patients, demonstrating that many of these patients succumb to their intercurrent medical illnesses. Another treatment option for selected medically ill patients is vaginal hysterectomy.

SYSTEMIC THERAPY

Patients with advanced or recurrent endometrial cancer are often treated with *cytotoxic chemotherapy*. A recent GOG trial has demonstrated that for patients with stage III or IV endometrial cancer, chemotherapy with doxorubicin and cisplatin is superior to whole-abdominal radiotherapy. Another GOG trial has demonstrated the superiority of doxorubicin, cisplatin, and paclitaxel (TAP) with filgrastim support over doxorubicin and cisplatin. This multiagent regimen was associated with significant toxicity, including thrombocytopenia, gastrointestinal problems, and neurotoxicity. A current GOG trial compares this regimen with the less toxic combination of carboplatin and paclitaxel.

Hormonal therapy is also an option for patients with advanced-stage disease. Both progestins and tamoxifen have been used. A recent study by Fiorica and coworkers demonstrated a median overall survival of 14 months in patients with advanced endometrial cancer treated with an alternating regimen of megestrol acetate and tamoxifen. Hormonal therapy tends to work best in patients with grade 1 endometrioid adenocarcinomas, which express estrogen and progesterone receptors. Progestational therapy is sometimes used as fertility-conserving surgery in young patients with complex endometrial hyperplasia with atypia or grade I endometrial cancers. Close monitoring is required to assure patients are having an appropriate response. The major side effect of hormonal therapy is thromboembolic disease.

INCIDENTAL DIAGNOSIS OF ENDOMETRIAL CANCER AT HYSTERECTOMY

For patients who undergo hysterectomy and have the unexpected diagnosis of endometrial cancer, there are three options: observation, reoperation for staging, or pelvic radiotherapy. Treatment decisions need to be individualized and will depend on the risk of nodal or extrauterine spread, which may be estimated from the tumor grade, depth of invasion, and evidence of lymphadenopathy on CT of the abdomen and pelvis. The patient's medical status and her willingness to undergo further surgery or radiotherapy must also be taken into account. Consultation with a gynecologic oncologist should be strongly considered.

POSTTREATMENT SURVEILLANCE

The appropriate follow-up for any malignancy is dependent on the pattern of recurrence. This will differ somewhat for type I and type II endometrial cancers. Aalders and associates evaluated 379 patients with recurrent endometrial cancer seen at the Norwegian Radium Hospital between 1960 and 1976. Local recurrence was observed in 50%, distant recurrence was observed in 29%, and both local and distant recurrence was observed in 21%. Patients who had received postoperative pelvic radiotherapy were much less likely to recur in the pelvis. One third of patients were diagnosed with recurrence within 1 year after the completion of therapy, and two thirds of patients were diagnosed with recurrence within 3 years.

There is no single accepted follow-up strategy for patients with endometrial cancer. Physicians have often recommended routine follow-up visits at 3- to 6-month intervals with vaginal cytology at each visit and an annual chest radiograph. Recent studies by multiple groups have demonstrated that this surveillance protocol is neither clinically nor cost effective. These studies demonstrate that 60% to 75% of patients will be symptomatic at the time of recurrence. Most patients with curable recurrences had vaginal bleeding from a vaginal lesion. Curable asymptomatic recurrences were uncommonly detected by routine screening.

Cooper and associates reported that among women with endometrial cancer, 430 Pap tests were required to detect one asymptomatic vaginal recurrence at an additional cost of $15,142 per asymptomatic recurrence detected. Berchuck and colleagues found that the salvage rate for patients with vaginal recurrences diagnosed by vaginal cytology alone was no different than that for women with a visible lesion. They also observed that no patient with an isolated pulmonary recurrence diagnosed by chest radiograph was salvaged. In a similar study from Canada by Shumsky and coworkers, no isolated vaginal recurrence was diagnosed by Pap test alone. Similar to the Duke study, no patient with pulmonary metastases diagnosed by chest x-ray was cured.

Despite the limited ability of routine follow-up to improve the outcomes of women with recurrent endometrial cancer, both patients and their physicians continue to favor some form of posttreatment surveillance. As emphasized by Berchuck and colleagues, continuing to be followed for some period of time by her oncologist and having a normal periodic exam likely provides some psychological reassurance to the patient. The focus should be on detection of vaginal recurrences, because most of these patients can be salvaged. Effective therapy is typically not available for patients who recur at distant sites.

Given these observations, routine surveillance for patients with endometrial cancer should include education of patients regarding the symptoms of recurrence, particularly vaginal bleeding, abdominopelvic or back pain, leg swelling, abdominal bloating, cough, or shortness of breath. Symptomatic patients should be instructed to report promptly for evaluation. The recent ACOG Practice Bulletin on the management of endometrial cancer suggests that women with endometrial cancer be seen in follow-up every 3 to 4 months for 2 to 3 years, then every 6 months. Berchuck and colleagues recommend biannual follow-up visits. Most authors agree that patients can return to routine annual well-woman care after 5 years. Each visit should include a thorough review of systems to evaluate for symptoms of recurrence and a focused physical exam, including lymph node survey, abdominal examination, and pelvic examination with speculum exam, bimanual exam, and rectovaginal exam. Routine surveillance with Pap testing and chest radiographs cannot currently be recommended. Other studies should be obtained as dictated by the findings of the patient's history and physical examination.

Certain groups may require modifications of this follow-up scheme. For example, patients with uterine papillary serous carcinoma are often followed with serial CA-125 determinations, similarly to patients with ovarian cancer. They are much more likely than patients with type I endometrial cancers to recur with peritoneal carcinomatosis. Patients who have been treated with radiation and/or chemotherapy may need more intensive follow-up to monitor them for long-term complications of their therapy. Again, there are no data to suggest that more intensive follow-up results in improved salvage rates.

FUTURE DIRECTIONS

As with all malignancies, the future will see increasing use of molecular staging to identify patients at risk for recurrence. This should allow for greater individualization of therapy. GOG is currently conducting a molecular staging study in endometrial cancer. Laparoscopic and robotic surgical techniques will continue to evolve. Complete lymphadenectomy may decrease in importance if sentinel lymph node techniques can be developed, as in melanoma and breast cancer. Chemotherapy is likely to play an increasing role in the therapy of advanced-stage and recurrent disease.

BEST SURGICAL PRACTICES

- Given that patients with endometrial cancer are often older and have multiple medical comorbidities, preoperative preparation is important. The preoperative history and physical examination should assess both the nature of the patient's presenting symptom and for occult cardiopulmonary and other medical illnesses. For patients with multiple medical comorbidities, preoperative cardiac, pulmonary, and anesthesia consultation should be considered. Extensive preoperative assessment for metastatic disease with CT, MRI, or PET is unnecessary.
- When beginning the hysterectomy, the bilateral uterine cornua are grasped with long Kelly or similar clamps, occluding the fallopian tubes. This allows manipulation of the uterus while preventing efflux of malignant cells via the tubes during the course of the hysterectomy. To avoid contaminating the pelvis with malignant cells from the uterus, a tenaculum, Leahy, or other perforating clamp should not be placed on the uterine fundus.
- In clamping the uterine artery and cardinal ligament pedicles, the clamp should be placed just against the cervix and not "rolled off" the cervix. The practicing of rolling the clamp off the cervix may cause the lateral cervix to be caught in the clamp, with risk of leaving residual cervix (and tumor) behind.
- Pre- and intraoperative assessment of tumor stage and grade have been shown to be inaccurate. Pelvic and paraaortic lymphadenectomy has been shown to have a therapeutic effect in patients with endometrial cancer. The results of full staging may change treatment recommendations in almost one third of patients. Thus, routine pelvic and paraaortic lymph node dissection should be considered for most patients with endometrial cancer. The use of postoperative,

adjuvant pelvic radiotherapy can best be guided by the performance of surgical staging.

- Laparoscopic hysterectomy and staging has been shown to be feasible for patients with endometrial cancer. Studies evaluating the outcomes of patients with endometrial cancer treated with the laparoscopic approach show decreased blood loss, shorter hospital stays, and equivalent recurrence and survival rates as compared with patients who undergo laparotomy.
- Uterine papillary serous carcinoma is a rare and aggressive histologic subtype of uterine cancer. It metastasizes early and often recurs in the upper abdomen with carcinomatosis. Surgical staging of uterine papillary serous carcinomas should be similar to that performed for ovarian cancer and should include hysterectomy, bilateral salpingo-oophorectomy, peritoneal washings, peritoneal biopsies, pelvic and paraortic lymph node dissection, and omentectomy.
- Most patients with recurrent endometrial cancer are symptomatic. Recurrences are rarely diagnosed based on routine studies, such as vaginal cytology or chest radiograph. These studies are not cost-effective. Routine follow-up for patients with endometrial cancer should include education of patients regarding symptoms of recurrence and a thorough history and physical examination—including a pelvic examination with speculum examination, bimanual examination, and rectovaginal examination—every 3 to 4 months for 2 to 3 years, then every 6 months.

Bibliography

Aalders JG, Abeler V, Kolstad P. Recurrent adenocarcinoma of the endometrium: a clinical and histopathological study of 379 patients. *Gynecol Oncol* 1984;17:85.

Amant F, Moerman P, Neven P, et al. Endometrial cancer. *Lancet* 2005;366:491.

Ambros RA, Kurman RJ. Identification of patients with stage I uterine endometrioid adenocarcinoma at high-risk of recurrence by DNA ploidy, myometrial invasion, and vascular invasion. *Gynecol Oncol* 1992;45:235.

American College of Obstetricians and Gynecologists. ACOG practice bulletin number 41: polycystic ovary syndrome. *Int J Gynaecol Obstet* 2003;80:335.

American College of Obstetricians and Gynecologists Committee on Gynecologic Practice. ACOG committee opinion number 336: tamoxifen and uterine cancer. *Obstet Gynecol* 2006;107:1475.

American College of Obstetricians and Gynecologists Committee on Gynecologic Practice. ACOG committee opinion number 337: noncontraceptive uses of the levonorgestrel intrauterine system. *Obstet Gynecol* 2006;107:1479.

American College of Obstetricians and Gynecologists Committee on Gynecologic Practice. ACOG committee opinion number 356: routine cancer screening. *Obstet Gynecol* 2006;108:1611.

American College of Obstetricians and Gynecologists Committee on Practice Bulletins-Gynecology. ACOG practice bulletin number 21: prevention of deep vein thrombosis and pulmonary embolism. *Am Fam Physician* 2001;63:2279.

American College of Obstetricians and Gynecologists Committee on Practice Bulletins-Gynecology. ACOG practice bulletin number 65: management of endometrial cancer. *Obstet Gynecol* 2005;106:413.

American College of Obstetricians and Gynecologists Committee on Practice Bulletins-Gynecology. ACOG practice bulletin number 74: antibiotic prophylaxis for gynecologic procedures. *Obstet Gynecol* 2006;108:225.

Anderson KE, Anderson E, Mink PJ, et al. Diabetes and endometrial cancer in the Iowa women's health study. *Cancer Epidemiol Biomarkers Prev* 2001;10:611.

Armstrong B, Doll R. Environmental factors and cancer incidence and mortality in different countries, with special reference to dietary practices. *Int J Cancer* 1975;15:617.

Ayabe T, Tsutsumi O, Sakai H, et al. Increased circulating levels of insulin-like growth factor-I and decreased circulating levels of insulin-like growth factor binding protein-1 in postmenopausal women with endometrial cancer. *Endocr J* 1997;44:419.

Ayhan A, Taskiran C, Celik C, et al. The long-term survival of women with surgical stage II endometrioid type endometrial cancer. *Gynecol Oncol* 2004;93:9.

Bahamondes L, Ribeiro-Huguet P, de Andrade KC, et al. Levonorgestrel-releasing intrauterine system (Mirena) as a therapy for endometrial hyperplasia and carcinoma. *Acta Obstet Gynecol Scand* 2003;82:580.

Barakat RR, Wong G, Curtin JP, et al. Tamoxifen use in breast cancer patients who subsequently develop corpus cancer is not associated with a higher incidence of adverse histologic features. *Gynecol Oncol* 1994;55:164.

Ben-Shachar I, Pavelka J, Cohn DE, et al. Surgical staging for patients presenting with grade 1 endometrial carcinoma. *Obstet Gynecol* 2005;105:487.

Ben-Yehuda OM, Kim YB, Leuchter RS. Does hysteroscopy improve upon the sensitivity of dilatation and curettage in the diagnosis of endometrial hyperplasia or carcinoma? *Gynecol Oncol* 1998;68:4.

Beral V, Bull D, Reeves G. Million Women Study Collaborators. Endometrial cancer and hormone-replacement therapy in the Million Women Study. *Lancet* 2005;365:1543.

Berchuck A, Anspach C, Evans AC, et al. Postsurgical surveillance of patients with FIGO stage I/II endometrial adenocarcinoma. *Gynecol Oncol* 1995;59:20.

Bokhman JV. Two pathogenetic types of endometrial carcinoma. *Gynecol Oncol* 1983;15:10.

Boronow RC, Morrow CP, Creasman WT, et al. Surgical staging in endometrial cancer: clinical-pathologic findings of a prospective study. *Obstet Gynecol* 1984;63:825.

Brinton LA, Berman ML, Mortel R, et al. Reproductive, menstrual, and medical risk factors for endometrial cancer: results from a case-control study. *Am J Obstet Gynecol* 1992;167:1317.

Bristow RE, Zahurak ML, Alexander CJ, et al. FIGO stage IIIC endometrial carcinoma: resection of macroscopic nodal disease and other determinants of survival. *Int J Gynecol Cancer* 2003;13:664.

Cancer and Steroid Hormone Study Group. Combination oral contraceptive use and the risk of endometrial cancer. The Cancer and Steroid Hormone Study of the Centers for Disease Control and the National Institute of Child Health and Human Development. *JAMA* 1987;257:796.

Castellsague X, Thompson WD, Dubrow R. Intrauterine contraception and the risk of endometrial cancer. *Int J Cancer* 1993;54:911.

Chan JK, Cheung MK, Huh WK, et al. Therapeutic role of lymph node resection in endometrioid corpus cancer: a study of 12,333 patients. *Cancer* 2006;107:823.

Chan JK, Lin YG, Monk BJ, et al. Vaginal hysterectomy as primary treatment of endometrial cancer in medically compromised women. *Obstet Gynecol* 2001;97:707.

Chan JK, Loizzi V, Youssef M, et al. Significance of comprehensive surgical staging in noninvasive papillary serous carcinoma of the endometrium. *Gynecol Oncol* 2003;90:181.

Chi DS, Welshinger M, Venkatraman ES, et al. The role of surgical cytoreduction in stage IV endometrial carcinoma. *Gynecol Oncol* 1997;67:56.

Chuang L, Burke TW, Tornos C, et al. Staging laparotomy for endometrial carcinoma: assessment of retroperitoneal nodes. *Gynecol Oncol* 1995;58: 189.

Clark TJ, Barton PM, Coomarasamy A, et al. Investigating postmenopausal bleeding for endometrial cancer: cost-effectiveness of initial diagnostic strategies. *BJOG* 2006;113:502.

Clarke-Pearson DL, DeLong E, Synan IS, et al. A controlled trial of two low-dose heparin regimens for the prevention of postoperative deep vein thrombosis. *Obstet Gynecol* 1990;75:684.

Clarke-Pearson DL, DeLong ER, Synan IS, et al. Variables associated with postoperative deep venous thrombosis: a prospective study of 411 gynecology patients and creation of a prognostic model. *Obstet Gynecol* 1987;69: 146.

Clarke-Pearson DL, Synan IS, Dodge R, et al. A randomized trial of low-dose heparin and intermittent pneumatic calf compression for the prevention of deep venous thrombosis after gynecologic oncology surgery. *Am J Obstet Gynecol* 1993;168:1146.

Clarke-Pearson DL, Synan IS, Hinshaw WM, et al. Prevention of postoperative venous thromboembolism by external pneumatic calf compression in patients with gynecologic malignancy. *Obstet Gynecol* 1984;63:92.

Clifford SL, Kaminetsky CP, Cirisano FD, et al. Racial disparity in overexpression of the p53 tumor suppressor gene in stage I endometrial cancer. *Am J Obstet Gynecol* 1997;176:S229.

Cooper AL, Dornfield-Finke JM, Banks HW, et al. Is cytologic screening an effective surveillance method for detection of vaginal recurrence of uterine cancer? *Obstet Gynecol* 2006;107:71.

Creasman WT, DeGeest K, DiSaia PJ, et al. Significance of true surgical pathologic staging: a Gynecologic Oncology Group study. *Am J Obstet Gynecol* 1999;181:31.

Creasman WT, Kohler MF, Odicino F, et al. Prognosis of papillary serous, clear cell, and grade 3 stage I carcinoma of the endometrium. *Gynecol Oncol* 2004;95:593.

Creasman WT, Morrow CP, Bundy BN, et al. Surgical pathologic spread patterns of endometrial cancer. A Gynecologic Oncology Group study. *Cancer* 1987;60:2035.

Creasman WT, Odicino F, Maisonneuve P, et al. Carcinoma of the corpus uteri. *J Epidemiol Biostat* 2001;6:45.

Creutzberg CL, van Putten WLJ, Koper PC, et al., for the PORTEC Study Group. The morbidity of treatment for patients with stage I endometrial cancer: results from a randomized trial. *Int J Radiat Oncol Biol Phys* 2001;51:1246.

Creutzberg CL, van Putten WLJ, Warlam-Rodenhuis CC, et al. Outcome of high-risk stage IC, grade 3, compared with stage I endometrial carcinoma patients: the postoperative radiation therapy in endometrial cancer trial. *J Clin Oncol* 2004;22:1234.

Dhar KK, NeedhiRajan T, Koslowski M, et al. Is levonorgestrel intrauterine system effective for treatment of early endometrial cancer? Report of four cases and review of the literature. *Gynecol Oncol* 2005;97:924.

Dijkhulzen FPHLJ, Mol BWJ, Brolmann HAM, et al. Diagnosis of patients with endometrial carcinoma and hyperplasia: a meta-analysis. *Cancer* 2000;89:1765.

Dove-Edwin I, Boks D, Goff S, et al. The outcome of endometrial carcinoma surveillance by ultrasound scan in women at risk of hereditary nonpolyposis colorectal carcinoma and familial colorectal carcinoma. *Cancer* 2002;94:1708.

Early Breast Cancer Trialists' Collaborative Group. Tamoxifen for early breast cancer: an overview of the randomized trials. *Lancet* 1998;351:1451.

Eltabbakh GH. Analysis of survival after laparoscopy in women with endometrial carcinoma. *Cancer* 2002;95:1894.

Eltabbakh GH. Effect of surgeon's experience on the surgical outcome of laparoscopic surgery for women with endometrial cancer. *Gynecol Oncol* 2000;78:58.

Eltabbakh GH, Shamonki MI, Moody JM, et al. Hysterectomy for obese women with endometrial cancer: laparoscopy or laparotomy? *Gynecol Oncol* 2000;78:329.

Eltabbakh GH, Shamonki J, Mount SL. Surgical stage, final grade, and survival of women with endometrial carcinoma whose preoperative endometrial biopsy shows well-differentiated tumors. *Gynecol Oncol* 2005;99:309.

Enriori CL, Reforzo-Membrives J. Peripheral aromatization as a risk factor for breast and endometrial cancer in postmenopausal women: a review. *Gynecol Oncol* 1984;17:1.

Epstein E, Ramirez A, Skoog L, et al. Dilatation and curettage fails to detect most focal lesions in the uterine cavity in women with postmenopausal bleeding. *Acta Obstet Gynecol Scand* 2001;80:1131.

Esteller M, Levine R, Baylin SB, et al. MLH1 promoter hypermethylation is associated with the microsatellite instability phenotype in sporadic endometrial carcinomas. *Oncogene* 1998;17:2413.

Faquin WC, Fitzgerald JT, Boynton KA, et al. Intratumoral genetic heterogeneity and progression of endometrioid type endometrial adenocarcinomas. *Gynecol Oncol* 2000;78:152.

Farrell T, Jones N, Owen P, et al. The significance of an "insufficient" Pipelle sample in the investigation of postmenopausal bleeding. *Acta Obstet Gynecol Scand* 1999;78:810.

Ferguson SE, Olshen AB, Levine DA, et al. Molecular profiling of endometrial cancers from African-American and Caucasian women. *Gynecol Oncol* 2006;101:209.

Fisher B, Costantino JP, Redmond CK, et al. Endometrial cancer in tamoxifen-treated breast cancer patients: findings from the National Surgical Adjuvant Breast and Bowel Project (NSABP) B-14. *J Natl Cancer Inst* 1994;86:527.

Fishman DA, Roberts KB, Chambers JT, et al. Radiation therapy as exclusive treatment for medically inoperable patients with stage I and II endometrioid carcinoma of the endometrium. *Gynecol Oncol* 1996;61:189.

Fleming GF, Burnetto VL, Cella D, et al. Phase III trail of doxorubicin plus cisplatin with or without paclitaxel plus filgrastim in advanced endometrial carcinoma: a Gynecologic Oncology Group study. *J Clin Oncol* 2004;22:2159.

Frumovitz M, Singh DK, Meyer L, et al. Predictors of final histology in patients with endometrial cancer. *Gynecol Oncol* 2004;95:463.

Frumovitz M, Slomovitz BM, Singh DK, et al. Frozen section analyses as predictors of lymphatic spread in patients with early stage uterine cancer. *J Am Coll Surg* 2004;199:388.

Furberg AS, Thune I. Metabolic abnormalities (hypertension, hyperglycemia and overweight), lifestyle (high energy intake and physical inactivity) and endometrial cancer risk in a Norwegian cohort. *Int J Cancer* 2003;104:669.

Gal D, Edman CD, Vellios F, et al. Long-term effect of megestrol acetate in the treatment of endometrial hyperplasia. *Am J Obstet Gynecol* 1983;146:316.

Gal D, Recio FO, Zamurovic D, et al. Lymphovascular space involvement—a prognostic indicator in endometrial cancer. *Gynecol Oncol* 1991;42:142.

Gemignani ML, Curtin JP, Zelmanovich J, et al. Laparoscopic-assisted vaginal hysterectomy for endometrial cancer: clinical outcomes and hospital charges. *Gynecol Oncol* 1999;73:5.

Goodman MT, Hankin JH, Wilkens LR, et al. Diet, body size, physical activity, and the risk of endometrial cancer. *Cancer Res* 1997;57:5077.

Goodman M, Wilkens LR, Hankin JH, et al. Association of soy and fiber consumption with the risk of endometrial cancer. *Am J Epidemiol* 1997;146:294.

Goff BA, Goodman A, Muntz HG, et al. Surgical stage IV endometrial carcinoma: a study of 47 cases. *Gynecol Oncol* 1994;52:237.

Goff BA, Kato D, Schmidt RA, et al. Uterine papillary serous carcinoma: patterns of metastatic spread. *Gynecol Oncol* 1994;54:264.

Goss PE. Emerging role of aromatase inhibitors in the adjuvant setting. *Am J Clin Oncol* 2003;26:S27.

Grady D, Gebretsadik T, Kerlikowske K, et al. Hormone replacement therapy and endometrial cancer risk: a meta-analysis. *Obstet Gynecol* 1995;85:304.

Granberg S, Wikland M, Karlsson B, et al. Endometrial stripe thickness as measured by endovaginal ultrasonography for identifying endometrial abnormality. *Am J Obstet Gynecol* 1991;164:47.

Gredmark T, Kvint S, Havel G, et al. Histopathological findings in women with postmenopausal bleeding. *BJOG* 1995;102:133.

Gupta JK, Chien PF, Voit D, et al. Ultrasonographic endometrial thickness for diagnosing endometrial pathology in women with postmenopausal bleeding: a meta-analysis. *Acta Obstet Gynecol Scand* 2002;81:799.

Hecht JL, Mutter GL. Molecular and pathologic aspects of endometrial carcinogenesis. *J Clin Oncol* 2006;24:4783.

Hendrickson MR, Ross J, Eifel P, et al. Uterine papillary serous carcinoma: a highly malignant form of endometrial adenocarcinoma. *Am J Surg Pathol* 1982;6:93.

Hicks ML, Phillips JL, Parham G, et al. The National Cancer Data Base report on endometrial carcinoma in African-American women. *Cancer* 1998;83:2629.

Hill DA, Weiss NS, Voigt LF, et al. Endometrial cancer in relation to intra-uterine device use. *Int J Cancer* 1997;70:278.

Hold I, Salimtschick M, Mouridsen HT. Tamoxifen treatment of advanced endometrial carcinoma. *Eur J Gynaecol Oncol* 1983;4:83.

Holub Z, Bartos P, Dorr A, et al. The role of laparoscopic hysterectomy and lymph node dissection in the treatment of endometrial cancer. *Eur J Gynaecol Oncol* 1999;20:268.

Holub Z, Jabor A, Bartos P, et al. Laparoscopic surgery for endometrial cancer: long-term results of a mulitcentric study. *Eur J Gynaecol Oncol* 2002;23:305.

Holub Z, Jabor A, Bartos P, et al. Laparoscopic surgery in women with endometrial cancer: the learning curve. *Eur J Obstet Gynecol Reprod Biol* 2003;107:195.

Homesley HD, Kadar N, Barrett RJ, et al. Selective pelvic and periaortic lymphadenectomy does not increase morbidity in surgical staging of endometrial cancer. *Am J Obstet Gynecol* 1992;167:1225.

Horn-Ross PL, John EM, Canchola AJ, et al. Phytoestrogens and endometrial cancer risk. *J Natl Cancer Inst* 2003;95:1158.

Hubacher D, Grimes DA. Noncontraceptive health benefits of intrauterine devices: a systematic review. *Obstet Gynecol Surv* 2002;57:120.

Hulka BS, Fowler WC Jr, Kaufman DG, et al. Estrogen and endometrial cancer: cases and two control groups from North Carolina. *Am J Obstet Gynecol* 1980;137:92.

Janda M, Gebski V, Forder P, et al. , LACE Trial Committee. Total laparoscopic versus open surgery for stage 1 endometrial cancer: the LACE randomized controlled trial. *Contemp Clin Trials* 2006;27:353.

Jemal A, Siegel R, Ward E, et al. Cancer Statistics, 2006. *CA Cancer J Clin* 2006;56:106.

Kasamatusu T, Onda T, Katsumata N, et al. Prognostic significance of positive peritoneal cytology in endometrial carcinoma confined to the uterus. *Br J Cancer* 2003;88:245.

Kelsey JL, Livolsi VA, Holford TR, et al. A case-control study of cancer of the endometrium. *Am J Epidemiol* 1982;116:333.

Kilgore LC, Partridge EE, Alvarez RD, et al. Adenocarcinoma of the endometrium: survival comparisons of patients with and without pelvic node sampling. *Gynecol Oncol* 1995;56:29.

Kodama S, Kase H, Tanaka K, et al. Multivariate analysis of prognostic factors in patients with endometrial cancer. *Int J Gynaecol Obstet* 1996;53:23.

Kornblith A, Walker J, Huang H, et al. Quality of life of patients in a randomized clinical trial of laparoscopy (scope) vs open laparotomy (open) for the surgical resection and staging of uterine cancer: a Gynecologic Oncology Group study. *Gynecol Oncol* 2006;101:S22(abst).

Kosary CL. FIGO stage, histology, histologic grade, age, and race as prognostic factors in determining survival for cancers of the female gynaecological system: an analysis of 1973-87 SEER cases of cancers of the endometrium, cervix, ovary, vulva, and vagina. *Semin Surg Oncol* 1994;10:31.

Kuoppala T, Tomas E, Heinonen PK. Clinical outcome and complications of laparoscopic surgery compared with traditional surgery in women with endometrial cancer. *Arch Gynecol Obstet* 2004;270:25.

Kurman RJ, Kaminski PF, Norris HJ. The behavior of endometrial hyperplasia: a long-term study of "untreated" hyperplasia in 170 patients. *Cancer* 1985;56:403.

Lambrou NC, Gomez-Marin O, Mirhashemi R, et al. Optimal surgical cytoreduction in patients with stage III and stage IV endometrial carcinoma: a study of morbidity and survival. *Gynecol Oncol* 2004;93:653.

Lentz SS, Brady MF, Major FJ, et al. High-dose megestrol acetate in advanced or recurrent endometrial carcinoma: a Gynecologic Oncology Group study. *J Clin Oncol* 1996;14:357.

Lesko SM, Rosenberg L, Kaufman DW, et al. Cigarette smoking and the risk of endometrial cancer. *N Engl J Med* 1985;313:593.

Lu KH, Broaddus RR. Gynecologic cancers in Lynch syndrome/HNPCC. *Fam Cancer* 2005;4:249.

Lu KH, Dinh M, Kohlmann W, et al. Gynecologic cancer as a "sentinel cancer" for women with hereditary nonpolyposis colorectal cancer syndrome. *Obstet Gynecol* 2005;105:569.

Lutman CV, Havrilesky LJ, Cragun JM, et al. Pelvic lymph node count is an important prognostic variable for FIGO stage I and II endometrial carcinoma with high-risk histology. *Gynecol Oncol* 2006;102:92.

Magrina JF. Outcomes of laparoscopic treatment for endometrial cancer. *Curr Opin Obstet Gynecol* 2005;17:343.

Magrina JF, Weaver AL. Laparoscopic treatment of endometrial cancer: five-year recurrence and survival rates. *Eur J Gynaecol Oncol* 2004;25:439.

Mansell H, Hertig AT. Granulosatheca cell tumors and endometrial carcinoma; a study of their relationship and a survey of 80 cases. *Obstet Gynecol* 1955;6:385.

Matias-Guiu X, Catasus L, Bussaglia E, et al. Molecular pathology of endometrial hyperplasia and carcinoma. *Hum Pathol* 2001;32:569.

Maxwell GL, Synan I, Dodge R, et al. Pneumatic compression versus low molecular weight heparin in gynecologic oncology surgery: a randomized trial. *Obstet Gynecol* 2001;98:989.

Maxwell GL, Tian C, Risinger J, et al. Racial disparity in survival among patients with advanced/recurrent endometrial adenocarcinoma: a Gynecologic Oncology Group study. *Cancer* 2006;107:2197.

Montz FJ, Bristow RE, Bovicellia A, et al. Intrauterine progesterone treatment of early endometrial cancer. *Am J Obstet Gynecol* 2002;186:651.

Moodley M, Roberts C. Clinical pathway for the evaluation of postmenopausal bleeding with an emphasis on endometrial cancer detection. *J Obstet Gynaecol* 2004;24:736.

Moradi T, Weiderpass E, Signorello LB, et al. Physical activity and postmenopausal cancer risk (Sweden). *Cancer Causes Control* 2000;11:829.

Morrow CP, Bundy B, Kurman R, et al. Relationship between surgical-pathological risk factors and outcome in clinical stages I and II carcinoma of the endometrium: a Gynecologic Oncology Group Study. *Gynecol Oncol* 1991;40:55.

Nelson G, Randall M, Sutton G, et al. FIGO stage IIIC endometrial carcinoma with metastases confined to pelvic lymph nodes: analysis of treatment outcomes, prognostic variables, and failure patterns following adjuvant radiation therapy. *Gynecol Oncol* 1999;75:211.

Obermair A, Manolitsas TP, Leung Y, et al. Total laparoscopic hysterectomy for endometrial cancer: patterns of recurrence and survival. *Gynecol Oncol* 2004;92:789.

Okaro E, Bourne T. Sporadic abnormal vaginal bleeding (intermenstrual, postcoital and postmenopausal bleeding). *Curr Opin Obstet Gynaecol* 2002;12:334.

Parazzini F, La Vecchia C, Moroni S. Intrauterine device use and risk of endometrial cancer. *Br J Cancer* 1994;70:672.

Parazzini F, LaVecchia C, Negri E, et al. Diabetes and endometrial cancer: an Italian case-control study. *Int J Cancer* 1999;81:539.

Parslov M, Lidegaard O, Klintorp S, et al. Risk factors among young women with endometrial cancer: a Danish case-control study. *Am J Obstet Gynecol* 2000;182:23.

Pillay OC, Te Fong LF, Crow JC, et al. The association between polycystic ovaries and endometrial cancer. *Hum Reprod* 2006;21:924.

Purdie DM, Green AC. Epidemiology of endometrial cancer. *Best Pract Res Clin Obstet Gynaecol* 2001;15:341.

Querleu D, Leblanc E, Cartron G, et al. Audit of preoperative and early complications of laparoscopic node dissection in 1000 gynecologic cancer patients. *Am J Obstet Gynecol* 2006;195:1287.

Quinn MA, Campbell JJ. Tamoxifen therapy in advanced/recurrent endometrial carcinoma. *Gynecol Oncol* 1989;32:1.

Randall ME, Filiaci VL, Muss H, et al. Randomized phase III trial of whole-abdominal irradiation versus doxorubicin and cisplatin chemotherapy in advanced endometrial carcinoma: a Gynecologic Oncology Group Study. *J Clin Oncol* 2006;24:36.

Randall TC, Armstrong K. Differences in treatment and outcome between African-American and white women with endometrial cancer. *J Clin Oncol* 2003;21:4200.

Randall TC, Kurman RJ. Progestin treatment of atypical hyperplasia and well-differentiated carcinoma of the endometrium in women under age 40. *Obstet Gynecol* 1997;90:434.

Reed SD, Voigt LF, Beresford SA, et al. Dose of progestin in postmenopausal-combined hormone therapy and risk of endometrial cancer. *Am J Obstet Gynecol* 2004;191:1146.

Reisinger SA, Staros, EF, Feld R, et al. Preoperative radiation therapy in clinical stage II endometrial carcinoma. *Gynecol Oncol* 1992;45:174.

Revel A, Tsafrir A, Anteby SO, et al. Does hysteroscopy produce intraperitoneal spread of endometrial cancer cells? *Obstet Gynecol Surv* 2004;59:280.

Rijcken FEM, Mourits MJE, Kleibeuker JH, et al. Gynecologic screening in hereditary nonpolyposis colorectal cancer. *Gynecol Oncol* 2003;91:74.

Rose PG, Cha SD, Tak WK, et al. Radiation therapy for surgically proven para-aortic node metastasis in endometrial cancer. *Int J Radiat Oncol Biol Phys* 1992;24:229.

Rosenblatt KA, Thomas DB. Intrauterine devices and endometrial cancer. The WHO Collaborative Study of Neoplasia and Steroid Contraceptives. *Contraception* 1996;54:329.

Rubatt JM, Slomovitz BM, Burke TW, et al. Development of metastatic endometrial endometrioid adenocarcinoma while on progestin therapy for endometrial hyperplasia. *Gynecol Oncol* 2005;99:472.

Salazar-Martinez E, Lazcano-Ponce EC, Gonzalez Lira-Lira G, et al. Reproductive factors of ovarian and endometrial cancer risk in a high fertility population in Mexico. *Cancer Res* 1999;59:3658.

Sartori E, Gadducci A, Landoni F, et al. Clinical behavior of 203 stage II endometrial cancer cases: the impact of primary surgical approach and of adjuvant radiation therapy. *Int J Gynecol Cancer* 2001;11:430.

Schimp VL, Ali-Fehmi R, Soloman LA, et al. The racial disparity in outcomes in endometrial cancer: could this be explained on a molecular level? *Gynecol Oncol* 2006;102:440.

Scholten AN, van Putten WLJ, Beerman H, et al., for the PORTEC Study Group. Postoperative radiotherapy for stage I endometrial carcinoma: long-term outcome of the randomized PORTEC trial with central pathology review. *Int J Radiat Oncol Biol Phys* 2005;63:834.

Scribner DR Jr, Mannel RS, Walker JL, et al. Cost analysis of laparoscopy versus laparotomy for early endometrial cancer. *Gynecol Oncol* 1999;75:460.

Scribner DR Jr, Walker JL, Johnson GA, et al. Laparoscopic pelvic and paraaortic lymph node dissection in the obese. *Gynecol Oncol* 2002;84:426.

Scribner DR Jr, Walker JL, Johnson GA, et al. Surgical management of early-stage endometrial cancer in the elderly: is laparoscopy feasible? *Gynecol Oncol* 2001;83:563.

Shapiro S, Kelly JP, Rosenberg L, et al. Risk of localized and widespread endometrial cancer in relation to recent and discontinued use of conjugated estrogens. *New Engl J Med* 1985;313:969.

Sherman ME, Bur ME, Kurman RJ. p53 in endometrial cancer and its putative precursors: evidence for diverse pathways of tumorigenesis. *Hum Pathol* 1995;26:1268.

Shumsky AG, Stuart GCE, Brasher PM, et al. An evaluation of routine follow-up for patients treated for endometrial carcinoma. *Gynecol Oncol* 1994;55:229.

Smith RA, Cokkinides V, Eyre HJ. American Cancer Society guidelines for the early detection of cancer, 2006. *CA Cancer J Clin* 2006;56:11.

Soler M, Shatenoud L, Negri E, et al. Hypertension and hormone-related neoplasms in women. *Hypertension* 1999;34:320.

Spirtos NM, Schlaerth JB, Gross GM, et al. Cost and quality-of-life analyses of surgery for early endometrial cancer: laparotomy versus laparoscopy. *Am J Obstet Gynecol* 1996;174:1795.

Stock RJ, Kanbour A. Prehysterectomy curettage. *Obstet Gynecol* 1975;45:537.

Stovall TG, Soloman SK, Ling FW. Endometrial sampling prior to hysterectomy. *Obstet Gynecol* 1989;73:405.

Straughn JM Jr, Huh WK, Kelly FJ, et al. Conservative management of stage I endometrial carcinoma after surgical staging. *Gynecol Oncol* 2001;84:194.

Straughn JM Jr, Huh WK, Orr JW, et al. Stage IC adenocarcinoma of the endometrium: survival comparisons of surgically staged patients with and without adjuvant therapy. *Gynecol Oncol* 2003;89:295.

Sturgeon SR, Brinton LA, Berman ML, et al. Intrauterine device use and endometrial cancer risk. *Int J Epidemiol* 1997;26:496.

Surveillance, Epidemiology and End Results (SEER) Program (www.seer.cancer.gov). SEER*Stat Database: Incidence-SEER 17 Regs Public Use, Nov 2005 Sub (1973-2003 varying), National Cancer Institute, DCCPS, Surveillance Research Program, Cancer Statistics Branch, released April 2006, based on the November 2005 submission.

Takeshima N, Nishida H, Tabata T, et al. Positive peritoneal cytology in endometrial cancer: enhancement of other prognostic indicators. *Gynecol Oncol* 2001;82:470.

Tao MH, Xu WH, Zheng W, et al. Oral contraceptive and IUD use and endometrial cancer: a population-based case-control study in Shanghai, China. *Int J Cancer* 2006;119:2142.

Terry PD, Rohan TE, Franceschi S, et al. Cigarette smoking and the risk of endometrial cancer. *Lancet Oncol* 2002;3:470.

Torrejon R, Fernandez-Alba JJ, Carnicer I, et al. The value of hysteroscopic exploration for abnormal uterine bleeding. *J Am Assoc Gynecol Laparosc* 1997;4:453.

Trimble CL, Kauderer J, Zaino R, et al. Concurrent endometrial carcinoma in women with a biopsy diagnosis of atypical endometrial hyperplasia: a Gynecologic Oncology Group study. *Cancer* 2006;106:812.

Viswanathan AN, Feskanich D, De Vivo I, et al. Smoking and the risk of endometrial cancer: results from the Nurses' Health Study. *Int J Cancer* 2005;114:996.

Walker JL, Mannel R, Piedmonte M, et al. Phase III trial of laparoscopy versus laparotomy for surgical resection and comprehensive surgical staging of uterine cancer: a Gynecologic Oncology Group study. *Gynecol Oncol* 2006;101:S11(abst).

Weiderpass E, Adami HO, Baron JA, et al. Risk of endometrial cancer following estrogen replacement with and without progestins. *J Natl Cancer Inst* 1999;91:1131.

Weiderpass E, Persson I, Adami HO, et al. Body size in different periods of life, diabetes mellitus, hypertension, and risk of postmenopausal endometrial cancer (Sweden). *Cancer Causes Control* 2000;11:185.

Weiss NS, Farewall VT, Szekely DR, et al. Oestrogens and endometrial cancer: effect of other risk factors on the association. *Maturitas* 1980;2:185.

Wickerham DL, Fisher B, Wolmark N, et al. Association of tamoxifen and uterine sarcoma. *J Clin Oncol* 2002;20:2758.

Wildemeersch D, Dhont M. Treatment of nonatypical and atypical endometrial hyperplasia with a levonorgestrel-releasing intrauterine system. *Am J Obstet Gynecol* 2003;188:1297.

Wood GP, Boronow RC. Endometrial adenocarcinoma and the polycystic ovary syndrome. *Am J Obstet Gynecol* 1976;124:140.

Word B, Gravlee LC, Wideman GL. The fallacy of simple uterine curettage. *Obstet Gynecol* 1958;12:642.

CHAPTER 49 ■ OVARIAN CANCER: ETIOLOGY, SCREENING, AND SURGERY

JOHN R. VAN NAGELL JR. AND DAVID M. GERSHENSON

DEFINITIONS

BRCA 1 gene—A tumor suppressor gene located on the long (q) arm of chromosome 17. Germline mutations in this gene are responsible for 80% to 90% of hereditary ovarian cancers.

BRCA 2 gene—A tumor suppressor gene located on the long (q) arm of chromosome 13. Germline mutations in this gene are responsible for 15% of hereditary cancers.

Genetic penetrance—The frequency with which patients with a known genetic abnormality demonstrate a phenotypic abnormality.

Hereditary breast–ovarian cancer syndrome (HBOC)—A syndrome characterized by multiple cases of early-onset (<50 years of age) breast and ovarian cancers. It is the most common of the familial ovarian cancer syndromes, making up 75% to 90% of all hereditary ovarian cancers.

Hereditary nonpolyposis colon cancer syndrome (HNPCC) or Lynch II syndrome—A syndrome characterized by early-onset (<50 years of age) proximal colon cancer associated with cancers of the ovary and endometrium. It is caused by a mutation in one of several mismatch repair, most commonly MLH1 and MSH2. It makes up approximately 5% to 10% of all hereditary ovarian cancers.

Hereditary site-specific ovarian cancer syndrome (HSSOC)—A syndrome characterized by multiple cases of early-onset (<50 years of age) ovarian cancer. It makes up approximately 5% of all hereditary ovarian cancers.

Intraperitoneal chemotherapy—Cytotoxic chemotherapy given intraperitoneally rather than intravenously. This is usually given via an intraperitoneal catheter in patients who have undergone optimal cytoreductive surgery.

Neoadjuvant chemotherapy—Chemotherapy given before definitive surgery to chemically debulk cancer with the intention of making future surgical efforts more successful and less complicated. Usually, several cycles of chemotherapy are given to women with advanced ovarian cancer who are poor surgical candidates because of their medical condition or perhaps the extent of disease. At the start of therapy, surgical debulking is planned if there is a response to chemotherapy, although surgery may not occur if the patient does not respond to chemotherapy or her medical condition fails to improve.

Optimal cytoreduction—Survival is related to the volume of residual cancer after initial surgery. It is preferable to remove as much tumor as possible. The definition of *optimal cytoreduction* has continued to change over the years and currently means surgical debulking so that the largest residual tumor mass is less than 1.0 or even 0.5 cm in diameter.

Ovarian tumor morphology indexing—A quantitative analysis relating tumor morphology from sonographically generated images to risk of malignancy.

Proteomics—Analysis of the expression, localization, function, and interaction of the proteins expressed by the genetic material of an organism.

Ovarian cancer is the leading cause of death from gynecologic malignancies in the United States. In 2006, more than 20,000 new cases of ovarian cancer was detected and more than 15,000 women would die from the disease. The lifetime risk for ovarian cancer in American women without a family history of the disease is 1 in 70 (1.4%). Because early ovarian cancer produces few specific symptoms, most women present with advanced-stage disease, for which the cost of treatment is high and the prognosis poor. Approximately 90% of malignant ovarian tumors in adults are of epithelial origin followed by sex cord–stromal tumors (6%) and germ-cell tumors (3%). Good surgery is a blend of good judgment and sound surgical technique. Much of this chapter is devoted to the natural history and results of various surgical and other treatment approaches for ovarian cancer. This background information provides the surgeon with the basis for clinical decision making concerning patient selection, choice of the right operation, and postoperative treatment recommendations. The operative techniques involved in surgery for ovarian cancer are illustrated in many of the other chapters in this text.

INCIDENCE AND RISK FACTORS

The incidence of ovarian cancer is highest in Sweden (19.6/100,000) and the United States (15.4/100,000), and lowest in Japan (10.1/100,000). In the United States, ovarian cancer incidence rates are highest in Caucasian women, intermediate in African American women, and lowest in Native American women.

Factors associated with an increase in ovarian cancer risk are age, nulliparity, and a family history of the disease. Ovarian cancer is rare before the age of 40, increases steadily thereafter, and peaks at ages 65 to 75. Parity is the most important nongenetic factor affecting risk for ovarian cancer (Table 49.1). Whittimore and colleagues analyzed 12 case-controlled studies in the United States and reported a significant risk reduction for ovarian cancer with each term pregnancy (odds ratio [OR] = 0.47). The risk of ovarian cancer decreased progressively with increasing numbers of pregnancies. Similarly, the use of oral contraceptives has been shown to reduce the risk of ovarian cancer. Ovarian cancer risk decreases approximately 11% per year of oral contraceptive use to a maximum of 46% after 5 years of use. These observations have led to the theory of "incessant ovulation" in the etiology of ovarian cancer.

TABLE 49.1

RISK FACTORS FOR OVARIAN CANCER

Factor	Odds ratio
Parity[a]	
Nulliparous	1.0
Parous	0.47
Oral contraceptive use[b]	
Never	1.0
2–5 years	0.73
Estrogen use[b]	
Never	1.0[c]
Ever	1.4
Clomid use[d]	
No	1.0
Yes	2.3
Tubal ligation[a]	
No	1.0
Yes	0.59
Hysterectomy[a]	
No	1.0
Yes	0.66
Talc use[e]	
No	1.0
Yes	1.5
Breast-feeding[a]	
No	1.0
Yes	0.73
Family History[f]	
1 first-degree relative with ovarian cancer	3.1
>2 first-degree relatives with ovarian cancer	4.6

[a]Whittemore AS, Harris R, Itnyre J. Collaborative Ovarian Cancer Group: characteristics relating to ovarian cancer risk, collaborative analysis of 12 U.S. case-control studies. II. Invasive epithelial ovarian cancers in white women. *Am J Epidemiol* 1992;136:1184.
[b]Riman T, Dickman PW, Nilsson S, et al. Hormone replacement therapy and the risk of invasive epithelial ovarian cancer in Swedish women. *J Natl Cancer Inst* 2002;94:497.
[c]Not significant.
[d]Rossing MA, Daling JR, Weiss NS, et al. Ovarian tumors in a cohort of infertile women. *N Engl J Med* 1994;331:771.
[e]Cook LS, Kamb ML, Weiss NS. Perineal powder exposure and risk of ovarian cancer. *Am J Epidemiol* 1997;145:459.
[f]Kerlikowske K, Brown JS, Grady DG. Should women with familial ovarian cancer undergo prophylactic oophorectomy? *Obstet Gynecol* 1992;80:700.

According to this theory, risk for epithelial ovarian cancer is related directly to the number of uninterrupted ovulatory cycles. With ovulation, the surface epithelium is ruptured and then undergoes rapid proliferation and repair. At the time of ovulation, there is invagination of the surface epithelium into the underlying stroma forming inclusion cysts. The epithelium lining these inclusion cysts then undergoes neoplastic transformation under the influence of oncogenic factors. The observation that early age of menarche and late menopause are associated with an increase in ovarian cancer risk is consistent with this theory, because both increase the number of ovulatory cycles.

A second theory of ovarian carcinogenesis is the retrograde menstruation hypothesis. According to this hypothesis, retrograde transportation of carcinogens from the uterus and lower genital tract through the fallopian tube to the ovary occurs at the time of menstruation. The protective effect of oral contraceptives is consistent with this hypothesis, because their use has been associated with a reduction in menstrual blood loss and therefore with decreased retrograde menstruation. Conversely, the observed increase in ovarian cancer risk associated with hormone replacement therapy (Table 49.1) may be mediated through the periods of abnormal uterine bleeding that occur with many hormonal regimens. This hypothesis is also supported by the known decrease in ovarian cancer risk in women who have undergone tubal ligation or hysterectomy, because these procedures prevent the ascent of potential oncogenic factors from the lower genital tract to the ovary.

A final hypothesis concerning the genesis of ovarian cancer is that exposure of ovarian epithelium to persistently high levels of pituitary gonadotropins results in neoplastic transformation. Follicle-stimulating hormone (FSH) has been shown to promote the growth of epithelial ovarian cancer cells *in vitro,* and this effect can be blocked by luteinizing hormone (LH). A corollary to this hypothesis is that elevated circulating gonadotropin levels promote estrogen biosynthesis in the ovarian stroma, which, in turn, causes abnormal proliferation of the adjacent epithelium. Breast-feeding, which has been reported to lower the risk of ovarian cancer, is associated with reduced serum concentrations of LH and estradiol. Pregnancy and the use of oral contraceptives presumably lower the risk of ovarian cancer by inhibiting pituitary secretion of gonadotropins. This theory also receives support from the observed increased risk of ovarian cancer in women taking fertility drugs because these drugs stimulate ovulation by increasing levels of FSH, particularly in the follicular phase of the cycle.

Perhaps the most important risk factor for epithelial ovarian cancer is a family history of the disease. The estimated odds ratio for the development of ovarian cancer in a woman with one first-degree relative who has ovarian cancer is 3.1 (95% CI = 2.1–4.5). This risk increases even further (OR 4.6 CI = 1.1–18.4) in a woman with two or more primary or secondary relatives who have ovarian cancer. These odds ratios translate to a lifetime risk for ovarian cancer of approximately 5% in a woman with one first-degree relative who has the disease and 7% in a woman with two or more relatives with the disease. It should be mentioned, however, that familial ovarian cancers make up a relatively small proportion of total ovarian cancer cases. Only 5% to 10% of ovarian cancer patients report having a positive family history of the disease.

Three familial ovarian cancer syndromes have been described. Hereditary breast–ovarian cancer syndrome (HBOC), hereditary site-specific ovarian cancer syndrome (HSSOC), and the hereditary nonpolyposis colon cancer syndrome (HNPCC). HBOC, the most common of the familial syndromes, is characterized by multiple cases of early-onset (<50 years of age) breast and ovarian cancers. This syndrome accounts for 75% to 90% of all hereditary ovarian cancer cases. HSSOC is manifested only by an increase in cases of early-onset ovarian cancer and makes up about 5% of hereditary ovarian cancers. Women with HSSOC are often younger and more commonly have tumors with serous histology than women with sporadic ovarian cancer. HNPCC, or Lynch syndrome type II, is characterized by a predominance of early-onset proximal colon cancer in association with cancers of the endometrium and ovary. HNPCC is often confirmed by a mutation in one of several mismatch-repair genes, in particular MLH1, MSH2, and MSH6. The estimated lifetime risk of ovarian cancer in women with HNPCC is 10% to 12%. These three familial ovarian cancer syndromes are inherited by autosomal dominant transmission through either maternal or paternal lineage. Therefore, the children of an affected parent have a 50% risk of inheriting the genetic abnormality.

Germline mutations in the BRCA1 or BRCA2 gene appear to account for most hereditary ovarian cancers. BRCA1 was identified in 1994 and is located on the long (q) arm of chromosome 17. BRCA1 is thought to be a tumor suppressor, because the normal copy of BRCA1 is always deleted in ovarian cancers that arise in women who inherit a mutant BRCA1 gene. It is estimated that germline mutations in BRCA1 are responsible for 80% to 90% of hereditary ovarian cancers. BRCA2 was identified in 1995 and is located on the long (q) arm of chromosome 13. In a recent report from the Breast Cancer Linkage Consortium, BRCA1 mutations were identified in 81% of ovarian cancer families, whereas BRCA2 mutations were detected in 14% of those families. Penetrance is variable (range 10%–50%) from one individual to another, and it is estimated that the lifetime risk of ovarian cancer is approximately 39% in BRCA1 carriers and 11% in BRCA2 carriers.

SIGNS AND SYMPTOMS

Although most reports indicate that patients with early-stage ovarian cancer have few symptoms, a recent national survey of 1,725 ovarian cancer patients provides evidence that many of these patients actually had symptoms that they or their primary health providers ignored. The most common symptoms of patients with stage I or II ovarian cancer were abdominal bloating or pain, indigestion, urinary frequency, and constipation. Because many of these symptoms are nonspecific, patients were unaware that they could be associated with ovarian cancer. As a result, 22% of patients ignored their symptoms entirely, and 30% reported that the wrong diagnosis was made. A pelvic examination was performed in only two thirds of patients, and 45% had a delay in diagnosis of more than 3 months. Patients with advanced disease commonly reported abdominal swelling, fatigue, and weight loss. In a subsequent study, four target symptoms were significantly more common in ovarian cancer patients before diagnosis than in age-matched control patients. These symptoms included abdominal pain (frequency 30%, OR 6.0), abdominal swelling (frequency 16.5%, OR 30), gastrointestinal symptoms (frequency 8.5%, OR 2.3), and pelvic pain (frequency 5.4%, OR 4.3). These observations emphasize the need for patient and physician education concerning the possible relationship of rather nonspecific abdominal symptoms to ovarian cancer. A high index of suspicion, coupled with pelvic ultrasound and CA-125 testing, may lead to the earlier diagnosis of ovarian cancer in selected patients with these symptoms.

Although vaginal bleeding is not commonly associated with ovarian cancer, it may be present in patients with metastatic involvement of the uterus. Likewise, endometrial hyperplasia and abnormal uterine bleeding can be caused by excess estrogen production from an ovarian stromal tumor. Ovarian cancer must be considered in a patient who presents with a pelvic mass and shortness of breath. A malignant pleural effusion from metastatic ovarian cancer is more common on the right side and is usually associated with dullness to percussion and decreased breath sounds. Finally, any patient with a clinically detected pelvic tumor on pelvic examination should undergo careful palpation of both groins to rule out inguinal lymphadenopathy secondary to metastatic disease.

EARLY DETECTION

It is now well documented that pelvic examination is inaccurate in assessing ovarian size, particularly in women who are postmenopausal or overweight. Most patients with ovarian cancer present with advanced disease, when survival is limited. As a result, there has been little improvement in overall prognosis of patients with ovarian cancer over the past 2 decades. According to data from the Surveillance, Epidemiology, and End Results (SEER) program database, the ovarian cancer mortality rate has decreased only from 9.3/100,000 in 1989 to 9.0/100,000 in 2002. Recent efforts to increase early detection of ovarian cancer have focused on screening asymptomatic women to detect ovarian cancer when it is still curable.

For screening to be effective, a disease should (a) be a major cause of mortality, (b) have a reasonably high prevalence in the screened population, (c) have a preclinical phase detectable by the screening test, and (d) be amenable to therapy, such that the survival rate of patients with early-stage disease is significantly higher than that of patients with advanced disease.

Ovarian cancer fulfills many of the prerequisites of a disease that should benefit from screening. First, it is a major cause of mortality in our population. As has been previously mentioned, more than 15,000 patients would die of ovarian cancer in the United States in 2006, making it the fourth most common cause of cancer death in American women. Although the prevalence of ovarian cancer in the general population is not high, it is more common in older women. According to SEER data, the incidence of ovarian cancer is age related and varies from approximately 20/100,000 in women from 40 to 50 years of age to 50/100,000 in women 60 to 70 years. It is even higher in women with a family history of the disease.

Knowledge concerning the duration of the preclinical phase of ovarian cancer is limited at best. Histologic transition from benign to borderline or malignant epithelium has been identified by light and electron microscopy in ovarian mucinous and serous cystadenocarcinomas. Likewise, transition from endometriosis to endometrioid ovarian carcinoma has been documented. These studies suggest that with time, certain benign ovarian tumors may undergo malignant transformation. Unfortunately, the frequency with which neoplastic transformation occurs in these tumors is unknown and is probably rare. Theoretically, the identification and removal of premalignant ovarian tumors, particularly in postmenopausal women, should decrease the subsequent occurrence of ovarian cancer.

Finally, there is little doubt that early-stage ovarian cancer is significantly more curable than late-stage disease. The 5-year survival of patients with stage I epithelial ovarian cancer is approximately 90%. In contrast, the 5-year survival of patients with stage III or IV epithelial ovarian cancer is only 20% to 25%, despite optimal surgery and combination chemotherapy. It has been estimated that if the 25% of ovarian cancer patients currently diagnosed with stage I tumors could be increased to 75% through early detection, the number of women dying from this disease could be halved.

The statistical definitions used in ovarian cancer screening are illustrated in Table 49.2. Characteristics of an optimal screening test include high sensitivity, high specificity, high positive predictive value (PPV), and high negative predictive value (NPV). In addition, the test should be easy to perform, time efficient, and well accepted by patients. An effective screening test should (a) decrease stage at detection, (b) decrease case-specific mortality, and (c) cause a statistically significant reduction in site-specific cancer mortality in the screened population.

TABLE 49.2

STATISTICAL DEFINITIONS IN OVARIAN CANCER SCREENING

	Screen	Findings
True positive (TP)	Positive	Ovarian cancer
False positive (FP)	Positive	No ovarian cancer
True negative (TN)	Negative	Absence of ovarian cancer for 1 year, confirmed by annual screening examination
False negative (FN)	Negative	Ovarian cancer within 1 year of normal screen

Sensitivity = (TP/TP + FN)
Specificity = (TN/TN + FP)
Positive Predictive Value (PPV) = TP/TP + FP
Negative Predictive Value (NPV) = TN/TN + FN

Finally, the screening test should be cost-effective, such that its use would reduce the overall cost of health care in the screened population.

At present, the two most effective screening methods for ovarian cancer are transvaginal sonography (TVS) and serum CA-125. TVS is usually performed using a standard ultrasound unit with a 5.0-mHz vaginal transducer. A complete screening examination takes 5 to 10 minutes and is painless. Each ovary is measured in three dimensions, and ovarian volume is calculated using the prolate ellipsoid formula ($L \times H \times W \times 0.523$). An ovarian volume >20 cm^3 in premenopausal women or >10 cm^3 in postmenopausal women is defined as abnormal. In addition, any solid or papillary projection from the tumor wall is considered abnormal.

A study evaluating ovarian cancer screening using TVS as the initial screening test was initiated at the University of Kentucky Medical Center in 1987. The current screening algorithm used at this center is illustrated in Figure 49.1. A woman with an abnormal screen is scheduled to have a repeat sonogram in 4 to 6 weeks. A woman with a persisting ovarian tumor at the time of the second screen is scheduled to have a serum CA-125 determination, tumor morphology indexing, color Doppler sonography, and proteomics. Following these studies, laparoscopic tumor removal is recommended. At the time of laparoscopy, the ovarian tumor is placed in an endocatch bag intraabdominally and removed through a midline subumbilical incision (Fig. 49.2). After removal, frozen section histologic examination is performed on all areas suspicious for malignancy. Patients with ovarian cancer on frozen section or patients with obvious metastatic disease at laparoscopy undergo immediate exploratory laparotomy with tumor debulking and staging. Using this algorithm, 25,327 asymptomatic women were screened from 1987 to 2002. Three hundred and sixty-four (1.4%) women with a persisting abnormality on TVS underwent surgical tumor removal. Forty-four of these patients were found to have primary ovarian cancer. Thirty-six (82%) had stage I or II disease, and all were cured after conventional therapy. The 5-year survival of patients with epithelial ovarian cancer detected by screening was 77%, which was significantly higher than that of patients who were not screened. Annual TVS screening was found to decrease stage at detection and reduce case-specific ovarian cancer mortality. The sensitivity of TVS was 0.850, and the specificity was 0.988. However, the PPV of TVS screening in detecting ovarian cancer was only 13.8%. Therefore, approximately eight benign ovarian tumors were removed for every ovarian cancer detected. Additional tests that can increase the PPV of TVS must be developed. One of the adjuvant methods capable of increasing the PPV of TVS screening is morphology indexing. Morphologic characteristics of ovarian tumors are related directly to the risk of malignancy. Unilocular cystic tumors are usually benign, whereas complex ovarian tumors with solid or papillary components are more often malignant. The addition of morphology indexing to TVS

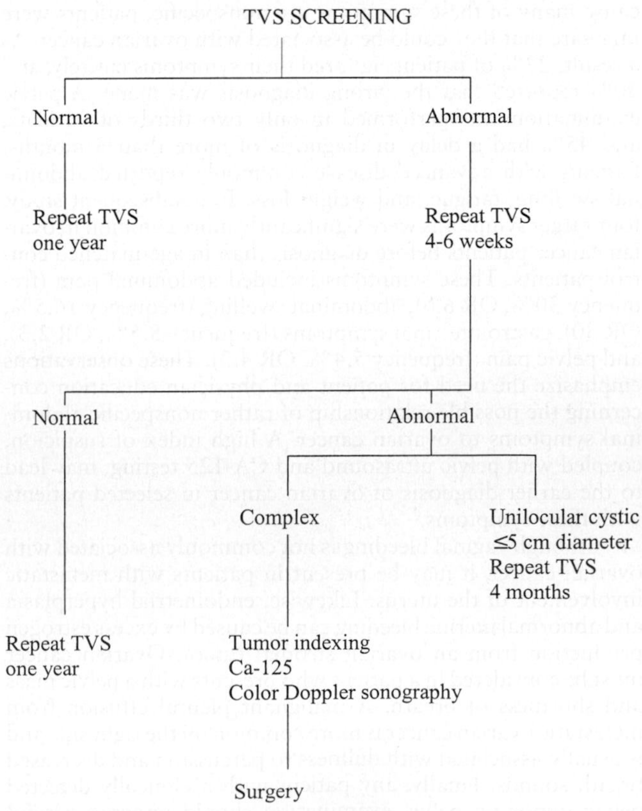

FIGURE 49.1. Ovarian cancer screening algorithm. University of Kentucky. TVS, transvaginal sonography.

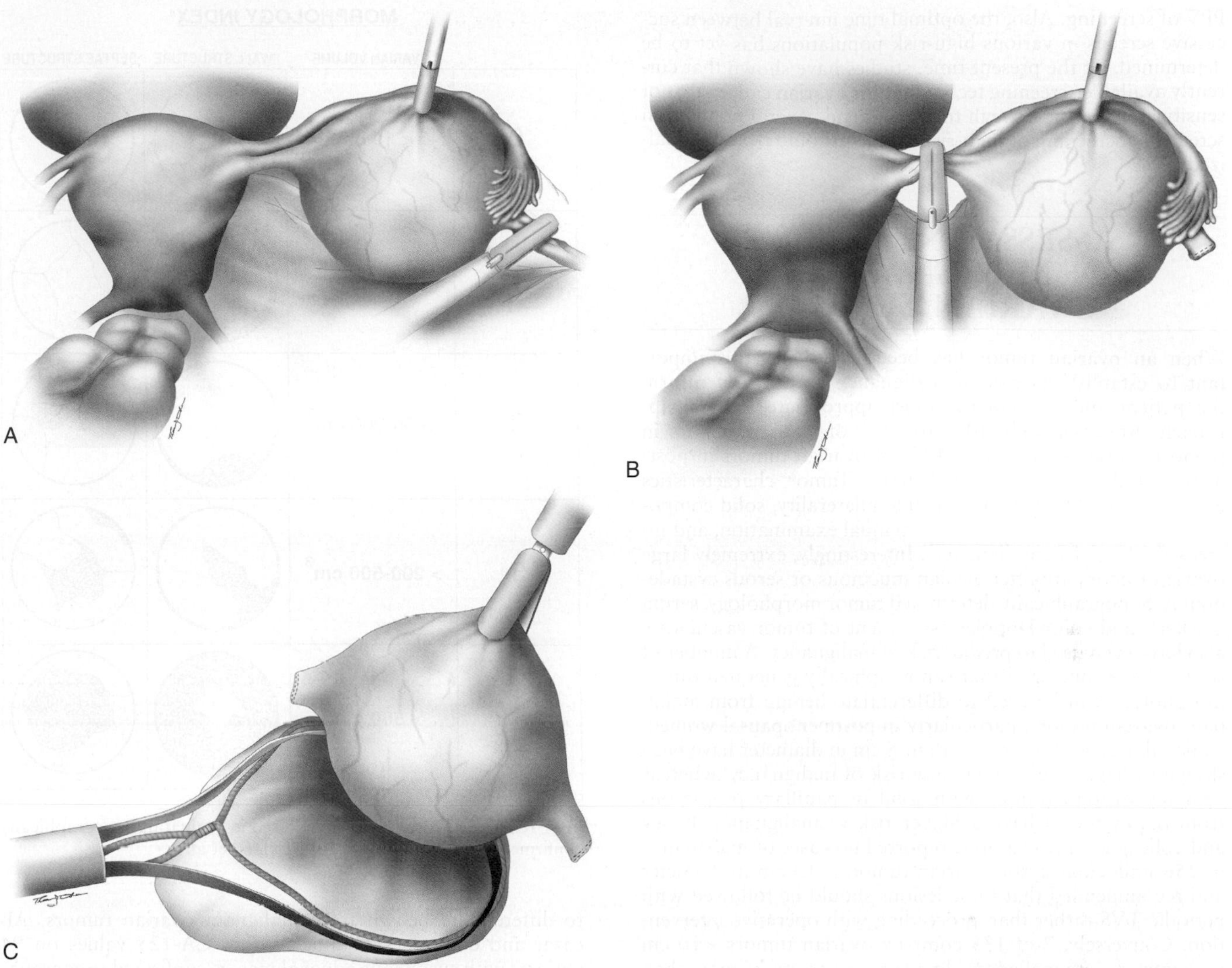

FIGURE 49.2. Laparoscopic removal of a right ovarian tumor. The infundibulopelvic and uteroovarian ligaments are stapled and transected. The ovarian tumor is placed in an endocatch bag and removed through a subumbilical incision.

in postmenopausal women has been reported to increase the PPV of sonographic screening.

CA-125 is an antigenic determinant on a high-molecular-weight glycoprotein recognized by a monoclonal antibody, OC-125. Despite repeated attempts, the gene encoding this molecule has not yet been cloned. CA-125 is expressed by epithelial ovarian cancers and is present in highest concentrations on the tumor cell surface. Although serum levels of this marker are elevated (>35 μ/mL) in as high as 80% of patients with advanced ovarian cancer, they are elevated in only 25% to 50% of patients with clinically detected stage I ovarian cancers. Likewise, serum CA-125 is elevated in patients with a number of benign ovarian conditions, such as endometriomas, inflammatory disease of the ovaries, and serous cystadenomas. Finally, this marker has been reported to be increased in a number of nongynecologic cancers, including cancers of the pancreas, breast, colon, and lung. Because many of the benign conditions producing elevated serum marker levels occur in younger women, the specificity of serum CA-125 is highest in postmenopausal women.

The efficacy of serum CA-125 as a screening method for ovarian cancer was evaluated in 22,000 asymptomatic postmenopausal women in England. Forty-one women (0.2%) had elevated (>30 μ/mL) serum CA-125 levels and underwent surgery. Eleven of these patients had ovarian cancer, but seven had advanced disease (stage III or IV). Eight additional patients developed ovarian cancer despite having a normal serum CA-125. A single serum CA-125 determination in this trial had a sensitivity of 58%, a specificity of 98.5%, and a PPV of 2%. When serum CA-125 was used as the initial screening method, early-stage cancers were missed, and stage at detection was not decreased appreciably. Subsequent studies have indicated that a rising trend in serum CA-125 levels over time is more predictive of ovarian cancer than a single elevated marker determination. Nevertheless, the lack of sensitivity of serum CA-125 in detecting early-stage ovarian cancer and its inability to lower stage at detection has limited its value as a screening method.

The challenge for future ovarian cancer detection trials is to combine TVS with serum markers and morphology indexing in an algorithm that improves the sensitivity, specificity, and

PPV of screening. Also, the optimal time interval between successive screens in various high-risk populations has yet to be determined. At the present time, studies have shown that currently available screening techniques for ovarian cancer are not sensitive or specific enough to recommend general population screening. Screening of high-risk women should be individualized.

ASSESSMENT OF RISK OF MALIGNANCY IN OVARIAN TUMORS

When an ovarian tumor has been identified, it is important to establish its risk of malignancy to properly inform the patient and to plan the most appropriate surgical approach. Approximately 10% to 15% of ovarian tumors in premenopausal women, and 40% of ovarian tumors in postmenopausal women, are malignant. Tumor characteristics associated with malignancy include bilaterality, solid composition, fixation in the pelvis on bimanual examination, and increased size (>10 cm diameter). Interestingly, extremely large ovarian tumors are often benign mucinous or serous cystadenomas. Sonographically determined tumor morphology, serum markers, and color Doppler assessment of tumor vasculature also have been used to predict risk of malignancy. A number of studies have concluded that sonographically generated tumor morphology can be used to differentiate benign from malignant ovarian tumors, particularly in postmenopausal women. Unilocular cystic tumors less than 5 cm in diameter have been shown to have an extremely low risk of malignancy, whereas complex ovarian tumors with solid or papillary projections from the cyst wall have a higher risk of malignancy. Bailey and colleagues, for example, reported no cases of malignancy in 256 unilocular cystic ovarian tumors <10 cm in diameter and recommended that these lesions should be followed with periodic TVS rather than proceeding with operative intervention. Conversely, 7 of 135 complex ovarian tumors <10 cm in diameter were malignant. In a subsequent study, more than 3,000 postmenopausal women with unilocular ovarian cysts <10 cm in diameter were followed with TVS at 6-month intervals for an average of 6 years. Approximately 70% of these cysts resolved spontaneously, and no patient developed ovarian cancer.

Using this reasoning, morphology indexes have been developed relating risk of malignancy to specific morphologic findings. The morphology index (MI) presently used in the University of Kentucky Ovarian Cancer Screening Trial was published initially by Ueland and colleagues and is illustrated in Figure 49.3. Both morphologic complexity and tumor volume, as calculated by the prolate ellipsoid formula, were related directly to the risk of malignancy. A point scale was constructed within each category, with total points per evaluation varying from 0 to 10. Risk of malignancy was assessed preoperatively in 442 ovarian tumors using this index. Morphologic abnormalities were easy to categorize, and interobserver variation was minimal. Risk of malignancy varied from 0.3% in ovarian tumors with a MI of <5 to 84% in tumors with a MI ≥8. Using a MI ≥5 as indicative of malignancy, the following statistical parameters were observed: sensitivity 0.981, specificity 0.808, PPV 0.409, and NPV 0.997. Therefore, morphologic indexing is a relatively accurate and cost-effective method to predict risk of malignancy in an ovarian tumor.

Serum biomarker levels have also been used both independently and in conjunction with sonographic findings as a means

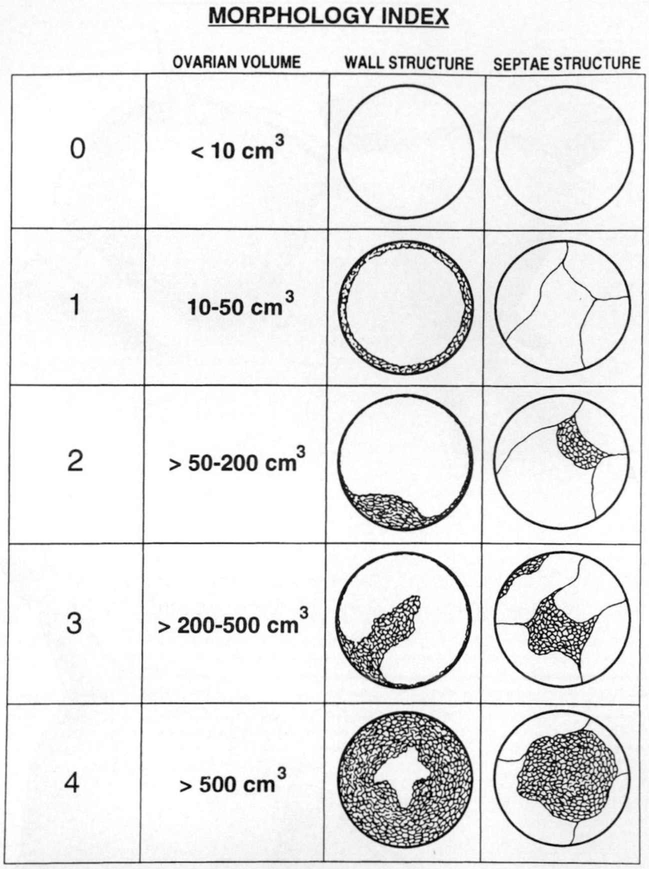

FIGURE 49.3. Morphology index used in evaluating sonographically confirmed ovarian tumors. (From: Ueland et al.)

to differentiate benign from malignant ovarian tumors. Alcazar and colleagues obtained serum CA-125 values on 94 patients with suspicious adnexal masses confirmed sonographically. A serum CA-125 value >35 μ/mL was designated as abnormal. Using this criterion, an elevated serum CA-125 in a postmenopausal woman with a sonographically confirmed ovarian tumor had a PPV for malignancy of 80%. The sensitivity and specificity of an elevated serum CA-125 were highest in postmenopausal women. In patients with an elevated serum CA-125, the presence of abnormal ovarian morphology significantly increased the risk of ovarian malignancy.

Recent data suggest that serial biomarker levels may be more effective than a single threshold value in distinguishing benign from malignant ovarian tumors. Generally, serum CA-125 values rise over time in patients with ovarian cancer, whereas they remain stable or decrease in patients with benign ovarian tumors. Using a risk calculation based on progressively rising serum CA-125 levels, Skates and colleagues were able to increase the sensitivity of ovarian cancer detection from 62% to 86%. Therefore, serial CA-125 determinations at 2- to 4-week intervals can be helpful in determining risk of malignancy in a sonographically confirmed ovarian tumor.

The use of color flow Doppler as a method to assess risk of malignancy in ovarian tumors is based on observed differences in resistance to blood flow between vessels supplying normal ovarian tissue and those associated with ovarian neoplasia. With tumor angiogenesis, there is an increase in the number and tortuosity of vessels. These vessels lack muscular intima and generally have low impedance to flow. Transvaginal color flow Doppler can be used to measure blood flow patterns within ovarian vessels.

In Doppler velocimetry, the flow velocity waveform obtained from a target vessel is evaluated according to standard parameters, pulsatility index (PI), and resistive index (RI). PI is calculated according to the formula: PI = S – D/A, where *S* is the maximum Doppler shift frequency, *D* is the minimum Doppler shift frequency, and *A* is the mean Doppler shift frequency during the cardiac cycle. RI is calculated according to the formula: RI = S – D/S. A PI of <1.0 and an RI of <0.4 are indicative of low impedance to flow and a high risk of malignancy. Using these criteria, Weiner and colleagues reported that vessels supplying ovarian malignancies had an abnormally low PI in 16 of 17 cases. In contrast, the PI of vessels supplying benign ovarian tumors was normal (≥1.0) in 35 of 36 cases. Other studies have confirmed that the mean PI and RI are lower in malignant and borderline ovarian tumors than in benign ovarian tumors. However, the overlap in values is such that preoperative color Doppler cannot be used as a reliable preoperative indicator of malignancy.

More recently, contrast-enhanced, three-dimensional power Doppler sonography has been shown to improve the visualization and diagnostic evaluation of tumor vascularity in complex adnexal masses. Intravascular contrast agents are used to enhance depiction of tumor vessels by providing a stronger Doppler signal. Image software systems are used to calculate the total power Doppler intensity for a designated region within each tumor. Preliminary studies suggest that this technology can be used to discriminate benign from malignant ovarian tumors. However, these methods are time-consuming and require sophisticated ultrasound equipment and sonographer skill. At present, Doppler flow studies are used as adjunctive tests in ovarian tumors suspected of being malignant on the basis of morphology indexing or serum marker patterns.

Proteomic profiling of serum using mass spectroscopy (surface-enhanced laser desorption and ionization) also has been proposed as a method to differentiate benign from malignant ovarian tumors. Basically, a population of proteins can be profiled according to the size and net electrical charge of the individual proteins. The discriminating proteomic pattern formed by a subset of proteins is defined by peak amplitude at key mass/charge positions along the spectrum. In 2002, Petricoin and associates, using this technology, reported a proteomic pattern that could discriminate ovarian cancer patients from normal controls or patients with benign gynecologic disease. Included in the ovarian cancer cases were 15 patients with stage I disease. Unfortunately, these initial results have proven difficult to reproduce, and several investigators have concluded that further work needs to be done before proteomic profiling can provide reproducible data from which to identify ovarian cancer.

Perhaps the most clinically valuable study concerning the differentiation of benign and malignant ovarian tumors was reported by Roman and colleagues. These investigators performed a prospective trial to evaluate the efficacy of pelvic examination, tumor markers, transvaginal gray scale sonography, and Doppler flow sonography in predicting ovarian malignancy. These tests were performed on 226 consecutive women before operative removal of an ovarian tumor. Positive findings included fixed or irregular consistency on pelvic examination, solid or papillary projections on TVS, a serum CA-125 >35 μ/m, and a PI <1.0 or a RI <0.4 on color Doppler. If all four indicators were positive in a postmenopausal woman, the risk for malignancy was 83%. In contrast, if all indicators were negative, 100% of postmenopausal women had benign ovarian tumors. Logistic regression analysis revealed that sonographically determined ovarian morphology and serum CA-125 were the most significant predictors of malignancy in the ovarian tumors of postmenopausal women. Spectral Doppler analysis of PI and RI did not improve diagnostic accuracy because of the overlap in values obtained between benign and malignant ovarian tumors.

Using morphologic indexing and serum markers, it is now possible to assess risk of malignancy in an ovarian mass and to plan accordingly. A recent analysis of national data has indicated that the highest survival of women with ovarian cancer occurred when a gynecologic oncologist was involved in their care. Therefore, patients with a high risk of ovarian malignancy on preoperative evaluation can be referred directly to a gynecologic oncologist.

PREOPERATIVE EVALUATION

Before operative intervention, each patient should undergo a thorough evaluation designed to determine the anatomic location, size, and morphology of the ovarian tumor, as well as possible sites of metastases. In addition, her general medical condition and ability to undergo a major surgical procedure should be established. All patients should undergo routine hematologic and biochemical testing. A chest x-ray provides valuable information concerning cardiac size, as well as the presence of pulmonary metastases or a pleural effusion. An electrocardiogram is indicated in all women older than age 40 or in a patient with specific signs or symptoms of cardiac disease.

As previously mentioned, TVS is the most accurate test in assessing ovarian tumor size and morphology. In selected patients with large ovarian tumors, it may be necessary to perform abdominal sonography as well as vaginal sonography to determine the full extent of the tumor. TVS is also valuable in identifying intrauterine tumor or occult ascites. A patient with an ovarian tumor and vaginal bleeding should undergo further evaluation to rule out coexisting endometrial cancer or a primary uterine cancer with spread to the ovaries.

In patients with an ovarian tumor confirmed by TVS, pelvic/abdominal computed tomography (CT) scanning with contrast may identify ureteral obstruction, retroperitoneal lymphadenopathy, omental disease, and peritoneal metastases. In a patient with ascites but no ovarian tumor, liver function studies should be performed to exclude cirrhosis or liver disease. Rarely, the presence of right heart failure and hepatic congestion will cause ascites. Although paracentesis is contraindicated in a patient with an ovarian tumor confirmed on sonography, it may be useful in a patient who presents with ascites and no evidence of an ovarian abnormality. The characteristics of malignant cells present in ascitic fluid may help identify the primary site of intraabdominal malignancy.

Common sites of nongynecologic cancer that spreads to the ovary include gastric malignancy, colonic carcinoma, and breast carcinoma. A careful history of physical examinations should arouse suspicion of other possible primary malignancies. Any such possibilities should be evaluated with appropriate ongoing studies and diagnostic evaluation, possibly including colonoscopy, upper gastrointestinal endoscopy, and/or mammography. A biopsy of a suspicious finding or easily accessible lymph node may clarify the diagnosis.

Finally, serum markers should be obtained according to the age and clinical findings of each patient (Table 49.3). Serum CA-125 and CEA often are elevated in patients with epithelial ovarian cancer, whereas serum alpha-fetoprotein, human chorionic gonadotropin, or lactate dehydrogenase are more

TABLE 49.3

SERUM MARKERS IN OVARIAN CANCER

Tumor histology	Serum marker
Epithelial ovarian cancer	CA-125
Mucinous cystadenocarcinoma	CEA
Endodermal sinus tumor	AFP
Embryonal cell carcinoma	hCG, AFP
Choriocarcinoma	hCG
Dysgerminoma	LDH-1, LDH-2
Granulosa cell tumor	Inhibin

AFP, alpha-fetoprotein; CEA, carcinoembryonic antigen; hCG, human chorionic gonadotropin; LDH, lactate dehydrogenase.

commonly increased in younger women with germ-cell ovarian malignancies. Serum inhibin is the most reliable marker in patients with ovarian granulosa cell tumors. The specific marker associated with each type of ovarian cancer is illustrated in Table 49.3. It is important to obtain a baseline serum marker value before surgery so that it can be used to monitor response to therapy.

PATTERNS OF SPREAD

Ovarian cancer spreads by (a) direct extension and exfoliation of tumor cells into the peritoneal cavity, (b) lymphatic metastases to regional and paraaortic lymph nodes, and (c) hematogenous dissemination (Fig. 49.4). The specific pattern of spread depends on the stage, cell type, and histologic differentiation of the tumor.

The earliest method of spread in epithelial ovarian cancer is by exfoliation of tumor cells from the ovarian surface. These cells migrate with the circulation of peritoneal fluid along the surfaces of the pelvic and mesenteric peritoneum. They also are carried cephalad in the paracolic spaces to the omentum and undersurface of the diaphragm. Spread to the right lung occurs through the transdiaphragmatic lymphatics in the right hemidiaphragm, often producing a right pleural effusion. Surface spread to the bowel and bladder is a common finding in advanced-stage ovarian cancer, but involvement of the bowel lumen or bladder mucosa is rare.

Lymphatic drainage from the ovary follows two pathways. The first involves lateral spread through the broad ligament to the pelvic lymph nodes. In patients with advanced-stage disease, there may be retrograde dissemination via the lymphatics of this pathway to the round ligament to the inguinal lymph

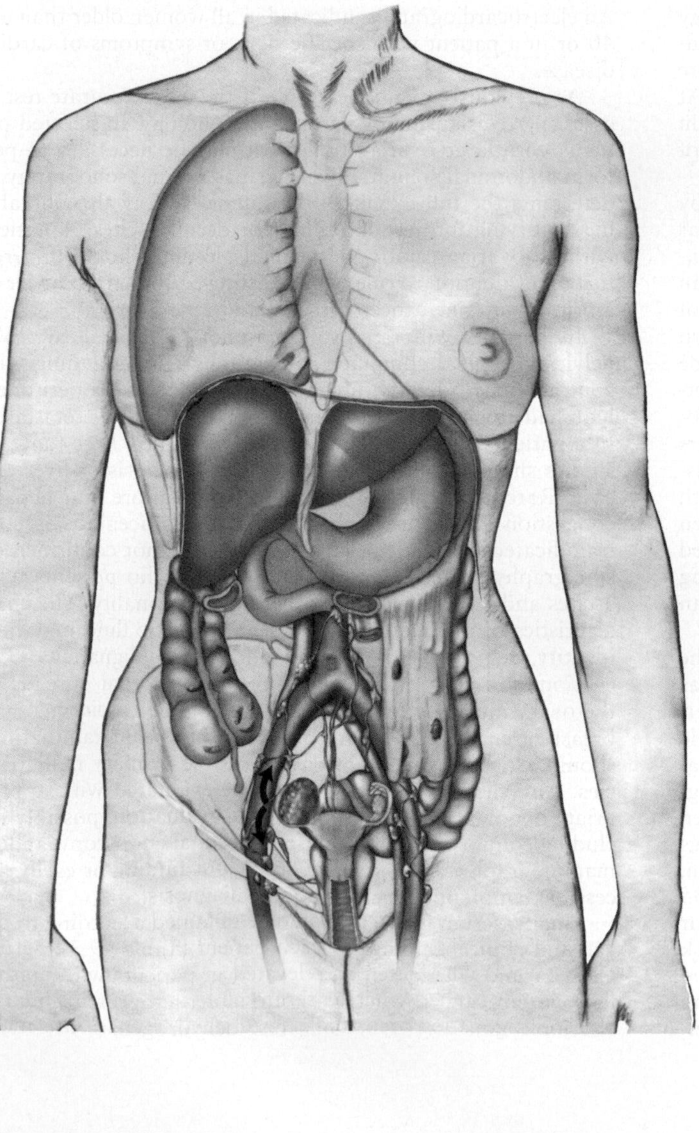

FIGURE 49.4. Patterns of spread of ovarian cancer.

TABLE 49.4

LYMPH NODAL METASTASES IN PATIENTS WITH CLINICALLY APPARENT STAGE I EPITHELIAL OVARIAN CANCER

Author	Patients	Pelvic lymph node metastases	Para-aortic lymph node metastases
Onda et al. (1996)	30	6 (18%)	5 (15%)
Carnino et al. (1997)	47	1 (4%)	0 (0%)
Burghardt et al. (1991)	20	3 (15%)	1 (5%)
Sakai et al. (1997)	46	1 (2%)	1 (2%)
Chen and Lee (1983)	11	1 (9%)	2 (18%)
Li et al. (2000)	91	9 (10%)	8 (9%)
Total	245	21 (9%)	17 (7%)

nodes. The second pathway of efferent lymphatic drainage follows the ovarian vein to the paracaval and paraaortic lymph nodes. Metastatic spread of ovarian cancer to lymph nodes is well documented even in early-stage disease (Table 49.4) and confirms that there may be separate pathways of dissemination to the pelvic and paraaortic lymph nodes. Cass and coworkers, for example, reported that 14 of 96 patients (15%) with disease visibly confined to one ovary had microscopic lymph node metastases. All 14 patients with nodal spread had poorly differentiated tumors. Isolated ipsilateral lymph node metastases occurred in five patients, and isolated contralateral lymph node metastases occurred in three patients. Pelvic lymph nodes were involved in six patients, paraaortic lymph nodes in five patients, and both in three patients. As expected, the frequency of lymph node metastases is related to stage of disease, cell type, and histologic differentiation of the tumor. Chen and Lee, for example, reported that the frequency of pelvic lymph node metastases increased from 9% in patients with clinically apparent stage I ovarian cancer to 33% in patients with stage IV disease. Similarly, the frequency of paraaortic lymph node involvement increased from 18% in patients with clinically apparent stage I disease to 67% in patients with stage IV disease. These findings are similar to those of Burghardt and colleagues, who noted lymph node metastases in 74% of patients with stage III or IV ovarian cancer. The incidence of lymph node metastases increased from 20% in well-differentiated ovarian cancers to 65% in poorly differentiated tumors and was higher in serous ovarian malignancies than in mucinous or endometrioid cancers.

Hematogenous spread of ovarian cancer to the parenchyma of the liver or lung is fortunately quite rare (<5%) at the time of initial diagnosis, but may occur, particularly in poorly differentiated tumors that become refractory to combination chemotherapy.

EXAMINATION OF OVARIAN TUMOR SPECIMENS AND HISTOLOGIC CLASSIFICATION

Ovarian tumor specimens should be described, fixed, and sectioned according to the guidelines established by the College of American Pathologists (CAP). Tumor should be classified histologically according to the World Health Organization classification and nomenclature of ovarian tumors (Table 49.5). Although there are numerous grading systems for ovarian cancers that use both architectural and nuclear features, it is recommended that four grades be used, with grade 4 (undifferentiated) applied to tumors with minimal or no differentiation. Recommendations concerning the use of special staining techniques or flow cytometry in establishing the correct histologic diagnosis of ovarian tumors are made in the CAP report. Immunohistochemical staining of ovarian tumors for cytokeratin 7 (CK7) and cytokeratin 20 (CK20) is helpful in differentiating primary mucinous ovarian carcinoma from colorectal adenocarcinoma that has metastasized to the ovary. Colorectal adenocarcinomas usually stain positively for CK20 and negatively for CK7. In contrast, ovarian carcinomas usually stain negatively for CK20 and positively for CK7.

PRIMARY SURGERY

Patterns of Care in Ovarian Cancer Surgery

All patients with suspected ovarian cancer should be referred to a gynecologic oncologist for evaluation and possible surgery. Unfortunately, in both Europe and the United States (where most of the outcomes studies have been conducted), too high a proportion of women with ovarian cancer are receiving substandard care. In a Norweigian study, Tingulstad and colleagues found that in advanced-stage ovarian cancer, patients who underwent primary surgery at teaching hospitals had significantly improved survival time compared with controls who underwent primary surgery at nonteaching hospitals. Two regional-based studies—one from Utah and the other from Maryland—have also indicated that a significant proportion of women with ovarian cancer are not receiving optimal treatment. Carney and associates found that less than 50% of ovarian cancer patients in Utah were cared for by a gynecologic oncologist. In addition, care by a gynecologic oncologist was associated with an apparent survival advantage. In the Maryland study, Bristow and coworkers found that the majority of ovarian cancer patients in Maryland were undergoing primary surgery in low-volume settings.

In a study of the SEER program database from 1991 and 1996, Harlan and colleagues found that comparing the two treatment periods, the majority of women with early-stage ovarian cancer did not receive guideline therapy in both periods, although the rate was improved in the 1996 cohort. For women with advanced-stage ovarian cancer, there was a higher rate of guideline therapy use but no improvement between 1991 and 1996—62.6% versus 62.3%. Goff and associates, surveying 10,432 women with ovarian cancer in nine states between 1999 and 2002, found that almost 50% of women with early-stage disease were not adequately staged, and in

TABLE 49.5

WORLD HEALTH ORGANIZATION HISTOLOGICAL CLASSIFICATION OF OVARIAN TUMORS

Surface epithelial-stromal tumors

- Serous tumors
  - Malignant
    - Adenocarcinoma
    - Surface papillary adenocarcinoma
    - Adenocarcinofibroma (malignant adenofibroma)
  - Borderline tumor
    - Papillary cystic tumor
    - Surface papillary tumor
    - Adenofibroma, cystadenofibroma
  - Benign
    - Cystadenoma
    - Surface papilloma
    - Adenofibroma and cystadenofibroma
- Mucinous tumors
  - Malignant
    - Adenocarcinoma
    - Adenocarcinofibroma (malignant adenofibroma)
  - Borderline tumor
    - Intestinal type
    - Endocervicallike
  - Benign
    - Cystadenoma
    - Adenofibroma and cystadenofibroma
  - Mucinous cystic tumor with mural nodules
  - Mucinous cystic tumor with pseudomyxoma peritonei
- Endometrioid tumors, including variants with squamous differentiation
  - Malignant
    - Adenocarcinoma, not otherwise specified
    - Adenocarcinofibroma (malignant adenofibroma)
    - Malignant mullerian mixed tumor (carcinosarcoma)
    - Adenosarcoma
    - Endometrioid stromal sarcoma (low grade)
    - Undifferentiated ovarian sarcoma
  - Borderline tumor
    - Cystic tumor
    - Adenofibroma and cystadenofibroma
  - Benign
    - Cystadenoma
    - Adenofibroma and cystadenofibroma
- Clear-cell tumors
  - Malignant
    - Adenocarcinoma
    - Adenocarcinofibroma (malignant adenofibroma)
  - Borderline tumor
    - Cystic tumor
    - Adenofibroma and cystadenofibroma
  - Benign
    - Cystadenofibroma
    - Adenofibroma and cystadenofibroma
- Transitional cell tumors
  - Malignant
    - Transitional cell tumor (non-Brenner type)
    - Malignant Brenner tumor
  - Borderline
    - Brenner tumor
      - Proliferating variant
  - Benign
    - Brenner tumor
      - Metaplastic variant
- Squamous cell tumors
  - Squamous cell carcinoma
  - Epidermoid cyst
- Mixed epithelial tumors (specify components)
  - Malignant
  - Borderline
  - Benign
- Undifferentiated and unclassified tumors
  - Undifferentiated carcinoma
  - Adenocarcinoma, not otherwise specified

Sex cord–stromal tumors

- Granulosa-stromal cell tumors
  - Granulosa cell tumor group
    - Adult granulosa cell tumor
    - Juvenile granulosa cell tumor
  - Thecoma-fibroma group
    - Thecoma, not otherwise specified
      - Typical
    - Luteinized
    - Fibroma
    - Cellular fibroma
    - Fibrosarcoma
    - Stromal tumor with mixed sex cord elements
    - Sclerosing stromal tumor
    - Signet-ring stromal tumor
    - Unclassified (fibrothecoma)
- Sertoli-stromal cell tumors
  - Sertoli-Leydig cell tumor group (androblastomas)
    - Well differentiated
    - Of intermediate differentiation
      - Variant with heterologous elements (specify type)
    - Poorly differentiated (sarcomatoid)
      - Variant with heterologous elements (specify type)
    - Retiform
      - Variant with heterologous elements (specify type)
  - Sertoli cell tumor
  - Stromal-Leydig cell tumor
  - Sex cord-stromal tumors of mixed or unclassified cell types
    - Sex cord tumor with annular tubules
    - Gynandroblastoma (specify components)
    - Sex cord–stromal tumor, unclassified
  - Steroid cell tumors
    - Stromal luteoma
    - Leydig cell tumor group
      - Hilus cell tumor
      - Leydig cell tumor, nonhilar type
      - Leydig cell tumor, not otherwise specified
    - Steroid cell tumor, not otherwise specified
      - Well differentiated
      - Malignant
  - Germ-cell tumors
  - Primitive germ-cell tumors
    - Dysgerminoma
    - Yolk sac tumor
      - Polyvesicular vitelline tumor
      - Glandular variant
      - Hepatoid variant
    - Embryonal carcinoma
    - Polyembryoma

TABLE 49.5

CONTINUED

Nongestational choriocarcinoma	Germ-cell sex cord–stromal tumors
Mixed germ-cell tumor (specify components)	Gonadoblastoma
Biphasic or triphasic teratoma	Variant with malignant germ-cell tumor
Immature teratoma	Mixed germ-cell/sex cord–stromal tumor
Mature teratoma	Variant with malignant germ-cell tumour
Solid	Tumors of the rete ovarii
Cystic	Adenocarcinoma
Dermoid cyst	Adenoma
Fetiform teratoma (homunculus)	Cystadenoma
Monodermal teratoma and somatic-type tumors associated with dermoid cysts	Cystadenofibroma
Thyroid tumor group	Miscellaneous tumors
Struma ovarii	Small-cell carcinoma, hypercalcemic type
Benign	Small-cell carcinoma, pulmonary type
Malignant (specify type)	Large-cell neuroendocrine carcinoma
Carcinoid group	Hepatoid carcinoma
Insular	Primary ovarian mesothelioma
Trabecular	Wilms tumor
Mucinous	Gestational choriocarcinoma
Strumal carcinoid	Hydatidiform mole
Mixed	Adenoid cystic carcinoma
Neuroectodermal tumor group	Basal cell tumor
Ependymoma	Ovarian wolffian tumor
Primitive neuroectodermal tumor	Paraganglioma
Medulloepithelioma	Myxoma
Glioblastoma multiforme	Soft tissue tumors not specific to the ovary
Others	Others
Carcinoma group	Tumorlike conditions
Squamous cell carcinoma	Luteoma of pregnancy
Adenocarcinoma	Stromal hyperthecosis
Others	Stromal hyperplasia
Melanocytic group	Fibromatosis
Malignant melanoma	Massive ovarian edema
Melanocytic naevus	Others
Sarcoma group (specify type)	Lymphoid and hematopoietic tumors
Sebaceous tumor group	Malignant lymphoma (specify type)
Sebaceous adenoma	Leukemia (specify type)
Sebaceous carcinoma	Plasmacytoma
Primary-type tumor group	Secondary tumors
Retinal anlage tumor group	
Others	

advanced-stage disease, aggressive cytoreductive procedures, such as intestinal resection and diaphragmatic debulking, were lower in low-volume hospitals. The totality of this information clearly underscores the need for improvement in patterns of referral.

Early-Stage Ovarian Cancer

Comprehensive Surgical Staging

Ovarian cancer is staged according to the International Federation of Gynecology and Obstetrics (FIGO) Staging System (Table 49.6) and is based on a thorough surgical evaluation of the primary ovarian tumor and its potential sites of metastatic spread (Table 49.7). Should preoperative evaluation suggest an area of extraabdominal or intrahepatic metastasis, fine needle aspiration or needle biopsy of this lesion should be performed. Because ovarian cancer frequently spreads to upper abdominal structures, a vertical midline abdominal incision is recommended. This incision should be extended high enough to remove the primary ovarian tumor and to evaluate the stomach, omentum, liver, and undersurface of the diaphragm. Rupture of a cystic ovarian malignancy is associated with a poorer prognosis, so the incision should be sufficient to allow excision of the primary tumor with its capsule intact. Once the abdomen has been opened, the following steps should be performed for adequate surgical staging:

1. The volume of ascitic fluid should be recorded, and a minimum of 25 mL should be sent for cytologic evaluation.
2. In the absence of ascites, separate saline washings should be obtained from the (a) pelvic cul-de-sac, (b) right paracolic space, (c) left paracolic space, and (d) undersurface of each hemidiaphragm. Approximately 100 mL of saline should

TABLE 49.6

FIGO STAGE GROUPING FOR PRIMARY CARCINOMA OF THE OVARY

Stage I	Growth limited to the ovaries.
Stage IA	Growth limited to one ovary; no ascites. No tumor on the external surface; capsule intact.
Stage IB	Growth limited to both ovaries; no ascites. No tumor on the external surface; capsules intact.
Stage IC[a]	Tumor either stage IA or IB but with tumor on the surface of one or both ovaries or with capsule ruptured or with ascites present containing malignant cells or with positive peritoneal washings.
Stage II	Growth involving one or both ovaries with pelvic extension.
Stage IIA	Extension and/or metastases to the uterus and/or tubes.
Stage IIB	Extension to other pelvic tissues.
Stage IIC[a]	Tumor either stage IIA or IIB but with tumor on the surface of one or both ovaries or with capsule(s) ruptured or with ascites present containing malignant cells or with positive peritoneal washings.
Stage III	Tumor involving one or both ovaries with peritoneal implants outside the pelvis and/or positive retroperitoneal or inguinal nodes. Superficial liver metastasis equals stage III. Tumor is limited to the true pelvis but with histologically verified malignant extension to small bowel or omentum.
Stage IIIA	Tumor grossly limited to the true pelvis with negative nodes but with histologically confirmed microscopic seeding of abdominal peritoneal surfaces.
Stage IIIB	Tumor of one or both ovaries with histologically confirmed implants of abdominal peritoneal surfaces, none exceeding 2 cm in diameter. Nodes negative.
Stage IIIC	Abdominal implants >2 cm in diameter and/or positive retroperitoneal or inguinal nodes.
Stage IV	Growth involving one or both ovaries with distant metastasis. If pleural effusion is present, there must be positive cytologic test results to allot a case to stage IV.

FIGO, International Federation of Obstetrics and Gynecology.
[a]To evaluate the impact on prognosis of the different criteria for allotting cases to stage IC or IIC, it would be of value to know whether rupture of the capsule was spontaneous or caused by the surgeon and whether the source of malignant cells detected was peritoneal washings or ascites.

be instilled in each of these areas, recovered, and sent for cytologic evaluation.

3. The ovarian tumor should be inspected, with particular attention to the presence of papillary excrescences on the surface or rupture of the capsule. The contralateral ovary and uterus should be examined for the presence of metastatic tumor. The pathways of ovarian tumor should be removed and sent for frozen-section examination. Removal of the opposite ovary and/or uterus are dependent on several factors and are discussed on the following pages.
4. Careful inspection and palpation of the peritoneal surfaces and intraabdominal viscera should be performed. This evaluation should be approached in a systematic fashion, beginning with the peritoneum of the cul-de-sac and small bowel mesentery. Inspection should continue with the ascending colon, liver, omentum, undersurface of the right and left hemidiaphragms, and stomach. Finally, the transverse colon, spleen, descending colon, and bladder peritoneum should be evaluated.
5. All areas suspicious for malignancy should be biopsied. In the absence of visible disease, biopsies should be taken of the cul-de-sac peritoneum, bladder peritoneum, both lateral pelvic walls, paracolic peritoneum bilaterally, and undersurface of the right hemidiaphragm. An infracolic omentectomy should be performed in patients with epithelial ovarian cancer and an omental wedge biopsy taken in patients with germ-cell or stromal tumors. Appendectomy should be performed in all patients with mucinous epithelial cancers involving the ovary. Primary appendiceal cancers, although rare, commonly spread to the ovaries and usually require right hemicolectomy as part of initial surgical staging.

TABLE 49.7

SURGICAL STAGING OF APPARENT EARLY-STAGE OVARIAN CANCER

Vertical midline incision
Evacuation of ascites or multiple cytologic washings
Complete abdominal inspection and palpation
Resection of ovaries, fallopian tubes, and uterus[a]
Omentectomy
Random peritoneal biopsies
Retroperitoneal lymph node sampling

[a]Exceptions may be made in selected patients who wish to preserve fertility.

6. As has been mentioned, ovarian cancer commonly spreads to both pelvic and paraaortic lymph nodes. Some patients with early-stage ovarian cancer have paraaortic lymph node metastases in the absence of pelvic lymph node spread. Therefore, these lymph node groups should be sampled separately in all patients. It is important that sampling include lymph nodes on the opposite side of the primary ovarian tumor, because isolated contralateral spread has been reported.
7. Finally, it should be emphasized that operative findings present at staging laparotomy must be carefully documented. Prognosis is related to the site and volume of metastatic tumor, as well as the amount of residual disease remaining after surgical debulking. Important data concerning the location and size of tumor metastases are often lost if the details concerning operative staging are not recorded.

Fertility-Sparing Surgery

Although the majority of ovarian malignancies occur in older women for whom bilateral salpingo-oophorectomy and hysterectomy are standard treatment, a significant subset of patients is young and can be managed more conservatively (Table 49.8). Conservative management is used here to denote surgery that preserves reproductive potential without compromising curability. With some exceptions, such a strategy may be applicable for women younger than 40 years who wish to bear children.

When contemplating surgery on a young patient with a suspected ovarian malignancy, it is important to discuss with her all possible operative findings and procedures and the long-term implications of the various options. If the patient is a child, the parents need to clearly understand this information.

In most instances, young patients have their initial surgery done outside major university hospitals or cancer centers. Common errors in surgical management include incomplete surgical staging and unnecessary bilateral salpingo-oophorectomy. In addition, some patients are mismanaged because of an error in the pathologic diagnosis of a rare ovarian neoplasm.

The optimal candidate for conservative surgical management is a young patient who has stage IA disease. If, on initial inspection, the suspected cancer is confined to one ovary, then unilateral salpingo-oophorectomy is appropriate. If the mass is thought to be benign, then ovarian cystectomy may be preferable. The specimen should be sent for frozen section examination. If malignancy is diagnosed, then appropriate staging biopsies should be performed, as discussed. If the contralateral ovary appears normal, it is recommended that it not be biopsied to avoid potential infertility caused by peritoneal adhesions or ovarian failure.

One should not rely too heavily on frozen section examination in making the decision to perform a hysterectomy and bilateral salpingo-oophorectomy. If the histologic diagnosis is in question, it is always preferable to wait for permanent section results for a young patient, even if this requires a repeat surgery.

The advent of *in vitro* fertilization technology should also have an impact on intraoperative management. Convention has dictated that if a bilateral salpingo-oophorectomy is necessary, a hysterectomy should also be performed. However, current technology for donor oocyte transfer and hormonal support allows a woman without ovaries to sustain a normal intrauterine pregnancy. Similarly, if the uterus and one ovary are resected because of tumor involvement, current techniques allow retrieval of oocytes from the patient's remaining ovary, *in vitro* fertilization with sperm from her male partner, and implantation of the embryo into a surrogate's uterus. Therefore, traditional guidelines concerning surgical management of ovarian cancer may no longer be applicable in selected young patients.

Approximately 50% to 70% of *malignant germ-cell tumors* are stage I. Except for dysgerminoma, in which the incidence of bilaterality is 10% to 15%, bilateral ovarian tumors are exceedingly rare. Such a finding almost always signifies advanced disease with metastatic spread from one ovary to the other or a mixed germ-cell tumor with a dysgerminoma component. Benign cystic teratoma is associated with malignant germ-cell tumors in 5% to 10% of cases and may occur in one or both ovaries. Therefore, unilateral salpingo-oophorectomy—preserving the contralateral ovary and uterus—combined with surgical staging can be performed in most patients with these neoplasms, even many with advanced-stage disease. If the contralateral ovary is enlarged, most likely it represents a benign cystic teratoma that can be managed with an ovarian cystectomy only. With the exception of stage IA pure dysgerminoma or stage IA, grade 1 immature teratoma, these patients require postoperative chemotherapy consisting of the combination of bleomycin, etoposide, and cisplatin (BEP). Several series have documented normal reproductive function in at least 80% of patients as well as pregnancies following fertility-sparing surgery and chemotherapy.

In the past few years, some investigators have advocated the practice of surgery alone for other categories of malignant germ-cell tumors, including stage IA, grade 2 and 3 immature teratomas, and stage IA yolk sac tumors. Such an approach, however, should be taken with caution; many experts would still consider it experimental. Nevertheless, there is a trend toward careful observation following surgery alone for most patients with stage I malignant ovarian germ-cell tumors. The Children's Oncology Group is currently conducting a clinical trial that includes postoperative surveillance for patients with stage I disease. Chemotherapy is initiated only for serum tumor marker elevation.

Most *sex cord–stromal tumors* are confined to the ovary. Stage I accounts for >50% (in some series as high as 100%) of granulosa cell tumors. More than 90% of Sertoli-Leydig cell tumors are stage IA. Bilaterality occurs in <5% of cases with either tumor type. Therefore, optimal surgical management of most patients with stromal tumors consists of unilateral adnexectomy combined with appropriate surgical staging. Endometrial biopsy or curettage also should be performed in any young patient whose uterus is preserved because 5% to 15% of patients with granulosa cell tumors develop endometrial cancer or hyperplasia. Postoperative therapy may be indicated for patients with metastatic disease or for selected patients with stage I disease (e.g., poorly differentiated Sertoli-Leydig cell tumor or granulosa cell tumor with rupture). The most commonly used regimens in this setting include either BEP or the combination of paclitaxel and carboplatin.

TABLE 49.8

CRITERIA FOR POTENTIAL FERTILITY-SPARING SURGERY IN OVARIAN CANCER PATIENTS

Patient desirous of preserving fertility
Patient and family consent and agree to close follow-up
No evidence of dysgenetic gonads
Specific situations:
Any unilateral malignant germ-cell tumor
Any unilateral sex cord–stromal tumor
Any unilateral borderline tumor
Stage IA invasive epithelial tumor

Approximately 10% to 15% of all ovarian neoplasms are of the *borderline or low malignant potential* classification. Although they were first described more than 70 years ago, only in the last few years have we begun to fully appreciate their biologic behavior. Approximately 33% to 60% of serous borderline tumors are limited to one ovary. Extraovarian spread is noted in approximately 20% to 30% of cases. Approximately 80% to 90% of mucinous borderline tumors are confined to one ovary. Both endometrioid and clear-cell borderline tumors are almost always stage I, and the vast majority are unilateral. For patients with borderline tumors seemingly confined to one ovary, appropriate surgical management includes unilateral salpingo-oophorectomy with surgical staging. The use of ovarian cystectomy instead of unilateral adnexectomy also has been reported, although some patients treated in this manner require repeat surgery for a recurrence of tumor in the same or opposite ovary. If bilateral borderline tumors are present, portions of one or both ovaries may be preserved with ovarian cystectomy, if feasible. Whatever the surgical approach, reported 5-year survival rates for patients with stage I borderline tumors treated with surgery alone are 95% or better.

For patients with borderline tumors and peritoneal implants, the optimal management remains controversial. However, surgical excision is the mainstay of treatment. After frozen-section confirmation of borderline tumor, an effort should be made to resect all gross disease. In addition, staging biopsies of peritoneal surfaces and lymph nodes are indicated, as are cytologic washings. However, there is no consensus regarding the extent of surgical staging required, particularly with regard to the need for lymphadenectomy. Even in the face of metastatic disease, a normal contralateral ovary may be preserved in young patients. In such cases, however, some recommend ovarian biopsy to assess for occult disease. In patients with advanced-stage serous disease, the incidence of bilateral tumors is approximately 75%. There are several reports detailing successful pregnancies following treatment in patients with borderline ovarian tumors.

The relapse risk for patients with peritoneal implants is related to the type: noninvasive versus invasive. For patients with noninvasive peritoneal implants, the lifetime risk is estimated to be at least 20%. For those with invasive peritoneal implants, the lifetime risk of relapse is estimated to be at least 50%. Consequently, postoperative platinum-based chemotherapy is recommended for the latter diagnosis by many groups. However, no study has demonstrated a survival benefit related to postoperative chemotherapy.

Invasive epithelial tumors account for approximately 70% of all ovarian malignancies. Despite the low overall survival rate associated with these tumors, selected young patients with stage I disease can be treated conservatively. The major factors that influence the selection process are histologic grade and bilaterality, in addition to stage. Serous tumors are bilateral in about 50% of cases. The incidence of bilaterality for mucinous tumors varies widely in reported series from as low as 5% to as high as 50%, but probably is no greater than 10% to 20%. Approximately 30% to 50% of endometrioid and clear-cell cancers are bilateral.

Several reports have detailed the reproductive outcomes of women with early-stage invasive epithelial ovarian cancer following treatment with fertility-sparing surgery with or without chemotherapy. In a multi-institutional retrospective review, Schilder and associates reported 52 patients with stage I invasive epithelial ovarian cancer treated with fertility-sparing surgery; 20 patients received adjuvant chemotherapy. Five patients developed recurrence 8 to 78 months after primary surgery, and nine patients required subsequent hysterectomy and contralateral oophorectomy for benign disease. Seventeen patients had 26 term deliveries and 5 spontaneous abortions.

Risk Assessment

To begin making decisions about which patients might benefit from postoperative or adjuvant therapy, one must categorize them based on risk of relapse. The risk of relapse is approximately 1% for patients with stage I borderline ovarian tumors; thus, adjuvant therapy is not recommended.

For women with stage IA or IB *sex cord–stromal tumors,* no adjuvant therapy is recommended because of the low risk of relapse. For those with stage IC disease, however, the level of risk remains uncertain; some studies suggest that tumor rupture or the presence of ascites is prognostic, whereas others do not.

All patients with early-stage malignant ovarian *germ-cell tumors*, except those with stage IA dysgerminoma or stage IA, grade 1 immature teratoma, require postoperative chemotherapy. As noted, there is some controversy about whether patients with stage IA yolk sac tumor or stage IA, grade 1 or 2 immature teratoma require adjuvant chemotherapy. Most experts in the United States favor treatment for such patients until such time as more information is available.

For patients with early-stage *epithelial ovarian cancer,* most experts currently accept a classification system of low and high risk (Table 49.9). Within the stage I category, histologic grade is the most powerful predictor of outcome. Patients with well-differentiated or grade 1 tumors have an excellent prognosis, with a 5-year survival rate of more than 90%. On the other hand, the 5-year survival rates for patients with grade 2 or 3 tumors are approximately 75% to 80% and 50% to 60%, respectively. Other factors that have been found to have prognostic significance include large-volume ascites, dense adherence, and clear-cell histology. Although older studies suggested that capsular rupture or excrescences may be associated with a worsened prognosis, more recent studies have found no independent influence of these features on prognosis. However, the issue of the influence of tumor rupture on prognosis remains controversial.

Therefore, low-risk early-stage epithelial ovarian cancer includes patients with the following factors: (a) stage IA or IB (intact capsule, no tumor excrescences, and no malignant ascites or negative peritoneal cytology) and (b) grade 1 or 2 disease. The standard treatment for this group of patients is surgery alone, and the 5-year survival is at least 95%. A controversy about whether grade 2 belongs in the low- or high-risk category remains unresolved; it is compounded by the lack of uniformity of grading systems.

TABLE 49.9

EARLY-STAGE EPITHELIAL OVARIAN CANCER RISK GROUPS

Low risk	High risk
Stage IA or IB, grade 1 and 2	Stage IA or IB, grade 3 Stage IC Tumor on external surface Ruptured capsule Ascites or positive peritoneal washing All stage II

High-risk early-stage epithelial ovarian cancer includes those patients with the following factors: (a) stages IC (ruptured capsule, tumor excrescences, positive peritoneal cytology, or malignant ascites) to II, (b) grade 3 disease, or (c) clear-cell histology. In some classification systems, dense adherence is also included in the high-risk category; however, in the view of many experts, this designation is simply a surrogate for stage II disease. This high-risk subset is thought to have a relapse risk in the range of 40% to 50% and is the focus of adjuvant therapy trials.

Persistent problems with incomplete surgical staging and interobserver variability in assigning histologic grade lead one to the realization that more objective and reliable methods would be desirable for assessment of risk in early-stage ovarian cancer. Currently, there is no universally accepted prognostic molecular biomarker. There are, however, reports of several putative or potential biomarkers. Among these are DNA ploidy, computerized morphometry, Ki-67, p53, and HER2/neu. Although none of the markers studied yet qualifies as prognostic, as technology advances, future studies will most certainly identify reliable biomarkers. Because there is no universal histologic grading system for epithelial ovarian cancer, investigators at M.D. Anderson Cancer Center recently reported a two-tier grading system for invasive serous carcinomas that emphasizes nuclear atypia rather than architecture, with mitotic count as a secondary feature. There is mounting evidence, both from genomic/molecular studies and clinical reports, supporting this low-grade/high-grade model.

Adjuvant Treatment

For patients with *malignant ovarian germ-cell tumors* who require adjuvant treatment, standard postoperative therapy consists of the combination of BEP. For patients with high-risk *early-stage sex cord–stromal tumors* (stage IC or II), there is no standard postoperative treatment. The most commonly used regimens include the BEP combination or the combination of paclitaxel and carboplatin.

Platinum-based chemotherapy has emerged as the standard treatment for patients with *early-stage epithelial ovarian cancer.* The optimal regimen and duration of therapy remains elusive. Bolis et al reported the results of two multicenter trials conducted by the Gruppo Italiano Collaborativo in Oncologia Ginecologica. A total of 271 patients were included in these two trials. Trial 1 compared single-agent cisplatin with observation in patients with stage IA and IB, grade 2 or 3. Trial 2 compared single-agent cisplatin with intraperitoneal chromic phosphate in patients with stages IA, grade 2, IB, grade 2, and IC disease. In both trials, although the cisplatin groups had a better disease-free survival, overall survival was not significantly different compared with the other arm. One possible explanation for these finding is that patients in the nonchemotherapy arm crossed over to cisplatin at time of relapse.

The Gynecologic Oncology Group (GOG) reported a randomized trial of cisplatin plus cyclophosphamide for three cycles versus intraperitoneal chromic phosphate in patients with high-risk early-stage ovarian cancer. With 204 evaluable patients randomized, relapse-free rates were 77% for the chemotherapy arm and 66% for the P^{32} arm. After adjusting for stage and histologic grade, the group receiving chemotherapy had a 29% decrement in estimated relapse. Chemotherapy was recommended as standard adjuvant therapy for this subset of patients because of the superior progression-free survival and the late bowel toxicity associated with P^{32}.

In a subsequent GOG trial, Bell and colleagues compared three versus six cycles of paclitaxel/carboplatin for patients with high-risk early-stage epithelial ovarian cancer. Although the recurrence rate associated with six cycles was 24% lower, the study was powered for a 50% or greater reduction in recurrence rate for six cycles. In addition, there was no difference in overall survival between the arms. In a recently completed GOG trial for early-stage disease, all patients initially received three cycles of paclitaxel/carboplatin and then were randomized between observation and 26 weekly doses of paclitaxel. Results of this trial are not yet available.

Two large European cooperative group trials in early-stage ovarian cancer were combined for analysis. Both the International Collaborative Ovarian Neoplasm 1 (ICON1) trial and the European Organisation for Research and Treatment of Cancer Collaborators—Adjuvant ChemoTherapy in Ovarian Neoplasm (EORTC-ACTION) trial randomized patients with early-stage epithelial ovarian cancer following surgery to observation versus platinum-based chemotherapy. Both overall survival and recurrence-free survival at 5 years were superior in the chemotherapy arm (82% vs. 74% and 76% vs. 65%, respectively).

Advanced-Stage Ovarian Cancer

Primary Cytoreductive Surgery

Cytoreductive or debulking surgery refers to a surgical procedure for which the goal is to reduce the amount of tumor as much as possible in a patient with metastatic ovarian cancer. Early studies suggested a relationship between the completeness of the surgery or the amount of residual tumor and survival. In a landmark paper, Griffiths demonstrated an inverse relationship between residual tumor diameter and survival; patients having residual disease less than 1.5 cm in diameter had a significantly improved survival compared with patients with bulky residual disease. Subsequent reports confirmed these findings. As our philosophy about cytoreductive surgery has evolved over the last 2 decades, *optimal debulking* has come to denote minimal residual disease less than or equal to 1.0 to 2.0 cm in greatest diameter; *suboptimal debulking* denotes bulky residual disease greater than 1.0 to 2.0 cm in diameter. Defining the extent of residual disease when dealing with tumor plaques on the peritoneal surfaces remains problematic. Furthermore, there is most certainly a lack of precision in measuring residual disease.

Cytoreductive surgery, of course, must be considered not in a vacuum but rather in the context of responsiveness of residual tumor to postoperative therapies. Both radiotherapy and chemotherapy trials have shown a higher response rate in patients with minimal residual disease. These observations are supported by basic studies that suggest that larger tumor masses have poorly perfused anoxic areas that are not accessible to cytotoxic agents. Furthermore, larger tumors may have a greater proportion of cells in the resting phase. These nonproliferating cells may be less sensitive to cytotoxic agents. Skipper espoused the fractional cell kill hypothesis, stating that the ability of chemotherapeutic agents to eradicate cancer cells depends on both the dose of drug and the number of cells present. A given dose of drug kills a constant fraction of cells with each exposure. However, certain factors—such as cell repair mechanisms, tumor heterogeneity, the fraction of cells in G0 phase, and the development of drug resistance—serve to counteract this process. Goldie and Coldman have shown that tumor cells have an intrinsic spontaneous mutation rate; larger tumors that go untreated for an extended period theoretically have a greater probability of containing cell populations resistant to anticancer agents. Therefore, even though patients with advanced ovarian cancer may undergo optimal debulking, the small residual tumor masses may still contain drug-resistant cells that preclude ultimate cure.

Several reports have described the accomplishment of optimal cytoreductive surgery in a high percentage of patients. The morbidity and mortality associated with cytoreductive surgery also have been analyzed. These studies generally reflect an operative mortality rate of less than 2%, a mean operating time of 3 to 5 hours, and a mean blood loss of approximately 500 to 1,500 mL. There is a wide range of postoperative complications, the most common of which are infection, hemorrhage (at times requiring reexploration), prolonged ileus, and cardiopulmonary problems. The primary question concerning the efficacy of primary cytoreductive surgery is whether improved survival is related more to the biology of the tumor or the skill and aggressiveness of the surgeon. In other words, are those tumors that can be debulked optimally also tumors that are less invasive, less infiltrative, and more indolent? Earlier studies do not suggest that this is the case. All demonstrated that patients who required extensive surgery to achieve minimal residual disease and those who had minimal disease at the outset had similar survival rates. More recent studies, however, suggest that patients with *de novo* minimal disease have a superior prognosis to those who are debulked to minimal disease, supporting the prognostic influence of substage categories within the stage III classification. Unfortunately, there are no randomized studies to resolve important issues in this area. Moreover, prospects for such studies are not good because of several factors, including deeply established biases, the multiplicity of associated prognostic factors, and the highly individualized nature of each procedure. In the meantime, the efficacy of cytoreductive surgery remains controversial. Better information will be required ultimately to define its role.

Studies indicate that optimal cytoreductive surgery may confer a survival advantage, even for patients with stage IV ovarian cancer. Four large retrospective reports noted that patients with stage IV disease who were optimally cytoreduced had a statistically superior survival to patients who were suboptimally cytoreduced (Table 49.10).

Exploration. The patient is placed in either the supine or semilithotomy or ski position, depending on the likelihood of a rectosigmoid resection. A vertical midline incision is employed and extended cephalad as much as necessary. On entering the abdomen, the initial steps outlined under surgical staging are followed. After evacuation of ascites, if present, and inspection and palpation, the size of the primary tumors(s) and size and extent of metastatic deposits should be noted.

During this initial phase of the operation, the surgeon must make an assessment of the feasibility of cytoreductive surgery. In a typical patient with advanced disease, the omentum may be totally replaced by tumor, and the pelvis may be filled with tumor, making it difficult or impossible for the surgeon to distinguish normal pelvic structures. Findings that may initially dissuade the surgeon from proceeding with aggressive tumor resection include extensive parenchymal hepatic involvement, massive diaphragmatic involvement, extensive infiltration of the small intestinal mesentery, or bulky nodal disease high in the paraaortic chain. On the other hand, even if minimal residual disease cannot be achieved, debulking of omental and pelvic masses may relieve production of ascites, reduce pressure on adjacent organs, and allow the patient increased comfort, at least temporarily. Moreover, intestinal resection still may be indicated for relief of impending or true obstruction.

Omentectomy. It is our preference to perform an omentectomy before focusing on the pelvis if the omentum is largely or completely replaced by tumor. If the omental tumor is adherent to the parietal peritoneum of the anterior abdominal wall, the pelvic structures, or loops of small intestine, it should be dissected from these structures. Once the omentum is mobilized and lifted cephalad, a dissection plane is developed between it and the serosa of the transverse colon, extending the dissection laterally in both directions (Fig. 49.5A). If the supracolic omentum is heavily involved with tumor and densely adherent to the transverse colon, it also may be necessary to establish a plane between the greater curvature of the stomach and the omentum by ligating the right and left gastroepiploic arteries and the individual gastric branches (Fig. 49.5B). Entrance into the lesser sac allows traction on the greater curvature of the stomach and facilitates exposure and transection of the gastric branches of the gastroepiploic arch. Occasionally, omental tumor may also involve the spleen or splenic hilum, necessitating splenectomy (see "Splenectomy").

Resection of Pelvic Tumor. Any adhesions of small intestine or cecum to the pelvic structures should be lysed. A self-retaining retractor then may be inserted and the bowel packed for adequate exposure. If normal pelvic spaces and planes are obliterated by tumor, then the retroperitoneal approach is preferred (Fig. 49.6). The lateral pelvic peritoneum is incised, and the incision is carried cephalad and caudad. As part of this maneuver, the round ligament is identified and ligated as well. The retroperitoneal space is thus entered and the

TABLE 49.10

EFFECT OF DEBULKING ON SURVIVAL IN STAGE IV OVARIAN CANCER

First author	Year	Surgical result	Patients	Optimal	Median survival	*p*
Curtin	1997	Optimal (<2 cm)	41	45%	40	0.01
		Suboptimal	51		18	
Liu	1997	Optimal (<2 cm)	14	30%	37	0.02
		Suboptimal	33		17	
Munkarah	1997	Optimal (<2 cm)	31	34%	25	0.02
		Suboptimal	61		15	
Bristow	1999	Optimal (≤1 cm)	25	30%	38	0.0004
		Suboptimal	59		10	

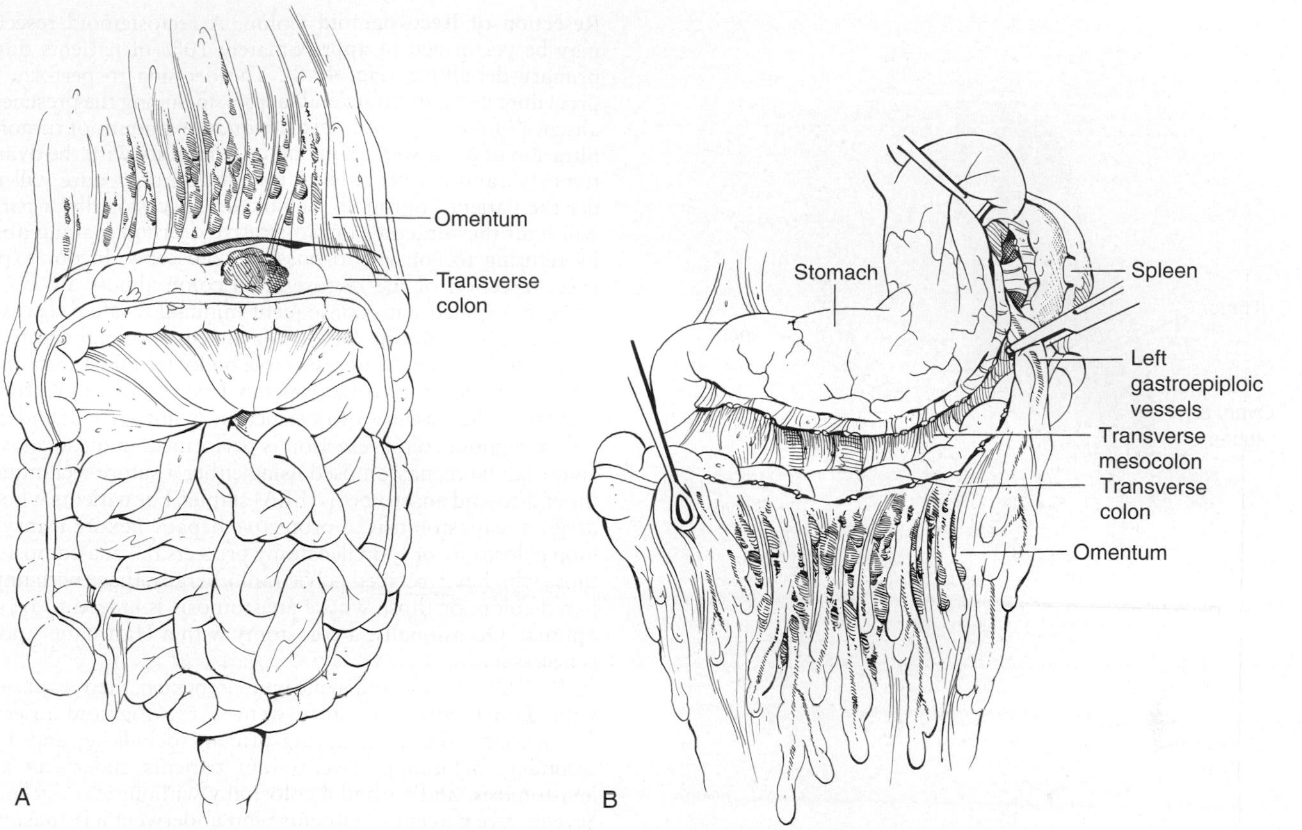

FIGURE 49.5. **A:** Omentectomy. Avascular dissection plane between omentum with metastatic ovarian tumor and transverse colon. **B:** Omentectomy. Dissection of omentum with tumor from stomach with ligation of gastric branches.

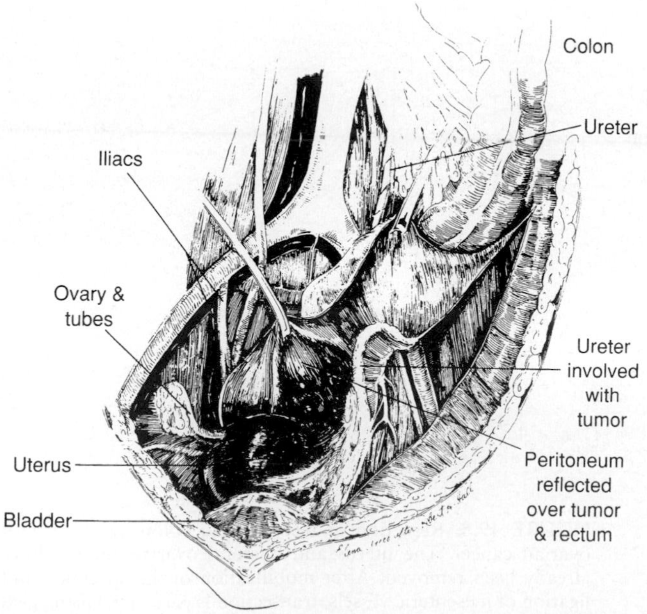

FIGURE 49.6. Retroperitoneal approach with lateral peritoneum incised, demonstrating the proximity of the left ovarian tumor to major pelvic vessels, the ureter, and the rectum.

structures—ureter, iliac vessels, and ovarian vessels—identified by using both sharp and blunt dissection. A suction tip is a very nice instrument for dissecting areolar tissue planes if used properly. Next, the ovarian vessels are ligated. The identical procedure is performed on the opposite side of the pelvis, and the tumor mass(es) is (are) mobilized medially.

If the ureters are densely adherent to the pelvic tumor, the surgeon may need to dissect them free, in some instances along the entire length of the pelvic portion of the ureter to the ureterovesical junction. In addition, the surgeon must establish a dissection plane between the sigmoid colon and the uterus and ovaries. This portion of the procedure may take considerable effort if this plane is obliterated by tumor. On the other hand, if the surgeon determines that such dissection is not feasible or that the wall of the colon is heavily infiltrated with tumor, resection of the rectosigmoid colon may be indicated (Fig. 49.7) (see "Resection of Rectosigmoid Colon"). Resection of the pelvic portion of the colon allows the surgeon access to the avascular retrorectal space. The uterus is dissected from the bladder as well. It is extremely rare for ovarian cancer to involve the bladder mucosa at the time of primary surgery, but the vesicouterine peritoneum may be heavily infiltrated. In such cases, resection of this area may be necessary, occasionally in conjunction with a partial cystectomy (see "Resection of the Urinary Tract"). Hysterectomy is then performed, the vagina is entered, and the mass is removed en bloc. In some instances, it may be necessary to ligate the uterine vessels at their origin rather than near the uterus if tumor is extensive in this area. Also, subtotal hysterectomy may be advisable if there is extensive unresectable tumor in the cul-de-sac.

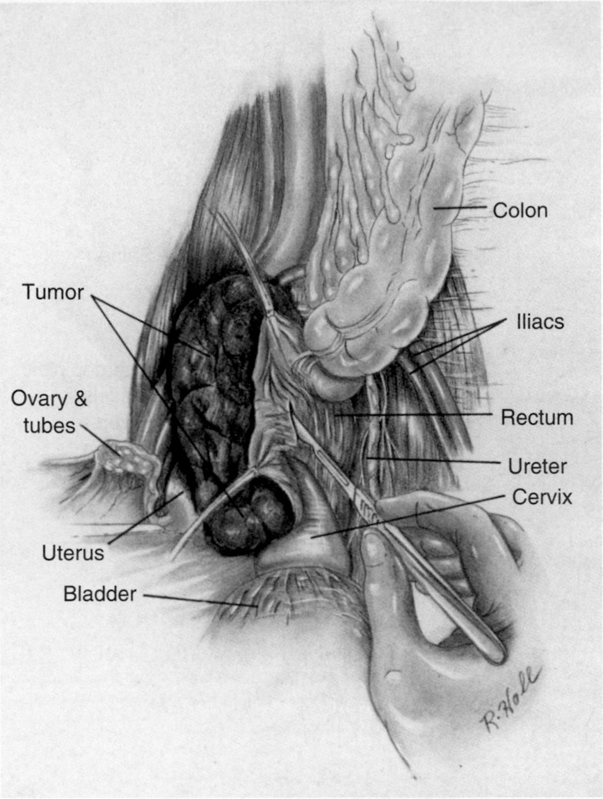

FIGURE 49.7. In the retroperitoneal approach, the proximity of the left ovarian tumor to the rectum is visualized before it is decided whether the tumor can be safely dissected from the rectum or resection of the rectosigmoid colon is required. (From Piver MS, Hempling RE. Ovarian cancer: etiology, screening, prophylactic oophorectomy, and surgery. In: Rock JA, Thompson JD. *Te Linde's Operative Gynecology.* 8th ed. Philadelphia: Lippincott Williams & Wilkins; 1997:1557.)

Resection of Rectosigmoid Colon. A rectosigmoid resection may be performed in approximately 10% of patients during primary debulking (Fig. 49.8). The decision to perform this procedure depends on several factors, including the presence or absence of rectosigmoid obstruction, the amount of tumor infiltration of the lower colon and its contiguity with the ovarian tumor(s), and the probability that such a procedure will render the patient "optimally debulked." Occasionally, a patient will limit the surgeon's intraoperative decision-making ability by refusing to consent to possible colostomy. In our experience, resection of the rectosigmoid colon almost always can be accomplished with consequent minimal residual disease in the pelvis; the limiting factor in achieving optimal cytoreduction, however, may be unresectable bulky residual tumor in the upper abdomen or retroperitoneum. In such cases, palliative resection in the absence of obstruction is not recommended. If a rectosigmoid colon resection is performed, in most cases the colon can be reanastomosed using either a suture technique or the end-to-end anastomosis (EEA) stapler. For patients who undergo a reanastomosis, a protective hepatic flexure transverse loop colostomy or loop ileostomy protects the anastomosis for those who have received pelvic radiotherapy, those with unprepared colon, or those whose anastomosis is judged to be suboptimal. Occasionally, a colostomy with a Hartmann's pouch is necessary.

In 1984, Berek and colleagues reported their experience with 35 patients who underwent a rectosigmoid resection for ovarian cancer, 22 during primary debulking and 13 at secondary debulking. Twenty-four patients underwent a reanastomosis, and 11 had a colostomy without reanastomosis. Seventy-five percent of patients who underwent a reanastomosis did not require a protective colostomy. Optimal cytoreduction (residual tumor <1.5 cm in diameter) was accomplished in 94% of patients undergoing primary surgery and 57% undergoing secondary surgery. Although major morbidity occurred in seven patients (20%), it was temporary in all except one, who developed an anastomotic stricture. There were no postoperative anastomotic leaks or pelvic abscesses.

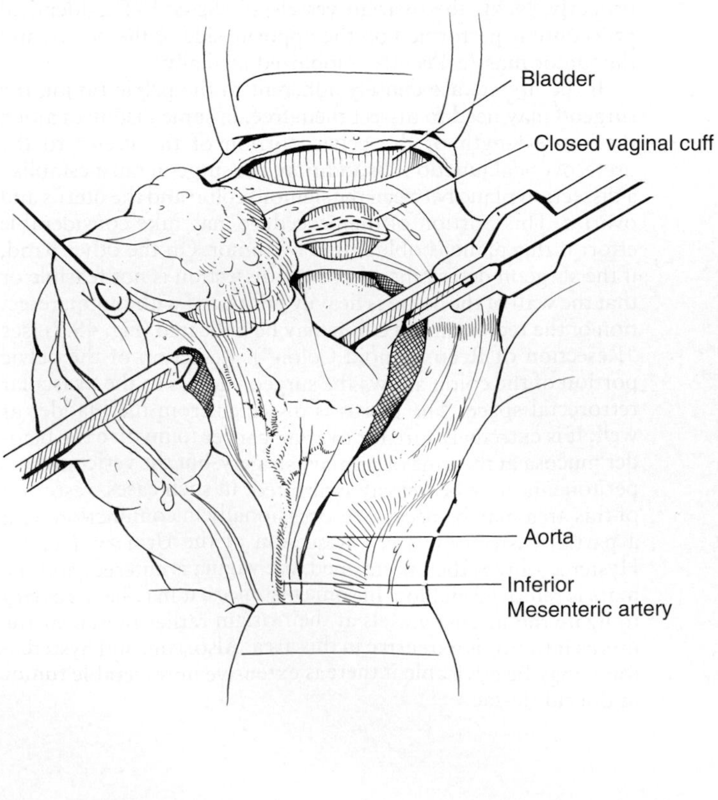

FIGURE 49.8. Resection of rectosigmoid colon involved with ovarian cancer. The uterus and bilateral ovarian tumors have already been removed. After mobilization of the specimen and ligation of mesenteric vessels, transection is performed using gastrointestinal anastomotic (GIA) stapling devices (or reticulating stapler for distal transection), and remainder of mesentery is ligated. Usually, reanastomosis using EEA stapler can be accomplished.

Soper and associates described 40 women who underwent rectosigmoid colon resection during cytoreductive surgery, 21 (53%) as part of a primary procedure and 19 (47%) as part of a secondary procedure. Residual disease was less than 1 cm in 54% of patients. A permanent colostomy was avoided in 78% of patients. Twenty-five percent of patients experienced major morbidity, including one patient who developed an anastomotic dehiscence and pelvic abscess requiring a colostomy. One patient (3%) died in the immediate postoperative period. Despite aggressive surgical resection and postoperative therapy, the median survival for the entire group was only 14.5 months. More recent studies have also confirmed the clinical observation that en bloc resection of the rectosigmoid colon during ovarian cancer surgery does result in a high rate of optimal or complete cytoreduction with acceptable morbidity.

Small Intestinal Resection. Although the small intestine is a common site of metastasis, both to the serosa and the mesentery, extensive tumor involvement is an uncommon finding at primary surgery. If the small intestine is extensively involved with tumor, it is usually in the terminal ileum. Occasionally, small intestinal obstruction, either partial or complete, is present at diagnosis. As noted, complete surgical staging includes careful examination of the entire length of the small intestine from the ligament of Treitz to the cecum. If, on exploration, loops of small intestine are adherent to the pelvic tumor, omental tumor, or other loops of intestine, then these adhesions should be lysed. Indications for small intestinal resection include obstruction or impending obstruction by tumor infiltrating the serosa and muscularis of a segment or a nonobstructing extensive lesion of the small intestine for which resection would result in minimal residual disease.

If the lesion involves the very terminal portion of the ileum, an ileocolectomy with resection of the cecum and portion of ascending colon adjacent to the small intestine may be necessary. Care should be taken to avoid the presence of tumor at the points of reanastomosis. The reanastomosis may be performed using either the suture or the stapling technique. In our experience and in the literature, small intestinal resection is indicated in approximately 5% to 10% of primary operations for ovarian cancer.

Resection of the Urinary Tract. Indications for ureteral resection or partial cystectomy are uncommon during cytoreductive surgery. If ureteral obstruction is noted preoperatively, it is almost always a result of ureteral compression rather than tumor infiltration. Although adherence of the ureter(s) to masses of ovarian cancer is not an unusual finding, the surgeon can almost always separate the ureter from the tumor using sharp dissection. If the distal ureter is resected as part of cytoreductive surgery, it usually can be reimplanted into the bladder. More commonly, the ureter may be injured during the course of debulking surgery. Depending on the site of injury, a primary reanastomosis, transureteroureterostomy, or ureteroneocystostomy may be indicated. In a report by Berek and associates, 16 of 848 patients (2%) underwent partial ureteral resection. Five patients had transureteroureterostomy, two had reanastomosis, and four had urinary diversion. Twelve of the operations were part of primary cytoreductive surgery, and four were part of secondary surgery. Nine of these 16 patients had evidence of ureteral obstruction on preoperative intravenous pyelograms.

On the other hand, tumor involvement of the peritoneum overlying the urinary bladder is not an uncommon finding during primary cytoreductive surgery. Occasionally, a partial cystectomy may be necessary to achieve optimal cytoreduction. In the series of Berek and associates, eight patients had a partial cystectomy for advanced ovarian cancer. Reconstruction necessitated ureteral reimplantation in two patients and an ileal conduit in one patient. If a partial cystotomy is indicated, we prefer a simple closure with two layers of chromic catgut suture, the inner layer as a continuous running suture and the outer layer as interrupted sutures.

In our experience, it is exceedingly rare to find involvement of the bladder mucosa with ovarian cancer at initial diagnosis. Such patients usually report hematuria in association with obvious massive disease. The definitive diagnosis can be made easily by preoperative cystoscopy.

Splenectomy. Splenectomy is indicated occasionally during primary cytoreductive surgery (Fig. 49.9). Various series report the incidence of splenectomy during primary cytoreductive surgery in 5% to 11% of cases of advanced ovarian cancer. In addition, the indications for splenectomy and the procedure itself have been described in case reports. Most commonly, the hilum of the spleen is involved with ovarian cancer in association with extensive omental involvement. Rarely, isolated splenic capsular involvement or even splenic parenchymal involvement may be found. In addition to tumor debulking, splenectomy also may be indicated during cytoreductive surgery because of a traction injury with avulsion of the splenic capsule during omentectomy or mobilization of the splenic flexure of the colon in association with descending colostomy or reanastomosis after rectosigmoid colon resection. If a splenic capsular avulsion injury does occur in the absence of tumor involvement, splenorrhaphy may be indicated before resorting to splenectomy.

In the series of Sonnendecker et al, five patients underwent splenectomy because of metastatic disease involving the spleen, one with parenchymal involvement, and one patient required splenectomy for capsular avulsion injury. In a report from M.D. Anderson Cancer Center, Morris and colleagues reported on 23 patients for whom the procedure was performed as part of cytoreductive surgery for advanced ovarian cancer. Splenectomy was planned preoperatively in only three of these patients. Seven patients had parenchymal involvement by tumor, 11 had capsular disease, and 5 had no pathologic involvement by tumor.

The methods of performing splenectomy during cytoreductive surgery may vary depending on the circumstances. Under controlled conditions (no uncontrolled hemorrhage), the surgeon may prefer to incise the gastrosplenic ligament, gain access to the lesser sac, and identify and ligate the splenic vessels as they run along the superior border of the pancreas. The spleen then can be mobilized by transecting its attachments to the colon, the left kidney, and the diaphragm. If hemorrhage is occurring or access to the lesser sac is limited by the distribution of tumor, the surgeon may prefer to first mobilize the spleen by dividing its peritoneal attachments while compressing the splenic vessels, and then ligate the splenic vessels using a posterior approach. The spleen is rotated anteriorly and medially in this technique.

Complications associated with splenectomy include hemorrhage, infection, thromboembolic phenomena, left-sided atelectasis or pneumonia, injury to the tail of the pancreas (with resultant pancreatic pseudocyst), or injury to the stomach (with resultant gastric fistula). Because of the risk of severe infection following splenectomy, the patient should receive perioperative antibiotic coverage and should be vaccinated with polyvalent pneumococcal, quadrivalent meningococcal, and hemophilus influenzae vaccines. We also prefer to insert a drain in the splenic bed postoperatively to diagnose early postoperative hemorrhage and reduce the infection rate.

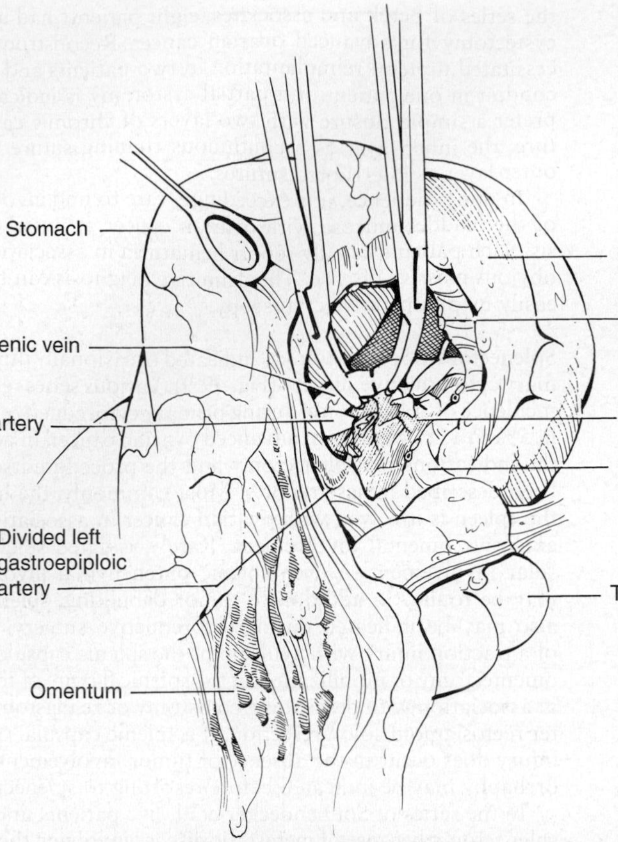

FIGURE 49.9. Splenectomy. Transection of splenic artery and vein along the superior border of the pancreas after access is gained to lesser sac with transection of gastrosplenic ligament.

Resection of Diaphragmatic Tumor. Several reports have described experience with resection of diaphragmatic metastatic deposits in patients with advanced ovarian cancer (Fig. 49.10). To gain access to the diaphragmatic surfaces, the abdominal incision is extended to just below the xiphoid process, and the liver is mobilized by transecting the entire falciform ligament and the coronary and triangular ligaments. After it is adequately exposed, the diaphragmatic tumor may be resected by stripping the peritoneum from the diaphragmatic muscle using sharp dissection with either Metzenbaum scissors or electrocautery. Alternative techniques of debulking in this area are discussed in the following. The anesthesiologist should be notified if the pleural cavity is entered. Defects in the diaphragm may be closed with interrupted sutures. If a large defect cannot be closed primarily or can be closed only under tension, then the defect may be closed using synthetic mesh. If the

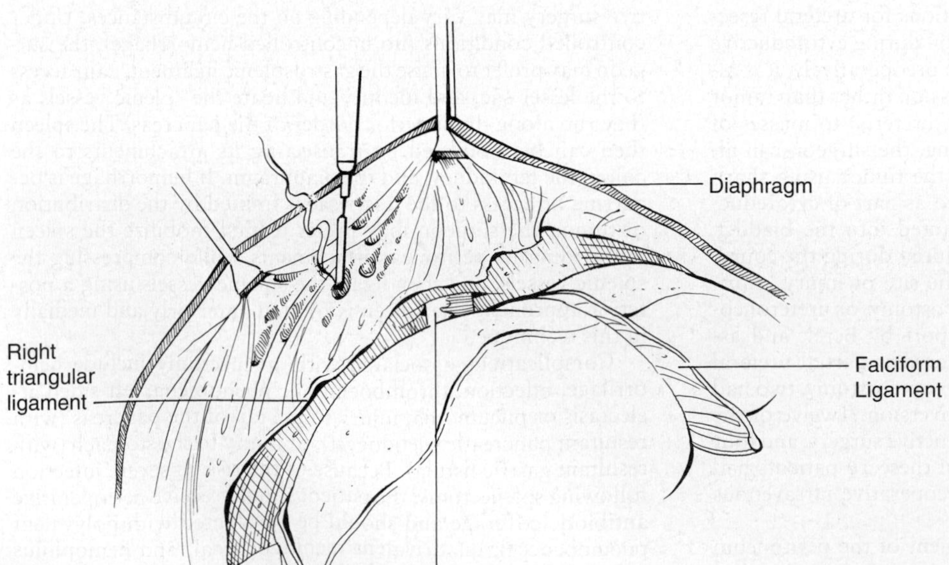

FIGURE 49.10. Ablation of subdiaphragmatic tumor implants with cautery after mobilization of liver. Sharp dissection, argon beam coagulator, or Cavitron ultrasonic surgical aspirator (CUSA) also may be used for the same purpose.

pleural cavity is entered, then a thoracostomy tube should be placed.

Possible complications associated with resection of diaphragmatic tumor include pneumothorax, hemorrhage from the phrenic arteries, infection, injury to the pericardial sac, and injury to such structures as the lung, the vena cava, or the phrenic nerves.

Whether aggressive resection of diaphragmatic metastases with associated potential complications is justified is unclear. Montz and coworkers reported that 13 of 14 patients with diaphragmatic tumor could be optimally debulked. The size of resected specimens ranged from 12 × 7 cm to 17 × 11 cm. Kapnick and colleagues found that tumors that penetrated the entire thickness of the diaphragm to involve the pleura were greater than or equal to 5.0 cm in diameter. Patients with tumors that penetrated the diaphragm had a median survival time of 8 months compared with a median survival time of 26 months for those patients without full-thickness diaphragmatic penetration by the tumor. Therefore, the assessment of the benefit of this procedure must await further studies.

In a review of the Mayo Clinic experience, Aletti and associates found that for the subgroup of 181 patients with ovarian cancer metastatic to the diaphragm, those who underwent diaphragm surgery had improved 5-year overall survival compared with those who did not (53% vs. 15%). In another recent study of 262 patients with stages IIIC to IV epithelial ovarian cancer, Eisenhauer and colleagues found that patients requiring extensive upper abdominal procedures to achieve optimal debulking demonstrated a similar initial response, progression-free survival, and overall survival to patients optimally debulked by standard surgical techniques.

Resection of Retroperitoneal Lymph Nodes. The initial retroperitoneal approach for cytoreductive surgery exposes the node-bearing areas. Lymph nodes are sampled as part of the staging technique, and every effort is extended to remove suspicious retroperitoneal nodes when the peritoneal cavity has been cleared of disease (Fig. 49.11). The benefit of radical resection of extensive retroperitoneal lymph node metastases also remains unclear. Burghardt and associates compared the survival of 70 patients with stage III ovarian cancer who had undergone radical pelvic lymphadenectomy with 40 patients with the same stage of disease treated without lymphadenectomy. The actuarial 5-year survival was superior for the former group: 53% versus 13%, respectively. In the reports of Wu and colleagues and Burghardt and associates, the role of pelvic and paraaortic lymphadenectomy at initial surgery for ovarian cancer is discussed, but there is no particular discussion of debulking of grossly enlarged retroperitoneal nodes. Benedetti-Panici and coworkers reported the findings of a prospective study on the feasibility and morbidity of radical paraaortic and pelvic lymphadenectomy in patients with gynecologic malignancies. They observed acceptable morbidity—principally hemorrhage, lymphocyst formation, and deep venous thrombosis—and no operative mortality. Scarabelli et al retrospectively evaluated the potential benefit on survival of systematic pelvic and paraaortic lymphadenectomy during both primary and secondary cytoreductive surgery in patients with stage IIIC or IV ovarian cancer. The previously untreated patients who underwent systematic lymphadenectomy had a significantly improved survival. The authors appropriately recommended a prospective randomized study to determine the efficacy of such an approach.

For patients with malignant germ-cell tumors, especially dysgerminoma, the advantages of debulking metastatic retroperitoneal nodes are even less apparent, because these tumors are generally much more sensitive to chemotherapy than are other ovarian tumors.

Until further information becomes available, it is probably reasonable to consider debulking enlarged retroperitoneal nodes if peritoneal metastases can be cytoreduced optimally, if there is no fixation to blood vessels, and if the surgeon believes that the procedure can be successfully accomplished without undue risk.

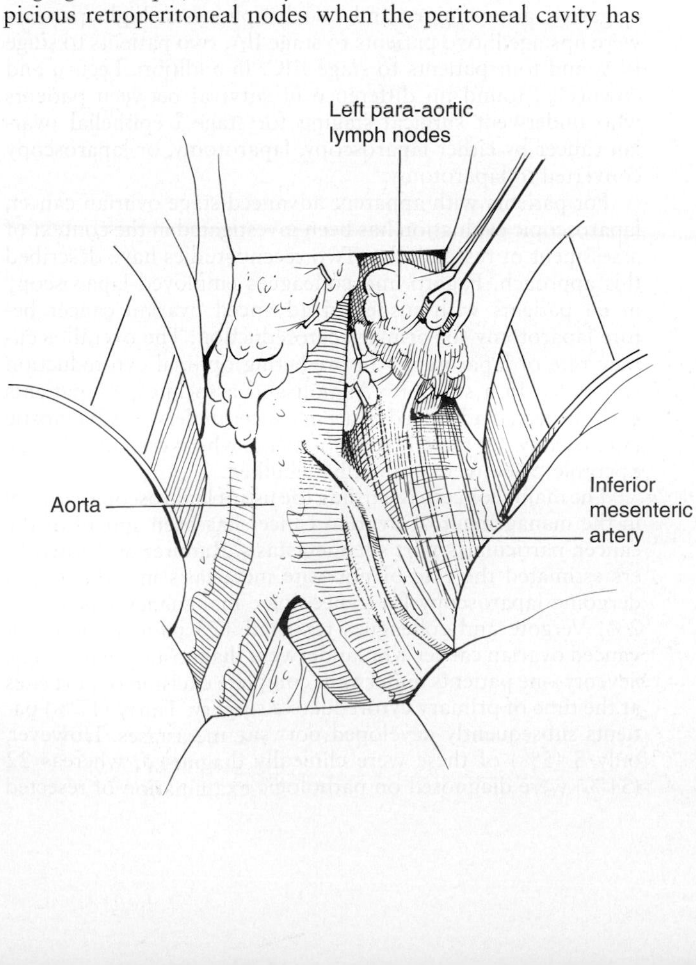

FIGURE 49.11. Retroperitoneal dissection of paraaortic lymph nodes involved with metastatic ovarian cancer.

Recently, the issue of systematic aortic and pelvic lymphadenectomy has come more to the forefront. Eisenkop and Spirtos reported on 100 patients with stage IIC to IV epithelial ovarian cancer who underwent a retroperitoneal lymph node dissection at the time of primary cytoreductive surgery. Sixty-six percent had positive lymph nodes. Five were microscopically positive, and 61 were macroscopically positive, of which 19 (31%) were positive by palpation, 16 (26%) were positive by inspection, and 26 (43%) were positive by dissection. On the other hand, there were 39 patients with negative or only microscopically positive nodes, and 15 of these patients (39%) were thought to have clinically positive nodes by the operating surgeon. The authors concluded that a significant proportion of patients had macroscopically positive lymph nodes that were detectable only after a dissection was in progress, and clinical impression of lymph node status was unreliable.

Morice and colleagues reported on 276 women with epithelial ovarian cancer who underwent systematic bilateral pelvic and paraaortic lymphadenectomy. The overall frequency of lymph node involvement was 44%. Pelvic and paraaortic lymph nodes were involved 30% and 40% of the time, respectively. In patients with apparent stage IA, IB, and IC disease, the rates of nodal involvement were 13%, 33%, and 38%, respectively. And, in their report of a large randomized clinical trial (N = 427 patients) comparing systematic pelvic and paraaortic lymphadenectomy versus resection of bulky lymph nodes only, Benedetti-Panici and colleagues found that systematic lymphadenectomy improves progression-free survival but not overall survival in women with optimally cytoreduced advanced ovarian cancer.

Additional Techniques for Cytoreductive Surgery. In the last few years, several reports described innovative techniques of debulking: the argon beam coagulator, the Cavitron ultrasonic surgical aspirator (CUSA), and various types of laser therapy.

The argon beam coagulator is an electrosurgical device that conducts current to tissue in a beam of inert argon gas. Brand and Pearlman reported the use of the argon beam coagulator for debulking in seven patients with advanced ovarian cancer. Areas treated using the device included the diaphragm, stomach, duodenum, small intestine, colon, liver capsule, peritoneum, bladder and ureters, vaginal apex and parametrium, iliac vessels, and abdominal wall. Four of the patients had no gross residual tumor, and three had residual masses of less than or equal to 2 to 3 mm in diameter. Bristow and Montz reported the use of the argon beam coagulator to facilitate cytoreduction in 31 patients and concluded that it is a useful adjunct to standard techniques and appears to significantly increase the feasibility of achieving optimal cytoreduction.

There have been several reports of the use of the CUSA for cytoreductive surgery. The CUSA combines tissue fragmentation, irrigation, and aspiration while dissecting tumor from blood vessels without injuring them. Adelson and associates described cytoreduction of tumors to less than 0.5 cm in 9 of 10 patients. The authors particularly noted that intestinal resections were avoided because of the use of the CUSA. Deppe et al reported on 11 patients who underwent optimal debulking using the CUSA. In other reports, the same authors described the utility of the CUSA in debulking diaphragmatic metastases and retroperitoneal lymph nodes. In the latter report, the authors were able to optimally resect extensive paraaortic and pelvic lymph node masses in five of six patients with advanced ovarian cancer. Two patients sustained lacerations of the inferior vena cava during the procedure.

Use of the neodymium-yttrium-aluminum-garnet (Nd-YAG) laser for the resection of intraabdominal tumors has been reported. Other reports of laser therapy for metastatic deposits of ovarian cancer undoubtedly will follow during the next few years.

The benefit of any of these new techniques for cytoreductive surgery remains unproved. Further studies will be necessary to elucidate their proper role.

Role of Laparoscopy in the Clinical Management of Ovarian Cancer

At present, the role of laparoscopy in the management of ovarian cancer is evolving. There are several clinical settings in which the potential for this surgical modality has been investigated: (a) primary surgery for early-stage ovarian cancer, (b) restaging of unstaged ovarian cancer, (c) primary cytoreductive surgery for advanced-stage ovarian cancer, (d) assessment of resectability, (e) intraperitoneal catheter placement, (f) second-look surgery, and (g) secondary cytoreductive surgery.

Chi and colleagues compared 20 patients who underwent surgical staging via a laparoscopic approach with 30 patients who underwent surgical staging via laparotomy for ovarian or fallopian tube cancer. They found no differences in body mass index, omental specimen size, and number of resected lymph nodes. The estimated blood loss and hospital stay were lower for laparoscopy patients, but operating time was longer. LeBlanc and associates performed laparoscopic restaging in 53 patients—42 early after initial surgery for ovarian or fallopian tube cancer and 11 for second-look surgery after primary chemotherapy. Of the 42 early restaging procedures, 41 were completed successfully. An average of 20 paraaortic lymph nodes and 14 pelvic lymph nodes were removed in these procedures. Complications included a hematoma from an inferior epigastric artery injury and two lymphocysts. Eight patients were upstaged: two patients to stage IIA, two patients to stage IIIA, and four patients to stage IIIC. In addition, Lecuru and coworkers found no difference in survival between patients who underwent surgical staging for stage I epithelial ovarian cancer by either laparoscopy, laparotomy, or laparoscopy converted to laparotomy.

For patients with apparent advanced-stage ovarian cancer, laparoscopic evaluation has been investigated in the context of assessment of resectability. Two recent studies have described this approach. Fagotti and colleagues employed laparoscopy in 64 patients with suspected advanced ovarian cancer before laparotomy for primary cytoreduction. The overall accuracy rate of laparoscopy in predicting optimal cytoreduction was 90%. In a study by Angioli and associates, 87 patients with suspected advanced ovarian cancer underwent diagnostic laparoscopy. Of the 53 (61%) patients who were judged to be operable, 96% were optimally debulked.

The major concern regarding the use of laparoscopic surgery in the management of ovarian cancer has been spread of the cancer, particularly port site metastasis. Ramirez and coworkers estimated the rate of port site metastasis in patients undergoing laparoscopy for gynecologic malignancies as 1% to 2%. Vergote and colleagues reported 173 patients with advanced ovarian cancer who underwent diagnostic laparoscopy. Seventy-one patients underwent complete excision of port sites at the time of primary cytoreductive surgery. Thirty (17%) patients subsequently developed port site metastases. However, only 8 (5%) of these were clinically diagnosed, whereas 22 (31%) were diagnosed on pathologic examination of resected port sites. All of the port-site metastases resolved during primary chemotherapy, and prognosis was not worsened by this finding.

Therefore, the role of laparoscopy is evolving. At present, the most useful settings for this approach appear to be primary surgery for apparent early-stage disease, restaging of apparent early-stage disease that is unstaged before referral, and assessment of resectability in patients with advanced-stage disease to determine whether primary cytoreductive surgery or neoadjuvant chemotherapy and interval debulking is preferable.

Primary Chemotherapy for Advanced Ovarian Cancer

For patients with advanced-stage *malignant ovarian germ-cell tumors,* the standard regimen is identical to that for patients with early-stage disease who require chemotherapy—the BEP regimen. The optimal number of cycles remains unknown, but for these patients with a potentially greater tumor burden than those with early-stage disease, four to six cycles may be required in some instances. Generally, administering two cycles following normalization of serum tumor markers may be a reasonable guide, although there are no definitive studies to support this practice.

For patients with advanced-stage *sex cord–stromal tumors,* platinum-based combination chemotherapy is generally recommended. As noted, the BEP combination regimen or the combination of paclitaxel/carboplatin are the most popular regimens in the United States.

For advanced-stage *epithelial ovarian cancer,* the combination of cisplatin and cyclophosphamide was the standard postoperative regimen throughout most of the 1980s and until the mid-1990s. Subsequently, based on encouraging results of phase II studies of paclitaxel in patients with refractory ovarian cancer, GOG initiated a randomized trial comparing the standard regimen of cyclophosphamide/cisplatin with the combination of paclitaxel/cisplatin in patients with suboptimally debulked advanced epithelial ovarian cancer. The findings of this study revealed a significant outcome advantage for the paclitaxel/cisplatin regimen in terms of progression-free survival and overall survival. A subsequent similar study conducted by a European consortium confirmed the results of the GOG study.

Subsequently, based on the results of a GOG phase I trial, GOG initiated a randomized study comparing paclitaxel/cisplatin with paclitaxel/carboplatin. In the latter regimen, paclitaxel was administered over 3 rather than 24 hours, as in the previous GOG study. Recent data from that study suggest that the paclitaxel/carboplatin regimen is equally efficacious and has a superior toxicity profile compared with the paclitaxel/cisplatin regimen. A study conducted by a German consortium (AGO) demonstrated similar results. Thus, because of its superior therapeutic index, the paclitaxel/carboplatin regimen has become the standard postoperative treatment for patients with advanced epithelial ovarian cancer.

Two other studies, however, have somewhat confused the issue. GOG reported the results of a phase III randomized study in which the 24-hour infusion paclitaxel and cisplatin regimen was compared with single-agent paclitaxel and single-agent cisplatin. Response with single-agent paclitaxel was significantly inferior, but overall survival was identical for all three arms of the study, probably because of significant crossover of patients on monotherapy to the other single agent. In another study conducted by the British Medical Research Council, the paclitaxel/carboplatin regimen was compared with a nonpaclitaxel regimen (either single-agent carboplatin or a combination of cyclophosphamide/doxorubicin/cisplatin). There was no difference in outcome between the two treatment arms with a relatively short follow-up time. However, approximately 20% of the patients in this trial had early-stage disease.

Vasey and colleagues conducted a phase III trial of docetaxel/carboplatin versus paclitaxel/carboplatin as first-line chemotherapy for stage IC to IV epithelial ovarian cancer and peritoneal cancer. A total of 1,077 patients were enrolled in the study. Although there were no differences in progression-free survival or overall survival between the two groups, the docetaxel/carboplatin regimen was associated with significantly less neurotoxicity but more myelotoxicity. GOG recently reported the preliminary results of their latest phase III trial in advanced ovarian cancer. This was a five-arm study that introduced three new drugs into first-line therapy as either three-drug combinations or sequential doublets, including liposomal doxorubicin, topotecan, and gemcitabine. The results indicated that no regimen demonstrated superiority to the control arm of paclitaxel/carboplatin.

Intraperitoneal chemotherapy also has been studied as primary treatment for patients with optimally cytoreduced advanced epithelial ovarian cancer. With the recent publication of GOG #172, three GOG studies have now demonstrated the benefits of intraperitoneal chemotherapy over intravenous chemotherapy in the treatment of this subgroup. In an intergroup study, the first such trial, 654 patients with less than 2 cm residual disease were randomized to receive intravenous cisplatin/cyclophosphamide versus intraperitoneal cisplatin plus intravenous cyclophosphamide. The median survival was significantly longer in the group receiving intraperitoneal cisplatin (49 months) than in the group receiving intravenous cisplatin (41 months). In addition, toxicity was worse in the intravenous group. The second GOG intraperitoneal study used intravenous versus intraperitoneal cisplatin as part of initial therapy. Patients on the intraperitoneal arm received an initial two cycles of moderate-dose systemic carboplatin. The results of that study showed a significant improvement in progression-free survival for the intraperitoneal arm but only a borderline effect on overall survival. Because of significant design flaws associated with each of these GOG studies, the role of intraperitoneal chemotherapy in the management of advanced ovarian cancer remained unclear.

In the most definitive trial to date, Armstrong and associates conducted a phase III trial comparing intravenous paclitaxel plus cisplatin versus intravenous paclitaxel and intraperitoneal cisplatin, with intraperitoneal paclitaxel on day 8. The median overall survival was significantly better for the intraperitoneal chemotherapy arm: 66 versus 50 months ($p = 0.03$). However, short-term quality of life and toxicity—principally fatigue, hematologic, gastrointestinal, metabolic, and neurological—were significantly worse in the intraperitoneal arm. Furthermore, only 42% of patients in the intraperitoneal chemotherapy arm were able to complete all six cycles of planned treatment. Nevertheless, this study has generated much renewed enthusiasm for the intraperitoneal chemotherapy approach, as well as controversy.

An article detailing the intraperitoneal catheter complications in the recent GOG trial was also published. Of the 119 patients in the intraperitoneal chemotherapy arm who were not able to complete six cycles of treatment, 34% discontinued therapy because of catheter complications, and 29% discontinued for noncatheter-related reasons. There also appeared to be an association between sigmoid resection and inability to initiate intraperitoneal chemotherapy.

Neoadjuvant Chemotherapy and Interval Cytoreductive Surgery

Over the past two decades, the concept of neoadjuvant chemotherapy followed by interval debulking (as a primary cytoreductive procedure after a few cycles of chemotherapy) has emerged. This approach began to be reported in the late 1970s for certain subsets of patients: patients who were referred to an oncologist after a surgical or nonsurgical biopsy or patients who initially were poor surgical candidates because of a debilitated state related to massive effusions or comorbid conditions. However, this approach has been proposed as a potential alternative for all patients with advanced epithelial ovarian cancer or for certain subsets, such as those predicted to be suboptimally resected. The potential advantage of such an approach is to operate on a patient with an improved nutritional status, a smaller tumor burden, and superior perioperative risk.

Although several studies have explored the concept of a surrogate marker of unresectability of advanced ovarian cancer, as evidenced by the outcome of bulky residual disease, this issue remains unresolved. If accurate, such a strategy could potentially avoid a suboptimal debulking with the associated morbidity. The principal focus has been on preoperative serum CA-125 or CT appearance of disease. Unfortunately, to date, neither has been accurate enough to be incorporated into standard care. Diagnostic laparoscopy has also been investigated as a tool for assessing respectability; this approach may ultimately prove to be the most practical and accurate method, but further study is indicated.

A number of retrospective series have reported the feasibility of neoadjuvant chemotherapy and interval debulking. Clinical observations from these reports indicate the following: (a) a high proportion (70%–80%) of patients treated with neoadjuvant chemotherapy have partial or complete responses before interval surgery; (b) a high proportion of patients so treated, possibly higher than with primary cytoreductive surgery, are optimally debulked with minimal residual disease; and (c) the surgical morbidity may be reduced compared with that associated with primary cytoreductive surgery. A European cooperative group is currently studying this approach in a randomized clinical trial. It is hoped that the results of this trial will elucidate the role of neoadjuvant chemotherapy and interval cytoreductive surgery.

SECONDARY SURGERY

Second-Look Laparotomy

Second-look laparotomy for evaluation of disease status following treatment for cancer of the colon was proposed initially by Wangensteen and associates in 1948. Beginning in the early 1960s, second-look laparotomy was used extensively in the management of ovarian cancer. The procedure continued to gain popularity as more ovarian cancer patients were treated with chemotherapy and fewer received radiotherapy. Since the mid-1980s, however, there has been increasing skepticism about the benefits of this procedure. Currently, second-look surgery is not part of the routine management of patients with any histologic type of ovarian cancer. Although it remains the most accurate method of assessing disease status at completion of primary chemotherapy, no study has demonstrated a survival benefit associated with the procedure. In addition to the lack of demonstrated survival benefit, second-look surgery is still not that precise; approximately 50% of patients with negative findings ultimately relapse. However, second-look surgery is still occasionally used if it is part of a clinical trial or if the findings would make a patient eligible for a subsequent clinical trial.

Most experts agree that the term *second-look surgery* should be restricted to an operation performed on a patient with no clinical evidence of persistent tumor for the purpose of determining disease status after a planned interval of treatment with chemotherapy. The term should not be applied to a surgical procedure performed in patients with clinical evidence of persistent or progressive disease for the primary purpose of debulking or treatment of complications.

The operative technique of second-look laparotomy has been well described. It is essentially identical to a staging laparotomy, as discussed previously. An adequate vertical midline abdominal incision is made. On entering the abdomen, cytologic washings from the pelvis, bilateral paracolic gutters, and subdiaphragmatic areas are obtained, and the entire contents of the peritoneal cavity are inspected and palpated. If obvious macroscopic tumor is present, then the procedure usually is limited. However, the extent of disease should be carefully determined, and a few biopsies should be taken for documentation of persistent disease (frozen as well as permanent section). If no obvious macroscopic disease is noted, then random biopsy specimens are taken routinely from the peritoneal surfaces, including the cul-de-sac, vesicouterine reflection, bilateral pelvic walls, bilateral paracolic gutters, and surfaces of the diaphragm. Omental biopsies and biopsies of the retroperitoneal lymph nodes also are performed. Lysis of adhesions is not uncommon in the process of performing these biopsies. Sites of previously documented tumor and adhesions should be carefully evaluated and generously sampled. An adequate procedure consists of a minimum of 20 to 30 biopsy specimens.

Of course, laparoscopy rather than laparotomy is an alternative for patients who undergo second-look surgery. Obvious advantages include better visualization of peritoneal surfaces as well as more rapid recovery and significantly reduced time in hospital. Both the "open" and "closed" techniques have been reported.

Findings at second-look surgery are classified as negative (grossly and pathologically negative), microscopically positive (grossly negative, pathologically positive), and macroscopically positive (grossly and pathologically positive). The clinical variables most consistently associated with findings at second-look surgery and survival afterward are histologic grade, amount of residual disease, and FIGO stage. Patients with minimal residual disease and early-stage disease have a greater probability of having negative findings at second-look laparotomy than do those with bulky residual disease or advanced-stage disease. Other variables found to correlate with second-look findings and subsequent survival in some of these studies are histologic type, type of chemotherapy, amount of disease found at the initial surgery, age, performance status, and peritoneal cytology status.

Findings in approximately 30% to 50% of patients with advanced ovarian cancer (and a smaller percentage of those with early-stage disease) will be macroscopically positive at second-look surgery. Approximately 20% of patients with advanced ovarian cancer who undergo second-look surgery have microscopically positive findings. Negative second-look surgery findings are noted in approximately 30% to 50% of patients with advanced ovarian cancer undergoing this procedure.

There is limited information in the literature regarding second-look surgery in patients with *malignant germ-cell tumors* and virtually no meaningful information about patients with *sex cord–stromal tumors.* In a review of the experience with second-look laparotomy in patients with malignant germ-cell tumors at M.D. Anderson Cancer Center, findings were negative in 52 of 53 such patients. One patient with negative findings subsequently experienced a relapse and died. Thirteen patients had biopsy-proven evidence of mature teratoma—so-called chemotherapeutic retroconversion—at second-look laparotomy; treatment was discontinued in all patients, and none developed a recurrence. Based on these observations, our group recommended limitation on the use of second-look laparotomy in this patient population as much as possible. Williams et al. reported the GOG experience, in which 117 patients with malignant germ-cell tumors underwent second-look laparotomy after treatment with platinum-based chemotherapy. Based on their findings, the authors concluded that patients with either completely resected tumor or advanced-stage incompletely resected tumor that does not contain elements of teratoma rarely, if ever, benefit from second-look laparotomy. They did recommend second-look surgery for patients with incompletely resected tumor that contains teratoma. However, a significant proportion of this latter subset of patients had clinically detectable tumor before second-look surgery. The procedure is not recommended for those patients with initially detectable levels of serum tumor markers, especially those with early-stage disease. Some patients with advanced disease, particularly those with initially undetectable serum tumor markers, continue to undergo second-look laparotomy. The issue of second-look surgery for patients with incompletely resected elements of teratoma remains unresolved. As better therapies are developed and refined, the procedure will inevitably become obsolete, except in unusual situations.

Secondary Cytoreductive Surgery

The term *secondary cytoreductive surgery* has no universal definition. It may denote cytoreductive surgery performed in one of several different settings: (a) in patients who are partial responders or nonresponders to primary chemotherapy, (b) in patients who have developed recurrent disease after receiving primary therapy and experience a prolonged disease-free interval off therapy (>6 months), (c) in patients who undergo a suboptimal debulking initially followed by three cycles of chemotherapy (so-called interval debulking), and, (d) in patients who have persistent macroscopic tumor at second-look laparotomy.

Tumors in these subgroups of ovarian cancer patients may have very different natural histories, principally defined by whether they are platinum resistant or platinum sensitive. For example, patients whose tumor progresses during first-line chemotherapy, whether progression is noted clinically or at second-look laparotomy, are by definition platinum resistant. Patients who have not yet received chemotherapy or are partial responders to chemotherapy (whether the response noted clinically or at second-look surgery) or who have developed recurrent disease after a prolonged interval off therapy may well be platinum sensitive. These subgroups may have very different survival rates based on their responsiveness to second-line chemotherapy after secondary cytoreductive surgery. Therefore, it is extremely important for studies designed to assess the impact of these various secondary procedures on survival rates to carefully define their study populations. Because of the lack of prospective randomized studies in this area, it is difficult if not impossible to draw any firm conclusions about the influence of secondary debulking in these settings. However, the principal setting for secondary cytoreductive surgery is for platinum-sensitive recurrent disease.

Secondary Cytoreductive Surgery for Recurrent Disease

Several retrospective studies have shown an improved survival for patients secondarily cytoreduced to small residual disease compared with patients who were not optimally cytoreduced. Optimal candidates for such a procedure appear to be those who are platinum sensitive. The longer the interval between completion of primary chemotherapy and the time of recurrence, the better the outcome. Results of published studies on secondary cytoreduction for recurrent ovarian cancer are summarized in Table 49.11. Clearly, the true value of debulking

TABLE 49.11

SURVIVAL AFTER SECONDARY CYTOREDUCTIVE SURGERY FOR RECURRENT EPITHELIAL OVARIAN CANCER

Study	Patients	Median survival (months)	Significance
Morris et al., 1988			
≤2 cm	17	18	$p = 0.2$
>2 cm	13	13	
Janicke et al., 1992			
None	14	29	
≤2 cm	12	9	$p = 0.004$
>2 cm	4	8	
Segna et al., 1993			
≤2 cm	61	27	$p = 0.0001$
>2 cm	39	9	
Vacarello et al., 1995			
<0.5 cm	14	NR	$p < 0.0001$
>0.5 cm	24	23	
Eisenkop et al., 1995			
Microscopic	87	44	$p = 0.007$
Macroscopic	19	19	
Gaducci et al., 2000			
Microscopic	17	37	$p = 0.04$
Macroscopic	13	19	
Tay et al., 2002			
None	30	38	
<1 cm	10	14.5	$p < 0.01$
>1 cm	6	11	
Zang et al., 2004			
None	11	NR	
≤1 cm	61	26	$p < 0.0001$
>1 cm	45	14.5	
Pfisterer et al., 2005			
Microscopic	133	45	$p < 0.0001$
Macroscopic	134	19	
Gungor et al., 2005			
Microscopic	34	19	$p = 0.007$
Macroscopic	10	9	
Chi et al., 2006			
≤0.5 cm	79	56	$p < 0.001$
>0.5 cm	73	27	
Harter et al., 2006			
None	133	45	$p < 0.0001$
≤1 cm	69	20	
>1 cm	65	2.0	

NR, not reported.

surgery for recurrent ovarian cancer can be assessed only by a prospective randomized study. GOG is in the process of planning such a study in the near future.

Chi and colleagues recently analyzed their experience with 153 evaluable patients who underwent secondary cytoreductive surgery for platinum-sensitive recurrent epithelial ovarian cancer. They confirmed previous observations that the longer the disease-free interval, the longer the survival time after secondary cytoreduction (30 months for disease-free interval of 6–12 months, 39 months for disease-free interval of 13–30 months, and 51 months for disease-free interval greater than 30 months). For patients who had residual disease less than or equal to 0.5 cm, the median survival was 56 months compared with a median survival of 27 months for those patients with residual disease greater than 0.5 cm. The authors further devised a set of recommendations for selection of candidates for secondary cytoreductive surgery based on the disease-free interval, the number of recurrence sites, and evidence of carcinomatosis.

Secondary Attempt at Cytoreductive Surgery after Suboptimal Debulking

The term *interval cytoreduction* has been used to describe two distinct entities: (a) a true secondary cytoreduction performed after primary cytoreduction that is suboptimal (with bulky residual disease remaining) and three cycles of chemotherapy, or (b) cytoreduction after a biopsy performed at surgery (by laparoscopy or laparotomy), fine needle aspiration, or paracentesis and a few (typically three) cycles of chemotherapy. The latter is really neoadjuvant chemotherapy followed by primary cytoreduction. These two entities have been confused and used interchangeably in the literature.

Several reports described secondary cytoreductive surgery as interval debulking after a suboptimal primary surgery and a few cycles of chemotherapy. Van der Burg and associates reported the findings of a large prospective randomized trial in which 278 patients with less than 1 cm residual tumor after primary cytoreductive surgery were enrolled. After three cycles of cisplatin cyclophosphamide chemotherapy, patients were randomized to receive either secondary cytoreductive surgery followed by three more cycles of chemotherapy or three more cycles of chemotherapy alone. Of the 140 patients randomized to the interval cytoreduction arm, 65% still had bulky tumor at the time of this secondary surgery. About 45% of these patients were able to be cytoreduced optimally. Both progression-free survival and overall survival were modestly improved in the interval cytoreduction group. GOG subsequently conducted a study with an identical study design in an effort to replicate the results of this European trial; however, the combination of paclitaxel/cisplatin was used rather than cyclophosphamide/cisplatin. Contrary to the findings of the European study, the addition of secondary cytoreductive surgery to postoperative chemotherapy did not improve either progression-free survival or overall survival. The explanation for the disparate results may lie in the less aggressive initial cytoreductive attempt with resultant larger residual tumor volumes by the European investigators. Based on these findings, this approach is not currently recommended.

MANAGEMENT OF INTESTINAL OBSTRUCTION

Approximately 25% of ovarian cancer patients develop intestinal obstruction in the terminal phase of their illness. One of the major dilemmas facing the gynecologic oncologist is whether to operate on a patient with refractory ovarian cancer and an intestinal obstruction. Although current information provides some guidelines, the decisions concerning the wisdom of surgical intervention and intraoperative management are based more on the art of the discipline and experience of the surgeon than on scientific criteria.

Signs and symptoms of intestinal obstruction resulting from ovarian cancer include nausea and vomiting, abdominal cramping, abdominal distention, and progressive constipation. In patients who have only partial obstruction, these symptoms and findings may be episodic and more subtle. Plain films of the abdomen may support the diagnosis. Dilatation of the small intestine and air fluid levels suggest involvement of the small bowel. Dilatation of the colon may characterize large bowel obstruction. In patients with early, partial obstruction, the radiographic findings may be nonspecific.

Although intestinal obstruction in patients with ovarian cancer may be caused by adhesions, progressive tumor usually is the inciting factor. Of course, if the patient has received abdominopelvic radiotherapy, obstruction that is due to adhesions should be considered. In our experience, and that of others, however, most cases of intestinal obstruction in ovarian cancer patients who have received prior radiotherapy are related primarily to tumor progression.

The site(s) of the obstruction may be solitary or multiple. In 5% to 10% of patients, there is simultaneous obstruction of the small and large bowel. Colon obstruction usually occurs in the area of the sigmoid colon because of growth of pelvic tumor and resultant extrinsic compression; occasionally there may be obstruction of more proximal segments. Small bowel obstruction is usually the result of adherence of loops of bowel by mesenteric or serosal tumor implants.

Once the appropriate evaluation is completed and the diagnosis of intestinal obstruction is made, the gynecologist should outline a plan of management. Many factors influence this decision, including age, the nutritional status and general condition of the patient, the amount of tumor present, the presence or absence of ascites, the options for postoperative salvage therapy, the attitude of the physician, and the wishes of the patient and her family. The decision of whether to operate or manage the patient nonoperatively is colored by the fact that surgery for patients with refractory ovarian cancer is associated with significant morbidity and mortality, the obstruction cannot be relieved in almost 20% of those undergoing surgery, and postoperative survival is disappointingly brief. In reported series, the serious complication rate has ranged from 28% to 49%, and the operative mortality rate is in the range of 12% to 16%. The median survival rate for patients who have undergone surgery is in the range of 3 to 5 months.

Although some investigators have used projected survival (usually >2 months) as a parameter to decide on type of management, such an indicator is too unpredictable. Krebs and Goplerud devised a scoring system for selection of patients for surgery that included patient age, nutritional status, amount of palpable tumor, presence of ascites, previous chemotherapy, and previous radiotherapy. Outcome seemed to correlate with the prognostic score. Clarke-Pearson and colleagues confirmed the influence of disease status, ascites, and nutritional status.

For initial management of a patient with small bowel obstruction, we prefer the insertion of a nasogastric tube rather than a long tube (Cantor, Miller-Abbott, or Dennis) for intestinal decompression. After extensive experience with both, we have found no advantage from the latter. Furthermore, long tubes are associated with considerably greater discomfort.

Long intestinal tubes seem to have the greatest success rate in patients with postoperative adhesions but are fairly ineffective in relieving obstruction resulting from cancer. In the study of Krebs and Goplerud, only 10% of patients had their obstruction relieved by tube decompression. In patients for whom no surgery is planned, we have extensively used the technique of percutaneous gastrostomy since 1984. This procedure has resulted in excellent palliation for terminal-stage ovarian cancer patients, avoiding the discomfort of the nasogastric tube and allowing the patient to be easily cared for at home in most cases. With such a device, the patient may even continue to eat, although the nutritional benefit is essentially nil.

Optimal preoperative preparation is desirable if a patient is judged to be a suitable candidate for surgical intervention. For patients with complete colonic obstruction or perforation of the small or large intestine, a surgical emergency exists unless the patient is in such poor condition that such an intervention is not feasible. In emergency cases, the patient should be stabilized with intravenous fluids and antibiotics before surgery. Emergency surgery is rarely indicated for patients with a small intestinal obstruction. It is preferable to optimize the patient's condition with nasogastric tube decompression and rehydration. In addition, a barium enema is usually indicated to rule out a coexisting colonic obstruction. If the patient is malnourished, then intravenous hyperalimentation may be indicated preoperatively. Ample information suggests that hyperalimentation places the patient in an anabolic state and reduces the incidence of postoperative morbidity; however, its effect on long-term survival is unclear.

Colonic obstruction usually is treated by performing a colostomy. The selection of the site of colostomy depends on the area of obstruction and the ability to find an adequate bowel segment free of cancer. Most commonly, a transverse loop colostomy is indicated in the presence of a descending colon or sigmoid colon obstruction. There is increasing experience with the use of colonic stents as a substitute for colostomy. Patient selection is key, because erosion of the colonic wall with perforation is a risk.

A number of options are available for small bowel obstruction, depending on the operative findings. Most commonly, there are multiple sites of obstruction in the terminal ileum, in which case an ileo-ascending colon bypass or ileo-transverse colon bypass is preferable. In such situations, it is usually both unwise and inappropriate to attempt resection and reanastomosis. If, on the other hand, there is an isolated area of obstruction, then a resection and reanastomosis may be indicated. The anastomosis may be either hand sewn using a two-layer technique or approximated with surgical staplers. We generally prefer the latter because of the time-saving aspect. Frequently, there may be extensive tumor with multiple areas of obstruction, making both bypass and resection impossible. A tube gastrostomy is indicated in such a situation, if possible. Procedures such as these are among the most demanding because of the meticulous, often tedious dissection required. Enterotomies are not uncommon and should be repaired as soon as they are identified. Complications of small intestinal procedures include wound infection, intraperitoneal abscess, sepsis, pneumonia, "blind loop syndrome," and enterocutaneous fistula.

BEST SURGICAL PRACTICES

- In the United States, more than 22,000 new cases of ovarian cancer are detected annually, and more than 16,000 women will die of the disease. The lifetime risk of ovarian cancer for a woman in the United States is 1/70. This risk increases to 5% in a woman with one first-degree relative who has ovarian cancer and to 7% if she has two or more relatives with the disease.
- There are three hereditary familial ovarian cancer syndromes: the hereditary breast–ovarian cancer syndrome (HBOC), the hereditary site-specific ovarian cancer syndrome (HSSOC), and the hereditary nonpolyposis colon cancer syndrome (HNPCC).
- Pelvic examination is inaccurate in assessing ovarian size and morphology, particularly in postmenopausal women and in women who are overweight.
- In a research study, ovarian cancer screening, using a combination of transvaginal sonography and serum biomarkers, results in a decrease in stage at detection and an increase in case-specific survival. However, it is not effective in detecting ovarian cancer in patients whose ovarian volume is normal. With present technology, ovarian cancer screening is not sensitive or specific enough to recommend general population screening. Screening of high-risk women should be individualized.
- Numerous studies have shown improved survival in both early- and advanced-stage ovarian cancer when the initial surgery has been done by a gynecologic oncologist. A careful evaluation of an adnexal mass using transvaginal ultrasound, serum CA-125, and, occasionally, supplemented by other imaging studies will usually identify the patient with a high risk of malignancy who should be referred for surgery by a gynecologic oncologist.
- Surgery for ovarian cancer includes both careful staging to document the extent of the disease and resection or debulking of the tumor. Careful attention to accurate and comprehensive staging is most important in early-stage disease, for which postoperative therapy decisions may depend on the findings and histopathologic diagnosis. In patients with advanced disease, maximum surgical debulking to less than 1 cm diameter of residual disease should be the goal.
- In some young women with ovarian cancer, fertility-sparing surgery is possible. In a woman with a lesion apparently confirmed to a single ovary (or rarely both ovaries) who desires future pregnancy, ovarian and uterine conservation should be discussed preoperatively. At surgery, a unilateral oophorectomy and careful staging should be done, but the opposite ovary is not biopsied if it appears normal. If the diagnosis or staging findings are uncertain, it is best to close and await a final review of the permanent sections on the staging studies. Reoperation is preferable to unnecessary radicality in a young woman in whom fertility is a concern.
- In women with advanced ovarian cancer, optimal cytoreduction to less than 1 cm residual disease—or even smaller—has clearly been shown to confer a survival advantage. This is true even in patients with stage IV disease. The techniques required to perform radical cytoreduction in ovarian cancer patients and the judgment to know when it is appropriate is a combination of skill and experience and is usually done by gynecologic oncologists operating in hospital with good teams of anesthesiologists, consultants, and critical care experts.
- Laparoscopic surgery for ovarian cancer is currently under investigation. Its role is uncertain at the present time.
- Postoperative chemotherapy is usually required for patients with ovarian cancer; in some cases, chemotherapy may be given before any definitive surgery. This is an important part of the management of ovarian cancer, but it is not addressed in this surgical textbook.

Bibliography

Adelson MD. Cytoreduction of diaphragmatic metastases using the Cavitron ultrasonic surgical aspirator. *Gynecol Oncol* 1991;41:1220.

Adelson MD, Baggish MS, Seifer DB, et al. Cytoreduction of ovarian cancer with the Cavitron ultrasonic surgical aspirator. *Obstet Gynecol* 1988;72:140.

Alberts DS, Liu PY, Hannigan EV, et al. Intraperitoneal cisplatin plus intravenous cyclophosphamide versus intravenous cisplatin plus intravenous cyclophosphamide for stage III ovarian cancer. *N Engl J Med* 1996;335:1950.

Alcazar JL, Errasti T, Zornoza A, et al. Transvaginal color Doppler ultrasonography and CA-125 in suspicious adnexal masses. *Int J Obstet Gynecol* 1999;66:255.

Allen DG, Baak J, Belpomme D, et al. Advanced epithelial ovarian cancer: 1993 consensus statement. *Ann Oncol* 1993;4(suppl 4):S83.

Aletti GD, Dowdy SC, Podratz KC, et al. Surgical treatment of diaphragm disease correlates with improved survival in optimally debulked advanced stage ovarian cancer. *Gynecol Oncol* 2006;100:283.

American Cancer Society. Cancer Facts and Figures, 2006. Atlanta: American Cancer Society; 2006.

Angioli R, Palaia I, Zullo MA, et al. Diagnostic open laparoscopy in the management of advanced ovarian cancer. *Gynecol Oncol* 2006;100:455.

Armstrong DK, Bundy B, Wenzel L, et al. Intraperitoneal cisplatin and paclitaxel in ovarian cancer. *N Engl J Med* 2006;354:34.

Aure JC, Hoeg K, Kalstad P. Clinical and histologic studies of ovarian carcinoma: long-term follow-up of 990 cases. *Obstet Gynecol* 1971;37:1.

Averette HE, Janicek MF, Menck HR. The national cancer data base report on ovarian cancer. *Cancer* 1995;76:1096.

Ayhan A, Gultekin M, Taskiran C, et al. Routine appendectomy in epithelial ovarian carcinoma: is it necessary? *Obstet Gynecol* 2005;105:719.

Baggerly K, Morris J, Edmonson S, et al. Signal in noise: evaluating reported reproducibility of serum proteomic tests for ovarian cancer. *J Natl Cancer Inst* 2005;97:307.

Bailey CL, Ueland FR, Land GL, et al. Malignant potential of small cystic ovarian tumors in postmenopausal women. *Gynecol Oncol* 1998;69:3.

Barnhill D, Hoskins W, Heller P, et al. The second-look surgical reassessment for epithelial ovarian carcinoma. *Gynecol Oncol* 1984;19:148.

Barnhill DR, Kurman RJ, Brady MF, et al. Preliminary analysis of the behavior of stage I ovarian serous tumors of low malignant potential: a Gynecologic Oncology Group study. *J Clin Oncol* 1995;13:2752.

Bast RC, Klug TL, St. John ER, et al. A radioimmunoassay using a monoclonal antibody to monitor the course of epithelial ovarian cancer. *N Engl J Med* 1983;308:883.

Bast RC, Xu FJK, Yu YH, et al. CA-125: the past and the future. *Int J Biol Markers* 1998;13:179.

Bell J, Brady MF, Young RC, et al. Randomized phase III trial of three versus six cycles of adjuvant carboplatin and paclitaxel in early stage epithelial ovarian carcinoma: a Gynecologic Oncology Group study. *Gynecol Oncol* 2006;102:432.

Benedetti-Panici GS, Scambia G, Baiocchi G, et al. Technique and feasibility of radical paraaortic and pelvic lymphadenectomy for gynecologic malignancies: a prospective study. *Int J Gynecol Cancer* 1991;1:133.

Benedetti-Panici P, Maggioni A, Hacker N, et al. Systematic aortic and pelvic lymphadenectomy versus resection of bulky nodes only in optimally debulked advanced ovarian cancer: a randomized clinical trial. *J Natl Cancer Inst* 2005;97:560.

Berchuck A, Schildkraut JM, Marks JR, et al. Managing hereditary ovarian cancer risk. *Cancer* 1999;86(suppl):1697.

Berek JS, Griffiths CT, Leventhal J. Laparoscopy for second-look evaluation in ovarian cancer. *Obstet Gynecol* 1981;58:192.

Berek JS, Hacker NF, Lagasse LD, et al. Lower urinary tract resection as part of cytoreductive surgery for ovarian cancer. *Gynecol Oncol* 1982;13:87.

Berek JS, Hacker NF, Lagasse LD. Rectosigmoid colectomy and reanastomosis to facilitate resection of primary and recurrent gynecologic cancer. *Obstet Gynecol* 1984;64:715.

Berek JS, Hacker NF, Lagasse LD, et al. Survival of patients following secondary cytoreductive surgery in ovarian cancer. *Obstet Gynecol* 1983;61:189.

Berek JS, Knapp RC, Malkasian GD, et al. CA-125 serum levels correlated with second-look operations among ovarian cancer patients. *Obstet Gynecol* 1986;67:685.

Blythe JG, Wahl TP. Debulking surgery: does it increase the quality of survival? *Gynecol Oncol* 1982;14:396.

Bolis G, Colombo N, Pecorelli S, et al. Adjuvant treatment for early epithelial ovarian cancer: results of two randomised clinical trials comparing cisplatin to no further treatment or chromic phosphate (^{32}P). *Ann Oncol* 1995;6:887.

Bonazzi C, Peccatori F, Colombo N, et al. Pure ovarian immature teratoma, a unique and curable disease: 10 years' experience of 32 prospectively treated patients. *Obstet Gynecol* 1994;84:598.

Bookman MA. GOG0182-ICON5: 5-arm phase III randomized trial of paclitaxel and carboplatin vs combinations with gemcitabine, PEG-liposomal doxorubicin, or topotecan in patients with advanced-stage epithelial ovarian or primary peritoneal carcinoma. *Proc Am Soc Clin Oncol* 2006;24:256s.

Bostwick DG, Tazelaar HD, Ballon SC, et al. Ovarian epithelial tumors of borderline malignancy: a clinical and pathologic study of 109 cases. *Cancer* 1986;58:2052.

Brand E, Pearlman N. Electrosurgical debulking of ovarian cancer: a new technique using the argon beam coagulator. *Gynecol Oncol* 1990;39:115.

Brand E, Wade ME, Lagasse LD. Resection of fixed pelvic tumors using the Nd:YAG laser. *J Surg Oncol* 1988;37:246.

Brenner D, Shaff M, Jones H, et al. Abdominopelvic computed tomography: evaluation in patients undergoing second-look laparotomy for ovarian carcinoma. *Obstet Gynecol* 1985;65:715.

Brewer M, Gershenson DM, Herzog CE, et al. Outcome and reproductive function after chemotherapy for ovarian dysgerminoma. *J Clin Oncol* 1999;17:2670.

Bristow RE, Chi DS. Platinum-based neoadjuvant chemotherapy and interval surgical cytoreduction for advanced ovarian cancer: a meta-analysis. *Gynecol Oncol* 2006;103:1070.

Bristow RE, Eisenhauer EL, Santillan A, et al. Delaying the primary surgical effort for advanced ovarian cancer: a systematic review of neoadjuvant chemotherapy and interval cytoreduction. *Gynecol Oncol* 2007;104:480.

Bristow RE, Montz FJ. Complete surgical cytoreduction of advanced ovarian carcinoma using the argon beam coagulator. *Gynecol Oncol* 2001;83:39.

Bristow RE, Montz FJ, Lagasse LD, et al. Survival impact of surgical cytoreduction in Stage IV epithelial ovarian cancer. *Gynecol Oncol* 1999;72:278.

Bristow RE, Zahurak ML, del Carmen MG, et al. Ovarian cancer surgery in Maryland: volume-based access to care. *Gynecol Oncol* 2004;93:353.

Brown CL, Dharmendra B, Barakat RR. Preserving fertility in patients with epithelial ovarian cancer (EOC): the role of conservative surgery in treatment of early-stage disease. *Gynecol Oncol* 2000;76:240(abst).

Brown J, Shvartsman H, Deavers M, et al. The activity of taxanes in the treatment of sex cord-stromal ovarian tumors. *J Clin Oncol* 2004;22:3517.

Burghardt E, Girardi F, Lahousen M, et al. Patterns of pelvic and paraaortic lymph node involvement in ovarian cancer. *Gynecol Oncol* 1991;40:103.

Burghardt E, Pickel H, Lahousen M, et al. Pelvic lymphadenectomy in operative treatment of ovarian cancer. *Am J Obstet Gynecol* 1986;155:15.

Carlson KJ, Skates SJ, Singer D. Screening for ovarian cancer. *Ann Intern Med* 1994;121:124.

Carney ME, Lancaster JM, Ford C, et al. A population-based study of patterns of care for ovarian cancer: Who is seen by a gynecologic oncologist and who is not? *Gynecol Oncol* 2002;84:36.

Carnino F, Fuda G, Ciccone G, et al. Significance of lymph node sampling in epithelial carcinoma of the ovary. *Gynecol Oncol* 1997;65:467.

Casagrande JT, Louie EW, Pike MC. Incessant ovulation and ovarian cancer. *Lancet* 1979;2:170.

Cass I, Li AJ, Runowicz CD, et al. Pattern of lymph node metastases in clinically unilateral stage I invasive epithelial ovarian carcinoma. *Gynecol Oncol* 2001;80:56.

Castaldo TW, Petrilli ES, Ballon SC, et al. Intestinal operations in patients with ovarian carcinoma. *Am J Obstet Gynecol* 1981;139:80.

Chaitin BA, Gershsenson DM, Evans HL. Mucinous tumors of the ovary: a clinicopathologic study of 70 cases. *Cancer* 1985;55:1958.

Chambers S, Chambers J, Kohorn E, et al. Evaluation of the role of second-look surgery in ovarian cancer. *Obstet Gynecol* 1988;72:404.

Chang J , Fryatt I, Ponder B, et al. A matched control study of familial epithelial ovarian cancer: patient characteristics, response to chemotherapy and outcome. *Ann Oncol* 1995;6:80.

Chen SS, Bochner R. Assessment of morbidity and mortality in primary cytoreductive surgery for advanced ovarian carcinoma. *Gynecol Oncol* 1985;20:190.

Chen SS, Lee L. Incidence of paraaortic and pelvic lymph node metastases in epithelial carcinoma of the ovary. *Gynecol Oncol* 1983;15:95.

Chi DS, Abu-Rustum NR, Sonoda Y, et al. The safety and efficacy of laparoscopic surgical staging of apparent stage I ovarian and fallopian tube cancers. *Am J Obstet Gynecol* 2005;192:1614.

Chi DS, McCaughty K, Diaz JP, et al. Guidelines and selection criteria for secondary cytoreductive surgery in patients with recurrent, platinum-sensitive epithelial ovarian carcinoma. *Cancer* 2006;106:1933.

Clarke-Pearson D, Bandy L, Dudzinski M, et al. Computed tomography in evaluation of patients with ovarian carcinoma in complete clinical remission: correlation with surgical-pathologic findings. *JAMA* 1986;255:627.

Clarke-Pearson DL, Chin NO, DeLong ER, et al. Surgical management of intestinal obstruction in ovarian cancer. *Gynecol Oncol* 1987;26:11.

Clarke-Pearson DL, DeLong ER, Chin NE, et al. Surgical management of intestinal obstruction in ovarian cancer. II. Analysis of factors associated with complications and survival. *Arch Surg* 1988;123:42.

Clayton RD, Obermair A, Hammond IG, et al. The western Australian experience of the use of en bloc resection of ovarian cancer with concomitant rectosigmoid colectomy. *Gynecol Oncol* 2002;84:53.
Cook LS, Kamb ML, Weiss NS. Perineal powder exposure and risk of ovarian cancer. *Am J Epidemiol* 1997;145:459.
Copeland L, Gershenson DM. Ovarian cancer recurrences in patients with no macroscopic tumor at second-look laparotomy. *Obstet Gynecol* 1986;68:873.
Copeland L, Gershenson D, Wharton JT, et al. Microscopic disease at second-look laparotomy in advanced ovarian cancer. *Cancer* 1985;55:472.
Copeland L, Silva E, Gershenson D, et al. The significance of mullerian inclusions found at second-look laparotomy in patients with epithelial ovarian neoplasms. *Obstet Gynecol* 1988;71:763.
Cramer DW, Welch WR. Determinants of ovarian cancer. Risk II. Inferences regarding pathogenesis. *J Natl Cancer Inst* 1983;71:717.
Creasman WT, Rutledge F. The prognostic value of peritoneal cytology in gynecologic malignant disease. *Am J Obstet Gynecol* 1971;110:773.
Curtin JP, Malik R, Venkatraman ES, et al. Stage IV ovarian cancer: impact of surgical debulking. *Gynecol Oncol* 1997;64:9.
Dark GG, Bower M, Newlands ES, et al. Surveillance policy for stage I ovarian germ cell tumors. *J Clin Oncol* 1997;15:620.
Dauplat J, Ferriere JP, Monique G, et al. Second-look laparotomy in managing epithelial ovarian carcinoma. *Cancer* 1986;57:1627.
Dembo AJ, Davy D, Stenwig AE, et al. Prognostic factors in patients with stage I epithelial ovarian cancer. *Obstet Gynecol* 1990;75:263.
Deppe G, Malviya VK, Boike G, et al. Use of Cavitron surgical aspirator for debulking of diaphragmatic metastases in patients with advanced carcinoma of the ovaries. *Surg Gynecol Obstet* 1989;168:455.
Deppe G, Malviya VK, Malone JM, et al. Debulking of pelvic and paraaortic lymph node metastases in ovarian cancer with the Cavitron ultrasonic surgical aspirator. *Obstet Gynecol* 1990;76:1140.
Deppe G, Zbella EA, Skogerson K, et al. The rare indication for splenectomy as part of cytoreductive surgery in ovarian cancer. *Gynecol Oncol* 1983;16:282.
DePriest DP, Banks ER, Powell DE, et al. Endometrioid carcinoma of the ovary and endometriosis: the association in postmenopausal women. *Gynecol Oncol* 1992;47:71.
DePriest P, Shenson D, Fried A, et al. Evaluation of CA-125 levels in differentiating malignant from benign tumors in patients with pelvic masses. *Obstet Gynecol* 1988;72:23.
DePriest P, Shenson D, Fried A, et al. A morphologic index based on sonographic findings in ovarian cancer. *Gynecol Oncol* 1993;51:7.
Di-Xia C, Schwartz PE, Xinguo L, et al. Evaluation of CA-125 levels in differentiating malignant from benign tumors in patients with pelvic masses. *Obstet Gynecol* 1988;72:23.
DuBois A, Lueck HJ, Meier W, et al. A randomized clinical trial of cisplatin/paclitaxel versus carboplatin/paclitaxel as first-line treatment of ovarian cancer. *J Natl Cancer Inst* 2003;95:1320.
Earle CC, Schrag D, Neville BA, et al. Effect of surgeon specialty on processes of care and outcomes for ovarian cancer patients. *J Natl Cancer Inst* 2006;98:172.
Easton DR, Bishop DT, Ford D. Genetic linkage analysis in familial breast and ovarian cancer: results in 214 families.The Breast Cancer Linkage Consortium. *Am J Hum Genet* 1993;52:678.
Einhorn N, Sjovak K, Knapp RC, et al. Prospective evaluations of serum CA-125 levels for early detection of ovarian cancer. *Obstet Gynecol* 1992; 8:14.
Eisenhauer EL, Abu-Rustum NR, Sonoda Y, et al. The addition of extensive upper abdominal surgery to achieve optimal cytoreduction improves survival in patients with stages IIIC-IV epithelial ovarian cancer. *Gynecol Oncol* 2006;103:1083.
Eisenkop SM, Friedman RL, Wang H-J. Secondary cytoreductive surgery for recurrent ovarian cancer. *Cancer* 1995;76:1606.
Eisenkop SM, Spirtos NM. The clinical significance of occult macroscopically positive retroperitoneal nodes in patients with epithelial ovarian cancer. *Gynecol Oncol* 2001;82:143.
Fagotti A, Fanfani F, Ludovisi M, et al. Role of laparoscopy to assess the chance of optimal cytoreductive surgery in advanced ovarian cancer: a pilot study. *Gynecol Oncol* 2005;96:729.
Fathalla MF. Incessant ovulation: a factor in ovarian neoplasia? [letter]. *Lancet* 1971;2:163.
Ferlay J, Bray P, Pisani P, et al. Globocan 2002: Cancer incidence mortality and prevalence worldwide. *IARC Cancer Base No. 5*. Lyon, France: IARC Press, 2004.
Fiorica JV, Hoffman MS, LaPolla JP, et al. The management of diaphragmatic lesions in ovarian carcinoma. *Obstet Gynecol* 1989;74:927.
Fleischer AC, Cullinan JA, Kepple DM, et al. Conventional and color Doppler transvaginal sonography of pelvic masses: a comparison of relative histologic specificities. *J Ultrasound Med* 1993;12:705.
Ford D, Easton DF. The genetics of breast and ovarian cancer. *Br J Cancer* 1995;72:805.
Ford D, Easton DF, Stratton M, et al. Genetic heterogeneity and penetrance analysis of the BRCA1 and BRCA2 genes in breast cancer families. The Breast Cancer Linkage Consortium. *Am J Hum Genet* 1998;62:676.
Friedman J, Weiss N. Second thoughts about second-look laparotomy in advanced ovarian cancer. *N Engl J Med* 1990;322:1079.
Gadducci A, Iacconi P, Cosio S, et al. Complete salvage surgical cytoreduction improves further survival of patients with late recurrent ovarian cancer. *Gynecol Oncol* 2000;79:344.
Gershenson DM. Conservative management of ovarian cancer. *Curr Probl Obstet Gynecol Fertil* 1994;27:165.
Gershenson DM. Management of early ovarian cancer: germ cell and sex cord-stromal tumors. *Gynecol Oncol* 1994;55:S62.
Gershenson DM. Update on malignant ovarian germ cell tumors. *Cancer* 1993;71:1581.
Gershenson DM, Copeland L, Del Junco G, et al. Second-look laparotomy in the management of malignant germ cell tumors of the ovary. *Obstet Gynecol* 1986;67:789.
Gershenson D, Copeland L, Wharton JT, et al. Prognosis of surgically determined complete responders in advanced ovarian cancer. *Cancer* 1985;55:1129.
Gershenson DM, Morris M, Burke TW, et al. Treatment of poor-prognosis sex cord-stromal tumors of the ovary with the combination of bleomycin, etoposide, and cis-platinum. *Obstet Gynecol* 1996;87:527.
Gershenson DM, Morris M, Cangir A, et al. Treatment of malignant germ cell tumors of the ovary with bleomycin, etoposide, and cisplatin. *J Clin Oncol* 1990;8:715.
Gershenson DM, Silva EG. Serous ovarian tumors of low malignant potential with peritoneal implants. *Cancer* 1990;65:578.
Gershenson DM, Silva EG, Levy L, et al. Ovarian serous borderline tumors with invasive peritoneal implants. *Cancer* 1998;82:1096.
Gershenson DM, Silva EG, Tortolero-Luna G, et al. Serous borderline tumors of the ovary with noninvasive peritoneal implants. *Cancer* 1998;83:2157.
Gertig DM, Hunter DJ, Cramer DW, et al. Ovarian carcinoma diagnosis: results of a national ovarian cancer survey. *Cancer* 2000;89:2068.
Gertig DM, Hunter DJ, Cramer DW, et al. Prospective study of talc use and ovarian cancer. *J Natl Cancer Inst* 2000;92:249.
Goff, BA, Mandel L, Muntz H, et al. Ovarian carcinoma diagnosis: results of a National Ovarian Cancer Survey. *Cancer* 2000;89:2068.
Goff BA, Matthews BJ, Wynn M, et al. Ovarian cancer: patterns of surgical care across the United States. *Gynecol Oncol* 2006;103:383.
Goldhirsch A, Triller J, Greiner R, et al. Computed tomography prior to second-look operation in advanced ovarian cancer. *Obstet Gynecol* 1983;62:630.
Goldie JH, Coldman AJ. A mathematical model for relating the drug sensitivity of tumors to their spontaneous mutation rate. *Cancer Treat Rep* 1979;63:1727.
Greenlee RT, Murray T, Bolden S, et al. Cancer statistics 2000. *Cancer* 2000;50:7.
Griffiths CT. Surgical resection of tumor bulk in the primary treatment of ovarian carcinoma: seminar on ovarian cancer. *J Natl Cancer Inst Monogr* 1975;42:101.
Griffiths CT, Parker LM, Fuller AF. Role of cytoreductive surgical treatment in the management of advanced ovarian cancer. *Cancer Treat Rep* 1979;63:235.
Gungor M, Ortac F, Arvas M, et al. The role of secondary cytoreductive surgery for recurrent ovarian cancer. *Gynecol Oncol* 2005;97:74.
Hacker NF, Berek JS, Lagasse LD, et al. Primary cytoreductive surgery for epithelial ovarian cancer. *Obstet Gynecol* 1983;61:413.
Hankinson SE. Prospective study of talc use and ovarian cancer. *J Natl Cancer Inst* 2000;92:249.
Hankinson SE, Colditz GA, Hunter DJ, et al. A quantitative assessment of oral contraceptive use and risk of ovarian cancer. *Obstet Gynecol* 1992;180: 708.
Harlan LC, Clegg LX, Trimble EL. Trends in surgery and chemotherapy for women diagnosed with ovarian cancer in the United States. *J Clin Oncol* 2003;21:3488.
Hart WR, Norris HJ. Borderline and malignant mucinous tumors of the ovary: histologic criteria and clinical behavior. *Cancer* 1973;31:1031.
Harter P, du Bois A, Hahmann M, et al. Surgery in recurrent ovarian cancer: the Arbeitsgemeinschaft Gynaekologische OnKologie (AGO) DESKTOP OVAR trial. *Ann Surg Oncol* 2006;13:1702.
Hartge P, Hoover R, McGowan L, et al. Menopause and ovarian cancer. *Am J Epidemiol* 1988;127:990.
Heintz APM, Hacker NF, Berek JS, et al. Cytoreductive surgery in ovarian carcinoma: feasibility and morbidity. *Obstet Gynecol* 1986;67:783.
Henriksen R, Runa K, Wilander E, et al. Expression and prognostic significance of platelet-derived growth factor and its receptors in epithelial ovarian neoplasms. *Cancer Res* 1993;53:4550.
Ho AG, Beller U, Speyer J, et al. A reassessment of the role of second-look laparotomy in advanced ovarian cancer. *J Clin Oncol* 1987;5:1316.
Homesley HD, Bundy BN, Hurteau JA, et al. Bleomycin, etoposide, and cisplatinum combination therapy of ovarian granulosa cell tumors and other stromal malignancies: a Gynecologic Oncology Group study. *Gynecol Oncol* 1999;72:131.
Hoskins W, Bundy B, Thigpen J, et al. The influence of initial surgery on progression-free interval (PFI) and survival (S) in optimal (<1 cm) stage III

epithelial ovarian cancer (EOC). Society of Gynecologic Oncologist Abstract. *Gynecol Oncol* 1992;45:76.
Hoskins WJ, Rubin SC, Dulaney E, et al. Influence of secondary cytoreduction at the time of second-look laparotomy on the survival of patients with epithelial ovarian carcinoma. *Gynecol Oncol* 1989;34:365.
Hulka BS. Cancer screening: degrees of proof and practical application. *Cancer* 1987;62:1776.
Hunter J, Andrews S, van Nagell, JR. Efficacy of a sonographic morphology index in identifying ovarian cancer: a multi-institutional investigation. *Gynecol Oncol* 1994;55:174.
Inciura A, Simavisius A, Juozaityte E, et al. Comparison of adjuvant and neoadjuvant chemotherapy in the management of advanced ovarian cancer: a retrospective study of 574 patients. *BMC Cancer* 2006;6:153.
International Collaborative Ovarian Neoplasm (ICON) Group. Paclitaxel plus carboplatin versus standard chemotherapy with either single-agent carboplatin or cyclophosphamide, doxorubicin, and cisplatin in women with ovarian cancer: the ICON3 randomized trial. *Lancet* 2002;360:505.
International Collaborative Ovarian Neoplasm 1 (ICON1) and European Organisation for Research and Treatment of Cancer Collaborators-Adjuvant Chemotherapy in Ovarian Neoplasms (EORTC-ACTION). International Collaborative Ovarian Neoplasm Trial 1 and Adjuvant Chemotherapy in Ovarian Neoplasm Trial: Two parallel randomized phase III trials of adjuvant chemotherapy in patients with early-stage ovarian carcinoma. *J Natl Cancer Inst* 2003;95:105.
International Federation of Gynecology and Obstetrics. FIGO staging for carcinoma of the ovary. In: Pecorelli S, ed. *Annual report on the results of treatment in gynecological cancer.* 24th ed. Milan, Italy: *J Epidemiol Biostat* (Italy) 2001;6(2).
International Federation of Gynecology and Obstetrics. FIGO staging for carcinoma of the ovary. In: Pettersson F, ed. *Annual report on the results of treatment in gynecological cancer.* 22nd ed. Stockholm, Sweden: 1997.
Jacob J, Gershenson DM, Morris M, et al. Neoadjuvant chemotherapy and interval debulking for advanced epithelial ovarian cancer. *Gynecol Oncol* 1991;42:146.
Jacobs I, Bast RC. The CA-125 tumour-associated antigen: a review of the literature. *Hum Reprod* 1989;4:1.
Jacobs I, Davies AP, Bridges J, et al. Prevalence screening for ovarian cancer in postmenopausal women by CA-125 measurement and ultrasonography. *Br Med J* 1993;306:1030.
Janicke F, Holscher M, Kuhn W, et al. Radical surgical procedure improves survival time in patients with recurrent ovarian cancer. *Cancer* 1992;70:2129.
Joyeux H, Szawlowski A, Saint-Aubert B, et al. Aggressive regional surgery for advanced ovarian carcinoma. *Cancer* 1986;57:142.
Kapnick SJ, Griffiths CG, Finkler NJ. Occult pleural involvement in stage III ovarian carcinoma: role of diaphragm resection. *Gynecol Oncol* 1990;39:135.
Kaunitz AM. Oral contraceptive health benefits: Perception versus reality. *Contraception* 1999;91:1131.
Kawai M, Kano K, Kikkawa F, et al. Transvaginal Doppler ultrasound with color flow imaging in the diagnosis of ovarian cancer. *Obstet Gynecol* 1992;79:163.
Keettel WX, Pixley EE, Buschbaum HJ. Experience with peritoneal cytology in the management of gynecologic malignancies. *Am J Obstet Gynecol* 1974;120:174.
Kerlikowske K, Brown JS, Grady DG. Should women with familial ovarian cancer undergo prophylactic oophorectomy? *Obstet Gynecol* 1992;80:700.
Knapp RC, Friedman EA. Aortic lymph node metastases in early ovarian cancer. *Am J Obstet Gynecol* 1974;119:1013.
Koch M, Gaedke H, Jenkins H. Family history of ovarian cancer patients: a case control study. *Int J Epidemiol* 1989;18:782.
Kohler MF, Kerns BM, Humphrey PA, et al. Mutation and overexpression of p53 in early-stage epithelial ovarian cancer. *Obstet Gynecol* 1993;81:643.
Krebs HB, Goplerud DR. The role of intestinal intubation in obstruction of the small intestine due to carcinoma of the ovary. *Surg Gynecol Obstet* 1984;158:467.
Krebs HB, Goplerud DR. Surgical management of bowel obstruction in advanced ovarian carcinoma. *Obstet Gynecol* 1983;61:327.
Kryscio RJ. The efficacy of transvaginal sonographic screening in asymptomatic women at risk for ovarian cancer. *Gynecol Oncol* 2000;77:350.
Kryscio RJ, van Nagell JR. A morphologic index based on sonographic findings in ovarian cancer. *Gynecol Oncol* 1993;51:7.
Kurjak A, Kupesic S, Anic T, et al. Three dimensional ultrasound and power Doppler improve the diagnosis of ovarian lesions. *Gynecol Oncol* 2000;76:28.
Kurjak A, Predanic M. New scoring system for prediction of ovarian malignancy based on transvaginal color Doppler sonography. *J Ultrasound Med* 1992;11:631.
Kurjak A, Schulman H, Zalud I, et al. Transvaginal ultrasound color flow and Doppler waveform of the postmenopausal adnexal mass. *Obstet Gynecol* 1992;80:917.
Larson JE, Podczaski ES, Manetta A, et al. Bowel obstruction in patients with ovarian carcinoma: analysis of prognostic factors. *Gynecol Oncol* 1989;35:61.
Lawton FG, Luesley D, Redman C, et al. Feasibility and outcome of complete secondary tumor resection for patients with advanced ovarian cancer. *J Surg Oncol* 1990;45:14.
LeBlanc E, Querleu D, Narducci F, et al. Laparoscopic staging of early stage invasive adnexal tumors: a 10-year experience. *Gynecol Oncol* 2004;94:624.
Lecuru F, Desfeux P, Camatte S, et al. Impact of initial surgical access on staging and survival of patients with stage I ovarian cancer. *Int J Gynecol Cancer* 2006;16:87.
Lele S, Piver MS. Interval laparoscopy as predictor of response to chemotherapy in ovarian carcinoma. *Obstet Gynecol* 1986;68:345.
Levine D, Gossink B, Wolf SI, et al. Simple adnexal cysts: the natural history in postmenopausal women. *Radiology* 1992;184:653.
Lewis MR, Deavers MT, Silva EG, et al. Ovarian involvement by metastatic colorectal adenocarcinoma. *Am J Surg Pathol* 2006;30:177.
Li A, Otero F, Funowica CD, et al. Pattern of lymph node metastases in apparent Stage IA invasive epithelial ovarian carcinomas. *Gynecol Oncol* 2000;76:239.
Lim-Tan SK, Cajigas HE, Scully RE. Ovarian cystectomy for serous borderline tumors: a follow-up study of 35 cases. *Obstet Gynecol* 1981;72:775.
Liotta L, Kohn E, Pertricoin E. Clinical proteomics: personalized molecular medicine. *JAMA* 2001;286:2211.
Liu PC, Benjamin I, Morgan MA, et al. Effect of surgical debulking on survival in stage IV ovarian cancer. *Gynecol Oncol* 1997;64:4.
Low JJH, Perrin LC, Crandon J, et al. Conservative surgery to preserve ovarian function in patients with malignant ovarian germ cell tumors: a review of 74 cases. *Cancer* 2000;89:391.
Lu JL, Zheng Y, Yuan J, et al. Decreased luteinizing hormone receptor in RNA expression in human ovarian epithelial cancer. *Gynecol Oncol* 2000;79:158.
Luesley D, Chan K, Fielding J, et al. Second-look laparotomy in the management of epithelial ovarian carcinoma: an evaluation of fifty cases. *Obstet Gynecol* 1984;64:421.
Luesley D, Chan K, Lawton F, et al. Survival after negative second-look laparotomy. *Eur J Surg Oncol* 1989;15:205.
Lund B, Jaconsen K, Rasch L, et al. Correlation of abdominal ultrasound and computed tomography scans with second- or third-look laparotomy in patients with ovarian carcinoma. *Gynecol Oncol* 1990;37:279.
Lund B, Williamson P. Prognostic factors for outcome of and survival after second-look laparotomy in patients with advanced ovarian carcinoma. *Obstet Gynecol* 1990;76:617.
Lynch HT, Harris RE, Guirgis HA, et al. Familial association of breast/ovarian carcinoma. *Cancer* 1978;41:1543.
Lynch HT, Lemon SJ, Karr B. Etiology natural history, management and molecular genetics of hereditary non-polyposis colorectal cancer (Lynch syndromes). *Cancer Epidemiol Biomarkers Prev* 1977;6:978.
Lynch HT, Watson P, Bewtra C. Hereditary ovarian cancer: heterogeneity in age at diagnosis. *Cancer* 1991;67:1460.
Malfetano JH. Splenectomy for optimal cytoreduction in ovarian cancer. *Gynecol Oncol* 1986;24:392.
Malkasian GD, Knapp RC, Zurawaski VR, et al. Preoperative evaluation of serum CA-125 levels in premenopausal and postmenopausal patients with pelvic masses: discrimination from malignant disease. *Am J Obstet Gynecol* 1988;159:341.
Malone JM, Koonce T, Larson DM, et al. Palliation of small bowel obstruction by percutaneous gastrostomy in patients with progressive ovarian carcinoma. *Obstet Gynecol* 1986;68:431.
Malpica A, Deavers M, Lu K, et al. Grading ovarian serous carcinoma using a two-tier system. *Am J Surg Path* 2004;28(4):496.
Mann W, Patsner B, Cohen H, et al. Preoperative serum CA-125 levels in patients with surgical stage I invasive ovarian adenocarcinoma. *J Natl Cancer Inst* 1988;80:208.
Marina NM, Cushing B, Giller R, et al. Complete surgical excision is effective treatment for children with immature teratomas with or without malignant elements: a Pediatric Oncology Group/Children's Cancer Group intergroup study. *J Clin Oncol* 1999;17:2137.
Markman M, Bundy B, Alberts DS, et al. Phase III trial of standard-dose intravenous cisplatin plus paclitaxel versus moderately high-dose carboplatin followed by intravenous paclitaxel and intraperitoneal cisplatin in small-volume stage III ovarian carcinoma: an intergroup study of the Gynecologic Oncology Group, Southwestern Oncology Group, and Eastern Cooperative Oncology Group. *J Clin Oncol* 2001;19:1001.
Marret H, Saugnet S, Giraudeau B, et al. Contrast-enhanced sonography helps in discrimination of benign from malignant adnexal masses. *J Ultrasound Med* 2004;23:1629.
Mazzeo F, Berliere M, Kerger J, et al. Neoadjuvant chemotherapy followed by surgery and adjuvant chemotherapy in patients with primarily unresectable, advanced-stage ovarian cancer. *Gynecol Oncol* 2003;90:163.
McGowan L, Lesher LP, Norris HJ, et al. Misstaging of ovarian cancer. *Obstet Gynecol* 1985;65:568.
McGuire WP, Hoskins WJ, Brady MF, et al. Cyclophosphamide and cis-platinum compared with paclitaxel and cisplatin in patients with stage III and stage IV ovarian cancer. *N Engl J Med* 1996;334:1.

McMahill HL, Calle EE, Koskinski AS, et al. Tubal ligation and fatal ovarian cancer in a large prospective cohort study. *Am J Epidemiol* 1997;145:349.
Miki Y, Swensen J, Shattuck-Eidens D, et al. A strong candidate for the breast ovarian cancer susceptibility gene BRCA1. *Science* 1994;266:66.
Miller D, Ballon S, Teng N, et al. A critical reassessment of second-look laparotomy in epithelial ovarian carcinoma. *Cancer* 1986;57:530.
Modesitt SC, Pavlik EJ, Ueland FR, et al. Risk of malignancy in unilocular ovarian cystic tumors less than 10 cms in diameter. *Obstet Gynecol* 2003;102:594.
Monga M, Carmichael JA, Shelley WE, et al. Surgery without adjuvant chemotherapy for early epithelial ovarian carcinoma after comprehensive surgical staging. *Gynecol Oncol* 1992;43:195.
Montz FJ, Schlaerth JB, Berek JS. Resection of diaphragmatic peritoneum and muscle: role in cytoreductive surgery for ovarian cancer. *Gynecol Oncol* 1989;35:338.
Morice P, Dubernard G, Rey A, et al. Results of interval debulking surgery compared with primary debulking surgery in advanced stage ovarian cancer. *J Am Coll Surg* 2003;197:955.
Morice P, Joulie F, Camatte S, et al. Lymph node involvement in epithelial ovarian cancer: analysis of 276 pelvic and paraaortic lymphadenectomies and surgical implications. *J Am Coll Surg* 2003;197:198.
Morice P, Wicart-Poque F, Rey A, et al. Results of conservative treatment in epithelial ovarian carcinoma. *Cancer* 2001;92:2412.
Morris M, Gershenson DM, Burke TW, et al. Splenectomy in gynecologic oncology: indications, complications, and technique. *Gynecol Oncol* 1991;43:118.
Morris RT, Gershenson DM, Silva EG, et al. Outcome and reproductive function after conservative surgery for borderline ovarian tumors. *Obstet Gynecol* 2000;95:541.
Morris M, Gershenson DM, Wharton JT. Secondary cytoreductive surgery in epithelial ovarian cancer: nonresponders to first-line therapy. *Gynecol Oncol* 1989;33:1.
Morris M, Gershenson DM, Wharton JT, et al. Secondary cytoreductive surgery for recurrent epithelial ovarian cancer. *Gynecol Oncol* 1989;34:334.
Morrow CP. An opinion in support of second-look surgery in ovarian cancer [Editorial]. *Gynecol Oncol* 2000;79:341.
Muggia FM, Braly PS, Brady MF, et al. Phase III randomized study of cis-platinum versus paclitaxel versus cis-platinum and paclitaxel in patients with suboptimal stage III or IV ovarian cancer: a Gynecologic Oncology Group study. *J Clin Oncol* 2000;18:106.
Muir C, Waterhouse J, Mack T, et al. *Cancer incidence in five continents IARC.* IARC Scientific Publication No. 88. Lyon, France: IARC Press; 1987:892.
Munkarah AR, Hallum AV, Morris M, et al. Prognostic significance of residual disease in patients with stage IV epithelial ovarian cancer. *Gynecol Oncol* 1997;64:13.
Munkarah A, Levenback C, Wolf JK, et al. Secondary cytoreductive surgery for localized intra-abdominal recurrences in epithelial ovarian cancer. *Gynecol Oncol* 2001;81:237.
Munoz KA, Harlan LC, Trimble EL. Patterns of care for women with ovarian cancer in the United States. *J Clin Oncol* 1997;15:3408.
Neijt JP, Huinink WW, van der Burg MEL, et al. Randomized trial comparing two combination chemotherapy regimens (CHAP-5 V CP) in advanced ovarian carcinoma. *J Clin Oncol* 1987;5:1157.
Nelson BE, Rosenfeld AT, Schwartz PE. Preoperative abdominopelvic computed tomographic prediction of optimal cytoreduction in epithelial ovarian carcinoma. *J Clin Oncol* 1993;11:166.
Nelson HD, Huffman LH, Rongwei F, et al. Genetic risk assessment and BRCA mutation testing for breast and ovarian cancer susceptibility: systematic evidence review for the U.S. Preventive Services Task Force. *Ann Intern Med* 2005;143:362.
Niloff JM, Bast RC, Schaetzl EM, et al. Predictive value of CA-125 antigen levels in second-look procedures for ovarian cancer. *Am J Obstet Gynecol* 1985;151:981.
Onda T, Yoshikawa H, Yokota H, et al. Assessment of metastases to aortic and pelvic lymph nodes in epithelial ovarian carcinoma. *Cancer* 1996;78:803.
Ozols R, Fisher R, Anderson T, et al. Peritoneoscopy in the management of ovarian cancer. *Am J Obstet Gynecol* 1981;140:611.
Ozols RF, Bundy BN, Greer BE, et al. Phase III trial of carboplatin and paclitaxel compared with cisplatin and paclitaxel in patients with optimally resected stage III ovarian cancer: a Gynecologic Oncology Group study. *J Clin Oncol* 2003;21:3194.
Parazzini F, Negri E, LaVecchia C, et al. Family history of reproductive cancers and ovarian cancer risk: an Italian case-control study. *Am J Epidemiol* 1992;135:35.
Park J-Y, Seo S-S, Kang S, et al. The benefits of low anterior en bloc resection as part of cytoreductive surgery for advanced primary and recurrent epithelial ovarian cancer patients outweigh morbidity concerns. *Gynecol Oncol* 2006;103:977.
Partridge EE, Gunter B, Gelder M, et al. The validity and significance of substages in advanced ovarian carcinoma. *Gynecol Oncol* 1993;48:236.
Patsner B, Orr J, Mann W, et al. Does serum CA-125 level prior to second-look laparotomy for invasive ovarian adenocarcinoma predict size of residual disease? *Gynecol Oncol* 1990;37:319.
Pavlik EJ, DePriest PD, Gallion HH, et al. Ovarian volume related to age. *Gynecol Oncol* 2000;77:410.
Petricoin EF, Ardekani AM, Hitt BA, et al. Use of proteomic patterns in serum to identify ovarian cancer. *Lancet* 2002;359:572.
Piccart MJ, Bertelsen K, James K, et al. Randomized intergroup trial of cisplatinum-paclitaxel versus cis-platinum-cyclophosphamide in women with advanced epithelial ovarian cancer: three-year results. *J Natl Cancer Inst* 2000;92:699.
Piver MS, Baker T. The potential for optimal (≤2 cm) cytoreductive surgery in advanced ovarian carcinoma at a tertiary medical center: a prospective study. *Gynecol Oncol* 1986;24:1.
Plentl AA, Friedman EA. Lymphatics of the ovary. In: *Lymphatic system of the female genitalia.* Philadelphia, London, Toronto: Sanders; 1971:173.
Podczaski E, Stevens C, Manetta A, et al. Use of second-look laparotomy in the management of patients with ovarian epithelial malignancies. *Gynecol Oncol* 1987;28:205.
Podratz K, Malkasian G, Hilton J, et al. Second-look laparotomy in ovarian cancer: evaluation of pathologic variables. *Am J Obstet Gynecol* 1985;152:230.
Podratz K, Malkasian G, Wieand H, et al. Recurrent disease after negative second-look laparotomy in stages III and IV ovarian carcinoma. *Gynecol Oncol* 1988;29:274.
Podratz KC, Schwarz MF, Wieand HS, et al. Evaluation of treatment and survival after positive second-look laparotomy. *Gynecol Oncol* 1988;31:9.
Prorok PC. Evaluation of screening programs for the early detection of cancer. *Natl Cancer Inst Statistical Textbook Monogr* 1984;51:267.
Puls LE, Powell DE, DePriest PD, et al. Transition from benign to malignant epithelium in mucinous and serous ovarian cystadenocarcinoma. *Gynecol Oncol* 1992;47:53.
Raju KS, McKinna JA, Barker GH, et al. Second-look operations in the planned management of advanced ovarian carcinoma. *Am J Obstet Gynecol* 1982;144:650.
Ramirez PT, Wolf JK, Levenback C. Laparoscopic port-site metastases: etiology and prevention. *Gynecol Oncol* 2003;91:179.
Ransohoff D. Lessons from controversy: ovarian cancer screening and serum proteomics. *J Natl Cancer Inst* 2005;97:315.
Reuter K, Griffin T, Hunter R. Comparison of abdominopelvic computed tomography results and findings at second-look laparotomy in ovarian carcinoma patients. *Cancer* 1989;63:1123.
Ries LAG, Eisner MP, Kosary CL, et al., eds. *SEER cancer statistics review, 1975-2002.* Bethesda, MD: National Cancer Institute, 2005.
Riman T, Dickman PW, Nilsson S, et al. Hormone replacement therapy and the risk of invasive epithelial ovarian cancer in Swedish women. *J Natl Cancer Inst* 2002;94:497.
Ripa R, Katballe N, Wikman FP, et al. Presymptomatic diagnosis using a deletion of a single codon in families with hereditary non-polyposis colorectal cancer. *Mutat Res* 2005;570:89.
Risch HA. Hormonal etiology of epithelial ovarian cancer, with a hypothesis concerning the role of androgens and progesterone. *J Natl Cancer Inst* 1998;90:1774.
Risch HA, Marrett LD, Howe GR. Parity, contraception, infertility, and the risk of epithelial ovarian cancer. *Am J Epidemiol* 1994;140:585.
Roberts W, Hodel K, Rich W, et al. Second-look laparotomy in the management of gynecologic malignancy. *Gynecol Oncol* 1982;13:345.
Roman LD, Muderspac LI, Stein SM, et al. Pelvic examination, tumor marker level and gray-scale and Doppler sonography in the prediction of pelvic cancer. *Obstet Gynecol* 1997;89:493.
Rose PG, Nerenstone S, Brady MF, et al. Secondary surgical cytoreduction for advanced ovarian carcinoma. *N Engl J Med* 2004;351:2489.
Rossing MA, Daling JR, Weiss NS, et al. Ovarian tumors in a cohort of infertile women. *N Engl J Med* 1994;331:771.
Rubin S, Hoskins W, Hakes T, et al. Recurrence after negative second-look laparotomy for ovarian cancer: analysis of risk factors. *Am J Obstet Gynecol* 1988;159:1094.
Rubin S, Hoskins W, Saigo P. Update on prognostic factors for recurrence following negative second-look laparotomy in ovarian cancer patients treated with platinum-based chemotherapy. *Gynecol Oncol* 1991;42:137.
Rubin SC, Hoskins WJ, Benjamin I, et al. Palliative surgery for intestinal obstruction in advanced ovarian cancer. *Gynecol Oncol* 1989;34:16.
Rubin SC, Wong GYC, Curtin JP, et al. Platinum-based chemotherapy of high-risk stage I epithelial ovarian cancer following comprehensive surgical staging. *Obstet Gynecol* 1993;82:143.
Russell P. The pathological assessment of ovarian neoplasms. I. Introduction to the common "epithelial" tumors and analysis of benign "epithelial" tumors. *Pathology* 1979;11:5.
Russell P, Merkur H. Proliferating ovarian "epithelial" tumours: a clinico-pathological analysis of 144 cases. *Aust N Z J Obstet Gynaecol* 1979;19:45.
Sakai K, Kamura T, Hirakawa T, et al. Relationship between pelvic lymph node involvement and other disease sites in patients with ovarian cancer. *Gynecol Oncol* 1997;65:164.
Sassone M, Timor-Tritsch I, Artner A, et al. Transvaginal sonographic characterization of ovarian disease: evaluation of a new scoring system to predict ovarian malignancy. *Obstet Gynecol* 1991;78:70.

Scarabelli C, Campagnutta E, Perin A, et al. La splenectomia enl trattameno chirurgico radicale del carcinoma ovarico. *Minerva Ginecol* 1985;37:37.
Scarabelli C, Gallo A, Carbone A, et al. Secondary cytoreductive surgery for patients with recurrent epithelial ovarian carcinoma. *Gynecol Oncol* 2001;83:504.
Scarabelli C, Gallo A, Zarrelli A, et al. Systematic pelvic and paraaortic lymphadenectomy during cytoreductive surgery in advanced ovarian cancer: potential benefit on survival. *Gynecol Oncol* 1995;56:328.
Schilder JM, Thompson AM, DePriest PD, et al. Outcome of reproductive age women with stage IA or IC invasive epithelial ovarian cancer treated with fertility-sparing surgery. *Gynecol Oncol* 2002: 87:1.
Schildkraut JM, Thompson WD. Familial ovarian cancer: a population-based case control study. *Am J Epidemiol* 1988;128:456.
Schneider VL, Schneider A, Reed KL, et al. Comparison of Doppler with two dimensional sonography and CA-125 for prediction of malignancy of pelvic masses. *Obstet Gynecol* 1993;81:983.
Schmeler K, Lynch HT, Chen LM, et al . Prophylactic surgery to reduce the risk of gynecologic cancers in the Lynch syndrome. *N Engl J Med* 2006;354:261.
Schwartz PE, Rutherford TJ, Chambers JT, et al. Neoadjuvant chemotherapy for advanced ovarian cancer: long-term survival. *Gynecol Oncol* 1999;72:93.
Schwartz P, Smith J. Second-look operations in ovarian cancer. *Am J Obstet Gynecol* 1980;138:1124.
Scully RE, Henson DE, Nielsen ML, et al. Ovary. Reporting on cancer specimens: protocols and case summaries. In: CAP Cancer Committee. *Cancer protocol manual.* 1998:1.
Scully RE, Hensen DE, Nielson ML, et al. Practice protocol for the examination of specimens removed from patients with ovarian tumors. *Arch Pathol Lab Med* 1995;199:1012.
SEER Cancer Statistics Review, 1973-1997. Bethesda, MD: National Cancer Institute, 1997.
Segna RA, Dottino PR, Mandeli JP, et al. Secondary cytoreduction for ovarian cancer following cis-platinum therapy. *J Clin Oncol* 1993;11:434.
Sevelda P, Dittrich C, Salzer H. Prognostic value of the rupture of the capsule in stage I epithelial ovarian carcinoma. *Gynecol Oncol* 1989;35:321.
Skates SJ, Feng J, Yin-Hua Y, et al. Toward an optimal algorithm for ovarian cancer screening with longitudinal tumor markers. *Cancer* 1995;76:2004.
Skates SJ, Manon U, MacDonald N, et al. Calculations of the risk of ovarian cancer from serial CA-125 values for preclinical detection in postmenopausal women. *J Clin Oncol* 2003;21:206s.
Skipper HE. Stepwise progress in the treatment of disseminated cancer. *Cancer* 1983;5:1773.
Slamon DJ, Godolphin W, Jones LA, et al. Studies of the HER-2/neu proto-oncogene in human breast and ovarian cancer. *Science* 1989;244:707.
Smirz L, Stehman F, Ulbright T, et al. Second-look laparotomy after chemotherapy in the management of ovarian malignancy. *Am J Obstet Gynecol* 1985;152:661.
Smith LH, Morris CR, Yasmeen S, et al. Ovarian cancer: can we make the clinical diagnosis earlier? *Cancer* 2005;104:1398.
Smith SA, Easton DF, Evans DG, et al. Allele losses in region 17 q12-21 in familial breast and ovarian cancer involving the wild-type chromosome. *Nat Genet* 1992;2:128.
Smith W, Day T, Smith J. The use of laparoscopy to determine the results of chemotherapy for ovarian cancer. *J Reprod Med* 1977;18:257.
Sonnendecker EW. Is routine second-look laparotomy for ovarian cancer justified? *Gynecol Oncol* 1988;31:249.
Sonnendecker EW, Guidozzi F, Margolius KA. Splenectomy during primary maximal cytoreductive surgery for epithelial ovarian cancer. *Gynecol Oncol* 1989;35:301.
Soper JT, Couchman G, Berchuck A, et al. The role of partial sigmoid colectomy for debulking epithelial ovarian carcinoma. *Gynecol Oncol* 1991;41: 239.
Stehman F, Calkins A, Wass J, et al. A comparison of findings at second-look laparotomy with preoperative computed tomography in patients with ovarian cancer. *Gynecol Oncol* 1988;29:37.
Stein S, Laifer-Narin S, Johnson MB, et al. Differentiation of benign and malignant adnexal masses: relative value of gray scale, color Doppler and spectral Doppler sonography. *Am J Radiol* 1995;164:381.
Stern J, Buscema J, Rosenshein N, et al. Can computed tomography substitute for second-look operation in ovarian carcinoma? *Gynecol Oncol* 1981; 11:82.
Stuart GC, Jeffries M, Stuart JL, et al. The changing role of "second-look" laparotomy in the management of epithelial carcinoma of the ovary. *Am J Obstet Gynecol* 1982;142:612.
Surwit E, Childers J, Atlas I, et al. Neoadjuvant chemotherapy for advanced ovarian cancer. *Int J Gynecol Cancer* 1996;6:356.
Tangir J, Zelterman D, Ma W, et al. Reproductive function after conservative surgery and chemotherapy for malignant germ cell tumors of the ovary. *Obstet Gynecol* 2003;101:251.
Tay E-H, Grant PT, Gebski V, et al. Secondary cytoreductive surgery for recurrent epithelial ovarian cancer. *Obstet Gynecol* 2002;99:1008.
Taylor JWK, Ramas I, Carter D, et al. Correlation of Doppler US tumor signals with neovascular morphologic features. *Radiology* 1988;166:157.
Tazelaar HD, Bostwick DG, Ballon SC, et al. Conservative treatment of borderline ovarian tumors. *Obstet Gynecol* 1985;66:417.
Tinelli R, Tinelli A, Tinelli FG, et al. Conservative surgery for borderline ovarian tumors: a review. *Gynecol Oncol* 2006;100:185.
Tingulstad S, Skjeldestad FE, Hagen B. The effect of centralization of primary surgery on survival in ovarian cancer patients. *Obstet Gynecol* 2003;102:499.
Tortolero-Luna G, Mitchell MF. The epidemiology of ovarian cancer. *J Cell Biochem Suppl* 1995;13:200.
Trimbos JB, Schueler JA, van Lent M, et al. Reasons for incomplete surgical staging in early ovarian carcinoma. *Gynecol Oncol* 1990;37:374.
Ueland FR, DePriest PD, DeSimone CP, et al. The accuracy of examination under anesthesia and transvaginal sonography in evaluating ovarian size. *Gynecol Oncol* 2005;99:400.
Ueland FR, DePriest PD, Pavlik EJ, et al. Preoperative differentiation of malignant from benign ovarian tumors: the efficacy of morphology indexing and Doppler flow sonography. *Gynecol Oncol* 2003;91:46.
Vacarello L, Rubin SC, Vlamis V, et al. Cytoreductive surgery in ovarian carcinoma patients with a documented previously complete surgical response. *Gynecol Oncol* 1995;57:61.
Valentin L, Sladkevicius P, Marsal, K. Limited contribution of Doppler velocimetry to the differential diagnosis of extra-uterine pelvic tumors. *Obstet Gynecol* 1994;83:425.
Van der Burg MEL, van Lent M, Buyse M, et al. The effect of debulking surgery after induction chemotherapy: on the prognosis in advanced epithelial ovarian cancer. *N Engl J Med* 1995;332:629.
van Nagell JR, DePriest PD, Reedy MB, et al. The efficacy of transvaginal sonographic screening in asymptomatic women at risk for ovarian cancer. *Gynecol Oncol* 2000;77:350.
van Nagell JR, Higgins RV, Donaldson ES, et al. Transvaginal sonography as a screening method for ovarian cancer: a report of the first 1000 cases screened. *Cancer* 1990;65:573.
Vasey PA, Jayson GC, Gordon A, et al. Phase III randomized trial of docetaxel-carboplatin versus paclitaxel-carboplatin as first-line chemotherapy for ovarian carcinoma. *J Natl Cancer Inst* 2004;96:1682.
Vasilev SA, Schlaerth JB, Canpean J, et al. Serum CA-125 levels in preoperative evaluation of ovarian masses. *Obstet Gynecol* 1988;71:751.
Vergote IB, Kaern J, Abeler VM, et al. Analysis of prognostic factors in stage I epithelial ovarian cancer: importance of degree of differentiation and deoxyribonucleic acid ploidy in predicting relapse. *Am J Obstet Gynecol* 1993;169:40.
Vergote I, Marquette S, Amant F, et al. Port-site metastases after open laparoscopy: a study in 173 patients with advanced ovarian cancer. *Int J Gynecol Cancer* 2005;15:776.
Vergote IB, Vergote-De Vos LN, Abeler VM, et al. Randomized trial comparing cis-platinum with radioactive phosphorus or whole-abdomen irradiation as adjuvant treatment of ovarian cancer. *Cancer* 1992;69:741.
Walker JL, Armstrong DK, Huang HQ, et al. Intraperitoneal catheter outcomes in a phase III trial of intravenous versus intraperitoneal chemotherapy in optimal stage III ovarian and primary peritoneal cancer: a Gynecologic Oncology Group study. *Gynecol Oncol* 2006;100:27.
Wangensteen OH, Lewis FJ, Tongen LA. The "second-look" in cancer surgery. *Lancet* 1951;71:303.
Webb M, Snyder J, Williams T, et al. Second-look laparotomy in ovarian cancer. *Gynecol Oncol* 1982;14:285.
Weiner Z, Thaler I, Beck D, et al. Differentiating malignant from benign ovarian tumors with transvaginal color flow imaging. *Obstet Gynecol* 1992;79:159.
Whittemore AS, Gong G, Itnyre J. Prevalence and contribution of BRCA1 mutations in breast cancer and ovarian cancer: results from three U.S. population-based case-control studies of ovarian cancer. *Am J Hum Genet* 1997;60: 496.
Whittemore AS, Harris R, Itnyre J. Collaborative Ovarian Cancer Group: characteristics relating to ovarian cancer risk, collaborative analysis of 12 U.S. case-control studies. II. Invasive epithelial ovarian cancers in white women. *Am J Epidemiol* 1992;136:1184.
Williams S, Blessing JA, Liao S, et al. Adjuvant therapy of ovarian germ cell tumors with cisplatin, etoposide, and bleomycin: a trial of the Gynecologic Oncology Group. *J Clin Oncol* 1994;12:701.
Williams SD, Blessing JA, DiSaia PJ, et al. Second-look laparotomy in ovarian germ cell tumors: the Gyneoclogic Oncology Group experience. *Gynecol Oncol* 1994;52:287.
Wiltshaw E, Raju KS, Dawson I. The role of cytoreductive surgery in advanced carcinoma of the ovary: an analysis of primary and second surgery. *BJOG* 1985;92:522.
Woods CH, Thompson EA. Transvaginal sonography as a screening method for ovarian cancer: a report of the first 1000 cases screened. *Cancer* 1990;65:573.
Wooster R, Bignell G, Lancaster J, et al. Identification of the breast cancer susceptibility gene BRCA2. *Nature* 1995;378:789.
World Health Organization Histological classification of ovarian tumours. In: Tavassoli FA, Devilee P, eds. *Pathology and genetics: tumors of the breast and female genital organs.* London: Oxford University Press; 2003:114.

World Health Organization histological classification of ovarian tumors. In: Scully RE, Young RH, Clement PB, eds. *Atlas of tumor pathology, tumors of the ovary, maldeveloped gonads, fallopian tube and broad ligament.* Bethesda, MD: AFIP; 1998:28.

Wu P-C, Qu J-Y, Lang J-H, et al. Lymph node metastasis of ovarian cancer: a preliminary survey of 74 cases of lymphadenectomy. *Am J Obstet Gynecol* 1986;155:1103.

Young RC. A second look at second-look laparotomy [editorial]. *J Clin Oncol* 1987;5:1311.

Young RC, Brady MF, Nieberg RM, et al. A randomized phase III trial of intraperitoneal ^{32}P or intravenous cyclophosphamide and cisplatin: a Gynecologic Oncology Group study. *J Clin Oncol* 2003;21:4350.

Young RC, Decker DG, Wharton JT, et al. Staging laparotomy in early ovarian cancer. *JAMA* 1983;250:3072.

Young RC, Walton LA, Ellenberg SS, et al. Adjuvant therapy in stage I and II epithelial ovarian cancer: results of two prospective randomized trials. *N Engl J Med* 1990;322:1021.

Zanetta G, Bonazzi C, Cantu MG, et al. Survival and reproductive function after treatment of malignant germ cell ovarian tumors. *J Clin Oncol* 2001;19:1015.

Zanetta G, Chiari S, Rota S, et al. Conservative surgery for stage I ovarian carcinoma in women of childbearing age. *BJOG* 1997;104:1030.

Zang R-Y, Li Z-T, Tang J, et al. Secondary cytoreductive surgery for patients with relapsed epithelial ovarian carcinoma: Who benefits? *Cancer* 2004;100:1152.

CHAPTER 50 ■ PELVIC EXENTERATION

THOMAS W. BURKE

DEFINITIONS

Anterior pelvic exenteration—Similar to a total exenteration, except the rectum is left intact. This procedure may be used for anterior pelvic recurrences, anterior vaginal cancers, or bladder or urethral tumors.

Posterior pelvic exenteration—Similar to a total exenteration, except the bladder, urethra, and distal ureters are left intact. This procedure may be suitable for posterior pelvic recurrences or some rectal lesions.

Total pelvic exenteration—Surgical removal of all the pelvic organs, including the uterus, cervix, tubes, ovaries, vagina, bladder, urethra, and distal rectum and anus. In most cases, a pelvic and paraaortic lymphadenectomy are also done.

Triad of trouble—Sometimes called the *terrible triad,* these signs and symptoms are usually indicators of pelvic sidewall involvement with tumor. The triad is composed of (i) unilateral ureteral obstruction, (ii) sciatic nerve pain, and (iii) unilateral leg edema.

Wet colostomy—An old practice of placing the ureters into the bowel just before it exits the abdomen via a colostomy. The urine and feces are passed via a single abdominal stoma. This technique was abandoned because of frequent pyelonephritis, electrolyte abnormalities, and very unpleasant stomal discharge.

It has been more than 50 years since Brunschwig introduced surgical evisceration as an option to control cancers within the pelvic organs. Initially, significant morbidity and mortality rates ranging from 50% to 70% were encountered. These rates have decreased dramatically, allowing the survival rate for those treated to increase substantially. The results of ultraradical pelvic surgery have been enhanced by a number of advances.

Improved surgical techniques and training have decreased operative time and blood loss and limited the extent of disfigurement. Perioperative morbidity has been reduced through the control of infection and the use of blood component therapy, improved anesthetic techniques, parenteral nutrition, and intensive care facilities managed by expert medical teams. Although pelvic exenteration is a formidable procedure, the 5-year survival rate is greater than 50% for appropriately targeted women (Table 50.1). Exenteration has become the treatment of choice for certain types of advanced or recurrent tumors of the pelvis, and it provides another chance at survival for women in whom primary therapy has failed.

Careful patient selection using a thorough and detailed approach to preoperative assessment is essential. Strict guidelines regarding the indications and contraindications for operability must be met. The adaptive ability of patients who survive is dramatic given the magnitude of anatomic and physiologic change associated with exenteration. However, those who die of their disease despite this heroic surgical effort commonly experience intractable pain from intestinal obstruction or distant metastases.

Many modifications of the Brunschwig procedure have been instituted since its introduction in 1948. The most significant modification was introduced in 1950 when Bricker developed and reported his classic ileal conduit technique. This technique provided an isolated conduit for urinary diversion, which became a replacement option for the traditional "wet colostomies" or ureterosigmoidostomy in which both stool and urine exited from a solitary stoma. The separation of urinary and fecal streams represented a huge advance in terms of reducing complication rates from infection. Despite the requirement for two stomas, this technique also achieved greater patient acceptance. Other more recent advances—such as continent urinary diversion, the use of automatic stapling devices for the gastrointestinal portion of the procedure, pelvic floor coverage, vaginal reconstruction, and low rectal anastomosis—also have improved the overall results and rehabilitation of patients.

Total pelvic exenteration encompasses removal of the genital organs (vagina, uterus, fallopian tubes, and ovaries) as well as the bladder and rectum. An isolated segment of bowel is used to construct a replacement urinary reservoir. A segment of small or large bowel or a combination of both may be considered. Modifications of the pelvic exenterative procedure include either an anterior or posterior exenteration or a total exenteration with a low rectal reanastomosis. Patients whose cancer is confined to the anterior pelvic structures are candidates for anterior exenteration, which removes the bladder and genital organs while leaving the gastrointestinal system intact. In this situation, a urinary conduit is developed from an isolated segment of bowel into which the ureters are anastomosed. For tumors limited to posterior structures, posterior exenteration can be used to remove the genital organs and rectum, allowing preservation of the urinary system. In selected patients who undergo a total pelvic exenteration, a low rectal anastomosis can be accomplished if the lower 6 to 10 cm of rectum is preserved. The end-to-end anastomosis (EEA) stapling device designed for this purpose is used to reconstruct the rectum low in the pelvis. Low anastomosis often requires a protective colostomy because the anastomosis has been constructed in an irradiated field. The colostomy can be reversed at a later date, eliminating one of the patient's stomas.

INDICATIONS AND CONTRAINDICATIONS

The decision-making process begins when the physician first sees the patient and takes her history. An initial diagnostic evaluation is obtained. If the patient appears to be a candidate for a pelvic exenterative procedure, she is referred to a gynecologic oncologist who is experienced in the evaluation and treatment of such patients. The best outcomes are achieved in patients who have centrally recurrent squamous cell carcinoma of the

TABLE 50.1

PERIOPERATIVE MORTALITY AND 5-YEAR SURVIVAL AFTER PELVIC EXENTERATION

Report	No. patients	Operative mortality (%)	5-year survival (%)
Parsons and Friedell (1964)	112	14	21
Brunschwig (1965)	535	16	20
Rutledge and Burns (1965)	108	17	29
Kiselow et al. (1967)	207	8	35
Symmonds et al. (1968)	118	12	26
Ketcham et al. (1970)	162	7	38
Brunschwig (1970)	225	8	19
Symmonds et al. (1975)	198	8	33
Rutledge et al. (1977)	296	13	48
Averrette et al. (1984)	92	24	37
Morley et al. (1989)	100	2	61
Shingleton et al. (1989)	143	6	50
Berek et al. (2005)	75	4	54

cervix or vagina. Exenteration may be appropriate for some women with advanced vulvar cancer when more conventional therapy has failed. In rare cases, patients with large vulvar carcinomas may require pelvic exenteration as primary treatment because of geographic spread of the disease to involve adjacent organs. Infrequently, a recurrent adenocarcinoma of the cervix or endometrium or a sarcoma in the pelvis may be isolated to the central pelvis and resectable by exenteration. Women with recurrent ovarian carcinomas are rarely candidates for exenterative resection because isolated pelvic recurrence is so unusual.

The primary indication for pelvic exenteration is recurrent or persistent squamous cell carcinoma of the cervix. This indication is most common because of the frequency of cervical cancer, and squamous cell lesions tend to spread by continuity and contiguity along tissue planes, often staying localized for long periods of time before metastasizing to more remote areas. The adjacent tissues—such as the bladder, urethra, and bowel—often are involved. Even when final pathologic examination shows no direct invasion of these adjacent organs, often it is not possible to obtain a satisfactory tumor-free margin in these previously irradiated, healing-impaired tissues without their removal. Consequently, control of the carcinoma cannot be achieved without their removal.

Total pelvic exenteration is the most common type of exenteration performed in most reported series. The more extensive resection ensures that an adequate margin beyond palpable disease is obtained. A philosophy of ensuring the widest margin of resection at the earliest possible moment is essential to obtaining a curative resection. The less extensive forms of radical pelvic surgery, such as radical hysterectomy, produce a higher incidence of treatment failure and an unacceptably high incidence of urinary or bowel fistulization because the pelvic tissues in the operative field have already been compromised by radiotherapy. Although some patients with focal recurrence can be curatively resected by radical hysterectomy or anterior or posterior exenteration, these approaches should be limited to patients with very small and well-defined recurrences.

Before the introduction of current diagnostic techniques, clinical evaluation of the patient and intravenous pyelography were the only methods available to assess whether the disease could be resected by exenteration. The so-called triad of trouble used in this assessment consisted of (a) an abnormal intravenous pyelogram demonstrating ureteral obstruction, (b) sciatic nerve distribution of pain suggesting neural sheath involvement at or near the lateral pelvic wall, and (c) lower-extremity edema, implying venous or lymphatic compromise of the iliac vessels. If none or one of these features were present, exploration to determine resectability was recommended. If two or more of these abnormalities were present, the patient's disease was considered unresectable. If there is any doubt whether the lesion can be resected, the patient should undergo exploratory surgery, because exenteration is often the patient's last opportunity for curative therapy.

Several diagnostic techniques can aid in assessing resectability in a patient who is believed to have central pelvic disease on clinical grounds. Evaluation of resectability is important from both a technical and psychological standpoint. A preoperative study that demonstrates the presence of nonresectable disease helps to avoid not only the morbidity of exploratory laparotomy, but also its attendant false hope for cure. There is a tremendous negative psychological impact on the patient when she is prepared preoperatively for the exenterative procedure only to be told postoperatively that she had an inoperable lesion.

Computed tomography (CT) or magnetic resonance imaging (MRI) can be most beneficial in assessing the presence of lateral pelvic wall invasion and unsuspected liver metastases as well as in further evaluation of the retroperitoneal lymph nodes. MRI is especially useful in locating tumor invasion at the pelvic wall.

Exenteration under anesthesia with transvaginal Tru-Cut needle biopsy can be used to evaluate a palpable pelvic mass at the lateral pelvic wall. These biopsies can differentiate between recurrent neoplasm and postirradiation fibrosis when thickened tissue is encountered throughout the pelvis. Fine-needle aspiration (FNA) of suspicious regional lymph nodes under CT scan guidance can be helpful in confirming unresectable metastases. McDonald and coworkers reported that FNA had an 85% accuracy rate in identifying positive nodes. Because the 5-year survival rate drops to 0% to 14% when the pelvic lymph nodes are positive, pelvic exenteration is unrewarding, and exploratory surgery is not recommended (Table 50.2). It

TABLE 50.2

EFFECT OF PELVIC LYMPH NODE METASTASIS ON SURVIVAL AFTER PELVIC EXENTERATION

Report	Negative nodes		Positive nodes	
	No. patients	5-year survival (%)	No. patients	5-year survival (%)
Barber and Jones (1971)	166	17	97	5
Creasman and Rutledge (1974)	29	27	14	14
Symmonds et al. (1975)	139	39	59	13
Averette et al. (1984)	92	—	6	0
Morley et al. (1989)	87	70	13	0
Shingleton et al. (1989)	106	—	10	10

must be remembered that a negative biopsy does not guarantee that cancer is not present, but merely that no cancer was identified at the focal point of the needle tip.

The final diagnostic decision concerning the operability of disease is made when the patient is examined under anesthesia and as the exploratory laparotomy is performed. Fixation of the tumor in the pelvis caused by recurrent disease extending to the pelvic sidewall, penetration of the tumor into the peritoneal cavity with dissemination of cells intraabdominally, and extrapelvic involvement of regional lymph nodes, omentum, liver, and other structures are all contraindications to the performance of pelvic exenteration with curative intent. These areas must be completely assessed by thorough palpation, visualization, and multiple frozen-section biopsies, when indicated. The use of the avascular paravesical and pararectal spaces can be helpful in evaluating the extent of the disease under these circumstances. Transection of the ureters and bowel commit the surgeon and the patient to exenteration. These components of the procedure should be delayed until resectability is confirmed. Incomplete resection with positive margins or metastatic disease is not curative and subjects the patient to an extended and difficult postoperative recovery without a realistic chance of long-term survival.

Pelvic exenteration is an appropriate therapeutic option for relatively few women with recurrent cancer. About one third of recurrences appear to be central pelvic failure by clinical examination. Of these, one half are excluded from surgical therapy when diagnostic studies reveal unresectable disease. About one half of women who undergo exploration for exenteration are found to have inoperable disease, and the procedure is aborted. Of those who undergo resection by exenteration, about one half obtain long-term survival and apparent cure (Fig. 50.1).

Pelvic exenteration is not considered a treatment of choice for primary disease except in a limited number of patients with carcinoma of the vulva and in selected patients with nongynecologic lesions that involve the bladder, urethra, or colon. In the past, stage IVA carcinoma of the cervix involving the bladder or rectum was treated in this manner; however, the results were not considered superior to those achieved by full-course pelvic radiotherapy. Exenteration has been abandoned as primary therapy for this lesion since Rutledge and Burns treated stage IV lesions with radiation therapy and showed an acceptable 28% survival rate. The same concept exists in regard to primary carcinoma of the vagina, for which radiation therapy is the preferred initial treatment. Current chemoradiation protocols with or without conservative surgery appear to provide results equivalent or superior to those obtained with exenteration for advanced tumors of the cervix, vulva, and vagina. Consequently, primary exenteration has become a rare operation.

Disease-free interval—the time from primary diagnosis to recurrence—is highly predictive of survival following exenteration. In all series, there is a direct relation between time from primary treatment to time of recurrence and survival: 5-year survival rate of greater than 90% has been reported when the disease-free interval was greater than 10 years, compared with a survival rate less than 50% when this interval was 1 year or less.

Pelvic exenteration occasionally may be indicated to manage severely damaged irradiated tissue in the pelvis. Many patients with radiation necrosis experience intractable pain, copious amounts of foul-smelling discharge, and both urinary and rectal fistulas from tissue necrosis. In many cases, symptoms can be relieved with urinary and/or bowel diversion procedures alone. *Palliative exenteration should be considered only in extreme cases in which more conservative approaches have failed.*

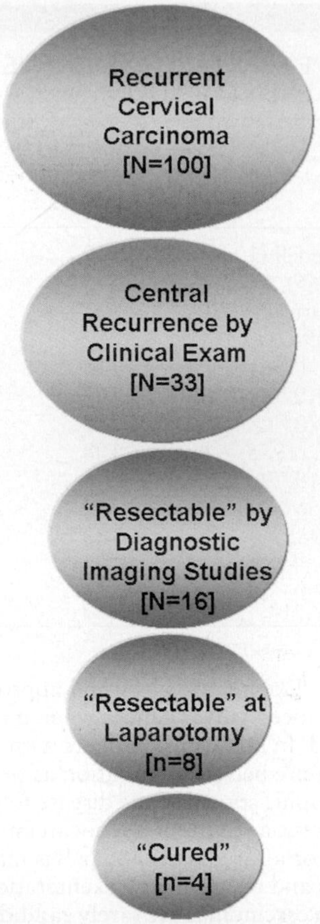

FIGURE 50.1. As women with recurrent disease undergo clinical, diagnostic, and surgical evaluation for possible exenteration, increasing numbers are determined not to be surgical candidates. One half of those who have their disease resected will obtain long-term survival.

Traditionally, the presence of recurrent or persistent adenocarcinoma of the female pelvic organs was a relative contraindication to exenterative therapy. These glandular lesions are more likely to disseminate through the hematologic or lymphatic routes and bypass the traditional, more orderly mode of spread seen with squamous tumors. However, small recent series suggest that exenteration can provide curative therapy for 30% to 50% of women with isolated central recurrence of adenocarcinoma of the endocervix and endometrium (Table 50.3). A diligent search for unresectable metastases must be performed before and during the operation. High tumor grade and short disease-free interval are correlated with decreasing chance of survival. Locally advanced or recurrent pelvic sarcoma, although rare, occasionally may be managed by pelvic exenteration.

Age, religious orientation, obesity, and medical and psychological alterations must be evaluated as potential contraindications to exenteration. Although life expectancy beyond 70 years for women who undergo this procedure steadily diminishes, this factor alone is not an absolute deterrent to this procedure. A number of patients older than 70 years have been treated successfully with return to fully functional status. Religious orientation is seldom a contraindication; however, the high likelihood of blood replacement requires that the patient be willing to accept transfusion of blood and blood products.

TABLE 50.3

PELVIC EXENTERATION OUTCOMES IN WOMEN WITH VULVAR OR ENDOMETRIAL CANCER

	Site	No. of patients	Morbidity (%)	5-year survival (%)
Phillips et al. (1981)	Vulva	12	85	45
Cavanagh and Shepherd (1982)	Vulva	13	—	50
Hopkins and Morley (1992)	Vulva	19	53	60
Miller et al. (1995)	Vulva	21	57	52
Morris et al. (1996)	Endometrium	20	60	45
Barakat et al. (1999)	Endometrium	44	80	20

Obesity is a relative contraindication to surgery. Most patients with recurrent cancer of the cervix have a protracted disease course and are rarely overweight. Obese patients present technical problems that further complicate an already difficult procedure, and they must be evaluated individually. Stomal construction can be difficult in these patients, operating time is prolonged, infection rates are increased, and pulmonary function may be compromised during the postoperative period.

Medical condition and psychological state are important factors in deciding whether some patients should undergo operation. Surgical risks must be weighed against the benefit of the procedure. The patient's willingness to actively participate in her recovery and her ability to adapt psychologically are key components to the success of resection. In most settings where exenteration is offered, there is no favorable alternative therapy. The patient must clearly understand the implications of her decision to seek or refuse exenteration. Although small, the risk of perioperative mortality with this operation is definite. Complications of some type are seen in 30% to 50% of cases.

The preoperative medical and anesthetic assessments of the cardiopulmonary, renal, and nutritional status of the patient must be thorough. Consultants with expertise in these areas must be available during the perioperative period. All patients require close surveillance in an intensive care unit postoperatively. Patients must also be psychologically prepared for the significant alterations in their excretory systems and their sexual function. These patients often benefit from counseling by an enterostomal therapist, psychologist, or psychiatrist before the operation. The consultant's aid in preparing the patient may be as important as the surgery itself. An informal discussion with another patient who has satisfactorily adjusted to the alterations of exenteration frequently is beneficial and should be considered.

The surgeon who undertakes pelvic exenterative therapy has responsibilities beyond the performance of surgery. The surgeon must consider the quality of life remaining for the patient after the operation, the long-term rehabilitation of the patient if the operation is successful, and the long-term terminal care of the patient if it is not.

EXENTERATION TECHNIQUE

Preoperative Preparation

The initial planning for pelvic exenteration begins in the outpatient office. A full discussion is undertaken with the patient before definitive surgery is planned. The complete operation—including the removal of the bladder, vagina, and rectum and the possible necessity of two ostomies—is fully outlined. Occasional patients cannot psychologically adjust to the concept of the operation and refuse further evaluation. Such decisions should be honored, and ongoing supportive care of the patient should be offered. For the patient who can psychologically commit to the removal of her pelvic viscera, a further discussion is undertaken to assess her desire for vaginal reconstruction, creation of a continent urinary diversion, and, potentially, low rectal reanastomosis.

Patients are admitted the day before surgery for bowel preparation and intravenous hydration and to be marked by the stomal therapist for ostomy placement. Arterial blood gas analysis is obtained routinely. For patients whose oxygen saturation is adequate, pulmonary function testing is not routinely performed. A central venous catheter should be placed during anesthetic induction to provide appropriate vascular access. Preoperative total parenteral nutrition is not used routinely unless the patient has a nutritional deficit. Intravenous prophylactic antibiotics are given on call to the operating room, and the patient is shaved just before surgery. Either subcutaneous heparin or sequential compression devices (SCDs) may be used for prophylaxis against deep venous thrombosis.

The patient is positioned for surgery using Allen stirrups. This position allows simultaneous access to the abdominal and perineal areas for bimanual assessment of the lesion intraoperatively and to facilitate the "double team" approach to operating transabdominally and transvaginally simultaneously. A two-team approach should be considered in all cases to shorten anesthetic time, reduce blood loss, and minimize fatigue of the surgical team. Rotation of members of the operative team in and out of the operating room allows for rest and refreshment and minimizes the chance of fatigue-related operator errors during the critical reconstructive phase of the operation.

Intraoperative Exploration

The abdomen is opened using a vertical midline incision. Although a transverse incision allows greater pelvic exposure and facilitates the lateral pelvic wall assessment, it limits the upper abdominal evaluation, aortic node dissection, and creation of continent urinary diversion (Fig. 50.2). On entry into the peritoneal cavity, the surgeon should carefully palpate all organs, surfaces, and lymph node areas. The liver is examined for evidence of metastatic disease. Cytologic washings and ascitic fluid, if present, can be recovered and sent for immediate cytologic analysis. Any areas that appear abnormal on the preoperative diagnostic studies are examined. Any questionable areas are biopsied and samples sent for frozen-section analysis. Abnormal nodal findings are similarly analyzed, with a specific focus on the pelvic, high common iliac, and paraaortic lymph nodes. Frozen-section support by a pathologist experienced in the evaluation and diagnosis of gynecologic cancers and irradiated tissue changes is absolutely essential.

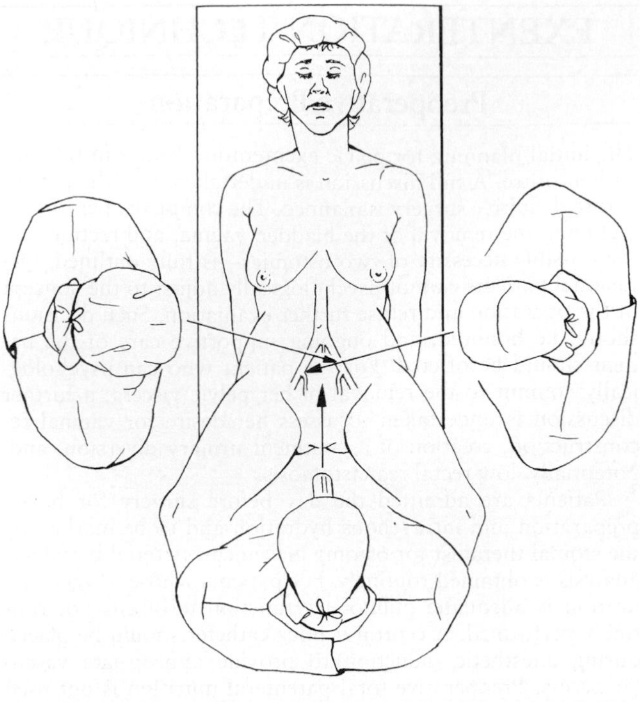

FIGURE 50.2. Use of the low lithotomy position and Allen stirrups allows three operating surgeons to have direct visual access to the abdominal cavity. This position also provides access for a second team to perform the perineal portion of the resection and the vaginal reconstruction while the upper team creates the urinary conduit and colostomy.

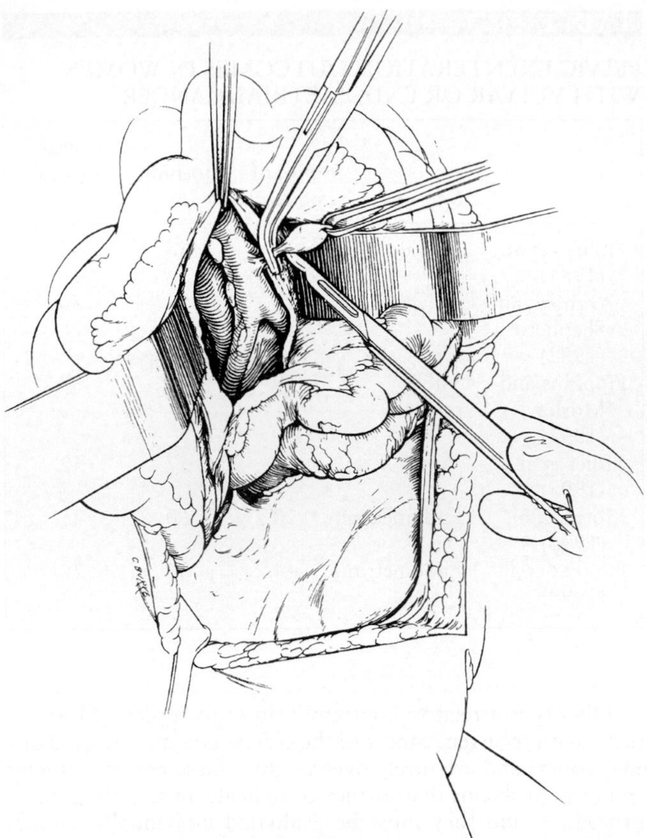

FIGURE 50.3. Lymph nodes are sampled by first incising the peritoneum overlying the aorta. Small vessels are ligated with hemoclips as the fat pad is elevated from the aorta fat pad over the inferior vena cava and should then be isolated in a similar manner. Great care must be used over the inferior vena cava to avoid injury to this thin-walled great vessel. Complete mobilization of the aorta is not necessary.

Paraaortic lymph node dissection is performed by initially incising the peritoneum over the lower aorta (Fig. 50.3) or right common iliac vessels. The area is carefully evaluated by visual and tactile examination. The lymph node dissection is begun at or just below the bifurcation of the aorta and proceeds cephalad. The lymphatic tissue is carefully freed from the aorta; hemoclips are used to ligate the small perforating vessels. Using gentle upward traction and sharp dissection, the surgeon can isolate the nodes to about the level of the inferior mesenteric artery. The uppermost pedicle is tied or ligated with an appropriate hemoclip. A similar dissection is performed over the anterior wall of the inferior vena cava to obtain lymph nodes located on the right side of the aorta. Squamous cell carcinoma of the cervix spreads in a stepwise manner; thus, extensive paraaortic node dissection to the level of the renal artery is not necessary. If the lower paraaortic tissue is negative for metastatic disease, none is found at a higher level. The high common iliac and pelvic lymph nodes are dissected similarly and evaluated. Dissection to the level of the renal vessels should be performed in patients with adenocarcinoma of the cervix or endometrium whose tumors have a less predictable pattern of lymphatic spread.

When this evaluation is completed and there are no contraindications to proceeding, the round ligaments are divided and the *pararectal and paravesical spaces* are opened. The paravesical space is developed by bluntly sweeping the bladder away from the pubic symphysis in the space of Retzius and continuing the dissection laterally, sweeping the bladder medially off the pelvic sidewall until the fibrovascular pedicles are encountered at the 4- and 8-o'clock positions. These fibrovascular pedicles, commonly referred to as "the web," contain the uterine artery and vein, the ureter, the base of the broad ligament extending from the upper vagina and cervix to the pelvic sidewall, and the superior hemorrhoidal vessels. One pelvic sidewall at a time should be evaluated. The round ligament is ligated and divided, and the peritoneum is incised over the iliopsoas muscle. This exposes the pararectal space, which is developed by bluntly freeing the medial leaf of the peritoneum with the attached ureter from its areolar attachment to the pelvic sidewall structures. When the pararectal space is fully developed, the fibrovascular pedicle can be palpated between the operator's thumb and index finger, allowing for evaluation of the pelvic sidewall. Any nodular or suspicious area in this region is biopsied and frozen section is obtained (Fig. 50.4). At this early stage in the operation, the mass of neoplasm should be movable. Free spaces should be present between the neoplasm and the pelvic sidewalls in both the paravesical and pararectal spaces. If the tumor mass is not freely movable, lateral invasion is likely, and a more extensive evaluation of resectability should be undertaken. Biopsy of the cardinal ligaments or lateral tumor spread at the pelvic sidewall should be taken for frozen section.

At this point in the operation, the patient has not been committed to an exenteration because neither the bowel nor the ureter has been transected. Once disease resectability has been confirmed and the decision to perform an exenteration is made, the specific type of procedure—total, posterior, or

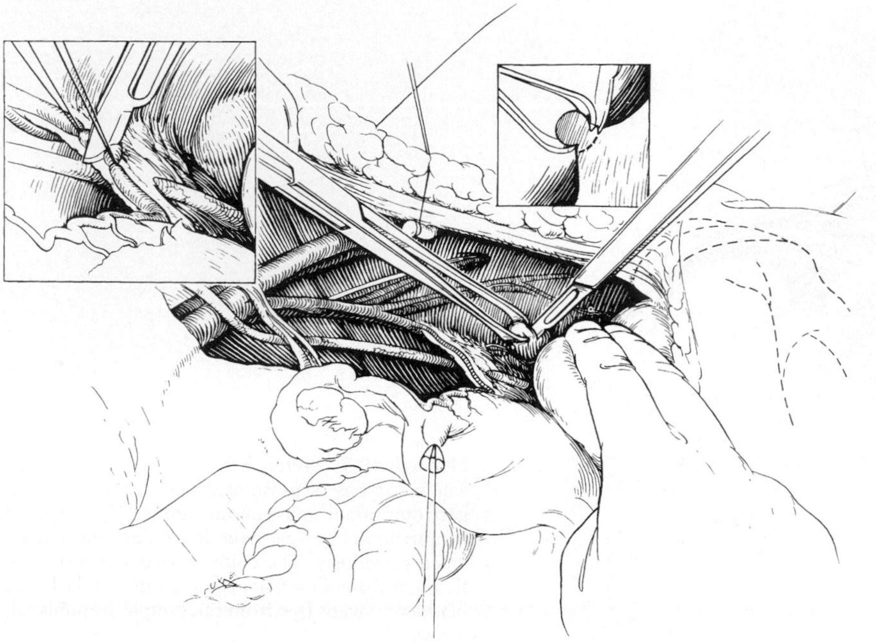

FIGURE 50.4. The pararectal and paravesical spaces have been developed. Thickened or suggestive areas of tumor extension to the sidewalls are sampled for frozen section analysis. The uterine artery is divided at its origin from the internal iliac and is tied with 2-0 silk.

anterior—must be chosen. The extent of the disease—including its involvement of the bladder, bowel, or both—must be estimated. If preoperative studies have shown involvement of the bladder or rectum, these organs must be removed. The surgeon must consider the possibility of microscopic disease that cannot be palpated or seen without magnification. The selected procedure must encompass the entire neoplasm with a margin of uninvolved tissue. Contraindications to pelvic exenteration include intraabdominal metastases, malignant cells in ascitic fluid, metastatic disease to regional lymph nodes, breakthrough of the tumor through the peritoneal surfaces, and presence of malignant disease at or beyond a surgically resected margin. The decision is made to perform the exenteration when all frozen-section reports are returned and are negative for metastatic disease.

Removal of the Specimen

An en bloc dissection of the pelvic tissue is undertaken by clamping and dividing the web of tissue at the pelvic sidewalls. Large pedicle clamps are used to clamp the tissue and control the bleeding from this area. The tissue is divided and ligated with suture, using either suture ligatures or large hemostatic clips. We prefer to clamp, divide, and ligate the uterine artery at the top of the web lateral to the ureter separately, allowing the dissection to continue along the pelvic sidewall. The ureters are freed from the medial leaf of the peritoneum with sharp dissection, clipped with large hemoclips, and transected as distally as possible. The proximal ureters distend during the remainder of this part of the procedure, facilitating their later anastomosis into the urinary conduit.

The sigmoid colon is divided using the gastrointestinal anastomotic (GIA) stapler. Before this division, small epiploic vessels are divided and tied. A free space is developed in the bowel mesentery just beneath the bowel wall. This allows introduction of either a bowel clamp or the stapler. The peritoneum overlying the mesentery is incised, exposing the vessels to the sigmoid colon. These are cross-clamped and tied. Transillumination of the vascular arcade leading to the bowel allows for preservation of the major blood supply, which consists of the sigmoidal and superior hemorrhoidal arteries arising from the inferior mesenteric artery, the middle hemorrhoidal arteries coming bilaterally from the hypogastric vessels, and the inferior hemorrhoidal vessels from the pudendal arteries. The sigmoidal artery usually is preserved, whereas the superior hemorrhoidal vessel is ligated.

When the sigmoid colon is divided and the superior hemorrhoidal vessel is clamped and divided, the sigmoid is detached from the sacrum, and a free space becomes apparent (Fig. 50.5). This is an avascular plane, and the dissection should be directed toward the colon and away from the sacrum. Using blunt dissection, the colon can be freed posteriorly to the levator ani muscles that compromise the lateral pelvic diaphragm. Care must be taken not to damage the sacral veins when dissecting the colon free in this area. If these sacral veins are torn, the resulting hemorrhage often is difficult to control. Attempts to clamp and ligate the sacral vessels are uniformly unsuccessful. Fine, absorbable figure-of-eight sutures or packing with the use of absorbable hemostatic substances may be more beneficial in these instances. Sterile thumbtacks placed directly into the sacrum also can be used to control this bleeding. The middle hemorrhoidal vessels are clamped, further freeing the pelvic specimen. These pedicles, entering from the 4- and 8-o'clock positions, are ligated with suture (Fig. 50.6).

As the pelvic diaphragm is approached abdominally, the second surgical team begins the perineal phase of the operation. The incision around the urethra, vagina, and rectum is outlined, and the dissection proceeds cephalad toward the pelvic diaphragm from below. These muscles are transected circumferentially, and the specimen is removed in toto through the pelvis. The pelvis is copiously irrigated, and hemostasis is achieved. The perineum is supported by approximating the levator muscles with absorbable sutures. If a bilateral myocutaneous graft is to be used for vaginal reconstruction, the second team begins "harvesting" the grafts while the team operating in the abdomen begins construction of the urinary conduit.

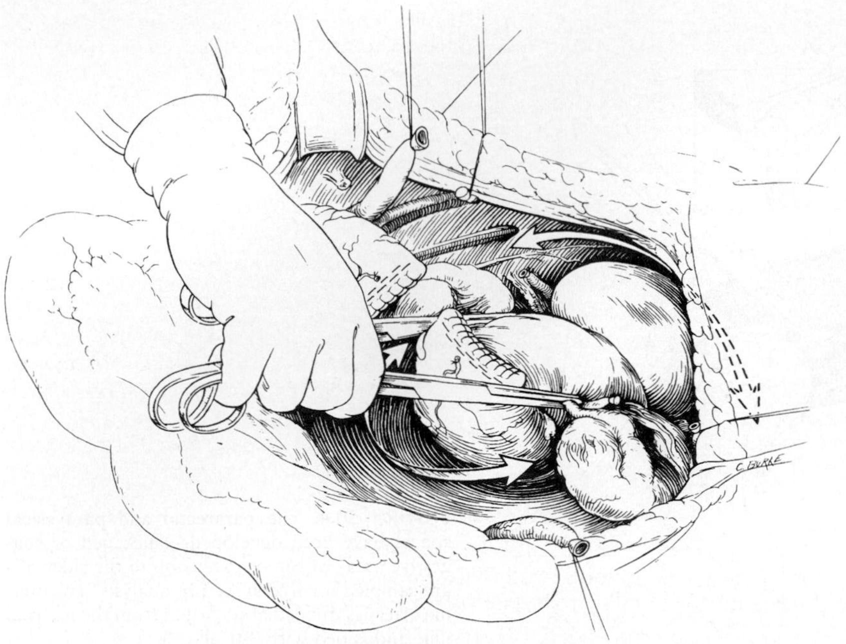

FIGURE 50.5. Ureters have been tied and divided. The colon has been isolated and divided with the gastrointestinal anastomotic stapler. The superior hemorrhoidal vessels have been clamped and divided previously. The colon is swept free by gentle blunt dissection from the sacrum. Similarly, the bladder is swept free from the symphysis pubis *(arrows)*.

Conduit Formation

We prefer either the continent urinary reservoir or the ileal conduit. About 15 cm of the terminal ileum is selected as the urinary conduit; it is divided with the GIA stapler. It is important to carefully estimate the length of the conduit segment. If the conduit is too short, stomal retraction and stenosis follows. An excessively long conduit can lead to stone formation or metabolic complications from fluid and electrolyte absorption across the bowel mucosa. In the obese patient, measurements for the conduit should be taken during the preoperative planning phase. In general, the conduit length should be 15 cm plus the thickness of the anterior abdominal wall when the patient is in the supine or standing position to account for the thickness of the patient's pannus. Alternatively, a segment of

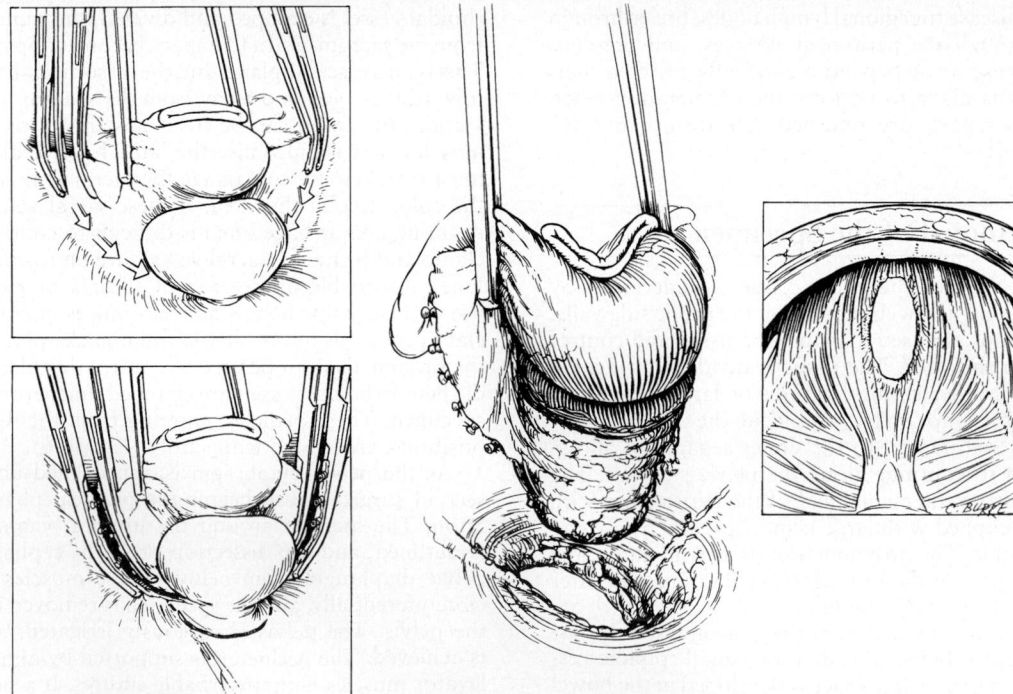

FIGURE 50.6. The fibrovascular pedicle (the "web") is progressively clamped and divided down to the pelvic floor. The perineal dissection is simultaneously performed with isolation and removal of the pelvic mass *in toto*.

sigmoid colon may be used. If a colostomy is to be done, this saves a small bowel anastomosis because an isolated segment of ileum is not needed for the conduit. If there is significant radiation injury to the bowel in the pelvis, a transverse colon conduit can be constructed.

The ureters are further freed along their routes using blunt and sharp dissection. Care should be taken to select an area of the ureter for anastomosis that is relatively free of radiation damage. The left ureter should be freed superiorly and tunneled through an avascular window in the bowel mesentery to reach the isolated segment of ileum. After an appropriate site is selected to ensure a tension-free anastomosis, the ureters are sutured to the bowel segment (Fig. 50.7). This site usually is 2 to 3 cm from the proximal end of the conduit. The site is opened sharply for about 1 cm. Some surgeons choose not to use stents; however, we routinely place a Silastic pediatric feeding tube through the lumen of the bowel and through the selected anastomotic site into the ureter. The stent is sutured to the bowel with fine absorbable suture passing through the bowel wall and the feeding tube. The ureter is then spatulated for a distance of about 4 to 5 mm. A full-thickness mucosa-to-mucosa anastomosis of the ureter to the antimesenteric border of the isolated segment of bowel is then performed using fine (3-0 or 4-0) absorbable suture. Six to ten interrupted sutures are used for the anastomosis. The ureter is anchored with long-acting absorbable suture to the underside of the conduit about 2 cm from the anastomosis to further reduce tension on the anastomosis. When the conduit is completed, the distal end is brought through the preselected site on the abdominal wall and, once positioned, is sutured to the peritoneum for stability. A "rosebud"-type stoma is fashioned to allow for ease of care and application of the urinary appliance. The proximal end of the conduit can be anchored to the sacral peritoneum to stabilize the unit.

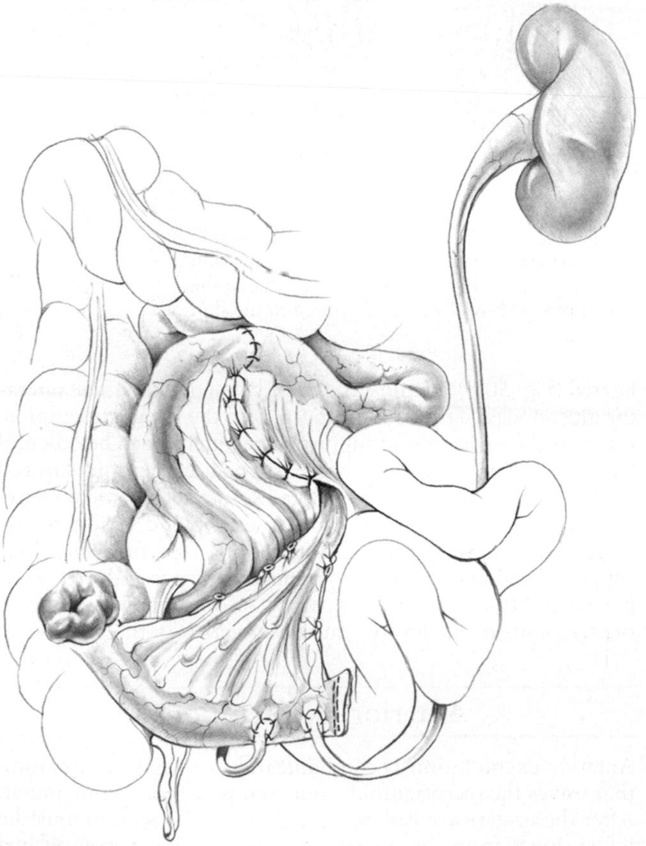

FIGURE 50.7. The ileal conduit is created by isolating a 15- to 20-cm segment of the distal ileum. The ureters are anastomosed near the closed end of the conduit. A "rosebud" stoma is constructed at the surface of the abdomen.

Continent Reservoir

The continent urinary conduit has gained increasing acceptance and now provides a legitimate alternative to the ileal conduit. This modification of the urinary diversion procedure requires serial catheterization but eliminates the need for an external appliance. Construction of the continent conduit is more complex but is a preferred option for appropriate patients.

The continent conduit is formed from the right colon and the proximal portion of the transverse colon as well as a distal part of the terminal ileum. The details of this technique are provided in Chapter 51. Once the continent urinary conduit has been developed, the terminal ileum is brought through the abdominal wall. This site should be preselected, and care must be taken to bring the terminal ileum straight through the layers of the abdominal wall so that catheterization is not impeded postoperatively. A kink or turn in the ileum may cause the patient to have difficulty with catheterization. Ureteral stents are placed at the time of ureteral implantation; these are brought through separate stab incisions in both the cecum and the abdominal wall. A Foley or 14 F red Robinson catheter is placed through the stoma, and the conduit drains dependently for about 10 to 20 days.

For all urinary diversions, an intravenous pyelogram or loopogram is obtained about 10 to 14 days postoperatively. If there is no urinary leakage, the ureteral stents can be removed. The patient is instructed on methods of appliance application (ileal conduit) or self-catheterization and irrigation (continent conduit).

Stoma Construction

The sites for urinary and fecal stomas, which are selected preoperatively by the stomal therapist, are marked on the abdomen using scratch marks or sterile methylene blue injections before the patient is draped. The urinary conduit is brought through the abdominal wall in the right lower quadrant, midway between the umbilicus and the anterior superior iliac spines, where a flat skin surface is available for attachment of the prosthesis. The sigmoid colostomy site is located in the left lower quadrant.

The abdominal wall aperture is prepared by removing a round segment, 2 to 3 cm in diameter, through its entire thickness to the level of the fascia. Skin, subcutaneous fat, and external oblique fascia must all be excised so that the flow of urine from the conduit is not obstructed. The urinary conduit is brought through the abdominal wall, and the serosa of the bowel is sutured to the peritoneum. The bowel mucosa is everted, creating a raised "rosebud" stoma, which projects over the abdominal wall. The stoma is fashioned with interrupted sutures of 3-0 delayed-absorbable suture, which passes initially through the dermis at the skin edge, then through the serosa and musculature of the adjacent bowel wall, and finally through the free margin of the bowel mucosa. When the sutures are tied, the mucosa is everted over the serosa of the bowel to produce a raised stoma that directs the urine away from the skin surface, thus reducing the chance for stricture and skin irritation.

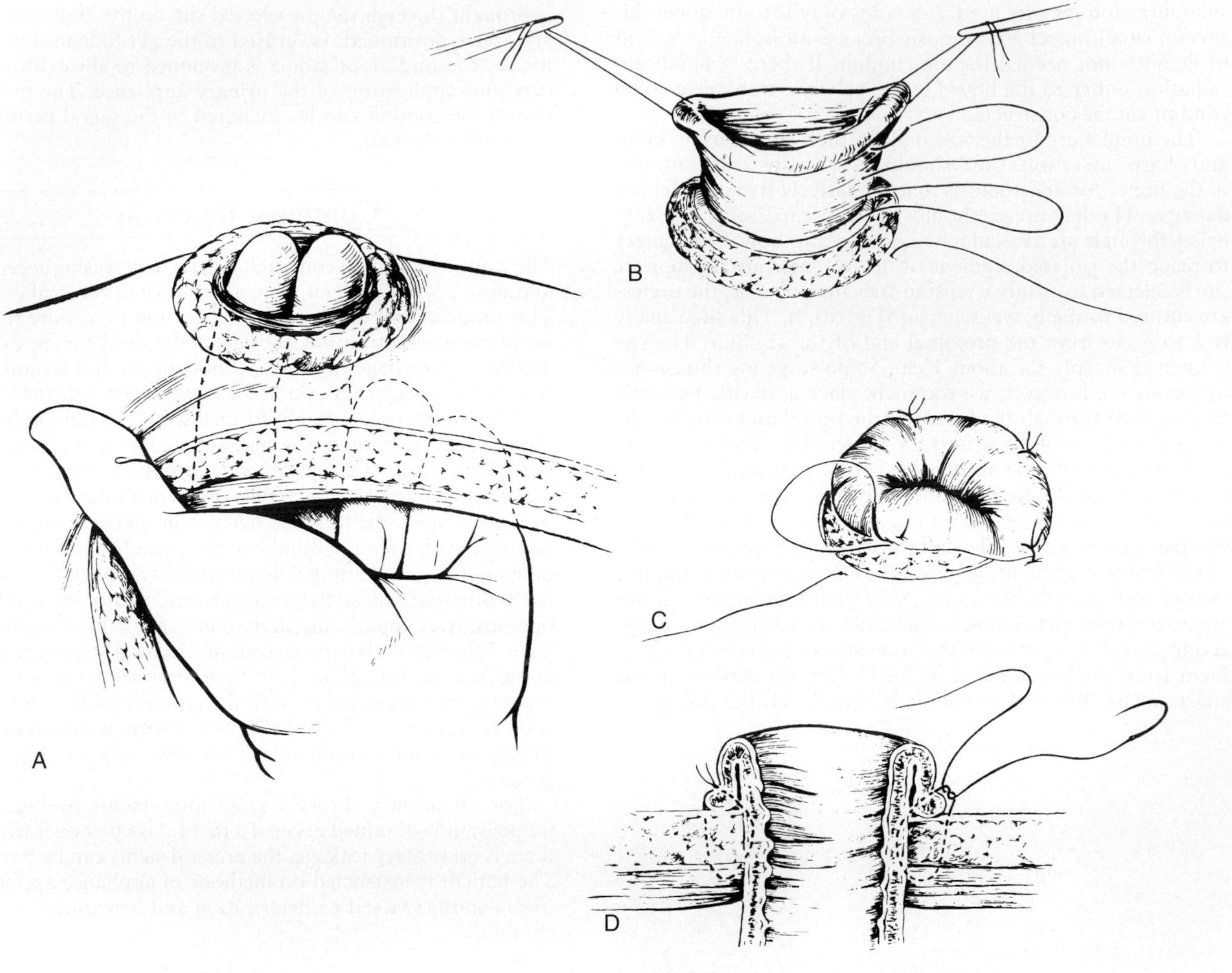

FIGURE 50.8. Technique for creating a bowel stoma that is elevated from the skin surface. This "rosebud" stoma is developed by excising a 3-cm circumferential segment of abdominal wall *(A)*, anchoring the skin margin with the adjacent wall of the exteriorized bowel *(B)*, and approximating the mucosal edge of the bowel to the skin *(C)*. The cross-sectional view demonstrates how the bowel wall is anchored to the skin margin to prevent retraction *(D)*.

Application of the urinary stoma bag also is facilitated by the raised opening.

The fecal stream is diverted through the left abdominal wall in a similar manner (Fig. 50.8). The free end of the sigmoid colon is brought through the abdominal wall to the skin through the previously marked site. If anatomically feasible, the colostomy bud should be placed below the waistline so that the colostomy bag is not constantly pulled on by the waistband of the patient's clothing. Stoma construction is accomplished as described in the preceding.

Pelvic Floor Coverage

Attention is then directed to the pelvic floor. If vaginal reconstruction has been done using myocutaneous flaps, these effectively fill the pelvis and bring in new blood supply. Coverage of this raw surface enhances hemostasis and minimizes the risks of bowel adhesions and subsequent obstruction. If no vaginal reconstruction is done, an omental J-flap is used for this purpose with satisfactory results. The omental attachment to the greater curvature of the stomach is isolated, transected, and ligated (Fig. 50.9). Hemostasis must be meticulous. The operator must preserve the blood supply from the left gastroepiploic artery as the major blood supply to the omentum. The omental flap can be laid into the pelvic basin as a carpet and sutured in place with absorbable interrupted sutures. The omental coverage of the pelvic floor provides "new" blood supply to the surgical site and enhances healing. Some type of pelvic floor support should be provided to minimize the possibility of vaginal evisceration. Usually, this can be accomplished by suturing the remnants of the levator muscles together in the midline.

Anterior Exenteration

Anterior exenteration is a modification of total exenteration that leaves the rectosigmoid colon and posterior vagina intact. After the ureters are isolated and divided, the rectum must be taken down from the posterior vagina. This is accomplished by incising the peritoneum along the rectovaginal peritoneal reflection. When this free space has been entered, the rectum can be bluntly dissected from the upper portion of the posterior vagina. It is freed laterally from the uterosacral ligament. The

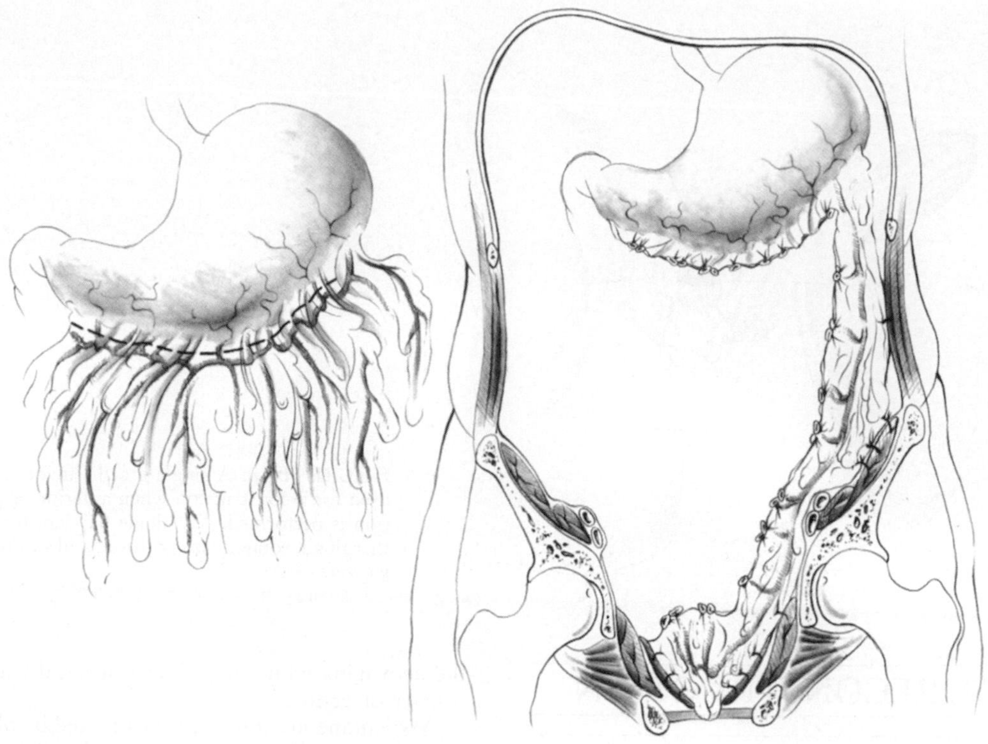

FIGURE 50.9. An omental "J-flap" can be developed by separating the right-sided portion of the omentum from the stomach and transverse colon. This pedicle then is positioned over the pelvic defect and loosely sutured in place.

uterosacral ligaments are clamped, divided, and ligated with sutures as close to the sacrum as possible. The procedure is carried down the pelvic sidewalls, similar to the procedure for total exenteration. Great care is taken to ensure that the rectum and its blood supply are not damaged. When the perineal phase is performed, the vagina is entered in its midportion and dissection connected into the upper portion of the rectovaginal septum. An ileal conduit is constructed as described. Alternatively, a continent reservoir can be created. A single gracilis myocutaneous flap can be used to replace the anterior vaginal wall.

Posterior Exenteration

Posterior exenteration is most often used for vulvar cancer and is also a modification of total exenteration. In this procedure, the uterovesical peritoneum is incised and the bladder is freed, using sharp and blunt dissection, from the cervix and vagina. After the uterine artery is ligated, the ureter must be dissected free down to the bladder. This is performed in a manner similar to that used for a radical hysterectomy. This allows for visualization of the ureter and frees it from the vagina. The web can be divided in a manner similar to that used for total exenteration. The ureter and bladder are preserved under direct visualization of these structures. The perineal phase retains the anterior vagina adjacent to the base of the bladder in the lowermost portion of the pelvis. The upper and posterior vagina are resected along with the rectosigmoid colon. An end sigmoid colostomy is created. A single gracilis myocutaneous flap can be used to replace the posterior vaginal wall and fill the surgical defect (Fig. 50.10). This is particularly useful because bladder prolapse is common following loss of the posterior support structures.

Total Exenteration with Low Rectal Reanastomosis

The lower 6 to 10 cm of rectum may be preserved in selected patients undergoing total pelvic exenteration. This depends on the location of the recurrent tumor. When this lower portion of the rectum is preserved, the sigmoid colon can be brought down and anastomosed to the rectal stump. This is greatly facilitated by use of the EEA stapler. In these patients, the colon has been previously divided using a GIA stapler proximally across the sigmoid and a TA-50 or reticulating stapler across the rectum. The staple line is cut off the sigmoid, and a running suture of 2-0 nylon or Prolene, starting on the outside, is placed on the open end of the sigmoid colon. The anvil of the EEA stapler is placed in the sigmoid, and the purse string is tied. The EEA stapler is introduced through the rectum and centered so that the spike can be advanced through or just above the staple line. The spike is removed, and the stem of the anvil is inserted. When the stapler is properly oriented, the two ends of the bowel are approximated, and the stapler is fired. When the stapler is removed, a "doughnut" of tissue from each end of the bowel should be present in the removed EEA stapler. The anastomosis is reinforced with interrupted sutures. A temporary diverting colostomy usually is necessary if the patient has been previously irradiated. Bowel continuity can be restored via colostomy closure in 3 to 6 months. This technique is illustrated in Chapter 43.

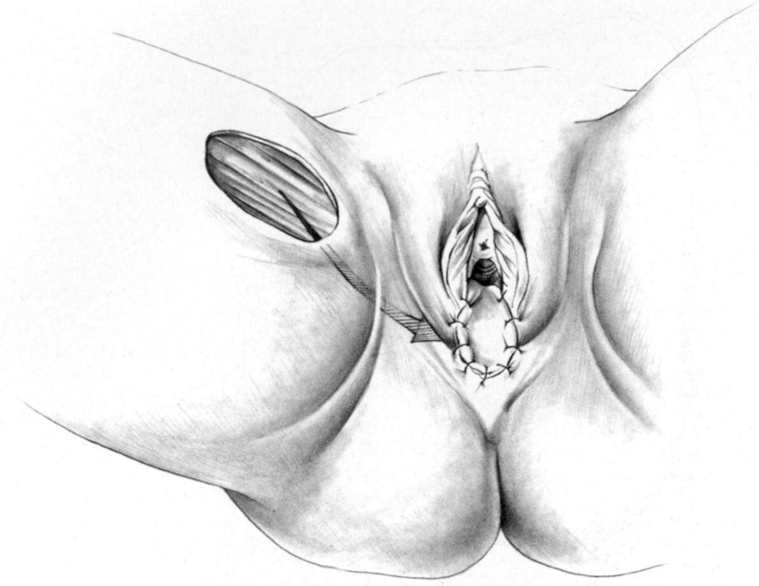

FIGURE 50.10. A single gracilis myocutaneous flap can be used for reconstruction when anterior or posterior exenteration is performed. The single flap can be harvested from either thigh, rotated into position, and sutured to the remaining vagina.

VAGINAL RECONSTRUCTION

Split-Thickness Skin Graft Vaginoplasty

The skin graft is taken from the buttocks or the posterior thigh as a split-thickness graft 10 to 15 cm in length at about 0.015 to 0.017 of an inch in thickness, using the air-powered dermatome. A vaginal stent is selected from commercially available supplies or fashioned from a foam obturator, the graft is sewn together over the obturator, and the visible end is sutured to the introitus. This technique is illustrated in Chapter 51. The patient is confined to bed for 3 days, and ambulation is allowed on the fourth or fifth day. The obturator is removed for the first time on about the fifth day, but may be left in place for up to 10 days. The patient leaves the obturator in place continuously for 4 to 6 months, removing it for cleaning and vaginal irrigation every day or so. It is worn at night for another 4 to 6 months to minimize the risk of stricture of the skin graft. A new obturator can be fashioned inexpensively by shaping a piece of foam rubber and covering it with a condom. The patient can attempt intercourse about 6 weeks after surgery. Skin grafts can provide an excellent result for vaginal reconstruction. Beemer and coworkers reported that 90% of their patients achieved satisfactory coitus.

Myocutaneous Gracilis Graft

The myocutaneous gracilis graft also can be used for creation of a neovagina. Some surgeons use the rectus abdominis myocutaneous graft to construct the neovagina. However, I believe that its abdominal donor site complicates stoma placement and so use the gracilis as our procedure of choice. Construction at the time of initial exenteration surgery is required. The advantages include immediate reconstruction of the vagina, and the tissue mass itself helps to fill the pelvic defect as well as introduce a new blood supply to the area. An obturator is not required to maintain patency. When this approach is chosen, it is best to have a second operating team harvest the grafts and construct the neovagina while the primary surgical team completes the urinary diversion.

Myocutaneous grafts are constructed by obtaining bilateral full-thickness muscle, adipose, and skin flaps. The initial incision is made in an elliptical manner along a line extending from the superior aspect of the symphysis pubis to the medial condyle of the femur. The overlying skin to be taken should measure 10 to 12 cm in length by 6 to 8 cm in width. The underlying gracilis muscle is identified separate from the adductor group and is divided using the cautery about 2 cm distal to the skin paddle. This muscle is mobilized toward the symphysis. The perforating vessels on the underside of the muscle are about 10 cm from the symphysis and should be dissected with the myocutaneous unit. When the muscle and overlying skin are fully mobilized, they are brought through a subcutaneous tunnel to the perineal defect. The posterior edges of the grafts from both sides are sutured together with absorbable interrupted sutures, followed by a similar approximation of the anterior edges. This graft is introduced (or inserted) into the pelvic cavity and sutured to the sacral periosteum or levator remnants with long-acting absorbable sutures. The opening to the new vaginal tube is sutured to the introitus with interrupted absorbable sutures (Fig. 50.11). The leg incisions are closed with skin staples. Jackson-Pratt drains are placed in the bed of each harvest site as well as in close proximity to the graft in the pelvis.

Postoperative Care

Patients are routinely admitted to the intensive care unit on completion of a pelvic exenteration. The continued oozing from the operative site with sequestration of fluids in the extravascular spaces causes significant fluid shifts; therefore, central venous pressure monitoring is essential. When left heart function and pulmonary function are adequate, a Swan-Ganz catheter is not routinely used. When ureteral stents are used, there is little chance of conduit obstruction from mucous plugging, and the urine output should accurately reflect kidney function. During the initial 24 hours after surgery, volume usually is replaced with crystalloid and blood products.

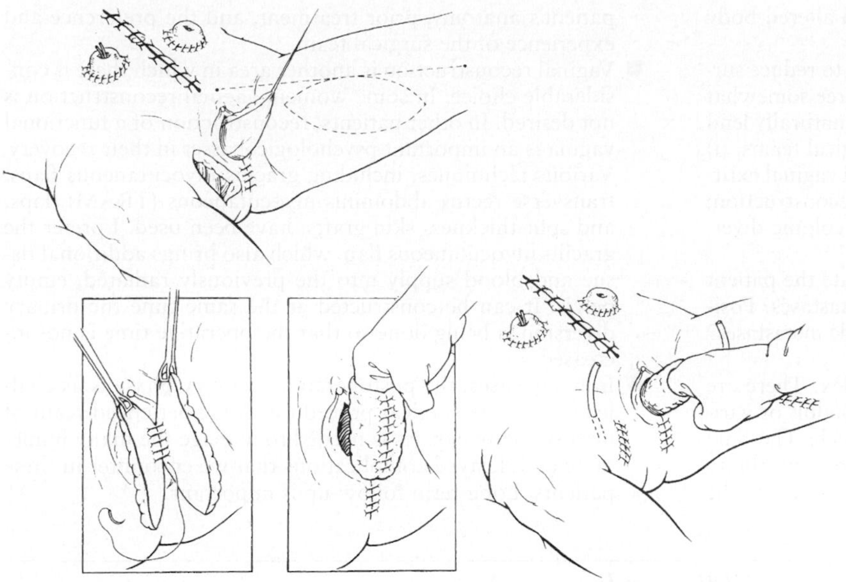

FIGURE 50.11. Full-thickness gracilis grafts, about 10 by 6 cm in dimension, are harvested from the medial thigh. They are tunneled through the thigh, sutured on themselves, and positioned in the pelvic cavity. The myocutaneous vaginoplasty is one of the alternative methods to a split-thickness skin graft vaginoplasty. Either one can be developed at the time of the pelvic exenteration.

Electrolytes and coagulation studies must be closely monitored, as well as calcium and magnesium levels. By the second to fourth postoperative day, the patient usually is ready to leave the intensive care unit. Hyperalimentation, which is started on the first postoperative day, is continued until the patient begins to have spontaneous bowel function. Intravenous antibiotics are continued for about 5 days. If vaginal reconstruction has not been performed or the perineum has not closed, the pelvic packing is changed daily after being left in place for the first 3 to 5 postoperative days.

Complications

The incidence of postoperative complications following pelvic exenteration is significant; complications occur in 30% to 50% of patients undergoing this procedure. The most common major complications after this operation primarily involve the urinary or gastrointestinal tracts and their reconstructions. Other complications include bleeding, infection, thromboembolism, and, some time later, stoma problems, such as stenosis, prolapse, and hernia.

The occurrence of ureteral stricture and urinary leakage at the ureterointestinal anastomotic site has significantly decreased with current techniques. Ureteral stricture, especially if ureteral obstruction coexists, must be corrected surgically without delay or a percutaneous nephrostomy done to preserve renal function. Most anastomotic leaks heal spontaneously without requiring surgical repair. Renal calculus formation does occur but can be reduced by avoiding exposed staple lines and permanent sutures in the conduit.

Intestinal obstruction occurs both as an early and a late complication of exenteration and continues to be a serious problem in 10% to 15% of cases. The incidence of this complication has been reduced by use of the omental J-flap to cover the raw pelvic surface at the level of the pelvic diaphragm. Most paralytic ileus problems seen in the postoperative period can be treated conservatively with traditional nasogastric decompression. Enteral fistulas are seen uncommonly but are more common when omental flap or vaginal reconstruction is not used. These fistulas may heal spontaneously with bowel rest and hyperalimentation.

Septicemia, which often originates as a urinary tract infection, usually responds to antibiotic therapy. Thromboembolic disease has become a less frequent postoperative complication since the use of low-dose heparin or SCDs began, even in the presence of a large denuded pelvic vault and exposed vessels. For wound and pelvic abscesses, CT-guided drainage, if feasible, is preferred to laparotomy.

The operative mortality rate related to pelvic exenterative surgery has improved dramatically since the 1970s. Earlier series reported a perioperative mortality rate ranging from 7% to 17%. In modern series, the reported mortality rate is less than 5% (Table 50.1).

BEST SURGICAL PRACTICES

- Pelvic exenteration is a technically challenging surgical procedure; but just as important, the postoperative care of these patients is extremely difficult from both a medical and psychological aspect. This operation and the care of these patients should be undertaken only by a well-trained and experienced team of specialists in a hospital staffed and equipped to manage the complex problems associated with the multiple organ systems involved in the ultraradical surgery, recovery, and rehabilitation.
- The main indication for pelvic exenteration is centrally recurrent cervical cancer after failure of primary radiation therapy. Occasionally, patients with vulvar, vaginal, or uterine cancer—and some patients with urologic or rectal cancer—may also be candidates. Women with cancer extending to the pelvic sidewall precluding a clear resection margin or those with metastatic disease are *not* candidates for exenteration. Occasionally, a patient with only anterior or posterior tumor involvement will be a suitable candidate for an *anterior* or *posterior* rather than the usual *total* pelvic exenteration.
- A very complete preoperative evaluation is necessary with all appropriate imaging studies to evaluate resectability. In addition, the patient must be evaluated medically and psychologically to be sure she can tolerate this extensive surgery

and will be able to deal with the stomas and altered body image postoperatively.

- Two or even three surgical teams may be used to reduce surgeon fatigue and operative time. There are three somewhat different phases of the surgical procedure that naturally lend themselves to the assignment of different surgical teams: (i) the pelvic extirpative part; (ii) the perineal and vaginal extirpative part and, where indicated, the vaginal reconstruction; and (iii) the construction of the urinary and colonic diversions.
- The initial phase of the operation is to evaluate the patient for resectability. Are there intraabdominal metastases? Positive washings? Pelvic or paraaortic lymph node metastases? Does the tumor extend to the pelvic walls?
- The choice of the urinary diversion is complex. There are several options, including an ileal or colon conduit or various modifications of a continent urinary pouch. The final decision will be based on the patient's desire and ability to manage a continent pouch or a conduit, as well as the patient's anatomy, prior treatment, and the preference and experience of the surgical team.
- Vaginal reconstruction is another area in which there is considerable choice. In some women, vaginal reconstruction is not desired. In other patients, reconstruction of a functional vagina is an important psychological asset in their recovery. Various techniques, including gracilis myocutaneous flaps, transverse rectus abdominis myocutaneous (TRAM) flaps, and split-thickness skin grafts, have been used. I prefer the gracilis myocutaneous flap, which also brings additional tissue and blood supply into the previously radiated, empty pelvis. It can be constructed at the same time the urinary diversion is being done so that the operative time is not increased.
- In many cases, the postoperative recovery phase is as challenging as the surgical procedure. An experienced team of intensive care experts is needed to manage the many immediate and delayed complications that we encounter in these patients. Long-term follow-up is important.

Bibliography

Anderson BL, Hacker NF. Psychosexual adjustment following pelvic exenteration. *Obstet Gynecol* 1983;61:331.

Averette HE, Lichtinger M, Seven BU, et al. Pelvic exenteration: a 15-year experience in a general metropolitan hospital. *Am J Obstet Gynecol* 1984;150:179.

Beemer W, Hopkins MP, Morley GW. Vaginal reconstruction in gynecologic oncology. *Obstet Gynecol* 1988;72:911.

Barakat RR, Goldman NA, Devendra AP, et al. Pelvic exenteration for recurrent endometrial cancer. *Gynecol Oncol* 1999;75:99.

Berek JS, Howe C, Lagasse LD, et al. Pelvic exenteration for recurrent gynecologic malignancy: Survival and morbidity analysis of the 45-year experience at UCLA. *Gynecol Oncol* 2005;99:153.

Bladou F, Houvnaeghel G, Delpero JR, et al. Incidence and management of major urinary complications after pelvic exenteration for gynecological malignancies. *J Surg Oncol* 1995;58:91.

Bricker EM. Bladder substitution for pelvic evisceration. *Surg Clin North Am* 1950;30:1511.

Brunschwig A. Complete excision of the pelvic viscera for advanced carcinoma. *Cancer* 1948;177.

Brunschwig A. What are the indications and results of pelvic exenteration? *JAMA* 1965;194:274.

Buchsbaum HJ, White AJ. Omental sling for management of pelvis floor following exenteration. *Am J Obstet Gynecol* 1973;117:407.

Burke TW, Morris M, Roh MS, et al. Perineal reconstruction using single gracilis myocutaneous flaps. *Gynecol Oncol* 1995;57:221.

Cavanagh D, Shepherd JH. The place of pelvic exenteration in the primary management of advanced carcinoma of the vulva. *Gynecol Oncol* 1982;13:318.

Copeland LJ, Hancock KC, Gershenson DM, et al. Gracilis myocutaneous vaginal reconstruction concurrent with total pelvic exenteration. *J Obstet Gynecol* 1989;150:1095.

Creasman WT, Rutledge F. Is positive pelvic lymphadenectomy a contraindication to radical surgery in recurrent cervical cancer? *Gynecol Oncol* 1974;2:482.

Hatch KD, Gelder MS, Soong SJ, et al. Pelvic exenteration with low rectal anastomosis: survival, complications and prognostic factors. *Gynecol Oncol* 1990;38:462.

Hopkins MP, Morley GW. Pelvic exenteration for the treatment of vulvar cancer. *Cancer* 1992;70:2835.

Ketcham AS, Deckers PJ, Sugarbaker EV, et al. Pelvic exenteration for carcinoma of the uterine cervix: a fifteen year experience. *Cancer* 1970;26:513.

Kiselow M, Butcher HR Jr, Bricker EM. Results of the radical surgical treatment of advanced pelvic cancer: a 15-year survey. *Ann Surg* 1967;166:428.

Lawhead RA Jr, Clark DG, Smith DH, et al. Pelvic exenteration for recurrent or persistent gynecologic malignancies: a 10-year review of the Memorial Sloan-Kettering Cancer Center experience (1972-1981). *Gynecol Oncol* 1989;33:279.

Matthews CM, Morris M, Burke TW, et al. Pelvic exenteration in the elderly patient. *Obstet Gynecol* 1992;79:773.

Miller B, Morris M, Gershenson DM, et al. Intestinal fistulae formation following pelvic exenteration: a review of the University of Texas M.D. Anderson Cancer Center experience, 1957–1990. *Gynecol Oncol* 1995;56:207.

Miller B, Morris M, Levenback C, et al. Pelvic exenteration for primary and recurrent vulvar cancer. *Gynecol Oncol* 1995;58:202.

Morley GW, Hopkins MP, Lindenauer SM, et al. Pelvic exenteration: University of Michigan 100 patients at five years. *Obstet Gynecol* 1989;74:934.

Morris M, Alvarez RD, Kinney WK, et al. Treatment of recurrent adenocarcinoma of the endometrium with pelvic exenteration. *Gynecol Oncol* 1996;60:288.

Parsons L, Friedell GH. Radical surgical treatment of cancer of cervix. *Proc Natl Cancer Conf* 1964;5:241.

Penalver MA, Bejany DE, Averette HE, et al. Continent urinary diversion in gynecology oncology. *Gynecol Oncol* 1989;34:274.

Popovich MJ, Hricak H, Sugimura K, et al. The role of MR imaging in determining surgical eligibility for pelvic exenteration. *AJR Am J Roentgenol* 1993;160:525.

Roos EJ, de Graeff A, van Eijekeren MA, et al. Quality of life after pelvic exenteration. *Gynecol Oncol* 2004;93:610.

Ramirez PT, Modesitt SC, Morris M, et al. Functional outcomes and complications of continent urinary diversions in patients with gynecologic malignancies. *Gynecol Oncol* 2002;85:295.

Ratliff CR, Gershenson DM, Morris M, et al. Sexual adjustment of patients undergoing gracilis myocutaneous flap vaginal reconstruction in conjunction with pelvic exenteration. *Cancer* 1996;78:2229.

Rutledge FN, Burns BC Jr. Pelvic exenteration. *Am J Obstet Gynecol* 1965;91:692.

Rutledge FN, McGuffee VB. Pelvic exenteration: prognostic significance of regional lymph node metastasis. *Gynecol Oncol* 1987;26:374.

Rutledge FN, Smith JP, Wharton JT, et al. Pelvic exenteration: analysis of 296 patients. *Am J Obstet Gynecol* 1977;129:881.

Salom EM, Mendez LE, Schey D, et al. Continent ileocolonic urinary reservoir (Miami pouch): the University of Miami experience over 15 years. *Am J Obstet Gynecol* 2004;190:994.

Shingleton HM, Soong SJ, Gelder MS, et al. Clinical and histopathologic factors predicting recurrence and survival after pelvic exenteration for cancer of the cervix. *Obstet Gynecol* 1989;73:1027.

Symmonds RE, Pratt JH, Webb MJ. Exenterative operations: experience with 198 patients. *Am J Obstet Gynecol* 1975;121:907.

Symmonds RE, Pratt JH, Welch JS. Exenterative operations. *Am J Obstet Gynecol* 1968;101:66.

Vera MI. Quality of life following pelvic exenteration. *Gynecol Oncol* 1981;12:355.

Webb MJ, Symmonds RE. Management of the pelvic floor after pelvic exenteration. *Obstet Gynecol* 1977;50:166.

CHAPTER 51 ■ SURGICAL RECONSTRUCTION OF THE PELVIS IN GYNECOLOGIC CANCER PATIENTS

LUIS E. MENDEZ AND MANUEL PENALVER

DEFINITIONS

Gluteal thigh flap—This flap is based on the gluteal muscle and the inferior gluteal artery. It should not be performed on a patient with a previous bilateral hypogastric artery ligation because compromise may occur.

Gracilis myocutaneous flap—A flap based on the gracilis muscle and overlying skin. The vascular supply is mainly based on the medial circumflex artery proximally. The distal muscle belly is supplied by minor vascular pedicles from the superficial femoral artery that can be sacrificed. Innervation is from the obturator nerve branches, resulting in a sensate flap.

Mechanical skin stretcher (SURE Closure)—A mechanized device that makes it possible to stretch skin in about 1 hour in the operating room to cover most defects.

Omental J-flap—A technique for revascularizing the pelvis after exenteration. The omentum is detached from the greater curvature of the stomach and brought down as a flap based on the left (or occasionally right) gastroepiploic artery. It is first sutured to the sacral promontory posteriorly, the public symphysis anteriorly, and pelvic walls laterally to form a pelvic lid.

Rectus abdominis myocutaneous flap—A flap based on the rectus abdominis muscle and overlying skin. The flap itself is based on the inferior epigastric artery and is taken from the supraumbilical portion of the laparotomy incision (vertically oriented). A unilateral rectus abdominis myocutaneous (RAM) flap is usually sufficient to repair large vulvar defects or create an adequate-sized neovagina. The horizontal diameter of the skin should be at least 10 to 12 cm wide to make a vagina that is about 4 cm in diameter.

Sigmoid neovagina—Use of an isolated sigmoid segment to construct a vagina after exenteration. The cardinal feature for use of an isolated segment of rectosigmoid colon is the integrity of the vascular supply of the colon via the superior hemorrhoidal artery.

The radical resection of pelvic malignancies to date remains an important procedure in the armamentarium of the gynecologic oncologist, despite significant advances in radiation therapy and chemotherapy. The trend toward minimization of surgical resective techniques has fared well for some patients in certain diseases, such as vulvar cancer. However, en bloc resection can be the only hope for survival for some women with certain advanced or recurrent gynecologic cancers. Contemporary techniques in reconstructive surgery should be used to restore these women to an acceptable quality of life. Reconstruction is the surgical challenge of this and future generations of pelvic surgeons. This surgical challenge has been addressed by other subspecialties, such as the oncologic surgical practices in head, neck, breast, and orthopedic surgery. It is imperative that pelvic surgeons begin to consider quality of life and the functional reintegration into society of the patients who undergo these radical surgical efforts.

This chapter reviews the techniques of reconstruction of a functional vagina, construction of an anatomically correct vulva, restoration of a functional rectum with elimination of colostomy, and construction of urostomy that allows for physiologic protection of the upper renal tracts and improves aesthetics as an alternative to the urine ostomy bag.

VAGINAL RECONSTRUCTION

Vaginal reconstruction has become a regular option presented to patients undergoing radical pelvic procedures. Vaginectomy, whether simple or radical, can be a primary procedure or a part of a more extirpative procedure, such as a pelvic exenteration. In addition, nonsurgical techniques such as radiation therapy can produce severe fibrosis or stenosis with the result of an essentially nonfunctional vagina.

With the advent of improved perioperative care and survival for radically resected patients, thoughts must extend to affording the patient acceptable sexual options. The loss of sexual gratification and function may be a devastating consequence to a woman even in the presence of a surgical cure. The oncologist has no way of knowing unless specific questions are presented to the patient as part of the routine preoperative history. The possibility of restoring a functional vagina may provide a woman with a tremendous source of psychological motivation in approaching her cancer therapy. It may alleviate some of the fears that she has toward her future psychosexual well-being as well as the domestic relationship with her partner. Physical sexual function, even though attempted, is not always successful. Depending on the procedure chosen and the commitment of the patient to maintain the neovagina, success rates of 80% are considered reasonable.

Besides its beneficial effects on psychosexual factors, reconstruction of the vagina after total pelvic exenteration has been shown to have a beneficial effect on wound healing, prevention of enteroperineal fistulae, and abscess or pelvic collection formation. The insertion of nonirradiated tissue in the previously radiated pelvis obliterates a great deal of dead space and provides a healthy vascular pedicle in an area with borderline blood supply resulting from extensive pelvic irradiation and radical resection.

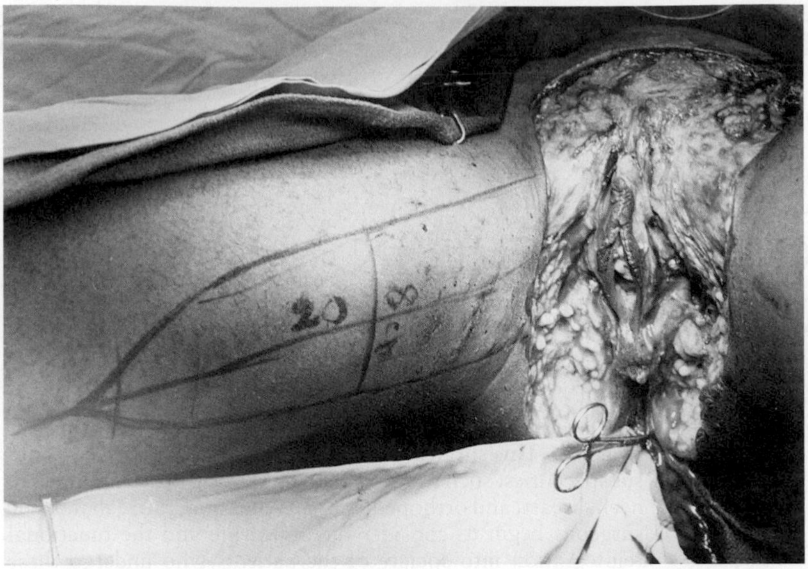

FIGURE 51.1. Vulva defect showing skin lines for gracilis myocutaneous flap.

Description of a neovagina using skin grafts attached to the colon posteriorly and bladder anteriorly supported by vaginal forms and stents was popularized by McIndoe and Banister as early as 1938. Techniques were also modified to use portions of the remaining viscera after less radical operations to fashion a neovagina. However, with the advent of ultraradical pelvic operations and the theory of en bloc resections to improve survival, it was evident that new efforts in reconstruction were needed. Classic reconstructive techniques that simply use skin grafts, as in the McIndoe procedure, are insufficient, because the supportive fasciae, rectum, bladder, and even pelvic floor have usually been extirpated.

Today there are various techniques to reconstruct the vagina. Some techniques, such as the pudendal thigh flap or the gluteal thigh flap, can be used for neovaginal construction. These are addressed in the section on vulvar reconstruction, where they are more commonly used. This section discusses the omental J-flap with skin graft, sigmoid neovagina, gracilis myocutaneous flap (GMF), and rectus abdominis flap.

Techniques for Vaginal Reconstruction

Gracilis Myocutaneous Flap

In the past, the GMF has been the workhorse of neovaginal reconstruction in patients who have had radical resections. The GMF was introduced by McGraw and colleagues in 1976 and had the immediate impact of decreasing perioperative morbidity and providing a potential for restoring coital function. The GMF is a versatile flap and has also been used for neovaginal and neovulvar reconstructions. However, it has not been without its problems. Initially, the GMF had rates of flap necrosis and prolapse as high as 65%. Techniques to anchor the neovagina and the trend to use smaller flaps have reduced this rate significantly to 13% to 37%. Infection is a problem and can complicate up to 37% of cases, but infection responds well to antibiotic therapy and local debridement if needed. Sexual adjustment has lagged and is reported to be significantly impaired in these women for various reasons, including the appearance of large inner thigh scars.

The GMF operation is begun with the patient in the dorsal supine position. The hips are abducted 45 degrees and flexed 30 degrees for exposure of the vulva, the knees are extended, and the feet are placed in gynecologic stirrups. This extended-knee position provides maximum visualization of the gracilis muscle and the overlying cutaneous skin.

The approximate upper limit for flap viability is 8 × 20 cm (Fig. 51.1). After determining the length and width of flap needed, the gracilis muscle is palpated from its origin on the pubic ramus to its insertion on the medial aspect of the knee. The extension of the knee aids in the palpation of the gracilis muscle and reduces the possibility of mistaking the sartorius muscle for the gracilis muscle. A line is drawn along the length of the gracilis muscle, and the skin island is marked carefully because only a 2- to 3-cm length of skin from the muscle edge will be supported (Fig. 51.2). The vascular supply is mainly based on the medial circumflex artery proximally. The distal muscle belly is supplied by minor vascular pedicles from the superficial femoral artery that can be sacrificed. Innervation is from the obturator nerve branches, resulting in a sensate flap.

An incision is made through the skin and subcutaneous tissue distally along the anterior border of the flap, down to the adductor longus fascia. It is extended along the line of the skin, outlining the paddle-shaped flap. Distally, at the edge of the flap, the gracilis is transected. We prefer to secure the muscle belly to the dermis with 3-0 synthetic absorbable suture to avoid shearing the flap. The vascular pedicle of the gracilis muscle is invested by the fascial layer that separates the adductor longus and adductor magnus muscles (Figs. 51.3 and 51.4). The surgical approach to the gracilis neurovascular bundle is made by reflecting the fascia to the adductor longus muscle. When the fascia is reflected, the adductor longus, adductor brevis, and the gracilis muscles are identified, exposing the vascular bundle of the gracilis muscle about 7 to 10 cm from the pubic ramus. The gracilis muscle is isolated and divided at its origin on the pubic ramus. At this point, the gracilis vascular pedicle is located by sterile Doppler ultrasound. Repeated use of sterile Doppler ultrasonography confirms the location of the blood supply to the muscle and ensures its protection. When the flaps from both legs have been adequately dissected and are ready for rotation, 1 to 3 g of intravenous fluorescein is administered. The flaps are exposed to an ultraviolet Wood's light in a darkened room.

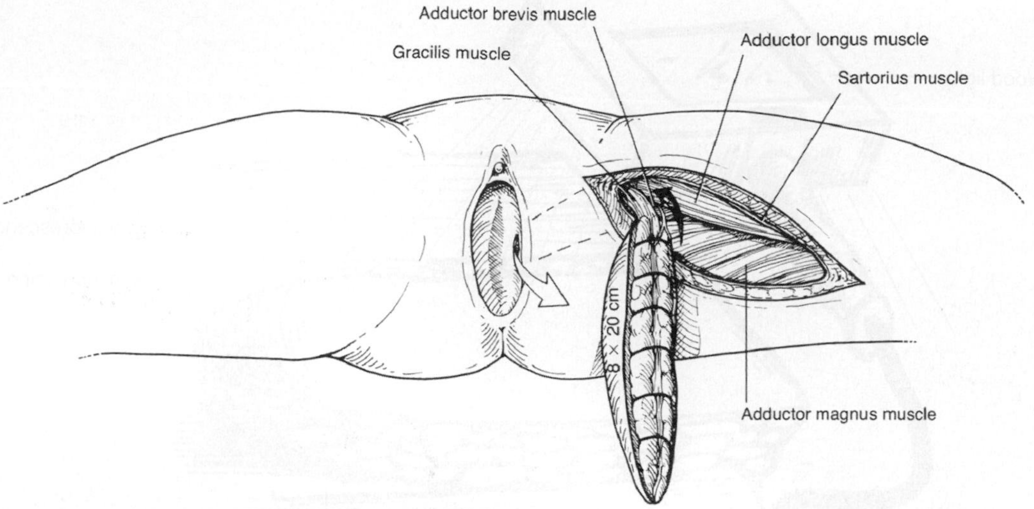

FIGURE 51.2. A mobilized gracilis myocutaneous flap. Note the 8- x 20-cm dimension and the critical muscle landmarks. (From: Gallup D, Talledo O. *Surgical atlas of gynecologic oncology.* Philadelphia: WB Saunders;1994:235, with permission.)

Nonviable areas of the flaps are demonstrated by their failure to fluoresce, and these areas are excised (Fig. 51.4). Each flap is rotated into position (or tunneled under a skin bridge if no vulvar defect is present) and either secured to cover one half of a vulvar defect or sutured together, tubularized, and inserted into the pelvic cavity to form the neovagina (Figs. 51.2, 51.5, and 51.6).

The remaining subcutaneous tissue of the defect is sutured to the subcutaneous tissue of the flap with interrupted 3-0 synthetic absorbable sutures if a vulvar defect is present. Otherwise, the flaps are tubularized and inserted into the empty pelvic cavity. Closed suction drains should be used at the harvest sites and the skin closed primarily. Sexual activity can commence after 6 to 8 weeks of recovery.

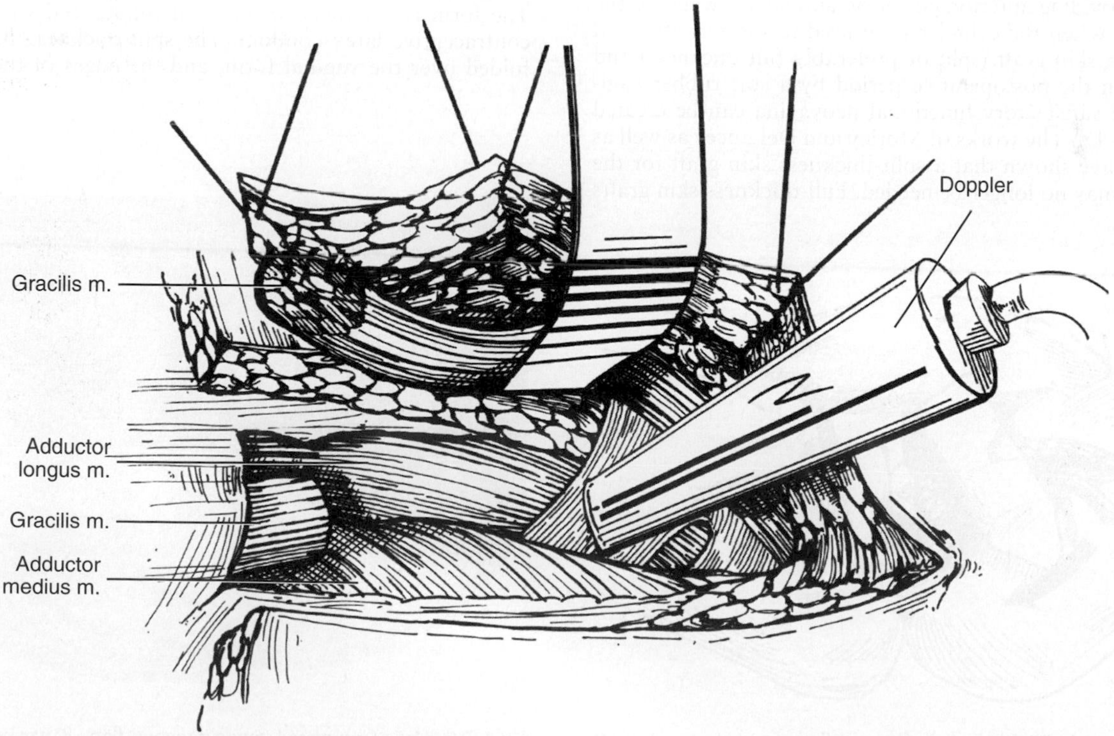

FIGURE 51.3. Gracilis myocutaneous flap. Doppler ultrasonography is used to confirm the neurovascular bundle emerging from the adductor longus (*Al*) and adductor magnus (*Am*) muscles. G, gracilis muscle.

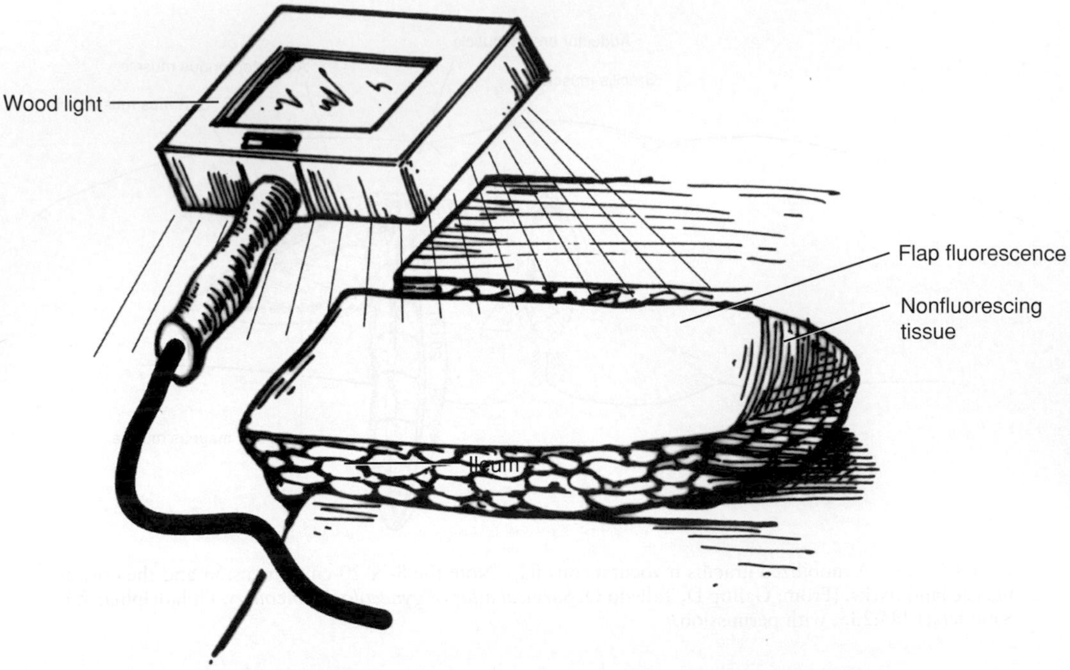

FIGURE 51.4. The Wood light focuses on a myocutaneous flap perfused with fluorescein dye. The avascular portion of the flap can be identified and excised.

Omental J-Flap with Split-Thickness Skin Graft

By modifying the omental flap that is normally used to close off the pelvic inlet after exenteration (Fig. 51.7A), with or without low coloproctostomy, the surgeon can create an omental cylinder, providing anterior, posterior, and lateral walls for the neovagina. When the cylinder is sutured to the introitus and lined with a skin graft (split or preferably full thickness) and expanded in the postoperative period by a soft rubber vaginal form, a satisfactory functional neovagina can be created (Fig. 51.7B–D). The works of Morley and DeLancey as well as Wheeless have shown that a split-thickness skin graft for the neovagina may no longer be needed. Full-thickness skin grafts work well for all neovaginal reconstructions. The full-thickness skin graft survives equally well as the split-thickness graft but has reduced the tendency to contract postoperatively compared with the split-thickness skin graft.

In Figure 51.7C, the skin graft is laid out on a vaginal form. The form is fashioned from foam rubber and stuffed into a contraceptive latex condom. The split-thickness skin graft is folded over the vaginal form, and the edges of the graft are

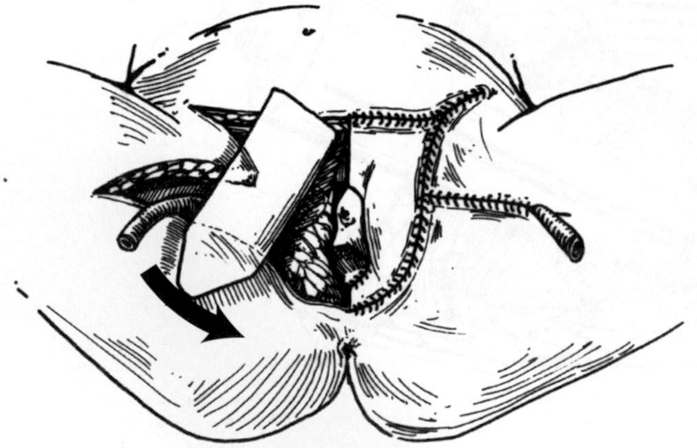

FIGURE 51.5. A: Bilateral myocutaneous flaps rotated into place. B: Completed neovulva.

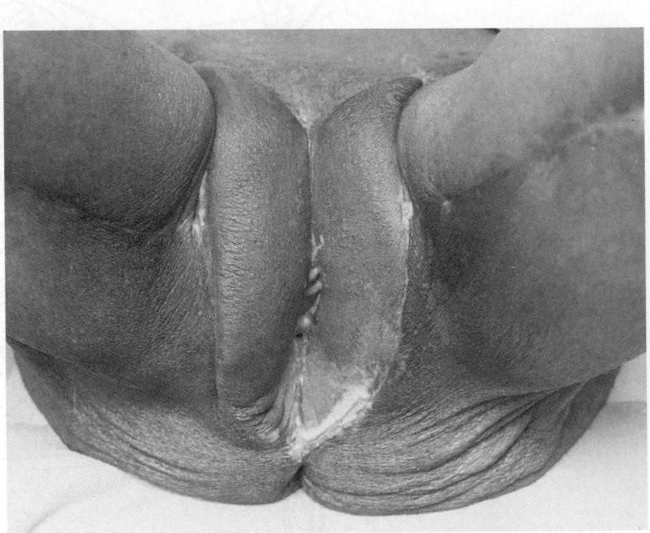

FIGURE 51.6. Completed myocutaneous flap, 8 weeks postoperatively.

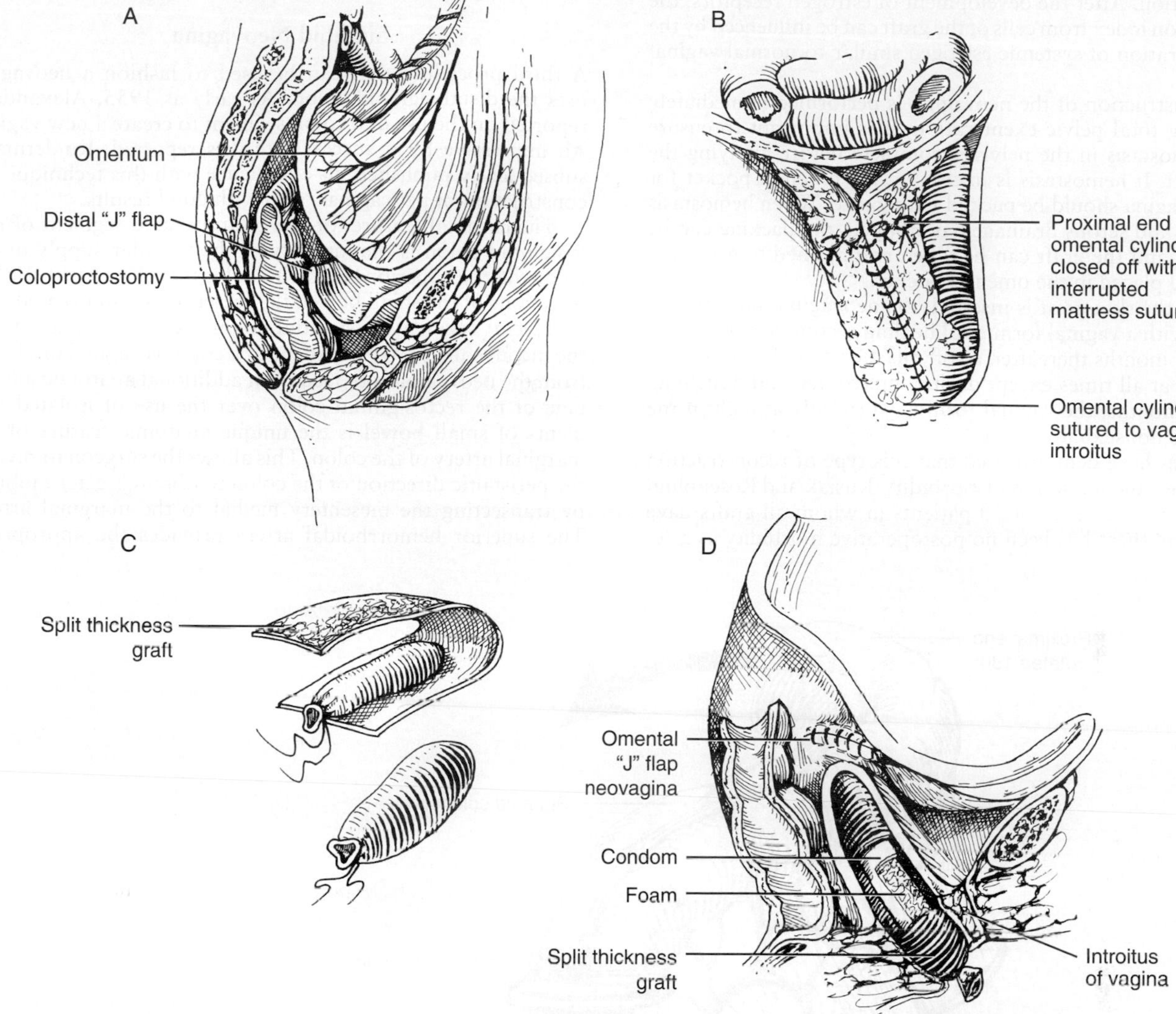

FIGURE 51.7. **A:** Drawing of the sagittal view of the pelvis after total exenteration. The colon has been reanastomosed to the rectum. The omentum has been taken off the stomach and brought into the pelvis as a J-flap for closing the pelvic inlet. The distal omentum of the J-flap is available for rolling into a cylinder, thus creating the walls of the neovagina. **B:** The distal omentum is rolled into a cylinder to be lined with a split-thickness skin graft. **C:** A foam rubber vaginal mold is covered with a condom. The split-thickness skin graft is sutured over the mold. **D:** Drawing of a sagittal view of the omental flap neovagina, lined with a split-thickness skin graft fashioned over a foam rubber vaginal mold covered with a condom.

sutured with a running 4-0 synthetic absorbable suture. The completed operation is shown in Figure 51.7D.

In Figure 51.7D, a sagittal section shows a patient who has undergone a total pelvic exenteration. The rectal stump was retained, and the descending colon was mobilized and brought down into the pelvis for a very low (below 6 cm) coloproctostomy. The omentum has been detached from the greater curvature of the stomach and brought down as a flap based on the left gastroepiploic artery. It is first sutured to the sacral promontory posteriorly, the pubic symphysis anteriorly, and pelvic walls laterally to form a pelvic lid. In patients who have insufficient omentum to form both the pelvic flap lid and walls of the neovagina, the omentum making the pelvic lid can be supplemented by the use of a sheet of synthetic, absorbable mesh.

The omentum, innervated by the vagus nerve, forms the wall of the neovagina. Normally, tugging or pulling on the omentum does not produce a sensation of pleasure that is associated with sexual intercourse; however, about 40% of the patients who have undergone this operation report that they experience sexual orgasm. Another possible physiologic change is the development of estrogen hormone receptors in the skin graft. The graft, taken from the skin on the buttocks or thigh, normally has no demonstrable hormone receptors. Once the skin is placed in the neovagina, the graft eventually becomes almost indistinguishable from normal vaginal mucosa on histologic examination. After the development of estrogen receptors, the maturation index from cells of the graft can be influenced by the administration of systemic estrogen similar to normal vaginal mucosa.

If construction of the neovagina is performed immediately following total pelvic exenteration, it is important to ensure that hemostasis in the pelvis is complete before applying the skin graft. If hemostasis is uncertain, the omental pocket for the neovagina should be packed with gauze. When hemostasis is secure and serous drainage has stopped, the packing can be removed and the graft can be taken and applied to a vaginal form and placed in the omental pocket.

After the skin graft is inserted, the neovagina must remain dilated with a vaginal form until healing is complete. For a period of 6 months thereafter, a soft Silastic vaginal form should be worn at all times except during intercourse and douching. After 6 months, the vaginal form is worn only at night if the patient is not sexually active.

Studies have demonstrated that this type of reconstruction works well and has minimal morbidity. Kusiak and Rosenblum have reported a series of 20 patients in whom all grafts have taken, and there has been no postoperative morbidity as a result of the neovagina. Up to 80% of patients have reported satisfactory vaginal function.

Sigmoid Neovagina

A third procedure that can be used to fashion a neovagina uses the distal sigmoid colon. As early as 1955, Alexandrov reported on the use of a colon segment to create a new vagina. An impressive 89% success rate was reported. Kindermann subsequently published his experience with this technique for construction of neovaginas, also with good results.

The cardinal feature for use of an isolated segment of rectosigmoid colon is the integrity of the vascular supply of the colon via the superior hemorrhoidal artery (Fig. 51.8). Unlike secretions of the small bowel, the secretions of an isolated (10- to 12-cm) segment of sigmoid colon are not copious. Thus, the inconvenience to the patient of a copious vaginal discharge from the neovagina is reduced. An additional anatomic advantage of the rectosigmoid colon over the use of isolated segments of small bowel is the unique anatomic feature of the marginal artery of the colon. This allows the surgeon to reverse the peristaltic direction of the colon to obtain greater mobility by transecting the mesentery medial to the marginal artery. The superior hemorrhoidal artery provides the appropriate

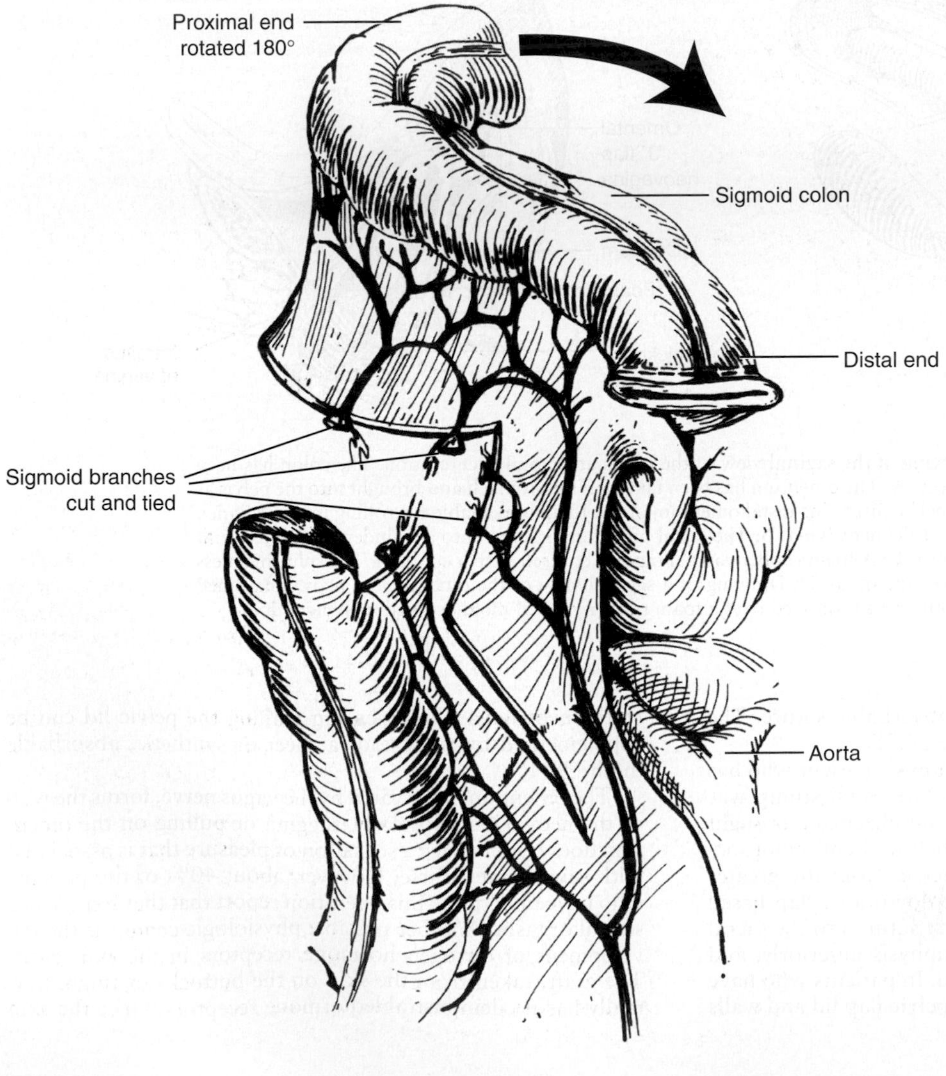

FIGURE 51.8. Colonic segment for a neovagina. The superhemorrhoidal artery is the blood supply to the colonic segment. The sigmoid neovagina must prolapse through the introitus.

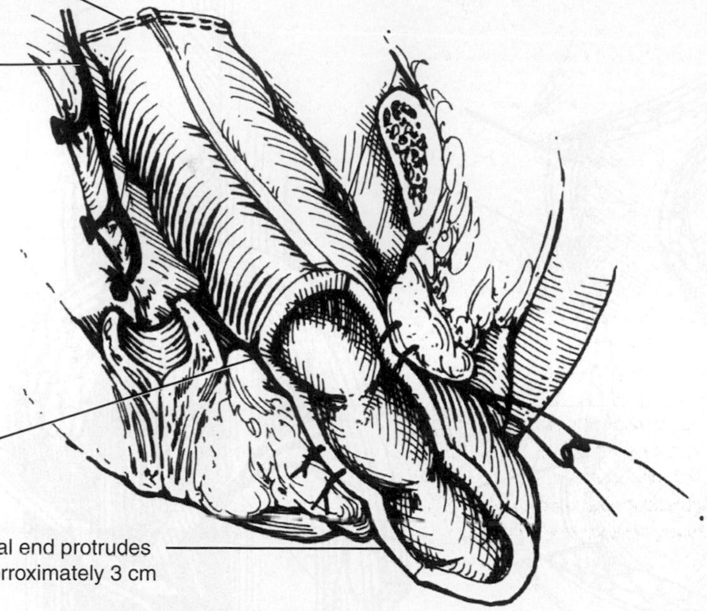

FIGURE 51.9. Prolapsed colon sutured to the vaginal introitus.

vascular supply to the colonic segment via the marginal artery. Thus, by bringing down the proximal segment of the isolated colon, it reaches the desired vaginal introitus without tension. The wall of the colon is sutured to the introitus with interrupted 3-0 synthetic absorbable sutures (Fig. 51.9). The colonic neovagina tends to retract postoperatively. Often, the prolapsed segment extending through the vaginal introitus retracts enough that it may not need to be trimmed 2 to 3 weeks postoperatively. If trimming is needed, it is a minor procedure requiring local anesthesia.

Results in most studies reveal adequate patient satisfaction and few complications. There are cases reported with persistent malodorous discharge. In rare cases, the transplanted colon segment can develop an invasive adenocarcinoma or even ulcerative colitis.

Rectus Abdominis Myocutaneous Flap

More recently the rectus abdominis myocutaneous (RAM) flap has come into widespread use for vaginal reconstruction. It is one of the most versatile myocutaneous flaps to date. The flap provides for a wide array of procedures, including vulvar reconstruction. It has a long pedicle, allowing for mobilization to most areas of groin, vagina, pelvis, and proximal thigh or even for contralateral procedures. Reports detailing the improved outcomes of these reconstructions when compared with other techniques are promising. The surgical procedure seems easier when compared with GMF, and there is a decreased incidence of flap necrosis and overall infection with the RAM flap. Both vertically oriented (VRAM) and transversely oriented (TRAM) flaps can be elevated to fit the specific needs of the surgeon.

The reported breakdown rate is 9% to 19%, better than with the GMF. Also, most studies report relatively few hernias or wound breakdowns with these flaps. The cosmetic benefits are obvious in that the same midline vertical abdominal incision used for laparotomy can be continued to outline the flap. This usually allows for easy primary skin closure, with or without mesh reinforcement of the fascia. A unilateral RAM flap is usually sufficient to repair large vulvar defects or create an adequate-sized neovagina. The horizontal diameter of the skin should be at least 10 to 12 cm wide to make a vagina that is about 4 cm in diameter.

There are some perioperative factors that may play a role in flap viability, such as obesity, diabetes, previous radiotherapy, smoking, and previous laparotomies. None of these factors seem to be absolute contraindications. However, a previous Maylard incision or one in which the inferior epigastric artery may be compromised is a contraindication because the flap is not viable without a reliable blood supply. Similar to the GMF, the RAM flap fills the pelvis with new blood supply and decreases dead space and postoperative pelvic infections. Prolapse is very uncommon with RAM flaps.

The flap itself is based on the inferior epigastric artery and is taken from the supraumbilical portion of the laparotomy incision (VRAM) (Fig. 51.10). Either a transverse or vertical skin island can be isolated, depending on the anatomy of the individual patient (Fig. 51.11). Average skin diameters can range up to 8 × 12 cm. The flap is outlined and the cutaneous portion is mobilized to the edge of the palpable muscle belly. The anterior rectus fascia and muscle belly are transected with electrocautery at the superior portion of the flap. Blood supply from the superior epigastric is interrupted without consequence as the flap survives from the inferior epigastric supply (Fig. 51.12). We always secure the cutaneous portion to the muscle belly with all our flaps to prevent shearing. After mobilization inferiorly, the anterior rectus sheath is incised, mindful of the vascular pedicle, to allow for mobility. Vascular integrity is confirmed with the intravenous administration of fluorescein and use of a Wood's lamp. The skin island is folded over itself and sutured to form a pouch that will function as the neovagina (Fig. 51.13). The unit is then brought into the pelvis and secured to the introitus using 3-0 interrupted delayed absorbable suture. A vaginal form is inserted and can be coated with a sulfa cream or a topical estrogen cream. Care must be taken to adequately mobilize the muscle belly to its insertion to eliminate tension. The donor site is usually closed without tension as part of the primary incision with permanent suture (nylon or polypropylene). If need

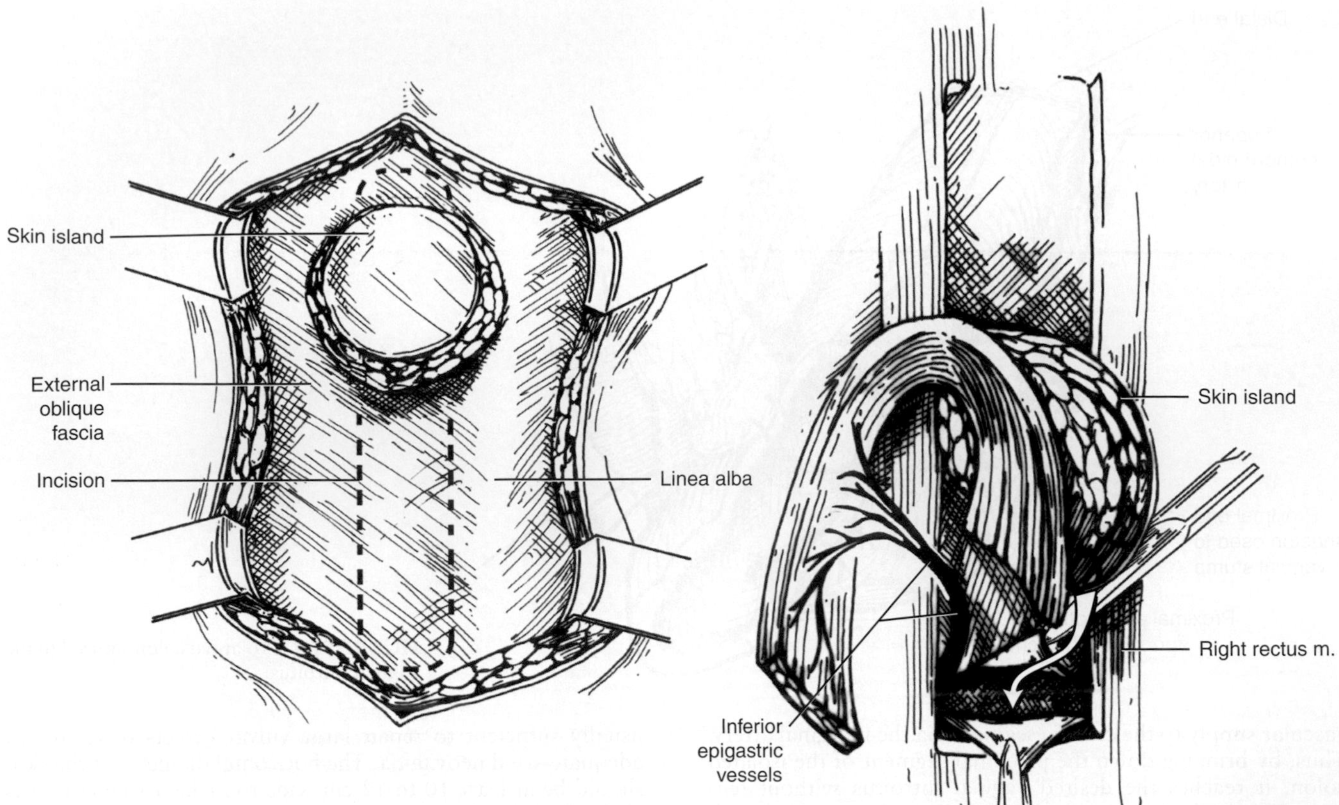

FIGURE 51.10. The vertical rectus abdominis flap. It is supplied inferiorly by the inferior epigastric artery and can be modified to fit the surgical defect and the patient's body habitus.

be, a synthetic mesh can be used to eliminate tension on the closures. Closed suction drains can be used if indicated. The vaginal form is removed from 5 to 7 days postsurgically, and the patient can attempt intercourse after 6 weeks.

The RAM family of myocutaneous flaps is becoming the procedure of choice for vulvovaginal reconstructive procedures in gynecologic oncology. Long-term sequelae of RAM flaps are few, and prolapse is greatly reduced. Carlson and colleagues reported on a pilot series in 1993 with 100% flap viability. Data are now available on longer-term follow-up of these patients. The authors published a 78% satisfaction rate of patients who underwent RAM reconstructions after pelvic exenteration.

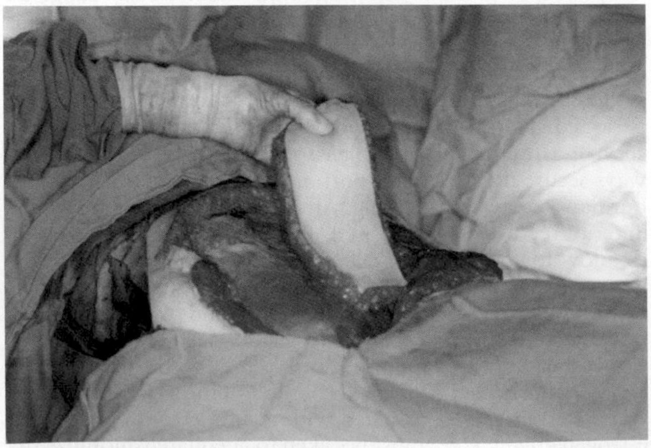

FIGURE 51.11. A vertical musculocutaneous segment isolated and elevated from the primary incision using rectus abdominis and overlying skin. See color version of figure.

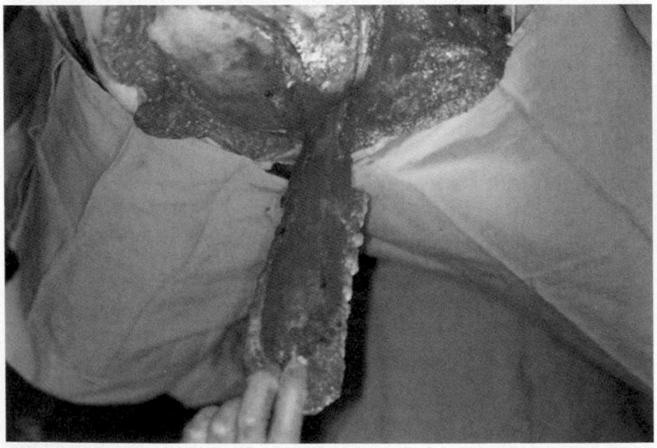

FIGURE 51.12. An elevated flap with the attached rectus abdominis muscle and supplying inferior epigastric pedicle.

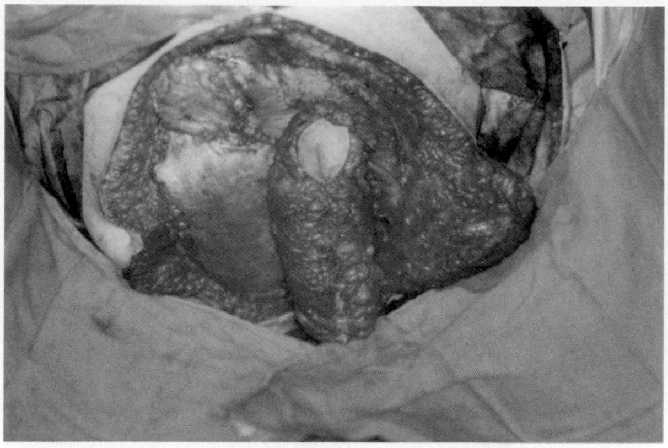

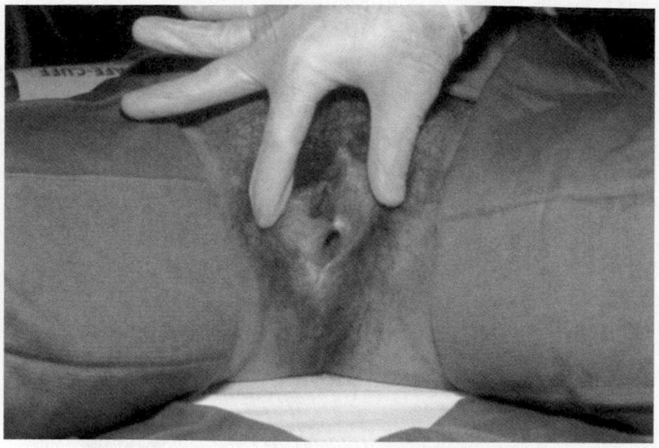

FIGURE 51.13. A: The vertically oriented rectus abdominis myocutaneous (VRAM) flap has been tubularized and is ready to be rotated into the pelvic cavity and secured to the introitus. **B:** A functional, well-healed VRAM neovagina.

Researchers at Duke University also found a 62% coitus rate 12 months after reconstruction in a similar cohort. Nonetheless, reports exist of squamous carcinomas of RAM neovaginas and perioperative complications, demanding that the utmost care be taken in developing this type of flap and in selecting the appropriate patient who will benefit from this extensive reconstructive procedure.

VULVAR RECONSTRUCTION

In the 1940s, the work of Taussig and Way demonstrated the efficacy of en bloc removal of the vulva, mons pubis, and inguinal lymph nodes from the anterior iliac spine to the adductor canal in patients with squamous cell carcinoma of the vulva. By using a more extensive dissection, pelvic surgeons have removed more tissue and thereby enhanced the probability of increased survival. This type of radical excision, however, has been complicated by problems associated with closure of large wounds—that is, difficulties involving postoperative necrosis of the suture line over the mons pubis and the inguinal and lateral vulvar skin (Fig. 51.14). Attempts have been made to redesign the incisions for radical vulvectomy to allow for adequate surgical margins and, at the same time, provide better primary healing of the incision with reduced necrosis. This includes the use of "separate incisions" to approach the primary tumor and the inguinofemoral lymph nodes. Nonetheless, resection of the primary tumor can result in defects necessitating extensive plastic reconstruction. Although these modifications of the original Way incision have allowed some improvement in the incidence of necrosis and pelvic contracture, many patients have had significant wound breakdown, requiring a split-thickness skin graft to cover the area that has become necrotic during the postoperative period. The hospital stay of these patients has been prolonged, awaiting acceptable healing of the wound. In addition, patients have developed severe perineal contractions with significant distortion of the bladder neck and urethra, resulting in incontinence of urine, perineal pain, pressure, and, in some cases, difficulty walking.

The ideal method of perineal reconstruction after a radical resection of the vulva should provide an immediate anatomic restoration and primary healing at the time of tumor resection. The neovulva should have as many of the anatomic characteristics of the original vulva as possible. The donor tissue ideally should be expendable from the donor site and transferable with minimal patient morbidity. Most radical vulvectomy operations can be closed primarily. Others can be closed with the assistance of the Z-plasty pedicle flaps advocated by Julian and Woodruff (Fig. 51.14) and by the other techniques described below. There are occasional perineal resections, however, that are so extensive that none of the cited techniques is adequate for primary closure. In these patients, myocutaneous flap is a means of primary closure. Efforts to reconstruct a radically resected vulva have been ongoing for decades. Many different techniques have been introduced, and each has a particular risk:benefit profile. With the refinement of surgical therapies for vulvar carcinoma, emphasis has shifted to the use of fasciocutaneous and local flaps for reconstruction. Nonetheless, in certain cases, the volume resected can only be reconstructed with a myocutaneous flap. This section describes split-thickness skin grafts, Z-plasty closures, the SURE Closure, V-Y advancement flaps, and the pudendal thigh flap. The gracilis and RAM flaps are discussed in the section on vaginal reconstruction. The myocutaneous flaps, however, continue to be the mainstay for vulvar reconstruction of very large defects.

Techniques for Vulvar Reconstruction

Split-Thickness Skin Graft

The use of the split-thickness skin graft for reconstruction of the vulva is not extensively described here. Most radical vulvar procedures resect deep to the perineal fascia, requiring a reconstruction that needs to provide greater thickness than that of a simple graft. However, in the case of an extensive simple or "skinning" vulvectomy, this technique alone can be adequate. The procedure for harvesting a graft is available in standard surgical texts. In brief, it involves taking a 0.35-mm (12/1,000 inch) split-thickness skin graft from an acceptable donor site with a dermatome and applying the split-thickness graft to the denuded area of the vulva. The margin of the graft is sutured to the margin of the defect with fine sutures, and a moist stent pack is used to ensure that the split-thickness skin graft is adequately pressed against the wound. Small pockets of serum can be aspirated by needle to allow the graft to lie flat over the denuded area. We have found the use of meshed grafts to be of particular value in large wounds in which the potential for infection and subgraft seroma collection can be significant. The small defects in the mesh allow adequate drainage of the wound while epithelization takes place. The physiologic and

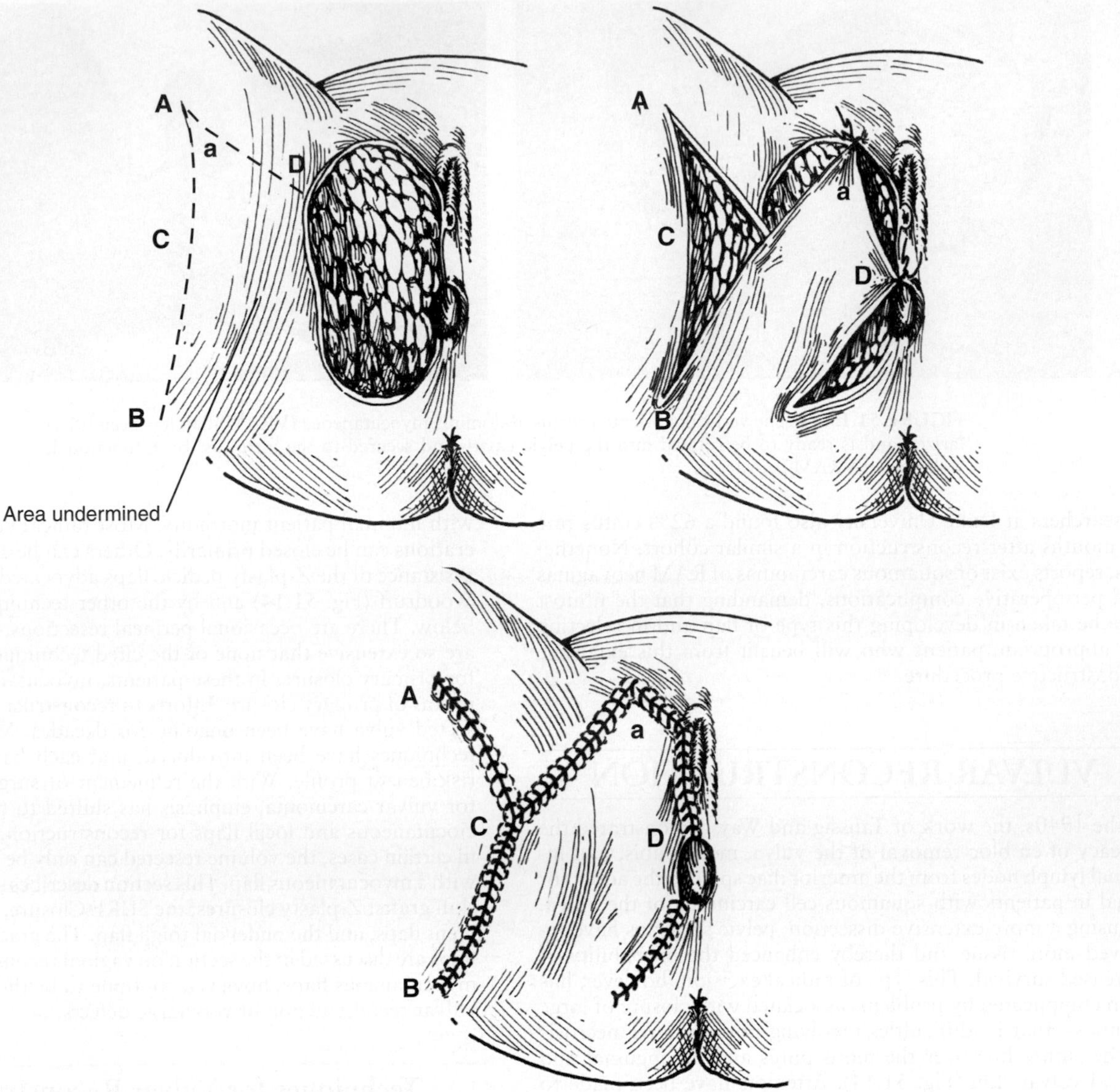

FIGURE 51.14. Vulvar flap. Note points *A* and *a*. When the flap is raised, point *a* moves to ventral portion of defect. Point *D* moves to posterior of the vagina.

logistic advantages of covering large, open wounds are well documented and are preferable to the long and costly process of granulation. Immobilization of the graft is an important key to success of the transplant.

Z-Plasty Full-Thickness Pedicle Flap

In cases in which primary closure of the vulvar wound cannot be performed without tension, the use of a pedicle flap, as advocated by Julian and Woodruff, has proven efficacious (Fig. 51.14). The flap is relatively easy to perform but must be well designed before making the actual incision for the flap. Particular attention should be given to the width of the base of the flap to ensure an adequate blood supply to the distal points of the flap. A general rule to follow is that 2 cm of base should be present for each 1 cm of length of the flap. After measuring the defect and translating these measurements into the appropriate size of flap needed, the future flap is marked along the designated lines with a surgical marker before the incisions are made. The incision should be full thickness, including epidermis, dermis, and subcutaneous fat, down to the fascia. The flap is rotated into position and sutured to the midline of the perineum without tension. Generally, it is difficult to rotate the flap beyond the midperineal line. If additional tissue is needed to close the contralateral vulvar defect, a flap is elevated from the opposite side and similarly sutured in the midline. The flap is sutured to the underlying fascia, covering the pubic rami, and to the incision line on the opposite side. Preferably, 3-0 synthetic absorbable suture is used. The suture in the skin margin should be fine synthetic monofilament suture, such as nylon or fine delayed absorbable suture. The medial margin of the flap is sutured to the margin of the vaginal mucosa with interrupted 2-0 synthetic absorbable sutures. A soft Silastic closed suction drain is placed under the flap, sutured into place, and placed to low suction. The remaining skin adjacent to the flap is brought into position to close the donor site and is sutured with a

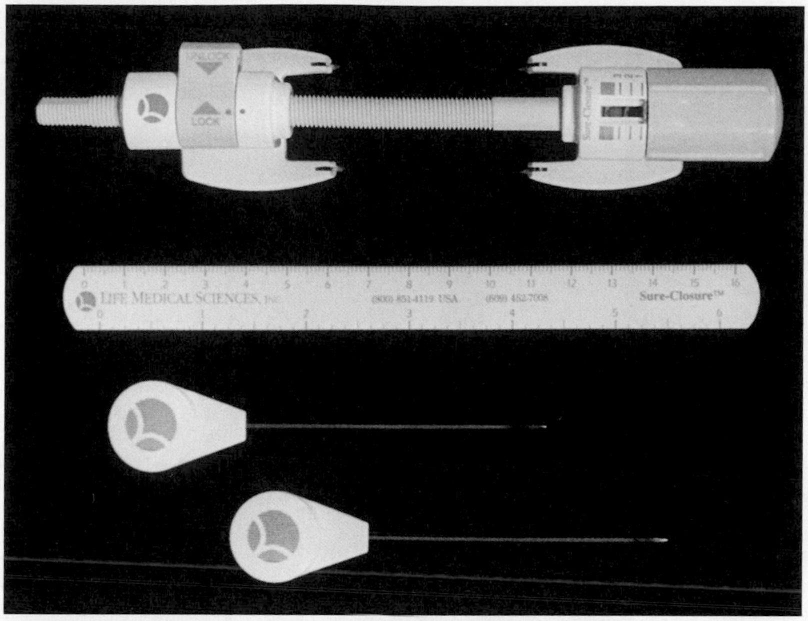

FIGURE 51.15. Mechanical skin stretcher instrument called the SURE Closure.

subcutaneous row of interrupted 3-0 synthetic absorbable sutures and 4-0 nylon sutures in the skin. The cardinal feature of successful healing of these flaps is positioning without tension. If they are under tension, separation occurs.

Modification of full-thickness pedicled flaps includes the gluteal thigh flap, which can incorporate a much larger skin paddle, depending on the inferior gluteal artery, and can range up to 8 × 20 cm. It should not be performed in a patient with a previous bilateral hypogastric artery ligation because compromise may occur.

Mechanical Skin Stretcher (SURE Closure)

A technique for closure of skin defects or to obtain a full-thickness skin graft for neovagina construction from donor site on the body is the mechanical skin stretcher (SURE Closure, Life Medical Sciences, Inc.) (Fig. 51.15). The skin, because of its viscoelastic properties, can be stretched significantly. (For example, the abdominal skin of a woman who is 40 weeks pregnant is significantly stretched.) Through the extensive work of Hirshowitz and Lindenbaum and through the mechanical engineering of the Life Medical Sciences, Inc., it is possible to stretch skin in about 1 hour in the operating room to cover most defects (Fig. 51.16). This device can have a significant role in pelvic surgery.

Large abdominal wall defects and certain vulvar defects may be closed without rotational flaps and split-thickness skin grafts. The application of the skin-stretching device to each margin of the large open abdominal defect allows stretching of the skin gradually over a 1-hour period under general anesthesia in the operating room such that the skin can be sutured without tension. Large abdominal skin defects can be closed primarily without skin grafting. Full-thickness skin grafts can be harvested for neovagina reconstruction without leaving a donor site scar. This device is worthy of the attention of all who perform extensive gynecologic surgery.

V-Y Advancement Flap

A simple sliding design for a skin flap that is dependent on random perfusion of perforating musculocutaneous arteries can reconstruct even moderately large vulvar defects. The upper inner thigh is the usual donor site for vulvar defects. Circulation to that area has been reported distally via a rich suprafascial plexus from gracilis and adductor musculocutaneous perforators and proximally from the external pudendal. Bilateral triangles can be drawn while the patient is in the dorsal lithotomy position. The incision is carried down to include subcutaneous fat. After mobilization, the flap is "slid" toward the defect and secured to the remaining vaginal mucosa or to each other, if needed. The original "V" incision is then closed as a "Y" (Fig. 51.17). With a good blood supply and adequate mobilization, the incidence of wound dehiscence is small. Closed suction drains should be placed and left for 7 to 10 days. Ambulation may begin after 3 days. In the interim, prophylactic antibiotics and thromboprophylaxis should be administered, as with most moderately extensive vulvar flaps.

The V-Y flap can be used for even larger reconstructions, as described by Tateo and associates, by transecting the gracilis toward the insertion and making it a type of sliding musculocutaneous flap after mobilization.

Gracilis and Rectus Abdominis Myocutaneous Flaps

The gracilis and RAM flaps are extremely versatile flaps, as described in the section on vaginal reconstruction. The same principles hold true for vulvar reconstruction in terms of elevating, rotating, and securing these flaps. The principal difference is that unilateral gracilis flaps can be used, depending on the vulvar defect, and no tubularization is necessary. Similar breakdown rates are seen with vulvar reconstruction as with vaginal reconstruction. We believe that the RAM flap continues to be a superior flap for all myocutaneous vulvovaginal reconstructions.

OPERATIONS TO PRESERVE URINARY CONTINENCE

Fecal and urinary diversions have been an essential part of total pelvic exenteration surgery. The early pioneer work of Brunschwig in total pelvic exenteration surgery used

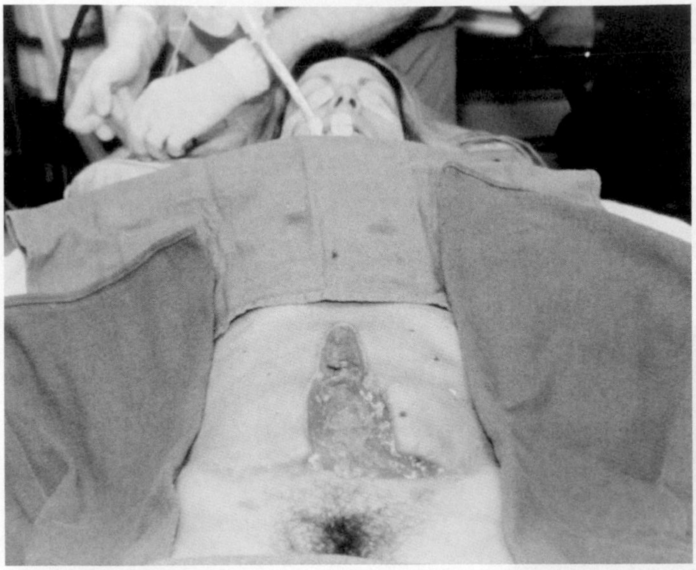
A

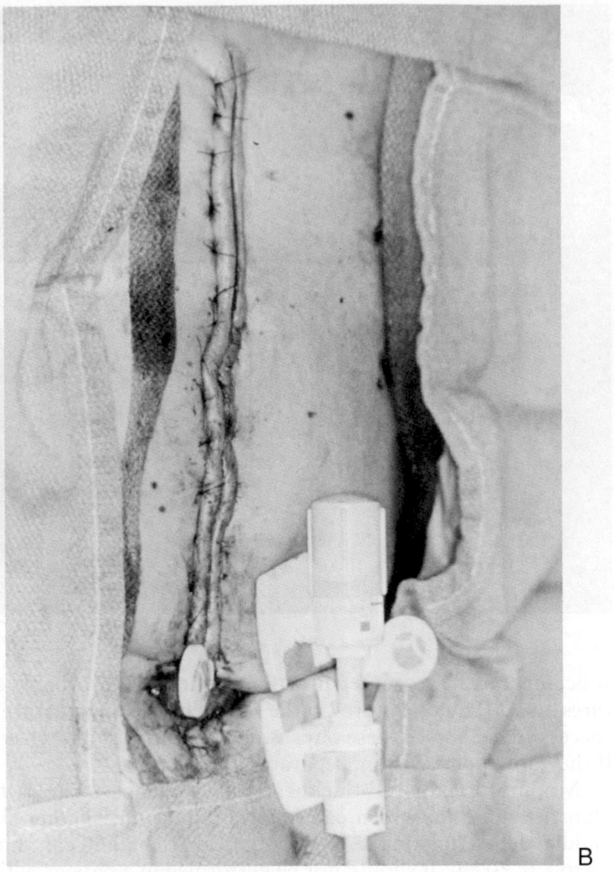
B

FIGURE 51.16. **A:** Photograph of an open abdominal wound to be closed with a skin stretcher instrument. **B:** Midline skin closed without tension. The transverse incision is stretched with the instrument before it is sutured.

ureterosigmoidostomy for urinary diversion (a "wet colostomy"). Reflux of fecal contaminated urine resulted in unacceptable rates of pyelonephritis and secondary renal deterioration. In 1950, Bricker introduced the isolated ileal loop urinary diversion. Later, the colonic loop modification was preferred by some operators. These two techniques have been the preferred techniques for urinary diversion for more than 40 years. Long-term follow-up of patients with isolated intestinal loop urinary diversion, however, has revealed a high incidence of ureteral stenosis and upper renal tract deterioration, especially in those patients who have had pelvic irradiation for gynecologic malignancies. In addition, negative quality-of-life issues secondary to the required urostomy bag—including its odor, reduced self-image, and reduced sexuality—make an alternative technique without a bag desirable. This section discusses the Kock pouch, which introduced the idea of a continent reservoir, and the Miami pouch, which is a newer continent ileocolonic reservoir that has become popular in gynecologic oncology. Each patient should be evaluated individually as to the type of reservoir best suited for her needs. The surgeon should consider the various types but should always perform the procedure that he or she is most comfortable with and that is best suited for the patient.

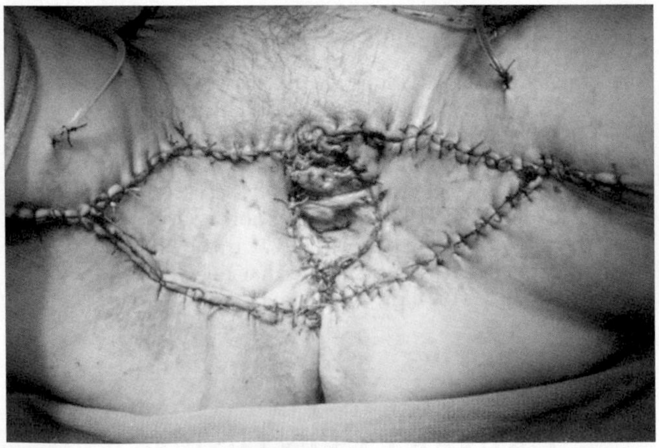

FIGURE 51.17. A completed V-Y flap used to reconstruct a patient who underwent radical vulvectomy. Notice the incision originally made as a "V" has been closed as a "Y." Closed suction drains are placed under the flaps to prevent fluid collections. See color version of figure.

Continent Urostomy Operations

There are unique pathologic and physiologic changes in pelvic organs after irradiation for gynecologic malignancies. The same levels of perioperative irradiation are not usually required for most urologic malignancies, such as carcinoma of the prostate and bladder. The pathophysiologic changes of irradiation-induced endarteritis, resulting in ischemia and later fibrosis, are not present in urinary diversions required for congenital anomalies. In selecting a continent, nonrefluxing urostomy that meets the physiologic requirements, several features must be considered. The ureteral intestinal anastomosis must be as free as possible from potential stricture formation that would result in hydronephrosis and eventual upper renal unit deterioration. Techniques that require the irradiated ureter to be buried in the muscular layers of irradiated colon to achieve the nonrefluxing feature of continent urostomy may be associated with a risk of stenosis and secondary hydronephrosis that is higher than acceptable. The integrity of the upper renal tracts remains to be evaluated in prospective, randomized trials between the incontinent urostomies and the ileoascending colonic variety of these operations. All continent urostomy pouches should have similar physiologic characteristics, including a low pouch pressure of less than 40 cmH_2O pressure, even at volumes greater than 500 mL. This reduces the chance of ureteral reflux and reduces the incidence of incontinence. Reflux and incontinence are reduced because, in the Kock pouch urostomy nipples, pressures are 90 cmH_2O. The use of small segments of irradiated large bowel in continent urostomies—that is, the Indiana pouch—may lead to unacceptable levels of pressure. This finding needs careful study with long-term follow-up.

The compliance of large bowel, especially after irradiation therapy, is less than that of small bowel. A larger segment of detubularized colon—that is, the entire ascending and proximal transverse colon (Miami pouch)—may overcome this problem and allow pressures within the pouch to remain at acceptable low levels. Patients should catheterize their continent pouches at least four times per day.

The continent urostomy is favored in gynecologic oncology patients for two reasons. First, medically, the continent urostomy should help prevent contaminated urine from refluxing into the kidney. This contaminated urine reflux sets up a chronic pyelonephritis. After a prolonged period of time, there could be deterioration of the upper renal units commonly associated with ileal or colonic loops. Second, quality of life is improved by elimination of the urinary bag with its attendant problems of awkwardness, odor, reduced self-image, and reduced sexuality.

Continent Urostomy with Ileal Reservoir (Kock Pouch)

The Kock pouch, developed by Nils Kock in 1982, was devised as a continent nonrefluxing urostomy. Modifications by Skinner improved the surgical technique and reduced the postoperative complications of the original Kock technique. This alternative to ileal or colonic loop urinary diversion should be considered by gynecologic oncologists. Skinner and coworkers have shown that construction of an internal reservoir suitable for urinary bladder replacement must provide (a) retention of 500 to 1,000 mL of fluid, (b) maintenance of low pressure after filling, (c) elimination of intermittent pressure spikes that produce reflux, (d) true continence day and night, (e) ease of catheterization, and (f) prevention of reflux.

The mucosa of the ileum in the wall of the pouch appears to adapt well to urine. The height of the villi of the ileal mucosa gradually decreases, and, in time, the mucosa becomes nearly flat, thereby proportionally reducing the absorption of electrolytes from the urine.

Prerequisites for constructing a continent urostomy include reasonable renal function (creatinine level <3.0 mg/dL), an adequate length of small bowel so that use of 80 cm of ileum taken out of the digestive tract does not result in significant short bowel syndrome, and a patient and her surgeon who are motivated for the procedure and who both understand the inherent risks (in irradiated bowel, an 8%–16% incidence of malfunction of the continent valve mechanism, necessitating additional surgery). When the pouch procedure is performed in conjunction with total pelvic exenteration, resection of the pelvic organs is performed first. For the conversion of an existing ileal or colon conduit to a continent urostomy, all the intraabdominal adhesions of the intestine must be taken down and the bowel inspected for enterotomies before initiating the Kock pouch continent urostomy.

Technique for Kock Pouch Continent Urostomies: Skinner Modification

As seen in Figure 51.18, knowledge and understanding of the anatomy of the terminal ileum and ascending colon and of the blood supply to these structures is essential for the success of the operation. The terminal ileum is transected about 16 cm from the ileocecal junction in the area of the avascular plane of Treves. To ensure mobility of the pouch, an incision is carried up the avascular plane of Treves for 25 to 30 cm. The ileocolic artery must be lateral to this incision, with the branches of the superior mesenteric artery medial to the incision.

The pouch requires 17 cm of ileum for the efferent nipple valve and bowel limb, two 22-cm segments of ileum for the pouch itself, and one 17-cm segment of ileum for the afferent bowel limb and nipple valve. As seen in Figure 51.19, 5 cm of proximal ileum is sacrificed to allow greater mobility of the completed pouch. The anterior wall of the pouch is opened with electrocautery. The posterior wall is sutured with two layers of synthetic absorbable suture (Fig. 51.19A).

The nipples are constructed by intussusception of the small intestine (Fig. 51.19B). Stapling the nipple intussusception with a TA-55 4.8-mm stapler to prevent deintussusception is a vital step in this procedure (Fig. 51.19C). The walls of the pouch are folded over and sutured in place to complete the pouch (Fig. 51.19D). The ureters are anastomosed to the afferent bowel limb over Silastic stents (Fig. 51.19E). The efferent bowel limb is tapered and brought through a defect in the umbilicus. The afferent bowel limb is anchored with suture near the promontory of the sacrum. The pouch itself is positioned in the pelvic inlet. The efferent bowel is tapered to the size of a 20-French catheter with a gastrointestinal anastomotic (GIA) stapler before it is exteriorized (Fig. 51.19F). The efferent system of the pouch requires a 30-French Medena catheter placed through the stoma and passed through the efferent nipple into the pouch for drainage of urine and intestinal mucus (Fig. 51.19G).

During the postoperative phase, all continent urostomies are protected by an adjacent, closed-suction drain placed in the area of the pouch. Leakage from pouch suture lines has been frequent, and, if not drained, a urinoma with septic abscess may occur. The catheter in the efferent limb and nipple and the closed suction drain can be removed 3 weeks postoperatively. Thereafter, the patient is trained by the enterostomal therapist in the technique of catheterizing the pouch. Three weeks postoperatively, endoscopy is performed on the pouch, the Silastic stents are removed from the ureters, and the pouch is tested for ureteral reflux as well as continence by filling the pouch with 200 mL of radiopaque contrast. An abdominal radiograph is obtained to observe reflux into the kidney. An intravenous pyelogram should be obtained after removal of the ureteral stents for baseline assessment of the kidney. Slight pyelocaliectasis (grade I) is not unusual in the postoperative period. For the first 3 weeks postoperatively, while the stents are in place, the patient is placed on a broad-spectrum antibiotic regimen.

Results of this procedure have been encouraging. In highly irradiated bowel, there is a higher percentage of nipple valve necrosis compared with the Kock and Skinner series that were predominately made up of nonirradiated patients. Long-term evaluation of upper renal tract deterioration in patients with

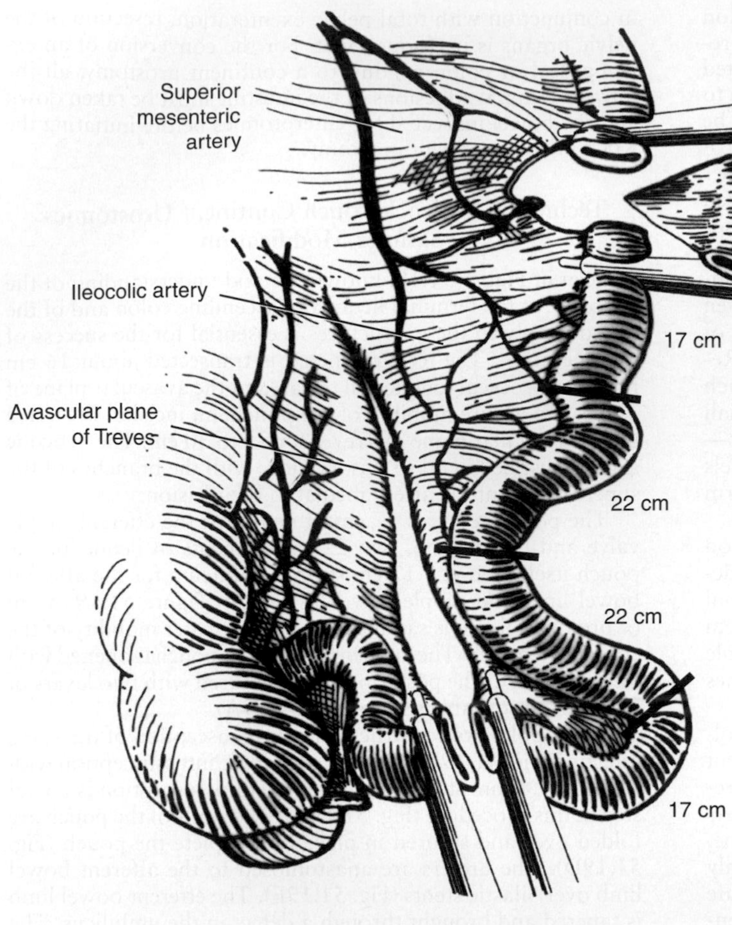

FIGURE 51.18. Anatomic drawing of the terminal ileum illustrating the avascular plane of Treves, the ileocolic artery, and the superior mesenteric artery. Note that the efferent system requires 17 cm of bowel, the Kock pouch requires two 22-cm segments of bowel, and the afferent system requires 17 cm of bowel. Five centimeters of intestine are resected to give additional mobility to the completed Kock pouch.

ileal and colonic loops compared with upper renal tract deterioration in patients with continent urostomies awaits further study. Early results reported by Skinner indicate a protective effect on the upper renal tracts secondary to a reduction of contaminated urinary reflux and its associated subclinical chronic pyelonephritis.

Ileocolic Continent Urostomy (Miami Pouch)

Another procedure for continent urostomies following removal of the bladder is the use of a small portion (10–15 cm) of terminal ileum, the ascending colon, and proximal transverse colon.

Earlier series of patients having a modification of this procedure—that is, the Indiana pouch—using irradiated bowel were discouraging because the amount of colon used was small (ascending colon only). The smaller segment of irradiated colon may result in higher pouch pressures and, therefore, greater ureteral reflux and incontinence. In a technique described at the University of Miami, modifications that used a larger segment of colon that included the entire ascending colon as well as the proximal portion of the transverse colon resulted in reduced pouch pressure, less reflux, and reduced incontinence (Fig. 51.20). The Miami pouch was developed by Bejany and Politano and was reported in 1988. The intention of the pouch was to improve the rate of urinary continence, allowing for both increased flexibility in reimplantation of the ureters and an adequate storage system. The alternative to the intussuscepted segment to prevent ureteral reflux was a nontunneled ureterocolonic anastomosis. Continence was achieved by reinforcing the ileocecal segment with three circumferential silk sutures, placed in a purse-string fashion, and tapering the distal segment of the ileum over a 14-French catheter. This technique created a low-pressure reservoir, high-pressure outlet to maximize continence.

The ileocolic continent urostomy (Miami pouch) does not require the intussusception of bowel to create the continent mechanism for the efferent system. A combination of the intact ileocecal valve, as well as reduction in the diameter of the lumen of the terminal ileum by tapering, elevates the pressure in the efferent system to about 80 to 90 cmH_2O. The pressure in the efferent system is higher than the pressure in the central pouch, which should be less than 40 cmH_2O. It is unclear whether patients who are continent after an ileocolic continent urostomy are continent secondary to an intact (competent) ileocecal valve or from the tapering of the terminal ileum. Furthermore, it is unclear which ureterocolic technique is the best for achieving a nonrefluxing anastomosis of the ureters to the colon. Further data are required to determine whether the traditional technique for achieving antireflux (i.e., embedding the ureter in the wall of the colon) prevents reflux because there is a naturally higher ureteral pressure compared with pouch pressure or because embedding the ureter in the wall of the colon elevates ureteral pressure to a level greater than the pouch. Stenosis at the ureteral anastomotic site can result in hydroureter and hydronephrosis. A benefit of the ileocolic continent urostomy technique is the elimination of the need for intussusception of the small bowel, as in the Kock pouch, to produce the continent afferent and efferent systems. Construction of an ileocolic

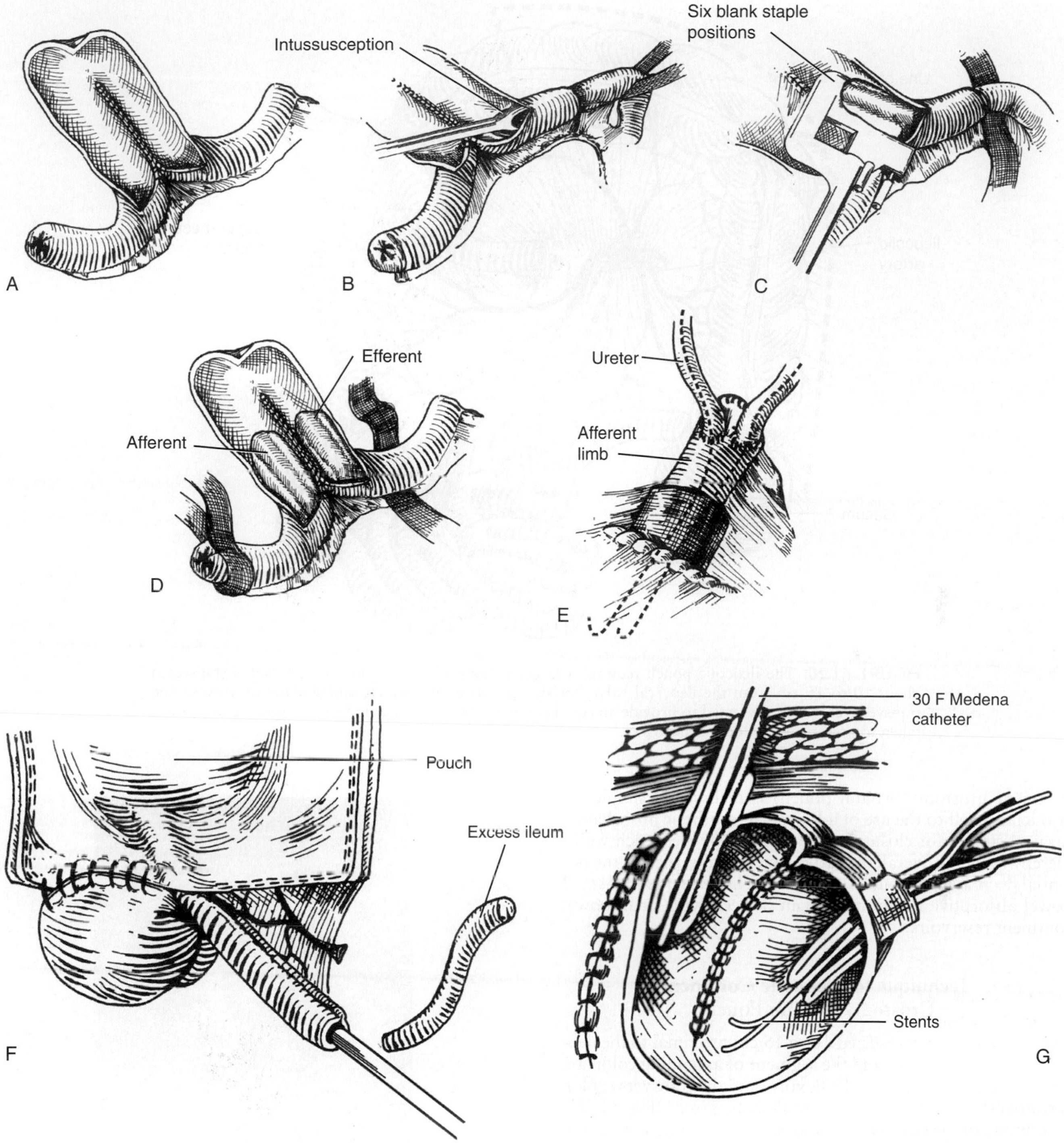

FIGURE 51.19. A: Drawing of Kock pouch opened. The posterior wall of the pouch is sutured with two layers of running synthetic absorbable suture. Efferent and afferent limbs are shown. **B:** Nipples are constructed by intussusception of the small intestine. **C:** The TA-55 4.8-mm stapler is used to staple the nipples at the 2- and 10-o'clock positions to prevent deintussusception. **D:** The completed pouch shows the efferent and afferent nipples constructed with their respective efferent and afferent bowel limbs. Strips of polyglycolic acid mesh have been inserted through the mesentery to be sutured adjacent to the intussusception to further reduce the incidence of deintussusception. The walls of the pouch are labeled B, B', A, A', C, and C'. These letters are connected to form the pouch. **E:** The ureters are anastomosed to the afferent bowel limb over the Silastic stents. **F:** The diameter of the lumen of the terminal ileum was reduced by applying the gastrointestinal anastomotic stapler over a number 14-French catheter used as a sizer. **G:** The completed pouch is positioned in the pelvic inlet. The efferent system of the pouch requires a number 24-French Medena catheter placed through the stoma and passed through the efferent nipple into the pouch for drainage of urine. The stoma is exteriorized at the umbilicus.

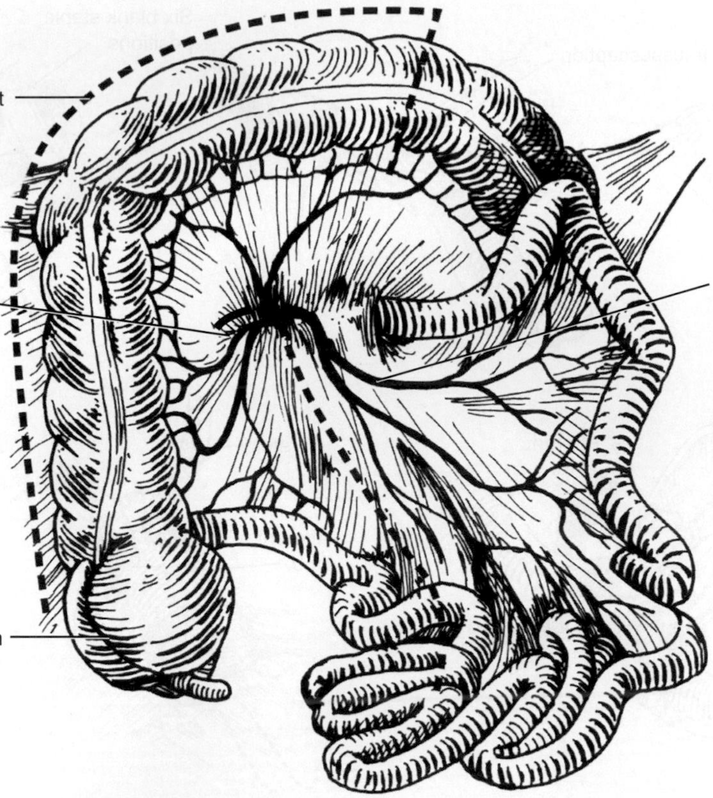

FIGURE 51.20. The ileocolic pouch requires a larger volume of colon. The small bowel is transected about 10 to 15 cm from the ileocecal valve. Incision is carried up the avascular plane of Treves. The transverse colon in transected to provide an equal segment of transverse colon to the right colon. Care is taken to preserve the middle colic artery.

continent urostomy (Miami pouch) is technically simpler. It also lends itself to the use of a Polysorb (synthetic absorbable) surgical stapler for closure of the margins of the pouch walls, thereby reducing overall operative time. Finally, there is the potential decreased morbidity by sparing a large segment of small bowel absorptive function that can be seen with small bowel continent reservoirs.

Technique for Ileocolic Continent Urostomy (Miami Pouch)

The distal ileum is transected 10 to 15 cm proximal to the ileocecal valve. The cecum and the segment of ascending colon are mobilized up to the right colic flexure, and the transverse colon is transected just distal to the middle colic artery (Fig. 51.21). Continuity of the bowel is restored with an ileotransverse colon anastomosis. If an appendectomy has not been performed, it should be done during the procedure. The colon is opened with cautery along the tenia and folded onto itself to create a U-shaped intestinal plate (Fig. 51.22). The legs of the "U" are anastomosed in a side-to-side fashion with absorbable staples or interrupted absorbable sutures to form the posterior wall of the reservoir (Fig. 51.23). This detubularizes the segment of bowel and reduces the potential for high pressure in the colon segment.

The left ureter is passed through the sigmoid mesocolon before entering the reservoir, unless the sigmoid colon has been removed. A mucosal incision is made to create a sulcus in which the ureters will be anastomosed. The distal ends of the ureters

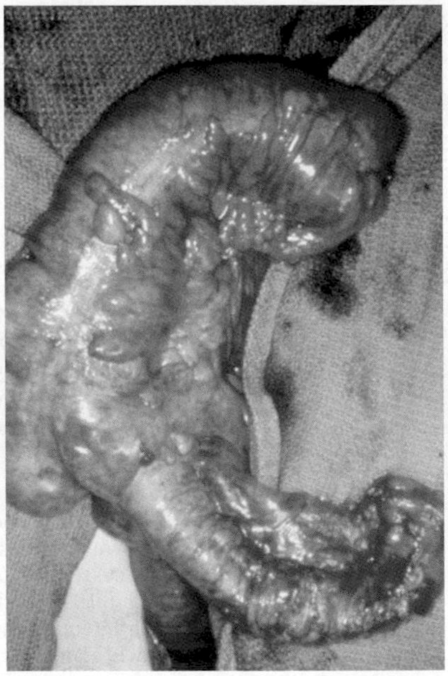

FIGURE 51.21. Pictured is the isolated segment of colon that will be used for construction of a Miami pouch. Approximately 10 to 15 cm of distal ileum are used, as are the entire ascending and half of the transverse colon. (From: Estape R, Mendez L, Angioli R, et al. Urinary diversion in gynecologic oncology. *Surg Clin North Am* 2001;81:787, with permission.)

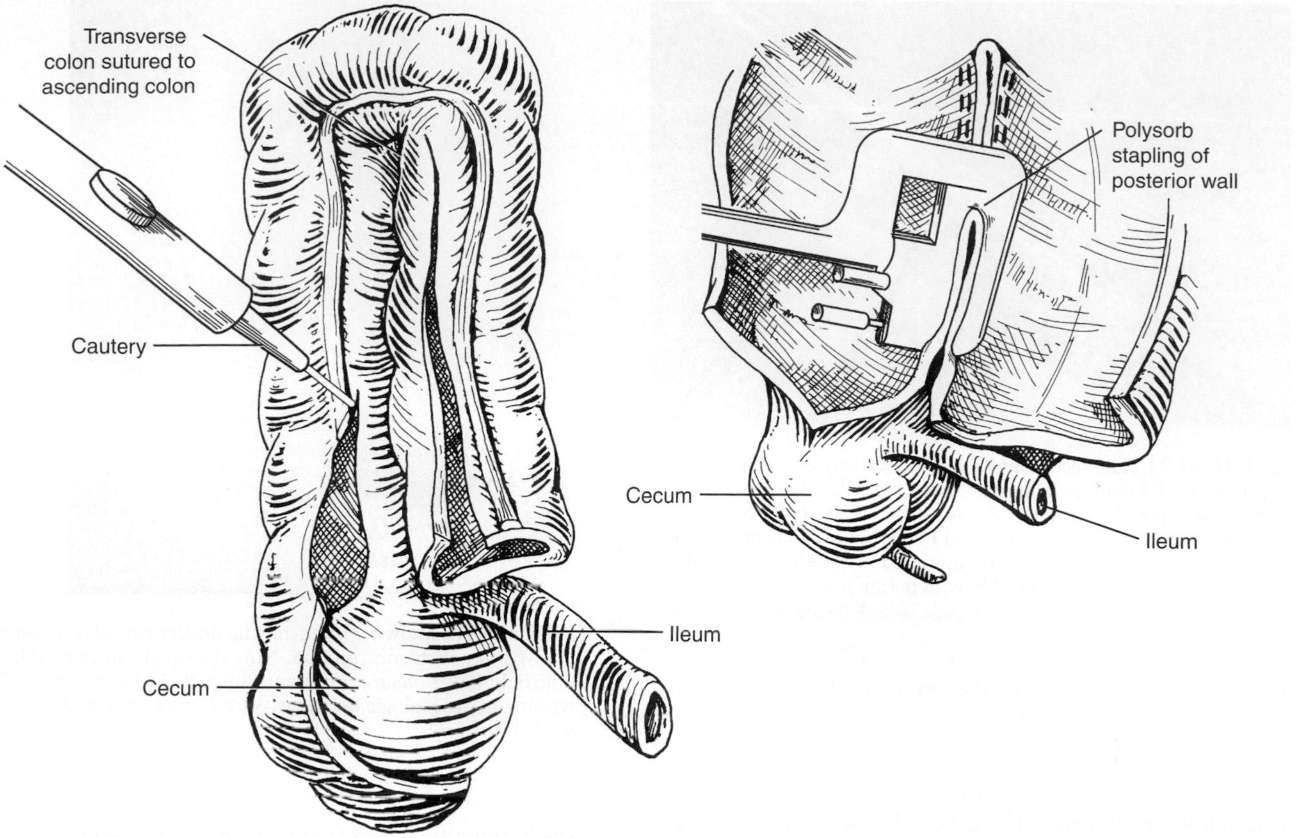

FIGURE 51.22. A: The transverse colon is brought along the side of the right colon. Interrupted sutures are placed in the adjacent segments of colon. A cautery is used to open the antimesenteric border of the transverse and right colon to the cecum. **B:** A TA-55 Polysorb stapler loaded with 0.6-mm staples is used to close the posterior wall of the opened pouch.

are spatulated and, with 4-0 polyglycolic acid sutures, anastomosed to the submucosal layers of the colon. The muscular wall of the colon and the low-pressure reservoir provide the antireflux mechanism. Extraluminally, the ureteral adventitia is fixed to the bowel serosa. The ureters are stented with 7-French single-J ureteral diversion stents that are secured distal to the ureterocolonic anastomosis with absorbable sutures; alternatively, double-J indwelling catheters may be used. The nontunneled ureteral anastomosis has worked well for us in the colon. Incidence of reflux and obstruction has been similar to that recorded with other forms of intestinal anastomosis.

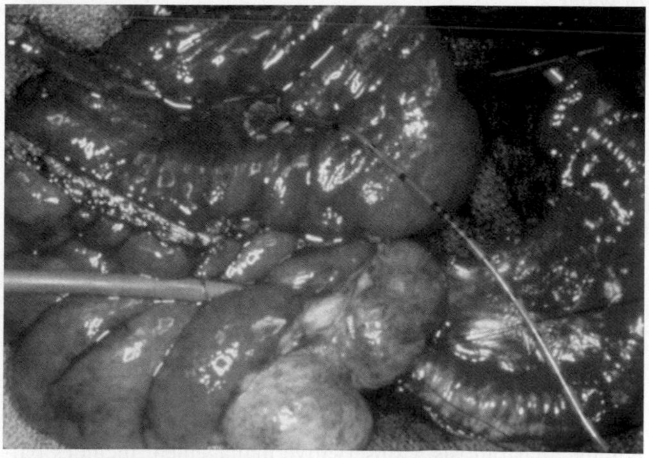

FIGURE 51.23. The opened segment of colon is brought together as a "U," and then the posterior wall is closed first. After this step, the ureters can be brought in to the pouch, secured to the mucosa, and catheterized, as seen here.

Tapering the segment of distal ileum and placing purse-string sutures at the level of the ileocecal valve helps create the continence mechanism. A 14-French rubber catheter is placed into the distal ileum. The ileum, with the rubber catheter in place, is clamped using four Babcock clamps on the mesenteric side. Allis clamps are placed on the antimesenteric border of the ileum and pulled to provide mild traction. A stapling instrument is applied to the ileum longitudinally between the Babcock and the Allis clamps to reduce the lumen diameter down to the underlying 14-French catheter (Fig. 51.24). This tapering is done to increase the pressure of this ileal segment and to provide continence by having a higher pressure than the colonic reservoir. Three purse-string sutures (0.5 cm apart) of 2-0 silk or polypropylene are placed in the seromuscular layer of the ileal segment at the level of the ileocecal valve to increase the final closure pressure and achieve urinary continence (Fig. 51.25). The tapered ileal segment is exteriorized as a stoma to the right lower quadrant of the abdomen for future self-catheterization by the patient.

The anterior wall of the reservoir is then closed with absorbable staples or suture in an interrupted fashion. The

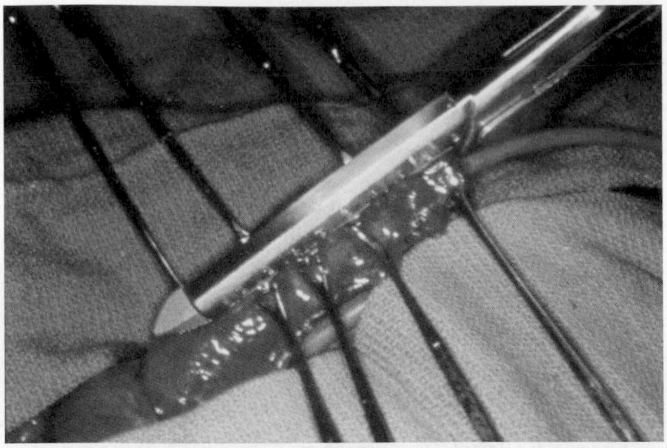

FIGURE 51.24. The second procedure to maintain continence when constructing a Miami pouch is tapering of the distal ileum. The ileal segment is tapered over a 14-French catheter. Care must be taken to taper the antimesenteric side so as not to disrupt blood supply. (From: Estape R, Mendez L, et al. Urinary diversion in gynecologic oncology. *Surg Clin North Am* 2001;81:788, with permission.)

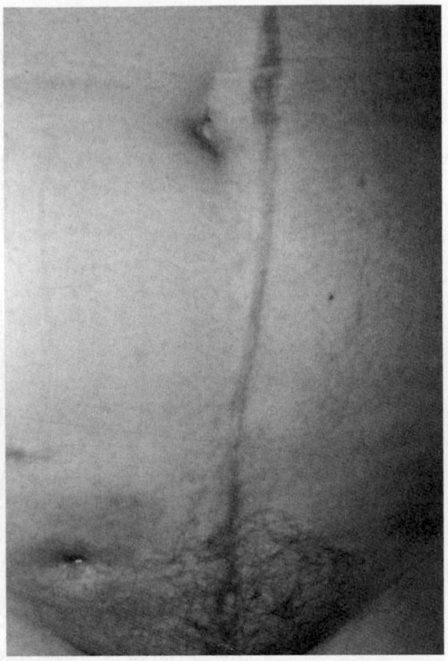

FIGURE 51.26. Shown is a patient who underwent pelvic exenteration with Miami pouch construction. Note the small catheterizable stoma in the right lower quadrant. (From: Estape R, Mendez L, et al. Urinary diversion in gynecologic oncology. *Surg Clin North Am* 2001;81:789, with permission.)

reservoir is secured to the abdominal wall peritoneum and the 14-French catheter and single-J stents are secured to the skin after stoma formation low in the right lower quadrant (Fig. 51.26).

Reinforcing the ileocecal valve is considered essential for maintaining continence. The ileocecal junction normally acts as a valve, thus preventing reflux of colonic contents into the lumen. If a urinary reservoir becomes distended, the ileocecal valve alone may not be sufficient to prevent leakage. By tapering the segment of the distal ileum and placing purse-string sutures at the ileocecal valve, the pressure of this segment of bowel exceeds the reservoir pressure at all times, thereby resulting in full continence.

Approximately 2 weeks after surgery, a contrast study of the reservoir and an intravenous urogram are performed to evaluate for leakage, reflux, or upper tract obstruction. If the radiographs show normal findings, the ureteral stents are removed, and the patient is taught to irrigate and catheterize the pouch. Initially, the patient catheterizes the stoma every 2 to 4 hours and irrigates it four times a day. The patient gradually decreases the frequency of catheterization and irrigation if continence and/or obstruction of the catheter by mucus is not a problem. Patients describe a feeling of fullness or slight cramping in the right lower quadrant, indicating the need to empty the reservoir. The average frequency of catheterization is five to six catheterizations in 24 hours. The time needed for emptying the reservoir is about $3\frac{1}{2}$ minutes. The amount of urine for each catheterization averages 365 mL (range, 250–500 mL). Urodynamic evaluation of the reservoir reveals that the basal pressure fluctuates between 10 and 20 cm of water, whereas in the tapered ileum it varies between 50 and 60 cm of water.

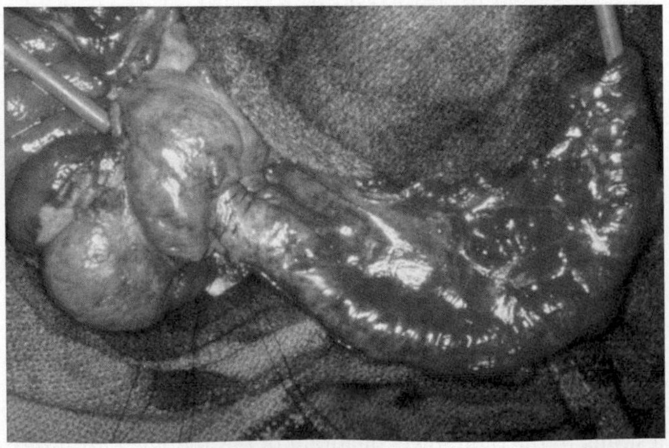

FIGURE 51.25. The continent feature of the efferent system is constructed by two separate surgical techniques. This drawing illustrates two purse-string sutures placed adjacent to the ileocecal junction.

We have reviewed the incidence and management of the urinary complications related to the creation of the Miami pouch at the Division of Gynecologic Oncology of the University of Miami. The majority of the patients who had urinary diversion—68 of 90 (76%)—underwent pelvic exenteration for recurrent cervical cancer, and the majority of these (93.5%) were previously irradiated. The most common complications of the 90 patients evaluated were urinary tract infection/pyelonephritis (40%), ureteral stricture/obstruction (20%), difficult catheterization (18%), and pouch leakage (14%). It is now clear that most of the complications related to the urinary diversion can be safely treated conservatively. Conservative treatment was efficacious in most of the urinary complications related to the creation of the Miami pouch. In this study, ureteral strictures were encountered in 10 patients (13%). All strictures were noted at the level of the ureterocolonic anastomosis. Conservative management includes balloon dilation, stent placement, and nephrostomy placement. Conservative treatment was successful in 8 of the 10 patients. Ureteral obstruction that was caused by stone formation was treated with lithotripsy in one patient; the other required surgical revision because of the dimension of the stones. Another five patients presented with ureteral obstruction, four of which cases were successfully managed conservatively. The total number of patients with stones was four (5.2%); only one, as previously mentioned, required surgical revision. Five patients developed a fistula with the Miami pouch; three of these cases were also managed conservatively.

We have recently reported our 15-year experience performing the Miami Pouch with favorable results. There was a 40% urinary tract infection rate and a 20% ureteral stricture rate; however, the rate of urinary continence in these patients was 93%.

Although complications related to the creation of the Miami pouch are not infrequent, early detection and conservative management are now recommended to manage the majority of these patients safely. Conservative management should be attempted whenever possible, but surgical intervention should not be delayed when indicated. The optimal management of these complications consists of multidisciplinary approach with the active participation of endoscopists, urologists, and radiologists.

In summary, the Miami Pouch continues to be an excellent choice for urinary reconstruction after radical resection for gynecologic cancer in the properly selected patient. With the advent of minimally invasive surgery being applied to radical pelvic resections and in certain cases even urinary reconstructions, we can expect the quality of life and recovery of these patients to continue to improve.

TECHNIQUES TO RESTORE RECTAL FUNCTION

In many gynecologic malignancies, resection of the rectosigmoid colon may be indicated to achieve optimal cure rates. In diseases ranging from primary ovarian cancer to recurrent cervical cancer, the rectosigmoid may need resection even with the anus for proper surgical management. In cases in which the anus is resected, the patient has few options except end colostomy. However, efforts have been made in patients who have rectal and anus-sparing procedures to improve the technical and functional results by reanastomosis. Metastasis of cervical cancer to the anus and lower rectum is rare. In 1954, Javert reported that the number of metastases of cervical carcinoma of the anus and rectum was less than 1%. Survival rates from sphincter-sparing supralevator pelvic exenteration procedures have not been statistically different from those in which the rectum is removed. Metastasis of ovarian cancer to the anus and lower rectum is also extremely rare. Therefore, in gynecologic oncology procedures, it seems reasonable to make every effort to retain the anus to preserve fecal continence and avoid permanent colostomy.

Rectosigmoid Colon Resection and "Straight" Colorectal Anastomosis

The first event that truly led to technically easier anastomosis operations was the widespread use of circular stapling devices in the 1980s. At first, fears existed that these stapled anastomoses would leak when compared with hand sewing. Studies of the double-staple line by Knight and Griffen confirmed the adequacy of the circular stapling device. The ability to resect tumors deep in the pelvis (>2 cm above the dentate line) with adequate margins (at least 2 cm) and perform a technically simple anastomosis procedure has spared many patients an undesirable end colostomy. This technique is described in Chapters 43 and 50.

The straight end-to-end colorectal anastomosis is not without its critics. Functional studies have revealed poor results with defecation disorders (leakage, urgency) in as many as 30% of patients, usually related to residual rectal length. Wheeless reported in 1987 on incontinence and dysfunction in gynecologic patients undergoing very low straight colorectal anastomoses. An unacceptably high 70% of patients reported more than four bowel movements per day, even 2 years after surgery. Some physiologic studies seem to indicate that the incontinence is due to damage of the internal anal sphincter. Introduction of any instrument transanally should be done with the utmost caution.

Frequency disorders, on the other hand, are a result of loss of rectal storage function. Many patients tend to improve over time, probably from an increased reservoir function of the remaining rectal stump; however, this adaptive period may last up to 2 years. For this reason, surgical options to improve functionality in patients undergoing rectosigmoid colon resection and anastomosis have been introduced with good results.

Colonic J-Pouch Reservoir for Very Low Coloproctostomy

Patients in whom a very low anterior resection of the colon was performed were frequently left with an end sigmoid colostomy and low Hartmann pouch. Historical attempts to reestablish continuity of the fecal stream in patients requiring very low anastomosis (<5 cm from anus) of the colon to the rectum at or below the level of the levator sling met with discouraging results.

Tenesmus and fecal frequency are common side effects of very low end-to-end coloproctostomy after very low rectosigmoid resection. The creation of a rectal J-pouch reservoir, even in irradiated colon and rectum, appears to restore the rectal ampullae bulb reservoir and is an effective method of substantially decreasing these troublesome symptoms.

As shown in Figure 51.27, the sigmoid colon is folded on itself with 5 to 7 cm extending into the afferent and efferent segments. A defect is opened in the bottom of the J-pouch, and the 10-cm in-line stapler with 4.8-mm staples is placed in both loops of the colon and fired. The end-to-end anastomosis (EEA) stapler is inserted through the rectum after two purse-string sutures are placed in the rectal stump and the bottom of the J-pouch. The EEA stapler is fired and the anastomosis is completed. The integrity of the anastomosis is tested by inserting a sigmoidoscope per anus, pumping air through the sigmoidoscope into the J-pouch, and observing all stapled sutured lines for air leaks under saline placed into the pelvis.

The problem of tenesmus and fecal frequency in very low anastomosis has been addressed by Lazorthes and coworkers in a study of 65 patients who underwent low anterior resection of the colon for rectal carcinoma. Forty of the 65 patients underwent end-to-end anastomosis at a mean distance of 2.3 cm from the anal verge, and 20 had construction of a rectal J-pouch reservoir with anastomosis to rectum at a mean distance of 1.4 cm from the anal verge. A statistically significant difference in the number of patients having fecal frequency was noted between the group with end-to-end anastomosis versus those having construction of a rectal J-pouch reservoir. A total of 60% of those with a J-pouch reservoir had one to two bowel movements per day versus 33% of those with an end-to-end

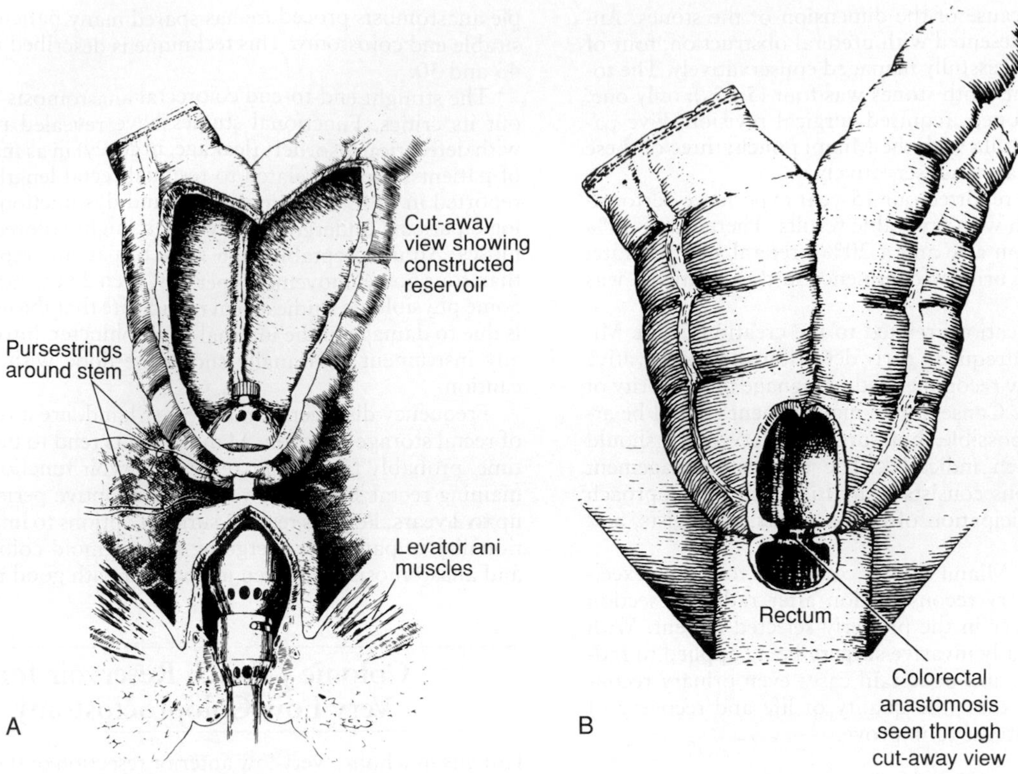

FIGURE 51.27. **A:** A cutaway view of the completed rectal J-pouch is shown positioned over the anus and rectal stump with the end-to-end anastomosis stapler inserted through the anus up the rectum. The anvil of the stapler has been inserted into the pouch, and two adjacent purse-string sutures are applied and tied around the central rod. The stapler is closed and activated. **B:** Completed rectal J-pouch coloproctostomy.

anastomosis. Fecal frequency in these patients is due to the surgical removal of the rectal ampullae, which acts as a low-pressure pouch that does not produce tenesmus until it is full. This improvement was ascribed to a manometrically confirmed and statistically significant higher maximum pressure and tolerable fecal volume in the neorectum of those patients with a neoreservoir (J-pouch) versus those having direct end-to-end anastomosis.

This is especially true in gynecologic oncology patients with irradiated rectosigmoid colons whose compliance is reduced. Therefore, the radius of the end-to-end anastomosis is small, and, under Laplace's law, the pressure becomes high. In the J-pouch, the radius is larger; therefore, the pressure is lower. There is little tenesmus, and fecal frequency is significantly reduced. A confirmatory study was published by Parc and colleagues, who reported on 30 patients who underwent low anterior resection and rectal J-pouch coloproctostomy. After surgery, the mean number of bowel movements in this group was 1.1 per day, and no patients reported tenesmus.

The use of this technique in patients undergoing surgery for gynecologic malignancy, particularly those whose condition has been previously treated with total pelvic irradiation and brachytherapy, has not been extensive. Some suggestion has been made that with the J-pouch there is a better blood supply, leading to a decreased incidence of anastomosis breakdown in patients with a history of pelvic radiotherapy.

The colonic J-pouch is not without complications itself. The principal shortcoming is incomplete emptying. Several studies have been directed at the limb length of the J-pouch. To minimize this problem, the consensus seems to be to construct a useful reservoir the limb length of 5 to 7 cm.

The issue of a protective colostomy or ileostomy when performing a colorectal anastomosis usually rears its ugly head at about this time. The literature at this time is unclear. Data in the colorectal literature suggest it is beneficial. However, data from our institution suggest, for patients undergoing pelvic exenteration, that the major risk factor for fistula formation or anastomotic breakdown is a history of pelvic radiotherapy, independent of the presence of a protective diversion. Indeed, 35% of previously irradiated patients will have an anastomotic breakdown (even with a proximal diversion) versus 7.5% in those with no history of radiotherapy.

In summary, colon J-pouches significantly improve the quality of life for patients, especially those patients who have irradiated bowel and in whom significant portions of the small bowel have been removed. It should be considered by all who perform gynecologic oncology surgery.

BEST SURGICAL PRACTICES

- Radical resection of pelvic malignancies or tissue injury from radiation may produce significant structural and functional pelvic or vulvar defects that need to be repaired by the gynecologic surgeon.
- Vaginal reconstruction: *Gracilis myocutaneous flaps* are the standard reconstruction technique for vaginal reconstruction after pelvic exenteration because they are bulky and fill the pelvic cavity with tissue and bring in new blood supply. An *omental J-flap with a split-thickness skin graft* can also be used, but this requires use of a vaginal stint or mold (for at least 6 months) to maintain patency. *Rectus abdominis*

flaps have also been used, but they cannot be constructed at the same time as the urinary and bowel diversions; thus, this technique prolongs the exenterative operation.

- Vulvar reconstruction: In most cases, even large vulvar defects can be closed primarily because of the loose skin of the vulva, thigh, and buttocks. The *Z-plasty full-thickness pedicle flap* is very useful and relatively easy to perform. The design of the flap is the most critical part of the procedure. As a rule, for every centimeter of flap length, the base must be 2 cm wide. Use of *V-Y advancement flaps split-thickness skin grafts* and various myocutaneous flaps may be helpful in some defects.
- Urinary tract reconstruction: Although an *ileal conduit* provides a relatively rapid technique with few complications for bladder replacement after exenteration, *continent urinary reservoirs* result in a more normal quality of life for the postoperative patient. We have had considerable experience with the *Miami pouch,* which uses a longer segment of colon to increase the size of the reservoir and a tapered segment of distal ileum resulting in good continence rates.
- Rectal reconstruction: When the anus and distal rectum can be preserved, several techniques to reestablish rectal continuity exist. The use of *end-to-end stapling devices* has allowed much more distal reanastomoses than was possible with hand-sewn anastomoses. In some patients, the loss of rectal storage function of the healthy sigmoid colon may lead to seepage, urgency, and incontinence. A *rectal J-pouch* may solve this problem. In all cases of low rectal anastomosis in a previously radiated pelvis, a temporary protective colostomy should be strongly considered.

ACKNOWLEDGMENT

We would like to acknowledge Clifford R. Wheeless Jr., MD, for his contributions to the current and prior editions of this chapter. Dr. Wheeless is a pioneer in the field of reconstructive gynecologic surgery, and his work has continued the rich tradition of the true pelvic surgeon.

Bibliography

Angioli R, Estape R, Cantuaria G, et al. Urinary complications of Miami pouch: trend of conservative management. *Am J Obstet Gynecol* 1998;179:343.

Angioli R, Panici PB, Mirhashemi R, et al. Continent urinary diversion and low colorectal anastomosis after pelvic exenteration: quality of life and complication risk. *Crit Rev Oncol Hematol* 2003;48(3):281.

Bejany DE, Politano VA. Stapled and nonstapled tapered distal ileum for construction of a continent colonic urinary reservoir. *J Urol* 1988;140:491.

Berek JS, Hacker NF, Lagasse LD. Delayed vaginal reconstruction in the fibrotic pelvis following radiation or previous reconstruction. *Obstet Gynecol* 1983;61:331.

Berek JS, Hacker NF, Lagasse LD. Vaginal reconstruction performed simultaneous with pelvic exenteration. *Obstet Gynecol* 1984;63:318.

Bricker EM. Symposium on clinical surgery: bladder substitution after pelvic evisceration. *Surg Clin North Am* 1950;30:1511.

Brown SR, Seow-Choen F. Preservation of rectal function after low anterior resection with formation of a neorectum. *Semin Surg Oncol* 2000;19:376.

Brunschwig A. Complete excision of the pelvic viscera for advanced carcinoma. *Cancer* 1948;1:177.

Burger RA, Riedmiller H, Friedberg V, et al. The ileocecal vagina. *Geburtshilfe Frauenheilkd* 1987;47:644.

Cain JM, Diamond A, Tamimi HK, et al. The morbidity and benefits of concurrent myocutaneous graft with pelvic exenteration. *Obstet Gynecol* 1989;74:185.

Carlson JW, Carter JR, Saltzman AK, et al. Gynecologic reconstruction with a rectus abdominis myocutaneous flap: an update. *Gynecol Oncol* 1996;61:364.

Carlson JW, Saltzman AK, Carter JR, et al. Recurrent squamous cell carcinoma in a rectus abdominis neovagina. *Gynecol Oncol* 1995;59:159.

Carlson JW, Soisson AP, Fowler JM, et al. Rectus abdominis myocutaneous flap for primary vaginal reconstruction. *Gynecol Oncol* 1993;51:323.

Copeland LJ, Hancock KC, Gershenson DM, et al. Gracilis myocutaneous vaginal reconstruction concurrent with total pelvic exenteration. *Am J Obstet Gynecol* 1989;160:1095.

Cormack GC, Lamberty BG. The blood supply of the thigh skin. *Plast Reconstr Surg* 1985;75:342.

Ferron G, Querleu D, Martel P, et al. Laparoscopy-assisted vaginal pelvic exenteration. *Gynecol Oncol* 2006;100(3):551.

Froese DP, Haggitt RC, Friend WG. Ulcerative colitis in the autotransplanted neovagina. *Gastroenterology* 1991;100:1749.

Gleeson NC, Baile W, Roberts WS, et al. Pudendal thigh fasciocutaneous flaps for vaginal reconstruction. *Gynecol Oncol* 1994;54:269.

Gleeson NC, Baile W, Roberts WS, et al. Surgical and psychosexual outcome following vaginal reconstruction with total pelvic exenteration. *Eur J Gynecol Oncol* 1994;15:88.

Hallbook O, Johansson K, Sjodahl R. Laser Doppler blood flow measurement in rectal resection for carcinoma-comparison between the straight and the colonic J pouch construction. *Br J Surg* 1996;83:389.

Harris WJ, Wheeless CR. Use of the end-to-end anastomosis stapling device in low colo-rectal anastomosis associated with radical gynecology surgery. *Gynecol Oncol* 1986;23:350.

Hartenbach EM, Saltzman AK, Carter JR, et al. Nonsurgical management strategies for the functional complications of ileocolonic continent urinary reservoirs. *Gynecol Oncol* 1995;56:127(abst).

Hida J, Yasutomi M, Maruyama T, et al. Functional outcome after low anterior resection with low anastomosis for rectal cancer using the colonic J pouch: prospective randomized study for determination of optimum pouch size. *Dis Colon Rectum* 1996;39:986.

Hida J, Yasutomi M, Maruyama T, et al. Indications for colonic J pouch reconstruction after anterior resection for rectal cancer. *Dis Colon Rectum* 1998;41:558.

Hirshowitz B, Lindenbaum E. A skin stretching device for harnessing of the visco-elastic properties of skin. *J Plast Reconstr Surg* 1993;92:260.

Ho YH, Tsang C, Tang CL, et al. Anal sphincter injuries from stapling instruments introduced transanally: randomized, controlled study with endoanal ultrasound and anorectal manometry. *Dis Colon Rectum* 2000;43:169.

Javert CT. Lymph nodes and lymph channels of the pelvis. In: Meigs JV, ed. *Surgical treatment of cancer of the cervix.* New York: Grune & Stratton; 1954.

Julian CG, Woodruff JD. Surgery of the vulva: vulvectomy. In: Ridley JH, ed. *Gynecologic surgery errors, safeguards, salvage.* Baltimore: Williams & Wilkins; 1974:256.

Jurado M, Bazan A, Elejabeitia J, et al. Primary vaginal and pelvic floor reconstruction at the time of pelvic exenteration: a study of morbidity. *Gynecol Oncol* 2000;77(2):293.

Kindermann G. The sigmoid vagina: experiences in the treatment of congenital absence or later loss of vagina. *Geburtshilfe Frauenheilkd* 1987;47:650.

Knight CD, Griffen FD. An improved technique for low anterior resection of the rectum using the EEA stapler. *Surgery* 1980;88:710.

Kock NG, Nilson AE, Nilsson LO, et al. Urinary diversion via continent ileal reservoir: clinical results of 12 patients. *Urology* 1982;128:469.

Kusiak JF, Rosenblum NG. Neovaginal reconstruction after exenteration using an omental flap and split-thickness skin graft. *Plast Reconstr Surg* 1996;97(4):775.

Lazorthes F, Fages P, Chiotasso P, et al. Resection of the rectum with construction of a colonic reservoir and colo-anal anastomosis for carcinoma of the rectum. *Br J Surg* 1986;73:136.

Licklider D, Mauffray O. Conventional urostomy vs continent urostomy. *Ostomy Wound Manage* 1991;34:26.

McCraw JB, Massey FM, Shanklin KD, et al. Vaginal reconstruction with gracilis myocutaneous flap. *Plast Reconstr Surg* 1976;58:176.

McIndoe AH, Banister JB. An operation for the care of congenital absence of the vagina. *Obstet Gynaecol Br Emp* 1938;45:490.

Mirhashemi R, Averette H, Estape R, et al. Low colorectal anastomosis following radical pelvic surgery: a risk factor analysis. *Am J Obstet Gynecol* 2000;183(6):1375.

Mirhashemi R, Averette HE, Lambrou N, et al. Vaginal reconstruction at the time of pelvic exenteration: a surgical and psychosexual analysis of techniques. *Gynecol Oncol* 2002;87(1):39.

Morley G, DeLancey JO. Full thickness skin graft vaginoplasty for treatment of the stenotic or foreshortened vagina. *Obstet Gynecol* 1991;77:485.

Orr JW, Shingleton HM, Hatch KD, et al. Urinary diversion in patients undergoing pelvic exenteration. *Am J Obstet Gynecol* 1982;142:883.

Pappalardo G, Toccaceli S, Dionisio P, et al. Preoperative and postoperative evaluation by manometric study of the anal sphincter after coloanal anastomosis for carcinoma. *Dis Colon Rectum* 1988;31:119.

Parc R, Tiret E, Frileaux P, et al. Resection and colo-anal anastomosis with colonic reservoir for rectal carcinoma. *Br J Surg* 1986;73:139.

Penalver MA, Angioli R, Mirhashemi R, et al. Management of early and late complications of ileocolonic continent urinary reservoir (Miami pouch). *Gynecol Oncol* 1998;69:185.

Pornel C, Castaigne D. Laparoscopic hand-assisted Miami pouch following laparoscopic anterior pelvic exenteration. *Gynecol Oncol* 2004;93(2):543.

Puntambekar S, Kudchadkar RJ, Gurjar AM, et al. Laparoscopic pelvic exenteration for advanced pelvic cancers: a review of 16 cases. *Gynecol Oncol* 2006;102(3):513.

Pursell SH, Day TG, Tobin TG. Distally based rectus abdominis flap for reconstruction in radical gynecologic procedures. *Gynecol Oncol* 1990;37:234.

Ratliff CR, Gershenson DM, Morris M, et al. Sexual adjustment of patients undergoing gracilis myocutaneous flap vaginal reconstruction in conjunction with pelvic exenteration. *Cancer* 1996;78:2229.

Rowland RG, Mitchell ME, Bihrle, et al. Indiana continent urinary reservoir. *J Urol* 1987;137:1136.

Salom EM, Mendez LE, Schey D, et al. Continent ileocolonic urinary reservoir (Miami pouch): the University of Miami experience over 15 years. *Am J Obstet Gynecol* 2004;190(4):994.

Schmidt JD, Buchsbaum HJ, Jacoby EC. Transverse colon conduit for supravesical urinary tract diversion. *Urology* 1976;8:542.

Skinner DG, Lieskovsky G, Boyd SD. Continuing experience in continent urinary diversion: the Kock pouch in 250 patients. Paper presented at American Urological Association; 1986; New York.

Skinner DG, Lieskovsky G, Boyd SD. Technique of creation of a continent internal ileal reservoir (Kock pouch) for urinary diversion. *Urol Clin North Am* 1984;11:741.

Smith HO, Genesen MC, Runowicz CD, et al. The rectus abdominis myocutaneous flap: modifications, complications and sexual function. *Cancer* 1998;83:510.

Soper JT, Berchuck A, Creasman WT, et al. Pelvic exenteration: factors associated with major surgical morbidity. *Gynecol Oncol* 1989;35:93.

Soper JT, Havrilesky LJ, Secord AA, et al. Rectus abdominis myocutaneous flaps for neovaginal reconstruction after radical pelvic surgery. *Int J Gynecol Cancer* 2005;15(3):542.

Tateo A, Tateo S, Bernasconi C, et al. Use of the V-Y flap for vulvar reconstruction. *Gynecol Oncol* 1996;62:203.

Taussig F. Primary cancer of the vulva, vagina and female urethra: five year results. *Surg Gynecol Obstet* 1935;60:477.

Tobin GR, Day TG. Vaginal and pelvic reconstruction with a distally based rectus abdominis and myocutaneous flaps. *Plast Reconstr Surg* 1988;81:62.

Valle G, Ferraris G. Use of the omentum to contain the intestines in pelvic exenteration. *Obstet Gynecol* 1969;33:772.

Wheeless CR. Recent advances in surgical reconstruction of the gynecologic cancer patient. *Curr Opin Obstet Gynecol* 1992;4:91.

Wheeless CR, Hempling RE. Rectal J pouch reservoir to decrease the frequency of tenesmus and defecation in low coloproctostomy. *Gynecol Oncol* 1989;35:136.

Williams NS, Price R, Johnston D. The long term effect of sphincter preserving operations for rectal carcinoma on the function of the anal sphincter in man. *Br J Surg* 1980;67:208.

■ QUESTIONS

CHAPTER 2

1. A legal document reflects that an adequate informal consent process has taken place.
   a. True
   b. False
2. An ethically valid informed consent requires that it be obtained through the voluntary authorization by a patient for a medical intervention.
   a. True
   b. False
3. An adverse surgical outcome is synonymous with negligence
   a. True
   b. False
4. The surgeon should document in the chart the alternatives to a selected procedure and indicate that they were each discussed with the patient before the procedure.
   a. True
   b. False
5. Competence of the patient is one of the core components required in the decision-making process.
   a. True
   b. False
6. An incorrect entry in a patient's chart should be corrected by a second entry without crossing out and initialing the erroneous entry.
   a. True
   b. False
7. Standard of care refers to a level of care that is generally thought to represent the norm.
   a. True
   b. False
8. The National Practitioners Data Bank receives and makes available data regarding infraction of practice standards.
   a. True
   b. False
9. The Health Insurance Portability and Accountability Act (HIPAA) establishes minimal national standards to ensure confidentiality of protected health information.
   a. True
   b. False
10. The Nuremberg Code establishes the need for voluntary consent of the patient.
    a. True
    b. False
11. Surgeons who choose to respect the wishes of a competent Jehovah's Witness patient to refuse blood products in the face of imminent exsanguination are, in general, protected from wrongful death liability.
    a. True
    b. False
12. A durable power of attorney for health care is a legal document in which a patient designates a specific individual to make health care decisions in the setting of loss of decisional capacity.
    a. True
    b. False

CHAPTER 3

1. Select the professional who should be responsible for answering patient's questions before she undergoes surgery:
   a. Office nurse who works with preoperative patients
   b. Ancillary personnel who has taken a course called "Preparing the Patient for Surgery"
   c. The patient's surgeon
   d. A trusted friend who has recently had the same procedure
2. In which of the following patients is an obliterative procedure indicated?
   a. A patient who is not sexually active
   b. An octogenarian
   c. An elderly widowed or divorced patient
   d. None of the above; age should not be a determinant
3. Which of the following questions should be answered for the patient before her surgery?
   a. How will surgery affect my sexuality?
   b. When can I safely resume sexual intercourse?
   c. What hormonal changes should I expect after surgery?
   d. Can I have ovarian cancer after my ovaries are surgically removed?
   e. Will I need hormone replacement therapy (HRT)?
   f. Is HRT safe?
   g. All of the above
4. What is a complete physician?
   a. A physician who has mastered and maintained his or her skills in the surgical arena
   b. One who keeps up to date by acquiring new skills
   c. One who is most well known in his community as a skilled surgeon
   d. A skilled surgeon who addresses his patient's psychological as well as physical needs
5. Which of the following should be considered "special needs" patients who require extra attention?
   a. Teenagers
   b. Patients from another culture
   c. A depressed patient
   d. The cancer patient
   e. The senior woman
   f. All of the above
6. Shaving the perineum preoperatively is:
   a. Always indicated before vaginal surgery
   b. Always indicated before abdominal surgery
   c. Decreases postoperative infections
   d. Indicated in the older patient

e. An outdated procedure that should no longer be performed routinely

7. Alleviating preoperative stress does the following:
   a. Releases endogenous opiates
   b. Has little or no effect on postoperative morbidity
   c. Has been shown to decrease the requirement for analgesics after surgery
   d. Wastes the time of the physician and personnel in the modern office

CHAPTER 4

1. The Standard of Care requires in most states in the United States that physicians must render the degree of care exercised by physicians under the same or similar circumstances in the:
   a. Community
   b. State
   c. Region
   d. Nation
2. An indirect cause-and-effect relationship must exist between the breach in the Standard of Care and the adverse outcome for malpractice to legally occur.
   a. True
   b. False
3. The ethical principles generally involved in providing adequate informed consent include:
   (1) Autonomy (2) Beneficence (3) Nonmaleficence (4) Justice
   a. 1 and 4
   b. 1 and 2
   c. 3 and 4
   d. 1, 2, 3, and 4
4. The primary purpose of a well-documented medical record is to:
   a. Protect the physician from a malpractice claim
   b. Provide adequate information to the patient's insurance company
   c. Communicate with members of the health care team
   d. Meet hospital requirements
5. The words___________ are medicolegally correct words to be use in describing, in a progress note or an operative note, an adverse event that might have occurred during an operative procedure:
   1. Unintentionally
   2. Inadvertently
   3. Accidentally
   4. Unfortunately
      a. 1 and 4
      b. 1 and 3
      c. 2 and 4
      d. None of the above
6. When a language barrier exists between the patient and physician, the physician is relieved of the ethical requirements to provide reasonable communication in providing informed consent.
   a. True
   b. False
7. The physician is protected from being sued for malpractice for an adverse outcome when the physician's managed care plan has denied the physician's patient access to studies or treatments recommended by the physician.
   a. True
   b. False
8. In preparation for and during a deposition, it is generally prudent for a physician to:
   1. Be unfamiliar with the office and hospital policies so that the plaintiff's attorney cannot question the physician about those areas
   2. Not attempt to educate his or her attorney about the medical facts of the case, because the insurance carrier would only use attorneys who are very knowledgeable about all the medical aspects of the case
   3. Always demand to be able to read and sign the deposition
   4. Be unfamiliar with the alternative forms of therapy that you might have used so that the plaintiff's attorney is unable to question you about them
      a. 1 and 2
      b. 1 and 4
      c. 3
      d. 2 and 4
9. During a trial, it is prudent for the physician to:
   1. Attend only those sessions where he or she has to give testimony to convey to the jury lack of concern about the matter
   2. Explain in complex medical terms the facts of the case so that the jury can be impressed with his or her medical knowledge
   3. Give the best educated guess to questions of which he or she is not completely sure of the answer
   4. Dress in a manner to convey to the jury that he or she is a rich and very successful physician
      a. 1 and 3
      b. 2 and 4
      c. 2 and 3
      d. None of the above
10. The emotional stress of a malpractice case has:
    a. Been equated to the loss of a loved one
    b. Resulted in symptoms of major depression in 40% of sued physicians
    c. Resulted in 8% of sued physicians having the onset of physical ailments of which one forth were life threatening
    d. All of the above

CHAPTER 5

1. Common electronic health record errors include which of the following?
   a. Entering and retrieving information
   b. Failure of software
   c. Communication and coordination of patient care processes
   d. Inability for physicians to learn how to navigate the programs
2. For resident education, Brazil requires which of the following?
   a. Weekends off
   b. 30 consecutive days off per year
   c. One day off in 5
   d. 10% of total work hours dedicated to educational activities
3. Regarding hospitalist programs, which of the following are true?
   a. The majority of clinical trials demonstrate decreased length of stay.
   b. These providers only work in hospitals.
   c. There are multiple models and work paradigms.

d. The providers work in isolation of the patients and other physicians until hospital discharge.

4. Pay-for-performance programs are:
 a. More effective when there is greater incentive
 b. More effective when the incentive applies to a larger percent of patients in the provider's practice
 c. Currently being evaluated by Center for Medicare and Medicaid Services (CMS)
 d. Uniformly effective
5. Which of the following are included in the Institute for Healthcare Improvement (IHI) 100,000 lives initiative?
 a. Deploying rapid response teams
 b. Prevention of surgical site infections
 c. Preventing adverse drug events through medication reconciliation
 d. Prevention of central line infections
6. Which of the following may be key issues with regards to implementing an electronic health record?
 a. Financing
 b. Establishing new workflows that optimize use of the HER
 c. Having adequate technical support
 d. Establishing a culture in the implementation setting that will allow for the necessary change
7. Which of the following are included in the current Accreditation Council for Graduate Medical Education (ACGME) 80-hour workweek regulations?
 a. 1 weekend off every 2 weeks
 b. Total duty hours should not exceed 80 hours when averaged over 4 weeks
 c. No more then 36 continuous patient care hours
 d. At least 10 hours of off time between worked shifts
8. The U.S. Preventative Task Force method of evaluating the evidence base for a research article:
 a. Is one of only several methods for ranking articles
 b. Gives a "B" recommendation when the data are based on limited or inconsistent scientific evidence
 c. Always is concordant with other ranking systems
 d. Is commonly used in obstetrics and gynecology for evaluating peer-reviewed literature

CHAPTER 6

1. Choose the *incorrect* statement.
 a. There has been a significant decrease in the number and types of major gynecologic cases.
 b. Financial constraints have dramatically affected the payment policies of the various payers of medical services.
 c. The surgical options available for various gynecologic symptoms have significantly narrowed because of mandatory precertification protocols.
 d. A decrease in the number of surgical cases has resulted from a better educated consumer.
 e. Decreased use of conservative medical management has increased the number of major surgical cases.
2. A decrease in the quality of gynecologic surgical training is due to:
 a. Changing residency curriculum
 b. Changing attitude and goals of residents
 c. Financial pressures on academicians
 d. Decreased funding in ob/gyn departments
 e. All of the above
3. Decreased time for resident educational activities results from which of the following?
 a. Increased departmental funding
 b. Decreased resident clinical responsibility
 c. Significantly increased ob/gyn knowledge base
 d. Decreased physical and emotional stress for residents
 e. Decreased medical-legal liability for surgeons who teach residents
4. Which of the following is required for the learning of surgical skills?
 a. Individual motivation and talent
 b. Dedicated time for practice
 c. Clarity, purpose, and imagination
 d. A skilled, caring, interested mentor
 e. All of the above
5. Which of the following is not an effective component of teaching surgical skills?
 a. Lectures, case presentations, and discussions
 b. Observing surgical videos
 c. Use of inanimate trainers and computer simulators
 d. Surgery on actual patients without supervision
 e. Human cadaveric dissections

CHAPTER 7

1. Which of the following structures is not considered part of the vulva?
 a. Mons
 b. Labia
 c. Clitoris
 d. Vestibule
 e. Anus
2. Choose the incorrect statement pertaining to the pudendal artery and nerve.
 a. The pudendal nerve provides only sensory innervation to the perineum.
 b. The pudendal nerve arises from the sacral plexus.
 c. The pudendal artery originates from the anterior division of the internal iliac artery.
 d. The nerve and vessels have three branches: clitoral, perineal, and inferior hemorrhoidal.
 e. The perineal branch of the pudendal artery is the largest of the three branches.
3. Choose the incorrect statement.
 a. Vulvar lymphatic channels lie medial to the labiocrural fold, establishing this as the lateral border of surgical resection.
 b. The clitoris never drains directly into the deep pelvic nodes.
 c. The superficial inguinal nodes lie in a T-shaped distribution 1 cm below the inguinal ligament.
 d. The deep inguinal nodes are found beneath the fascia cribrosa.
 e. Within the femoral triangle, the most medial structure is the femoral vein.
4. Choose the incorrect statement.
 a. The perineal membrane is a triangular sheet of fibromuscular tissue spanning the anterior half of the pelvic outlet.
 b. The perineal membrane attaches medially with the urethra, walls of the vagina, and the perineal body.
 c. The internal anal sphincter is indistinguishable from the external anal sphincter, and it lies just outside the external anal sphincter.

d. The levator ani muscles and their fascia are called the pelvic diaphragm.
e. The urogenital hiatus allows passage of the urethra, vagina, and rectum through the pelvic diaphragm.

5. Which of the following is a vaginal structure?
a. Anterior and posterior columns
b. Urethral carina
c. Anterior and posterior fornices
d. Lateral vaginal sulci
e. All of the above

6. Choose the incorrect statement.
a. In a woman of reproductive age, the uterine cervix is larger than the uterine corpus.
b. The muscle fibers of the uterine corpus are arranged in a complex diagonal crisscrossed pattern.
c. The cervix is divided into two portions: the portio vaginalis and the portio supravaginalis.
d. The external cervical os contains the transition from squamous to columnar epithelium.
e. The anterior portion of the uterine cervix is covered by the bladder.

7. Choose the correct statement.
a. The fallopian tubes are approximately 15 cm long.
b. The four portions of the fallopian tube from medial to lateral are the isthmus, interstitium, ampulla, and fimbriated end.
c. The outer layer of the tubal muscularis is composed of circular fibers, whereas the inner fibers are longitudinal.
d. The distal end of the fallopian tube is attached to the ovary by the fimbria ovarica.

8. Choose the incorrect statement.
a. The ovary attaches laterally to the pelvic sidewall with the infundibulopelvic ligament, which contains the ovarian vessels.
b. The ovary connects medially to the uterus with the uteroovarian ligament.
c. The normal ovary measures 7 cm long during reproductive life.
d. The ovary attaches to the broad ligament through the mesovarium.
e. Ovarian follicles, corpora lutea, and corpora albicantia are found within the ovarian cortex.

9. Choose the incorrect statement.
a. The blood supply of the upper adnexal structures comes from the ovarian arteries that arise from the aorta below the renal arteries.
b. The ovarian veins drain into the vena cava on the left and the renal vein on the right.
c. The uterine artery, which usually originates from the internal iliac artery, may have a common origin with the internal pudendal or vaginal arteries.
d. The uterine artery joins the uterus near the junction of the corpus and cervix.
e. The vagina receives blood supply from the uterine artery, vaginal artery, and the pudendal vessels.

10. Choose the incorrect statement pertaining to the ureter.
a. The ureter descends into the pelvis after passing over the bifurcation of the internal and external iliac arteries.
b. The ureter lies in a special connective tissue sheath within the medial leaf of the broad ligament.
c. The ureter crosses under the uterine artery in its course through the cardinal ligament.
d. The ureter lies approximately 3 cm from the anterolateral surface of the cervix.
e. The ureter receives blood supply from the common iliac, internal iliac, uterine, and vesical arteries.

CHAPTER 8

1. A preoperative evaluation of a patient with an uncomplicated gynecologic history and an uncomplicated medical or surgical status should include all of the following laboratory tests EXCEPT:
a. Electrocardiogram if older than 40 years
b. Pregnancy test if reproductive age, sexually active, not using contraception, or if using questionably effective contraception
c. Blood type and screen if the potential exists for a more than minimal surgical blood loss
d. Chemistry panel
e. Hematocrit or hemoglobin if older than 6 months

2. During the preoperative history, herbal therapy and dietary supplements should be questioned because of their potential adverse effects on surgical outcomes. These potential adverse effects may include:
a. Effect of anticoagulation
b. Effect on glycemic control
c. Effect on sedation
d. All of the above
e. None of the above

3. Pelvic surgery should always be preceded by a recent cytologic study of the cervix because:
a. A negative Papanicolaou smear always excludes the possibility of cervical, endocervical, or endometrial neoplasm.
b. Most preclinical malignancies of the cervix demonstrate significant gross lesions indicating the need for cytologic evaluation.
c. Patients with abnormal Papanicolaou smears showing repeated dysplasia should be evaluated by colposcopy and suspicious lesions biopsied before pelvic surgery.
d. A sampling of cells taken from the portio of the cervix is simple, inexpensive, and is indicative of cervical and endocervical pathology.
e. A finding of abnormal glandular cell dysplasia requires only an endocervical curettage for a complete evaluation.

4. In regards to the planning and accomplishment of gynecologic surgery on senior patients, which of the following statements is INCORRECT?
a. Senior gynecologic patients present with significantly greater health care problems.
b. Senior gynecologic patients are at increased risk during surgery.
c. Age is a relative contraindication for gynecologic surgery.
d. With appropriate evaluation and management, the risks of gynecologic surgery on senior patients can be reduced to a level not much greater than for premenopausal patients.
e. Age is not always an accurate indicator of organ function or malfunction.

5. Preoperative prophylactic antibiotics are recommended in which of the following gynecologic surgical procedures?
a. Ovarian cystectomy
b. Ectopic pregnancy
c. Uterine myomectomy
d. Tubal ligation
e. Vaginal and abdominal hysterectomy

6. Patients who are found during their preoperative examination to have bacterial vaginosis should be treated with:
a. Oral metronidazole for 7 days

b. Clindamycin vaginal cream for 7 days
c. Metronidazole vaginal gel for 5 days
d. a, b, or c
e. b or c

7. Patients receiving prophylactic antibiotics before gynecologic surgery should be given the antibiotic:
a. 6 hours before surgery
b. 1 to 2 hours before surgery, repeated once if the surgery lasts longer than 3 hours
c. 1 to 2 hours before surgery, repeated at 3 and 6 hours after the start of surgery
d. 6 hours before surgery, repeated again 1 to 2 hours before surgery
e. 6 hours before surgery, repeated every 6 hours for 2 days

8. A rectal examination, in combination with the abdominal-pelvic examination, offers all of the following EXCEPT:
a. A more complete assessment of the broad and uterosacral ligaments
b. A more effective assessment of the posterior bladder wall
c. A more complete assessment of the cul-de-sac of Douglas
d. A more effective assessment of the adnexa
e. A more effective assessment of the anal sphincter, anal canal, and lower rectum

9. All of the preoperative management actions are suggested in the preoperative care of gynecologic patients EXCEPT:
a. Discontinuation of the use of birth control pills 2 to 4 weeks before the planned gynecologic surgery
b. Immediate preoperative examination by the gynecologic surgeon and anesthesia assessment by an individual anesthesiologist or in the anesthesia preoperative clinic
c. Cleansing of the lower colon by a preoperative enema
d. Use of vaginal estrogen cream in postmenopausal women undergoing vaginal surgery
e. Use of gonadotropin-releasing hormone agonist for 2 to 3 months before hysteroscopic resection of submucous uterine leiomyoma

10. All of the following statements regarding preoperative patient preparation are true EXCEPT:
a. A full bowel prep should be carried out on all gynecologic surgeries.
b. Pelvic cleansing should be accomplished before all pelvic or abdominal surgeries.
c. Universal precautions should be used in all gynecologic surgeries.
d. Hepatitis B vaccination is recommended for all physicians accomplishing gynecologic surgeries.
e. In those gynecologic surgeries in which hair removal is deemed necessary, hair clipping, rather than hair shaving, is recommended just before surgery.

CHAPTER 9

1. Which form of pharmacologic venous thromboembolism(VTE) prophylaxis has the lowest rate of heparin-induced thrombocytopenia (HIT)?
2. What percentage of the Caucasian population has thrombophilia risk factors of factor V Leiden or G20210 A prothrombin gene mutation?
3. What risk factors are implicated in the development of postoperative atelectasis?
4. What are the five basic pathophysiologic mechanisms that cause hypoxemic respiratory failure?

CHAPTER 10

1. A preoperative evaluation of a patient with an uncomplicated gynecologic history and an uncomplicated medical or surgical status should include all of the following laboratory tests EXCEPT:
a. Electrocardiogram if older than 40 years
b. Pregnancy test if in the reproductive age, sexually active, not using contraception, or if using questionably effective contraception
c. Blood type and screen if the potential exists for a more than minimal surgical blood loss
d. Chemistry panel
e. Hematocrit or hemoglobin if older than 6 months

2. During the preoperative history, herbal therapy and dietary supplements should be questioned because of their potential adverse effects on surgical outcomes. These potential adverse effects may include
a. Effect of anticoagulation
b. Effect on glycemic control
c. Effect on sedation
d. All of the above
e. None of the above

3. Pelvic surgery should always be preceded by a recent cytologic study of the cervix because
a. A negative Papanicolaou smear always excludes the possibility of cervical, endocervical, or endometrial neoplasm
b. Most preclinical malignancies of the cervix demonstrate significant gross lesions indicating the need for cytologic evaluation
c. Patients with abnormal Papanicolaou smears showing repeated dysplasia should be evaluated by colposcopy and suspicious lesions biopsied before pelvic surgery
d. A sampling of cells taken from the portio of the cervix is simple, inexpensive, and is indicative of cervical and endocervical pathology
e. A finding of abnormal glandular cell dysplasia requires only an endocervical curettage for a complete evaluation

4. In regards to the planning and accomplishment of gynecologic surgery on senior patients, which of the following statements is INCORRECT
a. Senior gynecologic patients present with significantly greater health care problems
b. Senior gynecologic patients are at increased risk during surgery
c. Age is a relative contraindication for gynecologic surgery
d. With appropriate evaluation and management the risks of gynecologic surgery on senior patients can be reduced to a level not much greater than for premenopausal patients
e. Age is not always an accurate indicator of organ function or malfunction

5. Preoperative prophylactic antibiotics are recommended in which of the following gynecologic surgical procedures
a. Ovarian cystectomy
b. Ectopic pregnancy
c. Uterine myomectomy
d. Tubal ligation
e. Vaginal and abdominal hysterectomy

6. Patients receiving prophylactic antibiotics before gynecologic surgery should be given the antibiotic
   a. 6 hours before surgery
   b. 1-2 hours before surgery, repeated once if the surgery lasts longer than 3 hours
   c. 1-2 hours before surgery, repeated at 3 and 6 hours after the start of surgery
   d. 6 hours before surgery, repeated again 1–2 hours before surgery
   e. 6 hours before surgery, repeated every 6 hours for 2 days
7. A rectal examination, in combination with the abdominal-pelvic examination, offers all of the following EXCEPT
   a. A more complete assessment of the broad and uterosacral ligaments
   b. A more effective assessment of the posterior bladder wall
   c. A more complete assessment of the cul-de-sac of Douglas
   d. A more effective assessment of the adnexa
   e. A more effective assessment of the anal sphincter, anal canal, and lower rectum
8. All of the preoperative management actions are suggested in the preoperative care of gynecologic patients EXCEPT
   a. Discontinue the use of birth control pills 2 to 4 weeks before the planned gynecologic surgery
   b. Immediate preoperative examination by the gynecologic surgeon and anesthesia assessment by an individual anesthesiologist or in the anesthesia preoperative clinic
   c. Cleansing of the lower colon by a preoperative enema
   d. Use of vaginal estrogen cream in postmenopausal women undergoing vaginal surgery
   e. Use of gonadotropin-releasing hormone agonist for 2-3 months before hysteroscopic resection of submucous uterine leiomyoma
9. All of the following statements regarding preoperative patient preparation are true EXCEPT
   a. A full bowel prep should be carried out on all gynecologic surgeries
   b. Pelvic cleansing should be accomplished before all pelvic or abdominal surgeries
   c. Universal precautions should be used in all gynecologic surgeries
   d. Hepatitis B vaccination is recommended for all physicians accomplishing gynecologic surgeries
   e. In those gynecologic surgeries in which hair removal is deemed necessary, hair clipping, rather than hair shaving, is recommended just before surgery.

CHAPTER 11

1. Closing the subcutaneous space decreases the rate of superficial wound infection.
   a. True
   b. False
2. A 40-year-old woman is diagnosed by ultrasound with a left tuboovarian complex (6 × 6 cm). An open left salpingo-oophorectomy is performed without complications. On postoperative day 2, the patient reports pain at the incision site, and her temperature is noted to be 38.1° C (100.6° F). Examination and gentle probing of the wound show purulent drainage with an intact fascia. Along with antibiotic therapy, the next appropriate step in the management of this postoperative infection is:
   a. Return to the operating room for a thorough examination of the wound and fascial plane under general anesthesia.
   b. Open the wound widely to allow drainage and debridement of necrotic tissue, then cleanse the wound thoroughly with povidone-iodine before reclosing the wound.
   c. Open the wound widely and debride necrotic tissue, then insert a Penrose drain at the infected site before reclosing the wound.
   d. Open the wound widely to allow drainage and debridement of necrotic tissue, then apply wet-to-dry packing until the wound closes by secondary intention.
3. The most common site of surgical glove perforation during surgery is:
   a. Index finger of the left hand of the surgeon
   b. Index finger of the left hand of the first assistant
   c. Index finger of the right hand of the surgeon
   d. Index finger of the right hand of the first assistant
4. A 28-year-old woman was considered for prophylactic bilateral salpingo-oophorectomy (BSO) because of a strong family history of ovarian carcinoma and also personal history of positive BRCA1 gene. Her past medical history is significant for an allergy to penicillin. Which of the following AB regimens will be recommended for her prophylactic coverage?
   a. Metronidazole
   b. Levaquin
   c. Gentamycin
   d. Vancomycin
5. The recommended treatment for postoperative septic thrombophlebitis is:
   a. Heparin therapy until therapeutic International Normalized Ratio (INR), then continue Coumadin or Lovenox for at least 6 months
   b. Antibiotics plus heparin therapy until therapeutic INR, then continue Coumadin or Lovenox for at least 6 months
   c. Heparin and antibiotics for total of 7 to 10 days; no need for long-term anticoagulation therapy
   d. Antibiotics and heparin until afebrile for 24 to 48 hours, then discontinue antibiotics but continue anticoagulative therapy for at least 6 months

CHAPTER 12

1. Adult respiratory distress syndrome is characterized by:
   a. Narrowing of the alveolar-arterial O_2 gradient
   b. Supplemental oxygen usually able to maintain systemic oxygen saturation (arterial PaO_2 over 65 mm Hg)
   c. Intrapulmonary shunting
   d. Increased pulmonary compliance
   e. Increased functional residual capacity
2. Initial manifestations of early reversible shock include:
   a. Reduced cardiac output
   b. An increase in the systemic vascular resistance
   c. Cold, clammy skin
   d. Disorientation
   e. Oliguria
3. Platelet transfusion is indicated:
   a. For every 4 units of packed red cells transfused
   b. Whenever the platelet count falls below 50,000 μg/dL
   c. For persistent bleeding consistent with coagulopathy
   d. For platelet counts below 100,000 μg/dL before surgery

e. For persistent bleeding for coagulopathy following fresh frozen plasma replacement

4. At 5 to 12 μg/kg/min doses, dopamine has which of the following predominant effects?
   a. Maximizes cerebral, coronary artery, and renal blood flow
   b. α-adrenergic effects predominate
   c. β1-adrenergic effects predominate
   d. β2-adrenergic effects predominate
   e. Inotropic and vasoconstrictive effects
5. Which of the following characterizes dobutamine?
   a. Is an indirect acting inotropic agent
   b. Has both β1- and β2-adrenergic effects
   c. Reduces afterload by stimulation of β1-adrenergic receptors
   d. Increases O_2 consumption
   e. Causes clinically significant tachycardia
6. Following an uneventful total abdominal hysterectomy for symptomatic uterine leiomyomata, a 47-year-old, otherwise healthy patient is seen on morning rounds 24 hours after surgery. The estimated operative blood loss was approximately 1,500 mL. Current vital signs reveal that she is afebrile, has a blood pressure of 110/80 (consistent with her preoperative blood pressure); she does not appear to be in distress. Orthostatics reveal a positive tilt test. Her post-op hemoglobin, checked 24 hours after surgery, is 8 mg/dL. The best management initial treatment for this patient is:
   a. Packed red blood cells (1–2 units)
   b. Crystalloid infusion (1–2 L)
   c. Colloid solution (50–100 mL 25% albumin)
   d. Central venous catheterization
   e. Observation
7. A 22-year-old G0 presents to the emergency room with symptoms of diffuse abdominal pain. She reports that she was treated last year for pelvic inflammatory disease. On admission, her temperature is 38.4°C, her blood pressure is 100/65 mm Hg, and her heart rate is 90. Orthostatics reveal minimal change in blood pressure sitting and reclining. Abdominal examination reveals diffuse tenderness without rebound or guarding, and a bimanual exam reveals a left-sided mass. Laboratory investigation reveals a negative β-hCG titer; a white blood cell count is 21,000 with 90% mature segmental neutrophils. There is a 5-cm complex adnexal mass on ultrasound and no cul-de-sac fluid. Of the following, which is the most appropriate next step?
   a. Immediate intravenous antibiotics
   b. Immediate exploratory laparotomy
   c. Hospitalization
   d. Plain films of the abdomen and pelvis
   e. Blood and cervical cultures
8. Oliguric prerenal azotemia is characterized by:
   a. Hyponatremic hyperchloremic metabolic alkalosis
   b. Urine-plasma creatinine (40 mEq/L/24 hr
   c. Urine sodium excretion (20 mEq/L/24 hr
   d. Fractional excretion of sodium >1%
9. A 46-year-old woman underwent a difficult abdominal hysterectomy and bilateral salpingo-oophorectomy for endometriosis, and the estimated blood loss was 950 mL. Twenty-four hours later, she is anxious. Vital signs reveal a heart rate of 110 that increases to 125 on sitting, and her reclining blood pressure, 110/80 mm Hg, is 105/70 mm Hg in the sitting position. Over the past 8-hour shift, her urine output was 250 mL. These findings are most consistent with which class of shock?
   a. Class I
   b. Class II
   c. Class III
   d. Class IV
   e. Class V
10. Classically, the order of organ system loss in patients with multiorgan failure syndrome is:
    a. Lung, liver, gastrointestinal (GI), kidney
    b. Liver, lung, GI, kidney
    c. GI, kidney, liver, lung
    d. Kidney, GI, lung, liver
    e. Kidney, lung, liver, GI
11. Which of the following statements characterize the mechanism of action of an intact renin-angiotensinogen system?
    a. Angiotensin I is an active polypeptide.
    b. Angiotensin II is a potent vasoconstrictor.
    c. Aldosterone along with antidiuretic hormone promotes water and sodium excretion.
    d. Angiotensin II decreases venous return, stroke volume, and cardiac output.
    e. Increased sympathetic activation causes renin release.
12. A 58-year-old woman was admitted with fever and severe neutropenia 10 days after chemotherapy. Approximately 48 hours later, she continues to have a low-grade fever (37.9° C) and an absolute neutrophil count (ANC) of 500 mm^3. She has an indwelling vascular catheter, with no appreciable erythema or discharge around the catheter site. She is asymptomatic otherwise, and physical examination is unremarkable. Blood cultures are positive for Gram-positive cocci. What is the next logical step in her care?
    a. Empiric therapy with cefepime, ceftazidime, and imipenem
    b. Removal of the indwelling catheter
    c. Identification of etiology of the anaerobic organism before modifying antibiotic treatment
    d. Vancomycin antibiotic therapy
    e. Piperacillin-taxobactam antibiotic therapy
13. A 59-year-old patient 12 weeks after surgical staging, hysterectomy, and bilateral salpingo-oophorectomy is receiving cycle 2 of carboplatin and paclitaxel chemotherapy for stage III, grade 3 endometrial adenocarcinoma. Pretreatment complete blood count (CBC) reveals a serum Hb of 8.8 and hematocrit of 27 mg%. The patient has well-controlled hypertension and diabetes. Her blood pressure and pulse are in the normal range. She is able to perform most activities of daily living, but acknowledges chronic fatigue. In this clinical setting, the best first step in the management of her anemia is:
    a. Transfuse with 2 units of packed blood cells.
    b. Discontinue chemotherapy and begin pelvic radiation therapy.
    c. Initiate supplementation with oral folic acid and monthly B_{12} injections.
    d. Administer an erythropoietic stimulating agent.
    e. Give iron supplementation.

CHAPTER 13

1. What suture is the most appropriate for closure of first- and second-degree episiotomies?
   a. Plain catgut
   b. Chromic catgut

c. Polyglactin 910 Rapide
d. Polyglactin 910/Polyglycolic acid
e. There are no significant advantages of one of these sutures over the other.

2. What is the most common cause of fascial dehiscence?
a. Suture knot failure
b. Suture breakage
c. Suture pulling through fascia
d. Wound infection

CHAPTER 14

1. Which transverse abdominal incision is a muscle-cutting incision?
a. Pfannenstiel
b. Küstner
c. Maylard
d. Gridiron

2. The posterior rectus sheath, below the arcuate line, increases the strength of the anterior abdominal wall.
a. True
b. False

3. Which aponeuroses contribute to the posterior rectus sheath?
a. External and internal obliques
b. External oblique and transversalis
c. Internal oblique and transversalis
d. Transversalis and linea alba

4. If one used a Pfannenstiel incision to enter the abdomen for a gynecologic surgery, but found that the incision was inadequate for completion of that surgery, which is the best surgical option to improve visualization?
a. Transect the rectus muscles, similarly done when performing a Maylard incision.
b. Transect the rectus muscles at their insertion, similarly done when performing a Cherney incision.
c. Make a vertical incision, in the midline of the abdomen, bisecting the transverse skin incision and separating the rectus muscles.
d. Separate the anterior abdominal wall fascia from the overlying subcutaneous fat to the level of the umbilicus and make a vertical incision in the fascia, separating the rectus muscles, similarly done when performing a Küstner incision.

5. Which of the incisions listed below is *not* routinely used for an extraperitoneal approach to access the retroperitoneal structures?
a. Sunrise
b. J-shaped incision
c. Gridiron
d. Maylard

6. On average, how many days postoperatively does an evisceration occur?
a. 2
b. 4
c. 6
d. 8
e. 10

7. An inferior epigastric artery arises from which major vessel?
a. Internal iliac artery
b. External iliac artery
c. Femoral artery
d. Hypogastric artery

CHAPTER 15

1. To reduce the risk of unintentional burn when using monopolar electrosurgical devices, one should:
a. Use an energy current with a highly interrupted sinusoidal wave pattern (COAG).
b. Use a contemporary electrosurgical generator that uses a "floating ground" circuitry system.
c. Use a return electrode (ground) of large contact area to ensure a low-current density.
d. Use a higher voltage to concentrate the energy onto the intended tissue target.

2. To minimize risks of electrosurgical injury during laparoscopic surgery, all of the following practices are recommended EXCEPT:
a. If metal laparoscopic trocars are used, a plastic insulating collar should be used.
b. When changing from a flat-puddle electrode to a needle-point electrode, the power should be decreased.
c. With bipolar instruments, the CUT current should be used.
d. An in-line ammeter should be used with bipolar instruments to insure that coagulation of the tissue in the grasper is complete before the tissue bundle is cut.

3. While coagulating a small diameter bleeder clamped in a hemostat during an emergency laparotomy, the assistant surgeon's hand is burned where she holds the hemostats. This was due to:
a. Using CUT instead of COAG
b. A small hole in the assistant's glove
c. Using a return electrode with a low-current density
d. Activating the current before making contact with the clamp

4. Compared with desiccation, fulguration:
a. Is a desirable electrosurgical modality for venous bleeding, such as oozing from a muscle
b. Produces less necrosis and deep-tissue injury
c. Generates an energy current that avoids "spraying" of the tissue with electricity and injury to the adjacent structures
d. Is better for coaptive coagulation of an isolated bleeding vessel

5. When using a wire loop for a loop electrosurgical excision procedure (LEEP), all of the following are true EXCEPT:
a. Larger loop electrodes should be used with higher power settings to provide the same tissue effects as a smaller diameter loop.
b. Faster movement of the wire through the cervical tissue causes more thermal injury and makes it more difficult for the pathologist to interpret.
c. The power should be applied to the loop electrode before touching the cervical tissue.
d. During coagulation of bleeders in the cone bed, the ball electrode should not touch the tissue, allowing the sparks to arc to the surface.

CHAPTER 16

1. The following lasers can be transmitted through quartz fibers except:
a. Nd:YAG
b. CO_2
c. KTP
d. Ho:YAG

2. As the orbital distance of the electron from the nucleus of an atom increases, the energy level decreases.
   a. True
   b. False
3. Q-switching a laser produces the following except:
   a. Increase in pulse time
   b. Increase in peak power
   c. Minimalization of adjacent tissue effect
   d. Cutting of tissue with lower water content
4. One 1 joule equals 1 watt applied for 10 seconds.
   a. True
   b. False
5. Vaporization of tissue with laser occurs:
   a. Between 57°C and 100°C
   b. Above 100°C
   c. Above 100°F
   d. By conduction of the heat away from the laser impact site
6. Laser energy is unique in that it is uniform throughout the cross section diameter of the beam.
   a. True
   b. False
7. The most vulnerable organ to be damaged by laser is:
   a. Skin
   b. Eye
8. The best carbon dioxide laser backstop is:
   a. Glass
   b. Pyrex
   c. Quartz
   d. Water

CHAPTER 17

1. The most cost-effective trocar/sleeve system is which of the following?
   a. Reusable
   b. Disposable
   c. Reposable
   d. Suposable
2. The term *laser* is an acronym for light amplification by spontaneous emissions of radiation.
   a. True
   b. False
3. The inferior epigastric artery is a direct branch of what major blood vessel?
   a. Internal iliac artery
   b. External iliac artery
   c. Femoral artery
   d. Aorta
4. Which nerve injury is most commonly associated with placement of lateral trocars during laparoscopy?
   a. Obturator nerve
   b. Ilioinguinal nerve
   c. Sciatic nerve
   d. Lateral femoral cutaneous nerve
5. A 52-year-old woman presents to your office 1 week status post a difficult laparoscopic sacral colpopexy requiring 6 hours of surgery. A thorough history and physical exam reveal that she has an inability to dorsiflex or evert her foot. In addition, she has a loss of sensation to the lateral calf and dorsum of the foot. You find that she does have sensation in her toes and the plantar surface of her foot. Her injury is most consistent with which of the following?
   a. Injury to femoral nerve, excessive flexion of the hips with Allen stirrups
   b. Compression of the common peroneal nerve, compression by Allen stirrups
   c. Compression of the tibial nerve, compression by Allen stirrups
   d. Entrapment of pudendal nerve, sutures entrapping the nerve
6. The coagulation button on the cautery is actually an extremely "damped" or modified form of the cutting wave current.
   a. True
   b. False
7. The open technique for laparoscopy has been shown to result in a statistically significant decrease in deaths during laparoscopy when compared with the Veress needle technique.
   a. True
   b. False

CHAPTER 18

1. Choose the *incorrect* statement.
   a. Hysteroscopes are available with 0-degree straight on or 30-degree fore-oblique views.
   b. The telescope is composed of the eyepiece, the barrel, and the objective lens.
   c. Three types of light generators are available: tungsten, metal halide, and xenon.
   d. The tungsten light source is superior to other sources.
2. Choose the *incorrect* statement.
   a. The diagnostic hysteroscope is 4 to 5 mm in diameter.
   b. The operative hysteroscope is 15 mm in diameter.
   c. The operating electrodes include a ball, barrel, and cutting loop.
   d. Most resectoscopes are equipped with a 30-degree telescope.
3. Which of the following are available as accessory instruments for hysteroscopy?
   a. Grasping forceps
   b. Scissors
   c. Biopsy forceps
   d. Monopolar electrode
   e. All of the above
4. Which of the following is the distending medium of choice for office hysteroscopy?
   a. Carbon dioxide
   b. Hyskon
   c. Normal saline
   d. Glycine 1.5%
5. Which of the following should not be used with monopolar cautery?
   a. Carbon dioxide
   b. Hyskon
   c. Normal saline
   d. Glycine 1.5%
6. Which of the following should not be instilled in an amount greater than 500 mL because of its hyperosmotic activity?
   a. Carbon dioxide
   b. Hyskon
   c. Normal saline
   d. Glycine 1.5%

7. Because of its hypoosmolarity, while using which of the following should caution be taken when a fluid deficit of greater than or equal to 500 mL occurs?
   a. Carbon dioxide
   b. Hyskon
   c. Normal saline
   d. Glycine 1.5%
8. Choose the *incorrect* statement.
   a. Hysteroscopy should be performed during the luteal phase for best visualization of the endometrial cavity.
   b. Routine cervical dilatation should be avoided at the time of hysteroscopy.
   c. Uterine position should be determined by pelvic examination before beginning hysteroscopy.
   d. The hysteroscope should be advanced into the uterine cavity under direct visualization.
9. Simultaneous laparoscopy should be performed with all of the following hysteroscopic procedures EXCEPT:
   a. Metroplasty
   b. Resection of uterine synechiae
   c. Cannulation of the fallopian tube
   d. Endometrial ablation
10. Which is the most common complication of operative hysteroscopy?
   a. Infection
   b. Uterine perforation
   c. Carbon dioxide embolism
   d. Bleeding

CHAPTER 19

1. All of the following conditions increase the risk of intraoperative hemorrhage EXCEPT:
   a. Obesity
   b. Hepatitis B
   c. von Willibrand disease
   d. Pelvic malignancy
2. Which of the following is *not recommended* when trying to control significant bleeding in the area of the uterine artery at the time of hysterectomy?
   a. Use large figure-of-eight sutures so the suture will not cut through the tissue.
   b. Obtain good exposure with retraction, suction, and good lighting.
   c. Control the bleeding with pressure until adequate preparations have been made to identify and control the bleeding.
   d. Do a cystoscopy or open the bladder after controlling the bleeding to be sure the ureter has not been compromised.
3. Which of the following agents or techniques are *not* used to control pelvic bleeding?
   a. Microfibrillar collagen
   b. Fibrin glue
   c. Thumbtacks
   d. Lamellar platelets
4. The risk of which infection is *greatest* with blood transfusion?
   a. Hepatitis B
   b. Hepatitis C
   c. Human immunodeficiency virus (HIV)
   d. Human T-lymphotropic virus (HTLV)
5. Hypogastric artery ligation helps control pelvic bleeding by:
   a. Ligating the feeder vessels of the pelvic blood supply
   b. Reducing the pulse pressure
   c. Increasing pelvic thrombokinase
   d. Infarction of the uterus
6. The risk of fetal growth restriction is doubled in a pregnancy that occurs after bilateral hyopgastric artery ligation.
   a. True
   b. False
7. In a 150-lb. woman (68 kg), a 15% blood loss would be approximately 680 cc.
   a. True
   b. False
8. When using hypogastric artery ligation to control pelvic hemorrhage, all of the following are true EXCEPT:
   a. The right-angle clamp should be passed from lateral to medial under the artery.
   b. The hypogastric artery should be tied but not cut.
   c. Only the posterior division of the hypogastric artery should be ligated.
   d. The hypogastric arteries should be ligated bilaterally.
9. The risk of HIV infection due to blood transfusion in the United States is currently about:
   a. 1 in 2000
   b. 1 in 20,000
   c. 1 in 200,000
   d. 1 in 2 million
10. Venous bleeding is usually more easily controlled than arterial bleeding.
   a. True
   b. False

CHAPTER 20

1. What is the best therapy for a couple reporting infertility whose only finding is painless endometriosis in the female partner?
2. In a couple found to require *in vitro* fertilization (IVF) because of a male factor, it is found that the female partner age 35 has six intramural fibroids, the largest of which is 4 cm in diameter. Is pre-IVF treatment needed for these fibroids?
3. In a couple reporting infertility, it is found that the male partner has a sperm count of 1.5 million with 4% normal forms by the strict morphology classification. The female partner age 31 is found to have bilateral asymptomatic hydrosalpinges 2 cm in diameter. What therapy is required?
4. A female age 27 without children is found to have Hodgkin disease requiring intensive chemotherapy. What advice can a gynecologist offer her about options for preserving future reproduction?

CHAPTER 21

1. What is the most commonly isolated organisms in patients with pelvic inflammatory disease (PID)?
   a. *Escherichia coli*
   b. *Chlamydia trachomatis*
   c. *Neisseria gonorrhoeae*
   d. *Mycoplasma hominis*

2. Which of the following is NOT a contraindication to hysterosalpingography (HSG)?
   a. Possible pregnancy
   b. Undiagnosed uterine bleeding
   c. Lower genital tract infection
   d. Known tubal obstruction
3. Which of the following conditions can be managed by tubal cannulation?
   a. Tubal plugs
   b. Obliterative fibrosis
   c. Mild synechiae
   d. Cornual spasm
4. Patients with tubal factor infertility may achieve pregnancy through reconstructive surgery and/or IVF. Which is NOT an advantage of reconstructive surgery?
   a. Multiple cycles in which to achieve conception
   b. Opportunity to have more than one pregnancy
   c. Other pelvic factors that can be assessed, such as endometriosis
   d. Reduced risk of ectopic pregnancy
5. What is NOT a principle of microsurgical technique that minimizes tissue trauma?
   a. To use cautery during dissection to facilitate hemostasis
   b. To prevent foreign body contamination of the peritoneal cavity
   c. To minimize adjacent tissue damage
   d. To identify proper cleavage planes
6. Salpingostomy for cases of mild and moderate distal tubal disease is associated with excellent intrauterine pregnancy rates. What factor is considered in classifying tubal disease as mild, moderate, or severe?
   a. Proximal tubal thickness
   b. Endosalpingiosis of ampulla
   c. Presence of peritubal adhesions
   d. Nature of the tubal endothelium
7. What is a predictor of intrauterine pregnancy after tubotubal reanastomosis for reversal of sterilization?
   a. Duration of infertility
   b. Length of reconstructed tube
   c. Parity of woman
   d. History of PID

CHAPTER 22

1. Which of the following have been proposed as possible mechanisms for development of endometriosis?
   a. Retrograde menstruation and direct implantation
   b. Coelomic metaplasia
   c. Vascular dissemination
   d. Alterations in cellular immunity
   e. All of the above
2. Choose the incorrect statement.
   a. Laparoscopy provides inferior visualization of the posterior cul-de-sac compared with laparotomy.
   b. Conservative resection of endometriosis by laparotomy is most valuable in cases of extensive pelvic adhesions or endometriomas larger than 5 cm.
   c. Preoperative sigmoidoscopy and intravenous pyelography (IVP) are recommended in patients with symptoms suggestive of deeply invasive endometriosis.
   d. Surgery is successful in relieving pain symptoms in a high percentage of women and offers a better prognosis for pregnancy in cases of advanced disease.
3. Choose the correct statement.
   a. The classic triad associated with endometriosis includes infertility, dyspareunia, and dysmenorrhea.
   b. Pain typically does not correlate to steroid hormone fluctuations.
   c. Pain associated with endometriosis is only weakly associated to the depth of infiltration of the peritoneal surfaces.
   d. Surgical castration does not decrease pain in most patients.
4. Choose the correct statement.
   a. The rate of recurrence of pelvic pain and dysmenorrhea is equivalent for patients whose endometriomas are managed by cystectomy as compared with those undergoing fenestration and coagulation.
   b. Uterine suspension is efficacious as an adjunct in the treatment of endometriosis-associated pelvic pain.
   c. Presacral neurectomy, or division of the superior hypogastric plexus, is useful as an adjunctive procedure to reduce midline pelvic pain and dysmenorrhea in women with endometriosis.
   d. There is no difference in pain persistence or recurrence following laparoscopic resection or unipolar cauterization of endometriotic implants less than 1 cm in depth.
5. Choose the correct statement pertaining to the American Society for Reproductive Medicine (ASRM) classification of endometriosis.
   a. Endometriosis lesions are categorized as red, blue, and black. The percentage of surface involvement of each implant type is to be documented.
   b. The ASRM defines complete cul-de-sac obliteration as when no peritoneum is visible below the uterosacral ligaments.
   c. The classification system incorporates a scoring system for implants involving the intestinal and bladder serosa.
   d. Application of the classification system is very useful in predicting postoperative pain recurrence and fecundity rates.

CHAPTER 23

1. Match the diagnosis in Column A with the clinical finding in Column B.

A	B
1. Granuloma inguinale	a. Bubos
2. Chancroid	b. *Chlamydia trachomatis*
3. *Mulluscum contagiosum*	c. Donovan bodies
4. *Lymphogranuloma venereum*	d. Pox virus

2. A 58-year-old woman presents with the symptom of burning vulvar pain. Her exam shows an erythematous area involving the left posterior vulva, and biopsy confirms the diagnosis of Paget disease. You would recommend what therapy initially?
   a. Ultrapotent corticosteroid ointment (Clobetasol 0.05%)
   b. Topical testosterone cream (2%)
   c. Partial vulvectomy
   d. Total simple vulvectomy
3. A horseshoe-shaped perineoplasty excising the skin of the posterior vaginal introitus has been reported to effectively cure 75% to 90% of patients with vulvar vestibulitis.
   a. True
   b. False
4. A 35-year-old woman has a small 1.5-cm red area on the right anterior vulva. A 4-mm Key's punch biopsy is read as

vulvar intraepithelial neoplasia (VIN). Which of the following treatments is *not* appropriate?
a. CO_2 laser vaporization
b. Calverton Ultrasonic surgical aspirator (CUSA)
c. Simple vulvectomy
d. Wide local excision

CHAPTER 24

1. The hymen:
 a. Is usually imperforate during embryonic life
 b. Becomes patent when canalization of the most caudal portion of the vaginal plate at the urogenital sinus occurs
 c. Most frequently has a folded shape with an eccentric orifice in the newborn
 d. Is found to be imperforate in 1% of newborns
2. Choose the incorrect answer.
 a. Ambiguous external genitalia are remarkably constant in appearance regardless of etiology.
 b. Most patients have a high (suprasphincteric) urethral vaginal connection.
 c. Reconstruction must be timed properly to allow easy identification of all structures while preventing psychologic stress to the patient.
 d. Most hermaphrodites reared as girls do have a vagina or vaginal pouch.
3. Choose the incorrect answer.
 a. In the group of patients undergoing reconstruction of the external genitalia, 87% required further vaginal reconstructive surgery to allow intercourse.
 b. The most common long-term problem following reconstruction procedures is intravaginal stenosis.
 c. Vaginoplasty should be performed in infancy to prevent vaginal stenosis.
 d. In patients who underwent clitoridectomy, 29% reported no orgasms.
4. Classic bladder exstrophy is characterized by all of the following EXCEPT:
 a. Male-to-female ratio of 2:1
 b. Absence of anterior abdominal wall
 c. Absence of the posterior wall of the bladder exposing the ureteral orifices
 d. Poorly defined bladder neck and urethra
 e. Wide separation of the pubic symphysis
5. Other possible anomalies associated with bladder exstrophy include:
 a. Bifid clitoris
 b. Rectal prolapse
 c. Imperforate anus
 d. Renal agenesis
 e. All of the above
6. Choose the incorrect statement about vaginal carcinoma.
 a. The average age at presentation is 35 years.
 b. Vaginal carcinoma must meet specific International Federation of Obstetrics and Gynecology (FIGO) criteria to be considered a primary vaginal carcinoma.
 c. Vaginal carcinoma composes less than 2% of gynecologic malignancies.
 d. Clinicians must find the urethra, cervix, and vulva to be histologically negative to diagnose primary vaginal carcinoma.
7. Choose the incorrect statement about diethylstilbestrol (DES).
 a. DES is a nonsteroidal estrogenic hormone that was used in patients with a history of recurrent pregnancy loss until 1970.
 b. The incidence of vaginal adenocarcinoma in young women exposed to DES in utero is 0.14 to 1.4 pe 1,000.
 c. Seventy-five percent of women exposed to DES *in utero* have anatomic abnormalities.
 d. Vaginal adenosis has been found in 34% to 90% of women exposed to DES *in utero*.
8. Choose the incorrect answer pertaining to vaginal carcinoma.
 a. Stage 0 disease can be treated with surgery, carbon dioxide laser, or 5-fluorouracil cream.
 b. Stage 1 disease lesions can be treated with radiation therapy or total abdominal hysterectomy.
 c. Stage 2 or 3 lesions are treated with radiotherapy.
 d. Stage 4 lesions are treated with pelvic exenteration or radiotherapy.
9. Which of the following is not a possible cause of urethral diverticulum?
 a. *Neisseria gonorrhoeae* infection
 b. Trauma associated with childbirth
 c. Urethral stone
 d. Surgical trauma
 e. Infection of the Bartholin gland
10. Choose the incorrect answer.
 a. Dysuria, frequency, urgency, and hematuria occur in 85% to 90% of patients with urethral diverticula.
 b. Urethral diverticula frequently cause a palpable lump in the vagina.
 c. Most urethral diverticula are located in the proximal urethra.
 d. Urethral diverticula can be diagnosed with cystourethroscopy, positive pressure urethrography, or voiding cystourethrography.

CHAPTER 25

1. The müllerian anomalies associated with ipsilateral renal agenesis include all of the following EXCEPT:
 a. Unilateral vaginal obstruction
 b. Septate uterus
 c. Unilateral obstruction of a cavity of a double uterus
 d. Unicornuate uterus with a noncommunicating horn
2. Which of the following is true regarding vaginal development?
 a. The vagina develops from both the müllerian ducts and the urogenital sinus.
 b. A transverse septum is more common in the lower or distal vagina.
 c. Partial vaginal agenesis has a high incidence of associated renal anomalies.
 d. Abnormal development of the vagina never accompanies other anomalies.
3. All of the following are characteristics of women with müllerian agenesis EXCEPT:
 a. Genetic sex is female (XX)
 b. Congenital absence of a normal uterus and vagina
 c. Impaired ovarian function
 d. Frequent association of other anomalies, including skeletal, urologic, and renal

4. Evaluation of patients with müllerian agenesis should include all of the following EXCEPT:
   a. Psychologic support
   b. Genetic evaluation
   c. Ultrasonography or magnetic resonance imaging (MRI)
   d. Complete physical examination
   e. Laparoscopy
5. Which of these important issues in successful nonsurgical creation of a neovagina is true?
   a. Nonsurgical creation of a neovagina is not appropriate as a first-line approach.
   b. Greater than 90% patients have been shown to achieve anatomic and functional success by vaginal dilation.
   c. A "buddy" support system is not helpful in achieving success with vaginal dilation.
   d. Vaginal dilation should be initiated in any age patient, even in prepubertal girls.
6. According to Sir Archibald McIndoe, the important principles in successful surgical creation of a neovagina include all EXCEPT:
   a. Dissection of an adequate space between the rectum and bladder
   b. Inlay split-thickness skin grafting
   c. Continued and prolonged dilatation during the contractile phase of healing
   d. Adequate preoperative dilatation
7. Which of the following is true regarding cervical dysgenesis?
   a. Cervical agenesis is the most common müllerian anomaly.
   b. There is only one type of cervical dysgenesis.
   c. Creation of a passage between the uterus and vagina is a simple, highly successful procedure.
   d. Conservative management, with hormonal suppression of endometrial stimulation, is appropriate for young patients.
8. Lateral fusion disorders of the müllerian ducts include all of the following EXCEPT:
   a. Bicornuate uterus
   b. Septate uterus
   c. Didelphic uterus
   d. Rokitansky syndrome
9. The müllerian anomaly associated with the most reproductive success is:
   a. Septate uterus
   b. Bicornuate uterus
   c. Didelphic uterus
   d. Unicornuate uterus
10. Benefits of hysteroscopic resection of a uterine septum include all of the following EXCEPT:
   a. The potential for a vaginal delivery with future pregnancies
   b. A prolonged postoperative recovery period
   c. Similar success as an abdominal metroplasty
   d. That transcervical lysis may also be used to repair a complete septate uterus

CHAPTER 26

1. The most likely etiology of perimenarchal abnormal uterine bleeding is:
   a. Endometrial polyp
   b. Anovulatory bleeding
   c. Von Willebrand disease
   d. Endometrial hyperplasia
   e. Idiopathic thrombocytopenic purpura
2. Acute control of heavy abnormal uterine bleeding can be accomplished by all of the following except:
   a. Oral contraceptive pills
   b. Intravenous estogens
   c. Oral progestins
   d. Gonadotropin-releasing hormone (GnRH) analog injection
   e. Dilatation and curettage
3. Sonohysterography is best performed:
   a. During menstruation
   b. In the follicular phase
   c. Near ovulation
   d. In the luteal phase
   e. In anovulatory cycles
4. Hemostasis in a bleeding endometrium depends on which of the following?
   a. Thrombus plugs in superficial vessels
   b. Vasoconstriction of spiral arterioles
   c. Endometrial collapse with compression of bleeding vessels
   d. All of the above
5. A 26-year-old female patient reports menometrorrhagia unresponsive to oral contraceptive therapy. The best next step in her evaluation is:
   a. Endometrial biopsy
   b. Dilatation and curettage
   c. Sonohysterography
   d. MRI of pelvis
   e. Laparoscopy

CHAPTER 27

1. Techniques to reduce the likelihood of complications when the Veress needle is inserted into the abdominal cavity include all of the following EXCEPT:
   a. Directing the insertion of the needle in the midline toward the hollow of the sacrum or uterine fundus
   b. Elevating the abdominal wall before insertion
   c. Inserting the needle with the port closed
   d. Infiltration and aspiration of sterile fluid through the needle after insertion
   e. Elevating the abdominal wall after insertion to demonstrate negative intraperitoneal pressure
2. Which of the following methods of laparoscopic tubal occlusion would be most appropriate for a woman with thickened fallopian tubes or dense pelvic adhesions?
   a. Bipolar coagulation
   b. Spring clip application
   c. Filshie clip application
   d. Silicone rubber band application
3. Which of the following techniques for bipolar coagulation is least helpful in reducing the likelihood of pregnancy after the procedure?
   a. Avoiding coagulation of the proximal 2 cm of tube
   b. Coagulation of at least three contiguous areas
   c. Direct observation of tubal blanching and swelling
   d. Use of an optical flow meter
   e. Use of the cutting waveform

4. Which of the following conditions is less common in a woman who has undergone tubal sterilization than in a woman whose partner has undergone vasectomy?
   a. Ectopic pregnancy
   b. Hysterectomy
   c. Ovarian cancer
   d. Regret that sterilization was performed

CHAPTER 28

1. Gonadal primordia are of what embryologic developmental layer?
   a. Ectoderm
   b. Mesoderm
   c. Endoderm
   d. Trophectoderm
2. Which of the following is true regarding testicular determining factor?
   a. It is an HY cell surface antigen.
   b. It is located on the X chromosome.
   c. It is a growth factor.
   d. The bipotential gonad develops into a testicle through a default pathway because of the absence of testis-determining factor (TDF).
3. Meiosis begins at what gestational age (weeks)?
   a. 10
   b. 12
   c. 16
   d. 24
4. Which of the following is correct regarding ovarian nerve supply?
   a. It is parasympathetic only.
   b. It is sympathetic only.
   c. It contains both motor and sensory parasympathetic and sympathetic nerves.
   d. It is autonomic only.
5. Based on the Rotterdam Consensus for polycystic ovarian syndrome (PCOS), which of the following is true regarding PCOS?
   a. It is a clinical diagnosis.
   b. Criteria to establish the diagnosis include oligoovulation, clinical evidence for hyperandrogenemia, and polycystic-appearing ovaries on ultrasound.
   c. It begins in adolescence.
   d. All of the above

CHAPTER 29

1. When a patient reports pain in response to a gentle touch, this is an example of:
   a. Hyperalgesia
   b. Neuropathic pain
   c. Allodynia
   d. Myofascial pain
2. The prevailing theory of pain perception today is:
   a. Cartesian theory
   b. Neuromatrix theory
   c. Gate control theory
   d. Neuroplasticity theory
3. Irritable bowel syndrome, interstitial cystitis, and vulvar vestibulitis may all be examples of:
   a. Psychosomatic disorders
   b. Neuropathic pain
   c. Somatosensory disorders
   d. Immune deficiency disorders

CHAPTER 30

1. The Centers for Disease Control and Prevention (CDC) recommended treatment for patients hospitalized with pelvic inflammatory disease (PID) include:
   a. Intravenous metronidazole plus gentamicin
   b. Intravenous clindamycin plus gentamicin
   c. Intravenous ceftriaxone plus metronidazole
   d. Intravenous ceftriaxone plus oral ciprofloxacin
2. A young female patient with pelvic pain without an elevated white count or a fever cannot have PID.
   a. True
   b. False
3. The most common bacteria isolated from pus collected from the cul-de-sac in a woman with acute salpingitis is:
   a. *Neisseria gonorrhoeae*
   b. *Chlamydia trachomatis*
   c. *Trichomonas vaginalis*
   d. A polymicrobial mixture of aerobes and anaerobes
4. The CDC-recommended outpatient treatment regimens for PID include:
   a. Oral ciprofloxacin plus metronidazole
   b. Oral clindamycin plus doxycycline
   c. Intramuscular ceftriaxone plus oral metronidazole
   d. Oral ofloxacin plus metronidazole
5. Laparoscopic confirmation of PID does not need to be discussed or offered if a patient has had a previous appendectomy.
   a. True
   b. False

CHAPTER 31

1. Typical characteristics of uterine leiomyomata include all of the following EXCEPT:
   a. Typical locations are subserosal, submucosal, and intramural in nature.
   b. The most common change is hyaline degeneration.
   c. Red or carneous degeneration is never seen during pregnancy.
   d. A subserosal, pedunculated myoma may outgrow its blood supply.
2. Which degenerative changes are the least common?
   a. Hyaline degeneration
   b. Red or carneous degeneration
   c. Necrosis
   d. Sarcomatous degeneration
3. Which of the following is true regarding intravenous leiomyomatosis?
   a. The condition is quite common and may be found in as many as 50% patients with leiomyoma.
   b. The tumor behaves clinically as a benign entity.
   c. Wormlike extensions of tumor involve only the ovarian veins.
   d. The most common site of metastases is the brain.
4. In describing the clinical features of leiomyomata, it is important to remember that:
   a. Most leiomyomata are asymptomatic and may not require any treatment.

b. If the uterine size is believed to be greater than 12 weeks, a hysterectomy is recommended.
c. Most women will have an increase in symptomatology after menopause.

5. Hormonal management options for patients with a myomatous uterus may include all of the following EXCEPT:
   a. Mifepristone (RU486)
   b. Danazol
   c. GnRH analogues
   d. Oral contraceptives (30 to 35 pg ethinyl estradiol)
6. Which of the following is a true statement regarding hysteroscopic resection of submucous myomata?
   a. By combining the procedure with endometrial ablation, pregnancy rates are increased.
   b. Menorrhagia is only rarely controlled.
   c. It is recommended to combine laparoscopic guidance with the hysteroscopic procedure.
   d. Success rates are not dependent on the experience or skill of the surgeon.
7. Appropriate candidates for a laparoscopic myomectomy include which of the following?
   a. A postmenopausal patient with incidentally detected myomata on an annual examination
   b. A 34-year-old woman desiring future fertility with two intramural myomas each measuring 3 cm in diameter
   c. A 34-year-old woman desiring future fertility with two submucosal myomas each measuring 3 cm in diameter
   d. A 40-year-old woman who has completed childbearing with a 20-week-size uterus with multiple myomas
8. Methods to control intraoperative blood loss during an abdominal myomectomy may include all of the following EXCEPT:
   a. Preoperative treatment with oral contraceptive pills
   b. Local injection with vasoconstrictive agents
   c. Controlled induced hypotension
   d. Use of a uterine tourniquet
9. Postoperative morbidity commonly associated with an abdominal myomectomy includes all of the following EXCEPT:
   a. Significant blood loss
   b. Intraabdominal adhesion formation
   c. Febrile morbidity
   d. Pulmonary embolus
10. Which of the following statements is true regarding uterine artery embolization?
   a. Most patients report an improvement in menorrhagia and bulk-related symptoms.
   b. The overall success rate with an experienced team of providers is only about 25%.
   c. Less than 1% of patients develop postembolization syndrome with fever and malaise.
   d. The major complication rate approaches 50%.

CHAPTER 32A

1. Common indications for abdominal hysterectomy include all of the following EXCEPT:
   a. Endometriosis
   b. Leiomyoma
   c. Prolapse
   d. Malignancy
   e. Abnormal bleeding
2. The most common technique for hysterectomy in the United States is:
   a. Abdominal hysterectomy
   b. Vaginal hysterectomy
   c. Laparoscopically assisted vaginal hysterectomy
   d. Total laparoscopic hysterectomy
3. Which hysterectomy technique is associated with the fewest complications and most rapid return to full activity?
   a. Abdominal hysterectomy
   b. Vaginal hysterectomy
   c. Laparoscopically assisted vaginal hysterectomy
   d. Total laparoscopic hysterectomy
4. Compared with total abdominal hysterectomy, the documented advantages of supracervical (subtotal) hysterectomy include (check all that apply):
   a. Better postoperative sexual function
   b. A lower incidence of vaginal prolapse
   c. Shorter operative time
   d. Decreased risk of postoperative stress urinary incontinence
5. Bilateral oophorectomy at the time of hysterectomy reduces the risk of breast cancer.
   a. True
   b. False
6. To minimize bleeding, the bladder is dissected off the anterior cervix after the uterine vessels are clamped and ligated.
   a. True
   b. False
7. Ureteral injury is most commonly associated with all of the following EXCEPT:
   a. Previous tubal ligation
   b. Cervical fibroid
   c. Ovarian endometrioma
   d. Bleeding from the uterine artery pedicle
8. The risk of pelvic infections following abdominal hysterectomy has been shown to be reduced by which of these procedures? (Check all that apply).
   a. Vaginal douche with Betadine the night before surgery
   b. Shaving the pubic hair in the operating room before prepping the patient
   c. Prophylactic intravenous antibiotics within 1 hour before surgery
   d. Mechanical bowel prep the night before surgery
   e. Leaving the vaginal cuff open for drainage
9. In a subtotal abdominal hysterectomy, the uterine fundus is amputated *after* the uterine vessels have been ligated.
   a. True
   b. False
10. The mortality rate for abdominal hysterectomy in the United States is approximately:
   a. 1/100 hysterectomies
   b. 1/1,000 hysterectomies
   c. 1/10,000 hysterectomies
   d. 1/100,000 hysterectomies

CHAPTER 32B

1. Patients experience lower morbidity, less pain, more rapid recovery, more rapid return to normal activities, and consumption of fewer health care dollars and resources with what hysterectomy method?
   a. Laparoscopic assisted vaginal hysterectomy (LAVH)
   b. Abdominal hysterectomy

c. Total laparoscopic hysterectomy (TLH)
d. Laparoscopic supracervical hysterectomy (LSH)
e. Vaginal hysterectomy

2. The most limiting factor in selecting the vaginal approach to hysterectomy is:
a. Uterine size >280 g
b. Nulliparity
c. Bituberous diameter (8 cm
d. Comfort and preference with abdominal hysterectomy
e. Previous C-section

3. Skilled vaginal surgeons have reported successful vaginal oophorectomy associated with hysterectomy what percent of the time?
a. Less than10%
b. 15%–25%
c. 50%–65%
d. More than 90%

4. Adopting the National Guideline Clearinghouse guidelines for determining the route of hysterectomy for benign indications has increased the use of vaginal hysterectomy to what level?
a. 10%
b. 20%
c. 50%
d. 90%

5. All of the following techniques are recommended for decreasing the risk of ureteral injury during vaginal hysterectomy EXCEPT:
a. Dividing the uterine vessels
b. Dividing the cardinal ligament
c. Retracting the bladder anteriorly
d. Downward traction on the cervix

CHAPTER 32C

1. Prospective, randomized studies have shown that laparoscopic hysterectomies have which of the following significant advantages over total abdominal hysterectomy?
a. Fewer transfusions
b. Shorter operative time
c. Fewer complications
d. Shorter hospital stay

2. The difference between a laparoscopically assisted vaginal hysterectomy (LAVH) and a vaginally assisted laparoscopic hysterectomy (VALH) is:
a. The VALH is started vaginally.
b. The uterine vessels are secured laparoscopically in a VALH.
c. The uterus is removed vaginally with a VALH.
d. The tubes and ovaries cannot be removed with a VALH.

3. Studies have shown which of the following advantages for laparoscopic subtotal hysterectomy (compared with LAVH)?
a. Shorter operative time
b. Less postoperative urinary incontinence
c. Better sexual satisfaction postoperatively
d. Less vaginal prolapse postoperatively
e. All of the above

4. Maintenance of the pneumoperitoneum after colpotomy during a total laparoscopic hysterectomy (TLH) can be accomplished by all of the following techniques EXCEPT:
a. A McCartney tube®
b. KOH colpotomizer system®
c. The Vagiballoon®
d. Moistened laparotomy sponges

5. A large cervical fibroid might be a good indication for a vaginally assisted laparoscopic hysterectomy (VALH).
a. True
b. False

CHAPTER 33

1. In a patient who is hemodynamically stable with an incomplete or missed abortion, the most appropriate course of management is:
a. Expectant management
b. Surgical evacuation
c. Medical evacuation
d. All of the above

2. According to the Food and Drug Administration, medical abortion with mifepristone and misoprostol can be safely and effectively administered up to what gestational age?
a. 6 weeks
b. 7 weeks
c. 8 weeks
d. 9 weeks

3. Very early abortions cannot result in Rh sensitization.
a. True
b. False

CHAPTER 34

1. In order of decreasing frequency of incidence, rank the sites of ectopic implantation within the oviduct:
a. Fimbrial, ampullary, isthmus, interstitial
b. Ampullary, isthmic, fimbrial, interstitial
c. Ampullary, isthmic, interstitial, fimbrial
d. Interstitial, fimbrial, isthmic, ampullary

2. Which of the following diagnostic data in early pregnancy would be consistent with a nonviable (potential ectopic) pregnancy?
a. A random serum progesterone level of <5 ng/mL
b. A β-hCG rise of less than 50% in 2 days
c. Failure to visualize an intrauterine gestational sac by transvaginal ultrasonography when β-hCG titers are in excess of 2,000 mIU/mL
d. All of above

CHAPTER 35A

1. All of the following physiologic changes occur during pregnancy EXCEPT:
a. A decrease in gastric motility
b. An increase in pulmonary reserve
c. An increase in blood volume
d. A hypercoagulable state
e. An increase in renal blood flow

2. The rate of peripartum hysterectomy is increased as a result of:
a. A decrease in episiotomy rates
b. Increased safety of blood transfusion
c. An increased risk of placenta accreta
d. An increased request by patients

3. Which of the following complications are *not* increased with elective peripartum hysterectomy?
   a. Transfusion rate
   b. Bladder injuries
   c. Operation time
   d. Rate of infection
4. At the time of cesarean delivery for placenta accreta, the placenta is *not* removed.
   a. True
   b. False
5. At the time of a forceps delivery, an episiotomy reduces the risk of:
   a. Rectal sphincter tear
   b. Rectal mucosal injury
   c. Fetal brain injury
   d. Hemorrhage
   e. None of the above
6. Compared with a midline episiotomy, a mediolateral episiotomy is associated with all of the following EXCEPT:
   a. An increased risk of rectal sphincter tear
   b. More blood loss
   c. A higher level of postpartum pain
   d. A decreased risk of a fourth-degree laceration
   e. A more difficult repair
7. Current thinking suggests that dehiscence of an episiotomy should be repaired within 2 weeks of occurrence.
   a. True
   b. False

CHAPTER 35B

1. The most common ovarian neoplasm in pregnancy is:
   a. Papillary serous adenocarcinoma
   b. Embryonal carcinoma
   c. Dysgerminoma
   d. Benign cystic teratoma
2. The best management of a luteoma of pregnancy found at cesarean delivery is:
   a. Unilateral oophorectomy
   b. Biopsy only, no further surgery
   c. Unilateral oophorectomy, washings, staging biopsies
   d. Bilateral salpingo-oophorectomy, biopsies, hysterectomy, washings, staging biopsies
3. All of the following ovarian tumors can cause virilization in pregnancy EXCEPT:
   a. Hyperreactio luteinalis
   b. Sertoli-Leydig cell tumors
   c. Dysgerminoma
   d. Luteoma of pregnancy
4. A 26-year-old patient at 19 weeks of gestation has a pelvic ultrasound showing a 6-cm left adnexal complex mass with a pulsatility index of 1.4. There are no other abnormalities. The best management plan is:
   a. Repeat the ultrasound in 4 weeks.
   b. Schedule the patient for an ultrasound-guided cyst aspiration.
   c. Schedule the patient for a diagnostic laparoscopy.
   d. Schedule the patient for laparotomy with left oophorectomy and frozen section.
5. Evaluation of an adnexal mass during pregnancy should be evaluated by which of the following tests or exams?
   a. Serum CA-125
   b. Pelvic ultrasound
   c. Abdominal and pelvic computed tomography (CT) scan
   d. Positron emission tomography (PET scan)

CHAPTER 36A

1. The pelvic diaphragm is composed of all of the following muscles EXCEPT:
   a. Iliococcygeus
   b. Puborectalis
   c. Transversus perinei
   d. Pubococcygeus
2. The primary goal of defect-specific pelvic reconstructive surgery is to identify and reattach damaged endopelvic connective tissue to what central pelvic structure?
   a. Arcus tendineus fascia pelvis
   b. Sacrospinous ligament
   c. Levator plate
   d. Pericervical ring
3. Of the following factors, which is considered to be most important in the development of pelvic organ prolapse?
   a. Low estrogen levels
   b. Vaginal delivery
   c. Straining with defecation
   d. Coughing as a result of chronic lung disease
4. In both the Pelvic Organ Prolapse Quantification and Baden-Walker Halfway systems, what fixed anatomic reference point is used for measurements and grading?
   a. Ischial spine
   b. Vaginal introitus
   c. Cervix or apical vaginal vault
   d. Hymenal ring
5. Pelvic organ prolapse primarily affects:
   a. Longevity
   b. Quality of life
   c. The degree of pain a patient experiences

CHAPTER 36B

1. Anterior vaginal compartment defects include:
   a. Cystocele
   b. Paravaginal defects
   c. Urethroceles
   d. All of the above
2. Paravaginal defects create an abnormal connection between the:
   a. Vesicouterine and vesicocervical spaces
   b. Vesicovaginal and rectovaginal spaces
   c. Vesicovaginal and paravesical spaces
   d. Vesicouterine and prevesical spaces
3. Cystoceles are caused most frequently by:
   a. A general weakening of the pubocervical septum
   b. A transverse apical defect between the pericervical ring and the pubocervical septum
   c. Pressure from uterine prolapse
   d. Failure to perform Kegel exercises

CHAPTER 36C

1. Generally, where is the easiest place to identify the arcus tendineus fascia pelvis?
   a. The ischial spine
   b. Medial to the obturator foramen

c. At the attachment to the pubocervical fascias near the pelvic sidewall
d. The posterior aspect of the pubic bone

2. The bladder should not be dissected off the anterior vaginal wall during an open paravaginal defects repair because:
a. The bladder will lose support.
b. Troublesome bleeding may result.
c. The bladder will be denervated.
d. A midline defect in the anterior pelvic support will be created.

3. On examination, loss of the anterior, lateral vaginal sulcus is a sign of a paravaginal support defect.
a. True
b. False

4. In a vaginal repair of a paravaginal defect, sutures are:
a. Placed individually starting near the ischial spine
b. Absorbable to reduce the risk of infection
c. Tied individually starting with the suture nearest the vaginal apex
d. Placed through the sacrospinous ligament for support

5. Which of the following structures contributes to the "white line"?
a. Fascia of the iliopsoas muscle
b. Fascia of the puborectalis muscle
c. Fascia of the transversus perineal muscle
d. Fascia of the obturator internus muscle

CHAPTER 36D

1. In the last twenty-five years, the biggest change in surgery to treat pelvic organ prolapse is which of the following?
a. The change to site-specific defect repair
b. Advances in suture materials, antibiotics, and self-retaining retractors
c. The introduction of endoscopy to perform the surgery
d. The way it is taught in residency training programs

2. The underlying pathophysiology of pelvic organ prolapse is which of the following?
a. Inherent connective tissue weakness
b. Childbirth injury
c. Aging
d. All of the above

3. The most appropriate use of graft material in pelvic reconstructive surgery is for which of the following?
a. As a technique in primary surgery to reinforce a concomitant standard repair
b. To replace standard and site-specific reparative techniques
c. Only in sacrocolpopexy
d. In recurrent cases in which native pelvic tissues are weak

4. The most common complication of a synthetic mesh graft is which of the following?
a. Infection
b. Pain with intercourse
c. Mesh exposure
d. Vaginal stenosis

5. Which of the following statements regarding current pelvic reparative surgery techniques is true?
a. The best approach surgically is that which is least invasive.
b. Surgery by laparotomy is no longer indicated for pelvic organ prolapse.
c. Transvaginal reparative surgery produces a failure rate too great to make it a good technique.
d. It is one of the most common surgeries performed in women older than age 50 and has a high failure rate.

CHAPTER 36E

1. After performing a hysterectomy, to what ligament(s) should the vaginal apex be attached to minimize the risk of vaginal vault prolapse?
a. Round ligament
b. Cardinal and uterosacral ligaments
c. Uteroovarian ligament
d. Sacrospinous ligament

2. Which one of the following structures is at risk of injury during a McCall culdoplasty?
a. Sciatic nerve
b. Rectum
c. Internal iliac vein
d. Pudendal nerve

3. Which of the following structure(s) lie posterior to the ischia spine?
a. Pudendal nerve/vessels
b. Sciatic nerve
c. Hypogastric venous plexus
d. Inferior gluteal vessels

4. One of the late complications following sacrospinous ligament fixation is:
a. Uterine prolapse
b. Dyspareunia
c. Anterior vaginal wall prolapse
d. Medial thigh pain

5. All of the following procedures are performed as part of an abdominal sacral colpopexy EXCEPT:
a. Dissecting the peritoneum off the vagina
b. Attaching the mesh or graft to the vagina with nonabsorbable sutures
c. Suturing the mesh to the longitudinal ligament over the sacral promontory
d. Suturing the round ligaments to the anterior graft with nonabsorbable sutures

CHAPTER 36F

1. Pessaries are effective in the treatment of pelvic organ prolapse and should be considered for most patients.
a. True
b. False

2. Which of the following patient characteristics is associated with failure of successful pessary use?
a. Degree of pelvic organ prolapse
b. Vaginal mucosal atrophy
c. Wide vaginal introitus
d. Size of the genital hiatus

3. Which of the following pessaries is compatible with normal vaginal intercourse?
a. Gellhorn
b. Donut
c. Cube
d. Ring

4. All of the following are potential complications of pessary use EXCEPT:
   a. Increased difficulty with bowel movement
   b. Vaginal erosion
   c. Vaginal cancer
   d. Incarceration of the cervix
5. What is the most common reason a woman stops using her pessary?
   a. It keeps falling out.
   b. It does not improve her symptoms
   c. It hurts.
   d. It is difficult to remove.

CHAPTER 37

1. The dominant structure altering cause of stress urinary incontinence is thought to be:
   a. straining at stool
   b. obesity
   c. smoking
   d. *childbearing
   e. chronic cough
2. The most common pathophysiologic cause of stress incontinence is:
   a. hypermobile bladder neck
   b. intrinsic (urethral) sphincter deficiency
   c. combined hypermobile bladder neck and low urethral (closure) pressure
   d. *combined bladder neck hypermobility and intrinsic sphincter deficiency
   e. combined intrinsic sphincter deficiency and low leak point pressure
3. The basic evaluation for urinary incontinence requires all but one of the following:
   a. history
   b. urinalysis
   c. urolog summary (voiding diary)
   d. residual urine determination
   e. *cystometrogram
4. The following must be completed prior to initial management of stress urinary incontinence:
   a. cystometry
   b. urine culture
   c. *basic evaluation
   d. urodynamics
   e. Q-tip test
5. What is the least effective therapy for initial conservative management of pure stress urinary incontinence?
   a. pelvic floor muscle exercises
   b. bladder drills
   c. pessary
   d. *antimuscarinic medication
   e. biofeedback
6. What test is used to rule out detrusor overactivity incontinence?
   a. pressure voiding study
   b. uroflowmetry
   c. *cystometrogram
   d. leak point pressure
   e. urethral closure pressure profile
7. Which of the following procedures is the best recommendation for a primary approach for stress urinary incontinence?
   a. paravaginal defect repair
   b. periurethral collagen injection
   c. Kelly plication with anterior repair
   d. Pereyra procedure
   e. *suburethral sling
8. What is the main difference between a tension-free tape and a suburethral sling as performed today?
   a. indication for surgery
   b. cure rate
   c. *placement at midurethra
   d. placement without tension
   e. use of cystoscopy during placement
9. The 'gold standard' surgery for surgical correction of stress urinary incontinence is:
   a. sling procedure
   b. tension-free tape
   c. *retropubic urethropexy
   d. anterior colporrhaphy
   e. needle urethropexy
10. A positive Q-tip test is diagnostic for which of the following?
    a. overactive bladder
    b. stress urinary incontinence
    c. cystocele
    d. *mobile bladder neck
    e. urge incontinence

CHAPTER 38

1. The most common site of ureteral injury during pelvic surgery is:
   a. As the ureter transverses the tunnel of Wertheim
   b. Dorsal to the infundibulopelvic ligament near or at the pelvic brim
   c. At the cardinal ligament when the ureter passes under the uterine artery
   d. In the intramural portion of the ureter
2. The most important means to prevent ureteral injury is:
   a. Surgical knowledge of the location and anatomy the ureter
   b. Preoperative intravenous pyelogram
   c. Administration of intravenous indigo carmine during surgery
   d. Prophylactic ureteral stint placement
3. Following partial ureteral ligation, the preferred method of inserting a ureteral stint is:
   a. Ureterostomy
   b. Cystostomy
   c. Cystoscopy
   d. None of the above; no ureteral stint is indicated
4. The most common gynecologic surgical procedure during which the ureter is injured is:
   a. Total vaginal hysterectomy
   b. Bladder neck suspension
   c. Total abdominal hysterectomy
   d. Total laparoscopic hysterectomy
5. Uncomplicated total transection of the distal third of the ureter should be managed with:
   a. Primary repair over a ureteral stint
   b. Ureteroileal interposition
   c. Ureteroneocystomy with psoas hitch
   d. Ureteroureterostomy over ureteral stint

CHAPTER 39

1. Factors that may contribute to the formation of vesicovaginal fistula include all of the following except:
   a. Obstructed labor
   b. Pelvic radiation
   c. Tribal "gishiri" cuts to the vagina
   d. HIV infection
   e. Hysterectomy
2. Which of the following techniques of hysterectomy is most likely to result in vesicovaginal fistula?
   a. Laparoscopic
   b. Vaginal
   c. Abdominal
   d. Supracervical
3. Prolonged indwelling Foley catheter can predispose a patient to urethrovaginal fistula.
   a. True
   b. False
4. Vesicovaginal fistula as a complication of hysterectomy is most likely to be located:
   a. In the trigone near the ureteral orifices
   b. Superior to the interureteric ridge in the posterior bladder
   c. In the bladder dome
   d. At the bladder base proximal to the urethra
5. You are evaluating a patient in your office who had a TAH secondary to large uterine fibroids performed 4 years ago by one of your former partners who has since retired. She has occasional episodes of severe dysuria followed by hematuria that resolve after a few days without treatment. You review her operative note from her TAH, which notes that she sustained an intraoperative cystotomy that was repaired by mobilization of the tissue and tension-free multilayer closure with 3-0 silk suture. Her current symptoms are most likely secondary to:
   a. Recurrent urinary tract infections
   b. Poorly healed cystotomy with chronic intermittent wound separation
   c. Stone formation
   d. An occult vesicovaginal fistula
6. You are seeing a patient in the office 3 weeks after a laparoscopically assisted vaginal hysterectomy for small uterine fibroids and irregular bleeding. She reports an intermittent, watery discharge for the past 2 weeks. Exam of the vaginal apex shows no fistula, but a small amount of clear fluid is present. You fill the bladder with a dilute indigo carmine/saline solution and note no leakage on visualization of the vaginal apex with a speculum. Your next diagnostic test would be:
   a. Cystourethroscopy
   b. Intravenous urogram
   c. Insert a tampon in the vagina and have the patient walk around for 15 minutes
   d. Test the fluid for creatinine

CHAPTER 40

1. Vaginal birth may contribute to development of anal incontinence through damage to:
   a. The puborectalis muscle sling
   b. Pelvic enervation
   c. The anal sphincter complex
   d. a and c
   e. a, b, and c
2. The use of which of the following obstetrical practices are associated with anal sphincter disruption at the time of vaginal birth?
   a. Midline episiotomy
   b. Perineal massage
   c. Forceps delivery
   d. a and c
   e. a, b, and c
3. Which of the following anatomic structures are important in the woman to maintenance of continence of fecal material?
   a. External anal sphincter
   b. Puborectalis muscle
   c. Internal anal sphincter
   d. a and c
   e. a, b, and c
4. Which of the following testing modalities is the most cost-effective, accurate, and best tolerated by anally incontinent patients being investigated for the presence of a segmental anal sphincter defect?
   a. Pudendal nerve terminal motor latency (PNTML) testing
   b. Magnetic resonance imaging (MRI)
   c. Anal manometry
   d. Endoanal ultrasound
   e. Defecography
5. Patients undergoing sphincteroplasty and perineal reconstruction for anal incontinence should have a reasonable expectation of total continence postoperatively.
   a. True
   b. False

CHAPTER 41

1. Can the BRCA gene be transmitted from the paternal side of the family?
2. If the BRCA gene test is negative, does the patient need additional follow up?
3. If the patient has a normal mammogram in the face of a persistent mass, is it true that she doesn't need additional follow-up?
4. What prevention options are available to women at high risk?
5. What are the risk benefits of core needle biopsy (CNB) versus fine-needle aspiration (FNA)?
6. What risk-assessment model is most applicable in clinical practice?
7. What are the benefits of breast cancer risk assessment?
8. Stage II breast cancer includes tumors measuring 2 cm.
   a. True
   b. False
9. The majority of women with breast cancer have identifiable risk factors.
   a. True
   b. False

CHAPTER 42

1. Which of the following statements regarding the statistical nature of appendicitis is incorrect?
   a. The mortality rate of appendicitis with appropriate and timely treatment is less than 1%.
   b. Individuals have a 7% lifetime risk of developing appendicitis.
   c. With acute appendicitis, there is a 20% mean incidence

of perforation, during which the mortality rate increases to 5%.
d. The greatest incidence of appendicitis occurs in the third and fourth decades of life.
e. The overall mortality rate increases to 5% to 15% in the elderly population.

2. Which of the following definitions regarding diagnostic signs of appendicitis is incorrect?
a. McBurney's point: located at the junction of the middle and medial thirds of a line drawn from the umbilicus to right anterolateral spine
b. Rovsing sign: pain in the right lower quadrant when pressure is applied to the left lower quadrant
c. Psoas sign: increased pain in the abdomen as the right leg is extended at the hip when the patient is in the left lateral decubitus position
d. Obturator sign: increased pain in the right lower abdomen when passively flexing the hip

3. A 33-year-old G2P2 presents to the emergency room with right-sided abdominal pain and nausea. On exam, she is tender to palpation at McBurney's point with voluntary guarding, and her pelvic exam elicits pain on palpation of her right adnexa without note of an obvious mass. Her temperature is 99°F, her pulse is 88, and her blood pressure is 126/74. Labs reveal a WBC count of 9,400. CT scan suggests an appendiceal abscess. Given the below options, the best treatment plan at this point is:
a. Immediately, take the patient to the operating room for an emergency exploratory laparotomy and appendectomy.
b. Start intravenous fluids and a first-generation cephalosporin antibiotic, and consent the patient for a laparoscopic appendectomy to be performed in the morning.
c. Start intravenous fluids and broad-spectrum antibiotics with enteric organism coverage, keep the patient NPO, and keep the patient under close observation for progression of her illness.
d. Send the patient home with appendicitis precautions and a 14-day course of Levaquin and metronidazole.

4. A 28-year-old G2P1001 with a single intrauterine pregnancy at 16 weeks estimated gestational age has just been diagnosed with acute appendicitis and needs to undergo surgical intervention. Which of the following statements regarding appendicitis in pregnancy is correct?
a. Ectopic pregnancy excluded, appendicitis is responsible for 50% of cases of acute abdomen in pregnancy.
b. Premature labor and delivery are among most serious fetal risks, with up to 30% fetal mortality reported if perforation occurs.
c. Regardless of the duration of the pregnancy, a high midline incision should be used to remove the appendix.
d. Acute appendicitis occurs most often in the third trimester.
e. Because the increasing girth of the gravid uterus, infection from a perforated appendix is often walled off, decreasing the associated morbidity and mortality.

5. Which of the following is not an acceptable scenario in which to perform an incidental appendectomy?
a. A patient undergoing diagnostic laparoscopy for infertility who is found to have endometriosis implants along her appendix
b. A patient undergoing standard repeat cesarean section with tubal ligation
c. A patient undergoing a total abdominal hysterectomy and bilateral salpingo-oophorectomy for removal of a mucinous ovarian tumor
d. A patient undergoing laparoscopy for removal of right-sided tuboovarian abscess

CHAPTER 43

1. An 18-year-old nulliparous woman presents to your clinic for her annual exam. On exam there is a right adnexal mass that is about 5 × 5 cm. Ultrasonographically it is consistent with a dermoid cyst. Although without pain for the past several weeks, she has a history of right lower quadrant pain that has occurred intermittently over several years, and she has had guaiac positive stool in the past but none currently. She is taken to the operating room where she is found to have a dermoid, as expected, but is also found to have a diverticulum 9 cm in length arising from the antimesenteric border of the ileum 13 inches from the ileocecal valve. There is a slight thickening of the tip of the diverticulum, but the tissue otherwise appears totally healthy. Which of the following statements about the management of this case of Meckel's diverticulum is true?
a. The patient's symptoms have now resolved and the dermoid has been removed, so there is no need to remove the diverticulum, which likely will remain asymptomatic the patient's entire life.
b. The diverticulum should be removed because the patient has a history of symptoms that it may have caused, and it has slightly atypical features.
c. The diverticulum should be removed because any time a Meckel's diverticulum is discovered incidentally, it should be removed to prevent future complications.
d. The diverticulum should not be removed at this time, but if the patient has recurrent symptoms, she should be referred to general surgery for removal.

2. In which of the following patient(s) would sodium phosphate probably not be a good choice for a bowel prep?
a. A 26-year-old with systemic lupus erythematosus (SLE) who has end stage renal disease
b. A 54-year-old alcoholic with cirrhosis
c. A 64-year-old with stage IIB ovarian cancer
d. A 48-year-old with class II heart failure
e. A 35-year-old with diabetes with a hemoglobin A1C of 6.7

3. A patient is undergoing a laparoscopic tubal ligation. Upon insertion of the laparoscope, intraluminal bowel mucosa is seen, as well as reflux of enteric contents. Which of the following would be the best course of action?
a. Remove the trocar, convert to an open laparotomy, and repair the injury.
b. Leave to trocar in place, convert to an open laparotomy, and repair the injury.
c. Insert another trocar to confirm that bowel injury has occurred, then attempt to repair the injury laparoscopically.
d. Withdraw and reposition the trocar so that the injury is visible with the laparoscope, and then decide if laparoscopic repair is feasible.

4. A 37-year-old patient undergoes a laparoscopy for fulguration of endometriosis and is discharged the same day. Which of the following presentations would be most consistent with an electrosurgical injury that was unrecognized during surgery?
a. The patient presents to the ER 3 days postoperatively reporting nausea, vomiting, and fever.
b. The patient becomes hypotensive and tachycardic in the recovery room but responds to fluid boluses.

c. The patient presents to the ER on postop day one reporting worsening abdominal pain, fever, and constipation.
d. The patient calls the clinic 1 week postoperatively reporting nausea, vomiting, and diarrhea but denies fever.
e. The patient presents to clinic 1 month postoperatively reporting irregular bowel movements since surgery and continued abdominal pain.

5. Which of the following statement(s) regarding early feeding in patients who have undergone a bowel anastomosis are true?
   a. The rate of ileus is significantly higher in patients who are fed before passing flatus.
   b. The rate of anastomotic complications is significantly decreased by delaying feeding.
   c. Return of bowel function generally occurs at the same rate regardless of early or delayed feeding.
   d. Early feeding decreases the probable length of hospital stay.
   e. None of the above
6. Which of the following are the three most common reasons for bowel obstruction ?
   a. Adhesions
   b. Intestinal polyps
   c. Volvulus
   d. Hernias
   e. Malignancy
7. A 62-year-old patient undergoes a bowel resection. Because there is only 5 cm of rectum conserved, the decision is made to create a sigmoid J-pouch. Which of the following regarding the J-pouch is true?
   a. The patient is less likely to suffer from frequency, urgency, and incontinence of stool.
   b. The patient is less likely to have a sense of incomplete evacuation after bowel movements.
   c. Slight tension on the J-pouch will resolve over time and need not be a source of concern.
   d. Enemas should be avoided in patients who have had a J-pouch created.
8. A 34-year-old patient undergoes a TAH-BSO for leiomyomata. During the surgery, the small bowel sustains a thermal injury requiring resection of 4 cm of small bowel. The remaining bowel appears healthy. Which of the following types of anastomosis should probably not be used because of the higher potential for excessive luminal narrowing?
   a. End-to-end hand-sewn anastomosis
   b. Side-to-side hand-sewn anastomosis
   c. (True) end-to-end staple anastomosis
   d. Side-to-side staple anastomosis (functional end-to-end anastomosis)
9. A 38-year-old patient with a history severe endometriosis who is known to have extensive adhesive disease presents to the ER with abdominal pain. Physical exam and radiologic imaging lead to the diagnosis of small bowel obstruction. During surgery, which of the following characteristics of her injured bowel indicate viability most reliably? (Choose two.)
   a. Tissue color
   b. Bleeding from a cut edge
   c. Extent of edema
   d. Peristalsis
   e. Fluorescence of bowel wall under Wood's lamp 10 minutes after IV fluorescein
10. Designate whether each of the following statements is true or false.
    a. Intraluminal fluid collection in a complete obstruction is unlikely to exceed 2 L.
    b. Less than 20% of bowel injuries during gynecologic surgery occur during lysis of adhesions.
    c. Absent bowel sounds are usually indicative of ileus.
    d. Peristaltic waves causing pain every 12 minutes indicate a relatively high obstruction.
    e. Sodium phosphate generally provides better bowel prep for colonoscopy than polyethylene glycol.
    f. Stair-step air fluid levels from RLQ to LUQ is most consistent with adynamic ileus.
    g. The tissue edges on a bowel anastomosis should be everted.
    h. Colonic dysfunction following surgery usually resolves within 6 to 8 hours.

CHAPTER 44

1. How often do patients with documented colorectal cancer have a negative fecal hemoccult test?
   a. 10%
   b. 30%
   c. 50%
   d. 80%
2. The most common pelvic retroperitoneal mass related to the urinary tract is a:
   a. Lower ureteral carcinoma
   b. Urinoma
   c. Pelvic kidney
   d. Bladder diverticulum
3. Patients on broad-spectrum antibiotics and/or prolonged bowel preparations may have a prolonged prothrombin time.
   a. False
   b. True
4. Nongynecologic conditions most often seen by the gynecologist arise from what system or organ?
   a. Gastrointestinal
   b. Urinary tract
   c. Lymphatic system
   d. Orthopedic (muscle, bone)
5. Which is the most common neurogenic tumor that can arise in the pelvis and be mistaken as a gynecologic problem?
   a. Neurofibromas
   b. Asterocytoma
   c. Gelioblastoma
   d. Showanoma
6. At laparotomy, the finding of thickened mesentery with growth of mesenteric fat ("fat wrapping") around the circumference of leathery fibrotic bowel is pathognomonic of:
   a. Crohn disease
   b. Ulcerative colitis
   c. Tuberculosis
   d. Adenocarcinoma of small bowel
7. Of cancers metastatic to the ovary, which is the most common primary site?
   a. Colon
   b. Stomach
   c. Breast
   d. Uterus

CHAPTER 45

1. Which of the following is a recognized risk factor for vulvar malignancy?
   a. Diabetes
   b. Cigarette smoking
   c. Obesity
   d. Immunosuppression
2. You may consider omitting lymphadenectomy as part of the operative treatment for squamous cell vulvar carcinoma when:
   a. Lesion 1.5 cm diameter, less than 5 mm invasion
   b. Unilateral lesion, less than 5 mm invasion
   c. Any location, less than 1 mm invasion
   d. Unilateral lesion 1.3 cm diameter, 3 mm invasion
3. Which factor predisposes patients to develop local recurrence with squamous cell vulvar carcinoma?
   a. Midline location
   b. Enlarged inguinal nodes
   c. Close resection with margin less than 1 cm
   d. Poorly differentiated histology
4. The use of preoperative radiation therapy in patients with squamous cell vulvar carcinoma is most appropriate for:
   a. Patients with suspicious groin nodes
   b. Locally advanced disease or lesions encroaching on midline structures for which surgical removal is accompanied by significant morbidity
   c. Poorly differentiated histology type in stage 1 disease
   d. Multifocal lesions in stage 1 disease
5. When a woman has a Bartholin mass, what features would prompt you to consider biopsy or excision?
   a. Age younger than 40
   b. History of previous Bartholin abscess
   c. Failure to improve promptly with conservative therapy
   d. Negative culture
   e. Bilateral masses
6. The recurrence-free survival of patients with invasive squamous cell carcinoma of the vulva correlates most closely with:
   a. Tumor differentiation
   b. Tumor location
   c. Radiation tumor dose
   d. Pathologic status of the inguinal lymph nodes
   e. Age of the patient
7. The second most common histologic type of vulvar cancer is:
   a. Squamous cell carcinoma
   b. Melanoma
   c. Bartholin gland carcinoma
   d. Basal cell carcinoma
   e. Invasive Paget disease
8. Characteristics of Paget disease of the vulva include all the following EXCEPT:
   a. Presentation as a patchy, eczematous lesion
   b. The presence of underlying invasive disease in more than 90% of patients
   c. The development of another malignancy in about 25% of patients
   d. Histologic extension beyond that which is clinically apparent
   e. Tendency to occur in white postmenopausal women
9. Which of the following histologic types of vulvar cancer has the most favorable prognosis?
   a. Squamous cell carcinoma arising from a Bartholin gland
   b. Paget disease with an underlying apocrine gland adenocarcinoma
   c. Melanoma 4 mm in thickness
   d. Basal cell carcinoma
   e. Merkel cell carcinoma
10. Which of the following histologic variants of vulvar cancer is most likely to metastasize to the inguinal lymph nodes?
    a. Verrucous carcinoma
    b. Basosquamous carcinoma
    c. Warty carcinoma
    d. Carcinoma *in situ* with early stromal invasion
    e. Basal cell carcinoma

CHAPTER 46

1. Human papillomavirus (HPV) is the cause of at least 99% of all cervical cancers.
   a. True
   b. False
2. Based on studies of college-aged women in the United States, what percent of young women test positive for a cervical HPV infection during a 3- to 5-year interval?
   a. 10%
   b. 25%
   c. 50%
   d. 80%
   e. 100%
3. Effective screening for cervical cancer has been reported using each of the techniques EXCEPT:
   a. Cervical cytology
   b. Visual inspection with acetic acid
   c. Lugol's staining
   d. Colposcopy
   e. Computer-assisted cytology
4. A single Pap test, on average, would be able to pick up low-grade squamous intraepithelial lesion (LSIL) or worse in a screened patient what percent of the time?
   a. >95%
   b. 90%
   c. 80%
   d. 70%
   e. 50%
5. Recommended treatment for a 26-year-old woman in her first pregnancy at 24 weeks who has a colposcopically directed biopsy showing severe dysplasia at 1 o'clock is:
   a. Cryotherapy
   b. LEEP as an outpatient
   c. Cone biopsy in the operating room
   d. Cesarean section with cone biopsy at 36 weeks
   e. Follow-up with no treatment during pregnancy
6. How often will women with a biopsy diagnosis of mild cervical dysplasia resolve spontaneously with no treatment if followed for 24 months?
   a. 10%
   b. 25%
   c. 50%
   d. 75%
   e. 90% or more
7. All of the following are terms for abnormal colposcopic findings EXCEPT:
   a. Mosaic
   b. Metaplasia
   c. White epithelium

d. Punctation
e. Atypical vessels

8. Which of the following is the main advantage of LEEP over cryotherapy for the treatment of cervical intraepithelial neoplasia (CIN)?
a. It produces a specimen for histologic study.
b. It does not require expensive equipment.
c. It does not require general anesthesia.
d. It has a lower risk of premature labor in future pregnancies.
e. It requires less surgical skill and training.

9. HPV testing has been shown to be clinically effective for all of the following EXCEPT:
a. Triage of ASC-US Paps
b. Follow-up after LEEP
c. Cotesting with Pap for screening in women older than age 30
d. Identification of which patients with mild dysplasia need treatment

10. Traditional cold-knife cone biopsy under anesthesia is recommended by experts for which of the following two scenarios?
a. Cervical glandular lesions
b. Grossly visible cervical lesions
c. Lesions that extend into the canal
d. Suspected microinvasive lesions
e. Lesions greater than 2.0 cm in diameter

CHAPTER 47

1. A 3-cm cancer of the cervix with no signs of spread is probably:
a. Stage IA2
b. Microinvasive disease
c. Stage IB
d. Stage IIB

2. The most important determinant of prognosis of cervical cancer is:
a. Depth of invasion into the cervix
b. FIGO stage
c. Presence of lymph node metastasis
d. Histologic differentiation

3. The best rationale for choosing radical surgery over radiation for treatment of early-stage carcinoma of the cervix is:
a. Better survival with surgery
b. Fewer complications
c. Preservation of ovarian function
d. Decreased short-term recurrence

4. Which of the following tests is permitted for FIGO staging of cervical cancer?
a. Intravenous pyelogram
b. CT scans of abdomen and pelvis
c. Lymphangiogram
d. PET scan

5. Which of the avascular pelvic spaces lies immediately posterior to the cardinal ligament?
a. Space of Retzius
b. Pararectal space
c. Paravesical space
d. Rectovaginal space

6. In a classic type III radical hysterectomy, the uterine artery is ligated at which point?
a. Its origin from the hypogastric artery
b. Where it crosses over the ureter
c. 1 cm lateral to the uterus
d. As it enters the parametrial "web"

7. The most common late sequela of radical hysterectomy and pelvic lymphadenectomy is:
a. Vesicovaginal fistula
b. Numbness of the medial thigh
c. Leg edema
d. Bladder dysfunction

8. The most common symptom of early cervical cancer is:
a. Vaginal bleeding
b. Pelvic pressure/pain
c. Hematuria
d. Unilateral leg edema

9. In a radical vaginal hysterectomy, which step of the procedure is performed "blindly"?
a. Entry into the posterior cul de sac
b. Entry into the pararectal space
c. Entry into the paravesical space
d. Entry into the vesicouterine space

10. Following a radical vaginal trachelectomy for cervical cancer, what percentage of pregnancies reach the third trimester?
a. 25%–35%
b. 45%–55%
c. 65%–75%
d. More that 90%

CHAPTER 48

1. All of the following increase the risk of endometrial cancer EXCEPT:
a. Infertility
b. Tamoxifen use
c. Obesity
d. Cigarette smoking
e. Increasing age

2. A 65-year-old woman presents to your office with symptoms of vaginal spotting for the last 3 months. The next best step in her management is:
a. Office endometrial biopsy
b. D&C
c. Hysterectomy
d. Vaginal estrogen

3. A 53-year-old obese woman with diabetes and hypertension is diagnosed with grade 1 endometrioid adenocarcinoma of the endometrium. Her preoperative evaluation should include:
a. CA-125
b. CT of abdomen and pelvis
c. MRI of pelvis
d. PET scan
e. None of the above

4. Which of the following statements regarding surgery for endometrial cancer is correct?
a. Surgical staging for patients with uterine papillary serous carcinoma includes peritoneal washings and biopsies, pelvic and paraaortic lymph node dissection, and omentectomy.
b. When clamping the cardinal ligaments, it is important to include the lateral cervical tissues to decrease the risk of bleeding.

c. The survival of patients treated with laparoscopic surgery is significantly shorter than that of patients who undergo laparotomy
d. The fundus should be grasped with a tenaculum for manipulation of the uterus.
e. Debulking surgery does not improve survival in patients with advanced-stage endometrial cancer.

5. A 59-year-old woman presents for postoperative surveillance following surgery for stage IB, grade 1 endometrioid adenocarcinoma of the endometrium. Recurrent disease is most likely to be diagnosed by which of the following:
a. History and physical examination
b. Vaginal cytology
c. Chest x-ray
d. CT scan of abdomen and pelvis
e. CA-125

CHAPTER 49

1. A 23-year-old patient is diagnosed with a stage IA malignant ovarian germ-cell tumor. Which of the following would be the standard treatment?
a. Unilateral oophorectomy
b. Bilateral oophorectomy and hysterectomy
c. Unilateral oophorectomy followed by chemotherapy
d. Ovarian biopsy followed by chemotherapy
2. A 3-year-old patient is diagnosed with stage IB serous ovarian cancer, grade. Which of the following treatment regimens would generally be recommended with a 5-year survival of at least 95%?
a. Surgery followed with chemotherapy
b. Surgery alone
c. Surgery followed by pelvic radiation
d. Chemotherapy followed by surgery
3. Which of the following factors has not been shown to have prognostic significance in epithelial ovarian cancer?
a. Large volume ascites
b. Clear-cell histology
c. Capsular rupture
d. Histologic grade
4. You are consulted intraoperatively by a colleague who has a 33-year-old G2P0A2 patient diagnosed with endometrioid borderline tumor of the right ovary. The tumor appears to be confined to that ovary, which was 20 cm in diameter and was removed intact. The patient strongly desires to maintain her fertility. Which of the following treatments would you recommend?
a. Unilateral salpingo-oophorectomy with surgical staging
b. Unilateral salpingo-oophorectomy of the opposite ovary
c. Bilateral salpingo-oophorectomy without hysterectomy, with the possibility of donor oocyte pregnancy remaining
d. TAH-BSO with surgical staging
5. Several large studies have found that early ovarian cancer can be detected successfully using which of the following screening techniques?
a. Serum CA-125
b. Cul-de-sac aspiration cytology
c. BRCA1 genetic testing
d. Transvaginal pelvic ultrasound
6. Which of the following tumor markers is most often elevated in patients with ovarian granulosa cell tumors?
a. Serum inhibin
b. CA-125
c. AFP
d. β-hCG
7. Which of the following findings on color flow Doppler are consistent with a benign mass (as opposed to a possible malignant mass)?
a. Peripheral vasculature
b. Increased diastolic blood flow
c. Pulsatility index of >1
d. Resistive index of 0.2
8. A 56-year-old G3P3 patient presents for her annual exam with no symptoms. She experienced menopause at the age of 51 and has no complaints. She has been on combination hormone replacement therapy. Her mother died of metastatic cancer (unknown primary) at the age of 68. She is found on exam to have a mobile, firm, nontender right adnexal mass. Her bimanual and rectal exam have no other abnormal findings. An ultrasound shows a simple, unilocular cyst of the right ovary measuring 4 × 3 × 5 cm. Which of the following would be the best course of action?
a. Check a CA-125 level, and if normal, repeat the ultrasound in 3 months to determine if any change has occurred.
b. Assure the patient that everything looks all right and that she should return for her next annual exam in 1 year.
c. Recommend laparoscopy with laparoscopic RSO if the ovarian cyst looks benign.
d. Order a CT scan to reevaluate the findings seen on ultrasound.
9. What percentage of ovarian tumors in premenopausal women are malignant?
a. (10%
b. 10%–15%
c. 25%–50%
d. >75%
10. A 65-year-old G1P1A1 of Native American descent presents reporting bloating and weight loss for 6 months. Her mother is alive and well in her 80s. Her maternal aunt died of breast cancer at the age of 43. Her single pregnancy ended in spontaneous abortion at 10 weeks of gestation, and she was on birth control pills for 8 years over her life. Menarche had been at the age of 15 and menopause at the age of 56. Which of the following place the patient at increased risk of having ovarian cancer?
a. History of oral contraceptive use
b. Age of menarche (15)
c. Native American ethnicity
d. Nulliparity

CHAPTER 50

1. Which of the following is *not* a candidate for total pelvic exenteration?
a. A 36-year-old woman treated 1 year ago for stage IIIB cancer of the cervix with pelvic radiation and chemotherapy who now has a vesicovaginal and a rectovaginal fistula. Biopsies, exam, and imaging studies show no evidence of cancer.
b. A 65-year-old woman treated 20 months ago with pelvic radiation and chemotherapy for stage II squamous cell carcinoma of the anterior upper third of the vagina. She now has a 3-cm mass at the vaginal apex. Biopsy shows

recurrent carcinoma. On exam, the tumor does not extend to the pelvic sidewall, and imaging studies show no metastatic disease.
  c. A 48-year-old woman previously treated for stage IIIB cervical cancer who has biopsy-proven recurrence on the cervix, and on exam, the cervical mass extends to the right pelvic sidewall. However, an MRI shows tumor-free space between the central mass and the muscles of the right pelvis. There is no metastatic disease on imaging studies.
  d. A 56-year-old woman who was treated 15 months ago for stage IB2 squamous cell carcinoma of the cervix now has a biopsy-proven 1.0-cm recurrence in the cervix after previous pelvic radiation and chemotherapy. The mass is freely mobile. Her workup is negative except for a single 1.5-cm node in the low aortic area just above her previous radiation field. CT-guided FNA is positive for squamous cell carcinoma. There is no evidence of other metastatic disease.

2. Which of the following factors is *not* a relative contraindication to pelvic exenteration?
  a. Obesity
  b. Jehovah's Witness who will not accept blood products
  c. Inability to dress or care for herself because of mental or physical impairment
  d. Age older than 70
  e. Renal failure with a creatine higher than 1.5
3. All of the following clinical findings suggest that a patient's tumor will be unresectable EXCEPT:
  a. Unilateral leg edema
  b. Tumor causing a vesicovaginal fistula
  c. Sciatic nerve pain
  d. Unilateral ureteral obstruction
4. During a pelvic exenteration, all of the following pelvic spaces are used EXCEPT:
  a. Pouch of Douglas
  b. Space of Retzius
  c. Paravesical space
  d. Presacral space
  e. Pararectal space
5. Use of a myocutaneous flap for vaginal reconstruction during a pelvic exenteration has all of the following advantages EXCEPT:
  a. It brings in new blood supply to the pelvis.
  b. It fills in the pelvic defect.
  c. It does not require postoperative use of an obturator to maintain patency.
  d. It is technically quick and easy to perform.

CHAPTER 51

1. One technique for vaginal reconstruction after vaginectomy includes the omental J-flap with split-thickness skin graft (STSG). Which of the following is *not* considered a benefit of this technique?
  a. Psychosexual factors/satisfactory intercourse
  b. Prevention of enteroperineal fistulas
  c. Abscess collection
  d. Urinary continence
2. Incorporating which vessel is crucial to ensuring success of the sigmoid neovagina procedure?
  a. Inferior hemorrhoidal artery
  b. Superior hemorrhoidal artery
  c. Pudendal artery
  d. Dorsal clitoral artery
3. When identifying the structure for the gracilis myocutaneous flap, which muscle can be confused for the gracilis?
  a. Adductor longus
  b. Adductor brevis
  c. Adductor magnus
  d. Sartorius
4. When performing a rectus abdominis myocutaneous (RAM) flap, what is an absolute contraindication to the procedure?
  a. Previous Maylard incision
  b. Diabetes
  c. Obesity
  d. Previous radiotherapy
5. All of the following are considered disadvantages of the traditional vulvectomy except:
  a. Perineal contractions
  b. Distortion of the bladder neck/urethra leading to incontinence
  c. Increased risk of recurrence
  d. Wound breakdown
6. To ensure adequate closure with a Z-plasty pedicle flap, each of the following should be included *except*:
  a. Adequate blood supply
  b. A flap length 2 cm long and a base of 1 cm
  c. Full-thickness skin graft
  d. Rotation of the flap to the midperineal line
7. Physiologic characteristics of a continent urinary pouch are designed to prevent reflux, infection, and incontinence. Which describes the ideal situation for a continent urinary pouch?
  a. 40 cm H_20 pressure, 500 mL volume
  b. 80 cm H_20 pressure, 500 mL volume
  c. 80 cm H_20 pressure, 1,000 mL volume
  d. 40 cm H_20, 1,000 mL volume
8. The Kock pouch is suitable for urinary bladder replacement because it possesses features necessary for maintaining continence. These include all of the following except:
  a. Maintenance of low pressure after filling
  b. Prevention of reflux
  c. Retention of 1,000 to 1,500 mL of fluid
  d. Elimination of intermittent pressure spikes (promoting reflux)
9. Variations of the original Kock procedure have been designed that do not require intussusception of the bowel. One of these is the Miami pouch. In what way is it different from the Kock procedure?
  a. The distal terminal ileum is transected proximal to the ileocecal valve.
  b. Appendectomy is performed.
  c. The ureters are anastamosed directly into the muscular wall of the colon.
  d. Reinforcing the ileocecal valve by tapering the distal segment is essential for maintaining continence.
10. Rectosigmoid colon resection (RSC) can lead to several defecation disorders, including all of the following EXCEPT:
  a. Fecal incontinence
  b. Constipation
  c. Fecal urgency
  d. Tenesmus

ANSWERS

CHAPTER 2

1. b. False
2. a. True
3. b. False
4. a. True
5. a. True
6. b. False
7. a. True
8. a. True
9. a. True
10. a. True
11. a. True
12. a. True

CHAPTER 3

1. c. The patient's surgeon
2. d. None of the above; age should not be a determinant
3. g. All of the above
4. d. A skilled surgeon who addresses his patient's psychological as well as physical needs
5. f. All of the above
6. e. An outdated procedure that should no longer be performed routinely
7. a. Releases endogenous opiates
   and
   c. Has been shown to decrease the requirement for analgesics after surgery

CHAPTER 4

1. d. Nation
2. b. False
3. d. 1, 2, 3, and 4
4. c. Communicate with members of the health care team
5. d. None of the above
6. b. False
7. b. False
8. c. 3
9. d. None of the above
10. d. All of the above

CHAPTER 5

1. a. Entering and retrieving information
   c. Communication and coordination of patient care processes
2. b. 30 consecutive days off per year
   d. 10% of total work hours dedicated to educational activities
3. a. The majority of clinical trials demonstrate decreased length of stay.
   c. There are multiple models and work paradigms.
4. a. More effective when there is greater incentive
   b. More effective when the incentive applies to a larger percent of patients in the provider's practice
   c. Currently being evaluated by Center for Medicare and Medicaid Services (CMS)
5. a. Deploying rapid response teams
   b. Prevention of surgical site infections
   c. Preventing adverse drug events through medication reconciliation
   d. Prevention of central line infections
6. a. Financing
   b. Establishing new workflows that optimize use of the HER
   c. Having adequate technical support
   d. Establishing a culture in the implementation setting that will allow for the necessary change
7. b. Total duty hours should not exceed 80 hours when averaged over 4 weeks
   d. At least 10 hours of off time between worked shifts
8. b. Gives a "B" recommendation when the data are based on limited or inconsistent scientific evidence
   d. Is commonly used in obstetrics and gynecology for evaluating peer-reviewed literature

CHAPTER 6

1. e. Decreased use of conservative medical management has increased the number of major surgical cases.
2. e. All of the above
3. c. Significantly increased ob/gyn knowledge base

4. e. All of the above
5. e. Human cadaveric dissections

CHAPTER 7

1. e. Anus
2. a. The pudendal nerve provides only sensory innervation to the perineum.
3. b. The clitoris never drains directly into the deep pelvic nodes.
4. c. The internal anal sphincter is indistinguishable from the external anal sphincter and it lies just outside the external anal sphincter.
5. e. All of the above
6. a. In a woman of reproductive age, the uterine cervix is larger than the uterine corpus.
7. d. The distal end of the fallopian tube is attached to the ovary by the fimbria ovarica.
8. c. The normal ovary measures 7 cm long during reproductive life.
9. b. The ovarian veins drain into the vena cava on the left and the renal vein on the right.
10. d. The ureter lies approximately 3 cm from the anterolateral surface of the cervix.

CHAPTER 8

1. d. Chemistry panel
2. d. All of the above
3. c. Patients with abnormal Papanicolaou smears showing repeated dysplasia should be evaluated by colposcopy and suspicious lesions biopsied before pelvic surgery.
4. c. Age is a relative contraindication for gynecologic surgery.
5. e. Vaginal and abdominal hysterectomy
6. d. a, b, or c
7. b. 1 to 2 hours before surgery, repeated once if the surgery lasts longer than 3 hours
8. b. A more effective assessment of the posterior bladder wall
9. a. Discontinuation of the use of birth control pills 2 to 4 weeks before the planned gynecologic surgery
10. a. A full bowel prep should be carried out on all gynecologic surgeries.

CHAPTER 9

1. Low-molecular-weight heparin
2. 8%
3. Advanced age, obesity, intraperitoneal infections, prolonged anesthesia time, nasogastric tube placement, and a history of smoking
4. 1. Hypoventilation
   2. V/Q abnormalities
   3. Venous admixture
   4. Diffusion limitation
   5. Low inspired fraction of oxygen

CHAPTER 10

1. d. Chemistry panel
2. d. All of the above
3. c. Patients with abnormal Papanicolaou smears showing repeated dysplasia should be evaluated by colposcopy and suspicious lesions biopsied before pelvic surgery
4. c. Age is a relative contraindication for gynecologic surgery
5. e. Vaginal and abdominal hysterectomy
6. d. a, b, or c
7. b. 1–2 hours before surgery, repeated once if the surgery lasts longer than 3 hours
8. b. A more effective assessment of the posterior bladder wall
9. a. Discontinue the use of birth control pills 2 to 4 weeks before the planned gynecologic surgery
10. a. A full bowel prep should be carried out on all gynecologic surgeries

CHAPTER 11

1. b. False
2. d. Open the wound widely to allow drainage and debridement of necrotic tissue, then apply wet-to-dry packing until the wound closes by secondary intention.
3. a. Index finger of the left hand of the surgeon
4. a. Metronidazole
5. c. Heparin and antibiotics for total of 7 to 10 days; no need for long-term anticoagulation therapy

CHAPTER 12

1. c. Intrapulmonary shunting. Clinically, adult respiratory distress syndrome is characterized by intrapulmonary shunting, widening of alveolar-arterial O_2 gradient, and reduced pulmonary compliance and functional residual capacity. Although supplemental oxygen is used, arterial Pao_2 typically remains less than 65 mm Hg. In patients with significant pulmonary injury, hypoxemia is progressive despite adequate oxygen supplementation, and assisted mechanical ventilation is required.
2. e. Oliguria. For both hypovolemic and septic shock, oliguria is a manifestation of early early reversible shock and is also a clinical finding for patients with irreversible shock. Characteristics of late irreversible shock include a reduction in cardiac output, systemic vascular resistance, and cardiac index. Cold, clammy skin is present because of poor peripheral circulation, and disorientation or obtundation from decreased cerebral perfusion is present. In contrast, early reversible septic shock is characterized by an increase in cardiac output that is due to compensatory cardiac dilatation and sympathetic response; tachycardia is also present. Systemic vascular resistance is decreased but may be normal in the absence of hypotension. The skin is usually warm, secondary to an increase in cardiac output and peripheral vasodilatation and to the febrile response.
3. c. For persistent bleeding consistent with coagulopathy. Platelet transfusion is indicated intraoperatively whenever there is persistent bleeding consistent with coagulopathy. In general, 1 unit of platelets will increase the platelet count by 5000 to 10,000/mL. It is recommended that when

blood loss exceeds 25% of the total intravascular volume and is ongoing, or when there is bleeding consistent with coagulopathy, packed red blood cells are indicated in a 4:1 ratio with fresh frozen plasma. There are isolated reports of satisfactory outcome in asymptomatic patients with solid tumors who did not receive platelet transfusions in the absence of bleeding, unless the counts were below 10,000 ?g/dL. Depending on the bleeding risks, currently accepted indications for preoperative and intraoperative platelet transfusion include platelet counts of less than 50,000 mg/dL.

4. e. Inotropic and vasoconstrictive effects. Dopamine stimulates dopaminergic, β-adrenergic and β-adrenergic receptors. Dopamine is unique in that it stimulates these receptors in a dose-dependent fashion. At low doses (1–3 mg/kg/min), dopaminergic receptors are mainly affected. This results in preferential cerebral, renal, and mesenteric arterial vasodilatation. The net effect is an increase in urine output and blood flow to the brain and gastrointestinal tract without increasing the heart rate or significantly affecting blood pressure. In moderate doses (5–12 mg/kg/min), both β- and β-adrenergic receptors are affected. The effects are inotropic; that is, the effect is an increase in myocardial contractility, sinoatrial rate impulse conduction, and cardiac output. With increased myocardial contractility, myocardial oxygen consumption is increased with no compensatory increase in coronary blood flow. In a patient with a history of coronary artery disease, this effect could lead to myocardial ischemia. At high doses (20 mg/kg/min) ?-adrenergic effects predominate, resulting in severe generalized vasoconstriction, and the severity of vasoconstriction is similar to the effects of epinephrine or norepinephrine. Dopamine has little β2-adrenergic activity.
5. b. Has both β1- and β2-adrenergic effects. Dobutamine is a direct-acting inotropic agent that stimulates β1- and β2-adrenergic receptors. Its β2 effects reduce afterload and pulmonary congestion without increasing O_2 consumption or causing significant tachycardia. Because of these effects, dobutamine the drug of choice for the treatment of cardiogenic shock.
6. b. Crystalloid infusion (1–2 L). The most common types of shock in obstetrics and gynecology are hypovolemic and septic. A healthy, young patient who is otherwise asymptomatic and is tolerating a hemoglobin of 8 mg/dL may be managed adequately with crystalloid infusion and oral iron as soon as she is able to begin oral feeding. Blood transfusion is not indicated in this patient at this time. Although colloids such as 5% and 25% albumin and synthetic colloid preparations have been used in the past for volume replacement, the majority of studies have found no advantage of colloids over crystalloids in this clinical setting.

   When hemorrhagic shock is identified, the initial management consists of placement of a large-bore peripheral intravenous catheter and infusion of 1 to 2 L of an isotonic electrolyte solution. The rate of fluid administration is proportionate to the caliber and length of the catheter; thus, placement of a central venous catheter will not improve the rate of fluid administration. Furthermore, central venous catheterization carries a risk of pneumothorax and other life-threatening complications and is unnecessary in an otherwise healthy patient.
7. e. Blood and cervical cultures. In all probability, this patient has a tuboovarian abscess. In this young, nulliparous patient, to preserve fertility, aggressive intravenous antibiotic therapy specific for genital tract pathogens (chlamydia and anaerobes) is recommended. When the diagnosis of tuboovarian abscess is suspect, antibiotic therapy in the hospitalized setting is warranted, regardless of concerns for future fertility. Before initiation of intravenous antibiotics, a pelvic examination with appropriate cultures for gonorrhea and chlamydia should be performed and blood cultures obtained in a patient who is febrile and has a significant leukocytosis. Because this patient has no evidence of a perforated viscus, plain films for free air are not indicated at this time. If the patient does not respond to antibiotic therapy, exploratory laparotomy may be indicated, but the initial management should be intravenous antibiotics after obtaining appropriate cultures.
8. c. Urine sodium excretion <20 mEq/L/24 hr. Oliguric prerenal azotemia is an early reversible injury. It is characterized by urine-plasma creatinine ratio greater than 40 mEq/L/24 hr, a urine sodium excretion of less than 20 mEq/L/24 hr, a fractional excretion of sodium less than 1%, and a high urine osmolality (>500 mOsm). Patients can have normal, increased, or reduced serum sodium, depending on volume replacement and intake. Contraction alkalosis is characteristic of prolonged diuretic use. Characteristics of acute tubular necrosis, which results from prolonged hypoperfusion and cellular damage, is typically characterized by the loss of ability to concentrate urine. Osmolality of the urine is usually less than 350 mOsm.
9. b. Class II. Based on presenting signs and symptoms, hypovolemic shock is subdivided into four classes. Class I is generally characterized by blood loss of less than 750 mL, Class II with volume losses of 750 to 1,500 mL, and Class III with uncompensated blood or volume loss of more than 1,500 mL. Any volume loss may be associated with tachycardia, which can be a sympathomimetic response to pain or anxiety. In patients with less than 1,500 mL of volume loss, renal perfusion and urine output is typically maintained. The major clinical distinction between Class I and Class II hypovolemic shock is the presence of postural hypotension.
10. a. Lung, liver, GI, kidney. Multiorgan system dysfunction is a syndrome characterized by progressive manifestations of the systemic inflammatory response, even when there is no evidence of ongoing sepsis or insult. Mortality is high and depends on the number and severity of organ systems affected and patient reserve. This syndrome remains the predominant cause of death from shock in patients who appear to have received adequate resuscitation and who have no culture evidence of ongoing bacteremia. Classically, multiorgan failure affects the lungs first, followed by the liver, the gastrointestinal tract, and finally the kidneys, although clinical presentation is variable.
11. b. Angiotensin II is a potent vasoconstrictor. In response to hypovolemia, which results in decreased wall tension, decreased sodium, or increased sympathetic activation, renin is released from the juxtaglomerular cells. Renin converts angiotensinogen into angiotensin I, which is an inactive polypeptide. In the liver, angiotensin I is converted to angiotensin II. Angiotensin II is a potent vasoconstrictor that stimulates aldosterone release from the renal cortex. Aldosterone along with antidiuretic hormone promotes sodium and water retention. The net effect is an increase in venous return, stroke volume, cardiac output, and blood pressure.

12. d. Vancomycin antibiotic therapy. The best management of neutropenic patients depends on the underlying malignancy, prior prophylactic therapy, institutional/community drug resistance patterns, and patient risk factors. For this patient, empiric monotherapy with cefepime, ceftazidime, or imipenem should have been initiated before blood cultures were obtained. In this setting, the most likely infectious agent is staphylococcus. Therefore, vancomycin should be administered to this patient until culture results are obtained. Although indwelling catheters increase the risk of Gram-positive colonization from skin flora, the infection can often be treated without catheter removal. Piperacillin-taxobactam therapy is a cost-effective treatment for febrile neutropenic patients with hematological malignancies.
13. e. Give iron supplementation. Anemia is a common complication of cancer and cancer therapy. Because of alterations in tissue perfusion as well as immunological responses, significant anemia profoundly affects normal cellular and vascular physiology, impairing response to therapy and quality of life. Anemia preoperatively and postoperatively is an independent risk factor for postoperative infection, longer hospital stays, and death in noncardiac surgical patients. In several tumor models, anemia is a poor prognostic factor associated with poorer local control of disease and lower survival rates. Anemia leads to an increase in the tumor hypoxic fraction, with relative radioresistance resulting from impaired tumor oxygenation. The two most common reasons for anemia are iron deficiency and anemia of chronic disease. The patient described above is likely to have both true iron deficiency and inflammatory anemia. The best next step in the management of this patient is to determine relative iron stores; if serum ferritin levels are less than 30 nanograms per mL, iron therapy should be initiated. Although additional B_{12} and/or folic acid supplementation would be indicated for measurable deficits, vitamin deficiency is an uncommon cause for anemia in the adult patient with an intact gastrointestinal tract and a normal diet. Erythropoietin is the principal hematopoietic growth factor that regulates erythroid lineage cellular proliferation and differentiation. Erythropoietin is a pleotrophic cytokine that is proangiogenetic, with broad tissue-protective effects in diverse nonhematopoietic organs. Multiple trials demonstrate recombinant erythropoietin effectively reduces transfusion requirements and improves quality of life in cancer patients. However, erythropoietin does not reduce transfusion risks or correct anemia in the absence of sufficient iron stores. Therefore, administration of erythropoietic stimulating agents in conjunction with iron vitamin supplements is indicated for patients with anemia of chronic disease and mixed anemia. Red cell transfusion is indicated for acute symptomatic anemia, especially when blood loss is ongoing, for patients with comorbid conditions in which anemia increases the risk of ischemia, and in chronic symptomatic anemia unresponsive to erythropoietin and iron therapy. The choice of therapy (chemotherapy, radiation therapy, or both) is usually predicated by the stage of disease and tumor type. Changes in treatment are usually made based on response and toxicity.

CHAPTER 13

1. c. Polyglactin 910 Rapide. The well-vascularized, rapidly healing tissues of the vagina need support for only a short period of time after injury, suggesting the need for a rapidly absorbed suture. Multiple studies are now available that show significantly less postepisiotomy pain after repair with synthetic absorbable sutures compared with catgut sutures. This is believed to be caused by the intense inflammatory response produces by the gut sutures. Although use of longer delayed suture are also associated with less pain than catgut, the presence of suture material and knots has been associated with dyspareunia and pain after the postpartum period.
2. c. Suture pulling through fascia. Fascial dehiscence can be caused by multiple factors, including suture breakage, knot failure, and suture pulling through fascia, but the most common factor appears to be suture pulling through fascia. Wound infection may play a contributing factor in fascial dehiscence but is not a primary cause.

CHAPTER 14

1. c. Maylard
2. b. False. There is no posterior rectus sheath below the arcuate line.
3. c. Internal oblique and transversalis. The aponeuroses of the transversalis and the split aponeurosis of the internal oblique come together to form the posterior sheath of the rectus muscles above the arcuate line.
4. b. Transect the rectus muscles at their insertion, similarly done when performing a Cherney incision. Although one could use a Maylard, the risk of injury to the inferior epigastric vessels would be greater. Further, one would have to suture the muscle edges to the fascial edges to reapproximate the rectus muscle bellies. Given all of these pitfalls, the best option would be to transect the rectus muscles at their tendinous insertion into the pubic symphysis. Care must be taken to reattach the muscles to the tendon—not the periosteum of the pubic symphysis—at the completion of the procedure.
5. d. Maylard. The Maylard incision is used to enter the abdomen in a transperitoneal approach.
6. d. 8. Eviscerations usually occur from day 5 to 14 after the operation, with a mean of 8 days.
7. b. External iliac artery. The inferior epigastric artery arises from the external iliac artery. The superficial epigastric artery arises from the femoral artery. The hypogastric artery is another name for the internal iliac artery.

CHAPTER 15

1. c. Use a return electrode (ground) of large contact area to ensure a low-current density.
2. a. If metal laparoscopic trocars are used, a plastic insulating collar should be used.
3. d. Activating the current before making contact with the clamp.
4. a. Is a desirable electrosurgical modality for venous bleeding, such as oozing from a muscle.
5. b. Faster movement of the wire through the cervical tissue causes more thermal injury and makes it more difficult for the pathologist to interpret.

CHAPTER 16

1. b. CO_2
2. b. False

3. a. Increase in pulse time
4. b. False
5. b. Above 100°C
6. b. False
7. b. Eye
8. d. Water

CHAPTER 17

1. a. Reusable
2. a. True
3. b. External iliac artery
4. b. Ilioinguinal nerve
5. b. Compression of the common peroneal nerve, compression by Allen stirrups
6. a. True
7. b. False

CHAPTER 18

1. d. The tungsten light source is superior to other sources.
2. b. The operative hysteroscope is 15 mm in diameter.
3. e. All of the above
4. a. Carbon dioxide
5. c. Normal saline
6. b. Hyskon
7. d. Glycine 1.5%
8. a. Hysteroscopy should be performed during the luteal phase for best visualization of the endometrial cavity.
9. d. Endometrial ablation
10. d. Bleeding

CHAPTER 19

1. b. Hepatitis B
2. a. Use large figure-of-eight sutures so the suture will not cut through the tissue.
3. d. Lamellar platelets
4. a. Hepatitis B
5. b. Reducing the pulse pressure
6. b. False
7. a. True
8. c. Only the posterior division of the hypogastric artery should be ligated.
9. d. 1 in 2 million
10. b. False

CHAPTER 20

1. *In vitro* fertilization (IVF)
2. Yes
3. IVF with intracytoplasmic sperm injection (ICSI), salpingectomy before IVF
4. If married, cryopreservation of preembryos. If single, cryopreservation of oocytes or ovarian tissue; both procedures must be considered experimental.

CHAPTER 21

1. b. *Chlamydia trachomatis*
2. d. Known tubal obstruction
3. b. Obliterative fibrosis
4. d. Reduced risk of ectopic pregnancy
5. a. to use cautery during dissection to facilitate hemostasis
6. d. Nature of the tubal endothelium
7. b. Length of reconstructed tube

CHAPTER 22

1. e. All of the above
2. a. Laparoscopy provides inferior visualization of the posterior cul-de-sac compared with laparotomy.
3. a. The classic triad associated with endometriosis includes infertility, dyspareunia, and dysmenorrhea.
4. c. Presacral neurectomy, or division of the superior hypogastric plexus, is useful as an adjunctive procedure to reduce midline pelvic pain and dysmenorrhea in women with endometriosis.
5. b. The ASRM defines complete cul-de-sac obliteration as when no peritoneum is visible below the uterosacral ligaments.

CHAPTER 23

1. 1-c; 2-a; 3-d; 4-b
2. c. Partial vulvectomy
3. a. True
4. c. Simple vulvectomy

CHAPTER 24

1. b. Becomes patent when canalization of the most caudal portion of the vaginal plate at the urogenital sinus occurs
2. b. Most patients have a high (suprasphincteric) urethral vaginal connection.
3. c. Vaginoplasty should be performed in infancy to prevent vaginal stenosis.
4. c. Absence of the posterior wall of the bladder exposing the ureteral orifices
5. e. All of the above
6. a. The average age at presentation is 35 years.
7. c. Seventy-five percent of women exposed to DES *in utero* have anatomic abnormalities.
8. b. Stage 1 disease lesions can be treated with radiation therapy or total abdominal hysterectomy.
9. e. Infection of the Bartholin gland
10. c. Most urethral diverticula are located in the proximal urethra.

CHAPTER 25

1. b. Septate uterus
2. a. The vagina develops from both the müllerian ducts and the urogenital sinus.

3. c. Impaired ovarian function
4. e. Laparoscopy
5. b. Greater than 90% patients have been shown to achieve anatomic and functional success by vaginal dilation.
6. d. Adequate preoperative dilatation
7. d. Conservative management, with hormonal suppression of endometrial stimulation, is appropriate for young patients.
8. d. Rokitansky syndrome
9. c. Didelphic uterus
10. b. A prolonged postoperative recovery period

CHAPTER 26

1. b. Anovulatory bleeding
2. d. GnRH analog injection
3. b. In the follicular phase
4. d. All of the above
5. c. Sonohysterography

CHAPTER 27

1. c. Inserting the needle with the port closed. Careful attention to safety measures will reduce the likelihood of complications with Veress needle insertion. The needle should be inserted in the midline toward the hollow of the sacrum to avoid the major vessels laterally. The anterior abdominal wall should be elevated to avoid the dorsal vascular structures. The needle should be inserted with the port open and held to avoid occlusion of the spring mechanism of the inner safety obturator. Several techniques, including infiltration and aspiration of sterile fluid through the needle, can help to identify correct placement.
2. a. Bipolar coagulation. Both types of clips and the silicone rubber band are most likely to be effective if applied to normal fallopian tubes. Dense pelvic adhesions will decrease the likelihood that the tubes can be adequately mobilized for proper application of these methods. The presence of thickened or edematous tubes decreases the likelihood that the clip or band can adequately occlude the tube and increases the likelihood of tubal transection.
3. c. Direct observation of tubal blanching and swelling. Bipolar coagulation is highly effective with proper technique. Because thermal injury to the seromuscular layer of the tube can occur without adequate coagulation of the endosalpinx, visual end points for adequate coagulation are unreliable. The use of a cutting waveform with the power output at least 25 W against a 100-V load increase the likelihood of complete coagulation, and use of an optical flow meter assists in determining when coagulation has been adequate. Coagulation of at least three contiguous areas will enhance the likelihood that a sufficient amount of tube has been occluded, and avoiding the proximal isthmus is thought to decrease the risk of tuboperitoneal fistula formation.
4. c. Ovarian cancer. Women who undergo tubal sterilization are more likely than women whose partners undergo vasectomy to later experience an ectopic pregnancy and to undergo hysterectomy. They appear to be equally likely to experience regret after the procedure. For a reason that remains unclear, sterilized women are less likely to develop ovarian cancer than their nonsterilized counterparts.

CHAPTER 28

1. b. Mesoderm
2. a. It is an HY cell surface antigen.
3. b. 12
4. c. It contains both motor and sensory parasympathetic and sympathetic nerves.
5. d. All of the above

CHAPTER 29

1. c. Allodynia
2. b. Neuromatrix theory
3. c. Somatosensory disorders

CHAPTER 30

1. b. Intravenous clindamycin plus gentamicin
2. b. False
3. d. A polymicrobial mixture of aerobes and anaerobes
4. d. Oral ofloxacin plus metronidazole
5. b. False

CHAPTER 31

1. c. Red or carneous degeneration is never seen during pregnancy.
2. d. Sarcomatous degeneration
3. b. The tumor behaves clinically as a benign entity.
4. a. Most leiomyomata are asymptomatic and may not require any treatment.
5. b. Danazol
6. c. It is recommended to combine laparoscopic guidance with the hysteroscopic procedure.
7. b. A 34-year-old woman desiring future fertility with two intramural myomas each measuring 3 cm in diameter
8. a. Preoperative treatment with oral contraceptive pills
9. d. Pulmonary embolus
10. a. Most patients report an improvement in menorrhagia and bulk-related symptoms.

CHAPTER 32A

1. a. Prolapse
2. a. Abdominal hysterectomy
3. b. Vaginal hysterectomy
4. c. Shorter operative time
5. a. True
6. b. False

7. a. Previous tubal ligation
8. c. Prophylactic intravenous antibiotics within 1 hour before surgery
9. a. True
10. b. 1/1,000 hysterectomies

CHAPTER 32B

1. e. Vaginal hysterectomy
2. d. Nulliparity
3. d. More than 90%
4. d. 90%
5. a. Dividing the uterine vessels

CHAPTER 32C

1. d. Shorter hospital stay
2. b. The uterine vessels are secured laparoscopically in a VALH.
3. a. Shorter operative time
4. c. The Vagiballoon(r)
5. a. True

CHAPTER 33

1. d. All of the above. They are all appropriate management plans for the hemodynamically stable patient with incomplete abortion or missed abortion. Surgical management is more likely to result in completion than medical management, and medical management is more likely to result in completion than expectant management, but the inverse is true of costs incurred. Patient satisfaction can be seen with any of these management plans. Certainly in the face of severe anemia, hemodynamic instability, or infection, surgical evacuation should be performed. Without these, patient preference should be strongly considered.
2. b. 7 weeks. The FDA has approved mifepristone 600 mg orally followed by misoprostol orally 48 hours later up to 7 weeks for early medical abortion. Recent literature supports an alternative regimen that can be effective up to 9 weeks.
3. b. False. All abortions, spontaneous or induced, can result in Rh sensitization in an Rh-negative woman. All women with an abortion should be given anti-D immune globulin. 50 μg is sufficient before 12 weeks of gestation; 300 μg is necessary thereafter.

CHAPTER 34

1. b. Ampullary, isthmic, fimbrial, interstitial
2. d. All of above

CHAPTER 35A

1. b. An increase in pulmonary reserve
2. c. An increased risk of placenta accreta
3. d. Rate of infection
4. a. True
5. e. None of the above
6. a. An increased risk of rectal sphincter tear
7. a. True

CHAPTER 35B

1. d. Benign cystic teratoma
2. b. Biopsy only, no further surgery
3. c. Dysgerminoma
4. a. Repeat the ultrasound in 4 weeks.
5. b. Pelvic ultrasound

CHAPTER 36A

1. c. Transversus perinei
2. d. Pericervical ring
3. b. Vaginal delivery
4. d. Hymenal ring
5. b. Quality of life

CHAPTER 36B

1. d. All of the above
2. c. Vesicovaginal and paravesical spaces
3. b. A transverse apical defect between the pericervical ring and the pubocervical septum

CHAPTER 36C

1. d. The posterior aspect of the pubic bone
2. b. Troublesome bleeding may result.
3. a. True
4. a. Placed individually starting near the ischial spine
5. d. Fascia of the obturator internus muscle

CHAPTER 36D

1. a. The change to site-specific defect repair
2. d. All of the above
3. d. In recurrent cases in which native pelvic tissues are weak
4. c. Mesh exposure
5. d. It is one of the most common surgeries performed in women older than age 50 and has an unacceptably high failure rate.

CHAPTER 36E

1. b. Cardinal and uterosacral ligaments
2. b. Rectum
3. a. Pudendal nerve/vessels
4. c. Anterior vaginal wall prolapse
5. d. Suturing the round ligaments to the anterior graft with nonabsorbable sutures

CHAPTER 36F

1. a. True
2. c. Wide vaginal introitus
3. d. Ring
4. a. Increased difficulty with bowel movement
5. b. It does not improve her symptoms.

CHAPTER 37

1. d. Act to decrease intraurethral resistance
2. b. Has a retropubic passage
3. a. 85%
4. b. Q-tip straining angle of >40%
5. d. All of the above
6. d. Must perform a cystotomy to complete the procedure(s)

CHAPTER 38

1. c. At the cardinal ligament when the ureter passes under the uterine artery
2. a. Surgical knowledge of the location and anatomy the ureter
3. b. Cystostomy
4. c. Total abdominal hysterectomy
5. c. Ureteroneocystomy with psoas hitch

CHAPTER 39

1. d. HIV infection
2. a. Laparoscopic
3. a. True
4. b. Superior to the interureteric ridge in the posterior bladder
5. c. Stone formation
6. c. Insert a tampon in the vagina and have the patient walk around for 15 minutes

CHAPTER 40

1. e. a, b, and c
2. d. a and c
3. e. a, b, and c
4. d. Endoanal ultrasound
5. b. False

CHAPTER 41

1. Yes. Unlike sporadic breast cancers, which may be associated with primarily maternal family-history risk factors, BRCA can be transmitted from the paternal side of the family as well. One must take a detailed family history, including at least grandparents, parents, siblings, and children. A discussion of ancestry is important, as Ashkenazi Jewish ancestry evokes a higher risk and ascertaining the age at which relatives were diagnosed is critical in developing an accurate risk profile. You may see breast and early prostate cancers in male relatives as well as other nonreproductive cancers. The carrier relative may also be unaffected with disease at the time of review.
2. Yes. As inherited breast cancer (at this point) only accounts for 5% to 10% of breast cancers, once the gene is negative, the patient still remains at risk for the other 80% to 90% of sporadic breast cancers. We also have limited knowledge of other possible sources (undiscovered genes) for hereditary susceptibility to breast cancer. Thus, the patient should have, at minimum, mammographic, self-breast, and clinical breast examination (CBE) surveillance based on her age. And if familial breast cancer remains a concern, additional scrutiny may be warranted, including increased CBE. MRI testing is also currently showing promise in high-risk women, but additional studies are ongoing.
3. No. As mammograms have a 10% to 15% false-negative rate, a negative mammogram should not deter additional evaluation. Furthermore, the increased breast density noted in younger women portends an even higher false-negative rate.
4. Currently chemoprevention, prophylactic mastectomy/oophorectomy, lifestyle modification, and increased surveillance are risk-reducing options in women with high-risk characteristics. Decreased use of alcohol and tobacco in additional to early childbearing are options for women pursuing lifestyle modification. Initial prevention data indicating a nearly 50% reduction in breast cancer was based on tamoxifen prophylaxis. As tamoxifen has additional side effects (including but not limited to an increased risk of endometrial cancer and venous thromboembolism), raloxifene was reviewed, with promising information released in the Study of Tamoxifen and Raloxifene (STAR) trial indicating a similar risk-reduction benefit for raloxifene without the increased risk of endometrial cancer. The risk of venous thromboembolism (VTE), however, was increased, thus indicating the need for additional studies. Aromatase inhibitors are being studied in pending trials including STELLAR (Study of Letrozole and Raloxifene—accrual to begin in late 2006 or 2007) in postmenopausal women. Oral contraceptives have also been shown to decrease a women's risk for the development of ovarian cancer. This creates a quandary for women at increased risk for both ovarian and breast cancer.
5. CNBs provide a histologic sample rather than the cytologic sample of FNA. Thus, invasion past the basement membrane cannot (as a rule) be delineated, thereby decreasing one's ability to differentiate carcinoma *in situ* (CIS) from invasive cancer. Pathologists with significant experience in cytologic interpretation, however, may narrow this gap.
6. The Gail, Claus, and BRCAPRO are the most frequently used models in clinical practice. Of these, the Gail model is the only one that has been clinically validated. The risk for young women may be underestimated in both the Gail and Claus model. BRCA mutation carriers and those with paternal family history of breast cancer are underestimated in the Gail model. Moreover, the Gail model has not been validated in minority patients. The BRCAPRO model specifically focuses on genetic mutation risk. Thus, although each model has its advantages and limitations, it appears (from studies) that the Gail model may be most applicable. Also, it is assessable on the National Cancer Institute Web site.
7. Assessing an individual's risk for the development of breast cancer likely encourages awareness of breast cancer and breast cancer screening recommendations, provides a forum

for discussion and clarification of risk management (as women often overestimate their risk), and improves the overall quality of care as information is being released indicating differential effects of tamoxifen and breast-feeding in BRCA1 versus BRCA2 carriers. Thus, stratification is necessary to provide accurate information regarding risk reduction.

8. b. False. Tumors equal to 2 cm are considered stage I (i.e., tumor <2 cm). Another often-missed component is that tumors measuring 5 cm are considered stage II. Only those greater than 5 cm are considered stage III.
9. b. False. Actually, the majority of women with breast cancer have no identifiable risk factor other than sex and age.

CHAPTER 42

1. d. The greatest incidence of appendicitis occurs in the third and fourth decades of life.
2. a. McBurney's point: located at the junction of the middle and medial thirds of a line drawn from the umbilicus to right anterolateral spine
3. c. Start intravenous fluids and broad-spectrum antibiotics with enteric organism coverage, keep the patient NPO, and keep the patient under close observation for progression of her illness.
4. b. Premature labor and delivery are among most serious fetal risks, with up to 30% fetal mortality reported if perforation occurs.
5. b. A patient undergoing standard repeat cesarean section with tubal ligation

CHAPTER 43

1. b. The diverticulum should be removed because the patient has a history of symptoms that it may have caused, and it has slightly atypical features.
2. a. A 26 year old with SLE who has end-stage renal disease; b. A 54-year-old alcoholic with cirrhosis; and d. A 48 year old with class II heart failure
3. b. Leave the trocar in place, convert to an open laparotomy, and repair the injury.
4. a. The patient presents to the ER 3 days postoperatively reporting nausea, vomiting, and fever.
5. c. Return of bowel function generally occurs at the same rate regardless of early or delayed feeding.
6. a. Adhesions; d. Hernias; and e. Malignancy
7. b. The patient is less likely to have a sense of incomplete evacuation after bowel movements.
8. c. (True) end-to-end staple anastomosis
9. b. Bleeding from a cut edge; and e. Fluorescence of bowel wall under Wood's lamp 10 minutes after IV fluorescein
10. a. False; b. False; c. True; d. False; e. True; f. False; g. False; h. False

CHAPTER 44

1. c. 50%
2. c. Pelvic kidney
3. b. True
4. a. Gastrointestinal
5. a. Neurofibromas
6. a. Crohn disease
7. a. Colon

CHAPTER 45

1. d. Immunosuppression
2. c. Any location, less than 1 mm invasion
3. c. Close resection with margin less than 1 cm
4. b. Locally advanced disease or lesions encroaching on midline structures for which surgical removal is accompanied by significant morbidity
5. c. Failure to improve promptly with conservative therapy
6. d. Pathologic status of the inguinal lymph nodes
7. b. Melanoma
8. b. The presence of underlying invasive disease in more than 90% of patients
9. d. Basal cell carcinoma
10. b. Basosquamous carcinoma

CHAPTER 46

1. a. True
2. d. 80%
3. c. Lugol's staining
4. e. 50%
5. e. Follow-up with no treatment during pregnancy
6. c. 50%
7. b. Metaplasia
8. a. It produces a specimen for histologic study.
9. d. Identification of which patients with mild dysplasia need treatment
10. a and d. Cervical glandular lesions and suspected microinvasive lesions

CHAPTER 47

1. c. Stage IB
2. b. FIGO stage
3. c. Preservation of ovarian function
4. a. Intravenous pyelogram
5. b. Pararectal space
6. a. Its origin from the hypogastric artery
7. d. Bladder dysfunction
8. a. Vaginal bleeding
9. c. Entry into the paravesical space
10. c. 65%–75%

CHAPTER 48

1. d. Cigarette smoking
2. a. Office endometrial biopsy
3. e. None of the above

4. a. Surgical staging for patients with uterine papillary serous carcinoma includes peritoneal washings and biopsies, pelvic and paraaortic lymph node dissection, and omentectomy.
5. a. History and physical examination

CHAPTER 49

1. c. Unilateral oophorectomy followed by chemotherapy
2. b. Surgery alone
3. c. Capsular rupture
4. a. Unilateral salpingo-oophorectomy with surgical staging
5. d. Transvaginal pelvic ultrasound
6. a. Serum inhibin
7. a. Peripheral vasculature
8. a. Check a CA-125 level, and if normal, repeat the ultrasound in 3 months to determine if any change has occurred.
9. b. 10%–15%
10. d. Nulliparity

CHAPTER 50

1. d. A 56-year-old woman who was treated 15 months ago for stage IB2 squamous cell carcinoma of the cervix now has a biopsy-proven 1.0-cm recurrence in the cervix after previous pelvic radiation and chemotherapy. The mass is freely mobile. Her workup is negative except for a single 1.5-cm node in the low aortic area just above her previous radiation field. CT-guided FNA is positive for squamous cell carcinoma. There is no evidence of other metastatic disease.
2. d. Age older than 70
3. b. Tumor causing a vesicovaginal fistula
4. a. Pouch of Douglas
5. d. It is technically quick and easy to perform.

CHAPTER 51

1. d. Urinary continence
2. b. Superior hemorrhoidal artery
3. d. Sartorius
4. a. Previous Maylard incision
5. c. Increased risk of recurrence
6. b. A flap length 2 cm long and a base of 1 cm
7. b. 80 cm H_2O pressure, 500 mL volume
8. c. Retention of 1,000 to 1,500 mL of fluid
9. d. Reinforcing the ileocecal valve by tapering the distal segment is essential for maintaining continence.
10. b. Constipation

■ INDEX

Note: Page numbers followed by f indicate figures; t, tables.

B

J

K

M